Pharmacology and Therapeutics

Principles to Practice

ASSOCIATE EDITORS

EDITORIAL BOARD*

*All members of the Editorial Board are former presidents of the American Society for Clinical Pharmacology and Therapeutics (ASCPT).

Pharmacology and Therapeutics

Principles to Practice

Scott A. Waldman, MD, PhD, FCP

Past President, American Society for Clinical Pharmacology and Therapeutics
Samuel M.V. Hamilton Professor of Medicine
Professor of Pharmacology and Experimental Therapeutics and Medicine
Chair, Department of Pharmacology and Experimental Therapeutics
Director, Division of Clinical Pharmacology, Department of Medicine
Director, Gastrointestinal Malignancies Program, Kimmel Cancer Center
Director, NIH Training Program in "Clinical Pharmacology"
Thomas Jefferson University
Philadelphia, Pennsylvania

Andre Terzic, MD, PhD

Past President, American Society for Clinical Pharmacology and Therapeutics
Marriott Family Professor of Cardiovascular Research
Professor of Medicine and Pharmacology, Medical Genetics
Director, Marriott Heart Disease Research Program
Director, NIH Training Program in "Cardiovasology"
Mayo Clinic Associate Director for Research
Co-Director, Mayo Clinic Center for Individualized Medicine
Mayo Clinic
Rochester, Minnesota

SAUNDERS

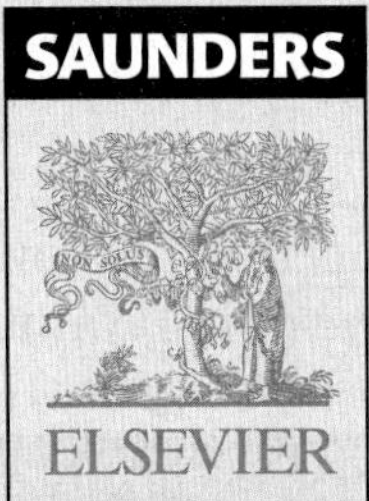

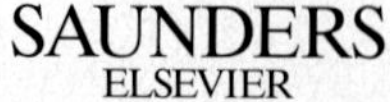

SAUNDERS
ELSEVIER

1600 John F. Kennedy Blvd.
Ste 1800
Philadelphia, PA 19103-2899

PHARMACOLOGY AND THERAPEUTICS: PRINCIPLES TO PRACTICE
ISBN: 978-1-4160-3291-5
Expert Consult: 978-1-4160-3291-5
Expert Consult Premium: 978-1-4160-6098-7

Notice

Knowledge and best practice in this field are constantly changing. As new research and experience broaden our knowledge, changes in practice, treatment and drug therapy may become necessary or appropriate. Readers are advised to check the most current information provided (i) on procedures featured or (ii) by the manufacturer of each product to be administered, to verify the recommended dose or formula, the method and duration of administration, and contraindications. It is the responsibility of the practitioner, relying on their own experience and knowledge of the patient, to make diagnoses, to determine dosages and the best treatment for each individual patient, and to take all appropriate safety precautions. To the fullest extent of the law, neither the Publisher nor the Editors assumes any liability for any injury and/or damage to persons or property arising out of or related to any use of the material contained in this book.

The Publisher

Library of Congress Cataloging-in-Publication Data
Pharmacology and therapeutics : principles to practice / [edited by] Scott A. Waldman, Andre Terzic.—1st ed.
p. ; cm.
ISBN 978-1-4160-3291-5
1. Pharmacology. 2. Chemotherapy. I. Waldman, Scott A. II. Terzic, Andre.
[DNLM: 1. Pharmacology, Clinical—methods. 2. Drug Therapy. QV 38 P53603 2008]
RM300.P5193 2008
615′.1—dc22
2007044208

Acquisitions Editor: Druanne Martin
Developmental Editor: Adrianne Brigido
Project Manager: Mary B. Stermel
Design Direction: Steven Stave
Text Designer: Ellen Zanolle
Editorial Assistant: John Ingram
Marketing Manager: Courtney Ingram

Printed in United States of America

Last digit is the print number: 9 8 7 6 5 4 3 2 1

To our mentors, who inspired the journey of discovery, championed the passions, and exposed the frontiers. To our colleagues, who enriched the path, multiplying the dimensions beyond imagination. To our institutions, which nurtured the nascent trajectory and fostered the ultimate destination. To the American Society of Clinical Pharmacology and Therapeutics and its Executive Director, Sharon Swan, who created a forum that crystallized interactions, driving us inexorably forward. To our Editor, Adrianne Brigido, without whom this book would not have been possible. To our families, who shared the ideals and enabled this extraordinary journey to progress every day.

CONTRIBUTORS

Darrell R. Abernethy, MD, PhD
Johns Hopkins University School of Medicine, Baltimore, Maryland; United States Pharmacopeia, Rockville, Maryland

Viola Andresen, MD
Israelitic Hospital, Hamburg, Germany

Arthur J. Atkinson, Jr., MD
Feinberg School of Medicine, Northwestern University, Chicago, Illinois

Michel Azizi, MD, PhD
Université Paris–Descartes; Hôpital Européen Georges Pompidou, Paris, France

Helen L. Baron, MD
Keck School of Medicine, University of Southern California, Los Angeles, California

Carol L. Beck, PharmD, PhD
Jefferson Medical College, Thomas Jefferson University, Philadelphia, Pennsylvania

Atta Behfar, MD, PhD
Mayo Clinic, Rochester, Minnesota

Rodney Bell, MD
Jefferson Medical College, Thomas Jefferson University, Philadelphia, Pennsylvania

Eduardo E. Benarroch, MD
Mayo Clinic College of Medicine; Mayo Clinic, Rochester, Minnesota

Neal L. Benowitz, MD
University of California, San Francisco; San Francisco General Hospital Medical Center, San Francisco, California

Wade Berrettini, MD, PhD
University of Pennsylvania School of Medicine, Philadelphia, Pennsylvania

Joseph S. Bertino, Jr., PharmD
College of Physicians and Surgeons, Columbia University, New York; Bertino Consulting, Schenectady, New York

Alfredo Bianchi, MD[†]
Clinica Malzoni, Agropoli; University of Salerno, Napoli, Italy

Michael J. Blake, PhD, MD
Ottumwa Pediatrics, Ottumwa, Iowa

Ann F. Bolger, MD, FACC, FAHA
University of California, San Francisco, School of Medicine; San Francisco General Hospital, San Francisco, California

Glenn D. Braunstein, MD
David Geffen School of Medicine at UCLA; Cedars-Sinai Medical Center, Los Angeles, California

David Brock, MD
Jefferson Medical College, Thomas Jefferson University; Thomas Jefferson University Hospital and Jefferson Hospital for Neuroscience, Philadelphia, Pennsylvania

Peter A. Calabresi, MD
Johns Hopkins Multiple Sclerosis Center, Johns Hopkins University School of Medicine, Baltimore, Maryland

Michael Camilleri, MD
Mayo Clinic College of Medicine; Mayo Clinic, Rochester, Minnesota

Mark Chaballa, PharmD
Thomas Jefferson University Hospital, Philadelphia, Pennsylvania

Omer Chaudhry, MD
Georgetown University, Washington, DC; Formerly University of Virginia, Charlottesville, Virginia

Doo-Sup Choi, PhD
Mayo Clinic College of Medicine, Rochester, Minnesota

Bart L. Clarke, MD
Mayo Clinic College of Medicine, Mayo Clinic, Rochester, Minnesota

Mary E. Dankert, BS
University of Pennsylvania, Philadelphia, Pennsylvania

Dawood Darbar, MB ChB, MD
Vanderbilt University School of Medicine; Vanderbilt University, Nashville, Tennessee

Mark Davis, MD
Mayo Clinic, Rochester, Minnesota

Daniel Deck, PharmD
University of California, San Francisco, School of Pharmacy; San Francisco General Hospital, San Francisco, California

Jan de Gans, MD, PhD
Center of Infection and Immunity, Academic Medical Center, University of Amsterdam, Amsterdam, The Netherlands

Joseph A. DeSimone, Jr., MD
Thomas Jefferson University, Philadelphia, Pennsylvania

Robert B. Diasio, MD
Mayo Clinic, Rochester, Minnesota

André Diedrich, MD, PhD
Vanderbilt University School of Medicine, Nashville, Tennessee

Darin D. Dougherty, MD
Massachusetts General Hospital; Harvard Medical School, Boston, Massachusetts

Laurence J. Egan, MD, FRCPI
National University of Ireland, Galway; Clinical Science Institute, University College Hospital Galway, Newcastle, Galway, Ireland

---

[†]Deceased

Claudine El-Beyrouty, PharmD
Jefferson Medical College, Thomas Jefferson University; Thomas Jefferson University Hospital, Philadelphia, Pennsylvania

Jean-Luc Elghozi, MD, PhD
Université Paris–Descartes; Hôpital Necker, Paris, France

Arthur M. Feldman, MD, PhD
Jefferson Medical College, Thomas Jefferson University, Philadelphia, Pennsylvania

Joanne Filicko-O'Hara, MD
Kimmel Cancer Center, Thomas Jefferson University; Thomas Jefferson University Hospital, Philadelphia, Pennsylvania

Charles W. Flexner, MD
Johns Hopkins University, Baltimore, Maryland

Neal Flomenberg, MD
Thomas Jefferson University, Philadelphia, Pennsylvania

Joseph F. Foss, MD
Cleveland Clinic, Cleveland, Ohio

Adam M. Frank, MD
Thomas Jefferson University Hospital, Philadelphia, Pennsylvania

Mark A. Frye, MD
Mayo Clinic College of Medicine, Rochester, Minnesota

Kishor Gandhi, MD, MPH
Thomas Jefferson University, Philadelphia, Pennsylvania

Joseph Genebriera, MD
Mayo Clinic, Rochester, Minnesota

William R. Gilliland, MD, MHPE
Uniformed Services University of the Health Sciences, Bethesda, Maryland

Jean Gray, CM, MD, FRCPC, LLD (Hon), DSc (Hon), FRCP (London)
Dalhousie University, Halifax, Nova Scotia, Canada

Benjamin M. Greenberg, MD, MHS
Johns Hopkins Encephalitis Center, Johns Hopkins Transverse Myelitis Center, Johns Hopkins University School of Medicine, Baltimore, Maryland

Naomi Gronich, MD
National Institute on Aging, National Institutes of Health, Baltimore, Maryland

Dolores Grosso, MSN, CRNP
Thomas Jefferson University Hospital, Philadelphia, Pennsylvania

Andrew R. Haas, MD, PhD
University of Pennsylvania; University of Pennsylvania Hospital, Philadelphia, Pennsylvania

Wael N. Haidar, MD
Mercy Hospitalists, Des Moines, Iowa

Christine A. Haller, MS, MD
Amgen Inc., South San Francisco, California

Daniel K. Hall-Flavin, MD
Mayo Clinic College of Medicine, Rochester, Minnesota

Lisa Hamaker, MD
Thomas Jefferson University Hospital, Philadelphia, Pennsylvania

William F. Harvey, MD
Boston University, Boston, Massachusetts

James W. Heitz, MD
Thomas Jefferson University, Philadelphia, Pennsylvania

Steven K. Herrine, MD
Jefferson Medical College, Thomas Jefferson University, Philadelphia, Pennsylvania

Raymond J. Hohl, MD, PhD
The University of Iowa, Iowa City, Iowa

Sarah A. Holstein, MD, PhD
The University of Iowa, Iowa City, Iowa

Dorothy Holt, PharmD
University of the Sciences in Philadelphia, Philadelphia College of Pharmacy; Thomas Jefferson University Hospital, Philadelphia, Pennsylvania

Linda S. Hostelley, BS
Merck Research Laboratories, West Point, Pennsylvania

Eric R. Houpt, MD
University of Virginia, Charlottesville, Virginia

Shiew-Mei Huang, PhD
Center for Drug Evaluation and Research, United States Food and Drug Administration, Silver Spring, Maryland

David J. Hunter, MBBS, PhD
Boston University; New England Baptist Hospital, Boston, Massachusetts

Serge Jabbour, MD, FACP, FACE
Jefferson Medical College, Thomas Jefferson University, and Thomas Jefferson University Hospital, Philadelphia, Pennsylvania

Robert M. Jacobson, MD
Mayo Clinic College of Medicine, Rochester, Minnesota

Arshad Jahangir, MD
Mayo Clinic, Rochester, Minnesota

Michael A. Jenike, MD
Harvard Medical School, Boston, Massachusetts

Kristine E. Johnson, MD
Johns Hopkins University School of Medicine, Baltimore, Maryland

Victor M. Karpyak, MD, PhD
Mayo Clinic College of Medicine, Rochester, Minnesota

Gregory L. Kearns, PharmD, PhD
University of Missouri–Kansas City; Children's Mercy Hospitals and Clinics, Kansas City, Missouri

Richard M. Keating, MD
The University of Chicago, Chicago, Illinois

Michael P. Keith, MD
Uniformed Services University of the Health Sciences; National Naval Medical Center, Bethesda, Maryland

Sundeep Khosla, MD
Mayo Clinic College of Medicine, Rochester, Minnesota

Julia Kirchheiner, MD, PhD
Institute of Pharmacology of Natural Products and Clinical Pharmacology, University of Ulm, Ulm, Germany

Walter J. Koch, PhD
Center for Translational Medicine, Thomas Jefferson University, Philadelphia, Pennsylvania

Bruce C. Kone, MD
University of Florida College of Medicine; Shands Hospital at the University of Florida, Gainesville, Florida

Walter K. Kraft, MD, MS
Thomas Jefferson University, Philadelphia, Pennsylvania

Robert F. Kushner, MD, MS
Feinberg School of Medicine, Northwestern University, Chicago, Illinois

Christine Laine, MD, MPH
Jefferson Medical College, Thomas Jefferson University; Annals of Internal Medicine, Philadelphia, Pennsylvania

Richard L. Lalonde, PharmD
Pfizer Global Research and Development, New London, Connecticut

Kiwon Lee, MD
College of Physicians and Surgeons, Columbia University, New York, New York

Teofilo Lee-Chiong, MD
National Jewish Medical and Research Center, and University of Colorado Health Sciences Center, Denver, Colorado

Frank T. Leone, MD, MS
University of Pennsylvania; Penn Lung Center, Penn Presbyterian Medical Center, Philadelphia, Pennsylvania

Lawrence J. Lesko, PhD
University of North Carolina, Chapel Hill, North Carolina; University of Florida, Gainesville, Florida; Center for Drug Evaluation and Research, United States Food and Drug Administration, Silver Spring, Maryland

Barbara A. Levey, MD
David Geffen School of Medicine, UCLA, Los Angeles, California

Lionel D. Lewis, MA, MB BCh, MD, FRCP (London)
Dartmouth Medical School and Dartmouth Hitchcock Medical Center, Lebanon, New Hampshire

Joseph Loscalzo, MD, PhD
Harvard Medical School; Brigham and Women's Hospital, Boston, Massachusetts

Anastasios Lymperopoulos, PharmD, MSc, PhD
Center for Translational Medicine, Thomas Jefferson University, Philadelphia, Pennsylvania

Joseph P. Lynch, III, MD
David Geffen School of Medicine at UCLA, Los Angeles, California

Christian Maaser, MD
University of Münster, Münster, Germany

Viqar Maria, MD
Michigan State University, East Lansing, Michigan

Paul E. Marik, MBBCh, FCP (SA), FRCP (C), FCCM, FCCP
Thomas Jefferson University; Thomas Jefferson University Hospital, Philadelphia, Pennsylvania

Marco A. Maurtua, MD
Cleveland Clinic Foundation College of Medicine of Case Western Reserve University; Cleveland Clinic, Cleveland, Ohio

Steven E. McKenzie, MD, PhD
Thomas Jefferson University, Philadelphia, Pennsylvania

Alex Mejia, MD
Thomas Jefferson University, Philadelphia, Pennsylvania

Michael C. Milone, MD, PhD
University of Pennsylvania School of Medicine; Hospital of the University of Pennsylvania, Philadelphia, Pennsylvania

Scott Mintzer, MD
Epilepsy Monitoring Unit and Epilepsy Surgery Program, Thomas Jefferson University, Philadelphia, Pennsylvania

Thomas P. Moyer, PhD
Mayo Clinic College of Medicine; Mayo Clinic, Rochester, Minnesota

David A. Mrazek, MD, FRCPsych
Mayo Clinic College of Medicine; Mayo Clinic, Rochester, Minnesota

Matthew S. Murphy, BMedSc, MB, BCh, BAO
National University of Ireland, Galway; University College Hospital Galway, Newcastle, Galway, Ireland

Filip Mussen, PhD
Merck Research Laboratories, Brussels, Belgium

Jasmine Nabi, MD
The University of Iowa, Iowa City, Iowa

Victor J. Navarro, MD
Thomas Jefferson University Hospital; Jefferson Medical College, Thomas Jefferson University, Philadelphia, Pennsylvania

Timothy J. Nelson, MD, PhD
Mayo Clinic, Rochester, Minnesota

Dionissios Neofytos, MD
Thomas Jefferson University Hospital, Philadelphia, Pennsylvania

Kathleen A. Neville, MD, MS
Children's Mercy Hospitals and Clinics, Kansas City, Missouri

Myaing Nyunt, MD, MPH
Johns Hopkins University School of Medicine, Baltimore, Maryland

Timothy O'Brien, MD, PhD
National University of Ireland, Galway; Regenerative Medicine Institute, National Centre for Biomedical Engineering Science, National University of Ireland, Galway; University College Hospital Galway, Newcastle, Galway, Ireland

Inna G. Ovsyannikova, PhD
Mayo Clinic College of Medicine, Rochester, Minnesota

Chi-Un Pae, MD, PhD
The Catholic University of Korea College of Medicine; Kangnam St. Mary's Hospital, Seoul, South Korea

James F. Pagel, MS, MD
Southern Colorado Residency Program, University of Colorado School of Medicine; Sleep Disorders Center of Southern Colorado, Parkview Episcopal Hospital, Pueblo, Colorado

Ashwin A. Patkar, MD
Duke University Medical Center, Durham, North Carolina

Kah Whye Peng, PhD
Mayo Clinic College of Medicine; Mayo Clinic, Rochester, Minnesota

Edith A. Perez, MD
Mayo Clinic, Jacksonville, Florida

Ronald C. Petersen, MD, PhD
Mayo Clinic College of Medicine, Rochester, Minnesota

Paul A. Pham, PharmD
Johns Hopkins University School of Medicine, Baltimore, Maryland

Jennifer M. Phillips, PhD
University of Pennsylvania, Philadelphia, Pennsylvania

Carissa Pineda, MD
Thomas Jefferson University Hospital; Jefferson Medical College, Thomas Jefferson University, Philadelphia, Pennsylvania

Mark R. Pittelkow, MD
Mayo Clinic College of Medicine, Rochester, Minnesota

Pierre-François Plouin, MD
Université Paris–Descartes; Hôpital Européen Georges Pompidou, Paris, France

Christopher V. Plowe, MD, MPH
Howard Hughes Medical Institute, Center for Vaccine Development, University of Maryland School of Medicine, Baltimore, Maryland

Gregory A. Poland, MD
Mayo Clinic School of Medicine, Rochester, Minnesota

Azad Raiesdana, MD
Harvard Medical School; Brigham and Women's Hospital, Boston, Massachusetts

John N. Ratchford, MD
Johns Hopkins Hospital, Baltimore, Maryland

Nandi J. Reddy, MD
Dartmouth Medical School and Norris Cotton Cancer Center, Lebanon, New Hampshire

Michael D. Reed, PharmD, FCCP, FCP
Children's Hospital Medical Center of Akron; Northeast Ohio Universities College of Medicine, Akron, Ohio

Douglas J. Rhee, MD
Harvard Medical School; Massachusetts Eye and Ear Infirmary, Boston, Massachusetts

Robert A. Rizza, MD
Mayo Clinic College of Medicine, Rochester, Minnesota

David Robertson, MD
General Clinical Research Center, Vanderbilt University Medical Center, Nashville, Tennessee

Dan M. Roden, MD
Oates Institute for Experimental Therapeutics, Vanderbilt University School of Medicine, Nashville, Tennessee

Anne M. Rompalo, MD, ScM
Johns Hopkins University School of Medicine, Baltimore, Maryland

Simona Rossi, MD
Jefferson Medical College, Thomas Jefferson University, Philadelphia, Pennsylvania

Vivek Roy, MD, FACP
Mayo Clinic; Mayo Clinic College of Medicine, Jacksonville, Florida

Stephen J. Russell, MD, PhD
Mayo Clinic College of Medicine; Mayo Clinic, Rochester, Minnesota

Steven Ryder, MD
Astellas Pharma Global Development, Inc., Deerfield, Illinois

Muhammad Wasif Saif, MD, MBBS
Yale Cancer Center, Yale University School of Medicine, New Haven, Connecticut

Rajiv Saini, MD
Weill Cornell Medical College; New York-Presbyterian Hospital, New York; Brookdale University Hospital and Medical Center, Brooklyn, New York

Kyoko Sato, MD
Vanderbilt University School of Medicine, Nashville, Tennessee

Kathryn M. Schak, MD
Mayo Clinic College of Medicine; Mayo Clinic, Rochester, Minnesota

Matthias Schwab, MD
Dr. Margarete Fischer-Bosch Institute of Clinical Pharmacology, Stuttgart; University Hospital, Tuebingen, Germany

Kumar Sharma, MD
Thomas Jefferson University Hospital; Center of Novel Therapies for Kidney Disease, Thomas Jefferson University, Philadelphia, Pennsylvania

Robert G. Sharrar, MD, MSc, DSc (Hon)
Merck Research Laboratories, West Point, Pennsylvania

Leslie M. Shaw, PhD
Clinical Toxicology Laboratory, University of Pennsylvania Medical Center, Philadelphia, Pennsylvania

Ludy Shih, MD
Harvard Medical School; Beth Israel Deaconess Medical Center, Boston, Massachusetts

Steven J. Siegel, MD, PhD
Translational Research Laboratory, University of Pennsylvania, Philadelphia, Pennsylvania

Peter A. Singer, MD
Keck School of Medicine, University of Southern California, Los Angeles, California

David R. Staskin, MD
New York-Presbyterian Hospital; Weill Cornell Medical College, New York, New York

Dale W. Stovall, MD
Virginia Commonwealth University Medical Center, Richmond, Virginia

Jerome F. Strauss, III, MD, PhD
School of Medicine, Virginia Commonwealth University, Richmond, Virginia

Paul V. Targonski, MD
Mayo Clinic College of Medicine, Rochester, Minnesota

Daniel Tarsy, MD
Harvard Medical School; Parkinson's Disease and Movement Disorders Center, Beth Israel Deaconess Medical Center, Boston, Massachusetts

William S. Tasman, MD
Wills Eye Institute, Thomas Jefferson Medical School, Philadelphia, Pennsylvania

Robert Temple, MD
Center for Drug Evaluation and Research, United States Food and Drug Administration, Silver Spring, Maryland

Andre Terzic, MD, PhD
Mayo Clinic, Rochester, Minnesota

John E. Tetzlaff, MD
Cleveland Clinic Lerner College of Medicine of Case Western Reserve University; Anesthesiology Institute, Cleveland Clinic, Cleveland, Ohio

Pritish K. Tosh, MD
Mayo Clinic College of Medicine, Rochester, Minnesota

Erev E. Tubb, MD
Thomas Jefferson University, Philadelphia, Pennsylvania

Kathleen Uhl, MD
Uniformed Services University of the Health Sciences, Bethesda, Maryland; United States Food and Drug Administration, Rockville, Maryland

Patrick Vallance, MD, FRCP, F Med Sci
GlaxoSmithKline, Greenford, Middlesex, United Kingdom

Diederik van de Beek, MD, PhD
Academic Medical Center, University of Amsterdam, Amsterdam, The Netherlands

Adrian Vella, MD, FRCP (Edin)
Mayo Clinic College of Medicine, Rochester, Minnesota

Eugene R. Viscusi, MD
Thomas Jefferson University, Philadelphia, Pennsylvania

John L. Wagner, MD
Merck Research Laboratories, Rahway, New Jersey; Thomas Jefferson University, Philadelphia, Pennsylvania

Scott A. Waldman, MD, PhD, FCP
Thomas Jefferson University, Philadelphia, Pennsylvania

Philip B. Wedegaertner, PhD
Thomas Jefferson University, Philadelphia, Pennsylvania

Alan J. Wein, MD, PhD (Hon)
University of Pennsylvania School of Medicine; Hospital of the University of Pennsylvania, Philadelphia, Pennsylvania

Ethan Weiner, MD
University of Connecticut School of Medicine, Farmington, Connecticut; Pfizer Global Research and Development, New London, Connecticut

Richard Weinshilboum, MD
Mayo Clinic, Rochester, Minnesota

Martijn Weisfelt, MD, PhD
Kennemer Gasthuis, Haarlem, The Netherlands

Lisa G. Winston, MD
University of California, San Francisco; San Francisco General Hospital, San Francisco, California

Run Yu, MD, PhD
David Geffen School of Medicine at UCLA; Carcinoid and Neuroendocrine Tumor Center, Cedars-Sinai Medical Center, Los Angeles, California

Ying Zhang, MD, PhD
Johns Hopkins Bloomberg School of Public Health, Baltimore, Maryland

PREFACE

From its earliest beginnings, the practice of medicine has encompassed patient management through intervention to prevent or treat disease. In turn, the principles of clinical therapeutics are rooted in fundamental pharmacology. Reflecting a continuous landscape without borders, pharmacology and therapeutics are at once intimately interrelated, recursively synergistic, and mutually reinforcing. This nexus of basic and clinical sciences has emerged as central to realizing the clinical value of advances in discovery sciences, driving translation at the laboratory bench to patient-directed practice. The biological and mechanistic diversity inherent in individuals and populations offers unprecedented opportunities to tailor further prevention and treatment, while minimizing off-target adverse events. Indeed, the close interdependence of basic and clinical pharmacological principles and their application to human therapeutics is the cornerstone required to realize the full potential of individualized therapy and the future of clinical care.

Beyond the interrelatedness of scientific principles, the diversity of mutually complementary approaches defines the practice of human therapeutics in the healthcare community worldwide. Students, scholars, and educators in human therapeutics approach the field from divergent practice perspectives with information requirements that emphasize different portions of a continuum of knowledge embodying drug discovery, development, regulation, and utilization. Discovery scientists seek insight into principles underlying the pharmacological basis of (patho)physiology to identify novel targets for therapeutic intervention. Drug development professionals translate discoveries in fundamental mechanisms of disease into safe and effective human therapy through clinical trials. Regulatory experts focus on mechanisms underlying drug actions, their adverse reactions, and their interactions in the context of heterogeneous populations to evaluate empirical data from human clinical trials and formulate objective decisions concerning the safety and efficacy of novel therapeutic agents. Clinicians and other health professionals apply the principles of basic pharmacology, the evidence base that supports specific therapeutic interventions, and an understanding of the principles and practice of clinical pharmacology to formulate and implement therapeutic algorithms that maximize efficacy of care, minimize adverse events, and optimize cost-effectiveness.

Collectively, the pharmacology and therapeutics continuum contributes directly to the value proposition of healthcare delivery. It is recognized that pharmacotherapy is the most cost-effective management tool in the clinical armamentarium. Beyond treatment of active disease, prevention is increasingly extended as a therapeutic paradigm to achieve sustained wellness and disease avoidance. As a prototype of success in public health, disease prophylaxis through immunization represents one of the capstone achievements of medicine in the last century, with a cost-effectiveness unmatched in other models of disease management. Looking forward, the revolution in regenerative medicine and therapeutic repair offers the opportunity to advance the management paradigm from palliation to cure, with the potential to transform the efficiency of disease resolution, shortening hospital stays and decreasing healthcare expenditures over the long-term. Thus, pharmacology and therapeutics is instrumental in realizing the clinical value of advances in the new biology, driving translation of discovery to personalized healthcare solutions.

The multidimensional texture of therapeutics draws from across all life sciences and provides a common thread through distinct patient management strategies. The strength and uniqueness of this contemporary model is rooted in its comprehensive systems approach, where the integrated development of pharmacological therapies enhanced by their companion diagnostics reflects the productivity of the discovery and development components, continuously surveyed and gated through feedback from regulatory and utilization processes. The pipeline of new products, along with the safety and efficacy of applied therapeutics, is thus dependent on the optimum linkage of the discovery engine with the high fidelity of fail-safe surveillance. The overarching goal of this continuum, defined by systems integration, is to achieve better clinical outcomes in patients and populations by ensuring the availability of innovative, effective, and safe therapeutic modalities.

Taken together, these considerations suggest the timeliness for a new textbook in human therapeutics that broadly integrates information over diverse disciplines to serve knowledge requirements across the continuum of practice. To fill this informational and conceptual gap, this new textbook integrates across three dimensions. First, concepts and information are presented in ever-increasing layers of complexity and integration. Next, there is integration across disciplines, wherein each therapeutic topic incorporates relevant information concerning biochemistry, physiology and pathophysiology, basic and clinical pharmacology, and clinical medicine. Lastly, there is integration across the continuum of practice, wherein each therapeutic topic incorporates relevant information or cross-references concerning discovery, development, regulatory considerations, and utilization. Importantly, where appropriate, each therapeutic topic presents specific recommendations for therapy according to guidelines for the standard of care and the critical evidence base that supports those recommendations, with appropriate citations to original literature. In the context of these three dimensions, each chapter in human therapeutics examines the fundamental principles of drug actions, the clinical pharmacology of specific agents, the evidence base supporting the efficacy of key therapeutic agents, practice guidelines for pharmacotherapy, and emerging paradigms for therapeutic intervention in the future. Integration in three dimensions optimizes assimilation of critical information by students and practitioners, permitting a "customized" approach to information acquisition, tailored to specific content requirements and learning platforms across the community of practices.

There are many who deserve acknowledgment, without whose efforts this textbook would not have been possible. Our Editorial Board represents a collection of key knowledge and opinion leaders in the fields of basic and clinical pharmacology and human therapeutics. They provided critical guidance and formative direction with respect to fundamental and applied pharmacological domains on which this textbook is focused. Associate Editors represent leaders in the field of human pharmacology and therapeutics who generously gave of their time to tirelessly review and edit each chapter in order to ensure the textbook met the highest standards of quality, accuracy, timeliness, and uniformity. The contributing Authors represent the backbone of the textbook. Many are colleagues, collaborators, and friends from around the world. All gave generously of their time to prepare and revise their chapters to realize the overarching vision for this textbook, and we take this opportunity to express our foremost gratitude for their scholarly contributions.

Moreover, we acknowledge Neal Benowitz, who had the foresight and confidence to recommend us to lead this project. Special thanks go to Kim Murphy, Publishing Director of Global Medicine, and Elsevier, who recognized a gap in the knowledge base of pharmacology and therapeutics, channeled the resources, and had the confidence in us to envision the project, assemble the team, and materialize the product. A special acknowledgment goes to our Editor, Adrianne Brigido, who has been the heart and soul of this project. With elegance, patience, extraordinary creativity, and aplomb she ensured the project maintained timelines, kept contributors on schedule, maintained production timetables, and filled gaps in conceptual and creative content. Special thanks to the American Society for Clinical Pharmacology and Therapeutics (ASCPT) and its Executive Director, Sharon Swan. Under

Sharon's direction, ASCPT has become a nucleus for the integration of basic and applied pharmacology, giving voice to the discipline of clinical pharmacology, and evolving the concepts across the continuum of drug discovery, development, regulation, and utilization that continue to nucleate the community of practice that embodies the science of therapeutics. Finally, we would like to acknowledge the contributions of our families. Tess, Jacob, Genevieve, and Zachary Waldman; and Carmen and Sofia Terzic provided continuous inspiration for this endeavor. We sincerely hope that their contributions accrue to the benefit of students and practitioners of pharmacology and therapeutics through this textbook.

Scott A. Waldman, MD, PhD, FCP; Philadelphia, Pennsylvania

Andre Terzic, MD, PhD; Rochester, Minnesota

Summer 2008

FOREWORD

Personalized therapy has emerged as the new frontier to realize the clinical value of advances in discovery sciences, driving translation of innovation to patient-centered practice. Modern biology provides the enabling platforms to customize patient-specific therapeutic strategies based on individual genetic makeup to predict, prevent, diagnose, and treat disease, advancing treatments beyond the traditional "one-size-fits-all" approach. The enormity of this challenge is apparent by considering that there are >25,000 genes in humans, and the information encoded therein is exponentially compounded by >100,000 splice variants of messenger RNA. Further, there are 15 million loci along the genome where a single base can differ between individuals or populations, contributing to the polygenic origins of disease. This diversity, further amplified by systems-wide epigenetic and posttranslational modifications, underscores the challenge of individualized therapy.

While daunting for such a complex matrix of information to be resolved, numerous therapeutic advantages come to mind. Identified subpopulations of patients with specific disorders within disease syndromes should permit improved therapeutic responses in smaller populations of patients in clinical trials and thereby reduce drug development costs. Specifically, individual designed therapy may also reduce side effects as well as healthcare costs.

The emergence of customized and personalized medicine as the envisioned future of healthcare, driven by the new biology, suggests the timeliness of a contemporary paradigm to maximize translation of pharmacology to human therapeutics. This paradigm bridges the traditional separation of basic and applied pharmacology. Hierarchically merging these core concepts with supporting principles in basic and clinical sciences forms a framework for defining individualized approaches to the patient, capitalizing on advances in medicine.

The Editors of ***Pharmacology and Therapeutics: Principles to Practice*** have captured that vision, providing a fully integrated curriculum directing the understanding of human therapeutics. This comprehensive textbook uniquely nucleates contemporary information across traditionally disparate domains providing a tool for knowledge acquisition and management. This dynamic synthesis enables clear conceptualization of therapeutics across the spectrum of fundamental and applied practice. Concepts are vertically organized, presented in increasing strata of complexity. Further, information is integrated across scientific disciplines, and therapeutic topics to incorporate concepts central to cell biology, biochemistry, physiology and pathophysiology, fundamental and applied pharmacology, and molecular and clinical medicine. Moreover, therapeutic topics incorporate concepts across the matrix of discovery, development, regulatory sciences, and utilization algorithms. Full integration across the continuum of practice is reflected by therapeutic recommendations formulated from recent practice guidelines for the standard of care and the evidence base that supports those recommendations.

I applaud the Editors for bringing together, between the covers of this first edition, a superb textbook bridging basic and clinical pharmacology, from classic principles to future concepts. This exciting textbook will be invaluable to students, scholars, and professionals across the practice in human therapeutics. My congratulations to the Editors for undertaking this enormous task of dedication, and for the outstanding result of those efforts.

Ferid Murad, MD, PhD

Nobel Laureate

Houston, Texas

Spring 2008

CONTENTS

Part I

Principles, 1

PHARMACOTHERAPEUTIC CONTINUUM: ENGINEERING THE FUTURE OF INDIVIDUALIZED MEDICINE, 3
Scott A. Waldman and Andre Terzic

SECTION 1 **Pharmacotherapeutic Continuum,** 7

1 DRUG DISCOVERY, 7
Patrick Vallance

2 DRUG DEVELOPMENT, 15
Steven Ryder and Ethan Weiner

3 REGULATIONS AND PHARMACOVIGILANCE, 29
Robert G. Sharrar, Linda S. Hostelley, and Filip Mussen

4 EVIDENCE-BASED DRUG UTILIZATION, 41
Christine Laine

SECTION 2 **Molecular Pharmacology,** 51

5 DRUG-RECEPTOR INTERACTIONS, 51
Scott A. Waldman

6 SIGNAL TRANSDUCTION, 67
Philip B. Wedegaertner

7 CELL CYCLE PHARMACOLOGY, ANTIPROLIFERATION, AND APOPTOSIS, 83
Sarah A. Holstein and Raymond J. Hohl

SECTION 3 **Systems Pharmacology,** 91

8 NEUROTRANSMITTERS, 91
Eduardo E. Benarroch

9 AUTONOMIC PHARMACOLOGY, 115
Anastasios Lymperopoulos and Walter J. Koch

10 FLUID AND ELECTROLYTE HOMEOSTASIS, 141
Bruce C. Kone

11 INFLAMMATION AND IMMUNOMODULATION, 157
Laurence J. Egan

12 PHARMACOBIOLOGY OF INFECTIONS, 173
Dionissios Neofytos, Claudine El-Beyrouty, and Joseph A. DeSimone, Jr.

SECTION 4 **Clinical Pharmacology,** 193

13 PHARMACOKINETICS, 193
Arthur J. Atkinson, Jr.

14 PHARMACODYNAMICS, 203
Richard L. Lalonde

15 PHARMACOGENETICS AND PHARMACOGENOMICS, 219
Richard Weinshilboum

16 HETEROGENEITY OF DRUG RESPONSES AND INDIVIDUALIZATION OF THERAPY, 225
Julia Kirchheiner and Matthias Schwab

17 PEDIATRIC PHARMACOLOGY, 239
Kathleen A. Neville, Michael J. Blake, Michael D. Reed, and Gregory L. Kearns

18 SEX DIFFERENCES IN PHARMACOLOGY, 251
Jean Gray

19 PHARMACOLOGY ACROSS THE AGING CONTINUUM, 257
Naomi Gronich and Darrell R. Abernethy

20 ADVERSE DRUG REACTIONS AND INTERACTIONS, 265
Shiew-Mei Huang, Lawrence J. Lesko, and Robert Temple

21 THERAPEUTIC DRUG MONITORING, 275
Michael C. Milone and Leslie M. Shaw

Part II

Practice, 289

SECTION 5 **Cardiovascular Therapeutics,** 291

22 HYPERTENSION, 291
Jean-Luc Elghozi, Michel Azizi, and Pierre-François Plouin

23 DYSLIPIDEMIAS, 303
Matthew S. Murphy and Timothy O'Brien

24 CORONARY ARTERY DISEASE, 321
Arshad Jahangir and Viqar Maria

25 RHYTHM DISORDERS, 367
Dawood Darbar and Dan M. Roden

26 HEART FAILURE, 389
Arthur M. Feldman

SECTION 6 **Pulmonary Therapeutics,** 401

27 PULMONARY ARTERIAL HYPERTENSION, 401
Azad Raiesdana and Joseph Loscalzo

28 ASTHMA AND CHRONIC OBSTRUCTIVE PULMONARY DISEASE, 417
Walter K. Kraft and Frank T. Leone

SECTION 7 **Renal Therapeutics,** 435

29 RENAL INSUFFICIENCY, 435
Kumar Sharma

30 VOIDING DYSFUNCTION, 445
Alan J. Wein, Rajiv Saini, and David R. Staskin

SECTION 8 **Gastroenterologic Therapeutics,** 457

31 ACID REFLUX AND ULCER DISEASE, 457
Alex Mejia and Walter K. Kraft

32 MOTILITY DISORDERS, 475
Michael Camilleri and Viola Andresen

33 INFLAMMATORY BOWEL DISEASES, 487
Laurence J. Egan and Christian Maaser

34 HEPATIC CIRRHOSIS, 505
Victor J. Navarro, Simona Rossi, and Steven K. Herrine

35 INFECTIOUS HEPATITIS, 527
Steven K. Herrine, Simona Rossi, and Victor J. Navarro

SECTION 9 **Endocrinologic Therapeutics,** 549

36 OBESITY AND NUTRITION, 549
Robert F. Kushner

37 DIABETES MELLITUS, 557
Robert A. Rizza and Adrian Vella

38 DISORDERS OF THE THYROID, 571
Helen L. Baron and Peter A. Singer

39 DISORDERS OF CALCIUM METABOLISM AND BONE MINERALIZATION, 587
Bart L. Clarke and Sundeep Khosla

40 DISORDERS OF THE HYPOTHALAMIC-PITUITARY AXIS, 611
Run Yu and Glenn D. Braunstein

41 ADRENAL DISORDERS, 623
Lisa Hamaker and Serge Jabbour

42 REPRODUCTIVE HEALTH, 631
Dale W. Stovall and Jerome F. Strauss, III

SECTION 10 **Neuropharmacologic Therapeutics,** 641

43 ALZHEIMER'S DISEASE AND DEMENTIAS, 641
Wael N. Haidar and Ronald C. Petersen

44 PARKINSON'S DISEASE, 651
Ludy Shih and Daniel Tarsy

45 SEIZURE DISORDERS, 663
Scott Mintzer

46 MULTIPLE SCLEROSIS, 685
Benjamin M. Greenberg, John N. Ratchford, and Peter A. Calabresi

47 DYSAUTONOMIAS, 703
Kyoko Sato, André Diedrich, and David Robertson

48 HEADACHE, 719
Alfredo Bianchi

49 STROKE, 743
Rodney Bell, Kiwon Lee, Carissa Pineda, and David Brock

SECTION 11 **Psychopharmacologic Therapeutics,** 753

50 OBSESSIVE-COMPULSIVE DISORDERS, 753
Darin D. Dougherty and Michael A. Jenike

51 ATTENTION-DEFICIT/HYPERACTIVITY DISORDER, 759
David A. Mrazek and Kathryn M. Schak

52 ANXIETY, 769
Chi-Un Pae and Ashwin A. Patkar

53 DEPRESSION AND BIPOLAR DISORDERS, 787
Wade Berrettini

54 PSYCHOSIS AND SCHIZOPHRENIA, 797
Steven J. Siegel, Mary E. Dankert, and Jennifer M. Phillips

55 DRUG ADDICTION, 817
Doo-Sup Choi, Victor M. Karpyak, Mark A. Frye, Daniel K. Hall-Flavin, and David A. Mrazek

56 NICOTINE DEPENDENCE, 837
Neal L. Benowitz

57 INSOMNIA (NARCOLEPSY)-RELATED DISORDERS, 849
Teofilo Lee-Chiong and James F. Pagel

SECTION 12 **Ophthalmologic Therapeutics,** 857

58 DRUGS IN OPHTHALMOLOGY, 857
Douglas J. Rhee and William S. Tasman

SECTION 13 **Anesthesia,** 863

59 LOCAL ANESTHESIA, 863
John E. Tetzlaff

60 GENERAL ANESTHESIA AND SEDATION, 873
Joseph F. Foss and Marco A. Maurtua

61 TREATMENT OF PAIN, 883
Kishor Gandhi, James W. Heitz, and Eugene R. Viscusi

SECTION 14 **Hematologic Therapeutics,** 895

62 ANEMIAS AND CYTOPENIAS, 895
Nandi J. Reddy and Lionel D. Lewis

63 DISORDERS OF HEMOSTASIS AND THROMBOSIS, 909
Erev E. Tubb and Steven E. McKenzie

SECTION 15 **Oncologic Therapeutics,** 921

64 LUNG CANCER, 921
Sarah A. Holstein and Raymond J. Hohl

65 BREAST CANCER, 933
Vivek Roy and Edith A. Perez

66 HEMATOLOGIC MALIGNANCIES, 945
Jasmine Nabi and Raymond J. Hohl

67 PROSTATE CANCER, 951
Sarah A. Holstein and Raymond J. Hohl

68 COLON CANCER, 959
Muhammad Wasif Saif and Robert B. Diasio

69 MELANOMA, 969
Jasmine Nabi and Raymond J. Hohl

SECTION 16 **Dermatologic Therapeutics,** 973

70 ACNE, 973
Joseph Genebriera and Mark Davis

71 PSORIASIS, 983
Mark R. Pittelkow and Joseph Genebriera

72 DERMATITIS, 1007
Mark Davis

SECTION 17 Rheumatologic Therapeutics, 1015

73 OSTEOARTHRITIS, 1015
William F. Harvey and David J. Hunter

74 RHEUMATOID ARTHRITIS, 1025
Richard M. Keating

75 GOUT, 1039
Michael P. Keith, William R. Gilliland, and Kathleen Uhl

76 SYSTEMIC LUPUS ERYTHEMATOSUS, 1047
William R. Gilliland, Michael P. Keith, and Kathleen Uhl

SECTION 18 Therapy of Infectious Diseases, 1063

77 INFLUENZA AND VIRAL RESPIRATORY INFECTIONS, 1063
Joseph P. Lynch, III

78 COMMUNITY-ACQUIRED PNEUMONIA, 1081
Andrew R. Haas and Paul E. Marik

79 TUBERCULOSIS, 1089
Ying Zhang

80 BACTERIAL MENINGITIS, 1109
Diederik van de Beek, Martijn Weisfelt, and Jan de Gans

81 ENDOCARDITIS, 1121
Lisa G. Winston, Daniel Deck, and Ann F. Bolger

82 MALARIA, 1141
Myaing Nyunt and Christopher V. Plowe

83 PROTOZOAN AND HELMINTHIC INFECTIONS, 1171
Eric R. Houpt and Omer Chaudhry

84 HIV INFECTIONS AND AIDS, 1187
Paul A. Pham and Charles W. Flexner

85 SEXUALLY TRANSMITTED DISEASES, 1201
Kristine E. Johnson and Anne M. Rompalo

SECTION 19 Practical Therapeutics, 1213

86 MEDICAL TOXICOLOGY AND ANTIDOTES, 1213
Thomas P. Moyer

87 OVER-THE-COUNTER MEDICATIONS, 1221
Barbara A. Levey

88 PRESCRIPTION AND ORDER WRITING, 1225
Carol L. Beck

89 PHARMACY AND THERAPEUTICS COMMITTEES AND THE HOSPITAL FORMULARY, 1233
Joseph S. Bertino, Jr.

SECTION 20 Emerging Therapeutics, 1237

90 COMPLEMENTARY AND ALTERNATIVE MEDICINE, NUTRACEUTICALS, AND DIETARY SUPPLEMENTS, 1237
Christine A. Haller

91 VACCINES, 1247
Paul V. Targonski, Inna G. Ovsyannikova, Pritish K. Tosh, Robert M. Jacobson, and Gregory A. Poland

92 TRANSPLANT MEDICINE, 1269
Mark Chaballa, Joanne Filicko-O'Hara, Dorothy Holt, Adam M. Frank, John L. Wagner, Dolores Grosso, and Neal Flomenberg

93 GENE THERAPY, 1295
Stephen J. Russell and Kah Whye Peng

94 REGENERATIVE MEDICINE AND STEM CELL THERAPEUTICS, 1317
Timothy J. Nelson, Atta Behfar, and Andre Terzic

INDEX, 1333

Part I

Principles

SECTION 1 Pharmacotherapeutic Continuum
1 Drug Discovery
2 Drug Development
3 Regulations and Pharmacovigilance
4 Evidence-Based Drug Utilization

SECTION 2 Molecular Pharmacology
5 Drug-Receptor Interactions
6 Signal Transduction
7 Cell Cycle Pharmacology, Antiproliferation, and Apoptosis

SECTION 3 Systems Pharmacology
8 Neurotransmitters
9 Autonomic Pharmacology
10 Fluid and Electrolyte Homeostasis
11 Inflammation and Immunomodulation
12 Pharmacobiology of Infections

SECTION 4 Clinical Pharmacology
13 Pharmacokinetics
14 Pharmacodynamics
15 Pharmacogenetics and Pharmacogenomics
16 Heterogeneity of Drug Responses and Individualization of Therapy
17 Pediatric Pharmacology
18 Sex Differences in Pharmacology
19 Pharmacology Across the Aging Continuum
20 Adverse Drug Reactions and Interactions
21 Therapeutic Drug Monitoring

PHARMACOTHERAPEUTIC CONTINUUM: ENGINEERING THE FUTURE OF INDIVIDUALIZED MEDICINE

Scott A. Waldman and Andre Terzic

Pharmacology and therapeutics, from principles to practice, constitute an essential biomedical discipline at the core of drug discovery science and patient care, integrating translational medicine to treat illness and preserve health.[1] *Pharmacology* comes from the ancient Greek words φάρμακον (*pharmakon*), or "drug," and λόγος (*logos*), or "knowledge." *Therapeutics,* from θεραπευτικός (*therapeutikos*), concerns the healing and curing of disease. Medical therapy has emerged from the earliest forms of treatment exemplified by empirical use of herbal remedies, animal extracts, and minerals.[2] Galen, considered a pioneer in the practice of pharmacology as early as 150 AD, recognized the importance of experimentation and theory in the rational use of medicines. In the 16th century, Paracelsus provided impetus to pharmacology by investigating active ingredients of therapeutic preparations, recognizing that the dose determines whether a compound is therapeutic or toxic.[3] Pharmacology evolved in the 19th century, with the work of Oswald Schmiedeberg, as a modern biomedical science applying principles of investigation to therapeutic contexts, making drug development possible. Over the next century, the science of human therapeutics rapidly advanced based on the expanding comprehension of disease mechanisms and identification of drug targets. Today, pharmacology is the cornerstone of the drug discovery and development process.[4] The genetic revolution has promoted to the forefront a novel concept at the heart of pharmacology and therapeutics—the right drug for the right target in the right patient and delivered at the right dose.[5] Indeed, in the 21st century, pharmacology and therapeutics are poised to apply individual genetic and molecular profiles to prognosis, prediction, cure, and prevention in pursuit of individualized health care[6] (Fig. 1).

Major advances in fundamental mechanisms underlying (patho)physiology over the past decades have generated a robust therapeutic armamentarium, exemplified by synthetic hormones, multigenerational antibiotics, and recombinant vaccines, offering effective interventions across a range of diseases.[7] The exponential ascent of the new biology has transformed the comprehension of human health and disease and revolutionized technology; redefining clinical pharmacology in the context of discovery and translation, and the role of the clinical pharmacologist as the bridge between the laboratory, the patient, and the population at large.[8,9] The integration of cross-disciplinary concepts emerging from discovery and driving therapeutic solutions has focused clinical pharmacology on the identification and deployment of tools for prognosis, prediction, cure, and, ultimately, prevention in a context of personalized medicine.[10] The promise of clinical pharmacology and its impact on the future of therapeutics, in the emerging areas of combinatorial pharmacogenetics, targeted interference with disease, and stem cell–based tissue repair and regeneration, to name a few, extends beyond individuals toward populations of all ages in need of individualized treatment for disease.[11-13] Indeed, the full potential of clinical pharmacology and therapeutics will only be achieved in the most global scope of world health.[14]

Modern pharmacology integrates across the spectrum of drug discovery, development, regulation, and utilization (Fig. 2). Discovery has been transformed by the integration of the enabling technologies of genomics, proteomics, metabolomics, molecular imaging, and applied systems biology, with concomitant advances in the curational sciences of bioinformatics, medical informatics, and biorepositories to resolve the molecular underpinnings of disease pathobiology.[15,16] The confluence of these synergistic technological platforms has provided the toolbox enabling the finest resolution of molecular elements underlying signaling pathways, effectors, and mediators central to normal physiology, and which are corrupted in disease.[17] The increased identification of these molecules and the concomitant mapping of their polygamous interactions offer insights that translate directly into targeted diagnostics and therapeutics, prognostic discriminators of disease variability, and predictors of treatment response subsets, refining the therapeutic objective at individual patient and population levels. It is anticipated that the continued elucidation of molecules and their interactions underlying pathobiology will provide the lexicon that ultimately must be translated to provide integrated diagnostic and therapeutic solutions for advanced patient management.[18]

Translation of fundamental pharmacologic principles at the bench into therapeutic modalities at the bedside has been based in the art of generalizing knowledge derived from preclinical and clinical trials to treatment guidelines in daily practice. Evidence-based medicine has emerged as an essential guide to patient management. While great inroads have been achieved in the science of therapeutics, the current challenges of today's pharmacotherapy include lack of specificity, interindividual variability, and off-target effects.[19] The sciences of molecular medicine have provided a powerful catalyst to generate integrated diagnostic and therapeutic platforms that can ultimately be tailored to the genetic and molecular profile of the individual patient to enhance specificity, reduce variability, and minimize adverse effects.[20] In this way, advances in molecular medicine are transforming the contemporary therapeutic continuum, including discovery through identification of specific therapeutic targets, development through subsetting patients and diseases, regulation through identifying pathways mediating off-target effects, and utilization through matching the patient to the optimal drug and dosing regimen.[21]

Beyond discovery of new diagnostic and therapeutic modalities, state-of-the-art technologies have provided tools to define dynamic disease states while exposing pathways of intervention. In this way, molecular medicine has advanced the identification of quantifiable measures predicting disease progression, susceptibility to therapy, and sensitivity to adverse drug reactions. These enabling platforms have opened a window on the molecular ontogeny of diverse disease syndromes, defining the spatiotemporal sequence of genetic and molecular alterations integrated at the systems level to form the mechanistic foundation from risk burden to development of overt disease.[22] Dissection of disease processes offers an unprecedented opportunity to identify and intervene in the earliest preclinical stages of disease, prior to irreversible disruption of tissue and decompensation of organ function. By resolving the intimate circuitry of processes that crystallize the biologic and pathophysiologic framework of drug action, molecular

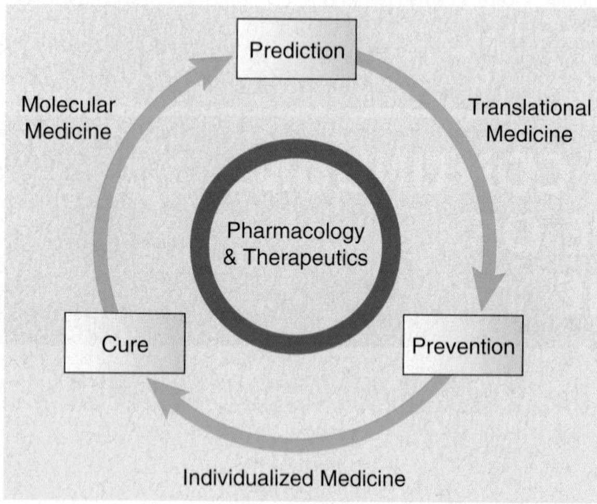

FIGURE 1 • Pharmacology and therapeutics, driven by advances in molecular, translational, and individualized medicine, have evolved into a multidisciplinary platform transforming the clinical enterprise, and enabling the application of evidenced-based customized solutions to achieve disease prediction, prevention, and cure.

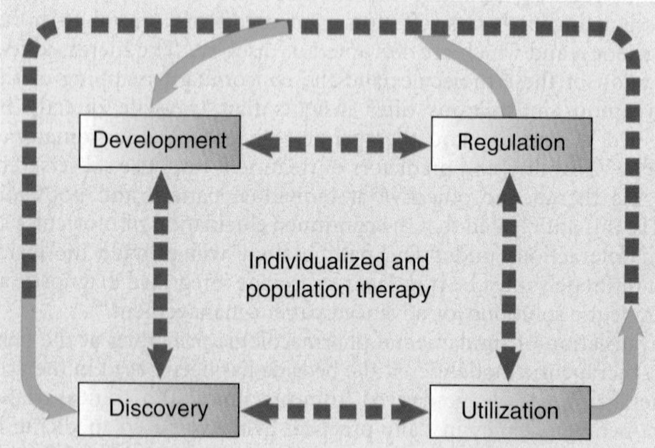

FIGURE 2 • The pharmacotherapeutic continuum encompasses the integrated modules of discovery, development, regulation, and utilization. Collectively, these processes are required for translation of molecular discoveries into safe and effective patient care at the levels of individuals and populations.

medicine has imposed evolutionary pressure transforming development and regulatory modules.

Molecular and genetic profiles sort patients into categories based on pathobiologic mechanisms providing predictive biomarkers, eliminating variability in drug responsiveness, thereby optimizing selection of patient populations to maximize the likelihood of success in critical-stage clinical trials. Conversely, metabolic genotyping and phenotyping identify patients with variable pharmacokinetics, placing them at greatest risk for adverse drug events, who therefore most benefit from dose adjustment to optimize safety.[23] Together, these previously unavailable technical and conceptual capabilities optimize therapeutics applied broadly across populations with inherent genetic and environmental variabilities, improving drug development success rates, return on research and development investment, and therapeutic efficacy, while reducing so-called idiosyncratic drug reactions and interactions, improving drug safety for each patient.

Insights into disease pathobiology and resultant innovations in target and biomarker identification and validation, prognostic and predictive patient subsetting, metabolic profiling, and target-based drug development and regulation—all directly emerging from the tools and concepts of molecular medicine—are rapidly transforming drug utilization in clinical practice. For example, insights gained from the dissection of the circuitry by which receptors for epidermal growth factor (EGF) regulate the growth and survival of cells and the corruption of those circuits in neoplasia established their role as key mechanism-based therapeutic targets in breast and lung cancer. In that regard, heterogeneity of expression motivated the integration of EGF receptor testing as a necessary prerequisite to subsetting patients with breast cancer to establish their eligibility to receive anti-EGF receptor monoclonal antibody therapy. Similarly, heterogeneity in mutations by tumors revealed the importance of profiling patients with lung cancer, to establish eligibility to receive small-molecule inhibitors of EGF receptors. Conversely, insights provided by metabolic profiling revealed the centrality of genetic polymorphisms in drug-metabolizing enzymes in mechanisms underlying life-threatening adverse drug responses in patients with solid tumors receiving irinotecan or those with leukemia receiving mercaptopurines.

While molecular medicine has revolutionized each node along the pharmacotherapeutic continuum to optimize the discovery, development, and implementation of therapeutic innovation, challenges remain in realizing the full potential in clinical uptake. Major challenges impeding implementation include the lack of evidence basis for clinical utility; unresolved issues with costs and coverage criteria; uncertainty of the regulatory pathway for the products of molecular medicine; and limitations in the specialized workforce and the science of health care delivery to integrate genomic-based technologies with clinical practice.[24] Additionally, these issues highlight previously unrecognized obstacles comprising legal liability and ethical challenges with respect to the application of the emerging molecular medicine armamentarium to patient care that will require solutions to maximize clinical uptake.[25] These challenges are highly related, since regulatory approval, payment, and clinical uptake are often predicated on the strength of the evidence about clinical utility and value.

These considerations notwithstanding, the revolution in molecular medicine has charted an unprecedented path for the development and application of novel diagnostic and therapeutic entities. The integrative role of clinical pharmacology in defining and implementing the pharmacotherapeutic continuum, and the unprecedented impact of molecular medicine at all stages along this continuum, integrates these two paradigms, placing them at the intersection of contemporary medical practice in the context of individual patients and populations. The promise that lies ahead is a transformation of diagnostic and therapeutic objectives from palliation to cure, ultimately achieving disease prediction and prevention, thereby engineering the future of individualized medicine to improve the value proposition and transform clinical practice.

REFERENCES

1. Waldman SA, Terzic MR, Terzic A. Molecular medicine hones therapeutic arts to science. Clin Pharmacol Ther 2007;82:343-347.
2. Vallance P, Smart TG. The future of pharmacology. Br J Pharmacol 2006;147:S304-S307.
3. Atkinson A, Lalonde R. Introduction of quantitative methods in pharmacology and clinical pharmacology: a historical overview. Clin Pharmacol Ther 2007;82:3-6.
4. Waldman SA, Christensen NB, Moore JE, Terzic A. Clinical pharmacology: the science of therapeutics. Clin Pharmacol Ther 2007;81:3-6.
5. Waldman SA, Terzic A. Individualized medicine and the imperative of global health. Clin Pharmacol Ther 2007;82:479-483.
6. Hood L, Heath JR, Phelps ME, Lin B. Systems biology and new technologies enable predictive and preventative medicine. Science 2004;306:640-643.
7. Waldman SA, Terzic A. Therapeutic targeting: a crucible for individualized medicine. Clin Pharmacol Ther 2008;83:651-654.
8. Honig PK. The value and future of clinical pharmacology. Clin Pharmacol Ther 2007;81:17-18.
9. Fitzgerald GA. Clinical pharmacology or translational medicine and therapeutics: reinvent or rebrand and expand? Clin Pharmacol Ther 2007;81:19-20.
10. Lesko LJ. Personalized medicine: elusive dream or imminent reality? Clin Pharmacol Ther 2007;81:807-816.
11. Pennisi E. Human genetic variation. Science 2007;318:1842-1843.
12. Giacomini KM, Brett CM, Altman RB, et al, for the Pharmacogenetics Research Network. The Pharmacogenetics Research Network: from SNP discovery to clinical drug response. Clin Pharmacol Ther 2007;81:328-345.
13. Piquette-Miller M, Grant DM. The art and science of personalized medicine. Clin Pharmacol Ther 2007;81:311-315.
14. Cortese DA. A vision of individualized medicine in the context of global health. Clin Pharmacol Ther 2007;82:491-493.

15. Hood L, Perlmutter RM. The impact of systems approaches on biological problems in drug discovery. Nat Biotechnol 2004;22:1215-1217.
16. Silver PA, Way JC. Molecular systems biology in drug development. Clin Pharmacol Ther 2007;82:586-590.
17. Waldman SA, Terzic A. Biomarkers in medicine: targeted diagnostics and therapeutics for individualized patient management. Biomarkers Med 2007;1:3-8.
18. Woodcock J. The prospects for "personalized medicine" in drug development and drug therapy. Clin Pharmacol Ther 2007;81:164-169.
19. Lesko LJ. Paving the critical path: how can clinical pharmacology help achieve the vision? Clin Pharmacol Ther 2007;81:170-177.
20. Wilson C, Schulz S, Waldman SA. Biomarker development, commercialization, and regulation: individualization of medicine lost in translation. Clin Pharmacol Ther 2007;81:153-155.
21. Wagner JA, Williams SA, Webster CJ. Biomarkers and surrogate end points for fit-for-purpose development and regulatory evaluation of new drugs. Clin Pharmacol Ther 2007;81:104-107.
22. Waldman SA, Terzic A. Translating microRNA discovery into clinical biomarkers in cancer. JAMA 2007;297:1921-1923.
23. Honig P. Benefit and risk assessment in drug development and utilization: a role for clinical pharmacology. Clin Pharmacol Ther 2007;82:109-112.
24. Buckman S, Huang SM, Murphy S. Medical product development and regulatory science for the 21st century: the critical path vision and its impact on health care. Clin Pharmacol Ther 2007;81:141-144.
25. Lee SS. The ethical implications of stratifying by race in pharmacogenomics. Clin Pharmacol Ther 2007;81:122-125.

1 DRUG DISCOVERY

Patrick Vallance

INTRODUCTION 7
WHAT MAKES A GOOD TARGET? 7
VALIDATING A TARGET 8
LEAD IDENTIFICATION 8
LEAD OPTIMIZATION 8
CLINICAL PHARMACOLOGY STUDIES 9
Testing the Concept 9
ALTERNATIVE APPROACHES—BIOPHARMACEUTICALS 13
GENETICS AND GENOMICS 14
CONCLUSIONS 14

INTRODUCTION

Drug discovery might better be termed *drug invention*. This inventive process starts with the decision about which target to work on and ends with a molecule that has achieved enough "proof of concept" to establish it as a potential new medicine. Traditionally, a drug is a small molecule with a molecular weight below 1000 that interferes with protein function, but of course in recent years, the number of exceptions to this model has increased. Large antibodies now form an important part of the therapeutic armamentarium, and small molecules may be directed at nonprotein targets.

WHAT MAKES A GOOD TARGET?

The first step of the process is to identify the target. The identification of a target may trigger a process that lasts 15 years or more and incurs very considerable expense. It is, therefore, probably the single most important decision made in drug discovery. Ideally, a target would be a single molecular entity in a pathway known to be of key importance in pathophysiology. It is worth considering target identification in relation to some of the key drugs in widespread clinical use. Professor Sir James Black[1] describes the process in his Nobel lecture. When he started his work on β-blockers, it was known that the onset of angina occurred when the heart rate increased in response to anxiety, emotion, or exercise. Adrenaline had been used as a provocation test, and it was recognized that heart rate increased when adrenaline stimulated subtypes of adrenoceptor on the heart. The target, therefore, was the β receptor, and the simple hypothesis was that blocking the receptor would slow the heart and thereby alter the threshold for onset of anginal symptoms. As Black put it, "I started at I.C.I. with a clear goal—I wanted to find a β-receptor antagonist. I expected this to reduce pulse rates at rest and during exercise and hoped that it would decrease the susceptibility of patients to angina pectoris." The important steps described in this simple tale are that (i) there was an understanding of the disease process, (ii) a key step in the disease symptomatology had been identified, and (iii) the physiology of the desired change was understood. A similar elegant story can be told for his identification of H_2 receptors as targets for ulcer healing. It might be argued in terms of target selection that the low-hanging fruit has been picked or that we have addressed simple command and control physiologic systems and are now tackling the more tricky areas of consensus or permissive modulation of complex processes, but the fundamental principles of target selection remain the same—understand the disease, understand the nature of the desired effect, and select a target in a key pathway to initiate the desired change: Easy to write and considerably more difficult to achieve.

A second consideration for target identification relates to the potential tractability of the target. Certain classes of target are considered intrinsically more likely to be "druggable" (amenable to chemistry that might ultimately lead to a compound with the properties of a medicine) than are others. For example, history indicates that seven transmembrane-spanning receptors (G protein–coupled receptors [GPCRs]) are good targets and identification of enzyme inhibitors is achievable, whereas finding enzyme activators may be tougher and disrupting protein-protein interaction with small molecules has been considered nigh on impossible, although this view is changing. Indeed, it is important to recognize that these are generalizations and that classes that once were seen as difficult, such as nuclear hormone receptors or kinases, have become tractable as an understanding of molecular structure and structure-activity relationships emerges.

The third consideration is a practical one related to assays. A robust, reproducible assay is essential. The approach to chemistry determines to some extent the nature of the required assay and vice versa. For high-throughput chemistry, an assay has to be scalable; for low-throughput iterative medicinal chemistry, more complex bioassays may be appropriate.

To what extent is the size of the potential market or the assessment of unmet medical need taken into account at this stage? No doubt this will vary depending on the priorities of the funder, but reality suggests that at this very early stage, it is usually possible to construct a plausible argument for pursuing a target if the scientific rationale is strong, an unmet patient need can be identified, and the target falls within the class of being druggable. Thus, the primary driver should be, and usually is, scientific opportunity coupled to an understanding of potential therapeutic outcome.

These processes of target identification hold true in principle today, but some things have changed. The molecular and genetic revolution identified hundreds of novel targets and many molecularly distinct subtypes of protein targets. In this approach, the molecular target can be clearly defined, but the function and its place in pathophysiology may remain obscure. This increase in molecular identification led to a change in paradigm in the 1990s, and it became fashionable to identify potential targets based on molecular convenience rather than clear pathophysiologic understanding. It also led for a while to the idea that a genetic association alone might provide justification for considering a protein sufficiently implicated in disease biology for it to become a drug target. Whereas genetic association can be a very important tool as part of developing a case for the pathophysiologic importance of a particular target, it paints only part of the picture. It is also important to remember that some targets important for drug action may not necessarily be implicated in the genetics of disease causation.

VALIDATING A TARGET

The ultimate validation of a target occurs in the clinic. The higher the degree of novelty of a target, the higher the degree of risk. To work on a fully validated target is in essence to set out to make a "me-too" medicine, because it means that there is already a medicine of proven efficacy based on that target. To work on a target identified as a protein with unknown function is to set out on a voyage of discovery with a very high risk of failure. In many instances, work starts on a target with some sort of biologic or clinical plausibility but with significant residual uncertainty. One approach is to identify partially validated targets (e.g., when a clinical "proof of concept" study has been published by a competitor) and then put a concerted effort to catch up or overtake—a fast-follower approach. Often, risk is reduced by selection of a novel target that nonetheless lies in a validated pathway. This involves pathway analysis and, increasingly, systems biology and bioinformatics to map out pathways, model integrated biology, and identify several points of potential interference. These approaches are likely to become increasingly important.

Confidence building at the early stages of drug discovery relies on multiple approaches. The process may be divided neatly, and rather artificially, into two: observational and interventional validation. Observational validation may be considered akin to circumstantial evidence in a court case. It could include analysis of expression or activity of the pathway or target of interest in cells, human tissues, or animal models of disease, gene association studies, and epidemiology. These observations may build a case, but they cannot deliver proof of causality. In contrast, interventional validation disrupts the target and directly probes validity, but it may have to do so in cells or animal models rather than in the clinic. Intervention may be through pharmacology, use of a tool compound, or through molecular tools. Genetically modified mice have been used to build confidence in a target, but of course, they have limitations in terms of species-specificity and the nature of the intervention. Interference with RNAi is increasingly used as a convenient way to disrupt pathways in human cells or animal models. The principles underlying target validation are

- Use multiple approaches.
- Use human cells and tissue where possible—ideally both diseased and healthy tissue.
- Glean as much information as possible from the clinic—from experimental medicine to observational epidemiology.
- Introduce interventional validation techniques as soon as possible.

The use of tool compounds to probe the validity of a pathway in the patients is still the exception rather than the rule but, if feasible, can provide considerable early confidence in the target. The readout might be some measure of pharmacodynamics or could be a demonstration of appropriate in vivo distribution with imaging techniques such as positron emission tomography (PET).

LEAD IDENTIFICATION

Once a target has been identified, the process of chemistry starts. The aim is to generate a lead molecule or, ideally, several chemically diverse lead series. The reason for starting with several different series is that structure-related unwanted effects or toxicity may be averted by switching series. Compounds must meet specific criteria in relation to potency (the strength of the interaction between the compound and the target), selectivity (the extent to which other targets are also affected), toxicity, and druggability. It is worth noting that when dealing with a novel target, toxicity of a molecule might be due to effects mediated through the desired pharmacologic effect on the target ("on-target" toxicity) or to effects on other pathways or molecules ("off-target" toxicity).

In some cases, the initial approach may be based on chemical modification of the natural ligand of a receptor or the substrate of an enzyme. However, in many cases, some form of screening will be undertaken looking for activities without a priori assumptions about the molecular scaffold. Whichever route is taken, it is necessary to design a robust and reproducible assay. Pharmaceutical companies have built up large collections of compounds, running into millions, and processes that allow automated robotic screening (Fig. 1-1). Several different screening approaches may be taken: high throughput across an entire collection, screening across a tailored library, or from specific subsets of compounds. Screening sets may be selectively enriched with compounds with a desired set of properties or may comprise only fragments from which full molecules can be synthesized. In large screening libraries, the initial "hit" needs to be identified and resynthesized and the positive result confirmed. Developing a lead molecule from the initial hit may not be straightforward. Some hits may not be druggable or may be promiscuous in their affinity for other targets. For others, crystal structure information about the target may help make rational modifications, or groups of chemists with "target-class expertise" may bring special insights into what will work and what will not. Starting with more than one lead series of diverse chemical structure increases the chance of ending up with a drug that will make it through the minefield that follows.

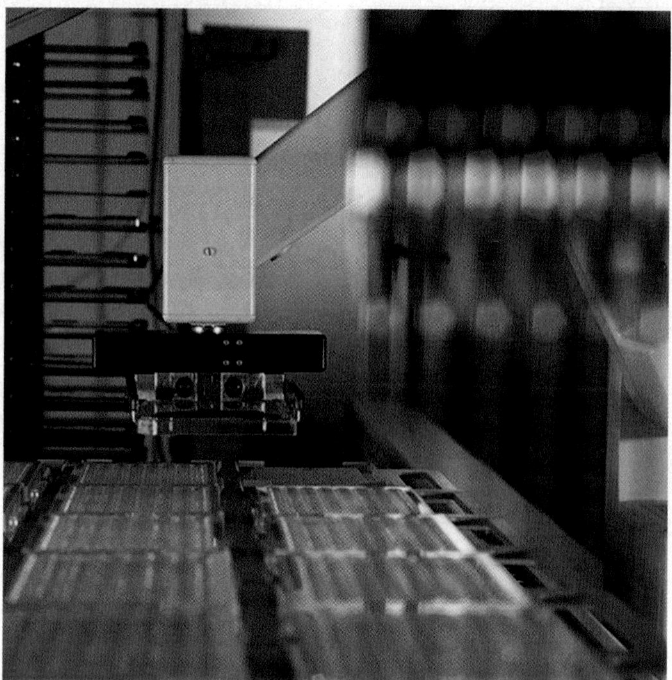

FIGURE 1-1 • **Robotic screening.**

LEAD OPTIMIZATION

Once a lead has been identified, the process of turning this into a drug candidate begins. In this iterative process, the medicinal chemist adjusts the molecule in response to information received from various forms of bioassay. The key questions addressed during lead optimization are

- Is the molecule potent and selective enough in bioassay and in vivo studies?
- Are there off-target effects that will cause problems?
- Are the pharmacokinetics likely to be suitable?
- Does the molecule get metabolized? Are there active or reactive metabolites? Are there liabilities for drug-drug interactions?
- Are there safety liabilities in the initial toxicologic studies?

This activity requires integration across several groups. Assay results from efficacy or safety studies are fed back to the chemist, and modifications to the molecule are made (Fig. 1-2). Often, there have to be trade-offs. Efficacy, toxicology, kinetics, and metabolism may not all pull in the same direction for the molecular scaffold. Despite this, it is clear that the greater the potency, the lower the potential risk of off-target effects become. It is now common for drugs to have low-nanomolar potency, and this itself should reduce the risk of unexpected toxicity unless these are mediated by binding to the target. It is usual for a molecule to be screened against a panel of other targets to assess the potential for unwanted effects.

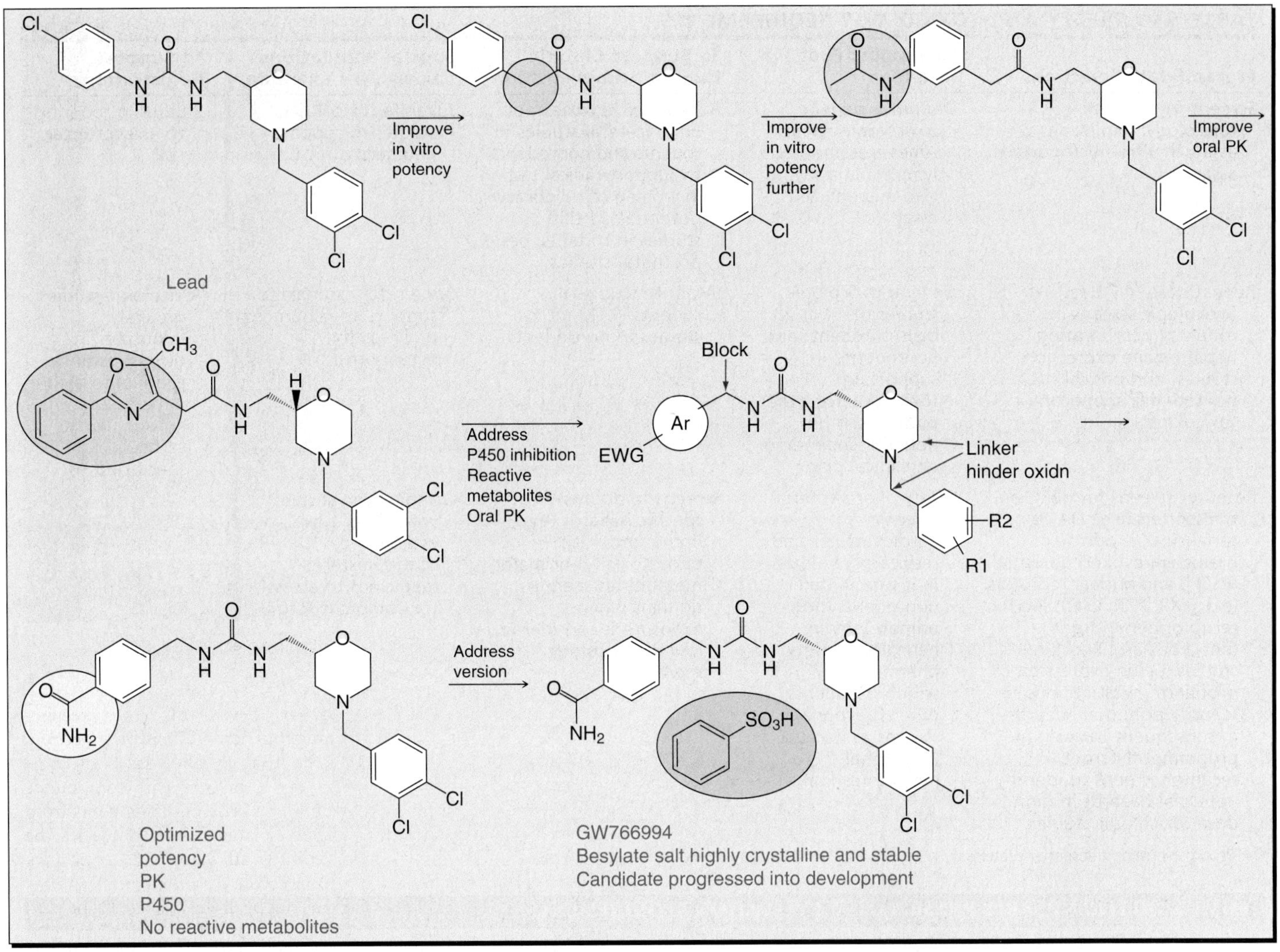

FIGURE 1-2 • Lead optimization. In the sequence shown, optimization included measures to increase potency, improve PK, and avoid problems of cytochrome P-450 interactions.

The science of safety assessment is advancing, and numerous assays and models are used to weed out unsuitable molecules and to flag potential problems to look for in the clinic (Table 1-1). As advances in bioinformatics allow more sophisticated modeling and searching of datasets, companies are trying to maximize the use of historical data to predict potential problems on the basis of the chemical structure and previous known toxicity. It is already known, for example, which features of a molecule increase the chance of finding an effect on QT interval prolongation through interaction with the hERG potassium channel.

The final set of considerations during this process of lead optimization are perhaps alien to the practicing doctor or academic, but are essential in the process of creating novel applicable therapeutics. The synthetic route may well be complex, and whereas this is not a problem for small-scale work, it has the capacity to kill a project. It must be possible to make an appropriate formulation, scale up synthesis, make reproducible and stable batches, and avoid problems such as the use of rare building blocks or controlled substances that will add undue complexity or cost to the eventual synthesis of the final product.

One thing is clear—you have to be an optimist to start on the path of drug discovery. Attrition rates are very high, and during these initial stages, there is considerable failure (Fig. 1-3). However, this stage of lead optimization and ensuring the best possible profile of the molecule as it enters the clinic for the first time is central to the process. The process comprises iterative cycles of improvement and a multidisciplinary approach involving chemists, biologists, toxicologists, and experts in drug metabolism and pharmacokinetics. It should also involve clinician scientists as they begin to plan the testing of the molecule in the clinic. Once a lead molecule has satisfied the drug discovery team that it has the desired properties, it is selected as a "candidate" and the clinical phase begins. Even though the nascent drug will now enter clinical studies, several longer-term toxicologic studies in animals will continue and an adverse read-out can terminate a project, even very late in clinical development.

CLINICAL PHARMACOLOGY STUDIES

Testing the Concept

Three main decision steps constitute the process of drug discovery—getting the target, selecting the best candidate molecule, and establishing a profile in the clinic. Just like the first two steps, this latter phase should not be considered a "process"; it should be thought of in terms of scientific experimentation. The "standardized" approach to clinical testing of a drug is shown in Figure 1-4, but for any drug candidate, key questions will need to be addressed in the clinic either to build confidence, inform the design of later-phase studies, or kill the drug. This is a major area for intelligent clinical pharmacology and experimental medicine. Increasingly with the recognition of important species differences, and with highly selective molecules that might have lower effect in animal models, entry to the clinic may come with somewhat incomplete information on the biologic effects. A key challenge

TABLE 1-1 SAFETY AND TOXICOLOGY REQUIREMENTS

Precandidate Selection	To Support First into Man	To Support Chronic Human Administration	Special Populations Various, for example:	To Support Registration
Screens for: Genetic toxicology; mini-Ames assay; in vitro micronucleus assay	*Definitive genetic toxicologic assays:* Ames test; mouse lymphoma assay; in vivo micronucleus assay	*Reproductive toxicology:* Embryo-fetal studies in rodents and nonrodents to support clinical testing in women of childbearing potential; fertility studies in rodents; peri-/postnatal studies	Juvenile toxicologic studies to support pediatric clinical trials	Studies in rodents to assess cancer risk
Repeat dose (4/7 days); toxicologic screens in rodents (incorporating hepatic gene expression studies) and possibly nonrodents; supporting toxicokinetics	*General toxicologic studies* of 14 or 28 days in rodents and nonrodents; supporting toxicokinetics; other options can be defined, depending on clinical plan	6-Month studies in rodents; 9-/12-month studies in nonrodents	Bone safety studies to support development of drugs for osteoporosis	Toxicologic studies on likely impurities in drug substance/product to assure patient safety and to clarify technical specifications
Receptor screens for hERG and transporters (e.g., OATPs), canalicular export (e.g., brainstem evoked potential [BSEP]) and nuclear receptors (e.g., FXR, PXR, CAR); specific receptor/gene target (knockout and knockin studies; tissue expression profiling) investigations to identify potential hazards in subsequent toxicology program; off-target receptor screens to identify potential hazards in high-dose toxicologic studies	*Safety pharmacology screens:* Cardiovascular and respiratory studies in instrumented nonrodents (dog or primate); Irwin neurologic safety pharmacology screen in rodents; other functional screens as necessary (e.g., renal, gastrointestinal)	Screens to address specific hazards (e.g., immunotoxicity, phototoxicity) or major metabolites seen in humans when exposure is considered low in toxicology species	Combination studies with other novel, or established, coadministered medicines to assess toxicologic synergy	

OATPs, organic anion transporter proteins.

BOX 1-1 DIFFERENT EARLY PHASE SAFETY EVALUATION REQUIREMENTS

1. Conventional—14-/28-day toxicologic studies
2. Screening Investigational New Drug (IND)
3. Exploratory IND (eIND)
4. Microdose clinical study (when pharmacologic effect is not anticipated)

It is worth noting that if an abbreviated package is used to fast-track to the clinic, there will be inevitable catch up required later on, and delays may occur during the progress to later phase studies and registration. The assessment of how much to do "experimentally" early on is a question of judgment based on the profile of the medicine and where the major risks lie. Of particular interest to the clinical pharmacologist or clinical experimentalist is the eIND. The potential use and limitations of this approach include

- eINDs support phase 1 clinical research, involve very limited human exposure and have no therapeutic or diagnostic intent.
- Dosing is limited to 7 days.
- The molecules evaluated in an eIND "are generally structurally related." This could preclude eINDs that are exploring effects at a common target through different mechanisms.
- The FDA specifically mentions the application of eIND principles in clinical settings involving serious diseases. It is possible that there is more latitude for creativity when working in these areas.
- An eIND cannot be transitioned into a traditional IND. A new submission is required, and this may add delays.
- Guidance emphasizes that eIND is intended for use in a limited number of subjects, limited dose/exposure levels (e.g., micro = 1/100th, 100X cover, 1/2 rodent AUC at no observed adverse effect level [NOAEL]) for a limited time (7 days).
- Up to 7 days of human dosing is supported by a 14-day rodent followed by a confirmatory nonrodent study.
- No definitive information is provided for the number of animals required in the confirmatory study, but the guidance states "but of sufficient number to rule out any toxicologically significant difference in sensitivity compared with rodent."

early in clinical investigation is to be sure that the drug molecule has the desired action, binds to the right target, and does so in a way that allows the clinical hypothesis to be tested. Failure to determine whether the drug has the desired binding and distribution characteristics means that all subsequent clinical investigation is fraught with problems of interpretation—particularly if the studies are negative. Whereas it is not possible to identify every eventuality, it is worth describing some possible approaches.

Microdosing allows administration of very small amounts of drug substance to test kinetic parameters. Although not infallible, it can be a useful technique if the primary go/no-go decision is critically dependent upon a certain pharmacokinetic profile. The advantage of using microdosing is that the toxicology package required is less than for conventional studies (Box 1-1), little drug substance is required, and it may be possible to take several molecules into humans in parallel and make the final decision on the preferred drug at this stage rather than at the usual candidate-selection stage. This approach may be particularly useful when the efficacy may be clear from the preclinical studies, but the kinetic properties in humans will ultimately determine therapeutic effect. Advances in imaging techniques have also enabled sophisticated approaches to establishing whether a molecule enters the brain or to assessing receptor occupancy at a given site (Fig. 1-5).

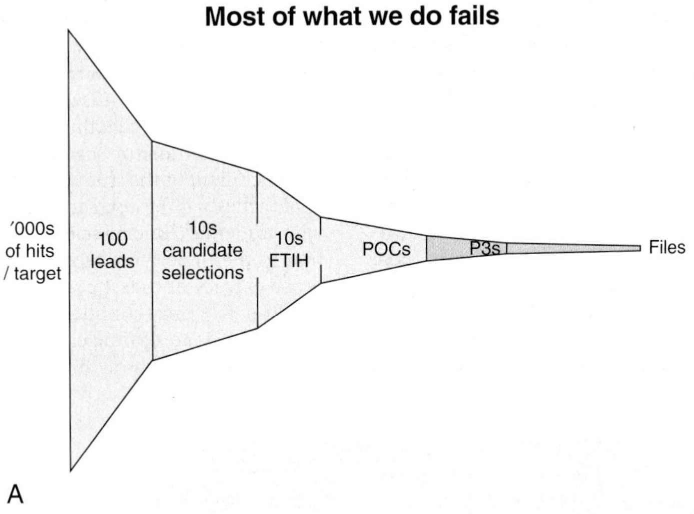

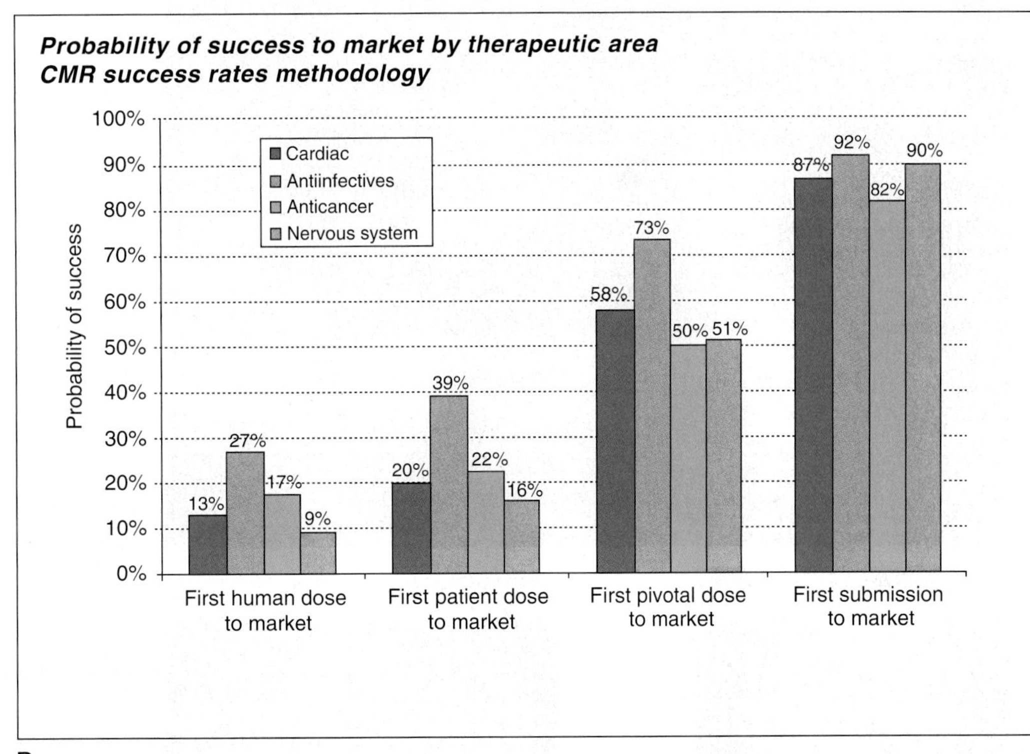

FIGURE 1-3 • Attrition across phases. A, Potential screening of many hundred targets narrows down. **B,** Note that early on in the process, the failure rate is high and fairly consistent across therapeutic areas. However, the more novel the target, the higher the likelihood of failure.

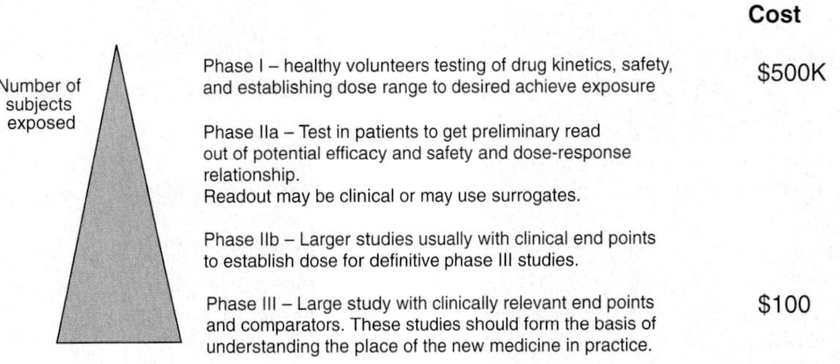

FIGURE 1-4 • "Conventional" path of clinical testing.

Often, however, the question will not be about kinetics but about dynamics. This is particularly true for drugs designed to affect novel targets. The key question for these novel drugs is whether there is a reason to believe that the drug will have the desired effect in humans. With advances in noninvasive imaging and sophisticated physiologic monitoring or use of biopsies, it is now possible to design studies that address the fundamental questions about mechanism of action and potential for therapeutic effect. Such studies may deviate from the usual practice in the pharmaceutical industry and require a more flexible approach to experimentation and study design. Fundamentally, these studies are more akin to laboratory or preclinical studies and require the same mindset. Examples might include the use of insulin clamps to test the effects of a compound on insulin sensitivity, the use of functional magnetic resonance imaging (fMRI) to establish the effects of a drug on an experimental psychological paradigm, or the use of specific phenotypic or genotypic subsets of patients or diseases to optimize the chance of detecting a positive signal. This latter approach might include selection of a rarer disease with a more clearly defined molecular and cellular pathology (e.g., the use of Muckle-Wells syndrome to test specific anti-inflammatory agents such as anti–interleukin-1 [anti-IL-1]), or enrichment of the study population by genotype. Such experimental approaches will be used increasingly, will require close collaboration with academic clinician scientists, and should link the clinical investigation to the underlying biologic rationale. Studies may be designed to probe efficacy or to test potential unwanted effects.

Ultimately, once confidence is gained about the likelihood of success and how best to optimize clinically relevant end points based on the biology of the pathway and the effects of the drug in experimental

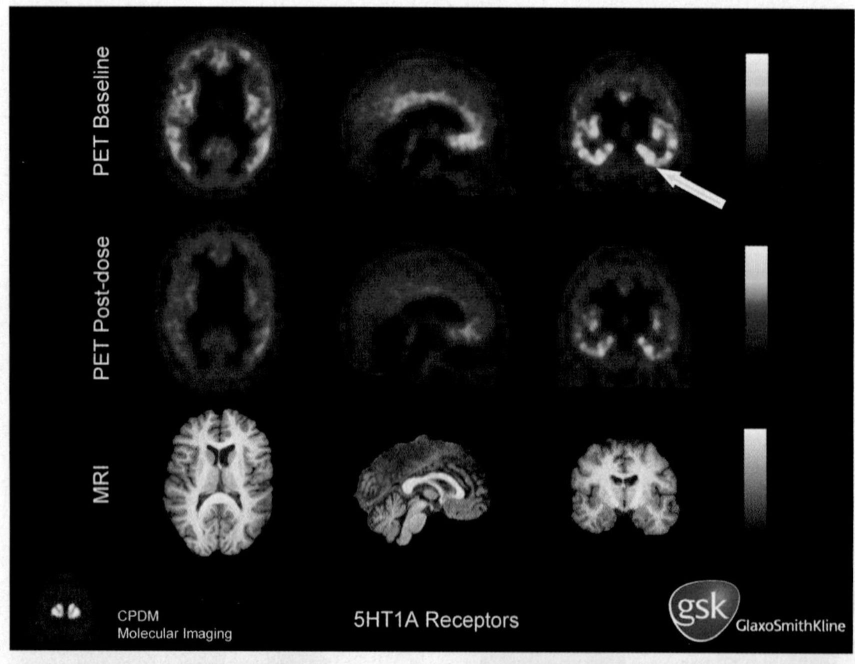

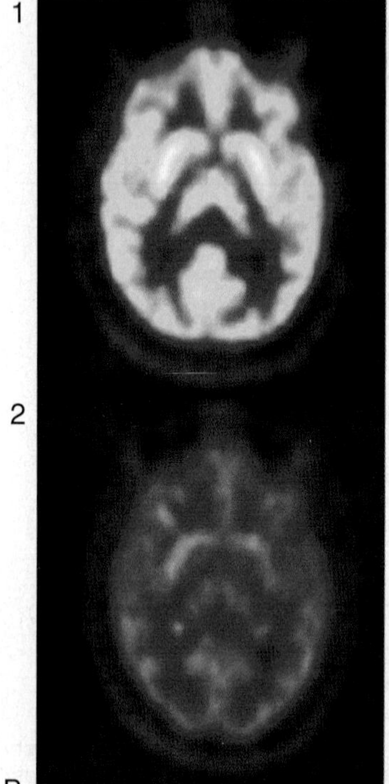

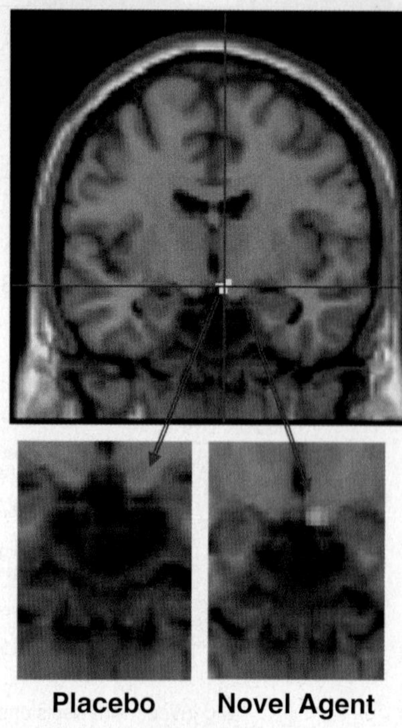

FIGURE 1-5 • **A,** Occupancy of serotonin 5HT1A receptors by a candidate drug. Transaxial (**left column**), sagittal (**middle column**), and coronal (**right column**) positron emission tomography images acquired after injection of the radiolabeled selective antagonist [^{11}C]WAY100635 in a human volunteer at baseline (**top row**) and 24 hr after oral administration of the candidate drug (**middle row**), with coregistered magnetic resonance imaging (MRI) scans (**bottom row**). PET images were obtained by summing activity distribution from 30 to 95 min postinjection, and were normalized to the injected dose. Under baseline conditions, the radiotracer distributed in areas rich in 5HT1A receptors, such as cortex and hippocampus (*arrow*). Pretreatment by the candidate drug reduced [^{11}C]WAY100635 specific binding by 35%, indicating that the candidate drug maintained significant occupancy of 5HT1A receptor at 24 hr postdose. **B,** Application of advanced imaging in drug development. A novel drug intended for cognitive enhancement was being developed. In an initial experimental medicine study, PET was used in healthy volunteers to predict an efficacious dose. Binding of a radioligand specific for the receptor target was measured in the brain of a healthy volunteer (*1*). At a range of doses in different volunteers, follow-up images were acquired after administration of the drug at different doses. The binding of the receptor-targeted radioligand was reduced as it was displaced by the drug (*2*). A dose-occupancy curve could then be defined. Using a dose defined as giving rise to sufficient receptor occupancy for potential biologic effect, a second experimental medicine study was performed using functional MRI (fMRI) with a paired associated learning memory task (*3*). Administration of the novel drug increased brain activity in the hippocampus, a brain region known to be involved in memory. This provides a pharmacodynamic signal and provides proof of biologic mechanism in humans. (**A** and **B,** courtesy of the Dr. M. Larvelle, GlaxoSmithKline Clinical Imaging Centre. **C,** courtesy of Dr. M. Mehta and Prof. S. Williams, Institute of Psychiatry, London.)

medicine, a high-quality clinical study can be designed. Again, there is an increasing use of adaptive trial designs to allow changes in approaches in response to results obtained and a Bayesian statistical approach to allow for prior expectation and inference to be accounted for at these early stages of probing a drug's potential. The key message is that at these early stages, particularly for novel drugs, the studies in the clinic are experiments and should be interpreted as such.

No section on clinical testing would be complete without a mention of biomarkers. The use of a biomarker in drug testing is not new. In Black's experiments,[1] a change in heart rate or an alteration in gastric pH were the biomarkers that signified likely therapeutic efficacy. The principle remains the same. A biomarker should be a measure of biologic activity that is relevant to the pathophysiology and the proposed mechanism of action of the drug. Just as in identification of a chemical, there are two broad approaches: A biomarker may emerge from a deep understanding of the biology and physiology, or it may be divined from a more industrialized approach such as non–hypothesis-driven proteomics or metabolomics. Whichever approach is taken, it is clear that unless the biomarker is truly related to the disease or the desired therapeutic effect, it is likely to be a misleading surrogate of effect or safety. In oncology studies, biomarkers are becoming increasingly important as drugs target highly specific pathways that are differentially expressed between tumors.

ALTERNATIVE APPROACHES—BIOPHARMACEUTICALS

Biopharmaceuticals have become mainstream and blockbuster—witness anti–tumor necrosis factor (anti-TNF), anti-CD20, and a plethora of new agents in the pipeline. For drug discovery, there are two main questions: For which targets/diseases does a biopharmaceutical approach make sense and what are the additional constraints on testing in humans. There are no hard and fast rules about when a target looks particularly amenable to taking an antibody-based approach, but it is worth considering the properties of antibodies that help define potential targets. Antibodies are large molecules, have much higher production costs than small molecules, may not access particular tissues or cells well, have high affinity and high specificity of binding, may invoke an immune response, and may have a prolonged half-life in the circulation. To date, antibodies have been very effective as antagonists of soluble factors such as cytokines, but it is clear that they may have much wider applications. If antibodies activate lytic processes, they may produce highly specific cell death and depletion as evidenced by B cell depletion therapy.

The testing of antibodies follows much the same route as that of small molecules, but there are additional considerations. In particular, prediction of dose may be difficult because there can be a very steep dose-response relationship, particularly if the antibody is activating rather than neutralizing. Because of the highly specific nature of antibody binding, there may also be very significant species differences in specificity and activation potential. Recent major problems with a superagonist for CD28 that stimulated a cytokine storm in healthy volunteers illustrated the potential for difficulty in predicting effects in humans and the need to proceed with appropriate caution based on the biology of the molecule. Next-generation antibody approaches include the use of antibody domains rather than the full molecule and the use of dual recognition sites to allow simultaneous binding of two target molecules with one antibody (Fig. 1-6).

Other biopharmaceutical approaches include the use of peptides. Of course, this is not new in medicine—insulin has been used for many

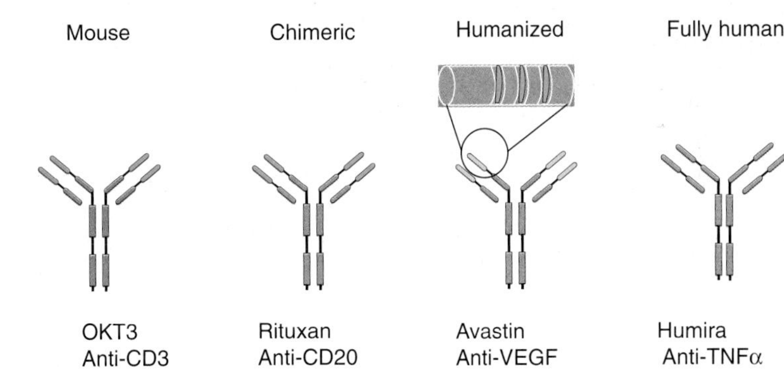

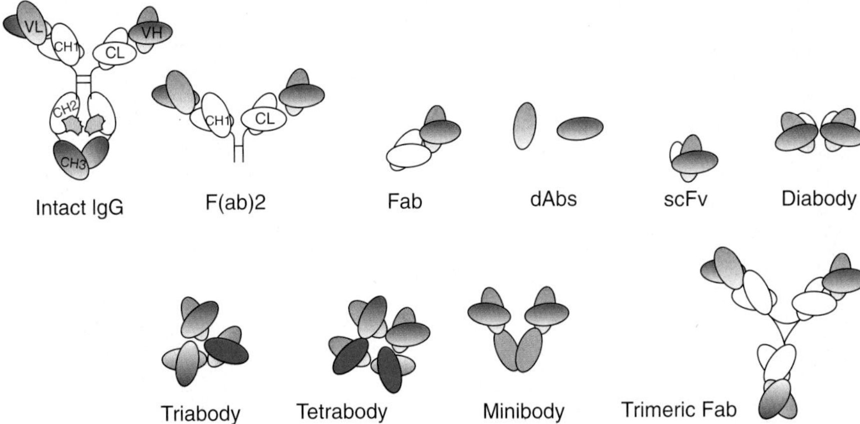

FIGURE 1-6 • Antibody approaches to therapeutics. The approach has moved from mouse antibodies through to fully humanized antibodies. Now engineered fragments containing combinations of the variable regions may offer the opportunity of reduced molecular weight, easier production, and binding to more than one target.

years. However, having been seen as unattractive as drug molecules, peptides are becoming more commonplace, and new routes of delivery or approaches to extend the half-life are favorably changing the perception of peptides as drug molecules. Finally, gene therapy is beginning to deliver in certain specialized areas, and the use of interfering RNA to silence RNA and thereby prevent protein synthesis holds promise.

GENETICS AND GENOMICS

Much has been written about the influence of genetic and genomic approaches on drug discovery. It is worth considering the different stages at which this information may apply. First, at the early stage of target identification, genetic disease association may give clues about potential targets or help build confidence in targets. Second, at the early phase of clinical drug testing, enriching the test population with individuals of a defined genotype may increase the size of a signal or improve signal-to-noise ratio. The same is also true, indeed perhaps more so, for the use of gene expression profiles in tumors for the potential identification of those most likely to respond. Third, if and when safety signals occur in the clinic, post-hoc analysis of genotype effects may help identify at-risk subjects or give specific insights into mechanisms. These approaches may aid the task of drug discovery, but this does not mean that they have direct clinical utility. In oncology, gene expression patterns or mutations within tumors are useful in determining response in the clinic, but the challenge for the use of common genetic variation (polymorphisms) in prediction of individuals who may show greater responses to a particular medicine or be at altered risk of side effects is to show sufficient predictability at the individual level as opposed to the population level. To date, most variants confer modest alterations of risk or benefit and do not alter risk-benefit relationships in a clinically useful way. It remains to be determined to what extent panels of variation across a range of genes will allow "personalization" of medicines.

CONCLUSIONS

Drug discovery is a high-risk, high-reward business that requires a multidisciplinary approach. Behind every successful drug, there are usually identifiable champions who have been prepared to stand by the drug through the tortuous route. The easiest decision at every stage of drug discovery is to kill the project, and there are usually reasons to consider doing so. Keen scientific judgment is required. The key elements are scientific and clinical insight, tenacity and passion, and at each stage, an understanding of experimental approach to answer defined questions. The optimal unit for drug discovery integrates the science of the various functions including chemistry, biology, clinical science, and toxicology.

REFERENCE

1. Black J. Drugs from emasculated hormones: the principles of syntopic antagonism. Available at http://nobelprize.org/nobel_prizes/medicine/laureates/1988/black-lecture.pdf.

FURTHER READING

Academy of Medical Sciences. Online Report Re: Safer Medicines. November 2005. Available at http://www.acmedsci.ac.uk/images/page/1132655880.pdf

Berry DA. Bayesian clinical trials. Nat Rev Drug Discov 2006;5(1):27-36.

Booth B, Zemmel R. Quest for the best. Nat Rev Drug Discov 2003;2:838-841.

Chapman K, Pullen N, Graham M, et al. Preclinical safety testing of monoclonal antibodies: the significance of species relevance. Nat Rev Drug Discov 2007;6(2):120-126.

Constable S, Johnson MR, Pirmohamed M. Pharmacogenetics in clinical practice: considerations for testing. Expert Rev Mol Diagn 2006;6(2):193-205.

Imming P, Sinning C, Meyer A. Drugs, their targets and the nature and number of drug targets. Nat Rev Drug Discov 2006;5(10):821-834.

Institute of Medicine Report: The Future of Drug Safety: Promoting and Protecting the Health of the Public. September 2006. Available at www.iom.edu

Lappin G, Kuhnz W, Jochemsen R, et al. Use of microdosing to predict pharmacokinetics at the therapeutic dose: experience with 5 drugs. Clin Pharmacol Ther 2006;80(3):203-215.

Lesko LJ, Woodcock J. Translation of pharmacogenomics and pharmacogenetics: a regulatory perspective. Nat Rev Drug Discov 2004;3(9):763-769.

Littman BH, Williams SA. The ultimate model organism: progress in experimental medicine. Nat Rev Drug Discov 2005;4(8):631-638.

Matthews PM, Honey GD, Bullmore ET. Applications of fMRI in translational medicine and clinical practice. Nat Rev Neurosci 2006;7(9):732-744.

Phillips KA, Van Bebber S, Issa AM. Diagnostics and biomarker development: priming the pipeline. Nat Rev Drug Discov 2006;5(6):463-469.

Roses AD, Saunders AM, Huang Y, et al. Complex disease-associated pharmacogenetics: drug efficacy, drug safety, and confirmation of a pathogenetic hypothesis (Alzheimer's disease). Pharmacogenomics J 2007;7(1):10-28.

2

DRUG DEVELOPMENT

Steven Ryder and Ethan Weiner

INTRODUCTION 15
THE DRUG DEVELOPMENT PROCESS 15
PRINCIPLES GUIDING THE PROCESS 18
DISCIPLINE- OR ACTIVITY-SPECIFIC GUIDANCE 21
Pharmaceutical Science 21
Nonclinical Safety Assessment 21
Clinical Research 21
DECISION-BASED CONTINUOUS DRUG DEVELOPMENT 23
Discovery 23
Candidate Nomination for Development 23
Proof of Mechanism 24
Proof of Concept 24
Proceed to Confirmatory Clinical Trials 24
Registration 24
Postapproval 24
SPECIAL TOPICS 25
Japan 25
Elderly, Pediatric, and Special Populations 25
Biologic Agents 26
Individual Assessment of Benefit-to-Risk 26
Orphan Drugs 27
SUMMARY AND CONCLUSIONS 27

INTRODUCTION

Drug development is the process of translating drug discoveries into new medical treatments. It begins with the planning of the program that (i) will explore and study the drug candidate, (ii) will determine whether it has the potential for becoming a new pharmaceutical treatment, (iii) provides the information allowing the entry of the drug into medical use, and (iv) continues to gather information on the drug product until it is superseded by a safer, more well-tolerated, or more effective treatment. The process builds information, and although it has stepwise milestones, it is continuous.

This review discusses the principles guiding the process, their application, and the ongoing improvement of the process. The chapter discusses the development process for drug therapeutics (small molecules and biologic agents) and does not specifically discuss the development process for medical procedures, devices or other nondrug (e.g., herbal) agents. It should be noted that whereas small molecules and biologics share much of the development process, biologics also have some specifically different issues, such as particular manufacturing issues or distinct issues around pharmacokinetics and pharmacodynamics. The chapter restricts itself to the development process for human therapeutics and does not discuss nonhuman (e.g., veterinary) drug development.

The goal of drug development is to acquire and refine the information necessary to determine the benefit-to-risk of using a potential new pharmaceutical as a medical treatment. The ability to investigate and establish the benefit-to-risk of a new medicine is at the heart of the development challenge, and the ability to effectively assess benefit-to-risk is directly linked to the ability to effectively plan, acquire, and analyze information. This is true in both nonclinical and clinical areas of study.

A rigorous scientific drug development process has allowed the introduction of a remarkable number of drug treatments, with an increasing amount of information and increasing precision in the determination of benefit and risk. To exemplify the incredible progress, it is worth reading the section from a 1951 medical text describing the medical treatment of vascular hypertension[1]:

- *Medical Therapy.* ANTIHYPERTENSIVE AND DEPRESSOR AGENTS. Tissue extracts, vegetable extracts, vaccines, hormones, nitrites, sedatives, pyrogens, phlebotomies, thiocyanates, and sympatholytic agents have all been administered for hypertensive disease, only to be abandoned.
- Within the therapeutic dosage range, the depressor activity of thiocyanates in experienced hands has been dubious. A number of deaths have occurred, even though the blood level has been carefully controlled. Serious toxic side effects, such as exfoliative dermatitis, have occurred. The use of thiocyanates for therapy of hypertension is to be discouraged except as a research procedure.
- The most powerful depressor substances belong to the *Veratrum viride* group of alkaloids. In the acute hypertensions (acute glomerulonephritis and toxemia of pregnancy), veratrum alkaloids have a real place in therapy. In chronic hypertension, on the other hand, the dosage that lowers blood pressure is usually about the same as that which produces nausea and vomiting. Until this serious side effect can be eliminated, there is no indication for their usage.

The text then goes on to describe dietary and surgical treatments in more lengthy sections.

The reader is invited to compare this discussion with the treatments currently available for hypertension, outlined in Chapter 27, Hypertension, or the antihypertensive treatment paradigm outlined in the *Seventh Joint National Committee on Prevention, Detection, Evaluation, and Treatment of High Blood Pressure* (JNC 7) report.[2] This report emphasizes that systemic blood pressure must be aggressively controlled, which usually requires multiple medications from among the many classes of effective and safe antihypertensive drugs: thiazide-type diuretics, angiotensin-converting enzyme inhibitors, angiotensin receptor blockers, calcium channel blockers, β-blockers, α-blockers, and others. In addition, each of these classes of antihypertensive drugs includes many different individual molecular entities, each with a specific pharmacokinetic, pharmacodynamic, efficacy, tolerance, and safety profile. This remarkable change in the antihypertensive pharmacopeia, and the corresponding change in many therapeutic areas, was enabled and allowed because of a constantly improving drug development process—beginning in the 1950s with the general introduction of the controlled clinical trial paradigm and continuing to the present with new adaptive study designs and data capture innovations. Along with these improvements in drug development, the response to the human immunodeficiency virus (HIV) epidemic, continued concern over personal safety and health, and a heightened awareness of drug withdrawals have increased the focus on drug development principles and many of its key issues.

THE DRUG DEVELOPMENT PROCESS

Since the mid-20th century, the drug development process has become more complex as understanding of the underlying biology has grown, as experience with the benefits and risks of previous generations of pharmaceuticals has been gained, and as the design and execution of clinical trials have been refined. The process itself has evolved from the traditional paradigm of discovery followed by phases I, II, III, and IV, to include a decision-based paradigm validating a specific pharmacology in humans and then seeking to confirm the effect of this pharmacology on specific end points. Key phases or decision steps in these paradigms follow:

Traditional drug development paradigm—key phases (Fig. 2-1):

- *Discovery:* Find chemical matter that has effects on a specific preclinical model or desired enzymatic or receptor target.
- *Phase I:* Test the drug in healthy volunteers primarily to determine pharmacokinetics and maximum tolerated dose. This phase usually involves up to approximately 100 healthy volunteer subjects, and the duration of study drug treatment is usually up to about 2 to 4 weeks.
- *Phase II:* Test the maximum tolerated dose in a specific disease, looking for a change in various clinical end points; then test lower doses, looking for the optimum balance of efficacy and adverse events. This phase usually involves up to about several hundred tightly defined subjects with the disease or condition of interest, and the duration of study drug treatment is usually up to several months.
- *Phase III:* Confirm the effect of the selected dose(s) on the selected clinical end points and accumulate sufficient safety data to rule out infrequent adverse events. This phase usually involves up to about several thousand more broadly defined subjects with the disease or condition of interest, and the duration of study drug treatment is usually up to many months to years. The exact specifications of the Phase III program leading to registration are generally agreed to by academic experts and regulatory agencies prior to its initiation, including a prespecification of both clinical and statistical success.
- *Phase IV:* Continue to acquire candidate information to address additional safety, tolerance, and efficacy issues and also to potentially supplement the initial approved medical indication and drug formulation with information supporting further indications or product formulations. Issues of tolerance and efficacy may be addressed. This phase usually involves up to several thousand more broadly defined subjects with the disease or condition of interest, and the duration of drug treatment up to many months to years. The exact specifications of the Phase IV program are typically agreed to by academic experts and regulatory agencies prior to the initial approval of the drug candidate.

Decision-based drug development paradigm—key decision steps (Fig. 2-2):

- *Candidate nomination for development:* Candidate nomination for development occurs at a time when the drug candidate has proven in vitro and in vivo pharmacology and meets rigorous standards of specificity and potency for the desired target. The candidate has also passed a battery of tests to ensure it has appropriate pharmaceutical and safety properties for further testing and administration to humans. In this paradigm, discovery is based on biology that identifies a receptor, enzyme, or other intermediary biologic system that, when stimulated or suppressed, offers the potential for therapeutic advantage compared with existing treatments.
- *Proof of mechanism (POM):* POM occurs when the appropriate pharmacology has been shown to take place in humans and an adequate pharmacokinetic and pharmacodynamic relationship has been demonstrated at doses well tolerated in humans.
- *Proof of concept (POC):* POC occurs once the drug candidate has shown desired effects with adequate safety and tolerability on either hard clinical end points (those that ultimately support registration of the product) in the intended disease state or surrogate end points, which are predictive of an ultimate effect upon the end points that can be registered. POC is not dependent upon the results of a single clinical trial but is based on the accumulated weight of evidence gathered to the decision time point.

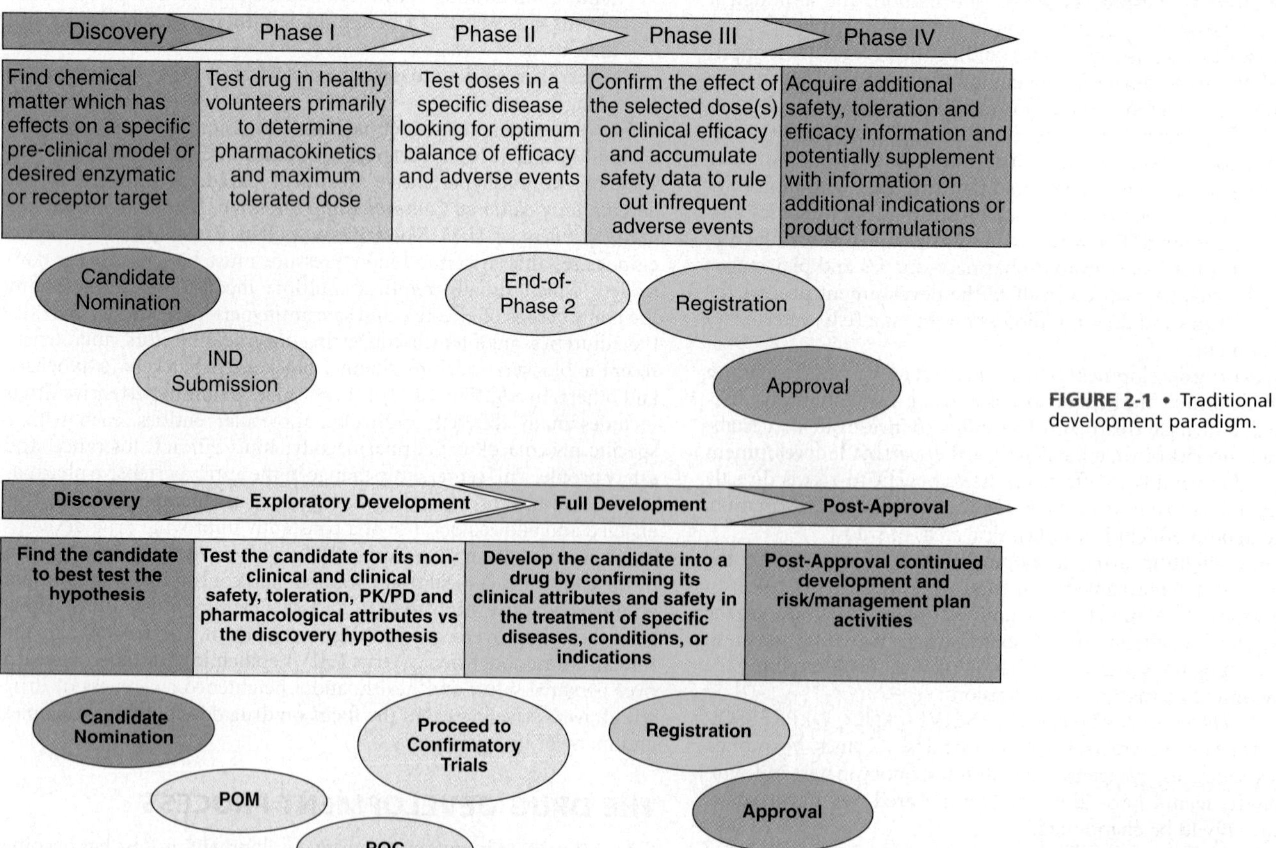

FIGURE 2-1 • Traditional drug development paradigm.

FIGURE 2-2 • Decision-based drug development paradigm.

- *Proceed to confirmatory clinical trials:* Drug development proceeds to confirmatory clinical trials when there is sufficient information to identify which doses are most likely to have a favorable efficacy, tolerance, and safety profile when used in a more broad-based population reflecting the patient population in which the development candidate would be used following approval.
- *Risk management plan (RMP):* The RMP for each development candidate is designed in collaboration with expert consultants and regulatory agencies and includes clinical trials designed to further acquire efficacy, safety, and tolerance about the development candidate beyond the time of first approval. The RMP is generally first prepared at the completion of the POC and continuously refined and updated as additional information is acquired.

This paradigm shift from a straight linear process, planning each phase for success, to a more decision-based process was driven by the continuing high failure rate of drug candidates since the late 1980s. One of the key issues of drug development is that despite advances in biology and exponential growth in research and development (R&D) spending since the late 1970s, the number of new molecular entities filed with and approved by regulatory agencies has remained generally constant at about 20 to 30 per year. Figure 2-3 shows the number of New Molecular Entity Drugs (NMEs) approved by the U.S. Food and Drug Administration (FDA) from 1945 through 2005.[3,4] Figure 2-3 also shows the R&D spending by member firms of the Pharmaceutical and Research Manufacturers of America from 1970 through 2005.[5] The rise in pharmaceutical R&D spending far outpaces any trend in the number of NMEs approved during this period.

Figure 2-4 shows drug candidate survival by traditional phase (I, II, III, and registration) of drug development, and Figure 2-5 shows the primary causes of failure. As anticipated, most attrition takes place early in development. Owing to improvement in in vivo and in vitro models of adverse effects on organ systems, improvements in genetic toxicology, and improvements in chemistry that allow the identification of potential small molecule toxicophores, development failures for toxicity have been on the decline, with only a small proportion of phase II/III failures due to infrequent but medically very significant (and usually idiosyncratic) safety events, such as fulminant hepatitis or blood dyscrasias. The bulk of failures currently occur in phase II (i.e.,

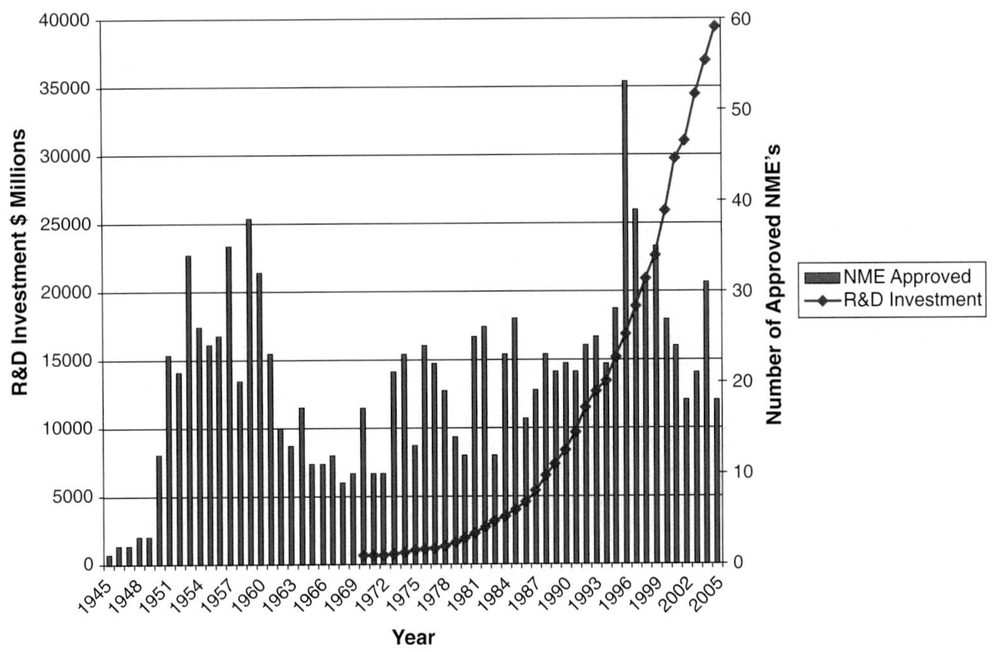

FIGURE 2-3 • New molecular entity new drug applications (NMEs) approved by the U.S. Food and Drug Administration (FDA) (1945-2005) and research and development (R&D) investment by Pharmaceutical and Research Manufacturers of America firms (1970-2005). (Adapted from Source for R&D Expenditure: Pharmaceutical Research and Manufacturers of America (PhRMA) Annual Report 2006. Source for NMEs approved http://www.fda.gov/cder/rdmt/default.htm [accessed September 19, 2006].)

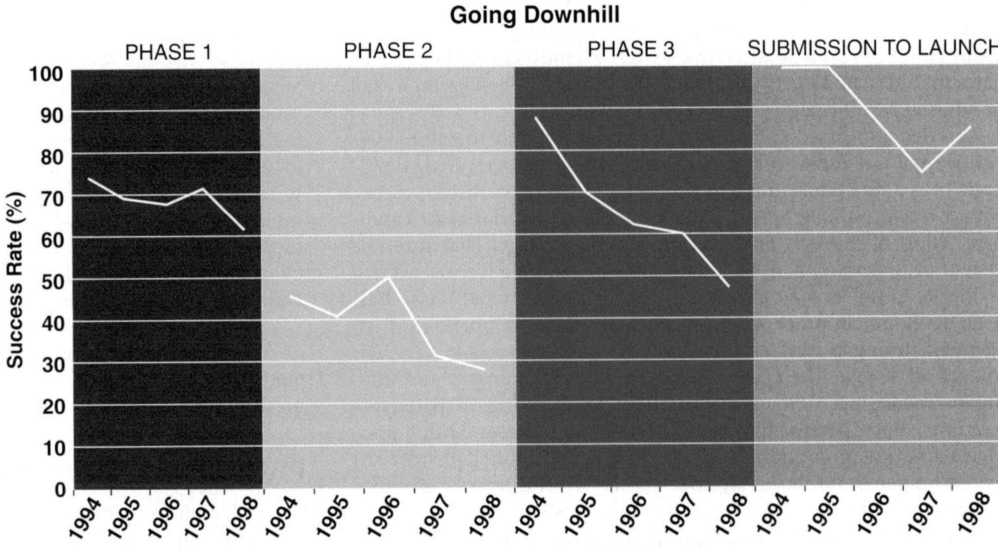

FIGURE 2-4 • Success rates according to traditional phase of drug development (1994-1998). (From Mervis J. Productivity counts—but the definition is key. Science 2005;309: 726–727.)

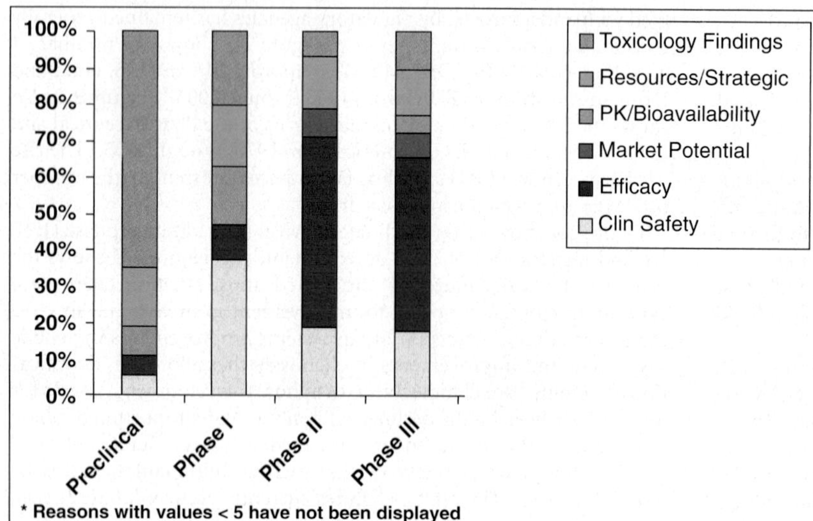

FIGURE 2-5 • Reasons for termination according to traditional phase of drug development (2001-2005). (Adapted from Arrowsmith and Mooney, personal communication. Pfizer Global Research and Development, 2006.)

before POC) because of failure to achieve efficacy. This reflects the exponential increase in knowledge about possible druggable targets. With many new targets, it is difficult to predict which will affect human disease. Few would have predicted, for instance, the profound effect of tumor necrosis factor-α (TNF-α) blockade on rheumatoid arthritis compared with the more modest effect seen with blockade of other cytokines (such as interleukin-1 [IL-1]) or chemokines, such as chemokine (C-C motif) receptor 2 (CCR-2). Furthermore, the great plasticity and redundancy of cellular processes can often allow a blocked step or receptor to be "bypassed" in the disease process. It is often impossible to predict which steps can be bypassed and which cannot.

In the traditional phase I-IV paradigm, a failure to show benefit in the target disease in phase II would leave doubt as to whether the failure was due to the drug target or to the drug candidate itself. A retrospective analysis of Phase II programs conducted at Pfizer Global Research and Development showed that the majority of failed development programs failed to fully assess the potential of the pharmacology in the disease state of interest (John Arrowsmith and George Mooney, personal communication). This resulted in the current focus on POM to establish, first, that the pharmacology is active in humans, followed by POC to establish whether the pharmacology is of benefit in the disease states of interest. In this way, many drugs are weeded out at the POM stage because of failure to affect the pharmacology in humans. These failures are used by drug discovery scientists to refine defects in the drug candidate that led to this failure. Thus, those drug candidates that achieve POM but fail to achieve POC can more clearly be deemed failure of the intended pharmacologic target to affect the disease. This information can then be used by discovery scientists to explore candidates for alternate targets. The few that survive can then go on to full or late-stage confirmatory clinical trial development.

This decision-based paradigm is important not only to enforce scientific rigor but also to ensure best use of R&D resources. Drug development is a time-consuming, highly complex, and expensive process, with a recent estimate of over $800 million per development candidate.[6] Most of this cost occurs at the post-POC stage. Therefore, the goal of drug development has changed from planning for success and trying to "push" every candidate through the traditional phase I-III drug development process until it fails, to a system of portfolio management, trying to test as many mechanisms as possible for their impact on disease. The decision-based paradigm emphasizes advancing to increasingly expansive development in a logical pattern—weeding out potentially toxic molecules, those with poor pharmaceutical properties, those not showing the required pharmacology in humans, and those not affecting the target disease or disorder before expanding the development process. This paradigm tests POM first, and POC second; only after achieving POC does the emphasis change from planning for early failure to planning for success and making the major investments that characterize full or late-stage confirmatory clinical trial development. Once POC is achieved and the prerequisite information for advanced development is obtained, then full development is initiated to confirm the efficacy hypothesis as definitively as possible and to establish a sufficiently large safety database to meaningfully assess benefit-to-risk at the time of registration.

The development process itself involves intricate detail at every step, to a degree often not realized even by investigators and scientists. Figure 2-6 shows the strategic high-level decision-based paradigm with two key decision points (POM and POC) and then "drills down" to a series of tactical subquestions, each of which requires multiple interconnected steps. POM and POC, for example, require a series of clinical trials, each dependent upon the other, each dependent on appropriate toxicology support, protocol generation, randomization procedures and study drug blinding, packaging of clinical supplies to good manufacturing practice standards, selection of investigators, and other activities. A further drill-down on a single one of these subquestions—a single clinical trial, for example—shows, in turn, many interdependent substeps. Figure 2-7 shows in detail one substep, the generation of a single protocol synopsis (encompassing key design elements of a single clinical trial protocol). This single substep, in turn, triggers many downstream trial-related processes, all of which make up the one "box" highlighted in Figure 2-6. When one considers that each box in the process display shown in Figure 2-6 contains a similar myriad of steps, the reason for the complexity, extended time frame, and cost of development becomes apparent.

Current development paradigms overlay the traditional phase I-IV paradigm with the decision-based paradigm, emphasizing the importance of acquiring decision-enabling information throughout the process. This enhanced paradigm provides a structure for understanding the necessary information and planning needs at each step. While identifying distinct steps and decision points in the drug development process, it is important to note that the process is continuous and builds upon acquired information. At all steps, the information is incremental, and feedback of key information to discovery scientists, pharmacologists, pharmaceutical science and drug safety professionals, and others is essential for furthering drug innovation.

Having taken a high-level look at what the process is intended to do, its overall form and complexity, we now look into the principles that guide the process and the complex interplay of subprocesses that make up drug development.

PRINCIPLES GUIDING THE PROCESS

The principles of drug development guide the process of acquiring candidate information effectively and efficiently while adhering to basic tenets of science, ethics, and law. Drug development is a scientific

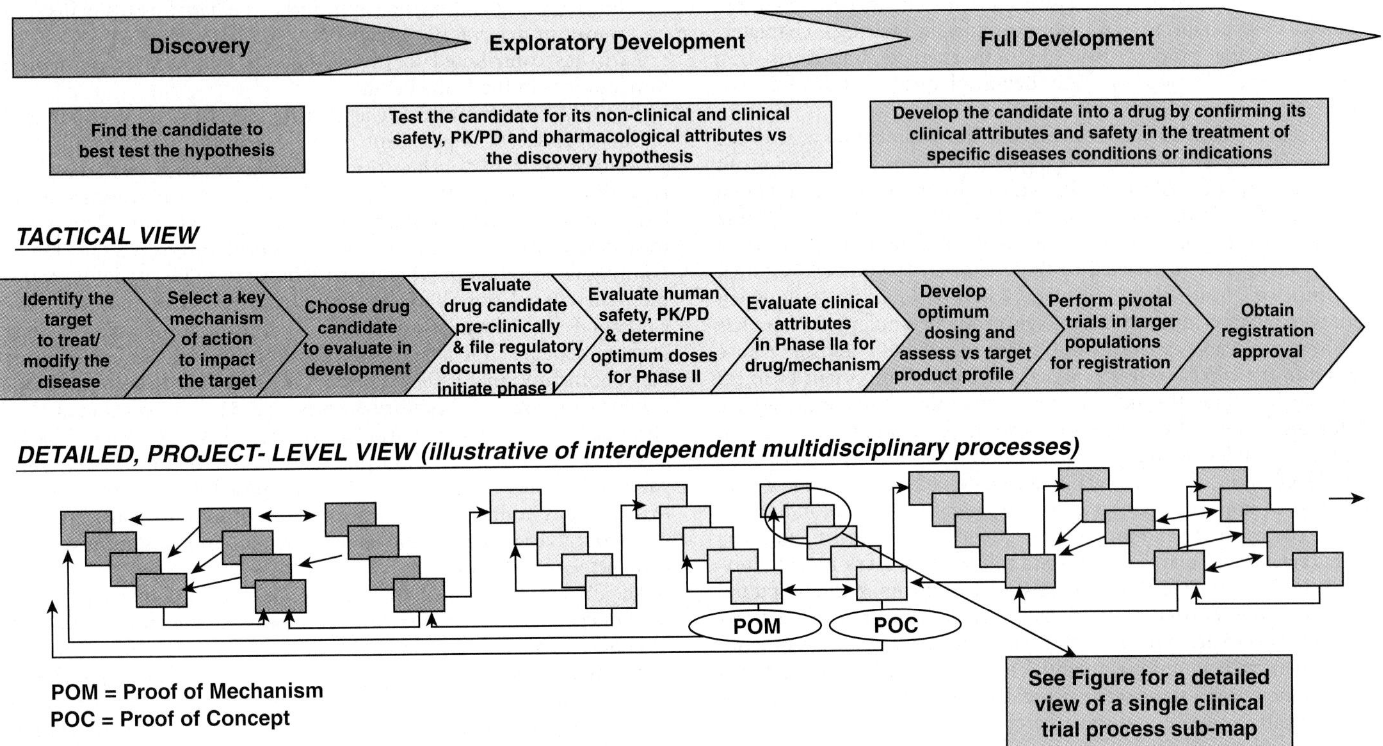

FIGURE 2-6 • Decision-based drug development: strategic, tactical, and detailed, project-level view.

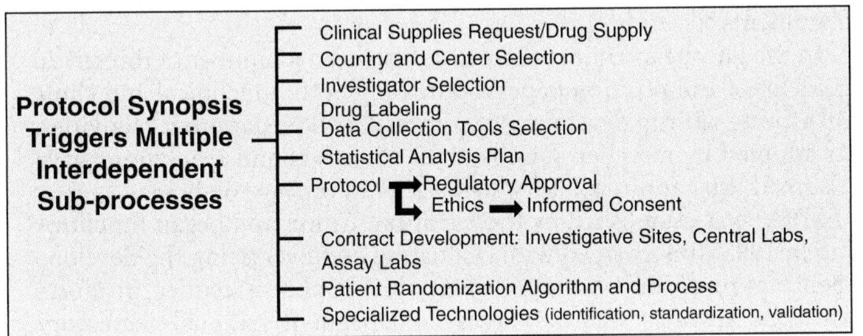

FIGURE 2-7 • View of a single clinical trial process substep: protocol synopsis-triggered activities.

process that adheres to the principles of scientific excellence and scientific integrity and that provides information that comes from the application of the scientific method. The process is based on a credible theory (e.g., that an identified physiologic pathway is involved in the pathogenesis and potential treatment of a medical disease or condition), uses the theory to predict a result (e.g., that a molecule displaying pharmacologic characteristics blocking or enhancing the physiologic pathway of interest will affect an end point associated with the condition or disease), and tests the prediction in well-planned, well-conducted, and well-analyzed experiments (e.g., both animal and then human clinical trials). Drug development is a primary example of applying an evidence-based, scientifically sound decision algorithm. The process should attempt to winnow out failures as early as possible while characterizing successful candidates in a planned and expanding manner. Along the way, scientific decisions will be made as credible and relevant information is gathered and applied to the current development candidate as well as to future development candidates.

Issues of integrity have been prominently noted in all fields of scientific endeavor. Scientific misconduct, including fraud and misrepresentation, has occurred in both nonclinical and clinical scientific research. Because clinical research involves human experimentation, it has been understandably especially scrutinized. These issues have led to an increasing emphasis on ensuring integrity through training, guidance, regulation, and law. Adhering to scientific integrity is mandatory for all professionals engaged in drug development, both nonclinical and clinical.

The development process must adhere to ethical guidance in the use of animals and humans in the research process. Ethical issues are of primary concern for a process as important and as clinically focused as drug development. As with scientific misconduct, ethical lapses have occurred in the conduct of clinical trials, both those conducted as part of a new drug development program and those conducted to enhance clinical knowledge of a disease or area of therapeutics. As with scientific integrity, adherence to ethical principles is mandatory. There have been several key reviews of fundamental ethical issues in the conduct of clinical research including ethical guidance issued by the U.S. Department of Health, Education, and Welfare (now the Department of Health and Human Services) in the Belmont Report,[7] the World Medical Association in the Declaration of Helsinki,[8] and the Council for International Organizations of Medical Sciences.[9] It is imperative that all clinical trial research be conducted with a respect for the rights and well-being of individuals, has an objective review of the proposed clinical research by an independent review body (e.g., institutional review boards, regulatory agencies), and has an ongoing assessment of risks and benefits as substantial new information becomes apparent (e.g., data safety monitoring boards for larger clinical trials with end points of mortality or significant morbidity).

The drug development process must adhere to applicable laws and regulations. Legal aspects to drug development may be grouped into three main categories: (i) protection of intellectual property; (ii) regulation of business activities; and (iii) regulation of R&D activities, regulatory submissions, drug approval, and postapproval activities.

Protection of intellectual property has become increasingly important owing to the expanding importance of nonbranded, generic drugs and the importance of proprietary invention throughout the discovery and development areas. As drug development has become more global in nature, intellectual property issues have become increasingly more global in their perspective and more complex in their legal characteristics. Intellectual property issues are important to consider as drug discovery and development are being planned, conducted, and analyzed.

Business regulations play a role in drug development because of the business nature of most sponsoring organizations, either for-profit organizations, such as most R&D-based pharmaceutical companies; not-for-profit organizations; or governmental institutions. These include a growing body of laws and regulations that range from rigid conflict of interest rules, such as those enacted by the U.S. National Institutes of Health, to the Federal Corrupt Practices Act, which addresses relationships with foreign government employees. There has also been noticeable expansion of the Healthcare and Fraud and Abuse Laws into the clinical research arena. Particularly important business regulations include the antitrust regulations that regulate the ability of for-profit competing firms to collaborate. As scientific consortia become necessary to address fundamental precompetitive areas such as the validation of biomarkers as surrogate end points or the determination of important genomic and proteomic markers of individual disease susceptibility and progression, attention to antitrust and other related regulations plays an important role in drug development. Publicly held firms, such as those whose stock ownership trades on public exchanges, must also adhere to securities regulations. These regulations generally govern areas such as information release in order to provide a level playing field among potential buyers and sellers of the firm's stock. Adherence to these security regulations plays an important role in information release and must be considered along with all other scientific and ethical principles. The importance of information from the standpoint of securities regulation is often tied to the materiality of the information, which is determined by its importance with respect to the financial worth of the particular organization. The results of an early POM clinical trial for a single drug candidate may be material from the standpoint of a small biotechnology firm and not material from the standpoint of a large R&D-based multinational pharmaceutical firm, which has many such projects ongoing simultaneously.

From the standpoint of drug development, the most influential of all legal considerations are the regulations governing R&D activities, regulatory submissions, drug approval, and postapproval activities. Although present throughout the world, these regulations have incrementally grown most noticeably in the United States and the European Union (E.U.). U.S. and E.U. regulations have, to a great extent, strongly influenced the global drug development process and continue to do so.

In the United States, the legal framework for the regulation of drug development, approval, and postapproval activities has been noticeably influenced by several Congressional acts, listed with highlights[10]:

- Food, Drug, and Cosmetic Act (1938)—established the requirement to prove safety prior to drug approval.
- Kefauver-Harris Amendment (1962)—established the requirement to prove efficacy by "adequate and well-controlled trials" prior to drug approval.
- Orphan Drug Act (1982)—facilitated the approval of drugs for orphan diseases, defined as diseases affecting fewer than 200,000 U.S. patients.
- Drug Price Competition and Patent Term Restoration Act (Waxman–Hatch) (1984)—facilitated the approval of generic drugs on the basis of bioequivalence.
- Prescription Drug User Fee Act (1992)—provided for user fees and the requirements for the FDA to meet targeted review timelines.
- FDA Modernization Act (1997)—provided for additional performance-related measures at the FDA and provided an extra 6 months of marketing exclusivity for products with complete pediatric data packages.
- Best Pharmaceuticals for Children Act (2002)—continued to provide an extra 6 months of marketing exclusivity for products with complete pediatric data packages.
- Pediatric Research Equity Act (2003)—required that applications for drug approval include appropriate pediatric assessments or a waiver or deferral from the FDA.

Each has contributed to the regulations that today govern drug development in the United States.

The FDA, an administrative arm of the Department of Health and Human Service (a department of the executive branch of the U.S. government), is the agency primarily charged with overseeing the regulation of drug R&D activities, regulatory submissions, drug approval, and postapproval activities in the United States. The previously noted and other Congressional Acts have authorized the FDA to issue regulations that provide the legal basis for these regulatory activities. These regulations have the strength of law and are codified in the Code of Federal Regulations (CFR).[11] Particularly pertinent to drug development are CFR Title 21, Part 50: Protection of Human Subjects; Part 56: Institutional Review Boards; Part 58: Good Laboratory Practice for Nonclinical Laboratory Studies; Part 312: Investigational New Drug Application; Part 314: Applications for FDA Approval to Market a New Drug; and Part 316: Orphan Drugs. As this text is being prepared, additional legislation has been proposed in the U.S. Congress to specifically address the issue of drug safety and drug safety reporting, clinical trial registration and reporting, and postapproval risk management activities.

The FDA has also issued draft and final guidance, points to consider, and other documents addressing a number of key issues pertinent to drug development for general as well as specific issues such as pediatric guidance, RMPs or good regulatory review practices. These also include guidance on the format and content of an Investigational New Drug Application (IND), which must be filed to initiate clinical research in the United States, and guidance on the format and content of nonclinical pharmacology/toxicology, chemistry, manufacturing and controls, human pharmacokinetics and bioavailability, and clinical and statistical sections of a New Drug Application (NDA). The FDA's web site contains a reference to a current listing of these documents.[12]

In the European Union, there have also been a number of directives, guidelines, and position papers addressing both nonclinical and clinical aspects of drug development, approval and postapproval activities. As adopted by member nations, these directives and regulations have assumed legal and regulatory status. The European Medicines Agency (EMEA) was established by the European Union and began functioning in 1995. It is charged with evaluating and overseeing the development, approval, and postapproval activities of pharmaceutical products for E.U. member states. Whereas independent national regulatory agencies continue to exist, the EMEA brings together the E.U. experience and offers consolidated views on relevant topics including centralized licensing applications. Numerous guidances and position papers have been issued by the EMEA, with a complete listing and reference maintained on its web site.[13]

Besides the United States and the European Union, a number of countries and corresponding regulatory agencies have established a legal and regulatory framework pertinent to drug development, with the issuance of guidances, position papers, and other relevant documents. In recognition of the large increase in laws, regulations, and guidance that pertained to drug development, the International Conference on Harmonisation of Technical Requirements for Registration of Pharmaceuticals for Human Use (ICH) was initiated in the early 1990s to harmonize the drug development regulatory guidances in the European Union, the United States, and Japan. ICH membership includes academic, regulatory, and pharmaceutical industry experts from the European Union, the United States, and Japan.[14] Six ICH conferences have been held, and many ICH guidelines have been issued on quality, safety, efficacy, and multidisciplinary topics, with the five-step process for implementation outlined by ICH for each of the three corresponding regions.[15]

Data privacy regulations also have an impact on clinical drug trials. The various national laws that implement the European Commission's Directive on Data Protection[16] and the U.S. Privacy Rule[17] enacted under the Health Insurance Portability and Accountability Act of 1996

(HIPAA) are examples of local regulations that directly or indirectly affect the conduct and reporting of clinical drug trials. These regulations and others worldwide have created a patchwork of inconsistent local rules that create logistical challenges for companies that conduct multinational drug trials. Particularly challenging are restrictions on the transnational flow of clinical data and on the use and disclosure of study data by the research sponsor. Appropriate application of general data privacy regulations to the unique requirements of clinical drug trials and the drug development process can, therefore, be difficult, and careful consideration must be given to ensuring that all appropriate standards are met for each clinical trial and development program. Informed consent of the study subject remains key to both protection of subject rights and the flexibility in the transfer, use, and disclosure of clinical data needed for drug development.

Familiarity and adherence to legislative acts, regulations, directives, guidances, and position papers—and to their corresponding operational consequences—are required for understanding and conducting drug development in the European Union, the United States, and Japan and on a global basis.

Overall, adhering to the general principles of science, ethics, and law allows the drug development process to evolve and improve as new technologies are introduced, new scientific discoveries are enabled, and new therapeutic challenges arise. Using the guidance and direction from these principles, new technologies and process improvements can be effectively incorporated into the drug development process.

DISCIPLINE- OR ACTIVITY-SPECIFIC GUIDANCE

Drug development is a complex scientific process involving many technical disciplines and many interdependent activities. Adherence to the principle of scientific excellence requires that each discipline and each activity be planned, conducted, analyzed, and reported to the highest level of excellence for each involved profession using state-of-the-art scientific guidance and methodology. Numerous scientific texts, guidances, and position papers continue to assist in achieving scientific excellence in drug development. Particularly relevant are the issuance of guidance and position papers by the EMEA,[13] the FDA,[12] and ICH.[15] Examples of disciplinary and activity areas and key guidance issues are noted in the following text.

Pharmaceutical Science

Pharmaceutical science is an important multidisciplinary area responsible for designing the synthetic pathway, the formulation, the manufacturing processes, and quality controls for the active pharmaceutical ingredient (API) and final dosage form (drug product) that will be available for use in medical practice. Key areas include designing a synthesis and process capable of producing APIs of high purity and a dosage form with appropriate and reliable in vivo performance. The manufacturability of the API and drug product at reasonable costs at commercial scale must also be assessed. Sensitive analytical methods are developed, validated, and used to measure key quality attributes such as potency, impurity levels, physical form, particle size, and in vitro release rate. Stability studies are conducted to establish appropriate storage conditions and shelf life for which the product will remain within acceptable quality specifications. All of these processes must be developed in compliance with many regulatory requirements, one example being the ICH guidance (Q7A) on "Good Manufacturing Practices" (GMPs), which has been adopted by both the FDA and the EMEA.[18]

In addition to the challenges presented by small molecule drug candidates, biologic drug products present a number of challenges as well. These include assessment of contaminants such as endotoxins, host cell proteins, and viral particles (if mammalian cell line derived), and comparability of biologic products following changes in the manufacturing process.

The importance of pharmaceutical sciences in allowing for successful drug development is often not appreciated. Many pharmaceutical products in current practice and development required extensive pharmaceutical sciences innovation in order to develop a usable drug product. For example, the intravenous administration of voriconazole, a novel antifungal therapy, required that the active drug be solubilized with an innovative new agent, sulphobutylether-β-cyclodextrin sodium.[19] Another pharmaceutical sciences innovation is the use of laser-drilled osmotic tablets to allow controlled release of the active pharmaceutical agent to provide daily dosing and improved tolerability, compliance, and efficacy. Other examples are the use of (i) spray-dried dispersions to increase absorption of poorly soluble compounds, (ii) slow-dissolving microspheres to limit gastric irritation and allow larger doses of drug to be orally administered, and (iii) transgenic animals to secrete therapeutic proteins in their milk, allowing for more economical manufacturing compared with that of tissue culture techniques.

Nonclinical Safety Assessment

Nonclinical safety assessment provides the indispensable foundation for the initiation and conduct of human drug testing. In vitro, in vivo, and animal safety testing are all essential parts of assessing safety before human testing. In silico modeling and in vitro testing still remain noticeably inadequate for this purpose. Key areas of concern include the design and assessment of safety pharmacology testing; the design and interpretation of genotoxicity, mutagenicity, and carcinogenicity testing; reproductive toxicology testing; animal pharmacokinetic and toxicokinetics; immunotoxicology; and other specialized safety areas such as assessment of ventricular repolarization. Guidance on the conduct of safety pharmacology studies for human pharmaceuticals, issued by ICH,[20] along with the codified Directives and Federal Regulations relating to good laboratory practice in the European Union[21,22] and the United States[23] direct the planning, conduct, and analysis of nonclinical studies for a drug development candidate.

Many pharmaceuticals have safety findings of note during their nonclinical safety assessments, with product labeling of many pharmaceuticals mentioning important nonclinical safety findings and their possible relevance to human use. Dedicated and expert review of these findings provides the essential knowledge that allows continued development of the candidate to capture the key information needed to further understand the safety issue and to support the candidate's benefit to risk assessment.

Clinical Research

Clinical research is at the center of the drug development process. Clinical research focuses on the planning, conduct, analysis, and reporting of clinical trial data. Clinical research enables the acquisition of the key clinical efficacy, safety, and tolerance data needed to establish the benefit-to-risk profile of a drug development candidate. Substantial recent focus has been on reviewing and improving the clinical trial process and on ensuring the proper treatment of clinical trial subjects. Development principles incorporate the principles of good clinical research conduct and good scientific data analysis and review. Many of these principles are outlined in the ICH Good Clinical Practice (GCP),[24] which is endorsed and implemented in the European Union[13] and the United States.[12] The guidance presents international ethical and scientific quality standards for designing, conducting, recording, and reporting trials that involve the participation of human subjects. Topics covered include

- Institutional Review Board/Independent Ethics Committee—responsibilities, composition, functions, operations, procedures, and records.
- Investigator—qualifications, resources, compliance, handling of investigational product(s), informed consent of trial subjects, records, and reports.
- Sponsor—trial management, data handling, record keeping, quality control/assurance, financing, monitoring, handling of safety information, and reporting obligations.

BOX 2-1 MORE FREQUENTLY AUDITED ASPECTS OF GOOD CLINICAL PRACTICE

Ethics Committees
- Ethics committee approvals
- Updates to ethics committees as the study is conducted
- Informed consent documented

Source Data Verification
- Patients can be verified
- Case report form data matches source documents
- Audit trail for all changes: who made them, why, when

Reporting of Serious Adverse Events
- To sponsors
- To ethics committees
- To regulatory authorities

Protocol Adherence
- To inclusion/exclusion criteria
- To scheduled activities, exams and procedures

- Clinical Trial Protocol—trial design and objective, selection and treatment of subjects, assessment of efficacy and safety, statistics, data handling, and clinical trial reporting.
- Investigator's Brochure—general considerations and contents for this document, which contains a summary of preclinical and clinical data known up to that point for use by investigators in clinical trials.
- Essential Documents—essential documents and their handling before, during, and after clinical trial conduct.

GCP regulations are enforced, patient rights are protected, sites are scrutinized, and data are carefully audited and verified. Box 2-1 presents some of the more frequently audited aspects of GCP compliance.

In addition to the topics covered in the GCP and related guidance, a number of contemporary topics in clinical research are important to consider in the planning and conduct of this key drug development activity.

- Statistical issues: Adherence to good statistical practices is essential during the planning, conduct, analysis, and reporting of clinical trials. Important topics include randomization, end point analytical procedures, and the handling and imputation of data derived from subjects noncompliant with the study protocol (e.g., dropouts or subjects who discontinue their participation in a clinical trial before it is completed). Statistical support is required for analysis of both efficacy and safety information and during all periods of drug development, nonclinical as well as clinical. All hypotheses to be tested by a confirmatory trial must have an a priori statistical analysis plan specifying, before data are analyzed, what changes in specific end points constitute proof of the hypothesis and what statistical methods will be used to reject the null hypothesis.
- Global conduct of clinical trials: The extent of clinical trial activity occurring in countries outside of the traditional European, North American, and Japanese regions has increased and is anticipated to continue to increase. This expanded theater of clinical trial activity has brought challenges to ensure that the conducted clinical research adheres to GCP and all related guidance and effectively supports drug development. Additional legal and regulatory frameworks must be considered, qualified investigators and investigative staff must be found, and the impact of new medical and cultural operating environments on clinical trial conduct and end point assessment must be considered. Educational efforts to train investigators and staff, efforts to ascertain the cross-cultural impact of end point assessment tools, efforts to understand the local medical practice, and efforts to support worldwide data collection are among many activities required by the expanded theater of clinical trial activity.
- Patient access to clinical trials and experimental drug therapy: Issues of patient access to both clinical trial participation and experimental study medication after completion of the clinical trial and outside of clinical trials have been extensively discussed and various perspectives presented. In the United States, both the legislative and the judiciary branches of government have become involved, and a number of legislative acts and judicial rulings have occurred.[25] Information on clinical trial activity should be available, and sponsors and investigators should clearly articulate their policy on experimental drug access as part of the informed consent process. Issues of patient access to the new drug treatment after participation in a clinical trial have special importance with the conduct of clinical trials in new geographic areas. Several organizations have endorsed the concept that clinical trials should be conducted only in geopolitical areas where the new drug development candidate is planned to be registered and made available for medical use.
- Placebo and active comparator: Use of placebo as a comparator arm of clinical trials has been questioned when studying medical diseases and conditions for which safe and effective therapies have been approved. Instead of placebo, it has been proposed that active comparators serve as the reference for an experimental drug candidate. Use of active comparator as the reference arm has a number of significant challenges, including statistical design of the trial to show noninferiority, or therapeutic equivalence, rather than superiority; the selection of a comparator agent suitable for the multiple medical practice environments in which modern global trials take place; the dose of the comparator agent; the duration of the trial; and the specific end point of the trial. Almost all NDAs do include comparative trial information supplementing placebo-controlled information. The ideal study design has been stated to be one including both a placebo and an active control arm: the placebo arm to provide the reference for the population and the active control to validate the experiment. Temple and Ellenberg[26,27] summarized the issues with use of placebo and concluded that use of placebo is essential both to establish the efficacy of a new drug development candidate and to prevent ineffective drugs from reaching medical usage, and it is permissible for limited durations of time during which additional morbidity caused by placebo usage would be minimal. Most drug development programs continue to depend on the use of placebo to establish the effectiveness of the drug candidate as well as provide a reference point for the establishment of drug-emergent safety and tolerance issues.
- Novel clinical trial designs: Several novel study designs have been introduced to support more efficient and effective drug development. One of the more advanced of these is the adaptive clinical trial design. Rather than conduct a trial using an inflexible, predetermined design (e.g., a rigid sample size and dose assignment), the adaptive clinical trial design uses a variety of approaches to adjust the study design (e.g., sample sizes and dose assignment) based on interim trial results. One type of adaptive design provides for starting the clinical trial with a very broad dose range and provides for a gradual narrowing (or "adaptation") of the dose based on interim reads of efficacy and tolerance data conducted using a predetermined algorithm. No study personnel are informed of interim results, and the dose adaptation is administered in a blinded fashion (e.g., dose assignments are blinded). Active discussion of using adaptive clinical trial design is ongoing. Importantly, the discussion highlights the importance of innovative clinical trial designs as tools to achieve more effective and efficient drug development.
- Use of biomarkers and surrogate end points: Consensus exists that a biomarker is a characteristic that is objectively measured and evaluated as an indicator of normal biologic processes, pathogenic processes, or pharmacologic responses to a therapeutic intervention.[28] Biomarkers play an important role in medical practice and in clinical research, aiding in the identification, diagnosis, staging, and treatment of affected individuals and individuals who may be at risk but do not yet exhibit symptoms. Commonly used

biomarkers include electrocardiograms, serum chemistries, bone mineral density measurements, pulmonary function tests, and other objective measurements. In contrast to the consensus around biomarkers, there are disparate views of which biomarkers can be called surrogate end points. Surrogacy is achieved when a biomarker is used to actually predict—in fact used in place of—a clinical end point and, operationally, can be used to demonstrate pharmaceutical utility for registration of a new drug.[28] Examples of biomarkers that have achieved surrogate status include blood pressure and low-density lipoprotein (LDL) cholesterol as surrogates for cardiovascular events, blood glucose as a surrogate for diabetic morbidity, and HIV viral load as a surrogate for subsequent HIV complications and survival. Examples of biomarkers that were shown, upon definitive testing, to be unrelated to clinical end points include premature ventricular contractions (PVCs), which were shown to be unrelated to sudden death (i.e., drugs that suppressed them increased mortality),[29] and improved exercise tolerance in patients with heart failure that did not correlate with improved longevity (i.e., drugs that improved exercise testing through phosphodiesterase inhibition actually shortened life).[30] Because of the length and size of the clinical trials needed to directly study clinical end points, biomarkers and clinical surrogates are increasingly important in drug development both in early exploratory development and in registration-supporting clinical trials. Breakthroughs in genomics, basic research, and combinatorial chemistry have resulted in an increasing number of new approaches and new chemicals to be studied as potential treatments for a number of diseases and conditions. Increasingly, these are chronic indolent diseases such as osteoarthritis or Alzheimer's disease in which a potential impact on the underlying disease state is seen only after months or years of treatment. This has put pressure on the clinical research activities to ascertain promptly and efficiently which approaches work and which do not. If clinical end point trials are required for the assessment of each new approach, especially for indolent and chronic diseases, the ability to provide informative feedback to discovery scientists will be very limited and will present an absolute roadblock in the translation of important bench breakthroughs to important new medicines for patients. The recognition of the need to advance the effective use of biomarkers and surrogate end points has been acknowledged, and a number of pathways to explore expanded use and validation of biomarkers and surrogate end points have been proposed. Because of the multiplicity of purposes, validation itself is not a black/white, single pathway process. Validation for exploratory development may be easier and require less than validation for regulatory approval. One general framework that can be customized was presented by Boissel and colleagues[31] and then further adapted by Espelande and associates.[32] The three proposed clinical criteria are practical, understandable, and actionable. They are (i) efficiency (the surrogate end point should be relatively easy to evaluate, precede the clinical end point, and require fewer resources), (ii) linkage (the relationship of the surrogate to the clinical end point should be understandable and should be established by clinical studies), and (iii) congruency (the surrogate should parallel estimates of risk and benefit compared with the clinical end point). Use of this framework may assist progress in the application and validation of biomarkers.

- Transparency of clinical study conduct and results: Transparency in both the conduct and the reporting of clinical trials has been an area of significant focus and concern. Discussion has centered on balancing the establishment of trust and the contribution to general scientific and medical knowledge with the intellectual property and proprietary concerns of investigators and sponsors of drug development. Discussion documents and statements have been issued[33-35] with general support that clinical trials should be registered prior to initiation of the study. One of the most common registries is the ClinicalTrials.gov registry provided by the U.S. National Library of Medicine of the National Institutes of Health (NIH).[36] ClinicalTrials.gov provides regularly updated information about federally and privately supported clinical research in human volunteers. ClinicalTrials.gov provides information about a trial's purpose, who may participate, locations, and phone numbers for more details. Subsequent to study conduct and analysis, there is general support for timely reporting of all clinical trial results. This may occur by scientific presentation, publication, or other publicly available release. One clinical trial results registry is the ClinicalStudyResults.org web site sponsored by the Pharmaceutical and Research Manufacturers of America.[37] This site is a central, widely accessible, web-based repository for clinical study results in a reader-friendly, standardized format. The intent of the database is to serve the valuable function of making clinical trial results for many marketed pharmaceuticals more transparent and to provide information to practicing physicians and their patients. Additional clinical trial result repositories include web sites sponsored by the U.S. National Cancer Institute as well as a number of individual pharmaceutical organizations.

DECISION-BASED CONTINUOUS DRUG DEVELOPMENT

Based firmly upon the general principles and the discipline- and activity-specific guidances, drug development proceeds to gather the information needed to understand the efficacy, safety, and tolerance of new development candidates. This understanding allows the continuous review of benefit to risk for the new candidate. Drug development begins with the initiation of a discovery program and concludes when the development candidate is superseded by better therapeutic alternatives. It is a planned process that at each stage and at key decision points notes the information that is needed and the activities that must be planned to gain the next informational increment. This section reviews the stepwise information needs and goals for key milestones in the drug development process.

Discovery

The initiation of a drug discovery program depends upon a firm medical knowledge of the relevant disease or disorder along with a solid knowledge of the chemical and biologic science that will provide the pharmacologic basis for the intervention. Understanding the medical disease or disorder is necessary in order to understand state-of-the-art treatment, the natural history of the illness or condition, and the resulting clinical significance of intervention. Medical disease knowledge is also needed to prepare the outline of a development plan. Relevant guidance documents and prior development plans, many of which have been outlined in publicly available regulatory documents, should be reviewed. Drug development begins during drug discovery, with an outline of the development pathway and the requirements for successful drug registration and approval. This is the stage at which the initial target product profile for the development candidate should be prepared, in order to provide a clear objective for candidate nomination and subsequent development. The target product profile is a compilation of key attributes that are expected of the drug candidate once development is complete including (i) indications to be treated, both at initial registration and at subsequent regulatory filings; (ii) clinical end points that will be used to achieve regulatory approval for those indications; (iii) anticipated key safety issues; (iv) benefits relative to existing drugs on the market; (v) the resulting benefit-to-risk statement based on (iii) and (iv); and (vi) the desired dosage form, route, and frequency of administration. It is against this target product profile that the drug candidate is constantly measured during the development process.

Candidate Nomination for Development

The nomination of a potential drug development candidate
a time when the drug candidate has proven in vitro and in
macology and meets rigorous standards of specificity and

the desired target. The candidate has also passed a battery of tests to ensure it has appropriate pharmaceutical and safety properties for further testing and, ultimately, administration to humans. Pharmacologic support exists that the characteristics featured in the target product profile could be achieved by the nominated candidate. In order to minimize candidate attrition, many key hurdles must be overcome before candidate nomination:

- Potency and selectivity have been established for the desired pharmacology both in vitro (using human and other relevant species laboratory systems) and in vivo. Undesired pharmacology has been looked at for using screening panels (with particular attention to effects on cardiac conduction).
- The pharmacokinetic and pharmacodynamic relationship in animal species has been established, and there is a suitable pharmacodynamic marker for human studies.
- Metabolic pathways and predicted clearance and distribution in humans are in a feasible range, and relationships between humans and other relevant species (such as those used to study pharmacology and toxicology) have been established for these parameters.
- Genetic toxicity has been assessed and found not to be an issue. In vivo tolerance in relevant animal models of pharmacology has shown no limiting toxicity or has demonstrated an acceptable therapeutic index.
- The drug candidate must be able to be adequately synthesized and scaled up at a reasonable cost of goods; if a small molecule, there must be no concerns with toxicophores.
- The candidate must be able to be formulated and have sufficient stability, solubility, and bioavailability to be a pharmaceutical agent.

Proof of Mechanism

POM occurs after the appropriate pharmacology has been shown to take place in humans and an adequate pharmacokinetic and pharmacodynamic relationship has been demonstrated at doses well tolerated in humans. To achieve POM, generally a small number (~50-100) of volunteers and patients with a restrictive definition of disease attributes will have been studied for periods of approximately 1 to 4 weeks.

Proof of Concept

POC occurs once the drug candidate has shown desired effects with adequate safety and tolerability on either hard clinical end points (those that ultimately support registration of the product) in the intended disease state or surrogate end points that are predictive of ultimate effect upon the registerable end points. POC is not dependent upon the results of a single clinical trial but is based on the accumulated weight of evidence gathered to the decision time point. To achieve POC, generally several hundred patients with a broader, but still restrictive, definition of disease attributes will have been studied for periods of approximately 4 to 24 weeks.

Proceed to Confirmatory Clinical Trials

Drug development proceeds to confirmatory clinical trials when there is sufficient information to identify the doses most likely to have a favorable efficacy, tolerance, and safety profile when used in a more broad-based population reflecting the patient population in which the development candidate would be used following approval. Prior to initiation of late-stage, confirmatory clinical trial development, known information includes

- Safety exposure in humans that is sufficient to identify tolerability and key safety issues other than rare events. Generally, this means that several hundred patients and volunteers have been exposed to the development candidate for several weeks to several months (depending on chronicity of intended use). RMPs for further characterizing safety in the period of confirmatory clinical trials and postapproval have been formulated, and the target product profile has been updated to incorporate these risks.
- Efficacy that has been characterized with statistically and clinically significant superiority demonstrated generally versus placebo in either a registrable end point or a reliable surrogate end point. Proposed registrable end points have been designed into plans for confirmatory clinical trial plans and are ready to be discussed with regulators.
- Pharmacokinetics, key drug interactions, and key metabolites that have been characterized and a justification for the dose(s) to be brought into late-stage development has been established.
- Key aspects of formulation, manufacturing, commercial scale-up that are identified and related activities are under way. Manufacture of the final commercial formulation is either complete (for use in confirmatory clinical trials) or well under way. An impurity control strategy is in place. Where possible, confirmatory trials should be conducted with the same formulation of the drug candidate that will be used for the marketed product.
- Critical appraisal of the characteristics of the drug development candidate compared with the target product profile, from scientific, regulatory, and medical use perspectives.

Generally, before confirmatory clinical trials begin, much of the preceding information and planning is summarized and discussed with regulators in the United States, the European Union, and Japan to ensure that the proposed late-stage development program, if successful, will meet requirements to establish benefit-to-risk and will allow registration of the development candidate. This often includes a detailed discussion of key end points in the confirmatory clinical trials, statistical testing to be used, the exact patient populations to be studied, and the anticipated size, diversity, and duration of treatment in the clinical trial database that will establish safety and tolerance in the target population.

Registration

The registration of a drug development candidate in order to obtain approval for medical use occurs when comprehensive and sufficient information is available to adequately assess the benefit-to-risk of using the product as described. This requires a firm and thorough understanding of the efficacy, safety, and tolerance profile of the candidate. Both regulation and guidance address the requirements for drug approval in the European Union, the United States, Japan, and other geopolitical regions. ICH guideline requirements stipulate that there be a minimum of 1500 subjects treated, with 100 treated for a year or more for chronic use agents.[38] Most current drug candidates, however, have much greater numbers of subjects treated and often 10-fold or more than the minimum number of subjects treated for 1 year at the time of registration. Replicated well-controlled clinical trials showing efficacy by preagreed criteria are generally required, with at least one set of studies for each claim. Most development programs include both placebo- and active-controlled trials. All regulatory agencies assess whether there is an adequately broad spectrum of disease represented (usually mild, moderate, and severe cases) and whether there are sufficient special populations included, such as the young, the elderly, and various ethnic and racial groups to allow generalization to the intended target population.

Regulatory review includes not only an assessment of efficacy and safety in humans but also a careful review of nonclinical pharmacology and toxicology. Reproductive toxicology is required for agents to be given to women of childbearing potential, and 2-year carcinogenicity studies in at least two animal species are required for chronic use drugs. Finally, there is a detailed assessment of pharmaceutics including manufacturing and formulation controls. Most drugs are not approved until manufacturing facilities have been inspected and key clinical trial sites have been audited for compliance to GMP and GCP, respectively.

Postapproval

An RMP for each development candidate is designed in collaboration with expert consultants and regulatory agencies and includes clinical

TABLE 2-1 PROBABILITY OF SEEING AN ADVERSE DRUG EVENT BASED ON ITS FREQUENCY AND THE SIZE OF THE CLINICAL SAFETY DATABASE

Frequency of the Event Rate (%)	Size of Safety Database	Probability of Seeing the Event at Least Once	Probability of Seeing the Event at Least Twice
1	500	0.993	0.96
0.50	500	0.918	0.713
	1,000	0.993	0.96
0.10	1,500	0.777	0.442
	3,000	0.95	0.801
0.01	6,000	0.451	0.122
	10,000	0.632	0.264
	20,000	0.865	0.594

Note: This table does not address whether the event is caused by the drug or just chance. It addresses only that the event will be observed. Much large numbers are needed to see whether the event rate is higher than expected if it is an event that occurs naturally in a non–study drug–treated population.

trials designed to further acquire efficacy, safety, and tolerance information about the development candidate, extending beyond the time of first approval. The RMP is generally first designed at the completion of POC and continuously refined as additional information is acquired. At the time of registration for approval, regulatory agencies expect that the information supported by the development program adequately addresses the safety, tolerance, and efficacy issues noted in the RMP, that the proposed labeling is consistent with it, and that a series of postapproval commitments are made consistent with the RMP. This latter aspect is particularly important because it is recognized that even a large well-conducted development program will be unable to detect rare adverse events. As shown in Table 2-1, even a submission database containing information from 10,000 subjects will have only approximately a 60% chance of detecting an adverse event of 1 in 10,000 and only approximately a 20% chance of seeing it twice (which is generally necessary to rule out a chance finding). Significant drug-related events (such as liver or bone marrow failure) that occur with a frequency of 1 in 10,000 or less, however, would significantly affect benefit-to-risk considerations and would probably restrict or eliminate use of the drug in all cases but those with very strong medical need. Further aspects of RMPs and pharmacovigilance are discussed in Chapter 3, Regulations and Pharmacovigilance.

SPECIAL TOPICS

Japan

Japan, after the United States, is the largest national user of pharmaceutical products. Although Japanese requirements for drug development and approval are becoming more aligned with those of the European Union and the United States through ICH, unique aspects to drug development projects seeking approval in Japan remain. Most of these are centered on the need for substantial data in Japanese study subjects. Historically, this meant that an entire clinical development program needed to be replicated in Japan in order to establish pharmacokinetics, dose response, efficacy, tolerance, and safety in Japanese subjects. Foreign data were, at best, supportive of this stand-alone program. With the advent of ICH, particularly ICH E5,[39] "bridging" strategies have become increasingly accepted by the Pharmaceutical and Medical Devices Agency (PMDA). As of 2003, about a quarter of all dossiers submitted to PMDA were based on bridging strategies.[40] Generally, these consist of single- and multiple-dose studies to establish similar pharmacokinetics between Japanese study subjects and those in the global database or to establish appropriate correction factors for weight (Japanese study subjects generally weigh 5-10 kg less than Westerners). In consultation with PMDA, a dose-response study is then generally conducted as a bridging study, which validates the remainder of the studies based on foreign data. This bridging study, usually of several hundred patients treated for several months for chronic conditions, establishes a tolerated, safe, and effective dose in Japanese patients. This is then bridged to the corresponding confirmatory global studies to provide confirmation of safety and efficacy of one or more doses. More recently, PMDA has accepted dossiers based on multicountry Asian studies, provided the database contains a sufficient number of Japanese subjects in order to confirm that safety, tolerance, and efficacy are similar in the subset of Japanese compared with that observed in the entire database. In essence, the Japanese subpopulation serves as the bridge to the larger study and to other non-Japanese studies in the dossier. More recently, both academics and regulators in Japan[40] have proposed a similar process using a global database with studies conducted in the European Union, the United States, and Japan, minimizing the need for unique studies in Japan and eliminating the need for a unique development plan exclusively for Japan. Whereas, to our knowledge, no pharmaceutical has been approved on this basis, it is anticipated that this practice will become commonplace in the future.

Elderly, Pediatric, and Special Populations

In planning and conducting drug development, it is important to ensure that adequate information has been obtained to allow benefit-to-risk determination in all appropriate populations. Depending on the disease or disorder under study, this may include the elderly, children, or other special groups. Depending on the inclusion/exclusion criteria of the clinical trials, adequate information from the main studies of the clinical program may not exist, and special studies may be needed. All of the principles and guidance that apply to the main development program also apply to development in elderly, pediatric, or other special populations.

Most diseases or disorders under study that occur in an adult population also occur in an elderly population—with elderly defined as aged 65 years or older. Most regulatory authorities recommend that elderly patients be included in the main drug development program, especially the confirmatory clinical trials, and that exclusion on the sole basis of age be used only when clinically necessary. Because elderly patients often have more concurrent medical illness and take more concomitant medications than younger patients, obtaining experience in the more broadly based confirmatory clinical trials provides the information needed to allow proper guidance in postapproval use of the drug. Interactions between the study drug and the concurrent medical illness or between the study drug and the concomitant medications can be assessed during these trials. As part of the assessment of the study drug, it is generally necessary to study the pharmacokinetic characteristics of the study drug in elderly subjects. This is especially appropriate in study drugs that are metabolized or excreted by the kidney or liver because hepatic and renal function declines with age. At the time of regulatory submission, current ICH guidance[4] requests a minimum of 100 elderly patients for diseases not unique but occurring in the elderly. For diseases mainly occurring in elderly (e.g., Alzheimer dementia), the main development program would predominantly include elderly subjects. Most regulatory authorities require that safety, tolerance, and efficacy information submitted at the time of product registration be separately presented for the elderly and the young. This allows a determination of whether the information provided in the application is adequate for review.

In addition to the elderly, it is essential that children have access to new drug treatments that offer substantial medical benefit and that use of the new drug treatment in children be based on solid information gained from application of the development process. The inclusion of pediatric patients in the drug development process, however, is more complicated than the inclusion of elderly patients. This is due to the ethical concerns around the inclusion of children as participants in experimental drug studies and the frequently different medical conditions or concerns present in children but not adults. Whereas it is realized that pediatric patients require clinical research data, it is also realized that they are a vulnerable population who must be protected from harm. The pediatric population includes a broad range of subjects. One classification is: neonates (aged <1 mo), infants (aged 1 mo-2 yr), children (aged 2-11 yr), and adolescents (aged 12-16/18 yr).[42] The physiology, medical conditions and concerns, social and cognitive abilities differ greatly among these groups. In planning pediatric drug development, it is essential to specifically identify the target group of patients that will benefit from the new treatment and clearly understand the medical condition and concerns of that population. A treatment bringing potential benefit to neonates will be developed differently from a treatment bringing benefit to adolescents. Each of the pediatric groups has some unique and some shared concerns.

Prior to the initiation of pediatric clinical research, it is necessary to ensure that there is adequate information from the nonclinical pharmacology and toxicology studies to support the initiation of clinical trials. Often, it is also necessary to ensure that there is information from the adult drug development program so that key safety and tolerance issues have been adequately characterized and POC for the drug under study has been established in the relevant disease or condition. The first clinical trials in pediatric patients are generally pharmacokinetic trials to determine the pharmacokinetic characteristics of the drug in the relevant pediatric groups (neonates, infants, children, and adolescents). For diseases with similar pathophysiology in pediatric and adult patients, this pharmacokinetic information may allow dose selection for further clinical trials on the basis of extrapolation.

Besides determining the pharmacokinetic characteristics, it is often necessary to develop a specific pediatric formulation in order to effectively dose pediatric patients. Medication compliance is a key issue with pediatric patients. Development and testing of an acceptable pediatric formulation may be a significant pharmaceutical science challenge and should be planned early in the development program.

In the United Stataes, the Pediatric Research Equity Act (PREA) of 2003 requires that all new drug and biologic applications for approval include information that allows an assessment of the use of the new drug or biologic in pediatric patients or that a waiver or deferral has been granted by the FDA. The FDA has issued specific guidance on compliance with the PREA.[43] Consideration of pediatric application of all new drug candidates should occur at the time of candidate nomination, before the initiation of any human clinical research. At this time, a pediatric development plan should be proposed that considers the medical need, the potential for the new drug to provide significant medical benefit, and the information required in order to initiate pediatric clinical trials. If the medical condition under study is not relevant to a pediatric population (e.g., Alzheimer dementia), then a waiver from pediatric development can be requested. If it is appropriate to obtain information from adults in order to best characterize safety and tolerance issues, then a deferral of pediatric development until after the initial registration for approval can be requested.

In addition to the PREA, current provisions of the Best Pharmaceutical for Children Act (BPCA) of 2002 provide an extra 6 months of marketing exclusivity for products with complete pediatric data packages. The contents of this complete data package are specified in a written request letter issued by the FDA.[44]

Obtaining informed consent directly and solely from pediatric patients is generally not legally or ethically permissible. Accordingly, this puts a special burden on the investigator, investigative staff, responsible institutional review board, and sponsor to ensure that informed consent is obtained from a parent or legal guardian following a full and understandable presentation of the risks and benefits of the research. Regulatory authorities, investigative review boards, or local law may also require the assent of a trial subject capable of understanding (often children aged 6-7 yr or above) and consent from older subjects such as adolescents.[45] A particular ethical challenge is posed by pharmacokinetic studies, which are essential to the safe development of drugs for children but which generally do not provide any potential benefit to the subject. Those responsible for pediatric research must additionally pay careful attention to even subtle coercion in either recruiting or retaining trial participants and their guardians.

Depending on the disease or condition under study, other special populations may exist in whom the new drug treatment would represent a significant improvement and who have not been included in the main development program. These could include populations with specific concurrent medical illness, such as congestive heart failure, in which a specific set of clinical trials may be indicated in order to obtain the information needed to assess benefit-to-risk. Identification of these special populations should occur early in the drug development process, program additions to address their needs planned, and discussions held with academic experts and regulatory authorities.

Biologic Agents

Most aspects of drug development for biologics are similar to those for small molecules. Clinical efficacy, tolerance, safety, and labeling claims are established using clinical trials of essentially the same design as would be used for small molecules seeking these claims. Differences, however, do exist in several areas, such as chemistry and manufacturing. Most biologics are made using cell culture or bacterial fermentation and, as large proteins, pose a unique set of manufacture and formulation issues, with cost of goods often a much more critical consideration than for small molecules.

Toxicology requirements are also different. In general, genetic toxicity testing is not helpful in risk assessment and is not required by regulatory agencies. Antibodies and several other classes of naturally occurring proteins do not require reproductive toxicology; however, this is offset by the failure of human proteins to be active in many toxicology species or by their tendency to be neutralized by anti-human antibodies to human molecules administered to toxicology species. Mechanism-related toxicology must often be explored using analogue proteins active in the relevant animal species. For many biologics, especially those affecting the immune system, such as immune-enhancing or -inhibiting antibodies, extensive immunotoxicologic testing is required to limit the risk of untoward effects such as cytokine release syndrome when the agent is given to humans. Monoclonal antibodies directed at novel T-cell, B-cell, or macrophage targets are particularly high risk in this regard. This became unfortunately apparent in the first-in-human clinical trials of TGN1412, a human anti-CD28 monoclonal antibody.[46] First-in-human study design for such agents will often call for extremely careful dose escalation and, frequently, dosing of single-subject cohorts with careful and extended observation. Because many biologic agents, particularly antibodies, have serum half-lives of several weeks, careful consideration must also be given to how long one dosing cohort needs to be observed before the next cohort can be dosed. Consideration must also be given to whether the risk of first-in-human dosing justifies the use of healthy volunteers or whether the agent is better given to patients with a disease state intended for treatment, who could derive benefit as well as tolerate risk from the administration of the biologic.[47]

Individual Assessment of Benefit-to-Risk

The U.S. Department of Health and Human Services Task Force on Risk Management noted that benefit-to-risk perspectives can depend on the viewpoint of the reviewer. Figure 2-8 is a graphic from the report showing that the FDA evaluates benefits/risks for the population, a provider evaluates it for a patient, and a patient evaluates it in terms of personal values. Refining and improving the ability to use medicines through a better assessment of individualized benefit and individualized risk is a generally recognized imperative in improving drug development. This includes not only using genomic, proteomic, or molecular biomarkers to look for predictors, correlates, or actual mediators of individual variation in risk and therapeutic response but also using clinically based assessments in determining variables affecting disease risk as well as the therapeutic risk—at the level of the individual patient. Examples include determining cardiovascular risk using a weighted multifactorial assessment[48-50] and using a measurement-based approach to guiding antidepressant therapy.[51] Improving the drug development process to allow for more individualized assessment of benefit-to-risk will require further defining relevant laboratory or clinical variables associated with disease onset and morbidity, improvement in individually based assessment tools, building individual benefit-to-risk assessment into dose selection, and emphasizing study designs that feature individual assessment of benefit-to-risk. These improvements will then provide the information needed to introduce individual assessment into clinical practice in an informed manner.

Orphan Drugs

The huge expense of drug development creates the public health concern that "orphan" drugs for rare diseases will not be developed in adequate numbers by the pharmaceutical industry in which there is little expectation of return on the large investment made. To offset this concern, legislation in the United States, the European Union, and Japan has provided special incentives for drugs intended to treat rare diseases. Each region stipulates that such drugs must be for serious diseases that either have no treatment or have treatments inferior to the one being developed. The specific definitions of orphan drugs for the three regions, as well as the incentives provided, are outlined in Table 2-2. In general, these incentives include market exclusivity for a period of 7 to 10 years, scientific advice by the regulatory agency, and possible aid in funding some of the research. The development plans for these diseases are expected to have the same rigor as for any other drug candidate, although allowances will generally be made for smaller sample sizes owing to the underlying rarity of the condition being treated. Since passage of the Orphan Drug Act in 1982 in the United States,[52] more than 200 orphan drugs have been brought to market.

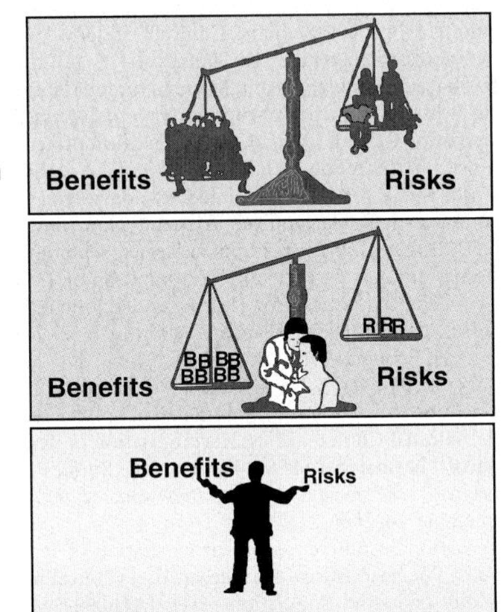

FIGURE 2-8 • Benefit-to-risk perspectives of the FDA, providers, and patients. (From Task Force on Risk Management. Part 1: Background-what are the risks and what is FDA's role in managing risk. In Managing the Risks from Medical Product Use, Creating a Risk Management Framework. U.S. Department of Health and Human Services and Food and Drug Administration, May 1999, pp 20–32.)

SUMMARY AND CONCLUSIONS

Modern drug development, the process by which a molecule with biologic effects in the laboratory is turned into a medication to treat human disease, is a long, arduous, and complex process.

Since the late 1960s, drug development has evolved greatly in sophistication and complexity from one of limited clinical trials in healthy volunteers and then patients to a process of hypothesis testing and confirmation: Is the agent adequately tolerated and can a pharmacokinetic and pharmacodynamic relationship be determined? Does this relationship have any impact in the relevant disease state at tolerated doses? Is this impact likely to be a medical advance over existing agents? Can the effects be confirmed in a larger, more broadly defined population, and can benefit-to-risk be adequately discerned in this larger population in order to support medical use of the drug?

If the answers to the second and third questions are encouraging, the approach shifts from attempting to show failure quickly to investing for success, although the likelihood that these latter questions will all have the positive answers required for approval still remains only about 50%. Throughout the process, the framing of the questions, especially the latter ones, is a cooperative effort among the sponsors, regulators, academic experts, and increasingly, other stakeholders including third-party payers, learned societies, and the public at large.

The process continues to evolve. In the future, even more transparency at each step of the decision-making process will be likely. As the cost and complexity of developing a successful candidate increases further, an ever-increasing reliance on biomarkers will occur to attempt to predict with short duration of treatment of a limited number of patients which drug candidates may ultimately have an impact on disease states after much longer treatment in many more patients. This will allow early elimination of unsuccessful candidates and focus further efforts on those with potential to be medical treatments.

Pharmacogenomics will increasingly inform this process by predicting which genetic subpopulations will respond best to certain

TABLE 2-2 ORPHAN DRUG LEGISLATION IN THE UNITED STATES, EUROPE, AND JAPAN

Region (Year of Legislation)	Definition of Orphan Drug	Incentives
United States (1982)	Disease in question affects <200,000 Americans or is too rare to achieve reasonable return on investment	• 7 years of market exclusivity for the orphan indication • Tax incentives • Grants to help fund clinical trials
European Union (2000)	Disease affects <5/10,000 people or is too rare to achieve reasonable return on investment	• Scientific advice by EMEA • 10 years of market exclusivity for the orphan indication • Tax incentives and possible funding to be provided by member states (varies by member state)
Japan (1993)	Serious diseases with <50,000 patients in Japan	• Priority consultation and review by regulatory agency • Up to 10 years of market exclusivity

EMEA, European Medicines Agency.

therapeutic agents. Although general use of "designer drugs" (defined as drugs specifically identified to an individual genomic type) is perhaps decades away, the use of genomic or proteomic markers to identify subsets of patients likely to have a preferential drug response is already influencing drug development and medical practice decision making.

By combining science from disciplines as diverse as chemistry, genomics, and clinical medicine with guidance from regulatory policy and law and, most importantly, with consideration for the needs of patients, the drug development process has produced profound advances in the medical therapeutics over the last 5 decades. Because it is an evolving process, it is poised to allow such advances to continue into the future.

REFERENCES

1. Dexter L. Vascular hypertension. In Cecil RL, Loeb RF (eds): Textbook of Medicine, 8th ed. Philadelphia: WB Saunders, 1951, pp 1077-1078.
2. U.S. National Heart, Lung, and Blood Institute. The Seventh Report of the Joint National Committee on Prevention, Detection, Evaluation, and Treatment of High Blood Pressure (JNC 7). Available at http://www.nhlbi.nih.gov/guidelines/hypertension/ (accessed September 10, 2006).
3. Schmid EF, Smith DA. Is declining innovation in the pharmaceutical industry a myth? Drug Disc Today 2005;10:1031-1039.
4. U.S. Food and Drug Administration. CDER drug and biologic approval reports. Available at http://www.fda.gov/cder/rdmt/default.htm (accessed October 14, 2006).
5. Pharmaceutical Research and Manufacturers of America. Pharmaceutical industry profile 2006. Available at: http://www.phrma.org (accessed October 14, 2006).
6. DiMasi JA, Hansen RW, Grabowski HG. The price of innovation: new estimates of drug development costs. J Health Econ 2003;22:151-185.
7. U.S. Department of Health, Education, and Welfare. The Belmont report. Available at http://www.hhs.gov/ohrp/humansubjects/guidance/belmont.htm (accessed September 10, 2006).
8. World Medical Association. The Declaration of Helsinki. Available at http://www.wma.net/e/policy/b3.htm (accessed September 10, 2006).
9. Council for International Organizations of Medical Sciences (CIOMS). International Ethical Guidelines for Biomedical Research Involving Human Subjects. Available at http://www.cioms.ch/guidelines_nov_2002_blurb.htm (accessed September 10, 2006).
10. U.S. Food and Drug Administration. Laws enforced by the FDA and related statutes. Available at http://www.fda.gov/opacom/laws/ (accessed September 11, 2006).
11. National Archives and Records Administration. Code of Federal Regulations: Title 21 Food and Drugs. Available at http://www.access.gpo.gov/cgi-bin/cfrassemble.cgi?title=200621 (accessed September 10, 2006).
12. U.S. Food and Drug Administration. Guidance documents. Available at http://www.fda.gov/cder/guidance/index.htm (accessed September 10, 2006).
13. European Medicines Agency. Regulatory guidance and procedures. Available at http://www.emea.europa.eu/sitemap.htm (accessed September 10, 2006).
14. International Conference on Harmonisation of Technical Requirements for Registration of Pharmaceuticals for Human Use. Home website. Available at http://www.ich.org (accessed September 10, 2006).
15. International Conference on Harmonisation of Technical Requirements for Registration of Pharmaceuticals for Human Use. ICH guidelines. Available at http://www.ich.org/cache/compo/276-254-1.html (accessed September 10, 2006).
16. Directive 95/46/EC on the protection of individuals with regard to the processing of personal data and on the free movement of such data. Available at http://ec.europa.eu/justice_home/fsj/privacy/law/index_en.htm (accessed November 21, 2006).
17. Standards for Privacy of Individually Identifiable Health Information, 45 CFR Parts 160, 162, and 164. Available at http://www.hhs.gov/ocr/hipaa/ (Accessed November 21, 2006).
18. International Conference on Harmonisation of Technical Requirements for Registration of Pharmaceuticals for Human Use. Guidance for industry: Q7A good manufacturing practice guidance for active pharmaceutical ingredients. Available at http://www.ich.org/LOB/media/MEDIA433.pdf (accessed September 10, 2006).
19. Tomaszewski K, Purkins L. The pharmacokinetics (PK) and safety of sulphobutylether-β-cyclodextrin (SBECD) [Abstract]. Intersci Conf Antimicrob Agents Chemother 2001;41:3.
20. International Conference on Harmonisation of Technical Requirements for Registration of Pharmaceuticals for Human Use. Guidance for industry: S7A safety pharmacology studies for human pharmaceuticals. Available at http://www.ich.org/LOB/media/MEDIA504.pdf (accessed September 10, 2006).
21. Official Journal of the European Union. Directive 2004/9/EC of the European Parliament and Council of 11 February 2004 on the inspection and verification of good laboratory practice (GLP) [codified version]. Available at http://europa.eu.int/eur-lex/pri/en/oj/dat/2004/l_050/l_05020040220en00280043.pdf (accessed September 10, 2006).
22. Official Journal of the European Union. Directive 2004/10/EC of the European Parliament and Council of 11 February 2004 on the harmonisation of laws, regulations and administrative provisions relating to the application of the principles of good laboratory practice and the verification of their applications for tests on chemical substances [codified version]. Available at http://europa.eu.int/eur-lex/pri/en/oj/dat/2004/l_050/l_05020040220en00440059.pdf (accessed September 10, 2006).
23. National Archives and Records Administration. Code of Federal Regulations: Title 21 Food and Drugs, Part 58: Good laboratory practice for nonclinical laboratory studies. Available at http://www.access.gpo.gov/nara/cfr/waisidx_06/21cfr58_06.html (accessed September 10, 2006).
24. International Conference on Harmonisation of Technical Requirements for Registration of Pharmaceuticals for Human Use. Guidelines for good clinical practice—E6(R1). Available at http://www.ich.org/LOB/media/MEDIA482.pdf (accessed September 10, 2006).
25. Okie S. Access before approval—a right to take experimental drugs? N Engl J Med 2006;355:437-438.
26. Temple R, Ellenberg S. Placebo-controlled trials and active-controlled trials in the evaluation of new treatments, Part 1: Ethical and scientific issues. Ann Intern Med 2000;133:455-463.
27. Ellenberg S, Temple R. Placebo-controlled trials and active-controlled trials in the evaluation of new treatments, Part 2: Practical issues and specific cases. Ann Intern Med 2000;133:464-470.
28. Biomarkers Definitions Working Group. Biomarkers and surrogate endpoints: preferred definitions and conceptual framework. Clin Pharm Ther 2001;69:89-95.
29. Echt DS, Liebson PR, Mitchell LB, et al. Mortality and morbidity in patients receiving encainide, flecainide, or placebo. The Cardiac Arrhythmia Suppression Trial. N Engl J Med 1991;324:781-788.
30. Packer M, Carver JR, Rodeheffer RJ, et al. Effect of oral milrinone on mortality in severe chronic heart failure. The PROMISE Study Research Group. N Engl J Med 1991;325:1468-1475.
31. Boissel JP, Collet JP, Moleur P, et al. Surrogate endpoints: a basis for a rational approach. Eur J Clin Pharmacol 1992;43:235-244.
32. Espeland MA, O'Leary DH, Terry JG, et al. Carotid intimal-media thickness as a surrogate for cardiovascular disease events in trials of HMG-CoA reductase inhibitors. Curr Control Trials Cardiovasc Med 2005;6:3-6.
33. World Health Organization. International Clinical Trial Registry Platform (ICTRP). Available at http://www.who.int/ictrp/en/ (accessed September 10, 2006).
34. Pharmaceutical Research and Manufacturers Association. Principles on conduct of clinical trials and communication of clinical trial results. Available at http://www.phrma.org/files/Clinical%20Trials.pdf (accessed September 10, 2006).
35. International Committee of Medical Journal Editors. Is this clinical trial fully registered? A statement from the International Committee of Medical Journal Editors. Available at http://www.icmje.org/clin_trialup.htm (accessed September 10, 2006).
36. National Library of Medicine. ClinicalTrials.gov. Available at: http://www.clinicaltrials.gov/ (accessed September 10, 2006).
37. Pharmaceutical Research and Manufacturers Association. Clinical study results. Available at http://www.clinicalstudyresults.org/ (accessed September 10, 2006).
38. International Conference on Harmonisation of Technical Requirements for Registration of Pharmaceuticals for Human Use. The extent of population exposure to assess clinical safety for drugs intended for long-term treatment of non–life threatening conditions. ICH Harmonized Tripartite Guideline (E1). Available at http://www.ich.org/LOB/media/MEDIA435.pdf (accessed September 17, 2006).
39. International Conference on Harmonisation of Technical Requirements for Registration of Pharmaceuticals for Human Use. Ethnic factors in the acceptability of foreign clinical data E5(R1). Available at http://www.ich.org/LOB/media/MEDIA481.pdf (accessed September 10, 2006).
40. Uyama Y, Shibata T, Nagai N, et al. Successful bridging strategy based on ICH E5 guideline for drugs approved in Japan. Clin Pharm Ther 2005;78:102-113.
41. International Conference on Harmonisation of Technical Requirements for Registration of Pharmaceuticals for Human Use. Studies in support of special populations: Geriatrics—E7. Available at http://www.ich.org/LOB/media/MEDIA483.pdf (accessed September 10, 2006).
42. International Conference on Harmonisation of Technical Requirements for Registration of Pharmaceuticals for Human Use: Clinical investigation of medicinal products in the pediatric population—E11. Available at http://www.ich.org/LOB/media/MEDIA487.pdf (Accessed September 10, 2006).
43. U.S. Food and Drug Administration. Guidance for industry: how to comply with the Pediatric Research Equity Act. Available at http://www.fda.gov/cder/guidance/6215dft.pdf (accessed September 10, 2006).
44. U.S. Food and Drug Administration. Guidance for industry: qualifying for pediatric exclusivity under section 505A of the Federal Food, Drug, and Cosmetic Act. Available at http://www.fda.gov/cder/guidance/2891fnl.pdf (accessed September 10, 2006).
45. Ross LF, Newburger JW, Saunders SP: Ethical issues in pediatric trials. Am Heart J 2001;142:233-236.
46. Suntharalingam G, Perry MR, Ward S, et al. Cytokine storm in a phase 1 trial of the anti-CD28 monoclonal antibody TGN1412. N Engl J Med 2006;355:1018-1028.
47. Association of the British Pharmaceutical Industry/BioIndustry Association. Early Stage Clinical Trial Taskforce—Joint ABPI/BIA Report. Available at http://www.abpi.org.uk/information/pdfs/BIAABPI_taskforce2.pdf#search=%22joint%20abpi%2Fbia%20report%22 (accessed September 11, 2006).
48. Assmann G, Cullen P, Schulte H. Simple scoring scheme for calculating the risk of acute coronary events based on the 10-year follow-up of the Prospective Cardiovascular Munster (PROCAM) study. Circulation 2002;105:310-315.
49. Conroy RM, Pyorala K, Fitzgerald AP, et al. Estimation of ten-year risk of fatal cardiovascular disease in Europe: the SCORE project. Eur Heart J 2003;24:987-1003.
50. Anderson KM, Wilson PW, Odell PM, et al. An updated coronary risk profile. A statement for health professionals. Circulation 2001;83:356-362.
51. Trivedi MH, Rush AJ, Wisniewski SR, et al. Evaluation of outcomes with citalopram for depression using measurement-based care in the STAR*D: implications for clinical practice. Am J Psychiatry 2006;163:28-40.
52. U.S. Food and Drug Administration: Office of Orphan Products Development. Available at http://www.fda.gov/orphan/ (accessed September 19, 2006).

3

REGULATIONS AND PHARMACOVIGILANCE

Robert G. Sharrar, Linda S. Hostelley, and Filip Mussen

INTRODUCTION 29
Benefit-Risk Assessment 29
REGULATORY AGENCIES 31
OTHER ORGANIZATIONS 32
COMPLIANCE 32
RISK-MANAGEMENT ACTIVITIES THROUGHOUT DRUG DEVELOPMENT 33
Phase I 33
Phase II 33
Phase III 33
Clinical Trials 33
Risk-Management Plans 34
Risk-Minimization Activities 35
Phase IV 35
Postmarketing Reporting Systems 35
Periodic Safety Update Reports 36
Passive Spontaneous Reporting 36
Individual Case Reports 38
Case Series 38
Disproportionality Analysis (Data Mining) 38
Epidemiologic Methods for Postauthorization Safety Studies 38
THE FUTURE OF PHARMACOVIGILANCE 39

INTRODUCTION

Regulatory agencies and pharmaceutical companies share a common interest, which is to provide the public with the safest, most effective medicines and vaccines possible. However, always remember that efficacy and safety are not absolute attributes and that no medical product is completely without risks. Regulatory agencies and pharmaceutical companies assess safety in the context of anticipated efficacy and throughout the lifecycle of the medical product. Whereas product safety and pharmacovigilance practices have received a great deal of attention in recent years, product safety has always been of utmost concern to pharmaceutical companies and regulatory agencies.

Drug development is a heavily regulated process. Regulatory agencies and other organizations throughout the world have issued laws, regulations, directives, and guidance documents to monitor all aspects of drug development, manufacturing, distribution, promotion, and use. These regulations apply to the pharmaceutical industry and clinical investigators who develop the drugs and to practitioners who use the drugs. This chapter describes the current regulations and guidelines that apply to pharmacovigilance and to monitoring product safety throughout the drug development process and marketed use of the product. Listings of some of these documents are shown in Tables 3-1 through 3-3. Although the focus of this chapter is on regulations and guidelines concerning the European Medicines Agency (EMEA) and the U.S. Food and Drug Administration (FDA), many of these principles apply to regulatory requirements throughout the world.

The World Health Organization (WHO) defines pharmacovigilance as "the science and activities related to the detection, assessment, understanding, and prevention of adverse drug effects or any other drug-related problem." It includes all observational (nonrandomized) postapproval scientific and data-gathering activities following the use of drugs in a population. Drug safety is normally described in terms of the drug's effect on a population. The word *pharmacovigilance* is derived from *pharmaco*, which means pertaining to a drug, and *vigilance*, which means watchfulness. Vigilance comes from the Latin word *vigil*, which means to stay awake during the normal hours of sleep, usually for a purpose.

Risk management, which consists of risk assessment and risk minimization, is the term used to describe the process for monitoring the safety profile of a drug.[1,2] *Risk assessment* consists of identifying and characterizing the nature, frequency, and severity of the risks associated with the use of a product. Risk assessment is performed throughout a product's life cycle from preclinical safety assessment, through clinical trials, and into the marketed environment. The goal of *risk minimization* is to minimize a drug's risk while preserving its benefits. Risk management is an iterative process of (i) assessing a product's benefit-risk balance, (ii) developing and implementing tools to minimize its risk while preserving its benefits, (iii) evaluating tool effectiveness and reassessing the benefit-risk balance, and (iv) making adjustments, as appropriate, to the risk minimization tools to further improve the benefit-risk balance.

Benefit-Risk Assessment

The decision to develop and approve a drug for use or to use a drug in a particular patient depends on the benefits derived from the drug compared with the risk or potential harm from the drug. The concept of benefit refers to the possibility of promoting or enhancing well-being in terms of improved symptoms, functioning, and/or prolonging life; the concept of risk refers to the possibility of suffering harm in terms of the seriousness of the outcome (death or disability) or the severity. Benefit and risk are also measured using different outcomes. Fundamentally, benefit and risk are evaluative terms that contain a value judgment in their meaning.[3] For example, clinical studies can show, within their limitations, that a drug has an effect and what the magnitude of that effect is across the population of patients studied. In most circumstances, clinical trials generally cannot determine the clinical relevance of that treatment effect. These types of questions are answered in the context of outcomes trials that can be long, large, expensive, and still not capable of addressing every possible clinical scenario. Thus, benefit-risk evaluations require superimposing evaluative judgments on the available efficacy and safety data.

Whereas regulatory agencies, pharmaceutical companies, payers, and other stakeholders conduct benefit-risk evaluations at the level of the patient population, physicians routinely make benefit-risk decisions for individual patients. In this respect, for an individual, the benefit-risk profile of a drug may be different from that for society at large. Furthermore, the willingness to accept risk varies from patient to patient. In general, patients with more serious diseases or with no alternative therapy are more willing to accept greater risk.

It is important to consider and weigh all available data when conducting a benefit-risk assessment. Efficacy data are derived from multiple clinical trials with different designs and endpoints. Similarly, safety data usually originate from multiple clinical trials, from spontaneous reporting, and from epidemiologic trials. As a result, for many drugs, a trade-off of multiple benefits versus multiple risks will be

TABLE 3-1 SELECTED REGULATIONS THAT PERTAIN TO PHARMACOVIGILANCE

EMEA
Rules Governing Medicinal Products in the European Union: Guidelines on Pharmacovigilance for Medicinal Products for Human Use, Vol. 9A. January 2007.
CHMP, Guidelines on Risk Management Systems for Medicinal Products for Human Use. November 2005. Doc. Ref. EMEA/CHMP/96268/2005.
Annex C. Template for EU Risk Management Plan (EU-RMP). Doc. Ref. EMEA/192632/2006.
2001/20/EC: European Clinical Trial Directive.
Report of the CHMP Working Group on Benefit-Risk Assessment Models and Methods. January 2007. Doc. Ref. EMEA/CHMP/15404/2007.
EV-EWG Guideline on the Use of Statistical Signal Detection Methods in the Eudravigilance Data Analysis System. November 2006. Doc. Ref. EMEA/106464/2006.
FDA
21 CFR 312.32 IND Safety Reports.
21 CFR 314.80 Postmarketing Reporting of Adverse Drug Experiences (Drugs).
21 CFR 600.80 Subpart D—Postmarketing Reporting of Adverse Experiences (Biologic Products).
21 CFR 803 Medical Device Reporting.
CBER
Guideline for the Format and Content of the Clinical and Statistical Sections of an Application, July 1988.
Guidance for Industry:
Premarketing Risk Assessment, March 2005.
Development and Use of Risk Minimization Action Plans, March 2005.
Good Pharmacovigilance Practices and Pharmacoepidemiologic Assessment, March 2005.

CBER, Center for Biologics Evaluation and Research; CHMP, Committee for Medicinal Products for Human Use; EMEA, European Medicines Agency; EU, European Union; EV-EWG, Eudravigilance Expert Working Group; FDA, U.S. Food and Drug Administration.

TABLE 3-2 SELECTED ICH GUIDELINES FOR PHARMACOVIGILANCE ACTIVITIES

Coding	Title	Status, Date
E1	The Extent of Population Exposure to Assess Clinical Safety for Drugs Intended for Long-Term Treatment of Non–Life-Threatening Conditions	Step 5, Oct. 1994
E2A	Clinical Safety Data Management: Definitions and Standards for Expedited Reporting	Step 5, Oct. 1994
E2B (R3)	Revision of the E2B (R2) ICH Guideline on Clinical Safety Data Management: Data Elements for Transmission of Individual Case Study Reports	Step 5/3, Nov. 2000 May 2005 (R3)
E2C (R1)	Clinical Safety Data Management: Periodic Safety Update Reports for Marketed Drugs Addendum to E2C	Step 5, Nov. 1996 Feb. 2003 (R1)
E2D	Postapproval Safety Data Management: Definitions and Standards for Expedited Reporting	Step 5, Nov. 2003
E2E	Pharmacovigilance Planning	Step 5, Nov. 2004
E6 (R1)	Good Clinical Practice: Consolidated Guidelines	Step 5, May 1996
E9	Statistical Principles for Clinical Trials	Step 5, Feb. 1998
E14	The Clinical Evaluation of QT/QTc Interval Prolongation and Proarrhythmic Potential for Nonantiarrhythmic Drugs	Step 5, May 2005

ICH, International Conference on Harmonization of Technical Requirements for the Registration of Pharmaceuticals for Human Use.

required. In this respect, the concept of risk drivers or dominant risks, which are the adverse effect(s) (AEs) that dominate the overall risk profile and carry the most weight, is important to note. In general, the Council for International Organizations of Medical Sciences (CIOMS) IV report[4] suggested that the three most often reported and the three most serious AEs should be considered as representatives for the risk profile of each medicine. Of equal importance is making explicit the uncertainties and evidential gaps with regard to the benefits and risks, which are usually caused by the limitations of clinical trials such as restrictions in the patient population, the number of patients in the trials, and the duration of the trials. An additional factor further complicating benefit-risk evaluations is that for some drugs, the benefits and risks are temporally offset (i.e., the benefits may be latent while the risks are constant over time): for example, the pronounced effect of statins on coronary heart disease over the long term versus the relatively small risk for myopathy that can appear within weeks to a few months. In contrast, for some drugs, such as oral contraceptives, the benefits are short term while the risks are long term.[5]

Several methods have been developed as tools to trade-off the benefits and risks of drugs. Within the scope of pharmacovigilance, the "Principle of Threes" model,[6] described in detail in the CIOMS IV report, is worth noting. This model establishes the concepts of seriousness, duration, and incidence as related to disease indication, disease amelioration by a medicine, and the AEs ascribed to the medicine. Each parameter is rated as high (3), medium (2), low (1), or absent (0). Most other models have been developed to determine the benefit-risk profile of drugs either in a specific therapeutic class or based on the efficacy and safety results from a single clinical trial. With regard to the latter category, one of the models frequently referred to is the Numbers Needed to Treat (NNT—the reciprocal of the absolute risk

TABLE 3-3 CIOMS PUBLICATIONS CONCERNING PRODUCT SAFETY AND PHARMACOVIGILANCE

CIOMS Number	Title	Comments
CIOMS I 1990	International Reporting of Adverse Drug Reactions	Standardized CIOMS reporting form
CIOMS II 1992	International Reporting of Periodic Drug-Safety Update Summaries	Established the standard for Periodic Safety Update Reports
CIOMS III 1999	Guidelines for Preparing Core Clinical-Safety Information on Drugs—Including New Proposals for Investigators Brochures (2nd ed.)	Harmonized Company Core Data Sheets and Core Safety Information
CIOMS IV 1998	Benefit-Risk Balance for Marketed Drugs: Evaluating Safety Signals	Established a methodology for doing benefit-risk
CIOMS V 2001	Current Challenges in Pharmacovigilance: Pragmatic Approaches	Discussed postmarketing surveillance issues
CIOMS VI 2005	Management of Safety Information from Clinical Trials	Discussed premarketing safety issues
CIOMS VII 2006	The Development Safety Update Report (DSUR): Harmonizing the Format and Content for Periodic Safety Reporting During Clinical Trials	Described a method for regular and timely updates on safety information during clinical trials

CIOMS, Council for International Organizations of Medical Sciences.

reduction due to a given therapy) versus Numbers Needed to Harm (NNH—the treatment effort expended before one patient experiences an adverse treatment–related outcome).[7]

An example of the use of NNTs is the following. In the Heart Protection Study (HPS), 20,536 patients with or without hyperlipidemia, who were at high risk of developing a major coronary event because of existing coronary heart disease (CHD), diabetes, history of stroke or other cerebrovascular disease, peripheral vascular disease, or hypertension, were treated either with simvastatin 40 mg/day ($N = 10,269$) or with placebo ($N = 10,267$) for a mean duration of 5 years.[8] Treatment with simvastatin 40 mg/day resulted in 587 (5.7%) deaths from CHD versus 707 (6.9%) with placebo, which represents an absolute risk reduction of 0.012 ($P = 0.0005$). This results in an NNT of 83 (1/0.012), or 83 patients with a baseline risk similar to those in the HPS trial who need to be treated with simvastatin 40 mg for a mean duration of 5 years in order to prevent one death from CHD. Because NNT is dependent on the baseline risk, for an individual patient the NNT must be converted by estimating that patient's susceptibility relative to the mean baseline risk in the clinical trial from which the NNT was calculated. This susceptibility can be expressed as a decimal fraction F, by which the reported NNT is divided. For example, if a patient is judged to be half as susceptible as the average patient in the example, $F = 0.5$ and $NNT/F = 83/0.5 = 166$.

Although other models have been developed to evaluate benefit-risk, most of these models share similar shortcomings. These include (i) difficulties in capturing multiple benefit attributes (e.g., multiple primary and/or secondary endpoints from a clinical trial) as well as risk attributes (e.g., multiple AEs, general risk estimates such as the incidence of serious AEs and the incidence of discontinuations owing to AEs), (ii) difficulties in incorporating data from multiple clinical trials, and (iii) nonvalidated methodology for converting the benefits and risks to the same scale. A Report of the Committee for Medicinal Products for Human Use (CHMP) Working Group (EMEA) on Benefit-Risk Assessment Models and Methods[9] recommended to the CHMP (i) using a structured and mainly qualitative benefit-risk approach, (ii) balancing and judging important findings in the specific therapeutic context, and (iii) describing uncertainties and quantifying their impact on the benefit-risk assessment. In addition, the working group also encouraged further research into the methodology of benefit-risk assessment.

REGULATORY AGENCIES

Most countries have agencies that regulate the manufacturing and distribution of pharmaceutical products. The three largest agencies are the U.S. Food and Drug Administration (FDA), the European Medicines Evaluation Agency (EMEA), and the Ministry of Health, Labour, and Welfare (MHLW) in Japan. Historically, these agencies developed at different times. The evolution of drug regulations in the United States has evolved to protect the health of the public and in response to past public health issues with marketed medical products.

Unsanitary food conditions, poisonous preservatives and dyes in food, and inappropriate and misleading claims of patented medicines led to the passage of the Pure Food and Drug Act in 1906, which prohibited the interstate commerce of mislabeled or adulterated drugs and food.[10] In 1937, more than 100 individuals died from renal failure after ingesting an elixir of sulfanilamide dissolved in ethylene glycol. This led to the passage of the Food, Drug, and Cosmetic Act (FD&CA) of 1938, which required that new drugs be tested for safety before marketing, that these safety data be submitted in a New Drug Application (NDA) to the FDA, and that drugs have adequate labeling for safe use. In response to the thalidomide tragedy, the Kefauver-Harris Amendment was enacted in 1962; it required manufacturers to prove that the drug was both safe and effective before marketing. This amendment also gave the FDA control over prescription drug advertising, required informed consent in clinical trials, and required FDA approval to conduct clinical trials based upon the results of animal toxicology studies.

Reporting of adverse experiences associated with the use of medicinal products began in the 1950s when the FDA, following the recognition that aplastic anemia was associated with the use of chloramphenicol, undertook a pilot study of adverse drug reaction reporting with the American Society of Hospital Pharmacists and the American Medical Association. Regulatory agencies in many countries developed regulations and guidelines for reporting information about suspected adverse drug reactions following the thalidomide tragedy. Additional amendments have been made to the Code of Federal Regulations (CFR) to regulate the reporting of adverse experiences associated with the use of a medicinal product.[11,12]

During the 1970s and 1980s, there was concern about the long process for drug approval, which caused a delay in patient access to drugs already approved in other countries and a delay in acquired immunodeficiency disease syndrome (AIDS) patients having more rapid access to promising therapies. Pharmaceutical companies were also concerned about the length of time it took the FDA to approve an NDA because of staff shortages. In response to these concerns, Congress passed the Prescription Drug User Fee Act (PDUFA) of 1992, which required drug and biologic manufacturers to pay fees to the FDA to help fund the evaluation of NDAs and supplements. Following this legislation, the number of approvals per year increased from 63 in 1991 to a high of 131 in 1996, and the median approval time decreased from about 24 months to 12 months from 1993 to 1998.[10] However, no PDUFA funds were allocated to postmarketing drug safety activities until PDUFA III was passed in 2002, when some funds were allocated for limited safety activities. However, the next version of PDUFA is expected to contain funds for product safety and postmarketing pharmacovigilance.

OTHER ORGANIZATIONS

During the 1960s and 1970s, regulatory agencies throughout the world developed a number of laws, regulations, and guidelines for assuring the quality, safety, and efficacy of marketed pharmaceutical products. At the same time, pharmaceutical companies were becoming more international and were developing a global market. Although the regulatory agencies had the same common goal, the different technical requirements in each country forced pharmaceutical companies to duplicate many time-consuming and expensive procedures to get a product approved for market.

The International Conference on Harmonization of Technical Requirements for the Registration of Pharmaceuticals for Human Use (ICH) was established in 1990 to improve, through harmonization, the process for developing and registering new medicinal products in Europe, Japan, and the United States.[13] The objective of the ICH is to establish harmonized guidelines for quality, safety, and efficacy for the development and regulation of medical products. ICH is composed of representatives from regulatory agencies and pharmaceutical companies, as equal partners. The six sponsors with voting members include regulators from the European Union (EU), the MHLW in Japan, and the FDA and representatives from the pharmaceutical companies through the European Federation of Pharmaceutical Industries and Associations (EFPIA), the Japan Pharmaceutical Manufacturers Association (JPMA), and the Pharmaceutical Research and Manufacturers of America (PhRMA). Nonvoting members, or ICH Observers, include WHO, Health Canada, and the European Free Trade Association (EFTA). The International Federation of Pharmaceutical Manufacturers & Associations (IFPMA) provides infrastructure support.

The ICH has a Steering Committee that charters an Expert Working Group (EWG), which is charged with developing a harmonization guideline to address a particular issue agreed upon by the voting members. The formal ICH procedure is a stepwise process. Step 1 is the agreed-upon final harmonized draft of the EWG. Step 2 is the sign off by the Steering Committee, which signifies acceptance for consultation by each of the six sponsors. Step 3 occurs when the three regulatory sponsors have commented on the document. The document is then returned to the EWG to harmonize the regulatory concerns before being submitted to the Steering Committee. Step 4 is reached when the Steering Committee agrees that there is scientific consensus on the technical issues. This occurs when the three regulatory bodies affirm that the guideline is recommended for adoption by the regulatory bodies of the three regions. Step 5 occurs when the guidelines are incorporated into national or internal procedures. More than 50 harmonized guidelines have been developed in the areas of product quality, safety, efficacy, and multidisciplinary topics. Table 3-2 lists the selective ICH guidelines pertaining to pharmacovigilance activities.

The ICH has been successful in achieving harmonization of technical guidelines concerning the quality, safety, and efficacy of medicinal products and on the format and content of registration applications. ICH guidelines have been adopted as regulations in the three ICH participating regions and in some non-ICH regions as well. ICH has been successful because its recommendations are based on scientific consensus between industry and regulatory experts and because of the commitment of the regulatory parties to implement the ICH tripartite: harmonized guidelines and recommendations. The Medical Dictionary for Regulatory Activities Terminology (MedDRA)[14] has been developed under the auspices of the ICH. This dictionary has standardized the terminology used to describe adverse experiences associated with the use of medicinal products in clinical trials and in the postmarketing environment.

CIOMS is an international, nongovernmental, nonprofit organization established in 1949 by WHO to facilitate and promote international activities in the field of biomedical sciences.[15] In 2003, the membership of CIOMS included 48 international member organizations and 18 national organizations, representing a substantial portion of the biomedical community and national academies of sciences and medical research councils. Two of its main programs include bioethics and drug development and use. It has issued the International Ethical Guidelines for Biomedical Research Involving Human Subjects and a number of publications containing recommendations on the assessment and monitoring of adverse drug reactions and pharmacogenetics (Table 3-3). Although CIOMS is not an official regulatory organization, many of its recommendations have been incorporated into official regulations.

COMPLIANCE

In order for a pharmaceutical company to market a drug, it must be compliant with all current regulations. Regulatory compliance ensures the proper communication of safety information between the market authorization holder (i.e., pharmaceutical company) and the regulators and enables the independent assessment by the regulatory agency of data received by the company. Regulatory agencies conduct routine pharmacovigilance inspections of pharmaceutical companies to ensure that adequate collection, verification, and reporting procedures for adverse experiences are in place, to ensure the timeliness of reporting, and to assess the latter compliance activities in the context of a company's overall ability to monitor the safety profile of its products.

In addition to routine pharmacovigilance inspections, regulatory agencies also conduct inspections of commercial and noncommercial investigator sites to ensure that the international standards established under the ICH E6: Good Clinical Practice (GCP): Consolidated Document (May 1996) have been met. Compliance with this standard ensures that the rights, safety, and well-being of clinical trial participants are protected and also ensures the integrity and quality of the clinical data. These GCP guidelines have been adopted and incorporated into regulations by the EMEA in Europe, the MHLW in Japan, and the FDA in the United States.

For example, the FDA has the authority to "have access and copy and verify any records and reports relating to a clinical investigation" conducted under an Investigational New Drug (IND) Application. Records under 21 CFR 312.58(a) include all regulatory files in the study binder (e.g., 15-day reports), all drug accountability records, informed consent, and all case report forms and ancillary laboratory/medical records (i.e., source of data). Site training records and qualifications of the staff as well as standard operating procedures describing the study-related activities must be available for examination by the FDA inspector at the time of an audit.

FDA's Division of Scientific Investigations (DSI) uses a sampling method to determine which sites and the number of sites to be inspected within a particular program for a pending NDA. Considerations will be given to investigators who are "high enrollers" for a program, sites with high dropout rates, sites with problematic histories, and sites for which a complaint has been received by DSI from a patient or staff member.

When an FDA inspector arrives at an investigational site, he or she shows a photo ID and gives a Notice of Inspection (FDA Form 482) to the clinical investigator. The FDA inspector should be accompanied by a site staff member at all times. The agency inspector should be limited to study-related information, including medical equipment. For routine FDA audits of clinical trial data, the principal investigator should be present. Refusal to permit a legally authorized inspection may lead to prosecution and/or arrest of the person refusing to cooperate.

At the completion of the inspection, the FDA inspector discusses the findings of the investigation. The final inspection results are classified according to the following categories: (i) No Action Indicated (NAI) (e.g., no compliance issues), (ii) Voluntary Action Indicated (VAI) (e.g., remedial actions are needed to correct identified deficiencies), or (iii) Official Action Indicated (OAI) (e.g., significant violations of regulations were identified that may result in enforcement action should the violations continue). If violations of FDA IND regulations were identified, an FDA Form 483 is issued. Investigators are expected to implement corrective action to any finding cited by the FDA and to document such action in a written response to the FDA. The final FDA Inspection Report (Establishment Inspection Report [EIR]) describes the site inspection in detail and is subject to further review by additional groups within the FDA. For egregious misconduct in the clinical trial arena, FDA has the ability to "debar" a clinical investigator and site staff from "providing any services" to a new drug product applicant.

RISK-MANAGEMENT ACTIVITIES THROUGHOUT DRUG DEVELOPMENT

Since 2004, regulatory agencies and other organizations have issued new laws, regulations, guidelines, and documents describing how risk-management activities should be conducted throughout the drug development process. This section consolidates and summarizes these documents into a reasonable approach to satisfying these requirements. ICH issued its E2E Guideline for Pharmacovigilance Planning in November 2004.[16] This has subsequently been adopted by the EMEA, FDA, and MHLW. A CHMP of the EMEA issued the European Union Clinical Trial Directive (EU CTD),[17] which became effective in May 2004, and the Guideline on Risk Management Systems for Medicinal Products for Human Use in November 2005.[2] When Congress reauthorized the PDUFA III in June 2002, it instructed the FDA to produce guidelines for industry on risk-management activities for drugs and biologic products. Accordingly, the FDA published three documents in March 2005 entitled (1) Premarketing Risk Assessment,[1] (2) Development and Use of Risk Minimization Action Plans,[18] and (3) Good Pharmacovigilance Practices and Pharmacoepidemiologic Assessment.[19]

Phase I

Phase I begins when clinical pharmacology studies are done in normal, healthy humans. Drug and food interaction studies are generally considered to be phase I studies even though they can be conducted at any time during the development of a new drug. With the initiation of the first Clinical Study Authorization for an investigational medicinal product, an annual safety report must be prepared and submitted in Europe and the United States.[17,20] A quarterly report, which is a line listing of all serious unexpected adverse experiences reported during the quarter, is submitted in countries where regulations permit aggregate reporting in place of or complementary to individual 15-day reports. This report is submitted to Institutional Review Boards (IRB) and Ethics Committees (EC) to keep them informed of serious adverse experiences that have occurred in clinical trials. The annual safety report is submitted to regulatory agencies and IRBs and contains a line listing of serious drug-related adverse experience reports, an aggregate analysis of these adverse experience reports, and a report on the subject's safety during clinical trials. This report contains an analysis of the evolving drug safety profile of the product, an evaluation of the benefit-risk of the product, and a discussion of any changes in the protocols or informed consent form that are necessary to protect the safety of the subjects.

Phase II

During phase II, proof of concept studies and dose-ranging studies are performed in patients with the disease process being treated. A team consisting of a clinical monitor, a safety physician, a regulatory liaison, a project manager, and others, as appropriate, is established to develop and execute a clinical development plan. Because consideration of patient safety is the most important first step in clinical development, CIOMS VI[21] recommended the early formation of a Safety Management Team. The team should consist of the clinical monitor, who has overall responsibility for the project including assessment of the benefit-risk profile of the product; a safety physician, who has the responsibility for identifying and evaluating risks relating to the product; a regulatory liaison, who advises the team on regulatory issues; and a project manager, who keeps track of the team's decisions, ensuring appropriate follow-up and completion of assigned tasks. Standard Operating Procedures should be in place to clearly define roles and responsibilities, to ensure the regular and timely review and evaluation of all available safety information in order to identify potential risks, and to assure consistent implementation of risk-minimization actions across protocols and study locations.

Phase III

Clinical Trials

Phase III studies are randomized, controlled clinical trials designed to demonstrate that a product is safe and effective for a specific indication in a specific population. The data collected during clinical trials are used by regulatory agencies to determine whether the benefit-risk is favorable so that the drug can be approved for marketing. The FDA's Guidance for Industry on Premarketing Risk Assessment[1] provides general recommendations concerning risk assessment during clinical trials. This guideline discusses the adequacy of assessment in terms of quantity of data (ensuring that enough patients were studied) and quality of the data (the appropriateness of the assessment performed, the patient population studied, and how the data were analyzed).

Data Monitoring Committees (DMC) are now used in many studies to monitor the clinical data collected to ensure the safety of the individuals participating in the trial and to make recommendations concerning the appropriateness of continuing the trial or the need to modify its scientific or procedural aspects.[22] A DMC should be composed of independent experts from the field of clinical medicine, biostatistics, epidemiology, pharmacology, ethics, and patient advocacy groups. DMCs are most useful in long-term multicenter, controlled trials that address severe and life-threatening conditions.

The size of the premarketing database depends on a number of factors specific to the product and to the population and condition being treated. Considerations on the size and overall duration of exposures required for new drugs are described in ICH E1.[23] In general, ICH E1 calls for approximately 1500 overall exposures, with 300 patients studied for 6 months and 100 patients exposed to the investigation product for 1 year. However, these requirements can vary greatly and can range from a few hundred for products to treat rare cancers to 70,000 for a vaccine that would be used in healthy children.[24] In general, a larger database is required for (1) a first-in-class new drug, (2) a new drug intended for long-term treatment for a non–life-threatening condition, (3) a product that could cause adverse events that increase in severity or frequency over time, (4) a product that is given to a healthy population for chemoprevention or vaccination, and (5) a product with safety issues identified in preclinical animal studies or clinical pharmacology studies. A smaller database may be acceptable for a product used to treat a life-threatening disease, especially when no alternative satisfactory treatment exists or for products used for a short period of time.

In general, most clinical trials are designed primarily to measure effectiveness, because one knows in advance what one wants to measure and the study is powered and a sample size is predetermined based on expected effect sizes and anticipated variability around endpoint measurements. However, the safety profile of a product generally cannot be known or predicted in advance. As such, safety is assessed by screening patients in a sensitive and broad fashion with frequent follow-up visits for AE assessments and clinical laboratory measurements. Clinical trials can identify common AEs associated with the use of the product. In some instances, pooling data from several clinical trials can be used to achieve a larger sample size to estimate the frequency of low-incidence events or to compare differences in rates between an exposed and an unexposed group. According to the rule of 3, if 0 events of interest occur in a clinical trial of 3000, one has excluded an adverse event that occurs at a rate of 1 in 1000 with 95% confidence.

The premarketing safety database should include a population sufficiently diverse to adequately represent the population that will use the drug in the marketplace. Clinical trials normally use a homogeneous population because it makes data interpretation easier. Only patients with obvious contraindications or other clinical considerations (pregnancy) should be excluded from clinical trials. Including the elderly and patients with concurrent conditions taking concomitant medications enhances the generalizability of the safety findings. This is, however, sometimes at odds with the desire to control variability in the efficacy assessments.

Because most clinical studies involve data from multiple trials at multiple sites, it is important to make certain that the quality of the data is uniform across sites. The studies should all use the same assessment methods, terminology, and standard terms for describing AEs to prevent distortion or obscuring of the safety data. The accuracy of coding used to identify safety signals should be evaluated to make certain that investigators are precisely communicating the severity or magnitude of the AE and that these events are being coded properly. Combining related coding terms or dividing the same event into many terms for analysis could either amplify a weak signal or obscure important toxicities.

Many factors must be considered when deciding how data should be analyzed in clinical trials. The temporal association between product exposure and the onset of an AE can be evaluated in a number of ways. Assessments of risk within discrete time intervals over the observation period (i.e., a hazard-rate curve) can be used to demonstrate changes in risk over time, whereas a life table or Kaplan-Meier curve can be used to evaluate events that do not occur at a constant rate with respect to time or for events in studies in which the size of the population at risk changes over time. It is important to determine the reasons why subjects drop out of clinical trials. If subjects withdraw from a study because of safety issues, they should be followed until the AE is resolved or stabilized. Regulatory agencies recommend that all subjects be followed until the end of the study to ascertain late safety events.[25, 26]

Long-term controlled (active comparator or placebo) safety studies may be necessary to detect increases in rates of events that are relatively common in the treated population (e.g., sudden death in patients with ischemic cardiac disease). A drug with a dose-related AE may require additional studies to determine whether a lower dose is effective. Certain kinds of side effects may not be detected or readily reported by patients without special attention and may require additional studies to determine whether the product has an effect on a patient's cognitive function, motor skills, and mood or on growth and development in a pediatric patient.

Pharmaceutical companies are also expected to assess and minimize the potential for medication errors that might be caused by the product's name, packaging, formulation, or labeling. NDAs for all new small-molecule drugs must include an evaluation of the product to determine whether it is associated with drug-related QTc prolongation; drug-related liver, kidney, or bone marrow toxicity; drug-drug interactions; and/or polymorphic metabolism.

Although randomized, controlled clinical trials are considered the "gold standard" for evaluating the efficacy and safety of a product, they have both strengths and limitations. One strength is that they have formal written protocols with randomization of subjects, which helps control for unknown confounders that may exist. They also have blinding of data and a concurrent control group. They collect large amounts of high-quality data on all subjects and can answer specific questions concerning common AEs and efficacy. However, clinical trials are limited because they normally involve a relatively small number of highly selected subjects who take the product for a relatively short period of time. Conversely, a marketed drug is given to a relatively large number of individuals (millions) for a longer period of time (years). Furthermore, many of these individuals have concurrent medical conditions and are on concurrent therapies.

Risk-Management Plans

Guidelines[2,16] have been developed to aid industry and regulators in planning for pharmacovigilance activities in the postmarketing environment. These guidelines were developed because information on safety is relatively limited at the time of authorization and because pharmacovigilance activities might be improved if they were more closely based on product-specific issues identified in product development. These guidelines want pharmaceutical companies to be focused and proactive in their pharmacovigilance activities. These guidelines describe a method for summarizing important safety issues and propose a structure for writing a risk-management plan (RMP). The development of the RMP takes place during phase III, and the plan is implemented when the product is marketed.

These documents are based on four underlying principles. The first is that pharmacovigilance activities should take place throughout the life cycle of the product. Therefore, safety physicians who were formerly experts in postmarketing pharmacovigilance should get involved earlier in the drug-development process. Second, pharmacovigilance requires effective collaboration between regulators and industry, and discussions about these activities should take place early in drug development. Third, pharmacovigilance should be a science-based approach to risk documentation and minimization. Pharmacovigilance activities should be designed to answer specific questions. Finally, pharmacovigilance activities should be applicable to all three ICH regions: Europe, Japan, and the United States.

An RMP is a description of a risk-management system. A risk-management system is a set of pharmacovigilance activities and interventions designed to identify, characterize, prevent, or minimize risks relating to medicinal products and to assess the effectiveness of those interventions. An RMP is now required with the application for a new marketing authorization for a new drug, a new indication in a new population, a change in the formulation of the product, or at the request of a regulatory agency.

An RMP contains two parts. Part I includes the Safety Specification (SS) and the Pharmacovigilance Plan (PVP). The SS is a summary of important identified and potential risks associated with the use of a medicinal product and important missing information that could affect the risk-benefit of the product or have implications for public health. The SS should discuss the evidence bearing on causality, severity, frequency, and reversibility of the AE and any information on risk factors or potential mechanisms that could explain the AE. The PVP proposes Safety Action Plans (SAPs) to address the safety concerns identified. Part II contains an evaluation of the need for risk-minimization activities, and if there is a need for additional (nonroutine) risk-minimization activity, a risk-minimization plan.

An identified risk is defined as an untoward occurrence for which there is adequate evidence of an association with the medicinal product, including an AE seen in preclinical studies and confirmed in clinical trials; an AE observed in clinical trials or epidemiologic studies for which the magnitude of the difference, compared with a comparator group, suggests a causal association; and for a marketed product, an AE seen in spontaneous reports, in which causality is suggested by frequency of reports, a temporal relationship, and biologic plausibility.

A potential risk is an untoward occurrence for which there is some basis for suspicion of an association with the medicinal product but this association has not been confirmed. This includes preclinical safety concerns that have not been observed or resolved in clinical studies; AEs observed in clinical trials or epidemiologic studies for which the magnitude of the difference, compared with a comparator group, raises a suspicion but is not large enough to suggest a causal association; an AE arising from spontaneous reports; or an AE associated with another product in the same class or that could be expected to occur based on the drug's mechanism of action.

Important identified or potential risks includes those that are frequent or serious and those that might also have an impact on the balance of benefits and risks of the medical product, which could cause the health care practitioner to modify treatment or use a lower dose. Important missing information is information about the safety of the product not available at the time of submission of a marketing application and that represents a limitation of the safety data with respect to predicting the safety of the product in the marketplace. The SS should discuss the population that will use the product, populations not studied in clinical trials, and the epidemiology of the disease process being treated. The discussion should include the incidence and prevalence of comorbid conditions and causes of mortality stratified by age, sex, and racial or ethnic origins. These data are important to help evaluate AEs that get reported in the marketed environment. The SS should also discuss drug-drug or drug-food interactions, the potential for overdose, transmission of an infectious agent, misuse for illegal purposes, medication error, off-label use, or off-label pediatric use.

The PVP is based on the SS and proposes actions to address the safety concerns identified. It includes a section that discusses the routine pharmacovigilance activities that are conducted for all products, enhanced pharmacovigilance activities to address the issues raised in the SS, and specific SAPs for safety concerns. Routine pharmacovigilance may be sufficient for medicinal products for which no special concerns have been identified. The objective of additional pharmacovigilance activities could be to further quantitate the risk of an AE in different populations, to determine whether the risk varies by dose or duration of therapy, or whether risk factors can be identified. An SAP should be developed for each safety signal identified, and it consists of a statement of the safety concern, the objectives of the proposed action(s), the action(s) proposed, the rationale for the proposed action(s), a description of how the safety concern and proposed action(s) will be monitored, and milestones for evaluation and reporting to regulatory agencies.

Risk-Minimization Activities

Risk minimization is a set of activities used to reduce the probability of an adverse reaction occurring or its severity, should it occur, while preserving its benefits.[2,18] An evaluation of the need for additional (nonroutine) risk-minimization activities should be performed for each safety signal identified. Routine risk-minimization activities include proper packaging and labeling of the product and adequate warnings or precautions in the product information material. Additional risk-minimization activities may be required when the AE is severe or preventable.

A *Risk Minimization Action Plan (RiskMAP)* is a term adopted by the FDA. A RiskMAP is a strategic safety program designed to meet specific goals and objectives in minimizing known risks while preserving the product's benefits. A goal is the achievement of a particular health outcome related to a known safety risk, for example, fetal exposure to drug X should not occur. Objectives are specific and measurable actions that result in processes or behavior changes that help achieve the goal, for example, pregnant women would not be able to get the drug. A risk-minimization tool is a process or system intended to minimize known risks and includes targeted education and outreach, reminder systems, and performance-linked access systems.

Targeted education and outreach are used to increase appropriate knowledge about safety concerns to modify the behavior of health care providers and consumers to prevent or mitigate the safety risk of concern. These include health care practitioner letters, training programs, and medication guides. Reminder systems are designed to prompt, remind, double-check, or guide physicians, pharmacists, and/or patients in prescribing, dispensing, receiving, or using a product in a way that minimizes risk. This includes the use of special consent forms, special data-collection systems, and special packaging. Performance-linked access systems link product access to required laboratory tests results or other documentation necessary for the safe and effective use of the product.

A RiskMAP should be designed to minimize the risk while maintaining the widest possible access to the product with the least burden to health care providers and consumers. It should be applicable to inpatient and outpatient use and in diverse locales. Caution should be taken to avoid unintended consequences by making it so difficult to access the drug that the patient either does not get the drug or seeks alternative sources of the product such as the Internet or counterfeit product. The RiskMAP should be monitored and its effectiveness evaluated on a regular basis to make certain it is achieving its goals or to assess whether it may no longer be required.

Phase IV

Phase IV is the postapproval phase in which the product is potentially used by expanded populations of patients for longer periods of time than originally studied. Consequently, it is not surprising that safety issues that were not seen in clinical trials may become apparent in the postmarketing environment. Postmarketing safety data collection and data from observational studies are critical for identifying a safety signal and for evaluating and characterizing a product's safety profile. A safety signal refers to an unusual occurrence of a particular AE in terms of either frequency (more than expected) or its distribution within a population (e.g., myocardial infarctions in young women). FDA's guideline on Good Pharmacovigilance Practices and Pharmacoepidemiologic Assessment provides guidance on (1) safety signal identification, (2) pharmacoepidemiologic assessment of observational data and safety signal interpretation, and (3) pharmacovigilance plan development.[19]

Postmarketing Reporting Systems

The main strategy for monitoring product safety in the marketed environment is the spontaneous AE reporting system, which in the United States includes AERS for drugs and biologics, VAERS for vaccines, and the Manufacturer and User Facility Device Experience Database (MAUDE) for medical devices. Other countries have similar systems. The FDA regulations governing postmarketing reporting are found in 21 CFR 314.80 for drugs, 21 CFR 600.80 for biologic products, and 21 CFR 803 for medical device reporting. Unlike the reporting requirements for INDs in which both investigator and sponsor have reporting obligations for AEs, the reporting postapproval is voluntary for everyone other than the NDA holder (i.e., sponsor/pharmaceutical company). In addition, AE reports postapproval can originate from multiple sources including health care professionals, sales representatives, patients, regulatory agencies, published literature, Internet, news media, and other pharmaceutical companies.

An AE is defined as any adverse experience associated with the use of a drug in humans, whether or not considered drug related.[11,12] A serious AE or reaction is any untoward medical occurrence that at any dose, results in death, is life-threatening, requires inpatient hospitalization or prolongation of existing hospitalization, results in present or significant disability or incapacity, or is a congenital anomaly or birth defect. Medical and scientific judgment should be exercised in deciding whether expedited reporting is appropriate in other situations, such as important medical events that may not be immediately life-threatening or result in death or hospitalization but may jeopardize the patient or may require intervention to prevent one of the other outcomes listed in the definition. These other medical events should also be considered serious. Examples of such events are intensive treatment in the emergency room or at home for an allergic bronchospasm, blood dyscrasias or convulsions that do not result in hospitalization, or development of drug dependency or drug abuse.

The second criteria, *expectedness*, refers to events that have been previously observed in clinical trials or the marketplace and not to what might be anticipated from the pharmacologic properties of the product. Expectedness means that the AEe term is listed in the product circulars or Confidential Investigator Brochure.

Unexpected means an adverse drug experience that is not listed in the current labeling for the drug and includes an event that may be symptomatically and pathophysiologically related to an event listed in the labeling but differs from the event because of greater severity. For example, hepatitis would not be considered expected if the package circular had only cited elevated transaminases.

Companies must set up procedures to ensure that AEs for marketed products arriving anywhere in the company reach the Product Safety Department within tight timelines (usually 1 to 2 business days). Staff trained in pharmacovigilance must be able to triage the AE reports, enter the report into the database, and evaluate it for the purpose of submitting the report to regulatory agencies. Postmarketing reports that are considered to be unexpected and serious and reports from clinical trials that are considered to be unexpected, serious, and

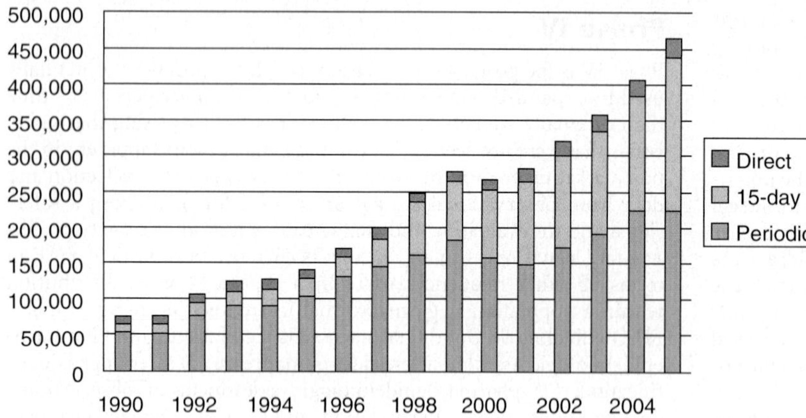

FIGURE 3-1 • Adverse event reporting system (AERS) report counts by type: 1990 through 2005. (From Green L: Food and Drug Administration, DIA 42nd Annual Meeting, June 2006.)

associated (a reasonable suspected, causal relationship to the medicinal product) must be submitted to regulatory agencies within 15 calendar days. Unexpected fatal or life-threatening AEs from clinical trials must be reported by telephone within 7 calendar days. It should be noted that causality assessment is required for AE reports from clinical trials. However, causality statements are not given to reports from the marketed environment. All nonserious reports are submitted to regulatory agencies on a periodic basis.

Figure 3-1 shows the number of AE reports submitted to the FDA from 1990 to 2005. The direct reports were submitted directly to the FDA. The periodic (nonserious and expected serious reports) and 15-day reports (serious unexpected reports) were submitted by pharmaceutical companies. Note the dramatic increase in serious unexpected reports that have occurred over this time period.

Periodic Safety Update Reports

The granting of marketing authorization for medicinal products ultimately results in the exposure of the public to potent pharmacologic and biologic agents that have the potential to both reduce and increase morbidity and mortality. Various ongoing processes are designed to assist interested parties in protecting the public health by facilitating the constant updating of the safety profiles of marketed drugs and vaccines. The systematic collection and analysis of safety data form the basis of these safety surveillance processes. Safety data collected by the manufacturer of the product are prioritized by regulations and laws for reporting to regulatory agencies. Safety information that is reported on a periodic basis, as opposed to serious individual reports on an expedited basis, is done so in the form of a Periodic Safety Update Report (PSUR).

The ICH E2C (R1) guideline, Clinical Safety Data Management: Periodic Safety Update Reports (PSUR) for Marketed Drugs, was approved in 1996 and updated in 2003.[27] The purpose of the PSUR is to periodically perform an overall safety evaluation of a product to determine whether there has been any change in the safety profile of the product following marketing authorization. PSURs are required at 6-month intervals for the first 2 years after marketing, then yearly for 2 years, and every 3 years after that. It contains a summary of any new safety issues identified during the time period covered by the PSUR and an update on the benefit-risk assessment of the product. The PSUR summarizes the market authorization status of the product, provides an estimate of the number of patients exposed to the product, and indicates whether any changes were made to the product package circulars. It also contains a tabular listing of all reported AEs from health care providers. The scheduling of PSURs at defined times following marketing authorization facilitates the reporting of the same information at the same time to multiple regulatory authorities. Routine pharmacovigilance activities also include analyzing data in response to specific queries from regulatory agencies and health care providers and evaluation of the AE information for consideration of a label change.

Passive Spontaneous Reporting

Table 3-4 describes the benefits and weaknesses of the types of data used to monitor product safety. The spontaneous AE reporting systems in the United States are voluntary, passive, incomplete reporting systems that contain AE reports submitted by health care providers or consumers directly to the manufacturer of the product or to the FDA. Reports of serious unexpected AEs from the medical literature are also added to the database. Reports are entered into the appropriate database using the verbatim terminology of the reporter. Because standard case definitions are not used for reporting purposes, the report may or may not reflect the correct clinical diagnosis. These databases contain reports that are temporally associated with the product and not necessarily causally related.

Because these spontaneous case reports of AEs are used to identify safety signals, every effort should be made to obtain complete and accurate data on all reports. In order for a report to be entered into the database, it should have an identifiable patient, an identifiable reporter, an identifiable product, and an AE. The characteristic of a quality pharmacovigilance report includes complete demographic data, a description of the AE with dates of onset and symptoms, relevant laboratory data to support the diagnosis, the clinical course of the event including therapeutic measures and outcome, suspected and concomitant therapy with dose and duration of treatment, past medical history and concurrent conditions, relevant family history of disease, and the presence of risk factors. Information about response to dechallenge and rechallenge should be noted.

These spontaneous reporting systems have limitations because of incomplete reporting of AEs, so there is not a good numerator; and an unknown number of individuals taking the drug, so there is not a good denominator. The degree of underreporting is not known and probably varies by the severity of the AE and by the length of time the product has been on the market. Therefore, it is not possible to calculate incidence rates from spontaneous reports. Instead, a reporting rate is frequently used, which is defined as the number of reported events divided by the estimated number of individuals taking the drug. This estimate could be obtained from drug distribution figures or from commercial drug utilization data sources. Furthermore, the database contains information only about people taking the medication so there are no data on a comparable control group. This reporting system is not good at detecting a small increase in a commonly occurring AEe in the general population, such as myocardial infarctions, or AEs that occur long after the drug was administered.

One of the strengths of the spontaneous reporting system is its ability to detect rare events (signal generation) following widespread use of the product in the general population. It contains information from a large number of health care providers on a large number of individuals receiving the product. If rare AEs occur in different parts of the country, and if health care providers take the time to report them, then the system would be presented with a cluster of cases that could be analyzed from an epidemiologic perspective. Furthermore,

TABLE 3-4 TYPES OF DATA USED TO MONITOR PRODUCT SAFETY

Type of Data	Benefits	Weakness	Comments
Passive spontaneous reports	Collects data from a large number of health care practitioners and patients who use the product in a real-world setting	Incomplete data, no control group; cannot be used to pick up a slight increase in a common background event or AEs that occur long after the drug was administered	Used to identify rare safety signals, observe safety profile of patients not included in clinical trials, and identify safety issues of concern
Individual case report	Can collect complete data	Hard to determine causality in an individual report	Look for reports of rechallenge positive, time to onset of AE, class effects, biologic plausibility, and confounders that could explain report
Case series	Can be developed from spontaneous reports	Case definition determines inclusion, no control group	Used to develop clinical spectrum of AE, to determine epidemiologic characteristics, and to identify risk factors
Disproportionality analysis	Statistical analysis that can be done on a large data set	Uses spontaneous AE reports, generates a large number of signals	Identifies a statistical association that needs to be further evaluated
Registries—exposure registries	Uses standardized questionnaire to collect data on individuals from different sources in a prospective fashion; can be done by industry	Expensive; no control group	Can follow patients over time to determine incidence rates and can be used for cohort studies
Registries—disease registries	Uses standardized questionnaire to collect data on individuals from different sources in a prospective fashion	Expensive; can be done only in an academic situation; industry does not have legal right to collect information on patients not using its products	Cases can be used for case-control studies
Active surveillance—sentinel sites	Can collect complete and accurate data; most efficient for institutional setting with dedicated reporting	Selection bias, small number of patients, and increased costs	Used to determine incidence rates and potential for abuse
Active surveillance—prescription event monitoring	Follow-up questionnaire sent to physician who prescribed the drug for a particular patient	Poor and incomplete response from physicians	Used to collect demographic data on patients using the product, indication for therapy, duration of therapy, reasons for discontinuation of drug, and more details on AE
Active surveillance—electronic databases include electronic medical records and claims databases	Can collect information on a large number of patients using a product, identify an appropriate comparison group, and measure drug utilization	Complicated, expensive, difficult to interpret; electronic medical records may not contain detailed information; claims databases require medical record review	Pharmacovigilance of the 21st century, but currently learning how to do it; need to validate the data; unknown pitfalls
Cross-sectional studies (surveys)—collect data on a population at a single point in time or for an interval of time	Relatively easy to do	Temporal relationship between exposure and outcome cannot be addressed.	Used to examine trends over time and to examine crude associations between exposure and outcome in ecologic analyses
Drug utilization studies (DUS)—describe how a drug is marketed, prescribed, and used in a population	Provides data on specific populations; can be used to determine denominator data	Lack of information on why product was used and on clinical outcome	Used to determine off-label use, potential for drug abuse, and response to regulatory actions
Cohort studies—follow a population at risk over time	Can evaluate multiple events, determine incidence rates, and examine safety concerns in a special population	Requires a large number of subjects; expensive; takes a long period of time; not good for rare outcomes; and needs an appropriate comparison group	May be retrospective or prospective depending on when the outcome of interest occurred in relation to when the study began; can be used to determine relative risk
Case-control studies—cases and controls are selected from the same source population	Relatively inexpensive; can be done in a short period of time; used to study rare events; can be stratified according to the population of interest	Studies only one event—the AE of interest; selection of control group may be difficult	Used to determine whether there is a possible association between a medicinal product and a specific AE and to identify possible risk factors; can determine odds ratio, which is an estimate of relative risk
Randomized clinical trials	High quality of data; good comparator group; can determine incidence rates	Cannot measure rare events; events that occur after a long period of time; expensive and time consuming	Used to determine incidence rates of common AEs, dose-response relationship, and drug-drug and drug-food interactions
Large simple trials	Patients randomized to treatment	Limited data collection and monitoring	Used to elucidate the benefit-risk profile of a product and to quantify the risk of a specific rare AE

AE, adverse experience.

these rare serious AEs could be studied in more detail to determine whether they are associated with the use of the product. Spontaneous reporting is also a good system for detecting rare drug-induced conditions, such as Stevens-Johnson syndrome, aplastic anemia, torsades de pointes, which have a low background rate. Another advantage of postmarketing surveillance is that it collects information on individuals who would not normally be included in clinical trials. An example would be the pregnancy registries that have been established to monitor the outcome of pregnancies in women who were inadvertently exposed to the product while pregnant. Perhaps the most important thing to learn from postmarketing surveillance is that it helps identify those issues of concern to health care providers using the products. If the health care provider reports it, it must be of concern to her or him because it represents a change in the patient's normal condition.

Individual Case Reports

A spontaneous AE reported in the marketed environment could have been caused by the drug in question, the underlying disease being treated, a concurrent illness, concurrent medications, or some other unknown factor. In an individual, it is very difficult to determine whether the AE was caused by a particular drug because there are few laboratory tests to prove an association. Oral polio vaccine has been shown to cause paralytic polio because some children developed paralysis after receiving the vaccine and an analysis of their cerebrospinal fluid has identified the presence of the vaccine strain of the poliovirus. If no laboratory tests prove an association, other criteria have to be used to determine whether there is a possible association between the product and the AE. These criteria include (1) the frequency of reports (i.e., the more reports, the more likely there is an association), (2) the timing of the AE (i.e., anaphylaxis occurring right after an injection, whereas cancer may require years of therapy before it occurs), (3) evidence of a positive rechallenge (i.e., the AEe goes away when the drug is stopped, but returns when the drug is restarted), (4) evidence of positive dechallenge (i.e., the AE goes away when the drug is discontinued), (5) consistency of the event with the established pharmacological/toxicologic effects of the product, (6) consistency of the event with the known effects of other products in the class, (7) evidence of other supporting evidence from preclinical studies, clinical trials, and/or pharmacoepidemiologic studies, and (8) absence of alternative explanations for the event.

In order to demonstrate that a particular AE is associated with a drug, one must be able to demonstrate that the AE is more common in a group of individuals taking the drug than in a comparable group of individuals not taking the drug. This epidemiologic approach requires more data. Furthermore, it does not identify which individual had the AE because of the drug. Reporting rates are frequently used to compare the frequency of AEs in a population taking the product with background incidence rates. Background incidence rates are obtained from the medical literature, from national health statistics, from large automated databases, or from epidemiologic studies. This comparison is weak because reporting rates are always lower owing to underreporting than background incidence rates in the population and because it is difficult to get rates in a comparable population.

Case Series

In addition to evaluating individual cases from the spontaneous reporting system, a case series can be assembled and clinical and epidemiologic data can be summarized to characterize the clinical description of the AE and any risk factor associated with its occurrence. Specifically, a case series can be used to describe the clinical and laboratory manifestation of the reported AE; the demographic characteristic of the patients who develop the AE; the dose, duration, and time interval between initiation of therapy and the onset of the AE; and risk factors such as comorbid conditions and concomitant medications.

Disproportionality Analysis (Data Mining)

Data mining is a disproportionality analysis that uses statistical or mathematical tools to identify safety signals (product-event combinations) that need to be evaluated.[28] The data mining methods described include the Multi-Item Gamma Poisson Shrinker (MGPS) algorithm,[29] the Proportional Reporting Ratio (PRR)[30] method, and the Bayesian Neural Network approach.[31] Data mining, utilizing a spontaneous AE reporting database, calculates the number of expected AEs that would occur based upon the proportionate reporting ratio for all of the other drugs in the database. It then compares this expected number with the actual observed number. The analysis can be refined by adjusting for age, year of reporting, or indication. A score (or statistic) generated by data mining quantifies the disproportionality between the observed and the expected values for a given product-event combination. A potential excess of AEs or safety signals can operationally be defined as any product-event combination with a score that exceeds a specified threshold. However, data mining is not a tool for establishing a causal association between a product and an AE.

One problem with data mining is that it generates a large number of signals that need to be evaluated to determine whether there is a possible association between an AE and a particular product. Data mining is a statistical analysis of spontaneous AE reports. When statistics are applied to a large number of events (multiplicity), signals emerge because of chance alone. The EMEA has recommended that when referring to statistical calculations devoid of any clinical context, the term *Signal of Disproportionate Reporting (SDR)* should be used.[32] Therefore, a clinical or medical interpretation of the data is mandatory. Because signal evaluation requires a great deal of resources (time, personnel, and money), it is important to establish criteria for signals that require further evaluation. Signals that require further evaluation are those that are biologically plausible based on the product's mechanism of action; those that are associated with other products in the same class, serious AEs, especially those that are rare in the general population; drug-interaction signals, and AEs associated with medication errors. The decision on what to do about an identified safety signal could range from a decision for no immediate action and continued monitoring, further assessment using complementary pharmacovigilance tools (e.g., formal pharmacoepidemiologic studies), labeling changes, or more significant regulatory actions.

Epidemiologic Methods for Postauthorization Safety Studies

Registries. A registry is an organized system for the standardized collection of data on individuals exposed to a particular product (drug registry) or with a particular disease (disease registry). Registries can follow patients over time, collect specific data that may not be available in other databases, and collect data from multiple sources. Exposure registries can be done by industry because they collect data on individuals using its product. However, they lack an internal appropriate control group. Pregnancy registries are useful for evaluating women inadvertently exposed to a product during their pregnancy and are used to determine pregnancy outcome incidence rates. Disease registries can be used to collect data on drug exposure and other factors associated with a clinical condition. They are normally done in academic centers and can be used to develop a case-control study. A registry should also have a formal written protocol describing its objectives; a review of the literature; its method for patient recruitment; the method of data collection, management, and analysis; and conditions under which the registry would be terminated.

Active Surveillance. Active surveillance can be established at preselected sentinel sites to ensure complete and accurate data on all AEs that occur. It is most efficient for products that are mainly used in institutional settings, such as hospitals or nursing homes, that provide an infrastructure for dedicated reporting. The weakness of this system includes a selection bias for the site, small number of patients, and increased costs.

Prescription Event Monitoring Systems have been developed in the United Kingdom and in Japan. They consist of patients who have received a drug from electronic prescription databases or automated health insurance claims. A follow-up questionnaire is sent to the prescribing physician requesting follow-up information on patient demographics, indication for treatment, duration of therapy, dosage, clinical events, and reasons for discontinuation. The weakness of the system is a poor response to the questionnaire.

Pharmacovigilance in the 21st century will include active surveillance using electronic databases to determine AEs associated with the use of a medicinal product, to identify a comparable comparative group not taking the product, and for drug utilization studies. This is now possible because of the establishment of linked large databases. However, it is expensive, complicated, and difficult to interpret and may lack some of the needed information. The data also needs to be validated by reviewing medical records. Because it is new, industry and regulators have to learn how to use these databases because there are unknown pitfalls.

Observational Studies. Important safety signals may need to be evaluated in nonrandomized, noninterventional, and nonexperimental observational studies, which include cross-sectional surveys, cohort studies, and case-control studies. The investigator simply observes and describes what is happening in the population receiving normal medical care. Pharmacoepidemiologic studies have a formal written protocol and a control group and are designed to test prespecified hypotheses concerning the risks associated with a drug exposure. The protocol should include a clearly stated study objective, a critical review of the literature, and a detailed description of the research methods, including the population to be studied, case definitions, the data source, the study size and statistical power calculations, and the methods for data collection, management, and analysis.[33] However, observational epidemiologic studies are subject to certain biases, such as effect modification and confounding by indication, that may make it difficult to interpret the results. Although epidemiologic methods are capable of detecting relative risks of 3 to 4, they are not good at detecting a modest increase in a relatively common background event such as myocardial infarction, strokes, or deaths. Randomized, controlled clinical trials are needed for this.[34]

Cross-sectional studies, which collect data on a population at a single point of time, are used to determine trends over time, possible associations between exposure to a product and outcome in ecologic analyses, and to collect drug utilization data. However, the temporal relationship between exposure and outcome cannot be determined in these surveys. Surveys can be used to assess the success of a RiskMAP and to evaluate the knowledge and practices of physicians, pharmacists, and patients concerning how the product should be used and what AEs need to be monitored. Surveys should have a formal written protocol describing the group to be surveyed, the projected sample size, and the method for data collection, management, and analysis.

Cohort studies follow an exposed and unexposed population over a long time period to determine outcomes in both populations. Because the at-risk population is known, incidence rates can be determined and a relative risk can be calculated. Although these studies can be used to determine all AEs associated with a product, they are difficult to do, require a large number of subjects, are expensive, and are not good for rare events. Prospective cohort studies follow a population forward in time to determine outcomes, whereas a retrospective cohort study looks backward at exposures and outcomes that occurred before the study began.

A case-control study compares exposure to a product in cases (patients with a particular AE) and controls selected from the same population. The difficult part of a case-control study is the selection of an appropriate control group. These studies can also be used to identify risk factors for developing the AE in question. An odds ratio, which is an estimate of the relative risk, can be determined. Case-control studies are relatively easy to do, can be done in a short period of time, require a smaller number of subjects, are relatively inexpensive, and are good for rare events.

Randomized clinical trials can be used to confirm possible associations between an AE and a medicinal product. These studies are of high quality because they randomize patients, have an appropriate control group, and collect high-quality data. However, they are costly, take time, and cannot be used for rare events or for events that occur a long time after the drug is administered. They can be used to quantitate the magnitude of the risk for common AEs and determine whether there is a dose-response relationship or drug-drug and drug-food interactions. Large simple trials, which randomize patients into treatment and control groups and collect limited data on a specific AE, can be used to quantitate the risk of a serious but relatively rare AE.

THE FUTURE OF PHARMACOVIGILANCE

The future of pharmacovigilance is linked closely with product development. As pharmaceutical companies develop new products that interfere with complex biochemical systems in the body, safety issues will undoubtedly occur. In order for a product to be marketed, it must be both effective and safe. In order for a health care provider and patient to derive the benefits of the product, they must know the safety profile of the product so that the product is used properly in the proper patient. Regulatory agencies and pharmaceutical companies are developing new guidance documents and tools for conducting pharmacovigilance activities.

In 2004 the FDA implemented its Drug Safety Initiative, which was to create a culture of openness, enhance oversight, and transparency in decision-making within the FDA. A Drug Safety Oversight Board was established in 2005 to identify, track, and oversee the management of important drug safety issues in the Center for Biologics Evaluation and Research (CBER) and to facilitate timely external communication of drug safety issues. A Drug Watch Web page was established in 2005 to improve communication with the public about emerging drug safety information. The goal is to help patients and health care professionals make informed decisions on the use of prescription drugs. The Institute of Medicine issued its report on The Future of Drug Safety: Promoting and Protecting the Health of the Public in 2006.[35] This report made a number of recommendations, which are currently being evaluated by the FDA.

Pharmaceutical companies are also developing new systems for evaluating product safety.[36] Electronic data capturing of all clinical trial data makes it easier to conduct systematic and regular assessments of all safety data from all clinical trials. Pooling data from clinical trials helps identify and quantitate less common AEs. New methods for screening patients for serious toxicities and new ways for determining background rates of AEs from electronic databases are being developed. There are commercially available tools for routinely performing a dysproportionality analysis on postmarketing reports and for evaluating the statistical signals identified. Their exact role in pharmacovigilance remains to be defined.

Regulatory agencies expect pharmaceutical companies to be proactive and focused in their approach to monitoring product safety. They also want pharmaceutical companies to have individuals dedicated to monitoring product safety and to be transparent about potential safety issues. The tools and processes used in pharmacovigilance are continually evolving because the technology to monitor product safety continues to evolve. It is clear that the world of pharmacovigilance has changed, is changing, and will continue to change in the years to come.

REFERENCES

1. U.S. Food and Drug Administration (FDA). Guidance for industry: premarketing risk assessment. March 2005. Available at http://www.fda.gov/cber/gdlns/premarkrisk.htm
2. European Medicines Agency (EMEA), Committee for Medicinal Products for Human Use (CHMP). Guidelines on risk management systems for medicinal products for human use. November 2005. Doc. Ref. EMEA/CHMP/96268/2005. Available at http://www.emea.eu.int/pdfs/human/euleg/9626805en.pdf
3. Veatch RM. Benefit/risk assessment: what patients can know that scientists cannot. Drug Inf J 1993;27:1021-1029.
4. Council for International Organizations of Medical Sciences (CIOMS). CIOMS IV: Benefit-risk balance for marketed drugs: evaluating safety signals. Geneva: CIOMS, 1998.
5. Herxheimer A. Benefit, risk and harm. Aust Prescr 2001;24:18.
6. Edwards R, Wiholm B-E, Martinez C. Concepts in risk-benefit assessment. A simple merit analysis of a medicine? Drug Saf 1996;15:1-7.
7. Mancini GBJ, Schulzer M. Reporting risks and benefits of therapy by use of the concepts of unqualified success and unmitigated failure; applications to highly cited trials in cardiovascular medicine. Circulation 1999;99:377-383.
8. Heart Protection Study Collaborative Group. MRC/BHF Heart protection study of cholesterol lowering with simvastatin in 20536 high-risk individuals: a randomised placebo-controlled trial. Lancet 2002;360:7-22.

9. European Medicines Agnecy (EMEA). Report of the CHMP working group on benefit-risk assessment models and methods. January 2007. Doc. Ref. EMEA/CHMP/15404/2007. Available at http://www.emea.europa.eu/pdfs/human/brmethods/1540407en.pdf
10. Hamilton D. FDA History Office, A brief history of the center for drug evaluation and research. 1997. Available at http://www.fda.gov/cber/about/history/default.htm
11. U.S. Food and Drug Administration (FDA). 21 CFR 314.80. Postmarketing reporting of adverse drug experiences (drugs). Available at http://www.accessdata.fda.gov/scripts/cdrh/cfdocs/cfcfr/CFRSearch.cfm?fr = 314.80
12. U.S. Food and Drug Administration (FDA). 21 CFR 600.80. Subpart D—reporting of adverse experiences (biologic products). Available at http://www.accessdata.fda.gov/scripts/cdrh/cfdocs/cfcfr/CFRSearch.cfm?fr = 600.80
13. International Conference on Harmonization of Technical Requirements for Registration of Pharmaceuticals for Human Use (ICH) web site. Available at http://www.ich.org/cache/compo/276-254-1.html
14. International Conference on Harmonization of Technical Requirements for Registration of Pharmaceuticals for Human Use (ICH). M5 Data Elements and Standards for Drug Dictionaries. Step 2 version, May 2005. Available at http://www.ich.org/cache/compo/276-254-1.html
15. Council for International Organizations of Medical Sciences (CIOMS) web site. Available at http://www.cioms.ch/
16. International Conference on Harmonization of Technical Requirements for Registration of Pharmaceuticals for Human Use (ICH). E2E Pharmacovigilance planning. November 2004. Available at http://www.ich.org/cache/compo/276-254-1.html
17. European Union Clinical Trial Directive 2001/20/EC. Official Journal of the European Communities L 121/34, 1.5.2001.
18. U.S. Food and Drug Administration (FDA). Guidance for industry: development and use of risk minimization plans. March 2005. Available at http://www.fda.gov/cder/guidance/6358fnl.htm
19. U.S. Food and Drug Adminstration (FDA). Guidance for industry: good pharmacovigilance practices and pharmacoepidemiologic assessment. March 2005. Available at http://www.fda.gov/cder/guidance/6359OCC.htm
20. U.S. Food and Drug Administration (FDA). 21 CFR 312.32. IND safety reports. Available at http://www.accessdata.fda.gov/scripts/cdrh/cfdocs/cfcfr/CFRSearch.cfm?fr = 312.32
21. Council for International Organizations of Medical Sciences (CIOMS). CIOMS VI: Management of safety information from clinical trials. Geneva: CIOMS, 2005.
22. Ellenberg S. Independent data monitoring committees: rationale, operations and controversies. Stat Med 2001;20:2573-2583.
23. International Conference on Harmonization of Technical Requirements for Registration of Pharmaceuticals for Human Use (ICH). E1 The extent of population exposure to assess clinical safety for drugs intended for long-term treatment of non–life-threatening conditions. October 1994. Available at http://www.ich.org/LOB/media/MEDIA435.pdf
24. Vesikari T, Madson D, Dennehy P, et al. Safety and efficacy of a pentavalent human-bovine reassortant rotavirus vaccine. N Engl J Med 2006;354:23-33.
25. International Conference on Harmonization of Technical Requirements for Registration of Pharmaceuticals for Human Use (ICH). E9 Statistical principles for clinical trials. February 1998. Available at http://www.ich.org/LOB/media/MEDIA485.pdf
26. U.S. Food and Drug Administration (FDA). Guidelines for the format and content of the clinical and statistical sections of an application. July 1988. Available at http://www.fda.gov/cder/guidance/statnda.pdf
27. International Conference on Harmonization of Technical Requirements for Registration of Pharmaceuticals for Human Use (ICH). E2C (R1) Clinical safety data management: periodic safety update reports (PSUR) for marketed drugs. November 1996 and updated in February 2003. Available at http://www.ich.org/LOB/media/MEDIA477.pdf
28. Almenoff J, Tonning JM, Gould AL, et al. Perspective on the use of data mining in pharmacovigilance. Drug Saf 2005;28:981-1007.
29. DuMouchel W. Bayesian data mining in large frequency tables, with an application to the FDA spontaneous reporting system. Am Stat 1999;53(3):177-202.
30. Evans SJW, Waller PC, Davis S. Use of proportional reporting ratios (PRRs) for signal generation from spontaneous adverse drug reaction reports. Pharmacoepidemiol Drug Saf 2001;10:483-486.
31. Bate A, Lindquist M, Edwards IR, et al. A Bayesian neural network method for adverse drug reaction signal generation. Eur J Clin Pharmacol 1998;54;315-321.
32. European Medicines Agency (EMEA). Eudravigilance Expert Working Group, Guideline on the use of statistical detection methods in the Eudravigilance Data Analysis System. November 2006. Doc. Ref. EMEA/106464/2006. Available at http://www.emea.europa.eu/pdfs/human/phvwp/10646406en.pdf
33. International Society for Pharmacoepidemiology. Guidelines for good pharmacoepidemiology practices (GPP). Revised August 2004. Available at www.pharmacoepi.org/resources/guidelines_08027.cfm
34. Temple R. Meta-analysis and epidemiologic studies in drug development and postmarketing surveillance. JAMA 1999;281(9);841-844.
35. Baciu A, Stratton K, Burke SP (eds). The future of drug safety: promoting and protecting the health of the public. Committee on the Assessment of the U.S. Drug Safety System, Institute of Medicine of the National Academies. Washington, DC: The National Academies Press, 2006.
36. Brewster W, Gibbs T, LaCroix K, et al. Evolving paradigms in pharmacovigilance. Curr Drug Saf 2006;1:127-134.

4

EVIDENCE-BASED DRUG UTILIZATION

Christine Laine

INTRODUCTION 41
FORMULATING GOOD CLINICAL QUESTIONS 41
GATHERING RELEVANT, COMPREHENSIVE EVIDENCE 42
Common Databases 42
Evaluating the Quality of Original Research Studies 44
What Was the Research Question or Study Objective? 44
What Was the Study Design? 45
What Outcomes (Endpoints) Did the Investigators Study and How Did They Measure Them? 46
What Intervention or Therapy Did the Investigators Study? 46
Did the Investigators Address Potential Confounders? 46
How Did the Investigators Sample/Select the Study Population? 46
Who Were the Study Subjects and Were They All Accounted for at the End of the Study? 46
Are the Results Clinically Significant? 46
How to Know a Good-Quality Review when You See One 46
GRADING EVIDENCE 47
UNDERSTANDING NUMERIC RESULTS FOR TRANSLATION INTO EVIDENCE-BASED PRACTICES 48
Risk 48
Comparing Risks 48
Statistical Significance 48
Measures of Precision 49
Number Needed to Treat (or Harm) 49
SUMMARY 49

"The deepest sin against the human mind is to believe without evidence."

Thomas H. Huxley, English biologist (1825-1895)

INTRODUCTION

To use medical therapeutics wisely, clinicians must be able to gather and interpret evidence about the effectiveness and safety of the interventions that they prescribe. In the 1990s, the evidence-based medicine movement was born of the increasing recognition that many medical practices that had become standard care were based more heavily on anecdote and opinion than on scientific observation.[1] Evidence-based medicine advocates a systematic approach to the search, selection, synthesis, evaluation, and dissemination of evidence to inform medical decision making. This chapter introduces the reader to the concepts underlying evidenced-based medicine. Although evidence-based medicine principles are relevant to all types of medical decisions (prevention, diagnosis, therapy, and prognosis), the focus here is on how one gathers and interprets evidence about therapies. The chapter serves as an anchor for understanding the requisite sections on the evidence basis for drug utilization that appear in each of the therapeutic-focused chapters of this book.

Sackett and colleagues proposed five steps essential to evidence-based practice (Box 4-1).[2] First, one must convert the need for information into a question. Second, one must gather the evidence available to inform the answer to this question. Third, one needs to evaluate the validity and quality of the evidence. Fourth, it is essential to integrate the evidence with clinical expertise and the unique characteristics and values of the patient to whom he or she wishes to apply the evidence. Last, Sackett and colleagues assert that practitioners of evidence-based medicine should close the loop by evaluating the effectiveness and efficiency of performance of the first four steps to improve the process when the next clinical question arises. In summary, the activities that make up evidence-based medicine include (in order) formulating a question, identifying and selecting evidence, appraising and synthesizing the evidence, applying the evidence to a particular patient, and evaluating the impact of the process.

In addition to reviewing the basic steps of an evidence-based approach to practice, this chapter provides information on some commonly used databases, reviews a practical framework for critical appraisal of original research reports, discusses what clinicians should look for in high-quality reviews about therapeutics, translates numeric results into concepts that clinicians can use, and provides an overview of some commonly used evidence rating systems. Readers who wish to delve more deeply into evidence-based medicine concepts should consult one of the excellent texts devoted to the topic.[2-5]

FORMULATING GOOD CLINICAL QUESTIONS

To make therapeutic decisions that are likely to benefit patients, clinicians need information about the effectiveness, safety, feasibility, and value of therapeutic interventions. Good clinical questions about therapeutics consider some or all of these issues.[6-8] In addition, to practice evidence-based medicine, one must ask questions that are sufficiently specific. Suppose that a physician is considering prescribing inhaled insulin for a patient and queries, "Does inhaled insulin work?" The answer to this question is clearly, "It depends." It depends on the outcomes one uses to define whether the therapy works, the therapies you compare it with, the kind of patient one is caring for, and the adverse effects the clinician and patient are willing to accept. "Does inhaled insulin work?" is too nonspecific a question to answer in a manner that will help the clinician treat the patient at hand. More helpful questions about therapeutics define the therapeutic goal (e.g., hemoglobin A1c below 7%), the alternatives considered (e.g., subcutaneous insulin or exanitide), the type of patient (e.g., an overweight patient with type 2 diabetes and poor glycemic control despite maximization of oral therapy), and any adverse effects the clinician and patients are not willing to accept (e.g., weight gain). The question becomes, "Would inhaled insulin or exanitide be a better treatment option for achieving hemoglobin A1c level less than 7% in an increasingly overweight patient with type 2 diabetes who has poor glycemic control despite maximization of oral therapy?" Articulating good clinical questions can be difficult, but it is an absolutely essential first task in searching for evidence-based answers. When questions are clinically relevant and sufficiently specific, the search for answers can be focused and the answers found will be more helpful in guiding clinical decision making.

GATHERING RELEVANT, COMPREHENSIVE EVIDENCE

Once one knows the question she or he is seeking to answer, the next step is to search for relevant, high-quality evidence to inform the answer. Two general categories of evidence—primary and secondary—are available to those who seek to practice evidence-based medicine. *Primary evidence* is raw evidence, meaning the reports of single studies that provide information relevant to a clinical question. One can think of primary evidence as the individual building blocks that make up a body of evidence. For many questions, these primary evidence blocks will be numerous and vary substantially in quality. Consequently, searching for, sorting, and stacking the blocks of raw evidence can be a daunting task. *Secondary evidence* is evidence that is the result of a process of a systematic evaluation that others have completed. Secondary evidence may take the form of prescreened and rated abstracts of individual studies, systematic reviews, meta-analyses, point-of-care decision aids, or practice guidelines. To return to the building block analogy, secondary evidence sources collect the blocks, filter out the faulty ones, and stack those that remain into a useful structure. Searching for evidence, whether primary or secondary, is a much less formidable undertaking today than it was before access to continuously updated, comprehensive, electronically searchable databases became ubiquitous. When the source is reliable and the methods of evaluation and synthesis transparent, secondary evidence can be especially valuable for busy clinicians.

BOX 4-1 THE BASIC STEPS TOWARD EVIDENCE-BASED PRACTICE

Formulate the clinical question
Gather evidence relevant to answering the question
Evaluate and synthesize the evidence
Integrate the evidence with clinical experience and patient factors
Evaluate the performance of the above steps and the impact on patient care

Common Databases

Familiarity with available databases is essential to those who seek to practice evidence-based medicine. A variety of databases of individual research reports (primary evidence) are available (Table 4-1). Those with access to medical librarians may find it useful to spend some time learning about efficient search strategies from these experienced professionals. Those without access to librarians might find it helpful to read about techniques for searching the literature before trying to tackle a search themselves.[3]

Of publicly available databases, MEDLINE (Medical Literature Analysis and Retrieval System Online) is the largest and the one most commonly used by clinicians and medical researchers. MEDLINE (www.ncbi.nlm.nih.gov/Pubmed) contains over 10 million biomedical references from nearly 5000 journals published in the United States and 70 other countries. Citations go back to 1996 and are continuously updated, with the addition of up to thousands of citations each week. MEDLINE content covers a wide range of health-related disciplines from bench to bedside. The U.S. National Library of Medicine (NLM) developed and maintains MEDLINE, which is available for free to anyone regardless of country of residence. The NLM examines the following critical elements when deciding which journals to index in MEDLINE: scope and coverage, quality of content, quality of editorial work and policies, production quality, type of content, and audience. Journals that the NLM considers for MEDLINE indexing are those that contain original research reports, clinical observations or case reports,

TABLE 4-1 EXAMPLES OF ELECTRONIC DATABASES OF PRIMARY EVIDENCE

Database	Content	Notes
MEDLINE http://www.nlm.nih.gov	Over 10 million biomedical references	• Covers nearly 5000 journals in 70 countries • Produced by the National Library of Medicine • Contains abstracts for many articles and links to full text sources • Free access through PubMed
AIDSLINE	Literature related to the biology, epidemiology, health care delivery, social and behavioral aspects of acquired immunodeficiency syndrome (AIDS), from 1980-2000	• Contained citations to journal articles, monographs, audiovisuals, journal articles, government reports, theses, AIDS newsletters (beginning with 1995 issues) and AIDS journals (beginning in 1995), and meeting abstracts from the International Conferences on AIDS and other meetings • Produced by the National Library of Medicine until 2001; since 2001, all journal article citations incorporated into MEDLINE • Free access
EMBASE	Pharmacologic and biomedical literature 1980–present	• Covers 4550 journals • Each record includes full citation and indexing terms; 80% have abstracts • Maintained by Elsevier • Specialty subsets are available
CINAHL http://www.cinahl.com	Nursing and allied health literature, 1982–present	• Contains citations and some abstracts and full text • Includes service to order full text
CURRENT CONTENTS http://www.isinet.com/	Multidisciplinary science	• Covers >8000 scholarly science journals, >2000 books, and selected conference proceedings and Internet documents • Produced by Thomson Scientific
Psyclit	Psychological literature 1800s–present	• Abstracts, not full text • Covers >2000 journals, books, dissertations, and other secondary publications • Maintained by the American Psychological Association
Cochrane Controlled Trials Register http://www.cochrane.org	Abstracts of clinical trials	• Contains nearly 500,000 records • Free access in some countries (not the United States)

reviews, statistical compilations, descriptions of methods or procedures, and analyses of philosophical, ethical, or social aspects of the health profession or biomedical science. Journals that do not contain any of these types of content—such as those that primarily abstract articles, provide news reports, or focus on matters relevant to a particular organization—generally do not appear in MEDLINE.

A useful feature of MEDLINE citations is the inclusion of links to sources at which users can access the full text of the articles cited. Some of these links provide access to full text at no cost to the user, such as for material archived in PubMed Central. PubMed Central is a digital archive of life sciences journal literature developed and managed by the National Institutes for Health's National Center for Biotechnology Information in the NLM. Participation by publishers in PubMed Central is voluntary, and journals must meet certain editorial standards to be included in the archive. For the many journals that do not participate in PubMed Central, MEDLINE links to journal and publisher web sites. At these sites, users can view articles for free or via "pay-per-view" mechanisms depending on the publishers' access policies. For articles not available on the web, the "Loansome Doc" feature in PubMed provides an electronic system for ordering copies of articles through the National Network of Libraries of Medicine.

Because some confusion exists among users, it is worth noting the differences between MEDLINE, MedlinePlus, PubMed (http://pubmed.gov), PubMed Central, and NLM Gateway (http://gateway.nlm.nih.gov). MedlinePlus (http://medlineplus.gov) is an NLM service that provides health information oriented to the lay public. Both PubMed and Gateway are electronic portals to MEDLINE and other NLM resources. Gateway is an electronic portal that the NLM initially released to the public in October 2000 to provide access to a variety of the NLM's information resources, including MEDLINE. Gateway is most useful to people who go to the NLM looking for information, but without a high level of knowledge of what is available through the library. Gateway allows the user to enter one query, but search in multiple retrieval systems. The results of Gateway searches are organized by type of information (bibliographic resources, consumer health resources, other information resources) rather than by database. Box 4-2 provides a list of resources accessible through NLM Gateway.

BOX 4-2 INFORMATION SOURCES ACCESSIBLE VIA NATIONAL LIBRARY OF MEDICINE'S GATEWAY

- MEDLINE/PubMed
- NLM Catalog—catalog information for books, serial titles, audiovisuals
- Bookshelf—full-text biomedical books
- TOXLINE Special—toxicology citations
- DART—Developmental and Reproductive Toxicology
- Meeting abstracts on HIV/AIDS, health services research, and space life sciences
- MedlinePlus—consumer health information
- ClinicalTrials.gov—information for the public about clinical trials
- DIRLINE—Directory of Health Organizations
- Genetics Home Reference—consumer information for genetic conditions
- Household Products Database
- HSRProj—health services research projects
- OMIM—Online Mendelian Inheritance in Man
- HSDB—Hazardous Substances Data Bank
- IRIS—Integrated Risk Information System
- ITER—International Toxicity Estimates for Risk
- GENE-TOX—Genetic Toxicology (Mutagenicity)
- CCRIS—Chemical Carcinogenesis Research Information System
- Profiles in Science—archives of several prominent biomedical scientists
- Document delivery through Loansome Doc
- UMLS—Metathesaurus

PubMed, another NLM portal, includes MEDLINE, OLDMEDLINE (references from before 1966), citations from indexed general science journals on topics unrelated to biomedicine, in-process citations that provide a record for an article before it is indexed with Medical Subject Headings (MeSH) and added to MEDLINE, and publisher-supplied citations that precede the date that a journal was selected for MEDLINE indexing. As stated previously, PubMed Central is the National Institutes of Health's voluntary electronic archive.

Clinicians interested in particular subsets of evidence may choose to search specialty databases that focus on a particular clinical area, and Table 4-1 lists some of these more focused databases. Much of what is contained in specialty databases is also included in MEDLINE. However, because of MEDLINE's broad scope, inexperienced users will often need to sift through considerable noise to find what they need. People who are interested in a specific area may encounter less noise in their search results when using a specialty database if one exists in their area of interest.

Because MEDLINE selects publications to index and then generally indexes the content of those publications without assessment of the quality of individual articles, presence in MEDLINE does not indicate that an article is a high-quality piece of evidence. For this reason, busy clinicians may find searching primary evidence sources to be frustrating and inefficient and may prefer to seek evidence from secondary evidence sources. In addition, when several studies of the same therapy for the same condition are available, a summative article that systematically reviews all of the available evidence is more likely to provide an accurate answer than any single study alone. For this reason, those seeking evidence-based answers should probably begin by searching for summative evidence first and resort to primary sources only when summaries are unavailable. Table 4-2 lists a sample of popular secondary evidence sources.

These sources vary considerably in form. Some, such as Up-to-Date and the American College Physicians' Physicians Information and Education Resource (PIER), are designed around clinical topics or modules with highly developed search features for easy use at point of care. Others, such as the Cochrane Library of Reviews or Evidence-Based Medicine Reviews, archive scholarly, summative articles such as systematic reviews, meta-analyses, and guidelines. Whereas much of this material generally will also appear on MEDLINE, users who are seeking summative evidence may find it more efficient to search databases that contain only reviews.

The Cochrane Library is a collection of several hundred systematic reviews (Cochrane Database of Systematic Reviews) and thousands of structured abstracts of randomized, controlled trials produced since 1993 by the Cochrane collaboration. The Cochrane Collaboration is an international network of medical professionals that produces systematic reviews of health care interventions and promotes the search for evidence in the form of clinical trials and other studies of interventions. A major effort of the Collaboration is the comprehensive identification of evidence, particularly randomized, controlled trials, about health care interventions. The group has been instrumental in the development of rigorous methodological standards for the conduct of systematic reviews and meta-analyses. The Cochrane Library is available by subscription, and many medical libraries subscribe to it. Published quarterly in CD-ROM and Internet versions, it includes all existing reviews, new reviews, and updates of previous reviews. The Cochrane web site (http://www.cochrane.org) provides free access to abstracts of the Cochrane reviews.

A third category of secondary evidence resources includes those that screen the literature and select for abstraction only that material that meets certain quality requirements. The most established of these resources is ACP Journal Club, which the American College of Physicians has published since 1991. Available bimonthly in print and in a continuously updated electronic form, ACP Journal Club editors carefully select original research and review articles from over 100 clinical journals through reliable application of explicit criteria for scientific merit, followed by assessment of relevance to medical practice by practicing clinicians. The publication includes lists of noted articles with abstracts and expert commentary accompanying those that receive the

TABLE 4-2 SAMPLE SOURCES FOR PREAPPRAISED EVIDENCE

Resource	Content	Notes
Cochrane Database of Reviews	Hundreds of systematic reviews and updates of reviews on the effectiveness and appropriateness of treatments (medications, surgery, education, etc.) in specific circumstances	• Published quarterly and available on CD-ROM and the Internet • Explore the evidence for and against • Full text available by subscription; abstracts and plain-language summaries are free
Evidence-Based Medicine Reviews http://www.ovid.com	Combines four evidence-based medicine resources: Cochrane Database of Systematic Reviews, The Database of Abstracts of Reviews of Effectiveness (DARE), Article reviews from ACP Journal Club, and the Cochrane Central Register of Controlled Trials	• Available through Ovid • Links to MEDLINE and some full text
American College of Physicians PIER: Physicians Information and Education Resource http://pier.acponline.org	PA Compendium of evidence-based clinical guidance presented electronically in a unique telegraphic format	• Designed for rapid access to clinical information at the point-of-care • 435 modules covering individual diseases, clinical presentations, and other topics • Rates strength of recommendations and each literature citation by evidence level • Peer reviewed and updated continually • Produced by and available from the American College of Physicians
Up-to-Date http://www.uptodate.com	Evidence-based clinical information resource available to clinicians on the Internet, CD-ROM, and Pocket PC	• Intended for use at the point-of-care • Nearly 3000 clinicians author the reviews • Referenced • Continuing Medical Education (CME) feature available • No commercial backing or sponsorship from any organization
ACP Journal Club http://www.acpjc.org	Screens, abstract, and provides commentary on selected studies and reviews	• Screens over 100 clinical journals with a focus on internal medicine • Rates quality and clinical relevance of selected articles • Continuously updated • Produced by McMaster University and available through the American College of Physicians

highest quality and importance ratings. ACP Journal Club is focused on internists, but an increasing number of similar publications are becoming available in other specialty areas. Many clinicians find subscription to these types of services helpful in keeping abreast of the current literature in their fields.

Evaluating the Quality of Original Research Studies

Once clinicians locate evidence, they need to be able to evaluate its validity, quality, and applicability to the clinical question they are trying to answer. This process of evaluation requires knowledge about study design and of systems for synthesizing and rating collections of evidence.

Being familiar with the evaluation of individual studies will also help readers better understand evidence summaries such as systematic reviews, meta-analyses, and clinical guidelines. The Evidence-Based Medicine Working Group has produced a series of practical guides for evaluating the medical literature.[5] These guides provide detailed assessment criteria for different types of studies (e.g., diagnosis, prognosis, therapy, harm, economic analyses, etc.) and are an excellent resource. The following focuses on a basic approach to critical assessment of studies about therapy.

Box 4-3 lists eight general questions applicable to almost any original research report about therapy. These questions can serve as a useful framework for determining whether a given study provides evidence useful to clinical decision making. By systematically addressing these questions, none of which requires statistical expertise to answer, even the inexperienced user of the medical literature can avoid becoming overwhelmed by the task of critical assessment.

BOX 4-3 EIGHT QUESTIONS TO ASK WHEN EVALUATING A STUDY ABOUT THERAPY

1. What was the **research question** or **study objective**?
2. What was the **study design**?
3. What **outcomes** (endpoints) did the investigators study and how did they measure them?
4. What **intervention** or **therapy** did the investigators study?
5. Did the investigators address potential **confounders**?
6. How did the investigators **sample/select** the study population?
7. Who were the **study subjects** and were they all accounted for at the end of the study?
8. Are the results **clinically significant**?

What Was the Research Question or Study Objective?

The first question to ask about a study is whether it actually addresses the clinical question you need to answer. Suppose that you are trying to answer the question posed earlier, "Would inhaled insulin or exanitide be a better treatment option for achieving hemoglobin A1c level less than 7% in an increasingly overweight patient with type 2 diabetes who has poor glycemic control despite maximization of oral therapy?" Your MEDLINE search yields a study that examines the effect on hemoglobin A1c of switching to inhaled insulin from subcutaneous insulin in a population of adults with type 1 diabetes and poor glycemic control. Although the study is about inhaled insulin and examines the endpoint you are interested in, its population and comparator treatment are entirely different from yours. You should waste no further time with this study. On occasion, you may have difficulty deciphering the objective of a study. When you do, you may also want to move on to the next study. A poorly stated objective often foreshadows a poorly executed study because a well-articulated question is the first step in good research.

What Was the Study Design?

Once you are certain that the study's objective corresponds closely enough to your clinical question, you need to determine the study design. Table 4-3 shows the hierarchy of study design and summarizes the advantages and disadvantages of each. In evidence-based medicine discussions, the *quality* of studies generally refers to the degree to which the study methods minimize the potential for bias. Features that minimize bias in studies of therapy include random assignment to study group, blinding of group assignment (especially important is that anyone involved in measuring study outcomes be unaware of which intervention patients received), selection of good comparison or control interventions, and complete follow-up of all participants. Empirical examinations have shown that three methodological features—randomization, concealment of randomization, and blinding of outcome assessment—most influence the degree of bias in studies of therapeutics.[9-11] The only study design that aims to meet all of these conditions is the randomized, controlled, double-blind trial. Consequently, such trials provide the strongest evidence about therapies. In fact, randomized, controlled trials are the only types that are experimental and the only type from which clinicians should draw conclusions about causal relationships between treatments and outcomes.

Why are randomized, controlled trials the best type of evidence about therapeutics? *Randomization* prevents conscious or unconscious assignment of patients to the group that the researchers or clinicians believe they are best suited to. Suppose that one wanted to compare an oral diabetes drug with a new injection drug. In a study that did not use random assignment, patients who were most likely to comply with injection might end up disproportionately assigned to the injection drug group. Because these patients were more compliant with injected therapy than the average patient, the study might provide a more favorable view of the effectiveness of this therapy than if injection-compliant and injection-adverse patients were equally distributed between the two groups. Random assignment prevents bias by balancing the distribution of both measured and unmeasured patient characteristics across the different study groups. Whenever treatment assignment is nonrandom, the possibility of bias exists because patient characteristics can influence which therapy they receive.

When evaluating randomized, controlled trials, evidence-based medicine practitioners should look to see that the researchers clearly describe the randomization methods, whether patients (and their clinicians and the researchers who measured outcomes) were effectively blinded to the type of therapy they were taking, and that all patients were analyzed in the group to which they were assigned. Details about these and other features of high-quality randomized trials are contained within the CONSORT (Consolidated Standards of Reporting Trials) recommendations.[12,13]

In descending order of evidence quality, observational study designs that one might encounter when searching for evidence about therapies include prospective cohort studies, retrospective cohort studies,

TABLE 4-3 HIERARCHY OF STUDY DESIGN

	Study Design	Description	Advantages	Disadvantages
STRONGEST ↑	Randomized, controlled trial	Randomly assigns participants to intervention and control/comparison groups, then follows them prospectively to measure outcomes	Distributes measured and unmeasured participant characteristics between the study groups	• Time consuming • Resource intensive • Patients often hesitant to consent to random assignment
	Nonrandomized, controlled trial	Nonrandomly assigns patients to intervention and control/comparison groups, then follows them prospectively to measure outcomes	Prospective outcome measurement is a strength	• Bias can result from nonrandom assignment • Patients more likely to respond to an intervention might be preferentially placed in that group
	Prospective cohort study	Assembles groups of patients—those who are receiving the intervention of interest and those who are receiving a comparison intervention—and follows them prospectively to measure outcomes	Prospective outcome assessment is a strength	• Bias results because patient clinical characteristics influence which intervention they receive • Confounding is often present
	Retrospective cohort study	Assembles groups of patients who have received the intervention of interest or a comparison intervention and retrospectively determines whether they had the outcome of interest	Can be concluded quickly because the outcomes have already occurred	• Bias results because patient clinical characteristics influence which intervention they receive • Confounding is often present • Retrospective measurement of outcomes often makes standard outcome assessment a challenge
	Case-control study	Assembles two groups of patients—one that has had the outcome of interest (cases) and one that has not (controls)—and then evaluates the proportion of each group that received a particular intervention	• Can be completed quickly because you do not have to wait for outcomes to occur • Useful in situations in which the outcome of interest is rare	• Bias can result from differential recollection of exposures among those who have and have not experienced the outcome
↓ WEAKEST	Case series	Descriptions of outcomes of a single patient or series of patients who received a particular treatment	• Useful in learning about adverse events • Hypothesis generating	• Absence of a comparison group and small numbers prohibit hypothesis testing

case-control studies, and case series or single case reports. None of these study designs are adequate to establish causality. The effect of postmenopausal hormone replacement therapy on prevention of cardiovascular disease in women is a recent, striking example of a therapeutic area in which careful randomized trials came to opposite conclusions on large bodies of observational studies.[14,15] However, whereas clinicians seeking to practice evidence-based medicine must be aware of the shortcomings of these study designs, observational studies are often the only type of evidence available to inform decision making. When integrating such studies into clinical decisions, the clinician must proceed cautiously and be aware of potential sources of bias. The questions in Box 4-3 can be particularly helpful in identifying potential sources of bias in observational studies.

What Outcomes (Endpoints) Did the Investigators Study and How Did They Measure Them?

The study will be helpful to you only if it studied an outcome that you and your patients consider important. The methods used to measure the outcome are also critical. High-quality studies employ consistent, replicable methods for measuring outcomes in all study participants. Further, those responsible for assessing outcomes should be unaware of patients' group assignments. Being blinded in this manner prevents them from biasing measurement to yield the results that they expected. For example, in a study that compared aspirin with placebo for the prevention of myocardial infarction among low-risk subjects, knowing that a patient received aspirin might tilt the outcome assessor from reading equivocal electrocardiographic (ECG) changes as signifying a myocardial infarction, and vice versa, in patients whom he or she knew were taking placebo.

What Intervention or Therapy Did the Investigators Study?

Before using a study to inform clinical decisions, you must be sure that the intervention studied is one that is available to you and acceptable to your patients. High-quality studies describe interventions in sufficient detail that interested readers can easily replicate them. With respect to pharmacologic agents, research reports should describe in detail the preparation, dose, methods of administration (including any counseling, education, or co-interventions that study participants might have received along with the study drug), and duration of therapy.

Did the Investigators Address Potential Confounders?

Confounders are factors other than the exposure/intervention that may affect the outcome of interest and that can be related to exposure/intervention. For example, in a study of the effects of caffeine on pregnancy outcomes, smoking might be a confounder if women who drank coffee were more likely to be smokers than were women who did not drink coffee. To see whether confounding might be an issue, readers should look for data on the baseline characteristics of the drug and comparison groups and check that they are similarly distributed between the treatment and the comparison groups, which will often be the case in at least moderately sized randomized, controlled trials.

How Did the Investigators Sample/Select the Study Population?

The method used to assemble the study population can introduce bias and affect the generalizability of study results. For example, if study subjects were selected in such a way that they were likely to be healthier or more adherent than people randomly selected from the general population, then the findings might not apply to the general population. The research reports should include sufficient detail about demographic and clinical characteristics to permit the reader to determine whether the results are likely to apply to her or his own patients.

Who Were the Study Subjects and Were They All Accounted for at the End of the Study?

If substantial numbers of study subjects drop out of the study and do not provide data on study endpoints, bias results. In most cases, the patients who drop out differ from those who remain in the study. As a rule of thumb, greater than 90% follow-up is good, 80% to 90% follow-up requires caution in interpreting the findings, and less than 80% follow-up indicates that you should refrain from drawing definitive conclusions from the study.[16]

Are the Results Clinically Significant?

Clinical significance relates to the importance of the outcomes measured and to the magnitude of the differences observed. If a study shows a statistically significant difference in an outcome that is unimportant to the patient, then the findings are not useful to the patient. An example of a statistically significant result that is not clinically significant is: Suppose a trial of a new cancer drug showed that the drug reduced tumor volume by half but had no effect on functional status or mortality (the outcomes the patient really cares about). With respect to the magnitude of the result, very large studies sometimes show that very small changes in the outcome of interest are statistically significant. For example, a large trial of a new blood pressure drug might show that patients who received the new drug had systolic blood pressure values that were 2 mm Hg less ($P < 0.05$) than those on the old drug. Although this result is statistically significant, a 2 mm Hg change in blood pressure is unlikely to justify use of the new drug, particularly if it is more expensive or more toxic than the old drug.

How to Know a Good-Quality Review When You See One

On occasion, clinicians may find themselves in a position of wanting or needing to personally and meticulously undertake all of these steps, such as when they are developing a clinical guideline or authoring a review. Most often, however, it is infeasible and inefficient for busy clinicians to gather, evaluate, and synthesize the primary evidence from scratch on their own. In such cases, clinicians can fill their information needs by seeking evidence that others have preappraised and/or synthesized. Thus, the following sections address the skills necessary for clinicians to be savvy users of preappraised evidence and evidence syntheses, which most often take the form of narrative reviews, systematic reviews, meta-analyses, and clinical guidelines.

Narrative reviews are historically the most prevalent type of review in the published literature, but they are generally the least helpful type of summary for clinicians seeking evidence to guide practice. Narrative reviews often address broad topic areas without describing in detail the methods the authors used to search, select, and synthesize evidence related to the topic. Consequently, it is difficult for readers to detect whether subtle or not so subtle biases have crept into the review.

Systematic reviews usually address one or a small number of focused questions and use rigorous, structured methods to search, select, evaluate, and synthesize the existing evidence to answer these questions. Whereas narrative reviews tend to lecture, systematic reviews attempt to educate the reader by describing the evidence.[17] Conducting high-quality systematic reviews is as demanding as conducting high-quality clinical research. Excellent, detailed resources are available to guide the preparation of evidence-based reviews, and readers who are participating in such activities should consult these resources.[18-22]

Some systematic reviews use meta-analysis to combine the findings of individual studies to arrive at more precise estimates of the true relationships between the interventions and the outcomes of interest. Quantitative estimates that sum large bodies of information into a single number can be very appealing, but meta-analysis is not always appropriate. Before quantitatively summarizing the results of a systematic review, the reviewers must carefully consider the appropriateness of pooling results. The more heterogeneous a body of evidence, the less appropriate pooling becomes.[23-25]

Clinical guidelines are summative articles that provide recommendations for patient care. Good-quality guidelines include systematic evidence summaries or are accompanied by systematic reviews or meta-analyses that represent the evidence base on which the guideline was developed.[26,27]

Evidence-based medicine practitioners should seek systematic evidence summaries.[28] Unsystematic approaches to selecting, evaluating, and synthesizing the evidence reduce the chances that a review will include all relevant evidence, recognize limitations of the evidence, or distinguish clearly between evidence and opinion. Systematic reviews are replicable because they describe the methods used to search, select, and evaluate the quality of studies related to a well-articulated question. However, even systematic reviews can fall short in execution. Clinicians seeking evidence for clinical decision making should look for the following features when deciding whether a review is sufficiently sound to justify integrating its findings into the care of their own patients.[17]

- The review should ask important, well-formulated questions and be organized to answer them.
- The review should include a methods section that contains details on bibliographic sources, dates of literature searches, types of studies that are most appropriate to address each question, and the critical appraisal and synthesis processes for evaluating and summarizing studies.
- The review should use search and selection strategies that yield the types of evidence best suited to answer the questions that are the focus of the review.
- The review should include evidence tables that present key features of studies to facilitate comparisons.
- The review should critique the quality of the literature such that readers can gain a clear understanding of the strengths and weaknesses of individual studies and the summative evidence.
- The review should synthesize the body of evidence rather than simply listing the results of individual studies, taking into account such variables as study design, study populations, tested strategies, and outcomes. Well-synthesized reviews summarize data with attention to amount, type, strength, and patterns of evidence and also attempt to explain inconsistent and conflicting evidence.
- The review should apply clinical judgment and critical appraisal of studies to help determine whether quantitative methods are appropriate to help summarize data, estimate a common effect, or evaluate heterogeneity across studies.
- When offering recommendations for clinical care, the review should articulate the quality of the evidence on which the recommendations are based.

GRADING EVIDENCE

A common and useful feature of many summative evidence-based medicine articles is the use of systems for rating or grading the quality of individual studies, the quality of a body of evidence, and/or the strength of recommendations. Frequently, recommendations receive numeric, letter, or descriptive (e.g., poor, moderate, high) grades to signify the strength of evidence on which the recommendation rests. Whereas such conventions have the potential to concisely convey the degree of confidence that clinicians should place in particular study or recommendation, the variety of different rating schemes in use can be dizzying and impedes effective communication about evidence-based medicine. Particularly confusing is the fact that the meaning of a grade of "poor" by one group does not necessarily correspond to "poor" by another group. In addition, a study of existing rating systems found low reproducibility of ratings within a given system.[29] Table 4-4 presents several commonly used evidence rating schemes.

TABLE 4-4 SAMPLE OF TAXONOMIES COMMONLY USED TO GRADE EVIDENCE

Taxonomy	Clinical Recommendations
GRADE	**High-quality evidence**: Further research is unlikely to change confidence in the estimate of effect. **Moderate-quality evidence**: Further research is likely to have an important influence on our confidence in any observed effects and might even change the estimate. **Low-quality evidence**: Further research is likely to have an important impact on the confidence in the estimate and is likely to change the estimate. **Very-low-quality evidence**: Any estimate of effect is very uncertain. **Strong recommendations**: These are supported by high-quality studies with consistent findings that occur across a spectrum of patients. **Weak recommendations**: These are based on weak studies with inconsistent results and substantial variation in outcomes according to patient characteristics
American Academy of Pediatrics	**Strong recommendation**: Anticipated benefits of the recommended action clearly exceed the harms, and the quality of the supporting evidence is excellent. In some clearly identified circumstances, strong recommendations may be made when high-quality evidence is impossible to obtain and the anticipated benefits strongly outweigh the harms. **Recommendation**: The anticipated benefits exceed the harms, but the quality of evidence is not as strong. In some clearly identified circumstances, recommendations may be made when high-quality evidence is impossible to obtain but the anticipated benefits outweigh the harms. **Option**: Either the quality of evidence is suspect or carefully performed studies have shown little clear advantage of one approach over another. **No recommendation**: There is a lack of pertinent published evidence, and the anticipated balance of benefits and harms is unclear.
USPSTF	**A**: Strongly recommends that clinicians provide the service to eligible patients; good evidence that the service improves important health outcomes and concludes that benefits substantially outweigh harms. **B**: Recommends that clinicians provide the service to eligible patients; at least fair evidence that the service improves important outcomes and that benefits outweigh harms. **C**: No recommendation for or against; at least fair evidence that the service can improve health outcomes but the balance of benefits and harms is too close to justify a general recommendation. **D**: Recommends against providing the service; at least fair evidence that the service is ineffective or that the harms outweigh the benefits. **I**: Evidence is insufficient to recommend for or against providing the service; evidence is lacking, conflicting, or of poor quality and cannot determine net of benefits and harms.
SORT (Strength of Recommendation Taxonomy)	**A level**: Based on consistent and good-quality patient-oriented evidence. **B-level**: Based on limited-quality or inconsistent patient-oriented evidence **C-level**: Based on consensus, opinion, usual practice, disease-oriented evidence, or case series.

USPSTF, United States Preventive Services Task Force.

In response to growing confusion and frustration related to inconsistencies in rating schemes, the Grading of Recommendations, Assessment, Development, and Evaluation (GRADE) Working Group has developed a new system and proposes that all parties use this new system when rating evidence.[30] The GRADE Working Group is a collaboration of people interested in improving evidence-based medicine grading systems. The GRADE system attempts to avoid some of the unnecessary complexity of other systems and addresses both the quality of evidence and the strength of recommendations. The GRADE Working Group characterizes *high-quality evidence* as being available when further research is unlikely to change confidence in the estimate of effect. *Moderate evidence* means that further research is likely to have an important influence on our confidence in any observed effects and might even change the estimate. *Low-quality evidence* indicates that further research is likely to have an important impact on the confidence in the estimate and is likely to change the estimate. *Very-low-quality evidence* indicates that any estimate of effect is very uncertain. In the GRADE system, recommendations are either strong or weak. *Strong recommendations* are supported by high-quality studies with consistent findings that occur across a spectrum of patients. *Weak recommendations* are based on weak studies with inconsistent results and substantial variation in outcomes according to patient characteristics. Other factors contributing to the strength of recommendations are the importance of treatment effects, precision of estimates of treatment effects, risks and burdens of therapy, costs, and the value that patients place on the outcome of interest.[31] A pilot study of the GRADE system suggests that the system balances simplicity with transparent consideration of all-important issues.[32]

UNDERSTANDING NUMERIC RESULTS FOR TRANSLATION INTO EVIDENCE-BASED PRACTICES

The translation of research results into helpful information for clinical decisions requires an understanding of the common expressions of numeric results in clinical studies.[33] These expressions include those that address frequency or risk of certain events, comparisons of frequency or risk in two or more groups, statistical significance, clinical significance, differentiation of definitively negative from inconclusive results, confounding, and clinically relevant measures of benefit and harm.

Risk

Risk is the probability that a particular event will occur. The concept of risk is important because clinicians and their patients want to know the chances that a particular outcome will occur if they implement a particular therapy. Consider the following scenario (Table 4-5). In a study of 1000 patients with a life-threatening illness, half are randomly assigned to receive drug A and half to receive placebo. The outcome of interest is death within 3 years. Among the 500 patients who received drug A, 50 died. In other words, the absolute risk of death with drug A is 50/500 or 0.10 (10%). *Absolute risks* are probabilities that vary between 0 (the event never occurs with a given treatment) and 1 (the event always occurs with a given treatment).

Comparing Risks

Absolute risks are informative, but clinicians and their patients need to compare risks in order to select one therapeutic option over another. These comparisons can take the form of ratios or differences. To return to the example of drug A, which demonstrated a risk of death of 10% among patients who received it. A 10% risk of death probably seems unacceptably high on first impression. However, this single risk estimate provides little useful clinical information without concomitant knowledge about the risk of death among patients who received placebo. To make informed decisions about whether to select drug A over no treatment, the clinician and patient need to know the relative risk of death with drug A compared with the risk of death on no therapy. Now suppose that of the 500 patients in the study who received placebo, 100 died. In other words, the absolute risk of death among patients on placebo was 100 ÷ 500 = 0.20 (20%). Thus, a death rate of 10% on drug A does not seem so bad. To express the difference between these two risks, one can use the risk difference or a risk ratio. The *risk difference* is the absolute difference between the risks: 0.20 − 0.10 = 0.10 (10%). *Relative risk* is the ratio of risk in one group compared with that in another or, in the case of our example, the relative risk of death on drug A compared with that on placebo is 0.10 ÷ 0.20 = 0.50 (50%). Knowledge of all of these risk expressions is important to those using study results to guide clinical decisions. The potential clinical significance of a risk ratio of 50% is very different if the absolute risks in the two groups compared were 10% and 20% (absolute risk difference = 10%) than if they were 1% and 2% (absolute risk difference = 1%). For a given relative risk (risk ratio), the absolute changes associated with therapy depend on the underlying frequency of the event in the population. The absolute risk difference becomes smaller as event rates become lower.[34]

Statistical Significance

Statistics enable one to estimate the probability that the observed or a greater degree of association between the dependent and independent variable would occur under the null hypothesis, which states that there is no difference between the groups. The *P*-value, the most common expression of statistical significance in health care research, is the probability that the difference observed could have occurred by chance if the groups were truly similar. Thus, a *P*-value less than 0.05 means there is less than a 5% probability that the results observed could have occurred by chance if there truly was no real difference between the two groups being compared. Convention alone has set the threshold for significance at 5%. In some cases, clinicians and patients might be willing to take action only with smaller *P*-values, especially if the therapy under consideration were very toxic or very expensive.

TABLE 4-5 UNDERSTANDING NUMERIC RESULTS

	New Drug	Old Drug
Number of patients in group	500	500
Number of cancer deaths	50	100
Number of patients who developed renal failure	0.15 (25%)	0.05 (5%)
Risk of death	50 ÷ 500 = 0.10 (10%)	100 ÷ 500 = 0.20 (20%)
Relative risk	0.10 ÷ 0.20 = 0.50 (50%)	
Absolute risk difference	0.20 − 0.10 = .10 (10%)	
Number needed to treat to prevent one cancer death	1 ÷ 0.10 = 10 For every 10 patients who receive the new drug, 1 death will be prevented	
Number needed to harm	1 ÷ (0.15 − 0.05) = 10 For every 10 patients who receive the new drug, 1 will experience renal failure	

Measures of Precision

When examining clinical studies, one must remember that the results are only estimates. The precision of these estimates depends on the amount of variation due to measurement error, sampling error, and random error. *Measurement error* is the variation due to measurement techniques. *Sampling error* is the variation that results from the number of study participants and the degree to which they represent the population of interest. Random error is a function of biologic variation in the outcome of interest. In order to know how confident one can be in using the estimates to guide clinical decisions, one must consider this precision. Commonly used statistical measures of variation include standard error, standard deviation, ranges, and confidence intervals. Of these, confidence intervals are the preferred method and best understood by clinicians.[35] *Confidence intervals* (CIs) are the range of values within which the estimate lies. The upper and lower boundaries of this interval are the confidence limits. A 95% CI means that if you repeated the experiment 100 times, 95% of the time the values would fall between the lower and the upper limits. The narrower the CI, the more confident you can be in the accuracy of the point estimate. CIs that accompany an estimate of the frequency of some characteristic or event in the study population provide useful descriptive information about the precision of that estimate.

Examination of confidence limits for estimated differences between groups or changes over time in one group are helpful in inferring the statistical and clinical significance of findings and in distinguishing truly negative studies from ones that are merely inconclusive.[36] The 95% CI relates to statistical significance at the $P < 0.05$ level. In general, a result is not statistically significant at the $P < 0.05$ level if the 95% CI for the estimate of the difference between groups (or between different measures in the same group over time) does not include 0. For example, if a study of a new weight-loss drug estimates the difference between baseline and 3-month weight as −7 pounds (95% CI, −15 to −0.05), then the difference between the groups is statistically significant at $P < 0.05$. However, if the estimate was −7 pounds (95% CI, −12 to +9), then the difference between the two weight-loss therapies is not statistically significant because 0 pounds (no difference in weight) is within the range of plausible values for the estimate. CIs are more informative than *P*-values because they provide information about the range within which the true value lies. Thus, examination of the confidence limits can help one interpret the clinical significance of observed results.[37] Because CIs provide information about the range of values that are consistent with the observed results, examination of the CI enables you to determine whether the range includes values that are clinically important. Returning to the previous example of the weight-loss drugs, a clinician and patient might decide that a drug is worth taking only if one can expect to lose at least 5 pounds, especially if the drug is associated with side effects or is expensive. If the study showed that the drug resulted in a mean of 4.7 pounds of weight loss, but the 95% CI went from −5.5 to −0.05 pounds, then despite the statistical significance of the findings, the clinician and patient might reasonably decide that the amount of weight loss is likely to be insufficient to be clinically important. In other words, although the results are statistically significant, they are not clinically significant.

CIs are also helpful in interpreting the significance of risk ratios. A risk ratio of 1 indicates that there is no difference in risk between groups. When the 95% CI for a risk ratio that compares two groups does not include 1, the results are significant at a level of $P < 0.05$.[36] Consider another hypothetical study of a new weight-loss drug. Suppose that the risk ratio for normalization of body mass index after 1 year on the drug was 2.1. That is, people who took the drug were more than twice as likely to achieve normal body mass index (BMI) at 1 year as those who took placebo. The 95% CI around the risk ratio 2.1 is 1.06-2.7. The interval does not include 1, so the difference between groups is statistically significant at $P < 0.05$. However, the confidence limit tells us that the risk ratio could be as close to 1 as 1.05, indicating that statistical significance of this finding is marginal, an important thing to know when considering prescribing the drug.

The literature contains numerous studies of therapy that report no statistical difference between groups. No statistical difference can mean one of two things: There is truly no clinically meaningful benefit of the drug or the study was too small to detect a clinically meaningful benefit that might actually exist. CIs can help the reader determine which of these situations they are dealing with. If the confidence limits exclude a clinically important effect, then the clinician can conclude that the study provides reasonable evidence that there truly is no important difference between the two groups. However, if the *P*-value is greater than 0.05, but the CI includes a clinically meaningful difference, then the study is inconclusive. Return to a hypothetical study of a new weight-loss drug. Suppose the clinician decides that a weight loss of 5% initial body weight is the minimal, clinically important amount of weight loss that would justify using the new drug. The study shows that the patients on the new drug lost an average 4% of initial body weight and the *P*-value was greater than 0.05. If the 95% confidence limits spanned from a 6.4% weight loss to a 2% weight gain, the study would be inconclusive because the 95% CI includes values at or greater than the minimal clinically important degree of weight loss (5% of initial body weight). However, if the study result was 3.6% (95% CI, 4.1% loss to 2% gain), it would be truly negative in that it conclusively excludes a clinically important result.

Number Needed to Treat (or Harm)

Many patients (and their clinicians, too) find it difficult to translate the numeric results of studies into meaningful information to inform decisions. Some find the concept of *number needed to treat* (NNT) more intuitive. The NNT is the number of patients that a clinician would need to treat with a given therapy to prevent one adverse outcome (or influence one positive outcome) over a specified period of time.[38] *Number needed to harm* (NNH) is the same concept applied to adverse effects of treatment. NNT is the reciprocal of the absolute risk reduction.[34] In the case of our example of drug A's effect on mortality compared with that of placebo, the absolute risk difference was $0.20 - 0.10 = 0.10$. The reciprocal of this value is $1 \div 0.10 = 10$. In other words, for every 10 patients treated, one could expect 1 fewer death to occur. This same concept can be used to describe harms. The NNH is simply the reciprocal of the risk difference in harms between the two study groups. If a study expresses the absolute risk difference as a proportion, then NNT can be calculated as 100 divided by the absolute risk reduction expressed as a proportion. In our example of drug A, the absolute risk reduction expressed as a proportion is 10%, 100 divided by 10 = 10, so either method yields the same NNT.

Although NNT and NNH are intuitively appealing, caution is necessary when using these concepts. First, one must understand that NNTs and NNHs are not precise estimates. As with any statistical estimate, the range of true values varies around the estimate. Sometimes, researchers will report CIs for NNTs and NNHs to address this concern. Second, one should refrain from applying NNTs and NNHs across conditions, particularly when the outcomes of interest are different. For example, the NNT to prevent one stroke cannot easily be compared with the NNT to prevent one migraine headache. In addition, one must consider the interval over which the outcomes were evaluated. You may have two interventions that have NNT of six to prevent one death; however, one study measured 30-day mortality whereas another measured mortality over a full year of follow-up. Last, the NNT estimates that come from studies assume the same relative risk difference regardless of an individual patient's baseline risk. In practice, however, the NNT may be different for patients based on their underlying risks for the outcome of interest.[34]

SUMMARY

To practice evidence-based medicine, clinicians must take the time to formulate clear clinical questions, be familiar with the sources of primary and secondary evidence likely to provide information relevant to these questions, and be facile with the criteria currently used to rate evidence and recommendations. In ending this brief introduction to evidence-based medicine, it is essential to emphasize that evidence should inform rather than dictate medical decisions.[39] In many situations, evidence alone will not lead to a good medical decision. For many therapeutic interventions, evidence is absent, sparse, equivocal, or even contradictory. Further, even when high-quality evidence from randomized, controlled trials or systematic reviews is available, clinicians must consider whether their patients have similar baseline risk for the outcomes studied (benefits and harms) as the study population. Second, clinicians must gather information about their patients' perceptions of and preferences for the potential benefits and harms of the therapy being considered. After gathering and interpreting the primary and secondary evidence that exists, clinicians must factor in their own experiences and patient preferences to make the best decisions about therapy for the individuals they care for.

REFERENCES

1. Evidence-Based Medicine Working Group. Evidence-based medicine. A new approach to teaching the practice of medicine. JAMA 1992;268:2420-2425.
2. Sackett DL, Straus SE, Richardson WS, et al (eds). Evidence-Based Medicine: How to Practice and Teach EBM. Edinburgh: Churchill Livingstone/Harcourt, 2000.
3. Greenlaugh T. How to Read a Paper: The Basics of Evidence-Based Medicine. London: BMJ Books, 2001.
4. Riegelman RK. Studying a Study and Testing a Test: How to Read the Medical Evidence. Philadelphia: Lippincott Williams & Wilkins, 2005.
5. Guyatt G, Rennie D (eds). Users' Guides to the Medical Literature: Essentials of Evidence-Based Practice. Chicago: AMA Press, 2002.
6. Haynes BR. Forming research questions. J Clin Epidemiol 2006;59(9):881-886.
7. Counsell C. Formulating questions and locating primary studies for inclusion in systematic reviews. Ann Intern Med 1997;127:380-387.
8. Richardson WS, Wilson MC, Nishikawa J, Hayward R. The well-built clinical question: a key to evidence-based decisions. ACP J Club 1995;123:A12-A13.
9. Schulz K, Chalmers I, Hayes RJ, Altman DG. Empirical evidence of bias. Dimensions of methodological quality associated with estimates of treatment effects in controlled clinical trials. JAMA 1995;273:408-412.
10. Sacks HS, Chalmers TC, Smith H Jr. Randomized versus historical assignment in controlled clinical trials. N Engl J Med 1983;309:1353-1357.
11. Chalmers TC, Celano P, Sacks HS, Smith H Jr. Bias in treatment assignment in controlled clinical trials. N Engl J Med 1983;309:1358-1361.
12. Moher D, Schulz KF, Altman D, et al. The CONSORT statement: revised recommendations for improving the quality of reports of parallel-group randomized controlled trials. Ann Intern Med 2001;134:657-662.
13. Altman D, Schulz KF, Moher D, for the CONSORT Group. The revised CONSORT statement for reporting randomized trials: explanation and elaboration. Ann Intern Med 2001;134:663-694.
14. Petitti DB. Some surprises, some answers, and more questions about hormone therapy: further findings from the Women's Health Initiative. JAMA 2005;294(2):245-246.
15. Rossouw JE, Anderson GL, Prentice RL, et al., and the Writing Group for the Women's Health Initiative Investigators. Risks and benefits of estrogen plus progestin in healthy postmenopausal women: principal results from the Women's Health Initiative randomized controlled trial. JAMA 2002;288(3):321-333.
16. Montori VM, Guyatt GH. Intention-to-treat principle. CMAJ 2001;165:1339-1341.
17. The Editors. Reviews: making sense of an often tangled skein of evidence. Ann Intern Med 2005;142:1019-1020.
18. Mulrow C, Cook D (eds). Systematic Reviews: Synthesis of Best Evidence for Health-Care Decisions. Philadelphia: American College of Physicians, 1998.
19. Chou R, Helfand M. Challenges in systematic reviews that assess treatment harms. Ann Intern Med 2005;142:1090-1099.
20. Hartling L, McAlister FA, Rowe BH, et al. Challenges in systematic reviews of therapeutic devices and procedures. Ann Intern Med 2005;142:1100-1111.
21. Santaguida PL, Helfand M, Raina P. Challenges in systematic reviews that evaluate drug efficacy or effectiveness. Ann Intern Med 2005;142:1066-1072.
22. Norris SL, Atkins D. Challenges in using nonrandomized studies in systematic reviews of treatment interventions. Ann Intern Med 2005;142:1112-1119.
23. Hatala R, Keitz S, Wyer P, Guyatt G, for the Evidence-Based Medicine Teaching Tips Working Group. Tips for learners of evidence-based medicine: 4. Assessing heterogeneity of primary studies in systematic reviews and whether to combine their results. CMAJ 2005;172:661-665.
24. Lau J, Ioannidis JPA, Schmid CH. Quantitative synthesis in systematic reviews. Ann Intern Med 1997;127:820-826.
25. Mulrow C, Langhorne P, Grimshaw J. Integrating heterogeneous pieces of evidence in systematic reviews. Ann Intern Med 1997;127:989-995.
26. Shiffman RN, Shekelle P, Overhage JM, et al. Standardized reporting of clinical practice guidelines: a proposal from the Conference on Guideline Standardization. Ann Intern Med 2003;139:493-498.
27. Cook DJ, Greengold NL, Ellrodt AG, Weingarten SR. The relation between systematic reviews and practice guidelines. Ann Intern Med 1997;127:210-216.
28. Mulrow C. Rationale for systematic reviews. BMJ 1994;309:597-599.
29. Atkins D, Eccles M, Flottorp S, et al., and the GRADE Working Group. Systems for grading the quality of evidence and the strength of recommendations: 1. Critical appraisal of existing approaches. BMC Health Serv Res 2004;4(1):38.
30. GRADE Working Group. Grading quality of evidence and strength of recommendations. BMJ 2004:328:1490-1494.
31. Guyatt G, Vist G, Falck-Ytter Y, et al. An emerging consensus on grading recommendations. ACP J Club 2006;144:A8-A9.
32. Atkins D, Briss PA, Eccles M, et al., and the GRADE Working Group. 2005. BMC Health Serv Res 5(1):25.
33. McQuay HJ, Moore RA. Using numerical results from systematic reviews in clinical practice. Ann Intern Med 1997;126:712-720.
34. Barrat A, Wyer P, Hatala R, et al., for the Evidence-Based Medicine Teaching Tips Working Group. Tips for learners of evidence-based medicine: 1. Relative risk reduction, absolute risk reduction, and number needed to treat. CMAJ 2004:171:353-358.
35. Montori VM, Kleinbart J, Newman TB, et al., for the Evidence-Based Medicine Teaching Tips Working Group. Tips for learners of evidence-based medicine: 2. Measures of precision (confidence intervals). CMAJ 2004:171:611-615.
36. Lange TA, Secic M. How to Report Statistics in Medicine. Philadelphia: American College of Physicians, 1997, pp. 55-63.
37. Goodman SSN, Berlin JA. The use of predicted confidence intervals when planning experiments and the misuse of power when interpreting results. Ann Intern Med 1994;121:200-206.
38. Cook RJ, Sackett DL. The number needed to treat: a clinically useful measure of treatment effect. BMJ 1995;310:452-454.
39. Straus SE, McAlister FA. Evidence-based medicine: a commentary on common criticisms. CMAJ 2000;163:837-841.

5 DRUG-RECEPTOR INTERACTIONS

Scott A. Waldman

PARAMETERS DETERMINING RESPONSES TO DRUGS 51
RECEPTORS 51
Receptor Properties Regulating Ligand Effects 52
Effector Mechanisms: Signal Transduction 52
Concentration and Receptor Occupancy 53
QUANTITATIVE RECEPTOR THEORY 54
Equilibrium Binding 54
Scatchard Analysis 56
Relationship of Ligand-Receptor Binding and Time: Kinetics 56
Dissociation 56
Association 57
Quantification of Association 57
Relationship of Kinetic and Equilibrium Receptor Occupancy 57
Quantification of Receptor Occupancy over Time 58
BEYOND LIGAND-RECEPTOR INTERACTIONS: THERAPEUTICS AND THE DOSE-RESPONSE RELATIONSHIP 59
Characteristics of the Concentration-Response Relationship of Drugs 59
Receptor Dynamics and the Concentration-Response Relationship 60
Receptor Dynamics 60
Receptor-Effector Coupling and Shape Factor 61
Relationship Between Intensity and Time Course of Drug Effects 62
AGONISTS AND ANTAGONISTS 63
POPULATION RESPONSES TO DRUGS AND INTERINDIVIDUAL VARIABILITY 64

PARAMETERS DETERMINING RESPONSES TO DRUGS

The response of a patient to an administered drug reflects the intersection of three key parameters (Fig. 5-1).[1,2] The *dose* of the drug is the specified quantity of therapeutic agent delivered to the patient, independent of the route of delivery (oral, intravenous, subcutaneous injection, inhalation, etc.). Doses are typically expressed as quantities (e.g., milligrams, milliliters), while the key parameter driving biologic and physiologic effects of drugs is the concentration (molarity) of drug presented to the site of action. The biochemical, pharmacologic, and clinical responses to a drug are directly proportional to the dose of drug administered: the larger the dose administered, the greater the response produced (*dose-response*).

Pharmacokinetics is the constellation of biochemical processes that convert the dose of drug administered to the final concentration of drug presented to the site of action.[3] For example, a drug administered orally dissolves in the stomach (dissolution), the dissolved particles go into solution (solubilization), followed by absorption across the gastric and intestinal mucosa into the portal circulation (absorption), where it is transported to the liver and undergoes first-pass metabolism. Once through the liver, drug is delivered to the systemic circulation, where it undergoes distribution to various compartments (intra/extracellular, intra/extravascular, lipid, water, etc.) based on its physicochemical characteristics. Further, distribution results in metabolism in various organs, including liver, lungs, and kidneys, which eliminates drug from the system. Moreover, drug can be eliminated through clearance mechanisms, including excretion through the kidney (urinary), biliary system (fecal), skin (sweat), and lungs (exhaled gases). These processes, which are integrated over time, ultimately define the concentration of drug presented to the site of action. Indeed, pharmacokinetics can be considered *what the body does to drugs*, and is explored in detail in Chapter 13 (Pharmacokinetics).

Finally, *pharmacodynamics* is the constellation of biochemical mechanisms translating the concentration of drug presented at the site of action into pharmacologic, cellular, tissue, and organismal responses. In contrast to pharmacokinetics, pharmacodynamics can be considered *what the drug does to the body*.[3] This chapter specifically focuses on the molecular and quantitative basis of pharmacodynamics and drug action. The theory and practice of pharmacodynamics applied to patient responses is examined in detail in Chapter 14 (Pharmacodynamics).

RECEPTORS

Cell processes and their regulation result from the interaction of molecules that transfer energy and information in a directed fashion to achieve an ultimate biologic outcome. In that context, drugs initiate their influence on cellular behavior through requisite interactions with receptors. Receptors are macromolecules involved in chemical signaling between and within cells, located at the cell surface or within the cytoplasm or nucleus. Activated receptors regulate biochemical processes, such as ion conductance, enzyme activities, gene transcription, and signal transduction. Molecules, including drugs, hormones, toxins, neurotransmitters, and other mediators that influence cell behavior (historically termed *autocoids*) that mediate their effects on cells by binding to receptors are known as *ligands*. Directionality of activity is *not* implied by these designations, and ligands may activate or inactivate a receptor, and activation may increase or decrease discrete cell functions.

Receptors represent one of the broadest classes of biologic molecules that share specific qualitative and quantitative functional characteristics and include representation from all categories of macromolecules. Proteins probably represent the largest and best characterized class of receptors and include classical hormone receptors, enzymes, ion channels, and structural elements. Carbohydrates also serve as receptors, exemplified by the saccharide moities of the GM_1 ganglioside that serve as receptors for cholera toxin and the heat-labile enterotoxin produced by diarrheagenic bacteria. The structure of DNA can be considered a receptor for cancer chemotherapeutic agents, including doxorubicin

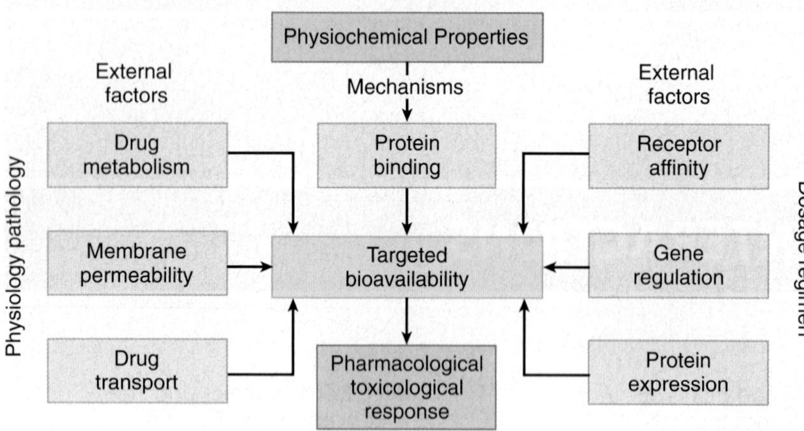

FIGURE 5-1 • Parameters defining the response of a patient to a drug. There is a direct relationship between how much drug a patient receives, the dose, and the magnitude of response (*dose-response*). Further, the drug must gain access to the target site of action, reflecting the interaction of the physicochemical properties of the drug and pharmacokinetic processes that define the final concentration of the drug (*what the body does to the drug*), including metabolism, transport, protein binding, and bioavailability. Moreover, the response is also dependent on the constellation of pharmacodynamic process that translate drug concentration into a cellular, tissue, organ, and organismal response (*what the drug does to the body*), including receptor binding and activation of downstream effector mechanisms. (From Chaurasia CS, Müller M, Bashaw ED, et al. AAPS-FDA Workshop White Paper: Microdialysis Principles, Application, and Regulatory Perspectives. Report From the Joint AAPS-FDA Workshop, November 4-5, 2005, Nashville, TN. AAPS J 2007;9[1].)

(Adriamycin), whose flat structure intercalates into the ordered planar arrays of purine and pyrimidine rings forming the core of the double helix, disrupting DNA replication. Moreover, the plasma membrane lipid bilayer can be considered a receptor for alcohol and inhalational anesthetics, which are highly lipophilic and selectively partition into the plasmalemma, disrupting membrane organization and the function of proteins residing therein, including other receptors and ion channels.

Receptor Properties Regulating Ligand Effects

Generally, receptors possess two cognate activities: ligand (drug) *binding* and activation of effector mechanisms or *agonism* (Box 5-1). It is noteworthy here that ligand binding can occur in the absence of agonism, the basis for the development of therapeutic *antagonists* that block the ability of specific receptors to produce deleterious signals in pathophysiology. For example, antihistamines bind to histamine receptors, without producing a downstream signal, blocking those receptors from activation with endogenous histamine and the resultant signs and symptoms of allergic reactions. However, binding is an absolute prerequisite for agonism or antagonism.

The concept of binding, and the quantitative relationships that ultimately evolved into the *dose/concentration-response relationship,* suggests that the magnitude of downstream pharmacologic effects produced by ligands is proportional to fractional *receptor occupancy.* There are two cardinal parameters central to the concepts of receptor occupancy: *affinity* and *specificity.* Affinity reflects the "attractiveness" of the ligand for the receptor. Conceptually, this can be envisioned as the strength of ligand-receptor interactions. Quantitatively, affinity defines the probability of receptor occupancy at a particular concentration of ligand. Specificity reflects the high complimentarity characterizing ligand-receptor interactions, conceptually analogous to the complimentarity between a lock and key. Specificity of ligand-receptor interactions and the resultant targeted downstream signaling events, in part, determines the orderly flow of information that directs structured biologic functions.

The information encoding affinity and specificity is contained in the chemical structure of the ligand and the complimentary binding site on the receptor. Indeed, the vast majority of drugs show a remarkably high correlation between structure, affinity, and specificity to produce pharmacologic effects. Thus the structure of the ligand has a profound effect on its activity (*structure-activity relationship*). Experimental evidence indicates that drugs interact with protein receptors that have specific three-dimensional shapes, generally requiring a minimum of three points of contact for binding. Small changes in the structure or composition of the drug can dramatically alter affinity and specificity.

With few exceptions, ligand-receptor interactions are *reversible,* a key feature of biologic systems mediating bidirectional regulation. Reversibility permits induction of downstream signaling events upon ligand-receptor *association* and receptor occupancy, but termination of those events upon ligand-receptor *dissociation.* All types of chemical forces, with the exception of covalent interactions, contribute to defining the affinity and specificity of reversible ligand-receptor interactions. Thus, acid and amine groups characterizing many ligands and their receptors, ionized at physiologic pH, produce ionic bonds and the attraction of opposite charges at the interface of complimentary interacting molecular surfaces. Polar interactions, including hydrogen bonding, are an extension of the attraction of opposite charges. Indeed, drug-receptor interactions essentially exchange the hydrogen bond between a drug molecule and surrounding water, with those at the receptor binding site. Hydrophobic bonds between nonpolar hydrocarbon groups at binding sites, directed at excluding water, while not highly specific, may be the strongest of the forces driving molecular interactions. Conversely, forces that decrease the stability of drug-receptor interactions include electrostatic repulsion of like charges and steric hindrance produced by three-dimensional features including repulsive electron clouds, inflexible chemical bonds, and bulky organic side chains.

BOX 5-1 SCHEMATIC REPRESENTATION OF BINDING AND EFFECTOR FUNCTIONS OF RECEPTORS

$$L + R \rightleftharpoons LR \longrightarrow \text{Effector mechanisms (Agonism)} \longrightarrow \text{Response}$$

- Free ligands (L) and receptors (R) interact to form ligand-receptor complexes (LR), reflecting the cognate binding function of receptors.
- Some ligands are agonists with intrinsic activity. For agonists, ligand-receptor interaction activates downstream effector mechanisms, producing a response.
- Other ligands may be antagonists, which exhibit the binding function but are devoid of intrinsic activity. Antagonists bind to receptors without activating them, inhibiting the ability of agonists to activate those receptors, essentially blocking their downstream signaling and response functions.

Effector Mechanisms: Signal Transduction

Once bound, a ligand induces an alteration in receptors resulting in initiation of effector cascades leading to a biologic response. Effector mechanisms permit the information contained in a ligand to be translated into a cellular response. This flow of information is called *signal transduction* and takes many forms within the cell.

Ligands bind to receptors that serve as transcriptional regulators, recognizing and binding to specific elements in the genome and alter-

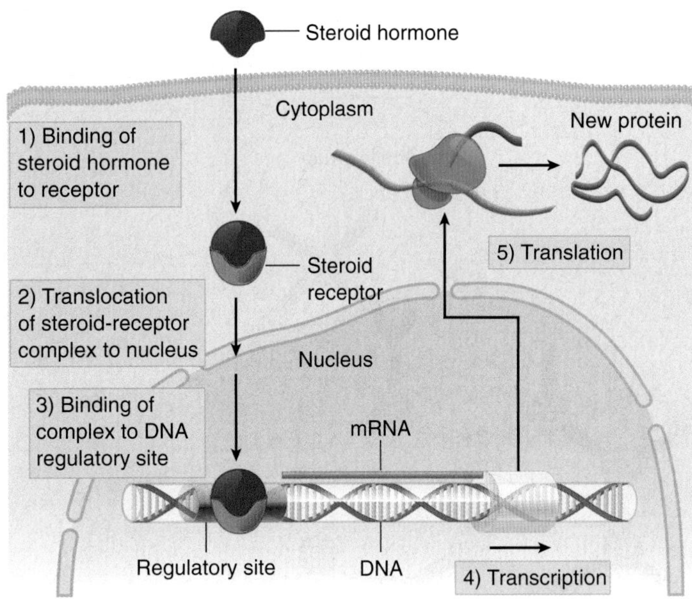

FIGURE 5-2 • Steroids and transcriptional regulation. Steroids bind to cytoplasmic receptors. The steroid and its receptor are then translocated to the nucleus, where the steroid-receptor complex serves as a transcription factor, binding to the promoter of target genes and inducing or repressing their transcription to messenger RNA (mRNA). The mRNA is processed and transported out of the nucleus into the cytoplasm, where it undergoes translation by ribosomes to new proteins. (Available at *http://www.rise.duke.edu/phr150/performance/howitworks.html*)

ing protein expression. Typically, binding of ligand increases association of receptors with those regulatory elements, increasing the transcription of the regulated genes and ultimately resulting in alterations in expression of proteins. This is exemplified by corticosteroids and their receptors[4] (Fig. 5-2).

Ligands bind to enzymes, altering their activity, which has direct effects on cell physiology. Nonsteroidal anti-inflammatory drugs, such as aspirin, interact with and inhibit cyclooxygenase, a key enzyme in the production of prostaglandins[5] (Fig. 5-3).

Ligands bind to ion channels and alter their conductance, which influences cell activity (Fig. 5-4). Calcium channel blockers interrupt intracellular calcium influx at the level of the plasma membrane, inducing vascular smooth muscle relaxation in hypertension and extracellular matrix remodeling in connective tissue diseases.[6]

Ligands bind to cell surface proteins and stimulate the production of a second signal molecule within the cell, which mediates the physiologic response of the cell. This downstream signal is termed a *second messenger.* These mechanisms underlie many of the physiologic responses mediated by endogenous ligands and are the best characterized mechanisms, to date. These mechanisms, which are explored in detail in Chapter 6 (Signal Transduction), include

- Receptors coupled to their downstream effectors through guanine nucleotide–binding proteins—for example, those that activate adenylyl cyclase, whose second messenger is cyclic AMP. These are exemplified by β-adrenergic receptors[7] (Fig. 5-5).
- Receptors that activate guanylyl cyclases, whose second messenger is cyclic GMP[8] (Fig. 5-6).
- Receptors that activate kinases—for example, growth factor receptors, which phosphorylate tyrosine residues of intracellular proteins[9] (Fig. 5-7).

Concentration and Receptor Occupancy

Integrated responses of cells, tissues, and organisms to ligands are directly proportional to the number of receptors occupied. Thus the more receptors occupied, the greater the response to the ligand, up to the point at which cell signaling mechanisms are saturated and cannot be further driven. In turn, the probability of receptor occupancy is directly related to the affinity for ligand. The relationship between receptor occupancy and ligand affinity is reflected by the importance of the concentration of ligand at the site of action for driving receptor responses. Indeed, the concentration of ligand at the site of action controls receptor occupancy and, ultimately, the resultant effect. The dependence of receptor occupancy and responses on the concentration of ligand forms the basis of the *concentration-response relationship,* one of the core principles of pharmacology underlying drug actions.

The relationship between the concentration of ligand and receptor occupancy is typically represented graphically (Fig. 5-8) with concentration plotted on the ordinate (*X* axis) and the measured effect (receptor binding, receptor occupancy) on the abscissa (*Y* axis). It is noteworthy that drug-receptor interactions are both concentration and time dependent and, here, responses are considered after the system has reached *equilibrium* and receptor occupancy is independent of time. These plots illustrate the cardinal characteristics of ligand-receptor interactions. Indeed, these interactions are concentration dependent, and increases in ligand concentration produce increases in receptor occupancy. Further, receptor occupancy is graded, and small increases in ligand concentration produce small increases in binding, while large changes in concentrations produce large increases in binding. Moreover, receptor occupancy is saturable. There is a concentration of ligand that produces 100% occupancy, beyond which further increases in ligand concentration produce no further increases in occupancy.

These graphical relationships can be represented as linear plots (see Fig. 5-8, left) or as log-linear plots (see Fig. 5-8, right) wherein ligand concentration is portrayed on the logarithmic axis. While linear plots produce a rectangular hyperbolic function defining Michaelis-Menten kinetics, log-linear plots produce the characteristic sigmoidal isotherm synonymous with the concentration-response relationship. Log-linear plots offer specific advantages, including facilitating direct comparisons of ligand-receptor interactions across a broad spectrum of affinities, and are generally the convention for graphical representation of concentration-response relationships.

The relationship between affinity, drug concentration, and receptor occupancy can be expressed by the *equilibrium dissociation constant* (K_d), the concentration of ligand that produces 50% receptor occupancy at equilibrium. The K_d is a direct expression of the affinity of the ligand-receptor complex. Indeed, when the affinity of the ligand-receptor complex is high, low concentrations of ligand are required to produce receptor occupancy, and the K_d is low. Conversely, when the affinity of the ligand-receptor complex is low, high concentrations of ligand are required to produce receptor occupancy, and the K_d is high. The K_d is a characteristic parameter for each ligand-receptor complex. Moreover, the K_d represents 50% receptor occupancy regardless of the number of receptors. Whether there are 10 receptors or 1 million

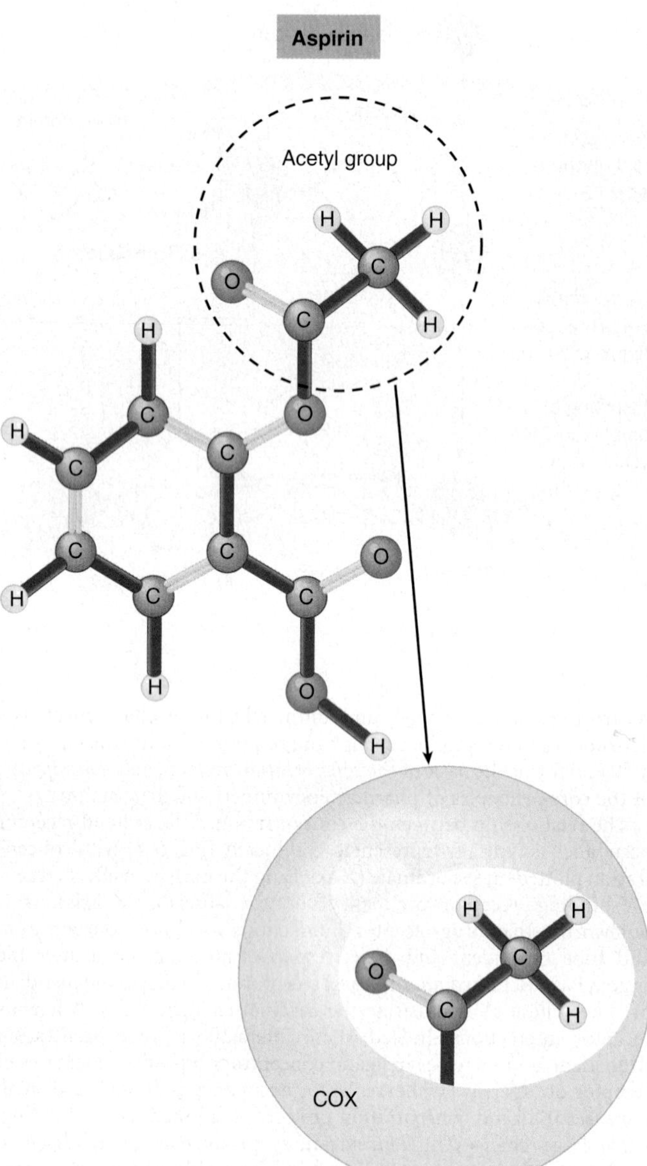

FIGURE 5-3 • Mechanism of action of aspirin. Aspirin nonselectively blocks both isoforms of cyclooxygenase, COX-1 and COX-2, which mediate ring closure and addition of oxygen to arachidonic acid to produce prostaglandins, principle mediators of fever, pain, swelling, and inflammation. The acetyl group on aspirin is hydrolyzed and then transferred to the alcohol group of serine on COX as an ester. This blocks the channel in the enzyme, and arachidonic acid cannot enter the active site to undergo catalytic conversion to prostaglandin. Acetylation of COX by aspirin is irreversible, permanently inactivating these enzyme molecules. Thus, recovery of prostaglandin synthesis requires production of new molecules of COX. (Available at *http://www.elmhurst.edu/~chm/vchembook/555prostagland.html*)

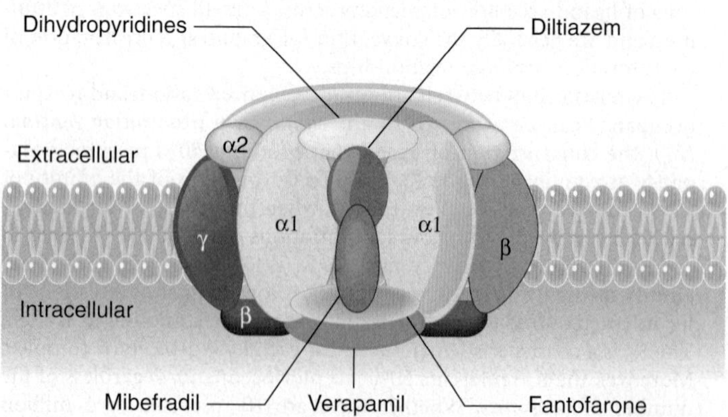

receptors, at the K_d concentration of ligand, 50% of the receptors are occupied at equilibrium.

QUANTITATIVE RECEPTOR THEORY

Equilibrium Binding[10,11]

Ligands and receptors bind to each other following the *Laws of Mass Action* (Box 5-2). The forward reaction is *bimolecular,* dependent on the concentrations of ligand and receptor, while the reverse reaction is *unimolecular,* dependent on the concentration of ligand-receptor complex only. This reaction can be considered at two general points in time (Fig. 5-9): approaching equilibrium (Fig. 5-9A) or at equilibrium (Fig. 5-9B).

At equilibrium, the *forward (association)* and *reverse (dissociation) reactions* have the same *rate* and are transferring the same quantities of materials in each direction. Thus at equilibrium there is no net increase or decrease in the concentrations of reactants or products. However, this is a dynamic state, and, although there is no net change in the concentrations of any element in the system, there is a constant transfer of reactants and products in each direction across the equilibrium. Indeed, if there is no net change in concentrations, but it is a dynamic condition, with materials exchanged in both directions, then it must be the case that the rates (amounts of material transferred/time) of the forward and reverse reactions are equal. If the system is perturbed by adding more reactants or products, there will be a period when forward and reverse reactions have different rates and different amounts of materials are transferred, driving the system to reestablish equilibrium. Equilibrium is established (or reestablished) in proportion to the concentration of reactants, including ligand ([L]) and receptor ([R]), and products, including bound or occupied (liganded) receptor ([LR]), and equilibrium constants, including k_{on} or $k_{association}$ and k_{off} or $k_{dissociation}$, as follows.

For a ligand-receptor system moving to equilibrium:

$$k_{on} \rightarrow k_{off}$$

$$[L] + [R] \rightarrow [LR] \rightarrow [L] + [R] \qquad \text{Eq. 5-1A}$$

Here, the rate of formation of [LR] = $[L][R]k_{on}$ while its rate of dissociation is $[LR]k_{off}$.

BOX 5-2 BINDING AND THE LAWS OF MASS ACTION

Ligand-receptor interactions obey the Laws of Mass Action:

$$L + R \underset{\text{Dissociation k-1}}{\overset{\text{Association k1}}{\rightleftharpoons}} LR$$

- The forward reaction is bimolecular, dependent on the concentrations of free ligands (L) and receptors (R), with a rate proportional to the association rate constant (k1).
- The reverse reaction is unimolecular, dependent on the concentrations of ligand-receptor complexes (LR) and proportional to the dissociation rate constant (k-1).

FIGURE 5-4 • Schematic overview of the drug interaction sites of calcium channel blockers (dihydropyridines, diltiazem, verapamil, fantofarone, mibefradil) with the L-type calcium channel. (From Sandmann S, Unger T. L- and T-type calcium channel blockade—the efficacy of the calcium channel antagonist mibefradil. J Clin Basic Cardiol 1999;2:187-201.)

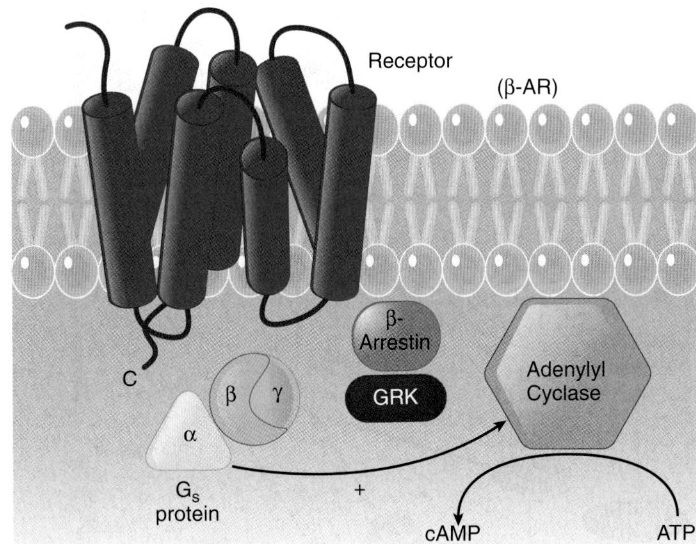

FIGURE 5-5 • G protein–coupled receptors. Upon ligand binding, β-adrenergic receptors (β-AR) bind to the heterotrimeric guanine nucleotide–binding protein Gs, inducing the exchange of GTP for GDP on the Gα subunit. Guanine nucleotide exchange induces dissociation of the α subunits from βγ subunits, the former of which activates adenylyl cyclase and the production of the second messenger cyclic AMP. Signaling is terminated by GTP hydrolysis by the Gα subunit, resulting in its occupation by GDP, promoting reassociation of the heterotrimeric αβγ complex and inactivation of adenylyl cyclase. Moreover, receptors are inactivated by phosphorylation by G protein–coupled receptor kinase (GRK) resulting in the binding of β-arrestin, producing receptor desensitization by preventing productive interaction with G proteins and inducing internalization.

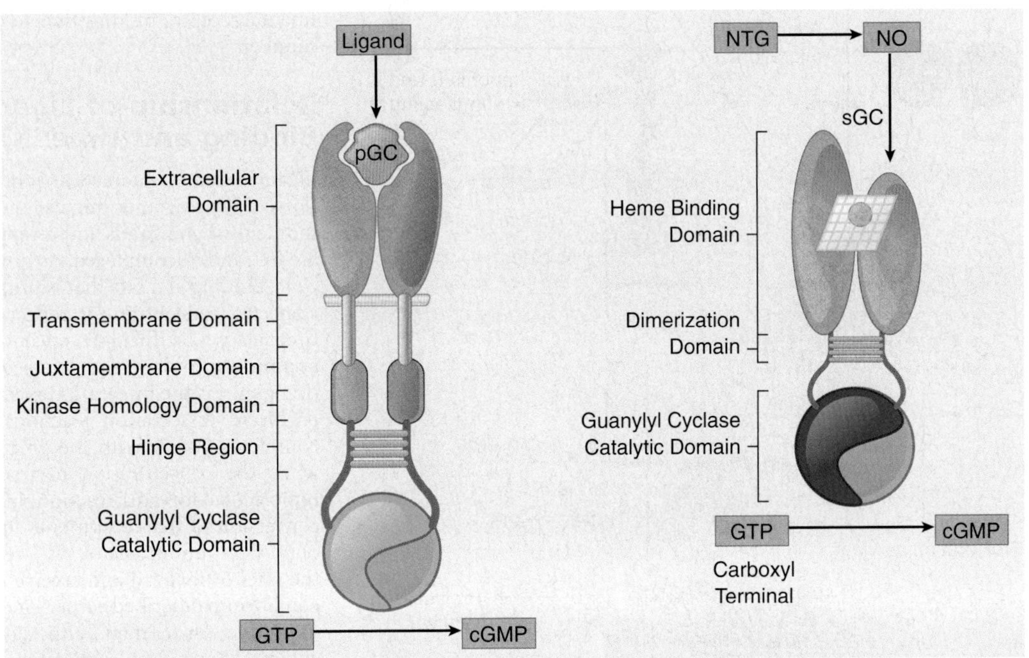

FIGURE 5-6 • Guanylyl cyclases and cyclic GMP. Guanylyl cyclases are a family of signaling molecules possessing canonical ligand-binding and catalytic domains. There are two principle subfamilies of these proteins, the membrane-bound, or particulate, isoforms and the cytosolic, or soluble, isoforms. Soluble guanylyl cyclases are heterodimers possessing a heme prosthetic group at the amino terminal that serves as the receptor for nitric oxide (NO). Particulate guanylyl cyclases are homodimeric transmembrane proteins possessing extracellular domains that bind specific peptide hormones and toxins. For both soluble and particulate guanylyl cyclases, ligand binding induces activation of the catalytic domains at the carboxyl terminal, which produces cyclic GMP. NTG, nitroglycerin.

At equilibrium:

$$[L][R]/[LR] = k_{off}/k_{on} = K_d \quad \text{Eq. 5-1B}$$

If the total concentration of receptors ($[R_T]$) = [R] + [LR], then:

$$[L][R_T - LR]/[LR] = K_d \quad \text{Eq. 5-1C}$$

which upon rearrangement yields:

$$[LR] = [R_T][L]/K_d + [L] \quad \text{Eq. 5-1D}$$

or

$$\text{Fractional receptor occupancy} = [LR]/R_T = [L]/K_d + [L] \quad \text{Eq. 5-1E}$$

Thus, once the binding parameters have been defined for ligand-receptor *equilibrium,* the number or proportion of total receptors occupied *at equilibrium* can be quantified. The significance of this concept is underscored by considering that the effect of a ligand, or drug, is proportional to the number of receptors occupied and eliciting that effect. Equation 5-1E highlights the fact that receptor occupancy is related to the ratio of the ligand concentration and the K_d.

- When the concentration of ligand is very low, below K_d, then receptor occupancy is linearly related to the ratio of the ligand concentration and the K_d. Thus, if the K_d is 10^{-9} M and the ligand concentration is 10^{-11} M, the proportion of receptors occupied is ~1%.
- When the concentration of ligand is near K_d, then receptor occupancy is related to the ratio of the ligand concentration and the K_d through a log-linear relationship. Thus, if the K_d is 10^{-9} M and the ligand concentration is 10^{-10} M, the proportion of receptors occupied is ~9%.
- When the concentration of ligand equals K_d, then 50% of receptors are occupied.
- When the concentration of ligand is much higher than K_d, then receptor occupancy is independent of ligand concentration (*zero order*) and all receptors are saturated (maximum binding, B_{max}). Thus, if the K_d is 10^{-9} M and the ligand concentration is 10^{-6} M, the proportion of receptors occupied is ~100%.

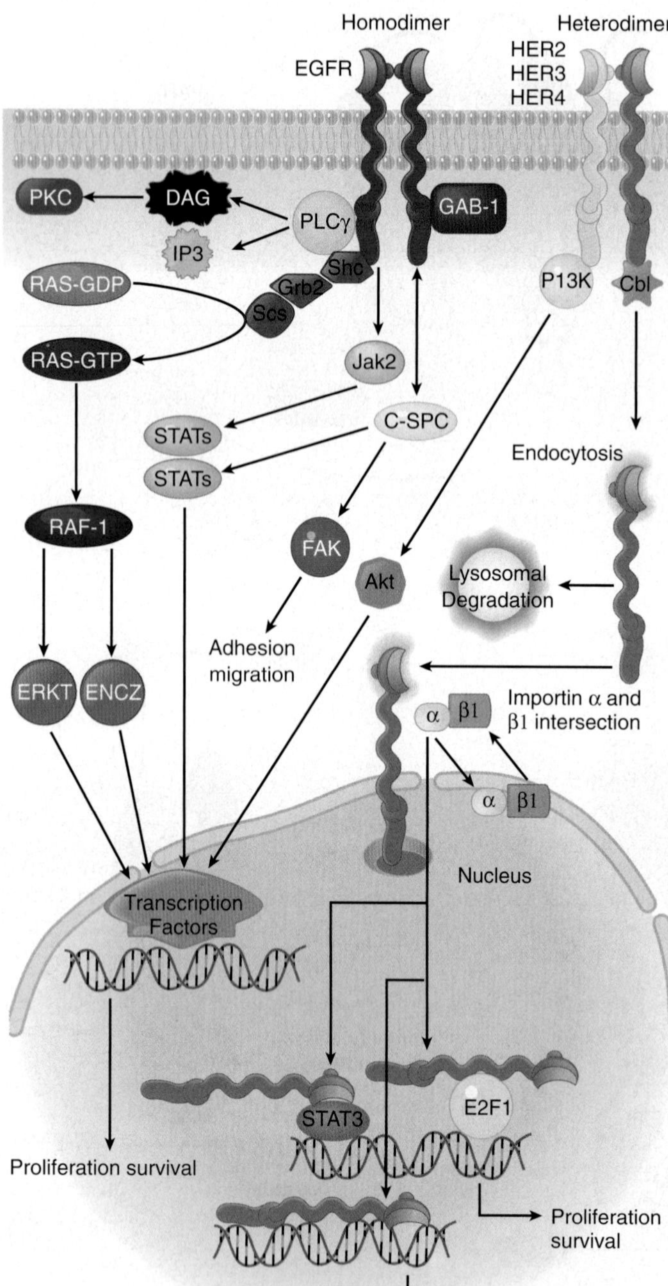

FIGURE 5-7 • Receptor tyrosine kinases. The epidermal growth factor receptor (EGFR) family of receptors are transmembrane proteins composed of an extracellular ligand-binding domain, a membrane-spanning domain, and a cytoplasmic domain that serves as the site of protein kinase activity. The intracellular domain of the EGFR family is highly conserved, with three recognizable sequence domains: the juxtamembrane region, the tyrosine kinase (TK) domain, and the carboxyl-terminal tail. Once the ligand binds to the extracellular domain, EGFR undergoes homodimerization or heterodimerization. Dimerization induces the activation of the TK domain, which leads to autophosphorylation of critical tyrosine residues on the cytoplasmic terminal. These tyrosine residues serve as attachment sites for a range of cellular docking proteins, activating a variety of downstream signaling cascades to affect gene transcription. Three signaling pathways downstream of EGFR have been identified: the Ras/Raf mitogen-activated protein (MAP) kinase, PI3K/Akt, and Jak2/STAT3 pathways.

Scatchard Analysis

In studies of receptors, the concentrations of ligand [L] and ligand-receptor complex [LR] can be quantified, but not the concentration of total receptors [R], because free, unbound (unliganded) receptors are silent in the system. Therefore, an extrapolation of the equations depicted above, derived by Scatchard, is employed to quantify ligand receptor affinities and receptor densities.[12]

From Eq. 5-1C, if $[L][R_T - LR]/[LR] = K_d$, then

$$[L][R_T - LR]/K_d = [LR] \qquad \text{Eq. 5-1F}$$

and, upon rearrangement:

$$[LR]/[L] = (-1/K_d)[LR] + R_T/K_d \qquad \text{Eq. 5-1G}$$

In its simplest form, a plot of the bound/free ligand ([LR]/[L]) versus bound ligand ([LR]) produces a linear isotherm with a negative slope of $(-1/K_d)$ and an *X*-intercept of R_T or B_{max} (Fig. 5-10). It should be apparent that ligand-receptor complexes with high affinities associated with low K_d's produce Scatchard plots with steep slopes. Conversely, ligand-receptor complexes with low affinities associated with high K_d's produce curves with shallow slopes. Moreover, the *X*-axis intercept represents the maximum number of binding sites (R_T, B_{max}) because this is the theoretical point at which binding occurs at infinite concentrations of ligand, the point at which all available receptors must be saturated. In more complex situations, ligands may bind to more than one receptor, or receptors with more than one affinity state, producing curvilinear plots, with slopes and associated intercepts representing the various constituent ligand-receptor interactions. Scatchard analysis is one of the standard methods for analyzing experimental receptor binding data to quantify ligand affinities and receptor number.

Relationship of Ligand-Receptor Binding and Time: Kinetics[10,11]

Ligand-receptor interaction is dependent not only on the concentrations of the reactants, but also on time (Fig. 5-11). Qualitatively, at the moment when ligands and receptors are mixed (time 0), all molecules are free and uncomplexed. As time elapses, ligands and receptors associate, binding at a rate that is proportional to their affinity and to their respective concentrations, reflecting the Laws of Mass Action. As more time elapses, sufficient concentrations of ligand-receptor complex accumulate to drive the reverse dissociation reaction. Thus, receptor occupancy is the integration over time of the forward association and backward dissociation reactions. Net formation of ligand-receptor complexes occurs with the greatest rates at the earliest time points, when the concentration of free receptors is greatest to drive the bimolecular forward reaction, but slows over time, reflecting the net conversion of free receptors to ligand-receptor complexes driving the opposing unimolecular reverse reaction. There is a time point at which the rates of forward and reverse reactions are equivalent, the point of equilibrium described earlier. At equilibrium, there is no net formation of products or reactants, although this is a dynamic process and ligand and receptor molecules continuously exchange across the equilibrium. At equilibrium, receptor occupancy is independent of time.

Dissociation

We start with a consideration of the time course of the dissociation of ligand-receptor complexes. This is a unimolecular reaction, dependent upon the concentration only of the ligand-receptor complex. In this regard, dissociation is a first-order phenomenon, with the rate of loss of ligand-receptor complexes being dependent only on the concentration of those complexes. Note that the linear graphical representation demonstrates a direct plot of the loss of ligand-receptor complexes from the system over time. The curve decreases in an exponential fashion and a semi-logarithmic plot is linear, characteristic of a system from which the fractional rate of loss is constant. That is, as time passes and there is dissociation and loss of ligand-receptor complexes from the system, the rate of loss of those complexes slows, reflecting the fact that the dissociation reaction is driven only by the concentration of ligand-receptor complexes.

While loss of complexes slows over time, the fractional rate of loss of complexes is a constant. Indeed, first-order reactions are characterized by a half-life, in which 50% of the reactants are lost regardless of how many complexes are present. For example, if the half-life of these

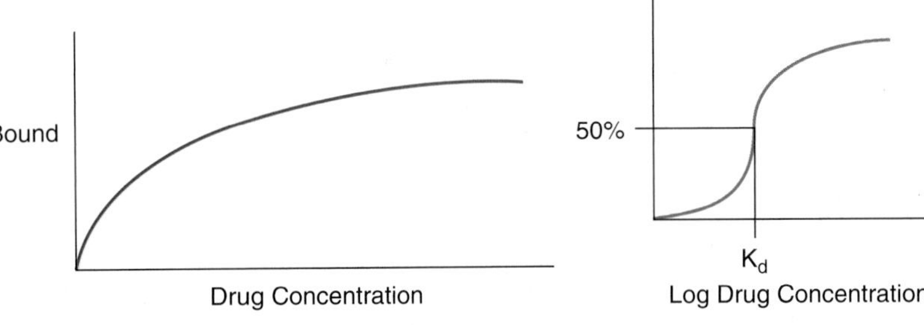

FIGURE 5-8 • Concentration dependence of ligand-receptor interactions. Ligand-receptor interactions are concentration dependent, graded, and saturable. Saturation (B_{max}) reflects the occupancy of virtually 100% of available receptors. The concentration of ligand yielding 50% receptor occupancy represents the equilibrium dissociation constant (K_d). The concentration-binding relationship can be portrayed graphically on a linear Michaelis-Menten plot **(left)** as a rectangular hyperbole, or as a log-linear plot **(right)**, which is the preferred convention.

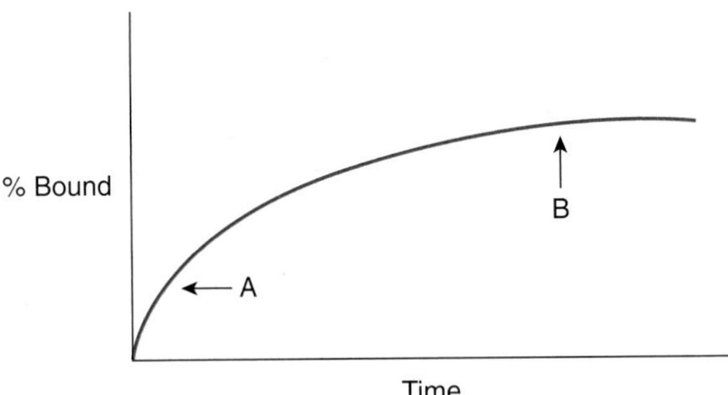

FIGURE 5-9 • Time course of ligand-receptor interactions. Ligands interact with their receptors in a time-dependent fashion, rapidly associating early, reflecting the highest concentrations of reactants comprising free ligand and free receptor **(A)**. As the reaction progresses, depletion of free reactants coupled with the accumulation of ligand-bound receptor, and the resulting dissociation reaction, slows the accumulation of ligand-receptor complexes. The time at which dissociation and association rates are equal and there is no net accumulation of reactants or products represents equilibrium **(B)**.

complexes is 5 minutes, and the initial number of complexes is 100, then after 5 minutes 50 complexes remain, after 10 minutes 25 complexes remain, after 15 minutes 12.5 complexes remain, and so on. However, if the starting amount is 1000 complexes, then after 5 minutes 500 complexes remain, after 10 minutes 250 complexes remain, and so on. Thus, for any ligand-receptor complex, there is a family of parallel log-linear dissociation plots with identical slopes. These are hallmark characteristics of a *first-order reaction* (dependent only on the concentration of one component) and the *slope of the semi-log plot is a direct measure of the dissociation rate constant* (k_d *or* k_{off}), with units of min^{-1} (Fig. 5-12).

Association

In contrast to dissociation, association is a bimolecular reaction, dependent upon the concentration of both ligand and receptor. Therefore, this is a *second-order phenomenon* and changes in ligand concentration alter the apparent rate of association. Note that this yields a family of association isotherms, reflecting increasing formation of ligand-receptor complexes, at different ligand concentrations (Fig. 5-13, left panel). All of these curves plateau at a time beyond which further receptor occupancy does not occur, reflecting equilibrium at that specific ligand concentration. Conceptually, it is important to realize that receptor occupancy represented by the plateau of these curves, at each ligand concentration, represents ligand concentration-specific receptor occupancy on the concentration-binding curves at equilibrium examined earlier (see Fig. 5-13, right panel). For example, the time course of association obtained with the K_d concentration of ligand yields a plateau that represents 50% receptor occupancy. Similarly, the time course of association with a concentration of ligand that is 100-fold higher than K_d yields a plateau that represents ~100% occupancy or saturation.

Quantification of the time course of receptor occupancy is typically performed under conditions in which there is a vast amount of ligand relative to the amount of receptor in the system. Under those conditions, receptor binding has an imperceptible effect on ligand concentration—there is no appreciable depletion of ligand. Thus ligand concentration is "constant," and the reaction is termed *pseudo–first order,* reflecting its dependence only on the change of free receptors in the system, at that specific ligand concentration. Indeed, these reactions can be expressed graphically as the rate of formation of occupied receptors, or loss of free receptors over time (Fig. 5-14). Here, loss of free receptors is calculated by subtracting the number of receptors occupied at a particular time from the maximum number of receptors that can be occupied at equilibrium at that specific ligand concentration ([Be – B]). Note that this curve decreases in an exponential fashion and, as for dissociation reactions, transformation to a semi-log coordinate system yields a linear association plot (see Fig. 5-14). However, unlike dissociation reactions, association reactions performed with increasing concentrations of ligand yield plots with increasing slopes, reflecting the second-order nature of these reactions.

Quantification of Association

The slope of the semi-log plot of association is a measure of the rate of formation of product ([B]) or disappearance of reactant ([Be – B]). It is linear because, at a fixed concentration of ligand, the rate of formation of ligand-receptor complexes is dependent upon the amount of free receptors remaining in the reaction. Therefore, this reaction is pseudo–first order. Unlike dissociation reactions, the slope here is *not* equivalent to the *association rate constant.* That is because the true association rate constant is independent of the ligand concentration, yet, as shown earlier, the rate of association in the system being examined is dependent upon the ligand concentration. Indeed, binding at three different ligand concentrations results in semi-log plots with three different slopes. In addition, the rate of product formation in this system does not only reflect association. Indeed, as the reaction progresses and product accumulates, there will be a measurable amount of *dissociation,* which will influence the amount of product formed. Thus the slope of the semi-log plot of association is the $k_{observed}$, with units of min^{-1}. The relationship of this constant to the association rate constant is

$$k_{observed} = [L]k_{association} + k_{dissociation} \qquad \text{Eq. 5-1H}$$

This is the equation describing the hybrid rate of association. It takes into consideration both the forward and backward reaction rates. Also, it takes into consideration the dependence of the measured association reaction on the ligand concentration, reflecting the fact that association is a second-order phenomenon. While three components of this equation can be experimentally quantified (k_{obs}, [L], and k_{diss}), k_{assoc} is calculated.

Example of Calculating $k_{association}$. Receptor studies demonstrate a $k_{obs} = 2 \times 10^{-2}\ min^{-1}$ at an $[L] = 10^{-10}$ M and a $k_{diss} = 1 \times 10^{-2}\ min^{-1}$. Since $k_{obs} = [L]k_{assoc} + k_{diss}$, then $2 \times 10^{-2}\ min^{-1} = (10^{-10}\ M)(k_{assoc}) + 1 \times 10^{-2}\ min^{-1}$, and $k_{assoc} = 1 \times 10^{8}\ M^{-1}\ min^{-1}$. Note that the association rate constant is second order, with units that include concentration ($M^{-1}\ min^{-1}$).

Relationship of Kinetic and Equilibrium Receptor Occupancy[10,11]

Association and dissociation rate constants are measures of the affinity of ligands and their receptors. Thus, a high k_{assoc} reflects accelerated

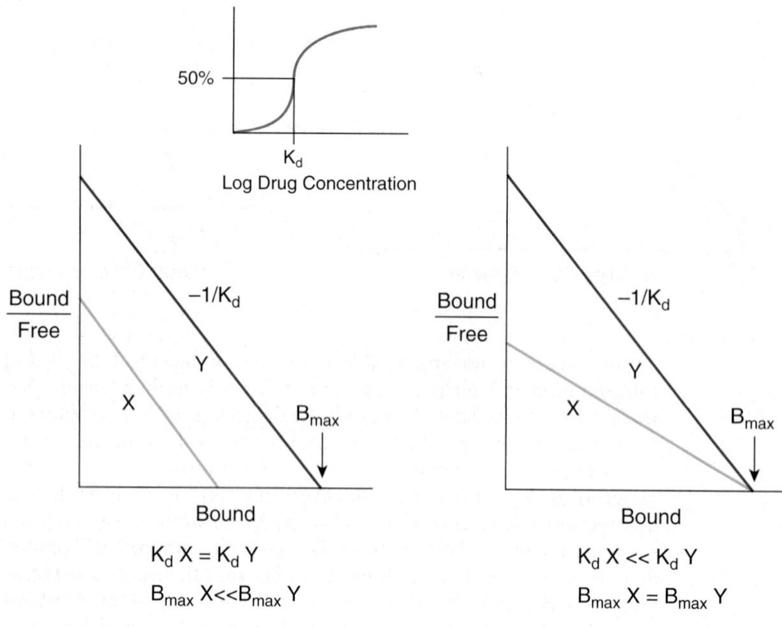

FIGURE 5-10 • Scatchard analyses of equilibrium ligand-receptor interactions. Receptor occupancy quantified at different ligand concentrations, typically employed to generate concentration-binding plots (**top**), are employed to calculate Bound/Free ligand (*Y* axis), which is plotted against Free ligand (*X* axis). Resulting plots have a characteristic slope that is $-1/K_d$, and an *X*-intercept of B_{max} or R_T. Ligands that have identical affinities for their receptors, but differ in their binding maxima, exhibit parallel slopes (**bottom left**). Ligands that have different affinities for their receptors, but identical binding maxima, diverge from a common *X*-axis intercept (**bottom right**). In the latter example, ligand Y has a greater affinity for its receptors compared to ligand X, reflected by a steeper slope due to a lower K_d.

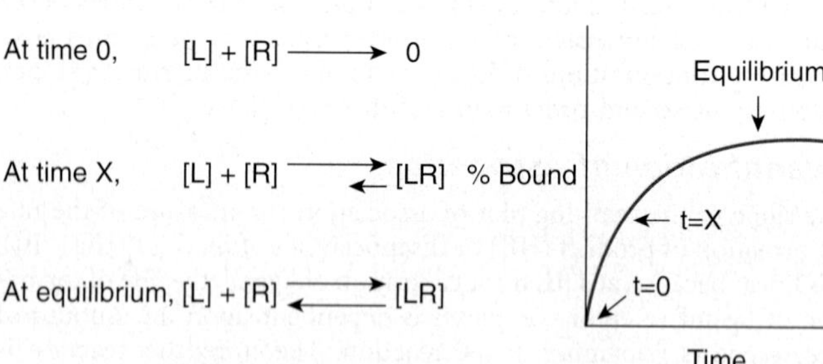

FIGURE 5-11 • Time dependence of ligand-receptor interactions. Receptor occupancy by ligand is a time-dependent phenomenon that obeys the Laws of Mass Action. At time zero, all ligand ([L]) and receptor ([R]) molecules are free and the association reaction is dominant, reflecting the maximum concentrations of the two reactants. As the reaction progresses (time X), the concentrations of ligand and receptors are reduced, reflecting the formation of product, ligand-receptor complexes ([LR]). The association reaction slows, reflecting reduced concentrations of reactants. In addition, there is a rate of dissociation, reflecting the accumulation of liganded receptors that drive the reverse reaction. A time is reached when the rates of association and dissociation are identical, a point at which there are no further changes in [L], [R], or [LR], which represents equilibrium.

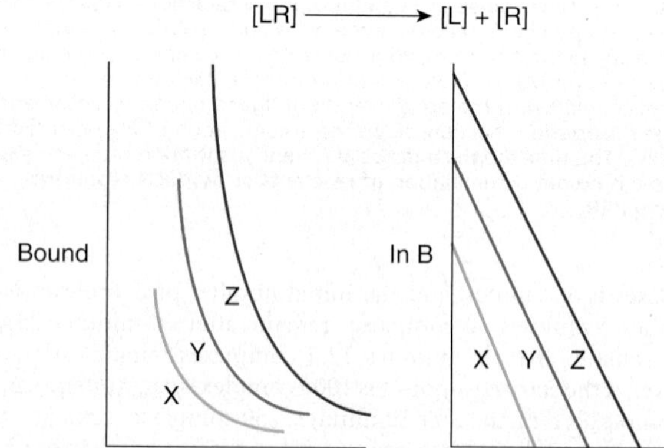

FIGURE 5-12 • Ligand-receptor dissociation. Ligand-receptor complex dissociation (**top**) is a first-order phenomenon, dependent only on the concentration of the complex. The time course of dissociation progresses with a constant rate of fractional loss directly proportional to the first-order dissociation rate constant, which has units of min^{-1}. This produces curvilinear isotherms of loss of bound receptors from the system over time (**bottom left**), which linearize upon log transformation (**bottom right**). The slopes of the log-linear plots represent $-d_{issociation}$, and a family of parallel isotherms represent dissociation reactions initiated with different concentrations of ligand-receptor complexes, all with identical dissociation rate constants.

formation of bound receptor, while a low k_{diss} reflects poor dissociation of bound receptor, both suggesting high affinity. Conversely, a low k_{assoc} reflects poor formation of bound receptor, while a high k_{diss} reflects rapid dissociation of ligand-receptor complexes, suggesting low affinity. These kinetic constants are related to the equilibrium measure of affinity (K_d) as follows:

$$KD = \frac{k_{diss}}{k_{assoc}} \quad \text{Eq. 5-1I}$$

Example of Comparing Equilibrium and Kinetic Determinations of Affinity. For receptors with $K_d = 10^{-9}$ M, $k_{assoc} = 1 \times 10^7\ M^{-1}\ min^{-1}$, and $k_{dissoc} = 1 \times 10^{-2}\ min^{-1}$, comparing kinetic and equilibrium affinity constants: $K_d = (1 \times 10^{-2})/(1 \times 10^7) = 10^{-9}$ M. Thus $K_{d\ (equilibrium)} = K_{d\ (kinetic)}$.

Quantification of Receptor Occupancy Over Time[10,11]

The number of receptors occupied is directly related to the effect produced, both the desired therapeutic effects and adverse, undesired effects. We have learned how to determine the proportion or number of receptors occupied at a given ligand concentration at equilibrium. However, we are rarely under equilibrium conditions when considering therapeutics, unless there is a constant intravenous infusion of drug and the serum concentration is at steady state. Rather, it is more often the case that ligand-receptor interactions are occurring under nonequilibrium conditions. How are the *number or proportion of receptors occupied* estimated when conditions are not at equilibrium? This is determined by the relationship demonstrated earlier for the observed rate of formation of ligand-receptor complexes. As described, this is an exponential phenomenon, which considers both the forward and reverse reactions and the ligand concentration and time at which the observation is made. Thus, the number of receptors bound or the proportion of total receptors bound at time *t* is

$$\text{Bound} = B_{equilibrium}(1 - e^{-k_{obs}t})$$

$$\text{Fractional occupancy} = \frac{\text{Bound}}{B_{max}} = \frac{B_{equilibrium}(1 - e^{-k_{obs}t})}{B_{max}} \quad \text{Eq. 5-1J}$$

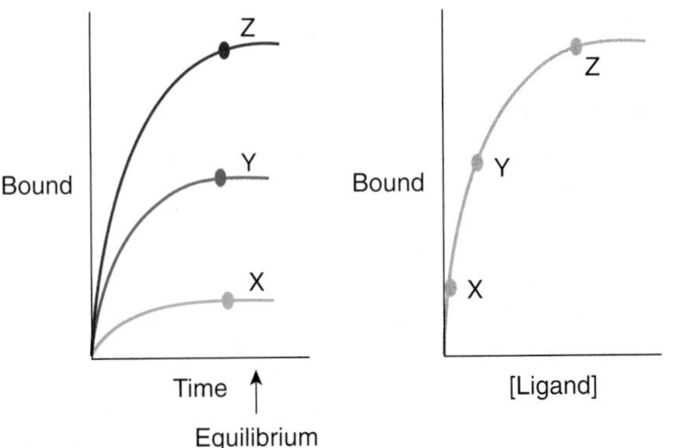

FIGURE 5-13 • Time course of association of ligands and receptors. The association reaction is bimolecular, dependent on the concentration of free ligands and receptors, and as such is a second-order reaction. Since ligand is typically in vast excess of receptors, binding does not influence ligand concentrations and, consequently, these reactions are pseudo–first order with respect to the concentration of receptors. Moreover, the observed association rate actually reflects the integration of forward and reverse reactions. Each initial concentration of ligand establishes a specific association time course, with a rate proportional to the ligand concentration and a plateau, representing equilibrium specific for that ligand concentration (**left**). Concentrations of ligand that are below K_d (*X*) result in a slower time course of association that reaches equilibrium at receptor occupancies below 50%. If this reaction is initiated with the K_d concentration of ligand (*Y*), then the association rate is faster, and at equilibrium 50% of receptors are occupied. If the reaction is initiated with a concentration of ligand in excess of the K_d, then the association rate is maximal and at equilibrium all available receptors are saturated (B_{max}). It is important to recognize here that the plateau regions of the time courses for association reactions represent equilibrium, when receptor occupancy becomes independent of time, and those plateaus represent discreet points along the concentration-binding curve (**right**).

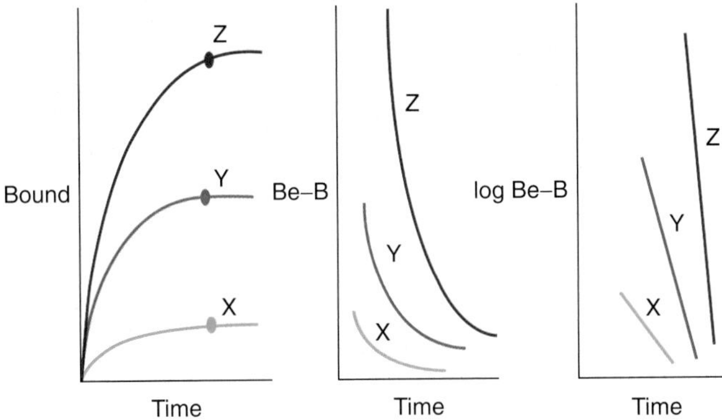

FIGURE 5-14 • Observed association rate. The time course of ligand-receptor formation at three different concentrations of ligand carried to equilibrium (**left**). Association can be quantified as loss of free receptors from the system (Be – B), where Be is the receptor occupancy at equilibrium at the specific ligand concentration and B represents the fraction of receptors bound at the specific time point. Association at different ligand concentrations produces individual plots of loss of free receptors (**middle**), which upon log transformation produce linear plots with differing slopes (**right**), reflecting the concentration dependence and second-order nature of the reaction. Moreover, association is a hybrid reaction, which integrates contributions from both forward and reverse reactions. Thus, the slopes of the log-linear plots represent the observed pseudo–first order concentration-specific association rate constant (k_{obs}), rather than the true second-order rate constant (k_{assoc}).

$B_{equilibrium}$ is calculated using the equilibrium binding equation. B_{max} is determined by equilibrium binding analysis employing the method of Scatchard.

Example of Calculating Receptor Occupancy under Nonequilibrium Conditions. Atrial natriuretic peptides (ANPs) are hormones that bind to a receptor, guanylyl cyclase A (GCA), and stimulate downstream signaling events in cells that produce an increase in cyclic GMP. The K_d for ANP and GCA is 10^{-9} M. However, induction of cyclic GMP accumulation in cells, measured over 15 minutes, exhibits a concentration-response relationship in which the concentration of ANP producing a half-maximum cyclic GMP response is 10^{-8} M. Why is the concentration producing a half-maximum response 10 times higher than the concentration producing 50% receptor occupancy? For this example, B_{max} = 1000 receptor sites, and $k_{obs} = 5 \times 10^{-2}$ min^{-1} at a ligand concentration of 10^{-9} M.

The answer is that equilibrium for ligand-receptor interaction is reached after ~120 minutes, while cyclic GMP accumulation is only measured at 15 minutes, which is insufficient time to permit 50% receptor occupancy at K_d. Indeed, a concentration of ligand that is 10 times higher than K_d is required in order to produce 50% receptor occupancy and cyclic GMP responses in 15 minutes. This principle can be demonstrated by the following calculation:

$$\text{At equilibrium, B} = [(10^{-8}\text{ M})(1000)]/(10^{-9}\text{ M}) + (10^{-8}\text{ M}) = 909\text{ sites}$$
$$\text{Fractional occupancy} = (909)(1 - e^{(-0.05)(15\text{ min})})/(1000)$$
$$= 48\%\text{ of the sites occupied}$$

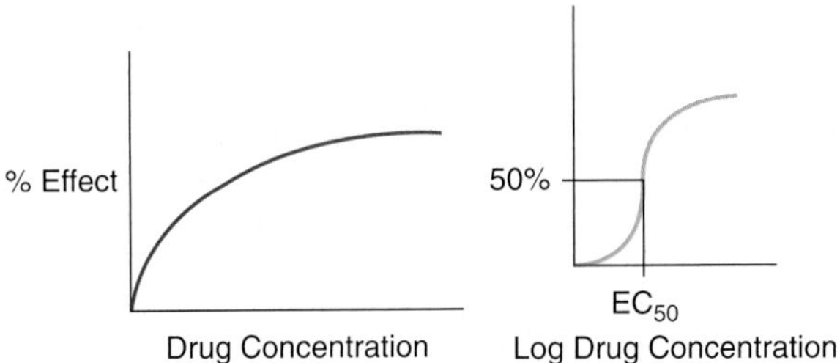

FIGURE 5-15 • Concentration dependence of drug responses. The concentration dependence of drug responses in part reflects occupancy of cognate receptors. Thus the concentration-response relationship exhibits characteristics that are analogous to ligand-receptor interactions. Indeed, drug responses are concentration dependent, graded, and saturable (E_{max}), reflecting the occupancy of all available receptors. These relationships can be portrayed as a Michaelis-Menten plot (**right**) or as a log-linear plot (**left**). The concentration of drug producing a half-maximum response is the EC_{50}.

BEYOND LIGAND-RECEPTOR INTERACTIONS: THERAPEUTICS AND THE DOSE-RESPONSE RELATIONSHIP

The quantitative and qualitative relationships concerning the behavior of receptors with respect to the concentration of ligand and time are the principles that underlie the behavior of drugs in humans. Certainly, the situation is more complex in a whole organism than in a test tube under ideal conditions. Nevertheless, the relationships developed previously directly pertain to the behavior of drugs in the whole organism. Recall that the effects of drugs are directly related to the occupancy of receptors. Therefore, at equilibrium, the intensity of the effects of a drug can be graphically represented as in Figure 5-15.

Here, the concentration of drug producing 50% of the maximum response is the EC_{50}, analogous to the K_d. Moreover, the maximum response produced at saturation by occupancy of 100% of the receptors (B_{max}) is E_{max}. By analogy with the concentration-binding relationship, the intensity of the effects of a drug can be quantified as:

$$\text{Intensity of effect} = \frac{[\text{Drug}][E_{max}]}{EC_{50} + [\text{Drug}]} \qquad \text{Eq. 5-1J}$$

This is the E_{max} *model* relating drug concentration to pharmacologic effect and has all the classical attributes of the ligand-receptor model, including being concentration or dose dependent, graded, and saturable. A detailed discussion of E_{max} models relating drug concentration and effects is provided in Chapter 14 (Pharmacodynamics).

Characteristics of the Concentration-Response Relationship of Drugs

$$L + R \rightarrow LR \rightarrow \text{Effector mechanisms} \rightarrow \text{Response}$$

The effects produced by a drug are dependent upon its ability to *bind* to the receptor and *activate effector mechanisms.* As discussed earlier for the general category of ligand-receptor interactions, the structural domains of the drug and receptor that mediate the induction of effector mechanisms can be separate and different from those mediating binding (again, the importance of structure to activity). Thus, one could conceive of drugs that bind well to their receptors but activate effector mechanisms poorly or not at all. This ability of a drug bound to its receptor to differentially activate downstream effector mechanisms reflects the *intrinsic activity* of the drug. Intrinsic activity reflects the property of a drug that determines the amount of biologic effect produced per unit of drug-receptor complex formed. Two agents combining with equivalent sets of receptors may not produce equal degrees of effect even if both agents are given in maximally effective doses; the agents differ in their intrinsic activities and the one producing the greater maximum effect has the greater intrinsic activity. As an example, meperidine and morphine combine with opiate receptors to produce analgesia, but, regardless of dose, the maximum degree of analgesia produced by morphine is greater than that produced by meperidine; morphine has the greater intrinsic activity. Like affinity, intrinsic activity depends on the physicochemical characteristics of both the drug and the receptor, but intrinsic activity and affinity can vary independently with changes in the drug molecule.

The relationship of drug concentration and biologic effect has characteristics of importance in addition to those described earlier for ligand-receptor interactions (Fig. 5-16). *Potency* refers to the concentrations of ligand required to yield an effect. Ligands with greater potency are required in lower concentrations to produce the same effects as those with lesser potency. This characteristic is related to the affinity of the ligand for binding to its receptor. *Efficacy* refers to the quantitative ability of a drug to produce a biologic effect. Drugs with greater efficacy produce greater biologic effects than those with lesser efficacy binding to the same receptor. This characteristic is related to the intrinsic activity of a drug and its ability to activate effector mechanisms once bound to the receptor. It is noteworthy that potency and efficacy are independent parameters, and drugs may be maximally efficacious but exhibit low potency.

Taking these concepts together, the ability of a drug to produce an effect can be defined using the E_{max} model as

$$\text{Intensity of effect} = \frac{(e)[\text{Drug}][\text{E}_{max}]}{\text{EC}_{50} + [\text{Drug}]} \qquad \text{Eq. 5-1K}$$

where the term *e* has been incorporated to reflect the intrinsic activity of the drug bound to the receptor. In this enhanced model of drug action, the ability of a drug to produce a physiologic effect is dependent on receptor occupancy, reflecting [Drug] and K_d, and the intrinsic ability of that drug to activate receptors once bound (*e*).

Receptor Dynamics and the Concentration-Response Relationship

To this point, the relationship between receptor occupancy and response has been considered simply: one ligand molecule occupies one receptor, which produces a response proportional to the total number of receptors occupied. In that model, 50% occupancy of receptors produces 50% of the maximum response. However, in reality the concentration-response relationship is rarely that straightforward. Rather, the response elicited by a ligand at a given concentration reflects receptor dynamics and the complex coupling characteristics of receptors to their downstream effectors.

Receptor Dynamics

Cells have the ability to respond to their environment by dynamically regulating the number of available receptors to ligands. For example, in heart failure, which is associated with a hyperadrenergic state to maintain cardiac output, cardiomyocytes dynamically respond to overstimulation by adrenergic ligands by down-regulating their β-adrenergic receptors.[13] Down-regulation reflects molecular mechanisms mediating receptor desensitization and internalization[14] (Fig. 5-17). Receptor desensitization is mediated by phosphorylation of ligand-stimulated receptors by β-adrenergic receptor kinase, one member of the family of G protein–coupled receptor kinases. Phosphorylation of β-adrenergic receptors induces binding of β-arrestin to phosphorylated residues, blocking the ability of these receptors to productively interact with and activate heterotrimeric G proteins, essentially rendering these receptors inactive (desensitized). Moreover, binding of β-arrestin triggers endocytosis and sequestration of phosphorylated receptors, removing them from the cell surface, rendering them inaccessible. The net result of this dynamic regulation is a reduction in the number of receptors available to interact with adrenergic agonists on each cardiomyocyte. Down-regulation decreases the maximum response produced by adrenergic ligands in those cells, reflecting the reduction in "responding units," rendering cells relatively insensitive to adrenergic stimulation (see Fig. 5-17). Clinically, these effects of β-adrenergic receptor desensitization, which interfere with the positive inotropic effects of endogenous catecholamines which can be beneficial in heart failure, is reversed by treating patients with antagonists of β-adrenergic receptors, which block their desensitization by endogenous ligands.[15]

Conversely, cells can dynamically upregulate their complement of specific receptors to increase their sensitivity to ligands. Here, cells create *spare receptors,* wherein only a fraction of the available receptors require engagement to provide a maximum response.[16] Spare receptors shift the apparent potency of ligand without altering maximum efficacy (Fig. 5-18). As an illustration (Fig. 5-19), if 100 receptors are required to maximally engage downstream effectors, then ligand concentrations at the K_d will produce 50% of the maximum effect by occupying 50 receptors. However, if the cell produces 400 spare receptors, so that there are now 500 available receptors for occupancy, then ligand concentrations that are 10-fold lower than K_d will occupy 50 receptors and produce a 50% maximum response, a gain in sensitivity of 10-fold. Further, if the cell produces 4900 spare receptors, so that there are now 5000 available receptors for occupancy, then ligand concentrations that are ~1/100 of the K_d will occupy 50 receptors and produce a 50% maximum response, a gain in sensitivity of 100-fold. These considerations underscore the concept that cells are not passive recipients of signals carried by ligands. Rather, they are dynamic units reacting to their environments to shape their sensitivity and responses to external signals.

In the context of these additional concepts, the model describing the ability of a drug to produce an effect can be further refined:

$$\text{Intensity of effect} = \frac{(f)(e)[\text{Drug}][\text{E}_{max}]}{\text{EC}_{50} + [\text{Drug}]} \qquad \text{Eq. 5-1L}$$

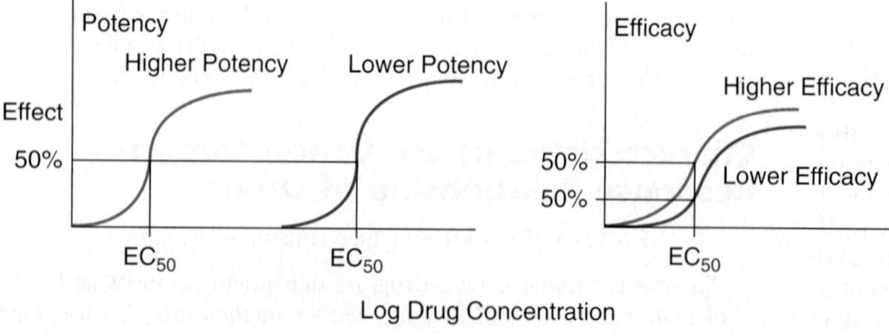

FIGURE 5-16 • Potency and efficacy. Drugs induce their responses in a concentration dependent, graded, and saturable fashion. Potency refers to the concentrations of ligand required to yield an effect. Ligands with greater potency are required in lower concentrations to produce the same effects as those with lesser potency. This characteristic is related to the affinity of the ligand for binding to its receptor. Efficacy refers to the quantitative ability of a drug to produce a biologic effect. Drugs with greater efficacy produce greater biologic effects than those with lesser efficacy binding to the same receptor. This characteristic is related to the intrinsic activity of a drug and its ability to activate effector mechanisms once bound to the receptor.

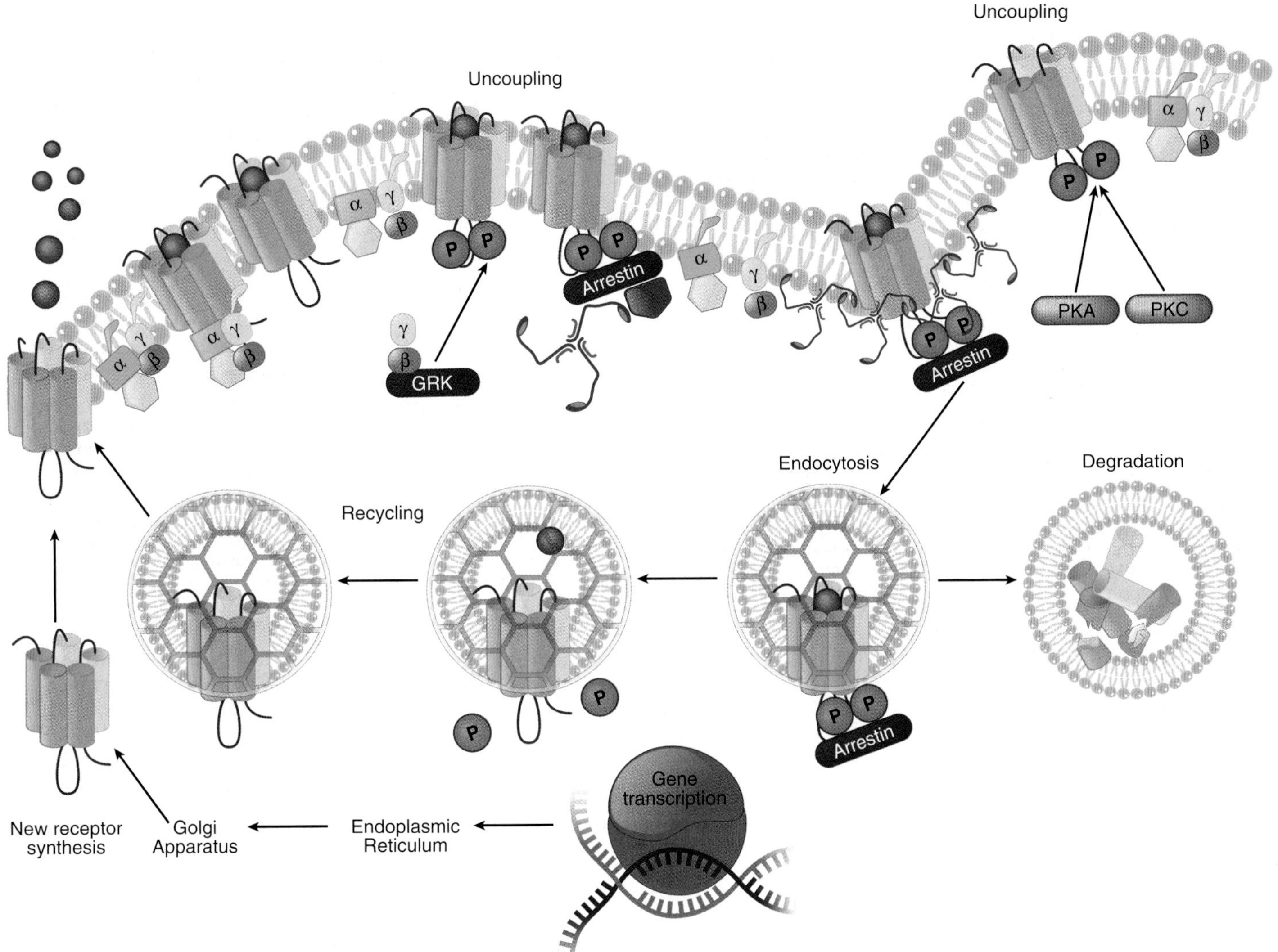

FIGURE 5-17 • G protein–coupled receptor dynamics. Regulation of G protein–coupled receptor signaling is effected by mechanisms that establish the number and responsiveness of receptors at the cell surface. Thus receptor uncoupling occurs as a result of G protein–coupled receptor kinase (GRK)–mediated phosphorylation of agonist-occupied receptor, which promotes arrestin binding to phosphorylated receptor, inhibiting receptor–G protein interactions. Arrestin binding to receptor also initiates internalization of receptors into clathrin-coated pits, after which receptors can traffic to lysosomes for degradation or be dephosphorylated and recycled back to the plasma membrane. (From Billington CK, Penn RB. Signaling and regulation of G protein-coupled receptors in airway smooth muscle. Respir Res 2003;4:2.)

where the term f has been incorporated to reflect amplification of potency from spare receptors.

Receptor-Effector Coupling and Shape Factor

Beyond the number of functional receptors available, ligand responses reflect the summation of multiple serial and parallel biochemical reactions that are triggered by ligand-receptor interactions across many tissues in the whole organism. In a responding system that has a linear relationship between occupancy and physiologic response, there is a direct proportionality between the degree of receptor activation and the generation of second messengers. This can be conceptualized as a small amount of receptor occupancy producing a small increase in the level of the second messenger inducing a small increase in physiologic response. In actuality, a small degree of receptor occupancy generates large increases in second messenger levels that, in turn, generate even larger physiologic responses. Signals are amplified at every step, transforming modest receptor occupancy into magnified physiologic response. Because the overall response is a summation and integration of these amplified reactions, the shape of the concentration-response curve may vary, reflecting deviation from linear receptor occupancy models of effect to nonlinear receptor-effector models.

The parts of a concentration-response curve include the initial linear phase, the 20% to 80% log-linear phase, and the plateau phase (Fig. 5-20). In the initial phase, there is linear increase in the response as the concentration of drug increases. In the log-linear phase, which comprises the middle 20% to 80%, there is a direct relationship between the log of the drug concentration and effect. In the plateau phase, there is little change in effect with large changes in drug concentration, reflecting the saturation of receptors in the system. Typically, the midphase 20% to 80% of the concentration-response curve is linear over a 16-fold range in concentration.

However, the integrated response to a drug may be "more rapid" so that responses exhibit larger increases per change in drug concentration (higher shape factor) (Fig. 5-21). Alternatively, responses may be "slower" so that responses exhibit smaller increases per change in drug concentration (smaller shape factor).

Most drugs have a shape factor between 1 and 3. When the shape factor (γ) = 1, then the semi-log relationship is linear from 20% to 80% over a 16-fold range of concentrations. When γ = 2, then the semi-log

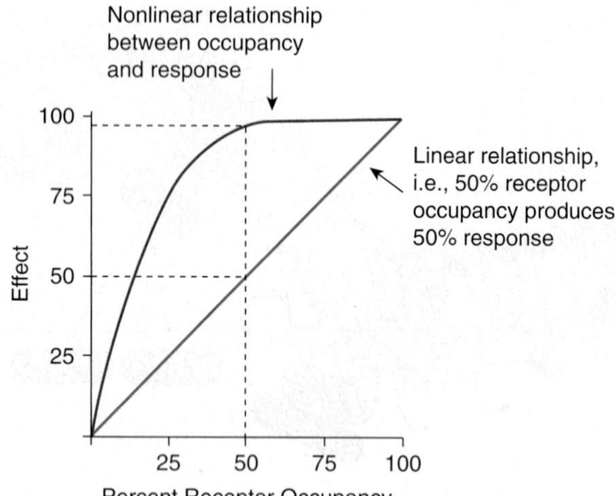

FIGURE 5-18 • Spare receptors. In most systems, the relationship between receptor occupancy and response is not linear but some function of receptor occupancy. This function is represented as hyperbolic curve, demonstrating that only a fraction, here 50%, of receptors require occupancy to produce a maximum response. This hyperbolic relationship between occupancy and response suggests that a fraction of receptors are "spare," in excess of those required for a full response.

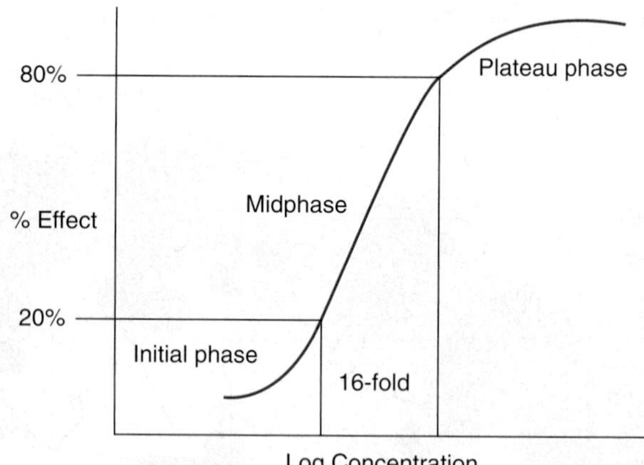

FIGURE 5-20 • Concentration-response curve. The parts of a concentration-response curve include the initial linear phase, the 20% to 80% log-linear phase, and the plateau phase. In the initial phase, there is linear increase in the response as the concentration of drug increases. In the log-linear phase, which comprises the middle 20% to 80%, there is a direct relationship between the log of the drug concentration and effect. In the plateau phase, there is little change in effect with large changes in drug concentration, reflecting the saturation of receptors in the system. Typically, the midphase 20% to 80% of the concentration-response curve is linear over a 16-fold range in concentration.

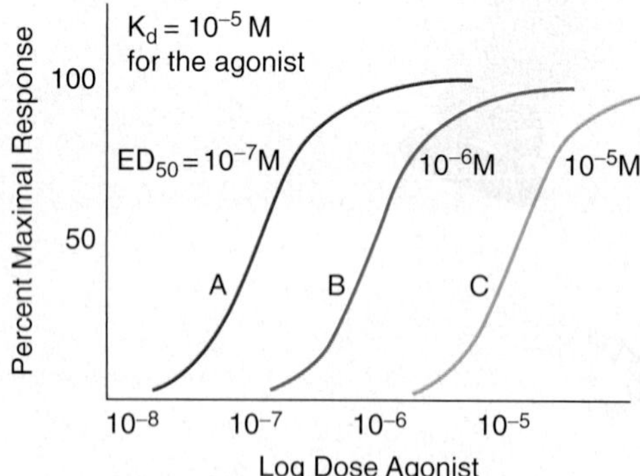

FIGURE 5-19 • Impact of spare receptors on the dose-response relationship. A, A one-to-one correspondence between receptor occupancy and the response indicates that there are few spare receptors. **B,** A 5-fold increase in the number of receptors in the system produces a 10-fold enhancement in the dose response. **C,** A 50-fold increase in receptors produces a 100-fold enhancement in the dose response. ED_{50}, dose of agonist producing 50% of the maximum responses.

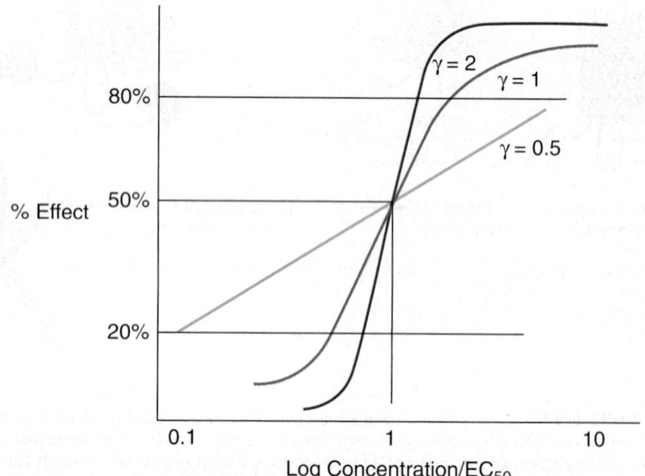

FIGURE 5-21 • Shape factor. Integrated response to a drug may be "rapid," reflecting high-amplification receptor-effector coupling, producing responses that exhibit large increases per change in drug concentration (higher shape factor). Alternatively, responses may be "slower," reflecting inefficient receptor-effector coupling or low amplification of downstream signals, producing responses that exhibit smaller increases per change in drug concentration (lower shape factor).

relationship is linear from 20% to 80% over a 4-fold range of concentrations. When $\gamma = 0.5$, then the semi-log relationship is linear from 20% to 80% over a 256-fold range of concentrations. Thus the relationship between drug concentration and effect becomes:

$$\text{Intensity of effect} = \frac{(f)(e)[\text{Drug}]^{\gamma}[\text{E}_{max}]}{\text{EC}_{50}{}^{\gamma} + [\text{Drug}]^{\gamma}} \qquad \text{Eq. 5-1M}$$

The impact of the shape factor on drug responses can be exemplified by considering a drug with an EC_{50} of 10^{-9} M. When $\gamma = 1$, then when [Drug] = 10^{-9} M, the percent of E_{max} = 50%; when [Drug] = 10^{-10} M, the percent of E_{max} = 9.1%; and when [Drug] = 10^{-8} M, the percent of E_{max} = 91%. However, when $\gamma = 2$, then when [Drug] = 10^{-9} M, the percent of E_{max} = 50%; when [Drug] = 10^{-10} M, the percent of E_{max} = 1%; and when [Drug] = 10^{-8} M, the percent of E_{max} = 99%.

Relationship Between Intensity and Time Course of Drug Effects

Again, the intensity of effect at any given moment reflects the number of receptors occupied, which is a function of the concentration of drug to which those receptors are exposed and the time of exposure. However, the concentration of drug in the serum is a function of a variety of pharmacokinetic mechanisms, including absorption, distribution, metabolism, and excretion. Typically, after peak concentrations of drug are achieved, the concentration of drug in the serum declines with a classic exponential time course.

As discussed previously, this decline is typical of a first-order phenomenon, the drug decreasing in the serum at a constant fraction per unit time. The semi-log plot of this phenomenon yields a linear plot with a slope that is the *elimination rate constant* (K_{elim}) (Fig. 5-22). The elimination rate constant is related to the half-life of the drug by the relationship:

$$K_{elim} = 0.693/t_{1/2}$$

Thus the time course of the intensity of the effect of a drug will depend upon the rate of decline of drug in the system (K_{elim}; $t_{1/2}$) and the binding characteristics of the drug and receptor (Fig. 5-23). If the drug

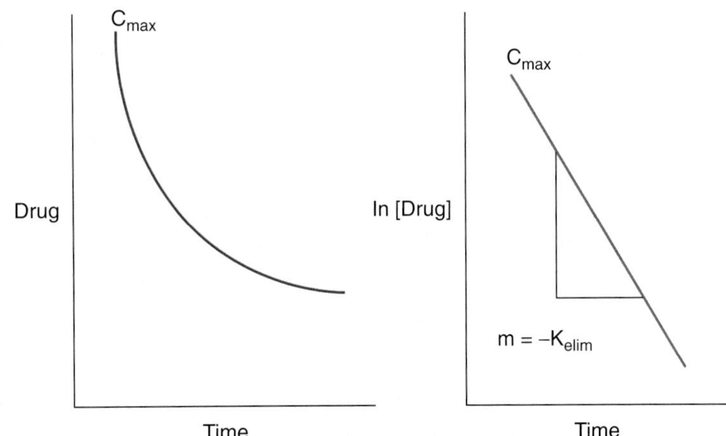

FIGURE 5-22 • Time course of drug elimination from the circulation. The concentration of drug in the serum reflects pharmacokinetic mechanisms including absorption, distribution, metabolism, and excretion. After peak concentrations of drug are achieved, the concentration of drug in the serum declines with an exponential time course (**left**): This decline is first-order and the drug decreases in the serum at a constant fraction per unit time. The semi-log plot of this phenomenon (**right**) yields a linear plot with a slope that is the elimination rate constant (K_{elim}).

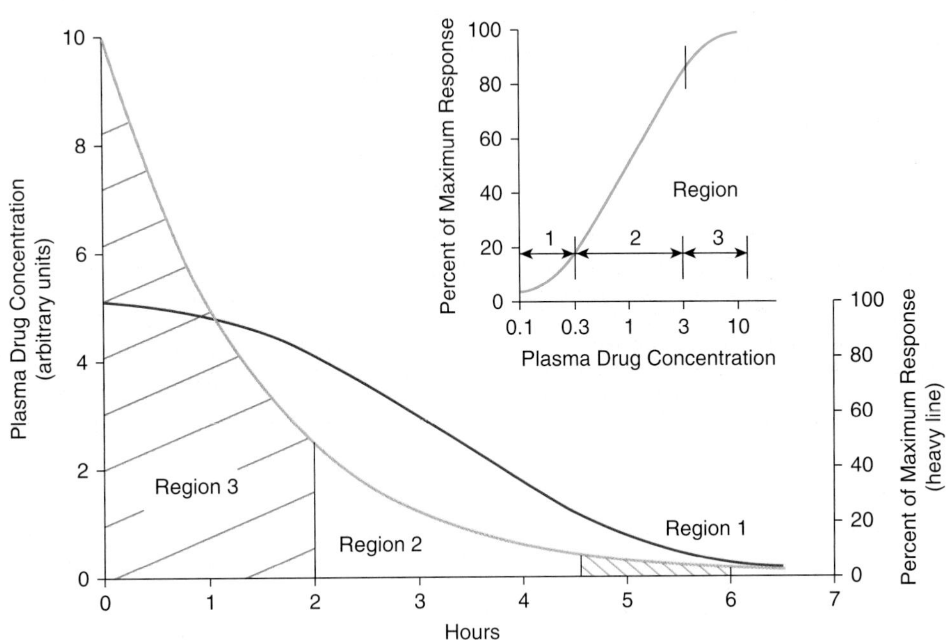

FIGURE 5-23 • Intensity and the time course of drug effects. The decline in intensity of pharmacologic effect with time after a single large dose has three parts corresponding to the regions of the concentration response curve. First, in region 3, the response remains almost maximal despite a 75% decrease in drug concentration, reflecting saturation of receptors at those concentrations and the zero-order character of the phenomenon. In region 2, the intensity of the response declines linearly with time, reflecting the log-linear decline of drug in the serum with time and the log-linear relationship of responses and drug concentration in this region. In region 1, responses parallel the decline of drug in the serum, reflecting the linear relationship between drug concentration and responses at these drug concentrations.

concentration is in region 3 (see Fig. 5-23), then receptors are saturated, and large changes in drug concentration will have minimal effects on the intensity of the effect. If the drug concentration is in region 2, then the intensity of the effect is proportional to the log of the drug concentration. If the drug concentration is in region 1, then the intensity of the effect is directly proportional to the drug concentration. A detailed discussion of the relationship between time, drug concentration, and responses is presented in Chapter 14 (Pharmacodynamics).

AGONISTS AND ANTAGONISTS[17-19]

Agonists occupy receptors and activate downstream effector mechanisms, producing a response. Conventional agonists increase the proportion of activated receptors while inverse agonists stabilize receptors in an inactive conformation and act similarly to competitive antagonists. Agonists can be classified as full or partial. Full agonists (e.g., epinephrine) produce a maximum biologic response and are maximally efficacious, independent of potency. Partial agonists (exemplified by opiate agonists, including pentazocine) produce less than 100% of the maximum biologic response, even at maximum receptor occupancy. *Antagonists* occupy receptors without activating downstream effector mechanisms, reflecting an absence of intrinsic activity. Antagonists can be classified as reversible or irreversible. Reversible antagonists, exemplified by antihistamines, readily dissociate from their receptor, while irreversible antagonists, such as phenoxybenzamine, form a stable covalent bond with their receptor. In competitive (reversible) antagonism, binding of the antagonist prevents binding of the agonist to receptors. In noncompetitive (irreversible) antagonism, agonist and antagonist can bind to receptors simultaneously, but antagonist binding reduces or prevents the action of the agonist. In competitive antagonism, a steady state forms among agonist, antagonist, and receptor that can be overcome (competed) by increasing the concentration of the agonist. In contrast, the covalent modification characterizing noncompetitive antagonists permanently inactivates receptors, removing them from the complement available to respond.

Agonists and antagonists produce characteristic quantitative alterations in the dose-response relationship that are diagnostic (Fig. 5-24). Agonists produce a response in the system characterized by an EC_{50} and full (E_{max}) or partial efficacy. Antagonists themselves do not produce a response; rather, their effects are revealed in the presence of agonists. Competitive antagonists shift the dose response to agonists to the right, characteristic of an apparent decrease in potency reflecting the reversibility of antagonism, without a change in efficacy. In contrast, noncompetitive antagonists covalently modify receptors and are irreversible, resulting in a loss of receptor units from the system, producing a decrease in maximum efficacy of agonists. However, the

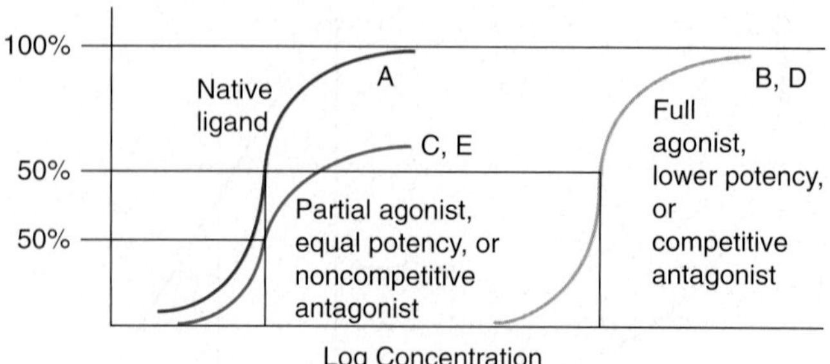

FIGURE 5-24 • Agonists and antagonists.

remaining receptor units possess the same affinity for drug, and agonist potency is characteristically unaffected by noncompetitive antagonists.

To illustrate these relationships, epinephrine is an adrenergic agonist, producing an increase in heart rate when β-adrenergic receptors in the heart are occupied. In an experimental model (animal, human), epinephrine can be infused intravenously to produce an increase in heart rate (see Fig. 5-24A). If increasing doses of epinephrine are infused sequentially, there is a dose-dependent and graded increase in heart rate to a maximum response (E_{max}), producing an EC_{50} characteristic for this drug. The structure of epinephrine can be modified to create new experimental agents that occupy the β-adrenergic receptor. One of these new agents produces an increase in heart rate to the E_{max} when infused into the model in a dose-dependent and graded fashion, although it exhibits an EC_{50} that is substantially higher than epinephrine (see Fig. 5-24B). Indeed, this is a full agonist with lower potency for β-adrenergic receptors compared to epinephrine. Another modified compound also produces a dose-dependent and graded increase in heart rate, with an EC_{50} that is comparable to epinephrine, but only ~75% of the E_{max} of epinephrine (see Fig. 5-24C). This compound is a partial agonist for the β-adrenergic receptor. A third compound produces no change in heart rate when infused into the model and is devoid of agonist activity. However, when the model first receives a dose of this new compound, followed by increasing doses of epinephrine, the new compound produces an apparent shift to the right of the epinephrine dose-response curve (see Fig. 5-24D). Here, it appears that the presence of the new agent increased the EC_{50} of epinephrine, decreasing its potency, without a change in E_{max}. These are the hallmark characteristics of a competitive antagonist. Finally, a new compound is created that also is devoid of agonist activity when infused into the model. However, when the model first receives a dose of this new compound, followed by increasing doses of epinephrine, the new compound produces a decrease in the maximum efficacy, without altering the EC_{50} of epinephrine, characteristic of a noncompetitive antagonist (see Fig. 5-24E).

POPULATION RESPONSES TO DRUGS AND INTERINDIVIDUAL VARIABILITY[20]

The ability to respond to a drug is influenced by genetic and environmental factors that create response variability among individuals in a population. Baseline receptor density and the efficiency of stimulus-response coupling mechanisms, which reflect genetic diversity, vary between individuals. Moreover, drugs, aging, mutations, and disease can increase (upregulate) or decrease (down-regulate) the number and binding affinity of receptors and/or their downstream effector mechanisms. For example, clonidine down-regulates α_2-adrenergic receptors, and rapid withdrawal can cause hypertensive crisis. Similarly, heart failure produces a chronic hyperadrenergic state resulting in tachyphylaxis and down-regulation of adrenergic receptors, producing resistance to the positive inotropic effects of catecholamines, which can benefit the failing heart.

In contrast to the previous discussion, which focused on drugs producing a graded effect in the individual, interindividual variability in

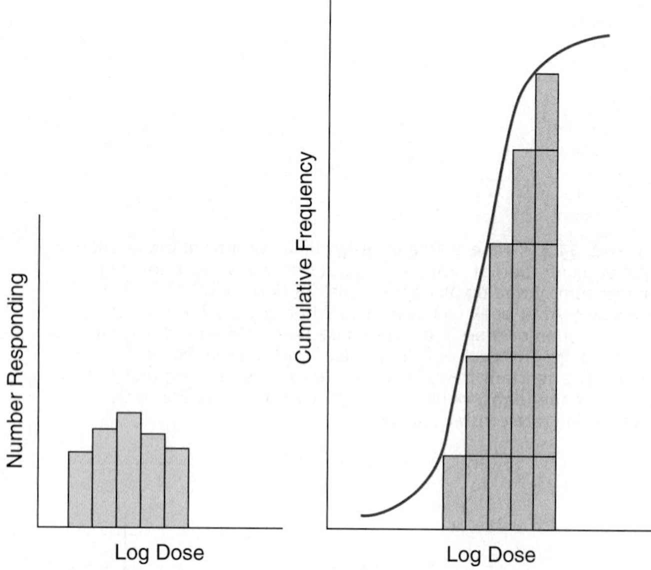

FIGURE 5-25 • Frequency (**left**) and cumulative frequency (**right**) distribution of drug responses in the population.

drug responsiveness across the population is measured as a quantal response. In this model, individuals are administered increasing concentrations of drug to elicit a fixed, predetermined quantal response. For example, returning to the earlier model, increasing doses of epinephrine could be infused into patients to determine the dose producing a 10-beat increase in heart rate. Here, there is no dose-dependent graded response. Generally, production of a response is normally distributed according to the log of the ligand concentration as a frequency distribution (Fig. 5-25). If these frequencies are summed at each concentration, a cumulative frequency distribution is produced. This cumulative frequency distribution expresses the pharmacodynamic variability in the population, rather than the concentration-dependent response to a ligand. Important therapeutic parameters derive from studies of ligand responses in populations and the resulting cumulative frequency distributions. The ED_{50} is the dose of drug producing the minimum response in 50% of the population. In contrast, the LD_{50} is the dose of drug producing death in 50% of the population (animal models). The LD_{50}/ED_{50} ratio is the *therapeutic index,* a measure of the safety of a therapeutic agent. Agents with a high therapeutic index, exemplified by the pencillins, exhibit a high margin of safety, since they produce a therapeutic effect at concentrations far below those producing lethal effects. In contrast, agents with a low therapeutic index, including digoxin and lithium, exhibit a narrow margin of safety, since the concentrations for therapeutic and lethal effects are closely overlapping.

REFERENCES

1. Chaurasia CS, Müller M, Bashaw ED, et al. AAPS-FDA Workshop White Paper: microdialysis principles, application and regulatory perspectives. Pharm Res 2007;24:1014-1025.
2. Chaurasia CS, Müller M, Bashaw ED, et al. AAPS-FDA Workshop White Paper: microdialysis principles, application, and regulatory perspectives. J Clin Pharmacol 2007;47:589-603.
3. Abdel-Rahman SM, Kauffman RE. The integration of pharmacokinetics and pharmacodynamics: understanding dose-response. Annu Rev Pharmacol Toxicol 2004;44:111-136.
4. Tata JR. Signalling through nuclear receptors. Nat Rev Mol Cell Biol 2002;3:702-710.
5. Kalgutkar AS, Crews BC, Rowlinson SW, et al. Aspirin-like molecules that covalently inactivate cyclooxygenase-2. Science 1998;280:1268-1270.
6. Abernethy DR, Schwartz JB. Calcium-antagonist drugs. N Engl J Med 1999;341:1447-1457.
7. Oldham WM, Hamm HE. Heterotrimeric G protein activation by G-protein-coupled receptors. Nat Rev Mol Cell Biol 2008;9:60-71.
8. Lucas KA, Pitari GM, Kazerounian S, et al. Guanylyl cyclases and signaling by cyclic GMP. Pharmacol Rev 2000;52:375-414.

9. Citri A, Yarden Y. EGF-ERBB signalling: towards the systems level. Nat Rev Mol Cell Biol 2006;7:505-516.
10. Molinoff PB, Wolfe BB, Weiland GA. Quantitative analysis of drug-receptor interactions: II. Determination of the properties of receptor subtypes. Life Sci 1981;29:427-443.
11. Weiland GA, Molinoff PB. Quantitative analysis of drug-receptor interactions: I. Determination of kinetic and equilibrium properties. Life Sci 1981;29:313-330.
12. van Zoelen EJ, Kramer RH, van Moerkerk HT, Veerkamp JH. The use of nonhomologous Scatchard analysis in the evaluation of ligand-protein interactions. Trends Pharmacol Sci 1998;19:487-490.
13. Feldman DS, Carnes CA, Abraham WT, Bristow MR. Mechanisms of disease: beta-adrenergic receptors—alterations in signal transduction and pharmacogenomics in heart failure. Nat Clin Pract Cardiovasc Med 2005;2:475-483.
14. Billington CK, Penn RB. Signaling and regulation of G protein-coupled receptors in airway smooth muscle. Respir Res 2003;4:2.
15. Foody JM, Farrell MH, Krumholz HM. β-Blocker therapy in heart failure: scientific review. JAMA 2002;287:883-889.
16. Homer LD, Nielsen TB. Spare receptors, partial agonists, and ternary complex model of drug action. Am J Physiol 1987;253:E114-E121.
17. Molinoff PB, Weiland GA, Heidenreich KA, et al. Interactions of agonists and antagonists with beta-adrenergic receptors. Adv Cyclic Nucleotide Res 1981;14:51-67.
18. Weiland GA, Minneman KP, Molinoff PB. Fundamental difference between the molecular interactions of agonists and antagonists with the beta-adrenergic receptor. Nature 1979;281:114-117.
19. Weiland GA, Minneman KP, Molinoff PB. Thermodynamics of agonist and antagonist interactions with mammalian beta-adrenergic receptors. Mol Pharmacol 1980;18:341-347.
20. Wilke RA, Reif DM, Moore JH. Combinatorial pharmacogenetics. Nat Rev Drug Discov 2005;4:911-918.

6

SIGNAL TRANSDUCTION

Philip B. Wedegaertner

INTRODUCTION 67
G PROTEIN–COUPLED RECEPTORS 68
HETEROTRIMERIC G PROTEINS 70
G PROTEIN EFFECTORS 71
ACs and cAMP 71
Phospholipase C 72
ENZYME-LINKED CELL-SURFACE RECEPTORS 73
PTK Receptors 73
PTP Receptors 75
Serine/Threonine Kinase Receptors 75
GC Receptors 75
OTHER CELL-SURFACE RECEPTOR SIGNALING PARADIGMS 76
Tyrosine Kinase–Associated Receptors 76
Cytokine Receptors and the Jak-STAT Pathway 76
Wnt/β-Catenin Signaling 76
Integrin Signaling 77
Ion Channels 77
NUCLEAR HORMONE RECEPTORS 78
INTRACELLULAR SIGNALING PATHWAYS 79
Ras Signaling 79
The Rho Family of Small GTPases 79
MAPK Signaling 79
Phosphatidylinositol 3-Kinase/Akt Signaling 80

INTRODUCTION

The term *signal transduction* refers to the cellular proteins and pathways through which a cell generates an output in response to the input of a ligand binding to a receptor. The typical signal transduction pathway is initiated by a small molecule binding to a receptor on the extracellular surface of a cell, although some receptors are located inside the cell. This ligand-receptor interaction promotes changes in the receptor that allow the receptor to interact with intracellular proteins or generate specific small molecules, or second messengers. These initial events propagate a "signal" that is conveyed through intracellular changes in protein-protein interactions, regulation of enzyme activity, and generation of new second messengers. Ligand binding to a receptor can initiate signal transduction, leading to rapid changes in cell function, such as regulation of ion flux, metabolism, and cell morphology; in addition, a signal transduction pathway often culminates in longer-term changes in gene expression.

Signaling by small molecule ligands can be considered in terms of the distances through which they act, and this is often referred to as *endocrine*, *paracrine*, or *autocrine signaling*. In endocrine signaling, hormones are generated in specialized endocrine cells; these ligands are then secreted into the bloodstream and transported throughout the body to numerous sites of action. Paracrine signaling refers to a ligand activating signaling only at nearby cells rather than diffusing long distances. An extreme example of this is in neurons, in which specialized synapses between a presynaptic and a postsynaptic cell ensure that a ligand, or neurotransmitter, is able to interact only with the target postsynaptic cell. In autocrine signaling, a cell produces a secreted ligand that activates receptors on the surface of that same cell or a group of identical cells.

The ligands are often thought of as circulating small molecules that interact with receptors located on the extracellular surface of cells. However, ligands can come in a variety of forms, and some ligands are able to penetrate the cell in order to bind to intracellular receptors. Extracellular ligands can be large proteins or enzymes. For example, the protease thrombin specifically cleaves a portion of an extracellular receptor, called the thrombin receptor, and this cleavage activates the receptor to initiate signaling. Some ligands are not able to diffuse but remain tethered to a cell. In this form of cell-to-cell communication, one cell containing a ligand molecule, typically a protein, on its extracellular surface must be in direct contact with another cell with an appropriate receptor on its extracellular surface. Most signaling ligands are hydrophilic and cannot cross a lipid bilayer to enter cells; thus, most ligands need to bind to receptors on the extracellular surface of cells. However, some important signaling ligands, such as steroid hormones, are hydrophobic, and in fact, they readily enter a cell where they specifically bind to intracellular receptors. Another example of a ligand that diffuses in and out of cells is the gas nitric oxide (NO). Lastly, not all ligands are produced inside the body; they can also take the form of environmental stimuli, such as photons of light and odorants, that have their own specific receptors.

Thus, ligands, the initiators of signal transduction, can take many forms. The receptors that the ligands bind to also come in a variety of types, with the common feature that receptors are always proteins.[1] The different types of receptors are discussed in some detail in this chapter. Briefly, receptors can be classified into several main types, including (i) G protein-coupled receptors (GPCRs) in which extracellular binding of a ligand allows the intracellular portion of the receptor to engage a set of proteins called G proteins; (ii) ion channels in which extracellular binding of ligand regulates the flow of specific ions through the channel that spans the cell's membrane; (iii) enzyme-linked receptors composed of an extracellular ligand-binding domain and an intracellular enzyme activity that is regulated by extracellular ligand binding; and (iv) nuclear receptors that are located entirely inside the cell and typically bind hydrophobic molecules such as steroids and also directly bind DNA to regulate transcription.

Although signal transduction is often thought of as simple linear pathways from extracellular ligand to intracellular responses, cells exquisitely organize and regulate the proteins involved in particular signaling pathways. In recent years, several key concepts common to most signaling pathways have emerged, and it is important to keep these in mind as different signaling pathways and components are discussed in this chapter. First, components of a signaling pathway are often organized into specific complexes. This clustering of certain signaling proteins can have important consequences in regulating the spatial and temporal characteristics of signal transduction. In this way, seemingly similar signal generations can have distinctly different responses, based on differences in the components of signaling complexes. Moreover, such organized signaling complexes present a therapeutic opportunity to develop drugs that would disrupt one particular branch of a pathway without disrupting other branches that might be considered as beneficial. Second, many intracellular signaling proteins are composed of multiple modular domains. These different domains can allow a single protein to carry out a number of diverse functions, either simultaneously or at different times, depending upon specific signaling inputs. For example, a single protein may have distinct domains that allow it to interact with specific membrane-bound organelles or interact with one or more additional proteins and have a specific enzyme activity. Third, signal transduction is a dynamic process. Many proteins rapidly and reversibly move from one subcellular location to another in response to activation of a particular signaling pathway. Fourth, activation of one signaling pathway by ligand binding to a receptor can affect the signaling properties of a different pathway activated by a completely different agonist binding to a completely different receptor. This concept is often referred to as *cross talk* among signaling pathways. The end result is that a ligand binding to a receptor can produce quite different signaling and physiologic responses depending on what other receptors are activated. Lastly, it has become more appreciated recently that just as important as turning on a signal transduction pathway is the cell's ability to turn off a signaling pathway. Many mechanisms are utilized to turn off or turn down a signaling response to ensure that a signal is generated only for the necessary duration. Failure to properly turn off a signaling response can have disastrous consequences leading to inappropriate signaling in numerous disease states, such as cancer and cardiac failure.

Although it is impossible to cover all important aspects of signal transduction in a single chapter, the goal of this chapter is to describe a number of signaling pathways and focus on specific examples that illustrate important concepts. Moreover, a majority of the emphasis of this chapter is placed on different types of receptor systems and events occurring just inside the cell after receptor activation. For the interested reader, a number of in-depth reviews are referenced throughout the chapter, and many books covering signal transduction in detail are available.[2]

G PROTEIN–COUPLED RECEPTORS

One of the largest families of proteins is the G protein–coupled receptor (GPCR) family, consisting of proteins encoded by over 800 genes.[3,4] GPCRs play critical roles in almost every physiologic function of the human body, and they are targets for a multitude of drugs. A major focus of this chapter is defining some of the basic mechanisms of how GPCRs are activated, how they are regulated, and what signaling pathways are engaged by agonist binding to a GPCR.

GPCRs consist of 7-transmembrane segments connected by extracellular and intracellular loops (Fig. 6-1); the membrane-spanning amino acids form helical structures, and therefore, GPCRs are sometimes called heptahelical receptors. A huge variety of extracellular ligands bind to and activate specific GPCRs, and these can be loosely divided into numerous categories based on their chemical characteristics, including

- Biogenic amines—small molecules such as adrenaline, serotonin, acetylcholine, dopamine, and histamine;
- Amino acids and ions—glutamate, γ-aminobutyric acid (GABA), and free Ca^{2+};
- Peptides and proteins—including peptide hormones such as follicle-stimulating hormone (FSH), luteinizing hormone (LH), thyroid-stimulating hormone (TSH), and angiotensin;
- Chemokines—a large family of small proteins with similar structures;
- Lipids and lipid-derived molecules—including lysophosphatidic acid (LPA), prostaglandins, and leukotrienes;
- Proteases—such as thrombin; and
- Environmental stimuli—such as photons of light, odorants, and tastes.

This is by no means an exhaustive list or a strict categorization of GPCR ligands, merely a listing to give some idea of the diversity of molecules that all produce their physiologic effects through binding to similarly structured GPCRs. Focusing on a few examples will highlight some differences and similarities in how an extracellular ligand activates a GPCR.

In simplified form, GPCRs can be considered to be in equilibrium between active and inactive states. In the absence of agonist, the equilibrium for most GPCRs would be shifted toward the inactive state to avoid constitutive signaling, although this equilibrium can vary depending upon the specific receptor. Binding of an agonist would shift the equilibrium of the GPCR to the active conformation, whereas an inverse agonist is defined as a ligand that strongly shifts the GPCR to the inactive conformation; an antagonist is a ligand that competes with an agonist for binding without shifting the equilibrium state of the GPCR. Almost all endogenous ligands, such as those listed previously, function as agonists, whereas many drugs are traditionally designed to be antagonists or inverse agonists. Very few examples of endogenous antagonists for GPCRs exist[5]; however, a number of allosteric modulators have been identified that function to change, or modulate, the effect of an agonist. This is an exciting area of current research that provides new opportunities for developing therapeutics that target GPCRs.[6] The remaining discussion of GPCR signaling in this chapter focuses on ligands that simply function as agonists to activate the receptor.

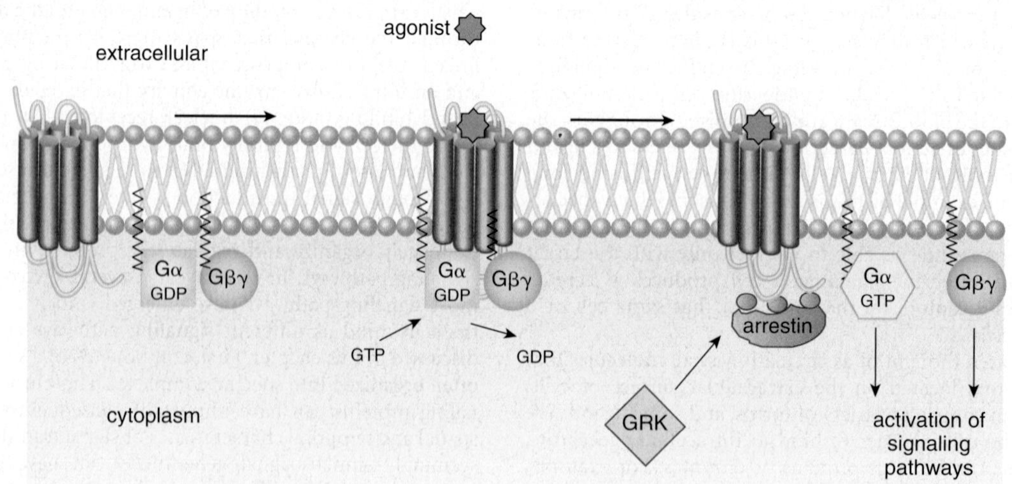

FIGURE 6-1 • G protein–coupled receptor (GPCR) signaling. As described in the chapter text, agonist binding to a GPCR induces an activating change that allows coupling to a heterotrimeric G protein. The agonist-activated GPCR stimulates guanine-nucleotide exchange (guanosine triphosphate [GTP] for guanosine diphosphate [GDP]) on the G protein Gα subunit. The activated Gα can dissociate from the Gβγ subunit, and both Gα and Gβγ are free to interact with and regulate downstream effector proteins. The activated GPCR is then phosphorylated by a GPCR kinase (GRK), and arrestin proteins are recruited to the phosphorylated GPCR to prevent further signaling. In addition, but not shown in this figure, arrestin can recruit additional proteins to initiate new signaling complexes or promote internalization of the receptor. The GPCR is shown as a single 7-transmembrane protein, but many GPCRs are likely to exist as homo- or heterodimers.

Most agonists activate GPCRs by binding either to the extracellular surface of the GPCR, often to a large *N*-terminal domain of a GPCR, or to a binding site within the transmembrane helices and located within the plane of the membrane.[7] Classic examples of the latter form of ligand-GPCR interaction are light-driven activation of the GPCR rhodopsin and biogenic amines binding to their cognate receptors. Numerous biochemical, spectroscopic, and mutagenetics studies have demonstrated that many small molecule agonists, such as ligands for adrenergic receptors, bind to a binding pocket formed by several transmembrane helices deep within the transmembrane bundle. In the case of rhodopsin, a chromophore, 11-*cis* retinal, is covalently bound to one of the transmembrane helices and is located within the transmembrane bundle similar to where small molecule agonists bind to other GPCRs. A single photon of light activates rhodopsin by causing a transition of the chromophore from the 11-*cis* to the all-*trans* form.

Other agonists activate their respective GPCRs by binding to the extracellular *N*-terminus and extracellular loop regions rather than intercalating into the transmembrane region. For example, glycoprotein hormones, such as LH, TSH, FSH, appear to bind to the *N*-terminal domains of GPCRs, and even Ca^{2+} and glutamate exert their effects by binding to a cleft in the large extracellular *N*-termini of the Ca^{2+} sensing receptor and metabotropic glutamate receptor, respectively. This latter mode of binding has been termed the *Venus flytrap module*. Binding of agonists to extracellular *N*-termini of GPCRs is likely to allow the agonist to also interact with extracellular loops that connect transmembrane helices or to promote an intramolecular interaction of the GPCR's *N*-terminal region with extracellular loops and/or transmembrane regions. A further example of unique agonist binding to a GPCR, that of thrombin's interaction with its GPCR, provides an interesting and illuminating example of the connection between a GPCR's extracellular *N*-terminus and its transmembrane regions. The protease thrombin specifically cleaves the extended *N*-terminus of the thrombin receptor, thus creating a new *N*-terminus for the GPCR. This newly exposed *N*-terminus is then able to intramolecularly interact with its extracellular loops and thereby function as a tethered ligand for activation of the thrombin receptor.[8]

Although agonists use varying mechanisms to bind different sites on GPCRs, it is likely that agonist binding results in a common mechanism of GPCR activation. The exact mechanism of GPCR activation is not fully understood, but a key event appears to be that agonist binding elicits a change in orientation of several of the transmembrane helices, which leads to a change at the intracellular surface of the GPCR.[9,10] These changes are believed to result in an optimal binding pocket for intracellular heterotrimeric G proteins. In addition, it has been recognized fairly recently that many, if not most, GPCRs are likely to exist as dimers, either homo- or heterodimers, and agonist binding may also influence the dimerization of a GPCR, thus contributing to the propagation of conformational changes to an intracellular binding site for G proteins and other signaling proteins.

After activation of a GPCR by agonist binding, the GPCR is able to productively interact with and activate heterotrimeric G proteins, which are composed of an α, a β, and a γ subunit.[11] Agonist-activated GPCR activates the G proteins by promoting the switch of the G protein α subunit (Gα) from the inactive guanosine diphosphate (GDP)–bound state to the active guanosine triphosphate (GTP)–bound state (see Fig. 6-1). This process is described in more detail in the next section. Moreover, the role of heterotrimeric G proteins in activating specific signaling responses and an understanding of how the G proteins are regulated is also discussed in some detail later, but first, it is important to consider how GPCRs themselves are further regulated after agonist binding.

In addition to transmitting a signal via activation of G proteins, agonist-activated GPCRs also undergo desensitization, internalization/trafficking, and the recruitment of additional signaling proteins. *Desensitization* refers to a diminished ability to respond to stimulation during prolonged stimulation, and desensitization of a GPCR can occur in several ways including loss of ability to interact with and activate a G protein, sequestration of the receptor such that it is no longer exposed to agonist, and loss of receptor by degradation. The classic example of GPCR desensitization involves phosphorylation by GPCR kinases (GRKs). Upon agonist activation of a GPCR, a GRK rapidly phosphorylates the activated GPCR at sites in the intracellular *C*-terminus or intracellular loops (see Fig. 6-1). The GRK family consists of seven members, GRKs 1-7. GRK1 and GRK7 are restricted to the retina where they regulate the GPCR rhodopsin; the other members are mostly ubiquitously expressed. GRKs display exquisite specificity for the agonist-activated forms of GPCRs, but how certain GRKs recognize only select GPCRs is still under investigation. The key consequence of phosphorylation of an activated GPCR by a GRK is that this phosphorylation promotes the recruitment to the GPCR of proteins known as arrestins (see Fig. 6-1). Only four forms of arrestins are present in humans, and two of those are retina specific. Binding of an arrestin protein to the GPCR "arrests" signaling by simply blocking the GPCR from interacting with a G protein; in this way, the signaling is turned off or desensitized even in the continued presence of stimulating agonist. This type of regulation is essential to prevent a signaling response from lasting too long. Although GRKs appear to play a major role in desensitizing GPCRs, other protein kinases are involved in feedback responses that not only desensitize a response but also function to promote switching to another response. For example, phosphorylation of the β_2-adrenergic receptor (β_2-AR) by protein kinase A (PKA) turns off the ability of β_2-AR to couple to the Gs class of G proteins and turns on the ability of β_2-AR to couple to the Gi class of G proteins. A critical concept to keep in mind is that many steps, that is, proteins, in a signaling pathway are subject to desensitization in order to tightly regulate the duration and spatial characteristics of a signaling response; such regulation of proteins other than GPCRs are discussed further in this chapter.

More recently, it has been recognized that in addition to arrestin's role in rapid GPCR desensitization by interacting with the activated receptor, arrestins are also key factors in longer-term regulation of GPCRs. One way they do this is by *recruiting* additional proteins, such as clathrin and the adaptor protein AP-2,[12,13] that mediate the *internalization*, or endocytosis, of GPCRs. Internalization is a common feature of agonist-activated GPCRs, and the best-characterized pathway is through clathrin-coated pit internalization, a mechanism used by many diverse cell-surface receptors. For GPCRs, the two major fates of the receptor after internalization are targeting to lysosomes for degradation or recycling back to the cell surface. Internalization and degradation of a particular GPCR provide a mechanism for preventing further signaling, at least until new receptors are made and replenished at the cell surface. Many internalized GPCRs are able to recycle back to cell surface. This recycling is somewhat slow, often on the order of 1 hour, but still, this is a faster way to restore the response to an agonist than the longer time it takes for a cell to synthesize new receptors. Although not completely understood, it appears that internalization of a GPCR is necessary for the receptor to undergo dephosphorylation and become competent for signaling again. Numerous cellular proteins interact with specific GPCRs to direct them to degradative or recycling pathways after internalization, and the details of how this trafficking is controlled for different GPCRs is an extremely active area of current research. Certainly, drugs that could affect the trafficking itinerary of a specific GPCR may have therapeutic potential.

GPCRs have been traditionally thought to carry out their signaling functions by activating heterotrimeric G proteins, and although this remains a major mode of action, it is now clear that GPCRs have G protein–independent signaling functions. Arrestin proteins can play a role in this process. Arrestin binding to the activated GPCR can recruit other proteins that are not involved in internalization but are required for initiating new signaling responses. An example of this is the demonstration that arrestin binding to activated GPCRs can recruit components of the mitogen-activated protein (MAP) kinase (MAPK) cascade, a group of protein kinases that transmit signals through serial phosphorylation (discussed further later in this chapter). This allows the activated GPCR to propagate a signal via the MAPK pathway that is independent of heterotrimeric G proteins. It appears that such a GPCR-arrestin-MAPK signaling complex can function at the plasma membrane or as an intracellular internalized complex. This ability to signal at different places in the cell reinforces a somewhat novel and important signal-transduction concept—events initiated by a cell surface receptor do not always occur at the plasma membrane, but instead may occur intracellularly with differing consequences for how the signal is ultimately interpreted by the cell. Proteins other than arrestins have also been identified that can serve as "scaffolds" to form a complex with a GPCR and other signaling proteins.[4] A number of GPCR-initiated signaling events that occur independently of G proteins have now been demonstrated, and it is clear that the repertoire of signaling responses generated by GPCRs is extremely diverse and still far from understood.

HETEROTRIMERIC G PROTEINS

Nonetheless, heterotrimeric G proteins are responsible for transmitting much of the signal from an agonist-activated GPCR. G proteins consist of Gα and Gβγ subunits and function as molecular switches by cycling, in a regulated manner, between GDP- and GTP-bound states. This is termed the *G protein cycle* (Fig. 6-2), and a great deal of work since the early 1980s has provided a detailed understanding of this cycle.[11] The inactive state consists of an αβγ heterotrimeric complex in which Gα is bound to GDP, while the active, and signaling competent, state consists of GTP-bound Gα dissociated from Gβγ. The G protein β and γ subunits are almost always found irreversibly bound to each other and, thus, are referred to as the *G protein βγ dimer* (Gβγ). For the most part, the heterotrimeric complex is unable to interact with and activate downstream proteins, that is, effectors, because the GDP-bound Gα is in a conformation that is not optimal for interacting with effector proteins and because the protein surfaces of Gα and Gβγ that interact with effectors are occluded when Gα and Gβγ are bound to each other. As mentioned previously, an agonist-bound GPCR serves as a guanine-nucleotide exchange factor to promote the release of GDP from Gα. The mechanistic details of the GPCR-catalyzed activation of G proteins remains to be fully elucidated, but the prevailing view is that agonist binding to a GPCR induces the formation of a binding pocket for a heterotrimeric G protein, and this interaction somehow stimulates the release of GDP from Gα. Once Gα is no longer bound to GDP, a molecule of GTP binds. A major factor in GTP binding is simply that the cellular concentration of GTP is much higher than that of GDP. After activation by a GPCR, GTP-bound Gα and Gβγ are free to interact with effector proteins, but this signaling is subsequently turned off and the heterotrimer returns to its inactive state. To accomplish this deactivation, Gα has intrinsic GTP hydrolysis activity that removes the third phosphate of GTP, thus converting Gα back to the GDP-bound form (see Fig. 6-2). The rate of GTP hydrolysis by Gα serves as a timer for determining the duration of G protein activation. For many cellular responses, researchers realized that the rate of GTP hydrolysis was too slow to be consistent with the rapid deactivation required in some G protein–signaling pathways, such as responding to light in the visual system and ion channel regulation by neurotransmitters. This conundrum led to the discovery of a family of proteins termed *regulators of G protein signaling* (RGS proteins). RGS proteins bind to an active Gα and greatly accelerate the ability of the Gα to hydrolyze GTP to rapidly deactivate G protein signaling. Thus, the G protein cycle functions as a tightly regulated molecular switch with an intrinsic timing device to carry out the transmission of a signal from an activated cell-surface receptor into an intracellular response.

Sixteen different Gα, 5 Gβ, and 12 Gγ proteins are encoded by the human genome. Whereas some of the subunits are restricted to specific cell types, many of them are ubiquitously expressed, suggesting a large number of possible αβγ combinations. Although it is not clear how many different combinations are actually formed and how different combinations affect signaling, it is clear that the Gα plays an important role in specifying interactions with select GPCRs and determining what signaling pathways are activated. Heterotrimeric G proteins are typically named based on the identity of the Gα.

The Gα are divided into four families based on amino sequence similarity and similarities in the effectors that are their direct targets. The α_s family consists of α_s and α_{olf}, a Gα involved in olfaction. The major effector for α_s is adenylyl cyclase (AC), an enzyme that generates the second messenger cyclic adenosine monophosphate (cAMP). α_s was originally named for its ability to stimulate cAMP production. The α_i family contains the most members, including α_{i1}, α_{i2}, α_{i3}, α_o, α_z, α_{t1}, α_{t2}, and α_{gust}. This family was originally named for the ability of several members to inhibit AC and, thus, lower the cell's concentration of cAMP and counteract the effects of α_s. However, it is now well known that members of the α_i family can regulate a number of different effectors. The most well studied of these are α_{t1} and α_{t2}, also known as transducins, which are found only in photoreceptor cells where they mediate vision by activating the enzyme cyclic guanosine monophosphate (cGMP) phosphodiesterase, after light-activation of the GPCR rhodopsin. The α_q family of Gα consists of α_q, α_{11}, α_{14}, and α_{16}. The best-characterized role for all four members of this family is their ability to activate the enzyme phospholipase C-β, which produces the second messengers diacylglycerol (DAG) and inositol 1,4,5-trisphosphate (IP_3). The last family of Gα is termed α_{12}, and it consists of two members α_{12} and α_{13}. A number of effectors for α_{12} and α_{13} have been determined. One particular α_{12} and α_{13} effector that has been the subject of much recent study is Rho guanine-nucleotide exchange factor (RhoGEF), which directly activates the so-called small GTPase Rho. This activation of Rho regulates several responses, including changes in the actin cytoskeleton that allow cell migration, cell shape changes, and cell division.

Although it was originally thought that Gα subunits were responsible for most of the signaling functions of G proteins and that Gβγ serve mostly to merely bind Gα, it is now clear that Gβγ can interact with and regulate numerous effector proteins.[14] For example, Gβγ are able to directly activate AC, phospholipase β (PLC-β), ion channels, and protein and lipid kinases. Interestingly, Gβγ regulate some of the same effectors that certain Gα regulate, for example, both α_q and Gβγ can activate PLC-β, indicating that in some situations Gα and Gβγ can potentiate the signaling of each other.

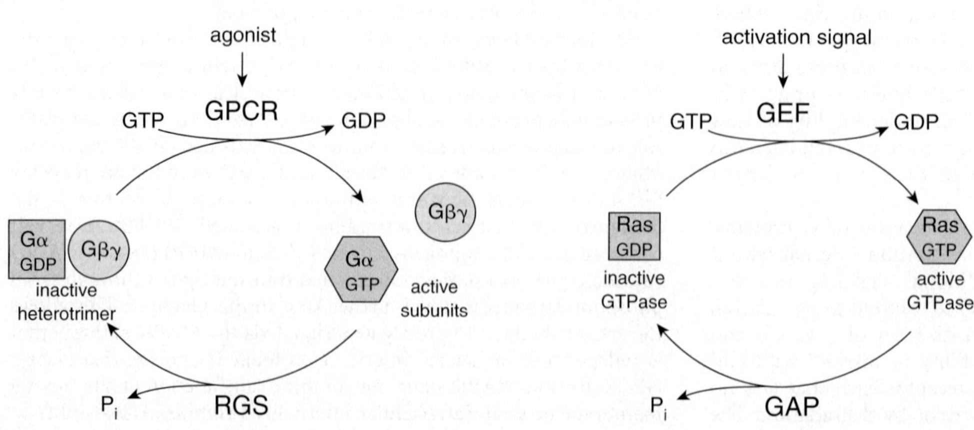

FIGURE 6-2 • The G protein cycle. Both heterotrimeric G proteins **(left)** and monomeric G proteins, also called small GTPases, of the Ras superfamily **(right)** undergo similar cycles of activation and inactivation that allow them to function as molecular switches, as further described in the chapter text.

Much research effort has been expended to identify which families of G proteins are activated by a particular GPCR, but a complete understanding of how a GPCR preferentially interacts with a select G protein family remains elusive. Some GPCRs predominantly couple to one G protein family. Conversely, many GPCRs couple to multiple G proteins. For example, the thrombin receptor couples to G12, Gq, and Gi heterotrimers. Moreover, the coupling of a GPCR to different G proteins can vary in different types of cells. In summary, the specific signaling pathways that are regulated and the ultimate physiologic response in a particular cell in response to an activated GPCR are a consequence of the combinatorial effect of the different G protein families that are activated and of the actions of both Gα and Gβγ.

G protein signaling is tightly regulated. After activation by a GPCR, the Gα hydrolyzes bound GTP to return to the inactive state, and this is facilitated in some cases by RGS proteins (see Fig. 6-2). More than 30 RGS proteins have been identified to date.[15-17] All RGS proteins have in common a ~120 amino acid RGS domain that can interact with Gα and function as a GTPase activating protein (GAP). Some RGS proteins consist of little more than the core RGS domain, whereas others are large, multidomain proteins. Thus, many RGS proteins not only directly regulate Gα but also serve to directly link G proteins to other critical signaling proteins, including GPCRs and downstream effectors. RGS proteins are an example of an important theme in signal transduction—key regulators of signaling pathways are proteins that can bind simultaneously to several proteins and, in doing so, bring together a complex of signaling proteins to efficiently regulate a signaling pathway spatially and temporally.

Another interesting family of G protein regulators has been identified. These proteins are termed *activators of G protein signaling* (AGS), and they have the common feature of being able to activate G proteins independently of GPCRs.[18] Just as it is now clear that GPCRs can activate certain signaling pathways in G protein–independent ways, it is also evident that G proteins can be activated in the absence of the typical agonist-activated GPCR.

An additional way in which G proteins are regulated is through their subcellular localization. Like many signaling proteins, G proteins are peripheral membrane proteins; they do not contain transmembrane segments that are embedded in a cellular membrane, but nonetheless, they spend much of their lifetime tightly attached to membranes. Membrane localization of G proteins, and numerous other signaling proteins, is absolutely essential for them to carry out their function. If they are not tightly bound to membranes, they cannot effectively interact with GPCRs at the cytoplasmic surface of the cell's plasma membrane. G proteins accomplish membrane localization owing to the fact that they have different lipids covalently attached to them. The three major lipid modifications of intracellular proteins are myristoylation, palmitoylation, and isoprenylation,[19] and all of these can contribute to G protein localization.[20] A particularly interesting modification is palmitoylation because it can be reversible. Palmitoylation occurs on most Gα, and activation of the Gα can lead to rapid depalmitoylation. This would have the result of decreasing the membrane attachment of the G protein. Although not as well studied as for GPCRs, G proteins can undergo reversible changes in membrane binding and move, or traffic, to diverse subcellular locations. The ability of some intracellular signaling proteins to move to different subcellular locations in response to extracellular activation of a receptor is another important theme in signal transduction.

G PROTEIN EFFECTORS

Activation of heterotrimeric G proteins leads to the activation of a number of intracellular effectors and signaling pathways. This section discusses two classic and important effectors, AC and PLC-β, and the signaling pathways they influence.

ACs and cAMP

Studies on the elucidation of the cAMP signaling pathway were responsible for numerous landmark discoveries in signal transduction. The identification of cAMP led to the concept of second messengers, and cAMP remains the prototypical second messenger. Studies on the generation of cAMP in response to epinephrine allowed the discovery of heterotrimeric G proteins. Studies on the target of cAMP led to discoveries of protein phosphorylation, and more recent discoveries on the spatial restriction of cAMP actions were instrumental in developing the concept of scaffolding, or anchoring, proteins.

ACs are a family of ten proteins that perform the function of converting cellular adenosine triphosphate (ATP) to cAMP (Fig. 6-3).[21] One form of AC, called sAC, is a soluble enzyme, but the remaining family members share a similar architecture of spanning the membrane 12 times with both the *N*- and the *C*-termini located intracellularly. The soluble sAC is not responsive to hormones and G proteins, and it plays a specific role in sperm maturation, motility and capacitation. Conversely, all the membrane forms of AC are directly regulated by G proteins and thus responsible for production of cAMP in response to extracellular agonists binding to GPCRs. Although the ACs span the plasma membrane multiple times, they do not appear to interact with any extracellular ligands nor do they function as channels to mediate communication between extracellular and intracellular environments. Instead, the membrane spanning appears to function merely as a way to localize AC to membranes, and the actual AC enzyme activity is located completely intracellular in two tandem domains. In fact, the intracellular AC domains can be produced in recombinant systems as soluble proteins without the transmembrane domains, and they can function as G protein–responsive ACs.

All membrane-bound ACs, that is, AC1-9, are activated by the Gα, α_s. Direct binding of the GPCR-activated GTP-bound α_s to the AC at the cytoplasmic surface of the plasma membrane promotes a structural rearrangement that activates the ability of AC to convert ATP to cAMP. Although AC1-9 are all activated by α_s, different forms of AC are subject to different inputs of additional regulation by other G protein subunits, and thus activation of different GPCRs can uniquely regulate cAMP signaling owing to distinct combinations of G proteins that are activated. α_i subunits are able to inhibit select forms of AC, primarily AC5 and AC6. Gβγ, which are dissociated from Gα in response to GPCR activation, can also regulate AC forms; AC2, 4, and 7 are stimulated by Gβγ, and AC1, 5, and 6 can be inhibited by Gβγ. Furthermore, several AC forms can be regulated by phosphorylation. One such phosphorylation is mediated by protein kinase C (PKC). Because PKC is activated by downstream second messengers generated in response to the activation of α_q (see PLC section, later), PKC phosphorylation of AC provides a mechanism for the additional G proteins, that is, the α_q family, to feed into regulation of cAMP production.

Much of the action of the second messenger cAMP is exerted through its binding to the cAMP-dependent protein kinase, also called protein kinase A (PKA). When the cellular levels of cAMP rise in response to activation of ACs, cAMP binds to inactive PKA, which is in the form of a tetramer of two cAMP-binding regulatory subunits and two catalytic subunits (R_2C_2). Upon two molecules of cAMP binding to each R subunit, two C subunits dissociate, and it is this dissociation from the R subunits that allows their activation. PKA is then free to phosphorylate any of a large number of protein substrates to generate physiologic responses.

cAMP was discovered as being the diffusible, nonprotein factor, that is, second messenger, that mediates the effects of epinephrine and glucagon on glycogen breakdown. Subsequently, this signaling pathway was clearly worked out such that it is now known that cAMP activates PKA, which phosphorylates another protein kinase called phosphorylase kinase, which in turn phosphorylates glycogen phosphorylase, which then becomes active to convert glycogen to glucose 1-phosphate. Depending upon the cell type and GPCRs that are activated, cAMP similarly mediates rapid changes in cell function by promoting PKA phosphorylation of key substrate proteins.

cAMP increases also often lead to changes in cell function on a slower timescale, and such changes are typically due to the induction of gene transcription. A common mechanism by which cAMP regulates gene expression is that the activated PKA (C subunit) can not only phosphorylate cytoplasmic proteins but can also directly move into the

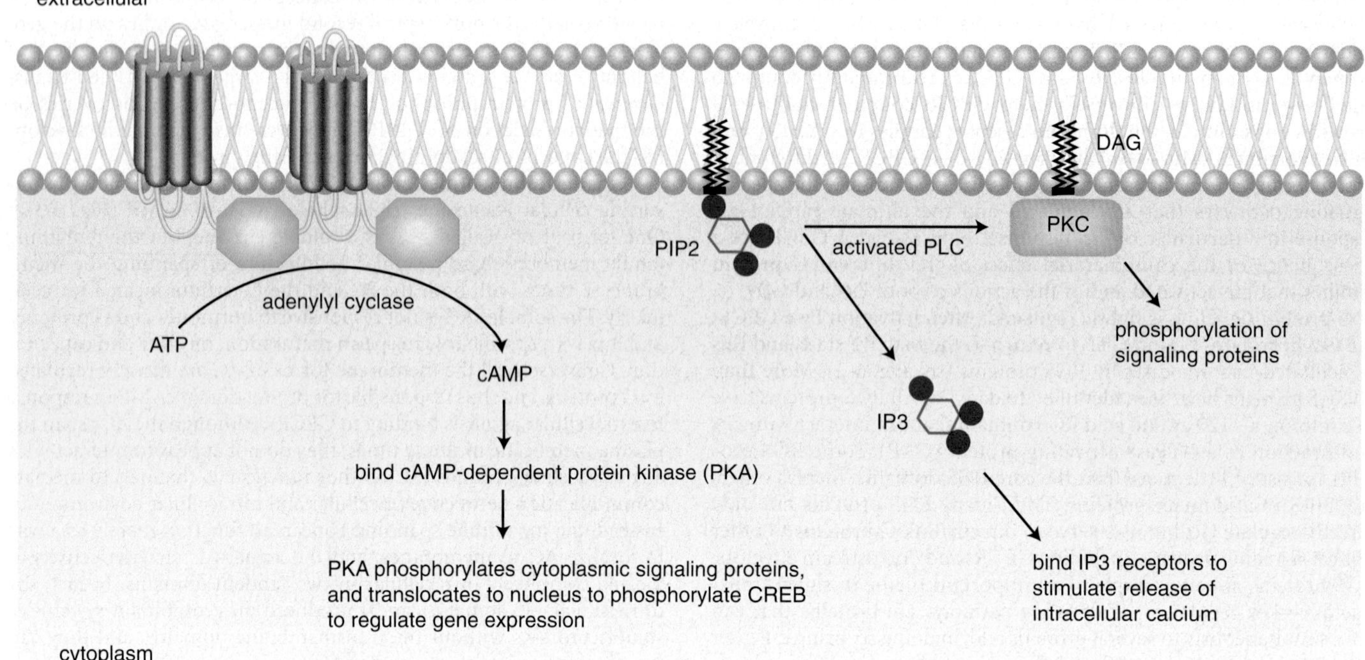

FIGURE 6-3 • Second messengers. This figure depicts two well-studied second messenger systems. **Left,** Adenylyl cyclases are primarily regulated by direct binding of activated heterotrimeric G protein subunits. The primary target of cAMP is PKA, but the guanine-nucleotide exchange factor Epac and cyclic nucleotide-gated ion channels are also regulated by cAMP binding. Not pictured, cAMP signaling is tightly regulated spatially and temporally by phosphodiesterases that degrade cAMP and anchoring/scaffolding proteins, as described in the chapter text. **Right,** Both GPCR and protein tyrosine kinase receptor signaling can activate phospholipase C (PLC) enzymes. Activated PLC cleaves the membrane constituent phosphatidylinositol 4,5-bisphosphate (PIP2) to generate the second messengers diacylglycerol (DAG) and inositol trisphosphate (IP3). PIP2 is depicted as two lipid chains buried in the membrane connected to the phosphorylated (*red circles*) inositol ring. Membrane-bound DAG binds and helps activate protein kinase C (PKC), and diffusible IP3 binds endoplasmic reticulum–localized receptors that regulate intracellular calcium release.

nucleus, where it phosphorylates a major regulator termed *cAMP response element–binding* (CREB) protein. Phosphorylated CREB binds to a specific DNA sequence termed the *cAMP response element* (CRE) and also recruits another nuclear protein, CREB-binding protein (CBP), a histone acetyltransferase. The end result is the induction of the expression of genes that contain the CRE regulatory sequence.

Although PKA is the major target that cAMP binds to, a couple of other important signaling proteins also directly bind cAMP. Cyclic nucleotide–gated (CNG) ion channels provide extremely rapid responses to cAMP and also cGMP (this cyclic nucleotide is discussed later in the chapter). CNG channels are nonselective cation channels found in a number of different cell types, including the heart and neurons.[22] Binding of cyclic nucleotides to an intracellular region of the CNG channel causes the channel to open, allowing the flow of cations, such as Ca^{2+} and Na^{+}, across the cell's membrane. In photoreceptor cells, cGMP binds to a CNG channel in the dark, allowing depolarization; however, light activation of the GPCR rhodopsin leads to rapid decreases in the cGMP concentration, resulting in closing of the CNG channel and hyperpolarization. Similarly, activation of olfactory GPCRs by odorants leads to an α_{olf}/AC-mediated increase in intracellular cAMP in olfactory neurons, resulting in cAMP binding to a CNG channel and depolarization of the cells. CNG channels play a number of other important roles, including regulating neurotransmitter release.

The most recently identified target of cAMP is a protein called *Epac*, for *exchange protein activated by cAMP*.[23-26] cAMP binding to Epac activates its guanine-nucleotide exchange activity, which is specifically responsible for activating Rap, a member of the Ras family of small GTPases. Epac has been shown to mediate the effects of cAMP in critical ways in a number of physiologic contexts, including cardiovascular function, neurotransmitter release, and insulin secretion. Moreover, Epac often works together with PKA to signal a cellular response to the second-messenger cAMP.

Like all signaling events, cAMP signaling is tightly regulated, and one critical way that this is accomplished is through the degradation of the cAMP molecule by a family of enzymes called *phosphodiesterases* (PDEs).[27] A large family of PDEs shares the common activity of inactivating cAMP, or cGMP, by cleaving the cyclic phosphate bond. The PDEs are essential for ensuring the proper duration of a cAMP signal. Their importance in a wide variety of physiologic responses is underscored by the number of drugs that have been developed to target PDEs. Caffeine was recognized early on to be an inhibitor of PDE activity, and PDE inhibitors have been developed or are being developed to treat heart failure, inflammation, erectile dysfunction, asthma, and central nervous system (CNS) disorders.

Another important way that cAMP signaling is regulated is through the formation of protein complexes that serve to restrict both the spatial and the temporal characteristics of cAMP signaling.[28] Although cAMP can be considered a freely diffusible second messenger, it has become clear that cAMP does not always diffuse throughout the cell and its effects are often restricted to discrete subcellular locations. The A kinase anchoring proteins (AKAPs) bind PKA and serve to localize PKA at specific sites within the cell. Often, AKAPs function to localize PKA near the site of cAMP generation, and thus, this AKAP-bound PKA will be preferentially activated, compared with PKAs localized in other subcellular localizations, promoting phosphorylation of only a select group of nearby substrates. Moreover, AKAPs can promote even more exquisite regulation of cAMP signaling by binding to other proteins, in addition to PKA. For example, some AKAPs can also interact with phosphatases or PDEs, critical regulators involved in turning off signaling. Such complexes thus provide tight control on the duration and location of signaling, and the formation of AKAP complexes composed of different components adds an important layer of specificity for cells to generate diverse responses from the increase of a common second messenger, cAMP.

Phospholipase C

Phosphoinositide–specific PLC enzymes (see Fig. 6-3) are responsible for hydrolyzing the membrane constituent phosphatidylinositol 4,5-

bisphosphate (PI 4,5-P_2, or simply PIP_2) to generate the important second messengers IP_3 and DAG that control intracellular Ca^{2+} levels and activation of PKC, respectively.[29,30] There are eleven PIP_2-specific PLCs, and they are divided into four families, based on amino acid sequence similarity and the proteins that activate them. In contrast to ACs, PLCs are not membrane-spanning proteins; they are typically soluble or loosely associated with membranes.

Members of the PLC-β family (PLC-β1-4) are directly activated by heterotrimeric G proteins and are thus considered one of the classic G protein effectors. GPCR-activated, that is, GTP-bound, Gα of the α_q family interact with PLC-βs at the cytoplasmic face of the plasma membrane. Although the activation mechanism is not completely understood, the binding of α_q greatly stimulates the ability of PLC-β to hydrolyze PIP_2. In addition to α_q family members, Gβγ can directly bind and activate PLC-β. A number of different combinations of Gβ and Gγ are capable of stimulation of PLC-β, and Gβγ preferentially activates the PLC-β2 and PLC-β3 isoforms. Thus, like AC, PLC-βs can be regulated by both Gα and Gβγ subunits of heterotrimeric G proteins. For example, GPCRs that do not activate Gq heterotrimers can still transmit a signal to activation of PLC-β through the release of Gβγ from other heterotrimers, such as Gi. This allows complex and combinatorial input into the regulation of this key enzyme.

The PLC-γ family consists of two members that are not responsive to G proteins. Instead, PLC-γ is activated by tyrosine kinase receptors (this family of receptors is discussed later). A unique feature of PLC-γ is the presence of an SH2 protein domain that allows it to directly bind to select proteins that have a phosphorylated tyrosine modification. This phosphotyrosine-mediated recruitment of cytoplasmic PLC-γ to the cytoplasmic surface of the plasma membrane is an important step in its activation. The other two family members are PLC-δ and PLC-ε; much less is known about these PLCs in terms of how they are regulated. However, recently, PLC-ε has been the subject of a great deal of research.[31] PLC-ε is able to detect and integrate inputs from a number of different pathways, including cAMP and tyrosine kinase signaling, and PLC-ε has important physiologic roles, such as in cardiovascular function.

Activated PLCs produce the extremely important and ubiquitous molecule IP_3 (see Fig. 6-3). PIP_2, a constituent of cellular membranes, contains two hydrophobic carbon chains embedded in the membrane and a phosphorylated inositol headgroup at the cytoplasmic surface of the membrane. Like all membrane lipid headgroups, the inositol headgroup is hydrophilic and accessible to cellular proteins. PLCs cleave off the headgroup, thus releasing IP_3, an inositol ring containing three phosphates, into the soluble cytoplasm environment of the cell. IP_3 then binds to IP_3 receptors that are located at intracellular membranes of the endoplasmic reticulum (ER) organelle. The activated IP_3 receptor then performs the important function of allowing the rapid release of Ca^{2+} from the ER into the cytoplasm. Thus, the second-messenger IP_3 induces the release of another second messenger, Ca^{2+}.[32] Almost all cells take advantage of Ca^{2+} signaling to carry out a wide variety of functions. Normally, the cytoplasmic concentration of Ca^{2+} is kept very low in a resting cell, but activation of IP_3 receptors, and plasma membrane Ca^{2+} channels that are activated by mechanisms other than IP_3, causes a rapid increase in the intracellular Ca^{2+} concentration. Ca^{2+} then regulates signaling by binding to several proteins, the most prominent of which is calmodulin. Upon Ca^{2+} binding, calmodulin undergoes a structural rearrangement that allows it to, in turn, bind and regulate other proteins. A family of Ca^{2+}/calmodulin-dependent protein kinases is a major target of calmodulin; these proteins then phosphorylate numerous substrate proteins in response to binding Ca^{2+}/calmodulin. Key aspects of Ca^{2+} signaling are that Ca^{2+} can also be removed from the cytoplasm very rapidly, making the effects quite transient, and that cells have developed mechanisms for generating numerous waves of intracellular Ca^{2+}. These waves and oscillations of Ca^{2+} play critical roles in development and neural function.

In addition to producing the soluble IP_3, activated PLCs also generate DAG, which is basically the dual-chain membrane lipid with the inositol ring removed, leaving only a small portion of the molecule accessible to intracellular proteins. However, members of a family of protein serine/threonine kinases called PKC specifically bind to and are activated by DAG. Thus, DAG can be considered a second messenger, albeit one that does not freely diffuse in the cell but instead remains localized to its membrane environment. Interestingly, PKCs also bind Ca^{2+}, and the binding of both DAG and Ca^{2+} together activate PKC so that it can phosphorylate key substrate proteins. Thus, in this case, both second messengers generated by PLCs ultimately activate the same target. In summary, PLCs are critical signaling intermediates that are activated by G proteins or other signaling pathways, depending on the PLC family. They hydrolyze the membrane constituent PIP_2 to generate second messengers. This pathway illustrates the importance of lipids in signal transduction and is one of several examples showing that not only are membrane phospholipids essential structural components of a cell, forming membranes to provide a physical barrier, but many lipids and their metabolites are also important signaling molecules.

ENZYME-LINKED CELL-SURFACE RECEPTORS

Many cell surface receptors consist of a large extracellular ligand-binding domain and a large intracellular enzyme domain connected by a single transmembrane segment (Fig. 6-4). Thus, ligand binding can directly activate the attached enzyme activity. This architecture is in contrast to GPCRs that have seven transmembrane helices and do not have a large intracellular domain. Agonist stimulation of GPCRs activate G proteins rather than activating an attached enzyme. Four major families of enzyme-linked cell surface receptors that are discussed later are protein tyrosine kinase (PTK) receptors, serine/threonine kinase receptors, guanylyl cyclases (GCs), and protein tyrosine phosphatases (PTPs).

PTK Receptors

PTK receptors constitute a large and important family of cell surface receptors. Fifty-eight genes in the human genome encode PTK receptors. Often generally referred to as *growth factor receptors*, most PTK receptors bind and are activated by extracellular protein factors, many of which have defined roles in cell growth and metabolism. PTK receptors can be subdivided into 20 subfamilies,[33] and some of the best-characterized subfamilies include

1. The epidermal growth factor (EGF) receptor family consists of four members involved in the development of epithelial tissues, and these receptors promote growth of numerous cell types. The ligand, EGF, was one of the first growth factors to be identified, along with nerve growth factor (NGF), based on an assay for accelerated eyelid opening in newborn mice.[34] In addition, the EGF receptor (EGFR) was the first PTK receptor to be identified.[35,36] Members of the EGFR family have been found to be amplified or mutated in a number of human cancers, and the cancer therapeutic Herceptin, a monoclonal antibody effective against breast cancer, targets a member of the EGFR family, ErbB2.
2. The insulin receptor subfamily consists of three members, including the insulin receptor and the insulin-like growth factor-1 receptor (IGF-1R), which play important roles in metabolic regulation and cell survival signaling, respectively. These receptors are unique among the PTK receptors in that they undergo processing that results in two disulfide-linked extracellular α subunits, and each α subunit is disulfide-linked to a β subunit that spans the membrane and contains the intracellular tyrosine kinase domain.
3. The platelet-derived growth factor (PDGF) receptor subfamily, which includes receptors for colony-stimulating factor-1 (CSF-1), plays important roles in the development of many cell types.
4. The vascular endothelial cell growth factor (VEGF) receptors are mainly expressed at the surface of endothelial cells, where they play critical roles in angiogenesis.

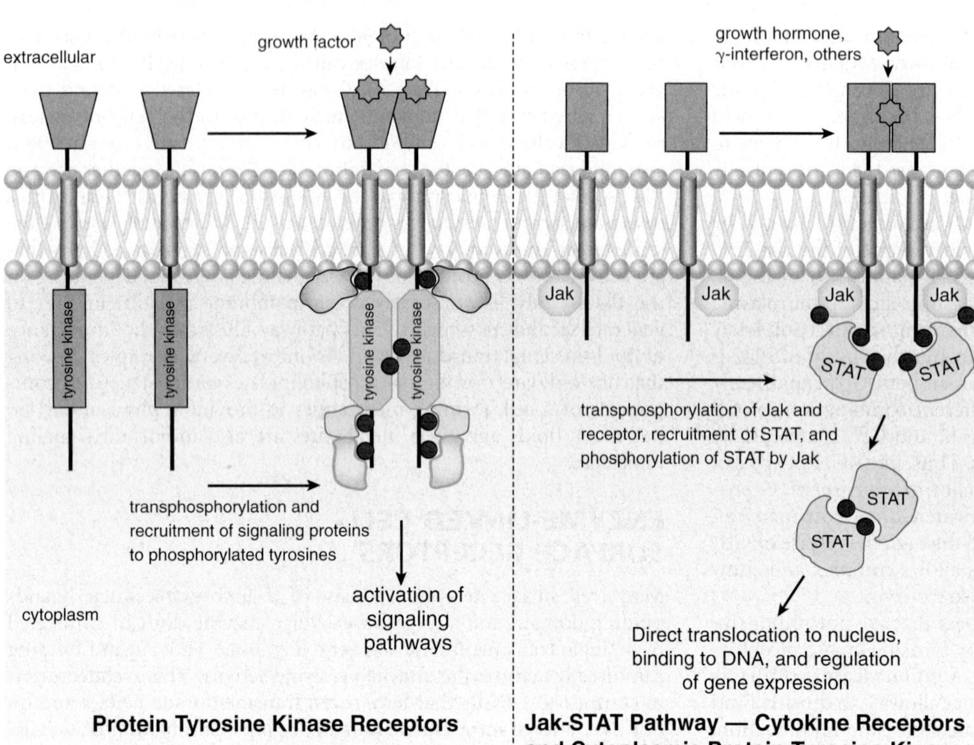

FIGURE 6-4 • Examples of tyrosine kinase signaling. Left, As described in the chapter text, growth factor binding to the extracellular domains of protein tyrosine kinase (PTK) receptors induces receptor dimerization and transphosphorylation. The tyrosine kinase can also phosphorylate other substrates. One important mode of signaling is that the phosphorylated tyrosines (*red circles*) on the activated receptor serve to bind specific proteins, often containing an SH2 domain. These new signaling complexes can generate a variety of signals. **Right,** In this example of signaling via cytoplasmic tyrosine kinases, a cytokine receptor does not have integral enzyme activity, but instead binds to a tyrosine kinase termed Jak. Activation of the receptor activates the associated Jak to promote transphosphorylation of Jaks and tyrosine phosphorylation of the receptor tail. The phosphorylated tyrosine (*red circle*) of the receptor recruits STAT, and STAT is then phosphorylated by Jak. Next, the STATs dissociate and dimerize by interacting with the phosphotyrosine of the partner STAT. This activated STAT dimer can then directly move into the nucleus, where it can bind DNA and regulate transcription of target genes.

5. The fibroblast growth factor (FGF) receptors are also important in angiogenesis and in the development of different cell types.
6. The neutrophin receptor family, also known as TrkA, B, and C, bind NGFs and play critical roles in neuron development and survival.
7. The Eph receptor subfamily has 14 members, making it the largest PTK receptor subfamily. Eph receptors play critical roles in neuronal guidance and also in angiogenesis and metastasis. A unique feature of Eph receptor signaling is that their ligands, termed ephrins, are themselves cell surface molecules. Thus, ephrin binding to an Eph receptor mediates direct cell-cell communication of neighboring cells, in contrast to signaling by circulating growth factors or hormones, such as insulin. Another interesting aspect of ephrin signaling has been termed reverse signaling. Not only does the ephrin ligand activate the tyrosine kinase-containing Eph receptor, but ephrin-Eph receptor interaction also stimulates signaling in the ephrin-containing cell. Although the ephrin ligand does not contain an intrinsic intracellular enzyme activity, interaction with Eph receptors promotes interaction of the intracellular tail of the ephrin protein with critical signaling proteins.

In addition to the seven subfamilies of PTK receptors outlined here, more subfamilies exist.

Most PTK receptors are thought to be activated by a similar mechanism. Ligand binding to the extracellular region of the receptor induces dimerization of the receptor. Dimerization activates the receptor by promoting autophosphorylation in *trans* of the intracellular tyrosine kinase domains (see Fig. 6-4). In this mechanism, dimerization induces proximity of the intracellular domains, allowing one tyrosine kinase domain to phosphorylate a tyrosine amino acid in the intracellular portion of the partner, and vice versa. The autophosphorylation can activate the tyrosine kinase activity and thereby stimulate the ability to phosphorylate tyrosine amino acids on additional downstream signaling proteins. In addition, autophosphorylation allows downstream signaling proteins to directly bind to the phosphorylated tyrosines of the receptor. SH2 domains have the ability to specifically bind to phosphorylated tyrosines, and proteins containing SH2 domains are often thus recruited to activated PTK receptors. Some of the key signaling proteins that are activated in this manner are discussed more later in this chapter. However, one group of proteins with SH2 domains are collectively referred to as *adaptor proteins*. Grb2 is one example. It consists of an SH2 domain and two SH3 domains. The SH2 domain binds to tyrosine phosphorylated proteins, and the SH3 domain, through its interaction with specific proline-containing sequences, binds to additional signaling proteins. In this way, Grb2 serves as a bridge or adaptor to link an activated receptor to downstream proteins. Another prominent example is insulin receptor substrate-1 (IRS-1), which plays a key role in mediating insulin and IGF-1R signaling. IRS-1 contains a phosphotyrosine-binding (PTB) domain, functionally similar to an SH2 domain, that mediates recruitment to activated insulin or IGF-1Rs. IRS-1 is then phosphorylated on multiple tyrosines, and those phosphotyrosines on IRS-1, in turn, can bind to and recruit a number of signaling proteins. The autophosphorylation-mediated recruitment of PTB and SH2 domain-containing proteins illustrates another important and common concept in signal transduction—activation of a protein, often through a covalent modification such as phosphorylation, can provide a docking site for other signaling proteins to promote the formation of a critical signaling complex.

The PTK receptors are regulated and deactivated through some of the similar mechanisms as discussed previously for GPCRs. Activated PTK receptors can undergo clathrin-mediated internalization. The inside of the endosomes, the membrane-bound vesicles that carry the internalized receptor, becomes acidified, resulting in dissociation of the ligand from the receptor. Like GPCRs, internalized PTK receptors can be recycled back to the cell surface to initiate more signaling or can be subject to degradation; the exact fate depends on the specific receptor and on the specific cell type. PTK receptors are also turned off by dephosphorylation. For example, a cytosolic tyrosine phosphatase termed SHP contains a SH2 domain that mediates recruitment to activated PTK receptors. The binding of SHP to the activated PTK receptor activates the tyrosine phosphatase activity and puts it in close proximity to dephosphorylate and thus deactivate the receptor. In addition, PTK receptors are subject to feedback regulation, and in fact, this is a common mechanism regulating numerous signaling proteins. As an example, several PTK receptors, including EGFRs, activate PKC through a series of signaling steps, and the activated PKC can phosphorylate and thereby inhibit, or turn down, the signaling ability of the receptor. Feedback regulation, in either a positive or a negative way, is another key concept to keep in mind when considering the regulation of a signaling pathway.

PTP Receptors

The PTPs constitute a large family of important signaling proteins,[37] and these are found in two main families, as cytoplasmic completely intracellular proteins and as membrane-spanning receptors. By virtue of their dephosphorylation activity of specifically removing phosphates attached to tyrosines, these proteins counteract the effects of tyrosine kinases. However, they should not be thought of as passive negative-signaling proteins. PTPs play essential signaling roles in coordinating signaling by other proteins, particularly PTK receptors, and controlling the rate and duration of a signaling response.

The PTP receptors possess an architecture similar to that of PTK receptors in that they have a large extracellular region followed by a single transmembrane segment connecting to a large intracellular region that contains the PTP enzyme activity. In spite of such receptor-like structure, surprisingly few ligands have been identified for the PTP receptors. A recent example is the identification of pleiotrophin, a soluble extracellular cytokine, as a ligand for the PTP receptor RPTPζ.[38] Pleiotrophin binding actually inhibits the PTP activity of RPTPζ, and studies with this ligand suggest that in some cases ligand binding to a PTP receptor would enhance tyrosine phosphorylation-mediated signaling by enhancing the tyrosine phosphorylation of specific substrates. Dimerization likely is important for PTP receptor regulation, but in contrast to dimerization-mediated activation of PTK receptors, it appears that dimerization serves to inhibit the PTP activity.

An exciting component of PTP regulation is reversible oxidation. Reactive oxygen species (ROS) not only are damaging molecules but have also been found to have discrete signaling functions,[39] and one key target is a cysteine at the active site of PTPs. For several PTPs, it has been demonstrated that this catalytic cysteine is particularly susceptible to modification by ROS, leading to inhibition of activity. An intriguing regulatory model has been suggested, involving the following steps:

1. Activation of tyrosine kinase signaling, for example, ligand activation of a PTK receptor, would induce localized production of ROS;
2. The ROS would oxidize the critical cysteines of nearby PTPs and thus result in PTP inhibition and enhanced tyrosine phosphorylation and signaling; and
3. The oxidation of PTPs is reversible, and then the PTP would be fully active and able to turn off signaling through dephosphorylation.

In summary, PTPs are key regulators of tyrosine kinase signaling, some of the PTPs function as cell surface receptors capable of regulation by extracellular ligands, and the PTPs are susceptible to many forms of regulation including reversible oxidation.

Serine/Threonine Kinase Receptors

The transforming growth factor β (TGFβ) receptors constitute another important family of enzyme-linked receptors. In this cell-surface family, a single transmembrane segment connects an extracellular ligand-binding domain to an intracellular serine/threonine protein kinase domain.[40] Thus, these receptors signal by transferring a phosphate from ATP to a serine or threonine amino acid in a substrate protein, rather than the tyrosine phosphorylation function of PTK receptors.

The TGFβ ligands constitute a large superfamily of more than 20 different human proteins that are subdivided into three families, TGFβ, activins, and bone morphogenetic proteins (BMP). These extracellular ligands control a wide variety of signaling pathways, including playing critical roles in embryogenesis and development. Some of the ligands function as graded morphogens in development, in that the fate of a cell in a developing organism depends on the concentration of ligand detected. A particular cell will have different signaling responses and an ultimate fate depending upon the cell's position in a concentration gradient of the ligand. TGFβ superfamily ligands also control numerous signaling responses in adult tissues, including proliferation of many cell types, and dysregulation can contribute to many disease states including cancer.

Twelve TGFβ receptors have been identified in mammals, and these receptors utilize a simple and elegant signaling mechanism. The TGFβ receptors are classified as type 1 or type 2; they are structurally similar, but only the type 1 receptors have a critical glycine- and serine-rich region, termed GS sequence, near the kinase domain. Ligand binding induces the formation of a heterotetrameric receptor complex, consisting of two type 1 and two type 2 receptors. The kinase domain of the type 2 receptors then phosphorylate serines in the GS sequence of the type 1 receptor, and this then activates the kinase domain of the type 1 receptors. The type 1 receptor then phosphorylates cytoplasmic proteins call Smads, a family of eight proteins and the only accepted substrates for the TGFβ receptors. After phosphorylation, Smads dissociate from the receptor, form a trimeric Smad complex, and move directly into the cell's nucleus. Once in the nucleus, the Smads function as transcription regulators, mediating the assembly of specific transcription factor complexes, with the end result of regulating the expression of key genes. Thus, basically a single protein transduces the signal from an activated cell-surface receptor to a transcriptional response. This is in striking contrast to signaling pathways initiated by other families of receptors that involve multiple steps, generation of second messengers, and multiple intracellular signaling proteins to generate the biologic response.

GC Receptors

Another variation on the theme of enzyme-linked receptors is provided by the guanylyl cyclase (GC) receptor family. As with the receptors described previously, GC receptors have a large ligand-binding extracellular domain connected via a single transmembrane segment to an intracellular domain with intrinsic enzyme activity. In contrast to the PTP, PTK, and TGFβ receptors, the GC receptors directly produce a diffusible small molecule second messenger, cGMP, rather than regulating the phosphorylation state of another protein.

There are seven different GC receptors, also referred to as membrane-bound GCs or particulate GCs (pGCs).[41,42] GC-A and GC-B are receptors for the natriuretic peptides, atrial natriuretic peptide (ANP), brain natriuretic peptide (BNP), and C-type natriuretic peptide (CNP). ANP is well known for its physiologic role in regulating blood pressure. GC-C is restricted to intestinal mucosal cells and has been identified as the receptor for the heat-stable enterotoxin produced by several bacteria, as well as the endogenous peptides guanylin and uroguanylin. Extracellular ligands have not been identified for the other GC receptor forms, including two retina-specific GCs, GC-E and GC-F, that are essential for signal transduction in the visual system.

GC receptors function as dimers, and they appear to exist as preformed homodimers, even in the absence of ligand. Binding of extracellular ligand to the dimeric GC receptor propagates a change, in a poorly understood manner, through the transmembrane region to activate the intracellular GC activity of the receptor and thus generate cGMP from GTP. The GC receptors utilize an interesting variation of phosphorylation-dependent desensitization to terminate signaling. In the inactive state, the GC receptor is phosphorylated on the intracellular domain, and this phosphorylation is necessary for ligand-dependent activation. However, ligand binding and GC activation then trigger dephosphorylation, leading to desensitization. Rephosphorylation returns the receptor to a state ready to be again activated by ligand. Thus, in contrast to GPCRs in which phosphorylation is a key part of desensitization, for the GC receptors dephosphorylation contributes to desensitization.

Activation of GC receptors causes increased intracellular concentration of cGMP, and the higher levels of cGMP activate various signaling proteins and pathways, leading to important physiologic responses that depend on the cell type. Similar to cAMP, many of the effects of cGMP are mediated through its binding to one of two cGMP-dependent protein kinases, also termed *protein kinase G* (PKG). Upon cGMP binding, PKG is activated to phosphorylate target proteins, only a limited number of which have been clearly identified. In vascular smooth muscle cells, cGMP binding to PKG promotes the ability of PKG to phosphorylate the IP_3 receptor and phospholamban, two key proteins in regulating levels of intracellular Ca^{2+}, ultimately leading to relaxation. Conversely, when ST binds to GC-G receptors in intestinal cells, the increased cGMP levels activate PKG, which in turn, phosphorylates the cystic fibrosis transmembrane conductance regulator (CFTR). This phosphorylation of CFTR leads to its persistent open state and an efflux of chloride ions from the cell, ultimately resulting in massive water transport into the lumen in the intestine and resulting in diarrhea. In addition to PKG, some effects of cGMP are mediated by its direct binding to CNG channels, as mentioned earlier for cAMP. Some CNG channels are more sensitive to cGMP versus cAMP and, thus, preferentially respond to increased levels of cGMP.

It is important to note here that in addition to the membrane-bound forms of GC, a soluble form (sGC) exists and plays critical physiologic roles. Most importantly, sGC is the main accepted receptor for NO gas. NO, which is produced by NO synthases in numerous cells, including nerve cells, is able to freely diffuse through cell membranes and activate sGC in neighboring cells. NO has a short lifetime, on the order of seconds, and thus, its actions are restricted to nearby cells, rather than being able to diffuse to distant cells in the body. sGC contains a bound Fe^{2+}-containing heme group, and NO binds directly to the heme causing a structural perturbation that results in activation of GC activity. One critical example of the importance of NO activation of sGC is that nitroglycerine's effects on the cardiovascular system can be explained because nitroglycerine is converted to NO, which then activates sGC in vascular smooth muscle cells, leading to relaxation and increased blood flow. Thus, sGC is an example of an intracellular receptor for a ligand, in this case a gas molecule, that can diffuse across membranes, thus circumventing the need for a cell-surface receptor. Another key example, discussed later, are the nuclear hormone receptors, intracellular proteins that bind hydrophobic steroid hormones.

OTHER CELL-SURFACE RECEPTOR SIGNALING PARADIGMS

Tyrosine Kinase–Associated Receptors

A number of cell-surface receptors activate intracellular cytoplasmic tyrosine kinases. In contrast to the PTK receptors, the tyrosine kinase is not an integral part of the receptor, but is instead a separate protein that is associated with the receptor. In general, tyrosine kinase–associated receptors have an extracellular ligand-binding domain connected through a single transmembrane domain to a small intracellular region that lacks enzyme activity but can interact with cytoplasmic tyrosine kinases.

The Src family, which includes Src, Fyn, Lyn, Yes, Lck, and Hck, is a major family of cytoplasmic tyrosine kinases. Src kinases are composed of several important parts, including

1. An *N*-terminal lipid modification that promotes association with the cytoplasmic surface of plasma membranes;
2. The catalytic kinase domain;
3. An SH2 domain that can specifically bind phosphotyrosine-containing sequences; and
4. An SH3 domain that binds specific proline-rich sequences.

Studies have revealed a general mechanism for activation of these kinases. They are kept in an inactive closed conformation by intramolecular interactions mediated by both the SH2 and the SH3 domains. The SH2 domain binds to a *C*-terminal phosphotyrosine in the same molecule, and thus, dephosphorylation is part of the activation mechanism that allows a more open conformation. In addition, phosphorylation of an activation loop is required, and this appears to be mediated by one Src phosphorylating another.

Immune cell signaling provides an important example of receptor signaling systems that utilize the Src kinases and other cytoplasmic tyrosine kinases.[43] In T-cell signaling, the Src kinase Lck is associated with the intracellular portion of CD4 or CD8, co-receptors for major histocompatibility complex (MHC)-peptide complexes on antigen presenting cells. The T-cell antigen receptor (TCR) is able to specifically recognize a MHC-peptide complex. When this happens, CD4 or CD8 assists by binding to a nonvariable region of the MHC. This initiates a TCR complex consisting of a number of membrane-bound proteins. Lck becomes activated, and in addition, another Src kinase, Fyn, is recruited to the complex. Then, both Lck and Fyn can phosphorylate specific tyrosine residues on the intracellular regions of components of the TCR complex. These phosphorylation sites are contained within specialized motifs called immunoreceptor tyrosine-based activation motifs (ITAMs). Next, the ITAMs serve as docking sites to recruit and activate members of another family of cytoplasmic tyrosine kinases, called the Syk family. In T-cell signaling, the Syk family kinase is termed ZAP-70. Activated ZAP-70 then phosphorylates additional proteins, such as the adaptors LAT and SLP-76, leading to the recruitment of additional proteins and activation of several signaling pathways necessary for ultimate T-cell activation. A similarly elaborate receptor network with associated tyrosine kinases is required for B-cell signaling.[44] Another example of cytoplasmic tyrosine kinase signaling is described in the next section.

Cytokine Receptors and the Jak-STAT Pathway

A large number of cytokine receptors are grouped together as a family based on the similarity in structure of their ligands, or cytokines, and on the similarity of their signaling mechanism.[45,46] Many of the cytokines—including a large number of interleukins and interferons, as well as erythropoietin, growth hormone, and prolactin—play major roles in regulating hematopoiesis and responses of the immune system. The receptors can consist of a single chain or two or three proteins together, in which the additional chains may function to modulate cytokine-ligand binding. The cytokine receptors have an extracellular ligand-binding domain, like all cell-surface receptors, connected to an intracellular domain by a single transmembrane helix. In contrast to other single transmembrane receptors, such as PTK, PTP, or TGFβ receptors, the intracellular domain of the cytokine receptors does not have intrinsic enzyme activity. Instead, the intracellular domains of the receptors bind to a cytoplasmic PTK of the Jak family (see Fig. 6-4). The role of ligand binding is to bring together, or dimerize, two receptors. This allows the associated Jaks to phosphorylate and activate each other. Thus, this activation mechanism is similar to that used by the PTK receptors, with the main difference that in the PTK receptors, the tyrosine kinase is part of the receptor whereas in the cytokine receptors, the tyrosine kinase is a distinct protein associated with the receptor. A major signaling pathway utilized by the cytokine receptors involves proteins called *signal transducers and activators of transcription* (STATs), a family of proteins that can move into the nucleus to regulate transcription. In this pathway, the activated Jaks then phosphorylate the intracellular domain of the receptor, and this phosphorylation serves to specifically recruit STATs that have an SH2 domain to bind the phosphorylated cytokine receptor. Next, the Jaks phosphorylate the recruited STATs, the STATs dissociate from the receptor, dimerize, and finally, move directly into the nucleus where they directly bind DNA and regulate transcription of target genes. Thus, cytokine receptor/Jak-STAT signaling has similarity to the TGFβ receptor signaling pathway in that a transcription factor is activated at the receptor and then proceeds to directly move into the nucleus, alleviating any requirement for cytoplasmic signaling intermediates.

Wnt/β-Catenin Signaling

The Wnt/β-catenin signaling pathway[47,48] is worth describing not only for its physiologic importance but also because it illustrates another key signal transduction concept—regulated degradation of a signaling protein can provide the switch to turn off or turn on a pathway. The Wnts are extracellular glycoproteins that have a major function of acting as morphogens, that is, ligands that function to specify the cell fates of neighboring cells during development of the organism. However, the Wnt signaling pathway not only functions during development but also has key roles in self-renewal of a variety of adult cells, including regulation of bone mass and maintenance of the epithelium of the small intestine. Disruptions of the Wnt/β-catenin pathway can have serious consequences, for example, promoting cancer of the colon.

The Wnt ligands bind to a family of Wnt receptors called *frizzleds* (Fz) and also must interact on the extracellular surface with a co-receptor, LRP. The Fz family of receptors are architecturally similar to GPCRs; they span the plasma membrane seven times with an extracellular *N*-terminus and an intracellular *C*-terminus. Most work on the Wnt pathway suggested that the Fz receptors do not require heterotrimeric G proteins to activate β-catenin, and thus Fz receptors are typically described as examples of GPCRs, or GPCR-like proteins, that signal independently of G proteins. However, several recent studies have implicated heterotrimeric G proteins in Fz receptor function[49,50]; the degree to which G proteins are required for Wnt signaling is still under active investigation. LRP stands for low-density lipoprotein (LDL) receptor-related protein; it is similar in structure to LDL receptor, which has an extracellular ligand-binding domain for LDL followed by a single transmembrane segment and a short intracellular region lacking in intrinsic enzyme activity. The Wnt ligand interacts with both Fz and LPR to activate signaling.

The key intracellular signaling intermediates are a protein called β-catenin and a protein complex responsible for regulating the degradation of β-catenin. In the absence of Wnt binding to Fz/LRP, β-catenin is constitutively phosphorylated by two serine/threonine kinases, glycogen synthase kinase-3β (GSK-3β) and casein kinase 1 (CK1), that are in a complex with other proteins, including axin and adenomatous polyposis coli (APC). The phosphorylation of β-catenin promotes its rapid degradation, thus keeping the pathway turned off by preventing accumulation of β-catenin. The protein complex is sometimes referred to as the *destruction complex* owing to its key role in mediating the destruction of β-catenin. Although the function of all members of the complex is not completely understood, their physiologic importance is underscored by the clear association of mutations in APC with colon cancer. Mutations in APC have been found in a large percentage of human colon cancers, and these APC mutants are defective in binding β-catenin. Because β-catenin does not bind well to APC and the destruction complex, β-catenin is not properly degraded. Instead, it accumulates and activates transcription of genes in an inappropriate manner that leads to uncontrolled cell proliferation and cancer.

When Wnt ligands bind to Fz/LRP, a protein termed *disheveled* (Dvl) is activated at the intracellular surface of the plasma membrane. The exact signaling sequence is not yet completely understood, but activation of Dvl involves its phosphorylation, paradoxically by GSK-3β and CK1, the kinases also responsible for shutting down this pathway. Activated Dvl then binds axin with the important result that phosphorylation of β-catenin is inhibited. In absence of its phosphorylation, β-catenin accumulates in the cytoplasm and then moves directly into the nucleus, where it activates transcription of several Wnt-responsive genes.

The pathway described previously, that relies on regulated degradation of β-catenin, is called the *canonical Wnt pathway*. Although less well understood, Wnt-activation of Fz receptors can also lead to signaling through other pathways that do not utilize β-catenin. These other mechanisms are called *noncanonical pathways*. Two noncanonical pathways both utilize the Dvl protein to regulate Ca^{2+} signaling and regulate changes in the actin cytoskeleton.[48]

Other important signaling pathways use regulated protein degradation as a signaling switch. One that has been rather well studied is the nuclear factor κB (NF-κB) pathway that functions in a number of inflammatory responses. For example, tumor necrosis factor (TNF) and interleukin-1 (IL-1) are two important proinflammatory cytokines that work through the NF-κB pathway. Binding of these cytokines to their cell-surface receptors leads to a series of protein aggregations and phosphorylations. The key switch is that in the inactive state, NF-κB is bound to an inhibitor called IκB, and this interaction prevents NF-κB from entering the nucleus. However, activation of the pathway leads to phosphorylation of IκB and its subsequent degradation. Then, NF-κB is no longer bound to IκB, and NF-κB moves into the nucleus to regulate the transcription of a large number of genes involved in the inflammatory response. In summary, for the NF-κB pathway, regulated protein degradation provides a critical switch in the turning on of signaling.

Integrin Signaling

Integrins are cell-surface receptors with a unique role in signal transduction. Unlike most cell-surface receptors, these receptors do not bind soluble ligands; instead, they specifically interact with extracellular matrix (ECM) proteins.[51] The ECM consists of a number of large secreted proteins, such as collagen, fibronectin, and laminin. These proteins form an extracellular network with a major role as structural support for surrounding cells. Integrins have large extracellular domains that specifically bind to different ECM proteins, connected by a single transmembrane domain to a small intracellular domain lacking in intrinsic enzyme activity. The intracellular region binds to a wide variety of proteins, but a major function is to bind to intracellular protein complexes that bind the actin cytoskeleton. In this way, integrins provide a link between the intracellular cytoskeleton, which provides structure to the inside of a cell, and the ECM, which provides structure on the outside. When integrins interact with the ECM, they cluster together, and the intracellular proteins they bind organize into complexes called *focal adhesions* that provide points of tight binding to the ECM.

In addition to forming structural linkages to the cytoskeleton, integrin binding to ECM proteins can also stimulate signaling inside the cell. Although many signaling pathways are directed toward ultimately regulating changes in gene expression, much of integrin signaling is confined to activating changes at focal adhesions. These very localized changes occur inside the cell but at or near the cytoplasmic surface of the plasma membrane, where there are contacts with the ECM just on the other side. A major player in integrin signaling is a tyrosine kinase called *focal adhesion kinase* (FAK); indeed, focal adhesions are very prominent sites of tyrosine phosphorylation. FAK-mediated tyrosine phosphorylation of a number of different substrate proteins allows a cell to respond to changes in the ECM by changing the composition of proteins involved in focal adhesions. One important physiologic function for focal adhesions is in cell migration. Many cells in the body need to migrate, for example, to heal wounds and to move to sites of infection. Migrating cells form large protrusions called *lamellipodia*, and focal adhesions function to allow these protrusions to tightly grip the underlying ECM. However, a moving cell must also be able to detach from the ECM in a regulated manner. Thus, changes in signaling within focal adhesions allow these dynamic changes. Moreover, integrins play an important role in unwanted forms of cell migration, such as metastasis of tumor cells.

Ion Channels

Ion channels are essential components of many cell types, but neurons and muscle cells strongly take advantage of these proteins. Ion channels are designed to serve as conduits between the extracellular environment and the cell's cytoplasm. They have the important properties of being able to selectively and rapidly let through inorganic ions, for example, Na^+, K^+, Cl^-, or Ca^{2+}, and they open and close (gated) in response to stimuli. When they open, select ions will flow down an electrochemical gradient. Several different stimuli—including changes in voltage across the membrane, extracellular ligands, and intracellular ligands—regulate, or gate, ion channels. The ion channels that can bind and be regulated by extracellular ligands thus can be considered as extracellular receptors. The ligands for this family of ion channels are neurotransmitters, and thus, these channels are often called *neurotransmitter-gated ion channels.*

The typical neurotransmitter-gated ion channel consists of five subunits, and each subunit consists of four connected transmembrane segments with the *N*-terminus and the *C*-terminus of the subunit both located extracellularly. The five subunits are arranged in the membrane in a circle to form a selective ion pore. The neurotransmitter-gated ion channels are divided into three families: (i) the nicotinic receptor family, including the glycine, serotonin, nicotinic acetylcholine, and $GABA_A$ receptors; (ii) the glutamate receptor family; and (iii) the ionotropic ATP receptors.[52] Neurotransmitter-gated ion channels can be excitatory or inhibitory. Excitatory neurotransmitters cause an opening of Na^+ channels that leads to a local depolarization across the membrane, which in turn, leads to opening of voltage-gated ion channels, further depolarization, and a resulting action potential to mediate electrical responses. Inhibitory neurotransmitters typically cause the opening of Cl^- or K^+ channels, and this decreases signaling by making it more difficult for the cell to depolarize the membrane.

Ion channels in general and neurotransmitter-gated ion channels in particular are extremely important targets for natural toxins and pharmacologic therapeutics. For example, neurotoxins in snake venom, such as α-bungarotoxin, and natural products from plants, such as curare, function by binding to and blocking the acetylcholine neurotransmitter-gated ion channel, causing loss of muscle function and paralysis. Moreover, many psychoactive drugs target neurotransmitter-gated ion channels directly or regulate the availability of the neurotransmitter ligand. Lastly, a number of inherited human diseases, including certain forms of epilepsy, have been linked to mutations in ion channels, including the neurotransmitter-gated ion channels, and, collectively these have been referred to as *channelopathies.*[52]

NUCLEAR HORMONE RECEPTORS

Although most signaling pathways are initiated by binding of a ligand to a receptor on the extracellular surface of a cell, some molecules interact with intracellular receptors by diffusing across the membrane barrier and thus directly moving from the extracellular milieu to the inside of cell. The nuclear hormone receptors represent the most prominent family of intracellular receptors. In principle, nuclear hormone receptor signaling is the simplest signal transduction pathway—the intracellular receptor is also the ultimate effector. The nuclear hormone receptors not only bind the hormone ligand but also are able to directly bind DNA and function as transcription factors to regulate gene expression.

The nuclear hormone receptors are also sometimes called the *steroid hormone receptors* because many of these receptors bind to cholesterol-derived steroid hormones, such as estradiol and testosterone. However, other ligands are not steroids. Nonetheless, the nuclear hormone receptors include intracellular receptors for many critical small molecules; the list includes estrogen, androgen, progesterone, glucocorticoid, mineralocorticoid, thyroid hormone, vitamin D, and retinoic acid receptors. Because the ligands are typically hydrophobic, many of them are associated with binding proteins to keep them soluble in the aqueous bloodstream.

These receptors all have a number of features in common (Fig. 6-5). First, they all have a common architecture that includes a ligand-binding domain, a DNA-binding domain, and a transactivation domain that allows the activated receptor to bind to other proteins of the transcriptional machinery. Second, these receptors are termed *nuclear hormone receptors* because their site of action is the nucleus where they bind DNA to regulate expression of subsets of genes. Interestingly, many of the nuclear hormone receptors also shuttle back and forth between the nucleus and the cytoplasm.[53] In absence of bound hormone, some of the receptors are predominantly located in the cytoplasm, whereas others are mostly nuclear. Thus, some ligands bind to cytoplasmic receptors, and then the activated receptors move into the nucleus, whereas other ligands diffuse into the nucleus before encountering their receptor. A third similarity of the nuclear hormone receptors is that when bound to ligand, they all bind DNA as dimers. In some cases, the receptors are homodimers, whereas others heterodimerize with other nuclear hormone receptors.

Ultimately, the physiologic response depends upon the set of genes whose expression is regulated in response to a ligand-activated nuclear receptor. In different cell types, different regulatory proteins may be available to interact with a particular receptor such that an activated receptor could regulate different sets of genes in different cells. Lastly, there are exceptions to the classic function of nuclear hormone receptors. Several hormones produce signal responses quite rapidly, and

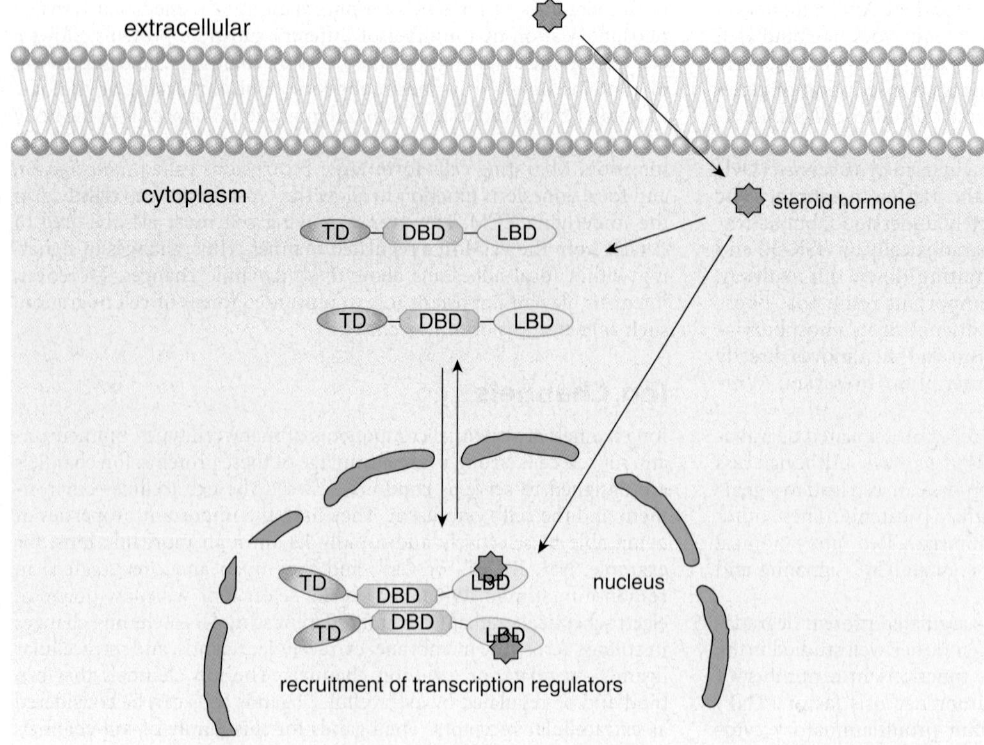

FIGURE 6-5 • Nuclear hormone receptors. In this mode of signaling, a hydrophobic ligand, such as a steroid hormone, can directly enter a cell to bind to nuclear hormone receptors. Hormone binding to the ligand-binding domain (LBD) can occur in the cytoplasm or the nucleus, depending on the receptor type. In general, hormone binding releases inhibitory proteins and induces dimerization of the receptor. This activated receptor moves into the nucleus, or is there already, where it directly binds DNA as a dimer through the DNA binding domains (DBD). The transactivation domain (TD) of the receptor can bind and recruit additional transcription factors to the DNA and, thus, regulate expression of target genes.

these rapid responses are incompatible with nuclear hormone receptor signaling solely mediated by changes in gene expression, which would take place on a timescale of hours.[54] Although many of these rapid (seconds or minutes) signaling responses are not well understood, it is clear that nuclear hormone receptors can interact with other signaling intermediaries to promote short-term changes such as phosphorylation. Another way that ligands such as steroid hormones can induce rapid signaling responses is by binding receptors other than the classic nuclear hormone receptors. For example, it has been recently demonstrated that estrogen can function as an agonist for a GPCR in addition to its nuclear hormone receptor.[55]

INTRACELLULAR SIGNALING PATHWAYS

A number of different signaling pathways connect activated receptors to intracellular changes in metabolism and nuclear changes in gene transcription, in addition to pathways described previously, such as cAMP and IP_3 signaling. This section highlights several well-studied pathways that connect multiple families of receptors to intracellular events.

Ras Signaling

Ras proteins are monomeric guanine-nucleotide binding proteins, often termed *small GTPases*, that play essential roles in cell differentiation and proliferation.[56,57] The term *Ras superfamily* is often used to describe a large family of over 100 members. The superfamily is divided into several groups including the Ras subfamily, containing approximately 12 members. Within the Ras subfamily are four classic and well-studied Ras proteins, termed *N-Ras*, *H-Ras*, *K-Ras4A*, and *K-Ras4B*, and indeed, these four are typically the subject when "Ras proteins" are discussed. The important role of these proteins is underscored by the multitude of findings showing that a large percentage of human tumors contain mutant forms of Ras, mostly K-Ras.

Ras proteins cycle between guanine-nucleotide bound states, binding to GDP in the inactive form and GTP in the active form (see Fig. 6-2). A family of guanine-nucleotide exchange factors (GEFs) promote the GDP-to-GTP transition. Ras proteins are also able to hydrolyze bound GTP to turn off and return to the GDP-bound state, although they do this very poorly by themselves and require interaction with a GTPase activating protein (GAP). Thus, Ras small GTPases (all members of the superfamily) function as molecular switches, identically to that described previously for the heterotrimeric G proteins. The key differences are that (i) Ras small GTPases are monomeric and do not require additional subunits, like $G\beta\gamma$; and (ii) the RasGEFs are intracellular signaling intermediates, rather than the cell-surface, extracellular ligand-binding GPCRs.

Ras small GTPases are typically associated with the cytoplasmic surface of the plasma membrane, or other intracellular membranes, owing to their modification by lipids, particularly the farnesyl or geranylgeranyl isoprenoid. In this way, they are also similar to the heterotrimeric G proteins and indeed many peripheral membrane-associated signaling proteins.[19,58] Ras is thus usually activated at a membrane location by a RasGEF. A number of different RasGEFs exist; almost all share the common feature of a domain that specifically activates Ras. Otherwise, the RasGEFs can be quite different, with various regions that allow them to detect and integrate a variety of signals. Thus, RasGEFs are responsible for recognizing signaling initiated by distinct cell-surface receptor systems and translating that into activation of Ras. One key signaling RasGEF is Sos, which is responsible for mediating PTK receptor activation of Ras. Sos contains a proline-rich region that allows it to bind to an SH3 domain of Grb2. Recall that Grb2 also has an SH2 domain that allows it to interact with specific phosphotyrosines on an activated PTK receptor, such as the EGFR. The end result is that the activation of a PTK receptor by an extracellular ligand can induce an intracellular complex of PTK receptor/Grb2/Sos that is now competent to directly activate Ras. Additional RasGEFs are activated and recruited to the plasma membrane through their ability to bind DAG and Ca^{2+}. In all cases, active Ras is then able to interact with a number of effector proteins to initiate intracellular signaling pathways. The most well-studied pathway that Ras activates is termed the *MAP kinase cascade*, a series of protein kinases that serially phosphorylate each other to eventually propagate a signal to nuclear changes in gene expression. In this pathway, the direct effector for Ras is the protein kinase Raf. Activated Ras recruits Raf to the membrane, where a signaling cascade is initiated; some details of MAP kinase cascades are discussed later. In addition, a small family of RasGAPs exists to turn off Ras signaling. These proteins also contain domains additional to the GAP domain; these other domains allow the GAPs to localize to specific protein complexes in order to turn off Ras signaling in a regulated manner, again emphasizing the point that both the activation and the deactivation of signaling proteins are tightly regulated.

The Rho Family of Small GTPases

The Rho family, consisting of approximately 20 members, is another subclass of the Ras superfamily of small GTPases. Although the Rho GTPases share a number of attributes with the Ras GTPases that were discussed previously, the Rho GTPases are briefly discussed here because they regulate unique and important signaling pathways.[59] Of particular interest, Rho GTPases are responsible for coupling activated cell-surface receptors to rapid changes in a cell's cytoskeleton architecture.

As described previously for Ras, Rho GTPases cycle between inactive GDP-bound states and active GTP-bound states. Families of RhoGEFs and RhoGAPs directly promote turn-on and turn-off, respectively. The RhoGEFs constitute an exceptionally large family of approximately 80 members, many of which were originally identified in screens for genes that would oncogenically transform cells. The RhoGEFs all have in common a domain that promotes GDP release from Rho GTPases, but they differ in that they are generally quite large proteins with multiple additional domains that allow them to detect inputs from a variety of receptors. For example, some RhoGEFs have SH2 domains that allow them to bind to phosphotyrosines and thus connect tyrosine kinase signaling to Rho activation, whereas another subgroup has RGS domains that allow them to directly bind to certain $G\alpha$.

When activated, Rho GTPases directly bind to a number of different effector proteins to regulate various responses, including development, cell proliferation, and cell differentiation. However, one unique aspect of Rho function is the ability to regulate changes in the actin cytoskeleton. The Rho GTPases can be further subdivided into three categories—Rho, Rac, and Cdc42—and each one can regulate different aspects of actin changes. Such changes in a cell's actin cytoskeleton are essential for a cell changing its shape, including retraction and extension of neurites, platelet shape changes, contraction of muscle cells, and migration of cells, both in normal processes, such as wound healing or movement of immune cells, and in disease states, such as metastasis of cancer cells. The Rho GTPases carry out their actin remodeling function by directly activating additional proteins that bind to actin. In migrating cells, Cdc42 can promote spiky extensions from cells called *filopodia*; these extensions are often a way for a cell to search out clues to its extracellular environment. Rac can promote the extension of large membrane protusions that allow the cell to move forward, and conversely, activated Rho stimulates large bundles of actin termed *stress fibers* that play roles in retraction of the trailing edge of the cell.

MAPK Signaling

MAPKs function in discrete modules to send signals from activated receptors to nuclear changes in gene expression. As the name implies, the MAPK pathway plays a fundamental role in transmitting signals for cell proliferation from mitogenic receptors, such as growth factor receptors.

The defining characteristic of MAPK signaling is a module of three protein kinases that sequentially phosphorylate and activate each other. In generic terms, a three-member MAPK module consists of a MAPK, a MAPK kinase (MAPKK), and a MAPK kinase kinase (MAPKKK). MAPK signaling can be separated into three basic modules, the extracellular signal-regulated kinase (ERK) pathway, the c-Jun *N*-terminal kinase (JNK) pathway, and the p38 MAPK pathway. The ERK module is the prototypical MAPK pathway, and the one activated by the small GTPase Ras. As described previously, activated Ras binds to and activates the protein kinase Raf, and this kinase serves as a MAPKKK, that is, the first kinase in the ERK module. Activated Raf then specifically phosphorylates a kinase termed MEK, for MAPK/ERK kinase. MEK, functioning as a MAPKK, then phosphorylates ERK. The MEKs are unique in that they can phosphorylate both a tyrosine and a threonine in a critical activation loop of ERK; this dual phosphorylation is essential for activation of ERK. After this sequential activation, the ERKs then are able to phosphorylate a number of different substrate proteins, but one of the major roles of activated ERK is to directly translocate from the cytoplasm into the nucleus, where it phosphorylates several transcription factors to ultimately regulate the expression of genes that regulate cell proliferation or differentiation.

Interestingly, activation of the same signaling pathway by different receptors can often cause different biologic responses, and the MAPK ERK module provides such an example. In pheochromocytoma PC12 cells, addition of EGF induces proliferation but NGF promotes differentiation instead of proliferation. However, both growth factors activate the same MAPK signaling pathway, leading to activation of ERK. The critical difference appears to be that EGF induces a rapid and strong but transient activation of ERK, whereas NGF promotes a slower but sustained activation of ERK.[60,61] This illustrates how mere differences in the time of activation of a signaling protein can be responsible for dramatically different, or even opposing, physiologic responses. Although it is not completely understood how the different kinetics of ERK activation occur, clearly EGF and NGF stimulation are differentially regulating key regulators of the MAPK pathway, such as scaffolding proteins and phosphatases.

The other two main MAPK modules differ from the ERK module in that the JNK and p38 MAPK modules typically are used to transduce stress, rather than mitogenic, signals. Some of the stresses that activate the JNK or p38 MAPK pathways include ultraviolet irradiation, heat shock, changes in osmolarity, inflammatory cytokines, and the septic shock–inducing bacterial endotoxin lipopolysaccharide. Although the actual MAPKKKs, MAPKKs, and MAPKs are different in each module, the basic function of sequential phosphorylation is preserved. Key differences are in the input and output from the MAPK module. For example, the JNK and p38 MAPK pathways are not typically activated by Ras but, instead, can be a result of the activation of other small GTPases, particularly Rac1 and Cdc42, members of the Rho family of small GTPases. In addition, JNK and p38 MAPK, the ultimate MAPKs in the JNK and p38 MAPK modules, respectively, phosphorylate different proteins compared with ERK in order to stimulate the appropriate transcriptional responses.

Another key characteristic of MAPK signaling is the presence of scaffolding proteins that can bind to all three members of a MAPK module. A number of different proteins can serve this scaffolding function. Keeping a MAPK module together via interaction with a scaffolding protein plays an important role in maintaining the exquisite specificity of a pathway; a MAPKKK will thus only phosphorylate a MAPKK that is in proximity in the same complex, and likewise for phosphorylation of the MAPK by the MAPKK. Moreover, different scaffolds can allow the same signaling proteins to be used to respond to different stimuli.

Phosphatidylinositol 3-Kinase/Akt Signaling

The phosphatidylinositol 3-kinase (PI3-K) pathway is another important and ubiquitous intracellular signaling pathway[62] that also illustrates the importance of the phospholipid membranes as key signaling components, as also described previosuly for PLC signaling. PI_3-Ks transfer a phosphate from ATP to the 3′ position of the six-member inositol ring of phosphatidylinositol (PI). Various phosphorylated forms of PI can be used as the substrate by PI3-K to generate the membrane lipids PI(3)-P, PI(3,4)-P_2, PI(3,5)-P_2, and PI(3,4,5)-P_2, and these lipids, containing a phosphate at the 3′ position, provide highly specific binding sites for recruiting to membranes and activating select signaling proteins. The PI_3-Ks are divided into three classes with class I being the most well understood in terms of coupling signals from activated receptors to intracellular responses. The two main lipid products generated by class I PI3-Ks are PI(3,4)-P_2 and PI(3,4,5)-P_2.

The class I PI_3-Ks are further divided into class IA and class IB based on how they are activated. The class IA PI_3-Ks consist of three proteins that associate with one of five different regulatory subunits. The regulatory subunits play critical roles in determining how the PI_3-K is activated. The regulatory subunits that associate with the class IA enzymes have the common feature of containing multiple SH2 domains that specifically bind to tyrosine phosphorylated proteins. Thus, the class IA PI_3-Ks are typically recruited to the cytoplasmic face of the plasma membrane by binding to specific phosphotyrosine-containing regions of activated PTK receptors or adapter proteins that have been phosphorylated by PTK receptors. Whereas the class IA PI_3-Ks predominantly function in coupling tyrosine kinase signaling to downstream responses, the class IB PI_3-Ks are activated in response to GPCR activation. In particular, Gβγ, released by GPCR activation of heterotrimeric G proteins, interacts with a regulatory subunit of the class IB PI_3-Ks and thus activates the PI3-K activity of the catalytic subunit.

As mentioned previously, PI_3-Ks signal by generating novel phosphatidylinositol lipid products, mainly PI(3,4)-P_2 and PI(3,4,5)-P_2. The main function of these lipids seems to be to provide a new binding site for certain proteins. Several well-described protein domains function to bind PI(3,4)-P_2 and/or PI(3,4,5)-P_2, and one such domain found in a multitude of signaling proteins is the pleckstrin homology (PH) domain. PH domain–containing proteins are thus often recruited to membrane sites of PI(3,4)-P_2 and/or PI(3,4,5)-P_2 generation; this membrane binding plays an important role in generating stable signaling complexes that further relay a signal down distinct pathways.

A prototypical PI(3,4,5)-P_2 responsive pathway is the Akt pathway. In this pathway, two protein kinases, PDK1 and Akt, have PH domains and are recruited to the plasma membrane in response to PI3-K activation. PDK1 and another protein kinase further activate Akt. Once activated, Akt can dissociate back into the cytoplasm, where it serves as a master regulator of a number of different pathways by phosphorylating many protein substrates. Physiologic responses regulated by Akt include cell proliferation, cell survival, and regulation of cell metabolism in insulin signaling. In cell survival, Akt activation leads to an inhibition of apoptosis, a cell's regulated death response. Akt plays this role by phosphorylating and inactivating key proteins such as the pro-apoptotic Bad protein and proteins that lead to enhanced expression of additional pro-apoptotic proteins. Enhanced Akt signaling is often found in cancer cells, and cancer cells use this activated Akt signaling to maintain survival and override the cell's mechanisms to terminate the cell.

The PI3-K pathway provides another excellent example of the importance of deactivation or turning off signaling. A protein termed PTEN is a phosphatase that removes the 3′ phosphate of PI(3,4)-P_2 and PI(3,4,5)-P_2 and thus counteracts the effect of PI3-K. In fact, the 3′ phosphorylated PI products are rather rare; in general it is believed that they are only present in membranes after a pulse of PI3-K activation. PTEN makes sure that PI(3,4)-P_2 and PI(3,4,5)-P_2 are not available for too long. PTEN's importance is underscored by the findings that its function is inactivated or decreased in a high percentage of tumors. Thus, PTEN is a tumor suppressor; its loss leads to longer-lived PI(3,4)-P_2 and PI(3,4,5)-P_2, which leads to overactive Akt signaling.

REFERENCES

1. Ben-Shlomo I, Yu Hsu S, Rauch R, et al. Signaling receptome: a genomic and evolutionary perspective of plasma membrane receptors involved in signal transduction. Sci STKE 2003;2003(187):RE9.
2. Bradshaw RA, Dennis EA (eds). Handbook of Cell Signaling. Philadelphia: Elsevier, 2003.
3. Marinissen MJ, Gutkind JS. G-protein-coupled receptors and signaling networks: emerging paradigms. Trends Pharmacol Sci 2001;22(7):368-376.

4. Pierce KL, Premont RT, Lefkowitz RJ. Seven-transmembrane receptors. Nat Rev Mol Cell Biol 2002;3(9):639-650.
5. Dinulescu DM, Cone RD. Agouti and agouti-related protein: analogies and contrasts. J Biol Chem 2000;275(10):6695-6698.
6. Kenakin T. Allosteric modulators: the new generation of receptor antagonist. Mol Interv 2004;4(4):222-229.
7. Kristiansen K. Molecular mechanisms of ligand binding, signaling, and regulation within the superfamily of G-protein-coupled receptors: molecular modeling and mutagenesis approaches to receptor structure and function. Pharmacol Ther 2004;103(1):21-80.
8. Vu TK, Hung DT, Wheaton VI, Coughlin SR. Molecular cloning of a functional thrombin receptor reveals a novel proteolytic mechanism of receptor activation. Cell 1991;64(6):1057-1068.
9. Palczewski K. G protein-coupled receptor rhodopsin. Annu Rev Biochem 2006;75:743-767.
10. Ridge KD, Palczewski K. Visual rhodopsin sees the light: structure and mechanism of G protein signaling. J Biol Chem 2007;282:9297–9301.
11. Cabrera-Vera TM, Vanhauwe J, Thomas TO, et al. Insights into G protein structure, function, and regulation. Endocr Rev 2003;24(6):765-781.
12. Goodman OB Jr, Krupnick JG, Santini F, et al. Beta-arrestin acts as a clathrin adaptor in endocytosis of the beta2-adrenergic receptor. Nature 1996;383(6599):447-450.
13. Laporte SA, Oakley RH, Zhang J, et al. The beta2-adrenergic receptor/betaarrestin complex recruits the clathrin adaptor AP-2 during endocytosis. Proc Natl Acad Sci U S A 1999;96(7):3712-3717.
14. Schwindinger WF, Robishaw JD. Heterotrimeric G-protein betagamma-dimers in growth and differentiation. Oncogene 2001;20(13):1653-1660.
15. Hollinger S, Hepler JR. Cellular regulation of RGS proteins: modulators and integrators of G protein signaling. Pharmacol Rev 2002;54(3):527-559.
16. Ross EM, Wilkie TM. GTPase-activating proteins for heterotrimeric G proteins: regulators of G protein signaling (RGS) and RGS-like proteins. Annu Rev Biochem 2000;69:795-827.
17. Chidiac P, Roy AA. Activity, regulation, and intracellular localization of RGS proteins. Receptors Channels 2003;9(3):135-147.
18. Blumer JB, Smrcka AV, Lanier SM. Mechanistic pathways and biological roles for receptor-independent activators of G-protein signaling. Pharmacol Ther 2006;113: 488-506.
19. Resh MD. Trafficking and signaling by fatty-acylated and prenylated proteins. Nat Chem Biol 2006;2(11):584-590.
20. Marrari Y, Crouthamel M, Irannejad R, Wedegaertner PB. Assembly and trafficking of heterotrimeric G proteins, Biochemistry 2007;46(26):7665-7677.
21. Sunahara RK, Taussig R. Isoforms of mammalian adenylyl cyclase: multiplicities of signaling. Mol Interv 2002;2(3):168-184.
22. Matulef K, Zagotta WN. Cyclic nucleotide-gated ion channels. Annu Rev Cell Dev Biol 2003;19:23-44.
23. Holz GG, Kang G, Harbeck M, et al. Cell physiology of cAMP sensor Epac. J Physiol 2006;577(Pt 1):5-15.
24. Schmidt M, Sand C, Jakobs KH, et al. Epac and the cardiovascular system. Curr Opin Pharmacol 2007;7:193-200.
25. Kawasaki H, Springett GM, Mochizuki N, et al. A family of cAMP-binding proteins that directly activate Rap1. Science 1998;282(5397):2275-2279.
26. de Rooij J, Zwartkruis FJ, Verheijen MH, et al. Epac is a Rap1 guanine-nucleotide-exchange factor directly activated by cyclic AMP. Nature 1998;396(6710):474-477.
27. Bender AT, Beavo JA. Cyclic nucleotide phosphodiesterases: molecular regulation to clinical use. Pharmacol Rev 2006;58(3):488-520.
28. Wong W, Scott JD. AKAP signalling complexes: focal points in space and time. Nat Rev Mol Cell Biol 2004;5(12):959-970.
29. Rebecchi MJ, Pentyala SN. Structure, function, and control of phosphoinositide-specific phospholipase C. Physiol Rev 2000;80(4):1291-1335.
30. Rhee SG. Regulation of phosphoinositide-specific phospholipase C. Annu Rev Biochem 2001;70:281-312.
31. Bunney TD, Katan M. Phospholipase C epsilon: linking second messengers and small GTPases. Trends Cell Biol 2006;16(12):640-648.
32. Berridge MJ, Bootman MD, Roderick HL. Calcium signalling: dynamics, homeostasis and remodelling. Nat Rev Mol Cell Biol 2003;4(7):517-529.
33. Blume-Jensen P, Hunter T. Oncogenic kinase signalling. Nature 2001;411(6835):355-365.
34. Edwin F, Wiepz GJ, Singh R, et al. A historical perspective of the EGF receptor and related systems. Methods Mol Biol 2006;327:1-24.
35. Ullrich A, Coussens L, Hayflick JS, et al. Human epidermal growth factor receptor cDNA sequence and aberrant expression of the amplified gene in A431 epidermoid carcinoma cells. Nature 1984;309(5967):418-425.
36. Lin CR, Chen WS, Kruiger W, et al. Expression cloning of human EGF receptor complementary DNA: gene amplification and three related messenger RNA products in A431 cells. Science 1984;224(4651):843-848.
37. Tonks NK. Protein tyrosine phosphatases: from genes, to function, to disease. Nat Rev Mol Cell Biol 2006;7(11):833-846.
38. Meng K, Rodriguez-Pena A, Dimitrov T, et al. Pleiotrophin signals increased tyrosine phosphorylation of beta beta-catenin through inactivation of the intrinsic catalytic activity of the receptor-type protein tyrosine phosphatase beta/zeta. Proc Natl Acad Sci U S A 2000;97(6):2603-2608.
39. Giles GI. The redox regulation of thiol dependent signaling pathways in cancer. Curr Pharm Des 2006;12(34):4427-4443.
40. Feng XH, Derynck R. Specificity and versatility in tgf-beta signaling through Smads. Annu Rev Cell Dev Biol 2005;21:659-693.
41. Lucas KA, Pitari GM, Kazerounian S, et al. Guanylyl cyclases and signaling by cyclic GMP. Pharmacol Rev 2000;52(3):375-414.
42. Padayatti PS, Pattanaik P, Ma X, van den Akker F. Structural insights into the regulation and the activation mechanism of mammalian guanylyl cyclases. Pharmacol Ther 2004;104(2):83-99.
43. Palacios EH, Weiss A. Function of the Src-family kinases, Lck and Fyn, in T-cell development and activation. Oncogene 2004;23(48):7990-8000.
44. Gauld SB, Cambier JC. Src-family kinases in B-cell development and signaling. Oncogene 2004;23(48):8001-8006.
45. Murray PJ. The JAK-STAT signaling pathway: input and output integration. J Immunol 2007;178(5):2623-2629.
46. Kisseleva T, Bhattacharya S, Braunstein J, Schindler CW. Signaling through the JAK/STAT pathway, recent advances and future challenges. Gene 2002;285(1-2):1-24.
47. Clevers H. Wnt/beta-catenin signaling in development and disease. Cell 2006;127(3): 469-480.
48. Montcouquiol M, Crenshaw EB 3rd, Kelley MW. Noncanonical Wnt signaling and neural polarity. Annu Rev Neurosci 2006;29:363-386.
49. Wang HY, Liu T, Malbon CC. Structure-function analysis of Frizzleds. Cell Signal 2006;18(7):934-941.
50. Katanaev VL, Ponzielli R, Semeriva M, Tomlinson A. Trimeric G protein-dependent frizzled signaling in Drosophila. Cell 2005;120(1):111-122.
51. van der Flier A, Sonnenberg A. Function and interactions of integrins. Cell Tissue Res 2001;305(3):285-298.
52. Kullmann DM. The neuronal channelopathies. Brain 2002;125(Pt 6):1177-1195.
53. Kumar S, Saradhi M, Chaturvedi NK, Tyagi RK. Intracellular localization and nucleo-cytoplasmic trafficking of steroid receptors: an overview. Mol Cell Endocrinol 2006;246(1-2):147-156.
54. Farach-Carson MC, Davis PJ. Steroid hormone interactions with target cells: cross talk between membrane and nuclear pathways. J Pharmacol Exp Ther 2003;307(3):839-845.
55. Prossnitz ER, Arterburn JB, Sklar LA. GPR30: A G protein-coupled receptor for estrogen. Mol Cell Endocrinol 2007;265-266:138-142.
56. Ehrhardt A, Ehrhardt GR, Guo X, Schrader JW. Ras and relatives—job sharing and networking keep an old family together. Exp Hematol 2002;30(10):1089-1106.
57. Plowman SJ, Hancock JF. Ras signaling from plasma membrane and endomembrane microdomains. Biochim Biophys Acta 2005;1746(3):274-283.
58. Smotrys JE, Linder ME. Palmitoylation of intracellular signaling proteins: regulation and function. Annu Rev Biochem 2004;73:559-587.
59. Jaffe AB, Hall A. Rho GTPases: biochemistry and biology. Annu Rev Cell Dev Biol 2005;21:247-269.
60. Marshall CJ. Specificity of receptor tyrosine kinase signaling: transient versus sustained extracellular signal-regulated kinase activation. Cell 1995;80(2):179-185.
61. Traverse S, Gomez N, Paterson H, et al. Sustained activation of the mitogen-activated protein (MAP) kinase cascade may be required for differentiation of PC12 cells. Comparison of the effects of nerve growth factor and epidermal growth factor. Biochem J 1992;288(Pt 2):351-355.
62. Engelman JA, Luo J, Cantley LC. The evolution of phosphatidylinositol 3-kinases as regulators of growth and metabolism. Nat Rev Genet 2006;7(8):606-619.

7

CELL CYCLE PHARMACOLOGY, ANTIPROLIFERATION, AND APOPTOSIS

Sarah A. Holstein and Raymond J. Hohl

INTRODUCTION 83
CELL CYCLE PHARMACOLOGY 83
S Phase 83
Antifolate Agents 83
Pyrimidine Analogues 83
Cytosine Arabinoside 84
Purine Analogues 84
M Phase 84
Vinca Alkaloids 84
Taxanes 84
Cyclin-Dependent Kinase Inhibitors 84
Specific cdk Inhibitors 84
Nonspecific cdk Inhibitors 84
ANTIPROLIFERATION 85
Growth Factor Receptor Inhibitors 85
Monoclonal Antibodies 85
Tyrosine Kinase Inhibitors 85
Ras Inhibitors 86
Raf Inhibitors 86
MEK Inhibitors 86
APOPTOSIS 86
The Intrinsic Pathway 86
Intrinsic Pathway Targets 86
The Extrinsic Pathway 87
Extrinsic Pathway Targets 87
Nuclear Factor-κB 88

INTRODUCTION

The application of pharmacologic agents to manipulate the cell cycle has broad application not only to cancer therapies but also to manipulate the immune system and more recently, when impregnated in intravascular stents, to treat vascular diseases. The first agents to intentionally disrupt cell proliferation were the nonspecific DNA-damaging agents, the alkylating agents. Nitrogen mustard was initially used as a chemical warfare agent in World War I, and it was only during the Second World War that its use as a chemotherapy agent was exploited by the pharmacology pioneers Louis Goodman and Alfred Gilman. Although the exact mechanisms by which DNA alkylation is cytotoxic are either obvious or increasingly complex depending upon individual perspectives, the comparatively nonspecific nature of the damage will exclude it from consideration in this chapter. The disease-specific chapters in this textbook will, however, highlight many of the alkylating agents as they have widespread clinical utility. The focus of this chapter is on the somewhat more specific agents that are known to interfere with cell cycling and signal transduction and to induce apoptosis. In this context, the reader is directed to Figures 7-1 through 7-3, which detail the cell cycle (Fig. 7-1), a common signal transduction pathway (Fig. 7-2), and the extrinsic and intrinsic apoptotic pathways (Fig. 7-3). Each of these figures is annotated with the agents or class of agents that predominantly affect their specific steps.

CELL CYCLE PHARMACOLOGY

Figure 7-1 displays the classic cell cycle with movement through growth phase 1 (G_1), the period of DNA synthesis (S), growth phase 2 (G_2), and the process of mitosis itself (M). The agents first used to intentionally affect this pathway generally targeted S and M phases.

S Phase

Antifolate Agents

Methotrexate inhibits dihydrofolate reductase and thus leads to disruption of DNA and RNA synthesis. The primary toxicities include cytopenias and mucositis; however, nephrotoxicity, interstitial nephritis, and hepatic dysfunction may occur. Low-dose methotrexate is used in a variety of rheumatologic disorders, including rheumatoid arthritis and psoriasis. Methotrexate has found widespread use as a chemotherapy agent, including non-Hodgkin's lymphoma, acute lymphoblastic leukemia, osteosarcoma, choriocarcinoma, and breast cancer. High-dose methotrexate is given with a leucovorin rescue to prevent severe toxicities. Methotrexate may also be given intrathecally and is of use in the management of meningeal carcinomatosis as well as meningeal leukemia or lymphoma.

More recently, pemetrexed, another antifolate agent, has been developed and is now used in clinical practice. This agent inhibits thymidylate synthase, dihydrofolate reductase, glycinamide ribonucleotide formyltransferase, and aminoimidazole carboxamide ribonucleotide formyltransferase, thus inhibiting purine and thymidine nucleotide synthesis.[1] This agent is given intravenously and undergoes minimal metabolism. Currently pemetrexed is used in the treatment of non–small cell lung cancer, bladder cancer, and mesothelioma. The use of pemetrexed in other malignancies is being explored.

Pyrimidine Analogues

5-Fluorouracil (5-FU) belongs to the class of halogenated pyrimidines. In order to be active, 5-FU must be converted to the nucleotide. 5-FU is incorporated into RNA, resulting in inhibition of RNA processing, as well as into DNA. In addition, 5-fluoro-2′-deoxyuridine-5′-phosphate inhibits thymidylate synthase. Resistance to 5-FU has been associated with decreased activity of enzymes required to activate 5-FU, amplification of thymidylate synthase,[2] or mutations in thymidylate synthase.[3] 5-FU is inactivated by dihydropyrimidine dehydrogenase, and deficiency of this enzyme has been associated with increased drug toxicity.[4,5] 5-FU remains the backbone of therapy for colorectal cancer. In addition, 5-FU is used in the treatment of other gastrointestinal malignancies, breast cancer, and head and neck cancer. 5-FU–containing regimens for colorectal cancer generally include the use of leucovorin, which is thought to improve formation of the complex with thymidylate synthase and to enhance clinical responses.

Capecitabine is an oral prodrug of 5-FU. Activation of capecitabine involves conversion to 5′-deoxy-5-fluorocytidine in the liver via carboxylesterase, followed by conversion to 5′-deoxy-5-fluorouridine in the liver and tumor tissues by cytidine deaminase, and then to 5-FU by thymidine phosphorylase in tumor tissues. Thus, in addition to having the advantage of being an oral medication, treatment with capecitabine is thought to lead to increased concentration in tumor tissues.[6] Like 5-FU, capecitabine has found clinical application in the treatment of colorectal cancer and breast cancer.

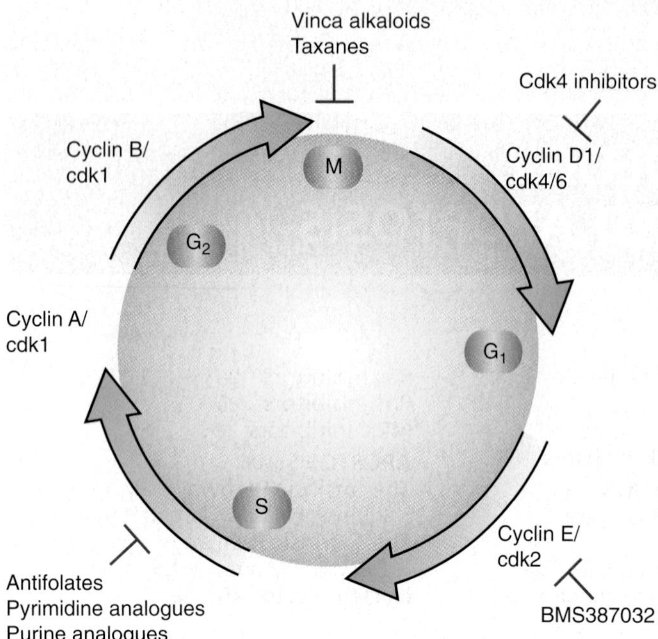

FIGURE 7-1 • The cell cycle.

Cytosine Arabinoside

Cytosine arabinoside (ara-C) is an analogue of 2′-deoxycytidine. Activation of ara-C requires conversion to ara-CMP, catalyzed by deoxycytidine kinase. Ara-CMP is then converted to ara-CDP, and then ara-CTP. Ara-CTP may become incorporated into DNA and will inhibit DNA synthesis.[7] Resistance to ara-C is achieved by decreased activity of deoxycytidine kinase or increased activity of cytidine deaminase, which converts ara-C to a nontoxic metabolite.[8] Ara-C remains the mainstay of therapy for acute leukemia.

Purine Analogues

Mercaptopurine is a purine analogue that inhibits DNA and RNA synthesis. It is a substrate for hypoxanthine-guanine phosphoribosyltransferase (HGPRT) and is converted to 6-thioinosine 5′-monophosphate (T-IMP). Accumulation of T-IMP leads to inhibition of conversion of inosine 5′-monophosphate to adenine and guanine nucleotides.[9] Mercaptopurine is also thought to be incorporated into DNA. Resistance to this agent is achieved by deficiency in HGPRT. Mercaptopurine is used in the treatment of acute lymphoblastic leukemia.

M Phase

Vinca Alkaloids

The vinca alkaloids, including vincristine, vinblastine, and vinorelbine, bind tubulin and block polymerization of microtubules.[10] This results in the disruption of the mitotic spindle. Vincristine is widely used in the treatment of non-Hodgkin's and Hodgkin's lymphoma, as well as acute lymphoblastic leukemia, primary brain tumors, rhabdomyosarcoma, and neuroblastoma. Peripheral neuropathy is often observed following repeated dosing. Vinblastine is employed in the management of Hodgkin's lymphoma and testicular cancer. Vinorelbine is predominantly used in non–small cell lung cancer.

Taxanes

Taxanes, like vinca alkaloids, bind microtubules and inhibit mitosis. Unlike the vinca alkaloids, however, taxanes promote microtubule formation, resulting in bundles of aberrant microtubules.[10] Paclitaxel, the first taxane identified, is now widely used in the treatment of breast cancer, non–small cell lung cancer, head and neck cancer, and ovarian cancer. Paclitaxel has poor solubility and must be administered in a polyethoxylated castor oil vehicle. The vehicle is responsible for hypersensitivity reactions that require premedication with dexamethasone and histamine blockers.[11] More recently, an albumin-bound form of paclitaxel, Abraxane, has been developed. Abraxane is currently approved for the use of relapsed or refractory breast cancer.[12] Docetaxel is a derivative of paclitaxel and is approved for the use of hormone-refractory metastatic prostate cancer, breast cancer, non–small cell lung cancer, gastric cancer, and head and neck cancer. Fluid retention induced by docetaxel may be prevented by corticosteroid use.

Cyclin-Dependent Kinase Inhibitors

The cell cycle is tightly regulated by the cyclin-dependent kinases (cdks). At least nine cdks have been identified thus far. The kinases are activated by cyclins. The Ink and Cip/Kip family of proteins serve as cdk inhibitors (ckis). The cdks phosphorylate members of the retinoblastoma (Rb) family. Rb binds to and sequesters E2F transcription factors, thus preventing activation of genes required for cell proliferation. Phosphorylation of Rb by cdks (specifically cyclin-D + cdk4/6 as well as cyclin-E + cdk2) in mid- to late G_1 phase leads to the release of E2F proteins, allowing for transcription of genes required for transition to S phase. Different cdks regulate other phases of the cell cycle. Cdks 1 and 2 with cyclin-A are responsible for S-phase progression, while cyclin-B + cdk1 allows for the G_2-M transition.

Alterations in expression and activity of cyclins/cdks/ckis have been found to be widespread in malignancies. The cki p16^{INK4A} may be inactivated by point mutation, gene deletion, or alteration in methylation patterns.[13] Amplification of cdk4 or the presence of mutated cdk4 that cannot bind p16^{INK4A} has also been reported.[14,15] Cyclin-D1 overexpression has been described in a variety of malignancies. Given the central role of the cdks in cell cycle progression, there has been interest in the development of agents that target the cdks as novel antineoplastic therapies.[16] Both specific and nonspecific cdk inhibitors are currently undergoing preclinical and clinical evaluation.

Specific cdk Inhibitors

R-roscovitine (CYC202, seliciclib) is an inhibitor of cdk1/cdk2/cdk5.[17] Preclinical studies have shown cell cycle arrest as well as induction of apoptosis.[18,19] This agent is orally bioavailable. In a Phase I trial, dose-limiting toxicities included fatigue, skin rash, hyponatremia, and hypokalemia.[20]

BMS 387032 is a potent cdk2 inhibitor.[21] A Phase I study evaluated the drug as both an intravenous infusion and an oral solution.[22] Average oral bioavailability was 19%, and the drug was well tolerated.[22]

A variety of cdk inhibitors are currently being studied in various preclinical settings, including the cdk4 inhibitor fascaplysin,[23] purvalanol,[24] SU9516,[25] and aloisines.[26]

Nonspecific cdk Inhibitors

Flavopiridol, a semisynthetic flavonoid, has been shown to induce cell cycle arrest at both G_1/S and G_2/M.[27] Further studies revealed reversible inhibition of cdks.[28,29] Crystal structure analysis has shown that flavopiridol binds to the ATP binding pocket.[30] Treatment of cells with flavopiridol has also been shown to lead to decreased transcription of cyclin-D1.[31] Induction of apoptosis by flavopiridol has been observed.[32] Synergistic effects with a variety of standard chemotherapy agents have been demonstrated, including paclitaxel, cytarabine, topotecan, doxorubicin, and etoposide.[33] In a Phase I clinical trial, the dose-limiting toxicity was gastrointestinal.[34] One patient with metastatic gastric cancer had a complete response. Phase II trials in metastatic hormone-refractory prostate cancer and metastatic non–small cell lung cancer failed to achieve objective responses.[35,36]

UCN-01 is an analogue of staurosporine, a nonspecific protein and tyrosine kinase inhibitor. UCN-01 has been shown to potently inhibit several protein kinase C isoenzymes.[37] In addition, UCN-01 can induce a G_1 arrest and abrogate a G_2 arrest, and may have effects on cdks by modulating upstream regulators.[38-41] A Phase I study evaluating a 72-hour continuous infusion was performed and showed dose-limiting toxicities of hyperglycemia with metabolic acidosis, nausea, and pulmonary dysfunction.[42] A Phase II study evaluating the combination of topotecan and UCN-01 in advanced ovarian cancer did not show significant activity.[43]

ANTIPROLIFERATION

The mitogen-activated protein kinase/extracellular signal–regulated kinase (MAPK/ERK) pathway is one of the key intracellular pathways regulating proliferation, differentiation, survival, adhesion, and angiogenesis (Fig. 7-2).[44] This pathway is activated by extracellular growth factors (including transforming growth factor-α, epidermal growth factor [EGF], and vascular endothelial growth factor [VEGF]) binding to their cell membrane receptors. Activation of the receptor then leads to activation of the small GTPase Ras. This, in turn, leads to the sequential phosphorylation and activation of a number of downstream kinases, including Raf, Mek, and MAPK. Ultimately, signals are relayed to the nucleus and changes in transcription occur. It has been estimated that this pathway is upregulated in approximately 30% of human cancer. Overexpression or activating mutations of EGF receptors, activating mutations of Ras, and activating mutations of Raf have all been described in human malignancies. Given the central role of this pathway in regulating proliferation, there has been intense interest in the development of inhibitors of this pathway as potential anticancer agents.[45]

Growth Factor Receptor Inhibitors

A number of EGF receptor inhibitors have been developed and are now being used to treat a variety of malignancies. These agents may be broadly classified into two groups: monoclonal antibodies directed against the ligand-binding domain of the receptors and orally bioavailable small-molecule tyrosine kinase inhibitors.

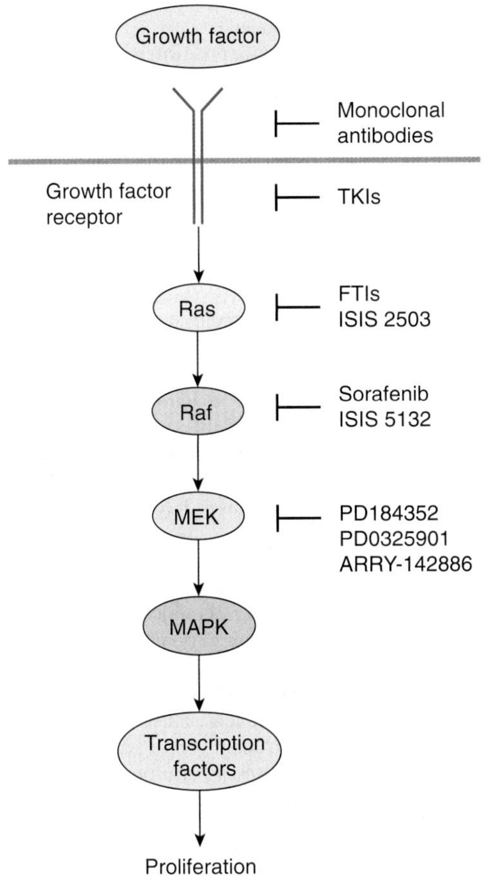

FIGURE 7-2 • The Ras-MAP kinase pathway.

Monoclonal Antibodies

Cetuximab is a recombinant human/mouse chimeric monoclonal antibody that binds the EGF receptor, competitively inhibiting the binding of ligands. Cetuximab is given as an intravenous injection once a week. A hypersensitivity reaction may occur during the infusion. Other toxicities include an acneiform skin rash, nausea, and hypomagnesemia. Cetuximab is now approved for the treatment of metastatic colorectal cancer as well as head and neck cancer. A Phase III trial in patients with recurrent or metastatic head and neck cancer compared cisplatin to cisplatin with cetuximab.[46] Overall response rate was improved; however, progression-free survival and overall survival were not significantly improved. Interestingly, in patients who developed a skin rash, there was a statistically significant improvement in survival. In another Phase III trial, patients with loco-regionally advanced head and neck cancer were randomized to radiation therapy alone versus radiation therapy with concurrent cetuximab.[47] The cetuximab arm achieved a significantly improved duration of locoregional control as well as overall survival. In a trial evaluating patients with metastatic colorectal cancer that was refractory to irinotecan, patients were randomized to cetuximab or cetuximab with irinotecan.[48] Crossover to cetuximab/irinotecan was allowed if disease progression occurred. Both response rate and median time to progression were improved in the combination arm. The use of cetuximab is also being evaluated in non–small cell lung cancer, glioblastoma multiforme, pancreatic cancer, gastric/gastroesophageal cancer, and hepatocellular cancer.

Panitumumab is a fully human monoclonal antibody that binds to the EGF receptor. It has been approved for the management of metastatic colorectal cancer. In a trial comparing panitumumab versus best supportive care in patients with metastatic colorectal cancer deemed to be chemorefractory, treatment with panitumumab yielded a 10% response rate and improved median progression-free survival time (8 weeks vs. 7.3 weeks).[49] Noted toxicities included skin rash, hypomagnesemia, and diarrhea.

Trastuzumab is a monoclonal antibody directed against human epidermal growth factor receptor 2 (HER2). HER2, also referred to as Her2/neu, is overexpressed in approximately 20% of breast cancers. Trastuzumab has been approved for the treatment of Her2/neu-positive breast cancer, in both the adjuvant and metastatic settings. In a randomized trial comparing 1 year of trastuzumab therapy versus observation following neoadjuvant or adjuvant chemotherapy for Her2/neu-positive breast cancer, patients who received trastuzumab had an improved disease-free survival at 2 years.[50]

Tyrosine Kinase Inhibitors

Gefitinib was the first anti-EGFR tyrosine kinase inhibitor to be approved by the U.S. Food and Drug Administration. Gefitinib inhibits epidermal growth factor receptor (EGFR) kinase, and to a lesser extent, HER2 kinase, activity. Data from Phase II studies evaluating the use of gefitinib in patients with advanced non–small cell lung cancer revealed response rates of approximately 19%.[51] However, Phase III trials comparing gemcitabine/cisplatin with gemcitabine/cisplatin/gefitinib,[52] or paclitaxel/carboplatin with paclitaxel/carboplatin/gefitinib,[53] showed no improvement in response rates or survival. It has been suggested that patients with activating mutations in EGFR may have increased sensitivity to gefitinib.[54] At this time, use of gefitinib is restricted to patients who have benefited from the agent.

Erlotinib was the second anti-EGFR tyrosine kinase inhibitor to be approved. Erlotinib potently inhibits EGFR, and to a lesser extent, HER2. Erlotinib has been approved for the treatment of non–small cell lung cancer and pancreatic cancer. As with gefitinib, Phase III trials evaluating the addition of erlotinib to standard chemotherapy regimens in non–small cell lung cancer have not yielded a survival advantage.[55,56] There did seem to be a correlation between development of a rash and response.[57] In a Phase III trial, patients with unresectable, locally advanced, or metastatic pancreatic cancer were randomized to gemcitabine with or without erlotinib.[58] Median overall survival was improved by a little over 1 week (6.24 vs. 5.91 months), a difference that was statistically significant. Erlotinib is also being evaluated in colorectal cancer, hepatocellular cancer, gastric/gastroesophageal cancer, glioblastoma multiforme, biliary cancer, mesothelioma, and prostate cancer.

Lapatinib is a dual kinase inhibitor that can target both EGFR and Her2/neu. Lapatinib is approved for use in combination with capecitabine in Her2/neu-positive breast cancer patients who have previously received trastuzumab. This is based on results of a Phase III trial that compared capecitabine with or without lapatinib.[59] The combination resulted in improved time to progression. Adverse effects of lapatinib include diarrhea, QTc prolongation, and left ventricular dysfunction.

Ras Inhibitors

Ras, like other members of the small GTPase superfamily, requires isoprenylation, a posttranslational modification, for proper membrane localization. Farnesyl protein transferase inhibitors (FTIs) have been developed as a mechanism to inhibit Ras function. It has been recognized that the activity of these agents may be secondary to effects on other isoprenylated targets as well. FTIs have been shown to have antiproliferative effects and to induce apoptosis in a variety of cancer cell lines.

Tipifarnib, an orally bioavailable agent, is one of the first FTIs to reach clinical trials. Phase I trials of this oral agent have shown myelotoxicity to be the dose-limiting toxicity.[60-62] Other Phase I trials have evaluated tipifarnib in combination with other agents, including gemcitabine/cisplatin,[63] irinotecan,[64] tamoxifen,[65] capecitabine,[66] docetaxel,[67] and imatinib.[68] Phase II studies have now been completed in non–small cell lung cancer,[69] pancreatic cancer,[70] breast cancer,[71] small cell lung cancer,[72] myelodysplastic syndrome,[73] urothelial transitional cell cancer,[74] colorectal cancer,[75] acute myeloid leukemia,[76] and myelofibrosis.[77] Interestingly, tipifarnib has also been shown to upregulate DR5 expression and augment apoptosis induced by tumor necrosis factor (TNF)–related apoptosis-inducing ligand (TRAIL).[78]

ISIS 2503 is a 20-base antisense oligonucleotide that targets H-ras. In preclinical studies, this agent has been shown to down-regulate H-ras expression.[79] In a Phase I trial involving patients with advanced malignancies, no dose-limiting toxicities were observed.[80] This drug was given as a continuous infusion (up to 10 mg/kg per day) for 14 days out of a 21-day cycle. Four of 23 patients had stabilization of disease. Levels of H-ras messenger RNA (mRNA) in peripheral blood lymphocytes were measured; however, no consistent decreases were observed.[80] In another Phase I study, patients received ISIS 2503 in combination with gemcitabine.[81] This combination was found to be well tolerated. In a Phase II trial, patients with metastatic or locally advanced pancreatic cancer received gemcitabine and ISIS 2503.[82] The response rate was 10%.

Raf Inhibitors

B-Raf mutations have been reported in malignant melanoma, papillary thyroid cancer, colorectal cancer, and non–small cell lung cancer. Sorafenib is an orally bioavailable agent that inhibits Raf kinase by competing with ATP in the kinase domain. While it does not inhibit EGFR, MAPK and ERK kinase (MEK), or MAPK, it does have activity against VEGF receptors, Flt-3, and platelet-derived growth factor receptor beta.[83] This drug has now been approved for the treatment of advanced renal cell cancer and hepatocellular cancer. Clinical trials are currently underway evaluating the use of sorafenib in a number of malignancies, including melanoma, prostate cancer, non–small cell lung cancer, and head and neck cancer. Dose-limiting toxicities have included hand-foot syndrome, diarrhea, and fatigue.

Raf has also been targeted using an antisense oligonucleotide approach. ISIS 5132 was designed to target Raf-1 mRNA. Preclinical studies did show evidence of down-regulation of Raf-1 activity and inhibition of tumor cell growth.[84] Phase I studies had inconsistent results with regard to changes in Raf-1 expression in peripheral mononuclear blood cells.[85,86] Phase II studies failed to yield responses, although in all studies there were patients who achieved stable disease.[87-90] These studies have raised the question as to whether this agent should be considered cytostatic.

MEK Inhibitors

Several MEK inhibitors have been developed and are currently undergoing preliminary clinical studies. These inhibitors are specific to MEK1 and MEK2, are noncompetitive with respect to ATP, and are orally active. PD184352 (CI-1040) has been evaluated in Phase I and Phase II trials. A Phase I study was able to demonstrate reduced levels of phosphorylated ERK1/2 in tumor samples.[91] Toxicities included diarrhea, asthenia, rash, and nausea/vomiting.[91] Subsequently, a Phase II trial was performed that evaluated this agent in patients with advanced breast, colon, non–small cell lung, and pancreatic cancer. No responses were observed.[92]

PD0325901 is a second-generation MEK inhibitor with a 50-fold increased potency against MEK and improved oral bioavailability.[93] Animal studies have shown marked inhibition of MAPK phosphorylation.[94] Phase I testing is currently underway. ARRY-142886 is another orally bioavailable agent that has been shown to specifically inhibit MEK 1/2[95] and to have activity in mouse xenograft models. This agent is also being evaluated in the Phase I setting.

APOPTOSIS

Apoptosis is the process by which cells undergo an orderly, programmed death. Apoptosis occurs during normal physiologic processes, including embryonic development and homeostasis of tissues. Dysregulation of apoptosis is a common theme in malignant cells. Many events can trigger apoptosis, including DNA damage, hypoxia, nutrient starvation, toxins, and oncogenic stresses. Virtually all traditional chemotherapy agents may induce apoptosis; however, this induction is more likely a response to generalized injury to the cell than to interaction with apoptosis-specific pathways. As research has provided greater detail regarding the key players in apoptosis pathways, new drug targets have been revealed.

Apoptosis may be induced by either the intrinsic or extrinsic pathway (Fig. 7-3). The intrinsic pathway is mediated by the mitochondria, while the extrinsic pathway depends on death receptor–mediated signaling. Key to both the intrinsic and extrinsic pathways are the caspases. These proteases are responsible for the orderly degradation of cellular components, leading to DNA fragmentation and membrane blebbing.

The Intrinsic Pathway

The intrinsic pathway may be activated by a variety of stressors, including DNA damage, which in turn, may be a consequence of chemotherapy agents. These signals activate p53, leading to the transcription of proapoptotic Bcl2 proteins such as PUMA and NOXA. BAK and BAX, also members of the Bcl2 family, are then activated, inducing release of cytochrome *c* from the mitochondria.[96] Cytochrome *c* may then interact with Apaf-1, leading to the activation of caspase 9. Finally, caspase 9 activates the effector caspases 3, 6, and 7.

Intrinsic Pathway Targets

It has been estimated that approximately half of solid tumors will have loss of function of p53. From a therapeutic standpoint, attempts have been made to restore p53 activity via adenoviral transfer in patients with malignancies.[97] Another approach has been the use of an adenovirus lacking E1Bp55, which allows for the selective replication of the virus in p53-deficient tumor cells. This adenovirus (ONYX-015) has been evaluated in Phase II trials involving patients with head and neck cancer.[98,99] This drug requires intratumoral expression, and, as with all adenoviral vectors, systemic delivery has been difficult. A third approach has involved an agent that is thought to stabilize p53 and rescue p53 mutants by restoring DNA-binding activity.[100] This agent, CP-31398, has been shown to induce apoptosis in human cancer cells.[101]

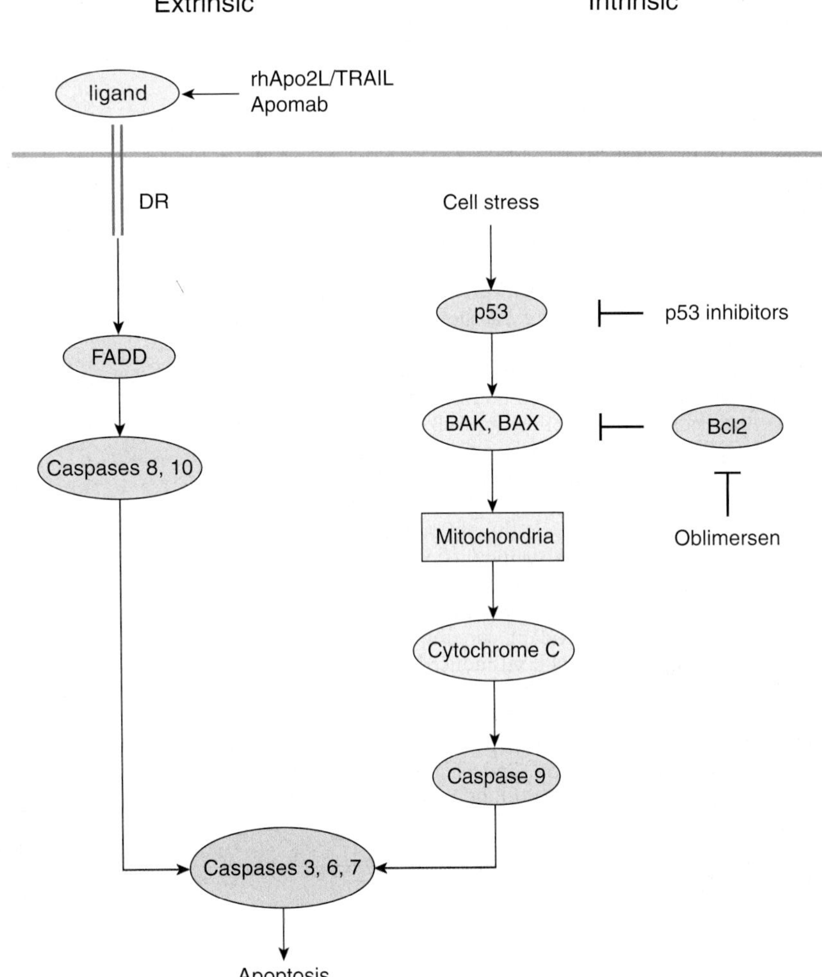

FIGURE 7-3 • **The extrinsic and intrinsic apoptosis pathways.**

Oblimersen, an 18-base oligodeoxynucleotide encoding antisense to the Bcl-2 genes, is currently being evaluated in a number of clinical trials. The antisense approach results in a decrease in Bcl-2 protein production by targeting the Bcl-2 mRNA for degradation. In a Phase III trial, patients with relapsed or refractory chronic lymphocytic leukemia (CLL) were randomized to fludarabine/cyclophosphamide with or without oblimersen (3 mg/kg per day as a 7-day continuous infusion).[102] The arm that received oblimersen had an improved response rate (17% complete response/nodular partial response [CR/nPR]) compared to the chemotherapy-only arm (7% CR/nPR).[102] In a Phase II trial, patients with advanced renal cell cancer received oblimersen (7 mg/kg per day as a 7-day continuous infusion) with α-interferon.[103] Only one patient had a partial response, and no changes in bcl-2 levels or Annexin/PI positivity were observed.[103] A Phase II trial in patients with acute myeloid leukemia in first relapse evaluated the combination of oblimersen with gemtuzumab.[104] The results from a Phase III trial evaluating standard induction chemotherapy with and without oblimersen in newly diagnosed acute myeloid leukemia are currently pending. Oblimersen is also being evaluated in hepatocellular cancer,[105] colorectal cancer,[106] hormone-refractory prostate cancer,[107,108] Waldenström's macroglobulinemia,[109] and melanoma.[110]

The Extrinsic Pathway

The extrinsic pathway of apoptosis is induced via binding of proapoptotic ligands to membrane receptors. The receptors are members of the TNF family. The ligands include Fas and TNFR1. Activation of the receptors results in recruitment of a death-inducing signaling complex (DISC). This complex recruits the Fas-associated death domain as well as procaspases 8 and 10. These caspases are activated, which in turn activates caspases 3, 6, and 7. Included among the proapoptotic ligands is TRAIL (also referred to as Apo2L/TRAIL).[111,112] TRAIL binds to the DR4 and DR5 receptors. TRAIL has been shown to induce apoptosis in transformed cells but to have less effect on normal cells.

Extrinsic Pathway Targets

Recently several approaches have been taken to target the extrinsic pathway in cancer cells. This is thought to be an attractive target, as this pathway is independent of p53. Thus, theoretically, cancer cells that are resistant to standard chemotherapy-induced effects on the intrinsic pathway might be sensitive to manipulation of the extrinsic pathway. Thus far, two agents have made their way to clinical trials: the recombinant human (rh) Apo2L/TRAIL and the human DR5 agonistic antibody Apomab.

Preclinical studies involving rhApo2L/TRAIL have shown that this agent induces apoptosis in human cancer cell lines and in mouse xenograft models.[113] The half-life of this agent is quite short (approximately 30 minutes in primates). There has been some evidence, based on preclinical studies, for the role of combining rhApo2L/TRAIL with standard chemotherapy agents. The combination of rhApo2L/TRAIL plus paclitaxel/carboplatin in a mouse xenograft model of non–small cell lung cancer resulted in tumor regression and improved survival.[114] In a pancreatic cancer mouse xenograft model, the combination of Apo2L/TRAIL with gemcitabine led to improved therapeutic efficacy.[115] Currently, there is an ongoing Phase I study involving rhApo2L/TRAIL in patients with advanced cancer.

Apomab has been shown to induce apoptosis in a variety of cancer cell lines. In xenograft models of human colorectal cancer, Apomab induced tumor regression. Results of an initial Phase I study indicated that the agent was well tolerated.[116] No objective responses were observed.

Nuclear Factor-κB

The nuclear factor-κB (NF-κB) pathway has been shown to be involved in the regulation of multiple cellular processes, including apoptosis, proliferation, differentiation, and stress response. NF-κB is a transcription factor that activates transcription of proteins such as a caspase 8 inhibitor (c-FLIP) and inhibitors of apoptosis proteins (IAPs). Overexpression and activation of NF-κB has been demonstrated in a variety of cancers.[117-119] Therefore, there has been interest in targeting the NF-κB pathway.

The naturally occurring rotenoid deguelin has been shown to decrease IκBα expression in B-CLL cells and to induce apoptosis.[120] Whether this is due to direct effects on IκB or is secondary to inhibition of PI3K/Akt signaling is unclear. Genistein, an isoflavonoid, has been shown to induce apoptosis and inhibit NF-κB activation.[121,122] Cell culture studies in breast cancer cells showed inactivation of NF-κB that appeared to be mediated via the Akt pathway.[123] There has been some interest in the ability of genistein to augment the activity of standard anticancer agents such as cisplatin, docetaxel, doxorubicin, gemcitabine, and CHOP (cyclophosphamide, doxorubicin, vincristine, prednisone).[124-126] The antioxidant curcumin has been reported to down-regulate NF-κB.[127] Paclitaxel-induced NF-κB activation was inhibited by curcumin in preclinical studies.[128] Also noted was a decreased incidence of metastatic disease in a breast cancer xenograft model.[128] Curcumin has also been shown to enhance the anticancer effects of gemcitabine, cisplatin, and doxorubicin.[129,130] Dehydroxymethylepoxyquinomicin is an NF-κB inhibitor[131] that has been shown to induce apoptosis.[132,133]

REFERENCES

1. Shih C, Chen VJ, Gossett LS, et al. LY231514, a pyrrolo[2,3-D]pyrimidine-based antifolate that inhibits multiple folate-requiring enzymes. Cancer Res 1997;57:1116-1123.
2. Washtien WL. Thymidylate synthetase levels as a factor in 5-fluorodeoxyuridine and methotrexate cytotoxicity in gastrointestinal tumor cells. Mol Pharmacol 1982;21:723-728.
3. Barbour KW, Berger SH, Berger FG. Single amino acid substitution defines a naturally occurring genetic variant of human thymidylate synthase. Mol Pharmacol 1990;37:515-518.
4. Harris BE, Carpenter JT, Diasio RB. Severe 5-fluorouracil toxicity secondary to dihydropyrimidine dehydrogenase deficiency: a potentially more common pharmacogenetic syndrome. Cancer 1991;68:499-501.
5. Lu Z, Zhang R, Diasio RB. Dihydropyrimidine dehydrogenase activity in human peripheral blood mononuclear cells and liver: population characteristics, newly identified deficient patients, and clinical implication in 5-fluorouracil chemotherapy. Cancer Res 1993;53:5433-5438.
6. Schuller J, Cassidy J, Dumont E, et al. Preferential activation of capecitabine in tumor following oral administration to colorectal cancer patients. Cancer Chemother Pharmacol 2000;45:291-297.
7. Mikita T, Beardsley GP. Functional consequences of the arabinosylcytosine structural lesion in DNA. Biochemistry 1988;27:4698-4705.
8. Cros E, Jordheim L, Dumontet C, Galmarini CM. Problems related to resistance to cytarabine in acute myeloid leukemia. Leuk Lymphoma 2004;45:1123-1132.
9. Davidson JD. Studies on the mechanism of action of 6-mercaptopurine in sensitive and resistant L1210 leukemia in vitro. Cancer Res 1960;20:225-232.
10. Dumontet C. Mechanisms of action and resistance to tubulin-binding agents. Expert Opin Investig Drugs 2000;9:779-788.
11. Gelderblom H, Verweij J, Nooter K, et al. The drawbacks and advantages of vehicle selection for drug formulation. Eur J Cancer 2001;37:1590-1598.
12. Henderson IC, Bhatia V. Nab-paclitaxel for breast cancer: a new formulation with an improved safety profile and greater efficacy. Expert Rev Anticancer Ther 2007;7:919-943.
13. Shapiro GI, Park JE, Edwards CD, et al. Multiple mechanisms of p16INK4A inactivation in non-small cell lung cancer cell lines. Cancer Res 1995;55:6200-6209.
14. He J, Allen JR, Collins VP, et al. CDK4 amplification is an alternative mechanism to *p16* gene homozygous deletion in glioma cell lines. Cancer Res 1994;54:5804-5807.
15. Wolfel T, Hauer M, Schneider J, et al. A p16INK4a-insensitive CDK4 mutant targeted by cytolytic T lymphocytes in a human melanoma. Science 1995;269:1281-1284.
16. Shapiro GI. Cyclin-dependent kinase pathways as targets for cancer treatment. J Clin Oncol 2006;24:1770-1783.
17. Meijer L, Borgne A, Mulner O, et al. Biochemical and cellular effects of roscovitine, a potent and selective inhibitor of the cyclin-dependent kinases cdc2, cdk2 and cdk5. Eur J Biochem 1997;243:527-536.
18. Alessi F, Quarta S, Savio M, et al. The cyclin-dependent kinase inhibitors olomoucine and roscovitine arrest human fibroblasts in G_1 phase by specific inhibition of CDK2 kinase activity. Exp Cell Res 1998;245:8-18.
19. McClue SJ, Blake D, Clarke R, et al. In vitro and in vivo antitumor properties of the cyclin dependent kinase inhibitor CYC202 (R-roscovitine). Int J Cancer 2002;102:463-468.
20. Benson C, White J, De Bono J, et al. A Phase I trial of the selective oral cyclin-dependent kinase inhibitor seliciclib (CYC202; R-Roscovitine), administered twice daily for 7 days every 21 days. Br J Cancer 2007;96:29-37.
21. Kim KS, Kimball SD, Misra RN, et al. Discovery of aminothiazole inhibitors of cyclin-dependent kinase 2: synthesis, X-ray crystallographic analysis, and biological activities. J Med Chem 2002;45:3905-3927.
22. Heath EI, Bible K, Martell RE, et al. A Phase 1 study of SNS-032 (formerly BMS-387032), a potent inhibitor of cyclin-dependent kinases 2, 7 and 9 administered as a single oral dose and weekly infusion in patients with metastatic refractory solid tumors. Invest New Drugs 2008;26:59-65.
23. Soni R, Muller L, Furet P, et al. Inhibition of cyclin-dependent kinase 4 (Cdk4) by fascaplysin, a marine natural product. Biochem Biophys Res Commun 2000;275:877-884.
24. Villerbu N, Gaben AM, Redeuilh G, Mester J. Cellular effects of purvalanol A: a specific inhibitor of cyclin-dependent kinase activities. Int J Cancer 2002;97:761-769.
25. Lane ME, Yu B, Rice A, et al. A novel cdk2-selective inhibitor, SU9516, induces apoptosis in colon carcinoma cells. Cancer Res 2001;61:6170-6177.
26. Mettey Y, Gompel M, Thomas V, et al. Aloisines, a new family of CDK/GSK-3 inhibitors: SAR study, crystal structure in complex with CDK2, enzyme selectivity, and cellular effects. J Med Chem 2003;46:222-236.
27. Kaur G, Stetler-Stevenson M, Sebers S, et al. Growth inhibition with reversible cell cycle arrest of carcinoma cells by flavone L86-8275. J Natl Cancer Inst 1992;84:1736-1740.
28. Losiewicz MD, Carlson BA, Kaur G, et al. Potent inhibition of CDC2 kinase activity by the flavonoid L86-8275. Biochem Biophys Res Commun 1994;201:589-595.
29. Carlson BA, Dubay MM, Sausville EA, et al. Flavopiridol induces G_1 arrest with inhibition of cyclin-dependent kinase (CDK) 2 and CDK4 in human breast carcinoma cells. Cancer Res 1996;56:2973-2978.
30. De Azevedo WF Jr, Mueller-Dieckmann HJ, Schulze-Gahmen U, et al. Structural basis for specificity and potency of a flavonoid inhibitor of human CDK2, a cell cycle kinase. Proc Natl Acad Sci U S A 1996;93:2735-2740.
31. Carlson B, Lahusen T, Singh S, et al. Down-regulation of cyclin D1 by transcriptional repression in MCF-7 human breast carcinoma cells induced by flavopiridol. Cancer Res 1999;59:4634-4641.
32. Parker BW, Kaur G, Nieves-Neira W, et al. Early induction of apoptosis in hematopoietic cell lines after exposure to flavopiridol. Blood 1998;91:458-465.
33. Bible KC, Kaufmann SH. Cytotoxic synergy between flavopiridol (NSC 649890, L86-8275) and various antineoplastic agents: the importance of sequence of administration. Cancer Res 1997;57:3375-3380.
34. Thomas JP, Tutsch KD, Cleary JF, et al. Phase I clinical and pharmacokinetic trial of the cyclin-dependent kinase inhibitor flavopiridol. Cancer Chemother Pharmacol 2002;50:465-472.
35. Liu G, Gandara DR, Lara PN Jr, et al. A Phase II trial of flavopiridol (NSC#649890) in patients with previously untreated metastatic androgen-independent prostate cancer. Clin Cancer Res 2004;10:924-928.
36. Shapiro GI, Supko JG, Patterson A, et al. A Phase II trial of the cyclin-dependent kinase inhibitor flavopiridol in patients with previously untreated stage IV non-small cell lung cancer. Clin Cancer Res 2001;7:1590-1599.
37. Seynaeve CM, Kazanietz MG, Blumberg PM, et al. Differential inhibition of protein kinase C isozymes by UCN-01, a staurosporine analogue. Mol Pharmacol 1994;45:1207-1214.
38. Seynaeve CM, Stetler-Stevenson M, Sebers S, et al. Cell cycle arrest and growth inhibition by the protein kinase antagonist UCN-01 in human breast carcinoma cells. Cancer Res 1993;53:2081-2086.
39. Yu L, Orlandi L, Wang P, et al. UCN-01 abrogates G_2 arrest through a Cdc2-dependent pathway that is associated with inactivation of the Wee1Hu kinase and activation of the Cdc25C phosphatase. J Biol Chem 1998;273:33455-33464.
40. Busby EC, Leistritz DF, Abraham RT, et al. The radiosensitizing agent 7-hydroxystaurosporine (UCN-01) inhibits the DNA damage checkpoint kinase hChk1. Cancer Res 2000;60:2108-2112.
41. Akiyama T, Yoshida T, Tsujita T, et al. G_1 phase accumulation induced by UCN-01 is associated with dephosphorylation of Rb and CDK2 proteins as well as induction of CDK inhibitor p21/Cip1/WAF1/Sdi1 in p53-mutated human epidermoid carcinoma A431 cells. Cancer Res 1997;57:1495-1501.
42. Sausville EA, Arbuck SG, Messmann R, et al. Phase I trial of 72-hour continuous infusion UCN-01 in patients with refractory neoplasms. J Clin Oncol 2001;19:2319-2333.
43. Welch S, Hirte HW, Carey MS, et al. UCN-01 in combination with topotecan in patients with advanced recurrent ovarian cancer: a study of the Princess Margaret Hospital Phase II consortium. Gynecol Oncol 2007;106:305-310.
44. Seger R, Krebs EG. The MAPK signaling cascade. FASEB J 1995;9:726-735.
45. Roberts PJ, Der CJ. Targeting the Raf-MEK-ERK mitogen-activated protein kinase cascade for the treatment of cancer. Oncogene 2007;26:3291-3310.
46. Burtness B, Goldwasser MA, Flood W, et al. Phase III randomized trial of cisplatin plus placebo compared with cisplatin plus cetuximab in metastatic/recurrent head and neck cancer: an Eastern Cooperative Oncology Group study. J Clin Oncol 2005;23:8646-8654.
47. Bonner JA, Harari PM, Giralt J, et al. Radiotherapy plus cetuximab for squamous-cell carcinoma of the head and neck. N Engl J Med 2006;354:567-578.

48. Cunningham D, Humblet Y, Siena S, et al. Cetuximab monotherapy and cetuximab plus irinotecan in irinotecan-refractory metastatic colorectal cancer. N Engl J Med 2004;351:337-345.
49. Van Cutsem E, Peeters M, Siena S, et al. Open-label Phase III trial of panitumumab plus best supportive care compared with best supportive care alone in patients with chemotherapy-refractory metastatic colorectal cancer. J Clin Oncol 2007;25:1658-1664.
50. Piccart-Gebhart MJ, Procter M, Leyland-Jones B, et al. Trastuzumab after adjuvant chemotherapy in HER2-positive breast cancer. N Engl J Med 2005;353:1659-1672.
51. Fukuoka M, Yano S, Giaccone G, et al. Multi-institutional randomized Phase II trial of gefitinib for previously treated patients with advanced non-small-cell lung cancer (The IDEAL 1 Trial) [corrected]. J Clin Oncol 2003;21:2237-2246.
52. Giaccone G, Herbst RS, Manegold C, et al. Gefitinib in combination with gemcitabine and cisplatin in advanced non-small-cell lung cancer: a Phase III trial—INTACT 1. J Clin Oncol 2004;22:777-784.
53. Herbst RS, Giaccone G, Schiller JH, et al. Gefitinib in combination with paclitaxel and carboplatin in advanced non-small-cell lung cancer: a Phase III trial—INTACT 2. J Clin Oncol 2004;22:785-794.
54. Lynch TJ, Bell DW, Sordella R, et al. Activating mutations in the epidermal growth factor receptor underlying responsiveness of non-small-cell lung cancer to gefitinib. N Engl J Med 2004;350:2129-2139.
55. Herbst RS, Prager D, Hermann R, et al. TRIBUTE: a Phase III trial of erlotinib hydrochloride (OSI-774) combined with carboplatin and paclitaxel chemotherapy in advanced non-small-cell lung cancer. J Clin Oncol 2005;23:5892-5899.
56. Gatzemeier U, Pluzanska A, Szczesna A, et al. Phase III study of erlotinib in combination with cisplatin and gemcitabine in advanced non-small-cell lung cancer: the Tarceva Lung Cancer Investigation Trial. J Clin Oncol 2007;25:1545-1552.
57. Wacker B, Nagrani T, Weinberg J, et al. Correlation between development of rash and efficacy in patients treated with the epidermal growth factor receptor tyrosine kinase inhibitor erlotinib in two large Phase III studies. Clin Cancer Res 2007;13:3913-3921.
58. Moore MJ, Goldstein D, Hamm J, et al. Erlotinib plus gemcitabine compared with gemcitabine alone in patients with advanced pancreatic cancer: a Phase III trial of the National Cancer Institute of Canada Clinical Trials Group. J Clin Oncol 2007;25:1960-1966.
59. Geyer CE, Forster J, Lindquist D, et al. Lapatinib plus capecitabine for HER2-positive advanced breast cancer. N Engl J Med 2006;355:2733-2743.
60. Zujewski J, Horak ID, Bol CJ, et al. Phase I and pharmacokinetic study of farnesyl protein transferase inhibitor R115777 in advanced cancer. J Clin Oncol 2000;18:927-941.
61. Punt CJ, van Maanen L, Bol CJ, et al. Phase I and pharmacokinetic study of the orally administered farnesyl transferase inhibitor R115777 in patients with advanced solid tumors. Anticancer Drugs 2001;12:193-197.
62. Crul M, de Klerk GJ, Swart M, et al. Phase I clinical and pharmacologic study of chronic oral administration of the farnesyl protein transferase inhibitor R115777 in advanced cancer. J Clin Oncol 2002;20:2726-2735.
63. Adjei AA, Croghan GA, Erlichman C, et al. A Phase I trial of the farnesyl protein transferase inhibitor R115777 in combination with gemcitabine and cisplatin in patients with advanced cancer. Clin Cancer Res 2003;9:2520-2526.
64. Cohen SJ, Gallo J, Lewis NL, et al. Phase I and pharmacokinetic study of the farnesyltransferase inhibitor R115777 in combination with irinotecan in patients with advanced cancer. Cancer Chemother Pharmacol 2004;53:513-518.
65. Lebowitz PF, Eng-Wong J, Widemann BC, et al. A Phase I trial and pharmacokinetic study of tipifarnib, a farnesyltransferase inhibitor, and tamoxifen in metastatic breast cancer. Clin Cancer Res 2005;11:1247-1252.
66. Gore L, Holden SN, Cohen RB, et al. A Phase I safety, pharmacological and biological study of the farnesyl protein transferase inhibitor, tipifarnib and capecitabine in advanced solid tumors. Ann Oncol 2006;17:1709-1717.
67. Awada A, Zhang S, Gil T, et al. A Phase I clinical and pharmacokinetic study of tipifarnib in combination with docetaxel in patients with advanced solid malignancies. Curr Med Res Opin 2007;23:991-1003.
68. Cortes J, Quintas-Cardama A, Garcia-Manero G, et al. Phase 1 study of tipifarnib in combination with imatinib for patients with chronic myelogenous leukemia in chronic phase after imatinib failure. Cancer 2007;110:2000-2006.
69. Adjei AA, Mauer A, Bruzek L, et al. Phase II study of the farnesyl transferase inhibitor R115777 in patients with advanced non-small-cell lung cancer. J Clin Oncol 2003;21:1760-1766.
70. Cohen SJ, Ho L, Ranganathan S, et al. Phase II and pharmacodynamic study of the farnesyltransferase inhibitor R115777 as initial therapy in patients with metastatic pancreatic adenocarcinoma. J Clin Oncol 2003;21:1301-1306.
71. Johnston SR, Hickish T, Ellis P, et al. Phase II study of the efficacy and tolerability of two dosing regimens of the farnesyl transferase inhibitor, R115777, in advanced breast cancer. J Clin Oncol 2003;21:2492-2499.
72. Heymach JV, Johnson DH, Khuri FR, et al. Phase II study of the farnesyl transferase inhibitor R115777 in patients with sensitive relapse small-cell lung cancer. Ann Oncol 2004;15:1187-1193.
73. Kurzrock R, Albitar M, Cortes JE, et al. Phase II study of R115777, a farnesyl transferase inhibitor, in myelodysplastic syndrome. J Clin Oncol 2004;22:1287-1292.
74. Rosenberg JE, von der Maase H, Seigne JD, et al. A Phase II trial of R115777, an oral farnesyl transferase inhibitor, in patients with advanced urothelial tract transitional cell carcinoma. Cancer 2005;103:2035-2041.
75. Whitehead RP, McCoy S, Macdonald JS, et al. Phase II trial of R115777 (NSC #70818) in patients with advanced colorectal cancer: a Southwest Oncology Group study. Invest New Drugs 2006;24:335-341.
76. Harousseau JL, Lancet JE, Reiffers J, et al. A Phase 2 study of the oral farnesyltransferase inhibitor tipifarnib in patients with refractory or relapsed acute myeloid leukemia. Blood 2007;109:5151-5156.
77. Mesa RA, Camoriano JK, Geyer SM, et al. A Phase II trial of tipifarnib in myelofibrosis: primary, post-polycythemia vera and post-essential thrombocythemia. Leukemia 2007;21:1964-1970.
78. Qiu Y, Liu X, Zou W, et al. The farnesyltransferase inhibitor R115777 up-regulates the expression of death receptor 5 and enhances TRAIL-induced apoptosis in human lung cancer cells. Cancer Res 2007;67:4973-4980.
79. Chen G, Oh S, Monia BP, Stacey DW. Antisense oligonucleotides demonstrate a dominant role of c-Ki-RAS proteins in regulating the proliferation of diploid human fibroblasts. J Biol Chem 1996;271:28259-28265.
80. Cunningham CC, Holmlund JT, Geary RS, et al. A Phase I trial of H-ras antisense oligonucleotide ISIS 2503 administered as a continuous intravenous infusion in patients with advanced carcinoma. Cancer 2001;92:1265-1271.
81. Adjei AA, Dy GK, Erlichman C, et al. A Phase I trial of ISIS 2503, an antisense inhibitor of H-ras, in combination with gemcitabine in patients with advanced cancer. Clin Cancer Res 2003;9:115-123.
82. Alberts SR, Schroeder M, Erlichman C, et al. Gemcitabine and ISIS-2503 for patients with locally advanced or metastatic pancreatic adenocarcinoma: a North Central Cancer Treatment Group Phase II trial. J Clin Oncol 2004;22:4944-4950.
83. Wilhelm SM, Carter C, Tang L, et al. BAY 43-9006 exhibits broad spectrum oral antitumor activity and targets the RAF/MEK/ERK pathway and receptor tyrosine kinases involved in tumor progression and angiogenesis. Cancer Res 2004;64:7099-7109.
84. Monia BP, Johnston JF, Geiger T, et al. Antitumor activity of a phosphorothioate antisense oligodeoxynucleotide targeted against C-raf kinase. Nat Med 1996;2:668-675.
85. Rudin CM, Holmlund J, Fleming GF, et al. Phase I trial of ISIS 5132, an antisense oligonucleotide inhibitor of c-raf-1, administered by 24-hour weekly infusion to patients with advanced cancer. Clin Cancer Res 2001;7:1214-1220.
86. Stevenson JP, Yao KS, Gallagher M, et al. Phase I clinical/pharmacokinetic and pharmacodynamic trial of the c-raf-1 antisense oligonucleotide ISIS 5132 (CGP 69846A). J Clin Oncol 1999;17:2227-2236.
87. Oza AM, Elit L, Swenerton K, et al. Phase II study of CGP 69846A (ISIS 5132) in recurrent epithelial ovarian cancer: an NCIC clinical trials group study (NCIC IND.116). Gynecol Oncol 2003;89:129-133.
88. Cripps MC, Figueredo AT, Oza AM, et al. Phase II randomized study of ISIS 3521 and ISIS 5132 in patients with locally advanced or metastatic colorectal cancer: a National Cancer Institute of Canada Clinical Trials Group study. Clin Cancer Res 2002;8:2188-2192.
89. Coudert B, Anthoney A, Fiedler W, et al. Phase II trial with ISIS 5132 in patients with small-cell (SCLC) and non-small cell (NSCLC) lung cancer: a European Organization for Research and Treatment of Cancer (EORTC) Early Clinical Studies Group report. Eur J Cancer 2001;37:2194-2198.
90. Tolcher AW, Reyno L, Venner PM, et al. A randomized Phase II and pharmacokinetic study of the antisense oligonucleotides ISIS 3521 and ISIS 5132 in patients with hormone-refractory prostate cancer. Clin Cancer Res 2002;8:2530-2535.
91. Lorusso PM, Adjei AA, Varterasian M, et al. Phase I and pharmacodynamic study of the oral MEK inhibitor CI-1040 in patients with advanced malignancies. J Clin Oncol 2005;23:5281-5293.
92. Rinehart J, Adjei AA, Lorusso PM, et al. Multicenter Phase II study of the oral MEK inhibitor, CI-1040, in patients with advanced non-small-cell lung, breast, colon, and pancreatic cancer. J Clin Oncol 2004;22:4456-4462.
93. Sebolt-Leopold JS, Merriman R, Omer C, et al. The biological profile of PD0325901: a second generation analog of CI-1040 with improved pharmaceutical potential. Proc Am Assoc Cancer Res 2004;45:925.
94. Brown AP, Carlson TC, Loi CM, Graziano MJ. Pharmacodynamic and toxicokinetic evaluation of the novel MEK inhibitor, PD0325901, in the rat following oral and intravenous administration. Cancer Chemother Pharmacol 2007;59:671-679.
95. Yeh TC, Marsh V, Bernat BA, et al. Biological characterization of ARRY-142886 (AZD6244), a potent, highly selective mitogen-activated protein kinase kinase 1/2 inhibitor. Clin Cancer Res 2007;13:1576-1583.
96. Cory S, Adams JM. The Bcl2 family: regulators of the cellular life-or-death switch. Nat Rev Cancer 2002;2:647-656.
97. Merritt JA, Roth JA, Logothetis CJ. Clinical evaluation of adenoviral-mediated p53 gene transfer: review of INGN 201 studies. Semin Oncol 2001;28:105-114.
98. Khuri FR, Nemunaitis J, Ganly I, et al. A controlled trial of intratumoral ONYX-015, a selectively-replicating adenovirus, in combination with cisplatin and 5-fluorouracil in patients with recurrent head and neck cancer. Nat Med 2000;6:879-885.
99. Nemunaitis J, Ganly I, Khuri F, et al. Selective replication and oncolysis in p53 mutant tumors with ONYX-015, an E1B-55kD gene-deleted adenovirus, in patients with advanced head and neck cancer: a Phase II trial. Cancer Res 2000;60:6359-6366.
100. Demma MJ, Wong S, Maxwell E, Dasmahapatra B. CP-31398 restores DNA-binding activity to mutant p53 in vitro but does not affect p53 homologs p63 and p73. J Biol Chem 2004;279:45887-45896.
101. Takimoto R, Wang W, Dicker DT, et al. The mutant p53-conformation modifying drug, CP-31398, can induce apoptosis of human cancer cells and can stabilize wild-type p53 protein. Cancer Biol Ther 2002;1:47-55.
102. O'Brien S, Moore JO, Boyd TE, et al. Randomized Phase III trial of fludarabine plus cyclophosphamide with or without oblimersen sodium (Bcl-2 antisense) in patients with relapsed or refractory chronic lymphocytic leukemia. J Clin Oncol 2007;25:1114-1120.

103. Margolin K, Synold TW, Lara P, et al. Oblimersen and alpha-interferon in metastatic renal cancer: a Phase II study of the California Cancer Consortium. J Cancer Res Clin Oncol 2007;133:705-711.
104. Moore J, Seiter K, Kolitz J, et al. A Phase II study of Bcl-2 antisense (oblimersen sodium) combined with gemtuzumab ozogamicin in older patients with acute myeloid leukemia in first relapse. Leuk Res 2006;30:777-783.
105. Knox JJ, Chen XE, Feld R, et al. A Phase I-II study of oblimersen sodium (G3139, Genasense) in combination with doxorubicin in advanced hepatocellular carcinoma (NCI # 5798). Invest New Drugs 2008;26:193-194.
106. Mita MM, Ochoa L, Rowinsky EK, et al. A Phase I, pharmacokinetic and biologic correlative study of oblimersen sodium (Genasense, G3139) and irinotecan in patients with metastatic colorectal cancer. Ann Oncol 2006;17:313-321.
107. Chi KN, Gleave ME, Klasa R, et al. A Phase I dose-finding study of combined treatment with an antisense Bcl-2 oligonucleotide (Genasense) and mitoxantrone in patients with metastatic hormone-refractory prostate cancer. Clin Cancer Res 2001;7:3920-3927.
108. Tolcher AW, Chi K, Kuhn J, et al. A Phase II, pharmacokinetic, and biological correlative study of oblimersen sodium and docetaxel in patients with hormone-refractory prostate cancer. Clin Cancer Res 2005;11:3854-3861.
109. Gertz MA, Geyer SM, Badros A, et al. Early results of a Phase I trial of oblimersen sodium for relapsed or refractory Waldenstrom's macroglobulinemia. Clin Lymphoma 2005;5:282-284.
110. Bedikian AY, Millward M, Pehamberger H, et al. Bcl-2 antisense (oblimersen sodium) plus dacarbazine in patients with advanced melanoma: the Oblimersen Melanoma Study Group. J Clin Oncol 2006;24:4738-4745.
111. Pitti RM, Marsters SA, Ruppert S, et al. Induction of apoptosis by Apo-2 ligand, a new member of the tumor necrosis factor cytokine family. J Biol Chem 1996;271:12687-12690.
112. Wiley SR, Schooley K, Smolak PJ, et al. Identification and characterization of a new member of the TNF family that induces apoptosis. Immunity 1995;3:673-682.
113. Ashkenazi A, Pai RC, Fong S, et al. Safety and antitumor activity of recombinant soluble Apo2 ligand. J Clin Invest 1999;104:155-162.
114. Jin H, Yang R, Fong S, et al. Apo2 ligand/tumor necrosis factor-related apoptosis-inducing ligand cooperates with chemotherapy to inhibit orthotopic lung tumor growth and improve survival. Cancer Res 2004;64:4900-4905.
115. Hylander BL, Pitoniak R, Penetrante RB, et al. The anti-tumor effect of Apo2L/TRAIL on patient pancreatic adenocarcinomas grown as xenografts in SCID mice. J Transl Med 2005;3:22.
116. Camidge D, Herbst RS, Gordon M, et al. A Phase I safety and pharmacokinetic study of apomab, a human DR5 agonist antibody, in patients with advanced cancer. J Clin Oncol 2007;25:3582.
117. Wang W, Abbruzzese JL, Evans DB, et al. The nuclear factor-kappa B RelA transcription factor is constitutively activated in human pancreatic adenocarcinoma cells. Clin Cancer Res 1999;5:119-127.
118. Sovak MA, Bellas RE, Kim DW, et al. Aberrant nuclear factor-kappaB/Rel expression and the pathogenesis of breast cancer. J Clin Invest 1997;100:2952-2960.
119. Shukla S, MacLennan GT, Fu P, et al. Nuclear factor-kappaB/p65 (Rel A) is constitutively activated in human prostate adenocarcinoma and correlates with disease progression. Neoplasia 2004;6:390-400.
120. Geeraerts B, Vanhoecke B, Vanden Berghe W, et al. Deguelin inhibits expression of IkappaBalpha protein and induces apoptosis of B-CLL cells in vitro. Leukemia 2007;21:1610-1618.
121. Davis JN, Kucuk O, Sarkar FH. Genistein inhibits NF-kappa B activation in prostate cancer cells. Nutr Cancer 1999;35:167-174.
122. Baxa DM, Yoshimura FK. Genistein reduces NF-kappa B in T lymphoma cells via a caspase-mediated cleavage of I kappa B alpha. Biochem Pharmacol 2003;66:1009-1018.
123. Gong L, Li Y, Nedeljkovic-Kurepa A, Sarkar FH. Inactivation of NF-kappaB by genistein is mediated via Akt signaling pathway in breast cancer cells. Oncogene 2003;22:4702-4709.
124. Li Y, Ellis KL, Ali S, et al. Apoptosis-inducing effect of chemotherapeutic agents is potentiated by soy isoflavone genistein, a natural inhibitor of NF-kappaB in BxPC-3 pancreatic cancer cell line. Pancreas 2004;28:e90-e95.
125. Mohammad RM, Banerjee S, Li Y, et al. Cisplatin-induced antitumor activity is potentiated by the soy isoflavone genistein in BxPC-3 pancreatic tumor xenografts. Cancer 2006;106:1260-1268.
126. Mohammad RM, Al-Katib A, Aboukameel A, et al. Genistein sensitizes diffuse large cell lymphoma to CHOP (cyclophosphamide, doxorubicin, vincristine, prednisone) chemotherapy. Mol Cancer Ther 2003;2:1361-1368.
127. Bharti AC, Donato N, Singh S, Aggarwal BB. Curcumin (diferuloylmethane) down-regulates the constitutive activation of nuclear factor-kappa B and IkappaBalpha kinase in human multiple myeloma cells, leading to suppression of proliferation and induction of apoptosis. Blood 2003;101:1053-1062.
128. Aggarwal BB, Shishodia S, Takada Y, et al. Curcumin suppresses the paclitaxel-induced nuclear factor-kappaB pathway in breast cancer cells and inhibits lung metastasis of human breast cancer in nude mice. Clin Cancer Res 2005;11:7490-7498.
129. Kunnumakkara AB, Guha S, Krishnan S, et al. Curcumin potentiates antitumor activity of gemcitabine in an orthotopic model of pancreatic cancer through suppression of proliferation, angiogenesis, and inhibition of nuclear factor-kappaB-regulated gene products. Cancer Res 2007;67:3853-3861.
130. Notarbartolo M, Poma P, Perri D, et al. Antitumor effects of curcumin, alone or in combination with cisplatin or doxorubicin, on human hepatic cancer cells: analysis of their possible relationship to changes in NF-κB activation levels and in IAP gene expression. Cancer Lett 2005;224:53-65.
131. Ariga A, Namekawa J, Matsumoto N, et al. Inhibition of tumor necrosis factor-alpha-induced nuclear translocation and activation of NF-kappa B by dehydroxymethylepoxyquinomicin. J Biol Chem 2002;277:24625-24630.
132. Starenki DV, Namba H, Saenko VA, et al. Induction of thyroid cancer cell apoptosis by a novel nuclear factor kappaB inhibitor, dehydroxymethylepoxyquinomicin. Clin Cancer Res 2004;10:6821-6829.
133. Horiguchi Y, Kuroda K, Nakashima J, et al. Antitumor effect of a novel nuclear factor-kappa B activation inhibitor in bladder cancer cells. Expert Rev Anticancer Ther 2003;3:793-798.

8

NEUROTRANSMITTERS

Eduardo E. Benarroch

INTRODUCTION 91
GENERAL PROCESS OF CHEMICAL NEUROTRANSMISSION 92
Presynaptic Events 92
Biosynthesis of Neurotransmitters 92
Storage in Synaptic Vesicles 92
Calcium-Dependent Exocytosis 93
Uptake of Neurotransmitters 93
Enzymatic Degradation 93
SYNAPTIC EFFECTS OF NEUROTRANSMITTERS 94
Classical Neurotransmission 94
Neurotransmitter-Gated Channels (Ionotropic Receptors) 94
Fast Synaptic Potentials 94
Desensitization and Allosteric Modulation of Ligand-Gated Receptors 94
Neuromodulation 94
GPCRs 94
Effects of GPCRs on Neuronal Function 95
Regulation of the GPCR Signal 95
Complexity of Neurochemical Signaling 95
Presynaptic Modulation 95
Multiple Effects of Single Neurotransmitters 95
Interactions among Neurotransmitters 95
Cotransmission 95
SPECIFIC NEUROTRANSMITTER SYSTEMS 96
Glutamate 96
Anatomic Distribution and Function 96
Biosynthesis, Storage, Release, Uptake, and Metabolism 96
iGluRs 96
mGluRs 97
Glutamatergic Neurotransmission as a Therapeutic Target 97
GABA and Glycine 98
Anatomic Distribution and Function 98
Biosynthesis, Storage, Release, Uptake, and Metabolism 98
$GABA_A$ Receptors 99
$GABA_B$ Receptors 99
Glycine as an Inhibitory Transmitter 99
GABAergic Neurotransmission as a Therapeutic Target 99
Acetylcholine 100
Anatomic Distribution and Function 100
Biosynthesis, Storage, and Metabolism 100
Nicotinic Receptors 100
Muscarinic Receptors 101
Cholinergic Transmission as a Therapeutic Target 102
Dopamine 103
Anatomic Organization and Function 103
Biosynthesis, Storage, Release, Reuptake, and Metabolism 103
Dopamine Receptors 104
Dopaminergic Neurotransmission as a Therapeutic Target 104
Norepinephrine 105
Anatomic Organization and Function 105
Biosynthesis, Storage, Release, Uptake, and Metabolism 105
Adrenergic Receptors (Adrenoceptors) 106
Adrenergic Transmission as a Therapeutic Target 107
Serotonin 108
Anatomic Organization and Function 108
Biosynthesis, Storage, Release, Reuptake, and Metabolism 108
Serotonin Receptors 108
Serotonergic Transmission as a Therapeutic Target 109
Histamine 109
Anatomic Organization and Function 109
Biosynthesis, Storage, and Metabolism 109
Histamine Receptors 109
Histaminergic System as a Therapeutic Target 109
Neuropeptides 110
Anatomic Localization 110
Synthesis, Release, and Metabolism 110
Neuropeptide Receptors 110
Peptidergic Neurotransmitter Systems as Therapeutic Targets 111
Other Neurochemical Transmitters 111
Purines 111
Nitric Oxide 111
Agmatine 111
Lipid Messengers 111
SUMMARY 112

INTRODUCTION

Chemical synapses provide the main mechanism of communication in the nervous system. Neurotransmitters released from synaptic vesicles located in presynaptic axon terminals act on a large variety of receptor molecules to elicit fast excitation or inhibition as well as slower modulatory effects on neuronal excitability and responsiveness to other neurotransmitters. In addition to electrophysiologic effects, chemical transmission triggers long-term effects on function, protein expression, and structure of the target cell. These effects are critical for dynamic, use-dependent, long-term changes in the efficacy and functional plasticity of synaptic transmission.

These interactions between the presynaptic and the postsynaptic events of chemical neurotransmission are bidirectional. Neurotransmitters affect their own release or that of another neurotransmitter. The postsynaptic cell may release diffusible retrograde messengers or growth factors that may affect the function and survival of the presynaptic cell. Some neurochemical signals may diffuse through the extracellular space. Astrocytes in the central nervous system (CNS) and Schwann cells in peripheral nervous system (PNS) have an integral role in signaling neural events. They contain neurotransmitter receptors and may also release neurochemical signals that affect synaptic events.

Chemical neurotransmission is a complex process that provides the nervous system with a great flexibility for information processing and functional plasticity. Every aspect of chemical neurotransmission involves critical molecules that are targets for pharmacologic manipulation. The aims of this chapter are to review the general principles of chemical neurotransmission, the main mechanisms of synthesis, storage, metabolism, reuptake, and synaptic effects of each of the main neurotransmitters, and the drugs that may affect each of these processes.

Neurotransmitters mediate chemical synaptic communication in the CNS and PNS. They include the amino acids L-glutamate, γ-aminobutyric acid (GABA), and glycine; acetylcholine (ACh); monoamines (catecholamines, serotonin, and histamine); neuropeptides; and purines. Other substances, such as nitric oxide (NO), lipid messengers, and steroids, may also act as chemical transmitters.

Chemical synaptic transmission is a complex process that involves several presynaptic and postsynaptic events (Fig. 8-1). Presynaptic events include synthesis, vesicular storage, exocytosis; presynaptic reuptake; and inactivation of the neurotransmitter. Postsynaptic events are mediated by ionotropic and metabotropic receptors, triggering fast synaptic potentials or slower modulatory signals, respectively.

The molecules involved in these presynaptic and postsynaptic events are targets for pharmacologic treatment of several disorders.

GENERAL PROCESS OF CHEMICAL NEUROTRANSMISSION

Presynaptic Events

The presynaptic events in chemical neurotransmission include synthesis and vesicular storage of the neurotransmitter; trafficking, docking, and priming of the synaptic vesicles in the presynaptic terminal; calcium (Ca^{2+})-dependent neurotransmitter release by exocytosis; endocytotic recycling of synaptic vesicles; and presynaptic reuptake and inactivation of the neurotransmitter[1] (Table 8-1).

Biosynthesis of Neurotransmitters

The amino acid neurotransmitters—L-glutamate, GABA, and glycine—and ACh originate, directly or indirectly, from the intermediate metabolism of glucose and Krebs cycle. The monoamine neurotransmitters, including *dopamine* (DA), *norepinephrine* (NE), *serotonin* (5-hydroxytryptamine, 5-HT), and *histamine* derive from essential dietary amino acid precursors via the activity of specific, rate-limiting enzymatic steps. The precursor for the biosynthesis of all catecholamines is L-tyrosine and that for the biosynthesis of serotonin is L-tryptophan. These amino acids pass across the blood-brain barrier (BBB) via a high-affinity neutral L-amino acid transporter, which also transports other large neutral L-amino acids, such as phenylalanine, valine, leucine, isoleucine, and methionine. Because there is a single neutral L-amino acid transporter, the different amino acids compete for their entrance to the brain. Plasma elevation of one amino acid may interfere with the BBB passage of others. This has important clinical implications, for example, in the case of competitive effects of dietary amino acids on absorption, and thus, therapeutic effects of L-dihydroxyphenylalanine (L-DOPA) in patients with Parkinson's disease.

Neuropeptides are synthesized from mRNA in the cell body. The specific steps for the biosynthesis of each of these neurotransmitters are described later in this chapter.

Storage in Synaptic Vesicles

Neurotransmitters are stored in different types of synaptic vesicles. Glutamate, GABA, glycine, and ACh are stored in small, clear vesicles, and monoamines are stored in intermediate-sized, dense-core vesicles. Both types of vesicles are loaded with the neurotransmitter

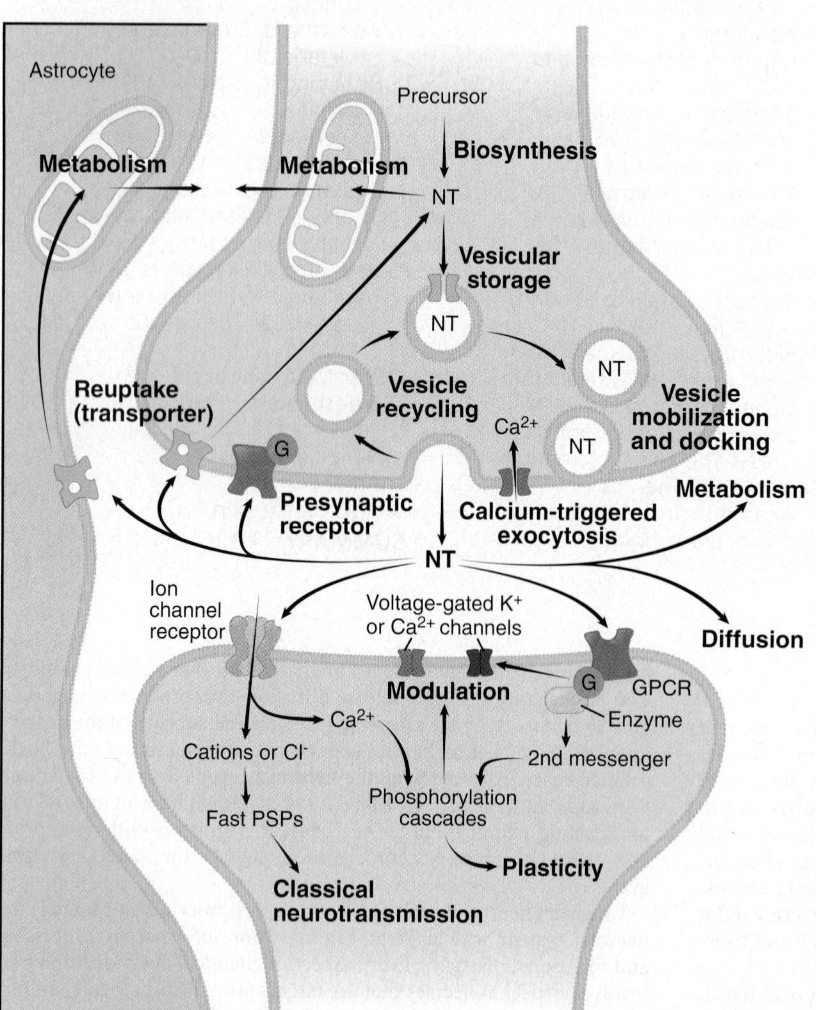

FIGURE 8-1 • Overview of the presynaptic and postsynaptic events of chemical neurotransmission. The presynaptic events include synthesis and vesicular storage of the neurotransmitter (NT); trafficking, docking, and priming of the synaptic vesicles in the presynaptic terminal; Ca^{2+}-dependent release by exocytosis; endocytotic recycling of synaptic vesicles; and presynaptic reuptake and inactivation of the neurotransmitter. The postsynaptic events are triggered by binding of the neurotransmitter to two classes of receptors: ligand-gated ion channels and G protein–coupled receptors (GPCR). Activation of ion channel receptors elicits rapid influx of cations or Cl^-, resulting in fast postsynaptic potentials (PSPs), referred to as classical neurotransmission, necessary for fast, precise transmission of neural information. Activation of GPCRs initiates transduction cascades that affect the function of K^+ and Ca^{2+} channels and other target proteins, which is called neuromodulation. Both types of receptors may trigger phosphorylation of target proteins, which may result in long-term synaptic plasticity. (Modified by permission from Benarroch EE. Basic Neurosciences with Clinical Applications. Philadelphia: Elsevier, 2005; Fig. 8-1.)

TABLE 8-1 SYNTHESIS, STORAGE, AND INACTIVATION OF THE MAIN NEUROTRANSMITTERS

Neurotransmitter	Precursor	Key Enzyme	Storage	Inactivation
L-Glutamate	α-KG Glutamine	GDH Glutaminase	VGLUT1-3	Reuptake (EAAT1-5)
GABA	L-Glutamate	GAD	VGAT	Reuptake (GAT) and GABA-T
Acetylcholine	Choline and acetyl CoA	Choline acetyltransferase	VAChT	Hydrolysis by AChE
Dopamine	L-Tyrosine	Tyrosine hydroxylase	VMAT2	Reuptake (DAT) followed by MAO_B and COMT
Norepinephrine	L-Tyrosine	Tyrosine hydroxylase and dopamine-β-hydroxylase	VMAT2	Reuptake (NET) followed by MAO and COMT
Serotonin	L-Tryptophan	Tryptophan hydroxylase	VMAT2	Reuptake (SERT) followed by MAO_A
Histamine	Histidine	Histidine decarboxylase	VMAT	Methyltransferase
Neuropeptides	Prepropeptide	Convertases	Secretory granule	Peptidases

Acetyl CoA, acetyl coenzyme-A; AChE, acetyl cholinesterase; α-KG, alpha-ketoglutarate; COMT, catechol-*O*-methyltransferase; DAT, dopamine transporter; EAAT, excitatory amino acid transporter; GABA, γ-aminobutyric acid; GABA-T, GABA transaminase; GAD, glutamic acid decarboxylase; GAT, GABA transporter; GDH, glutamate dehydrogenase; MAO, monoamine oxidase; NET, norepinephrine transporter; SERT, serotonin transporter; VAChT, vesicular acetylcholine transporter; VGAT, vesicular GABA transporter; VGLUT, vesicular glutamate transporter; VMAT, vesicular monoamine transporter.

at the nerve terminal. Vesicular storage of amino acids, ACh, and monoamines depends on specific *vesicular transporters* and is driven by an electrochemical gradient of H^+ across the vesicle membrane generated by the vacuolar adenosine triphosphate (ATP)–dependent proton pump. There are different vesicular transporters for glutamate (VGLUT1-3),[2] GABA and glycine (VGAT),[3] ACh (VAChT),[4] and monoamines (VMAT1 and VMAT2).[5]

In contrast to the classic neurotransmitters, which are synthesized and stored in synaptic vesicles at the synaptic terminals, neuropeptides are synthesized in the neuronal cell body, enter the secretory pathway, and are stored in large, dense-core vesicles that reach the synaptic terminal via fast axonal transport.[6]

Calcium-Dependent Exocytosis

Once loaded with the neurotransmitter, the synaptic vesicles undergo mobilization and docking at the presynaptic active zones, followed by priming for Ca^{2+}-triggered exocytosis. The specific sites for vesicle docking and fusion are the presynaptic *active zones*, which contain voltage-gated Ca^{2+} channels and other proteins involved in exocytosis.[7] The mobilization, docking, priming, and membrane fusion of the vesicles necessary for exocytosis are regulated by complex interactions between vesicle and presynaptic membrane proteins.[8] For example, synaptic vesicle docking to the active zone and vesicle priming for exocytosis depend critically on the proteins of the SNARE (soluble *N*-ethylmaleimide-sensitive factor attachment receptor) complex, formed by *synaptobrevin* (vesicular SNARE) and the presynaptic proteins *SNAP-25* (synaptosomal protein of 25 kD) and *syntaxin 1*. These SNARE complex proteins are the target of botulinum and tetanus toxins.[9,10]

The presynaptic voltage-gated Ca^{2+} channels involved in exocytosis are P/Q^- and the N channels. These channels are clustered in the active zones and open in response to depolarization triggered by arrival of the action potential, allowing a massive and transient Ca^{2+} influx.[11] The release of neuropeptides from large, dense-core vesicles is not restricted to the active zone and is triggered by high-frequency burst firing of the presynaptic neuron allowing Ca^{2+} influx via L channels present throughout the presynaptic membrane.[6]

Uptake of Neurotransmitters

The synaptic effects of a neurotransmitter are terminated by three mechanisms: uptake by presynaptic terminals or astrocytes; enzymatic metabolism; and diffusion out of the synaptic cleft. Uptake is the primary mechanism of inactivation of synaptic glutamate and the initial step in inactivation of GABA and monoamines. It is driven by the energy of the transmembrane Na^+ gradient maintained by the Na^+,K^+-ATPase and involves Na^+/ATP-dependent transporters present in the plasma membrane of presynaptic terminals or astrocytes. The ability of these specific carriers to concentrate neurotransmitters depends on the concurrent movement of Na^+. These transporters are members of two structurally and functionally distinct gene superfamilies. The family of Na^+/Cl^--dependent transporters includes the transporters for GABA (GAT1-3),[12] glycine (GLYT1-2),[13,14] and the monoamines dopamine (DAT), norepinephrine (NET), and serotonin (SERT).[15-17]

The second family includes the Na^+/K^+-dependent excitatory amino acid transporters (EAATs 1-5), involved in removal of glutamate from the synapses.[18,19] Transporters influence synaptic transmission not only by removal of the neurotransmitter signal from the synapses but also by eliciting changes in membrane potential of the presynaptic terminal. The influence of transporters in synaptic signaling depends on the density of expression and localization of the transporter in the plasma membrane and the intrinsic activity of the individual transporter, which is regulated by phosphorylation.

Transporters are also involved in carrier-mediated release, a Ca^{2+}-independent release of a cytoplasmic pool of neurotransmitter by a reversal of the transport mechanism. This occurs physiologically in some synapses or may be the consequence of the action of drugs that inhibit the Na^+,K^+-ATPase, such as ouabain, or displace the neurotransmitter from its vesicular storage or transporter binding sites. A typical example is amphetamine, which triggers nonvesicular release of DA, NE, and 5-HT. In pathologic conditions, carrier-mediated release is the manifestation of failure to maintain the Na^+ gradient owing to ATP depletion. A typical example is the carrier-mediated release of glutamate from the astrocytes in the setting of cerebral ischemia. Carrier-mediated release, combined with impaired reuptake, contributes to synaptic accumulation of glutamate in the synapse, triggering excitotoxic neuronal injury.[19]

Enzymatic Degradation

Enzymatic degradation is the main mechanism for termination of action of ACh and neuropeptides. ACh is rapidly inactivated by *acetyl cholinesterase* (AChE) present in the synaptic space or at the basal lamina of the neuromuscular junction.[20] Peptides are metabolized by extracellular *peptidases*.[6] After presynaptic or astrocytic uptake, GABA undergoes metabolism via *GABA transaminase* (GABA-T).

The monoamines (DA, NE, 5-HT, and histamine) are metabolized by *monoamine oxidases* (MAOs), located in the external mitochondrial membrane, and *methyltransferases* located in the cytosol. The two isoforms of MAO, MAO_A and MAO_B, are encoded by separate genes on the X chromosome.[21] MAO_A is located primarily in catecholaminergic neurons and preferentially oxidizes 5-HT; MAO_B is present in the striatum, serotonergic neurons and endothelial cells of the BBB, and metabolizes DA, NE, histamine, and tyramine (which are also substrates of MAO_A). The oxidative deamination reactions catalyzed by MAO generate hydrogen peroxide and ammonia, which may be potentially toxic to neurons. *Catechol-O-methyltransferase* (COMT) may act before or after the MAOs to generate the final metabolites of catecholamines. Whereas the enzymatic degradation of ACh terminates the synaptic effects of this neurotransmitter, the termination of the effects of catecholamines depends primarily on their uptake and dilution in the extracellular space.

SYNAPTIC EFFECTS OF NEUROTRANSMITTERS

The synaptic effects of neurotransmitters are triggered by their binding to two types of receptors: ligand-gated ion channel receptors (also called *ionotropic receptors*) and G protein–coupled receptors (GPCRs, or *metabotropic receptors*). Ion channel receptors allow rapid influx of cations or Cl^-, resulting in fast excitation or inhibition, respectively, of the postsynaptic neurons. This is called *classical neurotransmission.* Activation of GPCRs initiates multiple signal transduction cascades that affect the ion channels and other target proteins leading to changes in neuronal excitability and responsiveness to other synaptic stimuli This is referred to as *neuromodulation*.

Classical Neurotransmission

Classical neurotransmission provides a mechanism for rapid communication among neurons and is mediated by ionotropic receptors.

The summation of phasic excitatory and inhibitory postsynaptic potentials (EPSPs and IPSPs, respectively) and their interactions with intrinsic electrophysiologic properties of the neurons are the basic mechanisms of neuronal processing of information.

Neurotransmitter-Gated Channels (Ionotropic Receptors)

The ionotropic receptors belong to three superfamilies. The *cysteine (Cys)-loop superfamily* includes the *nicotinic* ACh receptor (nAChR) and the serotonin 5-HT_3 receptor, which are cation channels, and the $GABA_A$ and the glycine (GLYR-1) receptors, which are anion channels. The Cys-loop receptors are heteropentameric proteins formed by assembly of five subunits, each containing four transmembrane domains (M_1-M_4), and the M_2 domain forms the wall of the channel. The crystallographic structure of the prototype Cys-loop receptor, the nAChR, comprises an extracellular domain of mainly β-sheets, a channel domain of α-helices, and a cytoplasmic domain containing a large α-helix.[22] In these receptors, the ligand-binding domains are formed at the interface between α- and non–α-subunits. The presence of multiple subunit subtypes for each type of receptor provides for a large functional diversity.

The second superfamily of ion channel receptors is that of the ionotropic glutamate receptors (iGluRs).[23,24] These receptors are homo- or heteromeric assembles of four homologous subunits. Each subunit consists of an extracellular *N*-terminal domain, four hydrophobic regions, and an intracellular *C*-terminal domain.[25] Crystallographic studies reveal that these receptors have an amino-terminal domain; an agonist-binding domain, an ion-channel pore, and a cytoplasmic domain that vary in size among the different subtypes of iGluRs. The ligand-binding cores assemble as dimers, and an intact glutamate receptor (GluR) is believed to assemble as dimers of dimers.[23-25]

The third family of ionotropic receptors corresponds to the P_{2X} receptors, which are ATP-gated cation channels. These are homomeric or heteromeric proteins formed by the assembly of at least three of seven subunits (P_{2X1} to P_{2X7}). All subunits contain intracellular *N*- and *C*-termini, two transmembrane domains, and a relatively large extracellular ligand-binding loop.[26]

Neurotransmitter-gated ion channel receptors cluster at specialized postsynaptic sites that are closely apposed to the presynaptic active zones. This ensures rapid and precise intercellular signal transmission. Clustering of these receptors depends on interactions of some of their subunits with adaptor proteins as part of macromolecular complexes in which the receptors are coupled to transduction molecules and with submembrane cytoskeletal proteins.

Fast Synaptic Potentials

Binding of the neurotransmitter produces a change in the tridimensional conformation of the receptor protein, resulting in opening of the ion channel. Opening of ligand-gated cation channels, including the nicotinic, 5-HT_3, ionotropic glutamate, and P_{2X} receptors, allows rapid influx of Na^+, Ca^{2+}, eliciting rapid membrane depolarization (EPSPs). In contrast, the $GABA_A$ and the glycine receptors allow rapid inflow of Cl^-. In most adult neurons, this effect is inhibitory (fast IPSP), because it stabilizes the membrane at the equilibrium potential of Cl^- (−75 mV), thus blocking other synaptic responses (*shunt inhibition*).

Desensitization and Allosteric Modulation of Ligand-Gated Receptors

Ionotropic receptors undergo multiple conformational transitions and can exist in at least one of four interconvertible and functionally distinct states, closed, open, and two desensitized states, at any one time.[22] Binding of the neurotransmitter stabilizes the receptor in the open state, but the channels close when the neurotransmitter is still bound to the channel molecule. This process, called *desensitization*, produces a progressive depression of the synaptic responses to the agonist. The rate of desensitization and recovery varies with the type of ligand-gated channel. Ionotropic receptor molecules contain several intracellular phosphorylation sites, and their state of phosphorylation affects the expression, gating, kinetics, and internalization of these receptors. In addition, ionotropic receptors contain allosteric sites that critically affect receptor function.

Neuromodulation

Neuromodulation refers to the regulation of neuronal excitability and synaptic responsiveness to other extrinsic signals. Neuromodulation is the consequence of changes in ion channel function triggered by neurotransmitter binding of neurotransmitters to GPCRs.

GPCRs

The GPCRs constitute a large superfamily of receptors characterized structurally by a single polypeptide chain with seven α-helical transmembrane domains (I-VII) and are classified according to different criteria.[27-29] The GPCRs include the *metabotropic glutamate* receptors (mGluRs), *$GABA_B$* receptors, essentially all the receptors for monoamines, and the neuropeptide receptors. The GPCRs are coupled to heteromeric G proteins composed of α-, β-, and γ-subunits. Upon ligand binding, the receptor acts as a guanine nucleotide–exchanging factor that catalyzes the exchange of the Gα-subunit–bound guanosine diphosphate (GDP) for guanosine triphosphate (GTP). The active GTP-bound Gα-subunit dissociates from the β/γ complex. Both the Gα and the β/γ complex regulate effector proteins, including ion channels and enzymes, triggering second messenger pathways. The signal transduction pathways triggered by activation of GPCRs are discussed in Chapter 6, Signal Transduction, and only a few concepts are emphasized here.

The G proteins are classified into several subfamilies according to their α-subunit and transduction pathways. G_s proteins activate adenylyl cyclase, leading to production of cyclic adenosine monophosphate (cAMP). The primary effector of cAMP is activation of protein kinase A (PKA), which phosphorylates several membrane, cytoplasmic, cytoskeletal, and nuclear proteins, including ion channels and the transcription factor CREB (cAMP response element–binding protein). The actions of cAMP are terminated via its hydrolysis by cAMP phosphodiesterases (PDEs). The $G_{i/o}$ proteins, via their α-subunit, inhibit adenylyl cyclase and, via their β/γ complex, activate K^+ channels in the postsynaptic membrane and inhibit presynaptic N- and P/Q channels. The G_q proteins activate phospholipase Cβ (PLCβ), which hydrolyzes phosphatidylinositol biphosphate (PIP_2), resulting in production of diacylglycerol (DAG) and inositol triphosphate (IP_3). DAG activates protein kinase C (PKC), and IP_3 binds to IP_3 receptors in the endoplasmic reticulum, triggering Ca^{2+} release. Calcium binds to several effector proteins, including calmodulin (CaM), and the Ca^{2+}/CaM complex activates many effector proteins, including CaM kinases (CaMK) and nitric oxide synthase (NOS). G proteins may also activate phospholipase A_2, which acts on membrane phospholipids generating arachidonic acid (which gives rise to prostaglandins, leukotrienes, and endocannabinoids) and mitogen-activated protein kinases (MAPK). The kinases activated by these GPCR signals translocate to the nucleus and phosphorylate the CREB, activating gene expression. Some signal transduction pathways, unrelated to GPCRs, increase cytosolic levels of cyclic guanine monophosphate (cGMP). Membrane-bound guanylyl cyclases act as receptors for atrial and brain natriuretic peptides, and cytosolic guanylyl cyclase is activated by NO and carbon monoxide (CO).

Effects of GPCRs on Neuronal Function

Neurotransmitters, acting via GPCRs, may either increase or decrease specific voltage-gated or neurotransmitter-gated currents by several mechanisms.[30] These include α-guanosine triphosphate (α-GTP)-subunit activation of second messenger protein kinase cascades and ion channel phosphorylation, direct interaction of the β/γ complex with the ion channel, and activation of cyclic nucleotide-gated channels. The main targets are the voltage-gated K^+ and Ca^{2+} channels. Modulation of postsynaptic K^+ channels is a major mechanism to control the excitability and firing characteristics of a neuron because the multiplicity of K^+ currents "fine-tunes" the electrical output of the cell. One typical example of this effect is mediated by the β/γ-subunit of $G_{i/o}$, which directly activates inward rectifier K^+ channels (referred to as G protein–gated inward rectifier K^+ channels [GIRKS]), leading to decreases in neuronal excitability. In contrast, activations of some G_q-coupled receptors results in inhibition of K^+ currents, resulting in increased neuronal excitability.

Modulation of Ca^{2+} channels by GPCRs affect the ability of depolarizing currents to trigger or maintain bursts of action potentials in the postsynaptic neurons and regulate the presynaptic release of neurotransmitter. For example, receptors coupled with $G_{i/o}$, inhibit, via the β/γ-subunit-subunit, the presynaptic N- and P/Q-type Ca^{2+} channels responsible for exocytosis. By this mechanism, many presynaptic receptors inhibit neurotransmitter release.

Regulation of the GPCR Signal

The GPCR signal is turned off by several different mechanisms, including receptor desensitization, endocytosis, and down-regulation (see Chapter 6, Signal Transduction). *Receptor desensitization* occurs after short-term exposure to the agonist and involves phosphorylation of the receptor protein and uncoupling from the G protein. This involves G protein–receptor kinases that bind the β/γ-subunits of the G protein and functional cofactors called arrestins that bind to the phosphorylated receptor disrupt its coupling to the G protein and promote receptor endocytosis. Receptor down-regulation results from long-term continuous exposure of cells to the agonist and leads to a decrease in the total number of receptors as a consequence of enhanced receptor degradation, reduced receptor synthesis, or both. In contrast, decreased exposure to the agonist, either by receptor blockade or by denervation, may result in an increase in the number of postsynaptic receptors, a process called up-regulation. This results in a response to the agonist after denervation, a phenomenon called *denervation hypersensitivity*, which is prominent in the peripheral autonomic system (see Chapter 9, Autonomic Pharmacology).

Complexity of Neurochemical Signaling

Neurochemical signaling is a highly complex process owing to the high structural heterogeneity (protein isoforms) affecting the function of biosynthetic enzymes, transporters, receptors, and the homo- or hetero-oligomerization of GPCRs and the coexistence of different receptors and transported in "complexes" composed of several proteins. Receptor interactions or interactions between receptors and transporters located on the same plasma membrane increase this complexity. Studies of fresh human tissue provide insight into the functional pharmacology of these interactions.[31]

Presynaptic Modulation

The presynaptic terminals contain a large variety of ionotropic and metabotropic receptors, called *presynaptic receptors*, which regulate neurotransmitter release by affecting the probability of mobilization of synaptic vesicles, opening of presynaptic Ca^{2+} channels, or both. For example, activation of presynaptic nAChRs, increases Ca^{2+} influx and triggers exocytosis.

In many neurons, neurotransmitter release is regulated by presynaptic inhibitory GPCRs coupled to $G_{i/o}$ proteins that, via the β/γ complex, inhibit the N- or P/Q-channels. These presynaptic receptors may be activated by the neurotransmitter released from the same terminal (*presynaptic autoreceptors*), allowing a negative feedback modulation of synaptic neurotransmitter availability, or by a neurotransmitter released from neighboring terminals (heteroreceptor), allowing a cross-talk between neurochemical signals. There are also autoreceptors and heteroreceptors at the level of soma and dendrites, where they regulate excitability and firing of the neurons. This is an important mechanism regulating the monoaminergic neurons in the brainstem.

Multiple Effects of Single Neurotransmitters

A given neurotransmitter may have multiple actions in the nervous system, according to the subtype and localization of the receptor upon which it acts. For example, ACh, acting via postsynaptic nAChRs, elicits fast excitation of the target neurons such as the skeletal muscle or autonomic ganglion neurons; via presynaptic nAChRs, it increases release of DA in the striatum; via postsynaptic muscarinic M_1 receptors, it decreases K^+ conductances and increases excitability of cortical pyramidal neurons; and via presynaptic M_2 receptors, it inhibits its own release and release of other neurotransmitters. In addition, different neurotransmitters, acting via their respective receptors, may activate the same final transduction cascade and have the same effect on channel function.

Interactions among Neurotransmitters

There are abundant interactions among neurotransmitters at both postsynaptic and presynaptic levels.[31,32] In many areas of the CNS, excitatory synaptic boutons contact dendritic spines. At this level, glutamate, acting via excitatory inotropic and metabotropic receptors, elicits changes in dendritic Ca^{2+} concentrations that may lead to long-term changes in synaptic efficacy. The inhibitory effects of GABA on the neurons depend on the localization of the GABAergic synapse and the distribution of receptors. For example, GABAergic terminals on the axon hillock, the site of action potential generation, control the global output of the cell, whereas individual GABAergic terminals on the distal dendrites and dendritic spines exert a localized effect on and processing in synaptic microcircuits. ACh, monoamines, or neuropeptides exert an important neuromodulatory effect on central synaptic circuits. These neurochemicals are released from terminals of widely diverging axons of neurons located in restricted areas of the basal forebrain and brainstem. These neurochemical influences, acting via a variety of GPCRs, modulate the neuronal responsiveness to the fast excitatory or inhibitory synaptic inputs.

Cotransmission

There is evidence of cotransmission in many synapses of both the CNS and the PNS.[32] For example, several neuropeptides, ATP, or both, are present in many glutamatergic, GABAergic, cholinergic, and monoaminergic neurons, and may be coreleased with glutamate, GABA, and catecholamines in the hypothalamus and other areas of the CNS. There are also several examples of cotransmission in the PNS. For example, neuropeptide Y (NPY) and ATP coexist with NE in sympathetic terminals innervating the smooth muscle.

The physiologic significance of cotransmission is severalfold. Fast (classical) and slow (neuropeptides) cotransmitters are released in response to different firing patterns of neurons, may act at different targets, may presynaptically regulate the release of each other, may cooperate synergistically or participate in negative cross-talk at postsynaptic levels, or may act as trophic factors. For example, at the sympathetic neuroeffector junctions, NPY prevents presynaptic release of NE and potentiates the vasoconstrictor effect of NE on blood vessels.

The expression of cotransmitters in the nervous system is plastic and changes during development or in response to different stimuli.[32]

SPECIFIC NEUROTRANSMITTER SYSTEMS

Glutamate

Anatomic Distribution and Function

L-Glutamate is the primary excitatory neurotransmitter in the CNS. It mediates the excitatory influences of pyramidal neuron of the cerebral cortex on other cortical neurons, thalamus, striatum, brainstem nuclei, and motor nuclei of the brainstem and spinal cord. It is also the primary excitatory transmitter in the amygdala and hippocampal circuits, sensory relay nuclei, and central autonomic nuclei.

Glutamatergic neurotransmission has a critical role in sensory processing, motor control, emotion, and cognitive mechanisms, including memory. Glutamate has a critical role in mechanisms of synaptic plasticity during development, learning, and response to injury. In contrast, excessive glutamatergic activation results in neuronal and glial injury or death in the setting of hypoxia, ischemia, trauma, seizures, and neurodegenerative disorders. This is called *excitotoxicity* and involves several receptor mechanisms that lead to accumulation of intracellular Ca^{2+}, oxidative stress, and mitochondrial failure. A full discussion of these important topics is beyond the aims of this chapter.

Biosynthesis, Storage, Release, Uptake, and Metabolism

Glutamate is synthesized from α-ketoglutarate, an intermediary of the Krebs cycle, via a reversible reaction catalyzed by *glutamate dehydrogenase*, and by action of the *glutaminase*, which acts on glutamine derived from the astrocyte[33] (Fig. 8-2). Glutamate is stored by the action of specific vesicular carriers (VGLUT1-3). In some excitatory synapses, glutamate is costored with Zn^{2+} or with an *N-acetyl aspartylglutamate* (NAAG), a peptide that may be coreleased with glutamate and regulate excitatory neurotransmission.[34,35]

The synaptic levels of glutamate are regulated primarily by high-affinity, Na^+- and K^+-coupled EAATs 1-5.[18] The most important are EAAT2 and EAAT1, present in the astrocytes. Astroglial uptake has a key homeostatic role in maintaining low synaptic levels of glutamate, preventing its neurotoxic effects.[19]

iGluRs

Glutamate acts via iGluRs and mGluRs.[33] The iGluRs mediate fast excitation in the majority of synapses in the nervous system. Mammalian iGluRs consist of different combinations of 18 subunits that assemble to form four major families, the *AMPA* (α-amino-3-hydroxy-5-methyl-4-isoxazole propionic acid), *kainate*, *NMDA* (*N*-methyl-D-aspartate), and *delta* receptors.[36]

The AMPA receptors mediate most of the fast excitatory effects of glutamate in the CNS. AMPA receptors consist of GluR1 to GluR4 subunits, each consisting of an extracellular *N*-terminal domain, four hydrophobic regions (TM_1-TM_4), and an intracellular C-terminal

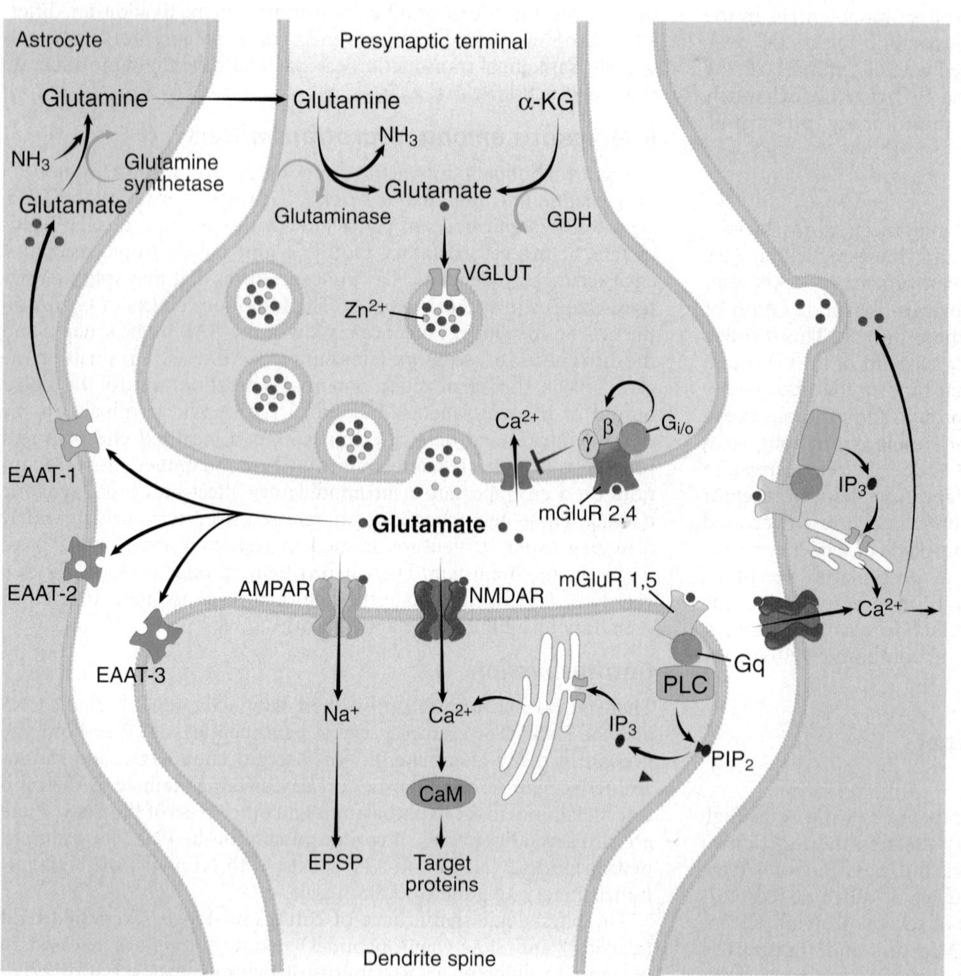

FIGURE 8-2 • Basic mechanisms of glutamatergic synaptic transmission. Glutamate derives from glutamine, by action of glutaminase and α-ketoglutarate (α-KG), by action of glutamate dehydrogenase (GDH). Glutamate is transported and stored via vesicular glutamate transporter (VGLUT) and is costored with Zn^{2+} in some synapses. Glutamate is rapidly cleared from the synaptic cleft by the excitatory amino acid transporters (EAATs), particularly EAAT-1 and EAAT-2 in astrocytes and EAAT-3 in neurons. The synaptic effects of glutamate are mediated by ionotropic and metabotropic receptors (mGluRs). Ionotropic receptors include the α-amino-3-hydroxy-5-methyl-4-isoxazole propionic acid receptor (AMPAR) and the *N*-methyl-d-aspartate receptor (NMDAR). The mGluRs are G protein–coupled receptors. Postsynaptic type I mGluRs are coupled to G_q and activate phospholipase C (PLC), resulting in hydrolysis of phosphatidylinositol biphosphate (PIP_2) to generate inositol triphosphate (IP_3) and diacylglycerol (DAG). Glutamate release is controlled by presynaptic inhibitory group II and III mGluRs, which reduce Ca^{2+} influx via *L*- and *N*-channels. CaM, calmodulin; EAAT, excitatory amino acid transporters; EPSP, excitatory postsynaptic potentials; PLC, phospholipase C. (Modified by permission from Benarroch E. Basic Neurosciences with Clinical Applications. Philadelphia: Elsevier, 2005; Fig. 10-1.)

domain.[25] TM2 forms an intracellular hairpin loop that contributes to the cation channel pore. The ion conductances and kinetics of AMPA receptors depend on their subunit composition. The presence of a GluR2 subunit confers AMPA receptors with a much higher permeability to Na^+ than Ca^{2+}. In the GluR2 subunit, the TM2 pore domain contains an mRNA editing site that allows a substitution of a glutamine (Q) by an arginine (R) residue, which results in a marked reduction of Ca^{2+} permeability. Although most AMPA receptors contain these edited GluR2 subunits, some neurons and glial cells contain AMPA receptors that either lack or have an unedited GluR2 subunit, and are therefore permeable to Ca^{2+}.[25] The TM3-TM4 loop of the AMPA receptor contains a flip/flop alternative splice region. The "flip" splice variants desensitize much slower than the "flop" variants and confer different sensitivity to allosteric modulators of the channel.[25] The appropriate targeting and clustering of the AMPA receptors at the postsynaptic sites, which depends on their interaction with several accessory proteins, is critical for the formation and maintenance of excitatory synapses. Phosphorylation of the AMPA receptor in res-ponse to synaptic activity has a major role in plasticity of excitatory synapses.[37,38]

The kainate (KA) receptors consist of tetrameric combinations of low-affinity GluR5, GluR6, or GluR7 subunits and high-affinity KA1 and KA2 subunits.[39] These receptors are, in general, more permeable to Na^+ than Ca^{2+} owing to the presence of a edited Q/R site in the GluR5, GluR6, and GluR7 subunits. KA receptors vary in their subunit composition and subcellular localization and may regulate activity of neuronal networks by several mechanisms. For example, presynaptic KA receptors control glutamate and GABA release, whereas postsynaptic KA receptors elicit fast excitatory responses and regulate neuronal excitability by inhibiting K^+ channels.

The NMDA receptors are heteromers formed by a common NR1 subunit and one or more of four types of NR2 subunits (NR2A, NR2B, NR2C, and NR2D) and, in some cases, an NR3 subunit.[40] All NMDA receptor complexes function as assemblies of two NR1 subunits in combination with at least one type of NR2 subunit.[41] The NMDA receptors are Ca^{2+} channels that have two unique characteristics: (i) their activation requires, in addition to binding of glutamate to an agonist site, the binding of glycine (or serine) to a modulatory site, and (ii) their channel is blocked by Mg^{2+} at resting membrane potential; this blockade is removed by depolarization.[41] Therefore, NMDA receptors act as "coincidence detectors" of three events—binding of glutamate, binding of glycine, and membrane depolarization. Several splice variants of NR1, NR2, and NR3 subunits are differentially distributed in the brain. The diverse subunit composition dramatically changes the pharmacologic properties of the NMDA receptor. The NR1 and NR2 subunits are structurally different, but both contain an identical pore-forming TM2 segment that serves as an ion selectivity filter and contributes to the Ca^{2+} permeability. The glutamate-binding site resides in the NR2 subunit, and the glycine-binding site is in a homologous region in the NR1 subunit. Endogenous D-serine, derived from astrocytes, mimics the activity of glycine as a positive allosteric modulator of the NMDA receptor.

Activation of NMDA receptors elicits an excitatory postsynaptic current with a much longer latency and slower decay than that elicited by AMPA receptor activation. The affinity of the receptor for glutamate, the time course of the NMDA current, and its sensitivity to Mg^{2+} blockade are influenced by the NR2 subunit subtype. Zinc, which may be coreleased with glutamate from some excitatory synapses, elicits a voltage-independent block of the NMDA receptor channel. The NMDA receptors are also inhibited by protons within the range of physiologic pH. NO inhibits the NMDA receptor channel by interaction with the cysteine sulfhydryl groups at a redox modulatory site of the receptor.

The endogenous polyamines spermidine and spermine produce both stimulatory and inhibitory effects on the NMDA receptor. *Agmatine*, a product of decarboxylation of arginine, is an endogenous polyamine that can block NMDA receptor–mediated responses. Agmatine is also an agonist of *imidazoline* receptors.

mGluRs

The mGluRs are GPCRs that are products of eight genes (mGluRs 1-8) and are classified into three main groups according to their amino acid sequence, transduction mechanisms, and distribution.[42] Group I receptors (mGluR1 and mGluR5) are mainly localized postsynaptically, are coupled to G_q proteins, and stimulate the phospholipase C/IP_3-Ca^{2+}/DAG pathway. Thus, activation of type I mGluRs potentiates the NMDA receptor–mediated increase in intracellular Ca^{2+}. Group II (mGluR2 and mGluR3) and group III (mGluR4, mGluR7, and mGluR8) are preferentially located in presynaptic terminals. In general, they are coupled to $G_{i/o}$ and inhibit adenylyl cyclase, activate K^+ currents, decreasing neuronal excitability, and inhibit presynaptic Ca^{2+} channels reducing release of glutamate, GABA, and other neurotransmitters.[42] NAAG, acting via presynaptic mGluR3 receptors, reduces release of glutamate and GABA.[43] The specific coupling of specific mGluRs with different intracellular transduction pathways depends on several interacting proteins.[42]

Glutamatergic Neurotransmission as a Therapeutic Target

Despite the marked interest and extensive research on pharmacologic manipulation of glutamatergic transmission for neuroprotection and management of several disorders, including stroke, epilepsy, dementia, pain, and psychiatric conditions, only a few drugs acting on glutamatergic mechanism are currently available for clinical use (Table 8-2). Drugs that inhibit glutamate release, such as *lamotrigine*, are currently used for treatment of seizures. β-lactam antibiotics (particularly ceftriaxone) increase EAAT2 expression and are neuroprotective both in vitro and in the superoxide dismutase (SOD) 1 mutant mice model of amyotrophic lateral sclerosis.[35] They have not been evaluated in this regard in humans.

The AMPA receptors are potential targets of several drugs, some of which are currently under investigation for application in treatment of Alzheimer's disease and other disorders.[44,45] *Ampakines* are centrally active positive allosteric modulators of the AMPA receptors that slow the deactivation and inactivation of the AMPA receptor.[46] The NMDA receptors are an attractive therapeutic target for treatment of conditions such as stroke, seizures, dementia, Parkinson's disease, pain, and schizophrenia.[47] *Ifenprodil*, an antagonist of NR2B containing NMDA

TABLE 8-2 DRUGS AFFECTING GLUTAMATERGIC TRANSMISSION

Target	Drug	Mechanism of Action	Therapeutic Use
Glutamate release	Lamotrigine	Inhibition	Seizures
AMPA receptor	Ampakines	Decrease inactivation	Alzheimer's disease?
NMDA receptor	Ketamine	Allosteric inhibition	Anesthesia
	Amantadine Memantine	Weak blocker Weak blocker	Parkinson's disease Alzheimer's disease
	Felbamate	Antagonist at the glycine allosteric site	Seizures

AMPA, α-amino-3-hydroxy-5-methyl-4-isoxazole propionic acid; NMDA, *N*-methyl-D-aspartate.

receptors, and open channel blockers, such as *ketamine* and *phencyclidine* (PCP), have neuroprotective and antinociceptive effects in experimental models, but their cognitive side effects prevent its utilization in humans. *Memantine* and *amantadine* are noncompetitive, low-affinity open-channel blockers. Memantine is currently used for treatment of Alzheimer's disease (see Chapter 43, Alzheimer's Disease and Dementias). Amantadine is used as adjuvant treatment of Parkinson's disease (see Chapter 44, Parkinson's Disease). *Felbamate*, a drug that blocks the glycine-binding site of the NMDA receptor, is a highly efficacious antepileptic drug, but it has limited clinical use because of the risk of inducing aplastic anemia (see Chapter 45, Seizure Disorders).

Positive and negative noncompetitive allosteric modulators of the mGluRs have emerged as agents with potential therapeutic potential for disorders such as pain, epilepsy, Parkinson's disease, anxiety, schizophrenia, and drug abuse.[48,49] Inhibition of the NAAG peptidase, increasing the availability of NAAG—which, acting via mGluR3 receptors, inhibits glutamate release—is investigated for potential applications in CNS injury, amyotrophic lateral sclerosis, pain, and schizophrenia.[34]

GABA and Glycine

Anatomic Distribution and Function

GABA is the most important inhibitory neurotransmitter in the CNS. It mediates inhibitory influences in the cerebral cortex, thalamus, basal ganglia, cerebellum, and motor and sensory nuclei of the brainstem and spinal cord. In most regions of the CNS, GABA is present in inhibitory local circuit neurons. GABA is also the primary transmitter of neurons of the striatum, globus pallidus, and Purkinje cells of the cerebellum. Thus, GABA has a critical role in regulating cortical excitability (and preventing seizures), sensory processing, and motor control. Glycine contributes to fast inhibitory transmission in the spinal cord and brainstem.

In the periphery, GABA is present in the endocrine pancreas and enteric nervous systems.

Biosynthesis, Storage, Release, Uptake, and Metabolism

GABA is produced by decarboxylation of L-glutamate by *glutamic acid decarboxylase* (GAD) (Fig. 8-3), which includes two isoforms, GAD_{65} (65 kDa) and GAD_{67} (67 kDa). The activity of GAD requires pyridoxal phosphate, a vitamin B_6 (pyridoxine) derivative. GABA is stored in flat, clear vesicles, by action of a specific vesicular transporter that also transports glycine (VGAT, also referred to as *vesicular inhibitory amino acid transporter*).[50]

Following release, the synaptic effects of GABA are terminated by its selective uptake via GAT, including GAT-1, located in presynaptic terminals; GAT-2, located in ependymal cells and choroid plexus; and GAT-3, located in astrocytes.[12] After uptake, GABA is metabolized by GABA-T to succinic semialdehyde, which, in the mitochondria, is metabolized by *succinic semialdehyde dehydrogenase* to succinic acid,

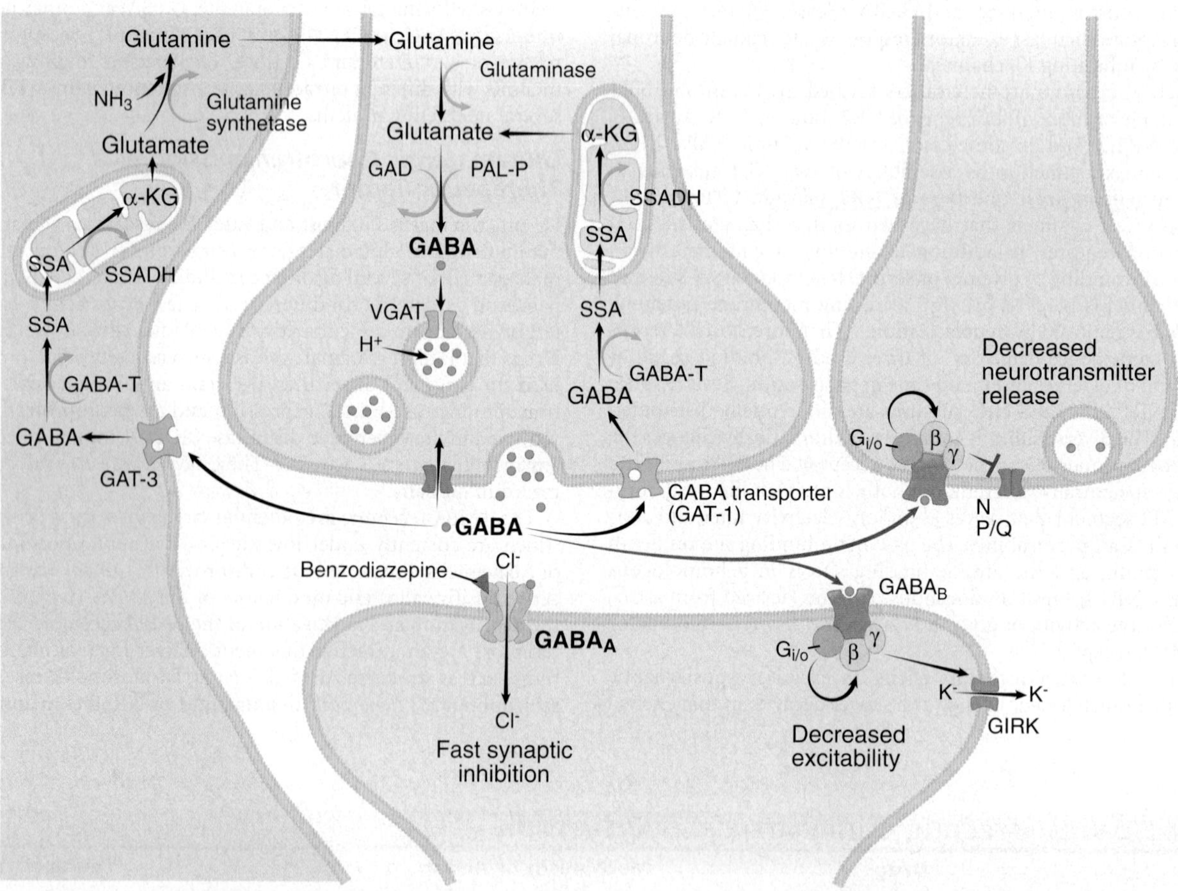

FIGURE 8-3 • Overview of γ-aminobutyric acid (GABA)ergic neurotransmission. GABA is produced by decarboxylation of L-glutamate by glutamic acid decarboxylase (GAD), which requires pyridoxal phosphate (PAL-P). GABA is stored by action of a specific vesicular transporter (VGAT) and undergoes uptake into GABAergic terminals and astrocytes via GABA transporters (GAT1 and GAT3). After uptake, GABA is metabolized by GABA-transaminase (GABA-T) to succinic semialdehyde (SSA), which is metabolized in the mitochondria by SSA dehydrogenase (SSADH) to succinic acid, which enters the Krebs cycle and gives rise to α-ketoglutarate (α-KG).

Astrocytes use L-glutamate to produce glutamine, by action of glutamine synthetase. The fast inhibitory effects of GABA are mediated by $GABA_A$ receptors, which are ligand-gated Cl^- channels that elicit fast inhibitory postsynaptic potentials and are allosterically activated by benzodiazepines and other modulators. The $GABA_B$ receptor is a G protein–coupled receptor that acts as a dimer and increases permeability to K^+ and decreases Ca^{2+} conductance. GIRK, G protein–activated inward-rectifying K^+ channel. (Modified by permission from Benarroch EE. Basic Neurosciences with Clinical Applications. Philadelphia: Elsevier, 2005; Fig. 11-1.)

which enters the Krebs cycle. Succinic semialdehyde can also be reduced to produce *γ-hydroxybutyrate* (GHB), which may also serve as a precursor of GABA.[51] Astrocytes, which actively take up glutamate, lack GAD and are therefore unable to resynthesize GABA. Instead, they use L-glutamate to produce glutamine, by action of *glutamine synthetase.* This enzyme is a specific marker for astrocytes and uses ammonia as a nitrogen donor; it therefore has a major role in ammonia detoxification in the CNS.

Glycine is a nonessential amino acid that is synthesized from glucose; its immediate precursor is L-serine, by action of *serine hydroxymethyltransferase.* After release, glycine undergoes presynaptic reuptake via the transporters *GLYT-1* and *GLYT-2* and is then catabolized by the *glycine-cleavage system* in the mitochondria.

GABA$_A$ Receptors

In the adult brain, GABA exerts primarily an inhibitory influence. The inhibitory effects of GABA are mediated by GABA$_A$ and GABA$_B$ receptors. Both classes of receptors mediate presynaptic and postsynaptic inhibition.

The GABA$_A$ receptors are Cl^- channels that belong to the Cys-loop superfamily of ligand-gated receptors.[52] A great diversity of GABA$_A$ receptor subtypes exists, each having distinct kinetic and pharmacologic properties and localization. This diversity is generated by different combinations of subunits. Based on their sequence homologies, these subunits are grouped into several families, α (α_1-α_6), β (β_1-β_3), γ (γ_1-γ_3) δ, ε, π, υ, and ρ (ρ_1-ρ_3).[52-56] Functional channels are pentameric heteromers. The most common subunit composition in the brain is two α_1-, two β_2-, and one γ_2-subunit. There is a regional specificity of distribution of GABA$_A$ receptor subtypes in the mature brain.

GABA binding occurs at the interface between the α- and the β-subunits and triggers opening of the intrinsic Cl^- channel. This leads to a rapid influx of Cl^-, which brings the membrane potential toward the equilibrium potential of Cl^-. This can lead to hyperpolarization, little or no change in membrane potential, or depolarization, according to the transmembrane Cl^- gradient.[57] The intracellular concentration of Cl^- is regulated by a neuronal K^+/Cl^- cotransporter, which in most adult neurons is responsible for extrusion of Cl^-, maintaining a low intracellular concentration, and allowing an influx of Cl^- upon GABA$_A$ receptor activation.[58] This leads to a classical hyperpolarizing fast IPSP resulting both from "shunting" of excitatory inputs owing to the large increase in membrane conductance (decreasing electrical resistance) and the hyperpolarizing effect of Cl^- influx. This inhibitory effect of GABA reduces the probability of generation of an action potential. Binding of GABA to the GABA$_A$ receptors is inhibited by competitive and noncompetitive antagonists, including *bicuculline* and *picrotoxin.* One important difference among the different subtypes of GABA$_A$ receptors is their sensitivity to the positive allosteric modulation by benzodiazepines. Receptors containing γ_2-subunits in association with α_1-α_3- or α_5-subunits, and two β_2-subunits have a *benzodiazepines-binding site.* Benzodiazepines are positive modulators of the receptors; they increase the opening frequency of the Cl^- channel elicited by GABA, without altering its single-channel conductance or opening duration. The presence of the γ_2-subunit also allows the receptors to cluster at the synapses, where they are activated by peak concentrations of synaptically released GABA, and generate fast, short-duration phasic inhibitory postsynaptic responses.

In contrast, GABA$_A$ receptors containing α_4-α_6-subunits, which combine with δ- instead of γ-subunits are expressed at extrasynaptic or perisynaptic sites, where they are activated by ambient extracellular GABA generated by spillover from the synapse, and mediate a tonic inhibitory influence regulating cell excitability. These δ-subunit–containing receptors are insensitive to benzodiazepines, but highly sensitive to modulation by steroids, including circulating estrogens and progesterone and *neurosteroids* derived from the astrocytes, as well as alcohol and general anesthetics.[56,57,59-61]

GABA$_B$ Receptors

The GABA$_B$ receptors form a separate class of GPCRs that function as heterodimers of a GABA$_B$ R1 and a GABA$_B$ R2 subunit, which interact via their *C*-terminus domains.[62,63] These receptors are coupled to $G_{i/o}$ transducing mechanisms. Postsynaptic GABA$_B$ receptor activation produces an increase in K^+ conductance, resulting in slow IPSPs. The effector channels are members of the GIRKs and the coupling involves the β/γ complex of the G protein. Presynaptic GABA$_B$ receptors, via this β/γ complex, decrease conductance of N- and P/Q-channels, thus inhibiting release of glutamate, monoamines, and neuropeptides. Somatodendritic and presynaptic GABA$_B$ autoreceptors may reduce GABA release from inhibitory interneurons. The GABA$_B$ receptors are also activated with low affinity by GHB, although this substance may also act via its own specific receptors.[51]

Glycine as an Inhibitory Transmitter

The inhibitory actions of glycine are mediated by the *GLYR-1,* a ligand-gated Cl^- channel that resembles the GABA$_A$ receptor. The GLYR-1 also has a pentameric structure consisting of α-, β-, and γ-subunits. It is activated not only by glycine but also by other amino acids, including β-alanine, taurine, L-alanine, L-serine, and proline. Activation of the GLYR-1 elicits fast inhibition. Unlike the GABA$_A$ receptor, responses to glycine are not blocked by bicuculline or allosterically potentiated by benzodiazepines. The inhibitory synaptic effects of glycine are specifically blocked by *strychnine.*

GABAergic Neurotransmission as a Therapeutic Target

Given the critical role of GABA in regulating excitability in the CNS, GABAergic transmission provides several pharmacologic targets for management of disorders such as seizures, pain, anxiety, and insomnia (Table 8-3). Drugs that increase availability of GABA at inhibitory synapses are used for treatment of epilepsy[64] (see Chapter 45, Seizure Disorders). *Valproate* is a broad-spectrum antiepileptic drug and the first-line drug for treatment of all types of primary generalized seizures. Valproate potentates GABAergic transmission via inhibition of GAT and by an effect on the benzodiazepine modulatory site of the GABA$_A$ receptor. *Tiagabine* is another inhibitor of GAT and is used as a second-line drug for partial seizure disorders. *Vigabatrin,* an inhibitor of GABA-T, is a potent antiepileptic drug, but it is not used in the United States owing to its side effects on the retina.

Benzodiazepines, which potentiate GABA$_A$ receptor–mediated inhibition, are used for management of seizures, anxiety, insomnia, spasticity, and stiff-man syndrome (see Chapters 45, Seizure Disorders; 52, Anxiety; and 57, Insomnia). Typical examples are *diazepam, lorazepam, clonazepam, alprazolam, triazolam,* and *midazolam.* The sedative-hypnotic effects of benzodiazepines involve α_1-subunit–containing GABA$_A$ receptors, whereas their anxiolytic effects are mediated by receptors containing α_2- or α_3-subunits.[65] Receptors containing the α_1-subunits also have high affinity for imidazopyridines, such as *zolpidem, zaleplone,* or *eszopliclone,* which are used clinically as hypnotics.[65] *Flumazenil* is an antagonist at the benzodiazepines-binding site of the receptor and prevents the positive modulatory effect of these drugs. This drug is used for treatment of benzodiazepine intoxication, hepatic encephalopathy, and a rare disorder called endozepine stupor. Barbiturates are also positive allosteric modulators of the GABA$_A$ receptors and have been used as general anesthetics (such as *thiopental*), hypnotics, and antiepileptic agents (typically *phenobarbital*).

Tonic GABAergic inhibitory receptors are the target of positive modulation by intravenous anesthetics, such as *etomidate* or *propofol,* or inhalational general anesthetics, such as *isoflurane.*[66] The presence of a β_3- or β_2-subunit is important for the action of general anesthetics. Receptors containing α_6-, $\beta_3\delta$-, and β_3-subunits are the main targets for the effects of *alcohol. Gaboxadol* acts via extrasynaptic tonic GABA receptors in the thalamus and has sleep-promoting effects.

Baclofen is a typical GABA$_B$ agonist that has central muscle-relaxant and analgesic properties by inhibition of neurotransmitter release in the dorsal horn and trigeminal nucleus. It is the drug of choice for spasticity associated with cerebral palsy and multiple sclerosis. Baclofen is also used as a second-line drug for treatment of trigeminal neuralgia.

TABLE 8-3 DRUGS AFFECTING GABAERGIC TRANSMISSION

Target	Drug	Mechanism of Action	Therapeutic Use
Presynaptic GABA transporter	Valproate	Blockade	Seizures Migraine
	Tiagabine	Blockade	Seizures
GABA-T	Vigabatrin	Blockade	Seizures
$GABA_A$ receptor	Diazepam Lorazepam Clonazepam Midazolam	Allosteric activation of γ2 subunit receptors	Anxiety, seizures Anxiety, seizures Seizures, myoclonus Gen An, SE
	Zolpidem Zaleplone Eszopliclone	Allosteric activation of α1 subunit receptors	Insomnia Insomnia Insomnia
	Propofol Isoflurane Alcohol	Allosteric activation of δ-subunit receptors	Gen An; SE Gen An, SE
	Barbiturates	Allosteric activators	Gen An, SE
	Flumazenil	Antagonist of the benzodiazepine site	Hepatic encephalopathy
$GABA_B$ receptor	Baclofen	Agonist	Spasticity Pain Dystonia

GABA, γ-aminobutyric acid; GABA-T, GABA transporter; Gen An, general anesthesia; SE, status epilepticus.

Acetylcholine

Anatomic Distribution and Function

Acetylcholine is an important neurotransmitter in both the CNS and the PNS. Cholinergic systems include (i) the spinal and brainstem somatic motor neurons innervating the skeletal muscle; (ii) the spinal and brainstem preganglionic neurons innervating the autonomic ganglia; (iii) parasympathetic ganglion neurons innervating the visceral organs; (iv) neurons of the basal forebrain (*septal area* and *nucleus basalis*) innervating the cerebral cortex; (v) neurons in the tegmentum of the pons and midbrain innervating the thalamus and the medulla; and (vi) local neurons in the striatum. Acetylcholine in the CNS has a critical role in mechanisms of attention and memory (see Chapter 43, Alzheimer's Disease and Dementias) and contributes to motor control. In the periphery, ACh mediates neuromuscular transmission and is the crucial neurotransmitter in a large number of autonomic functions (see Chapter 9, Autonomic Pharmacology).

Biosynthesis, Storage, and Metabolism

Acetylcholine is synthesized from acetyl coenzyme A (acetyl CoA) and choline by action of the *choline acetyltransferase* (ChAT)[67] (Fig. 8-4). This cytoplasmic enzyme is present in the synaptic terminals bound to the membrane of synaptic vesicles and is regulated by phosphorylation.[68] Although choline is in excess in the extracellular fluid, its availability for AChE synthesis at the presynaptic terminal depends on its presynaptic uptake via a high-affinity Na^+ and ATP-dependent *choline transporter* (ChT),[69] which is also highly regulated by depolarization phosphorylation.[70] Treatment with hemicoliniun-3, a drug that blocks ChT, leads to a decrease in ACh synthesis and release. Acetylcholine is concentrated in synaptic vesicles by action of a vesicular ACh transporter (VAChT), which is encoded by a gene contained within the ChAT gene locus on human chromosome 10.[71]

The synaptic actions of ACh are terminated by its hydrolysis by AChE.[20] This enzyme is present in neurons and in the basal lamina at the neuromuscular junction and exists in three isoforms that differ in solubility and membrane attachment.[72] AChE is a highly efficient enzyme, and its crystallographic structure has been recently unraveled. *Butyrylcholinesterase* (BuChE) is a serine hydrolase related to AchE, and it catalyzes the hydrolysis of esters of choline, including ACh. It is abundantly expressed in cell bodies and proximal dendrites of neurons of the amygdala, hippocampus, and thalamus as well as in glial and endothelial cells.

Nicotinic Receptors

The nicotinic ACh receptors (nAChRs) are ligand-gated cation channels of the Cys-loop family. They are permeable to Na^+, Ca^{2+}, and K^+, and their activation elicits membrane depolarization. Their crystallographic structure and functional domains have been recently reviewed.[22,73] To date, 17 nAChR channel subunits have been cloned. They include muscle-type subunits (α_1, β_1, δ, ε, and γ)[22] and neuronal-type subunits.[73,74] The ACh-binding site is located at the interface between the α- and the non–α-subunits. Binding of ACh produces large conformational changes in the α-subunits and opens the cation channel, resulting in rapid membrane depolarization. The type of α-subunit of the nAChR determines its relative permeability to Ca^{2+} with respect to Na^+ and the channel kinetics of activation and inactivation.

The muscle nAChR is composed of two α_1, and one each of β_1-, δ-, and ε- (in adult muscle), or γ- (in fetal muscle) subunits.[22] The neuronal type nAChRs, composed of only α- and β-subunits form a plethora of different subtypes. The α- (2-6) and β- (2-4) subunits form heteropentameric channels, with a prevalent stoichiometry $(\alpha)_2/(\beta)_3$.[73] The two main functional types of neuronal nAChRs are the ganglion-type receptor, composed of α_3/β_4-subunits, and the CNS neuronal type nAChR composed of α_4/β_2-subunits. The ganglion-type α_3/β_4-receptors have higher relative permeability to Ca^{2+} in relationship to Na^+ than the muscle nAChRs, and their activation elicits fast postsynaptic excitation in both sympathetic and parasympathetic ganglion cells (see Chapter 9, Autonomic Pharmacology). Central nAChRs (mostly α_4/β_2) are predominantly located presynaptically in dopaminergic, GABAergic, and other neuronal groups, and their activation elicits Ca^{2+} influx and neurotransmitter release.[74-76] However, some of these receptors are also present postsynaptically, eliciting fast depolarization of the target cells.[74] The α_7-α_9-subunits form homopentameric channels with a dramatically larger Ca^{2+} permeability and faster desensitization rates than the other nAChRs. Homomeric α_7 receptors typically localize in presynaptic glutamatergic terminals. The α_9- and α_9/α_{10} nAChRs have a mixed nicotinic/muscarinic pharmacologic profile and

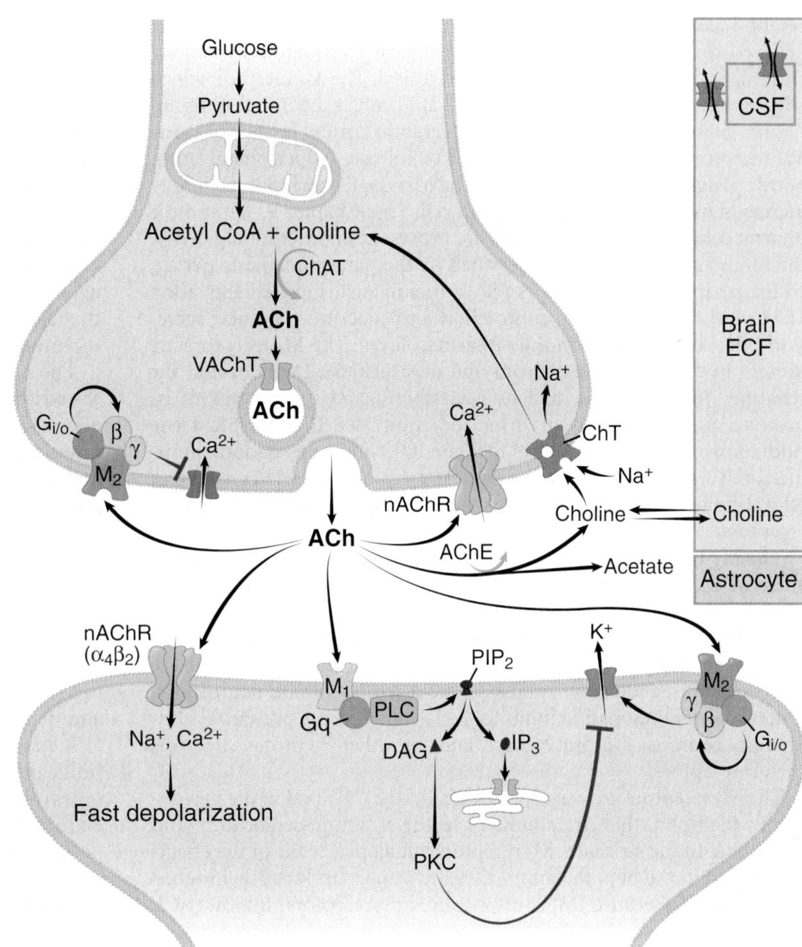

FIGURE 8-4 • Overview of cholinergic neurotransmission. Acetylcholine (*ACh*) is synthesized by the action of choline acetyltransferase (*ChAT*). The high-affinity uptake of choline uptake by the choline transporter (ChT) is a rate-limiting factor. ACh is concentrated in synaptic vesicles by action of a vesicular ACh transporter (VAChT), and its synaptic effects are terminated by acetylcholinesterase (AChE). ACh acts via nicotinic (nAChR) receptors and muscarinic M_1-type and M_2-type receptors. PLC, phospholipase C; PIP_2, phosphatidylinositol biphosphate; IP_3, inositol triphosphate; DAG, diacylglycerol; ECF, extracellular fluid; CSF, cerebrospinal fluid. (Modified by permission from Benarroch EE. Basic Neurosciences with Clinical Applications. Philadelphia: Elsevier, 2005; Fig. 23-2.)

are expressed in many tissues and organs, including the cochlear outer hair cells and some ganglia.

Like other ligand-gated channels, the nAChRs undergo multiple conformational transitions and can exist in at least one of four interconvertible and functionally distinct states, closed, open, and two (fast-onset and slow-onset) desensitized states, at any one time.[22] Although there is spontaneous (constitutive) opening of the nAChRs in the absence of an agonist, the probability of channel opening increases upon agonist binding to one site and is further dramatically increased by agonist occupation of the two binding sites of the receptor. Agonist binding stabilizes the active state, and antagonist binding stabilizes the resting state. After binding of the agonist, transient activation occurs followed by a slow desensitization. The resolution of the crystallographic structure of the nAChR and studies of the effects of mutations have allowed the definition of the critical sites and amino acids responsible for ACh binding, ion conductance, selectivity, gating, and desensitization of the receptor.[22,77]

The main agonist of the neuronal nAChRs that crosses the BBB is nicotine. The nicotinic agonist *epibatidine* has high specific affinity for the α_3- and α_4-subunits and allows identification of neuronal nAChRs. Homomeric α_7-receptors have high affinity for *α-bungarotoxin* and low affinity for ACh. Channel activators include galantamine (an anticholinesterase drug used for treatment of Alzheimer's disease) and Ca^{2+}. Therefore, L-type Ca^{2+} channel antagonists such as nifedipine and nimodipine can block agonist-induced activation of nAChRs, and this may have relevance in patients with neuromuscular transmission defects such as myasthenia gravis. Steroids, particularly progesterone, corticosterone, and dexamethasone, desensitize the nAChRs.

Long-term or repeated exposure to ACh or nicotine produces desensitization of the nAChR. The rates of activation and desensitization vary greatly among the different nAChR subtypes.[78] The muscle type nAChRs desensitize slowly but also have slow recovery from desensitization. The central neuronal type α_4/β_2 nAChRs are very prone to desensitization, whereas the ganglion-type α_3/β_4 receptors are moderately susceptible. Unlike other neurotransmitter receptors, the nAChRs undergo up-regulation on long-term exposure to nicotine or ACh. There are more ACh- and nicotine-binding sites in the brains of smokers than in those of nonsmokers. Desensitization, inactivation, and up-regulation are directly related to the duration of agonist exposure. These processes may provide the molecular basis of nicotine-induced tolerance and withdrawal symptoms in chronic smokers (see Chapter 55, Drug Addiction).

Muscarinic Receptors

The muscarinic receptors (mAChRs) are GPCRs that are present in virtually all organs and cell types. They are the most abundant ACh receptors in the brain. In the periphery, they are present in autonomic ganglia and in the targets in smooth muscle and exocrine glands (see Chapter 9, Autonomic Pharmacology). Muscarinic receptors have been divided into two major functional classes: M_1-like receptors (including M_1, M_3, and M_5) and M_2-like receptors (including M_2 and M_4).[79] Studies on mutant mice lacking one of each specific mAChR subtype have provided further insight into the functional role of each of these receptors.[80]

M_1 type receptors are coupled to G_q. Activation of M_1, M_3, and M_5 receptors elicit a G_q protein–triggered activation of PLC, and therefore the IP_3/DAG cascade, resulting in release of intracellular Ca^{2+} and activation of PKC, CaMKII, and MAPK. Activation of M_1-receptors elicits neuronal depolarization by inactivating the M current, a resting noninactivating K^+ current. The M_1 receptors are located postsynaptically and are most abundantly expressed in the forebrain, including the cerebral cortex, hippocampus, and striatum. These receptors are believed to be important for mechanisms of learning and memory, although other mAChRs may also be involved. The M_1 receptor, which triggers the MAPK pathway, may be important in neuronal differentiation, plasticity, and survival in the cerebral cortex. In the striatum, M_1 receptors may indirectly inhibit DA release. In peripheral autonomic ganglia, M_1 receptors inhibit the M-type K^+ currents, leading to increased excitability of the ganglion cells (see Chapter 9, Autonomic Pharmacology). The M_3 receptors are expressed in different regions of the brain and in all tissues innervated by the parasympathetic nerves. In the periphery, M_3 receptors play a role in ACh-induced activation of visceral smooth muscle contraction and exocrine glandular secretion (see Chapter 9, Autonomic Pharmacology). The M_5 receptors are present in dopaminergic neurons and may facilitate DA release in the striatum, including the nucleus accumbens, and may therefore be involved in mechanisms of drug addiction (see Chapter 55, Drug Addiction). M_5 receptors also mediate ACh-induced, endothelium-mediated vasodilatation of cerebral arteries and arterioles, whereas relaxation of extracranial vessels is mediated predominantly by the M_3 receptors.

The M_2-type receptors (M_2 and M_4) are coupled to G_i. They inhibit adenylyl cyclase via the $G\alpha$-subunit and, via direct membrane effect of the β/γ-subunits, activate GIRKs and inhibit presynaptic N- and P/Q-channels. Postsynaptic M_2-type receptors produce slow hyperpolarization and reduce excitability and firing frequency of the target neurons, and presynaptic M_2-type receptors inhibit neurotransmitter release. Presynaptic inhibitory M_2-receptors are present in cholinergic neurons (autoreceptors) and in other neuronal neurons (heteroreceptors).

The M_2 receptors are widely expressed in the CNS and in the periphery. In the brain, they are abundant in the striatum, cerebellum, and brainstem. In the striatum, M_2 receptors antagonize some of the effects of DA, and in the hypothalamus, they are important for ACh-induced hypothermia. Because M_2 presynaptic autoreceptors inhibit ACh release in the hippocampus and cerebral cortex, they may have a modulatory role in learning and memory processing.

In the periphery, M_2 are the most abundant receptors expressed in the heart and visceral smooth muscle (see Chapter 9, Autonomic Pharmacology). In the heart, M_2 receptors mediate the ACh-induced increase in GIRK current that reduces the rate of spontaneous depolarization and firing frequency of the sinus node. The M_2 receptors, which are more abundantly expressed than the M_3 receptors in the smooth muscle of the stomach, intestine, and bladder, elicit smooth muscle contraction via a G_i protein–mediated inhibition of adenylyl cyclase and cAMP production, thus antagonizing the sympathetically triggered smooth muscle relaxant effect of β-adrenergic receptors.

The M_4 receptors are primarily expressed in the CNS, particularly the striatum. They colocalize with D_1 DA receptors and antagonize the effects of DA but may also indirectly facilitate DA release. Overall, however, M_4 knock-out mice have increased basal locomotor activity, and therefore, blockade of M_4 receptors may be of benefit in patients with Parkinson disease or drug-induced parkinsonism. Both the M_2 and the M_4 receptors mediate spinal and supraspinal analgesia by central administration of muscarinic agonists.

Cholinergic Transmission as a Therapeutic Target

Cholinergic neurotransmission is the target of muscle relaxants and drugs used for treatment of myasthenia gravis, autonomic disorders, and dementia (Table 8-4).

Botulinum toxin inhibits ACh release at the neuromuscular junctions and is used to elicit muscle relaxation in patients with several types of dystonia (including spasmodic torticollis, blepharospasm, and adductor spastic dysphonia), spasticity, and other disorders. Because botulinum toxin also blocks ACh release at the sympathetic sudomotor terminals and parasympathetic terminals on other eccrine glands, it has been used for management of focal hyperhidrosis and sialorrhea.

TABLE 8-4 DRUGS AFFECTING CHOLINERGIC TRANSMISSION AND USE IN NEUROLOGIC DISEASE

Target	Drug	Mechanism of Action	Therapeutic Use
Acetylcholine release	Botulinum toxin	Inhibits SNARE complex for exocytosis	Focal dystonia Spasticity Hyperhidrosis Sialorrhea
Acetylcholinesterase	Pyridostigmine Neostigmine Edrophonium	Reversible inhibitors do not cross BBB	Myasthenia gravis Myasthenia gravis Myasthenia gravis
	Donepezil Rivastigmine Galantamine	Reversible inhibitors cross BBB	AD, DLB AD, DLB AD, DLB
Muscle nAChR	Vecuronium, Rocuronium, Atracuronium, Mivacurium	Blockade Blockade Blockade Blockade	Muscle relaxation Muscle relaxation Muscle relaxation Muscle relaxation
	Succinylcholine	Depolarizing agent	Muscle relaxation
Neuronal nAChR	Varenicline	Partial agonist of $\alpha_4\beta_2$	Nicotine addiction
Muscarinic receptors	Betanechol	Agonist	Gastroparesis Urinary retention
	Pilocarpine	Agonist	Acute-angle glaucoma
	Atropine Ipratropium Glycopyrrolate Oxybutynin Tolterodine Trihexyphenidyl Diphenhydramine	Blockade Blockade Blockade Blockade Blockade Blockade Blockade	Bradycardia COPD Hyperhidrosis Overactive bladder Overactive bladder Parkinson disease Acute dystonia

AD, Alzheimer disease; BBB, blood-brain barrier; COPD, chronic obstructive pulmonary disease; DLB, dementia with Lewy bodies; nAChR, nicotinic acetylcholine receptor; SNARE, soluble *N*-ethylmaleimide-sensitive factor attachment receptor.

It also has moderate efficacy in the treatment of migraine headache, by a still-undetermined mechanism.

The enzymatic degradation by AChE rapidly terminates the synaptic effects of ACh. Thus, drugs that inhibit AChE activity, known as *cholinesterase inhibitors* or anticholinesterase drugs, increase synaptic availability of this neurotransmitter. Reversible AChE inhibitors are quaternary compounds that bind the enzyme. They include *edophronium*, *neostigmine*, and *pyridostigmine*, which do not cross the BBB and are used for treatment of myasthenia gravis. Inhibition of AChE leads to rapid accumulation of ACh in the synaptic space and prolonged activation of muscle nAChRs. This could lead to desensitization of muscle nAChRs, resulting in worsening of weakness in myasthenia gravis. Reversible AChE inhibitors that cross the BBB, such as *donepezil*, *rivastigmine*, and *galantamine*, are used in Alzheimer's disease and dementia with Lewy bodies (see Chapter 43, Alzheimer's Disease and Dementias).

The main agonist of the neuronal nAChRs that crosses the BBB is *nicotine*, which has a stimulating and reinforcing effect. *Varenicline* is a partial agonist of the $\alpha_4\beta_2$ that has been evaluated against placebo and is efficacious for management of nicotine addiction[81] (see Chapter 55, Drug Addiction).

Muscle nicotinic receptors are the targets of blockade by drugs used as muscle relaxants in general anesthesia[82,83] (see Chapter 60, General Anesthesia and Sedation).

Muscarinic receptors are targets of multiple drugs. The typical muscarinic receptor blockers are the natural alkaloids *atropine*, which does not readily cross the BBB and, therefore, affects the PNS, and *scopolamine*, which crosses the BBB and blocks muscarinic transmission in both the CNS and the PNS. Muscarinic receptors are also blocked by several drugs used for treatment of neurologic and psychiatric disorders, and this accounts for important side effects of these drugs. Important examples include *amitriptyline* (antidepressant), *chlorpromazine* (neuroleptic), *diphenhydramine* (antihistaminic), and *trihexyphenidyl* (antiparkinsonian drug).

Some muscarinic antagonists, such as *oxybutynin*, *tolterodine*, *trospium*, *darifenacin*, and *solifenacin*, are used for management of overactive bladder. For a discussion of the use of cholinergic agonists and antagonists in autonomic disorders, see Chapter 9, Autonomic Pharmacology.

Dopamine

Anatomic Organization and Function

The main groups of dopaminergic neurons in the brain are located in the substantia nigra pars compacta (SNc), which innervates the striatum, and the ventral tegmental area of the midbrain, which innervates the limbic system and frontal and anterior cingulate cortices. These dopaminergic inputs provide reward signals that have a critical role in attention, behavioral drive, decision making, and selection of motor programs to achieve a behaviorally relevant goal.[84] Dopaminergic neurons in the infundibular nucleus of the hypothalamus tonically inhibit prolactin release. Dopaminergic neurons in the area postrema are involved in vomiting. Dopamine also exerts several peripheral effects on autonomic effectors (see Chapter 9, Autonomic Pharmacology).

Biosynthesis, Storage, Release, Reuptake, and Metabolism

The precursor for the biosynthesis of DA is L-tyrosine. The key and rate-limiting step of catecholamine biosynthesis is the conversion of L-tyrosine to L-DOPA by action of *tyrosine hydroxylase* (TH) (Fig. 8-5). This enzyme is regulated by phosphorylation[85] and allosterically con-

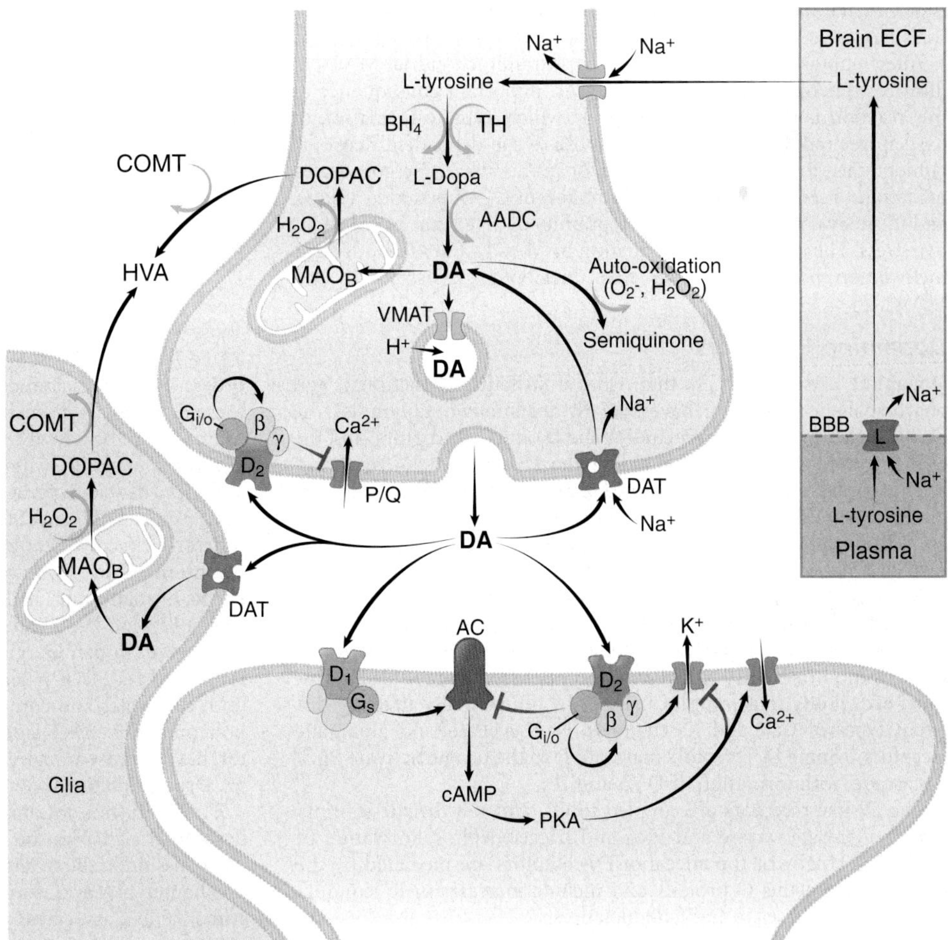

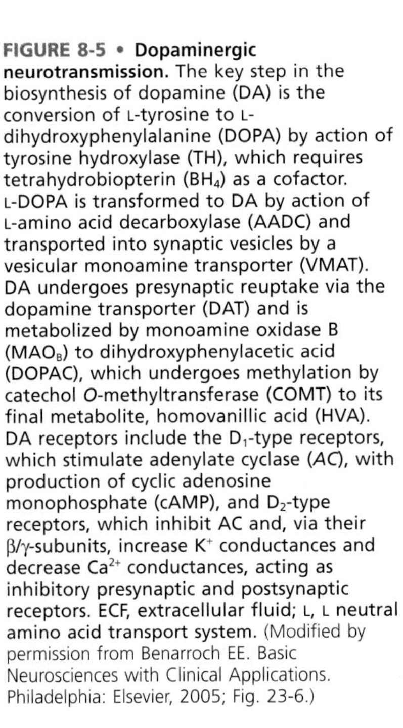

FIGURE 8-5 • Dopaminergic neurotransmission. The key step in the biosynthesis of dopamine (DA) is the conversion of L-tyrosine to L-dihydroxyphenylalanine (DOPA) by action of tyrosine hydroxylase (TH), which requires tetrahydrobiopterin (BH_4) as a cofactor. L-DOPA is transformed to DA by action of L-amino acid decarboxylase (AADC) and transported into synaptic vesicles by a vesicular monoamine transporter (VMAT). DA undergoes presynaptic reuptake via the dopamine transporter (DAT) and is metabolized by monoamine oxidase B (MAO_B) to dihydroxyphenylacetic acid (DOPAC), which undergoes methylation by catechol *O*-methyltransferase (COMT) to its final metabolite, homovanillic acid (HVA). DA receptors include the D_1-type receptors, which stimulate adenylate cyclase (*AC*), with production of cyclic adenosine monophosphate (cAMP), and D_2-type receptors, which inhibit AC and, via their β/γ-subunits, increase K^+ conductances and decrease Ca^{2+} conductances, acting as inhibitory presynaptic and postsynaptic receptors. ECF, extracellular fluid; L, L neutral amino acid transport system. (Modified by permission from Benarroch EE. Basic Neurosciences with Clinical Applications. Philadelphia: Elsevier, 2005; Fig. 23-6.)

trolled by feedback inhibition by its end products. Activity of TH requires molecular O_2 and *tetrahydrobiopterin* (BH_4) as a cofactor. *α-Methyl-p-tyrosine* is a competitive inhibitor of TH and thus blocks biosynthesis of all catecholamines.

L-DOPA is transformed to DA by action of *L-amino acid decarboxylase* (AADC), which requires pyridoxal phosphate, a vitamin B_6 derivative.[86] Dopamine is transported into synaptic vesicles via the VMAT2, coupled to the vesicular proton ATPase. Drugs such as *reserpine* and *tetrabenazine* specifically and irreversibly inhibit vesicular uptake and produce profound depletion of catecholamines (and serotonin). Drugs such as *tyramine, amphetamine,* and *methylphenidate* compete with endogenous catecholamines for the VAMT2 and displace them from their storage sites.

The synaptic effects of DA are terminated by their presynaptic reuptake via the DAT, encoded by the *DAT* gene, a gene on chromosome 5p15.3 in humans.[17,87,88] The DAT is inhibited by the psychostimulant drugs *cocaine* and *amphetamines.* Cocaine is a nonselective competitive inhibitor of all monoamine transporters (DAT, NET, and SERT). Amphetamine, methamphetamine (METH), and 3,4-methylene dioxymethamphetamine (MDMA) inhibit the DAT and the other monoamine transporters, but unlike cocaine, they are also substrates of these transporters. Amphetamines interact with the VMAT2 displacing DA from the synaptic vesicles, triggering the release of DA via reverse DAT mechanism.

Dopamine-like drugs have neurotoxic potential, leading to loss of dopaminergic axon terminals. This has been attributed to a reduction of capacity for DA vesicular storage via VMAT2, leading to accumulation of free dopamine, which could generate neurotoxic free radicals. The DAT also allows selective incorporation of neurotoxic substances that cause loss of dopaminergic neurons, including *6-hydroxydopamine* and *1-methyl-4-phenylpyridinium* (MPP^+), which is a product of metabolism of 1-methyl-4-phenyl-1,2,3,6-tetrahydropyridine (MPTP) by MAO_B in the astrocyte. Both drugs produce experimental models of Parkinson's disease (see Chapter 44, Parkinson's Disease).

After reuptake, DA is metabolized by intramitochondrial MAO_B to dihydroxyphenylacetic acid (DOPAC). An important consequence of this reaction is the generation of H_2O_2, which leads to formation of oxygen free radicals. This may predispose to age-dependent neuronal vulnerability to oxidative damage. Dopamine also undergoes autooxidation to semiquinones, with formation of O_2^- (superoxide anion), and this may contribute to the susceptibility of SNc neurons to oxidative stress. The product of DA oxidation by MAO_B, DOPAC, undergoes methylation by COMT to its final metabolite, *homovanillic acid* (HVA).

Dopamine Receptors

Dopamine acts via GPCRs that, from a structural, functional, and pharmacologic standpoint, have been divided into two subfamilies: the D_1-like receptor subfamily, including the D_1 and D_5 receptors, and the D_2-like receptor subfamily, including the D_2, D_3, and D_4 receptors. Phenotypic studies on mutants for each receptor have provided insight on the functions of these receptor subtypes.[89]

D_1-like receptors are coupled to G_s and stimulate adenylate cyclase, with production of cAMP and activation of PKA. The D_1 receptor–cAMP–PKA cascade results in phosphorylation of ion channels, pumps, transporters, and *DARPP-32* (dopamine- and cAMP-regulated phosphoprotein of 32 kDa), a phosphatase inhibitor. Both directly and via activation of DARPP-32, the D_1 receptor cascade modulates neuronal excitability in a complex manner by differentially affecting different types of Ca^{2+} and K^+ channels, Na,K-ATPase, and glutamate receptors.[90] Some D_1 receptors may couple to the G_q and activate PLC/PI cascade, with formation of DAG and IP_3.

The D_2-like receptors are coupled to $G_{i/o}$ and, via their α-subunit, inhibit adenylate cyclase and PKA and trigger dephosphorylation of DARPP-32. Many of the effects of D_2 receptors are mediated by the β/γ complex of this G protein, and include increases in K^+ conductances and decreases in Ca^{2+} conductances.

The DA receptors can be located postsynaptically, presynaptically, or extrasynaptically. Both D_1 and D_2-like receptors are present postsynaptically or extrasynaptically. The most abundant DA receptors in the caudate nucleus and putamen are D_1 and D_2 receptors. They are located postsynaptically in the neck of the spine of the medium-sized spiny GABAergic neurons, which are the output neurons in the striatum. At this level, these receptors may make homomeric complexes or heterodimeric complexes with other receptors, such as the AMPA, NMDA, $GABA_A$, and adenosine A_2 receptors.[91] These receptor mosaics may tune different effector mechanisms at the level of the postsynaptic membrane.

The D_2-like receptors act as somatodendritic and/or presynaptic inhibitory autoreceptors. Neurons of the SNc contain somatodendritic D_2 autoreceptors that mediate local inhibitory dendrodendritic interactions and presynaptic D_2 autoreceptors that inhibit DA release in the striatum. These receptors may also act as inhibitory presynaptic heteroreceptors. For example, DA, acting via presynaptic D_2 receptors, inhibits release of glutamate from cortical afferents to the striatum.

The D_3 and D_4 receptors are expressed primarily in limbic regions. For example, the D_3 receptors are concentrated in the nucleus accumbens (limbic striatum), hippocampus, and amygdala, and the D_4 receptors in the frontal cortex, amygdala, olfactory bulb, and hypothalamus. The D_5 receptors are mainly restricted to the olfactory tubercle and the hippocampal formation. All these areas receive dopaminergic inputs from neurons of the ventral tegmental area. These neurons differ from those of the SNc in various important features, including lack of somatodendritic D_2 receptors and higher expression of VMAT2 relative to DAT (which prevents accumulation of free DA in their terminals). These features are reflected by their higher basal activity and their lesser susceptibility of oxidative stress, which explain their relative sparing in early Parkinson disease.

Presynaptic and postsynaptic DA receptors undergo adaptive changes after prolonged exposure to DA agonists or antagonists. Presynaptic D_2 autoreceptors are more sensitive than postsynaptic D_2 receptors to dopaminergic agonists and more susceptible to desensitization after repeat exposure to DA agonists than the postsynaptic receptors.

Dopaminergic Neurotransmission as a Therapeutic Target

Given its multiple effects on attention, cognition, emotion, motor control, and endocrine regulation, the brain dopaminergic system is a therapeutic target for disorders such as schizophrenia (see Chapter 54, Psychosis and Schizophrenia), attention-deficit hyperactivity disorder (see Chapter 51, Attention-Deficit/Hyperactivity Disorders), substance abuse (see Chapter 55, Drug Addiction), Parkinson disease (see Chapter 44, Parkinson's Disease), and hyperprolactinemia (see Chapter 40, Disorders of Hypothalamic-Pituitary Axis). Because drug treatment of these disorders is discussed in other chapters of this book, only a few examples are briefly discussed here (Table 8-5).

Methylphenidate, which is used for treatment of narcolepsy and attention-deficit hyperactivity disorder, is a DAT inhibitor and also inhibits the NET and SERT. These multiple actions may explain its different effects on attention and hyperactivity[17] (see Chapter 51, Attention-Deficit/Hyperactivity Disorders), The initial reinforcing effects of many substances of abuse have been attributed to increased availability of DA in the striatum. Nicotine, via nAChRs, increases activity of dopaminergic neurons and DA release; amphetamines inhibits the VMAT2 (triggering nonsynaptic release of DA) and are both substrates and competitive antagonists of the DAT. Cocaine is a noncompetitive DAT antagonist. Conversely, *bupropion,* a DAT inhibitor, has been used for treatment of nicotine dependence (see Chapter 55, Drug Addiction).

The main (but not only) pathophysiologic mechanism for the manifestations of Parkinson's disease is impaired dopaminergic neurotransmission in the striatum. Management of this disorder is discussed in Chapter 44, Parkinson's Disease. The mainstay is *levodopa,* the precursor of DA, associated with an AADC inhibitor such as *carbidopa* or

TABLE 8-5 DRUGS AFFECTING DOPAMINERGIC TRANSMISSION

Target	Drug	Mechanism of Action	Therapeutic Use
Tyrosine hydroxylase	Alpha-methyl-*p* tyrosine	Competitive inhibition	Tardive dyskinesia
Dopa decarboxylase	Levodopa	Substrate	PD, DRD, RLS
	Carbidopa	Inhibitor	PD, DRD, RLS
	Benserazide	Inhibition	PD, DRD, RLS
VMAT2	Reserpine	Inhibition	Tardive dyskinesia
	Amphetamines	Inhibition	ADHD
DAT	Methylphenidate	Inhibition	Narcolepsy, ADHD
	Amphetamines	Inhibition	Narcolepsy, ADHD
	Bupropion	Inhibition	Depression Nicotine addiction
MAO_B	Selegiline Rasagiline	Inhibition	PD
Catechol-*O*-methyl transferase	Entacapone	Inhibition	PD
Dopamine receptors	Pramipexole	Non-ergot, D2 and D3 agonists	PD, RLS
	Ropinirole		PD, RLS
	Lisuride	D_2 agonist	PD
	Bromocriptine	D_2 agonist	PD, HyperProl
	Cabergoline	D_2 agonist	PD, HyperProl
	Haloperidol and Clozapine	D_2 antagonist	Psychosis, chorea
	Olanzapine	D_2/5-HT_2 blockade	Psychosis
	Risperidone	D_2/5-HT_2 blockade	Psychosis
	Sertindole	D_2/5-HT_2 blockade	Psychosis
	Ziprasidone	D_2/5-HT_2 blockade	Psychosis
	Aripiprazole	D_2/5-HT_2 blockade Partial D_2 agonist	Psychosis Psychosis
	Metoclopramide	Antagonist	Vomiting, GIMD
	Domperidone	Antagonist	Vomiting, GIMD

ADHD, attention-deficit/hyperactivity disorder; DAT, presynaptic dopamine transporter; DRD, dopa-responsive dystonia; GIMD, gastrointestinal motility disorders; 5-HT, 5-hydroxytryptamine; HyperProl, hyperprolactinemia; MAO_B, monoamine oxidase B; PD, Parkinson's disease; RLS, restless legs syndrome, VMAT2, vesicular monoamine transporter-2.

benserazide. Entacapone, a peripheral inhibitor of COMT, prevents the transformation of peripherally administered levodopa into 3-*O*-methyldopa. MAO_B inhibitors, such as *selegiline* and *rasagiline*, may for a short time delay the need for initiation of levodopa therapy in Parkinson disease and may have a neuroprotective effect. Direct dopaminergic agonists include the ergot derivatives *pergolide* (an agonist of D_1 and D_2 receptors), *bromocriptine*, and *lisuride* (which activate D_2 receptors). The most frequently used dopaminergic agonists are the nonergot derivatives *ropinirole* and *pramipexole*, which activate both D_2 and D_3 receptors. Potential side effects of all these drugs include peripheral effects (vomiting and orthostatic hypotension) and central effects (somnolence, dyskinesia, hallucinations, and pathologic gambling or other behavioral dyscontrol syndromes).

Drugs used for treatment of psychosis are discussed in Chapter 54, Psychosis and Schizophrenia. Classic antipsychotic drugs such as *chlorpromazine* and *haloperidol* are D_2 receptor antagonists. The new-generation agents, such as *clozapine*, *olanzapine*, *quetiapine*, *risperidone*, *sertindole*, and *ziprasidone*, are relatively more potent serotonin 5-HT_{2A} than D_2 receptor antagonists.[92] *Aripiprazole* is a partial D_2 receptor agonist. The distinct advantage of the novel, as opposed to classic, antipsychotic agents is their lower incidence of extrapyramidal side effects, including acute dystonia, parkinsonism, tardive dyskinesia, and neuroleptic malignant syndrome.

Antiemetic drugs, such as *metoclopramide* and *domperidone*, are potent D_2 antagonists. Domperidone does not cross the BBB and, therefore, lacks extrapyramidal side effects. Drugs that stimulate the D_2 receptors, such as bromocriptine, are used for management of prolactin-secreting tumors.

Norepinephrine

Anatomic Organization and Function

Norepinephrine is an important neurotransmitter in the brain and the sympathetic nervous system. In the brain, NE neurons form two anatomically segregated but functionally integrated systems, the locus ceruleus and the lateral tegmental system. The locus ceruleus provides the most abundant innervation of the brain and projects to the cerebral cortex, hippocampal formation, striatum, thalamus, cerebellum, and motor and sensory nuclei of the brainstem and spinal cord. Neurons of the lateral tegmental system, some of which may synthesize epinephrine, project to the amygdala, hypothalamus, and brainstem and spinal autonomic nuclei. The brain NE system has a critical role in mechanisms of attention in response to novel, potentially challenging stimuli and is involved in cortical arousal and central coordination of the endocrine and autonomic responses to stress. In the periphery, NE is the primary neurotransmitter of the sympathetic ganglion neurons, except those innervating the sweat glands. It elicits constriction, dilation of different vascular beds, cardiac stimulation, bronchodilation, relaxation of visceral smooth muscle, and a stimulation of the pupil dilator and bladder neck muscles (see Chapter 9, Autonomic Pharmacology).

Biosynthesis, Storage, Release, Uptake, and Metabolism

Norepinephrine and epinephrine, like DA, are synthesized from L-tyrosine by the rate-limiting action of TH, with formation of L-DOPA (Fig. 8-6). After incorporation in the synaptic vesicles, DA is converted

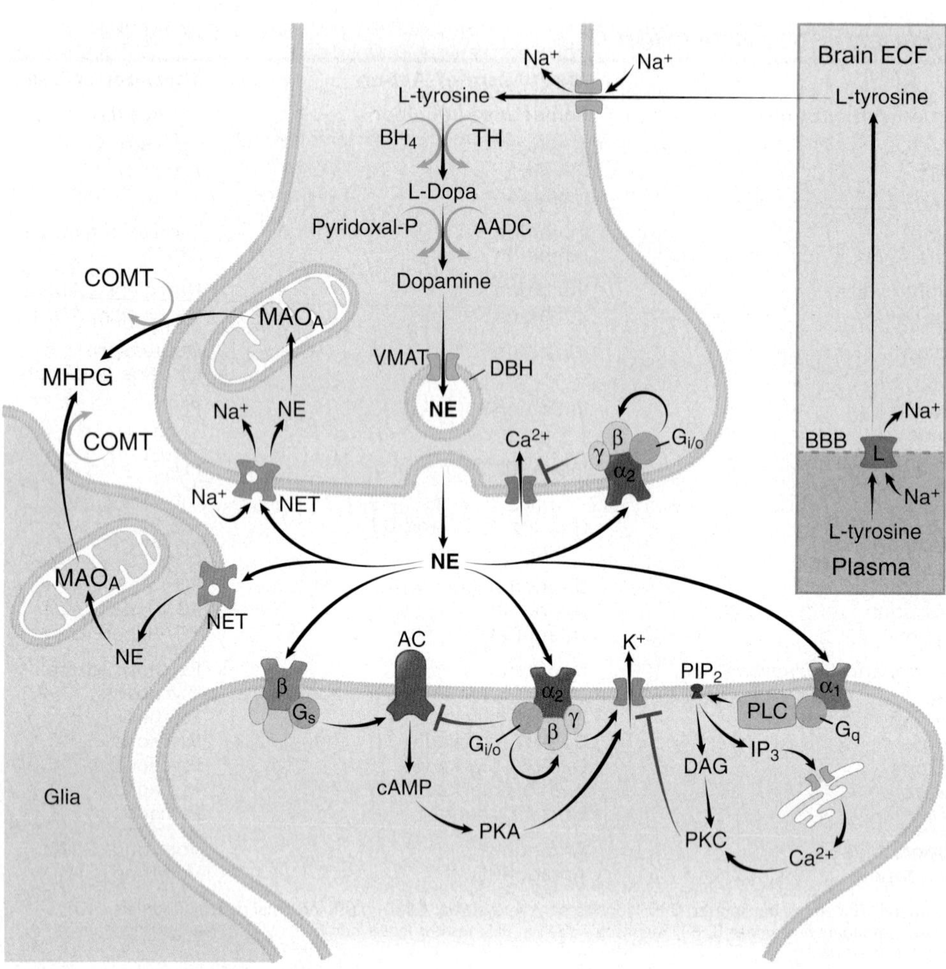

FIGURE 8-6 • Overview of central noradrenergic transmission. Norepinephrine (NE) is synthesized from L-tyrosine by the action of tyrosine hydroxylase (TH), with formation of L-dihydroxyphenylalanine (L-DOPA). L-DOPA is decarboxylated to dopamine (DA) by action of the L-amino acid decarboxylase (AADC). Dopamine-β-hydroxylase (DBH) converts DA into NE. Norepinephrine undergoes presynaptic reuptake via a selective norepinephrine transporter (NET) and is then metabolized via the combined action of monoamine oxidase A (MAO_A) and catechol-*O*-methyltransferase (COMT) to 3-methoxy, 4-hydroxyphenylglycol (MHPG). Norepinephrine and epinephrine act via α_1, α_2, and β receptors. The α_1 receptors activate the phospholipase C (PLC)-phosphatidyl inositol diphosphate (PIP_2) pathway, producing diacylglycerol (DAG), which activates protein kinase C (PKC), and inositol triphosphate (IP_3), which releases Ca^{2+} from intracellular stores. The α_2 receptors inhibit adenylyl cyclase (AC), open K^+ channels, and close Ca^{2+} channels. They act as inhibitory presynaptic autoreceptors. The β receptors stimulate the AC-cAMP-protein kinase A (PKA) pathway. BBB, blood-brain barrier; BH_4, tetrahydrobiopterin; L, L neutral amino acid transport system. (Modified by permission from Benarroch EE. Basic Neurosciences with Clinical Applications. Philadelphia: Elsevier, 2005; Fig. 23-12.)

into NE by action of *dopamine-β-hydroxylase* (DBH). Norepinephrine is stored in synaptic vesicles via the VMAT2. Epinephrine-synthesizing neurons contain *phenylethanolamine-N-methyltransferase* (PNMT), which transforms NE into epinephrine.

Presynaptic reuptake is the main mechanism of inactivation of NE. It involves a selective NET. Like the DAT, the NET transports amphetamines and is competitively inhibited by cocaine. Amphetamine-like drugs, as well as *tyramine*, elicit a translocation of NE from the synaptic vesicles to the cytosol, triggering nonexocytotic release via a reversal of the transport mechanism.

After neuronal uptake, NE undergoes metabolism by MAO_A and COMT. The main metabolite of NE in the CNS is *3-methoxy-4-hydroxyphenylglycol* (MHPG). The peripheral metabolism of NE is discussed in Chapter 9, Autonomic Pharmacology.

Adrenergic Receptors (Adrenoceptors)

Norepinephrine and epinephrine act via several types of GPCRs that are divided into three families: α_1, α_2, and β adrenoceptors, each encompassing different receptor subtypes with different effector mechanisms and distribution in the CNS and PNS. The functions of these receptors mediating the effects of NE as peripheral sympathetic neurotransmitters are discussed in Chapter 9, Autonomic Pharmacology. General concepts on their central effects are discussed here.

The α_1-adrenoceptors include the α_{1A}-, α_{1B}-, and α_{1D}-subtypes, encoded by genes on human chromosome 8, 5, and 20, respectively. These receptors are coupled to G_q and activate the PLCβ-IP_3-DAG cascade, resulting in Ca^{2+} release from intracellular stores and activation of PKC and CaMKII.[93] The α_1 adrenoceptors are predominantly excitatory, and in some cells, they decrease K^+ conductances. Activation of α_1 may also trigger arachidonic acid release, influx of Ca^{2+}, and activation of the MAPK cascade. The three α_1 adrenoceptor subtypes differ in their distribution, coupling efficiency, and susceptibility to desensitization.[94] In the CNS, α_1 adrenoceptors are located predominantly postsynaptically and are abundantly distributed in the targets of catecholaminergic neurons, including the cerebral cortex, hippocampus, thalamus, striatum, and hypothalamus. Somatodendritic α_{1A}-adrenoceptors are also present in the locus ceruleus and raphe nuclei, where they increase firing of noradrenergic and serotonergic neurons, respectively. In the periphery, α_1 adrenoceptors are present in visceral smooth muscle and are the primary type of adrenergic receptors (particularly the α_{1A}- and α_{1D}-subtypes) mediating sympathetically triggered muscle contraction. These receptors also regulate vascular smooth muscle growth.

The α_2 adrenoceptors (α_{2A}, α_{2B}, and α_{2C}) are coupled to $G_{i/o}$, and their transduction mechanisms include inhibition of adenylyl cyclase, opening of K^+ channels, and closing of Ca^{2+} channels. In the CNS, α_2 adrenoceptors mediate inhibitory presynaptic and postsynaptic effects. Inhibitory somatodendritic α_2 autoreceptors decrease firing of the noradrenergic neurons, and presynaptic α_2 autoreceptors inhibit NE release. Inhibitory α_2 heteroreceptors are located at somatodendritic and presynaptic levels in other neurons, including dopaminergic and serotonergic neurons, decreasing neuronal activity and neurotransmitter release at noradrenergic and serotonergic terminals. For example, presynaptic α_2 heteroreceptors decrease release of 5-HT in the frontal cortex. However, the majority of α_2 receptors in the brain are located postsynaptically at targets of the NE neurons.[95] In the central areas controlling cardiovascular function, α_{2A} adrenoceptors mediate sympathoinhibitory effects.[96]

The β-adrenoceptors include the β_1-, β_2-, and β_3-subtypes, which are encoded by three different genes on human chromosomes 10, 5, and 8, respectively.[97] β Adrenoceptors are coupled to G_s and stimulate the adenylate cyclase–cAMP–PKA pathway. Protein kinase A phosphorylates several substrates, including L-type Ca^{2+} channels, facilitating Ca^{2+} entry. In the CNS, β_2 adrenoceptors are distributed predominantly in supratentorial structures, and β_1 adrenoceptors are distributed in the cerebellum, brainstem, astrocytes, and blood vessels. In the brain, NE increases the signal-to-noise ratio in thalamic and cortical neurons. It reduces their baseline activity and increases their responsiveness to novel synaptic stimuli. These effects are mediated by the three types of adrenergic receptors. In cortical neurons, activation of β_2 adrenoceptors elicits a PKA-mediated phosphorylation and inhibition of a Ca^{2+}-activated K^+ channel, allowing a maintenance of cortical neuron discharge in response to a persistent stimulus. In the spinal cord, NE, acting via α_2 adrenoceptors, inhibits transmission of nociceptive inputs and polysynaptic nociceptive flexor reflexes.

Adrenergic Transmission as a Therapeutic Target

The noradrenergic (and serotonergic) systems have been implicated in the mechanism of depression and anxiety disorders and are the target for these conditions as well as peripheral autonomic disorders (Table 8-6). Several antidepressant drugs block the NET (see Chapter 53, Depression and Bipolar Disorders). These include some classic tricyclic antidepressants, such as *desipramine* and *nortriptyline* (which, to a lesser extent, also block the SERT), and the new antidepressant agents *venlafaxine* (which also blocks the SERT) and *reboxetine*. Another antidepressant, *mirtazapine*, blocks presynaptic α_2 adrenoceptors that inhibit release of NE or 5-HT. Drugs that inhibit MAO inhibitors increase synaptic NE (and 5-HT) availability. MAO_A is inhibited irreversibly by *clorgyline* and reversibly by *moclobemide*, and both MAO_A and MAO_B are irreversibly inhibited by *tranylcypromine* and *isocarboxazide*.

Inhibitory α_2 adrenoceptors in medullary sympathoexcitatory neurons are the target of agonists such as *clonidine* and *guanabenz*, which are used for treatment of hypertension (see Chapter 22, Hypertension). Clonidine, acting via α_2 adrenoceptors, also inhibits neurons of the locus ceruleus and is used for treatment of symptoms of opioid withdrawal, resulting in excessive locus ceruleus activity.

Peripheral noradrenergic transmission is the main target for drugs used for treatment of hypertension, hypotension, shock, heart failure, arrhythmias, asthma, glaucoma, and urinary symptoms in patients with benign prostatic hypertrophy (see Table 8-6). A comprehensive discussion of the drugs used for management of these conditions is beyond the scope of this chapter and is covered in Chapter 9, Autonomic Pharmacology.

TABLE 8-6 DRUGS AFFECTING ADRENERGIC TRANSMISSION

Target	Drug	Mechanism of Action	Therapeutic Use
L-Amino-acid-decarboxylase	L-threo-DOPS	Substrate	Orthostatic hypotension in DBH deficiency and other disorders
VMAT2	Reserpine	Inhibition	Tardive dyskinesia
	Amphetamines	Inhibition	ADHD
NET	Methylphenidate	Inhibition	Narcolepsy, ADHD
	Amphetamine	Inhibition	Narcolepsy, ADHD
	Reboxetine	Selective inhibition	Depression
	Venlafaxine	NET/SERT inhibition	Depression
	Desipramine	NET/SERT inhibition	Depression
	Nortriptyline	NET/SERT inhibition	Pain
	Duloxetine	NET/SERT inhibition	Pain
MAO_A	Clorgyline	Inhibition	Depression, anxiety
	Moclobemide	Inhibition	Depression, anxiety
	Tranylcypromine	Inhibition	Depression, anxiety
	Phenelzine	Inhibition	Depression, anxiety
$Alpha_1$ adrenoceptors	Midodrine	Agonist	Orthostatic hypotension
	Terazosin	Antagonist	BPH
	Tamsulosin	Antagonist	BPH
	Doxazosin	Antagonist	BPH
$Alpha_2$ adrenoceptors	Clonidine Dexmedetomidine	Agonist Agonist	Hypertension Opioid withdrawal Pain ADHD, TS Adjuvant of anesthesia
Beta adrenoceptors	Propranolol	Nonselective blockade	Tremor Migraine headache
	Acebutolol, atenolol, metoprolol, and others	Dose-dependent selective β_1 blockade	Tachyarrhythmias Congestive heart failure
	Labetalol	Nonselective β and α_1 blocker	Hypertensive emergencies
	Carvedilol	β_1 selective with an α_1 blocker	Heart failure
	Terbutaline	β_2 agonist	Airway obstruction
	Albuterol	β_2 agonist	Airway obstruction

ADHD, attention-deficit/hyperactivity disorder; BPH, benign prostatic hypertrophy; DBH, dopamine beta hydroxylase; L-threo-DOPS, L-threo-dihydroxyphenylserine; MAO_A, monoamine oxidase A; NET, norepinephrine transporter; SERT, serotonin transporter; TS, Tourette's syndrome; VMAT2, vesicular monoamine transporter-2.

Serotonin

Anatomic Organization and Function

The central serotonergic neurons are located in the raphe nuclei and adjacent reticular formation. The rostral raphe nuclei, located in the upper pons and midbrain, provide serotonergic innervation to the telencephalon and diencephalon and contribute inputs to the brainstem and cerebellum. The caudal raphe nuclei, located in the caudal pons and medulla, send descending projections to the brainstem and spinal cord. In the CNS, serotonin exerts a global homeostatic effect, including regulation of the sleep-wake cycle and modulation of pain and motor functions. Serotonin is also present in enterochromaffin neurons in the gut and initiates several reflexes via the enteric nervous system.

Biosynthesis, Storage, Release, Reuptake, and Metabolism

Serotonin is synthesized from L-tryptophan, via a rate-limiting step catalyzed by *tryptophan hydroxylase* with formation of 5-hydroxytryptophan (5-HTP) (Fig. 8-7). This enzyme has several features in common with TH, including requirement of molecular O_2 and BH_4 as cofactors. 5-HTP is converted to 5-HT via the nonspecific AADC. Serotonin is stored in synaptic vesicles by the action of VMATs. Serotonin undergoes presynaptic reuptake by action of a specific SERT encoded by a single gene on chromosome 17q. The SERT is the target of many drugs used for treatment of depression and anxiety disorders (see Chapter 53, Depression and Bipolar Disorders). The anorexigenic agent *fenfluramine* and MDMA (ecstasy) inhibits both the SERT and VMAT. This allows the accumulation of cytoplasmic 5-HT and triggers 5-HT release by a reverse transport mechanism. Serotonin is metabolized by MAO_A and its final metabolite, *5-hydroxyindoleacetic acid* (5-HIAA).

Serotonin Receptors

Of all neurotransmitters, 5-HT acts on the most diverse groups of receptors. There are, so far, seven families of 5-HT receptors identified ($5\text{-}HT_1$-$5\text{-}HT_7$), with at least 14 receptor subtypes.[98] With the exception of the $5\text{-}HT_3$ receptors, all the 5-HT receptor families so far cloned are members of the GPCR superfamily.

The $5\text{-}HT_1$ receptor family includes several members ($5\text{-}HT1_{A\text{-}E}$). In general, these receptors are coupled to $G_{i/o}$ and elicit, via its α-subunit, inhibition of adenylate cyclase, and via the β/γ-subunit, opening of inward-rectifying K^+ channels and closing of N- and P/Q-type Ca^{2+}

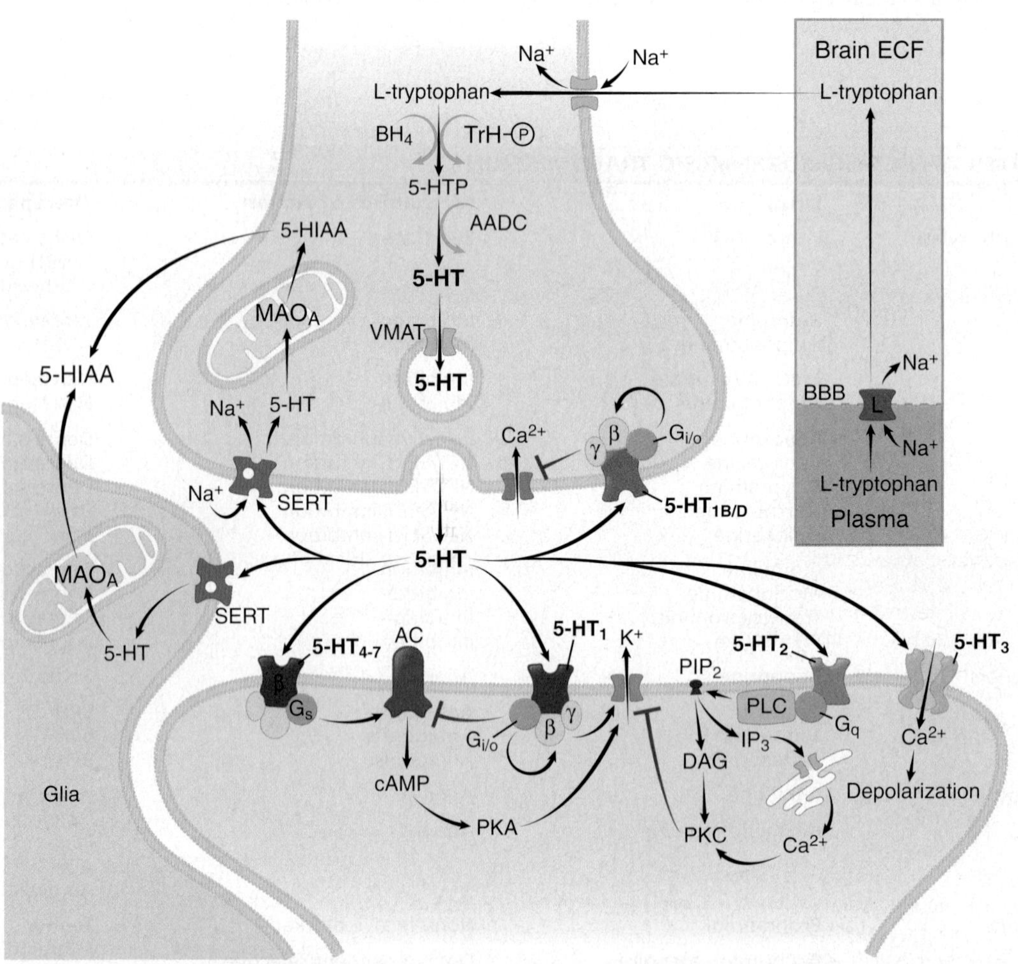

FIGURE 8-7 • Overview of serotonergic transmission. Serotonin (5-hydroxytryptamine, 5-HT) is synthesized from L-tryptophan by action of the tryptophan hydroxylase (TrH), with formation of 5-hydroxytryptophan (5-HTP), which is converted to 5-HT by action of the L-amino acid decarboxylase (AADC). Serotonin is stored in synaptic vesicles by action of a vesicular monoamine transporter (VMAT). After exocytosis, 5-HT undergoes presynaptic reuptake by action of a specific serotonin transporter (SERT) and is metabolized by monoamine oxidase A (MAO_A) to its final metabolite, 5-hydroxyindolacetic acid (5-HIAA). Serotonin acts via multiple families of receptors. Activation of $5\text{-}HT_1$ receptors inhibits adenylyl cyclase (AC), opens K^+ channels, and closes Ca^{2+} channels. Somatodendritic and presynaptic $5\text{-}HT_1$ receptors inhibit firing of the serotonergic neurons and 5-HT release or both. Activation of $5\text{-}HT_2$ receptors stimulates the phospholipase C (PLC)-phosphatidyl inositol diphosphate (PIP_2) pathway, producing diacylglycerol (DAG), which activates protein kinase C (PKC), and inositol triphosphate (IP_3), which releases Ca^{2+} from intracellular stores. The $5\text{-}HT_3$ receptor is cation channel highly permeable to Ca^{2+}. The α_2 receptors inhibit adenylyl cyclase (AC), open K^+ channels, and close Ca^{2+} channels. They act as inhibitory presynaptic autoreceptors. The $5\text{-}HT_4$, $5HT_6$, and $5\text{-}HT_7$ receptors stimulate the AC-cAMP-protein kinase A (PKA) pathway. BBB, blood-brain barrier; BH_4, tetrahydrobiopterin; L, L neutral amino acid transport system. (Modified by permission from Benarroch, EE. Basic Neurosciences with Clinical Applications. Philadelphia: Elsevier, 2005; Fig. 23-15.)

channels. The 5-HT_{1A} receptors are widely distributed throughout the CNS, particularly in the raphe nuclei and limbic areas. These receptors typically act as inhibitory somatodendritic or presynaptic receptors. Somatodendritic 5-HT_{1A} autoreceptors inhibit firing of the serotonergic raphe neurons, and 5-HT_{1A} heteroreceptors inhibit firing of the locus ceruleus. The 5-HT_{1A} receptors are also located postsynaptically at the target areas of serotonergic neurons. The hallucinogenic drug *lysergic acid diethylamide* (LSD) is one of the most effective 5-HT_{1A} agonists and suppresses firing of the raphe neurons. The 5-HT_{1D} receptors in humans (corresponding to the 5-HT_{1B} receptors in the rodent) are present in high density in the basal ganglia, limbic system, and frontal cortex. They are located in presynaptic terminals and act as inhibitory autoreceptors (inhibiting 5-HT release) or heteroreceptors (inhibiting release of other neurotransmitters, including glutamate, GABA, and substance P).

The 5-HT_2 receptor family includes the 5-HT_{2A}, 5-HT_{2B}, and 5-HT_{2C} receptors.[99] These receptors are coupled to G_q and stimulate the PLC-PIP_2 pathway, with production of DAG, and IP_3, leading to Ca^{2+} release from intracellular stores. Activation of 5-HT_2 receptors also decreases K^+ conductances, thus increasing neuronal excitability. 5-HT_2 receptors may also couple to phospholipase A_2. In general, 5-HT_2 receptors are located postsynaptically in the CNS, including the cerebral cortex, limbic system, and basal ganglia. In the cortex, they mediate neuronal depolarization by closing K^+ channels and increase GABA release from inhibitory neurons. The 5-HT_{2A} receptors are also present in cranial and spinal motoneurons, where they potentiate the excitatory effects of glutamate. In the periphery, 5-HT_{2A} receptors elicit contraction of the vascular smooth muscle and platelet aggregation. 5-HT_{2B} receptors are found in the cerebral cortex, cerebellum, caudate nucleus, amygdala, thalamus, hypothalamus, retina, and substantia nigra. The 5-HT_{2C} receptors are present in the striatum, substantia nigra, and choroid plexus.[100] Both the 5-HT_{2A} and the 5-HT_{2C} receptors are constitutively active in the absence of ligand.[101]

The 5-HT_3 receptors, unlike other monoamine receptors, are cation channels that belong to the Cys-loop family.[102] They are highly permeable to Ca^{2+}, and their activation elicits fast postsynaptic or presynaptic depolarization. In the brain, 5-HT_3 receptors are found postsynaptically in many neurons of the CNS, including those in the area postrema, where they activate release of DA, resulting in vomiting. These receptors also present in nociceptive afferents, where they may contribute to sensitization following injury.

The 5-HT_4, 5-HT_5, 5-HT_6, and 5-HT_7 receptors are coupled to G_s and stimulate the cAMP–PKA pathway. The 5-HT_4 receptors are highly concentrated in the striatum, substantia nigra, olfactory tubercle, and hippocampus. These receptors are also located on excitatory nerve terminals throughout the enteric nervous system and also have an important role in gastrointestinal tract motility (see Chapter 9, Autonomic Pharmacology). The 5-HT_7 receptors are present in the cerebral cortex, hippocampus, thalamus, and hypothalamus, and peripherally in the blood vessels and gut.[103]

Serotonergic Transmission as a Therapeutic Target

The serotonergic system is the target for drugs used in the management of a wide range of disorders, including depression, anxiety, psychosis, migraine headache, vomiting, and gastrointestinal dysmotility (Table 8-7). Evidence from functional neuroimaging studies indicates that the central serotonergic system is involved in disorders such as depression and anxiety disorders. Several drugs used for treatment of these disorders block 5-HT reuptake via the SERT (see Chapters 50, Obsessive-Compulsive Disorders; 51, Attention-Deficit/Hyperactivity Disorders; and 52, Anxiety). Important examples of selective SERT inhibitors include *fluoxetine, fluvoxamine, paroxetine, sertraline, citalopram,* and *escitalopram. Venlafaxine* inhibits both the SERT and the NET. This is also the case for some tricyclic antidepressants, such as *amitriptyline, nortriptyline, clomipramine,* and *protriptyline.* Some such as *trazodone, nefazodone,* and *mirtazapine* block the 5-HT_2 receptors.

Serotonergic neurotransmission is also a therapeutic target in management of anxiety and psychosis. *Buspirone* is a selective 5-HT_{1A} agonist that exerts a mild antianxiety effect without the sedative side effects of benzodiazepines. Several new-generation antipsychotic drugs, such as clozapine, risperidone, olanzapine, quetiapine, ziprasidone, and aripiprazole, have higher affinity for 5-HT_2 than D_2 receptors.

The serotonergic system has been implicated in the mechanism of migraine headaches. The most effective drugs for acute migraine attacks are *triptans* (including sumatriptan, rizatriptan, zolmitriptan, naratriptan, eletriptan, almotriptan, and frovatriptan). The triptans are agonists of presynaptic 5-$HT1_{B/D}$ receptors, decreasing release of glutamate and neuropeptides from nociceptive terminals at the trigeminal neurovascular junction and trigeminal nucleus caudalis (see Chapter 48, Headache). *Methysergide* and *cyproheptadine* are nonselective inhibitors of 5-HT_1 and 5-HT_2 receptors.

In the periphery, 5-HT_{2A} receptors elicit contraction of the vascular smooth muscle and platelet aggregation. Serotonergic mechanisms, via 5-HT_3 and 5-HT_4 receptors, have several important roles in control of gastrointestinal motility and have been implicated in gastrointestinal motility disorders (see Chapter 32, Motility Disorders). Activation of 5-HT_3 receptors in the area postrema, which lacks a BBB, triggers vomiting, possibly in part via local release of DA. The 5-HT_3 receptors have been implicated in emesis induced by chemotherapeutic agents. Therefore, 5-HT_3-5-HT_3 receptor antagonists such as *ondansetron, granisetron, alosetron, dolasetron,* and *palonosetron* are recommended for treatment of early vomiting induced by cyclophosphamide and other chemotherapeutic drugs.

Histamine

Anatomic Organization and Function

Histamine is synthesized by neurons located in the *tuberomammillary nucleus* of the hypothalamus. These cells send out many dendrites that may come into contact with the cerebrospinal fluid and project in a highly divergent fashion to the entire brain and spinal cord. The brain histamine system is important for mechanisms of arousal and participates in endocrine and autonomic control.

Biosynthesis, Storage, and Metabolism

Histamine is synthesized from the amino acid L-histidine by the enzyme *histidine decarboxylase.* This enzyme requires pyridoxal phosphate and shares some homologies with DOPA decarboxylase. Unlike other monoamines, histamine does not undergo presynaptic reuptake but may undergo uptake by astrocytes. In the brain, histamine undergoes methylation by the *histamine-N-methyltransferase* and is then metabolized by MAO_B to *methyl imidazoleacetic acid.*

Histamine Receptors

Histamine receptors are GPCRs and include three subtypes: H_1, H_2, and H_3.[104] The H_1 receptor is coupled to G_q and activates the IP_3/DAG transduction pathway, resulting in elevation of intracellular Ca^{2+} and PKC activation. Overall, these receptors mediate excitatory effects of histamine. There are high concentrations of H_1 in all areas involved in mechanisms of arousal, including the cerebral cortex, thalamus, cholinergic neurons of the basal forebrain and mesopontine tegmentum, locus ceruleus, and raphe nuclei. The H_2 receptors are coupled to G_s and activate cAMP production. The primary effects of H_2 receptor activation are neuronal depolarization and increased duration of the responses to excitatory inputs. The H_3 receptors are coupled to $G_{i/o}$ and act primarily as inhibitory somatodendritic and terminal receptors. These receptors also inhibit release of glutamate, GABA, ACh, DA, NE, 5-HT, and several neuropeptides.

Histaminergic System as a Therapeutic Target

Many drugs, including classic antihistaminics (such as *diphenhydramine*), tricyclic antidepressants (such as amitriptyline and doxepin), and first-generation antipsychotic drugs (such as chlorpromazine and promethazine), block central H_1 receptors, which results in increased somnolence, a common side effect of these drugs.

TABLE 8-7 DRUGS AFFECTING SEROTONERGIC TRANSMISSION

Target	Drug	Mechanism of Action	Therapeutic Use
SERT	Fluoxetine	SERT inhibitor	Depression, anxiety
	Fluvoxamine	SERT inhibitor	Depression, anxiety
	Sertraline	SERT inhibitor	Depression, anxiety
	Paroxetine	SERT inhibitor	Depression, anxiety
	Citalopram	SERT inhibitor	Depression, anxiety
	Escitalopram	SERT inhibitor	Depression, anxiety
	Amitryptiline	Blockade of SERT and NET	Depression, pain
	Duloxetine		Pain
	Venlafaxine		Depression
5-HT_1 receptors	Buspirone	5-HT1_A agonist	Anxiety
	Triptans	$5\text{-HT1}_{B/D}$ agonists	Migraine
5-HT_2 receptors	Cyproheptadine	5-HT_1 and 5-HT_2 receptor blockade	Serotonin syndrome
	Methysergide		Migraine
	Clozapine	Blockade	Psychosis
	Risperidone	Blockade	Psychosis
	Olanzapine	Blockade	Psychosis
	Quetiapine	Blockade	Psychosis
	Ziprasidone	Blockade	Psychosis
	Aripiprazole	Blockade	Psychosis
	Mirtazapine	Blockade, also blocks presynaptic α_2 receptors	Depression
	Trazodone	Blockade	Depression
	Neftazodone	Blockade	Depression
5-HT_3 receptor	Ondansetron	Blockade	ChemoT vomiting
	Granisetron	Blockade	ChemoT vomiting
	Alosetron	Blockade	ChemoT vomiting
	Dolasetron	Blockade	ChemoT vomiting
	Palonosetron	Blockade	ChemoT vomiting
5-HT_4 receptors	Cisapride	Agonist	GIMD
	Tegaserod	Agonist	GIMD
MAO_A	Clorgyline	Inhibition	Depression, anxiety
	Moclobemide	Inhibition	Depression, anxiety
	Tranylcypromine	Inhibition	Depression, anxiety
	Isocarboxazid	Inhibition	Depression, anxiety

ChemoT, chemotherapy-induced; GIMD, gastrointestinal motility disorder; 5-HT, 5-hydroxytryptamine; MAO_A, monoamine oxidase A; NET, norepinephrine transporter; SERT, serotonin transporter.

Neuropeptides

Neuropeptides include a large number of families that have a widespread but heterogeneous distribution in the CNS and PNS. They are involved in synaptic modulation, trophic influences, and vasomotor regulation. A comprehensive discussion of neuropeptides, their receptors, and functions is beyond the scope of this chapter. Only general features of neuropeptides as chemical transmitters are briefly reviewed here.

Anatomic Localization

In the CNS, neuropeptides are located in diffusely projecting neurons with cell bodies in the hypothalamus or brainstem or in local neurons distributed in virtually all brain regions and spinal cord. Neuropeptides are most abundant in the hypothalamus, limbic system (particularly the amygdala); peripheral nociceptive and visceral afferents; central pain control circuits, and central and peripheral autonomic pathways. In many central and peripheral neurons, neuropeptides colocalize with other neuropeptides, other neurotransmitters, or both.

Synthesis, Release, and Metabolism

Neuropeptides are synthesized in the neuronal cell body. Several families of genes give rise to peptide precursors that yield multiple copies of bioactive peptides.[6] Neuropeptides are first synthesized as a large precursor that is sequestered into the lumen of endoplasmic reticulum and then undergoes cleavage and posttranslational processing along the secretory pathway. The endoproteolytic cleavage via endoproteases called prohormone convertases is a limiting step in neuropeptide synthesis. Several mechanisms, including tissue-specific activation of transcription factors; alternative mRNA splicing; mRNA editing; differential proteolytic processing; and posttranslational modifications, account for the diversity of neuropeptide expression in the brain. Neuropeptides are contained in large, dense-core vesicles, reach the synaptic terminal via fast axonal transport, and are released during intense neuronal activation. Many nerve terminals contain both "classic" neurotransmitters (such as GABA, ACh, or NE) and neuropeptides. In these neurons, low-level neuronal activity triggers release of the classic neurotransmitter, and the neuropeptide is released in response to high-frequency or burst activity of the neuron.[32] Unlike monoamines and amino acids, neuropeptides do not undergo presynaptic reuptake. Their synaptic actions are terminated by their hydrolysis by extracellular peptidases, such as neutral endopeptidase and angiotensin-converting enzyme. In several peptidergic systems, the catabolic products of the secreted peptide may have a signal function, both presynaptically and in the target neuron.

Neuropeptide Receptors

Neuropeptides act via GPCRs and exert multiple effects, including modulation of synaptic transmission and trophic and vasomotor actions. For example, vasoactive intestinal polypeptide (VIP), calcitonin-gene related peptide (CGRP), and corticotrophin-releasing factor (CRF) act via receptors coupled with G_s, triggering the cAMP–PKA cascade. Opioid peptides, NPY, galanin, and somatostatin act via $G_{i/o}$-coupled receptors and inhibit adenylyl cyclase, increase K^+ currents, and inhibit Ca^{2+} currents. These receptors act as presynaptic inhibitory receptors or decrease excitability of the postsynaptic neuron. Substance P, acting via neurokinin-1 (NK1) receptors; arginine-vasopressin (AVP), acting via V_1 receptors; angiotensin 2, acting via angiotensin 1 (AT1) receptors; and hypocretin (also called orexin), acting via orexin-1 and orexin-2 receptors, activate G_q, resulting in inhibition of K^+ currents, activation of the IP_3/DAG cascade, release of intracellular Ca^{2+}, and activation of PKC.

Peptidergic Neurotransmitter Systems as Therapeutic Targets

Neuropeptides exert a potent control on endocrine, autonomic, sensory, motor, and behavioral functions, in many cases by interacting with other neurotransmitter systems. Many neuropeptides are critical for specific homeostatic functions. For example, CRF is critical for responses to stress, AVP for fluid homeostasis, angiotensin II for control of blood pressure and thirst, opioid peptides for central pain control, and hypocretin/orexin for control of the sleep cycle and food intake. Substance P and CGRP participate in transmission of pain and visceral inputs from primary afferents in the dorsal horn and brainstem. NPY is involved in control of emotional responses at the level of the amygdala, stimulation of food intake at the level of the hypothalamus, and modulation of release and response to NE. Many neuropeptides have vasomotor effects in both cerebral and peripheral blood vessels. Substance P, CGRP, VIP, natriuretic peptides, and bradykinin are vasodilators, and NPY, AVP, angiotensin II, and endothelin are vasoconstrictors.

The opioid system is a major pharmacologic target for management of pain (Chapter 61, Treatment of Pain), and the NPY, cholecystokinin, and CRF systems are potential targets for treatment of anxiety and stress-related disorders.[105] The most recent clinical application of neuropeptide pharmacology has been the introduction of the substance P NK-1 receptor antagonist *aprepitant* for the treatment of chemotherapeutic drug–induced emesis.[106,107]

Other Neurochemical Transmitters

Purines

ATP can act as a neurotransmitter in both the CNS and the PNS. ATP is costored in synaptic vesicles with other messengers, including ACh and NE, and is released with them in a frequency-dependent manner. ATP is hydrolyzed at its sites of release by a surface-bound membrane *ectoATP diphosphohydrolase* (ADPase) with production of adenosine monophosphate (AMP), and AMP is hydrolyzed by *ecto-5′nucleotidase* to produce *adenosine*. Both ATP and adenosine act as neurochemical signals by binding to *purinergic* receptors. These include P_1 or adenosine (A_1-A_3) receptors and P_2 receptors (P_{2X} and P_{2Y}) that respond primarily to ATP. Adenosine receptors are GPCRs that are blocked by xanthines, such as *caffeine*. The A_1 receptors are coupled to $G_{i/o}$ and inhibit adenylyl cyclase, increase K^+ currents, and decrease Ca^{2+} currents. Presynaptic A_1 receptors inhibit release of a variety of neurotransmitters, including glutamate, NE, and ACh. The A_2 receptors activate adenylyl cyclase and produce vasodilatation. Adenosine has been implicated in several physiologic roles, including promotion of sleep, motor control at the level of the basal ganglia, and coupling cerebral blood flow with energy demands. Adenosine may also have a neuroprotective role during hypoxia and ischemia and may protect against seizures by presynaptically inhibiting glutamate release.

The P_{2X} ($P_{2X1\text{-}2X7}$) receptors for ATP ligand-gated cation channels are permeable to Na^+ and Ca^{2+} and mediate fast excitatory neurotransmission. They are abundant in nociceptive afferents and visceral afferents, in sensory ganglia, and in vascular and visceral smooth muscles. P_{2X} receptors have been implicated in mechanisms of pain (see Chapter 61, Treatment of Pain) and control of gastrointestinal motility (see Chapters 9, Autonomic Pharmacology; and 32, Motility Disorders). The P_{2Y} receptors are linked to the IP_3/DAG pathway and are abundant in endothelial cells, where they mediate Ca^{2+}-dependent release of NO and endothelium-mediated vasodilatation. In the brain, they mediate the paracrine effects in communication between astrocytes.

Nitric Oxide

NO is a rapidly diffusible chemical transmitter in the CNS, PNS, and enteric nervous system. It is synthesized from arginine by the NOS. NOS includes neuronal and endothelial isoforms that are constitutively expressed and are activated by the Ca^{2+}/CaM complex in response to activation of several neurotransmitter receptors (including the NMDA, M_1, and NK-1 receptors) and an inducible isoform that is present in astrocytes and microglia, and is activated during inflammation. Synthesis of NO occurs throughout the brain, PNS, and enteric nervous system. NO does not act via membrane receptors. It activates cytoplasmic guanylate cyclase. Many effects of NO are mediated by cGMP, including endothelium-mediated vasodilatation and protein kinase G (PKG)–triggered phosphorylation of ion channels and receptors, modulating neuronal excitability, firing, neurotransmitter release, and receptor function. In addition to NO, *carbon monoxide* (CO) formed by the action of *heme oxygenase* may also act as a rapidly diffusible messenger that activates cGMP production.[108] CO may mediate nonadrenergic, noncholinergic inhibition of intestinal smooth muscle.

Agmatine

Agmatine derives from enzymatic decarboxylation of arginine by action of *arginine decarboxylase*. Agmatine may constitute an endogenous neurotransmitter in the brain.[109] It is stored in synaptic vesicles, released by exocytosis, and metabolized by *agmatinase*. Agmatine is one of the endogenous agonists of imidazoline receptors, which include I_1 and I_2 receptor subtypes. The I_1 receptors are located in the brainstem, including the rostral ventrolateral medulla, as well as in the hippocampus and prefrontal cortex and have high affinity for centrally acting antihypertensive drugs, including clonidine, moxonidine, and rimeldine.[110] The I_1 receptors may interact synergistically with the α_2 adrenoreceptors in the central regulation of cardiovascular function. The I_2 receptors constitute allosteric sites within the MAOs located in the external mitochondrial membrane. I_2 agonists act as allosteric inhibitors of both MAO_A and MAO_B. Agmatine has several effects, including blockade of NMDA, nicotinic, 5-HT_3, and ligand-gated Ca^{2+} channels; inhibition of inducible NOS; and facilitation of hormonal release. Agmatine crosses the BBB and may be of therapeutic value in neuroprotection, pain control, alcohol withdrawal, stress, and depression.

Lipid Messengers

Several neurotransmitters, either via GPCRs or by triggering Ca^{2+} influx, activate phospholipase A_2, which cleaves membrane phospholipids, with release of arachidonic acid (see Chapter 6, Signal Transduction). Arachidonic acid may regulate neuronal excitability via direct interactions with ion channels and is converted to biologically active metabolites, including *prostaglandins*, *leukotrienes*, and *endocannabinoids*. These lipid messengers are rapidly released from neurons and astrocytes and mediate autocrine and paracrine functions, including regulation of neuronal excitability and cerebral vasomotor tone and local blood flow.

The endocannabinoids, such as *anandamide*, are the endogenous ligands of the cannabinoid receptor. Anandamide binds CB_1 receptors and CB_2 receptors, which are GPCRs.[111] CB_1 receptors are coupled to $G_{i/o}$ that trigger inhibition of presynaptic Ca^{2+} channels and opening of inward-rectifying K^+ currents. The effects of anandamide in experimental animals mimic those of tetrahydrocannabinol and include analgesia, hypotension, hypothermia, antiemetic effects, endocrine effects, motor inhibition, and cognitive and behavioral changes. Anandamide also regulates the activity of the *vainilloid 1* (or TRPV1) receptor, a member of the transient receptor potential (TRP) family of channels that is highly permeable to Ca^{2+} and is present in primary nociceptive afferents. The TRPV1 receptor is activated by noxious or chemical stimuli, including heat, low pH, and, typically, by capsaicin. Anandamide binds to the intracellular portion of the TRPV1 channel, increasing the probability of channel opening and potentiating its response to other stimuli, particularly heat and protons.

SUMMARY

There are multiple neurotransmitter molecules in the CNS and PNS. They also have specific mechanisms of biosynthesis, storage, release, reuptake, and metabolism. Each neurotransmitter may exert multiple postsynaptic and presynaptic effects, via several subtypes of ion channel receptors and GPCR subtypes. A given synaptic terminal may release more than one neurotransmitter, and different neurotransmitters may interact via postsynaptic, presynaptic, and paracrine mechanisms to modify the responses of one another. This complexity of chemical synaptic transmission provides for a high degree of functional plasticity in the nervous system, including learning and functional repair following lesions. The increasing understanding of the molecular mechanisms underlying neurochemical transmission and their involvement by disease provides rationale for development of pharmacologic strategies for treatment of neurologic and psychiatric disorders.

REFERENCES

1. Fon EA, Edwards RH. Molecular mechanisms of neurotransmitter release. Muscle Nerve 2001;24(5):581-601.
2. Fremeau RT Jr, Voglmaier S, Seal RP, Edwards RH. VGLUTs define subsets of excitatory neurons and suggest novel roles for glutamate. Trends Neurosci 2004;27(2):98-103.
3. Chaudhry FA, Reimer RJ, Bellocchio EE, et al. The vesicular GABA transporter, VGAT, localizes to synaptic vesicles in sets of glycinergic as well as GABAergic neurons. J Neurosci 1998;18(23):9733-9750.
4. Parsons SM. Transport mechanisms in acetylcholine and monoamine storage. FASEB J 2000;14(15):2423-2434.
5. Finn JP 3rd, Edwards RH. Multiple residues contribute independently to differences in ligand recognition between vesicular monoamine transporters 1 and 2. J Biol Chem 1998;273(7):3943-3947.
6. Strand FL. Neuropeptides: general characteristics and neuropharmaceutical potential in treating CNS disorders. Prog Drug Res 2003;61:1-37.
7. Nudler S, Piriz J, Urbano FJ, et al. Ca^{2+} channels and synaptic transmission at the adult, neonatal, and P/Q-type deficient neuromuscular junction. Ann N Y Acad Sci 2003;998:11-17.
8. Sudhof TC. The synaptic vesicle cycle. Annu Rev Neurosci 2004;27:509-547.
9. Breidenbach MA, Brunger AT. New insights into clostridial neurotoxin-SNARE interactions. Trends Mol Med 2005;11(8):377-381.
10. Proux-Gillardeaux V, Rudge R, Galli T. The tetanus neurotoxin-sensitive and -insensitive routes to and from the plasma membrane: fast and slow pathways? Traffic 2005;6(5):366-373
11. Millan C, Sanchez-Prieto J. Differential coupling of N- and P/Q-type calcium channels to glutamate exocytosis in the rat cerebral cortex. Neurosci Lett 2002;330(1):29-32
12. Conti F, Minelli A, Melone M. GABA transporters in the mammalian cerebral cortex: localization, development and pathological implications. Brain Res Brain Res Rev 2004;45(3):196-212.
13. Betz H, Gomeza J, Armsen W, et al. Glycine transporters: essential regulators of synaptic transmission. Biochem Soc Trans 2006;34(Pt 1):55-58.
14. Aragon C, Lopez-Corcuera B. Glycine transporters: crucial roles of pharmacological interest revealed by gene deletion. Trends Pharmacol Sci 2005;26(6):283-286.
15. Rothman RB, Baumann MH. Monoamine transporters and psychostimulant drugs. Eur J Pharmacol 2003;479(1-3):23-40.
16. Gonzalez MI, Robinson MB. Neurotransmitter transporters: why dance with so many partners? Curr Opin Pharmacol 2004;4(1):30-35.
17. Elliott JM, Beveridge TJ. Psychostimulants and monoamine transporters: upsetting the balance. Curr Opin Pharmacol 2005;5(1):94-100.
18. Bridges RJ, Esslinger CS. The excitatory amino acid transporters: pharmacological insights on substrate and inhibitor specificity of the EAAT subtypes. Pharmacol Ther 2005;107(3):271-285.
19. Danbolt NC. Glutamate uptake. Prog Neurobiol 2001;65(1):1-105.
20. Silman I, Sussman JL. Acetylcholinesterase: "classical" and "non-classical" functions and pharmacology. Curr Opin Pharmacol 2005;5(3):293-302.
21. Youdim MB, Edmondson D, Tipton KF. The therapeutic potential of monoamine oxidase inhibitors. Nat Rev Neurosci 2006;7(4):295-309.
22. Sine SM, Engel AG. Recent advances in Cys-loop receptor structure and function. Nature 2006;440(7083):448-455.
23. Mayer ML. Glutamate receptors at atomic resolution. Nature 2006;440(7083):456-462.
24. Kristensen AS, Geballe MT, Snyder JP, Traynelis SF. Glutamate receptors: variation in structure-function coupling. Trends Pharmacol Sci 2006;27(2):65-69.
25. Palmer CL, Cotton L, Henley JM. The molecular pharmacology and cell biology of alpha-amino-3-hydroxy-5-methyl-4-isoxazolepropionic acid receptors. Pharmacol Rev 2005;57(2):253-277.
26. Stojilkovic SS, Tomic M, He ML, et al. Molecular dissection of purinergic P2X receptor channels. Ann N Y Acad Sci 2005;1048:116-130.
27. Kubo Y, Tateyama M. Towards a view of functioning dimeric metabotropic receptors. Curr Opin Neurobiol 2005;15(3):289-295.
28. Foord SM, Bonner TI, Neubig RR, et al. International Union of Pharmacology. XLVI. G protein-coupled receptor list. Pharmacol Rev 2005;57(2):279-288.
29. Schioth HB, Fredriksson R. The GRAFS classification system of G-protein coupled receptors in comparative perspective. Gen Comp Endocrinol 2005;142(1-2):94-101.
30. Wickman K, Clapham DE. Ion channel regulation by G proteins. Physiol Rev 1995;75(4):865-885.
31. Raiteri M. Functional pharmacology in human brain. Pharmacol Rev 2006;58(2):162-193.
32. Burnstock G. Cotransmission. Curr Opin Pharmacol 2004;4(1):47-52.
33. Foster AC, Kemp JA. Glutamate- and GABA-based CNS therapeutics. Curr Opin Pharmacol 2006;6(1):7-17.
34. Neale JH, Olszewski RT, Gehl LM, et al. The neurotransmitter *N*-acetylaspartylglutamate in models of pain, ALS, diabetic neuropathy, CNS injury and schizophrenia. Trends Pharmacol Sci 2005;26(9):477-484.
35. Dunlop J. Glutamate-based therapeutic approaches: targeting the glutamate transport system. Curr Opin Pharmacol 2006;6(1):103-107.
36. Mayer ML. Glutamate receptor ion channels. Curr Opin Neurobiol 2005;15(3):282-288.
37. Nicoll RA, Tomita S, Bredt DS. Auxiliary subunits assist AMPA-type glutamate receptors. Science 2006;311(5765):1253-1256.
38. Fukata Y, Tzingounis AV, Trinidad JC, et al. Molecular constituents of neuronal AMPA receptors. J Cell Biol 2005;169(3):399-404.
39. Jaskolski F, Coussen F, Mulle C. Subcellular localization and trafficking of kainate receptors. Trends Pharmacol Sci 2005;26(1):20-26.
40. Cull-Candy S, Brickley S, Farrant M. NMDA receptor subunits: diversity, development and disease. Curr Opin Neurobiol 2001;11(3):327-335.
41. Perin-Dureau F, Rachline J, Neyton J, Paoletti P. Mapping the binding site of the neuroprotectant ifenprodil on NMDA receptors. J Neurosci 2002;22(14):5955-5965.
42. Fagni L, Ango F, Perroy J, Bockaert J. Identification and functional roles of metabotropic glutamate receptor-interacting proteins. Semin Cell Dev Biol 2004;15(3):289-298.
43. Schoepp DD, Jane DE, Monn JA. Pharmacological agents acting at subtypes of metabotropic glutamate receptors. Neuropharmacology 1999;38(10):1431-1476.
44. O'Neill MJ, Bleakman D, Zimmerman DM, Nisenbaum ES. AMPA receptor potentiators for the treatment of CNS disorders. Curr Drug Targets CNS Neurol Disord 2004;3(3):181-194.
45. Stromgaard K, Mellor I. AMPA receptor ligands: synthetic and pharmacological studies of polyamines and polyamine toxins. Med Res Rev 2004;24(5):589-620.
46. Lynch G. Glutamate-based therapeutic approaches: ampakines. Curr Opin Pharmacol 2006;6(1):82-88.
47. Kemp JA, McKernan RM. NMDA receptor pathways as drug targets. Nat Neurosci 2002;5(Suppl):1039-1042.
48. Kew JN. Positive and negative allosteric modulation of metabotropic glutamate receptors: emerging therapeutic potential. Pharmacol Ther 2004;104(3):233-244.
49. Ritzen A, Mathiesen JM, Thomsen C. Molecular pharmacology and therapeutic prospects of metabotropic glutamate receptor allosteric modulators. Basic Clin Pharmacol Toxicol 2005;97(4):202-213.
50. Tunnicliff G. Membrane glycine transport proteins. J Biomed Sci 2003;10(1):30-36.
51. Crunelli V, Emri Z, Leresche N. Unravelling the brain targets of gamma-hydroxybutyric acid. Curr Opin Pharmacol 2006;6(1):44-52.
52. Wafford KA. $GABA_A$ receptor subtypes: any clues to the mechanism of benzodiazepine dependence? Curr Opin Pharmacol 2005;5(1):47-52.
53. Whiting PJ. GABA-A receptor subtypes in the brain: a paradigm for CNS drug discovery? Drug Discov Today 2003;8(10):445-450.
54. Mody I, Pearce RA. Diversity of inhibitory neurotransmission through GABA(A) receptors. Trends Neurosci 2004;27(9):569-575.
55. Sieghart W, Sperk G. Subunit composition, distribution and function of GABA(A) receptor subtypes. Curr Top Med Chem 2002;2(8):795-816.
56. Stell BM, Brickley SG, Tang CY, et al. Neuroactive steroids reduce neuronal excitability by selectively enhancing tonic inhibition mediated by delta subunit-containing $GABA_A$ receptors. Proc Natl Acad Sci U S A 2003;100(24):14439-14444.
57. Farrant M, Nusser Z. Variations on an inhibitory theme: phasic and tonic activation of GABA(A) receptors. Nat Rev Neurosci 2005;6(3):215-229.
58. Payne JA, Rivera C, Voipio J, Kaila K. Cation-chloride co-transporters in neuronal communication, development and trauma. Trends Neurosci 2003;26(4):199-206.
59. Belelli D, Lambert JJ. Neurosteroids: endogenous regulators of the GABA(A) receptor. Nat Rev Neurosci 2005;6(7):565-575.
60. Maguire JL, Stell BM, Rafizadeh M, Mody I. Ovarian cycle-linked changes in GABA(A) receptors mediating tonic inhibition alter seizure susceptibility and anxiety. Nat Neurosci 2005;8(6):797-804.
61. Wohlfarth KM, Bianchi MT, Macdonald RL. Enhanced neurosteroid potentiation of ternary GABA(A) receptors containing the delta subunit. J Neurosci 2002;22(5):1541-1549.
62. Bowery NG, Bettler B, Froestl W, et al. International Union of Pharmacology. XXXIII. Mammalian gamma-aminobutyric acid(B) receptors: structure and function. Pharmacol Rev 2002;54(2):247-264.
63. Bettler B, Kaupmann K, Mosbacher J, Gassmann M. Molecular structure and physiological functions of GABA(B) receptors. Physiol Rev 2004;84(3):835-867.

64. Sarup A, Larsson OM, Schousboe A. GABA transporters and GABA-transaminase as drug targets. Curr Drug Targets CNS Neurol Disord 2003;2(4):269-277.
65. Rudolph U, Mohler H. GABA-based therapeutic approaches: $GABA_A$ receptor subtype functions. Curr Opin Pharmacol 2006;6(1):18-23.
66. Hemmings HC Jr, Akabas MH, Goldstein PA, et al. Emerging molecular mechanisms of general anesthetic action. Trends Pharmacol Sci 2005;26(10):503-510.
67. Prado MA, Reis RA, Prado VF, et al. Regulation of acetylcholine synthesis and storage. Neurochem Int 2002;41(5):291-299.
68. Dobransky T, Rylett RJ. Functional regulation of choline acetyltransferase by phosphorylation. Neurochem Res 2003;28(3-4):537-542.
69. Okuda T, Haga T. High-affinity choline transporter. Neurochem Res 2003;28(3-4):483-488.
70. Sarter M, Parikh V. Choline transporters, cholinergic transmission and cognition. Nat Rev Neurosci 2005;6(1):48-56.
71. Shimojo M, Hersh LB. Regulation of the cholinergic gene locus by the repressor element-1 silencing transcription factor/neuron restrictive silencer factor (REST/NRSF). Life Sci 2004;74(18):2213-2225.
72. Meshorer E, Soreq H. Virtues and woes of AChE alternative splicing in stress-related neuropathologies. Trends Neurosci 2006;29(4):216-224.
73. Jensen AA, Frolund B, Liljefors T, Krogsgaard-Larsen P. Neuronal nicotinic acetylcholine receptors: structural revelations, target identifications, and therapeutic inspirations. J Med Chem 2005;48(15):4705-4745.
74. Paterson D, Nordberg A. Neuronal nicotinic receptors in the human brain. Prog Neurobiol 2000;61(1):75-111.
75. Wonnacott S. Presynaptic nicotinic ACh receptors. Trends Neurosci 1997;20(2):92-98.
76. Sher E, Chen Y, Sharples TJ, et al. Physiological roles of neuronal nicotinic receptor subtypes: new insights on the nicotinic modulation of neurotransmitter release, synaptic transmission and plasticity. Curr Top Med Chem 2004;4(3):283-297.
77. Miyazawa A, Fujiyoshi Y, Unwin N. Structure and gating mechanism of the acetylcholine receptor pore. Nature 2003;423(6943):949-955.
78. Giniatullin R, Nistri A, Yakel JL. Desensitization of nicotinic ACh receptors: shaping cholinergic signaling. Trends Neurosci 2005;28(7):371-378.
79. Caulfield MP, Birdsall NJ. International Union of Pharmacology. XVII. Classification of muscarinic acetylcholine receptors. Pharmacol Rev 1998;50(2):279-290.
80. Wess J. Muscarinic acetylcholine receptor knockout mice: novel phenotypes and clinical implications. Annu Rev Pharmacol Toxicol 2004;44:423-450.
81. Gonzales D, Rennard SI, Nides M, et al. Varenicline, an $alpha_4beta_2$ nicotinic acetylcholine receptor partial agonist, vs sustained-release bupropion and placebo for smoking cessation: a randomized controlled trial. JAMA 2006;296(1):47-55.
82. Flood P. The importance of myorelaxants in anesthesia. Curr Opin Pharmacol 2005;5(3):322-327.
83. Jonsson M, Dabrowski M, Gurley DA, et al. Activation and inhibition of human muscular and neuronal nicotinic acetylcholine receptors by succinylcholine. Anesthesiology 2006;104(4):724-733.
84. Wise RA. Dopamine, learning and motivation. Nat Rev Neurosci 2004;5(6):483-494.
85. Fujisawa H, Okuno S. Regulatory mechanism of tyrosine hydroxylase activity. Biochem Biophys Res Commun 2005;338(1):271-276.
86. Fiumara A, Brautigam C, Hyland K, et al. Aromatic L-amino acid decarboxylase deficiency with hyperdopaminuria. Clinical and laboratory findings in response to different therapies. Neuropediatrics 2002;33(4):203-208.
87. Bannon MJ. The dopamine transporter: role in neurotoxicity and human disease. Toxicol Appl Pharmacol 2005;204(3):355-360.
88. Sotnikova TD, Beaulieu JM, Gainetdinov RR, Caron MG. Molecular biology, pharmacology and functional role of the plasma membrane dopamine transporter. CNS Neurol Disord Drug Targets 2006;5(1):45-56.
89. Waddington JL, O'Tuathaigh C, O'Sullivan G, et al. Phenotypic studies on dopamine receptor subtype and associated signal transduction mutants: insights and challenges from 10 years at the psychopharmacology-molecular biology interface. Psychopharmacology (Berl) 2005;181(4):611-538.
90. Greengard P. The neurobiology of dopamine signaling. Biosci Rep 2001;21(3):247-269.
91. Agnati LF, Ferre S, Burioni R, et al. Existence and theoretical aspects of homomeric and heteromeric dopamine receptor complexes and their relevance for neurological diseases. Neuromolecular Med 2005;7(1-2):61-78.
92. Meltzer HY. What's atypical about atypical antipsychotic drugs? Curr Opin Pharmacol 2004;4(1):53-57.
93. Hawrylyshyn KA, Michelotti GA, Coge F, et al. Update on human alpha1-adrenoceptor subtype signaling and genomic organization. Trends Pharmacol Sci 2004;25(9):449-455.
94. Piascik MT, Perez DM. Alpha1-adrenergic receptors: new insights and directions. J Pharmacol Exp Ther 2001;298(2):403-410.
95. Arnsten AF, Li BM. Neurobiology of executive functions: catecholamine influences on prefrontal cortical functions. Biol Psychiatry 2005;57(11):1377-1384.
96. Kanagy NL. Alpha(2)-adrenergic receptor signalling in hypertension. Clin Sci (Lond) 2005;109(5):431-437.
97. Bylund DB, Eikenberg DC, Hieble JP, et al. International Union of Pharmacology nomenclature of adrenoceptors. Pharmacol Rev 1994;46(2):121-136.
98. Hoyer D, Hannon JP, Martin GR. Molecular, pharmacological and functional diversity of 5-HT receptors. Pharmacol Biochem Behav 2002;71(4):533-554.
99. Leysen JE. 5-HT2 receptors. Curr Drug Targets CNS Neurol Disord 2004;3(1):11-26.
100. Reynolds GP, Templeman LA, Zhang ZJ. The role of 5-HT2C receptor polymorphisms in the pharmacogenetics of antipsychotic drug treatment. Prog Neuropsychopharmacol Biol Psychiatry 2005;29(6):1021-1028.
101. Berg KA, Harvey JA, Spampinato U, Clarke WP. Physiological relevance of constitutive activity of 5-HT2A and 5-HT2C receptors. Trends Pharmacol Sci 2005;26(12):625-630.
102. Peters JA, Hales TG, Lambert JJ. Molecular determinants of single-channel conductance and ion selectivity in the Cys-loop family: insights from the 5-HT3 receptor. Trends Pharmacol Sci 2005;26(11):587-594.
103. Hedlund PB, Sutcliffe JG. Functional, molecular and pharmacological advances in 5-HT7 receptor research. Trends Pharmacol Sci 2004;25(9):481-486.
104. Haas H, Panula P. The role of histamine and the tuberomamillary nucleus in the nervous system. Nat Rev Neurosci 2003;4(2):121-130.
105. Holmes A, Heilig M, Rupniak NM, et al. Neuropeptide systems as novel therapeutic targets for depression and anxiety disorders. Trends Pharmacol Sci 2003;24(11):580-588.
106. Prommer E. Aprepitant (EMEND): the role of substance P in nausea and vomiting. J Pain Palliat Care Pharmacother 2005;19(3):31-39.
107. Kris MG, Hesketh PJ, Somerfield MR, et al. American Society of Clinical Oncology guideline for antiemetics in oncology: update 2006. J Clin Oncol 2006;24(18):2932-2947.
108. Boehning D, Snyder SH. Novel neural modulators. Annu Rev Neurosci 2003;26:105-131.
109. Reis DJ, Regunathan S. Is agmatine a novel transmitter in brain? Trends Pharmacol Sci 2000;21:187-193.
110. Bousquet P, Greney H, Bruban V, et al. I_1 imidazoline receptors involved in cardiovascular regulation: where are we and where are we going? Ann N Y Acad Sci 2003;1009:228-233.
111. Pertwee RG. Pharmacological actions of cannabinoids. Handb Exp Pharmacol 2005(168):1-51.

9

AUTONOMIC PHARMACOLOGY

Anastasios Lymperopoulos and Walter J. Koch

INTRODUCTION 115
FUNCTIONAL ORGANIZATION OF THE ANS 118
THE PARASYMPATHETIC NERVOUS SYSTEM 118
Anatomy 118
Neurotransmission 118
Cholinergic Receptors 119
Chemistry and Pharmacology of Acetylcholine and Cholinergic Agonists (Cholinomimetics) 119
Effects of Acetylcholine in Various Target Organs 120
Therapeutic Uses, Contraindications, and Interactions of Cholinergic Drugs 120
Cholinergic Agonists 120
Anticholinesterase Agents 120
Cholinergic Antagonists 121
Effects of Atropine and Other Antimuscarinics in Target Organs 121
Anti-Acetylcholinesterase Poisoning 123
Nicotinic Antagonists 123
Ganglionic Blockers 123
Neuromuscular Blockers 124
THE SYMPATHETIC NERVOUS SYSTEM 125
Anatomy 125
Neurotransmission 125
Receptors in the SNS 126
Dopaminergic Receptors 126
Adrenergic Receptors 126
Chemistry and Structure-Activity Relationships of Endogenous Catecholamines and Sympathomimetic Drugs 126
Effects of Catecholamines and Sympathomimetic Drugs in Various Target Organs 126
Cardiovascular Effects 126
Ophthalmic Effects 128
Respiratory Effects 128
Genitourinary Effects 129
Metabolic and Endocrine Effects 129
CNS Effects 129
Effects in Other Organs 129
Pharmacologic and Therapeutic Uses of Catecholamines and Sympathomimetic Agents 129
Epinephrine 129
Dopamine and Dopaminergic Agonists 130
Selective α_1AR Agonists 130
Selective α_2AR Agonists 130
Selective β_1AR Agonists 130
Selective β_2AR Agonists 130
Indirectly Acting Sympathomimetics 130
Other Sympathomimetics 131
Pharmacologic Properties of AR Antagonists (Sympatholytics) 131
αAR Antagonists (α-Blockers) 131
βAR Antagonists (β-Blockers) 132
NONADRENERGIC-NONCHOLINERGIC NEURONS 135
PHARMACOGENOMICS OF THE ANS 135
Cholinergic Receptor Polymorphisms 135
nAChR Polymorphisms 135
mAChR Polymorphisms 136
Polymorphisms and Mutations among ARs 136
α_1AR Polymorphisms 136
α_2AR Polymorphisms 136
βAR Polymorphisms 137

INTRODUCTION

The peripheral nervous system is divided into the somatic nervous system, which controls organs under voluntary control (mainly muscles), and the autonomic nervous system (ANS), which regulates individual organ function and homeostasis and, for the most part, is not subject to voluntary control. It is also known as the visceral or automatic system. The ANS is predominantly an efferent system transmitting impulses from the central nervous system (CNS) to peripheral organ systems. Its effects include control of heart rate and force of contraction, constriction and dilation of blood vessels, contraction and relaxation of smooth muscle in various organs, visual accommodation, pupillary size, and secretions from exocrine and endocrine glands. Autonomic nerves constitute all of the efferent fibers that leave the CNS, except those that innervate skeletal muscle. There are some afferent autonomic fibers (i.e., those that transmit information from the periphery to the CNS) that are concerned with the mediation of visceral sensation and the regulation of vasomotor and respiratory reflexes. For example, the baroreceptors and chemoreceptors in the carotid sinus and aortic arch are important in the control of heart rate, blood pressure, and respiratory activity. These afferent fibers are usually carried to the CNS by major autonomic nerves such as the vagus, splanchnic, or pelvic nerves, although afferent pain fibers from blood vessels may be carried by somatic nerves.

Reflex responses are also critical in the peripheral nervous system and involve autonomic efferent fibers that can cause contraction of smooth muscle in certain organs (e.g., blood vessels, eyes, lungs, bladder, gastrointestinal [GI] tract) and influence the function of the heart and glands. The efferent limbs of these reflexes may also involve the somatic nervous system (e.g., coughing and vomiting). Simple reflexes are circuited and controlled entirely within the organ concerned, whereas more complex reflexes are controlled by the higher autonomic centers in the CNS, such as in the hypothalamus.

The ANS is divided into two separate divisions, the **parasympathetic** and the **sympathetic** (SNS) nervous systems, on the basis of anatomic differences (Fig. 9-1). Both of these systems consist of myelinated preganglionic fibers, which make synaptic connections with unmyelinated postganglionic fibers, and these then innervate the effector organ. These synapses usually occur in clusters called **ganglia.** Most organs are innervated by fibers from both divisions of the ANS, and the influence is usually opposing (e.g., the vagus slows the heart, and the sympathetic nerves increase its rate and contractility), although it may also be parallel (e.g., the salivary glands). The responses of major effector organs to autonomic nerve impulses are summarized in Table 9-1.

The control of most bodily functions occurs primarily through the CNS and the peripheral nervous system (as well as the endocrine system). The regulation of organ function by the nervous systems is due to both electrical and chemical transmission via nerve fibers integrated into organ tissue. Fast-moving electrical impulses travel down the nerve, and in addition, nerve-to-nerve and nerve-to-tissue connections, called **synapses**, are present, which are the sites for chemical

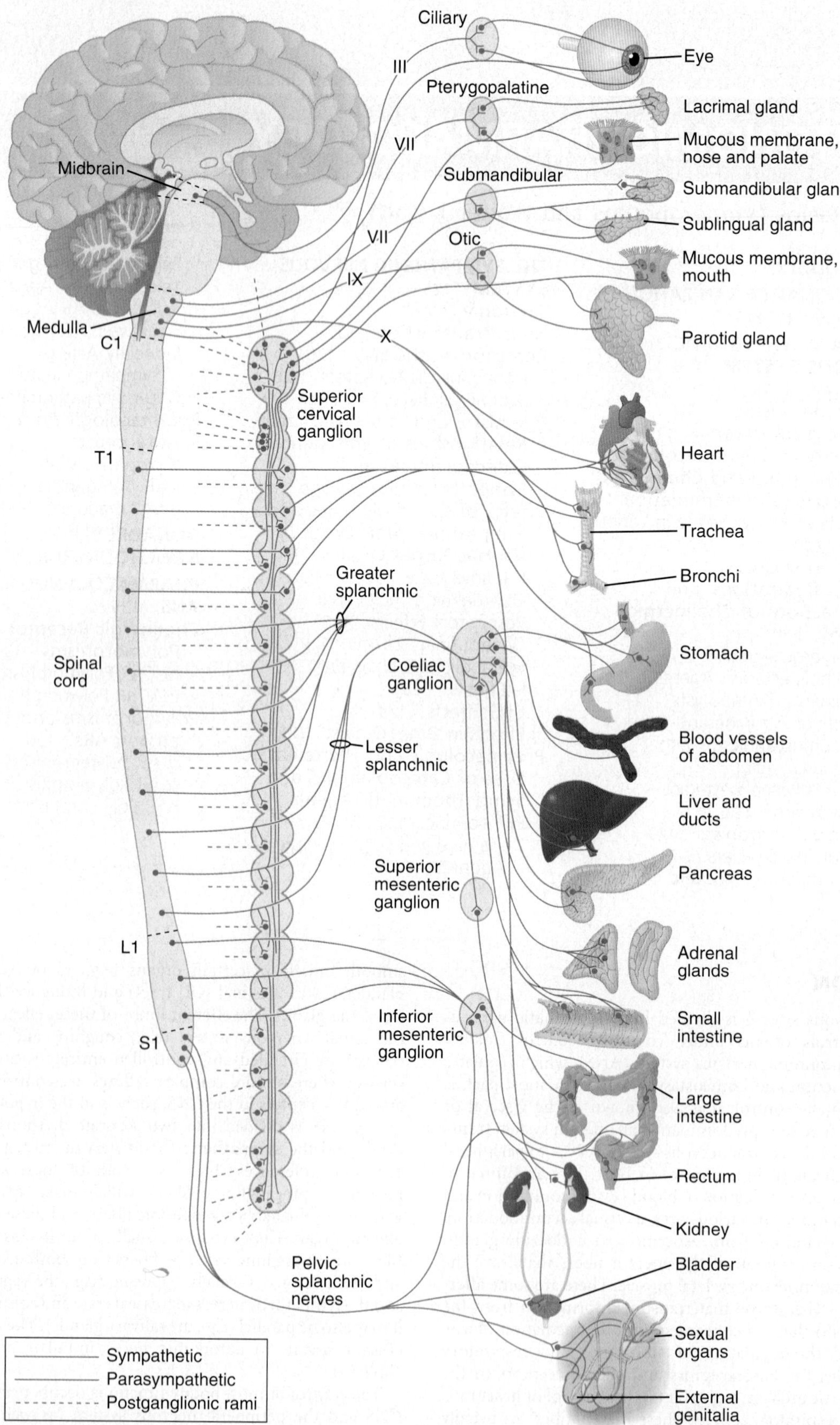

FIGURE 9-1 • Anatomic organization of the autonomic nervous system (ANS). (Adapted from Gray's Anatomy: The Anatomical Basis of Medicine and Surgery, 39th ed. New York: Churchill-Livingstone, 2004.)

TABLE 9-1 EFFECTS OF THE AUTONOMIC NERVOUS SYSTEM ON EFFECTOR ORGAN SYSTEMS

	Sympathetic Stimulation		***Parasympathetic Stimulation***	
Organ System	**Action**	**Receptor (Adrenergic)**	**Action**	**Receptor (Cholinergic)**
EYE				
Radial muscle of the iris	Contraction	α_1		
Circular muscle of the iris			Contraction	M_3
Ciliary muscle	Relaxation	β	Contraction (miosis)	M_3
HEART				
SA node	Acceleration of conduction	β_1, β_2	Slowing of conduction	M_2
AV node and ectopic pacemakers	Acceleration of conduction	β_1, β_2		
Contractility	Increase	β_1, β_2	Decrease (atrial muscle, minor effect)	M_2
VASCULATURE				
Cutaneous and splanchnic vascular smooth mucle	Contraction	α_1, α_2		
Skeletal muscle vessels	Vasodilation (direct effect in vascular smooth muscle)	β_2	Vasodilation (indirect effect through nitric oxide release from the vascular endothelium)	M_3
GASTROINTESTINAL TRACT				
Wall smooth muscle	Relaxation	α_2, β_2	Contraction	M_3
Sphincter smooth muscle	Contraction	α_1	Relaxation	M_3
Secretion			Increase	M_3
Myenteric plexus			Activation	M_1
GENITOURINARY TRACT				
Bladder wall smooth muscle	Relaxation	β_2	Contraction	M_3
Sphincter smooth muscle	Contraction	α_1	Relaxation	M_3
Uterine smooth muscle (pregnancy)	Relaxation	β_2	Contraction	M_3
Penis, seminal vesicles	Ejaculation	α	Erection	M
AIRWAYS				
Bronchiolar smooth muscle	Relaxation	β_2	Contraction	M_3
Bronchiolar mucus secretion			Activation	M_3
SKIN				
Pilomotor smooth muscle	Contraction	α		
SWEAT GLANDS				
Thermoregulatory	Increased secretions	M (cholinoceptor)		
Apocrine (stress-responsive)	Increased secretions	α		
INTERMEDIARY METABOLISM				
Liver	Gluconeogenesis and glycogenolysis	β, α		
Adipose tissue	Increased lipolysis	β_3		
Adipose tissue	Decreased lipolysis	α_2		
Pancreas	Insulin secretion	β_2		
Pancreas	Insulin secretion inhibition	α_2		
Kidney (juxtaglomerular apparatus)	Renin release	β_1		
ANS nerve endings	ACh release inhibition from cholinergic endings	α_2	Norepinephrine release inhibition from noradrenergic endings	M_1

Ach, acetylcholine; ANS, autonomic nervous system; AV, atrioventricular; SA, sinoatrial.

communication. Chemical transmission is carried out by small molecule neurotransmitters (see Chapter 8, Neurotransmitters) via diffusion across the synapse after release by presynaptic fibers. As part of the peripheral nervous system, the ANS regulates organ function involuntarily (outside of conscious control) and controls key visceral functions necessary for ordinary living.

The ANS communication system is organized with feed-forward and feedback circuits in place for a high degree of regulation. These are controlled primarily via pre- and postsynaptic receptors, transporters, and enzymes, membrane-embedded proteins that respond to and/or control the availability of neurotransmitters. Thus, these proteins regulate the overall function of the ANS and have historically been, and currently are, key targets for pharmacologic manipulation that have proved useful for the treatment of several maladies.

FUNCTIONAL ORGANIZATION OF THE ANS

In the brain, the two divisions of the ANS (parasympathetic nervous system and SNS) and the endocrine system are integrated with acetylcholine (ACh) along with sensory input from the CNS. The actions of the parasympathetic ANS usually leads to growth (anabolic actions), whereas the actions of the sympathetic ANS lead to energy expenditure in order for certain tasks to be performed ("fight or flight" response). For example, heart slowing and digestion stimulation by the parasympathetic system are typical energy-conserving actions, whereas cardiac stimulation, blood sugar elevation, and cutaneous vasoconstriction induced by the sympathetic system are actions that prime the organism for physical action.

Several important feedback inhibitory control mechanisms at the ANS nerve endings ensure accurate and consistent regulation of autonomic function. They can be broadly divided to presynaptic and postsynaptic (see later, and for additional details, see Chapter 9, Neurotransmitters). Autonomic receptors located presynaptically at ANS synapses are stimulated by the released neurotransmitter and regulate (inhibit or enhance) further neurotransmitter release.[1] These presynaptic receptors are called **autoreceptors**, because they respond to the very same neurotransmitter whose release is regulated. These receptors are exemplified by the presynaptic α_2-adrenergic receptors (ARs) that inhibit, and the presynaptic β_2ARs that facilitate norepinephrine (NE) release from adrenergic nerve terminals (see later and Chapter 8, Neurotransmitters). However, other presynaptic regulatory receptors exist that can be stimulated by neurotransmitters or endogenous chemicals and subsequently regulate the release of a different neurotransmitter.[1-3] These receptors are called **heteroreceptors** and important examples here are the presynaptic muscarinic M_2 cholinergic receptors, which are stimulated by ACh but inhibit NE release from adrenergic nerve terminals, and the presynaptic angiotensin II type 1 (AT_1) receptors that after stimulation by angiotensin II, facilitate NE release from adrenergic nerve terminals (see Chapter 8, Neurotransmitters, for a more detailed discussion of these neurotransmitters and their regulation).

Postsynaptic feedback regulatory mechanisms mainly involve the up- or down-regulation (increase or decrease of total cellular functional receptor number, respectively) of postsynaptic autonomic receptors located in the effector organs themselves. It is well established that chronic or repeated activation of these receptors leads to their down-regulation (decrease of their number) and chronic lack of activation, for example, upon denervation of some tissues, leads to up-regulation (increase of number) of autonomic receptors, resulting in a very enhanced sensitivity of the tissue to the action of the autonomic neurotransmitter upon subsequent stimulation (hence, the latter process is called **denervation supersensitivity**). Very important examples of denervation supersensitivity are the up-regulation of nicotinic cholinergic receptors (nAChRs) of the neuromuscular junction after surgical denervation, causing supersensitivity of the end plate to ACh stimulation (see later under "The Parasympathetic Nervous System" and "Neuromuscular Blockers" sections), and the supersensitivity of vascular smooth muscle and cardiac myocytes to adrenergic stimulation after administration of reserpine, an alkaloid that depletes NE stores in sympathetic nerve terminals that innervate these tissues (see Chapter 8, Neurotransmitters, for more details). The molecular mechanisms of these processes involve actions of intracellular kinases and other protein cofactors on ANS receptors, and their discussion is beyond the scope of this chapter. For a detailed discussion of these mechanisms, see Chapter 6, Signal Transduction.

THE PARASYMPATHETIC NERVOUS SYSTEM

Anatomy

The preganglionic outflow of the parasympathetic nervous system arises from the cell bodies of the motor nuclei of the cranial nerves III, VII, IX, and X in the brainstem and from the second, third, and fourth sacral segments of the spinal cord. It is, therefore, also known as the **craniosacral outflow**. The cranial nerves III, VII, and IX affect the pupil and salivary gland secretion, whereas the vagus nerve (X) carries fibers to the heart, lungs, stomach, upper intestine, and ureter. The sacral fibers form pelvic plexuses, which innervate the distal colon, rectum, bladder, and reproductive organs.

The preganglionic fibers themselves run quite close to the targeted organ that is innervated, and parasympathetic ganglia and synapses are always close to or within the organ, giving rise to relatively short postganglionic fibers that innervate the relevant tissue (Fig. 9-2). The ganglion cells can be either well organized (e.g., myenteric plexus of the intestine) or diffuse (e.g., bladder, blood vessels). As mentioned previously, these innervations of the parasympathetic nervous system generally function to conserve energy and maintain basic physiologic functions.

Neurotransmission

The chemical transmitter at both pre- and postganglionic synapses in the parasympathetic nervous system is ACh. Acetylcholine is also the neurotransmitter at sympathetic preganglionic synapses (thus, all autonomic ganglia), some sympathetic postganglionic synapses, the neuromuscular junction (somatic nervous system), and some sites in the CNS. Nerve fibers that release ACh from their endings are described as **cholinergic fibers** and include nerves integrating exocrine sweat glands (see later). Of note, ACh also has a direct vasodilator action on arterioles despite the absence of parasympathetic innervation. Choline acetyl transferase catalyzes the formation of ACh from choline and acetyl coenzyme A (acetyl-CoA). The latter is synthesized in the nerve terminal, and choline is taken up by active transport from the extracellular fluid within the nerve (see Chapter 8, Neurotransmitters).

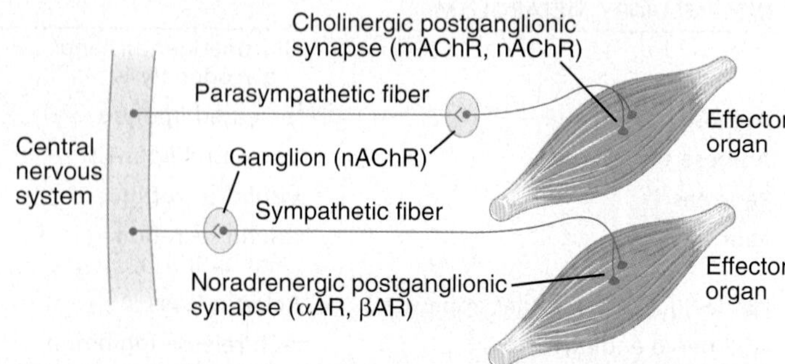

FIGURE 9-2 • Neuronal fibers of the ANS. See text for details. Note that the parasympathetic postganlionic fibers are so much shorter than the sympathetic ones that the parasympathetic ganglia are located very close to (or even, in some organs, inside) the wall of the innervated effector organ. The respective receptors at each autonomic synapse are also shown. Of note, at some particular effector organs, sympathetic fibers actually form cholinergic synapses releasing acetylcholine (Ach) on muscarinic cholinergic receptors (mAChRs) (e.g., salivary glands). αAR, alpha adrenoceptor; βAR, β-adrenoceptor; nAChR, nicotinic cholinergic receptor.

Acetylcholine is stored in synaptic vesicles, and is released in response to depolarization of the nerve terminal and a subsequent influx of Ca^{2+}. This Ca^{2+}-dependent release leads to a quantum of ACh available in the synapse and through diffusion; ACh activates receptors (see later) located on the pre- or postganglionic synaptic membrane.

Cholinergic Receptors

A number of different ACh receptors are distributed throughout the body, termed **cholinergic receptors** or **cholinoceptors**; they are broadly divided into two types: nicotinic (named after their high affinity for the alkaloid nicotine) and muscarinic (named after their high affinity for the alkaloid muscarine). These receptors are discussed in detail in Chapter 8, Neurotransmitters, and only a few key general features are discussed here. Nicotinic receptors are located primarily in autonomic ganglia, in the chromaffin cells of the adrenal medulla, and at the neuromuscular junctions.[4] Muscarinic receptors are localized in autonomic effector cells and are further subdivided into five different subgroups, M_1-M_5.[5] These receptors are members of the large family of G protein–coupled receptors (GPCRs) that have seven transmembrane-spanning domains and, upon agonist occupancy, undergo a conformational change that activates heterotrimeric G proteins and downstream signal transduction pathways (see Chapter 6, Signal Transduction). M_1 receptors appear to be localized to the CNS and perhaps parasympathetic ganglia (Table 9-2). Pirenzepine, a drug still under investigation for the treatment of gastroduodenal ulcers (see Chapter 31, Acid Reflux and Ulcer Disease), is a selective M_1-receptor antagonist.[6] M_2-receptors are the non-neuronal receptors of smooth muscle, cardiac muscle, and glandular epithelium. Bethanechol appears to be a selective agonist at M_2-receptors.

Muscarinic receptors can also be classified by their G protein coupling. M_1, M_3, and M_5 receptors couple to $G_{q/11}$ proteins, which trigger activation of phospholipase C and, therefore, downstream activation of the 1′,4′,5′-inositol triphosphate-diacylglycerol (IP_3-DAG) cascade, which ultimately results in Ca^{2+}-mediated activation of protein kinase C.[5] This signaling pathway can also lead to nitric oxide (NO) synthase activation and NO-mediated vasodilation (see Chapters 6, Signal Transduction; and 8, Neurotransmitters).[7,8] M_2 and M_4 receptors couple to $G_{i/o}$ proteins, which are pertussis toxin–sensitive G proteins (see Chapter 6, Signal Transduction) that can inhibit adenylyl cyclase, activate certain K^+ channels (e.g., G-protein regulated inwardly rectifying K^+ channels [GIRKs]) and inhibit voltage-dependent Ca^{2+} channels. Postsynaptic M_2 receptors, when activated, produce hyperpolarization, reducing excitability and firing frequency of target neurons, and presynaptic M_2 receptors inhibit neurotransmitter release. M_2 receptors are also present in cardiac atria, where they mediate slowing of sinus rhythm and electrical conduction (bradycardia).[9,10]

Chemistry and Pharmacology of Acetylcholine and Cholinergic Agonists (Cholinomimetics)

Acetylcholine action is terminated via its hydrolysis at the synaptic cleft by acetylcholinesterase (AChE) (see Chapter 8, Neurotransmitters). This enzyme is distinct from butyrylcholinesterase (BuChE), found in the plasma. Acetylcholine has virtually no clinical application owing to its rapid hydrolysis at the synaptic cleft by AChE and in the plasma by BuChE.[11] Consequently, numerous derivatives have been synthesized in attempts to provide drugs with longer durations of action and more receptor subtype–specific effects. Acetylcholine was first synthesized by Baeyer in 1867. Of the several hundred choline derivatives synthesized, only bethanechol, carbachol, and methacholine have been of any therapeutic use. Acetylcholine is the acetyl ester of choline, a quaternary ammonium derivative. The chemical structures of the important choline esters are given in Figure 9-3.

These small molecules differ from ACh in relative muscarinic or nicotinic activity and/or resistance to enzymatic hydrolysis. The degree

TABLE 9-2 MUSCARINIC CHOLINERGIC RECEPTOR SUBTYPES AND THEIR ANTAGONISTS

	M_1 Subtype	M_2 Subtype	M_3 Subtype
Localization	Nerves	Heart (atria), nerves	Glands, smooth muscle, vascular endothelium
Signal transduction	$G_{q/11}$-PLC, increase of IP_3-DAG	$G_{i/o}$, AC inhibition, K^+ channel activation	$G_{q/11}$-PLC, increase of IP_3-DAG
Primary physiologic effect	Neuronal depolarization-excitation, gastric acid secretion	Bradycardia, neuronal inhibition	Activation of secretions, vasodilation, bronchospasm, relaxation of smooth muscles
Selective antagonists	Pirenzepine, dicyclomine, telenzepine, trihexyphenidyl	Gallamine, methoctramine	Darifenacin, solifenacin

AC, adenylyl cyclase; DAG, diacylglycerol; IP_3, 1′,4′,5′, inositol triphosphate; PLC, phospholipase C.

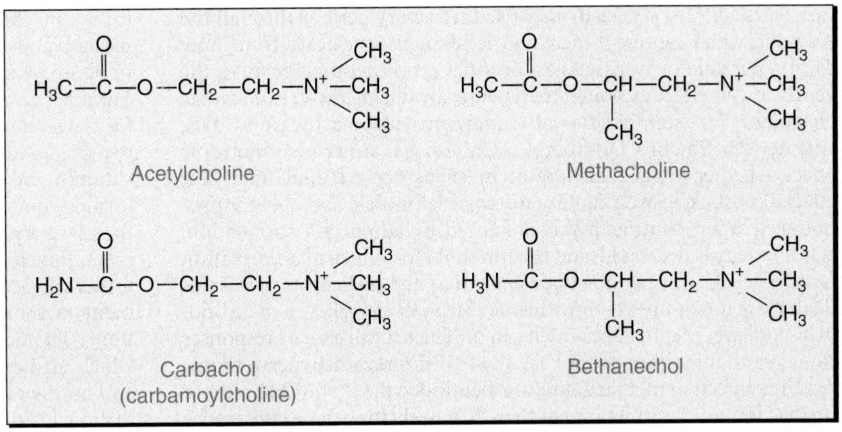

Acetylcholine

Methacholine

Carbachol (carbamoylcholine)

Bethanechol

FIGURE 9-3 • Chemical structures of acetylcholine and the most important of the other choline esters (cholinergic agonists, cholinomimetics).

of muscarinic activity decreases if the acetyl group is replaced; however, some substitutions result in resistance to hydrolysis. Carbachol, in which the acetyl group is replaced by a carbamoyl, has both muscarinic and nicotinic properties but is almost entirely resistant to hydrolysis by AChE or BuChE. Bethanechol is similarly resistant to hydrolysis; however, it possesses mainly muscarinic activity, as does methacholine, due to the β-methyl substitution. Although both carbachol and bethanechol possess muscarinic activity, their effects on the heart are minimal and their GI and genitourinary effects predominate. Methacholine, conversely, has predominantly cardiac effects; it is hydrolyzed by AChE, but at only one third of the ACh hydrolysis rate, and is resistant to BuChE.

Effects of Acetylcholine in Various Target Organs

Cardiovascular Effects. Acetylcholine has three primary effects upon the cardiovascular system[10]:

1. Vasodilation in almost all vascular beds, including pulmonary and coronary vessels.
2. Direct negative cardiac chronotropic effect.
3. Direct negative cardiac inotropic effect in atria.

In cardiac muscle, the effects of ACh are limited to atrial tissue because virtually no cholinergic receptors are expressed in ventricular muscle. Of note, the cardiovascular effects of ACh can be obscured by the ACh-mediated release of catecholamines (see Chapter 8, Neurotransmitters) and from dampening by the baroreceptor reflex. Although ACh is rarely given systemically, its cardiac effects are important because of the vagal involvement in the action of the cardiac glycosides and antiarrhythmic agents (see Chapters 25, Rhythm Disorders and 26, Heart Failure). Small ACh doses can cause a fall in blood pressure (hypotension) and reflex tachycardia; considerably larger doses are required to produce bradycardia via a direct action on the heart. If atropine, a muscarinic receptor blocker, is given prior to ACh, then a rise in blood pressure (hypertension) is seen owing to sympathoadrenal activation and ganglionic stimulation (effects mediated by the nicotinic receptors of ACh, which are unaffected by atropine).[12] Vasodilation is mediated by muscarinic receptors present in the vascular endothelium and not in vascular smooth muscle, which lacks parasympathetic innervation and is mediated by NO.[8,13-15] NO is produced in the endothelium in response to $G_{q/11}$-coupled muscarinic receptor activation and diffuses through to the smooth muscle of the vessel to produce relaxation.

Acetylcholine has actions on all types of specialized cardiac cells, as does the vagus nerve. Its cardiac effects are believed to be mediated by cardiac M_2 receptors.[9,10,16] Parasympathetic fibers are distributed extensively to the sinoatrial (SA) and atrioventricular (AV) nodes and the atrial muscle, but they display negligible innervation of the ventricles, ending predominantly on the His-Purkinje system. In the SA node, ACh decreases spontaneous depolarization by reducing the rate of phase 4 of the cardiac action potential and hyperpolarizing the resting cell membrane. In atrial muscle, ACh slows conduction, but it also reduces the action potential duration and the effective refractory period, therefore exacerbating atrial flutter or fibrillation from ectopic foci. These effects, especially increased refractory periods through the AV node, which represent increased vagal tone of the heart, contribute to the blockade of transmission of atrial proarrhythmic beats to the ventricles, an effect exploited therapeutically during the use of cardiac glycosides for suppression of supraventricular tachycardias (see Chapter 25, Rhythm Disorders). ACh also has a negative inotropic effect, whether applied directly or by vagus nerve stimulation. This effect almost exclusively applies to the atrial muscle and is more pronounced when contractility is enhanced by adrenergic stimulation. Automaticity is decreased, and the threshold for ventricular fibrillation is increased. Cardiac sympathetic and parasympathetic nerve terminals lie in close proximity and muscarinic receptors are believed to be both post- and presynaptic. Thus, ACh can modulate both cardiac responses to ACh and inhibition of the release of NE from cardiac nerve terminals. The effects of methacholine are identical to those of ACh; however, methacholine is far more potent than ACh in eliciting these effects. The cardiovascular effects of carbachol and bethanechol are less significant following subcutaneous (subQ) or oral doses as the effects consist of a small fall in diastolic blood pressure and a mild reflex tachycardia.

Gastrointestinal Effects. Acetylcholine and all the muscarinic agonists are capable of producing increased GI tract tone, motility, and secretion.[17] They also decrease the tone of sphincters, which may be accompanied by abdominal cramps, nausea and vomiting, and diarrhea.

Effects in Other Systems. Acetylcholine and related choline esters have various muscarinic receptor–mediated effects in various tissues (see Table 9-2). They increase ureteric peristalsis and cause detrusor contraction and trigonal and internal sphincter relaxation of the urinary bladder.[18-21] In the respiratory tract, they increase tracheobronchial secretions and bronchial tone and stimulate the carotid sinus and aortic body chemoreceptors, and they are thus used in tests of bronchial hyperactivity in asthmatics.[5,22] In the eye, they produce miosis, but the ensuing fall in intraocular pressure may be preceded by a transient rise, due to vasodilation and increased permeability of the vessels of the blood–aqueous humor barrier.[23,24] The effects at ganglia and the neuromuscular junctions of skeletal muscle (nicotinic receptor–mediated) are generally insignificant at therapeutic concentrations.[4]

Therapeutic Uses, Contraindications, and Interactions of Cholinergic Drugs

Cholinergic Agonists

Acetylcholine is used as an intraocular solution; carbachol is used intraocularly but also as a topical ophthalmic solution; and methacholine is rarely, if ever, used. Bethanechol is used in both tablet and injectable forms, as a urinary tract and GI tract stimulant (when there is no evidence of organ obstruction). The injectable forms are always administered subQ, not intramuscularly (IM). Pilocarpine, an alkaloid found in the leaves of the Pilocarpus shrubs of South America with predominantly muscarinic actions, is used topically to induce miosis for the treatment of glaucoma and the reversal of mydriasis.[23,24]

Acetylcholine and methacholine are hydrolyzed by cholinesterases; therefore, the concurrent administration of anti-AChE agents significantly enhances their effects. When administered prior to carbachol and bethanechol, anti-AChE agents produce only additive effects.[11] The muscarinic effects of these agents are competitively blocked by atropine. Epinephrine and other sympathomimetic amines counteract many of the muscarinic effects of these agents. The nicotinic actions at autonomic ganglia are blocked by hexamethonium, and their actions at the neuromuscular junction are antagonized by curare analogues.[4,25] The major contraindications to the use of these agents are asthma (because they cause bronchoconstriction),[22] ischemic heart disease (because they cause hypotension and lower coronary blood flow),[26] hyperthyroidism (because of increased risk of atrial flutter/fibrillation),[10] and peptic ulcer (because of increased gastric secretions).[17]

Anticholinesterase Agents

As discussed previously, two enzymes are capable of hydrolyzing choline esters (see Chapter 8, Neurotransmitters): AChE, which is found in cholinergic nerve fibers and in erythrocytes, but not in plasma, and BuChE, which is synthesized in the liver and also found in plasma, kidney, and the intestine.[27] The latter's physiologic action is unknown, and it is responsible for the hydrolysis of succinylcholine (see later) and the ester local anesthetics. Acetylcholinesterase exists in two classes of molecular forms: simple oligomers of a 70-kDa catalytic subunit, and elongated forms of complex molecular structures. The former contain a hydrophobic surface and are often associated with the plasma membrane, whereas the elongated forms consist of tetramers, linked by disulphide bonds to a filamentous structure. These forms are localized in the outer basal lamina of the synaptic cleft (basement membrane) and are primarily found at neuromuscular junctions. The active site of the enzyme consists of an anionic subsite, which attracts the positively charged quaternary ammonium group, and an esteratic subsite, which performs a nucleophilic attack on the carbonyl carbon atom of the substrate.[27]

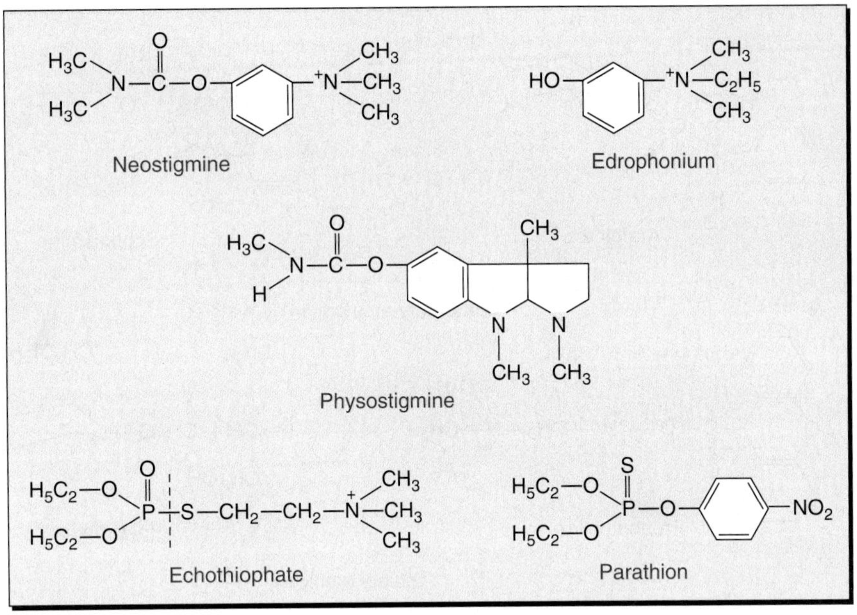

FIGURE 9-4 • Chemical structures of the most important anticholinesterase agents used in pharmacotherapy and of some representative organophosphate anticholinesterases.

The catalytic mechanism resembles other serine esterases, because the active site consists of a critical serine residue, whose hydroxyl group is activated by the imidazole side group, of an adjacent histidine residue.[11] The enzyme hydrolyzes ACh into choline and acetic acid, and the enzyme is regenerated upon termination of the reaction. The enzyme is very efficient, with a turnover rate of just 150 µsec. Acetylcholinesterase inhibitors (anti-AChEs) are quaternary ammonium compounds (Fig. 9-4) that inhibit the enzyme reversibly by binding the esteratic site (or another site termed *peripheral anionic site*).[11] Edrophonium binds reversibly and selectively to the active site. This reversible binding coupled with rapid renal elimination of the compound results in a short duration of action of edrophonium. Physostigmine and neostigmine, possessing a carbamoyl-ester linkage are hydrolyzed by AChE, but at a much slower rate. Both of these agents exist as cations at physiologic pH, thus enhancing their association with the active site. Physostigmine, existing in equilibrium with the nonionic species, readily crosses the blood-brain barrier. After binding AChE, the alcohol moiety is cleaved, giving rise to the carbamoylated enzyme, which is far more stable than the acetylated enzyme, with an in vivo duration of enzyme inhibition of 3 to 4 hours.[28]

Organophosphates, such as ecothiopate (see Fig. 9-4), serve as true hemi-substrates acting on the esteratic site, with the resultant phosphorylated enzyme being extremely stable, by means of their structural resemblance to the transition state of the acetyl-ester hydrolysis reaction. The stability of these complexes is enhanced by enzyme "aging," which refers to the biochemical process of one of the phosphonate alkyl groups of these complexes being lost, resulting in irreversibility of binding, thus necessitating new synthesis to regenerate the enzyme. Organophosphates are also termed *acid-transferring inhibitors*, in contrast to the reversible, competitive inhibitors such as edrophonium.[29]

Cholinergic Antagonists

Like agonists, cholinergic antagonists are subdivided into muscarinic and nicotinic antagonists, which are based on their specific receptor affinities. Antinicotinic agents comprise the ganglion-blockers and the neuromuscular junction blockers. Antimuscarinics act as classic "parasympatholytics," as they block the effects of activation of the parasympathetic nervous system. Naturally occurring alkaloids with antimuscarinic properties have been known for thousands of years as medicines, poisons, and cosmetics. The prototype of these alkaloids is atropine, also knows as hyoscyamine, the primary alkaloid found in the plant *Atropa belladonna* (deadly nightshade) and in *Datura stramonium* (jimsonweed, Jamestown weed, thorn apple). Scopolamine, or hyoscine, occurs in *Hyoscyamus niger* (henbane). The naturally occurring atropine is L(−)-hyoscyamine; however, clinically used atropine is racemic D,L(+,−)-hyoscyamine. The biologically active isomers of both atropine and scopolamine are the L(−)-isomers, and both are tertiary amine esters of tropic acid (Fig. 9-5). Various analogues with antimuscarinic effects have been synthesized. They are mainly used for their ophthalmic or CNS effects. Interestingly, many antihistaminics (H_1 histaminergic receptor blockers, see Chapter 11, Inflammation and Immunomodulation) and antidepressants (see Chapter 53, Depression and Bipolar Disorder) have similar structures and, consequently, anticholinergic properties. Quaternary ammonium antimuscarinic compounds (see Fig. 9-5) have also been synthesized, with pronounced peripheral and reduced CNS effects, because they exhibit minimal crossing of the blood-brain barrier owing to the positive charge of their molecules.

The natural alkaloids and tertiary amine compounds are well absorbed from the GI tract and conjunctival membranes. Scopolamine is also absorbed transdermally.[30] They are readily distributed into the CNS, especially scopolamine, which has the most potent central effects of all antimuscarinics. As expected, the quaternary ammonium antimuscarinics are minimally absorbed after oral administration owing to low lipid solubility. As for the clearance of these agents, atropine is rapidly cleared from the blood with a half-life of 2 hours. Its effects are short-lived in all organs except the eyes.[31]

Atropine and its congeners cause reversible blockade of muscarinic receptors of ACh, probably via binding with the amino acids of the receptor that are responsible for binding the nitrogen atom of ACh, thereby preventing ACh from binding and activating these receptors.[25] The tissues most sensitive to the actions of atropine are the exocrine glands (salivary, bronchial, sweat), and the least sensitive is the parietal cell lining of the stomach. Atropine blocks all muscarinic receptor subtypes, whereas the semisynthetic antimuscarinics display some subtype selectivity (see Table 9-2).

Effects of Atropine and Other Antimuscarinics in Target Organs

CNS Effects. Atropine has minimal stimulatory and long-lasting sedative effects in the brain, but scopolamine has more potent central effects, causing drowsiness and amnesia. At toxic doses, scopolamine causes agitation, excitement, hallucinations, and coma. Antimuscarinic agents reduce the Parkinson-related tremor, which is due to the relative excess of cholinergic activity going unopposed by the reduced dopaminergic activity of the basal ganglia in Parkinson's disease. For this reason, many antimuscarinics (e.g., benzotropine, trihexyphenidyl, biperiden) are used clinically in combination with levodopa and other

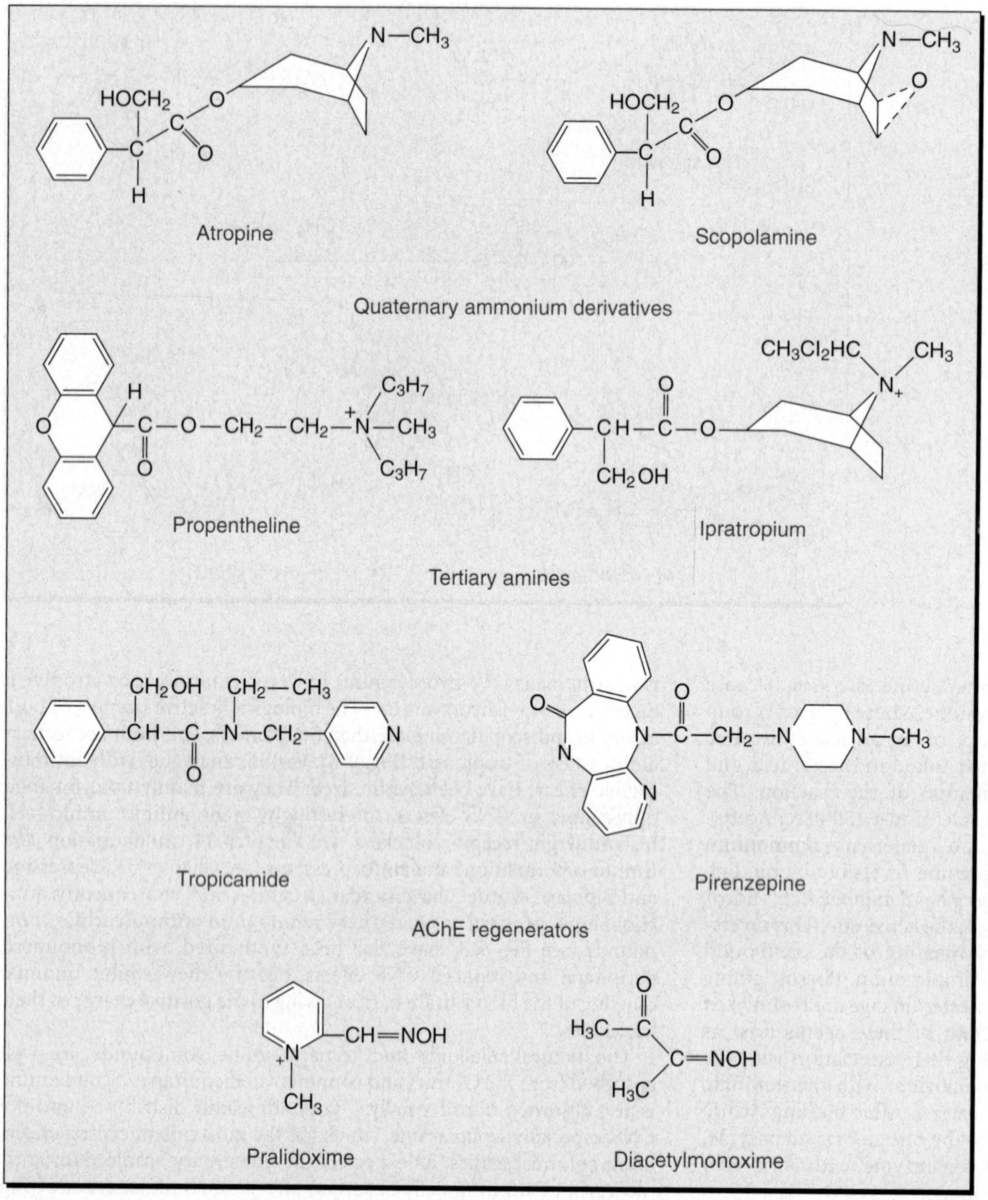

Atropine

Scopolamine

Quaternary ammonium derivatives

Propentheline

Ipratropium

Tertiary amines

Tropicamide

Pirenzepine

AChE regenerators

Pralidoxime

Diacetylmonoxime

FIGURE 9-5 • Chemical structures of various antimuscarinic agents and of the two most important cholinesterase regenerators.

dopaminergic agonists in symptomatic treatment of Parkinson's disease (see Chapter 44, Parkinson's Disease). Vestibular disorders, like motion sickness, involve muscarinic cholinergic discharge; therefore, they respond favorably to antimuscarinics.[5,30] Scopolamine is one of the oldest and most effective drugs at preventing or treating seasickness (and travel sickness in general) and is given by injection, orally, or as a transdermal patch.[30] Its main adverse effects are xerostomia (dry mouth) and sedation.

Ophthalmic Effects. mAChR activation results in contraction of the papillary constrictor muscle; therefore, atropine blocks this cholinergic effect, leaving the sympathetically mediated dilation of this muscle unopposed and, thus, causes mydriasis (pupil dilation). Dilated pupils were considered cosmetically pleasant during the Renaissance (in spite of the resulting extremely reduced visual acuity, see later); hence, the name "belladonna" ("beautiful woman" in Italian) was given to the plant from which eyedrops were made, containing high amounts of antimuscarinic alkaloids. In addition to mydriasis, antimuscarinics cause relaxation of the ciliary muscle of the eye, thus resulting in loss of the ability of the eye to accommodate (to focus for near vision), which is called *cycloplegia*. Owing to these actions, antimuscarinics can precipitate narrow-angle glaucoma and are contraindicated in this condition.[22,23] As with every exocrine gland secretion, they also reduce lacrimal secretion (causing dry eyes). Antimuscarinics are used topically as eyedrops or ophthalmic ointments to produce mydriasis and cycloplegia, which greatly facilitate eye and vision examination. If mydriasis without cycloplegia or short-lasting mydriasis is required, then α_1AR agonists, like phenylephrine, which cause transient mydriasis, are preferred.[22,23]

Cardiovascular Effects. As one could predict, the SA node effects of atropine are vagal pace slowing and relative tachycardia. Lower doses can cause initial bradycardia before the vagal block is manifest owing to presynaptic inhibition of ACh release from postganglionic vagal fibers.[10] However, central effects of atropine and scopolamine and the basal vagus activity regulating pulse interval and sinus rhythm might contribute to the effects of these drugs on cardiac sinus rhythm.[32] Atropine has the same effects on the AV node, where it can accelerate AV conduction and reduce the PR interval of the electrocardiogram (see Chapter 25, Rhythm Disorders). Because of blockade of the muscarinic receptors of the atrial muscle (mainly of the M_2 subtype), the propensity for atrial flutter and fibrillation is increased. Ventricular effects are negligible, because ventricular muscle lacks cholinergic innervation (see earlier).[9]

Blood vessels do not receive parasympathetic innervation, but ACh dilates arteries in the coronary circulation and in skeletal muscle vascular beds via activation of endothelial muscarinic receptors (mainly of the M_3 subtype), and this is readily blocked by atropine and related antimuscarinics.[33] The hemodynamic effects of atropine are minimal, because some tachycardia can be produced but blood pressure is unchanged. Upon cholinergic agonist administration, however, all the cardiovascular effects are readily blocked.

Effects in Other Organs. Atropine reduces the muscarinic receptor (mainly of the M_3 subtype)–mediated bronchoconstriction and bronchial secretions, an effect more pronounced in patients with pulmonary disease. This is why some antimuscarinics (e.g., ipratropium, tiotropium) are used in the form of aerosols for inhalation for asthma or chronic obstructive pulmonary disease (COPD), in conjunction with β_2AR agonists and other agents (see Chapter 28, Asthma and Chronic Obstructive Pulmonary Disease).[25,34] They are also used perioperatively prior to administration of inhalational (general) anesthetics to reduce bronchotracheal secretions and spasm. Atropine and its analogues suppress sweat gland thermoregulatory secretions by blockade of muscarinic receptors present in the sympathetic cholinergic fibers that innervate these glands. Therefore, they might cause temperature elevation (fever), especially at large doses.

Antimuscarinics reduce GI tract motility and secretions, thus causing delay of gastric emptying (an important effect if other drugs are coadministered) and reducing peristalsis (an important antidiarrheal effect), and markedly inhibit salivary gland secretions, causing severe dry mouth.[17,35] They can also cause transient intestinal paralysis. In combination with opioid antidiarrheal drugs, like diphenoxylate (Lomotil), they are given for traveler's diarrhea and GI hypermotility, although, in this combination, atropine is actually used as a deterrent against abuse of the opioid component (see Chapter 32, Motility Disorders). They also block gastric secretion to a lesser extent, and some more M_1 receptor subtype–selective antagonists (pirenzepine, telenzepine) with fewer adverse effects than atropine congeners have been developed for this purpose (they have some limited utility in peptic ulcer treatment in Europe, but not in the United States, where they are not on the market, see Chapter 31, Acid Reflux and Ulcer Disease).[6,17] Antimuscarinics also relax the smooth muscles of the bladder wall and ureters, slowing voiding, and inhibit sphincter relaxation, causing urinary retention. For these reasons, they are used for urinary urgency/incontinence (e.g., oxybutinin, tolterodine) and for relief of ureter spasms in urolithiasis, but they can precipitate pain and urinary retention in patients with prostate hypertrophy (see Chapter 30, Voiding Dysfunction).[18,36,37]

Adverse Effects and Contraindications of Antimuscarinics. Atropine and its congeners cause mydriasis and cycloplegia in the eyes (desirable therapeutic effects in ophthalmology but adverse effects when these drugs are given for some other indication), tachycardia, dry mouth, agitation, and hyperthermia (children are especially sensitive to temperature elevation by atropine). All these effects are treated symptomatically, because physostigmine or other AChE inhibitors that can be used to reverse these effects are rather more dangerous on their own than effective at reducing these adverse effects.[22,23] Poisoning with the quaternary ammonium antimuscarinic agents leads to ganglionic blockade and orthostatic hypotension without any central effects. Treatment of this, if required, involves administration of a quaternary ammonium anti-AChE, such as neostigmine, and sometimes phenylephrine might be needed to counteract the orthostatic hypotension.[38] All antimuscarinics are contraindicated in glaucoma, especially narrow-angle (or angle-closure) glaucoma, prostatic hyperplasia, peptic ulcer disease, and gastroesophageal reflux disease (GERD) (because they delay gastric emptying).

Anti-Acetylcholinesterase Poisoning

Both the muscarinic and the nicotinic effects of AChE inhibitors can be life-threatening; however, the nicotinic effects are very difficult to combat, because even agonism of nicotinic receptors, like antagonism, causes blockade of nicotinic transmission (see Chapter 8, Neurotransmitters).[38] Nevertheless, the muscarinic effects of anti-AChE poisoning can be effectively reversed by administration of antimuscarinics, most preferably atropine, provided that tertiary amine compounds (which readily penetrate the blood-brain barrier because they are uncharged and, hence, lipophilic) and not quaternary ammonium agents are used (which cannot pass into the CNS because of their charge, so they will leave the central effects of anti-AChE poisoning unaffected). Atropine sulfate is the antidote of choice, given intravenously (IV) at a dose of 1 to 2 mg every 10 minutes until signs of recovery appear. It has to be repeated several times to combat the long-lasting acute effects of the anti-AChE poison, which can last for at least 48 hours, so up to 1 g of atropine per day might need to be ingested to control a severe anti-AChE poisoning. Along with atropine, oxime agents, such as pralidoxime (2-PAM) and diacetylmonoxime (DAM), are given IV (1-2 g every 20-30 minutes).[39] These agents have the ability to hydrolyze the phosphoesteric bond between the organophosphate and the enzyme via the high affinity of their oxime groups for the electrophilic phosphorus atom of the organophosphates (see Fig. 9-5), thereby regenerating AChE.[38] In spite of the fact that if the enzyme complex is "aged" (see earlier), these agents are ineffective at regenerating the enzyme, some studies suggest that repeated administration of 2-PAM over a period of several days can be useful in severe poisoning.[40] In contrast, 2-PAM is completely useless in poisoning with carbamate AChE inhibitors. Unlike atropine, which is effective only at muscarinic sites, the oximes regenerate the enzyme at both muscarinic and nicotinic sites. However, 2-PAM carries a positive charge and, thus, cannot enter the CNS to reverse the central effects of anti-AChE poisoning, whereas DAM is highly lipophilic and can regenerate some of the CNS AChE.[41]

An alternative approach to combat anti-AChE poisoning is pretreatment with reversible AChE inhibitors like pyridostigmine or physostigmine, which prevents the nonreversible AChE inhibitor from binding the enzyme; this strategy is employed in situations in which chemical warfare–associated poisoning is anticipated. Again, atropine needs to be given concomitantly to counteract the muscarinic excess of the reversible anti-AChEs.[38]

Nicotinic Antagonists

As mentioned previously, nicotinic receptor antagonists consist of ganglion blockers and neuromuscular junction blockers.

Ganglionic Blockers

These agents block nAChRs at all autonomic ganglia (parasympathetic and sympathetic).[4,42] Therefore, they are able to suppress all autonomic outflow, but their lack of selectivity restricts their clinical use tremendously. All compounds in this class are synthetic amines, and their structural similarities with ACh are obvious (Fig. 9-6). Mecamylamine is a secondary amine with improved absorption from the GI tract. Decamethonium, a longer-chain analogue of hexamethonium, is a neuromuscular blocker (see later). Trimethaphan, which is inactive orally and given IV, blocks the nicotinic receptor and not the channel.[43] In contrast, hexamethonium appears to inhibit the channel operated by the nicotinic receptor, not the receptor per se. Ganglionic nicotinic receptors, like those of the neuromuscular junction (see later and Chapter 8, Neurotransmitters), can be subjected to both depolarizing and nondepolarizing blockade; however, currently used antiganglionics are nondepolarizing competitive blockers. Only mecamylamine, which is uncharged and lipophilic, crosses the blood-brain barrier and exerts central effects comprising sedation, tremor, and mental abnormalities.[44]

In the eye, these drugs cause cycloplegia and mild mydriasis (pupil dilation). In the cardiovascular system, they cause marked reduction of the sympathetically mediated vasomotor tone, peripheral arterial resistance, and venous return, resulting in severe postural hypotension. In the heart, they suppress contractility (sympatholytic effect) and cause mild tachycardia (muscarinolytic effect). In the GI tract, inhibition of secretion and motility occurs, precipitating constipation. Temperature-regulating sweating is blocked, but this does not lead to severe temperature elevation because it is offset by cutaneous vasodilation. Urination is inhibited and urinary retention might occur in men with

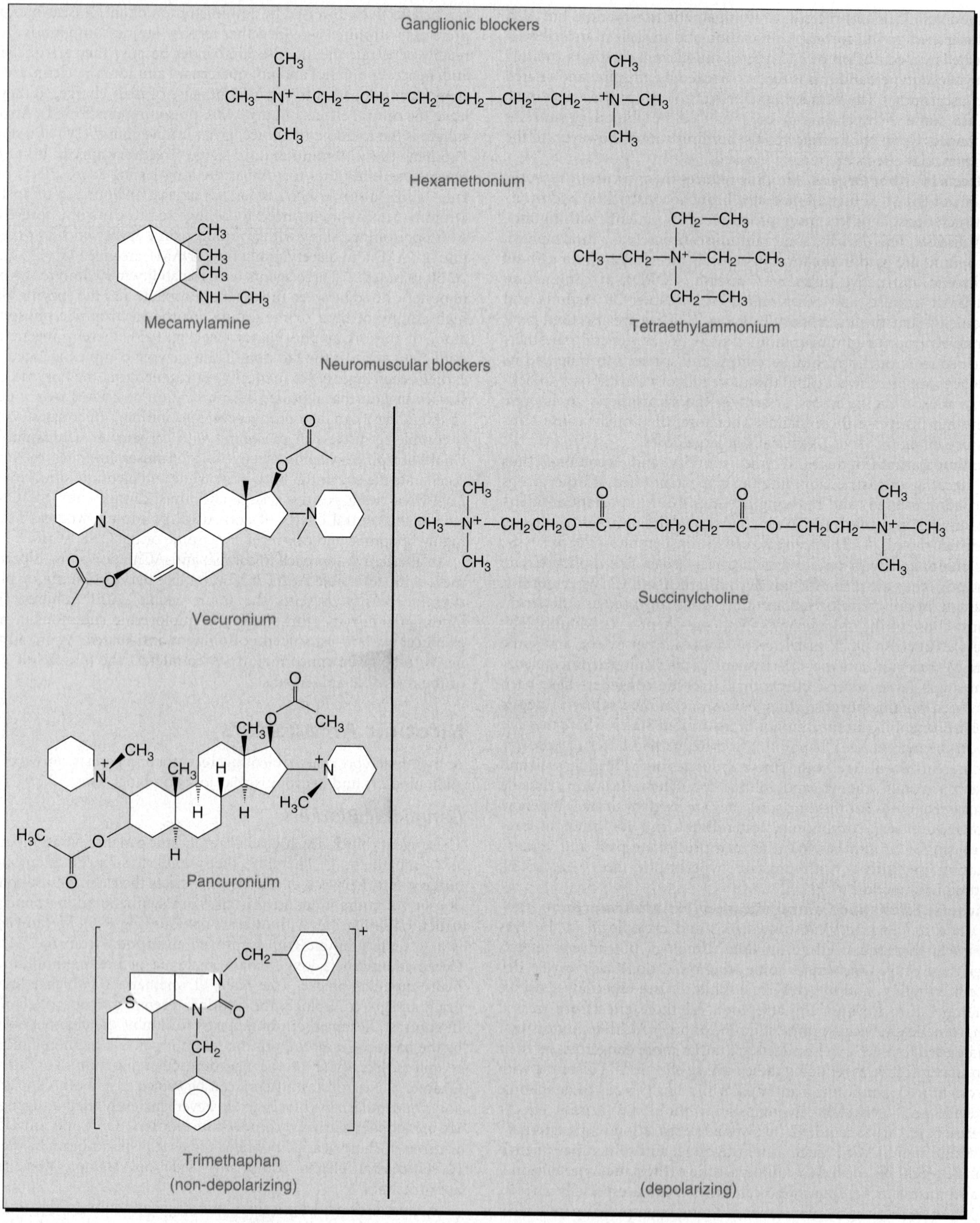

Ganglionic blockers

Hexamethonium

Mecamylamine

Tetraethylammonium

Neuromuscular blockers

Vecuronium

Succinylcholine

Pancuronium

Trimethaphan

(non-depolarizing)

(depolarizing)

FIGURE 9-6 • Chemical structures of the most important nicotinic antagonists.

prostatic hyperplasia. Sexual function is severely impaired because both erection (parasympathetic effect) and ejaculation (sympathetic effect) are inhibited. Mecamylamine is used experimentally to reduce nicotine cravings and assist smoking cessation.[44] Trimethaphan is sometimes used to control hypertensive crises due to aortic aneurysm or perioperatively in the neurosurgical setting.[43] The toxicity of these drugs comprises all these effects just described and precludes the use of these agents, except in acute cases.

Neuromuscular Blockers

During the 16th century, European explorers found that Native Americans were using an arrow poison (curare) that caused skeletal paralysis and death. The active ingredients of curare, D-tubocurarine, and its synthetic derivatives have since then revolutionized anesthesia and surgery. These compounds cause skeletal muscle relaxation and paralysis by blocking the action of ACh on its nicotinic receptors at the end plate (neuromuscular junction). This is achieved in two pharmacologically distinct ways[45]: (i) blockade of the nicotinic receptor of the innervated muscle preventing binding of ACh and subsequent depolarization of the muscle (pure, nondepolarizing antagonism), which is exerted by a subgroup of these drugs, with the prototype being D-tubocurarine, and (ii) excessive depolarizing activation of the receptor, which desensitizes the receptor over time and thus also produces nicotinic receptor blockade (see also Chapters 6, Signal Transduction; and 8, Neurotransmitters). The latter mechanism is exemplified by succinylcholine. All neuromuscular blockers resemble ACh structurally, and in fact, their structures seem to "connect two ACh molecules in one." All are polar and charged, because they contain quaternary ammonium groups, which render them unable to penetrate the blood-brain barrier, and thus, they lack central effects. They are also poorly absorbed orally (owing to low lipid solubility) and must be given parenterally.[24,46,47]

The most important nondepolarizing neuromuscular blockers are the isoquinoline derivatives atracurium, cisatracurium (the *cis* isomer of atracurium), mivacurium, doxacurium, and the steroid derivatives pancuronium, pipecuronium, rocuronium, and vecuronium. They differ in their duration of action, metabolism, and clearance.[48] The depolarizing neuromuscular blocker succinylcholine is readily degraded by plasma cholinesterase and, thus, has a very short duration of action (5-10 minutes only). Therefore, the activity of plasma cholinesterase is a critical regulator of the duration of succinylcholine's actions. Genetic variants of this enzyme exist that result in reduced or increased activity and can influence enormously the duration of neuromuscular blockade produced by succinylcholine. A test that measures the metabolizing activity of plasma cholinesterase is available based on dibucaine, a drug that inhibits the normal form of the enzyme far better than the abnormal, inactive variant form. The cardiovascular effects of these muscle blockers are minimal as they can cause mild hypotension through systemic histamine release, and pancuronium slightly increases heart rate and contractility via parasympathetic ganglionic blockade and NE release from adrenergic nerve terminals.[24] The depolarizing succinylcholine can cause cardiac arrhythmias, bradycardia, and decreased cardiac output by stimulating all nicotinic receptors of autonomic ganglia (parasympathetic and sympathetic) and also (indirectly) the atrial muscarinic M_2 receptors. These effects are effectively reversed by anticholinergics, such as atropine. Because neuromuscular blockers mediate histamine release, they can produce bronchoconstriction and bronchospasm. Rapacuronium does this through ACh release instead of histamine release, and it can be a significant adverse effect of this drug.[46] Succinylcholine can precipitate hyperkalemia under certain trauma conditions, occasionally resulting in life-threatening cardiac arrest, and it also raises intraocular pressure. Some of these drugs, especially rocuronium, have been associated with allergic reactions.[46] Neuromuscular blockers are used as adjuncts to anesthetics in surgical procedures, to assist in mechanical ventilation (they diminish airway muscle resistance and contractions, thus facilitating intubation), and to treat the peripheral spastic symptoms of seizures.[47]

These muscle blockers or relaxants display synergism in their activity with inhaled general anesthetics (see Chapter 60, General Anesthesia and Sedation) and with the aminoglycoside antibiotics (see Chapter 78, Community-Acquired Pneumonia), which block prejunctional Ca^{2+} channels responsible for release of ACh at the neuromuscular junction, thereby decreasing ACh availability at the end plate and potentiating neuromuscular blockade (they can also precipitate myasthenia gravis in this way). Myasthenia gravis and aging (associated with decreased drug clearance) greatly enhance the neuromuscular blockade produced by these agents, whereas conditions like burns and upper motor neuron diseases decrease the efficacy of nondepolarizing neuromuscular blockers, probably because of up-regulation of extrajunctional nicotinic receptors.[49] The effects of neuromuscular blockers are readily reversed by AChE inhibitors, such as edrophonium (short-acting) and neostigmine, which increase availability of ACh at the end plate to surmount the blockade of junctional nicotinic receptors.

THE SYMPATHETIC NERVOUS SYSTEM

Anatomy

The cell bodies of the sympathetic preganglionic fibers are in the lateral horns of the spinal segments T1-L2, the so-called thoracolumbar outflow. The preganglionic fibers travel a short distance in the mixed spinal nerve and then branch off as white rami (myelinated) to enter the sympathetic ganglia. These are mainly arranged in two paravertebral chains, which lie anterolateral to the vertebral bodies and extend from the cervical to the sacral region. They are called the *sympathetic ganglionic chains.* The short preganglionic fibers (unlike the long preganglionic fibers of the parasympathetic nervous system) that enter the chain make a synapse with a postsynaptic fiber either at the same dermatomal level or at a higher or lower level, and then the longer postganglionic fibers usually return to the adjacent spinal nerve via gray rami (unmyelinated) and are conveyed to the effector organ (see Fig. 9-2). At most postganglionic sympathetic endings, the chemical transmitter is NE (norepinephrine, noradrenaline), which is present in the presynaptic terminal as well as in the adrenal medulla (see later). In contrast, postganglionic sympathetic fibers in sweat glands release Ach, and this transmission is muscarinic.

Some preganglionic fibers do not synapse in the sympathetic chains but terminate in separate cervical or abdominal ganglia or travel in the greater splanchnic nerve and directly synapse with chromaffin cells of the adrenal medulla. As discussed previously, ACh is the neurotransmitter via a nicotinic receptor at the preganglionic synapse. The adrenal medulla is innervated by preganglionic fibers, and therefore, epinephrine (adrenaline) is released from the gland by stimulation of nicotinic ACh receptors, although some NE is also secreted.[4]

In contrast to the parasympathetic nervous system, the SNS enables the body to be prepared for fear, flight, or fight (see later). Sympathetic responses include an increase in heart rate, blood pressure, and cardiac output, a diversion of blood flow from the skin and splanchnic vessels to those supplying skeletal muscle, increased pupil size, bronchiolar dilation, contraction of sphincters, and metabolic changes such as the mobilization of fat and glycogen.

Neurotransmission

The pressor effects of suprarenal extracts were first demonstrated in 1895 by Oliver and Schäfer. The active principle was named epinephrine or adrenaline by Abel in 1899 and was first synthesized by Stolz and Dakin. Epinephrine and NE are catecholamines, and both are synthesized from the essential amino acid tyrosine by a series of steps that also includes the production of dopamine, which is another endogenous catecholamine. The terminal branches of the sympathetic postganglionic fibers have varicosities or swellings, giving them the appearance of a string of beads. These swellings form the synaptic contact with the effector organ and are also the site of synthesis and storage of NE. On the arrival of a nerve impulse, NE is released from granules in the presynaptic terminal into the synaptic cleft. The action of NE is terminated by diffusion from the site of action, reuptake back into the presynaptic nerve ending where it is inactivated by the enzyme monoamine oxidase (MAO) on the mitochondrial surface or metabolized locally by the enzyme catechol-*O*-methyl-transferase (COMT).

The synthesis and storage of catecholamines in the adrenal medulla are similar to those of sympathetic postganglionic nerve endings; however, owing to the presence of an additional enzyme termed *phenylethanolamine N-methyl transferase (PNMT)*, the majority of NE is converted to epinephrine. The adrenal medulla responds to nervous impulses in the sympathetic cholinergic preganglionic fibers by transforming the neural impulses into hormonal secretion. In situations involving physical or psychologic stress, much larger quantities are released. Overall, the actions of catecholamines are mediated by specific postsynaptic cell surface receptors (see later).

Receptors in the SNS

Dopaminergic Receptors

Dopamine is the third catecholamine produced endogenously in the body and produces its various biologic effects through its interactions with specific dopaminergic receptors (termed D_1-D_5) (see also Chapter 8, Neurotransmitters).[50] These receptors are particularly important in the CNS and in the splanchnic and renal vasculatures. D_1 and D_5 receptors couple to Gs proteins, resulting in adenylyl cyclase stimulation, and this relaxes renal vascular smooth muscle. D_2, D_3, and D_4 receptors couple to $G_{i/o}$ proteins and inhibit adenylyl cyclase and activate hyperpolarizing K^+ currents, thus modulating neurotransmission in the CNS.

Adrenergic Receptors

Dale and Berger (1910) studied a wide range of synthetic amines related to epinephrine and termed their physiologic actions *sympathomimetic*. They later discovered that cocaine or chronic denervation reduced the response to ephedrine and tyramine but not to epinephrine. Thus, it became evident that the differences between amines were not solely quantitative. Raymond Ahlquist in 1948, based on a series of experiments showing different activities of various sympathomimetic drugs (i.e., drugs that mimic the actions of the sympathetic catecholamines epinephrine and NE), proposed the existence of two different receptors for catecholamines, which he named α- and βARs.[51] αARs were those with increased affinity for epinephrine and NE and minimal affinity for isoproterenol, whereas βARs were characterized by their high affinity for isoproterenol and epinephrine and low affinity for NE. The advent of drugs that selectively blocked βARs (β-blockers) confirmed Ahlquist's suggested division of ARs and pharmacologic experiments that followed suggested the existence of more than one distinct subclass of these receptors. This experimentation and later molecular cloning led to the identification and characterization of three subfamilies of ARs: α_1-, α_2-, and βARs.[52] These can further be subdivided into three subtypes each. A more detailed discussion of ARs can be found in Chapter 8, Neurotransmitters, and only key features of the pharmacology of these receptors are outlined here.

αARs. Two major subfamilies of αARs exist: α_1- and α_2-ARs, identified based on their different affinities for a number of αAR antagonists such as prazosin (selective for α_1ARs) and yohimbine (selective for α_2ARs). Through laborious radioligand-binding experiments and, finally, molecular cloning of individual receptor genes, α_1ARs are now known to comprise three different subtypes: α_{1A}, α_{1B}, α_{1D}, whereas α_2ARs consist also of three different subtypes, designated α_{2A}, α_{2B}, α_{2C}.[53-56] Phenylephrine is the prototypic α_1AR-selective agonist, whereas clonidine and α-methyldopa are selective α_2AR agonists. Classically, α_1ARs couple to $G_{q/11}$ proteins and phosphoinositide hydrolysis, which results in contraction of smooth muscle (e.g., vasoconstriction, ureter and bladder sphincter constriction), whereas α_2ARs couple to $G_{i/o}$ proteins and inhibit adenylyl cyclase and activate hyperpolarizing K^+ currents, actions that can lead to inhibition of neuronal firing and neurotransmitter release in the CNS (see Chapters 6, Signal Transduction; and 8, Neurotransmitters, for more details).

βARs. Soon after the division of ARs into αARs and βARs, βARs were found to actually comprise at least two different receptor subtypes, designated β_1 and β_2, and were based on their different relative affinities for epinephrine and NE.[57] β_1ARs bind epinephrine and NE with equal affinity, whereas β_2ARs have a very high affinity for epinephrine but minimal affinity for NE. A third βAR subtype, β_3AR, originally identified in adipose tissue, displays higher affinity for NE than isoproterenol and minimal affinity for epinephrine. It is also unresponsive to classic β-blockers that antagonize β_1- and β_2ARs.[52] Dobutamine (see later) binds to β_1ARs with much higher affinity than to β_2ARs, while having no affinity for αARs. Dopamine and isoproterenol (isoprenaline) bind both β_1- and β_2ARs with equal affinity. In contrast, drugs like terbutaline, ritodrine, albuterol, metaproterenol, salmeterol, and formoterol are selective β_2AR agonists.

All three βARs are classically defined through their coupling to Gs proteins leading to activation of adenylyl cyclase. In cardiac muscle, this results in increased contractility and rate of contraction (positive inotropy and chronotropy) via cyclic adenosine monophosphate (cAMP) accumulation, whereas in smooth muscle, cAMP leads to muscle relaxation (vasodilation, bronchodilation, uterine muscle relaxation). β_2ARs and β_3ARs can also couple to Gi proteins and to inhibition of adenylyl cyclase under some circumstances, and β_3ARs have been shown to couple to NO synthase activation.[52] For a more detailed description of the signal transduction properties of these receptors, see Chapters 6, Signal Transduction; and 8, Neurotransmitters.

Chemistry and Structure-Activity Relationships of Endogenous Catecholamines and Sympathomimetic Drugs

3′,4′-Dihydroxy-phenylethylamine can be considered the backbone of all sympathomimetic drugs. The 3′,4′-dihydroxy-phenyl group is called *catechol*, and epinephrine, NE, and dopamine are all amines, thus the name *catecholamines* (Fig. 9-7). Substitutions made on the amino group, on the catechol ring, or on the α-carbon yield the large variety of sympathomimetic drugs available. These modifications have profound effects on the relative affinity of the resultant compound for α- versus βARs, on the potency at eliciting receptor activation, and on pharmacokinetic properties.

Substitution of the amino group with alkyl groups increases affinity for βARs versus αARs. In fact, the larger this alkyl group is, the greater the selectivity for βARs. Thus, epinephrine, which carries one methyl group on its terminal amino group, has increased activity at βARs (and especially β_2ARs) compared with NE, whose amino group is free (in fact, the prefix "nor" in the name of NE stands for exactly this feature of the molecule: it means "nitrogen without substitution group" in German). Isoproterenol, which carries a bulky isopropyl group on its amino group (see Fig. 9-7), is completely βAR-selective. β_2AR-selective agonists generally have large alkyl groups attached on the amino group.[58]

Substitution of one or both of the hydroxyl groups of the catechol ring, and especially of the 3′-OH group, leads to dramatic reductions in activity at adrenergic receptors. Conversely, these groups are the targets of the catecholamine metabolizing enzyme COMT (see Chapter 8, Neurotransmitters); therefore, absence of the catechol-OH groups increases bioavailability and duration of action. In addition, loss of catechol-OH groups increases the lipophilicity of the molecule, resulting in increased bioavailability upon oral administration and in increased distribution in the CNS (e.g., amphetamine, ephedrine, see Fig. 9-7).

Substitution of the α-carbon increases resistance to enzymatic oxidation by MAO (see Chapter 8, Neurotransmitters), which targets the β-OH group, prolonging the action of the drug. Of note, methyl substitution at the α-carbon yields compounds with enhanced indirect sympathomimetic activity (see Chapter 8, Neurotransmitters), that is, the ability to displace endogenous catecholamines from their storage sites in the noradrenergic nerves (e.g., ephedrine, amphetamine, see Fig. 9-7). Finally, the β-OH group is generally necessary for direct agonism of the ARs, although dopamine, which can activate βARs, lacks it.

Effects of Catecholamines and Sympathomimetic Drugs in Various Target Organs

Cardiovascular Effects

Catecholamines are important regulators of peripheral vascular resistance and venous capacitance. αARs increase arterial smooth muscle tone, whereas β_2ARs relax vascular smooth muscle. Skin and splanchnic vessels have mainly αARs and, thus, constrict in response to catecholamines, whereas skeletal muscle vessels have both α- and β_2ARs

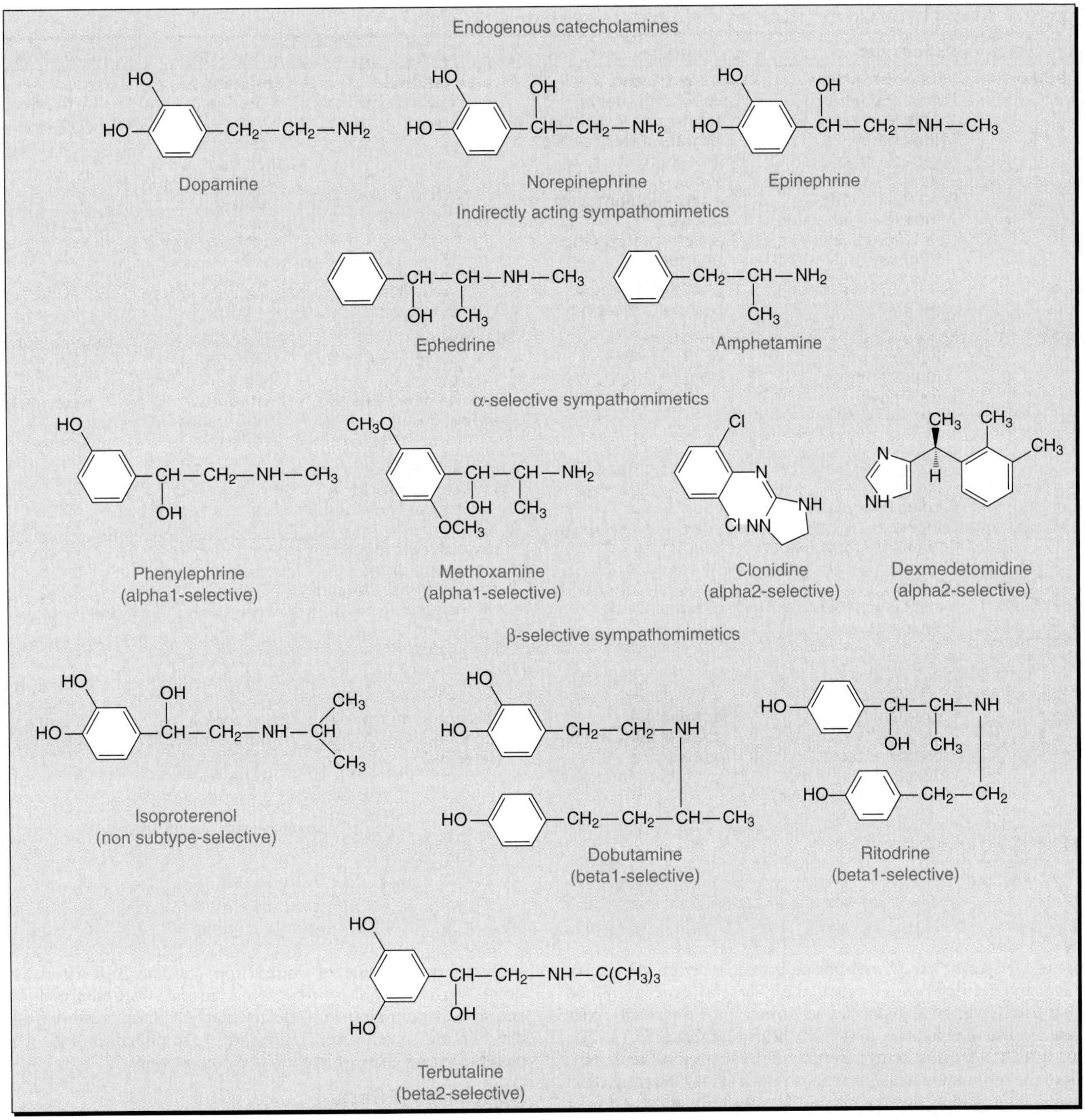

Endogenous catecholamines

Dopamine

Norepinephrine

Epinephrine

Indirectly acting sympathomimetics

Ephedrine

Amphetamine

α-selective sympathomimetics

Phenylephrine (alpha1-selective)

Methoxamine (alpha1-selective)

Clonidine (alpha2-selective)

Dexmedetomidine (alpha2-selective)

β-selective sympathomimetics

Isoproterenol (non subtype-selective)

Dobutamine (beta1-selective)

Ritodrine (beta1-selective)

Terbutaline (beta2-selective)

FIGURE 9-7 • Chemical structures of the endogenous catecholamines and various sympathomimetics.

and can either constrict or dilate, respectively, after catecholamine stimulation.[52] Renal, splanchnic, coronary, and cerebral vessels also have dopaminergic D_1 receptors, and they dilate in response to dopamine activation.[50] This mediates, in large part, the natriuresis (through increase of the resultant renal glomerular filtration rate) and the hypotension usually observed upon systemic administration of low doses of dopamine (the so-called "renal" dose of dopamine).

Endogenous catecholamines are extremely important in the regulation of cardiac contractile function primarily through their actions via cardiostimulatory βARs.[9,57,59,60] β_1ARs are the primary subtype in the heart, comprising 75% to 80% of total myocardial βARs. The remaining cardiac βARs are largely made up of β_2ARs, with a minor component of β_3ARs found in human myocardium. βAR activation results in increased pacemaker activity (at the SA node and in the Purkinje fibers) and conduction velocity at the AV node, whereas it decreases the refractory period. All these actions lead to positive chronotropy. Cardiac contractility is enhanced (positive inotropy), and relaxation is accelerated (positive lusitropy). The end result is a cardiomyocyte twitch response of increased tension but reduced duration. The intraventricular pressure of the intact heart rises and falls more rapidly, and the ejection time is decreased. These effects are clearer in the absence of reflexes to blood pressure changes. These normal reflexes usually confound the direct effects of catecholamines on the heart, and the resultant net effect on the heart depends on the relative balance between the actions of these reflexes and the direct actions of catecholamines on cardiac muscle.[57,60,61]

Catecholamines are among the most important regulators of systemic blood pressure. Their effects on blood pressure are a function of three parameters: (i) their direct effects on the heart; (ii) their effects on peripheral vascular resistance; and (iii) venous return (Table 9-3).

TABLE 9-3 PROPERTIES AND LIGANDS OF ADRENOCEPTOR SUBTYPES

	α_1 Subtype	α_2 Subtype	β_1 Subtype	β_2 Subtype	β_3 Subtype
Localization—effect	VSM—contraction Pupillary dilator muscle—contraction (mydriasis) Pilomotor smooth muscle—piloerection Prostate smooth muscle—contraction Heart—positive inotropy (mild effect)	Adrenergic and cholinergic nerve terminals—inhibition of transmitter release VSM—contraction (α_{2B} subtype) Fat cells—inhibition of lipolysis Platelets—aggregation (α_{2A} subtype)	Heart—positive inotropy, chronotropy, lusitropy	Respiratory, uterine SM and VSM—relaxation Skeletal muscle—activation of K^+ uptake Liver—glycogenolysis	Fat cells—activation of lipolysis
Signal transduction	$G_{q/11}$-PLC, increase of IP_3-DAG	$G_{i/o}$, AC inhibition, K^+ channel activation	G_s, AC activation	G_s, AC activation	G_s, AC activation
Agonists	Epinephrine, norepinephrine, phenylephrine (selective)	Epinephrine, norepinephrine, clonidine (selective)	Epinephrine, norepinephrine, isoproterenol, dobutamine (selective at low doses)	Epinephrine, isoproterenol, albuterol, ritodrine, terbutaline (selective)	Norepinephrine, isoproterenol, CGP 12177 (selective)
Cardiovascular responses to agonists	Vascular resistance increases in all beds Cardiac contractility increases slightly Cardiac HR drops (vagal reflex) CO drops Mean-systolic-diastolic BP increases	Vascular resistance increases in some beds No direct effects on the heart BP drops (centrally mediated inhibition of sympathetic outflow)	Vascular resistance drops in skeletal muscle, renal, splanchnic beds Total peripheral resistance drops Venous tone drops Cardiac contractility and HR increase significantly CO increases Mean-diastolic BP decreases	Systolic BP decreases slightly or does not change	
Antagonists	Phentolamine, phenoxybenzamine, prazosin, terazosin, doxazosin, alfuzosin, tamsulosin (selective)	Phentolamine, phenoxybenzamine, rauwolscine, yohimbine (selective)	Propranolol, metoprolol, atenolol, CGP 20712A (selective)	Propranolol, butoxamine, ICI 118551 (selective)	SR 59230A (selective)

AC, adenylyl cyclase; BP, blood pressure; CO, cardiac output; DAG, diacylglycerol; HR, heart rate; IP_3, 1′,4′,5′ inositol triphosphate; PLC, phospholipase C; SM, smooth muscle; VSM, vascular smooth muscle.

A pure α_1AR agonist like phenylephrine increases peripheral arterial resistance and decreases venous capacitance. Therefore, systemic blood pressure rises, which then evokes a baroreceptor-mediated reflex increase in vagal tone in order to slow the heart rate (Fig. 9-8). Cardiac output usually does not change, despite the reduction of heart rate, owing to the resultant increase in venous return (Frank-Starling effect on cardiac contractility, see Chapter 26, Heart Failure) and to a minor positive inotropic effect of direct cardiac α_1AR stimulation. These reflex responses are usually undetectable in hypotensive patients, in whom α_1AR agonists are given to normalize blood pressure.

Specific catecholamine responses follow the previously discussed characteristics. Epinephrine, which activates all ARs, is a very potent vasoconstrictor and cardiac stimulant. It raises systolic blood pressure (see Fig. 9-8 and Table 9-3) by increasing heart rate and force of contraction (cardiac βAR effect) and peripheral vascular resistance (α_1AR effect). However, it also dilates some peripheral vessels (mainly skeletal muscle vessels) via stimulation of β_2ARs; thus, it might actually decrease peripheral resistance and diastolic pressure. This skeletal muscle vessel dilation contributes to increased skeletal blood flow during exercise. Norepinephrine shares the activity of epinephrine at αARs but lacks significant β_2AR activity. Consequently, it increases peripheral resistance (via α_1ARs), heart rate, and force of contraction (cardiac β_1AR effect), thus raising both systolic and diastolic blood pressure. Vagal reflexes usually counteract the positive chronotropic but not inotropic effects of NE. A simple βAR agonist like isoproterenol (see Fig. 9-8 and Table 9-3) markedly increases cardiac output, contractility, and rate of contraction (cardiac βAR effects) while decreasing peripheral resistance by inducing β_2AR-mediated peripheral vasodilation. Therefore, the net effect on blood pressure is a fall in diastolic and mean arterial pressure in combination with a slight increase (or no change) in systolic blood pressure.[52,60,61]

Ophthalmic Effects

The pupillary dilator muscle of the iris expresses α_1ARs, which, when activated, can cause constriction of this muscle.[62,63] Therefore, sympathomimetics that activate α_1ARs such as phenylephrine cause mydriasis. Sympathomimetics are also important regulators of intraocular pressure, because α_1ARs promote the outflow of aqueous humor from the eye and βARs increase production of aqueous humor. This is why β-blockers are able to reduce intraocular pressure and are used for this purpose in the treatment of glaucoma (see later).[22,23]

Respiratory Effects

Bronchial smooth muscle expresses β_2ARs, which, when activated, cause relaxation resulting in bronchodilation. However, whereas it receives rich cholinergic innervation and is constantly under the stimulatory actions of ACh, bronchial smooth muscle lacks adrenergic innervation, and therefore, it appears to relax in response to circulating catecholamines (i.e., epinephrine). The vessels of the upper respiratory mucosa express α_1ARs and, when activated, cause constriction and mediate the nasal decongestant action of some sympathomimetics (see later).[61]

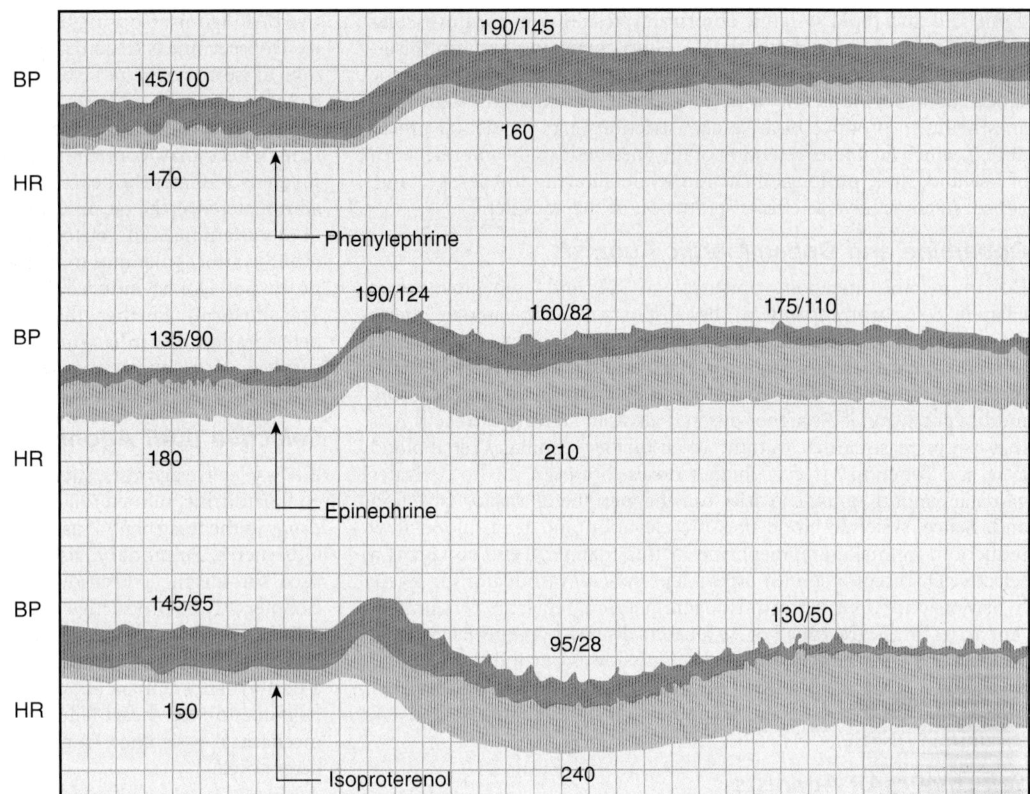

FIGURE 9-8 • Effects of an α_1-selective (phenylephrine), β-selective (isoproterenol), and nonselective (epinephrine) sympathomimetic on systemic blood pressure (BP) and heart rate (HR), given as an intravenous bolus injection to a dog. Reflexes are blunted but not eliminated in this anesthetized animal. (Adapted from Katzung BG. Basic and Clinical Pharmacology, 9th ed. New York: McGraw-Hill, 2004.)

Genitourinary Effects

Human uterine smooth muscle contains β_2ARs that promote relaxation after stimulation by an agonist. This effect is exploited clinically in pregnancy and preterm labor (see later). Bladder base, urethral sphincter, and prostate express α_1ARs (primarily the α_{1A} subtype in humans) that mediate contraction, thus, promoting urinary retention and contraction of the prostate. The latter can be particularly distressing upon concomitant prostate hypertrophy. α_1ARs present in the ductus deferens, seminal vesicles, and prostate are responsible for the process of ejaculation (with some contribution of purinergic and neuropeptide Y receptors).[18,64-66]

Metabolic and Endocrine Effects

Catecholamines play a central role in regulation of intermediary metabolism because they induce lipolysis in fat cells through β_3ARs causing release of free fatty acids and glycerol into the circulation.[67] This response is inhibited by activation of α_2ARs also present in fat cells. In the liver, glycogenolysis and release of glucose into the blood is promoted via βAR activation (resulting in hyperglycemia). At high concentrations, catecholamines can precipitate metabolic acidosis. In the pancreas, catecholamines induce (via β_2ARs) and inhibit (via α_2ARs) insulin secretion.[61,68] However, the main regulator of insulin secretion is plasma glucose levels, which are usually increased by the actions of catecholamines in the liver. βARs (primarily β_2ARs) promote the uptake of K^+ into cells through direct stimulation of the Na^+ pump (Na^+-K^+-ATPase). This can result in decreased extracellular K^+ and hypokalemia, which prevents the rise in plasma K^+ levels that usually occurs during stress or exercise. This effect also promotes repolarization of the hypoxic myocardium during cardiac arrest, which is one of the reasons for the emergency use of epinephrine in this setting.

In addition, catecholamines stimulate (via β_1ARs) and inhibit (via α_2ARs) renin secretion from the macula densa cells of the juxtaglomerular apparatus of the kidneys. Accordingly, they stimulate the renin-angiotensin-aldosterone system, which contributes greatly to systemic blood pressure elevation.[68] Catecholamines acting through β_2ARs also potently inhibit degranulation and histamine release from mast cells, which contributes significantly to the antiallergic and anti-anaphylactic reaction effects of epinephrine.[69]

CNS Effects

Endogenous catecholamines are relatively hydrophilic and, thus, cannot readily cross the blood-brain barrier to produce any significant CNS effects. However, their peripheral effects such as tachycardia and tremor resemble somatic signs of anxiety. Indirect-acting sympathomimetics, such as amphetamines, which can readily cross into the CNS, produce a variety of CNS effects, including, but not limited to, mild alerting, mood elevation, insomnia, euphoria, anorexia, and even psychosis.[70]

Effects in Other Organs

Catecholamines relax the GI smooth muscle through activation of α_2 and βARs. However, the α_2AR-mediated relaxation is predominant and is actually mediated indirectly via presynaptic inhibition of the release of ACh, serotonin, and other GI stimulatory hormones.[56,71] Through similar presynaptic mechanisms, activation of α_2ARs can also inhibit the salivary gland secretions (this is why α_2AR agonists like clonidine cause xerostomia, see later).[56,71] Stimulation of α_2ARs can also inhibit water and salt influx into the intestinal lumen. Sympathomimetics have no effect on thermoregulatory sweat glands because these are regulated by sympathetic cholinergic postganglionic fibers, that is, by ACh, see earlier under "Effects of Atropine and Other Antimuscarinics in Target Organs").

Pharmacologic and Therapeutic Uses of Catecholamines and Sympathomimetic Agents

Epinephrine

Epinephrine is the agent of choice for the initial acute treatment of anaphylactic shock and is given parenterally (and preferably IM, because subQ, and, to an even bigger extent, IV injection can lead to significant and rapid systemic absorption, resulting in cardiovascular complications, e.g., arrhythmias).[69] Glucocorticoids and antihistamines are also used as a second-line therapy for acute anaphylactic shock. Epinephrine is also used topically in combination with local anesthetics to produce local vasoconstriction (e.g., for dental procedures), which facilitates retention of the anesthetic in the intended area of use and, thus, prolongs its action while allowing for dosage (and, hence, systemic adverse effects) reduction of the anesthetic.

Dopamine and Dopaminergic Agonists

Dopamine, the metabolic precursor of NE and epinephrine (see Chapter 8, Neurotransmitters), has important cardiovascular effects depending on its systemic concentration. At low doses, as discussed previously, it causes vasodilation of renal and splanchnic vessels via D_1 receptors, thus increasing renal blood flow and function and causing mild hypotension.[50] At higher doses, it also can activate cardiac β_1ARs that can increase cardiac output, which further stimulates renal blood flow and function. At even higher doses, however, it also activates vascular smooth muscle α_1ARs causing peripheral vasoconstriction and, hence, systemic blood pressure elevation and renal blood flow reduction, mimicking epinephrine in this manner. Fenoldopam is a selective D_1-receptor agonist used as a peripheral vasodilator for severe hypertension.[72] Centrally acting dopaminergic agonists are very important drugs for the treatment of Parkinson's disease, hyperprolactinemia, and various GI disorders, but their discussion is beyond the scope of this chapter (they are discussed in detail in Chapters 32, Motility Disorders; 40, Disorders of the Hypothalamic-Pituitary Axis; and 44, Parkinson's Disease).

Selective α_1AR Agonists

Phenylephrine (etilephrine), midodrine, and methoxamine are selective α_1AR agonists, which cause peripheral vasoconstriction when administered and, thus, raise systemic blood pressure.[73] Accordingly, their main indication is for the treatment of orthostatic (postural) hypotension. Phenylephrine is also used for mydriasis and has recently been marketed for antiallergic nasal and ocular decongestion. Xylometazoline and oxymetazoline are αAR-selective agonists and their main use is in nasal decongestion by means of nasal mucosal vasoconstriction. Because it also possesses significant α_{2A}AR agonist activity, oxymetazoline can cause centrally mediated hypotension like clonidine does (see later).[59,74]

Selective α_2AR Agonists

Compounds selective for stimulating α_2ARs are important inhibitors of central sympathetic outflow to the periphery via inhibition of presynaptic release of NE, and this lowers systemic blood pressure. Of note, α_2AR agonists can also cause local vasoconstriction via direct stimulation of postsynaptic α_{2B}ARs present on vascular smooth muscle. Clonidine, methyldopa, guanfacine, guanabenz, moxonidine, and rilmenidine are the most important drugs in this class of agents; their main indication is treatment of systemic hypertension.[56,74] These drugs are discussed more thoroughly in Chapter 22, Hypertension. Clonidine is also used for treatment of opioid and alcohol withdrawal symptoms, for diminishing opioid and even nicotine dependence (it is sometimes used to facilitate smoking cessation), and for curbing menopause-associated hot flushes. However, its efficacy in all these indications has been debated. Dexmedetomidine is another centrally acting selective α_2AR agonist that, instead of being used for hypertension treatment, is used for the sedation of intubated and mechanically ventilated patients in the intensive care unit setting. Apraclonidine and brimonidine are selective α_2AR agonists that lower intraocular pressure and, accordingly, are used in glaucoma treatment.[74]

Selective β_1AR Agonists

Dobutamine is a relatively selective β_1AR agonist (although it can also activate β_2- and α_1ARs at higher doses) used as a positive inotropic agent to stimulate cardiac contractile function in acute decompensated heart failure (see later and Chapter 26, Heart Failure).[57,60] It is able to increase cardiac output with less reflex tachycardia than the nonselective βAR agonist isoproterenol because it lacks significant β_2AR activity. Dobutamine is structurally related to dopamine and consists of two optical isomers: the (+) isomer is a potent β_1AR agonist as well as an α_1AR antagonist; whereas the (−) isomer is a potent α_1AR agonist capable of producing peripheral vasoconstriction. The (+) isomer's latter effect may contribute to positive inotropic action because it further stimulates the heart in a reflex manner. Dobutamine is typically administered as the racemic mixture. The biggest limitations of the use of dobutamine and related positive inotropic agents are that they rapidly induce tolerance to their cardiostimulatory effects owing to the process of agonist-induced βAR desensitization (see Chapter 6, Signal Transduction). Further, they also increase the likelihood of clinical deterioration of cardiac function with decreased heart failure patient survival upon long-term use of these agents (see Chapter 26, Heart Failure).

Selective β_2AR Agonists

β_2AR-selective agonists, such as albuterol (or salbutamol), metaproterenol, ritodrine, salmeterol, formoterol, and terbutaline, are important drugs in the treatment of asthma (see Chapter 28, Asthma and Chronic Obstructive Pulmonary Disease).[75] They (especially ritodrine) are also used for uterine relaxation in order to delay premature labor (see Chapter 42, Reproductive Health). Clenbuterol is a selective β_2AR agonist that potently dilates vessels in skeletal muscle, increasing skeletal blood flow, and accordingly, has been used illegally by athletes as a performance-enhancing drug. This drug has been used experimentally in end-stage heart failure patients and those receiving ventricular mechanical assistance; some improvement in cardiac function has been noted.[76]

Indirectly Acting Sympathomimetics

Ephedrine is the main alkaloid of Ma-huang, an herbal medication deriving from the plant *Ephedra sinica*, which is found primarily in China. The herb Ma-huang has been used for therapeutic purposes for over 2 millennia. Because, like amphetamine, it lacks the two catechol ring OH groups (ephedrine is not a catecholamine), ephedrine has very good bioavailability and a long duration of action and can cross the blood-brain barrier, producing mild stimulatory CNS effects.[70] It has been used for asthma in the past (owing to βAR stimulation). However, its use in clinical pharmacotherapy is now obsolete. There are major safety concerns with ephedrine-like alkaloids, and nowadays only one of them, pseudoephedrine, an optical isomer of ephedrine, is used therapeutically in Western countries as a component of over-the-counter nasal decongestants (usually in combination with an antihistamine).

Amphetamine readily enters the CNS and is a potent CNS stimulant, increasing mood, alertness, and attention (initially) and decreasing appetite. However, tolerance readily develops to these actions, and amphetamine and its congeners carry a very high risk of abuse, although physical dependence (as with opioids) is probably not induced. Amphetamines are used for treatment of narcolepsy and of attention-deficit-hyperactivity disorder (the mixed sulfate salts of various amphetamines) (see Chapters 51, Attention-Deficit/Hyperactivity Disorders; and 57, Insomnia).[70,77] Methylphenidate, pemoline, and methamphetamine are similar to amphetamine in their pharmacologic actions and carry a similar big abuse potential (especially methamphetamine). 3′,4′-Methylenedioxymethamphetamine (MDMA), better known as "ecstasy," is a methamphetamine derivative and a popular street and party drug of abuse, that can result in deadly complications, especially if combined with alcohol (see Chapter 55, Drug Addiction). Methylphenidate and pemoline are used in attention-deficit hyperactivity disorder, in which, paradoxically, they appear to have some efficacy (see Chapter 51, Attention-Deficit/Hyperactivity Disorders).[70]

Modafinil, another CNS stimulant, activates central α_{1B}ARs, but its main effects appear mediated by the GABAergic, glutamatergic, and other CNS systems (see Chapters 8, Neurotransmitters; and 57, Insomnia). It is used as a CNS stimulant for narcolepsy. Phenylpropanolamine, a sympathomimetic drug that was used in the past as an anorexic agent (in combination with phentermine, the once-popular "phen-phen" over-the-counter drug) and also in nasal decongestants (in combination with antihistamines), was withdrawn from the market because it was associated with hemorrhagic strokes (probably due to resultant cerebral vasospasms).[70] For the mechanism of action of all these indirectly acting sympathomimetic drugs, see Chapter 8, Neurotransmitters.

Other Sympathomimetics

Cocaine, a semisynthetic derivative of an atropine-like alkaloid, inhibits NE and dopamine reuptake at synapses and, thus, enhances sympathetic and dopaminergic nerve activity, both in the brain and in the periphery (see Chapter 8, Neurotransmitters). It also causes vasoconstriction and tachycardia and has been used (now obsolete) as a local anesthetic. Currently, it remains a problematic recreational drug of abuse owing to its CNS stimulatory properties.[78]

Tyramine is found in fermented foods and drinks, such as cheese and wine, and is also normally produced in the body from tyrosine catabolism. Because it is readily metabolized by hepatic MAO upon oral administration (it undergoes significant first-pass metabolism, see Chapter 13, Pharmacokinetics), its oral bioavailability is low.[79] It causes release of catecholamines from their storage sites in the CNS (see Chapter 8, Neurotransmitters), thus producing significant CNS stimulatory sympathomimetic actions. These latter actions can be further enhanced upon concomitant inhibition of catecholamine metabolism (e.g., MAO inhibition). Therefore, patients taking MAO inhibitors (antidepressant drugs) must exert special caution not to ingest tyramine-containing foods and drinks because the combination of tyramine and MAO inhibitors can lead to significant sympathetic stimulation and hypertensive crisis (see Chapters 8, Neurotransmitters; and 53, Depression and Bipolar Disorder).

Pharmacologic Properties of AR Antagonists (Sympatholytics)

These agents bind to ARs and competitively antagonize the effects of catecholamines. Because the SNS is intimately involved in the modulation of a large number of homeostatic mechanisms, interference with its function impairs the capacity of the organism to generate appropriate physiologic responses to provocative or adverse environmental conditions. Therefore, many of the side effects of these agents are common to the group as a whole and include postural hypotension, sedation or depression, increased GI tract motility and diarrhea, impaired ejaculation/sexual dysfunction, and hypervolemia (increased blood volume with sodium retention). The first drug, synthesized in 1958, shown to produce selective AR blockade was dichloroisoproterenol for βARs. However, it was found to have partial βAR agonist activity and was, therefore, not used clinically. Propranolol, synthesized by Sir James Black and colleagues, was the first agent to come into widespread clinical use.[80] It is a highly potent, nonselective βAR antagonist with no intrinsic sympathomimetic activity (ISA). Because propranolol blocks both β_1ARs and β_2ARs, it could have mixed effects when β_1AR blockade was warranted or desired (such as for bronchoconstriction). Thus, cardioselective β_1AR blockers were searched for, and practolol was the first such agent. However, owing to toxicity involving epithelial structures after chronic use, this drug was abandoned. Currently, several nonselective and selective βAR antagonists are available. Medicinal chemistry has also led to a similar variety of selective and nonselective αAR blockers.

αAR Antagonists (α-Blockers)

Competitive and noncompetitive antagonists exist for αARs. Phenoxybenzamine and its congener, dibenamine, bind covalently to the α_1ARs, producing an irreversible (insurmountable) type of blockade (see Chapters 5, Drug-Receptor Interactions; and 14, Pharmacodynamics). Phentolamine, tolazoline, prazosin, and yohimbine bind reversibly to αARs and produce a competitive block that can be overcome by higher concentrations of agonists including local concentrations of endogenous catecholamines. These α-blockers differ markedly in their ability to block α_1ARs and α_2ARs. Prazosin is far more potent at α_1ARs, phenoxybenzamine is moderately selective for α_1ARs, phentolamine is nonselective, whereas yohimbine is a selective α_2AR antagonist. All of these agents in general can produce peripheral vasodilation by blocking postsynaptic α_1- and α_2ARs, thus lowering blood pressure and eliciting reflex increases in sympathetic tone. This reflex increase in sympathetic tone is actually more pronounced with yohimbine, because presynaptic α_2AR inhibition results in greater NE release from sympathetic nerve terminals. They also cause nasal congestion and facilitate the flow of urine by inhibiting α_1 receptors of the bladder base and the prostate.[81] The structures of some of the most commonly used α-blockers are given in Figure 9-9.

Specific αAR Blocking Agents—Effects and Uses. Phenoxybenzamine is a relatively selective α_1AR antagonist devoid of any agonist activity.[81] Its structure is closely related to the nitrogen mustards, and like the latter, the tertiary amine cyclizes to form a reactive ethyleniminium intermediate, which binds the receptor covalently and irreversibly. The formation of this reactive intermediate accounts for the delayed onset of action, even after IV administration. Importantly, the presence of catecholamine or another competitive α_1AR blocker can reduce the level of blockade achieved by simple competition, but once achieved, phenoxybenzamine blockade is unaffected by exposure to these agents. Onset of action is slow, peak effects not being seen until about 1 hour after IV administration (oral bioavailability is poor) and its half-life is approximately 24 hours, although demonstrable effects last for 3 to 4 days. The effects of daily administration are cumulative for nearly a week. Phenoxybenzamine causes significant reflex tachycardia owing to inhibition of the pressor peripheral vasoconstriction. In the CNS, phenoxybenzamine causes nausea and vomiting, motor excitability, hyperventilation, and convulsions, particularly with large doses injected rapidly IV. Usual doses also result in mild sedation. Phenoxybenzamine (and the nonselective α-blocker phentolamine, see later) is used clinically in the preoperative preparation of pheochromocytoma (tumor of the adrenal medulla) patients and in the long-term management of nonresectable pheochromocytomas (see Chapter 41, Adrenal Disorders). It can also be used for the management of transient hypertension during operative manipulation of the tumor. Oral phenoxybenzamine is the preferred drug in the first two situations, and a βAR antagonist is frequently also employed to block the excess stimulation to the heart during surgery.

Phentolamine and tolazoline are substituted imidazolines that produce a moderately effective αAR blockade, which is relatively transient.[81] Phentolamine is more potent in this respect. Given IV, these agents result in vasodilation, direct and reflex cardiac stimulation, tachycardia, and arrhythmias. In addition to being a nonselective α-blocker, phentolamine has important effects on other receptors such as serotonergic, histaminergic, and muscarinic receptors. Phentolamine and tolazoline have been used for the investigation of pheochromocytoma in the past. Nowadays, they are used perioperatively to manage the severe hypertension present during the removal of a pheochromocytoma tumor, as is phenoxybenzamine (see earlier). Phentolamine, in combination with the peripheral vasodilator papaverine (an opiate alkaloid), is used for treatment of erectile dysfunction in men via direct injection into the corpus carvenosum, because systemic absorption results in orthostatic hypotension. In case priapism develops, administration of a α_1AR agonist, such as phenylephrine, (or, alternatively, digoxin), might be required.[82]

Prazosin, terazosin, and doxazosin are quinazoline derivatives that are selective α_1AR antagonists (potency of prazosin at α_1ARs >1000-fold more than at α_2ARs). All are used for treatment of hypertension (see Chapter 22, Hypertension); the latter two are also used for benign prostatic hyperplasia.[64,73,83,84] Because they do not affect α_2ARs, the reflex tachycardia produced by these drugs is far less than that produced by nonselective α-blockers like phentolamine and phenoxybenzamine. However, they can produce significant reflex βAR-mediated effects that can counter their hypotensive actions. Moreover, they can produce postural hypotension by antagonizing α_1AR-mediated venoconstriction that prevents venous pooling and raises blood pressure when the patient assumes an upright position. Terazosin and

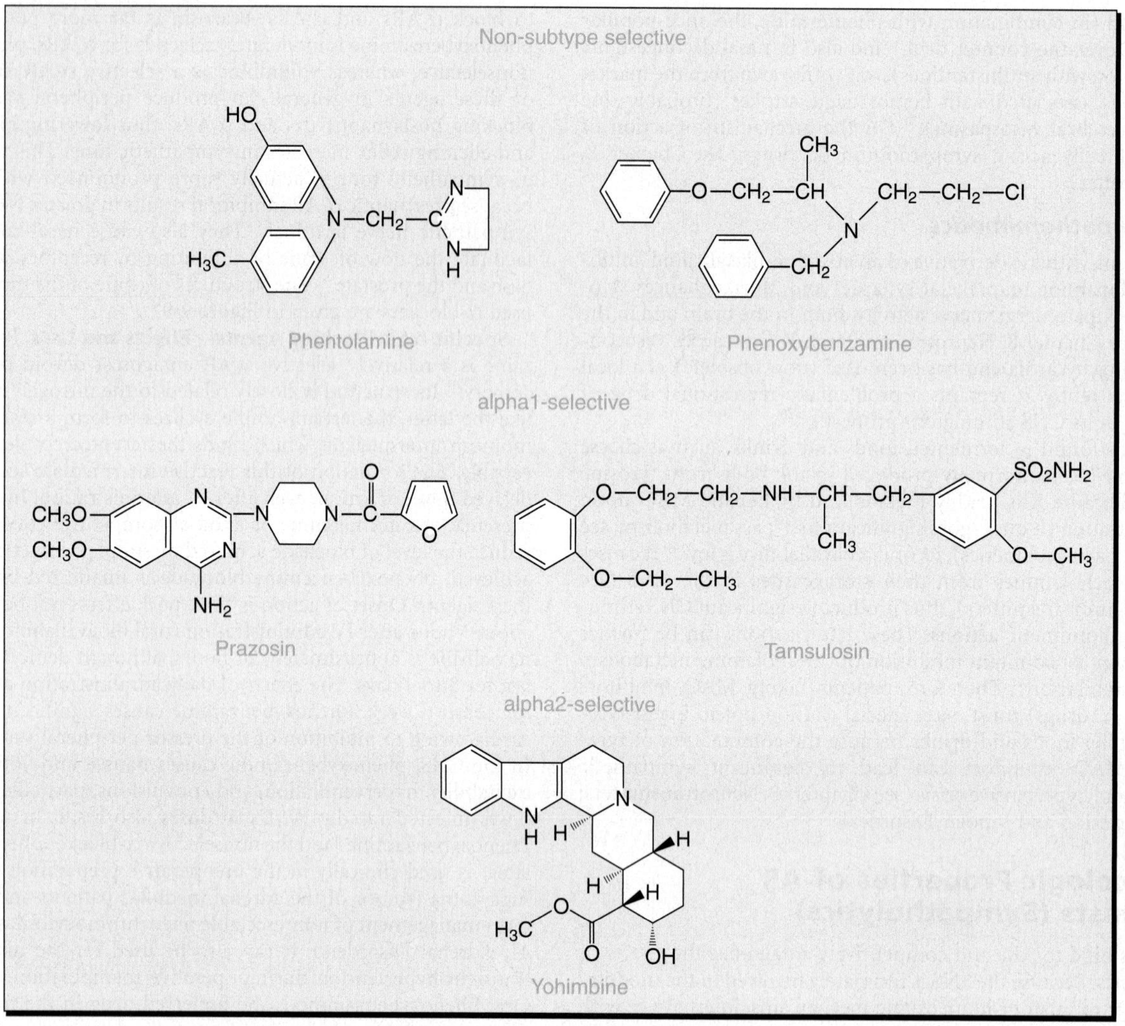

Non-subtype selective

Phentolamine

Phenoxybenzamine

alpha1-selective

Prazosin

Tamsulosin

alpha2-selective

Yohimbine

FIGURE 9-9 • Chemical structures of the most important α-adrenergic receptor blockers.

doxazosin have far longer durations of action than their older congener prazosin. Prazosin and phentolamine are also used occasionally for peripheral vascular disorders such as Raynaud's phenomenon, which is characterized by excessive peripheral vasospasm. However, they have been largely replaced by calcium channel blockers, which are far more efficacious for this indication.

Tamsulosin and alfuzosin are similar α_1AR selective antagonists that are efficacious in benign prostatic hypertrophy/hyperplasia.[85,86] Tamsulosin, in particular, displays further α_1AR subtype selectivity in that it has higher affinity for α_{1A}ARs and α_{1D}ARs than for α_{1B}ARs. For this reason, it purportedly inhibits selectively prostate smooth muscle contraction with very little effects on vascular smooth muscle contraction; thus, it causes less postural hypotension than do other selective α_1AR antagonists.[87]

Some neuroleptic drugs, such as haloperidol and chlorpromazine, which inhibit dopaminergic receptors in the brain, also block α_1ARs, which contributes to their hypotensive effects. Trazodone, an atypical antidepressant, also has α_1AR blocking properties (see Chapters 53, Depression and Bipolar Disorder; and 54, Psychosis and Schizophrenia). The ergot derivatives ergotamine and dihydroergotamine reversibly block α_1- and α_2ARs, but they also have important actions on other receptor systems (most prominently serotonergic receptors), which mediate their clinically significant effects.

There are few selective α_2AR blockers, and they have limited clinical utilities. The most important of these is yohimbine, an indole alkaloid, which also blocks serotonergic receptors. It has some limited utility in autonomic insufficiency disorders by promoting NE release via inhibition of presynaptic α_2ARs.[74] Mirtazapine, an atypical antidepressant (see Chapter 55, Depression and Bipolar Disorder), also has α_2AR blocking properties, which might contribute to its antidepressant actions.

βAR Antagonists (β-Blockers)

All available agents act by competitively blocking the effects of endogenous catecholamines and βAR agonists at βARs—that is, with a sufficiently high concentration of agonist, a full response is still possible; thus, the dose-response curve is shifted parallel to the right (surmountable blockade, see Chapters 5, Drug-Receptor Interactions; and 14, Pharmacodynamics). Most drugs in this class are neutral antagonists, that is, they occupy the receptor without eliciting any effects. Some drugs, however, are partial agonists, that is, they inhibit binding of endogenous catecholamines and full βAR agonists. However, in the absence of any agonist, they cause activation of the receptor, albeit to a smaller degree than that of endogenous and full agonists (see also Chapter 5, Drug-Receptor Interactions). In addition to partial agonism, some β-blockers have inverse agonist activity that, in the absence of endogenous agonists, promotes inactivation of receptor and shifts signaling outcomes in the negative direction instead of being neutral and simply blocking activation by β-agonists (Fig. 9-10).[88]

β-Blockers exist that have markedly different affinities for β_1- versus β_2ARs; however, these differences in affinity are relative and dose-dependent. Selective β_1AR blockers are not entirely specific because they will also block β_2ARs at higher concentrations. Importantly, this relative affinity is often sufficient because the use of β_1AR antagonists in patients with asthma is less likely to precipitate bronchospasm.

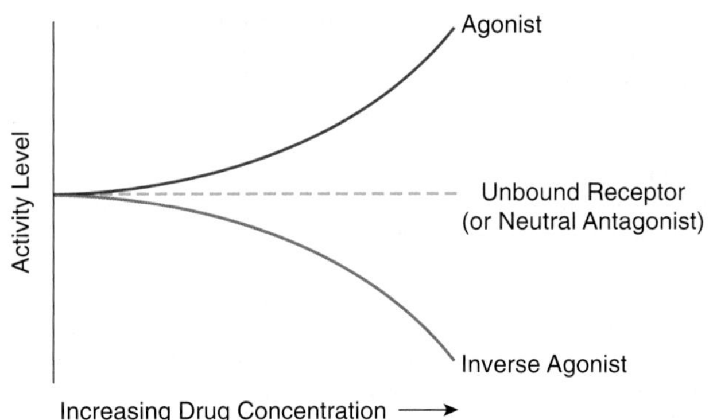

FIGURE 9-10 • Effects of agonists, inverse agonists (negative antagonists), or neutral antagonists on the activity of receptors.

However, in some patients at therapeutic doses, and probably in all patients at high doses, these agents will cause bronchoconstriction. In diabetics, nonselective agents may delay the recovery from hypoglycemia, whereas the selective agents are less likely to do so. In addition, severe bradycardia and elevated diastolic blood pressure have occurred in patients taking propranolol, but these effects are milder with selective agents. As discussed previously, some β-blockers have partial agonist activity (also known as ISA). These were initially believed to be preferable for heart disease because they would be less likely to be totally sympatholytic, since some low level of βAR stimulation may be good for patients with heart failure or cardiac dysfunction.[89] However, this has not been proved clinically, and in fact, these agents might actually be even more deleterious for heart failure patients in the long run owing to chronic βAR activation (see Chapter 26, Heart Failure). It was initially believed that agents lacking ISA would be more effective in the treatment of hyperthyroidism, but this has recently been disputed. The structures of some of the most commonly used β-blockers are given in Figure 9-11.

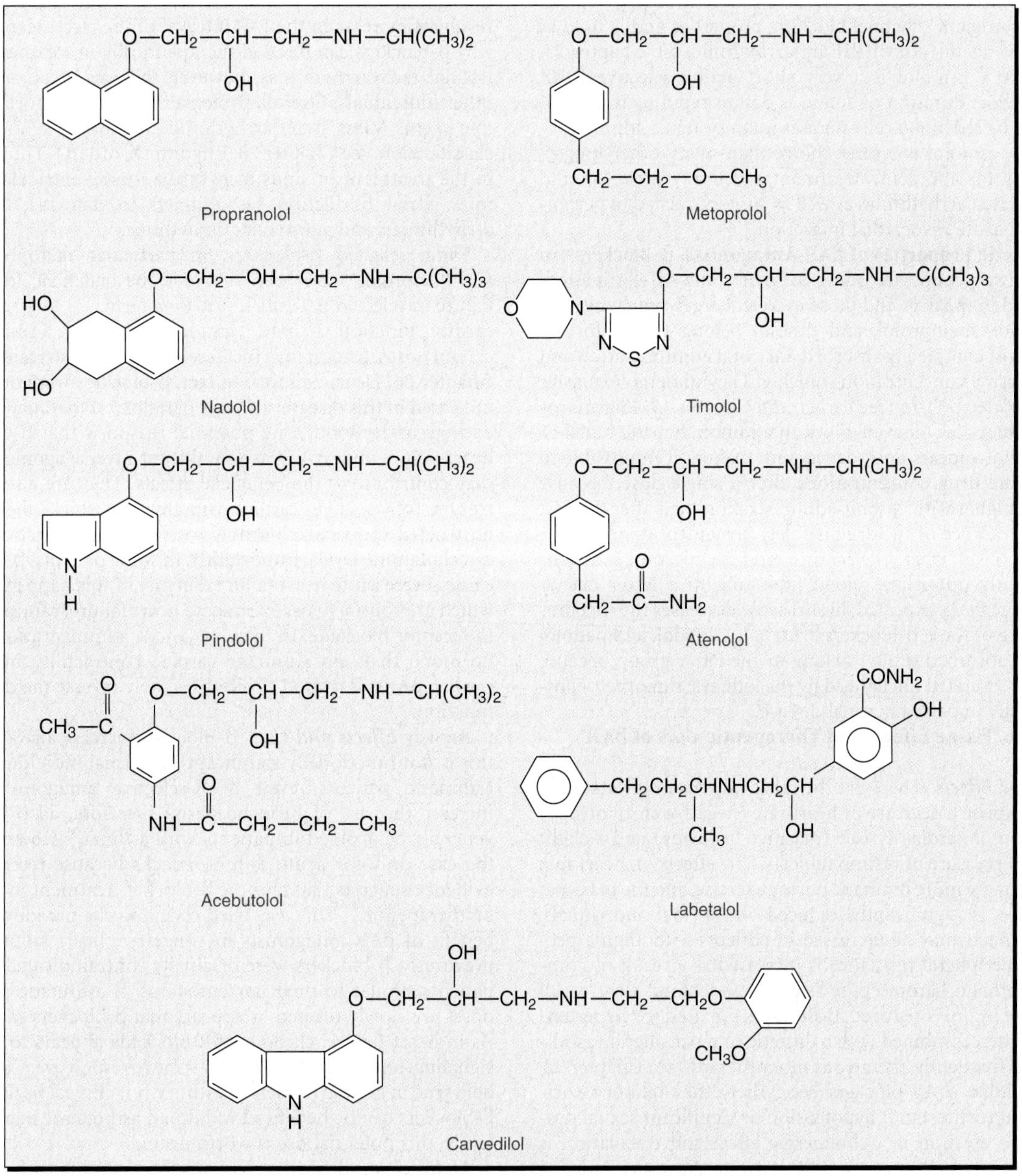

Propranolol

Metoprolol

Nadolol

Timolol

Pindolol

Atenolol

Acebutolol

Labetalol

Carvedilol

FIGURE 9-11 • Chemical structures of some of the most commonly used β-blockers.

Propranolol is the prototypical β-blocker. It has low and dose-dependent bioavailabilty owing to extensive first-pass metabolism in the liver (see later). Like propranolol, alprenolol is a nonselective βAR antagonist. Metoprolol, atenolol, betaxolol, acebutolol, and bisoprolol are selective β_1AR antagonists, which are preferable for patients with bronchoconstriction, diabetes, or peripheral vascular disease (because β_2ARs that are relatively spared mediate bronchodilation, insulin secretion, and peripheral vasodilation). Pindolol, acebutolol, carteolol, oxprenolol, and celiprolol are the β-blockers with ISA. Of those, celiprolol and acebutolol are also β_1AR-selective. Nadolol has a very long duration of action and is nonselective, like pindolol, carteolol, timolol (used mainly in glaucoma treatment), and labetalol. The latter has also α_1AR blocking properties and, because it also blocks βARs, can cause less reflex tachycardia than other α_1AR antagonists used for hypertension.[90]

Carvedilol and bucindolol are other nonselective β-blockers that can also block α_1ARs. These drugs also appear to have significant inverse agonist activity (especially carvedilol). Carvedilol in particular also has antioxidant and antiproliferative actions in vascular smooth muscle, which are adrenoceptor-independent.[91] These effects, along with its inverse agonism at βARs, might contribute to the clinical benefits of this drug in chronic heart failure. Sotalol is a nonselective β-blocker with additional cardiac K^+ channel blocking properties and is used as an antiarrhythmic agent (class II/III antiarrhythmic, see Chapter 25, Rhythm Disorders). Esmolol is a very short acting selective β_1AR antagonist. The short duration of action is due to rapid hydrolysis of its esteric linkage by red blood cell esterases upon systemic administration. Accordingly, esmolol is a safer choice than many other longer-acting β-blockers for the acute treatment of supraventricular and thyrotoxicosis-related arrhythmias as well as surgery-related hypertensive episodes and acute myocardial infarction.

Pharmacokinetic Properties of βAR Antagonists. β-Blockers can be divided into two groups according to their route of elimination: those metabolized in the liver and those excreted largely unchanged in urine. Propranolol, metoprolol, and timolol belong to the former group, being almost completely absorbed after oral administration and reaching peak plasma concentrations quickly. They undergo extensive first-pass hepatic metabolism (see earlier and Chapter 13, Pharmacokinetics), resulting in low bioavailability. In addition, hepatic metabolism of propranolol appears dose-dependent, making it impossible to predict steady-state drug concentrations after a single dose, because bioavailability is higher with chronic administration than after the first oral dose. Oral clearance of the drug is solely dependent upon intrinsic hepatic metabolism, whereas clearance after IV injection is dependent predominantly upon liver blood flow and, to a lesser extent, metabolizing capacity. As expected, liver disease decreases the metabolism and clearance of these β-blockers.[92] Atenolol, sotalol, and nadolol (which is poorly absorbed orally) belong to the latter group because they are primarily excreted unchanged by the kidneys; thus, their elimination is markedly impaired in renal disease.

Specific Organ/Tissue Effects and Therapeutic Uses of βAR Antagonists

Cardiovascular Effects. These are the most important effects of β-blockers and comprise a decrease of heart rate (negative chronotropy) with prolongation of cardiac systole (negative lusitropy) and a slight decrease in blood pressure of resting subjects. The effects on heart rate and cardiac output are more dramatic during exercise, and the maximal exercise tolerance is significantly reduced in normal individuals. However, these effects may be increased in patients with angina pectoris (see later). Peripheral resistance is increased as a result of compensatory sympathetic baroreceptor reflexes, and blood flow to all tissues, except the brain, is reduced. β-Blockers are used for hypertension treatment, often combined with a diuretic or a peripheral vasodilator, but are also frequently effective as monotherapy (see Chapter 22, Hypertension). Unlike α_1AR-blockers (see earlier), they are not associated with postural (orthostatic) hypotension or significant sexual dysfunction (because erection is a cholinergic effect and ejaculation is primarily an αAR effect). Moreover, reflex tachycardia is also reduced with βAR blockers, which is especially important when combined with vasodilators for hypertension. β_1AR-mediated renin release from the juxtaglomerular apparatus is also blocked after β_1AR selective and nonselective βAR blockade, and the Na^+ depletion–induced renin release is reduced. These effects contribute significantly to the blood pressure–lowering action of β-blockers and are more pronounced in individuals with elevated plasma renin activity.

β-Blockers are frequently used in the treatment of coronary artery disease (angina pectoris, ischemic heart disease).[93] The dose-dependent reduction of exercise-induced tachycardia and hypertension (i.e., cardiac workload) reduces oxygen demand and consumption of the heart and can limit cardiac ischemia (see Chapter 24, Coronary Artery Disease). β-Blockers have also been shown to decrease mortality and increase survival following myocardial infarction, possibly owing also to their antiarrhythmic action preventing ventricular fibrillation and "sudden death." In those trials in which therapy was started early, a reduction in infarct size was also demonstrated.

Ventricular dimensions and contractility are affected only minimally after βAR antagonist administration in normal resting individuals, but exercise-related contractility and exercise capacitance are reduced. They also block presynaptic neuronal β_2ARs, which facilitate NE release from sympathetic nerve terminals, thus decreasing neuronal release of this catecholamine.[1] β-Blockers also slow the AV conduction with a resultant increase in the P-R interval of the electrocardiogram. This is why β-blockers can be used therapeutically in treatment of supraventricular tachyarrhythmias; however, this can be an adverse effect for other individuals. Overall, β-blockers are very important antiarrhythmic agents (class II antiarrhythmics, according to Vaughan-Williams classification, see Chapter 25, Rhythm Disorders). Thus, they are useful in the treatment of sinus tachycardia, supraventricular tachyarrhythmias, atrial fibrillation (as adjuncts to digoxin), digoxin-induced arrhythmias, and ventricular arrhythmias.

Some selected β-blockers, in particular metoprolol, carvedilol, and bisoprolol, have been shown to be beneficial for chronic heart failure in selected patients in the long term.[94-96] Although they worsen cardiac function acutely, cautious long-term administration with careful dose titration may increase survival of heart failure patients (see Chapter 26, Heart Failure). In fact, β-blockers were originally contraindicated in this disease, and this paradoxical therapeutic benefit is not entirely understood. One potential reason is that β-blockers used in heart failure appear to have significant inverse agonist activity, which may contribute to the beneficial effects. They are also used in hypertrophic obstructive cardiomyopathy, in which they facilitate the obstructed ventricular outflow worsened by the actions of increased catecholamine levels. Importantly, in some patients, βAR blockade can cause severe acute heart failure. Further, if this happens, βAR agonists, which are routinely used for acute heart failure, cannot be used owing to receptor blockade. In these instances, administration of glucagon, a hormone that can stimulate cardiac contractility independently of cardiac βARs, is a good choice to acutely reverse the declining cardiac function.

Airway Effects and Uses. β-Blockers increase airway resistance, but this is not functionally significant in normal individuals. However, in asthmatic patients, even β_1AR-selective antagonists can severely increase the risk of bronchospasm; therefore, all β-blockers should generally be avoided in patients with asthma.[75] However, this may be the case only for acute asthma attacks because recent experimental evidence suggests that chronic β-blocker treatment in asthmatics may be therapeutic.[97] This was tried owing to the paradoxical therapeutic benefit of βAR antagonists in congestive heart failure (as discussed previously, β-blockers were originally contraindicated in heart failure patients similar to their current status in asthmatic patients), and if doses are slowly titrated, it appears that β-blockers may be beneficial. As in heart failure, chronic βAR blockade appears to "remodel" βAR signaling, and the system becomes more responsive. Currently, this has held true in animal models of asthma, but clinical trials to test whether β-blockers can be beneficial in human asthma are being planned; certainly, this potential use is worth noting.

Metabolism. β-Blockers considerably modify carbohydrate and fat metabolism.[68] They inhibit the catecholamine-induced lipolysis in adipose tissue, thus decreasing circulating free fatty acid levels. They reduce the hyperglycemic response to catecholamines inhibiting glycogenolysis in the heart, skeletal muscle, and liver. They do not affect plasma insulin or glucose levels in normal individuals or the rate and magnitude of hypoglycemia after insulin administration. However, they may prolong the subsequent recovery from hypoglycemia and prevent the rebound elevation of plasma glucose. Chronic administration of β-blockers has been associated with an unfavorable (in terms of coronary artery disease risk) decrease of the high-density lipoprotein–to–low-density lipoprotein (HDL/LDL) ratio. Agents with ISA appear to carry less risk to cause those lipid changes. The mechanism is unknown but likely involves effects of βARs on tissue sensitivity to insulin actions. Finally, β-blockers have been used for symptomatic treatment (primarily cardiovascular symptoms) of hyperthyroidism and in preparation for thyroid surgery (see Chapter 38, Disorders of the Thyroid).

Other Effects and Uses. Several β-blockers reduce intraocular pressure by decreasing production of aqueous humor in the eyes. This is why many of these agents have a prominent and very effective role in the treatment of glaucoma (see Chapter 58, Drugs in Ophthalmology).[22,23] Because of its lack of local anesthetic (membrane-stabilizing) effects, timolol is used topically for this indication. β-Blockers also block the catecholaminergic-mediated uterine relaxation.[64] Therefore, in a pregnant woman on β-blockers, β_2AR agonists are of no use to inhibit the uterine contractions of premature labor, and in this case, oxytocin-receptor antagonists (such as atosiban) that inhibit uterine contractions independently of βARs represent a good choice (see Chapter 42, Reproductive Health). Several β-blockers also have local anesthetic action (when used topically), also known as *membrane-stabilizing action*, which interestingly is related to weak Na^+ channel inhibition and not to specific βAR blockade.

Some β-blockers (propranolol, atenolol) are useful for preventing (but not acutely treating) migraine headaches (see Chapter 48, Headache). The mechanism for this is unknown. β-Blockers are also used in the treatment of portal hypertension (they reduce blood pressure within the portal vein) that can lead to variceal bleeding, for which the drugs of choice are somatostatin analogues (e.g., octreotide) and vasopressin analogues (e.g., desmopressin, terlipressin) (see Chapter 34, Hepatic Cirrhosis). Finally, β-blockers reduce sympathetically mediated skeletal tremors and anxiety, particularly performance-associated anxiety ("stage fright"), for which low doses of propranolol are particularly effective (see Chapter 52, Anxiety).[98]

Adverse Effects of βAR Antagonists. The most dramatic adverse effects of β-blockers are usually seen following the first dose, whereas further doses produce only relatively modest increases in the degree of blockade. Therefore, at-risk patients should be started on small doses, and slow dose titration should follow. This certainly must be done in heart failure because precipitation of ventricular dysfunction may occur acutely upon β-blocker administration in patients with compromised cardiac function owing to the negative inotropic action of these agents and to antagonism of the basal sympathetic tone of the heart. However, as detailed previously, dose titration can lead to beneficial therapeutic effects in heart failure patients. Likewise, as also discussed earlier, bronchospasm due to blockade of β_2ARs in bronchial smooth muscle can happen acutely in patients with asthma or chronic airway obstruction.

Peripheral vascular disease and Raynaud's phenomenon may be precipitated by βAR blockade, and therefore, calcium channel blockers are usually preferred in the treatment of these conditions. Of importance, β-blockers can mask the epinephrine-mediated warning signs of hypoglycemia in diabetic patients receiving antihyperglycemic treatment. Sweating, however, which is mediated by sympathetic cholinergic neurons (see earlier), may in fact be increased in a compensatory manner. Nonselective β-blockers may worsen the effects of hypoglycemia by increasing the rise in blood pressure; inhibiting catecholamine-mediated glycogenolysis and lipolysis, prolonging the period of hypoglycemia; and increasing the bradycardia. β_1AR-selective agents (e.g., metoprolol) might produce less marked hypoglycemic effects.[68] Finally, β-blockers also cause bradycardia (slowing of heart rate, negative chronotropic action), which should be considered an adverse effect necessitating drug discontinuation only in the presence of inadequate cardiac output.

Withdrawal Syndrome with β-Blockers. Following discontinuation of β-blockers, ventricular arrhythmias and severe angina resulting even in myocardial infarction and death might occur. These effects are postulated to be due to adrenergic supersensitivity mediated by βAR adaptive up-regulation (increase in receptor number) (see earlier, and Chapters 6, Signal Transduction; and 14, Pharmacodynamics). As expected, this phenomenon is less severe with agents with partial agonist activity (ISA), for example, pindolol. This is why discontinuation of β-blockers should be done gradually (preceded by slow dose tapering).

NONADRENERGIC-NONCHOLINERGIC NEURONS

Some autonomic effector tissues are innervated by fibers other than or in addition to cholinergic and/or adrenergic nerve fibers. These fibers are thus called *nonadrenergic-noncholinergic (NANC)*. Their transmitter substances are a variety of endogenous chemicals such as peptides (e.g., substance P, neuropeptide Y, calcitonin gene–related peptide [CGRP], cholecystokinin), purines (adenosine triphosphate, adenosine diphosphate), adenosine, and even the small molecule gases NO and carbon monoxide.[14,65,66,99-101] The fibers that innervate the gut wall are the richest NANC neurons in terms of chemical transmitter variety: NO, CGRP, enkephalins, serotonin, substance P, somatostatin, vasoactive intestinal polypeptide. These neurons comprise the so-called enteric nervous system (ENS), which is a semiautonomous nervous system integrating motor input from ANS outflow with sensory input back to the CNS.[35] The ENS is responsible for the synchronized impulses that promote propulsion of gut contents and GI contraction with concurrent sphincter relaxation. ENS fibers are activated by sensory input, release transmitter peptide locally in the sensory ending itself, and form branches that terminate back in autonomic ganglia. For a detailed discussion of these ENS and other NANC neuronal transmitter chemicals, see Chapter 8, Neurotransmitters.

PHARMACOGENOMICS OF THE ANS

With the initial completion of the Human Genome Project and the advancement of molecular biology in medicine, genetic factors influencing autonomic responses have been identified and found to have importance clinically. Mutations found naturally in receptor genes can have profound effects on physiology and, importantly, drug responses. Concerning pharmacology in the 21st century, it is now important to highlight and discuss what is known about genetic mutations and pharmacogenomics of the ANS. The cholinergic (muscarinic and nicotinic) and AR (α_1-, α_2-, and β-) subtypes that mediate the responses of the neurotransmitters of the ANS exhibit genetic variants with highly variable expression. Variants of muscarinic and α_1ARs are relatively rare, whereas α_2- and βAR subtype variants are quite common.[102] The largest amount of data available regards variants of these latter ARs in an effort to associate certain receptor genotypes, most commonly single nucleotide polymorphisms (SNPs), with particular phenotypes.

Cholinergic Receptor Polymorphisms

nAChR Polymorphisms

Numerous polymorphisms have been identified in the α3, α4, α5, α7, β2, and β4 subunits of the nAChR (Fig. 9-12). Some of the identified polymorphisms have been associated with neurologic disorders, including nocturnal frontal lobe epilepsy and schizophrenia; however, no evidence has been provided that such polymorphisms selectively alter ANS function.[103-108] Several mutations have been shown to alter receptor signaling properties experimentally in vitro. For example, a nonsynonymous coding SNP in the α4 subunit, Ser248Phe (C743T), located in the second transmembrane domain, exhibits faster

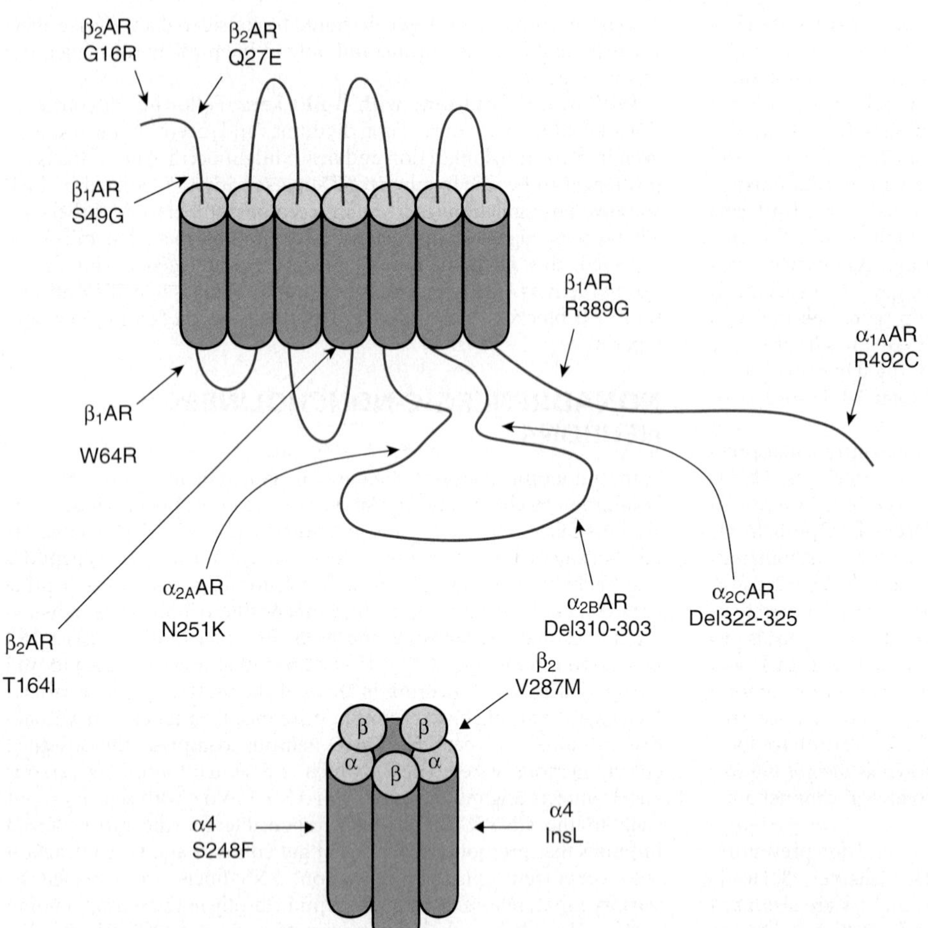

FIGURE 9-12 • Nonsynonymous polymorphisms in the protein-coding region of human autonomic receptor genes. **Top,** Adrenoceptor polymorphisms. **Bottom,** Nicotinic cholinergic receptor polymorphisms. See text for details. AR, adrenoceptor.

desensitization upon activation by ACh and slower recovery from the desensitized state compared with the wild-type receptor.

mAChR Polymorphisms

All five mAChR subtypes of the ANS appear to be highly conserved. However, recently, four SNPs were identified in the promoter region of the human M_3 receptor, which is largely expressed in airway smooth muscle.[109,110] No association with asthma was found, but there was a significant nonrandom transmission of haplotypes (see Chapter 15, Pharmacogenetics and Pharmacogenomics) to individuals with skin test reactivity to allergens, suggesting a role for this gene in atopic disorders.

Polymorphisms and Mutations among ARs

α_1AR Polymorphisms

A relatively common nonsynonymous variant (that changes the amino acid coded by mRNA), Arg492Cys (C1441T), has been identified for the human α_{1A}AR gene. The variation is localized in the carboxyl-terminal tail (see Fig. 9-12), but it has no apparent biochemical or signaling phenotype and shows no association with hypertension, clozapine-induced urinary incontinence, or benign prostatic hypertrophy.[102,111,112] However, a recent study of 16 young healthy male subjects suggested that the C genotype at position 492 has a longer P-R interval in their electrocardiogram. To date, no other highly frequent coding region nonsynonymous polymorphisms have been found in the other human α_1AR genes.

α_2AR Polymorphisms

Several polymorphisms and other mutations have been identified in the 5′-UTR (untranslated region), the coding region, and the 3′-UTR of the α_{2A}AR gene. Of these, the Asn251Lys (C753G) polymorphism located in the third intracellular loop alters function by enhancing agonist-promoted G protein (Gi) coupling (see Fig. 9-12). In the 3′-UTR, a restriction fragment length polymorphism (RFLP) with the restriction enzyme DraI has been identified. This DraI RFLP appears to be associated with hypertension, increased catecholamine-induced platelet aggregation (a α_{2A}AR-mediated effect), increased heart rate in response to lower body negative pressure, and decreased sodium excretion induced by immersion in thermal-neutral water. In a group of 147 hypertensive patients, the DraI RFLP polymorphism, although not associated with blood pressure or a family history of hypertension, was significantly associated with several measures indicative of altered lipid or glucose metabolism. Another α_{2A}AR polymorphism, −1291 C3G, located in the 5′-UTR of the gene, has been associated with abdominal fat accumulation in men and African American women, suggesting a role for α_{2A}ARs in determining the propensity to store abdominal fat, independent of total body fat.[111]

A polymorphism consisting of the deletion of three Glu residues (Glu301-Glu303) out of a highly acidic stretch of amino acids in the third intracellular loop of the human α_{2B}AR has been characterized (see Fig. 9-12). Studies with transfected cells revealed a decrease in agonist-promoted desensitization and phosphorylation of this deletion mutant variant compared with the wild-type receptor. This deletion polymorphism of the α_{2B}AR is more common in whites (31%) than in African Americans (12%) and is associated with increased risk for acute coronary events, decreased flow-mediated dilation of the brachial and carotid arteries (an indicator of subclinical atherosclerosis), but not with hypertension. In addition, this deletion polymorphism has been associated with blunted coronary blood flow increases in response to epinephrine infusion, nonthrombotic fatal (prehospital) acute myocardial infarction, increased risk for sudden cardiac death in white men, lower basal metabolic rate in obese subjects, increased body weight in nondiabetic subjects, and a significantly higher index of SNS activity and a lower index of parasympathetic nervous system activity. This latter alteration in ANS function may contribute to metabolic disorders. The Glu deletion polymorphism of the α_{2B}AR can also apparently interact with a Trp64Arg polymorphism of the β_3AR (see later), resulting in greater fat mass.[111]

A deletion variant has been found that lacks 12 nucleotides and 4 encoded amino acids (Gly-Ala-Gly-Pro; Del322-325 in the receptor protein sequence) in the third intracellular loop of the human α_{2C}AR (see Fig. 9-12). The polymorphism is much more common in African Americans than in whites. According to studies in heterologous in vitro systems, this deletion polymorphism confers a decrease in high-affinity agonist binding and in agonist-induced coupling to Gi proteins. Importantly, the combination of this α_{2C}AR deletion variant and a β_1AR polymorphism (Gly389Arg, see later) conferring increased function in vitro has been shown to significantly increase the risk of progression and the severity of heart failure in patient carriers. The working hypothesis is that the two variants would act synergistically to increase synaptic NE release and enhance receptor function at the cardiac myocytes, thereby increasing the risk for heart failure. Carriers of this α_{2C}AR deletion alone (especially African Americans) also appear to have increased risk for the development of heart failure.[102,111,112]

βAR Polymorphisms

β_1AR Polymorphisms. Two common coding SNPs have been reported for the β_1AR: Ser49Gly (A145G), located in the extracellular *N*-terminal domain (Gly allele frequency: 15% in whites and Asians, 30% in African Americans), and Arg389Gly (G1165C), located in the intracellular *C*-terminal domain (Gly allele frequency: 25% in whites and Asians, 40% in African Americans) (see Fig. 9-12). These two variations (Ser49Gly and Arg389Gly) are in linkage disequilibrium (see Chapter 15, Pharmacogenetics and Pharmacogenomics); that is, the Gly49Gly389 combination rarely occurs. The Gly49 variant yields higher basal and agonist-stimulated adenylyl cyclase activity and greater agonist-promoted down-regulation. The allelic distribution of the Ser49Gly polymorphism has been associated with long-term survival (decreased mortality risk in subjects with Gly49) of patients with congestive heart failure.[102,111,112] This finding may relate to results from in vitro studies that show increased desensitization and down-regulation of the Gly49 variant. However, contradictory data also exist showing the Ser49Gly polymorphism to be more frequently present in patients with idiopathic dilated cardiomyopathy (IDCM). Interestingly, a polymorphism in the 5′-UTR of the β_1AR located at nucleotide T2146C is in strong linkage disequilibrium with the Ser49Gly polymorphism and has also been associated with IDCM.

The Arg389 β_1AR polymorphism results in a gain of function receptor: enhanced coupling to Gs and increased adenylyl cyclase activity. However, in vivo studies have yielded inconsistent results for this variant. The Arg389Gly polymorphism has been associated with higher resting systolic and diastolic blood pressure in American individuals of European descent. Other researchers, however, found no impact of this polymorphism on exercise-induced, workload–dependent increases in heart rate or on resting heart rate. In contrast, individuals with symptomatic ischemic heart disease have been reported to show an association between the polymorphism and various hemodynamic measures, and individuals homozygous for Arg389 show larger decreases in blood pressure (but not heart rate) when treated with β-blockers. As discussed previously, the Arg389Gly polymorphism appears to have a synergistic effect with the Del322-325 α_{2C}AR polymorphism in promoting the progression of heart failure in African Americans. Finally, left ventricular mass, an important cardiovascular risk factor, has been shown to be associated with the Arg389Gly polymorphism because Gly389 individuals have greater left ventricular mass.[111]

β_2AR Polymorphisms. β_2ARs are highly polymorphic. Nine different SNPs have been identified in the coding region of the β_2AR, 4 of which are nonsynonymous: Arg16Gly, Gln27Glu, Val34Met, and Thr164Ile (see Fig. 9-12). Moreover, at least 9 variants have been identified in the 5′-UTR, some of which are in linkage disequilibrium with the Arg16Gly and Gln27Glu polymorphisms. Overall, 13 SNPs in the promoter and coding regions of the β_2AR gene were found; these are organized into 12 principal haplotypes, but of these, only 4 are relatively common.

The two major nonsynonymous SNPs in the β_2AR, Arg16Gly and Gln27Glu, are located in the extracellular amino terminus of the receptor (see Fig. 9-12).[102,111,112] They do not influence receptor binding or Gs coupling, but instead affect receptor desensitization. The Arg16Gly polymorphism leads to increased agonist-promoted down-regulation, whereas the Gln27Glu variant is resistant to down-regulation. The combination of Arg16Gly and Gln27Glu receptors resembles Arg16Gly alone, that is, displaying increased agonist-promoted down-regulation compared with the wild-type (Arg16, Gln27) β_2-AR. However, some recent findings with native human cells contrast with data from transfected cell systems and provide less consistent evidence that Gly16, alone or together with Glu27, is necessarily associated with greater desensitization or with a decrease in agonist-promoted responses. The Arg16 variant (especially in combination with Gln27) is associated with higher systolic blood pressure, in particular in subjects under the age of 50. It is well known that aging is associated with a decrease in β_2AR-mediated responses; thus, genetic variants in β_2ARs would be predicted to have a greater impact on physiology and pathophysiology in younger subjects. Heart failure patients homozygous for the Gln27 allele were less likely to respond to the β-blocker carvedilol than were those with the Glu27 allele. The Arg16Gly and Gln27Glu variants have been associated with obesity-related phenotypes and may be risk factors in obesity or the propensity to gain weight.

The Thr164Ile β_2AR polymorphism, located in the fourth transmembrane spanning domain, displays decreased functional coupling to G proteins (Gs) and, when overexpressed in the hearts of transgenic mice, shows decreased biochemical and physiologic activity.[111] Consistent with these findings, terbutaline-promoted inotropic and chronotropic responses are blunted in humans with the Ile164 variant. Thr164Ile carriers with congestive heart failure have significantly reduced survival and depressed exercise capacity, results consistent with studies in transgenic mice. The Thr164Ile variation has also been associated with obesity because freshly isolated subcutaneous fat cells that were heterozygous for Thr164Ile had a severalfold higher lipolytic EC50 of terbutaline compared with cells from homozygous Thr164 carriers.

β_3AR Polymorphisms. A SNP at nucleotide 827 (T to C) of the β_3AR gene results in a Trp64Arg substitution in the first intracellular loop of the receptor (see Fig. 9-12).[102,112] Additional variants have been identified at nucleotides 1856 (G to T) and 3139 (G to C) and are strongly associated with the Trp64Arg variation, comprising two haplotypes. Heterozygous Trp64Arg subjects show increased sensitivity to the increased blood pressure effects of infused NE and lower resting ANS activity compared with individuals homozygous for the Trp64 allele. Studies on the functional effects of the Trp64Arg β_3AR polymorphism in transfected cells have yielded variable results, with some showing no significant differences in agonist-binding properties or stimulation of cAMP, and some others showing decreased maximal cAMP accumulation in response to several agonists in transfected cells stably expressing Arg64 compared with Trp64 β_3AR. Of note, individuals homozygous for Arg64 secrete less insulin in response to glucose infusion and have higher fasting glucose levels compared with Trp64 homozygotes, effects that may contribute to the earlier onset of type 2 diabetes observed in individuals with the Arg64 allele. Some studies have found an association between the Trp64Arg polymorphism and obesity or type 2 diabetes, whereas others have not. As also mentioned previously, the Trp64Arg β_3AR and the α_{2B}AR Glu301-303 deletion variants interact, and when combined, these two variants are associated with greater fat mass and percentage of body fat in humans. Overall, it appears that the Trp64Arg β_3AR polymorphism can influence receptor function and, hence, lipid metabolism and perhaps onset or frequency of various metabolic disorders.

REFERENCES

1. Miller RJ. Presynaptic receptors. Annu Rev Pharmacol Toxicol 1998;38:201-227.
2. Schlicker E, Gothert M. Interactions between the presynaptic alpha$_2$-autoreceptor and presynaptic inhibitory heteroreceptors on noradrenergic neurons. Brain Res Bull 1998;47:129-132.
3. Slutsky I, et al. Presynaptic effects of muscarine on ACh release at the frog neuromuscular junction. J Physiol 1999;514:769-782.
4. Skok VI. Nicotinic acetylcholine receptors in autonomic ganglia. Auton Neurosci 2002;97:1-11.
5. Caulfield MP, Birdsall NJ. International Union of Pharmacology. XVII. Classification of muscarinic acetylcholine receptors. Pharmacol Rev 1998;50:279-290.
6. Doods HN, et al. Selectivity of muscarinic antagonists in radioligand and in vivo experiments for the putative M_1, M_2 and M_3 receptors. J Pharmacol Exp Ther 1987;242:257-262.
7. Furchgott RF. The role of endothelium in the responses of vascular smooth muscle to drugs. Annu Rev Pharmacol Toxicol 1984;24:175-197.
8. Moncada S, et al. Nitric oxide: physiology, pathophysiology, and pharmacology. Pharmacol Rev 1991;43:109-142.
9. Brodde OE, Michel MC. Adrenergic and muscarinic receptors in the human heart. Pharmacol Rev 1999;51:651-690.
10. Pappano AJ. Modulation of the heartbeat by the vagus nerve. In Zipes DP, Jalife J (eds): Cardiac Electrophysiology: From Cell to Bedside. Philadelphia: WB Saunders, 1995.
11. Hobbiger F. Pharmacology of anticholinesterase drugs. In Zaimis E (ed): Handbook of Experimental Pharmacology, Vol. 42: Neuromuscular Junction. New York: Springer, 1976.
12. Newton GE, et al. Muscarinic receptor modulation of basal and beta-adrenergic stimulated function of the failing human left ventricle. J Clin Invest 1996;98:2756-2763.
13. Toda N, Okamura T. The pharmacology of nitric oxide in the peripheral nervous system of blood vessels. Pharmacol Rev 2003;55:271-324.
14. Zanzinger J. Role of nitric oxide in the neural control of cardiovascular function. Cardiovasc Res 1999;43:639-649.
15. Furchgott RF, Zawadzki JV. The obligatory role of endothelial cells in the relaxation of arterial smooth muscle by acetylcholine. Nature 1980;288:373-376.
16. Gomeza J, et al. Pronounced pharmacologic deficits in M_2 muscarinic acetylcholine receptor knockout mice. Proc Natl Acad Sci U S A 1999;96:1692-1697.
17. Pfeiffer A, et al. Muscarinic receptors mediating acid secretion in isolated rat gastric parietal cells are of M3 type. Gastroenterology 1990;98:218-222.
18. Anderson KE. Pharmacology of lower urinary tract smooth muscles and penile erectile tissues. Pharmacol Rev 1993;45:253-308.
19. de Groat WC, Yoshimura N. Pharmacology of the lower urinary tract. Annu Rev Pharmacol Toxicol 2001;41:691-721.
20. Fetscher C, et al. M(3) muscarinic receptors mediate contraction of human urinary bladder. Br J Pharmacol 2002;136:641-643.
21. Noronha-Blob L, et al. Muscarinic receptors: relationships among phosphoinositide breakdown, adenylate cyclase inhibition, in vitro detrusor muscle contractions and in vivo cystometrogram studies in guinea pig bladder. J Pharmacol Exp Ther 1989;249:843-851.
22. Lee AM, et al. Selective muscarinic receptor antagonists for airway diseases. Curr Opin Pharmacol 2001;1:223-229.
23. Kanner E, Tsai JC. Glaucoma medications: use and safety in the elderly population. Drugs Aging 2006;23:321-332.
24. Alward WL. Medical management of glaucoma. N Engl J Med 1998;339:1298-1307.
25. Savarese JJ, et al. Pharmacology of muscle relaxants and their antagonists. In Miller RD (ed): Anesthesia, 5th ed. Philadelphia: Churchill-Livingstone, 2000.
26. Huikuri HV, Makikallio TH. Heart rate variability in ischemic heart disease. Auton Neurosci 2001;90:95-101.
27. Taylor P, Radic Z. The cholinesterases: from genes to proteins. Annu Rev Pharmacol Toxicol 1994;34:281-320.
28. Aquilonius SM, Hartvig P. Clinical pharmacokinetics of cholinesterase inhibitors. Clin Pharmacokinet 1986;11:236-249.
29. Abou-Donia MB, Lapadula DM. Mechanisms of organophosphorus ester-induced delayed neurotoxicity: type I and type II. Annu Rev Pharmacol Toxicol 1990;30:405-440.
30. Kranke P, et al. The efficacy and safety of transdermal scopolamine for the prevention of postoperative nausea and vomiting: a quantitative systematic review. Anesth Analg 2002;95:133-143.
31. Campbell SC. Clinical aspects of inhaled anticholinergic therapy. Respir Care 2000;45:864-867.
32. Médigue C, et al. Relationship between pulse interval and respiratory sinus arrhythmia: a time- and frequency-domain analysis of the effects of atropine. Pflugers Arch 2001;441:650-655.
33. Eglen RM, et al. Muscarinic receptor subtypes and smooth muscle function. Pharmacol Rev 1996;48:531-565.
34. Maesen FP, et al. Tiotropium bromide, a new long-acting antimuscarinic bronchodilator: a pharmacodynamic study in patients with chronic obstructive pulmonary disease (COPD). Dutch Study Group. Eur Respir J 1995;8:1506-1513.
35. Gershon MD, et al. Functional anatomy of the enteric nervous system. In Johnson LR (ed): Physiology of the Gastrointestinal Tract, 3rd ed. New York: Raven, 1994.
36. Chapple CR, et al. Muscarinic receptor subtypes and management of the overactive bladder. Urology 2002;60:82-88.
37. Andersson KE, Hedlund P. Pharmacologic perspective on the physiology of the lower urinary tract. Urology 2002;60:13-20.
38. Olson K. Mushrooms. In Olson K (ed): Poisoning and Drug Overdose, 3rd ed. New York: McGraw-Hill, 1998.
39. Farrar HC, et al. Use of continuous infusion of pralidoxime for treatment of organophosphate poisoning in children. J Pediatr 1990;116:658-661.
40. Solana RP, et al. Evaluation of a two-drug combination pretreatment against organophosphorus exposure. Toxicol Appl Pharmacol 1990;102:421-429.
41. Loke WK, et al. O-Substituted derivatives of pralidoxime: muscarinic properties and protection against soman effects in rats. Eur J Pharmacol 2002;442:279-287.
42. Rand MJ. Neuropharmacological effects of nicotine in relation to cholinergic mechanisms. Prog Brain Res 1989;79:3-11.
43. Petrides G, et al. Trimethaphan (Arfonad) control of hypertension and tachycardia during electroconvulsive therapy: a double-blind study. J Clin Anesth 1996;8:104-109.
44. Young JM, et al. Mecamylamine: new therapeutic uses and toxicity/risk profile. Clin Ther 2001;23:532-565.
45. Lee C. Structure, conformation, and action of neuromuscular blocking drugs. Br J Anaesth 2001;87:755-769.
46. Hunter JM. New neuromuscular blocking drugs. N Engl J Med 1995;332:1691-1699.
47. Meakin GH. Recent advances in myorelaxant therapy. Paediatr Anaesth 2001;11:523-531.
48. Atherton DP, Hunter JM. Clinical pharmacokinetics of the newer neuromuscular blocking drugs. Clin Pharmacokinet 1999;36:169-189.
49. Vincent A. Unravelling the pathogenesis of myasthenia gravis. Nat Rev Immunol 2002;2:797-804.
50. Missale C, et al. Dopamine receptors: from structure to function. Physiol Rev 1998;78:189-225.
51. Ahlquist RP. A study of the adrenotropic receptors. Am J Physiol 1948;153:586-600.
52. Bylund DB, et al. International Union of Pharmacology nomenclature of adrenoceptors. Pharmacol Rev 1994;46:121-136.
53. Graham RM, et al. Alpha 1-adrenergic receptor subtypes. Molecular structure, function, and signaling. Circ Res 1996;78:737-749.
54. Hieble JP, et al. International Union of Pharmacology. X. Recommendation for nomenclature of alpha 1-adrenoceptors: consensus update. Pharmacol Rev 1995;47:267-270.
55. Koshimizu T, et al. Recent progress in alpha 1-adrenoceptor pharmacology. Biol Pharm Bull 2002;25:401-408.
56. Philipp M, et al. Physiological significance of alpha(2)-adrenergic receptor subtype diversity: one receptor is not enough. Am J Physiol Regul Integr Comp Physiol 2002;283:R287-R295.
57. Post SR, et al. Beta-adrenergic receptors and receptor signaling in heart failure. Annu Rev Pharmacol Toxicol 1999;39:343-360.
58. Hoffman BB. Adrenoceptor-activating and other sympathomimetic drugs. In Katzung BG (ed): BG Katzung's Basic and Clinical Pharmacology, 9th ed. New York: Lange, 2004.
59. Brodde OE, et al. Presence, distribution and physiological function of adrenergic and muscarinic receptor subtypes in the human heart. Basic Res Cardiol 2001;96:528-538.
60. Rockman HA, et al. Seven-transmembrane-spanning receptors and heart function. Nature 2002;415:206-212.
61. Rohrer DK, Kobilka BK. Insights from in vivo modification of adrenergic receptor gene expression. Annu Rev Pharmacol Toxicol 1998;38:351-373.
62. Hieble JP, et al. International Union of Pharmacology. X. Recommendation for nomenclature of alpha 1-adrenoceptors: consensus update. Pharmacol Rev 1995;47:267-270.
63. Koshimizu T, et al. Recent progress in alpha 1-adrenoceptor pharmacology. Biol Pharm Bull 2002;25:401-408.
64. Ruffolo RR Jr, Hieble JP. Adrenoceptor pharmacology: urogenital applications. Eur Urol 1999;36:17-22.
65. Lundberg JM. Pharmacology of cotransmission in the autonomic nervous system: integrative aspects on amines, neuropeptides, adenosine triphosphate, amino acids and nitric oxide. Pharmacol Rev 1996;48:113-178.
66. McDonald A, et al. Contributions of alpha 1-adrenoceptors, alpha 2-adrenoceptors and P2x-purinoceptors to neurotransmission in several rabbit isolated blood vessels: role of neuronal uptake and autofeedback. Br J Pharmacol 1992;105:347-354.
67. Weyer C, et al. Development of beta 3-adrenoceptor agonists for the treatment of obesity and diabetes—an update. Diabetes Metab 1999;25:11-21.
68. Bernstein D. Cardiovascular and metabolic alterations in mice lacking beta1- and beta2-adrenergic receptors. Trends Cardiovasc Med 2002;12:287-294.
69. Ewan PW. Anaphylaxis. BMJ 1998;316:1442-1445.
70. Mitler MM, Hayduk R. Benefits and risks of pharmacotherapy for narcolepsy. Drug Saf 2002;25:791-809.
71. Trendelenburg A-U, et al. A study of presynaptic alpha2-autoreceptors in alpha2A/D-, alpha2B- and alpha2C-adrenoceptor-deficient mice. Naunyn Schmiedebergs Arch Pharmacol 2001;364:117-130.
72. Brogden RN, Markham A. Fenoldopam: a review of its pharmacodynamic and pharmacokinetic properties and intravenous clinical potential in the management of hypertensive urgencies and emergencies. Drugs 1997;54:634-650.
73. Jordan J. New trends in the treatment of orthostatic hypotension. Curr Hypertens Rep 2001;3:216-226.
74. Ruffolo RR Jr, et al. Pharmacologic and therapeutic applications of alpha 2-adrenoceptor subtypes. Annu Rev Pharmacol Toxicol 1993;33:243-279.
75. Spitzer WO, et al. The use of beta-agonists and the risk of death and near death from asthma. N Engl J Med 1992;326:501-506.

76. Birks EJ, et al. Left ventricular assist device and drug therapy for the reversal of heart failure. N Engl J Med 2006;355:1873-1884.
77. Bray GA. Use and abuse of appetite-suppressant drugs in the treatment of obesity. Ann Intern Med 1993;119:707-713.
78. Rocha BA, et al. Cocaine self-administration in dopamine-transporter knockout mice. Nat Neurosci 1998;1:132-137.
79. McCabe BJ. Dietary tyramine and other pressor amines in MAOI regimens: a review. J Am Diet Assoc 1986;86:1059-1064.
80. Black JW, et al. Comparison of some properties of pronethalol and propranolol. Br J Pharmacol Chemother 1965;25:577-591.
81. Ruffolo RR Jr, Hieble JP. Alpha-adrenoceptors. Pharmacol Ther 1994;61:1-64.
82. Becker AJ, et al. Oral phentolamine as treatment for erectile dysfunction. J Urol 1998;159:1214-1216.
83. Cooper KL, et al. Alpha-adrenoceptor antagonists in the treatment of benign prostatic hyperplasia. Drugs 1999;57:9-17.
84. Wilde MI, et al. Terazosin. A review of its pharmacodynamic and pharmacokinetic properties, and therapeutic potential in benign prostatic hyperplasia. Drugs Aging 1993;3:258-277.
85. Wilde MI, et al. Alfuzosin. A review of its pharmacodynamic and pharmacokinetic properties, and therapeutic potential in benign prostatic hyperplasia. Drugs 1993;45: 410-429.
86. Wilde MI, McTavish D. Tamsulosin. A review of its pharmacological properties and therapeutic potential in the management of symptomatic benign prostatic hyperplasia. Drugs 1996;52:883-898.
87. Harada K, et al. Comparison of the antagonistic activity of tamsulosin and doxazosin at vascular alpha 1-adrenoceptors in humans. Naunyn Schmiedebergs Arch Pharmacol 1996;354:557-561.
88. Bond RA, Ijzerman AP. Recent developments in constitutive receptor activity and inverse agonism, and their potential for GPCR drug discovery. Trends Pharmacol Sci 2006;27:92-96.
89. Fitzgerald JD. Do partial agonist beta-blockers have improved clinical utility? Cardiovasc Drugs Ther 1993;7:303-310.
90. van Zwieten PA. An overview of the pharmacodynamic properties and therapeutic potential of combined alpha- and beta-adrenoceptor antagonists. Drugs 1993;45:509-517.
91. Cheng J, et al. Carvedilol: molecular and cellular basis for its multifaceted therapeutic potential. Cardiovasc Drug Rev 2001;19:152-171.
92. Blaufarb I, et al. Beta-blockers. Drug interactions of clinical significance. Drug Saf 1995;13:359-370.
93. Freemantle N, et al. Beta blockade after myocardial infarction: systematic review and meta regression analysis. BMJ 1999;318:1730-1737.
94. Bristow M. Antiadrenergic therapy of chronic heart failure: surprises and new opportunities. Circulation 2003;107:1100-1102.
95. Cleland JG. Beta-blockers for heart failure: why, which, when, and where. Med Clin North Am 2003;87:339-371.
96. Teerlink JR, Massie BM. Beta-adrenergic blocker mortality trials in congestive heart failure. Am J Cardiol 1999;84:94R-102R.
97. Callaerts-Vegh Z, et al. Effects of acute and chronic administration of beta-adrenoceptor ligands on airway function in a murine model of asthma. Proc Natl Acad Sci U S A 2004;101:4948-4953.
98. Brantigan CO, et al. Effect of beta blockade and beta stimulation on stage fright. Am J Med 1982;72:88-94.
99. Boehm S, Kubista H. Fine tuning of sympathetic transmitter release via ionotropic and metabotropic presynaptic receptors. Pharmacol Rev 2002;54:43-99.
100. Burnstock G. Noradrenaline and ATP: cotransmitters and neuromodulators. J Physiol Pharmacol 1995;46:365-384.
101. Westfall DP, et al. ATP as a cotransmitter in sympathetic nerves and its inactivation by releasable enzymes. J Pharmacol Exp Ther 2002;303:439-444.
102. Kirstein SL, Insel PA. Autonomic nervous system pharmacogenomics: a progress report. Pharmacol Rev 2004;56:31-52.
103. Steinlein OK, et al. A missense mutation in the neuronal nicotinic acetylcholine receptor β4 subunit is associated with autosomal dominant nocturnal frontal lobe epilepsy. Nat Genet 1995;11:201-203.
104. Weiland S, et al. Neuronal nicotinic acetylcholine receptors: from the gene to the disease. Behav Brain Res 2000;113:43-56.
105. Duga S, et al. Characterization of the genomic structure of the human neuronal nicotinic acetylcholine receptor CHRNA5/A3/B4 gene cluster and identification of novel intragenic polymorphisms. J Hum Genet 2001;46:640-648.
106. Lev-Lehman E, et al. Characterization of the human β4 nAChR gene and polymorphisms in CHRNA3 and CHRNB4. J Hum Genet 2001;46:362-366.
107. Leonard S, et al. Association of promoter variants in the α7 nicotinic acetylcholine receptor subunit gene with an inhibitory deficit found in schizophrenia. Arch Gen Psychiatry 2002;59:1085-1096.
108. Lueders KK, et al. Genetic and functional analysis of single nucleotide polymorphisms in the β2-neuronal nicotinic acetylcholine receptor gene (CHRNB2). Nicotine Tob Res 2002;4:115-125.
109. Lucas JL, et al. Single nucleotide polymorphisms of the human M1 muscarinic acetylcholine receptor gene. AAPS PharmSci 2001;3:E31.
110. Donfack J, et al. Sequence variation in the promoter region of the cholinergic receptor muscarinic 3 gene and asthma and atopy. J Allergy Clin Immunol 2003;111:527-532.
111. Small KM, et al. Pharmacology and physiology of human adrenergic receptor polymorphisms. Annu Rev Pharmacol Toxicol 2003;43:381-411.
112. Flordellis C, et al. Pharmacogenomics of adrenoceptors. Pharmacogenomics 2004;5: 803-817.

10

FLUID AND ELECTROLYTE HOMEOSTASIS

Bruce C. Kone

INTRODUCTION 141
RENAL STRUCTURE AND ULTRASTRUCTURE 141
RENAL VASCULATURE, LYMPHATICS, AND INNERVATION 142
URINE FORMATION 142
Renal Blood Flow 142
Glomerular Filtration 143
Tubular Epithelial Transport Mechanisms 144
WATER BALANCE 145
Composition of Body Fluids 145
Water Handling along the Nephron 145
SODIUM BALANCE 146
Na^+ Handling along the Nephron 146
Responses to Changes in Extracellular Fluid Volume 146
POTASSIUM BALANCE 148
K^+ Distribution in Body Fluids 148
K^+ Handling along the Nephron 148
Responses to Changes in K^+ Intake 149
ACID-BASE BALANCE 149
Bicarbonate Reabsorption/Proton Secretion along the Nephron 149
CALCIUM BALANCE 150
Gastrointestinal and Renal Handling of Calcium 150
Responses to Changes in Ca^{2+} Balance 151
PHOSPHORUS BALANCE 152
Nephron Handling of P_i 152
Responses to Changes in P_i Balance 152
MAGNESIUM BALANCE 152
SECRETION OF ORGANIC ANIONS, CATIONS, PEPTIDES, AND NUCLEOTIDES 152
DIURETICS, AQUARETICS, AND NATRIURETICS: SITES AND MECHANISMS OF ACTIONS 153

INTRODUCTION

To meet the task of reabsorbing 99% of the 180 L of glomerular ultrafiltrate each day, the kidney fulfills several major functions to preserve fluid and electrolyte homeostasis. First, the organ regulates the excretion of several important inorganic and organic ions and participates in the regulation of acid-base balance. Second, the kidney works in an integrated manner with the cardiovascular and central nervous systems to regulate body fluid osmolality and volume. Third, the kidney excretes metabolic by-products and exogenous substances, including certain drugs. Finally, the kidney is an important endocrine organ, producing key hormones involved in the regulation of blood pressure, erythropoiesis, as well as sodium, potassium, calcium, phosphate, and bone metabolism. This reabsorption of solutes and water expends considerable metabolic energy; indeed, the kidney basally consumes about 10% of the total body oxygen to perform its work. This chapter examines the role of the kidney, and its coordination with other organ systems, in the maintenance of fluid and electrolyte balance.

RENAL STRUCTURE AND ULTRASTRUCTURE

The kidney parenchyma is divided into two major regions: the outer region, termed the *cortex*, in which the glomeruli reside, and the inner region, termed the *medulla*. The medulla is subdivided into 8 to 18 renal pyramids, whose bases begin at the corticomedullary junction and form an apex in a minor calyx of the papilla. The minor calyces drain into major calyces and then into the renal pelvis, which is an expanded region of the ureter. Smooth muscle contractions by the walls of the calyces, pelvis, and ureters drive the urine to the urinary bladder.

The functional unit of the kidney is the *nephron*. It consists of the renal corpuscle (containing the glomerulus and Bowman's capsule), the proximal tubule, Henle's loop, the distal tubule, and the collecting ducts (Fig. 10-1). The *proximal tubule* consists of initial convoluted segments (termed the *S1* and *S2 segments*) followed by a straight segment (termed the *S3 segment*) that descends toward the medulla. The proximal straight tubule then gives rise to the *thin descending limb of Henle*, which ends at a hairpin turn to become the *thin ascending limb of Henle* (in long-looped nephrons), which ascends through the medulla to form the *medullary* and *cortical thick ascending limbs of Henle*. The *macula densa*, a specialized portion of the cortical thick ascending limb, courses between the afferent and the efferent arterioles of the same nephron. The *distal tubule* begins after the macula densa segment and continues to the junction of two or more nephrons at the *cortical collecting duct*. The cortical collecting duct descends to become the *outer medullary collecting duct* and *inner medullary collecting duct*. Nephrons are further subdivided into superficial and juxtamedullary types. *Superficial nephrons* are characterized by glomeruli residing in the outer cortex, short Henle's loops, and efferent arterioles that branch into peritubular capillaries that enmesh neighboring nephrons. In contrast, *juxtamedullary nephrons* have glomeruli located in the cortex near its junction with the medulla, long Henle's loops that extend deep into the medulla, and efferent arterioles that form not only the peritubular capillary network but also the vasa recta. An overview of the functional properties of each of the nephron segments is presented in Figure 10-2.

The fenestrated endothelium of the glomerular capillaries together with the glomerular epithelium is anchored by the continuous glomerular basement membrane. The foot processes of the glomerular podocytes cover the outer segment of the capillary wall. The *glomerular filtration barrier* is formed by the fenestrae of the glomerular capillary endothelium, the glomerular basement membrane itself, and the podocyte foot processes.[1] The glomerular filtration barrier excludes molecules with molecular weight greater than 58,000 Da from passage. The net negative charge of the glomerular basement membrane tends to repel anionically charged proteins, such as albumin, and strongly influences glomerular permselectivity. The glomerular capillary network is anchored and organized around the mesangium, which comprised mesangial cells and extracellular matrix. The endothelium separates the glomerular capillary lumen from the mesangium, without an interposed glomerular basement membrane. The *juxtaglomerular apparatus*, a key participant in tubuloglomerular feedback, comprised

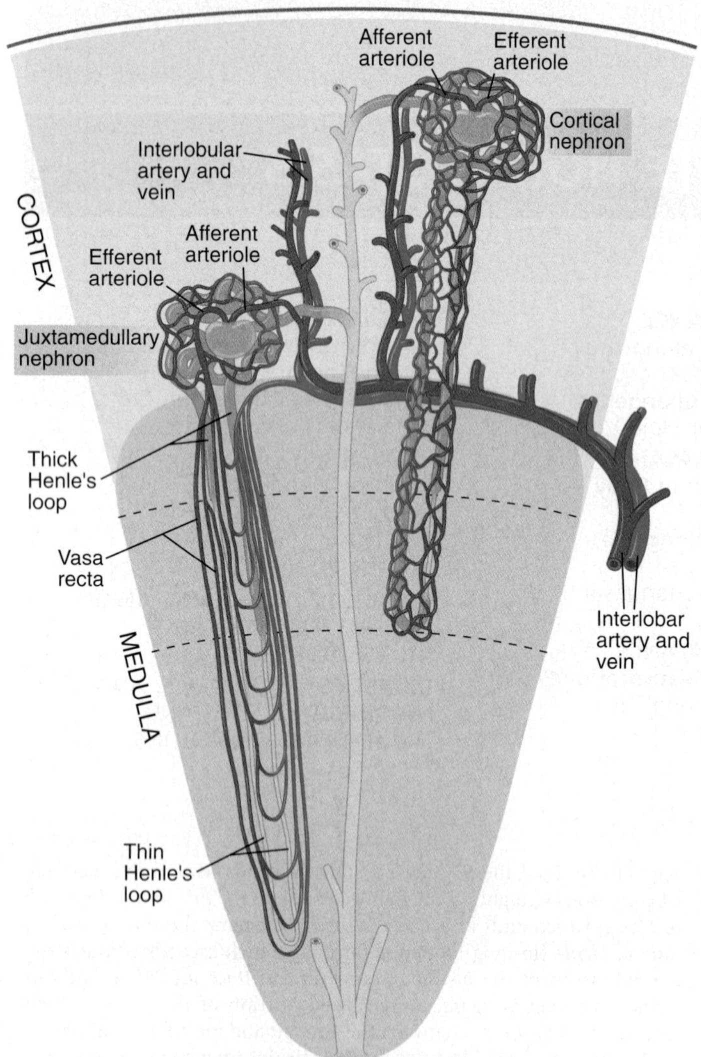

FIGURE 10-1 • Postglomerular circulation of superficial and juxtamedullary nephrons. Note that the efferent arteriole gives rise to the peritubular capillaries in both classes of nephrons and also the vasa recta in juxtamedullary nephrons. The vasa recta form capillary networks that surround the collecting ducts and ascending limbs of Henle's loop.

the macula densa, the extraglomerular mesangial cells, and the renin-producing granular cells of the afferent arteriole.[2]

RENAL VASCULATURE, LYMPHATICS, AND INNERVATION

The kidneys make up only 0.5% of the total body mass, yet they receive roughly 25% of the cardiac output. This high blood flow rate facilitates glomerular filtration. The blood flow is distributed principally to the renal cortex and diminishes progressively toward the medulla.[3] The renal arteries branch into interlobular arteries, which divide at the level of the corticomedullary junction to form the arcuate arteries. The arcuate arteries then branch into interlobar arteries, which divide into the afferent arterioles. The afferent arterioles give rise to the glomerular capillaries, which coalesce to form the efferent arteriole. The efferent arterioles become part of a second capillary network, the peritubular capillaries, which form a branching network surrounding the proximal tubules and successive nephron segments (see Fig. 10-1). The juxtamedullary efferent arterioles give rise to the descending vasa recta, which form a dense circuit of anastomosing, looping vessels that run parallel with Henle's loops to supply the outer and inner medulla with oxygen, nutrients, and substances for secretion to nephron segments and to return reabsorbed solutes and water to the systemic circulation. The venous system runs in parallel to the arterial vessels, with blood from the peritubular capillaries flowing sequentially through the stellate vein, the interlobular vein, arcuate vein, interlobar vein, and renal vein, which tracks beside the ureter. Blood from the ascending vasa recta enters the interlobular and arcuate veins.[4]

A network of lymphatic capillaries form superficially inside the renal capsule and more deeply between and around the renal vasculature.[5] The lymphatic networks inside the capsule and around the renal blood vessels drain into lymphatic channels coursing with the interlobular and arcuate blood vessels. The main lymph channels run in parallel with the main renal arteries and veins to drain into periaortic lymph nodes and lymph nodes near origin of the renal arteries. Whereas a few lymphatic capillaries are present in the renal parenchyma, associated with connective tissue, the glomeruli contain no lymphatics.

Sympathetic nerves, arising principally from the celiac plexus, innervate the kidney and are key regulators of renal blood flow (RBF), glomerular filtration rate (GFR), and tubule reabsorption of salt and water.[6] Adrenergic fibers travel adjacent to the smooth muscle cells of the interlobar, arcuate, and interlobular arteries and the afferent and efferent arterioles. Sympathetic nerves also innervate and can activate the renin-producing granular cells of the afferent arteriole, proximal tubule, Henle's loop, distal tubule, and collecting duct to regulate Na^+ reabsorption by these segments. Parasympathetic innervation to the kidney has not been described.

URINE FORMATION

Urine formation involves the integration of three processes: glomerular ultrafiltration, tubular reabsorption of solutes and water, and tubular secretion of endogenous and exogenous substances. Urine volume can have wide day-to-day variations, even in healthy individuals, depending on food and fluid intake and extrarenal fluid losses. The daily urine volume averages 1.5 L, but after exercise in heat, it may fall as low as 500 ml; and after excess fluid intake, it may reach 3 L or more. Within a given day, urine output is lowest in the early hours, maximal during the first few waking hours, and peaks after meals.

Renal Blood Flow

RBF represents the pressure difference between the renal artery and the renal vein, divided by the renal vascular resistance. RBF serves several critical functions: (i) it indirectly sets GFR; (ii) it delivers oxygen, nutrients, and hormones to renal cells and removes metabolic waste and reabsorbed fluid and solutes to the circulation; (iii) it modulates the reabsorptive rate of solute and water in the proximal tubule; (iv) it delivers substrates and drugs for urinary excretion; and (v) it contributes to urinary concentration and dilution. The relative changes in resistance of the afferent and/or efferent arterioles dictate the effects on renal blood flow and GFR.[7] RBF to each kidney is about 25% of the cardiac output (~600 ml/min) in resting individuals. About 90% of the total renal plasma flow (RPF) is directed to the cortex, about 9% to the outer medulla, with only 1% to the inner medulla and papilla. Metabolic, hormonal, and sympathetic nervous system influences govern the regional differences in blood flow across the renal parenchymal zones.

When the kidney is subjected to acute changes in blood pressure over the range of about 70 mm Hg to 180 mm Hg systolic blood pressure, renal RBF and GFR remain relatively constant through *autoregulation*, which insulates renal excretory function from fluctuations in blood pressure. Autoregulation is achieved by at least two mechanisms—a myogenic mechanism and tubuloglomerular feedback (TGF). A third mechanism, which is independent of TGF but slower than the myogenic response, is also operative, though its underlying regulatory mechanisms remain unclear.[4] The myogenic mechanism is a rapid (<10 sec), pressure-sensitive mechanism intrinsic to the vascular smooth muscle that responds to stretching by contracting.[4] Thus, elevations in arterial pressure stretch the renal afferent arteriole and the smooth muscle contracts, increasing resistance to the increased

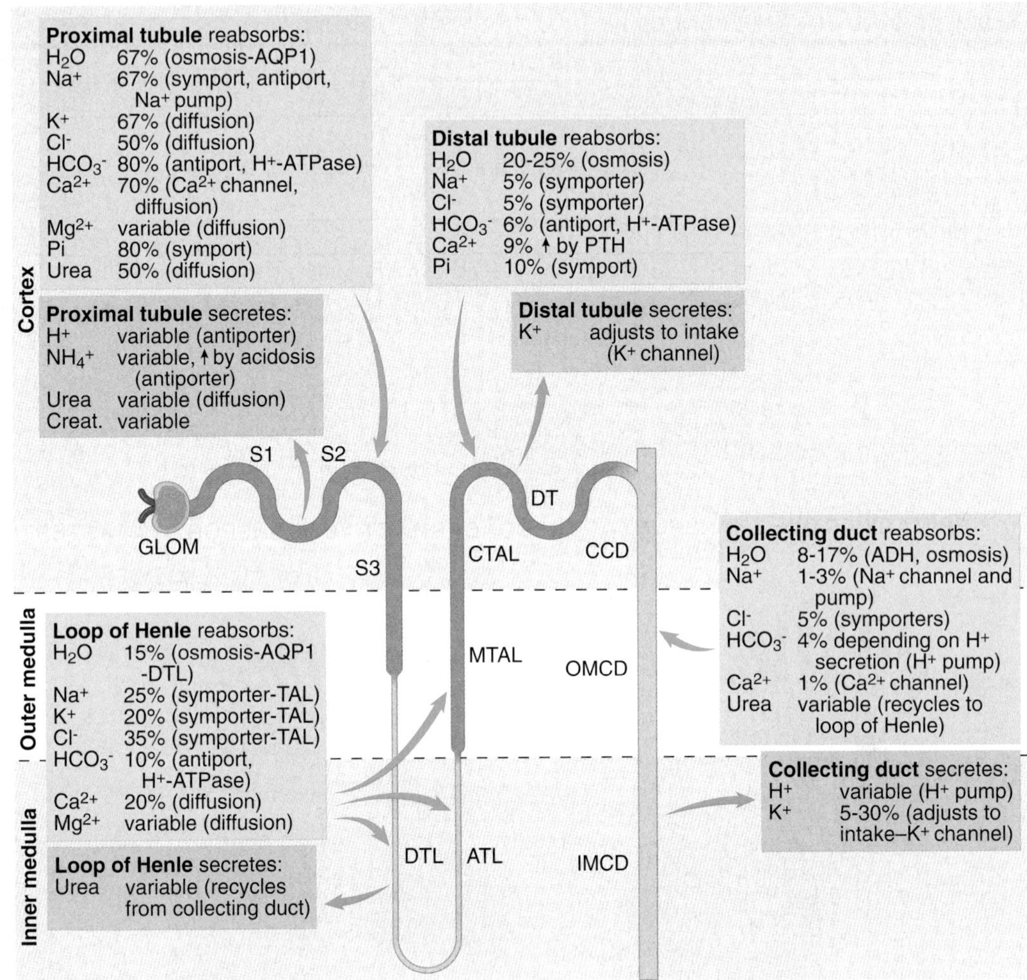

FIGURE 10-2 • Microanatomy and major segmental functions of an isolated nephron. The nephron is the functional unit of the kidney and consists of the renal corpuscle, proximal tubule, Henle's loop, distal tubule, and collecting system. The human kidney typically has more than 1 million nephrons, which function to filter and modify the blood to produce the final urine. Not drawn to scale. Each box depicts the major reabsorptive and secretory functions of the various nephron segments in handling ions, water, and inorganic and organic solutes. ATL, ascending thin limb of Henle; CCD, cortical collecting duct; CTAL, cortical thick ascending limb of Henle; DT, distal tubule; DTL, descending thin limb of Henle; GLOM, glomerulus; IMCD, inner medullary collecting duct; MTAL, medullary thick ascending limb of Henle; OMCD, outer medullary collecting duct; S1, S2, S3, segments of the proximal tubule.

arterial pressure so that RBF and GFR remain constant. Nitric oxide limits the strength, speed, and contribution of the myogenic response.[4] TGF is a process in which the macula densa senses the NaCl concentration (or another factor) in the tubular lumen and then transmits a paracrine signal to adjust, in an opposite manner, afferent arteriolar resistance and, thereby, GFR. Thus, enhanced NaCl delivery to the macula densa prompts these cells to increase NaCl uptake across the apical membrane via the Na^+-K^+-$2Cl^-$ (*NKCC2*) symporter, which increases the intracellular concentrations of adenosine triphosphate (ATP) and adenosine. ATP and adenosine bind to P2X and adenosine A1 receptors, respectively, in the membrane of afferent arteriolar smooth muscle cells, which increases intracellular Ca^{2+} concentrations and promotes vasoconstriction of the afferent arteriole.[8] ATP and adenosine also inhibit renin release by the granular cells of the afferent arterioles, thereby increasing afferent arteriolar tone and decreasing the renin release from granular cells. Further increases in luminal NaCl concentration stimulate nitric oxide release, which opposes the constrictor effect of adenosine, preventing excessive TGF vasoconstriction. Conversely, reduced NaCl delivery to the macula densa prompts vasodilation of the afferent arteriole so that RBF and GFR increase to normal levels.[9] Under resting conditions, the myogenic response contributes approximately 50% to overall RBF autoregulation, TGF 35% to 50%, and the third mechanism less than 15%. The relative contributions of these autoregulatory mechanisms dictates the amount and range of blood pressure fluctuations reaching the glomerular and postglomerular capillaries, and thus potentially affects glomerular filtration, tubular reabsorption, and medullary perfusion.

In addition to the myogenic response and TGF, sympathetic nerves, vasoconstrictor molecules, such as angiotensin II (Ang II) and endothelin, and vasodilator molecules, such as nitric oxide, bradykinin, and prostaglandins (particularly prostaglandins E_2 and I_2) act on the vascular tone of the afferent and efferent arterioles and thus contribute to the regulation of RBF (Table 10-1).[9] Angiotensin II plays a key role in the regulation of whole kidney blood flow, cortical and medullary blood flow, and renal autoregulation. Angiotensin II potently constricts both the afferent and the efferent arterioles, with responses modulated by paracrine and autocrine factors arising from endothelial cells and the macula densa. Factors that influence the vascular tone of the afferent and/or efferent arterioles or the TGF mechanism itself will cause alterations in GFR. Given the prime importance of Ang II, bradykinin, and prostaglandins in controlling vascular tone, pharmacologic interruption of these pathways with angiotensin-converting enzyme inhibitors, Ang II receptor antagonists, or cyclooxygenase inhibitors can disrupt autoregulation and the regulation of GFR.

Glomerular Filtration

The concentrations of ions and organic molecules in the glomerular ultrafiltrate are similar to those of plasma and essentially devoid of cells and proteins under normal conditions. The *filtration fraction*, the fraction of plasma entering the glomerulus that is actually filtered, is normally 15% to 20%, with the remaining plasma coursing on through the glomerular capillaries to the efferent arteriole and eventually returning to the circulation via the renal vein. Thus, for a typical RBF of 600 ml/min per kidney and GFR of roughly 120 ml/min, the filtration fraction is 0.2. Hydrostatic and oncotic pressures across the glomerular capillary membrane dictate the rate of ultrafiltration and, thus, GFR.[10] Because the ultrafiltrate is essentially protein-free as it arrives in Bowman's space, it contributes little oncotic pressure (P_{BS}), so that the glomerular capillary hydrostatic pressure (P_{GC}) is the only

TABLE 10-1 MAJOR INFLUENCES REGULATING RBF AND GFR

Hormone	Principal Stimulus	RBF Response	GFR Response
VASOCONSTRICTORS			
Ang II	↓ECV	↓	↓
Endothelin	↓ECV, Ang II, bradykinin, epinephrine, ↑stretch	↓	↓
Sympathetic nerves	↓ECV	↓	↓
VASODILATORS			
Nitric oxide	Bradykinin, acetylcholine, histamine, ↑shear stress, ATP	↑/no change	↑
Prostaglandins (PGE_1, PGE_2, PGI_2)	↓ECV, ↑shear stress, Ang II	↑	↑
Bradykinin	Prostaglandins, ↓ACE	↑	↑
ANP, BNP	↑ECV	↑	No change

ACE, angiotensin-converting enzyme; Ang II, angiotensin II; ANP, atrial natriuretic peptide; ATP, adenosine triphosphate; BNP, brain natriuretic peptide; ECV, extracellular fluid volume; GFR, glomerular filtration rate; PGE_1, prostaglandin E1; prostaglandin E_2; prostaglandin I_2; RBF, renal blood flow.

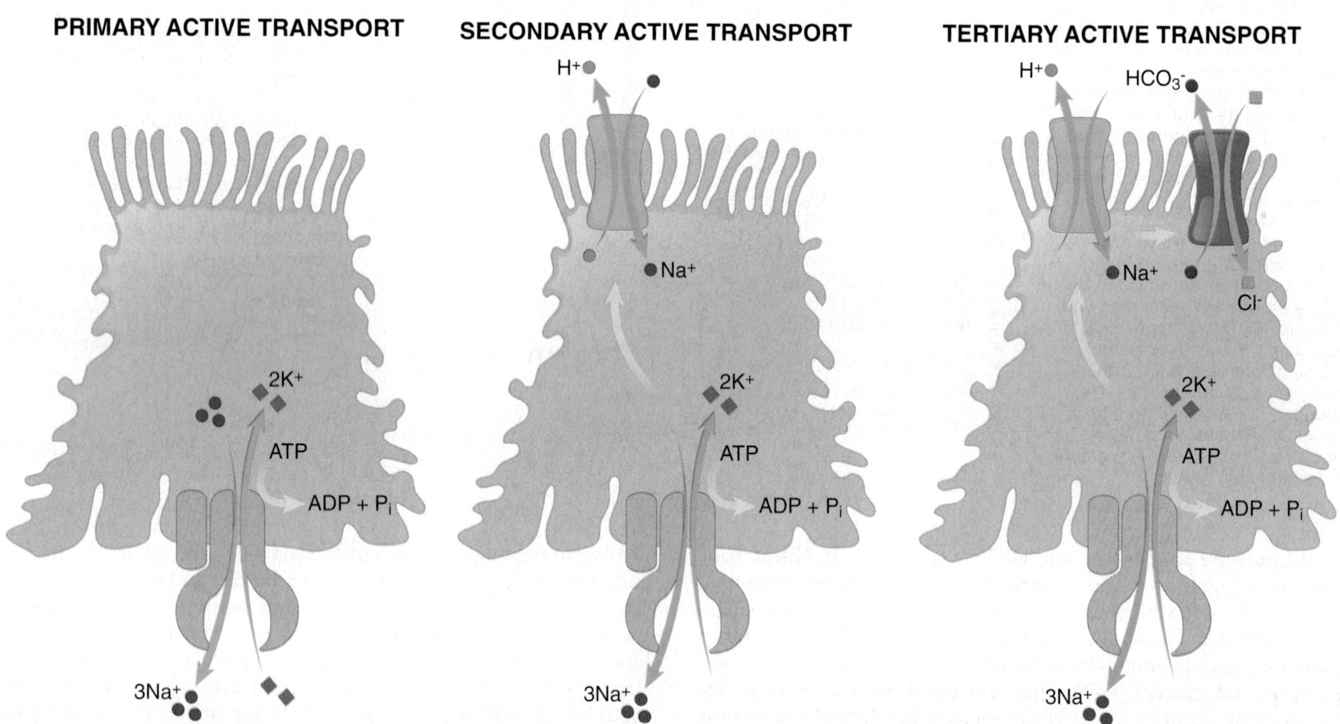

FIGURE 10-3 • Modes of active solute transport in renal epithelial cells. Models illustrate the different modes of active transport. Primary active transport (in this example, the Na^+,K^+-ATPase) uses adenosine triphosphate (ATP) hydrolysis to power the transport of solutes across the plasma membrane against their electrochemical gradients. Secondary active transport utilizes the energy inherent in the electrochemical gradient (in this case, the Na^+ gradient) generated by the primary active transporter to drive the influx or efflux of a coupled solute. Tertiary active transport couples the transport of a solute (in this example, Cl^-) to the gradient (in this example, H^+) created by the secondary active transport process.

driving force for filtration. It is opposed by the minor hydrostatic forces in Bowman's space (P_{BS}) and the oncotic pressure of the blood in the glomerular capillary (P_{GC}). These factors together with the glomerular capillary permeability (K_f, the product of the intrinsic permeability of the glomerular capillary and the glomerular capillary surface area available for filtration) are expressed in the equation for single-nephron GFR (SNGFR):

$$SNGFR = K_f\,[(P_{GC} - P_{BS}) - (P_{GC} - P_{BS})]$$

The net ultrafiltration pressure gradient, representing the difference between the hydrostatic and the oncotic pressure gradients, is greatest nearest the afferent arteriole, where the oncotic pressure is the lowest, and becomes progressively lower as the oncotic pressure increases along the glomerular capillaries to the efferent arteriole. In normal humans, alterations in P_{GC} resulting from changes in glomerular arteriolar resistance serve as the principal regulators of GFR.

Tubular Epithelial Transport Mechanisms

Because membranes are generally impermeable to ions distributed across them, ion pumps are used to interconvert chemical energy derived from ATP hydrolysis into electrochemical gradients to drive ion transport against a concentration gradient, in a process termed *primary active transport* (Fig. 10-3). In the kidney, the Na^+,K^+-ATPase is the primary mechanism for primary active transport, functioning to maintain the low concentration of Na^+ and high concentration of K^+ in the intracellular environment. In *secondary active transport*, solutes are transported along an electrochemical gradient, without direct energy consumption (Fig. 10-4). Thus, the energy stored in the steep Na^+ gradient generated by the Na^+,K^+-ATPase can direct Na^+-coupled transport of sugars, amino acids, and other solutes along the nephron. Finally, in *tertiary active transport*, the energy stored in the Na^+ gradi-

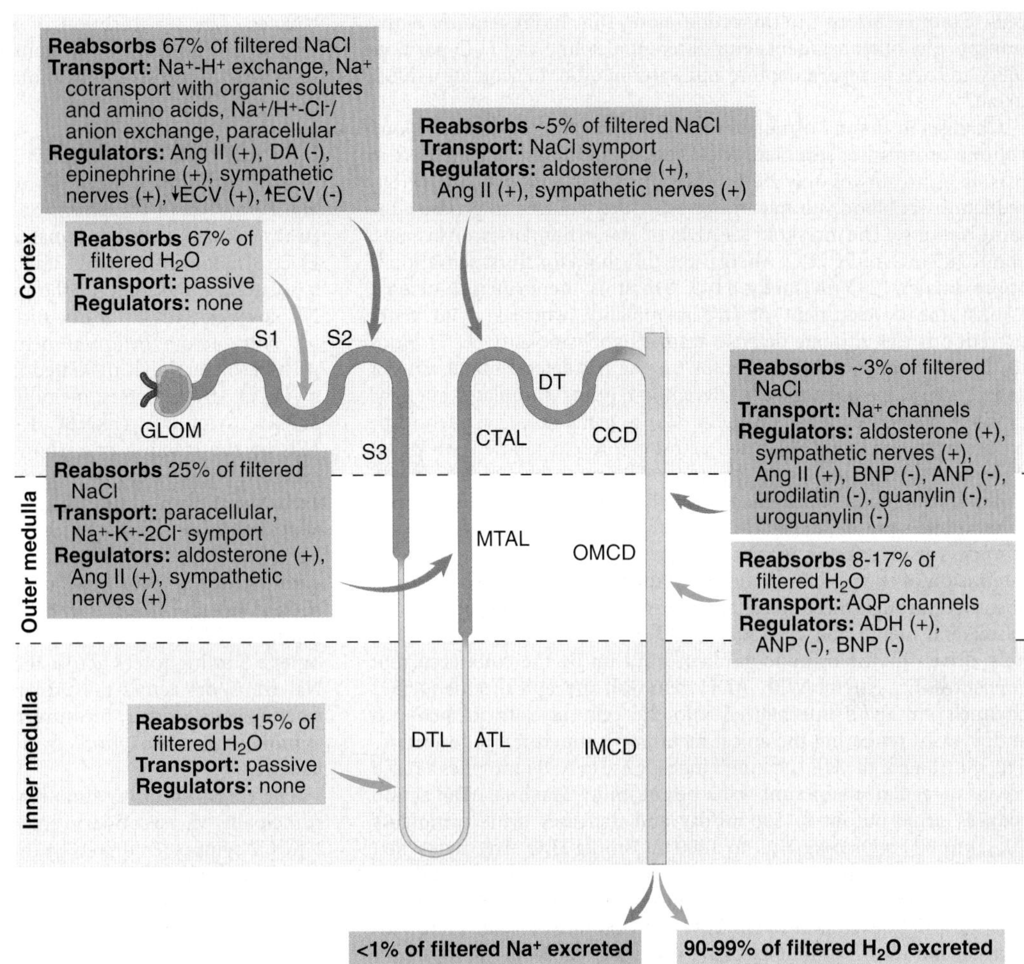

FIGURE 10-4 • Segmental sodium and water handling along the nephron. The percentage of filtered load reabsorbed, the mechanisms of Na entry across the apical membrane, and major regulatory hormones. (–), inhibition; (+), stimulation.

ent generated by the Na^+, K^+-ATPase can be indirectly used to drive the transport of other ions and organic molecules. For example, the Na^+/H^+ exchanger, a secondary active transporter driven by the transmembrane Na^+ gradient generated and maintained by the Na^+,K^+-ATPase, couples Na^+ influx with the H^+ efflux and is thus principally responsible for the existence of this H^+ gradient (see Fig. 10-3). This H^+ gradient can then drive the *tertiary active transport* of Cl^- across the brush border membrane via a Cl^-/HCO_3^- exchanger (see Fig. 10-3).

WATER BALANCE

Composition of Body Fluids

Under physiologic conditions, the osmolality of all body fluids is maintained within narrow limits (275-290 mOsm/kg H_2O) by appropriate changes in H_2O intake and excretion. H_2O balance is dependent on (i) access to H_2O and an intact thirst mechanism; (ii) extrarenal H_2O losses; (iii) appropriate renal excretion of solutes and H_2O; (iv) intact antidiuretic hormone (ADH) biosynthesis and release; and (v) appropriate collecting duct response. H_2O intake typically ranges from 1 to 5 L/day, depending on thirst, taste, habit, and physicians' prescriptions. H_2O excretion is regulated by factors that adjust renal excretion and by nonrenal losses (insensible, perspiratory, and gastrointestinal losses). Total body H_2O (TBW) constitutes approximately 50% of lean body mass (LBM) in women and approximately 60% in men, and it is distributed between intracellular (two thirds of TBW) and extracellular (one third of TBW) fluid compartments. Roughly one quarter of the extracellular fluid (ECF) is intravascular (plasma), and the remaining three quarters is primarily interstitial–lymph fluid. Because most cell membranes are freely permeable to water, osmotic equilibrium between the intracellular fluid (ICF) and the ECF is strictly maintained by appropriate fluid shifts between these compartments. The principal intracellular solutes are K^+, proteins, and inorganic phosphorus (P_i), whereas the major ECF solutes are Na^+, Cl^-, and HCO_3^-.

Water Handling along the Nephron

H_2O reabsorption is a highly integrated and regulated process that can vary between 0.3% and 15% of the amount filtered under physiologic conditions.[11] Under normal conditions, approximately 150 L of H_2O is freely filtered at the glomerulus each day. About two thirds of the filtered H_2O is passively reabsorbed in the proximal tubule, which expresses high levels of aquaporin-1 H_2O channels in the apical and basolateral membranes (see Fig. 10-4). The driving force for water reabsorption in this segment is the osmotic gradient across the tubule established by solute reabsorption. In contrast, medullary hypertonicity drives about 15% of the filtered H_2O reabsorbed along the descending limb of loop of Henle, which also expresses aquaporin-1 H_2O channels in the apical and basolateral membranes. Solutes, but not H_2O, are reabsorbed along the ascending limb and the distal tubule, so that these segments dilute the urine (see Fig. 10-4). The principal cells of the late distal tubule and collecting duct reabsorb variable amounts of the remaining H_2O via ADH-regulated aquaporin-2 H_2O channels in the apical membranes and aquaporin-3 and aquaporin-4 H_2O channels in the basolateral membranes. H_2O reabsoprtion along the length of the collecting duct is greatest in the cortex and least in the inner medulla, allowing maintenance of a hyperosmotic interstitium in the inner medulla. Countercurrent multiplication generates medullary hypertonicity in part by accumulation of NaCl reabsorbed by the NKCC2 cotransporter at the apical membrane of thick ascending limb cells. Countercurrent multiplication along thin limbs requires active transport by other segments and differential solute and H_2O permeability and acts to separate solute and water in order to generate a dilute urine.[12]

Changes in plasma osmolality and, to a much lesser degree, blood volume or pressure stimulate ADH release and thirst. An increase in plasma osmolality of only 2% to 3% elicits thirst, whereas 10% to 15% reductions in blood volume and pressure are required to produce the same response. The threshold for ADH release in humans is, on average, about 285 mOsm/kg H_2O, whereas the threshold for thirst sensation is approximately 295 mOsm/kg H_2O. Thirst is the principal defense against the development of hyperosmolality, whereas renal water excretion is the ultimate defense against hypoosmolality. ADH binds to the vasopressin-2 (V2) receptor on the basolateral membrane of collecting duct principal cells. Receptor-binding stimulates adenylyl cyclase via a stimulatory G protein (Gs) to generate cyclic adenosime monophosphate (cAMP), which activates protein kinase A to phosphorylate aquaporin-2 water channels. The molecular motor dynein drives the vesicles containing phosphorylated aquaporin-2 along microtubules toward the apical membrane, where soluble *N*-ethylmaleimide-sensitive factor attachment receptor (SNARE) proteins facilitate fusion of the vesicles in the apical membrane of the cell.[13] H_2O is absorbed through these apical aquaporin-2 channels and through the basolateral membrane via aquaporin-3 and aquaporin-4 H_2O channels, driven by the osmotic gradient built up by the countercurrent concentrating system. With ADH removal, the apical aquaporin-2 channels are again internalized into the cell via clathrin-mediated endocytosis, rendering the apical membrane impermeable to water.[13] The shuttling of the H_2O channels in response to ADH provides a rapid means to regulate membrane water permeability. Maximal ADH action reduces urine output to 500 ml/day and increases urine osmolality (U_{osm}) to 800 mOsm/kg H_2O to 1400 mOsm/kg H_2O. Any factor that impairs ADH synthesis or release, tubular responsiveness to ADH, or medullary hypertonicity will also limit urinary concentrating ability.

Appropriate excretion of an H_2O load requires (i) adequate glomerular filtration, without excessive proximal reabsorption, to deliver tubular fluid to the diluting segments of the nephron (ascending limb of Henle and early distal convoluted tubule); (ii) normal function of the diluting segments of the nephron; and (iii) suppression of ADH to prevent reabsorption of solute-free water in the collecting ducts. Excess renal H_2O losses are usually due to partial or complete failure to synthesize or secrete ADH (central diabetes insipidus) or due to diminished or absent renal response to its action (nephrogenic diabetes insipidus). These disorders are characterized by an inability to concentrate the urine maximally, the result of both ADH deficiency (or resistance) and washout of the medullary osmotic gradient by chronic polyuria. Patients with nephrogenic diabetes insipidus have impaired urinary concentrating ability despite maximal synthesis and release of ADH. Nephrogenic diabetes insipidus results from (i) a failure of the countercurrent mechanism to generate a hypertonic medullary and papillary interstitium and/or (ii) a failure of ADH to increase the water permeability of the collecting duct.[14] Nephrogenic diabetes insipidus may be congenital, but more commonly, it is an acquired disorder.

SODIUM BALANCE

Na^+ balance represents the net difference between intake (typically oral or intravenous) and excretion (primarily renal, gastrointestinal, and skin). Daily Na^+ intake averages 2 g to 6 g on a typical Western diet, but it varies by dietary access and habit, Na^+ appetite, and physicians' prescriptions. Na^+ excretion is regulated by factors that control renal and nonrenal losses. In healthy humans, approximately 25 mol/day of Na^+ is freely filtered at the glomerulus, with all but about 1% being reabsorbed along the length of the nephron. In the absence of pharmacologic interference, urinary excretion of Na^+ can vary between less than 0.1% and no more than 3% of the filtered load. Because spontaneous changes in GFR can dramatically alter the filtered load of Na^+, rapid adjustments in Na^+ reabsorption must occur along the nephron to prevent wide fluctuations in urinary Na^+ excretion and body Na^+ balance. The reabsorption of several important solutes is coupled directly or indirectly to Na^+ transport. Na^+ reabsorption varies inversely with arterial pressure, a phenomenon termed *pressure natriuresis*.[15]

Na^+ Handling along the Nephron

The proximal tubule reabsorbs about 65% of the filtered Na^+ (see Fig. 10-4). About two thirds of this Na^+ is reabsorbed across the cells (transcellular), with the remainder reabsorbed by paracellular routes. Electrochemical gradients established by the Na^+-K^+-ATPase in the basolateral membrane of the proximal tubule drive the transport of Na^+ coupled with H^+ or organic solutes.[16] The principal mechanism of Na^+ entry across the apical membrane is the Na^+-H^+ exchanger NHE3 with basolateral exit mediated in the first half of the proximal tubule by HCO_3^- transporters, including the Cl^--HCO_3^- (AE2) and the Na^+-$3HCO_3^-$ symporter (hkNBCe1, Fig. 10-5). HCO_3^- is generated in the cells by the reaction of carbon dioxide (CO_2) and H^+, facilitated by carbonic anhydrase. In the second half of the proximal tubule, Na^+-H^+ exchange is coupled to Cl^--anion exchange in the apical membrane to effect net NaCl uptake, with basolateral exit of Na^+ and Cl^- via the Na^+-K^+-ATPase and K^+-Cl^- cotransporter, respectively. The exact amounts of Na^+ reabsorbed are determined by many regulatory factors, such as glomerulotubular balance, Ang II, endothelin, sympathetic input, acid-base status parathyroid hormone (PTH), dopamine, and others. Starling forces across the peritubular capillaries also influence Na^+ transport across the proximal tubule. Increases in the filtration fraction cause oncotic pressure in the peritubular capillaries to increase, stimulating reabsorption, in a process known as *glomerulotubular balance*.[17,18]

The thick ascending limb reabsorbs about 25% of the filtered Na^+, principally via secondary active transport mediated by the apical NKCC2 symporter, driven by the Na^+-K^+-ATPase and facilitated by K^+ recycling to the NKCC2 symporter via the apical renal outer medulla potassium channel (ROMK) K^+ channel (see Figs. 10-4 and 10-5). Na^+-H^+ exchange also contributes to proximal tubule NaCl reabsorption. H_2O but not solute is reabsorbed from the thin descending limb of Henle's loop, increasing the luminal Na^+ concentration as the fluid descends to the tip of the loop. The thin and thick ascending limbs are impermeable to H_2O, so that Na^+ reabsorption in these segments reduces the osmolality ("dilutes") of the tubular fluid. The transport rate is determined by the Na^+ load and by several hormones and neurotransmitters, including prostaglandins, PTH, glucagon, calcitonin, ADH, and adrenaline.

The distal tubule reabsorbs about 4% to 5% of the remaining Na^+, but not H_2O, by the actions of the apical thiazide-sensitive NaCl cotransporter (NCCT) and the basolateral Na^+-K^+-ATPase (see Fig. 10-4). The rate of transport is again determined by the delivered load and by several hormones and neurotransmitters. The remaining 3% of filtered Na^+ is reabsorbed along the connecting tubule and collecting duct, with the apical epithelial Na^+ channel (ENaC) mediating Na^+ entry (see Figs. 10-4 and 10-5). Aldosterone, which is regulated directly by Ang II and by serum K^+ concentrations, governs Na^+ reabsorption along the second half of the distal convoluted tubule, the connecting tubule, and collecting duct (collectively termed the *aldosterone-sensitive distal nephron*) by stimulating ENaC abundance and/or activity and NCCT. Natriuretic peptides stimulate guanylyl cyclase along the collecting duct, generating cyclic guanosine monophosphate and inhibiting apical Na^+ channels in the collecting duct.

Responses to Changes in Extracellular Fluid Volume

During extracellular fluid volume (ECFV) contraction, baroreceptors trigger an increase in renal sympathetic nerve activity, which (i) vasoconstricts the afferent and efferent arterioles to reduce GFR; (ii) stimulates renin secretion by the juxtaglomerular cells, which ultimately increases circulating levels of Ang II and aldosterone, thereby stimulating Na^+ reabsorption; and (iii) stimulates ADH secretion, which promotes H_2O reabsorption by the collecting duct. Atrial natriuretic

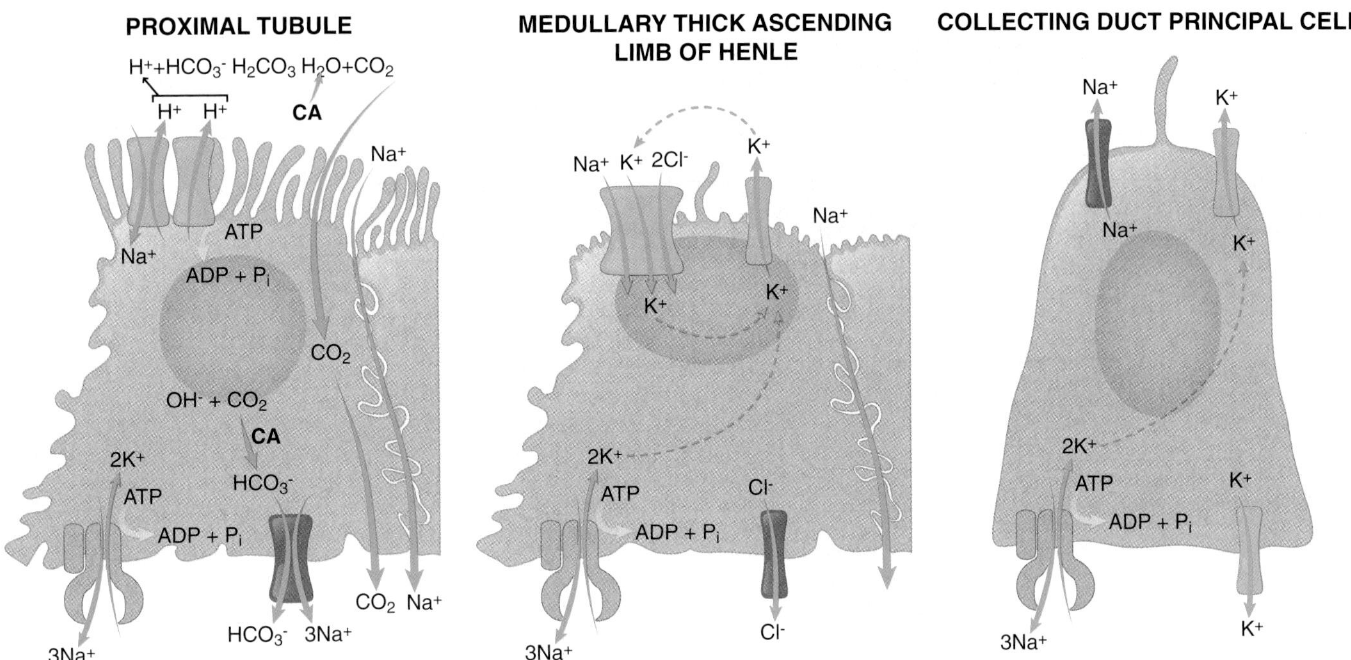

FIGURE 10-5 • Transport pathways involved in Na^+ and K^+ transport in the proximal tubule, medullary thick ascending limb of Henle, and cortical collecting duct. The principal transporters and enzymes involved in transepithelial Na^+ and K^+ transport and paracellular Na^+ transport in the three cell types. CA, carbonic anhydrase.

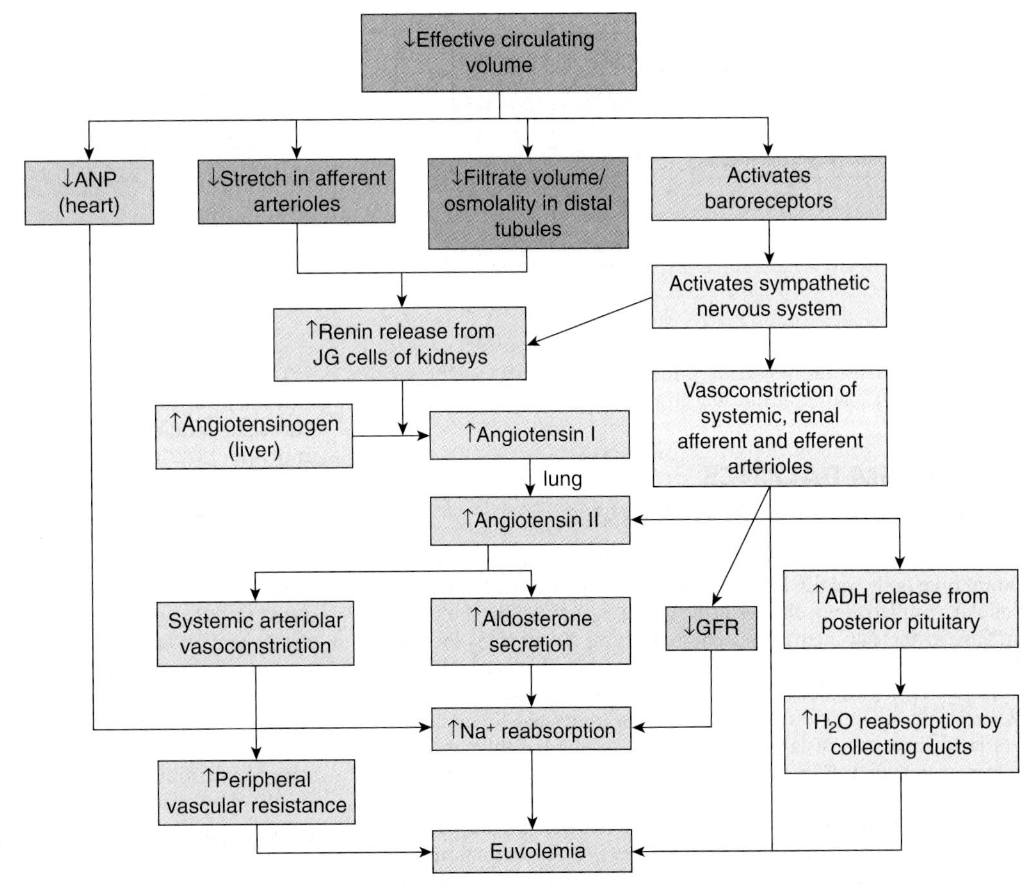

FIGURE 10-6 • Compensatory changes in renal sodium and water handling in response to a decrease in effective circulating volume (ECV). ADH, antidiuretic hormone; ANP, atrial natriuretic peptide; JG, juxtaglomerular cells of the afferent arteriole.

peptide (ANP) secretion is also inhibited. Collectively, these responses limit Na^+ and H_2O excretion to restore the ECFV to normal levels (Fig. 10-6). During ECFV expansion, renal sympathetic nerve activity is inhibited, and release of ANP and brain natriuretic peptide (BNP) from the heart and urodilatin from the distal tubules is stimulated. ANP has multiple effects, including (i) vasodilation of the afferent arterioles and vasoconstriction of the efferent arterioles to increase GFR and the filtered load of Na^+; (ii) inhibition of renin secretion by the afferent arteriole, thereby inhibiting Ang II production; (iii) inhibition of aldosterone secretion by the glomerulosa cells of the adrenal cortex; (iv) inhibition of apical Na^+ channel activity and thus Na^+ reabsorption in the medullary collecting duct; and (v) inhibition of

Principles: Systems Pharmacology

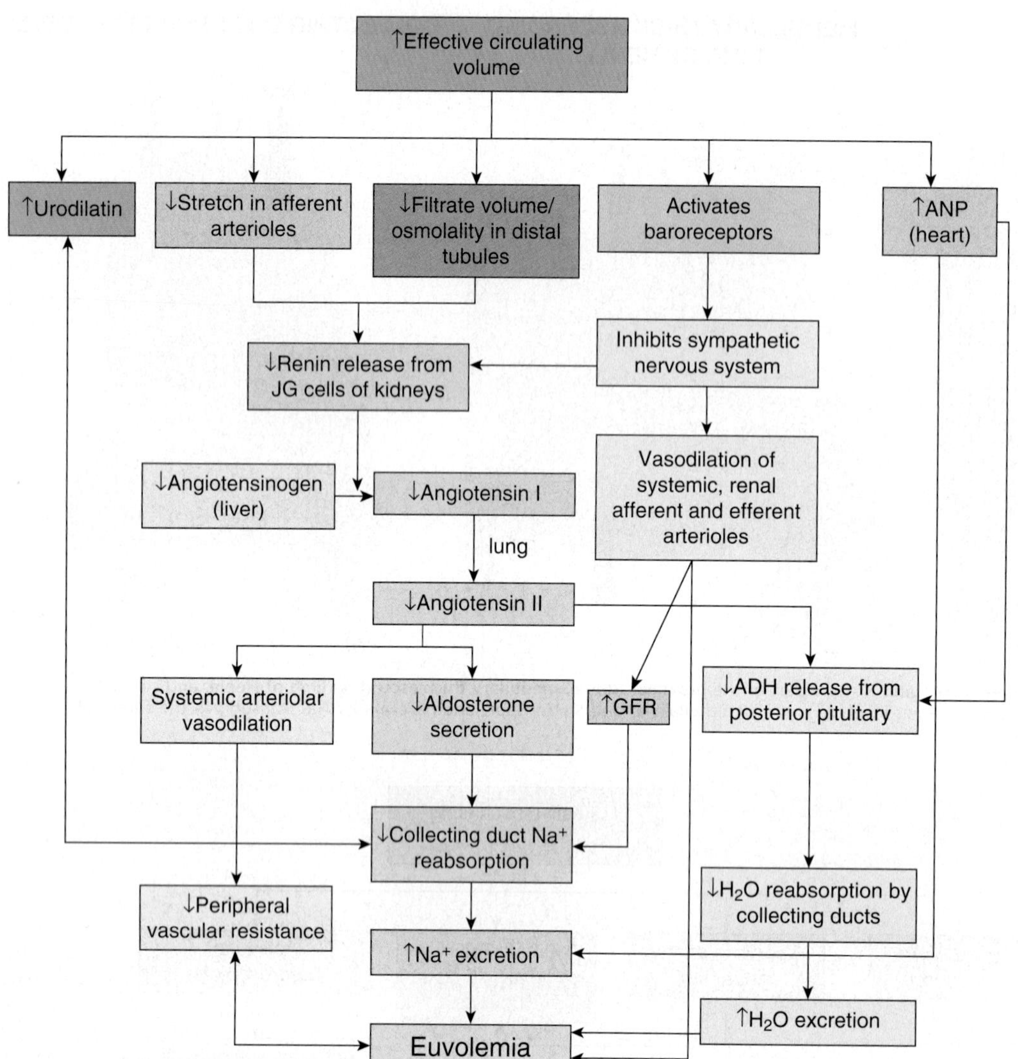

FIGURE 10-7 • Compensatory changes in renal sodium and water handling in response to an increase in effective circulating volume (ECV). ADH, antidiuretic hormone; ANP, atrial natriuretic peptide; JG, juxtaglomerular cells of the afferent arteriole.

ADH secretion by the posterior pituitary gland and, together with urodilatin, ADH action at the collecting tubule (Fig. 10-7).

POTASSIUM BALANCE

K+ Distribution in Body Fluids

The total body K+ content in humans is estimated to be approximately 50 mEq/kg body weight. Roughly 98% of K+ is distributed in the intracellular compartment, the result of active K+ uptake by the Na+-K+-ATPase in the cell membrane. The remaining 2% of K+ is located in the extracellular pool.[19] K+ intake based on a typical Western diet averages 70 mEq/day. Adolescents may consume larger amounts of K+, whereas elderly individuals may have more restricted K+ intake. Vegetarians who consume large amounts of K+–rich vegetables and fruits, may consume up to 275 mEq of K+ per day.[20] Urban white populations generally consume more K+ than their African-American counterparts.[21] Under normal conditions, excretion balances intake, with renal mechanisms accounting for 90% of excreted K+. The remaining 10% of K+ excretion occurs principally in the stool. Normal fecal K+ excretion averages about 9 mEq/day.[22] The bulk of intestinal K+ absorption, in K+–replete individuals, occurs in the small intestine, whereas the colon contributes little to net K+ absorption and secretion under basal conditions. K+ is absorbed or secreted mainly by passive mechanisms; the rectum and perhaps the sigmoid colon have the capacity to secrete actively K+, but the quantitative and physiologic significance of this active secretion is uncertain.

The internal K+ distribution needs to be tightly regulated, because movement of a mere 1% to 2% of K+ from the intracellular to the extracellular fluid compartment can result in a potentially fatal increase in plasma [K+]. Transcellular K+ redistribution can change the plasma K+ concentration without total body K+. Several hormones, including catecholamines, aldosterone, and insulin, promote increased Na+-K+-ATPase activity, net cellular K+ uptake, and hypokalemia. Metabolic alkalosis or alkalemia promotes net K+ uptake in exchange for the buffering effects of net H+ efflux. Conversely, metabolic acidosis produced by inorganic acids (e.g., HCl, H_2SO_4) promotes reciprocal H+ uptake and K+ efflux. In contrast, acute and chronic respiratory alkalosis or acidosis has only minor effects on intracellular : extracellular K+ balance and plasma [K+]. Increases in plasma osmolality cause cell volume reductions that elevate intracellular [K+], producing a driving force for K+ efflux and a resultant increase in plasma [K+]. Hypoosmolality has the opposite effect.

K+ Handling along the Nephron

The proximal tubule reabsorbs about 67% of the filtered K+, and the medullary thick ascending limb of Henle's loop reabsorbs another 20% as a constant fraction of the amount filtered (Fig. 10-8). In contrast, cells of the distal tubule and collecting duct have the dual ability to reabsorb and secrete K+, processes that are highly regulated by multiple hormones and other factors (see Fig. 10-8). Indeed, the principal mechanism for urinary K+ excretion is the action of principal cells of the distal tubule and collecting duct to secrete excess K+ from the blood

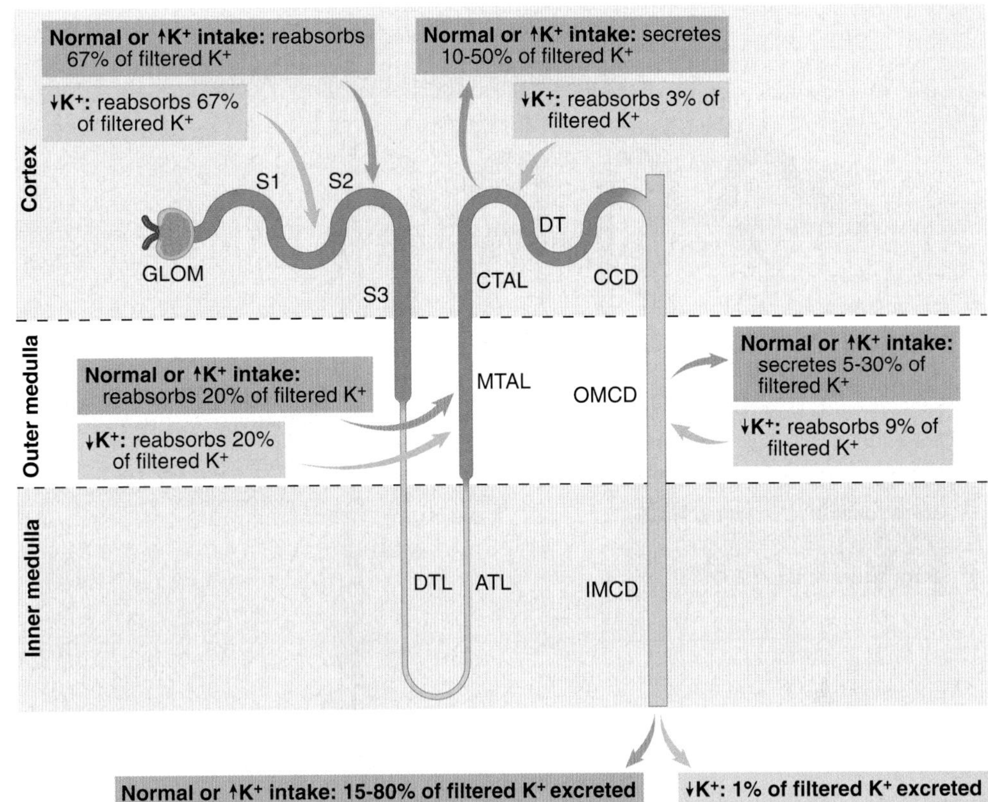

FIGURE 10-8 • Segmental potassium handling along the nephron under normal conditions and conditions of potassium excess or deficit. The magnitude of transport and key transport pathways and regulators.

into the tubular fluid.[23] ROMK (KCNJ1) K^+ channels in the apical membranes of principal cells are primarily responsible for determining K^+ permeability of the apical membrane and, hence, K^+ secretion (see Fig. 10-5). The activity and number of the apical ENaC Na^+ channels and basolateral Na^+-K^+-ATPase generate the electrochemical gradient favoring K^+ secretion through ROMK channels and are thus key regulatory steps in the process.

Responses to Changes in K^+ Intake

During states of K^+ deficiency, all but about 1% of the filtered K^+ is reclaimed (see Fig. 10-8), the result primarily of enhanced endocytosis of ROMK channels from the apical membrane of principal cells and consequent reductions in K^+ secretion by the distal tubule and collecting duct. In addition, intercalated cells of the outer and inner medullary collecting ducts may reabsorb K^+ to reclaim it before it is lost in the urine. Therefore, net transport of K^+ results from varying rates of K^+ secretion through principal cells and K^+ reabsorption through intercalated cells. Luminal, peritubular, and systemic factors regulate K^+ transport in these segments. Luminal factors include the rate of distal fluid and Na^+ delivery and the Na^+ and Cl^- concentrations in the fluid entering the distal tubule or cortical collecting duct.[23] Peritubular factors that affect net K^+ transport in these segments include changes in ion concentrations (K^+, H^+, and HCO_3^-) and hormones (aldosterone and ADH).[23] Systemic factors including K^+ intake, acid-base balance, adrenal steroid hormones, and ADH also regulate net K^+ transport.[23]

Excess K^+ intake results in increased plasma [K^+], which prompts (i) increased activity of the ROMK channel in the apical membrane of principal cells; (ii) inhibition of proximal tubule NaCl and H_2O reabsorption, thereby increasing distal tubule and collecting duct flow rate, a potent stimulus for K^+ secretion; and (iii) increased aldosterone secretion, which up-regulates the major components of K^+ secretion in principal cells (apical ROMK and Na^+ channels and basolateral Na^+K^+-ATPase). These concerted actions result in urinary excretion of the excess K^+.

ACID-BASE BALANCE

Normal humans on a Western diet of normal caloric intake will generate, through fat and carbohydrate metabolism, approximately 20,000 mEq of acid daily in the form of CO_2 eliminated by the lungs. Protein catabolism generates about 50 mEq to 60 mEq per day of inorganic, nonvolatile acids (e.g., sulfuric, phosphoric, or hydrochloric acids), which must be excreted by the kidney. In addition, the kidney must reclaim filtered HCO_3^- to maintain acid-base balance.

Bicarbonate Reabsorption/Proton Secretion along the Nephron

HCO_3^- reabsorption of the filtered load is virtually complete along the nephron under normal conditions[24] (Fig. 10-9). About 80% of the filtered load is reabsorbed in the proximal tubule in a process critically dependent on Na^+-H^+ exchanger NHE3 and carbonic anhydrase at the apical membrane. H^+ secreted into the lumen in exchange for Na^+ combines with filtered HCO_3^-, and it is converted via the action of carbonic anhydrase into CO_2 and H_2O (see Fig. 10-5). The CO_2 freely diffuses across the luminal membrane into the cell, where it is hydrated in the presence of carbonic anhydrase to H_2CO_3. The intracellular H_2CO_3 then dissociates into HCO_3^-, which is reabsorbed across the basolateral membrane, and H^+, which is secreted into the luminal fluid. Thus, the HCO_3^- actually reabsorbed is not that which was originally the filtrate, but the net effect is the same as if this were the case. Because of their interdependence, HCO_3^- reabsorption generally parallels the rate of proximal tubule Na^+ reabsorption. An H^+-ATPase in the apical membrane of proximal tubule participates in Na^+-independent HCO_3^- reabsorption. The thick ascending limb of Henle reabsorbs another 15% of filtered HCO_3^- by transport mechanisms similar to those operating in the proximal tubule (see Fig. 10-5).[25] The distal tubule and collecting duct reabsorb the small amount of HCO_3^- that escapes the more proximal segments.[26] A number of factors, including ECFV, Ang II, aldosterone, and plasma K^+ concentration, regulate HCO_3^- reabsorption along the nephron.

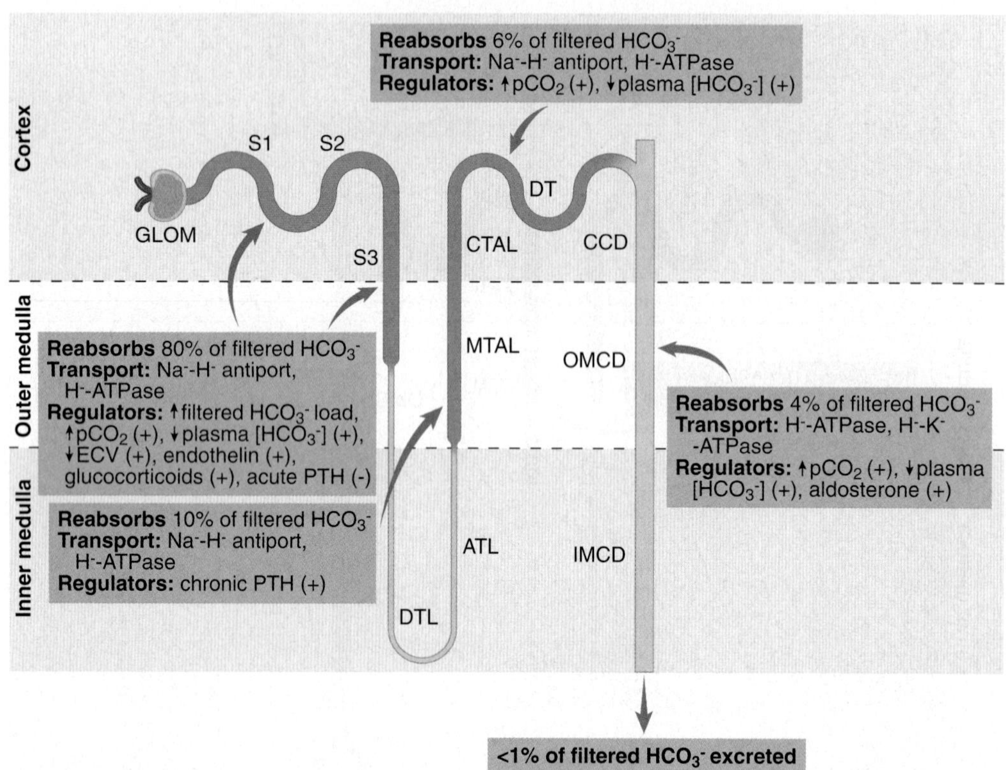

FIGURE 10-9 • Basal bicarbonate handling along the nephron. The key transport pathways and regulators.

Other bases besides HCO_3^- may buffer H^+ secreted into the distal tubules, and H^+ may combine with ammonia also secreted by the tubules. The principal non-HCO_3^- base in the tubular fluid is dibasic sodium phosphate (Na_2HPO_4), which can accept H^+ to form monobasic sodium phosphate (NaH_2PO_4). *Titratable acidity* of the urine refers to the amount of urinary H^+ buffered by bases such as HCO_3^- and phosphate. It is measured by titrating the urine with strong base until the pH of the plasma from which the filtrate is derived is reached.

Under physiologic conditions, about two thirds of the H^+ to be secreted in the urine is in the form of ammonium salts. To be appropriately excreted in urine, NH_4^+ must be synthesized by proximal tubular cells, secreted into the proximal tubular fluid, reabsorbed by the medullary thick ascending limb to be accumulated in the medullary interstitium, and finally secreted in medullary collecting ducts. Ammonia (NH_3) is absent from the plasma and glomerular ultrafiltrate but is formed, along with glutamic acid, from the hydrolysis of glutamine by the enzyme glutaminase. A further molecule of NH_3 arises from the deamination of glutamic acid to form glutaric acid, which is then metabolized. The NH_3 so formed passes into the lumen, where it combines with secreted H^+ to form NH_4^+, which, as a charged molecule, is then trapped in the lumen. The NH_4^+ is excreted in the urine as ammonium salts of excess anions (e.g., chloride, sulfate, and phosphate). Increasing acid accumulation stimulates production of NH_4^+ by the tubular cells. The rhesus glycoproteins RhBG and RhCG are expressed in the renal connecting segment and collecting duct and thought to mediate Na^+- and K^+-independent NH_4^+ transport. Electroneutral NH_4^+/H^+ exchange is also present in the collecting duct.[27] Key enzymes involved in ammoniagenesis (mitochondrial glutaminase and glutamate dehydrogenase) and gluconeogenesis (phosphoenolpyruvate carboxykinase) by the proximal tubule, the apical Na^+-K^+(NH_4^+)-$2Cl^-$ cotransporter of the medullary thick ascending limb, and the basolateral Na^+-K^+(NH_4^+)-$2Cl^-$ cotransporter of medullary collecting ducts are key steps in chronic adaptation to acid-base changes, and targets of regulation by acid pH and glucocorticoids.

Thus, H^+ secretion can be considered as the integration of three processes: reabsorption of filtered HCO_3^- in the proximal tubule, and in the distal nephron, formation of both monobasic phosphate and ammonium salts. Accordingly, the total tubular H^+ secretion represents the sum of the amount of HCO_3^- reabsorbed, the amount of titratable acid, and the amount of NH_4^+ excreted.

CALCIUM BALANCE

Ca^{2+} plays an important role in many vital biologic processes, including neurotransmission, muscle contraction, blood clotting, and is a key component of the extracellular matrix and bone. Overall Ca^{2+} balance is maintained by controlling the distribution of Ca^{2+} between bone and the ECF, net Ca^{2+} absorption by the intestine, and net Ca^{2+} excretion by the kidney. PTH, calcitriol, and to a lesser extent, calcitonin regulate the plasma [Ca^{2+}] by governing the Ca^{2+} distribution between bone and plasma (Fig. 10-10).

Gastrointestinal and Renal Handling of Calcium

The average dietary intake of Ca^{2+} is 1500 mg/day, and about 200 mg of this ingested Ca^{2+} is absorbed by the gastrointestinal tract (though this amount can triple when calcitriol levels increase) and matched by renal excretion. The 1300 mg/day of ingested Ca^{2+} that escapes gastrointestinal absorption is eliminated in the stool. In the intestinal epithelial cells, Ca^{2+} crosses the apical membrane via the Ca^{2+}-selective channel TRPV6 down a steep inward electrochemical gradient. In the cell, Ca^{2+} is bound to calbindin-D_{9K}, which ferries Ca^{2+} from the apical side to the basolateral side of the cell where the plasma membrane Ca^{2+}-ATPase (PMCA1b) extrudes Ca^{2+} into the blood compartment. Both calcitriol and dietary Ca^{2+} can independently regulate expression of the Ca^{2+} transport proteins[28] in the intestine (see Fig. 10-10).

Under normal conditions, 99% of the filtered Ca^{2+} is reabsorbed by the nephron. The proximal tubule reabsorbs 70% and the thick ascending limb of Henle an additional 20% of the filtered Ca^{2+} (Fig. 10-11). The distal tubule and collecting duct actively reabsorb about 9% and 1%, respectively. Transcellular Ca^{2+} reabsorption by the proximal tubule occurs via Ca^{2+} entry across the brush border membrane through a Ca^{2+}-permeable channel and Ca^{2+} exit across the basolateral membrane via the Ca^{2+}-ATPase. A substantial portion of Ca^{2+} reabsorption in the proximal tubule also occurs through paracellular path-

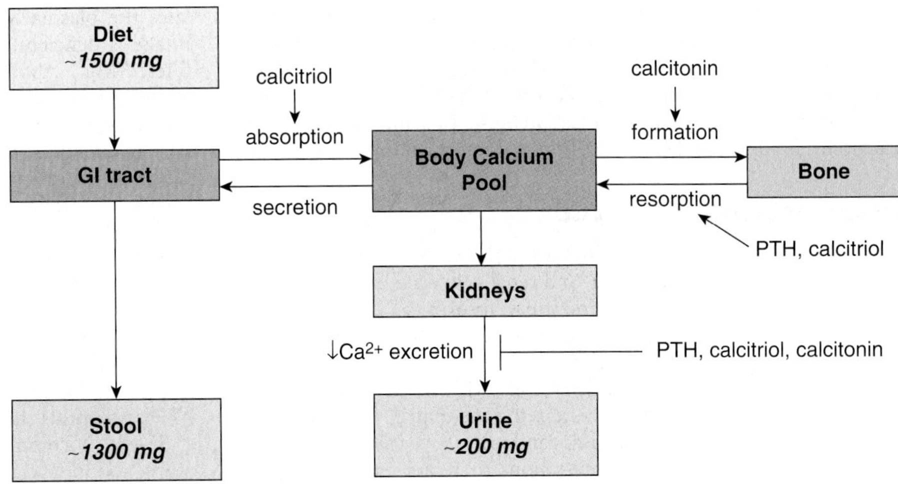

FIGURE 10-10 • Factors controlling body Ca^{2+} homeostasis. PTH, parathyroid hormone.

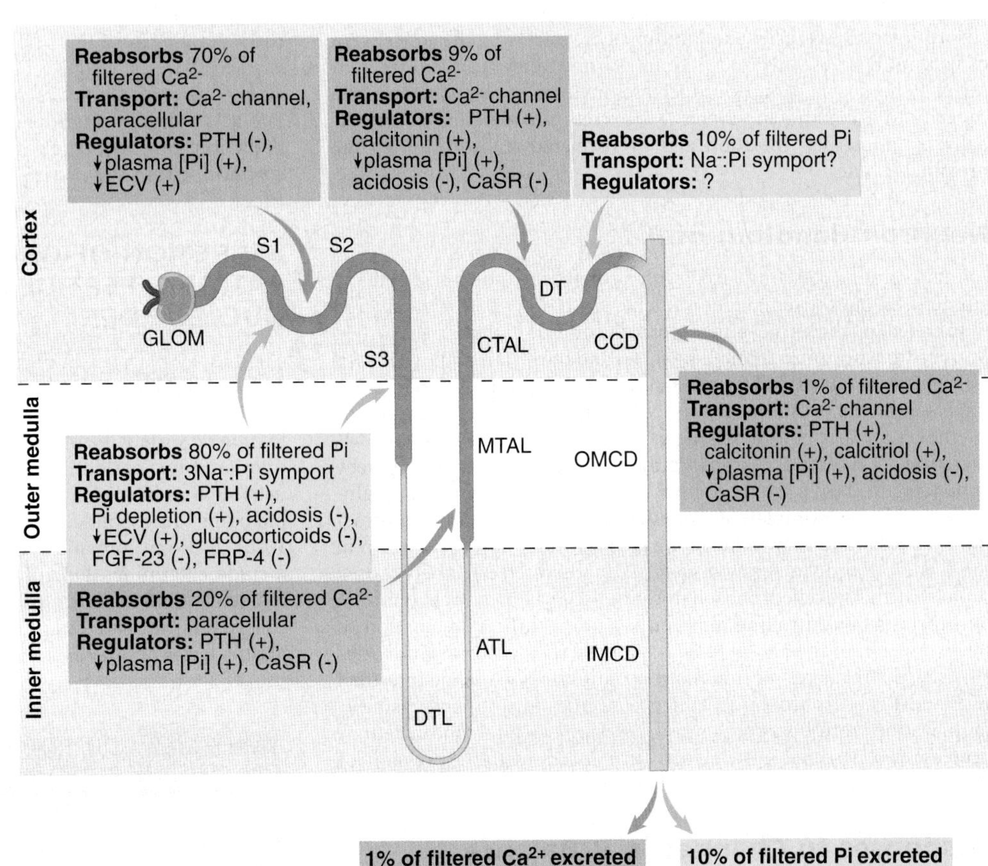

FIGURE 10-11 • **Calcium and phosphorus handling along the nephron.** The magnitude of transport and key transport pathways and regulators.

ways driven by solvent drag. In the thick ascending limb of Henle, Ca^{2+} reabsorption occurs by the paracellular pathway driven by the transepithelial electrochemical gradient for Ca^{2+} and regulated by the tight junction proteins claudin-16 and paracellin (PCLN-1).[29,30] Active Ca^{2+} reabsorption is restricted to the distal tubule and the connecting tubule. At the cellular level, Ca^{2+} enters these cells via the Ca^{2+}-selective channels TRPV5 and TRPV6, binds to calbindin, and is ferried from the apical side to the basolateral side where the $3Na^+$-Ca^{2+}-exchanger (NCX1) and the plasma membrane Ca^{2+}-ATPase (PMCA1b) extrude Ca^{2+} into the blood compartment.[31] PTH and vitamin D stimulate Ca^{2+} reabsorption in the thick ascending limb of Henle and distal tubule. ECFV status and acid-base balance also influence renal Ca^{2+} handling.

Various studies have demonstrated the regulatory roles of calcitriol, estrogens, PTH, and dietary Ca^{2+} in expression of the renal Ca^{2+} transport proteins. In addition, the Ca^{2+}-sensing receptor (CaSR)[32] in the thick ascending limb of Henle and distal tubule senses the Ca^{2+} demand and activates a cascade of pathways, eventually leading to the synthesis and release of calciotropic hormones, including calcitriol, PTH, and calcitonin. These hormones act in a paracrine fashion, efficiently regulating the previously described Ca^{2+} transport processes.[28]

Responses to Changes in Ca^{2+} Balance

Hypocalcemia stimulates the CaSR in parathyroid gland chief cells, which in turn activates PTH synthesis and release. PTH restores plasma

$[Ca^{2+}]$ levels by stimulating bone resorption, renal Ca^{2+} reabsorption, and calcitriol production, which promotes gastrointestinal and renal reabsorption of Ca^{2+} as well as Ca^{2+} release from the bone. Hypercalcemia stimulates the secretion of calcitonin, which blocks bone resorption and stimulates deposition of Ca^{2+} in bone. To a much lesser extent, calcitonin inhibits renal Ca^{2+} excretion and intestinal Ca^{2+} absorption.

PHOSPHORUS BALANCE

P_i is an important component of many cellular synthetic and metabolic reactions, skeletal mineralization, and renal acid excretion. P_i homeostasis is achieved by adjusting intestinal absorption, exchange with intracellular and bone storage pools, and renal tubular reabsorption. The skeleton represents the largest (85%) store of P_i, primarily complexed with Ca^{2+} in hydroxyapatite crystals, which constitute the main inorganic component of the mineralized bone matrix. About 15% of P_i is located in the intracellular fluid, and only 0.3% is in the extracellular fluid. Normal serum concentrations of P_i are relatively tightly regulated and range in adults from 2.5 mg/dl to 4.5 mg/dl. P_i values in children are substantially higher and vary with age (the younger the child, the higher the P_i). P_i is abundant in the diet, and intestinal absorption of P_i is efficient and minimally regulated by the active form of vitamin D, 1,25-dihydroxyvitamin D. The kidney is a major regulator of P_i homeostasis and can increase or decrease its P_i reabsorptive capacity to accommodate P_i need. P_i excretion is determined principally by glomerular filtration and by regulated reabsorption in the proximal tubule.

Nephron Handling of P_i

About 10% of P_i is complexed with protein and not filtered at the glomerulus, but the remainder is filtered, with only 10% of the filtered P_i excreted in the urine under normal conditions. P_i is reabsorbed primarily by the proximal tubule (~80%) and the distal tubule (~10%)[33] (see Fig. 10-11). Proximal tubule P_i reabsorption occurs by apical entry mediated by the brush border $3Na^+$-P_i symporter (NPT2a) and basolateral exit by a P_i-anion exchanger. PTH is the major regulator of P_i excretion. PTH inhibits P_i reabsorption by the proximal tubule, thereby enhancing urinary P_i excretion. Acidosis, volume expansion, and glucocorticoids also stimulate P_i excretion. In contrast, volume contraction, alkalosis, and growth hormone are known to limit P_i excretion in the urine.[33] Fibroblast growth factor-23 and secreted frizzled-related protein 4, the so-called phosphatonins, also play a central role in P_i homeostasis by controlling renal reabsorption through regulation of the expression of the $3Na^+$-P_i NT2a symporters.[34] In normal individuals, calcitriol regulates serum P_i concentrations by increasing intestinal Ca^{2+} and P_i absorption and, at high concentrations, by increasing P_i mobilization from bone.[35] This rise in serum calcium concentrations decreases PTH secretion, which in turn increases the expression of NPT2a.[36]

Responses to Changes in P_i Balance

Compensatory changes to restore P_i balance are tightly coupled to those of Ca^{2+}. Increases in P_i loading, PTH levels, ECFV all favor increased urinary P_i excretion, as do acidosis and glucocorticoids. In contrast, urinary P_i excretion is inhibited by decreased P_i stores, PTH levels, and ECF or with alkalosis or growth hormone excess. Hypophosphatemia is also a potent stimulus for the metabolism of calcifediol to calcitriol in the kidneys, which ultimately inhibits urinary P_i excretion and stimulates intestinal P_i absorption to restore plasma $[P_i]$.

MAGNESIUM BALANCE

Mg^{2+} is the second most common cation in the intracellular fluid and an important cofactor for important biologic processes, such as protein synthesis, cellular energy metabolism, and neuromuscular excitability. The balance of intestinal absorption and renal excretion tightly regulates the plasma Mg^{2+} concentration. In addition, when total Mg^{2+} intake is deficient, the kidney is capable of reabsorbing virtually all filtered Mg^{2+}. Approximately 80% of the total plasma Mg^{2+} is filtered at the glomerulus and subsequently reabsorbed in consecutive segments of the nephron.[37] The proximal tubule reabsorbs about 10% to 15% of the filtered Mg^{2+}, whereas the bulk (~60%) of filtered Mg^{2+} is reabsorbed in the cortical thick ascending limb via paracellular pathways by paracellin-1, a recently characterized tight junction protein that mediates renal epithelial Mg^{2+} and Ca^{2+} transport, driven by the transepithelial voltage.[38] The distal tubule reabsorbs the remaining 5% to 10% of filtered Mg^{2+} and serves as the final arbiter of urinary Mg^{2+} excretion. Apical Mg^{2+} entry is mediated by transient receptor potential (TRP) melastatin 6 (TRPM6) (and TRPM7), with extrusion across the basolateral membrane believed to occur via a Na^+/Mg^{2+} exchanger and/or ATP-dependent Mg^{2+} pump.[39] The γ-subunit of the Na^+-K^+-ATPase controls the transepithelial Mg^{2+} transport in this segment.[40]

Several hormones and nonhormonal factors influence renal Mg^{2+} reabsorption to variable extent in the cortical thick ascending limb of Henle and distal tubule. In states of dietary magnesium restriction, urinary Mg^{2+} excretion decreases through adaptation of magnesium transport in both the cortical thick ascending limb of Henle and the distal tubule. Elevation of plasma Mg^{2+} concentration is sensed by an extracellular Ca^{2+}/Mg^{2+}-sensing receptor located on the peritubular side of the cortical thick ascending limb of Henle and distal tubule cells and acts to inhibit Mg^{2+} reabsorption.[41] Metabolic acidosis, potassium depletion, or phosphate restriction results in diminished Mg^{2+} reabsorption within the cortical thick ascending limb of Henle and distal tubule.[38]

SECRETION OF ORGANIC ANIONS, CATIONS, PEPTIDES, AND NUCLEOTIDES

The kidney plays an important role in the elimination of numerous hydrophilic xenobiotics, including drugs, toxins, and endogenous compounds. The proximal tubule is the primary site of active transport for a wide variety of substrates, including organic anions/cations, peptides, and nucleosides. Anionic compounds include metabolic products, such as bile salts, urate, and oxalate, and commonly used drugs, including furosemide, penicillin, and hydrochlorothiazide (Table 10-2). Cationic organic molecules secreted by the proximal tubule include creatinine, dopamine, and epinephrine, as well as atropine, morphine, and other drugs (see Table 10-2). All organic compounds compete for the same transporter in the proximal tubule, so that high plasma levels of one organic ion can limit the secretion of the others.[42]

TABLE 10-2 SOME ORGANIC ANIONS AND CATIONS SECRETED BY THE PROXIMAL TUBULE

	Cations	Anions
Endogenous	Creatinine Dopamine Epinephrine Norepinephrine	cAMP, cGMP Ascorbate Folate Oxalate PGE_2, PGE_{2a} Urate Hippurates Bile salts
Drugs	Amiloride Cimetidine Quinine Procainamide Isoproterenol Morphine Atropine	NSAIDs Furosemide Bumetanide Hydrochlorothiazide Acetazolamide Salicylates Probenecid Penicillin

cAMP, cyclic adenosine monophosphate; cGMP, cyclic guanosine monophosphate; NSAIDs, nonsteroidal anti-inflammatory drugs; PGE_2, prostaglandin E_2; PGE_{2a}, prostaglandin E_{2a}.

The primary transporters of organic anions and cations on the basolateral membrane of proximal tubule cells are members of the organic anion transporter (OAT) (mainly OAT1 and OAT3) and organic cation transporter (OCT) families.[43] Gender, sex hormones, aging, diuretic therapy, and experimentally induced (in rats) hyperuricemia all influence the intrarenal expression patterns of certain OAT family members. The sulfate-anion antiporter 1 (SAT-1) may also contribute to organic anion transport at the basolateral membrane.[44] On the apical membrane of the proximal tubule, the multidrug-resistance–associated protein 2 (MRP2) functions as an efflux pump for more hydrophobic molecules and anionic conjugates.[45] Tubular reabsorption of peptide-like drugs such as β-lactam antibiotics and valacyclovir across the brush-border membranes appears to be mediated by two distinct H^+/peptide cotransporters: PEPT1 and PEPT2.[46] Along with drug-metabolizing enzymes, these transporters are important determinants of drug effectiveness and toxicity. A cDNA coding a new H^+/organic cation antiporter, human kidney-specific multidrug and toxin extrusion-2 (hMATE2-K), has been isolated from the human kidney and found to localize at the brush-border membranes of the proximal tubules.[47]

Several human urate transporters have recently been identified, including urate transporter-1 (URAT1), MRP2, OAT1, and OAT3.[48] URAT1 appears to be the central mediator of renal urate reabsorption and the target site for current and possibly future primary uricosuric agents.[49] URAT1 exhibits highly specific urate transport activity, exchanging this anion with others that are known to affect renal uric acid transport, including most endogenous organic anions and drug anions (e.g., the monocarboxylate metabolite of pyrazinamide).[50] URAT1 localizes selectively to the apical membrane of proximal tubule cell and mediates a non–voltage-dependent exchange. "Loss of function" mutations in the gene encoding URAT1 (*SLC22A12*) result in hypouricemia and hyperuricosuria in affected individuals.[51] Of clinical relevance, the uricosuric drugs probenecid, benzbromarone, sulfinpyrazone, and losartan potently suppress URAT1-mediated urate reabsorption by the proximal tubule.

A transport system for net transepithelial secretion of various hydrophobic organic anions has been described in the proximal tubule. This tertiary active transport process involves an organic anion/α-ketoglutarate exchange process in the basolateral membrane, Na^+-dicarboxylate cotransporters at both membranes, and an inwardly directed Na^+ gradient driving α-ketoglutarate uptake generated and maintained by the basolateral Na^+-K^+-ATPase. The transport of the organic anion into the cells against its electrochemical gradient occurs in exchange for α-ketoglutarate moving out of the cells down its electrochemical gradient. The outwardly directed gradient for α-ketoglutarate is maintained by metabolism and by transport into the cells by Na^+-dicarboxylate cotransporters. The inwardly Na^+ gradient–driving α-ketoglutarate uptake is in turn generated and maintained by the basolateral Na^+-K^+-ATPase. The basolateral organic acid/α-ketoglutarate exchange process appears to be regulated by peptide hormones, growth factors, and the autonomic nervous system.[52]

DIURETICS, AQUARETICS, AND NATRIURETICS: SITES AND MECHANISMS OF ACTIONS

A number of diuretic agents and other drugs target specific transport proteins or enzymes to effect their action (Table 10-3) (see also Chapters 22, Hypertension; and 26, Heart Failure). *Osmotic diuretics*, such as mannitol, inhibit fluid reabsorption by altering the osmotic driving forces along the nephron.[53] These agents are filtered at the glomerulus and are generally not reabsorbed by the tubules, so they remain in the tubular lumen to exert an osmotic pressure to oppose water reabsorption. This effect is most prominent in the segments that are constitutively water permeable (i.e., the proximal tubule and the thin descending limb of Henle). Other classes of diuretics act on specific membrane transport proteins or enzymes coupled to salt and water transport. *Carbonic anhydrase inhibitors* (i.e., acetazolamide), inhibit proximal Na^+ reabsorption. HCO_3^- reabsorption depends to a large extent on Na^+ (the Na-H exchanger in the proximal tubule apical membrane) (see Fig. 10-5).[54] This enzyme facilitates the formation of H^+ and HCO_3^- from CO_2 and H_2O. About one third of all proximal tubule Na^+ reabsorption is related to this process of HCO_3^- reabsorption. Carbonic anhydrase inhibitors inhibit only 5% to 10% of the filtered Na^+ load, in part because more distal segments, in particular the thick ascending limb, increase Na^+ reabsorption when Na^+ delivery is increased. *Loop diuretics* (e.g., furosemide, bumetanide, torsemide, ethacrynic acid) potently inhibit Na^+ absorption by blocking the NKCC2 cotransporter of the apical membrane of the thick ascending limb of Henle (see Fig. 10-5).[55] This action not only inhibits Na^+ reabsorption but also limits the kidney's ability both to concentrate and to dilute the urine. Loop diuretics promote an increase in Na^+ excretion that may reach 25% of the filtered load. The thick ascending limb is a major site of Ca^{2+} and Mg^{2+} reabsorption, processes that are dependent on normal Na^+ and Cl^- reabsorption. Therefore, loop diuretics increase urinary water, Na^+, K^+, Ca^{2+}, and Mg^{2+} excretion. *Thiazide diuretics* (e.g., chlorothiazide, metolazone, hydrochlorothiazide) inhibit Na^+

TABLE 10-3 DIURETICS, AQUARETICS, AND NATRIURETIC PEPTIDES: CLASSES AND MECHANISMS OF ACTIONS

Class	Site of Action	Mechanism inhibited	Filtered Na^+ Excreted in Urine (%)	Free H_2O Excretion	Free H_2O Reabsorption
Osmotic diuretics (e.g., mannitol)	Proximal tubule, TDL	Osmotic gradient for NaCl reabsorption	10	↑	↑
Carbonic anhydrase inhibitors (e.g., acetazolamide)	Proximal tubule	Na^+-H^+ exchange indirectly	5-10	↑	↑
Thiazide diuretics (e.g., hydrochlorothiazide)	Early distal tubule	NaCl cotransporter	5-10	↓	↓
Loop diuretics (e.g., furosemide)	TAL	Na^+-K^+-$2Cl^-$ cotransporter	20-25	↓	No change
Potassium-sparing diuretics [e.g., (a) amiloride, (b) spironalactone]	Collecting ducts	(a) Apical Na^+ channels; (b) aldosterone-stimulated Na^+ transport	1-2	No change	No change
Aquaretics (e.g., conivaptan)	Collecting ducts	Vasopressin V2 receptors	0	↑	↓
Natriuretic peptides (e.g., BNP)	Collecting ducts	cGMP-coupled Na^+ transport	2-3	↑	?

BNP, brain natriuretic peptide; cGMP, cyclic guanosine monophosphate; TAL, medullary thick ascending limb of Henle; TDL, thin descending limb of Henle.

reabsorption by blocking the NaCl cotransport in the apical membrane of the early distal tubule.[56] Thiazides also reduce the ability to dilute the urine, but because they do not interrupt the countercurrent multiplication system, they do not impair urinary concentration. Natriuresis with thiazides may approach 5% to 10% of the filtered load. By blocking sequential steps in Na^+ reabsorption along the nephron, the combined use of a loop diuretic and a thiazide diuretic results in even greater diuretic and natriuretic effect than either agent alone. *K^+-sparing diuretics* act on the late distal tubule and cortical collecting duct and work either by antagonizing aldosterone's action on the principal cells of the collecting duct (e.g., spironolactone), or by inhibiting apical membrane Na^+ channels in these cells (e.g., amiloride, triamterene) (see Fig. 10-5). Accordingly, these agents produce a natriuresis of only about 3% of the filtered load, but concomitantly inhibit K^+ secretion in the collecting duct and thereby limit urinary K^+ wasting.[57]

Because Na^+ is by far the most abundant cation present in proximal tubule fluid, it is the major cation that accompanies HCO_3^- out of the proximal tubule. When the increased Na^+ and HCO_3^- load reaches the distal nephron, Na^+ is largely reabsorbed; however, HCO_3^- is not reabsorbed. The distal nephron then secretes K^+ in exchange for the Na^+ that is reabsorbed. Hence, acetazolamide primarily causes an increase in urinary HCO_3^-, K^+, and water excretion.

The ability of a diuretic to promote urinary Na^+ excretion is dependent on the diuretic dose, the amount of Na^+ typically reabsorbed by the nephron segment it targets, and the capacity of more distal segments to compensate, by increasing reabsorption, for the excess amounts of Na^+. Most diuretics act at the apical membrane of the tubules to impair Na^+ entry mechanisms, so that there is a dose-dependent relationship between the rate of presentation of the diuretic to its site of action and the Na^+ absorption it inhibits. Loop diuretics are more potent than thiazide or K^+-sparing diuretics because they target a segment that reabsorbs much more Na^+. Finally, when counterregulatory responses of more distal segments are fully activated, as they are in congestive heart failure, for example, a given dose of loop diuretic will provoke less natriuresis than in normal subjects because of increased Na^+ reabsorption by the distal tubule and collecting duct. Provided the diuretic dose is constant, these counterregulatory responses typically lead to the establishment of a new steady state in which Na^+ intake balances Na^+ excretion within the first 2 weeks of diuretic therapy.[58] In general, fluid and electrolyte complications associated with diuretics occur within this adaptive 2-week period.

Vasopressin receptor antagonists are currently in late-stage clinical trials (lixivaptan, stavaptan, and tolvaptan) or have entered clinical use (conivaptan).[45] These agents are termed *aquaretics* because they promote free water diuresis without natriuresis or kaliuresis. Clinical trials have demonstrated that these antagonists increase free water excretion and serum sodium concentrations in patients with hyponatremia owing to the syndrome of inappropriate ADH secretion, refractory congestive heart failure, or cirrhosis.[59]

Recombinant human BNP, nesiritide, is approved in the United States for treatment of patients with acutely decompensated congestive heart failure who exhibit dyspnea at rest or with minimal activity.[60] In healthy volunteers, nesiritide maintains and perhaps even improves GFR, maintains RBF, and exerts modest diuretic and natriuretic effects. Direct tubular effects of BNP include inhibition of Ang II in the proximal tubules, vasopressin in the cortical collecting ducts, and Na^+ reabsorption in the medullary collecting duct. In some, but not all, studies, nesiritide has been shown to cause natriuresis and diuresis and to maintain GFR in patients with heart failure.[61]

REFERENCES

1. Kawachi H, Miyauchi N, Suzuki K, et al. Role of podocyte slit diaphragm as a filtration barrier. Nephrology (Carlton) 2006;11(4):274-281.
2. Peti-Peterdi J. Confocal imaging and function of the juxtaglomerular apparatus. Curr Opin Nephrol Hypertens 2005;14(1):53-57.
3. Fellner SK, Arendshorst WJ. Angiotensin II, reactive oxygen species, and Ca^{2+} signaling in afferent arterioles. Am J Physiol Renal Physiol 2005;289(5):F1012-F1019.
4. Just A, Arendshorst WJ. Dynamics and contribution of mechanisms mediating renal blood flow autoregulation. Am J Physiol Regul Integr Comp Physiol 2003;285(3): R619-R631.
5. Cockett AT. Lymphatic network of kidney. I. Anatomic and physiologic considerations. Urology 1977;9(2):125-129.
6. DiBona GF. Neural control of the kidney: functionally specific renal sympathetic nerve fibers. Am J Physiol Regul Integr Comp Physiol 2000;279(5):R1517-R1524.
7. Vallon V, Verkman AS, Schnermann J. Luminal hypotonicity in proximal tubules of aquaporin-1-knockout mice. Am J Physiol Renal Physiol 2000;278(6):F1030-F1033.
8. Peti-Peterdi J. Calcium wave of tubuloglomerular feedback. Am J Physiol Renal Physiol 2006;291(2):F473-F480.
9. Schnermann J, Levine DZ. Paracrine factors in tubuloglomerular feedback: adenosine, ATP, and nitric oxide. Annu Rev Physiol 2003;65:501-529.
10. Navar LG. Renal autoregulation: perspectives from whole kidney and single nephron studies. Am J Physiol 1978;234(5):F357-F370.
11. Verbalis JG. Whole-body volume regulation and escape from antidiuresis. Am J Med 2006;119(7 Suppl 1):S21-S29.
12. Pallone TL, Turner MR, Edwards A, Jamison RL. Countercurrent exchange in the renal medulla. Am J Physiol Regul Integr Comp Physiol 2003;284(5):R1153-R1175.
13. Frokiaer J, Nielsen S, Knepper MA. Molecular physiology of renal aquaporins and sodium transporters: exciting approaches to understand regulation of renal water handling. J Am Soc Nephrol 2005;16(10):2827-2879.
14. Robben JH, Knoers NV, Deen PM. Cell biological aspects of the vasopressin type-2 receptor and aquaporin 2 water channel in nephrogenic diabetes insipidus. Am J Physiol Renal Physiol 2006;291(2):F257-F270.
15. Evans RG, Majid DS, Eppel GA. Mechanisms mediating pressure natriuresis: what we know and what we need to find out. Clin Exp Pharmacol Physiol 2005;32(5-6):400-409.
16. Aronson PS. Ion exchangers mediating Na^+, HCO_3^- and Cl^- transport in the renal proximal tubule. J Nephrol 2006;19(Suppl 9):S3-S10.
17. Wang WH. Regulation of ROMK (Kir1.1) channels: new mechanisms and aspects. Am J Physiol Renal Physiol 2006;290(1):F14-F19.
18. Thomson SC, Deng A, Wead L, et al. An unexpected role for angiotensin II in the link between dietary salt and proximal reabsorption. J Clin Invest 2006;116(4):1110-1116.
19. Higham PD, Adams PC, Murray A, Campbell RW. Plasma potassium, serum magnesium and ventricular fibrillation: a prospective study. Q J Med 1993;86(9):609-617.
20. Ophir O, Peer G, Gilad J, et al. Low blood pressure in vegetarians: the possible role of potassium. Am J Clin Nutr 1983;37(5):755-762.
21. Adrogue HJ, Wesson DE. Role of dietary factors in the hypertension of African Americans. Semin Nephrol 1996;16(2):94-101.
22. Agarwal R, Afzalpurkar R, Fordtran JS. Pathophysiology of potassium absorption and secretion by the human intestine. Gastroenterology 1994;107(2):548-571.
23. Giebisch G, Hebert SC, Wang WH. New aspects of renal potassium transport. Pflugers Arch 2003;446(3):289-297.
24. Capasso G, Unwin R, Rizzo M, et al. Bicarbonate transport along the loop of Henle: molecular mechanisms and regulation. J Nephrol 2002;15(Suppl 5):S88-S96.
25. Good DW. The thick ascending limb as a site of renal bicarbonate reabsorption. Semin Nephrol 1993;13(2):225-235.
26. de Mello-Aires M, Malnic G. Distal tubule bicarbonate transport. J Nephrol 2002;15(Suppl 5):S97-S111.
27. Weiner ID. The Rh gene family and renal ammonium transport. Curr Opin Nephrol Hypertens 2004;13(5):533-540.
28. Ramasamy I. Recent advances in physiological calcium homeostasis. Clin Chem Lab Med 2006;44(3):237-273.
29. Kang JH, Choi HJ, Cho HY, et al. Familial hypomagnesemia with hypercalciuria and nephrocalcinosis associated with CLDN16 mutations. Pediatr Nephrol 2005;20(10): 1490-1493.
30. Ikari A, Hirai N, Shiroma M, et al. Association of paracellin-1 with ZO-1 augments the reabsorption of divalent cations in renal epithelial cells. J Biol Chem 2004;279(52):54826-54832.
31. Lambers TT, Bindels RJ, Hoenderop JG. Coordinated control of renal Ca^{2+} handling. Kidney Int 2006;69(4):650-654.
32. Desfleurs E, Wittner M, Simeone S, et al. Calcium-sensing receptor: regulation of electrolyte transport in the thick ascending limb of Henle's loop. Kidney Blood Press Res 1998;21(6):401-412.
33. Prie D, Beck L, Urena P, Friedlander G. Recent findings in phosphate homeostasis. Curr Opin Nephrol Hypertens 2005;14(4):318-324.
34. Berndt TJ, Schiavi S, Kumar R. "Phosphatonins" and the regulation of phosphorus homeostasis. Am J Physiol Renal Physiol 2005;289(6):F1170-F1182.
35. Portale AA, Halloran BP, Morris RC Jr. Physiologic regulation of the serum concentration of 1,25-dihydroxyvitamin D by phosphorus in normal men. J Clin Invest 1989;83(5):1494-1499.
36. Bacic D, Wagner CA, Hernando N, et al. Novel aspects in regulated expression of the renal type IIa Na/Pi-cotransporter. Kidney Int Suppl 2004;(91):S5-S12.
37. Dai LJ, Ritchie G, Kerstan D, et al. Magnesium transport in the renal distal convoluted tubule. Physiol Rev 2001;81(1):51-84.
38. Quamme GA, de Rouffignac C. Epithelial magnesium transport and regulation by the kidney. Front Biosci 2000;5:D694-D711.
39. Thebault S, Hoenderop JG, Bindels RJ. Epithelial Ca^{2+} and Mg^{2+} channels in kidney disease. Adv Chronic Kidney Dis 2006;13(2):110-117.
40. Meij IC, Koenderink JB, De Jong JC, et al. Dominant isolated renal magnesium loss is caused by misrouting of the Na^+,K^+-ATPase gamma-subunit. Ann N Y Acad Sci 2003;986:437-443.
41. Bapty BW, Dai LJ, Ritchie G, et al. Extracellular Mg^{2+}- and Ca^{2+}-sensing in mouse distal convoluted tubule cells. Kidney Int 1998;53(3):583-592.

42. Robertson EE, Rankin GO. Human renal organic anion transporters: characteristics and contributions to drug and drug metabolite excretion. Pharmacol Ther 2006; 109(3):399-412.
43. Sweet DH. Organic anion transporter (Slc22a) family members as mediators of toxicity. Toxicol Appl Pharmacol 2005;204(3):198-215.
44. Lee A, Beck L, Markovich D. The mouse sulfate anion transporter gene Sat1 (Slc26a1): cloning, tissue distribution, gene structure, functional characterization, and transcriptional regulation thyroid hormone. DNA Cell Biol 2003;22(1):19-31.
45. Maher JM, Slitt AL, Cherrington NJ, et al. Tissue distribution and hepatic and renal ontogeny of the multidrug resistance-associated protein (Mrp) family in mice. Drug Metab Dispos 2005;33(7):947-955.
46. Launay-Vacher V, Izzedine H, Karie S, et al. Renal tubular drug transporters. Nephron Physiol 2006;103(3):p97-p106.
47. Masuda S, Terada T, Yonezawa A, et al. Identification and functional characterization of a new human kidney-specific H^+/organic cation antiporter, kidney-specific multi-drug and toxin extrusion 2. J Am Soc Nephrol 2006;17(8):2127-2135.
48. Hediger MA, Johnson RJ, Miyazaki H, Endou H. Molecular physiology of urate transport. Physiology (Bethesda) 2005;20:125-133.
49. Enomoto A, Kimura H, Chairoungdua A, et al. Molecular identification of a renal urate anion exchanger that regulates blood urate levels. Nature 2002;417(6887):447-452.
50. Mount DB, Kwon CY, Zandi-Nejad K. Renal urate transport. Rheum Dis Clin North Am 2006;32(2):313-331, vi.
51. Ichida K, Hosoyamada M, Hisatome I, et al. Clinical and molecular analysis of patients with renal hypouricemia in Japan—influence of URAT1 gene on urinary urate excretion. J Am Soc Nephrol 2004;15(1):164-173.
52. Dantzler WH, Wright SH. The molecular and cellular physiology of basolateral organic anion transport in mammalian renal tubules. Biochim Biophys Acta 2003;1618(2):185-193.
53. Lang F. Osmotic diuresis. Ren Physiol 1987;10(3-4):160-173.
54. Brater DC. Pharmacology of diuretics. Am J Med Sci 2000;319(1):38-50.
55. Prandota J. Furosemide: progress in understanding its diuretic, anti-inflammatory, and bronchodilating mechanism of action, and use in the treatment of respiratory tract diseases. Am J Ther 2002;9(4):317-328.
56. Velazquez H. Thiazide diuretics. Ren Physiol 1987;10(3-4):184-197.
57. Puschett JB. Pharmacological classification and renal actions of diuretics. Cardiology 1994;84(Suppl 2):4-13.
58. Kim GH. Long-term adaptation of renal ion transporters to chronic diuretic treatment. Am J Nephrol 2004;24(6):595-605.
59. Verbalis JG. AVP receptor antagonists as aquaretics: review and assessment of clinical data. Cleve Clin J Med 2006;73(Suppl 3):S24-S33.
60. Abassi Z, Karram T, Ellaham S, et al. Implications of the natriuretic peptide system in the pathogenesis of heart failure: diagnostic and therapeutic importance. Pharmacol Ther 2004;102(3):223-241.
61. Houben AJ, van der Zander K, de Leeuw PW. Vascular and renal actions of brain natriuretic peptide in man: physiology and pharmacology. Fundam Clin Pharmacol 2005;19(4):411-419.

11

INFLAMMATION AND IMMUNOMODULATION

Laurence J. Egan

INTRODUCTION 157
The Immune System 157
Components 157
Barriers 157
Cells and Molecules 158
Structure and Function 158
THERAPEUTICS AND CLINICAL PHARMACOLOGY OF THE IMMUNE SYSTEM 159
Goals of Therapy 159
Therapeutics by Class 160
Corticosteroids 160
Thiopurines 161
Mycophenolate 163
Calcineurin Inhibitors 163
Mammalian Target of Rapamycin Inhibitors 164
Methotrexate 165
Cyclophosphamide 166
Antilymphocyte Immunoglobulins and Monoclonal Antibodies 166
Tumor Necrosis Factor-α Inhibitors 167
Inhibitors of Leukocyte Trafficking 168
Others 168
Biologic Therapeutics in Clinical Development 169

INTRODUCTION

The primary function of the mammalian immune system is to distinguish self from nonself. When nonself is recognized, effector mechanisms of the immune system are engaged; they act to eliminate that which has been recognized as nonself. In the context of human pharmacology, two distinct categories of clinical context exist in which therapeutic benefit can be gained from using drugs that modify the activity of the immune system (Table 11-1).

The first of these categories is a heterogeneous group of conditions in which primary dysregulation of the immune system causes disease. Examples of diseases in this category include autoimmune diseases such as rheumatoid arthritis and systemic lupus erythematosus. In such diseases, strong evidence exists that the normal control of the immune system is lost, resulting in the recognition of self as nonself.[1] This leads to activation of effector mechanisms of the immune system that damage certain tissues of the body in an effort to "eliminate" the mistakenly recognized tissues. Autoimmune diseases are characterized by the presence of circulating autoantibodies, immunoglobulins that react with self antigens. In addition to the classic autoimmune diseases, a large number of diseases also exists that lack the classic features of autoimmunity, but that are nevertheless characterized by an abnormal state of dysregulated overactivity of the immune system. The overactive immune system leads to chronic inflammation that damages tissues.[2] Examples of such chronic inflammatory diseases include inflammatory bowel diseases, seronegative arthritides, and chronic inflammatory skin diseases such as psoriasis and eczema. Certain allergic disorders, such as asthma, can manifest substantial chronic inflammation and can be treated with immunosuppressive drugs.

Drugs acting on the immune system are very useful in the second major clinical category that comprises two situations in which the immune system is appropriately activated but harms the patient. The first of these occurs in patients who have received allogeneic organ transplants in which immunosuppressive drugs are essential for the prevention and treatment of rejection of the transplanted allograft. Replacement of failed organs, including kidneys, liver, lungs, and hearts with healthy organs obtained from brain-dead donors or, in some cases, healthy relatives, is a highly effective way to treat patients with failure of those organs. However, because the transplanted organs express antigens that the immune system recognizes as nonself, they may be promptly rejected by the transplant recipients immune system unless immunosuppressive drugs are administered. The modern field of organ transplantation could not have progressed as it has without the development of highly effective immunosuppressant drugs.[3] The second clinical situation is graft-versus-host disease in allogeneic bone marrow transplant patients. In this condition, donor immune cells recognize antigens expressed by the recipient as nonself and mount an immune response against the recipient.[4] Immunosuppressive drugs are very useful in controlling graft-versus-host disease by suppressing activity of the donor immune cells.

The goal of this chapter is to describe the pharmacology of drugs used to treat autoimmune and chronic inflammatory diseases and of drugs used to prevent and treat allograft rejection and graft-versus-host disease. Initially, a brief overview of the components, organization, and function of the immune system is presented to provide a framework for understanding the points of action, at the molecular and cellular levels, of drugs acting on the immune system. This is followed by a detailed examination of the pharmacology of the individual drugs used to manipulate the human immune system. Because of extensive coverage in other chapters, the pharmacology of immunization and of allergy are not dealt with in this chapter, although both of these subjects involve the immune system.

The Immune System

Components

The immune system comprises physical barriers that separate the body from the environment, cells that survey the body for signs of infection or other abnormalities, other cells that carry out effector functions of the immune system, and the organs in which the cells function. The cells of the immune system carry out their highly specialized functions largely via the actions of specific molecules that they express.

Barriers

Epithelia separate the body from the environment, and by forming this specialized barrier, epithelia can be considered a component of the immune system. Epithelia are sheets of specialized cells that cover large surfaces of the body, and include the skin, the mucous membranes of the eye and oral cavity, the respiratory epithelium, and the gastrointestinal epithelium. Each of these different epithelia is uniquely structured to carry out the specific functions required of that part of the body. Thus, the skin is a multicellular layer that protects against physical injury and prevents excessive water evaporation. The respiratory epithelium contains a single layer of columnar epithelial cells arranged over a lamina propria that contains structural elements and many specialized immune cells. The epithelium of much of the gastrointestinal tract is specialized for the absorption of nutrients and fluids. Tight junctions block the passage of particles and microbes between

TABLE 11-1 CLINICAL USES OF IMMUNOSUPPRESSIVE DRUGS

Conditions with Dysregulated Activation of the Immune System	Conditions with Normal Activation of the Immune System
Autoimmune diseases	Allograft rejection
Chronic inflammatory diseases	Graft-versus-host disease
Allergic diseases	

cells of the single-layered epithelium of the small and large bowel, constituting an important element of the physical barrier separating the host from the environment of the lumen of the alimentary tract. Epithelial cells communicate information about the environment to specialized immune cells in the lamina propria.[5]

In addition to the physical barrier posed by the cells of the epithelium, other elements contribute to the maintenance of immunity at epithelial surfaces. Dendritic cells, specialized antigen-presenting cells, are found below the surface of the epithelium, where they sample the environment of the epithelium and possibly the external surface of the epithelium as well.[6] Plasma cells located in the lamina propria of the epithelium secrete antibodies, notably the secretory immunoglobulin A (IgA) subtype, that traverse the epithelial barrier. On the external surface of the epithelium, secretory IgA plays an important role in neutralizing potentially harmful microbes.

Cells and Molecules

The immune system contains several types of highly specialized cells. A detailed description of the current state of knowledge on those cells and the specialized molecules they express is beyond the scope of this chapter, but a brief overview of the main concepts is provided.

Neutrophils. Neutrophils are the most abundant type of leukocyte found in the blood. They are multinucleate and important in the phagocytosis of invading bacteria and their killing once ingested. Neutrophils are short-lived cells whose number in blood and in tissues can increase dramatically at times of infection, reflecting increased production and release from the bone marrow.

Monocytes and Macrophages. Monocytes are the circulating form of tissue macrophages. In tissues, macrophages are important both for phagocytosis and killing of bacteria and for the processing and presentation of antigens derived from invading microorganisms.

Eosinophils. Eosinophils contain densely eosinophilic granules and have important functions in the killing of antibody-coated parasites.

Mast Cells. Mast cells contain granules filled with the vasoactive mediator histamine. When mast cells degranulate, the released histamine causes capillaries in the vicinity to leak plasma and cells. They are important mediators of allergic reactions.

Dendritic Cells. Dendritic cells are the most highly differentiated cells specialized for antigen processing and presentation. They reside in many parts of the body where they uptake, process, and present antigens to lymphocytes. Dendritic cells have been termed *professional* antigen-presenting cells because this is their best-characterized function, in contrast with macrophages and B lymphocytes that can also present antigens but have additional important functions.

Lymphocytes. Lymphocytes are found in blood and in tissues and can be divided into two large categories: T lymphocytes that mature in the thymus and B lymphocytes that mature in the bone marrow. Lymphocytes are the cells that, through their expression of antigen-specific receptors, recognize foreign antigens.

Natural Killer Cells. Natural killer cells are similar to lymphocytes but do not express antigen receptors on their surface. They are capable of releasing lytic granules that can kill virus-infected cells.

Structure and Function

The body contains a variety of lymphoid organs that serve as the anatomic sites for much of the activity of the immune system. At these sites, cells and molecules of the immune system interact and orchestrate the subtle and complex activities involved in immune reactions.

Primary and Secondary Lymphoid Organs. The bone marrow is the site of production of most cells of the immune system. The cells derive from a pluripotent hematopoietic stem cell in the bone marrow and proceed down a pathway of differentiation resulting in the production of the active mature immune cells. B and T lymphocytes arise from a common lymphoid progenitor, whereas neutrophils, eosinophils, basophils, monocytes, and dendritic cells arise from a common myeloid precursor. Lymphocytes are released from the bone marrow and circulate in the blood. During development, B and T lymphocytes acquire the expression of a highly diverse repertoire of antigen receptors on their cell surface. The T-cell receptor is a complex multiprotein transmembrane receptor. The B-cell receptor is a form of transmembrane immunoglobulin. The diversity of the repertoire of these receptors is generated during lymphocyte development through a complex system of somatic gene rearrangements in gene segments that encode the antigen-binding portions of the receptors. In addition, somatic hypermutation of some segments of these genes can occur, adding even more diversity. The result of this process is that individual lymphocytes express slightly different antigen receptors on their surface, each receptor having different affinity for antigens.

After production in the bone marrow, lymphocytes are released into the circulation. Immature T lymphocytes home in to the thymus, whereas B lymphocytes return to the bone marrow. There, early in life, the immature T and B lymphocytes undergo a process of selection and maturation that results in the retention of lymphocytes that do not recognize self antigens and the elimination of those that do. The clonal selection hypothesis states that lymphocytes that express receptors having a high affinity for antigens that they encounter during maturation in the thymus and bone marrow are selected for elimination by apoptosis. In contrast, lymphocytes whose receptors do not encounter a high-affinity antigen survive. The result of this selection process is that only lymphocytes that express receptors for nonself antigens survive, whereas those that express receptors with high affinity for self are eliminated. This is the basis upon which the immune system can discriminate between self and nonself. Thereafter, B and T lymphocytes circulate in low numbers and as a diverse population of cells with a strikingly diverse repertoire of antigen receptors capable of recognizing a myriad of nonself antigens.

Secondary lymphoid organs include the lymph nodes, the spleen, and the mucosa-associated lymphoid structures. At these sites, immune cells interact with one another, which is essential for the proper functioning of the immune system.

Innate and Adaptive Immunity. The cells, tissues, and molecules of the immune system interact in certain functional paradigms that can be broadly described as *innate* and *adaptive (acquired) immunity*. Innate immunity refers to non–antigen-specific immune reactions, whereas adaptive immunity refers to antigen-specific reactions. A high degree of cross talk exists between innate and adaptive immune mechanisms. Key features of the innate and adaptive immune systems are contrasted in Table 11-2.

A typical immune reaction involves the activation of innate immune cells, such as neutrophils and tissue macrophages. Activation of those cells can occur by a number of mechanisms, but it typically involves the ligation of a pattern recognition receptor expressed in those cells by some factor derived from a microbial source. For example, many cells of the innate immune system express a type of pattern recognition receptor termed *toll-like receptors* on their cell surface.[7] Toll-like receptors can be activated by many different microbial ligands, such as lipopolysaccharide or flagellin. The activated phenotype is characterized by the secretion of cytokines, such as interleukin (IL)-1, tumor necrosis factor (TNF)-α, IL-6, chemokines such as IL-8, and other immune mediators such as eicosanoids. In summary, the innate immune reaction is a rapid, antigen-nonspecific early-defense mechanism whose primary role is in the prevention and containment of microbial infections.

The innate immune system is often sufficient to contain and prevent the spread of minor microbial infections. Nevertheless, the innate immune system often activates the adaptive immune system, which is required for the resolution of many infections. Cells such as dendritic cells and macrophages engulf invading microbes, kill them, and process their proteins into small peptides. Most virus-infected cells can process peptides derived from viral proteins expressed in those cells. The microbial-derived peptides are then expressed on the surface of those antigen-presenting cells in the context of major histocompatibility complex molecules.

The adaptive immune response is triggered when those peptides are recognized by antigen-specific receptors expressed on the surface of B and T lymphocytes. A B or T lymphocyte becomes activated by a high-affinity interaction between its receptor and an antigen, leading to a cascade of molecular events within the lymphocyte. Important among these is the induced expression of IL-2, a cytokine that promotes the expansion of activated lymphocytes. In this way, even rare cells within a diverse population of lymphocytes have the capability of massive clonal expansion that is essential for them to carry out their acquired immune functions. For proper activation of T lymphocytes, in addition to acquiring an activation signal through the T-cell receptor, those cells also require activation through costimulatory receptors, the most important of which is CD28. The proper activation of B lymphocytes also requires two signals. The first comes from the B-cell receptor after its engagement with a high-affinity antigen; the second usually comes from adjacent T lymphocytes in the form of secreted cytokines.

TABLE 11-2 INNATE AND ADAPTIVE IMMUNE SYSTEMS CONTRASTED

	Innate	Adaptive
Receptors	Pattern recognition receptors	T-cell and B-cell receptors
Receptor specificity	Low	High
Receptor diversity	Low	High
Reactions	Fast (minutes to hours)	Slow (days)
Memory	No	Yes
Main cells	Macrophages, neutrophils, natural killer cells	Lymphocytes

Once activated, lymphocytes act to control infections by a number of mechanisms, including the direct killing of virus-infected cells and the activation of adjacent cells such as macrophages that can engulf and kill microorganisms. The effective triggering of adaptive immune mechanisms can usually be detected by testing the blood for antibodies specific for antigens of the infecting microorganism. For example, in the clinical setting, it is possible to diagnose infectious diseases such as hepatitis and human immunodeficiency virus by the presence of circulating antibodies against antigens of those viruses.

THERAPEUTICS AND CLINICAL PHARMACOLOGY OF THE IMMUNE SYSTEM

Goals of Therapy

Drugs acting on the immune system are used to treat many different diseases affecting diverse organs of the body, with highly variable symptoms resulting from those diseases. Therefore, one cannot comprehensively list a common set of therapeutic goals for drugs affecting the immune system. Nevertheless, two general principles can be stated:

- The drug must achieve effective blockade of pathogenic immune mechanisms.
- The drug should not impair normal immunity to the point that the patient is exposed to significantly greater risk of infections.

Few diseases of the immune system exhibit specific pathogenic mechanisms that allow the introduction of highly selective drugs that block that abnormal mechanism without significantly affecting normal immune functions. Moreover, for most immunosuppressive drugs, common toxicities like the development of opportunistic infections are a direct extension of the pharmacologic activity of the drug. Therefore, toxicity of these drugs is often dose-related and cannot be uncoupled from desirable pharmacologic effects. One approach to mitigate this problem has been the use of cocktails of two or three immunosuppressants at doses at which the individual drugs rarely cause toxicity. This clinical strategy is effective at minimizing specific side effects of those drugs, but common side effects, such as elevated risk of opportunistic infections, can in fact be worsened by polypharmacy.[8]

Table 11-3 lists important immune system–active drugs and their molecular targets.

TABLE 11-3 IMMUNE SYSTEM DRUGS AND THEIR MOLECULAR AND CELLULAR TARGETS

Drug	Molecular Target	Cellular Target	Pharmacologic Effects
Corticosteroids	Glucocorticoid receptor	Numerous: lymphocytes, macrophages, endothelial cells, etc.	↓ Expression proinflammatory molecules
Thiopurines	DNA/RNA synthesis	Lymphocytes	↓ Proliferation, ↑ apoptosis of lymphocytes
Methotrexate	Dihydrofolate reductase	Lymphocytes	↓ Proliferation, ↑ apoptosis of lymphocytes
Mycophenolate	Inosine monophosphate dehydrogenase	Lymphocytes	↓ Proliferation, ↑ apoptosis of lymphocytes
Cyclosporine and tacrolimus	Calcineurin	Lymphocytes	↓ IL-2 production and lymphocyte proliferation
Sirolimus	mTOR	Lymphocytes	↓ Proliferation, ↑ apoptosis of lymphocytes
Cyclophosphamide	DNA	Lymphocytes	↑ Apoptosis of lymphocytes
Antilymphocyte globulins	Cell surface–expressed proteins	Lymphocytes	↓ Survival of lymphocytes
OKT3	CD3	Lymphocytes	↓ Survival of lymphocytes
Basiliximab, daclizumab	IL-2 receptor	Lymphocytes	↓ Proliferation of lymphocytes
Infliximab, adalimumab, etanercept	TNFα	Numerous: lymphocytes, macrophages, etc.	↓ Proinflammatory signaling, ↑ apoptosis of target cells
Natalizumab	α4 Integrin	Activated monocytes, lymphocytes	↓ Extravasation of target cells

mTOR, mammalian target of rapamycin; OKT3, ornithine ketoacid transaminase; TNFα, tumor necrosis factor-α.

Therapeutics by Class

Corticosteroids

When cortisone was first purified and later tested as a therapeutic by Kendall and Hench of the Mayo Clinic and Reichstein of Basel University Switzerland, winning them the Nobel Prize in 1950, early clinical experience with this drug in the treatment of rheumatoid arthritis produced dramatic beneficial results.[9] However, initial enthusiasm for cortisone decreased after it was realized that long-term use caused considerable side effects. In clinical practice to this day, the optimum use of corticosteroids requires striking a careful balance between the powerful anti-inflammatory actions of these drugs and their potential to cause serious morbidity, especially with long-term high-dose usage.

Pharmacokinetics and Metabolism. Many different corticosteroids are used in clinical practice. Most of these are synthetic structural analogues of the endogenous corticosteroid cortisol (hydrocortisone). Others are structurally unrelated, but share the key pharmacologic property of binding to and activating glucocorticoid receptors. Many corticosteroids also bind, albeit with lower affinity, to mineralocorticoid receptors. The level of affinity of a particular corticosteroid for the glucocorticoid versus the mineralocorticoid receptor determines its potency as analogues of the endogenous hormones cortisol or aldosterone. Most clinically useful corticosteroids have much greater activity at glucocorticoid than at mineralocorticoid receptors and thus have high metabolic activity and low salt-retaining activity.

Corticosteroids can be administered by many routes, including oral, intravenous, and topical to the skin, eyes, airways, nose, and gastrointestinal tract. Corticosteroids are lipophilic and generally well absorbed. Most corticosteroids are active drugs, although prednisone, a commonly used corticosteroid, is a prodrug metabolically activated to prednisolone. Topically administered corticosteroids can exert their pharmacologic action at the site of the administration. For example, inhaled corticosteroids that act topically on the respiratory mucosa exert anti-inflammatory actions on immune cells and possibly epithelial cells located in the epithelium or submucosa of the small airways. In contrast, systemically administered corticosteroids, such as oral or intravenous preparations, must first be absorbed into the bloodstream and distributed to the site of action. Corticosteroids circulate bound to corticosteroid-binding globulin. The unbound fraction of corticosteroid is free to traverse the plasma membrane of all cell types, which is required for pharmacologic activity. The typical half-life of systemically administered corticosteroids is 2 or 3 hours,[10] but their pharmacologic activity often lasts much longer because of the profound changes that these drugs exert on gene expression profiles within their target cells.

Corticosteroids are metabolized in the liver, and orally administered corticosteroids undergo significant first-pass metabolism.

Mechanism of Action. At the molecular level, the mechanism of action of corticosteroids has been well elucidated (Fig. 11-1).[11] After traversing the plasma membrane, the steroid encounters its receptor, which is expressed in the cytoplasm of most cells. The immunosuppressive effects of corticosteroids are mediated by their engagement of glucorticoid receptors. The corticosteroid-glucocorticoid receptor complex dissociates from heat-shock protein chaperones and migrates into the nucleus. Corticosteroid-glucocorticoid receptor complexes are active transcription factors, capable of dramatically altering the expression of target genes. Genes responsive to active glucocorticoid receptors contain specific nucleotide sequences in promoter or enhancer regions termed *glucocorticoid response elements*. For some of these genes, binding of corticosteroid-glucocorticoid receptor complexes results in the increased transcription of those genes, leading to the increased expression of the encoded protein. The expression of some genes may be decreased by these complexes.

Some alternative mechanisms of altered gene expression have been attributed to corticosteroids. One of these centers on the ability of active glucocorticoid receptors to antagonize the activities of proinflammatory transcription factors, such as nuclear factor-κB and AP-1.[12-14] In one version of this model, direct physical interaction occurs between active glucocorticoid receptors and the proinflammatory transcription factor, which impairs the ability of that transcription factor to induce expression of its target genes. In another version of this model, active glucocorticoid receptors compete with proinflammatory transcription factors for limiting amounts of essential nuclear coactivators of transcription, such as Creb binding protein and p300. This results in a decreased capacity of the proinflammatory transcription factors to effectively engage the transcription initiation complex and up-regulate expression of their target genes. The extent to which

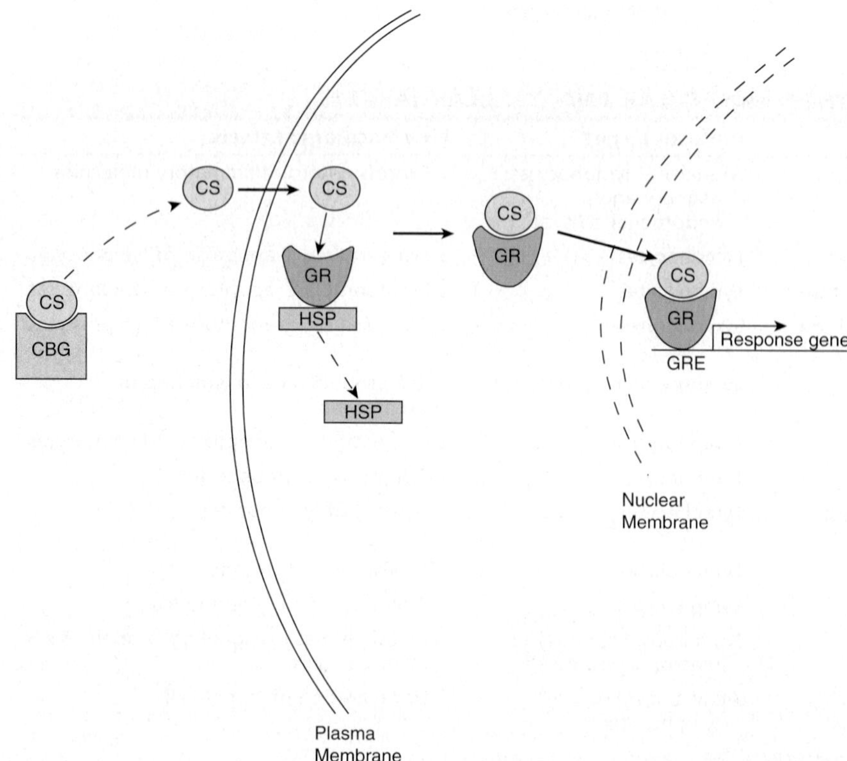

FIGURE 11-1 • Mechanism of action of corticosteroids. Corticosteroids (CS) circulate bound extensively to corticosteroid-binding globulin (CBG). Free CS diffuses across the plasma membrane of all cells. In the cytoplasm, CS binds to corticosteroid receptors, most importantly, the glucocorticoid receptor (GR). GRs are retained in the cytoplasm through their interaction with heat shock proteins (HSP), and this interaction is disrupted by the binding of CS to GR. The CS-GR complex, free of HSP, translocates to the nucleus and can bind to glucocorticoid response elements (GREs) located in the promoter and enhancer regions of response genes. The binding of the CS-GR complex to the GREs can increase or decrease the transcription of the response gene, depending on a host of additional factors.

these alternative molecular mechanisms of action of corticosteroids contribute to their immunosuppressive properties is not known.

Overall, the net effect of alterations in gene expression following corticosteroid treatment results in a down-regulated immune response. In this sense, the effects of corticosteroids are nonspecific in that no single gene target appears to mediate the immunosuppressant properties of the drugs, but rather reflects the aggregate effect of many alterations in cellular physiology. Many different cell types express glucocorticoid receptors and, thus, are pharmacologic targets of corticosteroids. The immunosuppressive effects of these drugs are probably mediated by their effects on active immune cells, such as lymphocytes and macrophages. However, it is also possible that the immunosuppressant properties of corticosteroids depend in part on effects these drugs have on other nonimmune cell types such as fibroblasts, epithelial cells, or endothelial cells.

Toxicity. The clinical utility of corticosteroids is severely compromised by the occurrence of predictable dose- and exposure-dependent adverse effects. These effects are mediated by glucocorticoid receptors. Therefore, it has not yet been possible to uncouple adverse effects of corticosteroids from desired pharmacologic effects.

Acutely, corticosteroids can cause psychosis[15] and impaired immunity, resulting in increased risks of opportunistic infections.[16] Blood glucose elevates, plasma cholesterol rises, and especially with corticosteroids that activate mineralocorticoid receptors resulting in salt retention, blood pressure can be elevated. Higher doses of corticosteroids are more likely to cause these acute side effects.

The chronic adverse effects of corticosteroids produce a clinical picture termed *Cushing's syndrome*, which is easily recognizable and essentially the same as that produced by excessive production of endogenous corticosteroids. Features of this syndrome include weight gain, moon face, osteoporosis, reduced growth, and cataracts. The greater the cumulative dose of corticosteroids, the greater the likelihood that these chronic adverse effects will occur.[17]

What strategies are effective in reducing long-term corticosteroid side effects? Most important is the avoidance or minimization of systemic corticosteroid exposure. Many diseases, such as asthma, allergic rhinitis, dermatitis, uveitis, and Crohn's disease, can be effectively treated using topical, poorly absorbed corticosteroids. Side effects with these agents are minimal, although with years of inhaled corticosteroid therapy for asthma, cataracts may be caused.[18] When systemic corticosteroids must be administered, use of the lowest effective dose for the shortest time period is recommended. One general strategy that helps to achieve this goal is to combine corticosteroids with other safer immunosuppressants, allowing the gradual reduction of corticosteroid. Such a strategy is commonly employed in transplant recipients and patients with chronic inflammatory diseases like inflammatory bowel disease.[19] Finally, certain specific adverse effects such as osteoporosis can be mitigated by administration of calcium supplements, vitamin D, and antiresorbtive drugs.[20,21]

Because exogenous corticosteroids inhibit pituitary secretion of adrenocorticotropic hormone (ACTH), chronic corticosteroid therapy results in significant suppression of adrenal function. Therefore, if chronic systemic corticosteroid therapy is abruptly discontinued, an adrenal insufficiency crisis can ensue. This problem can be avoided by the gradual lowering of corticosteroid dose in patients on chronic therapy, allowing resumption of ACTH secretion and recovery of normal adrenal function. If clinical uncertainty exists about adrenal function in a corticosteroid-treated patient, it is useful to perform an ACTH stimulation test to measure basal and induced capacity of adrenal glands to secrete cortisol. Because of the potential gravity of adrenal insufficiency, especially at times of stress such as trauma or surgery, many surgeons administer a large dose of corticosteroid in the perioperative period to patients who have recently been treated with such drugs.[22]

Clinical Uses. Corticosteroids are used to treat a wide variety of immune-related disorders and allergic disorders. These include inflammatory arthritides,[23] inflammatory bowel diseases,[24,25] asthma,[26] inflammatory skin diseases, and allergic rhinitis. Corticosteroids are also used in the prevention and treatment of allograft rejection[27] and in the management of graft-versus-host disease.[28]

Thiopurines

The most important thiopurines in clinical use as immunosuppressants are azathioprine (AZA) and 6-mercaptopurine (6-MP). Both drugs are purine nucleoside analogues that interfere with the normal synthesis of DNA. 6-Mercaptopurine was first synthesized by Elion and Hitchings, and later, the imidazolyl derivative AZA was developed.[29] 6-Thioguanine (6-TG) is another member of this class that has been used successfully in leukemia and chronic inflammatory diseases such as Crohn's disease. However, the development of nodular hyperplasia of the liver has severely limited the utility of 6-TG.[30,31]

Pharmacokinetics and Metabolism. Azathioprine and 6-MP are both administered orally. They are well absorbed from the gastrointestinal tract, and after absorption,[32] AZA is rapidly converted to 6-MP in a nonenzymatic reaction when the drug is exposed to nucleophiles (Fig. 11-2). The pharmacologic activity of AZA is essentially the same

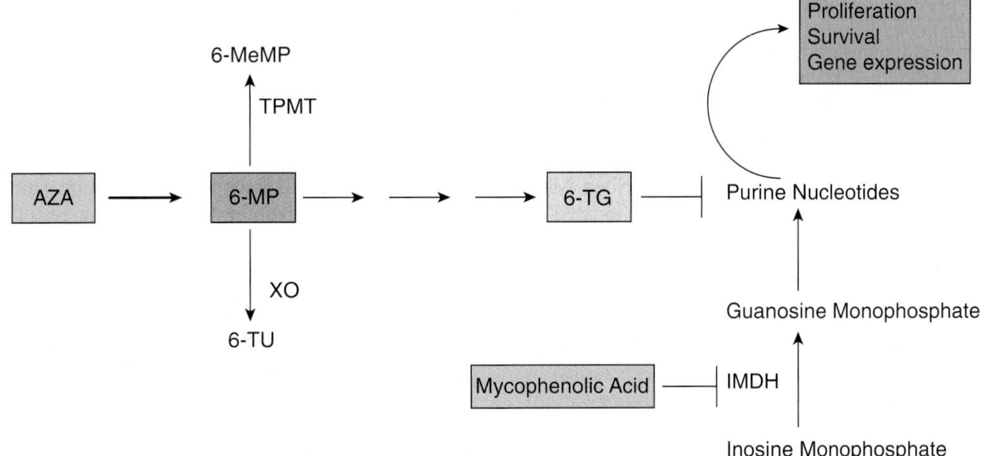

FIGURE 11-2 • Metabolism and action of thiopurines and mycophenolate. Azathioprine (AZA) is nonenzymatically converted to 6-mercaptopurine (6-MP). 6-MP can be converted to the pharmacologically inactive metabolites 6-methyl-mercaptopurine (6-MeMP) or 6-thiouric acid (6-TU) by thiopurine methyltransferase (TPMT) and xanthine oxidase (XO), respectively. 6-MP can also enter another metabolic pathway that leads to the production of the pharmacologically active 6-thioguanine (6-TG) metabolites. 6-TG metabolites block purine nucleotide biosynthesis. Mycophenolate inhibits inosine monophosphate dehydrogenase (IMDH), a key enzyme in the biosynthetic pathway of guanosine. Therefore, both thiopurines and mycophenolate result in a cellular deficiency of purine nucleotides, especially in lymphocytes. This deficiency is accompanied by an inhibition of lymphocyte proliferation, survival, and gene expression.

as that of 6-MP, and therefore, AZA can be considered a prodrug of 6-MP. The pharmacologic effects of thiopurines appear to depend not on 6-MP, but on the 6-TG nucleotide metabolites. As illustrated in Figure 11-2, 6-MP can enter a metabolic pathway that is initially catalyzed by hypoxanthine phosphoribosyl transferase, eventually leading to the production of 6-TG nucleotides.

The plasma half-life of thiopurines is quite short, between 1 and 2 hours, but active 6-TG nucleotides accumulate intracellularly, resulting in a longer duration of pharmacologic activity. Because of this, once-daily dosing is adequate. Azathioprine is usually administered at a dose of 2.5 mg/kg per day, and 6-MP at 1.5 mg/kg per day.

Clinical experience with thiopurines indicates that these drugs begin to exert their beneficial effects only long after initiating therapy. For example, in the treatment of inflammatory bowel disease, beneficial effects were absent in short-term clinical trials.[33,34] However, in longer trials, clear benefits of thiopurine therapy were seen.[35] Most clinicians who use thiopurines advise patients to expect a 2- or 3-month delay before the onset of beneficial effects. In an effort to hasten the onset of action of thiopurines, one group of investigators administered an intravenous loading dose of AZA equivalent to 1 month's cumulative oral dose. Although the initial pilot study of this approach was promising, the placebo-controlled trial failed to establish any benefit of an intravenous loading dose of AZA.[36]

In addition to metabolic activation into 6-TG nucleotides, 6-MP can also enter two other well-characterized metabolic pathways, leading to the production of different metabolites. One pathway is catalyzed by xanthine oxidase, leading to the production of 6-thiouric acid. This metabolite does not have any known active pharmacologic effects. Another pathway is metabolized by thiopurine methyltransferase (TPMT), leading to the production of 6-methylmercaptopurine. This metabolite does not contribute to the beneficial pharmacologic effects of thiopurines, but has been associated with the hepatotoxicity of these agents.[37]

The complex metabolic pathways of thiopurines constitute the basis for important drug interactions and pharmacogenetic influences on these agents. One important drug interaction is between allopurinol, a xanthine oxidase inhibitor, and 6-MP or azathioprine.[38] In this drug interaction, allopurinol, by inhibiting xanthine oxidase activity, effectively closes that metabolic pathway to 6-MP. As a result, 6-MP is shunted into the other metabolic pathways available to it. This results in increased production of active 6-TG nucleotides. Therefore, the coadministration of allopurinol along with a thiopurine results in a quite dramatic increase in potency of the thiopurine, which frequently causes excessive pharmacologic activity, which may lead to myelosuppression.[39] If allopurinol must be coadministered with a thiopurine, it is usual to decrease the dose of thiopurine to approximately 25% of the standard amount.

Enzymes in the metabolic pathway of thiopurines are subject to strong pharmacogenetic influences. The best studied of these is TPMT, the enzyme involved in the conversion of 6-MP into 6-methylmercaptopurine.[40] The gene encoding thiopurine methyltransferase is located on chromosome 6, contains 10 exons, and is highly polymorphic.[41] At least 20 mutant or variant alleles of this gene have been described. Most of these variations are single nucleotide polymorphisms located in coding regions of the gene. In addition, some single nucleotide polymorphisms have been noted in introns and outside the open reading frame, and a variable number tandem repeat has been described in the promoter of TPMT. Thiopurine methyltransferase protein encoded off variant alleles appears to undergo proteasomal degradation more rapidly than the wild-type protein.[42] This leads to the expression of lower enzymatic activity in people who harbor one or more variant alleles of TPMT.

Population studies of TPMT activity have revealed a trimodal pattern of distribution.[43] Approximately 90% of individuals have high TPMT activity, corresponding to two wild-type alleles; and approximately 10% of people have intermediate TPMT activity, corresponding to one wild-type and one variant allele. Approximately 1 in 300 individuals has very low or absent TPMT activity, corresponding to two variant low-activity alleles. The activity of TPMT can be assayed in red blood cells based on the conversion of 6-MP into 6-methylmercaptopurine. At the genetic level, common single nucleotide polymorphisms in the TPMT gene can be detected using allele-specific polymerase chain reaction.

Because TPMT catalyxes the conversion of 6-MP into a metabolite that does not contribute to the pharmacologic activity of thiopurines, low activity of this enzyme appears to shunt more 6-MP into the pathway, leading to the production of the active 6-TG nucleotide metabolites. This results in a higher incidence of excessive pharmacologic activity, manifest commonly as leukopenia, in thiopurine-treated individuals who have one or two variant thiopurine methyltranferase alleles.[44] Indeed, the rare individuals who have no detectable TPMT activity are at very high risk for developing early leukopenia during thiopurine treatment.[45] For this reason, it is advisable to check TPMT activity in individuals in whom one is planning to start AZA or 6-MP. It is usual to administer half of the usual dose in individuals found to have TPMT activity in the intermediate range, and to avoid these drugs altogether in individuals with no detectable TPMT activity.[46]

Recently, a number of published studies have sought to assess the utility of therapeutic drug monitoring as a guide to the clinical use of thiopurines. These studies rely primarily on the measurement of 6-TG nucleotide concentrations in blood. Some of these studies have shown that a 6-TG nucleotide concentration cut-off point can be identified, above which clinical responses are more likely than when concentrations are below the cut-off.[47,48] These intriguing findings have not been replicated in all series in which they were studied.[49] Nevertheless, the data do suggest that the production of 6-TG nucleotides is a valid biomarker of the therapeutic efficacy of thiopurines.[50] A number of studies have carried this observation forward and increased the dose of thiopurines in an attempt to get 6-TG nucleotide concentrations into the putative therapeutic range. However, for reasons that are not well understood, the elevation of thiopurine doses above normal was not accompanied by reliable increases of 6-TG nucleotide concentrations or the improvement of clinical responses.[37] In fact, many patients whose thiopurine dose was increased developed hepatotoxicity, probably related to increased concentrations of 6-methylmercaptopurine. As a result of these studies, the utility of measuring 6-TG nucleotide concentrations is limited, but may be useful in patients in whom poor compliance is suspected.

One intriguing approach toward improving the clinical utility of thiopurines involves the coadministration of allopurinol. In populations of thiopurine-treated patients, one can define a subset of patients in whom, despite administration of standard doses of thiopurines, 6-TG nucleotide concentrations remain low. In such patients, by reducing thiopurine dose to 25% of the standard dose and coadministering allopurinol, it has been possible to elevate 6-TG nucleotide concentrations and lower 6-methylmercaptopurine concentrations.[51] Such an outcome would be predicted to be highly beneficial in minimizing hepatotoxicity and improving the efficacy of these drugs. Indeed, early clinical reports indicate that in some patients, such a therapeutic maneuver is beneficial.[52]

Mechanism of Action. During DNA synthesis in patients treated with thiopurines, 6-TG triphosphate becomes incorporated into DNA. This impairs cell proliferation and may result in the apoptosis of actively dividing cells, especially lymphocytes during an adaptive immune response.[53] As a consequence of impaired lymphocyte proliferation and survival under conditions of thiopurine treatment, acquired immune reactions are significantly impaired.

More recently, an alternative mechanism of action of AZA has been proposed. 6-Thioguanine triphosphate has been shown to block the activity of Vav, a guanine nucleotide exchange factor. In the setting of lymphocyte activation, defective Vav activity under thiopurine treatment results in apoptosis.[54] Whatever the precise biochemical mechanism of action of thiopurines, it is clear that treatment with these agents impairs the proliferation of lymphocytes and induces their apoptosis, especially under conditions of activation during an immune response. In addition to these effects on lymphocyte numbers, thiopurines also appear to inhibit the secretion of proinflammatory cytokines by lymphocytes.[55]

Toxicity. Allergy to thiopurines is relatively common, and up to 25% of patients started on one such drug cannot tolerate it, because of either allergy or another form of intolerance. Typical allergic reactions are skin rash, fever, or abdominal pain.[56] In some patients, pancreatitis develops.[57] More minor gastrointestinal intolerance, such as nausea, is also relatively common. In patients who experience intolerances such as gastrointestinal upset or headache on AZA, switching to 6-MP can sometimes help.[58] However, more major allergic reactions such as fever, rash, or pancreatitis cannot be managed by switching from AZA to 6-MP. Thiopurines have also been associated with significant hepatotoxicity, including peliosis and nodular regenerative hyperplasia.

Because of the possibility of bone marrow suppression during thiopurine therapy,[59] it is appropriate not only to check TPMT activity prior to initiating therapy but also to periodically monitor for the development of leukopenia. Initially, this is best done every week. Once the patient has been stabilized on thiopurine therapy and leukopenia has not developed, the frequency of blood test monitoring can be reduced. However, it is important to note that leukopenia can develop in patients maintained on a stable dose of thiopurine many years after initiating such therapy.[45] Therefore, this monitoring must be carried out indefinitely. It is also prudent to check liver biochemical tests at the same time as blood count monitoring, because of the possibility of hepatotoxicity.

Chronic thiopurine therapy can be associated with significant adversity. Because of their immunosuppressive properties, thiopurines are associated with an increased risk of opportunistic infections.[56,59,60] The most common infections that are noted in thiopurine-treated patients are viral infections such as Epstein-Barr virus, cytomegalovirus, and herpesvirus infections.[8] Chronic thiopurine therapy has also been associated with an increased risk of lymphoma.[61] Although controversial, a meta-analysis supported the notion that chronic thiopurine therapy increases the risk of lymphoma by about fourfold over disease controls.[62] Most of these lymphomas appear to be related to Epstein-Barr virus infection, resembling posttransplantation lymphoproliferative disorders.[63]

Clinical Uses. Azathioprine and 6-MP have very similar pharmacologic effects and are used interchangeably, albeit at different doses. These drugs are in widespread use for inflammatory bowel diseases,[46] autoimmune hepatitis,[64] inflammatory arthritides, and the prevention of renal allograft rejection.[65]

Mycophenolate

Mycophenolate was developed as an alternative to AZA for the prevention of transplanted solid organ rejection.[66] Two versions of this drug are currently used: mycophenolate mofetil and enteric-coated mycophenolate sodium. After absorption, these drugs are converted into mycophenolic acid, the active metabolite.[67] This conversion is catalyzed by esterases present in the intestinal epithelium and liver. Mycophenolic acid has an elimination half-life of approximately 18 hours and is usually administered twice daily. For the chronic prophylaxis of allograft rejection, usual doses range from 720 mg to 1.5 g twice daily of mycophenolate mofetil or mycophenolate sodium.

Mycophenolic acid is a selective uncompetitive reversible inhibitor of inosine monophosphate dehydrogenase, a key enzyme in the de novo production of guanosine nucleotide[68] (see Fig. 11-2). Deficiency of guanosine exerts a profound antiproliferative effect on lymphocytes, resulting in impairment of acquired immune responses. Selectivity for lymphocytes is believed to lie in the fact that other cell types can utilize salvage pathways for purine nucleotide production, whereas lymphocytes do not appear to use such pathways.[69]

Side effects of mycophenolate are dose-related. The most troublesome side effect is gastrointestinal upset, manifest as gastritis and diarrhea.[70] Gastrointestinal investigations have revealed an inflammatory bowel disease–like clinical picture in some patients suffering from mycophenolate-induced diarrhea. Treatment of this problem is difficult and usually requires lowering the dose of mycophenolate or discontinuing it. This increases the risk of rejection. Some patients who are taking mycophenolate mofetil may note a reduction in gastrointestinal symptoms when switched to enteric-coated mycophenolate sodium.[71] When mycophenolate is stopped, it is usual to substitute AZA. Other side effects include leukopenia, hyperglycemia, and dizziness.

Mycophenolate is used in the prevention of renal allograft rejection.

Calcineurin Inhibitors

The success of modern solid organ transplantation could not have been achieved without the development of two drugs that are potent inhibitors of T-lymphocyte activation.[3] The first to be developed was cyclosporine, followed by tacrolimus. Although these two drugs are structurally unrelated—cyclosporine is a fungal peptide, whereas tacrolimus is structurally related to macrolide antibiotics—they share an essentially identical molecular mechanism of action. Considerable overlap is also present in their toxicities, suggesting that their pharmacologic actions can probably not be uncoupled from many of the toxicities associated with their use.

Pharmacokinetics and Metabolism. Cyclosporine was discovered by the Sandoz Chemical Company in fungi isolated from soil samples. It consists of 11 amino acids arranged in a cyclic polypeptide and has a lipophilic configuration resulting in poor water solubility. Cyclosporine is available in two oral preparations and is also prepared for intravenous administration. The absorption of orally administered standard formulation cyclosporine is quite variable, with bioavailability ranging to 20% to 50%.[72] Erratic inter- and intraindividual bioavailability is a limitation of cyclosporine that may underlie some dose-related toxicities. A microemulsion formulation of cyclosporine has been developed that has less erratic and slightly higher bioavailability than the standard oral preparation.[73] After an oral dose, cyclosporine blood concentrations peak after 1½ to 2 hours. The bioavailability of cyclosporine is affected by food, and patients taking cyclosporine long term should be counseled to take the drug at regular daily times in relationship to food intake.[74] After absorption, cyclosporine is widely distributed and has a high volume of distribution, up to 5 L/kg.

Cyclosporine undergoes extensive metabolism by the cytochrome P (CYP)-450 system, especially the 3A4 isoform. CYP3A4 activity in intestinal epithelial cells and in the liver is responsible for extensive first-pass metabolism of cyclosporine.[75] Cyclosporine metabolites, of which there are many, have low pharmacologic activity.

Metabolism of cyclosporine by CYP3A4 results in a significant potential for drug interactions. Inhibitors or high-affinity substrates for CYP3A4, when coadministered with cyclosporine, tend to elevate cyclosporine blood concentrations. Grapefruit juice, which contains a substance that inhibits CYP3A4 in intestinal epithelial cells, is well documented as a cause of dramatic elevations in cyclosporine blood concentrations.[76,77] Patients taking cyclosporine must be advised not to take grapefruit or grapefruit juice, and care must be exercised if any other CYP3A4 substrates are coadministered. Drugs known to elevate cyclosporine blood concentrations include imidazole antifungals, erythromycin, and some calcium channel blockers.

Because of marked variability in blood cyclosporine levels, it can be useful to monitor blood cyclosporine concentrations, both during intravenous administration and during chronic oral therapy. Two widely used assay systems for measuring blood cyclosporine concentrations exist: radioimmunoassay and high-pressure liquid chromatography.[78] These two assay methodologies produce significantly different blood cyclosporine concentrations, so it is important for physicians to interpret blood results in the context of the specific assay being used.[79] During intravenous administration, steady state blood cyclosporine levels can be checked. During oral therapy, when the drug is commonly given twice daily, it is somewhat controversial as to whether blood levels should be measured at the trough time point immediately before another dose or 2 hours after a preceding dose.[80] Both strategies have advantages and disadvantages. The trough level does not correlate well with the area under the blood concentration time curve, but is useful for detecting high levels that might be associated with toxicity. The 2-hour postdose estimation correlates better with the area under the curve than the trough level does but can be misleading in patients with delayed gastric emptying. In practice, once the patient has been stabilized on a dose of oral cyclosporine, there may be little benefit in regular checking of blood levels unless the clinical situation changes significantly.

Tacrolimus, also known as FK506, is the other clinically important calcineurin inhibitor. Cyclosporine and tacrolimus are not interchangeable in individual patients, and variations in bioavailability and administration rather than significant differences in mechanisms of action underlie this difference. Tacrolimus can be administered orally or intravenously. Absorption from the gastrointestinal tract is variable, and bioavailability ranges from 15% to 20%.[52,81] After absorption, tacrolimus is widely distributed and is metabolized in the liver by members of the CYP3A family. Blood concentration monitoring is useful to individualize dose.[82]

Mechanism of Action. The pharmacologic mechanisms of action of cyclosporine and tacrolimus have been extensively characterized[83] (Fig. 11-3). Cyclosporine diffuses across the plasma membrane and binds to cyclophilin, a specific cyclosporine-binding protein. The cyclosporine-cyclophilin complex binds to and inactivates the cytoplasmic phosphatase calcineurin. The phosphatase activity of calcineurin is required for the activation of nuclear factor of activated T cell (NFAT), a critical transcription factor. NFAT is mobilized during the activation program of T lymphocytes after those lymphocytes have received appropriate stimulation through the T-cell receptor and a coreceptor.[84] This results in the activation of calcineurin, which dephosphorylates NFAT, the latter posttranslational modification being an essential step in the nuclear translocation of NFAT. In the nucleus, NFAT increases the expression of a number of T-lymphocyte activation genes, most notably the gene encoding IL-2.[85] Interleukin-2 is a key T-lymphocyte growth factor required for clonal expansion of T lymphocytes during adaptive immune responses. By blocking this program, cyclosporine effectively abrogates normal adaptive immune responses.

The molecular mechanism of action of tacrolimus closely parallels that of cyclosporine. Tacrolimus diffuses across the plasma membrane and binds to FK-binding protein, an immunophilin similar to cyclophilin. The tacrolimus–FK-binding protein complex inhibits calcineurin, in the same way that the cyclosporine-cyclophilin complex does.[83]

A number of other biochemical mechanisms have been attributed to calcineurin inhibitors such as inhibition of some nuclear factor-κB (NF-κB)–containing proteins[86] and also increasing the expression of transforming growth factor-β. However, these alternative mechanisms are probably less important than the classic mechanism involving inhibition of IL-2 production.

Toxicity. Side effects are quite common with cyclosporine therapy, and most of these are dose-related. Important toxicities include renal dysfunction, tremor, hirsutism, hypertension, and dyslipidemia. The development of nephrotoxicity is a particular concern in patients who have had a renal transplantation.[87] Hypertension is closely linked to the development of renal dysfunction and occurs in as many as 50% of cyclosporine-treated patients. At high cyclosporine blood levels, seizures can occur owing to a direct toxic effect of cyclosporine on central nervous system electrical activity. One study has suggested that malnutrition, assessed as low blood cholesterol levels, is a predictor of cyclosporine neurotoxicity.[88] The administration of potent immunosuppressants such as cyclosporine, particularly when used along with other immune-suppressing drugs like corticosteroids or thiopurines, does increase the risk of opportunistic infections. Indeed, many clinical series of cyclosporine-treated patients contain examples of patients who died as a result of infections of unusual severity or infections with microorganisms that rarely cause disease in immunocompetent individuals.[89] Therefore, it is important to counsel patients extensively about early warning signs of serious infections and also to appropriately administer immunizations. Cyclosporine increases the risk of squamous cell skin cancers[90] and lymphoproliferative disorders.

Side effects of tacrolimus are quite common and include nephrotoxicity, neurotoxicity, hypertension, and diabetes. Unlike cyclosporine, tacrolimus does not cause dyslipidemia. However, the potential for opportunistic infections with tacrolimus is similar to that seen with cyclosporine.

Clinical Uses. Calcineurin inhibitors are used extensively in the prevention of rejection of transplanted allogeneic kidneys, livers, hearts, lungs, small intestine, and pancreas.[91,92] Cyclosporine and tacrolimus have also been used in the treatment of severely active chronic inflammatory diseases, notably inflammatory bowel diseases.[93] Tacrolimus ointment is useful in the management of chronic eczema.[94]

Mammalian Target of Rapamycin Inhibitors

Rapamycin, also known as sirolimus, is the best-studied inhibitor of the mammalian target of rapamycin. Sirolimus is a fungal metabolite that is a member of the macrolide antibiotic family and was originally developed as a potential antifungal agent. This drug is useful as an immunosuppressant, particularly in the setting of renal transplanta-

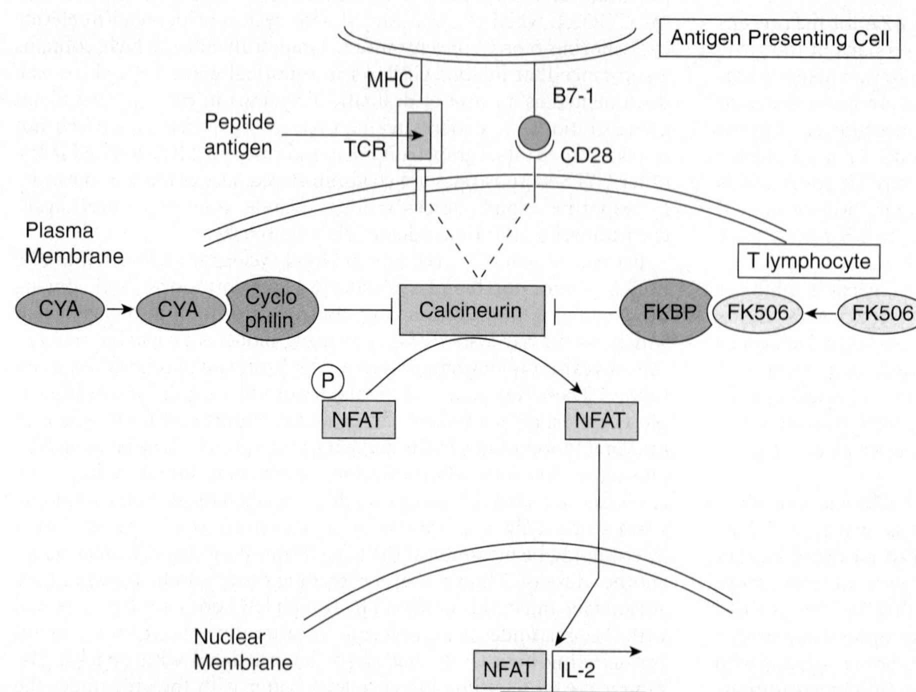

FIGURE 11-3 • Mechanism of action of calcineurin inhibitors. T lymphocyte activation is triggered by signals from the T-cell receptor (TCR) and a costimulatory signal receptor (CD28), when they are engaged by appropriate stimuli from antigen-presenting cells. This triggers a cascade of intracellular signaling that leads to the activation of calcineurin, a cytoplasmic phosphatase. Calcineurin dephosphorylates nuclear factor of activated T cell (NFAT), an event essential for the translocation of that transcription factor into the nucleus. Nuclear NFAT dramatically increases expression of the interleukin-2 (IL-2) gene leading to increased expression of IL-2, a growth factor essential for T-lymphocyte expansion and function during adaptive immune responses. Cyclosporine (CYA) binds to cyclophilin, and tacrolimus (FK506) binds to FK-binding protein (FKBP), both cytoplasmic immunophilin proteins. When bound by their ligand, immunophilins block the activity of calcineurin, preventing NFAT dephosphorylation and IL-2 expression.

tion because it appears to have less renal toxicity than the calcineurin inhibitors.[95]

Sirolimus is administered orally but has low bioavailability, approximately 15%. The half-life of elimination is long, about 2 to 3 days, and metabolism is mainly via CYP3A4.[96]

Sirolimus acts by binding to an intracellular receptor, FKBP12.[97] Lymphocytes appear to be the main target cells for the immunosuppressive effects, although it is likely that sirolimus also affects nonimmune cells. The sirolimus-FKBP12 complex binds to and inhibits the mammalian target of rapamycin complex in lymphocytes, which reduces sensitivity to the activating effects of IL-2.[98] As a result, the proliferation of lymphocytes is markedly reduced by sirolimus, and this effect impairs acquired immune responses, resulting in immunosuppression.

The main advantage of sirolimus over calcineurin inhibitors is its lack of nephrotoxicity.[99] However, sirolimus does possess some unique and significant toxicity. Most notable is an adverse effect on wound healing that has prompted many transplant centers to delay introduction of sirolimus until postoperative wounds have healed.[100]

The precise role of sirolimus in the prevention of renal allograft rejection is not yet known, but it has been evaluated as an alternative to both calcineurin inhibitors and antimetabolites (thiopurines and mycophenolate).[101] Additional studies will be needed to determine the optimum role for this drug.

Everolimus is another inhibitor of the mammalian target of rapamycin that is similar in mode of action to sirolimus. It may have additional vascular protective properties and, for this reason, has been developed in particular for the prevention of cardiac allograft rejection.[102] Early clinical results appear promising, but confirmatory studies are needed.

Methotrexate

Methotrexate (MTX) is a classic antimetabolite drug developed initially as a treatment for leukemia. Methotrexate is still used in the treatment of a number of cancers, but has emerged in the 1970s and 1980s as an important immunosuppressant.

Pharmacokinetics and Metabolism. Methotrexate can be administered orally, and bioavailability is good, especially at doses of 15 mg or lower.[103] Above this dose, bioavailability reduces to less than 50%, possibly because of adverse effects of MTX on the epithelial lining of the small intestine, which impair absorption of the drug.[104,105] Methotrexate can also be administered intramuscularly or subcutaneously with almost 100% bioavailability.[106] In cancer chemotherapy, MTX is administered intravenously, but this route is usually reserved for the high doses used in some regimens. After administration, MTX is widely distributed, and within 24 hours, approximately 90% of the drug is excreted unchanged in the urine. A minor metabolite, 7-hydroxy-methotrexate is produced in the liver. The plasma elimination half-life of MTX is approximately 4 hours. However, a slow terminal phase of elimination can be observed when the drug is administered weekly.[106] This slow phase of elimination is believed to result from the release of drug from pools of MTX that become stored intracellularly as polyglutamate derivatives. This fact is believed to underlie the long-term beneficial effects of MTX as an immunosuppressant when it is administered only once weekly. After initiating weekly MTX therapy, intracellular MTX levels, as measured in erythrocytes, gradually accumulate to reach a plateau after about 6 weeks.[107] The beneficial effects of MTX take approximately 4 to 6 weeks to begin, suggesting that intracellular drug concentrations are an important determinant of efficacy.

Mechanism of Action. The classic biochemical mechanism of action of MTX is the competitive inhibition of dihydrofolate reductase with respect to dihydrofolate as substrate (Fig. 11-4). The inhibition of dihydrofolate reductase impairs the intracellular synthesis of fully reduced folate cofactors. Tetrahydrofolate, the product of dihydrofolate reductase, is necessary for many essential biosynthetic reactions, for example, those producing purine nucleotides and thymidylate. Deficiency of these metabolic intermediates impairs DNA synthesis and cell division. Compared with MTX, the polyglutamate derivatives appear to have inhibitory actions at additional steps in purine metabolism, notably the inhibition of thymidylate synthase.

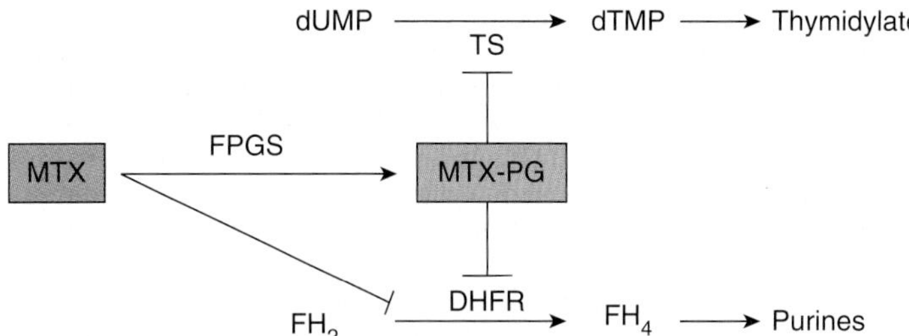

FIGURE 11-4 • Mechanism of action of methotrexate. Methotrexate is a substrate for folylpolyglutamate synthase (FPGS), which conjugates the parent drug with polyglutamate moieties that greatly increase intracellular retention of the drug. Therefore, long-lived polyglutamate derivatives (MTX-PG) accumulate. MTX-PG inhibits dihydrofolate reductase (DHFR), the key enzyme in the production of fully reduced folate cofactors (FH_4). Deficiency of FH_4 impairs de novo synthesis of purine nucleosides. MTX-PG also inhibits thymidylate synthase (TS), the enzyme that converts (dUMP) to thymidine-5′-phosphate (dTMP), resulting in deficiency of thymidylate. These effects are associated with decreased lymphocyte proliferation and increased apoptosis.

Methotrexate renders target cells, particularly lymphocytes, more susceptible to undergoing apoptosis during cellular activation.[108] This is probably the relevant cellular event that mediates the immunosuppressive properties of this drug. In addition to immunosuppression, the antiproliferative effects of MTX might be an added advantage of this drug in the treatment of psoriasis, a disease in which hyperproliferation of keratinocytes is a feature.

Toxicity. Many patients with chronic inflammatory diseases under treatment with MTX tolerate the drug very well when it is administered at low doses, for example 7.5 mg to 15 mg once a week. Some patients experience transient nausea after the weekly dose, but this is rarely troublesome.[107,109] Slightly higher doses, for example, 25 mg/wk can cause more problematic nausea. Because of its antiproliferative effects, MTX can cause gastrointestinal toxicity at least in part related to the inhibition of the normal proliferation of gastrointestinal epithelial crypt cells, which are among the fastest proliferating cells in the body. Similarly, alopecia or cytopenias can occur and reflect the antiproliferative effects of MTX on hair follicles and bone marrow.

Hepatotoxicity is a significant problem with MTX. Several well-conducted studies in patients with arthritis or psoriasis who were receiving chronic weekly MTX demonstrated a cumulative dose-dependent occurrence of hepatotoxicity.[110,111] Hepatotoxicity can range from minor elevation of serum aminotransferase activity to cirrhosis and liver failure. Elevation of aminotransferase activity appears to be dose-related and can be managed by lowering the dose of MTX. The precise histologic correlate of elevated aminotransferase activity during chronic MTX therapy is not certain. However, many chronic MTX-treated patients have developed hepatic fibrosis or cirrhosis without antecedent dramatic abnormalities of liver biochemical tests. This fact has prompted some to recommend serial liver biopsy in all MTX-treated patients to screen for the development of irreversible liver damage.[112] However, the usefulness of serial liver biopsy is not universally accepted,[113] with some reports failing to find any evidence of progressive liver damage with increasing cumulative doses of MTX.[114] Moreover, the absolute risk of permanent liver damage by MTX appears to be low and can be mitigated by the judicious use of this drug in carefully selected patients. Known risk factors for the development of serious liver toxicity during MTX treatment include prior liver disease of any type, especially nonalcoholic fatty liver disease or alcoholic liver disease.[115] Methotrexate should probably be avoided in such patients, and all patients on chronic MTX therapy should avoid alcohol. Patients with metabolic syndrome and type 2 diabetes mellitus, who commonly have fatty liver disease, should be monitored especially closely for the development of significant liver abnormalities or should avoid MTX use altogether.

Allergy to MTX is rare, but a small number of patients develop idiopathic pneumonitis.[116] This is manifest clinically as dyspnea and cough. Pulmonary evaluation reveals interstitial lung infiltrates and a restrictive lung defect. If MTX is stopped early during this process, the changes are probably reversible.[117] Because of its immunosuppressant properties, MTX does appear to somewhat increase the risk of opportunistic infections.[118] The absolute risk conferred by MTX for such infections is not known.

The coadministration of folic acid at the same time as a weekly MTX dose has been advocated as a means of minimizing the toxicity of this drug without compromising its clinical efficacy.[119] The precise mechanism of how MTX toxicity might be minimized by the coadministration of folic acid without losing efficacy as an immunosuppressant is not known, but this practice has been widely adopted.

Methotrexate has established teratogenic and abortifacient properties and should not be used in pregnant women or women at risk of becoming pregnant.[120]

Before beginning MTX therapy, pregnancy should be excluded, liver biochemical tests should be checked, and a blood count should be obtained. During therapy, monthly or 2-monthly liver biochemical tests and blood counts should be checked. The persistent elevation of serum aminotransferase activity to more than twice normal or the development of bone marrow suppression are indications to lower the dose or stop MTX.

Clinical Uses. Methotrexate is an important drug in the management of chronic inflammatory arthritides,[121] psoriasis,[122] and some types of inflammatory bowel disease.[109]

Cyclophosphamide

Cyclophosphamide is an alkylating agent and one of the most active immunosuppressive agents available. The clinical utility of cyclophosphamide is limited by quite marked toxicity, so this drug is utilized only in aggressive inflammatory or autoimmune diseases that cannot be controlled with safer agents.

Pharmacokinetics and Metabolism. Cyclophosphamide can be administered orally or intravenously. In the liver, this drug is converted to aldophosphoramide and a bladder-toxic metabolite acrolein. Aldophosphoramide is converted to phosphoramide mustard, the active metabolite. Active and inactive metabolites are eliminated unchanged in the urine.

Mechanism of Action. The active metabolites of cyclophosphamide alkylate cellular macromolecules, creating covalent linkages that prevent their dissociation.[123] The most important target is probably DNA, because the alkylation of DNA prevents cell division and also perturbs gene expression. After cyclophosphamide treatment, lymphocyte count and function are markedly reduced.[124]

Toxicity. Cyclophosphamide is a potent suppressor of bone marrow and can cause significant cytopenias. This can lead to the complications of bleeding and opportunistic infections.[125] This drug is also toxic to male and female gonads, and many patients are rendered infertile after cyclophosphamide therapy.[126] Malignancies, especially lymphomas, are more common in patients who have undergone cyclophosphamide treatment.[127] Acrolein, a metabolite of cyclophosphamide, is toxic to the bladder, causing cystitis, and later bladder cancer can develop.[128] Sodium 2-mercaptoethane sulfonate (MESNA) is used to prevent cyclophosphamide bladder toxicity.

Clinical Uses. Cyclophosphamide is used to treat certain types of glomerulonephritis and systemic vasculitides.

Antilymphocyte Immunoglobulins and Monoclonal Antibodies

A series of polyclonal and monoclonal antibody therapeutics has been developed to prevent and treat acute rejection of transplanted allografts. These antibody preparations target molecules expressed on the surface of lymphocytes, especially T lymphocytes. The rationale for targeting T lymphocytes to prevent rejection lies in the fact that recognition of transplanted organs as nonself depends on the recognition of donor-derived peptides by host T lymphocytes as foreign, leading to the subsequent activation of those cells, and development of an adaptive immune response. Therefore, T lymphocytes are critical to the development of rejection reactions. The different agents discussed in this section are administered intravenously, usually in the critical early posttransplant period or at the time of acute rejection. Many different dosing regimens and combinations with other drugs have been tested. The different forms of antilymphocyte antibodies are illustrated in Figure 11-5.

Polyclonal antithymocyte globulin was developed by immunizing horses or rabbits with human thymocytes and purifying gammaglobulins from serum. These preparations contain antibodies reactive against many different antigens expressed on the surface of lymphocytes. The polyclonal sera prepared from those animals are used at the time of allograft implantation and afterward to prevent early acute rejection.[129] The administration of antithymocyte globulins results in profound killing of host lymphocytes. In addition to antilymphocyte effects, polyclonal antithymocyte globulins can cause neutropenia and thrombocytopenia, leading to opportunistic infections and bleeding risk.[130,131] Several different dosing regimens are used for polyclonal antithymocyte globulins in kidney transplant recipients.

Ornithine ketoacid transaminase (OKT3), also known as monomurab-CD3, is the first monoclonal antibody developed using biotechnology to be used in humans.[132] This murine antibody targets the CD3 component of the T-lymphocyte receptor on the surface of T cells. This

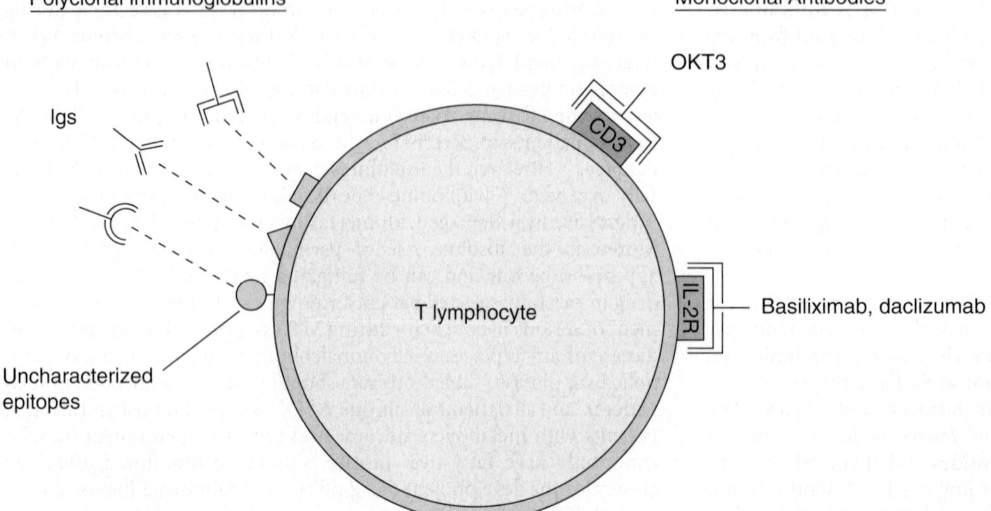

FIGURE 11-5 • Mechanism of action of antilymphocyte antibodies. Polyclonal immunoglobulins (Ig) are raised in horses or rabbits by inoculation with human thymocytes or lymphocytes. Gammaglobulins are purified from serum of the animals and the Igs contained in the preparation are diverse in their recognition of a large array of uncharacterized epitopes that were expressed on the surface of cells used for inoculation. Monoclonal antilymphocyte antibodies have been engineered to recognize a single epitope on the surface of lymphocytes. Thus, ornithine ketoacid transaminase (OKT3) binds to CD3, and basiliximab and daclizumab bind to the interleukin-2 receptor (IL-2R).

leads to the killing of those cells, which profoundly impairs lymphocyte-dependent immune reactions.[133,134] OKT3 causes a cytokine release syndrome with the first dose, which manifests clinically as fever, often with rigors, vomiting, wheezing, and hypotension.[135] This is caused by the sudden release of large amounts of cytokines from lymphocytes killed by OKT3 soon after administration. Cytokine release syndrome can be minimized by pretreatment with methylprednisolone, antihistamines, and acetaminophen. Additional adverse effects of OKT3 include susceptibility to opportunistic infections, especially with viruses such as cytomegalovirus and Epstein-Barr virus.[136] In the long-term, doses of OKT3 have been associated with posttransplantation lymphoproliferative disease, a form of lymphoma caused by Epstein-Barr virus.[137]

Because of the pivotal importance of IL-2 in the development of robust adaptive immune responses, strategies to inhibit signaling by this cytokine have been developed. In addition to the effects of drugs such as cyclosporine, FK506, and sirolimus that inhibit IL-2 at the intracellular signaling level, monoclonal antibodies that target and neutralize the IL-2 receptor have proved clinically effective. Basiliximab is a chimeric mouse/human anti-IL-2 receptor monoclonal antibody. This agent effectively blocks IL-2–stimulated T lymphocyte proliferation and markedly dampens acquired immune responses.[138] One notable limitation with this antibody is the fact that patients who receive subsequent doses some time (months) after the initial dose appear to be at high risk for hypersensitivity-type infusion reactions.[139] This is likely to be due to the formation of antichimeric antibodies after the initial dose. Daclizumab is another anti-IL-2 receptor chimeric mouse/human monoclonal antibody.[140] Daclizumab has been evaluated for the prevention of renal allograft rejection and is approved for such use.

Antilymphocyte immunoglobulins and monoclonal antibodies are used to prevent and treat rejection of allogeneic solid organ transplants.[141-144]

Tumor Necrosis Factor-α Inhibitors

TNFα is a pivotal proinflammatory cytokine. The concentration of TNFα is elevated in inflamed tissues in many chronic inflammatory diseases such as rheumatoid arthritis and inflammatory bowel disease. This cytokine exerts profound effects on cells that express specific receptors on their cell surface, resulting in the activation of immune mechanisms in those cells.[145] The production of TNFα is a highly regulated process, and cell types that are involved in the production of large amounts of TNFα in chronic inflammatory diseases include activated monocytes and macrophages, lymphocytes, and probably a variety of other nonimmune cells such as fibroblasts, endothelial cells, and epithelial cells.

The engagement of TNFα with its receptors initiates cascades of intracellular signaling events that result in activation of a number of pivotal proinflammatory transcription factors such as NF-κB and activating protein 1 (AP1).[146] The activated forms of these transcription factors increase the expression of many genes whose encoded proteins promote inflammation. Genes known to be up-regulated by TNFα include proinflammatory cytokines, chemokines, nitric oxide synthase, and cyclooxygenase-2. For these reasons, TNFα plays a central and pivotal role in many inflammatory responses. It is less clear whether TNFα plays an important role in adaptive immune responses.

Several approaches have been undertaken to block the biologic actions of TNFα. Thalidomide is a small molecule that appears to decrease the secretion of TNFα from cells, but by unclear mechanisms.[147] Teratogenicity has severely limited the usefulness of this drug. More recently, several so-called biologic agents have been developed to specifically block the activity of TNFα (Fig. 11-6). Three such agents are currently licensed for use, and several others are in clinical development.

Infliximab. Initially termed cA2, infliximab is a chimeric mouse-human monoclonal antibody against TNFα.[148] Infliximab contains human constant and murine variable regions. This antibody was found to be beneficial in patients with inflammatory arthritis[149,150] and with inflammatory bowel disease.[151-153] Infliximab is administered intravenously, usually as a 2-hour infusion. The elimination half-life is approximately 10 days, and the maximum serum concentration is in the region of 100 mg/L at typical doses of 3 mg/kg to 5 mg/kg. Infliximab is detectable in blood for approximately 8 weeks after administration of usual doses, and clinical studies suggest that the presence of detectable trough infliximab concentrations is associated with good clinical outcomes.[154,155] Common practice is to administer three doses over the initial 6 weeks of therapy followed by infusions every 8 weeks, if continuous therapy is appropriate.

Infliximab binds to human TNFα with a dissociation constant of 10^{-10} M. As a result of this high-affinity interaction, the biologic activities of TNFα are effectively neutralized by infliximab.[156] Notably, infliximab can bind to both the soluble and the membrane-associated forms of TNFα. When this drug binds membrane-associated TNFα, it activates caspase cascades within cells, leading to their apoptosis.[157,158]

Most patients tolerate infliximab quite well. Early clinical experience with infliximab was positive, but when patients who had initially received this drug in clinical trials, often as a single dose, were retreated several years later after the drug was approved, infusion reactions were quite common. These reactions are classified as anaphylactoid-type and appear to be a consequence of IgE-mediated mast cell degranulation.[159] Infusion reactions typically manifest as hypotension, fever, nausea, and shortness of breath. They can be managed by stopping the infusion or, if mild, by slowing the rate of the infusion. Some practitioners advocate pretreatment with an antihistamine and the administration of a single intravenous dose of corticosteroid such as hydrocortisone 100 mg to prevent infusion reactions. Rarely, patients have experienced life-threatening reactions during infliximab infusions.[160] Serum sickness–like reactions have also been reported in

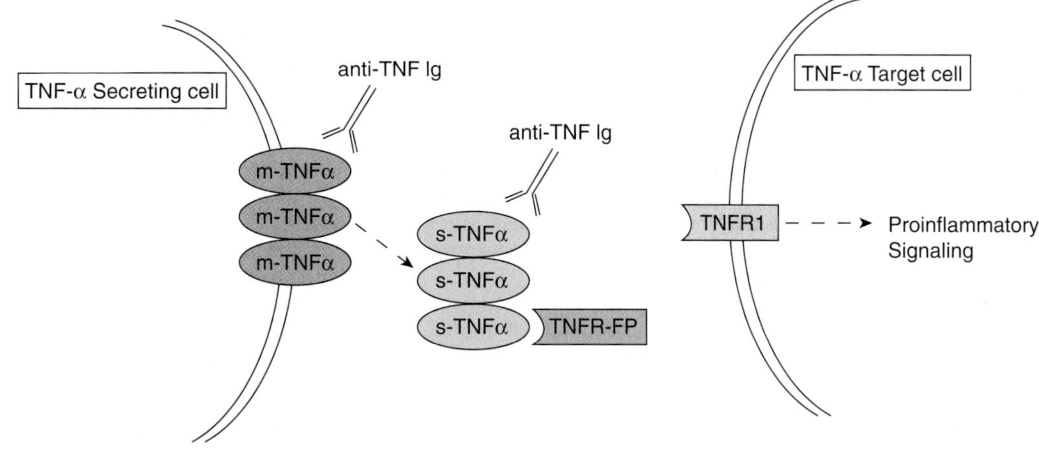

FIGURE 11-6 • Mechanism of action of anti-tumor necrosis factor-α (TNFα) agents. TNFα is produced by cells and initially expressed as a membrane-associated cytokine (m-TNF). TNFα can be shed into the extracellular matrix as soluble cytokine (s-TNF). Antibodies to TNFα, such as infliximab and adalimumab, can bind to both m-TNF and s-TNF, neutralizing their biologic activity. The binding of those antibodies to m-TNF may also induce apoptosis of the expressing cells. Etanercept, a soluble TNF-receptor fusion protein (TNFR-FP), also neutralizes s-TNF but does not bind avidly to m-TNF or induce apoptosis of expressing cells.

which patients experienced arthralgias and/or skin eruptions 3 to 4 days after an infliximab infusion. Two strategies have been proposed to minimize the likelihood of the development of immune responses to infliximab. First, some recommend the continuous, rather than intermittent, use of infliximab, with maintenance infusions being given usually every 8 weeks. This is because the rate of formation of antibodies against infliximab, which mediate infusion reactions, appears to be lower in patients who receive the drug on a continuous rather than episodic basis.[159] Second, the use of a concomitant immunosuppressant such as a thiopurine or MTX also appears to be associated with lower rates of antibody formation. Finally, one study suggested that the administration of intravenous hydrocortisone before infliximab infusions reduces the likelihood of antibody formation.[161]

Infliximab, in common with other anti-TNFα agents, has been strongly associated with the development of active tuberculosis.[162] Most likely, this is because TNFα is required for effective granuloma formation, which is necessary for the containment of intracellular pathogens such as *Mycobacterium tuberculosis*. When TNFα activity is strongly neutralized, granulomas appear to disintegrate, allowing the reactivation of latent tuberculosis. Therefore, it is essential that for all patients in whom anti-TNFα therapy is planned, the possibility of latent tuberculosis must first be excluded. Usually, this is done by administering a tuberculin skin test. Patients with reactions greater than 5 mm should be treated with isoniazid and rifampicin for 6 months. It is also usual to obtain a chest x-ray to exclude the possibility of radiographic evidence of tuberculosis.

In addition to tuberculosis, infliximab has also been associated with active infection by other intracellular pathogens, notably histoplasmosis.[163] It is also possible, but less certain, that infliximab may increase the risk of other sorts of opportunistic infections. In particular, the risk of opportunistic infection with infliximab is probably increased by the concomitant use of other immune-suppressing drugs.

Infliximab use has not been definitively linked with an increased risk of cancer. Nevertheless, a rare and very aggressive form of lymphoma, hepatosplenic T-cell lymphoma, has been reported in a number of children who received infliximab.[164] The majority of these children were also receiving AZA or 6-MP, and at present, it is not clear whether there is a causal association between infliximab and the occurrence of these lymphomas.

A number of quite rare neurologic problems have also been associated with infliximab. Most notable of these is the development of central nervous system demyelinating disease that resembles multiple sclerosis.[165] Moreover, infliximab was tested as a therapy for multiple sclerosis but was abandoned because of the apparent worsening of the disease.[166] Therefore, anti-TNFα agents such as infliximab should not be administered to any patient with known or suspected multiple sclerosis. It is possible that the observed cases of central nervous system demyelination after anti-TNFα treatment may, in fact, represent the unmasking of latent or early multiple sclerosis in susceptible individuals. Infliximab use has also been associated with peripheral neuropathy in a small number of cases. Patients with advanced heart failure, New York Heart Association class 3 or 4, should not receive infliximab because of reports of worsening cardiac failure.

Adalimumab. Adalimumab is a fully human IgG1 monoclonal anti-TNFα antibody. Adalimumab is administered subcutaneously, usually once every 2 weeks. Subcutaneous administration provides bioavailability of approximately 60%, and the terminal half-life of elimination is about 2 weeks. Steady state serum concentrations after subcutaneous administration are reached after about 5 or 6 days. Adalimumab binds to TNFα in both the soluble and the membrane-associated forms. This binding effectively neutralizes the biologic activity of TNFα. Moreover, when adalimumab binds membrane-associated TNFα, it appears to produce the apoptosis of those cells.[167]

Side effects of adalimumab are similar to those of infliximab, with the exception of infusion reactions. The development of immunogenicity to adalimumab may be less than with infliximab, because this antibody is fully humanized, as opposed to human-mouse chimeric. Compared with chimeric antibodies, it is possible that the absence of any murine protein in fully human antibodies such as adalimumab may decrease the likelihood of the development of immunogenicity. However, this point has not yet been proved. Some patients do note soreness and itch at the site of adalimumab injections, but this can be minimized by the use of antihistamines.

Other side effects, including increased risk of infections and central nervous system demyelination, are similar to those occurring with infliximab.[168]

Etanercept. Etanercept is a soluble TNFα receptor fusion protein that effectively neutralizes the biologic activity of TNFα. This protein consists of two molecules of the p75 TNFα receptor linked by the Fc portion of IgG. Etanercept resides in the body far longer than nonfusion protein or native TNFα receptors, and the dimeric structure is important for effective neutralization of TNFα.[169] Etanercept is administered by subcutaneous injections once or twice weekly. The mechanism of action appears to relate to the neutralization of secreted, but not membrane-associated, TNFα by preventing binding of the cytokine to its receptor. After administration, the drug has a half-life of elimination of approximately 5 days. Peak concentrations are reached about 3 days after an injection. Infusion reactions or injection site reactions are not common.

Other side effects, including increased risk of infections and central nervous system demyelination, are similar to those occurring with infliximab.

TNFα inhibitors are used to treat inflammatory arthritides, inflammatory bowel diseases, psoriasis, and numerous other more rare inflammatory disorders.

Inhibitors of Leukocyte Trafficking

Because of the necessity for leukocytes to emigrate from blood vessels into tissues to exert their functions in immune responses, a recent approach to immunosuppression has been the development of drugs to inhibit leukocyte extravasation. The drug that has progressed clinically with most success in this group is a humanized monoclonal antibody against the α_4 integrin subunit, natalizumab.[170] α_4 Integrin is expressed on activated lymphocytes and monocytes in the circulation. This integrin is required for efficient extravasation of those cells and is mediated by interaction with vascular cell adhesion molecule-1, which is expressed on endothelial cells. Administration of natalizumab results in the retention within the vasculature of circulating white blood cells that express α_4 integrins.[171] Monocytes and lymphocytes are most notably affected by natalizumab, but eosinophils and basophils are also affected. Because of the blockade of extravasation, the accumulation of activated monocytes and lymphocytes at sites of inflammation is diminished by natalizumab. It is also possible that natalizumab blocks the interaction of α4 integrin–expressing cells in inflamed tissues with ligand expressed at those sites.

Natalizumab is administered by intravenous injection every 4 weeks. The dose of 300 mg has demonstrated efficacy. The most important toxicity that has been observed is the development of progressive multifocal leukoencephalopathy.[172-175] This is a rare, fatal neurodegenerative brain disease linked to reactivation of latent JC virus infection. Three such cases developed in approximately 2000 patients who received natalixumab in clinical trials of this drug for multiple sclerosis or Crohn's disease. Because of this toxicity, natalizumab use is reserved for patients with severe disease for whom other therapies are not effective. In addition to progressive multifocal leukoencephalopathy, natalizumab is associated with increased risk of infections such as respiratory and gastrointestinal tract pathogens.

Natalizumab is used to treat multiple sclerosis refractory to other agents.[176,177] Large clinical trials have also established the efficacy of natalizumab for Crohn's disease,[178] but progressive multifocal leukoencephalopathy has prevented the use of natalizumab in such patients to date.

Others

Leflunomide is a unique agent that is an inhibitor of de novo pyrimidine biosynthesis. After oral ingestion, this drug undergoes metabolic activation in the liver to form a malononitrilamide derivative. This

TABLE 11-4 BIOLOGIC THERAPEUTICS IN CLINICAL DEVELOPMENT THAT ACT ON THE IMMUNE SYSTEM

Agent	Target	Type of Biologic	Intended Use
Visilizumab	CD3	Humanized MAb	Ulcerative colitis
Fontolizumab	Interferon-γ	Humanized MAb	Crohn's disease
ABT-874/J695	IL-12	Humanized MAb	Crohn's disease
Certolizumab pegol	TNFα	Pegylated MAb fragment	Crohn's disease
MLN02	α4β7 Integrin	Humanized MAb	Ulcerative colitis, Crohn's disease
Tocilizumab	IL-6 receptor	Humanized MAb	Rheumatoid arthritis, ulcerative colitis
Golimumab	TNFα	Fully human MAb	Rheumatoid arthritis, Crohn's disease
Abatacept	CD80/86	CTLA4-Ig fusion protein	Graft-versus-host disease, rheumatoid arthritis
Belatacept	CD80/86	CTLA4-Ig fusion protein	Transplant rejection
Mesenchymal stem cells	Unknown	Donor-derived human cells	Graft-versus-host disease, Crohn's disease

CTLA4-Ig, cytotoxic T-lymphocyte-associated protein 4-immunoglobulin; IL, interleukin; MAb, monoclonal antibody; TNFα, tumor necrosis factor-α.

metabolite inhibits dihydro-oratate-dehydrogenase, which is the rate-limiting enzyme for pyrimidine biosynthesis during DNA replication at the time of cell division. Rapidly cycling activated lymphocytes appear to be sensitive to the antiproliferative effects of leflunomide, which probably underlies this drug's immunosuppressant properties. Gastrointestinal disturbances and hepatotoxicity limit the usefulness of leflunomide. Clinical uses of leflunomide include rheumatoid arthritis[179] and psoriatic arthritis, and it is being evaluated for the prevention of allograft rejection.

Rituximab is a chimeric mouse/human monoclonal antibody against CD20, a specific antigen expressed on the surface of B lymphocytes during their differentiation from the pre–B-cell stage through maturation. The expression of CD20 is lost in differentiated plasma cells. Rituximab binds CD20 with high affinity and results in marked depletion of B lymphocytes. This drug is important in the treatment of B-cell non-Hodgkins lymphomas, but it has also been increasingly used in rheumatoid arthritis.[180]

Anakinra is recombinant human IL-1 receptor antagonist. This agent, like the endogenous form, binds to but does not activate the IL-1 receptor and effectively competes with IL-1 for those receptors. Administration of recombinant human IL-1 receptor antagonist is effective anti-inflammatory therapy and is useful in the treatment of rheumatoid arthritis.[181]

Biologic Therapeutics in Clinical Development

Fuelled by advances in the capability of the biotechnology industry to produce recombinant proteins and engineered monoclonal antibodies, many new biological agents that target the immune system have been developed since the late 1990s. A variety of technologies have been used to discover molecules amenable to targeting using monoclonal antibodies. The majority of such drug targets are cell surface–expressed proteins or secreted proteins that regulate immunity. At the same time that biologic agents have become a rich form of novel therapeutic agents, new immune system–active small molecule drugs have been less numerous. Monoclonal antibody therapeutics have several inherent benefits, including long duration of action and specificity of targeting. However, these benefits are offset by high costs of production, the requirement for parenteral administration, and the potential for immunogenicity. Table 11-4 provides a list of some biologic antibodies, currently in clinical development, that target the immune system.

REFERENCES

1. Smith HR, Steinberg AD. Autoimmunity—a perspective. Annu Rev Immunol 1983;1:175-210.
2. McInnes IB, Schett G. Cytokines in the pathogenesis of rheumatoid arthritis. Nat Rev Immunol 2007;7:429-442.
3. Groth CG, Brent LB, Calne RY, et al. Historic landmarks in clinical transplantation: conclusions from the consensus conference at the University of California, Los Angeles. World J Surg 2000;24:834-843.
4. Shlomchik WD. Graft-versus-host disease. Nat Rev Immunol 2007;7:340-352.
5. Neutra MR, Mantis NJ, Kraehenbuhl JP. Collaboration of epithelial cells with organized mucosal lymphoid tissues. Nat Immunol 2001;2:1004-1009.
6. Niess JH, Brand S, Gu X, et al. CX3CR1-mediated dendritic cell access to the intestinal lumen and bacterial clearance. Science 2005;307:254-258.
7. Janeway CA Jr, Medzhitov R. Innate immune recognition. Annu Rev Immunol 2002;20:197-216.
8. Toruner M, Loftus EV Jr, Colombel JF, et al. Risk factors for opportunistic infections in inflammatory bowel diseases: a case-control study. Gastroenterology 2006;130: A-71.
9. Hench PS, Kendall EC, Slocumb CH, Polley HF. Effects of cortisone acetate and pituitary ACTH on rheumatoid arthritis, rheumatic fever and certain other conditions. Arch Med Interna 1950;85:545-666.
10. Frey BM, Frey FJ. Clinical pharmacokinetics of prednisone and prednisolone. Clin Pharmacokinet 1990;19:126-146.
11. Rhen T, Cidlowski JA. Antiinflammatory action of glucocorticoids—new mechanisms for old drugs. N Engl J Med 2005;353:1711-1723.
12. De Bosscher K, Schmitz ML, Vanden Berghe W, et al. Glucocorticoid-mediated repression of nuclear factor-kappaB-dependent transcription involves direct interference with transactivation. Proc Natl Acad Sci U S A 1997;94:13504-13509.
13. Doucas V, Shi Y, Miyamoto S, et al. Cytoplasmic catalytic subunit of protein kinase A mediates cross-repression by NF-kappa B and the glucocorticoid receptor. Proc Natl Acad Sci U S A 2000;97:11893-11898.
14. Vanden Berghe W, Francesconi E, De Bosscher K, et al. Dissociated glucocorticoids with anti-inflammatory potential repress interleukin-6 gene expression by a nuclear factor-kappaB-dependent mechanism. Mol Pharmacol 1999;56:797-806.
15. Warrington TP, Bostwick JM. Psychiatric adverse effects of corticosteroids. Mayo Clin Proc 2006;81:1361-1367.
16. Lionakis MS, Kontoyiannis DP. Glucocorticoids and invasive fungal infections. Lancet 2003;362:1828-1838.
17. van Staa TP, Leufkens HG, Cooper C. The epidemiology of corticosteroid-induced osteoporosis: a meta-analysis. Osteoporos Int 2002;13:777-787.
18. Jick SS, Vasilakis-Scaramozza C, Maier WC. The risk of cataract among users of inhaled steroids. Epidemiology 2001;12:229-234.
19. Markowitz J, Grancher K, Kohn N, et al. A multicenter trial of 6-mercaptopurine and prednisone in children with newly diagnosed Crohn's disease. Gastroenterology 2000;119:895-902.
20. Homik J, Cranney A, Shea B, et al. Bisphosphonates for steroid induced osteoporosis. Cochrane Database Syst Rev 2000:CD001347.
21. Homik J, Suarez-Almazor ME, Shea B, et al. Calcium and vitamin D for corticosteroid-induced osteoporosis. Cochrane Database Syst Rev 2000:CD000952.
22. Axelrod L. Perioperative management of patients treated with glucocorticoids. Endocrinol Metab Clin North Am 2003;32:367-383.
23. Kirwan JR, Bijlsma JW, Boers M, Shea BJ. Effects of glucocorticoids on radiological progression in rheumatoid arthritis. Cochrane Database Syst Rev 2007:CD006356.
24. Egan LJ, Sandborn WJ. Advances in the treatment of Crohn's disease. Gastroenterology 2004;126:1574-1581.
25. Hanauer SB. Medical therapy for ulcerative colitis 2004. Gastroenterology 2004;126:1582-1592.
26. Adams NP, Bestall JB, Malouf R, et al. Inhaled beclomethasone versus placebo for chronic asthma. Cochrane Database Syst Rev 2005:CD002738.
27. Wiesner RH, Ludwig J, Krom RA, et al. Treatment of early cellular rejection following liver transplantation with intravenous methylprednisolone. The effect of dose on response. Transplantation 1994;58:1053-1056.
28. Chao NJ, Schmidt GM, Niland JC, et al. Cyclosporine, methotrexate, and prednisone compared with cyclosporine and prednisone for prophylaxis of acute graft-versus-host disease. N Engl J Med 1993;329:1225-1230.
29. Hitchings GH, Elion GB, Falco EA, et al. Studies on analogs of purines and pyrimidines. Ann N Y Acad Sci 1950;52:1318-1335.

30. Dubinsky MC, Vasiliauskas EA, Singh H, et al. 6-Thioguanine can cause serious liver injury in inflammatory bowel disease patients. Gastroenterology 2003;125:298-303.
31. Vora A, Mitchell CD, Lennard L, et al. Toxicity and efficacy of 6-thioguanine versus 6-mercaptopurine in childhood lymphoblastic leukaemia: a randomised trial. Lancet 2006;368:1339-1348.
32. Lin SN, Jessup K, Floyd M, et al. Quantitation of plasma azathioprine and 6-mercaptopurine levels in renal transplant patients. Transplantation 1980;29:290-294.
33. Rhodes J, Bainton D, Beck P, Campbell H. Controlled trial of azathioprine in Crohn's disease. Lancet 1971;2:1273-1276.
34. Summers RW, Switz DM, Sessions JT Jr, et al. National Cooperative Crohn's Disease Study: results of drug treatment. Gastroenterology 1979;77:847-869.
35. Candy S, Wright J, Gerber M, et al. A controlled double blind study of azathioprine in the management of Crohn's disease. Gut 1995;37:674-678.
36. Sandborn WJ, Tremaine WJ, Wolf DC, et al. Lack of effect of intravenous administration on time to respond to azathioprine for steroid-treated Crohn's disease. North American Azathioprine Study Group. Gastroenterology 1999;117:527-535.
37. Dubinsky MC, Yang H, Hassard PV, et al. 6-MP metabolite profiles provide a biochemical explanation for 6-MP resistance in patients with inflammatory bowel disease. Gastroenterology 2002;122:904-915.
38. Prager D, Rosman M, Bertino JR. Azathioprine and allopurinol [Letter]. Ann Intern Med 1974;80:427.
39. Zazgornik J, Kopsa H, Schmidt P, et al. Increased danger of bone marrow damage in simultaneous azathioprine-allopurinol therapy. Int J Clin Pharmacol Ther Toxicol 1981;19:96-97.
40. Weinshilboum R. Methyltransferase pharmacogenetics. Pharmacol Ther 1989;43:77-90.
41. Wang L, Weinshilboum R. Thiopurine *S*-methyltransferase pharmacogenetics: insights, challenges and future directions. Oncogene 2006;25:1629-1638.
42. Wang L, Nguyen TV, McLaughlin RW, et al. Human thiopurine *S*-methyltransferase pharmacogenetics: variant allozyme misfolding and aggresome formation. Proc Natl Acad Sci U S A 2005;102:9394-9399.
43. Tinel M, Berson A, Pessayre D, et al. Pharmacogenetics of human erythrocyte thiopurine methyltransferase activity in a French population. Br J Clin Pharmacol 1991;32:729-734.
44. Lennard L, Van Loon JA, Lilleyman JS, Weinshilboum RM. Thiopurine pharmacogenetics in leukemia: correlation of erythrocyte thiopurine methyltransferase activity and 6-thioguanine nucleotide concentrations. Clin Pharmacol Ther 1987;41:18-25.
45. Colombel JF, Ferrari N, Debuysere H, et al. Genotypic analysis of thiopurine *S*-methyltransferase in patients with Crohn's disease and severe myelosuppression during azathioprine therapy. Gastroenterology 2000;118:1025-1030.
46. Lichtenstein GR, Abreu MT, Cohen R, Tremaine W. American Gastroenterological Association Institute technical review on corticosteroids, immunomodulators, and infliximab in inflammatory bowel disease. Gastroenterology 2006;130:940-987.
47. Cuffari C, Theoret Y, Latour S, Seidman G. 6-Mercaptopurine metabolism in Crohn's disease: correlation with efficacy and toxicity. Gut 1996;39:401-406.
48. Dubinsky MC, Lamothe S, Yang HY, et al. Pharmacogenomics and metabolite measurement for 6-mercaptopurine therapy in inflammatory bowel disease. Gastroenterology 2000;118:705-713.
49. Lowry PW, Franklin CL, Weaver AL, et al. Measurement of thiopurine methyltransferase activity and azathioprine metabolites in patients with inflammatory bowel disease. Gut 2001;49:665-670.
50. Osterman MT, Kundu R, Lichtenstein GR, Lewis JD. Association of 6-thioguanine nucleotide levels and inflammatory bowel disease activity: a meta-analysis. Gastroenterology 2006;130:1047-1053.
51. Sparrow MP, Hande SA, Friedman S, et al. Allopurinol safely and effectively optimizes tioguanine metabolites in inflammatory bowel disease patients not responding to azathioprine and mercaptopurine. Aliment Pharmacol Ther 2005;22:441-446.
52. Staatz CE, Tett SE. Clinical pharmacokinetics and pharmacodynamics of mycophenolate in solid organ transplant recipients. Clin Pharmacokinet 2007;46:13-58.
53. Quemeneur L, Gerland LM, Flacher M, et al. Differential control of cell cycle, proliferation, and survival of primary T lymphocytes by purine and pyrimidine nucleotides. J Immunol 2003;170:4986-4995.
54. Tiede I, Fritz G, Strand S, et al. CD28-dependent Rac1 activation is the molecular target of azathioprine in primary human CD4+ T lymphocytes. J Clin Invest 2003;111:1133-1145.
55. Thomas CW, Myhre GM, Tschumper R, et al. Selective inhibition of inflammatory gene expression in activated T lymphocytes: a mechanism of immune suppression by thiopurines. J Pharmacol Exp Ther 2005;312:537-545.
56. Korelitz BI, Zlatanic J, Goel F, Fuller S. Allergic reactions to 6-mercaptopurine during treatment of inflammatory bowel disease. J Clin Gastroenterol 1999;28:341-344.
57. Haber CJ, Meltzer SJ, Present DH, Korelitz BI. Nature and course of pancreatitis caused by 6-mercaptopurine in the treatment of inflammatory bowel disease. Gastroenterology 1986;91:982-986.
58. Boulton-Jones JR, Pritchard K, Mahmoud AA. The use of 6-mercaptopurine in patients with inflammatory bowel disease after failure of azathioprine therapy. Aliment Pharmacol Ther 2000;14:1561-1565.
59. Present DH, Meltzer SJ, Krumholz MP, et al. 6-Mercaptopurine in the management of inflammatory bowel disease: short- and long-term toxicity. Ann Intern Med 1989;111:641-649.
60. Pearson DC, May GR, Fick GH, Sutherland LR. Azathioprine and 6-mercaptopurine in Crohn disease. A meta-analysis. Ann Intern Med 1995;123:132-142.
61. Farrell RJ, Ang Y, Kileen P, et al. Increased incidence of non-Hodgkin's lymphoma in inflammatory bowel disease patients on immunosuppressive therapy but overall risk is low. Gut 2000;47:514-519.
62. Kandiel A, Fraser AG, Korelitz BI, et al. Increased risk of lymphoma among inflammatory bowel disease patients treated with azathioprine and 6-mercaptopurine. Gut 2005;54:1121-1125.
63. Dayharsh GA, Loftus EV Jr, Sandborn WJ, et al. Epstein-Barr virus–positive lymphoma in patients with inflammatory bowel disease treated with azathioprine or 6-mercaptopurine. Gastroenterology 2002;122:72-77.
64. Montano Loza AJ, Czaja AJ. Current therapy for autoimmune hepatitis. Nat Clin Pract Gastroenterol Hepatol 2007;4:202-214.
65. Bergan S, Rugstad HE, Bentdal O, et al. Monitored high-dose azathioprine treatment reduces acute rejection episodes after renal transplantation. Transplantation 1998;66:334-339.
66. Allison AC, Eugui EM. Immunosuppressive and other effects of mycophenolic acid and an ester prodrug, mycophenolate mofetil. Immunol Rev 1993;136:5-28.
67. Allison AC, Eugui EM. Mycophenolate mofetil and its mechanisms of action. Immunopharmacology 2000;47:85-118.
68. Langman LJ, Shapiro AM, Lakey JR, et al. Pharmacodynamic assessment of mycophenolic acid–induced immunosuppression by measurement of inosine monophosphate dehydrogenase activity in a canine model. Transplantation 1996;61:87-92.
69. Allison AC, Eugui EM. Preferential suppression of lymphocyte proliferation by mycophenolic acid and predicted long-term effects of mycophenolate mofetil in transplantation. Transplant Proc 1994;26:3205-3210.
70. Behrend M. Adverse gastrointestinal effects of mycophenolate mofetil: aetiology, incidence and management. Drug Saf 2001;24:645-663.
71. Budde K, Glander P, Kramer BK, et al. Conversion from mycophenolate mofetil to enteric-coated mycophenolate sodium in maintenance renal transplant recipients receiving tacrolimus: clinical, pharmacokinetic, and pharmacodynamic outcomes. Transplantation 2007;83:417-424.
72. Cyclosporine. Pharmacokinetics. Transplant Proc 1983;15:2401-2456.
73. Ritschel WA, Adolph S, Ritschel GB, Schroeder T. Improvement of peroral absorption of cyclosporine A by microemulsions. Methods Find Exp Clin Pharmacol 1990;12:127-134.
74. Ptachcinski RJ, Venkataramanan R, Rosenthal JT, et al. The effect of food on cyclosporine absorption. Transplantation 1985;40:174-176.
75. Kolars JC, Awni WM, Merion RM, Watkins PB. First-pass metabolism of cyclosporin by the gut. Lancet 1991;338:1488-1490.
76. Ducharme MP, Provenzano R, Dehoorne-Smith M, Edwards DJ. Trough concentrations of cyclosporine in blood following administration with grapefruit juice. Br J Clin Pharmacol 1993;36:457-459.
77. Hollander AA, van Rooij J, Lentjes GW, et al. The effect of grapefruit juice on cyclosporine and prednisone metabolism in transplant patients. Clin Pharmacol Ther 1995;57:318-324.
78. Kivisto KT. A review of assay methods for cyclosporin. Clinical implications. Clin Pharmacokinet 1992;23:173-190.
79. Holt DW. Therapeutic drug monitoring of immunosuppressive drugs in kidney transplantation. Curr Opin Nephrol Hypertens 2002;11:657-663.
80. Kahan BD, Keown P, Levy GA, Johnston A. Therapeutic drug monitoring of immunosuppressant drugs in clinical practice. Clin Ther 2002;24:330-350; discussion 329.
81. Venkataramanan R, Jain A, Warty VW, et al. Pharmacokinetics of FK 506 following oral administration: a comparison of FK 506 and cyclosporine. Transplant Proc 1991;23:931-933.
82. Oellerich M, Armstrong VW. The role of therapeutic drug monitoring in individualizing immunosuppressive drug therapy: recent developments. Ther Drug Monit 2006;28:720-725.
83. Liu J, Farmer JD Jr, Lane WS, et al. Calcineurin is a common target of cyclophilin-cyclosporin A and FKBP-FK506 complexes. Cell 1991;66:807-815.
84. Clipstone NA, Crabtree GR. Identification of calcineurin as a key signalling enzyme in T-lymphocyte activation. Nature 1992;357:695-697.
85. Macian F. NFAT proteins: key regulators of T-cell development and function. Nat Rev Immunol 2005;5:472-484.
86. Kalli K, Huntoon C, Bell M, McKean DJ. Mechanism responsible for T-cell antigen receptor- and CD28- or interleukin 1 (IL-1) receptor-initiated regulation of IL-2 gene expression by NF-kappaB. Mol Cell Biol 1998;18:3140-3148.
87. Morozumi K, Takeda A, Uchida K, Mihatsch MJ. Cyclosporine nephrotoxicity: how does it affect renal allograft function and transplant morphology? Transplant Proc 2004;36:251S-256S.
88. de Groen PC, Aksamit AJ, Rakela J, et al. Central nervous system toxicity after liver transplantation. The role of cyclosporine and cholesterol. N Engl J Med 1987;317:861-866.
89. Singh N. Infectious complications in organ transplant recipients with the use of calcineurin-inhibitor agent-based immunosuppressive regimens. Curr Opin Infect Dis 2005;18:342-345.
90. Otley CC, Pittelkow MR. Skin cancer in liver transplant recipients. Liver Transpl 2000;6:253-262.
91. Haddad EM, McAlister VC, Renouf E, et al. Cyclosporin versus tacrolimus for liver transplanted patients. Cochrane Database Syst Rev 2006:CD005161.
92. Webster A, Woodroffe RC, Taylor RS, et al. Tacrolimus versus cyclosporin as primary immunosuppression for kidney transplant recipients. Cochrane Database Syst Rev 2005:CD003961.
93. Garcia-Lopez S, Gomollon-Garcia F, Perez-Gisbert J. Cyclosporine in the treatment of severe attack of ulcerative colitis: a systematic review. Gastroenterol Hepatol 2005;28:607-614.
94. Thestrup-Pedersen K. Tacrolimus treatment of atopic eczema/dermatitis syndrome. Curr Opin Allergy Clin Immunol 2003;3:359-362.
95. Knight RJ, Kahan BD. The place of sirolimus in kidney transplantation: can we reduce calcineurin inhibitor renal toxicity? Kidney Int 2006;70:994-999.

96. Johnson EM, Zimmerman J, Duderstadt K, et al. A randomized, double-blind, placebo-controlled study of the safety, tolerance, and preliminary pharmacokinetics of ascending single doses of orally administered sirolimus (rapamycin) in stable renal transplant recipients. Transplant Proc 1996;28:987.
97. Galat A, Lane WS, Standaert RF, Schreiber SL. A rapamycin-selective 25-kDa immunophilin. Biochemistry 1992;31:2427-2434.
98. Dumont FJ, Staruch MJ, Koprak SL, et al. Distinct mechanisms of suppression of murine T cell activation by the related macrolides FK-506 and rapamycin. J Immunol 1990;144:251-258.
99. Morales JM, Wramner L, Kreis H, et al. Sirolimus does not exhibit nephrotoxicity compared to cyclosporine in renal transplant recipients. Am J Transplant 2002;2:436-442.
100. Valente JF, Hricik D, Weigel K, et al. Comparison of sirolimus vs. mycophenolate mofetil on surgical complications and wound healing in adult kidney transplantation. Am J Transplant 2003;3:1128-1134.
101. Webster AC, Lee VW, Chapman JR, Craig JC. Target of rapamycin inhibitors (TOR-I; sirolimus and everolimus) for primary immunosuppression in kidney transplant recipients. Cochrane Database Syst Rev 2006:CD004290.
102. Eisen HJ, Tuzcu EM, Dorent R, et al. Everolimus for the prevention of allograft rejection and vasculopathy in cardiac-transplant recipients. N Engl J Med 2003;349:847-858.
103. Bischoff KB, Dedrick RL, Zaharko DS, Longstreth JA. Methotrexate pharmacokinetics. J Pharm Sci 1971;60:1128-1133.
104. Trier JS. Morphologic alterations induced by methotrexate in the mucosa of human proximal intestine. II. Electron microscopic observations. Gastroenterology 1962; 43:407-424.
105. Trier JS. Morphologic alterations induced by methotrexate in the mucosa of human proximal intestine. I. Serial observations by light microscopy. Gastroenterology 1962;42:295-305.
106. Egan LJ, Sandborn WJ, Mays DC, et al. Systemic and intestinal pharmacokinetics of methotrexate in patients with inflammatory bowel disease. Clin Pharmacol Ther 1999;65:29-39.
107. Egan LJ, Sandborn WJ, Tremaine WJ, et al. A randomized dose-response and pharmacokinetic study of methotrexate for refractory inflammatory Crohn's disease and ulcerative colitis. Aliment Pharmacol Ther 1999;13:1597-1604.
108. Genestier L, Paillot R, Fournel S, et al. Immunosuppressive properties of methotrexate: apoptosis and clonal deletion of activated peripheral T cells. J Clin Invest 1998;102:322-328.
109. Feagan BG, Fedorak RN, Irvine EJ, et al. A comparison of methotrexate with placebo for the maintenance of remission in Crohn's disease. North American Crohn's Study Group Investigators. N Engl J Med 2000;342:1627-1632.
110. Roenigk HH Jr, Bergfeld WF, St. Jacques R, et al. Hepatotoxicity of methotrexate in the treatment of psoriasis. Arch Dermatol 1971;103:250-261.
111. Tobias H, Auerbach R. Hepatotoxicity of long-term methotrexate therapy for psoriasis. Arch Intern Med 1973;132:391-396.
112. Kremer JM, Alarcon GS, Lightfoot RW Jr, et al. Methotrexate for rheumatoid arthritis. Suggested guidelines for monitoring liver toxicity. American College of Rheumatology. Arthritis Rheum 1994;37:316-328.
113. Boffa MJ, Chalmers RJ, Haboubi NY, et al. Sequential liver biopsies during long-term methotrexate treatment for psoriasis: a reappraisal. Br J Dermatol 1995;133:774-778.
114. Te HS, Schiano TD, Kuan SF, et al. Hepatic effects of long-term methotrexate use in the treatment of inflammatory bowel disease. Am J Gastroenterol 2000;95:3150-3156.
115. Berends MA, Snoek J, de Jong EM, et al. Liver injury in long-term methotrexate treatment in psoriasis is relatively infrequent. Aliment Pharmacol Ther 2006;24:805-811.
116. Whitcomb ME, Schwarz MI, Tormey DC. Methotrexate pneumonitis: case report and review of the literature. Thorax 1972;27:636-639.
117. Salaffi F, Manganelli P, Carotti M, et al. Methotrexate-induced pneumonitis in patients with rheumatoid arthritis and psoriatic arthritis: report of five cases and review of the literature. Clin Rheumatol 1997;16:296-304.
118. Boerbooms AM, Kerstens PJ, van Loenhout JW, et al. Infections during low-dose methotrexate treatment in rheumatoid arthritis. Semin Arthritis Rheum 1995;24:411-421.
119. van Ede AE, Laan RF, Rood MJ, et al. Effect of folic or folinic acid supplementation on the toxicity and efficacy of methotrexate in rheumatoid arthritis: a forty-eight week, multicenter, randomized, double-blind, placebo-controlled study. Arthritis Rheum 2001;44:1515-1524.
120. Lloyd ME, Carr M, McElhatton P, et al. The effects of methotrexate on pregnancy, fertility and lactation. QJM 1999;92:551-563.
121. Silverman E, Mouy R, Spiegel L, et al. Leflunomide or methotrexate for juvenile rheumatoid arthritis. N Engl J Med 2005;352:1655-1666.
122. Heydendael VM, Spuls PI, Opmeer BC, et al. Methotrexate versus cyclosporine in moderate-to-severe chronic plaque psoriasis. N Engl J Med 2003;349:658-665.
123. Hall AG, Tilby MJ. Mechanisms of action of, and modes of resistance to, alkylating agents used in the treatment of haematological malignancies. Blood Rev 1992;6:163-173.
124. McCune WJ, Golbus J, Zeldes W, et al. Clinical and immunologic effects of monthly administration of intravenous cyclophosphamide in severe systemic lupus erythematosus. N Engl J Med 1988;318:1423-1431.
125. Pryor BD, Bologna SG, Kahl LE. Risk factors for serious infection during treatment with cyclophosphamide and high-dose corticosteroids for systemic lupus erythematosus. Arthritis Rheum 1996;39:1475-1482.
126. Watson AR, Rance CP, Bain J. Long term effects of cyclophosphamide on testicular function. Br Med J (Clin Res Ed) 1985;291:1457-1460.
127. Radis CD, Kahl LE, Baker GL, et al. Effects of cyclophosphamide on the development of malignancy and on long-term survival of patients with rheumatoid arthritis. A 20-year follow-up study. Arthritis Rheum 1995;38:1120-1127.
128. Talar-Williams C, Hijazi YM, Walther MM, et al. Cyclophosphamide-induced cystitis and bladder cancer in patients with Wegener granulomatosis. Ann Intern Med 1996;124:477-484.
129. Kashiwagi N, Brantigan CO, Brettschneider L, et al. Clinical reactions and serologic changes after the administration of heterologous antilymphocyte globulin to human recipients of renal homografts. Ann Intern Med 1968;68:275-286.
130. Najarian JS, Simmons RL. The clinical use of antilymphocyte globulin. N Engl J Med 1971;285:158-166.
131. Sell S. Antilymphocytic antibody: effects in experimental animals and problems in human use. Ann Intern Med 1969;71:177-196.
132. Van Wauwe JP, De Mey JR, Goossens JG. OKT3: a monoclonal anti-human T lymphocyte antibody with potent mitogenic properties. J Immunol 1980;124:2708-2713.
133. Janssen O, Wesselborg S, Kabelitz D. Immunosuppression by OKT3—induction of programmed cell death (apoptosis) as a possible mechanism of action. Transplantation 1992;53:233-234.
134. Wesselborg S, Janssen O, Kabelitz D. Induction of activation-driven death (apoptosis) in activated but not resting peripheral blood T cells. J Immunol 1993;150:4338-4345.
135. Jeyarajah DR, Thistlethwaite JR Jr. General aspects of cytokine-release syndrome: timing and incidence of symptoms. Transplant Proc 1993;25:16-20.
136. Morgan JD, Horsburgh T, Simpson A, et al. Cytomegalovirus infection during OKT3 treatment for renal allograft rejection. Transplant Proc 1992;24:2634-2635.
137. Raymond E, Tricottet V, Samuel D, et al. Epstein-Barr virus–related localized hepatic lymphoproliferative disorders after liver transplantation. Cancer 1995;76:1344-1351.
138. Nashan B, Moore R, Amlot P, et al. Randomised trial of basiliximab versus placebo for control of acute cellular rejection in renal allograft recipients. CHIB 201 International Study Group. Lancet 1997;350:1193-1198.
139. Baudouin V, Crusiaux A, Haddad E, et al. Anaphylactic shock caused by immunoglobulin E sensitization after retreatment with the chimeric anti-interleukin-2 receptor monoclonal antibody basiliximab. Transplantation 2003;76:459-463.
140. Vincenti F, Kirkman R, Light S, et al. Interleukin-2-receptor blockade with daclizumab to prevent acute rejection in renal transplantation. Daclizumab Triple Therapy Study Group. N Engl J Med 1998;338:161-165.
141. Ringe B, Moritz M, Zeldin G, Soriano H. What is the best immunosuppression in living donor liver transplantation? Transplant Proc 2005;37:2169-2171.
142. Sandrini S. Use of IL-2 receptor antagonists to reduce delayed graft function following renal transplantation: a review. Clin Transplant 2005;19:705-710.
143. Vincenti F, de Andres A, Becker T, et al. Interleukin-2 receptor antagonist induction in modern immunosuppression regimens for renal transplant recipients. Transpl Int 2006;19:446-457.
144. Webster A, Pankhurst T, Rinaldi F, et al. Polyclonal and monoclonal antibodies for treating acute rejection episodes in kidney transplant recipients. Cochrane Database Syst Rev 2006:CD004756.
145. Aggarwal BB. Signalling pathways of the TNF superfamily: a double-edged sword. Nat Rev Immunol 2003;3:745-756.
146. Karin M, Lin A. NF-kappaB at the crossroads of life and death. Nat Immunol 2002;3:221-227.
147. Klausner JD, Freedman VH, Kaplan G. Thalidomide as an anti-TNF-alpha inhibitor: implications for clinical use. Clin Immunol Immunopathol 1996;81:219-223.
148. Knight DM, Trinh H, Le J, et al. Construction and initial characterization of a mouse-human chimeric anti-TNF antibody. Mol Immunol 1993;30:1443-1453.
149. Elliott MJ, Maini RN, Feldmann M, et al. Randomised double-blind comparison of chimeric monoclonal antibody to tumour necrosis factor alpha (cA2) versus placebo in rheumatoid arthritis. Lancet 1994;344:1105-1110.
150. Elliott MJ, Maini RN, Feldmann M, et al. Repeated therapy with monoclonal antibody to tumour necrosis factor alpha (cA2) in patients with rheumatoid arthritis. Lancet 1994;344:1125-1127.
151. Hanauer SB, Feagan BG, Lichtenstein GR, et al. Maintenance infliximab for Crohn's disease: the ACCENT I randomised trial. Lancet 2002;359:1541-1549.
152. Present DH, Rutgeerts P, Targan S, et al. Infliximab for the treatment of fistulas in patients with Crohn's disease. N Engl J Med 1999;340:1398-1405.
153. Targan SR, Hanauer SB, van Deventer SJ, et al. A short-term study of chimeric monoclonal antibody cA2 to tumor necrosis factor alpha for Crohn's disease. Crohn's Disease cA2 Study Group. N Engl J Med 1997;337:1029-1035.
154. Bendtzen K, Geborek P, Svenson M, et al. Individualized monitoring of drug bioavailability and immunogenicity in rheumatoid arthritis patients treated with the tumor necrosis factor alpha inhibitor infliximab. Arthritis Rheum 2006;54:3782-3789.
155. Maser EA, Villela R, Silverberg MS, Greenberg GR. Association of trough serum infliximab to clinical outcome after scheduled maintenance treatment for Crohn's disease. Clin Gastroenterol Hepatol 2006;4:1248-1254.
156. Siegel SA, Shealy DJ, Nakada MT, et al. The mouse/human chimeric monoclonal antibody cA2 neutralizes TNF in vitro and protects transgenic mice from cachexia and TNF lethality in vivo. Cytokine 1995;7:15-25.
157. Lugering A, Schmidt M, Lugering N, et al. Infliximab induces apoptosis in monocytes from patients with chronic active Crohn's disease by using a caspase-dependent pathway. Gastroenterology 2001;121:1145-1157.
158. Mitoma H, Horiuchi T, Hatta N, et al. Infliximab induces potent anti-inflammatory responses by outside-to-inside signals through transmembrane TNF-alpha. Gastroenterology 2005;128:376-392.
159. Mayer L, Young Y. Infusion reactions and their management. Gastroenterol Clin North Am 2006;35:857-866.

160. Riegert-Johnson DL, Godfrey JA, Myers JL, et al. Delayed hypersensitivity reaction and acute respiratory distress syndrome following infliximab infusion. Inflamm Bowel Dis 2002;8:186-191.
161. Farrell RJ, Alsahli M, Jeen YT, et al. Intravenous hydrocortisone premedication reduces antibodies to infliximab in Crohn's disease: a randomized controlled trial. Gastroenterology 2003;124:917-924.
162. Keane J, Gershon S, Wise RP, et al. Tuberculosis associated with infliximab, a tumor necrosis factor alpha-neutralizing agent. N Engl J Med 2001;345:1098-1104.
163. Colombel JF, Loftus EV Jr, Tremaine WJ, et al. The safety profile of infliximab in patients with Crohn's disease: the Mayo clinic experience in 500 patients. Gastroenterology 2004;126:19-31.
164. Mackey AC, Green L, Liang LC, et al. Hepatosplenic T cell lymphoma associated with infliximab use in young patients treated for inflammatory bowel disease. J Pediatr Gastroenterol Nutr 2007;44:265-267.
165. Thomas CW Jr, Weinshenker BG, Sandborn WJ. Demyelination during anti-tumor necrosis factor alpha therapy with infliximab for Crohn's disease. Inflamm Bowel Dis 2004;10:28-31.
166. van Oosten BW, Barkhof F, Truyen L, et al. Increased MRI activity and immune activation in two multiple sclerosis patients treated with the monoclonal anti-tumor necrosis factor antibody cA2. Neurology 1996;47:1531-1534.
167. Shen C, Van Assche G, Rutgeerts P, Ceuppens JL. Caspase activation and apoptosis induction by adalimumab: demonstration in vitro and in vivo in a chimeric mouse model. Inflamm Bowel Dis 2006;12:22-28.
168. Schiff MH, Burmester GR, Kent JD, et al. Safety analyses of adalimumab (HUMIRA) in global clinical trials and US postmarketing surveillance of patients with rheumatoid arthritis. Ann Rheum Dis 2006;65:889-894.
169. Suffredini AF, Reda D, Banks SM, et al. Effects of recombinant dimeric TNF receptor on human inflammatory responses following intravenous endotoxin administration. J Immunol 1995;155:5038-5045.
170. Rice GP, Hartung HP, Calabresi PA. Anti-alpha4 integrin therapy for multiple sclerosis: mechanisms and rationale. Neurology 2005;64:1336-1342.
171. Ghosh S, Goldin E, Gordon FH, et al. Natalizumab for active Crohn's disease. N Engl J Med 2003;348:24-32.
172. Yousry TA, Major EO, Ryschkewitsch C, et al. Evaluation of patients treated with natalizumab for progressive multifocal leukoencephalopathy. N Engl J Med 2006;354:924-933.
173. Van Assche G, Van Ranst M, Sciot R, et al. Progressive multifocal leukoencephalopathy after natalizumab therapy for Crohn's disease. N Engl J Med 2005;353:362-368.
174. Kleinschmidt-DeMasters BK, Tyler KL. Progressive multifocal leukoencephalopathy complicating treatment with natalizumab and interferon beta-1a for multiple sclerosis. N Engl J Med 2005;353:369-374.
175. Langer-Gould A, Atlas SW, Green AJ, et al. Progressive multifocal leukoencephalopathy in a patient treated with natalizumab. N Engl J Med 2005;353:375-381.
176. Rudick RA, Stuart WH, Calabresi PA, et al. Natalizumab plus interferon beta-1a for relapsing multiple sclerosis. N Engl J Med 2006;354:911-923.
177. Polman CH, O'Connor PW, Havrdova E, et al. A randomized, placebo-controlled trial of natalizumab for relapsing multiple sclerosis. N Engl J Med 2006;354:899-910.
178. Sandborn WJ, Colombel JF, Enns R, et al. Natalizumab induction and maintenance therapy for Crohn's disease. N Engl J Med 2005;353:1912-1925.
179. Kalden JR, Antoni C, Alvaro-Gracia JM, et al. Use of combination of leflunomide with biological agents in treatment of rheumatoid arthritis. J Rheumatol 2005;32:1620-1631.
180. Smolen JS, Keystone EC, Emery P, et al. Consensus statement on the use of rituximab in patients with rheumatoid arthritis. Ann Rheum Dis 2007;66:143-150.
181. Cohen SB. The use of anakinra, an interleukin-1 receptor antagonist, in the treatment of rheumatoid arthritis. Rheum Dis Clin North Am 2004;30:vii, 365-380.

12

PHARMACOBIOLOGY OF INFECTIONS

Dionissios Neofytos, Claudine El-Beyrouty, and Joseph A. DeSimone, Jr.

INTRODUCTION 173
Principles of Antimicrobial Therapy 173
ANTIBACTERIAL AGENTS 174
Mechanism of Action 175
Pharmacokinetics and Pharmacodynamics 176
Spectrum of Activity and Indications 177
Adverse Events 178
Resistance 178
ANTIFUNGAL AGENTS 179
Mechanism of Action 180
Pharmacokinetics and Pharmacodynamics 180
Spectrum of Activity and Indications 181
Adverse Events 182
Resistance 182
Topical Antifungal Agents 183
ANTIVIRAL AGENTS 183
Pharmacobiology 184
Pharmacokinetics 185
Mechanisms of Action 186
Drugs for Human Herpesviruses 186
Drugs for Hepatitis B 187
Drugs for Hepatitis C 187
Drug for Influenza 187
Spectrums of Activity 187
Indications 188
Adverse Effects 188
Resistance 190

INTRODUCTION

This chapter is a review of the three major classes of antimicrobial agents: antibacterial, antifungal, and antiviral. We discuss the importance of pharmacokinetics (PK), pharmacodynamics (PD), and mechanisms of action of the most frequently administered antimicrobial agents in clinical practice. In addition, pertinent information on their antimicrobial spectrum of activity, major indications, and adverse events are presented.

Antimycobacterial, antiretroviral, antiparasitic, and locally administered antimicrobial agents are not discussed in this chapter. For more information on any of these agents, we refer the reader to the particular chapters on each agent.

Principles of Antimicrobial Therapy

Proper selection of antimicrobial agents is based on a number of factors. Specific spectrums of activity, toxicities, and drug interactions of individual agents are discussed in the rest of this chapter. The PK and PD of antimicrobials play a significant role in both the selection of an agent and the optimization of a dosing regimen.[1] *Pharmacodynamics*, specifically for antimicrobial agents, is the interaction of drugs and microbes. Basic PK and PD principles are reviewed in this section.

Most anti-infective agents can be classified as bacteriostatic or bactericidal, though it is unlikely that any agent is purely bacteriostatic or bactericidal. By definition, a *bacteriostatic agent* prevents growth of bacteria, keeping them in the stationary phase of growth. *Bactericidal agents* kill more than 99.9% of bacteria found in an inoculum. In reality, often bacteriostatic agents kill some bacteria but less than the 99.9% required to be defined as bactericidal. Conversely, many bactericidal agents do not result in the death of every organism, especially in infections with a large inoculum of bacteria. The clinical importance of bactericidal action being better than bacteriostatic action has not been proved.[2] The few clinical situations in which bactericidal activity is believed to be necessary include endocarditis secondary to cardiac vegetations with high concentrations of organism/gram of tissue and a slow rate of growth requiring high doses of prolonged therapy to kill any dormant bacteria once they start to divide; meningitis due to the need to eradicate the infection as soon as possible and the poor immune competence of the central nervous system; and neutropenia due to the immunocompromised status of the host.

Empirical therapy with antimicrobial agents takes into account the suspected pathogen and the likelihood of resistance as well as patient characteristics. The use of two antimicrobial agents as empirical therapy is based on both the principle of synergistic killing as well as broadening the spectrum of organism coverage. *Synergy* is defined as two agents demonstrating greater than additive activity.

Antimicrobial susceptibility testing is used to help de-escalate therapy to a narrower-spectrum agent. Quantitative susceptibility testing using twofold dilutions of antimicrobial agents in a liquid culture medium is the "gold standard." The lowest concentration of an antibacterial agent that inhibits visible growth is called the *minimum inhibitory concentration (MIC)*. Subcultures of samples obtained from clear tubes are made on a medium free of antibacterial agents and reincubated for an additional 18 to 24 hours to determine the *minimum bactericidal concentration (MBC)*. The MBC is the lowest concentration of an antibacterial agent that either totally prevents growth or results in a greater than 99.9% decrease in the initial inoculum.[1,2]

Once an agent is selected based on known or suspected pathogen, the drug must be delivered to the site of infection. Effective treatment depends on the concentration of the anti-infective agents being in excess of the MIC at the site of infection. This is especially vital when host defenses are limited (e.g., by valvular vegetations or in immunocompromised patients).[1] Pharmacokinetic principles can be used to predict the antimicrobial effect or PD response. Most antimicrobials can be classified into one of two PD categories: *time-dependent activity* in which bacteria are killed at the same rate and to the same extent once the threshold concentration is reached; and *concentration-dependent activity* in which the rate and extent of killing increases progressively with higher antibacterial concentrations.[2] Concentration-dependent PD are best described by measuring peak concentration (Cmax)–to–MIC ratios. There is a correlation of Cmax/MIC ratios of greater than 8 to 10 with antimicrobial efficacy. Resistance is noted when values for Cmax/MIC fall to less than 3:1. Higher doses of some antibacterials, such as aminoglycosides, have been implemented to attain these goals. Time-dependent agents are evaluated by time above MIC, percentage of day, or percentage of dosing interval greater than MIC. Improved mortality rates have been documented when serum concentrations remain above the MIC for 40% or more of the dosing interval.[3] This target can be achieved by giving frequent daily doses or continuous infusions. Another parameter used to integrate PK and PD is the area under the inhibitory curve (AUIC), which represents the ratio of the antibiotic area under the concentration time curve in 24 hours (AUC_{24}) to the organism's MIC. An AUIC of at least 125 should be targeted to avoid resistance, especially in gram-negative

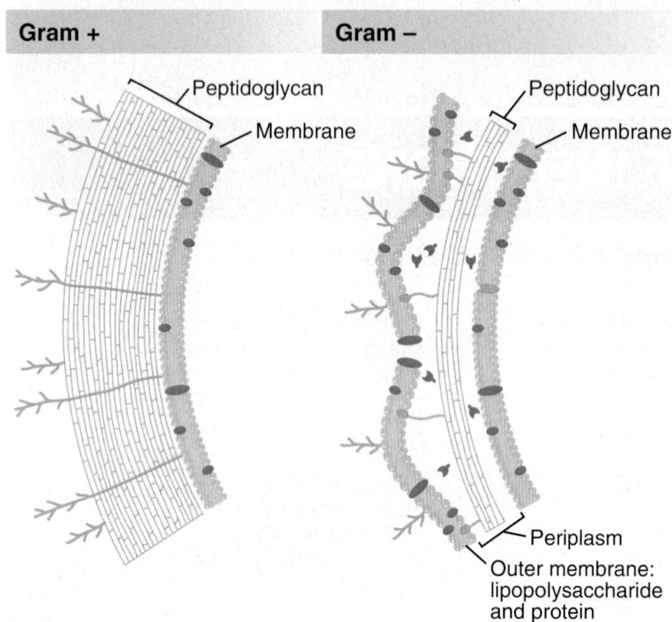

FIGURE 12-1 • Structure of bacterial cell wall and membrane. (Adapted from www-micro.msb.le.ac.uk)

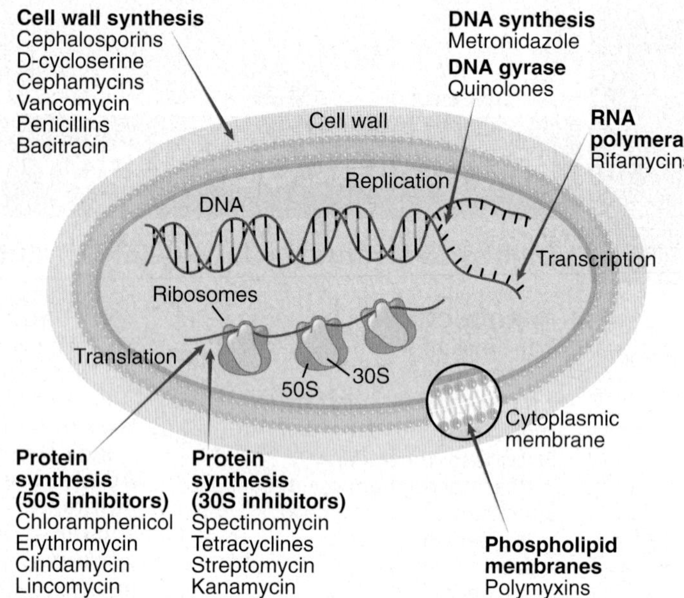

FIGURE 12-2 • Bacterial sites of action of different antibacterial agents. (Adapted from www.wiley.com/.../index.html)

bacteria. For newer antimicrobial agents with longer half-lives, the distinction between concentration- and time-dependent agents is less important.[3] Antimicrobial agents exhibiting a postantibiotic effect, in which persistent suppression of bacterial growth occurs after drug levels have fallen below the MIC, may also be dosed less frequently.[1]

Resistance to antibiotics can result from the normal genetics of the pathogen (called *inherent resistance*) or when pathogens have spontaneously mutated or received resistance genes through horizontal transfer (*acquired resistance*). Selective pressure, such as overuse or misuse of antibiotics, is one factor that leads to the emergence and spread of resistance.[4] Optimizing the PD principles described previously, by selecting agents that meet PD targets and using them at optimum doses, can help to ensure eradication of infection and reduce the chance of resistance developing.

ANTIBACTERIAL AGENTS

Antibacterial agents represent the vast majority of antimicrobial drugs. This is a reflection of the common encounter of bacterial infections and their devastating consequences if left untreated. The most commonly used systemic antibacterial agents are summarized in Tables 12-1 and 12-2.

Bacteria can be classified by shape (cocci, bacteria, spirochetes), cell wall presence and properties (gram-positive vs. gram-negative), and growth requirements (aerobic vs. anaerobic, extracellular vs. intracellular).[5] Other classification systems may use the presence of a capsule (e.g., encapsulated bacteria) or spores (e.g., spore-forming bacteria). The major components of bacteria include the cell wall, cell membrane, cytoplasm, and nucleoid. All bacteria, except *Mycoplasma* spp., are surrounded by a cell wall, which includes an outer membrane and an inner layer of peptidoglycan. A staining procedure (Gram stain) colors the cell wall; this is the basis on which bacteria are classified as gram-positive or gram-negative. This classification is of major clinical importance for the identification of bacteria and the initial selection of the appropriate antimicrobial agent.

As illustrated in Figure 12-1, gram-positive bacteria have a thicker peptidoglycan layer than that of gram-negative bacteria, which have an outer membrane surrounding a thin layer of peptidoglycan. Enzymes (e.g., β-lactamases) that inactivate certain antibacterial agents are located in the periplasmic space existing between the outer membrane and the cell membrane of gram-negative bacteria. The cytoplasmic membrane of bacteria is a phospholipid bilayer that surrounds the cytoplasm and the nucleoid. This represents potential target sites for a variety of available antimicrobial agents (Fig. 12-2). All β-lactams and the glycopeptides act on the cell wall, whereas daptomycin and the polymyxins target the cell membrane.[6] Macrolides, tetracyclines, aminoglycosides, and lincosamides inhibit protein syn-

TABLE 12-1 MOST FREQUENTLY ADMINISTERED SYSTEMIC ANTIBACTERIAL AGENTS

Class	Antibacterial Agent
β-Lactams*	Penicillins, cephalosporins, monobactams, carbapenems
Glycopeptides	Vancomycin
Lipopeptides	Daptomycin
Polymyxins	Colistin
Aminoglycosides†	Streptomycin, gentamicin, tobramycin, amikacin, neomycin
Tetracyclines	Tetracycline, doxycycline, minocycline, tigecycline
Macrolides	Erythromycin, clarithromycin, azithromycin
Lincosamides	Clindamycin, lincomycin
Ketolides	Telithromycin
Streptogramins	Quinupristin and dalfopristin
Fluoroquinolones	Ciprofloxacin, levofloxacin, moxifloxacin, gatifloxacin, gemifloxacin, ofloxacin
Rifamycins	Rifampin, rifabutin, rifapentine, rifaximin
Oxazolidinones	Linezolid
Sulfonamides and trimethoprim	Sulfamethoxazole, sulfadiazine, sulfisoxazole, trimethoprim
Nitroimidazoles	Metronidazole
Nitrofurans	Nitrofurantoin
Chloramphenicol	Chloramphenicol

*For more information on β-lactams, refer to Table 12-2.
†Other aminoglycosides approved by the U.S. Food and Drug Administration (FDA) are kanamycin, paromomycin, netilmicin, and spectinomycin.

TABLE 12-2 MOST FREQUENTLY ADMINISTERED SYSTEMIC β-LACTAMS

	Intravenously Administered				
	Natural	**Penicillinase-Resistant**	**Aminopenicillins**	**Carboxypenicillins**	**Ureidopenicillins**
PENICILLINS	Penicillin G	Nafcillin	Ampicillin	Ticarcillin	Azlocillin Mezlocillin Piperacillin
	First Generation	**Second Generation**	**Third Generation**	**Fourth Generation**	
CEPHALOSPORINS	Cefazolin	Cefuroxime Cefotetan Cefoxitin	Ceftriaxone Cefotaxime Ceftazidime Cefoperazone	Cefepime	
MONOBACTAMS	Aztreonam				
CARBAPENEMS	Imipenem-cilastatin, meropenem, ertapenem, doripenem				

	Orally Administered		
	Natural	**Penicillinase-Resistant**	**Aminopenicillins**
PENICILLINS	Penicillin V	Oxacillin, cloxacillin, dicloxacillin	Amoxicillin
	First Generation	**Second Generation**	**Third Generation**
CEPHALOSPORINS	Cefadroxil, cephalexin, cephradine	Cefaclor, cefuroxime axetil, Loracarbef	Cefdinir, cefixime, cefpodoxime, ceftibuten

thesis by acting on the ribosomes. Nucleic acid synthesis may be inhibited by agents such as the fluoroquinolones, sulfonamides, and rifamycins.

Antibacterial agents can be classified based on their mechanism of action, antibacterial spectrum, PD and PK properties, and route of administration. In clinical practice, it is important to know which antibacterial agents are bactericidal (agents that kill bacteria) and which are bacteriostatic (agents that inhibit bacterial growth but do not kill them). For life-threatening infections (e.g., meningitis, endocarditis), when rapid and effective killing of bacteria is required, bactericidal agents are preferred.

In this chapter, a brief review of the most important systemically administered antibacterial agents, including their mechanism of action, PD and PK properties, antibacterial spectrum, major indications, and adverse events, are presented. Antimycobacterial and locally administered antibacterial agents are not discussed. For more information, we refer the reader to the particular chapters on each agent.

Mechanism of Action

All β-lactams bind to and inhibit certain enzymes, called *penicillin-binding proteins (PBPs)*, located on the bacterial cell membrane. These enzymes are responsible for the cross-linking of peptidoglycan, which is the final step for the synthesis of bacterial cell wall. Inhibition of cell wall synthesis leads to cell death by osmotic rupture, a property that makes β-lactams bactericidal agents. However, β-lactams are bactericidal only when bacteria grow and peptidoglycan is produced; they are bacteriostatic during the stationary phase of bacteria. Notably, different types of PBPs exist and β-lactams have different affinities for certain PBPs. Bacteria can produce enzymes called β-lactamases that disrupt the β-lactam ring and subsequently destroy the drug. Some of these enzymes can be inactivated by certain compounds, the β-lactamase inhibitors, which bind to β-lactamases as a suicide substrate. β-Lactamase inhibitors are weak antibiotics and can be combined with other β-lactams as fixed preparations. Three β-lactamase inhibitors currently used are clavulanic acid, sulbactam, and tazobactam (Table 12-3).

TABLE 12-3 COMBINATION DRUGS OF β-LACTAMS AND β-LACTAMASE INHIBITORS

β-Lactam	**β-Lactamase Inhibitor**	**Form of Administration**
Amoxicillin	Clavulanic acid	PO
Ampicillin	Sulbactam	IV
Piperacillin	Tazobactam	IV
Ticarcillin	Sulbactam	IV

IV, intravenous; PO, per os (oral).

Glycopeptides (e.g., vancomycin) inhibit the synthesis of cell wall by binding to peptidoglycan precursors (murein monomers) and forming a stable complex, which cannot be further incorporated into the growing peptidoglycan. Lipopeptides (e.g., daptomycin) exert their action by destabilizing the cell membrane through a calcium-dependent mechanism, whereas polymyxins disrupt the phospholipids of the bacterial cell membrane; they can both lead to rapid cell death.

Bacterial ribosomes have two different subunits, 50S and 30S. Aminoglycosides bind to messenger RNA (mRNA), whereas tetracyclines reversibly bind to transfer RNA (tRNA), both on the 30S subunit. Although aminoglycosides may have a bactericidal effect, the exact mechanism remains unclear. Chloramphenicol, macrolides, and lincosamides bind to the 50S ribosomal subunit. Whereas lincosamides act by blocking the formation of peptide bonds at an earlier stage, macrolides inhibit the peptide chain elongation by dissociation of the peptidyl-tRNA from the ribosome. The mechanism of action of ketolides closely resembles that of macrolides, but the former show a higher binding affinity for the 50S subunit. Notably, macrolides and ketolides may directly inhibit the synthesis of the 50S ribosomal subunit. Inhibition of the synthesis of the bacterial ribosomal 70S unit is achieved by oxazolidinones.

The fluoroquinolones inhibit bacterial DNA synthesis by binding to DNA gyrase and topoisomerase IV, which are their principal targets for gram-positive and gram-negative organisms, respectively. Para-aminobenzoic acid (PABA) binds to a pteridine compound to form dihydropteroate, which is converted to tetrahydropteroate by dihydrofolate reductase. The latter is the precursor of folic acid, purines, and DNA. Sulfonamides and trimethoprim inhibit the synthesis of dihydropteroate and tetrahydropteroic acid, respectively. Rifamycins selectively inhibit the bacterial RNA polymerase and subsequently block mRNA synthesis. Although metronidazole is one of the most commonly used antibacterial agents, its mechanism of action is still not fully understood. After entering the cell, metronidazole produces free radicals that may subsequently interact and disrupt the bacterial nucleic acid.

Pharmacokinetics and Pharmacodynamics

Antibiotics are metabolized and eliminated through different pathways and have different degrees of protein binding and absorption. The route of administration of an antibacterial agent depends on its absorption, the severity of the infection treated, and the functional state of the patient. The oral route is commonly preferred for the treatment of mild-to-moderate infections in the outpatient setting, provided the patient is able to swallow and absorb the administered drug. Certain agents are poorly, if at all, absorbed when orally administered (e.g., penicillin G, ampicillin). Fluoroquinolones and the oxazolidinones are well absorbed and attain high blood levels, administered either orally or intravenously.[7] Thus, the excellent bioavailability after oral administration of the fluoroquinolones can obviate the need for intravenous administration in certain cases. When vancomycin is administered orally, it is not absorbed but has local activity within the gut lumen. This property makes it an appealing agent for the treatment of colitis caused by *Clostridium difficile*. Parenteral administration is recommended for the treatment of moderate-to-severe infections, when higher doses and concentrations of the prescribed antibacterial agent in the blood are required. Certain antimicrobial agents (e.g., penicillin G, carbapenems, aminoglycosides, glycopeptides) are administered intravenously in severely ill patients with a life-threatening infection (e.g., endocarditis, meningitis) or patients who cannot take oral drugs. Intramuscular administration of an antibacterial agent may be applied in patients with poor intravenous access or when a prolonged treatment course is required, and therapeutic drug levels can be maintained by weekly or monthly intramuscular injections. Penicillin may be given intramuscularly for the treatment of most cases of syphilis or for prophylaxis in cases of rheumatic fever. Similarly, intramuscular administration of ceftriaxone or spectinomycin can be used for the treatment of gonorrhea.

Certain body compartments, such as bone, vitreous fluid, and prostate gland, are not easily accessible for most antibiotics. Penicillin G and the third-generation cephalosporins minimally penetrate the cerebrospinal fluid (CSF) barrier. However, in cases of meningeal inflammation (e.g., meningitis), the penetration of these agents is significantly enhanced. Protein binding is essential for the penetration and distribution of an antibacterial agent into various tissues. Traditionally, only the free compound of each antimicrobial is considered to be active. Vancomycin is heavily protein-bound, which decreases the ability of the drug to effectively enter certain body compartments and also decreases the concentration of the unbound drug in sites such as the meninges or the lung alveoli.[8,9] In contrast, linezolid is minimally protein-bound and penetrates and attains high free drug concentrations in most human tissues.[10]

Based on properties of their metabolism and elimination, antibacterial agents can be administered once or more than once daily. Certain agents, such as β-lactams with time-dependent killing characteristics, should be administered at shorter intervals or even as a continuous infusion in cases of serious infections, that is, to maintain a higher than the MIC of the antibacterial agent for a prolonged period of time. In contrast, concentration-dependent antibacterial agents (e.g., daptomycin, telithromycin, metronidazole) are more effective when achieving high initial concentrations. Thus, once-daily administration of aminoglycosides and fluoroquinolones ascertains more rapid and efficient killing of susceptible bacteria.

Coadministration of other compounds may affect the absorption and metabolism of certain antimicrobial agents. Notably, tetracyclines should not be administered with milk products, antacids, or iron supplements, because these agents decrease their absorption. Similarly, fluoroquinolones should not be administered with antacids and antihistamine agents. The disulfiram reaction can be observed in patients treated with metronidazole who consume alcohol.[11] Antibacterial agents may be inactivated when interacting with certain body compartments. Imipenem is inactivated by dihydropeptidase I, an enzyme located on the membrane of the proximal renal tubules. This is prevented by coadministration of imipenem with cilastatin, which binds to and inactivates this enzyme. Similarly, daptomycin is not active in the lungs, where it is inactivated by surfactant.

Most antibacterial agents are metabolized and eliminated via the kidneys and need to be dose-adjusted when administered to patients with renal impairment (Table 12-4). Creatinine clearance levels have traditionally been used to dose-adjust certain antimicrobial agents and minimize the potential for antibiotic-related toxicities. Inappropriate dosing in patients with decreased creatinine clearance may lead to toxic serum drug levels with variable clinical outcomes. Higher than normal serum levels of penicillins and imipenem may result in seizures; of aminoglycosides and polymyxins may result in renal toxicity; of daptomycin may result in high phosphokinase levels and muscle aches. Patients who require hemodialysis should be carefully managed; reference to appropriate guides regarding administration and dosing of antibacterial agents is strongly recommended.

Some antimicrobial agents (e.g., macrolides, lincosamides, chloramphenicol) are metabolized in the liver. Impaired liver function may result in high serum levels of these drugs and potential toxicities. Metabolism through the cytochrome P-450 (CYP) system is of major

TABLE 12-4 ANTIBACTERIAL AGENTS THAT DO OR DO NOT REQUIRE RENAL DOSE ADJUSTMENT

Antibacterial Agent	Creatinine Clearance (mg/dl)	Antibacterial Agent	Creatinine Clearance (mg/dl)
Penicillin	<50	Vancomycin	<50
Ampicillin/amoxicillin	<50	Daptomycin	<50
Piperacillin/ticarcillin	<50	Colistin	<50
Cefazolin	<50	Fluoroquinolones	<50
Cefuroxime, cefotetan, cefoxitin	<50	Trimethoprim and sulfonamides	<50
Cefotaxime, ceftazidime	<50	Tetracycline	<50
Cefepime	<50	Nitrofurantoin	<50*
Aztreonam	<50	Macrolides	<30
Imipenem-cilastatin, meropenem, ertapenem	<50	Metronidazole	<10
Amikacin, gentamicin, tobramycin, streptomycin	<90		
Nafcillin, cefoperazone, ceftriaxone, moxifloxacin, doxycycline[†]			

*Use not recommended for impaired renal function.
[†]Agents are not renally metabolized; no dose adjustment required.

importance. Rifamycins, rifampin in particular, are strong inducers of the CYP3A metabolic pathway, resulting in lower levels of all coadministered drugs metabolized through the same system. Careful review of the patient's drug list is recommended prior to prescribing such agents.

Spectrum of Activity and Indications

Antibacterial efficacy requires binding of drugs at the site of action. Bacterial characteristics may differ significantly, which makes them susceptible or intrinsically resistant to different antibacterials. None of the β-lactams is active against methicillin-resistant *Staphylococcus aureus* (MRSA). Penicillins are active against *Enterococcus* spp. but not bactericidal unless coadministered with other agents, such as aminoglycosides. Penicillin G is the drug of choice for the treatment of infections caused by penicillin-susceptible *Staphylococcus aureus, Streptococcus pneumoniae, Streptococcus viridans, Neisseria meningitidis*, certain *Clostridia* spp., and *Treponema pallidum*. Group A β-hemolytic *Streptococcus* remains highly susceptible to penicillin. *S. aureus* became rapidly resistant to penicillin by producing penicillinases, which can cleave the penicillin molecule. Thus, penicillinase-resistant penicillins were produced (e.g., nafcillin) and used for the treatment of infections with methicillin-sensitive *S. aureus* (MSSA) strains. Penicillins are not active against any of the gram-negative rods; thus, aminopenicillins were produced for the treatment of infections caused by the Enterobacteriaceae. Aminopenicillins are not active against *Pseudomonas* spp., which resulted in the advent of carboxypenicillins and ureidopenicillins. Notably, ticarcillin lacks predictable activity against *Enterococcus* and *Klebsiella* spp., but it is the only β-lactam with some activity against *Stenotrophomonas maltophilia*, a common pathogen in the intensive care unit (ICU) setting. A combination of a β-lactam and a β-lactamase inhibitor is frequently used in clinical practice, when broad antibacterial coverage is required and concerns about β-lactamase production exist. Tazobactam has intrinsic activity against *Acinetobacter* spp., which may be of some clinical importance in critically ill patients in the ICU setting.

As a general rule, none of the cephalosporins has any activity against *Enterococcus* and MRSA spp. First-generation cephalosporins are active against most gram-positive cocci and some of the Enterobacteriaceae. The gram-negative spectrum of second-generation cephalosporins is broader, including *Haemophilus influenzae* and *Enterobacter* spp., whereas their activity against gram-positive bacteria is more limited. Cephamycins are the only cephalosporins active against *Bacteroides* spp., and cefoxitin is commonly used perioperatively in cases of abdominal or pelvic surgery. Most gram-negative organisms, including *Pseudomonas* spp., are susceptible to most third-generation cephalosporins. Ceftazidime has traditionally been the drug of choice against *Pseudomonas aeruginosa*, particularly in cases of meningitis. Ceftriaxone and cefotaxime are active against susceptible or intermediate-susceptible–to–penicillin strains of *S. pneumoniae*. They are recommended for the empirical treatment of meningitis and meningitis caused by *N. meningitides* or β-lactamase–positive *H. influenzae.*[12] Ceftriaxone is also the treatment of choice for gonorrhea and some forms of Lyme disease. Cefepime is the only fourth-generation cephalosporin approved by the U.S. Food and Drug Administration (FDA). Its spectrum of activity is similar to that of third-generation cephalosporins, including *S. pneumoniae* and *Pseudomonas* spp.

Monobactams have no activity against any gram-positive or anaerobic organisms. Aztreonam is the only agent used from this group, and it is highly active against most gram-negative organisms, including *P. aeruginosa*. As there is no cross-allergenicity between aztreonam and other β-lactams, it may be used in patients who are allergic to penicillin and have a significant gram-negative infection. However, patients allergic to ceftazidime may develop an allergic reaction to aztreonam, because the two agents share a similar side chain. Carbapenems are active against most gram-positive and -negative aerobic and anaerobic organisms, with the exception of MRSA, vancomycin-resistant *Enterococcus* spp. (VRE), *Stenotrophomonas maltophilia, Burkholderia cepacia*, and some *Corynebacterium* spp. Notably, ertapenem is not active against *Pseudomonas* spp. In addition, penicillins, cephamycins, carbapenems, and combinations of β-lactam and β-lactamase inhibitors are active against most gram-positive and gram-negative anaerobic organisms.

Colistin is used against infections caused by multidrug-resistant *Acinetobacter* spp. Vancomycin is active against most aerobic and anaerobic gram-positive organisms, including MRSA and most *Streptococcus* spp. *Enterococci* are commonly susceptible to vancomycin, which is always bacteriostatic against these organisms. Notably, *Lactobacillus* and *Erysipelothrix* spp. may be resistant to vancomycin. Certain *Enterococcus* spp., such as *E. faecium*, may develop resistance to glycopeptides, commonly referred to as VRE. Daptomycin and linezolid are active against gram-positive organisms, including MRSA and VRE. Quinupristin-dalfopristin is active against most gram-positive and some gram-negative organisms. This combination drug is bactericidal, unless resistance develops against one of its compounds, in which case it demonstrates bacteriostatic activity only.[13] In clinical practice, quinupristin-dalfopristin is preserved for infections caused by drug-resistant gram-positive organisms, including VRE. Notably, this agent is not active against *E. faecalis.*

All agents acting at the ribosomal level can theoretically be used for the treatment of an infection caused by any organism that contains ribosomes, assuming the drugs can get into the bacterial cell. Aminoglycosides are primarily used against strictly aerobic gram-negative organisms, including *Pseudomonas* spp. They may also be used synergistically with other antibiotics, primarily β-lactams, for the treatment of serious infections (e.g., endocarditis) with MRSA or *Enterococcus* spp.[14] Notably, streptomycin is the drug of choice for the treatment of certain zoonoses, caused by *Francisella tularensis*,[15] *Yersinia pestis*,[16] and in combination with other agents in cases of infections caused by *Brucella* spp.[17] moreover, streptomycin is active against *Mycobacterium tuberculosis*, and amikacin may be used in combination with other agents for the treatment of infections with atypical mycobacteria. Finally, paromomycin is active against certain protozoa.

Tetracyclines have a broad spectrum of activity, including extracellular and intracellular bacteria, spirochetes and *Mycoplasma* spp. Doxycycline is recommended for the treatment of uncomplicated Lyme disease,[18] ehrlichiosis,[19] Rocky Mountain spotted fever, other rickettsioses, and infections caused by *Chlamydia* and *Mycoplasma* spp. Tigecycline may be additionally active against *Stenotrophomonas maltophilia, Acinetobacter* spp., and VRE. Macrolides are used for the treatment of respiratory infections caused by *Chlamydia, Mycoplasma*, and *Legionella* spp. Clarithromycin is used in combination with other agents in the management of infections with *Helicobacter pylori* and *Mycobacterium avium* complex. Macrolides may also be used in patients allergic to penicillin, treated against organisms susceptible to macrolides. Telithromycin can be active against macrolide-resistant strains of *S. pneumoniae.*[20]

Ciprofloxacin and levofloxacin are predominantly active against most aerobic gram-negatives, including *P. aeruginosa*. Moxifloxacin and gatifloxacin have a broader antibacterial spectrum, including some streptococci, staphylococci, and anaerobes, but their activity against *Pseudomonas* spp. is significantly weakened. Notably, gemifloxacin is the most active fluoroquinolone against *S. pneumoniae*. Fluoroquinolones have activity against certain atypical organisms, including *Chlamydia, Mycoplasma*, and *Legionella* spp. With the exception of moxifloxacin, fluoroquinolones are frequently used in the treatment of urinary tract infections and prostatitis. Ofloxacin and levofloxacin can be used for the treatment of pelvic inflammatory disease, and in addition to ciprofloxacin, they may be used as alternative regimens for the treatment of uncomplicated gonorrhea. Levofloxacin and moxifloxacin can be used in cases of community-acquired pneumonia. Finally, certain fluoroquinolones are active against *M. tuberculosis* and some atypical mycobacteria.

Rifampin is frequently administered in combination with other agents for the treatment of infections with MRSA (e.g., infective endocarditis in patients with a prosthetic heart valve), *Brucella* spp., *Francisella tularensis*, and *M. tuberculosis*. Owing to the fast development of high-level resistance if used alone, monotherapy with rifampin should be avoided; it may be administered alone only in cases of meningococcal prophylaxis. Sulfonamides and trimethoprim are primarily used in the treatment of urinary tract infections. They are the antibacterial agents of choice for infections with *Pneumocystis jirovecii*, *Nocardia* spp., and *Stenotrophomonas maltophilia*.

Clindamycin and metronidazole have been considered the agents of choice for anaerobic infections. Most *Clostridium* and *Bacteroides* spp. are susceptible to clindamycin. Moreover, this agent may be used in the treatment of skin and soft tissue infections (including those caused by MRSA) and in combination with penicillin G in cases of serious infections with *Streptococcus pyogenes*. Finally, clindamycin may be used in combination with other agents in certain cases of toxoplasmosis and malaria. Metronidazole has activity against *Clostridium*, *Fusobacterium*, *Prevotella*, and most *Bacteroides* spp. It may be used for the treatment of *Clostridium difficile* colitis and in combination with other agents for the eradication of *H. pylori*. It is also the preferred agent for the treatment of bacterial vaginosis and infections caused by *Entamoeba* spp. and *Trichomonas vaginalis*.

Adverse Events

The most common adverse reactions of antibacterial agents are illustrated in detail in Table 12-5. β-Lactams have been associated with a rash, hives, or anaphylactic shock. These reactions are most commonly observed with penicillins. Patients with a severe allergy to penicillin are at higher risk to develop similar reactions if treated with cephalosporins.[21] Most β-lactams, when administered for a prolonged period of time, may cause bone marrow toxicity that presents as neutropenia and/or thrombocytopenia. Aminoglycosides have traditionally been associated with reversible renal toxicity and, rarely, irreversible ototoxicity. Case reports of reversible neutropenia and thrombocytopenia attributed to long courses and higher drug levels of vancomycin have also been reported. Notably, when vancomycin is administered rapidly, flushing and a macular rash on the neck and upper trunk may be observed. This "red man" syndrome is related to the infusion rate and is fully reversible upon discontinuation of the antibiotic. Tetracyclines can cause irreversible bone pigmentation that appears as dark-colored gums and may permanently stain the teeth if given during pregnancy or childhood. Minocycline has been associated with a systemic lupus erythematosus–like syndrome and central nervous system toxicities, such as dizziness, vertigo, and pseudotumor cerebri. Antibiotic-related diarrhea due to *C. difficile* has been associated with various antibacterial agents, in particular aminopenicillins, cephalosporins, clindamycin, and fluoroquinolones.[22] Linezolid should be cautiously administered to patients taking selective serotonin receptor inhibitors; coadministration can rarely lead to the serotonin syndrome, characterized by tachycardia, hyperthermia, and muscle rigidity. Antibacterial agents that should be avoided during pregnancy; their potential toxicities are summarized in Table 12-6.

TABLE 12-5 MOST FREQUENT ADVERSE EFFECTS OF ANTIBACTERIAL AGENTS

Antibacterial Agent	Adverse Reactions
β-Lactams	Rash/anaphylaxis, serum sickness, diarrhea, hemolytic anemia
Penicillin	CNS toxicities, seizures (at high doses)
Nafcillin/oxacillin	Interstitial nephritis/hepatitis
Ureidopenicillins	Seizures, hemorrhagic diathesis, hypokalemia
Ceftriaxone	Cholelithiasis
Cefamandole, cefotetan	Hemorrhagic diathesis
Imipenem	CNS toxicities, seizures
Vancomycin	Ototoxicity, neutropenia, thrombocytopenia
Daptomycin	Muscle aches
Colistin	Renal impairment, neutropenia, thrombocytopenia, neurotoxicity
Aminoglycosides	Renal impairment, hearing deficits, neuromuscular blockade
Doxycycline	Photosensitivity, teeth and gums discoloration
Tigecycline	Nausea/vomiting
Macrolides (erythromycin > newer)	Abdominal pain, nausea/vomiting, QT-prolongation, hearing loss
Telithromycin	Liver toxicity, QT-prolongation, visual disturbances
Clindamycin	Diarrhea, rash, liver toxicity
Streptogramins	Arthralgias/myalgias, phlebitis, bone marrow toxicity
Moxifloxacin	QT-prolongation
Gemifloxacin	Rash (age and gender dependent)
Rifampin	Liver toxicity, uveitis, SLE-like syndrome, orange secretions
Linezolid	Bone marrow toxicity, neuropathy
Metronidazole	Metallic taste, peripheral neuropathy disulfiram reaction
Sulfonamides and trimethoprim	Renal impairment, hyperkalemia and hyperuricemia, pancytopenia, rash/ Stevens-Johnson syndrome
Chloramphenicol	Bone marrow toxicity, optic neuritis
Nitrofurantoin	Interstitial pneumonitis

CNS, central nervous system; SLE, systemic lupus erythematosus.

Resistance

Bacteria may be intrinsically resistant to certain antibacterial agents. For example, nafcillin cannot penetrate the outer membrane of gram-negative organisms. Furthermore, bacteria can develop resistance to antibacterial agents through a variety of mechanisms, including decreased penetration, efflux pump altered target sites, and inactivation by enzymes[5] (Fig. 12-3).

Gram-negative bacteria form water-filled channels, called porins, in their outer membrane, through which certain antibacterial agents may pass into the cell. If these porins are lost, the entry of antibiotics, such as the aminoglycosides or carbapenems, into the cell is impaired and resistance develops; loss of the D2-porin makes *P. aeruginosa* resistant to imipenem. Alterations in the energy-dependent mechanism of entry of aminoglycosides through the cell membrane of gram-negative bacteria may confer resistance. Antibacterial agents may be driven outside the bacterial cell through an efflux mechanism, which is the most common mechanism of resistance for tetracyclines. This may also be observed in macrolides, streptogramins, lincosamides, and aminoglycosides.

Gram-positive organisms may become resistant to vancomycin by altering the drug's target on the bacterial cell wall. Vancomycin normally binds to a D-alanine-D-alanine terminus in the peptidoglycan precursors. Mutations on a plasmid carrying the VanA gene of enterococci may lead to an altered binding protein that confers resistance to glycopeptides. The most common genotype of enterococcal resistance to vancomycin, type A, leads to a D-alanine-D-lactate terminus, resulting in decreased affinity for vancomycin.[6] This plasmid may be transferred to other organisms, including *S. pyogenes* and, more recently. MRSA. Alterations of PBPs consist of decreased affinity for β-lactams, decreased expression of PBPs, or induction of new PBPs with decreased affinity. This mechanism of resistance may be observed in organisms such as *S. pneumoniae* and *S. aureus*. Alteration of ribosomal target sites is the most common resistance mechanism for macrolides, streptogramins, and lincosamides, whereas DNA gyrase changes may confer resistance to quinolones.

Inactivation of β-lactam antibiotics by β-lactamases may be chromosomal (encoded on the bacterial chromosome) and plasmid or transposon mediated.[6] Most chromosomal β-lactamases are inducible, that is, they may be produced in the presence of an antibacterial agent. Bacteria such as *Proteus*, *Citrobacter*, *Enterobacter*, and *Serratia* spp., when exposed to cephalosporins, may produce an inducible chromosomal β-lactamase. Most plasmid-mediated β-lactamases are constitutive and traditionally confer resistance to penicillins and first- and second-generation cephalosporins. Bacteria such as *Escherichia coli* and *Klebsiella pneumoniae* have been found to produce extended-spectrum β-lactamases (ESBL) that confer resistance to third- and fourth-generation cephalosporins and aztreonam.[23] These organisms remain susceptible in vitro to the cephamycins and β-lactam/β-lactamase inhibitor combinations. In the clinical setting, infections with organisms producing ESBLs should be treated with a carbapenem, until more data are available.

ANTIFUNGAL AGENTS

Since the introduction of amphotericin B in 1959, significant progress has been made in the field of antifungal therapy. Currently, 14 systemically administered antifungal agents are approved by the FDA (Table 12-7).[6] Many of these newer agents offer advantages over older antifungal medications in terms of spectrum of activity, PK, and safety.

TABLE 12-6 ANTIBACTERIAL AGENTS CONTRAINDICATED DURING PREGNANCY

Antibacterial Agent	Adverse Effect
Aminoglycosides	Ototoxicity
Tetracyclines	Teeth and gums discoloration, limb abnormalities, bone growth inhibition
Erythromycin	Hepatitis
Sulfonamides*	Hemolytic anemia, kernicterus
Fluoroquinolones	Cartilage abnormalities
Metronidazole	Possible teratogenicity
Rifampin	Possible teratogenicity
Trimethoprim	Possible teratogenicity
Nitrofurantoin	Hemolytic anemia
Chloramphenicol	Gray baby syndrome

*In babies with glucose-6-phosphate dehydrogenase deficiency.

Fungi are eukaryotic organisms. They have a cytoplasmic cell membrane composed of ergosterol and zymosterol. The cell membrane is surrounded by a fungal cell wall composed of mannoproteins, chitin, and glucans (β-(1→3)-glucan, and β-(1→6)-glucan) (Fig. 12-4). Fungi are classically divided into three forms: yeasts, molds, and dimorphic fungi. Yeasts, such as *Candida* spp., are round organisms that reproduce by asexual budding. Molds, such as *Aspergillus* spp., are composed of tubular structures known as hyphae and grow by branching. Hyphae are often described as septate (with divisions) or nonseptate (without divisions). The dimorphic fungi, such as *Histoplasma capsulatum*, exist as molds in the environment and grow as yeasts at body temperature.

Higher incidence rates of invasive fungal infections (IFIs) have recently been reported. The overall incidence of candidemia has increased significantly, and *Candida* spp. are currently the fourth most common cause of bloodstream infections in the hospital setting. The

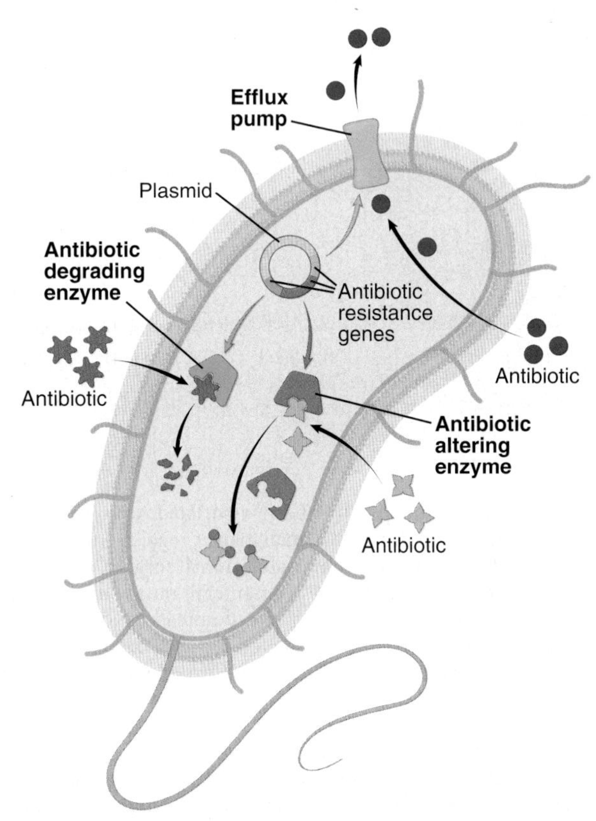

FIGURE 12-3 • Mechanisms of bacterial resistance. (Adapted from www.scq.ubc.ca/.../08/ResistanceMechanisms.gif)

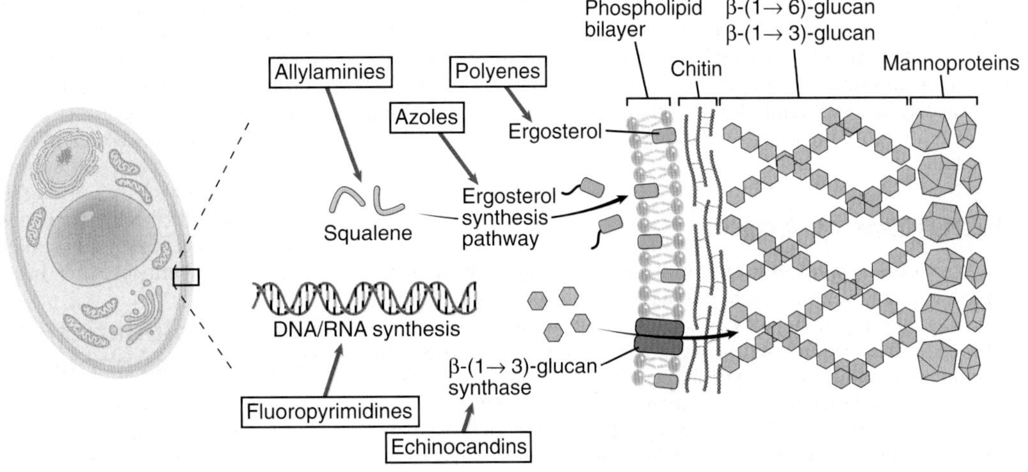

FIGURE 12-4 • Fungal cell membrane and cell wall synthesis and targets of systemic antifungal agents. (From Dodds Ashley ES, Lewis R, Lewis JS, et al. Pharmacology of systemic antifungal agents. Clin Infect Dis 2006;43[Suppl 1]:S28, S39.)

TABLE 12-7 AVAILABLE FORMULATIONS AND ADULT REGULAR DOSING OF ANTIFUNGAL AGENTS

Agent	Formulation	Dose
Amphotericin B deoxycholate	Powder for reconstitution 50 mg Oral suspension 100 mg (1 ml)	0.3-1.5 mg/kg/day
Amphotericin B lipid complex	Suspension 5 mg/ml (20 ml)	3-5 mg/kg/day
Liposomal amphotericin B	Powder for reconstitution 50 mg	3-5 mg/kg/day
Amphotericin B colloidal dispersion	Powder for reconstitution 50 mg, 100 mg	3-5 mg/kg/day
Nystatin	Capsule/tablet Suspension Cream/ointment Powder Vaginal tablet	500,000 units 100,000 units/ml (5 ml, 60 ml, 480 ml) 100,000 units/g (15 g, 30 g) 100,000 units/g (15 g, 30 g, 60 g) 100,000 units
Ketoconazole	Tablets 200 mg Shampoo 1% Cream 2%	200-800 mg/day Twice weekly Once or twice daily
Fluconazole	Tablets 50 mg, 100 mg, 150 mg, 200 mg Powder for oral suspension 10 mg/ml, 40 mg/ml Infusion 2 mg/ml (100 ml, 200 ml)	200-800 mg/day 200-800 mg/day 200-800 mg/day
Itraconazole	Capsule 100 mg Oral solution 100 mg/10 ml (150 ml)	200-400 mg/day 200-400 mg/day
Voriconazole	Tablet 50 mg, 200 mg Powder for oral suspension 200 mg/5 ml (70 ml) Powder for reconstitution 200 mg	100-300 mg q12h 100-300 mg q12h 4-6 mg/kg q12h
Posaconazole	Oral suspension (40 mg/ml, 105 ml)	200 mg q8h
Caspofungin	Powder for reconstitution 50 mg, 70 mg	70 mg/day × 1; 50 mg/day
Micafungin	Powder for reconstitution 50 mg	50-150 mg/day
Anidulafungin	Powder for reconstitution 50 mg	200 mg/day × 1; 100 mg/day
Flucytosine	Capsule 250 mg, 500 mg	50-150 mg/kg/day

development of candidemia has been associated with several risk factors, including premature birth, malignancy, renal failure requiring hemodialysis, disease severity, intra-abdominal surgery, presence of intravenous central catheters, total parenteral nutrition, or use of broad-spectrum antibiotic agents.[24] The widespread use of fluconazole and the administration of antifungals for prophylaxis or preemptive therapy in specific patient populations have brought about epidemiologic changes in rates of infection due to certain *Candida* spp.[24] Higher rates of candidemia in the outpatient setting have recently been reported as well.[25] Moreover, the increasing number of patients who require medical immunosuppression, such as solid organ and hematopoietic stem cell transplant recipients, has led to more frequent IFIs caused by molds. *Aspergillus* spp. remain the most common cause of IFIs in severely immunosuppressed hosts. However, the previously less common molds, such as *Fusarium* spp., *Scedosporium* spp., and the zygomycetes, may be increasing in frequency in this patient population.[26]

The increased incidence and changing epidemiology of IFIs in the hospital and community setting have prompted the aggressive development of antifungal agents. A brief review of the major systemic antifungal agents, including their mechanisms of action, metabolism, susceptibility profiles, recommendations for use, and adverse effects, is presented.

Mechanism of Action

Four main classes of systemic antifungal agents are currently available: polyenes, azoles, echinocandins, and pyrimidine analogues. The mechanisms of action of these agents include disruption of the cell membrane (polyenes, azoles) or cell wall synthesis (echinocandins) and blocking of DNA synthesis (pyrimidine analogues) (see Fig. 12-4).

Polyenes (amphotericin B, nystatin, and pimaricin) act directly on the fungal cell membrane. They bind to ergosterol and increase membrane permeability for several electrolytes, ultimately leading to cell death. In 1959, 4 years after amphotericin B was isolated from *Streptomyces nodosus*, amphotericin B deoxycholate (conventional amphotericin B [CAB]) became the first systemic antifungal agent. More than 30 years later, three lipid-related formulations of amphotericin were licensed: amphotericin B lipid complex (ABLC) in 1995, amphotericin B colloidal dispersion (ABCD) in 1996, and liposomal amphotericin B (L-AMB) in 1997.

The azole antifungals inhibit C-14α demethylation of lanosterole, resulting in the accumulation of C-14α methylsterols and decreased ergosterol concentration. Thus, the fungal cell membrane cannot be maintained, as a result of lower ergosterol production. Since 1979, when ketoconazole was licensed, several newer azoles, the triazoles (i.e., fluconazole, voriconazole), have been marketed. Fluconazole, one of the most commonly used antifungal agents, was licensed in 1990, followed by itraconazole in 1992, and voriconazole in 2002. Posaconazole is a new, broad-spectrum triazole, approved by the FDA in 2006. The echinocandins exert their antifungal activity by inhibiting the production of β-(1→3)-glucan. Thus, they inhibit the synthesis and disrupt the integrity of the fungal cell wall. Currently, three echinocandins are licensed: caspofungin, micafungin, and anidulafungin.

Flucytosine (5-FCt) is the fluorine analogue of cytosine. It was originally designed as an antitumor agent but was found to have antifungal properties and was subsequently licensed in 1972, solely as an antifungal agent. It is activated by deamination to 5-fluorouracil (5-FU) in the fungal cell and is subsequently converted into 5-fluorodeoxyuridylic acid monophosphate. This noncompetitive inhibitor of thymidylate synthetase then interferes with fungal DNA synthesis.

Pharmacokinetics and Pharmacodynamics

All amphotericin B products are poorly absorbed when administered orally. They are highly protein-bound (≥95%), and therefore, their concentration in the CSF after systemic administration is minimal.[27]

However, amphotericin B has been validated for the treatment of fungal infections in the central nervous system (CNS) and is the drug of choice for the treatment of cryptococcal and coccidioidal meningitis. Although the metabolism of amphotericin B is not fully understood, no dose adjustment is necessary for patients with impaired hepatic or renal impairment. The lipid-associated formulations of amphotericin B are frequently used interchangeably. However, concentrations in different organs and compartments may slightly differ among different lipid-associated formulations. Notably, L-AMB attains higher concentrations in the plasma than that of the other lipid formulations.[28] In vitro susceptibility differences against *Aspergillus* spp. between amphotericin B formulations have also been reported.[29]

All azoles are lipophilic and can be administered orally with satisfactory bioavailability. Ketoconazole and itraconazole are highly protein bound and, thus, attain high concentrations in fatty tissues and low concentrations in the CSF.[27] Fluconazole and voriconazole are minimally protein-bound (voriconazole > fluconazole) and, thus, can attain high concentrations in the CSF. Except for fluconazole, which is minimally metabolized and excreted almost unchanged in the urine, all azoles are metabolized through the liver.[27] The dose of fluconazole should be reduced when the calculated creatinine clearance is less than 50 ml/min. The intravenous cyclodextrin-based solutions of itraconazole and voriconazole should be avoided when the creatinine clearance is less than 30 ml/min and less than 50 ml/min, respectively. Itraconazole is available as a capsule, a cyclodextrin-based oral suspension, and an intravenous formulation. Absorption of the oral formulations of the drug varies based on the formulation and the stomach content. Voriconazole is readily absorbed on an empty stomach and is metabolized in the liver. Genetic polymorphisms in CYP 2C19 between different ethnicities may affect the metabolism of voriconazole, occasionally leading to fourfold higher serum concentrations. However, dose adjustments are not currently recommended. Posaconazole is available only as an oral solution and should be administered with food or a high-lipid nutritional supplement for optimal absorption.

Echinocandins are available only as intravenous preparations. They are highly protein bound and, therefore, have minimal CSF and vitreal penetration.[27] Caspofungin is metabolized hepatically, and its maintenance dose should be adjusted to 35 mg/day in patients with moderate hepatic insufficiency. Micafungin is hepatically metabolized but does not require adjustment for mild-to-moderate hepatic dysfunction. However, micafungin has not been studied in patients with severe hepatic impairment. Anidulafungin is the only echinocandin not metabolized by the liver. It undergoes extrahepatic, nonenzymatic metabolism and, thus, does not require dose adjustment in the setting of hepatic insufficiency.

Flucytosine is available in readily absorbed oral capsules, and its minimal protein binding leads to high concentrations in the CSF, aqueous humor, joints, and bone. Dose adjustment is recommended when the creatinine clearance is less than 40 ml/min. In patients with renal impairment, monitoring of serum 5-FCt levels is recommended twice per week.

Spectrum of Activity and Indications

Most of the yeasts and molds identified clinically are susceptible to amphotericin B. Intrinsic resistance to amphotericin B has been described for *Candida lusitaniae*, *Trichosporon* spp., *Aspergillus terreus*, *Scedosporium prolificans*, and occasionally, *Scedosporium apiospermum* and *Fusarium* spps.

The azoles were initially licensed for the treatment of yeast infections, but with the advent of broader-spectrum agents, namely itraconazole, voriconazole and posaconazole, the spectrum of activity has significantly broadened. Ketoconazole and fluconazole are active against most *Candida* spp., *Cryptococcus neoformans*, *Coccidioides immitis*, *Histoplasma capsulatum*, and *Blastomyces dermatidis*. *Candida krusei* is intrinsically resistant to fluconazole, and higher fluconazole MICs have been increasingly reported for *Candida glabrata* isolates. Notably, both agents have no activity against *Aspergillus* spp. and other molds. Itraconazole and voriconazole are additionally active against *Aspergillus* spp. Moreover, other molds, such as *Fusarium* spp. and *Scedosporium* spp., may be susceptible to voriconazole. Voriconazole is not considered active against the zygomycetes group of molds. Most yeasts and molds, including the zygomycetes, are susceptible to posaconazole.

Echinocandins are active against most yeasts and are fungistatic for *Aspergillus* spp. *Cryptococcus* and *Trichosporon* spp. do not possess β-(1→3)-glucan in their cell wall, and thus, these organisms are intrinsically resistant to all echinocandins. Echinocandins are not active against molds other than *Aspergillus* spp. and show higher MICs for *Candida parapsilosis* and *Candida guilliermondii*. However, given the serum concentrations that can be achieved with standard dosing, most *C. parapsilosis* isolates remain susceptible to this class of agents.[30] Flucytosine is active against *Candida* spp. and *Cryptococcus neoformans*, but it should not be used alone for the treatment of these pathogens.

Amphotericin B has traditionally been considered the drug of choice for severe IFIs, including mucormycosis, as well as disseminated or invasive infections of the central nervous system. CAB is indicated for use in the treatment of esophageal and systemic candidiasis, cryptococcal meningitis, invasive endemic mycoses, and mold infections. The advent of the lipid-associated formulations of amphotericin B has had a significant impact on the treatment of IFIs in patients unable to tolerate CAB. These agents may be used instead of CAB if CAB cannot be tolerated in patients with renal impairment or in patients who have failed treatment with CAB. However, the significantly higher cost of these agents may be a limiting factor in their widespread use. Based on similarities in their spectrum and metabolic profile, lipid-associated formulations of amphotericin B are occasionally used interchangeably with CAB in clinical practice. Notably, there are not enough data from randomized, prospective trials to support such use for most IFIs.

L-AMB was found to be superior to CAB solely when studied for the treatment of invasive histoplasmosis in patients with acquired immunodeficiency syndrome (AIDS).[31] Randomized, prospective studies showed noninferiority of L-AMB to CAB in the treatment of patients with cryptococcal meningitis and febrile neutropenia.[32,33] Similarly, in a randomized, double-blind, prospective trial, L-AMB and ABLC were found to have similar success rates in the treatment of patients with febrile neutropenia.[34] Finally, ABCD was found to be comparable with CAB in efficacy for the treatment of invasive aspergillosis and rhinocerebral mucormycosis.[35,36]

Amphotericin B has also been used intrathecally in cases of coccidioidal meningitis, intraocularly in fungal endophthalmitis, locally in fungal peritonitis, or as bladder irrigations for patients with candiduria, but more data are required to support its use in these settings.

Since the newer triazoles were made available, the use of ketoconazole has been limited as a result of its limited spectrum and adverse reactions. It may be used in the treatment of mucocutaneous candidiasis, mild forms of endemic mycoses, and cutaneous dermatophytoses. Fluconazole is approved for use in patients with mucocutaneous and systemic candidiasis, cryptococcal and coccidioidal meningitis, and for antifungal prophylaxis in hematopoietic stem cell transplant recipients and patients with AIDS. Fluconazole's proven efficacy, ease of administration, and minimal adverse reactions make it an appealing agent for the treatment of candidemia. Comparable efficacy of fluconazole to amphotericin B has been shown in nonneutropenic patients with candidemia.[37,38] Notably, scattered data for the treatment of candidemia in neutropenic patients are available. In cases of *C. glabrata*—when the MIC–to–fluconazole ratio is greater than 16 mcg/ml or not available—and *C. krusei* fungemia, it would be prudent to use another agent (e.g., echinocandin, amphotericin B).[39]

Itraconazole is indicated for the treatment of endemic mycoses (histoplasmosis, coccidioidomycosis, blastomycosis) and as salvage treatment for aspergillosis. Itraconazole has been validated as a prophylactic agent in neutropenic patients and hematopoietic stem cell transplant recipients in multiple studies.[40,41] It may also be used as secondary prophylaxis in human immunodeficiency virus (HIV)–positive patients with disseminated histoplasmosis.

Voriconazole was found to be more effective than CAB for the treatment of invasive aspergillosis in an international, multicenter, randomized, open-label trial in hematopoietic stem cell transplant recipients and patients with hematologic malignancies.[42] Based on the results of this study, voriconazole is currently the drug of choice for the treatment of invasive aspergillosis. It should be noted that voriconazole has been compared with lipid-associated formulations of amphotericin B as salvage treatment only for invasive aspergillosis.[43] Voriconazole may also be used for the treatment of fusariosis and scedosporiosis and as empirical antifungal treatment in patients with febrile neutropenia.[44,45]

Use of posaconazole has been reported in the treatment of oropharyngeal candidiasis and fusariosis and as salvage treatment in aspergillosis and mucormycosis.[46] When compared with fluconazole as prophylaxis for neutropenic patients with hematologic malignancy or hematopoietic stem cell transplant recipients with severe graft-versus-host-disease, posaconazole was associated with a significantly decreased incidence of IFIs with *Aspergillus* spp.[47,48] Its extended spectrum of activity, including the zygomycetes, ease of administration, and safe profile will probably make posaconazole an appealing prophylactic and therapeutic agent in the hematopoietic stem cell transplant setting.

Caspofungin is used for the treatment of esophageal and systemic candidiasis and as empirical antifungal treatment in patients with febrile neutropenia.[49] It has also been used as salvage therapy in the treatment of invasive aspergillosis, either alone or in combination.[50] Prospective, randomized, double-blinded trials to evaluate caspofungin (or echinocandins) as first-line or combination treatment for invasive aspergillosis should be performed before any further treatment recommendations can be made. Micafungin has indications for use in esophageal candidiasis and as prophylaxis in hematopoietic stem cell transplant recipients. Data coming from a randomized, prospective trial comparing micafungin with L-AMB for the treatment of invasive candidiasis showed comparable efficacy between the two agents. Micafungin is not currently licensed in the United States for use in patients with invasive candidiasis. Anidulafungin is the only echinocandin studied against fluconazole in a randomized, double-blind trial for the treatment of invasive candidiasis. Based on the results of this study, anidulafungin was approved by the FDA for the treatment of candidemia in 2006. Certain *Candida* spp., such as *C. parapsilosis*, have been associated with higher MICs against echinocandins. However, based on the available limited data, treatment failures of *C. parapsilosis* IFIs with echinocandins have not been reported. When 5-FCt is used alone, resistance to this agent may emerge. Thus, 5-FCt is currently recommended for combination treatment with amphotericin B in cryptococcal meningitis.

TABLE 12-8 DRUG INTERACTIONS WITH AZOLES

AGENTS THAT DECREASE AZOLES LEVELS	KET	FLU	ITR	VOR
Rifampin, isoniazid	+	+	+	+
Phenytoin, carbamazepine, phenobarbital	+	±	+	+
Didanosine, H_2 antagonists, proton pump inhibitors	+	–	+	–
Efavirenz	–	–	–	+
Ritonavir	+	–	–	+
AGENTS THAT INCREASE AZOLES LEVELS				
Sulfonylureas	–	+	–	–
Cyclosporine	–	+	–	–
Theophylline	–	+	–	–
INCREASED BY AZOLES DRUG LEVELS				
Warfarin	+	+	+	+
Phenytoin, carbamazepine	+	+	+	+
Cyclosporine, tacrolimus	+	+	+	+
Triazolam, midazolam	+	+	+	+
Lovastatin, simvastatin, atorvastatin	+	+	+	+
Digitalis, quinidine	+	+	+	+
Calcium channel blockers	+	+	+	+
Glipizide, glyburide, pioglitazone, rosiglitazone	+	+	+	+
Zidovudine	–	+	–	–
Ritonavir and other protease inhibitors	+	–	+	–
Terfinadine, astemizole, cisapride	+	+	+	+

FLU, fluconazole; ITR, itraconazole; KET, ketoconazole; VOR, voriconazole.

Adverse Events

Amphotericin B interacts with cholesterol on human cell membranes, leading to several toxicities that may significantly limit its use. CAB has traditionally been associated with nephrotoxicity, decreased glomerular and renal tubular blood flow, azotemia, and electrolyte imbalance. Infusion-related reactions, such as chills, fever, tachypnea, and myalgias, are commonly encountered within 10 to 20 minutes after administration of CAB. In addition, thrombophlebitis at the site of infusion may occur, particularly if a peripheral venous catheter is used. Lipid-associated amphotericin B formulations share less infusion-related reactions and lower rates of nephrotoxicity. However, administration of L-AMB has been associated with chest pain and dyspnea; abdominal, flank, or lower extremities pain; or flushing and urticaria. Fever and hypoxia have also been reported after treatment with ABLC and ABCD.

The most frequently encountered adverse reactions of ketoconazole are nausea, vomiting, and decreased appetite. Decreased testosterone and cortisol levels have been reported, resulting in gynecomastia, oligospermia, and menstrual irregularities. In addition, ketoconazole has been associated with a reversible reduction in testosterone- and/or adrenocorticotropic-related cortisol response. The most serious, but quite rare, side effect of ketoconazole is liver toxicity that ranges from asymptomatic elevation of liver function tests to fulminant liver failure. With the exception of reversible alopecia and mild elevation of transaminases, fluconazole lacks other significant toxicities and is an overall well-tolerated agent.

The presence of cyclodextrin in the oral formulation of itraconazole may cause severe gastrointestinal complaints (nausea, diarrhea). Itraconazole has been associated with a triad of hypokalemia, hypertension, and edema and with a negative inotropic effect. Use of voriconazole has been associated with mild elevation of liver enzymes and the development of a phototoxicity rash. Visual disturbances, in the form of color changes, blurred vision, bright colors, or photophobia, have been reported in patients treated with voriconazole. This effect usually appears 30 minutes after drug administration, but it is mild and transient. It should be noted that all azoles are metabolized to some degree by CYP450 and are also reversible inhibitors of CYP enzymes. Thus, significant drug interactions of all azoles exist and should be carefully reviewed when prescribing (Table 12-8).

Echinocandins are generally well-tolerated agents, but infusion-related reactions have been encountered. Common adverse effects of 5-FCt include nausea, vomiting, diarrhea, and rash. Flucytosine may affect the bone marrow, leading to leukopenia and thrombocytopenia. In cases of renal impairment (e.g., coadministration with amphotericin B), higher levels of 5-FCt may lead to potentiation of its toxicities.

Resistance

Fungi may be or become insensitive to an antifungal agent, leading to intrinsic or secondary resistance respectively. The increasing incidence of IFIs and extensive use of antifungal agents, preemptively and therapeutically, has led to higher rates of resistance. Primary or intrinsic resistance is characterized by resistance of an organism to a certain drug it has never been exposed to, such as the resistance of *C. krusei* to fluconazole or *Candida lusitaniae* to amphotericin B. Fungi may also develop secondary resistance to certain drugs as a result of repeated or prolonged exposure to that agent. Emerging resistance to amphotericin B has been associated with changes in the plasma membrane composition. Fungi may become resistant to azoles by alterations in the efflux or influx pumps and target enzymes. Finally, echinocandins may become inactive by an alteration of the β-glucan synthase of the fungal cell wall.

Based on data obtained from the Artemis Disk Antifungal Surveillance Program (1997-2003), most *C. albicans*, *C. parapsilosis*, *Candida tropicalis*, and *C. lusitaniae* isolates remain susceptible to fluconazole.[51] However, increasing resistance to fluconazole of *C. glabrata* and *C. guilliermondii* has been noted.[51] For fluconazole-resistant *C. glabrata* isolates, cross-resistance with other azoles (e.g., itraconazole, voriconazole) has been extensively reported. Recently, reports have noted increasing resistance to amphotericin B with isolates of *C. glabrata*, *C. krusei*, and the South African clade of *C. albicans*. Echinocandins are uniformly active against most *Candida* spp., but elevated MICs have been reported for *C. parapsilosis* and *C. guilliermondii*. Cross-resistance among different agents in this class is well documented as well. *Aspergillus terreus* shows intrinsic resistance to amphotericin B, but limited data are available concerning molds and antifungal susceptibility.

Susceptibility testing of fungi against antifungal agents is a significant adjunct in the treatment of IFIs. New developments in antifungal susceptibility testing have recently been accomplished. Most progress has been made in validating susceptibility testing for yeasts, *Candida* spp. in particular. The Clinical and Laboratory Standards Institute (CLSI) Subcommittee on Antifungal Susceptibility Testing has validated two methods—the broth dilution and the disk diffusion—for resistance testing of yeasts to antifungal agents.[52]

Notably, interpretive breakpoints have been reported only for *Candida* spp. against fluconazole, itraconazole, voriconazole, and 5-FCt. The E-test method (AB Biodisk) is one of the most commonly used commercial test systems for antifungal susceptibility. It is available for several antifungal agents, including amphotericin B, fluconazole, voriconazole, itraconazole, posaconazole, and caspofungin. It is more helpful than broth dilution testing in assessing the activity of amphotericin B against *Candida* spp. and *C. neoformans* because of the narrow MIC range obtained by broth dilution.

Topical Antifungal Agents

For the treatment of mucosal, skin, and nail fungal infections, several systemic or locally applied antifungal compounds can be used. The most commonly administered topical antifungal agents and their major indications and formulations are illustrated in Table 12-9.

ANTIVIRAL AGENTS

The development of antiviral agents initially progressed slowly owing to failures of early antiviral drugs to selectively inhibit virus versus human cells.[53] The first agent evaluated for treatment of human herpesvirus (HHV) was idoxuridine, which was found to be too toxic for systemic use. However, once molecular events unique to virus replication were identified, virus-specific targets were designed. Today's targets of antiviral therapy are viral enzymes and proteins that affect the assembly of the virus.[54] Vidarabine was one of several nucleoside derivatives being developed as anticancer agents during the 1960s, when it was determined that several humanherpes viruses were sensitive to this agent. At the time, low therapeutic : toxic ratios were considered inevitable for antivirals. Vidarabine produced lower toxicity at therapeutic concentrations compared with other purine/pyrimidine analogues being studied. This effect was due to its preferential effect on viral rather than cellular DNA synthesis.[55] The current era of effective specific antiviral therapy began with acyclovir.[54] Acyclovir was

TABLE 12-9 TOPICAL ANTIFUNGAL AGENTS

Agent	Indication	Formulation
POLYENES		
Nystatin	Mucocutaneous, oral and vaginal candidiasis	Capsule, cream, ointment, powder Suspension, Oral & vaginal tablets
Pimaricin	Keratomycosis	Ophthalmic suspension (2.5% and 5%)
AZOLES		
Miconazole	Vulvovaginal candidiasis, tinea infections	Cream, liquid spray, ointment, powder Suppository, Tablet, Tincture
Clotrimazole	Dermatophytosis, cutaneous and vaginal candidiasis	Cream 1%, solution 1%, vaginal cream and tablet, troche
Butoconazole	Vulvovaginal candidiasis	Cream vaginal 2%
Econazole	Cutaneous candidiasis, tinea infections	Cream 1%
Oxiconazole	Tinea infections	Cream 1%, lotion 1%
Sulconazole	Tinea infections	Cream 1%, solution 1%
Terconazole	Vulvovaginal candidiasis	Vaginal cream and suppositories (0.4% and 0.8%)
Tioconazole	Vulvovaginal candidiasis	Vaginal ointment 6.5%
GRISEOFULVIN	Dermatophytosis	Oral suspension 125 mg/5 ml, tablet
ALLYLAMINES		
Terbinafine	Onychomycosis, tinea infections	Cream 1% (12 g), solution 1% (30 ml), tablet 250 mg
Amorolfine	Onychomycosis	Nail lacquer
Naftifine	Dermatophytosis	Cream and gel 1%
Butenafine	Dermatophytosis	Cream 1%
CICLOPIROX	Onychomycosis, tinea infections, Cutaneous candidiasis, seborrheic dermatitis	Cream/gel 0.77%, shampoo 1% (120 ml) Solution (nail lacquer) 8%, solution as olamine 0.77%
BUTENAFINE	Tinea infections	Cream 1%
TOLNAFTATE	Tinea infections	Aerosol liquid and powder 1%, cream 1%, powder 1% Solution 1%, swab 1%

discovered in 1974 and was the first effective antiviral drug to be used extensively.[56] Since then, over a dozen antiviral agents have become available (Table 12-10), excluding those used for treatment of HIV-1 (see Chapter 84, HIV Infection and AIDS).

In immunocompetent patients, the goals for use of antivirals are to decrease the severity of the illness and prevent complications while decreasing the rate of transmission of the virus. In patients with chronic viral infections, antivirals are used to prevent damage to organs such as the liver. Antivirals are used in four distinct ways: as prophylaxis to prevent virus acquisition; as suppression to keep viral replication low enough to prevent damage; as preemptive therapy triggered by quantitative evidence of infection before symptoms present; and as treatment of overt disease.[53] This section focuses on the currently used antiviral agents for common viruses such as HHVs, including herpes simplex virus 1 and 2 (HSV 1 and 2), cytomegalovirus (CMV), varicella-zoster virus (VZV), as well as influenza and hepatitis B and C (HBV and HCV).

Pharmacobiology

Viruses are obligate intracellular pathogens dependent on host-cell function. Currently, three main steps of the viral life cycle serve as targets of therapy. First is the interference of attachment between the virus and the host cell membrane and prevention of entry of the virus into the host cell. Second is the inhibition of transcription or translation at various steps. Third is the interference with viral assembly. All of these stages occur only in actively replicating viruses rather than latent viruses (Fig. 12-5). The antivirals that target each of these stages in specific viruses are discussed.

In the HHVs (HSV 1 and 2, CMV, EBV, VZV), one of the main targets of therapy is the viral DNA polymerase. This enzyme is essential for replication. Its role is to incorporate nucleotide triphosphates onto the end of an elongated DNA chain. For HBV, the major target is the virally encoded reverse transcriptase enzyme, which transcribes viral RNA into DNA during late stages of the replication cycle. HCV

TABLE 12-10 ANTIVIRALS USED FOR HUMAN HERPESVIRUSES*

Antiviral Drug	Mechanism of Action	Viruses Targeted
Acyclovir	Guanosine analogue; inhibits viral DNA polymerase	**HSV, VZV,** CMV, EBV
Valacyclovir	Same as acyclovir	**HSV, VZV,** CMV
Famciclovir	Same as penciclovir	**HSV, VZV**
Penciclovir	Guanosine analogue; inhibits viral DNA polymerase	HSV
Ganciclovir	Guanosine analogue; inhibits viral DNA polymerase	**Cytomegalovirus,** HSV, VZV, EBV, HHV 8
Valganciclovir	Same as ganciclovir	**CMV**
Foscarnet	Inhibits viral DNA polymerase by binding to pyrophosphate binding site	CMV, **acyclovir-resistant HSV, acyclovir-resistant VZV**
Cidofovir	Cytosine nucleotide analogue; inhibits viral DNA polymerase	Adenovirus, polyomavirus, papillomavirus, and poxvirus; retains activity against **thymidine kinase–negative HSV** and **phosphotransferase-negative CMV,** which are mutant viruses resistant to acyclovir and ganciclovir.

*Indications for which drug is the agent of choice are in bold type.
CMV, cytomegalovirus; EBV, Epstein-Barr virus; HHV, human herpesvirus; HSV, herpes simplex virus; VZV, varicella-zoster virus.

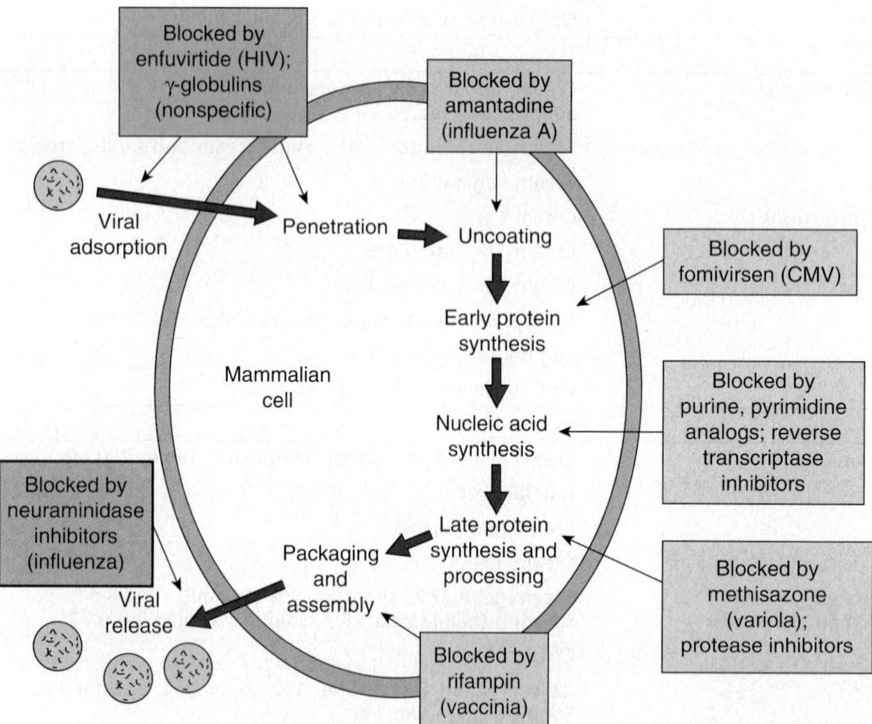

FIGURE 12-5 • Example of sites of antiviral action (From Safrin S. Antiviral agents. In Katzung BG [ed]. Basic and Clinical Pharmacology, 10th ed. New York: McGraw Hill, 2004.)

is an RNA virus that relies on an RNA-dependent RNA polymerase for replication. This enzyme lacks a proofreading function, resulting in diverse quasispecies within an infected person. This makes targeted therapy challenging.[57] The enzyme is currently one of the few targets of therapy for HCV in use today.

Treatment for influenza currently targets two steps in the viral life cycle: fusion of the virus to the host cell and budding of the virus from the host cell. Two proteins are involved in fusion of the virus to the host. The first is the membrane protein M2, which is responsible for uncoating of the virus and release of nucleic acid from the infectious virus into the cell.[55] The second is viral hemagglutinin (HA), which mediates entry of the virus into cells by fusion of viral envelope with cell membrane.[54] Budding, or cell-to-cell spread of the virus, depends on neuraminidase, a glycoprotein found in the viral envelope. Neuraminidase removes cellular receptors that bind the other major influenza surface enzyme, HA, a process essential for virus cell fusion. Interference with neuraminidase activity inhibits the escape of the influenza virus from the infected cell.[56]

Pharmacokinetics

Pharmacokinetic factors play a key role in the selection of an appropriate antiviral agent (Table 12-11). Vidarabine is poorly soluble and requires intravenous administration with large volumes of fluid.[58] Acyclovir is orally bioavailable (10%-20%) and is used in both oral and intravenous forms. It is the only member of this family of drugs available in intravenous form. Acyclovir is primarily renally eliminated with 80% of the drug that reaches the systemic circulation found unchanged in the urine. Dosage adjustments are recommended for patients with renal impairment or those on dialysis. Valacyclovir is the L-valyl ester of acyclovir. It is converted to acyclovir by the enzyme valacyclovir hydrolase found in the gastrointestinal tract and liver. It is available only in an oral dosage form. However, the oral bioavailability is three to five times that of acyclovir. Therefore, it may be dosed less frequently than acyclovir. Famciclovir is metabolized to penciclovir by deacetylation in the gastrointestinal tract, blood, and liver. The intracellular half-life of the active drug, penciclovir triphosphate, is long, allowing less frequent dosing. Penciclovir itself cannot be administered orally owing to its poor bioavailabiity. It is available only in topical form. Famciclovir is eliminated via the kidneys and requires dosage adjustment in patients with renal impairment. Ganciclovir is available in both oral and intravenous forms. Oral ganciclovir has a bioavailability of only 8% to 9%, thus preventing its use for the treatment of CMV. It was originally used for prophylaxis of CMV but has been replaced by the prodrug valganciclovir. Valganciclovir is an L-valyl ester of ganciclovir that is rapidly metabolized to ganciclovir following oral administration. Because of its enhanced bioavailability (60%), it is preferred over oral ganciclovir. Ganciclovir is primarily eliminated as active drug in the urine (91%), requiring dose adjustment in patients with renal impairment. Foscarnet must be given intravenously. It is not metabolized, and the active drug is eliminated by glomerular filtration and tubular secretion. Cidofovir is available in intravenous form only and is significantly eliminated by the kidneys.

Ribavirin is degraded in the gastrointestinal tract and liver. Aerosolized ribavirin is absorbed systemically. Lamivudine has an excellent bioavailability and a 5- to 7-hour half-life, which allows once-daily dosing for HBV. All of the HBV nucleoside analogues have good bioavailability, although entecavir requires administration with food. All require dose adjustment in patients with renal impairment. Interferons are not orally bioavailable and need to be given by intramuscular or subcutaneous injection. A polyethylene glycol moiety is attached to interferon (pegylated interferon) and decreases clearance and increases half-life, requiring less frequent dosing.

Amantadine and rimantidine are both available in oral form only. Amantadine peak plasma concentrations are three times higher in patients older than 60 years than in younger adults, and the half-life is 12 hours longer in this group. The drug is primarily eliminated by tubular secretion of the active compound, and thus, it is likely that the higher levels in older patients are due to impaired renal function. Rimantidine is 75% metabolized in the liver through hydroxylation, and doses should be decreased in older patients owing to diminished hepatic function. Interferons are not orally bioavailable and need to be given by either intramuscular or subcutaneous routes. Zanamavir is given by aerosolized form because it is rapidly cleared from the plasma if given systemically. Four percent to 17% of inhaled doses are absorbed systemically. Oseltamivir has a 75% oral bioavailability, and 94% of the active drug is renally excreted. Dose adjustment is required in patients with impaired renal function.

TABLE 12-11 SELECTED PHARMACOKINETIC PROPERTIES OF DRUGS USED FOR HUMAN HERPESVIRUSES

Drug	Dosage Forms Available and Usual Doses	Bioavailability	Metabolism
Acyclovir	PO: 400 mg 5 × day orolabial; 400 tid genital herpes IV: 10 mg/kg q8h encephalitis Topical: 5% cream 5 × day orolabial	10-20%	Renal excretion: 62%-91% Renal clearance decreases with reduced renal function
Valacyclovir	PO: 1 g bid genital herpes/mucocutaneous	54%	Renal excretion: <1% valacyclovir; 40%-50% acyclovir
Famciclovir	PO: 125-500 mg PO bid	77%	Excretion: famciclovir, fecal: 27%; penciclovir, renal: 60%-65%
Penciclovir	Topical: 1% cream q2h while awake	1.5%	Approximately 70% of a dose excreted unchanged in the urine; however, IV form not available in United States
Ganciclovir	PO: 1 g tid prophylaxis IV: 5 mg/kg q12h treatment Ophthalmic insert: 4.5 mg q 5-8 mo	8%-9%	Little to no metabolism; renal excretion: 100% unchanged drug
Valganciclovir	PO: 900 mg bid treatment; 900 mg qd prophylaxis	60%	Hepatic and intestinal metabolism by esterases; hydrolysis to active metabolite: ganciclovir; renal excretion: primarily as ganciclovir
Foscarnet	IV: 40 mg/kg IV q8h herpes	0%	Renal excretion: 73%-94%
	90 mg/kg IV q12h CMV		Eliminated almost exclusively as unchanged drug via glomerular filtration
Cidofovir	IV: 5 mg/kg IV q wk × 2 followed by 5 mg/kg q 2 wk	0%	80% excreted unchanged in urine

bid, twice a day; CMV, cytomegalovirus; IV, intravenous; PO, per os (oral); q, every; tid, three times a day.

Mechanisms of Action

Drugs for Human Herpesviruses

The mechanism of action of all drugs used against HHVs is inhibition of viral synthesis of DNA.[58] The majority of the drugs used fall into the family of nucleoside analogues. Nucleoside analogues bear a resemblance to the naturally occurring nucleosides adenosine, thymidine, guanine, and cytidine.[59] Vidarabine was the original purine analogue, although it is no longer used systemically. Acyclovir is the representative agent in this class, which also includes ganciclovir, famciclovir, penciclovir, valacyclovir, valganciclovir, and cidofovir. All of these agents are converted to mono-, di-, and triphosphate forms by cellular kinases, viral kinases, or both.[60] Acyclovir is an analogue of deoxyguanosine. Two different enzymes are involved in the antiviral activity of acyclovir. Viral and cellular thymidine kinases are responsible for the conversion of acyclovir to its active form (Fig. 12-6). The first step to convert acyclovir to a monophosphate is carried out by thymidine kinase induced in cells infected with HCV or VZV or by phosphotransferase produced by CMV. Cellular enzymes add the next two phosphate steps.[58,61] The viral DNA polymerase is the target of acyclovir's activity.[60] It inhibits the synthesis of viral DNA by competing with deoxyguanosine triphosphate as a substrate for viral DNA polymerase. Once inserted, DNA synthesis stops (Fig. 12-7). The effect is irreversible, and acyclovir is considered a "suicide inhibitor" because it inactivates the DNA polymerase.[53,54] Acyclovir inhibits herpes DNA polymerase 30 times more than human alpha polymerase. Valacyclovir is a prodrug of acyclovir and is converted to acyclovir after absorption. Penciclovir has a mechanism of action similar to that of acyclovir, but it is not an obligate DNA chain terminator. Famciclovir is converted to penciclovir after oral administration. Hence, all four drugs are guanosine nucleoside analogues and share a common requirement for phosphorylation by thymidine kinase.

Ganciclovir serves as a nucleoside analogue of guanine. It is converted to ganciclovir monophosphate by viral-encoded phosphotransferase. Unlike acyclovir, it does not cause absolute DNA chain termination.[53,54] As a ganciclovir prodrug, valganciclovir has the same mechanism of action. Cidofovir is a cytosine nucleotide analogue that does not require viral enzymes for phosphorylation.

The second major class for HHVs are the analogues of pyrophosphate, of which foscarnet is the only currently used agent. Unlike the nucleoside analogues, foscarnet does not require phosphorylation to become active and, therefore, does not rely on viral or cellular enzymes. It inhibits the viral DNA polymerases by binding to the

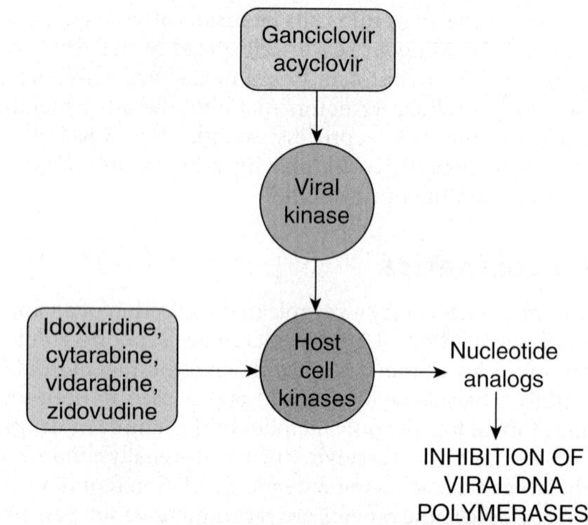

FIGURE 12-6 • Antiviral actions of purine and pyrimidine analogues. **Ganciclovir and acyclovir are phosphorylated first by viral kinase. The monophosphate products and the drugs shown to the left are then phosphorylated by host cell kinases to the nucleotide analogues that inhibit viral replication.** (From Safrin S. Antiviral agents. In Katzung BG [ed]. Basic and Clinical Pharmacology, 10th ed. New York: McGraw Hill, 2004.)

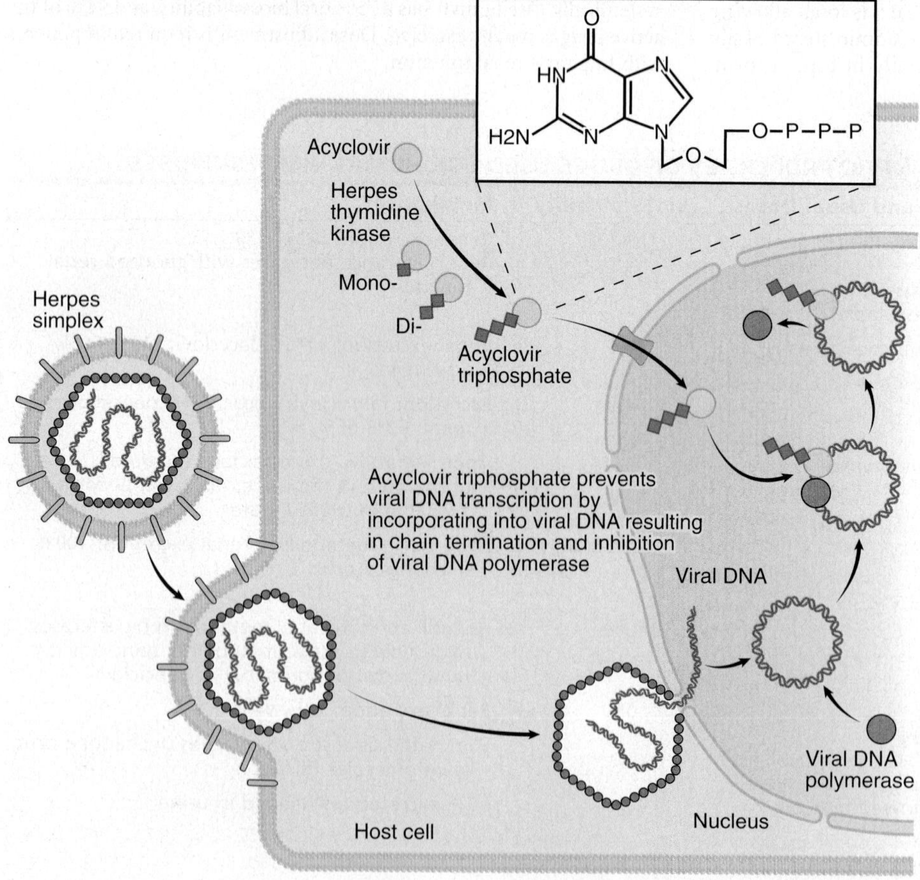

FIGURE 12-7 • Example of image to create to illustrate mechanism of action of acyclovir. (From Balfour HH Jr. Antiviral drugs. N Engl J Med 1999;340[16]:1262.)

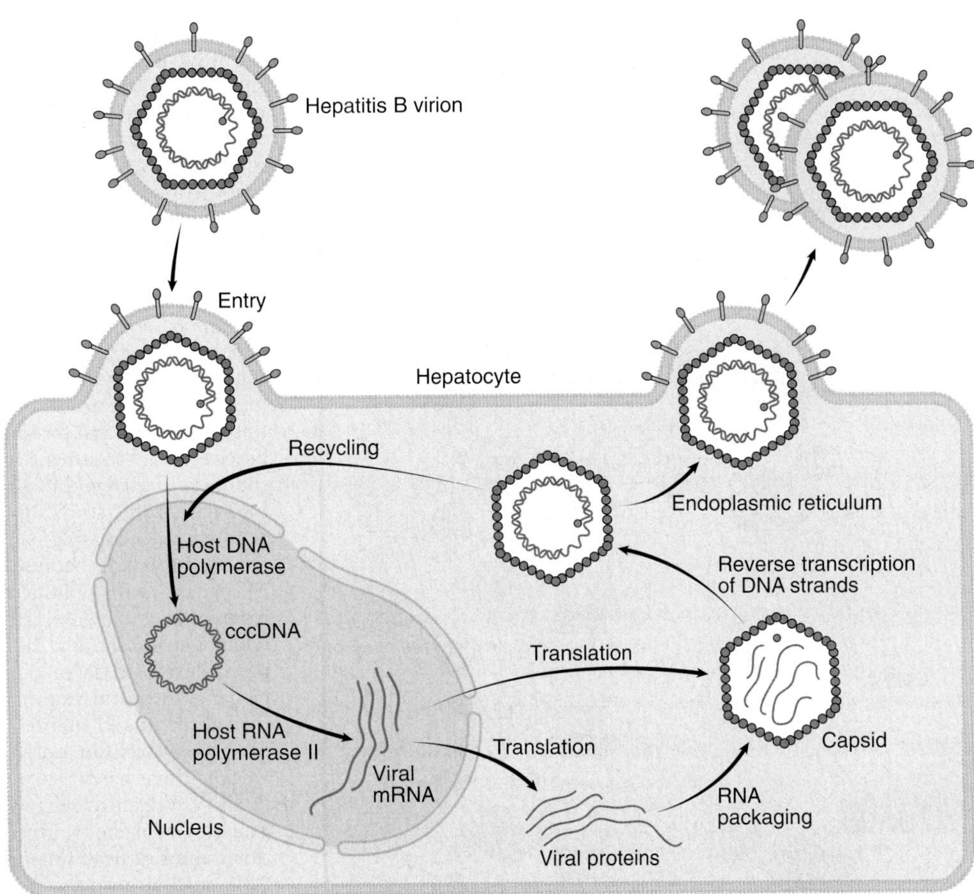

FIGURE 12-8 • Replication of hepatitis B virus. (From Younger HM, Bathgate AJ, Hayes PC. Nucleoside analogues for the treatment of chronic hepatitis B [Review article]. Aliment Pharmacol Ther 2004;20[11-12]:1214.)

site integral to the release of pyrophosphate product of DNA synthesis.[60] It forms a complex with DNA polymerase at its pyrophosphate-binding site, preventing cleavage of pyrophosphate from nucleoside triphosphate. The result is blockade of further primer template extension.[53,58]

Drugs for Hepatitis B

Nucleoside analogues are also used in the treatment of the hepatitis viruses in which they exert their antiviral effect through integration into HBV DNA.[59] Lamivudine is a cytidine analogue that is metabolized intracellulary to lamivudine triphosphate. It inhibits the HBV DNA polymerase (as well as HIV reverse transcriptase; see Chapter 84, HIV Infection and AIDS), which reverse transcribes an RNA intermediate to synthesize a DNA strand (Fig. 12-8).[53,59] It competes with cytidine triphosphate for incorporation into HBV polymerase DNA, causing immediate DNA chain termination (Fig. 12-9).[59] Adefovir is an analogue of the nucleotide adenosine. It contains a phosphate group and, thus, requires only one final phosphorylation step before competing with adenosine for integration into HBV DNA. Entecavir is a deoxyguanosine analogue with a mechanism similar to that of lamivudine and adefovir. The addition to this class is telbivudine, a synthetic thymidine nucleoside analogue.

Drugs for Hepatitis C

Ribavirin is a guanosine analogue that is intracellularly phosphorylated to a triphosphate. It interferes with viral transcription by acting as a substrate mimic for misincorporation by viral polymerase. Other proposed mechanisms of action include inhibition of the kinase responsible for synthesis of guanosine triphosphate; enhancement of T-cell immunity; and error catastrophe (stimulation of transcription errors).[53,58,62] Interferons are natural glycoproteins with antiviral activity. Unlike the nucleoside analogues, they are not directly virucidal or virustatic.[58] Their mechanism of action is believed to be the induction of cellular enzymes that interfere with synthesis of viral proteins. Commercial preparations are made in bacteria by recombinant DNA techniques. These products inhibit viral RNA transcription and translation by augmenting cellular immune function.

Drug for Influenza

Amantadine and rimantidine inhibit the replication of the influenza A virus by blocking the viral M2 protein ion channel established by influenza A to allow virion to fuse with cell membrane and enter the cell. The result is reduced ability of this protein to effect viral uncoating and pH regulation.[53,56] The release of nucleic acid from infectious virus into cell is prevented.[55] The neuraminidase inhibitors zanamavir and oseltamivir prevent the action of neuraminidase, which cleaves the cellular receptor to which newly formed particles are attached. Without the action of neuraminidase, the escape of the influenza virus from the infected cell is inhibited. The inhibitors mimic the natural substrate, fitting into the active site (Fig. 12-10).[63]

Spectrums of Activity

The original antiviral vidarabine was active against the HHVs as well as influenza and some RNA viruses. However, today, it is not used systemically. Acyclovir is active against the HHVs, with preferential activity against HSV 1 and 2, EBV, and VZV. Much higher concentrations of acyclovir are required for suppression of CMV. This is believed to be due to the lack of thymidine kinase in CMV.[58] The related compounds of valacyclovir, famciclovir, and penciclovir share the same spectrum of activity. Ganciclovir and valganciclovir are better substrates for the phosphotransferase enzyme found in CMV and have a longer intracellular half-life than acyclovir. For these reasons, they are more active against CMV. They offer no advantage to acyclovir in the treatment of HSV 1 and 2, EBV, and VZV.[53] Foscarnet is active against all of the HHVs, as well as HIV and HBV. Cidofo-

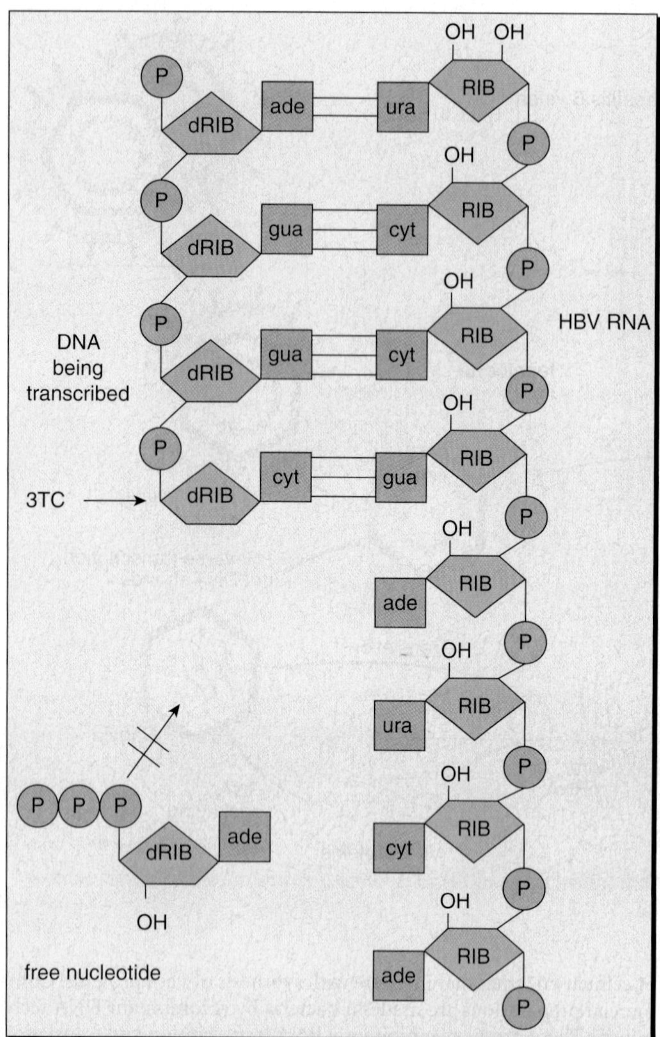

FIGURE 12-9 • Mechanism of action of lamivudine in hepatitis B. ade, adenosine; cyt, cytosine; dRIB, D-ribose; gua, guanosine; 3TC, lamivudine; p, phosphate; thy, thymidine; ura, uracil.

vir is active against all of the HHVs, including CMV, HSV, and VZV. Common or adverse effects of antiviral agents are summarized in Table 12-12.[64]

Many of the reverse transcriptase inhibitors that showed activity against HIV were evaluated against HBV. Unfortunately, many were found to be active in vitro but not in vivo or were too toxic.[56] Lamivudine, entecavir, adefovir, and telbivudine have all been approved for use in HBV. Lamivudine is also used as part of a highly active antiretroviral regimen for HIV-1.

Ribavirin also possesses broad activity against a number of DNA and RNA viruses including parainfluenza, mumps, measles, HSV, adenoviruses, HCV, and coxsackieviruses.[58] The interferons are active against papillomaviruses, HHV 8 (Kaposi's sarcoma), and HCV.

Amantadine and rimantadine have intrinsic activity against influenza A only. Their effectiveness has become limited by resistance. However, the neuraminidase inhibitors, zanamavir and oseltamivir, are active against both strains of influenza A and B as well as some strains of avian influenza.[63]

Indications

Acyclovir, famciclovir, and valacyclovir are all indicated for the treatment of genital herpes (see Table 12-10). Drug treatment was shown in clinical trials to speed healing of lesions and decrease the duration of pain. For mucocutaneous herpes, immunocompromised patients should be treated to accelerate healing. In immunocompetent patients, the need for treatment is questionable because the symptoms are short-lived. Penciclovir is approved for orofacial herpes in immunocompetent patients. However, application is necessary every 2 hours while awake to decrease healing time by 0.7 day.[65] For neonatal herpes, intravenous acyclovir is indicated followed by a prolonged course of oral therapy. Herpes encephalitis requires treatment with intravenous acyclovir for at least 21 days to reduce the possibility of late relapses. Relapses were reported in patients treated for only 10 days. Prophylaxis with acyclovir in bone marrow transplant or kidney transplant patients has been found to decrease reactivation of herpes. For chickenpox in immunocompetent adults, treatment with acyclovir, valacyclovir, or famciclovir—if started within 24 hours of the appearance of the rash—can decrease the duration and severity of symptoms by 25%. Treatment is also recommended for pregnant women in the second and third trimesters and for immunocompromised children. Similarly, for herpes zoster, treatment with acyclovir, famciclovir, or valacyclovir should be started within 72 hours of onset of rash to accelerate healing by 2 days. Some studies found valacyclovir to be more effective than acyclovir at decreasing pain. Treatment should be offered to patients older than 50 years because of their high risk of postherpetic neuralgia. All patients with ophthalmic zoster should be treated. For patients resistant to acyclovir, foscarnet has been shown to be superior to vidarabine in clinical trials. Although acyclovir was initially studied for the prophylaxis of CMV in kidney transplant patients, it has been replaced by ganciclovir and valganciclovir. Intravenous ganciclovir is used for the treatment and suppression of CMV. Oral ganciclovir can be used for prophylaxis but not treatment owing to its low bioavailability. Valganciclovir has largely replaced oral ganciclovir for the prophylaxis of CMV. Valganciclovir was shown to be as effective as intravenous ganciclovir for the treatment and duration of CMV retinitis.[65] Ganciclovir and foscarnet were found to be equivalent for the treatment of CMV in clinical trials.[53] Foscarnet can cause less hematologic toxicity when used in allogeneic stem cell transplants.[65] Cidofovir is an additional alternative for CMV disease in patients who cannot tolerate ganciclovir.

Pegylated interferon and ribavirin are the treatments of choice for chronic HCV. Combination therapy provides sustained viral responses of 54% to 63% and is clinically synergistic.[62,65] Lamivudine has been shown to reduce HBV DNA levels, normalize serum transaminases, and improve histologic indices in patients with both hepatitis B early antigen (HBeAg)–positive and –negative disease. Serconversion rates of 50% are reached within 5 years. However, owing to the extensive development of resistance, lamivudine as chronic monotherapy is not ideal.[59] In studies comparing adefovir with placebo, patients with both HbeAg-negative and -positive chronic HBV had significant histologic, virologic, and biochemical improvement. It is indicated for treatment-naïve as well as lamivudine-experienced patients.[66,67] Entecavir was compared with lamivudine in both HbeAg-negative and -positive chronic HBV patients and was found to have statistically significantly better rates of histologic improvement and virologic response.[65,68] It also is indicated for both treatment-experienced and -naïve patients. Telbivudine was compared with lamivudine and adefovir in clinical trials with positive findings. It is indicated for chronic HBV. The current reverse transcriptase inhibitors for HBV are used to suppress rather than clear the infection, and a rebound effect in HBV replication is observed with all of them once withdrawn.[56]

Current Centers for Disease Control and Prevention guidelines recommend against the use of rimantidine/amantadine for either treatment or prophylaxis owing to high rates of resistance. Oseltamivir is effective for decreasing the duration of both influenza A and B if started within 36 hours of the onset of symptoms. Zanamavir must be started within 2 days. Both can be used for the treatment and prophylaxis of influenza A and B.[69]

Adverse Effects

The currently used antiviral agents are associated with fewer toxicities owing to their selectivity for viral rather than cellular molecular targets

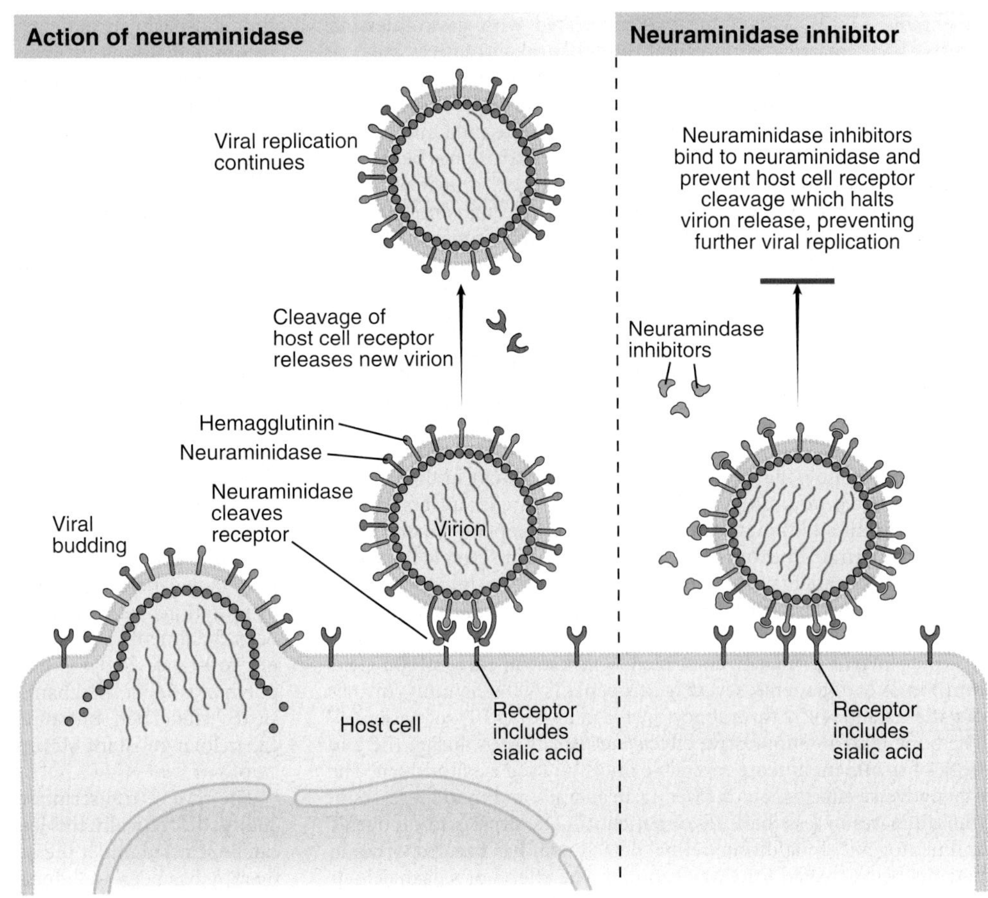

FIGURE 12-10 • Mechanism of action of neuraminidase inhibitors. A, The action of neuraminidase in the continued replication of virions in influenza infection. **B,** The replication is blocked by neuraminidase inhibitors, which prevent virions from being released from the surface of infected cells.

TABLE 12-12 COMMON OR SEVERE ADVERSE EFFECTS OF ANTIVIRAL AGENTS

Drug	Adverse Effect	Management
Acyclovir	Reversible nephropathy	Hydration; reduce dose in patients with impaired creatinine clearance
	Encephalopathy	Discontinue drug
Valacyclovir	Same as acyclovir	Same as acyclovir
	Thrombotic micrangiopathy	Discontinue drug
Famciclovir	None	
Penciclovir	None	
Ganciclovir	Bone marrow suppression	Reduce dose or discontinue drug, administer granulocyte growth factors
Valganciclovir	Same as ganciclovir	Same as ganciclovir
Foscarnet	Renal insufficiency	Hydrate with saline before administration; monitor renal function; reduce dosage in renal impairment
	Electrolyte imbalance	Monitor serum electrolytes twice weekly; provide replacement as needed
	Nausea and vomiting	Effect of electrolyte imbalance
Cidofovir	Nephrotoxicity, metabolic acidosis	Intravenous saline loading and oral probenicid before and after each dose
	Neutropenia	Granulocyte colony-stimulating factor
Ribavirin	Anemia	Reduce dose
Lamivudine, adefovir, entecavir, telbivudine	Lactic acidosis and server hepatomegaly with steatosis	Discontinue drug
Amantadine/rimantadine	Central nervous system dysfunction	Reduce dose by 50% in elderly patients
Zanamavir	Bronchospasm	Avoid in patients with reactive airway disease
Oseltamivir	Nausea/vomiting	Take with food
Interferon alfa	Influenza-like symptoms	Reduce or withhold dose temporarily
	Central nervous system dysfunction	Reduce or withhold dose temporarily

(see Table 12-12). Vidarabine was associated with gastrointestinal effects, bone marrow suppression, and neurologic effects such as peripheral neuropathy, altered mental status, agitation, coma, and seizures.[58] Acyclovir is well tolerated, as are most of its related compounds. Intravenous acyclovir is associated with inflammation or phlebitis at the infusion site. A reversible renal toxicity has been associated with use of the intravenous form in 5% to 10% of patients. Risk factors for the development of renal toxicity include high doses at rapid infusion rates, dehydration, and preexisting renal impairment. The cause is the precipitation and crystallization of the drug in the renal tubules, which may be prevented with adequate intravenous hydration. Renal toxicity has not been associated with the oral dosage form. Neurologic effects including confusion, delirium, lethargy, tremors, and seizures have been reported in 1% of patients and are associated with high serum concentrations (>25 mcg/ml). The other adverse effects, including nausea, vomiting, lightheadedness, diaphoresis, and rash, are mild.[58] The manufacturer advises to avoid the drug in pregnancy; however, data show that women treated with acyclovir in the first trimester reported no problems. Valacyclovir has similar adverse effects to acyclovir. In addition, thrombotic thrombocytopenic purpura and hemolytic uremic syndrome have been reported in severely immunocompromised patients who received valacyclovir for long periods of time. Famciclovir is well tolerated and causes headache, nausea, and diarrhea.

Ganciclovir is primarily associated with neutropenia (<1000 cells/mm^3) in 38% of patients, severe neutropenia (<500 cells/mm^3) in 16% of patients, and severe thrombocytopenia in less than 10% of patients.[69] The bone marrow suppressive effects are usually seen during the 2nd week of treatment and are reversible once the drug is withdrawn. The other adverse effects include fever, rash, anemia, and mild increases in transaminases in less than 2% of patients.[58] The drug is carcinogenic and teratogenic. In addition, retinal detachment has been reported in patients being treated for CMV retinitis. The effects of valganciclovir are similar to those of ganciclovir. Foscarnet causes nephrotoxicity in 25% of patients. The effect is reversible and can be minimized by adjusting doses, saline-loading patients, and maintaining adequate hydration. The other adverse effects are anemia, hypo- and hyperphosphatemia, hypo- and hypercalcemia, and seizures.[58] Cidofovir is associated with several severe adverse effects, and 25% of patients have been shown to discontinue the drug secondary to these effects. Patients experience nephrotoxicity, neutropenia, and metabolic acidosis. To help prevent the nephrotoxicity, patients should be given intravenous saline loading and oral probenicid before and after each dose.[69]

Ribavirin is teratogenic and is contraindicated in pregnancy. The best-documented adverse effect is a dose-dependent anemia that develops in most patients. Other adverse effects include increased bilirubin, uveitis, nausea, headache, and lethargy. The aerosolized form is well tolerated.[58] The interferons are known to cause an "influenza-like syndrome" especially during the 1st week of therapy. Patients experience fever and myalgias. Other adverse effects include headache, diarrhea, and alopecia.[58] Patients should also be advised of weight loss, psychiatric syndromes such as depression, anxiety, and emotional lability as well as the production of auto-antibodies and exacerbation/induction of autoimmune diseases.[65,69] Lamivudine causes headache, nausea, and dizziness. There have been reports of pancreatitis, primarily in children.[69] Adefovir was initially studied at higher doses for HIV and found to cause renal toxicity. The lower doses used for hepatitis are less likely to cause azotemia and renal tubular dysfunction. Another risk factor is preexisting renal impairment.[65] Entecavir and telbivudine both have mild adverse effect profiles.

Amantadine displays primarily central nervous system effects, including nervousness, anxiety, lightheadedness, confusion, and insomnia. These are especially prominent in elderly patients. Milder adverse effects such as nausea, anorexia, urinary retention, rash, and peripheral edema have also been reported.[69] Rimantidine produces gastrointestinal complaints similar to those of amantadine but has a lower risk of central nervous system effect.[69] Zanamavir has caused nasal and throat discomfort in its aerosolized form and can cause bronchospasm in patients with reactive airway disease. The current recommendations are to avoid the drug in these patients.[69] Oseltamivir is well tolerated with mild effects of nausea and vomiting, which can be reduced if it is taken with food.[69]

Resistance

Clinical resistance to acyclovir is defined as progression of mucocutaneous HSV lesions despite therapy. This has most often been reported in immunocompromised patients after prolonged courses of acyclovir in the setting of drug-induced immunosuppression.[60] There are two main mechanisms of resistance to acyclovir. The first is an alteration or deletion of the gene for thymidine kinase. This leads to resistance to acyclovir, famciclovir, valacyclovir, and ganciclovir but not to foscarnet, which does not require phosphorylation. The second, less frequently documented, mechanism of resistance is an alteration of DNA polymerase, which leads to resistance to the entire acyclovir family of drugs as well as to foscarnet.[58,70] These strains may be susceptible to cidofovir. Ganciclovir resistance in CMV is also believed to be due to a decrease in phosphorylation.[58,70] Mutations have been noted in the gene that codes for the phosphotransferase enzyme required to phosphorylate ganciclovir to its active form. Resistance can also be caused by mutations in the DNA polymerase. Cross-resistance to cidofovir has been documented, but these strains will respond to foscarnet. Foscarnet resistance in HSV has been localized to mutation in the DNA polymerase gene. Mechanisms of resistance to cidofovir have not been clearly elucidated, but an altered DNA polymerase has been noted in ganciclovir-resistant strains of CMV with reduced susceptibility to cidofovir.[71]

The reverse transcriptase enzyme in hepatitis B lacks proofreading ability; theoretically, this leads to quasispecies in each individual, which can be selected under pressure of drug therapy. Resistance to anti-HBV therapy has been well documented. Studies show that after 5 years of therapy with lamivudine, 70% of patients have detectable mutations of the reverse transcriptase gene.[59] Resistance with adefovir is much lower at 4% after 3 years of therapy.[59] Entecavir resistance was not documented in the clinical trials.[61,68] The adefovir, entecavir, and telbivudine studies show a benefit to using these agents in patients already resistant to lamivudine.[59,68] Resistance to ribavirin in HCV is still rare, but resistant strains have been shown to possess a mutation in the viral polymerase.

Strains of influenza A with mutations in the amino acid sequence of the M2 protein possess resistance to amantadine and rimantidine. The large majority of influenza A isolates possesses mutations correlated with resistance to amantadine/rimantidine.[72] Development of resistance to the neuraminidase inhibitors is much rarer. Neuraminidase mutations lead to a functionally defective enzyme. Overall reported rates of resistance to both zanamavir and oseltamivir are below 1%.[63]

REFERENCES

1. Hessen M, Kaye D. Principles of use of antibacterial agents. Infect Dis Clin North Am 2004;18:435-450.
2. Pankey GA, Sabath LD. Clinical relevance of bacteriostatic versus bactericidal mechanisms of action in the treatment of gram positive bacterial infections. Clin Infect Dis 2004;38:864-870.
3. Schentag JJ, Gilliland KK, Paladino JA. What have we learned from pharmacokinetic and pharmacodynamic theories? Clin Infect Dis 2001;32(Suppl 1):S39-S46.
4. Rybak MJ. Resistance to antimicrobial agents: An update. Pharmacotherapy 2004;24(12 Pt 2):203S-215S.
5. Levinson W, Jawetz E. Medical Microbiology and Immunology, 4th ed, Vol. 1. Stamford, CT: Appleton & Lange, 1996, pp 423-523.
6. Rex JH, Stevens DA. Systemic antifungal agents. In Mandell GL, Bennett JE, Dolin RD (eds): Principles and Practice of Infectious Diseases, 6th ed. Philadelphia: Elsevier, 2006, pp 502-514.
7. Lode H, Hoffken G, Boeckk M, et al. Quinolone pharmacokinetics and metabolism. J Antimicrob Chemother 1990;26(Suppl B):41-49.
8. Moellering RC Jr, Krogstad DJ, Greenblatt DJ. Pharmacokinetics of vancomycin in normal subjects and in patients with reduced renal function. Rev Infect Dis 1981;3(Suppl):S230-S235.
9. Cruciani M, Gatti G, Lazzarini L, et al. Penetration of vancomycin into human lung tissue. J Antimicrob Chemother 1996;38(5):865-869.

10. Lovering AM, Zhang J, Bannister GC, et al. Penetration of linezolid into bone, fat, muscle and haematoma of patients undergoing routine hip replacement. J Antimicrob Chemother 2002;50(1):73-77.
11. Alexander I. "Alcohol-antabuse" syndrome in patients receiving metronidazole during gynaecological treatment. Br J Clin Pract 1985;39(7):292-293.
12. Tunkel AR, Hartman BJ, Kaplan SL, et al. Practice guidelines for the management of bacterial meningitis. Clin Infect Dis 2004;39(9):1267-1284.
13. Leclercq R, Dutka-Malen S, Brisson-Noel A, et al. Resistance of enterococci to aminoglycosides and glycopeptides. Clin Infect Dis 1992;15(3):495-501.
14. Baddour LM, Wilson WR, Bayer AS, et al. Infective endocarditis: Diagnosis, antimicrobial therapy, and management of complications: a statement for healthcare professionals from the Committee on Rheumatic Fever, Endocarditis, and Kawasaki Disease, Council on Cardiovascular Disease in the Young, and the Councils on Clinical Cardiology, Stroke, and Cardiovascular Surgery and Anesthesia, American Heart Association: endorsed by the Infectious Diseases Society of America. Circulation 2005;111(23): e394-e434.
15. Enderlin G, Morales L, Jacobs RF, Cross JT. Streptomycin and alternative agents for the treatment of tularemia: review of the literature. Clin Infect Dis 1994;19(1):42-47.
16. Butler T, Levin J, Linh NN, et al. *Yersinia pestis* infection in vietnam. II. Quantiative blood cultures and detection of endotoxin in the cerebrospinal fluid of patients with meningitis. J Infect Dis 1976;133(5):493-499.
17. Ariza J, Gudiol F, Pallares R, et al. Treatment of human brucellosis with doxycycline plus rifampin or doxycycline plus streptomycin. A randomized, double-blind study. Ann Intern Med 1992;117(1):25-30.
18. Wormser GP, Nadelman RB, Dattwyler RJ, et al. Practice guidelines for the treatment of lyme disease. The Infectious Diseases Society of America. Clin Infect Dis 2000;31(Suppl 1):1-14.
19. Fishbein DB, Dawson JE, Robinson LE. Human ehrlichiosis in the United States, 1985 to 1990. Ann Intern Med 1994;120(9):736-743.
20. Jalava J, Kataja J, Seppala H, Huovinen P. In vitro activities of the novel ketolide telithromycin (HMR 3647) against erythromycin-resistant streptococcus species. Antimicrob Agents Chemother 2001;45(3):789-793.
21. Kelkar PS, Li JT. Cephalosporin allergy. N Engl J Med 2001;345(11):804-809.
22. Bartlett JG. The new epidemic of *Clostridium difficile*-associated enteric disease [Narrative review]. Ann Intern Med 2006;145(10):758-764.
23. Pfaller MA, Segreti J. Overview of the epidemiological profile and laboratory detection of extended-spectrum beta-lactamases. Clin Infect Dis 2006;42(Suppl 4):S153-S163.
24. Nucci M, Marr KA. Emerging fungal diseases. Clin Infect Dis 2005;41(4):521-526.
25. Sofair AN, Lyon GM, Huie-White S, et al. Epidemiology of community-onset candidemia in Connecticut and Maryland. Clin Infect Dis 2006;43(1):32-39.
26. Marr KA, Carter RA, Crippa F, et al. Epidemiology and outcome of mould infections in hematopoietic stem cell transplant recipients. Clin Infect Dis 2002;34(7):909-917.
27. Dodds Ashley ES, Lewis R, Lewis JS, et al. Pharmacology of systemic antifungal agents. Clin Infect Dis 2006;43(Suppl 1):S28, S39.
28. Sperry PJ, Cua DJ, Wetzel SA, Adler-Moore JP. Antimicrobial activity of AmBisome and non-liposomal amphotericin B following uptake of *Candida glabrata* by murine epidermal Langerhans cells. Med Mycol 1998;36(3):135-141.
29. Oakley KL, Moore CB, Denning DW. Comparison of in vitro activity of liposomal nystatin against aspergillus species with those of nystatin, amphotericin B (AB) deoxycholate, AB colloidal dispersion, liposomal AB, AB lipid complex, and itraconazole. Antimicrob Agents Chemother 1999;43(5):1264-1266.
30. Kartsonis N, Killar J, Mixson L, et al. Caspofungin susceptibility testing of isolates from patients with esophageal candidiasis or invasive candidiasis: relationship of MIC to treatment outcome. Antimicrob Agents Chemother 2005;49(9):3616-3623.
31. Johnson PC, Wheat LJ, Cloud GA, et al. Safety and efficacy of liposomal amphotericin B compared with conventional amphotericin B for induction therapy of histoplasmosis in patients with AIDS. Ann Intern Med 2002;137(2):105-109.
32. Walsh TJ, Finberg RW, Arndt C, et al. Liposomal amphotericin B for empirical therapy in patients with persistent fever and neutropenia. National Institute of Allergy and Infectious Diseases Mycoses Study Group. N Engl J Med 1999;340(10):764-771.
33. Prentice HG, Hann IM, Herbrecht R, et al. A randomized comparison of liposomal versus conventional amphotericin B for the treatment of pyrexia of unknown origin in neutropenic patients. Br J Haematol 1997;98(3):711-718.
34. Wingard JR, White MH, Anaissie E, et al. A randomized, double-blind comparative trial evaluating the safety of liposomal amphotericin B versus amphotericin B lipid complex in the empirical treatment of febrile neutropenia. L Amph/ABLC Collaborative Study Group. Clin Infect Dis 2000;31(5):1155-1163.
35. White MH, Anaissie EJ, Kusne S, et al. Amphotericin B colloidal dispersion vs. amphotericin B as therapy for invasive aspergillosis. Clin Infect Dis 1997;24(4):635-642.
36. Bowden R, Chandrasekar P, White MH, et al. A double-blind, randomized, controlled trial of amphotericin B colloidal dispersion versus amphotericin B for treatment of invasive aspergillosis in immunocompromised patients. Clin Infect Dis 2002;35(4):359-366.
37. Rex JH, Bennett JE, Sugar AM, et al. A randomized trial comparing fluconazole with amphotericin B for the treatment of candidemia in patients without neutropenia. Candidemia Study Group and the National Institute. N Engl J Med 1994;331(20):1325-1330.
38. Rex JH, Pappas PG, Karchmer AW, et al. A randomized and blinded multicenter trial of high-dose fluconazole plus placebo versus fluconazole plus amphotericin B as therapy for candidemia and its consequences in nonneutropenic subjects. Clin Infect Dis 2003;36(10):1221-1228.
39. Pappas PG, Rex JH, Sobel JD, et al. Guidelines for treatment of candidiasis. Clin Infect Dis 2004;38(2):161-189.
40. Huijgens PC, Simoons-Smit AM, van Loenen AC, et al. Fluconazole versus itraconazole for the prevention of fungal infections in haemato-oncology. J Clin Pathol 1999;52(5):376-380.
41. Marr KA, Crippa F, Leisenring W, et al. Itraconazole versus fluconazole for prevention of fungal infections in patients receiving allogeneic stem cell transplants. Blood 2004;103(4):1527-1533.
42. Herbrecht R, Denning DW, Patterson TF, et al. Voriconazole versus amphotericin B for primary therapy of invasive aspergillosis. N Engl J Med 2002;347(6):408-415.
43. Patterson TF, Boucher HW, Herbrecht R, et al. Strategy of following voriconazole versus amphotericin B therapy with other licensed antifungal therapy for primary treatment of invasive aspergillosis: impact of other therapies on outcome. Clin Infect Dis 2005;41(10):1448-1452.
44. Walsh TJ, Lutsar I, Driscoll T, et al. Voriconazole in the treatment of aspergillosis, scedosporiosis and other invasive fungal infections in children. Pediatr Infect Dis J 2002;21(3):240-248.
45. Walsh TJ, Pappas P, Winston DJ, et al. Voriconazole compared with liposomal amphotericin B for empirical antifungal therapy in patients with neutropenia and persistent fever. N Engl J Med 2002;346(4):225-234.
46. Raad II, Hachem RY, Herbrecht R, et al. Posaconazole as salvage treatment for invasive fusariosis in patients with underlying hematologic malignancy and other conditions. Clin Infect Dis 2006;42(10):1398-1403.
47. Ullmann AJ, Lipton JH, Vesole DH, et al. Posaconazole or fluconazole for prophylaxis in severe graft-versus-host disease. N Engl J Med 2007;356(4):335-347.
48. Cornely OA, Maertens J, Winston DJ, et al. Posaconazole vs. fluconazole or itraconazole prophylaxis in patients with neutropenia. N Engl J Med 2007;356(4):348-359.
49. Mora-Duarte J, Betts R, Rotstein C, et al. Comparison of caspofungin and amphotericin B for invasive candidiasis. N Engl J Med 2002;347(25):2020-2029.
50. Marr KA, Boeckh M, Carter RA, et al. Combination antifungal therapy for invasive aspergillosis. Clin Infect Dis 2004;39(6):797-802.
51. Pfaller MA, Diekema DJ, Rinaldi MG, et al. Results from the ARTEMIS DISK Global Antifungal Surveillance Study: a 6.5-year analysis of susceptibilities of candida and other yeast species to fluconazole and voriconazole by standardized disk diffusion testing. J Clin Microbiol 2005;43(12):5848-5859.
52. National Committee for Clinical Laboratory Standards. Methods for Antifungal Disk Diffusion Susceptibility Testing of Yeasts: Approved Guideline, M44-A. Wayne, PA, National Committee for Clinical Laboratory Standards, 2004.
53. Balfour HH Jr. Antiviral drugs. N Engl J Med 1999;340(16):1255-1268.
54. Crumpacker CS II. Molecular targets of antiviral therapy. N Engl J Med 1989;321(3):163-172.
55. Hirsch MS, Swartz MN. Drug therapy: antiviral agents (first of two parts). N Engl J Med 1980;302(16):903-907.
56. Kinchington D. Recent advances in antiviral therapy. J Clin Pathol 1999;52(2): 89-94.
57. Lauer GM, Walker BD. Hepatitis C virus infection. N Engl J Med 2001;345(1): 41-52.
58. Keating MR. Antiviral agents. Mayo Clin Proc 1992;67(2):160-178.
59. Younger HM, Bathgate AJ, Hayes PC. Nucleoside analogues for the treatment of chronic hepatitis B [Review article]. Aliment Pharmacol Ther 2004;20(11-12):1211-1230.
60. Laufer DS, Starr SE. Resistance to antivirals. Pediatr Clin North Am 1995;42(3):583-599.
61. Chang TT, Gish RG, de Man R, et al. A comparison of entecavir and lamivudine for HBeAg-positive chronic hepatitis B. N Engl J Med 2006;354(10):1001-1010.
62. Lau JY, Tam RC, Liang TJ, Hong Z. Mechanism of action of ribavirin in the combination treatment of chronic HCV infection. Hepatology 2002;35(5):1002-1009.
63. Moscona A. Neuraminidase inhibitors for influenza. N Engl J Med 2005;353(13):1363-1373.
64. Kendle JB, Fan-Havard P. Cidofovir in the treatment of cytomegaloviral disease. Ann Pharmacother 1998;32(11):1181-1192.
65. Drugs for non-HIV viral infections. Med Lett 2005;3(32):23-32.
66. Hadziyannis SJ, Tassopoulos NC, Heathcote EJ, et al. Adefovir dipivoxil for the treatment of hepatitis B e antigen-negative chronic hepatitis B. N Engl J Med 2003;348(9):800-807.
67. Marcellin P, Chang TT, Lim SG, et al. Adefovir dipivoxil for the treatment of hepatitis B e antigen-positive chronic hepatitis B. N Engl J Med 2003;348(9):808-816.
68. Lai CL, Shouval D, Lok AS, et al. Entecavir versus lamivudine for patients with HBeAg-negative chronic hepatitis B. N Engl J Med 2006;354(10):1011-1020.
69. Drugs for non-HIV viral infections. Med Lett 2002;44(1123):9-16.
70. Crumpacker CS. Mechanism of action of foscarnet against viral polymerases. Am J Med 1992;92(2A):3S-7S.
71. Erice A. Resistance of human cytomegalovirus to antiviral drugs. Clin Microbiol Rev 1999;12(2):286-297.
72. Bright RA, Shay DK, Shu B, et al. Adamantane resistance among influenza A viruses isolated early during the 2005-2006 influenza season in the United States. JAMA 2006;295(8):891-894.

13

PHARMACOKINETICS

Arthur J. Atkinson, Jr.

INTRODUCTION 193
BASIC PHARMACOKINETIC CONCEPTS 193
Initiation of Drug Therapy—Concept of Apparent Distribution Volume 193
Effect of Protein Binding on Apparent Volume of Distribution 194
Effect of Tissue Binding on Apparent Volume of Distribution 194
Continuation of Drug Therapy (Concepts of Elimination Half-Life and Clearance) 195
Elimination Half-Life 195
Elimination Clearance 195
Drug Cumulation and the Plateau Principle 197
Drug Absorption—Concept of Bioavailability 197
Bioavailability 199
ADDITIONAL PHARMACOKINETIC CONCEPTS 199
Nonlinear Elimination Kinetics 199
Multicompartmental Models of Drug Distribution 200
Clinical Consequences of Drug Distribution Kinetics 200
PHARMACOKINETIC EFFECTS OF RENAL AND HEPATIC IMPAIRMENT 200
Pharmacokinetic Effects of Impaired Kidney Function 201
Pharmacokinetic Effects of Impaired Liver Function 201
Restrictively Eliminated Drugs 202
Nonrestrictively Eliminated Drugs 202

"All things are poison and not without poison; only the dose makes a thing not a poison."

Paracelsus (1493-1541)[1]

INTRODUCTION

Pharmacokinetics has been defined as the quantitative analysis of the processes of drug absorption, distribution, and elimination. As such, it links drug dose to its concentration in biologic fluids and, for most drugs, determines the intensity and time course of drug action. *Pharmacodynamics* (Chapter 14, Pharmacodynamics) deals with the mechanism of drug action that links these drug concentrations to their pharmacologic effects. Interindividual differences in pharmacokinetics and pharmacodynamics are both responsible for the variation in patient response encountered when standard drug doses are administered. Thus, an understanding of both is required if patients are to received appropriately individualized drug therapy.

The relationship between drug concentrations in plasma, serum, or blood and the pharmacologic response of a patient—the *concentration-response* relationship—is usually less variable than the *dose-response* relationship. This reflects the fact that individual variation in the pharmacokinetic processes of drug absorption, distribution, and elimination affects dose-response relationships but not the relationship between the free (nonprotein-bound) drug in plasma water and the intensity of effect (Fig. 13-1). Accordingly, periodic measurement of blood or plasma drug concentrations has become routine for some drugs that have only a small safety margin between therapeutic and toxic doses or effects that are not easy to assess clinically. This is discussed further in Chapter 21, Therapeutic Monitoring.

BASIC PHARMACOKINETIC CONCEPTS

Widmark[2] conducted the first pharmacokinetic studies in 1919, using a single compartment open model to characterize drug distribution, elimination, and cumulation. A schematic of this model incorporating the primary pharmacokinetic parameters of *distribution volume* (V_d) and *elimination clearance* (CL_E) is shown in Figure 13-2.

Pharmacokinetics provides the scientific basis for dose regimen design and dose selection, those essential processes that have long been recognized as essential to convert drugs from poisons to therapeutically useful agents (see quotation at beginning of text). The model shown in Figure 13-2 is adequate for most clinical applications of pharmacokinetics and is used in the context of its relevance to dose regimen design to illustrate the basic concepts of distribution volume, elimination clearance, and *elimination half-life* ($t_{1/2}$). Because pharmacokinetics is quantitative, it is inescapably mathematical. Although full understanding of pharmacokinetic theory requires a grasp of calculus, we demonstrate that most clinical applications fortunately entail only simple algebraic calculations.

Initiation of Drug Therapy—Concept of Apparent Distribution Volume

In Figure 13-2, drug concentration (C) is represented as uniform throughout the body, so that its apparent volume of distribution is defined by the equation

$$V_d = X/C \qquad (13\text{-}1)$$

where X is the total body drug content. This volume can be estimated either from the drug concentration change resulting from administration of a drug dose or from removal of a measured amount of drug by hemodialysis or hemoperfusion. As can be seen from this equation, the concept of distribution volume is clinically useful because it defines the relationship between the plasma concentration of a drug, which relates to its pharmacologic action, and the total amount of drug in the body, which is a function of the rates of drug administration and elimination.

One way of estimating the apparent distribution volume of a drug is from a plot of its plasma concentrations after administration of a drug dose. For example, a plot of expected digoxin plasma concentrations resulting from intravenous administration of a dose of this drug is shown in Figure 13-3. Inspection of the log plasma level–versus–time curve indicates that concentrations of this drug do not distribute throughout the body instantaneously in a kinetically uniform fashion.

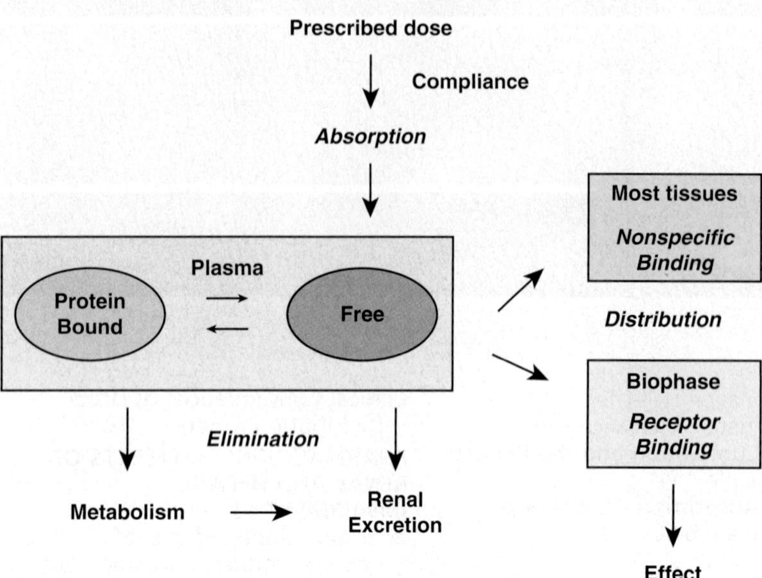

FIGURE 13-1 • Diagram of factors that account for variability in observed effects when standard drug doses are prescribed. Some of this variability can be compensated for by using plasma concentration measurements to guide dose adjustments. (From Atkinson AJ Jr. Clinical pharmacokinetics. In Atkinson AJ Jr, Abernethy DR, Daniels CE, et al [eds]: Principles of Clinical Pharmacology, 2nd ed. San Diego: Elsevier, 2007.)

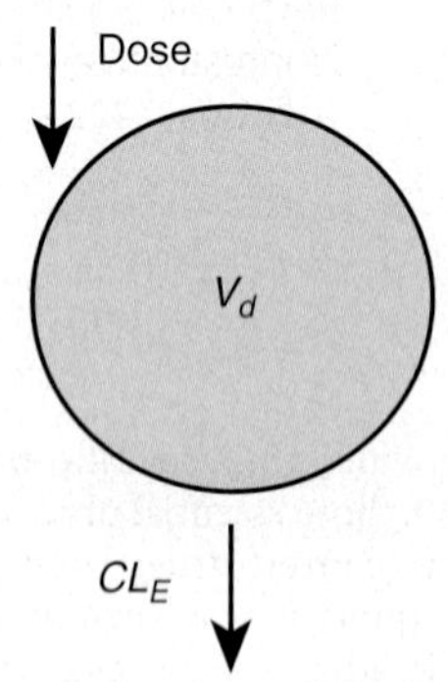

FIGURE 13-2 • Diagram of a single compartment model in which the primary kinetic parameters are the apparent distribution volume of the compartment (V_d) and the elimination clearance (CL_E).

The curve eventually becomes a straight (technically "log-linear") line on the graph; this part of the curve is termed the *elimination phase.* Back-extrapolation of this line to time 0 provides an estimate of the hypothetical drug concentration (C_0) that would have occurred if the digoxin dose had distributed instantaneously throughout the body. As shown in Figure 13-3, the administered dose (D) and C_0 can be substituted into Equation 13-1 to calculate an apparent distribution volume designated $V_{d(extrap.)}$.

$$V_{d(extrap.)} = D/C_0 \qquad (13\text{-}2)$$

The initial part of the plasma concentration–versus–time curve, in which concentrations lie above the back-extrapolated elimination phase line, is termed the *distribution phase* and reflects the fact that distribution equilibrium is reached only slowly after a digoxin dose is administered. This is a consequence of the underlying *multicompartmental* nature of digoxin distribution from the intravascular space to peripheral tissue compartments. Although estimates of apparent distribution volume are based on the assumption that drug binding in tissues and in plasma are equal, digoxin has a much higher binding affinity for peripheral compartment tissues than for plasma. This accounts for the fact that its apparent distribution volume is much larger than physiologic body compartments.

Digoxin is typical of most drugs in that its apparent volume of distribution does not correspond to physiologic body fluid spaces. However, some drugs and other compounds have distribution volumes that are physiologically identifiable. Thus, the distribution volumes of inulin and quaternary neuromuscular blocking drugs approximate expected values for extracellular fluid (ECF) space. Also, the distribution volumes of urea, ethyl alcohol, and caffeine provide reliable estimates of total body water (TBW).[3]

Effect of Protein Binding on Apparent Volume of Distribution

Binding to plasma proteins acts to reduce estimates of apparent distribution volume when they are based on total (bound + free) rather than unbound (free) drug concentrations. Because "plasma" proteins distribute throughout ECF, the distribution volume of highly protein bound drugs exceeds plasma volume and approximates ECF in many cases.[3] For example, thyroxine is 99.97% protein bound and its distribution volume of 0.15 L/kg[4] approximates ECF estimates of 0.16 ± 0.01 L/kg made with inulin.[5] Distribution volumes generally exceed ECF for uncharged drugs that are less tightly protein bound to plasma proteins. For example, the nonprotein-bound fraction of theophylline, a methylxanthine chemically similar to caffeine, distributes in TBW. The relationship between the extent of plasma protein binding and the theophylline distribution volume is shown in Figure 13-4 and is given by the following equation:

$$V_d = ECF + f_U\,(TBW - ECF) \qquad (13\text{-}3)$$

where f_U is the fraction of unbound theophylline that can be measured in plasma samples.[6] An additional correction has been proposed because interstitial fluid protein concentrations are less than those in plasma.[7] However, this correction does not account for the heterogeneous nature of interstitial fluid composition and entails additional complexity that may not be warranted.[3]

Effect of Tissue Binding on Apparent Volume of Distribution

Many drugs have distribution volumes greater than expected values for TBW, or larger than ECF, despite extensive binding to plasma proteins. The extensive tissue binding of these drugs increases their apparent distribution volume, as indicated by the following modification of Equation 13-3:

$$V_d = ECF + \Phi f_U\,(TBW - ECF) \qquad (13\text{-}4)$$

where (Φ) is a parameter characterizing tissue-binding affinity. For many drugs, the extent of tissue binding is related to their distribution coefficient (D_{oct}), a coefficient that takes into account drug lipophilicity and extent of ionization at physiologic pH.[8] In Figure 13-5, published experimentally determined values for log D_{oct} are compared with estimates of log Φ. For example, digoxin is a neutral compound that incorporates a lipophilic steroid moiety (aglycone) but is relatively

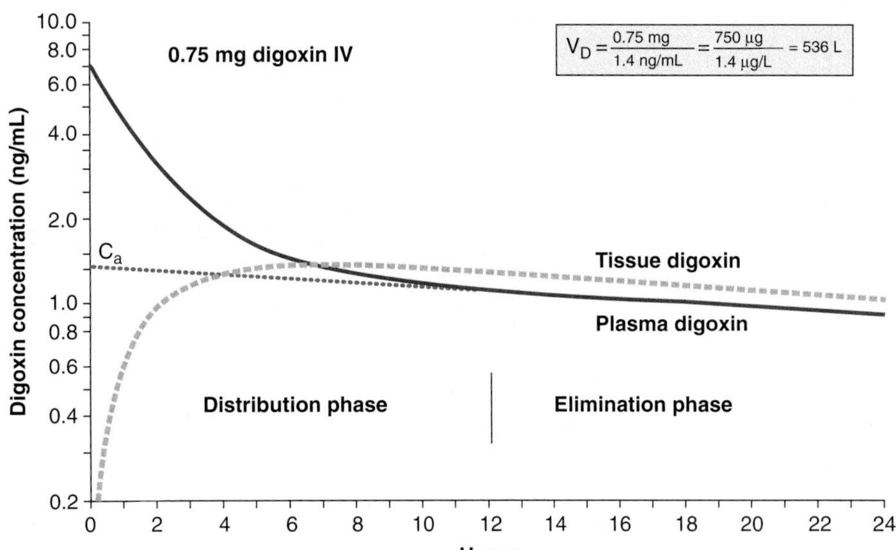

FIGURE 13-3 • Simulation of plasma (*solid line*) and tissue (*broken line*) digoxin concentrations after intravenous administration of a 0.75-mg loading dose to a 70-kg patient with normal renal function. C_0 is estimated by back extrapolation (*dotted line*) of elimination-phase plasma concentrations. V_d is calculated by dividing the administered drug dose by this estimate of C_0, as shown. Tissue concentrations are referenced to the apparent distribution volume of a peripheral compartment that represents tissue distribution. (From Atkinson AJ Jr, Kushner W. Clinical pharmacokinetics. Annu Rev Pharmacol Toxicol 1979;19:105-127.)

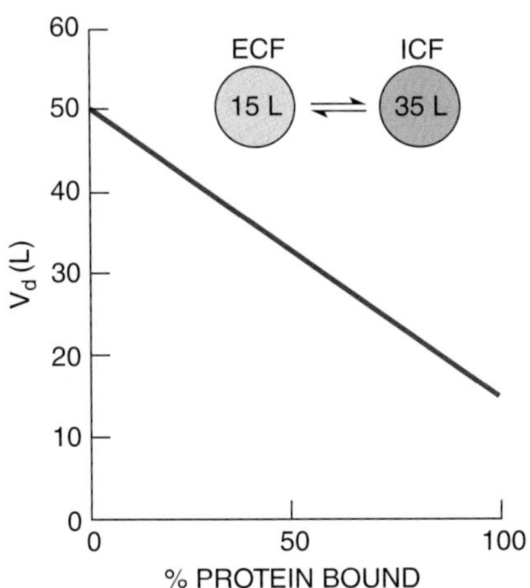

FIGURE 13-4 • Analysis of theophylline V_d in terms of protein binding, extracellular fluid (ECF), and intracellular fluid (ICF) components of total body water (TBW) in a hypothetical 70-kg subject. Theophylline is normally 40% bound, so its V_d approximates 35 L or 0.5 L/kg. (From Atkinson AJ Jr, Ruo TI, Frederiksen MC. Physiological basis of multicompartmental models of drug distribution. Trends Pharmacol Sci 1991;12:96-101.)

polar because three glycoside (sugar) groups are attached to it. It also binds very tightly to the enzyme Na/K-ATPase that is present in most body tissues. Because digoxin is only 25% bound to plasma proteins ($f_U = 0.75$), Equation 13-4 can be used to estimate that the 536-L distribution volume of this drug corresponds to a Φ value of 20, consistent with the relationship between lipophilicity and tissue partitioning shown in Figure 13-5.

Continuation of Drug Therapy (Concepts of Elimination Half-Life and Clearance)

Maintenance of a sustained therapeutic effect usually necessitates administering repeated drug doses to replace the amount of drug that has been excreted or metabolized during the *dosing interval.* A *steady state* is reached when the amount of drug that is eliminated during a dosing interval is equal to the dosing rate. Because the elimination of most drugs interval is a *first-order* process, the rate of drug elimination is directly proportional to the drug concentration in plasma. This is fortunate because it enables their elimination to be characterized by both an *elimination half-life* and an *elimination clearance* and results in the fact that changes in dose result in directly proportionate changes in drug concentration, a property referred to as *dose proportionality.*

Elimination Half-Life

It is convenient to characterize the elimination of drugs with first-order elimination rates by their *elimination half-life,* the time required for half an administered drug dose to be eliminated. For example, when therapy is initiated by giving a loading dose to rapidly achieve therapeutic drug concentrations, it is often practical to continue by administering half the loading dose at an interval of one elimination half-life. This enables drug elimination to be balanced by drug administration, thus maintaining therapeutic efficacy from the onset of therapy. However, digoxin has an elimination half-life of 1.6 days in patients with normal renal function, so it is inconvenient to administer digoxin at this interval. Thus, it is customary to initiate maintenance therapy in patients with normal renal function by administering daily digoxin doses equal to one third of the required loading dose.

Elimination Clearance

Elimination clearance is the primary pharmacokinetic parameter that characterizes drug elimination by first-order kinetics. The term *clearance* was first introduced in renal physiology to describe the proportional relationship between the rate of urea excretion by the kidneys and the concentration of urea in blood.[9] Currently, creatinine clearance (CL_{CR}) is used to evaluate renal function and is calculated from the following equation:

$$CL_{CR} = UV/P \qquad (13\text{-}5)$$

where U is the concentration of creatinine excreted over a certain period of time in a measured volume of urine (V) and P is the serum concentration of creatinine. This is really a first-order differential equation because UV is simply the rate at which creatinine is being excreted in urine (dE/dt). Hence,

$$dE/dt = CL_{CR} \cdot P \qquad (13\text{-}6)$$

We can then write the following equation to describe the rate of change of creatinine in the body (dX/dt):

$$dX/dt = I - CL_{CR} \cdot P \qquad (13\text{-}7)$$

Here I is the rate of *synthesis* of creatinine in the body and $CL_{CR} \cdot P$ is the rate of creatinine *elimination.* By definition, these rates are equal at steady state and there is no change in the total body content of creatinine (dX/dt = 0), so:

$$P = I/CL_{CR} \qquad (13\text{-}8)$$

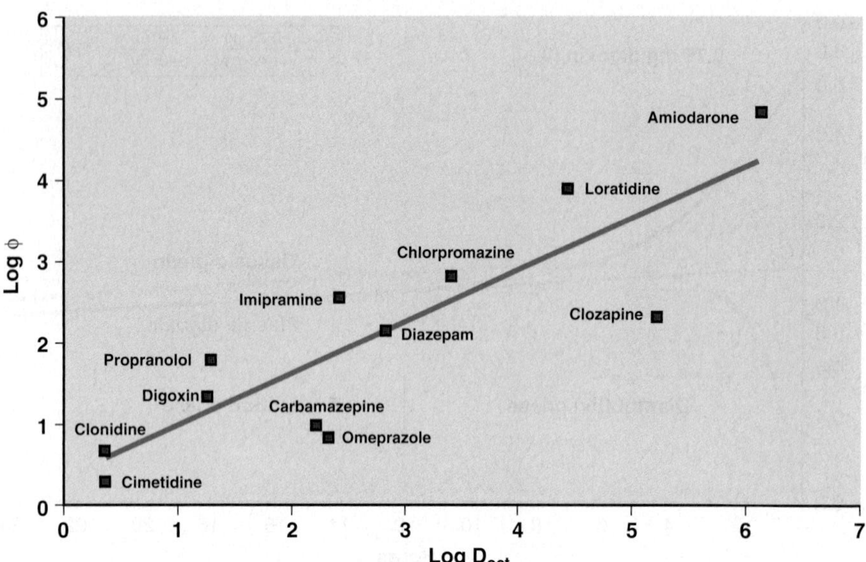

FIGURE 13-5 • Relationship between lipophilicity, estimated from D_{oct}, and tissue/plasma partition ratio (Φ) for several commonly used drugs. (From Atkinson AJ Jr. Compartmental analysis of drug distribution. In Atkinson AJ Jr, Abernethy DR, Daniels CE, et al [eds]: Principles of Clinical Pharmacology, 2nd ed. San Diego: Elsevier, 2007.)

This equation explains why it is hazardous to estimate the status of renal function solely from serum creatinine results in patients who have a reduced muscle mass and a decline in creatinine synthesis rate. For example, renal function and excretion of drugs may be markedly impaired in elderly patients, but it is not unusual for their serum creatinine concentration to remain within normal limits because their rate of creatinine synthesis is substantially reduced.

The same approach applied to the intravenous infusion of drugs yields an analogous equation for the eventual steady state drug concentration (C_{ss}):

$$C_{ss} = I/CL_E \tag{13-9}$$

where the drug infusion rate is given by I and CL_E is the elimination clearance of the drug. When intermittent parenteral doses are administered at a dosing interval of τ, the corresponding equation is:

$$\bar{C}_{ss} = \frac{Dose/\tau}{CL_E} \tag{13-10}$$

where C_{ss} is the mean concentration during the dosing interval. Because intermittent administration results in a continuing fluctuation between maximum ("peak") and minimum ("trough") drug levels, only a quasi–steady state is reached. But unless attention is focused on these peak and trough levels, no distinction is generally made in clinical pharmacokinetics between the true steady state that is reached with a continuous intravenous infusion and the quasi–steady state that results from intermittent drug administration.

Equations 13-9 and 13-10 are the most important equations in clinical pharmacokinetics because they specify a directly proportionate relationship between drug dose and steady state plasma concentration for drugs that are eliminated by first-order kinetics. This provides a straightforward guide to plasma concentration–based dose adjustment for these drugs. Thus, plasma levels are doubled when the dose is doubled and halved when the dose is halved. These equations also stipulate that the steady state concentration is determined only by the maintenance dose and elimination clearance. The distribution volume and the loading dose do not appear in the equations and they do not affect the eventual steady state concentration.

In contrast to elimination clearance, elimination half-life ($t_{1/2}$) is not a primary pharmacokinetic parameter because it is determined by distribution volume as well as by elimination clearance.

$$t_{1/2} = \frac{0.693\ V_{d(area)}}{CL_E} \tag{13-11}$$

The value of V_d in this equation is not $V_{d(extrap.)}$ but represents a second estimate of distribution volume, referred to as $V_{d(area)}$ or $V_{d(\beta)}$, that is generally estimated from measured elimination half-life and clearance. The similarity of these two distribution volume estimates reflects the extent to which drug distribution is accurately described by the single compartment model shown in Figure 13-2.

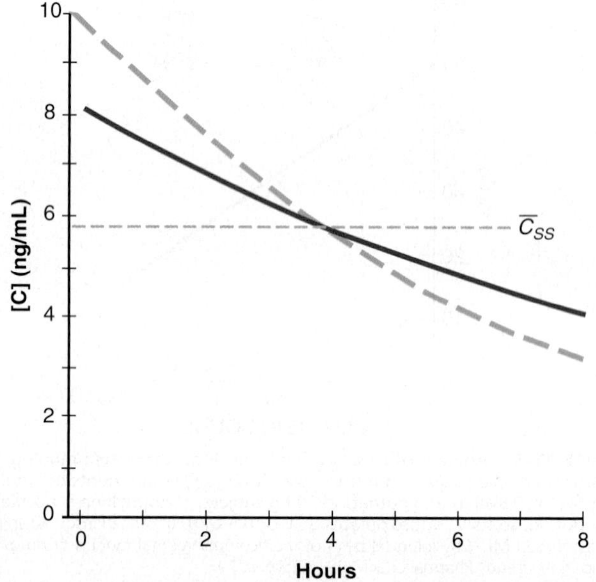

FIGURE 13-6 • Plasma concentrations after repeated administration of the same drug dose to two hypothetical patients whose elimination clearance is the same but whose distribution volumes differ. The patients have the same $\bar{C}_{SS}$, but the larger distribution volume results in lower peak and higher trough plasma levels (*solid line*) than when the distribution volume is smaller (*broken line*). (From Atkinson AJ Jr. Clinical pharmacokinetics. In Atkinson AJ Jr, Abernethy DR, Daniels CE, et al [eds]: Principles of Clinical Pharmacology, 2nd ed. San Diego: Elsevier, 2007.)

Figure 13-6 illustrates how differences in distribution volume affect elimination half-life and peak and trough plasma concentrations when the same drug dose is given to two patients with the same elimination clearance. If these patients were given the same nightly dose of a sedative-hypnotic drug for insomnia, $\bar{C}_{ss}$ would be the same for both. However, the patient with the larger distribution volume might not obtain high-enough plasma levels to fall asleep at night and would have a prolonged elimination half-life, resulting in an elevated plasma level that might cause drowsiness in the morning.

Drug Cumulation and the Plateau Principle

A consequence of first-order elimination kinetics is that a constant fraction of the total drug in the body will be eliminated in a given time interval. Thus, if there is no urgency in establishing a therapeutic effect, an initial loading dose can be omitted and maintenance doses will provide drug concentrations that reach 90% of the eventual steady state drug concentration in a period of time equal to 3.3 elimination half-lives. The increase in drug concentrations with repeated drug doses is referred to as *cumulation*, and Gaddum[10] provided a rigorous mathematical analysis of the time course and extent of this process, establishing what is termed the *plateau principle*. However, a brute-force example will provide considerable insight into the nature of this process.

Let us take as an example a case in which we omit the 0.75-mg digoxin loading dose shown in Figure 13-3, termed the *digitalizing dose* in clinical practice, and simply begin therapy with a 0.25 mg/day maintenance dose. If the patient has normal renal function, approximately one third of the total amount of digoxin present in the body will be eliminated each day and two thirds will remain when the next daily dose is administered. As shown in Scheme 13-1, the patient will have digoxin body stores of 0.66 mg just after the fifth daily dose (3.3×1.6 day half-life = 5.3 days). This is 88% of the total body stores that would have been provided by a 0.75-mg loading dose.

The *bottom broken line* in Figure 13-7 shows the time course of digoxin cumulation in this patient and illustrates the important point that digoxin concentrations approach only asymptomatically the steady state that would be reached if digoxin loading and maintenance doses were perfectly matched (*solid line*). The figure also emphasizes the important point that *the eventual steady state level is determined only by the maintenance dose*, regardless of the size of the loading dose. In fact, administration of an inappropriately high digitalizing dose only subjects patients to an interval of added risk without achieving a permanent increase in the extent of digitalization. However, when a high loading dose is administered to control ventricular rate in patients with atrial fibrillation or flutter, a higher than usual maintenance dose also will be required.

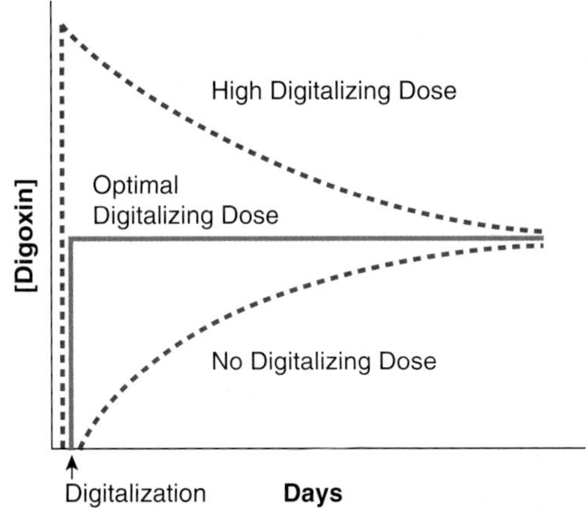

FIGURE 13-7 • Expected digoxin plasma concentrations after administering perfectly matched loading and maintenance doses (*solid line*), no initial loading dose (*bottom broken line*), or a loading dose that is large in relation to the subsequent maintenance dose (upper broken line). (From Atkinson AJ Jr. Clinical pharmacokinetics. In Atkinson AJ Jr, Abernethy DR, Daniels CE, et al [eds]: Principles of Clinical Pharmacology, 2nd ed. San Diego: Elsevier, 2007.)

Eventual steady state drug concentrations at any time during a dosing interval can be predicted from concentrations measured at the corresponding time after the initial drug dose simply by multiplying them by the *cumulation factor (CF):*

$$CF = \frac{1}{1 - e^{-k\tau}} \tag{13-12}$$

where k is the elimination rate constant for the drug, defined as ln 2/ elimination half-life, and τ is the dosing interval.

Drug Absorption—Concept of Bioavailability

A large number of factors can affect the rate and extent of absorption of an oral drug dose. These are summarized in Figure 13-8. Biopharmaceutic factors include drug solubility and formulation characteristics that affect the rate of drug disintegration and dissolution. From the physiologic standpoint, passive nonionic diffusion is the mechanism by which most drugs are absorbed once they are in solution, but specialized small intestine transport systems are involved in the absorption of some drugs.[11]

Absorption by passive diffusion is primarily determined by the molecular size and shape, degree of ionization, and lipid solubility of a drug. Classic explanations of the rate and extent of drug absorption have been based on the pH-partition hypothesis. According to this hypothesis, weakly acidic drugs that are largely unionized and lipid-soluble in acid medium should be absorbed best by the stomach. Conversely, weakly basic drugs should be absorbed primarily from the more alkaline contents of the small intestine. Absorption would be negligible for drugs that are permanently ionized, such as quaternary ammonium compounds. Actually, the stomach is not a major site for the absorption of even acidic drugs because the surface area of the intestinal mucosa is so much greater than that of the stomach; this more than compensates for the decreased absorption rate per unit area. Therefore, the rate of gastric emptying becomes a prime determinant of the rate of drug absorption and is a major contributing factor to the delay that occurs between the time of drug administration and its first appearance in the systemic circulation.

Slow gastric emptying not only retards drug absorption but also may lead to less complete absorption of some drugs. Thus, feeding and concurrent administration of drugs that modify gastric motility may affect drug absorption. For example, penicillin is degraded under acid conditions, and levodopa is decarboxylated by enzymes in the gastric mucosa. Accordingly, patients should be advised to take these medications before meals. Conversely, the prolonged gastric residence time that follows feeding may be needed to optimize the bioavailability of saquinavir and other drugs that either are poorly soluble or are prepared in formulations that have a slow rate of disintegration.

SCHEME 13-1

.25 x 2/3 = .17	Dose #1
+.25	Dose #2
.42 x 2/3 = .28	
+.25	Dose #3
.53 x 2/3 = .36	
+.25	Dose #4
.61 x 2/3 = .41	
+.25	Dose #5
.66 x 2/3 = .44	
+.25	Dose #6
.69 x 2/3 = .46	
+.25	Dose #7
.71	

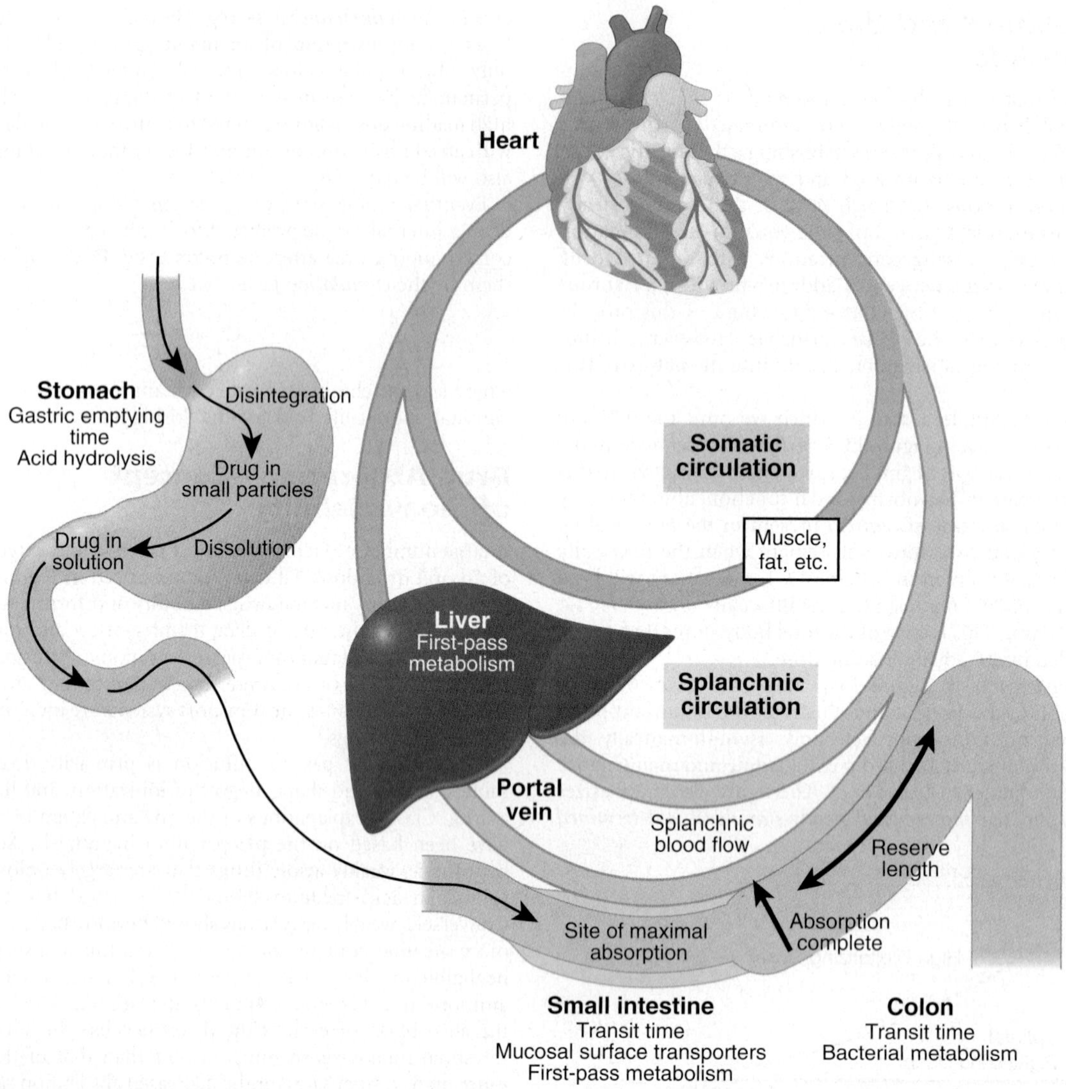

Heart
Stomach
Gastric emptying time
Acid hydrolysis
Disintegration
Drug in small particles
Drug in solution
Dissolution
Somatic circulation
Muscle, fat, etc.
Liver
First-pass metabolism
Splanchnic circulation
Portal vein
Splanchnic blood flow
Reserve length
Absorption complete
Site of maximal absorption
Small intestine
Transit time
Mucosal surface transporters
First-pass metabolism
Colon
Transit time
Bacterial metabolism

FIGURE 13-8 • Summary of biopharmaceutic and physiologic processes that affect the rate and extent of absorption of an orally administered drug dose. Further explanation is provided in the text. (From Atkinson AJ Jr. Drug absorption and bioavailability. In Atkinson AJ Jr, Abernethy DR, Daniels CE, et al [eds]: Principles of Clinical Pharmacology, 2nd ed. San Diego: Elsevier, 2007.)

Transit through the small intestine averages 3 ± 1 hours (± standard error [SE]), is similar for large and small particles, and is not significantly affected by fasting or fed state. Reductions in small intestinal transit time may reduce the absorption of compounds that either are relatively insoluble or are administered as extended-release formulations that have an absorption window with little reserve length. *Reserve length* is defined as the anatomic length over which absorption of a particular drug can occur minus the length at which absorption is complete (see Fig. 13-8). Digoxin is an important example of a compound that has marginal reserve length. Manninen and colleagues[12] showed that changes in small bowel motility affect the extent of digoxin absorption, decreasing digoxin absorption when it is coadministered with metoclopramide and increasing absorption when an atropinic was given shortly before the digoxin dose. Drug-drug and food-drug interactions not only can affect gastrointestinal motility but also can have a direct effect on drug absorption, as is discussed in Chapter 20, Adverse Drug Reactions and Interactions. Mucosal integrity of the small intestine also may affect the bioavailability of drugs that have little reserve length. Splanchnic blood flow can affect the rate and extent of drug absorption, but few clinical studies have been designed to demonstrate its significance.

Even after they are absorbed, drugs can be extruded by P-glycoprotein in the small intestine or metabolized before reaching the systemic

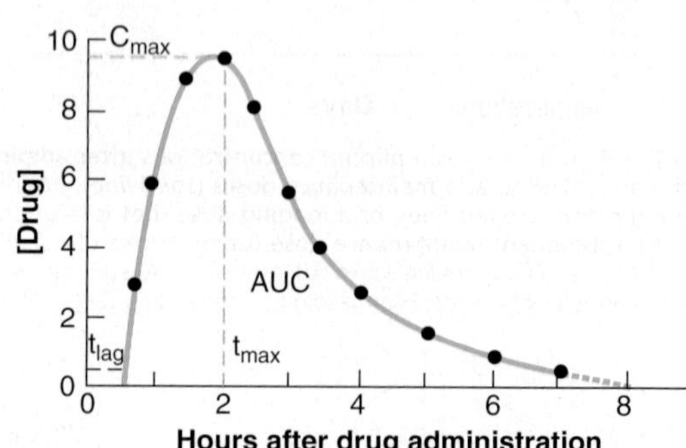

FIGURE 13-9 • Hypothetical plasma concentration–vs.–time curve after a single oral drug dose. Calculation of the area under the plasma level–vs.–time curve (AUC) requires extrapolation of the elimination phase curve beyond the last measurable plasma concentration, as shown by the *broken line*. (From Atkinson AJ Jr. Drug absorption and bioavailability. In Atkinson AJ Jr, Abernethy DR, Daniels CE, et al [eds]: Principles of Clinical Pharmacology, 2nd ed. San Diego: Elsevier, 2007.)

circulation. This *first-pass metabolism* occurs either within the intestinal mucosa or after delivery by the portal circulation to the liver. Cytochrome P-450 (CYP) 3A4 is primarily responsible for the intestinal metabolism of drugs and other xenobiotics and is strategically placed at the apex of intestinal villi. Hepatic first-pass metabolism of a number of drugs has been well studied and, in many cases, reflects the activity of CYP450 enzymes. Morphine, organic nitrates, propranolol, lidocaine, and cyclosporine are some commonly used drugs that have extensive first-pass metabolism or intestinal P-glycoprotein transport. As a result, effective oral doses of these drugs are substantially higher than intravenously administered doses.

Bioavailability

Bioavailability is the term most often used to characterize drug absorption. Koch-Weser[13] defined bioavailability as the relative *amount* of a drug administered in a pharmaceutical product that enters the systemic circulation in an unchanged form and the *rate* at which this occurs. This definition implies that a comparison is being made. *Absolute bioavailability* refers to a comparison between an oral and an intravenous formulation of a drug, which by definition, has 100% bioavailability. *Relative bioavailability* refers to a comparison made between two different oral formulations. As shown in Figure 13-9, the bioavailability of a drug is usually characterized in terms of the maximum drug concentration in plasma (C_{max}), the time needed to reach this maximum (t_{max}), and the area under the plasma or serum-concentration–versus–time curve (AUC). Biopharmaceutic factors and gastric emptying generally account for an initial lag period (t_{lag}) that occurs before drug concentrations are measurable in plasma.

The AUC measured after administration of a drug dose is related to the extent of drug absorption in the following way. By analogy with the first-order differential equation describing creatinine clearance (Eq. 13-6), the equation that describes the rate of drug elimination from a single compartment model is:

$$dE/dt = CL_E \cdot C \qquad (13\text{-}13)$$

where dE/dt is the rate of drug elimination, CL_E is the elimination clearance, and C is the concentration of drug in the compartment. Separating variables and integrating yields the result:

$$E = CL_E \int_0^{\infty} C\,dt \qquad (13\text{-}14)$$

where E is the total amount of drug eliminated in infinite time. By mass balance, E also equals the total amount of the drug dose that is absorbed. The integral is simply the AUC. Thus, for an oral drug dose (D_{oral}):

$$D_{oral} \cdot F = CL \cdot AUC_{oral} \qquad (13\text{-}15)$$

where F is the fraction of the dose that is absorbed and AUC_{oral} is the AUC resulting from the administered oral dose.

Absolute bioavailability most often is measured by sequentially administering single intravenous and oral doses (D_{IV} and D_{oral}) of a drug and comparing their respective AUCs. The extent to which the oral dose is absorbed can be calculated by modifying Equation 13-5 as follows:

$$\%\,Absorption = \frac{CL_E \cdot D_{IV} \cdot AUC_{oral}}{CL_E \cdot D_{oral} \cdot AUC_{IV}} \times 100 = \frac{D_{IV} \cdot AUC_{oral}}{D_{oral} \cdot AUC_{IV}} \times 100 \qquad (13\text{-}16)$$

The assumption usually is made that the elimination clearance remains the same in the interval between drug doses. This problem can be circumvented by administering an intravenous dose of the stable isotope–labeled drug intravenously at the same time that the test formulation of unlabeled drug is given orally.[14]

Relative bioavailability is assessed using an equation analogous to Equation 13-16, and two oral formulations of a drug are generally regarded as being *bioequivalent* if the 90% confidence interval of the ratios of the estimates of AUC and C_{max} for the test and reference formulations lies within a preestablished bioequivalence limit, usually 80% to 125%.[15] Although *therapeutic equivalence* is assured if two formulations are bioequivalent, the therapeutic equivalence of two bioinequivalent formulations can be judged only within a specific clinical context.[13] For example, we ordinarily treat streptococcal throat infections with a penicillin dose many times greater than that needed for therapeutic efficacy, so a formulation having half the bioavailability of the usual formulation would still be therapeutically equivalent.

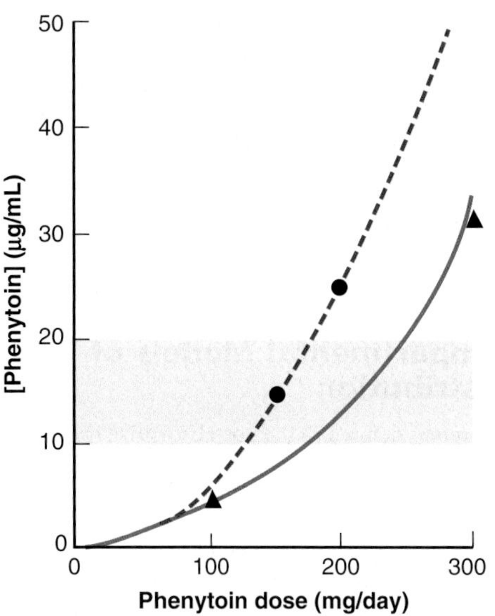

FIGURE 13-10 • The *lines* show the relationship between dose and steady state plasma phenytoin concentrations predicted for two patients based on the measured steady state plasma concentrations shown by the *solid circles* and *triangles*. The *shaded area* shows the usual range of therapeutically effective phenytoin plasma concentrations, which in these patients, who both became toxic after initial treatment with the usual dose of 300 mg/day, is traversed by a dose increment of less than 100 mg/day. (From Atkinson AJ Jr. Clinical pharmacokinetics. Med Clin North Am 1974;58:1037-1049.)

ADDITIONAL PHARMACOKINETIC CONCEPTS

Although the assumption of first-order elimination kinetics and the single compartment distribution model shown in Figure 13-2 are adequate for most clinical applications of pharmacokinetics, there are important exceptions in which nonlinear elimination kinetics and multicompartmental models of drug distribution are needed.

Nonlinear Elimination Kinetics

For drugs eliminated by first-order kinetics, the relationship between dosing rate and steady state plasma concentration is linear and is given by rearranging Equation 13-10 as follows:

$$Dose/\tau = CL_E \cdot \bar{C}_{ss} \qquad (13\text{-}17)$$

Phenytoin is a widely used anticonvulsant that has nonlinear elimination kinetics. The primary pathway of its elimination entails initial metabolism to form 5-(*p*-parahydroxyphenyl)-5-phenylhydantoin (*p*-HPPH), followed by glucuronide conjugation. The metabolism of this drug follows *Michaelis-Menten* kinetics because the microsomal enzyme system that forms *p*-HPPH is partially saturated at phenytoin concentrations of 10 mcg/ml to 20 mcg/ml that are therapeutically effective. The result is that phenytoin is a drug that does not exhibit *dose proportionality*, and plasma concentrations rise hyperbolically as dosage is increased (Fig. 13-10). This nonproportional relationship between phenytoin dose and plasma level complicates patient management and undoubtedly contributes to the high incidence of adverse reactions in patients treated with this drug.

For phenytoin, the equation corresponding to Equation 13-17 is:

$$Dose/\tau = \frac{V_{max}}{K_m + \bar{C}_{ss}} \cdot \bar{C}_{ss} \qquad (13\text{-}18)$$

where V_{max} is the maximum rate of drug metabolism and K_m is the apparent Michaelis-Menten constant for the enzymatic metabolism of phenytoin. Even though many drugs in common clinical use are eliminated by drug metabolizing enzymes, relatively few of them have Michaelis-Menten elimination kinetics (e.g., aspirin and ethyl alcohol). The reason for this is that K_m for most drugs is much greater than $\bar{C}_{ss}$. Hence for most drugs, $\bar{C}_{ss}$ can be ignored in the denominator of Equation 13-8 and this equation reduces to:

$$\text{Dose}/\tau = \frac{V_{max}}{K_m} \cdot \bar{C}_{ss} \tag{13-19}$$

where the ratio V_{max}/K_m is equivalent to CL_E in Equation 13-17.

Multicompartmental Models of Drug Distribution

Drug distribution is defined as the postabsorptive transfer of drug from one location in the body to another. The single compartment model shown in Figure 13-2 is obviously inadequate to analyze the kinetics of drug distribution, and multicompartmental models are required. For example, the three-compartment model shown in Figure 13-11 has been used to analyze the distribution kinetics of inulin and urea, previously described as physiologic markers for ECF and TBW.[5] The central compartment of the model represents intravascular space. Two peripheral compartments are needed because transcapillary exchange between the intravascular and the interstitial fluid spaces is kinetically heterogeneous, occurring rapidly across fenestrated and discontinuous capillaries that are located primarily in the splanchnic vascular bed but more slowly across less porous capillaries that have a continuous basement membrane and are located primarily in skeletal muscle and other somatic tissues.[16] The rate of transfer of compounds between compartments is characterized by a parameter termed *intercompartmental clearance* that is volume-independent and mathematically analogous to elimination clearance. In this model, transcapillary exchange is the rate-limiting step in the distribution of both inulin and urea and their intercompartmental clearance (CL_I) is a function of both the blood flow (Q) and the capillary surface area–permeability coefficient (P · S) of each compartment.[5]

$$CL_I = Q(1 - e^{-P \cdot S/Q}) \tag{13-20}$$

As in this case, drug distribution is usually a symmetrically reversible process and requires no input of energy. However, in some cases, receptor-mediated endocytosis and carrier-mediated active transport are important in either increasing or limiting the extent of drug distribution.

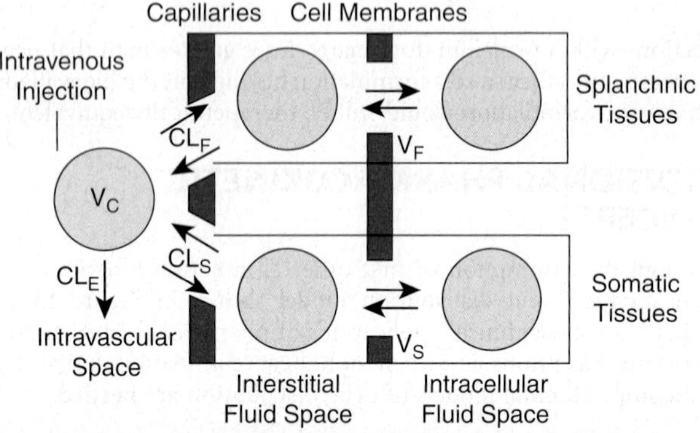

FIGURE 13-11 • Multicompartmental model of the kinetics of inulin and urea distribution and elimination. After injection into a central compartment corresponding to intravascular space (V_C), both compounds distribute to rapidly (V_F) and slowly (V_S) equilibrating peripheral compartments (*rectangles*), at rates of transcapillary exchange that are characterized by intercompartmental clearances CL_F and CL_S. These peripheral compartments contain both interstitial and intracellular fluid components, but transfer of urea between them is too rapid to be distinguished kinetically. Inulin is limited in its distribution to the interstitial fluid components of the peripheral compartments. (From Odeh YK, Wang Z, Ruo TI, et al. Simultaneous analysis of inulin and $^{15}N_2$-urea kinetics in humans. Clin Pharmacol Ther 1993;53:419-425.)

Clinical Consequences of Drug Distribution Kinetics

The kinetics of drug distribution can either delay the onset of action of some drugs or be primarily responsible for terminating the action of other drugs. Thus, drug distribution delays the onset of insulin-stimulated glucose uptake by skeletal muscle and of both the inotropic and the chronotropic actions of digoxin, which parallel the time course of tissue distribution shown in Figure 13-3. For this reason, digoxin plasma levels do not reflect the cardiac effects of this drug until 6 hours have elapsed after an administered dose and an elimination phase has been reached in which plasma levels are proportionate to tissue levels. Conversely, the short duration of pharmacologic action after administration of bolus intravenous doses of thiopental or lidocaine reflects the redistribution of these drugs from rapidly equilibrating tissues, which contain the site of drug action, termed the *biophase*, to skeletal muscle and other tissues that are pharmacologically inert. Drug elimination is responsible for the fall in gentamicin concentration seen in the interval between drug doses (Fig. 13-12).[17] In this case, the distribution phase *follows* the elimination phase, a situation referred to as *flip-flop kinetics*. In addition, the distribution phase reflects renal uptake of gentamicin by receptor-mediated endocytosis, a process that leads to the nephrotoxicity of this drug. Because this uptake process is saturable, gentamicin exhibits *dose-regimen dependency* in that gentamicin is less nephrotoxic when a large dose is administered at a 24-hour interval than when the same total dose is partitioned into smaller doses given more frequently.

PHARMACOKINETIC EFFECTS OF RENAL AND HEPATIC IMPAIRMENT

Later chapters deal specifically with the individualization of drug therapy and with the special challenges posed by pharmacotherapy of pediatric and elderly patients. Pharmacokinetic principles play a central role in these areas and are particularly important in treating

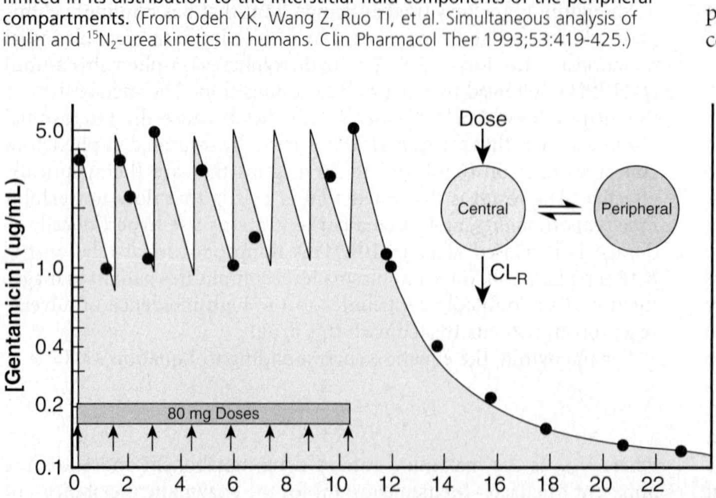

FIGURE 13-12 • Serum gentamicin concentrations measured in a patient during and after a 10.5-day course of therapy (80 mg q 36 hr). Data were analyzed with the two-compartment model shown in the figure. The half-life of serum levels during therapy primarily reflects renal elimination. The terminal half-life seen after therapy was stopped is the actual distribution phase. (From Schentag JJ, Jusko WJ, Plaut ME, et al. Tissue persistence of gentamicin in man. JAMA 1977;238:327-329. With permission of the American Medical Association.)

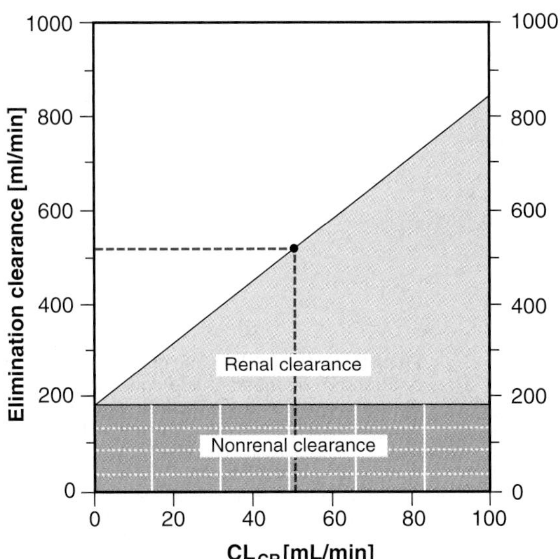

FIGURE 13-13 • Nomogram for estimating cimetidine elimination clearance (CL_E) for a 70-kg patient with impaired renal function. The right-hand ordinate indicates cimetidine CL_E measured in young adults with normal renal function, and the left-hand ordinate indicates expected cimetidine CL_E in a functionally anephric patient, based on the fact that 23% of an administered dose is eliminated by nonrenal routes in normal subjects. The *heavy line* connecting these points can be used to estimate cimetidine CL_E from creatinine clearance (CL_{CR}). For example, a 70-kg patient with CL_{CR} of 50 ml/min (*large dot*) would be expected to have a cimetidine CL_E of 517 ml/min and to respond satisfactorily to doses that are 60% of those recommended for patients with normal renal function. (From Atkinson AJ Jr, Craig RM. Therapy of peptic ulcer disease. In Molinoff PB [ed]: Peptic Ulcer Disease. Mechanisms and Management. Rutherford, NJ: Healthpress, 1990, pp. 83-112.)

patients with impaired kidney function or liver disease. Because drug elimination pathways operate in parallel, the elimination clearance of many drugs consists of additive renal (CL_R) and nonrenal (CL_{NR}) components, such that:

$$CL_E = CL_R + CL_{NR} \tag{13-21}$$

Nonrenal clearance is usually equated with hepatic drug metabolism but could include metabolism by other organs, hemodialysis, and other means of drug elimination.

Pharmacokinetic Effects of Impaired Kidney Function

Creatinine clearance is routinely used in clinical practice to evaluate renal function and can be calculated from Equation 13-5 on the basis of measured creatinine concentrations in blood and urine samples. More frequently, it is estimated for adults from the Cockcroft and Gault equation.[18] For men, creatinine clearance can be estimated from this equation as follows:

$$CL_{CR}\,(\text{mL/min}) = \frac{(140-\text{age})(\text{weight in kg})}{72(\text{serum creatinine in mg/dL})} \tag{13-22}$$

For women, this estimate should be reduced by 15%. Although this equation provides a reasonable estimate of creatinine clearance, it overestimates true glomerular filtration rate (GFR) as measured by inulin clearance because creatinine is secreted by the renal tubule as well as filtered at the glomerulus.

Dettli[19] proposed that the additive property of *elimination rate constants* provides a way of either using Equation 13-21 or constructing nomograms to estimate appropriate dose reductions for patients with impaired renal function. This approach can also be used to estimate *elimination clearance*, as illustrated by the nomogram shown in Figure 13-13. The reliability of the Dettli method of predicting drug clearance depends on the two assumptions that CL_E declines in a linear fashion with CL_{CR} and that the nonrenal clearance of the drug remains constant when renal function is impaired. Even though CL_{CR} primarily reflects GFR, it serves as a rough guide to the renal clearance of drugs that have extensive renal tubular secretion or reabsorption because CL_R usually declines fairly linearly with reductions in CL_{CR}. This is a consequence of the glomerulotubular balance that is maintained in damaged nephrons by intrinsic tubule and peritubular capillary adaptations that parallel reductions in single nephron GFR.

Glomerular filtration affects all drugs of small molecular size and is *restrictive* in the sense that it is limited by drug binding to plasma proteins.

$$\text{Drug filtration rate} = \text{GFR} \times f_u \times C \tag{13-23}$$

Conversely, renal tubular secretion is *nonrestrictive* because both protein-bound and free drug concentrations in plasma are available for elimination. For example, para-aminohippurate is so rapidly eliminated by renal tubular secretion that its clearance is used as a measure of renal blood flow. In general, it can be inferred that there is net renal tubular secretion of a drug if CL_R exceeds drug filtration rate and that there is net renal tubular absorption if CL_R is less than drug filtration rate.

Most drugs are not excreted unchanged by the kidneys but are first converted to metabolites that are then excreted. Renal failure may retard the excretion of these metabolites, some of which have important pharmacologic activity, and may also affect certain drug metabolic pathways. Whereas impaired renal function generally has no effect on drug oxidation or glucuronide conjugation, it results in markedly reduced CL_{NR} for drugs metabolized by acetylation (e.g., procainamide) and some tissue peptidases (e.g., insulin). These constitute important exceptions to Dettli's second assumption. Impaired renal function is also associated with a decrease in the extent to which acidic, but not basic, drugs bind to plasma proteins and in the extent of tissue binding of digoxin.

Pharmacokinetic Effects of Impaired Liver Function

Usually, hepatic clearance is equated with nonrenal clearance and is calculated from Equation 13-21 as total body clearance (CL_E) minus renal clearance (CL_R). In one model of hepatic drug clearance, the factors that affect hepatic clearance (CL_H) include blood flow to the liver (Q), the fraction of drug not bound to plasma proteins (f_u), and intrinsic clearance (CL_{int}). These affect hepatic clearance as follows[20]:

$$CL_H = Q\left[\frac{f_u\,CL_{int}}{Q + f_u\,CL_{int}}\right] \tag{13-24}$$

Hepatic intrinsic clearance is simply the clearance that would be observed in the absence of blood flow and protein binding restrictions. The terms within the brackets are referred to as the *extraction ratio (ER)*.

Two limiting cases arise when $f_u\,CL_{int} << Q$ and when $f_u\,CL_{int} >> Q$.[21] In the first case, Equation 13-24 can be simplified to:

$$CL_H = f_u\,CL_{int} \tag{13-25}$$

Hepatic clearance is termed *restrictive* in this case, because it is limited by protein binding. This situation is analogous to the elimination of drugs by glomerular filtration. Drugs that are restrictively eliminated have extraction ratios less than 0.3.

When $f_u\,CL_{int} >> Q$, Equation 13-24 can be reduced to:

$$CL_H = Q \tag{13-26}$$

In this case, hepatic clearance is *flow limited*, similar to the renal tubular excretion of para-aminohippurate. Because protein binding does not affect their clearance, drugs whose hepatic clearance is flow limited are said to be *nonrestrictively* eliminated and have extraction ratios greater than 0.7. Nonrestrictively eliminated drugs exhibit extensive first-pass metabolism that is a consequence of their high hepatic extraction ratios. Equation 13-26 actually reflects the limiting case in which no orally absorbed drug would pass through the liver to the systemic circulation (i.e., ER = 1).

Unfortunately, the parameters of Equation 13-24 are not accessible to routine clinical measurement, and there is no simple test analogous to creatinine clearance that can be used to assess liver function. As a result, the Pugh modification of Child's classification of liver disease

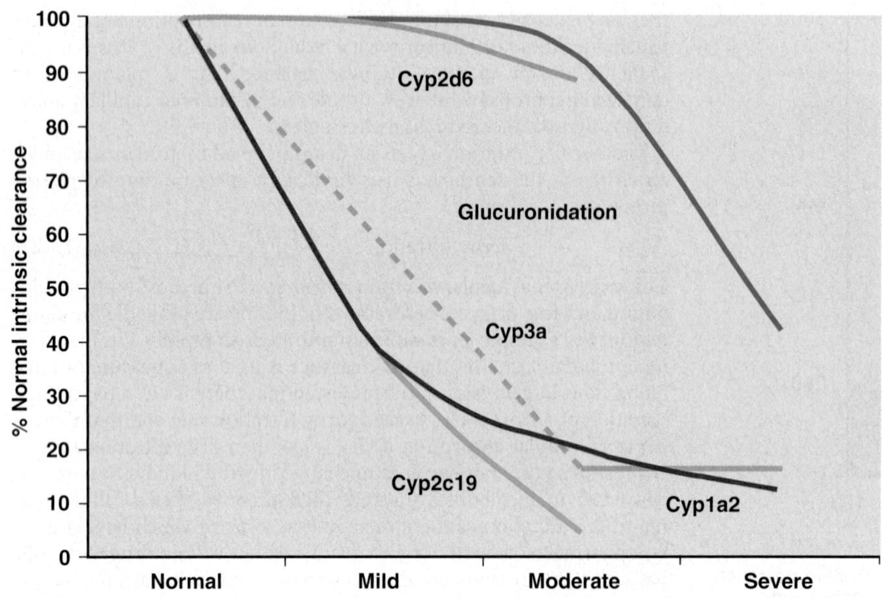

FIGURE 13-14 • Schematic diagram showing the relationship between Child-Pugh stages of liver disease severity and the intrinsic clearance of drugs mediated by specific cytochrome P-450 (CYP) metabolic pathways. The erythromycin breath test was used to assess hepatic CYP3A in a study in which no patients with mild liver disease were included and results in patients with moderate and severe liver disease were combined. (From Atkinson AJ Jr. Pharmacokinetic effects of liver disease. In Atkinson AJ Jr, Abernethy DR, Daniels CE, et al [eds]: Principles of Clinical Pharmacology, 2nd ed. San Diego: Elsevier, 2007.)

severity is used most commonly in studies designed to formulate drug-dosing recommendations for patients with liver disease.[22]

Restrictively Eliminated Drugs

Because protein binding reduces the hepatic clearance of restrictively eliminated drugs, the hypoalbuminemia that results from severe liver disease will decrease the protein binding of these drugs and increase their hepatic clearance. The hepatic clearance of these drugs will also be increased by the decreased protein binding that accompanies impaired renal function and some drug interactions. Although this will result in a decreased *total* drug concentration, steady state *free* concentrations will not be increased unless intrinsic clearance is also reduced. Because pharmacologic effects are related to free rather than total drug concentrations, reductions in protein binding will be of little consequence unless the decrease in total drug concentration prompts an inappropriate dose increase, as sometimes occurs with phenytoin.

Evaluation of drug intrinsic clearance is complicated by the fact that different metabolic pathways differ in the extent to which they are impaired as liver function deteriorates. This is demonstrated in Figure 13-14, in which probe drugs for several metabolic pathways were administered to normal subjects and to patients with liver disease. However, even when the metabolic pathway for a given drug is known, prediction of hepatic drug clearance in individual patients would be complicated by the effects of pharmacogenetic variation, variability in extent of enzyme induction, and drug interactions.

Nonrestrictively Eliminated Drugs

Although reduced protein binding will not affect the clearance or total plasma concentration of nonrestrictively eliminated drugs, it will increase the plasma concentration of free drug. This may increase the intensity of pharmacologic effect observed at a given total drug concentration. Liver cirrhosis not only decreases total liver blood flow but also results in extrahepatic and intrahepatic shunts that further reduce the effective perfusion of drug-metabolizing hepatocytes. Both these changes have a major effect on the clearance of nonrestrictively eliminated drugs. In addition, shunting results in markedly increased first-pass metabolism and increased bioavailability of nonrestrictively eliminated drugs but has little effect on the bioavailability of restrictively eliminated drugs because their first-pass hepatic metabolism is minimal.

Cirrhosis affects drug metabolism more than any other form of liver disease and may decrease the intrinsic clearance of drugs that are nonrestrictively eliminated in subjects with normal liver function to the extent that hepatic clearance no longer approximates hepatic blood flow. In this case, hepatic clearance is determined to a significant extent by intrinsic clearance, as described by Equation 13-24. The effects of liver disease on all of the parameters of Equation 13-24 also need to be considered for the few drugs that have intermediate extraction ratios between 0.3 and 0.7.

REFERENCES

1. Krieger WC. Foreword on paracelsus-dose response. In Krieger WC (ed): Handbook of Pesticide Toxicology. New York: Academic Press, 2001. Available at http://www.mindfully.org/Pesticide/Paracelsus-Dose-ToxicologyOct01.htm (Accessed June 21, 2006).
2. Widmark EMP. Studies in the concentration of indifferent narcotics in blood and tissues. Acta Med Scand 1919;52:87-164.
3. Atkinson AJ Jr, Ruo TI, Frederiksen MC. Physiological basis of multicompartmental models of drug distribution. Trends Pharmacol Sci 1991;12:96-101.
4. Larsen PR, Atkinson AJ Jr, Wellman HN, et al. The effect of diphenylhydantoin on thyroxine metabolism in man. J Clin Invest 1970;49:1266-1279.
5. Odeh YK, Wang Z, Ruo TI, et al. Simultaneous analysis of inulin and $^{15}N_2$-urea kinetics in humans. Clin Pharmacol Ther 1993;53:419-425.
6. Frederiksen MC, Ruo TI, Chow MJ, et al. Theophylline pharmacokinetics in pregnancy. Clin Pharmacol Ther 1986;40:321-328.
7. Øie S, Tozer TN. Effect of altered plasma protein binding on apparent volume of distribution. J Pharm Sci 1979;68:1203-1205.
8. Lombardo F, Shalaeva MY, Tupper KA, et al. ElogD$_{oct}$: a tool for lipophilicity determination in drug discovery. 2. Basic and neutral compounds. J Med Chem 2001;44:2490-2497.
9. Möller E, McIntosh JF, Van Slyke DD. Studies of urea excretion. II. Relationship between urine volume and the rate of urea excretion in normal adults. J Clin Invest 1929;6:427-465.
10. Gaddum JH. Repeated doses of drugs. Nature 1944;153:494.
11. Tsuji A, Tamai I. Carrier-mediated intestinal transport of drugs. Pharm Res 1996;13:963-977.
12. Manninen V, Melin J, Apajalahti A, et al. Altered absorption of digoxin in patients given propantheline and metoclopramide. Lancet 1973;1:398-399.
13. Koch-Weser J. Bioavailability of drugs. N Engl J Med 1974;291:233-237, 503-506.
14. Atkinson AJ Jr, Ruo TI, Piergies AA, et al. Pharmacokinetics of *N*-acetylprocainamide in patients profiled with a stable isotope method. Clin Pharmacol Ther 1989;46:182-189.
15. Patnaik RN, Lesko LJ, Chen ML, et al. Individual bioequivalence: new concepts in the statistical assessment of bioequivalence metrics. Clin Pharmacokinet 1997;33:1-6.
16. Atkinson AJ Jr, Ruo TI, Frederiksen MC. Physiological basis of multicompartmental models of drug distribution. Trends Pharmacol Sci 1991;12:96-101.
17. Schentag JJ, Jusko WJ, Plaut ME, et al. Tissue persistence of gentamicin in man. JAMA 1977;238:327-329.
18. Cockroft DW, Gault MH. Prediction of creatinine clearance from serum creatinine. Nephron 1976;16:31-41.
19. Dettli L. Individualization of drug dosage in patients with renal disease. Med Clin North Am 1974;58:977-985.
20. Rowland M, Benet LZ, Graham GG. Clearance concepts in pharmacokinetics. J Pharmacokinet Biopharm 1973;1:123-136.
21. Wilkinson GR, Shand DG. A physiological approach to hepatic drug clearance. Clin Pharmacol Ther 1975;18:377-390.
22. CDER, CBER. Pharmacokinetics in patients with impaired hepatic function: study design, data analysis, and impact on dosing and labeling. Guidance for Industry. Rockville, MD: FDA, 2003. Available at http://www.fda.gov/cder/guidance/3625fnl.pdf (Accessed June 21, 2006).

14

PHARMACODYNAMICS

Richard L. Lalonde

INTRODUCTION 203
PHARMACODYNAMIC PRINCIPLES BASED ON DRUG AND RECEPTOR INTERACTIONS 203
PHARMACODYNAMIC MODELS 204
Sigmoid E_{max} Model 204
E_{max} Model 205
Linear Model 205
Logarithmic Models 205
Operational Model of Drug Action 206
TIME COURSE OF PHARMACOLOGIC RESPONSE 206
Direct Reversible Effects 207
Equilibration Delays 208
Indirect Effects and Turnover Models 209
Transduction Steps and Transit Compartment Models 212
Irreversible Effects 213
Effects on Production of Natural Cells 213
Dose-Response-Time Data: Pharmacodynamic Modeling without Drug Concentrations 214
NONCONTINUOUS PHARMACODYNAMIC MEASURES 214
PHARMACODYNAMICS OF DRUG COMBINATIONS 214
TIME-DEPENDENT PHARMACODYNAMICS 215
Tolerance 215
Sensitization 216
PHARMACODYNAMICS AND DISEASE PROGRESSION MODELS 216

INTRODUCTION

Pharmacodynamics is broadly defined as the biologic effects resulting from the interaction between drugs and biologic systems.[1] A simple and useful distinction is to think of pharmacodynamics as "what the drug does to the body" whereas pharmacokinetics (see Chapter 13, Pharmacokinetics) is "what the body does to the drug." Figure 14-1 is a very simplified illustration of how pharmacokinetics and pharmacodynamics determine the observed pharmacologic effects of a drug.[1] Figure 14-1 also illustrates why pharmacokinetics and pharmacodynamics are often linked. The relationship between drug dose and biologic fluid concentration is most useful when it is also linked to a pharmacologic effect that is associated with a particular concentration. Similarly, the pharmacologic response by itself does not provide information about some very important determinants of that response (e.g., relationship between the dose and the time course of drug concentrations in plasma or other tissues). Appropriate linking of pharmacokinetic and pharmacodynamic principles provides a rational basis to understand the impact of different dosage regimens on the time course of pharmacologic response.[2,3]

The relationship between drug concentration and the observed pharmacologic response depends on the mechanism by which a drug exerts its effect. The response may be the result of a direct reversible effect, which may be mediated through binding with a specific receptor (e.g., β-adrenoceptor blockers). For these drugs, there will be a relatively simple and direct relationship between drug concentration and pharmacologic effect. The response to other drugs will be through an indirect effect. The best example is warfarin, which blocks the synthesis of vitamin K–dependent clotting factors but has no effect on the degradation of these same factors. In this case, drug concentrations may be related to clotting factor synthesis but only indirectly related to the observed anticoagulant effect.[4] Although most pharmacologic effects are reversible, certain drugs have an irreversible effect. Examples of drugs with irreversible effects include acetylsalicylic acid (ASA) (on platelet aggregation), omeprazole, bactericidal antibiotics, and some antineoplastic agents. Other physiologic processes (e.g., production rate and degradation rate of enzymes, hormones, cells) need to be taken into account in order to properly understand the time course of response to these drugs. The development of a variety of more physiologic and mechanistic methods for the evaluation of pharmacodynamic data has been a particularly important development since the 1990s.

PHARMACODYNAMIC PRINCIPLES BASED ON DRUG AND RECEPTOR INTERACTIONS

The relationship between drug dose or concentrations and pharmacologic response can often be described using models derived from the law of mass action.[5] Let R represent the concentration of available or unoccupied receptors; C, the drug concentration available at the receptor site; and RC, the concentration of drug-receptor complex. If drug binding to the receptor is reversible as

$$R + C \xrightarrow{k_{on}} RC \xrightarrow{k_{off}} R + C \tag{14-1}$$

then at equilibrium

$$\frac{[R][C]}{[RC]} = \frac{k_{off}}{k_{on}} = K_d \tag{14-2}$$

where k_{on} is the association constant for the drug and receptor, k_{off} is the dissociation constant for the drug-receptor complex, and K_d is the equilibrium dissociation constant. If RT equals the total concentration of receptors, then RT = R + RC. If we solve for R, the concentration of receptors not bound to any drug, and substitute in Equation 14-2, we obtain

$$\frac{[R_T - RC][C]}{[RC]} = K_d \tag{14-3}$$

which can be rearranged to give

$$[RC] = \frac{[R_T][C]}{K_d + [C]} \tag{14-4}$$

If pharmacologic effect (E) is assumed to be a function (f) of the number or concentration of occupied receptors (RC) this results in

$$E = f[RC] = f\left[\frac{[R_T][C]}{K_d + [C]}\right] \tag{14-5}$$

The most commonly used pharmacodynamic models described in the next section are based on Equation 14-5 and different assumptions about the shape of the relationship between E and RC.

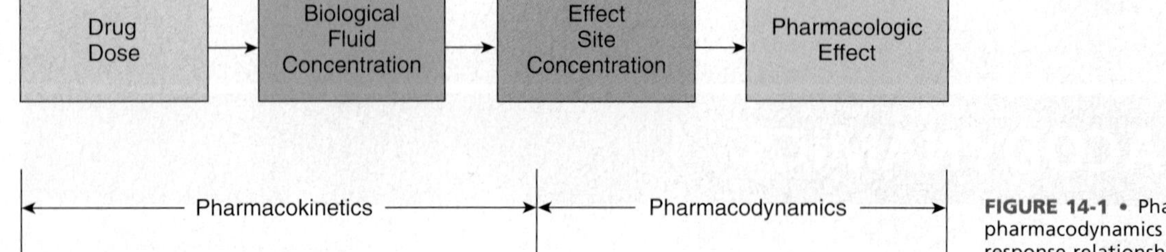

FIGURE 14-1 • Pharmacokinetics and pharmacodynamics as determinants of the dose-response relationship.

PHARMACODYNAMIC MODELS

The simplest form of Equation 14-5 is to assume a linear relationship (i.e., f is a constant) between pharmacologic effect (E) and the concentration of drug-receptor complex (RC). This is also known as the *receptor occupancy assumption*. Under this assumption, the maximum effect (E_{max}) is directly proportional to R_T because the right side of Equation 14-5 will approach $f[R_T]$ at very high drug concentrations. This yields the key relationship

$$E = \frac{E_{max}[C]}{K_d + [C]} \quad (14\text{-}6)$$

If n drug molecules bind to each receptor site, then Equation 14-6 can be modified as

$$E = \frac{E_{max}[C]^n}{K_d + [C]^n} \quad (14\text{-}7)$$

where Kd is the equilibrium dissociation constant for the interaction of n molecules with one receptor. In addition to the receptor occupancy assumption, other assumptions are made in the derivation and usual application of Equations 14-6 and 14-7. First, it is commonly assumed that a negligible amount of drug is bound to the receptor relative to the total amount of drug (C_T), so that the concentration of drug not bound to the receptor (C), as used in the previous equations, is approximated by C_T. Response is also often assumed to be independent of time (i.e., no development of tolerance or sensitization).

The hyperbolic function described by Equation 14-6 has been found very useful to describe a multitude of dose/concentration-effect relationships. It is intuitively appealing because the function predicts no effect in the absence of drug and a maximum effect as the dose or concentration approaches infinity. The more general Equation 14-7 has also been widely used, often empirically, without any specific knowledge of the number of molecules that bind to a specific receptor (i.e., value of n). Similar equations and models have been used to describe a variety of biochemical processes (e.g., protein binding, enzyme kinetics). The Michaelis-Menten equation, which relates the rate of a chemical reaction to the concentration of substrate, the maximum velocity (V_{max}), and the Michaelis constant (K_m), is in the form of Equation 14-6. The equation is also analogous to the Langmuir adsorption isotherm used to describe the adsorption of gases to solid surfaces.[6] In 1926, Clark[7] may have been the first investigator to have used this type of pharmacodynamic model to evaluate the effects of drugs. He studied the effects of acetylcholine on isolated frog muscles and used a rearrangement of Equation 14-7 to describe the relationship between drug concentration and pharmacologic effect. The association of oxygen and hemoglobin was described by Hill[8] in 1910 using the equation

$$\%\,\text{saturation of hemoglobin} = \frac{100K[C]^n}{1 + K[C]^n} \quad (14\text{-}8)$$

where C is oxygen tension, K and n are parameters of the model, and 100 represents the maximum saturation when the latter is expressed as a percentage. Equation 14-8 can be rearranged to the form of Equation 14-7 (K in Eq. 14-8 is equivalent to $1/K_d$ in Eq. 14-7) and is often called the *Hill equation*. Based on the previous discussion, it should be evident that many pharmacodynamic concepts and principles have their roots in a rather broad range of scientific disciplines. The mathematical relationships are relatively simple and can be derived by application of principles that have been widely recognized since the early 1900s.[5,9,10]

Pharmacodynamic models relate effect site concentrations and pharmacologic response. Whenever plasma or other tissue concentrations are used in pharmacodynamic models, the inherent assumption is that these concentrations are in equilibrium with those at the effect site. This may be difficult to validate when dealing with clinical data and may necessitate the use of more complex pharmacodynamic models that are linked to pharmacokinetic models. The most widely used pharmacodynamic models are described briefly in the following sections.[1,11-13]

Sigmoid E_{max} Model

The Hill equation, rearranged in the form of Equation 14-7, has been proposed as a useful model to describe the in vivo relationship between dose/concentration and pharmacologic effect for many different drugs.[11-13] The equation can be modified as

$$E = \frac{E_{max}[C]^n}{EC_{50}^n + [C]^n} \quad (14\text{-}9)$$

where C is the drug concentration and EC_{50} is the "effective" concentration that produces half of the maximum effect attributable to the drug (E_{max}). The only difference from Equation 14-7 is that the parameter K_d is replaced with EC_{50}^n. This particular version is often called the *sigmoid E_{max} model* and is conceptually simpler because it includes a parameter, EC_{50}, that is more relevant in clinical pharmacology. Although Equation 14-9 can be derived based on drug and receptor interaction principles, one must be cautious in attributing any particular meaning to certain parameters when the model is applied to in vivo pharmacodynamic data. This should not detract from using the model if it provides a relatively simple method to describe and predict pharmacologic response. Therefore, the sigmoid E_{max} model and other similar models must often be regarded as empirical mathematical functions that describe the shape of the concentration-effect relationship for a particular drug. In this context, n can be considered a parameter that determines the sigmoid shape of the relationship (Fig. 14-2). If n equals 1, a simple hyperbolic function will result (see "E_{max} Model," later). When n is greater than 1, the function becomes more sigmoid in shape with a steeper slope in its central region. Conversely, when n is less than 1, the curve is steeper at low concentrations but more shallow at higher concentrations.

Practical and ethical considerations may prevent exploration of high enough doses to approach E_{max}. This will be evident when, upon inspection of the concentration-effect data, there is no apparent plateau in response. In such cases, the sigmoid E_{max} model parameter estimates are likely to be biased and imprecise.[14] Furthermore, the experimental data may not allow adequate estimation of n, or its value may be close to unity. In these cases, simpler models (see later under "E_{max} Model" and "Linear Models") should be considered.

The sigmoid E_{max} model, as defined previously, predicts that the effect will be 0 when the concentration is 0. When evaluating certain responses (e.g., blood pressure, white blood cell count), there is a

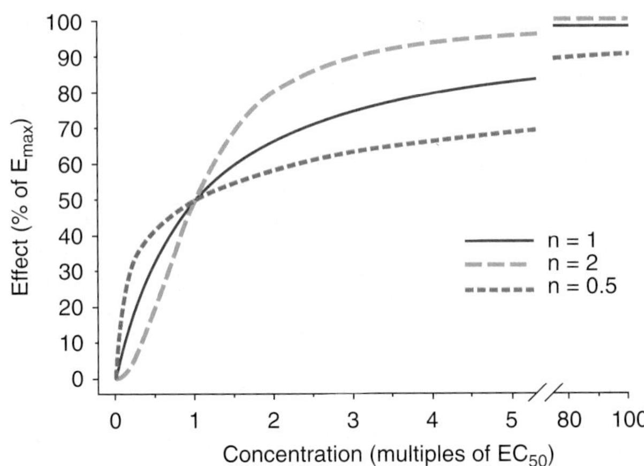

FIGURE 14-2 • The effect of the exponent (n) on the shape of the sigmoid E_{max} concentration-effect relationship. A hyperbolic function or E_{max} model is the result when n = 1.

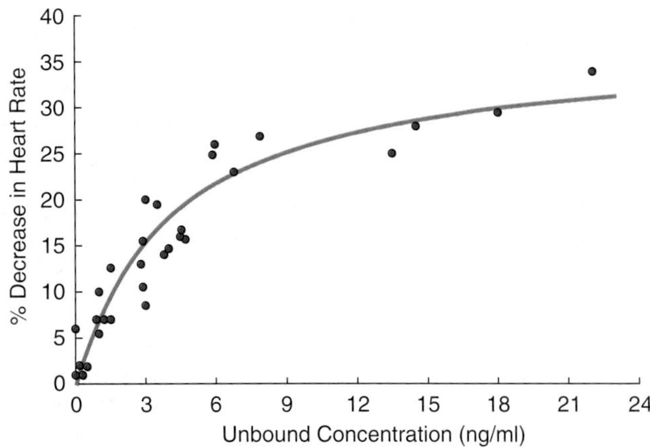

FIGURE 14-3 • The relationship between unbound propranolol serum concentrations and the inhibition of tachycardia after a standard treadmill exercise in one subject. The *solid line* is the E_{max} model fit to the data. (From Lalonde RL, Straka RJ, Pieper JA, et al. Propranolol pharmacodynamic modeling using unbound and total concentrations in healthy volunteers. J Pharmacokinet Biopharm 1987;15:569-582. With kind permission from Springer Science +Business Media.)

baseline effect in the absence of drug that must be incorporated into the model. In such cases, the following modification can be used:

$$E = E_0 + \frac{E_{max}[C]^n}{EC_{50}^n + [C]^n} \qquad (14\text{-}10)$$

The only new parameter is E_0, which is the baseline effect measured in the absence of drug.

In other cases, the effect of the drug may be the inhibition of a physiologic response such as the lowering of heart rate with a β-blocker. In those circumstances, the sigmoid E_{max} equation is subtracted from the baseline effect.

$$E = E_0 - \frac{E_{max}[C]^n}{EC_{50}^n + [C]^n} \qquad (14\text{-}11)$$

If the pharmacologic effect is an inhibition, then E_{max} and EC_{50} are often renamed I_{max} (maximum inhibition) and IC_{50} (concentration that produces 50% inhibition), respectively. If the maximum effect is total inhibition of the baseline response, then E_{max} and E_0 will have the same value, and there will be one less parameter in Equation 14-11.

E_{max} Model

The E_{max} model can be considered a submodel of the sigmoid E_{max} model when n = 1 or a modification of Equation 14-6 with EC_{50} substituted for K_d, as follows:

$$E = \frac{E_{max}[C]}{EC_{50} + [C]} \qquad (14\text{-}12)$$

All parameters are the same as defined previously. As discussed earlier for the sigmoid E_{max} model, the E_{max} model can be modified to evaluate data with a baseline effect or an inhibitory effect. Equation 14-12 is based on the interaction of a single drug molecule with a receptor site, but the same caution must be used in giving meaning to the parameters as that applied to the use of the sigmoid E_{max} model. The E_{max} model will describe a typical hyperbolic concentration-effect relationship with no effect in the absence of drug and a maximum effect (E_{max}) when concentrations approach infinity. These attributes of the E_{max} model may appear self-evident, but they differentiate it from the log-linear model, which historically has been very commonly used (see "Logarithmic Models").

The E_{max} model has been described as obeying the "law of diminishing returns" because of the smaller increments in pharmacologic response as concentrations increase (see Fig. 14-2). This concept is also illustrated by the relationship between propranolol unbound serum concentrations and the percent inhibition of exercise heart rate (Fig. 14-3).[15] The mean E_{max} estimated in this study was 33.5% and reflects the adrenergic component of exercise-induced tachycardia. Based on the mean EC_{50} value of 1.7 ng/ml (18 ng/ml for total propranolol), four fifths of E_{max} will be achieved at unbound concentrations of 6.8 ng/ml or total concentrations of 72 ng/ml. Relatively little additional β-blockade is produced if concentrations are increased further. This supports the clinical observation that very high doses are not generally needed for the treatment of exercise-induced angina. Conversely, at concentrations well below the EC_{50}, there is a near linear relationship between effect and concentrations. This is the basis for the linear model discussed in the next section.

Linear Model

Concentration versus effect relationships may often be described using a simple linear model, particularly if only a limited range of concentrations is evaluated. The linear model can be considered a submodel of the E_{max} model when C is much less than EC_{50}. The E_{max} model then simplifies to the following relationship:

$$E = S[C] \qquad (14\text{-}13)$$

where S is a slope parameter that will approach the value of E_{max}/EC_{50}. At low concentrations relative to EC_{50}, E_{max} and EC_{50} cannot be estimated independently but the slope or ratio of E_{max}/EC_{50} can be estimated. The linear model will predict no effect when concentrations are 0, but its major limitation is that it predicts that pharmacologic response will increase indefinitely as concentrations increase. The absence of a maximum effect goes against some widely accepted principles of pharmacodynamics and is not consistent with clinical observations for many drugs. Like the E_{max} and sigmoid E_{max} models, the linear model can be modified to evaluate data with a baseline effect [$E = E_0 + S(C)$] or inhibition of a baseline effect [$E = E_0 - S(C)$].

Logarithmic Models

In his landmark more than over 80 years ago, Clark[7] described the advantages of the logarithmic transformation of an equation that is actually a rearrangement of Equation 14-7. He used the relationship:

$$\log\left(\frac{E}{E_{max} - E}\right) = \log K + n\log[C] \qquad (14\text{-}14)$$

where all parameters are as previously defined except that K is equivalent to $1/K_d$ in Equation 14-7. This allows all parameters of the sigmoid E_{max} model or Hill equation to be determined by simple graphic methods or linear regression. However, a different and empirical log-linear model has traditionally been used by scientists for more than 60 years. This method relates the logarithm of the concentration to the effect as follows:

$$E = S\log[C] + A \tag{14-15}$$

where A is a constant with no clear biologic significance, S is a slope parameter, and E and C are the same as defined for previous models. The log-linear method will effectively compress the scale of the abscissa and facilitate graphic representation of the wide range of concentrations (or doses) typically used with in vitro or animal studies. Another attribute of the log-linear model is that it will linearize the typical E_{max} or sigmoid E_{max} concentration-effect relationship when the observed effects range from 20% to 80% of the maximum response. In the past, this was particularly useful to scientists because such results could then be analyzed by simple linear regression, and it allowed the comparison of slopes and concentration (or dose) ratios to assess relative potency and competitive inhibition. However, this is no longer a significant advantage with the widespread availability of nonlinear regression software.

Several inherent disadvantages to the log-linear model are evident upon inspection of Equation 14-15. There is no maximum effect predicted at very high concentrations, and an effect cannot be predicted when the concentration is 0 because of the logarithmic function. Furthermore, if an apparent maximum effect is not clearly determined by the observations, then it is difficult or impossible to conclude that specific parts of the data fall between 20% and 80% of the maximum effect. These limitations notwithstanding, the log-linear model has been used successfully by numerous investigators to describe in vivo pharmacodynamic data including the landmark study of the time course of warfarin's anticoagulation effect by Nagashima and colleagues.[4]

Despite the widespread use of the log-linear model in the past, no biologic basis exists for such a transformation of the concentration data. Although the range from 20% to 80% of maximum effect may be important, one must question the use of a model that cannot be applied to data that describe a significant portion of the concentration-effect relationship. Observations will likely deviate from the predictions of the log-linear model at concentrations well below or well above the EC_{50} and lead to errors in predicting the time course of pharmacologic effect.[16] Therefore, the E_{max} or sigmoid E_{max} models, which can describe the whole concentration-effect relationship, should be used whenever possible.

Operational Model of Drug Action

The various pharmacodynamic models described previously are based on the assumption of a direct proportionality between pharmacologic effect and the number of occupied receptors (i.e., f in Equation 14-5 is a constant). However, experimental data have demonstrated that this assumption is not valid in many biologic systems. These systems are said to have "spare receptors" because near-maximum responses are produced with much less than maximal receptor occupancy. The operational model of agonism described by Black and Leff[17] addresses this problem and has several other interesting characteristics. They proposed a hyperbolic function to relate receptor occupancy and pharmacologic effect (f in Equation 14-5) as shown by

$$E = \frac{E_{max:system}[RC]}{K_E + [RC]} \tag{14-16}$$

where $E_{max:system}$ refers to the maximum effect achievable in the system and K_E is the concentration of occupied receptors required to produce half of $E_{max:system}$. The new term $E_{max:system}$ is used to distinguish between the maximum effect possible in a particular system or tissue and the maximum effect that can be achieved with different agonists (E_{max}), the latter depending on the efficacy of different agonists (see later). Substituting the right side of Equation 14-4 for RC in Equation 14-16 yields the full operational model of agonism as shown by

$$E = \frac{E_{max:system}[R_T][C]}{K_d K_E + ([R_T] + K_E)[C]} \tag{14-17}$$

All the symbols are as defined previously. A new drug efficacy parameter (τ) can be defined as

$$\tau = \frac{[R_T]}{K_E} \tag{14-18}$$

and represents the ratio of the total concentration of receptors (R_T) to the concentration of occupied receptors needed to produce half of $E_{max:system}$. Thus τ is a measure of the efficiency of the transduction of occupied receptors into a pharmacologic effect. It can be readily seen from Equation 14-16 that pharmacologic effects approaching $E_{max:system}$ could be achieved at relatively low concentrations of occupied receptors (RC) if K_E is relatively low (i.e., τ is relatively high). Substitution of Equation 14-18 into Equation 14-17 and rearranging produces a function that is expressed in terms of the efficacy parameter τ:

$$E = \frac{E_{max:system}\tau[C]}{K_d + [C] + [C]\tau} \tag{14-19}$$

Figure 14-4 illustrates how the relationship between drug concentration and the observed pharmacologic effect is dependent on the relationship between drug concentration and receptor occupancy as well as on the underlying relationship between receptor occupancy and pharmacologic effect. Flatter or steeper relationships between pharmacologic effect and receptor occupancy can also be accommodated with the inclusion of an exponential term in Equations 14-16, 14-17, and 14-19.[17,18]

The operational model of agonism has some interesting characteristics because it helps differentiate between properties of the drug (i.e., receptor affinity, intrinsic efficacy) and properties of the system (i.e., receptor density, $E_{max:system}$) and how the two come together to produce the observed concentration-effect relationship. For example, inspection of Equation 14-19 reveals that at drug concentrations much greater than K_d, the maximum effect produced by a particular drug (E_{max}) is actually dependent on both system and drug parameters, as

$$E_{max} = E_{max:system}\frac{\tau}{\tau + 1} \tag{14-20}$$

Therefore, a drug with high efficacy (τ) will produce an E_{max} approaching the maximum effect possible in the particular system, whereas a drug with low efficacy may produce an E_{max} that is only a small fraction of the maximum response possible for the system. Furthermore, it helps explain how a drug can be a full, partial, or "silent" agonist at the same receptor in different tissues because of tissue differences in R_T and/or relationship between E and RC.[17,19] Excellent examples were reported by Van der Graaf and coworkers[18,19] with the effect of various adenosine A_1 receptor agonists. Jonker and associates[20] also used this model to describe the effect of dofetilide on QT interval prolongation in humans and to link the response to in vitro blockade of potassium channels. The operational model of agonism reflects the important trend to more mechanistic models as we gain new knowledge about the steps involved in generating a particular pharmacologic response. These models help provide a better scientific basis for extrapolation from in vitro data to in vivo drug effects.

When no information on receptor binding is available, the operational model of agonism essentially collapses to the simpler E_{max}-type models. In the following sections, the discussion typically focuses on E_{max}-type models, but it should be understood that the operational model of agonism could be substituted for the E_{max} model whenever appropriate.

TIME COURSE OF PHARMACOLOGIC RESPONSE

The time course of pharmacologic response depends on the mechanism by which a drug exerts its effect. Drugs that have a direct and reversible effect will have a time course of pharmacologic response that is a relatively simple function of the drug's pharmacokinetics. However, drugs that have an indirect effect will have a time course of response that will be a more complex function of not only the pharmacokinetics of the drug but also the turnover rate of the intermediary that is

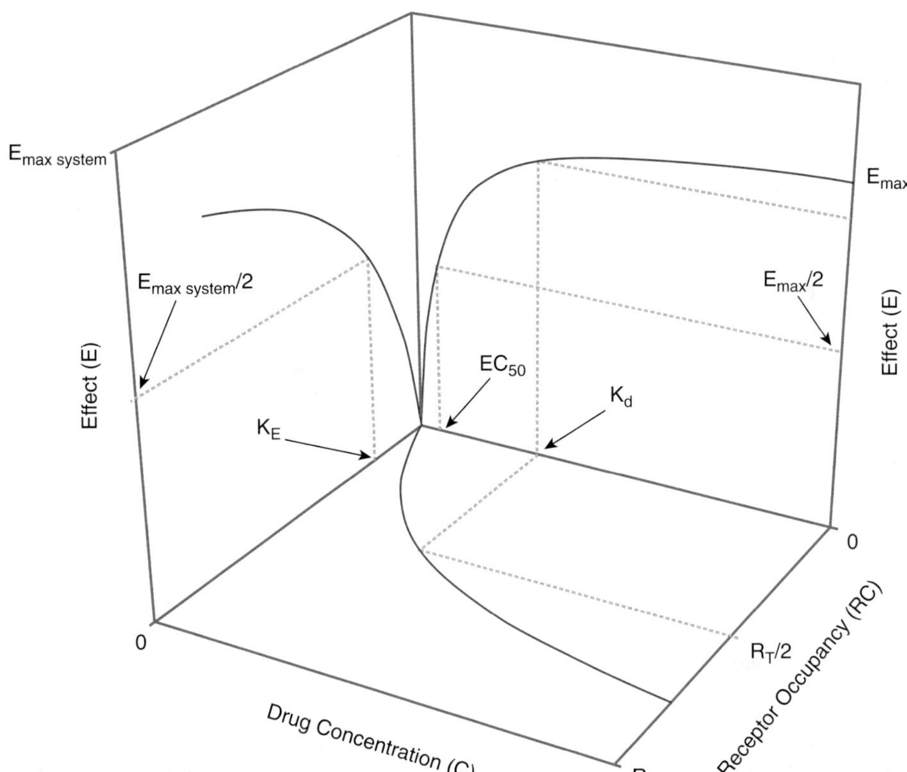

FIGURE 14-4 • Schematic diagram of the operational model of drug action shows the relationship between drug concentration (C), receptor occupancy in terms of the receptor-drug complex (RC), and effect (E). The example is for a drug with relatively high efficacy as shown by a relatively low concentration of occupied receptors (K_E) needed to produce half of the maximum effect possible for the system ($E_{max: system}$). The drug concentration (K_d) yields 50% receptor occupancy ($R_T/2$) but produces an effect that is close to the maximum possible effect for the drug (E_{max}). The drug concentration (EC_{50}) needed to produce an effect half of E_{max} is significantly lower than the drug concentration needed to produce 50% receptor occupancy. (From Black JW, Leff P. Operational models of pharmacological agonism. Proc R Soc Lond 1983;220 B:141-162.)

affected by the drug (e.g., vitamin K–dependent clotting factors for the anticoagulant effect of warfarin). Drugs that act irreversibly have a time course of response that is largely dependent on the turnover of the target. For example, ASA irreversibly inhibits platelet membrane cyclooxygenase and results in impaired platelet aggregation for the life of the platelet, long after the drug has been eliminated from the body. Furthermore, equilibration delays between drug in plasma and the site of drug action as well as postreceptor transduction mechanisms may also affect the time course of drug response. The following sections discuss the factors that affect the time course of pharmacologic response based on an understanding of the mechanism of drug action and link this information to pharmacokinetics.

Direct Reversible Effects

Pharmacodynamic models generally relate drug concentration at the "effect site" to pharmacologic response. However, effect-site concentrations are typically not measured in clinical studies, and thus, investigators often make the assumption that drug concentrations measured in plasma (or other tissue) are in equilibrium with those at the effect site. It is important to emphasize that it is not necessary to assume that plasma concentrations are equal to effect-site concentrations but that they are in direct proportion to the effect-site concentrations. The simplest example would be to relate observed drug concentrations with observed responses measured at the same time. The propranolol concentration-effect data in Figure 14-3 are an example of this approach and are, therefore, independent of any other assumptions about the pharmacokinetics of the drug.

In order to describe and understand the time course of drug response, it is necessary to link appropriate pharmacokinetic and pharmacodynamic models that adequately describe the concentration-time data and the concentration-effect data, respectively. The simplest method is to relate pharmacologic effects to the central compartment concentrations in the pharmacokinetic model. Therefore, the concentration (C) term in the various pharmacodynamic models described earlier is replaced by the equation that describes the plasma concentration-time profile for the drug. The use of a pharmacokinetic model eliminates the need to measure concentration and effect at the same time because the predicted concentration can be used. Levy[21,22] was probably the first to use these principles to describe the time course of pharmacologic effect. Based on the time course of muscle strength after tubocurarine administration, he used a one-compartment pharmacokinetic model with first-order elimination and the log-linear pharmacodynamic model to explain that pharmacologic effects would decline as a linear function of time. However, these predictions will hold only for that range of pharmacologic effect where there is a linear relationship between the logarithm of the concentration and effect (about 20% to 80% of E_{max}). As indicated previously, these predictions will be in error at concentrations that lead to responses that are above or below this range.[16]

Duration of effect implies that there is a specific level of pharmacologic response that is of particular interest (e.g., lowering of diastolic blood pressure to 90 mm Hg). If the plasma concentration (assuming equilibration with the site of action) that produces this effect is known, then the duration of action can be predicted based simply on the pharmacokinetic model and will be independent of any pharmacodynamic model. Thus, after intravenous bolus administration and assuming a monoexponential decline in concentration, the time to reach a certain threshold concentration will be determined by the dose (or initial drug concentration) and the half-life. In this case, the duration of action of a particular drug will be proportional to the logarithm of the dose. Thus, increasing the dose is a relatively inefficient way to extend the duration of action of a drug.

A more complete description of the time course of pharmacologic effect may be obtained if the pharmacokinetic model is linked to the E_{max} or sigmoid E_{max} model, as first described in 1968 by Wagner.[11] Integration of these pharmacodynamic and pharmacokinetic principles can help explain the (expected) common observation of a discrepancy between the time course of plasma concentrations and the pharmacologic effects. Figure 14-5 was generated to illustrate this point for a typical drug with first-order elimination and an E_{max} model to describe the concentration-effect relationship. In order to make the figure more generally applicable, concentrations are in multiples of EC_{50}, time is in terms of half-life, and the effect is expressed as a

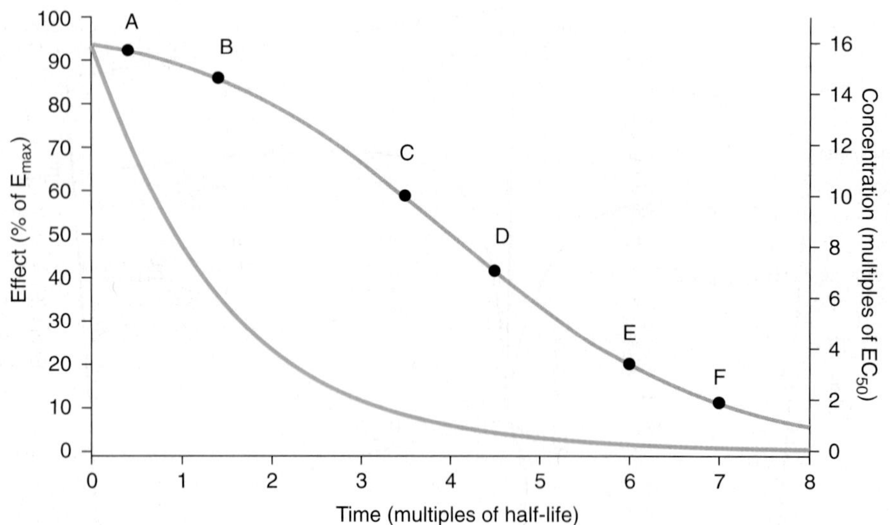

FIGURE 14-5 • Simulated time course of pharmacologic effect based on the E_{max} model (*yellow line*). The simulation was done assuming first-order decline in drug concentration (*green line*) and no delay in observed effect. The initial concentration is 16 × EC_{50}, and the time axis is in terms of the drug's terminal half-life. There is 1 half-life between points A and B, C and D, and E and F. At concentrations far exceeding the EC_{50}, a 50% decrease in concentration leads to only a small change in effect from 92.4% **(A)** to 85.8% **(B)** of E_{max}. It will take 4 half-lives for the initial effect to decline by one half, thus emphasizing how the "apparent pharmacodynamic half-life" is much longer than the "pharmacokinetic half-life." At concentrations approximating the EC_{50}, the effect declines as a linear function of time, from 58.6% **(C)** to 41.4% **(D)** of E_{max}. More than 1.7 half-lives are still necessary for the effect to decline by one half. Finally, at concentrations below 0.25 × EC_{50}, the effect declines from 20.0% **(E)** to 11.1% **(F)** of E_{max} and approximates the first-order rate of decline in concentration. (From Lalonde RL, Straka RJ, Pieper JA, et al. Propranolol pharmacodynamic modeling using unbound and total concentrations in healthy volunteers. J Pharmacokinet Biopharm 1987;15:569-582. With kind permission from Springer Science+Business Media.)

percentage of E_{max}. Two important points are obvious upon inspection of Figure 14-5. First, there is a clear discrepancy between the rate of decline of concentrations and the rate of decline of pharmacologic effect. Second, the rate of decline of effect is not constant but varies depending on the concentration range. Despite a steady first-order decline in concentrations, pharmacologic effect is relatively constant when concentrations are well above the EC_{50}. This would be expected based on receptor theory whenever there are more than enough drug molecules to occupy most receptors even if the drug concentration is reduced by one half. Within the range from 80% of E_{max} (4 × EC_{50}) to 20% of E_{max} (0.25 × EC_{50}), pharmacologic effect will decline as a linear function of time, as predicted by Levy.[21] At concentrations well below the EC_{50}, there is a nearly linear relationship between concentration and effect (see "Linear model," earlier); consequently, pharmacologic response declines in parallel (first-order) with the same half-life as drug concentrations. Therefore, it should be emphasized that there is no such parameter as the "pharmacodynamic half-life" of a particular drug because the rate of decline in pharmacologic effect varies based on the concentration. Actually, the term *half-life* is applicable only for a first-order process, which, in the particular case of pharmacologic response, occurs only when concentrations are very small relative to the EC_{50}. These principles can be used to explain some common clinical observations. Propranolol, for example, can maintain its cardiac β-blocking effect for a time period that greatly exceeds its half-life because typical doses will achieve drug concentrations that greatly exceed the EC_{50}.[23] A similar approach can be used to compare the extent of pharmacologic response with different dosage regimens. Based on the E_{max} and one-compartment pharmacokinetic models, Wagner[11] calculated the area under the effect-time curve (AUC_e) as a measure of the total pharmacologic response over 24 hours and the impact of changing the dosing interval while keeping the total daily dose constant. He demonstrated that the AUC_e over 24 hours progressively increased as the same total daily dose was administered over progressively shorter dosing intervals. These results are expected based on the continuously decreasing slope of the E_{max} model (Eq. 14-12) as concentrations increase (see Fig. 14-3). The greater fluctuations associated with once-daily administration will lead to higher peak concentrations, but these will not produce proportionately higher pharmacologic effects. Therefore, the increased pharmacologic response at the higher concentrations will not fully compensate for the decreased response at the lower concentrations, and there will be a net decrease in AUC_e over 24 hours with once-daily administration. The extent of the increase in AUC_e with shorter dosing intervals will depend on the EC_{50} relative to the observed concentrations. When concentrations greatly exceed the EC_{50}, the increase in AUC_e will be less than when the concentrations approach the EC_{50} because of the change in the slope of the concentration-effect relationship (see Fig. 14-3). A similar argument can be used to explain why the difference in AUC_e for inhibition of exercise-induced tachycardia produced by sustained-release capsules and immediate-release tablets of propranolol was much less than the twofold difference in the AUC for drug concentration.[23] The same concepts also explain the greater diuretic response with loop diuretics administered by continuous infusion versus intermittent doses in healthy subjects,[24] patients with renal impairment[25] and patients with heart failure.[26] Alvan and colleagues[27] extensively discussed the concept of efficiency (pharmacologic effect per unit of drug concentration) for pharmacodynamics based on these principles.

Equilibration Delays

The time course of certain pharmacologic effects may lag behind plasma drug concentrations. This occasionally leads to an erroneous conclusion that there is no relationship between drug concentration and pharmacologic response. However, a more mechanistic approach to pharmacodynamics often provides a biologic basis for the delay in drug response. A possible explanation for a lag in pharmacologic response is an equilibration delay between the drug concentration in plasma and at the site of drug action. Other causes of a lag in response such as indirect effects and transduction steps are discussed later in the sections on "Indirect Effects and Turnover Models" and "Transduction Steps and Transit Compartment Models," respectively.

A lag between plasma drug concentrations and response will generally be evident upon inspection of the data as a function of time. Another approach is to plot the plasma concentration-effect data and connecting the points in time sequence in order to show the characteristic counterclockwise loop or hysteresis. The term *hysteresis* is used to mean "late" in the sense that a particular concentration, late after a dose, will produce a greater effect than the same concentration measured earlier. A counterclockwise loop may indicate an indirect response, delays due to transduction processes, increased sensitivity (e.g., up-regulation of receptors), formation of an active metabolite if the ratio of metabolite to parent drug increases with time, or an equilibration delay between plasma concentrations and the concentrations at the effect site. The biologic basis for any observed delay in response should be investigated thoroughly so that the method or model selected to evaluate the data will, as much as possible, reflect the mechanism of drug action.

Equilibration delays can be avoided if the concentration-effect relationship is evaluated under steady state conditions (e.g., continuous intravenous infusions). However, this is not always feasible. Another approach is to account for the delay observed in non–steady state experiments using appropriate pharmacokinetic-pharmacodynamic models. For example, Wagner and coworkers[28] demonstrated that the

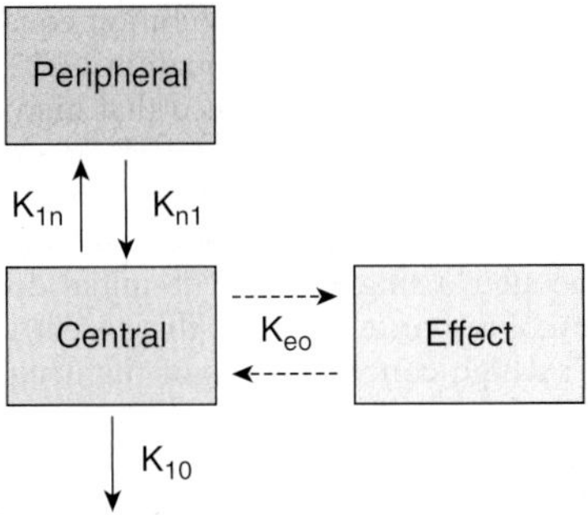

FIGURE 14-6 • Schematic representation of an effect compartment model linked to a typical pharmacokinetic model. (Based on Sheiner LB, Stanski DR, Vozeh S, et al. Simultaneous modeling of pharmacokinetics and pharmacodynamics: application to D-tubucurarine. Clin Pharmacol Ther 1979;25:358-371.)

effects of lysergic acid diethylamide (LSD) on mental performance were more closely related to the predicted peripheral pharmacokinetic compartment drug concentrations than to plasma concentrations. A similar approach was used to describe the delay in the inotropic effects of digoxin.[29] Some drawbacks exist to the use of peripheral pharmacokinetic compartment concentrations to describe concentration-effect relationships. There is no reason to expect that the effect-site concentrations must have the same time course as any pharmacokinetic compartment identified from measurement of plasma concentrations. If the pharmacologic effect site receives only a small amount of drug, then there will be no measurable effect on drug disposition in plasma or the particular pharmacokinetic model necessary to describe drug disposition. It may simply be a coincidence if the effect site happens to have a similar time course of drug concentration as a particular peripheral compartment that represents a type of weighted average of several different tissues/organs. Furthermore, a peripheral compartment approach can be used only for multicompartmental drugs, despite the fact that equilibration delays can occur with drugs that exhibit apparent one-compartment characteristics.

A completely different approach is to use the time course of pharmacologic effect itself to estimate the equilibration rate with the effect site. From concepts originally described by Segre,[30] Sheiner and colleagues[31] developed a method commonly called the *effect compartment* or *link model* (Fig. 14-6). The central compartment of the pharmacokinetic model is linked to a hypothetical effect compartment. The exact form of the pharmacokinetic model is irrelevant as long as it adequately describes the central compartment concentrations. The rate of equilibration with the effect compartment is determined by the rate out of that compartment (k_{eo}), much like the time to reach steady state in pharmacokinetics is determined by the elimination rate constant. It is assumed that a negligible amount of drug enters the effect compartment, and consequently, the effect compartment does not alter the plasma concentration-time curve. The following simple differential equation is used to describe the equilibration delay between plasma and the effect compartment:

$$\frac{dC_e}{dt} = k_{eo}(C - C_e) \quad (14\text{-}21)$$

where dC_e/dt is the rate of change of the hypothetical drug concentration in the effect compartment (C_e), k_{eo} is the rate of equilibration with the effect compartment, and C is the drug concentration in the central compartment of the pharmacokinetic model. C_e can be substituted for concentration (C) in the various pharmacodynamic models described previously. Although the actual value of the rate constant into the effect compartment is irrelevant, it is convenient to set it equal to the rate out of the effect compartment (i.e., k_{eo}). The result is that C_e is then expressed in terms of equivalent central (plasma) compartment concentrations at steady state.

The various pharmacodynamic models described previously assume that there is an equilibrium between the concentrations that are measured (usually in plasma) and the corresponding concentrations at the effect site. This assumption is not required with the effect compartment approach because the onset of pharmacologic effect itself is used to estimate the theoretical concentration at the effect site. With the use of a suitable estimation method, a pharmacokinetic model can first be fitted to the plasma concentration-time data, and then these parameters can be used as constants in the pharmacokinetic-pharmacodynamic model to estimate the remaining parameters. Alternatively, both the pharmacokinetic and the pharmacodynamic models can be fitted simultaneously.[32,33] "Nonparametric" methods that make fewer assumptions about the structure of the pharmacokinetic or pharmacodynamic models have also been used to estimate equilibration delays with an effect compartment.[34,35]

The magnitude of k_{eo} will depend on the extent of the delay in pharmacologic response relative to plasma concentrations. A long delay will be associated with a small k_{eo} and a long equilibration half-life. Conversely, whenever k_{eo} is relatively large, the time course of the effect compartment concentrations will parallel concentrations in plasma. In such cases, there will be no hysteresis due to equilibration delays, and plasma concentrations can be used as input for the various pharmacodynamic models. If k_{eo} approaches the value of the rate constant from a peripheral compartment to the central compartment (k_{n1} in Fig. 14-6), then the effect compartment concentrations will parallel those in the peripheral pharmacokinetic compartment. Therefore, the use of a peripheral pharmacokinetic compartment concentration to account for a delay in response, as discussed previously, will only be appropriate when k_{eo} happens to be equal or nearly equal to a particular k_{n1}.

The effect compartment method is particularly helpful when dealing with lags in response that are due to equilibration delays or at least when there is a basis to expect an equilibration delay with the site of action. Investigators have also used the effect compartment approach empirically to account for a lag in response due to unknown causes. For example, there is a significant delay in the effect of tacrine on cognitive improvement in patients with Alzheimer's disease. Holford and Peace[36] used an effect compartment approach to estimate the "equilibration" half-time of 3 weeks for this response. However, the authors acknowledged that this long equilibration half-time is not due to the time it takes for the drug to inhibit cholinesterase in the brain but rather to other unknown causes downstream from the effect on cholinesterase. Appropriate caution is necessary when using models empirically before attributing a particular physiologic meaning to a parameter. Careful investigations under different experimental conditions (e.g., range of doses, repeated or continuous drug administration, measuring onset and offset of response), whenever feasible, will help to test the appropriateness of a model and give more confidence in the predictions from the model. Other approaches in addition to the effect compartment model can account for delays in response and may be more appropriate depending on the mechanism of drug action (e.g., see later under "Indirect Effects and Turnover Models").

Indirect Effects and Turnover Models

There has been an important trend since the early 1990s away from empirical models and toward more mechanistic pharmacodynamic models that include components of one or more physiologic processes. This is particularly evident with the increasing use of indirect pharmacodynamic response models.[37-39] Approximately 40 years ago, however, Nagashima and colleagues[4] used an indirect response model to evaluate warfarin's hypoprothrombinemic effects. The hypoprothrombinemic effect is determined by both synthesis and degradation of clotting factors, yet warfarin will affect only the rate of synthesis. Thus, although peak plasma concentrations of warfarin occur within a few hours after an oral dose, the maximum hypoprothrombinemic effect will not be evident for a few days.

Daneyka and coworkers[37] more recently proposed four general models of indirect pharmacologic response. The basic structure of these models is illustrated in Figure 14-7. Indirect effects may result from the inhibition or stimulation of either the production or the elimination of a response variable (e.g., clotting factors). Typical pharmacodynamic models such as the E_{max} model (or other pharmacodynamic models discussed previously) may be used to describe the stimulatory or inhibitory effect. Differential equations are used to then describe the change in response variable, which will also take into account the time course of drug concentrations. For example, the following equation describes the rate of change in response variable (dR/dt) for model I in Figure 14-7.

$$\frac{dR}{dt} = k_{in}\left(1 - \frac{I_{max}C}{IC_{50} + C}\right) - k_{out}R \qquad (14\text{-}22)$$

where k_{in} is the zero-order rate constant for the production/synthesis of response R, k_{out} is the first-order rate constant for the loss or degradation of response, C is the drug concentration as a function of time from an appropriate pharmacokinetic model, I_{max} is the maximum fractional inhibition that can be produced by the drug, and IC_{50} is the drug concentration that will produce inhibition equal to 50% of I_{max}. Models I and II from Figure 14-7 and Equation 14-22 are often shown without the I_{max} parameter if it is assumed that high drug concentrations completely inhibit k_{in}, which effectively means that I_{max} is 1. Figure 14-8 illustrates how inhibition of the production of the response variable will lead to a decline and subsequent increase in response variable over time after a single dose. The initial decline reflects the rate of elimination of response when the drug is present. If k_{in} is completely inhibited by high concentrations of the drug, then the initial rate of decline will approach k_{out} R (i.e., a plot of ln R versus time will have a slope of $-k_{out}$). As drug concentrations decrease over time, there is progressively less inhibition of production, and consequently, the response variable increases. Eventually, when the drug effect is absent, the response measure will return to its baseline or predrug level, based on the assumption that the physiologic parameters do not change over time. The baseline response measure (Ro) is equal to k_{in}/k_{out} and reflects

Pharmacodynamic Models of Indirect Response

I. Inhibition of k_{in}

k_{in} → Response (R) → k_{out}

IC_{50}

$$\frac{dR}{dt} = k_{in}\,(1 - \frac{I_{max}\,C}{IC_{50} + C}) - k_{out}\,R$$

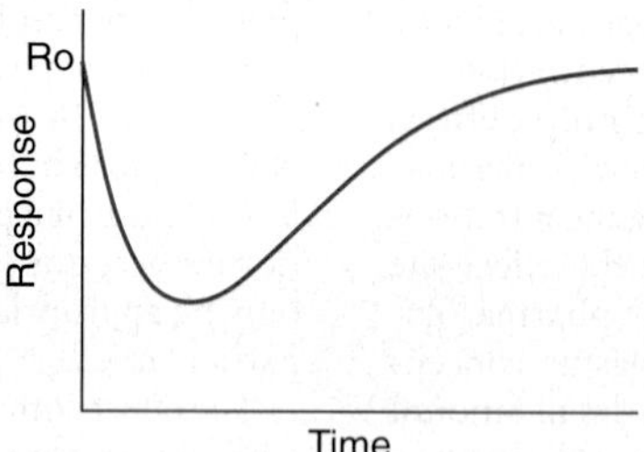

II. Inhibition of k_{out}

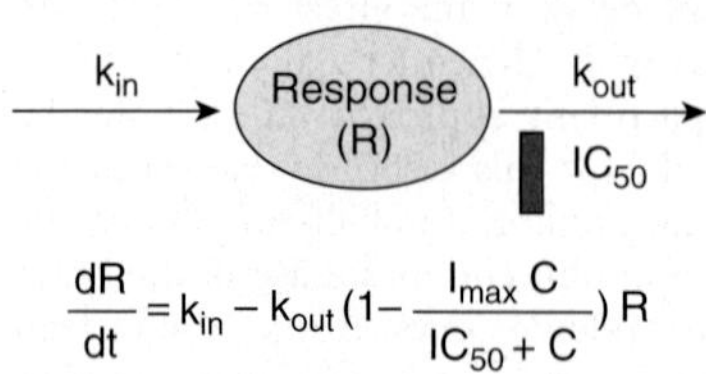

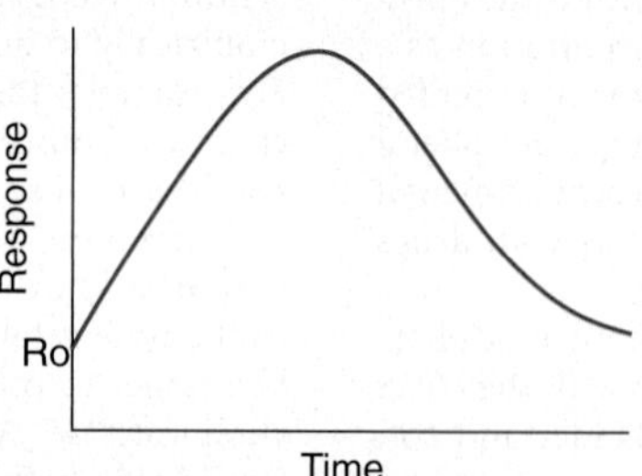

III. Stimulation of k_{in}

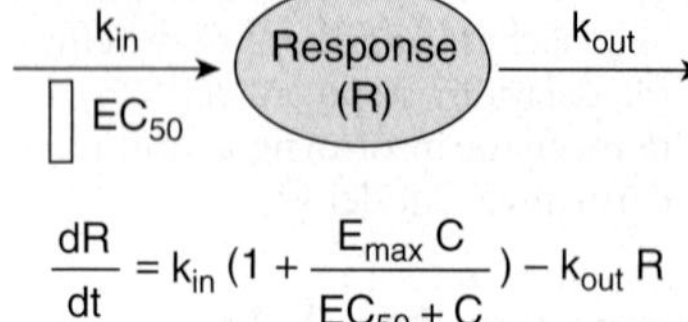

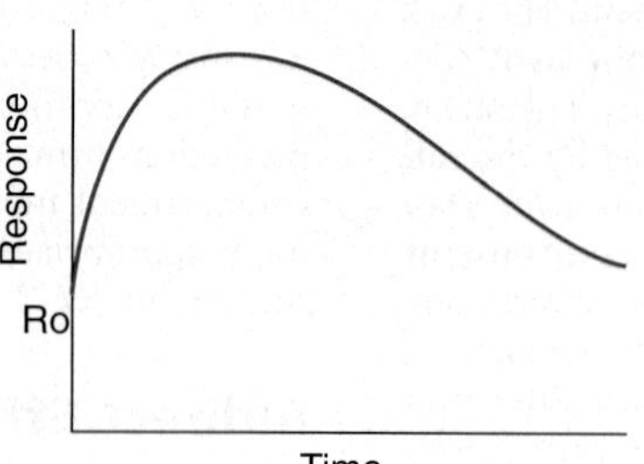

IV. Stimulation of k_{out}

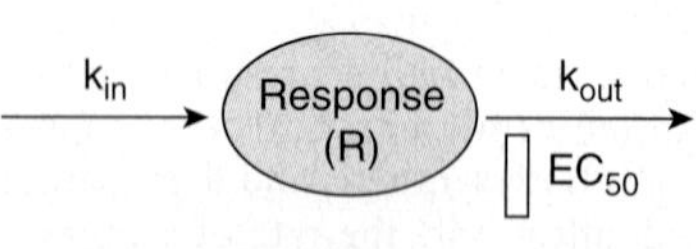

$$\frac{dR}{dt} = k_{in} - k_{out}\,(1 + \frac{E_{max}\,C}{EC_{50} + C})\,R$$

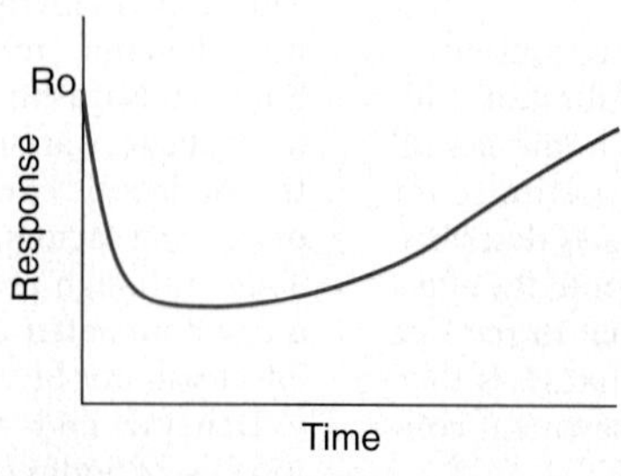

KEY EC_{50} Stimulation IC_{50} Inhibition

FIGURE 14-7 • Four basic indirect response models characterized by either inhibition or stimulation of the rate of production or elimination of the response variable. Symbols are defined in the text. The shapes of the response versus time profiles are depicted for each model. (From Daneyka NL, Garg V, Jusko WJ. Comparison of four basic models of indirect pharmacologic response. J Pharmacokinet Biopharm 1993;21:457-478.)

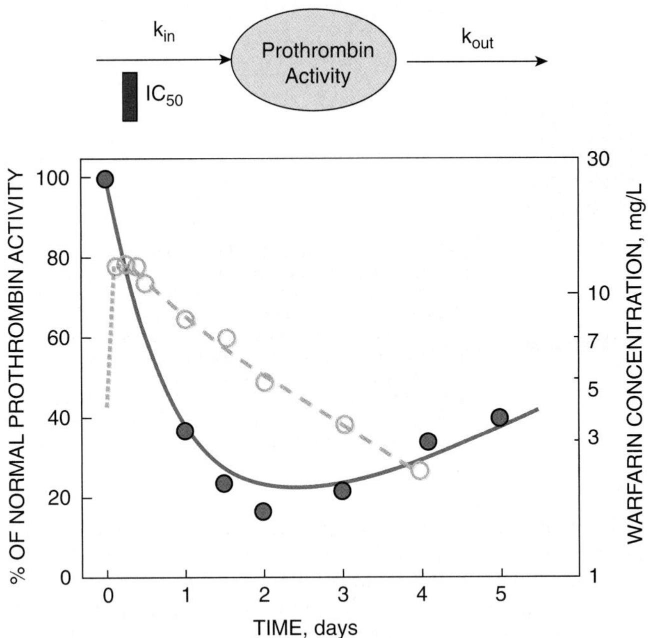

FIGURE 14-8 • Indirect response model shows the relationship between warfarin concentrations (*open circles*) and prothrombin complex activity (*solid circles*) after an oral dose of 1.5 mg/kg of sodium warfarin. The *solid line* is the fit of the indirect response model to the data. (From Jusko WJ, Ko HC. Physiologic indirect response models characterize diverse type of pharmacodynamic effects. Clin Pharmacol Ther 1994;56:406-419; based on data from Nagashima R, O'Reilly RA, Levy G. Kinetics of pharmacologic response in man: the anticoagulant action of warfarin. Clin Pharmacol Ther 1969;10:22-35.)

a steady state between production and elimination of the response variable in the absence of drug. Typical patterns of response over time for the different indirect pharmacodynamic response models are shown in Figure 14-7.

Jusko and Ko[38] demonstrated that the previously discussed basic models can describe the time course of response to diverse types of pharmacologic effects, such as the effects of aldose reductase inhibitors on red blood cell sorbitol concentrations, methylprednisolone on cell trafficking and plasma cortisol concentration, cholinesterase inhibitors on muscle response in myasthenia gravis, terbutaline on bronchodilation and plasma potassium concentration, furosemide on diuresis, and cimetidine on prolactin plasma concentration. In each case, maximum effects occur after peak drug concentrations. The indirect response model, like the effect compartment model, will therefore help account for a lag between drug concentration and response. Figure 14-9 illustrates the similarities and a key difference between the effect compartment model and indirect response model I. The time of maximum effect (lowest value in this particular case) for the indirect response model will occur at progressively later times as doses are increased. This occurs because it takes progressively longer for the rate of production to exceed the rate of loss as doses are increased because adequate drug concentrations will be present to inhibit k_{in} for a longer period of time. An increase in the time of maximum effect with increasing dose is characteristic of all four indirect response models, albeit to different extents.[37,40,41] Conversely, the effect compartment model predicts that maximum effects will occur at exactly the same time after different doses because the time of maximum effect is dependent only on k_{eo}, a parameter that does not depend on dose (see Fig. 14-9).

The difference in the time course of pharmacologic response can be relatively minor between models, as evidenced by Figure 14-9. Selection of an appropriate model should be based on the mechanism of action of the drug. Evaluation of the time course of response after different doses will also be a useful method to differentiate between the effect compartment and the indirect response models. The characteristics of the four indirect response models shown in Figure 14-7 and the impact of changes in dose and drug properties (IC_{50}, EC_{50}, I_{max}, E_{max}) have been reported.[40-42] Similarities and differences between the effect compartment and the indirect response models have been discussed extensively.[43-45]

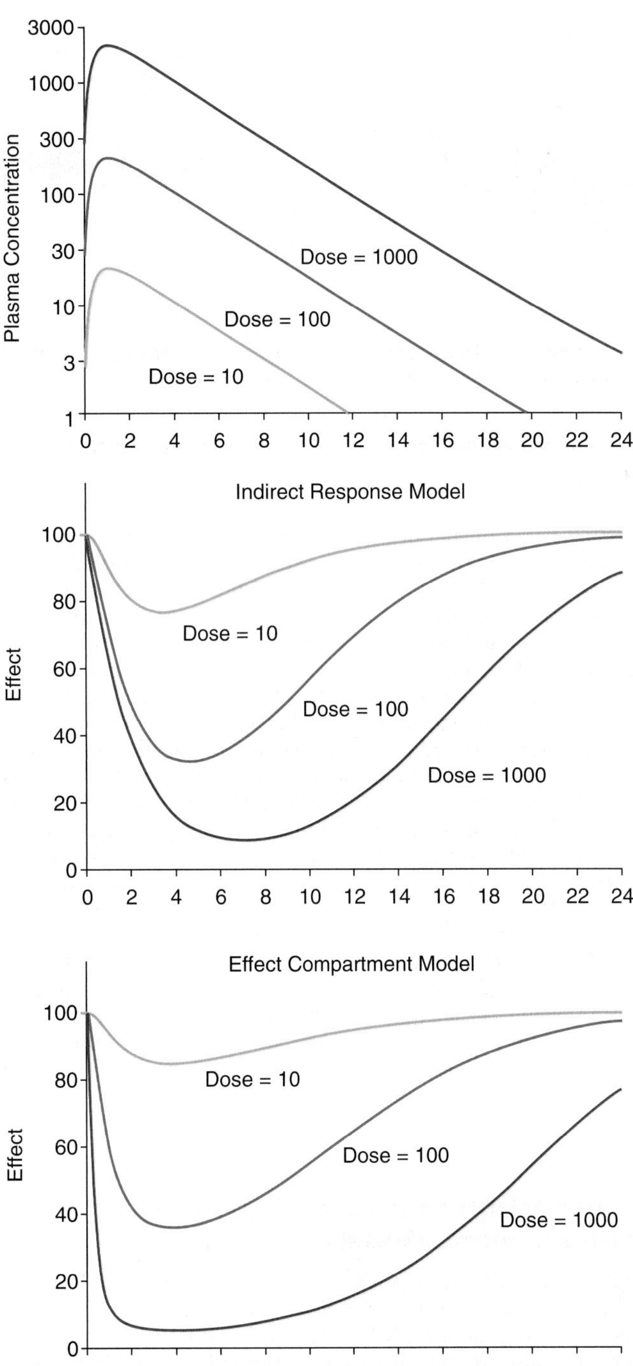

FIGURE 14-9 • Simulated concentration-time relationship (**top panel**) and effect-time relationships for the indirect response model I (**middle panel**) and effect compartment model (**bottom panel**). The time of peak (minimum in this case) response increases with dose for the indirect response model but is independent of dose for the effect compartment model.

More complex versions of the models previously discussed may be necessary to describe certain pharmacodynamic responses. For example, instead of a simple zero-order k_{in}, a circadian function may be necessary to account for different rates of synthesis at different times of day. Kong and associates[46] used this approach to evaluate the effect of methylprednisolone on plasma cortisol concentrations. The inhibition/stimulation effect may require a sigmoid E_{max}-type function or a

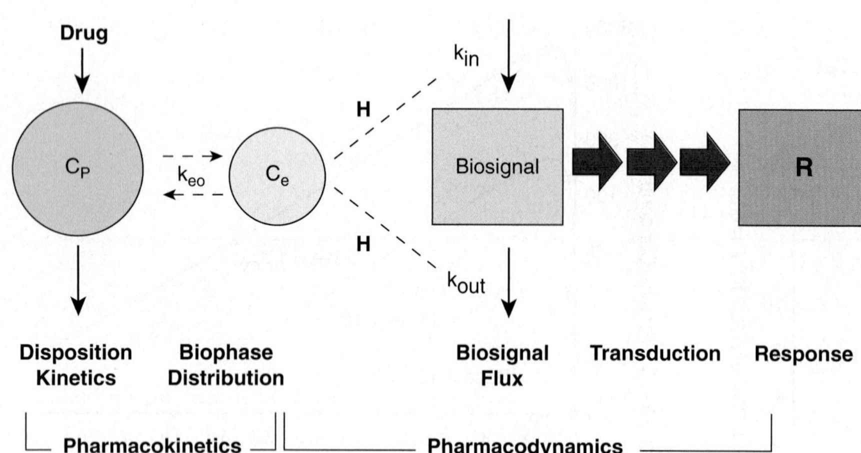

FIGURE 14-10 • Integrated pharmacokinetic and pharmacodynamic model. Determinants of drug action include pharmacokinetics, distribution to the biophase (k_{eo}), inhibition or stimulation (H) of production (k_{in}) or removal (k_{out}) of a mediator biosignal and signal transduction. (From Jusko WJ, Ko HC, Ebling WF. Convergence of direct and indirect pharmacodynamic response models. J Pharmacokinet Biopharm 1995;23:5-8. With kind permission from Springer Science+Business Media.)

function based on the operational model of drug action described previously. Complex models that reflect the gene-mediated mechanism of action of corticosteroids have been used with animal data.[47] The general model shown in Figure 14-10[44] combines some of the elements of various models discussed previously to describe the steps involved in the generation of a pharmacodynamic response. Figure 14-10 illustrates how drug distribution to an effect site, drug effects on a mediator or biosignal, and transduction of the biosignal into a response may be needed to describe the time course of pharmacologic response. The mechanistic model in Figure 14-10 can be contrasted with the very simple Figure 14-1. It should be emphasized that inclusion of all the different elements in Figure 14-10 is typically not required because certain steps are relatively fast and, thus, are not rate limiting. For example, a relatively high k_{eo} value means that equilibration with the effect site will be very rapid, and thus, plasma concentration may be sufficient to relate to response. A relatively high k_{out} means that the drug will appear to have a direct effect on the mediator or biosignal. Finally, signal transduction may be rapid relative to other steps in Figure 14-10 and, thus, will not have a significant impact on the time course of response (see the next section on "Transduction Steps and Transit Compartment Models"). However, the figure illustrates the possible elements that may need to be taken into account depending on the characteristic of a particular system and the mechanism of action of the drug.

Transduction Steps and Transit Compartment Models

Advances in molecular biology and molecular pharmacology have helped to better understand the steps involved in producing a pharmacodynamic response after a drug binds to a particular receptor. Signal transduction may involve gene transcription, second messengers, protein phosphorylation, activation of ionic channels, and other processes before the ultimate response is generated. These steps may require enough time that delays will be evident between drug-receptor binding and the observed pharmacologic effect. For example, delays of a few hours have been observed with corticosteroids induction of hepatic tyrosine aminotransferase.[48] Transit compartments have been proposed to account for time-dependent signal transduction.[49,50] Although transit compartments have typically been applied to animal models with extensive measurements of the different steps in the cascade leading to the observed pharmacologic response,[47] relatively simple models have been successfully applied to describe the time course of pharmacodynamic response in humans.[50] One example is the following relationship:

$$R + C \Leftrightarrow RC \overset{\varepsilon}{\cdots\cdots} E^* \xrightarrow{\tau_1} E \xrightarrow{\tau_2} \qquad (14\text{-}23)$$

where R is the concentration of unoccupied receptors, C is the drug concentration available at the receptor, RC is the concentration of drug-receptor complex, ε is the efficacy of the drug, E* is the biosignal that results from the drug-receptor interaction, E is the observed pharmacologic effect, and τ_1 and τ_2 are transit times. The transit times τ_1 and τ_2 are equivalent to the reciprocal of the first-order rate constants for the production and loss, respectively, of the observed effect E. The following equation describes the rate of change in effect using the transit compartment model shown in Equation 14-23.

$$\frac{dE}{dt} = \frac{1}{\tau_1} E^* - \frac{1}{\tau_2} E \qquad (14\text{-}24)$$

If the biosignal that results from the drug-receptor interaction is described using the E_{max} model and assuming that the transit times are equal ($\tau_1 = \tau_2$), then the following equation is obtained.

$$\frac{dE}{dt} = \frac{1}{\tau}\left(\frac{E_{max} C}{EC_{50} + C}\right) - \frac{1}{\tau} E \qquad (14\text{-}25)$$

where parameters are as defined previously. Note that plasma drug concentrations will often be used as a surrogate for C (as previously discussed, this assumes that plasma drug concentrations are in direct proportion but not necessarily equal to the drug concentrations at the receptor site). This particular model, with the addition of a baseline effect, was used to describe the time course of bronchodilation after terbutaline administration.[50] More than one transit compartment may be necessary to account for the delay in the observed pharmacologic effect. Thus, one or more additional compartments can be added before the observed pharmacologic effect in Equation 14-23 and will necessitate an equivalent number of additional differential equations. A common transit time can be used for the different compartments. The impact of adding more transit compartments on the time course of response is shown in Figure 14-11. The time course of response to interferon alfa-n3 was described using a model with three transit compartments and accounted for the delay of approximately 18 hours between peak drug plasma concentrations and peak response.[50]

The transit compartment approach should be considered when delays in pharmacologic response are believed to be due to time-dependent signal transduction. Although the effect compartment model has been used extensively to account for delays in response, distribution delays between plasma and the site of action are not expected for many drugs that work through receptors that are readily accessible on cell membranes, particularly after extravascular administration of drugs that typically results in a gradual change in plasma drug concentrations over time. Very long delays in response, as described previously with interferon alfa-n3, are most likely not due to distribution to the site of action but rather to postreceptor mechanisms. If there is specific prior information on time-dependent signal transduction or actual measurement of second messengers/intermediaries, then transit compartments may prove very useful and reflect the mechanism of drug action.[47,48] Wider application of these models may help better understand the factors that contribute to variability in

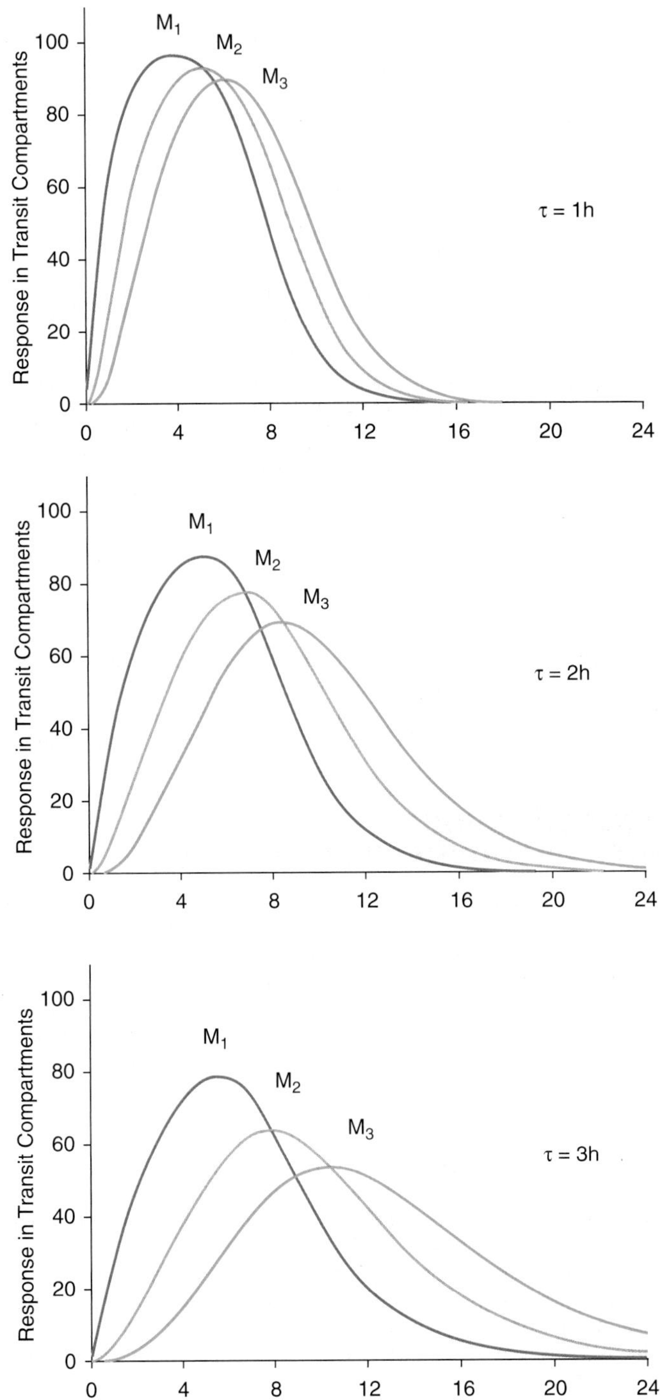

FIGURE 14-11 • The effect of transit time on signal transduction in a series of three compartments. The **upper, middle,** and **lower graphs** are for transit times of 1, 2 and 3 hours, respectively. (From Sun YN, Jusko WJ. Transit compartments versus gamma distribution function to model signal transduction in pharmacodynamics. J Pharm Sci 1998;87:732-737.)

transit times. However, incomplete understanding of the cause of delays in certain pharmacodynamic effects means that transit compartment models will often be used empirically. Appropriate caution is then necessary in interpreting the meaning of the estimates for transit times.

Different modifications of the transit compartment model have been proposed. An exponent can be added on certain compartment terms (e.g., E* in Eq. 14-24) to reflect amplification or diminution of the transduction process.[49] An exponent greater than 1 will amplify the signal whereas an exponent less than 1 will reduce it. Different transit times may be used for different compartments to account for specific rate-limiting cascade steps. Elements of other pharmacodynamic models may also be added if there is evidence of distribution delays to the site of action (i.e., effect compartment) or drug effect based on the operational model of drug action (i.e., Eq. 14-17). It should also be noted that the time course of pharmacodynamic response predicted using certain transit compartment models and indirect response models may be similar or even identical under some circumstances.[50]

Irreversible Effects

All pharmacodynamic models discussed so far apply to drugs that have reversible effects and, thus, relatively fast association/dissociation between drug and receptor. However, several drugs have irreversible effects. ASA and omeprazole are two very commonly used drugs that have irreversible effects on platelet aggregation and gastric acid secretion, respectively. The time course of response to drugs with irreversible effects is more dependent on the turnover of the target than on the pharmacokinetics of the drugs. Covalent acetylation of platelet membrane cyclooxygenase by ASA leads to an irreversible effect on platelet aggregation. Because platelets do not synthesize new proteins, the effect lasts for the lifespan of the platelet (7 to 10 days). Thus, only small doses of ASA (80 mg to 325 mg) administered once a day are adequate to produce an important effect on platelet aggregation and clinical benefit in patients with various cardiovascular diseases.

Omeprazole produces an irreversible effect on H^+,K^+-ATPase (proton pump) in parietal cells. The resulting inhibition of gastric acid secretion may last more than 24 hours, even though the drug has a half-life in plasma of less than 1 hour. In this case, the duration of effect depends on the turnover of H^+,K^+-ATPase. Äbelö and colleagues[51] proposed the turnover model in Figure 14-12 to describe the time course of gastric acid secretion after omeprazole administration. Mechanistic elements, based on previous information about the mechanism of drug action and turnover of proton pumps, were included in the model. Irreversible inhibition of H^+,K^+-ATPase by omeprazole was captured as an increased rate of loss of response (k_{ome} in Fig. 14-12). A precursor pool of H^+,K^+-ATPase that reflects a reserve of inactive proton pumps was included in the model (see also later under "Effects on Production of Natural Cells"). After initial exposure to omeprazole and inhibition of active proton pumps, the precursor pool provides newly activated proton pumps. Then, with continued drug exposure, the precursor pool becomes depleted and new proton pumps must come from de novo synthesis. The rate of accumulation of new proton pumps is relatively slow and explains the prolonged duration of action observed with chronic dosing. The model was used to describe the time course of inhibition of gastric acid secretion after both short-term and long-term omeprazole administration.[51]

Bactericidal antibiotics and certain antineoplastic agents cause cell death after the drugs are incorporated into cellular biochemical processes. Models were previously proposed to evaluate tumor cell response to cell-cycle–specific and nonphase-specific drugs.[52,53] These models were modified by Gibaldi and Perrier[54] and are actually similar to the model proposed in Figure 14-6, with the exception that the effect compartment includes variables to account for tumor cell number, tumor cell turnover, and the number of cells in a specific cycle that may be sensitive to a drug effect.

Effects on Production of Natural Cells

Drugs like erythropoietin and granulocyte colony-stimulating factor (G-CSF) produce an effect by stimulating the production of cells. The time course of response to these agents is therefore dependent on the life span of the cells affected. Pharmacodynamic models, based on the mechanism of action and life span of the cells, have been proposed to describe the response to such drugs.[55-57] Krzyzanski and coworkers[56] used various modifications of indirect response models to describe the

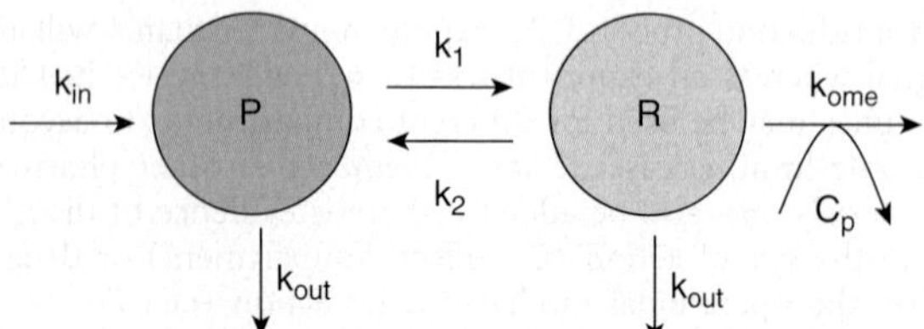

FIGURE 14-12 • Schematic representation of the turnover model used to describe the irreversible effects of omeprazole on gastric acid secretion. P is the precursor pool of inactive proton pumps, R is the pool of active proton pumps, k_{ome} is the second-order rate constant for the irreversible effect of omeprazole on proton pumps, Cp is the plasma omeprazole concentration, k_{in} is the zero-order production rate of P, k_{out} is the first-order rate of degradation, k_1 and k_2 are intercompartmental rate constants. (From Äbelö A, Eriksson UG, Karlsson MO, et al. A turnover model of the irreversible inhibition of gastric acid secretion by omeprazole in the dog. J Pharmacol Exp Ther 2000;295:662-669.)

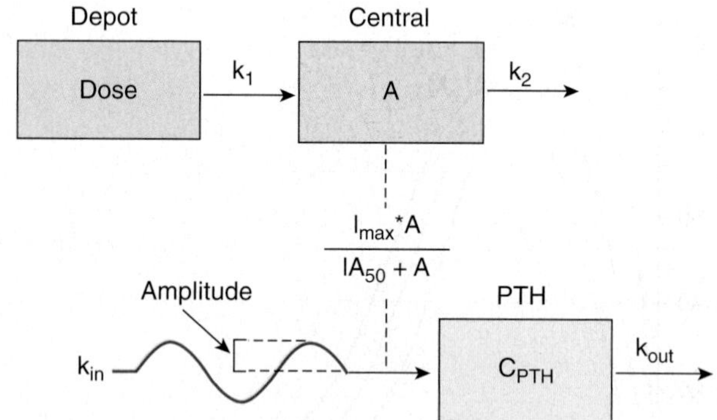

FIGURE 14-13 • Pharmacodynamic modeling without drug concentration. The response (PTH plasma concentration) is a function of its rate of production (k_{in}) with a circadian rhythm, rate of elimination (k_{out}), and the inhibition of secretion by the drug. A is the amount of drug, I_{max} is the maximum effect of the drug, IA_{50} is the amount of drug that will produce an effect equal to 50% of I_{max}, k_1 and k_2 are the first-order rate constants for input and output of active drug to the site of action, respectively. (From Lalonde RL, Gaudreault J, Karhu DA, et al. Mixed-effects modeling of the pharmacodynamic response to the calcimimetic agent R-568. Clin Pharmacol Ther 1999;65:40-49.)

time course of neutrophil response to G-CSF, platelet response to thrombopoietin, and reticulocyte response to erythropoietin. A key feature of these models is that the rate of loss of response (i.e., number of cells/ml) is not a first-order process like typical indirect response models but rather is based on the estimated life span of the cells. A precursor pool, similar to that shown in Figure 14-12, was necessary in some cases to account for the delay of 2 or more days between drug administration and increased cells in the circulation. This is consistent with the time needed for precursor cells (e.g., megakaryocytes) to mature and eventually release their products (e.g., platelets) in the circulation.

Dose-Response-Time Data: Pharmacodynamic Modeling without Drug Concentrations

The time course of pharmacologic response provides useful information about the pharmacokinetics (i.e., time course of availability at the site of action) and pharmacodynamics (i.e., relationship between drug at the site of action and response) of a drug, even if drug concentration data are not available.[58,59] Pharmacodynamic modeling without drug concentration is possible, based on the dose-response-time data.[60,61] Bragg and associates[60] used this approach to explain how the time course of paralysis after vecuronium administration can be different for respiratory muscles versus other muscles. Lalonde and colleagues[62] used a similar approach to evaluate the effects of a calcium receptor agonist on parathyroid hormone (PTH) concentration in plasma, based on the model shown in Figure 14-13. Agonists at calcium receptors on the parathyroid cells cause a decrease in PTH secretion and could therefore be beneficial for patients with hyperparathyroidism. The model in Figure 14-13 includes elements of an indirect response model with circadian variability in the rate of PTH secretion. A one-compartment model with first-order input and output was used to describe the time course of drug in the central compartment, which was assumed to be in equilibrium with the site of action. Plasma drug concentrations were not available, and therefore, the "pharmacokinetic" compartment is in terms of amount (same scale as dose). An inhibitory E_{max} model was used to describe the effect of drug on PTH secretion, and the observed response was PTH plasma concentration. The model adequately described the time course of PTH response after administration of a wide range of doses. Although the IC_{50} cannot be estimated without drug concentrations, estimation of IA_{50} (amount of drug that produces a response equal to 50% of I_{max}) is possible. The product of IA_{50} and the rate constant (k_2) is the dosing rate of drug necessary to produce mean steady state amounts of drug that will inhibit PTH secretion by 50% of I_{max}. The model also allows predictions of the time course of PTH response with different dosage regimens based on the model parameter estimates and the turnover of PTH in plasma.

The modeling of dose-response-time data provides insight into the underlying factors that alter the observed time course of response. The approach may be helpful whenever drug concentrations are not available but generally requires a lot of pharmacologic effect data to properly estimate the model parameters. Extrapolations beyond the conditions of the study should be done with caution, given the assumptions of the model.

NONCONTINUOUS PHARMACODYNAMIC MEASURES

Although most pharmacologic effects are continuous, many important measures of pharmacodynamic response and clinical outcome are not. Noncontinuous measures include ordered categorical data (e.g., pain scale using mild, moderate, severe), nonordered categorical data (e.g., sleep stages), counts or frequencies (e.g., number of seizures per week), and time to event or survival (e.g., time to an adverse event). Typical methods of data analysis used for continuous data are not suitable for these noncontinuous measures. An added complication is encountered when noncontinuous data are measured repeatedly over time in the same individuals. A series of important advances have allowed investigators to better evaluate various types of noncontinuous data, including repeated measures data, using nonlinear mixed-effects modeling methods. A detailed presentation of these concepts and examples is beyond the scope of this discussion. The reader is referred to the following references for further information concerning the evaluation of noncontinuous pharmacodynamic data: ordered categorical data including censoring when patients drop out[63,64]; counts or frequency[65,66]; time to (repeated) occurrence of an event[67]; and nonordered categorical data.[68]

PHARMACODYNAMICS OF DRUG COMBINATIONS

The pharmacologic response of drug combinations was discussed in the classic reviews by Ariens and Simonis.[9,10] If two drugs act at different sites to produce a similar pharmacologic effect, then the overall pharmacologic response can be described as the sum of two functions such as the linear, E_{max}, or sigmoid E_{max} models. In this case, each drug has its own pharmacodynamic parameters (e.g., E_{max}, EC_{50}) that are best determined after administration of the individual agents. Synergism or antagonism will be evident if pharmacologic response to the drug combination is different from that predicted by the simple addition of the individual concentration-effect relationships.[69]

Many drugs act at the same type of receptors and, consequently, will compete for access to those receptors. Just as the interaction between a drug molecule and a receptor was used as the basis to develop Equations 14-1 to 14-6 and the E_{max} model (Eq. 14-12), the following relationship can be developed if two different drug molecules competitively bind with a common receptor[9]:

$$E_{A+B} = \frac{E_{max_A} C_A}{EC_{50_A}\left(1+\frac{C_B}{EC_{50_B}}\right)+C_A} + \frac{E_{max_B} C_B}{EC_{50_B}\left(1+\frac{C_A}{EC_{50A}}\right)+C_B} \quad (14\text{-}26)$$

where the subscripts A and B refer to the two different drugs, E_{A+B} is the combined effect of the two drugs, and the remaining parameters are as defined previously. This relationship will describe the combined effects of two agonists when their pharmacologic responses are mediated through a single receptor (e.g., isoproterenol and epinephrine with β-adrenoceptors). Equation 14-26 can also be modified if more than one molecule of each drug binds to each receptor or more than two drugs competitively bind to the same receptor. If E_{maxB} is significantly less than E_{maxA}, then drug B is said to be a partial agonist. When this occurs, E_{A+B} may be greater or less than the effect of each drug alone, depending on the concentrations of the two agents. Similarly, drug B may have no intrinsic activity when it binds to the receptor ($E_{max} = 0$) and will be considered a competitive antagonist. In such a case, Equation 14-26 will simplify to the following relationship:

$$E_{A+B} = \frac{E_{max_A} C_A}{EC_{50_A}\left(1+\frac{C_B}{IC_{50_B}}\right)+C_A} \quad (14\text{-}27)$$

Compared with the E_{max} model (Eq. 14-12), the net effect of antagonist B is to cause a shift in the agonist A concentration-effect relationship and increase the apparent agonist EC_{50} value because EC_{50A} is multiplied by the term $(1 + C_B/IC_{50B})$. Therefore, low antagonist concentrations relative to its IC_{50} will cause little change in the agonist concentration-effect relationship. The effect of the antagonist will become more apparent as its concentrations approach or exceed its IC_{50}. The maximum effect of the agonist is not affected by the antagonist (when C_A is very large, $E_{A+B} = E_{maxA}$), which is characteristic of competitive antagonism. A model based on Equation 14-27 combined with an effect compartment was used by Jonkers and associates[70] to describe the hypokalemic response to terbutaline and its inhibition by β-blockers.

Equation 14-27 is greatly simplified if the concentration of agonist is adjusted to produce the same pharmacologic response in both the presence and the absence of antagonist. The following relationship is then obtained:

$$\frac{C_A^*}{C_A} - 1 = \frac{C_B}{IC_{50_B}} \quad (14\text{-}28)$$

where C_A^* is the concentration of agonist in the presence of antagonist and C_A is the concentration of agonist in the absence of antagonist. The ratio on the left side of Equation 14-28 is often called the *concentration ratio*, or *dose ratio* if only doses are known. The concentration or dose ratio is a measure of the shift in the concentration-response or dose-response relationship produced by the antagonist. The advantage of Equation 14-28 is that the IC_{50} of an antagonist can be determined if the concentration of antagonist is known, even without knowledge of the EC_{50} of the agonist. As stated previously, it is assumed that concentrations measured in plasma are in equilibrium with those at the effect site. This approach was used in clinical pharmacodynamic studies to determine the IC_{50} of β-blockers with isoproterenol as the agonist and to evaluate the effects of age, stereoselective disposition, and protein binding on the sensitivity (IC_{50}) to propranolol.[71-73] Figure 14-14 shows an example of the isoproterenol dose-response relationship in the presence and absence of propranolol. The 30-fold increase in the dose of isoproterenol required to produce the same heart rate response during propranolol administration is one of the clearest demonstrations of competitive antagonism in a clinical study. Although the combined effects of β-agonists and β-antagonists have been commonly studied in clinical pharmacodynamic investigations, the principles previously discussed will apply to any drug combinations that act through a common receptor.

TIME-DEPENDENT PHARMACODYNAMICS

Tolerance

The various methods described thus far assume that the effect site concentration-effect relationship does not vary over time (i.e., the pharmacodynamic parameters are constant). Therefore, the effect compartment method assumes that the lag between drug concentration and effect is due only to an equilibration delay between plasma and effect site and that a certain effect site concentration will lead to the same pharmacologic effect at any time after the dose. However, numerous pharmacologic examples exist in which this assumption is clearly erroneous. *Tolerance*, defined as a decrease in pharmacologic response after prolonged exposure to a drug, has been demonstrated with glyceryl trinitrate, morphine, dobutamine, nicotine, cocaine, and the benzodiazepines, to name a few examples.[74] This type of functional tolerance is differentiated from metabolic tolerance due to auto-induction of drug metabolism.

Tolerance will lead to clockwise loop or proteresis[75] in the concentration-effect data if the points are connected in time sequence. Thus, concentrations late after the dose will produce a lesser effect than that of the same concentrations earlier after the dose. Proteresis also can occur if an inhibitory metabolite is produced and there is an increase in the metabolite–to–parent drug ratio over time, or when the effect site equilibrates with arterial blood drug concentrations faster than does the concentration at the sampling site (e.g., forearm venous blood).[76] Generally, tolerance can result from a down-

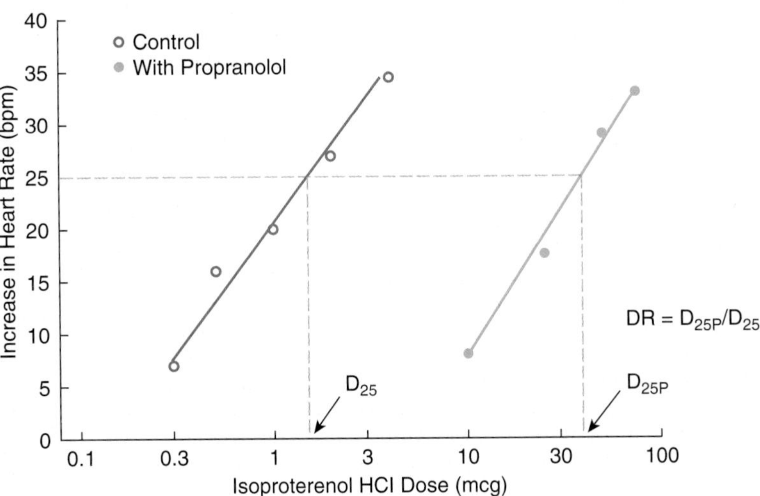

FIGURE 14-14 • Isoproterenol log dose-response relationship before and during a continuous infusion of propranolol in one subject. The ratio of doses to produce a specific increase in heart rate (DR) is used to calculate the in vivo IC_{50} of propranolol. (From Tenero DM, Bottorff MB, Burlew BS, et al. Altered beta-adrenergic sensitivity and protein binding to l-propranolol in the elderly. J Cardiovasc Pharmacol 1990;16:702-705.)

regulation of receptors (decreased number), a decreased affinity between the drug and the receptor, a decrease in receptor-generated response despite drug-receptor binding, or neurohormonal responses that may counteract the primary effect of a drug. Depending on the mechanism, tolerance can develop acutely (minutes to hours) or chronically (days to weeks). Several different pharmacodynamic methods have been proposed to describe the development of tolerance with modification of some of the models described earlier.[74] For example, the E_{max} model can be modified to include a time-dependent exponential decrease in E_{max} (i.e., $E_{max} \times e^{-kt}$, down-regulation of receptors) or increase in EC_{50} (i.e., $EC_{50} \times e^{kt}$, decreased affinity), where k is a constant that governs the rate of development of tolerance and t is time of exposure to the drug. A disadvantage of these modifications is that they predict that drug effect will disappear entirely if drug administration is maintained long enough. Another approach is to have a change in E_{max} (or EC_{50}) to a lower (higher) plateau and thus only partially decrease drug response. These methods use time but ignore the extent of drug exposure as a factor in the development of tolerance.

Porchet et al.[77] proposed a more versatile method to describe the development of acute tolerance to the effects of nicotine on heart rate. The investigators postulated the generation of a hypothetical substance (e.g., metabolite of nicotine) that acts as an antagonist of the effects of nicotine. The hypothetical antagonist production is driven by the plasma concentration of the parent drug (nicotine), and the amount of antagonist accumulates in a compartment linked to the central compartment for nicotine. This tolerance compartment model is analogous to the effect compartment model in Figure 14-6, and the equilibration between the plasma and the tolerance compartments is determined by a differential equation analogous to Equation 14-21. There are important advantages with this approach compared with the other tolerance models described earlier. Tolerance development is not simply a function of time; rather, it is dependent on the intensity (concentration, time) of drug exposure and also the time since drug exposure stopped (for the decrease in tolerance). Porchet et al.[77] used this model to demonstrate that the half-life of tolerance development to the chronotropic effects of nicotine was 35 minutes. The model correctly predicted not only the development of tolerance but also the decrease in tolerance when the interval between nicotine administrations was extended.

Various modifications of the tolerance compartment approach previously discussed have been used to describe the tolerance to the effects of morphine.[74] Tolerance models based on indirect response[78] and adaptive pool models[79] have also been described for furosemide and morphine, respectively. Gardmark et al.[74] reviewed the differences and interchangeability between several different pharmacodynamic models of tolerance.

Sensitization

Sensitization, defined as an increase in pharmacologic response with time at the same effect site concentration, can occur when there is an up-regulation of receptors. When sensitization occurs quickly, a counterclockwise loop or hysteresis in the concentration-effect data will be evident, although, as discussed previously, there are several other possible explanations for such hysteresis. Examples of up-regulation include surgical denervation and antagonist blockade of receptors for an extended period. The best clinical example may be the up-regulation of β-adrenoceptors and increase in adenylate cyclase activity after chronic administration of β-blockers, which result in hypersensitivity to catecholamines after sudden withdrawal of the antagonist.[80] Lima and colleagues[81] proposed a method to describe the time course of adrenergic responsiveness both during and after sudden withdrawal of propranolol. The model correctly predicted peak chronotropic hypersensitivity to isoproterenol 48 hours after abrupt withdrawal of propranolol. Furthermore, the model demonstrated that the time course of hypersensitivity was dependent on the differences in the rates of decline of propranolol (or other antagonist) concentrations and β-adrenoceptor density.

PHARMACODYNAMICS AND DISEASE PROGRESSION MODELS

The baseline effect for a particular physiologic response is typically evaluated using a model similar to Equation 14-10, where E_0 is the baseline effect and is assumed to be constant over time. However, many physiologic responses change over time, even without therapeutic intervention. There is now increased attention to the development of disease models that account for changes over time in physiologic parameters as well as the impact of different therapeutic interventions at different steps in the disease model.[82,83] This is particularly important for drugs used to treat chronic diseases such as Alzheimer's disease, diabetes mellitus, and rheumatoid arthritis. A modification of Equation 14-10 can be used to differentiate the effects of disease progression versus the effects of the drug over time, as follows:

$$E = E_0 + \frac{E_{max}[C]^n}{EC_{50}^n + [C]^n} = \text{disease progression} + \text{drug effect} \quad (14\text{-}29)$$

In order to account for disease progression, E_0 is replaced with a suitable function that describes disease progression over time. The simplest example would be a linear model with a slope to account for disease progression over time, as was used to evaluate the effects of tacrine in patients with Alzheimer's disease.[36] These models are more commonly applied to relatively large clinical trials from long-term studies. They require the use of mixed-effect models to properly account for observations that come from different individuals versus repeated observations in the same individual over the duration of the clinical trial. The components of Equation 14-29 can be modified to account for placebo effects, time-dependent effects of drug, and the impact of different patient characteristics on drug response and disease progression. Drug effects on disease progression can be classified in two main categories. The first category is for drugs providing symptomatic relief but not altering the underlying process of disease progression. The second is for drugs having a protective effect and altering the time course of disease severity (e.g., slope of the disease progression over time). Some recent examples have been reported for the treatment of Parkinson's disease[84] and type 2 diabetes.[85] These drug and disease models represent an important development and the way of the future as scientists integrate knowledge of system biology, pathophysiology, molecular biology, molecular pharmacology, and pharmacogenomics into increasingly complex but more predictive pharmacodynamic models.

REFERENCES

1. Holford NHG, Sheiner LB. Pharmacokinetic and pharmacodynamic modeling in vivo. CRC Crit Rev Bioeng 1981;5:273-322.
2. Lalonde RL. Pharmacodynamics. In Burton ME, Shaw LM, Evans WE, Schentag JJ (eds): Applied Pharmacokinetics and Pharmacodynamics: Principles of Therapeutic Drug Monitoring, 4th ed. Philadelphia: Williams & Wilkins, 2005, pp 60-81.
3. Csajka C, Verotta D. Pharmacokinetic-pharmacodynamic modelling: history and perspectives. J Pharmacokinet Pharmacodyn 2006;33:227-279.
4. Nagashima R, O'Reilly RA, Levy G. Kinetics of pharmacologic response in man: the anticoagulant action of warfarin. Clin Pharmacol Ther 1969;10:22-35.
5. Kenakin T (ed). Pharmacologic Analysis of Drug-Receptor Interaction, 3rd ed. Philadelphia: Lippincott-Raven, 1997.
6. Langmuir I. The adsorption of gases on plane surfaces of glass, mica, and platinum. J Am Chem Soc 1918;40:1361-1403.
7. Clark AJ. The reaction between acetylcholine and muscle cells. J Physiol 1926;61:530-546.
8. Hill AV. The possible effects of the aggregation of the molecules of hemoglobin on its dissociation curves. J Physiol 1910;40:iv-vii.
9. Ariens EJ, Simonis AM. A molecular basis of drug action. J Pharm Pharmacol 1964;16:137-157.
10. Ariens EJ, Simonis AM. A molecular basis for drug action. The interaction of one or more drugs with different receptors. J Pharm Pharmacol 1964;16:289-312.
11. Wagner JG. Kinetics of pharmacologic response. J Theor Biol 1968;20:173-201.
12. Holford NHG, Sheiner LB. Kinetics of pharmacologic response. Pharmacol Ther 1982;16:141-166.
13. Holford NHG, Sheiner LG. Understanding the dose-effect relationship: clinical application of pharmacokinetic-pharmacodynamic models. Clin Pharmacokinet 1981;6:429-453.
14. Dutta S, Matsumoto Y, Ebling WF. Is it possible to estimate the parameters of the sigmoid E_{max} model with truncated data typical of clinical studies? J Pharm Sci 1996;85:232-239.

15. Lalonde RL, Straka RJ, Pieper JA, et al. Propranolol pharmacodynamic modeling using unbound and total concentrations in healthy volunteers. J Pharmacokinet Biopharm 1987;15:569-582.
16. Platzer R, Galeazzi RL, Niederberger W, et al. Simultaneous modeling of bopindolol kinetics and dynamics. Clin Pharmacol Ther 1984;36:5-13.
17. Black JW, Leff P. Operational models of pharmacological agonism. Proc R Soc Lond 1983;220 B:141-162.
18. Van der Graaf PH, Van Schaick EA, Mathot RAA, et al. Mechanism-based pharmacokinetic-pharmacodynamic modeling of the effects of N^6-cyclopentyladenosine analogs on heart rate in rat. Estimation of in vivo operational affinity and efficacy at adenosine A_1 receptors. J Pharmacol Exp Ther 1997;283:809-816.
19. Van der Graaf PH, Van Schaick EA, Visser ASG, et al. Mechanism-based pharmacokinetic-pharmacodynamic modeling of antilipolytic affects of adenosine A_1 receptor agonists in rats: prediction of tissue-dependent efficacy in vivo. J Pharmacol Exp Ther 1999;290:702-709.
20. Jonker DM, Kenna LA, Leishman D, et al. A pharmacokinetic-pharmacodynamic model for the quantitative prediction of dofetilide QT prolongation from human ether-a-go-go-related gene current inhibition data. Clin Pharmacol Ther 2005;77:572-582.
21. Levy G. Relationship between rate of elimination of tubocurarine and rate of decline of its pharmacological activity. Br J Anaesth 1964;36:694-695.
22. Levy G. Kinetics of pharmacologic response. Clin Pharmacol Ther 1966;7:362-372.
23. Lalonde RL, Pieper JA, Straka RJ, et al. Pharmacokinetics and pharmacodynamics of propranolol after single doses and at steady state. Eur J Clin Pharmacol 1987;33: 315-318.
24. Van Meyel JJ, Smits P, Russel FG, et al. Diuretic efficiency of furosemide during continuous administration versus bolus injection in healthy volunteers. Clin Pharmacol Ther 1992;51:440-444.
25. Rudy DW, Voelker JR, Greene PK, et al. Loop diuretics for chronic renal insufficiency: a continuous infusion is more efficacious than bolus therapy. Ann Inten Med 1991;115:360-366.
26. Ferguson JA, Sundblad KJ, Becker PK, et al. Role of duration of diuretic effect in preventing sodium retention. Clin Pharmacol Ther 1997;62:203-208.
27. Alvan G, Paintaud G, Wakelkamp M. The efficiency concept in pharmacodynamics. Clin Pharmacokinet 1999;36:375-389.
28. Wagner JG, Aghajanian GK, Bing OH. Correlation of performance test scores with tissue concentration of lysergic acid diethylamide in human subjects. Clin Pharmacol Ther 1968;9:635-638.
29. Kramer WG, Kolibash AJ, Lewis RP, et al. Pharmacokinetics of digoxin: relationship between response intensity and predicted compartmental drug levels in man. J Pharmacokinet Biopharm 1979;7:47-61.
30. Segre G. Kinetics of interaction between drugs and biological systems. II. Farmaco 1968;23:906-918.
31. Sheiner LB, Stanski DR, Vozeh S, et al. Simultaneous modeling of pharmacokinetics and pharmacodynamics: application to D-tubocurarine. Clin Pharmacol Ther 1979; 25:358-371.
32. Zhang L, Beal SL, Sheiner LB. Simultaneous vs. sequential analysis for population PK/PD data I: best-case performance. J Pharmacokinet Pharmacodyn 2003;30:387-404.
33. Zhang L, Beal SL, Sheiner LB. Simultaneous vs. sequential analysis for population PK/PD data II: robustness of methods. J Pharmacokinet Pharmacodyn 2003;30:405-416.
34. Fuseau E, Sheiner LB. Simultaneous modeling of pharmacokinetics and pharmacodynamics with a nonparametric pharmacodynamic model. Clin Pharmacol Ther 1984;35:733-741.
35. Unadkat JD, Bartha F, Sheiner LB. Simultaneous modeling of pharmacokinetics and pharmacodynamics with nonparametric kinetic and dynamic models. Clin Pharmacol Ther 1986;40:86-93.
36. Holford NHG, Peace KE. Results and validation of a population pharmacodynamic model for cognitive effects in Alzheimer patients treated with tacrine. Proc Natl Acad Sci U S A 1992;89:11471-11475.
37. Daneyka NL, Garg V, Jusko WJ: Comparison of four basic models of indirect pharmacologic response. J Pharmacokinet Biopharm 1993;21:457-478.
38. Jusko WJ, Ko HC. Physiologic indirect response models characterize diverse type of pharmacodynamic effects. Clin Pharmacol Ther 1994;56:406-419.
39. Levy G. Mechanism-based pharmacodynamic modeling. Clin Pharmacol Ther 1994; 56:356-358.
40. Sharma A, Jusko WJ. Characterization of four basic models of indirect pharmacodynamic responses. J Pharmacokinet Biopharm 1996;24:611-635.
41. Krzyzanski W, Jusko WJ. Mathematical formalism for the properties of four basic models of indirect pharmacodynamic responses. J Pharmacokinet Biopharm 1997; 25:107-123.
42. Krzyzanski W, Jusko WJ. Indirect pharmacodynamic models for responses with multicompartmental distribution or polyexponential disposition. J Pharmacokinet Pharmacodyn 2001;28:57-78.
43. Verotta D, Sheiner L. A general conceptual model for non-steady state pharmacokinetic/pharmacodynamic data. J Pharmacokinet Biopharm 1995;23:1-4, 9-10.
44. Jusko WJ, Ko HC, Ebling WF. Convergence of direct and indirect pharmacodynamic response models. J Pharmacokinet Biopharm 1995;23:5-8.
45. Sheiner LB, Verotta D. Further notes on physiologic indirect response models. Clin Pharmacol Ther 1995;58:238-240.
46. Kong AN, Ludwig EA, Slaughter RL. Pharmacokinetics and pharmacodynamic modeling of direct suppression effect of methylprednisolone on serum cortisol and blood histamine in human subjects. Clin Pharmacol Ther 1989;46:616-628.
47. Ramakrishnan R, DuBois DC, Almon RR, et al. Fifth-generation model for corticosteroid pharmacodynamics: application to steady-state receptor down-regulation and enzyme induction patterns during seven-day continuous infusion of methylprednisolone in rats. J Pharmacokinet Pharmacodyn 2002;29:1-24.
48. Sun YN, DuBois DC, Almon RR, et al. Fourth generation model for corticosteroid pharmacodynamics: a model for methylprednisolone effects on receptor/gene-mediated glucocorticoid receptoer down-regulation and tyrosine aminotransferase induction in rat liver. J Pharmacokinet Biopharm 1998;26:289-317.
49. Sun YN, Jusko WJ. Transit compartments versus gamma distribution function to model signal transduction in pharmacodynamics. J Pharm Sci 1998;87:732-737.
50. Mager DE, Jusko WJ. Pharmacodynamic modeling of time-dependent transduction systems. Clin Pharmacol Ther 2001;70:210-216.
51. Äbelö A, Eriksson UG, Karlsson MO, et al. A turnover model of the irreversible inhibition of gastric acid secretion by omeprazole in the dog. J Pharmacol Exp Ther 2000;295:662-669.
52. Jusko WJ. Pharmacodynamics of chemotherapeutic effects: dose-time-response relationships for phase-nonspecific agents. J Pharm Sci 1971;60:892-895.
53. Jusko WJ. A pharmacodynamic model for cell-cycle-specific chemotherapeutic agents. J Pharmacokinet Biopharm 1973;1:175-200.
54. Gibaldi M, Perrier D. Pharmacokinetics, 2nd ed. New York: Marcel Dekker, 1982, pp 254-265.
55. Uehlinger DE, Gotch FA, Sheiner LB. A pharmacodynamic model of erythropoietin therapy for uremic anemia. Clin Pharmacol Ther 1992;51:76-89.
56. Krzyzanski W, Ramakrishnan R, Jusko WJ. Basic pharmacodynamic models for agents that alter production of natural cells. J Pharmacokinet Biopharm 1999;27:467-489.
57. Krzyzanski W, Woo S, Jusko WJ. Pharmacodynamic models for agents that alter production of natural cells with various distribution of lifespans. J Pharmacokinet Pharmacodyn 2006;33:125-166.
58. Smolen VR. Theoretical and computational basis for drug bioavailability determinations using pharmacological data 1: general considerations and procedures. J Pharmacokinet Biopharm 1976;4:337-353.
59. Verotta D, Sheiner LB. Semiparametric analysis of non-steady-state pharmacodynamic data. J Pharmacokinet Biopharm 1991;19:691-712.
60. Bragg P, Fisher DM, Shi J, et al. Comparison of twitch depression of the adductor pollicis and the respiratory muscles. Anesthesiology 1994;80:310-319.
61. Gabrielsson J, Jusko WJ, Alari L. Modeling of dose-response-time data: four examples of estimating the turnover parameters and generating kinetic functions from response profiles. Biopharm Drug Dispos 2000;21:41-52.
62. Lalonde RL, Gaudreault J, Karhu DA, et al. Mixed-effects modeling of the pharmacodynamic response to the calcimimetic agent R-568. Clin Pharmacol Ther 1999;65:40-49.
63. Sheiner LB. A new approach to the analysis of analgesic drug trials, illustrated with bromfenac data. Clin Pharmacol Ther 1994;56:309-322.
64. Sheiner LB, Beal SL, Dunne A. Analysis of nonrandomly censored ordered categorical longitudinal data from analgesic trials. J Am Stat Assoc 1997;92:1235-1255.
65. Gupta SK, Sathyan G, Lindemulder EA, et al. Quantitative characterization of therapeutic index: application of mixed-effects modeling to evaluate oxybutynin dose-efficacy and dose-side effect relationships. Clin Pharmacol Ther 1999;65:672-684.
66. Miller R, Frame B, Corrigan BW, et al. Exposure-response analysis of pregabalin add-on treatment of patients with refractory partial seizures. Clin Pharmacol Ther 2003;73:491-505.
67. Cox EH, Veyrat-Follet C, Beal SL, et al. A population pharmacokinetic-pharmacodynamic analysis of repeated measures time-to-event pharmacodynamic responses: the antiemetic effect of ondansetron. J Pharmacokinet Biopharm 1999;27:625-644.
68. Karlsson MO, Schoemaker RC, Kemp B, et al. A pharmacodynamic Markov mixed-effects model for the effect of temazepam on sleep. Clin Pharmacol Ther 200;68:175-188.
69. Mandema JW, Hermann D, Wang W, et al. Model-based development of gemcabene, a new lipid-altering agent. AAPS J 2005;7:E513-E522 (http://www.aapsj.org/).
70. Jonkers R, van Boxtel CJ, Koopmans RP, et al. A nonsteady-state agonist antagonist interaction model using plasma potassium concentrations to quantify the beta-2 selectivity of beta blockers. J Pharmacol Exp Ther 1989;249:297-302.
71. Cleaveland CR, Rangno RE, Shand DG. A standardized isoproterenol sensitivity test. The effects of sinus arrhythmia, atropine and propranolol. Arch Intern Med 1972; 130:47-52.
72. Vestal RE, Wood AJ, Shand DG. Reduced beta-adrenoceptor sensitivity in the elderly. Clin Pharmacol Ther 1979;26:181-186.
73. Tenero DM, Bottorff MB, Burlew BS, et al. Altered beta-adrenergic sensitivity and protein binding to I-propranolol in the elderly. J Cardiovasc Pharmacol 1990;16:702-707.
74. Gardmark M, Brynne L, Hammarlund-Udenaes M, et al. Interchangeability and predictive performance of empirical tolerance models. Clin Pharmacokinet 1999;36:145-167.
75. Girard P, Boissel JP. Clockwise hysteresis or proteresis. J Pharmacokinet Biopharm 1989;17:401-402.
76. Porchet HC, Benowitz NL, Sheiner LB, et al. Apparent tolerance to the acute effect of nicotine: results in part from distribution kinetics. J Clin Invest 1988;244:231-236.
77. Porchet HC, Benowitz NL, Sheiner LB. Pharmacodynamic modeling of tolerance: application to nicotine. J Pharmacol Exp Ther 1988;244:231-236.
78. Wakelkamp M, Alvan G, Gabrielsson J, et al. Pharmacodynamic modeling of furosemide tolerance after multiple intravenous administration. Clin Pharmacol Ther 1996; 60:75-88.
79. Gardmark M, Karlsson MO, Jonsson F, et al. Morphine-3-glucuronide has a minor effect on morphine antiniciception. Pharmacodynamic modeling. J Pharm Sci 1998; 87:813-820.
80. van der Meiracker AH, Man in't Veld AJ, Boomsma F, et al. Hemodynamic and beta-adrenergic receptor adaptation during long-term beta-adrenoceptor blockade. Circulation 1989;80:903-914.

81. Lima JJ, Krukemyer JJ, Boudoulas H. Drug- or hormone-induced adaptation: model of adrenergic hypersensitivity. J Pharmacokinet Biopharm 1989;17:347-364.
82. Chan PLS, Holford NHG. Drug treatment effects on disease progression. Annu Rev Pharmacol Toxicol 2001;41:625-659.
83. Post TM, Freijer JI, DeJongh J, et al. Disease system analysis: basic disease progression models in degenerative disease. Pharm Res 2005;22:1038-1049.
84. Holford NHG, Chan PLS, Nutt JG, et al. Disease progression and pharmacodynamics in Parkinson disease—evidence for functional protection with levodopa and other treatments. J Pharmacokinet Pharmacodyn 2006;33:281-311.
85. de Winter W, DeJongh J, Post T, et al. A mechanism-based disease progression model for comparison of long-term effects of pioglitazone, metformin and gliclazide on disease processes underlying type 2 diabetes mellitus. J Pharmacokinet Pharmacodyn 2006;33:313-343.

15

PHARMACOGENETICS AND PHARMACOGENOMICS

Richard Weinshilboum

INTRODUCTION 219
PHARMACOGENETICS AND PHARMACOGENOMICS: DEVELOPMENT 219
PHARMACOGENOMICS: CLINICAL APPLICATION 220
PHARMACOGENOMICS: BEYOND METABOLISM TO PATHWAYS 222
CONCLUSIONS 223

INTRODUCTION

Pharmacogenetics and pharmacogenomics have developed as a result of the union of two "revolutions." A therapeutic revolution in the development of potent and specific drugs occurred during the latter half of the 20th century and continues in the 21st.[1] At the same time, a genomic revolution occurred and continues to occur at an accelerating pace.[2,3] As a result of the therapeutic revolution—as demonstrated throughout this textbook—diseases that range from childhood leukemia to hypertension and from depression to viral infections have been cured or controlled for the first time in human history. However, because the drugs described in this textbook are both potent and effective, advances in molecular pharmacology require that we develop ways to maximize drug efficacy, to minimize drug toxicity, and to select for therapy only those patients who might respond to a specific drug. A variety of factors that include patient age, sex, underlying disease, and the administration of other drugs can result in variations in drug response. However, during the past half century, it has become clear that inheritance is also an important factor. That realization led to the birth of pharmacogenetics.

The incorporation into pharmacogenetics of the dramatic advances in human genomics that occurred in the late 20th century has resulted in the evolution of pharmacogenetics into pharmacogenomics. Pharmacogenomics has many definitions, but a transition from the study of monogenic to polygenic traits, from individual polymorphisms in a few genes to haplotypes (all of the sequence variation across a gene) as applied within pathways, together with the integration of genomic science into studies of drug response—culminating in genome-wide studies—are hallmarks of that evolutionary process. Pharmacogenetic-pharmacogenomic effects are often classified as those that alter factors that influence the concentration of a drug reaching its target, so-called pharmacokinetic factors, and those that involve the target itself or signaling downstream from the target, so-called pharmacodynamic factors. When a drug is administered, it must be absorbed, distributed to its site of action, interact with its target(s), undergo metabolism, and be excreted. Absorption, distribution, metabolism, and excretion can all influence pharmacokinetics, and it is these processes, especially drug metabolism, that were first studied from a pharmacogenetic perspective. However, it has become clear that genetic variation can also occur in drug targets, or in signaling cascades downstream from those targets; that is, that pharmacodynamics can also be influenced by inheritance, as described subsequently for the anticoagulant drug warfarin.[4-6]

In this chapter, we briefly review the process by which our understanding of pharmacogenetics and pharmacogenomics has developed; beginning with monogenic (mendelian) traits that influence pharmacokinetics. We then highlight an example of pharmacogenomics that involves both pharmacokinetic and pharmacodynamic factors, ending with a brief description of genome-wide approaches currently being applied to pharmacogenetics and pharmacogenomics. We also mention the integration of pharmacogenetics and pharmacogenomics into regulatory science and challenges associated with "translating" this science into the clinic to help individualize drug therapy. Therefore, the subsequent discussion begins with a brief description of the development of pharmacogenetics and pharmacogenomics and its initial focus on simple monogenic traits, most often traits involving drug metabolism; then moves to polygenic traits that involve both pharmacokinetic and pharmacodynamic factors; and ends with a brief description of recent attempts to use genome-wide techniques to study the contribution of inheritance to drug response. The importance of the pharmaceutical and biotechnology industries and of regulatory agencies such as the U.S. Food and Drug Administration (FDA) in the translation of pharmacogenetics and pharmacogenomics into the clinic are also mentioned.[7]

Pharmacogenetics and pharmacogenomics involve study of the role of inheritance in individual variation in drug response.[8] Therefore, pharmacogenetics and pharmacogenomics represent an important aspect of our attempt to "individualize" drug therapy. Drug response phenotypes can vary from potentially life-threatening adverse drug reactions at one end of the spectrum to equally serious lack of therapeutic efficacy at the other. Obviously, it is important to avoid both ends of this spectrum. Pharmacogenetic studies began half a century ago with a focus on relatively simple monogenic, mendelian traits, often involving inherited variation in drug metabolism.[9] That variation resulted in either lack of the desired drug effect or the occurrence of adverse drug reactions. Recent studies have increasingly addressed variation in genes encoding entire "pathways" of proteins that influence both pharmacokinetics—factors that determine the concentration of drug reaching its target(s)—and pharmacodynamics, the drug target itself and signaling downstream from the target.[8] Experimental approaches that survey the entire genome are also being applied in an attempt to understand inherited variation in drug response. As a result, pharmacogenetics has gradually evolved into pharmacogenomics with the convergence of advances in molecular pharmacology and equally rapid advances in genomic science. Today, pharmacogenomics is already being used in the clinic to individualize drug therapy, and it is also being incorporated into the drug development process as well as governmental regulation of drug use.

PHARMACOGENETICS AND PHARMACOGENOMICS: DEVELOPMENT

The conceptual basis for pharmacogenomics can be traced to Sir Archeobald Garrod's "Inborne Factors in Disease," in which he speculated that inheritance might alter drug response.[10] That speculation took on practical reality in the 1950s and 1960s when a series of monogenic traits—traits associated with inherited variation in drug

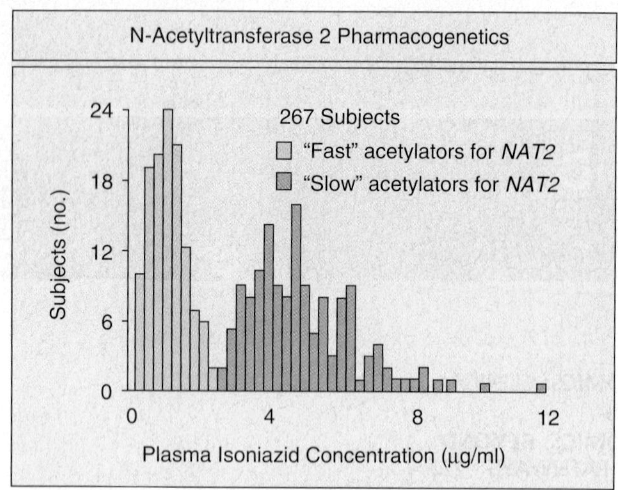

FIGURE 15-1 • *N*-Acetyltransferase 2 pharmacogenetics. Plasma concentrations of isoniazid in 267 subjects 6 hours after the administration of an identical oral dose of the drug. (Modified from Price Evans DA, Manley KA, McKusick VA: Genetic control of isoniazid metabolism in man. Br Med J 1960;2:485-491.)

metabolism—were reported. Those examples began with the observation of striking differences among patients in their response to "standard" drug doses, often coupled with large variations in plasma or urinary drug or drug metabolite concentrations. Two classic examples involved inherited variation in the enzymatic hydrolysis of the short-acting muscle relaxant succinylcholine in a reaction catalyzed by the enzyme butyrylcholinesterase (BCHE; pseudocholinesterase)[9,11] and the enzymatic acetylation of drugs such as the antituberculosis drug isoniazid.[12] Both of these examples behaved as monogenic traits, both involved pharmacokinetic variation, variation due to inherited differences in drug metabolism, and both were due to genetic variation in the enzyme catalyzing the reaction.

Isoniazid was one of the first effective antituberculosis drugs.[13] Plasma concentrations of isoniazid showed a "biomodal" frequency distribution after the administration of identical doses of drug to large numbers of subjects (Fig. 15-1).[12] This trait was shown by segregation analysis to be inherited and to result from genetic variation in metabolism, in this case, *N*-acetylation catalyzed by the enzyme *N*-acetyltransferase 2 (NAT2). We now know that the bimodal frequency distribution shown in Figure 15-1 is due to genetic polymorphisms in the *NAT2* gene, polymorphisms that influence the pharmacokinetics of drugs as disparate as isoniazid, the antihypertensive agent hydralazine, and the antiarrhythmic drug procainamide.[14,15] Subjects who are genetically "slow" acetylators for hydralazine and procainamide have increased risk for the occurrence of autoimmune disorders after exposure to these drugs.[16,17] Isoniazid continues to be used to treat tuberculosis, and hydralazine, although used only rarely to treat hypertension other than in patients with preeclampsia,[18] has recently reemerged as one of two active ingredients, together with isosorbide dinitrate, in BiDil.[19] BiDil is a combination drug recently approved for the treatment of patients with serious congestive heart failure. However, the FDA approved BiDil only for use in patients of African ancestry,[20] presumably because of an ethnic-dependent genetic difference in drug response.

At the same time that early examples of monogenic variation in drug response such as those represented by isoniazid *N*-acetylation and succinylcholine hydrolysis were discovered, it was also demonstrated that plasma drug half-life values in monozygotic and dizygotic twin pairs could demonstrate a high degree of heritability.[21] All of these observations served as a stimulus for the discovery of many additional examples of pharmacogenetics, most often involving drug metabolism, in the second half of the 20th century. Those examples continued to originate mainly from clinical observations, and they were often studied by either administering a "probe drug" to a group of subjects and measuring plasma and/or urinary drug or metabolite concentrations or by directly assaying a drug-metabolizing enzyme activity in an easily accessible tissue source such as the red blood cell (RBC) (e.g., a series of methyltransferase enzymes). This overall approach involved the application of the only research strategy available at that time, a phenotype-to-genotype approach analogous to the strategy applied throughout human genetics at that time. Two "prototypic" examples of that era, examples that have become "icons" of pharmacogenetics—both of which also bridge the transition from biochemical to molecular pharmacogenetics and both of which are widely applied clinically today—are the cytochrome P450 2D6 (*CYP2D6*) and the thiopurine *S*-methyltransferase (*TPMT*) genetic polymorphisms. Once again, both of these genetic polymorphisms involved drug metabolism.

PHARMACOGENOMICS: CLINICAL APPLICATION

The *CYP2D6* and *TPMT* genetic polymorphisms, one involving a gene encoding a phase I and the other a phase II drug-metabolizing enzyme, serve to illustrate the importance of monogenic, Mendelian traits in our evolving appreciation of the role of inheritance in individual variation in drug response phenotypes. Both of these examples have recently been the subject of FDA public hearings on pharmacogenetics (see http://www.fda.gov); as a result, pharmacogenetic information for these enzymes has now been incorporated into drug labeling. In addition, testing for these two pharmacogenetic traits is widely available and is being applied clinically. As described in detail elsewhere in this volume, the cytochromes P-450 (CYPs) are a family of microsomal drug-metabolizing enzymes, and CYP2D6 is the member of that family that has been studied most intensively from a pharmacogenomic perspective. Probe drugs were used extensively to study *CYP2D6* genetic variation. As mentioned previously, probe drugs are substrates for the enzyme of interest that are administered to a large number of subjects, and urinary or blood drug or metabolite concentrations are measured as "markers" for genetic variation in drug metabolism and effect. A drug that has been used widely for that purpose with *CYP2D6* is the antihypertensive agent debrisoquine.[22] The frequency distribution of debrisoquine *metabolic ratio*, the ratio of the parent drug to oxidized metabolite, is shown in Figure 15-2A.[23] This frequency distribution includes a group of debrisoquine *poor metabolizers (PMs)*, shown, counterintuitively, at the far right of the figure; a group of *extensive metabolizers (EMs)*; and a small group of *ultrarapid metabolizers (UMs)*, some of whom have been shown to have multiple copies of the *CYP2D6* gene.[24]

CYP2D6 catalyzes the biotransformation of scores of drugs, including tricyclic antidepressants such as nortriptyline and antihypertensive β-adrenoceptor blockers such as metoprolol.[25] *CYP2D6* is also required to metabolically activate the prodrug codeine to form its active analgesic metabolite morphine.[26,27] Therefore, *CYP2D6* PMs have excessive drug effect when treated with standard doses of drugs such as metoprolol that are inactivated by this enzyme, whereas codeine is relatively ineffective in PMs because it requires *CYP2D6*-catalyzed metabolism to form its active metabolite morphine. Conversely, UM subjects display an inadequate therapeutic response after treatment with standard doses of drugs inactivated by *CYP2D6*, but those subjects can be "overdosed" with codeine.[28] This latter situation has resulted in respiratory arrest after treatment with standard cough-suppressant doses of codeine.[28] Equally dramatic is the relative lack of therapeutic efficacy for the estrogen receptor antagonist tamoxifen in women with breast cancer who are *CYP2D6* PMs. Tamoxifen, like codeine, is a prodrug. The parent drug is a poor estrogen receptor antagonist and requires *CYP2D6*-catalyzed hydroxylation to form a metabolite that is a potent estrogen receptor antagonist.[29] Women who are *CYP2D6* PMs have an increased incidence of breast cancer recurrence when treated with tamoxifen.[29] Table 15-1 lists selected examples of clinically relevant applications of pharmacogenetics, including the role of *CYP2D6* in codeine and tamoxifen clinical effect.

The cloning and characterization of the *CYP2D6* cDNA and gene made it possible to determine molecular mechanisms responsible for

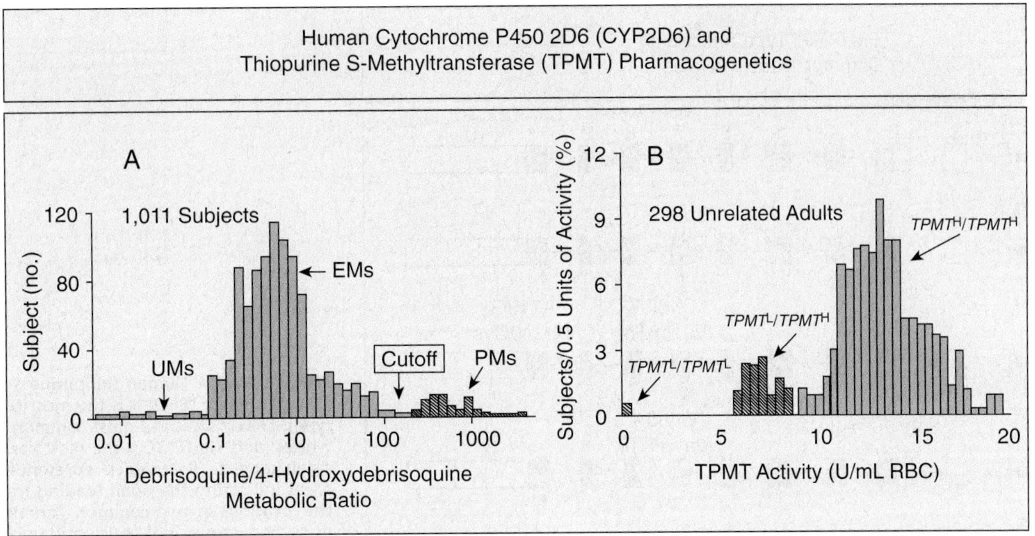

FIGURE 15-2 • A, Cytochrome P450 (CYP) 2D6 pharmacogenetics. B, Thiopurine *S*-methyltransferase (TPMT) pharmacogenetics. A, The ratio of urinary debrisoquine to its metabolite 4-hydroxydebrisoquine in 1011 Swedish subjects. "Cutoff" is the demarcation between poor metabolizers (PMs) and extensive metabolizers (EMs). UM, ultrarapid metabolizer. **B,** Red blood cell (RBC) TPMT activity in 298 randomly selected white subjects. Presumed genotypes for the TPMT genetic polymorphism are also shown. $TPMT^L$ and $TPMT^H$ ("low" and "high," respectively) were allele designations used before the molecular basis of the TPMT polymorphism was established. (**A,** Modified from Bertilsson L, Lou YQ, Du YL, et al. Pronounced differences between native Chinese and Swedish populations in the polymorphic hydroxylations of debrisoquin and S-mephenytoin. Clin Pharmacol Ther 1992;51:388-397 [published erratum appears in Clin Pharmacol Ther 1994;55:648]. **B,** Modified from Weinshilboum RM, Sladek SL. Mercaptopurine pharmacogenetics: monogenic inheritance of erythrocyte thiopurine methyltransferase activity. Am J Hum Genet 1980;32:651-662.)

TABLE 15-1 CLINICAL APPLICATIONS OF PHARMACOGENOMICS

Gene(s)*	Drug Examples	Clinical Effect
CYP2D6	Codeine	PMs: lack of analgesia UMs: excessive morphine effect
	Tamoxifen†	PMs: lack of therapeutic efficacy
TPMT	6-Mercaptopurine†	TPMT*3A homozygotes: profound myelosuppression
	Azathioprine†	TPMT*3A homozygotes: profound myelosuppression
UGT1A1	Irinotecan†	UGT1A1*28 homozygotes: severe diarrhea and myelosuppression
CYP2C9 *VKORC1*	Warfarin†	Hemorrhage risk

*Genes encoding genetically polymorphic enzymes (CYP2D6, TPMT, UGT1A1, and CYP2C9) and drug targets (VKORC1) are listed.
†The U.S. Food and Drug Administration (FDA) has held public hearings with regard to the inclusion of pharmacogenomic information in labeling for the drug indicated.
CYP, cytochrome P; PMs, poor metabolizers; TMPT, thiopurine *S*-methyltransferase; UMs, ultrarapid metabolizers; VKORC1, vitamin K epoxide reductase complex 1.

genetic variation in *CYP2D6*-catalyzed drug metabolism. Those mechanisms include nonsynonymous single nucleotide polymorphisms (SNPs) that alter the encoded amino acid sequence and are associated with decreased enzyme activity, gene deletion, and—as mentioned previously—gene duplications in UMs, with some subjects having up to 13 active copies of this gene.[24] Although *CYP2D6* duplication occurs relatively infrequently among Northern Europeans, in East Africa the frequency of alleles with *CYP2D6* duplication can be as high as 29%.[30] Another clinically important example of pharmacogenetics that developed in parallel with *CYP2D6* was that involving TPMT, a phase II drug-metabolizing enzyme.

TPMT catalyzes the *S*-methylation of thiopurine drugs such as 6-mercaptopurine and azathioprine.[31] These cytotoxic and immunosuppressive drugs are used to treat acute lymphoblastic leukemia of childhood, inflammatory bowel disease, and organ transplant recipients.[32] Although thiopurines are very useful drugs, they have a narrow therapeutic index (i.e., the difference between the dose of drug required to achieve the desired therapeutic effect and that causing toxicity is relatively small). The most serious thiopurine-induced toxicity is life-threatening myelosuppression (bone marrow suppression).[32] The most common variant allele for *TPMT* in whites, with a frequency of approximately 5%, is *TPMT*3A*, an allele predominantly responsible for the trimodal frequency distribution of level of RBC TPMT activity that is shown in Figure 15-2B.[33,34] The level of TPMT activity in the RBC reflects the relative level of this drug-metabolizing enzyme activity in other human tissues.[31] The gene encoding *TPMT*3A* has two nonsynonymous SNPs, one in exon 7 and another in exon 10 (Fig. 15-3). As just mentioned for *CYP2D6*, there are also striking ethnic differences in frequencies of *TPMT* variant alleles. For example, *TPMT*3A* is rarely, if ever, observed in East Asian populations, but *TPMT*3C*, with only the exon 10 SNP (see Fig. 15-3) and with less dramatic functional consequences, is the most common variant allele in East Asia, with a frequency of approximately 2%.[31,35] Subjects homozygous for *TPMT*3A* are at greatly increased risk for life-threatening myelosuppression when treated with standard doses of thiopurine drugs because they are unable to metabolize these drugs by *S*-methylation; so they are "overdosed" at standard doses (see Table 15-1).[35] These patients can be treated with approximately one tenth to one fifteenth the standard dose, but even then, they require careful monitoring to avoid life-threatening myelosuppression. Because of its clinical importance, TPMT was the first example selected by the FDA for public hearings on the inclusion of pharmacogenetic information in drug labeling. For the same reason, testing for common TPMT genetic polymorphisms is widely applied clinically. TPMT has also served as a "model system" to help us understand how the inherited alteration in only two amino acids (see Fig. 15-3) in this enzyme can result in a virtual lack of TPMT protein in human tissues. In this case—and in many other examples—the variant protein is made, but it is rapidly degraded through a ubiquitin-proteasome–mediated process.[31,36,37]

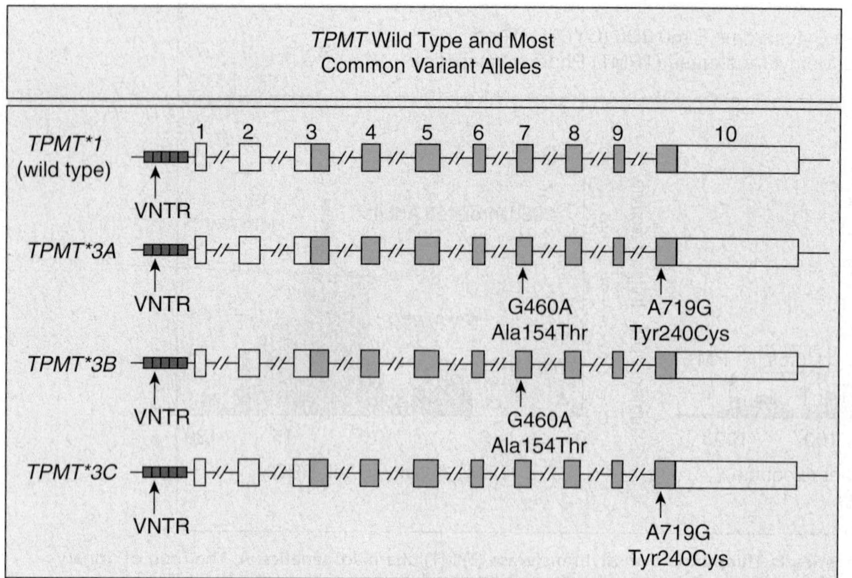

FIGURE 15-3 • Human thiopurine *S*-methyltransferase (TPMT) alleles. TPMT*1 is the most common allele (wild-type); TPMT*3A is the most common variant allele in whites; and TPMT*3C is the most variant allele in East Asian subjects. *Rectangles* represent exons, with *dark areas* indicating the open reading frame. *Arrows* indicate the locations of two common, functionally significant nonsynonymous single nucleotide polymorphisms (SNPs) as well as a 5′-flanking region variable number of tandem repeats (VNTR).

Other phase II, conjugating drug-metabolizing enzymes also display common, clinically relevant pharmacogenetic variation. For example, the second drug for which the FDA held public hearings on pharmacogenetics was the anticancer agent irinotecan. There is a common, functionally significant variable number of tandem repeats in the "TATA box" of the *UGT1A1* gene. Subjects with seven rather than six of these TA repeats have decreased ability to drive *UGT1A1* transcription.[38] This is a common variant, so approximately 10% to 15% of white subjects are homozygous for the 7 TA variant (*UGT1A1*28*) associated with decreased transcription.[38] Because *UGT1A1* catalyzes the glucuronidation of bilirubin, these subjects have mild unconjugated hyperbilirubinemia—a generally benign condition referred to medically as *Gilbert's syndrome.* However, if they are treated with standard doses of irinotecan, these subjects will be overdosed and are at increased risk for the development of serious diarrhea and myelosuppression (see Table 15-1).[39] Clinical testing for the *UGT1A1*28* variant allele, like that for the *TPMT*3A* variant allele, is now increasingly available in clinical settings.

TPMT, CYP2D6, and *UGT1A1* all represent examples of the potentially important role of genetic variation in individual differences in drug metabolism and drug effect. *CYP2D6* and *TPMT* have been studied intensively for decades, so their clinical consequences and the underlying molecular mechanisms responsible are well understood. Another, much more recent example of the clinical importance of pharmacogenetics involves the widely used anticoagulant drug warfarin. Warfarin is a valuable and effective drug, but like the thiopurines, it has a narrow therapeutic index. Warfarin pharmacogenomics illustrates the expansion of this discipline beyond genetic variation in drug metabolism to include variation in the drug target, pharmacodynamics, and demonstrates that more than one gene can be involved in altering the effect of a single drug.

PHARMACOGENETICS: BEYOND METABOLISM TO PATHWAYS

Warfarin is the most widely prescribed oral anticoagulant in North America and in many European countries.[4] In the United States, more than 20 million prescriptions are written for warfarin each year.[4] However, in spite of the availability of a laboratory test (the International Normalized Ratio [INR]) that is used universally to follow its effect on coagulation, serious adverse reactions—involving both hemorrhage and coagulation—continue to complicate warfarin therapy. Warfarin is a racemic mixture, and "S-warfarin" is three to five times more potent than "R-warfarin" as an anticoagulant, has a shorter half-life, and is metabolized predominantly by a genetically polymorphic CYP isoform, CYP2C9. Two common *CYP2C9* nonsynonymous SNPs are associated with striking reductions in the level of enzyme activity as compared with the wild-type *CYP2C9* allele.[40] It has been known since the mid 1990s that patients who required a "low" dose of warfarin after dosage adjustment based on INR values more often carried one or more of the common *CYP2C9* variant alleles than randomly selected subjects did. Those subjects also had an increased risk of hemorrhage during warfarin therapy.[40] However, these pharmacokinetic-pharmacogenetic observations failed to explain most of the variation in final dose of warfarin in patients anticoagulated with this important but potentially dangerous drug. Therefore, when the molecular target for coumadin-based anticoagulant drugs such as warfarin was identified in 2004,[41,42] the gene encoding that target, vitamin K epoxide reductase complex 1 (*VKORC1*), was resequenced, and variant haplotypes for the gene were evaluated for their possible effect on warfarin anticoagulation. Those studies showed that genetic variation in *VKORC1* also played an important role in variation in drug response. A series of studies showed from 30% to 50% of the total variation in final warfarin dose could be predicted by genotyping for *CYP2C9* and *VKORC1* (Table 15-2).[4-6] It should be emphasized that inheritance is not the only factor responsible for differences among patients in warfarin response, because age and the intake of food containing vitamin K (e.g., green leafy vegetables) also contributes to that variation. The current status of warfarin pharmacogenomics is illustrated schematically in Figure 15-4, which shows that both pharmacokinetic (*CYP2C9*) and pharmacodynamic (*VKORC1*) pharmacogenomics contribute to individual differences in the warfarin anticoagulant response. The example presented by warfarin represents an evolving model of polygenic pharmacogenomics that will probably be observed with increasing frequency in the future.

TABLE 15-2 WARFARIN PHARMACOGENOMICS*

Study	*VKORC1*	*CYP2C9*
Wadelius et al, 2005[6]	~30%	~12%
Rieder et al, 2005[4]	~25%	~6%-10%
Sconce et al, 2005[5]	~15%	~18%

*The proportion of variance in warfarin dose accounted for by single nucleotide polymorphisms (SNPs) or haplotypes in vitamin K epoxide reductase complex 1 (*VKORC1*) or cytochrome P450 2C9 (*CYP2C9*).

As the focus of pharmacogenomics moves to "pathways" that include genes encoding drug-metabolizing enzymes and transporters that might influence the final concentration of a drug that reaches its

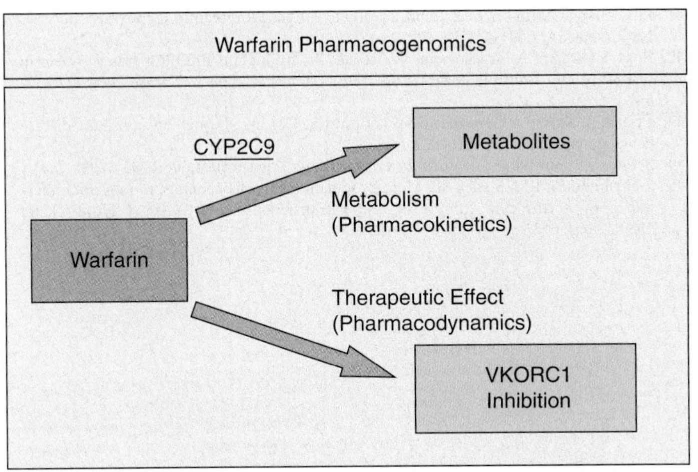

FIGURE 15-4 • Warfarin pharmacogenomics. Schematic representation of pharmacokinetic (CYP2C9-dependent) and pharmacodynamic (VKORC1-dependent) pharmacogenomic factors that influence final warfarin dose. (From Weinshilboum RM, Wang L. Pharmacogenetics and pharmacogenomics: development, science, and translation. Annu Rev Genomics Hum Genet 2006;7:223-245.)

target(s)—together with genes encoding the drug target and proteins involved in signaling cascades downstream from that target—the relatively "simple" examples represented by *CYP2D6* and *TPMT* will probably prove to be relatively unusual. In addition, the application of new research techniques such as "genome-wide association studies" will make it possible to query the entire range of genetic variation across the entire human genome that contributes to individual variation in drug response phenotypes.[43] Finally, as the clinical importance of pharmacogenomics is demonstrated by *CYP2D6, TPMT, UGT1A1, CYP2C9,* and *VKORC1*—and many other examples—pharmacogenomics is increasingly being incorporated into drug development and the actions of regulatory agencies such as the FDA. In addition, the pharmaceutical and biotechnology industry is also slowly moving away from the "blockbuster" drug, "one size fits all,"[44] mentality to incorporate pharmacogenomics into their business models.

CONCLUSIONS

Pharmacogenetics and pharmacogenomics represent an important aspect of the movement toward more highly individualized medicine—in this case, individualized drug selection and dosing. Although a variety of factors other than inheritance result in differences among patients in their response to drug therapy, the past half century has produced overwhelming evidence that genetics is an important factor responsible for variation in the occurrence of adverse drug reactions or the failure of individual patients to achieve the desired therapeutic response when treated with "standard" doses of a drug. Striking examples such as those represented by monogenic traits such as *CYP2D6* and *TPMT* illustrated the potential importance of inheritance for variation in drug response. However, warfarin pharmacogenomics represents an example of the effects of multiple genes that will probably be discovered with increasing frequency to influence variation in response to most drugs. In the future, as increasingly rich genomic information becomes available to physicians, a major challenge will be the integration of that information into evidence-based approaches that will make it possible to move toward the goal of truly individualized drug therapy.

REFERENCES

1. Weinshilboum RM, Wang L. Pharmacogenetics and pharmacogenomics: development, science, and translation. Annu Rev Genomics Hum Genet 2006;7:223-245.
2. Kalow W. Pharmacogenetics: Heredity and the Response to Drugs. Philadelphia, London: WB Saunders, 1962.
3. Weinshilboum RM. The therapeutic revolution. Clin Pharmacol Ther 1987;42:481-484.
4. Lander ES, Linton LM, Birren B, et al. Initial sequencing and analysis of the human genome. Nature 2001;409:860-921 [published errata appears in Nature 2001;411:720; 412:565].
5. Venter JC, Adams MD, Myers EW, et al. The sequence of the human genome. Science 2001;291:1304-1351 [published errata appears in Science 2001;292:1838].
6. Rieder MJ, Reiner AP, Gage BF, et al. Effect of VKORC1 haplotypes on transcriptional regulation and warfarin dose. N Engl J Med 2005;352:2285-2293.
7. Sconce EA, Khan TI, Wynne HA, et al. The impact of CYP2C9 and VKORC1 genetic polymorphism and patient characteristics upon warfarin dose requirements: proposal for a new dosing regimen. Blood 2005;106:2329-2333.
8. Wadelius M, Chen LY, Downes K, et al. Common VKORC1 and GGCX polymorphisms associated with warfarin dose. Pharmacogenomics J 2005;5:262-270.
9. U.S. Department of Health and Human Services, Food and Drug Administration, Center for Drug Evaluation and Research, Center for Biologics Evaluation and Research, Center for Devices and Radiological Health. "Draft" Guidance for Industry: Pharmacogenomics Data Submissions. In November 2003.
10. Scriver CR, Childs B. Garrod's Inborn Factors in Disease. New York: Oxford University Press, 1989.
11. Kalow W, Gunn DR. The relationship between dose of succinylcholine and duration of apnea in man. J Pharmacol Exp Ther 1957;120:203-214.
12. Price Evans DA, Manley KA, McKusick VA. Genetic control of isoniazid metabolism in man. Br Med J 1960;2:485-491.
13. Weber WW. The Acetylator Genes and Drug Response. New York: Oxford University Press, 1987.
14. Reidenberg MM, Drayer DE, Levy M, Warner H. Polymorphic acetylation of procainamide in man. Clin Pharmacol Ther 1975;17:722-730.
15. Timbrell JA, Harland SJ, Facchini V. Polymorphic acetylation of hydralazine. Clin Pharmacol Ther 1980;28:350-355.
16. Perry HM Jr, Tan EM, Carmody S, Sakamoto A. Relationship of acetyl transferase activity to antinuclear antibodies and toxic symptoms in hypertensive patients treated with hydralazine. J Lab Clin Med 1970;76:114-125.
17. Woosley RL, Drayer DE, Reidenberg MM, et al. Effect of acetylator phenotype on the rate at which procainamide induces antinuclear and the lupus syndrome. N Engl J Med 1978;298:1157-1159.
18. Belfort MA, Anthony J, Saade GR, et al. A comparison of magnesium sulfate and nimodipine for the prevention of eclampsia. N Engl J Med 2003;348:304-311.
19. Taylor AL, Ziesche S, Yancy C, et al. A-AHFT: combination of isosorbide dinitrate and hydralazine in blacks with heart failure. N Engl J Med 2004;351:2049-2057.
20. Branca MA. BiDil raises questions about race as a marker. Nat Rev Drug Discov 2005;4:615-616.
21. Vesell ES, Page JG. Genetic control of drug levels in man: antipyrine. Science 1968;161:72-73.
22. Mahgoub A, Idle JR, Dring LG, et al. Polymorphic hydroxylation of debrisoquine in man. Lancet 1977;2:584-586.
23. Bertilsson L, Lou YQ, Du YL, et al. Pronounced differences between native Chinese and Swedish populations in the polymorphic hydroxylations of debrisoquin and *S*-mephenytoin. Clin Pharmacol Ther 1992;51:388-397 [published erratum appears in Clin Pharmacol Ther 1994;55:648].
24. Johansson I, Lundqvist E, Bertilsson L, et al. Inherited amplification of an active gene in the cytochrome P450 CYP2D locus as a cause of ultrarapid metabolism of debrisoquine. Proc Natl Acad Sci U S A 1993;90:11825-11829.
25. Kroemer HK, Eichelbaum M. "It's the genes, stupid." Molecular bases and clinical consequences of genetic cytochrome P450 2D6 polymorphism. Life Sci 1995;56:2285-2298.
26. Mortimer O, Persson K, Ladona MG, et al. Polymorphic formation of morphine from codeine in poor and extensive metabolizers of dextromethorphan: relationship to the presence of immunoidentified cytochrome P-450IID1. Clin Pharmacol Ther 1990;47:27-35.
27. Sindrup SH, Brosen K. The pharmacogenetics of codeine hypoalgesia. Pharmacogenetics 1995;5:335-346.
28. Gasche Y, Daali Y, Fathi M, et al. Codeine intoxication associated with ultrarapid CYP2D6 metabolism. N Engl J Med 2004;351:2827-2831.
29. Goetz MP, Knox SK, Suman VJ, et al. The impact of cytochrome P450 2D6 metabolism in women receiving adjuvant tamoxifen. Breast Cancer Res Treat 2007;101:113-121.
30. Aklillu E, Persson I, Bertilsson L, et al. Frequent distribution of ultrarapid metabolizers of debrisoquine in the Ethiopian population carrying duplicated and multiduplicated functional CYP2D6 alleles. J Pharmacol Exp Ther 1996;278:441-446.
31. Wang L, Weinshilboum RM. Thiopurine *S*-methyltransferase (TPMT) pharmacogenetics: insights, challenges and future directions. Oncogene Rev 2006;25:1629-1938.
32. Lennard L. The clinical pharmacology of 6-mercaptopurine. Eur J Clin Pharmacol 1992;43:329-339.
33. Szumlanski C, Otterness D, Her C, et al. Thiopurine methyltransferase pharmacogenetics: human gene cloning and characterization of a common polymorphism. DNA Cell Biol 1996;15:17-30.
34. Tai H-L, Krynetski EY, Yates CR, et al. Thiopurine *S*-methyltransferase deficiency: two nucleotide transitions define the most prevalent mutant allele associated with loss of catalytic activity in Caucasians. Am J Hum Genet 1996;58:694-702.
35. Collie-Duguid ESR, Pritchard SC, Powrie RH, et al. The frequency and distribution of thiopurine methyltransferase alleles in Caucasian and Asian populations. Pharmacogenetics 1998;9:37-42.
36. Tai H-L, Krynetski EY, Schuetz EG, et al. Enhanced proteolysis of thiopurine *S*-methyltransferase (TPMT) encoded by mutant alleles in humans (TPMT*3A, TPMT*2): mechanisms for the genetic polymorphism of TPMT activity. Proc Natl Acad Sci U S A 1997;94:6444-6449.

37. Wang L, Sullivan W, Toft D, Weinshilboum R. Thiopurine *S*-methyltransferase pharmacogenetics: chaperone protein association and allozyme degradation. Pharmacogenetics 2003;13:555-564.
38. Bosma PJ, Chowdhury JR, Bakker C, et al. The genetic basis of the reduced expression of bilirubin UDP-glucuronosyltransferase 1 in Gilbert's syndrome. N Engl J Med 1995;333:1171-1175.
39. Iyer L, Das S, Janisch L, et al. UGT1A1*28 polymorphism as a determinant of irinotecan disposition and toxicity. Pharmacogenomics J 2002;2:43-47.
40. Aithal GP, Day CP, Kesteven PJ, Daly AK. Association of polymorphisms in the cytochrome P450 CYP2C9 with warfarin dose requirement and risk of bleeding complications. Lancet 1999;353:717-719.
41. Li T, Chang CY, Jin DY, et al. Identification of the gene for vitamin K epoxide reductase. Nature 2004;427:541-544.
42. Rost S, Fregin A, Ivaskevicius V, et al. Mutations in VKORC1 cause warfarin resistance and multiple coagulation factor deficiency type 2. Nature 2004;427:537-541.
43. Couzin J, Kaiser J. Genome-wide association. Closing the net on common disease genes. Science 2007;316:820-822.
44. Service RF. Surviving the blockbuster syndrome. Science 2004;303:1796-1799.
45. Weinshilboum RM, Sladek SL. Mercaptopurine pharmacogenetics: monogenic inheritance of erythrocyte thiopurine methyltransferase activity. Am J Hum Genet 1980;32:651-662.

16

HETEROGENEITY OF DRUG RESPONSES AND INDIVIDUALIZATION OF THERAPY*

Julia Kirchheiner and Matthias Schwab

INTRODUCTION 225
GENETIC VARIABILITY AND CONSEQUENCES FOR DRUG RESPONSE AND SAFETY 226
Genetic Polymorphisms on the Pharmacokinetic Part of Drug Action 226
Genetic Polymorphisms on the Pharmacodynamic Part of Drug Action 227
GENOTYPE-BASED DOSING 228
Limitations of Pharmacogenetic Dose Adjustments 229
CLINICAL IMPLICATIONS OF PHARMACOGENETIC TESTING 229
Depression 229
Cardiovascular Disease 230
β-Blockers 230
Vitamin K Antagonists 230
Ulcer Disease and Proton Pump Inhibitors 231
Pain Treatment: NSAIDs 231
Malignant Diseases 231
Tamoxifen 231
Thiopurines 232
5-Fluorouracil 233
Irinotecan 233
PHARMACOGENETIC STUDY DESIGNS 234
CONCLUSION 234

INTRODUCTION

The response of individual patients to the same drug given in the same dose varies considerably for many substances. Many patients will experience the desired drug effect, some may suffer from well-known adverse drug reactions, others may experience no effects, and very rarely, a patient will die from severe side effects. It is currently difficult for physicians to prescribe the optimal drug in the optimal dose for each patient, because prediction of a patient's response to any one specific drug is rarely possible. For instance, according to a study on the incidence of adverse drug effects in hospitalized patients, about 6.7% of all hospitalizations are due to severe adverse drug reactions (ADRs); 0.37% end in death.[1] ADRs are the fifth leading cause of death in the United States, directly after coronary heart disease, cancer, stroke, and lung diseases and even before accidents, diabetes mellitus, and pneumonia. The ADR-related costs are estimated between $1.4 billion and $4 billion in the United States per year.[1] For Europe, similar data are published,[2] and more recently, the burden of ADRs was investigated in a prospective analysis of 18,820 patients aged 16 years and older admitted over 6 months to two large general hospitals in Merseyside, U.K.[3] The prevalence was 6.5%, with the ADRs directly leading to the admission in 80% of cases. The overall fatality was 0.15%.

To understand why individual patients respond differently to drugs, it is helpful to envisage the progress of a particular drug from its administration to its observed effect. The effect of a drug will depend first on its systemic concentration and its concentration at the drug target. The systemic concentration of a drug depends on several pharmacokinetic factors, commonly referred to by the acronym ADME (drug absorption, distribution, metabolism, and elimination). It has long been known that a wide variety of individual patient factors may influence the pharmacokinetics of a drug and must, therefore, be taken into account when determining dosage for a given patient. Drug concentration at its target will, in many cases, represent a mere fraction of the systemic concentration. Active transport processes, however, may influence local target concentrations; for example, the blood-brain barrier is an important determinant of drug concentration in the cerebrospinal fluid. It has become increasingly clear that hereditary variances in drug-metabolizing enzymes and drug transporters can exert considerable influence on drug concentrations. However, in addition to inherited variants, many other factors (e.g., age, sex, weight, body fat, alcohol consumption, concomitant drugs, nutritional status, liver and renal function, cardiovascular function, and environmental pollutants) are known to influence the pharmacokinetics of drugs.

The second crucial determinant of an observed drug effect is the response of the drug target to a given drug concentration. Differences in activity or gene expression, sometimes caused by hereditary variants, have been discovered and characterized in receptors, drug transporters, ion channels, lipoproteins, coagulation factors, and many other factors involved in immune response, cell development, cell cycle control, and other functions that significantly influence the manifestation and course of diseases. Many of these polymorphic structures are at the same time targets of specific drugs and can thus potentially influence the effect specific drug concentration will exert at the drug target.

The individual reaction toward a given drug varies a lot between the individuals and may depend on many factors such as age, sex, weight, body fat, concomitant drugs, nutritional status, and liver and renal function. However, for many drugs, pharmacogenetic polymorphisms are known to affect biotransformation and clinical outcome. This chapter focuses on the clinical importance of this inherited variability in drug response, which depends on allele frequency and the effect size of the clinical outcome parameters. Further, it depends on the therapeutic range of the drug that is affected, on predictability of drug response, and on duration until onset of therapeutic efficacy. Consequences arising from genotyping might include adjustment of dose according to genotype, choice of therapeutic strategy, or even choice of drug. Clinical application of pharmacogenetics is first used within the field of cancer therapy and antidepressant drug treatment. Thiopurines are catalyzed by the polymorphically expressed enzyme thiopurine *S*-methyltransferase (TPMT), leading to exaggerated high levels of active metabolites and subsequent pancytopenia in cases of TPMT deficiency and standard dosage. Tamoxifen, which is widely used for treatment of breast cancer, is metabolized via the polymorphic cytochrome P-450 (CYP) enzymes CYP2D6; evidence suggests that therapeutic efficacy of tamoxifen depends strongly on pharmacogenetics. Moreover, pharmacokinetics of many tricyclic antidepressant drugs (TCAs), some selective serotonin reuptake inhibitors (SSRIs), and other antidepressant drugs is significantly altered by genetic polymorphisms. However, controversy still exists on whether therapeutic

*This manuscript is supported by the Robert-Bosch Foundation, Stuttgart, Germany.

efficacy may be improved and/or adverse events can be prevented by genetically driven adjustment of drug dosage.

Thus, pharmacogenetics is one important factor to individualizing drug treatment according to the patients' genetic make-up. Pharmacogenetic-based dose adjustment can be derived from pharmacokinetic data with the aim of obtaining equal drug concentrations in each individual. Routine application of pharmacogenetic dosing in clinical practice requires prospective validation. For instance, a controlled clinical trial with one arm receiving genotype-based dose adjustments and the other arm receiving therapy as usual will elucidate the benefit of pharmacogenomics-based individualization of certain drug therapies.

GENETIC VARIABILITY AND CONSEQUENCES FOR DRUG RESPONSE AND SAFETY

The aim of this chapter is to summarize the contribution of major genetic factors to explain heterogeneity of drug response and individualization of therapy. Pharmacogenetics aims to explain the genetic variability in drug response.[4] One of the major tasks is to optimally adapt the choice and amount of a drug to the individual need of a patient and, therefore, to prevent overdosing with the risk of ADRs.

Genetic variability influences drug effects from absorption of the drug and complete elimination.[4] Figure 16-1 depicts the molecular sites of genetic variability with their impact on variability in drug response. Genetic variability exists at the pharmacokinetic part of drug action (ADME) as well as at the pharmacodynamic side of drug action. Many enzymes involved in drug metabolism carry genetic variants (polymorphism) that can decrease enzyme activity or even lead to complete deficiency.[5] In heterozygous carriers of genetic variants, the effects are between homozygous and carriers of the wild-type. Variants in genes of drug transport influence drug disposition and entrance into body compartments. Genetic variants in drug targets such as receptor molecules or intracellular structures of signal transduction and gene regulation directly and indirectly influence drug response.

In the future, the genetic background of drug response will be studied extensively owing to the modern technologies of high-throughput genotyping. This knowledge will serve to improve drug development as well as individual drug therapy.

Genetic polymorphisms in molecules involved in drug action are often the same that also influence the course and susceptibility of illness.[6] Thus, genetic information about disease susceptibility and individual drug response will lead to a much more precise diagnosis and therapeutic strategy.

Genetic Polymorphisms on the Pharmacokinetic Part of Drug Action

Pharmacogenetic variants in enzymes of drug metabolism lead to differences in pharmacokinetic parameters such as higher or lower blood or tissue concentrations of a drug and its metabolites. Pharmacokinetic parameters of drug action that are affected by genetic variability are plasma concentrations, clearance, volume of distribution, elimination half-life, and the area under the plasma concentration time curve (AUC).

Table 16-1 presents important enzymes, known to be genetically polymorphic, involved in drug metabolism. The so-called phase I reactions in biotransformation are small molecular modifications such as oxidations and reductions and are mostly mediated by the enzyme family of the CYP enzymes. Five members of this family, CYP3A4, CYP2D6, CYP2C19, CYP2C9 and CYP1A2, are responsible for the major part of drug metabolism.[7] For CYP2D6 and CYP2C19, genetic polymorphisms are known to lead to complete deficiency of the enzyme.[8-10] CYP2C9 has genetic polymorphisms that largely decrease enzyme activity.[11] Recently, CYP2B6 was identified to be highly polymorphically expressed.[12] The interindividual variability of CYP3A4 activity has not yet been explained by genetic mechanisms.[13,14]

Genetic polymorphisms within CYP enzymes mainly affect pharmacokinetics of drugs that are substrates for those enzymes. Those differences in drug metabolism, exposition, and elimination lead to differences in drug response as well as to an altered risk for ADRs. Accumulation of a metabolite that is not further metabolized because of a lack of enzyme activity might lead to differential pharmacologic effects or even to toxic events.

However, CYP enzymes are not the only factors in drug metabolism; physiologic substrates metabolized by those enzymes (e.g., most steroid hormones or arachidonic acid) and genetic polymorphisms also play a role in biotransformation of drugs. This is why genetic polymor-

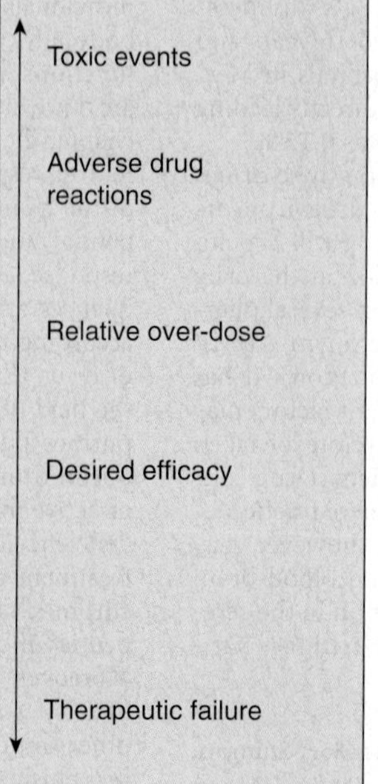

FIGURE 16-1 • Interplay of genetic variability in molecules of drug metabolism and elimination versus pharmacodynamic structures.

TABLE 16-1 IMPORTANT ENZYMES OF XENOBIOTIC METABOLISM THAT ARE GENETICALLY POLYMORPHIC

	Functional Effect of Polymorphism	Frequency of Homozygous Carriers in the White Population (%)	Drugs Metabolized by This Enzyme
PHASE I			
Cytochrome P-450 (CYP) 1A2	High inducibility	46%	Clozapine, imipramine, caffeine, lidocaine, paracetamol, theophylline
CYP2A6	Reduced activity	1%	Fadrazole, halothane, losigamone, nicotine, tegafure
CYP2B6	Reduced activity	2%	Bupropion, propofol, efavirenz
CYP2C8	Reduced activity	1.7%	Carbamazepine, cerivastatin, paclitaxel, pioglitazone, rosiglitazone, tolbutamide, verapamil, warfarin
CYP2C9	Reduced activity	1%-3%	Celecoxib, clopidogrel, diclofenac, fluvastatin, glyburide, ibuprofen, losartan, phenprocoumon, phenytoin, piroxicam, sildenafil, tolbutamide, torasemide, warfarin
CYP2C19	Deficient activity	3%	Diazepam, lansoprazole, omeprazole, pantoprazole, proguanil, propranolol, rabeprazol
CYP2D6	Deficient activity and extremely high activity caused by gene duplication	7% 2%-3%	Ajmaline, amitriptyline, carvedilol, codeine, flecainide, fluoxetine, galanthamine, haloperidol, metoprolol, mexiletine, ondansetron, propafenon, tamoxifen, timolol, tropisetrone
CYP3A4, CYP3A5, CYP3A7	Slightly decreased activity (?) Expression of CYP3A7 in the adult	Several rare mutations	Quinidine, cyclosporine, cortisol, dapsone, diltiazem, erythromycin, lidocaine, midazolam, nifedipine, paclitaxel, sildenafil, simvastatin, tacrolimus, triazolam, verapamil, zolpidem
Flavine-dependent monooxygenase 3 (FMO3)	Reduced activity	9%	Perazine, sulindac, albendazole, benzydamine
Butyrylcholinesterase (BCHE)	Reduced activity	0.03%	Succinylcholine
Dihydropyrimidinedehydrogenase (DPYD)	Reduced activity	<1%	5-Fluorouracil
PHASE II			
Arylamine-*N*-acetyltransferase 2 (NAT2)	Slow acetylation	55%	Isoniazide, hydralazine, sulfonamides, procainamide, dapsone
Uridine-diphosphate-glucuronosyltransferase 1A1 (UGT1A1)	Reduced activity	10.9%	Irinotecan
Glutathione-*S*-transferase M1 (GSTM1)	Deficient activity	55%	Disposition for bladder cancer
Catechol-*O*-methyltransferase (COMT)	Reduced activity	25%	Estrogen, L-dopa, α-methyldopa, amphetamine
Thiopurine *S*-methyltransferase (TPMT)	Deficient activity	0.3%	Azathioprine, 6-mercaptopurine

phisms within CYP enzymes have also been shown to be associated with risk for certain diseases such as hypertension and cancer.[15,16]

The clinical importance of genetic variants depends on the allele frequency but also on the effect size of the clinical outcome parameter. Further, it depends on the therapeutic range and safety of the drug because pharmacokinetic changes might not be important for each drug but may be especially important for drugs that have to be carefully monitored because of a small dose range for response and a high risk for ADRs. The importance of genotyping is larger in drug therapies in which the individual response can be badly predicted. For example, in antidepressant drug therapy, 30% of the patients will not respond sufficiently to drug therapy, and therapeutic effects are first expected after 2 weeks of drug intake. In this case, all factors possibly predicting individual drug response are important to know (e.g., the actual metabolic activity measured by therapeutic drug monitoring, previous treatment success, and genetic factors involved in drug targets), and genetically caused differences in drug metabolizing enzyme activity might be one important point to consider in order to optimize treatment before failure.

Consequences arising from genotyping might include adjustment of dose according to genotype, choice of therapeutic strategy, or even a different drug.

Genetic Polymorphisms on the Pharmacodynamic Part of Drug Action

Genetic variability in the drug targets as receptors or molecules of signal transduction can affect the effect and tolerability of drugs.

As an example, the β_2-adrenoreceptor taking part in vasoregulation and bronchodilation carries two point mutations, Arg16Gly and

TABLE 16-2 POLYMORPH GENES WITH INFLUENCE ON THE DRUG EFFECT AT THE RECEPTOR OR AT THE GOAL STRUCTURE

Gene	Example	Clinical Effects	Reference
β_2-Adrenoceptor (ADRB2)	Albuterol, isoproterenol	Differences in bronchodilation Tachyphylaxia, desensitization and effect depending on genotype	17-19
Dopamine transporter (DAT1)	L-Dopa	Occurrence of psychosis or dyskinesia	145
5-Lipoxygenase (ALOX5)	Zileutone	No antiasthmatic effects in carriers of the tandem repeat	146
Apolipoprotein E (APOE)	Tacrine	Effective only in APOE negative patients with M. Alzheimer	147
O-6-Methylguanin-DNA-methyltransferase (MGMT)	Alkylating substances	Methylation of the promoter influences therapy response in patients with glioma	148
Voltage-dependent potassium channel type 2 (KCNE2)	Sulfamethoxazole, procainamide, oxatomide	Drug-induced long QT syndrome in carriers of the variant	149
Glycoprotein IIIa (ITGB3)	Platelet aggregation inhibitors (aspirin, abciximab)	Smaller effects in carriers of *PLA2*	150-152
Cholesterylestertransfer protein (CETP)	Pravastatin	Protective effect against artherosclerosis in carriers of *B1B1* genotype	153
α-Adducine (ADD1)	Hydrochloro-thiazide	Stronger hypotensive effect in carriers of *460Gly/Trp*	154
Angiotensin-converting enzyme (ACE)	Enalaprilate	Stronger effects in carriers of the insertion	155

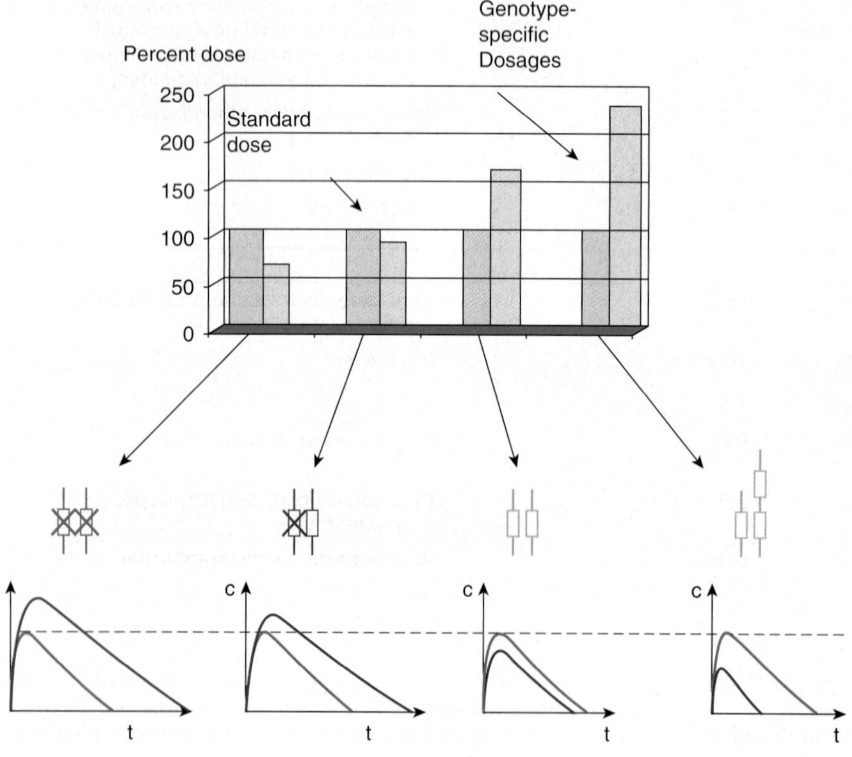

FIGURE 16-2 • Principle of calculation of genotype-based dose adjustments based upon differences in pharmacokinetic parameters such as clearance and area under the plasma concentration time curve (AUC). The theoretical dosages for genetically caused subgroups of poor, intermediate, extensive, and ultrarapid metabolizers are depicted as schematic genotype-specific dosages in order to obtain equal plasma concentration time courses.

Gln27Glu, influencing the effects of β_2-adrenoceptor agonists on vasodilation and bronchodilation.[17-19] Further genetic polymorphisms influencing drug effects are shown in Table 16-2.

GENOTYPE-BASED DOSING

Genetically caused variability in drug metabolism is reflected in differences in clearance, half-life, and maximal plasma concentrations. These pharmacokinetic differences are highly replicable and can be considered in genotype-based dose adjustments. These dose adjustments can be calculated according to the principles of bioequivalence under consideration of special circumstances such as linearity of pharmacokinetics, activity of metabolites, and dose range of the underlying studies. Methods for extracting dose adjustments from pharmacokinetic data in dependence of genotypes have been developed and are published elsewhere.[20-22]

Differences in pharmacokinetic parameters such as oral clearances could then be overcome by adjustment of the drug dose. Figure 16-2

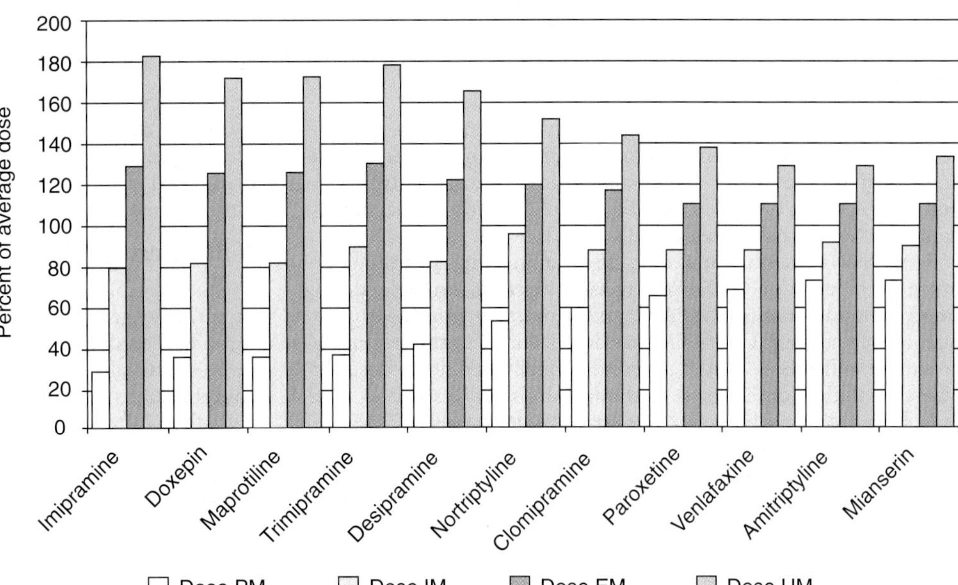

FIGURE 16-3 • *CYP2D6* genotype-dependent quantitative changes in pharmacokinetics of antidepressant drugs expressed as percent dose adaptations. CYP2D6 poor metabolizers (PM; *white*), intermediate metabolizers (IM; *light gray*), extensive metabolizers (EM; *dark gray*), ultrarapid metabolizers (UM; *black*). Dose adaptations are based on an average dose of 100% and are aimed for the white population. Data from studies in Asiatic or African or other populations were not incorporated because PM data are lacking. (Dose adaptations were calculated as described in Kirchheiner J, Nickchen K, Bauer M, et al. Pharmacogenetics of antidepressants and antipsychotics: the contribution of allelic variations to the phenotype of drug response. Mol Psychiatry 2004;9:442-473.)

depicts the theoretical dosages for different genotypes predicting high, ultrahigh, intermediate, or slow metabolic activity derived from the difference plasma concentration courses as schematic genotype-specific dosages. These theoretical dose adjustments make sense for those kinds of drug therapies in which a similar plasma concentration time course also leads to similar clinical effects. For some drugs, plasma concentrations correlate poorly with clinical efficacy, and empirical dose-finding rather than drug concentrations is used to avoid ADRs.

Figure 16-3 presents the differences in mean oral clearance between carriers of none, one, two, and more active *CYP2D6* genes expressed as percentages of dose adjustments for antidepressants. In this figure, the huge differences between the single substrate in extent of *CYP2D6*-mediated variability in clearance is visible, and it has to be decided, for each single substance, whether a genotype-based dose adjustment might be clinically important.

Limitations of Pharmacogenetic Dose Adjustments

When calculating quantitative dose adjustments from pharmacokinetic data depending on genotypes, several points have been taken into account:

- Often, metabolites exist with their own pharmacologic activity, either therapeutic activity or ADRs. Thus, if metabolites exist in considerable concentrations in plasma, this should be acknowledged in the dosing adjustments either by summarizing to the whole active drug compound or by deciding to give no dose adjustment or to recommend a change in drug choice (if metabolites are generated that have potential for ADRs).
- The sample size and power of the existing data have to be large enough to derive dose adjustments. Data on carriers of homozygous variations should at least be available. Further, the dose range of the studies from which dose adjustments are derived should be in the clinical range. Often, this is not the case because many studies are being done in healthy volunteers at lower doses. However, dose recommendations cannot be extrapolated automatically to the dose range used in patients.
- Comedication must be considered. Different genotypes lead to different consequences from interacting substances. For example, a genetically caused poor metabolizer (PM) cannot be increased or decreased in enzyme activity by substances that are inductors or inhibitors of an enzyme. In contrast, extensive (EMs) or ultrarapid metabolizers (UMs) can convert to phenotypically PMs by strong enzyme inhibitors. Thus, genotype-based dose adjustments have to be weighed against changes in phenotype caused, for example, by comedication.

Prospective validation of genotype-based dose adjustments is necessary, and several studies are now being performed comparing therapy with pharmacogenetic diagnostics with *therapy as usual* in a randomized, controlled fashion.

CLINICAL IMPLICATIONS OF PHARMACOGENETIC TESTING

Next, some examples are presented on fields in which enough pharmacogenetic data are available to derive dosing adjustments and in which compensation for differences in drug exposition can be expected to positively influence therapeutic outcome.

Depression

Pharmacotherapy of depression, one of the major psychiatric disorders, is characterized by long duration of drug therapy, relatively narrow therapeutic index, and poor predictability of individual response. About 30% of all patients with depression do not respond sufficiently to the first antidepressant drug given.[23] Failure to respond to antidepressant drug therapy as well as intolerable side effects not only determines personal suffering to individuals and their families but also imposes considerable costs on society. At present, there is no possibility of reliably predicting an individual's response probability before onset of a certain drug treatment.

The group of TCAs undergoes similar biotransformation in the liver with *CYP2D6* catalyzing hydroxylation or demethylation reactions.[24] *CYP2D6* is characterized by a high interindividual variability in catalytic activity, mainly caused by genetic polymorphisms.[25] The respective phenotype determined by *CYP2D6* genotype is predicted by the number of functional *CYP2D6* alleles, so that the presence of two, one, or no functional *CYP2D6* gene copies results in phenotype of, respectively, rapid metabolizer or EM, intermediate metabolizer (IM), and slow metabolizers or PMs.[9,26] Furthermore, inheritance of three or more functional alleles by gene duplication or gene amplification determines the UM phenotype showing higher-than-average enzymatic activity.[9,26,27]

PMs of *CYP2D6* have largely (≥50%) decreased clearances, which were reported for amitriptyline, clomipramine, desipramine, imipramine, nortriptyline, doxepin, and trimipramine.[28]

Individuals to whom TCAs are prescribed could benefit from *CYP2D6* genotyping if the dose is adjusted for the group of PMs and UMs of *CYP2D6*.

In addition to CYP2D6, another highly polymorphic enzyme, CYP2C19, also takes part in biotransformation of some TCAs such as amitriptyline, imipramine, and clomipramine.[29] Thus, genotyping for both CYP2D6 and CYP2C19 might be useful for optimization of antidepressant drug treatment, especially with TCAs.[30]

Some SSRIs such as fluoxetine, fluvoxamine, and paroxetine are potent inhibitors of CYP2D6 activity. Therefore, multiple dosing causes autoinhibition of CYP2D6, and conversion from EM to PM phenotype and from UM to EM was described.[31,32] In the case of fluvoxamine, differences in AUCs were described after single doses,[33,34] whereas multiple doses result in similar AUCs in PMs and in EMs, indicating a strong inhibitory effect on CYP2D6 in EMs.[35]

In paroxetine treatment, even if it is also a CYP2D6 inhibitor, twofold higher AUCs of the drug were observed in CYP2D6 PMs than in EMs after multiple doses.[36] In another study, one UM carrying at least three functional *CYP2D6* gene copies had undetectable drug concentrations.[32] In contrast, no influences of *CYP2D6* polymorphisms on pharmacokinetic parameters of sertraline and citalopram have been observed. Moclobemide, sertraline, and citalopram are metabolized by CYP2C19 as well, and differences in AUCs in CYP2C19 PMs were about twofold (moclobemide and citalopram) or less (sertraline).[37-39]

Thus, in conclusion, within the group of SSRIs, CYP inhibition poses a problem for drug interaction, but the *CYP2D6* gene polymorphism has less effect, and *CYP2D6*-based dose adjustments do not seem to be useful for this group of antidepressants (with the exception of paroxetine).

For mirtazapine, it could be shown that the *CYP2D6* genotype had a significant influence on the variability in the plasma concentration; however, when comparing UMs to EMs, the magnitude of concentration differences was only moderate.[40]

CYP2D6 is responsible for the transformation of venlafaxine to the equipotent *O*-desmethyl-venlafaxine.[41-44] However, a higher risk for cardiotoxic events might exist in PMs because cases of severe arrhythmia have been reported in four patients treated with venlafaxine who were all PMs according to CYP2D6.[45]

The *CYP2D6* polymorphism seems to have no major influence on metabolism of nefazodone, moclobemide, reboxetine, and trazodone.[46-49]

Differences in pharmacokinetic parameters caused by genetic polymorphisms affect the outcome and the risk of ADRs of antidepressants, which has been shown in several studies. In a German study evaluating the effect of *CYP2D6* genotype on ADRs and nonresponse during treatment with CYP2D6-dependent antidepressants, PMs and UMs were significantly overrepresented as compared with the control population, respectively, in the group of patients suffering from ADRs (fourfold) and nonresponders (fivefold).[50] At the same time, Grasmader and colleagues[51] did not find any influence of *CYP2D6* and *CYP2C19* genotype on antidepressant drug response, although the incidence of relevant side effects tended to be higher in PMs of CYP2D6. Furthermore, a prospective 1-year clinical study of 100 psychiatric inpatients suggested a trend toward longer duration of hospital stay and higher treatment costs in UMs and PMs of CYP2D6.[52]

Thus, in conclusion for treatment with antidepressants, considerable evidence indicates, first of all, that *CYP2D6* and, to a lower extent, *CYP2C19* polymorphisms affect pharmacokinetics of several antidepressants and possibly affect therapeutic outcome and ADRs. The usefulness of genotyping procedures in depressed patients, however, has not been confirmed in prospective clinical trials; therefore, this approach is currently limited to a few hospitals and to some patients with adverse or lacking therapeutic effects. Nevertheless, with the recent approval of the pharmacogenetic test assessing for both polymorphic genes *CYP2D6* and *CYP2C19* by the U.S. Food and Drug Administration (FDA), it could be expected that a new era of personalized therapy of depression is beginning.

Cardiovascular Disease

Cardiovascular diseases are the major cause of morbidity and mortality in the developed countries. Clinical implications resulting from genetic polymorphisms in drug metabolism are discussed for some drugs used in the therapy of cardiovascular diseases, such as some β-blockers and sartans.

β-Blockers

For metoprolol, one of the most often prescribed β-blockers, the role of *CYP2D6* genetic polymorphisms in its pharmacokinetics seems to be well established. *CYP2D6* catalyzes *O*-demethylation and, even more specifically, α-hydroxylation of the drug.[53] Metoprolol plasma concentrations as well as effects on heart rate correlated significantly with the *CYP2D6* metabolic phenotype.[53,54] We described effects of *CYP2D6* genotype on pharmacokinetics of metoprolol and heart rate.[55] In UMs carrying the *CYP2D6* gene duplication, total clearance of metoprolol was about 100% higher compared with the EMs as the reference group (367 vs. 168 L/h). These pharmacokinetic differences were reflected in pharmacodynamics such that the reduction of exercise-induced heart rate by metoprolol in the UM group was only about half of that observed in the EMs.

On the basis of the considerable impact of the *CYP2D6* polymorphism on the disposition of *CYP2D6* substrates, it has often been suggested that *CYP2D6* PMs are more susceptible to adverse effects than are EMs at standard doses of metoprolol.[56-58] For instance, the *CYP2D6* PM genotype was overrepresented among 24 patients with severe metoprolol-associated ADRs in a retrospective study.[56] However, metoprolol is well tolerated in the majority of patients with cardiovascular diseases. The effect of β-blockers on quality of life in hypertensive patients has not been extensively studied. In a prospective, 6-week, multicenter study including 121 patients treated with metoprolol, the *CYP2D6* genotype–derived phenotype was not significantly associated with a propensity for ADRs to develop during treatment.[59] The wide therapeutic range of metoprolol may explain why it is well tolerated in the majority of *CYP2D6* PMs and IMs despite severalfold higher plasma concentrations.

Another β-blocker, the racemate carvedilol, which has been approved as adjunctive therapy in the treatment of heart failure, is known to be stereoselectively metabolized by CYP enzymes.[60] *CYP2D6* polymorphism has been shown to alter the stereoselective disposition of carvedilol with PMs demonstrating an impaired clearance of the R-enantiomer, thus being affected by a more pronounced α_1-blockade that might outweigh the beneficial β_1-blocking effects.[61] Hence, *CYP2D6* genotyping might predict therapeutic outcome in cardiac-insufficient patients treated with carvedilol. However, inhibition of CYP2D6 metabolism by administration of fluoxetine in EMs led to significant changes in plasma pharmacokinetics in favor of the R-enantiomer without any effects on blood pressure and heart rate, which casts doubt on the clinical significance of the *CYP2D6* genotype for the use of carvedilol in antihypertensive therapy.[62]

In summary, *CYP2D6* genotyping might be beneficial, if at all, for long-term treatment with metoprolol in indications such as heart failure or in patients postmyocardial infarction in whom no surrogate parameter such as blood pressure is available to predict long-term efficacy.

Vitamin K Antagonists

The S-enantiomers of all three vitamin K antagonists, acenocoumarol, phenprocoumon, and warfarin, are substrates of CYP2C9. Warfarin is mainly prescribed in North America and Asia, whereas acenocoumarol and phenprocoumon are more commonly used in Europe. Both *CYP2C9* alleles, *CYP2C9*2* and **3*, have substantial effect on the intrinsic clearance of (S)-warfarin.[63-66] For acenocoumarol, heterozygous carriers of *CYP2C9*3* had only 40% of the clearance measured in *CYP2C9*1/*1* carriers, whereas differences in International Normalized Ratio (INR) between these two groups resulted in a mean daily dose that was 70% that of wild-type patients in **1/*3* carriers.[67-71] Many clinical studies reported a higher risk for ADRs, especially bleeding complications, in patients at the beginning of treatment with oral anticoagulants.[72]

The vitamin K antagonistic effects of the coumarin derivatives are mediated by inhibition of the vitamin K epoxide reductase.[73] The required dosage of vitamin K antagonists to achieve target level of anticoagulation largely depends on the activity of the vitamin K epoxide reductase. About 25% of variability in warfarin dose was shown to be explained by the vitamin K epoxide reductase complex 1 (VKORC1) haplotypes with one single functional single nucleotide polymorphism (SNP) being responsible for the differences in gene expression.[74,75] The mean daily dose requirement of phenprocoumon differs largely depending on the G-1639A polymorphism of VKORC1, with GG carriers requiring more than twice of the mean dose than AA carriers.[76] Owing to the lower dose requirement in AA carriers, those individuals had a higher risk for bleeding even if the INR values were stable. For acenocoumarol, the –1639AA genotype is the major risk factor for overanticoagulation, with an odds ratio of 10.5 [3.3-34.1], and predisposes to larger INR variations.[77,78]

In addition to dosing according to INR, the FDA insert in the drug labeling of warfarin recommends genotyping for *CYP2C9* and *VCORC1* prior to the onset of anticoagulant therapy.

Ulcer Disease and Proton Pump Inhibitors

Proton pump inhibitors (PPIs), such as omeprazole, esomeprazole, lansoprazole, pantoprazole, and rabeprazole, are commonly prescribed in combination with antibiotics for *Helicobacter pylori* eradication and in patients with peptic ulcer as well as in gastroduodenal reflux disease. These agents undergo extensive presystemic biotransformation in the liver with the involvement of genetically polymorphic *CYP2C19*.[79,80] *CYP2C19*2* and *CYP2C19*3* are the most common nonfunctional alleles responsible for the majority of PM phenotypes of CYP2C19.[8]

Andersson and associates[81] observed that in PMs of mephenytoin (a model substrate of CYP2C19), the AUC for omeprazole, lansoprazole, and pantoprazole at steady state was fivefold higher than that for EMs, indicating that approximately 80% of the dose for all three PPIs is metabolized by CYP2C19. For different PPIs, drug exposures, which were defined with AUC values, were 3 to 13 times higher in PMs and about 2 to 4 times higher in heterozygous EMs than in homozygous EMs of CYP2C19.[79] At the same time, the elevation of intragastric pH as a pharmacodynamic response to PPIs could be shown to be related directly to the respective AUC, and a much higher pH can be monitored over 24 hours after the administration of PPIs in PMs than in EMs.[79]

In a systematic review on pharmacogenetic studies with PPIs, Chong and coworkers[82] evaluated the effects of *CYP2C19* genetic polymorphism on the clinical outcomes, that is, *H. pylori* eradication rates upon therapy with these drugs. The results of most studies supported the hypothesis that eradication rates vary with *CYP2C19* genotype and that PMs have a significantly better efficacy of PPIs.

Furuta and colleagues[83] showed that eradication rates of *H. pylori* within triple therapy comprising PPI, clarithromycin, and amoxicillin were 72.7%, 92.1%, and 97.8% in *CYP2C19* EMs, IMs, and PMs, respectively. The authors concluded that the *CYP2C19* genotype seems to be one of the important factors associated with the cure rates of *H. pylori* infections with the PPI-based therapy.[83] Moreover, these authors[84] conducted a prospective clinical study showing in a randomized prospective way that *CYP2C19* genotyping provides a cost-effective benefit in *H. pylori* eradication treatment.

The role of *CYP2C19* polymorphism for eradication of *H. pylori* was also studied in the white population. However, in contrast to the Asian population, the prevalence of PM of *CYP2C19* in whites is much lower (i.e., about 2.8% vs. 21.3%, respectively) in whites and Japanese.[85] We could show significant differences considering efficacy of lansoprazole-based quadruple therapy between white patients carrying wild-type alleles one and two *CYP2C19* defect alleles with cure rates of 80.2%, 97.8%, and 100% in the respective groups.[80]

Treatment of gastroesophageal reflux disease (GERD) demands long-term application of PPIs. Two retrospective analyses in Japanese patients showed that the healing rate of GERD using lansoprazole was 20% to 40% higher in PMs or IMs compared with EMs of CYP2C19 and that PMs even benefit in prevention of relapse of GERD.[86-88]

In summary, according to the results of numerous clinical studies, *CYP2C19* polymorphism is an important factor affecting pharmacokinetics of most PPIs, values of intragastric pH, and eradication rates of *H. pylori*. Therefore, in our opinion, genotyping for *CYP2C19* polymorphisms, first of all in the Asian populations, characterized by a high prevalence of defect *CYP2C19* alleles, could be recommended. The natural consequence of this approach could be higher dosages in the group of EMs and/or adjusted treatment regimen. Only prospective controlled clinical trials could show if the patients might benefit from such individually tailored therapy.

Pain Treatment: NSAIDs

One large field in which the *CYP2C9* polymorphism plays a role is treatment with nonsteroidal anti-inflammatory drugs (NSAIDs). At least 16 different registered NSAIDs are currently known to be at least partially metabolized via CYP2C9. These include aceclofenac, acetylsalicylic acid, azapropazone, celecoxib, diclofenac, flurbiprofen, ibuprofen, indomethacin, lornoxicam, mefenamic acid, meloxicam, naproxen, phenylbutazone, piroxicam, suprofen, and tenoxicam.[89] There were significant intergenotypic differences in the pharmacokinetics of celecoxib, flurbiprofen, ibuprofen, and tenoxicam, which could be translated into dose recommendations based upon *CYP2C9* genotype. Celecoxib has been one of the first drugs for which the manufacturer's drug information recommends caution when administering celecoxib to "poor metabolizers of CYP2C9 substrates" because they might have abnormally high plasma levels (Celebrex drug information, Searle Pfizer, Chicago, USA).

In contrast, the relative contribution of CYP2C9 to the pharmacokinetics of diclofenac was found to be independent of *CYP2C9* polymorphisms in several clinical studies.[90-93]

Figure 16-4 depicts the mean differences in oral clearance of NSAIDs for several *CYP2C9* genotypes that could be directly translated into dose adjustments with carriers of the *CYP2C9*1/*1* genotype getting 100% of the dose, and adjustments made for the other genotypes according to the differences in oral clearance. The data of the single studies have been taken from Kirchheiner and coworkers.[20]

Malignant Diseases

Most anticancer drugs are characterized by a very narrow therapeutic index and severe consequences of over- or underdosing in the form of life-threatening ADRs or treatment failure, respectively. Polymorphisms in genes encoding drug metabolizing enzymes (DMEs) are considered to be an important factor contributing to individual drug response in patients undergoing chemotherapy.

Tamoxifen

The clinical benefit of the antiestrogen tamoxifen for the treatment of estrogen receptor (ER)–positive breast cancer has been evident since the late 1970s,[94] but 30% to 50% of patients with adjuvant tamoxifen therapy relapse or die. Several lines of evidence suggest that the metabolites 4-hydroxy tamoxifen (4-OH-TAM) and 4-hydroxy-*N*-desmethyl tamoxifen (endoxifen) are the active therapeutic moieties because, compared with the parent drug, these two metabolites have an up to 100-fold higher potency in terms of binding to ER.[95] CYP2D6 is one of the key enzymes for the formation of 4-OH-TAM and endoxifen,[96] and CYP2D6 PMs have been shown to have very low endoxifen plasma levels[97] and nonfavorable clinical outcomes.[98] Of note, between 15% and 20% of European patient populations carry genetic *CYP2D6* variants associated with a pronounced impairment in the formation of antiestrogenic tamoxifen metabolites. We recently investigated the role

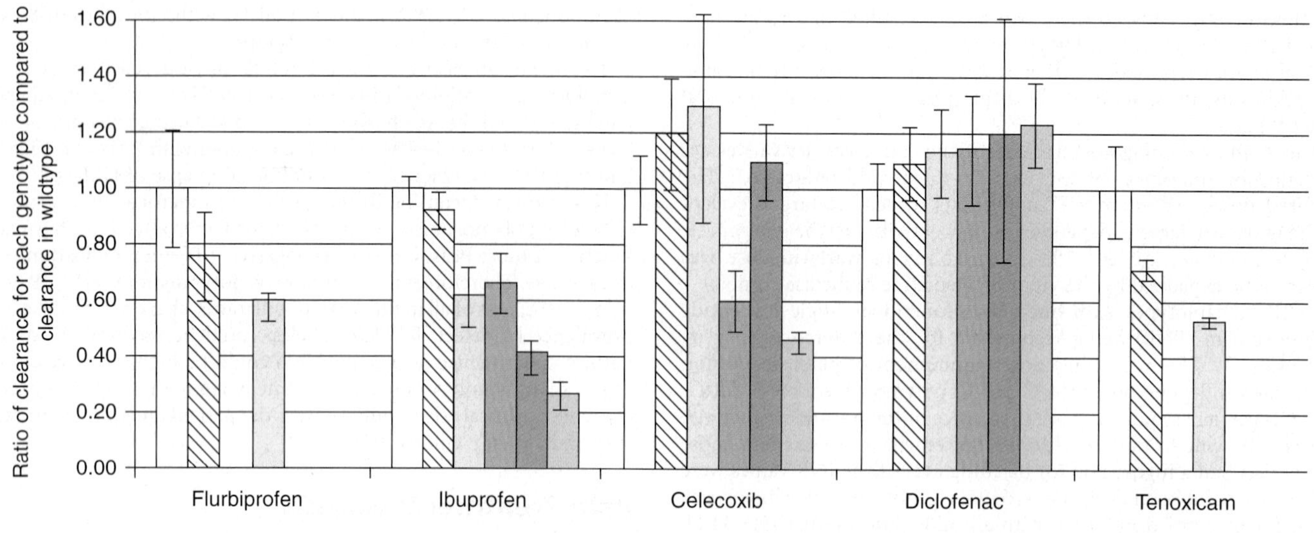

FIGURE 16-4 • Differences in oral clearances of nonsteroidal anti-inflammatory drugs based on *CYP2C9* genotype in whites. The ratios $Cl_{genotype}/Cl_{wildtype}$ are depicted. The variability of the data from the different studies is shown as *error bars* depicting the standard deviations of the means for each genotype. (Data of clinical studies are taken from Kirchheiner J, Brockmoller J. Clinical consequences of cytochrome P450 2C9 polymorphisms. Clin Pharmacol Ther 2005;77:1-16.)

of *CYP2D6* variants in the outcome of adjuvant tamoxifen therapy through a comprehensive *CYP2D6* PM and IM genotyping approach.[99] In addition *CYP3A5*, *CYP2B6*, *CYP2C9*, and *CYP2C19* variants were analyzed because these enzymes contribute to the formation of antiestrogenic metabolites. Tamoxifen-treated patients carrying the *CYP2D6* alleles **4*, **5*, **10*, and **41* associated with impaired formation of antiestrogenic metabolites had significantly more recurrences, shorter relapse-free time (hazard ratio [HR] = 2.24; 95% confidence interval [CI], 1.16-4.33; $P = 0.02$), and worse event-free survival (HR = 1.89; 95% CI, 1.10-3.25; $P = 0.02$) compared with carriers of functional alleles. Moreover, the first genetic evidence for the *CYP2C19*17* polymorphism[100] as a putative supplementary biomarker for the classification of patients with favorable treatment outcome was reported. Patients with the *CYP2C19* high enzyme activity promoter variant **17* had a more favorable clinical outcome (HR = 0.45; 95% CI, 0.21-0.92; $P = 0.03$) than carriers of **1*, **2*, and **3* alleles. *CYP2C19* contributes to tamoxifen metabolism toward the antiestrogenic metabolite 4-OH-TAM with in vitro activities similar to those of *CYP2D6*.[95,96] This study supported the feasibility of treatment outcome prediction for tamoxifen based on the patients' genetic constitution. In the absence of any other significant genotype-outcome relationship of the tested bioactivation enzymes, our study puts emphasis on *CYP2D6* and *CYP2C19* as tamoxifen-predictive markers.

Although our study and those by Goetz and associates[98,101] identified the genetic *CYP2D6* status as an independent predictor for the outcome of tamoxifen treatment in women with early breast cancer, others did not observe this relationship.[102,103] Beyond that, it is important to note that the studies of others were limited to *CYP2D6*4* and the infrequent **6* allele, whereas we[99] extended the assessment of a decreased *CYP2D6* metabolizer status with predicted low endoxifen levels from 6% to 15% by additional testing for the gene deletion allele **5* and combined IM and PM genotype analysis, which considerably increased the power of our study.

Altogether these findings are particularly important in light of the current debate on the effectiveness of tamoxifen for postmenopausal women with hormone receptor–positive breast cancer. Randomized trials demonstrated that, for instance, the administration of an aromatase inhibitor after 5 years of tamoxifen[104] significantly prolongs disease-free and overall survival. Because the definition of patient groups with nonfavorable and favorable tamoxifen treatment appears to be feasible through a priori genetic assessment of *CYP2D6* and possibly *CYP2C19* metabolism, and given the long-term experience of tamoxifen as a safe and effective antihormonal treatment, we suggest using these assets toward a refinement of choice and/or sequencing of hormonal therapy in prospective clinical trials.

Thiopurines

Thiopurines, such as 6-mercaptopurine and thioguanine, are largely used in the treatment of acute leukemias, whereas autoimmune diseases and chronic inflammatory bowel diseases are common fields of application for azathioprine.[105] The major underlying mode of action in treatment of leukemia is suggested to be the incorporation of the active metabolites 6-thioguanine nucleotides (6-TGN) into DNA and RNA, thereby inhibiting replication, DNA repair mechanisms, and protein synthesis.[106] The cytosolic enzyme TPMT as well as xanthin oxidase (XO) are the predominant catabolic enzymes in the metabolism of thiopurines. Whereas TPMT, which catalyzes the *S*-adenosyl-L-methionine–dependent *S*-methylation of 6-mercaptourine (6-MP) and its metabolites, is expressed ubiquitously in humans (e.g., in the intestine, liver, red blood cells [RBCs], and white blood cells), XO is not expressed in hematopoietic tissue. Therefore, TPMT-dependent methylation is critical in white blood cells, leading to an enhanced cytotoxic effect in patients with low TPMT activity. In 1980, Weinshilboum and Sladek[107] first reported on a trimodal frequency distribution of TPMT activity with about 10% IMs and 1 out of 300 homozygous for the trait with very low/undetectable TPMT activity. To date, 24 mutant alleles responsible for variation in TPMT enzyme activity have been described, and most of these alleles are characterized by one or more nonsynonymous SNPs, resulting in decrease or loss of enzyme activity.[108] In several independent studies, *TPMT* genotype showed excellent concordance with TPMT phenotype, and the most comprehensive analysis was conducted by Schaeffeler and colleagues[109] including 1214 healthy white blood donors. The overall concordance rate between TPMT phenotype and genotype was 98.4% and specificity, sensitivity, and positive and negative predictive power of the genotyping test were estimated to be higher than 90%. Of importance, three issues with regard to TPMT activity and thiopurine therapy in leukemic patients have to be addressed here. First, children with leukemia frequently may require RBC transfusions owing to bone marrow insufficiency inherent with the disease. Transfused donor RBCs may bias TPMT activity measurements, and therefore, TPMT phenotyping is limited.[110] Second, in patients with leukemia, TPMT activity may also be biased by an older age of RBCs. In the course of leukemia, RBC production is decreasing, leading to relatively older RBC populations with lower TPMT activity.[111] Third, physicians should be aware that some drugs that may be coadministered might have a potential influence on TPMT activity. Such interactions with TPMT activity have been described in ex vivo experiments for aminosalicylates, diuretics, and NSAIDs.[112-114] Patients with TPMT deficiency treated with standard doses of azathioprine/6-MP are at high risk to develop severe myelosuppression within a few weeks after commencing drug therapy independent from the underlying disease (e.g., childhood leukemia, inflammatory bowel disease).[115-117] This can be explained by an 8- to 15-fold increase of 6-TGN levels in RBCs compared with wild-type patients subsequently leading to an exaggerated cytotoxic effect. Moreover, an increased risk for hematotoxicity in *TPMT* heterozygous subjects receiving standard thiopurine therapy is also well known from patients with childhood acute lymphoblastic leukemia (ALL) and rheumatologic diseases.[118,119] Thus, dose adjustment, at least in TPMT-deficient patients, is required with an initial dose reduction to 10% to 15% of the standard dose as exemplarily shown for patients with ALL and Crohn's disease.[120,121] Moreover, it was also demonstrated that TPMT phenotype or genotype influences effectiveness of therapy. Low TPMT activity has been associated with higher 6-TGN levels and improved survival whereas high TPMT activity was associated with lower 6-TGN concentrations and an increased relapse risk.[122] The German ALL BFM Study Group recently reported on the association of *TPMT* genotype and minimal residual disease (MRD) in 810 children with childhood ALL,[123] indicating a significant impact of *TPMT* genotype on MRD after administration of 6-MP in the early course of childhood ALL. This may provide a rationale for genotype-based adaptation of 6-MP dosing in the early course of childhood ALL, provided that the described observations will translate into improved long-term outcome.

In conclusion, present genotyping or phenotyping strategies predict, with high accuracy, individuals deficient with respect to TPMT and should routinely precede onset of therapy with thiopurine-derived drugs in order to minimize life-threatening and cost-intensive myelotoxic adverse events. Besides, for 6-MP, the FDA has recently implemented respective pharmacogenetic data considering the impact of the polymorphic *TPMT* on severe toxicity as well as availability of genotypic and phenotypic testing into the product label.[124]

In addition, thiopurines are an excellent example that genetic and nongenetic factors are important factors to explain the heterogeneity of drug response including ADRs. Concomitant treatment with the XO inhibitor allopurinol without dose adjustment of azathioprine/6-MP is highly critical, because thiopurines are catalyzed by XO. Thus, allopurinol will increase the oral bioavailability (systemic drug exposure) of 6-MP by a factor of five,[125] consequently leading to severe pancytopenia in the absence of TPMT polymorphism.[126] Thus, as recommended by the manufacturer, a reduction of azathiopurine/6-MP to 25% of the daily standard doses under allopurinol comedication is required.

5-Fluorouracil

Following administration, 5-fluorouacil (5-FU) undergoes complex anabolic and catabolic biotransformations that play an eminent role for both antitumor activity and toxicity. Whereas the effectiveness of 5-FU depends on its bioactivation, resulting in 5-fluoronucleotides that interfere with normal DNA and RNA function preferentially in cancer cells, over 80% of a given dose is rapidly metabolized by dihydropyrimidine dehydrogenase (DPD), the rate-limiting enzyme of pyrimidine catabolism, to the inactive 5-fluoro-5,6-dihydrouracil.[127] A potential role of DPD as a factor determining 5-FU toxicity was initially suggested by Diasio and coworkers[128] who could show complete deficiency of DPD enzyme activity in a patient with the rare familial metabolic disorder pyrimidinemia who had developed severe neurotoxicity during 5-FU treatment and by later studies showing correlation between lymphocyte DPD activity and 5-FU clearance.[129,130] Numerous genetic variants in the corresponding *DPYD* gene were described, including the most common variant, a G to A change in the 5′-splice recognition site of intron 14 (exon 14–skipping mutation), which leads to a corresponding mRNA-lacking exon 14 and an enzymatically deficient enzyme.[130,131] In addition to DPYD mutations, other patient characteristics including age and sex have also been suggested to influence 5-FU clearance, and female patients experience 5-FU toxicity more frequently and more severely than men.[132] Other polymorphic candidate genes considered as potential factors for 5-FU toxicity include the thymidylate synthase (TYMS), which is strongly inhibited by 5-FU as well as methylenetetrahydrofolate reductase (MTHFR), which forms the reduced folate cofactor essential for TYMS inhibition.[133] Application of 5-FU is restricted by a narrow therapeutic index and could be complicated by severe toxicity of World Health Organization (WHO) grades III-IV with symptoms like mucositis and granulocytopenia. Moreover, severe adverse events have also been observed with capecitabine, which is the orally available prodrug of 5-FU.[134] Three percent to 5% of whites have been reported to show a reduced DPD enzymatic activity, potentially leading to severe 5-FU–related toxicity in cancer patients.[135] However, measuring individual DPD activity in peripheral mononuclear blood cells does not provide a valid phenotyping approach because the correlation with hepatic DPD activity and 5-FU pharmacokinetics is poor.[136,137]

Although polymorphisms within the human DPD gene (*DPYD*) have been associated with DPD deficiency and severe 5-FU–related toxicity in cancer patients, the predictive value of genotyping for severe toxicity in cancer patients receiving 5-FU is still unknown because only retrospective studies are published.[130] Screening for known mutations in a cohort of cancer patients undergoing 5-FU chemotherapy explained the low DPD activity phenotype in only 17% of all cases, and the sole carrier of the exon 14–skipping mutation was inconspicuous with regard to enzyme activity.[135] Nevertheless, to identify patients at increased risk for severe 5-FU–induced toxicity, routine screening for the exon 14–skipping mutation before onset of chemotherapy has been recommended.[138] To this end, the sample sizes of the previous studies were virtually too small to dare a valid estimation of the clinical value of *DPYD* genotyping in order to prevent 5-FU–related toxicity; further elucidation in large prospective studies is needed. However, data from the so far largest prospective study on 5-FU toxicity implicate that pharmacogenetic testing for DPD *2A in patients might be of limited value due to the low sensitivity of 5.5%.[138a]

Irinotecan

Recently, much attention has been paid to the importance of pharmacogenetic polymorphisms in uridine diphosphate glucuronosyltransferase (UGT) and its role in toxicity and therapeutic response in cancer patients undergoing treatment with the potent antitumor agent irinotecan. SN-38, the active metabolite of irinotecan and topoisomerase I inhibitor, is glucuronidated to its inactive form by UGT1A1, the UGT isoform, which is also responsible for glucuronidation of bilirubin. Several variant alleles leading to reduced enzymatic UGT1A1 activity have been identified in the *UGT1A1* gene. These polymorphisms become manifest as unconjugated hyperbilirubinemias in the form of Crigler-Najjar or Gilbert's syndromes as well as in patients treated with irinotecan; they result in reduced SN-38 glucuronidation rates.[137] For *UGT1A1* genetic variations, major interethnic differences have been shown; whereas *UGT1A1*28* promoter polymorphism (TA repeat in the promoter) is quite common in the white population, *UGT1A1*6* and *UGT1A1*27*, situated in the coding region of *UGT1A1*, are found mainly in Asians.[139]

The impact of *UGT1A1* polymorphisms on irinotecan toxicity, which is characterized by severe diarrhea and neutropenia, has been studied in several retrospective as well as prospective studies. It could be shown that presence of common *UGT1A1* mutant alleles, even in heterozygous carriers, changed significantly the disposition of irinotecan causing severe toxicity in patients.[139-141] Consecutively, genotyping for *UGT1A1* polymorphisms prior to therapy with irinotecan was recommended for patients of all ethnic groups. If *UGT1A1* genotyping is not possible, measurement of the total bilirubin level was proposed as an easy surrogate parameter for prediction of life-threatening toxicity due to irinotecan[113]; however, the usefulness of this approach should definitely be confirmed in further clinical trials. Finally, given the cumulative evidence, the FDA has approved a new labeling for irinotecan in favor of *UGT1A1*28* genotyping, which reflects the prevalence of the *UGT1A1*28* allele in European Americans. A reduced initial dose of irinotecan has been recommended for homozygous carriers of this variant allele because they are at increased risk for neutropenia (FDA, http://www.fda.gov).

In summary, importance of individually tailored medicine for cancer patients seems to be of critical importance for developing safe and effective chemotherapy. Even if genetically polymorphic DMEs are not the only factor contributing to the wide interindividual variation in toxicity and efficacy of anticancer drugs, the recent implementation of the pharmacogenetic data to the product labels of 6-MP and irinotecan could be assessed as milestones in oncology and pharmacogenetics.[142] However, successful implementation of pharmacogenetic tests in cancer patients would depend on the thorough analysis of clinical benefits and cost-effectiveness of this approach.

In conclusion, differences in pharmacokinetic parameters caused by *CYP* polymorphisms could be overcome by adjustment of the drug dose. The potential clinical benefit of dose adjustment according to genotype differences in pharmacokinetics is not evident. For some drugs, plasma concentrations correlate poorly with clinical efficacy, and empirical dose finding rather than drug concentrations is used to avoid ADRs.

Thus, the list of drugs for which *CYP*-genotype–specific dose reductions may be clinically useful has been restricted to those with a clear relationship between genotype and effect. At the moment, this probably is the case for tamoxifen, warfarin, acenocoumarol, TCAs, some NSAIDs for long-term use, and thiopurines.

Nevertheless, before routine genotyping can be incorporated into the clinical setting, the benefits of genotype-based therapeutic recommendations have to be tested by a prospective, randomized, controlled clinical trial.

PHARMACOGENETIC STUDY DESIGNS

Before a pharmacogenetic polymorphism can be routinely considered in drug development and in drug treatment, it has to be extensively characterized. This includes functional studies in vitro; after that, its functional impact on pharmacokinetics or pharmacodynamics has to be studied in controlled clinical trials in healthy volunteers, and its medical impact on drug efficacy and adverse effects has to be studied in patients measuring clinical end points. Thus, the functional validation of the impact of a pharmacogenetic variant is similar to the clinical part of new drug development. Different types of study designs evaluate the medical impact of genetic variability in drug treatment and the potential for improving therapy by genotyping. Consideration of the most valid study design, which is most frequently the double-blinded, randomized, controlled clinical trial, is self-evident in the mainstream of drug development but not necessarily in the accompanying pharmacogenomic research (Fig. 16-5).

One study type frequently used in pharmacogenetic research is the so-called panel study. In this design, volunteers are included in the study after genotyping, and as far as possible, participants are selected with the aim of getting equal sample sizes for each genotype group to be studied. Preselecting genotypes enables studying a sufficient number of individuals even of the more rare genotypes without having to include high numbers of carriers of the frequent genotypes. Of course, prior to such volunteer studies, a genotype selection screening will have to take place, which would also reveal the population frequencies of the genotypes of interest. The aim of such studies cannot be representative elucidation of the population impact of genetic variability, but the aim is to find out, in a very short time and with high statistical significance, what the consequences of genetic variability in humans are.

A cohort study in all patients receiving a certain drug treatment coupled with subsequent analysis for the differences in therapeutic outcomes related to genotype is among the most valid study designs possible in pharmacogenetic research. This approach usually requires a relatively large sample size but is feasible as a pharmacogenetic add-on study to clinical phase 2 and phase 3 trials. If informed consent for genotyping can be obtained from all patients in the clinical trial, there is relatively little selection bias and the data are representative for the treatment with this respective drug. From these kinds of cohort studies, the true relative risk for nonresponse or adverse effects based on genetic variation, as well as the health economic value of genotyping, can be estimated with reasonable validity. Currently, these studies are mostly performed as add-on studies. Investigators and readers of such studies have to be aware of a possible selection bias if only a fraction of less than 80% of the main study population participates in the pharmacogenetic study.

In the pharmacogenetic analysis of rare adverse events, a case-control design study in which patients with a certain clinical outcome (e.g., a specific type of adverse event or nonresponse) are compared with appropriate controls that do not have such an outcome is often the only existing feasible approach. In this study design, the so-called odds ratios as indicators of the strength of genotype effects can be calculated. A case-control study may often be an appropriate clinical research method in safety-related pharmacogenetic research, but this also bears the risk of several types of bias.[143] Despite these limitations, a formal and correctly performed case-control study may often be the best and only existing feasible study design because prospective cohort or controlled trials would require inclusion of 100,000 or more subjects if we want to analyze adverse events with frequencies of 1 : 5000 or less, and studies with so many participants are only rarely possible.

A randomized, controlled, clinical trial is generally considered as the most valid design[144] and provides the most stringent proof-of-concept for pharmacogenetics-based optimization of drug therapy. Such valid studies on pharmacogenetic diagnostics will be relatively expensive, and it is apparently difficult to find sponsors. Drug companies have low interest in sponsoring such studies because they are mostly interested in providing their drug to the largest patient population possible (one-dose-fits-all principle). The diagnostics industry, which has great interest in developing new pharmacogenetics diagnostic tests (PGDx) tests, often has insufficient resources to sponsor major clinical trials. The governmental agencies, finally, are often in favor of sponsoring basic research. Last but not least, the clinicians prefer to abstain from the large amount of new pharmacogenomic information because it appears to be an additional burden and complication of the already complex therapeutic decision networks.

Codevelopment of a new drug to be applied in combination with a pharmacogenetic diagnostic test is an additional option for drug therapy in the future. Optimally, the pivotal study in this case would be a three-armed randomized, controlled trial: a first arm with conventional therapy or placebo, a second arm with the new drug without pharmacogenetics test, and a third arm with the new drug with pharmacogenetics test. Diagnostic codevelopment already has been successfully realized for the modern molecularly targeted cancer therapies such as herceptin, which is only indicated in patients who have been tested positive for *Her2* overexpression.

CONCLUSION

This chapter outlines the major hereditary factors that determine an individual patient's response to drugs. Consideration is given to the effects of these factors on pharmacokinetic and pharmacodynamic processes. It is known that crucial enzymes of phase I (e.g., CYP2C9, CYP2C19, and CYP2D6) and phase II (e.g., TPMT, UGT1A1) drug metabolism are subject to genetic polymorphism, which may in turn lead to reduced or totally absent enzyme activity—and that these differences in enzyme activity contribute substantially to the interindividual differences in drug concentrations. In parallel with the ongoing elucidation of the genetic basis of diseases is an increasing awareness of the possible uses of genetic information to subdivide previously homogenous conditions into subgroups that respond differently to drugs or to identify individuals at risk of "idiosyncratic" adverse responses, not predictable on the basis of the known pharmacology of the drug.

Despite a number of promising examples, the use of genotype information in drug prescribing is still in its infancy. The implementation of pharmacogenetics into clinical practice, like other new procedures, must be subject to clinical trials. Increasingly, the clinical trials that form part of drug development are designed by pharmaceutical companies with the collection and analysis of genotype information in

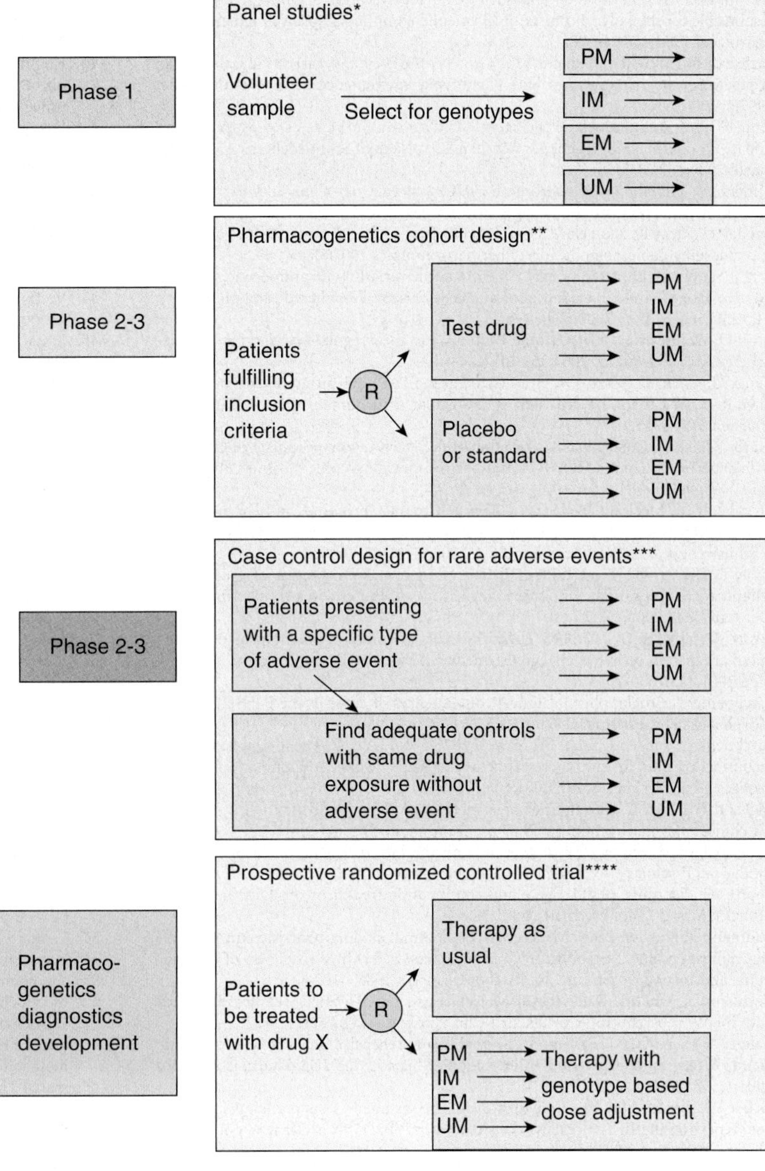

FIGURE 16-5 • Optimal study designs for pharmacogenetic studies on CYP2D6 polymorphism. In phase I studies, a panel of healthy volunteers selected owing to their genotypes is the most powerful study design for analyses of in vivo effects of specific genotypes. A small sample size of homozygous and heterozygous carriers of genetic variants generates maximum statistical power to prove genotype effects. A case-control design is most favorable for studying adverse drug effects: Patients presenting a certain phenotype with regard to adverse drug effects are compared with matched controls of patients with the same drug treatment not resulting in this adverse effect. This design allows estimate of the relative risk for getting an adverse drug effect in a specific genotype. Finally, the design of a randomized, controlled, prospective trial for proof-of-concept of a pharmacogenetic test in combination with a therapeutic recommendation is presented. In this case, the conventional therapy (one-dose-fits-all) is compared with the pharmacogenetics-based individualized treatment including genotype-specific dosing or treatment recommendations. This design allows a final estimate of the cost-benefit relationship between pharmacogenetic individualized and conventional treatment and will result in the number needed to genotype in order to improve drug treatment and decrease costs. (Modified from Kirchheiner J, Fuhr U, Brockmöller J. Pharmacogenetics-based therapeutic recommendations—ready for clinical practice? Nat Rev Drug Disc 2005;4:639-647.)

mind. It may be possible to identify genotype response relationships at an early stage such that the drug is marketed with appropriate recommendations. There is a need for well-conducted studies after licensing of a drug and as part of postmarketing surveillance to detect associations as well as to establish and test the validity and usefulness of the pharmacogenetic approach. By necessity, the tailoring of drug treatment in this way requires the collection of sensitive information from the patient.

REFERENCES

1. Lazarou J, Pomeranz BH, Corey PN. Incidence of adverse drug reactions in hospitalized patients: a meta-analysis of prospective studies. JAMA 1998;279:1200-1205.
2. Schneeweiss S, Hasford J, Gottler M, et al. Admissions caused by adverse drug events to internal medicine and emergency departments in hospitals: a longitudinal population-based study. Eur J Clin Pharmacol 2002;58:285-291.
3. Pirmohamed M, James S, Meakin S, et al. Adverse drug reactions as cause of admission to hospital: prospective analysis of 18,820 patients. BMJ 2004;329:15-19.
4. Evans WE, McLeod HL. Pharmacogenomics—drug disposition, drug targets, and side effects. N Engl J Med 2003;348:538-549.
5. Evans WE, Relling MV. Pharmacogenomics: translating functional genomics into rational therapeutics. Science 1999;286:487-491.
6. Lindpaintner K. Pharmacogenetics and the future of medical practice. J Mol Med 2003;81:141-153.
7. Shimada T, Yamazaki H, Mimura M, et al. Interindividual variations in human liver cytochrome P-450 enzymes involved in the oxidation of drugs, carcinogens and toxic chemicals: studies with liver microsomes of 30 Japanese and 30 Caucasians. J Pharmacol Exp Ther 1994;270:414-423.

8. De Morais SMF, Wilkinson GR, Blaisdell J, et al. Identification of a new genetic defect responsible for the polymorphism of (S)-mephenytoin metabolism in Japanese. Mol Pharmacol 1994;46:594-598.
9. Sachse C, Brockmöller J, Bauer S, et al. Cytochrome P450 2D6 variants in a Caucasian population: allele frequencies and phenotypic consequences. Am J Hum Genet 1997;60:284-295.
10. Zanger UM, Raimundo S, Eichelbaum M. Cytochrome P450 2D6: overview and update on pharmacology, genetics, biochemistry. Naunyn Schmiedebergs Arch Pharmacol 2004;369:23-37.
11. Miners JO, Birkett DJ. Cytochrome P4502C9: an enzyme of major importance in human drug metabolism. Br J Clin Pharmacol 1998;45:525-538.
12. Zanger U, Klein K, Saussele T, et al. Polymorphic CYP2B6: molecular mechanisms and emerging clinical significance. Pharmacogenomics 2007;8:743-759.
13. Sata F, Sapone A, Elizondo G, et al. CYP3A4 allelic variants with amino acid substitutions in exons 7 and 12: evidence for an allelic variant with altered catalytic activity. Clin Pharmacol Ther 2000;67:48-56.
14. Burk O, Wojnowski L. Cytochrome P450 3A and their regulation. Naunyn Schmiedebergs Arch Pharmacol 2004;369:105-124.
15. Jiang JG, Chen CL, Card JW, et al. Cytochrome P450 2J2 promotes the neoplastic phenotype of carcinoma cells and is up-regulated in human tumors. Cancer Res 2005;65:4707-4715.
16. Mayer B, Lieb W, Gotz A, et al. Association of the T8590C polymorphism of CYP4A11 with hypertension in the MONICA Augsburg echocardiographic substudy. Hypertension 2005;46:766-771.
17. Drysdale CM, McGraw DW, Stack CB, et al. Complex promoter and coding region beta 2-adrenergic receptor haplotypes alter receptor expression and predict in vivo responsiveness. Proc Natl Acad Sci U S A 2000;97:10483-10488.
18. Israel E, Drazen JM, Liggett SB, et al. The effect of polymorphisms of the beta(2)-adrenergic receptor on the response to regular use of albuterol in asthma. Am J Respir Crit Care Med 2000;162:75-80.
19. Dishy V, Sofowora GG, Xie HG, et al. The effect of common polymorphisms of the beta2-adrenergic receptor on agonist-mediated vascular desensitization. N Engl J Med 2001;345:1030-1035.
20. Kirchheiner J, Brockmoller J. Clinical consequences of cytochrome P450 2C9 polymorphisms. Clin Pharmacol Ther 2005;77:1-16.
21. Kirchheiner J, Brøsen K, Dahl ML, et al. CYP2D6 and CYP2C19 genotype-based dose recommendations for antidepressants: a first step towards subpopulation-specific dosages. Acta Psychiatr Scand 2001;104:173-192.
22. McLeod HL, Siva C. The thiopurine *S*-methyltransferase gene locus—implications for clinical pharmacogenomics. Pharmacogenomics 2002;3:89-98.
23. Bauer M, Whybrow PC, Angst J, et al., and the World Federation of Societies of Biological Psychiatry (WFSBP). Guidelines for biological treatment of unipolar depressive disorders, part 1: acute and continuation treatment of major depressive disorder. World J Biol Psychiatry 2002;3:5-43.
24. Baumann P, Jonzier Perey M, Koeb L, et al. Amitriptyline pharmacokinetics and clinical response: II. Metabolic polymorphism assessed by hydroxylation of debrisoquine and mephenytoin. Int Clin Psychopharmacol 1986;1:102-112.
25. Bertilsson L, Dahl ML, Dalen P, et al. Molecular genetics of CYP2D6: clinical relevance with focus on psychotropic drugs. Br J Clin Pharmacol 2002;53:111-122.
26. Zanger UM, Fischer J, Raimundo S, et al. Comprehensive analysis of the genetic factors determining expression and function of hepatic CYP2D6. Pharmacogenetics 2001;11:573-585.
27. Griese EU, Zanger UM, Brudermanns U, et al. Assessment of the predictive power of genotypes for the in-vivo catalytic function of CYP2D6 in a German population. Pharmacogenetics 1998;8:15-26.
28. Kirchheiner J, Nickchen K, Bauer M, et al. Pharmacogenetics of antidepressants and antipsychotics: the contribution of allelic variations to the phenotype of drug response. Mol Psychiatry 2004;9:442-473.
29. Brøsen K, Gram LF. Pharmacokinetic and clinical significance of genetic variability in psychotropic drug metabolism. Psychopharmacol Ser 1989;7:192-200.
30. Steimer W, Zopf K, von Amelunxen S, et al. Amitriptyline or not, that is the question: pharmacogenetic testing of CYP2D6 and CYP2C19 identifies patients with low or high risk for side effects in amitriptyline therapy. Clin Chem 2005;51:376-385.
31. Laine K, Tybring G, Hartter S, et al. Inhibition of cytochrome P4502D6 activity with paroxetine normalizes the ultrarapid metabolizer phenotype as measured by nortriptyline pharmacokinetics and the debrisoquin test. Clin Pharmacol Ther 2001;70:327-335.
32. Lam YW, Gaedigk A, Ereshefsky L, et al. CYP2D6 inhibition by selective serotonin reuptake inhibitors: analysis of achievable steady-state plasma concentrations and the effect of ultrarapid metabolism at CYP2D6. Pharmacotherapy 2002;22:1001-1006.
33. Carrillo JA, Dahl ML, Svensson JO, et al. Disposition of fluvoxamine in humans is determined by the polymorphic CYP2D6 and also by the CYP1A2 activity. Clin Pharmacol Ther 1996;60:183-190.
34. Spigset O, Granberg K, Hagg S, et al. Relationship between fluvoxamine pharmacokinetics and CYP2D6/CYP2C19 phenotype polymorphisms. Eur J Clin Pharmacol 1997;52:129-133.
35. Spigset O, Granberg K, Hagg S, et al. Non-linear fluvoxamine disposition. Br J Clin Pharmacol 1998;45:257-263.
36. Sindrup SH, Brøsen K, Gram LF. Pharmacokinetics of the selective serotonin reuptake inhibitor paroxetine: nonlinearity and relation to the sparteine oxidation polymorphism. Clin Pharmacol Ther 1992;51:288-295.
37. Gram LF, Guentert TW, Grange S, et al. Moclobemide, a substrate of CYP2C19 and an inhibitor of CYP2C19, CYP2D6, and CYP1A2: a panel study. Clin Pharmacol Ther 1995;57:670-677.
38. Wang JH, Liu ZQ, Wang W, et al. Pharmacokinetics of sertraline in relation to genetic polymorphism of CYP2C19. Clin Pharmacol Ther 2001;70:42-47.
39. Sindrup SH, Brøsen K, Hansen MG, et al. Pharmacokinetics of citalopram in relation to the sparteine and the mephenytoin oxidation polymorphisms. Ther Drug Monit 1993;15:11-17.
40. Kirchheiner J, Henckel HB, Meineke I, et al. Impact of the CYP2D6 ultrarapid metabolizer genotype on mirtazapine pharmacokinetics and adverse events in healthy volunteers. J Clin Psychopharmacol 2004;24:647-652.
41. Fukuda T, Yamamoto I, Nishida Y, et al. Effect of the CYP2D6*10 genotype on venlafaxine pharmacokinetics in healthy adult volunteers. Br J Clin Pharmacol 1999; 47:450-453.
42. Fukuda T, Nishida Y, Zhou Q, et al. The impact of the CYP2D6 and CYP2C19 genotypes on venlafaxine pharmacokinetics in a Japanese population. Eur J Clin Pharmacol 2000;56:175-180.
43. Otton SV, Ball SE, Cheung SW, et al. Venlafaxine oxidation in vitro is catalysed by CYP2D6. Br J Clin Pharmacol 1996;41:149-156.
44. Veefkind AH, Haffmans PM, Hoencamp E. Venlafaxine serum levels and CYP2D6 genotype. Ther Drug Monit 2000;22:202-208.
45. Lessard E, Yessine M, Hamelin B, et al. Influence of CYP2D6 activity on the disposition and cardiovascular toxicity of the antidepressant agent venlafaxine in humans. Pharmacogenetics 1999;9:435-443.
46. Barbhaiya RH, Buch AB, Greene DS. Single and multiple dose pharmacokinetics of nefazodone in subjects classified as extensive and poor metabolizers of dextromethorphan. Br J Clin Pharmacol 1996;42:573-581.
47. Dostert P, Benedetti MS, Poggesi I. Review of the pharmacokinetics and metabolism of reboxetine, a selective noradrenaline reuptake inhibitor. Eur Neuropsychopharmacol 1997;7(Suppl 1):S23-S35; discussion S71-S73.
48. Faucette SR, Hawke RL, Shord SS, et al. Evaluation of the contribution of cytochrome P450 3A4 to human liver microsomal bupropion hydroxylation. Drug Metab Dispos 2001;29:1123-1129.
49. Schoerlin MP, Blouin RA, Pfefen JP, et al. Comparison of the pharmacokinetics of moclobemide in poor and efficient metabolizers of debrisoquine. Acta Psychiatr Scand Suppl 1990;360:98-100.
50. Rau T, Wohlleben G, Wuttke H, et al. CYP2D6 genotype: impact on adverse effects and nonresponse during treatment with antidepressants—a pilot study. Clin Pharmacol Ther 2004;75:386-393.
51. Grasmader K, Verwohlt PL, Rietschel M, et al. Impact of polymorphisms of cytochrome-P450 isoenzymes 2C9, 2C19 and 2D6 on plasma concentrations and clinical effects of antidepressants in a naturalistic clinical setting. Eur J Clin Pharmacol 2004;60:329-336.
52. Kawanishi C, Lundgren S, Agren H, et al. Increased incidence of CYP2D6 gene duplication in patients with persistent mood disorders: ultrarapid metabolism of antidepressants as a cause of nonresponse. A pilot study. Eur J Clin Pharmacol 2004;59:803-807.
53. Lennard MS, Silas JH, Freestone S, et al. Oxidation phenotype—a major determinant of metoprolol metabolism and response. N Engl J Med 1982;307:1558-1560.
54. Lennard MS, Silas JH, Freestone S, et al. Defective metabolism of metoprolol in poor hydroxylators of debrisoquine. Br J Clin Pharmacol 1982;14:301-303.
55. Kirchheiner J, Heesch C, Bauer S, et al. Impact of the ultrarapid metabolizer genotype of cytochrome P450 2D6 on metoprolol pharmacokinetics and pharmacodynamics. Clin Pharmacol Ther 2004;76:302-312.
56. Wuttke H, Rau T, Heide R, et al. Increased frequency of cytochrome P450 2D6 poor metabolizers among patients with metoprolol-associated adverse effects. Clin Pharmacol Ther 2002;72:429-437.
57. Rau T, Heide R, Bergmann K, et al. Effect of the CYP2D6 genotype on metoprolol metabolism persists during long-term treatment. Pharmacogenetics 2002;12:465-472.
58. Zineh I, Beitelshees AL, Gaedigk A, et al. Pharmacokinetics and CYP2D6 genotypes do not predict metoprolol adverse events or efficacy in hypertension. Clin Pharmacol Ther 2004;76:536-544.
59. Fux R, Morike K, Prohmer AM, et al. Impact of CYP2D6 genotype on adverse effects during treatment with metoprolol: a prospective clinical study. Clin Pharmacol Ther 2005;78:378-387.
60. Neugebauer G, Neubert P. Metabolism of carvedilol in man. Eur J Drug Metab Pharmacokinet 1991;16:257-260.
61. Zhou HH, Wood AJ. Stereoselective disposition of carvedilol is determined by CYP2D6. Clin Pharmacol Ther 1995;57:518-524.
62. Graff DW, Williamson KM, Pieper JA, et al. Effect of fluoxetine on carvedilol pharmacokinetics, CYP2D6 activity, and autonomic balance in heart failure patients. J Clin Pharmacol 2001;41:97-106.
63. Takahashi H, Kashima T, Nomoto S, et al. Comparisons between in-vitro and in-vivo metabolism of (S)-warfarin: catalytic activities of cDNA-expressed CYP2C9, its Leu359 variant and their mixture versus unbound clearance in patients with the corresponding CYP2C9 genotypes. Pharmacogenetics 1998;8:365-373.
64. Takahashi H, Kashima T, Nomizo Y, et al. Metabolism of warfarin enantiomers in Japanese patients with heart disease having different CYP2C9 and CYP2C19 genotypes. Clin Pharmacol Ther 1998;63:519-528.
65. Scordo MG, Pengo V, Spina E, et al. Influence of CYP2C9 and CYP2C19 genetic polymorphisms on warfarin maintenance dose and metabolic clearance. Clin Pharmacol Ther 2002;72:702-710.
66. Loebstein R, Yonath H, Peleg D, et al. Interindividual variability in sensitivity to warfarin—nature or nurture? Clin Pharmacol Ther 2001;70:159-164.
67. Verstuyft C, Morin S, Robert A, et al. Early acenocoumarol overanticoagulation among cytochrome P450 2C9 poor metabolizers. Pharmacogenetics 2001;11:735-737.
68. Thijssen HH, Ritzen B. Acenocoumarol pharmacokinetics in relation to cytochrome P450 2C9 genotype. Clin Pharmacol Ther 2003;74:61-68.

69. Thijssen HH, Drittij MJ, Vervoort LM, et al. Altered pharmacokinetics of R- and S-acenocoumarol in a subject heterozygous for CYP2C9*3. Clin Pharmacol Ther 2001;70:292-298.
70. Visser LE, Vliet M, Schaik RHN, et al. The risk of overanticoagulation in patients with cytochrome P450 2C9*2 and CYP2C9*3 alleles on acenocoumarol or phenprocoumon. Pharmacogenetics 2004;14:27-33.
71. Tassies D, Freire C, Pijoan J, et al. Pharmacogenetics of acenocoumarol: cytochrome P450 CYP2C9 polymorphisms influence dose requirements and stability of anticoagulation. Haematologica 2002;87:1185-1191.
72. Visser LE, Schaik RH, Vliet M, et al. The risk of bleeding complications in patients with cytochrome P450 CYP2C9*2 or CYP2C9*3 alleles on acenocoumarol or phenprocoumon. Thromb Haemost 2004;92:61-66.
73. Rost S, Fregin A, Ivaskevicius V, et al. Mutations in VKORC1 cause warfarin resistance and multiple coagulation factor deficiency type 2. Nature 2004;427:537-541.
74. Geisen C, Watzka M, Sittinger K, et al. VKORC1 haplotypes and their impact on the inter-individual and inter-ethnical variability of oral anticoagulation. Thromb Haemost 2005;94:773-779.
75. Rieder MJ, Reiner AP, Gage BF, et al. Effect of VKORC1 haplotypes on transcriptional regulation and warfarin dose. N Engl J Med 2005;352:2285-2293.
76. Reitsma PH, van der Heijden JF, Groot AP, et al. A C1173T dimorphism in the VKORC1 gene determines coumarin sensitivity and bleeding risk. PLoS Med 2005;2: e312.
77. Osman A, Enstrom C, Arbring K, et al. Main haplotypes and mutational analysis of vitamin K epoxide reductase (VKORC1) in a Swedish population: a retrospective analysis of case records. J Thromb Haemost 2006;4:1723-1729.
78. Quteineh L, Verstuyft C, Descot C, et al. Vitamin K epoxide reductase (VKORC1) genetic polymorphism is associated to oral anticoagulant overdose. Thromb Haemost 2005;94:690-691.
79. Klotz U, Schwab M, Treiber G. CYP2C19 polymorphism and proton pump inhibitors. Basic Clin Pharmacol Toxicol 2004;95:2-8.
80. Schwab M, Schaeffeler E, Klotz U, et al. CYP2C19 polymorphism is a major predictor of treatment failure in white patients by use of lansoprazole-based quadruple therapy for eradication of *Helicobacter pylori*. Clin Pharmacol Ther 2004;76:201-209.
81. Andersson T, Holmberg J, Rohss K, et al. Pharmacokinetics and effect on caffeine metabolism of the proton pump inhibitors, omeprazole, lansoprazole, and pantoprazole. Br J Clin Pharmacol 1998;45:369-375.
82. Chong SA, Tan EC, Tan CH, et al. Polymorphisms of dopamine receptors and tardive dyskinesia among Chinese patients with schizophrenia. Am J Med Genet 2003;116:51-54.
83. Furuta T, Shirai N, Takashima M, et al. Effects of genotypic differences in CYP2C19 status on cure rates for *Helicobacter pylori* infection by dual therapy with rabeprazole plus amoxicillin. Pharmacogenetics 2001;11:341-348.
84. Furuta T, Shirai N, Kodaira M, et al. Pharmacogenomics-based tailored versus standard therapeutic regimen for eradication of *H. pylori*. Clin Pharmacol Ther 2007; 81:521-528.
85. Wedlund PJ. The CYP2C19 enzyme polymorphism. Pharmacology 2000;61:174-183.
86. Furuta T, Shirai N, Watanabe F, et al. Effect of cytochrome P4502C19 genotypic differences on cure rates for gastroesophageal reflux disease by lansoprazole. Clin Pharmacol Ther 2002;72:453-460.
87. Kawamura M, Ohara S, Koike T, et al. The effects of lansoprazole on erosive reflux oesophagitis are influenced by CYP2C19 polymorphism. Aliment Pharmacol Ther 2003;17:965-973.
88. Kawamura M, Ohara S, Koike T, et al. Cytochrome P450 2C19 polymorphism influences the preventive effect of lansoprazole on the recurrence of erosive reflux esophagitis. J Gastroenterol Hepatol 2007;22:222-226.
89. Rendic S. Summary of information on human CYP enzymes: human P450 metabolism data. Drug Metab Rev 2002;34:83-448.
90. Brenner SS, Herrlinger C, Dilger K, et al. Influence of age and cytochrome P450 2C9 genotype on the steady-state disposition of diclofenac and celecoxib. Clin Pharmacokinet 2003;42:283-292.
91. Dorado P, Berecz R, Norberto MJ, et al. CYP2C9 genotypes and diclofenac metabolism in Spanish healthy volunteers. Eur J Clin Pharmacol 2003;59:221-225.
92. Kirchheiner J, Meineke I, Steinbach N, et al. Pharmacokinetics of diclofenac and inhibition of cyclooxygenases 1 and 2: no dependence from the CYP2C9 genetic polymorphism in humans. Br J Clin Pharmacol 2003;55:51-61.
93. Yasar Ü, Eliasson E, Forslund-Bergengren C, et al. The role of CYP2C9 genotype in the metabolism of diclofenac in vivo and in vitro. Pharmacol Toxicol 2001;89: 106.
94. Early Breast Cancer Trialists' Collaborative Group. Tamoxifen for early breast cancer: an overview of the randomised trials. Lancet 1998;351:1451-1467.
95. Desta Z, Ward BA, Soukhova NV, et al. Comprehensive evaluation of tamoxifen sequential biotransformation by the human cytochrome P450 system in vitro: prominent roles for CYP3A and CYP2D6. J Pharmacol Exp Ther 2004;310:1062-1075.
96. Coller JK, Krebsfaenger N, Klein K, et al. The influence of CYP2B6, CYP2C9 and CYP2D6 genotypes on the formation of the potent antioestrogen Z-4-hydroxy-tamoxifen in human liver. Br J Clin Pharmacol 2002;54:157-167.
97. Borges S, Desta Z, Li L, et al. Quantitative effect of CYP2D6 genotype and inhibitors on tamoxifen metabolism: implication for optimization of breast cancer treatment. Clin Pharmacol Ther 2006;80:61-74.
98. Goetz MP, Knox SK, Suman VJ, et al. The impact of cytochrome P450 2D6 metabolism in women receiving adjuvant tamoxifen. Breast Cancer Res Treat 2007;101:113-121.
99. Schroth W, Antoniadou L, Fritz P, et al. Breast cancer treatment outcome with adjuvant tamoxifen relative to patient CYP2D6 and CYP2C19 genotypes. J Clin Oncol 2007;25:5147-5149.
100. Sim SC, Risinger C, Dahl ML, et al. A common novel CYP2C19 gene variant causes ultrarapid drug metabolism relevant for the drug response to proton pump inhibitors and antidepressants. Clin Pharmacol Ther 2006;79:103-113.
101. Goetz MP, Rae JM, Suman VJ, et al. Pharmacogenetics of tamoxifen biotransformation is associated with clinical outcomes of efficacy and hot flashes. J Clin Oncol 2005;23:9312-9318.
102. Nowell SA, Ahn J, Rae JM, et al. Association of genetic variation in tamoxifen-metabolizing enzymes with overall survival and recurrence of disease in breast cancer patients. Breast Cancer Res Treat 2005;91:249-258.
103. Wegman PP, Wingren S. CYP2D6 variants and the prediction of tamoxifen response in randomized patients: author response. Breast Cancer Res 2005;7:E7.
104. Goss PE, Ingle JN, Martino S, et al. Randomized trial of letrozole following tamoxifen as extended adjuvant therapy in receptor-positive breast cancer: updated findings from NCIC CTG MA.17. J Natl Cancer Inst 2005;97:1262-1271.
105. Teml A, Schaeffeler E, Herrlinger KR, et al. Thiopurine treatment in inflammatory bowel disease: clinical pharmacology and implication of pharmacogenetically guided dosing. Clin Pharmacokinet 2007;46:187-208.
106. Somerville L, Krynetski EY, Krynetskaia NF, et al. Structure and dynamics of thioguanine-modified duplex DNA. J Biol Chem 2003;278:1005-1011.
107. Weinshilboum RM, Sladek SL. Mercaptopurine pharmacogenetics: monogenic inheritance of erythrocyte thiopurine methyltransferase activity. Am J Hum Genet 1980; 32:651-662.
108. Schaeffeler E, Eichelbaum M, Reinisch W, et al. Three novel thiopurine *S*-methyltransferase allelic variants (TPMT*20, *21, *22)—association with decreased enzyme function. Hum Mutat 2006;27:976.
109. Schaeffeler E, Fischer C, Brockmeier D, et al. Comprehensive analysis of thiopurine *S*-methyltransferase phenotype-genotype correlation in a large population of German-Caucasians and identification of novel TPMT variants. Pharmacogenetics 2004;14:407-417.
110. Schwab M, Schaeffeler E, Marx C, et al. Shortcoming in the diagnosis of TPMT deficiency in a patient with Crohn's disease using phenotyping only. Gastroenterology 2001;121:498-499.
111. Lennard L, Chew TS, Lilleyman JS. Human thiopurine methyltransferase activity varies with red blood cell age. Br J Clin Pharmacol 2001;52:539-546.
112. Xin HW, Fischer C, Schwab M, et al. Thiopurine *S*-methyltransferase as a target for drug interactions. Eur J Clin Pharmacol 2005;61:395-398.
113. Xin H, Fischer C, Schwab M, et al. Effects of aminosalicylates on thiopurine *S*-methyltransferase activity: an ex vivo study in patients with inflammatory bowel disease. Aliment Pharmacol Ther 2005;21:1105-1109.
114. Dilger K, Schaeffeler E, Lukas M, et al. Monitoring of thiopurine methyltransferase activity in postsurgical patients with Crohn's disease during 1 year of treatment with azathioprine or mesalazine. Ther Drug Monit 2007;29:1-5.
115. Evans WE, Hon YY, Bomgaars L, et al. Preponderance of thiopurine *S*-methyltransferase deficiency and heterozygosity among patients intolerant to mercaptopurine or azathioprine. J Clin Oncol 2001;19:2293-2301.
116. Colombel JF, Ferrari N, Debuysere H, et al. Genotypic analysis of thiopurine *S*-methyltransferase in patients with Crohn's disease and severe myelosuppression during azathioprine therapy. Gastroenterology 2000;118:1025-1030.
117. Sebbag L, Boucher P, Davelu P, et al. Thiopurine *S*-methyltransferase gene polymorphism is predictive of azathioprine-induced myelosuppression in heart transplant recipients. Transplantation 2000;69:1524-1527.
118. Relling MV, Hancock ML, Rivera GK, et al. Mercaptopurine therapy intolerance and heterozygosity at the thiopurine *S*-methyltransferase gene locus. J Natl Cancer Inst 1999;91:2001-2008.
119. Black AJ, McLeod HL, Capell HA, et al. Thiopurine methyltransferase genotype predicts therapy-limiting severe toxicity from azathioprine. Ann Intern Med 1998; 129:716-718.
120. Evans WE, Rodman JH, Relling MV, et al. Concept of maximum tolerated systemic exposure and its application to phase I-II studies of anticancer drugs. Med Pediatr Oncol 1991;19:153-159.
121. Kaskas BA, Louis E, Hindorf U, et al. Safe treatment of thiopurine *S*-methyltransferase deficient Crohn's disease patients with azathioprine. Gut 2003;52:140-142.
122. Lennard L, Lilleyman JS, Van Loon J, et al. Genetic variation in response to 6-mercaptopurine for childhood acute lymphoblastic leukaemia. Lancet 1990;336:225-229.
123. Stanulla M, Schaeffeler E, Flohr T, et al. Thiopurine methyltransferase (TPMT) genotype and early treatment response to mercaptopurine in childhood acute lymphoblastic leukemia. Jama 2005;293:1485-1489.
124. Maitland ML, Vasisht K, Ratain MJ. TPMT, UGT1A1 and DPYD: genotyping to ensure safer cancer therapy? Trends Pharmacol Sci 2006;27:432-437.
125. Zimm S, Collins JM, O'Neill D, et al. Inhibition of first-pass metabolism in cancer chemotherapy: interaction of 6-mercaptopurine and allopurinol. Clin Pharmacol Ther 1983;34:810-817.
126. Kennedy DT, Hayney MS, Lake KD. Azathioprine and allopurinol: the price of an avoidable drug interaction. Ann Pharmacother 1996;30:951-954.
127. Heggie GD, Sommadossi JP, Cross DS, et al. Clinical pharmacokinetics of 5-fluorouracil and its metabolites in plasma, urine, and bile. Cancer Res 1987;47: 2203-2206.
128. Diasio RB, Beavers TL, Carpenter JT. Familial deficiency of dihydropyrimidine dehydrogenase. Biochemical basis for familial pyrimidinemia and severe 5-fluorouracil–induced toxicity. J Clin Invest 1988;81:47-51.
129. Etienne MC, Lagrange JL, Dassonville O, et al. Population study of dihydropyrimidine dehydrogenase in cancer patients. J Clin Oncol 1994;12:2248-2253.
130. Soong R, Diasio RB. Advances and challenges in fluoropyrimidine pharmacogenomics and pharmacogenetics. Pharmacogenomics 2005;6:835-847.

131. Morel A, Boisdron-Celle M, Fey L, et al. Clinical relevance of different dihydropyrimidine dehydrogenase gene single nucleotide polymorphisms on 5-fluorouracil tolerance. Mol Cancer Ther 2006;5:2895-2904.
132. Chansky K, Benedetti J, Macdonald JS. Differences in toxicity between men and women treated with 5-fluorouracil therapy for colorectal carcinoma. Cancer 2005; 103:1165-1171.
133. Robien K, Boynton A, Ulrich CM. Pharmacogenetics of folate-related drug targets in cancer treatment. Pharmacogenomics 2005;6:673-689.
134. Frickhofen N, Beck FJ, Jung B, et al. Capecitabine can induce acute coronary syndrome similar to 5-fluorouracil. Ann Oncol 2002;13:797-801.
135. Collie-Duguid ES, Etienne MC, Milano G, et al. Known variant DPYD alleles do not explain DPD deficiency in cancer patients. Pharmacogenetics 2000;10:217-223.
136. Fleming RA, Milano G, Thyss A, et al. Correlation between dihydropyrimidine dehydrogenase activity in peripheral mononuclear cells and systemic clearance of fluorouracil in cancer patients. Cancer Res 1992;52:2899-2902.
137. Van Kuilenburg AB, Van Lenthe H, Tromp A, et al. Pitfalls in the diagnosis of patients with a partial dihydropyrimidine dehydrogenase deficiency. Clin Chem 2000;46:9-17.
138. van Kuilenburg AB, Baars JW, Meinsma R, et al. Lethal 5-fluorouracil toxicity associated with a novel mutation in the dihydropyrimidine dehydrogenase gene. Ann Oncol 2003;14:341-342.
138a. Schwab M, Zanger UM, Marx C, et al. for the German 5-FU Toxicity Study Group. Role of genetic and nongenetic factors for fluorouracil treatment-related severe toxicity: a prospective clinical trial by the German 5-FU Toxicity Study Group. J Clin Oncol 2008;26:2131-2138.
139. Sai K, Saeki M, Saito Y, et al. UGT1A1 haplotypes associated with reduced glucuronidation and increased serum bilirubin in irinotecan-administered Japanese patients with cancer. Clin Pharmacol Ther 2004;75:501-515.
140. Innocenti F, Iyer L, Ratain MJ. Pharmacogenetics of anticancer agents: lessons from amonafide and irinotecan. Drug Metab Dispos 2001;29:596-600.
141. Araki K, Fujita K, Ando Y, et al. Pharmacogenetic impact of polymorphisms in the coding region of the UGT1A1 gene on SN-38 glucuronidation in Japanese patients with cancer. Cancer Sci 2006;97:1255-1259.
142. Innocenti F, Undevia SD, Iyer L, et al. Genetic variants in the UDP-glucuronosyltransferase 1A1 gene predict the risk of severe neutropenia of irinotecan. J Clin Oncol 2004;22:1382-1388.
143. Rothman K, Greenland S. Modern Epidemiology, 2nd ed. Philadelphia: Lippincott Williams & Wilkins, 1998.
144. Patsopoulos NA, Analatos AA, Ioannidis JP. Relative citation impact of various study designs in the health sciences. JAMA 2005;293:2362-2366.
145. Kaiser R, Hofer A, Grapengiesser A, et al. L-Dopa–induced adverse effects in PD and dopamine transporter gene polymorphism. Neurology 2003;60:1750-1755.
146. Drazen JM, Yandava CN, Dube L, et al. Pharmacogenetic association between ALOX5 promoter genotype and the response to anti-asthma treatment. Nat Genet 1999; 22:168-170.
147. Poirier J, Delisle MC, Quirion R, et al. Apolipoprotein E4 allele as a predictor of cholinergic deficits and treatment outcome in Alzheimer disease. Proc Natl Acad Sci U S A 1995;92:12260-12264.
148. Esteller M, Garcia-Foncillas J, Andion E, et al. Inactivation of the DNA-repair gene MGMT and the clinical response of gliomas to alkylating agents. N Engl J Med 2000;343:1350-1354.
149. Sesti F, Abbott GW, Wei J, et al. A common polymorphism associated with antibiotic-induced cardiac arrhythmia. Proc Natl Acad Sci U S A 2000;97:10613-10618.
150. Cooke GE, Bray PF, Hamlington JD, et al. PlA2 polymorphism and efficacy of aspirin. Lancet 1998;351:1253.
151. Michelson AD, Furman MI, Goldschmidt-Clermont P, et al. Platelet GP IIIa Pl(A) polymorphisms display different sensitivities to agonists. Circulation 2000;101:1013-1018.
152. Wheeler GL, Braden GA, Bray PF, et al. Reduced inhibition by abciximab in platelets with the PlA2 polymorphism. Am Heart J 2002;143:76-82.
153. Kuivenhoven JA, Jukema JW, Zwinderman AH, et al. The role of a common variant of the cholesteryl ester transfer protein gene in the progression of coronary atherosclerosis. The Regression Growth Evaluation Statin Study Group. N Engl J Med 1998;338:86-93.
154. Cusi D, Barlassina C, Azzani T, et al. Polymorphisms of alpha-adducin and salt sensitivity in patients with essential hypertension. Lancet 1997;349:1353-1357.
155. Ueda S, Meredith PA, Morton JJ, et al. ACE (I/D) genotype as a predictor of the magnitude and duration of the response to an ACE inhibitor drug (enalaprilat) in humans. Circulation 1998;98:2148-2153.

17

PEDIATRIC PHARMACOLOGY*

Kathleen A. Neville, Michael J. Blake, Michael D. Reed, and Gregory L. Kearns

INTRODUCTION 239
DEVELOPMENTAL DIFFERENCES IN DRUG DISPOSITION 239
Drug Absorption 239
Drug Distribution and Plasma Protein Binding 241
Drug Transporters 242
Drug Metabolism 242
Phase I Enzymes 243
Phase II Enzymes 243
Renal Elimination 243
AGE-RELATED CHANGES IN DRUG RESPONSE 244
PEDIATRIC DOSE AND REGIMEN SELECTION 244
OTHER CONSIDERATIONS IN PHARMACOLOGIC TREATMENT OF CHILDREN 245
Drug Formulation and Route of Administration 245
Oral Drug Administration 245
Parenteral Drug Administration 245
Other Routes for Drug Administration 246
Adherence and Compliance: Practical Considerations 246
Adverse Drug Reactions 246
Special Considerations of Pediatric Clinical Pharmacology Research 247
CONCLUSION 248

INTRODUCTION

More than 100 years ago, Dr. Abraham Jacobi, the father of American pediatrics, recognized the importance of and need for age-appropriate pharmacotherapy and wrote, "pediatrics does not deal with miniature men and women, with reduced doses and the same class of disease in smaller bodies, but . . . has its own independent range and horizon. . . ."[1,2] By age 5 years, 95% of children have been prescribed medications, with an average of 8.5 prescriptions and 5.5 different medications and with the greatest number of prescriptions given to children between the ages of 7 and 12 months of age.[3] During the past several decades, our increasing understanding of human ontogeny has led to the realization that developmental changes greatly influence drug disposition and response, thereby necessitating age-dependent dose adjustments.[4]

Human growth and development consists of a continuum of biologic events that includes somatic growth, neurobehavioral maturation, and eventual reproduction. The impact of these developmental changes in drug biodisposition is largely related to changes in body composition (e.g., body water content, plasma protein concentrations) and function of organs important in metabolism (e.g., the liver) and excretion (e.g., the kidney).[4] During the first decade of life, these changes are dynamic and can be nonlinear and discordant, making standardized dosing inadequate for effective drug dosing across the span of childhood. Consequently, "dosing equations" that have been used in the past have been largely abandoned and replaced by choice of drug dose as a function of either body weight (BW; mg/kg) or body surface area (BSA; mg/m^2). Although such guidelines are generally adequate for initiating therapy, they may not be sufficient for sustained or chronic treatment because significant developmental variation in pharmacokinetics and/or pharmacodynamics can occur both within a given patient and between patients. Therefore, safe and effective drug therapy for children requires a fundamental and integrative understanding of how ontogeny influences drug disposition and action (Fig. 17-1).

Over the past 50 years, pediatric clinical pharmacology has evolved from an area of special emphasis to a subdiscipline of clinical pharmacology of particular importance to the medical care of pediatric patients. The large amount of knowledge generated during this time in the area of developmental pharmacology and therapeutics precludes the presentation of a comprehensive treatise in this chapter. Rather, it is the intention of the authors to provide readers with a "primer" on pediatric clinical pharmacology that will be sufficient to produce a solid foundation for further inquiry and also to provide the important fundamentals upon which sound therapeutic decision making in pediatrics can be based.

DEVELOPMENTAL DIFFERENCES IN DRUG DISPOSITION

Drug Absorption

As in adults, drugs can be administered to pediatric patients by a variety of routes. The majority of drugs administered to children are given either orally (the most common route), rectally, or percutaneously. Developmental changes can alter absorption of drugs delivered by any of these routes. For any drug, absorption is the result of a drug's ability to overcome chemical, physical, mechanical, and biologic barriers. Age-related changes in the absorptive surfaces (e.g., gastrointestinal tract, skin, pulmonary tree) can markedly influence the rate and/or extent of drug bioavailability (Table 17-1).

For drugs that are orally administered, the rate and extent of gastrointestinal (GI) absorption are primarily dependent upon (i) pH-dependent passive diffusion and (ii) motility of both the stomach and the small intestine.[4] Variations in GI intraluminal pH can directly affect the amount of drug available for absorption through its influence on both drug stability and degree of ionization. At birth, the gastric pH drops from approximately 7 to 3 within the first few hours of life. It then rises and remains elevated (pH > 4) during the neonatal period as a result of reductions in both basal acid output and volume of gastric secretions.[2,5,6] Adult values are not reached until 20 to 30 months of age.[4] The result is that oral bioavailability for acid-labile compounds is increased and oral bioavailability for weak acids is decreased in neonates compared with levels in adults.[2]

Gastric and intestinal motility also influence absorption because they are the primary determinants of the rate at which drugs are distributed along the mucosal surface of the small intestine. Although few studies have systematically evaluated the effect of developmental changes in motility on drug absorption in infants and children, it is known that there is a marked increase in gastric emptying during the first week of life[2,7,8] and that intestinal motor activity matures through

*The authors gratefully acknowledge the contributions made by Dr. J. Steven Leeder and the support of this work by grant #U 01 HD31313-14 (G.L.K.), Pediatric Pharmacology Research Unit Network, National Institute of Child Health and Human Development, Bethesda, MD.

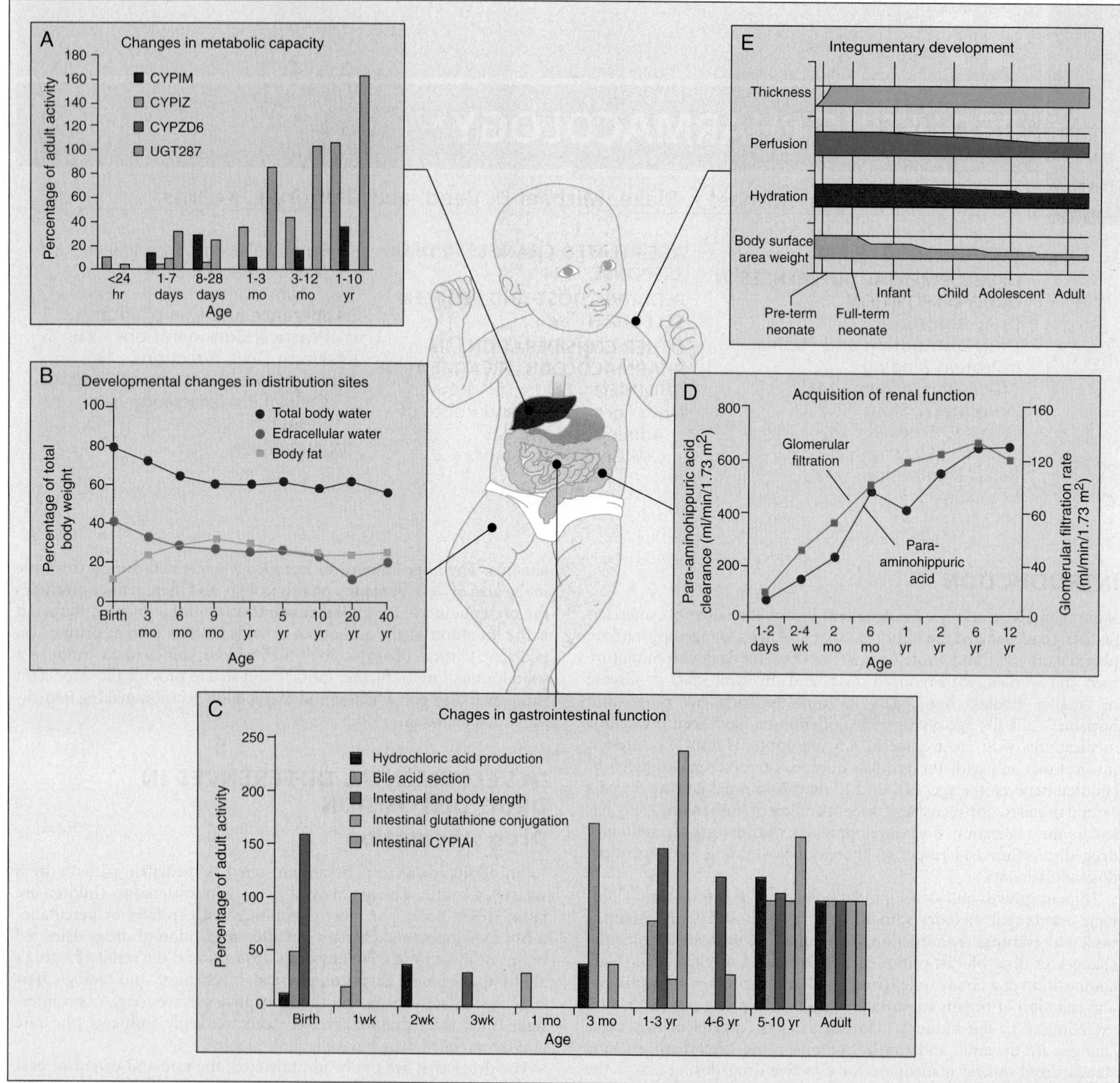

FIGURE 17-1 • Developmental changes in physiologic factors that influence drug disposition in infants, children, and adolescents. Physiologic changes in multiple organs and organ systems during development are responsible for age-related differences in drug disposition. **A,** The activity of many cytochrome P-450 (CYP) isoforms and a single glucuronosyltransferase (UGT) isoform is markedly diminished during the first 2 months of life. In addition, the acquisition of adult activity over time is enzyme- and isoform-specific. **B,** Age-dependent changes in body composition, which influence the apparent volume of distribution for drugs. Infants in the first 6 months of life have markedly expanded total body water and extracellular water, expressed as a percentage of total body weight, as compared with older infants and adults. **C,** Age-dependent changes in both the structure and the function of the gastrointestinal tract. As with hepatic drug-metabolizing enzymes (**A**), the activity of CYP1A1 in the intestine is low during early life. **D,** The effect of postnatal development on the processes of active tubular secretion—represented by the clearance of para-aminohippuric acid and the glomerular filtration rate, both of which approximate adult activity by 6 to 12 months of age. **E,** Age dependence in the thickness, extent of perfusion, and extent of hydration of the skin and the relative size of the skin-surface area (reflected by the ratio of body surface area to body weight). Although skin thickness is similar in infants and adults, the extent of perfusion and hydration diminishes from infancy to adulthood. (**A-D,** Data adapted from references 5, 6, 15, 19, 26, 29, 36, 39, 42, 44, 69, 70-75. Reprinted by permission from Kearns GL, Abdel-Rahman SM, Alander SW, et al. Developmental pharmacology—drug disposition, action, and therapy in infants and children. N Engl J Med 2003;349:1157-1167.)

infancy such that by approximately 4 months of age, the absorption of nutrient macromolecules (subject to both passive and active transport) appears to have matured.[9] Therefore, the rate at which most drugs are absorbed is slower in neonates and young infants relative to older infants and children. Consequently, the time to achieve maximum plasma concentrations is prolonged.

Whereas it is generally assumed that intestinal surface area is reduced in early life, average intestinal length as a percentage of adult values exceeds other anthropometric measurements, with villous formation beginning at 8 weeks of gestation and maturing by week 20. Therefore, it is unlikely that smaller surface areas in the small intestine contribute to reduced absorption. Instead, age-associated changes in splanchnic

TABLE 17-1 SUMMARY OF IMPORTANT FACTORS THAT INFLUENCE DRUG ABSORPTION IN NEONATES, INFANTS, AND CHILDREN

	Neonates*	Infants*	Children*
PHYSIOLOGIC ALTERATION			
Gastric emptying time	Irregular	Slightly increased	Increased
Gastric pH	>5	4-2	Adult pattern
Intestinal motility	Reduced	Increased	Slightly increased
Intestinal surface area	Reduced	Near adult pattern	Adult pattern
Microbial colonization	Reduced	Near adult pattern	Adult pattern
Biliary function	Immature	Near adult pattern	Adult pattern
Muscular blood flow	Reduced	Increased	Adult pattern
Skin permeability	Increased	Increased	Near adult pattern
POSSIBLE PHARMACOKINETIC CONSEQUENCES			
Oral absorption	Erratic—reduced	↑ Rate	Near adult pattern
Intramuscular absorption	Variable	Increased	Adult pattern
Percutaneous absorption	Increased	Increased	Near adult pattern
Rectal absorption	Very efficient	Efficient	Near adult pattern
Presystemic clearance	<Adult pattern	>Adult pattern	>Adult pattern (↑ rate)

*Direction of alteration given relative to expected normal adult patterns.
Adapted from Morselli PL.[76] Reprinted by permission from Ritschel WA, Kearns GL. *Handbook of Basic Pharmacokinetics . . . Including Clinical Applications,* 6th edition. Washington, DC: American Pharmacists Association, 2006, table 24-1, © 2004 by the American Pharmacists Association.

blood flow that occur in the first 2 to 3 weeks of life likely influence absorption rates by altering the concentration gradient that occurs across the intestinal mucosa.[2,10-14] Immaturity of the intestinal mucosa leading to increased permeability, high levels of β-glucuronidase activity, and variability of microbial colonization in the gut also plays a role in intestinal drug absorption.[4]

The rate at which orally administered drugs are absorbed is also influenced by a drug's individual biochemical properties and is generally slower in neonates and young infants relative to older infants and children, resulting in a prolonged time to achieve maximum plasma concentrations.[2] For example, the ability to solubilize and subsequently absorb lipophilic drugs is dependent on developmental changes in biliary function. Specifically, immaturity in conjugation and/or transport of bile salts into the intestinal lumen results in low intraduodenal levels despite blood levels that exceed those of adults.[2,15,16]

Developmental differences in the activity of intestinal drug-metabolizing enzymes (DMEs) and efflux transporters can markedly alter orally administered drug bioavailability.[17] Studies suggest that epoxide hydrolase and glutathione peroxidase activities demonstrate little age dependence in contrast to intestinal cytochrome P-450 (CYP) 1A1 activity, which increases with age.[18] Interestingly, these studies also suggest that a reduction in glutathione-*S*-transferase activity occurs from infancy through early adolescence, as illustrated by reduced oral clearance of busulfan, a substrate for this enzyme.[19] Developmental expression of the efflux transporter P-glycoprotein (MDR1) in the human intestine may also influence the oral bioavailability (presystemic clearance) of drugs that are substrates for this protein. As reported by Fakhoury and colleagues,[20] CYP3A protein was uniformly present in samples of human small intestine by 6 months of age, whereas in younger infants, it was not present in all samples. Currently, the functional significance of these findings relative to the ontogeny of intestinal P-glycoprotein in humans is not known.

The bioavailability of rectally administered drugs (e.g., diazepam and acetaminophen) is related to both translocation across the rectal mucosa and clearance by DMEs in the liver.[4] The enhanced bioavailability for extensively metabolized compounds administered rectally in neonates and very young infants is likely due to developmental immaturity in hepatic metabolism rather than to enhanced mucosal translocation. However, infants have a greater number of high-amplitude pulsatile contractions in the rectum that can enhance expulsion of solid dosage forms[21] and effectively decrease absorption of drugs, necessitating that rigorous procedures be in place to ensure full dose administration.[22-24]

Absorption of cutaneously and percutaneously administered drugs can differ in neonates and young children when compared with that in adults for several reasons. First, the ratio of total BSA to body mass in infants and young children far exceeds that of adults. Consequently, relative systemic exposure to drugs applied topically (e.g., corticosteroids, antihistamines, antiseptics) to infants and children may exceed that in adults.[2,25,26] Enhanced percutaneous absorption during infancy occurs as a result of a thinner stratum corneum[27] as well as differences in perfusion and hydration of the epidermis when compared with those of adults.[28,29] These factors may lead to systemic toxicity with seemingly small amounts of drug administration during the first year of life. Drugs known to cause systemic toxicity include diphenhydramine, lidocaine, isopropyl alcohol, lindane, corticosteroids, and hexachlorophene.[4]

In contrast to drugs administered topically, the bioavailability of drugs administered intramuscularly may be reduced in neonates when compared with that in older infants and children. Generally, intramuscular (IM) absorption of drugs in the neonate is low and erratic, with the rate largely dependent on the chemical properties of the drug and the maturational stage of the neonate.[4] Relatively decreased muscular blood flow and inefficient muscular contractions, which are responsible for drug dispersion, act to reduce the rate of IM drug absorption in neonates.[4,30] An increased percentage of water per unit of muscle mass also contributes to reduced bioavailability of drugs administered by the IM route. However, the influence of these factors may be offset by the relative increase in skeletal muscle capillary density observed in infants as compared with that in older children,[31] resulting in more efficient IM drug absorption for particular agents (e.g., amikacin, cephalothin).[32,33] Generally speaking, the IM route is not used routinely for parenteral drug administration to infants and young children, with the exception of situations in which very intermittent dosing is required (e.g., one-time administration of an antimicrobial agent) or when therapy must be instituted before vascular access can be established.

Drug Distribution and Plasma Protein Binding

Marked changes in body composition occur during development. These changes alter the physiologic spaces into which drugs distribute.

TABLE 17-2 ONTOGENIC INFLUENCES OF PLASMA DRUG PROTEIN BINDING AND DRUG DISTRIBUTION IN NEONATES, INFANTS, AND CHILDREN

	Neonates*	Infants*	Children*
PHYSIOLOGIC ALTERATION			
Plasma albumin concentration	Reduced	Near normal	Near adult pattern
Fetal albumin concentration	Present	Absent	Absent
Total protein concentration	Reduced	Decreased	Near adult pattern
Total globulin concentration	Reduced	Decreased	Near adult pattern
Serum bilirubin	Increased	Normal	Normal adult pattern
Serum free fatty acids	Increased	Normal	Normal adult pattern
Blood pH	7.1-7.3	7.4 (normal)	7.4 (normal)
Adipose tissue	Scarce (↑ CNS)	Reduced	Generally reduced
Total body water	Increased	Increased	Near adult pattern
Extracellular water	Increased	Increased	Near adult pattern
Endogenous maternal substances (ligands)	Present	Absent	Absent
POSSIBLE PHARMACOKINETIC CONSEQUENCES			
Free drug fraction	Increased	Increased	Slightly increased
Apparent volume of distribution			
Hydrophilic drugs	Increased	Increased	Slightly increased
Hydrophobic drugs	Reduced	Reduced	Slightly decreased
Tissue : plasma ratio	Increased	Increased	Slightly increased

*Direction of alteration given relative to expected normal adult patterns.
CNS, central nervous system.
Adapted from Morselli PL.[76] Reprinted by permission from Ritschel WA, Kearns GL. *Handbook of Basic Pharmacokinetics . . . Including Clinical Applications*, 6th edition. Washington, DC: American Pharmacists Association, 2006, table 24-2, © 2004 by the American Pharmacists Association.

The most dynamic changes occur during the first year of life, with the exception of total body fat whose greatest change occurs between ages 10 and 20 years (in males, body fat is reduced by approximately 50%; in females, it decreases from approximately 28% to approximately 25% during that time period).[4]

Neonates and young infants have larger extracellular and total body water compartments, and their adipose tissue has significantly higher water content than that of older children and adults. These alterations produce lower plasma concentrations for a given dose of hydrophilic drugs that distribute primarily into these respective compartments. Conversely, lipophilic drugs that are distributed primarily within tissue are less affected by age-related influences on the apparent volume of distribution.[2,4] Despite the fact that body fat content during the first 3 months of life is low relative to other periods of development, the lipid content of the developing central nervous system (CNS) is quite high and confers a risk for adverse effects associated with administration of lipophilic compounds (e.g., propanolol). In addition, limited neonatal data suggest that passive drug diffusion into the CNS increases between 28 and 39 weeks of gestational age. Furthermore, animal studies suggest that changes in blood flow and pore density (rather than pore size) contribute to increases in CNS drug permeability observed in neonates and young infants, although these data have not been systematically evaluated in humans.[2,4,34]

Variations in the composition and amount of circulating plasma proteins (e.g., albumin and α_1 acid-glycoprotein) also influence the distribution of highly bound drugs. Neonates and young infants have a smaller amount of plasma protein than do older children and adults. This causes an increase in the free fraction of drug that is bioavailable. The greater proportion of α-fetoprotein (which has reduced binding affinity for weak acids) versus adult albumin and relatively increased levels of endogenous substances (e.g., bilirubin, free fatty acids) capable of displacing drug from albumin binding sites in the neonatal period may also contribute to higher free fractions of highly protein-bound drugs. Reduced plasma-binding protein associated with absolute and relative differences in the sizes of various physiologic compartments often influences both the apparent volume of distribution for many drugs and their localization in tissue. Consequently, the apparent volume of distribution for small-molecular-weight compounds that are not highly bound to plasma proteins is influenced more by age-related changes in total body water, whereas the apparent volume of distribution of drugs that are extensively bound to plasma proteins or tissues is better associated with age-related changes in body composition and binding affinity. Other factors associated with development and/or disease such as variability in regional blood flow, organ perfusion, permeability of cell membranes, changes in acid-base balance, and cardiac output can also influence drug binding and/or distribution (Table 17-2).

Drug Transporters

Whereas a substantial portion of drug distribution is the result of simple passive diffusion along concentration gradients and binding of drug to tissue components, transmembrane drug transporters also play a key role in drug distribution because they are capable of producing a functional barrier. Relatively little is known about the ontogeny of drug transporters despite documented differences in the handling of drugs among neonates, children, and adults. P-glycoprotein, a member of the adenosine triphosphate (ATP)–binding cassette (ABC) transporter family, is an efflux transporter that can expel toxins and xenobiotics from cells. Limited data regarding the ontogeny of P-glycoprotein expression exist for humans. However, a study of post-mortem infants of 23 to 42 weeks' gestation suggests that whereas localization patterns are similar to those of adults during late gestation and at term, levels of expression are lower than those of adults.[35]

Drug Metabolism

Generally, activities of DMEs are reduced to a varying degree in the neonate when compared with those of adults for both phase I (primarily oxidation) and phase II (conjugation) reactions (Table 17-3). For some DMEs, distinct patterns of isoform-specific developmental changes exist.[36,37] In fact, some polymorphically expressed DMEs display discordant genotype/phenotype relationships during develop-

TABLE 17-3 DRUG METABOLISM IN NEONATES, INFANTS, AND CHILDREN

	Neonates*	Infants*	Children*
PHYSIOLOGIC ALTERATION			
Liver : body weight ratio	Increased	Increased	Slightly increased
Cytochrome P-450 activity	Reduced	Increased	Slightly increased
Blood esterase activity	Reduced	Normal (by 12 mo)	Adult pattern
Hepatic blood flow	Reduced	Increased	Near adult pattern
Phase II enzyme activity	Reduced	Increased	Near adult pattern
POSSIBLE PHARMACOKINETIC CONSEQUENCES			
Metabolic rates	Reduced	Increased	Near adult pattern†
Presystemic clearance	Reduced	Increased	Near adult pattern
Total body clearance	Reduced	Increased	Near adult pattern†
Inducibility of drug-metabolizing enzymes	More evident	Slightly increased	Near adult pattern†

*Direction of alteration given relative to expected normal adult patterns.
†Denotes assumption of adult pattern of activity after the conclusion of puberty. The activity of all drug-metabolizing enzymes is generally higher before than after puberty.
Adapted from Morselli PL.[76] Reprinted by permission from Ritschel WA, Kearns GL. *Handbook of Basic Pharmacokinetics . . . Including Clinical Applications*, 6th edition. Washington, DC: American Pharmacists Association, 2006, table 24-1, © 2004 by the American Pharmacists Association.

ment. Hence, age-related changes in DME activity can lead to significant drug toxicity or lack of efficacy, making age-appropriate dosing regimens essential for many drugs commonly used in neonates, young infants, and children.

Whereas the disposition of drugs metabolized by phase I and phase II DMEs varies widely, the age-dependent increase in plasma clearance in children under 10 years compared with that in adults is consistent and confers relatively higher weight-based (i.e., mg/kg) dose requirements. The mechanism(s) underlying these age-related increases in plasma drug clearance remains largely unknown. However, it is unlikely that higher drug clearance in infants and young children can be attributed solely to a disproportionately greater liver mass, given that the weight of the liver as a percentage of total body mass reaches maximum values between 1 and 3 years of age. Clinically, the significance of developmentally associated increases in DME activity are related to associated changes in plasma drug clearance (see later).

Phase I Enzymes

Development has a profound effect on the expression of phase I enzymes. Insight into the ontogeny of drug metabolism is most often derived from pharmacokinetic studies of drugs that are substrates for specific CYP isoforms. For example, midazolam plasma clearance following parenteral administration of the drug primarily reflects hepatic CYP3A4/5 activity. CYP2C9 and, to a lesser extent, CYP2C19 are primarily responsible for phenytoin biotransformation, whereas CYP2C9 and CYP2C8 are responsible for the metabolism of nonsteroidal anti-inflammatory agents given to neonates to pharmacologically close a patent ductus arteriosus (e.g., indomethacin, ibuprofen) and to older infants and children for the treatment of pain and/or fever. Caffeine and theophylline, drugs both commonly prescribed to neonates and young infants for the treatment of apnea of prematurity, are substrates for CYP1A2 whose plasma clearance serves as a surrogate "marker" for the ontogeny of this DME.

Distinct postnatal patterns of isoform-specific developmental CYP expression have been observed between DMEs. CYP3A7 is the predominant CYP3A isoform expressed in fetal liver, and it is functionally active and inducible during gestation. CYP3A7 expression peaks shortly after birth and then declines, such that it is absent by 1 to 4 weeks of age. Interestingly, approximately 5% of individuals have persistent expression of CYP3A7, even when CYP3A4 predominates. CYP2D6 is low to absent in fetal liver, but it is present at 1 week of age. It reaches approximately 20% of adult activity by 1 month of age and full adult activity by approximately 12 months. CYP3A4 reaches approximately 30% to 40% of adult activity by 1 month of age and full activity by 6 months of age. Interestingly, CYP3A4 activity may exceed that of adult levels between 1 and 4 years of age, with persistence of the increased activity until after puberty. CYP2C enzymes (CYP2C9 and CYP2C19) have low activity in the first 2 to 4 weeks of life and reach adult levels by approximately 6 months. Activity of these enzymes may also exceed adult levels during childhood, with persistence of greater than adult levels until after puberty. CYP1A2 is the last hepatic CYP to be acquired, with significant expression not appearing until 1 to 3 months of life and increased expression at 1 to 2 years of age, with decreases to adult levels of expression after puberty.[2,4]

Phase II Enzymes

The ontogeny of conjugation reactions (i.e., phase II enzymes) is less well established than that for phase I enzymes. It is known that individual glucuronosyl transferase (UGT) isoforms have unique maturational profiles with tangible pharmacokinetic consequences. Glucuronidation of morphine (a UGT2B7 substrate) can be detected in premature infants as young as 24 weeks' gestational age, but the proportions of morphine 3-glucuronide and morphine 6-glucuronide change with increasing age and birth weight.[38] Morphine's plasma clearance is positively correlated with gestational age and increases approximately fourfold between 27 and 40 weeks' gestational age. Given the changes in both proportion of morphine glucuronide metabolites and clearance, increased doses are required to maintain effective analgesia in neonates.[39-41] Glucuronidation of acetaminophen (a substrate for UGT1A6 and, to a lesser extent, UGT1A9) is another example of important age-related changes in phase II drug metabolism. Metabolism of acetaminophen is impaired in newborns and young children relative to that in adolescents and adults.[42] Whereas age-related changes in metabolism that result in toxicity are well described and historically embodied by the tragic gray baby syndrome caused by chloramphenicol, more modern examples continue to illustrate the importance of taking age into account when considering drugs that undergo phase II metabolism. For example, it has been shown that the oral clearance of zidovudine (a UGT2B7 substrate) is reduced in infants when compared with older children and that this lower clearance leads to increased zidovudine exposure, which contributes to increased hematologic toxicity in these patients.[43]

Renal Elimination

Renal function, more than any other organ system, depends on gestational age and postnatal adaptations. Renal function begins to mature early during fetal organogenesis and is complete by early childhood. Increases in glomerular filtration rate (GFR) result from both nephrogenesis, a process that is completed by 36 weeks of gestation, and

TABLE 17-4 RENAL FUNCTION IN NEONATES, INFANTS, AND CHILDREN

	Neonates*	Infants*	Children*
PHYSIOLOGIC ALTERATION			
Kidney : body weight ratio	Increased	Increased	Near adult values
Glomerular filtration rate	Reduced	Normal (by 12 mo)	Normal adult values
Active tubular secretion	Reduced	Near normal	Normal adult values†
Active tubular reabsorption	Reduced	Near normal	Normal adult values
Proteins present in urine	Present (30%)	Low to absent	Normally absent
Urinary acidification capacity	Low	Normal (by 1 mo)	Normal adult activity
Urine output (ml/hr/kg)	3-6	2-4	1-3
Urine concentrating capacity	Reduced	Near normal	Normal adult values
POSSIBLE PHARMACOKINETIC CONSEQUENCES			
Active drug excretion	Reduced	Near normal	Normal adult pattern
Passive drug excretion	Reduced to increased	Increased	Normal adult pattern
Excretion of basic drugs	Increased	Increased	Near normal

*Direction of alteration given relative to expected normal adult patterns.
†Denotes slight increase in excretion rate for basic compounds.
Adapted from Morselli PL.[76] Reprinted by permission from Ritschel WA, Kearns GL. *Handbook of Basic Pharmacokinetics . . . Including Clinical Applications*, 6th edition. Washington, DC: American Pharmacists Association, 2006, table 24-6, © 2004 by the American Pharmacists Association.

changes in renal and intrarenal blood flow.[44] GFRs vary widely among different postconceptional ages and range from approximately 2 ml/min/1.73 m^2 to 4 ml/min/1.73 m^2 in term neonates to a low of 0.6 ml/min/1.73 m^2 to 0.8 ml/min/1.73 m^2 in preterm neonates. The GFR increases rapidly during the first 2 weeks of life and then more slowly until adult values are reached by 8 to 12 months.[45,46] Age affects not only GFR but also tubular secretion, which is immature at birth and reaches adult capacity during the first year of life.

Developmental changes that occur in renal function are better characterized than any other organ system (Table 17-4). Renal function can significantly alter the plasma clearance of compounds that are renally eliminated and is a major determinant of drug-dosing regimens in children. Failure to account for the ontogeny of renal function and adjust dosing regimens accordingly can result in potentially toxic serum concentrations. For example, a starting gentamicin dosage interval of 12 hours in infants of any gestational age, or a starting dosage interval of 24 hours for infants of less than 30 weeks' gestational age, has been shown to lead to serum gentamicin trough levels in the toxic range.[47] It is important to note that use of some medications concomitantly (i.e., betamethasone and indomethacin) may cause alteration of the normal pattern of renal maturation in the neonate.[48] Therefore, both maturation and effects of treatment with regard to renal function are important considerations when determining appropriate drug treatments in neonates and infants.

AGE-RELATED CHANGES IN DRUG RESPONSE

Although it is generally accepted that development can alter drug action and response, there is a relative lack of information describing the impact of human ontogeny on overall pharmacodynamic effects and the relationship between individual drugs and their receptors. As discussed previously, a multitude of drugs exist for which developmental differences in pharmacodynamics occur as a consequence of alterations in absorption, distribution, metabolism, and/or elimination. However, data also support true age-dependent differences in pharmacologic targets for drug action (e.g., warfarin, cyclosporine) or in the plasma concentration versus effect relationship (e.g., midazolam).[49-52] In addition, whereas it is known that pharmacogenetic determinants may directly affect drug metabolism, evidence now suggests that pharmacogenetic determinants of drug action may also contribute to age-dependent differences in response and in the creation of adverse events (e.g., increased hepatotoxicity of valproic acid in young infants).[53-55] Clearly, any assessment of pharmacodynamics in pediatric patients must consider that ontogeny can influence drug effect (both efficacy and toxicity) not only through its effects on drug disposition but also through its direct effects on drug response.

PEDIATRIC DOSE AND REGIMEN SELECTION

Most current age-specific dosing requirements are based on the known influence of ontogeny on drug disposition.[56] As illustrated in Figure 17-1, developmental changes in physiology produce many of the age-associated changes in drug absorption, distribution, metabolism, and excretion that collectively result in altered pharmacokinetics and, therefore, serve as the determinants of age-specific drug dose requirements. Current gaps in our knowledge (e.g., incomplete developmental profiles for hepatic and extrahepatic DMEs, lack of knowledge with regard to expression of drug transporters that may influence drug clearance and/or bioavailability) prevent the use of simple formulas and/or allometric scaling for effective pediatric dose prediction.[2,57] Such approaches may have some potential clinical utility in children older than 8 years of age and adolescents whose organ function and body composition approximates that of young adults, but in general, these methods have limited utility in very young infants and children in whom ontogeny produces dramatic differences in drug disposition.

Age-specific dosing regimens for selected drugs commonly employed in pediatric therapy based on age-dependent differences in drug disposition illustrate this point. For specific drugs, dramatic differences in both dose and dose interval selection when compared with "standard" adult doses are evident. For drugs whose plasma concentrations are routinely measured clinically (e.g., aminoglycosides, digoxin, methylxanthines, anticonvulsants, methotrexate, cyclosporine, tacrolimus, mycophenolate mofetil), or for whom pharmacokinetic characteristics were defined in pediatric patients during the drug development process, individualization of treatment based on patient-derived and, in selected instances, population-estimated pharmacokinetic parameters is easily achieved. However, in the absence of such pharmacokinetic data and/or established pediatric dosing guidelines, alternate methods must often be employed.

To date, more than 20 different approaches for pediatric dose selection have been published.[4] As discussed previously, the majority of these utilize either BW or BSA to reflect the developmental changes of either body composition or the organ function required for drug clearance. Selection based on BW or BSA will generally produce similar relationships between drug dose and resultant plasma concentration, except for those drugs whose apparent volume of distribution (V_d) corresponds to the extracellular fluid pool (i.e., $V_d < 0.3$ L/kg), in which a BSA-based approach is preferable. In contrast, for drugs whose apparent V_d exceeds the extracellular fluid space (i.e., >0.3 L/kg), a BW-based approach for dose selection is preferable and, as a result, is the approach most frequently used for dosing in pediatrics.

When the pediatric dose for a given drug is not known, these principles can be used to best approximate a proper dose for the initiation of treatment. Ritschel and Kearns[4] described an approach to determine dose in infants that is illustrated by the following equations:

$$\text{Infant dose (if } V_d < 0.3 \text{ L/kg)} = (\text{infant BSA in m}^2/1.73 \text{ m}^2) * \text{adult dose}$$

$$\text{Infant dose (if } V_d \geq 0.3 \text{ L/kg)} = (\text{infant BW in kg}/70 \text{ kg}) * \text{adult dose}$$

This approach is useful only for selection of dose size and does not offer information regarding dosing interval because the equations contain no specific variable that describes potential age-associated differences in drug clearance. It is also important to note that this approach assumes that the body height and BW of a given child are appropriate (i.e., normal) for age and there are no abnormalities in body composition (e.g., edema, ascites).

In neonates and young infants, the dosing interval for drugs with significant (i.e., >50%) renal elimination by glomerular filtration can be approximated by estimation of the apparent elimination half-life ($t_{1/2}$) of the drug at a given point in development by using the following equations:

$$k_{el\ infant} = k_{el\ adult}\ (\{[(GFR_{infant}/GFR_{adult}) - 1]*F_{el}\} + 1)$$

$$T_{1/2\ infant} = 0.693/k_{el\ infant}$$

where k_{el} represents the average terminal apparent terminal elimination rate constant, GFR is an estimate of the GFR (which can be obtained from either a creatinine clearance determination or age-related normal values), and F_{el} is the fraction of drug excreted unchanged in the urine.

OTHER CONSIDERATIONS IN PHARMACOLOGIC TREATMENT OF CHILDREN

Drug Formulation and Route of Administration

One of the more unique challenges in pediatric pharmacotherapeutics, which is rarely if ever a concern in older patients, is the drug formulation itself. Despite the increasing sensitivity for the need to study drugs in children before they are used in children and to have available "pediatric-friendly" formulations, these benefits sadly are available for only a small portion of the drugs commonly used in pediatrics.

Oral Drug Administration

One of the principal determinants of oral drug administration in children is the ability to actually get the drug into the body. Oral formulations are often expelled by children because of poor taste and texture. This is a significant issue, especially when considering that taste sensation differs as a consequence of development and on an interindividual basis. Whereas solid oral formulations such as tablets and capsules offer a stable and convenient method of administration in adults, these are not easily administered to the majority of infants and children owing to their inability to easily and safely swallow such a formulation. Hence, these formulations offer significantly limited ability for dose titration and dosing flexibility. In some instances, limitations of flexibility in dosing produced by compressed tablets and/or capsules have been more recently addressed by the introduction of titratable, rapidly dissolving oral tablets and transmucosal delivery systems. Because more accurate dosing can be achieved by liquid formulations, these remain the preferred formulation for oral drug administration in infants and young children. However, palatability of these formulations is of paramount importance in order to ultimately achieve successful drug administration in children.

Administration of liquid medications is not without problems and can pose a significant risk if the device for administering the medication is not used properly or if the dosage given is not measured accurately for the patient's age or weight. Inaccurate dosing can occur when a caregiver uses a dosing cup from a different bottle of medication, misreads the directions, uses a tableware teaspoon or tablespoon to measure the medication, or misreads the markings on a dosing cup. The low cost and convenience of hypodermic syringes has prompted many physicians and pharmacists to dispense them with liquid medications in order to improve accuracy. However, since 1988, the U.S. Food and Drug Administration (FDA) has received several reports of children swallowing or choking on the plastic caps of syringes used to give liquid medication.[58] Finally, accuracy in drug administration associated with oral liquid formulations can also be compromised by physicochemical factors (e.g., drug precipitation, degradation), especially when storage conditions and/or labeled stability information is discounted.

Parenteral Drug Administration

For the sick pediatric patient, drugs are usually administered by the intravenous (IV) route, which poses challenges not perceived from adult experience. Age-associated changes in body composition and, in particular, body fat distribution can complicate location of a peripheral vein suitable for cannula insertion, as can a marked reduction in the internal diameter of the blood vessels. In addition, the common use of topical anesthetics prior to needle insertion often leads to vasoconstriction, which further increases the degree of difficulty for successful catheter placement.

Inability to establish vascular access for drug administration to sick infants and children produces a scenario often used to validate the need for IM drug administration, a route that should be reserved for use only in those children in whom vascular access is completely unavailable and this route is used only until vascular access can be reestablished. In addition, disease-induced modifications in peripheral blood flow that may result in poor absorption from the muscular bed consequent to impaired local distribution of the drug and translocation into the vasculature may compromise the efficiency of this alternate route.

An underappreciated complicating issue for parenteral drug administration to infants is the relative lack of formulations in concentrations suitable for IV administration. Physiologic limitations such as a low (as compared with adults) intravascular blood volume and reduced diameter of peripheral veins make the use of IV formulations created for administration to adult patients problematic in infants and, in particular, in neonates. Errors consequent to improper dilution of adult formulations necessary to ensure appropriate osmolarity and volume for IV administration (the most common resulting in a 10-fold overdose) are not uncommon. For example, morphine, a drug commonly used in neonates, infants, and children, is commonly available in an 8-mg/ml concentration. A usual 0.1-mg/kg morphine dose for a 1-kg infant using this formulation would require a nurse or pharmacist to accurately withdraw 0.013 ml and administer it into a length of IV tubing with a dead space volume that may exceed that of the dose by 100-fold. In this situation, accuracy of dose and infusion time can be significantly compromised.

Although underdosing is often a serious problem when attempting to administer these very small volumes, overdoses also occur owing to inaccurate extemporaneous dilutions. Moreover, attempts to compensate for the volumes present within the IV tubing further predispose the patient to receive an incorrect, possibly unsafe, dose. Whenever such concentrated drug formulations are the only source for use, appropriate alteration of the stock parenteral solution should be performed and manufactured by the pharmacy department. One additional step to foster avoidance of such dose errors is the use of standard dilutions that all practitioners are aware of and using standardized approaches for IV drug administration that minimize complications associated with unrealized drug dilution and errant infusion times (e.g., pediatric syringe pumps attached to low-volume tubing). Until pediatric formulations for parenteral drug administration become as commonly available as they are for older patients, the need for special extemporaneous preparations will continue. The importance of these formulation manipulations cannot be overemphasized when considering the increasing potency of many newer drugs in which even small errors in dose calculation can lead to devastating results.

Other Routes for Drug Administration

Neonates, infants, children, and adolescents with certain pulmonary conditions (e.g., reactive airway disease, viral-induced bronchiolitis, asthma, cystic fibrosis) frequently receive drugs (e.g., corticosteroids, β-adrenergic agonists, antimicrobial agents, mucolytic drugs) via inhalation. The pulmonary surface area in pediatric patients of all ages is a very effective, easily traversable barrier for drug absorption. As in adults, rate-limiting factors for pulmonary drug absorption include physicochemical factors associated with the drug and delivery system (e.g., particle size, diffusion coefficient, chemical stability of drug molecule in the lung) and physical factors that influence intrapulmonary drug disposition (e.g., active vs. passive drug delivery to the tracheobronchial tree, respiratory minute volume, internal airway diameter); many of which are developmentally determined. For drugs formulated for delivery using a metered-dose inhaler (either drug powder or suspended particles using a carrier gas), developmental factors (e.g., incoordination of device actuation with inhalation, inability to follow instructions for clearing of airway, and passive inhalation with actuation of delivery device) either prevent their use (such as in infants and small children) or limit the bioavailability of the drug to be administered. In these instances, specific devices (e.g., masks, spacer chambers) and/or methods of delivery (e.g., continuous aerosolization via mask) can be used to improve the efficiency of drug delivery and, thereby, drug efficacy.

In pediatric patients, percutaneous drug administration is generally reserved for agents intended to produce a local effect within the dermis. As denoted previously (see "Drug Absorption"), development has an impact on the barrier of the skin that, if not recognized and controlled for with proper drug administration techniques, can produce situations in which systemic toxicity can result. Similar therapeutic challenges occur when transmucosal routes (e.g., buccal, sublingual, rectal) are used for drug administration. Specifically, unpredictable systemic bioavailability may complicate treatment consequent to variability in the rate and/or extent of drug absorption. As a consequence, transmucosal drug administration to pediatric patients is no longer widely used as a matter of convenience but, rather, when the condition of the patient does not enable drug administration by the oral or the parenteral routes.

Finally, direct intraosseous drug administration via puncture of the tibia is occasionally used in infants and small children for administration of drugs and, occasionally, crystalloid fluids given acutely during resuscitation efforts. It is particularly useful when vascular access sufficient for drug administration cannot be immediately accomplished. As reflected by the information contained in Table 17-5, the onset of drug action by this route is comparable with that seen following IV administration.

TABLE 17-5 RELATIVE ONSET OF ACTION AS A CONSEQUENCE OF DRUG ADMINISTRATION ROUTE

Route of Administration	Time until Effect
Intravenous	30-60 sec
Intraosseous	30-60 sec
Inhalation	2-3 min
Sublingual	3-5 min
Intramuscular	10-20 min
Subcutaneous	15-30 min
Rectal	5-30 min
Ingestion	30-90 min
Transdermal (topical)	Variable (min–hr)

Adapted from www.gov.mb.ca/health/ems/guidelines/A2.pdf

Adherence and Compliance: Practical Considerations

Beyond proper individualization of drug dose based on developmental considerations, the influence of concomitant disease/treatment and the selection of the proper drug formulation, the success of drug treatment in a pediatric patient depends, as in adults, upon successful administration of the drug. Physical and cognitive immaturity makes the infant and the child a dependent creature in almost all respects, including those related to therapeutic drug administration. Until a child reaches an age at which they can physically self-administer a drug in an accurate, proficient fashion and can mentally assume responsibility for same (generally from 7 to 14 years of age, depending on the individual child), compliance with a drug regimen becomes the responsibility of an adult. In a hospital environment, compliance is ensured through the actions of physicians, nurses, and pharmacists who, collectively through an integrated system of medical care, assume this responsibility. Upon discharge, the responsibility is transferred to parents/guardians or other adult caregivers in an environment that is generally nonmedical. At this juncture, therapeutic compliance morphs into adherence as defined by the potential for conflicting demands (e.g., multiple adult caregivers; different external environments such as home, daycare, school; parents tending to the needs of multiple children) to introduce variability (anticipated and unpredictable) in drug administration. Whether treatment is for a self-limiting (e.g., antibiotic administration) or chronic (e.g., asthma, diabetes) condition, challenges to therapeutic adherence have the potential to serve as rate-limiting events in the determination of drug safety and efficacy in infants and young children.

In contrast to the period encompassing infancy and childhood, adolescence poses its own unique challenges to therapeutic adherence. During this period, psychosocial maturation almost always lags behind physical maturation. Development of cognitive and physical skills in most adolescents enables them to self-administer a prescribed medication in a proper manner with little to no supervision. However, psychodynamic issues experienced by a substantial number of adolescents (e.g., complete understanding of the ramifications of undertreatment, disease progression and/or roles of disease prevention and/or health maintenance; perceptions of immortality and the associated lack of need for treatment; disorganized patterns of thinking capable of confounding treatment schedules; defiant/oppositional behavior toward authority figures) can often precipitate therapeutic failure, through either undertreatment or overtreatment, the latter occasionally leading to drug toxicity.

Unfortunately, the only maneuver that can be used to facilitate therapeutic compliance and adherence in the pediatric patient is the combination of vigilance (on behalf of all caregivers) and repetitive education coupled with positive reinforcement. When children reach the age of assent (i.e., generally by 7 years of age in children who have normal neurobehavioral development), they have the beginning level of cognitive ability sufficient to engender understanding about their medical condition(s) and how effective treatment can be used to improve their life. Through diligent efforts placed toward patient education and reeducation, older children and adolescents can assume a level of responsibility for active partnership in their overall medical management, one that will mature as educational efforts, driven by a shared desire for an optimal outcome, are regularly made.

Adverse Drug Reactions

Approved product labeling for marketed drug products in the United States and many countries throughout the world contains information describing the incidence of adverse drug reactions (ADRs). As recently denoted by Shah and coworkers,[59] off-label drug use in pediatric patients ranges from 36% to 92% throughout much of the world; a consequence of the fact that the vast majority of drugs (i.e., 50%-70% of approved products in the Unites States) are not sufficiently studied in pediatric patients to accurately profile age-specific dosing requirements (based on specific knowledge of how development influences the dose-concentration-effect relationship) and/or adverse event profiles.[60] Thus, much of the accumulated information and presumed knowledge regarding ADRs and their incidence is derived from experience in adult patients.

Despite the paucity of data concerning pediatric ADRs, they represent a significant health concern. A meta-analysis of 17 published reports of pediatric ADRs concluded (i) the overall incidence of ADRs in outpatient children was approximately 1.5%; (ii) 2.1% of admissions to children's hospitals were due to ADRs, with 39% of these being potentially life-threatening; and (iii) in hospitalized children, the incidence of ADRs was much higher, 9.5% (95% confidence interval, 6.8%-12.3%), with 12.3% of those reactions classified as severe.[61] These estimates almost certainly underestimate the true incidence of ADRs in children because there is no standard reporting system for ADRs and available primary data are derived from assessments conducted in individual pediatric hospitals. As a consequence, approximately 95% of ADRs in pediatric patients appear to be not reported,[62] thereby making a systematic assessment of causality next to impossible.

Recent data from a national surveillance of emergency departments in the United States (21,298 ADRs reports from 701,547 individuals) demonstrated that the overall incidence of ADRs in children 0 to 4 years of age (3.8%) was more than double that seen at any other time from the period of birth through adolescence.[63] Common things being common, many of the ADRs reported for infants and young children are associated with drug classes commonly used to treat such patients (e.g., antimicrobial agents, antipyretics) and, with the general exception of accidental drug overdose, frequently manifest as hypersensitivity reactions. In contrast, there are several potentially serious idiosyncratic ADRs that have a greater frequency in infants and children than in adults. As previously reviewed by Leeder,[55] developmental differences in drug biotransformation may predispose infants and young children to certain ADRs, causing their incidence to be higher than that observed in adults. For example, antenatal exposure to selective serotonin reuptake inhibitors (SSRIs) may produce symptoms compatible with serotonin toxicity in neonates consequent to developmentally determined low CYP2D6 activity during the first 2 weeks of life.[64] The incidence of fatal hepatotoxicity associated with valproic acid (VPA) given as part of multidrug therapy to treat childhood seizures is highest in children less than 2 years of age (~1 : 500) as compared with that in young adults (~1 : 39,000). Whereas the nature of this particular ADR is arguably multifactorial (e.g., endogenous glutathione pool, activity and inducibility of multiple DMEs), enhanced CYP2C9 activity in infants and young children appears to be associated with greater formation of the potentially hepatotoxic 4-ene-VPA metabolite.

Special Considerations of Pediatric Clinical Pharmacology Research

Historically, children have been categorized as a vulnerable population requiring targeted protection and had, therefore, generally been excluded from participation in investigational research. Drug dosing requirements and effects in pediatric patients cannot be simply extrapolated and/or accurately simulated from data obtained during the course of adult studies owing to developmental differences in pharmacokinetics and pharmacodynamics. Simply stated, an adult is not an acceptable pharmacologic surrogate for an infant or a child.

In both the United States and the European Union, regulations exist mandating that drugs being developed for the treatment of diseases in pediatric patients be evaluated in these target populations to specifically determine age-appropriate dose, characterize exposure-response relationships, and examine drug tolerability/safety.[65] This has produced a renaissance in pediatric clinical pharmacology and, with respect to drug development, has given children a priority and stature that is no different from those of adults—which has been long overdue and is well deserved.[66] Prior to the institution of these regulations, much of the knowledge concerning drug disposition and action across the pediatric spectrum was derived from investigations conducted outside of the formal drug development process. The accumulated knowledge of how ontogeny influences both pharmacokinetics and pharmacodynamics can now be used to guide the design of ethical and rational clinical drug trials in neonates, infants, children, and adolescents[67]—a testimonial for the value of applying the principles of clinical pharmacology to pediatrics. In some real measure, the use of pharmacokinetics and pharmacogenetics to individualize drug therapy for age provides proof-of-concept for individualized medicine.

The application of clinical pharmacology principles (e.g., pharmacokinetics, pharmacogenetics, pharmacodynamics) to the study of drugs in pediatrics is, in most respects, similar to what must be done in adults. What is different are the approaches and, in some instances, the "restrictions" superimposed by facets of normal human development; examples of which are illustrated in the following paragraphs.

Given the invasiveness and risk of trauma and infection, the use of an indwelling catheter or intermittent catheterization cannot be justified for routine studies in healthy children. Thus, pharmacokinetic studies in pediatrics are generally performed in patients who have a condition in which the test article either is used therapeutically (off-label) or, ostensibly, could be used if the drug were licensed for a pediatric indication. The requirement for repeated blood sampling to support pharmacokinetic studies is generally addressed by the use of an indwelling venous catheter (as opposed to repeated venipuncture, which continues to be used in adult volunteer subjects in phase I drug studies). To begin, venipuncture is generally technically more challenging in children than in adults and requires study nurses or phlebotomists skilled in blood sampling from this age group. The mere suggestion of a procedure involving a needle can prompt a variety of behavioral and emotional responses in a child. Although the application of local anesthetic agents to the site of catheter insertion can minimize discomfort associated with puncture of the skin, it does not completely ablate the responses (e.g., crying, extremity movement) to this procedure. The frequent heightened emotional response to pain in children often elicits a sympathetic guilt in parents and study personnel that may be difficult to cope with. Consequently, few parents will tolerate more than one or two attempts at venous access before reconsidering their permission.

Developmental changes in circulating blood volume produce limitations on the quantity of blood that can be removed to support a pharmacokinetic investigation in a pediatric patient. Generally speaking, blood volume removed to support a given study (e.g., samples for quantification of drug/metabolites, safety monitoring, genotyping) may not exceed 3% of the estimated circulating blood volume (Table 17-6) over a 6-week period. Nontherapeutic phlebotomy to support study objectives should be further limited in patients with anemia or low cardiac output. This restriction may limit the number of serial blood samples obtained for pharmacokinetic studies or the quantity

TABLE 17-6 ESTIMATED BLOOD VOLUME BASED ON AGE

Age	Blood Volume (ml/kg)
Preterm infants	90
Term newborns/neonates	85
Infants 1 mo-1 yr of age	80
Toddlers ≤3 yr	75
Older children and teenagers	65

Adapted from Linderkamp O, Versmold HT, Riegel KP, Betke K. Estimation and prediction of blood volume in infants and children. Eur J Pediatr 1977;125:227-234.

of sample obtained at any one time. Fewer blood samples may limit the ability of pharmacokinetic models to predict blood concentrations, whereas less sample volume requires that analytic methods be modified (e.g., use of high performance liquid chromatography with tandem mass spectrometry [HPLC/MS/MS] as opposed to less sensitive methods for drug/metabolite measurement) to accommodate small quantities. These variables, mostly unique to pediatric practice, underscore the importance of applying optimal blood sampling methodologies whenever developing a pharmacokinetic study in infants/young children and in children.

In contrast to phase I and phase II studies conducted in adult subjects, accomplishing these same goals in a pediatric cohort is often considerably more costly in terms of time and capital investment needed to complete a drug development program. So that the impact of age (development) can be adequately characterized in the face of anticipated normal variability in pharmacokinetics and/or pharmacodynamics, a sufficient number of pediatric patients across the developmental continuum must be included in the study design.[67] In addition, pediatric patients (and in particular, infants and small children) must be studied in an environment ideally suited to address their unique medical and psychosocial needs—generally a pediatric clinic and/or hospital as opposed to a unit designed to house healthy adults. Consequently, studying drugs in children costs significantly more than in adults because three to four times the number of studies must be conducted to cover the developmental continuum that occurs from neonates and infants through childhood and adolescence.[68]

Studies involving the quantitation of drugs/metabolites from urine specimens can also provide insights into the impact of development on drug disposition. Activities of certain DMEs can be assessed in vivo by administration of drugs that pharmacologically serve as "probe substrates" for specific enzymes. In adults, postdose urine samples can usually be generated on demand. In infants and young children who do not already have indwelling urinary catheters placed for medical reasons, the collection of an accurate, quantitative urine collection can be extremely difficult, if not impossible. In children, toilet training does not typically occur before age 2 (a critical time for the development of DME expression and activity) and is highly variable between individual children. Even episodic urinary incontinence will invalidate a quantitative urine collection necessary to determine renal drug clearance and/or extent of renal drug/metabolite excretion. Not only is the use of adhesive urine collection bags cumbersome for parents but also, if the bag is not properly sealed, loss of sample is significant. In addition, repeated application of these devices to young infants can cause excoriation of the perineum, with associated discomfort and increased risk of infection. Similarly, the use of cotton balls or other absorbent materials placed between the infant and the diaper poses similar complications for handling and storage by parents and for contamination by fecal material. Temporal and environmental factors contribute additional problems to sample acquisition and degradation. Whereas postvoid urine samples from adults can be collected immediately and either processed or stored, this is not routinely possible in infants and small children. Urine remains in the diapers at near body temperature for varying lengths of time before the diaper is changed. Heat-labile drugs and metabolites or compounds that degrade spontaneously over time may be adversely affected. Assay procedures must be validated to account for possible differences in conditions to which samples may be exposed. Therefore, alternative methods for sample acquisition are needed.

CONCLUSION

The past decade has brought about a reawakening in pediatric clinical pharmacology with rapid growth in research and new opportunities for therapeutic advances. Using available data and existing technology, study protocols can be designed in an age-appropriate manner to ensure appropriate recruitment strategies; avoid unrealistic, unsafe, or unnecessary study components; afford the least invasive study procedures possible; and produce data that are as robust and useful as those produced from adult clinical trials.[67] Proof-of-concept abounds for the value of integrating pharmacokinetics, pharmacodynamics, and pharmacogenetics as applied to the principles and practice of clinical pharmacology in pediatrics. Future integration of functional genomics that link disease, drug, and treatment variables in the context of predictive models will continue to improve the efficacy and safety of drug treatment in pediatric patients. The success of integrating clinical pharmacology into pediatrics and the resultant knowledge have truly transformed the child from a "therapeutic orphan" into a citizen of prominent standing, entitled to the benefits of drug therapy that accrue as a result of careful and complete evaluation. It is essential that the ultimate goal to provide infants and children with safe and effective drug therapy remain in the forefront of clinical pharmacology.

REFERENCES

1. Halpern S. The social dynamic of professionalism. In American Pediatrics. Berkeley, CA: University of California Press, 1988, p 52.
2. Kearns GL, Abdel-Rahman SM, Alander SW, et al. Developmental pharmacology—drug disposition, action, and therapy in infants and children. N Engl J Med 2003;349(12):1157-1167.
3. Loebstein R, Koren G. Clinical pharmacology and therapeutic drug monitoring in neonates and children. Pediatr Rev 1998;19(12):423-428.
4. Ritschel WA, Kearns GL. Pediatric pharmacokinetics. In Ritschel WA, Kearns GL (eds): Handbook of Basic Pharmacokinetics Including Clinical Applications. Washington, DC: American Pharmacists Association, 2004, pp 227-239.
5. Agunod M, Yamaguchi N, Lopez R, et al. Correlative study of hydrochloric acid, pepsin, and intrinsic factor secretion in newborns and infants. Am J Dig Dis 1969;14(6):400-414.
6. Rodbro P, Krasilnikoff PA, Christiansen PM. Parietal cell secretory function in early childhood. Scand J Gastroenterol 1967;2(3):209-213.
7. Gupta M, Brans YW. Gastric retention in neonates. Pediatrics 1978;62(1):26-29.
8. Ittmann PI, Amarnath R, Berseth CL. Maturation of antroduodenal motor activity in preterm and term infants. Dig Dis Sci 1992;37(1):14-19.
9. Heimann G. Enteral absorption and bioavailability in children in relation to age. Eur J Clin Pharmacol 1980;18(1):43-50.
10. Weaver LT, Austin S, Cole TJ. Small intestinal length: a factor essential for gut adaptation. Gut 1991;32(11):1321-1323.
11. Grand RJ, Watkins JB, Torti FM. Development of the human gastrointestinal tract. A review. Gastroenterology 1976;70(5 pt 1):790-810.
12. Martinussen M, Brubakk AM, Linker DT, et al. Mesenteric blood flow velocity and its relation to circulatory adaptation during the first week of life in healthy term infants. Pediatr Res 1994;36(3):334-339.
13. Martinussen M, Brubakk AM, Vik T, Yao AC. Mesenteric blood flow velocity and its relation to transitional circulatory adaptation in appropriate for gestational age preterm infants. Pediatr Res 1996;39(2):275-280.
14. Yanowitz TD, Yao AC, Pettigrew KD, et al. Postnatal hemodynamic changes in very-low-birthweight infants. J Appl Physiol 1999;87(1):370-380.
15. Poley JR, Dower JC, Owen CA Jr, Stickler GB. Bile acids in infants and children. J Lab Clin Med 1964;63:838-846.
16. Suchy FJ, Balistreri WF, Heubi JE, et al. Physiologic cholestasis: elevation of the primary serum bile acid concentrations in normal infants. Gastroenterology 1981; 80(5 pt 1):1037-1041.
17. Hall SD, Thummel KE, Watkins PB, et al. Molecular and physical mechanisms of first-pass extraction. Drug Metab Dispos 1999;27(2):161-166.
18. Stahlberg MR, Hietanen E, Maki M. Mucosal biotransformation rates in the small intestine of children. Gut 1988;29(8):1058-1063.
19. Gibbs JP, Liacouras CA, Baldassano RN, Slattery JT. Up-regulation of glutathione *S*-transferase activity in enterocytes of young children. Drug Metab Dispos 1999; 27(12):1466-1469.
20. Fakhoury M, Litalien C, Medard Y, et al. Localization and mRNA expression of CYP3A and P-glycoprotein in human duodenum as a function of age. Drug Metab Dispos 2005;33(11):1603-1607.
21. Di Lorenzo C, Flores AF, Hyman PE. Age-related changes in colon motility. J Pediatr 1995;127(4):593-596.
22. Coulthard KP, Nielson HW, Schroder M, et al. Relative bioavailability and plasma paracetamol profiles of Panadol suppositories in children. J Paediatr Child Health 1998;34(5):425-431.
23. Stratchunsky LS, Nazarov AD, Firsov AA, Petrachenkova NA. Age dependence of erythromycin rectal bioavailability in children. Eur J Drug Metab Pharmacokinet 1991;spec no 3:321-323.
24. van Lingen RA, Deinum JT, Quak JM, et al. Pharmacokinetics and metabolism of rectally administered paracetamol in preterm neonates. Arch Dis Child Fetal Neonatal Ed 1999;80(1):F59-F63.
25. Amato M, Huppi P, Isenschmid M, Schneider H. Developmental aspects of percutaneous caffeine absorption in premature infants. Am J Perinatol 1992;9(5-6): 431-434.
26. West DP, Worobec S, Solomon LM. Pharmacology and toxicology of infant skin. J Invest Dermatol 1981;76(3):147-150.
27. Rutter N. Percutaneous drug absorption in the newborn: hazards and uses. Clin Perinatol 1987;14(4):911-930.
28. Fluhr JW, Pfisterer S, Gloor M. Direct comparison of skin physiology in children and adults with bioengineering methods. Pediatr Dermatol 2000;17(6):436-439.

29. Okah FA, Wickett RR, Pickens WL, Hoath SB. Surface electrical capacitance as a noninvasive bedside measure of epidermal barrier maturation in the newborn infant. Pediatrics 1995;96(4 pt 1):688-692.
30. Greenblatt DJ, Koch-Weser J. Intramuscular injection of drugs. N Engl J Med 1976;295(10):542-546.
31. Carry MR, Ringel SP, Starcevich JM. Distribution of capillaries in normal and diseased human skeletal muscle. Muscle Nerve 1986;9(5):445-454.
32. Kafetzis DA, Sinaniotis CA, Papadatos CJ, Kosmidis J. Pharmacokinetics of amikacin in infants and pre-school children. Acta Paediatr Scand 1979;68(3):419-422.
33. Sheng KT, Huang NN, Promadhattavedi V. Serum concentrations of cephalothin in infants and children and placental transmission of the antibiotic. Antimicrob Agents Chemother (Bethesda) 1964;10:200-206.
34. Painter MJ, Pippenger C, Wasterlain C, et al. Phenobarbital and phenytoin in neonatal seizures: metabolism and tissue distribution. Neurology 1981;31(9):1107-1112.
35. Tsai C, Ahdab-Barmada M, Daood MJ, Watchko JF. P-Glycoprotein expression in the developing human central nervous system: cellular and tissue localization. Pediatr Res 2001;47:436A.
36. Hines RN, McCarver DG. The ontogeny of human drug-metabolizing enzymes: phase I oxidative enzymes. J Pharmacol Exp Ther 2002;300(2):355-360.
37. McCarver DG, Hines RN. The ontogeny of human drug-metabolizing enzymes: phase II conjugation enzymes and regulatory mechanisms. J Pharmacol Exp Ther 2002;300(2):361-366.
38. Hartley R, Green M, Quinn MW, et al. Development of morphine glucuronidation in premature neonates. Biol Neonate 1994;66(1):1-9.
39. Barrett DA, Barker DP, Rutter N, et al. Morphine, morphine-6-glucuronide and morphine-3-glucuronide pharmacokinetics in newborn infants receiving diamorphine infusions. Br J Clin Pharmacol 1996;41(6):531-537.
40. Saarenmaa E, Neuvonen PJ, Rosenberg P, Fellman V. Morphine clearance and effects in newborn infants in relation to gestational age. Clin Pharmacol Ther 2000;68(2):160-166.
41. Scott CS, Riggs KW, Ling EW, et al. Morphine pharmacokinetics and pain assessment in premature newborns. J Pediatr 1999;135(4):423-429.
42. Miller RP, Roberts RJ, Fischer LJ. Acetaminophen elimination kinetics in neonates, children, and adults. Clin Pharmacol Ther 1976;19(3):284-294.
43. Capparelli EV, Englund JA, Connor JD, et al. Population pharmacokinetics and pharmacodynamics of zidovudine in HIV-infected infants and children. J Clin Pharmacol 2003;43(2):133-140.
44. Robillard J, Guillery E, Petershack J. Renal function during fetal life. In Barratt TM, Avner ED, Harmon WE (eds): Pediatric Nephrology. Baltimore: Lippincott Williams & Wilkins, 1999, pp 21-37.
45. Arant BS Jr. Developmental patterns of renal functional maturation compared in the human neonate. J Pediatr 1978;92(5):705-712.
46. van den Anker JN, Schoemaker RC, Hop WC, et al. Ceftazidime pharmacokinetics in preterm infants: effects of renal function and gestational age. Clin Pharmacol Ther 1995;58(6):650-659.
47. Davies MW, Cartwright DW. Gentamicin dosage intervals in neonates: longer dosage interval—less toxicity. J Paediatr Child Health 1998;34(6):577-580.
48. van den Anker JN, Hop WC, de Groot R, et al. Effects of prenatal exposure to betamethasone and indomethacin on the glomerular filtration rate in the preterm infant. Pediatr Res 1994;36(5):578-581.
49. Marshall J, Rodarte A, Blumer J, et al. Pediatric pharmacodynamics of midazolam oral syrup. Pediatric Pharmacology Research Unit Network. J Clin Pharmacol 2000; 40(6):578-589.
50. Marshall JD, Kearns GL. Developmental pharmacodynamics of cyclosporine. Clin Pharmacol Ther 1999;66(1):66-75.
51. Takahashi H, Ishikawa S, Nomoto S, et al. Developmental changes in pharmacokinetics and pharmacodynamics of warfarin enantiomers in Japanese children. Clin Pharmacol Ther 2000;68(5):541-555.
52. deWildt NN, Kearns GL, Sie SD, et al. Pharmacodynamics of intravenous and oral midazolam in preterm infants. Clin Drug Invest 2003;23:27-38.
53. Pui CH, Campana D, Evans WE. Childhood acute lymphoblastic leukaemia—current status and future perspectives. Lancet Oncol 2001;2(10):597-607.
54. Silverman ES, Liggett SB, Gelfand EW, et al. The pharmacogenetics of asthma: a candidate gene approach. Pharmacogenomics J 2001;1(1):27-37.
55. Leeder JS. Ontogeny of drug-metabolizing enzymes and its influence on the pathogenesis of adverse drug reactions in children. Curr Ther Res 2001;62:900-912.
56. Kearns GL. Impact of developmental pharmacology on pediatric study design: overcoming the challenges. J Allergy Clin Immunol 2000;106(3 suppl):S128-S138.
57. Alcorn J, McNamara PJ. Ontogeny of hepatic and renal systemic clearance pathways in infants: part II. Clin Pharmacokinet 2002;41(13):1077-1094.
58. Rheinstein PH. Avoiding problems with liquid medications and dosing devices. Am Fam Physician 1994;50(8):1771-1772.
59. Shah SS, Hall M, Goodman DM, et al. Off-label drug use in hospitalized children. Arch Pediatr Adolesc Med 2007;161(3):282-290.
60. Roberts R, Rodriguez W, Murphy D, Crescenzi T. Pediatric drug labeling: improving the safety and efficacy of pediatric therapies. JAMA 2003;290(7):905-911.
61. Impicciatore P, Choonara I, Clarkson A, et al. Incidence of adverse drug reactions in paediatric in/out-patients: a systematic review and meta-analysis of prospective studies. Br J Clin Pharmacol 2001;52(1):77-83.
62. Carleton BC, Smith MA, Gelin MN, Heathcote SC. Paediatric adverse drug reaction reporting: understanding and future directions. Can J Clin Pharmacol 2007;14(1): e45-e57.
63. Budnitz DS, Pollock DA, Weidenbach KN, et al. National surveillance of emergency department visits for outpatient adverse drug events. JAMA 2006;296(15):1858-1866.
64. Blake MJ, Gaedigk A, Pearce RE, et al. Ontogeny of dextromethorphan *O*- and *N*-demethylation in the first year of life. Clin Pharmacol Ther 2007;81(4):510-516.
65. Ward RM, Kauffman R. Future of pediatric therapeutics: reauthorization of BPCA and PREA. Clin Pharmacol Ther 2007;81(4):477-479.
66. Kearns GL, Ritschel WA, Wilson JT, Spielberg SP. Clinical pharmacology: a discipline called to action for maternal and child health. Clin Pharmacol Ther 2007;81(4):463-468.
67. Abdel-Rahman SM, Reed MD, Wells TG, Kearns GL. Considerations in the rational design and conduct of phase I/II pediatric clinical trials: avoiding the problems and pitfalls. Clin Pharmacol Ther 2007;81(4):483-494.
68. Gilman JT, Gal P. Pharmacokinetic and pharmacodynamic data collection in children and neonates. A quiet frontier. Clin Pharmacokinet 1992;23(1):1-9.
69. Friis-Hansen B. Water distribution in the foetus and newborn infant. Acta Paediatr Scand Suppl 1983;305:7-11.
70. Young WS, Lietman PS. Chloramphenicol glucuronyl transferase: assay, ontogeny and inducibility. J Pharmacol Exp Ther 1978;204(1):203-211.
71. Treluyer JM, Jacqz-Aigrain E, Alvarez F, Cresteil T. Expression of CYP2D6 in developing human liver. Eur J Biochem 1991;202(2):583-588.
72. Kinirons MT, O'Shea D, Kim RB, et al. Failure of erythromycin breath test to correlate with midazolam clearance as a probe of cytochrome P4503A. Clin Pharmacol Ther 1999;66(3):224-231.
73. Pynnonen S, Sillanpaa M, Frey H, Iisalo E. Carbamazepine and its 10,11-epoxide in children and adults with epilepsy. Eur J Clin Pharmacol 1977;11(2):129-133.
74. Aranda JV, Collinge JM, Zinman R, Watters G. Maturation of caffeine elimination in infancy. Arch Dis Child 1979;54(12):946-949.
75. Murry DJ, Crom WR, Reddick WE, et al. Liver volume as a determinant of drug clearance in children and adolescents. Drug Metab Dispos 1995;23(10):1110-1116.
76. Morselli PL. Development of physiological variables important for drug kinetics. In Morselli PL, Pippenger CE, Penry JK (eds): Antiepileptic Drug Therapy in Pediatrics. New York: Raven, 1983, pp 1-12.
77. Linderkamp O, Versmold HT, Riegel KP, Betke K. Estimation and prediction of blood volume in infants and children. Eur J Pediatr 1977;125:227-234.

18

SEX DIFFERENCES IN PHARMACOLOGY

Jean Gray

INTRODUCTION 251
BIOLOGIC DIFFERENCES BETWEEN MALES AND FEMALES 251
DISEASE DIFFERENCES 251
PHARMACOLOGIC DIFFERENCES 252
Pharmacokinetics 252
Pharmacodynamics 253
Cardiovascular Therapy 253
Psychiatric Therapy 253
Gastrointestinal Disease 253
HIV Infection 253
Adverse Drug Reactions 253
Hormonal Effects 254
Menstrual Cycle in Women 254
Oral Contraceptives 254
Pregnancy 254
Menopause 255
Andropause 255
CONCLUSIONS 255

INTRODUCTION

Being male or female is a basic human variable that affects health, illness, and response to treatment throughout the life span.[1] *Sex* describes the biologic and physiologic characteristics that define males and females and serves as the defining term in this chapter. *Gender* refers to the individual's self-representation as masculine or feminine and is shaped by environment and experience. The biologic characteristics of sex do not differ among different cultures, whereas aspects of gender can vary greatly.

BIOLOGIC DIFFERENCES BETWEEN MALES AND FEMALES

Males and females differ at the molecular, cellular, and whole organism level.[2] For example, males have a Y chromosome, and females do not. Females have two X chromosomes, males have one. Only females have a paternal X chromosome. Female cells inactivate one X chromosome by random methylation, resulting in the production of a ball of genetically inert DNA known as the *Barr body*. Recent analysis of gene expression differences in four tissues of female and male mice—liver, adipose, muscle, and brain—demonstrate substantial sexually dimorphic expression, particularly in liver and adipose tissue.[3] Mitochondria are present in both female and male cells but derive exclusively from the mother.

Both sexes make the same steroid hormones but in markedly different quantities.[4] Androgen serves as the building block for estrogen synthesis. The male testis synthesizes large quantities of testosterone daily but virtually no estrogen, whereas the female ovary converts almost all androgen produced into estradiol. Many cells contain aromatase, the enzyme that converts androgen to estrogen, but only some tissues contain 5-alpha reductase that converts testosterone to its more potent metabolite dihydrotestosterone (Fig. 18-1).

Cellular responses to sex steroids require an intracellular receptor. Androgens interact with a single receptor, whereas there are two estrogen receptors, estrogen α and estrogen β, that are variably expressed in different tissues.

Secondary sexual characteristics reflect this interplay of genetics, hormones, and physiology. Men display muscularity, deep voices, facial hair, growth of the prostate gland, phallic growth, almost continuous and life-long spermatogenesis, sex drive, and erectile function under the influence of testosterone. Puberty brings estrogen-mediated breast development, cyclic fertility, and menstrual flow to women.

DISEASE DIFFERENCES

Most diseases demonstrate little predilection for females or males but a few do demonstrate that women and men have different risks for and manifestations of illness and respond differently to treatment. A few examples are cited here.

Some diseases are more common in one sex. For example, systemic lupus erythematosus, the most common of the autoimmune diseases, has a lifetime female : male ratio of 9 : 1.[5] Multiple sclerosis affects twice as many females as males.[6] Sex hormonal status may explain why the prevalence of migraine headache is similar in boys and girls before puberty but is threefold higher in postpubertal females than in males.[7] Idiopathic pulmonary hypertension occurs three times more frequently in females than males, also suggesting an influence of sex hormones on pulmonary vascular reactivity.[8]

Manifestations of a disease may be different in men and women. In the field of mental health,[9] women are more likely than men to become depressed, but men are more severely affected by schizophrenia. Females experience more anxiety, whereas males exhibit more antisocial behavior. Most addicts and alcoholics are males, but females have more eating disorders. Females attempt suicide more frequently than males, but men are more successful in their attempts. Attention-deficit/hyperactivity disorder (ADHD) is diagnosed far more frequently in boys and results in hyperactivity in boys and passive inattention in girls.[10] Although differences in pain sensitivity between men and women may be partly due to psychosocial factors, laboratory studies in humans have demonstrated sex differences in sensitivity to noxious stimuli, suggesting an underlying biologic mechanism.[11]

Cardiovascular disease is a major cause of morbidity and mortality for both men and women but occurs uncommonly in premenopausal women. Sex differences in the molecular and cellular physiology of the cardiovascular system have been noted, as have variations in the availability of and response to therapy between males and females.[12]

Sex differences in hemoglobin and hematocrit levels are well-known in healthy individuals and have resulted in sex-specific normative laboratory values. Lower hemoglobin levels in women may be related to the relative lack of androgens and the inhibitory effect of estrogens on hemoglobin responsiveness to erythropoietin. Women tolerate lower hemoglobin levels better than men do, even in disease states such as chronic renal failure.[13]

Lung cancer, currently the leading cause of cancer death in North America in both men and women, appears to be a biologically different disease in women.[14] Female smokers tend to develop adenocarcinoma, male smokers develop squamous cell carcinoma. Nonsmokers who develop lung cancer are 2.5 times more likely to be female than male. Breast cancer, long studied as a female disease, also occurs in males, but men have not been included in clinical trials, resulting in a relative absence of information about appropriate treatment regimens for males.[15]

Endogenous sex hormones appear to differentially modulate glycemic status and risk of type 2 diabetes in men and women. High

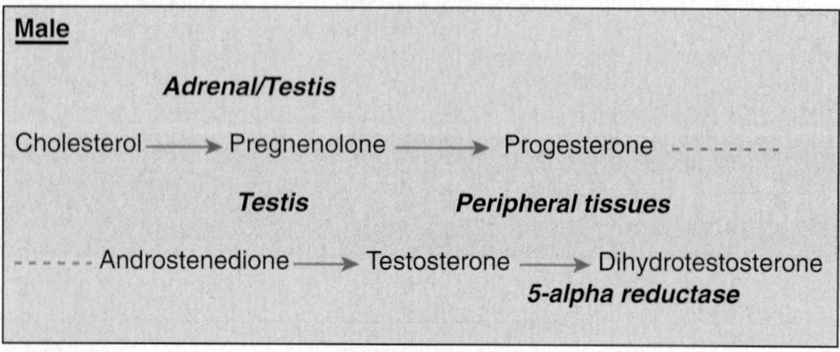

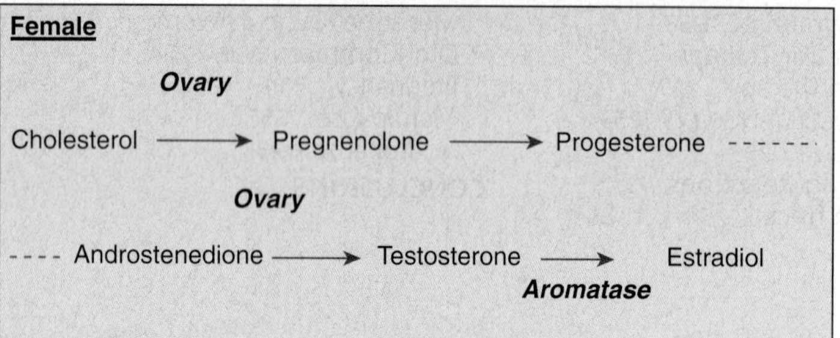

FIGURE 18-1 • **Biosynthesis of gonadal hormones.**

testosterone levels are associated with higher risk of type 2 diabetes in women but with a lower risk in men.[16]

Understanding the genetic, hormonal, and treatment-responsiveness differences between males and females is an important area of research at the present time but will provide meaningful information only if all genetic and genomic studies published include information on the sex of the animals or cells that served as the source of genetic material.

PHARMACOLOGIC DIFFERENCES

Sex-specific differences that can influence drug response include a lower body mass index and smaller organ size in females than in males, resulting in larger volumes of distribution in males. Women have a higher proportion of body fat, which can influence the volume of distribution of lipophilic drugs. The distribution of tissue water fluctuates during the menstrual cycle, resulting in salt and water retention in females. Glomerular filtration rates and creatinine clearances are lower in women, whereas increased muscle mass and metabolism in males augment creatinine clearance.[17]

Pharmacokinetics (Table 18-1)

Oral drug absorption is influenced by diet (women tend to eat more fruits and vegetables that are higher in fiber, whereas consumption of meat, fat, and cholesterol is higher in men), rate of gastric emptying (slower in women), intestinal micro-organisms, intestinal transit time, drug-metabolizing enzymes within the gut wall, and gastrointestinal drug transporters. The primary drug-metabolizing enzyme located in the intestine is cytochrome P-450 3A4 (CYP3A4). Using midazolam as a probe, females show higher drug bioavailability compared with males and greater effects of inhibition of this gut enzyme.[18] Studies of the drug transporter P-glycoprotein in gut mucosa have not demonstrated any clear sex differences.[19] **Transdermal drug absorption**, despite the sex differences in fat distribution, results in similar drug concentrations in women and men.[20] **Inhalational absorption** comparative studies are limited to aerosolized ribavirin and cyclosporine and suggest lower bioavailability in women than in men, probably related to lower tidal volumes in women.[21,22]

Women have a lower **volume of distribution** of alcohol than do men, resulting in greater initial concentrations and increased effect for a given dose consumed. Men, conversely, have a lower volume of distribution for diazepam, leading to a decreased duration of effect and a lower elimination time than those of women.[23] Binding of drugs to plasma proteins shows some sex differences, but the results are inconsistent.[17]

TABLE 18-1 PHARMACOKINETIC SEX DIFFERENCES

	Men > Women	Men = Women	Women > Men
ABSORPTION			
Oral			+
Transdermal		+	
Inhalational	+		
DISTRIBUTION VOLUME			
Water soluble	+		
Lipophilic			+
RENAL CLEARANCE	+		
HEPATIC METABOLISM			
Phase I clearance			
CYP1A	+		
CYP2D6		+	
CYP2C19		+	
CYP2C9		+	
CYP2E1	+		
CYP3A			+
Phase II clearance	+		

CYP, cytochrome P-450.

Renal clearance of most drugs should show a sex-related difference because glomerular filtration rate (GFR), on average, is higher in men than in women as are some aspects of renal tubular secretion. Men produce more creatinine than do women, so sex must always be considered when calculating GFR from creatinine clearance and when calculating dosage for drugs such as the aminoglycosides, cephalosporins, digoxin, or fluoroquinolones that are excreted by the kidneys. Tubular secretion of cations is higher in men than in women, and inhibitors of renal secretion, such as quinine and quinidine, have more impact in males than in females.[17]

Hepatic drug metabolism occurs in two phases. Phase I metabolism includes oxidation, reduction, and hydrolysis and is largely carried out by CYP450 isozymes.[17,24] CYP1A activity, as measured by clearance of olanzapine and clozapine, is higher in males than in females, although ethnic differences, hormone replacement therapy (HRT), and oral contraceptives (OCs) appear to eliminate the sex effect. Sex differences have also been demonstrated for CYP2D6 activity, although the results are inconsistent. For example, dextromethorphan and metoprolol are cleared faster in men than in women with the extensive metabolizer phenotype. Sertraline is cleared more slowly in men, whereas desipramine is cleared more slowly in women. Propranolol clearance is lower in men than in women in both white and Chinese recipients. Using mephenytoin or (R)-mephobarbital as probes, no sex differences have been noted in CYP2C19 activity. CYP2C9 also does not appear to demonstrate sex differences, but CYP2E1 activity, measured using chlorzoxazone metabolism, is higher in men than in women.

The hepatic CYP3A family metabolizes the largest number of drugs and endogenous substrates and shows inconsistent sex difference in activity. Age influences hepatic blood flow and interacts with sex to affect CYP3A function.[25] Young women have higher clearance rates of oral triazolam than young men. Women have a higher clearance of both intravenous and oral nimodipine than do men at all ages. After multiple doses of nefazodone, elderly women have lower clearance rates than elderly men, but trazodone showed no sex-dependent changes in either young or elderly groups. Inconsistent or no sex differences have been found for verapamil, 3-hydroxy-3-methylglutaryl coenzyme A (HMG-CoA) reductase inhibitors (statins), buspirone, cocaine, and lidocaine.[25] Intriguingly, CYP3A4 expression in a large collection of surgical liver samples showed twofold higher levels of both the enzyme and CYP3A4 messenger RNA in female compared with male samples as well as a corresponding 50% increase in the CYP3A4-dependent *N*-dealkylation of verapamil in the female samples.[26]

Phase II metabolism involves the processes of conjugation including glucuronidation, sulfation, acetylation, methylation, and glutathione conjugation. In general, these processes all proceed more rapidly in males than in females.

The study of the influence of sex on pharmacokinetics is still relatively new and is only just beginning to identify interesting sex-based variability.

Pharmacodynamics

Individual responses to drugs do demonstrate sex differences and are of clinical significance. Sex-based variability in response is being identified as the numbers of women enrolled in clinical trials increases. Where differences have been identified, it is unclear whether receptors or other aspects of drug response are involved.

Cardiovascular Therapy

Aspirin has long been one of the cornerstones of cardiovascular and cerebrovascular secondary prevention strategies. In the treatment of acute myocardial infarction and in the secondary prevention of cardiovascular disease in both men and women, aspirin is effective. Recent studies of the role of aspirin in the primary prevention of cardiovascular disease, however, have shown a clear sex difference. Women have a reduced risk of ischemic stroke with aspirin therapy but little cardiac benefit, whereas men have a reduced risk of acute myocardial infarction but no significant benefit for the prevention of stroke.[27,28] The risk of bleeding is similar in both men and women. Antiplatelet agents such as clopidogrel do not appear to have any sex-specific effects.

Other cardiovascular therapies also show a sex difference in response,[29] although insufficient women were included in early clinical trials to allow sex-specific analysis for some established therapies (e.g., β-blocker therapy in the secondary prevention of myocardial infarction). The use of β-blockers in the management of congestive heart failure demonstrates a greater benefit for men than for women. Similarly, angiotensin-converting enzyme inhibitors (ACE-I) in heart failure appear less effective in women than in men. Women with asymptomatic left ventricular dysfunction do not experience either improved morbidity or mortality when treated with ACE-I but men do. The role of ACE-I in the primary and secondary prevention of cardiovascular disease appears similar for men and for women. No sex-specific differences have been noted for angiotensin II antagonists or for the aldosterone receptor blockers spironolactone and eplerenone. Similarly, major trials with adequate numbers of women show no sex-specific differences in response to calcium channel blocking agents or statins.

Digoxin demonstrated a distinct sex-specific difference in the Digitalis Investigation Group (DIG) trial in a post-hoc analysis.[30] Women experienced significantly elevated mortality on digoxin compared with placebo therapy, possibly as a consequence of excessive dosage, because women demonstrated higher blood levels of digoxin than did men. Other antiarrhythmic drugs also show different outcomes in men and women. Women have a higher risk of experiencing an acquired long QT syndrome. Class I and III antiarrhythmics, including ibutilide, D,L-sotalol, D-sotalol, dofetilide, and amiodarone show a higher incidence of torsades de pointes tachycardia in women.[29]

Psychiatric Therapy

Sex differences have been observed with drugs for the treatment of psychiatric disease, but it is not clear whether the effects are secondary to differences in pharmacokinetics or pharmacodynamics. For example, young women seem to respond better than men to psychotropic agents but experience more severe side effects. Depressed men respond better to tricyclic antidepressants than do women, who experience better outcomes from monoamine oxidase inhibitors than do men. Women have a greater response to selective serotonin reuptake inhibitors (SSRIs) than do men, and sertraline has been approved by the U.S. Food and Drug Administration (FDA) for the treatment of posttraumatic stress disorder *in women* but not in men.[1] Women and men who smoke marijuana experience similar levels of intoxication, but women report more dizziness than men and experience a greater drop in blood pressure.[31]

Gastrointestinal Disease

Functional gastrointestinal disorders are more prevalent in women than in men. Painful irritable bowel syndrome occurs in both men and women, but women experience more non–pain-associated symptoms such as constipation, bloating, and extraintestinal manifestations. The 5-hydroxytryptamine (5-HT)3 antagonist alosetron is indicated *only* for women with severe, chronic irritable bowel symptoms. The 5-HT4 agonist tegaserod has been approved for the treatment of chronic constipation in both women and men under the age of 65, but clinical trials suggest better efficacy in women than in men.[32]

HIV Infection

Pharmacodynamic sex differences have not been extensively studied in human immunodeficiency virus (HIV)–associated disease, but some evidence suggests that women have a more favorable response to highly active antiretroviral therapy (HAART) than do men. Women tend to have greater CD4 cell increases than do men and fewer acquired immunodeficiency disease (AIDS)–related illnesses and hospitalizations while on HAART therapy.[33,34]

Adverse Drug Reactions

More reports of adverse drug effects involve women than men. Reasons for such results include frequency of prescription (women visit physicians and receive more drugs than men), inadequate adjustment of dosage for smaller women, or increased susceptibility of women to adverse drug reactions. For example, female sex is a risk factor for prolonged QT interval and potentially fatal arrhythmias.[35] Three of the drugs removed from the U.S. market between 1997 and 2000 (terfenadine, astemizole, and cisapride) caused lethal cardiac arrhythmias in young women more frequently than in young men.[23] Frequency of prescriptions to women is the probable reason why the appetite suppressants fenfluramine and dexfenfluramine were associated with fibrotic cardiac valvular disease more frequently in women than in men. Several of the drugs used in the treatment of HIV (e.g., nucleoside reverse transcriptase inhibitors [NRTI], nevirapine) have been reported to have a higher rate of adverse events in women than in men, possibly on the basis of inadequate dosage adjustments for differing body sizes and the potential for drug interactions with OCs.[33]

Hormonal Effects

Menstrual Cycle in Women

Hormonal fluctuations within the menstrual cycle may be a cause of documented sex differences in the pharmacokinetics and pharmacodynamics of drugs. Some diseases show fluctuation during the menstrual cycle, suggesting that variations in renal, cardiovascular, hematologic, and immune systems all undergo regular cyclic changes. Most clinical pharmacologic studies of menstrual cycle effects on either pharmacokinetics or pharmacodynamics include small numbers of women, do not exclude anovulatory cycles, and follow the subjects through very few cycles.[36]

Drug absorption and distribution are not influenced by hormonal cycling. Drug metabolism studies suggest that CYP1A2 activity does not vary during the menstrual cycle, nor does CYP2A6, using nicotine and cotinine as substrates. In most studies, CYP2C9 does not show cyclic variability, although a group of patients with epilepsy experiencing a high frequency of seizures during the menstrual phase of the menstrual cycle had lower phenytoin concentrations and higher oral clearance during menses. Using omeprazole as a probe, CYP2C19 activity shows no cycle effects.[37] CYP2D6 activity may be mildly increased in the luteal phase of the cycle but is definitely increased during pregnancy. A number of CYP3A4 substrates have been studied and show no changes in clearance during the menstrual cycle.[38]

Oral Contraceptives (Table 18-2)

Hormonal contraceptives include combined estrogen-progestin, estrogen-only, and progesterone-only preparations. Many studies of the impact of OCs on pharmacokinetics have used volunteers taking OCs and have not considered the effect of each of these differing classes of hormonal contraceptives. Ethinyl estradiol (the major estrogenic compound used in OCs) is metabolized by CYP3A4, and the modest inhibition in CYP3A4 activity by OCs may reflect competitive inhibition.

Most studies indicate that OCs inhibit oxidative drug metabolism. For example, OCs have been associated with decreased clearance of drugs metabolized by CYP1A2 (caffeine, theophylline), CYP3A4 (prednisone, prednisolone, alprazolam, triazolam), and CYP2C19 (omeprazole, mephenytoin, diazepam) as well as increased conjugation including glucuronidation (lorazepam, temazepam, acetaminophen) and glycine (salicylate).[39]

A practical example of the impact of OCs on drug metabolism is found in smoking-cessation treatment. Success rates with nicotine replacement therapy are lower in women than in men, and higher doses of nicotine gum are required to suppress nicotine withdrawal symptoms in women. Enhanced metabolism of nicotine has been demonstrated in women on OCs and could be one explanation of these results.[39]

Drug interactions with OCs are also important for several treatment programs. For example, almost all protease inhibitors (PI) and non-NRTIs used in the treatment of HIV/AIDS have significant interactions with OCs. The only PI with which concurrent use of OCs is safe and effective is indinavir. Indinavir, atazanavir, and efavirenz are known to increase estradiol and norethindrone levels substantially (increasing the risk of thromboembolism), and ritonavir, nelfinavir, and lopinavir markedly reduce estradiol levels, requiring the use of other contraceptive techniques to avoid pregnancy.[33]

There are currently no studies of drug interactions with newer methods of hormonal contraceptive delivery methods such as patches, depot preparations, vaginal rings, and emergency contraception.

TABLE 18-2 CLINICALLY IMPORTANT INTERACTIONS WITH ORAL CONTRACEPTIVES

CONSIDER USING ALTERNATIVE CONTRACEPTION: OC FAILURE
Case Reports: Mechanism Unknown
Antifungals: Griseofulvin, ketoconazole, fluconazole, itraconazole
Anticonvulsants: Ethosuximide, topiramate
Antimicrobials: Trimethoprim, tetracyclines, cotrimoxazole, metronidazole
Increased Drug Clearance
Anticonvulsants: Carbamazepine, felbamate, oxcarbazepine, phenytoin, primidone
Note: Gabapentin does not appear to interact with combination OCs
Antimicrobials: Rifabutin, rifampin, erythromycin
HIV therapy: Ritonavir, nelfinavir, lopinavir, nevirapine
Note: Indinavir does not appear to interact with combination OCs
Herbal therapy: St. John's wort
Reduced Enterohepatic Recirculation
Antibiotics: Penicillins (ampicillin, oxacillin, penicillin V), cephalosporins
OC EFFECT ON OTHER DRUGS
Decreased Drug Clearance
Coumarin anticoagulants: Warfarin, phenprocoumon
Benzodiazepines: Oxazepam, temazepam, lorazepam, triazolam, alprazolam
Note: Midazolam does not appear to interact with combination OCs
Corticosteroids: Prednisolone
Tricyclic antidepressants
β-Blockers: Metoprolol, propranolol
Monoamine oxidase inhibitors: Selegiline
Phenothiazines: Chlorpromazine
Increased Drug Clearance
Narcotics: Morphine
HIV therapy: Amprenavir, fosamprenavir

HIV, human immunodeficiency virus; OC, oral contraceptives.
Compiled from Lexi-Comp Online available at http://online.lexicom; and The Medical Letter on Drugs and Therapeutics Handbook of Adverse Drug Interactions Software 2006. Available at http://www.medletter.com.

Pregnancy

Proper prescribing during pregnancy is a challenge because the physiologic changes of pregnancy result in altered pharmacokinetics of drugs, and every effort must be made to ensure maximal safety to the fetus while, at the same time, providing therapeutic benefit to the mother.

Physiologic changes during pregnancy include changes in total body weight and body fat composition, delayed gastric emptying and prolonged gastrointestinal transit time, increased extracellular fluid and total body water, increased cardiac output and elevated maternal heart rate, as well as increased GFR. Clearance rates of drugs generally increase during pregnancy owing to enhanced renal and hepatic elimination (e.g., digoxin, phenytoin), although some drugs have reduced clearance rates (e.g., theophylline). CYP2A6 and CYP2D6 activities are both induced by pregnancy.

Fear of the teratogenic potential of drugs often results in discontinuation of treatment prior to or early in conception. Untreated diseases, such as asthma or depression, can lead to poor fetal outcomes. For example, about half of women who discontinue antidepressant treatment prior to conception experience a relapse of their depressive illness during pregnancy, necessitating resumption of treatment.[40]

The fetus is vulnerable to the effect of drugs during three phases of pregnancy. Exposure during the *earliest phase* from conception until somite formation can result in death and miscarriage or intact survival. The totipotential embryonic cells are capable of repair, provided drug exposure is not continued. The *embryonic period*, from 18 to 60 days, is one of considerable fetal vulnerability because this is the phase in which organogenesis begins. Exposure to teratogens during this period has the greatest likelihood of fetal structural abnormalities. Drug exposure during the *fetal phase*, from the end of the embryonic phase until term, can affect fetal growth or the size or function of an organ.

Possible teratogens include D-penicillamine, diazepam, efavirenz, and methimazole. Proven teratogens in humans are alcohol (fetal alcohol syndrome), ACE-I and angiotensin II inhibitors,[41] carbamazepine, chemotherapeutic agents, cocaine, systemic corticosteroids, coumarin anticoagulants, diethylstilbestrol, folic acid antagonists (methotrexate), hydantoins (phenytoin), lithium, misoprostol, retinoids, tetracyclines, thalidomide, and valproic acid.[42]

Continuation of drug therapy during pregnancy can result in a neonatal withdrawal syndrome. For example, continuation of SSRIs such as citalopram throughout pregnancy is associated with an increased incidence of poor neonatal adaptation syndrome characterized by neonatal irritability, respiratory difficulty, constant crying, jitteriness, increased muscle tone, eating and sleeping difficulties, seizures, hypoglycemia, and jaundice.[43] Maintenance of maternal health is critical to successful pregnancy outcome, but awareness of the possibility of neonatal withdrawal should guide management of the child as well.

Most drugs taken by the mother are excreted into breast milk, but the likelihood of infant exposure is influenced by the pharmacokinetic properties of the drug in the infant and the mother, milk composition, the amount of milk consumed, and the infant's suckling pattern. Drugs to be used with caution during breast-feeding include antineoplastic drugs, ergot alkaloids, lithium, drugs of abuse, gold, OCs, phenobarbital, radioactive compounds, and iodine-containing compounds.[44]

Multiple sources can assist health care providers in assessing reproductive toxicities from drug exposures.[45,46] For example, the online REPRORISK system available from Micromedex, Inc., contains electronic versions of four teratogen information databases. These periodically updated, scientifically reviewed resources critically evaluate the literature regarding human and animal pregnancy drug exposures. Other sources of information are the comprehensive multidisciplinary Teratogen Information Services (TIS) located in the United States and Canada, which provide patient counseling and risk assessments regarding potential teratogenic exposures (www.otispregnancy.org). Many TIS, such as MotherRisk (www.motherisk.org) employ genetic counselors, who are excellent resources for pre- and postconception counseling. The National Society of Genetic Counselors (www.nsgc.org) can also locate genetic counselors in most geographic regions in the United States.

Menopause

As ovarian function declines, levels of estrogen fall. Women now begin to experience cardiovascular and cerebrovascular disease at rates comparable with those of men. For many years, HRT was considered to extend the cardioprotective effect of ovarian estrogen production beyond the cessation of menses. Reports from several large scale placebo-controlled trials (e.g., the Women's Health Initiative[47]) showing increased cardiovascular disease, increased breast cancer risk, and increased thromboembolic disease during estrogen therapy have resulted in current recommendations *not* to use HRT. These results are discordant with previous observational studies in humans and trials in animals suggesting that estrogen compounds are cardioprotective. Some experts believe the timing of estrogen therapy is critical (observational studies followed women who initiated HRT in the perimenopausal period, whereas the Women's Health Initiative and other trials recruited women who were older and more advanced in menopause). The development of more cardiospecific selective estrogen-receptor modulators (SERMs) is proceeding because first-generation SERMs, such as raloxifene, have not demonstrated cardiovascular benefit.[48,49]

Estrogen is also the key regulating signal for bone remodeling. When estrogen levels fall during the menopause, osteoblasts demonstrate diminished function but osteoclasts continue to remove bone mineral and break down collagen. Women lose 1% to 2% of their bone mineral density per year around the menopause. Genetics, race, small body build, number of pregnancies, and lifestyle are also contributing risk factors. Bisphosphonates and SERMs provide stabilized bone mineral

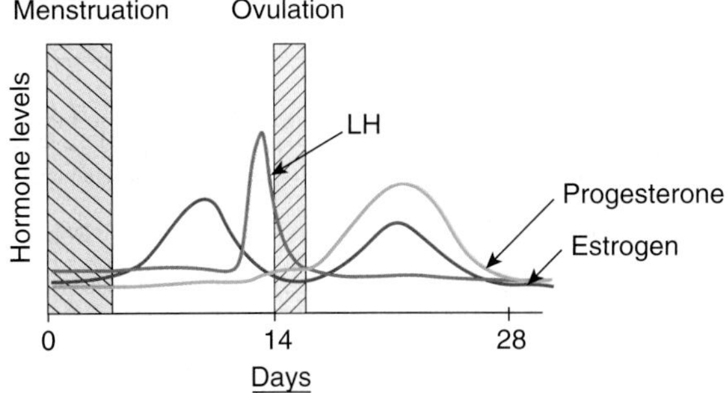

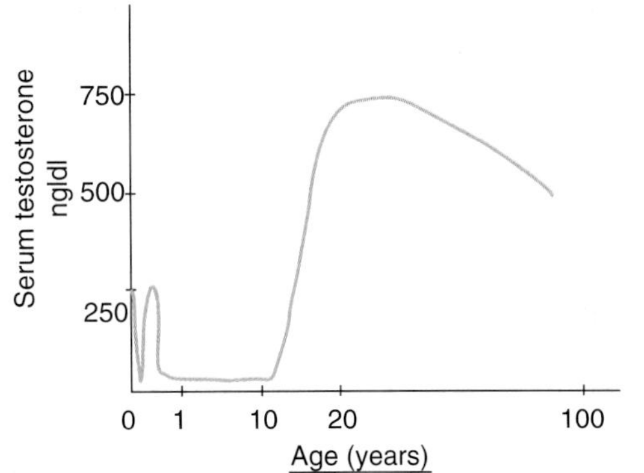

FIGURE 18-2 • Hormonal cycles in men and women.

density and a reduced likelihood of vertebral and possibly long bone fractures in postmenopausal women.[50,51]

Andropause

As men age, a constellation of changes in sexual function, testosterone production, and psychological problems are noted. This combination of problems is often referred to as *manopause* or *andropause*, although the existence of such a phase in the male life cycle is still being debated.[52] Unlike the dramatic changes in hormonal production that women experience, the age-related changes in reproductive hormones in men are subtle and occur gradually (Fig. 18-2). Several studies have shown that testosterone levels decline gradually at a rate of about 1% a year from the age of 19. Changes in the hypothalamic-pituitary-gonadal axis and a decline in adrenal androgen production contribute to reduced testosterone levels. In addition, the conversion of testosterone to dihydrotestosterone declines with age, in part because of down-regulation of 5α-reductase activity and increased estrogen production. The impact of these hormonal changes on disease manifestation and drug clearance is a topic of current research interest.[25]

Despite the major concerns about the relative absence of women from major clinical trials in the past, there are some obvious areas in which males have not been studied adequately. For example, there is insufficient evidence to guide treatment of osteoporosis[53] or breast cancer in males.[15] Both of these diseases do occur in men, but enrollment in clinical trials has been limited.

CONCLUSIONS

Men and women are different! Attention to these differences, both in disease presentation and in drug treatment, is a relatively new area of research, but one with some interesting outcomes. Development in the understanding of these sex differences has been dramatic since the 1990s and should continue to evolve rapidly in the future. Both basic and clinical research must include adequate numbers of male and female animals or subjects to permit appropriate determination of the impact of sex on drug effects. Regulatory statutes and clinical practice guidelines must insist on reviewing data on both male and female subjects. Vive la difference!

REFERENCES

1. Wizemann TM, Pardue ML (eds). Exploring the Biological Contributions to Human Health: Does Sex Matter? Washington, DC: National Academy Press, 2001.
2. Sex and Gender Course. Available at http://sexandgendercourse.od.nih.gov (accessed August 22, 2006).
3. Yang X, Schadt EE, Wang S, et al. Tissue-specific expression and regulation of sexually dimorphic genes in mice. Genome Res 2006;16:995-1004.
4. Federman DD. The biology of sex differences. N Engl J Med 2006;354:1507-1514.
5. Ackerman LS. Sex hormones and the genesis of autoimmunity. Arch Dermatol 2006;142:371-376.
6. El-Etr M, Vukusic S, Gignoux L, et al. Steroid hormones in multiple sclerosis. J Neurol Sci 2005;233:49-54.
7. Ashkenazi A, Silberstein SD. Hormone-related headache: pathophysiology and treatment. CNS Drugs 2006;20:125-141.
8. Smith AM, Jones RD, Channer KS. The influence of sex hormones on pulmonary vascular reactivity: possible vasodilator therapies for the treatment of pulmonary hypertension. Curr Vasc Pharmacol 2006;4:9-15.
9. Holden C. Sex and the suffering brain. Science 2005;308:1574-1577.
10. Staller J, Faraone SV. Attention-deficit hyperactivity disorder in girls: epidemiology and management. CNS Drugs 2006;20:107-123.
11. Wiesenfeld-Hallin Z. Sex differences in pain perception. Gend Med 2005;2:127-145.
12. Mendelsohn ME, Karas RH. Molecular and cellular basis of cardiovascular gender differences. Science 2005;308:1583-1587.
13. Duncan JA, Levin A. Sex, hemoglobin and kidney disease: new perspectives. Eur J Clin Invest 2005;35(Suppl 3):52-57.
14. Patel JD. Lung cancer in women. J Clin Oncol 2005;23:3212-3218.
15. Fentiman IS, Fourquet A, Hortobagyi GN. Male breast cancer. Lancet 2006;367:595-604.
16. Ding EL, Song Y, Malik VS, Liu S. Sex differences of endogenous sex hormones and risk of type 2 diabetes: A systematic review and meta-analysis. JAMA 2006;295:1288-1299.
17. Schwartz JB. The influence of sex on pharmacokinetics. Clin Pharmacokinet 2003; 42:107-121.
18. Gorski J, Jones D, Haehner-Daniels B, et al. The contribution of intestinal and hepatic CYP3A to the interaction between midazolam and clarithromycin. Clin Pharmacol Ther 1998;64:133-143.
19. Kim R, Leake B, Choo E, et al. Identification of functionally variant MDR1 alleles among European Americans and African Americans. Clin Pharmacol Ther 2001;70:189-199.
20. Dias V, Tendler B, Oparil S, et al. Clinical experience with transdermal clonidine in African-American and Hispanic-American patients with hypertension: evaluation from a 12-week prospective, open label clinical trial in community-based clinics. Am J Ther 1999;6:19-24.
21. Knight V, Yu C, Gilbert B, Divine GW. Estimating the dosage of ribavirin aerosol according to age and other variables. J Infect Dis 1988;158:443-447.
22. Rohatagi S, Calic F, Harding N, et al. Pharmacokinetics, pharmacodynamics, and safety of inhaled cyclosporine A (AD1628) after single and repeated administration in healthy male and female subjects and asthmatic patients. J Clin Pharmacol 2000;40:1211-1226.
23. Understanding pharmacokinetics and pharmacodynamics: sex-related differences. Lesson 5. Sex and Gender Course. Available at http://sexandgendercourse.od.nih.gov/lesson5 (accessed August 22, 2006).
24. Wilkinson GR. Drug metabolism and variability among patients in drug response. N Engl J Med 2005;352:2211-2221.
25. Cotreau MM, von Moltke LL, Greenblatt DJ. The influence of age and sex on the clearance of cytochrome P4503A substrates. Clin Pharmacokin 2005;44:33-60.
26. Wolbold R, Klein K, Burk O, et al. Sex is a major determinant of CYP3A4 expression in human liver. Hepatology 2003;38:978-988.
27. Ridker PM, Cook NR, Lee IM, et al. A randomized trial of low-dose aspirin in the primary prevention of cardiovascular disease in women. N Engl J Med 2005;352:1293-1304.
28. Berger JS, Roncalgioni MC, Avanzini F, et al. Aspirin for the primary prevention of cardiovascular events in women and men: A sex-specific meta-analysis of randomized controlled trials. JAMA 2006;295:306-313.
29. Jochmann N, Stangl K, Garbe E, et al. Female-specific aspects in the pharmacotherapy of chronic cardiovascular diseases. Eur Heart J 2005;26:1585-1595.
30. Rathore SS, Wang Y, Krumholz HM. Sex-based differences in the effect of digoxin for the treatment of heart failure. N Engl J Med 2002;347:1404-1411.
31. Craft RM. Sex differences in behavioral effects of cannabinoids. Life Sci 2005;77:2471-2478.
32. Chang L, Toner BB, Fukudo S, et al. Gender, age, society, culture, and the patient's perspective in the functional gastrointestinal disorders. Gastroenterology 2006;130:1435-1446.
33. Clark RA, Squires KE. Gender-specific considerations in the antiretroviral management of HIV-infected women. Expert Rev Anti Infect Ther 2005;3:213-227.
34. Ofotokun I. Sex differences in the pharmacologic effects of antiretroviral drugs: potential roles of drug transporters and phase 1 and 2 metabolizing enzymes. Top HIV Med 2005;13:79-83.
35. Priori SG, Schwartz PJ, Napolitano C, et al. Risk stratification in the long-QT syndrome. N Engl J Med 2003;348:1866-1874.
36. Kashuba ADM, Nafziger AN. Physiological changes during the menstrual cycle and their effects on the pharmacokinetics and pharmacodynamics of drugs. Clin Pharmacokinet 1998;34:203-218.
37. Laine K, Tybring G, Bertilsson L. No sex-related differences but significant inhibition by oral contraceptives of CYP2C19 activity as measured by the probe drugs mephenytoin and omeprazole in healthy Swedish white subjects. Clin Pharmacol Ther 2000; 68:151-159.
38. Hukkanen J, Gourlay SG, Kenkare S, Benowitz NL. Influence of menstrual cycle on cytochrome P450 2A6 activity and cardiovascular effects of nicotine. Clin Pharmacol Ther 2005;77:159-169.
39. Benowitz NL, Lessov-Schlaggar CN, Swan GE, Jacob P. Female sex and oral contraceptive use accelerate nicotine metabolism. Clin Pharmacol Ther 2006;79:480-488.
40. Cohen LS, Altshuler LL, Harlow BL, et al. Relapse of major depression during pregnancy in women who maintain or discontinue antidepressant treatment. JAMA 2006;295:499-507.
41. Cooper WO, Hernandez-Diaz S, Arbogast PG, et al. Major congenital malformations after first-trimester exposure to ACE inhibitors. N Engl J Med 2006;354:2443-2451.
42. Diav-Citrin O, Koren G. Drug exposure during pregnancy and lactation. In Gray J (ed): Therapeutic Choices, 4th ed. Ottawa, Ontario: Canadian Pharmacists Association, 2003, pp 1215-1224.
43. Sivojelezova A, Shuhaiber S, Sarkissian L, et al. Citalopram use in pregnancy: prospective comparative evaluation of pregnancy and fetal outcome. Am J Obstet Gynecol 2005;193:2004-2009.
44. Uhl K, Kennedy DL, Kweder SL. Accurate information on drug effects on pregnancy is crucial. Am Fam Physician 2003;67:700-701.
45. Uhl K, Kennedy DL, Kweder SL. Information on medication use in pregnancy. Am Fam Physician 2003;67:2476-2478.
46. Ito S. Drug therapy for breast-feeding women. N Engl J Med 2000;343:118-126.
47. Writing Group for the Women's Health Initiative Investigators. Risk and benefits of estrogen plus progestin in healthy menopausal women: principal results from the Women's Health Initiative Randomized Controlled Trial. JAMA 2002;288:321-333.
48. Barrett-Connor E, Mosca L, Collins P, et al., for the Raloxifene Use for the Heart (RUTH) Trial Investigators. Effects of raloxifene on cardiovascular events and breast cancer in postmenopausal women. N Engl J Med 2006;355:125-137.
49. Vogelvang TE, van der Mooren MJ, Mijatovic V, Kenemans P. Emerging selective estrogen receptor modulators: special focus on effects on coronary heart disease in postmenopausal women. Drugs 2006;66:191-221.
50. Cranney A, Wells G, Willan A, et al. The Osteoporosis Methodology Group and the Osteoporosis Research Advisory Group. Meta-analysis of alendronate for the treatment of post-menopausal women. Endocr Rev 2002;23:508-516.
51. Cranney A, Tugwell P, Zytaruk N, et al. The Osteoporosis Methodology Group, and the Osteoporosis Research Advisory Group. Meta-analysis of raloxifene for the prevention and treatment of postmenopausal osteoporosis. Endocr Rev 2002;23:524-528.
52. Mooradian AD, Korenman SG. Management of the cardinal features of andropause. Am J Ther 2006;13:145-160.
53. Sawka AM, Papaioannou A, Adachi JD, et al. Does alendronate reduce the risk of fracture in men? A meta-analysis incorporating prior knowledge of anti-fracture efficacy in women. BMC Musculoskel Disord 2005;6:39-51.
54. Lexi-Comp Online. Available at http://online.lexi.com (accessed August 31, 2006).
55. The Medical Letter on Drugs and Therapeutics Handbook of Adverse Drug Interactions Software 2006. Available at http://www.medletter.com (accessed August 31, 2006).

19

PHARMACOLOGY ACROSS THE AGING CONTINUUM

Naomi Gronich and Darrell R. Abernethy

INTRODUCTION 257
AGE-RELATED CHANGES IN PHARMACOKINETICS 257
Drug Absorption 257
Drug Distribution 258
Drug Metabolism 258
Drug Elimination 259
AGE EFFECTS ON DRUG PHARMACODYNAMICS 259
Central Nervous System 259
Dopaminergic 259
Serotonergic 259
Cholinergic 260
Adrenergic 260
GABAergic 260
Opiates 261
Cardiovascular System 261
β-Adrenergic 261
α-Adrenergic 261
Baroreflex Responsiveness 261
Renin-Angiotensin-Aldosterone Axis 261
Cardiac and Vascular Structure/Function 261
Cardiovascular Drug Disposition and Response with Increased Age 262
Adrenergic Drugs 262
ADVERSE EFFECTS OF DRUG EXPOSURE IN OLDER PATIENTS 262
CONCLUSION 263

INTRODUCTION

The older patient represents an increasingly large part of the population that is exposed to pharmacotherapy. In the United States, individuals over the age of 65 were estimated to have spent $50 billion on prescription drugs in 2002. This represents 33% of the total prescription drug expenditure that year, at a time that this group was only 12.6% of the total population.[1] Multiple concurrent disease processes are the hallmark of the older patient, with an individual commonly being diagnosed with different combinations of arthritis, hypertension, coronary heart disease and/or congestive heart failure, osteoporosis, cancer, and prostate disease. A group of older women living in the community had an average of three concurrent diseases.[2] A group of older men cared for by the U.S. Veterans Administration had an average of four concurrent diseases.[3] In addition, a subset of older patients are frail, a syndrome characterized by weakness, weight loss, slow walking speed, fatigue, and low activity level. Frailty may coexist with disease diagnoses, but it is independent from them.[4] Therefore, it is not surprising that utilization of medicines in the older patient is greater than that seen in a younger patient population. The effectiveness of drug therapy for many of these diseases in older patients is as great as for a younger patient population, leading to the need for multiple drugs for multiple diseases.[5-8] At the same time, exposure of the older patient to multiple medications (polypharmacy) has been associated with decreased functional status and increased morbidity and mortality. This is particularly true for medications that impair central nervous system (CNS) functions such as attention and cognition. Sedative-hypnotics, antidepressants, and drugs with anticholinergic effects have been particularly associated with increased risk of falls, hip fracture, and impaired cognitive function.[9,10] The challenge is to provide the older patient with drugs for their illnesses for which there is known benefit, while protecting them from unnecessary and/or excessive drug exposure for which there is known harm.

The older patient is often defined in terms of chronologic age, although this is an imperfect descriptor of physiologic age, with physiologic age the more important predictor of changes in drug disposition and effect. A usual approach is to stratify the older patient group into "young-old" (aged 65-75 years), "old" (aged 75-85 years), and "old-old" (aged 85 and over). Information characterizing drug disposition (pharmacokinetics) and effect (pharmacodynamics) with respect to age has generally been developed in the young-old and old with very limited information in the old-old. In addition, most of the data from clinical studies has been obtained from relatively healthy individuals. Studies in animal and cellular models for aging have provided useful information to help determine whether or not extrapolating clinical study findings in younger and healthier individuals to the older and more ill is appropriate. That being said, study of the old-old and those with multiple concurrent illnesses is in an early phase with quite limited data,[11,12] and it is unclear how appropriate it is to apply published information to the old-old with multiple illnesses.

The disposition of and response to drugs in older individuals compared with younger individuals are rarely qualitatively different; however, these are often quantitatively different, with respect to both pharmacokinetics and pharmacodynamics. An understanding of the physiologic and pathologic changes in the older patient that relate to altered drug disposition and effect is fundamental to understanding how to administer effective pharmacotherapy to this patient group.

AGE-RELATED CHANGES IN PHARMACOKINETICS

Drug Absorption

Gastrointestinal. Decreased intestinal motility and blood flow occur with advancing age, and decreased gastric acid secretion has in the past been considered an age-related phenomenon; however, more recent information indicates that this occurs only in patients with atrophic gastritis. This may include no more than 11% of the aged population with only 5% to 6% with gastric pH above 4.5.[13,14] Absorption of most drugs from the gastrointestinal tract does not change in advanced age.[15] Absorption of drugs such as ketoconazole that require an acidic gastric environment (pH < 5.0) for absorption may be decreased in the subset of older patients with severe atrophic gastritis. In addition to absorptive processes, some drugs undergo presystemic elimination due to metabolism at the intestinal wall, blockade of absorption by intestinal wall drug transporters, or a combination of the two processes. The role of age in these processes has not been well described; however, for a few drugs (verapamil,[16] labetalol,[17] sustained release diltiazem,[18] and ciprofloxacin[19]) increased bioavailability following oral administration has been reported.

Transdermal. Skin aging is characterized by decreases in keratinocyte proliferative capacity and impaired capacity to undergo repair of the epidermal barrier following injury. This is associated with delayed lipid reaccumulation and prolonged time of increased permeability to both water-soluble and fat-soluble substances.[20,21] Transdermal administration of medications such as the opioid fentanyl, estrogen, testosterone, the corticosteroids, scopolamine, and clonidine is widely practiced; however, few data exist about the effect of age on the rate or extent of absorption. Transdermal absorption of the more hydrophilic drugs (e.g., hydrocortisone) has been shown to be reduced in older individuals, whereas that of testosterone and estradiol was not.[22]

Parenteral. Medications are often administered subcutaneously or intramuscularly; however, from a very limited database, drug absorption from an intramuscular injection may not change appreciably with age.[23,24]

Drug Distribution

Changes in body composition with age include decreased muscle mass and increased total body fat in both men and women. Though somewhat variable, in nonobese individuals, total body fat is 10% to 20% of total body weight in men and 20% to 30% in women. In older individuals, this increases to 20% to 30% total body fat in men and 30% to 40% total body fat in women. For overweight and obese individuals, the proportion of total body fat's contribution to total body weight is correlated with the degree of obesity; therefore, the proportion of total body weight that is fat is greater than that noted previously. Fat-soluble drugs such as diazepam have much greater distribution in older and obese individuals, whereas non–fat-soluble drugs such as aminoglycoside antibiotics have decreased total body distribution in older and obese individuals. The pharmacokinetic consequence is shown in this relationship:

$$\text{Elimination half-life}\left(t_{1/2}\right)=\frac{0.693V_{\text{area}}}{\text{Clearance}}$$

Thus, drug elimination half-life increases in direct proportion to drug distribution volume in the absence of any change in systemic drug clearance. The implication for therapy is that in instances of increased drug distribution (e.g., diazepam in older or obese individuals), both drug accumulation during chronic dosing and drug elimination after cessation of dosing will be prolonged; however, in the absence of a change in drug clearance, there will be no difference in steady-state drug concentration at a given drug dose.[25] Drug distribution across physiologic barriers in the body such as the blood-brain barrier has not been well studied in older compared with younger individuals.

Drug Metabolism

The major routes of drug biotransformation to active or inactive metabolites may be categorized as phase 1 (oxidative, degradative) and phase 2 (synthetic) pathways. The phase 1 pathways are nearly all mediated by the membrane-bound cytochromes P-450 (CYP), with the notable exception being cytosolic alcohol dehydrogenase. The phase 2 pathways include the glucuronyl transferases, sulfotransferases, and acetyltransferases. The major site of drug metabolism is the liver; however, for some phase 1 pathway drugs, the intestinal wall contributes to the metabolic process. Other organs including the kidneys, lungs, and adipose tissue may contribute to the biotransformation of selected drugs. These extrahepatic sites of drug metabolism are of limited importance quantitatively except in the case of the intestinal wall for some phase 1 pathway drugs and the kidneys for some peptide drugs (Fig. 19-1). Many of the pathways of drug metabolism are mediated by enzymes that have genetic variants that markedly decrease or increase their rate of drug metabolism; however; these are described in Chapter 17 (Heterogenity of Drug Responses and Individualization of Therapy) and are not discussed here because a number of clinical studies have shown that the frequency of these genetic variants does not change with aging.

Liver volume decreases by 20% to 40% over the adult human lifespan. Cellular components that prominently change are decreased

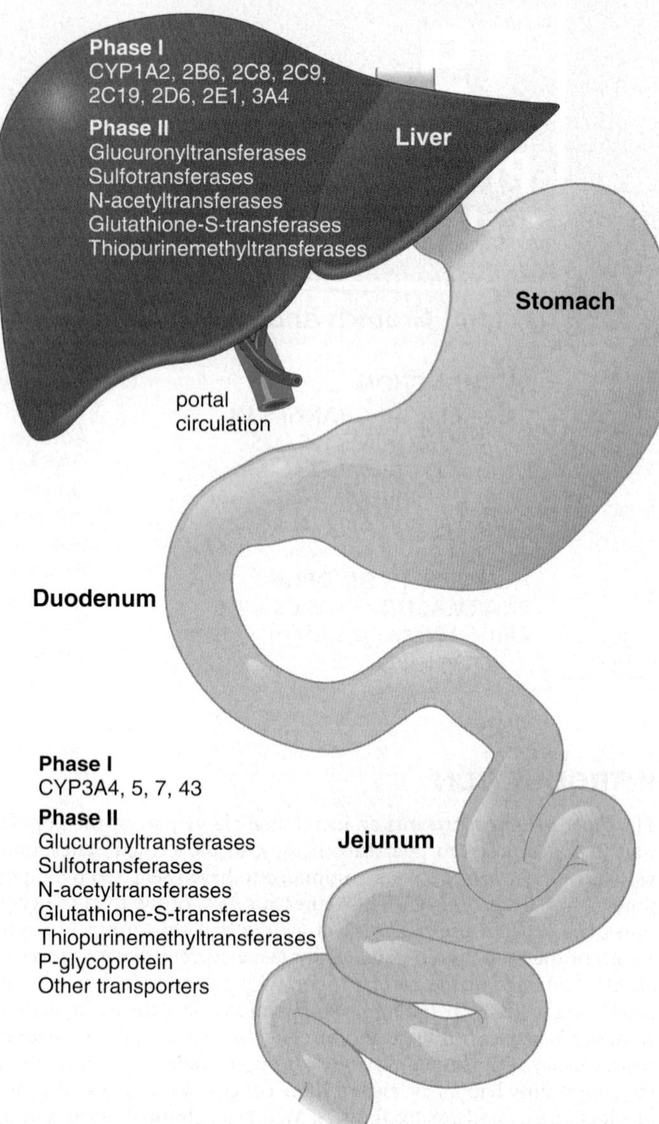

FIGURE 19-1 • The major site of drug metabolism is the liver; however, for some phase 1 pathway drugs, the intestinal wall contributes to the metabolic process.

surface area of the smooth endoplasmic reticulum, thickening of the hepatic sinusoidal endothelium, and decrease in the fenestrations (pores) of the hepatic sinusoidal endothelium. The amount and/or activity of enzymes of drug metabolism may not change with advanced age. The physiologic consequences of the structural changes are decreased hepatic blood flow and decreases in the organelle in which the phase 1 and phase 2 drug biotransformation enzymes reside (smooth endoplasmic reticulum).[26,27]

Age Effects on Drug Metabolism. Phase 1 drug biotransformations are variably decreased in aging, with drugs that are substrates for CYP3A enzymes most completely studied.[28] The isoforms of CYP3A (CYP3A4, CYP3A5, CYP3A7, and CYP3A43) make up about 30% of the total CYP activity in the liver and 70% of the total intestinal CYP activity. The CYP3A isoforms are structurally quite similar, have considerable overlap in their capacity to catalyze drug substrates, and are variably present among individuals. For those reasons, they are often considered as a group. Other CYP enzymes that catalyze drug metabolism include CYP1A2, CYP2B6, CYP2C8, CYP2C9, CYP2C19, CYP2D6, and CYP2E1. The drugs that are substrates for each of these phase 1 enzymes can be found at www.Drug-Interactions.com. The CYP3A enzymes metabolize many clinically important drugs, and their disposition and effects have been most extensively studied in older individuals. The relevant pharmacokinetic parameter that links drug dose and exposure is clearance as shown in the equation:

$$\text{Steady state drug concentration} = \frac{\text{drug infusion rate (dose/unit time)}}{\text{Clearance}}$$

Intravenous administration of a drug that has hepatic blood flow limited clearance gives an estimate of hepatic drug clearance, whereas oral administration is more reflective of intestinal wall drug clearance.[29] Hepatic CYP drug clearance has been studied in older individuals for a large number of drugs and is decreased 10% to 40% for most drugs studied. Intestinal wall drug clearance has not been well studied in older individuals. It should be noted that these studies are nearly all in the young-old and old, generally conducted in individuals without significant illness. In contrast, studies in old and old-old frail and nursing home patients suggest that clearance for at least two CYP3A substrates, amlodipine and erythromycin, is not changed as a function of age or comorbid illness.[11,12] Future studies are needed to reconcile these apparently different findings.

Drug Elimination

Renal Aging. The major organ of drug elimination is the kidney. Structural changes over the adult lifespan in the kidney include decrease in weight by as much as one third, with the loss primarily in the renal cortex. This results in decreases in both number and size of renal glomeruli and decreased blood flow to the remaining glomeruli owing to shunting of blood from afferent to efferent arterioles. These structural changes result in a progressive age-related decrease in glomerular filtration rate (GFR) with the loss quite variable, however, in the range of 0.5 ml/min/yr to 1.0 ml/min/yr. This decrease may be accentuated with concurrent congestive heart failure and concurrent renal disease. Renal filtration fraction increases with age owing to a relatively greater decrease in renal plasma flow than in GFR.[30] Within the kidney, angiotensin II–mediated vasoconstriction is maintained with age; however, endothelium-mediated vascular relaxation is impaired. Circulating atrial natriuretic factor is increased in older individuals, which may result in suppressed renal renin release and the relatively low renin state seen in older patients with hypertension.

Age Effects on Renal Drug Elimination. Renal drug clearance rather closely follows GFR, even for drugs that undergo renal tubular reabsorption or secretion. Therefore, for drugs that undergo renal clearance without prior metabolism such as the aminoglycoside antibiotics, lithium, and penicillin, an estimate of GFR gives a reasonable proportional estimate of drug clearance. This estimate is commonly made using the Cockroft-Gault equation,[31] which incorporates age, weight, and approximate changes in muscle mass as represented by serum creatinine in the following equation.

$$\text{Creatinine clearance (ml/min)} = \frac{(140 - \text{age})(\text{weight in kg})}{72(\text{serum creatinine in mg/dl})}$$

For women, the result is multiplied by 0.85.

For drugs that undergo metabolism prior to renal elimination, impaired renal function may result in accumulation of the metabolite in proportion to the decrease in glomerular filtration. An example of this is lorazepam, a benzodiazepine anxiolytic drug that undergoes phase 2 biotransformation (glucuronidation) with the glucuronide metabolite undergoing renal elimination. With progressive renal dysfunction, patients being treated with lorazepam have extensive accumulation of the metabolite lorazepam glucuronide.[32] This is of importance only if the metabolite has pharmacologic activity (not the case for lorazepam) or it is unstable and can be hydrolyzed back to the active drug (e.g., clofibrate glucuronide).[33] This is dependent on the glucuronide linkage with ether glucuronides (as in the case of lorazepam), generally stable in blood, and ester glucuronides (as in the case of clofibrate), undergoing hydrolysis to re-form the parent drug.

AGE EFFECTS ON DRUG PHARMACODYNAMICS

Central Nervous System

A number of neurotransmitter systems figure importantly in drug action in the CNS, including dopaminergic, serotonergic, cholinergic, noradrenergic, GABAergic, and opiate systems. It is useful to characterize age-related changes in these systems and then place them into the context of known disease-related changes and of drug responses to treat such illnesses in older patients. General age-related structural and functional changes in the brain are progressive volume loss, particularly in the prefrontal cortex; slowing of mental processing that may be multifactorial; and more widespread brain activation occurring to accomplish the same task as in younger individuals.[34]

Dopaminergic

Both dopamine D_1 and D_2 receptors decrease in number with advancing age in the absence of neurologic disease.[35,36] These decreases are most notable anatomically in the caudate nucleus and putamen and are associated with impairments in motor function (D_1) and in motor function and measures of mental flexibility and attention (D_2). Such findings may in part explain the susceptibility of older individuals to extrapyramidal disorders and impaired attention/cognition.

Neuroleptic Drug Disposition and Response in Aging

Pharmacokinetics. As a group, the phenothiazines, butyrophenones, and atypical neuroleptics undergo phase 1 biotransformation. In many cases, the specific CYP enzymes have not been well characterized. Clearance is somewhat decreased in older patients; therefore, a lower dose is required to achieve the same extent of drug exposure. Some examples follow. Risperidone and its active metabolite total concentration, after adjusting to the daily dose, are higher in older people, with linear increase in plasma concentration of about 35% with every decade of life starting after the age of 40.[37] Olanzapine plasma concentration corrected to weight and dose is about 10% higher per every 10 years of age.[38] Haloperidol plasma concentration corrected to dose and weight is also higher in older subjects.[39]

Pharmacodynamics. Neuroleptic drugs are generally characterized in the context of their capacity to block brain dopaminergic D_2 activity; however, it is clear that these drugs act at multiple brain receptors including serotonergic 5HT2, dopaminergic D_1 and D_4, muscarinic cholinergic, α-adrenergic and histaminergic H_1. The dopaminergic hypothesis of schizophrenia has evolved over time to include alterations in serotonergic, glutamatergic, and GABAergic systems in addition to enhanced dopaminergic function.[40] Therefore, it is difficult to ascribe age- and/or disease-related changes in a single one of these systems to an age-related change in therapeutic effect. Treatment of psychosis in older patients is effective, with risperidone and olanzapine having both similar efficacy and similar side effects as compared with those in younger patients. Similar studies indicate haloperidol is also efficacious in older patients.[41] For patients with dementia, the conventional and the atypical antipsychotics probably are similar[42] and may provide little or no benefit to patients.[43] In addition to their use for the treatment of psychotic illness, these drugs are used for the treatment of agitated dementia; however, their role for the treatment of patients with dementia is unclear, and their use is not recommended routinely unless significant risk or distress exists.[43,44] All of these drugs are associated with increased risk of sudden death in older patients, with the cause of death likely to be cardiac arrhythmia.[45] Drug-induced parkinsonism and tardive dyskinesia, owing to dopamine receptor blockade, occur more frequently in older than in younger patients.[46]

Serotonergic

Age-related decreases in the brain of the serotonin $5HT_{1A}$ receptor in various brain regions[47] and the $5HT_{2A}$ receptor in limbic and paralimbic brain regions in women[48] with little or no age-related change in the serotonin reuptake pump have been noted, with these changes accentuated in Alzheimer's disease. The serotonergic hypothesis for depression states that at least some components of major depression are associated with impaired brain serotonergic function; this has provided the rationale for the use of serotonin reuptake inhibitors for the treatment of depression.

Pharmacokinetics. As a group, the antidepressant drugs undergo CYP-mediated phase 1 biotransformation with elimination of active and inactive metabolites. As such, clearance is somewhat decreased in older patients, such that higher drug exposure occurs at a given chronic dosage. For example, citalopram was found to have a 30% longer half-life in elderly men and women.[49] Mirtazapine exposure is greater in older individuals at the same dose and has about a 50% longer elimination half-life.[50] Each of these findings indicates that at a given dose for the antidepressant drugs somewhat greater drug exposure will occur in older patients. It is unclear how age changes the efficacy or toxicity of the antidepressant drugs. Therefore, in general, the same drug exposure for all patients is the therapeutic goal, with decreased doses required to achieve the desired exposure in older patients.

Cholinergic

Brain cholinergic function in older individuals has been implicated in impairments in memory and cognition, with impairments in cholinergic function accentuated in patients with Alzheimer's and other dementias. In animal models, decreases in muscarinic cholinergic (M_1) receptors in the forebrain and other brain regions, altered acetylcholinesterase enzyme, and altered M_1 receptor–stimulated phosphoinositide hydrolysis have been reported.[51-53] How these findings relate to older humans and their cognitive function is uncertain; however, blockade of central muscarinic cholinergic function by scopolamine or atropine does create deficits in memory and learning in humans. The current cholinesterase inhibitor treatments for Alzheimer's disease are based on a hypothesis that this disease is associated with a selective loss of CNS cholinergic neurons and function. The limited clinical effectiveness of such drugs (e.g., donepezil) may be due to the loss of cholinergic neurons, therefore lack of presence of acetylcholine, or the observed central cholinergic deficit is not central to the pathogenesis of the disease.

Pharmacokinetics. The cholinesterase inhibitors tacrine, donepezil, and galantamine undergo phase 1 biotransformation via multiple CYP enzymes, CYP1A2 and CYP2D6 in the case of tacrine and CYP2D6 and CYP3A4 in the case of donepezil and galantamine. In contrast, rivastigmine is hydrolyzed by cholinesterase prior to sulfate conjugation and/or demethylation with renal excretion of the metabolites. Modest age-related changes in the distribution and clearance of these drugs have been reported; however, the changes are not of a magnitude to require a change in doses as a function of patient age.[54]

Pharmacodynamics. The effectiveness of these drugs for the treatment of Alzheimer's disease is limited, and there is little information to suggest that this changes with advancing patient age.

Adrenergic

CNS sympathetic outflow in subcortical suprabulbar regions is increased with age, and this has been associated with a state of generalized adrenergic activation.[55] Central α-adrenoceptors are not changed with age; however, central β-adrenoceptors are reduced, similar to what has been seen in the peripheral adrenergic nervous system. Age-related change in norepinephrine presynaptic reuptake, the site of action of some antidepressant drugs, has not been well defined.

Pharmacokinetics/Pharmacodynamics. Many of the tricyclic antidepressants have some selectivity for inhibition of norepinephrine reuptake. These drugs as a group undergo phase 1 CYP enzyme–mediated biotransformation, often to active metabolites. The CYP isoenzymes involved include CYP3A, CYP2D6, and CYP1A2. As with other classes of drugs, clearance is impaired by 10% to 40% in older individuals, with, for example, imipramine and desipramine.[56] For drugs with some therapeutic concentration range identified (e.g., nortriptyline), there is no evidence for differences in efficacy between younger and older depressed patients, indicating that somewhat lower doses may be appropriate in older patients to achieve the same plasma concentration and, by inference, the same therapeutic effect.

TABLE 19-1 AVERAGE CHANGES IN APPARENT ORAL CLEARANCE OF OLDER AND NEWER AEDS IN ELDERLY PATIENTS*

Drug	Effect of Old Age on Drug Clearance	Route of Clearance
Carbamazepine	Decrease by 25%-40%	CYP3A4
Felbamate	Decrease by 10%-20%	
Gabapentin	Decrease by about 30%-50%	Renal
Lamotrigine	Decrease by about 35%	Glucuronidation
Levetiracetam	Decrease by about 20%-40%	Renal
Oxcarbazepine	Decrease by 25%-35%†	Glucuronidation
Phenobarbital	Decrease by about 20%	CYP2C9, 2C19
Phenytoin	Decrease by about 25%‡	CYP2C9, 2C19
Tiagabine	Decrease by about 30%	CYP3A4
Topiramate	Decrease by 20%	Renal
Valproic acid	Decrease by about 40%§	Glucuronidation
Vigabatrin	Decrease by 50%-85%‖	Renal
Zonisamide	No data	CYP3A4

*Interindividual variation may be considerable in relation to age and other factors.
†Data refer to the active metabolite monohydroxycarbazepine.
‡Decrease in clearance of unbound drug may be greater.
§Decrease in unbound drug clearance. Clearance of total (unbound + protein-bound drug) may not change.
‖These patients, who had various pathologies, were preselected to cover a wide range of impaired renal function.
CYP, cytochrome P-450.
Modified from Perucca E, Berlowitz D, Birnbaum A, et al. Pharmacological and clinical aspects of antiepileptic drug use in the elderly. Epilepsy Res 2006;685:549-563. Reprinted with permission.

GABAergic

The role of aging in the function of brain γ-aminobutyric acid (GABA) neurotransmitter systems is not described. Many widely used classes of drugs, including barbiturates, benzodiazepines, and other antiepileptics such as gabapentin, have a chloride ion channel modulated by the $GABA_A$ receptor as the primary target for their pharmacologic effects. The synaptic inhibition caused by GABA is increased with exposure to such drugs. Other antiepileptic drugs commonly used in older patients have different mechanisms of action. For example, phenytoin promotes an inactivated state of voltage-activated sodium channels.

Pharmacokinetics. Disposition of a number of antiepileptic drugs in older versus younger patients is summarized in Table 19-1. Benzodiazepines such as diazepam and lorazepam, frequently used for the treatment of status epilepticus, and clonazepam and clorazepate, used for longer-term treatment of seizure disorders, have well-described increased effects in older patients. As noted, these drugs act by increasing synaptic inhibition caused by $GABA_A$ receptors, with a specific "benzodiazepine receptor" subunit on the chloride channel activated by GABA. Diazepam, clonazepam, and clorazepate undergo phase 1 biotransformation by CYP enzymes, and diazepam, the most studied, has an approximately 30% decrease in clearance in older individuals. Lorazepam is metabolized by glucuronidation, a phase 2 pathway, and its clearance is not altered with advancing age. Other benzodiazepines used as sedative-hypnotics (e.g., chlordiazepoxide) and for conscious sedation (e.g., midazolam) undergo phase 1 biotransformation and have decreased clearance in older individuals.[58,59] Similarly, zolpidem, a nonbenzodiazepine that exerts its sedative-hypnotic effect via increased synaptic inhibition through $GABA_A$ receptors, the same mechanism as that of benzodiazepines, has an approximately 50% decrease in clearance in older individuals.[60]

Pharmacodynamics. The efficacy and toxicity of antiepileptic drugs as a group have not been well studied in older patients. Benzodiazepines have increased sedative effect at a given drug exposure.[61] The combination of somewhat impaired clearance, resulting in greater drug exposure at a given dose, and increased sensitivity at the same exposure in older individuals may in part explain the potential for severe adverse events such as hip fracture associated with benzodiazepine sedative-hypnotics.[62]

Opiates

Few data describe age-related changes in μ, κ, or σ opiate receptors and their function in humans. In human frontal cortex, pentazocine binding (a partial μ receptor agonist and a κ agonist) is decreased with advancing age.[63] It is uncertain how such structural alterations relate to function of the endogenous opioid system in relationship to aging. However opiate and opioid drugs have considerable importance in the treatment of pain and for use during anesthesia in clinical medicine. Therefore, clinical study of many of these drugs in older individuals has been undertaken.

Pharmacokinetics. The clearance of morphine, fentanyl, and alfentanyl change little with age.[64,65] Morphine is metabolized to active glucuronide metabolites (phase 2 metabolism), whereas fentanyl and alfentanyl undergo oxidative demethylations (phase 1 metabolism).

Pharmacodynamics. Using electroencephalogram spectral edge as a measure of CNS depression during anesthesia with fentanyl, alfentanyl, and remifentanyl,[65,66] older individuals are more sensitive than younger individuals to these μ opiate receptor agonists. In contrast, using respiratory depression as a measure of drug effect, sensitivity to morphine was no different between younger and older individuals.[67]

Cardiovascular System

Many neurotransmitter systems and local hormones—including β-adrenergic, α-adrenergic, cholinergic, renin-angiotensin-aldosterone, natriuretic peptides, and endothelin—are essential for maintenance of cardiovascular homeostasis. In addition, integrated sympathetic and parasympathetic systems regulate baroreflex function. Many of these systems are important therapeutic targets for the treatment of cardiovascular disease. The structure of both heart and blood vessels contributes to maintenance of cardiovascular homeostasis as well. An understanding of age and age-/disease-related changes in these systems and structures that affect pharmacologic responses may be useful for optimal treatment of cardiovascular diseases, the leading cause of death in the United States and other developed countries.

β-Adrenergic

Both β_1- and β_2-adrenergic responses are decreased with advancing age. The mechanism for this is not well understood; however, a number of postreceptor events have been studied in detail.[68] The decline in β_1-adrenergic responsiveness results in decreased tachycardic response in response to sympathetic stimulation. The decline in β_2-adrenergic responsiveness results in a relative state of peripheral vascular constriction owing to loss of β_2-adrenergic vasorelaxation.[69] A generalized state of relative sympathetic activation in older individuals[70] may be a response to the decreased adrenergic responses seen with age or the decreased responsiveness may be the result of relative sympathetic activation. Mechanisms for the increased basal sympathetic function with advancing age are not well enough understood to determine the proximate factor.

α-Adrenergic

α_1-Adrenergic vasoconstrictor responses are impaired in older individuals.[71] This is not the case for all peripheral arterial vasoconstrictor responses because, in the same individuals, angiotensin II–mediated vasoconstriction was not changed with age.

Baroreflex Responsiveness

The vagally mediated baroreflex suppresses heart rate with increases in blood pressure, and conversely, with decrease in blood pressure as occurs with upright posture, suppression of vagal activity results in increased heart rate. In older individuals, loss of baroreflex function leads to impaired control, or buffering, of blood pressure when arterial vasoconstriction or vasodilation occurs.[72,73] The impairment in baroreflex function is increased in patients with hypertension.

TABLE 19-2 PHARMACODYNAMICS

System	Receptor	Receptor Subtypes	Number/ Binding
	Receptor Changes with Age		
CNS*	Dopaminergic	D_1	↓
		D_2	↓
	Serotonergic	$5HT_{1A}$	↓
		$5HT_{2A}$	↓ In women
		M_1	↓
	Cholinergic	α	↔
	Adrenergic	β	↓
			?
	GABAergic	μ, κ	↓
	Opiates	σ	?
			Response
CVS†	β-Adrenergic	β_1	↓
		β_2	↓
	α-Adrenergic	α_1	↓
	Integrated Function Changes with Age		
	Baroreflex responsiveness		↓
	Renin-angiotensin-aldosterone axis		↓ Plasma renin activity

*A number of neurotransmitter systems figure importantly in drug action in the CNS. This action might change as a result of age-related decreases in receptor number or function.

†Neurotransmitter systems and local hormones are essential for maintenance of cardiovascular homeostasis. In addition, integrated sympathetic and parasympathetic systems regulate baroreflex function. Many of these systems are important therapeutic targets for the treatment of cardiovascular disease, and the decrease in their level or response with age might influence the effect of drugs.

CNS, central nervous system; CVS, cardiovascular system; D, dopamine; 5HT, 5-hydroxytryptamine (serotonin); M, muscarinic; ↓, reduced; ↔, not changed; ?, not known.

Renin-Angiotensin-Aldosterone Axis

Plasma renin activity is decreased with advancing age. Therefore, older individuals may have less contribution to basal vascular tone by angiotensin II. This leads to decreased stimulus for aldosterone secretion with increased age and may have a role in the increased prevalence of hyporeninemic hypoaldosteronism in older individuals.[74,75] The changes in receptor function and humoral responses that occur with age are summarized in Table 19-2.

Cardiac and Vascular Structure/Function

Left ventricular cardiac wall thickness increases with age. This occurs with increased myocyte size, decreased myocyte numbers, and increased collagen deposition. This results in left ventricular "stiffness" and is associated with decreased early diastolic filling and increased dependence of late diastolic filling on effective atrial contraction. In addition to this structural change, in animal models, cardiomyocyte sarcoplasmic reticulum (SR) calcium reuptake is slowed owing to decreased expression of the SR calcium ATPase.[76] Resting cardiac output does not change with age; however, at maximal exercise, cardiac output is decreased in healthy older versus younger individuals.[77] These changes in cardiac function are increased in patients with hypertension.

Arterial structure changes with age as well, with increased vascular intimal thickness in large elastic vessels such as the aorta and the carotid artery. The thickness is associated with decreased distensibility. The carotid intimal layer may increase as much as two to three times when comparing individuals aged 20 and 90. This is in part due to

BOX 19-1 SOME NARROW THERAPEUTIC INDEX DRUGS THAT REQUIRE DOWNWARD DOSE ADJUSTMENT IN OLDER PATIENTS

Decreased Renal Clearance
- Lithium
- Digoxin
- Aminoglycosides
- Vancomycin

Decreased Phase 1 Biotransformation
- Thiopental
- Opioids in anesthesia
- Benzodiazepines
- Theophylline
- Lidocaine

increased collagen and ground substance deposition.[78] Endothelium-mediated vascular relaxation is also impaired with increasing age.[79] All of these changes are increased in patients with hypertension, diabetes, and hyperlipidemia.

Cardiovascular Drug Disposition and Response with Increased Age

As previously noted, drugs that undergo phase 1 biotransformation may have some decrease in clearance in older individuals (Box 19-1), those that have phase 2–mediated inactivation have little or no change with increased age, and those that have renal clearance as a means of inactivation have decreased drug clearance that is in parallel with decreased GFR. Drugs with high clearance that is a function of hepatic blood flow (e.g., lidocaine) also have decreased clearance in older individuals.[80] However, for cardiovascular drugs, which generally have a rather wide therapeutic index, age-related change in drug effect is much more related to the interface of cardiovascular pathophysiologic change with age and drug response. An exception to this is digoxin, a drug that has 60% to 70% renal elimination and the remainder by nonrenal mechanisms. Decreased digoxin clearance in older individuals requires downward dose adjustment owing to its low therapeutic index[81] (see Box 19-1).

Adrenergic Drugs

β-Adrenergic Antagonists. β-Adrenergic antagonists are widely used in older patients for the treatment of angina, hypertension, and congestive heart failure. These drugs may have less effectiveness for the treatment of hypertension in older patients, probably owing to the decreased role of β-adrenergic function in the maintenance of cardiovascular homeostasis with advancing age. No information exists about age-related change in effectiveness of these drugs for the treatment of angina and congestive heart failure; however, they are effective when evaluated in older patients with these illnesses.[7] A subgroup, the α_1 β-adrenergic antagonists labetalol and carvedilol may cause greater postural change in blood pressure (orthostatic hypotension) in older hypertensive patients, probably owing to the drugs' impaired ability to increase heart rate and cardiac output in response to the α_1-adrenergic–mediated peripheral vasodilation caused by these drugs.[82]

β-Adrenergic Agonists. Older patients with asthma and chronic obstructive pulmonary disease may often be treated with β_2-adrenergic agonists such as albuterol, terbutaline, or sabutamol. As a group, these drugs are not totally selective for β_2-adrenergic receptors and cause some increase in heart rate owing to β_1-adrenergic agonist effects. Older patients have less tachycardia when exposed to these drugs owing to impaired capacity for β_1-adrenergic stimulation.[83] Tremor, another prominent side effect of these drugs, has not been well studied in younger and older patients.

α-Adrenergic Antagonists. α-Adrenergic antagonists such as terazosin are often used for the treatment of urinary outflow obstruction due to benign prostatic hypertrophy in older men and have been suggested as particularly useful for individuals who have both hypertension and prostatic hypertrophy. The decrease in peripheral vascular resistance caused by α_1-adrenergic blockade results in sympathetic activation and reflex tachycardia with increased cardiac output to maintain vital organ perfusion. Older patients have less response to the sympathetic activation due to impaired β_1-adrenergic function, and in addition, impaired baroreflex function that also limits increased heart rate. The result is increased postural change in blood pressure.[84]

Calcium Antagonist Drugs. Calcium antagonist drugs for the treatment of hypertension, angina, and supraventricular arrhythmias are extensively used in older patients. They decrease blood pressure by peripheral vasodilation due to blockade of vascular L-type calcium channels; however, they are associated with less reflex tachycardia than are other peripheral vasodilators, probably as a result of cardiac sinus node suppression. Amlodipine, a prototype calcium antagonist used for hypertension, decreases blood pressure in older patients to the same extent as in younger patients with the same drug exposure.[85] Verapamil and diltiazem, drugs with more prominent sinus node suppression and atrioventricular conduction delay than amlodipine and other dihydropyridine drugs in the class, paradoxically cause less decrease in atrioventricular conduction in older than in younger patients; however, the mechanism is not clear.[86,87]

Angiotensin Blockade. Angiotensin-converting enzyme inhibitors (ACEIs) and angiotensin receptor blockers (ARBs) are used for the treatment of hypertension and congestive heart failure by decreasing angiotensin II effect, via inhibition of formation by the ACEI and receptor blockade by the ARB. The effect of ACEI, may be in part due to enhanced bradykinin-mediated vasodilation as well. These drugs may be less effective for the treatment of hypertension in older patients, probably owing to the relative decrease in the role of renin-angiotensin-aldosterone axis function in the maintenance of blood pressure with increased age. There are no data with respect to their use in the treatment of congestive heart failure in older versus younger patients. However, to the extent they have been evaluated in older patients, they decrease heart failure–related mortality just as well as in younger patients.[6]

Diuretics. Thiazide and thiazide-like drugs are used for the treatment of hypertension, and in older patients without severely impaired renal function, they are at least as, if not more, effective in older and in younger patients. This is probably related to sodium retention being an important component of hypertension in older patients as contrasted to vasoconstriction in younger patients. Such statements apply to patient populations, with each individual patient having a relatively unique hypertensive phenotype. Large hypertension treatment trials have clearly shown thiazide-type diuretics to be as effective as or more effective than other classes of antihypertensive drugs in older patients.[88-90]

ADVERSE EFFECTS OF DRUG EXPOSURE IN OLDER PATIENTS

The multiple illnesses that may benefit from drug treatment in older individuals often result in the administration of many concurrent drugs. A survey of nursing homes in the Los Angeles area indicated a mean of eight concurrent medicines across a broad sample.[91] However, a number of studies conducted in the outpatient, inpatient, and extended care settings showed that the likelihood of an adverse drug reaction is directly related to the number of concomitant medications an older patient receives.[92-94] Drugs with anticholinergic and sedative effects may be particularly implicated. Examples include impaired cognitive function with exposure to drugs with anticholinergic effects, increased risk of falls with exposure to antidepressants and benzodiazepines, and increased risk of hip fracture in older patients who receive benzodiazepines.[9,10] Therefore, it is essential that for each drug treatment considered for the older patient, the risks of treatment as well as the benefits be considered. Frequently, drugs with anticholinergic and sedative effects are prescribed for nonspecific indications or for indications for which there is little evidence of effectiveness (e.g.,

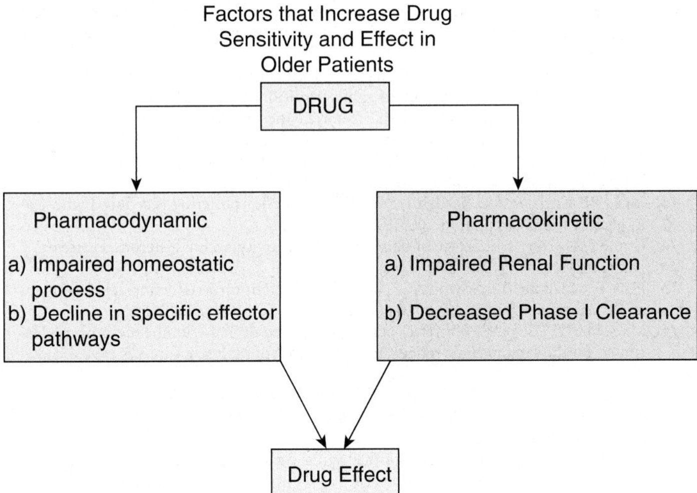

FIGURE 19-2 • Factors that increase drug sensitivity and effect in older patients.

the use of neuroleptics for the treatment of agitation in patients with Alzheimer's disease).[43,44] It is particularly important to avoid such practices in older patients.

Some specific drug exposures have been particularly associated with drug toxicity in older patients, with the mechanisms not well understood. Warfarin oral anticoagulant therapy is indicated for the treatment of venous thromboembolism and atrial fibrillation in older patients, and risk of bleeding is substantially increased with increasing patient age.[95] ACEI therapy for the treatment of congestive heart failure is clearly efficacious in older patients[6]; however, it is associated with increased risk of hyperkalemia.[96] This is perhaps due to drug effect superimposed on the depressed renin-angiotensin-aldosterone axis and resulting predisposition to hyporeninemic hypoaldosteronism. Nonsteroidal anti-inflammatory drug treatment is useful for the treatment of arthritis; however, it is associated with increased likelihood of gastrointestinal bleeding.[97] This is somewhat, although not completely, abolished with the use of cyclooxygenase-2 selective inhibitors and is increased with concomitant low-dose aspirin treatment commonly used in older patients for prevention of cardiovascular events.[98] The increased likelihood of gastrointestinal bleeding may be related to decreased gastroduodenal mucosal prostaglandins in older individuals.[99] Finally, older patients have markedly increased susceptibility to cardiac arrhythmia and seizure with theophylline treatment[100]; this has resulted in limited use of this treatment for lung disease with associated bronchospasm in older patients.

CONCLUSION

Use of multiple medications in older patients with multiple coexisting illnesses that can be effectively treated is a common situation, and the older patient should not have effective therapies withheld owing to fear of adverse drug effect. However, the pharmacokinetic and pharmacodynamic changes that occur on a background of aging pathophysiology generally result in the older patient having a narrowed therapeutic index for nearly any drug exposure (Fig. 19-2). This is increased when multiple medications are administered at the same time. Therefore, before administration of any drug treatment to the older patient, there should be clear evidence for therapeutic efficacy and the risk-benefit relationship carefully considered.

REFERENCES

1. Agency for Healthcare Research and Quality; Prescription medicines—mean and median expenses per person with expense and distribution of expenses by source of payment: United States 2002. Published Dec. 23, 2004; revised Sept. 30, 2005.
2. Fried LP, Bandeen-Roche K, et al, for the Women's Health in Aging Study Collaborative Research Group. Association of comorbidity with disability in older women: The Women's Health and Aging Study. J Clin Epidemiol 1999;32:27-37.
3. Selim AJ, Berlowitz DR, Fincke G, et al. The health status of elderly veteran enrollees in the Veterans Health Administration. J Am Geriatr Soc 2004;52:1271-1276.
4. Walston J, Hadley EC, Ferrucci L, et al. Research agenda for frailty in older adults: towards a better understanding of physiology and etiology: summary from the American Geriatrics Society/National Institute on Aging research conference on frailty in older adults. J Am Geriatr Soc 2006;54:991-1001.
5. Mangoni AA, Jackson SHD. The implications of a growing evidence base for drug use in elderly patients. Part 1. Statins for primary and secondary cardiovascular prevention. Br J Clin Pharmacol 2006;61:494-501.
6. Mangoni AA, Jackson SHD. The implications of a growing evidence base for drug use in elderly patients. Part 2. ACE inhibitors and angiotensin receptor blockers in heart failure and high cardiovascular risk patents. Br J Clin Pharmacol 2006;61:502-512.
7. Mangoni AA, Jackson SHD. The implications of a growing evidence base for drug use in elderly patients. Part 3. β-Adrenoceptor blockers in heart failure and thrombolytics in acute myocardial infarction. Br J Clin Pharmacol 2006;61:513-520.
8. Dhesi JK, Allain TJ, Mangoni AA, Jackson SHD. The implications of a growing evidence base for drug use in elderly patients. Part 4. Vitamin D and bisphosphonates for fractures and osteoporosis. Br J Clin Pharmacol 2006;61:521-528.
9. Ray WA, Griffin MR, Schaffner W, et al. Psychotropic drug use and the risk of hip fracture. N Engl J Med 1987;316:363-369.
10. Hanlon JT, Horner RD, Schmader KE, et al. Benzodiazepine use and cognitive function among community-dwelling elderly. Clin Pharmacol Ther 1998;64:684-692.
11. Kang D, Verotta D, Schwartz JB. Population analyses of amlodipine in patients living in the community and patients living in nursing homes. Clin Pharmacol Ther 2006;79:114-124.
12. Schwartz JB. Erythromycin breath test results in elderly, very elderly, and frail elderly persons. Clin Pharmacol Ther 2006;79:440-448.
13. Hurwitz A, Brady DA, Schaal SE, et al. Gastric acidity in older adults. JAMA 1979; 278:659-662.
14. Hurwitz A, Ruhl CE, Kimler BF, et al. Gastric function in the elderly: effect on absorption of ketoconazole. J Clin Pharmacol 2003;43:996-1002.
15. Castleden CM, Volans CN, Raymond K. The effect of ageing on drug absorption from the gut. Age Ageing 1977;6:138-143.
16. Storstein L, Larsen A, Midtbo K, Saevareid L. Pharmacokinetics of calcium blockers in patients with renal insufficiency and in geriatric patients. Acta Med Scand Suppl 1984;681:25-30.
17. Kelly JG, McGarry K, O'Malley K, O'Brien ET. Bioavailability of labetalol increases with age. Br J Clin Pharmacol 1982;14:304-305.
18. Bianchetti G, Billy S, Ascalone V, et al. Multicenter studies on the pharmacokinetic profile of sustained release oral diltiazem (300 mg) after once a day repeated administration: influence of age. Int J Clin Pharmacol Ther 1996;195-201.
19. Ljungberg B, Nilsson-Ehle I. Pharmacokinetics of ciprofloxacin in the elderly: increased oral bioavailability and reduced renal clearance. Eur J Clin Microbiol Infect Dis 1989;8:515-520.
20. Ghadially R, Brown BE, Sequeira-Martin SM, et al. The aged epidermal permeability barrier. Structural, functional, and lipid biochemical abnormalities in humans and a senescent murine model. J Clin Invest 1995;95:2281-2290.
21. Yaar M, Gilchrest BA. Ageing and photoageing of keratinocytes and melanocytes. Clin Exp Dermatol 2001;26:583-591.
22. Roskos KV, Maibach HI, Guy RH. The effect of aging on percutaneous absorption in man. J Pharmacokinet Biopharm 1989;17:617-630.
23. Divoll M, Greenblatt DJ, Ochs HR, Shader RI. Absolute bioavailability of oral and intramuscular diazepam. Anesth Analg 1983;62:1-8.
24. Holazo AA, Winkler MB, Patel IH. Effects of age, gender and oral contraceptives on intramuscular midazolam pharmacokinetics. J Clin Pharmacol 1988;28:1040-1045.
25. Abernethy DR, Greenblatt DJ. Drug disposition in obese humans. An update. Clin Pharmacokinet 1986;11:199-213.
26. Schmucker DL. Age-related changes in liver structure and function: implications for disease? Exp Gerontol 2005;40:650-659.
27. McLean AJ, Le Couteur DG. Aging biology and geriatric clinical pharmacology. Pharmacol Rev 2004;56:163-184.
28. Cotreau MM, von Moltke LL, Greenblatt DJ. The influence of age and sex on the clearance of cytochrome P4503A substrates. Clin Pharmacokinet 2005;44:33-60.
29. Wu C-Y, Benet LZ, Herbert MF, et al. Differentiation of absorption and first-pass gut and hepatic metabolism in humans: studies with cyclosporine. Clin Pharmacol Ther 1995;58:492-497.
30. Davies DF, Shock NW. Age changes in glomerular filtration rate, effective renal plasma flow, and tubular excretory capacity in adult males. J Clin Invest 1950;29:496-507.
31. Cockcroft DW, Gault MH. Prediction of creatinine clearance from serum creatinine. Nephron 1976;16:31-41.
32. Verbeeck R, Tjandramaga TB, Verberckmoes R, DeScheffer PJ. Biotransformation and excretion of lorazepam in patients with chronic renal failure. Br J Clin Pharmacol 1976;3:1033-1039.
33. Meffin PJ, Zilm DM, Veenendaal JR. Reduced clofibric acid clearance in renal dysfunction is due to a futile cycle. J Pharmacol Exp Ther 1983;227:732-738.
34. Raz N. Aging of the brain and its impact on cognitive performance: integration of structural and functional findings. In Craik FIM, Salthouse TA (eds): The Handbook of Aging and Cognition, 2nd ed. Mahwah, NJ: Lawrence Erlbaum Associates, 2000, pp 1-90.
35. Rinne JO, Lonnberg P, Marjamaki P. Age-dependent decline in human brain dopamine D_1 and D_2 receptors. Brain Res 1990;508:349-352.

36. Volkow ND, Gur RC, Wang GJ, et al. Association between decline in brain activity with age and cognitive and motor impairment in health individuals. Am J Psychiatr 1998;155:344-349.
37. Aichhorn W, Weiss U, Marksteiner J, et al. Influence of age and gender on risperidone plasma concentrations. J Psychopharmacol 2005;19:395-401.
38. Weiss U, Marksteiner J, Kemmler G, et al. Effects of age and sex on olanzapine plasma concentrations. J Clin Psychopharmacol 2005;25:570-574.
39. Ohara K, Tanabu S, Ishibashi K, et al. Effects of age and the CYP2D6*10 allele on the plasma haloperidol concentration/dose ratio. Prog Neuropsychopharmacol Biol Psychiatr 2003;27:347-350.
40. Carlsson A, Waters N, Holm-Waters S, et al. Interactions between monoamines, glutamate, and GABA in schizophrenia: new evidence. Annu Rev Pharmacol Toxicol 2001;41:237-260.
41. Marriott RG, Neil W, Waddingham S. Antipsychotic medication for elderly people with schizophrenia. Cochrane Database Syst Rev 2006;25:CD005580.
42. Verhey FR, Vorkaaik M, Lougberg R, Olanzapine-Haloperidol in Dementia Study Group. Olanzapine versus haloperidol in the treatment of agitation in elderly patients with dementia: results of a random controlled double-blind trial. Dement Geriatr Cogn Disord 2006;21:1-8.
43. Schneider LS, Tariof PN, Dagerman KS, et al, for the CATIE-AE Study Group. Effectiveness of atypical antipsychotic drugs in patients with Alzheimer's Disease. N Engl J Med 2006;355:1525-1538.
44. Ballard C, Waite J. The effectiveness of atypical antipsychotics for the treatment of aggression and psychosis in Alzheimer's disease. Cochrane Database Syst Rev 2006;25: CD003476.
45. Wang PS, Schneeweiss S, Avorn J, et al. Risk of death in elderly users of conventional vs. atypical antipsychotic medications. N Engl J Med 2005;353:2335-2341.
46. Caligiuri M, Lacro JP, Jeste DV. Incidence and predictors of drug-induced parkinsonism in older psychiatric patients treated with very low doses of neuroleptics. J Clin Psychopharmacol 1999;19:322-328.
47. Meltzer CC, Smith G, Price JC, et al. Reduced binding of [18F] altanserin to serotonin type 2A receptors in aging: persistence of effect after partial volume correction. Brain Res 1998;813:167-171.
48. Costes N, Merlet I, Ostrowsky K, et al. A ^{18}F-MPPF PET normative database of 5-HT$_{1A}$ receptor binding in men and women over aging. J Nucl Med 2005;46:1980-1989.
49. Gutierrez M, Abramowitz W. Steady-state pharmacokinetics of citalopram in young and elderly subjects. Pharmacotherapy 2000;20:1441-1447.
50. Timmer CJ, Sitsen JM, Delbressine LP. Clinical pharmacokinetics of mirtazapine. Clin Pharmacokinet 2000;38:461-474.
51. Ayyagari PV, Gerber M, Joseph JA, Crews FT. Uncoupling of muscarinic cholinergic phosphoinositide signals in senescent cerebral cortical and hippocampal membranes. Neurochem Int 1998;32:107-115.
52. Freund CO. Cholinergic receptor loss in brains of aging mice. Life Sci 1980;26:371-375.
53. Pedigo NW, Polk DM. Reduced muscarinic receptor plasticity in frontal cortex of aged rats after chronic administration of cholinergic drugs. Life Sci 1985;37:1443-1449.
54. Jann MW, Shirley KL, Small GW. Clinical pharmacokinetics and pharmacodynamics of cholinesterase inhibitors. Clin Pharmacokinet 2002;41:719-739.
55. Esler M, Hasting J, Lambert G, et al. The influence of aging on the human sympathetic nervous system and brain norepinephrine turnover. Am J Physiol 2002;282:R909-R916.
56. Abernethy DR, Greenblatt DJ, Shader RI. Imipramine and desipramine disposition in the elderly. J Pharmacol Exp Ther 1985;232:183-188.
57. Perucca E, Berlowitz D, Birnbaum A, et al. Pharmacological and clinical aspects of antiepileptic drug use in the elderly. Epilepsy Res 2006;685:549-563.
58. Greenblatt DJ, Shader RI, Abernethy DR. Drug therapy: current status of benzodiazepines. N Engl J Med 1983;309:354-358, 410-416.
59. Greenblatt DJ, Abernethy DR, Locniskar A, et al. Effect of age, gender, and obesity on midazolam kinetics. Anesthesiology 1984;61:27-35.
60. Olubodun JO, Ochs HR, von Moltke LL, et al. Pharmacokinetic properties of zolpidem in elderly and young adults: possible modulation by testosterone in men. Br J Clin Pharmacol 2003;56:297-304.
61. Jacobs JR, Reves JG, Marty J, et al. Aging increases pharmacodynamic sensitivity to the hypnotic effects of midazolam. Anesth Analg 1995;80:143-148.
62. Ray WA, Griffin MR, Downey W. Benzodiazepines of long and short elimination half-life and the risk of hip fracture. JAMA 1989;262:3303-3307.
63. Kornhuber J, Schoppmeyer K, Bendig C, Riederer P. Characterization of [^{3}H]-pentazocine binding sites in post-mortem human frontal cortex. J Neural Transm 1996;103:45-53.
64. Owen JA, Sitar DS, Berger L, et al. Age-related morphine kinetics. Clin Pharmacol Ther 1983;34:364-368.
65. Scott JC, Stanski DR. Decreased fentanyl and alfentamil dose requirements with age. A simultaneous pharmacokinetic and pharmacodynamic evaluation. J Pharmacol Exp Ther 1987;240:159-165.
66. Minto CF, Schnider TW, Egan TD, et al. Influence of age and gender on the pharmacokinetics and pharmacodynamics of remifentanil: I. Model development. Anesthesiology 1997;86:10-23.
67. Arunasalam K, Davenport HT, Painter S, Jones JG. Ventilatory response to morphine in young and old subjects. Anaesthesia 1983;38:529-533.
68. Schutzer WE, Mader SL. Age-related changes in vascular adrenergic signaling: clinical and mechanistic implications. Ageing Res Rev 2003;2:169-190.
69. Pan HYM, Hoffman BB, Porsche RA, Blaschke TF. Decline in beta-adrenergic receptor-mediated vascular relaxation with aging in man. J Pharmacol Exp Ther 1986;239:802-807.
70. Seals DR, Dinenno FA. Collateral damage: cardiovascular consequences of chronic sympathetic activation with human aging. Am J Physiol 2004;287:H1895-H1905.
71. Hogikyan RV, Supiano MA. Arterial α-adrenergic responsiveness is decreased and SNS activity is increased in older humans. Am J Physiol 1994;266:E717-E724.
72. Gribbin B, Pickering TG, Sleight R, Peto R. Effect of age and high blood pressure on baroreflex sensitivity in man. Circ Res 1971;29:424-431.
73. Jones PP, Christen DD, Jordan J, Seals DR. Baroreflex buffering is reduced with age in healthy men. Circulation 2003;107:1770-1774.
74. Crane MG, Harris JJ. Effect of aging on renin activity and aldosterone excretion. J Lab Clin Med 1976;87:947-959.
75. Hall JE, Coleman TG, Guyton AC. The renin-angiotension system: normal physiology and changes in older hypertensives. J Am Geriatr Soc 1989;37:801-813.
76. Maciel LMZ, Poliker R, Rohrer D, et al. Age-induced decreases in the messenger RNA coding for the sarcoplasmic reticulum Ca^{2+}-ATPase of rat heart. Circ Res 1990;67:230-234.
77. Lakatta EG, Levy D. Arterial and cardiac aging: Major share holders in cardiovascular disease enterprises. Part II. The aging heart in health: links to heart disease. Circulation 2003;107:346-354.
78. Lakatta EG, Levy D. Arterial and cardiac aging: major shareholders in cardiovascular disease enterprises. Part I. Aging arteries: a "set up" for vascular disease. Circulation 2003;107:139-146.
79. Andrawis NS, Jones DS, Abernethy DR. Aging is associated with endothelial dysfunction in the human forearm vasculature. J Am Geriatr Soc 2000;48:193-198.
80. Abernethy DR, Greenblatt DJ. Impairment of lidocaine clearance in elderly male patients. J Cardiovasc Pharmacol 1983;5:1093-1096.
81. Cusack B, Kelly J, O'Malley K, et al. Digoxin in the elderly: pharmacokinetic consequences of old age. Clin Pharmacol Ther 1979;25:772-776.
82. Abernethy DR, Schwartz JB, Plachetka JR, et al. Comparison in young and elderly patients of pharmacodymanics and disposition of labetalol in systemic hypertension. Am J Cardiol 1987;60:697-702.
83. Vestal RE, Wood AJJ, Shand DG. Reduced beta-adrenoceptor sensitivity in the elderly. Clin Pharmacol Ther 1979;26:181-186.
84. Hosmane BS, Maurath CJ, Jordan DC, Laddu A. Effect of age and dose on the incidence of adverse events in the treatment of hypertension in patients receiving terazosin. J Clin Pharmacol 1992;32:434-443.
85. Abernethy DR, Gutkowska J, Winterbottom LM. Effects of amlodipine, a long-acting dihydropridine calcium antagonist, in aging hypertension: pharmacodynamics in relation to disposition. Clin Pharmacol Ther 1990;48:76-86.
86. Abernethy DR, Schwartz JB, Todd EL, et al. Verapamil pharmacodynamics and disposition in young versus elderly hypertensive patients. Ann Intern Med 1986;105:329-336.
87. Schwartz JB, Abernethy DR. Responses to intravenous and oral diltiazem in elderly versus younger patients with systemic hypertension. Am J Cardiol 1987;59:1111-1117.
88. SHEP Cooperative Research Group. Prevention of stroke by antihypertensive drug treatment in older persons with isolated systolic hypertension: final results of the Systolic Hypertension in the Elderly Program (SHEP). JAMA 1991;265:3255-3264.
89. Insua JT, Sacks HS, Lau T-S, et al. Drug treatment of hypertension in the elderly: a meta-analysis. Ann Intern Med 1994;121:355-362.
90. The ALLHAT Officers and Coordinators for the ALLHAT Collaborative Research Group. Major outcomes in high-risk hypertensive patients randomized to angiotensin-converting enzyme inhibitor or calcium channel blocker vs. diuretic: the Antihypertensive and Lipid-Lowering Treatment to Prevent Heart Attack Trial (ALLHAT). JAMA 2002;288:2981-2997.
91. Beers MH, Ouslander JG, Fingold SF, et al. Inappropriate medication prescribing in skilled nursing facilities. Ann Intern Med 1992;117:684-689.
92. Smith JW, Seidl LG, Cluff LE. Studies of the epidemiology of adverse drug reactions. V. Clinical factors influencing susceptibility. Ann Intern Med 1966;65:629-640.
93. Hutchinson TA, Flegel KM, Kramer MS, et al. Frequency, severity and risk factors for adverse drug reactions in adult outpatients. J Chronic Dis 1986;533-542.
94. Gurwitz JH, Field TS, Avorn J, et al. Incidence and preventability of adverse drug events in the nursing home setting. Am J Med 2000;109:87-94.
95. Pautas E, Gonin-Thibault I, Debray M, et al. Haemorrhagic complications of vitamin K antagonists in the elderly: risk factors and management. Drugs Aging 2006;23:13-25.
96. Reardon LC, Macpherson DS. Hyperkalemia in outpatients using angiotensin converting enzyme inhibitors. Arch Intern Med 1998;158:26-32.
97. Gabriel SE, Jaakkimainen L, Bombardier C. Risk for serious gastrointestinal complications related to use of nonsteroidal anti-inflammatory drugs. Ann Intern Med 1991; 115:787-796.
98. Dubois RW, Melmed GY, Henning JM, Bernal M. Risk of upper gastrointestinal injury and events in patients treated with cyclooxygenase (COX)-1/COX-2 nonsteroidal anti-inflammatory drugs (NSAIDs), COX-2 selective NSAIDs, and gastroprotective cotherapy: an appraisal of the literature. J Clin Rheumatol 2004;10:178-189.
99. Cryer B, Lee E, Feldman M. Factors influencing gastroduodenal mucosal prostaglandin concentrations: roles of smoking and aging. Ann Intern Med 1992;116:636-640.
100. Shannon M, Lovejoy FH. The influence of age vs. peak serum concentration on life-threatening events after chronic theophylline intoxication. Arch Intern Med 1990; 150:2045-2048.

20

ADVERSE DRUG REACTIONS AND INTERACTIONS

Shiew-Mei Huang, Lawrence J. Lesko, and Robert Temple

INTRODUCTION 265
CASE 1: TERFENADINE AND KETOCONAZOLE INTERACTION 265
Discussion 266
CASE 2: LOVASTATIN AND GRAPEFRUIT JUICE INTERACTION 269
Discussion 269
CASE 3: CYCLOSPORINE AND ST. JOHN'S WORT INTERACTION 269
Discussion 269
CASE 4: TAMOXIFEN AND CYP2D6 INHIBITION 269
Discussion 270
CASE 5: CLARITHROMYCIN AND DIGOXIN 270
Discussion 270
CASE 6: REPAGLINIDE WITH GEMFIBROZIL AND ITRACONAZOLE 270
Discussion 270
SUMMARY 270
CONCLUSION 271

INTRODUCTION

New drugs have provided major benefits to the public, significantly reducing cardiovascular morbidity and mortality; improving survival in a wide range of malignancies; treating significant neurologic and psychiatric disorders; modifying the course of a variety of tenacious, debilitating diseases like Crohn's disease, rheumatoid arthritis, and psoriasis; and providing relief for a wide range of symptomatic conditions. But drugs also cause a wide range of serious adverse drug reactions (ADRs), contributing, according to at least one estimate, to 100,000 deaths annually[1] and to millions of episodes of discomfort or injury. Some of these ADRs are the results of inappropriate use of drugs, inadequate monitoring, and other preventable causes. Others are *idiosyncratic*, a term generally used to mean unpredictable and, thus, by implication, unavoidable. With the emergence of pharmacogenomics, the hope is that it will, in fact, become possible to identify people at risk for ADRs by examining genetic or proteomic predictors of risk so that these patients can be given alternative therapies or treated in ways, such as by using lower doses, that avoid the risk.

One cause of ADRs—those resulting from drug-drug interactions—has, since the mid 1990s, become far more manageable than in the past. These have been identified as contributing as much as 4% of preventable ADRs.[2] Some of these interactions can be pharmacologic (potassium supplements plus aldosterone antagonists cause hyperkalemia; QT prolongers plus hypokalemia resulting from diuretics cause torsades de pointes arrhythmias; sildenafil plus organic nitrates cause hypotension), but many more involve pharmacokinetic interactions: one drug altering the excretion or metabolism of another leading to toxic blood levels, equivalent to a drug overdose or, in some cases, to serious underdosing.

The U.S. Food and Drug Administration (FDA) has issued guidance to industry on the best practices for studying potential pharmacokinetic (PK) drug interactions for New Molecular Entity Drugs (NMEs) prior to approval.[3-6] These PK interactions can result in patients receiving much larger exposures (≥2 times) than those intended by the prescriber. Most important PK interactions occur when one drug inhibits the metabolism of another drug via the cytochrome P-450 (CYP) enzyme system. The potential for such interactions can be anticipated by understanding the metabolism of a new drug (is it CYP mediated and to what extent?) and its ability to inhibit or induce CYP enzymes. When such potential for interaction is discovered, the extent of the interaction is evaluated using model compounds to characterize the effect of these interactions on blood levels of the concomitantly used drugs. More specific information on the evaluation of drug interactions during drug development can be found on the FDA website[5,6]: http://www.fda.gov/cder/drug/drugInteractions/default.htm. A patient educational module describing different interaction mechanisms is also available.[7] Approved package inserts of drug products[8] have sections describing drug metabolism and PK interactions and (if necessary) steps needed to avoid problems. Labels generally will not describe every potential drug interaction, however, so that the practitioner must be aware of how a drug's metabolism and inhibition/induction ability can lead to potential interactions.

This chapter is intended to illustrate the general principles underlying assessment and understanding of PK drug-drug interactions through a series of case studies and clinical scenarios. It does not provide a complete list of all drug interactions because the list is constantly expanding and can be found on electronic drug interactions databases; the more important drug interactions will be described in package inserts. The chapter is intended to remind physicians of the need to be cognizant of the potential for a drug to act as a "substrate" for an interacting drug (i.e., have its metabolism and/or transport altered by concomitant therapy) or as an inhibitor or inducer of metabolism and/or transport of some other drug the patient is receiving.

Although drug interactions have long been recognized, experience with terfenadine in 1990 was a "wake-up call," because it showed how a very benign drug could become lethal through a drug interaction.

CASE 1: TERFENADINE AND KETOCONAZOLE INTERACTION[9]

A 39-year-old woman was admitted to the hospital for episodes of syncope and light-headedness. She was taking the recommended dose of terfenadine (60 mg bid) in addition to cefaclor (250 mg tid), ketoconazole (200 mg bid), and medroxyprogesterone. On admission, her corrected QT interval (QTc) was 655 msec. All medications were discontinued, and continuous cardiac monitoring was initiated. She experienced several paroxysmal episodes of palpitations, dyspnea, and near syncope associated with torsades de pointes 10 hours after admission. Her terfenadine level in serum collected on admission was 57 ng/ml. The QTc gradually decreased to 429 msec 7 days later.

Terfenadine is extensively metabolized by a CYP enzyme, CYP3A, to various metabolites, including the active metabolite fexofenadine. After oral administration of a typical 60-mg dose of terfenadine, only trace amounts of terfenadine can be found in the systemic circulation (<10 ng/ml), so that the patient has at least a sixfold increase when terfenadine is given with a strong CYP3A inhibitor such as ketoconazole, itraconazole, erythromycin, or mibefradil. Terfenadine metabolism is markedly reduced, and blood concentrations of unmetabolized terfenadine are increased substantially. The unchanged terfenadine is a powerful inhibitor of the HERG channel and causes substantial prolongation of the QTc,[10] in some cases causing torsades de pointes–type ventricular tachycardia. Cases of ventricular tachycardia have also occurred in patients with comorbid liver diseases that impeded metabolism of terfenadine.[11]

Discussion

The desirable and undesirable effects of a drug usually arise from its concentration at its sites of action; these are usually reflected in the blood concentration, which is determined by the amount administered (dose) and how the drug is then handled by the body: absorption, distribution, metabolism, and excretion. Elimination of a drug and its metabolites occurs either by metabolism, usually by the liver or gut mucosa, or by excretion, usually by the kidneys and liver. Figure 20-1 depicts how a drug given orally may be subject to first-pass metabolism and transport in the enterocyte and hepatocyte.[11]

Hepatic elimination can occur by excretion into the bile, but for many drugs, the liver metabolizes the drug, primarily by the CYP family of enzymes located in the hepatic endoplasmic reticulum. Non-CYP enzyme systems, such as *N*-acetyl and glucuronosyl transferases, can also be important. Some hepatic enzymes (such as CYP2D6) are subject to genetic variability (some people lack the enzyme activity); all of them can be inhibited by medications; and some can be inhibited by foods such as grapefruit juice. Other factors, including the presence or absence of disease, can also alter hepatic and intestinal drug metabolism. Whereas most of these factors are relatively stable over time, concomitant medications can alter metabolism abruptly and are of particular concern because they can affect a patient whose drug dose has been carefully titrated and assessed.

CYP3A is the major component of liver and intestinal CYP enzymes, representing more than half of the total hepatic activity and almost half of intestinal CYP activity (Fig. 20-2).[12] More than 50% of marketed drugs are metabolized by this enzyme.

CYP3A4 in the intestine contributes to low bioavailability of drugs metabolized by that enzyme in the gastrointestinal tract. Therefore, inhibition increases the maximum plasma concentration (C_{max}). The area under the plasma concentration-time curve (AUC) will be increased as well because more drug reaches the circulation, but these gastrointestinal effects do not alter the drug's half-life. Drugs with little first-pass effect in the gastrointestinal tract that depend on hepatic metabolism for elimination, in contrast, can have a greatly increased half-life; the AUC can increase dramatically, and, with drug accumulation, there can be a significant effect on C_{max}.

The magnitude of the effect of interactions will depend on the % contribution of the CYP3A pathway to overall clearance. Figure 20-3 shows the increase in one of the parameters for systemic exposure (AUC) when various drugs were given with ketoconazole, a strong CYP3A inhibitor. The AUC of midazolam, which is cleared almost entirely by CYP3A metabolism, was increased 16-fold, whereas ritonavir was only minimally increased, about 2-fold.[13] Midazolam would therefore be considered a "sensitive" substrate; ritonavir would not. The magnitude of the effect of midazolam with CYP3A inhibitors also depends on the potency of CYP3A inhibition. For example, although ketoconazole increased midazolam's AUC 16-fold, cimetidine or ranitidine, two weaker CYP3A inhibitors, increased midazolam's AUC by less than 2-fold.[13] The magnitude of an interaction thus depends on the substrate, specifically how important the inhibited pathway is to its elimination, and the potency of the inhibitor. The clinical implications of any given interaction depend on the therapeutic ratio of the

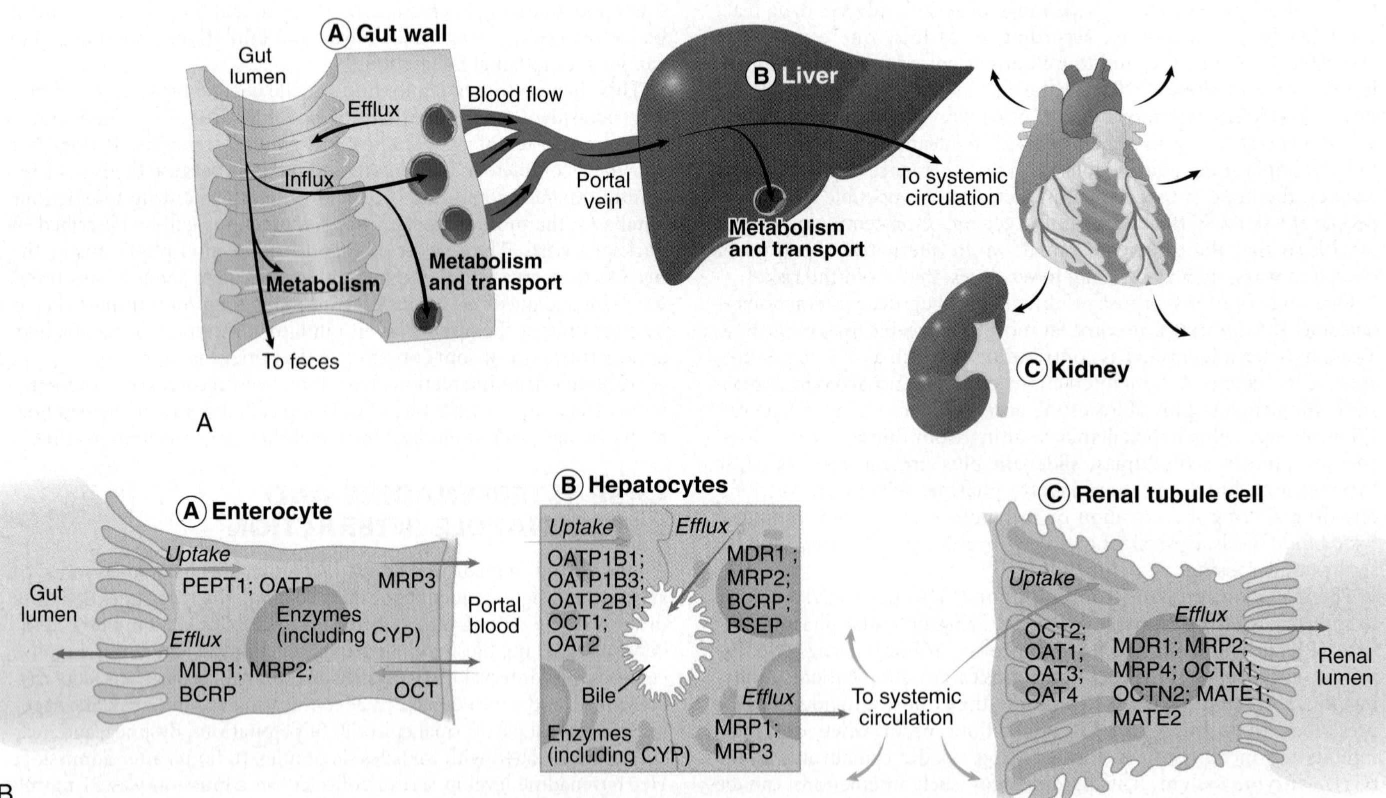

FIGURE 20-1 • An orally administered drug is absorbed through the gut wall and may be subject to metabolism and transport before it reaches the liver, where it can be further metabolized and transported prior to entering the systemic circulation. The efflux and uptake transporters with high expressions in the gut wall (A), liver (B), and kidney (C) are indicated. (For additional efflux and uptake transporters, see Fig. 20-4 and Table 20-4.) BCRP, breast cancer resistance protein; BSEP, bile salt export pump; MDR1, multidrug resistance (P-gp, P-glycoprotein); MRP, multidrug resistance–related protein; OAT, organic anion transporter; OATP, organic anion transporting peptide; OCT, organic cation transporter; PEPT, peptide transporter.

substrate drug. Thus, a 2-fold increase in a narrow therapeutic ratio drug could be a concern, whereas it would not be a problem for a drug, such as loratadine, with little dose-related toxicity. In the course of drug development, new drugs are characterized by their metabolic pathways and then by the importance of each pathway (i.e., whether it is a sensitive substrate). For any important pathway (generally at least 20% of clearance), a strong inhibitor will be used in a clinical study to seek the largest possible interaction with the substrate. Depending on the result, weaker inhibitors may also be tested.

Table 20-1 lists substrates, inhibitors, and inducers of various CYP enzymes.[3-6] When a drug is found to be a sensitive CYP3A substrate and the exposure-response data indicate that there is potential toxicity from the large induced increase in exposure, it can be concluded that the drug should not be used with strong CYP3A inhibitors. In that case, the labeling will say this and will include a list of strong CYP3A inhibitors (Table 20-2), including inhibitors that may not have been evaluated clinically for their interactions with this drug. For example, eletriptan is a sensitive CYP3A substrate (Table 20-3).[5,6] Ketoconazole increased its AUC and C_{max} by eight- and fourfold, respectively. The labeling of eletriptan includes the following statement: "it should not be used within at least 72 hours with potent CYP3A inhibitors . . . ketoconazole, itraconazole, ritonavir, nelfinavir, nefazodone, clarithromycin."[14] Although only ketoconazole was studied, the interaction result would be similar with any strong CYP3A4 inhibitor. The advice

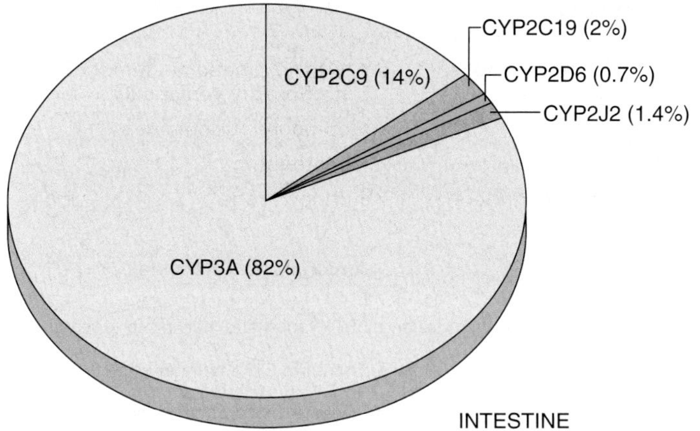

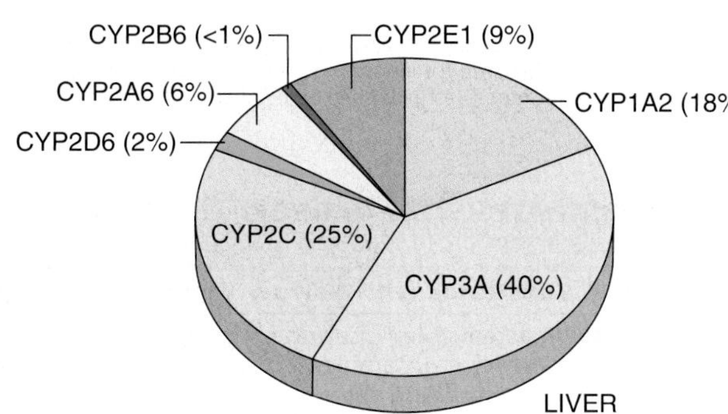

FIGURE 20-2 • The average human proximal small intestinal and hepatic P450 pies. The percent contributions of individual P450 enzymes are based on total immunoquantified P450 content. (From Paine MF, Hart HL, Ludington SS, et al: The human intestinal cytochrome P450 "pie". Drug Metab Disp 2006;34:880-886.)

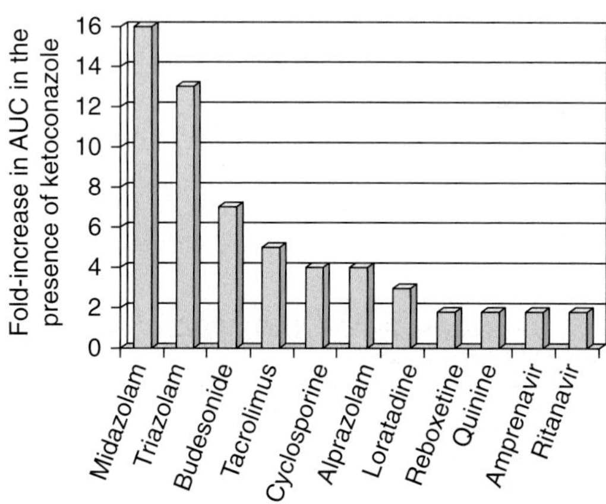

FIGURE 20-3 • The fold-increase in plasma area under the plasma-time curve (AUC) of various cytochrome P-450 (CYP) 3A substrates when coadministered with ketoconazole. (Adapted from Huang S-M. Clinical drug-drug interactions. In Krishna R [ed]: Pharmacokinetic Applications in Drug Development. Kluwer Academic/Plenum, 2003.)

TABLE 20-1 EXAMPLES OF IN VIVO SUBSTRATE, INHIBITOR, AND INDUCER FOR SPECIFIC CYP ENZYMES RECOMMENDED FOR STUDY (ORAL ADMINISTRATION)*

CYP	Substrate	Inhibitor	Inducer
1A2	Theophylline, caffeine	Fluvoxamine	Smoking
2B6	Efavirenz, bupropion		Rifampin
2C8	Repaglinide, rosiglitazone	Gemfibrozil	Rifampin
2C9	Warfarin, tolbutamide	Fluconazole, amiodarone	Rifampin
2C19	Omeprazole, esoprazole, lansoprazole, pantoprazole	Fluvoxamine, moclobemide, omeprazole	Rifampin
2D6	Desipramine, dextromethorphan, atomoxetine	Paroxetine, quinidine, fluoxetine	None identified
2E1	Chlorzoxazone	Disulfirum	Ethanol
3A4/3A5	Midazolam, buspirone, felodipine, lovastatin, eletriptan, sildenafil, simvastatin, triazolam	Atazanavir, clarithromycin, indinavir, itraconazole, ketoconazole, nefazodone, nelfinavir, ritonavir, saquinavir, telithromycin	Rifampin, carbamazepine

**Note:* Substrates for any particular CYP enzyme listed in this table are those with plasma AUC values increased by 2-fold or higher when coadministered with inhibitors of that CYP enzyme; for CYP3A, only those with plasma AUC increased by 5-fold or higher (sensitive substrates) are listed. Inhibitors listed are those that increase plasma AUC values of substrates for that CYP enzyme by 2-fold or higher. For CYP3A inhibitors, only those that increase AUC of CYP3A substrates by 5-fold or higher (strong inhibitors) are listed. Inducers listed are those that decrease plasma AUC values of substrates for that CYP enzyme by 30% or higher. [Note that this is not an exhaustive list. For an updated list, see http://www.fda.gov/cder/drug/drugInteractions/default.htm]

AUC, area under the plasma-time curve; CYP, cytochrome P-450.

Adapted from Huang S-M, Temple R, Throckmorton DC, Lesko L. Drug-drug interactions: study design, data analysis and implications for dosing recommendations. Clin Pharmacol Ther 2007;81:298-304; U.S. Food and Drug Administration (FDA). Drug development and drug interactions. Available at http://www.fda.gov/cder/drug/druglnteractions/default.htm (accessed October 20, 2006); and U.S. Food and Drug Administration (FDA). Guidance for industry: drug interaction studies—study design, data analysis, and implications for dosing and labeling. Available at http://www.fda.gov/cder/guidance/index.htm; Draft published September 2006. Available at http://www.fda.gov/cder/guidance/6695dft.pdf (accessed October 20, 2006).

TABLE 20-2 CLASSIFICATION OF CYP INHIBITORS*

CYP	Strong Inhibitors	Moderate Inhibitors	Weak Inhibitors
	>5-Fold Increase in AUC	>2 but <5-Fold Increase in AUC	>1.25 but <2-Fold Increase in AUC
3A	Atazanavir, clarithromycin, indinavir, itraconazole, ketoconazole, nefazodone, nelfinavir, ritonavir, saquinavir, telithromycin	Amprenavir, aprepitant, diltiazem, erythromycin, fluconazole, fosamprenavir, grapefruit juice,[†] verapamil	Cimetidine
1A2	Fluvoxamine	Ciprofloxacin, mexiletine, propafenone, zileuton	Acyclovir, cimetidine, famotidine, norfloxacin, verapamil
2B6			Clopidogrel, ticlopidine
2C8		Gemfibrozil	Trimethoprim
2C9		Amiodarone, fluconazole, oxandrolone	Sulfinpyrazone
2C19	Fluvoxamine	Moclobemide, omeprazole	
2D6	Fluoxetine, paroxetine, quinidine	Duloxetine, terbinafine	Amiodarone, sertraline

**Note:*
- A *strong inhibitor* is one that causes a ≥5-fold increase in the plasma AUC values or more than an 80% decrease in clearance of CYP substrates (not limited to sensitive CYP substrate) in clinical evaluations.
- A *moderate inhibitor* is one that causes a ≥2- but a <5-fold increase in the AUC values or a 50%–80% decrease in clearance of sensitive CYP substrates when the inhibitor was given at the highest approved dose and the shortest dosing interval in clinical evaluations.
- A *weak inhibitor* is one that causes a ≥1.25- but a <2-fold increase in the AUC values or a 20%–50% decrease in clearance of sensitive CYP substrates when the inhibitor was given at the highest approved dose and the shortest dosing interval in clinical evaluations.
- This is not an exhaustive list. For an updated list, see http://www.fda.gov/cder/drug/drugInteractions/default.htm

[†]The effect of grapefruit juice varies widely.

AUC, area under the plasma-time curve; CYP, cytochrome P-450.

Adapted from Huang S-M, Temple R, Throckmorton DC, Lesko L. Drug-drug interactions: study design, data analysis and implications for dosing recommendations. Clin Pharmacol Ther 2007;81:298-304; U.S. Food and Drug Administration (FDA). Drug development and drug interactions. Available at http://www.fda.gov/cder/drug/drugInteractions/default.htm (accessed October 20, 2006); and U.S. Food and Drug Administration (FDA). Guidance for industry: drug interaction studies—study design, data analysis, and implications for dosing and labeling. Available at http://www.fda.gov/cder/guidance/index.htm; Draft published September 2006. Available at http://www.fda.gov/cder/guidance/6695dft.pdf (accessed October 20, 2006).

TABLE 20-3 EXAMPLES OF SENSITIVE CYP SUBSTRATES OR CYP SUBSTRATES WITH NARROW THERAPEUTIC RANGE*

CYP	Sensitive CYP3A Substrates[†]	CYP3A Substrates with Narrow Therapeutic Range[‡]
3A	Budesonide, buspirone, eplerenone, eletriptan, felodipine, fluticasone, lovastatin, midazolam, saquinavir, sildenafil, simvastatin, triazolam, vardenafil	Alfentanil, astemizole,[§] cisapride,[§] cyclosporine, diergotamine, ergotamine, fentanyl, pimozide, quinidine, sirolimus, tacrolimus, terfenadine[§]
1A2	Duloxetine, alosetron	Theophylline, tizanidine
2B6	Bupropion, efavirenz	
2C8	Repaglinide	Paclitaxel
2C9		Warfarin, phenytoin
2C19	Omeprazole	*S*-mephenytoin
2D6	Desipramine	Thioridazine

*Note that this is not an exhaustive list. For an updated list, see http://www.fda.gov/cder/drug/drugInteractions/default.htm

[†]Refers to drugs whose plasma AUC values have been shown to increase 5-fold or higher when coadministered with a known CYP inhibitor.

[‡]Refers to drugs whose exposure-response indicates that increases in their exposure levels by the concomitant use of CYP inhibitors may lead to serious safety concerns (e.g., torsades de pointes).

[§]Not available in the United States.

AUC, area under the plasma-time curve; CYP, cytochrome P-450.

Adapted from Huang S-M, Temple R, Throckmorton DC, Lesko L. Drug-drug interactions: study design, data analysis and implications for dosing recommendations. Clin Pharmacol Ther 2007;81:298-304; U.S. Food and Drug Administration (FDA). Drug development and drug interactions. Available at http://www.fda.gov/cder/drug/drugInteractions/default.htm (accessed October 20, 2006); and U.S. Food and Drug Administration (FDA). Guidance for industry: drug interaction studies—study design, data analysis, and implications for dosing and labeling. Available at http://www.fda.gov/cder/guidance/index.htm; Draft published September 2006. Available at http://www.fda.gov/cder/guidance/6695dft.pdf (accessed October 20, 2006).

to avoid itraconazole, ritonavir, nelfinavir, nefazodone, and clarithromycin was based on the interaction data with ketoconazole. Similarly, if a drug has been determined to be a strong inhibitor of CYP3A, it does not need to be tested with all CYP3A substrates to warn about an interaction with "sensitive CYP3A substrates" or "CYP3A substrates with narrow therapeutic range." The labeling of telithromycin (Ketek) has the following statement: "telithromycin is a strong inhibitor of the cytochrome P450 3A4 system. . . . Use of simvastatin, lovastatin, or atorvastatin concomitantly with KETEK should be avoided. . . . The use of KETEK is contraindicated with cisapride, pimozide."[15] The interaction information for lovastatin/atorvastatin and pimozide was extrapolated from data from simvastatin and cisapride, respectively. Box 20-1 lists lessons learned from Case 1.

BOX 20-1 LESSONS FROM CASE 1

Understanding a drug's clearance pathways, especially metabolic pathways, is the first step in assessing how coadministered drugs may affect its safe and effective use.

Drugs primarily metabolized by cytochrome P-450 (CYP) 3A enzymes will have increased exposure when coadministered with drugs that are CYP3A inhibitors, leading to increased pharmacologic effects with potentially untoward effects. The likelihood of adverse consequence will depend on the extent of the increase in exposure from the drug interaction and the relationship between the exposure and the effect.

CASE 2: LOVASTATIN AND GRAPEFRUIT JUICE INTERACTION[16]

A 60-year-old male with hypertension, chronic lower extremity venous stasis/edema, renal insufficiency, non–insulin-dependent diabetes mellitus, and a familial history of hyperlipidemia was receiving lovastatin (40-mg tablet bid) for 5 to 10 years, as well as gemfibrozil (600 mg bid), amlodipine, and an oral hypoglycemic agent. Early in the year, the patient's creatinine was 3.5 mg/dl. In October, the patient began drinking grapefruit juice in the morning for the first time in his life. During this time, the patient denied any strenuous exercise. Two weeks later, the patient was in so much pain that he went to an emergency room, where his creatine phosphokinase was greater than 40,000 U/L. He was admitted to the hospital with a diagnosis of rhabdomyolysis. Therapy with lovastatin and gemfibrozil was discontinued. During that time, his creatinine increased to about 5.0 mg/dl. The patient was discharged from the hospital after approximately 1 week. The physician believed that the patient's rhabdomyolysis was caused by the interaction of the grapefruit juice with lovastatin and gemfibrozil and told the patient to avoid grapefruit juice.

Both lovastatin and gemfibrozil are known to cause dose-related muscle pain and rhabdomyolysis. Grapefruit juice inhibits the metabolism of lovastatin, resulting in very high concentrations of lovastatin; the combination of gemfibrozil, which can itself cause muscle damage, and the high exposure to lovastatin led to rhabdomyolysis in this patient. This is recognized in current labeling for several "statins." For example, the "Warnings/Precautions" section of labeling for simvastatin states that "The use of simvastatin concomitantly with the potent CYP3A4 inhibitors itraconazole, ketoconazole, erythromycin, clarithromycin, telithromycin, human immunodeficiency virus protease inhibitors, nefazodone, or large quantities of grapefruit juice (>1 quart daily) should be avoided."[17]

Discussion

Foods and dietary supplements can affect drug metabolism in ways similar to concomitant drug treatment. Grapefruit juice contains furanocoumarins, including bergamottin and 6′,7′-dihydroxybergamottin (DHB),[18] both of which inhibit CYP3A. Lovastatin is a sensitive CYP3A substrate, and coingestion with grapefruit juice has been shown to increase the exposure of lovastatin 10- to 20-fold.[19] Most interactions are not of this magnitude, but currently 35 drug products have grapefruit juice interactions that are discussed in labeling, about half based on clinical trial data, the rest based on case reports or mechanistic expectations.[20] The labeling may describe the interactions, warn about them (sometimes in a Box Warning), or contraindicate concomitant use.[21]

Grapefruit juice is considered a moderate CYP3A inhibitor,[4,5] but its effect on CYP3A is variable and can be affected by many factors, including variables that are difficult to control, such as the source, brand, lot-to-lot variation of the same brand, and the preparation procedure (including the extent of dilution by consumers using frozen concentrates) of the grapefruit juice.

BOX 20-2 LESSONS FROM CASES 2 AND 3

Juices and dietary supplements can interfere with the metabolism and/or transport of drugs.[32]

Depending on what is known about a drug's exposure-response relationship,[3,33] interactions of a drug with other drugs can sometimes be ignored, can sometimes be addressed by dose adjustments of one or both of the coadministered drugs, and can always be managed by avoiding concomitant use. Because the components of juices and dietary supplements are present in unpredictable amounts, an important interaction with juices or dietary supplements can be addressed only by avoiding their concomitant use.

Recent studies have shown that grapefruit juice decreases the plasma concentrations of fexofenadine, possibly owing to the inhibition of an uptake transporter, organic anion transporting peptide (OATP).[22] The labeling of fexofenadine states that "Fruit juices such as grapefruit, orange and apple may reduce the bioavailability and exposure of fexofenadine . . . to maximize the effects of fexofenadine, it is recommended that Allegra . . . should be taken with water" (FDA labeling).[23] Box 20-2 lists lessons learned from Cases 2 and 3.

CASE 3: CYCLOSPORINE AND ST. JOHN'S WORT INTERACTION[24]

A 50-year-old patient was given cyclosporine after a heart transplant. Her plasma concentration of cyclosporine had been stable. She began to take St. John's wort a year after the transplant; within 1 week, her cyclosporine levels had dropped from approximately 200 ng/ml to less than 100 ng/ml and she developed grade 3 rejection (ISHT3A). After she stopped taking St. John's wort, her cyclosporine level increased to 200 ng/ml within 1 week.

St. John's wort is a CYP3A and P-glycoprotein (P-gp) inducer. Cyclosporine is a substrate of CYP3A and P-gp. The concomitant use of St. John's wort and cyclosporine increased the metabolism of cyclosporine, resulting in decreased plasma concentration and diminished efficacy.

Discussion

St. John's wort products contain hyperforin, which has been shown to be an inducer of CYP3A in vitro[25] and in vivo.[26,27] In addition, St. John's wort also induces P-gp and other CYP enzymes.[28,29] St. John's wort products are standardized with respect to their hypericin content, but the hyperforin content varies greatly among products,[30] and the absorption of hyperforin, as with many dietary supplements, has not been well defined. The effect of St. John's wort on drugs that are CYP3A substrates is therefore highly variable. Many drugs that are substrates of CYP3A and whose plasma concentration and effectiveness would be reduced when coadministered with CYP3A inducers have warnings about their use with such inducers, including St. John's wort. For example, imatinib labeling states that "Co-medications that induce CYP3A4 (e.g., dexamethasone, phenytoin, carbamazepine, rifampin, phenobarbital or St. John's wort) may significantly reduce exposure to Gleevec. . . . In patients where rifampin or other CYP3A4 inducers are indicated, alternative therapeutic agents with less enzyme induction potential should be considered."[31] Many of the oral contraceptive products carry warnings on coadministration with St. John's wort.[20] Box 20-2 lists lessons learned from Cases 2 and 3.

CASE 4: TAMOXIFEN AND CYP2D6 INHIBITION*

A 48-year-old woman, recently diagnosed with estrogen receptor + (ER+) ductal carcinoma of the breast, telephoned a health care provider about a research article she had read on the Internet. The new research indicated that individuals deficient in CYP2D6 had a high probability of early breast cancer recurrence if treated by tamoxifen hormonal therapy. She had been receiving tamoxifen, with notable hot flashes, and was receiving an antidepressant for this. Although she could not remember the name of the antidepressant, she knew that some of them were CYP2D6 inhibitors. She wanted to be advised to go back to her oncologist to have the oncologist change her to an aromatase inhibitor.

Tamoxifen is metabolized by CYP2D6 to one of its active metabolites. Deficiency in the CYP2D6 enzyme (either because of genetic CYP2D6 deficiency or because of coadministration of a CYP2D6 inhibitor) may decrease production of the active metabolite and decrease the efficacy of tamoxifen.

---

*Dennis Okane, personal communication, Annual Meeting of the American College of Clinical Pharmacology; September 26, 2006, Boston, MA.

Discussion

The patient's concern was well founded. One of the active metabolites of tamoxifen, *N*-desmethyl-4-hydroxy-tamoxifen (endoxifen), is produced via CYP2D6.[34] CYP2D6 deficiency has been shown to reduce relapse-free survival and disease-free survival in breast cancer patients taking tamoxifen,[35] and a drug that inhibits CYP2D6 would be expected to have a similar effect. Breast cancer patients on tamoxifen are often prescribed selective serotonine reuptake inhibitor (SSRI) antidepressants, such as paroxetine, to ameliorate hot flashes (off-label use) caused by tamoxifen. Some SSRI antidepressants, including fluoxetine and paroxetine, are strong CYP2D6 inhibitors,[4,5] will cause a patient to become a poor metabolizer of CYP2D6, and decrease the plasma concentrations of endoxifen.[34,35] These drugs should be avoided in favor of alternatives that are not strong CYP2D6 inhibitors.

CASE 5: CLARITHROMYCIN AND DIGOXIN[36]

A 7-year study of Ontario residents aged 66 years old or older treated with digoxin showed that those admitted to hospital with digoxin toxicity (n = 1051) were about 12 times more likely to have been treated with clarithromycin than those who have not.

Only a small fraction of digoxin is metabolized, so clarithromycin's CYP3A inhibition does not explain the toxicity. Elimination of digoxin is predominantly renal, although in adult volunteers, about a quarter of serum digoxin is eliminated through the intestinal lumen, excreted in bile, or secreted directly into the lumen by P-gp. The elevated digoxin concentrations that have been reported in patients receiving clarithromycin and digoxin concomitantly result from inhibition of intestinal and renal P-gp by clarithromycin, sometimes resulting in digoxin toxicity, including potentially fatal arrhythmias.[37]

Discussion

A number of important human drug transporters have been identified; they can be expressed at the apical or basal side of the epithelial cells in various tissues. Most drug transporters belong to two superfamilies, adenosine triphosphate (ATP)–binding cassette (ABC) and solute-linked carrier (SLC), including both cellular uptake and efflux transporters as shown in Figure 20-4.[38] Numerous polymorphisms have been identified in transporter genes, and allele frequencies have been determined in various populations.[39] Unlike polymorphisms observed for major drug-metabolizing enzymes and their effects on drug disposition,[40] the clinical relevance of transporter genetic variations is less well established. The most studied is the P-gp (multidrug resistance [MDR1]) transporter,[41] but the reports on effects of genetic variations have been inconsistent and, in some cases, conflicting.[42]

The P-gp efflux transporter is mainly, although not exclusively, present on the apical side of epithelial cells, and its modulations can affect the intestinal absorption of some drugs, as well as biliary and renal clearance, brain uptake, and access of drugs to various tissues (see Fig. 20-4). For example, modulation of MDR1 expression in tumor tissues can affect access to the tumor, and modulation of expression in the placenta can affect access to the fetus. Box 20-3 lists lessons learned from Case 5.

BOX 20-3 LESSONS FROM CASE 5

Concomitant administration of an inhibitor of a transporter can cause significant drug interactions.

Drugs that inhibit P-glycoprotein (P-gp) and increase digoxin concentrations include quinidine and clarithromycin. Conversely, drugs that induce P-gp and decrease digoxin concentrations include rifampin and St. John's wort. Table 20-4 lists some of the major human transporters and known substrates, inhibitors, and inducers.

CASE 6: REPAGLINIDE WITH GEMFIBROZIL AND ITRACONAZOLE[43]

In a randomized crossover study, 12 healthy volunteers received either 600 mg gemfibrozil, 100 mg itraconazole (first dose, 200 mg), both gemfibrozil and itraconazole, or placebo twice daily for 3 days. On day 3, they ingested a 0.25-mg dose of repaglinide. The AUC of repaglinide increased 19-fold when taken with itraconazole and gemfibrozil together. When taken with itraconazole or gemfibrozil separately, in contrast, repaglinide plasma levels increased only 1.4- and 8.1-fold, respectively.

Gemfibrozil and itraconazole inhibit repaglinide metabolism mediated via CYP2C8 and CYP3A, respectively. The combined inhibition led to the enormous increase in the repaglinide plasma concentration, because each inhibitor interfered with the principal remaining metabolic pathway left unaffected by the other drug.

Discussion

Repaglinide is primarily eliminated by metabolism, mainly by CYP2C8 and CYP3A. Inhibition of the single CYP2C8 pathway by a strong inhibitor of CYP2C8, gemfibrozil, increased the AUC 8.1-fold, whereas inhibition of the single CYP3A pathway by a strong inhibitor of CYP3A, itraconazole, increased the AUC 1.4-fold. Additional studies indicated that the gemfibrozil and its glucuronide inhibit the organic anion transporting peptide 1B1 (OATP1B1 or SLCO1B1)[44] in addition to inhibiting CYP2C8.[45] This case illustrates the potentially large effects when two major metabolic pathways are inhibited, as well as the complex interplay between metabolism and transporter-based mechanisms of drug interaction. The labeling of Prandin (repaglinide) indicates that "Caution should be used in patients already on Prandin and gemfibrozil—blood glucose levels should be monitored and Prandin dose adjustment may be needed. Rare post-marketing events of serious hypoglycemia have been reported in patients taking Prandin and gemfibrozil together. Gemfibrozil and itraconazole had a synergistic metabolic inhibitory effect on Prandin. Therefore, patients taking Prandin and gemfibrozil should not take itraconazole."[46]

A similar synergistic inhibitory effect on loperamide by the coadministration of gemfibrozil and itraconazole has been observed, with a 12.6-fold increase in loperamide AUC when the three drugs were coadministered, whereas itraconazole and gemfibrozil increased the loperamide AUC 3.8- and 2.2-fold, respectively.[47] Box 20-4 lists lessons learned from Case 6.

SUMMARY

The six cases illustrate drug interactions that can result in either adverse events or loss of efficacy of coadministered drugs. Drug interactions can also, with proper planning, be of therapeutic value. An early example (in the 1940s) was the use of probenecid to decrease the renal excretion and prolong the half-life of penicillins.[48] Probenecid is also used with cidofovir to decrease the latter's renal toxicity. Probenecid is a potent organic anion transporter (OAT) inhibitor, and recent studies show that its interactions appear to involve renal transport via that transporter.[49] Other successful cases of coadministration of interacting drugs include the recent development of NMEs that are substrates of CYP3A and are used with a CYP3A inhibitor to allow use of

BOX 20-4 LESSONS FROM CASE 6

Results of multiple drug interactions can be greater than would be predicted from single component interaction studies; with both major metabolic pathways inhibited, there is little ability to clear the drug left and a metabolite of a drug may contribute to the inhibition (or induction) of the enzymes and/or transporters being affected by the parent compound, resulting in larger than expected inhibition (or induction).

lower doses of the NMEs; thus, ritonavir is used to increase the systemic exposure of lopinavir (10- to 20-fold increase) and tipranavir (29-fold increase).[50,51] The labeling of Kaletra (lopinavir/ritonavir) and Aptivus (tipranavir) indicates that each is to be used with ritonavir. One potential problem with such approaches is that the inhibitor will affect the exposure of any other concomitant drug that is a substrate for the inhibited CYP or transporter.

CONCLUSION

Of the adverse effects that occur when drugs are used,[52,53] those resulting from drug interactions should be avoidable with appropriate evaluation, determination, and education. These adverse effects can be troublesome because they occur in patients who seem stable on therapy, that is, after the initial period of close observation when a therapy is initiated. They can also be quite serious. Increased anticoagulation from warfarin and digoxin toxicity are possible consequences of drug interactions, and it is striking that several important drugs—terfenadine, mibefradil, astemizole, cisapride, and cerivastatin—have been removed from the market at least partly because of drug-drug interactions.[54,55]

Many factors need to be considered when determining the impact of a drug's propensity to interact pharmacokinetically with other drugs on its development and ultimate marketing approval: the severity of the potential ADRs, the likelihood of concomitant use, the disease being treated, the availability of alternative therapy, the value of treatment, and whether the interaction can be properly managed. Thus, in the context of a non–life-threatening condition for which safe and effective alternative therapies exist, a drug that shows significant cardiac toxicity when taken with a CYP3A inhibitor would have a weak argu-

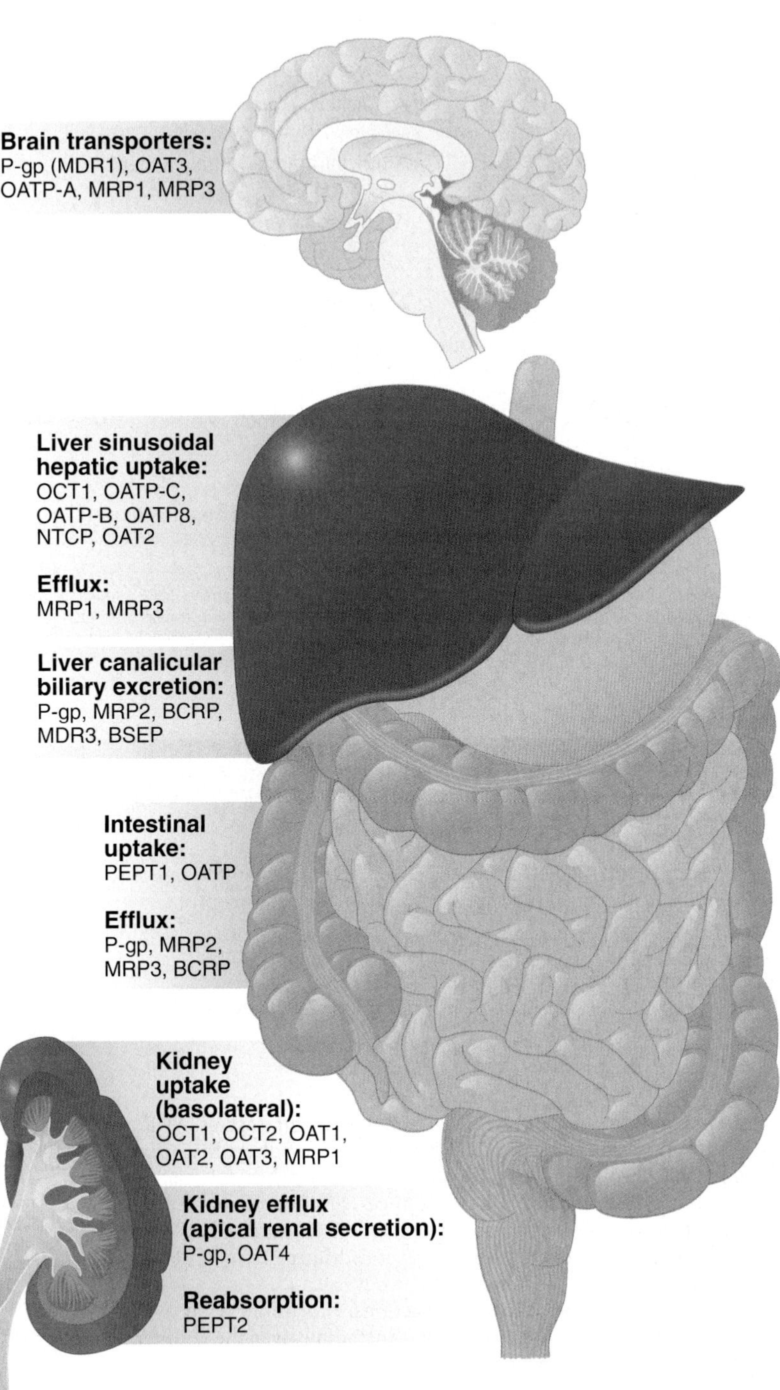

FIGURE 20-4 • Tissue localization of transporters and their role in drug disposition. ABC, adenosine triphosphate (ATP)–binding cassette transporter superfamily; BCRP, breast cancer resistance protein; BSEP, bile salt export pump; MDR, multidrug resistance; MRP, multidrug resistance–related protein; NTCP, sodium taurocholate cotransporting polypeptide; OAT, organic anion transporter; OATP, organic anion transporting peptide; OCT, organic cation transporter; PEPT, peptide transporter; P-gp, p-glycoprotein; SLC, solute-linked carrier transporter family; SLCO, solute-linked carrier organic anion transporter family. [OATP-A = SLC21A3; OATP-C = OATP1B1 = SLCO1B1; OATP8 = SLCO1B3; OATP-B = SLCO2B1; NTCP = SLC6A8; P-gp = MDR1 = ABCB1; PEPT1 = SLC15A1; MRP1 = ABCC1; MRP2 = ABCC2; MRP3 = ABCC3; BCRP = ABCG2; OCT1 = SLC22A1; OCT2 = SLC22A2; OCT3 = SLC22A3; OAT1 = SLC22A6; OAT2 = SLC22A7; OAT3 = SLC22A8]. (See also Table 20-4.) (Adapted from Zhang L, Strong JM, Wei Q, et al. Scientific perspective on drug transporters and their role in drug interactions. Mol Pharmacol 2006;3:62-69.)

TABLE 20-4 MAJOR HUMAN TRANSPORTERS*

Gene	Aliases	Drug Substrate	Inhibitor	Inducer
ABCB1	P-gp, MDR1	Digoxin, fexofenadine, indinavir, vincristine, colchicine, topotecan, paclitaxel	Ritonavir, cyclosporine, verapamil, erythromycin, ketoconazole, itraconazole, quinidine	Rifampin, St John's wort
ABCB4	MDR3	Digoxin, paclitaxel, vinblastine		
ABCB11	BSEP	Vinblastine		
ABCC1	MRP1	Adefovir, indinavir		
ABCC2	MRP2, CMOAT	Indinavir, cisplatin	Cyclosporine	
ABCC3	MRP3, CMOAT2	Etoposide, methotrexate, tenoposide		
ABCG2	BCRP	Daunorubicin, doxorubicin, topotecan, rosuvastatin, sulfasalazine	Gefitinib	
SLCO1B1	OATP1B1, OATP-C OATP2	Rifampin, rosuvastatin, methotrexate, pravastatin, thyroxine	Cyclosporine, rifampin	
SLC15A1	PEPT1	Ampicillin, amoxicillin, captopril, valacyclovir		
SLC15A2	PEPT2	Ampicillin, amoxicillin, captopril, valacyclovir		
SLC22A1	OCT1	Acyclovir, amantadine, desipramine, ganciclovir, metformin	Disopyramide, midazolam, phenformin, phenoxy-benzamine, quinidine, quinine, ritonavir, verapamil	
SLC22A2	OCT2	Amantadine, cimetidine, memantine	Desipramine, phenoxy-benzamine, quinine	
SLC22A3	OCT3	Cimetidine	Desipramine, prazosin, phenoxy-benzamine	
SLC22A6	OAT1	Acyclovir, adefovir, methotrexate, zidovudine	Probenecid, cefadroxil, cefamandole, cefazolin	
SLC22A7	OAT2	Zidovudine		
SLC22A8	OAT3	Cimetidine, methotrexate, zidovudine	Probenecid, cefadroxil, cefamandole, cefazolin	

*Note that this is not an exhaustive list. For an updated list, see http://www.fda.gov/cder/drug/drugInteractions/default.htm

ABC, adenosine triphosphate (ATP)–binding cassette transporter superfamily; BCRP, breast cancer resistance protein; BSEP, bile salt export pump; MDR, multidrug resistance; MRP, multidrug resistance–related protein; OAT, organic anion transporter; OCT, organic cation transporter; P-gp, P-glycoprotein; SLC, solute-linked carrier transporter family; SLCO, solute-linked carrier organic anion transporter family.

BOX 20-5 INTERACTING DRUG PAIRS AND THE MECHANISMS OF INTERACTIONS

Case 1: Terfenadine–ketoconazole (cytochrome P-450 [CYP] 3A inhibition)
Case 2: Lovastatin–grapefruit juice (intestinal CYP3A inhibition)
Case 3: Cyclosporine–St. John's wort (CYP3A and P-glycoprotein [P-gp] induction)
Case 4: Tamoxifen–CYP2D6 inhibitor (CYP2D6 inhibition)
Case 5: Digoxin–clarithromycin (P-gp inhibition)
Case 6: Repaglinide–gemfibrozil/itraconazole (CYP2C8/CYP3A & OATP1B1 inhibition)

ment for approval. In contrast, even a potential for serious ADRs resulting from drug interactions can be tolerated for drugs that treat severe or life-threatening conditions, particularly when alternative treatments are not available. In these instances, close attention to labeling and other aspects of risk management would be expected.

In this chapter, we have discussed several drug pairs in order to illustrate various types of interactions (Box 20-5).

To prevent serious drug-drug interactions, practitioners need to know ALL of a patient's medications—including over-the-counter products, dietary supplements, and special food products, including juices, that the patients currently take or regularly consume—before prescribing an additional drug. Understanding of the underlying mechanisms of interactions and using available tools (electronic prescribing, electronic patient data management) can minimize the risks of ADRs resulting from drug-drug interactions.

REFERENCES

1. Lazarou J, Pomeranz BH, Corey PN. Incidence of adverse drug reactions in hospitalized patients: a meta-analysis of prospective studies. JAMA 1998;279:1200-1205.
2. Raschetti R, Morgutti M, Menniti-Ippolito F, et al. Suspected adverse drug events requiring emergency department visits or hospital admissions. Eur J Clin Pharmacol 1999;54:959-963.
3. Huang S-M, Temple R, Throckmorton DC, Lesko L. Drug-drug interactions: study design, data analysis and implications for dosing recommendations. Clin Pharmacol Ther 2007;81:298-304.
4. Huang S-M, Strong J, Zhang L, et al. New era in drug interaction evaluation: US FDA update on CYP enzymes, transporters and the guidance process, J Clin Pharmacol 2008;48:662-670.
5. U.S. Food and Drug Administration (FDA). Drug development and drug interactions. Available at http://www.fda.gov/cder/drug/drugInteractions/default.htm (accessed October 20, 2006).
6. U.S. Food and Drug Administration (FDA). Guidance for industry: drug interaction studies—study design, data analysis, and implications for dosing and labeling. Available at http://www.fda.gov/cder/guidance/index.htm; Draft published September 2006. Available at http://www.fda.gov/cder/guidance/6695dft.pdf (accessed October 20, 2006).
7. U.S. Food and Drug Administration (FDA). Available at http://www.fda.gov/cder/drug/drugreactions (accessed October 20, 2006).
8. Drugs @ FDA. Available at http://www.accessdata.fda.gov/scripts/cder/drugsatfda/ (accessed October 20, 2006).

9. Monahan BP, Ferguson CL, Killeavy ES, et al. Torsades de pointes occurring in association with terfenadine use. JAMA 1990;264:2788-2790.
10. Honig PK, Wortham DC, Zamani K, et al. Terfenadine-ketoconazole interaction. Pharmacokinetic and electrocardiographic consequences. JAMA 1993;269:1513-1518.
11. Shaffer D, Singer S, Korvick J, Honig P. Concomitant risk factors in reports of torsades de pointes associated with macrolide use: review of the United States Food and Drug Administration Adverse Event Reporting System. Clin Infect Dis 2002;35:197-200.
12. Paine MF, Hart HL, Ludington SS, et al. The human intestinal cytochrome P450 "pie." Drug Metab Dispos 2006;34:880-886.
13. Huang S-M. Clinical drug-drug interactions. In Krishna R (ed): Pharmacokinetic Applications in Drug Development. London: Kluwer Academic/Plenum, 2003.
14. Relpax (eletriptan). Electronic PDR. Label updated March 2005. Available at http://www.thomsonhc.com/pdrel/librarian/PFDefaultActionId/pdrcommon.IndexSearchTranslator (accessed October 26, 2006).
15. Ketek (kelithromycin) labeling. Label updated June 2006. Drugs @ FDA. Available at http://www.fda.gov/cder/foi/label/2006/021144s011lbl.pdf (accessed October 26, 2006).
16. Piazza-Hepp T. Grapefruit juice interaction reports from FDA's post-marketing adverse event reporting system. In Lam F, Huang S-M, Hall S (eds): Herbal Supplements and Drug Interactions. New York: Taylor & Francis, 2006.
17. Zocor (simvastatin) labeling. Updated August 2005. Drugs @ FDA. Available at http://www.fda.gov/cder/foi/label/2005/019766s069lbl.pdf (accessed October 26, 2006).
18. Paine MF, Widmer WW, Hart HL, et al. A furanocoumarin-free grapefruit juice establishes furanocoumarins as the mediators of the grapefruit juice–felodipine interaction. Am J Clin Nutr 2006;83:1097-1105.
19. Kantola T, Kivisto KT, Neuvonen PJ. Grapefruit juice greatly increases serum concentrations of lovastatin and lovastatin acid. Clin Pharmacol Ther 1998;63:397-402.
20. Huang S-M, Temple R, Lesko LJ. Drug-drug, drug-dietary supplement, and drug-citrus fruit and other food interactions—labeling implications. In Lam F, Huang S-M, Hall S (eds): Herbal Supplements and Drug Interactions. New York: Taylor & Francis, 2006.
21. Neoral (cyclosporine) labeling. Updated March 2006. Drugs @ FDA. Available at http://www.fda.gov/cder/foi/label/2006/050715s024,050716s025lbl.pdf (accessed October 26, 2006).
22. Dresser GK, Kim RB, Bailey DG. Effect of grapefruit juice volume on the reduction of fexofenadine bioavailability: possible role of organic anion transporting polypeptides. Clin Pharmacol Ther 2005;77:170-177.
23. Allegra (fexofenadine) labeling. Updated October 2005. Drugs @ FDA. Available at http://www.fda.gov/cder/foi/label/2005/020872s015lbl.pdf (accessed October 26, 2006).
24. Ruschitzka F, Meier PJ, Turina M, et al. Acute heart transplant rejection due to Saint John's wort. Lancet 2000;355:548-549.
25. Moore LB, Goodwin B, Jones SA, et al. St. John's wort induces hepatic drug metabolism through activation of the pregnane X receptor. Proc Natl Acad Sci U S A 2000;97:7500-7502.
26. Hall SD, Wang Z, Huang SM, et al. The interaction between St John's wort and an oral contraceptive. Clin Pharmacol Ther 2003;74:525-535.
27. Wang Z, Gorski JC, Hamman MA, et al. The effects of St John's wort (*Hypericum perforatum*) on human cytochrome P450 activity. Clin Pharmacol Ther 2001;70:317-326.
28. Perloff MD, von Moltke LL, Stormer E, et al. J. Saint John's wort: an in vitro analysis of P-glycoprotein induction due to extended exposure. Br J Pharmacol 2001;134:1601-1608.
29. Komoroski BJ, Zhang S, Cai H, et al. Induction and inhibition of cytochromes P450 by the St. John's wort constituent hyperforin in human hepatocyte cultures. Drug Metab Dispos 2004;32:512-518.
30. Wurglics M, Westerhoff K, Kaunzinger A, et al. Comparison of German St. John's wort products according to hyperforin and total hypericin content. J Am Pharm Assoc (Wash) 2001;41:560-566.
31. Gleevec (imatinib) labeling. Label updated March 2005. Electronic PDR. Available at http://www.thomsonhc.com/pdrel/librarian/PFDefaultActionId/pdrcommon.IndexSearchTranslator (accessed October 26, 2006).
32. Huang S-M, Hall SD, Watkins P, et al. Drug interactions with herbal products & grapefruit juice: a conference report. Clin Pharmacol Ther 2004;75:1-12.
33. Huang S-M, Lesko LJ. Drug-drug, drug-dietary supplement and drug-citrus fruit and other food interactions—what have we learned? J Clin Pharmacol 2004;44:559-569.
34. Jin Y, Desta Z, Stearns V, et al. CYP2D6 genotype, antidepressant use, and tamoxifen metabolism during adjuvant breast cancer treatment. J Natl Cancer Inst 2005;97:30-39.
35. Goetz MP, Knox SK, Suman VJ, et al. The impact of cytochrome P450 2D6 metabolism in women receiving adjuvant tamoxifen. Breast Cancer Res Treat 2007;101:113-121.
36. Juurlink DN, Mamdani M, Kopp A, et al. Drug-drug interactions among elderly patients hospitalized for drug toxicity. JAMA 2003;289:1652-1658.
37. Digoxin labeling. Label updated August 2004. Drugs @ FDA. Available at http://www.fda.gov/cder/foi/label/2004/21648lbl.pdf (accessed October 26, 2006).
38. Zhang L, Strong JM, Wei Q, et al. Scientific perspective on drug transporters and their role in drug interactions. Mol Pharmacol 2006;3:62-69.
39. Ho RH, Kim RB. Transporters and drug therapy: implications for drug disposition and disease. Clin Pharmacol Ther 2005;78:260-277.
40. Andresson T, Flockhart DA, Goldstein DB, et al. Drug metabolizing enzymes—clinical utility of pharmacogenomic test. Clin Pharmacol Ther 2005;78:559-581.
41. Marzolini C, Paus E, Buclin T, Kim RB. Polymorphisms in human MDR1 (P-glycoprotein): recent advances and clinical relevance. Clin Pharmacol Ther 2004;75:13-33.
42. Chinn LS, Kroetz DL. ABCB1 pharmacogenetics: progress, pitfalls and promise. Clin Pharmacol Ther 2007;81:265.
43. Niemi M, Backman JT, Neuvonen M, Neuvonen PJ. Effects of gemfibrozil, itraconazole, and their combination on the pharmacokinetics and pharmacodynamics of repaglinide: potentially hazardous interaction between gemfibrozil and repaglinide. Diabetologia 2003;46:347-351. Epub: 2003;Feb 27.
44. Shitara Y, Hirano M, Sato H, Sugiyama Y. Gemfibrozil and its glucuronide inhibit the organic anion transporting polypeptide 2 (OATP2/OATP1B1:SLC21A6)–mediated hepatic uptake and CYP2C8-mediated metabolism of cerivastatin: analysis of the mechanism of the clinically relevant drug-drug interaction between cerivastatin and gemfibrozil. J Pharmacol Exp Ther 2004;311:228-236. Epub: 2004;Jun 11.
45. Ogilvie BW, Zhang D, Li W, et al. Glucuronidation converts gemfibrozil to a potent, metabolism-dependent inhibitor of CYP2C8: implications for drug-drug interactions. Drug Metab Dispos 2006;34:191-197. Epub: 2005;Nov 18.
46. Prandin (repalinide) labeling. February 2005 version. Drugs @ FDA. Available at http://www.fda.gov/cder/foi/label/2005/20741s022lbl.pdf (accessed October 26, 2006).
47. Niemi M, Tornio A, Pasanen MK, et al. Itraconazole, gemfibrozil and their combination markedly raise the plasma concentrations of loperamide. Eur J Clin Pharmacol 2006;62:463-472. Epub: 2006;Apr 27.
48. Barza M, Weinstein L. Pharmacokinetics of the penicillins in man. Clin Pharmacokin 1976;1:297-308.
49. Burckhardt BC, Burckhardt G. Transport of organic anions across the basolateral membrane of proximal tubule cells [Review]. Rev Physiol Biochem Pharmacol 2003;146:95-158. Epub: 2003;Jan 30.
50. Kaletra (lopinavir/ritonavir) labeling. April 2005 version. Drugs @ FDA Available at http://www.fda.gov/cder/foi/label/2005/021226s016lbl.pdf (accessed October 26, 2006).
51. Aptivus (tipranavir) labeling. August 2006 version. Drugs @ FDA. Available at http://www.fda.gov/cder/foi/label/2006/021814s001s002lbl.pdf (accessed October 26, 2006).
52. Pirmohamed M, James S, Meakin S, et al. Adverse drug reactions as cause of admission to hospital: prospective analysis of 18,820 patients. BMJ 2004;329(7456):15-19.
53. Budnitz DS, Pollock DA, Weidenbach KN, et al. National surveillance of emergency department visits for outpatient adverse drug events. JAMA 2006;296:1858-1866.
54. Friedman MA, Woodcock J, Lumpkin MM, et al. The safety of newly approved medicines: do recent market removals mean there is a problem? JAMA 1999;281:1728-1734.
55. Huang SM, Miller M, Toigo T, et al. Evaluation of drugs in women: Regulatory perspective. In Legato M (ed): Principles of Gender-Specific Medicine, Section 11: Drug Metabolism/Clinical Pharmacology (Schwartz J, sect ed). San Diego: Academic, 2004, pp 848-859.

21

THERAPEUTIC DRUG MONITORING

Michael C. Milone and Leslie M. Shaw

INTRODUCTION 275
RATIONALE FOR THERAPEUTIC DRUG MONITORING 275
CONCEPT OF A "THERAPEUTIC RANGE" 276
Preanalytic Factors That Affect TDM Results 277
Accuracy of the Dose Delivered 277
Accuracy of the Sampling Time 277
Collection and Transport of TDM Specimens 277
MEASURING DRUGS IN THE LABORATORY 277
ASSESSING TEST PERFORMANCE 278
Precision 278
Accuracy 278
Selectivity 279
ANALYTIC METHODS: PRINCIPLES AND PRACTICE 279
Antibody-Based Analytic Methods 279
Chromatography-Based Analytic Methods 279
TDM IN CLINICAL PRACTICE 282
Drug Concentration Monitoring as a Clinical Diagnostic Test 282
Drug Concentration Monitoring as a Risk Reduction Tool 282
Methotrexate 282
Forecasting Optimal Dosing Based on Concentration Data 283
Importance of a Pharmacokinetic Model 283
Linear Dose Adjustment Using a Single Concentration 283
Dose Prediction 284
THE CLINICAL PHARMACOKINETICS SERVICE 285
BIOMARKERS AND THE FUTURE OF TDM 285
CONCLUSIONS 286

INTRODUCTION

Natural substances and synthetic chemicals, which we call "drugs," have been used for millennia to prevent, diagnose, or treat disease. The recognition of both desirable and toxic effects of drugs and the relationship of these effects to dose is also hardly a new concept. However, the application of careful scientific study to the use of drugs only began in the past century. Through these studies, we have gained a significant understanding of the effects that many drugs have on the individual (see Chapter 14, Pharmacodynamics) and the effects of the individual on these drugs (see Chapter 13, Pharmacokinetics). This has led to numerous advances in drug design, formulation, and dosing that attempt to maximize the efficacy and minimize the toxicity of drug therapy. Despite our improved understanding, many of the drugs in current use today still possess significant poisonous attributes that limit their clinical utility.

Along with the great strides made in pharmacology, advances in the area of analytic chemistry and laboratory medicine have made it possible to measure almost all drugs in biologic samples with a high degree of specificity and sensitivity. These developments have now made it possible to apply pharmacokinetic and pharmacodynamic principles to drug dosing in individual patients by assessing the quantity of drug in their bodily fluids, most often in serum or whole blood. This area of medicine, often referred to as therapeutic drug monitoring (TDM) or applied pharmacokinetics, has expanded rapidly over the past 3 decades, yielding significant improvements in patient care. It has become an integral part of drug therapy for many pharmaceuticals. Table 21-1 provides a list of drugs for which TDM is commonly used.

Successful application of TDM to individualize drug therapy, however, requires that the health care practitioner has a solid understanding of a drug's pharmacology and the benefits and limitations of serum drug concentrations or the pharmacokinetic parameters estimated from them. This chapter provides an overview of the rationale behind monitored drug therapy, the methods used to measure drugs in clinical specimens, and the application of this information to individualize a patient's drug therapy. The reader is also referred to the literature and some recent texts[1,2] devoted to the subject of TDM for more detailed, up-to-date discussions of specific drugs and the role of TDM in their use.

RATIONALE FOR THERAPEUTIC DRUG MONITORING

As Paracelsus, the often-quoted father of toxicology, recognized over 500 years ago, all substances are poisonous: It is simply a matter of quantity. For many drugs with a very high toxic : therapeutic dose ratio, the quantity of drug that is required for clinical efficacy is quite different from that required for toxicity. Penicillin provides a classic example wherein the dose of penicillin necessary to produce toxicity is so far above effective doses typically used in clinical practice that dose-related toxicity is never observed. In contrast, several drugs in clinical use today exhibit a relatively low toxic : therapeutic dose ratio (the therapeutic index). Choosing an appropriate dose a priori for many of these drugs can be quite difficult due to significant inter- and intrapatient variability in pharmacokinetic and pharmacodynamic behavior. The ability to use these drugs without harming the patient can be rather challenging. For many of these drugs, monitoring the blood or serum concentration during therapy has shown utility in maximizing efficacy and minimizing toxicity.[3-10]

While unpredictable pharmacokinetic and pharmacodynamic behaviors of a drug are important factors in support of TDM, these factors alone do not necessarily warrant concentration monitoring of drug therapy. Antihypertensive drugs possess significant variability in their pharmacokinetic and pharmacodynamic behavior due to numerous factors, including age, comorbid disease, associated organ dysfunction, and genetics.[11] This variability can lead to widely disparate dose requirements for maintenance of adequate blood pressure control in patients. However, the pharmacodynamic effect of blood pressure reduction is easily monitored, permitting adjustment of dose without the need for concentration monitoring despite the low toxic : therapeutic dose ratio for many of these drugs. In contrast, the use of immunosuppressant drugs for the control of organ transplant rejection is much more difficult to monitor clinically. A patient could receive a dose that is sub- or supratherapeutic for weeks before the consequences of acute organ rejection or life-threatening infection are recognized.[12]

TABLE 21-1 COMMONLY MONITORED DRUGS AND TYPICAL THERAPEUTIC RANGES*

Drug	Method	Therapeutic Range
Antiarrhythmics		
Lidocaine	Immunoassay	1.5-5.0 mg/L
Procainamide	Immunoassay	4-10 mg/L 5-30 mg/L (procainamide + NAPA)
Antibiotics		
Amikacin	Immunoassay	C_0 <8 mg/L C_{max}: 40-60 mg/L (once daily) C_{max}: 20-30 mg/L (traditional)
Gentamicin	Immunoassay	C_0 <2 mg/L C_{max}: 10-20 mg/L (once daily) C_{max}: 5-10 mg/L (traditional)
Tobramycin	Immunoassay	C_0 <2 mg/L C_{max}: 10-20 mg/L (once daily) C_{max}: 5-10 mg/L (traditional)
Vancomycin	Immunoassay	C_0: 5-20 mg/L; C_{max}: 20-40 mg/L
Anticancer agents		
Methotrexate	Immunoassay	Protocol dependent
Busulfan	GC-MS	Protocol dependent
Antiepileptic drugs		
Carbamazepine	Immunoassay	4-10 mg/L or 6-12 mg/L[†]
Phenobarbital	Immunoassay	10-40 mg/L
Phenytoin	Immunoassay	10-20 mg/L (total) 1-2 mg/L (free)
Valproic acid	Immunoassay	50-100 mg/L (total)
Caffeine	Immunoassay	10-30 mg/L
Digoxin	Immunoassay	0.9-2 mcg/L
Immunosuppressive drugs		
Cyclosporine	HPLC-UV	Varies by organ and time posttransplantation
Tacrolimus (FK506)	LC-MS/MS	Varies by organ and time posttransplantation
Mycophenolic acid	HPLC-UV	1-3.5 mg/L (with cyclosporine) 1.8-4.5 mg/L (with tacrolimus)
Rapamycin	LC-MS/MS	4-12 mcg/L
Lithium	AAS	0.5-1.2 mmol/L
Theophylline	Immunoassay	10-20 mg/L; 5-10 mg/L (neonates)

*Typical ranges are those used at the Hospital of the University of Pennsylvania.
†When used as single agent.
AAS, atomic absorption spectrophotometry; C_0, trough concentration; C_{max}, mean peak concentration; GC-MS, gas chromatography–mass spectrometry; HPLC-UV, high-performance liquid chromatography–ultraviolet; LC-MS/MS, liquid chromatography–mass spectrometry/mass spectroscopy; NAPA, *N*-acetyl procainamide.

In this latter situation, concentration monitoring may improve care by enhancing the efficacy and limiting the toxicity of drug therapy.

TDM may also play a useful role in monitoring adherence to drug therapy. The frequency of nonadherence to drug therapy is highly variable depending upon a number of factors, including the frequency of drug dosing, complexity of the drug regimen, and side effects of a drug. Even in highly motivated patient populations such as organ transplant recipients, nonadherence to immunosuppressant drug therapy is reported to occur with rates of greater than 20%.[13-16] This nonadherence can be very difficult to detect, and persistently low drug concentrations may provide a strong indicator of this serious situation.

CONCEPT OF A "THERAPEUTIC RANGE"

The relationship between serum drug concentration and clinical outcome forms the basis for TDM. Figure 21-1 illustrates a theoretical dose-response relationship for a drug likely to benefit from concentration monitoring. A plausible therapeutic range is highlighted. One of the most common interpretative errors encountered regarding therapeutic ranges is presumption that a concentration within this range will ensure treatment success in the absence of toxicity, and concentrations outside this range will not; however, as shown for our theoretical drug in Figure 21-1, the probability of success and toxicity is a continuum across different concentrations. These probabilities are maximized and minimized, respectively, within the therapeutic range. Nevertheless, therapeutic success can certainly occur at concentrations below the therapeutic range, as exemplified by the patient with epilepsy who attains excellent seizure control with a phenytoin concentration of 7 mg/L (typical therapeutic range for phenytoin is 10 to 20 mg/L). Success may also be achieved in a portion of treated patients by concentrations above the therapeutic range without associated toxicity. Experienced users of TDM generally recognize the probalistic nature of these relationships, and weigh the risks and potential benefits of drug concentrations in the context of the clinical situation using the therapeutic range as a guide.

Another limitation to the strict application of therapeutic ranges for drugs is the reality that these ranges are generally based upon population data from drug therapy trials. The application of these population-based ranges to an individual therefore assumes similarity to the studied population. Differences in metabolism, physiology, and/or the underlying disease process can all alter these relationships, leading to unexpected and undesirable results. Phenytoin used for seizure control illustrates one potential pitfall. A fairly good relationship exists between non–protein-bound (unbound or free) serum phenytoin concentration and seizure control. However, the presence of either concomitant kidney or liver disease significantly reduces phenytoin binding to albumin.[17,17a] Because phenytoin is restrictively eliminated, a given phenytoin dose results in lower total (bound plus free) phenytoin levels in these patients, even though free phenytoin levels are comparable. As

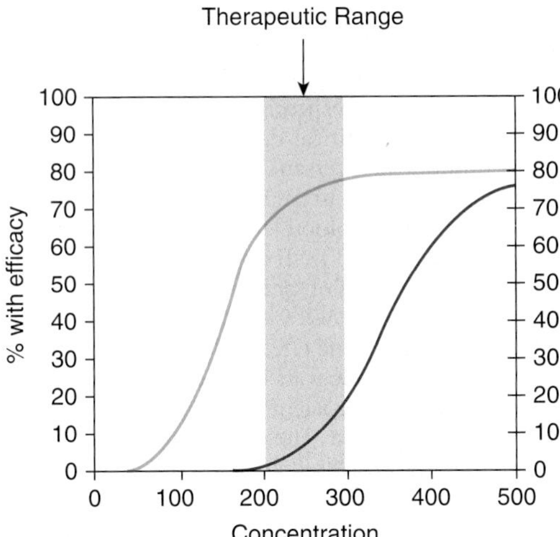

FIGURE 21-1 • Concept of a therapeutic range.

a result, individuals with kidney or liver disease are at significantly higher risk of toxicity at total serum phenytoin concentrations that are appropriate for most other individuals. The recognition of this problem has led to the development of methods for measuring free drug concentrations. Therefore, there is a need for caution in applying population-based relationships to individual patients who may not be represented by the population used for defining the therapeutic range.

Preanalytic Factors That Affect TDM Results

The ability to provide accurate, useful TDM data depends upon many factors that relate to the laboratory methods used to perform the drug concentration measurement. However, there are several preanalytic factors that affect the result of a TDM test and its interpretation that are independent of the laboratory methods used. For example, unlike laboratory procedures, which are performed under highly standardized operating procedures, collection and transport of blood specimens to the laboratory are much less standardized. Nevertheless, these factors are critically important to the validity and utility of the drug monitoring data, and failure to recognize their importance could even be detrimental to the care of a patient. Some important preanalytic factors include accuracy of the dose delivered and the sampling time, and collection and transport of TDM specimens.

Accuracy of the Dose Delivered

Drug dose is an important variable in all pharmacokinetic models used for individualized drug dosing, and its accuracy is critical to interpretation of TDM data. However, it cannot be assumed that the dose delivered to an individual patient is always the desired dose. In some cases, some commercial drug formulations have been inexact.[18] Inaccurate delivery of dose due to human error or loss during administration (e.g., adsorption to components of infusion system) can also lead to inaccurate dosing of patients. These potential sources of dosing error should always be considered during pharmacotherapy, but these errors may be especially important for narrow therapeutic index drugs that are the typical candidates for concentration monitoring.

Accuracy of the Sampling Time

Time is an important variable in most models of applied pharmacokinetics. Most calculations involve this variable or assume it—for example, mean peak concentration (C_{max}) or trough concentration (C_0) measurements. Many of the models used in applied pharmacokinetics for dose adjustment also assume that concentration measurements are made during steady state conditions. Accuracy in the timing of sample collection in relation to dosing and the accuracy in recording of this time are absolutely essential to the usefulness of TDM data. Unfortunately, errors in the timing occur with significant frequency. Estimates indicate that as many as 78% of all TDM specimens are collected at inappropriate times or without time of collection recorded.[19] Unfortunately, verification of accurate collection times is often difficult or impossible. Prediction algorithms such as bayesian methods reduce the overall effect of incorrect sample timing. However, appropriate care and effort should always be taken to ensure that accepted TDM sampling protocols are followed.

Collection and Transport of TDM Specimens

Following collection of a blood specimen, drug/metabolite concentrations in the specimen may change over time. These changes occur through a variety of mechanisms, including compound decomposition, interactions with other sample constituents, and/or adsorption by the storage container. Often this instability can be limited through special procedures such as rapid separation of the blood component to be analyzed (e.g., plasma separation), collection/storage tube selection (e.g., empty collection tubes compared with serum separator tubes), and cold temperature storage (e.g., 4° C or −20° C). Anticoagulants and other additives to collection containers can also have effects on TDM data through analytic interference with the laboratory method. Therefore, concentration monitoring data should be cautiously interpreted when deviations from standard sample collection practices are used.

MEASURING DRUGS IN THE LABORATORY

Analytic methods used for the quantitative analysis of samples can be classified into three categories based upon their performance characteristics. The most accurate and precise methods are termed definitive methods. The International Union of Pure and Applied Chemistry (IUPAC) defines these methods as:

A method of exceptional scientific status which is sufficiently accurate to stand alone in the determination of a given property for the certification of a reference material. Such a method must have a firm theoretical foundation so that systematic error is negligible relative to the intended use. Analyte masses (amounts) or concentrations must be measured directly in terms of the base units of measurements, or indirectly related through sound theoretical equations. Definitive methods, together with Certified Reference Materials, are primary means for transferring accuracy—i.e. establishing traceability.[20]

Definitive methods are generally very time consuming and expensive techniques (e.g., isotope dilution–mass spectrometry) that are not practical for general use in a clinical laboratory. Rather, these techniques are relegated to laboratories such as those of the National Institute of Standards and Technology (NIST) that produce certified standard reference material (SRM) that is used by other laboratories for calibration of other analytic systems. In contrast to definitive methods, reference methods are those analytic methods possessing "small, estimated inaccuracies relative to the end use requirement."[20] These methods are still somewhat complex, expensive, and time consuming, but they are generally more easily established by most experienced laboratories. Importantly, the accuracy of reference methods should be demonstrated through direct comparison to definitive methods or a certified standard SRM. With the exception of anticonvulsants, SRMs unfortunately do not exist for most drugs measured in the clinical TDM laboratory, leading to potential problems in testing agreement across different laboratories. Finally, most clinical laboratories do not perform either definitive or reference methods for drug concentration monitoring. Rather, they perform a myriad of "routine" tests that are adequate for clinical use. These methods do not display the performance characteristics required of reference or definitive methods.

It is imperative that producers and consumers of TDM data understand the unique principles and performance characteristics of each test they use. Without a thorough understanding of these aspects of drug monitoring, significant errors in test interpretation may occur that may not only negate the beneficial effects of monitored drug therapy, but could also be detrimental to the care and well-being of patients.

ASSESSING TEST PERFORMANCE

Accurate, precise, and reliable analytic methods are essential for the successful application of TDM. Unfortunately, all analytic measurements are subject to error. This error falls into two principle components, random error and systematic error (also known as bias). Recognition of analytic error, its magnitude, and its causes is paramount to understanding the performance characteristics of clinical drug monitoring tests. The most important criteria to consider in assessing the performance of any analytic method, including those of the TDM laboratory, include precision, accuracy, and selectivity.

Precision

Assay precision refers to how close assay results will be with repeated measurements of the same sample. Figure 21-2 shows hypothetical results for three different testing platforms (A, B, and C) for a single sample analyzed repeatedly. Platforms A and C demonstrate the same mean value; however, as revealed by the dispersion in the data, platform A exhibits much greater assay precision compared with platform C. This precision is dependent upon the random error that exists within any analytic system. The cause(s) of random error are largely unknown and uncontrollable. Some factors that might contribute to random error in measurements include uncontrollable factors such as voltage or temperature fluctuations, variability in sample preparation such as during extraction, and human error. The most common way to quantify assay precision is using a calculated ratio termed the *coefficient of variation* (CV):

$$CV = \sigma_x/\bar{x} \times 100$$

where σ_x is the standard deviation of a series of repeated measurements and $\bar{x}$ is the mean of these measurements. Generally, a CV of 3% to 6% is considered to be ideal for most clinical assays. However, the variability in repeated measurement tends to increase as sample concentrations approach the extreme values for any method. While most laboratories strive to meet the ideal of a very low CV, this is not always possible. In reality, the CV of some clinical TDM tests exceeds 10%. The U.S. Food and Drug Administration (FDA) has published a guidance document indicating that a CV of less than 15% be considered the standard precision for bioanalytic drug assays, with an acceptable CV as high as 20% at the lower limit of quantitation.[21]

While this degree of assay precision may be adequate for some clinical TDM tests, some critical-dose drugs clearly require greater precision. The immunosuppressant tacrolimus illustrates this point. When first introduced for the prevention of renal transplant rejection, available data suggested that blood tacrolimus levels in the range of 10 to 20 ng/ml were ideal. The MEIA-II microparticle enzyme immunoassay developed for monitoring of tacrolimus blood concentrations has fairly good precision, with a CV less than 10%, within this therapeutic range. Over the past decade, the effects of tacrolimus, within this concentration range, on renal allograft function were better appreciated, and new immunosuppressive agents such as mycophenolate mofetil and sirolimus were introduced. The target range for blood tacrolimus levels has subsequently decreased for patients in some centers to a range as low as 5 to 8 ng/ml in an effort to reduce the adverse effects of these drugs when combined with other immunosuppressive agents. While the MEIA-II assay displays adequate precision in the former therapeutic range, the CV for this assay in the newer, lower target range is reported to be as high as 19%. At this level of precision, approximately one of every five individuals with a measured value of 6 ng/ml will actually have a level below 5 ng/ml. Given the potentially serious consequences of a subtherapeutic tacrolimus concentration, this error clearly limits the usefulness of this assay within this lower target range. This example highlights the need to consider assay precision and the useful analytic range in the interpretation of TDM data.

Accuracy

Accuracy refers to the closeness of the average measured drug concentration to the "true" concentration of a drug. While a method may demonstrate a high degree of precision, measurement of a specimen may still deviate from the "true" value due to systematic error or bias. The hypothetical example of Figure 21-2 illustrates this point. Methods A and B have identical assay precision. Nonetheless, method B systematically provides higher concentrations with a mean value that is 20% higher than method A. The most common cause of a systematic error is a nonstandardized calibrator. If the calibrator used to establish a standard curve for an assay deviates from the "true" mean, then all measurements made by an instrument using this calibrator will deviate accordingly. The development of SRM helps to eliminate bias across

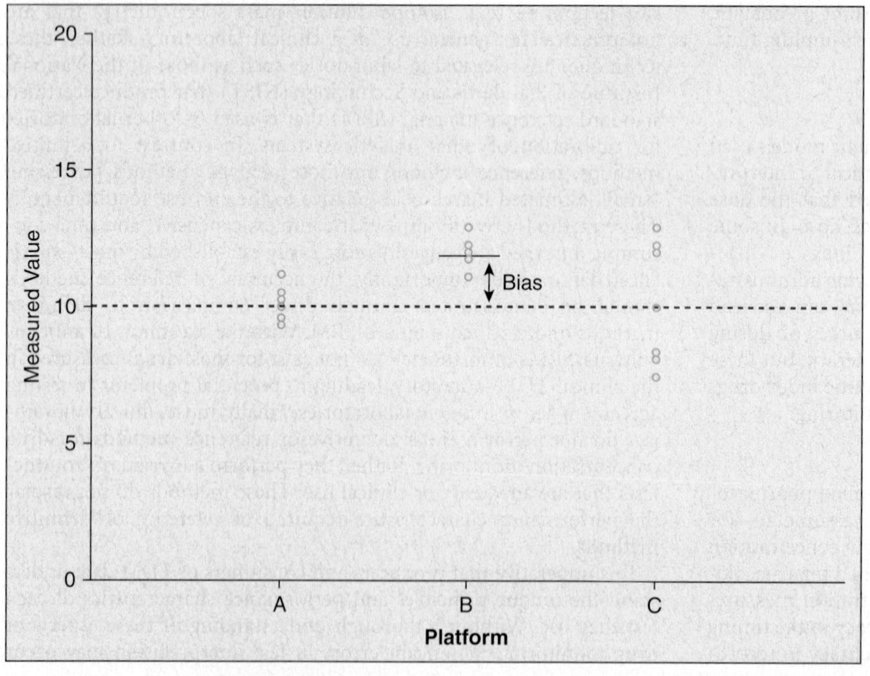

FIGURE 21-2 • Accuracy and precision of an analytic method.

different labs due to variant calibrator material. Studies performed in the 1970s to assess the interlaboratory variability in TDM for antiepileptic drugs demonstrated that approximately half of laboratories reported results in excess of 1 standard deviation of the mean result obtained by five reference laboratories.[22] This study contributed greatly to the development of a reference standard for these drugs that is now available from NIST. Nevertheless, even with standardized calibrators, bias may be introduced in other ways as well, such as calibrator decomposition, inaccurate measurement devices, sample compositional differences that affect analysis, and assay specificity (see section on Selectivity later).

While precision is easily quantified and controlled in the clinical laboratory, changes in test accuracy are often insidious, especially when they relate to outside effects such as inaccurate calibrator material. All clinical laboratories participate in external proficiency testing in which a set of samples are tested across the different laboratories performing the same test even though different test platforms may be used. This testing may uncover important bias, especially when assays demonstrate high precision and SRM is used for calibration. Despite external proficiency testing, significant, unrecognized bias still makes its way into testing. Therefore, consideration of this important test characteristic, especially in the context of testing across different laboratories, is therefore critical and cannot be overemphasized.

Selectivity

The ability of a given method to detect a compound of interest among many potential substances present in a sample is vital to the reliability and usefulness of any analytic test. This is particularly important for TDM tests since many drugs are structurally related, including to some endogenously produced compounds.[23,24] Most drugs are also extensively metabolized through a number of different pathways of biotransformation. These metabolites are often similar to the parent compound in structure, but pharmacologic activity is variable. Tacrolimus again provides a useful example. The MEIA-II immunoassay for tacrolimus demonstrates similar reactivity toward tacrolimus and two of its metabolites, 15-desmethyl-tacrolimus and 31-desmethyl-tacrolimus (Fig. 21-3). Although both metabolites are detected equally, the 15-desmethyl metabolite exhibits little immunosuppressive activity, whereas the 31-desmethyl metabolite exhibits equal immunosuppressive activity when compared to that of tacrolimus. These metabolites are generally low in abundance in most patients; however, alterations in metabolism due to liver dysfunction can lead to their accumulation, complicating TDM interpretation. Since selectivity often differs greatly across platforms, this important performance characteristic must be understood when interpreting TDM results, especially when different laboratories perform testing.

ANALYTIC METHODS: PRINCIPLES AND PRACTICE

Techniques based upon antibody binding, collectively referred to as immunoassays, and chromatography-based methods comprise the vast majority of testing methods. In addition, chromatographic techniques can often serve as reference methods as well, being used in a routine fashion when testing volume is not very large. Given the importance of these analytic techniques and the likelihood of encountering these assay platforms in routine TDM, they are the focus of this section. A more in-depth discussion of these common techniques and less common techniques are provided by some of the many exellent reference texts available, such as the text by Burtis.[25]

Antibody-Based Analytic Methods

The use of antibodies in laboratory testing has evolved greatly since the development of the first immunoassay in the 1950s by Rosalyn Yalow and Solomon Berson. The success of these assays rests upon several features of antibodies that make them ideal reagents for quantitative assays in clinical laboratories. These features include (i) the high degree of specificity exhibited by antibodies toward diverse compounds; (ii) the high affinity of antibodies for their antigenic targets (dissociation constant $>10^{-9}$); (iii) the relative ease of generating large quantities of antibodies to most chemical and biologic substances; and (iv) their remarkable structural stability, permitting an assortment of chemical modifications that contribute to their analytic usefulness.

Fundamentally, all immunoassays strive to measure the abundance of antigen bound to antibody. The original radioimmunoassay developed by Yalow and Berson for the measurement of insulin in serum used insulin-specific antibodies that were immobilized onto glass tubes.[26] Insulin conjugated to radioactive iodine (^{121}I) was then added to these tubes along with a serum sample. After allowing the competitive binding process to reach equilibrium, the free insulin, both conjugated and nonconjugated, was washed away and the bound, radioactively labeled insulin was then measured. The insulin concentration present in the serum sample could then be determined by its inverse relationship to the measured radioactivity. This assay would be characterized today as a competitive, heterogeneous immunoassay since it relies on the competitive binding process and requires the physical separation of bound from free antigen (or antibody). Molecular biology and ingenuity have given rise to many novel immunoassay testing platforms that include both competitive and noncompetitive designs. Due to the commercial drive to produce high-throughput, relatively "hands-free" testing, successful methods for performing immunoassays that do not require physical separation of the antigen-antibody complex, termed *homogeneous immunoassays,* have been developed.

The cloned enzyme donor immunoassay (CEDIA; Microgenics Corporation) provides one of many examples of a competitive, homogeneous immunoassay design that has been successfully applied in clinical laboratories.[27] In this immunoassay design, the first to use recombinant DNA technology, the cloned bacterial enzyme β-galactosidase is split into two fragments termed the *enzyme donor* (ED) and the *enzyme acceptor* (EA) fragments (Fig. 21-4). The ED fragment is conjugated to the drug. When free, the ED-drug conjugate can associate with the EA fragment to reconstitute full enzymatic activity; however, this association is blocked by drug-specific antibody when bound to the ED-drug conjugate. As a result, enzyme activity is restored as free drug present in a sample competes with the ED-drug conjugate. This enzymatic activity is assessed by conversion of the substrate chlorophenol red–β-galactoside into chlorophenol red. This reaction product is then easily measured by absorbance of light at 570 and 660 nm. Other homogeneous immunoassay designs include the enzyme-multiplied immunoassay technique (EMIT) and the fluorescence polarization immunoassay (FPIA). Commonly encountered heterogeneous immunoassay platforms include the microparticle enzyme immunoassay (MEIA) and enzyme-linked immunosorbent assay (ELISA). Although homogeneous assay designs are somewhat easier to automate, they are generally more susceptible to sample matrix interferences. Heterogeneous assays, in contrast, remove much of the interfering substances during the extensive washing steps at the cost of more labor and difficulty in automation.

Chromatography-Based Analytic Methods

Chromatography-based methods of analysis all strive to accomplish the same goal, separation of a compound of interest from the complex mixture of a biologic sample such as plasma. Once this separation is accomplished, a variety of methods are then used to measure the compound of interest as it leaves the chromatographic system. Chromatographic separation is almost universally accomplished through the differential partitioning of compounds between a flowing carrier gas or liquid, termed the *mobile phase,* and a nonmoving, immiscible liquid or solid, termed the *stationary phase* (Fig. 21-5). Following separation, detection of compounds leaving the chromatography system can be accomplished through a variety of techniques that take advantage of the physical and/or chemical properties of the target compound (e.g., ion formation, light absorbance). Analytic specificity is achieved

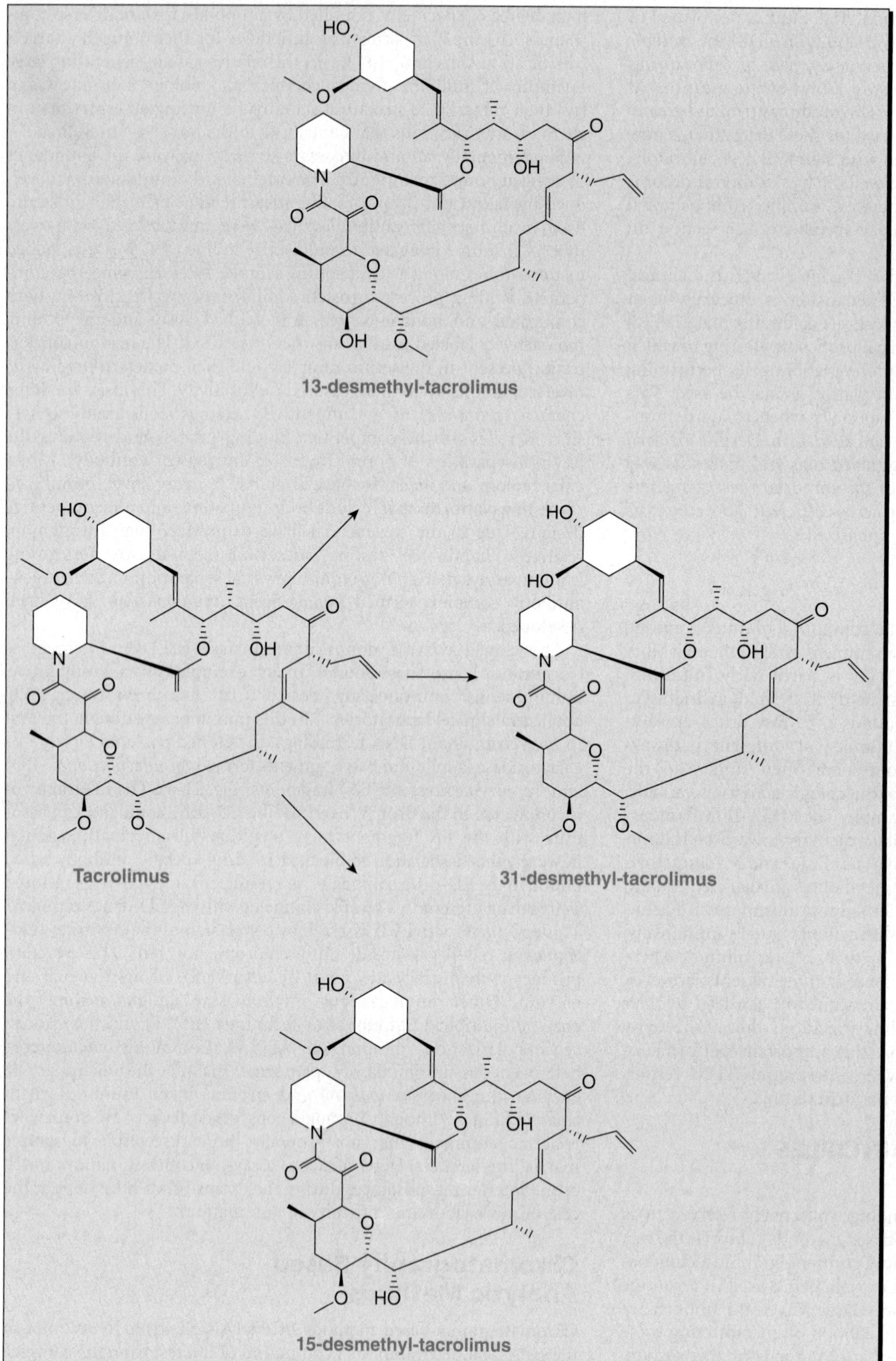

FIGURE 21-3 • Metabolism of tacrolimus.

by these methods through the unique time required for a compound to pass through a chromatographic system (known as the retention time). The retention time and adequacy of separation depend upon a number of factors, including the chemical nature of the compounds of interest, the physical and chemical properties of the stationary and mobile phases of the chromatographic system, the flow rate of the mobile phase, and the temperature of the system. Control of these factors is therefore critical to the success of chromatography.

Although retention time provides a great deal of specificity, additional specificity is often required, especially when analyzing the complex samples of the clinical laboratory. Use of ultraviolet or visible light absorbance at multiple wavelengths through a photodiode array is one method of increasing analytic specificity. In situations requiring the highest degree of specificity, the highly specific chemical identification afforded by mass spectrometry can be combined with the separation power of chromatography (both gas and liquid) to produce

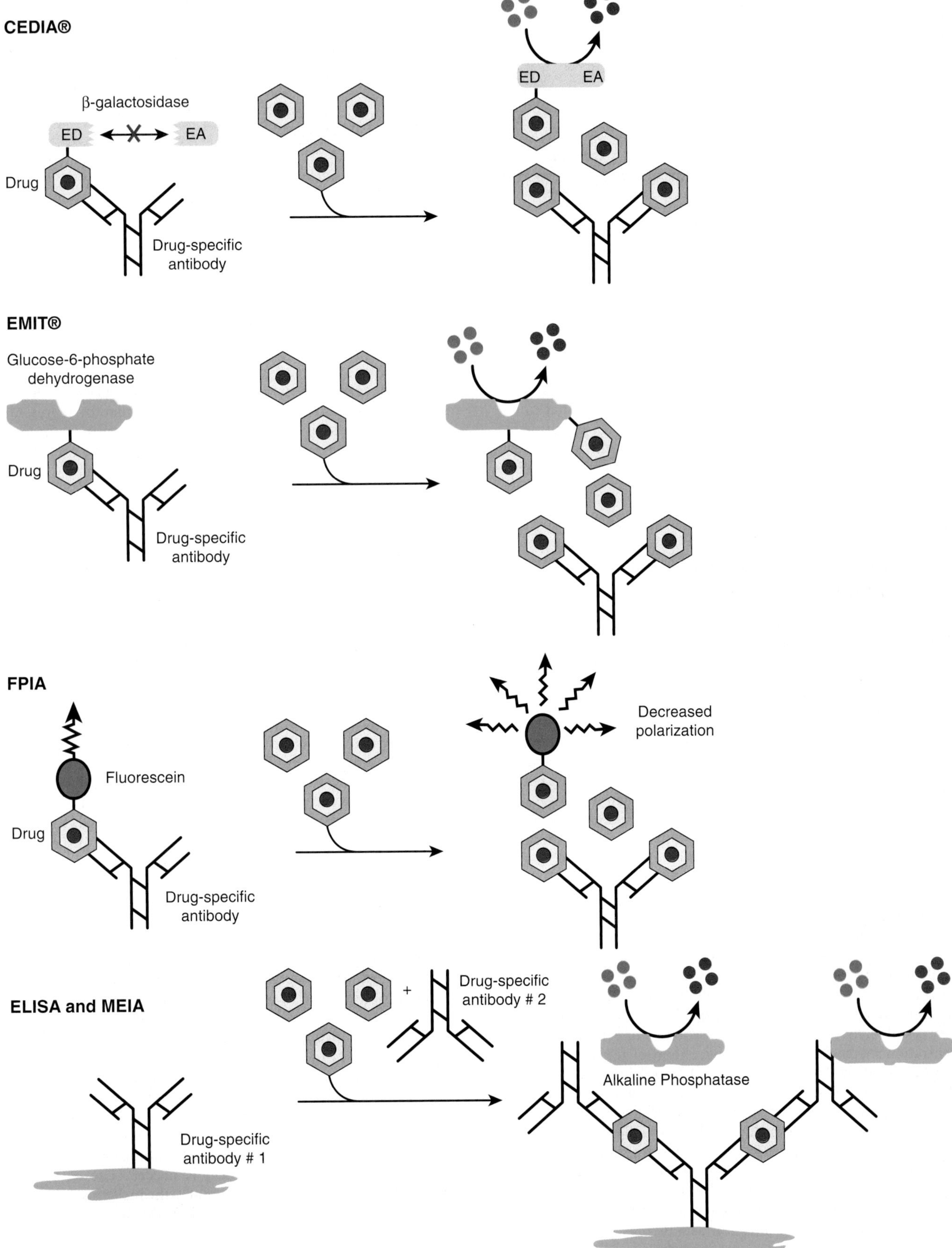

FIGURE 21-4 • Common immunoassay designs.

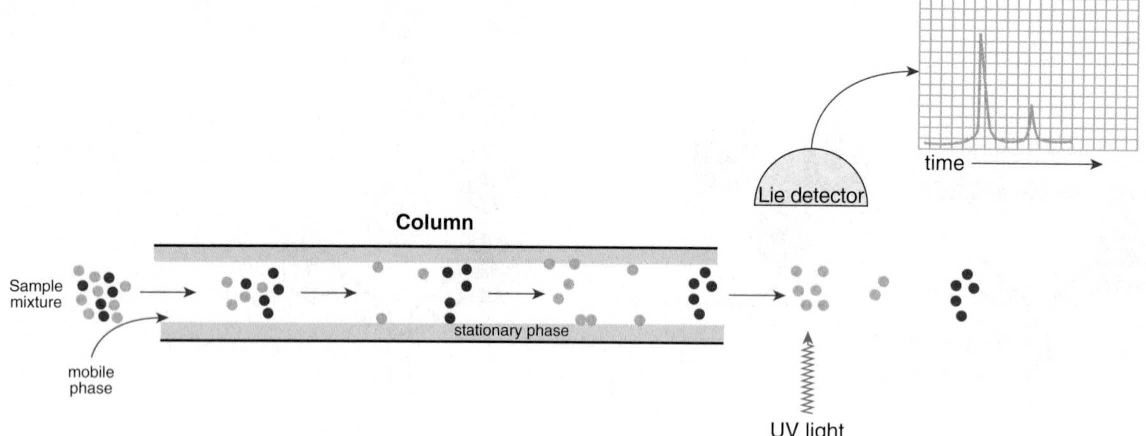

FIGURE 21-5 • Sample analysis by chromatography.

methods that also have high sensitivity. The increasing availability of these methods has greatly broadened the array of analytes that can be measured in the clinical laboratory; however, the cost of instrumentation and high level of technical skill required to operate these instruments generally restricts these analytic methods to highly specialized reference laboratories.

TDM IN CLINICAL PRACTICE

Drug Concentration Monitoring as a Clinical Diagnostic Test

Drug concentration monitoring performs many roles in modern-day clinical practice. In one of its primary roles, drug concentration monitoring serves as an important diagnostic tool in the clinical evaluation of patients treated with critical-dose drugs. Presented with a patient experiencing signs and symptoms consistent with drug toxicity, the presence of a concentration in a range associated with toxicity may lend significant support to the diagnosis of toxicity. In contrast, minimal observed response to drug therapy may be a consequence of either insufficient drug exposure or true resistance to the drug's effects. Distinguishing these two explanations for inadequate response is of critical importance since approaches are very different—increase in dose for the first case versus discontinuation of the drug in the latter case.

Regardless of use, the clinical sensitivity and specificity of a drug concentration measurement (not to be confused with the analytic sensitivity and specificity) for prediction of outcome, either efficacy or toxicity, must be understood for appropriate interpretation of the data. As discussed in the previous section on the concept of a therapeutic range, the average pharmacodynamic relationship for a drug does not generally apply to every patient. Thus, while a concentration of phenytoin greater than the upper limit of the therapeutic range (i.e., 20 mg/L) is associated with increased risk of toxicity, the likelihood of toxicity is still relatively low at values close to this upper "limit." As the concentration increases, so does the likelihood of toxicity. A similar scenario exists at the lower limit of the therapeutic range. Thus, the positive predictive value (or negative predictive value) for toxicity or resistance to therapy is dependent upon the pretest probability that a particular patient is experiencing toxicity or therapeutic failure. Attempts at formalizing this diagnostic using decision analysis have been proposed; however, in most cases, the concentration data are applied by the clinical team in a subjective manner. Regardless, a thorough understanding of the toxicity and efficacy relationship is essential to interpretation of drug concentration data used as a diagnostic test.

Drug Concentration Monitoring as a Risk Reduction Tool

Although useful as a diagnostic test, there are other ways in which TDM has potential to improve drug therapy by preventing toxicity and maximizing efficacy. For example, the use of TDM in high-dose methotrexate (MTX) with leucovorin "rescue" therapy represents one of the simplest, yet highly effective, approaches to using concentration monitoring to improve the safety and efficacy of drug therapy.

Methotrexate

Methotrexate (4-amino-10-methylpteroylglutamic acid) is an antimetabolite that is used in the treatment of a range of neoplastic and non-neoplastic disorders. For many indications, MTX is administered as low-dose, oral therapy for prolonged periods of time, such as in rheumatoid arthritis. Studies in the late 1960s and early 1970s demonstrated that the severe, life-threatening toxicity of MTX is dependent upon not only the magnitude of the dose or serum concentration reached with a particular dose, but also upon the duration of exposure to concentrations of MTX above a toxic threshold level. Thus, short-term exposures to very high concentrations of MTX permit beneficial uptake of the drug into cells and compartments unaffected by lower doses of MTX, provided the unwanted toxic effects of MTX are countered sufficiently with the reduced folate leucovorin (folinic acid, citrovorum factor) (for an in-depth discussion and review, see Chabner and Longo[28]). This "rescue" therapy with leucovorin permits treatment with MTX doses that would otherwise be lethal, and renders the therapy relatively free of toxicity; however, use of high-dose therapy with leucovorin rescue is not without its challenges. Insufficient leucovorin therapy following high-dose MTX can lead to significant, irreversible toxicity and a fatal outcome.[29]

Although most individuals eliminate MTX fairly predictably, MTX elimination is prolonged in a subset of individuals, placing them at increased risk of severe toxicity and/or death from insufficient leucovorin rescue therapy. Monitoring serum MTX concentration has therefore become an integral component of high-dose MTX treatment. Regimens for high-dose MTX treatment vary in the dose and duration of MTX infusions; however, the approach to using MTX serum concentration monitoring is generally similar. Leucovorin therapy is usually initiated 24 to 48 hours after the start of MTX. Methotrexate levels, most commonly determined using simple, rapid immunoassay techniques, are typically measured beginning 24 hours after the start of the MTX infusion and daily thereafter. Leucovorin dose is adjusted according to measured drug concentrations and established nomograms until the MTX level falls below a 50-nmol/L threshold concentration when no further leucovorin is needed. Use of this simple concentration-monitoring scheme reduces the incidence of severe, life-threatening toxicity from high-dose MTX therapy,[4,30-36] and demonstrates the tremendous impact that a TDM program can have on drug therapy.

Although the results with MTX are significant, this mode of monitoring is unusual. Overall, a TDM program primarily reduces risk by functioning as a feedback control system or "thermostat" for optimizing drug therapy, referred to as the target concentration strategy (Fig. 21-6). This strategy aims to regulate a drug's future concentration

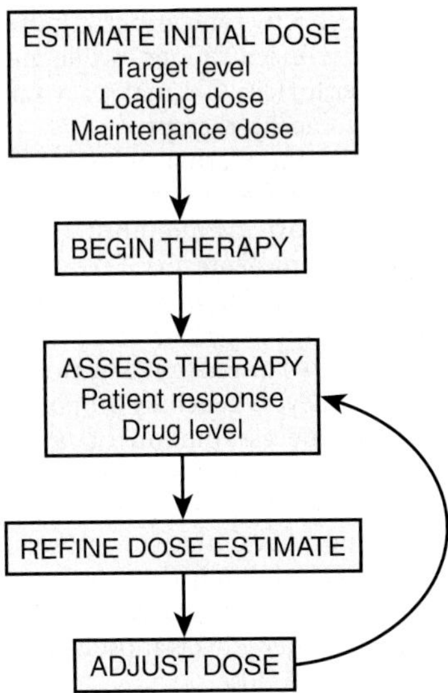

FIGURE 21-6 • Adaptive control approach to therapeutic drug monitoring. (Adapted from Atkinson AJ. Principles of Clinical Pharmacology, 2nd ed. Boston: Academic Press, 2007.)

within a target range that maximizes the likelihood of therapeutic success and minimizes the likelihood of failure by using past drug concentration measurements to adapt dosing. In most cases, the adequacy of therapy is difficult to assess for monitored drugs due to the discrete, time-dependent nature of their primary pharmacodynamic end points (e.g., occurrence of transplanted organ rejection, occurrence of a seizure). Provided a good relationship exists between the drug concentration and outcome, concentration serves as a useful surrogate end point that can be used to optimize therapy. High-dose busulfan therapy represents another example of risk reduction; in this case, risk reduction is accomplished through regulating drug concentration.

Forecasting Optimal Dosing Based on Concentration Data

Given data on drug concentrations in a particular patient, how does one proceed to adjust dosing to achieve the goal of reaching and maintaining a new targeted drug concentration? No single monitoring approach will work for every drug. Numerous strategies have been developed to achieve this goal. The best possible strategy for a particular drug will depend upon a number of factors that include the nature of the drug dosing regimen (e.g., single-dose therapy such as anticancer agents or chronic therapy such as lithium maintenance therapy for bipolar disorder), the pharmacokinetic and pharmacodynamic behavior of the drug and the required precision of control. The urgency of achieving adequate control, and other practical issues such as the timing of physician office hours, also have a significant influence on the way that various drugs are monitored.

Importance of a Pharmacokinetic Model

Regardless of the approach, successful TDM requires a pharmacokinetic model. Without a model, dose adjustment would amount to little more than a patient-specific experiment that could produce disastrous results, as illustrated by the drug phenytoin. The antiseizure activity and toxicity of phenytoin is related to serum concentration; however, the therapeutic index of this drug, like other antiepileptic drugs, is narrow. Unlike most drugs, the relationship between dose and steady state concentration (C_{ss}) for phenytoin is nonlinear (see Fig. 13-10 in Chapter 13, Pharmacokinetics). In an individual taking 300 mg/day with a C_{ss} of 10 mg/L, an empirical dose increase of as little as 100 mg/day may lead to a serum C_{ss} above 30 mg/L and likely toxicity (see Chapter 13, Pharmacokinetics).

As described in Chapter 13 (Pharmacokinetics), models vary in their complexity. The most commonly used pharmacokinetic model in clinical TDM is the one-compartment model with first-order (linear) kinetics of drug elimination. Nevertheless, it must be recognized that even more complex pharmacokinetic models are merely approximate descriptions of a drug's behavior in vivo in mathematical terms. Statistician George Box said it best: "Essentially, all models are wrong, but some are useful." The useful pharmacokinetic models are those that permit predictions of serum drug concentrations associated with dosage changes with a clinically acceptable degree of error. A one-compartment, first-order kinetic model accomplishes this for most clinically used drugs; however, in addition to appropriate model specification, the accuracy of model predictions is still affected by many other factors, including laboratory errors, sample collection errors (e.g., timing), and unexpected altered physiology. Busulfan illustrates some of the benefits of pharmacokinetic model–based approaches to dose adjustment.

Busulfan. High-dose busulfan is often used as part of the preparative regimen for hematopoietic stem cell transplantation (HSCT). Clinical use of busulfan is complicated by significant interpatient variability in pharmacokinetic behavior, with reported CVs of 23%[37] and 25%[38] for the oral and intravenous formulations, respectively. Age, obesity, underlying disease, and organ dysfunction also exert a significant influence on observed clearance for busulfan. Children under the age of 6 typically display more than twice the average clearance of 2.5 ml/min per kilogram reported for adults.[39,40] The observed variability in the pharmacokinetic behavior of busulfan is relevant because several studies have identified a pharmacodynamic relationship between exposure to busulfan and both its toxicity and efficacy. Exposure to busulfan is typically estimated by measurement of several plasma concentrations over a 6-hour dose interval. This exposure is generally expressed as either area under the concentration-time curve (AUC) (in mmol*min/ml) or mean C_{ss}, which is easily derived from the AUC (in ng*min/ml) by dividing this quantity by the dose interval in minutes. The risk of toxicity due to busulfan (veno-occlusive disease or pulmonary toxicity) appears to rise significantly with a mean C_{ss} of greater than 900 to 1025 ng/ml.[41-44] In contrast, the risk of relapse in patients undergoing HSCT for chronic myeloid leukemia rises substantially with a mean C_{ss} of less than 917 ng/ml, indicating that a very narrow therapeutic range of exposure exists for this drug.[45]

Control of busulfan exposure within this tight range requires an accurate and precise estimate of exposure. In order to achieve this level of accuracy and precision, a pharmacokinetic study using extensive sampling is typically required. Early approaches used noncompartmental analysis with estimation of AUC using the trapezoidal rule. Although this approach was effective, fitting the concentration data to a one-compartment, first-order pharmacokinetic model by nonlinear regression has become the preferred method for estimating the mean C_{ss} or AUC for a dose interval. Dosing of busulfan is usually every 6 hours over 4 days for a total of 16 doses. As a result, a study is typically performed following the first dose, and the results are promptly reported in order to effect a dose adjustment as early as possible in the course of the treatment regimen; however, the completion and reporting of a busulfan pharmacokinetic study is not a simple task. A variety of chromatographic methods are used for measurement of busulfan in plasma, with gas chromatography–mass spectrometry generally the preferred method. Given the complexity of this analytic method, on-site testing is not always available. Sample extraction and analysis also usually require several hours to complete for a single patient. Nevertheless, using the above-described TDM approach with dose adjustment, exposures that are within less than 10% of the target exposure are possible, and toxicity can be avoided without a compromise in efficacy.[41,42,44-46]

Linear Dose Adjustment Using a Single Concentration

Although the intense sampling approach used for busulfan provides an excellent degree of precision in the estimation of AUC for this drug, this approach is hardly amenable to TDM of all, but the most toxic and narrow therapeutic index drugs. More commonly, a single measured drug concentration is used to forecast drug dose due to the simplicity of obtaining this information in a clinical setting. The timing of collection varies, and depends to a great extent on the pharmacokinetic behavior of a drug. Drugs that display a very long half-life tend to exhibit relatively small variations in concentration during a dosing interval. Thus, once distributional equilibrium has been achieved, a concentration measured anytime during the dosing interval may be used (e.g., >6 hr after dosing for digoxin). In contrast, drugs that display a relatively short half-life (e.g., aminoglycoside antibiotics) tend to exhibit wide variations in concentration during the dose interval. In these cases, a more precisely timed concentration measurement is typically performed, such as a predose/trough (C_0) or peak (C_{max}) concentration measured at the end of intravenous infusion. The basis for this approach is the expectation that a single, appropriately timed concentration of a drug can be used to predict concentrations at other times during the dosing interval and, more importantly, the outcome of therapy. When these concentrations are not measured under steady state conditions, the drug's elimination half-life can be estimated from paired concentration measurements made during the initial dosing interval and the cumulation factor used to estimate eventual steady state levels (see Equation 13-12 in Chapter 13, Pharmacokinetics).

An important assumption used in this monitoring approach is direct proportionality of concentration to dose—the superposition principle. This assumption is only valid when the pharmacokinetic behavior of the drug is well described by a linear kinetic model. Although this is the case for many of the critical-dose drugs that are monitored, such as the aminoglycoside antibiotics and lithium, phenytoin is an important example of a drug that is eliminated by nonlinear kinetics (see Fig. 13-10 in Chapter 13, Pharmacokinetics). In this case, steady state concentrations measured at two different dose levels are needed to estimate the Michaelis-Menten parameters that characterize phenytoin elimination kinetics. Finally, these approaches are highly susceptible to error associated with preanalytic and analytic sources leading to poor precision in estimation.

Lithium. A group I metal, lithium shares chemical properties with sodium and potassium, and has a history of clinical use that dates back to the 19th century for the treatment of gout. Toxicity associated with its use eventually led to its disappearance from clinical medicine. It was resurrected in the 1940s as a possible salt substitute for individuals on a sodium-restricted diet; however, numerous cases of severe toxicity and death occurred, terminating this use as well.[47,48] Fortunately, lithium was again explored as a drug by John Cade, an Australian psychiatrist, who reported in 1949 that it had utility for the treatment of bipolar disorder[49] (see Chapter 53, Depression and Bipolar Disorder). Significant concerns of toxicity precluded its FDA approval for treatment of bipolar disorder for an additional 20 years. Currently, lithium is an important part of the drug armamentarium for the treatment of bipolar disorder.

Lithium is formulated predominantly as capsules containing lithium carbonate, although a lithium citrate liquid formulation is also available. The bioavailability of both preparations is virtually 100%; however, absorption is more rapid for the citrate compared with the carbonate form. The distribution of lithium is slow, and takes as long as 10 hours to reach completion. Lithium distributes primarily into the aqueous compartments of the body with little appreciable protein binding, and it dispays an apparent volume of distribution at steady state of 0.66 L/kg with a CV of 25%. Urinary excretion accounts for greater than 95% of Li^+ elimination. Li^+ is freely filterable by the glomerulus, similar to Na^+ and K^+, but approximately 80% of the filtered Li^+ is reabsorbed along with Na^+. Thus, Li^+ clearance is approximately 20% of creatinine clearance and the elimination half-life of serum Li^+ is approximately 22 hours. As a result, alterations in glomerular filtration rate (GFR) that occur secondary to age, drugs such as angiotensin-converting enzyme inhibitors, and disease have a significant impact on Li^+ clearance. States of reduced Na^+ clearance such as hypovolemia also reduce Li^+ clearance due both to reduced GFR and increased Na^+ and Li^+ reabsorption by the kidney. All of these factors lead to significant pharmacokinetic variability, both among different individuals, and occasionally within an individual. The relationship between serum Li^+ concentration and pharmacologic response has been examined for prophylactic therapy in bipolar disorder through several prospective concentration-controlled studies (see Sproule[50] for a detailed review of these studies). The general conclusion of these studies is that a serum Li^+ concentration above 0.7 mEq/ml is likely to be most effective; however, lithium may be effective at concentrations as low as 0.4 mEq/ml. In addition, higher concentrations, while more effective, also appear to produce greater toxicity (i.e., nausea, vomiting, tremor) that may lead to poorer adherence to therapy.[51]

Since lithium has significant pharmacokinetic variability and a very narrow therapeutic index but a clear concentration-response relationship for both efficacy and toxicity, monitoring serum Li^+ concentrations has become standard clinical practice. Several different approaches have been advocated for utilization of Li^+ concentration data in dose adjustment, but all rely on the superposition principle that is characteristic of drugs with linear elimination kinetics.[52] Since the rate of clearance of Li^+ via the kidneys is generally proportional to the lithium concentration in serum, the assumption of first-order elimination kinetics is fairly well supported for this drug. Thus, a 20% increase in dose should translate into a 20% increase in the serum Li^+ concentration at steady state.The optimal timing for measuring an individual's serum Li^+ concentration is commonly considered to be 10 to 12 hours after a dose, after the distribution phase has been completed. In patients on a twice-daily dosing regimen, this is most easily done immediately prior to the patient's morning dose.

Dose Prediction

One of the major pitfalls to the use of a single, timed drug level for the adjustment of drug dosing is the potential error associated with forecasting based upon a single measurement. In addition, patients are often treated with drugs during times when physiology is quite variable, such as the critically ill patient with an infection receiving an aminoglycoside antibiotic. Under these circumstances, a single concentration measurement usually does not possess sufficient information content to assess the adequacy of exposure or forecast future drug concentrations with dose changes.

Zaske-Sawchuk Method. In order to improve the precision of dose estimating based upon a monitored drug concentration, several pharmacokinetic-based methods have been developed to estimate patient-specific pharmacokinetic parameters utilizing two or more drug concentrations. The first-described and most simple of these methods as referred to as the Zaske-Sawchuk method.[53] Aminoglycosides have a narrow therapeutic index, and the major limitation to their use is renal and cochlear toxicity. The incidence of nephrotoxicity has been reported to range from approximately 2% to as high as 58% depending upon the patient populations evaluated and the criteria used to define changes in renal function. Ototoxicity is reported to occur in 2% to 10% of patients receiving aminoglycoside therapy. Toxicity is associated with several factors, including treatment duration, the average daily dose, peak drug concentration, and trough (predose) concentration. Unfortunately, the distribution and elimination of aminoglycoside antibiotics are variable among different individuals, precluding accurate prediction of drug concentration based upon dose alone[54-56] and therefore necessitating the use of TDM to individualize drug dosing.

Several retrospective studies have documented the correlation between gentamicin serum concentrations and clinical efficacy.[3,8,57-59] In all cases, C_{max} was found to be significantly correlated with treatment success. In addition to its correlation with efficacy, C_{max} also correlates with aminoglycoside toxicity. In a retrospective study that evaluated all of the patients who received gentamicin during clinical trials from 1962 to 1969, approximately half of the patients displaying ototoxicity (10 of 19 patients) had a serum gentamicin C_{max} of 8 mg/ml or higher, with 70% of patients who experienced toxicity demonstrating a C_{max} of 16 to 40 mg/ml.[60] A similar association was reported for amikacin with C_{max} greater than 32 mg/ml. While the C_{max} of aminoglycoside antibiotics correlates well with efficacy and ototoxicity, half of the patients with ototoxicity identified in this study still had serum concentrations less than 8 mg/ml. These patients therefore experienced toxicity despite serum concentrations within the targeted "therapeutic range" that is generally used for these drugs.

In addition to C_{max}, trough concentrations (C_0) for aminoglycoside antibiotics are also associated with toxicity, as revealed by a study showing that 36% of patients with C_0 greater than 2 mg/ml were found to have a rise in serum creatinine concentrations indicative of nephrotoxicity, whereas no patient with a C_0 less than 2 mg/ml developed a significant change in renal function.[61] While these retrospective data lend support to the hypothesis that allowing C_0 to fall below 2 mg/ml would significantly reduce the risk of nephrotoxicity from these drugs, the possibility that these elevated trough concentrations are merely a consequence of renal damage attributable to aminoglycoside use rather than its cause is equally plausible. A prospective trial comparing concentration-guided conventional aminoglycoside therapy to fixed, once-daily dosing revealed that toxicity was lower in the concentration-guided, conventional dosing study group, supporting that the retrospectively defined targets for C_{max} and C_0 are appropriate.[62]

Bayesian Methods. Although the Zaske-Sawchuk method has significantly improved the precision of therapy with aminoglycoside antibiotics and other drugs, numerous limitations still exist. Multiple concentration measurements are generally required for adequate confidence in parameter estimation, and many data are wasted. More importantly, multiple concentration measurements ignore prior information regarding parameter estimates that have been derived from prior population studies, as well as prior studies performed in a patient under evaluation.

Improved methods of parameter estimation that utilize Bayes' theorem have been developed in an attempt to overcome some of these limitations. Although beyond the scope of this chapter, Bayes' theorem provides a theoretical framework to relate the parameter estimates that are made from a set of concentration data to any prior information about these parameters. As a result, bayesian methods permit incorporation of prior concentration and parameter information into the estimation process. Numerous studies have demonstrated the improvement in precision of concentration control for many drugs, often with less available data; however, the question of whether bayesian methods improve clinical outcomes over simpler approaches still remains.

THE CLINICAL PHARMACOKINETICS SERVICE

Implementation of an effective TDM program typically involves several different disciplines within a health delivery system. These include physicians, nursing staff, the clinical laboratory, and often a clinical pharmacokinetics service generally composed of pharmacists with specialized expertise in applied pharmacokinetics. While some simple formulas and nomograms have been developed to help guide clinicians in applying TDM data, many of the approaches to TDM are complex, requiring thorough understanding of the principles underlying the approaches. This has led to the establishment in many health care systems of clinical pharmacokinetics services, which have been shown to improve clinical outcomes and reduce health care costs.[63,64] These integrated clinical services often provide 24-hour consultation on individualized drug therapy, and they have become a vital part of care in many settings, such as solid organ transplantation and oncology.

BIOMARKERS AND THE FUTURE OF TDM

The technological advances of the 1970s and 1980s in analytic measurement of drugs drove a revolution in our understanding of pharmacokinetics and the ways in which drugs are used, especially those with a low therapeutic index. The recent rise in genomics and proteomics technology has now set the stage for groundbreaking advances in our understanding of the pharmacokinetic and pharmacodynamic behavior of low therapeutic index drugs. It is anticipated that TDM over the next decade will progress from traditional pharmacokinetic approaches to more integrated pharmacokinetic-pharmacodynamic monitoring approaches that fine-tune a drug regimen through incorporation of newly identified genetic and protein biomarkers. The goals will remain the same: finding the right drug and regimen for a patient. The tools are simply evolving.

The use of biomarkers in the individualization of drug therapy is not a new concept. Creatinine is a well-known biomarker of GFR; estimated creatinine clearance is one of the most widely used biomarkers in medicine. Since renal clearance mechanisms play important roles in the elimination of many drugs, creatinine clearance estimates are valuable in determining the initial starting dose for critical-dose drugs such as the aminoglycoside antibiotics. Increases in serum creatinine are also a useful toxicity biomarker for nephrotoxic agents, such as the aminoglycoside antibiotics, tacrolimus, and cyclosporin A. Empirical

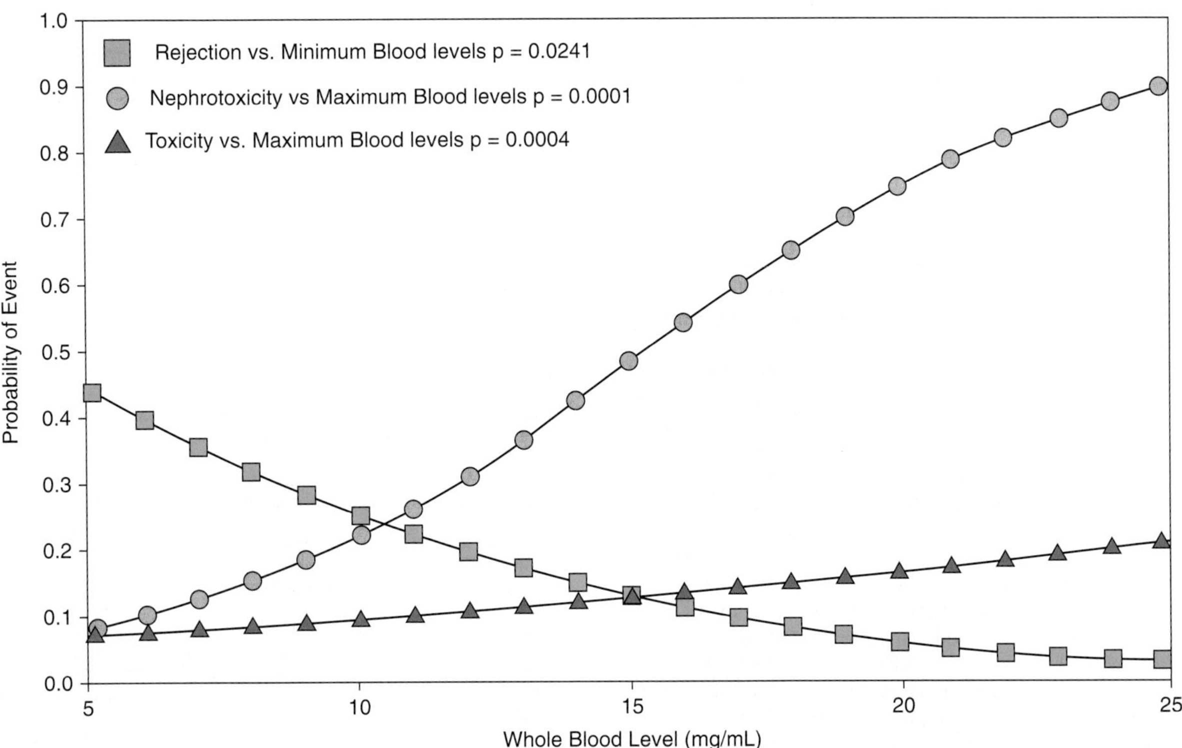

FIGURE 21-7 • The pharmacodynamics of tacrolimus in renal transplantation. (Adapted from Venkataramanan R, Shaw LM, Sarkozi L. Clinical utility of monitoring tacrolimus blood concentrations in liver transplant patients. J Clin Pharmacol 2001;41:542-551.)

modification of dosing based upon changes in serum creatinine along with serum concentration data plays an important part in the TDM for these drugs. Biomarkers are also widely used in the assessment of drug efficacy, such as blood glucose concentration and glycosylated hemoglobin for hypoglycemic agents or low-density lipoprotein cholesterol for statins.

Nevertheless, useful biomarkers are nonexistent for most drugs used in clinical practice, and an important challenge in TDM remains the identification of individualized therapeutic ranges. As discussed in the previous sections, most of the concentration ranges targeted for monitored drug therapy are derived from population-based outcome studies. Figure 21-7 illustrates the pharmacodynamic relationship for a population of kidney transplant recipients on tacrolimus. As is evident from the data, some individuals can tolerate relatively high concentrations of tacrolimus with minimal evidence of renal toxicity. Other patients may show a decline in renal function at concentrations below the targeted therapeutic range. In these patients, drug concentrations are typically modified downward using serum creatinine measurements as a guide. Unfortunately, efficacy is much more difficult to determine in a treated individual.

Several groups have sought biomarkers of effective immunosuppression to aid in individualizing therapy with immunosuppressive drugs. The ImmuKnow (Cylex, Columbia, MD) immune cell function assay, an FDA 510k cleared assay, attempts to assess cell-mediated immunity by measuring the production of ATP in $CD4^+$ cells following mitogen activation using a luciferase-based reaction.[65] Evaluation of this biomarker assay in a cohort of 155 healthy adults and 127 solid organ transplant recipients revealed that immune responsiveness of transplant recipients as assessed by the ImmuKnow assay is significantly reduced; however, significant overlap in the assay results for these two populations are evident. Interestingly, no correlation between the results of the ImmuKnow assay and tacrolimus trough concentrations was observed in this study.[66] Other assays also aimed at assessment of global immune function in transplant recipients have been described, including flow cytometric evaluation of cellular activation markers on immune cells, in vivo and in vitro cytokine levels, and cellular proliferation assays (for review, see Oellerich et al.[67]). More direct pharmacodynamic assays for the immunosuppressant mycophenolic acid (MPA) have been developed that measure the activity of inosine-5′-monophosphate dehydrogenase (IMPDH), the enzyme targeted by this drug.[68-70] Evaluation of healthy individuals using one of these assays reveals that IMPDH activity in human blood mononuclear cells is highly variable (34% to 45% CV), yet significant inhibition of activity is observed in transplant recipients following a single dose of the drug.[68,71] Interestingly, a follow-up study using this assay found that patients with low IMPDH activity before transplantation had a higher likelihood of requiring a dose reduction of mycophenolate mofetil (CellCept).[71] This result suggests that measurement of IMPDH may be helpful in defining an individualized therapeutic range for patients on MPA immunosuppression. Nevertheless, much work remains to determine whether any of these assays will help to individualize immunosuppressive drug therapy.

Another challenge that may be aided by biomarkers is the reality that patient response to drug therapy often cannot be determined until after one or more doses have been administered. This results in many failed regimens, sometimes with disastrous outcomes. Since genetics clearly plays important roles in both the pharmacokinetic and pharmacodynamic behavior of drugs, genetic biomarkers may provide a predictive basis for better initial selection of agents and dosing regimens that may minimize adverse effects and maximize therapeutic efficacy. The recent identification of genetic polymorphisms that impact the pharmacokinetics and pharmacodynamics of drugs such as antipsychotics,[72] warfarin,[73,74] and irinotecan[75] demonstrates the potential of this area. A recent study using microarray profiling of tumors to identify "transcriptional signatures" that distinguish tumors responsive to particular chemotherapeutic agents illustrates how advances in genomics and proteomics offer new and exciting opportunities for biomarker discovery and greater personalization of pharmacotherapy.[76]

CONCLUSIONS

A considerable body of published clinical study data exists that provides a strong foundation for individualizing drug therapy based on pharmacokinetic/pharmacodynamic data. Although delivery of fully personalized medicine is not yet possible, the advent of genomics, metabanomics, and the various other "-omics" technologies is rapidly expanding our understanding of the causes of human variation, especially in the area of pharmacology. This understanding is vital if we are going to build on current practice and deliver truly personalized medicine to our patients. The importance and significance of the contributions of each member of the multidisciplinary team (patient, physician, pharmacist, laboratorian, phlebotomist) to the best practice of therapeutic drug monitoring cannot be overstated, and the essential contribution of accurate and timely patient-specific information in an electronic form to facilitate patient-specific dosing should be very obvious to every prescriber in an era that has higher expectations of the health care delivery system.

REFERENCES

1. Burton ME, Shaw LM, Schentag JJ, Evans WE. Applied Pharmacokinetics & Pharmacodynamics: Principles of Therapeutic Drug Monitoring, 4th ed. Baltimore: Lippincott Williams & Wilkins, 2006.
2. Schumacher GE. Therapeutic Drug Monitoring. Norwalk, CT: Appleton & Lange, 1995.
3. Deziel-Evans LM, Murphy JE, Job ML. Correlation of pharmacokinetic indices with therapeutic outcome in patients receiving aminoglycosides. Clin Pharm 1986;5:319-324.
4. Evans WE, Crom WR, Abromowitch M, et al. Clinical pharmacodynamics of high-dose methotrexate in acute lymphocytic leukemia: identification of a relation between concentration and effect. N Engl J Med 1986;314:471-477.
5. Froscher W, Eichelbaum M, Gugler R, et al. A prospective randomised trial on the effect of monitoring plasma anticonvulsant levels in epilepsy. J Neurol 1981;224:193-201.
6. Gram LF. Plasma level monitoring of tricyclic antidepressants: methodological and pharmacokinetic considerations. Commun Psychopharmacol 1978;2:373-380.
7. Kragh S, Hansen CE, Baastrup PC, Hvidberg EF. Therapeutic control of plasma concentrations and long-term effect of nortriptyline in recurrent affective disorders. Pharmakopsychiatr Neuropsychopharmakol 1976;9:178-182.
8. Moore RD, Smith CR, Lietman PS. Association of aminoglycoside plasma levels with therapeutic outcome in gram-negative pneumonia. Am J Med 1984;77:657-662.
9. van Gelder T, Hilbrands LB, Vanrenterghem Y, et al. A randomized double-blind, multicenter plasma concentration controlled study of the safety and efficacy of oral mycophenolate mofetil for the prevention of acute rejection after kidney transplantation. Transplantation 1999;68:261-266.
10. Vozeh S, Kewitz G, Perruchoud A, et al. Theophylline serum concentration and therapeutic effect in severe acute bronchial obstruction: the optimal use of intravenously administered aminophylline. Am Rev Respir Dis 1982;125:181-184.
11. Frishman WH, Alwarshetty M. Beta-adrenergic blockers in systemic hypertension: pharmacokinetic considerations related to the current guidelines. Clin Pharmacokinet 2002;41:505-516.
12. Shaw LM, Kaplan B, Kaufman D. Toxic effects of immunosuppressive drugs: mechanisms and strategies for controlling them. Clin Chem 1996;42:1316-1321.
13. De Geest S, Borgermans L, Gemoets H, et al. Incidence, determinants, and consequences of subclinical noncompliance with immunosuppressive therapy in renal transplant recipients. Transplantation 1995;59:340-347.
14. Denhaerynck K, Steiger J, Bock A, et al. Prevalence and risk factors of non-adherence with immunosuppressive medication in kidney transplant patients. Am J Transplant 2007;7:108-116.
15. Kiley DJ, Lam CS, Pollak R. A study of treatment compliance following kidney transplantation. Transplantation 1993;55:51-56.
16. Russell CL, Conn VS, Ashbaugh C, et al. Medication adherence patterns in adult renal transplant recipients. Res Nurs Health 2006;29:521-532.
17. Hooper WD, Bochner F, Eadie MJ, Tyrer JH. Plasma protein binding of diphenylhydantoin: effects of sex hormones, renal and hepatic disease. Clin Pharmacol Ther 1974;15:276-282.

17a. Shoeman DW, Azarnoff DL. The alteration of plasma proteins in uremia as reflected in their ability to bind digitoxin and diphenylhydantoin. Pharmacology 1972;7:169-177.

18. Manninen V, Korhonen A. Inequal digoxin tablets [Letter]. Lancet 1973;2:1268.
19. D'Angio RG, Stevenson JG, Lively BT, Morgan JE. Therapeutic drug monitoring: improved performance through education intervention. Ther Drug Monit 1990;12:173-181.
20. McNaught AD, Wilkinson A. IUPAC Compendium of Chemical Terminology—The Gold Book, 2nd ed. Cambridge, England: Royal Society of Chemistry, 1997.
21. U.S. Food and Drug Administration. Guidance for Industry: Bioanalytical Method Validation. Center for Drug Evaluation, 2001. Available at *http://www.fda.gov/CDER/GUIDANCE/4252fnl.htm*
22. Pippenger CE, Penry JK, White BG, et al. Interlaboratory variability in determination of plasma antiepileptic drug concentrations. Arch Neurol 1976;33:351-355.
23. Shaikh IM, Lau BW, Siegfried BA, Valdes R Jr. Isolation of digoxin-like immunoreactive factors from mammalian adrenal cortex. J Biol Chem 1991;266:13672-13678.

24. Jortani SA, Valdes R Jr. Digoxin and its related endogenous factors. Crit Rev Clin Lab Sci 1997;34:225-274.
25. Burtis CA. Tietz Fundamentals of Clinical Chemistry, 6th ed. St. Louis: Elsevier Saunders, 2007.
26. Yalow RS, Berson SA. Assay of plasma insulin in human subjects by immunological methods. Nature 1959;184(Suppl 21):1648-1649.
27. Henderson DR, Friedman SB, Harris JD, et al. CEDIA, a new homogeneous immunoassay system. Clin Chem 1986;32:1637-1641.
28. Chabner B, Longo DL. Cancer Chemotherapy and Biotherapy: Principles and Practice, 4th ed. Philadelphia: Lippincott Williams & Wilkins, 2006.
29. Woods RL, Fox RM, Tattersall MH. Methotrexate treatment of squamous-cell head and neck cancers: dose-response evaluation. Br Med J (Clin Res Ed) 1981;282:600-602.
30. Delepine N, Delepine G, Cornille H, et al. Dose escalation with pharmacokinetics monitoring in methotrexate chemotherapy of osteosarcoma. Anticancer Res 1995;15:489-494.
31. Delepine N, Delepine G, Jasmin C, et al. Importance of age and methotrexate dosage: prognosis in children and young adults with high-grade osteosarcomas. Biomed Pharmacother 1988;42:257-262.
32. Evans WE, Pratt CB, Taylor RH, et al. Pharmacokinetic monitoring of high-dose methotrexate: early recognition of high-risk patients. Cancer Chemother Pharmacol 1979;3:161-166.
33. Evans WE, Relling MV, Rodman JH, et al. Conventional compared with individualized chemotherapy for childhood acute lymphoblastic leukemia. N Engl J Med 1998;338:499-505.
34. Isacoff WH, Morrison PF, Aroesty J, et al. Pharmacokinetics of high-dose methotrexate with citrovorum factor rescue. Cancer Treat Rep 1977;61:1665-1674.
35. Nirenberg A, Mosende C, Mehta BM, et al. High-dose methotrexate with citrovorum factor rescue: predictive value of serum methotrexate concentrations and corrective measures to avert toxicity. Cancer Treat Rep 1977;61:779-783.
36. Stoller RG, Hande KR, Jacobs SA, et al. Use of plasma pharmacokinetics to predict and prevent methotrexate toxicity. N Engl J Med 1977;297:630-634.
37. Gibbs JP, Gooley T, Corneau B, et al. The impact of obesity and disease on busulfan oral clearance in adults. Blood 1999;93:4436-4440.
38. Busulfex Product Information. Fremont, CA: PDL BioPharma, 2007.
39. Slattery JT, Risler LJ. Therapeutic monitoring of busulfan in hematopoietic stem cell transplantation. Ther Drug Monit 1998;20:543-549.
40. Vassal G, Fischer A, Challine D, et al. Busulfan disposition below the age of three: alteration in children with lysosomal storage disease. Blood 1993;82:1030-1034.
41. Dix SP, Wingard JR, Mullins RE, et al. Association of busulfan area under the curve with veno-occlusive disease following BMT. Bone Marrow Transplant 1996;17:225-230.
42. Grochow LB. Busulfan disposition: the role of therapeutic monitoring in bone marrow transplantation induction regimens. Semin Oncol 1993;20:18-25; quiz 26.
43. Grochow LB, Jones RJ, Brundrett RB, et al. Pharmacokinetics of busulfan: correlation with veno-occlusive disease in patients undergoing bone marrow transplantation. Cancer Chemother Pharmacol 1989;25:55-61.
44. Slattery JT, Sanders JE, Buckner CD, et al. Graft-rejection and toxicity following bone marrow transplantation in relation to busulfan pharmacokinetics. Bone Marrow Transplant 1995;16:31-42.
45. Slattery JT, Clift RA, Buckner CD, et al. Marrow transplantation for chronic myeloid leukemia: the influence of plasma busulfan levels on the outcome of transplantation. Blood 1997;89:3055-3060.
46. Bolinger AM, Zangwill AB, Slattery JT, et al. Target dose adjustment of busulfan in pediatric patients undergoing bone marrow transplantation. Bone Marrow Transplant 2001;28:1013-1018.
47. Hanlon LW, Romaine M, Gilroy FJ. Lithium chloride as a substitute for sodium chloride in the diet. J Am Med Assoc 1949;139:688-692.
48. Talbott JH. Use of lithium salts as a substitute for sodium chloride. AMA Arch Intern Med 1950;85:1-10.
49. Cade JFJ. Lithium salts in the treatment of psychotic excitement. Med J Aust 1949;2:349-352.
50. Sproule B. Lithium in bipolar disorder: can drug concentrations predict therapeutic effect? Clin Pharmacokinet 2002;41:639-660.
51. Gelenberg AJ, Kane JM, Keller MB, et al. Comparison of standard and low serum levels of lithium for maintenance treatment of bipolar disorder. N Engl J Med 1989;321:1489-1493.
52. Gibaldi M, Perrier D. Pharmacokinetics, 2nd ed. New York: Marcel Dekker, 1982.
53. Sawchuk RJ, Zaske DE. Pharmacokinetics of dosing regimens which utilize multiple intravenous infusions: gentamicin in burn patients. J Pharmacokinet Biopharm 1976;4:183-195.
54. Kaye D, Levison ME, Labovitz ED. The unpredictability of serum concentrations of gentamicin: pharmacokinetics of gentamicin in patients with normal and abnormal renal function. J Infect Dis 1974;130:150-154.
55. Barza M, Brown RB, Shen D, et al. Predictability of blood levels of gentamicin in man. J Infect Dis 1975;132:165-174.
56. Gyselynck AM, Forrey A, Cutler R. Pharmacokinetics of gentamicin: distribution and plasma and renal clearance. J Infect Dis 1971;124(Suppl):S70-S76.
57. Noone P, Parsons TM, Pattison JR, et al. Experience in monitoring gentamicin therapy during treatment of serious gram-negative sepsis. Br Med J 1974;1:477-481.
58. Anderson ET, Young LS, Hewitt WL. Simultaneous antibiotic levels in "breakthrough" gram-negative rod bacteremia. Am J Med 1976;61:493-497.
59. Moore RD, Lietman PS, Smith CR. Clinical response to aminoglycoside therapy: importance of the ratio of peak concentration to minimal inhibitory concentration. J Infect Dis 1987;155:93-99.
60. Jackson GG, Arcieri G. Ototoxicity of gentamicin in man: a survey and controlled analysis of clinical experience in the United States. J Infect Dis 1971;124(Suppl):S130-S137.
61. Dahlgren JG, Anderson ET, Hewitt WL. Gentamicin blood levels: a guide to nephrotoxicity. Antimicrob Agents Chemother 1975;8:58-62.
62. Bartal C, Danon A, Schlaeffer F, et al. Pharmacokinetic dosing of aminoglycosides: a controlled trial. Am J Med 2003;114:194-198.
63. Whiting B, Kelman AW, Bryson SM, et al. Clinical pharmacokinetics: a comprehensive system for therapeutic drug monitoring and prescribing. Br Med J (Clin Res Ed) 1984;288:541-545.
64. Destache CJ. Clinical and economic benefits of a clinical pharmacokinetic service: 1987 versus 1992 data. Med Interface 1994;7:84-86, 89-90.
65. Wier ML. Methods for measurement of lymphocyte function. Washington, DC: U.S. Patent Office, 1998.
66. Kowalski R, Post D, Schneider MC, et al. Immune cell function testing: an adjunct to therapeutic drug monitoring in transplant patient management. Clin Transplant 2003;17:77-88.
67. Oellerich M, Barten MJ, Armstrong VW. Biomarkers: the link between therapeutic drug monitoring and pharmacodynamics. Ther Drug Monit 2006;28:35-38.
68. Glander P, Braun KP, Hambach P, et al. Non-radioactive determination of inosine 5′-monophosphate dehydrogenase (IMPDH) in peripheral mononuclear cells. Clin Biochem 2001;34:543-549.
69. Langman LJ, LeGatt DF, Yatscoff RW. Pharmacodynamic assessment of mycophenolic acid-induced immunosuppression by measuring IMP dehydrogenase activity. Clin Chem 1995;41:295-299.
70. Albrecht W, Storck M, Pfetsch E, et al. Development and application of a high-performance liquid chromatography-based assay for determination of the activity of inosine 5′-monophosphate dehydrogenase in whole blood and isolated mononuclear cells. Ther Drug Monit 2000;22:283-294.
71. Glander P, Hambach P, Braun KP, et al. Pre-transplant inosine monophosphate dehydrogenase activity is associated with clinical outcome after renal transplantation. Am J Transplant 2004;4:2045-2051.
72. Malhotra AK, Murphy GM Jr., Kennedy JL. Pharmacogenetics of psychotropic drug response. Am J Psychiatry 2004;161:780-796.
73. Rieder MJ, Reiner AP, Gage BF, et al. Effect of VKORC1 haplotypes on transcriptional regulation and warfarin dose. N Engl J Med 2005;352:2285-2293.
74. Higashi MK, Veenstra DL, Kondo LM, et al. Association between CYP2C9 genetic variants and anticoagulation-related outcomes during warfarin therapy. JAMA 2002;287:1690-1698.
75. Innocenti F, Undevia SD, Iyer L, et al. Genetic variants in the UDP-glucuronosyltransferase 1A1 gene predict the risk of severe neutropenia of irinotecan. J Clin Oncol 2004;22:1382-1388.
76. Potti A, Dressman HK, Bild A, et al. Genomic signatures to guide the use of chemotherapeutics. Nat Med 2006;12:1294-1300.

Part II

Practice

SECTION 5 Cardiovascular Therapeutics
22 Hypertension
23 Dyslipidemias
24 Coronary Artery Disease
25 Rhythm Disorders
26 Heart Failure

SECTION 6 Pulmonary Therapeutics
27 Pulmonary Arterial Hypertension
28 Asthma and Chronic Obstructive Pulmonary Disease

SECTION 7 Renal Therapeutics
29 Renal Insufficiency
30 Voiding Dysfunction

SECTION 8 Gastroenterologic Therapeutics
31 Acid Reflux and Ulcer Disease
32 Motility Disorders
33 Inflammatory Bowel Diseases
34 Hepatic Cirrhosis
35 Infectious Hepatitis

SECTION 9 Endocrinologic Therapeutics
36 Obesity and Nutrition
37 Diabetes Mellitus
38 Disorders of the Thyroid
39 Disorders of Calcium Metabolism and Bone Mineralization
40 Disorders of the Hypothalamic-Pituitary Axis
41 Adrenal Disorders
42 Reproductive Health

SECTION 10 Neuropharmacologic Therapeutics
43 Alzheimer's Disease and Dementias
44 Parkinson's Disease
45 Seizure Disorders
46 Multiple Sclerosis
47 Dysautonomias
48 Headache
49 Stroke

SECTION 11 Psychopharmacologic Therapeutics
50 Obsessive-Compulsive Disorders
51 Attention-Deficit/Hyperactivity Disorder
52 Anxiety
53 Depression and Bipolar Disorders
54 Psychosis and Schizophrenia
55 Drug Addiction
56 Nicotine Dependence
57 Insomnia (Narcolepsy)-Related Disorders

SECTION 12 Ophthalmologic Therapeutics
58 Drugs in Ophthalmology

SECTION 13 Anesthesia
59 Local Anesthesia
60 General Anesthesia and Sedation
61 Treatment of Pain

SECTION 14 Hematologic Therapeutics
62 Anemias and Cytopenias
63 Disorders of Hemostasis and Thrombosis

SECTION 15 Oncologic Therapeutics
64 Lung Cancer
65 Breast Cancer
66 Hematologic Malignancies
67 Prostate Cancer
68 Colon Cancer
69 Melanoma

SECTION 16 Dermatologic Therapeutics
70 Acne
71 Psoriasis
72 Dermatitis

SECTION 17 Rheumatologic Therapeutics
73 Osteoarthritis
74 Rheumatoid Arthritis
75 Gout
76 Systemic Lupus Erythematosus

SECTION 18 Therapy of Infectious Diseases
77 Influenza and Viral Respiratory Infections
78 Community-Acquired Pneumonia
79 Tuberculosis
80 Bacterial Meningitis
81 Endocarditis
82 Malaria
83 Protozoan and Helminthic Infections
84 HIV Infection and AIDS
85 Sexually Transmitted Diseases

SECTION 19 Practical Therapeutics
86 Medical Toxicology and Antidotes
87 Over-the-Counter Medications
88 Prescription and Order Writing
89 Pharmacy and Therapeutics Committees and The Hospital Formulary

SECTION 20 Emerging Therapeutics
90 Complementary and Alternative Medicine, Nutraceuticals, and Dietary Supplements
91 Vaccines
92 Transplant Medicine
93 Gene Therapy
94 Regenerative Medicine and Stem Cell Therapeutics

22

HYPERTENSION

Jean-Luc Elghozi, Michel Azizi, and Pierre-François Plouin

INTRODUCTION 291
EPIDEMIOLOGY 291
Hypertension as a Modifiable Risk Factor 291
Definition and Prevalence of Hypertension 291
PATHOPHYSIOLOGY OF HYPERTENSION 292
Genetic Factors 292
Acquired Factors 292
Hemodynamic Aspects 292
The Kidney and Ionic Metabolism 292
Vascular Anomalies 293
Neural and Hormonal Control 293
Vascular Reactivity 294
Hyperinsulinism, Insulin Resistant, and Primary Hypertension 294
SECONDARY HYPERTENSION AND REVERSIBLE HYPERTENSION 294
Monogenic Hypertension 294
Iatrogenic Hypertension 295
Alcohol 295
Oral Contraceptives 295
Licorice 295
Sympathomimetics 295
Corticosteroids and Nonsteroidal Anti-Inflammatory Drugs 295
Agents Rarely Involved 295
Hypertension with Renal Artery Stenosis 295
Adrenal Hypertension 295
Primary Hyperaldosteronism 295
Pheochromocytoma 296
Cushing's Syndrome 296
Rare Causes of Reversible Hypertension 296
THERAPEUTIC APPROACH AND PATIENT FOLLOW-UP 296
Decision Thresholds and Delays in the Decision to Treat 296
Nonpharmacologic Measures or Lifestyle Modifications 296
Pharmacologic Treatment 296
Results from Clinical Trials 296
Choice of Initial Drug Therapy 297
Classes of Antihypertensive Drugs 297
Synergistic Associations 298
Associated Treatments 298
BP Goals 298
Resistant Hypertension 299
Strategy of Hypertension Care Outside of an Emergency 299
Hypertensive Emergencies 299

INTRODUCTION

Hypertension is a worldwide disorder which affects more than one in every six adults. It is a major cause of cardiovascular mortality in all countries. Hypertension also is a major risk factor in atherosclerotic complications and is recognized as a foremost cause of morbidity, especially in the increasingly important and numerous elderly population. A development of great importance to world health has been the demonstration that many of the major complications associated with hypertension are preventable by antihypertensive drug treatment. The present chapter has a major emphasis on pathophysiological mechanisms of hypertension and relates the clinical pharmacological and therapeutic aspects to these.

EPIDEMIOLOGY

Hypertension as a Modifiable Risk Factor

Arterial hypertension is defined by chronically elevated blood pressure (BP). It was the first quantifiable condition, identified in surveys on mortality by an American insurance company, that showed a statistical relation between the initial BP and the subsequent risk of cerebral stroke, cardiac failure, and myocardial infarction. In the 40- to 69-year-old age group, a 20 mm Hg increase in systolic BP or a 10 mm Hg increase in diastolic BP is associated with more than double the risk of mortality from stroke and double the risk of mortality from myocardial infarction or other cardiovascular complications (e.g., cardiac failure, aneurysms).[1] Controlled trials have shown that the cardiovascular risk associated with hypertension is largely reversible by treatment.[2]

Definition and Prevalence of Hypertension

The risk of cardiovascular complication is as increased as BP is high and as reduced as BP is low; the risk is a continuing function of BP. Consequently, it is artificial to distinguish one hypertensive population from another normotensive one because these two populations are in continuum. Nevertheless, this artifice is necessary in clinical practice, which addresses individuals and not groups.

As for all quantifiable disease states (another example being hypercholesterolemia), the prevalence of hypertension depends on the method of measurement and the diagnostic threshold. The reference method to measure BP is a clinical measurement—a measure obtained by a doctor or a nurse using a mercury sphygmomanometer or an automatic validated monitor. Exposure to a startle reaction in an isolated measurement transitorily elevates BP and can lead to an overestimation of the prevalence of hypertension in the population. The current recommendations underline the necessity of repeated measurements over several consultations and separated by some months (when the first measurement is a systolic BP of 140-179 mm Hg or a diastolic BP of 90-109 mm Hg) or over several days (in rarer cases in which the initial BP is 180/110 mm Hg or higher).

The artifice, consisting of an agreed threshold of BP to diagnose hypertension, has a direct influence on the prevalence of hypertension diagnosed. In the 1980s, this threshold was 160/95 mm Hg. Currently, it is an average BP, established by repeated clinical measurements, of 140/90 mm Hg or higher. In the American population during the Third National Health and Nutrition Examination Survey (NHANES III) inquiry, the prevalence of hypertension in men aged 18 to 74 years was 14.7% or 22.8%, according to those who used either the 160/95 mm Hg or the 140/90 mm Hg threshold, which were modified over the course of the inquiry.[3] Current conventions have determined the prevalence of hypertension in the Western adult population to be 20% or greater. The reduction in the diagnostic threshold of hypertension and the increased apparent prevalence are not the consequence of arbitrary inflation. They are justified by the demonstrated benefit of antihypertensive treatment in terms of cardiovascular prevention, at least in certain subgroups of patients, from the threshold of 140/90 mm Hg.

The alternatives to isolated clinical measurements (ambulatory measurements over 12 or 24 hr or at-home self-measurements allowing for at least four measurements each day over a minimum of 4 days) are currently being evaluated. According to these measurements, for diurnal values, the threshold for diagnosis of hypertension is 135/85 mm Hg. However, the threshold for justifying the start of treatment has not yet been determined.

PATHOPHYSIOLOGY OF HYPERTENSION

Genetic Factors

Predisposition to primary (or essential) hypertension is established by BP familial resemblance and the high level of concordance between monozygotic twins. Around 30% of individual BP variation is genetically determined. Some rare forms of hypertension are monogenic, but the predisposition to essential hypertension (EH) is polygenic. Among the genes possibly implicated are those encoding for angiotensinogen, alpha-adducin, or the angiotensin II AT_1 receptor.[4] The polygenic character of EH has led to the development of genetically determined experimental models of hypertension by selecting for hypertensive animals from consecutive crosses. From their youngest age, the Japanese strain of spontaneously hypertensive rats (SHRs) has a higher BP than their strain of reference; this is similar to clinical observations of elevated BP in children of hypertensive parents. The effect on target organs is detected early, and an increased risk of cardiovascular mortality characterizes this strain. Thus, the numerous studies necessary for the comprehension of this phenomenon observed in humans have been realized in these animals. Before antihypertensive drugs were used in humans, they were tested experimentally in SHRs.[5]

Acquired Factors

Multiple concurrent anomalies raise BP, and EH must be considered a multifactorial disease. This notion, developed by Irvine Page (Fig. 22-1), explains why it is misleading to search for one cause of EH.[6] To optimize antihypertensive treatment, it is more appropriate to search for predominant alterations.

Hemodynamic Aspects

Poiseuille's law states that the mean BP is equal to the product of cardiac output times the total peripheral resistance. An increase in cardiac output is frequently observed in young people with hypertension. Over time, this cardiac output normalizes, and an increase in peripheral resistance maintains the elevation in BP. It has been suggested that the initial anomaly of EH is increased cardiac output. Increased cardiac output would be responsible for an increased tissue perfusion. An autoregulatory process would then decrease this perfusion by increasing arteriolar resistance. This is being debated today; the consensus is that there is a default in vasomotor control, including an endothelial dysfunction.[7] This anomaly translates into a more marked increase of vascular resistance in response to a vasoconstrictor constraint (e.g., the cold) and, similarly, a failure of vasodilation (e.g., to acetylcholine) than is seen in normotensive subjects. A decrease in total blood volume is observed in stable adult EH, which is explained by a reduced compliance of the arterial and venous system.

The Kidney and Ionic Metabolism

The kidney plays a determining role in the occurrence of EH. Replacing the kidneys of a genetically hypertensive animal with those of a normotensive animal corrects the EH of the recipient. Similarly, a kidney transplant from an animal with a genetic predisposition to EH (before hypertension even develops) to a normotensive recipient confers this predisposition to EH, associated with salt and water retention, to the latter. Renal blood flow is significantly reduced as early as the onset of EH. The increased renal resistance largely surpasses the increased resistance of other vascular beds in the advanced stage of EH, suggesting an anomaly in the renal vessels. The glomerular filtration rate is normal in the early phase of EH but decreases over time. The nature of intrinsic renal alteration in EH remains to be determined. An anomaly of sodium excretion, a deficit of vasodilator hormones, or an excess of pressor hormones is suggested. A reduction in the surface area of glomeruli could contribute to EH; this reduction would be associated with an increased sensitivity to salt. The anomaly of sodium excretion could also be of renal tubular origin.

Anomalies of Sodium Excretion. In humans, as in other mammals, salt intake leads to EH only if the capacity of renal excretion is altered.[8] In normal humans, the possibility of excretion extrapolated from experimental data is close to 200 g/day. This excretion capacity is reduced only in cases of reduced nephron capacity or when the sodium

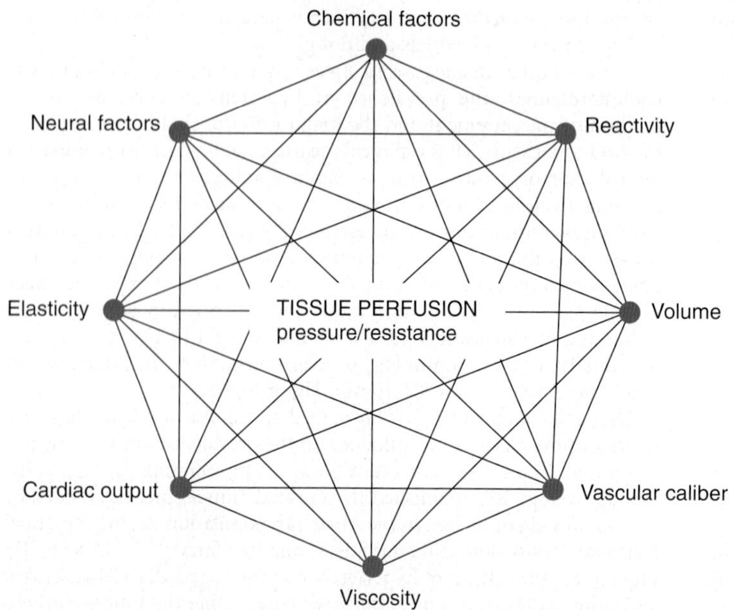

FIGURE 22-1 • Page's mosaic theory of hypertension. (Adapted from Page IH. The mosaic theory of arterial hypertension—its interpretation. Perspect Biol Med 1967;10:325–333.)

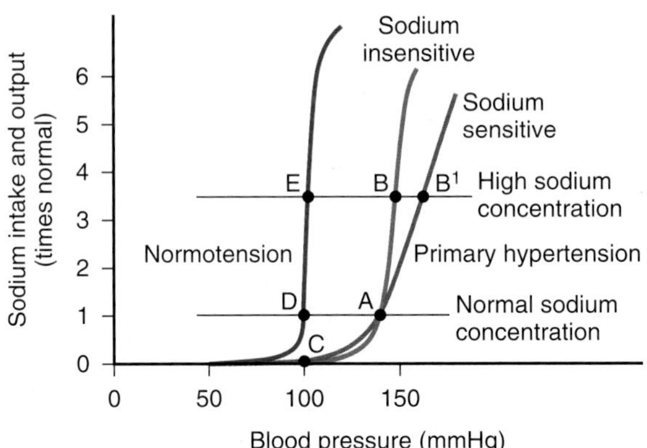

FIGURE 22-2 • Pressure-natriuresis curve. (Adapted from Guyton AC, Coleman TG, Young DB, et al. Salt balance and long-term blood pressure control. Annu Rev Med 1980;31:15-27.)

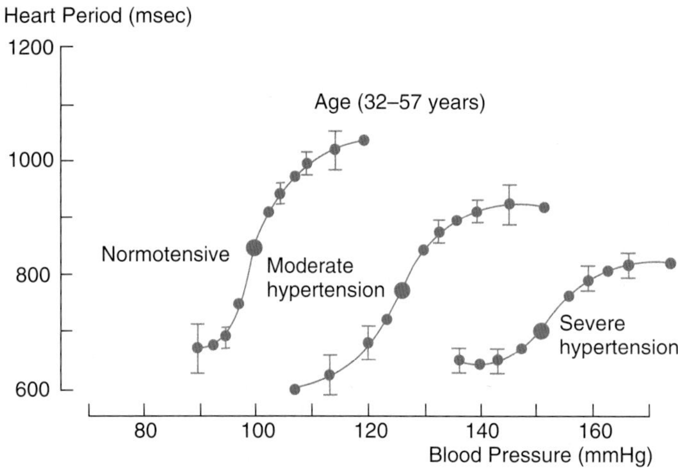

FIGURE 22-3 • Baroreflex sensitivity and the level of BP. (Adapted from Korner PI, West MJ, Shaw J, Uther JB. "Steady-state" properties of the baroreceptor-heart rate reflex in essential hypertension in man. Clin Exp Pharmacol Physiol 1974;1:65-76.)

intake is increased in conjunction with the addition of a mineralocorticoid (as with the experimental model associating deoxycorticosterone acetate, unilateral nephrectomy, and salty drinking water). An excessive intake of salt is not sufficient to cause hypertension. However, this does not prevent the observable positive relationship between BP and the intake of sodium in the general population. It is estimated that a reduction of sodium intake of 100 mmol/day (6 g/day; a population like ours consumes, on average, 10 g/day) prevents an increase of 9 mm Hg between the ages of 25 and 55.

A particular sensitivity to salt can lead to increased BP in response to increased sodium intake. Dahl salt-sensitive rats have this tendency, with vasoconstriction resulting from an increase in sodium intake, whereas salt-insensitive rats respond by vasodilation. This susceptibility to salt is also found in certain people with EH; a substantial reduction in sodium content may be effective. The genetic basis of this susceptibility is yet to be determined. Nevertheless, people with EH can eliminate acute sodium loading more rapidly than normal subjects can. This difference in people with EH is explained by a marked decrease in sympathetic tone (of reflex origin) in response to sodium loading and by the secretion of atrial natriuretic peptide (ANP).

Pressure-Natriuresis Curve. Blood volume is reduced more in EH than in normotension because of a reduction in arterial and especially venous vascular compliance. Nevertheless, the blood volume in people with hypertension remains ill adapted and too high for the level of BP. In the end, this relative increase in blood volume causes natriuresis. The pressure-natriuresis curve of EH is shifted to the right in relation to that of normotensive subjects such that the level of BP required to balance the excretion of sodium with the intake of sodium is elevated (Fig. 22-2).

This displacement of the pressure-natriuresis curve could be due to neural-hormonal factors (catecholamines, vasopressin, angiotensin II, mineralocorticoids) or an intrinsic renal default (potentially implicating nitric oxide [NO]). Thus, hypertension compensates only for a default in sodium excretion.[9] Figure 22-2 shows the difference in the curve according to whether the subject is resistant or sensitive to salt. When a subject is sensitive to salt, the increase in BP required to excrete excessive salt is significant and results in a weak pressure-natriuresis gradient. Therefore, to induce hypertension, a circulatory anomaly must, in parallel, reduce the capacity of sodium excretion (which results in a shift toward the right of the pressure-natriuresis curve). Conversely, to be effective, antihypertensive treatment must shift this curve toward the left.

Metabolism of Potassium, Calcium, and Magnesium Ions. Potassium supplementation moderately lowers BP by different mechanisms: a direct vasodilator effect, a direct or an indirect natriuretic effect (implying an increase in the synthesis of renal kallikrenin, itself responsible for the synthesis of bradykinin, a vasodilator and natriuretic peptide), and an increased sensitivity of arterial baroreceptors. Calcium deficiency has a deleterious role in hypertension, particularly in groups at risk (people sensitive to salt with hypertension, older people with hypertension, African Americans, pregnant women, diabetic patients, and alcoholics). Calcium intake enhances the secretion of a vasodilator peptide, calcitonin gene–related peptide (CGRP), and reduces the secretion of a parathyroid pressor factor. The reduction of extracellular magnesium provokes vasoconstriction and potentiates the pressor effects of angiotensin II and noradrenalin.

Vascular Anomalies

Primary hypertension is characterized by a rarefaction of microvessels and the thickening of arteries and arteriolar tissue. This thickening arises from an increase in volume (hypertrophy) and number (hyperplasia) of smooth muscle cells, combined with an increase in the extracellular matrix, particularly collagen, which causes rigidity.[10] These anomalies raise peripheral resistance, decreasing the vascular lumen and increasing the reactivity to vasoconstrictor stimuli.[11] They also affect the large arterial trunks (e.g., aorta, radial artery). Lowering arterial distensibility results in a limitation of the buffering function of the large trunks during systole. Moreover, the speed of pulse waves increases if the arteries are more rigid and the wave reflections occur more prematurely, which in itself adds to some systolic elevation in BP. These early alterations depend on a combination of factors: sympathetic hyperactivity, trophic effects of angiotensin II, and genetic predisposition.

Neural and Hormonal Control

Sympathetic Nervous System and Baroreflex Anomalies. The sympathetic nervous system is involved in the development of EH.[8,12] Early renal sympathetic denervation slows the appearance of hypertension in SHRs and increases sodium excretion but does not affect BP in adult SHRs. In addition, in humans, adrenaline increases BP by facilitating noradrenergic transmission through activation of β-adrenergic receptors situated on sympathetic terminals and in contact with the arterioles. This mechanism contributes to increased arterial resistance and constitutes one of the mechanisms affected by antihypertensive β-blockers. Sympathetic nervous discharge is elevated in EH, and the pharmacologic lowering of sympathetic activity translates into a proportional lowering of BP. Elevated pressure is accompanied by a readjustment of the baroreflex to a higher setpoint, which maintains short-term regulation of BP. However, a decrease in sensitivity of the baroreflex limits the capacity of the organism to compensate for sharp changes in BP[13] (Fig. 22-3). This observation could reflect an altered transduction in nervous discharges to distention, due to the changing mechanical properties of the artery walls in barosensitive zones (carotid sinus, aortic arch). The so-called low-pressure baroreflex, involving cardiopulmonary baroreceptors of the low-pressure system, is stimulated by a reduced vascular compliance in EH. This phenomenon tends to oppose sympathetic hyperactivity.

The Renin-Angiotensin System and Other Vasoconstrictors. The renin-angiotensin system (RAS) plays a major role in the physiologic regulation of BP and hydromineral metabolism. An increase in renin secretion, the enzyme that generates angiotensin I from angiotensinogen, can induce hypertension.[14] Nevertheless, plasma concentrations of renin measured during the course of EH are continuously distributed. Certain people with hypertension have elevated renin (high-renin hypertension) and are more sensitive to RAS blockers. Conversely, low levels of renin can be the consequence of an increase in volume related to excess mineralocorticoid secretion, explaining the marked effect of aldosterone antagonists. The hypertensive response to diuretics is also marked in this subpopulation. Blocking the RAS with angiotensin-converting enzyme (ACE) inhibitors and angiotensin receptor antagonists (ARAs) has become a major therapeutic approach in medicine. ACE inhibitors are used to test the hypothesis that the RAS participates in the regulation of BP dependent on sodium balance and can have a particular vasculotoxic role. Numerous mechanisms can contribute to the beneficial effects of RAS blockers: neutralization of the hemodynamic effect of angiotensin II and of its tissue effects on the generation of growth factors, free radicals, and fibrosis mediators.

Other vasoconstricting agents such as vasopressin, endothelin, thromboxane A_2, and serotonin may play a role in the development of hypertension or severe hypertension. Their role in maintaining the BP elevated in EH is not dominant.

Vasodilation Systems. Urinary excretion of kallikrein is reduced in EH. A failure in the synthesis of vasodilator prostaglandins (prostaglandin E_2 [PGE_2], prostacyclin) is also observed in EH. However, a causal link between these observations and hypertension has not been demonstrated. An acute secretion of ANP can be observed in EH, which reflects a compensatory mechanism of hypertension. It results from an increased arterial distention due to decreased peripheral venous compliance. Conversely, the response to an acute arterial distention is not accompanied by a sufficient secretion of ANP. Brain natriuretic peptide is reduced in EH, even before the onset of hypertension. Renal dopaminergic deficits have been associated with hypersensitivity to exogenous dopamine, which induces increases in renal blood flow, glomerular filtration, and sodium excretion in EH than is seen in normotensive subjects. CGRP is a vasodilator (as discussed previously). Adrenomedullin, principally of adrenal medullar origin, has a structural similarity to CGRP. It provokes vasodilation by direct effects on specific receptors linked with cyclic adenosine monophosphate (cAMP) and indirectly by stimulation of NO synthesis.

Vascular Reactivity

The imbalance between vasodilation and vasoconstriction systems has not been clearly established. However, an anomaly of vascular reactivity is implicated. Secondary structural alterations to this increase in BP thicken vascular walls and amplify this reactivity.

Functional Modification of Smooth Muscle Fibers. Ionic transport anomalies have been described in EH, owing to the heterogeneity of populations and investigatory techniques. Alterations of several ionic transporters may reflect a global alteration of membranes affecting phospholipids. The function of cellular calcium expelling calcium-ATPase would then be reduced in hypertension. An anomaly of Na^+-K^+-Ca^{2+} cotransport would also result. The Na^+-K^+-ATPase pump would be inhibited by an ouabain-like circulating factor, which generates a vascular fiber hypercontractility. This blockade in effect increases intracellular sodium, which decreases the sodium/calcium exchange and increases cytosolic calcium concentration, the source of the contraction.

Endothelium-Dependent Vasomotricity Anomalies. In EH, a decrease in brachial arterial vasodilation can be observed, induced by either acetylcholine or an increase in flow. This fault is found again in experimental models of hypertension and correlates with the level of BP. In rats having undergone aortic coarctation, the endothelium-dependent vasodilation is preserved following stenosis, implying that this anomaly is more of a consequence than a cause of hypertension. Nevertheless, less NO is produced by the endothelium in EH, favoring vasoconstriction.

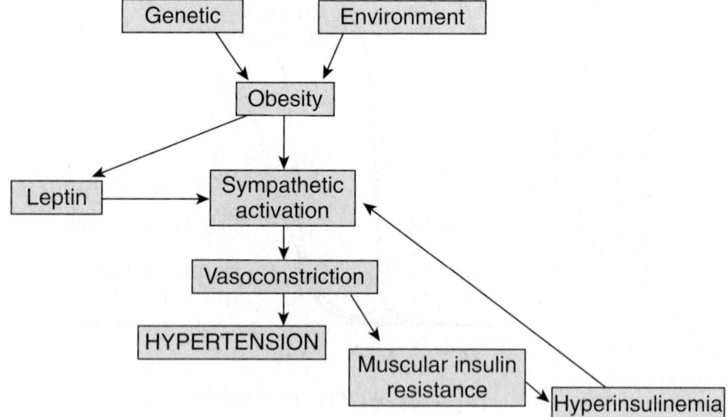

FIGURE 22-4 • Links to arterial hypertension in obesity.

Different factors generating vasoconstriction involve the endothelium. Endothelin is a powerful vasoconstrictor, but its secretion is not clearly increased in hypertension and is reserved more for conditions of "endothelial stress" (e.g., septic shock). In vasoconstriction, PGH_2, an endothelial vasoconstrictor, is produced in excess and contributes to the unbalancing of endothelial function. PGH_2 adds to platelet activation, resulting in accumulated aggregation to the endothelium. Serotonin, a powerful platelet vasoconstrictor, has also been proposed to play a role in EH. Normalization of BP with antihypertensive drugs restores endothelial function and vasomotricity.

Hyperinsulinism, Insulin Resistant, and Primary Hypertension (Fig. 22-4)

Hyperinsulinism associated with being overweight (metabolic syndrome) can precede EH.[15] Correction through weight reduction or the administration of somatostatin (blocking the secretion of insulin) lowers BP. At the same time, a correction of vasomotor function is noticed. This insulin resistance may be the consequence of chronic sympathetic activation. Sympathetic activation generates vasoconstriction and, secondarily, a thickening of arterioles, which leads to less muscle perfusion. Consequently, muscle use of glucose is reduced because fast-contracting fibers become less sensitive to insulin owing to β-adrenergic hyperactivity. The pancreas responds by acute secretion of insulin. Sympathetic activation observed in the obese patient could, in certain cases, result from a cerebral action of leptin, secreted in excess by adipocytes.[16]

SECONDARY HYPERTENSION AND REVERSIBLE HYPERTENSION

In a minority of cases, hypertension is the sign of an underlying renal, renovascular, or adrenal disease. Cases of secondary hypertension have a determined cause but are not necessarily reversible. The most frequent cases are linked to irreversible nephropathies—glomerulopathies, polycystic kidneys, and other nephropathies with renal failure. Some nephropathies are spontaneously reversible (acute postinfectious glomerulonephritis) or due to specific treatment (rapidly progressing glomerulonephritis sensitive to corticotherapy possibly combined with immunosuppressor treatment). In practice, however, cases of potentially reversible hypertension are forms for which specific treatment exists.

A potentially reversible hypertension is not necessarily reversed by specific treatment, either from the failure of the procedure or because the hypertension persists despite the success of the procedure. Probability of recovery is linked to age; the level of success decreases with increased age.[17]

Monogenic Hypertension

Other than monogenic diseases with pheochromocytoma (see later), these exceptional cases, often diagnosed in childhood, are not discussed here: deficits in 11β- or 17α-hydroxylases, apparent mineralocorticoid excess, family hyperaldosteronism, and Liddle and Gordon syndromes.

Iatrogenic Hypertension

Certain substances have a direct pressor effect; others reduce the efficacy of antihypertensives and can induce resistance to treatment. A systematic search for their presence is necessary. Diagnosis and treatment of iatrogenic hypertension require removing the exposure to pressor agents whenever possible.

Alcohol

Excessive consumption of alcohol (more than two alcoholic drinks per day) is liable to induce elevated BP, resistance to treatment, or poor compliance. This increases the risk of stroke. It can also lead to a significant calcium increase, induce obesity, and aggravate diabetes. Otherwise, severe hypertension can appear during sudden alcohol withdrawal, but this recedes in several days if the intake of alcoholic drinks is gradually reduced.

Oral Contraceptives

Surveillance of BP while the patient is taking contraceptive estrogens should be systematic. This method of contraception includes a weak but detectable elevation of BP, which generally stays within normal limits. Some patients, in particular those who are overweight or have a family history of hypertension, develop hypertension. Conversely, cases of preeclampsia or hypertension during pregnancy are not related to the development of hypertension while the patient is on the pill. An association with renal anomalies probably increases susceptibility to hypertension. Therefore, it is possible to detect renal arterial fibromuscular dysplasia or a segmented renal hypoplasia in patients who develop severe hypertension while on synthetic estrogen treatment. Hormone replacement therapy using natural estrogen (17β-estradiol) does not lead to hypertension.

Licorice

Some ice creams, sweets, and beverages without alcohol contain licorice, which can raise BP with significant consumption. Licorice inhibits type 2 11β-hydroxysteroid dehydrogenase, which converts cortisol into cortisone. Normally, this enzyme protects the mineralocorticoid receptor, sensitive to cortisol but not to cortisone. In the case of licorice consumption or of a genetic enzyme deficiency (syndrome of apparent mineralcorticoid excess), cortisol stimulates the mineralocorticoid receptor and induces hypertension with hypokalemia and low renin and low aldosterone levels.

Sympathomimetics

Sympathomimetics, in the form of nasal decongestants or anorectics, are liable to acutely or chronically elevate BP. They can interact with antihypertensive treatment and induce resistance to treatment.

Corticosteroids and Nonsteroidal Anti-Inflammatory Drugs

Corticosteroids induce an elevation in BP by stimulating the mineralocorticoid receptor, which provokes hypertension with a hypokalemic tendency. BP measurement is part of systematic assessment of patients treated with these agents. Nonsteroidal anti-inflammatory drugs (NSAIDs) do not directly increase BP but rather reduce the efficiency of diuretics, β-blockers, and RAS blockers.

Agents Rarely Involved

Immunosuppressors (ciclosporine, tacrolimus), with or without corticosteroids, increase BP in 50% to 80% of patients. When cyclosporine alone is used in situations other than transplantations, hypertension appears in 25% to 30% of patients. An increase in BP is linked to a peripheral vasoconstriction, which induces a decrease in glomerular filtration and an increase in sodium reabsorption. Recombinant human erythropoietin increases BP in 18% to 45% of patients with end-stage renal disease. Hypertension is provoked by an increase in systemic vascular resistance and is not correlated with hematocrit or viscosity. Consumption of cocaine should be considered in patients seen in emergency departments with hypertension in the presence of tachycardia, dilated pupils, and an alteration of higher functions or convulsion. Other substances (e.g., anabolic steroids, lead, bromocriptine and other derivatives of ergot alkaloids, monoamine oxidase inhibitors [after ingestion of small amounts of normally harmless pressor amines in foods], or other antidepressants that may interfere with BP control of patients with hypertension) can induce an elevated BP by inducing changes in BP and orthostatic hypotension.

Hypertension is also emerging as one of the most common side effects of treatment with angiogenesis inhibitors—such as anti–vascular endothelial cell growth factor (VEGF) antibodies (bevacizumab) and tyrosine kinase inhibitors of VEGF—used in metastatic colorectal and renal carcinomas.[18]

Hypertension with Renal Artery Stenosis

Renal artery stenosis may be responsible for hypertension if it reduces luminal diameter by at least 50%. All renal artery stenoses do not necessarily lead to a reversible hypertension, and the term *renovascular hypertension* is reserved for hypertension with renal artery stenosis that can be reversed by revascularization. Therapeutic methods include revascularization, antihypertensive drugs, drugs to treat dyslipidemia, and antiplatelet agents.

Revascularization is accomplished by angioplasty with or without an endoprothesis (stent) and reconstructive surgery. Angioplasty reduces BP and allows a reduction in the intensity of treatment. Recovery (e.g., normotension without treatment) is frequent in renal artery stenosis with fibromuscular dysplasia. Recovery is infrequent in cases of atherosclerotic stenosis, which accounts for the large frequency of intrarenal vessel changes and chronic glomerular changes linked to the duration of the hypertension or diabetes. Moreover, these patients often consequently have extrarenal, notably coronary, vascular lesions, which require specific medical treatment. Therefore, angioplasty of atherosclerotic stenosis is recommended in (i) cases of failed medical treatments (hypertension resistant to treatment; discussed later), (ii) hypertension complicated with acute pulmonary edema, (iii) patients in whom renal function spontaneously deteriorates, or (iv) patients treated with ACE inhibitors.[19]

Adrenal Hypertension

Adrenal hypertension is the consequence of a tumor or hyperplasia with hypersecretion of aldosterone (primary hyperaldosteronism with idiopathic hyperplasia or Conn's adenoma), of catecholamines (pheochromocytoma), or cortisol (Cushing's syndrome).

Primary Hyperaldosteronism[20]

The prevalence of primary hyperaldosteronism is around 6%, about half of which are Conn's adenomas. These benign tumors are no larger than 20 mm in diameter and exclusively secrete aldosterone. Other primary hyperaldosteronism adenomas are mainly bilateral hyperplasia requiring continuous medication. Detection of primary hyperaldosteronism at the time of the initial assessment relies on measuring potassium levels, recommended in all patients with hypertension. Primary hyperaldosteronism is associated with hypokalemia in only about half of all cases but can lead to resistant hypertension. Resistance to treatment is the second reason to search for primary hyperaldosteronism.

The diagnosis of primary hyperaldosteronism relies on the determination of both aldosterone and renin. Spironolactone must be stopped for at least 6 weeks; diuretics, β-blockers, or RAS blockers should be stopped for at least 15 days. If necessary, treatment can be replaced with central antihypertensive drugs, α-blockers, or calcium channel antagonists. In the case of hypokalemia, potassium supplementation is given to avoid cardiac hyperexcitability and facilitate diagnosis. Indeed, a significant hypokalemia can partially inhibit aldosterone secretion and make the biologic profile less relevant. Sodium is lost in primary hyperaldosteronism; thus, edema is present in this condition. Natriuresis reflects sodium intake in the same way that kaliuresis reflects potassium intake. Sodium consumption is usually superior to that of potassium; therefore, the Na : K ratio is not inverted.

The biologic signature of primary hyperaldosteronism is elevated plasma or urinary aldosterone in the presence of low renin (plasma renin activity or plasma concentration of active renin), with an increase in the aldosterone : renin ratio.

The distinction between adenoma and hyperplasia frequently relies on imaging. If Conn's adenoma is confirmed, surgical removal is possible. However, the hypertension is not always completely reversible.

Pheochromocytoma

Pheochromocytoma is a tumor that secretes catecholamines and derives from the adrenal medulla or other sympathetic ganglions. The most frequent clue for pheochromocytoma is hypertension, recognizable by its variability, a tendency toward orthostatic hypertension, and an association with hyperglycemia. Patients with hypertension who report headache, sweating, and palpitations and those in whom hypertension is paroxysmal or associated with diabetes without weight gain should be tested for pheochromocytoma.

Diagnosis relies on the measurement of plasma or urinary metanephrines. Imaging specifies the number of tumors, their location, and their relationship while also detecting possible metastasis. Surgical treatment is always advised because of the potential risk, even if the reversion to hypertension is unpredictable, notably when age increases.

Cushing's Syndrome

Cushing's syndrome is rarely revealed by hypertension. The investigation and treatment of the variety of syndromes in adrenocorticotropic hormone (ACTH)–dependent and ACTH-independent Cushing's syndrome are beyond the scope of this chapter.

Rare Causes of Reversible Hypertension

Some cases of hypertension are associated with acromegaly and are removed by hypophysectomy. Hypertension is often found in hypothyroid and hyperparathyroid conditions, but the treatment of these conditions does not lead to recovery from hypertension.

Scars from a reflux nephropathy lead to hypertension in 10% to 20% of patients, which may progress to renal failure. Repeated infections justify treating reflux, but this rarely leads to improved BP. Resection of a small kidney caused by congenital hypoplasia is advised only if the scintigraphy scan reveals negligible kidney function and the treatment is justified by the prevention of infection. Hydronephrosis accompanies hypertension in a minority of cases. Functional preservation is the priority; an improvement in BP can be increasingly achieved, if the secretion of renin is lateralized. Lastly, renin-dependent hypertension has been reported in association with renal tuberculosis, fibrosis encapsulation of the kidney resulting from hematoma or infection, voluminous cysts, and certain cancers of the kidney.

Renin tumors develop from the juxtaglomerular apparatus and secrete prorenin and active renin. Hypertension is reversible by surgery if paraneoplastic secretion is not involved.

Finally, several cases of neurogenic hypertension have been reported resulting from tumoral or neurovascular compression of the cardiovascular centers of the medulla oblongata. Neurogenic hypertension compares with sinoaortic denervation (after cervical radiotherapy or intervention with the two carotid bifurcations), which leads to major instability of BP through loss of baroreflex control.[21]

In conclusion, in a minority of cases, secondary hypertension can lead to treatment with the potential for recovery. These cases include iatrogenic hypertension, if withdrawal from exposure is possible; hypertension associated with fibrodysplasic renal artery stenosis and in some patients with atherosclerotic renal artery stenosis; and about half the cases of hypertension associated with adrenal tumors. Surgery or angioplasty should be discussed on a case-by-case basis; however, the expected BP benefit is often compromised by age.

THERAPEUTIC APPROACH AND PATIENT FOLLOW-UP

Decision Thresholds and Delays in the Decision to Treat

The benefits of treating hypertension for prevention of cardiovascular and renal complications have largely been demonstrated. In clinical trials, antihypertensive therapy has been associated with reductions in stroke, averaging 35% to 40%; in myocardial infarction, averaging 20% to 25%; and in heart failure, of 50%.

Current recommendations advise rapid initiation of treatment with antihypertensive medication in patients with a diastolic BP of 180 mm Hg or greater and/or a systolic BP of 110 mm Hg or greater after several days of surveillance to confirm the consistency of high BP levels.[22] In all other cases, lifestyle measures are initiated for a 3-month to 1-year period with BP regularly monitored at 3-month intervals. This surveillance period allows for strict evaluation of the average BP levels of an individual patient and the evaluation of possibly associated cardiovascular and/or renal risk factors. At the end of the surveillance period, the decision to treat is based on BP level criteria and associated cardiovascular risk factors (age, male sex, obesity, physical inactivity, smoking, diabetes, hypercholesterolemia), target organ damage (left ventricular hypertrophy, renal failure, micro/macroproteinuria, grade III or IV hypertensive retinopathy, atherosclerotic plaques), and associated clinical conditions (diabetes, coronary heart disease, cerebrovascular disease, peripheral artery disease, renal disease) affecting the prognosis.

Nonpharmacologic Measures or Lifestyle Modifications

Weight loss induced by reducing calorie intake and following a low-fat diet, reducing alcohol intake, increasing exercise, reducing salt intake, and increasing potassium are among the lifestyle measures that can reduce, although modestly, BP in hypertensive patients.[23] These measures should be continued even when an antihypertensive treatment has been initiated. Encouraging current smokers to quit smoking is of primary importance to reduce global cardiovascular risk. Moreover, weight reduction, dietary manipulation, and physical activity reduce the incidence of type 2 diabetes, and a low-saturated-fat diet reduces dyslipidemia.

Pharmacologic Treatment

Results from Clinical Trials

More than 100 medications are used to treat hypertension, grouped into four major, most frequently used classes (diuretics, β-blockers, calcium channel blockers, and RAS blockers) and three other classes (α-blockers, centrally acting antihypertensive drugs, and vasodilators). These drugs have been marketed at doses selected to achieve a similar fall in BP.

The initial uncertainty about the comparative effects of the four most frequently used BP-lowering treatments on major cardiovascular events was refuted by the Blood Pressure Lowering Treatment Trialist's Collaboration overview of 29 randomized trials including 162,341 hypertensive patients followed up from 2.0 to 8.4 years (700,000 patient-years).[24] This overview showed that (i) treatment with any commonly used regimen reduces the risk of total major cardiovascular events compared with that of placebo and (ii) greater reductions in BP produce larger reductions in risk, indicating that BP lowering is a major component of the benefit conferred by the different classes of drugs.

Although no significant differences were demonstrated in total major cardiovascular events between ACE inhibitors, calcium channel blockers, diuretics, or β-blockers, some differences were observed between drug classes in their effects on specific cardiovascular outcomes:

1. Treatments based on ACE inhibitors/ARAs or on diuretics or β-blockers were more effective at preventing heart failure than those based on calcium channel blockers.

2. For coronary heart disease, there was no trend toward a lesser efficacy of calcium channel blockers compared with diuretics, β-blockers, or ACE inhibitors.
3. Calcium channel blockers demonstrated a trend toward greater reductions in stroke risk.

Data from subsequent trials and overviews showed

1. The effects of the different BP-lowering regimens on major cardiovascular events was comparable in patients with or without diabetes in a follow-up overview by the Blood Pressure Lowering Treatment Trialist's Collaboration.[25]
2. The importance of prompt BP control in hypertensive patients at high cardiovascular risk was emphasized in both the Valsartan Antihypertensive Long-term Use Evaluation (VALUE)[26] and the Anglo-Scandinavian Cardiac Outcomes Trial—Blood Pressure Lowering Arm (ASCOT-BPLA)[27] studies.
3. The results of the VALUE trial[26] (amlodipine-based treatment vs. valsartan-based treatment in 15,000 high-risk patients with hypertension), the International Verapamil SR/Trandolapril Study (INVEST)[27] (verapamil-based vs. atenolol-based treatments in 22,500 patients with hypertension and coronary heart disease), the A Coronary disease Trial Investigating Outcome with Nifedipine GITS (ACTION) trial[28] (nifedipine GastroIntestinal Therapeutic System (GITS) vs. placebo in 7500 patients with established coronary artery disease), and the ASCOT trial[29] (amlodipine-based vs. atenolol-based treatment in 19,000 patients with hypertension and three or more other cardiovascular risk factors) reinforced the results of the Blood Pressure Lowering Treatment Trialist's Collaboration overview[25] on the beneficial effects of calcium channel blockers on major cardiovascular events, especially stroke incidence.
4. The ASCOT study[29] provided comparative data on mortality or morbidity to guide selection of optimal combinations. This trial showed that in high-risk hypertensive patients, an amlodipine-perindopril regimen did not differ from an atenolol-bendroflumethiazide regimen for reducing nonfatal myocardial infraction and fatal coronary events, but it was better at reducing all-cause morality, total stroke, all coronary events, total cardiovascular events and procedures, and cardiovascular mortality. This difference is in part due to a difference of 2.7/1.9 mm Hg in clinical BP and, above all, a difference in central aortic systolic BP of 4.3 mm Hg (95% confidence interval [CI], 3.3-5.4) and in central aortic pulse pressure of 3.0 mm Hg (95% CI, 2.1-3.9) derived from radial artery applanation tonometry measures and pulse wave analysis in favor of the amlodipine-perindopril regimen.[30]
5. ACE inhibitors or ARAs have been shown to decrease the risk of developing new-onset type 2 diabetes in individual trials and in a meta-analysis.[31]
6. The role of β-blockers as initial therapy in hypertensive patients who do not have a compelling indication, such as coronary heart disease and congestive heart failure, has been reappraised. These drugs (especially atenolol) have been shown to be less effective than other drugs at preventing major cardiovascular events, especially stroke.[32] They also have an unfavorable metabolic profile and can induce the development of diabetes, especially when used in combination with diuretics.

Choice of Initial Drug Therapy

The World Health Organization (WHO)[22] recommends determining the initial treatment for an individual patient according to associated clinical conditions and contraindications, as indicated in Tables 22-1 and 22-2. The subsequent adjustment to treatment takes into consideration the BP-lowering effect of the initially selected class of antihypertensive drug and the possible appearance of undesirable side effects. According to the WHO recommendations "For the majority of patients without a compelling indication for another class of drug, a low dose of a diuretic should be considered as the first choice of therapy on the basis of comparative trial data, availability and cost." The importance of cost consideration will be minimized in the coming years because most of the antihypertensive drugs will become generics.

TABLE 22-1 FIRST-CHOICE DRUGS

Compelling Indications	Drugs
Elderly with isolated systolic hypertension	Diuretic DHP CCB
Renal disease	
Diabetic nephropathy type 1	ACEI
Diabetic nephropathy type 2	ARA
Nondiabetic nephropathy	ACEI
Cardiac disease	
Post–myocardial infarction	ACEI, ARA, β-blocker
Left ventricular dysfunction	ACEI
CHF (diuretics almost always included)	ACEI, ARA, β-blocker
Left ventricular hypertrophy	ARA
Cerebrovascular disease	Diuretic or ACEI + diuretic

ACEI, angiotensin-converting enzyme inhibitor; ARA, angiotensin receptor antagonist; CHF, congestive heart failure; DHP CCB, dihydropyridine calcium channel blocker.

Adapted from Whitworth JA. 2003 World Health Organization (WHO)/International Society of Hypertension (ISH) statement on management of hypertension. J Hypertension 2003;21:1983-1992.

TABLE 22-2 CONTRAINDICATIONS OF ANTIHYPERTENSIVE DRUGS

Drug	Contraindications
ACEI, ARA	Pregnancy Bilateral renal artery stenosis Hyperkalemia
β-Blockers	High-degree heart block Severe bradycardia < 50/min Obstructive airways disease Raynaud's phenomenon
Diuretics	Gout
Non–DHP CCB	High-degree heart block Severe bradycardia < 50/min

ACEI, angiotensin-converting enzyme inhibitor; ARA, angiotensin receptor antagonist; DHP CCB, dihydropyridine calcium channel blocker.

Adapted from Whitworth JA. 2003 World Health Organization (WHO)/International Society of Hypertension (ISH) statement on management of hypertension. J Hypertension 2003;21:1983-1992.

Certain drugs may also be chosen for other reasons: a diuretic or calcium channel blocker used as monotherapy may lower BP more in African Americans and older patients than an ACE inhibitor, a β-blocker, or an α-blocker. Although not specifically recommended by the WHO, a low-dose combination antihypertensive therapy may also be used as initial treatment because of its antihypertensive additive efficacy, which is not counterbalanced by an increase in adverse effects.[33]

Finally, considerations on the choice of initial drug therapy must be balanced with the fact that a large proportion of patients, especially the elderly with isolated systolic hypertension or those with diabetes or chronic nephropathy, will need multiple drug regimens with two or more antihypertensive drugs to achieve BP control (as many as 30% of patients will need three or more antihypertensive drugs).

Classes of Antihypertensive Drugs

Diuretics. Diuretics have been used since the late 1960s. They are low cost and recommended as the first choice in hypertension treatment. The three types of diuretics are loop diuretics, thiazides and related diuretics, and potassium-sparing diuretics (sodium-amiloride–sensitive channel blockers and aldosterone antagonists). Diuretics inhibit sodium reabsorption from the renal tubular lumen, and their antihypertensive efficacy depends on their natriuretic effect. Diuretics can be administered once daily. They should be part of any combined antihypertensive therapy. In the case of renal failure (glomerular filtration rate <30 ml/min), only loop diuretics conserve their natriuretic and antihypertensive efficacy.

Adverse lipid metabolic and glycemic effects have been shown in short-term studies using high doses of diuretics, especially combined with β-blockers. Hypokalemia is a frequent dose-dependent adverse effect of thiazides and loop diuretics, but it can be prevented by a combination with a potassium-sparing diuretic or an RAS blocker. The active metabolite of spironolactone can cause dose-dependent specific adverse effects such as gynecomastia in men and intermenstrual or postmenopausal bleeding in women.

β-Blockers. In the short term, β-blockers lead to a decrease in cardiac output and heart rate and an increase in peripheral resistance. They also decrease renin secretion. In the long term, peripheral resistance decreases, contributing to the decrease in BP. The compelling indications for using β-blockers in hypertensive patients are coronary heart disease and congestive heart failure. β-Blockers should not be interrupted suddenly in patients with coronary heart disease. β-Blockers can mask certain clinical signs of hypoglycemia in diabetic patients.

RAS Blockers: ACE Inhibitors and ARAs. ACE inhibitors block the generation of the vasoconstrictor and antinatriuretic peptide angiotensin II and the degradation of a vasodilator and natriuretic peptide, bradykinin. Whereas ACE inhibitors limit the production of angiotensin II, ARAs directly block the AT_1 angiotensin II receptors. ARAs have an antihypertensive efficacy comparable with that of ACE inhibitors.

Blockade of the RAS with ACE inhibitors or ARAs has become one of the most successful therapeutic approaches in medicine. Considerable evidence shows that this treatment reduces BP, left ventricular mass, and proteinuria. RAS blockade decreases cardiovascular morbidity and mortality in patients with chronic heart failure and left ventricular systolic dysfunction and after myocardial infarction. RAS blockers retard the progression of renal insufficiency in type 1 (ACE inhibitors) and type 2 (ARAs) diabetes mellitus and nondiabetic chronic renal disease. Finally, a high dose of an ACE inhibitor administered in the evening reduces the rate of death, cardiac events, and stroke in patients with a high cardiovascular risk at baseline.

The principal adverse effect of ACE inhibitors is a dry cough (5%-10%). A very rare but serious secondary effect is angioneurotic edema. ACE inhibitors are contraindicated in patients with records of hereditary angioneurotic edema and Quincke's edema. ARAs are very well tolerated and have a placebo-like tolerability profile. They offer a therapeutic alternative to patients with a dry cough who are taking ACE inhibitors or have a contraindication to ACE inhibitors.

The introduction of RAS blockers should be done carefully when renal function is altered because of sodium depletion or use of a diuretic and in elderly patients. In this case, administering a lower dose and testing serum creatinine and potassium are recommended. An elevation in creatinine while taking an RAS blocker requires searching for the presence of renal artery stenosis. RAS blockers are contraindicated during pregnancy.

Calcium Channel Blockers. Calcium channel blockers have a vasodilator action that inhibits calcium flow at the level of the membrane of contractile cells. This vasodilation leads to a decrease in peripheral resistance and a decrease in BP. Short-acting dihydropyridines induce sympathetic reflex stimulation. This heterogeneous class includes short-acting dihydropyridines (which should no longer be used as antihypertensive drugs), long-acting dihydropyridines, such as amlodipine, and two other subclasses, verapamil and diltiazem.

Dihydropyridines are contraindicated or ill advised during pregnancy. Verapamil and diltiazem are contraindicated in sick sinus syndrome, supraventricular conduction irregularities, and heart failure. The most frequent undesirable effects are peripheral edema (not sensitive to diuretics), headache, and flush. With verapamil, specific undesirable effects are constipation, bradycardia, and atrioventricular heart block. With verapamil and diltiazem, myocardial contractile function is reduced.

Other Classes

α-Blockers. The antihypertensive action of α-blockers results from a selective antagonism of postsynaptic peripheral α_1-adrenergic receptors. Their principal adverse effects are orthostatic hypotension and sodium retention. Short-acting drugs can also provoke severe hypotension at administration of the first dose, especially in patients receiving vasodilator or diuretic treatment and in those with heart failure. There are no outcome data for these drugs. In the Antihypertensive and Lipid-Lowering treatment to prevent Heart Attack Trial (ALLHAT),[34] the doxazosin arm was prematurely interrupted because of an increased risk of congestive heart failure over that with diuretics.

Centrally Acting Antihypertensive Drugs. The central inhibition of the sympathetic system is achieved by stimulation of α_2-adrenergic receptors and specific imidazoline receptors. Centrally acting antihypertensive drugs are specific agonists of α_2-adrenergic receptors (α-methyldopa converted to α-methylnoradrenaline), specific agonists of imidazoline receptors (rilmenidine, monoxidine), and mixed agonists (clonidine). These drugs have no proven efficacy in cardiovascular disease prevention. Clonidine has a sedative effect; can provoke constipation and dryness of the mouth and the eyes; and induces a risk of severe rebound hypertension after treatment is stopped, linked to hypersecretion of catecholamines. Imidazoline receptor agonists are better tolerated.

Peripheral Vasodilators. Peripheral vasodilators are no longer used. They act directly at the level of arteriolar or venous vascular smooth muscle cells. They either generate NO, inducing relaxation by stimulating the guanylate cyclase–cyclic guanosine monophosphate (cGMP) pathway (nitroprusside, hydralazine), or activate potassium channels (diazoxide, minoxidil). The principal adverse effects are pulsating headache, sodium retention, tachycardia, and increased cardiac output (by reflex sympathetic and RAS activation). These drugs must be prescribed in combination with diuretics and β-blockers. Minoxidil provokes the development of hypertrichosis.

Synergistic Associations

The percentage of patients responding to a single antihypertensive drug is around 50% to 60%. The average reduction in BP observed with a monotherapy in patients with an initial BP of 160/95 mm Hg is 7 mm Hg to 13 mm Hg in systolic BP and 4 mm Hg to 8 mm Hg in diastolic BP. The Hypertension Optimal Treatment (HOT) study[35] showed that 70% of patients needed at least a double therapy to reach a target diastolic BP below 90 mm Hg. Figures are even worse for the systolic BP target (140 mm Hg).

Combination therapy is achieved by either adding antihypertensive drugs with synergistic antihypertensive effects or using fixed-dose combination treatments. The recommended combinations are

- Double therapy: ACE inhibitor + diuretic; ARA + diuretic; ACE inhibitor + calcium channel blocker; ARA + calcium channel blocker; β-blocker + diuretic; β-blocker + dihydropyridine.
- Triple therapy: calcium channel blocker + ACE inhibitor + diuretic; calcium channel blocker + β-blocker + diuretic

Associated Treatments

Prescription of Statins. In hypertensive patients with a high cardiovascular risk (multiple risk factors or the presence of overt cardiovascular disease), the prescription of a statin reduces the incidence of infarction by 36% and of stroke by 30%, even in the presence of BP well controlled with antihypertensives.

Prescription of Aspirin. In the absence of compelling indications (multiple risk factors or the presence of overt cardiovascular disease), the benefit of aspirin at low doses in patients with hypertension should be put in balance with the risk of bleeding. Aspirin should not be prescribed while hypertension is well controlled.

BP Goals

The general objective fixed by the WHO[22] is to reduce systolic BP to less than 140 mm Hg and diastolic BP to less than 90 mm Hg. In the particular case of patients with hypertension and diabetes, the objective is stricter, to less than 130 mm Hg for systolic BP and to 80 mm Hg or less for diastolic BP. In patients with renal failure, the objective is to reduce BP to less than 130/80 mm Hg and proteinuria to less than 0.5 g/24 hr. Finally, in those over 80 years, the objective is to reduce systolic BP to less than 150 mm Hg and to avoid orthostatic hypotension.

Resistant Hypertension

Hypertension resistant to treatment is defined by a systolic BP equal to or greater than 140 mm Hg or a diastolic BP equal to or greater than 90 mm Hg despite triple therapy including a diuretic at effective doses. This justifies a specialist consultation to distinguish resistant hypertension from an overestimation of BP levels, to ensure an adequate prescription and patient compliance. In the case of failure to effect a change in BP, the etiologic enquiry is revisited.

A frequent cause of the overestimation of BP levels occurs in patients with large or bulky arms. The inflatable cuff must constrict at least two thirds of the arm circumference for the measurement to be valid. Another cause of overestimation is an alarm reaction induced by "white coat hypertension." Certain patients with well-controlled BP in daily life have an elevated BP at the doctor's office. These cases are distinguished by the absence of visceral complications and confirmed by self-measurement at home or by measuring ambulatory BP.

Abandoning all or part of treatment is a frequent result of pseudoresistance. This is often associated with young age, moderate hypertension, males, lower socioeconomic group, and consumption of alcohol and/or tobacco. Otherwise, an antihypertensive prescription at insufficient dosages, poor compliance, or poor absorption linked to the simultaneous prescription of antacids can be responsible for poor BP control. Medical interference—taking a contraceptive pill containing a synthetic progesterone, NSAIDs, cyclosporine, erythropoietin, sympathomimetics, ergot alkaloids, and glucocorticoids—can be responsible for resistant hypertension.

Having distinguished these false-resistant causes, an etiologic enquiry should search for renal artery stenosis or adrenal disease.

If the EH is confirmed, and after dismissing alcohol exposure or medication interfering with BP, an attempt is made to improve compliance by simplifying dosages, educating the patient, and increasing therapy. The therapy should obey simple rules:

1. Medications are used at full dose.
2. Reinforcing the diuretic component is often necessary, especially in the case of renal failure (in this last case, an increasing dose of loop diuretics is used).
3. A change to quadritherapy may be necessary (e.g., with a diuretic, a β-blocker, a calcium channel blocker, and an ACE inhibitor).

Strategy of Hypertension Care Outside of an Emergency

Strategy of hypertension care outside of an emergency is summarized in Figure 22-5.

Hypertensive Emergencies

Hypertensive emergencies result from certain acute elevations in BP that cause an immediate risk of vital complications or disability. These emergencies often consist of neurovascular emergencies—frequent

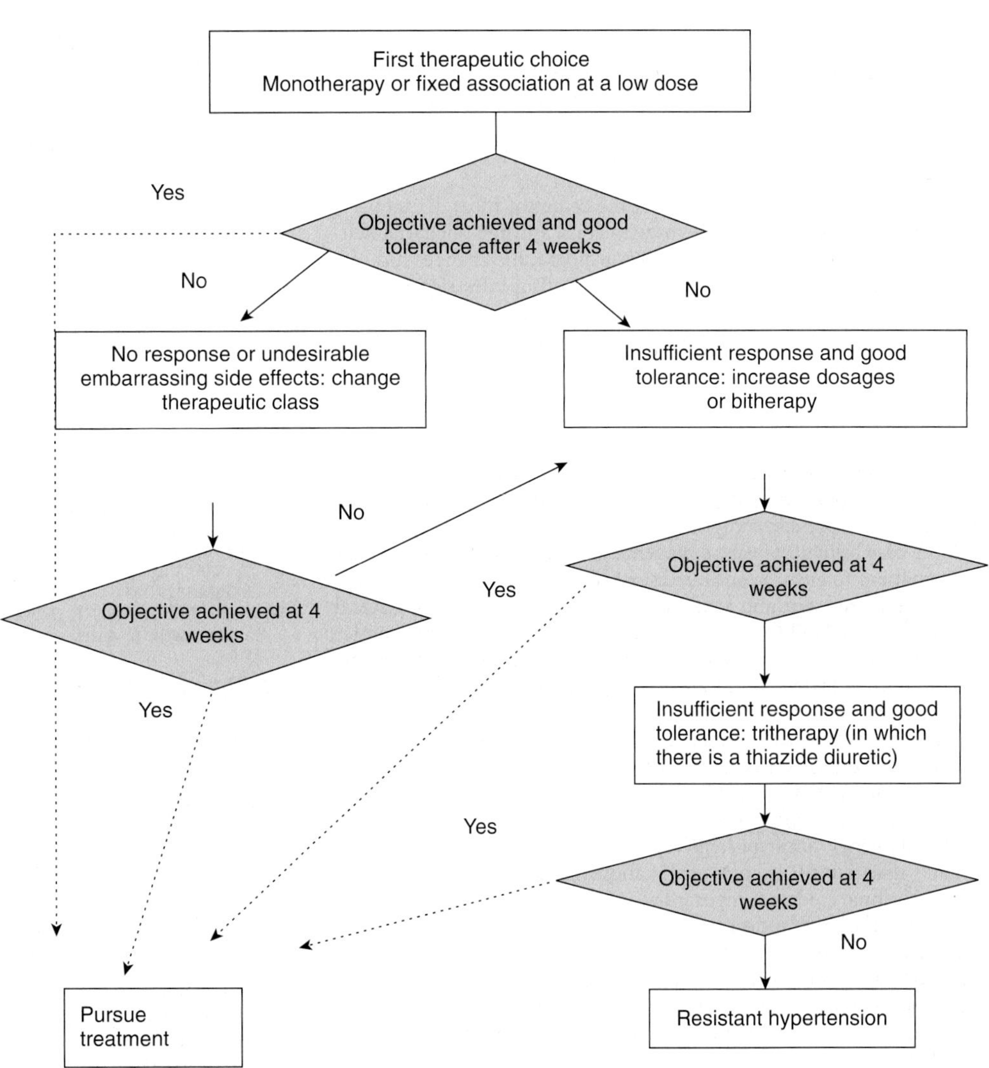

FIGURE 22-5 • Example of a strategy to manage hypertension. (Adapted from Halimi JM. Management of adults with essential hypertension—2005 update. Report from the Haute Autorité de Santé.)

Practice: Cardiovascular Therapeutics

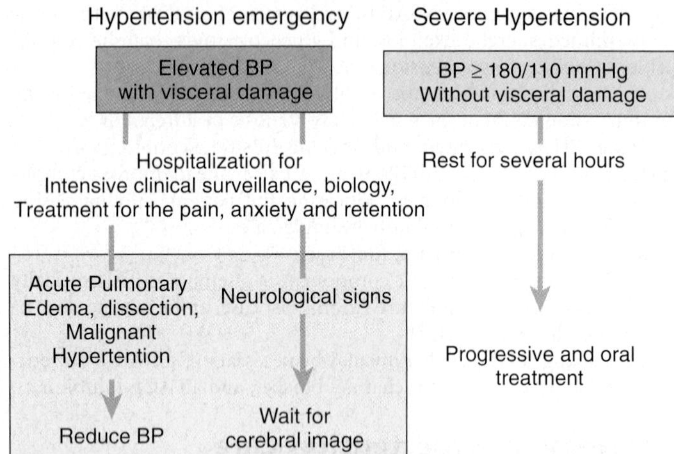

FIGURE 22-6 • Decision diagram in the case of acute elevation of arterial blood pressure.

brief periods of increased BP with focal neurologic deficit—that expose patients to death or severe disability, but in which the risk of rapid reduction of BP could be greater than no attempt to lower BP. BP elevations without immediate visceral damage, in the particular case of severe or grade 3 hypertension, should be distinguished from real hypertensive emergencies because their excessive treatment is not useful and sometimes dangerous. Figure 22-6 demonstrates that elements of decision are the presence or absence of visceral damage among the real emergencies. Neurovascular cases are distinguished from other causes: myocardial infarction with frequent brief periods of increased BP; acute pulmonary edema; acute aortic dissection; malignant hypertension; and encephalopathic hypertension. (Eclampsia, which is part of hypertensive emergencies, is not covered in this chapter.)

The search for visceral damage is at the center of these decisions. A focal neurologic deficit or problems with consciousness suggest a neurovascular emergency. Pain and electrocardiographic changes indicate an infarction; orthopnea and bilateral crepitating rales signify acute pulmonary edema; violent thoracoabdominal pain, diastolic murmur, anisotension, and pulse abolition relate to aortic dissection. A recent period of headache with thirst, weight loss, and decreased visual acuity suggests a malignant hypertension to be confirmed by eye fundus examination (hemorrhage, exudates, or papillary edema). Information about therapeutic context is obtained from the patient or the family. Does the patient take medications; if so, which? Will ceasing any of the medications expose the patient to rebound effects (clonidine)? Does the patient take pressor compounds?

In the case of hypertensive emergencies, the first step is to hospitalize the patient to ensure continued surveillance of BP and neurologic, cardiac, and renal state and to administer specific treatment for visceral damage. The availability of a brain computerized tomographic scanner or, better still, a magnetic resonance imaging scanner, is essential in the case of neurologic deficit. In the case of a suspected myocardial infarction or aortic dissection, the patient is transferred to a hospital that provides intensive cardiac care and/or cardiovascular surgery.

While waiting for transfer, no treatment should be given to reduce BP if the patient has a neurologic deficit, because this treatment can be undertaken only after cerebral imaging.

An emergency antihypertensive drug is administered only if the patient's diastolic BP is consistently above 120 mm Hg with signs of acute pulmonary edema, myocardial infarction, or aortic dissection. Sublingual administration of nifedipine in hypertensive emergencies is no longer authorized. When the patient arrives at the hospital, a semicontinuous surveillance of BP should be undertaken. Stress, pain, and urine retention can elevate BP and should be treated. Without delay, urine examination with a dipstick, electrocardiographic studies, and blood samples to measure electrolytes and renal function, and if necessary, a measure of cardiac enzymes or aortic echography are obtained. In the presence of a neurologic deficit, a cerebral image should urgently be performed and a neurologic vascular consultation performed to facilitate the careful reduction of BP (in case of hemorrhage) or to prevent any attempt to lower BP (in case of ischemia). In the absence of a neurologic deficit, antihypertensive treatment is administered intravenously. Diuretics are reserved for acute pulmonary edema treatment and are rapidly followed by an injectable derivative of nitroglycerine. Strictly speaking, antihypertensives are administered by electric syringe. The most adapted products are those in which output can be precisely adjusted according to BP obtained (e.g., injectable nicardipine). Normal BP should not be sought. The recommended objective is no more than a 25% reduction in average BP within 2 hours, then a gradual reduction toward 160/100 mm Hg in 2 to 6 hours. After rectifying the urgent situation, an oral antihypertensive drug should generally be prescribed. This is done only in the case of elevated BP without immediate visceral damage.

REFERENCES

1. Lewington S, Clarke R, Qizilbash N, et al. Age-specific relevance of usual blood pressure to vascular mortality: a meta-analysis of individual data for one million adults in 61 prospective studies. Lancet 2002;360:1903-1913.
2. Staessen JA, Wang JG, Thijs L. Cardiovascular protection and blood pressure reduction: a meta-analysis. Lancet 2001;358:1305-1315.
3. Burt VL, Cutler JA, Higgins M, et al. Trends in the prevalence, awareness, treatment, and control of hypertension in the adult US population. Data from the Health Examination surveys, 1960 to 1991. Hypertension 1995;26:60-69.
4. Corvol P, Persu A, Gimenez-Roqueplo AP, Jeunemaitre X. Seven lessons from two candidate genes in human essential hypertension: angiotensinogen and epithelial sodium channel. Hypertension 1999;33:1324-1331.
5. Lerman LO, Chade AR, Sica V, Napoli C. Animal models of hypertension: an overview. J Lab Clin Med 2005;146:160-173.
6. Page IH. The mosaic theory 32 years later. Hypertension 1982;4:177.
7. Thuillez C, Richard V. Targeting endothelial dysfunction in hypertensive subjects. J Hum Hypertens 2005;19(suppl 1):S21-S25.
8. DiBona GF. Sympathetic nervous system and the kidney in hypertension. Curr Opin Nephrol Hypertens 2002;11:197-200.
9. Guyton AC, Coleman TG, Young DB, et al. Salt balance and long-term blood pressure control. Annu Rev Med 1980;31:15-27.
10. Folkow B. The haemodynamic consequences of adaptive structural changes of the resistance vessels in hypertension. Clin Sci 1971;41:1-12.
11. Laurent S, Vanhoutte P, Cavero I, et al. The arterial wall: a new pharmacological and therapeutic target. Fundam Clin Pharmacol 1996;10:243-257.
12. Guyenet PG. The sympathetic control of blood pressure. Nat Rev Neurosci 2006;7:335-346.
13. Korner PI, West MJ, Shaw J, Uther JB. "Steady-state" properties of the baroreceptor-heart rate reflex in essential hypertension in man. Clin Exp Pharmacol Physiol 1974;1:65-76.
14. Persson PB. The kidney and hypertension. Am J Physiol Regul Integr Comp Physiol 2003;284:R1176-R1178.
15. Safar ME, Thomas F, Blacher J, et al. Metabolic syndrome and age-related progression of aortic stiffness. J Am Coll Cardiol 2006;47:72-75.
16. Rahmouni K, Correia ML, Haynes WG, Mark AL. Obesity-associated hypertension: new insights into mechanisms. Hypertension 2005;45:9-14.
17. Streeten DH, Anderson GH Jr, Wagner S. Effect of age on response of secondary hypertension to specific treatment. Am J Hypertens 1990;3:360-365.
18. Sica DA. Angiogenesis inhibitors and hypertension: an emerging issue. J Clin Oncol 2006;24:1329-1331.
19. Plouin PF, Rossignol P, Bobrie G. Atherosclerotic renal artery stenosis: to treat conservatively, to dilate, to stent, or to operate? J Am Soc Nephrol 2001;12:2190-2196.
20. Stewart PM. Mineralocorticoid hypertension. Lancet 1999;353:1341-1347.
21. Elghozi JL, Girard A, Ribstein J. L'insuffisance du baroréflexe: un cas exceptionnel de variabilité tensionnelle extrême. Rev Med Interne 2001;22:1261-1268.
22. Whitworth JA. 2003 World Health Organization (WHO)/International Society of Hypertension (ISH) statement on management of hypertension. J Hypertens 2003;21:1983-1992.
23. Dickinson HO, Mason JM, Nicolson DJ, et al. Lifestyle interventions to reduce raised blood pressure: a systematic review of randomized controlled trials. J Hypertens 2006;24:215-233.
24. Turnbull F. Effects of different blood-pressure-lowering regimens on major cardiovascular events: results of prospectively-designed overviews of randomised trials. Lancet 2003;362:1527-1535.
25. Turnbull F, Neal B, Algert C, et al. Effects of different blood pressure-lowering regimens on major cardiovascular events in individuals with and without diabetes mellitus: results of prospectively designed overviews of randomized trials. Arch Intern Med 2005;165:1410-1419.
26. Julius S, Kjeldsen SE, Weber M, et al. Outcomes in hypertensive patients at high cardiovascular risk treated with regimens based on valsartan or amlodipine: the VALUE randomised trial. Lancet 2004;363:2022-2031.

27. Pepine CJ, Handberg EM, Cooper-DeHoff RM, et al. A calcium antagonist vs a non-calcium antagonist hypertension treatment strategy for patients with coronary artery disease. The International Verapamil-Trandolapril Study (INVEST): a randomized controlled trial. JAMA 2003;290:2805-2816.
28. Poole-Wilson PA, Lubsen J, Kirwan BA, et al. Effect of long-acting nifedipine on mortality and cardiovascular morbidity in patients with stable angina requiring treatment (ACTION trial): randomised controlled trial. Lancet 2004;364:849-857.
29. Dahlof B, Sever PS, Poulter NR, et al. Prevention of cardiovascular events with an antihypertensive regimen of amlodipine adding perindopril as required versus atenolol adding bendroflumethiazide as required, in the Anglo-Scandinavian Cardiac Outcomes Trial-Blood Pressure Lowering Arm (ASCOT-BPLA): a multicentre randomised controlled trial. Lancet 2005;366:895-906.
30. Williams B, Lacy PS, Thom SM, et al. Differential impact of blood pressure-lowering drugs on central aortic pressure and clinical outcomes: principal results of the Conduit Artery Function Evaluation (CAFE) study. Circulation 2006;113:1213-1225.
31. Gillespie EL, White CM, Kardas M, et al. The impact of ACE inhibitors or angiotensin II type 1 receptor blockers on the development of new-onset type 2 diabetes. Diabetes Care 2005;28:2261-2266.
32. Lindholm LH, Carlberg B, Samuelsson O. Should beta blockers remain first choice in the treatment of primary hypertension? A meta-analysis. Lancet 2005;366:1545-1553.
33. Chalmers J, Castaigne A, Morgan T, Chastang C. Long-term efficacy of a new, fixed, very-low-dose angiotensin-converting enzyme-inhibitor/diuretic combination as first-line therapy in elderly hypertensive patients. J Hypertens 2000;18:327-337.
34. Pressel SL, Davis BR, Wright JT, et al. Operational aspects of terminating the doxazosin arm of The Antihypertensive and Lipid Lowering Treatment to Prevent Heart Attack Trial (ALLHAT). Control Clin Trials 2001;22:29-41.
35. Hansson L, Zanchetti A. The Hypertension Optimal Treatment (HOT) Study: 24-month data on blood pressure and tolerability. Blood Press 1997;6:313-317.

23

DYSLIPIDEMIAS

Matthew S. Murphy and Timothy O'Brien

INTRODUCTION 303
LIPOPROTEIN PHYSIOLOGY 303
Exogenous Pathway 303
Endogenous Pathway 303
Reverse Cholesterol Transport 305
PATHOPHYSIOLOGY 305
Atherosclerosis 305
LDL Cholesterol as Cardiovascular Risk Marker 305
Other Lipid Cardiovascular Risk Factors 306
Nonlipid Risk Factors 306
Emerging Risk Factors 306
CLASSIFICATION OF LIPOPROTEIN DISORDERS 306
Primary Lipoprotein Disorders 306
Primary (Genetic) Hyperlipoproteinemias 307
Primary Hypolipoproteinemia 308
Abetalipoproteinemia and Hypobetalipoproteinemia 308
Secondary Dyslipidemia 308
GOALS OF THERAPY AND THERAPEUTIC APPROACH 308
Adult Treatment Panel III Guidelines 309
THERAPEUTIC AGENTS 309
HMG CoA Reductase Inhibitors 309
Mechanism of Action of HMG CoA Reductase Inhibitors 309
Pleiotropic Effects of HMG CoA Reductase Inhibitors 310
Pharmacokinetics 311
Adverse Events 311
Pharmacogenetics 312
Therapeutic Use 312
Bile Acid Sequestrants 312
Cholesterol Absorption Inhibitors 313
Niacin 313
Omega-3 Fatty Acids 314
Fibrates 314
Other Therapies 315
Therapeutic Lifestyle Changes 315
Plant Sterols 315
Surgery 315
Rimonabant 315
Orlistat 315
Sibrutamine 315
EMERGING THERAPIES 316
CETP Inhibitors 316
MTP Inhibitors 316
ACAT Inhibitors 316
Bile Acid Transport Inhibitors 316
LXR Agonists 316
Gene Therapy 316
SUMMARY 316

INTRODUCTION

Atherosclerosis is a leading cause of death in the developed world and is becoming the leading cause of mortality globally.[1] It is the most common cause of coronary artery disease, peripheral vascular disease, and cerebrovascular disease. Dyslipidemia is a modifiable risk factor for atherosclerosis and is second in magnitude only to tobacco smoking in this respect.[2] Treatment for dyslipidemia is proven to be effective in primary and secondary prevention of ischemic heart disease and is also of benefit in other atherosclerotic diseases.[3] Despite the effectiveness of therapy in individual patients, the global burden of mortality from ischemic heart disease is predicted to double from 1990 to 2020.[4]

LIPOPROTEIN PHYSIOLOGY

Lipoproteins are spherical particles with lipid and protein components. The lipoprotein has an outer layer containing phospholipids and other polar lipids, free cholesterol, proteins (termed *apolipoproteins*), and a central core of hydrophobic lipids (mostly triglycerides and cholesterol esters). One exception to this is nascent, or newly formed, high-density lipoprotein (HDL), which is a discoid lipid bilayer because it lacks a central hydrophobic lipid core, which it gains as it matures.

Exogenous Pathway

The products of lipid digestion are absorbed from the intestinal micelles by the intestinal enterocyte (Fig. 23-1). Intestinal cholesterol is absorbed by the sterol transporter, Niemann-Pick C1–like 1 (NPC1L1) transporter, which is located in the brush border of the small intestine and is responsible for the jejunal uptake of cholesterol and other phytosterols.[5] Free cholesterol is esterified by acyl coenzymeA:cholesterol acyltransferase 2 (ACAT2) to cholestryl esters. Lecithin and triglycerides are also produced from the products of lipid digestion. Triglycerides, phospholipids, and cholesteryl esters are combined with apolipoprotein B48 (apoB48) and form chylomicrons that are secreted into the lymph. The transfer of triglyceride is mediated by microsomal triglyceride transfer protein (MTP), an essential enzyme in lipoprotein assembly. ApoB48 is unique to chylomicrons. ApoB48 arises from a posttranslational modification of ApoB mRNA, which causes in a single nucleotide substitution that results in introduction of a stop codon at position 48 in a process known as *apo B mRNA editing*.[6] Nascent, newly formed chylomicrons also receive apolipoprotein C (apoC-I, apoC-II, apoC-III) from HDL particles. Chylomicrons also have apolipoprotein E (apoE) as a surface component, possibly received from HDL.

Lipoprotein lipase is found on the vascular endothelium in tissues with high requirement for triglycerides; adipose tissue, skeletal muscle, cardiac muscle, and in lactating women, breast. It releases triglycerides from lipoproteins, hydrolyzing them into free fatty acids and glycerol. After chylomicrons receive apoC-II, they are capable of activating lipoprotein lipase. After triglyceride hydrolysis, chylomicrons become smaller and transfer surface components (such as free cholesterol, apoC and phospholipids) to HDL (Fig. 23-2). The particle formed as a result of this process, the chylomicron remnant, contains apoE and apoB48 on the surface. Hepatic removal of chylomicron remnants is mediated by apoE, inhibited by apoC-III, and mediated via the low-density lipoprotein (LDL) receptor. There is an alternative pathway for removal of chylomicron remnants via the LDL receptor–related protein (LRP) pathway. The triglyceride content in the chylomicron remnant is further hydrolyzed by hepatic lipase (HL).

Endogenous Pathway

The liver produces very low density lipoprotein (VLDL) as a triglyceride-rich lipoprotein expressing apoB100, apoC-I, apoC-II, apoC-III,

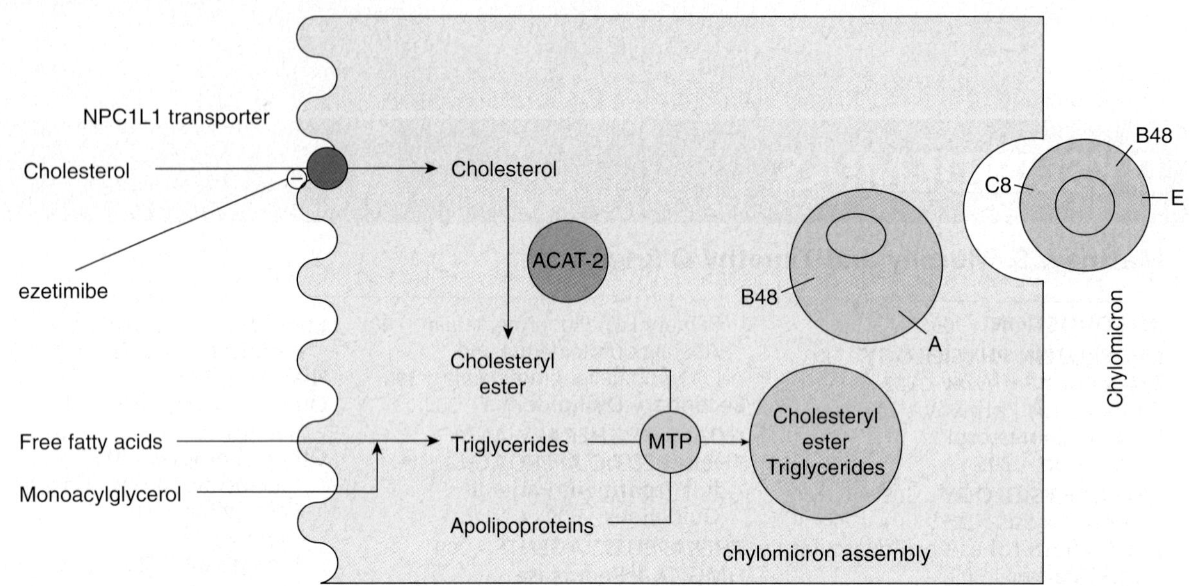

FIGURE 23-1 • Simplified schematic figure of cholesterol absorption and chylomicron assembly in the intestinal enterocyte. Free cholesterol is absorbed by Niemann-Pick C1–like 1 (NPC1L1) transporter and subsequently esterified by acyl coenzyme A: cholesterol acyltransferase 2 (ACAT2) to hydrophobic cholesteryl esters. Triglycerides are absorbed as free fatty acids and monoacylglycerol, which are the products of digestion, and subsequently reassembled. Chylomicrons are assembled in a two-step process under the action of microsomal triglyceride transfer protein (MTP) and secreted into the lymph.

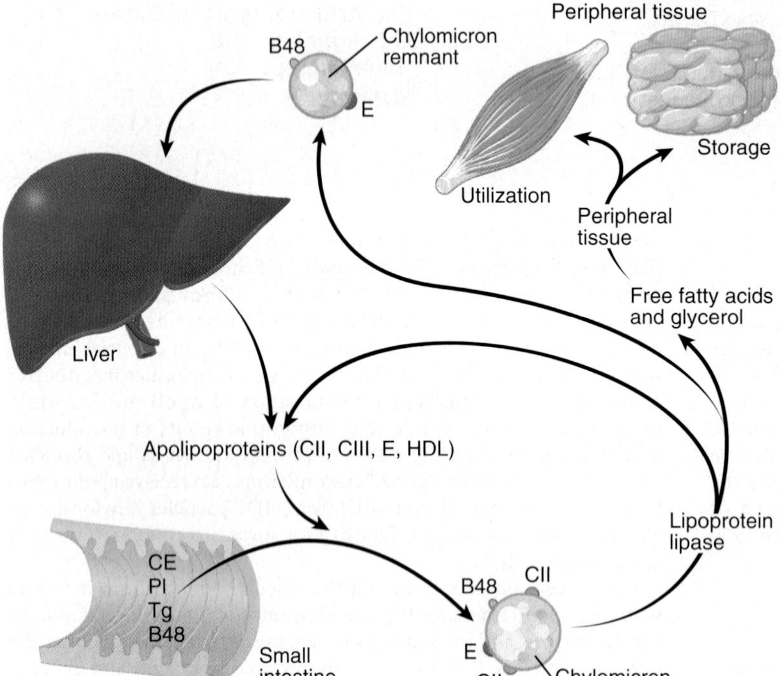

FIGURE 23-2 • Transport and metabolism of chylomicron and chylomicron remnants. The triglyceride content of chylomicrons is hydrolyzed by lipoprotein lipase into free fatty acids and glycerol; these are taken up by peripheral tissues. Consequently, chylomicrons become smaller and lose surface components. The cholesteryl ester–rich remnant of this process is removed by the liver, predominantly by a pathway mediated by apolipoprotein E. B48, apolipoprotein B48; C I, apolipoprotein C I; C II, apolipoprotein CII; C III, apolipoprotein C III; CE, cholesteryl ester; E, apolipoprotein E; FFA, free fatty acids; HDL, high-density lipoprotein; Pl, phospholipid; Tg, triglyceride.

and apoE (Fig. 23-3). Triglycerides are transferred to the nascent VLDL particle by MTP. Cholesterol is transferred from the liver into VLDL particles as free cholesterol. This is subsequently converted into cholesteryl esters as it circulates by HDL-associated ACAT2. Plasma VLDL is subject to metabolism by lipoprotein lipase, which leads to triglyceride hydrolysis. The triglyceride-poor remnant of the VLDL particle formed as a result of this process is called intermediate-density lipoprotein (IDL). Approximately half the IDL is subject to further triglyceride hydrolysis by lipoprotein lipase, forming LDL with loss of apoC to HDL. The remaining IDL is removed by the liver. ApoE is intimately involved in triglyceride metabolism and is found on the triglyceride-rich lipoproteins; chylomicrons, chylomicron remnants, VLDL, and IDL. The apoE-associated lipoprotein fraction of IDL and chylomicron remnants is often referred to as *β-VLDL.*

LDL is largely produced from IDL. LDL particles are cholesterol-rich lipoproteins that express apoB100 and bind predominantly to the LDL receptor facilitating their clearance. The major site of LDL receptor expression is the liver, the major site of LDL catabolism. The LDL particle bound to its receptor is internalized and degraded. Intracellular cholesterol interacts with sterol regulator element-binding proteins (SREBP) that negatively inhibits the transcription of the LDL receptor, thus modulating intracellular cholesterol concentrations. Non–LDL receptor–mediated pathways are responsible for minor amounts of LDL catabolism. Oxidation of LDL particles increases atherogenicity and may result in uptake by macrophages via the scavenger receptor resulting in foam cell formation, an early stage in the development of an atherosclerotic plaque. Uptake by this pathway, in contrast to the LDL receptor, is not down-regulated when intracellular

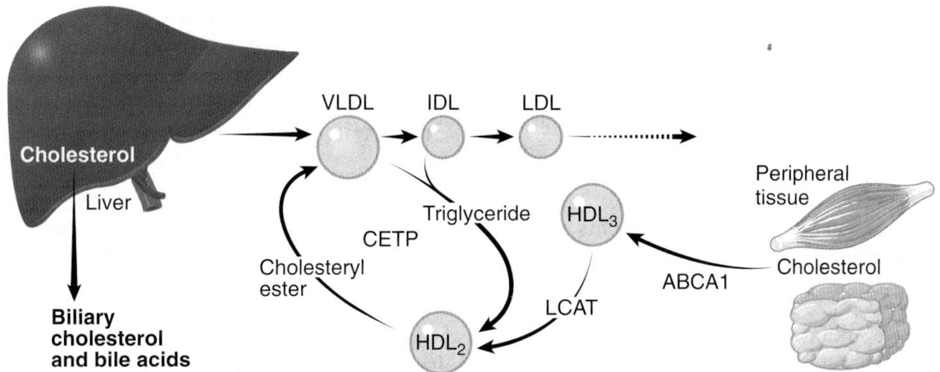

FIGURE 23-3 • Simplified schematic of transport and metabolism of endogenous-derived lipids from liver to peripheral tissues. Very low density lipoprotein (VLDL) is assembled by the hepatocyte in a two-step process and secreted into the circulation. VLDL is metabolized by lipoprotein lipase, and the triglyceride is hydrolyzed into free fatty acids (FFA), and glycerol, which is taken up by peripheral tissue. Approximately half of these triglyceride-poor remnants are catabolized by the liver. The remainder are converted to low-density lipoprotein (LDL) with loss of apolipoproteins C and E. LDL is cleared by the liver after binding to the LDL receptor or by other non-LDL receptor–mediated pathways. B100, apolipoprotein B100; C I, apolipoprotein C I; C II, apolipoprotein C II; C III, apolipoprotein C III; E, apolipoprotein E; HL, hepatic lipase; IDL, intermediate-density lipoprotein.

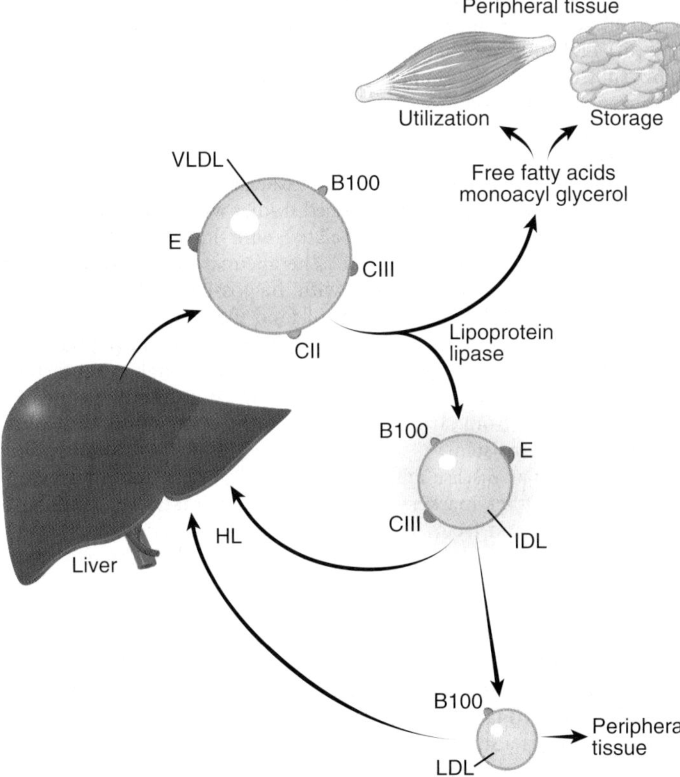

FIGURE 23-4 • Simplified schematic of reverse cholesterol transport. Free cholesterol is transferred from peripheral cells to newly formed high-density lipoprotein (HDL) by adenosine triphosphate (ATP)–binding cassette A1 (ABCA1) to form HDL_3. This cholesterol is esterified by lecithin:cholesterol acyl transferase (LCAT) to cholesteryl ester, forming HDL_2. Cholesteryl ester transfer protein (CETP) exchanges these cholesteryl esters with triglycerides (Tg) from apolipoprotein B lipoproteins. Cholesteryl ester–enriched apoB lipoproteins and the remnant HDL_1 are metabolized by the liver. IDL, intermediate-density lipoprotein; LDL, low-density lipoprotein; VLDL, very low density lipoprotein.

cholesterol levels increase. Levels of oxidized LDL are closely correlated with atherosclerosis.[7]

Reverse Cholesterol Transport

Reverse cholesterol transport, mediated by HDL particles, refers to the transfer of lipid from tissues to the liver (Fig. 23-4). Nascent HDL, sometimes referred to as pre-β1 HDL, is a discoid lipid bilayer that becomes spherical as it acquires a hydrophobic lipid core of predominantly cholesteryl esters. The cell membrane shuttle protein adenosine triphosphate (ATP)–binding cassette A1 (ABCA1) facilitates the transfer of free cholesterol from cells to the HDL particle. Two proteins are central to reverse cholesterol transport; lecithin:cholesterol acyl transferase (LCAT), which is responsible for esterification of free cholesterol within the HDL particle, and cholesteryl ester transfer protein (CETP), which mediates bidirectional transfer of cholesteryl ester and triglycerides between HDL and apoB lipoproteins. The net effect of inhibition of CETP is to raise HDL cholesterol.[8] As the newly formed HDL_3 particle gains cholesteryl esters, it matures into HDL_2 and expresses apoA-II in addition to apoA-I. CETP mediates the transfer of cholestryl esters from the mature HDL_2 to apoB lipoproteins, VLDL, IDL, LDL, and chylomicrons. A number of enzymes, such as paraoxonase, associated with HDL protect HDL and LDL from oxidation. During episodes of acute inflammation, this protective mechanism can be overwhelmed. Free cholesterol and cholesteryl esters are handled by the liver by a number of pathways—uptake of apoB lipoproteins enriched with cholesteryl esters by CETP, uptake and internalization of HDL lipoproteins, and selective uptake of cholesteryl esters and free cholesterol by hepatic scavenger receptor BI (SRBI) and hepatic lipase (HL).

PATHOPHYSIOLOGY

Atherosclerosis

Atherosclerosis is a progressive disease process that primarily affects large elastic arteries (such as the aorta, carotid, and iliac arteries) and large and medium-sized muscular arteries (such as the coronary and popliteal arteries). The earliest pathologic abnormalities are fatty streaks, composed of lipid-filled foam cells, and extracellular lipid deposition, seen in the arteries of pediatric subjects at postmortem.[9] It is generally believed that these evolve into a fibrous plaque that ultimately becomes organized. With time, these fibrous plaques become mature atherosclerotic plaques with a lipid core.

Atherosclerosis is a progressive disease, and although the plaque may occupy an increasing percentage of the lumen of the artery, it generally is not associated with clinical symptoms until stenosis approaches 70% or greater. Plaque rupture is a more acute phenomenon that can lead to an abrupt reduction in blood flow; this is the likely etiology in the majority of myocardial infarctions.[10] One of the major determinants of both the initiation of vessel damage and the rate of development of the atherosclerotic lesion seems to be plasma levels of key lipoprotein particles.

LDL Cholesterol as Cardiovascular Risk Marker

Epidemiologic studies have established the relationship between LDL cholesterol and cardiovascular risk. This relationship is similar for both primary onset and secondary recurrence of a major cardiovascular event. The relationship was initially described for total cholesterol, of which LDL cholesterol is a major component, and has subsequently been described for LDL cholesterol.[11,12] Whereas, initially, it was believed that a threshold LDL cholesterol level existed above which the risk of cardiovascular disease risk increased, it is becoming more evident that there is no threshold. In populations in which there are very low levels of cholesterol (LDL < 100 mg/dl), there is a low but definite prevalence of cardiovascular disease. Further insights into the relationship of LDL cholesterol and cardiovascular disease risk are seen in clinical trials of LDL cholesterol–lowering therapies. Lowering LDL cholesterol has been shown to reduce cardiovascular disease outcomes in primary and secondary prevention studies.

Other Lipid Cardiovascular Risk Factors

Other traditional lipid risk factors for cardiovascular disease are elevated triglycerides,[13] low HDL,[14] and elevated non-HDL cholesterol.[15] One particular lipoprotein profile associated with atherosclerosis is the combination characterized by elevated triglycerides, borderline high LDL cholesterol, small dense LDL particles, and reduced HDL cholesterol.[16] Often, each component is marginally abnormal, with the cumulative effect being a markedly increased cardiovascular disease risk. This profile, termed *atherogenic dyslipidemia*, is associated with a threefold increased risk of cardiovascular disease and is approximately three times more common in patients with diabetes mellitus. Atherogenic dyslipidemia is a component of the American Heart Association/National Heart, Lung, and Blood Institute (AHA/NHLBI) definition of the metabolic syndrome.[17]

Prospective epidemiologic studies show a positive correlation between serum triglyceride measurements and the subsequent incidence of cardiovascular disease in univariate analysis.[13] Elevated triglycerides are commonly associated with other cardiovascular risk factors. When the data are subject to multivariate analysis, the relative risk attributed to triglycerides is diminished and possibly abolished.[18,19] Clinical trials using triglyceride-lowering drugs have shown a reduction in cardiovascular events in primary and secondary studies, but because these drugs have effects on many lipoproteins, the role of triglyceride lowering per se remains unclear.

Low HDL cholesterol is a well-established independent and predictive risk factor for cardiovascular disease. An inverse relationship exists between HDL cholesterol and cardiovascular disease risk in both men and women. Whereas there is evidence that HDL may be directly antiatherogenic, as with triglycerides, HDL level also correlates with other atherosclerotic influences. Low HDL is a component of the metabolic syndrome and a marker for insulin resistance. There is also an inverse relationship between HDL cholesterol and triglycerides. Drugs that elevate HDL are associated with improved cardiovascular risk outcomes, but these drugs have effects on other lipoproteins, making the individual contribution of raising HDL cholesterol difficult to dissect. Apolipoprotein A-I (apoA-I) is the major apolipoprotein associated with HDL. The plasma concentration of apoA-I is closely and inversely correlated with cardiovascular risk. HDL is also involved in mitigating the pathogenic risk of LDL, in particular the inflammatory effects of LDL on the vasculature.[20]

Non-HDL cholesterol is calculated as the difference between total and HDL cholesterol. It is a measure of apoB containing lipoproteins; VLDL, IDL, and LDL, including small dense LDL. Non-HDL cholesterol appears to be particularly useful as a cardiovascular risk marker in those with combined dyslipidemia with triglycerides greater than 200 mg/dl.[21] ApoB measurement has also shown this protein to be a strong predictor of cardiovascular events; it may in itself become a primary therapeutic target.[22,23]

Nonlipid Risk Factors

Nonmodifiable risk factors for cardiovascular disease are age, male sex, and a family history of premature cardiovascular disease. Modifiable risk factors are hypertension, cigarette smoking, diabetes mellitus, overweight/obesity, physical inactivity, and diets with a high intake of saturated fats and cholesterol.[24]

Emerging Risk Factors

There is considerable interest in enhancing the identification of those at risk of onset or progression of atherosclerotic disease. There are many emerging risk factors which may enhance risk prediction but the role of measurement remains an area of active investigation.[25,26]

Lipoprotein(a) (Lp[a]) is a modified lipoprotein particle with a covalent binding of apoB100 and specific apolipoprotein apo(a). Serum concentrations of apo(a) correlate closely with cardiovascular disease risk among white populations.[27] Apoprotein (a) is structurally related to plasiminogen and appears to interfere with endothelium-mediated fibrinolysis.[28] Nicotinic acid, estrogen therapy, and LDL apheresis are effective modulators of Lp(a). Recent data suggest the atherogenic nature of Lp(a) may be related to oxidation of the particle.[29] Among black populations, Lp(a) measurements are generally twice those in white populations; however, the association of Lp(a) or apo(a) and cardiovascular disease is less robust.[30,31]

Small dense LDL appears to be generated by intravascular remodeling of VLDL after interaction with lipoprotein lipase, HL, and CETP. This subfraction of LDL appears to be particularly atherogenic and is prone to oxidation. Nicotinic acid derivatives and fibrates convert small LDL particles into more buoyant, less atherogenic LDL particles.[32,33]

Elevated levels of homocysteine are associated with cardiovascular disease in prospective population-based studies with increased rates of cardiovascular disease and is associated with impaired endothelial function and a procoagulant state.[34] Therapeutic options to decrease homocysteine are dietary folic acid with the possible addition of vitamins B_6 and B_{12}. Folate fortification of food in the United States has been shown to reduce the average homocysteine level in the population and to halve the percentage of the population with a high homocysteine level.[35] There is some evidence for a reduction in the incidence and/or mortality from stroke with folate supplementation, although the data are inconsistent.[34,36] C-reactive protein (CRP) is a biomarker for cardiovascular disease and correlates with adverse cardiovascular outcomes.[27,37] Other markers, erythrocyte sedimentation rate (ESR), and von Willebrand factor have shown weaker correlations with cardiovascular disease risk. In addition, therapies that have been shown to modulate cardiovascular disease risk have also been shown to modulate CRP in primary and secondary prevention studies.[38] Many other potential risk markers for cardiovascular disease are under investigation, either individually or in combination, for example, apoB : apoA-I ratio.[26] Early detection of atherosclerosis using techniques such as detection of coronary calcium by ultrafast computed tomographic (CT) scanning is also of interest.[26]

CLASSIFICATION OF LIPOPROTEIN DISORDERS

Primary disorders of lipoproteins have been classified by Fredrickson/World Health Organization (WHO) based on the lipoprotein classes present in excess (Table 23-1). To summarize; type Ia is associated with elevations of chylomicrons, type IIa with elevation of LDL particles, type IIb with elevation of LDL and VLDL, type III with elevated remnant particles (β-VLDL), type IV with elevation of VLDL, and type V with elevation of VLDL and chylomicrons. It is crucial to rule out secondary causes of hyperlipidemia such as hypothyroidism, drugs, diabetes mellitus, and renal dysfunction, which are discussed in this chapter.

Primary Lipoprotein Disorders

In this section, we discuss primary (genetic) lipoprotein disorders including familial hypercholesterolemia (FH), autosomal recessive hypercholesterolemia (ARH), familial combined hyperlipidemia

TABLE 23-1 WHO CLASSIFICATION OF HYPERLIPOPROTEINEMIA

Type	Lipoprotein Increased	Lipid Increased
I	Chylomicrons	Triglycerides
IIa	LDL	Cholesterol
IIb	LDL and VLDL	Cholesterol and triglycerides
III	β-VLDL (IDL and chylomicron remnants)	Cholesterol and triglycerides
IV	VLDL	Triglycerides
V	Chylomicrons and VLDL	Cholesterol and triglycerides

IDL, intermediate-density lipoprotein; LDL, low-density lipoprotein; VLDL, very low density lipoprotein.

(FCHL), polygenic hypercholesterolemia, familial dysbetalipoproteinemia, and familial hypertriglyceridemia. Primary lipoprotein disorders in which a relative deficiency of certain lipoproteins exists are also discussed.

Primary (Genetic) Hyperlipoproteinemias

Familial Hypercholesterolemia (FH). FH was first described by Muller in 1938. It is characterized by increased plasma levels of total and LDL cholesterol, tendinous xanthomata, and premature coronary heart disease (CHD). It is inherited as an autosomal dominant disorder with homozygotes having a more severe phenotype than heterozygotes. FH can result from mutations in the LDL receptor (LDL-R) gene. An identical phenotype is also seen with mutations in the *apoB-100* gene and also with mutations in the proprotein convertase subtilisin/kexin type 9 (PCSK9) gene.[39] The LDL-R gene is located in chromosome 19 (19p13.1-p13.3) with over 800 associated mutations in the LDL-R gene identified. Homozygous FH is the most severe form of FH, with a prevalence of approximately 1 in 100,000. It is characterized by development of cutaneous xanthomata in childhood, premature atherosclerosis and without treatment, patients may die before age 30. Total cholesterol is typically greater than 600 mg/dl. Atherosclerotic cardiovascular disease in childhood is frequent, often requiring invasive coronary intervention. By adolescence, atheromatous deposits on the aortic root may lead to aortic stenosis. Current therapeutic options include LDL apheresis and use of high doses of 3-hydroxy-3-methylglutaryl coenzyme A (HMG CoA) reductase inhibitors in combination with bile acid sequestrants, ezetimibe, or niacin.[40,41] Liver transplantation has also been used to treat this condition; in rare instances, combined liver and heart transplantation has been performed.[42]

The frequency of heterozygous FH is typically 1 in 500, but this can vary in specific geographic populations owing to the "founder effect." The phenotypic expression of heterozygous FH is variable. Certain LDL-R mutations are associated with a more severe phenotype. Typically, the total cholesterol is 350 mg/dl to 450 mg/dl. Usually, triglycerides are normal, resulting in a type IIa pattern, but rarely, triglycerides can be elevated, giving a type IIb pattern. In those individuals with elevated triglycerides, HDL may also be lower. Untreated by the age of 65, 85% of affected males and 50% of affected females with FH will have a major coronary event. Screening for FH is based on diagnostic criteria using family history and measured cholesterol.[41] Screening for FH by genetic testing is difficult owing to the large number of genetic mutations associated with FH. However, a study has shown analysis by gene array to be reproducible, highly specific, and sensitive.[43]

Autosomal Recessive Hypercholesterolemia (ARH). ARH results from a monogenetic mutation in the ARH protein gene on chromosome 1 (1p35-36) that modulates internalization of LDL and causes a tissue-specific defect in LDL removal.[44] The phenotype, described in 1999, has many similarities with autosomal dominant homozygous FH with huge xanthomata and premature atherosclerosis; however, its phenotype is less severe. Pharmacologic drug therapy is important and often more successful than in homozyg-ous FH, with up to a 60% reduction in LDL seen with bile acid sequestrants.[45,46]

Familial Combined Hyperlipidemia (FCHL). FCHL is one of the most common primary dyslipidemias, with a prevalence of 1% to 2%.[47] The typical lipoprotein profile is of elevated cholesterol and/or elevated triglyceride levels, elevated apoB, and a preponderance of small dense LDL. In addition, there may be elevations in VLDL particles and decreases in HDL and apoA-I.[48] The phenotype is often type IIb, sometimes type Iia, and less commonly, type IV. These phenotypes of FCHL often vary over time. FCHL is estimated to account for up to 10% of premature atherosclerosis cases.[49] It is a genetically heterogeneous disease with multiple gene loci under investigation.[50] The two major genes implicated in FCHL are one that relates to apoB-100 secretion and another that influences small dense LDL.[51,52]

Common (Polygenic) Hypercholesterolemia. The most common cause of isolated hypercholesterolemia appears to be polygenic with evidence for an interaction between a number of genetic defects and the environment leading to possible overproduction of VLDL and conversion to LDL. Obesity and a diet high in saturated fat and cholesterol are associated with this accumulation of LDL cholesterol overwhelming the clearance of LDL. Expression of the phenotype of polygenic hypercholesterolemia and the associated development of atherosclerosis may be delayed many decades, in contrast to the early presentation of FH and ARH.

The presence of Achilles tendon xanthomata is specific for FH and can be a clinically useful factor to distinguish FH from polygenic hypercholesterolemia and other genetic hyperlipoproteinemias.[53] Tendon xanthomata also can occur in cerebrotendinous xanthomatosis and phytosterolemia; however, these are rare metabolic disorders. Cerebrotendinous xanthomatosis caused by mutations in the sterol 27-hydroxylase gene are associated with elevated cholestanol levels and secondary accumulation of cholestanol in brain, lens, tendons, and other tissues. In phytosterolemia, also called β-sitosterolemia, there is a failure to regulate intestinal absorption of plant sterols and a decrease in biliary excretion of sterols. Subsequent deposition of these sterols in tendons and other tissues occurs. Phytosterolemia (β-sitosterolemia) is associated with aggressive atherosclerosis.[54]

Familial Dysbetalipoproteinemia (Remnant Removal Disease). Familial dysbetalipoproteinemia (remnant removal disease) is associated with type III hyperlipoproteinemia and is characterized by increased levels of chylomicron remnants and IDL, collectively known as β-VLDL. Polymorphisms of the apoE gene locus, typically homozygosity for apoε2, lead to the deficient clearance of β-VLDL. Ninety percent of patients with type III hyperlipoproteinemia are homozygous for apoε2, with the bulk of the remainder being heterozygous apoε2/apoε3 or apoε2/apoε4. However, not all individuals with apoε2 have type III hyperlipoproteinemia, and frequently, a secondary cause such as hypothyroidism may unmask the condition (Box 23-1). Type III hyperlipoproteinemia has a clinical phenotype of striate palmar xanthomata and tuberoeruptive xanthomata. It is associated with accelerated atherosclerosis in all vascular beds with a strong predilection for peripheral vascular disease. Biochemically, elevations in both total cholesterol and triglycerides are often elevated to similar extents.

Familial Hypertriglyceridemia. Hypertriglyceridemia may occur either as a primary (familial) or, more commonly, as a secondary disorder consequent to another disorder (Box 23-2). Type I hyperlipoproteinemia is associated with severe fasting hypertriglyceridemia (>1000 mg/dl) and with an excess of chylomicrons. In the absence of a secondary cause, primary severe hypertriglyceridemia is often familial with an autosomal recessive inheritance. It is commonly due to a defect in lipoprotein lipase leading to a reduced clearance of chylomicrons and, usually, of VLDL.[55] It is rarely due to a deficiency in apoC-II.[55] It usually presents in childhood. However, it commonly changes phenotype to a type V hyperlipoproteinemic pattern with a rise in VLDL later in life. Physical signs in severe hypertriglyceridemia are tuberoeruptive xanthomata, hepatosplenomegaly, and lipidemia retinalis. Severe hypertriglyceridemia (>1000 mg/dl) is associated with pancreatitis. Reduction of triglyceride to less than 1000 mg/dl reduces the incidence of pancreatitis. This can often be achieved with a combination of avoidance of known causes of secondary hypertriglyceri-

BOX 23-1 SECONDARY CAUSES OF HYPERCHOLESTEROLEMIA

Hypothyroidism
Obstructive liver disease
Nephrotic syndrome
Anorexia nervosa
Acute intermittent prophyria
Drugs
- Progestogens
- Cyclosporine
- Thiazides

BOX 23-2 SECONDARY CAUSES OF HYPERTRIGLYCERIDEMIA

Obesity	Drugs
Diabetes mellitus	Estrogen
Chronic renal failure	Isoretinoin
Alcohol	β-Adrenergic antagonists
Glycogen storage disorders	Glucocorticoids
Ileal bypass surgery	Bile acid sequestrants
Lipodystrophy	Thiazides
Pregnancy	Protease inhibitors
Acute hepatitis	
Monoclonal gammopathies	
Multiple myeloma	
Lymphomas	
Stress	
Sepsis	
Systemic lupus erythematosus	

demia, where possible, and of dietary and pharmacologic therapy. Plasmapheresis may be useful as an adjuvant therapy.[56]

Type IV hyperlipoproteinemia is often referred to as moderate hypertriglyceridemia. The typical lipid profile is of an elevated triglyceride measurement typically 200 mg/dl to 900 mg/dl with a total cholesterol not exceeding 200 mg/dl. Type IV hyperlipoproteinemia is associated with diabetes mellitus and excess alcohol intake.

Primary Hypolipoproteinemia

Primary hypoalphalipoproteinemias are a heterogeneous group of disorders. Single gene mutations account for a minority of these. Tangier disease is an autosomal recessively inherited lipoprotein disorder associated with a mutation of the ABCA1 transporter, which is involved in the transfer of cholesterol and phospholipids to the apoA-containing nascent HDL lipoprotein particle. The consequence of this mutation is intracellular accumulation of cholesteryl ester, especially in macrophages and other reticuloendothelial cells, forming foam cells, low HDL, and aggressive atherosclerosis. Clinical features of Tangier disease include large yellow-orange tonsils, neuropathies, splenomegaly, hepatomegaly, and ocular abnormalities. Homozygotes have a virtual absence of plasma HDL and apoA-I, decreased LDL, and hypertriglyceridemia (>300 mg/dl). Homozygotes have a 30-fold increased risk of cardiovascular disease. Heterozygotes have a less severe phenotype. Study of this disease has led to insights into the function to the ABCA1 transporter. Peroxime proliferator activator receptor γ (PPARγ) agonists, liver X receptor (LXR) agonists, and retinoid X receptor (RXR) agonists appear to favorably modulate ABCA1.[57]

Familial LCAT Deficiency. Familial LCAT deficiency (FLD) is a hereditary primary lipoprotein disorder with autosomal recessive inheritance. LCAT is an enzyme involved in reverse cholesterol transport. Its primary role is in the formation and maturation of HDL particles, and it is responsible for esterification of free cholesterol within the HDL particle. It also has some cholesterol esterification activity in apoB-containing LDL.[58] LCAT deficiency is associated with low HDL levels. Clinical features are corneal opacities, anemia, and renal disease. A less severe phenotype in which there is a partial LCAT deficiency is fish eye disease (FED). In FLD, LCAT catalytic activity is completely lacking, whereas in FED, the mutant LCAT lacks activity on HDL particles but esterifies cholesterol to apoB-containing lipoproteins.[59,60] Lipoproteins are affected with lower HDL, apoA-I, apo A-II, apoB, higher triglycerides, and similar LDL concentrations compared with those in control populations.[60] It is unclear whether there is an increased risk of cardiovascular disease in LCAT deficiency, but recent evidence suggests this to be the case.[61]

Other Hypolipoproteinemias. A small number of patients with defective HDL production due to mutations in the apoA-I gene on chromosome 11 have been described. Homozygotes are characterized by very low HDL cholesterol, and they develop clinically significant atherosclerotic heart disease between the ages of 25 and 50 years.[62] ApoA-IMilano is an apoA-I polymorphism associated with low HDL levels. However, this mutation appears to be protective against atherosclerosis.[63] Recombinant apoA-IMilano, other forms of apoA-I and apoA-I mimetics show promise as therapeutic agents against atherosclerotic disease.[64,65]

Abetalipoproteinemia and Hypobetalipoproteinemia

Abetalipoproteinemia is a disorder of lipoprotein metabolism caused by mutations in MTP. It is characterized by an absence of apoB-containing lipoproteins. Consequently, there is a deficiency of fat-soluble vitamins with associated acanthosis, spinocerebellar degeneration, and atypical retinitis pigmentosa. Inheritance is autosomal recessive. Supplementation with fat-soluble vitamins, in particular vitamin E, can arrest progression of neuropathy.[66]

Familial hypobetalipoproteinemia (FHBL) is a hereditary disorder of lipoprotein metabolism characterized by very low levels of apoB-100 with an estimated prevalence of 0.1% to 1.9%. Consequently, levels of VLDL, IDL, and LDL are very low, and this condition is associated with low levels of cardiovascular disease.[67] Inheritance is autosomal dominant. Homozygous FHBL has a similar phenotype to abetalipoproteinemia and also requires supplementation with fat-soluble vitamins.[68]

Secondary Dyslipidemia

Significant dyslipidemia may occur as a consequence of other disorders and most commonly presents with either a type V or a type IV pattern. Likewise, primary disorders outlined previously may be exacerbated by these conditions. Some of the more common causes of secondary dyslipidemia are diabetes mellitus, hypothyroidism, and obesity. Therapeutic agents such as β-adrenergic antagonists, thiazide diuretics, retinoic acid derivatives, estrogens, androgens, and glucocorticoids may also cause a secondary dyslipidemia. Alcohol may also cause a secondary dyslipidemia. All of these conditions should be considered in patients presenting with dyslipidemia.

GOALS OF THERAPY AND THERAPEUTIC APPROACH

The goals of therapy for dyslipidemia are to reduce the burden of diseases secondary to this disorder—atherosclerosis resulting in coronary artery disease, cerebrovascular disease, peripheral vascular disease, and other diseases such as pancreatitis in patients with severe hypertriglyceridemia. Lipid-lowering therapy is effective and reduces cardiovascular risk in primary and secondary prevention.[3]

The guiding principle of therapy for dyslipidemia is that the intensity of the intervention is proportionate to the associated cardiovascular risk. In addition to treating cardiovascular risk factors, all other risk factors present should be targeted (Box 23-3).

Many guidelines are available for the prevention of cardiovascular disease—the National Cholesterol Program's Adult Treatment Panel (ATP III),[24] Joint Task Force of European and Other Societies on cardiovascular disease prevention in clinical practice,[69] the Joint British Societies' guidelines on prevention of cardiovascular disease in clinical

BOX 23-3 NONLIPID RISK FACTORS FOR CHD

Hypertension
Cigarette smoking
Thrombogenic/hemostatic state
Diabetes mellitus
Obesity
Physical inactivity
Atherogenic diet
Age
Male sex
Family history of premature CHD

CHD, coronary heart disease.
Based on Grundy SM, Cleeman JI, Merz CN, et al. Implications of recent clinical trials for the National Cholesterol Education Program Adult Treatment Panel III Guidelines. J Am Coll Cardiol 2004;44:720-732; and Stone NJ, Bilek S, Rosenbaum S. Recent National Cholesterol Education Program Adult Treatment Panel III update: adjustments and options. Am J Cardiol 2005;96(4A):53E-59E.

practice (JBS 2).[70] Although some variation exists between guidelines, there is a concordance among all sets of guidelines in the emphasis on cardiovascular disease, global risk assessment, and the establishment of treatment targets. Guidelines must be considered dynamic and undoubtedly will change over time as risk factors (both traditional and emerging) are considered, as risk prediction models are reassessed, and as the results of clinical trials become available.[25,71]

Adult Treatment Panel III Guidelines

ATP III guidelines were published in 2001,[72] with the full report published in 2002.[24] This was an updated report in an ongoing process.[73,74] The basic principle underlying the guidelines for cholesterol-lowering intervention is that the intensity of treatment is directly related to the degree of risk for CHD events, with more aggressive goals for those at highest risk. The risk is stratified according to the presence of CHD (or a CHD risk equivalent) and the number of CHD risk factors present. In those without CHD (or CHD risk equivalent) but with multiple CHD risk factors, calculation of 10-year cardiovascular risk is used to set goals.

In ATP III, CHD is defined as symptomatic ischemic heart disease, including myocardial infarction, stable or unstable angina, demonstrated myocardial ischemia by noninvasive testing, and history of coronary artery procedures. CHD risk equivalents are found in those patients with noncoronary forms of clinical atherosclerotic disease—for example, peripheral arterial disease, abdominal aortic aneurysm, carotid artery disease (symptomatic [e.g., transient ischemic attack or stroke of carotid origin] or >50% stenosis on angiography or ultrasound)—and likely other forms of clinical atherosclerotic disease (e.g., renal artery disease). Diabetes mellitus or the presence of multiple cardiovascular risk factors and a predicted 10-year risk for CHD greater than 20% are also considered a CHD risk equivalent.

The major independent risk factors are cigarette smoking, hypertension (blood pressure [BP] ≥ 140/90 mm Hg or on antihypertensive medication), low HDL cholesterol (<40 mg/dl), family history of premature CHD (CHD in male first-degree relative < 55 yr; CHD in female first-degree relative < 65 yr) or age (men ≥ 45 yr; women ≥ 55 yr). If a person has high HDL cholesterol (≥60 mg/dl), one risk factor is subtracted from the count. In the ATP III guidelines, risk assessment for determining 10-year risk is carried out according to Framingham risk scoring.

ATP III recommends a two-step approach to cholesterol management. Priority goes to attaining the goal for LDL cholesterol; thereafter emphasis shifts to management of the metabolic syndrome and other lipid risk factors (e.g., hypertriglyceridemia and low HDL cholesterol). The first step in management is to initiate therapeutic lifestyle changes (TLC), which involves (i) reduced intake of saturated fats and cholesterol, (ii) therapeutic dietary options to enhance LDL lowering (plant stanols/sterols and increased viscous fiber), (iii) weight control, and (iv) increased physical activity. TLC is recommended for all patients, and guidelines on TLC were updated recently.[75] In those with the highest degree of risk and the lowest LDL cholesterol goal, it may be appropriate to initiate simultaneous commencement of therapeutic lifestyle change and drug therapy and to begin pharmacotherapy at the first visit. In others, after an appropriate trial of dietary therapy to reduce LDL cholesterol (~3 mo), two additional therapeutic decisions may be required. First, if the LDL cholesterol goal has not been achieved, consideration may be given to initiating drug therapy. Second, if the metabolic syndrome is present, additional lifestyle changes (i.e., weight reduction and increased physical activity) will be needed. Later, if lifestyle therapies do not alleviate the metabolic syndrome, drug therapy for treatment of the metabolic risk factors may be required.

After publication of major clinical trials,[76-80] revisions to the ATP III guidelines were suggested (Table 23-2).[21] These studies confirmed that the relationship between LDL cholesterol and the risk of a cardiovascular event was robust and curvilinear in nature. Two studies in particular demonstrated benefit in reducing LDL cholesterol below the ATP III goal in high-risk patient populations, especially those with additional risk factors.[81] For these patients, a new category, termed *very high risk*, was proposed. These patients have established cardiovascular disease plus (i) multiple major risk factors (especially diabetes mellitus), (ii) severe and poorly controlled risk factors (especially continued cigarette smoking), (iii) multiple risk factors of the metabolic syndrome, and (iv) acute coronary syndromes. For this patient category, LDL cholesterol goal was 100 mg/dl with an optional goal of 70 mg/dl.[21] An additional consideration, if drug therapy is needed, is to prescribe a dose of a drug to reduce LDL cholesterol by 30% to 40% to achieve a significant cardiovascular risk reduction. For high-risk patients with LDL cholesterol of 100 mg/dl to 129 mg/dl, a reduction in LDL cholesterol of 30% to 40% and not merely a target LDL cholesterol less than 100 mg/dl should be the goal. The advice for moderately high-risk patients with a 10-year risk of 10% to 20% and two or more risk factors, an optional goal of 100 mg/dl was supported by clinical trial evidence. For patients with lower risk categories, there was no change from the 2001 guidelines.

The initial choice of drug therapy to achieve the primary goal of lowering LDL cholesterol for the majority of patients is an HMG CoA reductase inhibitor (statin). Addition of either bile acid sequestrants or nicotinic acid derivative was suggested if LDL cholesterol target was not achieved. For those with atherogenic dyslipidemia, use of a fibrate, nicotinic acid, or other agents is suggested to correct non-LDL lipoprotein abnormalities.

THERAPEUTIC AGENTS

HMG CoA Reductase Inhibitors

Competitive inhibitors of HMG CoA reductase inhibitors, often termed *statins*, reduce the synthesis of intracellular cholesterol. The prototypical HMG CoA reductase inhibitor, mevastatin, was identified in 1971 and led to development of this class of drugs.[82] Lovastatin, pravastatin, and simvastatin were approved in 1990 and subsequently followed to market by fluvastatin, cerivastatin, atorvastatin, pitavastatin, and rosuvastatin (cerivastatin was later withdrawn).[83] The efficacy of HMG CoA reductase inhibitors in reducing LDL cholesterol is well documented. High-potency statins—atorvastatin, simvastatin and rosuvastatin—also have a moderate effect in lowering triglyceride levels but are ineffective in cases of severe hypertriglyceridemia associated with chylomicronemia.

Mechanism of Action of HMG CoA Reductase Inhibitors

HMG CoA reductase inhibitors bind reversibly to HMG CoA reductase and inhibit the catalytic enzyme that regulates the conversion of HMG CoA to mevalonate, the rate-limiting step in cholesterol biosynthesis. This leads to a decrease in intracellular cholesterol level in hepatocytes. In response to a reduction in intracellular cholesterol, increased expression of the LDL-R gene is induced by removing SREBP-mediated

TABLE 23-2 CLINICAL RISK CATEGORIES, LDL CHOLESTEROL GOALS, AND THRESHOLDS

Risk Category	LDL Cholesterol Goal	LDL Cholesterol Threshold to Initiate Drug Therapy	LDL Cholesterol Threshold to Initiate TLC	Comment
Very high risk Presence of CHD* or CHD risk equivalent† or 10-yr CV risk > 20%‡ AND Multiple or severe and poorly controlled risk factors§	<100 mg/dl <70 mg/dl (optional)	≥100 mg/dl ≥70 mg/dl	≥100 mg/dl ≥70 mg/dl	If high triglycerides present, secondary goal is non-HDL < 100 mg/dl
High risk Presence of CHD* or CHD risk equivalent† or 10-yr CV risk > 20%‡	<100 mg/dl	≥100 mg/dl	≥100 mg/dl	
Moderately high risk Two or more risk factors‖ 10-yr CV risk 10%-20%‡	<130 mg/dl <100 mg/dl (optional)	≥130 mg/dl ≥100 mg/dl	≥130 mg/dl ≥100 mg/dl	If starting drug therapy, use dose that would be expected to reduce LDL cholesterol by 30%-40%
Moderate risk Two or more risk factors‖ 10-yr CV risk < 10%‡	<130 mg/dl	≥160 mg/dl	≥130 mg/dl	
Low risk Zero or 1 risk factor	<160 mg/dl	≥190 mg/dl	≥160 mg/dl	

*Coronary heart disease (CHD) is defined as symptomatic ischemic heart disease, including myocardial infarction, stable or unstable angina, demonstrated myocardial ischemia by noninvasive testing, and history of coronary artery procedures.

†CHD risk equivalents are those with noncoronary forms of clinical atherosclerotic disease—e.g., peripheral arterial disease, abdominal aortic aneurysm, carotid artery disease (symptomatic [e.g., transient ischemic attack or stroke of carotid origin] or >50% stenosis on angiography or ultrasound)—and likely other forms of clinical atherosclerotic disease (e.g., renal artery disease) or diabetes mellitus or a person with multiple risk factors and a predicted 10-yr risk for CHD > 20%.

‡10-yr cardiovascular (CV) risk calculator available at www.nhlbi.nih.gov/guidelines/cholesterol

§Factors to consider are (i) multiple major risk factors, especially diabetes; (ii) severe and poorly controlled risk factors, especially continued cigarette smoking; (iii) multiple risk factors of the metabolic syndrome, especially triglycerides ≥ 200 mg/dl plus non–high-density lipoprotein (HDL) cholesterol ≥ 130 mg/dl with low HDL cholesterol < 40 mg/dl; and (iv) acute coronary syndromes.

‖Risk factors counted are cigarette smoking, hypertension (BP ≥ 140/90 mm Hg or on antihypertensive medication), low HDL cholesterol (<40 mg/dl), family history of premature CHD (CHD in male first-degree relative <55 yr; CHD in female first-degree relative < 65 yr) or age (men ≥ 45 yr; women ≥ 55 yr). If a person has a high HDL cholesterol (≥60 mg/dl), one risk factor is subtracted from the count.

BP, blood pressure; LDL, low-density lipoprotein; TLC, total lifestyle changes.

Based on updated Grundy SM, Cleeman JI, Merz CN, et al. Implications of recent clinical trials for the National Cholesterol Education Program Adult Treatment Panel III Guidelines. J Am Coll Cardiol 2004;44:720-732; and Stone NJ, Bilek S, Rosenbaum S. Recent National Cholesterol Education Program Adult Treatment Panel III update: adjustments and options. Am J Cardiol 2005;96(4A):53E-59E.

inhibition of LDL-R transcription. This results in increased surface expression of LDL-Rs with increased clearance of apoB- and apoE-containing lipoproteins, particularly LDL particles. ApoB is present on LDL, VLDL, and IDL, and clearance of these particles is increased after the introduction of HMG CoA reductase therapy. LDL-Rs also bind apoE, so likewise, there is increased clearance of apoE-containing lipoproteins; VLDL, IDL, and chylomicron remnants. Statins may directly reduce VLDL production.[84] In addition, it appears that statins may reduce the assembly and secretion of apoB-containing lipoproteins.[85] The ability of statins to reduce both LDL and VLDL lipoproteins in patients with type 2 diabetes mellitus makes them particularly useful to treat the characteristic dyslipidemia in this patient population, which is characterized by overproduction of apoB-expressing lipoproteins.[86] Although a decrease in triglycerides may be seen, triglycerides may remain above target and require further therapy.

Statins also have modest effects on HDL cholesterol, typically increasing HDL by 5% to 10%, but this was not seen in all studies.[87,88] Statins may exert this effect on HDL through PPARα, leading to increased expression of apoA-I and increased production of HDL, with additional decreases in triglyceride-rich lipoprotein particles and a decrease in CETP activity.[8,89] Rosuvastatin and simvastatin may have a modest effect over other statins to elevate HDL.[87,90-93]

Pleiotropic Effects of HMG CoA Reductase Inhibitors

Much debate exists in the literature as to whether the effects of statin therapy on reducing cardiovascular disease and mortality are solely due to LDL cholesterol lowering. Clinical trials have shown that lipid-lowering therapy results in substantially greater reduction in cardiovascular events than would be expected from the modest angiographic changes observed in regression trials, and additional effects on plaque stabilization seem likely. Several studies suggest that lipoproteins may contribute to the development of atherosclerosis by initiating and sustaining the inflammatory response in the vessel wall. Early use of atorvastatin in acute coronary syndromes leads to a reduction in recurrent coronary events as early as 16 weeks.[94] Likewise, a study comparing high-dose atorvastatin with standard-dose pravastatin found an early reduction in the composite endpoint of all-cause mortality, nonfatal myocardial infarction, unstable angina requiring hospitalization, revascularization procedures, or cerebrovascular events within 180 days, with separation of the curves seen within 3 weeks that may represent an effect on atherosclerotic plaque stability.[80] The extent of the benefit afforded by the 80-mg dose of atorvastatin is in keeping with what would be expected on the basis of the greater degree of lipid lowering compared with pravastatin 40 mg once daily. This is consistent with a similar improvement in outcomes with a similar decrease in LDL cholesterol in the Heart Protection Study.[76]

Putative mechanisms of this early reduction in cardiovascular outcomes are due to a reduction in isoprenoids, intermediary metabolites of cholesterol, that are involved in regulation of smooth muscle and endothelial cell physiology. Statins have been shown to enhance endothelial function. Studies have also demonstrated rapid changes in plaque morphology within months of starting statin therapy with less lipid, oxidized LDL, cyclooxygenase 2, metalloproteinase activity, fewer T cells and macrophages, and more collagen found in atherosclerotic plaques.[95,96] These changes may represent the mechanism by which

TABLE 23-3 PHARMACOKINETIC PROPERTIES OF STATINS BASED ON 40-MG DOSE[132,228,229]

Statin	Origin	Lipophilic	CYP-450 Metabolism (Major)	Half-Life ($T_{½}$) (hr)	Metabolites
Atorvastatin	Synthetic	Yes	CYP3A4	15-30	Active
Fluvastatin	Synthetic	Yes	CYP2C9	0.5-2.3	Inactive
Lovastatin	Fungal	Yes	CYP3A4	2.9	Active
Pravastatin	Fungal	No	Sulfation	1.3-2.8	Inactive
Rosuvastatin	Synthetic	No	CYP2C9	20.8	Active (minor)
Simvastatin	Fungal	Yes	CYP3A4	2-3	Active

CYP-450, cytochrome P-450.
Based on Schmitz G, Langmann T. Pharmacogenomics of cholesterol-lowering therapy. Vascul Pharmacol 2006;44:75-89; Mason RP, Walter MF, Day CA, et al. Intermolecular differences of 3-hydroxy-3-methylglutaryl coenzyme A reductase inhibitors contribute to distinct pharmacologic and pleiotropic actions. Am J Cardiol 2005;96(5A):11F-23F; and Corsini A, Bellosta S, Baetta R, et al. New insights into the pharmacodynamic and pharmacokinetic properties of statins. Pharmacol Ther 1999;84:413-428.

statin therapy leads to plaque stabilization and an improvement in endothelial homeostasis. Similar pleiotrophic effects may also be seen with other medications (e.g., fibrates, angiotensin-converting enzyme inhibitors, and angiotensin receptor blockers).[97]

HMG CoA reductase inhibitors also have anti-inflammatory and immunomodulatory effects and have been shown to reduce plasma fibrinogen levels, plasma viscosity, and CRP and to increase activation of nitric oxide synthase. CRP is a well-described marker of cardiovascular disease, and the balance of published information supports a role of CRP in endothelial dysfunction, vascular remodeling, and atherothrombosis. Elevated CRP levels are considered a nontraditional cardiovascular disease risk factor, with many prospective studies confirming a significant association between CRP levels and cardiovascular disease.[38] Statins have been shown to reduce CRP concentrations.[98] Whether this is a direct effect or due to an LDL-lowering effect and subsequent reduction of lipoprotein-mediated inflammation is unclear. In intervention studies, concomitant reduction of both LDL and CRP with statin therapy resulted in a greater benefit in cardiovascular endpoints.[99,100] These studies also demonstrated a greater correlation between reduction in cardiovascular events and on-drug CRP levels than LDL cholesterol.[99] Statins may also alter the atherogenicity of LDL by reducing oxidized LDL cholesterol through an increased activity of paraoxonase. This enzyme catalyzes the hydrolysis of oxidized phospholipids on LDL particles.[8]

Pharmacokinetics

Lovastatin, pravastatin, and simvastatin are derived from fungal metabolites, whereas atorvastatin, fluvastatin, and rosuvastatin are synthetic compounds. The pharmacokinetic properties of statins is summarized in Table 23-3. Lovastatin and simvastatin are lactone prodrugs activated in the liver to their active forms. All statins are subject to first-pass metabolism. Rosuvastatin and pravastatin are considered hydrophilic (or lipophobic), whereas the others (atorvastatin, fluvastatin, lovastatin and simvastatin) are considered lipophilic. Lipophilic statins enter the liver by diffusion, whereas hydrophilic statins enter the liver via the organic anion transporter protein 2 (OATP2). Statins, with the exception of pravastatin, are metabolized by cytochrome P-450 (CYP) V3A4 or CYP2C9. CYP2C8 significantly metabolizes simvastatin, lovastatin, atorvastatin, and fluvastatin but has little or no effect on pravastatin or rosuvastatin.[101] The metabolites of statins also have some HMG CoA reductase inhibitory activity. Statins and their metabolites, with the exception of pravastatin, are highly protein bound with greater than 95% bound to plasma proteins.[102]

Adverse Events

Serious adverse events associated with statin use are rare cases of liver failure and rhabdomyolysis.[103] Lesser degrees of liver and muscle dysfunction may also occur.[104] Other side effects include rash, thrombocytopenic purpura, peripheral neuropathy, insomnia, and poor concentration. One recent case-control study found that an increase in lymphoma incidence may be associated with statin use.[105] All statins are contraindicated in pregnancy and lactation.

Hepatotoxicity and Liver Function Test Monitoring. Reports of liver failure are rare.[106] Abnormal liver function tests (mild-to-moderate elevations in aspartate transaminase [AST] or alanine transaminase [ALT]) are seen in approximately 0.5% to 2.0% of patients using statins. Liver function tests should be checked at baseline and repeated at 4 to 6 weeks after initiation of a statin, any significant change in dose of a statin, or initiation of any medication with potential interactions (e.g., other lipid-lowering medications). Otherwise, liver function tests should be performed annually.[107] Early concerns in relation to noncardiovascular mortality with statin therapy have not been substantiated in many subsequent large studies, and the risk is generally now considered to be equal to that of placebo.[108,109]

Musculoskeletal Side Effects. All statins are associated with musculoskeletal side effects, including rhabdomyolysis, myositis, and other rarer conditions (e.g., polymyositis and tendon rupture). Myalgias are more common and can occur in up to 5% of patients on statins.

Rhabdomyolysis. Rhabdomyolysis can present in a variety of ways, and a high index of suspicion is necessary. The most common presentations of rhabdomyolysis are a flu-like syndrome, diffuse myalgia, muscle tenderness, weakness, progression of low back pain, and fatigue. Rhabdomyolysis, defined as muscle symptoms (pain, tenderness, or weakness) and an elevated creatinine phosphokinase greater than 10 times the upper limit of normal with an elevated creatinine level (usually consistent with a pigment-induced nephropathy), is one of the major adverse effects associated with statin therapy.[110] Although rare, it has a case mortality of 10%. Statin-related rhabdomyolysis has led to the voluntary withdrawal of cerivastatin from the world market. When cerivastatin is excluded from analyses, the incidence of statin-induced rhabdomyolysis in randomized, controlled clinical trials is low. One large study found that the incidence of rhabdomyolysis requiring hospitalization in patients on statin monotherapy was approximately 0.44 cases per 10,000 patient-years of use.[111] In the same study, the relative risk of rhabdomyolysis is markedly increased when statins are combined with fibrates; this therapy resulted in a 12-fold increased risk of this side effect. The relative risk of rhabdomyolysis with fibrate monotherapy is approximately 5-fold more common than with statin monotherapy.[111] One mechanism for this drug-drug interaction is via a fibrate-induced increase in circulating concentrations of statins by inhibiting glucuronidation. The risk of rhabdomyolysis is also increased when statins are combined with niacin and cyclosporine or when they are used in the presence of renal impairment.[112]

Rhabdomyolysis is a class effect of statin drugs, but differences in lipophilicity and cytochrome metabolism may, in theory, lead to different risks of rhabdomyolysis and other musculoskeletal adverse events. Hydrophilic agents such as rosuvastatin and pravastatin may have a reduced risk of this complication. In contrast, lipophilic statins impair the function of skeletal muscle mitochondria more than hydrophilic agents.[113] Statins, with the exception of pravastatin, are metabolized by CYP3A4 or CYP2C9. Drugs that inhibit CYP3A4 or CYP2C9 can increase statin levels in the bloodstream and increase the risk of toxicity. Intestinal CYP3A4 is irreversibly inactivated by grapefruit, and there is potential for a drug-diet interaction in this situation.[114]

Pomegranate juice also inhibits CYP3A4. Although rosuvastatin is not metabolized by CYP3A4, rhabdomyolysis has been reported with a combination of rosuvastatin, ezetimibe, and pomegranate juice.[115] CYP2C8 significantly metabolizes simvastatin, lovastatin, atorvastatin, and fluvastatin but has little or no effect on pravastatin or rosuvastatin.[101] Gemfibrozil is the single most common drug associated with statin-related myopathy and rhabdomyolysis. Gemfibrozil inhibits the uptake of statin by OATP2, leading to increased plasma statin levels. It also has effects on the glucuronidation of most statins and alters their bioavailability. There is no clear consensus in the literature supporting the relative safety of one statin over another.[111,116,117]

Statins should be withdrawn immediately in all patients in whom rhabdomyolysis is suspected. Evidence of muscle damage may be identified by the presence of myoglobinuria. Rhabdomyolysis leads to release of intracellular contents and can eventually lead to complications such as cardiac arrest or arrhythmias, acute renal failure, or compartment syndrome. Treatment is focused on withdrawal of the causative agent(s), correcting electrolyte abnormalities, treating hypovolemia and hypotension, and preventing dehydration.

Other risk factors for statin-related rhabdomyolysis include age greater than 80 years; multisystem disease, especially renal or hepatic dysfunction; hypothyroidism; hypertriglyceridemia; excessive alcohol consumption; heavy exercise; and certain drug combinations.[116] Certain genetic mutations also may predispose individuals to statin-induced rhabdomyolysis. Case-control studies have identified carriers for carnitine palmitoyltransferase II deficiency, carriers for McArdle disease, and homozygotes for myoadenylate deaminase deficiency to be at increased risk.[118] Studies show that a high proportion of patients who have a history of statin-related rhabdomyolysis develop symptoms when challenged with an alternative statin.[119]

Myositis and Other Myopathies. Myositis is defined as muscle symptoms with any elevation of creatine phosphokinase (CPK) without an elevation in creatinine levels, which is seen in rhabdomyolysis. Myositis is considered significant if there is an elevation in CPK greater than 10 times the upper limit of normal.[104,110] Myositis is much more common than rhabdomyolysis and occurs in approximately 0.1% to 0.5% of patients on statin monotherapy in randomized, controlled trials. It is characterized by the onset of generalized myalgia with concomitant symptoms of weakness and fatigue. Myalgia is defined as muscle ache or weakness without elevations in CPK. This can occur in up to 5% of patients on statin therapy. Mild myalgias without features of muscle inflammation or rhabdomyolysis do not necessarily require discontinuation of therapy if it is tolerated by the patient. There have been isolated reports of polymyositis,[120] dermatomyositis,[121] and tendinopathy.[122]

Pharmacogenetics

There is evidence that polymorphisms in certain genes can predict the efficacy of statin therapy. These include HMG CoA reductase,[123] apoE,[124] CETP,[125] HL,[126] apoA-I,[127] LDL-R,[128] and ADAMTS-1 metalloproteinase.[129] It has been demonstrated that certain single nucleotide polymorphisms (SNP) in the HMG CoA reductase gene are associated with a greater response to statin therapy.[123] These may reflect genetic influences on lipoprotein metabolism, which may account for apparent differences in therapeutic efficacy rather than gene-drug interactions.[130,131] Further study of pharmacogenetics will extend this list of genes and, in time, may lead to microarray analysis to target effective treatment in terms of maximizing efficacy and reducing adverse events of statin therapy.[132]

Therapeutic Use

Statins are licensed for the treatment of hypercholesterolemia. There is a robust evidence base for the use of statins in the primary and secondary prevention of cardiovascular disease. For every statin, there is a dose range and a dose-dependent LDL cholesterol reduction (Table 23-4). The dose and choice of statin depend on the degree of LDL cholesterol reduction required to get to target. The choice of statins may also be influenced by the presence of hypertriglyceridemia. These agents should not be used to treat severe hypertriglyceridemia. However, high-potency statins such as atorvastatin, simvastatin, and rosuvastatin can reduce triglyceride levels and may yield additional benefit in mild-to-moderate hypertriglyceridemia. Other considerations that may influence prescribing choice include concomitant medication usage (e.g., pravastatin and cyclosporine). All statins are given once daily and, with the exception of atorvastatin and rosuvastatin, should be given in the evening.

Bile Acid Sequestrants

Bile acid sequestrants, also termed bile acid–binding resins, are nonabsorbable positively charged anion exchange resins that bind negatively charged bile acids. This prevents absorption of bile acids in the terminal ileum interrupting enterohepatic recirculation of bile acids. It is estimated that bile acid sequestrants reduce the pool of bile acids by 40%. Synthesis of bile acids from cholesterol in the liver is increased to replenish the pool, resulting in decreased intracellular cholesterol concentrations and an increase in LDL-R expression. In parallel, there is an increase in cholesterol synthesis de novo with up-regulation of the enzymes involved in cholesterol synthesis including HMG-CoA reductase. Bile acid sequestrant use may increase triglyceride levels. This rise is typically trivial and not usually of clinical significance except in patients with underlying hypertriglyceridemia. Use of bile acid sequestrants typically leads to a reduction in LDL cholesterol levels of 15% to 26%.[133] Although bile acid sequestrants are not absorbed, they may interfere with the absorption of some drugs. Side effects are gastrointestinal disturbance, constipation, and myalgia. Transient elevations in liver function tests are described; these are usually mild and self-limiting. Levels of fat-soluble vitamins such as A, D, E, and K rarely may decrease during bile acid sequestrant therapy with cholestyramine and colestipol; during long-term therapy, monitoring of vitamin levels and supplementation may be required.[134-136] Colesevelam, a newer bile acid sequestrant, does not appear to have this effect on vitamin levels despite having a higher specificity for binding bile acids.[137] Maximum doses of cholestyramine and colestipol

TABLE 23-4 AVERAGE PERCENTAGE REDUCTION IN LDL ACCORDING TO STATIN AND DOSE

	Dose				
Statin	**5 mg (% Reduction)**	**10 mg (% Reduction)**	**20 mg (% Reduction)**	**40 mg (% Reduction)**	**80 mg (% Reduction)**
Atorvastatin	31	37	43	49	55
Fluvastatin	10	15	21	27	33
Lovastatin		21	29	37	45
Pravastatin	15	20	24	29	33
Rosuvastatin	38	43	48	53	58
Simvastatin	23	27	32	37	42

LDL, low-density lipoprotein.
From Paramsothy P, Knopp R. Management of dyslipidaemias. Heart 2006;92:1529-1534.

TABLE 23-5 AVAILABLE BILE ACID SEQUESTRANTS

Agent	Daily Dose Range (g)	Mean LDL Lowering (% across Dose Range)
Cholestyramine	12-24	9-28
Colestipol	5-30	5-26
Colesevelam	3.75-4.375	15-19

are generally not well tolerated, with side effects of bloating and dyspepsia seen more commonly with these bile acid sequestrants than with colesevelam.

Three commonly used bile acid sequestrants are cholestyramine, colestipol, and the newer agent colesevelam (Table 23-5). Both cholestyramine and colestipol are packaged as powders and need to be mixed with liquid before consumption. Suspension of the powder in liquid many hours before consumption may reduce symptoms of bloating and dyspepsia. The usual dose of cholestyramine is 12 g to 24 g daily either in a single dose or divided in two doses daily, starting with a single dose of 4 g daily and gradual titration of the dose. The dose of colestipol is 5 g to 30 g taken once or twice daily. Colesevelam is a specifically engineered bile acid sequestrant with a greater affinity and capacity for binding bile acids.[138] Recently published data confirm colesevelam is an effective LDL cholesterol–lowering agent without a concomitant increase in plasma triglycerides.[139,140] Colesevelam is packaged as a tablet with 625 mg of active agent and usually prescribed at a dose of 3.75 g (6 tablets) daily either in a single or divided dose with meals. When combined with a statin, a lower dose of 2.5 g may be used though a dose of 3.75 g may be optimal. Maximum daily dose is 4.375 g. Colesevelam appears to be better tolerated than the traditional bile acid sequestrants.

Owing to the complementary actions of bile acid sequestrants and statins, they are often used in combination. Whereas doubling the dose of statin results in a further reduction of LDL cholesterol levels, the addition of cholestyramine to a statin reduces LDL cholesterol by a greater degree.[141] Bile acid sequestrants may also be used with niacin, fibrates, and ezetimibe.[142-144]

Cholesterol Absorption Inhibitors

Ezetimibe is a member of a new class of lipid-lowering compounds that selectively inhibit the intestinal absorption of cholesterol and related plant sterols. The molecular target of ezetimibe is the sterol transporter NPC1L1, which is located in the brush border of the small intestine and is responsible for the jejunal uptake of cholesterol and other phytosterols (see Fig. 23-1).[5] It inhibits the intestinal absorption of cholesterol by about 50%, but it does not inhibit the absorption of triglycerides, fatty acids, vitamins A and D, bile acids, or ethinyl estradiol.[145] It is taken orally and metabolized in the small intestine and the liver to the active compound ezetimibe glucuronide, which is subsequently secreted in the bile with significant enterohepatic circulation prolonging the half-life of ezetimibe (22 hr), allowing once-daily administration. The net effect of ezetimibe monotherapy is to reduce LDL cholesterol by 18%, reduce triglyceride levels by 4%, and increase HDL cholesterol by 1%.[146] Its route of elimination is largely fecal. There may be a compensatory increase in cholesterol synthesis in the liver, which can be inhibited by use of a statin, thus providing a rationale for combination therapy with ezetimibe and a statin.[147]

Ezetimibe has been studied most often in combination with statin therapy with no change in the plasma levels of statins.[145] There is typically a reduction in LDL cholesterol of 15% to 35% when ezetimibe is added to any statin at any dose, which is greater than the effect seen with a doubling of the dose of statin. The effect of ezetimibe has also been studied in homozygous FH. Addition of ezetimibe 10 mg to high-dose statin therapy reduced LDL cholesterol by an additional 20% and triglycerides by an additional 10%.[148]

The recommended dose of ezetimibe is 10 mg once daily. It is licensed for the treatment of primary hypercholesterolemia as an adjunct to dietary measures and statin therapy and the treatment of homozygous FH. It can be used as monotherapy in those patients in whom a statin is contraindicated or not tolerated. It is also licensed as an adjunct to dietary measures in homozygous sitosterolemia, a rare genetic disorder associated with abnormal plant sterol absorption associated with tendon and tuberous xanthomata and accelerated and premature atherosclerosis.[149] Side effects are gastrointestinal disturbances; headache, fatigue, and myalgia. Less common side effects are hypersensitivity reactions including rash and angioedema, hepatitis, pancreatitis, cholelithiasis, cholecystitis, and thrombocytopenia. Adverse events with myalgia, raised creatine kinase, myopathy, and rhabdomyolysis are described. Most of the reported cases of rhabdomyolysis were in patients on concomitant statin therapy. Any patient initiating this therapy, especially in combination with a statin therapy, should be specifically advised of this side effect and asked to seek medical attention if muscle pain, tenderness, or weakness develop. Like statins, ezetimibe is also contraindicated in pregnancy and lactation, an important consideration in women of childbearing age.

An interaction between ezetimibe and cholestyramine reduces the bioavailability of ezetimibe. However, even with this decreased bioavailability, addition of ezetimibe may further reduce cholesterol levels.[150] Ezetimibe may increase cyclosporine levels; it should be used with caution in patients on this agent.[145]

Niacin

Niacin, a vitamin of the B complex, is one of the more potent HDL cholesterol–modifying drugs available, with a primary mechanism of action to decrease adipocyte lipolysis by inhibiting triglyceride lipase.[151] It typically increases HDL cholesterol by 30% to 40% with concomitant reductions in LDL cholesterol and triglycerides of 20% to 30% and 35% to 45%, respectively. The increase in HDL cholesterol is associated with an increase in apoA-1 and an increase in the HDL_2:HDL_3 ratio. Niacin also causes a decrease in apoB-100, an apolipoprotein associated with VLDL, LDL, and Lp(a). Niacin has a preferential effect in reducing the highly atherogenic small dense LDL particles.[152] Niacin monotherapy has been shown to reduce nonfatal myocardial infarction and mortality.[153] It has also been shown to have benefit in combination with other lipid-lowering therapies, as detailed later.

Niacin is one of the drugs that has been available for many decades to treat dyslipidemia, but use of the agent has been limited by side effects.[32] The most common side effects are flushing and dyspepsia. These tend to occur when niacin is initiated or when there is an increase in dose and seem to abate after 2 weeks on a stable dose. Symptoms can recur if a dose of niacin is missed. Flushing can be associated with consumption of alcohol or hot beverages (e.g., coffee). Flushing can be minimized by starting at a low dose and taking niacin after a meal. Flushing and its associated pruritus appear to be prostaglandin related and may be alleviated by aspirin or nonsteroidal anti-inflammatory drugs taken 30 minutes prior to niacin. Dyspepsia is also less likely if niacin is taken after a meal. Hepatotoxicity has been described with niacin, with rare cases of fulminant hepatic necrosis reported.[154] Regular monitoring of liver function tests should be performed in all patients on this drug. Hepatotoxicity may manifest as a substantial decline in LDL cholesterol; any patient with a reduction in LDL cholesterol of greater than 50% should undergo assessment of liver function.[155] Rhabdomyolysis can also occur with combinations of niacin and statin therapy; patients on this combination should be specifically advised of this side effect and told to seek medical attention if they develop muscle pain, tenderness, or weakness. Other side effects are headache, dry skin, acanthosis nigricans, and diarrhea. Peptic ulcer disease and gout are relative contraindications to niacin use because it may exacerbate both conditions. Niacin may also exacerbate insulin resistance; in patients with diabetes mellitus, worsening glycemia may occur and its use should be restricted.

Niacin is currently available in standard and extended-release preparations. In the standard preparation, often termed *crystalline niacin*, the initial dose is 100 mg to 200 mg three times daily, gradually increasing the dose over 2 to 4 weeks to 1 g to 2 g three times daily. In the extended-release preparation the initial dose is 375 mg once daily for the first week, increasing to 500 mg for the second week, 750 mg for the third week, 1 g for the fourth week; if necessary, the dose can be further increased to a maximum of 2 g administered once daily. The extended-release preparation should be taken at night to minimize side effects. The standard and extended-release preparations are not interchangeable, and then changing from one preparation to another, the starting dose should be low and titrated as per the recommended protocol for that preparation.

The addition of niacin to a statin is an effective combination therapy. The combination may be particularly useful in patients on a statin in whom the HDL cholesterol remains low. A fixed-dose combination of extended-release niacin and lovastatin has been shown to have greater LDL cholesterol– and triglyceride-lowering and HDL cholesterol elevation than either drug alone. The net effect of a combination of 2 g of niacin and 40 mg of lovastatin is to lower LDL cholesterol by 42% and triglyceride by 44% and to increase HDL cholesterol by 30%.[156] Similar benefits have been seen with combinations of niacin and other statins.[157]

Niacin can also be used in combination with other lipid-lowering therapies. The combination of niacin and clofibrate has been shown to reduce total and cardiovascular mortality by 26% and 35%, respectively, in men with previous myocardial infarction.[142] The combination of niacin and bile acid sequestrants has also been shown to be an effective combination. Niacin and colestipol combination therapy raised HDL cholesterol by 43%, lowered LDL cholesterol by 32%, and resulted in regression of atherosclerosis.[158] This effect was also seen in a study in men with a history of coronary bypass grafting.[159]

Omega-3 Fatty Acids

Omega-3 fatty acids can be used as a treatment for hypertriglyceridemia as an adjunct to diet in type IV hyperlipidemia and with statin therapy for type IIb hyperlipidemia. Diets that lead to high consumption of long-chain omega-3 fatty acids, also termed n-3 polyunsaturated fatty acids, are associated in epidemiologic studies with a low prevalence of coronary artery disease.[160,161] Omega-3 fatty acids lead to a reduction in triglycerides largely through an effect of reducing VLDL particle synthesis. They may be associated with cardioprotection through a number of additional mechanisms such as a reduction of arterial blood pressure and heart rate, acting as an antiarrhythmic with membrane-stabilizing effects, reducing thrombosis through effects on platelet function and coagulation factors, stabilizing plaque, favorably modifying endothelial function, moderating insulin resistance, and reducing inflammation.[162,163] Omega-3 fatty acids are typically subdivided into two groups, those with long chains (e.g., eicosapentaenoic acid [EPA] and docasapentaenoic acid [DPA]) and those with short chains (e.g., α linolenic acid [ALA]), which may be converted to a variable degree into longer-chain omega-3 fatty acids. Omega-3 fatty acids are found in oily fish or fish oils and in some green plants.

Omega-3 fatty acids are available either as omega-3 acid ethyl esters of EPA and DPA or as purified omega-3 marine triglycerides, essentially a concentrated fish oil containing EPA and DPA. The most common side effects with these medications are nausea, dyspepsia, and bloating. Less common side effects are taste disturbances, dizziness, and hypersensitivity reactions; rarely, hepatic disorders, headache, hyperglycemia, acne, and rash have been described. Owing to effects on hemostasis, these compounds should be used with caution in patients on warfarin. Commercial preparations are standardized and allow for dose titration. The therapeutic effects of these compounds have been studied as dietary supplements, most commonly as a capsule, and as an intervention with dietary advice.

Omega-3 fatty acids, given as a capsule with 1.0 g of omega-3 fatty acids in patients post–myocardial infarction, have been shown to reduce all-cause mortality, cardiovascular mortality, and sudden death.[164] The measured reduction in triglycerides (~5%) is not considered to be sufficient to completely explain this mortality benefit, and it may represent an antiarrhythmic effect of omega-3 fatty acids. Subsequent analyses demonstrate a benefit of omega-3 fatty acids in most randomized, controlled trials.[165,166] However, another meta-analysis of studies on the effects of omega-3 fatty acids concluded that both long-chain and short-chain omega-3 fatty acids failed to demonstrate any favorable change in combined cardiovascular events.[167] They may be used as adjuvant treatment in secondary prevention after myocardial infarction in addition to other standard therapy (e.g., statins, antiplatelet agents, β-adrenergic antagonists, angiotensin-converting enzyme inhibitors).

Omega-3 fatty acids are available as omega-3-acid ethyl esters and omega-3 marine triglycerides. Omega-3-acid ethyl esters are packaged in 1-g capsules containing 460 mg EPA ethyl esters and 380 mg docosahexaenoic (DHA) ethyl esters. The dose for secondary prevention post–myocardial infarction is 1 capsule a day. The dose for the treatment of hypertriglyceridemia is 2 to 4 capsules a day. Omega-3 marine triglycerides are licensed for the treatment of hypertriglyceridemia and are packaged as 1-g capsules containing 170 mg EPA and 115 mg DHA. The dose is 5 capsules twice daily. A liquid preparation of omega-3 marine triglycerides is also available.

TABLE 23-6 DOSES OF FIBRATES

Fibrate	Daily Dose Range (mg)
Bezafibrate	400-600
Ciprofibrate	100
Clofibrate	1000-2000
Fenofibrate (non-micronized)	200-400
Gemfibrozil	900-1500

Fibrates

Fibrates are a class of drugs, derived from fibric acid, comprising five drugs: clofibrate, gemfibrozil, bezafibrate, ciprofibrate, and fenofibrate (Table 23-6). Treatment with a fibrate reduces LDL cholesterol by 5% to 20%, increases HDL cholesterol by 10% to 15%, and decreases triglycerides by 20% to 50%.[168] This profile makes them attractive for the treatment of mixed dyslipidemia. It is now widely considered that fibrates act as agonists of PPARα. Clinical studies have shown a reduction in cardiovascular mortality and atherosclerotic progression using these agents.[21] Fibrates are efficacious in lowering triglycerides and have a proven role in the management of severe hypertriglyceridemia in reducing the risk of pancreatitis. Fibrates are suitable in combination with statins and bile acid sequestrants. Side effects of fibrate therapy include myopathy, elevation in liver transaminases, cholelithiasis, and pancreatitis. They can also be used to prevent pancreatitis in severe hypertriglyceridemia. Monitoring of liver function tests every 3 months for the first year of fibrate therapy and annually thereafter is advised.

Myopathy and rhabdomyolysis may occur with the use of all fibrates but in particular with gemfibrozil.[169] Myopathy is typically seen in patients on combination therapy with a statin but may also be seen with fibrate monotherapy with gemfibrozil or fenofibrate. Gemfibrozil interacts with statin glucuronidation, which is not seen with fenofibrate, which leads to elevations in statin levels and an increased risk of myopathy. Fenofibrate does not interfere with the metabolism of statins, and thus, the risk of myopathy may be less when a statin is used in combination with this agent.[170,171] Patients on fibrate therapy should be advised to seek medical attention if they experience unexplained muscle pain, tenderness, or weakness. Fibrate therapy should be stopped immediately in all patients with elevated CPK. Fibrates can be given with bile acid sequestrants; however, they should be taken at least 2 hours before or more than 6 hours after the bile acid sequestrant.

Gemfibrozil is a nonhalogenated fibrate, which chemically differentiates it from other fibrates. Gemfibrozil is usually given in a dose of

900 mg to 1200 mg a day in two divided doses with a maximum daily dose of 1500 mg. Gemfibrozil has demonstrated significant improvement in cardiovascular outcomes, but the mechanism of this improvement is not clear. A large primary prevention study, the Helsinki Heart Study, demonstrated a 34% reduction in combined cardiac death and nonfatal myocardial infarction with gemfibrozil in patients with hypercholesterolemia with or without hypertriglyceridemia, with a greater reduction seen in those with diabetes mellitus and severe dyslipidemia (68% and 71%, respectively).[172] Recent long-term data confirmed the durability of this benefit.[173] Another study has shown the benefit of gemfibrozil in patients with coronary artery disease who have a low HDL cholesterol (≤40 mg/dl) and a relatively normal LDL cholesterol (≤140 mg/dl), with a 22% reduction in the primary endpoint of cardiac death and nonfatal myocardial infarction.[174] Patients with greater increases in HDL cholesterol showed most benefit. Whereas the measured LDL cholesterol did not change, a subsequent study showed that gemfibrozil increased LDL particle size, which correlated with improved cardiovascular outcomes.[33]

Fenofibrate is a fibrate with once daily dosing. The dose for the non-micronized preparation is 200 to 400 mg daily. 67 mg of the micronized preparation is equivalent to 100 mg of the non-micronized preparation and is commonly given in a usual dose range of up to 200 mg daily and a licensed maximum dose of 267 mg daily for severe hypertriglyceridemia. In patients with hypercholesterolemia, fenofibrate typically causes a decrease in LDL cholesterol of 20% to 30% and an increase in HDL cholesterol of 10% to 30%. In patients with hypertriglyceridemia, triglyceride levels decrease by 40% to 55%. In time, regression of xanthomata is described in patients with severe hypertriglyceridemia. In patients at high risk of CHD with high triglycerides and low HDL cholesterol, especially those with diabetes mellitus or features of the metabolic syndrome, fenofibrate reduces cardiovascular risk.[175] In angiographic studies in patients with diabetes mellitus, fenofibrate reduced angiographic progression of coronary artery disease.[176] In a large randomized, placebo-controlled trial in patients with type 2 diabetes mellitus, fenofibrate failed to show a significant reduction in the primary endpoint of nonfatal myocardial infarction and coronary heart death, although it did show a reduction in the secondary endpoint of nonfatal myocardial infarction.[177] Fenofibrate also has a mild uricosuric effect, which may be of additional benefit in the one fifth of patients with dyslipidemia who have elevations of urate. The bioavailability of fenofibrate is not altered by the bile acid sequestrant colesevelam.[178]

Bezafibrate is taken in a standard preparation at a dose of 200 mg three times daily or in a modified-release preparation of 400 mg once daily. Ciprofibrate has a profile similar to that of other second-generation fibrates and is taken at a dose of 100 mg daily. Clofibrate, the prototypical fibrate, has a dose range of 1000 mg to 2000 mg daily in divided doses.

Other Therapies

Therapeutic Lifestyle Changes

Weight loss of 5% to 10% has been shown to have benefits on cardiovascular risks, in particular in high-risk populations, and the benefits are presumed to be greater when healthier weight is maintained for long periods.[179] In overweight and obese individuals, weight loss achieved with most interventions over 1 to 2 years leads to improvements in triglyceride levels. Improvements in total cholesterol, HDL cholesterol, and LDL cholesterol have been reported in studies using dietary interventions combined with exercise.[180] Notwithstanding the difficulties associated with trials in dietary therapy, there is a reasonable evidence base that dietary therapy may influence lipoprotein metabolism and reduce cardiovascular disease rates.[181] Specific dietary recommendations that have been shown to influence cardiovascular disease rates in clinical trials include replacing saturated fat with polyunsaturated vegetable oils, use of a Mediterranean-style diet after myocardial infarction,[182] and use of fish oil after myocardial infarction.[75] Dietary changes are to be considered as part of thera-peutic lifestyle change with recently published guidelines detailing targets and encouraging the limitation of saturated fat to less than 7% of energy and daily cholesterol intake to less than 300 mg/day.[75]

Plant Sterols

Plant sterols, also known as phytosterols, and stanols, saturated derivatives of plant sterols, are effective at lowering LDL cholesterol levels by up to 15% and are a therapeutic option in addition to diet and lifestyle modification for individuals with hypercholesterolemia.[183-185] The mechanism of action of these agents appears to be the inhibition of intestinal cholesterol absorption and enhancement of LDL-R expression by reducing intracellular cholesterol levels.[186] Maximum effects with plant sterols are seen with intakes of 2 g/day.[187] Plant sterols are currently available in a wide variety of foods, drinks, and soft gel capsules.

Surgery

Surgery is a potential therapy for hypercholesterolemia. Partial ileal bypass has been shown to have dramatic effects on dyslipidemia. One large study in patients with an established first myocardial infarction demonstrated reductions in total cholesterol (23%) and LDL cholesterol (37%) and increases in HDL cholesterol (4%) and triglycerides (20%) compared with placebo.[188,189] In longer-term follow-up of this secondary prevention trial, there was a reduction in overall mortality, CHD death, and atherosclerotic endpoints of non-fatal myocardial infarction, coronary revascularization procedures, and onset of peripheral vascular disease but not cerebrovascular events.[190,191] Side effects of the procedure include diarrhea, renal calculi, gallstones, and intestinal obstruction.

The effects of bariatric surgery for obesity have less clear-cut benefits on dyslipidemia. Bariatric surgery and its consequent weight loss have been shown to improve hypertriglyceridemia and decreased HDL cholesterol. However, analyses of randomized, controlled trials of bariatric surgery demonstrate that LDL cholesterol may not benefit from surgically induced weight loss,[192] in particular when statins are not used.[193] However, bariatric surgery was shown to reduce cardiovascular mortality.

Rimonabant

Rimonabant has shown promise in the therapeutic approach to atherogenic dyslipidemia by modulating glucose tolerance, raising HDL and reducing triglycerides, and decreasing waist circumference (see Chapter 36).[194] Placebo-controlled trials in patients who were obese (body mass index [BMI] > 30) or overweight (BMI > 27) with hypertension and/or dyslipidemia with rimonabant 20 mg have demonstrated increases in HDL and reductions in triglycerides[195-197] with greater effects after longer duration of therapy.[197] Rimonabant has not been demonstrated to decrease LDL cholesterol in studies to date. HDL cholesterol levels increased by 10 mg/dl (+20%) from baseline, and triglycerides decreased by 18 mg/dl (−3%) from baseline. The extent of these changes was greater than expected from weight loss alone. Similar changes in lipoproteins with rimonabant therapy were seen in those with diabetes mellitus.[180] Side effects of rimonabant are nausea, vomiting, diarrhea, headache, dizziness, and anxiety. Rimonabant is contraindicated in patients with depression and is not recommended for those on antidepressant medication.

Orlistat

Orlistat is an inhibitor of pancreatic, gastric, and carboxylester lipase enzymes, which consequently results in a decreased intestinal absorption of fat. It is an effective therapy for obesity and has favorable effects on the lipid profile. Orlistat, compared with placebo, typically lowers LDL cholesterol, elevates HDL cholesterol, and may be associated with a small decrease in triglycerides.[198,199] These effects are seen in all obese patients, including those with diabetes mellitus.[200]

Sibrutamine

Sibrutamine has favorable effects on the dyslipidemic profile associated with obesity (see Chapter 36). Compared with placebo, sibutramine has no effect on LDL cholesterol, but it typically elevates HDL cholesterol and reduces triglycerides.[198]

EMERGING THERAPIES

CETP Inhibitors

Cholesteryl ester transport protein (CETP) is a plasma glycoprotein that mediates the transfer of cholesteryl esters from HDL particles to VLDL and LDL particles in exchange for triglyceride (see Fig. 23-4). These triglyceride-laden HDL particles are subsequently catabolized by HL in the liver. A second effect of CETP is to mediate the conversion of HDL_2 to HDL_3.[201] JJT-705 is the prototypical CETP inhibitor. Phase III trials have shown this agent to increase HDL cholesterol levels with concomitant reductions in LDL cholesterol and triglycerides. Trials of torcetrapib, another CETP inhibitor, have recently been stopped owing to an increase of mortality and cardiovascular events in those who received a combination of torcetrapib and statin.[202] CETP inhibition raises HDL cholesterol in a dose-dependent fashion, and on the higher doses tested, CETP inhibitors had the effect of approximately doubling HDL cholesterol, an increase superior to that seen with current therapies.[203] Animal studies with JJT-705 have shown regression of atherosclerosis.[204] However, CETP is influenced by genetic and environmental factors, and these may influence the effectiveness of these agents in individual patients. In particular, the influence of severe hypertriglyceridemia may potentially reverse the antiatherogenic effect of CETP inhibition; this needs to be further investigated.

MTP Inhibitors

Microsomal triglyceride transfer protein (MTP) is found in the endoplasmic reticulum and is primarily involved in the assembly and secretion of VLDL and chylomicrons (see Fig. 23-1). It is responsible for the incorporation of triglycerides into the nascent apoB-containing lipoprotein particles. Mutations in the MTP gene result in abetalipoproteinemia, an autosomal recessive condition associated with profound hypocholesterolemia and hypotriglyceridemia. Prototypical MTP inhibitors currently undergoing phase I and phase II trials have been shown to have potent LDL cholesterol– and triglyceride-lowering effects.[205] The enzyme may also be targeted as a therapy for obesity.

ACAT Inhibitors

Acyl-coenyzme A : cholesterol transferase (ACAT), also known as sterol *o*-acyltransferase, converts cholesterol into cholesteryl esters, an important step in intestinal absorption of cholesterol and the assembly and secretion of apoB-containing lipoproteins. ACAT exists in two isoforms. ACAT1 is expressed in almost all cell types and there is evidence suggesting it plays a role in foam cell formation.[204] ACAT2 is limited to small intestine enterocytes and hepatocytes. It functions to provide cholestryl esters for incorporation into chylomicrons and VLDL, respectively (see Fig. 23-1).[206] ACAT2 inhibitors may lower intestinal cholesterol absorption and have profound effects on lipoprotein metabolism and atherosclerosis.[207] The utility of these agents has been limited by poor bioavailability and adrenotoxicity.

Bile Acid Transport Inhibitors

The therapeutic use of bile acid–binding resins is well developed. Specific inhibitors of bile acid transport in the ileum prevent reuptake of bile acids and reduce enterohepatic circulation. This has a similar effect to that observed with bile acid sequestrants in the liver with increased conversion of cholesterol to bile acids and up-regulation of the LDL-R in the hepatocyte. Specific bile acid transport inhibitors as well as novel bile acid sequestrants are under investigation at present.[208]

LXR Agonists

Liver X receptors (LXRs) (LXRα, LXRβ) are sterol-responsive cholesterol sensors and modulate cholesterol transport and metabolism, glucose metabolism, and inflammation.[209] LXRs associated with retinol X receptors (RXRs) bind sterols, which leads to increased transcription of cholesterol 7α-hydroxylase, a rate-limiting enzyme in bile acid synthesis.[133] The relevance of these effects for the development of cardiovascular disease is clear from studies showing that LXR agonists inhibit atherosclerosis in animal models. Nonspecific LXR agonists, however, are associated with elevation of triglyceride levels, and further studies of this potential novel therapy are required.

Other potential therapies under investigation include farnesoid X receptor antagonists[210] and berberine, a compound isolated from a Chinese herb Huanglian, *Coptis chinensis*, that modulates LDL receptor expression in the liver and has been shown in clinical studies to lower LDL by 25%.[211]

Gene Therapy

FH is a severe monogenetic cause of hypercholesterolemia. In the most severe form of the disease, specifically homozygous FH, pharmacotherapy is often unsatisfactory. A combination of LDL apheresis performed every 1 to 2 weeks and statin therapy has shown some success,[212] as have high-dose statins in combination with ezetimibe.[148] Increasing LDL-R activity by gene therapy is a potential therapy for this disorder.[213,214] Preliminary data show this to be a potential and effective therapy in animal models.[215] Phase I studies in human subjects of ex vivo gene therapy for homozygous FH have been performed, but there is still no evidence of the utility of this therapy in humans.[216,217] Other potential targets under study as potential targets for gene therapy are lipoprotein lipase,[218] apoE,[219] apoA-I,[220] *ABCA1*,[221] LCAT,[222] endothelial lipase,[223] macrophage scavenger receptor type A-I,[224] interleukin-10,[225] and paraoxonase-1.[226]

SUMMARY

The following treatment approach is suggested and based on the updated ATP III and other guidelines.[21,72,75,81,227] The first step is to determine the patient risk category and treatment goals. Therapeutic lifestyle change (TLC) refers to a balanced caloric intake and physical activity to achieve and maintain a healthy body weight; a diet rich in fruit, vegetables, viscous fiber, and oily fish and low in saturated fat (<7% energy), *trans*-fat (<1%), cholesterol (300 mg/day), added sugars and salt; and if alcohol is consumed, it should be in moderation.[75] Addition of plant sterols is considered part of TLC. Simultaneous commencement of TLC and drug therapy should be considered in those with severe hypercholesterolemia in which dietary change cannot achieve primary LDL target or for those with CHD or a CHD risk equivalent in which dietary change cannot achieve primary LDL target. Otherwise, drug therapy is considered after a trial of TLC.

The initial choice of drug therapy for the majority of patients with hypercholesterolemia will be an HMG CoA reductase inhibitor. The initial dose should be sufficient to be likely to achieve the LDL cholesterol goal. If this goal is not achieved, two options exist. The first is to increase the dose of the statin that will result in approximately a further 6% reduction in LDL cholesterol levels. The second is to use combination therapy. The concomitant presence of hypertriglyceridemia would favor addition of ezetimibe, fibrate, niacin, or omega-3-fatty acids. In patients with hypertriglyceridemia, bile acid sequestrants are relatively contraindicated. In isolated hypercholesterolemia, combination therapy with bile acid sequestrants, ezetimibe, or niacin should be considered.

In those patients at very high cardiovascular risk, the optional LDL target may be difficult to achieve; however, it is generally possible to achieve at least a 50% reduction in LDL cholesterol with high-potency statins or drug combinations.[227] Treatment of the elderly, similar to that for the general population is advised with due consideration of comorbidities and other therapies.[69,72]

In patients with diabetes mellitus, treatment of elevated LDL cholesterol is no different from that in the general population except for two additional considerations. First, the goals for LDL are lower than in those without diabetes mellitus. Second, other lipoprotein abnormalities are more common (e.g., high triglycerides and/or low HDL).

Whereas combination therapy may be warranted to address these abnormalities, large-scale studies addressing this issue have not been performed.

REFERENCES

1. Yach D, Leeder SR, Bell J, et al. Global chronic diseases. Science 2005;307(5708): 317.
2. Yusuf S, Hawken S, Ounpuu S, et al. Effect of potentially modifiable risk factors associated with myocardial infarction in 52 countries (the INTERHEART study): case-control study. Lancet 2004;364(9438):937-952.
3. Costa J, Borges M, David C, et al. Efficacy of lipid lowering drug treatment for diabetic and non-diabetic patients: meta-analysis of randomised controlled trials. BMJ 2006;332(7550):1115-1124.
4. Yusuf S, Reddy S, Ounpuu S, et al. Global burden of cardiovascular diseases: part I: general considerations, the epidemiologic transition, risk factors, and impact of urbanization. Circulation 2001;104:2746-2753.
5. Sudhop T, von Bergmann K. Cholesterol absorption inhibitors for the treatment of hypercholesterolaemia. Drugs 2002;62:2333-2347.
6. Davidson NO. Apolipoprotein B mRNA editing: a key controlling element targeting fats to proper tissue. Ann Med 1993;25:539-543.
7. Graner M, Kahri J, Nakano T, et al. Impact of postprandial lipaemia on low-density lipoprotein (LDL) size and oxidized LDL in patients with coronary artery disease. Eur J Clin Invest 2006;36:764-770.
8. Kassai A, Illyes L, Mirdamadi HZ, et al. The effect of atorvastatin therapy on lecithin: cholesterol acyltransferase, cholesteryl ester transfer protein and the antioxidant paraoxonase. Clin Biochem 2007;40:1-5.
9. Ross R. Atherosclerosis—an inflammatory disease. N Engl J Med 1999;340:115-126.
10. Naghavi M, Libby P, Falk E, et al. From vulnerable plaque to vulnerable patient: a call for new definitions and risk assessment strategies: Part I. Circulation 2003;108:1664-1672.
11. Gordon T, Castelli WP, Hjortland MC, et al. Diabetes, blood lipids, and the role of obesity in coronary heart disease risk for women. The Framingham study. Ann Intern Med 1977;87:393-397.
12. Pekkanen J, Linn S, Heiss G, et al. Ten-year mortality from cardiovascular disease in relation to cholesterol level among men with and without preexisting cardiovascular disease. N Engl J Med 1990;322:1700-1707.
13. Austin MA, Hokanson JE, Edwards KL. Hypertriglyceridemia as a cardiovascular risk factor. Am J Cardiol 1998;81(4A):7B-12B.
14. Gordon DJ, Probstfield JL, Garrison RJ, et al. High-density lipoprotein cholesterol and cardiovascular disease. Four prospective American studies. Circulation 1989;79:8-15.
15. Cui Y, Blumenthal RS, Flaws JA, et al. Non–high-density lipoprotein cholesterol level as a predictor of cardiovascular disease mortality. Arch Intern Med 2001;161:1413-1419.
16. Grundy SM. Does a diagnosis of metabolic syndrome have value in clinical practice? Am J Clin Nutr 2006;83:1248-1251.
17. Grundy SM, Cleeman JI, Daniels SR, et al. Diagnosis and management of the metabolic syndrome: an American Heart Association/National Heart, Lung, and Blood Institute Scientific Statement. Circulation 2005;112:2735-2752.
18. Shai I, Rimm EB, Hankinson SE, et al. Multivariate assessment of lipid parameters as predictors of coronary heart disease among postmenopausal women: potential implications for clinical guidelines. Circulation 2004;110:2824-2830.
19. Hokanson JE, Austin MA. Plasma triglyceride level is a risk factor for cardiovascular disease independent of high-density lipoprotein cholesterol level: a meta-analysis of population-based prospective studies. J Cardiovasc Risk 1996;3:213-219.
20. Navab M, Anantharamaiah GM, Reddy ST, et al. Mechanisms of disease: proatherogenic HDL—an evolving field. Nat Clin Pract Endocrinol Metab 2006;2:504-511.
21. Grundy SM, Cleeman JI, Merz CN, et al. Implications of recent clinical trials for the National Cholesterol Education Program Adult Treatment Panel III Guidelines. J Am Coll Cardiol 2004;44:720-732.
22. Barter PJ, Ballantyne CM, Carmena R, et al. Apo B versus cholesterol in estimating cardiovascular risk and in guiding therapy: report of the thirty-person/ten-country panel. J Intern Med 2006;259:247-258.
23. Pischon T, Girman CJ, Sacks FM, et al. Non–high-density lipoprotein cholesterol and apolipoprotein B in the prediction of coronary heart disease in men. Circulation 2005;112:3375-3383.
24. Third Report of the National Cholesterol Education Program (NCEP) Expert Panel on Detection, Evaluation, and Treatment of High Blood Cholesterol in Adults (Adult Treatment Panel III) final report. Circulation 2002;106:3143-3421.
25. Folsom AR, Chambless LE, Ballantyne CM, et al. An assessment of incremental coronary risk prediction using C-reactive protein and other novel risk markers: the Atherosclerosis Risk in Communities study. Arch Intern Med 2006;166:1368-1373.
26. Vasan RS. Biomarkers of cardiovascular disease: molecular basis and practical considerations. Circulation 2006;113:2335-2362.
27. Danesh J, Collins R, Peto R. Lipoprotein(a) and coronary heart disease. Meta-analysis of prospective studies. Circulation 2000;102:1082-1085.
28. Deb A, Caplice NM. Lipoprotein(a): new insights into mechanisms of atherogenesis and thrombosis. Clin Cardiol 2004;27:258-264.
29. Tsimikas S, Brilakis ES, Miller ER, et al. Oxidized phospholipids, Lp(a) lipoprotein, and coronary artery disease. N Engl J Med 2005;353:46-57.
30. Albert MA, Torres J, Glynn RJ, et al. Perspective on selected issues in cardiovascular disease research with a focus on black Americans. Circulation 2004;110:e7-e12.
31. Guerra R, Yu Z, Marcovina S, et al. Lipoprotein(a) and apolipoprotein(a) isoforms: no association with coronary artery calcification in the Dallas Heart Study. Circulation 2005;111:1471-1479.
32. Meyers CD, Kamanna VS, Kashyap ML. Niacin therapy in atherosclerosis. Curr Opin Lipidol 2004;15:659-665.
33. Otvos JD, Collins D, Freedman DS, et al. Low-density lipoprotein and high-density lipoprotein particle subclasses predict coronary events and are favorably changed by gemfibrozil therapy in the Veterans Affairs High-Density Lipoprotein Intervention Trial. Circulation 2006;113:1556-1563.
34. Bonaa KH, Njolstad I, Ueland PM, et al. Homocysteine lowering and cardiovascular events after acute myocardial infarction. N Engl J Med 2006;354:1578-1588.
35. Jacques PF, Selhub J, Bostom AG, et al. The effect of folic acid fortification on plasma folate and total homocysteine concentrations. N Engl J Med 1999;340:1449-1454.
36. Lonn E, Yusuf S, Arnold MJ, et al. Homocysteine lowering with folic acid and B vitamins in vascular disease. N Engl J Med 2006;354:1567-1577.
37. Pearson TA, Mensah GA, Alexander RW, et al. Markers of inflammation and cardiovascular disease: application to clinical and public health practice: a statement for healthcare professionals from the Centers for Disease Control and Prevention and the American Heart Association. Circulation 2003;107:499-511.
38. Scirica BM, Morrow DA. Is C-reactive protein an innocent bystander or proatherogenic culprit? The verdict is still out. Circulation 2006;113:2128-2134; discussion 2151.
39. Sun XM, Eden ER, Tosi I, et al. Evidence for effect of mutant PCSK9 on apolipoprotein B secretion as the cause of unusually severe dominant hypercholesterolaemia. Hum Mol Genet 2005;14:1161-1169.
40. Naoumova RP, Thompson GR, Soutar AK. Current management of severe homozygous hypercholesterolaemias. Curr Opin Lipidol 2004;15:413-422.
41. Civeira F. Guidelines for the diagnosis and management of heterozygous familial hypercholesterolemia. Atherosclerosis 2004;173:55-68.
42. Bilheimer DW, Goldstein JL, Grundy SM, et al. Liver transplantation to provide low-density-lipoprotein receptors and lower plasma cholesterol in a child with homozygous familial hypercholesterolemia. N Engl J Med 1984;311:1658-1664.
43. Tejedor D, Castillo S, Mozas P, et al. Reliable low-density DNA array based on allele-specific probes for detection of 118 mutations causing familial hypercholesterolemia. Clin Chem 2005;51:1137-1144.
44. Sirinian MI, Belleudi F, Campagna F, et al. Adaptor protein ARH is recruited to the plasma membrane by low density lipoprotein (LDL) binding and modulates endocytosis of the LDL/LDL receptor complex in hepatocytes. J Biol Chem 2005;280:38416-38423.
45. Naoumova RP, Neuwirth C, Lee P, et al. Autosomal recessive hypercholesterolaemia: long-term follow up and response to treatment. Atherosclerosis 2004;174:165-172.
46. Zuliani G, Arca M, Signore A, et al. Characterization of a new form of inherited hypercholesterolemia: familial recessive hypercholesterolemia. Arterioscler Thromb Vasc Biol 1999;19:802-809.
47. Goldstein JL, Schrott HG, Hazzard WR, et al. Hyperlipidemia in coronary heart disease. II. Genetic analysis of lipid levels in 176 families and delineation of a new inherited disorder, combined hyperlipidemia. J Clin Invest 1973;52:1544-1568.
48. Zambon A, Brown BG, Deeb SS, et al. Genetics of apolipoprotein B and apolipoprotein AI and premature coronary artery disease. J Intern Med 2006;259:473-480.
49. Brunzell JD, Schrott HG, Motulsky AG, et al. Myocardial infarction in the familial forms of hypertriglyceridemia. Metabolism 1976;25:313-320.
50. Shoulders CC, Jones EL, Naoumova RP. Genetics of familial combined hyperlipidemia and risk of coronary heart disease. Hum Mol Genet 2004;13(spec no 1):R149-R160.
51. Jarvik GP, Brunzell JD, Austin MA, et al. Genetic predictors of FCHL in four large pedigrees. Influence of ApoB level major locus predicted genotype and LDL subclass phenotype. Arterioscler Thromb 1994;14:1687-1694.
52. Ayyobi AF, McGladdery SH, McNeely MJ, et al. Small, dense LDL and elevated apolipoprotein B are the common characteristics for the three major lipid phenotypes of familial combined hyperlipidemia. Arterioscler Thromb Vasc Biol 2003;23:1289-1294.
53. Junyent M, Gilabert R, Zambon D, et al. The use of Achilles tendon sonography to distinguish familial hypercholesterolemia from other genetic dyslipidemias. Arterioscler Thromb Vasc Biol 2005;25:2203-2208.
54. Patel MD, Thompson PD. Phytosterols and vascular disease. Atherosclerosis 2006;186:12-19.
55. Reina M, Brunzell JD, Deeb SS. Molecular basis of familial chylomicronemia: mutations in the lipoprotein lipase and apolipoprotein C-II genes. J Lipid Res 1992;33:1823-1832.
56. Iskandar SB, Olive KE. Plasmapheresis as an adjuvant therapy for hypertriglyceridemia-induced pancreatitis. Am J Med Sci 2004;328:290-294.
57. Oram JF, Heinecke JW. ATP-binding cassette transporter A1: a cell cholesterol exporter that protects against cardiovascular disease. Physiol Rev 2005;85:1343-1372.
58. Vanloo B, Peelman F, Deschuymere K, et al. Relationship between structure and biochemical phenotype of lecithin: cholesterol acyltransferase (LCAT) mutants causing fish-eye disease. J Lipid Res 2000;41:752-761.
59. Kuivenhoven JA, Pritchard H, Hill J, et al. The molecular pathology of lecithin: cholesterol acyltransferase (LCAT) deficiency syndromes. J Lipid Res 1997;38:191-205.
60. Calabresi L, Pisciotta L, Costantin A, et al. The molecular basis of lecithin: cholesterol acyltransferase deficiency syndromes: a comprehensive study of molecular and biochemical findings in 13 unrelated Italian families. Arterioscler Thromb Vasc Biol 2005;25:1972-1978.
61. Hovingh GK, Hutten BA, Holleboom AG, et al. Compromised LCAT function is associated with increased atherosclerosis. Circulation 2005;112:879-884.
62. Dammerman M, Breslow JL. Genetic basis of lipoprotein disorders. Circulation 1995;91:505-512.
63. Duffy D, Rader DJ. Emerging therapies targeting high-density lipoprotein metabolism and reverse cholesterol transport. Circulation 2006;113:1140-1150.

64. Calabresi L, Sirtori CR, Paoletti R, et al. Recombinant apolipoprotein A-IMilano for the treatment of cardiovascular diseases. Curr Atheroscler Rep 2006;8:163-167.
65. Navab M, Anantharamaiah GM, Reddy ST, et al. Apolipoprotein A-I mimetic peptides and their role in atherosclerosis prevention. Nat Clin Pract Cardiovasc Med 2006;3:540-547.
66. Wang J, Hegele RA. Microsomal triglyceride transfer protein (MTP) gene mutations in Canadian subjects with abetalipoproteinemia. Hum Mutat 2000;15:294-295.
67. Sankatsing RR, Fouchier SW, de Haan S, et al. Hepatic and cardiovascular consequences of familial hypobetalipoproteinemia. Arterioscler Thromb Vasc Biol 2005;25:1979-1984.
68. Linton MF, Farese RV Jr, Young SG. Familial hypobetalipoproteinemia. J Lipid Res 1993;34:521-541.
69. De Backer G, Ambrosioni E, Borch-Johnsen K, et al. European guidelines on cardiovascular disease prevention in clinical practice. Third Joint Task Force of European and Other Societies on Cardiovascular Disease Prevention in Clinical Practice. Eur Heart J 2003;24:1601-1610.
70. JBS 2: Joint British Societies' guidelines on prevention of cardiovascular disease in clinical practice. Heart 2005;91(suppl 5):v1-v52.
71. Thompson JB, Rivera JJ, Blumenthal RS, et al. Primary prevention for patients with intermediate Framingham risk scores. Curr Cardiol Rep 2006;8:261-266.
72. The Third Report of The National Cholesterol Education Program (NCEP) Expert Panel on Detection, Evaluation, And Treatment of High Blood Cholesterol In Adults (Adult Treatment Panel III). Executive summary. JAMA 2001;285:2486-2497.
73. National Cholesterol Education Program. Second Report of the Expert Panel on Detection, Evaluation, and Treatment of High Blood Cholesterol in Adults (Adult Treatment Panel II). Circulation 1994;89:1333-1445.
74. National Cholesterol Education Program. Report of the Expert Panel on Population Strategies for Blood Cholesterol Reduction: executive summary. National Heart, Lung and Blood Institute, National Institutes of Health. Arch Intern Med 1991;151:1071-1084.
75. Lichtenstein AH, Appel LJ, Brands M, et al. Diet and lifestyle recommendations revision 2006: a scientific statement from the American Heart Association Nutrition Committee. Circulation 2006;114:82-96.
76. MRC/BHF Heart Protection Study of cholesterol lowering with simvastatin in 20,536 high-risk individuals: a randomised placebo-controlled trial. Lancet 2002;360(9326):7-22.
77. Shepherd J, Blauw GJ, Murphy MB, et al. Pravastatin in elderly individuals at risk of vascular disease (PROSPER): a randomised controlled trial. Lancet 2002;360(9346): 1623-1630.
78. Major outcomes in moderately hypercholesterolemic, hypertensive patients randomized to pravastatin vs usual care: The Antihypertensive and Lipid-Lowering Treatment to Prevent Heart Attack Trial (ALLHAT-LLT). JAMA 2002;288:2998-3007.
79. Sever PS, Dahlof B, Poulter NR, et al. Prevention of coronary and stroke events with atorvastatin in hypertensive patients who have average or lower-than-average cholesterol concentrations, in the Anglo-Scandinavian Cardiac Outcomes Trial—Lipid Lowering Arm (ASCOT-LLA): a multicentre randomised controlled trial. Lancet 2003;361(9364):1149-1158.
80. Cannon CP, Braunwald E, McCabe CH, et al. Intensive versus moderate lipid lowering with statins after acute coronary syndromes. N Engl J Med 2004;350:1495-1504.
81. Stone NJ, Bilek S, Rosenbaum S. Recent National Cholesterol Education Program Adult Treatment Panel III update: adjustments and options. Am J Cardiol 2005;96(4A):53E-59E.
82. Endo A, Kuroda M, Tsujita Y. ML-236A, ML-236B, and ML-236C, new inhibitors of cholesterogenesis produced by *Penicillium citrinium*. J Antibiot (Tokyo) 1976;29:1346-1348.
83. Rutishauser J. The role of statins in clinical medicine—LDL-cholesterol lowering and beyond. Swiss Med Wkly 2006;136(3-4):41-49.
84. Myerson M, Ngai C, Jones J, et al. Treatment with high-dose simvastatin reduces secretion of apolipoprotein B-lipoproteins in patients with diabetic dyslipidemia. J Lipid Res 2005;46:2735-2744.
85. Chapman MJ, Caslake M, Packard C, et al. New dimension of statin action on ApoB atherogenicity. Clin Cardiol 2003;26(1 suppl 1):I7-I10.
86. Ginsberg HN. Efficacy and mechanisms of action of statins in the treatment of diabetic dyslipidemia [Review]. J Clin Endocrinol Metab 2006;91:383-392.
87. Edwards JE, Moore RA. Statins in hypercholesterolaemia: a dose-specific meta-analysis of lipid changes in randomised, double blind trials. BMC Fam Pract 2003;4:18.
88. Mikhailidis DP, Wierzbicki AS. HDL-cholesterol and the treatment of coronary heart disease: contrasting effects of atorvastatin and simvastatin. Curr Med Res Opin 2000;16:139-146.
89. Schaefer EJ, Asztalos BF. The effects of statins on high-density lipoproteins. Curr Atheroscler Rep 2006;8:41-49.
90. Cheng JW. Rosuvastatin in the management of hyperlipidemia. Clin Ther 2004;26:1368-1387.
91. Jones PH, Davidson MH, Stein EA, et al. Comparison of the efficacy and safety of rosuvastatin versus atorvastatin, simvastatin, and pravastatin across doses (STELLAR* Trial). Am J Cardiol 2003;92:152-160.
92. Crouse JR 3rd, Frohlich J, Ose L, et al. Effects of high doses of simvastatin and atorvastatin on high-density lipoprotein cholesterol and apolipoprotein A-I. Am J Cardiol 1999;83:1476-1477, A1477.
93. Heinonen TM, Stein E, Weiss SR, et al. The lipid-lowering effects of atorvastatin, a new HMG-CoA reductase inhibitor: results of a randomized, double-masked study. Clin Ther 1996;18:853-863.
94. Schwartz GG, Olsson AG, Ezekowitz MD, et al. Effects of atorvastatin on early recurrent ischemic events in acute coronary syndromes: the MIRACL study: a randomized controlled trial. JAMA 2001;285:1711-1718.
95. Crisby M, Nordin-Fredriksson G, Shah PK, et al. Pravastatin treatment increases collagen content and decreases lipid content, inflammation, metalloproteinases, and cell death in human carotid plaques: implications for plaque stabilization. Circulation 2001;103:926-933.
96. Martin-Ventura JL, Blanco-Colio LM, Gomez-Hernandez A, et al. Intensive treatment with atorvastatin reduces inflammation in mononuclear cells and human atherosclerotic lesions in one month. Stroke 2005;36:1796-1800.
97. Libby P, Aikawa M. Stabilization of atherosclerotic plaques: new mechanisms and clinical targets. Nat Med 2002;8:1257-1262.
98. Balk EM, Lau J, Goudas LC, et al. Effects of statins on nonlipid serum markers associated with cardiovascular disease: a systematic review. Ann Intern Med 2003;139:670-682.
99. Ridker PM, Cannon CP, Morrow D, et al. C-reactive protein levels and outcomes after statin therapy. N Engl J Med 2005;352:20-28.
100. de Lemos JA, Blazing MA, Wiviott SD, et al. Early intensive vs a delayed conservative simvastatin strategy in patients with acute coronary syndromes: phase Z of the A to Z trial. JAMA 2004;292:1307-1316.
101. Tornio A, Pasanen MK, Laitila J, et al. Comparison of 3-hydroxy-3-methylglutaryl coenzyme A (HMG-CoA) reductase inhibitors (statins) as inhibitors of cytochrome P450 2C8. Basic Clin Pharmacol Toxicol 2005;97:104-108.
102. Lennernas H, Fager G. Pharmacodynamics and pharmacokinetics of the HMG-CoA reductase inhibitors. Similarities and differences. Clin Pharmacokinet 1997;32:403-425.
103. Omar MA, Wilson JP. FDA adverse event reports on statin-associated rhabdomyolysis. Ann Pharmacother 2002;36:288-295.
104. Thompson PD, Clarkson P, Karas RH. Statin-associated myopathy. JAMA 2003;289: 1681-1690.
105. Iwata H, Matsuo K, Hara S, et al. Use of hydroxy-methyl-glutaryl coenzyme A reductase inhibitors is associated with risk of lymphoid malignancies. Cancer Sci 2006;97:133-138.
106. Law M, Rudnicka AR. Statin safety: a systematic review. Am J Cardiol 2006;97(8A):52C-60C.
107. Smellie WS. Testing pitfalls and summary of guidance in lipid management. BMJ 2006(7558);333:83-86.
108. LaRosa JC, Hunninghake D, Bush D, et al. The cholesterol facts. A summary of the evidence relating dietary fats, serum cholesterol, and coronary heart disease. A joint statement by the American Heart Association and the National Heart, Lung, and Blood Institute. The Task Force on Cholesterol Issues, American Heart Association. Circulation 1990;81:1721-1733.
109. Shepherd J, Cobbe SM, Ford I, et al. Prevention of coronary heart disease with pravastatin in men with hypercholesterolemia. West of Scotland Coronary Prevention Study Group. N Engl J Med 1995;333:1301-1307.
110. Pasternak RC, Smith SC Jr, Bairey-Merz CN, et al. ACC/AHA/NHLBI clinical advisory on the use and safety of statins. J Am Coll Cardiol 2002;40:567-572.
111. Graham DJ, Staffa JA, Shatin D, et al. Incidence of hospitalized rhabdomyolysis in patients treated with lipid-lowering drugs. JAMA 2004;292:2585-2590.
112. Ballantyne CM, Corsini A, Davidson MH, et al. Risk for myopathy with statin therapy in high-risk patients. Arch Intern Med 2003;163:553-564.
113. Kaufmann P, Torok M, Zahno A, et al. Toxicity of statins on rat skeletal muscle mitochondria. Cell Mol Life Sci 2006;63:2415-2425.
114. Bailey DG, Dresser GK. Interactions between grapefruit juice and cardiovascular drugs. Am J Cardiovasc Drugs 2004;4:281-297.
115. Sorokin AV, Duncan B, Panetta R, et al. Rhabdomyolysis associated with pomegranate juice consumption. Am J Cardiol 2006;98:705-706.
116. Antons KA, Williams CD, Baker SK, et al. Clinical perspectives of statin-induced rhabdomyolysis. Am J Med 2006;119:400-409.
117. Cziraky MJ, Willey VJ, McKenney JM, et al. Statin safety: an assessment using an administrative claims database. Am J Cardiol 2006;97(8A):61C-68C.
118. Vladutiu GD, Simmons Z, Isackson PJ, et al. Genetic risk factors associated with lipid-lowering drug-induced myopathies. Muscle Nerve 2006;34:153-162.
119. Golomb BA. Implications of statin adverse effects in the elderly. Expert Opin Drug Saf 2005;4:389-397.
120. Riesco-Eizaguirre G, Arpa-Gutierrez FJ, Gutierrez M, et al. [Severe polymyositis with simvastatin use]. Rev Neurol 2003;37:934-936.
121. Zuech P, Pauwels C, Duthoit C, et al. [Pravastatin-induced dermatomyositis]. Rev Med Interne 2005;26:897-902.
122. Chazerain P, Hayem G, Hamza S, et al. Four cases of tendinopathy in patients on statin therapy. Joint Bone Spine 2001;68:430-433.
123. Chasman DI, Posada D, Subrahmanyan L, et al. Pharmacogenetic study of statin therapy and cholesterol reduction. JAMA 2004;291:2821-2827.
124. Gerdes LU, Gerdes C, Kervinen K, et al. The apolipoprotein epsilon4 allele determines prognosis and the effect on prognosis of simvastatin in survivors of myocardial infarction : a substudy of the Scandinavian Simvastatin Survival Study. Circulation 2000;101:1366-1371.
125. Carlquist JF, Muhlestein JB, Horne BD, et al. The cholesteryl ester transfer protein Taq1B gene polymorphism predicts clinical benefit of statin therapy in patients with significant coronary artery disease. Am Heart J 2003;146:1007-1014.
126. Lahoz C, Pena R, Mostaza JM, et al. The -514C/T polymorphism of the hepatic lipase gene significantly modulates the HDL-cholesterol response to statin treatment. Atherosclerosis 2005;182:129-134.
127. Lahoz C, Pena R, Mostaza JM, et al. Apo A-I promoter polymorphism influences basal HDL-cholesterol and its response to pravastatin therapy. Atherosclerosis 2003;168:289-295.
128. Lahoz C, Pena R, Mostaza JM, et al. Baseline levels of low-density lipoprotein cholesterol and lipoprotein (a) and the AvaII polymorphism of the low-density lipopro-

tein receptor gene influence the response of low-density lipoprotein cholesterol to pravastatin treatment. Metabolism 2005;54:741-747.
129. Sabatine MS, Seidman JG, Seidman CE. Cardiovascular genomics. Circulation 2006;113:e450-e455.
130. Boekholdt SM, Sacks FM, Jukema JW, et al. Cholesteryl ester transfer protein TaqIB variant, high-density lipoprotein cholesterol levels, cardiovascular risk, and efficacy of pravastatin treatment: individual patient meta-analysis of 13,677 subjects. Circulation 2005;111:278-287.
131. Humphries SE, Hingorani A. Pharmacogenetics: progress, pitfalls and clinical potential for coronary heart disease. Vascul Pharmacol 2006;44:119-125.
132. Schmitz G, Langmann T. Pharmacogenomics of cholesterol-lowering therapy. Vascul Pharmacol 2006;44:75-89.
133. Insull W Jr. Clinical utility of bile acid sequestrants in the treatment of dyslipidemia: a scientific review. South Med J 2006;99:257-273.
134. West RJ, Lloyd JK. The effect of cholestyramine on intestinal absorption. Gut 1975;16:93-98.
135. Saraux H, Offret H, Levy VG. [Severe amblyopia caused by vitamin A deficiency induced by prolonged cholestyramine treatment]. Bull Soc Ophtalmol Fr 1980;80(4-5):367-368.
136. Vroonhof K, van Rijn HJ, van Hattum J. Vitamin K deficiency and bleeding after long-term use of cholestyramine. Neth J Med 2003;61:19-21.
137. Melian EB, Plosker GL. Colesevelam. Am J Cardiovasc Drugs 2001;1:141-146; discussion 147-148.
138. Davidson MH, Dillon MA, Gordon B, et al. Colesevelam hydrochloride (cholestagel): a new, potent bile acid sequestrant associated with a low incidence of gastrointestinal side effects. Arch Intern Med 1999;159:1893-1900.
139. Devaraj S, Autret B, Jialal I. Effects of colesevelam hydrochloride (WelChol) on biomarkers of inflammation in patients with mild hypercholesterolemia. Am J Cardiol 2006;98:641-643.
140. Bays HE, Davidson M, Jones MR, et al. Effects of colesevelam hydrochloride on low-density lipoprotein cholesterol and high-sensitivity C-reactive protein when added to statins in patients with hypercholesterolemia. Am J Cardiol 2006;97:1198-1205.
141. Sprecher DL, Abrams J, Allen JW, et al. Low-dose combined therapy with fluvastatin and cholestyramine in hyperlipidemic patients. Ann Intern Med 1994;120:537-543.
142. Carlson LA, Rosenhamer G. Reduction of mortality in the Stockholm Ischaemic Heart Disease Secondary Prevention Study by combined treatment with clofibrate and nicotinic acid. Acta Med Scand 1988;223:405-418.
143. McKenney J, Jones M, Abby S. Safety and efficacy of colesevelam hydrochloride in combination with fenofibrate for the treatment of mixed hyperlipidemia. Curr Med Res Opin 2005;21:1403-1412.
144. Armani A, Toth PP. Colesevelam hydrochloride in the management of dyslipidemia. Expert Rev Cardiovasc Ther 2006;4:283-291.
145. Kosoglou T, Statkevich P, Johnson-Levonas AO, et al. Ezetimibe: a review of its metabolism, pharmacokinetics and drug interactions. Clin Pharmacokinet 2005;44:467-494.
146. Knopp RH, Gitter H, Truitt T, et al. Effects of ezetimibe, a new cholesterol absorption inhibitor, on plasma lipids in patients with primary hypercholesterolemia. Eur Heart J 2003;24:729-741.
147. Gylling H, Miettinen TA. Drug-induced effects on cholesterol catabolism and bile acids. Curr Opin Investig Drugs 2006;7:214-218.
148. Gagne C, Gaudet D, Bruckert E. Efficacy and safety of ezetimibe coadministered with atorvastatin or simvastatin in patients with homozygous familial hypercholesterolemia. Circulation 2002;105:2469-2475.
149. Salen G, von Bergmann K, Lutjohann D, et al. Ezetimibe effectively reduces plasma plant sterols in patients with sitosterolemia. Circulation 2004;109:966-971.
150. Xydakis AM, Guyton JR, Chiou P, et al. Effectiveness and tolerability of ezetimibe add-on therapy to a bile acid resin-based regimen for hypercholesterolemia. Am J Cardiol 2004;94:795-797.
151. Tunaru S, Kero J, Schaub A, et al. PUMA-G and HM74 are receptors for nicotinic acid and mediate its anti-lipolytic effect. Nat Med 2003;9:352-355.
152. Guyton JR. Extended-release niacin for modifying the lipoprotein profile. Expert Opin Pharmacother 2004;5:1385-1398.
153. Canner PL, Berge KG, Wenger NK, et al. Fifteen-year mortality in Coronary Drug Project patients: long-term benefit with niacin. J Am Coll Cardiol 1986;8:1245-1255.
154. Mullin GE, Greenson JK, Mitchell MC. Fulminant hepatic failure after ingestion of sustained-release nicotinic acid. Ann Intern Med 1989;111:253-255.
155. Tato F, Vega GL, Grundy SM. Effects of crystalline nicotinic acid–induced hepatic dysfunction on serum low-density lipoprotein cholesterol and lecithin cholesteryl acyl transferase. Am J Cardiol 1998;81:805-807.
156. Hunninghake DB, McGovern ME, Koren M, et al. A dose-ranging study of a new, once-daily, dual-component drug product containing niacin extended-release and lovastatin. Clin Cardiol 2003;26:112-118.
157. Brown BG, Zhao XQ, Chait A, et al. Simvastatin and niacin, antioxidant vitamins, or the combination for the prevention of coronary disease. N Engl J Med 2001;345:1583-1592.
158. Brown G, Albers JJ, Fisher LD, et al. Regression of coronary artery disease as a result of intensive lipid-lowering therapy in men with high levels of apolipoprotein B. N Engl J Med 1990;323:1289-1298.
159. Blankenhorn DH, Nessim SA, Johnson RL, et al. Beneficial effects of combined colestipol-niacin therapy on coronary atherosclerosis and coronary venous bypass grafts. JAMA 1987;257:3233-3240.
160. Din JN, Newby DE, Flapan AD. Omega 3 fatty acids and cardiovascular disease—fishing for a natural treatment. BMJ 2004;328(7430):30-35.
161. Zhang J, Sasaki S, Amano K, et al. Fish consumption and mortality from all causes, ischemic heart disease, and stroke: an ecological study. Prev Med 1999;28:520-529.
162. Thies F, Garry JM, Yaqoob P, et al. Association of n-3 polyunsaturated fatty acids with stability of atherosclerotic plaques: a randomised controlled trial. Lancet 2003;361(9356):477-485.
163. Bhatnagar D, Durrington PN. Omega-3 fatty acids: their role in the prevention and treatment of atherosclerosis related risk factors and complications. Int J Clin Pract 2003;57:305-314.
164. Marchioli R, Barzi F, Bomba E, et al. Early protection against sudden death by n-3 polyunsaturated fatty acids after myocardial infarction: time-course analysis of the results of the Gruppo Italiano per lo Studio della Sopravvivenza nell'Infarto Miocardico (GISSI)-Prevenzione. Circulation 2002;105:1897-1903.
165. He K, Song Y, Daviglus ML, et al. Accumulated evidence on fish consumption and coronary heart disease mortality: a meta-analysis of cohort studies. Circulation 2004;109:2705-2711.
166. Wang C, Harris WS, Chung M, et al. n-3 Fatty acids from fish or fish-oil supplements, but not alpha-linolenic acid, benefit cardiovascular disease outcomes in primary- and secondary-prevention studies: a systematic review. Am J Clin Nutr 2006;84:5-17.
167. Hooper L, Thompson RL, Harrison RA, et al. Risks and benefits of omega 3 fats for mortality, cardiovascular disease, and cancer: systematic review. BMJ 2006;332(7544):752-760.
168. Chapman MJ. Beyond the statins: new therapeutic perspectives in cardiovascular disease prevention. Cardiovasc Drugs Ther 2005;19:135-139.
169. Jacobson TA, Zimmerman FH. Fibrates in combination with statins in the management of dyslipidemia. J Clin Hypertens (Greenwich) 2006;8:35-41; quiz 42-33.
170. Pan WJ, Gustavson LE, Achari R, et al. Lack of a clinically significant pharmacokinetic interaction between fenofibrate and pravastatin in healthy volunteers. J Clin Pharmacol 2000;40:316-323.
171. Prueksaritanont T, Tang C, Qiu Y, et al. Effects of fibrates on metabolism of statins in human hepatocytes. Drug Metab Dispos 2002;30:1280-1287.
172. Frick MH, Elo O, Haapa K, et al. Helsinki Heart Study: primary-prevention trial with gemfibrozil in middle-aged men with dyslipidemia. Safety of treatment, changes in risk factors, and incidence of coronary heart disease. N Engl J Med 1987;317:1237-1245.
173. Tenkanen L, Manttari M, Kovanen PT, et al. Gemfibrozil in the treatment of dyslipidemia: an 18-year mortality follow-up of the Helsinki Heart Study. Arch Intern Med 2006;166:743-748.
174. Rubins HB, Robins SJ, Collins D, et al. Gemfibrozil for the secondary prevention of coronary heart disease in men with low levels of high-density lipoprotein cholesterol. Veterans Affairs High-Density Lipoprotein Cholesterol Intervention Trial Study Group. N Engl J Med 1999;341:410-418.
175. Robins SJ, Rubins HB, Faas FH, et al. Insulin resistance and cardiovascular events with low HDL cholesterol: the Veterans Affairs HDL Intervention Trial (VA-HIT). Diabetes Care 2003;26:1513-1517.
176. DAIS Investigators. Effect of fenofibrate on progression of coronary-artery disease in type 2 diabetes: the Diabetes Atherosclerosis Intervention Study, a randomised study. Lancet 2001;357(9260):905-910.
177. Keech A, Simes RJ, Barter P, et al. Effects of long-term fenofibrate therapy on cardiovascular events in 9795 people with type 2 diabetes mellitus (the FIELD study): randomised controlled trial. Lancet 2005;366(9500):1849-1861.
178. Jones MR, Baker BA, Mathew P. Effect of colesevelam HCl on single-dose fenofibrate pharmacokinetics. Clin Pharmacokinet 2004;43:943-950.
179. Douketis JD, Macie C, Thabane L, et al. Systematic review of long-term weight loss studies in obese adults: clinical significance and applicability to clinical practice. Int J Obes (Lond) 2005;29:1153-1167.
180. Gadde KM, Allison DB. Cannabinoid-1 receptor antagonist, rimonabant, for management of obesity and related risks. Circulation 2006;114:974-984.
181. Sacks FM, Katan M. Randomized clinical trials on the effects of dietary fat and carbohydrate on plasma lipoproteins and cardiovascular disease. Am J Med 2002;113(suppl 9B):13S-24S.
182. de Lorgeril M, Renaud S, Mamelle N, et al. Mediterranean alpha-linolenic acid–rich diet in secondary prevention of coronary heart disease. Lancet 1994;343(8911):1454-1459.
183. Nguyen TT. The cholesterol-lowering action of plant stanol esters. J Nutr 1999;129:2109-2112.
184. Devaraj S, Jialal I. The role of dietary supplementation with plant sterols and stanols in the prevention of cardiovascular disease. Nutr Rev 2006;64(7 pt 1):348-354.
185. Moruisi KG, Oosthuizen W, Opperman AM. Phytosterols/stanols lower cholesterol concentrations in familial hypercholesterolemic subjects: a systematic review with meta-analysis. J Am Coll Nutr 2006;25:41-48.
186. Plat J, Mensink RP. Plant stanol and sterol esters in the control of blood cholesterol levels: mechanism and safety aspects. Am J Cardiol 2005;96(1A):15D-22D.
187. Grundy SM. Stanol esters as a component of maximal dietary therapy in the National Cholesterol Education Program Adult Treatment Panel III report. Am J Cardiol 2005;96(1A):47D-50D.
188. Buchwald H, Matts JP, Fitch LL, et al. Program on the Surgical Control of the Hyperlipidemias (POSCH): design and methodology. POSCH Group. J Clin Epidemiol 1989;42:1111-1127.
189. Buchwald H, Varco RL, Matts JP, et al. Effect of partial ileal bypass surgery on mortality and morbidity from coronary heart disease in patients with hypercholesterolemia. Report of the Program on the Surgical Control of the Hyperlipidemias (POSCH). N Engl J Med 1990;323:946-955.
190. Buchwald H, Varco RL, Boen JR, et al. Effective lipid modification by partial ileal bypass reduced long-term coronary heart disease mortality and morbidity: five-year posttrial follow-up report from the POSCH. Program on the Surgical Control of the Hyperlipidemias. Arch Intern Med 1998;158:1253-1261.
191. Buchwald H, Williams SE, Matts JP, et al. Overall mortality in the program on the surgical control of the hyperlipidemias. J Am Coll Surg 2002;195:327-331.

192. Mango VL, Frishman WH. Physiologic, psychologic, and metabolic consequences of bariatric surgery. Cardiol Rev 2006;14:232-237.
193. Buchwald H, Avidor Y, Braunwald E, et al. Bariatric surgery: a systematic review and meta-analysis. JAMA 2004;292:1724-1737.
194. Vinik AI. The metabolic basis of atherogenic dyslipidemia. Clin Cornerstone 2005;7(2-3):27-35.
195. Van Gaal LF, Rissanen AM, Scheen AJ, et al. Effects of the cannabinoid-1 receptor blocker rimonabant on weight reduction and cardiovascular risk factors in overweight patients: 1-year experience from the RIO-Europe study. Lancet 2005; 365(9468):1389-1397.
196. Despres JP, Golay A, Sjostrom L. Effects of rimonabant on metabolic risk factors in overweight patients with dyslipidemia. N Engl J Med 2005;353:2121-2134.
197. Pi-Sunyer FX, Aronne LJ, Heshmati HM, et al. Effect of rimonabant, a cannabinoid-1 receptor blocker, on weight and cardiometabolic risk factors in overweight or obese patients: RIO-North America: a randomized controlled trial. JAMA 2006;295:761-775.
198. Padwal R, Li SK, Lau DC. Long-term pharmacotherapy for obesity and overweight. Cochrane Database Syst Rev 2004(3):CD004094.
199. Hollander PA, Elbein SC, Hirsch IB, et al. Role of orlistat in the treatment of obese patients with type 2 diabetes. A 1-year randomized double-blind study. Diabetes Care 1998;21:1288-1294.
200. Hutton B, Fergusson D. Changes in body weight and serum lipid profile in obese patients treated with orlistat in addition to a hypocaloric diet: a systematic review of randomized clinical trials. Am J Clin Nutr 2004;80:1461-1468.
201. Forrester JS, Makkar R, Shah PK. Increasing high-density lipoprotein cholesterol in dyslipidemia by cholesteryl ester transfer protein inhibition: an update for clinicians. Circulation 2005;111:1847-1854.
202. Barter PJ, Caulfield M, Eriksson M, et al. Effects of torcetrapib in patients at high risk for coronary events. N Engl J Med 2007;357:2109-2122.
203. Clark RW. Raising high-density lipoprotein with cholesteryl ester transfer protein inhibitors. Curr Opin Pharmacol 2006;6:162-168.
204. Evans M, Roberts A, Davies S, et al. Medical lipid-regulating therapy: current evidence, ongoing trials and future developments. Drugs 2004;64:1181-1196.
205. Chandler CE, Wilder DE, Pettini JL, et al. CP-346086: an MTP inhibitor that lowers plasma cholesterol and triglycerides in experimental animals and in humans. J Lipid Res 2003;44:1887-1901.
206. Rudel LL, Lee RG, Parini P. ACAT2 is a target for treatment of coronary heart disease associated with hypercholesterolemia. Arterioscler Thromb Vasc Biol 2005;25:1112-1118.
207. Leon C, Hill JS, Wasan KM. Potential role of acyl-coenzyme A:cholesterol transferase (ACAT) inhibitors as hypolipidemic and antiatherosclerosis drugs. Pharm Res 2005;22:1578-1588.
208. Kramer W, Glombik H. Bile acid reabsorption inhibitors (BARI): novel hypolipidemic drugs. Curr Med Chem 2006;13:997-1016.
209. Tontonoz P, Mangelsdorf DJ. Liver X receptor signaling pathways in cardiovascular disease. Mol Endocrinol 2003;17:985-993.
210. Urizar NL, Liverman AB, Dodds DT, et al. A natural product that lowers cholesterol as an antagonist ligand for FXR. Science 2002;296(5573):1703-1706.
211. Kong W, Wei J, Abidi P, et al. Berberine is a novel cholesterol-lowering drug working through a unique mechanism distinct from statins. Nat Med 2004;10:1344-1351.
212. Masaki N, Tatami R, Kumamoto T, et al. Ten-year follow-up of familial hypercholesterolemia patients after intensive cholesterol-lowering therapy. Int Heart J 2005; 46:833-843.
213. Rader DJ. Gene therapy for familial hypercholesterolemia. Nutr Metab Cardiovasc Dis 2001;11(suppl 5):40-44.
214. Broedl UC, Rader DJ. Gene therapy for lipoprotein disorders. Expert Opin Biol Ther 2005;5:1029-1038.
215. Lebherz C, Gao G, Louboutin JP, et al. Gene therapy with novel adeno-associated virus vectors substantially diminishes atherosclerosis in a murine model of familial hypercholesterolemia. J Gene Med 2004;6:663-672.
216. Grossman M, Raper SE, Kozarsky K, et al. Successful ex vivo gene therapy directed to liver in a patient with familial hypercholesterolaemia. Nat Genet 1994;6(4):335-341.
217. Grossman M, Rader DJ, Muller DW, et al. A pilot study of ex vivo gene therapy for homozygous familial hypercholesterolaemia. Nat Med 1995;1(11):1148-1154.
218. Zsigmond E, Kobayashi K, Tzung KW, et al. Adenovirus-mediated gene transfer of human lipoprotein lipase ameliorates the hyperlipidemias associated with apolipoprotein E and LDL receptor deficiencies in mice. Hum Gene Ther 1997;8(16):1921-1933.
219. Tsukamoto K, Tangirala R, Chun SH, et al. Rapid regression of atherosclerosis induced by liver-directed gene transfer of ApoE in ApoE-deficient mice. Arterioscler Thromb Vasc Biol 1999;19:2162-2170.
220. Belalcazar LM, Merched A, Carr B, et al. Long-term stable expression of human apolipoprotein A-I mediated by helper-dependent adenovirus gene transfer inhibits atherosclerosis progression and remodels atherosclerotic plaques in a mouse model of familial hypercholesterolemia. Circulation 2003;107:2726-2732.
221. Wellington CL, Brunham LR, Zhou S, et al. Alterations of plasma lipids in mice via adenoviral-mediated hepatic overexpression of human ABCA1. J Lipid Res 2003;44:1470-1480.
222. Mertens A, Verhamme P, Bielicki JK, et al. Increased low-density lipoprotein oxidation and impaired high-density lipoprotein antioxidant defense are associated with increased macrophage homing and atherosclerosis in dyslipidemic obese mice: LCAT gene transfer decreases atherosclerosis. Circulation 2003;107:1640-1646.
223. Ishida T, Choi S, Kundu RK, et al. Endothelial lipase is a major determinant of HDL level. J Clin Invest 2003;111:347-355.
224. Jalkanen J, Leppanen P, Pajusola K, et al. Adeno-associated virus-mediated gene transfer of a secreted decoy human macrophage scavenger receptor reduces atherosclerotic lesion formation in LDL receptor knockout mice. Mol Ther 2003;8:903-910.
225. Liu Y, Li D, Chen J, et al. Inhibition of atherogenesis in LDLR knockout mice by systemic delivery of adeno-associated virus type 2-hIL-10. Atherosclerosis 2006;188: 19-27.
226. Bradshaw G, Gutierrez A, Miyake JH, et al. Facilitated replacement of Kupffer cells expressing a paraoxonase-1 transgene is essential for ameliorating atherosclerosis in mice. Proc Natl Acad Sci U S A 2005;102:11029-11034.
227. Smith SC Jr, Allen J, Blair SN, et al. AHA/ACC guidelines for secondary prevention for patients with coronary and other atherosclerotic vascular disease: 2006 update endorsed by the National Heart, Lung, and Blood Institute. J Am Coll Cardiol 2006;47:2130-2139.
228. Mason RP, Walter MF, Day CA, et al. Intermolecular differences of 3-hydroxy-3-methylglutaryl coenzyme A reductase inhibitors contribute to distinct pharmacologic and pleiotropic actions. Am J Cardiol 2005;96(5A):11F-23F.
229. Corsini A, Bellosta S, Baetta R, et al. New insights into the pharmacodynamic and pharmacokinetic properties of statins. Pharmacol Ther 1999;84:413-428.
230. Paramsothy P, Knopp R. Management of dyslipidaemias. Heart 2006;92:1529-1534.

24

CORONARY ARTERY DISEASE

Arshad Jahangir and Viqar Maria

OVERVIEW 321
PATHOPHYSIOLOGY 321
Pathobiology of Coronary Atherosclerosis 321
Pathophysiology of Acute Coronary Syndrome 322
Pathophysiology of Post-MI Cardiac Remodeling 323
THERAPEUTICS AND CLINICAL PHARMACOLOGY 324
Clinical Spectrum of Coronary Atherosclerosis 324
Management of CAD 324
Primary Prevention of CHD 324
Management of Chronic Stable Angina 325
Management of UA and NSTEMI 325
Management of STEMI 325
THERAPEUTICS BY CLASS 325
Antiplatelet Agents 325
Thromboxane Inhibitors 328
ADP Receptor Antagonists: Thienopyridines 330
Glycoprotein IIb/IIIa Receptor Antagonists 333
Other Antiplatelet Agents 335
Novel Antiplatelet Agents under Investigation 335
Antithrombotic Agents (Anticoagulants) 335
Antithrombins 335
Factor Xa Inhibitors 339
Direct Thrombin Inhibitors 339
Fibrinolytic Agents 340
Anti-ischemic Agents 343
Nitrates 343
β-Adrenergic Receptor Antagonists 345
Calcium Channel Blockers 351
Nitric Oxide Donors Under Investigation 353
Other Anti-ischemic Agents 353
Inhibitors of the Renin-Angiotensin-Aldosterone System 354
Mechanism of Action 355
Pharmacokinetics 355
Therapeutic Considerations 355
Adverse Effects, Precautions, and Contraindications 357
Lipid-Lowering Agents 358
Management of Dyslipidemias 358
Emerging Targets and Therapeutics 361

OVERVIEW

Cardiovascular diseases are the leading cause of mortality, accounting for approximately 30% of all deaths worldwide and 37% of deaths in the United States each year.[1] More than 15 million people in the United States have coronary heart disease (CHD). Of these, half experience angina pectoris, and more than 7 million suffer acute myocardial infarction (MI), with 700,000 new and 500,000 recurrent MIs per year. Approximately 40% of all who suffer an MI die prematurely, with approximately 479,000 coronary deaths every year. The first coronary presentation for women is more likely to be angina, compared to MI in men. The annual CHD event rates in women following menopause, however, increase two- to threefold over premenopausal rates (<1% per year).[2] A progressive decline in the age-adjusted CHD fatality rate has been achieved over the last 5 decades. However, the proportion of deaths that are sudden and unexpected continues to be high, accounting for more than half of all coronary deaths. The direct and indirect costs for the care of patients with CHD and associated disability were greater than $431 billion in 2007, more than for any other diagnostic category in the United States.[2,3] With the rapid growth in the elderly population and the increases in obesity and metabolic syndrome, the prevalence of CHD is expected to rise, and it is crucial to aggressively pursue strategies to modify risk factors for coronary atherosclerosis, and recognize the disease early with timely interventions to relieve symptoms of myocardial ischemia and prevent complications of acute infarction or chronic remodeling.[4]

PATHOPHYSIOLOGY

Pathobiology of Coronary Atherosclerosis

The normal myocardial perfusion is regulated by the heart's requirements for oxygen, with the ability of the coronary vascular bed to change its resistance and blood flow to meet the increased demand for O_2 and nutrients with exercise and emotional stress. With coronary artery disease (CAD), atherosclerosis builds up within the vascular wall due to an accumulation of lipids that initially alters endothelial function, disrupting normal regulation of vascular tone, anticoagulant surface, and protection against inflammatory cells.[3] Loss of these protective responses results in inappropriate vasoconstriction and predisposition to adhesion of blood cells, platelet aggregation, and activation of luminal clotting. Coronary atherosclerosis may start in early years of life and progress over years before symptoms of chronic angina or acute coronary syndrome (ACS) develop. Major risk factors that accelerate atherosclerosis include high plasma low-density lipoprotein cholesterol (LDL-C), low plasma high-density lipoprotein cholesterol (HDL-C), cigarette smoking, hypertension, chronic kidney disease, and diabetes mellitus. With progression of coronary atherosclerosis, there is segmental collection of subintimal fat, smooth muscle cells, fibroblasts, and intercellular matrix forming atherosclerotic plaques that reduce luminal diameter (Figs. 24-1 and 24-2). Once vascular cross-sectional area is reduced by these stenoses by greater than 70%, blood flow increase with cardiac work is restricted and myocardial nutrient demands are unmet, causing ischemia manifesting as angina pectoris during exertion, emotional stress, or tachycardia.[3] With progression of atherosclerosis and reduction in luminal area by ≥80%, blood flow is reduced even at rest, causing myocardial ischemia, particularly with any change in vessel caliber due to vasomotion, coronary spasm (Prinzmetal's angina), or platelet plugs that further compromise the critical balance between oxygen supply and demand, precipitating myocardial ischemia.[3,5] Fissuring, erosion, hemorrhage, or thrombosis within or around the atherosclerotic plaque destabilizes the flow by suddenly worsening luminal narrowing, reducing coronary blood flow and precipitating myocardial ischemia and unstable angina (UA) or acute MI (see Fig. 24-1). Gradual narrowing of the coronary vascular diameter and myocardial ischemia result in the development of collateral vessels, which can provide adequate blood flow to maintain the viability and function of the myocardium at rest but not with increased demand during stress.[3,5,6] A reduction in the blood oxygen-carrying capacity with severe anemia or carboxyhemoglobinemia may also disturb the balance between myocardial O_2 demand and supply, espe-

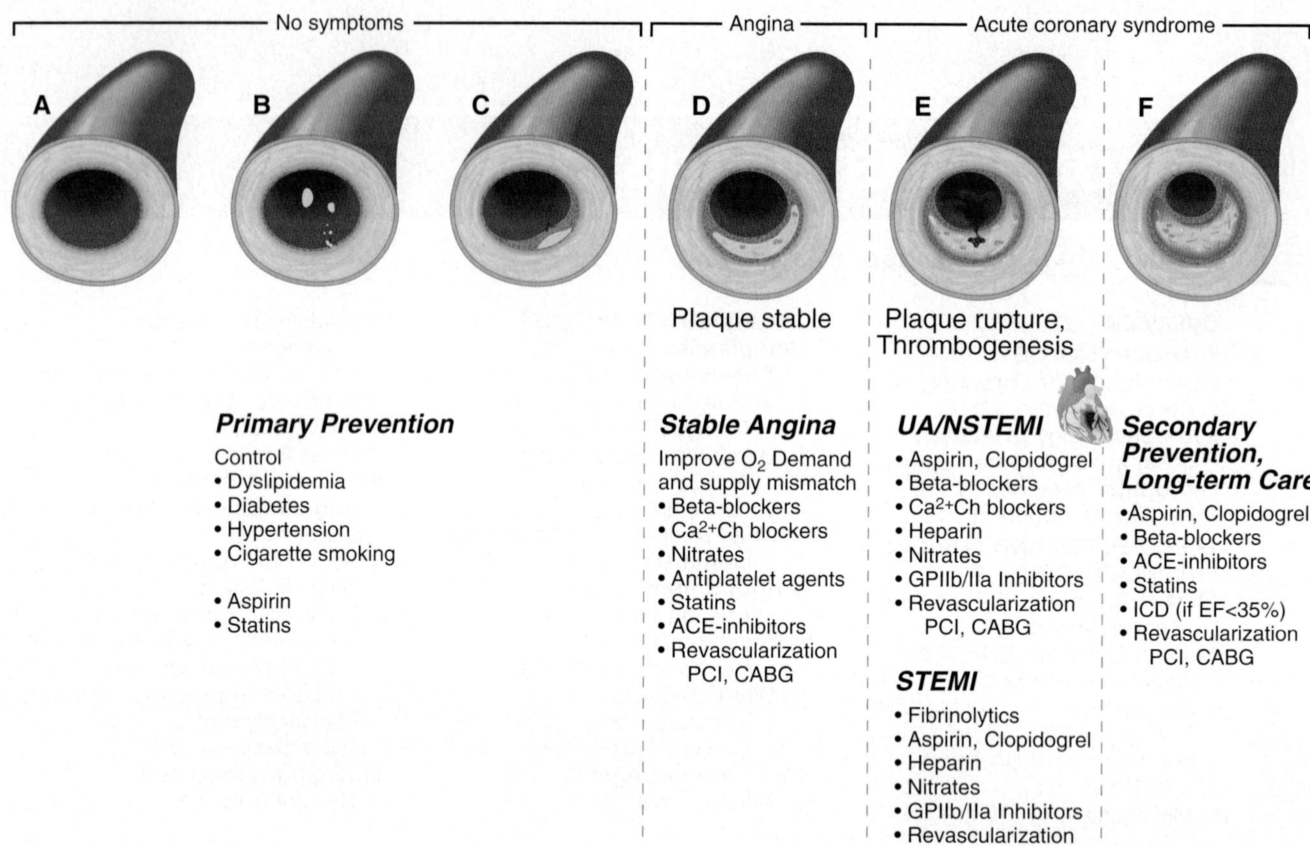

FIGURE 24-1 • **Progression of coronary artery disease from normal to advanced organized plaque, with therapeutic approaches for each stage of the disease.** Coronary arteries progresses from normal vascular wall (*a*), to initial lesion with intimal lipid deposition (*b*), to intimal thickening with smooth muscle cell proliferation (*c*), to stable fibrofatty plaque (*d*), to unstable plaque with disruption of the fibrous cap resulting in acute coronary syndrome and unstable angina (UA) due to platelet activation and thrombogenesis, producing vascular occlusion and myocardial infarction (MI) with or without ST-segment elevation on ECG (*e*). This may be followed by thrombus resorption, collagen accumulation, and smooth muscle cell growth. The spectrum of the management of coronary artery disease extends from primary prevention strategies to reduce risk factors associated with accelerated atherosclerosis to correction of myocardial O_2 demand-supply mismatch by interventions that decrease myocardial workload, prevent progression of coronary stenosis, recruit collateral vessels to improve flow to the ischemic area, and prevent vessel clogging by inhibiting platelets or by coronary artery revascularization. Thrombolytics, antithrombotics, and antiplatelet agents are used to restore flow to the ischemic area by preventing thrombus extension and promoting thrombus lysis, or flow is mechanically restored by catheter-based or surgical revascularization. Secondary prevention involves modification of factors reducing progression of atherosclerosis and instability of plaque. Long-term management also includes interventions to prevent adverse remodeling of the damaged heart. ACE, angiotensin-converting enzyme; GP, glycoprotein; NSTEMI, non–ST-elevation MI; STEMI, ST-elevation MI.

cially in patients with CAD or those with severe ventricular hypertrophy precipitating myocardial ischemia.

With limitation in coronary flow during stress, cardiac ischemia in the atherosclerotic territory results in transient regional biochemical, electrical, and mechanical disturbances, which are more intense within the endocardium than the epicardium.[3,5,6] Sudden occlusion of a coronary artery results in contractile failure or electrical instability that may result in heart block or tachyarrhythmias causing cardiac arrest.[3,5,6] When ischemia is transient, myocardial injury is reversible and may cause angina pectoris, at times associated with repolarization changes on electrocardiogram (ECG) evidenced by T-wave inversion or ST-segment depression. With prolonged (≥20 minutes) ischemia, MI results and, depending on endocardial versus transmural necrosis, may cause ST-segment depression or elevation, respectively, on the ECG.

Pathophysiology of Acute Coronary Syndrome

ACS results from sudden occlusion of a coronary artery and, depending on the extent of myocardial ischemia, results in UA or MI without or with ST-segment elevation (non–ST-elevation MI [NSTEMI] or ST-elevation MI [STEMI], respectively) on ECG. Gradual narrowing of the coronary arteries allow development of collateral vessels that can perfuse myocardium despite complete occlusion of the epicardial vessel, thus preventing myocardial necrosis.[3,5,6] Conversely, sudden coronary artery occlusion by a thrombus precipitated by erosion or rupture of the fibrous cap of a lipid-laden, macrophage- and inflammatory cell–rich "vulnerable" plaque (see Fig. 24-2) results in platelet activation, adhesion, and aggregation that generate thrombin. Thrombin further stimulates platelets and generates fibrin, which cross-links to form the backbone of the thrombus. In addition to activating the clotting system, thrombin also activates fibrinolysis by inducing production and release of tissue plasminogen activator (tPA) from endothelial cells, which activates plasminogen to plasmin bound to fibrin. Plasmin then degrades fibrin, resulting in partial or complete dissolution of the thrombus, thus preventing MI or limiting necrosis with spontaneous reperfusion of the infarct artery. In the majority of patients, however, occlusion of the infarct artery by thrombus persist in the first 6 to 12 hours while the affected myocardial zone is undergoing necrosis (Fig. 24-3).

Interruption of nutrients and oxygen supply with coronary occlusion precipitates MI. Within 15 minutes of perfusion loss, a wave front of necrosis spreads from the endocardium toward the epicardium, resulting in myocardial loss, if left uninterrupted, results in transmural muscle loss (see Fig. 24-3).[4] The extent of infarction is modulated by the presence of collateral flow, O_2 demand, and spontaneous fibrinolysis that may extend the window for myocardial salvage with acute reperfusion therapy. Coronary thrombus may be documented angiographically in 90% of patients with STEMI and 35% to 75% of patients with UA/NSTEMI, but only 1% with stable angina. Therefore, both antithrombin and antiplatelet therapy becomes essential in all patients with an ACS but not necessarily for patients with stable angina, which benefits from anti-ischemic therapy, whereas pharmacologic or catheter-based reperfusion therapy is required in those with persistent ST-segment elevation (see Fig. 24-1).

Pathophysiology of Post-MI Cardiac Remodeling

Following MI, the left ventricle goes through a complex remodeling process with progressive changes in cavity size, wall thickness, and overall geometry. The necrotic myocardium experiences dilation and thinning due to infarct expansion, while noninfarcted segments undergo compensatory hypertrophy as a result of activation of local signaling pathways and generalized neurohumoral system response. Adrenergic and renin-angiotensin-aldosterone system (RAAS) activation plays an important role in post-MI ventricular remodeling. Inhibition of the endogenously active neurohumoral system, including adrenergic and RAAS activation, and prevention of myocardial decompensation and electrical instability thus become cornerstones of chronic therapy after MI.[7]

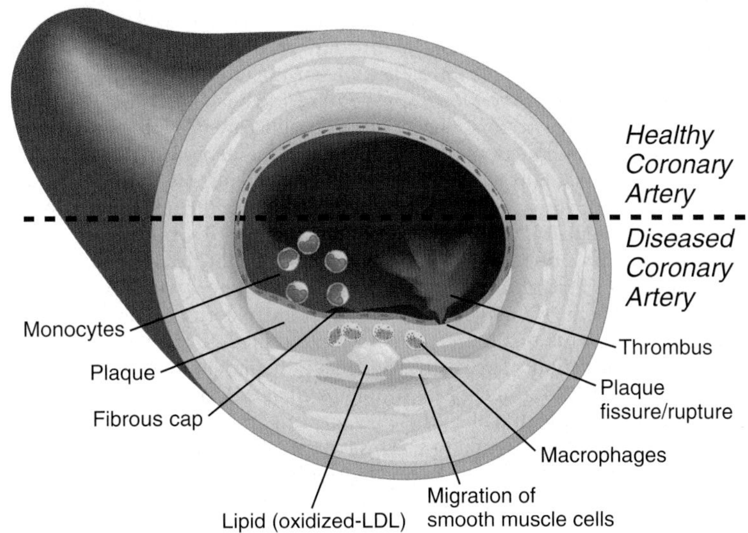

FIGURE 24-2 • Schematic diagram illustrating normal healthy coronary artery and diseased coronary artery with plaque rupture and acute thrombosis.

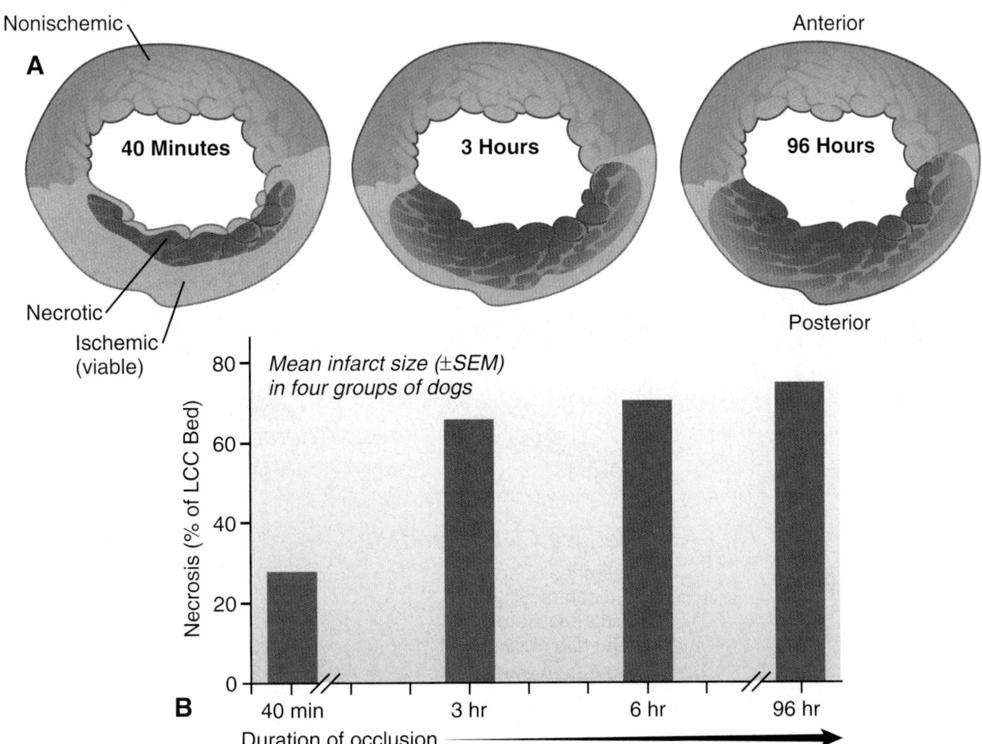

FIGURE 24-3 • Progression of cell death versus time after experimental occlusion of the coronary artery. A, Necrosis occurs first in the subendocardial region of the myocardium. With extension of the occlusion time, a wave front of cell death moves from the subendocardial zone across the wall to involve progressively more of the transmural thickness of the ischemic zone. **B,** Infarct size variation with increasing duration of coronary occlusion. Infarct size dramatically increases from 40 minutes to 3 hours; however, there is very little increase between 3 and 6 hours and between 6 and 96 hours of coronary artery occlusion. (From Reimer KA, Jennings RB. The "wave front phenomenon" of myocardial ischemic cell death: II. Transmural progression of necrosis with the framework of ischemic bed size [myocardium at risk] and collateral flow. Lab Invest 1979;40:633-644.)

THERAPEUTICS AND CLINICAL PHARMACOLOGY

Clinical Spectrum of Coronary Artherosclerosis

Patients with coronary artery atherosclerosis may have a wide spectrum of presentation, ranging from asymptomatic disease to stable chronic exertional angina or acute MI due to abrupt plaque rupture. The underlying substrate in typical **stable angina** is fixed atherosclerotic narrowing of coronary arteries that are unable to dilate to meet cardiac workload with increase in heart rate, contractility, or wall stress, resulting in myocardial ischemia with oxygen supply and demand mismatch (Fig. 24-4). Typical angina is experienced as a squeezing, substernal discomfort or pressure sensation, often with radiation to the left shoulder, arm, jaw, or epigastrium, usually precipitated by exertion or emotional stress and relieved by rest or use of nitroglycerin. Angina pectoris may occur in a stable pattern with exertion for years or become unstable with increase in frequency, duration, or severity or onset at rest. Altered vessel tone with episodic focal or diffuse coronary vasospasm may result in **variant** or **Prinzmetal's angina**. UA or acute MI may result from sudden atherosclerotic plaque rupture that may present with chest pain, dyspnea, light-headedness, heart failure, or arrhythmias. One third of patients who develop MI may not survive the acute ischemic event, with the majority of deaths occurring within the first 2 hours after symptom onset, usually from ventricular fibrillation.[8] For many, sudden death may be the initial manifestation of CHD. Thirty percent to 50% of all MIs may be clinically unrecognized, with half of these being silent and the remainder presenting with atypical symptoms.[9] This is particularly the case in the elderly, women, diabetics, and those with prior heart failure. The diagnosis of MI is delayed in these patients, and they are less likely to receive timely treatment, increasing the likelihood of death and disability.[9] Although ischemia may be silent or have atypical symptoms, the risk of subsequent mortality in these MI patients is not different from those with recognized symptoms,[3] and a high index of suspicion for MI should be maintained so as not to delay initiation of treatment.

Management of CAD

Based on a thorough review of the available scientific evidence, the American College of Cardiology (ACC) and the American Heart Association (AHA) have published practice guidelines reflecting a consensus of expert opinion for the management of patients with CAD.[3,5-7] The aims of these guidelines are to improve the effectiveness of patient care, optimize outcomes, and reduce overall cost of care by focusing resources on the most effective strategies. A classification of recommendations providing an estimate of the size of the treatment effect and level of evidence grades estimating certainty of the treatment effect are provided, as summarized in Box 24-1, to help health care providers in clinical decision making.

Primary Prevention of CHD

Major risk factors that accelerate atherosclerosis, including high LDL-C, low HDL-C, other dyslipidemias, cigarette smoking, hypertension, and diabetes mellitus, should be screened and followed at regular intervals (3 to 5 years). In patients who have two or more major risk factors for CHD or CHD risk equivalent, such as diabetes mellitus, peripheral vascular disease, chronic kidney disease, or 10-year risk of coronary event greater than 20% should be aggressively managed with lifestyle modification and medications to prevent or slow the progression of CAD (primary prevention) or reduce the risk of an acute coronary event in those who have CHD (secondary prevention).

Diets low in saturated fat and cholesterol, high in fiber, and rich in vegetables, fruits, and whole grains should be encouraged, with addition of statins or other drugs to obtain appropriate levels for lipid management.[10] Blood glucose level should be managed, and hypertension should be treated with diet along with a regular aerobic exercise

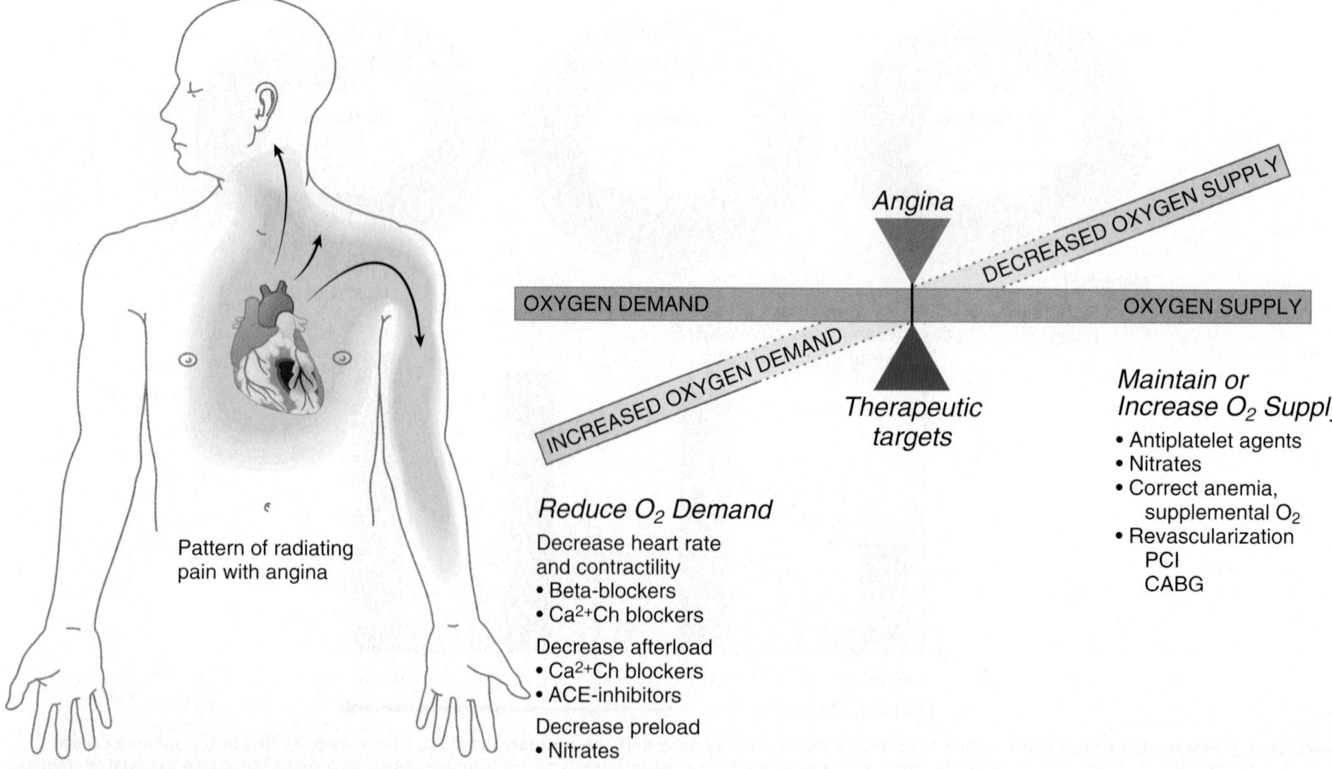

FIGURE 24-4 • Pathophysiologic approach to the management of angina pectoris by reduction of myocardial ischemia by improving myocardial oxygen (O_2) demand-supply mismatch. This may be achieved by decreasing cardiac oxygen demand by reduction in heart rate, ventricular contractility, or wall stress or by prevention of coronary blood flow limitation, thus preventing angina experienced as a squeezing substernal discomfort or pressure sensation, often with radiation to the left shoulder, arm, jaw, or epigastrium precipitated by exertion or emotional stress.

Practice: Cardiovascular Therapeutics

BOX 24-1 ACC/AHA GUIDELINES CLASSIFICATION OF RECOMMENDATIONS AND LEVEL OF EVIDENCE

Classification of Recommendations

Class I: There is evidence and/or general agreement that the given treatment is beneficial, useful, and effective. **Benefit >>> Risk.**

Class II: There is conflicting evidence and/or a divergence of opinion about the usefulness/efficacy of treatment.

- **Class IIa:** Weight of evidence/opinion is in favor of usefulness/efficacy. **Benefit >> Risk.**
- **Class IIb:** Usefulness/efficacy is less well established by evidence/opinion. **Benefit ≥ Risk.**

Class III: There is evidence and/or general agreement that the treatment is not useful/effective and in some cases may be harmful. **Risk ≥ Benefit**

Level of Evidence

A: Data derived from multiple randomized clinical trials or meta-analyses.

B: Data derived from a single randomized trial, or nonrandomized studies.

C: Only consensus opinion of experts, case studies, or standard-of-care.

program and antihypertensive medication, such as thiazide diuretics, angiotensin-converting enzyme (ACE) inhibitors, angiotensin receptor blockers (ARBs), β-blockers, or long-acting calcium channel blockers. Smoking cessation should be advised strongly and support provided in terms of counseling and pharmacotherapy with nicotine replacement or withdrawal-relieving medication such as bupropion.[3] Aspirin prophylaxis (75 to 162 mg/day) is likely to benefit patients whose 10-year risk of CHD is ≥6% and should be considered.

Management of Chronic Stable Angina

Specific treatment of angina is directed toward improving myocardial oxygen supply, reducing myocardial oxygen demand, and treating precipitating factors or concurrent disorders (e.g., hypertension, anemia) that may exacerbate ischemia (see Fig. 24-1). The selection of an effective regimen is based on the acuity and severity of symptoms, the presence of associated disease (e.g., pulmonary or renal), and the patient's age and activity level. Because the etiology of myocardial ischemia is often multifactorial, a combination of agents with different mechanisms of action frequently is more effective than monotherapy. The major pharmacologic agents used in the treatment of angina include nitrovasodilators, β-adrenergic receptor antagonists, Ca^{2+} channel antagonists, and antiplatelet agents as well as hydroxymethylglutaryl coenzyme A (HMG-CoA) reductase inhibitors, which may have a role in stabilizing the vulnerable plaque. The antianginal agents improve the balance of myocardial oxygen supply and demand, increasing supply by dilating the coronary vasculature or decreasing demand by reducing cardiac work (see Fig. 24-4).

Management of UA and NSTEMI

Hemodynamically stable patients with recurrent symptoms suggestive of ACS, ST-segment changes on ECG, or cardiac biomarkers indicative of myocardial injury should be hospitalized with continuous rhythm monitoring. Hemodynamically unstable patients or those with continuous ischemic symptoms should be monitored in a coronary care unit with facilities to perform defibrillation quickly if needed. Unless contraindicated, aspirin, a β-blocker, heparin, and a glycoprotein (GP) IIb/IIIa inhibitor should be administered to all patients (see Fig. 24-1). Clopidogrel should be administered to all patients with UA/NSTEMI, whether managed with a conservative or an invasive strategy requiring percutaneous coronary intervention (PCI) (Fig. 24-5), but should be deferred until the coronary anatomy is defined because of the bleeding risk if an urgent coronary artery bypass graft (CABG) is required. Based on risk factors, a decision regarding invasive or conservative strategy should be made. An "early invasive approach" should be considered for all patients with recurrent ischemia, ST-segment depression, elevated troponin levels, heart failure, diabetes, or life-threatening cardiac arrhythmias. If PCI is intended, a 300- to 600-mg loading dose of clopidogrel should be given (Box 24-2).[11] The "initial conservative strategy" is appropriate for low-risk patients, with angiography reserved for those with recurrent ischemia, depressed ventricular function on imaging, or a high-risk stress test (see Fig. 24-5).[6]

Management of STEMI

The mortality and morbidity from MI can be reduced significantly by shortening the time to definitive treatment by increasing awareness of symptom recognition, early activation of the Emergency Medical Services system, and delivery of care without delay. If no improvement in symptoms occurs after 5 minutes of onset or administration of sublingual nitroglycerin, medical attention should be sought. If MI is suspected, non–enteric-coated aspirin (162 to 325 mg) should be administered (chewed) unless its use is contraindicated (Fig. 24-6).[11] In patients with aspirin allergy, clopidogrel or ticlopidine may be substituted (see Box 24-2). Supplemental oxygen should be initiated in all patients for the first 6 hours and continued in those with arterial oxygen saturation less than 90%.[12] Oxygen may limit ischemic myocardial injury and reduce ST-segment elevation[13]; however, excess oxygen can result in systemic vasoconstriction and thus oxygen should not be continued routinely beyond 6 hours.[12] Cardiac monitoring should be initiated and emergency resuscitation equipment should be available, including a defibrillator. In patients with ongoing ischemic pain, sublingual nitroglycerin (0.4 mg) should be administered every 5 minutes for a total of three doses and intravenous nitroglycerin initiated in those with persistent ischemic discomfort, hypertension, or pulmonary congestion. Morphine sulfate (2 to 4 mg intravenously [IV] with increments of 2 to 8 mg at 5- to 15-minute intervals) should be given (see Fig. 24-6) to relieve pain and reduce anxiety,[3,5] apprehension, and endogenous release of catecholamines and sympathetic activation.

A 12-lead ECG should be performed within 10 minutes to identify patients with ST-segment elevation, who can benefit from reperfusion therapy.[14] Based on the time from the onset of symptoms, evidence of STEMI, risk of bleeding, presence of cardiogenic shock, and the time required for transport to a skilled PCI laboratory, the decision regarding reperfusion strategy with thrombolytics versus primary PCI should be made within the next 10 minutes, with the goal to achieve a door-to-needle time of less than 30 minutes for fibrinolytic therapy, and a door-to-balloon time of less than 90 minutes for PCI (see Fig. 24-6).[15] Fibrinolytic therapy, when initiated early (particularly within 2 hours of symptom onset), has the greatest benefit, with a trend toward lower 30-day mortality than primary PCI.[3] Primary PCI has the distinct advantage of lower bleeding rates than fibrinolytic therapy, and achieves higher blood flow rates in the infarct-related artery. A meta-analysis of 23 randomized trials documented a benefit from primary PCI on both short-term and longer term mortality and morbidity.[3] Patients with STEMI who have cardiogenic shock or are at high risk of dying, such as those with severe heart failure or contraindications to fibrinolytic therapy, should undergo cardiac catheterization and rapid revascularization with PCI or CABG if it can be performed within 18 hours of onset of shock (see Fig. 24-6).[16] In the absence of ST-segment elevation, benefits of fibrinolytic therapy for patients with normal ECG, nonspecific changes, or ST-segment depression (except for posterior wall injury) have not been documented, and it is not recommended. Irrespective of concomitant fibrinolytic therapy or performance of primary PCI, a β-blocker should be administered early, either orally (Class I indication) or intravenously (Class IIa indication), to those patients without a contraindication, especially if tachycardia or hypertension is present.[5,17]

THERAPEUTICS BY CLASS

Antiplatelet Agents

Antiplatelet therapy in patients with atherosclerotic vascular disease reduces nonfatal MI by one third, nonfatal stroke by one quarter, and

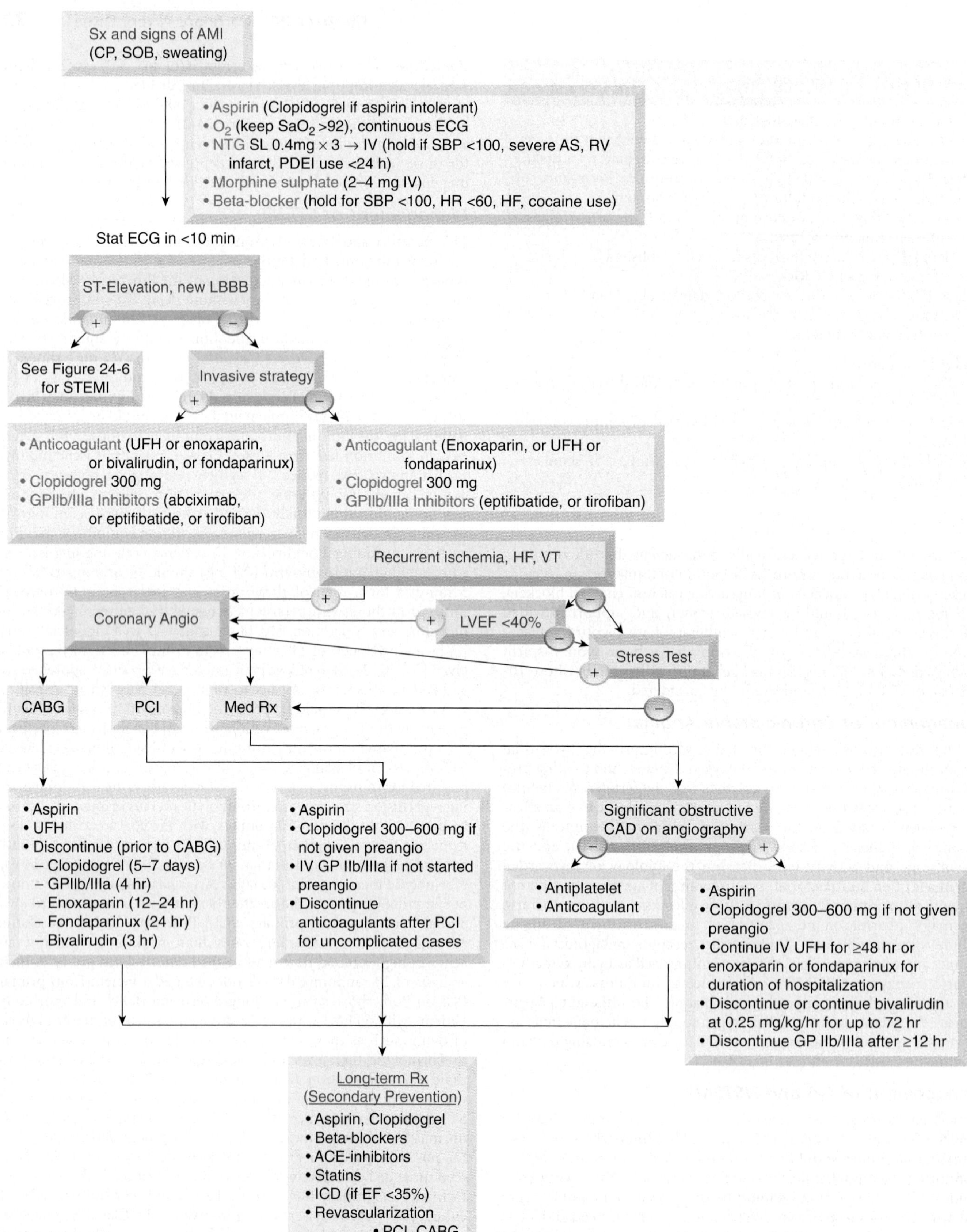

FIGURE 24-5 • Management of UA/NSTEMI based on the 2007 ACC/AHA recommendations. AMI, acute myocardial infarction; AS, aortic stenosis; CABG, coronary artery bypass graft; CAD, coronary artery disease; CP, chest pain; GP, glycoprotein; HF, heart failure; HR, heart rate; IV, intravenous; LBBB, left bundle branch block; LVEF, left ventricular ejection fraction; Med Rx, medical treatment; NTG, nitroglycerin; PCI, percutaneous intervention; PDEI, phosphodiesterase inhibitor; RV, right ventricle; SBP, systolic blood pressure; SL, sublingual; SOB, shortness of breath; STEMI, ST-segment elevation myocardial infarction; UFH, unfractionated heparin; VT, ventricular tachycardia. (Adapted from Anderson JL, Adams CD, Antman EM, et al. ACC/AHA 2007 guidelines for the management of patients with unstable angina/non ST-elevation myocardial infarction: a report of the American College of Cardiology/American Heart Association Task Force on Practice Guidelines (Writing Committee to Revise the 2002 Guidelines for the Management of Patients with Unstable Angina/Non ST-Elevation Myocardial Infarction); developed in collaboration with the American College of Emergency Physicians, the Society for Cardiovascular Angiography and Interventions, and the Society of Thoracic Surgeons; endorsed by the American Association of Cardiovascular and Pulmonary Rehabilitation and the Society for Academic Emergency Medicine. J Am Coll Cardiol 2007;50:e1-e157.)

BOX 24-2 RECOMMENDATIONS FOR THERAPY WITH ANTIPLATELET AGENTS IN CORONARY ARTERY DISEASE

Class I

Aspirin

- **Chronic stable angina:** Unless contraindicated, ***aspirin*** at 75 to 162 mg/day and continued indefinitely (LoE: A).
- **STEMI or UA/NSTEMI:** Unless contraindicated, ***aspirin*** (chewed) at 162 mg (LoE: A) to 325 mg (LoE: C) with acute MI and then continued at 75 to 162 mg/day indefinitely (LoE: A) in the absence of allergy.

Clopidogrel or Ticlodipine

- **STEMI or UA/NSTEMI:** In the absence of contraindication, ***clopidogrel*** at 75 mg/day or ***ticlodipine*** when aspirin is contraindicated or not tolerated (LoE: A).

Dual Antiplatelet Therapy

- **UA/NSTEMI**
  - With *initial noninvasive strategy*, ***aspirin*** and ***anticoagulant*** therapy as soon as possible (300 mg) and continued (75 mg/day) ≥1 month (LoE: A) and ideally up to 1 year (LoE: B).
  - With *initial invasive strategy*, ***aspirin*** and additional antiplatelet therapy with either ***clopidogrel*** *or* an IV ***GP IIb/IIIa inhibitor*** before diagnostic angiography (LoE: A). Abciximab is indicated only if there is no appreciable delay to angiography and PCI is likely to be performed; otherwise, IV eptifibatide or tirofiban is preferred (LoE: B).
  - *With PCI and bare-metal stents* (BMSs), ***aspirin*** (162 to 325 mg/day) for ≥1 month (LoE: B), then indefinitely (75 to 162 mg/day) (LoE: A), plus ***clopidogrel*** (75 mg/day) for ≥1 month and ideally 1 year (unless increased risk of bleeding; then it should be given for minimum of 2 weeks) (LoE: B).
  - *With PCI and drug-eluting stents* (DESs), ***aspirin*** (162 to 325 mg/day) for ≥3 months after sirolimus-eluting stent and 6 months after paclitaxel-eluting stent, then continued (75 to 162 mg/day) indefinitely (LoE: B), plus ***clopidogrel*** (75 mg/day) for ≥1 year (LoE: B).
- **STEMI**
  - After diagnostic catheterization in patients for whom *PCI is planned*, ***clopidogrel*** should be started and continued for ≥1 month (ideally 12 months) after BMS implantation and for ≥12 months after DES implantation if not at high risk for bleeding (LoE: B).
  - ***Clopidogrel*** (75 mg/day) orally should be *added to* ***aspirin*** *regardless of reperfusion therapy* (LoE: A) and continued for ≥14 days (LoE: B).
- **CABG**
  - In patients taking ***clopidogrel*** in whom *CABG is planned*, the drug should be withheld for at least 5 days, and preferably 7 days, unless the urgency for revascularization outweighs the risks of excess bleeding (LoE: B).

Class IIa

- **UA/NSTEMI**
  - In patients selected for *initial invasive strategy*, it is reasonable to initiate antiplatelet therapy with both ***clopidogrel*** and an IV ***GP IIb/IIIa inhibitor*** (LoE: B). Abciximab is indicated only if there is no appreciable delay to angiography and PCI is likely to be performed; otherwise, IV eptifibatide or tirofiban is the preferred choice of GP IIb/IIIa inhibitor (LoE: B).
  - In patients selected for *initial invasive strategy*, but who have *recurrent ischemic discomfort* with ***clopidogrel, aspirin***, and ***anticoagulant*** therapy, it is reasonable to add a ***GP IIb/IIIa*** antagonist before diagnostic angiography (LoE: C).
  - In patients selected for *initial invasive strategy*, it is reasonable to omit upstream administration of an IV GP IIb/IIIa antagonist before diagnostic angiography if ***bivalirudin*** is selected as the anticoagulant and at least 300 mg of ***clopidogrel*** was administered at least 6 hours earlier than planned catheterization or PCI (LoE: B).
  - In patients with *concerns regarding risk of bleeding*, a lower initial ***aspirin*** dose (75 to 162 mg) after PCI is reasonable (LoE: C).
- **STEMI**
  - In patients *<75 years of age regardless of reperfusion therapy*, it is reasonable to administer an oral loading dose of ***clopidogrel*** 300 mg (LoE: C).
  - *Long-term maintenance therapy* (1 year) with ***clopidogrel*** (75 mg/day orally) is reasonable regardless of whether patients undergo reperfusion therapy.
  - ***Clopidogrel*** is probably indicated in patients *receiving fibrinolytic therapy who are unable to take aspirin* because of hypersensitivity or major GI intolerance (LoE: C).

Class IIb

- **UA/NSTEMI**
  - In patients selected for *initial invasive strategy*, but who have *recurrent ischemic discomfort* with ***clopidogrel***, ***aspirin***, and ***anticoagulant*** therapy, it is reasonable to add a ***GP IIb/IIIa*** antagonist before diagnostic angiography (LoE: C).
  - In patients selected for *initial invasive strategy*, it may be reasonable to add ***eptifibatide*** or ***tirofiban*** to ***anticoagulant*** and ***oral antiplatelet*** therapy (LoE: B).
- **STEMI or UA/NSTEMI**
  - In patients *after DES placement*, ***clopidogrel*** (75 mg) may be continued beyond 1 year (LoE: B).

Class III

- **UA/NSTEMI**
  - ***Abciximab*** should *not be administered* to patients in whom *PCI is not planned* (LoE: A).
  - ***Dipyridamole*** is *not recommended* as an antiplatelet agent in *post-MI patients* (LoE: A).

CABG, coronary artery bypass graft; GI, gastrointestinal; GP, glycoprotein; IV, intravenous; LoE, level of evidence; MI, myocardial infarction; NSTEMI, non–ST-elevation myocardial infarction; PCI, percutaneous coronary intervention; STEMI, ST-elevation myocardial infarction; UA, unstable angina.

vascular mortality by one sixth.[11,18] Various antiplatelet agents have been developed that act at different sites to prevent platelet activation, adhesion, or aggregation and initiation of the clotting cascade as summarized in Figure 24-7. Endothelial injury promotes platelet activation and adhesion by exposure to subendothelial collagen and release of von Willebrand factor (vWF), a multimeric glycoprotein (GP) synthesized in the endothelial cells and megakaryocytes.[16] Platelets contain specific GP receptors on their membranes that bind to vWF (GP Ib/IX/V and GP IIb/IIIa), subendothelial collagen (GP Ia/IIa, GP IV, and GP VI), and fibrinogen (GP IIb/IIIa), as well as receptors for adenosine 5′-diphosphate (ADP) ($P2Y_1$ and $P2Y_{12}$) and thrombin (PAR1, PAR3, and PAR4) (Figs. 24-7 and 24-8). Stimulation of these receptors results in platelet activation and promotes adhesion by binding to vWF (see Fig. 24-7). GP or ADP receptor activation stimulates inositol triphosphate formation and release of calcium from the endoplasmic reticulum, which leads to activation of phospholipases and cyclooxygenase (COX) that causes phospholipid breakdown, thromboxane A_2 formation, and activation of actin-myosin contractile proteins. Contraction of platelets and/or mechanical shear stress causes conformational changes in platelets that expose the GP IIb/IIIa and Ib receptors that mediate the final common pathway of platelet aggregation by increasing binding with vWF, fibrinogen, thrombin, and thrombospondin, enhancing adhesion of circulating platelets to each other and those adhered to the vessel wall (see Fig. 24-7). Release of 5-hydroxytryptamine (serotonin), platelet factor 4, and β-thromboglobulin further promotes platelet aggregation and vasoconstriction that leads to vascular stasis and thrombosis by binding of coagulation factors such as factor Va and VIIIa. Antiplatelet agents, by preventing platelet activa-

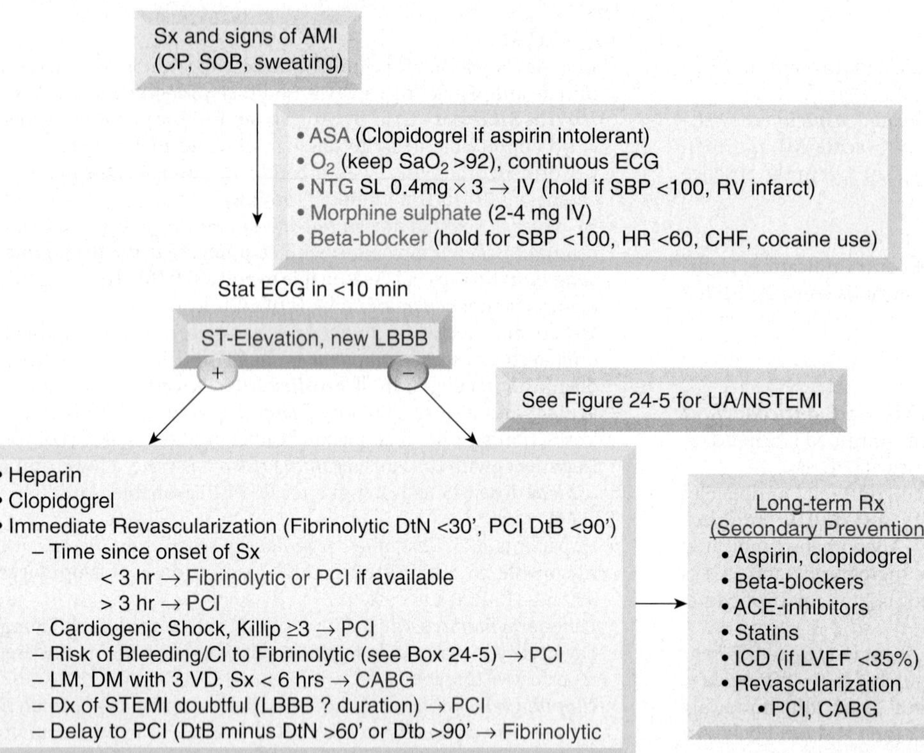

FIGURE 24-6 • Management of STEMI based on the 2007 ACC/AHA recommendations. 3VD, three-vessel disease; CI, contraindication; DM, diabetes mellitus; DtB, door to balloon time in minutes; DtN, door to needle time in minutes; GP, glycoprotein; HF, heart failure; ICD, implantable cardioverter-defibrillator; IV, intravenous; LBBB, left bundle branch block; LM, left main; LVEF, left ventricular ejection fraction; NTG, nitroglycerin; UA/NSTEMI, unstable angina/non–ST-elevation myocardial infarction; UFH, unfractionated heparin; VT, ventricular tachycardia. (From Antman EM, Hand M, Armstrong PW, et al. 2007 Focused Update of the ACC/AHA 2004 Guidelines for the Management of Patients with ST-Elevation Myocardial Infarction: a report of the American College of Cardiology/American Heart Association Task Force on Practice Guidelines; developed in collaboration with the Canadian Cardiovascular Society; endorsed by the American Academy of Family Physicians: 2007 Writing Group to Review New Evidence and Update the ACC/AHA 2004 Guidelines for the Management of Patients with ST-Elevation Myocardial Infarction, Writing on Behalf of the 2004 Writing Committee. Circulation 2008;117:296-329.)

tion, adhesion, and aggregation and release of vasoactive substances and growth factors, reduce the risk of arterial thrombosis and vasoconstriction (see Figs. 24-7 and 24-8). Based on their site of action, these agents are divided into thromboxane inhibitors, ADP receptor antagonists, and GP IIb/IIIa receptor antagonists. The current recommendations by the ACC and AHA for the use of antiplatelet agents in CAD, along with the level of evidence for their use, are summarized in Box 24-2.

Thromboxane Inhibitors

Aspirin (Acetylsalicylic Acid). The bark and leaves of the willow tree have been in use to relieve pain and fever for more than 2500 years, but pure "salicin" crystals were isolated initially in 1828 by Johann Buchner. Acetylsalicylic acid was later (1853) prepared by Charles Frederic Gerhardt, and its mechanism of action through suppression of prostaglandins and thromboxanes was first demonstrated in 1971 by John Robert Vane, who was awarded Nobel Prize in Physiology and Medicine in 1982. The U.S. Food and Drug Administration (FDA) approved aspirin for secondary prevention of MI in 1985.

Mechanism of Action. Aspirin blocks production of thromboxane A_2 by irreversibly acetylating a serine residue near the active site of platelet cyclooxygenase-1 (COX-1), and thus reduces platelet aggregation and vasoconstriction mediated by thromboxane (see Fig. 24-8). Platelets are anucleated and have limited capacity for new protein synthesis; therefore, irreversible inhibition of COX-1 by aspirin is permanent, lasting for the lifespan of platelets (7 to 10 days). Aspirin is a relatively weak antiplatelet agent, and only blocks platelet aggregation in response to stimulation by thromboxane. Therefore, platelet activation by other agonists (see Fig. 24-8)—especially thrombin, which acts directly on the GP IIb/IIIa or ADP receptors, bypassing the thromboxane pathway—can easily overcome its inhibitory effect.[19] Aspirin also has feeble anti-inflammatory effects due to weak inhibition of COX-2, the isoform that produces prostaglandins contributing to the inflammatory response.

Pharmacokinetics. The rate of absorption of aspirin after oral administration depends on its dosage, the presence of food, gastric pH, use of antacids, gut motility, and drug formulation. Enteric-coated aspirin is absorbed erratically, while non–enteric-coated formulations are absorbed more readily from the buccal mucosa, with a rapid inhibitory effect on thromboxane that is unrelated to serum concentrations. Aspirin is eliminated by zero-order pharmacokinetics, with a constant rate of elimination regardless of plasma concentration. Renal excretion is dependent upon urinary pH, with increased clearance on alkalinization of the urine, a feature helpful in the management of aspirin overdose.

Therapeutic Considerations. Aspirin is beneficial in the prevention and treatment of CHD, and unless a contraindication exists, all patients at any stage of symptomatic ischemic heart disease or with a prior cardiovascular event should be considered for aspirin therapy because of its antiplatelet effects, which on average reduce the risk of any further vascular event by about one fourth.[11] In a meta-analysis of 287 studies involving 135,000 patients, the beneficial effects of aspirin in patients with angina pectoris and after MI, stroke, and CABG surgery was demonstrated.[11] Aspirin reduced the risk of MI or sudden death in those with angina pectoris by 34%, in those with UA by 46%, in those with coronary angioplasty by 53%, and in those with prior MI, stroke or transient ischemic attack, atrial fibrillation, or peripheral arterial disease by 22% to 25%, compared to placebo.[20] In women, prophylactic low-dose aspirin therapy was associated with a reduced risk of overall and ischemic stroke, but not with reduction of risk of MI or death from cardiovascular causes, indicating sex-related differences in its efficacy.[21] When aspirin is used for primary prevention in those patients at low to moderate risk, there are almost as many disabling strokes and major bleeds as MIs prevented: five nonfatal MIs were avoided for every 1000 patients treated for 5 years at a risk of one excess disabling stroke and two to four serious gastrointestinal (GI) bleeds requiring transfusions.[3,22] Thus, the benefit of aspirin outweighs the risk in those patients in whom it is used for secondary prevention, but not for primary prophylaxis,[21,23] in which case aspirin should be reserved for only high-risk individuals or men with elevated C-reactive protein levels.[24]

For patients presenting with symptoms of ACS, non–enteric-coated aspirin (162 to 325 mg) is preferred and should be chewed for more

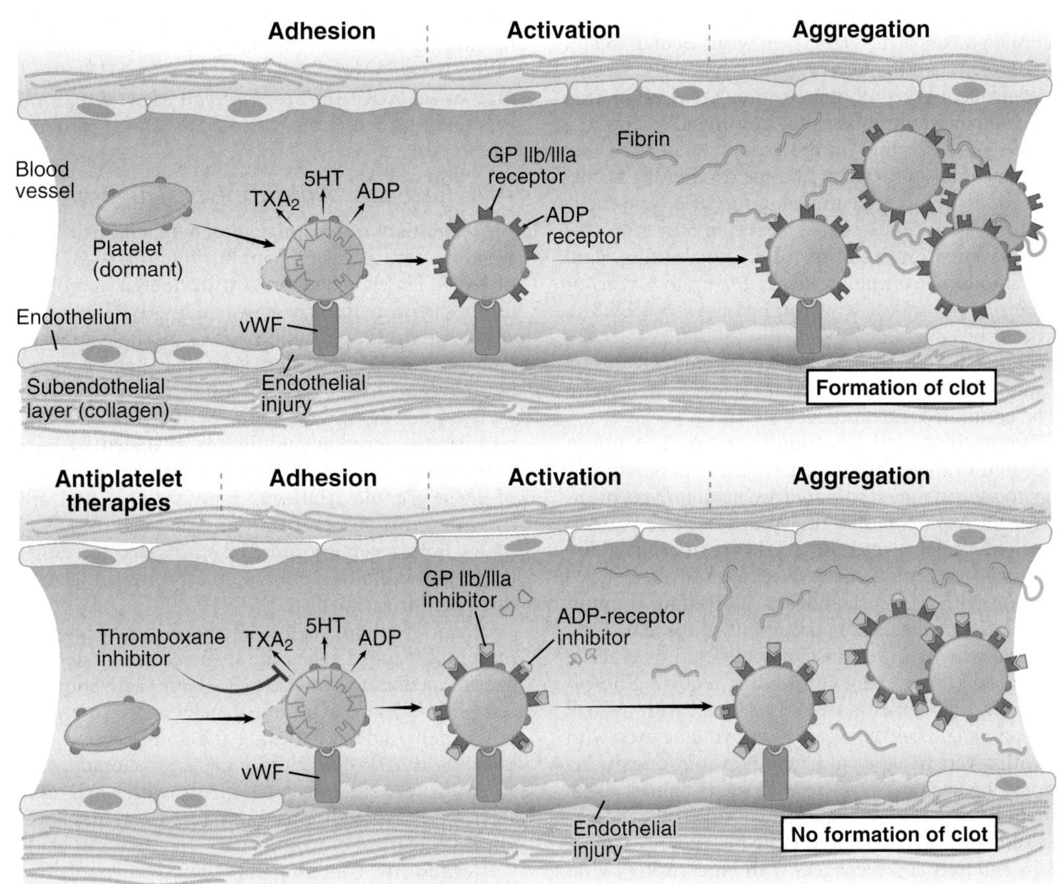

FIGURE 24-7 • Pathophysiology of platelet activation, adhesion, and aggregation and antiplatelet therapy. Endothelial injury promotes platelet activation and adhesion by exposure to subendothelial collagen and binding of the platelet to von Willebrand factor (vWF) through glycoprotein (GP) Ia and Ib receptors, respectively. This results in activation of phospholipases and cyclooxygenase, increasing thromboxane A_2 formation, and release of adenosine diphosphate (ADP), serotonin (5HT), platelet factor 4, and other mediators that stimulate GP or ADP receptors and signal transduction pathways within platelets, all of which ultimately converge on the platelet receptor GP IIb/IIIa, binding and cross-linking activated GP IIb/IIIa on adjacent platelets by plasma fibrinogen or vWf as the final common pathway to platelet aggregation and coronary thrombosis. Antiplatelet agents acting at various points of this activation-aggregation cascade as thromboxane inhibitors, ADP receptor inhibitors, and GP IIb/IIIa inhibitors reduce risk of arterial thrombosis.

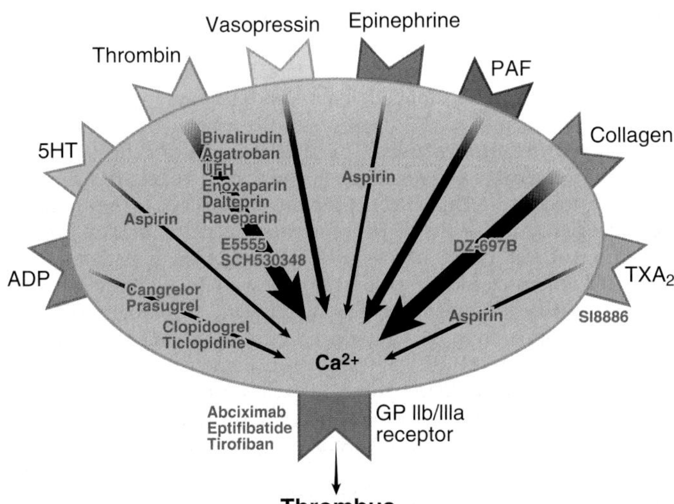

FIGURE 24-8 • Platelet glycoprotein (GP) IIb/IIIa activation as the final common pathway of platelet activation and aggregation predisposing to coronary thrombosis and antiplatelet therapy. Clinically available (*red*) and investigational (*blue*) antiplatelet agents that prevent platelet activation-aggregation by inhibiting the effect of various platelet activators, including collagen, thrombin, ADP, thromboxane A_2, epinephrine, serotonin (5HT), and GP IIb/IIIa receptor, reducing risk of arterial thrombosis. The width of the arrow indicates the intensity of action.

rapid buccal absorption and inhibition of thromboxane A_2 compared to enteric-coated aspirin, which is absorbed erratically.[25] Aspirin suppositories (300 mg) can be used safely in those patients with severe nausea, vomiting, or known upper GI disorders. In patients with aspirin allergy, clopidogrel or ticlopidine may be substituted (see Box 24-2).[26] The efficacy of prompt use of aspirin in evolving MI on reduction in mortality was demonstrated in the Second International Study of Infarct Survival (ISIS-2),[13] with an absolute risk difference in 35-day mortality of 2.4% and a relative risk reduction of 23% compared with placebo.[27] In combination with streptokinase, the effect was even more pronounced, with absolute risk difference in mortality of 5.2% (relative risk reduction, 42%), with reduction in coronary reocclusion and recurrent ischemic events after thrombolytic therapy with streptokinase or alteplase.[28] This led to the recommendation that aspirin should be initiated immediately if the diagnosis of ACS is suspected.[3,28,29]

In the absence of data from large trials of different durations of antiplatelet treatment in patients with established CHD or in primary prevention of high-risk individuals, it seems reasonable to continue aspirin therapy indefinitely at a daily dosage of 75 to 162 mg unless side effects develop.[30] The recommendation for low-dose aspirin comes from the analysis of data from the Clopidogrel in Unstable angina to prevent Recurrent ischemic Events (CURE) trial[31] indicating no difference in the rate of thrombotic events according to aspirin dose, but a dose-dependent increase in major bleeding in those patients receiving higher doses of aspirin: 2.0% with less than 100 mg/day, 2.3% with 100 to 200 mg/day, and 4.0% with greater than 200 mg/day.[30]

In patients undergoing PCI and stenting, pretreatment with aspirin and acute unfractionated heparin (UFH), low-molecular-weight heparin (LMWH), or other antiplatelet agents is strongly recommended to help prevent acute thrombotic closure.[30] A combination therapy with aspirin and clopidogrel should be continued for up to 1 month to 1 year or longer depending on the type of stent used (see Box 24-2). A maintenance dose of aspirin 162 to 325 mg/day is currently recommended for 1 month after implantation of a bare-metal stent and for 3 months (for sirolimus-coated stents) to 6 months (for paclitaxel-coated stents) after implantation of a drug-eluting stent (DES).[30] Clopidogrel should be continued ideally for up to 1 year for those with a bare-metal stent and at least for 1 year with a DES in patients with low risk of bleeding.[30]

In patients undergoing CABG surgery, aspirin should be started within 48 hours of surgery, which reduces total mortality by about two thirds, and should be continued indefinitely.[11]

Adverse Effects, Precautions, and Contraindications. The use of aspirin is contraindicated in those individuals with a hypersensitivity to salicylates. Allergy to aspirin may result in hives, nasal polyps, bronchospasm, or anaphylaxis. Aspirin should be avoided in those patients with active bleeding, hemophilia, severe untreated hypertension, active peptic ulcer, or serious GI or genitourinary bleeding. Adverse effects such as gastric irritation with dyspepsia, nausea, ulceration, tinnitus, hearing loss, and interstitial nephritis may occur with chronic use, but the incidence is reduced when a lower dose or a buffered or enteric-coated preparation is used (Table 24-1). GI bleeding requiring hospitalization occurs in 2 per 1000 patients treated per year, with a small increase in risk of hemorrhagic stroke.[11] Aspirin needs to be used with caution in patients with severe hepatic failure, and sodium-containing buffered aspirin should be avoided in those with heart failure. Renal functional impairment or uric acid increase may occur in the elderly, and blood uric acid and creatinine may need to be monitored. Aspirin should be avoided in children and teenagers with chickenpox or flu symptoms due to an increased risk of Reye's syndrome.

Drug Interactions. The risk of bleeding increases with concurrent use of aspirin with warfarin, especially if higher doses are used. The risk of aspirin-induced GI bleed is increased by concomitant use of nonsteroidal anti-inflammatory drugs (NSAIDs), corticosteroids, or alcohol. Because of a diminishment of the cardioprotective effect of aspirin by ibuprofen,[18] which has been associated with limitation of aspirin's access to its acetylation site in platelet COX-1, these drugs should not be taken together and an alternate NSAID, such as diclofenac, should be substituted or ibuprofen given at least 30 minutes before or 8 hours after aspirin administration. An interaction between ACE inhibitors and aspirin producing a negative impact on renal hemodynamics as a result of their opposing effects on prostaglandins synthesis (aspirin inhibiting, ACE inhibitors increasing) has been proposed, with reduction in prostaglandin-mediated decrease in arterial pressure by ACE inhibitors and increase in sodium and water retention.[3] The decrease in the beneficial effect of ACE inhibitors on MI and mortality by aspirin is controversial, with significant reduction demonstrated in some but not in other analyses.[3] This interaction does not appear to interfere significantly with the clinical benefits of therapy with either agent in chronic heart failure, or for postinfarct protection or high-risk prevention.[3] When used together with an ACE inhibitor, the dose of aspirin should be kept low, especially in heart failure patients.

The efficacy of aspirin may be reduced by antacids, which alter the pH of the stomach and its absorption, as well as by phenobarbital, phenytoin, and rifampin through induction of the hepatic enzymes metabolizing aspirin. Aspirin may increase the effect of oral hypoglycemic agents and insulin and reduce the efficacy of uricosuric drugs such as sulfinpyrazone and probenecid. The excretion of uric acid may decrease with concomitant use of aspirin and thiazides, which can precipitate gout.

Dosing. The lowest dose of aspirin that retains efficacy without increasing GI or bleeding risk should be used. Daily aspirin at 80 mg completely blocks platelet aggregation induced by COX-1[3]; however, the full antithrombotic effect takes up to 2 days to manifest. In a meta-analysis of 287 trials, the reduction in vascular events was comparable for doses of 75 to 150 mg daily and 160 to 325 mg daily; however, doses of less than 75 mg/day had less benefit.[3] Therefore, the recent guidelines by the ACC/AHA recommend use of a 162- to 324-mg daily dose for initial presentation with ACS, with a maintenance dose of 75 to 162 mg daily (see Box 24-2).[3]

ADP Receptor Antagonists: Thienopyridines

Mechanism of Action. Clopidogrel and ticlodipine are two thienopyridine derivatives that inhibit binding of ADP to its receptors on platelets. Platelets contain two purinergic receptors, $P2Y_1$ and $P2Y_{12}$, on their surface that are activated by ADP binding. The $P2Y_1$ receptor couples to the G_q-phospholipase C–inositol triphosphate–Ca^{2+} pathway and induces a change in platelet shape and aggregation when stimulated by ADP. The $P2Y_{12}$ receptor, through G_i coupling and adenylyl cyclase inhibition, reduces the cyclic AMP (cAMP) level and activate platelets by deceasing inhibition mediated by cAMP.[3] Activation of these receptors by ADP increases platelet aggregation and the release of dense granule, ADP, serotonin, factor 4, and other vasoactive and thrombogenic substances, promoting thrombosis (see Figs. 24-7 and 24-8). Both receptors must be stimulated to result in platelet activation,[32] and inhibition of either receptor is sufficient to block activation through this mechanism.

Thienopyridines act by directly and irreversibly inhibiting the $P2Y_{12}$ receptor for the platelets' life span, reducing their activation and aggregation mediated by ADP-dependent activation of the GP IIb/IIIa complex. They also inhibit platelet aggregation induced by agonists other than ADP by blocking the amplification of platelet activation by released ADP. Both clopidogrel and ticlopidine are approved for use as antiplatelet therapy in patients with CAD and, when added to aspirin, have an additional inhibitory effect on platelet aggregation that improves clinical outcomes.[33]

Clopidogrel. Clopidogrel (Plavix) is currently the preferred thienopyridine antiplatelet agent because of its extensive evidence base, rapid onset of action, and better safety profile than ticlodipine, which is associated with liver and blood abnormalities. It was approved by the FDA in 1997 for use in ACS.

Pharmacokinetics. Clopidogrel is rapidly absorbed after oral administration. Clopidogrel is an inactive prodrug that is oxidized by the hepatic and intestinal cytochrome P-450 (CYP) 3A4 isoenzyme into the active metabolite. The elimination half-life of the main circulating metabolite is 8 hours. It is extensively metabolized by the liver and requires no renal dose adjustment. An oral loading dose of 600 mg clopidogrel achieves maximal inhibition of platelets in 2 hours, whereas a 300-mg loading dose requires 24 to 48 hours.[34] Kinetics of clopidogrel are nonlinear, with a markedly decreased clearance on repeated dosing. When dosing is stopped, it takes about 5 days for the effect on platelets to wear off.

Therapeutic Considerations. The platelet-inhibitory effect of clopidogrel is irreversible and requires a loading dose to effectively shorten the time to achieve this effect. Clopidogrel appears to have added benefit when given with aspirin as dual antiplatelet therapy for the reduction of risk of MI, stroke, or vascular death in patients with advanced atherosclerotic disease and those with ACS with or without PCI or stenting.[20,35-37] Aspirin (325 mg/day) and clopidogrel (75 mg/day) were compared in the Clopidogrel vs. ASA in Patients at Risk of Ischemic Events (CAPRIE)[3,23] trial, which demonstrated the overall safety profile of clopidogrel and a 9% relative risk reduction of the combined end point of ischemic stroke, MI, or vascular death.

Clopidogrel should be administered to all patients with UA/NSTEMI, whether managed with a conservative or an invasive strategy requiring PCI (see Fig. 24-5 and Box 24-2). Since the bleeding risk increases after urgent CABG, clopidogrel may need to be held until the coronary anatomy is defined. In the CHARISMA[37] study, addition of clopidogrel to low-dose aspirin in patients either with evident cardiovascular disease or with multiple risk factors increased bleeding without reduction in outcome events. These results are in sharp contrast with a large body of data that demonstrate a beneficial effect of adding clopidogrel to aspirin in ACS or following PCI and stenting.

TABLE 24-1 SIDE EFFECTS OF ANTIPLATELET AGENTS AND ANTICOAGULANTS*

Drug	Toxic Side Effects	General Side Effects	Hypersensitivity	Safe Use in Pregnancy
Aspirin	Reye's syndrome (children), bleeding, **GI ulceration,** renal toxicity, pulmonary edema, blood dyscrasias	Tinnitus and hearing changes, minor bleeding, hemolytic anemia, **gastritis**	Bronchospasm, urticaria, angioedema, vasomotor rhinitis, anaphylaxis, shock, purpura, hemorrhagic vasculitis, erythema multiforme, Stevens-Johnson syndrome, Lyell's syndrome	Yes (C)—no increased risk in large cohort studies
Abciximab	**Bleeding, thrombocytopenia,** hypotension	Pain, sweating	Unknown (none reported with chimeric form); rare with reexposure	Unknown (C)
Clopidogrel	**Hemorrhage**, skin reactions, gastric ulceration	**Gastritis,** fatigue, flulike syndrome, myalgias	Allergic reactions (necrosis, ischemic)	Unknown (B)
Dipyridamole	Bleeding, myocardial infarction, chest pain, partial seizure	ST-segment abnormalities, GI, dizziness, rash, dyspnea, syncope	Allergic reactions reported (skin)	Unknown (C)
Eptifibatide	Hemorrhage, hypotension, **thrombocytopenia**	Minor bleeding		Unknown (B)
Fibrinolytics	Hemorrhage, hemorrhagic stroke, transient hypotensive reactions with streptokinase, embolic phenomena, reperfusion arrhythmias	Phlebitis at site (streptokinase)	Most associated with streptokinase (history of prior exposure to *Streptococcus* spp.), Guillain-Barré syndrome, hemolysis, anaphylactic shock, pyrexia, skin rash, angioedema, bronchospasm, ARDS	Yes (urokinase) (B); others unknown (C)
Low-molecular-weight heparin	Hemorrhage, **thrombocytopenia** (type I [mild] and type II [severe] but lower incidence than UFH; **cross-reactive with UFH-induced events)**	Same as for UFH	Same as for UFH	Yes (B)
(Protamine)[†]	Noncardiogenic pulmonary edema	**Hypotension (with too-rapid infusion rates)**	Flushing, urticaria, wheezing, angioedema and hypotension, anaphylaxis, bronchospasm or shock **(IgE or IgG mediated if prior exposure to protamine zinc insulin injections)**	Unknown (C)
Ticlopidine	Hemorrhage, hematologic disorders (**leukopenia, agranulocytosis, thrombocytopenia and pancytopenia** [reversible], thrombotic thrombocytopenia [some lethal cases]), hepatitis	Skin rashes, severe chronic diarrhea	Rashes (immunogenically mediated unknown)	Unknown (B)
Tirofiban	Hemorrhage, **thrombocytopenia**	Mild bleeding, edema, pain, CNS	Not reported, no repeat exposure information available	(B)
Unfractionated heparin (UFH)	**HIT** type I (mild) and type II (severe), syndrome of thrombohemorrhagic complications (see Hypersensitivity), hypotension, emboli	Delayed wound healing, osteoporosis (chronic therapy), minor bleeding, hypoaldosteronism, priapism	Urticaria, conjunctivitis, rhinitis, asthma, cyanosis, tachypnea, fever, angioneurotic edema, anaphylactic shock Rarely—hemorrhagic skin necrosis, vasospastic reactions	Chronic administration: osteopenia for mother (B)
Warfarin	Hemorrhage, hemorrhagic skin necrosis, fetal toxicity Rare—cholestatic hepatitis	Vasodilation, cholesterol embolization ("purple toe or glove syndrome")	Maculopapular rashes, pruritic purpuritic skin eruptions	No (X) (warfarin): embryopathy, especially in first trimester

***Boldface** type signifies more prevalence or more severe reactions.

[†]Protamine is used to reverse the effect of heparin and is not an antiplatelet or anticoagulant agent.

ARDS, acute respiratory distress syndrome; B, C, X, U.S. Food and Drug Administration pregnancy safety categories; CNS, central nervous system effects; GI, gastrointestinal effects; HIT, heparin-induced thrombocytopenia; IgE, immunoglobulin E; IgG, immunoglobulin G.

Modified from Ou NN, Oyen LJ, Murphy JG, Jahangir A. *In* Murphy JG, Lloyd MA (eds): Mayo Clinic Cardiology: Concise Textbook, 3rd ed. Rochester: Mayo Clinic Scientific Press/Informa Healthcare, 2007, pp. 1291-1308.

In patients with UA/NSTEMI in whom a noninterventional medical approach is planned, clopidogrel 300 mg should be given initially, followed by a 75-mg daily dose for at least 1 month and ideally up to 1 year.[17] In the Clopidogrel in Unstable angina to prevent Recurrent ischemic Events (CURE) trial,[31] a favorable outcome with a clopidogrel-aspirin combination was demonstrated for an average of 9 months and up to 1 year.[3]

In patients with UA/NSTEMI undergoing PCI, clopidogrel (300 to 600 mg) should be given with aspirin before the coronary intervention and continued (75 mg daily) for at least 1 month (see Box 24-2) and ideally for up to 1 year for those patients receiving a bare-metal stent and at least for 1 year with a DES.[30] DESs with the antiproliferative action of sirolimus or paclitaxel have consistently been shown to reduce stent restenosis, but the associated delay in endothelialization predisposes to late (>3 to 6 months) or very late (>1 year) thrombosis after stent placement[30] and therefore require dual antiplatelet therapy with clopidogrel for at least 1 year and aspirin indefinitely.[30]

In patients with STEMI, clopidogrel 75 mg/day should be added to aspirin in those who have not received reperfusion therapy or who were initially treated with fibrinolytic therapy and continued for at least 14 days, as a beneficial effect was demonstrated in the COMMIT-CCS-2[38] and CLARITY-TIMI 28[39] studies. A loading dose of clopidogrel 300 mg followed by 75 mg/day is reasonable and should be continued for a year in those patients under 75 years of age, but in elderly patients (>75 years) the efficacy and safety of the loading dose is not known.[3] No data are available from clinical trials regarding long-term clopidogrel treatment in STEMI patients, and the recommendations for its use are mostly extrapolated from data from patients with UA/NSTEMI, and those undergoing PCI. In the TIMI 28 trial,[39] all patients with STEMI received a fibrinolytic agent within 12 hours of symptoms onset, with coronary angiography after 2 to 8 days to assess late patency of the infarct-related artery and with PCI in more than half. Addition of clopidogrel (300 mg) within 45 minutes of the start of fibrinolytic therapy and then 75 mg daily was associated with a significant reduction in the rate of occlusion of an infarct-related artery and reduction in the incidence of recurrent MI, cardiovascular death, or stroke after PCI when compared to a placebo-treated group, without significant increase in major or minor bleeding.[3] In a mega-trial conducted in Chinese patients with acute MI, clopidogrel administration (75 mg daily without a loading dose) along with aspirin (162 mg daily) within 12 hours of onset of symptoms significantly reduced death, reinfarction, or stroke without excess major bleeding compared to the placebo group. Clopidogrel was most effective in those who received it within 6 hours of onset.[38]

Adverse Effects, Precautions, and Contraindications. Clopidogrel, although structurally similar to ticlopidine, seems to be safer, with a low risk of myelotoxicity (neutropenia or thrombocytopenia). The incidence of GI adverse effects is similar to aspirin. Rash, pruritus, purpura, and diarrhea may occur (see Table 24-1). Risk of serious bleeding is increased, and it should not be given to patients who are actively bleeding or have peptic ulcer or history of intracranial hemorrhage. It should be withheld for 5 to 7 days before elective CABG surgery. In patients with a history of GI bleed, drugs to minimize the risk of recurrent bleeding, such as proton-pump inhibitors, should be considered.[3,40]

Aspirin and Clopidogrel Resistance. Resistance to the antiplatelet effect of aspirin and clopidogrel is increasingly recognized. Resistance is defined either as the failure of aspirin or clopidogrel to prevent individuals from clinical thrombotic complications or as the failure to produce an expected response on a laboratory measurement of platelet activation or aggregation. Some degree of aspirin resistance with a recurrent vascular event, despite adequate therapeutic dose, may affect up to 50% of patients.[3,25,26,35,41,42] Long-term risk of death, MI, or stroke may increase threefold in those with inadequate platelet inhibition and clinical unresponsiveness.[43] The mechanisms of such resistance remain to be fully elucidated but are believed to be a combination of clinical, cellular, genetic, and other factors, or including platelet GP polymorphisms,[44] reduction in bioavailability due to inadequate dosage or noncompliance, rapid production of new platelets, activation of platelets by pathways other than the thromboxane pathway (see Fig. 24-8), and enhanced inflammatory activity with increased expression of COX-2 that is not strongly inhibited by aspirin. The optimal therapeutic approach to patients with aspirin hyporesponsiveness remains to be determined, but clopidogrel could be considered.[3]

Considerable interpatient variability also exists for sensitivity to clopidogrel, with increased risk of ischemic events in those with reduced responsiveness. The mechanisms underlying diminished responsiveness to clopidogrel, which must be distinguished from noncompliance, are not fully understood, but variation in absorption, generation of the active metabolite, genetic polymorphisms involving the $P2Y_{12}$ receptor, and drug interactions are responsible. An increase in the dose may be required to achieve platelet inhibition.[35,45,46]

Drug Interactions. The risk of bleeding increases with concomitant use of clopidogrel with other antiplatelet agents, including aspirin, NSAIDs, or anticoagulants such as warfarin. Clopidogrel is a prodrug converted to its active metabolite predominantly by the CYP3A4 isoenzyme, and therefore its antiplatelet effect could be perturbed by modulators of CYP3A4 activity. Lipophilic statins such as atorvastatin that also utilize the CYP3A4 substrate (but not pravastatin or rosuvastatin) have been shown to competitively inhibit clopidogrel activation,[47] raising concerns regarding the efficacy of clopidogrel in patients using concomitant statins. Clinical studies, however, have not shown any significant clopidogrel-statin adverse interactions.[3] This could be due to alternative CYP isoenzymes (e.g., 3A5, 2C9, 2C19, 2B6, or 1A2) that may become more relevant in patients concomitantly treated with multiple CYP3A4-metabolized drugs.[3] At this time there are no convincing data for withholding lipophilic statins in clopidogrel-treated patients[30,48-50]; however, given potential concerns, higher doses of concomitant CYP3A4 inhibitors should be used cautiously in patients recovering from ACS or those who recently received DESs.[30]

Dosing. A loading dose of 300 mg or 600 mg clopidogrel in the setting of ACS and PCI and/or stenting is recommended, followed by a maintenance dose of 75 mg/day for at least 1 month and ideally for up to 1 year for those with a bare-metal stent and at least for 1 year for those with a DES. No dose adjustment for maintenance therapy is needed for those patients with renal impairment or elderly patients.

Ticlodipine. Ticlodipine (Ticlid) is a prodrug that requires conversion to the active thiol metabolite by the hepatic CYP enzyme system. Its use is limited because of myelotoxicity and the risk of thrombotic thrombocytopenic purpura (TTP), and it has largely been replaced by clopidogrel.

Pharmacokinetics. Ticlodipine is readily absorbed after oral administration, with peak plasma levels at 2 hours. Maximum inhibition of platelet aggregation occurs after 4 to 7 days but can be achieved quickly by oral loading. It is largely metabolized by the liver, followed by renal excretion. The elimination follows a nonlinear pharmacokinetics, and clearance decreases markedly on repeated dosing and with advancing age. The plasma half-life on constant dosing is 4 to 5 days.

Therapeutic Considerations. Ticlodipine has been used successfully for the secondary prevention of stroke, transient ischemic attack, or MI and for the prevention of stent closure and graft occlusion.[30] Despite a decrease in platelet function in patients with chronic stable angina, unlike aspirin, ticlodipine was not shown to decrease adverse cardiovascular events in these patients.[51] Currently, ticlodipine is recommended as an alternate to aspirin or clopidogrel when these drugs are contraindicated or poorly tolerated due to side effects, or as adjunctive therapy with aspirin to reduce stent thrombosis (see Box 24-2). In patients undergoing coronary artery stenting, treatment must begin 3 days prior to the procedure, or alternatively ticlodipine must be given as a loading dose of 500 mg at the time of the procedure and continued for 2 to 4 weeks.

Adverse Effects, Precautions, and Contraindications. The major side effect of ticlodipine is neutropenia, which occurs in 2.4% of patients and usually resolves within 1 to 3 weeks of discontinuation of therapy, but very rarely may be fatal. TTP occurs in approximately 0.01% of patients and could be life threatening, requiring immediate plasma exchange. Minor bleeding may occur in up to 10%. Skin rashes, liver toxicity, diarrhea, abdominal pain, nausea, and vomiting may occur. Ticlodipine should not be used in patients with liver impairment, bleeding disorders, neutropenia, thrombocytopenia, or a past history of TTP. The neutropenia occurs within the first 3 months of treatment, and therefore a complete blood count with a differential should be obtained before starting treatment, and every 2 weeks for the first 3 months of therapy.

Drug Interactions. Ticlodipine is an inhibitor of CYP, and inhibits the metabolism of other drugs that are metabolized by this system. Ticlodipine clearance is reduced by concomitant treatment with cimetidine. Corticosteroids may reduce the effect on bleeding time.

Dosing. A loading dose of 500 mg ticlodipine orally followed by a maintenance dose of 250 mg twice per day with food to lessen intolerance and to increase absorption is recommended for at least 1 month and ideally up to 1 year for patients with a bare-metal stent and at least 1 year in those with a DES implantation.

Glycoprotein IIb/IIIa Receptor Antagonists

The GP IIb/IIIa (αIIbβ3) receptor belongs to a large family of receptors called integrins, which are heterodimeric cell surface proteins that play important roles in cell adhesion.[3] Unlike other integrins, GP IIb/IIIa has a limited tissue distribution, being found only on cells of the megakaryocytic lineage. These receptors constitute one of the most abundant proteins on the surface of platelets, with some 80,000 copies per quiescent platelet and are the major platelet surface receptor involved in platelet aggregation. Collagen, ADP, and thrombin act as strong platelet activators by stimulating the transfer of the GP IIb/IIIa found in the alpha granules of unstimulated platelets to the platelet surface (see Fig. 24-7), thereby increasing de novo expression and activation of the GP IIb/IIIa receptors on the platelet surface, possibly through a conformational change (see Fig. 24-8). Activated GP IIb/IIIa in turn acts as a receptor for soluble fibrinogen, vWF, vitronectin, and fibronectin. The tripeptide arginine-glycine–aspartic acid (RGD) sequence of the fibrinogen molecule is recognized by the GP receptor. Binding of fibrinogen and vWF leads to platelet aggregation by cross-linking GP IIb/IIIa on the surfaces of adjacent activated platelets (see Fig. 24-7). Platelet activation by thrombin and collagen leads to redistribution of phosphatidylserine from the inner to the outer surface of the platelet membrane, which provides the surface for binding of coagulation factor Va and VIIIa that in turn facilitate conversion of prothrombin (factor II) to thrombin (IIa) by factor Xa, and factor X to Xa by factor IXa (Fig. 24-9).

Drugs that inhibit the platelet GP IIb/IIIa receptor are effective antiplatelet agents.[11,52] Currently three GP IIb/IIIa antagonists—abciximab, eptifibatide, and tirofiban—are approved for use in patients with CAD. Their development arose from the understanding of Glanzmann thrombasthenia, a condition in which the GP IIb/IIIa receptor is lacking and the platelets fail to aggregate in response to agonists. The RGD sequence of the fibrinogen formed the basis for the molecular structure of eptifibatide and tirofiban.[53]

Mechanism of Action. Glycoprotein IIb/IIIa receptor activation results in binding of the circulating fibrinogen to the activated platelets and cross-linking of adjacent platelets to create a platelet-fibrinogen complex. Inhibition of the receptor activation by antiplatelet agents and GP IIb/IIIa antagonists prevents thrombus formation (see Figs. 24-7 and 24-8) by inhibiting binding of the fibrinogen and vWF to platelets, the final common pathway for platelet aggregation through these receptors, and has become an important therapeutic target for the management of ACS and ischemic complications of PCI and stenting (see Box 24-2). Each of the three approved platelet GP IIb/IIIa inhibitors (abciximab, tirofiban, and eptifibatide) has been shown to reduce myocardial injury in the setting of coronary intervention and in ACS (Fig. 24-10).

Pharmacokinetics

Abciximab. Abciximab (ReoPro) is a chimeric monoclonal antibody against the GP IIb/IIIa receptor. It consists of a murine variable portion of the Fab fragment combined with the human constant region. It was the first GP IIb/IIIa inhibitor approved by the FDA (in 1994). It blocks large molecules from binding to the receptor by steric hindrance and conformational changes. Its action can be reversed by repeated platelet transfusions.

Abciximab has a plasma half-life of about 10 minutes. Inhibition of platelet aggregation is maximal at 2 hours after a bolus injection, and

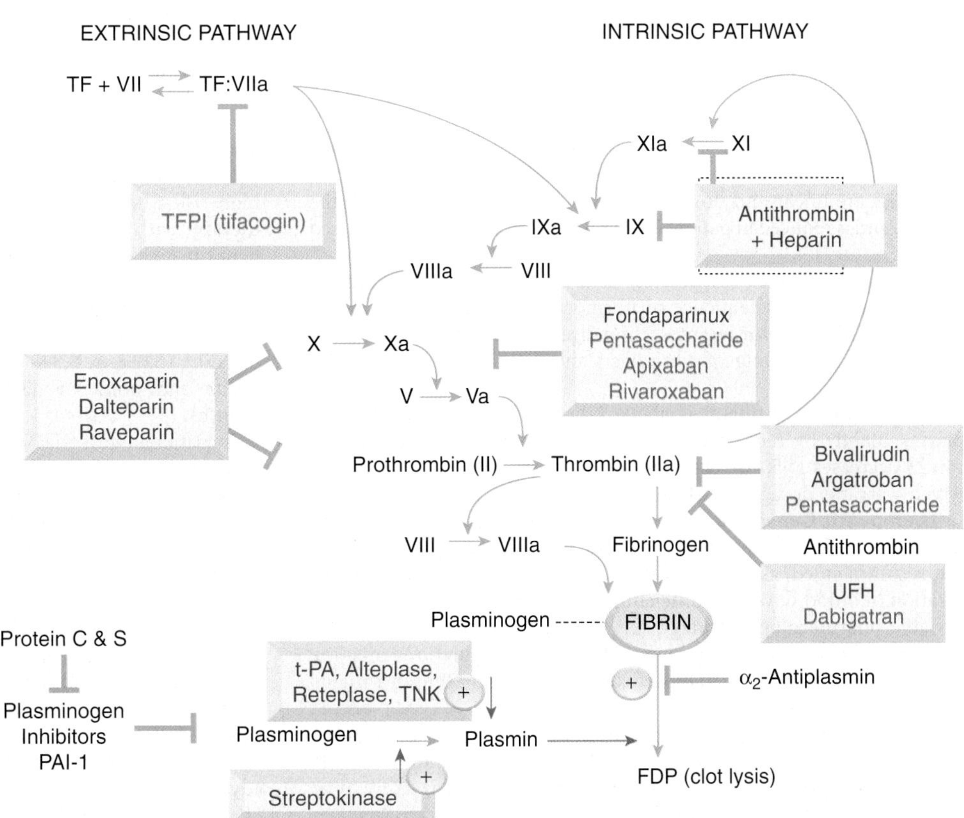

FIGURE 24-9 • Site of action of antithrombotic and fibrinolytic agents on the extrinsic and intrinsic pathways of coagulation and fibrinolysis. Clinically available and investigational drugs are shown in *red* and *blue*, respectively. rt-PA, reteplase; UFH, unfractionated heparin.

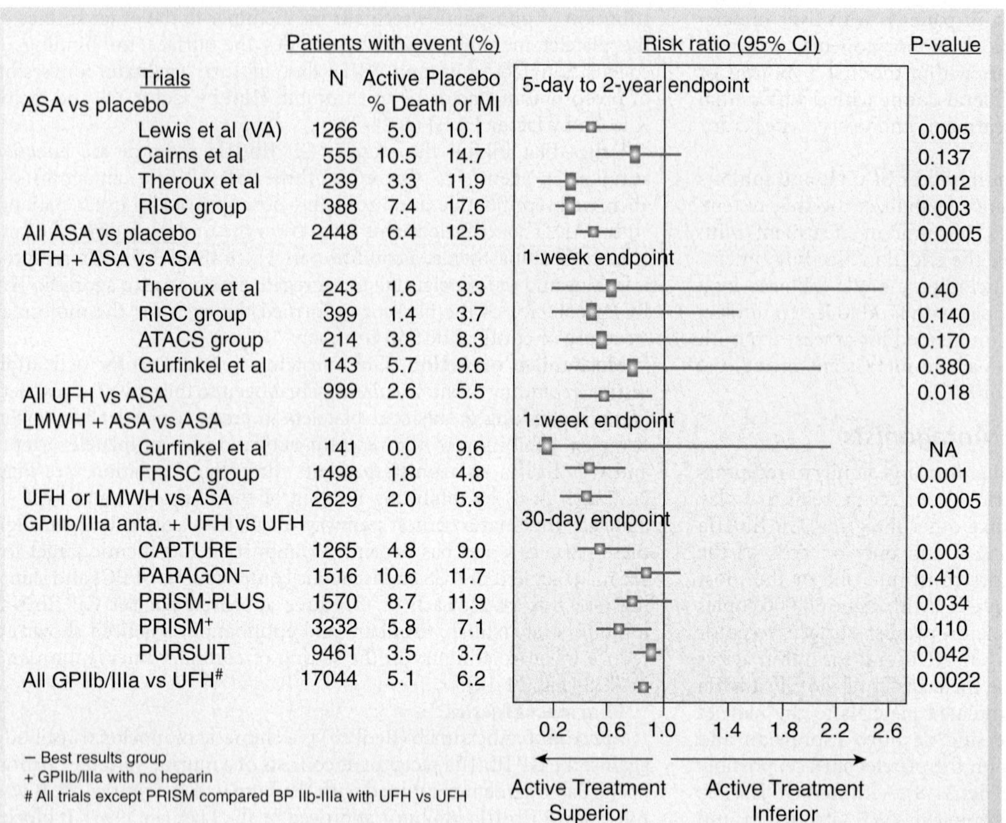

FIGURE 24-10 • Summary of trials of antithrombotic therapy in unstable angina. Meta-analysis of randomized trials in unstable angina/non–ST-segment-elevation myocardial infarction that have compared aspirin (ASA) with placebo, the combination of unfractionated heparin (UFH) and ASA with ASA alone, the combination of a low-molecular-weight heparin (LMWH) and ASA with ASA alone, and the combination of a platelet glycoprotein (GP) IIb/IIIa antagonist (anta.), UFH (hep.), and ASA with UFH plus ASA. The relative risk (RR) values, 95% confidence intervals (CIs), and probability value for each trial are shown. The timing of the end point (death or MI) varied. Results with the platelet GP IIb/IIIa antagonists are reported at the 30-day time point. Incremental gain is observed from single therapy with ASA to double therapy with ASA and UFH and to triple antithrombotic therapy with ASA, UFH, and a platelet GP IIb/IIIa antagonist. In the CAPTURE trial, nearly all patients underwent percutaneous coronary intervention after 20 to 24 hours per study design. (From Fuster V, Alexander RW, O'Rourke RA, et al. Hurst's The Heart, 11th ed. New York: McGraw-Hill, 2004.)

returns to almost normal at 12 hours. However, the antibody is transmitted to new platelets and can be detected for about 2 weeks in a platelet-bound state after the initial administration.[3]

Eptifibatide. Eptifibatide (Integrilin) is a synthetic cyclic heptapeptide based on the 73–amino acid sequence compound barbourin, a constituent of southeastern pigmy rattlesnake venom. Barbourin is highly selective, with affinity only for GP IIb/IIIa.[54] It contains the Lys-Gly-Asp sequence and inhibits the fibrinogen binding site on the GP IIb/IIIa receptor.

The half-life of eptifibatide is 2 to 3 hours, and platelet aggregation returns to normal in 4 to 8 hours after discontinuation.[3] The pharmacokinetics are linear and dose proportional. Clearance is through the kidneys and is reduced in patients with renal insufficiency and advanced age.[3]

Tirofiban. Tirofiban (Aggrastat) is a highly specific nonpeptide mimetic of the RGD sequence of fibrinogen[3] that reversibly inhibits the GP IIb/IIIa receptor by interacting directly with the RGD binding site,[3] inhibiting binding of fibrinogen and vWF to the GP IIb/IIIa receptor.[10]

The half-life of tirofiban is about 2 hours. It is cleared from the plasma mainly by renal excretion, and the plasma clearance significantly decreases (>50%) with renal insufficiency and in the elderly, which warrants dosage adjustment.

Therapeutic Considerations. Isolated use of a GP IIb/IIIa inhibitor as the sole means of reperfusion without a fibrinolytic agent or PCI is not recommended, as clinical studies have not shown significant restoration of blood flow in a sufficient proportion of patients to make it a viable pharmacologic strategy. GP IIb/IIIa antagonists are recommended to be used in conjunction with PCI or fibrinolytic agents (see Box 24-2).[3] Abciximab is a highly effective antiplatelet agent in patients selected for an invasive strategy for ACS with UA/NSTEMI[3] and is given intravenously over a short period to tide the patient through the acute phase of the syndrome or to cover the PCI. It is indicated only if there is no appreciable delay to angiography and PCI is likely to be performed; otherwise, IV eptifibatide or tirofiban is preferred (see Box 24-2). The GPIIb/IIIa inhibitors are used in conjunction with aspirin and heparin (either enoxaparin or low-dose IV UFH) controlled by activated partial thromboplastin times (aPTTs) or activated clotting times (ACTs). If PCI is not planned, abciximab should not be used because of the lack of benefit and risk of bleeding as shown in the GUSTO-IV-ACS study.[55] The patients most likely to benefit are those undergoing early PCI with ST-segment changes on ECG at admission, those already on aspirin therapy, diabetics, and those with abnormal troponin levels and intracoronary thrombus.[3,56] In those patients at lower risk, there is no evidence of benefit. In the TACTICS trial[53] in patients with UA, tirofiban with PCI was better than tirofiban alone in high-risk patients. In a study on patients receiving triple antiplatelet therapy with aspirin, clopidogrel, and a GP IIb/IIIa inhibitor plus heparin, abciximab was compared with tirofiban in patients undergoing PCI for ACS or stable angina.[53] Abciximab was found to be more effective in inhibiting platelet activity than tirofiban, with greater reduction in MI at 30 days (5.4% vs. 6.9%) and a slight excess of minor bleeding (5.6% vs. 3.3% with tirofiban) but no difference in the composite end point of death, MI, or urgent revascularization at 6 months.

In patients with STEMI who are treated with fibrinolytics, the GP IIb/IIIa blockers in combination do not reduce mortality, yet bleeding is clearly increased.[3] In patients with STEMI undergoing primary PCI and stenting, initial reperfusion might improve with abciximab, with recanalization of the infarct-related artery; however, long-term outcomes were not different in the Intracoronary Stenting and Antithrombotic Regimen-2 (ISAR-2)[56] and the CADILLAC trials.[3,57] Recent analysis indicates that the use of abciximab or other GP IIb/IIIa inhibitors during primary PCI is beneficial (see Fig. 24-10).[5,17] Clinical trials with the oral GP IIb/IIIa inhibitor have had negative or neutral results, and only IV administration is recommended (see Box 24-2).

Adverse Effects, Precautions, and Contraindications. Major adverse effects of GP IIb/IIIa inhibitors include the risk of bleeding (1% to 4%), especially at the arterial access site when there is cardiac catheterization and thrombocytopenia (3% to 5%).[5,17] Arterial access site care after PCI and close monitoring of ACT and platelet count are required.[5,17] If thrombocytopenia occurs (2.5% to 6% with abciximab vs. 1.1% to 1.9% with eptifibatide or tirofiban), platelet aggregation returns to 50% of baseline within 1 day in most patients. For eptifibatide and tirofiban, dosage adjustment is required for renal insufficiency. These agents should not be used in patients with a history of bleeding diathesis, active bleeding within 30 days, thrombocytopenia, severe hypertension (>200/110 mm Hg), major surgery within less than 6 weeks, stroke within less than 30 days, or any history of hemorrhagic stroke.[5,17,30]

Dosing. Abciximab is administered intravenously as a 0.25-mg/kg bolus dose followed by continuous infusion of 10 mcg/min (or a weight-adjusted infusion of 0.125 mcg/kg per minute to a maximum of 10 mcg/min).[6]

The usual dose of eptifibatide is a 180-mcg/kg bolus followed by a 2-mcg/kg per minute infusion for up to 96 hours.[6]

Tirofiban is administered at an initial rate of 0.4 mcg/kg per minute for 30 minutes, followed by 0.1 mcg/kg per minute for 48 hours. Patients with severe renal insufficiency (creatinine clearance <30 ml/min) should receive half the dose.[6]

Other Antiplatelet Agents

Sulfinpyrazone, like aspirin, inhibits COX but is more expensive and requires multiple daily dosing without any significant benefit in patients already on aspirin. Similarly, dipyridamole, cilostazol, prostacyclin, prostacyclin analogues, thromboxane synthase blockers, and thromboxane A_2 receptor antagonists were not advantageous over aspirin in ACS and are not recommended.[5,17] In contrast, clopidogrel or ticlodipine had additive effects to aspirin with reduction in clinical cardiac events.[6]

Dipyridamole is a pyrimido-pyrimidine derivative that has antiplatelet and antithrombotic effects due to an increase in platelet cAMP level by inhibition of phosphodiesterase and activation of adenylate cyclase, as well as vasodilatory effects on coronary resistance vessels due to inhibition of uptake of adenosine from vascular endothelium and erythrocytes. It can enhance exercise-induced myocardial ischemia in patients with stable angina, and should not be used as an antiplatelet agent (see Box 24-2). Long-acting dipyridamole, however, when combined with aspirin, helped reduce recurrent stroke.[58,59]

Novel Antiplatelet Agents under Investigation

Several antiplatelet agents targeting different enzymes or receptors involved in the activation, adhesion, and aggregation of platelets are currently under investigation, as summarized in Figure 24-8.

Antithrombotic Agents (Anticoagulants)

Thrombosis results from a complex process initiated by endothelial or platelet injury and involves interactions between blood cells, particularly platelets and proteins of the coagulation system. The conversion of prothrombin to thrombin is a crucial step in the coagulation process, which may occur through activation of what have been classically described as extrinsic or intrinsic pathways (see Fig. 24-9). Tissue or endothelial injury or plaque rupture in patients with CAD exposes tissue factor, a cell surface glycoprotein that forms a complex with and activates clotting factor VII. Activated factor VIIa then promotes the activation of factor X to Xa, both directly and indirectly by activating factor IX (see Fig. 24-9). Factor Xa converts prothrombin (factor II) to thrombin (factor IIa). The intrinsic coagulation pathway involves a series of interactions (see Fig. 24-9) that lead to activation of factor IX (forming IXa), that in turn activates factor X to Xa, which then acts on prothrombin to form thrombin. Thrombin in turn promotes activation of factors Va and VIIIa, and conversion of fibrinogen (factor I) to fibrin (factor Ia), which is cross-linked by factor XIIIa that binds to additional platelet surfaces, stabilizing the thrombus. Coagulation is further amplified with thrombus propagation by activation of more platelets and clotting proteins. Thrombin, in addition to activating the clotting system, also activates fibrinolysis by inducing production and release of tissue plasminogen activator (tPA) from endothelial cells. Binding of tPA and plasminogen to fibrin results in conversion of plasminogen to plasmin, which degrades fibrin, resulting in partial or complete dissolution of thrombus (see Fig. 24-9). Clotting is restricted by several other proteins, including antithrombin, tissue factor pathway inhibitors, and activated proteins C and S (see Fig. 24-9).

In patients with ACS and STEMI, thrombin generation is a pivotal event resulting in myocardial ischemia and infarction, and inhibition of the coagulation cascade at single or multiple positions is essential for the acute management of these patients to establish and maintain patency of the culprit artery. Several drugs that inhibit the coagulation pathway or potentiate the effect of anticoagulants in the blood have been shown to effectively prevent or reduce damage related to acute coronary thrombosis. This includes drugs that target antithrombin, clotting factor Xa, direct thrombin inhibitors, and fibrinolytic pathways.

Antithrombins

Unfractionated Heparin. UFH is a heterogeneous mixture of mucopolysaccharide chains of molecular weights ranging from 10,000 to 30,000 Da (Table 24-2). UFH has complex effects on the coagulation

TABLE 24-2 PROPERTIES OF ANTICOAGULANTS

Drug	Unfractionated Heparin	Low-Molecular-Weight Heparins	Direct Thrombin Inhibitors
Molecular weight	10,000-30,000	4000-6500	2200
Route of administration	Intravenous	Subcutaneous	Intravenous
Bioavailability	+	++	+++
Half-life (min)	30-60	120-180	25-35
Inactivated by heparinases	+++	+	–
Renal clearance	++	+++	++
Dose adjustments	Frequent, adjusted by aPTT	Fixed, weight adjusted	Fixed, weight adjusted
Anticoagulant effects	Factor Xa = IIa	Factor Xa >> IIa	Factor IIa
Antithrombin dependent	–	++	–
Inactivates clot-bound thrombin	–	–	++
Inhibits platelet function	+++	++	+++
Risk of HIT	+++	+	–
Liver toxicity (↑ liver enzymes)	++	+	–

Intensity of effect from none to intense indicated by the signs –, +, ++, +++.
aPTT, activated partial thromboplastin time; HIT, heparin-induced thrombocytopenia.

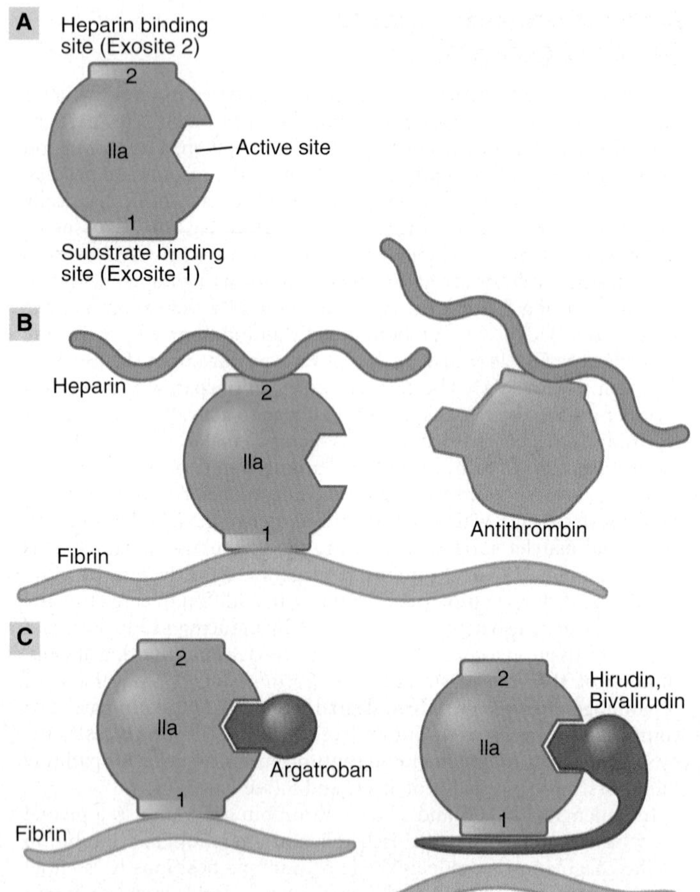

FIGURE 24-11 • Thrombin (IIa) and direct thrombin inhibitor interactions. **A,** Thrombin possesses an active site and two positively charged exosites. Exosite 1 serves as the substrate (fibrin) binding site while exosite 2 binds heparin. **B,** With simultaneous binding of both heparin and fibrin to thrombin, antithrombin (AT)–bound heparin cannot bind to thrombin to form a ternary heparin-thrombin-AT complex, thus demonstrating heparin's inability to inhibit clot-bound thrombin. **C,** Univalent inhibitors, such as argatroban, inhibit fibrin-bound thrombin without displacing thrombin from fibrin. Bivalent inhibitors, such as hirudin and bivalirudin, displace thrombin from fibrin during the inactivation process.

system, blood vessels, and platelets, preventing thrombus propagation without lysing existing thrombi.[60]

Mechanism of Action. UFH exerts its anticoagulant effect by binding to antithrombin (at its pentasaccharide recognition site) and thrombin, forming a ternary complex (Fig. 24-11) that, by inducing a conformational change, accelerates the action of antithrombin (a serine protease) to inactivate thrombin, factor IXa, and factor Xa. UFH also inhibit platelet activation by thrombin and vWF. The heparin-antithrombin-thrombin ternary complex can be formed only by pentasaccharide-containing heparin chains composed of at least 18 saccharide units. Most of the chains of UFH are ≥18 saccharide units long compared to LMWH, which contains fewer chains of sufficient length to bind to both antithrombin and thrombin, and therefore UFH has equivalent activity against factor Xa and thrombin, while LMWH has greater activity against factor Xa.

Pharmacokinetics. UFH is not absorbed from the GI tract and requires parenteral administration. After IV or subcutaneous injection, it is extensively bound to plasma proteins with variable plasma half-life depending on the dose and route of administration, ranging from 1 to 6 hours (average 1.5). The half-life is slightly prolonged in patients with renal impairment, decreased in those with pulmonary embolism, and either increased or decreased in those with liver disorders. UFH is excreted in the urine, mainly as metabolites, but after large doses up to 50% may be excreted unchanged. It does not cross the placenta. There is marked variability in anticoagulant response,[61] requiring monitoring of its anticoagulant effect with the aPTT, a test that is sensitive to the inhibitory effects of UFH on thrombin (factor IIa), factor Xa, and factor IXa.

Therapeutic Considerations. The rapid onset of action of UFH on the coagulation system after IV administration makes it an essential part of the management of patients with ACS and STEMI. In patients presenting with UA/NSTEMI, UFH should be added to aspirin.[61] An IV bolus of 60 to 70 units/kg should be administered, followed by a 12- to 15-unit/kg infusion adjusted to maintain an aPTT of 1.5 to 2.0 times baseline (~50 to 70 seconds) and continued for 2 to 7 days.[62]

In patients with STEMI treated with thrombolytics or primary PCI, UFH is recommended as a Class I indication (Box 24-3).[63] The recommendations for the use of UFH depend on the type of fibrinolytic agent chosen. The use of IV UFH appears to result in higher rates of infarct-related artery perfusion in conjunction with alteplase.[61] In patients treated with alteplase, reteplase, or tenecteplase, UFH should be administered as a 60-unit/kg IV bolus (maximum 4000 units) followed by a 12-unit/kg per hour (maximum 1000 units/hr) infusion adjusted to maintain the aPTT at 1.5 to 2.0 times control (~50 to 70 seconds).[61] The incidences of death, stroke, reinfarction, and bleeding were lowest in the aPTT range of 50 to 70 seconds (1.5 to 2.0 times control),[64] while higher aPTTs increased the risk of cerebral bleeding without conferring any survival advantage and should be avoided.[65]

In patients with STEMI receiving nonspecific fibrinolytic agents (streptokinase, anistreplase, and urokinase) that produce a systemic coagulopathy (due to depletion of factors V and VIII and production of fibrinogen degradation products; see Fig. 24-9), IV UFH should be reserved for those at high risk for systemic emboli, such as patients with large or anterior MI, atrial fibrillation, previous embolus, or known left ventricular (LV) thrombus. In a meta-analysis of clinical trials enrolling a total of 68,000 patients comparing subcutaneous UFH with no routine heparin in conjunction with nonspecific fibrinolytic agents, it was demonstrated that 5 lives were saved per 1000 patients treated with UFH in addition to the fibrinolytic.[3]

Although no placebo-controlled trials with UFH have been performed in patients undergoing primary PCI for STEMI, UFH (70 to 100 units/kg in the absence of GP IIb/IIIa and 50 to 70 units/kg when GP IIb/IIIa is used) is indicated because of the risk of acute thrombotic closure (see Box 24-3). During primary PCI, UFH dose titration in the cardiac catheterization laboratory should be adjusted by the ACT because the level of anticoagulation required is beyond the range measured accurately by the aPTT.[5,17] The target ACT is recommended to be 250 to 300 seconds in the absence of GP IIb/IIIa inhibition and 200 to 250 seconds with a GP IIb/IIIa inhibitor. Platelet counts should be monitored daily to assess for heparin-induced thrombocytopenia (HIT).[66]

The optimal duration of anticoagulation with UFH remains undefined. With limited evidence supporting benefits of prolonged infusion to reduce ischemic complications, and concerns regarding bleeding or HIT with prolonged exposure, routine UFH infusions should be limited to 48 hours, unless clinical considerations dictate longer use.[5,17] Concern has also been raised regarding abrupt discontinuation of UFH due to the presence of a high-risk period for recurrent thrombosis (heparin rebound) with increased thrombin activity.[67] It may be prudent to reduce UFH infusions gradually, by half within 6 hours and then discontinuing over the subsequent 12 hours.[30]

Adverse Effects, Precautions, and Contraindications. Bleeding and mild thrombocytopenia are common adverse effects (10%).[30] The risk of serious bleeding increases when UFH is used in conjunction with fibrinolytic therapy, and the recommended dose of UFH should not be exceeded. The risk of hemorrhage is higher in patients with bleeding disorders, hepatic disease, or GI ulcerative lesions. HIT is usually asymptomatic and transient (HIT type 1). However, rarely (~0.2% to 3%) there is an immune-mediated potentially fatal syndrome in which the immunoglobulins bridge platelets, causing both thrombocytopenia and risk of thrombosis (HIT type 2).[66] This can occur shortly after initiation of UFH or, rarely, later (after 5 to 19 days). If the platelet count drops below 100,000, a test for HIT should be obtained and the

BOX 24-3 RECOMMENDATIONS FOR THERAPY WITH ANTICOAGULANTS IN CORONARY ARTERY DISEASE

Class I

UA/NSTEMI

- ***Anticoagulant*** therapy should be added to ***antiplatelet*** therapy immediately.
- For patients selected for *conservative strategy*, ***enoxaparin*** or ***UFH*** (LoE: A) or ***fondaparinux*** (LoE: B) have established efficacy.
- For patients selected for *conservative strategy* with *increased risk of bleeding*, ***fondaparinux*** is preferable (LoE: B).
- For patients selected for *invasive strategy*, regimens with established efficacy at a
  - LoE: A include ***enoxaparin*** and ***UFH***
  - LoE: B include ***bivalirudin*** and ***fondaparinux***

STEMI (also see Box 24-4):

- For patients undergoing *reperfusion with fibrinolytics*, ***anticoagulant*** therapy should be administered for a minimum of 48 hours (LoE: C) and preferably for the duration of hospitalization (up to 8 days). (For >48 hours' use, regimens other than UFH are recommended because of the risk of heparin-induced thrombocytopenia [LoE: A].)
  - ***UFH*** 60 units/kg IV (max. 4000 units) followed by 12 units/kg per hour IV (max. 1000 units/hr), adjusted to maintain aPTT at 1.5 to 2.0 times control (~50 to 70 seconds) (LoE: C), *or*
  - ***Enoxaparin*** (provided the serum creatinine is <2.5 mg/dl in men and 2.0 mg/dl in women). For patients *less than 75 years of age:* 30-mg IV bolus followed at 15 minutes with 1.0 mg/kg subQ injection repeated every 12 hours. For patients *75 years of age or older:* no IV bolus is required; subQ dose is reduced to 0.75 mg/kg every 12 hours.
  - If the *creatinine clearance is less than 30 ml/min*, subQ enoxapirin dose is reduced to 1.0 mg/kg every 24 hours (LoE: A).
  - ***Fondaparinux*** (provided the serum creatinine is <3.0 mg/dl): initial dose is 2.5 mg IV, then 2.5 mg subQ once daily (LoE: B).
- For patients undergoing *primary PCI*, ***anticoagulant*** therapy should be continued
  - For those with *prior treatment with* ***UFH***, administer additional boluses of ***UFH*** as needed to support PCI, taking into account whether ***GP IIb/IIIa receptor antagonists*** have been administered (LoE: C). ***Bivalirudin*** may also be used (LoE: C).
  - For those with *prior treatment with* ***enoxaparin***, if the last subQ dose was given less than 8 hours ago, no additional enoxaparin should be given. If the last subQ dose was given between 8 and 12 hours ago, ***enoxaparin*** IV 0.3 mg/kg should be given (LoE: B).
- For patients with *prior treatment with* ***fondaparinux***, additional IV ***anticoagulant*** possessing anti–factor IIa activity should be used, taking into account whether ***GP IIb/IIIa receptor antagonists*** have been administered (LoE: C).

Class IIa

UA/NSTEMI

- For patients selected for *conservative strategy*, ***enoxaparin*** or ***fondaparinux*** is preferable to UFH, unless CABG is planned in less than 24 hours (LoE: B).

STEMI

- For patients *not undergoing reperfusion therapy*, ***anticoagulant*** therapy (non-UFH regimen) for the duration of the index hospitalization (up to 8 days) (LoE: B).
  - ***LMWH*** (LoE: C) or ***fondaparinux*** (LoE: B) using the same dosing regimens as for patients who receive fibrinolytic therapy.

Class III

STEMI

- Because of the risk of catheter thrombosis, ***fondaparinux*** *should not be used as the sole anticoagulant to support PCI.* An additional anticoagulant with anti–factor IIa activity should be administered (LoE: C).

aPTT, activated partial thromboplastin time; CABG, coronary artery bypass graft; GP, glycoprotein; IV, intravenous; LoE, level of evidence; LMWH, low-molecular-weight heparin; NSTEMI, non–ST-elevation myocardial infarction; PCI, percutaneous coronary intervention; STEMI, ST-elevation myocardial infarction; subQ, subcutaneous; UA, unstable angina; UFH, unfractionated heparin.

patient monitored for thrombotic complications.[66] All UFH, including that used to flush IV lines, should be immediately discontinued and, if acute anticoagulation is needed, a direct thrombin inhibitor (either bivalirudin or argatroban) used (see Box 24-3). Daily hematocrit and platelet measurements are recommended during UFH therapy. Heparin is derived from animal tissue, and occasionally causes allergy. Heparin may cause hyperkalemia due to inhibition of aldosterone secretion and, with long-term therapy, rarely causes osteoporosis (see Table 24-1).

Drug Interactions. The risk of bleeding with UFH is increased when used with oral anticoagulants (warfarin), antiplatelet drugs (e.g., aspirin, clopidogrel, dipyridamole), NSAIDs, dextrans, thrombolytics, and high doses of penicillins.

Dosing. The dose-effect relationship is difficult to predict because UFH is a heterogeneous group of molecules extracted by a variety of procedures with variable strength from batch to batch, and also has variable binding to plasma proteins, endothelial cells, and macrophages. A weight-adjusted dosing regimen provides more predictable anticoagulation than the fixed-dose regimen. An initial bolus of 60 to 70 units/kg (maximum 4000 units), followed by an initial infusion of 12 to 15 units/kg per hour (maximum 1000 units/hr) and then adjusted to maintain the aPTT at 1.5 to 2.0 times control (approximately 50 to 70 seconds), has been recommended.[6]

The use of nomograms results in fewer subtherapeutic aPTTs and less bleeding. The infusion rate should be decreased by 50% if the aPTT is greater than or equal to three times, and by 25% if two to three times, the control values. If the aPTT is less than 1.5 times the control, the infusion should be increased by 25% to a maximum rate of 2500 IU/hr. During PCI in the cardiac catheterization laboratory, UFH dose titration should be adjusted by the ACT because the level of anticoagulation required is beyond the range measured accurately by aPTT. The target ACT is recommended to be between 250 and 300 seconds in the absence of GP IIb/IIIa inhibition and 200 to 250 seconds when UFH is administered in conjunction with a GP IIb/IIIa inhibitor.[5,17]

Overdose. Heparin overdosage is treated by discontinuing the infusion and, if clinically required, administering protamine sulfate (1 mg for every 100 units of UFH given in the preceding 4 hours) as a slow infusion of no more than 50 mg in any 10-minute period.[30]

Low-Molecular-Weight Heparins. LMWHs are about one third of the molecular weight of UFH and differ from UFH in their pharmacokinetics and relative inhibitory activity against factor Xa and thrombin (see Table 24-2).

Mechanism of Action. The LMWHs, like UFH, enhance the action of antithrombin but have a higher ratio of anti–factor Xa to antithrombin (anti–factor IIa) activity (see Fig. 24-9). Approximately 25% to 30% of LMWH preparations contain the crucial greater-than-18 pentasaccharide–containing chains that are needed to bind to both antithrombin and thrombin and inactivate thrombin and factor Xa (see Fig. 24-11), while they contain more chains with less than 18 saccharide units that inactivate factor Xa but not thrombin. LMWHs have less effect on platelet aggregation than does UFH. They have no significant effect on blood coagulation tests such as aPTT, and therapeutic effect may be monitored by measurement of plasma anti–factor Xa activity, which is not routinely done due to a more predictable effect of LMWH.

Pharmacokinetics. Different LMWH preparations are available with molecular weights ranging from 4000 to 6500 Da, with differences in pharmacokinetic and pharmacodynamic profiles (see Table 24-2).

They have greater bioavailability, less binding to plasma protein and endothelial cells, dose-independent clearance more through the kidneys, and a longer plasma half-life than UFH. The level of anticoagulation is more predictable and sustained, with once- or twice-a-day subcutaneous administration and no requirement for laboratory monitoring of activity. The ratios of anti–factor Xa to anti–factor IIa (Xa : IIa) vary between various LMWH preparations, ranging from 3 : 1 with enoxaparin to 2 : 1 with dalteparin.[68]

Enoxaparin is rapidly and almost completely absorbed after subcutaneous injection, with a bioavailability of about 100%. Peak plasma activity is reached within 1 to 5 hours. The elimination half-life is about 4 to 5 hours, but anti–factor Xa activity persists for up to 24 hours after a 40-mg dose. Enoxaparin is metabolized in the liver and excreted in the urine as unchanged drug and metabolites, with prolongation of elimination in patients with renal impairment.[30]

Dalteparin is almost completely absorbed after subcutaneous administration, with a bioavailability of about 87%. Peak plasma activity is reached in about 4 hours, with a terminal half-life of 2 hours after IV and 3 to 5 hours after subcutaneous injection. It is excreted via the kidneys, with prolongation of the half-life with renal impairment.[30]

The bioavailability of reviparin sodium after subcutaneous administration is about 95%, with peak plasma concentration achieved in 3 hours and an elimination half-life of about 3 hours; it is mainly excreted in the urine.[30]

Therapeutic Considerations. Subcutaneous LMWHs are an alternative to UFH for treatment of patients with ACS and STEMI, and current recommendations for their use are summarized in Box 24-3. Because of convenience, more predictable anticoagulant effect, no need for routine monitoring of anticoagulation, and lower incidence of HIT, LMWH is in general preferred to UFH.[66] Most clinical trials have used enoxaparin, and little information is available about other LWMHs; the data from the enoxaparin trial cannot be extrapolated due to differences between various LMWHs. When compared to UFH, equivalence or superiority of LMWH in clinical outcomes in the management of patients with ACS was demonstrated in several but not all trials.[6] In patients with UA/NSTEMI in the ESSENCE and TIMI 11B trials, the reduction in the combined end points of death, MI, and urgent revascularization was greater in the enoxaparin compared to UFH group. Similarly, in a meta-analysis, reduction in death or MI at days 8 and 43 was better in the enoxaparin compared to the UFH group.[69] In high-risk patients with ACS undergoing PCI, the primary composite end point of death or MI at 30 days was, however, not different between the groups receiving UFH or enoxaparin in the Superior Yield of the New Strategy of Enoxaparin, Revascularization and Glycoprotein IIb/IIIa Inhibitors (SYNERGY) trial,[43] with increased risk of bleeding in the enoxaparin group. In the Safety and Efficacy of Enoxaparin in Percutaneous Coronary Intervention Patients trial (STEEPLE),[70] less bleeding and similar efficacy with enoxaparin compared to UFH in patients undergoing nonemergent PCI was demonstrated.

In patients with STEMI undergoing fibrinolytic therapy, full-dose tenecteplase with enoxaparin emerged as the most promising reperfusion regimen, reducing the combined end point of 30-day mortality, in-hospital reinfarction, or ischemia in the Assessment of the Safety and Efficacy of New Thrombolytic regimens (ASSENT-3) trial[71] compared to full-dose tenecteplase plus UFH or half-dose tenecteplase with UFH and abciximab. However, the risk of serious bleeding was increased in the ASSENT-3 Plus[34] and the ExTRACT-TIMI 25[72] trials, particularly in the elderly, indicating a need for further studies to define bleeding risks of high-risk patients including the elderly, women, low-body-weight patients, and those with renal dysfunction. A small increase in the risk of bleeding was also demonstrated with reviparin in patients with STEMI within 15 minutes of thrombolytic therapy that also reduced the composite outcome of death, MI, or recurrent ischemia at 7 days compared to placebo.[73] Use of an anticoagulant with fibrinolytic therapy in patients with STEMI is recommended (Box 24-4; see Box 24-3) based on the benefits demonstrated by enoxaparin, reviparin, and fondaparinux started in different trials concurrently with fibrinolytic agents.[5,17] Enoxaparin appears to be safe when used in combination with eptifibatide or tirofiban during PCI.[5,6]

BOX 24-4 RECOMMENDATIONS FOR USE OF ANTITHROMBINS AS ANCILLARY THERAPY TO REPERFUSION THERAPY IN PATIENTS WITH STEMI

Unfractionated Heparin (UFH)

Class I

- In patients with **STEMI** undergoing
  - *PCI or surgical revascularization* (LoE: C).
  - *Reperfusion therapy* with ***alteplase***, ***reteplase***, or ***tenecteplase***: IV 60-unit/kg bolus (max. 4000 units) followed by 12-unit/kg per hour infusion (max. 1000 units/hr) adjusted to maintain aPTT at 1.5 to 2.0 times control (~50 to 70 seconds) (LoE: C).
  - *Reperfusion* with ***nonselective fibrinolytic agents*** (streptokinase, anistreplase, or urokinase) who are at high risk for systemic emboli (large or anterior MI, atrial fibrillation, previous embolus, or known LV thrombus) (LoE: B).
  - Platelet counts should be monitored daily in patients given UFH (LoE: C).

Class IIb

- In patients with **STEMI** undergoing *reperfusion therapy* with ***streptokinase*** (LoE: B).

Low-Molecular-Weight Heparin (LMWH)

Class IIb

- In patients with **STEMI** undergoing *fibrinolytic therapy*, as an alternative to UFH for patients *less than 75 years of age without significant renal dysfunction* (serum creatinine <2.5 mg/dl in men or 2.0 mg/dl in women). ***Enoxaparin*** (30-mg IV bolus followed by 1.0-mg/kg subQ injection every 12 hours until hospital discharge) used in combination with full-dose ***tenecteplase*** is the most comprehensively studied regimen in patients less than 75 years of age (LoE: B).

Class III

- In patients with **STEMI** undergoing fibrinolytic therapy, ***LMWH*** *should not be used as alternative to UFH* for those
  - 75 years of age or older (LoE: B).
  - less than 75 years of age but with serum creatinine greater than 2.5 mg/dl in men or 2.0 mg/dl in women (LoE: B).

Bivalirudin

Class IIa

- In patients with *known heparin-induced thrombocytopenia*, it is reasonable to consider bivalirudin as an alternative to heparin in conjunction with ***streptokinase***.
  - IV 0.25-mg/kg ***bivalirudin*** bolus followed by 0.5-mg/kg per hour infusion for the first 12 hours and then 0.25 mg/kg per hour for 36 hours (LoE: B).

aPTT, activated partial thromboplastin time; IV, intravenous; LoE, level of evidence; LV, left ventricular; MI, myocardial infarction; PCI, percutaneous coronary intervention; STEMI, ST-elevation myocardial infarction; subQ, subcutaneous.

Adverse Effects, Precautions, and Contraindications. LMWHs should not be given to patients who have developed thrombocytopenia with heparin, had prior major bleeding, or are at very high risk of bleeding (see Table 24-1). Plasma anti–factor Xa activity may need to be monitored in patients with active bleeding or those at increased risk of bleeding with renal impairment, those with extremes of body weight, the elderly, particularly women, or those on concomitant therapy with clopidogrel, NSAIDs, or warfarin. Plasma potassium concentrations should be monitored in all patients with risk factors for hyperkalemia if LMWH is administered long term. The anticoagulant effect of LMWH is less effectively reversed with protamine than that of UFH, with protamine neutralizing the antithrombin effect but only partially neutralizing the anti–factor Xa effect.

Drug Interactions. LMWH should be used with caution with oral anticoagulants or antiplatelet agents, such as aspirin, NSAIDs, and dipyridamole.

Dosing. The dosing for various anticoagulants are summarized in Box 24-3.

Factor Xa Inhibitors

Fondaparinux. Fondaparinux is a synthetic pentasaccharide that is an antithrombin-dependent indirect inhibitor of factor Xa. Like LMWH, fondaparinux differs from UFH in terms of decreased plasma protein binding, dose-independent clearance, a longer half-life that results in more predictable and sustained anticoagulation with fixed-dose and once-a-day subcutaneous administration, and no need for laboratory monitoring of anticoagulation activity.

Mechanism of Action. Fondaparinux selectively binds and potentiates the antithrombin-mediated neutralization of factor Xa, inhibiting the multiplier effects of the downstream coagulation reactions, thus interrupting thrombin formation and development of thrombus (see Fig. 24-9). At the recommended dose, fondaparinux does not affect fibrinolytic activity, inactivate thrombin (factor IIa), or affect platelet function.

Pharmacokinetics. Fondaparinux is rapidly and completely absorbed after subcutaneous injection, with 100% bioavailability. The peak steady state plasma concentration is reached in 3 hours, and the elimination half-life is 17 hours with primarily renal clearance.

Therapeutic Considerations. Fondaparinux has been shown to be as effective as UFH or enoxaparin in reducing clinical outcomes in patients with ACS. In patients presenting with UA/NSTEMI, fondaparinux was an effective alternative to enoxaparin in the Organization for the Assessment of Strategies for Ischemic Syndromes–5 (OASIS-5) trial, with similar outcomes for the primary composite end points of death, MI, and need for revascularization and improved efficacy in reducing stroke, with much less major bleeding than enoxaparin.[74] In patients with UA/NSTEMI selected for a conservative strategy, regimens using enoxaparin, UFH, or fondaparinux have established efficacy, with enoxaparin or fondaparinux preferable to UFH as anticoagulant therapy, unless CABG is planned within 24 hours, and fondaparinux preferable in those with increased risk of bleeding (see Box 24-3). In patients with UA/NSTEMI selected for an invasive strategy, anticoagulant therapy with UFH, enoxaparin, bivalirudin, or fondaparinux should be added to antiplatelet drugs (see Fig. 24-5).

In patients presenting with STEMI, use of 7 to 8 days of fondaparinux (2.5 mg daily) resulted in a relative risk reduction of 14% and 18% in death or reinfarction at 30 days, respectively, compared to UFH for less than 48 hours or placebo in the OASIS-6 trial, with a trend toward fewer major bleeds, but no benefit in patients who underwent primary PCI.[47] In patients with STEMI treated with fibrinolytics (alteplase), no difference in coronary patency at 90 minutes with a trend toward less reocclusion and more major bleeding was observed in those treated with IV followed by subcutaneous fondaparinux compared to UFH (see Box 24-4).[5,17] In patients undergoing primary PCI, no advantage of fondaparinux was observed with an excess of catheter thrombosis, indicating the need for an additional anticoagulant with anti–factor IIa activity, such as UFH, to support PCI.[5,17]

Adverse Effects, Precautions, and Contraindications. An increased rate of catheter thrombosis was observed with fondaparinux during PCI, which likely results from lack of any effect of factor Xa inhibitors when used alone against thrombin that is already formed or freshly generated, and an additional anticoagulant with anti–factor IIa activity, such as UFH, should be used to support PCI. Thrombocytopenia can occur, and platelet counts should be monitored.[5,17]

Bleeding risk increases with fondaparinux, particularly in patients with impaired renal function. In cases of major bleeding, fondaparinux needs to be discontinued and fresh frozen plasma administered to replenish coagulation factors. Protamine is ineffective in reversing the anticoagulant effect of direct thrombin inhibitors and fondaparinux because of lack of a protamine-binding domain.

Drug Interactions. No significant effect on pharmacokinetics or pharmacodynamics was observed when fondaparinux was used concomitantly in the short term with warfarin, aspirin, piroxicam, and digoxin. Fondaparinux does not markedly inhibit common CYP enzymes. Patients should be monitored closely for risk of bleeding during fondaparinux use with other anticoagulants and antiplatelet agents.[30]

Dosing. Fondaparinux is administered as a 2.5-mg daily dose. Its anticoagulant activity does not need to be monitored routinely.

Direct Thrombin Inhibitors

Three direct thrombin inhibitors—bivalirudin, hirudin, and argatroban—have been evaluated as alternatives to heparin during PCI.

Mechanism of Action. These agents directly inhibit soluble and clot-bound thrombin in an antithrombin-independent manner and are more potent than UFH (see Fig. 24-11). They have high specificity and potency for thrombin inhibition by binding directly to the anion-binding and the catalytic sites of thrombin, and prevent thrombin-mediated platelet activation and aggregation.[68]

Pharmacokinetics

Bivalirudin. Bivalirudin (Hirulog, Angiomax) is a synthetic analogue of hirudin that binds reversibly to thrombin—as opposed to hirudin, which inhibits thrombin irreversibly—thus improving its safety profile. Of the available direct thrombin inhibitors, it is the most studied agent in patients undergoing PCI.

After IV administration, the plasma half-life is approximately 25 minutes in patients with normal renal function. Bivalirudin is partly metabolized and partly excreted by the kidney, with prolongation of half-life in patients with renal impairment. It does not bind to plasma proteins and is removed by hemodialysis.

Argatroban. Argatroban is hepatically metabolized by CYP3A4/5 isoenzymes, with active metabolites that have weaker anticoagulant effect than argatroban. Steady state levels are attained within 1 to 3 hours. The terminal elimination half-life ranges between 40 and 50 minutes.

Therapeutic Considerations. Direct thrombin inhibitors are more effective than UFH in ACS, but carry a higher risk of major bleeding, except for bivalirudin. Bivalirudin has been shown to reduce ischemic complications after PCI at rates similar to those with combined UFH and GP IIb/IIIa inhibition, with reduced rates of major and minor bleeding complications.

Bivalirudin has not been tested in patients with UA/NSTEMI selected for a noninvasive strategy and hence cannot be recommended at this time. With PCI, bivalirudin is associated with less bleeding and outcomes similar to those in patients treated with UFH and GP IIb/IIIa antagonists. In patients with UA or post-MI angina undergoing coronary angioplasty without stents or GP IIb/IIIa inhibitors, bivalirudin had an efficacy similar to UFH in reducing death, MI, and need for emergency CABG surgery, with less major bleeding.[68] The safety of combining a GP IIb/IIIa blocker and bivalirudin in elective coronary stenting was demonstrated in the Comparison of Abciximab Complications with Hirulog for Ischemic Events Trial (CACHET)[75] pilot study, the Randomized Evaluation in PCI Linking Angiomax to reduced Clinical Events (REPLACE-2) trial,[76] and the Acute Catheterization and Urgent Intervention Triage Strategy (ACUITY)[77] trial to reduce ischemic complications and major bleeding. In patients with ACS who undergo early invasive management, the ACUITY trial supports the use of bivalirudin given before PCI (0.75 mg/kg) and continued (1.75 mg/hr) for the duration of the procedure as a cost-effective substitute for UFH plus a GP IIb/IIIa inhibitor, in particular if patients are pretreated with clopidogrel (see Box 24-3).[60,77] In the HERO-2 trial,[78] bivalirudin added to streptokinase in patients presenting with STEMI reduced the rate of reinfarction compared with UFH, but at the cost of increased bleeding. To clarify the role of bivalirudin in patients with STEMI, further studies are needed. Given the lower rate of bleeding complications in the majority of studies, bivalirudin may be particularly useful for patients at high risk of bleeding, such as the elderly or those with renal insufficiency.

Hirudin was evaluated in patients with UA undergoing PCI in the HELVETICA trial and, despite reduction in early ischemic events compared to UFH, the primary outcome of event-free survival at 7 months between those receiving both IV and subcutaneous hirudin, IV hirudin only, and UFH was not different.[79]

Argatroban use in patients with HIT undergoing PCI,[66] compared with historical control subjects with HIT, reduced the incidence of the composite end points of all-cause death, all-cause amputation, or new thrombosis. Bivalirudin or argatroban is recommended (see Boxes 24-3 and 24-4) as an alternative antithrombotic treatment to heparin during PCI for patients with HIT or those at risk for developing it.[17,19]

Adverse Effects, Precautions, and Contraindications. Direct thrombin inhibitors should be used with caution in patients with hepatic or renal impairment. The infusion dose of bivalirudin should be reduced in patients with renal impairment, and the ACT should be monitored.

Drug Interactions. Use of direct thrombin inhibitors with thrombolytics, oral anticoagulants, or drugs that affect platelet function may increase the risk of bleeding, particularly in the elderly.

Dosing. Bivalirudin may be used as a 0.75-mg/kg IV bolus followed by a 1.75-mg/kg per hour infusion for up to 4 hours, and then 0.2 mg/kg per hour for up to 20 hours if required.

Argatroban may be initiated at 2 mcg/kg per minute IV, with subsequent adjustments to be guided by the aPTT.

Fibrinolytic Agents

Reperfusion Therapy. Following coronary artery occlusion by a thrombus, spontaneous dissolution of the clot may occur by activation of the endogenous fibrinolytic system (see Fig. 24-9), but in the majority of patients the thrombus persists in the first 6 to 12 hours after onset of symptoms while myocardial necrosis proceeds. Restoration of flow in the infarct artery can be achieved by pharmacologic means, PCI, or surgery. Time to restoration of flow in the infarct artery is a critical determinant of MI size, and short- and long-term outcomes and timely use of some reperfusion therapy is more important than the choice of therapy. Ischemia persisting for more than 30 minutes results in irreversible cell damage (see Fig. 24-3). Reperfusion within 90 minutes may salvage 50% of the myocardium at risk and correlates with a mortality reduction at 30 days. After 4 to 6 hours of ischemia, minimum myocardium can be saved unless collaterals are present or ischemic preconditioning has occurred.

The efficacy of fibrinolytics in lysing thrombus decreases with the passage of time, with maximum efficacy achieved if administered within the first 2 hours of symptom onset, which can occasionally abort MI and improve survival. A ≤ 30-minute door-to-needle time is therefore the goal for thrombolysis in every patient with STEMI. Primary PCI should be considered in those patients with delayed presentation or when the estimated mortality with fibrinolysis is high from cardiogenic shock, hemodynamic instability, or increased risk of major bleeding (see Fig. 24-6). Despite restoration of blood flow with revascularization in the infarct artery, perfusion to the infarct area may still be sluggish due to microvascular injury and reperfusion damage that results in platelet activation, embolization, reactive oxygen species generation, and cellular edema. Therefore, with reperfusion therapy, adjunctive and ancillary treatment to minimize platelet activation, thrombus extension, inflammation, and oxidative damage to diminish further myocardial loss should be instituted.

The goals of reperfusion therapy are to achieve early patency of the infarct artery and salvage myocardium with preservation of myocardial functional and electrical stability to lower mortality. Early reperfusion can be achieved by either fibrinolysis or PCI. Various fibrinolytic agents are available (Table 24-3), all of which convert plasminogen into active plasmin.

Mechanism of Action. Clot dissolution by fibrinolytic agents is mediated by activation of the inactive plasminogen to its active form plasmin, which takes place when plasminogen binds to fibrin in the presence of a plasminogen activator (see Fig. 24-9). Plasmin then degrades fibrin clots and hydrolyzes other coagulation proteins, including factors II, V, VIII, and XII. As fibrin is lysed, plasmin is released that is inhibited by α_2-antiplasmin to prevent development of a systemic lytic state. tPA secreted from endothelial cells binds to fibrin and thus activates plasminogen bound to fibrin much more rapidly than circulating plasminogen; therefore, the fibrinolytic action of tPA is fibrin specific (see Fig. 24-9).

There are two types of fibrinolytic agents:

1. Fibrin specific: alteplase, reteplase, and tenecteplase, which act by promoting tPA-mediated conversion of fibrin-bound plasminogen to plasmin.
2. Fibrin nonspecific: streptokinase, anistreplase, and urokinase, which activate endogenous plasminogen indirectly by forming a complex with circulating unbound fibrinogen that becomes an active enzyme to convert plasminogen to plasmin (see Fig. 24-9). Streptokinase may also increase circulating levels of activated protein C, which enhances clot lysis.

Properties of different fibrinolytic agents are summarized in Table 24-3.

Pharmacokinetics

Reteplase (Alteplase). Reteplase (Retavase) is a deletion mutant of alteplase. Based on fibrinolytic activity, reteplase is reported to have an initial half-life of about 14 minutes and a terminal half-life of 1.6 hours in patients with acute MI.[30]

Tenecteplase (TNK-tPA). Tenecteplase is a genetically engineered mutant of native tPA with amino acid substitutions at three sites, which result in decreased plasma clearance, a longer half-life, increased

TABLE 24-3 PROPERTIES OF FIBRINOLYTIC AGENTS

	Streptokinase	Alteplase	Reteplase	Tenecteplase (TNK-tPA)
Dose and duration	1.5 million units over 30-60 min	Up to 100 mg in 90 min (Bolus 15 mg, then 0.75 mg/kg for 30 min [max 50 mg], then 0.5 mg/kg for 60 min [max 35 mg])	10 units × 2 each over 2 min	30-50 mg, by weight: 30 mg for <60 kg; 35 mg for 60-69 kg; 40 mg for 70-79 kg; 45 mg for 80-89 kg; 50 mg ≥ 90 kg
Bolus	–	–	+	+
Half-life (min)	23	<5	13-15	20
Systemic fibrinogen depletion	Marked	Mild	Moderate	Minimal
Fibrin selective	–	+	+	+
Fibrinogen breakdown	++++	++	?	++
Early heparin	±	+	+	+
Hypotension	++	–	–	–
Allergic reactions	++	–	–	–

Intensity of effect from none to intense indicated by the signs –, ±, +, ++, ++++.
?, unknown.

fibrin specificity, and resistance to plasminogen activator inhibitor-1. After IV administration, tenecteplase has a biphasic clearance from plasma, with an initial half-life of 20 to 24 minutes and a terminal-phase half-life of 90 to 130 minutes. It is cleared mainly by hepatic metabolism.[30]

Streptokinase. Streptokinase (Streptase) is derived from streptococci. After IV or subcutaneous administration, it is rapidly cleared with biphasic elimination, with an initial more rapid phase due to binding of specific antibodies. A half-life of 23 minutes has been reported for the streptokinase-activator complex.[30]

Anistreplase. Anistreplase (Eminase) is cleared from plasma more slowly than streptokinase, with a fibrinolytic half-life of about 90 minutes. It is metabolized to the plasminogen-streptokinase complex at a steady rate.[30]

Urokinase. After IV infusion, urokinase (Abbokinase) is cleared rapidly from the circulation by the liver. A plasma half-life of up to 20 minutes has been reported.[30]

Therapeutic Considerations. The potential for benefit with fibrinolytic therapy on mortality and clinical and functional end points is observed when given within 12 hours of symptom onset, with greatest benefit within the first 2 hours and in patients with anterior wall STEMI, diabetes, hypotension (systolic <100 mm Hg), or tachycardia (heart rate >100 bpm) (Fig. 24-12). The absolute benefit is less with inferior wall STEMI, except for the subgroup with associated right ventricular (RV) infarction. The presence of symptoms of MI within 12 hours and ST-segment elevation of greater than 0.1 mV in two contiguous leads or a tall R wave with ST-segment depression in precordial leads V_1–V_4, indicative of a posterior wall MI, or new left

Presentation features	Percent of patients dead: Fibrinolytic	Percent of patients dead: Control	Stratified statistics: O – E	Stratified statistics: Variance
ECG				
BBB	18.7%	23.6%	–24.5	83.3
ST elev, anterior	13.2%	16.9%	–122.0	420.6
ST elev, inferior	7.5%	8.4%	–27.1	237.4
ST elev, other	10.6%	13.4%	–42.1	159.6
ST depression	15.2%	13.8%	12.9	108.7
Other abnormality	5.2%	5.8%	–9.6	103.2
Normal	3.0%	2.3%	3.4	12.9
Hours from onset				
0–1	9.5%	13.0%	–29.3	83.3
2–3	8.2%	10.7%	–100.2	354.8
4–6	9.7%	11.5%	–78.5	387.6
7–12	11.1%	12.7%	–51.5	336.7
13–24	10.0%	10.5%	–11.1	212.6
Age (years)				
< 55	3.4%	4.6%	–45.9	155.6
55–64	7.2%	8.9%	–86.3	360.0
65–74	13.5%	16.1%	–113.7	533.0
75 +	24.3%	25.3%	–12.6	266.6
Gender				
Male	8.2%	10.1%	–208.1	928.0
Female	14.1%	16.0%	–62.2	436.8
Systolic BP (mmHg)				
< 100	28.9%	35.1%	–38.7	132.2
100–149	9.6%	11.5%	–168.9	850.0
150–174	7.2%	8.7%	–59.2	290.0
175 +	7.2%	8.2%	–10.8	74.1
Heart rate				
< 80	7.2%	8.5%	–83.2	464.9
80–99	9.2%	11.3%	–65.8	287.2
100 +	17.4%	20.7%	–51.7	238.6
Prior MI				
Yes	12.5%	14.1%	–43.7	322.4
No	8.9%	10.9%	–288.5	1001.9
Diabetes				
Yes	13.6%	17.3%	–41.4	145.7
No	8.7%	10.2%	–142.6	830.4
ALL PATIENTS	2820/29315 9.6%	3357/29285 11.5%	–269.5	1377.4

Odds ratio & CIs: Fibrinolytic better | Control better

18% SD 2 odds reduction
2P < 0.00001

0.5 1.0 1.5

FIGURE 24-12 • Proportional effects of fibrinolytic therapy on mortality during days 0 to 35 subdivided by presentation features. "Observed minus expected" (O–E) number of events among fibrinolytic-allocated patients (and its variance) is given for subdivisions of presentation features, stratified by trial. This is used to calculate the odds ratios (ORs) of death among patients allocated to fibrinolytic therapy versus that among those allocated as controls. ORs (*blue squares* with areas proportional to amount of "statistical information" contributed by the trials") are plotted with their 99% confidence intervals (CIs; *horizontal lines*). *Squares* to left of the solid vertical line indicate benefit (significant at $P < 0.01$ only where entire CI is to left of *vertical line*). Overall result and 95% CI represented by *diamond*, with overall proportional reduction in the odds of death and statistical significance given alongside. Chi-square tests for evidence of heterogeneity of, or trends in, size of ORs in subdivisions of each presentation feature are also given. (From Indications for fibrinolytic therapy in suspected acute myocardial infarction: collaborative overview of early mortality and major morbidity results from all randomised trials of more than 1000 patients. Fibrinolytic Therapy Trialists' (FTT) Collaborative Group. Lancet 1994;343:311-322.)

bundle branch block on ECG are conditions for which fibrinolytic therapy should be considered if no contraindication (Box 24-5) to its use is present. Patients with UA/NSTEMI, or those with STEMI who are asymptomatic with initial symptoms beginning more than 24 hours earlier, should not be considered for fibrinolytic therapy.

Randomized controlled trials of fibrinolytic therapy have demonstrated a survival benefit of initiating fibrinolytic therapy as early as possible after onset of ischemic symptoms. Mortality reduction from fibrinolytic therapy is greatest during the "golden" first hour after symptom onset (see Fig. 24-12); thereafter, a decline in benefit of approximately 1.6 lives per 1000 patients treated is seen per 1-hour delay.[54] Despite such strong evidence for benefit, reperfusion therapy continues to be underutilized and often is not administered soon after presentation.[54]

The choice of fibrinolytic agent may depend on a patient's risk of complications such as intracranial or other major bleeding, myocardial area at risk, time since symptom onset, availability of fibrinolytic agent, and local expertise. Accelerated alteplase and reteplase, when administered with IV heparin in patients with STEMI in the GUSTO-I[80] and GUSTO-III trials, were more effective than streptokinase in restoring early arterial patency, but were more expensive and associated with a slightly greater risk of intracranial hemorrhage (ICH).[81,82] Thus, in patients at low risk of ICH with a large area of injury or an anterior infarction who present early after symptom onset, alteplase or reteplase may have a better cost : benefit ratio.[3] Because of antigenic response to streptokinase, its reuse should be avoided, preferably indefinitely, because of a high prevalence of potentially neutralizing antibody titers. In patients at highest risk (approximately 10% of patients), including those with cardiogenic shock or heart failure, primary PCI should be considered.[3] Adjunctive antiplatelet and anticoagulant combination therapy with fibrinolytics (Fig. 24-13; see Box 24-4) is considered for

BOX 24-5 CONTRAINDICATIONS TO THE USE OF FIBRINOLYTIC THERAPY

Absolute

- Any prior intracranial hemorrhage
- Known structural cerebral vascular lesion (e.g., arteriovenous malformation)
- Known malignant intracranial neoplasm (primary or metastatic)
- Ischemic stroke within less than 3 months **EXCEPT** acute ischemic stroke within less than 3 hours
- Suspected aortic dissection
- Active bleeding or bleeding diathesis
- Significant closed-head or facial trauma within less than 3 months

Relative

- Severe uncontrolled hypertension
- History of prior ischemic stroke within greater than 3 months, dementia, or known intracranial pathology
- Traumatic or prolonged (>10 minutes) cardiopulmonary resuscitation or major surgery (within <3 weeks)
- Recent (<2 to 4 weeks) internal bleeding
- Noncompressible vascular punctures
- Prior exposure (>5 days ago) or allergic reaction to streptokinase/anistreplase
- Pregnancy
- Active peptic ulcer
- Current use of anticoagulants

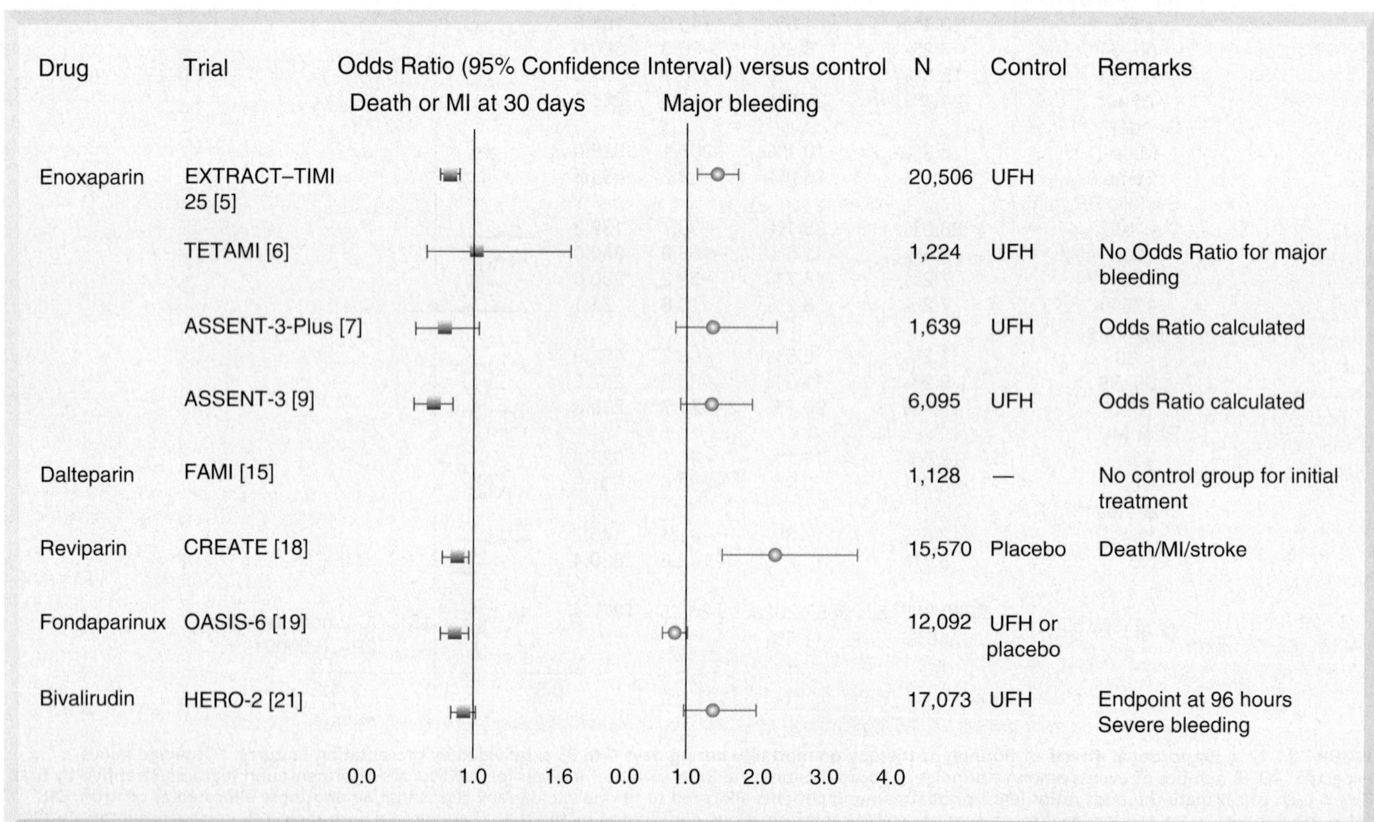

FIGURE 24-13 • Clinical outcomes of trials with anticoagulants including more than 1000 STEMI patients. Please note that trials are not directly comparable due to differences in trial design. (From Gurm HS, Eagle KA. Use of anticoagulants in ST-segment elevation myocardial infarction patients: a focus on low-molecular-weight heparin. Cardiovasc Drugs Ther, 2008;22:59-69.)

improvement in reperfusion flow, prevention of reinfarction, and other complications in high-risk STEMI patients such as those with anterior MI with no risk factors for bleeding (see "Antiplatelet Agents" and "Antithrombotic Agents [Anticoagulants]" sections). When combination therapy is used, the dose of fibrinolytic agent is reduced by 50%.

Facilitated PCI. Facilitated PCI refers to a strategy of planned immediate PCI after administration of an initial pharmacologic regimen intended to reduce thrombus burden and improve coronary patency before the procedure, thereby helping to avoid the adverse effects of long delays to PCI. Fibrinolytic agents, UFH, GP IIb/IIIa inhibitors, and the combination of a GP IIb/IIIa inhibitor with a reduced-dose (50% dose) fibrinolytic agent have been tested. Despite suggestions that earlier time to reperfusion, lower infarct artery thrombus burden, and better flow rates were achieved, major clinical trials of facilitated PCI (ASSENT-4 PCI)[83] and trials reported at the European Society of Cardiology Congress in 2007 (FINESSE and CARESS AMI) have not demonstrated any benefit in reducing infarct size or improving outcomes (death, heart failure, or shock), and facilitated PCI is currently not recommended.

Rescue PCI. Rescue angioplasty may be beneficial in patients with continuing pain or hemodynamic instability, or if very early fibrinolysis appears to have failed.[17] Some degree of resistance of thrombi to lysis can be expected in perhaps 10% to 15% of patients; the causes may include deep fissuring or rupture of the plaque or the presence of platelet-rich thrombus, which is very resistant to lysis. Adjunctive therapy with GP IIb/IIIa antagonists may enhance the safety and clinical outcome of rescue angioplasty.

Adverse Effects, Precautions, and Contraindications. Major bleeding complications of fibrinolytic therapy primarily include ICH and other moderate to severe bleeding that may or may not require transfusion. The excess risk of ICH occurs predominantly within the first day of therapy and appears to be limited to elderly patients (>75 years of age).[17] Fibrinolytic, anticoagulant, and antiplatelet therapies should be immediately discontinued and protamine sulfate and fresh frozen plasma administered to reverse the actions of heparin and replenish coagulation factors.

Invasive procedures, including intramuscular injections, should be avoided during and immediately before and after fibrinolytic administration. Gentamicin sensitivity is a specific exclusion for alteplase therapy, because gentamicin is used in the preparation of alteplase.[3] Allergic reactions and hypotension are more common with streptokinase, and it should not be used after a recent streptococcal infection or previous streptokinase use because of a high prevalence of potentially neutralizing antibody titers.[3]

Absolute and relative contraindications to the use of fibrinolytics are summarized in Box 24-5. They should not be given in pregnancy, particularly in the first 18 weeks, because of the risk of placental separation. Menstruation is not a contraindication.

Drug Interactions. Oral anticoagulants, heparin, and antiplatelet drugs may increase the risk of hemorrhage. The risk may also be increased with dextrans, and with other drugs that affect coagulation or platelet function. Heparin must not be given through the same IV line because of physical incompatibility.

Dosing. The dosing for commonly used fibrinolytic agents are summarized in Table 24-3.

Anti-ischemic Agents

The anti-ischemic drugs can be grouped as follows:

1. Nitrates
2. β-Adrenergic receptor antagonists
3. Calcium channel blockers
4. Nitric oxide donors
5. Ranolazine
6. Trimetazidine
7. Potassium channel openers
8. Specific bradycardic agents

Nitrates

Organic nitrates are the most commonly used anti-ischemic drugs in cardiovascular medicine.[84,85]

Mechanism of Action. Nitrates are nitric oxide (NO) donors that relax vascular smooth muscles by an endothelial-independent pathway acting through a soluble guanylate cyclase–mediated increase in cyclic guanosine monophosphate (cGMP) production, which relaxes smooth muscle cells by reduction in cytosolic calcium (Fig. 24-14). Nitrates act as anti-ischemic agents by relaxation of normal and atherosclerotic epicardial coronary arteries and arterioles (>100 μm) that improve blood flow, relieve spontaneous and exercise-induced coronary spasm, and promote dilation of collateral vessels, improving blood flow to the ischemic region and subepicardial-to-subendocardial flow redistribution. In addition, cardiac workload is reduced by decrease in preload (predominantly) and to some extent afterload, thus limiting myocardial oxygen demand, ischemia, and infarct size.[3]

The decrease in myocardial oxygen demand is in part offset by reflex increases in heart rate and contractility, which counteract the reductions in oxygen consumption unless a β-blocker is concurrently administered. Inhibition of platelet aggregation also occurs with nitroglycerin, but the clinical significance of this action is not well defined.

Pharmacokinetics. Nitrates are readily absorbed from the mucous membranes, skin, and GI tract; therefore various preparations with different routes of administration are available for clinical use. They have a large apparent volume of distribution and are taken up by smooth muscle cells, and the nitrate group is cleaved to inorganic nitrite and then to NO. This reaction requires the presence of cysteine or another thiol (see Fig. 24-14).

Sublingual nitroglycerin is available as tablets or a metered-dose spray. Peak pharmacologic action occurs within 2 minutes and continues for approximately 30 minutes.

Topical 2% nitroglycerin ointment applied to the skin has onset of action within 30 minutes and activity may last for over 24 hours with the timed-release preparation.

Intravenous nitroglycerin rapidly disappears from the blood with a half-life of only a few minutes, and is cleared by extrahepatic mechanisms and metabolism in the liver by glutathione–organic nitrate reductase that converts the parent molecule to longer acting and active dinitrates and mononitrates (see Fig. 24-14). The dinitrates are less potent vasodilators than glyceryl trinitrate and mononitrates.

Long-Acting Nitrates. Isosorbide 5-mononitrate has high bioavailability, as it does not undergo first-pass hepatic metabolism, with a half-life of 4 to 6 hours with renal excretion. Isosorbide dinitrate undergoes first-pass metabolism in the liver and is converted to the active mononitrates, with a slight delay in antianginal action (~4 minutes).

Therapeutic Considerations. In patients with stable or mixed angina, nitroglycerin (sublingually or as spray) relieves symptoms usually within minutes, and is recommended for the immediate relief of angina or for prophylaxis to avoid ischemic episodes before planned exercise, while long-acting preparations are indicated for reduction of symptoms when β-blockers are contraindicated or not successful (Box 24-6). The beneficial effect of sublingual (0.3 to 0.6 mg), topical, or oral (5 mg isosorbide dinitrate) nitrovasodilators as initial antianginal and anti-ischemic therapy, with improvement in symptoms, extent of myocardial perfusion defects, and exercise tolerance in patients with severe coronary atherosclerotic disease and endothelial dysfunction, has been demonstrated.[3] All long-acting nitrates appear to be equally effective when a sufficient nitrate-free interval is provided. Therapeutic effect is apparent within 1 to 3 minutes of IV or sublingual administration and within 30 to 60 minutes of transdermal patch application, lasting for 3 to 5 minutes for IV, 30 to 60 minutes for sublingual, and up to 8 hours for oral doses and transdermal patches. Tolerance develops during sustained therapy, but can be minimized with the use of rapid-release preparations, given twice daily in an eccentric pattern with doses spaced by 7 hours.[85,86]

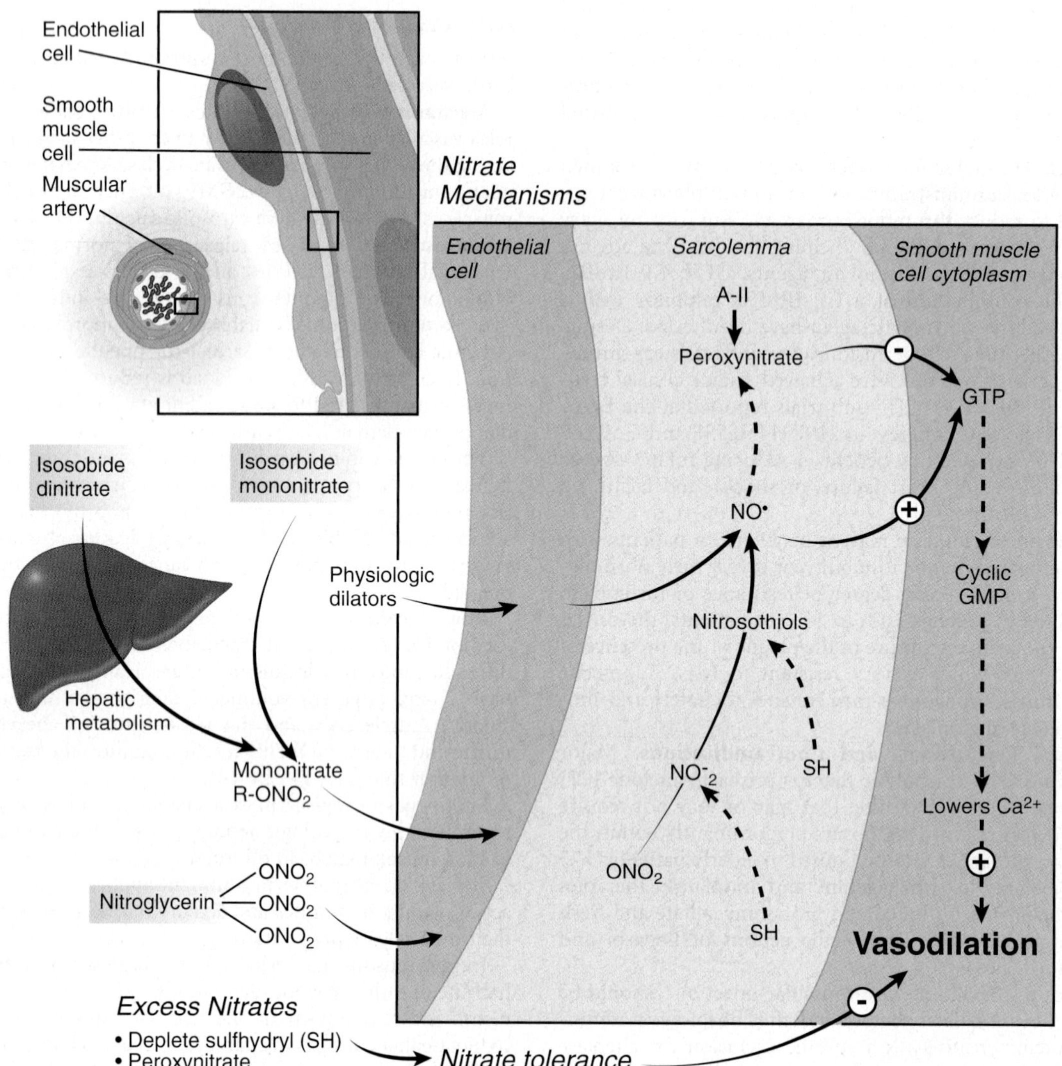

FIGURE 24-14 • Effects of nitrates in generating NO• and stimulating guanylate cyclase to cause vasodilation. Note role of cysteine cascade in stimulating guanylate cyclase. Previously SH depletion was thought to explain nitrate tolerance. Current emphasis is on the generation of peroxynitrite, which in turn inhibits the conversion of GTP to cyclic GMP. Note that mononitrates bypass hepatic metabolism. GMP, guanosine monophosphate; GTP, guanosine triphosphate; SH, sulfhydryl. (From Opie LH, Gersh BJ. Drugs for the Heart: Textbook with Online Updates, 6th ed. Amsterdam: Elsevier, 2004.)

In patients with variant or Prinzmetal's angina with vasospastic disease or in those who develop coronary spasm during angiography, nitroglycerin is highly effective in relieving the coronary spasm.[6]

In patients with UA/NSTEMI or STEMI with ongoing ischemic symptoms, nitroglycerin (0.4 mg) sublingually should be administered promptly. In the absence of symptom relief, the patient should be transferred to a medical care facility, while an additional two doses at 5-minute intervals can be considered in stable patients. For patients with persistent ischemia, heart failure, or hypertension after UA/NSTEMI or STEMI, IV nitroglycerin (5 to 10 mcg/min) should be initiated in the hospital (see Box 24-6), with gradual titration by 5 to 20 mcg/min every 5 to 10 minutes (up to 200 mcg/min) until symptoms are relieved or mean arterial blood pressure is reduced by 10% of baseline level in normotensives and up to 30% for hypertensives but not hypotensives (those with a systolic pressure of <90 mm Hg or a drop of ≥30 mm Hg below baseline). Tolerance to the hemodynamic effects of nitrates may develop after 24 hours of continuous therapy, requiring an increase in the infusion rate to maintain efficacy. After the relief of ischemia and symptom control, nitroglycerin infusion should be tapered over several hours to prevent exacerbation of ischemia with abrupt discontinuation. Beyond the first 48 hours after STEMI, nitrates are useful for the treatment of patients with recurrent angina or persistent heart failure if their use does not preclude therapy with β-blockers or ACE inhibitors. In the absence of continued or recurrent angina or heart failure after STEMI, continued use of nitroglycerin may be helpful, although the benefit is likely to be small and is not well established.[3]

Although routinely used, there are no randomized placebo-controlled trials of nitrate therapy in patients with UA/NSTEMI to assess its efficacy on mortality reduction, symptom relief, or decrease in cardiac events. In patients with STEMI, a pooled analysis of more than 80,000 patients treated with nitrate-like preparations used acutely and continued subsequently in 22 trials, including the ISIS-4[87] and GISSI-3[88] trials, revealed only a modest reduction in mortality compared to control. Nitrates should not be administered to STEMI or UA/NSTEMI patients with hypotension (systolic blood pressure <90 mm Hg or ≥30 mm Hg below baseline), severe bradycardia (<50 bpm), tachycardia (>100 bpm) in the absence of symptomatic heart failure, RV infarction, or those who have used a phosphodiesterase inhibitor for erectile dysfunction within the preceding 24 to 48 hours (see Box 24-6).[6] Patients with RV infarction are particularly dependent on adequate RV preload to maintain cardiac output and may experience hypotension during administration of nitrates.[6]

BOX 24-6 RECOMMENDATIONS FOR THERAPY WITH NITRATES IN CORONARY ARTERY DISEASE

Class I

- Sublingual ***nitroglycerin*** or nitroglycerin spray for the *immediate relief of angina* (LoE: B).
- ***Long-acting nitrates*** as initial therapy for reduction of *angina when β-blockers are contraindicated or not successful* (LoE: B).
- In patients presenting with **STEMI** or **UA/NSTEMI** with *ongoing ischemic symptoms*, ***nitroglycerin*** 0.4 mg sublingually every 5 minutes for three doses should be given, followed by assessment for IV nitroglycerin (LoE: C).
- For patients with *persistent ischemia, heart failure, or hypertension* after ***STEMI*** or **UA/NSTEMI,** use IV ***nitroglycerin*** for first 48 hours (LoE: B).
- IV, oral, or topical ***nitrates*** are useful beyond the first 48 hours after **STEMI** for treatment of *recurrent angina or persistent heart failure* if their use does not preclude therapy with β-blockers or ACE inhibitors (LoE: B).

Class IIb

- Continued use of nitrate therapy *more than 24 to 48 hours after MI in the absence of continued or recurrent angina or heart failure* may be helpful, although the benefit is likely to be small and is not well established in contemporary practice (LoE: B).

Class III

- Nitrates should *not be administered* to **STEMI** or **UA/NSTEMI** patients with systolic BP less than 90 mm Hg or ≥30 mm Hg below baseline, severe bradycardia (<50 bpm), tachycardia (>100 bpm) in the absence of symptomatic heart failure, or right ventricular infarction (LoE: C).
- Nitroglycerin or other nitrates should *not be administered* to patients with **STEMI** or **UA/NSTEMI** who had received a phosphodiesterase inhibitor for erectile dysfunction within 24 hours (sildenafil) or 48 hours (tadalafil) of use. The suitable time for the administration of nitrates after vardenafil has not been determined (LoE: C).

ACE, angiotensin-converting enzyme; BP, blood pressure; bpm, beats per minute; IV, intravenous; LoE, level of evidence; MI, myocardial infarction; NSTEMI, non–ST-elevation myocardial infarction; STEMI, ST-elevation myocardial infarction; UA, unstable angina.

In patients with cocaine-induced STEMI or UA/NSTEMI, nitroglycerin and calcium channel blockers are recommended as they effectively reverse cocaine-induced hypertension, vasoconstriction, and tachycardia.[3]

In patients with acute or chronic heart failure, nitrate therapy is useful for the relief of symptoms with preload reduction, particularly in those with pulmonary congestion. In patients with severe heart failure who cannot tolerate an ACE inhibitor, a nitrate-hydralazine combination should be used[3] as the combination therapy has been shown to be better than placebo in decreasing mortality.[6] In moderate to severe (New York Heart Association [NYHA] classes III and IV) heart failure patients of African descent, a hydralazine–isosorbide dinitrate combination should be added to standard therapy based on the results of the African-American Heart Failure Trial (A-HeFT)[89] demonstrating a significant reduction in mortality and heart failure hospitalizations and improved quality-of-life scores compared to those treated with standard care.

Adverse Effects, Precautions, and Contraindications. A common side effect of nitrates is the development of headache and flushing (Table 24-4) with sublingual administration and at the start of therapy with long-acting formulations, which may be dose limiting. Concomitant treatment with aspirin may help. Hypotension is also common with initiation of nitrates, particularly in volume-depleted patients, those on diuretics, or those with RV failure, and initiation of a low-dose IV nitroglycerin infusion with gradual dose titration in response to arterial pressure should be considered. In patients with suspected RV infarction or in those who have used a phosphodiesterase inhibitor for erectile dysfunction within the last 24 hours (48 hours for tadalafil), nitrates should not be administered (see Box 24-6) as the hypotensive effects of nitrates could be potentiated by NO increasing cGMP.[6,90]

Nitroglycerin and nitrates are relatively contraindicated in patients with hypertrophic obstructive cardiomyopathy, because nitrates can increase LV outflow tract obstruction and severity of mitral regurgitation, precipitating presyncope or syncope. Similarly, in patients with severe aortic valve stenosis, nitroglycerin should be avoided.[3]

Nitrate tolerance, resulting in reduced therapeutic response, may occur with all nitrate preparations presumably through depletion of sulfhydryl groups in the vessel wall and inhibition of NO synthase and vascular mitochondrial superoxide and/or peroxynitrite production. A nitrate-free interval of at least 10 to 12 hours can enhance treatment efficacy. When nitrates cannot be discontinued, even for a short time, higher doses may be required to compensate for nitrate tolerance.

Other rare side effects include halitosis with sublingual nitrates. Methemoglobinemia may occur with prolonged high-dose therapy and requires discontinuation of nitrates and at times IV methylene blue (1 to 2 mg/kg over 5 minutes). Nitroglycerin tablets may lose efficacy with time and should be kept in airtight containers. Nitrate sprays are inflammable.

Drug Interactions. Hypotension can be exaggerated by use of nitrates with diuretics, hydralazine, ACE inhibitors, calcium channel blockers, β-blockers, or phosphodiesterase-5 inhibitors. Phosphodiesterase degrades cGMP, which mediates the vascular smooth muscle relaxation by NO. Therefore, phosphodiesterase inhibitors particularly potentiate the hypotensive effects of nitrates due to exaggerated vasodilation and refractory hypotension, and MI or even death may occur. Nitrates should not be administered to patients who have used a phosphodiesterase inhibitor for erectile dysfunction in the prior 24 to 48 hours.[90] In cases of refractory hypotension with inadvertent use of nitrates with phosphodiesterase inhibitors, an α-adrenergic agonist or norepinephrine should be considered.[3]

Dosing. Sublingual nitroglycerin 0.4 mg should be administered for angina and repeated at 5-minute intervals for three doses if symptoms persist.

Topical nitroglycerin ointment, applied to the skin as a 1- to 2-inch measured dose every 4 to 6 hours, or 7.5 to 10 mg/12-hr skin patches, removed after 12 hours, can be used for patients unable to take oral medications.

Intravenous nitroglycerin can be initiated at 5 to 10 mcg/min with increases of 5 to 20 mcg/min until symptoms are relieved or mean arterial blood pressure is reduced by 10% of baseline level in normotensives and by up to 30% for hypertensive patients, but not below systolic pressure of 90 mm Hg or a drop of ≥30 mm Hg below baseline.

Long-Acting Nitrates. Sustained-release isosorbide 5-mononitrate permits once-daily (120 to 240 mg) dosing. Isosorbide dinitrate is administered at 30 mg at 7 A.M. and 1 P.M., with a 12-hour nitrate-free interval to avoid the development of nitrate tolerance.

β-Adrenergic Receptor Antagonists

Sir James Black, who was awarded the 1988 Nobel Price in Medicine, initially designed β-adrenergic receptor blockers, which revolutionized the medical management of angina pectoris. His work led to the development of propranolol, the prototype β-blocker.

Mechanism of Action. β-Blockers competitively inhibit catecholamine effects at the β-adrenergic receptors, preventing catecholamine-mediated increase in myocardial contractility (negative inotropic effect) and in heart rate through sinus node automaticity (negative chronotropic effect) and conduction over the atrioventricular (AV) node (negative dromotropic effect). They also decrease systolic blood pressure. Thus, overall cardiac workload and oxygen consumption are reduced, an effect that is beneficial in patients with CHD by reducing frequency of ischemic symptoms, myocardial wall stress, infarct size, and electrophysiologic instability. Slowing of heart rate providing longer diastolic time also helps improve subendocardial myocardial perfusion. Most of the β-blockers in clinical use are *pure antagonists*;

TABLE 24-4 CARDIAC DRUG SIDE EFFECTS*

Drug	Toxic Side Effects	General Side Effects	Hypersensitivity	Safe Use in Pregnancy
Angiotensin II antagonists	Hypotension, **renal failure, hyperkalemia**	Headache	Hepatitis, angioedema (rare, cross reaction with ACE inhibitor)	No (D)
ACE inhibitors	Renal failure, hypotension, hyperkalemia, hepatitis	**Cough**, skin rashes, taste disturbance	**Angioedema**, skin rash, bone marrow suppression, hepatitis, alveolitis	No (D)
β-Blockers	**Bradycardia, bronchospasm, hypotension**, heart failure	Raynaud's phenomenon, impotence, increased serum glucose/lipid levels	None	Yes (B, C)†
Calcium channel blockers‡	**Hypotension, end-organ ischemia ("steal syndrome")—nifedipine IR, bradycardia with verapamil or diltiazem**	Dizziness, flushing, peripheral edema, constipation, postural hypotension, taste disturbances	Verapamil, nifedipine, diltiazem: skin eruption, liver and kidney function defects, fever, eosinophilia, lymphadenopathy, maculopapular rash	Unknown (C)
Digoxin	Cardiovascular (**heart block**, ectopic proarrhythmias, ventricular extra beats, ventricular tachycardia, **paroxysmal atrial tachycardia**)	GI (anorexia, nausea, vomiting, diarrhea) CNS (drowsiness, dizziness, confusion, **vision abnormalities**, photophobia) with toxicity	Rare: thrombocytopenia, rash	May be used therapeutically for fetal arrhythmias (C)
Loop diuretics	Dehydration, pancreatitis, jaundice, **deafness (high dose)**, thrombocytopenia, **gout**	Dizziness, postural hypotension, hyponatremia, hypokalemia	Interstitial nephritis, skin reactions (erythema multiforme, Stevens-Johnson syndrome, tissue necrosis)	Use with caution (C)
Nitrates	**Hypotension**, transient ischemic attacks, peripheral edema, methemoglobinemia	**Headache**, flushing, palpitations	Contact irritation, allergic contact dermatitis	Unknown (C)
Potassium-sparing diuretics§	**Hyperkalemia**, dehydration	Rashes, **gynecomastia in men** (spironolactone) and breast enlargement/soreness in women§	Skin reactions	Unknown, amiloride (B)

***Boldface** type signifies more prevalence or more severe reactions.
†Metoprolol, atenolol, and labetalol may be used in late pregnancy (JNC VII).
‡Unproven association with internal malignancy.
§Possible association with breast carcinoma and antiandrogenic effect.
ACE, angiotensin-converting enzyme; B, C, D, U.S. Food and Drug Administration pregnancy safety categories; CNS, central nervous system effects; GI, gastrointestinal effects; IR, immediate release; JNC VII, recommendations of the Seventh Joint National Committee on Hypertension.
Modified from Ou NN, Oyen LJ, Murphy JG, Jahangir A. *In* Murphy JG, Lloyd MA (eds): Mayo Clinic Cardiology: Concise Textbook, 3rd ed. Rochester: Mayo Clinic Scientific Press/Informa Healthcare, 2007, pp. 1291-1308.

that is, by occupying a β receptor, they prevent the receptor from being stimulated by agonists. Some β-blockers (pindolol and acebutolol), are *partial agonists*; that is, in addition to β-blockade, they also possess *intrinsic sympathomimetic activity*, which causes weak β-adrenergic activation. New-generation β-blockers, such as carvedilol, labetalol, and bucindolol, have additional α-adrenergic receptor blockade causing vasodilation. Carvedilol and its metabolites are also cardioprotective by their antioxidant and antiproliferative effects, inhibiting free radical–induced activation of transcription factors and programmed cell death. D-Propranolol and carvedilol have additional quinidine-like membrane-stabilizing (class I antiarrhythmic) effects, whereas D-sotalol also possesses class III antiarrhythmic properties. Some of the clinical effects of individual β-blockers may be due to effects independent of β-adrenergic blockade; therefore, these drugs should not be considered interchangeable for all applications.

Pharmacokinetics. The pharmacokinetics of various β-adrenergic blockers is summarized in Table 24-5. Most β-blockers are well absorbed after oral administration, with peak concentration occurring 1 to 3 hours after ingestion. β-Blockers exhibit different degrees of protein binding and lipid solubility (Fig. 24-15; see Table 24-5). Lipid-soluble β-blockers, such as propranolol and metoprolol, are primarily metabolized by the liver and have relatively shorter plasma half-lives compared to hydrophilic β-blockers, such as atenolol and nadolol, which are cleared by the kidney and tend to have longer plasma half-lives. The elimination half-life of β-blockers varies from 9 minutes for esmolol to 24 hours for nadolol. At lower concentrations, β-blockers exhibit various degrees of cardiac selectivity (i.e., affinity for β_1 versus β_2 receptors), but this selectivity can be overcome if large doses are used.

Therapeutic Considerations. The ACC/AHA guidelines for the use of β-blockers in patients with CHD are summarized in Box 24-7.

In patients with chronic stable angina, β-blockers reduce the frequency of anginal episodes and improve exercise tolerance. With nitrates and antiplatelet agents (aspirin and/or clopidogrel), β-blockers form the standard treatment for effort and mixed angina. The treatment is usually initiated with a β-blocker and a nitrate or a calcium channel blocker and then continued as combined triple therapy for additive effects while monitoring for adverse side effects. When used alone, β-blockers are superior to nitrates and calcium channel blockers in reducing angina symptoms as well as episodes of silent ischemia.[91] All β-blockers are potentially equally effective in angina pectoris, and in patients who do not have concomitant disease, any of the β-blockers could be used. A meta-analysis of large multicenter clinical trials demonstrated the beneficial effect of β-blockers in delaying ischemic

TABLE 24-5 PHARMACOKINETICS OF β-ADRENERGIC RECEPTOR ANTAGONISTS

	Bioavailability (%)	Protein Binding (%)	Time to Peak Action after Oral Intake (hr)	Elimination Half-Life (hr)	Route of Major Elimination
Acebutolol	70	25	3-8	3-10	Hepatic (renal)
Bucindolol			0.5-1.6	2-7	Hepatic
Carvedilol	30	95	1.0-1.5	7-10	Hepatic
Labetalol	30	50	2-4 (5 min IV)	3-6	Hepatic (renal)
Metoprolol	50	10	1-2	3-6	Hepatic
Timolol	50	10	1-2	4-5	Hepatic
Propranolol	35	90	1-2	3-5	Hepatic
Esmolol	(100 IV)	55	(2-5 min IV)	9 min	Blood esterase (renal)
Atenolol	50	15	2-4 (10 min IV)	6-9	Renal
Bisoprolol	80	30	2-4	9-12	Renal (hepatic)
Nadolol	30	30	3-4	14-24	Renal
Pindolol	90	55	1-3	3-4	Renal (hepatic)
Sotalol	100	0	2-4	10-15	Renal

IV, intravenous.

Beta-Blockers

	Relative β_1 Selectivity	β_1 Blockade Potency Ratio (Propranolol=1.0)	Lipid Solubility	Intrinsic Sympathomimetic Activity	Other Effects	Other Antiarrhythmic Class Effect
Cardioselective						
Acebutalol	+	0.3	+	$+\beta_1$		I
Atenolol	++	1.0	–	–		–
Bisoprolol	+	5–10	+			–
Esmolol	++	0.03	+	–		–
Metoprolol	++	1.0	++	–		I
Noncardioselective						
Bucindolol		3.0	+	+	α_1 block	
Carvedilol		2–4	+	–	α_1 block antioxidant	I
Labetalol		0.3	++	β_2	α_1 block	I
Nadolol		1.0	–	–		–
Pindolol		6.0	++	++		I
Propranolol		1.0	+++	–		I
Timolol		6.0	+	±		
Sotalol		0.3	–	–		III

FIGURE 24-15 • β-Blockers: relative cardioselectivity, potency, lipid solubility intrinsic sympathomimetic activity, and membrane-stabilizing properties. +, low; ++, moderate; +++, high; ISA, intrinsic sympathomimetic activity; I, class I antiarrhythmic effect or sodium channel blockade; III, class III or potassium channel blockade.

threshold and reducing angina aggravation and the onset of angina during exercise, yet reduction in new MI or death in patients with chronic stable angina who do not have a previous MI has not been demonstrated.[3] Performance during exercise stress testing for the diagnosis of suspected CAD may be influenced by the use of β-blockers, which reduce the sensitivity of the test to detect myocardial ischemia, but β-blockers should not be discontinued abruptly in these patients. In patients with pure vasospastic (Prinzmetal's) angina, β-blockers may increase coronary spasm from unopposed α-adrenergic activity and are therefore not indicated.

In patients with UA/NSTEMI, insufficient data from randomized trials are available to fully assess the efficacy of β-blockers in the acute or chronic phase, but the proven efficacy in patients with STEMI, congestive heart failure, and angina and pathophysiologic considerations have led to the recommendation for their use in ACS (see Box 24-7). In patients presenting acutely with UA/NSTEMI, IV β-blocker therapy should be reserved for only those with ongoing rest pain, especially with tachycardia or hypertension, and should be avoided in those with heart failure, hemodynamic instability, or other contraindications (see Box 24-7). There are no comparative studies in this setting between different β-blockers; therefore, patients with a favorable pharmacokinetics and side effect profile should be selected, while avoiding those with intrinsic sympathomimetic activity. The duration of benefit with long-term oral therapy is uncertain and likely varies with the extent of revascularization and LV dysfunction.[92] In patients with compensated heart failure or LV systolic dysfunction, oral β-blockers should be initiated before hospital discharge, with a gradual titration scheme long term.[92] An overview of initial double-blind, randomized trials of β-blocker therapy in patients with threatening or evolving MI conducted prior to the routine use of aspirin, clopidogrel, heparin, GP IIb/IIIa inhibitors, and revascularization suggested an approximately 13% reduction in the risk of progression to MI, but the effect on mortality could not be assessed due to the limited statistical power.[92] In a pooled analysis of GP IIb/IIIa receptor blockers in patients

BOX 24-7 RECOMMENDATIONS FOR THERAPY WITH β-BLOCKERS IN CORONARY ARTERY DISEASE

Class I

- Start and continue indefinitely in all patients with **STEMI, UA/NSTEMI,** or **LV dysfunction** with or without heart failure symptoms, *unless contraindicated* (LoE: A).
- In patients *recovering from* **UA/NSTEMI** or **STEMI** with *moderate to severe LV failure*, β-blocker should be initiated with a gradual titration scheme (LoE: B).
- ***Oral β-blockers*** should be *initiated in the first 24 hours* of **STEMI** and **UA/NSTEMI** in patients who do not have any of the following (LoE: B):
  - signs of heart failure
  - evidence of a low output state
  - risk for cardiogenic shock (age >70 years, systolic BP < 120 mm Hg, heart rate >110 or <60 bpm, and increased time since onset of symptoms)
  - other relative contraindications to β blockade (PR interval >0.24 seconds, second- or third-degree heart block, active asthma, or reactive airways disease)
- Patients with *early contraindications within the first 24 hours of* **STEMI** should be re-evaluated for candidacy for β-blocker therapy as secondary prevention (LoE: C).

Class IIa

- It is reasonable to prescribe β-blockers in patients *recovering from* **UA/NSTEMI** *with low-risk profile* (normal LV function, revascularized, no high-risk features) in the absence of absolute contraindications (LoE: B).
- It is reasonable to give an ***IV β-blocker*** in **STEMI** and **UA/NSTEMI** patients at the time of presentation who are *hypertensive* and do not have any of the following (LoE: B):
  - signs of heart failure
  - evidence of a low output state
  - risk for cardiogenic shock (age >70 years, systolic BP < 120 mm Hg, heart rate >110 or <60 bpm, and increased time since onset of symptoms)
  - other relative contraindications to β blockade (PR interval >0.24 seconds, second- or third-degree heart block, active asthma, or reactive airways disease)

Class III

- ***IV β-blockers*** should *not be administered* to **STEMI** patients who have any of the following (LoE: A):
  - signs of heart failure
  - evidence of a low output state
  - risk for cardiogenic shock (age >70 years, systolic BP < 120 mm Hg, heart rate >110 or <60 bpm, and increased time since onset of symptoms)
  - other relative contraindications to β blockade (PR interval >0.24 seconds, second- or third-degree heart block, active asthma, or reactive airways disease)

BP, blood pressure; bpm, beats per minute; IV, intravenous; LoE, level of evidence; LV, left ventricular; NSTEMI, non–ST-elevation myocardial infarction; STEMI, ST-elevation myocardial infarction; UA, unstable angina.

undergoing PCI for ACS, however, the protective effect of β-blocker therapy on mortality at 30 days and 6 months was demonstrated.

In patients presenting with STEMI, β-blockers should be initiated early in the course unless contraindicated and continued in the absence of adverse effects (see Box 24-7). The early administration of β-blockers during the acute phase, with or without concomitant fibrinolytic therapy, decreases the risk of sudden death, reinfarction, and recurrent ischemia.[93] In patients with suspected MI not receiving fibrinolytic therapy, the immediate IV administration of a β-blocker followed by an oral maintenance β-blocker in the Atenolol in ISIS-I and the Metoprolol in Acute Myocardial Infarction (MIAMI) trials significantly reduced short-term mortality compared with those given placebo.[94,95] A meta-analysis of trials from the prefibrinolytic era (>24,000 patients receiving β-blockers in the convalescent phase) showed a reduction in mortality at 7 days (14% relative risk reduction) and long term (23% relative risk reduction) (Fig. 24-16). The mortality difference was evident early (within 24 hours) and was sustained. The mechanism for this is unclear but may be related to the prevention of cardiac rupture and ventricular arrhythmias.[3] It is reasonable to administer IV β-blocker therapy within 24 hours of hospitalization for STEMI when hypertension is present and the patient is not at an increased risk of cardiogenic shock based on the risk factors as defined in Box 24-7. Patients with sinus tachycardia or atrial fibrillation should have LV function assessed before administration of IV β-blockers. After 24 hours, in patients who are free of contraindications, oral β-blockers should be continued indefinitely in those at high risk (low ejection fraction and heart failure), with gradual dose titration.

In STEMI patients receiving concomitant fibrinolytic therapy, IV administration of β-blockers in the absence of contraindications to their use reduced reinfarction and recurrent ischemia in earlier trials. However, in those presenting with STEMI and heart failure or hemodynamic instability, an early IV β-blocker is not recommended (see Box 24-7). The benefits of early use of IV β-blockers were not confirmed in recent trials.[5,6,96] In the COMMIT study, a large trial of mostly STEMI (93%) patients, no overall survival benefit was demonstrated by early IV followed by oral metoprolol.[96] A modest reduction in reinfarction and ventricular fibrillation by β-blocker therapy was counterbalanced by an increase in cardiogenic shock in those presenting with early heart failure, hemodynamic instability, or risk factors for shock (time delay, higher Killip class, older age, female sex, hypotension, tachycardia, and previous hypertension). A moderate net benefit was present in those who were relatively stable and at low risk of shock. Early (<24 hours) oral β-blocker therapy is recommended for patients not at high risk for complications, especially with ongoing pain, tachycardia, or hypertension (see Box 24-7). Patients with contraindications within the first 24 hours of STEMI should be re-evaluated for candidacy for β-blocker therapy as secondary prevention.

In patients with STEMI undergoing PCI, randomized trials of β-blocker therapy have not been performed. However, such therapy seems reasonable as its beneficial effect was documented in the Carvedilol Post-Infarct Survival Controlled Evaluation (CAPRICORN), which included patients undergoing revascularization with either PCI or thrombolytics.[97]

In high-risk patients surviving MI, the chronic long-term use of β-blockers for secondary prophylaxis or symptom control in those with recurrent ischemia, a large or anterior infarct, ventricular dysfunction, or cardiac arrhythmias decreases all-cause mortality, sudden death, and reinfarction by about 25%. These beneficial effects have been shown in patients who did or did not receive concomitant fibrinolytic therapy (see Fig. 24-16) and are of special benefit in those with ongoing or recurrent ischemia, infarct extension, or tachyarrhythmias.[3] In those with bradycardia or mild to moderate heart failure, a β-blocker should be initiated after 24 to 48 hours of freedom from such a relative contraindication. Propranolol, atenolol, timolol, metoprolol, and carvedilol have been shown to be effective in reducing sudden and nonsudden cardiac death, an effect that is more striking in the setting of reduced LV function.[3] The beneficial effects of β-blockers in post-MI patients with asymptomatic LV dysfunction appear to be additive to those of ACE inhibitors in reducing the risk of cardiovascular mortality by 30% and development of heart failure by 21%.[3] The benefits of β-blockers are greatest in the first year after MI compared with the second and third years with ACE inhibitors.[3] The beneficial survival effect is maintained in post-MI patients with coexisting diabetes mellitus and heart failure. The nonselective β-blockers without intrinsic sympathomimetic activity appear to have a larger effect on mortality reduction than selective β-blockers. The mechanism of protection by β blockade in these patients is not clear and may be related to electrophysiologic and anti-ischemic effects.

In low-risk patients surviving MI (without previous infarction, anterior infarction, advanced age, ventricular dysrhythmias, or ventricular dysfunction), long-term prognosis is good, and it is not clear whether

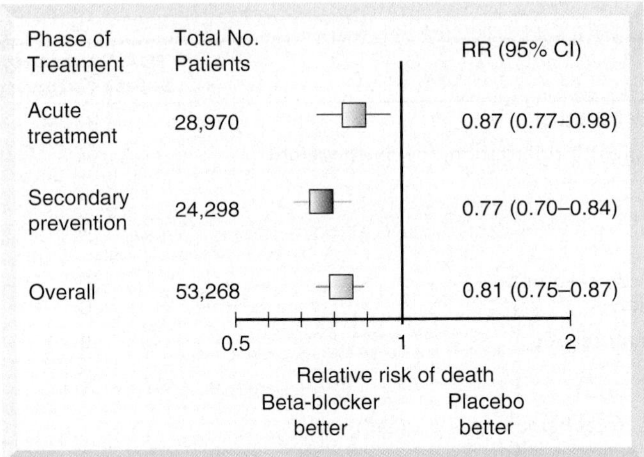

FIGURE 24-16 • Summary of data from meta-analysis of trials of β-blocker therapy from the prefibrinolytic era in patients with myocardial infarction. CI, confidence interval; No., number; RR, relative risk. (From Antman EM, Braunwald E. Acute myocardial infarction. *In* Braunwald E, Zipes DP, Libby P [eds]: Heart Disease: A Textbook of Cardiovascular Medicine, 6th ed. Philadelphia: WB Saunders, 2001, p 1168.)

BOX 24-8 CONTRAINDICATIONS TO β-BLOCKER THERAPY

Absolute

- Severe bradycardia
- Severe conduction system disease (sinus node dysfunction or high-grade AV block)
- Overt ventricular failure
- Severe asthma or active bronchospasm
- Severe peripheral vascular disease with rest ischemia
- Severe depression

Relative

- PR interval greater than 0.24 seconds
- Systolic arterial pressure less than 100 mm Hg
- Signs of peripheral hypoperfusion
- Raynaud's phenomenon
- Pure vasospastic angina
- Insulin-dependent diabetes mellitus with frequent hypoglycemic reactions
- Mild asthma or severe COPD
- Excessive fatigue
- Hyperlipidemia
- Impotence
- Pregnancy

AV, atrioventricular; COPD, chronic obstructive pulmonary disease.

adding β-blockers to their therapy improves outcome. However, because β-blockers are well tolerated and have several potential beneficial effects, their use in this low-risk patient population is also recommended (see Box 24-7). Therapy with β-blockers should be continued for at least 2 to 3 years following MI and longer if well tolerated, although long-term data are lacking. Despite the proven value of β-blocker use in secondary prevention in post-MI patients, these agents are still underused and should be considered for all patients after infarction, unless clearly contraindicated (Box 24-8).

In patients with cocaine-induced STEMI or UA/NSTEMI, β-blockers should be avoided due to concern regarding β blockade–mediated coronary arterial vasoconstriction. Calcium channel blockers and nitroglycerin are preferred as they can reverse cocaine-induced coronary arterial vasoconstriction, hypertension, or tachycardia.[3]

In patients with congestive heart failure, β-blockers (metoprolol, carvedilol, and bucindolol) attenuate the detrimental effects of the activation of the sympathetic nervous system and the chronic hyperadrenergic state. The collective experience from more than 10,000 patients with heart failure participating in more than 20 published placebo-controlled clinical trials documents their beneficial effects on hemodynamics, ventricular function, symptoms, overall well-being, and quality of life, along with reduction in the risk of worsening heart failure, death, and hospitalization.[3] A reduction in the risk of mortality in patients with heart failure has been demonstrated with nonselective vasodilating (carvedilol) and β_1-selective (metoprolol and bisoprolol) β-blockers.[92] When switching treatment from one β-blocker to another, improvement of LV function in patients with heart failure is maintained. The time course of improvement of LV function by β blockade exceeds 12 months of therapy, irrespective of the β-blocker used. These effects are thought to occur through the prevention of catecholamine toxicity and improved myocardial energetics. β-Blockers are more likely to have an effect on patients with severe heart failure who have greater sympathetic activation and a higher resting heart rate than on patients with slower heart rates.

Heart failure patients with preserved systolic function, low heart rates (<65 bpm), or low systolic blood pressure (<85 mm Hg) and those with decompensated heart failure or NYHA class IV symptoms either were not recruited or represented only a small proportion of the patients enrolled in clinical trials; therefore, data regarding efficacy and safety in these patients are not available. In those with decompensated heart failure, systolic blood pressure less than 80 mm Hg, or signs of peripheral hypoperfusion or dependence on intravenous inotropic agents, β-blockers should not be used. Otherwise, β-blockers (only carvedilol and long-acting metoprolol are approved in the United States) should be prescribed to all patients with stable heart failure unless a contraindication to their use is present (see Box 24-8).

In patients with diastolic ventricular dysfunction with preserved systolic function, such as the elderly, hypertensives, or those with hypertropic cardiomyopathy, β-blockers are beneficial in reducing symptoms of heart failure by slowing the heart rate and improving ventricular filling and stroke volume, especially with development of atrial fibrillation with rapid ventricular rate response or myocardial ischemia.

Adverse Effects, Precautions, and Contraindications. The absolute and relative contraindications to β-blocker use are summarized in Box 24-8. Most of the cardiac side effects of β-blockers are related to their negative chronotropic, dromotropic, and inotropic properties, causing sinus bradycardia or AV conduction block in patients with sinus node dysfunction or conduction disease. In patients with ventricular systolic dysfunction, heart failure may occur; however, with proper dose titration and monitoring, β-blockers are beneficial in the long term. In patients with ischemic heart disease, abrupt discontinuation of β-blockers after chronic use should be avoided to prevent myocardial ischemia (withdrawal syndrome) because of possible rebound hypersensitivity to physiologic adrenergic stimulation with "up-regulation" of the number of β-adrenergic receptors during chronic blockade. β-Blockers should not be administered to patients with STEMI precipitated by cocaine use because of the risk of exacerbating coronary spasm. Other adverse effects, particularly with a nonselective β-blocker, include bronchospasm in patients with a history of asthma, easy fatigability, decreased exercise capacity, sedation, sleep disturbances, hallucination, depression, and rarely psychotic reactions. Impotence and worsening of symptoms due to severe peripheral vascular or vasospastic disorders may occur.

Because of the overall beneficial effects of β-blockers in diabetic patients, their use should not be avoided due to concerns regarding masking of hypoglycemia symptoms in those requiring insulin therapy or exacerbation of glucose intolerance or insulin resistance. In liver disease or low-output states, the dose of hepatically metabolized drugs (see Table 24-5) should be decreased; sotalol, atenolol, and nadolol dosing needs to be adjusted in patients with renal impairment. The safety of β-blocker use during pregnancy has not been well established, and the potential benefit should be weighed against the risk to the fetus (low birth weight) (Table 24-6).

Drug Interactions. β-Blockers should be used with caution in conjunction with drugs that slow conduction (digitalis and calcium

TABLE 24-6 CARDIOVASCULAR DRUGS IN PREGNANCY

Drug Class	Adverse Fetal Effects	FDA Pregnancy Safety Category
ACE inhibitors/ARBs	Fetal abnormalities, renal defects, may be lethal	D
β-Blockers	Bradycardia, neonatal hypoglycemia, growth retardation, low birth weight	C
Ca^{2+} channel blockers	? Fetal abnormalities	C
Digoxin	—	C
Diuretics		
Furosemide	Electrolyte imbalance, increased fetal urine output	C
Thiazide	? Birth defects, bone marrow depression	D
Nitrates	None (may be useful in delaying premature labor)	B
Anticoagulants		D
Heparin	(preferable anticoagulant)	
Warfarin	Birth defects, fetal warfarin syndrome, fetal hemorrhage or death	
Lipid-lowering drugs		
Statins	Toxic	X
Gemfibrozil	? Birth defects	C
Cholestyramine		B

ACE, angiotensin-converting enzyme; ARBs, angiotensin II receptor blockers; FDA, U.S. Food and Drug Administration.
Modified from Ou NN, Oyen LJ, Murphy JG, Jahangir A. *In* Murphy JG, Lloyd MA (eds): Mayo Clinic Cardiology: Concise Textbook, 3rd ed. Rochester: Mayo Clinic Scientific Press/Informa Healthcare, 2007, pp. 1291-1308.

channel blockers) and those that have negative inotropic effects (calcium channel blockers and disopyramide). Levels of hepatically metabolized β-blockers (propranolol, metoprolol, carvedilol, labetalol) are increased by cimetidine and verapamil. β-Blockers, by decreasing hepatic flow, may affect blood levels of drugs such as lidocaine that are primarily metabolized in the liver.

Dosing. All β-blockers have about the same antianginal and anti-ischemic efficacy at comparable doses, and no one agent is superior to others at equipotent doses. The usual daily dosages of various β-blockers are summarized in Table 24-7.

In patients presenting acutely with STEMI or UA/NSTEMI, unless contraindicated (see Box 24-8), metoprolol may be given in 5-mg increments by slow IV administration (over 1 to 2 minutes), repeated every 5 minutes for a total dose of 15 mg, followed in 15 minutes by oral therapy at 25 to 50 mg every 6 hours for 48 hours and then a maintenance dose of up to 100 mg twice daily. The dose may need to be adjusted to reduce the heart rate to 55 to 60 bpm at rest and to limit the increase in heart rate during exercise to less than 75% of the rate response associated with onset of ischemia (or <100 bpm). In an individual patient, ancillary properties such as β_1-adrenergic receptor selectivity, lipid solubility, vasodilation, intrinsic sympathomimetic activity, longer half-life, and cost may affect selection of one agent over the others. Cardioselective agents are preferable in patients with chronic lung disease and insulin-requiring diabetes mellitus.

When β-blockers are used in patients with a history of heart failure, treatment should be started at a low dose and titrated up slowly to the maximum tolerated dose. The patient should be monitored closely for changes in heart rate, blood pressure, and weight gain because severe bradycardia, hypotension, or worsening heart failure could be precipitated during initiation of β blockade. Every effort should be made to achieve the target doses shown to be effective in major clinical trials. It may be more than 2 to 3 months before any improvement in heart failure is noticed, so lack of symptomatic improvement should not lead to discontinuation of therapy because the risk of disease progression, future clinical deterioration, and major clinical events, including sudden death, is reduced. In cases in which cardiac decompensation occurs but is associated with only mild to moderate symptoms, the dose up-titration should be delayed for 2 to 4 weeks and the schedule of diuretics and ACE inhibitors adjusted.

In patients with a history of fluid retention, β-blockers should not be prescribed without diuretics to avoid fluid retention that can accompany the initiation of therapy. General fatigue, weakness, or sense of lassitude may develop but usually resolves spontaneously within several weeks. If severe symptoms result, β-blockers should either be decreased by 50% (for pulmonary edema) or held (for cardiogenic shock) and intravenous inotropes whose effects are mediated independently of the β receptor (such as a phosphodiesterase inhibitor, preferentially milrinone) or vasodilators (nitroprusside or nitroglycerin) used. If β-blocker therapy is discontinued temporarily, it could be started at the previous dose if held for less than 3 days or at one-half the previous dose if held between 3 and 7 days and then

TABLE 24-7 USUAL DAILY DOSAGE OF β-ADRENERGIC AGENTS

	Usual Daily Dosage*	Dose Reduction with Renal Impairment
Acebutolol	200-600 mg q12h	Y
Atenolol	50-100 (up to 200 mg) daily	
Betaxolol	10-20 mg/day	
Bisoprolol	2.5-10 mg daily	
Carvedilol	12.5-25 mg q12h	
Esmolol	IV: LD 500 mcg/kg over 1 min; then 50-300 mcg/kg/min	Y
Labetalol	100 mg q12h (up to 400 mg twice daily) IV: 20 mg over 2 min, add 40 and 80 mg at 10-min interval Infusion: 2 mg/min	
Metoprolol	50-200 mg q12h IV: 5 mg × 3 at 2-min intervals	
Nadolol	40-80 mg (up to 240 mg) daily	Y
Pindolol	2.5-7.5 mg 3 times daily	Y
Propranolol	80-160 mg q12h (extended release) IV: 1 mg/min (up to 6 mg)	
Timolol	10-30 mg q12h	
Sotalol	80-240 mg q12h (for arrhythmias)	Y

*All doses are for oral preparation, unless indicated.
IV, intravenously, LD, loading dose; Y, yes.

resumed and up-titrated as before. If discontinued for more than 7 days, treatment should be resumed at the initial dose and up-titrated as before.

Overdose. In overdose, β-blockers may cause central nervous system depression and potentiate hypotension, hypoglycemia, and bronchospasm. In a life-threatening situation with β-blocker overdose or toxicity or untoward effects such as excessive bradycardia, AV block, or hypotension, the adverse cardiac effects may be counteracted with infusion of glucagon (100 mcg/kg over 1 minute, then 1 to 5 mg/hr), isoproterenol (up to 0.10 mcg/kg per minute), or high-dose dobutamine (15 mcg/kg per minute). The IV administration of atropine should be tried for symptomatic bradycardia, and a temporary pacemaker may be needed in refractory cases.

Calcium Channel Blockers

Calcium channel blockers are a heterogeneous group of drugs that can be chemically classified into dihydropyridines (DHPs) and non-DHPs. DHPs exhibit greater selectivity for vascular smooth muscle, whereas the non-DHPs have additional inhibitory effects on the sinoatrial and AV nodes. Examples of calcium channel blockers include

- Dihydropyridines: nifedipine, amlodipine, felodipine, isradipine, nicardipine, nisoldipine, nimodipine
- Non-dihydropyridines
  - Phenylalkylamine: verapamil
  - Benzothiazepine: diltiazem

Mechanism of Action. Calcium channel blockers bind in a voltage-dependent manner to specific receptors on the alpha subunit of the voltage-gated L-type calcium channels. This results in marked reduction in calcium influx into the cells, causing relaxation of vascular smooth muscle (vasodilation) and decreased excitability of nodal tissue (bradycardia, AV conduction delay) and myocardial contractility (negative inotropy). They have an antianginal effect due to direct coronary vasodilation and ventricular afterload reduction with decrease in peripheral vascular resistance. Under physiologic conditions, DHPs are more selective for vascular smooth muscle cells and are potent vasodilators with fewer cardiac depressant and electrophysiologic effects than verapamil or diltiazem. However, in the presence of myocardial disease and/or β-adrenergic blockers, DHPs can also have significant cardiac depressant effects. Short-acting DHPs are potent vasodilators that can abruptly decrease blood pressure, causing reflex adrenergic activation and sinus tachycardia. Verapamil and diltiazem, in contrast, have depressant effect on cardiac nodal tissue and myocardium, thus decreasing the sinus rate, AV nodal conduction, and myocardial contractility. Calcium channel blockers may have a direct anti atherosclerotic action, limiting the progression of coronary atherosclerosis. This is believed to occur through an NO-mediated mechanism, but the extent and clinical importance of this effect have yet to be established.

Pharmacokinetics. The pharmacokinetic properties of most common calcium channel blockers are summarized in Table 24-8. Most clinically used calcium channel blockers are absorbed completely after oral administration but have high first-pass liver metabolism that reduces their bioavailability. The time to peak concentration and plasma half-life is short, except for newer generation calcium channel blockers such as amlodipine, which has a prolonged effect with a plasma half-life of 35 to 50 hours. Most of these agents are bound extensively to plasma proteins. Metabolites of diltiazem and verapamil are also biologically active and have additional ion channel–blocking properties. Plasma drug concentrations are not routinely measured during therapy.

Therapeutic Considerations. Indications for the use of calcium channel blockers in patients with CHD are summarized in Box 24-9.

In patients with chronic stable angina, calcium channel blockers (verapamil or diltiazem) are indicated for the relief of symptoms when initial treatment with β-blockers is not successful, is contraindicated, or leads to unacceptable side effects, or as combination therapy with β-blockers and nitrates (see Box 24-9). For combination therapy, slow-release DHPs or new-generation, long-acting DHPs are preferred.[7] All calcium channel blockers are potent coronary vasodilators and inhibit exercise-induced coronary vasoconstriction, increasing the exercise time to onset of angina or ischemia. In addition, verapamil and diltiazem decrease myocardial oxygen requirement by reducing myocardial contractility, heart rate, cardiac afterload, and ventricular wall stress. Slowing of the heart rate also increases diastolic coronary blood flow, thus limiting myocardial ischemia. Heart rate–slowing calcium channel blockers are effective in the treatment of exertional or exercise-induced angina, decreasing the number of anginal attacks and nitroglycerin tablet consumption, increasing maximal exercise time, and decreasing exercise-induced ST-segment depression.[7] Studies comparing β-blockers with calcium antagonists have reported equal efficacy in controlling stable angina.[7] Short-acting DHP calcium antagonists have the potential to aggravate myocardial ischemia due to reflex adrenergic activation that increases heart rate and cardiac workload, increasing the risk of adverse cardiac events, and should be avoided unless concomitantly given with a β-blocker. In patients with Prinzmetal's or variant angina or those with cardiovascular syndrome X or a history of rest and nocturnal angina suggestive of vasospasm, DHP calcium channel blockers (with long-acting nitrates) are especially effective in relieving and preventing coronary artery spasm and angina symptoms.[7]

In patients with UA/NSTEMI, despite well-established anti-ischemic properties, calcium channel blockers do not reduce mortality. Several clinical trials and a meta-analysis of 24 trials using a short-acting calcium channel antagonist in MI have indicated a detrimental effect on long-term survival. Several explanations for this detrimental effect have been given, including hypotension with a reduction in coronary perfusion pressure, disproportionate dilation of the coronary arteries adjacent to the ischemic area (steal phenomenon), and reflex tachycardia increasing the myocardial oxygen demand due to activation of the sympathetic nervous system. In patients with UA/NSTEMI without complicating pulmonary congestion or ventricular dysfunction, a non-significant reduction in the incidence of reinfarction and the combined

Practice: Cardiovascular Therapeutics

TABLE 24-8 PHARMACOKINETICS OF ORAL CALCIUM CHANNEL BLOCKERS

	Bioavailability (%)	Protein Binding (%)	Onset of Action after Oral Intake (hr)	Time to Peak Concentration (hr)	Plasma Half-Life (hr)	Route of Major Elimination
Verapamil	20-35	90	1	1-2	5-12	Renal, hepatic
Diltiazem	40-65	80	1	1-3	5-7	Hepatic
Amlodipine	65-90	97	1-2	6-12	35-50	Hepatic
Felodipine	15-20	99	1-2	2-5	11-16	Hepatic, renal
Isradipine	15-25	95	0.5	1-2	8	Hepatic, renal
Nicardipine	35	95	0.5	1-2	9	Hepatic, renal
Nifedipine (SR)	45-70	95	0.5	2-6	6-11	Hepatic
Nimodipine	13	95		1	8-9	Hepatic

SR, sustained release.

BOX 24-9 RECOMMENDATIONS FOR THERAPY WITH CALCIUM CHANNEL BLOCKERS IN CORONARY ARTERY DISEASE

Class I

- In patients with **chronic stable angina** and **UA/NSTEMI**, ***verapamil*** or ***diltiazem*** for *reduction of symptoms* when initial treatment with β-blockers is not successful, is contraindicated, or leads to unacceptable side effects (LoE: B).
- In patients with **ST-segment elevation or depression** that accompanies *ischemia after cocaine use* (LoE: C).
- In patients with **variant angina** whose coronary angiogram shows *no or nonobstructive coronary artery lesions* (LoE: B).
- In patients with **cardiovascular syndrome X**, alone or in combination with ***nitrates*** and ***β-blockers*** (LoE: B).

Class IIa

- ***Long-acting nondihydropyridine calcium channel blockers*** are reasonable for use in **UA/NSTEMI** patients for *recurrent ischemia in the absence of contraindications* after ***β-blockers*** and ***nitrates*** have been fully used (LoE: C).
- ***Verapamil*** or ***diltiazem*** is reasonable for patients with **STEMI** in whom *β-blockers are ineffective or contraindicated* for relief of ongoing ischemia or control of a rapid ventricular rate response with atrial fibrillation or flutter in the absence of HF, LV dysfunction, or AV block (LoE: C).
- Can be beneficial for patients with **normal ECGs** or **minimal ST-segment deviation** suggestive of *ischemia after cocaine use* (LoE: C).

Class IIb

- ***Extended-release nondihydropyridine calcium channel blockers*** may be considered *instead of a β-blocker* in patients with **UA/NSTEMI** (LoE: B).
- ***Immediate-release dihydropyridine calcium channel blockers***, in the presence of *adequate β blockade*, may be considered in patients with **UA/NSTEMI** with *ongoing ischemic symptoms or hypertension* (LoE: B).

Class III

- ***Diltiazem*** and ***verapamil*** are *contraindicated* in patients with **STEMI** and associated systolic LV dysfunction and CHF (LoE: A).
- ***Immediate-release dihydropyridine calcium channel blockers*** are *contraindicated* in treatment of **STEMI** because of the reflex sympathetic activation, tachycardia, and hypotension associated with their use (LoE: B).
- ***Immediate-release dihydropyridine calcium channel blockers*** should *not be administered* to patients with **UA/NSTEMI** in the absence of a β-blocker (LoE: A).

AV, atrioventricular; CHF, congestive heart failure; ECG, electrocardiogram; HF, heart failure; LoE, level of evidence; LV, left ventricular; NSTEMI, non–ST-elevation myocardial infarction; STEMI, ST-elevation myocardial infarction; UA, unstable angina.

end points of reinfarction and death has been observed with the heart rate–slowing calcium channel blockers diltiazem and verapamil.[6] Therefore, when β-blockers cannot be used, and in the absence of clinically significant LV dysfunction, heart rate–slowing calcium channel blockers (verapamil or diltiazem) can be used for relief of ongoing ischemia or control of a rapid ventricular rate response with atrial fibrillation or flutter (see Box 24-9).[6] When combined with a β-blocker for refractory ischemic symptoms, extra caution should be used as heart failure or bradyarrhythmia could be induced; therefore, in patients with heart failure or LV dysfunction, they should not be used (see Box 24-9).[6]

In patients with ST-segment elevation or depression that accompanies ischemia after cocaine use, calcium channel blockers are indicated to reverse cocaine-mediated vasoconstriction, hypertension, or tachyarrhythmia.

BOX 24-10 RELATIVE CONTRAINDICATIONS TO USE OF CALCIUM CHANNEL BLOCKERS

- Overt ventricular failure
- Severe sinus node dysfunction
- Severe conduction system disease
- Wolff-Parkinson-White syndrome
- Wide complex tachycardia of unknown cause
- Digitalis toxicity
- Severe aortic stenosis
- Hypertrophic obstructive cardiomyopathy (dihydropyridines)
- Hypotension
- Severe constipation (verapamil)
- Known hypersensitivity
- Pregnancy
- Post–myocardial infarction or angina at rest (short-acting dihydropyridines in the absence of β blockade)

Adverse Effects, Precautions, and Contraindications. Adverse effects due to calcium channel blockers are mainly the result of vasodilation (dizziness, headache, flushing, and ankle swelling) and a decrease in heart rate and blood pressure (fatigue and lassitude) (see Table 24-4). Dizziness and flushing are less common with the sustained-release formulations or DHPs with a long plasma half-life. The ankle edema likely results from increased hydrostatic pressure due to precapillary dilation and reflex postcapillary constriction. Calcium channel blockers can cause or aggravate gastroesophageal reflux due to the inhibition of lower esophageal sphincter contraction. Constipation is common with verapamil. Occasionally, skin reaction and gingival swelling may occur. These effects are mild and dose dependent.

Calcium channel blockers should be avoided or used cautiously in conditions summarized in Box 24-10. In patients with underlying sinus node or conduction system disease, verapamil and diltiazem may cause profound slowing of the heart rate and heart block, which may be exacerbated by the concomitant use of digoxin or β-blockers. In patients with significant ventricular systolic dysfunction, calcium channel blockers can precipitate heart failure and should be avoided. Short-acting nifedipine increases the incidence of MI and should not be used orally or sublingually for urgent reduction of elevated blood pressure. In patients with wide complex tachycardia not definitively known to be supraventricular in origin, calcium channel blockers are contraindicated because they may precipitate hemodynamic collapse in those patients with ventricular tachycardia or Wolff-Parkinson-White syndrome. A concern regarding a possible link between the use of calcium channel blockers and cancer was not supported in recent studies.[6]

Drug Interactions. Drug-drug interactions are common with the use of calcium channel blockers. Verapamil increases the concentration of digoxin due to inhibition of P-glycoprotein drug transporter in the kidneys and liver. Sinus node– and AV node–slowing agents (digoxin, β-blockers) and negative inotropic agents (disopyramide, β-blockers) may increase the negative chronotropic, dromotropic, and inotropic effects of verapamil and diltiazem and may result in symptomatic bradycardia, heart block, or congestive heart failure. Concomitant calcium administration may prevent the hypotensive response to intravenous calcium channel blockers. In patients with digitalis toxicity, verapamil is contraindicated because it can increase the blood level of digoxin and lead to complete heart block. Calcium channel blockers inhibit the hepatic CYP3A4 isoenzyme, and therefore potentially increase blood levels of most statins, carbamazepine, cyclosporine, theophylline, and sildenafil. Cimetidine increases the bioavailability of calcium channel blockers. Grapefruit juice also inhibits the metabolism of felodipine and DHPs.

Dosing. The usual dosages of commonly used calcium channel blockers are given in Table 24-9.

TABLE 24-9 USUAL DAILY DOSAGE OF CALCIUM CHANNEL BLOCKERS

	Usual Dosage*
Verapamil	240-480 mg/day *For PSVT:* IV 5-10 mg over 2 min, repeat in 10 min; then 0.005 mg/kg/min for 30-60 min
Diltiazem	120-360 mg/day *For PSVT:* IV 0.25 mg/kg over 2 min, then 0.35 mg/kg over 2 min; then 5- to 15-mg/hr infusion
Amlodipine	5-10 mg once daily
Felodipine SR	5-10 mg once daily
Isradipine	2.5-10 mg q12h
Nicardipine SR	30-60 mg twice daily IV: 5-15 mg/hr
Nifedipine SR	30-90 mg/day
Nimodipine	60 mg every 4 hr for 21 days (for subarachnoid hemorrhage)

*All doses are for oral preparation, unless indicated.
IV, intravenously, PSVT, paroxysmal supraventricular tachycardia; SR, sustained release formulation.

Overdose and Toxicity. In life-threatening situations due to overdose or toxicity of calcium channel blockers, intravenous calcium gluconate (1 to 2 g) or calcium chloride (0.5 to 1 mg) should be used. Managing combined myocardial depression and hypotension with calcium channel blocker toxicity is difficult. Positive inotropic agents (dobutamine, dopamine), vasoconstrictive catecholamines (norepinephrine, dopamine), or glucagon (5 to 10 mg for hypotension) with repeated doses of calcium may be necessary. Intravenous atropine or isoproterenol and a temporary pacemaker might be needed for AV block.

Nitric Oxide Donors Under Investigation

Apart from nitrates, there are a group of other drugs that act as NO donors and as an anti-anginal drugs.

Molsidomine and Its Metabolites. Molsidomine is the endogenous precursor of the NO donor 3-morpholinosydnonomine (SIN-1), which has been shown to stimulate soluble guanylate cyclase activity by an NO-mediated pathway in blood vessels, causing vasodilation, as well as through activation of potassium channels. Molsidomine has a slower onset and longer duration of action than conventional nitrates due to the relatively slow rate of conversion to SIN-1. SIN-1 itself has a rapid onset and short duration of action. However, molsidomine and SIN-1 do not appear to induce tolerance and are not cross-tolerant with conventional nitrates.

Molsidomine and SIN-1 are therapeutic alternatives to traditional organic nitrates in stable angina, coronary vasospasm, and heart failure with the benefit of avoiding tolerance. However, large-scale trials have failed to show any benefit of molsidomine on survival following MI. Continuous chronic administration might offer other benefits, especially through inhibition of platelet activation. SIN-1 has been shown to protect against thrombotic occlusion of blood vessels following balloon angioplasty. SIN-1 has also been shown to have beneficial effects in reperfusion injury, reducing neutrophil sequestration and vascular resistance as well as preserving endothelial function.

Diazeniumdiolates (NONOates). These are a group of novel NO donor drugs. They are stable in the solid form and decompose spontaneously in solution to generate up to 2 NO radicals per molecule, capable of stimulating soluble guanylate cyclase in a number of biologic systems. Preclinical studies have already identified a number of potential applications for NONOates, particularly in cardiovascular disease. In addition to the cardiovascular system, NONOates have been found to cause bronchodilation, perhaps through both cGMP-dependent and -independent pathways. These compounds have also been shown to have relaxant effects in cervical smooth muscle, perhaps indicating therapeutic applications in parturition.[98]

S-Nitrosothiols. S-Nitrosothiols constitute another class of newer NO donor drugs. Nitrosothiols decompose spontaneously in solution to their disulfide form, generating NO in the process, and present a potential alternative to current NO donors, particularly as they do not appear to engender vascular tolerance. Of the endogenous S-nitrosothiols (SNOs) that might prove therapeutically beneficial, GSNO is the most promising on account of its relative stability in solution. Exogenous GSNO has been shown to have several potentially beneficial cardiovascular effects, including an inhibitory effect on platelet activation following balloon angioplasty and in patients with acute MI and UA.[98]

Mesoionic Oxatriazole Derivatives. Mesoionic oxatriazole derivatives constitute another class of NO donor drugs whose biologic action is mediated through spontaneous NO generation on dissolution. These drugs show a full range of NO-mediated actions, including vasodilation, inhibition of platelet aggregation, antibacterial activity, inhibition of neutrophil function, inhibition of smooth muscle cell proliferation, and prevention of oxidation of lipoproteins. Like many other novel NO donors, the therapeutic potential of these drugs in cardiovascular medicine is yet to be fully explored.[98]

Other Anti-ischemic Agents

Ranolazine. Ranolazine is a piperazine derivative that was recently approved for the treatment of patients with chronic angina who have not achieved an adequate response with other antianginal drugs.[99] Several mechanisms of its action have been proposed.[100] At clinically relevant concentrations, ranolazine inhibits the slowly inactivating component of the sodium current (late INa) in the heart, decreasing the deleterious effects associated with the intracellular sodium and calcium overload that accompany and probably promote myocardial ischemia. At higher concentrations, ranolazine has been shown to have partial fatty acid oxidase inhibitor activity, shifting ATP production away from fatty acid oxidation in favor of glucose oxidation. Because more oxygen is needed to phosphorylate a given amount of ATP during fatty acid oxidation than during carbohydrate oxidation, the ranolazine-induced shift in substrate utilization reduces oxygen demand without decreasing the ability of the tissue to do work. However, this effect occurs at higher concentrations and is unlikely to be the primary mechanism for clinical efficacy. Ranolazine is also shown to protect the heart from H_2O_2-induced mechanical and metabolic alterations, which may contribute to its cardioprotective effect against ischemia-reperfusion damage. Ranolazine has also been shown to attenuate the ischemia-induced increase in myocardial α_1-adrenoreceptors that are responsible for cardiac contractile force and the resistance of the coronary arteries and systemic blood vessels, leading to an imbalance between the myocardial oxygen supply and demand.

Ranolazine improves exercise tolerance and reduces the frequency of angina attacks in patients with ischemic heart disease.[100,101] In placebo-controlled studies in chronic angina patients, ranolazine increased treadmill exercise parameters without associated changes in rest or exercise heart rates or decreases in rest or exercise blood pressures. Statistically significant increases in exercise times were only observed, however, after doses of greater than 240 mg, when ranolazine plasma concentrations were near their peak. There was no evidence for antianginal efficacy 8 or 12 hours after any dose. These studies suggested a potential for ranolazine as an antianginal drug but indicated that the immediate-release formulation was impractical because of the short duration of its effect. Ranolazine, despite a small QTc-prolonging effect on ECG, appeared to be safe and well tolerated in short-term, placebo-controlled trials. In the Monotherapy Assessment of Ranolazine In Stable Angina (MARISA) and Combination Assessment of Ranolazine In Stable Angina (CARISA) Phase III clinical trials, the beneficial effect of ranolazine as an antianginal drug in chronic stable angina was demonstrated.[99,102]

In patients with UA/NSTEMI in the recent Metabolic Efficiency With Ranolazine for Less Ischemia in Non-ST-Elevation Acute Coronary Syndromes (MERLIN-TIMI 36) trial, the addition of ranolazine to standard treatment for ACS was not effective in reducing major cardiovascular events (cardiovascular death, MI, or recurrent ischemia) without significant adverse effect during a median of 1 year of treatment.[100] A 13% relative reduction in the risk of recurrent ischemia, fewer increases in other antianginal therapy, and reduction in the frequency of arrhythmias detected by Holter monitor recording during the first 7 days after randomization were reported. Thus, ranolazine appears to be safe for symptom relief after UA/NSTEMI, but it does not appear to improve the underlying disease substrate.[100]

Currently, ranolazine is indicated alone or in combination with amlodipine, β-blockers, or nitrates for the treatment of chronic angina that has failed to respond to standard antianginal therapy. The recommended initial dose is 500 mg orally twice daily, to a maximum of 1000 mg twice daily. The adverse effects of ranolazine include headache, dizziness, and asthenia. It is contraindicated in patients with prolonged QT intervals and should be used cautiously with other repolarization-prolonging drugs.

Trimetazidine. Trimetazidine is a novel antianginal drug that has been shown to act at different levels of the sequence of cellular events that appear during ischemia.[103] It partially reduces fatty acid beta oxidation secondary to the selective inhibition of the mitochondrial enzyme 3-ketoacyl coenzyme A thiolase.[104] This results in a shift of cardiac metabolism from fatty acids to glucose oxidation, which in turn restores ATP production and protects the heart from ischemia-related damage. Numerous experimental studies have demonstrated the anti-ischemic properties of trimetazidine and have proposed the clinical use of this drug in myocardial ischemia, either as first-line monotherapy or in combination with classic antianginal drugs. The anti-ischemic effect of trimetazidine, which can be observed at doses devoid of any hemodynamic action, improves postischemic recovery during reperfusion. The antianginal efficacy of trimetazidine has been proven in monotherapy in comparison with reference drugs and in addition to hemodynamic agents in patients with a positive exercise test and angina symptoms despite monotherapy with a β-blocker or a calcium antagonist.

Trimetazidine is well tolerated anti-ischemic agent that, in addition to providing symptom relief and functional improvement in patients with angina pectoris, has a cytoprotective action during ischemia. The drug is suggested to be suitable for initial use as monotherapy in patients with angina pectoris and, because of its different mechanism of action, as adjunctive therapy in those with symptoms not sufficiently controlled by nitrates, β-blockers, or calcium channel blockers. The TIGER study provided evidence of the clinical value of trimetazidine in elderly coronary patients who are resistant to hemodynamic therapy.[105] The absence of clinically significant reported drug interactions with trimetazidine is of particular value in using this drug.[103,105]

Potassium Channel Openers. Potassium channel openers are chemically diverse agents that target ATP-sensitive potassium (K_{ATP}) channels that link membrane electrical excitability with changes in cellular energetic state.[106,107] K_{ATP} channels protect the heart during myocardial ischemia, and act as molecular mediators of the adaptive response to distress.[108,109] The various potassium channel openers used in cardiovascular medicine are nicorandil, pinacidil, and cromakalim, but none is currently approved in the United States for the treatment of CHD.[106]

Potassium channel openers have proven useful in limiting myocardial dysfunction under conditions of ischemia-reperfusion and heart failure through direct actions on the myocardium.[106,107] This protective action exploits the essential role of K_{ATP} channels in cardiac stress adaptation, ranging from preservation of contractile performance under imposed load to myocardial salvage following ischemic challenge. The benefit of potassium channel openers apparently stems from prevention of intracellular calcium overload, as opening of plasma membrane K_{ATP} channels shortens the action potential duration, limiting cellular injury by preserving cellular energetics and ultimately cell survival by additional mitochondrial effects. In addition, through regulation of vascular smooth muscle, they are also potent vasodilators. Nicorandil also reduces preload and afterload, enhances cardiac endothelial NO synthase expression, and has antiplatelet, fibrinolytic, and antioxidant properties.[110] Unlike nitroglycerin, no development of tolerance to the antianginal effect of nicorandil has been reported.[61]

In patients with ischemic heart disease, the value of potassium channel openers in protecting the myocardium is clinically best documented with nicorandil for the management of both stable angina and UA with minimum adverse effects.[61] In placebo-controlled, single- and double-blind studies of patients with stable angina pectoris, nicorandil attenuated effort and rest angina, prolonged the time to onset of angina or ischemic ECG changes, and prolonged duration of exercise. In a multicenter trial enrolling more than 5000 subjects with stable angina pectoris, long-term use of nicorandil was associated with reduction in cardiovascular events and the combined end points of death, MI, and hospitalization due to chest pain.[63]

In patients with UA, nicorandil, when added to aggressive antianginal treatment, reduces transient myocardial ischemia and arrhythmias when compared to placebo.[61,106] Nicorandil improves ischemia-induced regional wall motion abnormalities as well as perfusion in infarct-related areas. In patients undergoing angioplasty, nicorandil preconditions the heart, improves coronary hemodynamics, dilates stenotic and nonstenotic segments, and ameliorates the "no-reflow" phenomenon. Intravenous nicorandil, in conjunction with coronary angioplasty, preserves microvascular integrity and myocardial viability in patients with acute MI. Nicorandil is an effective antianginal agent at a dose of 10 to 40 mg twice a day, controlling stable chronic angina in 70% to 80% of patients.[61] The response to nicorandil is maintained for 12 hours, with an efficacy that compares favorably with that of nitrates, β-adrenergic receptor antagonists, and calcium channel blockers. The main side effects include headache, GI disturbances, mucosal ulceration, and dizziness. No adverse interaction has been reported in patients on oral anticoagulants.

Specific Bradycardic Agents. Specific bradycardic agents are a novel group of drugs that selectively inhibit the If current (pacemaker current) in the sinoatrial node, reducing the rate of diastolic depolarization and heart rate without affecting AV node conduction, ventricular refractoriness, myocardial contractility, or systemic hemodynamics.[111] A number of specific bradycardic agents have been developed, including zatebradine, alinidine, falipamil, and ivabradine, but the only drug that is currently under clinical evaluation is ivabradine. By reducing heart rate, specific bradycardic agents improve myocardial oxygen demand-supply mismatch and are useful for the management of stable angina pectoris. In animal models, specific bradycardiac agents limit exercise-induced tachycardia in the absence of any inotropic or dromotropic effects.[111]

Phase II studies conducted in patients with stable angina confirmed the specific heart rate–slowing effect of ivabradine at rest and during exercise with anti-ischemic and antianginal efficacy.[112,113] Ivabradine (not available in the United States) was approved by the European Medicines Agency in 2005 for the symptomatic treatment of stable angina pectoris in patients with normal sinus rhythm who have a contraindication or intolerance to β-blockers.[111] It has been shown to be noninferior to the β-blocker atenolol and the calcium channel blocker amlodipine for this indication. A dose of 5 mg (2.5 mg in elderly patients) twice daily is recommended initially; after 1 month, it is recommended to increase the dose to 7.5 mg twice daily to get the optimal efficacy linked to heart rate reduction.[111] Visual disturbances due to blockade of the If current in the retina, headache, and dizziness may occur. Ivabradine is contraindicated in patients with sinus node dysfunction and should be used cautiously with CYP3A4-inhibiting drugs such as ketoconazole, macrolide antibiotics, and antiretroviral drugs.[111]

Inhibitors of the Renin-Angiotensin-Aldosterone System

The RAAS plays a major role in cardiovascular pathology, with angiotensin II and aldosterone contributing to maladaptive post-MI remodeling of the heart. Angiotensin converting enzyme (ACE) inhibitors act on the enzyme that generates angiotensin II, whereas ARBs inhibit the angiotensin II receptor (AT1 subtype) and aldosterone receptor antagonists block the effect of aldosterone. They are beneficial in improving survival after MI by preventing adverse ventricular remodeling and in primary and secondary protection from cardiovascular disease, particularly in diabetics.

Mechanism of Action

ACE inhibitors act as competitive antagonists of ACE, preventing conversion of angiotensin I to angiotensin II and the breakdown of bradykinin. Decreased angiotensin II formation and increased bradykinin levels that stimulate prostaglandin synthesis result in reduction of afterload, blood pressure lowering, aldosterone reduction, natriuresis, preservation of serum potassium levels, reduction in cardiac fibrosis, and improvement in endothelial function.[114] ACE inhibitors also have indirect antiadrenergic effects by reducing angiotensin II–mediated release of norepinephrine from adrenergic terminal neurons, as well as central and ganglionic transmission. They reduce plasminogen activator inhibitor-1, thus enhancing fibrinolysis, and confer a preconditioning-like protection, acting via bradykinin BK2 receptor activation.[114,115]

ARBs directly block the AT1 receptor and the adverse effects of angiotensin II, which mediates vasoconstriction, myocyte hypertrophy,[6] and antinatriuresis. The advantage of ARBs over ACE inhibitors is avoidance of bradykinin-related adverse effects, with a lower incidence of cough and angioedema and possibly hormonal "escape" due to hyperreninemia and increase in angiotensin II with chronic ACE inhibition.

Pharmacokinetics

Please see Chapter 26 (Heart Failure) for a detailed description of the pharmacology of inhibitors of the RAAS. Here we summarize therapeutic uses in CAD.

ACE inhibitors can be classified into three broad groups based on chemical structure (Table 24-10). Based on their pharmacokinetics, ACE inhibitors can be classified (Table 24-11)[116] as

1. Active compounds that have additional active metabolites (e.g., captopril)
2. Prodrugs that are active only after conversion to diacid by hepatic metabolism (e.g., enalapril)
3. Nonmetabolized, water-soluble compounds excreted unchanged by the kidneys (e.g., lisinopril)

Many ACE inhibitors are prodrugs that are 100 to 1000 times less potent than the active molecules but have a much better oral bioavailability. There appears to be little advantage to any one agent over others, but since some drugs have been better tested for specific situations in a major outcome trial, they are more likely to be used, unless they have an inconvenient dosage schedule (short-acting captopril) or side effect profile (neutropenia with SH group–containing captopril). Lisinopril, being water soluble, has simple pharmacokinetics with no liver transformation and renal excretion, making it an easy drug to use without risk of hepatic pharmacokinetic interactions.

The role of pharmacogenomics with regard to ACE inhibitors is not very clear at this moment. Some studies have shown a correlation between the known ACE polymorphisms (ACE insertion/deletion, angiotensinogen [M235T], and angiotensin II receptor subtype 1 [573C/T]) and ACE inhibitor therapy, while others have shown no such relationship.[117,118] More studies in this field, perhaps with discovery of other gene polymorphisms that may be involved, are needed.

Therapeutic Considerations

Recommendations for therapy with inhibitors of the RAAS in patients with CHD are summarized in Box 24-11 and those for heart failure in Chapter 26 (Heart Failure). Major outcome trials of RAAS are summarized in Table 24-12.

ACE inhibitors are not direct antianginal agents, but have an indirect anti-ischemic effect on myocardial oxygen demand by reduction in the afterload and adrenergic activation[119] as well as improvement in blood flow by restoration of endothelial function and vasodilation.[120] In

TABLE 24-10 ACE INHIBITOR CLASSIFICATION ACCORDING TO CHEMICAL STRUCTURE

Chemical Structure	Drugs
Sulfhydryl-containing	Captopril, fentiapril,* pivalopril,* zofenopril,* alacepril*
Dicarboxyl-containing	Enalapril, lisinopril, benazepril, quinapril, moexipril, ramipril, trandolapril, spirapril,* perindopril, pentopril,* cilazapril*
Phosphorus-containing	Fosinopril

*Drugs not approved for use in the United States.

TABLE 24-11 SUMMARY OF PHARMACOLOGIC PROPERTIES, CLINICAL INDICATIONS, AND DOSES OF ACE INHIBITORS

Drug	Zinc Ligand	Active Drug	Elimination Half-Life (hr)	Dose	Post-MI or HF Target Dose in Large Trials
CLASS I: CAPTOPRIL-LIKE					
Captopril	Sulfhydryl	Captopril	4-6	25-50 mg × 3	50 mg × 3
CLASS II: PRODRUGS					
Benazepril	Carboxyl	Benazeprilat	11	10-40 mg in 1-2 doses	Not established
Cilazepril	Carboxyl	Cilazeprilat	9	2.5-5 mg × 1	Not established
Enalapril	Carboxyl	Enalaprilat	6; 11 (accum)	5-20 mg in 1-2 doses	10 mg × 2
Fosinopril	Phosphoryl	Fosinoprilat	12	10-80 mg × 1 or × 2	Not established
Perindopril	Carboxyl	Perindoprilat	3-10	4-8 mg × 1	Not established
Quinapril	Carboxyl	Quinaprilat	1.8	10-80 mg in 1-2 doses	Not established
Ramipril	Carboxyl	Ramiprilat	13-17	2.5-10 mg in 1-2 doses	5 mg × 2
Spirapril	Carboxyl	Spiraprilat	<2	3-6 mg in 1 dose	Not established
Trandolapril	Carboxyl	Trandoprilat	10	0.5-4 mg × 1, then 4 mg × 2	4 mg × 1
CLASS III: WATER-SOLUBLE					
Lisinopril	Carboxyl	Lisinopril	7; 12 (accum)	10-40 mg × 1	10-35 mg × 1

accum, accumulation half-life; HF, heart failure; MI, myocardial infarction.
From Opie LH, Gersh BJ. Drugs for the Heart: Textbook with Online Updates, 6th ed. Amsterdam: Elsevier, 2004.

TABLE 24-12 MAJOR OUTCOME TRIALS OF RAAS INHIBITORS

RAAS Blocker	Risk Prevention	HTN	Chronic HF	HF Post-MI	AMI, Early Phase	Diabetic Nephropathy	Chronic Renal Disease
ANGIOTENSIN-CONVERTING ENZYME (ACE) INHIBITORS							
Captopril		+ CAPP		++ SAVE		++ (type 1 diabetes)	+
Enalapril		++ ANBP2	++ SOLVD,V-HeFT, CONSENSUS				+
Lisinopril		+ ALLHAT	+ ATLAS		++ GISSI		
Perindopril	++ EUROPA						
Ramipril	++ HOPE			++ AIRE		+ MICROHOPE	++ REIN, AASK
Trandolapril	++ PEACE	+ INVEST		++ TRACE			
ANGIOTENSIN II RECEPTOR BLOCKERS (ARBS)							
Candesartan			++ CHARM				
Irbesartan						++ IDNT, IRMA	
Losartan		++ (with LVH) LIFE	ELITE 1 & 2 (dose too low)	OPTIMAAL (dose too low)		++ RENAAL	
Valsartan	? VALUE		++ VAL Heft	++ VALIANT			
ALDOSTERONE ANTAGONISTS							
Spironolactone			++ RALES				
Eplerenone				++ EPHESUS			

++, strongly indicated; +, indicated.
AMI, acute myocardial infarction; HF, heart failure; HTN, hypertension; LVH, left ventricular hypertrophy; MI, myocardial infarction; RAAS, renin-angiotensin-aldosterone inhibitors.
From Opie LH, Gersh BJ. Drugs for the Heart: Textbook with Online Updates, 6th ed. Amsterdam: Elsevier, 2004.

patients with recent MI and LV systolic dysfunction with and without overt heart failure, ACE inhibitors attenuate LV remodeling and reduce the risk of subsequent MI and mortality, as demonstrated in the ISIS-4, GISSI-3, and SMILE trials (see Table 24-12).[87,88,121] The proportional benefit of ACE inhibitor therapy is highest in higher risk subgroups, including patients with previous infarction, heart failure, depressed LV ejection fraction, and tachycardia.

In high-risk patients with CAD even with preserved LV function, ACE inhibitors improve survival.[122-125] This protective effect is most likely a class effect as reduction in MI and mortality was demonstrated by different ACE inhibitors in several trials, including SAVE (captopril),[126] SOLVD (enalapril),[127] HOPE (ramipril),[128] and EUROPA (perindopril).[129] In the Heart Outcomes Prevention Evaluation (HOPE) study, a decrease in mortality (cardiovascular death by 37%), and vascular events (MI by 22%, stroke by 33%, nephropathy by 24%) was reported with the long-term use of ramipril in moderate-risk patients with CAD, many with preserved LV function, as well as in patients without symptoms but at high risk of developing CHD.[128] Similar beneficial effects were reported in the EUropean trial on Reduction Of cardiac events with Perindopril in patients with stable coronary Artery disease (EUROPA) study.[129] Ramipril shifts the fibrinolytic balance toward lysis after an MI, with reduction in plasminogen activator inhibitor-1 antigen levels and activity that may account for the reduced risk of MI in clinical trials.[130] In the long term, the need for coronary revascularization procedures also appears to be reduced.[128] Therefore, unless contraindicated, ACE inhibitors should be administered to all high-risk patients with CAD (see Box 24-11), particularly diabetics and those with LV dysfunction with or without overt heart failure.[92] The beneficial effect of ACE inhibitors extends over the long term, and they should be administered indefinitely unless side effects preclude their use.[92,123] Within the first 24 hours of STEMI, intravenous ACE inhibitors should not be given because of the risk of hypotension (see Box 24-11),[5] but they should be administered as routine therapy for secondary prevention, particularly in diabetics without severe renal disease.

ARBs should be substituted in patients who have indications for the use of ACE inhibitors (those with hypertension, heart failure, or LV dysfunction) but are unable to tolerate them due to adverse effects (see Box 24-11).[5] The use of ARBs after STEMI has not been explored as much as ACE inhibitors, but in patients with MI complicated by LV systolic dysfunction, use of valsartan was as effective as captopril in patients at high risk for cardiovascular events after MI.[131] Similarly, in the Candesartan in Heart failure Assessment in Reduction of Mortality (CHARM) study, candesartan treatment reduced cardiovascular deaths and hospital admissions of patients with chronic heart failure, including post-MI patients.[132]

In post-MI patients with ventricular dysfunction and heart failure, aldosterone receptor blockade is recommended (see Box 24-11) in those without significant renal dysfunction (serum creatinine ≤2.5 mg/dl in men and ≤2.0 mg/dl in women) or hyperkalemia (serum potassium ≤5.0 mEq/L).[5] In patients with heart failure with LV dysfunction, including those after MI, spironolactone in the Randomized ALdactone Evaluation Study (RALES) and eplerenone in the Eplerenone Post-Acute Myocardial Infarction Heart Failure Efficacy and Survival Study (EPHESUS), when added to standard therapy including an ACE inhibitor, decreased both morbidity and mortality.[133,134]

BOX 24-11 RECOMMENDATIONS FOR THERAPY WITH INHIBITORS OF THE RENIN-ANGIOTENSIN-ALDOSTERONE SYSTEM IN CORONARY ARTERY DISEASE

Class I

- ***ACE inhibitors*** should be continued indefinitely in all patients with *LVEF ≤ 40%* and in those with *hypertension, diabetes, or chronic kidney disease* unless contraindicated (LoE: A).
- ***ACE inhibitors*** should be started and continued indefinitely in patients with **chronic stable angina** or those recovering from **UA/NSTEMI** or **STEMI** who are *not lower risk* (lower risk defined as those with normal LVEF in whom cardiovascular risk factors are well controlled and revascularization has been performed), unless contraindicated (LoE: A).
- ***Angiotensin receptor blockers*** are recommended for patients with **chronic stable angina** or those recovering from **UA/NSTEMI** or **STEMI** who have *hypertension*, have *indications for but are intolerant of ACE inhibitors*, have *HF*, or have *LVEF ≤ 40%* (LoE: A).
- ***Aldosterone blockade*** is recommended for use in **post-MI** patients *without significant renal dysfunction* (creatinine clearance >30 ml/min) *or hyperkalemia* (potassium ≤5 mEq/L) who are *already receiving therapeutic doses* of an ***ACE inhibitor*** and a ***β-blocker***, have *LVEF ≤ 40%*, and have *diabetes or HF* (LoE: A).

Class IIa

- It is reasonable to use ***ACE inhibitors*** in lower risk patients with **chronic stable angina** (LoE: B), **UA/NSTEMI** (LoE: A), or **STEMI** (LoE: B) with *mildly reduced or normal LVEF* in whom *cardiovascular risk factors are well controlled and revascularization has been performed*, unless contraindicated.
- An ***angiotensin receptor blocker*** can be useful as an alternative to ACE inhibitors in **UA/NSTEMI** patients who *do not tolerate ACE inhibitors*, provided there are clinical or radiologic signs of HF and LVEF ≤ 40% (LoE: B).

Class IIb

- ***Angiotensin receptor blockers*** may be considered in combination with ***ACE inhibitors*** for *HF due to LV systolic dysfunction* (LoE: B).
- The combination of an ***ACE inhibitor*** and an ***angiotensin receptor blocker*** may be considered in the long-term management of patients with **chronic stable angina** or those recovering from **UA/NSTEMI** with *HF and LVEF ≤ 40% despite conventional therapy* including an ACE inhibitor or an angiotensin receptor blocker alone (LoE: B).

Class III

- IV ***ACE inhibitors*** should *not be given* to patients within the first 24 hours of **STEMI** because of the risk of hypotension (a possible exception may be patients with refractory hypertension) (LoE: B).

ACE, angiotensin-converting enzyme; HF, heart failure; IV, intravenous; LoE, level of evidence; LV, left ventricular; LVEF, left ventricular ejection fraction; MI, myocardial infarction; NSTEMI, non–ST-elevation myocardial infarction; STEMI, ST-elevation myocardial infarction; UA, unstable angina.

Adverse Effects, Precautions, and Contraindications

Cough is common with the use of ACE inhibitors, with incidence as high as 10% to 20%, occurring more commonly in women than men and usually developing between 1 week and 6 months after initiation of therapy.[135] Increased production of bradykinin and prostaglandins probably are responsible. A change to an ARB may be required in those with persistent cough. Postural hypotension may occur, particularly at high doses or in patients on multiple medications for heart failure control that alter intravascular volume and vascular tone. Dose reduction of ACE inhibitors or other medications may reduce orthostatic symptoms. Hypotension is common; however; in general; as long as orthostatic symptoms do not occur, the absolute blood pressure is not crucial and many patients do well with systolic pressures of 80 to 90 mm Hg. Hyperkalemia may occur when ACE inhibitors are given with potassium-sparing diuretics or in the presence of renal failure.

Transient renal dysfunction may occur with hypotension, especially in the elderly and those with severe heart failure, hyponatremia and volume depletion, or underlying renal disease. A slight stable increase in serum creatinine after the introduction of an ACE inhibitor should not limit its use, and an early decrease in glomerular filtration rate, hypotension, and hyperkalemia can be managed without discontinuation of the agent. In patients with renal insufficiency (serum creatinine >1.4 mg/dl) treated with ACE inhibitors, progression of renal disease slows down in the long run. ACE inhibitor therapy, however, should be discontinued if serum creatinine rises above 30% of the baseline during the first 2 months after initiation or if hyperkalemia (serum potassium ≥5.6 mmol/L) develops. Irreversible renal failure may occur with bilateral renal stenosis. Captopril may cause taste disturbance, rash, neutropenia, and proteinuria. During chronic ACE inhibition, reactive hyperreninemia occurs with re-emergence of circulating angiotensin II and aldosterone and decreases the efficacy of ACE inhibitors. Leukocyte counts with differential, electrolytes, and creatinine should be obtained during the first 3 months of therapy. The dose should be adjusted in patients with renal impairment.

Contradictions to use of ACE inhibitors include known allergy or hypersensitivity, bilateral renal artery stenosis, history of angioedema, and pregnancy. Angioedema, although rare (0.3% to 1.6% in African Americans) can be life threatening and requires immediate discontinuation of the ACE inhibitor, but ARBs can be substituted. ACE inhibitors have been assigned to FDA pregnancy category D (see Table 24-6). Category D drugs are those for which evidence indicates risk to the human fetus based on adverse reaction from data collected in investigational or marketing experience or studies in humans. The use of ACE inhibitors is contraindicated during the second and third trimesters of pregnancy because of the risk of fetal hypotension, anuria, and renal failure, sometimes associated with fetal malformations or death.[136] Recent evidence also implicates first-trimester exposure to ACE inhibitors in increased teratogenic risk.[137] ACE inhibitors should not be used in women planning to conceive. In women of childbearing age, ACE inhibitors should only be given after careful counseling and consideration of individual risks and benefits. When pregnancy is detected, ACE inhibitors should be discontinued as soon as possible and fetal development should be monitored regularly.

Drug Interactions

Concomitant use of ACE inhibitors with potassium-sparing diuretics, potassium supplements, NSAIDs, and β-blockers, especially in patients with renal impairment, may result in hyperkalemia, and necessitates careful monitoring of the serum potassium level.[30] The safety and efficacy of low doses of spironolactone, when carefully added to ACE inhibitors in patients with severe heart failure, have been demonstrated in the RALES study.[134] Antacids may reduce the bioavailability of ACE inhibitors; capsaicin may worsen ACE inhibitor–induced cough; and NSAIDs may reduce the antihypertensive effect of ACE inhibitors and should be avoided. The impact of aspirin on the beneficial effect of ACE inhibitors on MI and mortality is controversial, but does not appear to significantly interfere with the clinical benefits of therapy with either agent in chronic heart failure or post-MI protection.[138,139] When used together with an ACE inhibitor, the dose of aspirin should be kept low, especially in heart failure patients. ACE inhibitors may increase plasma levels of digoxin and lithium and may increase hypersensitivity reactions to allopurinol. Plasma levels of digoxin or lithium should be monitored when these drugs are given concurrently with ACE inhibitors.

Dosing

The starting and target doses of commonly used ACE inhibitors, ARBs, and aldosterone antagonists are summarized in Table 24-11.

Lipid-Lowering Agents

Elevated total cholesterol level has been linked to the development of CAD, mainly due to increased LDL-C, but also associated with other lipid abnormalities. A 2% to 3% increase in risk for coronary events has been estimated for every 1% increase in LDL-C level, and for every 1% reduction in total cholesterol, a 2% to 3% reduction in fatal and nonfatal coronary events was reported in earlier lipid-lowering trials using bile-acid sequestrants (cholestyramine), fibric acid derivatives (gemfibrozil and clofibrate), or niacin.[140,141] With active lipid-lowering therapy, a decrease in progression and stabilization of coronary atherosclerotic plaque with reduction in adverse clinical events has been demonstrated. Reduction in total cholesterol levels with lipid-lowering drugs was associated with significant reductions in total and CHD mortality (Table 24-13, Fig. 24-17). In patients without and with established CAD, recent clinical trials with several HMG-CoA reductase inhibitors (statins), which effectively lower LDL-C levels, have confirmed a protective effect of these agents on reduction in adverse ischemic events, including overall and CHD mortality in both men and women and the elderly (Table 24-14, Fig. 24-18). The benefits of lipid-lowering therapy are observed even in patients with minimal elevation of LDL-C level (CARE study)[142] or in the lowest baseline quartile of LDL-C level (4S study).[143]

Major primary and secondary prevention statin trials with baseline cholesterol levels and long-term major significant outcomes are summarized in Table 24-14 and Figure 24-19. The largest of these trials, the Heart Protection Study,[144] enrolled more than 20,000 men and women age 40 to 80 years with coronary or other vascular disease, diabetes, and/or hypertension. Over 5 years' mean follow-up, total mortality (the primary end point), was reduced by approximately 25% in the simvastatin-treated group (40 mg) compared to placebo, including in women, elderly patients (>75 years old), diabetics, and those with baseline LDL-C of less than 100 mg/dl. Despite LDL-C reduction, arteriographic progression of coronary disease may continue in many patients (25% to 60%), even with the most aggressive LDL-C–lowering treatments. In 25% of patients who have recovered from STEMI, low HDL-C may be present in the absence of elevated total cholesterol level.[5] Maximum benefit may require management of other atherogenic risk factors and lipid abnormalities, including elevated non–HDL-C and low HDL-C.

Management of Dyslipidemias

The major classes of drugs for consideration are (Table 24-15)

- HMG-CoA reductase inhibitors (statins)—atorvastatin, fluvastatin, lovastatin, pravastatin, rosuvastatin, simvastatin
- Fibric acid derivatives (fibrates)—gemfibrozil, fenofibrate, clofibrate
- Bile acid sequestrants—cholestyramine, colestipol, colesevelam
- Nicotinic acid—niacin

These drugs provide benefit in patients across the entire spectrum of cholesterol levels, primarily by reducing levels of LDL-C. Please see Chapter 23 (Dyslipidemias) for a detailed description of the pharmacology of individual lipid-lowering drugs and their therapeutic considerations, adverse effects, and contraindications to use (Table 24-16). In this section we have summarized the management of dyslipidemias depending on the risk factors for or presence of CAD and baseline LDL-C, HDL-C, non–HDL-C, and triglyceride levels.

Elevated Total Cholesterol and LDL-C. In patients with moderately high risk with two or more CHD risk factors or established CAD, nonpharmaceutical management for LDL-C levels greater than 100 mg/dl and drug treatment for LDL-C levels greater than 130 mg/dl are warranted, with the goal to maintain LDL-C level less than 100 mg/dl. For patients with LDL-C levels between 101 and 129 mg/dl, lifestyle changes and/or drug therapies to lower LDL-C need to be intensified, along with emphasis on dietary restriction (calories, saturated fat, and trans-fat), weight reduction, increased physical activity, increase in soluble fiber (10 to 25 g/day) and plant stanols/sterols (2 g/day), and use of statins or other lipid-lowering agents (Box 24-12). The intensity of the treatment must be sufficient to achieve a reduction in LDL-C levels to less than 100 mg/dl and ideally less than 70 mg/dl.[140] When the less-than 70-mg/dL target is chosen, the dose of statins should be increased gradually to determine a patient's response and tolerance. If the target LDL-C level cannot be achieved because of a high baseline LDL-C, LDL-C reductions of at least greater than 50% should be considered with combination therapy.[7]

For those patients who need lipid-lowering drugs, the statins have the best outcome evidence supporting their use and should be the mainstay of treatment (see Box 24-12). Control of other lipid or non-lipid risk factors also needs to be considered, including use of nicotinic acid or fibric acid for elevated triglyceride or low HDL-C levels. In all patients with established CHD, a complete blood lipid profile should be determined.[7] In patients with acute MI, the timing of blood collection for the determination of lipid profile is important, and unless obtained within 24 hours of the onset of symptoms, should be delayed because LDL-C levels begin to decrease and are significantly reduced by 48 hours and remain so for many weeks.[3]

In patients with ACS, the risk for recurrent coronary events is high and should be reduced by intensive LDL-lowering therapy.[145,146] Treatment with statins initiated during hospitalization with ACS significantly reduces clinical events, including recurrent ischemia, nonfatal

TABLE 24-13 PROPERTIES AND EFFECT OF HMG-COA REDUCTASE INHIBITORS ON LIPID PROFILE AND CV END POINT

Characteristics	Atorvastatin (Lipitor)	Fluvastatin (Lescol)	Lovastatin (Mevacor)	Pravastatin (Pravachol)	Rosuvastatin (Crestor)	Simvastatin (Zocor)
Dose (mg/day) Starting→Max	10→80	20→80	20→80	40→80	10→40	20→80
Metabolism	Hepatic, CYP3A4	Hepatic, CYP2C9	Hepatic, CYP3A4	Hepatic, (sulfation, oxidation, isomerization)	Hepatic, CYP2C9	Hepatic, CYP3A4
Renal excretion of absorbed dose %	<2	<6	10	20	28	13
Dose reduction in renal failure	–	–	+	+	+	+
LDL reduction % at max dose	↓60	↓36	↓40	↓37	↓63	↓47
HDL increase % at max dose	↑5	↑5.6	↑9.5	↑13	↑10	↑8
CV end point ↓	+	Probable	+	+ (↓ mortality)	No data	+ (↓ mortality)

CV, cardiovascular; CYP, cytochrome P-450; HDL, high-density lipoprotein; LDL, low-density lipoprotein; –, no; +, yes.

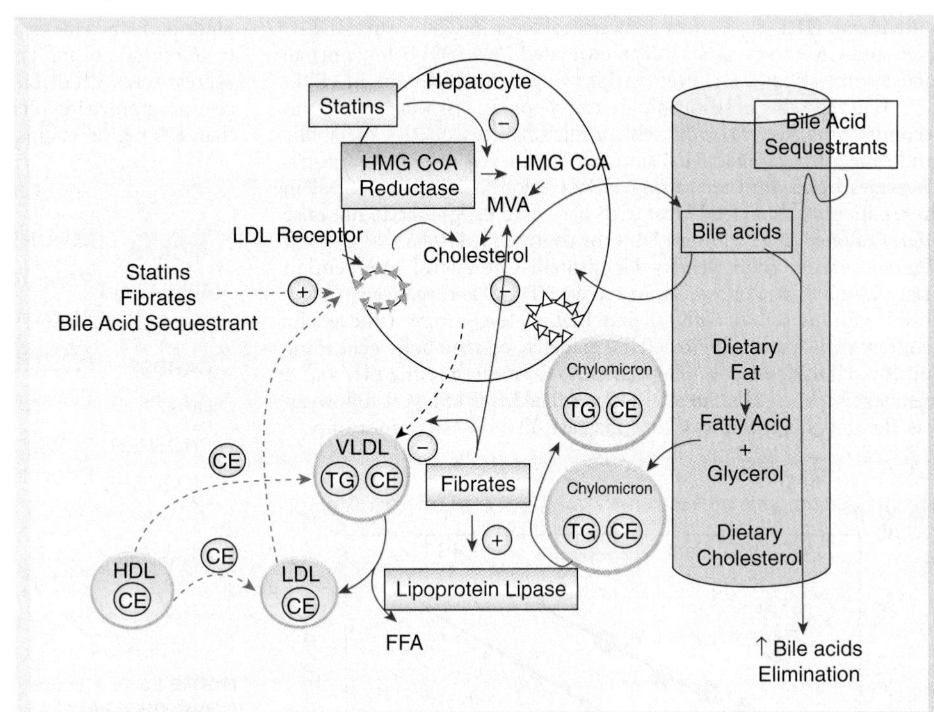

FIGURE 24-17 • Lipid-lowering therapy affecting cholesterol synthesis and transport. CE, cholesteryl ester; FFA, free fatty acid; HMG CoA, hydroxymethylglutaryl coenzyme A; MVA, mevalonic acid; TG, triglyceride.

TABLE 24-14 MAJOR SECONDARY AND PRIMARY PREVENTION TRIAL OF HMG COA REDUCTASE INHIBITORS

Trial	Statin (Dose)	Duration (yr)	LDL (% Reduction)	Events	Events % (Comparator)	Events % (Statin)	Absolute Risk Reduction (%)
SECONDARY PREVENTION TRIALS							
HPS[144]	Simvastatin, 40 mg	5	30	Death Vascular death Total MI	14.7 9.1 11.8	12.9 7.6 8.7	1.8 1.5 3.1
PROSPER[167]	Pravastatin, 40 mg	3.2	34	CHD death or nonfatal MI	12.2	10.1	2.1
LIPID[168]	Pravastatin, 40 mg	5	28	Death AMI	14.1 10.3	11.0 7.4	3.1 2.9
CARE[142]	Pravastatin, 40 mg	5	32	Fatal or nonfatal MI	13.2	10.2	3.0
4S[143]	Simvastatin, 20 or 40 mg	5.4	34	Total mortality MI + CHD death	11.5 22.6	8.2 15.9	3.3 30
PRIMARY PREVENTION TRIALS							
ASCOT-LLA[169]	Atorvastatin,10 mg	3.3	35	Nonfatal MI + CHD death	3.0	1.9	1.1
AFCAPS[170]	Lovastatin, 20 or 40 mg	5	25	CAD death	0.5	0.3	0.2
WOSCOPS[171]	Pravastatin, 40 mg	5	26	Death Primary end point	4.1 7.5	3.2 5.3	0.9 2.2

AMI, acute myocardial infarction; CAD, coronary artery disease; CHD, congestive heart disease; LDL, low-density lipoprotein; MI, myocardial infarction.

MI, and stroke.[3] All patients admitted to the hospital for UA/NSTEMI or STEMI should be treated with the LDL-C targeted to less than 70 mg/dl.[6] Choice of drug and dosage should be guided by measurement of LDL-C, triglyceride, and HDL-C levels. If the baseline LDL-C level is higher, a high dose of statin or the combination of a standard dose of a statin with a bile acid sequestrant, nicotinic acid, or fibrates may be required for those with high triglycerides (>200 mg/dl) or low HDL-C (<40 mg/dl).[140,141]

Elevated Non–HDL-C. Non–HDL-C is highly correlated with atherogenic triglycerides and total apolipoprotein B, the major apolipoprotein of all atherogenic lipoproteins, which strongly predicts severity of coronary atherosclerosis and CHD events.[140] In persons with high triglyceride levels (>200 mg/dl), non–HDL-C (total cholesterol minus HDL-C), or the sum of LDL-C and very-low-density cholesterol, is a target of lipid-lowering therapy with the goal to keep non–HDL-C less than 100 mg/dl in high-risk patients.[140]

Reduced HDL-C. A strong inverse association between HDL-C levels and CAD risk exists, with an estimated 2% to 3% below normal increase in risk for CHD events with every 1-mg/dl decline in HDL-C.[147] Whether this relationship is causal or an association due to accompanying adverse cardiac risk profile (diabetes, obesity, metabolic syndrome, physical inactivity, smoking, high levels of LDL-C and triglycerides), and whether raising HDL-C alone will be beneficial in these patients, is not clear. Most trials have used drugs that do not raise HDL-C alone but also lower LDL-C or triglyceride levels. In the recent Veterans Affairs High-Density Lipoprotein Cholesterol Intervention Trial (VA-HIT) trial, however, increased HDL-C and reduced triglycerides without significantly altered LDL-C levels were achieved by gemfibrozil in patients with CHD, diabetes, or metabolic syndrome and low HDL-C without elevated LDL-C (mean 112 mg/dl), and a relative reduction (22%) in fatal and nonfatal MI over 5-year follow-up was demonstrated without any increase in non-CHD mortality.[148]

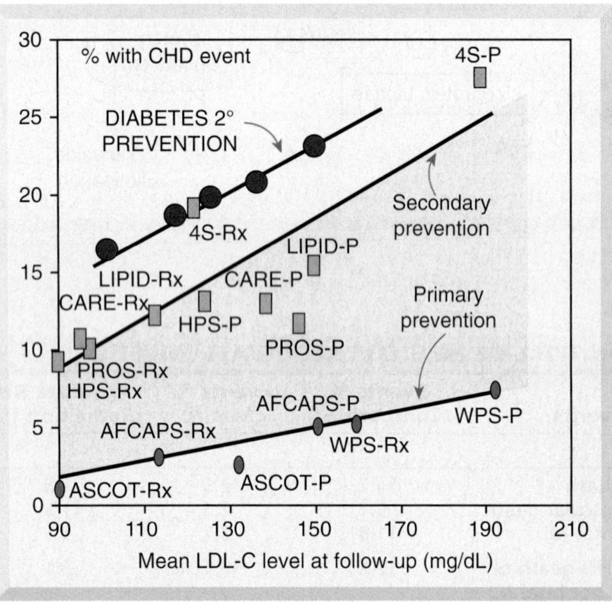

FIGURE 24-18 • Primary and secondary prevention statin trials with mean LDL-C levels and CHD events. (From Opie LH, Gersh BJ. Drugs for the Heart: Textbook with Online Updates, 6th ed. Amsterdam: Elsevier, 2004.)

Since patients with established coronary disease and low HDL-C (<35 to 40 mg/dl) are at high risk for coronary events, they should be treated aggressively with dietary modification, weight loss, and a regular exercise program with pharmacologic reduction in LDL-C levels to less than 100 mg/dl (statins) and in non–HDL-C levels to less than 130 mg/

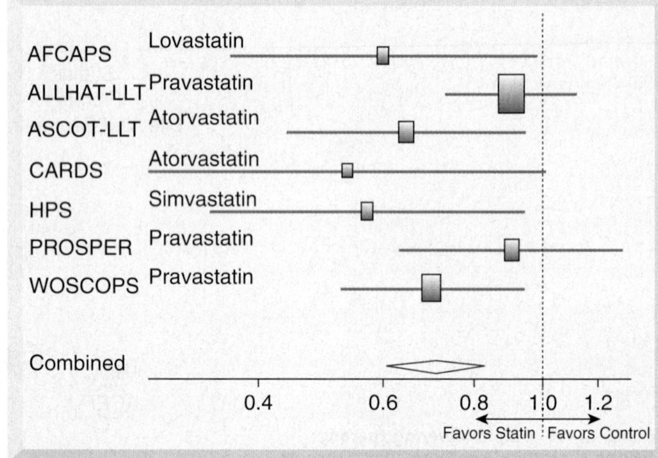

FIGURE 24-19 • Primary and secondary prevention statin trials with relative risk ratios of major coronary events and 95% confidence intervals. (Adapted from Thavendiranathan P, Bagai A, Brookhart MA, Choudry NK. Primary prevention of cardiovascular diseases with statin therapy: a meta-analysis of randomized controlled trials. Arch Intern Med 2006;166:2307-2313.)

TABLE 24-15 LIPID-LOWERING DRUG CLASSES WITH THEIR IMPACT ON LIPID PROFILE

	% Reduction		
Drug Class	**LDL**	**HDL**	**Triglycerides**
HMG-CoA reductase inhibitors	↓18-55%	↑5-15%	↓7-30%
Fibric acid derivatives	↓5-20%	↑10-35%	↓20-50%
Bile acid sequestrants	↓15-30%	↑3-5%	↔ or ↑
Nicotinic acid	↓5-25%	↑15-35%	↓20-50%

HDL, high-density lipoprotein; HMG-CoA, hydroxymethylglutaryl coenzyme A; LDL, low-density lipoprotein.

TABLE 24-16 ADVERSE EFFECTS OF LIPID-LOWERING DRUGS*

Drug	Toxic Side Effects	General Side Effects	Hypersensitivity	Safe Use in Pregnancy
Binding resins	None	GI, increased triglycerides, **vitamin deficiency (fat-soluble vitamins)**	Possible	May bind fat-soluble vitamins (B)
Fibrates	Rhabdomyolysis (rare), hepatitis (rare), renal failure	GI, diuretic (clofibrate), leukopenia, **cholecystitis**, cholelithiasis, rash (photosensitivity)	Arthritis, vasculitis; Stevens-Johnson syndrome (clofibrate)	Safety is unknown (C)
HMG-CoA reductase inhibitors	Rhabdomyolysis (rare), hepatitis (rare), pancreatitis, **proteinuria (rosuvastatin)**	GI, CNS, **myositis, myalgia, increased serum transaminases (liver)**, conjunctivitis	LLS, rash (lichenoid eruption), arthralgia, thrombocytopenia	Do not use: reports of birth defects (X)
Nicotinic acid derivatives	Hepatitis, rhabdomyolysis (rare), coronary steal, hypotension, lactic acidosis	Ocular changes, decreased vision, **rash (itching and flushing,** acanthosis nigricans, exfoliation, brown pigmentation), GI, CNS, **hyperglycemia, gout**	Rash (not determined to be allergic-mediated)	(A); not "toxic" in usual doses for lipid therapy

***Boldface** type signifies more prevalence or more severe reactions.

A, B, C, X, U.S. Food and Drug Administration pregnancy safety categories; CNS, central nervous system effects; GI, gastrointestinal effects; HMG-CoA, hydroxymethylglutaryl coenzyme A; LLS, lupus-like syndrome.

Modified from Ou NN, Oyen LJ, Murphy JG, Jahangir A. *In* Murphy JG, Lloyd MA (eds): Mayo Clinic Cardiology: Concise Textbook, 3rd ed. Rochester: Mayo Clinic Scientific Press/Informa Healthcare, 2007, pp. 1291-1308.

BOX 24-12 RECOMMENDATIONS FOR THERAPY WITH LIPID-LOWERING AGENTS

Class I

- If **LDL-C is ≥100 mg/dl,** ***LDL-lowering drug therapy*** should be initiated (LoE: A) or intensified (LoE: A) in addition to therapeutic lifestyle changes.
- If **TG is ≥500 mg/dl,** therapeutic options to lower the TG level to reduce the risk of pancreatitis are ***nicotinic acid (niacin)*** and ***fibric acid derivatives*** (fenofibrate, gemfibrozil); these should be initiated before LDL-C–lowering therapy. The goal is to achieve non–HDL-C less than 130 mg/dl if possible, and LDL-C should be treated to goal after TG-lowering therapy (LoE: C).
- ***Drug combinations*** are beneficial for patients on lipid-lowering therapy who are *unable to achieve LDL-C less than 100 mg/dl* (LoE: C).
- ***Statins,*** in the absence of contraindications, regardless of baseline cholesterol and diet modification, should be given to **post-MI** patients, including post-revascularization patients (LoE: A).
- Therapeutic options to reduce non–HDL-C are recommended, including *more intense LDL-C–lowering therapy* (LoE: B).

Class IIa

- Adding ***plant stanols/sterols*** (2 g/day) and/or ***viscous fiber*** (>10 g/day) is reasonable to further lower LDL-C (LoE: A).
- Reduction of *LDL-C to less than 70 mg/dl* or ***high-dose statin*** therapy is reasonable (LoE: A).
- ***Fibrate*** therapy as a therapeutic option can be useful to reduce non–HDL-C (after LDL-C–lowering therapy) (LoE: B).
- If LDL-C less than 70 mg/dl is the chosen target, consider *drug titration* to achieve this level to minimize side effects and cost (LoE: C).
- When LDL-C less than 70 mg/dl is not achievable because of *high baseline LDL-C levels,* it is generally possible to achieve reductions of greater than 50% in LDL-C levels by either ***statins*** or LDL-C–lowering ***drug combinations*** (LoE: C).
- ***Nicotinic acid (niacin)*** and ***fibric acid derivatives*** (fenofibrate, gemfibrozil) can be useful as therapeutic options (after LDL-C–lowering therapy) for *HDL-C less than 40 mg/dl* (LoE: B).
- ***Nicotinic acid (niacin)*** and ***fibric acid derivatives*** (fenofibrate, gemfibrozil) can be useful as therapeutic options (after LDL-C–lowering therapy) for *TG greater than 200 mg/dl* (LoE: B).

Class IIb

- For all patients, encouraging consumption of ***ω-3 fatty acids*** in the form of fish or in capsule form (1 g/day) for risk reduction may be reasonable. For treatment of *elevated TG,* higher doses (2 to 4 g/day) are usually necessary for risk reduction (LoE: B).

HDL-C, high-density lipoprotein cholesterol; LDL-C, low-density lipoprotein cholesterol; LoE, level of evidence; MI, myocardial infarction; TG, triglycerides.

dl and an increase in HDL-C levels by fibrates or nicotinic acid.[140,141] The Adult Treatment Panel III of the National Cholesterol Education Program does not specify a goal for HDL raising as the evidence from clinical trials to reduce risk, although suggestive, is insufficient to specify a goal of therapy.

The cholesteryl ester transfer protein (CETP) is a plasma glycoprotein that plays a critical role in the reverse cholesterol transport pathway and recycling of HDL particles. Mutations in the CETP gene with reduced CETP activity have been associated with high HDL levels and reduced cardiovascular risk,[149] while elevated CETP levels correlate with low HDL-C levels, progression of coronary atherosclerosis, and responsiveness to statin therapy.[150] Early human trials with CETP inhibitors such as torcetrapib and JTT-705 demonstrated a beneficial effect with significant increase in HDL-C and modest reduction in LDL-C levels. Despite these beneficial effects on the lipid profile, torcetrapib therapy when added to atorvastatin was associated with increased mortality and cardiac events along with increase in blood pressure, aldosterone level, and electrolyte abnormalities.[151] It is not clear whether these results, which led to the early termination of the Investigation of Lipid Level Management to Understand its Impact in Atherosclerotic Events (ILLUMINATE) trial, were due to inhibition of CETP or to off-target effects of the drug, and this needs to be further clarified.[151]

Elevated Triglycerides. Elevated triglyceride levels increases CHD risk mainly due to association with other factors, including diabetes, obesity, hypertension, abnormalities in hemostatic factors, and high LDL-C and low HDL-C levels, but also have an independent effect. Patients with elevated triglycerides (>200 mg/dl) should be treated by dietary modification, alcohol reduction, smoking cessation, weight loss, regular exercise, and pharmacologic means. Risk of pancreatitis increases with triglyceride levels greater than 500 mg/dl, which should be aggressively treated (see Box 24-12). Drugs that can lower triglycerides include gemfibrozil and other fibrate derivatives, nicotinic acid, and to a lesser degree statins. In the Helsinki Heart Study, gemfibrozil reduced triglycerides levels by 35% and LDL-C levels by 11%, while raising HDL-C levels by 11%, with a 34% reduction in CHD events over 5 years.[152] Gemfibrozil was more beneficial in diabetics, obese persons, and subjects with high triglyceride and low HDL-C levels than in the treated group as a whole.[141,152] It is not clear at this time whether treatment directed at high triglyceride levels alone reduces risk for CHD events.

ω-3 Fatty acid therapy (1 to 2 g/day) is reasonable for reduction of risk of CAD and in patients with elevated triglyceride levels (see Box 24-12).

Emerging Targets and Therapeutics

Strategies to protect the heart against ischemic injury currently involve early reperfusion following coronary occlusion (fibrinolytics, antithrombotics, or PCI) or interventions that reduce energy demands during ischemia with drugs and preventive therapies to reduce atherosclerotic burden and progression (see Fig. 24-4 and Box 24-13). In addition to these established therapeutic strategies, activation of endogenous protective responses can increase myocardial tolerance to ischemia-reperfusion injury.[153] Two major endogenous protective responses, ischemic preconditioning and postconditioning, have been identified in the heart.[153-155] Ischemic preconditioning is one of the most powerful endogenous cardioprotective mechanisms, whereby transient nonlethal ischemic events render the myocardium resistant to subsequent prolonged ischemia, limiting infarct size and myocardial mechanical and electrical dysfunction following reperfusion.[154] Brief repetitive interruptions in blood flow in the early minutes of reperfusion (postconditioning) is also cardioprotective against reperfusion injury by limiting infarct size.[156,157]

Insights into mechanisms underlying endogenous cardioprotective responses have resulted in the exploration of novel therapeutic avenues (Fig. 24-20). This includes administration or promotion of endogenous production of cardioprotective adenosine, NO, or opioids that trigger protective signal transduction pathways.[158] Similarly, drugs that directly activate or increase the synthesis of cardioprotective proteins may enhance tolerance of the heart against injury (see Fig. 24-20). These drugs include potassium channel openers,[106] volatile anesthetics,[159] and various agonists of G protein–coupled receptors.[160] Stem cells in the heart or in the peripheral tissues have also been shown to increase the potential to differentiate into myocardial, endothelial, and vascular tissue and are being considered for cell-based therapies as a strategy to replace damaged myocardium and/or promote endogenous cardioprotective responses.[161,162] The efficacy of such therapy to improve long-term clinical outcomes and safety in humans[163] needs to be further evaluated in randomized clinical trials. Interventions that target signaling cascades or receptors that restore endogenous cardioprotective responses with exercise, caloric restriction, or ischemic pre- or postconditioning responses are all potential strategies that need to be systematically studied in humans to identify their beneficial effect in reducing morbidity and mortality in patients with ischemic heart disease.[158,164-166]

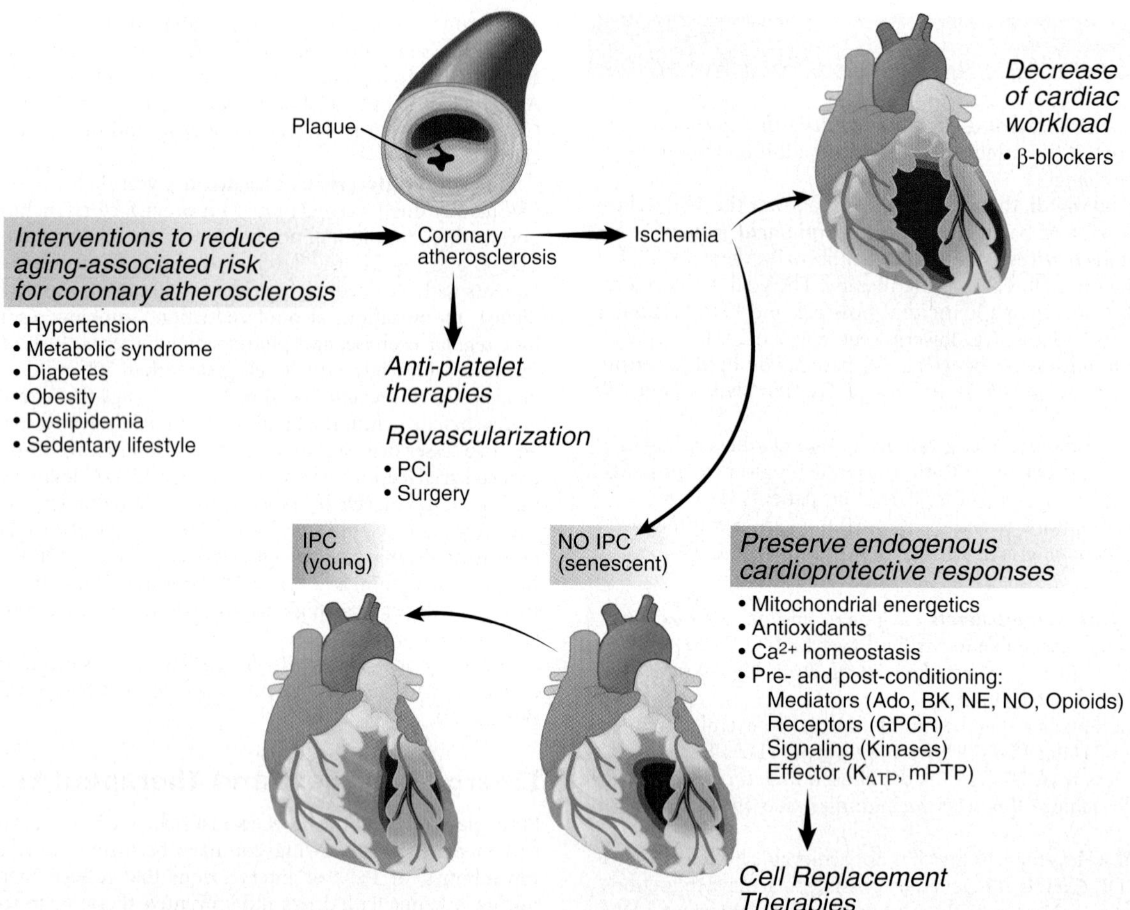

FIGURE 24-20 • Strategies to reduce risk for coronary atherosclerosis, limit myocardial ischemia, and salvage myocardium by restoration of endogenous cardioprotective responses during stress. Interventions to control risk factors for coronary atherosclerosis, reduce cardiac work load or improve O_2 supply, and targeting pathways of cardioprotection and cell therapies for myocardial repair/replacement are all strategies to limit myocardial dysfunction in patients with coronary heart disease. Ado, adenosine; BK, bradykinin; GPCR, G protein–coupled receptors; IPC, ischemic preconditioning; K_{ATP}, ATP-sensitive K channel; NE, norepinephrine; NO, nitric oxide; MPTP, mitochondrial permeability transition pore; PCI, percutaneous coronary intervention; RNS, reactive nitrogen species; ROS, reactive oxygen species. (From Jahangir A, Sagar S, Terzic A. Aging and cardioprotection. J Appl Physiol 2007;103:2120-2128.)

BOX 24-13 ACC/AHA RECOMMENDATION CLASS AND LEVEL OF EVIDENCE FOR CARDIOVASCULAR DRUGS

		Indication Class/Level of Evidence		
Agent	**Drug Indication**	**Stable Angina**	**UA/NSTEMI**	**STEMI**
Aspirin	Antiplatelet effect	I/A	I/A	I/A
Clopidogrel or ticlodipine	Antiplatelet effect when aspirin is contraindicated	I/A	I/A	I/A
Aspirin and clopidogrel	Dual antiplatelet effect	—	I/B	I/B
β-Blockers	Anti-ischemic	I/A	I/B	I/A
ACE inhibitors	EF < 40% or heart failure	I/A	I/A, IIa/A	I/A
Calcium channel blockers	Antianginal	I/B	I/B	I/B
Nitrates	Antianginal	I/B	I/C	I/C
Dipyridamole	Antiplatelet	III/A	III/A	III/A
Statins	LDL-C > 70 mg/dl	Ia	Ia	Ia
Fibrates	HDL-C < 40 mg/dl	IIa/B	IIa/B	IIa/B
Niacin	HDL-C < 40 mg/dl	IIa/B	IIa/B	IIa/B
Niacin or fibrate	Triglycerides >200 mg/dl	IIa/B	IIa/B	IIa/B
Omega-3 fatty acids	Triglycerides >200 mg/dl	IIb	IIb	IIb

ACE, angiotensin-converting enzyme; EF, ejection fraction; HDL-C, high-density lipoprotein cholesterol; LDL-C, low-density lipoprotein cholesterol; NSTEMI, non–ST-elevation myocardial infarction; STEMI, ST-elevation myocardial infarction; UA, unstable angina.

REFERENCES

1. World Health Organization. World Health Statistics 2006. Geneva: World Health Organization, 2006. Available at *http://www.who.int/whosis/whostat2006.pdf*
2. Rosamond W, Flegal K, Furie K, et al. Heart disease and stroke statistics 2008 update: a report from the American Heart Association Statistics Committee and Stroke Statistics Subcommittee. Circulation 2008;117:e25-e146.
3. Antman EM, Anbe DT, Armstrong PW, et al. ACC/AHA guidelines for the management of patients with ST-elevation myocardial infarction: a report of the American College of Cardiology/American Heart Association Task Force on Practice Guidelines (Committee to Revise the 1999 Guidelines for the Management of Patients with Acute Myocardial Infarction). Circulation 2004;110:e82-e292.
4. Reimer KA, Jennings RB. The "wavefront phenomenon" of myocardial ischemic cell death. II. Transmural progression of necrosis within the framework of ischemic

bed size (myocardium at risk) and collateral flow. Lab Invest 1979;40:633-644.

5. Antman EM, Hand M, Armstrong PW, et al. 2007 Focused Update of the ACC/AHA 2004 Guidelines for the Management of Patients with ST-Elevation Myocardial Infarction: a report of the American College of Cardiology/American Heart Association Task Force on Practice Guidelines; developed in collaboration with the Canadian Cardiovascular Society; endorsed by the American Academy of Family Physicians: 2007 Writing Group to Review New Evidence and Update the ACC/AHA 2004 Guidelines for the Management of Patients with ST-Elevation Myocardial Infarction, Writing on Behalf of the 2004 Writing Committee. Circulation 2008;117:296-329.
6. Anderson JL, Adams CD, Antman EM, et al. ACC/AHA 2007 guidelines for the management of patients with unstable angina/non ST-elevation myocardial infarction: a report of the American College of Cardiology/American Heart Association Task Force on Practice Guidelines (Writing Committee to Revise the 2002 Guidelines for the Management of Patients with Unstable Angina/Non ST-Elevation Myocardial Infarction); developed in collaboration with the American College of Emergency Physicians, the Society for Cardiovascular Angiography and Interventions, and the Society of Thoracic Surgeons; endorsed by the American Association of Cardiovascular and Pulmonary Rehabilitation and the Society for Academic Emergency Medicine. Circulation 2007;116:e148-e304.
7. Gibbons RJ, Abrams J, Chatterjee K, et al. ACC/AHA 2002 guideline update for the management of patients with chronic stable angina—summary article: a report of the American College of Cardiology/American Heart Association Task Force on Practice Guidelines (Committee on the Management of Patients with Chronic Stable Angina). Circulation 2003;107:149-158.
8. Cummins RO, Ornato JP, Thies WH, et al. Improving survival from sudden cardiac arrest: the "chain of survival" concept. A statement for health professionals from the Advanced Cardiac Life Support Subcommittee and the Emergency Cardiac Care Committee, American Heart Association. Circulation 1991;83:1832-1847.
9. Sheifer SE, Manolio TA, Gersh BJ. Unrecognized myocardial infarction. Ann Intern Med 2001;135:801-811.
10. Antman EM, Braunwald E. Acute myocardial infarction. *In* Braunwald E, Zipes DP, Libby P (eds): Heart Disease: A Textbook of Cardiovascular Medicine, 6th ed. Philadelphia: WB Saunders, 2001, pp 1114-1251.
11. Collaborative meta-analysis of randomised trials of antiplatelet therapy for prevention of death, myocardial infarction, and stroke in high risk patients. BMJ 2002;324:71-86.
12. Maroko PR, Radvany P, Braunwald E, et al. Reduction of infarct size by oxygen inhalation following acute coronary occlusion. Circulation 1975;52:360-368.
13. Randomised trial of intravenous streptokinase, oral aspirin, both, or neither among 17,187 cases of suspected acute myocardial infarction: ISIS-2. ISIS-2 (Second International Study of Infarct Survival) Collaborative Group. Lancet 1988;2:349-360.
14. Menown IB, Mackenzie G, Adgey AA. Optimizing the initial 12-lead electrocardiographic diagnosis of acute myocardial infarction. Eur Heart J 2000;21:275-283.
15. Roux S, Christeller S, Ludin E. Effects of aspirin on coronary reocclusion and recurrent ischemia after thrombolysis: a meta-analysis. J Am Coll Cardiol 1992;19:671-677.
16. Collaborative overview of randomised trials of antiplatelet therapy—I: Prevention of death, myocardial infarction, and stroke by prolonged antiplatelet therapy in various categories of patients. Antiplatelet Trialists' Collaboration. BMJ 1994;308:81-106.
17. King SB 3rd, Smith SC Jr, Hirshfeld JW Jr, et al. 2007 Focused Update of the ACC/AHA/SCAI 2005 Guideline Update for Percutaneous Coronary Intervention: a report of the American College of Cardiology/American Heart Association Task Force on Practice Guidelines: 2007 Writing Group to Review New Evidence and Update the ACC/AHA/SCAI 2005 Guideline Update for Percutaneous Coronary Intervention, Writing on Behalf of the 2005 Writing Committee. Circulation 2008;117:261-295.
18. MacDonald TM, Wei L. Effect of ibuprofen on cardioprotective effect of aspirin. Lancet 2003;361:573-574.
19. Smith SC Jr, Feldman TE, Hirshfeld JW Jr, et al. ACC/AHA/SCAI 2005 Guideline Update for Percutaneous Coronary Intervention-Summary Article: a report of the American College of Cardiology/American Heart Association Task Force on Practice Guidelines (ACC/AHA/SCAI Writing Committee to Update the 2001 Guidelines for Percutaneous Coronary Intervention). J Am Coll Cardiol 2006;47:216-235.
20. The Clopidogrel in Unstable Angina to Prevent Recurrent Events Trial I: effects of clopidogrel in addition to aspirin in patients with acute coronary syndromes without ST-segment elevation. N Engl J Med 2001;345:494-502.
21. Ridker PM, Cook NR, Lee IM, et al. A randomized trial of low-dose aspirin in the primary prevention of cardiovascular disease in women. N Engl J Med 2005;352:1293-1304.
22. Fleming T, Nissen SE, Borer JS, et al. Report from the 100th Cardiovascular and Renal Drugs Advisory Committee meeting: U.S. Food and Drug Administration, December 8-9, 2003, Gaithersburg, MD. Circulation 2004;109:e9004-e9005.
23. A randomised, blinded, trial of Clopidogrel versus Aspirin in Patients at Risk of Ischaemic Events (CAPRIE). CAPRIE Steering Committee. Lancet 1996;348:1329-1339.
24. Ridker PM, Cushman M, Stampfer MJ, et al. Inflammation, aspirin, and the risk of cardiovascular disease in apparently healthy men. N Engl J Med 1997;336:973-979.
25. Mason PJ, Jacobs AK, Freedman JE. Aspirin resistance and atherothrombotic disease. J Am Coll Cardiol 2005;46:986-993.
26. Hankey GJ, Eikelboom JW. Aspirin resistance. Lancet 2006;367:606-617.
27. Angiolillo DJ, Fernandez-Ortiz A, Bernardo E, et al. Variability in individual responsiveness to clopidogrel: clinical implications, management, and future perspectives. J Am Coll Cardiol 2007;49:1505-1516.
28. Steinhubl SR, Moliterno DJ. The role of the platelet in the pathogenesis of atherothrombosis. Am J Cardiovasc Drugs 2005;5:399-408.
29. Coller BS. Platelets and thrombolytic therapy. N Engl J Med 1990;322:33-42.
30. Physicians Desk Reference Electronic Library, Version 5.1 (Intranet). Montvale, NJ: Thomson Healthcare, 2008.
31. Fox KA, Mehta SR, Peters R, et al. Benefits and risks of the combination of clopidogrel and aspirin in patients undergoing surgical revascularization for non-ST-elevation acute coronary syndrome: the Clopidogrel in Unstable angina to prevent Recurrent ischemic Events (CURE) trial. Circulation 2004;110:1202-1208.
32. Jin J, Kunapuli SP. Coactivation of two different G protein-coupled receptors is essential for ADP-induced platelet aggregation. Proc Natl Acad Sci U S A 1998;95:8070-8074.
33. Antman EM, Cohen M, McCabe C, et al. Enoxaparin is superior to unfractionated heparin for preventing clinical events at 1-year follow-up of TIMI 11B and ESSENCE. Eur Heart J 2002;23:308-314.
34. Wallentin L, Goldstein P, Armstrong PW, et al. Efficacy and safety of tenecteplase in combination with the low-molecular-weight heparin enoxaparin or unfractionated heparin in the prehospital setting: the Assessment of the Safety and Efficacy of a New Thrombolytic regimen (ASSENT)-3 PLUS randomized trial in acute myocardial infarction. Circulation 2003;108:135-142.
35. Lev EI, Patel RT, Maresh KJ, et al. Aspirin and clopidogrel drug response in patients undergoing percutaneous coronary intervention: the role of dual drug resistance. J Am Coll Cardiol 2006;47:27-33.
36. Gurbel PA, Bliden KP, Zaman KA, et al. Clopidogrel loading with eptifibatide to arrest the reactivity of platelets: results of the Clopidogrel Loading with Eptifibatide to Arrest the Reactivity of Platelets (CLEAR PLATELETS) study. Circulation 2005;111:1153-1159.
37. Bhatt DL, Fox KA, Hacke W, et al. Clopidogrel and aspirin versus aspirin alone for the prevention of atherothrombotic events. N Engl J Med 2006;354:1706-1717.
38. Chen ZM, Jiang LX, Chen YP, et al. Addition of clopidogrel to aspirin in 45,852 patients with acute myocardial infarction: randomised placebo-controlled trial. Lancet 2005;366:1607-1621.
39. Sabatine MS, Cannon CP, Gibson CM, et al. Addition of clopidogrel to aspirin and fibrinolytic therapy for myocardial infarction with ST-segment elevation. N Engl J Med 2005;352:1179-1189.
40. Leontiadis GI, Sharma VK, Howden CW. Systematic review and meta-analysis of proton pump inhibitor therapy in peptic ulcer bleeding. BMJ 2005;330:568.
41. Bhatt DL. Aspirin resistance: more than just a laboratory curiosity. J Am Coll Cardiol 2004;43:1127-1129.
42. Maree AO, Cox D, Fitzgerald DJ. Drug insight: aspirin resistance—fact or fashion? Nat Clin Pract Cardiovasc Med 2007;4:E1; author reply E2.
43. Ferguson JJ, Califf RM, Antman EM, et al. Enoxaparin vs unfractionated heparin in high-risk patients with non-ST-segment elevation acute coronary syndromes managed with an intended early invasive strategy: primary results of the SYNERGY randomized trial. JAMA 2004;292:45-54.
44. Lev EI, Patel RT, Guthikonda S, et al. Genetic polymorphisms of the platelet receptors $P2Y_{12}$, $P2Y_1$ and GP IIIa and response to aspirin and clopidogrel. Thromb Res 2007;119:355-360.
45. Serebruany VL, Steinhubl SR, Berger PB, et al. Variability in platelet responsiveness to clopidogrel among 544 individuals. J Am Coll Cardiol 2005;45:246-251.
46. Lau WC, Gurbel PA, Watkins PB, et al. Contribution of hepatic cytochrome P450 3A4 metabolic activity to the phenomenon of clopidogrel resistance. Circulation 2004;109:166-171.
47. Yusuf S, Mehta SR, Chrolavicius S, et al. Effects of fondaparinux on mortality and reinfarction in patients with acute ST-segment elevation myocardial infarction: the OASIS-6 randomized trial. JAMA 2006;295:1519-1530.
48. Neubauer H, Gunesdogan B, Hanefeld C, et al. Lipophilic statins interfere with the inhibitory effects of clopidogrel on platelet function—a flow cytometry study. Eur Heart J 2003;24:1744-1749.
49. Angiolillo DJ, Alfonso F. Clopidogrel-statin interaction: myth or reality? J Am Coll Cardiol 2007;50:296-298.
50. Mukherjee D, Kline-Rogers E, Fang J, et al. Lack of clopidogrel-CYP3A4 statin interaction in patients with acute coronary syndrome. Heart 2005;91:23-26.
51. Balsano F, Rizzon P, Violi F, et al. Antiplatelet treatment with ticlopidine in unstable angina: a controlled multicenter clinical trial. The Studio della Ticlopidina nell'Angina Instabile Group. Circulation 1990;82:17-26.
52. Topol EJ, Byzova TV, Plow EF. Platelet GPIIb-IIIa blockers. Lancet 1999;353:227-231.
53. Mukherjee D, Roffi M. Current strategies with high-dose tirofiban. Expert Opin Drug Metab Toxicol 2007;3:275-280.
54. Boersma E, Maas AC, Deckers JW, et al. Early thrombolytic treatment in acute myocardial infarction: reappraisal of the golden hour. Lancet 1996;348:771-775.
55. Simoons ML. Effect of glycoprotein IIb/IIIa receptor blocker abciximab on outcome in patients with acute coronary syndromes without early coronary revascularisation: the GUSTO IV-ACS randomised trial. Lancet 2001;357:1915-1924.
56. Montalescot G, Antoniucci D, Kastrati A, et al. Abciximab in primary coronary stenting of ST-elevation myocardial infarction: a European meta-analysis on individual patients' data with long-term follow-up. Eur Heart J 2007;28:443-449.
57. Tcheng JE, Kandzari DE, Grines CL, et al. Benefits and risks of abciximab use in primary angioplasty for acute myocardial infarction: the Controlled Abciximab and Device Investigation to Lower Late Angioplasty Complications (CADILLAC) trial. Circulation 2003;108:1316-1323.
58. Halkes PH, van Gijn J, Kappelle LJ, et al. Aspirin plus dipyridamole versus aspirin alone after cerebral ischaemia of arterial origin (ESPRIT): randomised controlled trial. Lancet 2006;367:1665-1673.
59. Norrving B. Dipyridamole with aspirin for secondary stroke prevention. Lancet 2006;367:1638-1639.

60. Stone GW, McLaurin BT, Cox DA, et al. Bivalirudin for patients with acute coronary syndromes. N Engl J Med 2006;355:2203-2216.
61. Simpson D, Wellington K. Nicorandil: a review of its use in the management of stable angina pectoris, including high-risk patients. Drugs 2004;64:1941-1955.
62. Markham A, Plosker GL, Goa KL. Nicorandil: an updated review of its use in ischaemic heart disease with emphasis on its cardioprotective effects. Drugs 2000;60:955-974.
63. Trial to show the Impact Of Nicorandil in Angina (IONA): design, methodology, and management. Heart 2001;85:E9.
64. Bucchi A, Baruscotti M, DiFrancesco D. Current-dependent block of rabbit sino-atrial node I_f channels by ivabradine. J Gen Physiol 2002;120:1-13.
65. Savelieva I, Camm AJ. Novel I_f current inhibitor ivabradine: safety considerations. Adv Cardiol 2006;43:79-96.
66. Castelli R, Cassinerio E, Cappellini MD, et al. Heparin induced thrombocytopenia: pathogenetic, clinical, diagnostic and therapeutic aspects. Cardiovasc Hematol Disord Drug Targets 2007;7:153-162.
67. Granger CB, Miller JM, Bovill EG, et al. Rebound increase in thrombin generation and activity after cessation of intravenous heparin in patients with acute coronary syndromes. Circulation 1995;91:1929-1935.
68. Gurm HS, Eagle KA. Use of anticoagulants in ST-segment elevation myocardial infarction patients: a focus on low-molecular-weight heparin. Cardiovasc Drugs Ther 2008;22:59-69.
69. Antman EM, Cohen M, Radley D, et al. Assessment of the treatment effect of enoxaparin for unstable angina/non-Q-wave myocardial infarction: TIMI 11B-ESSENCE meta-analysis. Circulation 1999;100:1602-1608.
70. Montalescot G, White HD, Gallo R, et al. Enoxaparin versus unfractionated heparin in elective percutaneous coronary intervention. N Engl J Med 2006;355:1006-1017.
71. Efficacy and safety of tenecteplase in combination with enoxaparin, abciximab, or unfractionated heparin: the ASSENT-3 randomised trial in acute myocardial infarction. Lancet 2001;358:605-613.
72. Antman EM, Morrow DA, McCabe CH, et al. Enoxaparin versus unfractionated heparin with fibrinolysis for ST-elevation myocardial infarction. N Engl J Med 2006;354:1477-1488.
73. Yusuf S, Mehta SR, Xie C, et al. Effects of reviparin, a low-molecular-weight heparin, on mortality, reinfarction, and strokes in patients with acute myocardial infarction presenting with ST-segment elevation. JAMA 2005;293:427-435.
74. Mehta SR, Granger CB, Eikelboom JW, et al. Efficacy and safety of fondaparinux versus enoxaparin in patients with acute coronary syndromes undergoing percutaneous coronary intervention: results from the OASIS-5 trial. J Am Coll Cardiol 2007;50:1742-1751.
75. Lincoff AM, Kleiman NS, Kottke-Marchant K, et al. Bivalirudin with planned or provisional abciximab versus low-dose heparin and abciximab during percutaneous coronary revascularization: results of the Comparison of Abciximab Complications with Hirulog for ischemic Events Trial (CACHET). Am Heart J 2002;143:847-853.
76. Lincoff AM, Bittl JA, Harrington RA, et al. Bivalirudin and provisional glycoprotein IIb/IIIa blockade compared with heparin and planned glycoprotein IIb/IIIa blockade during percutaneous coronary intervention: REPLACE-2 randomized trial. JAMA 2003;289:853-863.
77. Stone GW, Ware JH, Bertrand ME, et al. Antithrombotic strategies in patients with acute coronary syndromes undergoing early invasive management: one-year results from the ACUITY trial. JAMA 2007;298:2497-2506.
78. White H. Thrombin-specific anticoagulation with bivalirudin versus heparin in patients receiving fibrinolytic therapy for acute myocardial infarction: the HERO-2 randomised trial. Lancet 2001;358:1855-1863.
79. Serruys PW, Herrman J-PR, Simon R, et al. A comparison of hirudin with heparin in the prevention of restenosis after coronary angioplasty. N Engl J Med 1995;333:757-764.
80. Lee KL, Woodlief LH, Topol EJ, et al. Predictors of 30-day mortality in the era of reperfusion for acute myocardial infarction: results from an international trial of 41,021 patients. GUSTO-I Investigators. Circulation 1995;91:1659-1668.
81. White HD, Barbash GI, Califf RM, et al. Age and outcome with contemporary thrombolytic therapy: results from the GUSTO-I trial. Global Utilization of Streptokinase and TPA for Occluded coronary arteries trial. Circulation 1996;94:1826-1833.
82. Giugliano RP, McCabe CH, Antman EM, et al. Lower-dose heparin with fibrinolysis is associated with lower rates of intracranial hemorrhage. Am Heart J 2001;141:742-750.
83. Primary versus tenecteplase-facilitated percutaneous coronary intervention in patients with ST-segment elevation acute myocardial infarction (ASSENT-4 PCI): randomised trial. Lancet 2006;367:569-578.
84. Thadani U, Ripley TL. Side effects of using nitrates to treat heart failure and the acute coronary syndromes, unstable angina and acute myocardial infarction. Expert Opin Drug Saf 2007;6:385-396.
85. Munzel T, Daiber A, Mulsch A. Explaining the phenomenon of nitrate tolerance. Circ Res 2005;97:618-628.
86. Abrams J. How to use nitrates. Cardiovasc Drugs Ther 2002;16:511-514.
87. ISIS-4: a randomised factorial trial assessing early oral captopril, oral mononitrate, and intravenous magnesium sulphate in 58,050 patients with suspected acute myocardial infarction. ISIS-4 (Fourth International Study of Infarct Survival) Collaborative Group. Lancet 1995;345:669-685.
88. GISSI-3: effects of lisinopril and transdermal glyceryl trinitrate singly and together on 6-week mortality and ventricular function after acute myocardial infarction. Gruppo Italiano per lo Studio della Sopravvivenza nell'Infarto miocardico. Lancet 1994;343:1115-1122.
89. Taylor AL, Ziesche S, Yancy C, et al. Combination of isosorbide dinitrate and hydralazine in blacks with heart failure. N Engl J Med 2004;351:2049-2057.
90. Cheitlin MD, Hutter AM Jr, Brindis RG, et al. ACC/AHA expert consensus document: use of sildenafil (Viagra) in patients with cardiovascular disease. American College of Cardiology/American Heart Association. J Am Coll Cardiol 1999;33:273-282.
91. Pepine CJ, Cohn PF, Deedwania PC, et al. Effects of treatment on outcome in mildly symptomatic patients with ischemia during daily life. The Atenolol Silent Ischemia Study (ASIST). Circulation 1994;90:762-768.
92. Hunt SA, Abraham WT, Chin MH, et al. ACC/AHA 2005 Guideline Update for the Diagnosis and Management of Chronic Heart Failure in the Adult: a report of the American College of Cardiology/American Heart Association Task Force on Practice Guidelines (Writing Committee to Update the 2001 Guidelines for the Evaluation and Management of Heart Failure); developed in collaboration with the American College of Chest Physicians and the International Society for Heart and Lung Transplantation; endorsed by the Heart Rhythm Society. Circulation 2005;112:e154-e235.
93. Held C, Hjemdahl P, Rehnqvist N, et al. Fibrinolytic variables and cardiovascular prognosis in patients with stable angina pectoris treated with verapamil or metoprolol: results from the Angina Prognosis study in Stockholm. Circulation 1997;95:2380-2386.
94. Metoprolol in acute myocardial infarction: patient population. The MIAMI Trial Research Group. Am J Cardiol 1985;56:10G-14G.
95. Randomised trial of intravenous atenolol among 16 027 cases of suspected acute myocardial infarction: ISIS-1. First International Study of Infarct Survival Collaborative Group. Lancet 1986;2:57-66.
96. Chen ZM, Pan HC, Chen YP, et al. Early intravenous then oral metoprolol in 45,852 patients with acute myocardial infarction: randomised placebo-controlled trial. Lancet 2005;366:1622-1632.
97. Dargie HJ. Effect of carvedilol on outcome after myocardial infarction in patients with left-ventricular dysfunction: the CAPRICORN randomised trial. Lancet 2001; 357:1385-1390.
98. Miller MR, Megson IL. Recent developments in nitric oxide donor drugs. Br J Pharmacol 2007;151:305-321.
99. Chaitman BR, Skettino SL, Parker JO, et al. Anti-ischemic effects and long-term survival during ranolazine monotherapy in patients with chronic severe angina. J Am Coll Cardiol 2004;43:1375-1382.
100. Morrow DA, Scirica BM, Karwatowska-Prokopczuk E, et al. Effects of ranolazine on recurrent cardiovascular events in patients with non-ST-elevation acute coronary syndromes: the MERLIN-TIMI 36 randomized trial. JAMA 2007;297:1775-1783.
101. Siddiqui MA, Keam SJ. Spotlight on ranolazine in chronic stable angina pectoris. Am J Cardiovasc Drugs 2006;6:357-359.
102. Chaitman BR, Pepine CJ, Parker JO, et al. Effects of ranolazine with atenolol, amlodipine, or diltiazem on exercise tolerance and angina frequency in patients with severe chronic angina: a randomized controlled trial. JAMA 2004;291:309-316.
103. Marzilli M. Does trimetazidine prevent myocardial injury after percutaneous coronary intervention? Nat Clin Pract Cardiovasc Med 2008;5:16-17.
104. Stanley WC, Marzilli M. Metabolic therapy in the treatment of ischaemic heart disease: the pharmacology of trimetazidine. Fundam Clin Pharmacol 2003;17:133-145.
105. Kolbel F, Bada V. Trimetazidine in geriatric patients with stable angina pectoris: the TIGER study. Int J Clin Pract 2003;57:867-870.
106. Jahangir A, Terzic A. K(ATP) channel therapeutics at the bedside. J Mol Cell Cardiol 2005;39:99-112.
107. Zingman LV, Alekseev AE, Hodgson-Zingman DM, et al. ATP-sensitive potassium channels: metabolic sensing and cardioprotection. J Appl Physiol 2007;103:1888-1893.
108. Gross ER, Hsu AK, Gross GJ. Delayed cardioprotection afforded by the glycogen synthase kinase 3 inhibitor SB-216763 occurs via a KATP and MPTP-dependent mechanism at reperfusion. Am J Physiol Heart Circ Physiol 2008;294:H1497-H1500.
109. John SA, Weiss JN, Xie LH, et al. Molecular mechanism for ATP-dependent closure of the K^+ channel Kir6.2. J Physiol (Lond) 2003;552:23-34.
110. Jahangir A, Terzic A, Shen WK. Potassium channel openers: therapeutic potential in cardiology and medicine. Expert Opin Pharmacother 2001;2:1995-2010.
111. Savelieva I, Camm AJ. I_f inhibition with ivabradine: electrophysiological effects and safety. Drug Saf 2008;31:95-107.
112. Borer JS, Fox K, Jaillon P, et al. Antianginal and antiischemic effects of ivabradine, an I_f inhibitor, in stable angina: a randomized, double-blind, multicentered, placebo-controlled trial. Circulation 2003;107:817-823.
113. Lopez-Bescos L, Filipova S, Martos R. Long-term safety and efficacy of ivabradine in patients with chronic stable angina. Cardiology 2007;108:387-396.
114. Morris SD, Yellon DM. Angiotensin-converting enzyme inhibitors potentiate preconditioning through bradykinin B2 receptor activation in human heart. J Am Coll Cardiol 1997;29:1599-1606.
115. Pretorius M, Murphey LJ, McFarlane JA, et al. Angiotensin-converting enzyme inhibition alters the fibrinolytic response to cardiopulmonary bypass. Circulation 2003; 108:3079-3083.
116. Opie LH, Gersh BJ. Drugs for the Heart: Textbook with Online Updates, 6th ed. Amsterdam: Elsevier, 2004.
117. Schelleman H, Klungel OH, Witteman JC, et al. Angiotensinogen M235T polymorphism and the risk of myocardial infarction and stroke among hypertensive patients on ACE-inhibitors or beta-blockers. Eur J Hum Genet 2007;15:478-484.
118. Schelleman H, Klungel OH, Witteman JC, et al. Pharmacogenetic interactions of three candidate gene polymorphisms with ACE-inhibitors or beta-blockers and the risk of atherosclerosis. Br J Clin Pharmacol 2007;64:57-66.
119. Prasad A, Mincemoyer R, Quyyumi AA. Anti-ischemic effects of angiotensin-converting enzyme inhibition in hypertension. J Am Coll Cardiol 2001;38:1116-1122.

120. Pepine CJ, Rouleau JL, Annis K, et al. Effects of angiotensin-converting enzyme inhibition on transient ischemia: the Quinapril Anti-ischemia and Symptoms of Angina Reduction (QUASAR) trial. J Am Coll Cardiol 2003;42:2049-2059.
121. Ambrosioni E, Borghi C, Magnani B. The effect of the angiotensin-converting-enzyme inhibitor zofenopril on mortality and morbidity after anterior myocardial infarction. The Survival of Myocardial Infarction Long-term Evaluation (SMILE) Study Investigators. N Engl J Med 1995;332:80-85.
122. Effect of ramipril on mortality and morbidity of survivors of acute myocardial infarction with clinical evidence of heart failure. The Acute Infarction Ramipril Efficacy (AIRE) Study Investigators. Lancet 1993;342:821-828.
123. Kober L, Torp-Pedersen C, Carlsen JE, et al. A clinical trial of the angiotensin-converting-enzyme inhibitor trandolapril in patients with left ventricular dysfunction after myocardial infarction. Trandolapril Cardiac Evaluation (TRACE) Study Group. N Engl J Med 1995;333:1670-1676.
124. Latini R, Tognoni G, Maggioni AP, et al. Clinical effects of early angiotensin-converting enzyme inhibitor treatment for acute myocardial infarction are similar in the presence and absence of aspirin: systematic overview of individual data from 96,712 randomized patients. Angiotensin-Converting Enzyme Inhibitor Myocardial Infarction Collaborative Group. J Am Coll Cardiol 2000;35:1801-1807.
125. Al-Mallah MH, Tleyjeh IM, Abdel-Latif AA, et al. Angiotensin-converting enzyme inhibitors in coronary artery disease and preserved left ventricular systolic function: a systematic review and meta-analysis of randomized controlled trials. J Am Coll Cardiol 2006;47:1576-1583.
126. Pfeffer MA, Braunwald E, Moye LA, et al. Effect of captopril on mortality and morbidity in patients with left ventricular dysfunction after myocardial infarction: results of the Survival and Ventricular Enlargement Trial. The SAVE Investigators. N Engl J Med 1992;327:669-677.
127. Effect of enalapril on mortality and the development of heart failure in asymptomatic patients with reduced left ventricular ejection fractions. The SOLVD Investigators. N Engl J Med 1992;327:685-691.
128. Yusuf S, Sleight P, Pogue J, et al. Effects of an angiotensin-converting-enzyme inhibitor, ramipril, on cardiovascular events in high-risk patients. The Heart Outcomes Prevention Evaluation Study Investigators. N Engl J Med 2000;342:145-153.
129. Fox KM. Efficacy of perindopril in reduction of cardiovascular events among patients with stable coronary artery disease: randomised, double-blind, placebo-controlled, multicentre trial (the EUROPA study). Lancet 2003;362:782-788.
130. Wagner A, Herkner H, Schreiber W, et al. Ramipril prior to thrombolysis attenuates the early increase of PAI-1 in patients with acute myocardial infarction. Thromb Haemost 2002;88:180-185.
131. Solomon SD, Skali H, Anavekar NS, et al. Changes in ventricular size and function in patients treated with valsartan, captopril, or both after myocardial infarction. Circulation 2005;111:3411-3419.
132. Yusuf S, Pfeffer MA, Swedberg K, et al. Effects of candesartan in patients with chronic heart failure and preserved left-ventricular ejection fraction: the CHARM-Preserved Trial. Lancet 2003;362:777-781.
133. Pitt B, Remme W, Zannad F, et al. Eplerenone, a selective aldosterone blocker, in patients with left ventricular dysfunction after myocardial infarction. N Engl J Med 2003;348:1309-1321.
134. Pitt B, Zannad F, Remme WJ, et al. The effect of spironolactone on morbidity and mortality in patients with severe heart failure. Randomized Aldactone Evaluation Study Investigators. N Engl J Med 1999;341:709-717.
135. Laurence L, Brunton P (eds). Goodman & Gilman's The Pharmacological Basis of Therapeutics, 11th ed. New York: McGraw-Hill, 2006.
136. Friedman JM. ACE inhibitors and congenital anomalies. N Engl J Med 2006;354:2498-2500.
137. Cooper WO, Hernandez-Diaz S, Arbogast PG, et al. Major congenital malformations after first-trimester exposure to ACE inhibitors. N Engl J Med 2006;354:2443-2451.
138. Teo KK, Yusuf S, Pfeffer M, et al. Effects of long-term treatment with angiotensin-converting-enzyme inhibitors in the presence or absence of aspirin: a systematic review. Lancet 2002;360:1037-1043.
139. Barbash IM, Goldbourt U, Gottlieb S, et al. Possible interaction between aspirin and ACE inhibitors: update on unresolved controversy. Congest Heart Fail 2000;6:313-318.
140. Grundy SM, Cleeman JI, Merz CN, et al. Implications of recent clinical trials for the National Cholesterol Education Program Adult Treatment Panel III guidelines. Circulation 2004;110:227-239.
141. Third Report of the National Cholesterol Education Program (NCEP) Expert Panel on Detection, Evaluation, and Treatment of High Blood Cholesterol in Adults (Adult Treatment Panel III) final report. Circulation 2002;106:3143-3421.
142. Sacks FM, Pfeffer MA, Moye LA, et al. The effect of pravastatin on coronary events after myocardial infarction in patients with average cholesterol levels. Cholesterol and Recurrent Events Trial investigators. N Engl J Med 1996;335:1001-1009.
143. Randomised trial of cholesterol lowering in 4444 patients with coronary heart disease: the Scandinavian Simvastatin Survival Study (4S). Lancet 1994;344:1383-1389.
144. MRC/BHF Heart Protection Study of cholesterol lowering with simvastatin in 20,536 high-risk individuals: a randomised placebo-controlled trial. Lancet 2002;360:7-22.
145. Schwartz GG, Olsson AG, Ezekowitz MD, et al. Effects of atorvastatin on early recurrent ischemic events in acute coronary syndromes: the MIRACL study: a randomized controlled trial. JAMA 2001;285:1711-1718.
146. Arntz HR, Agrawal R, Wunderlich W, et al. Beneficial effects of pravastatin (+/- colestyramine/niacin) initiated immediately after a coronary event (the randomized Lipid-Coronary Artery Disease [L-CAD] Study). Am J Cardiol 2000;86:1293-1298.
147. Gordon DJ, Probstfield JL, Garrison RJ, et al. High-density lipoprotein cholesterol and cardiovascular disease: four prospective American studies. Circulation 1989;79:8-15.
148. Robins SJ, Collins D, Wittes JT, et al. Relation of gemfibrozil treatment and lipid levels with major coronary events. VA-HIT: a randomized controlled trial. JAMA 2001; 285:1585-1591.
149. Barzilai N, Atzmon G, Schechter C, et al. Unique lipoprotein phenotype and genotype associated with exceptional longevity. JAMA 2003;290:2030-2040.
150. Klerkx AH, de Grooth GJ, Zwinderman AH, et al. Cholesteryl ester transfer protein concentration is associated with progression of atherosclerosis and response to pravastatin in men with coronary artery disease (REGRESS). Eur J Clin Invest 2004;34:21-28.
151. Barter PJ, Caulfield M, Eriksson M, et al. Effects of torcetrapib in patients at high risk for coronary events. N Engl J Med 2007;357:2109-2122.
152. Frick MH, Elo O, Haapa K, et al. Helsinki Heart Study: primary-prevention trial with gemfibrozil in middle-aged men with dyslipidemia. Safety of treatment, changes in risk factors, and incidence of coronary heart disease. N Engl J Med 1987;317:1237-1245.
153. Jahangir A, Sagar S, Terzic A. Aging and cardioprotection. J Appl Physiol 2007;103:2120-2128.
154. Murry CE, Jennings RB, Reimer KA. Preconditioning with ischemia: a delay of lethal cell injury in ischemic myocardium. Circulation 1986;74:1124-1136.
155. Zhao ZQ, Corvera JS, Halkos ME, et al. Inhibition of myocardial injury by ischemic postconditioning during reperfusion: comparison with ischemic preconditioning. Am J Physiol Heart Circ Physiol 2003;285:H579-H588.
156. Gross GJ, Auchampach JA. Reperfusion injury: does it exist? J Mol Cell Cardiol 2007;42:12-18.
157. Kloner RA, Rezkalla SH. Preconditioning, postconditioning and their application to clinical cardiology. Cardiovasc Res 2006;70:297-307.
158. Bolli R. Preconditioning: a paradigm shift in the biology of myocardial ischemia. Am J Physiol Heart Circ Physiol 2007;292:H19-H27.
159. Riess ML, Stowe DF, Warltier DC. Cardiac pharmacological preconditioning with volatile anesthetics: from bench to bedside? Am J Physiol Heart Circ Physiol 2004;286: H1603-H1607.
160. Bolli R, Li QH, Tang XL, et al. The late phase of preconditioning and its natural clinical application—gene therapy. Heart Fail Rev 2007;12:189-199.
161. Ballard VL, Edelberg JM. Stem cells and the regeneration of the aging cardiovascular system. Circ Res 2007;100:1116-1127.
162. Behfar A, Perez-Terzic C, Faustino RS, et al. Cardiopoietic programming of embryonic stem cells for tumor-free heart repair. J Exp Med 2007;204:405-420.
163. Assmus B, Honold J, Schachinger V, et al. Transcoronary transplantation of progenitor cells after myocardial infarction. N Engl J Med 2006;355:1222-1232.
164. Chen Q, Camara AK, Stowe DF, et al. Modulation of electron transport protects cardiac mitochondria and decreases myocardial injury during ischemia and reperfusion. Am J Physiol Cell Physiol 2007;292:C137-C147.
165. Downey JM, Davis AM, Cohen MV. Signaling pathways in ischemic preconditioning. Heart Fail Rev 2007;12:181-188.
166. Lim SY, Davidson SM, Hausenloy DJ, Yellon DM. Preconditioning and postconditioning: the essential role of the mitochondrial permeability transition pore. Cardiovasc Res 2007;75:530-535.
167. Shepherd J, Blauw GJ, Murphy MB, et al. Pravastatin in elderly individuals at risk of vascular disease (PROSPER): a randomised controlled trial. Lancet 2002;360:1623-1630.
168. The Long-Term Intervention with Pravastatin in Ischemic Disease (LIPID) Study Group. Prevention of cardiovascular events and death with pravastatin in patients with coronary heart disease and a broad range of initial cholesterol levels. N Engl J Med 1998;339:1349-1357.
169. Sever PS, Dahlöf B, Poulter NR, et al. Prevention of coronary and stroke events with atorvastatin in hypertensive patients who have average or lower-than-average cholesterol concentrations, in the Anglo-Scandinavian Cardiac Outcomes Trial–Lipid Lowering Arm (ASCOT-LLA): a multicentre randomised controlled trial. Lancet 2003;361:1149-1158.
170. Downs JR, Clearfield M, Weis S, et al. Primary prevention of acute coronary events with lovastatin in men and women with average cholesterol levels: results of AFCAPS/TexCAPS. Air Force/Texas Coronary Atherosclerosis Prevention Study. JAMA 1998;279:1615-1622.
171. Shepherd J, Cobbe SM, Ford I, et al. Prevention of coronary heart disease with pravastatin in men with hypercholesterolemia. West of Scotland Coronary Prevention Study Group. N Engl J Med 1995;333:1301-1307.

25

RHYTHM DISORDERS

Dawood Darbar and Dan M. Roden*

INTRODUCTION 367
ARRHYTHMIAS: MECHANISMS 367
Normal Cardiac Excitation 367
Cellular Mechanism of Clinical Arrhythmias 369
Enhanced/Abnormal Automaticity 369
Triggered Automaticity 369
Reentry 369
PRINCIPLES OF ANTIARRHYTHMIC THERAPY 369
Benefit Should Outweigh Risk 369
Mechanism-Based Approaches 370
Classification of Antiarrhythmic Drugs 371
Drug-Channel Interactions 372
Pharmacokinetic Principles 372
Cytochrome P-450s and Other Drug-Elimination Molecules 373
APPROACH TO THE PATIENT WITH ARRHYTHMIAS 374
Symptoms Associated with Arrhythmias 374
Evaluation of Antiarrhythmic Therapy 374
Noncardiac Adverse Effects of Antiarrhythmic Drugs 374
The Problem of Proarrhythmia 375
Digitalis Toxicity 375
Proarrhythmias Due to QT Prolongation 375
Proarrhythmias Due to Sodium Channel Block 376
NONPHARMACOLOGIC THERAPY OF ARRHYTHMIAS 377
THERAPY FOR SPECIFIC ARRHYTHMIAS 378
Evidence-Based Guidelines for Selecting Drugs in Specific Arrhythmias 378
Guidelines for Management of SVT 378
Short-Term Therapy 378
Long-Term Therapy 379
Guidelines for Drug Therapy of AF 379
Ventricular Arrhythmias and Cardiac Arrest 379
SUMMARY OF IMPORTANT PROPERTIES OF INDIVIDUAL DRUGS 380
Adenosine 380
Amiodarone 380
Disopyramide 381
Dofetilide 381
Flecainide 382
Ibutilide 382
Lidocaine 382
Mexiletine 382
Procainamide 382
Propafenone 383
Quinidine 383
Sotalol 383
β-Blockers as Antiarrhythmic Agents 383
Antiarrhythmic Effects of Calcium Channel Blockers 384
Digoxin 384
Magnesium 384
EMERGING TARGETS AND THERAPEUTICS 384
New Molecular Targets for Treating Arrhythmias 384
T-type Ca^{2+} Channels 384
Modulation of Intracellular Ca^{2+} 385
Tissue-Specific Channel Blockers 385
Targeting Signaling Pathways for Treatment of Arrhythmias 385

INTRODUCTION

Antiarrhythmic therapy has progressed from a handful of poorly tolerated, relatively ineffective drugs with incompletely understood mechanisms of action to a more rational selection of drug and other therapies based on an improved understanding of risks and benefits derived from clinical trials as well as mechanistic studies. Although antiarrhythmics have improved, like many other drugs, they produce widely divergent actions in patients. The spectrum of responses range from suppression of highly symptomatic arrhythmias to inefficacy to provocation of life-threatening arrhythmias by the drugs themselves. The elucidation of the mechanisms underlying this striking variability in drug response has been useful not only for improving therapy with available antiarrhythmic drugs but also for delineating further mechanistic insights into arrhythmogenesis and new therapies. Indeed, the development of any new drug entity with modest efficacy and yet not characterized by proarrhythmia or other side effects would represent a major advance in therapy of arrhythmias. Whether such drugs could, or should, supplant increasingly sophisticated nonpharmacologic therapies is not yet clear.

In this chapter, we discuss the major mechanisms of arrhythmias and describe specific therapies directed at treatment of various arrhythmias. The study of the variability in antiarrhythmic drug actions has elucidated principles broadly applicable to pharmacotherapy, involving the genetics of drug responses, the role of active metabolites in drug therapy, and general principles in mechanisms of adverse drug responses. Nonpharmacologic therapies are curative for many arrhythmias (such as atrioventricular [AV] nodal reentry or atrial flutter), and recently, tremendous progress has been made in catheter ablation for the commonest arrhythmia in clinical practice, atrial fibrillation (AF). However, it remains to be determined whether such an approach can be applied to the majority of patients with this condition. Another area in which it is difficult to envision pharmacologic therapy being superior to nonpharmacologic approaches is in the use of implantable cardioverter-defibrillator (ICD) devices in the prevention of sudden cardiac death in high-risk patients.

ARRHYTHMIAS: MECHANISMS

Normal Cardiac Excitation

In the normal heart, the specialized pacemaker tissue of the sinus node, located in the high right atrium at its junction with the superior vena cava, depolarizes rhythmically, usually at a rate of 60 to 80 times per minute. Impulses are then propagated rapidly from the sinus node throughout the atria, causing atrial systole and propelling atrial blood through the mitral and tricuspid valves into the ventricles (Fig. 25-1). On the surface electrocardiogram (ECG), atrial depolarization is inscribed as the P-wave. The wave of impulses then enters the AV node

*Supported in part by grants from the United States Public Health Service (UO1 HL65962 and HL075266).

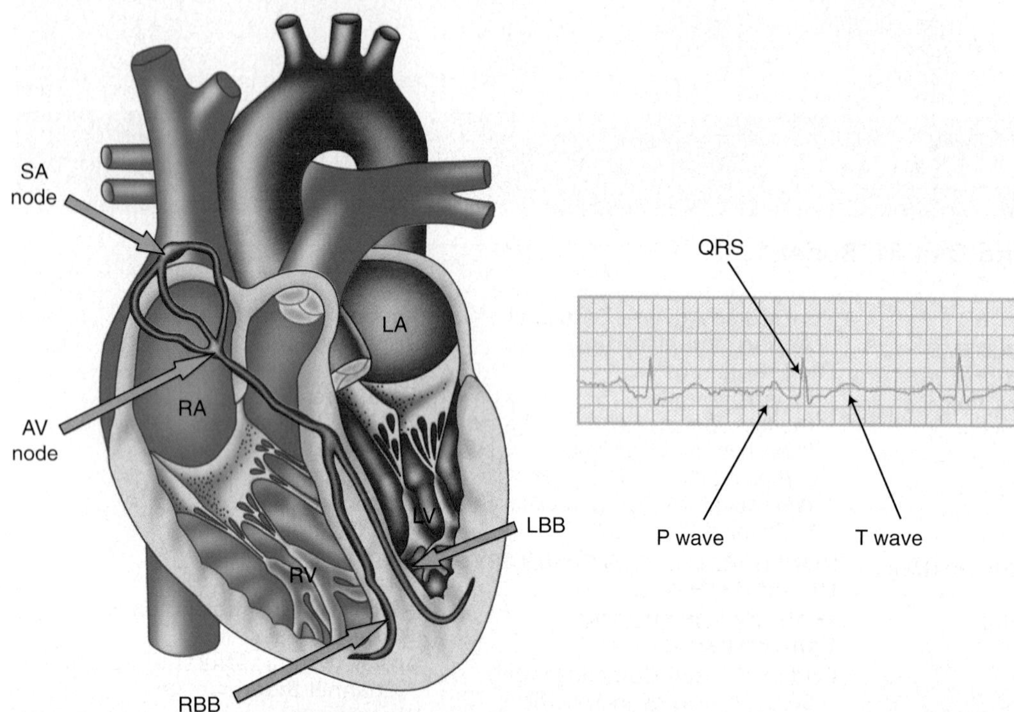

FIGURE 25-1 • Normal impulse propagation in the heart. Impulses arise in the sinoatrial (SA) node and propagate through the left and right atria (LA, RA), the atrioventricular (AV) node, and then the right and left bundle branches (RBB, LBB) of the conducting system. The normal electrocardiogram (ECG) is inscribed as a result of this normal propagation. LV, left ventricle; RV, right ventricle.

located in the lower atrial septum. Conduction in the AV node is considerably slower than elsewhere in the heart, and 150 msec to 200 msec elapses before the propagating wave front emerges from the AV node and enters the specialized conduction system of the ventricles. The passage of impulses in the specialized conduction system of the heart—whose fibers are located in the subendocardium of both ventricles—is extremely rapid, and activation of the ventricles then proceeds from subendocardial conducting system fibers transmurally to the epicardium, inscribing the QRS complex of the ECG. After depolarization, ventricular cells repolarize, inscribing the T-wave of the normal ECG. The time from QRS onset to the end of the T-wave (QT interval) is frequently used as a measurement of repolarization (action potential duration) in individual cells in the ventricle.

An *arrhythmia* is defined as any deviation from the previous description of a normal heart beat. Such deviations may arise because the heart rate is faster or slower than normal, although the activation sequence described previously is intact (sinus tachycardia and sinus bradycardia, respectively). Impulse propagation may also fail, most commonly in or below the AV node, causing heart block or bundle branch block. Single or multiple beats arising from sites other than the sinus node (i.e., ectopic beats) may excite the heart prematurely and in abnormal sequence. Ectopic beats arising in the atrium are called *atrial premature contractions* (APCs) and in the ventricle, *premature ventricular contractions* (PVCs). These may occur as isolated beats or consecutively, in which case they are called atrial tachycardia (AT) and ventricular tachycardia (VT), respectively.

The fundamental cellular event correlate of normal electrical activity in the whole heart is the cardiac action potential. The configuration and duration of action potentials vary in different regions of the heart (atrium, ventricle, sinus node, AV node, etc.) even under physiologic conditions. With disease, action potential durations and configurations diverge even further, and these changes are believed to cause or contribute to some arrhythmias. The crucial molecular events that control the changes in transmembrane voltage that occur during a cardiac action potential are ion currents flowing across the membrane of heart cells during excitation and recovery from excitation. Ion currents flow across specific pore-forming protein complexes called "ion channels." An ion channel opens and closes according to stimuli such as changes in voltage, and the coordinated activity of multiple ion channels results in the cardiac action potential (Fig. 25-2). Most

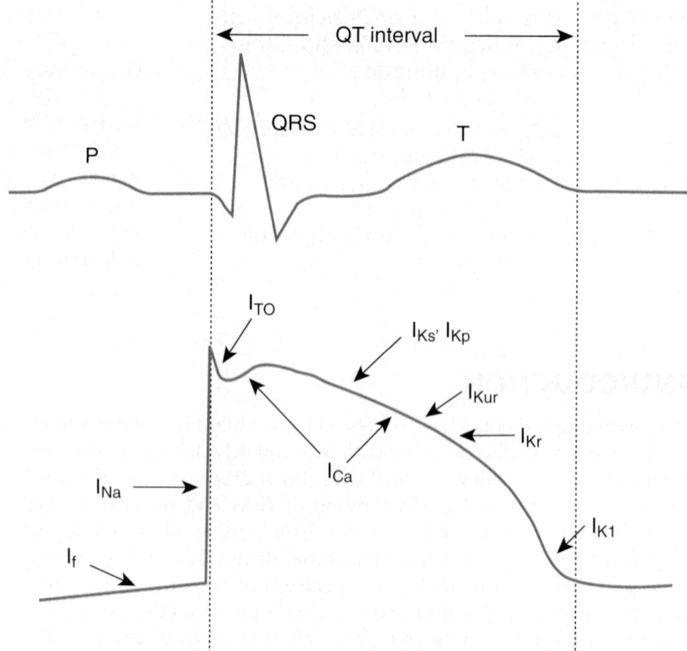

FIGURE 25-2 • Relationship between the surface electrocardiogram (ECG) (top) and the ventricular action potential (bottom). The QRS complex of the ECG corresponds to ventricular depolarization (action potential upstroke), whereas the QT interval is determined by the duration of the action potential. Ion currents move through pore-forming membrane proteins, termed *ion channels.* Sodium and calcium currents move into the cells to depolarize them, and potassium currents move out of cells and repolarize them. Multiple potassium currents have been identified, and each plays a prominent role during specific portions of the action potential as shown. Ion current amplitudes vary as a function of such factors as antiarrhythmic drugs, adrenergic tone, heart rate, location of the cell in the heart, and disease. As a consequence, there is substantial cell-to-cell variability not only in the shape but also in the duration of individual action potentials, because these are determined by the integrated behavior of the all-membrane currents.

contemporary drugs used in the treatment of arrhythmias have one or more cardiac ion currents as their major mechanism of action block.

Cellular Mechanism of Clinical Arrhythmias

The three major cellular mechanisms responsible for tachyarrhythmias are enhanced automaticity, triggered automaticity, and reentry.[1]

Enhanced/Abnormal Automaticity

Automaticity is the property of a cell to initiate an impulse spontaneously, without the need for prior stimulation; automaticity is normal in the sinus node and certain other cardiac cells. In enhanced or abnormal automaticity, propagation of the impulse wave originates from cell(s) outside the sinus node that are undergoing spontaneous depolarization at a rate faster than in the sinus node.

Triggered Automaticity

Triggered automaticity refers to spontaneous beat(s) whose appearance depends on previous normal beats. The cellular correlates of triggered automaticity are afterdepolarizations: depolarizations in the cardiac action potential that occur before or after full repolarization of the cell, early afterdepolarizations (EADs) or delayed afterdepolarizations (DADs), respectively (Fig. 25-3). EADs have been commonly implicated for the lengthened repolarization time and ventricular arrhythmias associated with the congenital and acquired forms of the long QT syndrome (LQTS). Arrhythmias due to intracellular calcium overload (e.g., with digitalis intoxication or in certain congenital arrhythmia syndromes such as catecholaminergic polymorphic VT) are believed to arise as a result of DADs and are often exacerbated by antecedent rapid sinus rates (Table 25-1).

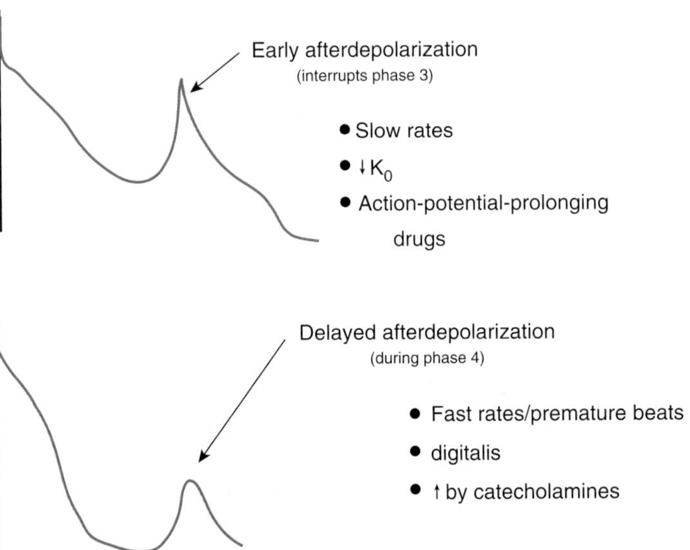

FIGURE 25-3 Contrasting appearances and basic and clinical features of early and delayed afterdepolarizations.

Reentry

Electrical activity during each normal cardiac cycle begins in the sinus node and continues until the entire heart has been activated. Each cell becomes activated in turn, and the cardiac impulse dies out when action potentials in all cells have returned to rest. If, however, a group of fibers not activated during the initial wave of depolarization recovers excitability in time to be discharged before the impulse dies out, they may serve as a link to reexcite areas that were just discharged and have now recovered from the initial depolarization. This latter situation is known as "reentry."

The formal requirements for reentry are that two points are connected by more than one conduction pathway and that these pathways have different electrophysiologic properties. One good example is the AV reentrant tachycardia occurring in the Wolff-Parkinson-White (WPW) syndrome (Fig. 25-4). Subjects with WPW are born with accessory pathway(s), or bypass tracts, connecting the atrium and the ventricle in addition to the normal AV node (i.e., atria and ventricles are connected by two pathways). During sinus rhythm, AV conduction occurs via both the AV node and the accessory pathway, resulting in the typical short PR interval and delta wave characteristic of preexcitation (see Fig. 25-4). If conduction block occurs in the bypass tract, impulses can propagate from the atrium to the ventricle via the AV node and then reenter the atrium via the accessory pathway (or, rarely, vice versa). Reentrant excitation can also occur in anatomically fixed circuits within and around the AV node (AV nodal reentrant tachycardia), at the rim of a healed myocardial infarction (MI; monomorphic VT), and within the atrium (atrial flutter). In yet other cases, reentrant excitation can occur not because of anatomically fixed pathways but because contiguous fibers exhibit functionally different electrophysiologic properties caused by local differences in transmembrane action potential. Dispersion of excitability and/or refractoriness creates an electrophysiologic milieu that promotes initiation and maintenance of reentry. In such cases a reentrant pathway is not fixed, and multiple reentrant circuits may meander around the atria (AF) or the ventricle (VF).

PRINCIPLES OF ANTIARRHYTHMIC THERAPY

Benefit Should Outweigh Risk

The benefits of antiarrhythmic drug therapy are clearly evident in the acute setting, when a patient presents with a highly symptomatic, often sustained, arrhythmia that drug therapy terminates rapidly. In this setting, symptomatic benefits are obvious, and the risk is minimized because patients are monitored and exposed to the drug for only a brief period of time.

By contrast, with chronic therapy, the balance between benefit and risk is more difficult to evaluate. Chronic therapy in a patient with heart disease may be beneficial initially but efficacy may be lost with time owing to a changing electrophysiologic milieu (substrate). Indeed, in virtually all clinical trials, chronic antiarrhythmic therapy is partially effective in preventing recurrence of tachycardia. Furthermore, the consequences of arrhythmia recurrence are clinically important (varying from recurrent hospitalization to death), and the risk of

TABLE 25-1 CONTRASTING EARLY AND DELAYED AFTERDEPOLARIZATIONS

	Early Afterdepolarizations	Delayed Afterdepolarizations
Inciters	QT-prolonging drugs	Digitalis, catecholamines
Exaggerated by	Slow heart rates, hypokalemia	Rapid rates
Blunted by	Rapid rates, K^+, Mg^{2+}	Ca^{2+} channel block
Mechanism(s)	Net increase in inward plateau current	Intracellular Ca^{2+} overload
Putative clinical rhythm	Torsades de pointes	Digoxin toxicity; ischemia; some genetic syndromes (catecholaminergic ventricular tachycardia)

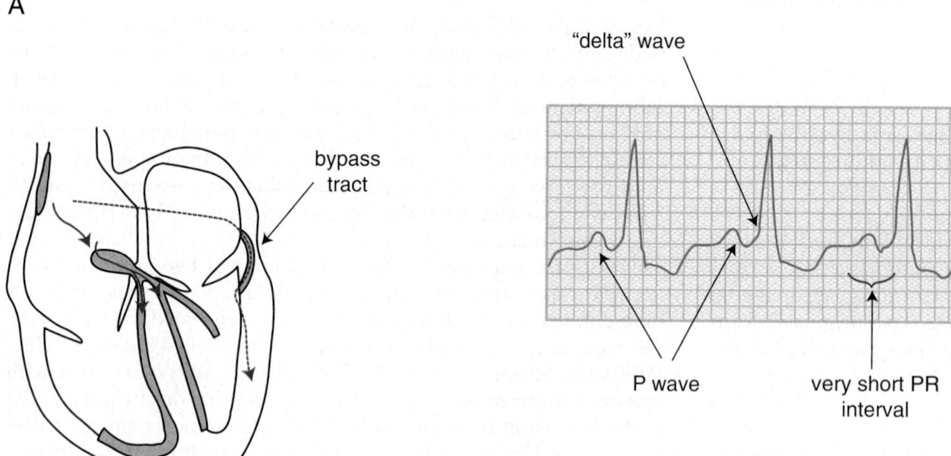

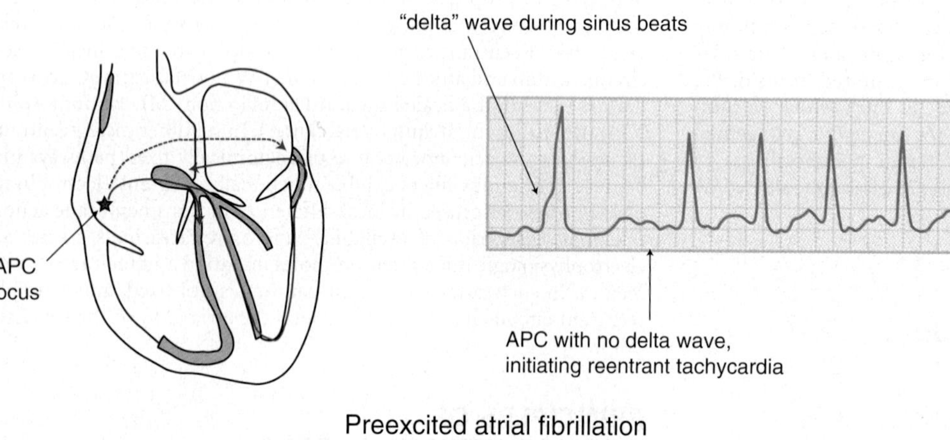

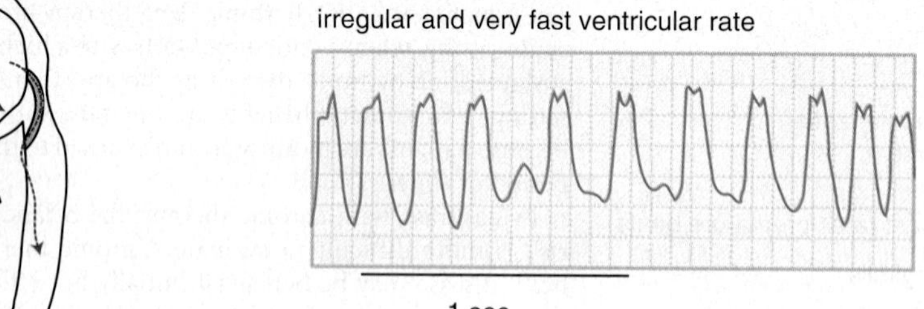

FIGURE 25-4 • Mechanisms in the Wolff-Parkinson-White (WPW) syndrome. A, Pathways for cardiac depolarization during sinus rhythm. In addition to the normal pathways (shown in Fig. 25-1), there is an accessory pathway that bypasses the atrioventricular (AV) node. Therefore, during sinus rhythm, a portion of the ventricle is activated prematurely, which accounts for the short PR interval and the delta wave. **B,** Initiation of AV reentry in WPW. An atrial premature complex (APC) fails to propagate in the bypass tract but continues to conduct through the AV node, leading to longer PR interval and no delta wave. However, the propagating wavefront can reenter the atrium via the bypass tract and thus initiate sustained AV reentry (see text for more details). **C,** Occasionally, patients with WPW develop atrial fibrillation. AV conduction can then take place across the bypass tract and result in a bizarre appearance of the QRS complexes and a very rapid heart rate (can be >300/min). Although preexcited atrial fibrillation is rare, it is important to recognize because drugs commonly used to treat supraventricular tachycardias (verapamil, digoxin) can be fatal in this syndrome.

serious adverse effects appears to increase over time. Therefore, in contemporary antiarrhythmic therapy, drugs retain a primary role in the acute termination of arrhythmias and in selected chronic arrhythmia settings, notably AF, in which arrhythmia recurrence may not be catastrophic. By contrast, device-based and ablative therapies are more desirable from a risk-benefit point of view in other settings (e.g., VT) in which antiarrhythmic drugs have assumed a secondary role. However, as ablative therapies for AF continue to evolve, it is possible that drugs may assume a secondary role here as well. Nevertheless, the development of new drug therapies for AF that are highly effective and, more importantly, safe during chronic therapy is also highly desirable.

Mechanism-Based Approaches

One universal principle of pharmacologic therapy is that the best treatment is that targeted specifically to disease mechanisms. In arrhythmia therapy, a good example is cure of arrhythmias in the WPW syndrome by bypass tract ablation. As our understanding of the molecular and cellular basis of arrhythmias has evolved, so too has the list of arrhythmias for which specific mechanisms have been defined, and therefore, specific antiarrhythmic drug therapies may be indicated (Table 25-2). Thus, the role of adrenergic triggering in right ventricular outflow tract (RVOT) VT makes β-blockers a rational, mechanism-based therapy. Recognition of the critical role of slow conduction within the AV node

TABLE 25-2 MECHANISM-BASED ANTIARRHYTHMIC DRUG THERAPY

Arrhythmia	Mechanism-Based Therapy*	Mechanism Targeted
AV nodal reentry AV reentry	Adenosine Verapamil	Macro-reentry utilizing the AV node
Outflow tract VT	β-Blockers Verapamil, diltiazem	Adrenergically driven
Fascicular VT	β-Blockers Verapamil, diltiazem	Reentry within the His-Purkinje system
Torsades de pointes due to drugs or bradyarrhythmias	Pacing Isoproterenol K^+ supplementation to 4.5 mEq/L-5 mEq/L	I_{Kr} block leading to bradycardia-dependent early afterdepolarizations and unstable intraventricular reentry due to heterogeneity of repolarization
Congenital long QT syndrome, type 1	β-Blockers; other antisympathetic maneuvers (stellate ganglionectomy)	Failure of the adrenergically activated K^+ current I_{Ks} to maintain action potentials short during adrenergic activation
Congenital long QT syndrome, type 2	K^+ supplementation to 4.5 mEq/L-5 mEq/L	Abnormal action potential prolongation and heterogeneity due to loss of I_{Kr} function
Congenital long QT syndrome, type 3	Sodium channel block (mexiletine, flecainide)	Abnormal action potential prolongation and heterogeneity due to increased inward sodium current during the action potential plateau
Brugada syndrome	I_{TO} block (possibly quinidine)	Increased heterogeneity of action repolarization due to loss of sodium channel function and maintained I_{TO}
AF, VF, or T-wave oversensing in short QT syndrome	Quinidine, sotalol	Increased outward current, leading to shortened action potentials, due to abnormally increased I_{Ks}, I_{Kr}, or I_{KI}.
Catecholaminergic polymorphic VT	β-Blockers	Leaky SR leading to afterdepolarization-mediated arrhythmias with heart rate increases due to adrenergic stimulation

*Other therapies may be effective such as magnesium for torsades de pointes but are not listed here because their mechanisms of action are not clearly defined.
AF, atrial fibrillation; AV, atrioventricular; I_{KI}, inward rectifier potassium current; I_{Kr}, rapid component of the delayed rectifier potassium current; I_{Ks}, slow component delayed rectifier potassium current; I_{Kur}, ultrarapid rectifier potassium current; SR, sarcoplasmic reticulum; VF, ventricular fibrillation; VT, ventricular tachycardia.

or orthodromic reciprocating tachycardia makes adenosine a rational, mechanism-based choice of therapy for the acute termination of these arrhythmias. The recent advances in our understanding of molecular mechanisms in specific rare genetic syndromes may also prompt consideration of specific mechanism-based therapies—although the numbers of patients evaluated are small, and very often the agents available are not specific.

Unfortunately, for most common arrhythmias, such as VT associated with myocardial disease or AF, arrhythmia mechanisms have been difficult to define, and so the choice of drug therapy remains "empiric." In such settings, drugs shown by clinical experience or controlled trials to be effective often target multiple mechanisms, including modifying the arrhythmia-prone substrate or inhibiting known or putative trigger(s) of arrhythmias. Because specific mechanisms for many arrhythmias have not been well defined, the expectation that all patients with AF or VT will respond to therapy in a similar fashion assumes that underlying mechanisms are homogeneous across patients. However, as genetic, molecular, and cellular studies continue to demonstrate, this assumption is largely unfounded. Therefore, the incomplete efficacy of drugs in treating these arrhythmias, which appear to represent a spectrum of arrhythmias mechanisms, is perhaps not unexpected.

Large clinical trials provide the best evidence for choosing among drug therapies and dosages in settings like AF and VT. The use of evidence-based principles should be complemented by consideration of patient-specific characteristics that may make one drug more or less desirable than others. Thus, a remote history of MI would argue against the use of sodium channel blockers in a patient with AF, owing to the risk of proarrhythmia.

Classification of Antiarrhythmic Drugs

Several approaches have been proposed to classify drugs used for treatment of cardiac arrhythmias. The earliest schemes classified drugs into classes based on shared efficacies and toxicities. Some antiarrhythmic drugs share important electrophysiologic properties—notably block of sodium channels or of the rapid component of the delayed rectifier potassium current (I_{Kr}) (the common mechanism underlying QT prolongation)—and these can provide the basis for predicting shared or "class" actions including toxicities (Table 25-3). Block or enhancement of other ionic currents—such as the slow component of the delayed rectifier potassium component (I_{Ks}), the transient outward current (I_{TO}), or acetylcholine-activated current ($I_{K\text{-}Ach}$)—may also contribute to clinical drug actions in some cases and are not usually considered in broad classification schemes.

An alternative approach is to classify not drugs but rather the key electrophysiologic mechanisms involved in arrhythmogenesis, thereby allowing specific drugs to be chosen to target these. This approach, adopted by the "Sicilian gambit" investigators, is nicely exemplified by the definition of new molecular mechanisms in congenital arrhythmia syndromes and the way in which these then lead naturally to mechanism-based therapies. An evolving understanding of the molecular and cellular basis of arrhythmias should allow a more rational choice of key molecules(s) whose targeting is likely to be safe and effective in the therapy of a particular arrhythmia.

The term *antiarrhythmic drugs* has traditionally been taken to include drugs targeting ion channels in cardiac myocytes (sodium channel blockers, calcium channel blockers, and QT-prolonging drugs, generally potassium channel blockers), β-adrenergic receptor blockers, and a series of drugs with diverse mechanisms used primarily for the therapy of arrhythmias, such as digoxin, amiodarone, magnesium, and adenosine. However, recent studies have demonstrated that other widely used cardiovascular therapies, such as angiotensin-converting enzyme and 3-hydroxy-3-methylglutaryl coenzyme A (HMG CoA) reductase inhibitors may also exert important antiarrhythmic effects. Such effects may include not only reduction of sudden cardiac death (SCD), an arrhythmic event that represents the final common pathway for many potential disease pathways, but also prevention of AF. These

TABLE 25-3 EXPECTED EFFECTS OF BLOCKING ANTIARRHYTHMIC DRUG TARGETS IN THE HEART

Ionic Target	Blocking Drugs	Effect of Therapeutic Doses on Normal ECG	Cardiac Toxicity of Excess Block	Extracardiac Toxicity
Sodium channel	Amiodarone Quinidine Procainamide Disopyramide Cibenzoline Pilsicainide Propafenone Flecainide Lidocaine* Mexiletine*	QRS prolongation, exaggerated at high concentration and/or fast sinus rates PR prolongation	Slow atrial flutter, occasionally with 1:1 AV conduction Bradyarrhythmias Increased pacing threshold Increased energy requirement for defibrillation More frequent episodes of reentrant VT or SVT	Exacerbation of myasthenia gravis
L-Type calcium channels†	Verapamil Diltiazem	Sinus rate slowing; PR interval prolongation	Bradyarrhythmias AV nodal block Depressed contractility	Peripheral edema
Rapid component of the delayed rectifier potassium current (I_{Kr})‡	Amiodarone‡ Quinidine Procainamide§ Disopyramide Dofetilide Sotalol Ibutilide	QT interval prolongation (sinus bradycardia may also occur)	Torsades de pointes	
β-Adrenergic receptors	β-Blockers, including sotalol Propafenone‖ Amiodarone‖	Sinus rate slowing; PR interval prolongation	Bradyarrhythmias AV nodal block Depressed contractility (acutely)	Fatigue Sleep difficulties Erectile dysfunction Bronchospasm Depression

*Lidocaine and mexiletine have faster rates of onset and offset of binding to the channel and so tend to exhibit fewer of the effects (such as QRS prolongation) listed for other blockers.

†Many other drugs such as dihydropyridines like nifedipine and amlodipine, block *L*-type calcium channels but not in myocardium; their effects on cardiac electrophysiology generally reflect sympathetic activation due to peripheral vasodilation.

‡I_{Kr} block is also the mechanism whereby many "noncardiovascular" drugs prolong QT interval and cause torsades de pointes. Other drugs such as flecainide and verapamil also block I_{Kr} but have such potent effects on inward currents (Na^+ or Ca^{2+}) that the clinical effects of I_{Kr} block—QT prolongation and torsades de pointes risk—are not seen. Similarly, torsades de pointes is rare with amiodarone.

§QT prolongation during procainamide therapy is often due to accumulation of the active metabolite *N*-acetylprocainamide (NAPA), which does not block cardiac sodium channels.

‖The β-blocking properties of propafenone are most evident clinically at high concentrations of the parent drug in individuals deficient in cytochrome P-450 (CYP) 2D6 activity on a genetic basis or due to concomitant drug therapy. Unlike many drugs that competitively block β-receptors, amiodarone exhibits antiadrenergic properties by noncompetitive blockade, reducing the number of receptors available for occupancy by agonists such as adrenaline.

AV, atrioventricular; ECG, electrocardiogram; SVT, supraventricular tachycardia; VT, ventricular tachycardia.

studies not only provide new potential therapies but also implicate new signaling pathways in the pathogenesis of arrhythmias and, therefore, as potential new targets for the development of effective antiarrhythmic interventions. The pharmacologic properties of these nontraditional "antiarrhythmic agents" are discussed later in this chapter.

AF is the commonest arrhythmia for which drugs remain primary therapy, but the efficacy of currently available drugs is disappointing. As a result, the role of nonpharmacologic therapies for AF continues to evolve, and new drugs are currently in development. Some (like azimilide or dronedarone) seem similar to available agents in that they target multiple potassium channels including I_{Kr} and I_{Ks}. Others are reported to target atrial-specific channels (including an ultrarapid rectifier potassium current [I_{Kur}]) or receptors. Experimental studies have suggested that manipulation of activated phosphorylation pathways or of abnormal intracellular calcium homeostasis could also provide antiarrhythmic effects in AF and other settings.[2] It is possible that new drugs targeting these mechanisms could affect overall management of AF.

Drug-Channel Interactions

Experimental studies even prior to the cloning era indicated that ion channels, the targets of antiarrhythmic drugs, have specific drug-binding sites. Further, drug binding to these "receptor" sites on the channels to modify their function was found to be modulated by the "state" of the channel (open, closed, or inactivated). These observations led to formulation of the modulated receptor hypothesis to analyze drug-channel interactions. More contemporary studies have demonstrated the existence of specific drug-binding sites on ion channel proteins, and the interaction of drugs with these sites can be modulated by channel protein conformation (or state). In some cases, ion channels are blocked by direct binding in the pore region (a common mechanism for most I_{Kr} blockers), whereas in others, drug binding to other regions of the protein alters its function, an "allosteric" effect.

Most sodium channel blocking drugs inhibit open or inactivated states of the channel; hence, during each cardiac cycle, they associate with and block channels, and then dissociate during diastole, ultimately reaching a steady state level of block. If the heart rate is increased, there is less time for dissociation, so channel block is enhanced. Furthermore, the rate of dissociation from the channel varies among drugs. For drugs like lidocaine with "fast-off" kinetics, very little block occurs even at fast rates. In contrast, with "slow-off" drugs, like flecainide, block accumulates even at physiologic rates. Because sodium channel block slows intraventricular conduction, it prolongs QRS duration on the surface ECG. This explains why QRS widening is apparent at normal heart rates during flecainide (but not lidocaine) therapy, and why it widens further if the heart rate is increased. In addition, because conduction slowing promotes reentry, slowing conduction by the drug at faster rates may explain cases of flecainide-induced VT during exercise.[3]

Pharmacokinetic Principles

One important mechanism underlying variability in response to antiarrhythmic drugs is variability in pharmacokinetics, the result of the

TABLE 25-4 ANTIARRHYTHMIC DRUGS ELIMINATED BY A SINGLE PATHWAY

Drug	Pathway	Blocking Drugs	Inducing Drugs
Digoxin	Excretion by P-glycoprotein	Amiodarone Quinidine Cyclosporine Erythromycin Ketoconazole Itraconazole	Rifampicin St. John's wort
Propafenone	Metabolism by CYP2D6*	Quinidine Many antidepressants	
Procainamide	Metabolism by *N*-acetylation*		

*Clinically important variation in drug elimination can also be due to common genetic variants.
CYP, cytochrome P-450.

processes of drug absorption, distribution, metabolism, and elimination. Variability in pharmacokinetics contributes substantially to variability in efficacy or toxicity when there is a narrow therapeutic window (the margin between dosages and plasma concentrations that are associated with efficacy and those associated with toxicity) and when the drug is metabolized or excreted by a single pathway. These criteria apply to many antiarrhythmic drugs. Sotalol and dofetilide are examples of drugs with narrow therapeutic windows, and the risk of toxicity—namely, torsades de pointes—increases for both agents with increasing dosages. In addition, both drugs are largely excreted by a single pathway, renal excretion. As a result, drug dosages need to be adjusted in renal failure to avoid increased risk of torsades de pointes. By contrast, whereas the toxicity of flecainide is also concentration-dependent, the drug has two major routes of elimination—renal excretion and hepatic metabolism. Thus, impaired metabolism or renal dysfunction alone does not generally alter response to the drug; although rare cases of flecainide toxicity due to inhibited drug metabolism in a patient with renal dysfunction have been reported. Table 25-4 identifies drugs with narrow therapeutic windows, eliminated by a single pathway, and lists circumstances under which the meeting of these two clinical conditions can result in serious and often unexpected drug toxicity.

Cytochrome P-450s and Other Drug-Elimination Molecules

Drug metabolism, elimination, and disposition are accomplished by specific gene products, most commonly drug-metabolizing enzymes (primarily members of the cytochrome P-450 [CYP] superfamily) and drug-transport molecules. DNA variants that alter the activity of these proteins are increasingly well recognized; although some exert only subtle effects on protein function, in other cases, an individual patient may totally lack enzymatic activity. This is especially important if the affected pathway is critical for elimination of a drug with a narrow therapeutic margin. Furthermore, concomitant drug therapy can modulate the activity of the drug-metabolizing and -transport molecules. In most cases, such drug interactions result in inhibition of the elimination pathway. Occasionally, however, concomitant drug therapy can induce expression of drug metabolism and, thus, accelerate elimination. Under this circumstance, an increase in the drug dosage may be required to maintain a therapeutic effect.

The major drug-metabolizing enzymes for antiarrhythmic drugs are CYP2D6, CYP2C9, and CYP3A4/5. Approximately 5% to 10% of whites and African Americans are homozygous for loss of function alleles in CYP2D6. these individuals totally lack enzymatic activity and are designated "poor metabolizers" (PMs). CYP2D6 PMs have markedly decreased propafenone clearance and accumulate the parent drug to plasma concentrations high enough to produce clinically significant β-blockade; as a result, asthma can be a risk in these subjects. Similarly, CYP2D6 PMs also have higher concentrations of timolol and metoprolol. Propafenone and quinidine are CYP2D6 inhibitors and may, therefore, alter the effects of these CYP2D6 substrates.

CYP2C9 is the enzyme primarily responsible for the metabolism of warfarin's active *S*-enantiomer. Reduction of function of CYP2C9 alleles has been described, and homozygous individuals appear to be at very high risk for bleeding complications, even at very low dosages. Amiodarone is a potent CYP2C9 inhibitor, and dosages of warfarin must, therefore, be adjusted downward with amiodarone therapy.

CYP3A4/5 are two closely related enzymes that are the most abundant cytochromes in the liver (and in other sites, such as enterocytes) and are responsible for the metabolism of the majority of currently used antiarrhythmic drugs including quinidine, disopyramide, propafenone, and dofetilide. Individuals totally lacking CYP3A activity have not been described, although the activity has substantial interindividual variability. However, CYP3A activity can be almost totally inhibited by concomitant drug therapy, notably with certain azole antifungals (ketoconazole), macrolide antibiotics (erythromycin), human immunodeficiency virus (HIV) protease inhibitors (ritonavir), amiodarone, diltiazem, verapamil, and large doses of grapefruit juice. CYP3A activity can also be induced by rifampin, phenytoin, and St. John's wort; reduction in plasma concentrations and loss of drug effects can occur under these conditions. Inhibition of CYP3A-mediated elimination by these drug interactions was the major cause of terfenadine accumulation in plasma, leading to cases of torsades de pointes that eventually prompted the drug's withdrawal from the market.

N-Acetyltransferase (NAT) activity is responsible for the elimination of procainamide. There are two NAT genes, *NAT1* and *NAT2*. *NAT1* is expressed in all individuals, but loss of functional alleles has been reported in *NAT2*. As a result, patients can be divided into rapid and slow acetylators (there are no nonacetylators). Slow acetylators have a higher incidence of procainamide-induced lupus syndrome during chronic therapy.[4]

In addition to metabolizing enzymes, transport across biologic membranes is another crucial determinant of drug disposition that has received increasing attention since the mid 1990s. The multisubstrate efflux carrier P-glycoprotein is the most well studied to date in terms of cardiovascular drugs. P-Glycoprotein is the product of the multidrug resistance 1 (*MDR1; ABCB1*) gene and is a member of the ABCB subfamily of adenosine triphosphate (ATP)–binding cassette (ABC) transmembrane proteins that have been implicated with drug resistance in cancer. P-Glycoprotein is expressed not only in drug-resistant cancer cells but also in many organs such as the gut and kidney, where it plays an important role in distribution and elimination. It acts as an efflux pump in the gut, preventing the entry of toxic compounds; in the liver and kidney, it serves to remove xenobiotics from the circulation. Although P-glycoprotein substrates are diverse, there is considerable overlap between the substrates transported by P-glycoprotein and those metabolized by CYP3A4/5. One important role for P-glycoprotein in cardiovascular medicine is that it transports cardiac glycosides. A synonymous single nucleotide polymorphism in exon 26 (C3435T) in the *MDR1* gene has been associated with expression of the transporter and variable digoxin concentration.[5] Furthermore, correlation of the *MDR1* genotype and digoxin uptake in vivo has been described.[6]

Many drugs (e.g., amiodarone, quinidine, verapamil, itraconazole, cyclosporine, and erythromycin) inhibit P-glycoprotein activity; their use with digoxin can lead to increased digoxin plasma concentrations and toxicity.[7]

APPROACH TO THE PATIENT WITH ARRHYTHMIAS

Symptoms Associated with Arrhythmias

Treatment for arrhythmias is undertaken either to suppress symptoms or to prevent morbidity or mortality associated with the arrhythmia. The most common symptoms associated with arrhythmias are palpitations (a feeling of the heart beating rapidly or irregularly), lightheadedness, dizziness, and/or transient loss of consciousness (syncope). Palpitations are most often associated with APCs, PVCs, or AF. The severity of symptoms associated with arrhythmias is often related to the extent of underlying heart disease. For example, patients with AV nodal reentrant tachycardia or AV reentrant tachycardia (who generally have otherwise normal hearts) may have heart rates in excess of 250 beats per minute (bpm) and yet may note only lightheadedness or palpitations. By contrast, patients with sustained monomorphic VT in the setting of advanced underlying heart disease due to remote MI may have slower tachycardia rates but may nevertheless present with more severe symptoms such as recurrent syncope due to severe hypotension without even premonitory palpitations. The most extreme example of this is the syndrome of SCD, which kills 300,000 to 400,000 Americans each year; in over half the cases, coronary heart disease has not previously been recognized clinically, and SCD is the first symptom. In most cases, SCD is caused by VF culminating in ineffective contractile function; the patient will die within minutes unless effective cardiopulmonary resuscitation is initiated.

In AF, the AV node is bombarded with multiple impulses, and the ventricular rate is often very rapid (150-180 bpm in an untreated patient), with symptoms such as dyspnea, chest pain, and palpitations. In patients with WPW syndrome, the development of AF can result in extremely rapid ventricular rates because the ventricle may be excited not only via the AV node but also via the AV connection through the accessory pathway (see Fig. 25-4). Although this arrhythmia (called "preexcited AF") is rare, it is critical to recognize because drugs, such as digitalis or diltiazem, usually used to slow the ventricular response rate in AF have been associated with paradoxical increases in ventricular rate and the development of VF in this special rare setting. Deaths in patients with WPW syndrome are probably attributable to this mechanism.

Patients with AT (in which an automatic focus fires repetitively at rapid rates, resulting in heart rates of 150-200 bpm) may present with symptoms of heart failure with no specific arrhythmia symptoms such as palpitations. In such cases of "tachycardia-induced cardiomyopathy," normal contractile function may return after several weeks of suppression of the arrhythmia. Similarly, advanced contractile dysfunction can also be seen in patients with a form of AV reentrant tachycardia (called "permanent junctional reciprocating tachycardia") associated with a slowly retrograde-only conducting accessory pathway, and the occasional patient with persistent AF or atrial flutter with rapid rates.

Patients with severe symptoms due to recurrent or ongoing arrhythmias can and should be treated. However, in patients with milder symptoms (e.g., palpitations due to APCs or PVCs), many treatments may confer risk; indeed in these patients, the risk of therapy may exceed any potential benefits, and therapy should be deferred. In patients who are asymptomatic, currently available data, described later, indicate that therapy should not be undertaken except in very specialized instances (e.g., tachycardia-induced cardiomyopathy). Some studies, however, indicate that certain arrhythmias (e.g., PVCs) that occur in patients with advanced heart disease are a marker for an increased risk for SCD due to VF. Thus, further studies, such as an electrophysiology study, may be needed to evaluate the risk of developing these more serious arrhythmias in such patients.

Evaluation of Antiarrhythmic Therapy

As with all forms of therapy, clinicians using antiarrhythmic therapies must ensure that the potential benefits of treatments outweigh the potential risks. One way to achieve this is by establishing the correct arrhythmia diagnosis and selecting the most appropriate treatment. Risk can be minimized by appropriate dose selection based on formal pharmacokinetic principles, appropriate drug selection to reduce adverse effects, and maneuvers to minimize the risk of proarrhythmia.

The best commonly used available tool for appropriate arrhythmia diagnosis is the 12-lead ECG. This may allow distinction of, for example, supraventricular from ventricular arrhythmias. Although the ECG in these arrhythmias may occasionally resemble each other, the distinction is clinically important because treatments directed at supraventricular tachycardia (SVT) (e.g., intravenous verapamil) can result in hemodynamic collapse if the arrhythmia is actually VT. In addition, diagnostic criteria have been developed for specific forms of VT and for subtypes of SVT, including AV reentrant tachycardia and AV nodal reentrant tachycardia. This information can be useful not only in selection of drug therapy but also in guiding nonpharmacologic approaches, described further later. Another tool available for assessing risk of arrhythmias is the signal-averaged ECG (SAECG), designed to detect slow conduction that is the substrate for reentrant ventricular arrhythmias in patients with a remote history of MI or myocardial scar. Microvolt T-wave alternans (MTWA) is the most recent non-invasive tool that has been proposed to identify patients at high risk of ventricular arrhythmias. However, the extent to which SAECG and MTWA supply additional information beyond that obtained from validated predictors of risk, such as ejection fraction, is controversial; currently neither test is widely used as a means to risk-stratify patients at risk for ventricular arrhythmias.

In patients presenting with intermittent symptoms such as palpitations or lightheadedness, a diagnosis should be established before initiating drug therapy. If symptoms are frequent, a 24- or 48-hour continuous recording of cardiac rhythm (Holter monitor) can often help in establishing the diagnosis. Conversely, if the symptoms are more sporadic, patient-activated or automatic "event recorders," which can record cardiac rhythm at specific times over weeks or months, should be considered. For patients with rare (one or two times per year) but disabling symptoms (e.g., syncope), an implantable loop recorder should be considered, particularly if the other tools have failed to establish a diagnosis. Tilt-table testing can also be used to investigate vasovagal and other forms of syncope. However, the sensitivity and specificity of the technique are unclear. Ultimately, a clinically occurring sustained tachyarrhythmia can sometimes be reproduced (and their symptoms and response to therapy can be evaluated) during programmed electrical stimulation of the heart, which includes pacing and recording from specific intracardiac sites using electrode catheters. However, "nonclinical" arrhythmias, to which the patient may not be susceptible in ordinary life, may also be elicited by these techniques.

Noncardiac Adverse Effects of Antiarrhythmic Drugs

Many antiarrhythmic drugs commonly cause noncardiac adverse effects, and this can have an important impact on the selection of antiarrhythmic therapy. For example, disopyramide exerts prominent anticholinergic effects, which may include not only dry mouth and constipation but also increased intraocular pressure and urinary hesitancy. Consequently, disopyramide should not be used in patients with glaucoma or prostatism. Another problem with noncardiac adverse effects of antiarrhythmic drugs is the potential to cause diagnostic confusion. For example, a relatively common adverse effect during long-term use of procainamide is the development of drug-induced lupus syndrome. Because this can manifest as arthralgias and arthritis, use of procainamide in patients with rheumatoid arthritis would be inadvisable as it would be difficult to establish whether a flare-up of symptoms was due to the drug or to the underlying disease. Similarly,

TABLE 25-5 ADVERSE EFFECTS OF ANTIARRHYTHMIC DRUGS

Drug	Major Adverse Effects	Underlying Disease in which Potential for Drug Toxicity Creates Relative Contraindication
Adenosine	Chest discomfort Prolonged asystole Precipitate atrial fibrillation	Asthma Accessory bypass tract Underlying conduction disease
Amiodarone	Pulmonary fibrosis Liver dysfunction Peripheral neuropathy Thyroid dysfunction, photosensitivity, corneal deposits Bradyarrhythmias	Lung disease Advanced liver disease Preexisting neuropathy Underlying conduction disease
β-Blockers	Adverse effects secondary to β-blockade	Asthma, insulin-dependent diabetes with symptomatic hypoglycemia
Calcium channel blockers	Congestive heart failure AV block	Underlying conduction system disease LV dysfunction
Digoxin	Bradyarrhythmias and tachyarrhythmias AV block	Renal failure Underlying conduction disease
Disopyramide	Congestive heart failure Torsades de pointes Urinary retention Increased intraocular pressure	LV dysfunction Baseline QT prolongation, hypokalemia Prostatism Glaucoma
Dofetilide	Torsades de pointes	Renal failure QT prolongation, hypokalemia
Flecainide	Increased mortality post-MI	Coronary artery disease
Ibutilide	Torsades de pointes	Baseline QT prolongation, hypokalemia
Lidocaine, mexiletine	Tremors Seizures	Seizure disorder
Procainamide	Lupus-like syndrome Agranulocytosis	Chronic arthritis Preexisting blood dyscrasia
Propafenone	Bronchospasm Congestive heart failure Bradyarrhythmias	Asthma LV dysfunction Conduction system disease
Quinidine	Diarrhea Torsades de pointes	Chronic gastrointestinal disease Baseline QT prolongation
Sotalol	Side effects secondary to β-blockade (e.g., bronchospasm) Torsades de pointes	Asthma, insulin-dependent diabetes with symptomatic hypoglycemia Baseline QT prolongation, risk factors for torsades de pointes

AV, atrioventricular; LV, left ventricular; MI, myocardial infarction.

the use of amiodarone in patients with lung disease is undesirable because it might cause diagnostic confusion when patients present with increasing shortness of breath and dyspnea. Common noncardiac adverse effects of antiarrhythmic drugs are listed in Table 25-5.

The Problem of Proarrhythmia

The recognition that drugs designed to suppress arrhythmias can, in some patients, actually increase arrhythmias or provoke new ones is probably the single most important factor governing the selection and use of antiarrhythmic therapy. For example, not only are drugs incompletely effective at preventing VF, but they may also increase the risk of sudden death in some patients. Therefore, many clinicians choose to use nonpharmacologic therapy, rather than drugs, as primary therapy in such patients. Proarrhythmia is not attributable to a single mechanism. Rather, multiple proarrhythmia syndromes have now been elucidated, and these are detailed in Table 25-6. Treatment of these proarrhythmia syndromes includes early recognition, withdrawal of the offending agents, and specific mechanism-based therapies, described later.

Digitalis Toxicity

The drug first associated with the development of abnormal rhythms was probably digitalis. Although intoxication with digitalis glycosides can produce virtually any arrhythmia, certain arrhythmias should raise a particular suspicion. These include ectopic rhythms such as atrial tachycardia or PVCs (believed to be due to DAD-related triggered automaticity with sinus slowing or AV nodal block) owing to the drug's indirect vagomimetic effects. The major mechanism underlying digoxin toxicity is related to inhibition of P-glycoprotein activity by drugs such as amiodarone, quinidine, verapamil, and the azole antifungal agents. For asymptomatic arrhythmias due to digitalis toxicity, discontinuation of the drug and observation are probably sufficient. For more advanced cases, the therapy of choice is antidigoxin antibodies. Very occasionally, temporary pacing may be required.

Proarrhythmias Due to QT Prolongation

In some patients, therapy with action potential–prolonging drugs such as sotalol, quinidine, dofetilide, or ibutilide can be associated with marked prolongation of the QT interval and induction of a morphologically distinctive polymorphic VT, torsades de pointes. Torsades de pointes can also occur during treatment with noncardiovascular drugs, including terfenadine, cisapride, haloperidol, and thioridazine.[8] Many such cases are attributable to inhibition of drug elimination—and thus accumulation of drug to unusually high plasma concentrations—often due to coadministration of CYP3A4 inhibitors. Occasional cases are also unrelated to drug therapy and can be attributed to the syndrome of congenital LQTS, marked bradyarrhythmias, hypokalemia, recent

TABLE 25-6 PROARRHYTHMIA SYNDROMES AND THEIR MANAGEMENT

Syndrome	Mechanism	Clinical Presentations	Therapy*
Digitalis intoxication	Na-K-ATPase inhibition → intracellular calcium overload	Ectopic activity, with suppressed sinus and AV nodal function Atrial or junctional tachycardia Bidirectional VT	Mild: observe; possible temporary pacing Serious: antidigoxin antibody
Torsades de pointes	I_{Kr} block	Pause-dependent polymorphic VT, with QT prolongation and deformity	Mild: magnesium Serious: pacing, isoproterenol
Sodium channel blocker toxicity	Block of cardiac sodium channels, often exacerbated by underlying tachycardia or ischemia	Increased pacing or defibrillation threshold Atrial flutter slowing with 1:1 AV conduction Frequent or difficult to cardiovert monomorphic or polymorphic VT Incessant SVT Increased death rate during long-term therapy after myocardial infarction	Mild: no therapy or heart rate slowing (β-blocker) Serious: IV sodium bicarbonate
β-Blocker withdrawal	Upregulation of receptor number with chronic therapy; withdrawal → more receptors available for agonist	Sinus tachycardia, other sympathetically mediated arrhythmia, hypertension	β-Blocker
Ventricular fibrillation	Multiple drug-related mechanisms: 1. Digitalis in manifest preexcitation with atrial fibrillation 2. Coronary vasoconstriction (many drugs: cocaine, ergot) 3. Inappropriate use of verapamil for sustained VT	VF	No specific therapy beyond drug withdrawal and resuscitation
Calcium channel blocker toxicity	Calcium channel blocker excess, often in overdose	Hypotension, bradycardia, AV block	Temporary pacing, IV calcium

*Therapy in all cases consists of recognition, withdrawal of the offending agent(s), and correction of any other potential exacerbating conditions (hypokalemia, hypoxia, myocardial ischemia). "Mild" refers to minimally symptomatic patients, whereas "serious" refers to those with recurrent destabilizing arrhythmias.
AV, atrioventricular; I_{Kr}, rapid component of the delayed rectifier potassium component; IV, intravenous; SVT, supraventricular tachycardia; VF, ventricular fibrillation; VT, ventricular tachycardia.

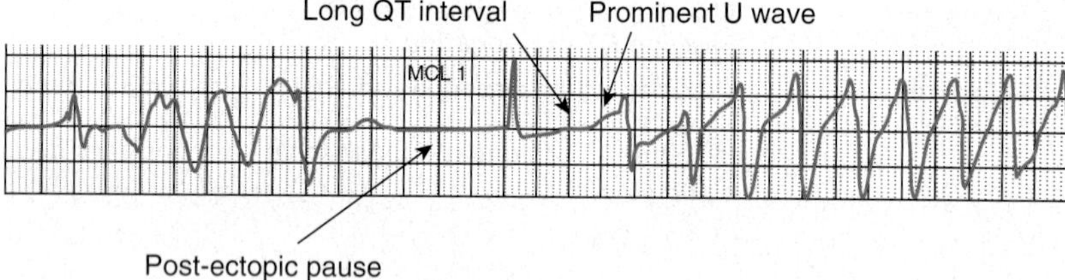

FIGURE 25-5 • Torsades de pointes in a patient receiving sotalol. This telemetry strip shows a couple of ectopic beats followed by a pause and a postpause sinus beat with a remarkably long and deformed QTU interval. The tachycardia starts after this U wave. This pattern of pause dependence and QTU changes is typical for drug-induced torsades de pointes.

conversion from AF, or acute central nervous system injury.[8] Drugs associated with torsades de pointes appear to block a single, specific cardiac potassium current, termed I_{Kr}. Mutations in genes that encode the channel responsible for I_{Kr} are now recognized as a cause of congenital LQTS—a disease associated with QT prolongation, torsades de pointes, and SCD.

Risk factors for torsades de pointes include female gender, hypokalemia, bradycardia, and high drug dosages or plasma concentrations of drugs listed previously.[8] An exception is quinidine, in which the reaction can occur with the first dose at "subtherapeutic" plasma concentrations. Other data suggest that advanced heart failure, recent conversion from AF, and very rapid intravenous administration of drug can also trigger an episode of torsades de pointes.[9] Uncontrolled clinical trials suggest that potassium supplementation (to a concentration above 4.5 mEq/L) and intravenous magnesium should be the first approaches to therapy, because they are relatively simple and unlikely to cause harm. If these are ineffective, maneuvers to increase the heart rate to greater than 90 bpm are usually effective in the acute setting; this can be accomplished either by isoproterenol or by temporary ventricular pacing.

Most recognized cases of torsades de pointes occur shortly after starting culprit drug(s). However, a specific I_{Kr} blocker, the dextrorotatory isomer of sotalol (D-sotalol), was found in Survival With Oral D-Sotalol (SWORD), a large study with a Cardiac Arrhythmia Suppression Trial (CAST; discussed later)–like design,[10] to increase long-term mortality compared with that of placebo in patients judged to be at risk for SCD.[11] Because the drug is not a sodium channel blocker, a mechanism different from that in CAST seems likely. Torsades de pointes occurring during chronic long-term outpatient treatment is one leading possibility (Fig. 25-5).

Proarrhythmias Due to Sodium Channel Block

Sodium channel block is a common mechanism underlying many well-described proarrhythmia syndromes. First, in patients with atrial flutter, sodium channel block can slow the flutter rate (e.g., from 300/min to 200/min). When the atrial flutter rate is 300/min, the usual AV nodal response is 2:1 block—that is, a ventricular rate of 150/min. However, when the flutter rate slows to 180/min to 200/min, 1:1 AV nodal conduction can occur with a paradoxical increase in ventricular rate that was not seen before the drug was administered. Because the effects of sodium channel block increase at fast rates, patients with this syndrome often present with wide QRS complexes, making the distinction from VT difficult. Treatment includes drugs such as calcium channel blockers to increase the degree of AV nodal block.

Second, slow conduction in the edges of an old MI plays a prominent role in the pathogenesis and maintenance of sustained monomorphic VT. The use of sodium channel blockers can, in some patients, increase the frequency of episodes of this arrhythmia, likely by further slowing conduction. β-Blockers have been effective in some cases, possibly by slowing sinus rate and thereby decreasing the extent of sodium channel block. In addition, some data suggest that intravenous sodium (as bicarbonate) may be useful in treating this form of proarrhythmia.

Third, sodium channel block reduces excitability of the heart. In patients with pacemakers or ICDs, increased output of the devices may be required for effective function. Rarely, ventricular arrhythmias occurring in the presence of sodium channel blockers cannot be effectively terminated by internal or external direct current cardioversion, and deaths have been reported. For this and other reasons, management of patients with ICDs is best left to specialized clinical electrophysiologists.

Fourth, sodium channel blockers can increase mortality during long-term treatment. This was established by the CAST, a landmark study that tested, in a placebo-controlled, randomized, double-blind fashion, the then-prevailing wisdom that suppression of PVCs in patients convalescing from an MI would reduce the incidence of sudden death.[10] In CAST, patients with PVCs and a recent MI were randomly assigned to one of three sodium channel blocker therapies, which was then titrated to the dose that appeared to suppress PVCs on a 24-hour Holter monitor. Once the effective dose and drug were established, patients were randomly assigned to continue drug or placebo. Remarkably, mortality among patients randomized to drug was two to three times that among those randomized to placebo. The mechanism underlying this striking, and previously undefined, effect of sodium channel block remains uncertain. However, conduction slowing with an increased risk of sustained ventricular arrhythmias (including VF) seems a plausible explanation. It has been argued that other sodium channel blockers may not produce the same effect as the three drugs tested in CAST (encainide [no longer available], flecainide, and moricizine). However, preclinical data suggest this may be a class action of sodium channel block, and other less well-designed studies with mexiletine and with disopyramide showed a similar trend to increased mortality. Perhaps the most important implications of CAST were the recognition that "surrogate" endpoints (in this case, PVCs as a surrogate for arrhythmic death) should be used with extreme caution in clinical medicine unless well validated, and that physicians should recognize that their own biases, which so often drive therapy in areas in which data are not available, may be erroneous.

More recently, it has become apparent that administration of sodium channel blockers to patients with the Brugada syndrome (an inherited arrhythmia syndrome associated with SCD) not only may elicit an unusual pathognomic ECG phenotype but also may rarely induce VF (Fig. 25-6).[12,13] It is likely that SCD in these patients is probably related to induction of VF, usually during sleep. The latter is analogous to the situation of a patient with subclinical LQTS in whom administration of an I_{Kr}-blocker exposes the genetic defect.

NONPHARMACOLOGIC THERAPY OF ARRHYTHMIAS

Chronic or recurrent symptomatic bradyarrhythmias are treated with permanent pacemakers. Transient bradyarrhythmias, such as those occurring in the setting of digitalis toxicity or MI, may occasionally respond to temporizing measures such as isoproterenol or atropine, but temporary pacemakers may also be required. Specific indications for temporary or permanent pacemaker insertion are outlined in published guidelines.[14]

In the 1970s, surgical procedures were developed to section accessory AV connections and thereby to cure patients with the WPW syndrome and frequently recurring and life-threatening arrhythmias. In the late 1980s, techniques were developed to allow permanent interruption of such accessory pathways via radiofrequency (RF) energy applied through catheters advanced to specific locations in the heart. These procedures cause minimal discomfort, often do not require general anesthesia, and require minimal inpatient hospitalization. Radiofrequency catheter ablation techniques have had a dramatic impact on the approach to the treatment of a variety of cardiac arrhythmias. This is especially evident in the case of WPW syndrome and AV nodal reentrant tachycardia, in which RF catheter ablation of accessory pathways and AV nodal slow pathways has become first-line therapy. More recently, RF catheter ablation has been applied successfully in patients with ATs and atrial flutter. However, catheter ablation of more complex arrhythmias including many forms of intra-atrial reentry, many VTs, and AF continues to pose a major challenge. Arrhythmias for which ablation is most effective (accessory pathways, AV nodal reentrant tachycardia, typical atrial flutter, RVOT VT) depend primarily on anatomically well-defined substrates. Accordingly, approaches to mapping and ablation of these arrhythmias are anatomically directed (e.g., accessory pathways along the annuli, outflow tract for RVOT VT), if not completely determined by anatomic location (AV nodal reentrant tachycardia, typical atrial flutter). Improvements in catheter-based mapping of cardiac chambers and imaging, however, may facilitate further advances in our understanding and treatment of more complex cardiac arrhythmias.

Recent advances in our understanding of AF have led to development of catheter ablation techniques that could feasibly achieve a cure for AF. Catheter ablation for AF was first reported in the early 1990s and stemmed from the success of the surgical Maze procedure, a surgical method based on mapping studies of animal and human AF reported to successfully control AF in more than 90% of selected cases.[15] A key advance has been recognition that the pulmonary veins are a common source of arrhythmogenic foci with abnormal automaticity that induce paroxysmal AF.[16] Modifications of the Maze procedure (Maze III) involve encircling the pulmonary veins, and they may prevent initiation of AF by isolating such potentially arrhythmogenic foci. Surgeons currently tend to use the procedure for patients who have drug-refractory AF undergoing surgery for concomitant cardiac disease (frequently mitral valve disease). Given the success of the surgical approach, several ablation strategies have been designed. Ablation of these foci eliminates or reduces the frequency of recurrent AF in

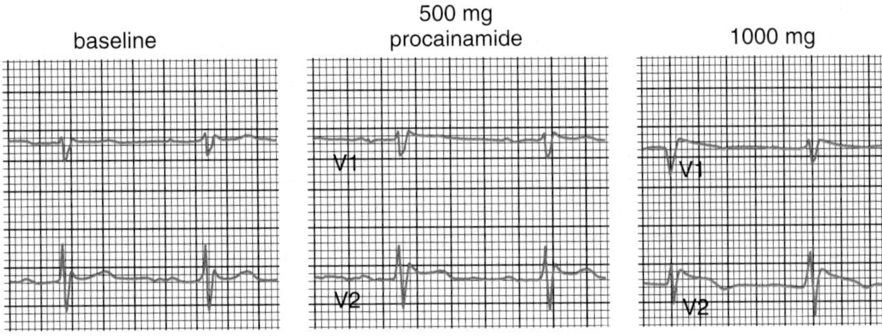

FIGURE 25-6 • Unmasking of Brugada syndrome by intravenous infusion of a sodium channel blocker (procainamide). On the baseline tracings, the ST-T segments in leads V1 and V2 are unremarkable. After administration of 500 mg of procainamide, a persistent ST elevation ("saddleback") pattern develops but the "coved"-type ST-segment elevation, pathognomic for Brugada syndrome, becomes apparent only after 1000 mg of procainamide has been administered.

more than 60% of patients, although there is still a small recurrence rate following the procedure, necessitating the need for antiarrhythmic drugs. In a recent small randomized trial, pulmonary vein isolation with RF ablation was compared with antiarrhythmic drug therapy as initial treatment for symptomatic AF.[17] After 1 year of follow-up, the patients who underwent pulmonary vein isolation had better outcomes in terms of AF recurrences and hospitalizations, as well as a better quality of life at 6 months. The substantial enthusiasm for pulmonary vein isolation needs to be tempered by the potential for rare but serious complications (such as pulmonary vein stenosis, cardiac perforation, or stroke) and by other outcome data reporting that at the 6-month follow-up period, only 54% and 82% of patients remained free from arrhythmia-related symptoms after circumferential pulmonary vein ablation and after segmental pulmonary vein ablation, respectively.[18] Although catheter-directed ablation of AF represents a substantial achievement promising better therapy for a large number of patients at present resistant to pharmacologic or electrical conversion to sinus rhythm, the limited available studies suggest that this approach offers benefit to selected patients with AF. Furthermore, these studies do not provide convincing evidence of optimum catheter positioning or absolute rate of treatment success.[19] For now, pulmonary vein isolation may best be considered for patients resistant to pharmacologic treatment, especially those who are younger and have lone AF.

Another strategy—RF ablation of the AV node and permanent pacing—has also been used for symptomatic relief in patients with medically refractory paroxysmal AF. In a meta-analysis of 21 studies (n = 1181 patients),[20] significant improvements in quality of life and clinical outcome measures occurred after ablation and pacing therapy, and the calculated 1-year total and sudden death mortality rates were 6.3% and 2.0%, respectively.

The ICD is widely used nonpharmacologic therapy for patients who have survived an episode of VT or VF (secondary prevention) or in some groups judged to be at high risk for these arrhythmias (primary prevention). The ICD device is placed, like a pacemaker, subcutaneously in the pectoral region and is connected by a specialized lead to the right ventricular endocardium. The device senses cardiac rhythm. Should a very fast tachycardia (e.g., VT/VF) occur, the device can initiate pacing (antitachycardia pacing) and/or defibrillating therapies to "rescue" the patient. Pacing therapies are preferred because they are painless, whereas shocks are painful. Currently available devices are very sophisticated, offering features such as programmability of the characteristics of tachycardia to be treated, algorithms for discrimination of SVT and VT/VF, antibradycardia pacing, and storage (with retrieval capability by telemetry) of electrical signals corresponding to abnormal rhythms. These devices are increasingly used for prophylaxis against sudden death due to arrhythmias. ICDs improve survival compared with antiarrhythmic drugs (mainly amiodarone) in patients resuscitated from cardiac arrest or sustained VT.[21] In asymptomatic patients with coronary artery disease judged to be at high risk for sudden death because of low ejection fraction and/or arrhythmias inducible by programmed electrical stimulation of the heart, three trials have now shown lower mortality in those with ICDs compared with those receiving conventional medical therapy with or without antiarrhythmic drugs.[22-24] Similar trends have been observed among patients with nonischemic dilated cardiomyopathy.[25,26] "Biventricular" ICDs, which pace the left and right ventricles simultaneously, improve symptoms and survival in patients with advanced heart failure.[27]

As with drug therapy for arrhythmias, nonpharmacologic therapies do have recognized risks. The risks of RF catheter ablation include cardiac perforation, damage to the AV node (with a subsequent need for a permanent pacemaker), and formation of intracardiac thrombi with subsequent embolization. In experienced hands, these risks are very small. First-generation ICDs, implanted in the mid-1980s, included a 2% operative mortality, because placement of those devices required thoracotomy. With current-generation devices, mortality should be near zero. The major complications related to ICD placement and therapy include infection (which usually requires removal of the whole system), lead failures (which usually manifest as ICD shock(s) when the underlying rhythm is normal), and inappropriate shock(s) because of supraventricular arrhythmias such as sinus tachycardia or AF with a rapid ventricular response.

THERAPY FOR SPECIFIC ARRHYTHMIAS

Evidence-Based Guidelines for Selecting Drugs in Specific Arrhythmias

National and international societies have formulated guidelines for management of specific arrhythmias.[19,28,29] Guideline documents provide extensive summaries of available evidence on outcomes in controlled clinical trials and other settings, with summarized levels of recommendations and graded levels of evidence. Whereas choice of antiarrhythmic drugs remains an art in some patients, use of the guidelines and the evidence that goes into formulating them in clinical practice should result in more rational and improved therapy. Classification of recommendations are scaled from class I (strong) to class III (do not use); class IIa and IIb recommendations are reserved for therapies that may in some situations be more or less desirable. Each recommendation is accompanied by a level of evidence ranging from A for evidence derived from multiple controlled clinical trials to C for anecdotal evidence and expert opinion. Joint American College of Cardiology/American Heart Association/European Society of Cardiology (ACC/AHA/ESC) Practice Guidelines were published in 2003 for acute and chronic therapy of SVT.[28] More recently, guidelines for the management of AF[19] and ventricular arrhythmias and SCD[29] were published. The major points of these documents are summarized here and in the accompanying tables and figures; the documents themselves include very extensive literature annotation and discussion for the rationale for choice of therapy in each clinical situation.

Guidelines for Management of SVT[28]

SVT refers to paroxysmal tachyarrhythmias, which require atrial or AV nodal tissue, or both, for their initiation and maintenance. SVTs are often recurrent, occasionally persistent, and a frequent cause of visits to emergency rooms and primary care physicians. Most types of SVTs have a reentry mechanism, and they are classified according to the location of the reentry circuit. Approximately 60% of cases of SVT are due to an AV nodal reentry circuit, and about 30% are due to an AV reentry circuit mediated by an accessory pathway. AT accounts for about 10% of cases and often has a focal origin. However, paroxysmal or persistent AT occurring long after cardiac surgery that involved a large atrial incision is usually caused by an intra-atrial reentry mechanism. Sinus node reentry tachycardia, inappropriate sinus tachycardia, ectopic junctional tachycardia, and nonparoxysmal junctional tachycardia are rare.

SVTs are not usually associated with structural heart disease, although exceptions occur (e.g., the presence of accessory pathways associated with hypertrophic cardiomyopathy or Ebstein's anomaly and ATs in patients with congenital or acquired heart disease). Typically reentry arrhythmias are induced by premature atrial or ventricular ectopic beats, and precipitating factors, such as excessive caffeine intake or use of alcohol or recreational drugs, can increase the risk of recurrence. Many of these features are useful in distinguishing SVTs from other tachyarrhythmias.

Short-Term Therapy

Most regular narrow-complex SVTs will respond to intravenous administration of AV nodal–blocking drugs, and adenosine is preferred over calcium channel blockers (verapamil or diltiazem) or β-blockers (esmolol, metoprolol, propranolol) because of its rapid onset and offset of action. Failure to terminate a regular narrow complex with these agents suggests an alternate diagnosis, such as inappropriate sinus tachycardia or AT. Other drugs whose intravenous administration can be useful include amiodarone and digoxin. In patients with a regular wide-complex tachycardia, efforts should be made to distinguish SVT from VT. In most settings, it is prudent to treat wide-complex tachycardia of unknown origin as VT. Procainamide, sotalol, amiodarone, and lidocaine can be used in this setting. In children, SVT is more likely and options may be different. In patients with poor left ventricular performance, amiodarone or lidocaine is preferred.

Long-Term Therapy

The risk of recurrence after a single episode of SVT is not well known, and a single episode is not an indication for long-term therapy. For patients with recurrent symptoms, options for long-term treatment include medication and ablation therapy. For those in whom chronic drug therapy is entertained, many agents have been used with success: verapamil, diltiazem, β-blockers, sotalol, and amiodarone, and in patients with relatively preserved left ventricular function, flecainide and propafenone. Digoxin is also occasionally effective. However, digoxin, verapamil, and diltiazem are contraindicated in patients with manifest preexcitation, because they increase the risk of ventricular rate acceleration and VF. In this situation, flecainide, propafenone, sotalol, amiodarone, and β-blockers are preferred.

The pharmacologic management of ATs has not been well evaluated in controlled trials. Depending on the mechanism causing the arrhythmia, β-blockers, calcium channel blockers, sodium channel blockers, and I_{Kr} blockers may reduce or eliminate symptoms.

Guidelines for Drug Therapy of AF[19]

Management strategies in AF include rate control and rhythm control as well as anticoagulation. For short-term control of rapid ventricular rate response, intravenous verapamil, diltiazem, esmolol, and metoprolol are the drugs of choice. Digoxin is generally less effective and is most useful in the setting of concomitant heart failure, but it is contraindicated in patients with manifest accessory pathway conduction (ventricular preexcitation). Oral therapy for long-term rate control includes the same drugs, with the addition of amiodarone.

Drugs can be used to pharmacologically convert AF to sinus rhythm, especially if the arrhythmia has been present for a short duration, that is, less than 7 days. Decisions to proceed to pharmacologic or electrical cardioversion are heavily dependent on the clinical circumstances and, in particular, the need for anticoagulation. Drugs with proven efficacy for acute conversion of AF include dofetilide, flecainide, propafenone, ibutilide, and amiodarone. Disopyramide, quinidine, and procainamide are second-line agents. However, digoxin and sotalol should not be used for acute conversion of AF. The "pill in the pocket" approach may be useful for patients with relatively infrequent episodes (e.g., 1/mo) of highly symptomatic AF and structurally normal hearts.[30] In this setting, single, large doses of propafenone or flecainide have been used successfully to effect pharmacologic cardioversion. In patients who have responded under monitored conditions to this approach, the drugs to be used for acute termination of further episodes of AF may then be prescribed. Risks include hypotension and precipitation of atrial flutter with 1 : 1 AV conduction; however, the risk of the latter can be minimized by administration of an AV nodal blocking agent 30 minutes prior to taking the antiarrhythmic drug.

The choice of drug to maintain sinus rhythm is governed largely by the presence and type of underlying heart disease (Fig. 25-7). Notably, even the most effective of drugs has a significant recurrence rate (30%-50% over a year). As a result, many recommend continuing therapy in a patient with rare recurrences on an otherwise well-tolerated drug regimen. In patients with no evidence of heart disease, as assessed by history, physical examination, ECG, and echocardiogram, flecainide, propafenone, or sotalol is the drug of first choice. Amiodarone and dofetilide may also be considered; disopyramide, procainamide, and quinidine are rarely used.

In patients with heart failure, the strongest evidence supports the use of amiodarone or dofetilide.[31] In patients with coronary disease, sotalol, amiodarone, or dofetilide is preferred, followed by consideration of disopyramide, procainamide, or quinidine. Flecainide and propafenone are contraindicated in patients with coronary disease. Patients with hypertension present a particular management problem because this is a very common coexisting condition in AF. If hypertension has resulted in severe left ventricular hypertrophy (LVH), amiodarone is the drug of choice. There are few other pharmacologic options for maintenance of sinus rhythm. If LVH is mild (LV wall thickness < 1.4 cm), some authorities will entertain use of flecainide and propafenone, although this is controversial.

Ventricular Arrhythmias and Cardiac Arrest

Acute management of patients with cardiac arrest follows structured flowcharts and cardiac life support guidelines, including confirmation of the arrhythmia, airway management, and cardiopulmonary resuscitation. Drugs that may be useful in pulseless electrical activity or asystole include epinephrine, atropine, and sodium bicarbonate. For VF or pulseless VT, prompt defibrillation is the first intervention. If this fails, intubation and cardiopulmonary resuscitation are initiated. Drugs of first choice in this setting include epinephrine (1 mg intravenously repeated every 3-5 min) or vasopressin (40 units, once). If

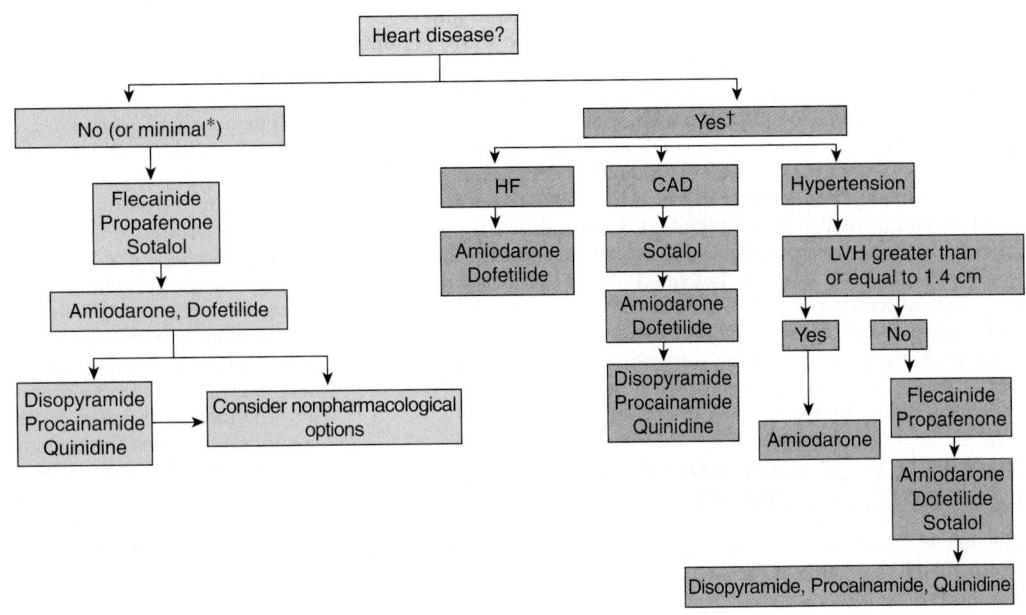

FIGURE 25-7 Flow chart for selecting among drugs to maintain sinus rhythm in patients with atrial fibrillation (see text for details). LVH, left ventricular hypertrophy.

further defibrillating shocks are ineffective, epinephrine, sodium bicarbonate, and/or antiarrhythmics can be attempted. Antiarrhythmics useful in this situation may include amiodarone, lidocaine, magnesium, and procainamide. In randomized trials, survival to hospitalization is superior with amiodarone than with lidocaine, although survival to hospital discharge is no different.[32,33]

Asymptomatic ventricular arrhythmias are not an indication for chronic therapy, regardless of the etiology. Patients with symptomatic ventricular ectopy may occasionally be highly symptomatic, and β-blockers are preferred as initial therapy. If these are ineffective, propafenone or flecainide may be entertained in the absence of underlying heart disease. If such ectopy has characteristics of a RVOT origin, calcium channel blockers may also be considered. Patients with outflow tract tachycardia or fascicular tachycardia can be managed with β-blockers or calcium channel blockers, although ablation is increasingly the preferred primary approach.

Symptomatic ventricular ectopy or nonsustained VT can also arise in patients with virtually any type of structural heart disease or with a mutation (often in genes encoding ion channels) resulting in a structurally normal heart with serious arrhythmia, a cardiac ion channelopathy. In these situations, ICDs may be used to manage the problem of sudden death risk, but drugs are often required to manage symptoms and are often needed if ICD shocks are frequent. In patients with coronary disease, amiodarone and sotalol are the drugs of choice, and flecainide and propafenone are contraindicated. Randomized, controlled trials have shown reduced ICD discharges with sotalol[33] and with the investigational agent azimilide,[34] but not with dofetilide.[35]

Another situation in which antiarrhythmic drugs may be considered is in a patient in whom an ICD would ordinarily be used, but for some reason (e.g., age, concomitant disease, ICD infection) is not. In this setting, amiodarone has been used as a "gold standard." although well-controlled clinical trial data attesting to its efficacy are lacking. A meta-analysis of its effects in placebo-controlled trials in the post-MI setting suggests modest benefit, and this may add to long-recognized benefits of β-blockers in this setting.[36] By contrast, in the Sudden Cardiac Death-Heart Failure Trial (SCD-HeFT), amiodarone appeared to increase mortality compared with that in placebo among patients with class III heart failure.[26] Nevertheless, amiodarone continues to be used in this setting, in part because other drugs appear at least equally ineffective and are probably more likely to cause serious proarrhythmia.

The increasing recognition of individual syndromes of genetically determined arrhythmias, and elucidation of their potential mechanisms at the molecular and cellular levels, has, in turn, led to proposals for "unusual therapies" in some of these settings (see Table 25-2). In the congenital LQTS, β-blockers continue to be recommended as first-line therapy for patients known to be mutation carriers, although some data suggest that β-blockers are less effective in the LQT2 and LQT3 subtypes of the disease.[37] In the LQT3 form of the disease, sodium channel block with mexiletine or flecainide may be a useful adjunct,[38] although flecainide may increase the risk of proarrhythmia if Brugada syndrome–type physiology is also present.[39] Similarly, I_{TO} block using quinidine may be useful in patients with Brugada syndrome, particularly in the setting of ICD storm.[40] Quinidine has also been used in the congenital short QT syndrome, in which it appears to normalize QT duration and to reduce the amplitude of very peaked T waves.[41] The latter action may be especially useful in patients with the short QT syndrome and ICDs, in whom double counting of the peaked T waves may lead to inappropriate ICD discharges.[42] Patients with catecholaminergic polymorphic VT are best treated with β-blockers.[43] Among those with hypertrophic cardiomyopathy, amiodarone has frequently been used both to reduce the incidence of nonsustained VT and to prevent AF with rapid ventricular responses.[44]

SUMMARY OF IMPORTANT PROPERTIES OF INDIVIDUAL DRUGS

The following section describes key pharmacologic agents used for the treatment of arrhythmias as well as their pharmacologic properties and common usage.

Adenosine

Pharmacology. Adenosine is a naturally occurring nucleoside whose effects are mediated by interaction with specific adenosine receptors. In the heart, this action produces a decrease in calcium channel current and activation of a G-protein–regulated potassium channel, likely the same channel as that activated by acetylcholine ($I_{K\text{-}ACh}$). The net result of these actions is action potential shortening in atrium and hyperpolarization of the nodal cells resulting in AV nodal conduction slowing or block.

Pharmacokinetics. Adenosine is eliminated from the circulation in seconds by rapid uptake into cells and inactivation by adenosine deaminase. Dipyridamole inhibits cellular uptake and thus exaggerates adenosine effects. Methylxanthines including theophylline and caffeine block adenosine receptors and so may blunt the drug's effects.

Use. Rapid bolus intravenous administration of adenosine produces transient AV nodal block, which terminates arrhythmias using the AV node as a portion of their circuit such as AV nodal reentry or AV reentry. In atrial arrhythmias, transient AV nodal block may be useful in differentiating arrhythmia mechanism by unmasking continuous atrial tachyarrhythmia despite AV block and establishing the diagnosis. Outflow tract and fascicular VTs, occurring in the normal heart, may also be terminated by adenosine. However, common forms of VT observed in patients with myocardial disease are adenosine-resistant. Induction of AV block by adenosine may be useful in establishing the diagnosis. Because of its extremely rapid elimination rate, adenosine is unique among antiarrhythmic (and most other) drugs in that it must be administered as a very rapid intravenous bolus, preferably through a large venous or central line. Slower intravenous infusions of adenosine are used in other settings (e.g., neurosurgery) to produce controlled hypotension or during assessment for cardiac perfusion defect in conjunction with nuclear imaging studies. ATP is also available in some countries for intravenous administration to terminate SVT; it acts by rapid degradation to adenosine.

Adverse Effects. Adenosine has supplanted other pharmacotherapy for acute termination of SVT because its actions dissipate rapidly, making side effects only transient. Most patients feel a sense of air hunger and nonspecific chest discomfort with administration of adenosine; bronchospasm can rarely occur.[45] Asystole that follows administration of the drug and termination of the arrhythmia may last several seconds; prolonged asystole requiring resuscitation has been reported after cardiac transplant.[46] By activating potassium current in the atrium, adenosine shortens atrial refractory period and may thereby precipitate AF. This is unusual, but if the patient has an accessory pathway, very rapid ventricular responses can be elicited. Adenosine should be avoided in those with known preexcitation or WPW syndrome.[47]

Amiodarone

Pharmacology. Amiodarone is a nonspecific antiarrhythmic agent, interacting with multiple ion channels, cell surface receptors, and other molecules to block their function. The drug is unusually lipophilic; this accounts for its unusual pharmacologic effects, including its very slow uptake and elimination. Whereas the onset of many of the drug's electrophysiologic effects are slow, some actions can be manifest on acute exposure. Antiadrenergic actions tend to be prominent early, and changes in refractoriness may take longer to be apparent. In animal experiments, amiodarone administration appears to alter steady state transcript levels of mRNAs encoding multiple ion channels.[48] Thus, the drug likely produces both acute and chronic effects by interacting with ion channels and other molecular targets and may, in addition, "remodel" the heart through an effect on transcription.

Amiodarone blocks multiple potassium channels, including I_{Kr} that results in prolongation of refractoriness and QT interval. In addition, amiodarone is a sodium channel blocker, interacting primarily with inactivated states of the channel.[49] This effect, and its calcium channel blocking effect, may underlie its ability to inhibit afterdepolarizations in vitro; this, in turn, may be important in explaining the strikingly low incidence of torsades de pointes despite the marked QT prolongation. It has antiadrenergic effects. However, unlike traditional β-blockers, the drug acts as a noncompetitive antagonist; the number of β receptors available during chronic amiodarone therapy is reduced, but the drug does not compete for access to those receptors with agonists such as norepinephrine. Amiodarone is a potent inhibitor of many drug-metabolizing enzymes and drug transporters, notably CYP3A4, CYP2C9, and P-glycoprotein.

Pharmacokinetics. Amiodarone is 30% to 50% bioavailable, so intravenous doses are smaller than oral ones. The drug undergoes CYP3A4-mediated metabolism to desethylamiodarone, an active metabolite. Amiodarone is eliminated extraordinarily slowly, with a terminal phase elimination half-life measured in weeks to months. Thus, the time for the drug to achieve true steady state may be as long as a year. For this reason, loading regimens are required when amiodarone is initiated, and dosages can often be reduced progressively during long-term therapy.

Use. Intravenous amiodarone has emerged as a drug of choice for a wide range of arrhythmias. It is superior to comparator drugs (procainamide or bretylium [an older drug that is no longer available]) in life-threatening recurrent VT or VF and may be especially useful in polymorphic VT caused by active myocardial ischemia.[50,51] In patients with out-of-hospital cardiac arrest, survival to hospital admission is improved with intravenous amiodarone compared with standard therapy.[52] Therefore, intravenous amiodarone has supplanted lidocaine as the drug of choice in many cardiac arrest situations. Intravenous amiodarone can convert AF to sinus rhythm (although with a time delay compared with other drugs) but, unlike many other antiarrhythmics, slows the ventricular response rate in AF. It has been used successfully for rate control in postoperative junctional ectopic tachycardia in children.

Chronic amiodarone is used as adjunctive therapy to reduce recurrence of VT in patients with ICD, as primary therapy for ventricular arrhythmias, and as therapy for AF and atrial flutter. In each setting, the goal of therapy is to achieve an early drug effect by administration of relatively large doses (800 mg-1200 mg daily) and to taper these over several days or weeks to maintenance dosages. Thus, in a patient with very frequent ICD discharges, a reasonable regimen might start with 1200 mg daily for several days and taper to 400 mg daily over several weeks. Conversely, in patients with AF, where the indication is less pressing, one regimen is 800 mg daily for a week and then chronic therapy with 200 mg (or eventually less) daily.

Adverse Effects. Intravenous amiodarone can cause phlebitis and severe cellulitis if extravasated. For this reason, it is preferable to administer the drug through a large-bore venous or central line. Hypotension is common. Marked QT prolongation and torsades de pointes can occur. During chronic oral therapy, PR, QRS, and QT intervals are all prolonged. Despite QT prolongation, torsades de pointes is exceedingly unusual during amiodarone therapy; the likely explanation is that the drug includes, among its many pharmacologic actions, block of inward currents that prevent initiation of torsades de pointes.[53] Amiodarone does not generally produce major depression of ventricular performance, an advantage over other antiarrhythmic drugs.

The major forms of amiodarone toxicity during chronic therapy involve extracardiac tissue. The most feared toxicity is pulmonary fibrosis. The cardinal laboratory manifestation of amiodarone toxicity is reduction in pulmonary diffusion capacity for carbon monoxide (DL_{co}). Pulmonary toxicity does appear to be dose-related and is unusual (but not unheard of) during chronic therapy with doses at or below 200 mg daily. Routine surveillance with chest x-rays and pulmonary function studies have been advocated as a method to detect early amiodarone toxicity, but the efficacy of these maneuvers is not established. Once pulmonary toxicity is suspected, further diagnostic workup may include lung biopsy, right heart catheterization (to eliminate a role for concomitant heart failure), and gallium scanning. None of these is specific, and biopsy often reveals foam cells but cannot make a definitive diagnosis of toxicity. If toxicity is strongly suspected, the drug should be withdrawn. Corticosteroids have been used, but their efficacy is not certain. Death from pulmonary insufficiency can occur. Underlying pulmonary disease may be a risk factor, and patients often seem to manifest amiodarone pulmonary toxicity following a separate incident of lung injury owing to heart failure exacerbation, pneumonia, or general anesthesia.

Corneal microdeposits are ubiquitous during chronic amiodarone therapy but rarely interfere with vision; halos around lights at night may be one complaint. Much more rarely, the drug has been associated with optic neuritis. Liver function is often abnormal and, rarely, may progress to cirrhosis. Peripheral neuropathy can be severe. Photosensitivity is common, and patients should be warned to use sunscreen and wear broad-brimmed hats. Both hypo- and hyperthyroidism can occur; hypothyroidism requires thyroid supplementation, and hyperthyroidism—which can present as worsened arrhythmias—may require thyroid ablation or withdrawal of amiodarone. Because of the potential for toxicity, chest x-rays, thyroid function studies, and liver function tests have been recommended every 6 to 12 months even in the absence of symptoms.[54]

Disopyramide

Pharmacology. Disopyramide is a sodium channel blocker with onset and offset kinetics similar to those of quinidine. It also prolongs QT interval by blocking the potassium channel. Disopyramide exerts prominent anti-inotropic and anticholinergic effects at clinical dosages.

Pharmacokinetics. Disopyramide is eliminated by hepatic metabolism and renal excretion. The elimination pathways are induced by phenytoin, suggesting participation by CYP3A4 and/or P-glycoprotein. The drug is administered as a racemate; the enantiomers are equally potent as sodium channel blockers, but only one, *S*-disopyramide, prolongs action potentials in vitro. The drug is variably bound to plasma proteins within the therapeutic range, and its binding is saturable; as a result, monitoring plasma concentrations of total drug is not useful.

Use. Disopyramide is used as second- or third-line therapy for atrial arrhythmias. Its anticholinergic actions make it suitable for patients with vagally mediated AF. Its negative inotropic effects may also be useful in management of patients with hypertrophic cardiomyopathy and dynamic left ventricular outflow tract obstruction. In addition, it may occasionally be used in patients with neurocardiogenic syncope.

Adverse Effects. Torsades de pointes, exacerbation of heart failure, and anticholinergic effects (constipation, urinary retention, glaucoma, dry eyes and mouth) can all occur. In a post-MI prophylaxis trial in the mid 1980s (prior to CAST), disopyramide tended to increase mortality.[55]

Dofetilide

Pharmacology. Dofetilide is a potent and specific blocker of I_{Kr}, with no other significant pharmacologic actions. As a result, the drug produces QT prolongation. Torsades de pointes is its only significant toxicity.

Pharmacokinetics. Dofetilide is excreted largely by renal excretion and, to a small extent, by CYP3A4-mediated metabolism. Its elimination half-life (10 hr) allows twice-daily dosing. Certain drugs, including cimetidine, verapamil, ketoconazole, trimethoprim-sulfamethoxazole, and hydrochlorothiazide, appear to inhibit dofetilide elimination and are contraindicated because they may thereby increase QT prolongation and the risk of torsades de pointes.

Use. Oral administration of dofetilide is effective in pharmacologic conversion of AF in about 30% of cases at 0.5 mg twice daily, the highest recommended dose, with reduced efficacy at lower doses. The drug also reduces recurrence of AF after restoration of sinus rhythm. Dofetilide reduces rehospitalization for heart failure, an effect that may be attributable to maintenance of sinus rhythm in patients with AF.[31] Placebo-controlled trials have failed to demonstrate efficacy of the drug in reducing the frequency of episodes of paroxysmal AF or in reducing episodes of VT or ICD discharges.

Adverse Effects. Data on torsades de pointes incidence are available from large trials in which the drug was initiated with in-hospital monitoring. In the Danish Investigations of Arrhythmia and Mortality on Dofetilide (DIAMOND) studies, dofetilide was compared with placebo in patients convalescing from MI and in those with recent hospitalization for heart failure.[56,57] In the heart failure arm, the incidence of torsades de pointes was 3%, and some cases were fatal. In the post-MI group, the incidence was lower, 1%. Because of the risk of torsades de pointes, the drug can be prescribed in the United States only by practitioners certified in its use. The drug is initiated in the hospital and is unique among antiarrhythmics in that the starting dose, 0.5 mg twice daily, is the highest allowable; downward dose adjustments are made if the QT interval is excessively long or if renal function is impaired. The drug should not be used in patients with advanced renal failure.

Flecainide

Pharmacology. Flecainide is a potent sodium channel blocker, with slow onset and offset kinetics. PR and QRS widening are usual. It also blocks I_{Kr}, although reports of torsades de pointes are exceedingly rare.[58]

Pharmacokinetics. Flecainide is eliminated with a half-life of 10 to 17 hours by hepatic metabolism by CYP2D6 and by renal excretion. Defects in either pathway are generally well tolerated if the alternate pathway is unperturbed. Occasional patients with CYP2D6 deficiency (owing to genetic factors or interactions with inhibiting drugs) and concomitant renal failure can develop flecainide toxicity.[59] Flecainide is usually administered twice daily. In children 1 to 12 years of age (but not younger), elimination half-life is reduced (8 hr), often requiring dosing three times daily. Milk blocks flecainide absorption, and therefore, toxicity may result from removal of milk products from the diet.

Uses. Flecainide is effective in restoring and maintaining sinus rhythm in patients with AF and SVT.

Adverse Effects. Flecainide increased mortality after MI in the CAST study[10] and, therefore, is generally contraindicated in patients with coronary artery disease and, by extension, in those with advanced structural heart disease. The drug can depress left ventricular performance and precipitate or exacerbate heart failure. Flecainide can organize atrial electrical activity during AF to produce atrial flutter with 1:1 AV conduction. It can increase pacing and defibrillating thresholds and exacerbate VT.

Ibutilide

Ibutilide is an I_{Kr} blocker that may also prolong QT interval by enhancing sodium entry during the action potential plateau phase. The channel through which this entry occurs has not been well delineated.[60,61] Intravenous ibutilide is effective in converting AF or atrial flutter to sinus rhythm.[62] It is more effective in flutter than in fibrillation and in recent onset than in chronic arrhythmias. Cardioversion after ibutilide administration can help maintain sinus rhythm in those in whom cardioversion alone is ineffective.[63] The drug is administered as an intravenous bolus (1 mg over 10 min, which can be repeated 10 min later) and is subsequently eliminated by hepatic metabolism. Peak pharmacologic effects coincide roughly with the end of the infusion. The elimination half-life is 4 to 6 hours; therefore, patients should be observed for at least 4 hours after administration of the drug. The major adverse effect is torsades de pointes. Ibutilide can be safely used in patients receiving chronic amiodarone therapy.[64] Ibutilide is also effective in patients with AF and rapid ventricular responses due to antegrade accessory pathway conduction. In this setting, it not only can convert AF but also slows conduction down the bypass tract.[65]

Lidocaine

Pharmacology. Lidocaine is a sodium channel blocker with fast-on/fast-off kinetics. It does not generally produce significant effects on the ECG.

Pharmacokinetics. After intravenous administration of a bolus of lidocaine, plasma concentrations decline biexponentially. The first phase is rapid, with a half-life of 8 minutes, and is attributed to rapid distribution of the drug from plasma to the periphery. After distribution, the drug is eliminated by hepatic metabolism, with a half-life of approximately 2 hours. Thus, after initiation of a lidocaine maintenance infusion, steady state plasma concentrations are approached in 8 to 10 hours (4-5 elimination half-lives).

Drug concentration in plasma is a reasonable guide to efficacy. To rapidly achieve therapeutic plasma concentrations, a loading regimen of 3 mg/kg to 4 mg/kg is generally required. Administration as a single large bolus runs a high risk of central nervous system toxicity, notably seizures, so the loading regimen should be administered as a rapid infusion or a series of smaller intravenous boluses (e.g., 100 mg, followed by 50 mg 5-10 min later, followed by a further 50 mg 5-10 min later). If the target arrhythmia is ongoing and suppressed by lidocaine loading, then a maintenance infusion is appropriate; however, if the target arrhythmia persists after lidocaine loading, a maintenance infusion is unlikely to add any efficacy. A maintenance infusion of 1 mg/kg to 4 mg/kg will achieve therapeutic plasma concentrations of 2 mcg/ml to 5 mcg/ml.

In heart failure, the central volume of distribution is contracted and clearance is reduced; accordingly, the size of both the loading regimen and the maintenance infusion should be reduced. In liver disease, clearance is reduced, therefore, a lower maintenance infusion rate is required. Lidocaine dosage does not need to be adjusted in patients with renal failure.

Use. Lidocaine is used intravenously to acutely suppress symptomatic or life-threatening ventricular arrhythmias.

Adverse Effects. Lidocaine can cause bradyarrhythmias. Prophylactic lidocaine was shown to prevent VF in acute MI in the 1970s.[66] However, overall mortality appears to be unaffected or may increase.[67] Accordingly, the drug is no longer used for this indication.

Lidocaine is cleared by CYP3A4-mediated hepatic metabolism to metabolites that exert modest antiarrhythmic effects and may mediate some of the central nervous system toxicity. Extraction of the drug is nearly complete during a single pass through the liver, which explains why lidocaine is not administered orally. Propranolol and cimetidine reduce lidocaine clearance; therefore, lower infusion rates may be required.

Mexiletine

Mexiletine is a lidocaine analogue that can be administered orally. It is occasionally useful when added to other drugs (amiodarone, quinidine, sotalol) in patients with symptomatic VT.[68] Mexiletine tended to increase mortality in a post-MI trial. In addition, mexiletine has been proposed to be useful for the congenital LQTS, notably in the type 3 form (sodium channel–linked) subtype, in which it may directly block the plateau sodium current that causes QT prolongation.[69]

Mexiletine is eliminated by hepatic metabolism and is generally administered three times daily. Side effects such as tremor and nausea are common and may be reduced by administering the drug with food, which decreases the peak plasma concentrations without affecting overall absorption. Another lidocaine analogue, tocainide, with similar electrophysiologic effects but eliminated primarily by renal excretion, is no longer available because of bone marrow depression.

Procainamide

Pharmacology. The major effect of procainamide is sodium channel block, with relatively rapid onset and offset kinetics. QT prolongation is also evident during procainamide therapy, and at least some of this effect reflects generation of an active metabolite, *N*-acetylprocainamide (NAPA), which is a weak I_{Kr} blocker that does not block sodium channels. PR, QRS, and QT prolongation are seen during procainamide therapy. The drug has ganglionic blocking properties, so hypotension during intravenous infusion is common.

Pharmacokinetics. Procainamide is eliminated by renal excretion and by *N*-acetylation to NAPA; as discussed earlier, this metabolism is in part genetically determined. Its elimination half-life is short, 3 to 4 hours, whereas that of NAPA is somewhat longer (8-12 hr). As a result of this rapid elimination—and a narrow margin between concentrations required to produce efficacy and those producing toxicity—chronic oral therapy requires very frequent dosing or the use of sustained-release formulations. NAPA is eliminated by renal excretion. In renal failure, accumulation of either parent or metabolite can occur, depending in part on acetylator phenotype.

Monitoring procainamide plasma concentrations should be used to ensure that concentrations of the parent drug remain in the 4-mcg/ml to 8-mcg/ml range. Procainamide concentrations above 10 mcg/ml appear to carry a risk of marked QRS widening and potential arrhythmia exacerbation. NAPA concentrations greater than 20 mcg/ml appear to carry a higher risk of torsades de pointes.

Uses. Intravenous procainamide can be effective in suppressing symptomatic or life-threatening ventricular arrhythmias. It can also be effective in converting AF to sinus rhythm and can slow ventricular rate in patients presenting with preexcited AF and rapid ventricular responses. Procainamide is administered as an intravenous loading dose; one reasonable regimen is 15 mg/kg (approximately 1 g in an adult), administered over 50 minutes. Maintenance infusion rates are 30 mcg/kg/min to 60 mcg/kg/min (1-4 mg/min in an adult). The drug is not well tolerated during chronic therapy, although occasional patients (e.g., those with highly symptomatic and drug-resistant ventricular arrhythmias) may be considered for therapy.

Adverse Effects. During intravenous administration, the major adverse effect of procainamide is hypotension. Marked QRS widening and QT prolongation with torsades de pointes can also occur, particularly if plasma concentrations of the parent drug or the metabolite, respectively, are elevated. Adverse effects during chronic therapy are common and include anorexia, nausea, electrocardiographic toxicity (discussed previously), agranulocytosis, and the drug-induced lupus syndrome.

Propafenone

Pharmacology. Propafenone is a potent sodium channel blocker with slow onset and offset kinetics. Propafenone is also a β-blocker in vitro, and this effect can be observed at high plasma concentrations in human subjects.

Pharmacokinetics. Propafenone is eliminated by CYP2D6. As a result, PMs and individuals receiving CYP2D6 inhibitors develop high plasma concentrations and increased risk of adverse effects, including bronchospasm and bradycardia. A sustained-release formulation allows twice-daily dosing.

Uses. Propafenone is effective in restoring and maintaining sinus rhythm in patients with AF and SVT.

Adverse Effects. Propafenone has not been formally tested in patients after MI. Therefore, it is generally contraindicated in patients who have coronary disease and those with advanced structural heart disease. Other adverse effects include depressed left ventricular performance, exacerbation of heart failure, atrial flutter with 1 : 1 AV conduction, and increased pacing and defibrillation thresholds.

Quinidine

Pharmacology. Quinidine is a component of an antimalarial extract from the bark of the cinchona plant and was developed as an antiarrhythmic by Wenckebach just after the First World War. It blocks the sodium current channel and multiple potassium currents, including I_{Kr}, I_{Ks}, and I_{TO}. Its kinetics of interaction with the sodium channel are intermediate between those of lidocaine and those of flecainide. I_{Kr} block can occur at very low concentrations. In vitro, low quinidine concentrations prolong action potentials, and this effect is blunted at higher concentrations, likely reflecting an additional effect of sodium channel block.[70]

Quinidine is an α-adrenergic receptor blocker and can thereby produce hypotension when administered intravenously. It has vagolytic actions and can enhance AV nodal conduction during atrial flutter. It is a very potent inhibitor of CYP2D6, exerting this pharmacologic action at dosages as low as 5 mg; low-dose quinidine has actually been used in combination with CYP2D6 substrates to increase and make more uniform the plasma concentrations. Quinidine is also an inhibitor of P-glycoprotein and, as a result, decreases digoxin clearance, increasing its serum concentrations and risk of toxicity.[71]

Pharmacokinetics. Quinidine is eliminated by CYP3A4-mediated hepatic metabolism, with a half-life of 6 to 12 hours. Metabolites have some pharmacologic activity, but none is more potent than the parent drug. Maintaining plasma concentrations between 1.5 mcg/ml and 5 mcg/ml has been a useful way of reducing dose-related toxicity. Quinidine reduces clearance of many other drugs by its effect on CYP2D6 and P-glycoprotein. In addition, quinidine metabolism is subject to variability owing to coadministration of drugs that inhibit or enhance CYP3A4 activity.

Uses. Quinidine can be effective in atrial and ventricular arrhythmias. It has also been used in some congenital arrhythmia syndromes such as the Brugada syndrome and the short QT syndrome (see Table 25-1).

Adverse Effects. Quinidine is not well tolerated and, therefore, is not used as first-line therapy. It frequently causes gastrointestinal upset (diarrhea or nausea); the mechanism is unknown. Torsades de pointes occurs in 1% to 5% of patients in most series. Quinidine causes a number of immunologic adverse effects, notably thrombocytopenia or hemolytic anemia.

Sotalol

Pharmacology. Sotalol is a nonselective β-blocker with additional I_{Kr} blocking effects, resulting in sinus bradycardia and PR and QT prolongation.

Pharmacokinetics. Sotalol is eliminated by renal excretion of unchanged drug, with a half-life of 6 to 12 hours. Dosages must be adjusted downward in patients with renal failure.

Uses. Sotalol is effective in atrial and ventricular arrhythmias. The drug is available for oral administration in the United States; an intravenous formulation is available in other parts of the world.

Adverse Effects. Major adverse effects are those related to β blockade (bradycardia) and prolongation of the QT interval with a risk of torsades de pointes (0.5%-3.3% in controlled trials). The drug must be started in the hospital and cardiac rhythm closely monitored. Hypokalemia, hypomagnesemia, bradycardia, and high drug doses (except with quinidine) increase the risk of torsades de pointes with all QT-prolonging drugs.[8]

β-Blockers as Antiarrhythmic Agents

Pharmacology. Epinephrine and norepinephrine are physiologic agonists at α- and β-adrenergic receptors. Available β-blockers compete with these physiologic agonists for access to β-adrenergic receptors and thereby blunt agonist activity. During chronic therapy, receptor up-regulation can occur. β_1-Receptors mediate tachycardia and increase contractility in normal hearts, although in heart failure, there may be an increased contribution by β_2 receptors. β_2-Agonists produce arterial vasodilation. Acute antiarrhythmic effects are mediated primarily by β_1 receptor antagonism, although during chronic therapy, especially in patients with advanced heart disease, β-blockers produce multiple beneficial effects, not all of whose underlying physiologic mechanisms are yet understood. Many available β-blockers produce a number of other effects such as α-adrenergic blockade, antioxidant effects, and "membrane stabilization" (sodium channel block) that may contribute to antiarrhythmic actions. β-Blockade inhibits VF due to acute myocardial ischemia in animal models. Most available β-blockers are administered once or twice a day. Some undergo predominant hepatic metabolism (e.g., propranolol), whereas others are eliminated by renal excretion of unchanged drug (e.g., nadolol, atenolol). Metoprolol, timolol, and carvedilol are metabolized by CYP2D6, and excess pharmacologic effects can be observed in subjects with defective CYP2D6 activity on a genetic basis or due to drug interactions.[72-74]

Uses. β-Blockers can control the ventricular rate in AF or atrial flutter, terminate paroxysmal SVT and occasional VT, notably in those patients with idiopathic forms. They are also safer, although somewhat less effective, than other drugs for suppression of symptomatic PVCs. β-Blockers, except those with intrinsic sympathomimetic activity, decrease both short- and long-term mortality after acute MI and are now indicated, particularly carvedilol (and metoprolol), for patients with heart failure.[75] β-Blockers are first-line therapy for all forms of congenital LQTS; some data suggest they may be especially useful in the LQT1 form.[76]

Adverse Effects. β-Blockers can produce hypotension, excess bradycardia, and AV block in susceptible individuals. Exacerbation of heart failure can occur, although β-blockers are beneficial in the long term when appropriately titrated in patients with heart failure.

Antiarrhythmic Effects of Calcium Channel Blockers

Verapamil and diltiazem block *L*-type calcium channels, prolong AV nodal refractoriness, and are effective in terminating SVT and slowing the ventricular rate in AF or atrial flutter. They are also useful in treating rare patients with idiopathic ventricular arrhythmias in structurally normal hearts. The drugs can be administered intravenously for acute arrhythmia management and orally for long-term therapy. Their intravenous use can be complicated by hypotension or bradycardia, especially with concurrent use of other cardiodepressant drugs, in patients with underlying heart disease, and in those with sustained VT.[77] During chronic oral therapy, constipation is common with verapamil, and peripheral edema can occur with both agents. Currently available dihydropyridine calcium channel blockers have no antiarrhythmic activity in usual doses. Either diltiazem or verapamil can raise serum digoxin levels, and both interact with many other drugs, including β-blockers.

Digoxin

Pharmacology. Digoxin is a high-potency inhibitor of sodium potassium adenosine triphosphatase (ATPase). In heart cells, this action, in turn, increases sodium-calcium exchange and increases intracellular calcium concentration. These actions are responsible for the drug's positive inotropic effects and likely also mediate some of its proarrhythmic actions. A second major effect produced by digoxin is increased vagal activity, which underlies the drug's sinus and AV nodal slowing properties.

Pharmacokinetics. Digoxin is eliminated slowly primarily by renal excretion. With an elimination half-life of 36 hours in normal individuals, steady state is approached in 7 to 10 days. Intravenous loading doses will transiently produce very high plasma concentrations, but distribution into peripheral tissues is required for the drug to produce its effect; this can be delayed for several hours. Other forms of digitalis glycoside have been, and continue to be, used in some parts of the world, and these may be eliminated by other routes. Digitoxin is eliminated primarily by hepatic metabolism.

Uses. Digoxin is used as adjunctive therapy for rate control of AF or atrial flutter, particularly in patients with heart failure. Addition of a second agent (β-blocker or calcium channel blocker) is frequently required to maintain rate control during exertion. Digoxin, like verapamil and diltiazem, is contraindicated for use in AF in patients with WPW syndrome.

Adverse Effects. The hallmark of excess digitalis is arrhythmias, which often have features of both enhanced automaticity and inhibition of sinus and AV nodal function. Junctional tachycardia or paroxysmal atrial tachycardia with AV block are characteristic, as are isolated ventricular arrhythmias. Neurologic symptoms, such as confusion and visual disturbances, occur during chronic toxicity, particularly in the elderly. With suicidal ingestion, digoxin produces striking and difficult-to-manage hyperkalemia, with accompanying asystole. Management of mild digoxin toxicity consists of drug withdrawal and observation of the patient. Temporary pacing may occasionally be required. With more serious forms of toxicity, antidigoxin antibodies are indicated. These can be highly effective, even in patients presenting with cardiac arrest.[78] Serum digoxin concentrations are artifactually elevated after administration of the antibody.

Magnesium

Uses. When serum magnesium is low, arrhythmias (including torsades de pointes) can occur and can be effectively suppressed by restoring normal magnesium. Intravenous magnesium sulfate can also be effective for some arrhythmias (torsades de pointes, digitalis toxicity) even in the absence of hypomagnesemia. Excess magnesium causes hypermagnesemia with areflexia and respiratory suppression.

EMERGING TARGETS AND THERAPEUTICS[79]

Cardiac arrhythmias are a leading cause of morbidity and mortality in many developed countries. Despite intense investigation, the cellular mechanisms for most cardiac arrhythmias have not been clearly established. As a consequence, drug therapy for most forms of atrial and ventricular arrhythmias remains largely empirical and ineffective, leading to increased use of nonpharmacologic therapies. Clearly, new approaches to the prevention and treatment of cardiac arrhythmias are needed. However, evolving knowledge about the molecular mechanisms of cardiac arrhythmias provides innovative strategies for discovering new cardiac antiarrhythmic drugs. Here, we review the development of new compounds on the verge of clinical use and other approaches that hold promise for future drug development.

New Molecular Targets for Treating Arrhythmias

An increasingly recognized link in the pathway between an initial molecular lesion and the manifestation of an arrhythmia is the process known as "electrical remodeling." This is the cascade of events that translates a molecular stimulus to a transiently, semipermanently, or permanently altered substrate that, with an appropriate trigger, then develops arrhythmias. This process has a variety of potentially deleterious clinical consequences, and its prevention is a potentially attractive therapeutic option. Electrical remodeling plays an important role in the maintenance and recurrence of AF, and studies have shown that Ca^{2+} may be an important mediator of these changes.

T-*Type* Ca^{2+} *Channels*

T-Type Ca^{2+} channels represent one potential target for treatment of arrhythmias. These channels have different physiologic and molecular properties than those of *L*-type Ca^{2+} channels and are expressed in a number of tissues including blood vessels, conduction system (including sinoatrial node and Purkinje cells), kidneys, and adrenal glands. They may have a role in atrial arrhythmias and are also believed to be involved in cardiac pacing (sinoatrial node). However, they appear to play no role in the working myocardium. Most of the data on tissue selectivity of *T*-type Ca^{2+} channels comes from clinical experience with mibefradil, a partial *T*-type Ca^{2+} channel antagonist. Mibefradil inhibits both *T*-type and *L*-type Ca^{2+} channels with some selectivity for *T*-type over *L*-type channels. It is also a potent inhibitor of a number of common drug-metabolizing enzymes (2D6, 3A4) and is an I_{Kr} blocker. Mibefradil was first approved in 1997 for hypertension, angina pectoris, and congestive heart failure but was withdrawn from the market a year later because of drug interactions owing to its inhibition of multiple CYP isoforms. Because the reasons for withdrawal were unrelated to *T*-type antagonism, the role of these channels in various tissues awaits better characterization and more selective drugs.

Modulation of Intracellular Ca^{2+}

Calcium overload is an important mediator in the pathogenesis of arrhythmias. The sarcoplasmic reticulum (SR) plays an important role in buffering the levels of free calcium during diastole. During systole, the ryanodine receptor on the SR releases Ca^{2+}, thereby initiating contraction. The Ca^{2+} release is modulated by protein kinase (PK)–mediated phosphorylation, which causes the dissociation of the tacrolimus (FK-506)-binding protein (FKBP12.6), promoting Ca^{2+} release from the SR and cardiac contractility. Increased phosphorylation of the cardiac ryanodine receptor (RyR2) has been reported in heart failure and with exercise, and mutations in the *RyR2* receptor gene have been associated with a rare arrhythmia called "catecholaminergic polymorphic VT."[80] It has been proposed that the mutations, or hyperphosporylation of the channel in heart failure or in AF, reduce the affinity of FKBP12.6 for RyR2, leading to abnormal leak of Ca^{2+} from the SR and resulting in DADs, which can trigger fatal ventricular arrhythmias.[81] Ryanodine and flanarizine, both inhibitors of SR Ca^{2+} handling, prevent some arrhythmias.[82] Stabilization of FKBP12.6 binding to the RyR2 receptor with a small molecule may not only inhibit triggered activity associated with the hyperadrenergic states but also reduce remodeling associated with Ca^{2+} overload. The recent discovery of the small molecule JTV519 that stabilizes the interaction between FKB12.6 and the RyR2 receptor represents a possible therapeutic breakthrough for treatment of Ca^{2+} overload–associated arrhythmias.[83]

Afterdepolarizations are associated with sympathetic nervous activation through protein kinase A (PKA) activity. β-Adrenoreceptor antagonists, which are now well recognized to reduce sudden cardiac death risk, prevent agonist-mediated increases in PKA activity.[84] An association between triggered arrhythmias and activation of other protein kinases (notably Ca^{2+}/calmodulin-dependent protein kinase II [CaMKII]) suggests that kinase inhibition may be antiarrhythmic. CaMKII activity increases during action potential prolongation, and CaMKII inhibition prevents DADs without shortening action potential duration in isolated hearts.[85] Recently, chronic CaMKII inhibition in mouse heart has been shown to prevent hypertrophy, arrhythmias, and sudden death after coronary occlusion.[86] These findings suggest that if appropriate subtype targets could be achieved, CaMKII inhibition may be a novel approach for antiarrhythmic therapy.[87]

Tissue-Specific Channel Blockers

One approach to increasing the efficacy and reducing the risks of fatal ventricular proarrhythmia of ion channel blocking drugs is the development of atrium-specific drugs. One potential molecular target is the potassium channel gene *KCNA5* (*Kv1.5*) whose expression underlies the I_{Kur}. In humans, *KCNA5* expression is much greater in atrium than in ventricle, and I_{Kur} is readily recorded in atrium but not in ventricle. The novel atrial-selective I_{Kur} blockers S1185, S9947, S20951, and RSD1235 show marked prolongation of left atrial refractoriness.[88] Furthermore, a recent study showed that AVE0118, a blocker of potassium currents activated early in the atrial APD (I_{Kur} as well as I_{TO}) not only markedly prolonged the atrial refractory period during AF but also did so without affecting QT duration in remodeled atria of goats. However, the functional roles of *KCNA5* in other tissues in which it is highly expressed (e.g., smooth muscle) are not well understood; and therefore, whether appropriate efficacy and safety might be achieved with blockers of this channel in humans remains to be determined. Moreover, loss-of-function mutations in KCNA5 have recently been linked to familial AF,[89] so I_{Kur} block remains to be established as an anti-AF intervention.

Targeting Signaling Pathways for Treatment of Arrhythmias

Large randomized clinical trials have described striking effects on sudden death of several interventions not yet developed as targeting arrhythmia triggers or substrates. Gruppo Italiano per lo Studio della Sopravvivenza nell'Infarto Miocardico-Prevenzione (GISSI-Provenzione)[90] prospectively evaluated the effect of n-3 polyunsaturated fatty acid (fish oil) supplementation in more than 11,000 patients with recent (<3 mo) acute MI and found a 53% reduction in sudden death at 4 months. Similar unexpected large effects of "nonarrhythmic" drugs on sudden death have been seen in trials of angiotensin-converting enzyme inhibitors,[91] HMG CoA reductase inhibitors (statins),[92] and aldosterone receptor antagonists.[93] Although an overall beneficial effect on plaque stability and the progression of coronary disease may underlie these drug actions, a direct modulatory effect on heretofore poorly understood signaling pathways that generate the arrhythmic substrate is a hypothesis requiring further evaluation. Further understanding of the way in which these pathways affect arrhythmogenesis may point to entirely new and specific antiarrhythmic therapies.

Along similar lines, studies point to oxidant stress as a common feature of AF, and it has been proposed that ascorbate and specific antioxidant treatments may have a role in prevention of AF.[94-96] Nutritional factors may also play an important role in the pathophysiology of AF. Consumption of broiled or baked fish has been associated with lower incidence of AF,[97] and it is noteworthy that fish and fish-derived n-3 fatty acid have a potent anti-inflammatory effect. Retrospective studies suggest that angiotensin-converting enzyme inhibitor therapy is associated with a lower incidence of AF, and a placebo-controlled trial found a similar beneficial effect of adding the angiotensin receptor blocker irbesartan to amiodarone.[98,99] Inhibition of the renin-angiotensin-aldosterone system appears to prevent the development of AF by suppressing electrical and structural cardiac remodeling.

REFERENCES

1. Zipes DP. Mechanisms of clinical arrhythmias. J Cardiovasc Electrophysiol 2003;14:902-912.
2. Vest JA, Wehrens XH, Reiken SR, et al. Defective cardiac ryanodine receptor regulation during atrial fibrillation. Circulation 2005;111:2025-2032.
3. Ranger S, Talajic M, Lemery R, et al. Amplification of flecainide-induced ventricular conduction slowing by exercise. A potentially significant clinical consequence of use-dependent sodium channel blockade. Circulation 1989;79:1000-1006.
4. Woosley RL, Drayer DE, Reidenberg MM, et al. Effect of acetylator phenotype on the rate at which procainamide induces antinuclear antibodies and the lupus syndrome. N Engl J Med 1978;298:1157-1159.
5. Hoffmeyer S, Burk O, von Richter O, et al. Functional polymorphisms of the human multidrug-resistance gene: multiple sequence variations and correlation of one allele with P-glycoprotein expression and activity in vivo. Proc Natl Acad Sci U S A 2000;97:3473-3478.
6. Verstuyft C, Schwab M, Schaeffeler E, et al. Digoxin pharmacokinetics and MDR1 genetic polymorphisms. Eur J Clin Pharmacol 2003;58:809-812.
7. Kim RB. Drugs as P-glycoprotein substrates, inhibitors, and inducers. Drug Metab Rev 2002;34:47-54.
8. Roden DM. Drug-induced prolongation of the QT interval. N Engl J Med 2004;350:1013-1022.
9. Choy AM, Darbar D, Dell'Orto S, et al. Exaggerated QT prolongation after cardioversion of atrial fibrillation. J Am Coll Cardiol 1999;34:396-401.
10. The Cardiac Arrhythmia Suppression Trial (CAST) Investigators. Preliminary report: effect of encainide and flecainide on mortality in a randomized trial of arrhythmia suppression after myocardial infarction. N Engl J Med 1989;321:406-412.
11. Waldo AL, Camm AJ, deRuyter H, et al., and The SWORD Investigators. Survival With Oral D-Sotalol. Effect of D-sotalol on mortality in patients with left ventricular dysfunction after recent and remote myocardial infarction. Lancet 1996;348:7-12.
12. Brugada R, Brugada J, Antzelevitch C, et al. Sodium channel blockers identify risk for sudden death in patients with ST-segment elevation and right bundle branch block but structurally normal hearts. Circulation 2000;101:510-515.
13. Darbar D, Yang T, Churchwell K, et al. Unmasking of Brugada syndrome by lithium. Circulation 2005;112:1527-1531.
14. Gregoratos G, Abrams J, Epstein AE, et al. ACC/AHA/NASPE 2002 guideline update for implantation of cardiac pacemakers and antiarrhythmia devices: summary article. A report of the American College of Cardiology/American Heart Association Task Force on Practice Guidelines (ACC/AHA/NASPE Committee to Update the 1998 Pacemaker Guidelines). J Cardiovasc Electrophysiol 2002;13:1183-1199.
15. Damiano RJ Jr, Gaynor SL, Bailey M, et al. The long-term outcome of patients with coronary disease and atrial fibrillation undergoing the Cox maze procedure. J Thorac Cardiovasc Surg 2003;126:2016-2021.
16. Haissaguerre M, Jais P, Shah DC, et al. Spontaneous initiation of atrial fibrillation by ectopic beats originating in the pulmonary veins. N Engl J Med 1998;339:659-666.
17. Wazni O, Martin DO, Marrouche NF, et al. C reactive protein concentration and recurrence of atrial fibrillation after electrical cardioversion. Heart 2005;91:1303-1305.
18. Karch MR, Zrenner B, Deisenhofer I, et al. Freedom from atrial tachyarrhythmias after catheter ablation of atrial fibrillation: a randomized comparison between 2 current ablation strategies. Circulation 2005;111:2875-2880.
19. Fuster V, Ryden LE, Cannom DS, et al. ACC/AHA/ESC 2006 guidelines for the management of patients with atrial fibrillation: a report of the American College of Cardiology/American Heart Association Task Force on Practice Guidelines and the European

Society of Cardiology Committee for Practice Guidelines (Writing Committee to Revise the 2001 Guidelines for the Management of Patients With Atrial Fibrillation): developed in collaboration with the European Heart Rhythm Association and the Heart Rhythm Society. Circulation 2006;114:e257-e354.
20. Wood MA, Brown-Mahoney C, Kay GN, et al. Clinical outcomes after ablation and pacing therapy for atrial fibrillation. Circulation 2000;101:1138-1144.
21. The Antiarrhythmics versus Implantable Defibrillators (AVID) Investigators. A comparison of antiarrhythmic-drug therapy with implantable defibrillators in patients resuscitated from near-fatal ventricular arrhythmias. N Engl J Med 1997;337:1576-1583.
22. Moss AJ, Hall WJ, Cannom DS, et al., and the Multicenter Automatic Defibrillator Implantation Trial Investigators. Improved survival with an implanted defibrillator in patients with coronary disease at high risk for ventricular arrhythmia. N Engl J Med 1996;335:1933-1940.
23. Buxton AE, Lee KL, Fisher JD, et al., and the Multicenter Unsustained Tachycardia Trial Investigators. A randomized study of the prevention of sudden death in patients with coronary artery disease. N Engl J Med 1999;341:1882-1890.
24. Moss AJ, Zareba W, Hall WJ, et al. Prophylactic implantation of a defibrillator in patients with myocardial infarction and reduced ejection fraction. N Engl J Med 2002;346:877-883.
25. Kadish A, Dyer A, Daubert JP, et al. Prophylactic defibrillator implantation in patients with nonischemic dilated cardiomyopathy. N Engl J Med 2004;350:2151-2158.
26. Bardy GH, Lee KL, Mark DB, et al. Amiodarone or an implantable cardioverter-defibrillator for congestive heart failure. N Engl J Med 2005;352:225-237.
27. Bristow MR, Saxon LA, Boehmer J, et al. Cardiac-resynchronization therapy with or without an implantable defibrillator in advanced chronic heart failure. N Engl J Med 2004;350:2140-2150.
28. Blomstrom-Lundqvist C, Scheinman MM, Aliot EM, et al. ACC/AHA/ESC guidelines for the management of patients with supraventricular arrhythmias—executive summary: a report of the American College of Cardiology/American Heart Association Task Force on Practice Guidelines and the European Society of Cardiology Committee for Practice Guidelines (Writing Committee to Develop Guidelines for the Management of Patients With Supraventricular Arrhythmias). Circulation 2003;108:1871-1909.
29. Zipes DP, Camm AJ, Borggrefe M, et al. ACC/AHA/ESC 2006 guidelines for management of patients with ventricular arrhythmias and the prevention of sudden cardiac death: a report of the American College of Cardiology/American Heart Association Task Force and the European Society of Cardiology Committee for Practice Guidelines (Writing Committee to Develop Guidelines for Management of Patients With Ventricular Arrhythmias and the Prevention of Sudden Cardiac Death): developed in collaboration with the European Heart Rhythm Association and the Heart Rhythm Society. Circulation 2006;114:e385-e484.
30. Alboni P, Botto GL, Baldi N, et al. Outpatient treatment of recent-onset atrial fibrillation with the "pill-in-the-pocket" approach. N Engl J Med 2004;351:2384-2391.
31. Torp-Pedersen C, Moller M, Bloch-Thomsen PE, et al., and the Danish Investigations of Arrhythmia and Mortality on Dofetilide Study Group. Dofetilide in patients with congestive heart failure and left ventricular dysfunction. N Engl J Med 1999;341:857-865.
32. Kudenchuk PJ, Cobb LA, Copass MK, et al. Amiodarone for resuscitation after out-of-hospital cardiac arrest due to ventricular fibrillation. N Engl J Med 1999;341:871-878.
33. Pacifico A, Hohnloser SH, Williams JH, et al., and the D,L-Sotalol Implantable Cardioverter-Defibrillator Study Group. Prevention of implantable-defibrillator shocks by treatment with sotalol. N Engl J Med 1999;340:1855-1862.
34. Dorian P, Borggrefe M, Al-Khalidi HR, et al. Placebo-controlled, randomized clinical trial of azimilide for prevention of ventricular tachyarrhythmias in patients with an implantable cardioverter defibrillator. Circulation 2004;110:3646-3654.
35. Mazur A, Anderson ME, Bonney S, et al. Pause-dependent polymorphic ventricular tachycardia during long-term treatment with dofetilide: a placebo-controlled, implantable cardioverter-defibrillator-based evaluation. J Am Coll Cardiol 2001;37:1100-1105.
36. Boutitie F, Boissel JP, Connolly SJ, et al., and The EMIAT and CAMIAT Investigators. Amiodarone interaction with beta-blockers: analysis of the merged EMIAT (European Myocardial Infarct Amiodarone Trial) and CAMIAT (Canadian Amiodarone Myocardial Infarction Trial) databases. Circulation 1999;99:2268-2275.
37. Priori SG, Napolitano C, Schwartz PJ, et al. Association of long QT syndrome loci and cardiac events among patients treated with beta-blockers. JAMA 2004;292:1341-1344.
38. Priori SG, Napolitano C, Cantu F, et al. Differential response to Na^+ channel blockade, beta-adrenergic stimulation, and rapid pacing in a cellular model mimicking the SCN5A and HERG defects present in the long-QT syndrome. Circ Res 1996;78:1009-1015.
39. Benhorin J, Taub R, Goldmit M, et al. Effects of flecainide in patients with new SCN5A mutation: mutation-specific therapy for long-QT syndrome? Circulation 2000;101:1698-1706.
40. Belhassen B, Glick A, Viskin S. Efficacy of quinidine in high-risk patients with Brugada syndrome. Circulation 2004;110:1731-1737.
41. Gaita F, Giustetto C, Bianchi F, et al. Short QT syndrome: pharmacological treatment. J Am Coll Cardiol 2004;43:1494-1499.
42. Schimpf R, Giustetto C, Gaita F, et al. Congenital short QT syndrome and implantable cardioverter defibrillator treatment. J Cardiovasc Electrophysiol 2003;14:1273-1277.
43. Sumitomo N, Harada K, Nagashima M, et al. Catecholaminergic polymorphic ventricular tachycardia: electrocardiographic characteristics and optimal therapeutic strategies to prevent sudden death. Heart 2003;89:66-70.
44. Stewart JT, McKenna WJ. Management of arrhythmias in hypertrophic cardiomyopathy. Cardiovasc Drugs Ther 1994;8:95-99.
45. DeGroff CG, Silka MJ. Bronchospasm after intravenous administration of adenosine in a patient with asthma. J Pediatr 1994;125:822-823.
46. Crosson JE, Etheridge SP, Milstein S, et al. Therapeutic and diagnostic utility of adenosine during tachycardia evaluation in children. Am J Cardiol 1994;74:155-160.
47. Exner DV, Muzyka T, Gillis AM. Proarrhythmia in patients with the Wolff-Parkinson-White syndrome after standard doses of intravenous adenosine. Ann Intern Med 1995;122:351-352.
48. Le Bouter S, El Harchi A, Marionneau C, et al. Long-term amiodarone administration remodels expression of ion channel transcripts in the mouse heart. Circulation 2004;110:3028-3035.
49. Mason JW, Hondeghem LM, Katzung BG. Block of inactivated sodium channels and of depolarization-induced automaticity in guinea pig papillary muscle by amiodarone. Circ Res 1984;55:278-285.
50. Wolfe CL, Nibley C, Bhandari A, et al. Polymorphous ventricular tachycardia associated with acute myocardial infarction. Circulation 1991;84:1543-1551.
51. Kowey PR, Levine JH, Herre JM, et al., and The Intravenous Amiodarone Multicenter Investigators Group. Randomized, double-blind comparison of intravenous amiodarone and bretylium in the treatment of patients with recurrent, hemodynamically destabilizing ventricular tachycardia or fibrillation. Circulation 1995;92:3255-3263.
52. Dorian P, Paquette M, Newman D, et al. Quality of life improves with treatment in the Canadian Trial of Atrial Fibrillation. Am Heart J 2002;143:984-990.
53. Lazzara R. Amiodarone and torsade de pointes. Ann Intern Med 1989;111:549-551.
54. Goldschlager N, Epstein AE, Naccarelli G, et al. Practical guidelines for clinicians who treat patients with amiodarone. Practice Guidelines Subcommittee, North American Society of Pacing and Electrophysiology. Arch Intern Med 2000;160:1741-1748.
55. U.K. Rythmodan Multicentre Study Group. Oral disopyramide after admission to hospital with suspected acute myocardial infarction. Postgrad Med J 1984;60:98-107.
56. Kober L, Bloch Thomsen PE, Moller M, et al. Effect of dofetilide in patients with recent myocardial infarction and left-ventricular dysfunction: a randomised trial. Lancet 2000;356:2052-2058.
57. Pedersen OD, Bagger H, Keller N, et al. Efficacy of dofetilide in the treatment of atrial fibrillation-flutter in patients with reduced left ventricular function: a Danish investigation of arrhythmia and mortality on dofetilide (diamond) substudy. Circulation 2001;104:292-296.
58. Follmer CH, Colatsky TJ. Block of delayed rectifier potassium current, IK, by flecainide and E-4031 in cat ventricular myocytes. Circulation 1990;82:289-293.
59. Evers J, Eichelbaum M, Kroemer HK. Unpredictability of flecainide plasma concentrations in patients with renal failure: relationship to side effects and sudden death? Ther Drug Monit 1994;16:349-351.
60. Lee KS, Lee EW. Ionic mechanism of ibutilide in human atrium: evidence for a drug-induced Na^+ current through a nifedipine inhibited inward channel. J Pharmacol Exp Ther 1998;286:9-22.
61. Yang T, Snyders DJ, Roden DM. Ibutilide, a methanesulfonanilide antiarrhythmic, is a potent blocker of the rapidly activating delayed rectifier K^+ current (IKr) in AT-1 cells. Concentration-, time-, voltage-, and use-dependent effects. Circulation 1995;91:1799-1806.
62. Stambler BS, Wood MA, Ellenbogen KA, et al., and the Ibutilide Repeat Dose Study Investigators. Efficacy and safety of repeated intravenous doses of ibutilide for rapid conversion of atrial flutter or fibrillation. Circulation 1996;94:1613-1621.
63. Oral H, Souza JJ, Michaud GF, et al. Facilitating transthoracic cardioversion of atrial fibrillation with ibutilide pretreatment. N Engl J Med 1999;340:1849-1854.
64. Glatter K, Yang Y, Chatterjee K, et al. Chemical cardioversion of atrial fibrillation or flutter with ibutilide in patients receiving amiodarone therapy. Circulation 2001;103:253-257.
65. Glatter KA, Dorostkar PC, Yang Y, et al. Electrophysiological effects of ibutilide in patients with accessory pathways. Circulation 2001;104:1933-1939.
66. Lie KI, Wellens HJ, van Capelle FJ, et al. Lidocaine in the prevention of primary ventricular fibrillation. A double-blind, randomized study of 212 consecutive patients. N Engl J Med 1974;291:1324-1326.
67. MacMahon S, Collins R, Peto R, et al. Effects of prophylactic lidocaine in suspected acute myocardial infarction. An overview of results from the randomized, controlled trials. JAMA 1988;260:1910-1916.
68. Impact Research Group. International Mexiletine and Placebo Antiarrhythmic Coronary Trial: I. Report on arrhythmia and other findings. J Am Coll Cardiol 1984;4:1148-1163.
69. Wang DW, Yazawa K, Makita N, et al. Pharmacological targeting of long QT mutant sodium channels. J Clin Invest 1997;99:1714-1720.
70. Antzelevitch C, Shimizu W, Yan GX, et al. The M cell: its contribution to the ECG and to normal and abnormal electrical function of the heart. J Cardiovasc Electrophysiol 1999;10:1124-1152.
71. Fromm MF, Kim RB, Stein CM, et al. Inhibition of P-glycoprotein–mediated drug transport: a unifying mechanism to explain the interaction between digoxin and quinidine. Circulation 1999;99:552-557.
72. Lennard MS, Silas JH, Freestone S, et al. Oxidation phenotype—a major determinant of metoprolol metabolism and response. N Engl J Med 1982;307:1558-1560.
73. Edeki TI, He H, Wood AJ. Pharmacogenetic explanation for excessive beta-blockade following timolol eye drops. Potential for oral-ophthalmic drug interaction. JAMA 1995;274:1611-1613.
74. Zhou HH, Wood AJ. Stereoselective disposition of carvedilol is determined by CYP2D6. Clin Pharmacol Ther 1995;57:518-524.
75. Poole-Wilson PA, Swedberg K, Cleland JG, et al. Comparison of carvedilol and metoprolol on clinical outcomes in patients with chronic heart failure in the Carvedilol or Metoprolol European Trial (COMET): randomised controlled trial. Lancet 2003;362:7-13.
76. Fenichel RR, Malik M, Antzelevitch C, et al. Drug-induced torsades de pointes and implications for drug development. J Cardiovasc Electrophysiol 2004;15:475-495.
77. Cannom DS, Prystowsky EN. Management of ventricular arrhythmias: detection, drugs, and devices. JAMA 1999;281:172-179.

78. Antman EM, Wenger TL, Butler VP Jr, et al. Treatment of 150 cases of life-threatening digitalis intoxication with digoxin-specific Fab antibody fragments. Final report of a multicenter study. Circulation 1990;81:1744-1752.
79. Darbar D, Roden DM. Future of antiarrhythmic drugs. Curr Opin Cardiol 2006;21:361-367.
80. Priori SG, Napolitano C, Tiso N, et al. Mutations in the cardiac ryanodine receptor gene (hRyR2) underlie catecholaminergic polymorphic ventricular tachycardia. Circulation 2001;103:196-200.
81. Fozzard HA. Afterdepolarizations and triggered activity. Basic Res Cardiol 1992;87(suppl 2):105-113.
82. Marban E, Robinson SW, Wier WG. Mechanisms of arrhythmogenic delayed and early afterdepolarizations in ferret ventricular muscle. J Clin Invest 1986;78:1185-1192.
83. Wehrens XH, Lehnart SE, Reiken SR, et al. Protection from cardiac arrhythmia through ryanodine receptor-stabilizing protein calstabin 2. Science 2004;304:292-296.
84. Kendall MJ, Lynch KP, Hjalmarson A, Kjekshus J. Beta-blockers and sudden cardiac death. Ann Intern Med 1995;123:358-367.
85. Anderson ME, Braun AP, Wu Y, et al. KN-93, an inhibitor of multifunctional Ca^{++}/calmodulin-dependent protein kinase, decreases early afterdepolarizations in rabbit heart. J Pharmacol Exp Ther 1998;287:996-1006.
86. Zhang R, Khoo MS, Wu Y, et al. Calmodulin kinase II inhibition protects against structural heart disease. Nat Med 2005;11:409-417.
87. Anderson ME. Calmodulin kinase signaling in heart: an intriguing candidate target for therapy of myocardial dysfunction and arrhythmias. Pharmacol Ther 2005;106:39-55.
88. Knobloch K, Brendel J, Peukert S, et al. Electrophysiological and antiarrhythmic effects of the novel I(Kur) channel blockers, S9947 and S20951, on left vs. right pig atrium in vivo in comparison with the I(Kr) blockers dofetilide, azimilide, d,l-sotalol and ibutilide. Naunyn Schmiedebergs Arch Pharmacol 2002;366:482-487.
89. Olson TM, Alekseev AE, Liu XK, et al. Kv1.5 channelopathy due to *KCNA5* loss-of-function mutation causes human atrial filbrillation. Hum Mol Genet 2006;15:2185-2191.
90. Marchioli R, Barzi F, Bomba E, et al. Early protection against sudden death by n-3 polyunsaturated fatty acids after myocardial infarction: time-course analysis of the results of the Gruppo Italiano per lo Studio della Sopravvivenza nell'Infarto Miocardico (GISSI)-Prevenzione. Circulation 2002;105:1897-1903.
91. Yusuf S, Sleight P, Pogue J, et al., and The Heart Outcomes Prevention Evaluation Study Investigators. Effects of an angiotensin-converting-enzyme inhibitor, ramipril, on cardiovascular events in high-risk patients. N Engl J Med 2000;342:145-153.
92. Mitchell LB, Powell JL, Gillis AM, et al. Are lipid-lowering drugs also antiarrhythmic drugs? An analysis of the Antiarrhythmics versus Implantable Defibrillators (AVID) trial. J Am Coll Cardiol 2003;42:81-87.
93. Pitt B, Zannad F, Remme WJ, et al., and the Randomized Aldactone Evaluation Study Investigators. The effect of spironolactone on morbidity and mortality in patients with severe heart failure. N Engl J Med 1999;341:709-717.
94. Chung MK, Martin DO, Sprecher D, et al. C-reactive protein elevation in patients with atrial arrhythmias: inflammatory mechanisms and persistence of atrial fibrillation. Circulation 2001;104:2886-2891.
95. Carnes CA, Chung MK, Nakayama T, et al. Ascorbate attenuates atrial pacing-induced peroxynitrite formation and electrical remodeling and decreases the incidence of postoperative atrial fibrillation. Circ Res 2001;89:E32-E38.
96. Mihm MJ, Yu F, Carnes CA, et al. Impaired myofibrillar energetics and oxidative injury during human atrial fibrillation. Circulation 2001;104:174-180.
97. Mozaffarian D, Psaty BM, Rimm EB, et al. Fish intake and risk of incident atrial fibrillation. Circulation 2004;110:368-373.
98. Madrid AH, Bueno MG, Rebollo JM, et al. Use of irbesartan to maintain sinus rhythm in patients with long-lasting persistent atrial fibrillation: a prospective and randomized study. Circulation 2002;106:331-336.
99. Healey JS, Baranchuk A, Crystal E, et al. Prevention of atrial fibrillation with angiotensin-converting enzyme inhibitors and angiotensin receptor blockers: a meta-analysis. J Am Coll Cardiol 2005;45:1832-1839.

26

HEART FAILURE

Arthur M. Feldman

INTRODUCTION 389
PATHOPHYSIOLOGY 389
THERAPEUTICS AND CLINICAL PHARMACOLOGY 389
Goals of Therapy 389
Therapeutics by Class 389
β-Blockers 389
ACE Inhibitors 390
Angiotensin II Receptor Blockers 392
Aldosterone Receptor Blockers 394
Digoxin 395
Diuretics 395
Vasodilators 395
Inotropes 396
Calcium Sensitizers 396
Calcium Channel Blockers 397
Anticoagulation 398
SUMMARY 398

INTRODUCTION

Heart failure (HF) has 5 million victims in the United States alone.[1] It occurs equally in men and women and is more prevalent among African Americans, Hispanics, and American Indians than among whites. About 75% of these individuals are older than 65. Each year, nearly 1 million people are hospitalized with congestive HF, 30% to 60% of who are "readmits." The congestive HF death rate has increased by 35% in the past quarter century. The incidence of HF is increasing as our population ages and as the lives of our cardiac patients are extended by our interventions and innovative therapeutics. In spite of our advancement in treatments for coronary artery disease (CAD), the damage to the myocardium leads to HF. In addition, the high rate of obesity in America has escalated the incidence of diabetes and high blood pressure, increasing the risk of CAD and HF. Despite improvements in therapy, the mortality rate in patients with HF has remained unacceptably high.[2]

PATHOPHYSIOLOGY

Myocardial damage regardless of etiology can cause a decrease in cardiac output, which stimulates a cascade of events dictated by the sympathetic nervous system and renin-angiotensin-aldosterone system (RAAS) in order to restore cardiac output and supply enough oxygen to meet the increasing demands. The main mechanism of action focuses on increasing preload and decreasing afterload and, to some extent, increasing contractility to allow for forward flow.

Since the 1970s, when β-blockers and angiotensin-converting enzyme (ACE) inhibitors were first introduced, investigators have learned more about the pathophysiology of systolic function in HF patients. During an exacerbation of HF, the neurohormonal system is activated to help with the process of compensation. Chronic activation of the neurohormonal system has a significant impact on disease progression. As a result, the neurohormonal system has provided a key target for pharmacologic therapy in patients with HF secondary to systolic dysfunction. These targets include the RAAS as well as the sympathetic nervous system.

THERAPEUTICS AND CLINICAL PHARMACOLOGY

Goals of Therapy

The goals of pharmacologic therapy in HF patients are to improve symptoms, slow or reverse deterioration in myocardial function, and reduce mortality. The treatment of the decompensated heart requires targeting all the neurohormonal axes activated by the failing heart. Therefore, the foundation of HF therapy lies with ACE inhibitors and β-blockers, which have been clinically proven to improve symptoms and mortality. Symptomatic relief, however, is best addressed with diuretics. Other treatment strategies, including the use of inotropic agents to improve pump function, and investigational therapies must also be considered to alleviate HF symptoms in some patients.

Therapeutics by Class

β-Blockers work by inhibiting the effects of the sympathetic nervous system, including vasoconstriction, increase in heart rate and contractility, and direct cardiotoxicity mediated by the increase in neurohormonal activity and the vicious cycle of HF.

Two classes of drugs, the *ACE inhibitors* and the *angiotensin II receptor blockers* (ARBs), suppress the activity of angiotensin II, the major effector hormone of the RAAS. As noted in Figure 26-1, ACE inhibitors and ARBs have different sites of action. They both play a role in decreasing preload (decreasing salt and water retention) and afterload (inhibiting vasoconstriction).

The ACE inhibitors competitively inhibit the nonspecific enzyme kininase II, which converts inactive angiotensin I to active angiotensin II. This is the major pathway, although not the only pathway for the production of angiotensin II. Angiotensin II stimulates aldosterone, which leads to salt and water retention. Kininase II also metabolizes bradykinin to inactive degradation products. Both of these effects contribute to the actions of ACE inhibitors.

The ARBs selectively block the interaction of angiotensin II with the AT1 receptors. The AT1 receptors are responsible for all the major actions of angiotensin II, including vasoconstriction, salt and water retention, and cell growth and proliferation.

Aldosterone receptor blockers decrease preload by blocking the receptors and thereby blocking water and salt retention.

Diuretics also work on preload by decreasing intravascular volume. *Vasodilators* decrease both afterload and preload by vasodilation, which in turn decreases strain on the myocytes, thereby impeding the progression of adverse remodeling.

β-Blockers

Symptomatic HF results in neurohormonal activation as a means of early compensation. The increase in sympathetic activity may have deleterious effects, and a number of trials have shown that blockade of β-adrenergic receptors leads to symptomatic improvement and enhanced survival in many patients with HF.[3] As a result of this compelling evidence, β-blockers are now considered an important component of standard therapy in HF. This is an important shift, since

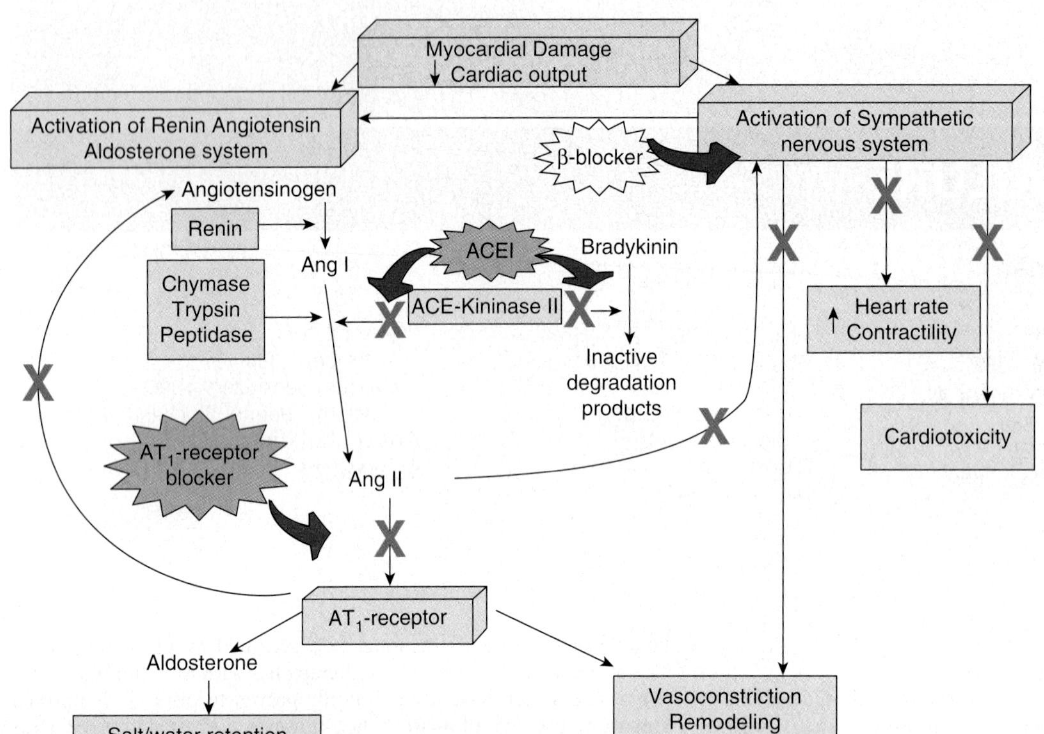

FIGURE 26-1 • The pathophysiology of heart failure. (From Willenheimer R, Dahlöf B, Rydberg E, Erhardt L. AT1-receptor blockers in hypertension and heart failure: clinical experience and future directions. Eur Heart J 1999;20:997-1008.)

β-blockers were previously considered contraindicated in patients with HF because of their negative inotropic activity. The beneficial effect of β-blockers in HF is due to many factors including reduction in catecholamines, which are directly toxic to the myocytes; up-regulation in β_1 receptors allowing for better contractility; and reduction in myocardial oxygen consumption.[4] The chronic simulation of β receptors leads to a decrease in heart rate variability, increased arrhythmias, myocardial cell toxicity, and remodeling. After initial observations suggesting a survival benefit with β-blockers in HF,[5] a number of major trials confirmed this benefit with several β-blockers (metoprolol, carvedilol, and bisoprolol) in selected patients with HF.

The first randomized controlled trial to assess the effects of β-blocker therapy on morbidity and/or mortality was the Metoprolol in Dilated Cardiomyopathy (MDC) study, which demonstrated a reduction in death or the need for cardiac transplantation in 383 patients with New York Heart Association (NYHA) functional class II-III heart failure (Table 26-1). This was followed in 1996 by the U.S. Carvedilol trials demonstrating in 1094 patients that the use of the nonselective β-blocker carvedilol was associated with a reduction in mortality and an improvement in quality of life and decreased disease progression.[6] Subsequently, the Cardiac Insufficiency Bisoprolol Study (CIBIS II)[7] tested the efficacy of the second-generation β_1 receptor–selective β-blocker bisoprolol, in NYHA class III-IV patients with ischemic and nonischemic cardiomyopathy. The study was stopped early due to the demonstrated improvement in morbidity and mortality. Metoprolol and carvedilol have also been shown to reduce all-cause mortality in the Metoprolol Randomized Intervention Trial in Heart Failure (MERIT-HF)[8] and the Carvedilol Prospective Randomized Cumulative Survival (COPERNICUS) trial,[9] respectively. MERIT-HF enrolled class II-III patients, whereas the COPERNICUS trial, which mainly enrolled class IV patients, was the largest study to demonstrate mortality benefit in patients with severe chronic HF.

The Carvedilol or Metoprolol European Trial (COMET)[10] that compared both drugs sparked a huge controversy. It enrolled patients in 15 European countries. Most patients were NYHA class II-III with an ejection fraction less than 36%. Patients were randomized to metoprolol or carvedilol. The average doses used in the study were carvedilol 21 mg twice daily and metoprolol 43 mg twice daily. The study showed 5.7% better absolute survival in carvedilol-treated patients over 5 years. However, the metoprolol dose used was not the dose that showed benefit in the MDC trial[11] or the extended-release form used in the MERIT-HF trial. Therefore, it is argued that, in order to compare the benefit of these agents, the study dose that proved benefit should have been used.

All of these trials were performed with background ACE inhibitors and diuretics; therefore, the benefit seems to be an additive effect. The CIBIS III trial has recently shown that starting treatment of congestive HF with a β-blocker (bisoprolol), followed by the addition of an ACE inhibitor (enalapril), is as effective and well tolerated as starting with an ACE inhibitor.[12] In these trials, β-blockers not only reduced all-cause mortality by 35% but also reduced cardiovascular mortality, sudden death, and hospitalizations. In addition to that, they have been shown to improve NYHA functional class.

Indeed, long-term therapy with a β-blocker has been shown to improve myocardial function and structural geometry, modify the expression of genes that are maladaptively altered in the failing human heart,[13] and improve cardiac metabolism.[14] However, an interesting finding is that many patients do not respond to β-blocker therapy. This failure to respond may be predicted by the presence of polymorphisms in the β_1 and β_2 receptor genes that alter the ability of the receptor to bind with ligand or to activate adenylyl cyclase.[15] This hypothesis will be tested in an upcoming study that may lead to genetic analysis of individual patients before attempting β-blocker therapy.

The use of β-blockers for the therapy of patients with symptomatic or asymptomatic HF is a class I recommendation (Table 26-2). That is, they should be used for treatment of clinically stable patients with left ventricular systolic dysfunction and mild to moderate HF symptoms (NYHA class II-III) who are on standard therapy (ACE inhibitors, diuretics as needed, and digoxin).[16] β-Blockers should be initiated at low doses and uptitrated slowly to target doses if the patient remains clinically stable (Box 26-1).

ACE Inhibitors

The RAAS is activated by the hemodynamic changes that accompany cardiac dysfunction. Angiotensinogen, produced by the liver, is converted to angiotensin I by renin, produced in the kidney. Angiotensin

TABLE 26-1 β-BLOCKER THERAPY IN HEART FAILURE

Study	Design	Results
MDC: Metoprolol in Dilated Cardiompathy	• 383 nonischemic patients • NYHA class II-III HF • EF < 40% • 18 mo • Short-acting **metoprolol** (100 mg/day) vs. placebo	• 34% risk reduction • Improved EF • Reduction in transplant listing
CIBIS I: Cardiac Insufficiency Bisoprolol Study	• 641 ischemic or nonischemic patients • NYHA class III-IV HF: 3 yr • **Bisoprolol** (5 mg/day) vs. placebo	• Reduced hospitalizations • Improved NYHA functional class
U.S. Carvedilol Heart Failure Study	• 1094 ischemic and nonischemic patients • NYHA class II-III HF • EF < 35% • **Carvedilol** (25-50 mg bid) vs. placebo	• 65% lower risk of death • Reduced risk of cardiac hospitalization • Trial was stopped early
New Zealand Carvedilol Trial	• 415 patients • NYHA class II-IV HF • EF < 45% • 19 mo • **Carvedilol** (25 mg bid) vs. placebo	• 21% reduction in death and hospitalization
CIBIS II: Cardiac Insufficiency Bisoprolol Study	• 2647 ischemic and nonischemic patients • NYHA class III-IV HF • EF < 35% • **Bisoprolol** (10 mg/day) vs placebo	• 33% reduction in all-cause mortality • Decreased heart-related deaths • Decreased heart-related hospitalizations
MERIT-HF: Metoprolol CR/XL Randomized Intervention Trial in Heart Failure	• 3991 ischemic and nonischemic patients • NYHA class II-III HF • EF < 35% • **Metoprolol XL** vs. placebo	• 34% reduction in all-cause mortality • 32% reduction in HF hospitalization • Study stopped early
COPERNICUS: Carvedilol Prospective Randomized Cumulative Survival Study	• 2289 ischemic and nonischemic patients • NYHA class IV HF • EF 25% • **Carvedilol** vs. placebo	• 35% reduction in mortality • 24% reduction in combined risk of death or hospitalization • Study stopped early
BEST: Beta-blocker Evaluation Survival Trial	• 2708 patients • NYHA class III-IV HF • EF < 30% • **Bucindolol** (50-100 mg bid) vs. placebo	• No difference in all-cause mortality • Decreased heart-related deaths • Study stopped early
COMET: Carvedilol or Metoprolol European Trial	• 3029 patients • NYHA class II-III • EF < 35% • Metoprolol (5-50 mg bid) vs. **carvedilol** (3.125-25 mg bid)	• 5.7% better 5-yr absolute survival

bid, twice daily; EF, ejection fraction; HF, heart failure; NYHA, New York Heart Association; XL, extended release.

TABLE 26-2 β-BLOCKERS

Drug	Initial Dose	Target Dose
Carvedilol (Coreg)	3.125 mg bid	<188 pounds: raise to 25 mg bid >187 pounds: raise to 50 mg bid
Metoprolol extended release (Toprol XL)	12.5 mg daily, class III-IV 25 mg daily, class I-II	200 mg regardless of body weight
Bisoprolol (Zebeta)	Start at 2.5 mg daily	10 mg regardless of body weight

bid, twice daily.

BOX 26-1 β-BLOCKERS: CLASS SIDE EFFECTS

- **Most common:** tiredness and sleep disturbance (nightmares), cold hands and feet
- **Less common:** impotence, dizziness, wheezing, digestive tract problems, skin rashes, dry eyes

I is then converted to angiotensin II by ACE. Angiotensin II stimulates production of renin by the kidney.[17] Angiotensin II has a variety of effects that include direct vasoconstriction, increased sympathetic discharge, increased sodium reabsorption in the proximal tubule, the release of aldosterone, synthesis of extracellular matrix proteins in the heart, and increased expression of cardiac proto-oncogenes and growth factors. Additionally, it was noted that the beneficial effects of ACE inhibitors were due in part to their effects on bradykinin activation and subsequent nitric oxide release as ACE inhibitors block the breakdown of bradykinin. While the effects of activating the RAAS are beneficial during settings of acute blood loss or hemodynamic compromise, chronic activation augments cardiac afterload and increases adverse cardiac remodeling, and thus facilitates the progression of HF and feeds into a vicious cycle. There is a direct relationship between circulating levels of angiotensin II and mortality in patients with HF.[18] Two therapeutic modalities have proven useful in blunting the renin-angiotensin system: the ACE inhibitors and, more recently, the angiotensin II receptor antagonists.

The Captopril Multicenter Trial was the first major ACE inhibitor trial to show a benefit in patients with HF. In this trial, patients randomized to captopril demonstrated increased exercise tolerance and improved symptoms when compared with those randomized to placebo.[19] A subsequent trial, the Captopril-Digoxin Multicenter Study, found that captopril and digoxin were superior to placebo but indistinguishable from one another.[20] A large number of newer ACE inhibitors underwent clinical evaluation beginning in 1985, showing a significant mortality benefit (Table 26-3). Enalapril was shown to decrease mortality in patients with NYHA class IV HF in the Cooperative North Scandinavian Enalapril Survival Study (CONSENSUS).[21] The treatment arm of the Studies of Left Ventricular Dysfunction (SOLVD) trial[22] demonstrated a mortality benefit in less severe HF, while the SOLVD prevention arm demonstrated that the use of an ACE inhibitor could decrease hospitalizations and thus disease progression in a group of patients with decreased left ventricular function but without symptoms of HF.[23]

The Survival and Ventricular Enlargement (SAVE) study[24] and the Trandolapril Cardiac Evaluation (TRACE) study[25] demonstrated that the salutary benefits of ACE inhibition could also be seen in post–myocardial infarction (MI) patients with left ventricular dysfunction. Ramipril showed reduction in cardiovascular events, including cardiovascular death, stroke, and MI, in a group of patients with high cardiovascular risk but without systolic dysfunction in the Heart Outcomes Prevention Evaluation (HOPE) study.[26] In the EUROPA trial, perindopril demonstrated a reduction in cardiovascular risk in a low-risk population with stable coronary heart disease and no HF.[27]

Although ACE inhibitors are well tolerated in patients with HF, common side effects can include a dry cough (in 5% of patients) that usually develops after 1 week to 6 months of therapy (Box 26-2). Patients should also be counseled to avoid the use of nonsteroidal anti-inflammatory drugs in combination with ACE inhibitors as these can attenuate the favorable effects of the drug in addition to causing renal dysfunction and electrolyte imbalance.[28] An attempt should be made to titrate ACE inhibitors to doses that are comparable with those used in clinical trials, as a high-dose lisinopril group had fewer HF hospitalizations than a low-dose group in the ATLAS trial.[29]

ACE inhibitors relieve symptoms, improve NYHA functional class, and decrease the combined risk of death and hospitalization. Their major benefits include decreased ventricular remodeling and prolonged survival. Therefore, they are a class I recommendation for the treatment of all patients with asymptomatic or symptomatic HF[16] (Table 26-4).

Angiotensin II Receptor Blockers

Two types of angiotensin II receptors are known: angiotensin II type 1 (AT1) receptors and angiotensin II type 2 (AT2) receptors. It appears that the AT1 receptor mediates vasoconstriction, aldosterone secretion,

BOX 26-2 ACE INHIBITORS: CLASS SIDE EFFECTS

- **Most common:** cough, elevated potassium, low blood pressure, dizziness, headache, drowsiness, weakness, abnormal taste (metallic taste), and rash.
- The **most serious**, but rare, side effects of ACE inhibitors are kidney failure and allergic reactions (angioedema).
- ACE inhibitors are not prescribed for pregnant patients because they may cause birth defects.

ACE, angiotensin-converting enzyme.

TABLE 26-3 ACE INHIBITOR THERAPY IN HEART FAILURE

Study	Design	Results
CONSENSUS: Cooperative North Scandinavian Enalapril Survival Study	• 253 ischemic and nonischemic patients • NYHA class IV HF • **Enalapril** or placebo	• 27% reduction in all-cause mortality
SOLVD Treatment Trial: Studies of Left Ventricular Dysfunction	• 2569 patients • EF < 35% • **Enalapril** vs. placebo	• Lower all-cause death (16%) • Reduced HF hospitalization (26%)
SOLVD Prevention Trial: Studies of Left Ventricular Dysfunction	• 4228 ischemic and nonischemic patients • EF < 35% • **Enalapril** or placebo	• No effect on all-cause mortality • Lower HF hospitalizations (36%) • Lower combined risk of death and hospitalization (20%)
SAVE: Survival and Ventricular Enlargement Trial	• 231 recent MI patients • EF < 40% • Placebo or **captopril**	• Decreased all-cause mortality (19%) • Decreased risk of HF (22%)
TRACE: Trandolapril Cardiac Evaluation Study	• 1749 recent MI patients • EF < 35% • Placebo or **trandolapril**	• Decreased all-cause mortality (22%) and risk of HF (29%)

ACE, angiotensin-converting enzyme; EF, ejection fraction; HF, heart failure; MI, myocardial infarction; NYHA, New York Heart Association.

TABLE 26-4 ACE INHIBITORS

Drug	Initial Dose	Target Dose	Max Dose
Lisinopril (Prinivil or Zestril)	5 mg once daily	20 mg once daily	40 mg daily
Fosinopril sodium (Monopril)	10 mg once daily 5 mg if weak kidneys	40 mg once daily	
Enalapril maleate (Vasotec)	2.5 mg bid	20 mg bid	40 mg bid
Benazepril (Lotensin)	5 mg once daily on diuretic 10 mg once daily, no diuretic	40 mg/day: one 40-mg dose or two 20-mg doses	
Quinapril (Accupril)	5 mg bid 2.5 mg bid if weak kidneys	20 mg bid	
Ramipril (Altace)	1.25-2.5 mg bid	10 mg bid	

ACE, angiotensin-converting enzyme; bid, twice daily.

and vasopressin secretion. The AT2 receptor mediates antiproliferation effects, cell differentiation, tissue repair, and apoptosis. Therefore, it was hypothesized that selective blockade of the AT1 receptor might have benefits when compared to blockade of both receptors or of angiotensin II; the current blockers have greater than 1000-fold better affinity to AT1. While an AT1 receptor blocker (ARB) might not be as beneficial as an ACE inhibitor alone in the therapy of patients with HF, it was hypothesized that the combination of an ACE and an ARB might have added benefits. Based on these theoretical conclusions, a group of large-scale clinical trials were carried out to evaluate the beneficial effects of ARBs both as alternatives to ACE inhibitors and in combination with an ACE inhibitor (Table 26-5).

The Evaluation of Losartan in the Elderly II (ELITE II) study compared the effects of captopril with losartan in patients with HF.[30] Blocking the AT1 receptor was not superior to ACE inhibition; indeed, ACE inhibitors appeared to be somewhat superior to ARBs. The Val-HeFT[31] and the CHARM-Added[32] trials evaluated the effects of adding ARBs to an ACE inhibitor in patients with HF. In Val-HeFT, the addition of the ARB valsartan to the treatment of patients not receiving an ACE inhibitor resulted in a decrease in morbidity and mortality.[33] However, when valsartan was added to an ACE inhibitor, the addition of the ARB did not influence outcomes. In addition, patients receiving triple therapy with an ACE inhibitor, an ARB, and a β-blocker had an increased mortality. By contrast, in the CHARM-Added trial, there was a small but significant difference in the number of patients who either died or were hospitalized for HF in the group that received the ARB candesartan (38% of patients in the candesartan group had an event, whereas 42% of the patients in the placebo group experienced a primary outcome event).[34] Furthermore, the concomitant use of a β-blocker with an ACE inhibitor and candesartan did not appear to influence mortality as it had in Val-HeFT. However, both Val-HeFT and CHARM-Alternative[34] clearly demonstrated that ARBs could serve as an alternative for an ACE inhibitor. However, patients on an ARB were more likely to stop the drug for renal dysfunction, hyperkalemia, and hypotension compared with placebo in the Val-HeFT trial (Box 26-3). Furthermore, angioedema and renal dysfunction still occurred in some patients who had experienced them on an ACE inhibitor. The VALIANT trial compared the effects of the ARB valsartan, the ACE inhibitor captopril, and the combination of valsartan and captopril in patients with evidence of left ventricular dysfunction and HF following an MI.[35] Valsartan and captopril proved equivalent in their ability to influence mortality, while patients receiving both drugs had the most adverse events.

Taken together, the clinical trials data on ARBs suggest that they are a useful class of drugs in the treatment of patients with chronic HF and of high-risk post-MI patients (Table 26-6). Because ACE inhibitors are substantially lower in cost and because there is a much greater amount of experience with these drugs, they remain the drug of choice. The addition of an ARB to an ACE inhibitor is not recommended in post-MI patients; it may be considered in patients with chronic HF

BOX 26-3 ANGIOTENSIN II RECEPTOR BLOCKERS (ARBs): CLASS SIDE EFFECTS

- **Most common:** cough, elevated potassium levels, low blood pressure, dizziness, headache, drowsiness, diarrhea, abnormal taste sensation (metallic or salty taste), and rash.
- Compared to ACE inhibitors, cough occurs less often with ARBs.
- The **most serious**, but rare, side effects are kidney failure, liver failure, allergic reactions, a decrease in white blood cells, and angioedema.
- ARBs are not prescribed for pregnant patients because they may cause birth defects.

ACE, angiotensin-converting enzyme.

TABLE 26-5 ANGIOTENSIN II RECEPTOR BLOCKER THERAPY IN HEART FAILURE

Study	Design	Results
Val-HeFT: Valsartan in Heart Failure Trial	• 5010 patients • NYHA class II-IV HF • EF < 40% • On background therapy* • **Valsartan** or placebo	• 13.3% decrease in combined morbidity and mortality • Fewer HF hospitalizations
CHARM-Alternative: Candesartan in Heart Failure: Assessment of Reduction in Mortality and Morbidity	• 2028 patients • EF < 41% • ACE intolerance • **Candesartan** vs. placebo	• 23% relative risk reduction in HF deaths and hospitalization
CHARM-Added	• 2500 patients • EF < 41% • On ACE inhibitors • **Candesartan** added	• 15% relative risk reduction of heart failure death or HF hospitalization
CHARM-Preserved	• 3023 patients • EF > 40% • **Candesartan** vs. placebo	• No difference in risk of heart-related death • Fewer hospitalized for HF

*Background therapy: diuretics, digoxin, ACE inhibitor.
ACE, angiotensin-converting enzyme; EF, ejection fraction; HF, heart failure; NYHA, New York Heart Association.

TABLE 26-6 ANGIOTENSIN II RECEPTOR BLOCKERS IN HEART FAILURE

Drug	Initial Dose	Target Dose
Losartan (Cozaar)	25 mg bid or 50 mg daily 12.5 mg bid or 25 mg daily if weak liver function	50 mg bid
Candesartan (Atacand)	4-8 mg once daily	32 mg daily
Valsartan (Diovan)	80 mg once daily	160 mg daily 80 mg once daily if weak liver function
Ibesartan (Avapro)	150 mg once daily	300 mg daily

bid, twice daily.

TABLE 26-7 ALDOSTERONE RECEPTOR BLOCKER THERAPY IN HEART FAILURE

Study	Design	Results
RALES: Randomized Aldactone Evaluation Study[38]	• NYHA class III-IV HF • EF < 35% • On ACE inhibitor • **Aldactone** vs. placebo	• 30% relative reduction in risk of all-cause death and HF hospitalization
EPHESUS: Eplerenone Post AMI Heart Failure Efficacy and Survival[40]	• 6632 post-MI patients • NYHA class III-IV • EF < 40% • Standard drug therapy* *plus* • **Eplerenone** or placebo	• 15% fewer overall deaths • 21% fewer sudden cardiac deaths • 15% decrease in hospitalizations for HF
REMODEL study (Pfizer A6141078)	• 210 patients • EF < 35% • NYHA class II-III • **Eplerenone** vs. placebo	• Results of study are pending

*Standard/background therapy: diuretics, digoxin, ACE inhibitor.
ACE, angiotensin-converting enzyme; EF, ejection fraction; HF, heart failure; MI, myocardial infarction; NYHA, New York Heart Association.

who continue to be symptomatic on appropriate doses of ACE inhibitors and β-blockers or who have uncontrolled hypertension.

ARBs have hemodynamic actions similar to ACE inhibitors, but they have not been shown to be more effective. They lower blood pressure, improve exercise capacity, and lower norepinephrine levels. Based on the previously mentioned trials, the ARB candesartan has been approved to be added to ACE inhibitor therapy for treating NYHA class II-IV HF patients with an ejection fraction of less than 40%. They are also recommended as an alternative for patients who are ACE inhibitor intolerant. The addition of an ARB to conventional therapy (ACE inhibitors, β-blockers, diuretics as needed, and digoxin) in patients who are persistently symptomatic with reduced left ventricular ejection fraction (LVEF) is also recommended.[16] However, it is not clear whether an aldosterone inhibitor should be added before or after the addition of an ARB, and there are potential adverse consequences of treating HF patients with four neurohormonal blockers (ACE inhibitors, β-blockers, aldosterone antagonists, and ARBs) concomitantly.

Aldosterone Receptor Blockers

Aldosterone is produced by the adrenal glands through both renin-angiotensin and potassium signaling. Aldosterone acts through mineralocorticoid receptors and has two mechanisms of action: it increases the transcription of target genes via intracellular receptors and effects rapid changes in second-messenger signaling. Raised levels of aldosterone effect changes in salt and water retention, vasoconstriction, and up-regulation of inflammatory mediators resulting in cytokine production and myocyte necrosis; increased levels also stimulate the growth of fibroblasts and the synthesis of collagen and increase the aggregation and activation of platelets.[36] Elevations of aldosterone are associated with an increased mortality in patients with HF.[37] In view of the prognostic role of aldosterone levels in patients with HF and the finding that it activates pathways associated with maladaptive remodeling in the heart and HF disease progression, investigators hypothesized that aldosterone antagonists might have a beneficial effect in patients with HF. This hypothesis was strengthened by the finding that ACE inhibitors did not adequately suppress levels of aldosterone in patients with HF.

In the late 1950s, spironolactone, an aldosterone receptor competitive antagonist was first developed for the treatment of hypertension. This drug was first evaluated in a large multicenter clinical trial called the RALES trial.[38] Spironolactone increased the probability of survival, with a 30% reduction in the primary end point of all-cause mortality over a mean follow-up of 24 months (Table 26-7). All patients were receiving concomitant therapy with an ACE inhibitor and a loop diuretic. Patients with serum creatinine concentrations of more than 2.5 mg/dl or a serum potassium concentration of more than 5.0 mmol/L were excluded from the study. The major side effect of spironolactone, gynecomastia, was reported in 10% of the study patients. Unfortunately, only 10% of the patients in the RALES trial were receiving a β-blocker. Thus, it was not clear whether spironolactone would have benefited patients receiving β-blocker therapy.

TABLE 26-8 ALDOSTERONE RECEPTOR BLOCKERS

Drug	Initial Dose	Target Dose
Spironolactone (Aldactone)	25 mg once daily	25 mg once daily
Eplerenone (Inspra)	25 mg once daily	50 mg once daily

BOX 26-4 ALDOSTERONE RECEPTOR BLOCKERS: CLASS SIDE EFFECTS

- **Most common:** elevated potassium levels, breast tissue growth (gynecomastia) in males (spironolactone)
- **Less common:** headache, dizziness, diarrhea, stomach pain, nausea

Eplerenone, a selective aldosterone receptor antagonist, was developed in order to obviate the effect of gynecomastia. Eplerenone had 1000-fold less binding to the androgen receptor and 100-fold less binding to the progesterone receptor while having only a mild reduction in binding to the mineralocorticoid receptor.[39] In the Eplerenone Post-Acute Myocardial Infarction Survival and Efficacy Study (EPHESUS),[40] 6632 patients with an ejection fraction of less than 40% were randomized to placebo or eplerenone following an acute MI. Eplerenone was associated with a 15% reduction in all-cause mortality and a 13% reduction in death or hospitalization for cardiovascular causes. There was also a significant reduction in the rate of sudden death from cardiac causes. However, severe hyperkalemia was increased in the eplerenone group.

Based on these studies, aldosterone receptor blockers are among the class I recommendations for NYHA class III-IV patients[16] (Table 26-8). Patients must be monitored for potassium increase and renal function (Box 26-4). Many clinicians now recommend low-dose spironolactone (25 mg/day) in patients with recent or current symptoms of HF at rest despite the use of ACE inhibitors, diuretics, digoxin, and a β-blocker.[16] Eplerenone, in contrast, has been recommended for use in patients with left ventricular systolic dysfunction and evidence of HF following an MI.[41] Overuse of spironolactone has been associated with hyperkalemia as well as with hyperkalemia-associated increases in morbidity and mortality.[42] The role of aldosterone antagonism and specifically of eplerenone is presently being evaluated in a multicenter randomized and controlled trial of patients with NYHA class II-III heart failure called the REMODEL trial. The results of this study may impact our use of both eplerenone and aldosterone antagonists in general.

Digoxin

Digitalis is the oldest agent that continues to be used in current clinical practice in cardiology. Despite its history, the role of digoxin in the treatment of HF remains controversial (Box 26-5). Digoxin works by inhibiting sodium/potassium ATPase, which leads to an increase in intracellular sodium-calcium exchange resulting in increased intracellular calcium and leading to increased contractility. Despite the controversy surrounding the benefit of digoxin, it is commonly used, in part because it is easy to use in combination with other HF therapies and it is inexpensive.

PROVED was a placebo-controlled digoxin withdrawal study. This study enrolled patients in sinus rhythm with reduced systolic left ventricular function and stable HF symptoms who were receiving digoxin and diuretics (Table 26-9). The digoxin group had lower incidences of worsening HF and hospitalization for HF. This group also had lower blood urea nitrogen and creatinine levels, a higher LVEF, and a better exercise capacity. Patients in whom digoxin was discontinued had a twofold increase in worsening HF and a decrease in both exercise capacity and LVEF.[43] The RADIANCE trial evaluated patients with NYHA class II-III heart failure and LVEFs of 35% or less in normal sinus rhythm who were clinically stable and revealed that digoxin discontinuation was associated with a sixfold increase in worsening HF.[44]

A collective analysis of the RADIANCE and PROVED trials suggested that triple therapy with digoxin, an ACE inhibitor, and a diuretic was associated with the lowest risk of worsening HF. The rate of progression of HF was 19% among patients treated with digoxin and diuretics, 25% in those treated with ACE inhibitors and diuretics, and 39% among patients receiving diuretics alone. Use of digoxin therapy in patients with stable HF would result in a significant net annual savings.[45,46] In the DIG trial, patients with LVEFs of 45% or less were randomly assigned to digoxin or placebo, in addition to diuretics and ACE inhibitors. Digoxin had no effect on total mortality rates, but reduced the overall number of hospitalizations or deaths caused by worsening HF.[47]

BOX 26-5 DIGOXIN SIDE EFFECTS

- **Most common:** nausea, vomiting, heart rhythm disturbances, kidney dysfunction, and electrolyte abnormalities.
- These side effects are generally a result of elevated blood levels.

TABLE 26-9 DIGOXIN THERAPY IN HEART FAILURE

Study	Design	Results
PROVED	• 88 stable HF patients • NSR • 12 wk • Digoxin & diuretics	Digoxin discontinuation → • Worsening HF • Decreased exercise capacity • Decreased EF
RADIANCE	• 178 stable HF patients • NSR • Digoxin, diuretics, & ACEI • 12 wk	Digoxin discontinuation → • Worsening HF
DIG—main	• 6800 HF patients • EF < 45% • Digoxin vs. placebo • On ACEI & diuretics	Digoxin • No effect on mortality • Reduced HF hospitalization • Reduced HF death

ACEI, angiotensin-converting enzyme inhibitor; EF, ejection fraction; HF, heart failure; NSR, normal sinus rhythm.

Diuretics

Although there have been no large randomized trials to evaluate the effects of diuretics on morbidity and mortality, they remain a potent option in the management of the volume overload symptoms of HF.[16] These drugs decrease preload and are usually associated with symptomatic improvement. The dose of diuretics in patients with chronic HF is highly individualized. The removal of edema and congestion in response to diuretics should take place gradually, because rapid mobilization of extravascular fluid may result in significant metabolic abnormalities that may worsen the HF state, such as contraction alkalosis, hyponatremia, hypokalemia, increased blood urea nitrogen and creatinine, and hypomagnesemia. Once fluid retention has resolved, treatment with diuretics should be maintained to prevent recurrent edema, which may require frequent adjustments to the dose given.[48]

Potential side effects of diuretics include dehydration, electrolyte abnormalities (particularly low potassium levels), hearing disturbances, and low blood pressure. It is important for patients to prevent low potassium levels by taking supplements, when appropriate. Such electrolyte disturbances may make patients susceptible to serious heart rhythm disturbances.

Vasodilators

Vasodilators decrease preload and afterload by dilating both arterial and venous blood vessels. Vasodilators have been shown to slow ventricular remodeling and HF progression. In the Veterans Administration Heart Failure Trial I (V-HEFT-I),[49] HF patients on digoxin and diuretics were shown to have a mortality benefit from adding the combination of hydralazine plus isosorbide dinitrate versus placebo (Table 26-10). In V-HEFT-II,[50] the hydralazine–isosorbide dinitrate combination was compared to enalapril. The enalapril arm showed a larger reduction in mortality. In the African-American Heart Failure Trial (A-HEFT),[51] patients with NYHA class III-IV HF who identified themselves as black (of African descent) were randomized to either

TABLE 26-10 VASODILATOR THERAPY IN HEART FAILURE

Study	Design	Results
V-HEFT-I: Veterans Administration Heart Failure Trial I	• 642 males with HF • All on digoxin and diuretics • Placebo vs. prazosin vs. combined **hydralazine/isosorbide dinitrate**	• No effect with prazosin or placebo • Lower 2-year mortality in hydralazine/isosorbide dinitrate
V-HEFT-II: Veterans Administration Heart Failure Trial II	• 804 men • NYHA class II-III HF • **Enalapril** vs. hydralazine/isosorbide	• 28% decrease in mortality • Mortality benefit due to decrease in sudden death
A-HEFT: African-American Heart Failure Trial	• 1050 patients • NYHA class III-IV • Placebo vs. **isosorbide dinitrate** (20-40 mg tid) plus **hydralazine** (37.5-75 mg tid)	• Lower mortality (6.2% vs. 10.2%)

HF, heart failure; NYHA, New York Heart Association; tid, three times daily.

placebo or a fixed-dose combination of isosorbide dinitrate plus hydralazine. The trial was terminated early because of a significantly lower mortality rate in the nitrate plus hydralazine arm, with a lower rate of first hospitalizations for HF and greater improvement in quality of life.

The 2005 American College of Cardiology (ACC)/American Heart Association (AHA) guidelines made no reference to race, and suggested that hydralazine and a nitrate might be added in patients with persistent HF symptoms on an ACE inhibitor and β-blocker, or those who cannot tolerate an ACE inhibitor or ARB[16] (Box 26-6 and Table 26-11).

Inotropes

Increasing cardiac contractility has long been considered an attractive therapeutic goal in HF. Although inotropic agents may improve hemodynamic parameters and relieve symptoms, their acute, intermittent, and continuous administration has been associated with increased mortality in a variety of trials.[52,53] Nonetheless, inotropes can play an important role in the care of patients with acute class IV symptoms or in those who require palliation for symptoms that cannot be alleviated by routine pharmacologic therapy. Approximately 14% of the patients in ADHERE were treated with ≥1 acute infusions of inotropic agents (dobutamine 6%, dopamine 6%, and milrinone 3%) in the hospital.[54]

Milrinone. Milrinone is a cyclic AMP–specific phosphodiesterase (PDE) inhibitor that can produce both positive inotropic effects and vasodilation independent of β_1-adrenergic receptor stimulation in the cardiovascular system. Milrinone was approved for short-term intravenous use in the late 1980s. The use of oral milrinone as a continuous treatment has been shown to increase mortality,[55] but its intravenous use has been studied in a few randomized controlled trials.

Anderson and colleagues studied the effects of short-term use of intravenous milrinone and found that it provided symptomatic relief compared with placebo. However, there was also a tendency toward increased ventricular arrhythmias associated with the use of milrinone.[56,57] The OPTIME-CHF[52] investigators randomized patients admitted with an exacerbation of systolic HF with NYHA class III-IV and an LVEF less than 0.40 to study the effect of short-term milrinone infusion (Table 26-12). The study concluded that there were no significant differences between the treatment and placebo groups for the number of days hospitalized within the 60-day period, the number of rehospitalizations, the length of initial stay, in-hospital mortality, or 60-day mortality. There were more incidents of sustained hypotension, atrial fibrillation, atrial flutter, ventricular tachycardia, and ventricular fibrillation in the treatment group.

Despite the increased risk of arrhythmias (Box 26-7), milrinone has improved the functional capacity and a sense of well-being in end-stage heart failure patients. Moreover, it has been instrumental in patients awaiting orthotropic heart transplantation. The homodynamic effects of PDEs have been shown to be unaffected and possibly enhanced in patients on concurrent β-blocker therapy.[60]

Dobutamine. Dobutamine is a direct-acting inotropic agent whose primary activity results from stimulation of the β_1 receptors of the heart, producing chronotropic and mild vasodilator effects (Box 26-8). The clinical trials in the field of inotropes are not many and overall did not show any mortality benefit. The DICE trial found no improvement in functional status and a nonsignificant trend toward decreased hospitalization[61] (Table 26-13). A meta-analysis by Thackray and colleagues calculated an odds ratio of 1.5 (95% confidence interval, 0.51 to 3.92) for all-cause mortality in the dobutamine group compared with the control group.[53]

Calcium Sensitizers

Calcium sensitizers enhance myocardial response to a given concentration of calcium without increasing the actual concentration.[67] Several compounds have been identified that increase the sensitivity of the myocardial contractile apparatus to calcium, causing an increase in tension development and myocardial contractility.

Administration of pimobendan to patients with HF resulted in increases in stroke volume and cardiac index and reductions in left ventricular end-diastolic pressure, systemic vascular resistance, and mean arterial pressure.[68] In two randomized, placebo-controlled trials

BOX 26-6 VASODILATORS: CLASS SIDE EFFECTS

- **Most common:** dizziness, drowsiness, light-headedness, headache, constipation, loss of appetite

TABLE 26-11 VASODILATORS

Drug	Initial Dose	Target Dose
Isosorbide dinitrate	20 mg tid	20-40 mg tid
Hydralazine	37.5 mg tid	37.5-75 mg tid

tid, three times daily.

BOX 26-7 MILRINONE SIDE EFFECTS

- **Most common:** headache, chest pain, slight fever, increased risk of arrhythmias

BOX 26-8 DOBUTAMINE SIDE EFFECTS

- **Most common:** headache, nausea or vomiting, restlessness, muscle cramps or weakness, chest pain, dizziness, palpitations, rash

TABLE 26-12 MILRINONE THERAPY IN HEART FAILURE

OPTIME-CHF Investigators	Design	Results
Felker et al.[53]	• 951 patients • 2 mo • 48-72 hr at 0.5 mcg/kg/min	• Ischemic heart disease • Worse outcomes for death and hospitalization
Cuffe et al.[59]	• 951 patients • 2 mo • 48 hr at 0.5 mcg/kg/min	• No significant difference in hospital stay or 60-day mortality
Seino et al.[60]	• 52 patients • 50 mcg/kg loading dose • 6 hr at 0.5 mcg/kg/min	• Decreased PAOP, RAP • Increased SV • 16% ventricular arrhythmias
Anderson et al.[57]	• 31 patients • 50 mcg/kg loading dose • 1 hr at 0.5 mcg/kg/min	• Increased CI, SV • Decreased PCWP, SVR, MAP

CI, cardiac index; MAP, mean arterial pressure; PAOP, pulmonary artery occlusion pressure; PCWP, pulmonary capillary wedge pressure; RAP, right atrial pressure; SV, stroke volume; SVR, systemic vascular resistance.

TABLE 26-13 DOBUTAMINE THERAPY IN HEART FAILURE

DICE Trial Investigators	Design	Results
Oliva et al.[62]	• 38 patients • F/U 8 wk: CI • F/U 6 mo: other outcomes • Infusion: 48 hr/wk for 6 mo	• No significant increase in mortality
Elis et al.[63]	• 119 patients • F/U until death • Infusion: 24 hr/2 wk for 6 wk, then 24 hr/3 wk for 6 mo	• No difference in number of hospitalizations or survival
Adamopoulos et al.[64]	• 20 patients • F/U 6 wk • Infusion: to raise HR to 70%-80% max. for 30 min/day × 4 days/wk for 3 wk	• No significant arrhythmias
Erlemeier et al.[65]	• 20 patients • F/U 3 days • Infusion: 24 hr/8 days over 4 wk with at least 3 days in between	• No difference in mortality
Dies et al.[66]	• 60 patients • F/U 8 wk • Infusion: 48 hr/wk for 24 wk	• Substantial increase in mortality
Leier et al.[67]	• 26 patients • F/U 24 wk • Infusion: 4 hr/wk for 24 wk	• No significant change in CI or EF

CI, cardiac index; EF, ejection fraction; F/U, follow-up; HR, heart rate.

TABLE 26-14 CALCIUM CHANNEL BLOCKER THERAPY IN HEART FAILURE

Study	Design	Results
PRAISE I: Prospective Randomized Amlodipine Survival Evaluation	• 1153 patients • NYHA class III-IV HF • EF < 30% • **Amlodipine** vs. placebo • On background therapy*	• Nonsignificant 16% reduction in all-cause mortality • Less hypertension and angina symptoms • Survival benefit in patients with NICM
PRAISE II	• 1650 patients • Nonischemic • **Amlodipine** vs. placebo	• No mortality benefit • No improvement in quality of life, or NYHA functional class

*Background therapy: diuretics, digoxin, ACE inhibitor.
ACE, angiotensin-converting enzyme; EF, ejection fraction; HF, heart failure; NICM, nonischemic cardiomyopathy; NYHA, New York Heart Association.

of patients treated with digoxin, diuretics, and ACE inhibitors, short-term administration of oral pimobendan resulted in improvements in exercise duration and quality of life.[69] The long-term safety and efficacy of this drug are not known.

Levosimendan works via a dual mechanism of action, which enhances cardiac contractility and vasodilation without affecting intracellular free calcium, and so should have reduced proarrhythmic potential. It can be administered intravenously, which makes it a therapeutic option for acute decompensated congestive HF. Several studies have evaluated the efficacy of levosimendan in patients with HF.[70,71] The LIDO trial compared the short-term hemodynamic effects of a 24-hour intravenous infusion of levosimendan with dobutamine in 203 patients with severe, deteriorating HF, acute HF, or HF after coronary artery bypass grafting.[72] The hemodynamic end point (35% increase in cardiac index and 25% reduction in pulmonary capillary wedge pressure at 24 hours) was more frequently achieved with levosimendan than dobutamine (28% vs. 15%). The long-term effects of levosimendan are less well established, but a benefit has been suggested.

Several studies are ongoing that will further define the short- and long-term impact of levosimendan therapy. Levosimendan currently remains investigational in the United States.[73]

Calcium Channel Blockers

Calcium channel blockers reduce peripheral vasoconstriction and thereby reduce left ventricular afterload; they therefore might be expected to benefit HF patients with systolic dysfunction. However, these agents also have negative inotropic activity, and several studies demonstrated clinical deterioration in patients treated with nifedipine and diltiazem. As a result, these drugs have generally been avoided in patients with systolic HF, even for the treatment of coexisting angina or hypertension.[74] The second-generation calcium channel blockers amlodipine and felodipine have little or no negative inotropic activity at the usual therapeutic doses, and may be better tolerated than the other calcium channel blockers for hypertension and angina treatment in patients with HF.[75] The Prospective Randomized Amlodipine Survival Evaluation (PRAISE) trial[76] established the safety profile of amlodipine for the treatment of patients with left ventricular dysfunction with a history of angina or hypertension, but the mortality benefit it showed for patients with nonischemic cardiomyopathy was disproved in the PRAISE II trial.[77] In PRAISE II, no difference in mortality was observed, and no benefit in exercise tolerance, quality of life, or NYHA class was demonstrated (Box 26-9 and Table 26-14).

The lack of benefit of calcium channel blockers in patients with HF was confirmed by the results of these studies in addition to other trials

BOX 26-9 CALCIUM CHANNEL BLOCKERS: CLASS SIDE EFFECTS

- **Most common:** headache, edema of the lower extremities
- **Less common:** dizziness, flushing, fatigue, nausea, palpitations

with different calcium channel blockers. These agents do not improve exercise tolerance, quality of life, or survival.[78] Therefore, the use of calcium channel blockers in patients with HF was not recommended by the ACC/AHA.[16] Amlodipine and felodipine are safe and well tolerated in patients with HF and can be used for the treatment of hypertension or angina.[16] Nevertheless, ACE inhibitors and β-blockers should be given first in patients with hypertension.

Anticoagulation

Patients with HF are at risk for thrombosis and thromboemboli secondary to stasis in the dilated hypokinetic left ventricle. There are no controlled trials of warfarin or other antithrombotic agents in patients with HF. However, the ACC/AHA task force recommends warfarin therapy in patients with HF who have experienced a previous embolic event or who have paroxysmal or chronic atrial fibrillation or atrial flutter.[16] It is not clear how anticoagulants should be prescribed in patients with HF who do not have these indications. Warfarin therapy may be of benefit in selected stable patients in sinus rhythm with an LVEF below 35% and in those with evidence of a left ventricular thrombus. Possible side effects of anticoagulation are bleeding and necrosis (gangrene) of the skin. Bleeding can occur in any organ or tissue.

SUMMARY

Patients with congestive HF tend to have extremely poor quality of life and a prognostic outlook that is comparable to many forms of cancer.[79] Repetitive hospitalizations are a major health problem in this population, with noncompliance being the main reason for hospitalizations. Evidence-based therapy of HF improves symptoms and mortality, yet many HF patients are not receiving optimum medical therapy. This has led to an increasing interest in the role of multidisciplinary programs that optimize the management of HF patients and push for better compliance, in addition to tailoring clinically proven regimens for all HF patients. Mechanical devices that resynchronize the damaged ventricle to create a more forceful contractile force, along with devices that may temporarily take over the pumping function of the heart, are all a part of the complex treatment algorithm required to manage the advanced chronic HF patient. In spite of all therapeutic interventions, the pool of HF patients continues to grow. Unfortunately, all pharmacologic measures and device interventions that currently exist are not capable of halting this process, but they can help alleviate symptoms to some extent.

REFERENCES

1. American Heart Association. Heart Disease and Stroke Statistics: 2004 Update. Dallas: American Heart Association, 2004.
2. Ho KK, Pinsky JL, Kannel WB, Levy D. The epidemiology of heart failure: the Framingham Study. J Am Coll Cardiol 1993;22:6A.
3. Sackner-Bernstein JD, Mancini DM. Rationale for treatment of patients with chronic heart failure with adrenergic blockade. JAMA 1995;274:1462.
4. Bristow MR. β-Adrenergic receptor blockade in chronic heart failure. Circulation 2000;101:558.
5. Swedberg K, Waagstein F, Hjalmarson A, Wallentin I. Prolongation of survival in congestive cardiomyopathy by beta receptor blockade. Lancet 1979;1:1374.
6. Colucci WS, Packer M, Bristow MR, et al. US Carvedilol Heart Failure Study. Circulation 1996;94:2800-2806.
7. The CIBIS II Scientific Committee. Design of the Cardiac Insufficiency Bisoprolol Study II (CIBIS II). Fundam Clin Pharmacol 1997;11:138-142.
8. MERIT-HF Study Group. Effect of metoprolol CR/XL in chronic heart failure: Metoprolol CR/XL Randomized Intervention Trial in Congestive Heart Failure (MERIT-HF). Lancet 1999;353:2001-2009.
9. Packer M, Coats AJ, Fowler MB. Effect of carvedilol on survival in severe chronic heart failure. N Engl J Med 2001;344:1651-1658.
10. Poole-Wilson PA, Swedberg K, Cleland JG. Comparison of carvedilol and metoprolol on clinical outcomes in patients with chronic heart failure in the Carvedilol Or Metoprolol European Trial (COMET): randomized controlled trial. Lancet 2003;362:7-13.
11. Waagstein F. Beneficial effects of metoprolol in idiopathic dilated cardiomyopathy. Metoprolol in Dilated Cardiomyopathy (MDC) Trial Study Group. Lancet 1993;342:1441-1449.
12. Willenheimer R, Erdmann E, Follath F. Comparison of treatment initiation with bisoprolol vs. enalapril in chronic heart failure patients: rationale and design of CIBIS III. Eur J Heart Fail 2004;6:493-500.
13. Lowes BD, Gilbert EM, Abraham WT, et al. Myocardial gene expression in dilated cardiomyopathy treated with beta-blocking agents. N Engl J Med 2002;46:1357-1365.
14. Ventura-Clapier R, Garnier A, Veksler V. Energy metabolism in heart failure. J Physiol (Lond) 2003:555:1-13.
15. Liggett SB. β_2-Adrenergic receptor pharmacogenetics. Am J Respir Crit Care Med 2000;161:197-201.
16. Hunt SA, Baker DW, Chin MH, et al. ACC/AHA guidelines for the evaluation and management of chronic heart failure in the adult: executive summary. A report of the American College of Cardiology/American Heart Association Task Force on Practice Guidelines (Committee to Revise the 1995 Guidelines for the Evaluation and Management of Heart Failure). Circulation 2001;104:2996-3007.
17. Brunton L, Lazo J, Parker K (eds). Goodman & Gilman's The Pharmacological Basis of Therapeutics, 11th ed. New York: McGraw-Hill, 2006.
18. Lee AF, MacFadyen RJ, Struthers AD. Neurohormonal reactivation in heart failure patients on chronic ACE inhibitor therapy: a longitudinal study. Eur J Heart Fail 1999;1:401-406.
19. A placebo-controlled trial of captopril in refractory chronic congestive heart failure. Captopril Multicenter Research Group. J Am Coll Cardiol 1983;2:755-763.
20. Comparative effects of therapy with captopril and digoxin in patients with mild to moderate heart failure. The Captopril-Digoxin Multicenter Research Group. JAMA 1988;259:539.
21. The CONSENSUS Trial Study Group. Effects of enalapril on survival in patients with reduced left ventricular ejection fractions and congestive heart failure. N Engl J Med 1987;316:1429-1435.
22. The SOLVD Investigators. Effect of enalapril on survival in patients with reduced left ventricular ejection fractions and congestive heart failure. N Engl J Med 1991;325:293-302.
23. The SOLVD Investigators. Effect of enalapril on mortality and the development of heart failure in asymptomatic patients with reduced left ventricular ejection fractions. N Engl J Med 1992;327:685-691.
24. Pfeffer MA, Braunwald E, Moye LA. Effect of captopril on mortality and morbidity in patients with left ventricular dysfunction after myocardial infarction: results of the Survival And Ventricular Enlargement Trial. The SAVE investigators. N Engl J Med 1992;327:669-677.
25. Rober L, Torp-Pedersen C, Carlesen JE. A clinical trial of the angiotensin-converting enzyme inhibitor trandolapril in patients with left ventricular dysfunction after myocardial infarction. Trandolapril Cardiac Evaluation (TRACE) Study group. N Engl J Med 1995;333:1670-1676.
26. Yusuf S, Sleight P, Pogue J, et al. Effects of an angiotensin-converting enzyme inhibitor, ramipril, on cardiovascular events in high-risk patients. The Heart Outcomes Prevention Evaluation Study Investigators. N Engl J Med 2000;342:145-153.
27. Efficacy of perindopril in reduction of cardiovascular events among patients with stable coronary artery disease: randomised, double-blind, placebo-controlled, multicentre trial (the EUROPA study). The EURopean trial On reduction of cardiac events with Perindopril in stable coronary Artery disease Investigators. Lancet 2003;362:782-788.
28. Packer M. Adaptive and maladaptive actions of angiotensin II in patients with severe congestive heart failure. Am J Kidney Dis 1987;10:66-73.
29. Schwartz JS, Wang YR, Cleland JGF, et al. for the ATLAS Study Group. High-versus low-dose angiotensin converting enzyme inhibitor therapy in the treatment of heart failure: an economic analysis of the Assessment of Treatment with Lisinopril And Survival (ATLAS) Trial. Am J Manag Care 2003;9:417-424.
30. Pitt B, Poole-Wilson PA, Segal R, et al. for the ELITE II Investigators. Effect of losartan compared with captopril on mortality in patients with symptomatic heart failure: randomised trial—the Losartan Heart Failure Survival Study ELITE II. Lancet 2000;355:1582-1587.
31. Maggioni AP, Anand I, Gottlieb SO, et al. Effects of valsartan on morbidity and mortality in patients with heart failure not receiving angiotensin-converting enzyme inhibitors. J Am Coll Cardiol 2002;40:1414-1421.
32. McMurray JJ, Ostergren J, Swedberg K. Effects of candesartan in patients with chronic heart failure and reduced left-ventricular systolic function taking angiotensin-converting enzyme inhibitors: the CHARM-Added trial. Lancet 2003;362:767-771.
33. Cohn JN, Tognoni G, for the Valsartan Heart Failure Trial Investigators. Randomized trial of the angiotensin-receptor blocker valsartan in chronic heart failure. N Engl J Med 2001;345:1667-1675.
34. Granger CB, McMurray JJ, Yusuf S, et al. for the CHARM Investigators and Committees. Effects of candesartan in patients with chronic heart failure and reduced left-ventricular systolic function intolerant to angiotensin-converting enzyme inhibitors: the CHARM-Alternative trial. Lancet 2003;362:772-776.
35. Velazquez EJ, Pfeffer MA, McMurray JV, et al. VALsartan In Acute myocardial iNfarcTion (VALIANT) trial: baseline characteristics in context. Eur J Heart Fail 2003;5:537-544.
36. Bozkurt B. Aldosterone antagonism in the pharmacologic management of chronic heart failure. *In* Feldman AM (ed): Heart Failure: Pharmacologic Management. New York: Wiley-Blackwell, 2006.
37. Swedberg K, Eneroth P, Kjekshus J, Wilhelmsen L. Hormones regulating cardiovascular function in patients with severe congestive heart failure and their relation to mortality. CONSENSUS Trial Study Group. Circulation 1990;82:1730-1736.
38. Pitt B, Zannad F, Remme WJ. The effect of spironolactone on morbidity and mortality in patients with severe heart failure. Randomized Aldactone Evaluation Study Investigators. N Engl J Med 1999;341:709-717.
39. de Gasparo M, Joss U, Ramjoue HP, et al. Three new epoxy-spirolactone derivatives: characterization in vivo and in vitro. J Pharmacol Exp Ther 1987;240:650-656.
40. Pitt B, Remme WJ, Zannad F. Eplerenone, a selective aldosterone blocker, in patients with left ventricular dysfunction after myocardial infarction. N Engl J Med 2003; 348:1309-1321.

41. Antman EM, Anbe DI, Armstrong PW, et al. Management of patients with STEMI: ACC/AHA guidelines for the management of patients with ST-Elevation Myocardial Infarction—executive summary. A report of the American College of Cardiology/ American Heart Association Task Force on Practice Guidelines (Writing Committee to Revise the 1999 guidelines for the management of patients with acute myocardial infarction). J Am Coll Cardiol 2004;44:671-719.
42. Juurlink DN, Mamdani MM, Lee DS, et al. Rates of hyperkalemia after publication of the Randomized Aldactone Evaluation Study. N Engl J Med 2004;351:543-551.
43. Uretsky BF, Young JB, Shahidi FE, et al. Randomized study assessing the effect of digoxin withdrawal in patients with mild to moderate chronic congestive heart failure: results of the PROVED trial. PROVED Investigative Group. J Am Coll Cardiol 1993;22:955-962.
44. Packer M, Gheorghiade M, Young JB, et al. for the RADIANCE Study. Withdrawal of digoxin from patients with chronic heart failure treated with angiotensin-converting enzyme inhibitors: RADIANCE Study. N Engl J Med 1993;329:1-7.
45. Young JB, Gheorghiade M, Uretsky BF, et al. Superiority of "triple" drug therapy in heart failure: insights from the PROVED and RADIANCE trials. Prospective Randomized Study of Ventricular Function and Efficacy of Digoxin, Randomized Assessment of Digoxin and Inhibitors of Angiotensin-Converting Enzyme. J Am Coll Cardiol 1998;32:686-692.
46. Ward RE, Gheorghiade M, Young JB, Uretsky B. Economic outcomes of withdrawal of digoxin therapy in adult patients with stable congestive heart failure. J Am Coll Cardiol 1995;26:93-101.
47. Digitalis Investigation Group. The effect of digoxin on mortality and morbidity in patients with heart failure: the Digitalis Investigation Group. N Engl J Med 1997;336: 525-533.
48. Gheorghiade M, Cody RJ, Francis GS, et al. Current medical therapy for advanced heart failure. Am Heart J 1998;135;S231-S248.
49. Cohn JN, Archibald DG, Ziesche S, et al. Effect of vasodilator therapy on mortality in chronic congestive heart failure: results of a Veterans Administration Cooperative Study. N Engl J Med 1986;314:1547.
50. Cohn JN, Johnson G, Ziesche S, et al. A comparison of enalapril with hydralazine-isosorbide dinitrate in the treatment of chronic congestive heart failure: Vasodilator-Heart Failure Trial II. N Engl J Med 1991;325:303-310.
51. Taylor AL, Ziesche S, Yancy C, et al. Combination of isosorbide dinitrate and hydralazine in blacks with heart failure. N Engl J Med 2004;351:2049.
52. Felker GM, Benza RL, Chandler AB, et al. Heart failure etiology and response to milrinone in decompensated heart failure: results from the OPTIME-CHF study. J Am Coll Cardiol 2003;41:997-1003.
53. Thackray S, Easthaugh J, Freemantle N, Cleland JG. The effectiveness and relative effectiveness of intravenous inotropic drugs acting through the adrenergic pathway in patients with heart failure: a meta-regression analysis. Eur J Heart Fail 2002;4:515-529.
57. ADHERE Scientific Advisory Committee, Study Group, and Investigators, Fonarow GC, Yancy CW, Heywood JT. Adherence to heart failure quality-of-care indicators in US hospitals: analysis of the ADHERE registry. Arch Intern Med 2005;165:1469-1477.
55. Packer M, Carver JR, Rodeheffer RJ, et al. for the PROMISE Study Research Group. Effect of oral milrinone on mortality in severe chronic heart failure. N Engl J Med 1991;325:1468-1475.
56. Anderson JL. Hemodynamic and clinical benefits with intravenous milrinone in severe chronic heart failure: results of a multicenter study in the United States. Am Heart J 1991;121:1956-1964.
57. Anderson JL, Baim DS, Fein SA, et al. Efficacy and safety of sustained (48 hour) intravenous infusions of milrinone in patients with severe congestive heart failure: a multicenter study. J Am Coll Cardiol 1987;9:711-722.
58. Cuffe MS, Calif RM, Adams KF Jr. Short-term intravenous milrinone for acute exacerbation of chronic heart failure: a randomized controlled trial. JAMA 2002;287:1541-1547.
59. Seino Y, Momomura S, Takano T, et al. for the Japan Intravenous Milrinone Investigators. Multicenter, double-blind study of intravenous milrinone for patients with acute heart failure in Japan. Crit Care Med 1996;24:1490-1497.
60. Metra M, Nodari S, D'Aloia A, et al. Beta-blocker therapy influences the hemodynamic response to inotropic agents in patients with heart failure: a randomized comparison of dobutamine and enoximone before and after chronic treatment with metoprolol or carvedilol. J Am Coll Cardiol 2002;40:1248-1258.
61. Oliva F, Latini R, Politi A, et al. Intermittent 6-month low-dose dobutamine infusion in severe heart failure: DICE multicenter trial. Am Heart J 1999;138:247-253.
62. Elis A, Bental T, Kimchi O, et al. Intermittent dobutamine treatment in patients with chronic refractory congestive heart failure: a randomized, double-blind, placebo-controlled study. Clin Pharmacol Ther 1998;63:682-685.
63. Adamopoulos S, Piepoli M, Qiang F, et al. Effects of pulsed beta-stimulant therapy on beta-adrenoceptors and chronotropic responsiveness in chronic heart failure. Lancet 1995;345:930.
64. Erlemeier HH, Kupper W, Bleifeld W. Intermittent infusion of dobutamine in the therapy of severe congestive heart failure: long-term effects and lack of tolerance. Cardiovasc Drugs Ther 1992;6:391-398.
65. Dies F, Krell MJ, Whitlow P. Intermittent dobutamine in ambulatory outpatients with chronic cardiac failure. Circulation 1986;74(Suppl II):II-38.
66. Leier CV, Heban PT, Huss P. Comparative systemic and regional hemodynamic effects of dopamine and dobutamine in patients with cardiomyopathic heart failure. Circulation 1981;63:1279-1285.
67. Kass DA, Solaro RJ. Mechanisms and use of calcium-sensitizing agents in the failing heart. Circulation 2006;113:305.
68. Katz SD, Kubo SH, Jessup M, et al. A multicenter, randomized, double-blind, placebo-controlled trial of pimobendan, a new cardiotonic and vasodilator agent, in patients with severe congestive heart failure. Am Heart J 1992;123:95.
69. Kubo SH, Gollub S, Bourge R, et al. Beneficial effects of pimobendan on exercise tolerance and quality of life in patients with heart failure: results of a multicenter trial. Circulation 1992;85:942.
70. Slawsky MT, Colucci WS, Gottleib SS, et al. on behalf of the Study Investigators. Acute hemodynamic and clinical effects of levosimendan in patients with severe heart failure. Circulation 2000;102:2222.
71. Nieminen MS, Akkila J, Hasenfuss G, et al. Hemodynamic and neurohumoral effects of continuous infusion of levosimendan in patients with congestive heart failure. J Am Coll Cardiol 2000;36:1903.
72. Follath F, Cleland JG, Just H, et al. Efficacy and safety of intravenous levosimendan compared with dobutamine in severe low-output heart failure (the LIDO study): a randomised double-blind trial. Lancet 2002;360:196.
73. De Luca L, Colucci WS, Nieminen MS, et al. Evidence-based use of levosimendan in different clinical settings. Eur Heart J 2006;27:1908.
74. Elkayam U, Amin J, Mahra A, et al. A prospective, randomized, double-blind crossover study to compare the efficacy and safety of chronic nifedipine therapy with that of isosorbide dinitrate and their combination in the treatment of chronic CHF. Circulation 1990;82:1954.
75. Littler WA, Sheridan DJ. Placebo controlled trial of felodipine in patients with mild to moderate heart failure. UK Study Group. Br Heart J 1995;73:428.
76. Packer M, O'Conner CM, Ghali JK, et al. Effect of amlodipine on morbidity and mortality in severe chronic heart failure. N Engl J Med 1996;335:1107.
77. O'Connor CM, Carson PE, Miller AB, et al. Effect of amlodipine on mode of death among patients with advanced heart failure in the PRAISE trial. Prospective Randomized Amlodipine Survival Evaluation. Am J Cardiol 1998;82:881.
78. Udelson JE, DeAbate CA, Berk M, et al. Effects of amlodipine on exercise tolerance, quality of life, and left ventricular function in patients with heart failure from left ventricular systolic dysfunction. Am Heart J 2000;139:503.
79. Stewart S, MacIntyre K, Hole DA, et al. More malignant than cancer? Five-year survival following a first admission for heart failure in Scotland. Eur J Heart Fail 2001;3:315-322.

27 PULMONARY ARTERIAL HYPERTENSION

Azad Raiesdana and Joseph Loscalzo

OVERVIEW 401
INTRODUCTION 401
Clinical Presentation and Diagnosis 401
Etiology 402
Assessment of Disease Severity 402
Natural History and Survival 403
Targets of Therapy 403
PATHOPHYSIOLOGY 403
Cellular Mechanisms 403
Cellular Proliferation 403
Vasoconstriction 403
Thrombosis 404
Molecular Mechanisms 404
Endothelin 404
Serotonin (5-HT) 404
Nitric Oxide 406
Prostacyclin 406
Vasoactive Intestinal Peptide 406
Genetic Factors 406
Bone Morphogenetic Protein Receptor II 406
Activin-Like Kinase Type-1 406
Serotonin (5-Hydroxytryptamine) Transporter 406
Environmental Risk Factors 407
Associated Conditions 407
THERAPEUTICS AND CLINICAL PHARMACOLOGY 407
Goals of Therapy 407
Lifestyle Modification 407
Conventional Measures 408
Therapeutics by Class 408
Calcium Channel Blockers 408
Prostanoids 408
Endothelin Receptor Antagonists 409
Nitric Oxide and Phosphodiesterase Inhibitors 410
Combination Therapy 411
Interventional and Surgical Therapies 411
Transplantation 411
Therapeutic Approach 411
Emerging Targets and Therapeutics 411

OVERVIEW

Pulmonary arterial hypertension (PAH) is a disease of the small pulmonary arteries characterized by vascular narrowing and increased pulmonary vascular resistance, which eventually leads to right ventricular failure. Vasoconstriction, vascular proliferation, remodeling of the pulmonary vessels, and thrombosis are all contributing factors to the increased vascular resistance seen in this disease.[1-3] PAH develops as a sporadic disease (idiopathic), as an inherited disorder (familial), or in association with certain conditions such as collagen vascular diseases, portal hypertension, human immunodeficiency virus (HIV) infection, congenital systemic-to-pulmonary shunts, ingestion of drugs or dietary products, or persistent fetal circulation.[3-5] The pathogenesis of PAH is a complicated, multifactorial process, and it seems doubtful that any one factor alone is sufficient to activate the necessary pathways leading to the development of this disease. Rather, clinically apparent PAH most likely develops after a second insult occurs in an individual who is already susceptible owing to genetic factors, environmental exposures, or acquired disorders.[6]

Currently, there is no cure for PAH, but several novel therapeutic options are now available that can improve symptoms and increase survival. Within the past 10 years, significant advances in the treatment of PAH have occurred, specifically medical therapies targeting specific pathways that are believed to play pathogenic roles in the development of this condition. Despite these advancements, PAH still remains a serious, life-threatening disease, and a thorough understanding of therapeutic options is critical to the optimal management of patients with this disorder.

INTRODUCTION

PAH is a disease of the small pulmonary arteries (muscular pulmonary arteries and arterioles) characterized by vascular narrowing and increased pulmonary vascular resistance, which eventually leads to right ventricular failure. Vasoconstriction, vascular proliferation, remodeling of the pulmonary vessels, and thrombosis all contribute to the increased vascular resistance seen in this disease.[1-3] PAH refers to conditions that share common isolated elevations in pulmonary arterial pressure. Hemodynamically, it is defined as a sustained mean pulmonary arterial pressure greater than 25 mm Hg in the setting of normal or reduced cardiac output and normal mean pulmonary capillary wedge pressure (<15 mm Hg).[7-9]

Previously, pulmonary hypertension was classified as either primary or secondary based on the presence or absence of identifiable causes or risk factors.[10,11] It has become clear, however, that certain conditions formerly categorized as secondary pulmonary hypertension have histopathologic lesions and clinical features resembling those observed in primary pulmonary hypertension. For this reason, in 2003 an international meeting of experts adopted the current World Health Organization (WHO) classification scheme for pulmonary hypertension. Based on pathologic features, mechanism of disease, and response to therapeutic intervention, pulmonary hypertensive diseases were placed into five groups: 1) pulmonary arterial hypertension; 2) pulmonary hypertension with left heart disease; 3) pulmonary hypertension associated with lung diseases and/or hypoxemia; 4) pulmonary hypertension due to chronic thrombotic and/or embolic disease, and 5) a miscellaneous category (Box 27-1).[12,13] Based on the revised classification system, PAH (group 1) is categorized as sporadic disease (idiopathic), an inherited disorder (familial), or associated with certain conditions, including collagen vascular diseases, congenital systemic-to-pulmonary shunts, portal hypertension, HIV infection, ingestion of drugs or dietary products, and persistent fetal circulation.[3-5]

Clinical Presentation and Diagnosis

Although symptoms of PAH are often nonspecific and may mimic common disorders, most patients are diagnosed as a result of an evaluation initiated because of a symptomatic complaint. Exertional

The authors wish to thank Ms. Stephanie Tribuna for expert secretarial assistance.

BOX 27-1 THE REVISED WORLD HEALTH ORGANIZATION CLASSIFICATION OF PULMONARY HYPERTENSION

Group 1. Pulmonary Arterial Hypertension*
Idiopathic
Familial
Associated conditions:
- Collagen vascular disease
- Congenital systemic-to-pulmonary shunts (large, small, repaired, or nonrepaired)
- Portal hypertension
- Human immunodeficiency virus disease
- Drugs and toxins (anorexigens, rapeseed oil, L-tryptophan, methamphetamine, and cocaine)
- Other (thyroid disorders, glycogen storage disease, Gaucher's disease, hereditary hemorrhagic telangiectasia, hemoglobinopathies, myleoproliferative disorders, and splenectomy)

Associated with significant venous or capillary involvement
- Pulmonary veno-occlusive disease
- Pulmonary capillary hemangiomatosis

Persistent pulmonary hypertension of the newborn

Group 2. Pulmonary Hypertension with Left Heart Disease†
Left-sided atrial or ventricular heart disease
Left-sided valvular heart disease

Group 3. Pulmonary Hypertension Associated with Lung Diseases and/or Hypoxemia†
Chronic obstructive pulmonary disease
Interstitial lung disease
Sleep-disordered breathing
Alveolar hypoventilation disorders
Long-term exposure to high altitudes
Developmental abnormalities

Group 4. Pulmonary Hypertension due to Chronic Thrombotic or Embolic Disease†
Thromboembolic obstruction of proximal pulmonary arteries
Thromboembolic obstruction of distal pulmonary arteries
Pulmonary embolism (tumor, parasites, foreign material)

Group 5. Miscellaneous†
Sarcoidosis
Pulmonary Langerhans cell histiocytosis
Lymphangiomatosis
Compression of pulmonary vessels (adenopathy, tumor, fibrosing mediastinitis)

*WHO group 1 comprises a group of conditions with common clinical and pathophysiologic characterisitics known collectively as pulmonary arterial hypertension (PAH).
†WHO groups 2 through 5 are a heterogenous group of disorders for which treatment is typically directed at the underlying process rather than the PAH.

dyspnea is the most commonly encountered symptom of PAH, although symptoms such as fatigue or weakness, angina, syncope, or peripheral edema may also be present. The disorder is occasionally discovered during screening of an asymptomatic high-risk population. Screening with Doppler echocardiography is advised in individuals with a known genetic mutation that is associated with PAH, or if the individual under consideration has a first-degree relative with idiopathic pulmonary arterial hypertension (IPAH). In addition, individuals with scleroderma, congenital heart disease, systemic-to-pulmonary shunts, or portal hypertension undergoing evaluation for liver transplant should be screened.[10]

A diagnostic strategy of testing should be employed to determine if the patient's symptoms are due to PAH and, if so, the underlying etiology. The initial assessment in detecting PAH should include a physical examination, chest radiograph, electrocardiogram, and transthoracic echocardiogram, including a Doppler assessment. Despite use of these various testing modalities, Doppler echocardiography is typically the first test with results that firmly suggest the diagnosis of PAH.[14] Doppler echocardiography is able to estimate the pulmonary artery systolic pressure noninvasively, although a right heart catheterization is ultimately needed for definitive diagnosis and is often used to assess severity and prognosis, and to guide initial therapy. In addition to an assessment of pulmonary arterial pressures, transthoracic echocardiography provides an assessment of right ventricular size and function (a critical determinate of prognosis in patients with pulmonary hypertension) as well as potential etiologies or contributory factors, including left-sided disease, valvular disease, or intracardiac shunts. Confirmation of suspected PAH by right heart catheterization is warranted prior to beginning an extensive evaluation to determine an underlying etiology or prognosis.

Etiology

Certain tests are essential in the evaluation of PAH to establish an underlying etiology, determine severity and prognosis, and choose an initial treatment strategy. Initial serologic testing may include antinuclear antibody titer, HIV serology, complete blood count with a platelet count, liver function tests, and antiphospholipid antibody levels.[10,15] Pulmonary function testing should be performed to exclude or characterize the contribution of underlying obstructive or restrictive disease to the overall pathophysiology of the pulmonary hypertension. This testing also helps to quantify the extent of hypoxemia (potentially due to ventilation-perfusion mismatch, right-to-left cardiac shunt, or intrapulmonary shunting), diffusion capacity abnormalities (potentially due to systemic sclerosis), and restrictive disease (potentially due to IPAH or chronic thromboembolic pulmonary arterial hypertension [CTEPH]).[10,16-18]

Since CTEPH is a potentially curable cause of PAH, ventilation-perfusion (V/Q) lung scintigraphy should be performed in all individuals in whom chronic pulmonary embolism (PE) is suspected. The V/Q scan in patients with chronic PE typically shows at least one segmental-sized perfusion defect. If the V/Q scan is equivocal and there is a high level of suspicion for chronic PE or a need to define a suspected embolism, additional testing, such as contrast-enhanced spiral (or helical) computed tomography (CT), high-resolution CT, or pulmonary angiography, should be performed.[19-22] Spiral CT has a sensitivity of greater than 85% to 90% for the detection of central pulmonary embolism, which is visualized as complete occlusion of pulmonary arteries, eccentric filling defects, recanalization, stenosis, or webs. High-resolution CT provides detailed views of the lung parenchyma and may allow for diagnosis of pulmonary fibrosis as another contributing cause of pulmonary hypertension.[23,24] Magnetic resonance imaging is increasingly used in patients with PAH for the evaluation of pathologic and functional changes of both the heart and pulmonary circulation, but additional experience is needed before it is used routinely in the assessment of PAH.[25] Pulmonary angiography, the definitive test for the diagnosis and preoperative assessment of patients with thromboembolic pulmonary hypertension, allows for localization and determination of the exact type of pulmonary artery obstruction.[26]

Assessment of Disease Severity

After diagnosis and classification of PAH, assessment of functional exercise capacity should be undertaken to evaluate disease severity. The two most commonly used exercise tests for patients with pulmonary hypertension are the 6-minute walk test (6MWT) and cardiopulmonary exercise testing (CPET) with gas exchange measurements. These tests determine baseline functional capacity, which is used initially to guide therapy and assess prognosis, and later in the course of the disease to follow response to therapy.

For the 6MWT, patients are asked to walk as far as possible in 6 minutes. This submaximal exercise test determines functional capacity for patients who are incapable of undergoing maximal exercise testing.

BOX 27-2 WORLD HEALTH ORGANIZATION FUNCTIONAL CLASSIFICATION OF PULMONARY ARTERIAL HYPERTENSION

Class I: Pulmonary arterial hypertension without limitation in physical activity; normal physical activity does not cause increased dyspnea, fatigue, chest pain, or near syncope

Class II: Pulmonary arterial hypertension with mild limitation of physical activity; no discomfort at rest, but normal physical activity causes increased dyspnea, fatigue, chest pain, or near syncope

Class III: Pulmonary arterial hypertension with marked limitation of physical activity; no discomfort at rest, but less than ordinary physical activity causes increased dyspnea, fatigue, chest pain, or near syncope

Class IV: Pulmonary arterial hypertension with an inability to perform any physical activity without symptoms; signs of right heart failure; dyspnea, fatigue, or both may be present even at rest, and discomfort is increased by any physical activity

Adapted from Barst R, McGoon M, Torbicki A, et al. Diagnosis and differential assessment of pulmonary arterial hypertension. J Am Coll Cardiol 2004;43:40S-47S.

In patients with IPAH, the 6MWT result is predictive of survival and correlates inversely with New York Heart Association (NYHA)/WHO functional status severity (Box 27-2). A recent study observed an 18% mortality risk reduction for each additional 50 m walked during the 6MWT.[27-29] Moreover, the 6MWT is a critical factor used in all PAH treatment trials to determine clinical response. CPET is a measure of ventilation and pulmonary gas exchange during exercise, and often provides an objective evaluation of functional capacity that is independent of effort. The peak oxygen consumption or the anaerobic or lactic acid threshold in submaximal exercise provides an estimate of the magnitude of exercise limitation in individuals with PAH.[30]

Natural History and Survival

Prior to the development of recent therapies, the clinical course of IPAH followed a fairly rapid progression from right ventricular failure to death. In earlier prospective trials, PAH patients had 1-, 3-, and 5-year survival rates of 68% to 77%, 40% to 56%, and 22% to 38%, respectively. Patients with connective tissue disease-associated PAH tend to have a worse prognosis, whereas patients with PAH due to congenital systemic-to-pulmonary shunts tend to have a slower progression of disease and longer survival. Indicators of a poor prognosis include a history of right heart failure, NYHA/WHO functional class III or IV, elevated right atrial pressure, decreased cardiac output, elevated pulmonary vascular resistance (PVR), and low mixed venous oxygen saturation.[31,32]

Targets of Therapy

Currently, there is no cure for PAH, but several therapeutic options targeted to specific molecular mechanisms are now available. Treatment has vastly improved over the past decade and now not only offers patients symptom relief, but also often prolongs their survival. Yet, the selection of the most appropriate therapy is complex, and requires familiarity with the disease process, evidence from treatment trials, complicated drug delivery systems and dosing regimens, and drug side effects and complications. The mainstay of current therapy consists of the use of a combination of agents, which may include supplemental oxygen, diuretics, anticoagulants, calcium channel blockers, prostanoids, endothelin receptor antagonists, phosphodiesterase-5 inhibitors, and interventional and surgical procedures. The etiology and severity level of PAH determine the therapeutic approach (Fig. 27-1).

PATHOPHYSIOLOGY

The pathogenesis of PAH is a complicated, multifactorial process. It seems doubtful that any one factor alone is sufficient to activate the necessary pathways leading to the development of this vascular disease. Rather, clinically apparent PAH most likely develops after a second insult occurs in an individual who is already susceptible owing to genetic factors, environmental exposures, or acquired disorders. Thus, an understanding of the interaction of these risk factors is critical to identifying possible pathogenic mechanisms and defining the spectrum of disease[6] (Fig. 27-2).

Cellular Mechanisms

The primary vascular changes leading to increased vascular resistance in PAH are vasoconstriction, remodeling of the pulmonary vascular wall, and thrombosis. Pulmonary vasoconstriction, one of the earliest components of the pulmonary hypertensive process, is most likely due to an abnormal expression of vascular smooth muscle potassium channels or endothelial dysfunction. Excessive vasoconstriction causes an alteration in cell proliferation, coagulation, and production of growth factors and vasoactive substances. Chronic impairment in the production of these vascular cell mediators ultimately results in a homeostatic imbalance that affects vascular tone and promotes vascular remodeling.[2,33]

Cellular Proliferation

Endothelial cell dysfunction resulting from hypoxia, shear stress, inflammation, or a response to drugs or toxins in the setting of genetic susceptibility results in disorganized proliferation of endothelial cells, which leads to the formation of plexiform lesions (i.e., focal proliferation of endothelial channels lined by myofibroblasts, smooth muscle cells, and connective tissue matrix) (Fig. 27-3).[2,34] Defects in growth-suppressive genes, including transforming growth factor-β (TGF-β) receptor-2, have been reported in plexiform lesions in patients with IPAH.[35] Owing to an abnormal angiogenic response to hypoxia, endothelial cells within the plexiform lesions tend to overexpress vascular endothelial growth factor (VEGF) and its receptor, VEGF receptor-2, which leads to clonal expansion of these endothelial cells.[2,34-37] Endothelial dysfunction also leads to chronically impaired production of vasodilators such as nitric oxide (NO) and prostacyclin, along with overexpression of vasoconstrictors such as endothelin (ET)-1.[38]

Pulmonary vascular remodeling is the characteristic pathologic change of PAH. Remodeling, which occurs in all layers of the vessel wall, includes hypertrophy and hyperplasia of smooth muscle cells, and is often stimulated by either physical stress (mechanical stretch and shear stress) or chemical stress (hypoxia, viral infection, vasoactive mediators, and growth factors) to the vessel.[39,40] Smooth muscle cell hyperplasia results in the extension of proximal smooth muscle into distal, nonmuscular vessels. The formation of a layer of myofibroblasts and extracellular matrix (collagen and elastin) in the vessel, and the differentiation and migration of fibroblasts from the adventia to the media, contribute to the remodeling process. Patients with PAH may have an imbalance in the rate of proliferation and apoptosis resulting in thickened, obstructive pulmonary arteries.[6,41,42]

Vasoconstriction

Pulmonary vasoconstriction is thought to be an early component of the pulmonary hypertensive process. Excessive vasoconstriction is associated with abnormal function or expression of potassium channels and endothelial dysfunction leading to chronically impaired production of vasodilators, such as NO and prostacyclin, and prolonged overexpression of vasoconstrictors, such as ET-1.[2,43] This homeostatic imbalance results in altered vascular tone and promotion of vascular remodeling. Hypoxia inhibits voltage-gated potassium channels (K_v), causing membrane depolarization and an increase in calcium channels, which raise cytosolic calcium, thereby promoting vasoconstriction. In PAH, K_v1.5 channels are down-regulated.[6,44] It is unclear whether this abnormality is genetic or acquired; however, it is clear that anorexigens directly inhibit K_v1.5 and K_v2.2 channels. Augmenting K_v pathways should cause pulmonary vasodilation and promote regression of pulmonary remodeling. Certain drugs, including dichloroacetate and sildenafil, may enhance the expression and function of these potassium channels.[6,45]

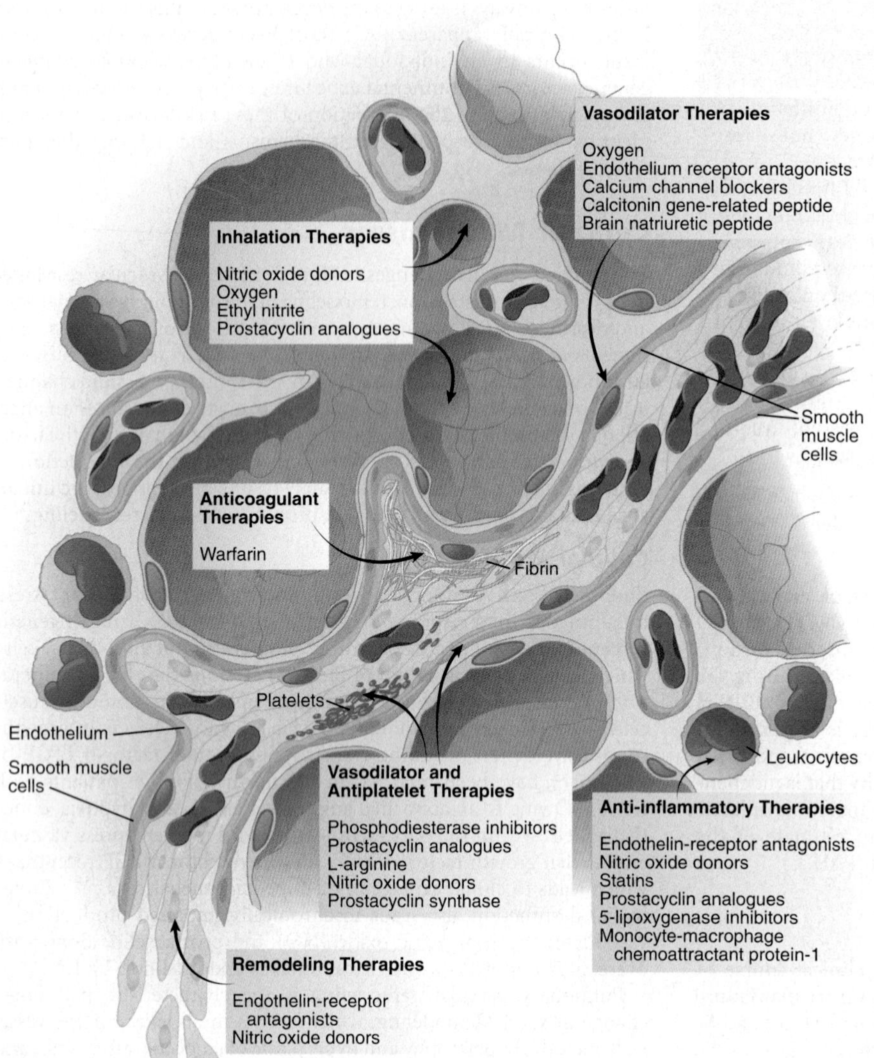

FIGURE 27-1 • Therapeutic approaches to pulmonary hypertension. A model pulmonary arteriolar system and alveolus are illustrated, with the sites of action of each of six major classes of agents indicated. Pulmonary vascular smooth muscle cells are indicated in *orange*, platelets in *purple*, leukocytes in *blue* with pale nuclei, and fibrin as *tan* strands. (From Farber HW, Loscalzo J. Pulmonary arterial hypertension. N Engl J Med 2004;351:1655-1665. Copyright © 1990 Massachusetts Medical Society. All rights reserved.)

Thrombosis

Although it still remains unclear whether thrombotic lesions and platelet dysfunction are causes or consequences of PAH, they remain potentially important processes in the disease. Procoagulant activity and fibrinolytic functions of pulmonary endothelium are altered in PAH and lead to continuous intravascular thrombosis with elevated plasma levels of fibrinopeptide A, D-dimer, von Willebrand factor, and plasminogen activator inhibitor type 1. In situ pulmonary artery thrombosis may be initiated or aggravated by abnormalities in the clotting cascade, injury to the vessel wall, or platelet dysfunction resulting in the release of various procoagulants and vasoactive and mitogenic mediators.[6,46]

Molecular Mechanisms

Dysfunctional pulmonary artery endothelial cells, such as those observed in individuals with IPAH, have decreased production of prostacyclin[47] and endogenous NO[43,48] with increased production of ET-1.[49-51] This imbalance promotes vasoconstriction and proliferation of smooth muscle cells in the pulmonary arteries (see Fig. 27-3).

Endothelin

Endothelins, a family of 21–amino acid peptides, play a major role in the regulation of vascular tone. In patients with PAH, endothelin levels are elevated and clearance of endothelin in the pulmonary vasculature is reduced.[50,52] ET-1, a direct vasoconstrictor, also stimulates cellular proliferation of vascular smooth muscle cells, induces fibrosis, and acts as a proinflammatory mediator by enhancing the expression of adhesion molecules.[53-56] ET-1 is typically secreted from the luminal side of the endothelial cells toward adjacent smooth muscle cells, which contain specific endothelin receptors.[57] Two endothelin receptors, endothelin-A (ET_A) and endothelin-B (ET_B), have been identified.[55-58] Activation of ET_A receptors induces vasoconstriction and proliferation of vascular smooth muscle cells, while ET_B receptors mediate pulmonary endothelin clearance and induce vasodilation through increased production of NO and prostacyclin.[58]

Serotonin (5-HT)

In addition, pulmonary artery smooth muscle cells in IPAH have a strong proliferative response to serum serotonin (5-hydroxytryptamine [5-HT]) owing to an overexpression of the 5-HT transporter.[59,60] In several studies, individuals with IPAH were found to have decreased levels of vasoactive intestinal polypeptide (VIP) in the serum and lungs,[61] elevated levels of plasma 5-HT,[59] reduced expression of prostacyclin and NO synthase,[43,62] and up-regulation of ET_B receptors[63,64] on smooth muscle cells, all of which contribute to the general vasoconstriction response. Overall, the homeostatic imbalance that occurs in PAH favors vasoconstriction, endothelial cell proliferation, and thrombosis.

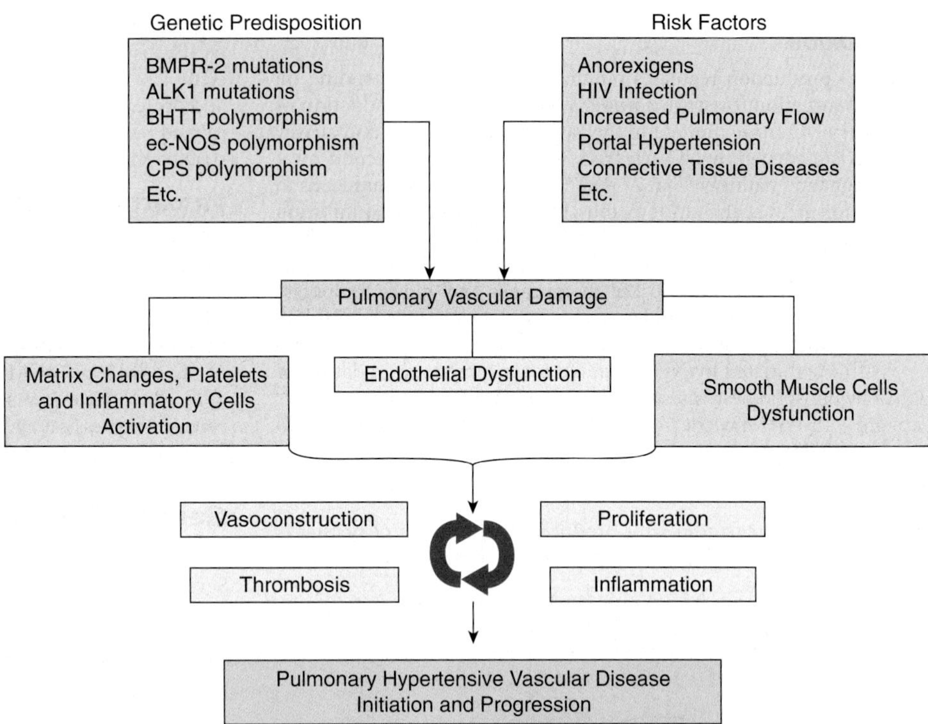

FIGURE 27-2 • Pulmonary arterial hypertension: potential pathogenetic and pathobiologic mechanisms. ALK 1, activin-receptor-like kinase 1 gene; BMPR-2, bone morphogenetic protein receptor type-2 gene; CPS, carbamylphosphate synthetase gene; 5-HTT, serotonin transporter gene; ec-NOS, nitric oxide synthase gene. (From The Task Force on Diagnosis and Treatment of Pulmonary Arterial Hypertension of the European Society of Cardiology. Guidelines on diagnosis and treatment of pulmonary arterial hypertension. Eur Heart J 2004;25:2243-2278.)

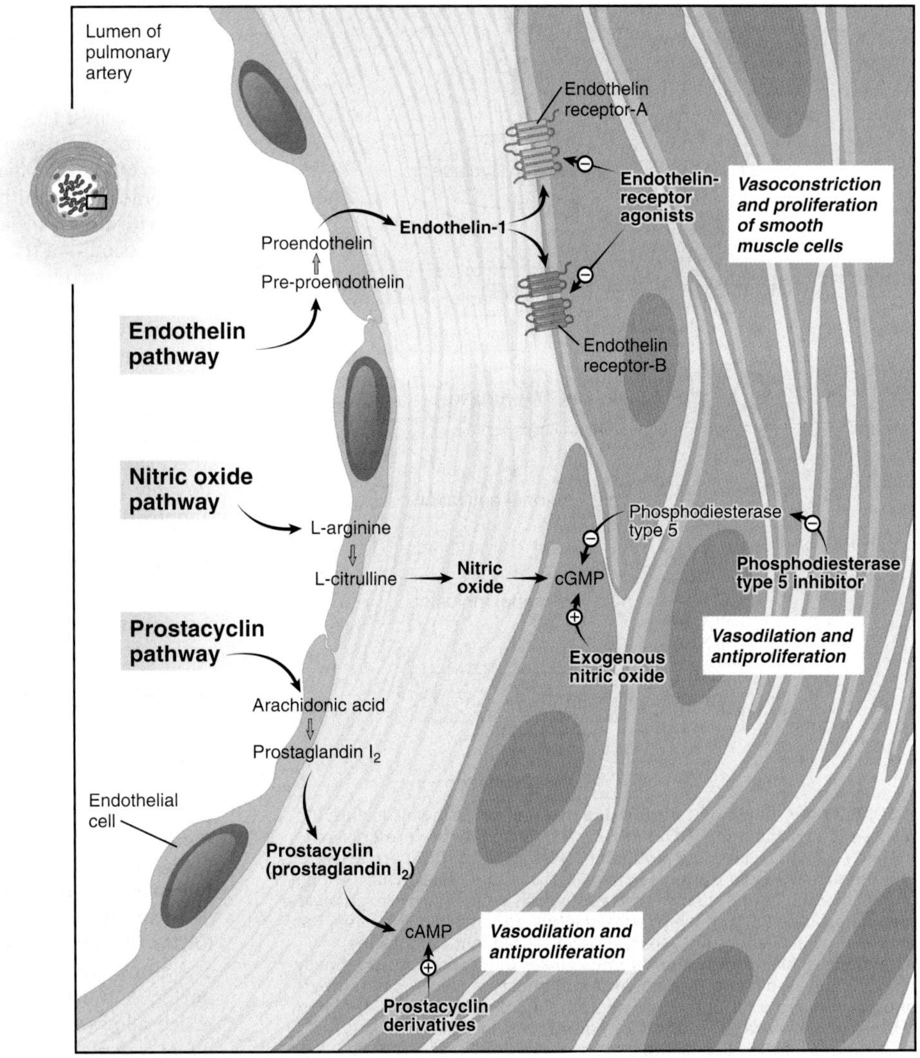

Lumen of pulmonary artery

Endothelin receptor-A

Endothelin-receptor agonists

Vasoconstriction and proliferation of smooth muscle cells

Endothelin-1

Proendothelin

Pre-proendothelin

Endothelin pathway

Endothelin receptor-B

Nitric oxide pathway

L-arginine

L-citrulline

Nitric oxide

cGMP

Phosphodiesterase type 5

Phosphodiesterase type 5 inhibitor

Exogenous nitric oxide

Vasodilation and antiproliferation

Prostacyclin pathway

Arachidonic acid

Prostaglandin I_2

Endothelial cell

Prostacyclin (prostaglandin I_2)

cAMP

Vasodilation and antiproliferation

Prostacyclin derivatives

FIGURE 27-3 • Molecular mechanisms that target therapies for pulmonary arterial hypertension. Three major pathways involved in abnormal proliferation and contraction of the smooth muscle cells of the pulmonary artery in patients with pulmonary arterial hypertension are shown. These pathways correspond to important therapeutic targets in this condition and play a role in determining which of four classes of drugs—endothelin-receptor antagonists, nitric oxide, phosphodiesterase type 5 inhibitors, and prostacyclin derivatives—will be used. At the top of the figure, a transverse section of a small pulmonary artery (<500 μm in diameter) from a patient with severe pulmonary arterial hypertension shows intimal proliferation and marked medial hypertrophy. Dysfunctional pulmonary artery endothelial cells (*blue*) have decreased production of prostacyclin and endogenous nitric oxide, with an increased production of endothelin-1—a condition promoting vasoconstriction and proliferation of smooth muscle cells in the pulmonary arteries (*red*). Current or emerging therapies interfere with specific targets in smooth muscle cells in the pulmonary arteries. In addition to their actions on smooth muscle cells, prostacyclin derivatives and nitric oxide have several other properties, including antiplatelet effects. *Plus signs* denote an increase in the intracellular concentration; *minus signs* denote blockage of a receptor, inhibition of an enzyme, or a decrease in the intracellular concentration. cGMP, cyclic guanosine monophosphate. (From Humbert M, Sitbon O, Simonneau G. Treatment of pulmonary arterial hypertension. N Engl J Med 2004;351:1425-1436.)

Nitric Oxide

Local NO production regulates pulmonary perfusion, depending on alveolar ventilation to assure optimal V/Q distribution. Production of pulmonary NO from arginine in the vascular endothelium and airway epithelia is mediated by NO synthase, which is part of a second messenger signaling pathway (Fig. 27-4).[65,67] This complex system leads to vasodilation in vascular smooth muscle cells, and platelet inhibition principally through production of cyclic guanosine monophosphate (cGMP), which activates cGMP kinase. Activation of this enzyme opens potassium channels on cell membranes and allows for potassium efflux, membrane depolarization, calcium channel inhibition, and diminished activation of the contractile apparatus. The vasodilatory pathway initiated by NO is limited by enzymatic degradation of cGMP by phosphodiesterases (PDEs), a superfamily of 11 enzymes.[68-70] Patients with PAH have decreased NO synthase expression leading to vasoconstriction.[42]

Prostacyclin

Prostacyclin (prostaglandin I_2) is produced by the action of prostacyclin synthase on arachidonic acid in endothelial cells. Acting through a cyclic adenosine monophosphate (cAMP)-dependent pathway, prostacyclin is an important pulmonary vasodilator. This endogenous molecule also inhibits the proliferation of vascular smooth muscle cells and decreases platelet aggregation. In PAH, prostacyclin synthase activity and prostacyclin levels are diminished, while levels of the vasoconstrictor thromboxane are increased.[61,64]

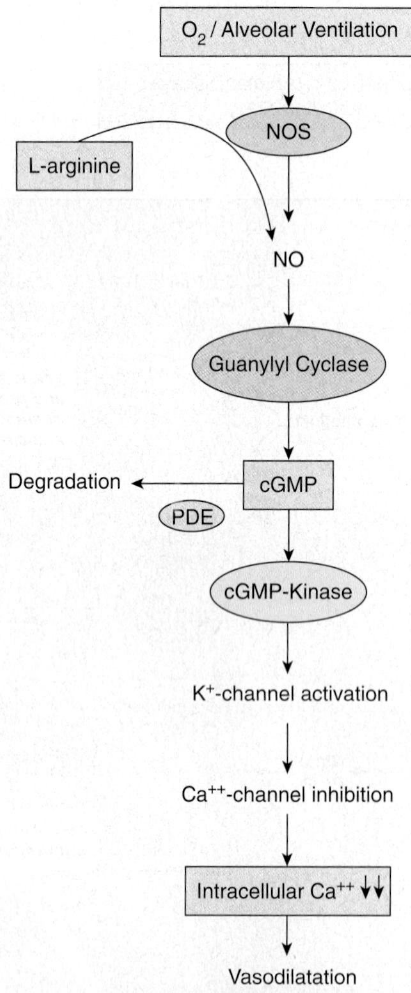

FIGURE 27-4 • Scheme of nitric oxide metabolism pathway. In this diagram, the nitric oxide (NO) pathway is depicted. In the presence of oxygen (O_2) and/or alveolar ventilation, NO synthases (NOS) are activated and produce NO from L-arginine via L-citrulline. The NO activates soluble and membrane-bound guanylyl cyclases, which synthesize cyclic guanylate monophosphate (cGMP), which subsequently activates cGMP kinase. This enzyme—by activation of K^+ channels and subsequent Ca^{2+} channel inhibition—evokes a reduction of intracellular Ca^{2+} concentration, finally resulting in vasodilation. The downstream effects of NO are limited by phosphodiesterase (PDE)-induced degradation of cGMP. (From Ghofani HA, Pepke-Zaba J, Barbera JA, et al. Nitric oxide pathway and phosphodiesterase inhibitors in pulmonary arterial hypertension. J Am Coll Cardiol 2004;43:68S-72S.)

Vasoactive Intestinal Polypeptide

VIP is a neuropeptide that functions as a potent systemic and pulmonary vasodilator and an inhibitor of platelet aggregation and smooth muscle cell proliferation. VIP acts through two receptor subtypes, VPAC-1 and VPAC-2, which are coupled to adenylyl cyclase and expressed in the pulmonary vasculature. Stimulation of the receptors leads to activation of the cAMP and cGMP pathways. A recent study found that patients with IPAH have low serum concentration of the neuropeptide and elevated expression and binding activity of its receptors in pulmonary artery smooth muscle cells, which reflects VIP deficiency.[53,54,71]

Genetic Factors

The familial form of PAH occurs in approximately 6% of all cases.[10] Several genotypes have been confirmed to be associated with the occurrence of PAH.

Bone Morphogenetic Protein Receptor II

Recently, mutations in two receptors of the TGF-β family have been identified in the majority of cases of inherited (familial) PAH.[72] The TGF-β family consists of the TGF-β isoforms, the bone morphogenetic proteins, activins, and growth and differentiation factors. These molecules have diverse roles in a wide variety of physiologic processes, such as smooth muscle cell proliferation and differentiation, immunity, and inflammation.[73,74]

Mutations in the gene encoding for the bone morphogenetic protein receptor type 2 (BMPR2), which normally modulates the growth and survival of vascular smooth muscle cells,[75] are present in approximately 50% to 60% of familial cases of PAH and in 10% to 30% of idiopathic or sporadic cases. Although some of the sporadic cases may be associated with de novo mutations, the majority are likely due to familial transmission of a truncated or point mutation with a low penetrance. The gene encoding for BMPR2 has been localized to chromosome 2q33, and more than 45 different mutations have been identified in patients with familial PAH.[76-79] Inheritance occurs in an autosomal dominant pattern with highly variable and incomplete expression, female predominance, and genetic anticipation (i.e., with each successive generation, clinical disease develops earlier and in a more severe form).[80] Exonic mutations of the gene encoding for BMPR2 most likely affect signal transduction in pulmonary vascular smooth muscle cells, possibly leading to an alteration in the mechanisms responsible for apoptosis with subsequent cellular proliferation.[81]

Activin-Like Kinase Type-1

Mutations in another TGF-β family member, activin-like kinase type 1 receptor on endothelial cells, have been found in a minority of patients with hereditary hemorrhagic telangiectasia and coexistent PAH.[82]

Serotonin (5-Hydroxytryptamine) Transporter

Serotonin, a neuropeptide produced in the pulmonary vasculature and stored in platelets, is one of the best studied modifiers of pulmonary hypertension.[79] Activity of the 5-HT transporter is associated with proliferation of pulmonary artery smooth muscle cells. Anorexigens interact with the serotonin transporter and cause release of 5-HT from platelets, thereby increasing free circulating levels and inhibiting its reuptake.[83,84] Patients with PAH exhibit elevated plasma levels of 5-HT, and exposure to fenfluramine derivatives results in an increased risk for the development of PAH.

A single gene on chromosome 17q11.2 encodes for the 5-HT transporter. A functional polymorphism in the gene's promoter region, which allows for increased expression of the transporter and subsequent vascular smooth cell proliferation, is more prevalent in individuals with IPAH than controls. Additionally, the polymorphism contributes to differences in the level of hypoxia-induced 5-HT expression and may affect susceptibility to hypoxic pulmonary hypertension.[53,85]

Environmental Risk Factors

Environmental factors, such as use of appetite-suppressant or stimulant drugs and chronic hypoxia, may be one step in the pathway leading to the development or progression of PAH. IPAH is 7.5 times more likely to occur in individuals using anorexigenic agents, such as fenfluramine, for greater than 6 months. Although the incidence of PAH increases with the duration of use of fenfluramine, increased pulmonary arterial pressure was observed after only a limited exposure time, approximately 3 to 4 weeks.[35,38,86,87] It has also been suggested that stimulant use, including methamphetamine and cocaine, may be associated with an increased risk of PAH, but no conclusive studies have confirmed that these drugs are clearly risk factors.[88] Although chronic hypoxia is probably not a crucial risk factor for the development of PAH, it may contribute to disease progression through the mechanism of pulmonary arterial vasoconstriction and subsequent vascular remodeling.[89,90]

Associated Conditions

Several associated or coexisting conditions have been identified with an increased prevalence of PAH. Some of the strongest evidence exists for the following conditions: scleroderma (especially limited scleroderma), infection with HIV or human herpesvirus, portal hypertension, thrombocytosis, hemoglobinopathies, and hereditary hemorrhagic telangiectasia (Osler-Weber-Rendu disease).[3] Hereditary hemorrhagic telangiectasia is an autosomal dominant disorder characterized by the presence of multiple arteriovenous malformations, particularly in the pulmonary, hepatic, and cerebral circulations.[91,92] The association between chronic myeloproliferative disorders and PAH may be the result of splenectomy, portal hypertension, chemotherapy-induced pulmonary veno-occlusive disease, or pulmonary parenchymal infiltration with hematopoietic cells. Hemodynamic studies have demonstrated that PAH exists in 2% to 5% of patients with cirrhosis and in approximately 6% of patients undergoing assessment for liver transplantation.[93-95]

THERAPEUTICS AND CLINICAL PHARMACOLOGY

Goals of Therapy

Current treatment of PAH is based on a growing understanding of the pathogenesis of the disorder. Insight into the roles of vasoconstriction and vascular remodeling as causes of increased pulmonary vascular resistance has stimulated trials of treatment, first with vasodilators and more recently with agents that reverse vascular remodeling. The numerous clinical trials performed recently in PAH allow for the adoption of evidence-based therapy. Box 27-3 provides the grading system used to determine the level of evidence for each treatment and each therapeutic recommendation. The grading systems are based on the number of favorable controlled clinical trials performed with a given medication.[96] The efficacy and regulatory status of selected treatments can be found in Table 27-1.[96]

Lifestyle Modification

Owing to the lack of data, most of the following lifestyle recommendations are based on expert opinion. Patients with PAH must be careful since they are more likely to develop cardiopulmonary symptoms with relatively normal activities. Heavy physical activity or isotonic exercise may cause exertional syncope; thus, patients are encouraged to participate in only low-level aerobic exercise, such as walking. They should avoid high altitudes because of the possibility of hypoxic vasoconstriction, and may require supplemental oxygen when traveling by airplane. Since excess sodium intake may predispose patients to right-sided heart failure, they should restrict their intake to less than 2400 mg daily. In terms of prevention, patients need to receive immunizations against influenza and pneumonia and avoid vasoconstricting sinus or cold medication and anorexigens.[70]

Pregnancy and labor place an increased demand on the cardiopulmonary system in patients with PAH and result in a maternal mortal-

TABLE 27-1 GRADING OF EVIDENCE FOR EFFICACY AND REGULATORY APPROVAL STATUS OF SELECTED TREATMENTS*

Treatment	Number of RCTs	Grade of Rec.	Level of Evidence	Regulatory Approval	Type of PAH	NYHA/WHO FC
Oral anticoagulants	0	IIa/IIb	C	—	—	—
Diuretics	0	I	C	—	—	—
Digoxin	0	IIb	C	—	—	—
Oxygen	0	C	C	—	—	—
Calcium channel blockers	0	C	C	—	—	—
Epoprostenol	3	A	A	Europe USA, Canada	IPAH PAH–CTD	III-IV
Treprostinil	2	B	B	USA	PAH	II-IV
Iloprost	2	B	B/C	Europe, Australia New Zealand	IPAH PAH–CTD CTEPH	III-IV
Beraprost	2	B	B	Japan, Korea	IPAH	II-IV
Bosentan	2	A	A	Europe USA, Canada	PAH	III III-IV
Sitaxsentan	2	B	B	Europe, Canada	PAH	II-IV
Ambrisentan	1	C	C	USA, Europe	PAH	II-III
Sildenafil	1	I	A	USA	PAH	III-IV

*Committee Practice Guidelines of the European Society of Cardiology in 2004.[96]

CTD, connective tissue disease; CTEPH, chronic thromobembolic pulmonary hypertension; FC, functional class; IPAH, idiopathic pulmonary arterial hypertension; NYHA, New York Heart Association; PAH, pulmonary arterial hypertension; RCTs, randomized controlled trials; Rec., recommendation; WHO, World Health Organization.

BOX 27-3 LEVELS OF EVIDENCE AND CLASSES FOR STUDIES*

Levels of Evidence for Efficacy

Grade A: Data derived from multiple randomized clinical trials or meta-analyses

Grade B: Data derived from single randomized clinical trial or large nonrandomized studies

Grade C: Consensus of opinion of the experts and/or small studies, retrospective studies, registries

Classes of Recommendations

Class I: Evidence and/or general agreement that a given diagnostic procedure/treatment is beneficial, useful, and effective

Class II: Conflicting evidence and/or a divergence of opinion about the usefulness/efficacy of the treatment

- **Class IIa:** Weight of evidence/opinion is in favor of usefulness/efficacy
- **Class IIb:** Usefulness/efficacy is less well established by evidence/opinion

Class III: Evidence of general agreement that the treatment is not useful/effective and in some cases may be harmful

*Committee Practice Guidelines of the European Society of Cardiology in 2004.[96]

ity risk of 30% to 50%; thus, pregnancy is contraindicated in these patients. Safe and effective contraception is therefore recommended in all women of childbearing age with pulmonary hypertension. Usually, either dual barrier method contraception or progesterone-only oral contraceptives, in women without a history of thromboembolic disease, are the recommended forms of birth control for these patients. Estrogen-containing contraceptives are not recommended as they may lead to an increased risk of venous thromboembolism.[13,32] In addition, endothelin receptor antagonists, commonly prescribed for PAH, are teratogenic.

Conventional Measures

Initial therapy is often directed at the underlying causes or contributing factors, such as the use of supplemental oxygen for hypoxemia, continuous positive airway pressure with supplemental oxygen for obstructive sleep apnea, or anticoagulation and potential thromboendartectomy for PAH due to chronic thromboembolic disease. Following the identification and treatment of underlying disorders and contributing factors, specific therapy to address the effects of PAH, such as vasoconstriction, vascular proliferation, remodeling of the pulmonary vessels, and thrombosis, should be considered in all PAH patients.[1-3]

Anticoagulation with warfarin in patients with IPAH is based on two small studies, one retrospective and one prospective, that reported improved 3-year survival rates of 21% to 49% and 31% to 47%.[24,26] There is no evidence of a difference in anticoagulation efficacy for different functional classes of PAH, and the use of anticoagulation is controversial in patients with PAH due to scleroderma or congenital heart disease owing to lack of efficacy data and the theoretical increased risks of gastrointestinal bleeding in patients with scleroderma and of hemoptysis in congenital heart disease patients. Owing to the increased risk of catheter-associated thrombosis, all patients receiving long-term intravenous (IV) epoprostenol treatment generally receive anticoagulation in the absence of contraindications. Current consensus suggests a target international normalized ratio of 1.5 to 2.5 for IPAH patients on anticoagulation.[27,28]

Patients with evidence of right heart failure frequently benefit from the use of diuretics. The exact class and dose of diuretic is left to the discretion of the treating physician since trial data are lacking, although twice-daily loop diuretics are the norm. The use of digoxin in patients with isolated right ventricular failure remains controversial since digoxin appears to be most beneficial in patients with cor pulmonale or atrial fibrillation. Short-term intravenous use of digoxin in idiopathic disease may improve cardiac output and decrease the circulating levels of norepinephrine, although studies have not been conducted to evaluate the effect of its long-term administration.[29,30] There are no consistent data concerning long-term use of supplemental oxygen in PAH, but since chronic hypoxemia may cause vasoconstriction, supplemental oxygen is routinely used to maintain oxygen saturation above 90%.[32] The use of supplemental oxygen is more controversial in patients with significant right-to-left shunts due to congenital heart disease with Eisenmenger physiology, but its use may decrease the need for phlebotomy and reduce potential neurologic complications.[95]

Therapeutics by Class

Calcium Channel Blockers

Smooth muscle cell hypertrophy and pulmonary artery vasoconstriction contribute to the pathogenesis of PAH.[2,26] A small, prospective, nonrandomized trial of patients with IPAH demonstrated that those patients who responded to short-acting vasodilators had improved 1-, 3-, and 5-year survival with long-term use of calcium channel blockers as compared to nonresponders. Therefore, despite evidence from a randomized controlled trial, general consensus dictates that it is prudent for patients with IPAH to undergo an acute vasodilator challenge within the catheterization laboratory using short-acting agents, such as IV epoprostenol, adenosine, or inhaled NO, to identify which patients might benefit from long-term use of a calcium channel blocker. The development of acute pulmonary edema in response to acute vasodilator study suggests the presence of pulmonary veno-occlusive disease or pulmonary capillary hemangiomatosis, and is a contraindication to chronic vasodilator therapy. A positive short-term response to vasodilators is defined as at least a 10 mm Hg decrease in mean pulmonary arterial pressure to 40 mm Hg or less, with normal or increased cardiac output. Only approximately 10% to 15% of patients with IPAH will meet these criteria. Of those patients started on long-term therapy, about one half will maintain a sustained hemodynamic (measured at 3 months) and functional (NYHA/WHO functional class I or II) improvement.[27-29]

Calcium channel blockers with negative inotropic effects, such as verapamil, should be avoided. Depending on the patient's baseline heart rate, nifedipine, diltiazem, and amlodipine are the most frequently used calcium channel blocking agents. If a patient does not improve to functional class I or II with calcium channel blocker therapy, an alternate therapy should be initiated. The effects of high-dose calcium channel blockers on other types of pulmonary arterial hypertension have not yet been clearly demonstrated.[30]

Prostanoids

Prostacyclin, a metabolite of arachidonic acid, is endogenously produced by vascular endothelium, inhibits platelet aggregation, and is a potent vasodilator in both pulmonary and systemic circulations. In patients with PAH, the ratio of prostacyclin to the potent vasoconstrictor thromboxane is decreased[96] and their lung tissue exhibits decreased expression of prostacyclin synthase,[97] suggesting that inadequate prostacyclin synthesis may contribute to the etiology of PAH. Exogenously administered prostanoid analogues, such as IV epoprostenol, subcutaneous (subQ) treprostinil, inhaled iloprost, and oral beraprost, are used in patients with moderately severe to severe PAH to help overcome the adverse effects of decreased endogenously produced prostacyclin (Table 27-2).

Epoprostenol. The efficacy of IV epoprostenol was initially studied in a 12-week, prospective, multicenter, randomized, controlled, open-label trial comparing continuously infused epoprostenol plus conventional therapy (oral vasodilators and anticoagulation) to conventional therapy alone in 81 patients with NYHA functional class III and IV idiopathic PAH. When compared to conventional therapy alone, continuous IV infusion of epoprostenol improved symptoms and exercise capacity, increased cardiac output, and decreased PVR. In patients with scleroderma-associated PAH, treatment with IV epoprostenol as compared to conventional therapy improved exercise capacity and cardio-

TABLE 27-2 PROSTANOID THERAPY

	Drug Name (Trade Name)			
	Epoprostenol (Flolan)	**Treprostinil (Remodulin)**	**Iloprost (Ventavis)**	**Beraprost**
Mode of delivery	Continuous IV infusion	IV and subQ	IV and inhalation	Oral
Beginning dose (interval)	2-4 ng/kg/min (continuous infusion)	1.25 ng/kg/min (continuous infusion)	2.5 mcg per dose (6-9 times/day)	80 mcg per dose (4 times/day)
Optimal dosing range (interval)	25-40 ng/kg/min (continuous infusion)	25-40 ng/kg/min (continuous infusion)	5 mcg/dose (via nebulizer, 6-9 times/day)	—
Half-life	5 min	3 hr	20-25 min	35-40 min
Contraindications	Dominant left-to-right shunt	—	—	—
Drug interactions	Anticoagulants*	Anticoagulants,* diuretics,† antihypertensives†	Anticoagulants,* antihypertensives†	
Side effects	Flushing, headache, jaw pain, diarrhea, nausea, rash, myalgias	Headache, diarrhea, flushing, jaw and foot pain, local site reaction	Cough, headache, flushing, syncope	Symptoms consistent with systemic vasodilation
Pregnancy category	B	B	C	—
Annual cost	$72,000	$93,000	$50,000	—

*Increased risk of bleeding when coadministered with prostanoids.
†Prostanoids may increase the hypotensive effect of diuretics and antihypertensive medication.
IV, intravenous; subQ, subcutaneous.

pulmonary hemodynamics at 12 weeks.[32,97,98] The beneficial effects of this therapy may be sustained for several years in many patients with IPAH.[99-102] Improvements with epoprostenol have also been reported in patients who had PAH associated with congenital left-to-right shunts, portal hypertension, and HIV infection.[103-105]

More recent studies have examined the effect of epoprostenol treatment on long-term survival rates and attempted to determine the factors associated with survival in patients with IPAH. In a study of 162 IPAH patients, treatment with epoprostenol resulted in significantly greater survival rates at 1, 2, and 3 years (87.8%, 76.3%, and 62.8%, respectively) as compared to historical controls (58.9%, 46.3%, and 35.4%, respectively). Predictors of survival after the first year of treatment included functional class and improvement in mean pulmonary artery pressure, exercise tolerance, and cardiac index.[102] In a slightly larger trial of IPAH patients treated with epoprostenol, predictors of survival at 5 years depended on the severity of disease at baseline and the response to 3 months of epoprostenol therapy.[99,101]

With a half-life of less than 6 minutes, epoprostenol requires constant IV infusion, and abrupt or inadvertent discontinuation leads to rebound worsening of pulmonary hypertension and symptomatic deterioration. Common, dose-dependent side effects include flushing, headache, jaw and lower extremity muscular pain, diarrhea, nausea, and rash.[97,99,102] Complications of chronic IV therapy with epoprostenol include line-related infections, catheter-associated venous thrombosis, thrombocytopenia, and ascites. Epoprostenol is approved for patients with idiopathic or scleroderma-associated PAH with NYHA/WHO functional class III or IV, but its use is usually reserved for patients with advanced disease who have failed oral therapy.[106]

Treprostinil. As a result of the complications associated with long-term IV therapy of epoprostenol, other prostacyclin analogues with alternate delivery systems have been developed. Treprostinil is a stable prostacyclin analogue with a half-life of approximately 3 hours, which allows for subQ or IV administration. The side effects are similar to those of epoprostenol with the addition of infusion site pain and erythema when delivered subQ; often the site pain limits this mode of delivery. Both IV and subQ formulations are approved by the U.S. Food and Drug Administration (FDA) for treatment of PAH with NYHA/WHO functional class II, III, or IV.

After an initial trial demonstrated that treprostinil could be administered safely and effectively as a subQ agent in an outpatient setting, enrollment began in a large, international, placebo-controlled trial assessing the efficacy of subQ treprostinil treatment in patients with PAH (IPAH or PAH associated with connective tissue disease or congenital systemic-to-pulmonary shunts). Significant hemodynamic improvement in mean right atrial pressure, mean pulmonary arterial pressure, cardiac index, and PVR was observed with treprostinil therapy. Although significant improvement was also observed in exercise capacity and symptoms in patients treated with treprostinil for 3 months, the improvement was relatively modest compared to prior trials with IV epoprostenol. Most likely, the less significant improvement with treprostinil was related to the trial's broad entry criteria, which included patients with NYHA/WHO functional class II and with PAH due to congenital systemic-to-pulmonary shunts.[106,107] Investigational trials of inhaled and oral formulations of treprostinil are ongoing.

Iloprost. Iloprost, an inhaled prostacyclin analogue, has been shown to improve exercise capacity and hemodynamic pulmonary variables in both 3-month and 1-year open, uncontrolled studies. Side effects included coughing, flushing, headache, and syncope. A larger 3-month, randomized, double-blind, placebo-controlled European trial with inhaled iloprost in patients with IPAH (NYHA/WHO functional class III and IV), PAH associated with collagen vascular disease, or CTEPH demonstrated an improvement in exercise capacity, NYHA functional class, and quality of life. When compared to baseline, hemodynamic variables were improved at 3 months when measured after iloprost inhalation, but disappeared 60 to 90 minutes after inhalation unless repeated. Therefore, owing to the drug's short half-life (20 to 25 minutes), 6 to 9 inhalations are required per day, with each inhalation taking 5 to 15 minutes' duration. Inhaled iloprost is FDA approved for use in patients with NYHA/WHO functional class III or IV.[108-110]

Beraprost. Beraprost is an orally active prostacyclin analogue that reaches peak concentration after 30 minutes with a half-life of 35 to 40 minutes. Two randomized, double-blind, placebo-controlled trials in patients in NYHA/WHO functional class II and III with PAH of various etiologies demonstrated improved exercise capacity after 3 and 6 months of beraprost therapy,[108] but not after 9 or 12 months.[109] The beneficial effects of beraprost may attenuate with time. Currently, beraprost is approved for use in Korea and Japan.

Endothelin Receptor Antagonists (Table 27-3)

Endothelins, a family of 21–amino acid peptides, play a major role in the regulation of vascular tone. In addition to exerting a direct vaso-

TABLE 27-3 ENDOTHELIN RECEPTOR ANTAGONISTS

	Drug Name (Trade Name)		
	Bosentan (Tracleer)	**Sitaxsentan**	**Ambrisentan**
Mechanism of elimination	Liver	Liver	Liver
Mode of delivery	Oral	Oral	Oral
Beginning dose (interval)	62.5 mg (2 times/day)	50-100 mg (once/day)	5 mg (once/day)
Dosing range (interval)	125 mg (2 times/day)	—	10 mg (once/day)
Half-life	5 hr	5-7 hr	—
Contraindications	Glyburide,* cyclosporin A*	—	—
Drug interactions	Drug inhibitors of CYP450†	Warfarin‡	
Side effects	Flushing, headache, liver function abnormalities, anemia, peripheral edema	Headache, peripheral edema, nausea, nasal congestion, dizziness, liver function abnormalities	Cough, headache, flushing, syncope
Pregnancy category	X	—	X
Monitoring	Monthly: aminotransferases and pregnancy test Every 3 months: hemoglobin	—	Monthly: aminotransferases and pregnancy test Every 3 months: hemoglobin
Annual cost	$39,105	—	—

*Glyburide increased the risk of elevated aminotransferases when taken with bosentan. Cyclosporine increased the serum level of bosentan when coadministered.
†Toxicity may increase when administered concomitantly with inhibitors of the cytochrome P-450 (CYP450) system.
‡Increased risk of bleeding when coadministered with sitaxsentan.

constrictor effect, ET-1 stimulates cellular proliferation of vascular smooth muscle cells, induces fibrosis, and acts as a proinflammatory mediator by enhancing the expression of adhesion molecules.[53-55] ET-1 from cultured endothelial cells is typically secreted from the luminal side of the cells toward adjacent smooth muscle cells, which contain specific endothelin receptors.[57]

Two endothelin receptors—ET_A receptors, which are located on pulmonary vascular smooth muscle cells, and ET_B receptors, which are expressed on both pulmonary vascular endothelial cells and smooth muscle cells—have been identified.[55,56,58] Activation of ET_A receptors induces vasoconstriction and proliferation of vascular smooth muscle cells, while ET_B receptors mediate pulmonary endothelin clearance and induce vasodilation through increased production of NO and prostacyclin.[58] ET_B receptors may, under some circumstances, contribute to vasoconstriction through receptors located on vascular smooth muscle cells. These vasoconstrictive actions may become more pronounced in the setting of PAH through the up-regulation of ET_B receptors.[63,64] Patients with IPAH have been found to have higher serum levels and arterial-to-venous ratios of ET-1. Patients with PAH due to congenital heart disease exhibit increased levels of ET_A receptor density and circulating serum levels of ET-1, which occasionally decrease after corrective cardiac surgery.[51,111]

Bosentan. Bosentan, an orally active dual endothelin receptor antagonist, has been studied in patients with idiopathic and scleroderma-associated PAH. This agent blocks both ET_A and ET_B receptor activity. Two, large, randomized, multicenter trials[112,113] led the FDA to approve bosentan for the treatment of PAH patients with functional class III or IV. The initial trial[112] of bosentan demonstrated a statistically significant improvement in the bosentan group as compared to placebo in 6MWT and pulmonary hemodynamics after 12 weeks of therapy. A larger second trial[113] showed improvement in cardiopulmonary hemodynamic variables, exercise capacity, and time to clinical worsening.

This agent is, however, associated with asymptomatic, dose-dependent hepatic aminotransferase elevations in some patients. Elevations up to eight times the upper limit of normal occurred in 3% of patients taking the 125-mg dose.[113] Additional potential side effects include anemia, edema, teratogenicity, male infertility, and testicular atrophy. Liver function tests need to be performed monthly owing to this potential of liver toxicity. In addition, hemoglobin/hematocrit should be monitored every 3 months, and a pregnancy test in women of childbearing age should be performed monthly.[70,113] Studies on long-term efficacy have demonstrated sustained improvement in functional class and pulmonary hemodynamics for at least 1 year and increased survival at 3 years.[114,115] Investigational trials of bosentan in PAH patients with functional class II and PAH associated with sickle cell disease and CTEPH are ongoing.

Sitaxsentan. Sitaxsentan, a selective, orally active ET_A receptor antagonist, has been studied in two placebo-controlled trials. The initial trial enrolled 178 patients with functional class II, III, or IV IPAH, connective tissue disease–associated PAH, or congenital heart disease–associated PAH. Patients received daily doses of either 100 mg or 300 mg of sitaxsentan. Both dosages improved exercise capacity as measured by 6MWT, functional class, and hemodynamics (PVR and cardiac index) after 12 weeks. The most common side effects observed in the study included headache, peripheral edema, nausea, nasal congestion, and dizziness. Participants in the trial also experienced elevated hepatic aminotransferases (up to >3 times the upper limit of normal in 5% of patients taking the 100-mg dose and 21% of patients taking the 300-mg dose). Owing to the unacceptably high incidence of elevated hepatic enzymes with the 300-mg dose, it was discontinued and a subsequent trial studied only 50-mg and 100-mg dosages. After a period of 18 weeks, patients taking 100 mg of sitaxsentan demonstrated an increased exercise capacity, whereas this improvement was not significant in the 50-mg group. The potential for interaction with warfarin metabolism is an issue for patients on both therapies. Sitaxsentan is currently under review by the FDA.[112,116]

Ambrisentan. Ambrisentan, another selective ET_A receptor antagonist, has recently been approved in the United States for the treatment of PAH. In the ARIES-I study of 202 patients with idiopathic PAH or PAH associated with connective tissue disease, ambrisentan improved 6MWD, symptoms, and brain natriuretic peptide level compared to placebo. Like the other endothelin receptor antagonists, ambrisentan predisposes to peripheral edema and nasal congestion. However, ambrisentan appears to have a greatly reduced incidence of hepatic enzyme elevations, although the FDA still mandates monthly liver function testing. Further trials are ongoing, including a study in patients with group 3 PAH (in the setting of lung diseases).[112,116]

Nitric Oxide and Phosphodiesterase Inhibitors

Nitric oxide is a potent vasodilator, platelet inhibitor, and antiproliferative agent, and it acts on the vascular smooth muscle cells by stimulating guanylyl cyclase, which leads to increased production of intracellular cGMP. The vasodilatory effects of intracellular cGMP are

TABLE 27-4 PHOSPHODIESTERASE

	Sildenafil (Revatio)
Mode of delivery	Oral
Beginning dose (interval)	20 mg (3 times/day)
Dosing range (interval)	20 mg (3 times/day)
Half-life	2-4 hr
Contraindications	Nitrates
Drug interactions	α-Blockers, ketoconazole, erythromycin, cimetidine
Side effects	Headaches, flushing, dyspepsia, nasal congestion, epistaxis
Pregnancy category	B
Annual cost	$9,360

relatively short lived because of its rapid degradation by PDEs. PDE-5 gene expression and activity are increased in the pulmonary vasculature in patients with chronic pulmonary hypertension.[15,68,117]

Sildenafil. Sildenafil, an erectile dysfunction medication, is a highly specific PDE-5 inhibitor that acutely reduces pulmonary artery pressure in patients with PAH and both augments and prolongs the effects of inhaled NO.[118] In the first double-blind, placebo-controlled study of sildenafil, 278 PAH patients (IPAH or PAH related to connective tissue disease or repaired congenital heart disease) were randomized to receive either 20-, 40-, or 80-mg doses of sildenafil three times per day. All three dosage groups demonstrated an increased 6MWT distance at 12 weeks, and, of the 222 patients who continued therapy for 1 year, this improvement was sustained. Most patients who continued therapy with active drug for 1 year were increased to 80 mg three times per day. Side effects included headache, flushing, dyspepsia, and epistaxis. In 2005, sildenafil was approved for use in patients with functional class III or IV PAH at a dose of 20 mg three times daily (Table 27-4).[119] Studies of other phosphodiesterase inhibitors (e.g., tadalafil) are ongoing in PAH.

Combination Therapy

With the development of therapeutic agents with different mechanisms of action, considerable interest has developed in the possibility of combination therapy. The goal of combination therapy would be to maximize efficacy while minimizing toxicity. A small placebo-controlled trial examined the effect of adding bosentan or a placebo to IV epoprostenol therapy in patients with IPAH or PAH related to connective tissue disease (functional class III or IV). The trial failed to show any significant difference with the combination therapy.[120] Preliminary studies suggest that the pulmonary antihypertensive effects of sildenafil may enhance and prolong the effects of inhaled iloprost.[121] Owing to the different mechanisms of action of currently approved therapies, it is likely that combination therapies will provide at least additive benefit in functional improvement and, perhaps, survival. Further studies need to be performed before combination therapy is a standard treatment option for PAH.

Interventional and Surgical Therapies

Different interventional and surgical techniques have been developed over the past 20 years to treat PAH. The main interventions include atrial septostomy, pulmonary endarterectomy, and lung transplantation. Graded balloon dilation atrial septostomy is indicated in patients with persistent right ventricular heart failure and/or recurrent syncope who have failed conventional medical therapy and have no other therapeutic options or are awaiting lung transplantation.[122,123] Atrial septostomy creates a right-to-left shunt that increases cardiac output, augments systemic oxygen transport, reduces afterload, and improves right ventricular failure. This procedure has been performed mainly in patients with IPAH with an overall procedure-related mortality of 5.4%.[124] In most studies, exercise endurance and the symptoms and signs of right ventricular heart failure improve after atrial septostomy, but the impact on long-term survival is unknown.[124,125]

Transplantation

For patients who do not respond to conventional therapy, transplantation should be considered. Since the waiting time for transplantation is usually of long duration, patients who have not responded to IV epoprostenol therapy as determined by right heart catheterization have a guarded prognosis and should proceed to transplantation evaluation.[99,101] Serial 6MWTs and CPET may be useful in determining the appropriate timing for transplantation. Patients with a 6MWT distance of less than 332 m have a 1-year mortality of 40%, and patients with a peak oxygen uptake of 10.4 ml/kg per minute and a peak systolic blood pressure of 120 mm Hg have a 1-year mortality of 50% and 70%, respectively. Only 23% of patients survive for 1 year if both peak oxygen uptake and peak blood pressure values are reduced.[19,125]

Transplantation procedures currently being performed in patients with PAH include single-lung, bilateral-lung, and heart-lung transplantation. No randomized trials have been performed to evaluate the relative efficacy of different transplantation procedures, so significant debate and practice variability exist between individual centers.[126,127] Single-lung transplantation is more readily available, is an easier procedure to perform, and usually requires less ischemic and cardiopulmonary bypass time, but has an increased chance of V/Q mismatch and reperfusion injury.[126-128] Yet, despite the potentially large V/Q imbalance with single-lung transplantation, early 30-day survival rates have been similar to those observed for bilateral-lung transplantation. Although not statistically significant, increased posttransplantation survival rates have been observed in bilateral-lung transplantation recipients registered in the International Society for Heart and Lung Transplantation database. This survival advantage in posttransplantation IPAH patients was observed at all time points up to 9 years. Initially by providing better overall lung function, bilateral-lung transplantation may be protective against common manifestations of chronic rejection. A survival benefit of heart-lung transplantation over single-lung or bilateral-lung transplantation has not been clearly elucidated.[129,130]

Therapeutic Approach

Therapy for PAH has been recently addressed in detail in major consensus documents,[96] which provide an evidence-based therapeutic algorithm (Fig. 27-5). The algorithms are restricted to patients with WHO functional class III or IV because they represent the largest population included in controlled clinical trials. In addition, the different treatments have been evaluated mainly in sporadic IPAH patients and in patients with PAH associated with scleroderma or anorexigen use. Extrapolation of these recommendations to the other PAH subgroups should be done with caution. Both uncontrolled and controlled clinical trials with different medications and procedures are reviewed, graded, and compared in order to define an efficacy-to–side effect ratio for each treatment.

Emerging Targets and Therapeutics

There are at least five potentially promising and novel treatments that have been studied in animal models and human tissue. All the therapies appear to prevent and reduce pulmonary arterial medial hyperplasia through their antiproliferative and/or proapoptotic effects: serotonin transporter inhibitors by blocking serotonin uptake; dichloroacetate by activating K_v channels; simvastatin by preventing activation of small guanosine triphosphatases (GTPases); imatinib (STI571) by preventing phosphorylation of the platelet-derived growth factor (PDGF) receptor; and Bay58-2667 and Bay41-2272 by stimulating or activating guanylyl cyclase.

Serotonin, a known systemic vasodilator and pulmonary vasoconstrictor, is one of the more promising therapeutic targets because of its known actions in pulmonary artery endothelial and smooth muscle

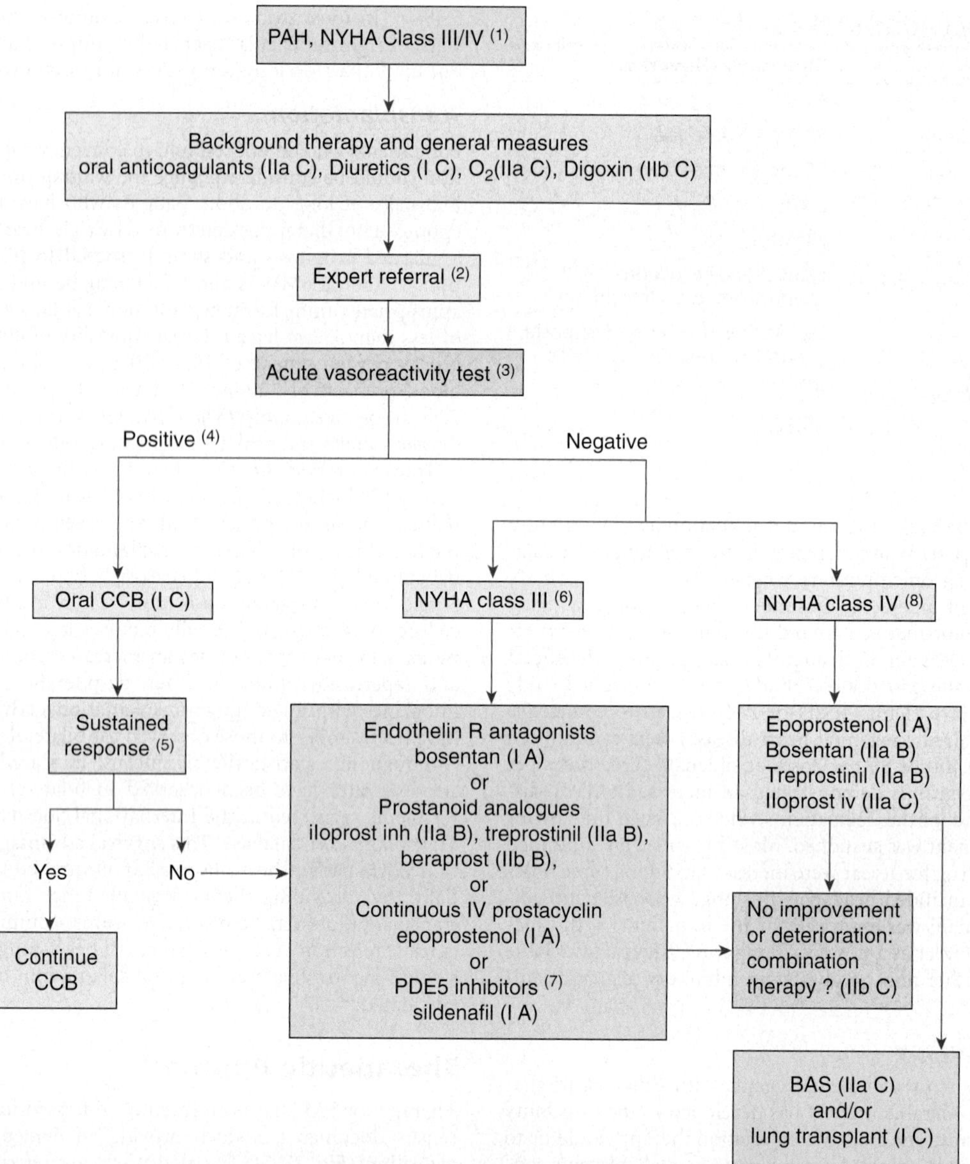

FIGURE 27-5 • Evidence-based treatment algorithm. (1) The algorithm is restricted to patient in NYHA functional class III or IV because they represent the largest population included in controlled clinical trials. For NYHA class I or II, very few data are available. In addition, the different treatments have been evaluated mainly in sporadic idiopathic pulmonary arterial hypertension (IPAH) patients, and in PAH associated with scleroderma or anorexigen use. Extrapolation of these recommendations to the other PAH subgroups should be done with caution. (2) Due to the complexity of the acute vasoreactivity tests, and of the treatment options available, it is strongly recommended that consideration be given to referral of patients with PAH to a specialized center. (3) Acute vasoreactivity test should be performed in all patients with PAH even if the greater incidence of positive response is achieved in patients with IPAH and PAH associated with anorexigen use. (4) A positive acute response to vasodilators is defined as a fall in mean pulmonary artery pressure of at least 10 mm Hg up to ≤40 mm Hg, with an increased or unchanged cardiac output during acute challenge with inhaled NO, iv epoprostenol, or iv adenosine. (5) Sustained response to CCB is defined as patients being in NYHA functional class I or II with near-normal hemodynamics after several months of treatment. (6) In patients in NYHA functional class III, first-line therapy may include oral endothelin receptor antagonists, chronic IV epoprostenol, or prostanoid analogues. (7) At the time of writing, sildenafil is not approved for PAH by any regulatory agency. (8) Most experts consider that NYHA functional class IV patients in unstable condition should be treated with iv epoprostenol (survival improvement, worldwide experience, and rapidity of action). A, B, and C grading are according to Box 27-3. CCB, calcium channel blockers; inh, inhaled; iv, continuous intravenous; PDE, phophodiesterase; R, receptors. (From The Task Force on Diagnosis and Treatment of Pulmonary Arterial Hypertension of the European Society of Cardiology. Guidelines on diagnosis and treatment of pulmonary arterial hypertension. Eur Heart J 2004;25:2243-2278.)

cells. It has been shown to cause acute vasoconstriction in pulmonary arteries in both rodents and humans through interactions with 5-$HT_{1B/1D}$ and 5-HT_{2A} receptors. 5-HT also has been strongly implicated in pulmonary vascular remodeling by directly promoting smooth muscle hypertrophy and hyperplasia. In cultured rat pulmonary artery smooth muscle cells, fluoxetine and paroxetine, selective serotonin transporter gene (5-HTT) inhibitors, blocked 5-HTT expression and mitogenic response to serotonin. Similar results were seen in cultured human pulmonary artery smooth muscle cells.[58,131-134]

Another common pathway mediating both vasoconstriction and vascular remodeling is the pulmonary artery smooth muscle cell cytosolic calcium ion concentration. Increased calcium stimulates smooth muscle cell contraction and proliferation. Cellular movement of calcium is controlled by K_v channels, which are sensitive to hypoxia. Dichloroacetate, an inhibitor of mitochondrial pyruvate dehydrogenase kinase, has been shown to increase potassium current in ischemic rat cardiac cells, which led to decreased vasoconstriction. Therefore, by up-regulating potassium channels through multiple signaling pathways, dichloroacetate might be able to reverse vascular remodeling.[135-139]

An additional potential therapeutic target for the prevention and treatment of PAH is the use of simvastatin, a hydroxymethylglutaryl-coenzyme A reductase inhibitor. By competitively inhibiting the synthesis of the cholesterol precursor molecule mevalonate and the intermediate isoprenoid molecules, simvastatin causes an accumulation of inactive GTPases in the cytosol that will attenuate vascular smooth muscle proliferation. These statin drugs may also have beneficial effects in PAH by up-regulating endothelial NO synthesis. Due to the promising animal study results that demonstrated a decrease in hypoxia-induced PAH in chronically hypoxic rats, an open-label observational study of simvastatin in patients with varying types of PAH was undertaken. Patients received 20 to 80 mg of the simvastatin daily and, over 3 months, the majority of patients showed an improvement in cardiopulmonary hemodynamic parameters and exercise capacity.[140-144]

Progression of PAH is associated with increased proliferation and migration of pulmonary vascular smooth muscle cells. PDGF, a potent mitogen and chemoattractant for smooth muscle cells, has been shown to be an important contributor to the development and progression of PAH. Expression of the PDGF receptor was found to be significantly increased in the lung tissue of patients with PAH. Daily treatment with imatinib (STI571), a PDGF receptor antagonist, was shown to reduce right heart hypertrophy, improve cardiac output, reverse pulmonary vessel proliferation, and improve survival in rats with monocrotaline-induced PAH. Similar results were observed in chronically hypoxic mice, which were treated with imatinib after development of PAH. Most likely, the PDGF-inhibitory capacity of imatinib occurs through prevention of phosphorylation of the PDGF receptor and subsequent suppression of the downstream signaling pathways.[145-148] Emerging case reports of left ventricular dysfunction in some patients receiving imatinib for malignancies raise concern for its suitability for the treatment of PAH, in which right ventricular dysfunction is such a major feature.

Chronic hypoxia causes structural and functional changes in the pulmonary arterial vasculature leading to increased vasomotor tone and the chronic remodeling of resistant vessels in PAH. NO, which is synthesized by endothelial NO synthase, is a potent vasodilator and considered to play an important role in regulating pulmonary vascular tone through the regulation of soluble guanylate cyclase (sGC), which synthesizes cGMP. Bay41-2272, a compound that stimulates sGC directly and enhances the sensitivity of sGC to NO, was shown to partially reverse the structural changes induced by hypoxia and monocrotaline in both rats and mice with PAH. It has also been shown to augment the vasodilative response to inhaled NO in acute pulmonary hypertension in lambs. Another compound, Bay58-2667, which activates sGC in its oxidized or heme-free form, showed similar results in mice and rats with PAH. Most likely the reversal in systolic pulmonary artery pressure and right heart hypertrophy is due to increased levels of cGMP that lead to acute vasodilation and antiaggregation and chronic vascular remodeling.[6,149-152]

Current treatment of PAH is evolving based on an understanding of the complicated and multifactorial pathogenesis of the disease. Yet, despite the major advances in the treatment of PAH, it still remains a disorder with high morbidity and mortality, making it all the more important to continue to focus on new potential pathways that might lead to novel future therapies.

REFERENCES

1. Runo JR, Loyd JE. Primary pulmonary hypertension. Lancet 2003;361:1533-1544.
2. Voelkel NF, Tuder RM, Weir EK. Pathophysiology of primary pulmonary hypertension. In Rubin LJ, Rich S (eds): Primary Pulmonary Hypertension: Lung Biology in Health and Disease. New York: Marcel Dekker, 1997, pp. 83-129.
3. Simonneau G, Galie N, Rubin LJ, et al. Clinical classification of pulmonary hypertension. J Am Coll Cardiol 2004;43:5S-12S.
4. Pietra GG, Capron F, Stewart S, et al. Pathologic assessment of vasculopathies in pulmonary hypertension. J Am Coll Cardiol 2004;43:25S-32S.
5. Pietra GC. The pathology of primary pulmonary hypertension. In Rubin LJ, Rich S (eds): Primary Pulmonary Hypertension: Lung Biology in Health and Disease. New York: Marcel Dekker, 1997, pp 19-61.
6. Humbert M, Morrell NW, Archer SL, et al. Cellular and molecular pathobiology of pulmonary arterial hypertension. J Am Coll Cardiol 2004;43:13S-24S.
7. Rubin LJ. Primary pulmonary hypertension. N Engl J Med 1997;336:111-117.
8. McGoon M, Gutterman D, Steen V, et al. Screening, early detection and diagnosis of pulmonary arterial hypertension: ACCP evidence-based clinical practice guideline. Chest 2004;126(1 Suppl):14S-34S.
9. Gaine SP, Rubin LJ. Primary pulmonary hypertension. Lancet 1998;352:719-725.
10. Rich S, Dantzker DR, Ayres SM, et al. Primary pulmonary hypertension: a national prospective study. Ann Intern Med 1987;107:216-223.
11. Barst RJ. Medical therapy of pulmonary hypertension: an overview of treatment and goals. Clin Chest Med 2001;22:509-515.
12. Fishman AP. Clinical classification of pulmonary hypertension. Clin Chest Med 2001;22:385-391.
13. Humbert M, Nunes H, Sitbon O, et al. Risk factors for pulmonary arterial hypertension. Clin Chest Med 2001;22:459-475.
14. Steen V, Medsger TA Jr. Predictors of isolated pulmonary hypertension in patients with systemic sclerosis and limited cutaneous involvement. Arthritis Rheum 2003;48:516-522.
15. Azarian R, Wartski M, Collignon MA, et al. Lung perfusion scans and hemodynamics in acute and chronic pulmonary embolism. J Nucl Med 1997;38:980-983.
16. Worsley DF, Palevsky HI, Alavi A. Ventilation-perfusion lung scanning in the evaluation of pulmonary hypertension. J Nucl Med 1994;35:793-796.
17. D'Alonzo GE, Bower JS, Dantzker DR. Differentiation of patients with pulmonary and thromboembolic pulmonary hypertension. Chest 1984;85:457-461.
18. Moser KM, Auger WR, Fedullo PF. Chronic major-vessel thromboembolic pulmonary hypertension. Circulation 1990;81:1735-1743.
19. Miyamoto S, Nagaya N, Satoh T, et al. Clinical correlates and prognostic significance of six-minute walk test in patients with primary pulmonary hypertension: comparison with cardiopulmonary exercise testing. Am J Respir Crit Care Med 2000;161:487-492.
20. Rubin LJ, Badesch DB. Evaluation and management of the patient with pulmonary arterial hypertension. Ann Intern Med 2005;143:282-293.
21. Paciocco G, Martinez F, Bossone E, et al. Oxygen desaturation on the six-minute walk test and mortality in untreated primary pulmonary hypertension. Eur Respir J 2001;17:647-652.
22. Hoeper MM, Oudiz RJ, Peacock A, et al. Endpoints and clinical trial designs in pulmonary arterial hypertension: clinical and regulatory perspectives. J Am Coll Cardiol 2004;43:48S-55S.
23. Humbert M, Sitbon O, Simonneau G. Treatment of pulmonary arterial hypertension. N Engl J Med 2004;351:1425-1436.
24. Fuster V, Steele PM, Edwards WD, et al. Primary pulmonary hypertension: natural history and the importance of thrombosis. Circulation 1984;70:580-587.
25. Ley S, Krietner KF, Fink C, et al. Assessment of pulmonary hypertension by CT and MR imaging. Eur Radiol 2004;14:359-368.
26. Rich S, Kaufmann E, Levy PS. The effect of high doses of calcium-channel blockers on survival in primary pulmonary hypertension. N Engl J Med 1992;327:76-81.
27. Rich S, Brundage BH. High-dose calcium channel-blocking therapy for primary pulmonary hypertension: evidence for long-term reduction in pulmonary arterial pressure and regression of right ventricular hypertrophy. Circulation 1987;76:135-141.
28. Raffy O, Azarian R, Brenot F, et al. Clinical significance of the pulmonary vasodilator response during short-term infusion of prostacyclin in primary pulmonary hypertension. Circulation 1996;93:484-488.
29. Barst RJ, Maislin G, Fishman AP. Vasodilator therapy for primary pulmonary hypertension in children. Circulation 1999;99:1197-1208.
30. Nootens M, Kaufmann E, Rich S. Short-term effectiveness of nifedipine in secondary pulmonary hypertension. Am J Cardiol 1993;71:1475-1476.
31. Owens GR, Fino GJ, Herbert DL, et al. Pulmonary function in systemic sclerosis: comparison of CREST syndrome variant with diffuse scleroderma. Chest 1983;84:546-550.
32. Rubin LJ, Mendoza J, Hood M, et al. Treatment of primary pulmonary hypertension with continuous intravenous prostacyclin (epoprostenol): results of a randomized trial. Ann Intern Med 1990;112:485-491.
33. Jeffery TK, Morrell NW. Molecular and cellular basis of pulmonary vascular remodeling in pulmonary hypertension. Prog Cardiovasc Dis 2002;45:173-202.
34. Cool CD, Stewart JS, Werahera P, et al. Three-dimensional reconstruction of pulmonary arteries in plexiform pulmonary hypertension using cell-specific markers: evidence for a dynamic and heterogeneous process of pulmonary endothelial cell growth. Am J Pathol 1999;155:411-419.
35. Abenhaim L, Moride Y, Brenot F, et al. Appetite-suppressant drugs and the risk of primary pulmonary hypertension. N Engl J Med 1996;335:609-616.
36. Tuder RM, Flook BE, Voelkel NF. Increased gene expression for VEGF and the VEGF receptors KDR/Flk and Flt in lungs exposed to acute or chronic hypoxia: modulation of gene expression by nitric oxide. J Clin Invest 1995;95:1798-1807.
37. Yeager ME, Halley GR, Golpon HA, et al. Microsatellite instability of endothelial cell growth and apoptosis genes within plexiform lesions in primary pulmonary hypertension. Circ Res 2001;88:e2-e11.
38. Simonneau G, Fartoukh M, Sitbon O, et al. Primary pulmonary hypertension associated with the use of fenfluramine derivatives. Chest 1998;114(Suppl 3):195S-199S.
39. Martin KB, Klinger JR, Rounds SIS. Pulmonary arterial hypertension: new insights and new hope. Respirology 2006;11:6-17.
40. Chazova I, Loyd JE, Zhdanov VS, et al. Pulmonary artery adventitial changes and venous involvement in primary pulmonary hypertension. Am J Pathol 1995;146:389-397.
41. Stenmark KR, Gerasimovskaya E, Nemenoff RA, et al. Hypoxic activation of adventitial fibroblasts: role in vascular remodeling. Chest 2002;122:326S-334S.
42. Davie NJ, Crossno JT Jr, Frid MG, et al. Hypoxia-induced artery adventitial remodeling and neovascularization: contribution of progenitor cells. Am J Physiol Lung Cell Mol Physiol 2004;286:L668-L678.

43. Giaid A, Saleh D. Reduced expression of endothelial nitric oxide synthase in the lungs of patients with pulmonary hypertension. N Engl J Med 1995;333:214-221.
44. Yuan JX, Wang J, Juhaszova M, et al. Attenuated K^+ channel gene transcription in primary pulmonary hypertension. Lancet 1998;351:726-727.
45. Weir EK, Reeve HL, Huang JMC, et al. Anorexic agents aminorex, fenfluramine, and dexfenfluramine inhibit potassium current in rat pulmonary vascular smooth muscle and cause pulmonary vasoconstriction. Circulation 1996;94:2216-2220.
46. Herve P, Humbert M, Sitbon O, et al. Pathobiology of pulmonary hypertension: the role of platelets and thrombosis. Clin Chest Med 2001;22:451-458.
47. Christman BW, McPherson CD, Newman JH, et al. An imbalance between the excretion of thromboxane and prostacyclin metabolites in pulmonary hypertension. N Engl J Med 1992;327:70-75.
48. McQuillan LP, Leung GK, Marsden PA, et al. Hypoxia inhibits expression of eNOS via transcriptional and posttranscriptional mechanisms. Am J Physiol Heart Circ Physiol 1994;267:H1921-H1927.
49. Allen SW, Chatfield BA, Koppenhafer SA, et al. Circulating immunoreactive endothelin-1 in children with pulmonary hypertension: association with acute hypoxic pulmonary vasoreactivity. Am Rev Respir Dis 1993;148:519-522.
50. Giaid A, Yanagisawa M, Langleben D, et al. Expression of endothelin-1 in the lungs of patients with pulmonary hypertension. N Engl J Med 1993;328:1732-1739.
51. Vincent JA, Ross RD, Kassab J, et al. Relation of elevated plasma endothelin in congenital heart disease to increased pulmonary blood flow. Am J Cardiol 1993;71: 1204-1207.
52. Stewart DJ, Levy RD, Cernacek P, et al. Increased plasma endothelin-1 in pulmonary hypertension: marker or mediator of disease? Ann Intern Med 1991;114:464-469.
53. Yanagisawa M, Kurihara H, Kimura S, et al. A novel potent vasoconstrictor peptide produced by vascular endothelial cells. Nature 1988;332:411-415.
54. Hirata Y, Takagi Y, Fukuda Y, et al. Endothelin is a potent mitogen for rat vascular smooth muscle cells. Artherosclerosis 1989;78:225-228.
55. Fagan KA, McMutry IF, Rodman DM. Role of endothelin-1 in lung disease. Respir Res 2001;2:90-101.
56. DiCarlo VS, Chen SJ, Meng QC, et al. ETA-receptor antagonist prevents and reverses chronic hypoxia-induced pulmonary hypertension in rat. Am J Physiol Lung Cell Mol Physiol 1995;269:L690-L697.
57. Yoshimoto S, Ishizaki Y, Sasaki T, et al. Effect of carbon dioxide and oxygen on endothelin production by cultured porcine cerebral endothelial cells. Stroke 1991;22:378-383.
58. Benigni A, Remuzzi G. Endothelin antagonists. Lancet 1999;353:133-138.
59. Lee SL, Wang WW, Lanzillo JJ, et al. Serotonin produces both hyperplasia and hypertrophy of bovine pulmonary artery smooth muscle cells in culture. Am J Physiol Lung Cell Mol Physiol 1994;266:L46-L52.
60. Herve P, Launay JM, Scrobohaci ML, et al. Increased plasma serotonin in primary pulmonary hypertension. Am J Med 1995;99:249-254.
61. Petkov V, Mosgoeller W, Ziesche R, et al. Vasoactive intestinal peptide as a new drug for treatment of primary pulmonary hypertension. J Clin Invest 2003;111:1339-1346.
62. Tuder RM, Cool CD, Geraci MW, et al. Prostacyclin synthase expression is decreased in lungs from patients with severe pulmonary hypertension. Am J Respir Crit Care Med 1999;159:1925-1932.
63. Dupuis J, Jasmin JF, Prie S, et al. Importance of local production of endothelin-1 and of the ET_B receptor in the regulation of pulmonary vascular tone. Pulm Pharmacol Ther 2000;13:135-140.
64. Kuc R, Davenport A. Endothelin-A receptors in human aorta and pulmonary arteries are downregulated in patients with cardiovascular disease: an adaptive response to increased levels of endothelin-1? J Cardiovasc Pharmacol 2000;36(Suppl 1):S377-S379.
65. German Z, Chambliss KL, Pace MC, et al. Molecular basis of cell-specific endothelial nitric-oxide synthase expression in airway epithelium. J Biol Chem 2000;275:8133-8139.
66. Ghofani HA, Pepke-Zaba J, Barbera JA, et al. Nitric oxide pathway and phosphodiesterase inhibitors in pulmonary arterial hypertension. J Am Coll Cardiol 2004;43:68S-72S.
67. Ide H, Nakano H, Ogasa T, et al. Regulation of pulmonary circulation by alveolar oxygen tension via airway nitric oxide. J Appl Physiol 1999;87:1629-1636.
68. Beavo JA. Cyclic nucleotide phosphodiesterases: functional implications of multiple isoforms. Physiol Rev 1995;75:725-748.
69. Ahn HS, Foster M, Cable M, et al. Ca/CaM-stimulated and cGMP-specific phosphodiesterases in vascular and non-vascular tissues. Adv Exp Med Biol 1991;308:191-197.
70. McLaughlin VV, McGoon MD. Pulmonary arterial hypertension. Circulation 2006;114:1417-1431.
71. Maruno K, Absood A, Said SI. VIP inhibits basal and histamine-stimulated proliferation of human airway smooth muscle cells. Am J Physiol Lung Cell Mol Physiol 1995;268:L1047-L1051.
72. Loscalzo J. Genetic clues to the cause of primary pulmonary hypertension. N Engl J Med 2001;345:367-371.
73. Massague J, Chen YG. Controlling TGF-beta signaling. Genes Dev 2000;14:627-644.
74. Shi Y, Massague J. Mechanisms of TGF-beta signaling from cell membrane to the nucleus. Cell 2003;113:685-700.
75. Stewart DJ. Bone morphogenetic protein receptor-2 and pulmonary arterial hypertension: unraveling a riddle inside an enigma? Circ Res 2005;96:1033-1035.
76. Lane KB, Machado RD, Pauciulo MW, et al. Heterozygous germ-line mutations in BMPR2, encoding a TGF-β receptor, cause familial primary pulmonary hypertension. The International PPH Consortium. Nat Genet 2000;26:81-84.
77. Thomson JR, Machado RD, Pauciulo MW, et al. Sporadic primary pulmonary hypertension is associated with germline mutations of the gene encoding BMPR-II, a receptor member of the TGF-β family. J Med Genet 2000;37:741-745.
78. Newman JH, Wheeler L, Lane KB, et al. Mutation in the gene for bone morphogenetic protein receptor II as a cause of primary pulmonary hypertension in a large kindred. N Engl J Med 2001;345:319-324.
79. Newman JH, Trembath RC, Morse JA, et al. Genetic basis of pulmonary arterial hypertension: current understanding and future directions. J Am Coll Cardiol 2004;43:33S-39S.
80. Loyd JE, Butler MG, Foroud TM, et al. Genetic anticipation and abnormal gender ratio at birth in familial primary pulmonary hypertension. Am J Respir Crit Care Med 1995;152:93-97.
81. Farber HW, Loscalzo J. Pulmonary arterial hypertension. N Engl J Med 2004;351:1655-1665.
82. Deng Z, Morse JH, Slager SL, et al. Familial primary pulmonary hypertension (gene *PPH1*) is caused by mutations in the bone morphogenetic protein receptor-II gene. Am J Hum Genet 2000;67:737-744.
83. Eddahibi S, Humbert M, Fadel E, et al. Serotonin transporter overexpression is responsible for pulmonary artery smooth muscle hyperplasia in primary pulmonary hypertension. J Clin Invest 2001;108:1141-1150.
84. MacLean MR, Herve P, Eddahibi S, et al. 5-Hydroxytryptamine and the pulmonary circulation: receptors, transporters and relevance to pulmonary arterial hypertension. Br J Pharmacol 2000;131:161-168.
85. Eddahibi S, Chaouat A, Morrell N, et al. Polymorphism of the serotonin transporter gene and pulmonary hypertension in chronic obstructive pulmonary disease. Circulation 2003;108:1839-1844.
86. Mark EJ, Patalas ED, Chang HT, et al. Fatal pulmonary hypertension associated with short-term use of fenfluramine and phenteramine. N Engl J Med 1997;337:602-606.
87. Rich S, Rubin L, Walker AL, et al. Anorexigens and pulmonary hypertension in the United States: results from the Surveillance of North American Pulmonary Hypertension. Chest 2000;117:870-874.
88. Albertson TE, Walby WF, Derlet RW. Stimulant-induced pulmonary toxicity. Chest 1995;108:1140-1149.
89. Dumas JP, Bardou M, Goirand F, Dumas M. Hypoxic pulmonary vasoconstriction. Gen Pharmacol 1999;33:289-297.
90. Sweeney M, Yuan JX. Hypoxic pulmonary vasoconstriction: role of voltage-gated potassium channels. Respir Res 2000;1:40-48.
91. Trembath RC, Thomson JR, Machado RD, et al. Clinical and molecular genetic features of pulmonary hypertension in patients with hereditary hemorrhagic telangiectasia. N Engl J Med 2001;345:325-334.
92. Chaouat A, Coulet F, Favre C, et al. Endoglin germline mutation in a patient with hereditary haemorrhagic telangiectasia and dexfenfluramine associated pulmonary arterial hypertension. Thorax 2004;59:446-448.
93. Marvin K, Spellberg RD. Pulmonary hypertension secondary to thrombocytosis in a patient with myeloid metaplasia. Chest 1993;103:642-644.
94. Rostagno C, Prisco D, Abbate R, et al. Pulmonary hypertension associated with long-standing thrombocytosis. Chest 1991;99:1303-1305.
95. Sandoval J, Aguirre JS, Pulido T, et al. Nocturnal oxygen therapy in patients with Eisenmenger syndrome. Am J Respir Crit Care Med 2001;164:1682-1687.
96. The Task Force on Diagnosis and Treatment of Pulmonary Arterial Hypertension of the European Society of Cardiology. Guidelines on diagnosis and treatment of pulmonary arterial hypertension. Eur Heart J 2004;25:2243-2278.
97. Barst RJ, Rubin LJ, Long WA, et al. A comparison of continuous intravenous epoprostenol (prostacyclin) with conventional therapy for primary pulmonary hypertension. The Primary Pulmonary Hypertension Study Group. N Engl J Med 1996;334: 296-302.
98. Badesch DB, Tapson VF, McGoon MD, et al. Continuous intravenous epoprostenol for pulmonary hypertension due to the scleroderma spectrum of disease: a randomized, controlled trial. Ann Intern Med 2000;132:425-434.
99. Stibon O, Humbert M, Nunes H, et al. Long-term intravenous epoprostenol infusion in primary pulmonary hypertension: prognostic factors and survival. J Am Coll Cardiol 2002;40:780-788.
100. Barst RJ, Rubin LJ, McGoon MD, et al. Survival in primary pulmonary hypertension with long-term continuous intravenous prostacyclin. Ann Intern Med 1994;121:409-415.
101. Shapiro SM, Oudiz RJ, Cao T, et al. Primary pulmonary hypertension: improved long-term effects and survival with continuous intravenous epoprostenol infusion. J Am Coll Cardiol 1997;30:343-349.
102. McLaughlin VV, Shillington A, Rich S. Survival in primary pulmonary hypertension: the impact of epoprostenol therapy. Circulation 2002;106:1477-1482.
103. Rosenzweig EB, Kerstein D, Barst RJ. Long-term prostacyclin for pulmonary hypertension with associated congenital heart defects. Circulation 1999;99:1858-1865.
104. Kuo PC, Johnson LB, Plotkin JS, et al. Continuous intravenous infusion of epoprostenol for the treatment of portopulmonary hypertension. Transplantation 1997;63: 604-606.
105. Aquilar RV, Farber HW. Epoprostenol (prostacyclin) therapy in HIV-associated pulmonary hypertension. Am J Respir Crit Care Med 2000;162:1846-1850.
106. Badesch DB, McLaughlin VV, Delcroix M, et al. Prostanoid therapy for pulmonary arterial hypertension. J Am Coll Cardiol 2004;43:56S-61S.
107. Simonneau G, Barst RJ, Galie N, et al. Continuous subcutaneous infusion of treprostinil, a prostacyclin analogue, in patients with pulmonary arterial hypertension: a double-blind randomized, placebo-controlled trial. Am J Respir Crit Care Med 2002;165:800-804.

108. Olschewski H, Ghofrani HA, Schmehl T, et al. Inhaled iloprost to treat severe pulmonary hypertension: an uncontrolled trial. German PPH Study Group. Ann Intern Med 2000;132:435-443.
109. Hoeper MM, Schwarze M, Ehlerding S, et al. Long-term treatment of primary pulmonary hypertension with aerosolized iloprost, a prostacyclin analogue. N Engl J Med 2000;342:1866-1870.
110. Olschewski H, Simonneau G, Galie N, et al. Inhaled iloprost for severe pulmonary hypertension. N Engl J Med 2002;347:322-329.
111. Ishikawa S, Miyauchi T, Sakai S, et al. Elevated levels of plasma endothelin-1 in young patients with pulmonary hypertension caused by congenital heart disease are decreased after successful surgical repair. J Thorac Cardiovasc Surg 1995;110:271-273.
112. Barst RJ, Langleben D, Frost A, et al. Sitaxsentan therapy for pulmonary arterial hypertension. Am J Respir Crit Care Med 2004;169:441-447.
113. Beavo JA, Reifsnyder DH. Primary sequence of cyclic nucleotide phosphodiesterase isozymes and the design of selective inhibitors. Trends Pharmacol Sci 1990;11:150-155.
114. Sitbon O, Badesch DB, Channick RN, et al. Effects of the dual endothelin antagonist bosentan in patients with pulmonary arterial hypertension: a 1-year follow-up study. Chest 2003;124:247-254.
115. McLaughlin V, Sitbon O, Rubin LJ, et al. The effect of first-line bosentan on survival in patients with primary pulmonary hypertension. Am J Respir Crit Care Med 2003;167:A442.
116. Barst R, Langleben D, Badesch D, et al. Treatment of pulmonary arterial hypertension with the selective endothelin-A receptor antagonist sitaxsentan. J Am Coll Cardiol 2006;47:2049-2056.
117. Braner DA, Fineman JR, Chang R, et al. M&B 22948, a cGMP phosphodiesterase inhibitor, is a pulmonary vasodilator in lambs. Am J Physiol Heart Circ Physiol 1993;264:H252-H258.
118. Michalakis E, Tymchak W, Lien D, et al. Oral sildenafil is an effective and specific pulmonary vasodilator in patients with pulmonary arterial hypertension: comparison with inhaled nitric oxide. Circulation 2002;105:2398-2403.
119. Galie N, Ghofani HA, Torbicki A, et al. Sildenafil citrate therapy for pulmonary arterial hypertension. N Engl J Med 2005;353:2148-2157.
120. Humbert M, Barst RJ, Robbins IM, et al. Combination of bosentan with epoprostenol in pulmonary arterial hypertension: BREATHE-2. Eur Respir J 2004;24:353-359.
121. Ghofrani HA, Wiedemann R, Rose F, et al. Combination therapy with oral sildenafil and inhaled iloprost for severe pulmonary hypertension. Ann Intern Med 2002;136:515-522.
122. Rothman A, Slansky MS, Lucas VW, et al. Atrial septostomy as a bridge to lung transplantation in patients with severe pulmonary hypertension. Am J Cardiol 1999;84:682-686.
123. Sandoval J, Rothman A, Pulido T. Atrial septostomy for pulmonary hypertension. Clin Chest Med 2001;22:547-560.
124. Sandoval J, Gaspar J, Pulido T, et al. Graded balloon dilation atrial septostomy in severe primary pulmonary hypertension: a therapeutic alternative for patients nonresponsive to vasodilator treatment. J Am Coll Cardiol 1998;32:297-304.
125. Wensel R, Opitz CF, Anker SD, et al. Assessment of survival in patients with primary pulmonary hypertension: importance of cardiopulmonary exercise testing. Circulation 2002;106:319-324.
126. Doyle RL, McCrory D, Channick RN, et al. Surgical treatments/interventions for pulmonary arterial hypertension: ACCP evidence-based clinical practice guidelines. Chest 2004;126:63S-71S.
127. Pielsticker EJ, Martinez FJ, Rubenfire M. Lung and heart-lung transplant practice patterns in pulmonary hypertension centers. J Heart Lung Transplant 2001;20:1297-1304.
128. Boujoukos AJ, Martich GD, Vega JD, et al. Reperfusion injury in single lung transplant recipients with pulmonary hypertension and emphysema. J Heart Lung Transplant 1997;16:439-448.
129. Hertz MI, Mohacsi PJ, Taylor DO, et al. The registry of the International Society for Heart and Lung Transplantation: introduction to the twentieth official reports. J Heart Lung Transplant 2003;22:610-615.
130. Bando K, Armitage JM, Paradis IL, et al. Indications for and results of single, bilateral, and heart-lung transplantation for pulmonary hypertension. J Thorac Cardiovasc Surg 1994;108:1056-1065.
131. MacLean MR, Clayton RA, Templeton AG, et al. Evidence for 5-HT1-like receptor-mediated vasoconstriction in human pulmonary artery. Br J Pharmacol 1996;119:277-282.
132. MacLean MR, Sweeney G, Baird M, et al. 5-Hydroxytryptamine receptors mediating vasoconstriction in pulmonary arteries from control and pulmonary hypertensive rats. Br J Pharmacol 1996;119:917-930.
133. Marcos E, Adnot S, Pham MH, et al. Serotonin transporter inhibitors protect against hypoxic pulmonary hypertension. Am J Respir Crit Care Med 2003;168:487-493.
134. Pitt BR, Weng W, Steve AR, et al. Serotonin increases DNA synthesis in rat proximal and distal pulmonary vascular smooth muscle cells in culture. Am J Physiol Lung Cell Mol Physiol 1994;266:L178-L186.
135. Mauban JRH, Remillard CV, Yuan JX-J. Hypoxic pulmonary vasoconstriction: role of ion channels. J Appl Pysiol 2005;98:415-420.
136. Large WA. Receptor-operated $Ca2^+$ permeable nonselective cation channels in vascular smooth muscle: a physiologic perspective. J Cardiovasc Electrophysiol 2002;13:493-501.
137. Stacpoole PW. The pharmacology of dichloroacetate. Metabolism 1989;38:1124-1144.
138. Rozanski GJ, Xu Z, Zhang K, et al. Altered K^+ current of ventricular myocytes in rats with chronic myocardial infarction. Am J Physiol Heart Circ Physiol 1998;274:H259-H265.
139. Yuan XJ, Wang J, Juhaszova M, et al. Attenuated K^+ channel gene transcription in primary pulmonary hypertension. Lancet 1998;351:726-727.
140. Takemoto M, Liao JK. Pleiotrophic effects of 3-hydroxy-3-methylglutaryl coenzyme A reductase inhibitor. Arterioscler Thromb Vasc Biol 2001;21:1712-1719.
141. Laufs U, Marra D, Node K, et al. 3-Hydroxy-3-methylglutaryl-CoA reductase inhibitors attenuate vascular smooth muscle proliferation by preventing rhoGTPase-induced down-regulation of p27Kipl. J Biol Chem 1999;274:21926-21931.
142. Walter DH, Dimmeler S, Zeiher AM. Effects of statins on endothelium and endothelial progenitor cell recruitment. Semin Vasc Med 2004;4:385-393.
143. Girgis RE, Li D, Zhan X, et al. Attenuation of chronic hypoxic pulmonary hypertension by simvastatin. Am J Physiol Heart Circ Physiol 2003;285:H938-H945.
144. Kao PN. Simvastatin treatment of pulmonary hypertension: an observational case series. Chest 2005;127:1446-1452.
145. Balasubramaniam V, LeCras TD, Ivy DD, et al. Role of platelet-derived growth factor in vascular remodeling during pulmonary hypertension in the ovine fetus. Am J Physiol Lung Cell Mol Physiol 2003;284:L826-L833.
146. Yu Y, Sweeney M, Zhang S, et al. PDGF stimulates pulmonary vascular smooth muscle cell proliferation by upregulating TRPC6 expression. Am J Physiol Cell Physiol 2003;284:C316-C330.
147. Humbert M, Monti G, Fartoukh M, et al. Platelet-derived growth factor expression in primary pulmonary hypertension: comparison of HIV seropositive and HIV seronegative patients. Eur Respir J 1998;11:554-559.
148. Schermuly RT, Dony E, Ghofrani HA, et al. Reversal of experimental pulmonary hypertension by PDGF inhibition. J Clin Invest 2005;115:2811-2821.
149. Boerrigter G, Costello-Boerrigter LC, Cataliotti A, et al. Cardiorenal and humoral properties of a novel direct soluble guanylate cyclase stimulator BAY 41-2272 in experimental congestive heart failure. Circulation 2003;107:686-689.
150. Evgenov OV, Ichinose F, Evgenov NV, et al. Soluble guanylate cyclase activator reverses acute pulmonary hypertension and augments the pulmonary vasodilator response to inhaled nitric oxide in awake lambs. Circulation 2004:110:2253-2259.
151. Stasch JP, Schmidt P, Alonso-Alija C, et al. NO- and haem-independent activation of soluble guanylyl cyclase: molecular basis and cardiovascular implications of a new pharmacological principle. Br J Pharmacol 2002;136:773-783.
152. Dumitrascu R, Weissmann N, Ghofrani H, et al. Activation of soluble guanylate cyclase reverses experimental pulmonary hypertension and vascular remodeling. Circulation 2006;113:286-295.

28

ASTHMA AND CHRONIC OBSTRUCTIVE PULMONARY DISEASE

Walter K. Kraft and Frank T. Leone

INTRODUCTION 417
PHYSIOLOGY 417
PATHOPHYSIOLOGY 419
Cell Types Involved in Inflammation 419
Mediators of Inflammation 419
DISEASE CHARACTERISTICS AND CLASSIFICATION 419
THERAPEUTICS AND CLINICAL PHARMACOLOGY 420
Goals of Therapy 420
Specific Agents 420
β-Agonists 420
Anticholinergics 423
Corticosteroids 424
Leukotriene Modifiers 426
Chromones 428
Xanthines 428
INTEGRATED PHARMACOTHERAPEUTIC APPROACH TO THE ASTHMATIC OR COPD PATIENT 429
Special Populations 430
Pregnancy 430
Pediatrics 430
Alternative Therapies 430
Novel Targets 430

INTRODUCTION

Asthma is a disease of reversible airflow obstruction manifested by wheezing, breathlessness, chest tightness, and cough. Mucosal edema and airway lumen obstruction by mucus contribute to this process, particularly in severe disease, but the primary mechanism underlying airflow obstruction is bronchial smooth muscle contraction with hyperresponsiveness and exaggerated responses to environmental stimuli. Symptoms can be persistent or intermittent and can aggressively worsen in an acute exacerbation (Table 28-1). Signs and symptoms primarily reflect inflammation, and long-term disease control relies on its continuous suppression. Pharmacotherapy of the asthmatic patient encompasses a two-pronged approach employing drugs that cause bronchorelaxation for immediate symptomatic relief paired with those that attenuate the inflammation that mediates bronchial hyperresponsiveness.

The syndrome complex characterizing asthma shares features with chronic obstructive pulmonary disease (COPD). Besides having differing etiologies from patients with asthma, COPD patients have varying degrees of irreversible airflow obstruction, based upon loss of parenchyma (emphysema) and a decreased capacity for gas exchange, coupled with small airway obstructive bronchiolitis. Many patients will exhibit overlap in obstructive lung disease phenotype, such as irreversible decline in lung function in some asthmatics or modest reversibility of airflow obstruction in COPD patients. In that context, asthma encompasses numerous subtypes that manifest many of the same symptoms and pathophysiology but differ in etiology, presentation, and response to treatment.[1] Subtypes include exercise- or aspirin-induced, cough variant, occupational and environmental, adult-onset and childhood, all with varying degrees of severity (Table 28-2). This heterogeneity, in part, reflects different patterns of expression of inflammatory mediators, genetic variability, and environmental exposure. Despite these differences, a consensus exists for a unified treatment based upon disease severity. Clearly identifiable clinical subtypes have long been recognized in COPD. There is some treatment overlap with asthma, though with some differences based upon pathophysiology and concomitant medical illnesses. Unless otherwise specified, treatments discussed in this chapter apply to both asthma and COPD.

PHYSIOLOGY

Pulmonary ventilation is analogous to a bellows device, in which contraction of muscles that surround the thorax—primarily the diaphragm and external intercostal muscles—expands the chest wall and generates negative intrathoracic pressure, filling the lungs with air during inspiration. Relaxation of these muscles, coupled with the elastic recoil of the lung, mediates the passive outflow of air under conditions of normal breathing. Within the lung, individual airways are surrounded by smooth muscle. These muscles contract and narrow the lumen in the presence of low carbon dioxide (CO_2) partial pressures or upon exposure to chemical and mechanical irritants. Endogenous triggers of airway constriction include histamine, leukotrienes, and thromboxane, as well as other ligands such as serotonin and acetylcholine. In contrast, bronchodilation is induced by activation of the sympathetic nervous system or by local decreases in the partial pressure of oxygen (O_2).

Baseline airway tone is governed by a circadian pattern, with highest tone at night and during early morning hours, which, in part, underlies the clinical observation of worsening asthmatic symptoms in the predawn hours. Overall control of bronchial airway tone is mediated by the autonomic nervous system (Fig. 28-1). It should be noted that asthma and COPD are not disorders of dysfunctional autonomic control in lungs, though the importance of this system as a therapeutic target is demonstrated by the dramatic clinical efficacy of sympathetic agonists and muscarinic antagonists. The parasympathetic system primarily controls bronchial tone under usual conditions. Of the five identified muscarinic receptor subtypes,[2] M_1, M_2, and M_3 are expressed in lung. M_3 richly innervates smooth muscle mostly in larger airways,[3] and its activation induces bronchoconstriction.[4] Also, preganglionic vagus nerve cholinergic innervation is primarily located in larger airways, although local nonvagal release of acetylcholine occurs in the face of an inflammatory stimulus in other parts of the lung.[5] Of significance, asthma generally affects smaller, rather than larger, airways.[6] M_2 serves as an inhibitory autoreceptor in a feedback loop to modulate basal tone. In the setting of asthmatic inflammation, especially eosinophil-mediated cytokine release, loss of M_2 inhibitory function likely contributes to bronchial constriction.[7]

TABLE 28-1 ASTHMA DISEASE SEVERITY STRATIFICATION AND TREATMENT OUTLINE

Severity	Symptoms	Nocturnal Symptoms	Lung Function	Treatment
Mild intermittent	Symptoms ≤ twice a week Normal PEF when asymptomatic Exacerbations brief; intensity may vary Nighttime symptoms	≤ Twice a month	FEV_1 or PEF ≥80% predicted FEV_1/FVC ratio normal	SABA
Mild persistent	Symptoms < twice a week but < once a day Exacerbations may affect activity	> Twice a month	FEV_1 or PEF ≥80% predicted FEV_1/FVC ratio normal	Low dose ICS (alternate: LTI or mast cell stabilizer)
Moderate persistent	Daily symptoms and daily use of inhaled SABA Exacerbations affect activity Exacerbations ≥ twice a week; may last days.	> Once a week	FEV_1 or PEF >60% to <80% predicted FEV_1/FVC ratio reduced 5%	Low dose ICS + LABA or medium dose ICS (alternate: low dose ICS + LTI)
Severe persistent	Continual symptoms that limit physical activity Frequent exacerbations	Frequent	FEV_1 or PEF ≤ 60% predicted FEV_1/FVC ratio reduced > 5%	Medium dose ICS + LABA (alternate: medium dose ICS + LTI) If not controlled, high dose ICS + LABA and consider oral corticosteroids at lowest possible dose and/or omalizumab (for patients with allergies).

FEV_1, forced expiratory volume in one minute; FVC, forced vital capacity; ICS, inhaled corticosteroid; LABA, long acting beta agonist; LTI, leukotriene inhibitor; PEF, peak expiratory flow; SABA, short acting beta agonist.
Adapted from NAEPP Expert Panel Report 3: Guidelines for the Diagnosis and Management of Asthma, 2007.

TABLE 28-2 COPD SEVERITY STRATIFICATION AND TREATMENT OUTLINE

Stage: Severity	Lung Function	Intervention
1: Mild	FEV_1/FVC < 70% predicted FEV_1 ≥ 80% predicted	Add short-acting bronchodilator (as needed) Reduce risk factors (smoking cessation and immunization)
2: Moderate	FEV_1/FVC < 70% predicted 50% predicted ≤ FEV_1 ≤ 80% predicted	Add treatment with one or more long-acting bronchodilators Add rehabilitation
3: Severe	FEV_1/FVC < 70% predicted 30% predicted ≤ FEV_1 ≤ 50% predicted	Add inhaled corticosteroids if repeated exacerbations
4: Very severe	FEV_1/FVC < 70% predicted FEV_1 ≤ 30% predicted or FEV_1 ≤ 50% predicted with chronic respiratory failure	Add long-term oxygen therapy

COPD, chronic obstructive pulmonary disease; FEV_1, forced expiratory volume in 1 min; FVC, functional vital capacity.
Adapted from Global Initiative for Chronic Obstructive Lung Disease, Global Strategy for the Diagnosis, Management, and Prevention of Chronic Obstructive Pulmonary Disease, 2006.

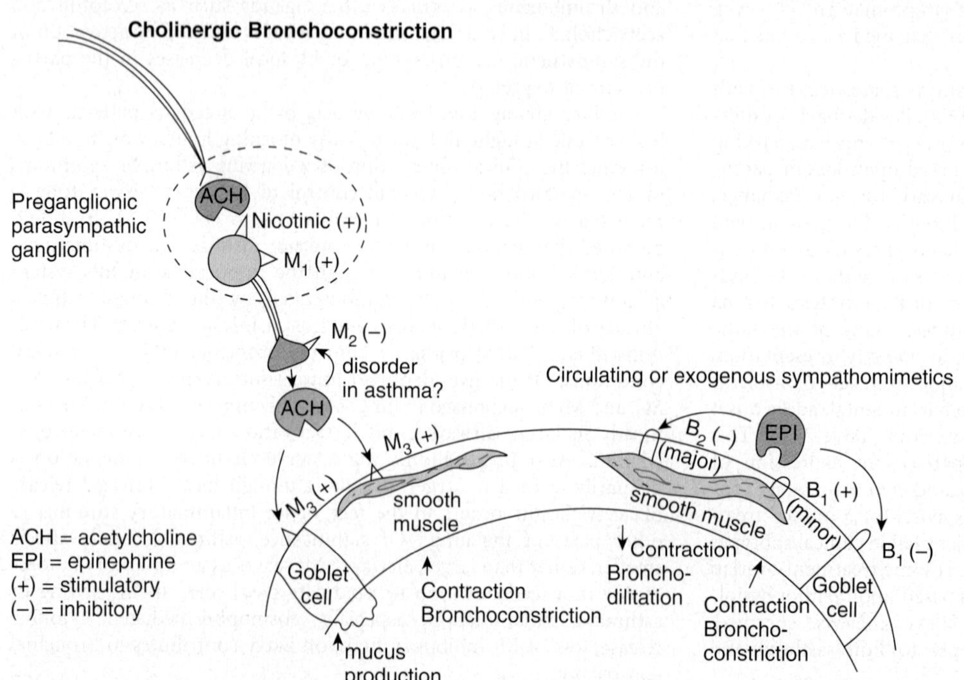

FIGURE 28-1 • Normal control of bronchial tone.

Sympathetic control of bronchial tone is mediated by the β_2-adrenergic receptors, whose activation induces intracellular signaling through heterotrimeric G proteins. In human lung, the ratio of β_1- to β_2-adrenergic receptors is approximately 3:1,[8] with β_1 receptors localized to submucosal glands. β_2 receptors are more widely distributed on bronchial and vascular smooth muscle and epithelium, in addition to localization on submucosal glands. Activation of the β_2 receptor on airway smooth muscle leads to bronchodilation of large and small airways. In contrast to the cholinergic system, direct sympathetic innervation of smooth muscle is limited and β_2 receptors expressed by bronchial smooth muscle respond primarily to circulating endogenous agonists. Airway dilation by sympathetic innervation reflects a physiologic require-ment for increased cardiopulmonary activity (e.g., in "fight or flight" states) associated with elevated sympathetic tone and circulating epinephrine.

PATHOPHYSIOLOGY

Asthma is often a disease of waxing and waning intensity, with exacerbation of symptoms often following exposure to an inducing stimulus (e.g., an allergen, cold air, or a viral respiratory infection). The primary perturbations within the lung during an acute asthmatic exacerbation include bronchial hyperreactivity with airway constriction, mucus secretion, and peribronchial edema. These factors increase intra-alveolar and intrathoracic pressure and resistance to expiratory flow, associated with characteristic signs, including expiratory wheezes, and symptoms, including dyspnea and cough. The etiology of these changes is the inflammatory cascade, which follows a predictable pattern during an acute exacerbation. However, the disease often involves longer-term subacute inflammation, especially in poorly controlled asthma. Although cellular changes and symptoms are reversible between episodes or with adequate anti-inflammatory treatment, asthmatic lungs exhibit remodeling, with increased bronchial smooth muscle density and the presence of subepithelial fibrosis. The degree to which remodeling occurs varies between patients, and its precise relationship to inflammation, long-term decline in lung function, and prevention with treatment remains unclear.[9]

Like asthmatics, COPD patients also are subject to acute worsening of airflow obstruction. However, the disease is characterized by significantly less reversibility of obstruction between acute exacerbations. The expiratory outflow obstruction is also mediated by inflammation causing small airway obstruction, as well as a characteristic destruction of lung parenchyma called *emphysema*. This process causes loss of recoil in the lung and collapse of airways, obstructing the outflow of air during exhalation as well as causing disturbances in gas exchange not typically seen in asthma. The limited regenerative properties of the lung lead to the chronic and fixed nature of airflow obstruction.

Cell Types Involved in Inflammation

Inflammation is present in mild, moderate, and severe asthma. The cell types that contribute to asthmatic inflammation are protean. The most important include mast cells, T lymphocytes, eosinophils, and immunoglobulin E (IgE)–producing B lymphocytes. In addition, neutrophils, basophils, and macrophages are involved, as well as cell types not previously considered to be mediators of inflammation, such as bronchial epithelial cells, endothelial cells, smooth muscle cells, and myofibroblasts. All of these cell types can secrete mediators that propagate the asthmatic process. Moreover, T helper lymphocytes (Th) have two phenotypes—Th1 cells associated with cell-mediated immunity and Th2 cells associated with allergic responses—and a perturbation in their balance may be a key element in the etiology of asthma. The lower incidence of asthma in the developing world and in children who attend day care centers suggests that exposure to infectious diseases at a young age may protect against the development of asthma. This process, known as the "hygiene hypothesis," may reflect a shift in the balance of Th to a Th2 phenotype. At the cellular level, Th2 coordinate asthmatic inflammation, primarily by the production of cytokines such as interleukin (IL)-3, -4, -5, -6, -10 and -13 that direct cell recruitment and responses. Eosinophils drive the asthmatic inflammatory process, and infiltration of airways by these cells is common in both acute and chronic asthma. Eosinophils appear to play an especially important role in mild to moderate asthma. Neutrophils play a larger role in severe, near-fatal, and steroid-resistant asthma relative to milder forms and in smokers.[10] Recruitment of neutrophils is mediated primarily by epithelial cell–derived IL-8 and leukotrienes.[11] Neutrophilic inflammation is generally resistant to attenuation by corticosteroids.

Atopy—allergic responses and IgE production to aeroallergens—is a common feature in asthma, particularly in asthma with an onset in childhood. Of asthmatic patients, approximately 90% suffer from allergic rhinitis.[12] An inhaled allergen binds and cross-links two mast cell–bound IgE molecules, leading to immediate degranulation of preformed mediators, such as histamine and tryptase, and the synthesis of new mediators such a leukotriene C4 (LTC_4) and prostaglandin D_2 (PGD_2). Levels of IgE antibodies have been correlated with severity of disease. There are, however, individuals with asthma without evidence of allergy. The molecular mechanisms underlying the inflammatory process in these "intrinsic asthmatic" patients appears similar to that in atopic asthmatics,[13] including the involvement of IgE.[14] In addition, the pulmonary inflammation is often persistent in atopic asthmatics, even in the absence of ongoing exposure to allergen. The precise relationship between asthma and allergic rhinitis has yet to be fully elucidated, but there is considerable overlap with respect to incidence and cell types mediating inflammatory processes. Indeed, an allergen challenge administered only in the nose or lung will cause inflammatory changes in the reciprocal unchallenged organ, demonstrating a unifying systemic basis for etiology and treatment and highlighting the importance of anti-inflammatory therapy in the entire airway.

In contrast to asthma, the cell types mediating COPD include primarily neutrophils, macrophages, and CD8+ T cells (Tc1). Exposure to tobacco and biomass smoke (generally from cooking fires in the developing world) is a strong driver of this divergent inflammatory process. A key concept is a disruption of the normal balance of proteases and antiproteases. The increase in serine and cysteine proteases and matrix metalloproteinases, coupled with decreased antiproteases, results in the characteristic tissue loss of COPD. The disease generally affects distal more than proximal airways relative to asthma, and the inflammatory process is less responsive to corticosteroids. Whereas these differences in the inflammatory milieu are characteristic of the general phenotypes, there is overlap in inflammatory mechanisms. Inflammation in asthmatic smokers and those with severe asthma shares many of the characteristics of COPD and, accordingly, some of the same responses to treatment.

Mediators of Inflammation

More than 100 mediators of inflammation have been identified in patients with obstructive lung diseases[15] including amine- and lipid-derived mediators, peptides, cytokines, chemokines, small molecules, and proteases. These mediators can increase bronchial reactivity, cause plasma leak, increase mucus secretion, activate neurons, induce sloughing of the airway epithelium, and induce fibrosis, all of which contribute to the characteristic symptoms. In addition, other mediators recruit inflammatory cells to continue this process. In asthma, eotaxin, IL-4, IL-5, and IL-13 predominate, whereas in COPD, IL-8, tumor necrosis factor-α (TNF-α), IL-1β, and IL-6 play key roles. The complexity of interactions between cell types and mediators accounts for the observation that drugs targeting one mediator alone will generally not control obstructive symptoms as well as drugs that affect multiple cell types and mediators.

DISEASE CHARACTERISTICS AND CLASSIFICATION

No single diagnostic criterion defines either asthma or COPD. Expiratory wheezing is common in both, but it is neither sensitive nor specific for diagnosis. Common symptoms include cough, difficulty in breathing, and recurrent chest tightness. In asthma, these symptoms are usually variable, intermittent, and often worse at night and after exercise; viral infections; or exposure to animal dander, cold air, or other environmental factors. An objective assessment of airflow obstruction can be obtained by spirometry, specifically, the volume of air exhaled in 1 second, the *forced expiratory volume* (FEV_1), and the *forced vital capacity* (FVC), the amount of air exhaled after maximal inhalation. Characteristic features of obstruction include a decreased FEV_1 and a decreased FEV_1/FVC ratio. In asthma, these can be normal in between symptomatic exacerbations. Obstruction is characteristically reversed by drugs that act as bronchodilators, and generally diffusion capacity, measured clinically by the use of inhaled carbon monoxide (DLco), is normal. Also, patients with asthma demonstrate airflow obstruction after inhalation of histamine or the cholinergic agonist methacholine at lower concentrations than do nonasthmatics (Box 28-1). COPD, in contrast, has a component of fixed obstruction, minimal improvement with bronchodilators, and impaired diffusion capacity. Peak expiratory flow (PEF) is often used as a surrogate for spirometry, because measurement of flow is easier to obtain than that of volume and can be easily performed by patients. The use of spirometry aids not only in the diagnosis of asthma and COPD but also in stratification of disease severity and assessment of response to treatment. The proper identification and stratification of patients based upon disease severity is a critical element driving treatment choices and is an absolute requirement for quality asthma care (see Tables 28-1 and 28-2).[16] Patients classified at any level of severity can have mild, moderate, or severe acute exacerbations. Some patients with intermittent asthma can experience severe acute exacerbations separated by long periods of normal lung function and no symptoms.

BOX 28-1 INHALED DELIVERY OF DRUGS

Chronic obstructive pulmonary disease (COPD) has systematic effects, but the primary pathology is limited to the airways. Asthma is a disease limited to the airways. Drug delivery by inhalation has the advantage of maximizing local concentration of drug to the organ of interest and minimizing systemic drug exposure. Systemic drug exposure generally provides little in the way of efficacy but is responsible for the majority of drug-associated adverse effects. Some drugs, such as the chromones and anticholinergics, are efficacious only by the inhaled route. Others, such as the leukotriene modifiers, have limited nonpulmonary targets and are thus better suited for oral administration. β-Agonists are available in both inhaled and systemic forms, but are more preferably administered by the inhaled route. The same is true of corticosteroids, with the exception of an acute exacerbation. In this case the doses delivered by inhalation are inadequate and systemic administration is required.

Unlike volatile anesthetics, which are true gases dosed in partial pressures, inhaled drugs for obstructive lung disease delivered are solutions or suspensions that are aerosolized into small inhaled droplets, or are dry particulate powders. Solutions can be nebulized using pressured air or an ultrasonic piezoelectric element. A mist of droplets is generated that is passively inhaled with normal tidal breathing. Droplet or powder size is an important determinant of the degree to which a drug is deposited in the lung. The ideal size for drug deposition is between 1 μm and 5 μm. Smaller particles are generally exhaled, whereas larger droplets are deposited in the oropharynx.

Whereas patients often subjectively feel that the nebulized delivery of drug provides superior symptom relief, direct comparisons between delivery devices in aggregate have shown little difference in terms of therapeutic efficacy. This does not suggest that the choice of a device does not matter in the individual patient, because operator characteristics and training are critical for proper technique.[17] Whereas studies comparing devices were conducted in individuals who had demonstrated proficiency in the use of a particular device, in actual practice, device choices should be individualized. Pediatric or demented patients and those with poor hand-eye coordination are more appropriate candidates for nebulized therapy, which require less operator intervention. Conversely, metered-dose inhaler (MDI) devices are convenient and cost effective and have demonstrated excellent clinical outcomes, even in the setting of acute asthma in the emergency department.

THERAPEUTICS AND CLINICAL PHARMACOLOGY

Goals of Therapy

The specific goals of pharmacologic therapy in the patient with asthma and COPD are improvement in the hallmark symptoms and a reduction in the rate of exacerbations. Another goal is improvement in lung function, specifically FEV_1 and PEF. Optimal therapy combines control of inflammation with shorter-term control of symptoms. The more prominent *quick-relief medications* are those that relax bronchial smooth muscle (bronchodilators) and provide symptomatic relief but do not decrease the inflammatory process at the root of the asthmatic response. These drugs are used in conjunction with *long-term control medications,* which provide long-term control of asthma but do not produce immediate symptom relief. Anti-inflammatory drugs reduce markers of airway inflammation in airway tissue or secretions. These changes ultimately lead to a decrease in airway responsiveness. Corticosteroids offer the most efficacious long-term control in asthma because they provide broad anti-inflammatory effects involving multiple cell types, whereas other therapies target specific mediators (such as the leukotrienes) or specific cell types and functions (such as the inhibition of mediator release from mast cells). Bronchodilators with long half-lives can also serve as controller medications, but they do not control underlying inflammation.

Specific Agents

β-Agonists

Background. Activation of β_2 receptors in the lung provides therapeutic benefit in obstructive lung diseases primarily by relaxation of constricted bronchial smooth muscle. Moreover, β_2-agonists prevent bronchoconstriction when delivered prior to exposure to an allergic or chemical trigger, a process known as *bronchoprotection*. The sympathomimetic alkaloids ephedrine and pseudoephedrine from the plant *ma huang* have been used in traditional Chinese medicine for respiratory ailments for 2000 years.[18] The development of modern specific β_2-agonists is a historical example of medicinal chemists exploiting the structure-activity relationship to improve agonist specificity for a pharmacologic target. A review of the sympathetic nervous system is covered in Chapter 8, Autonomic Pharmacology. Sympathomimetic agents were introduced into the therapeutic armamentarium at the beginning of the 20th century with the subcutaneous administration of epinephrine.[19] In addition to β_2-mediated therapeutic effects, epinephrine use is associated with tachycardia, hypertension, and arrhythmias owing to systemic activation of α and β_1 receptors. Development of the β-specific drug isoproterenol in the 1940s was a therapeutic advance, and indeed, characterization of its effects were important in the subsequent identification of α and β receptor subtypes. Target specificity increased in the 1960s with the development of the β_2-specific agonists albuterol[20] (known outside of the United States as salbutamol) and terbutaline.[21] Both are noncatechol derivatives of epinephrine, resulting from substitutions around the benzene ring. This structure confers resistance to the endogenous metabolic enzyme catechol-O-methyltransferase (COMT), resulting in a prolonged duration of action characterizing these compounds. Subsequently developed short-acting β_2 agonists as well as a specific *R* enantiomer (levalbuterol) have not offered major advantages over albuterol, and this drug remains the prototypic β_2-agonist. More recently, agents with longer durations of action, including salmeterol and formoterol, or improved receptor specificity, including levalbuterol, have been developed (Fig. 28-2). Whether these newer agents offer any therapeutic advantage remains to be defined. A list of commonly used β-agonists is presented in Table 28-3.

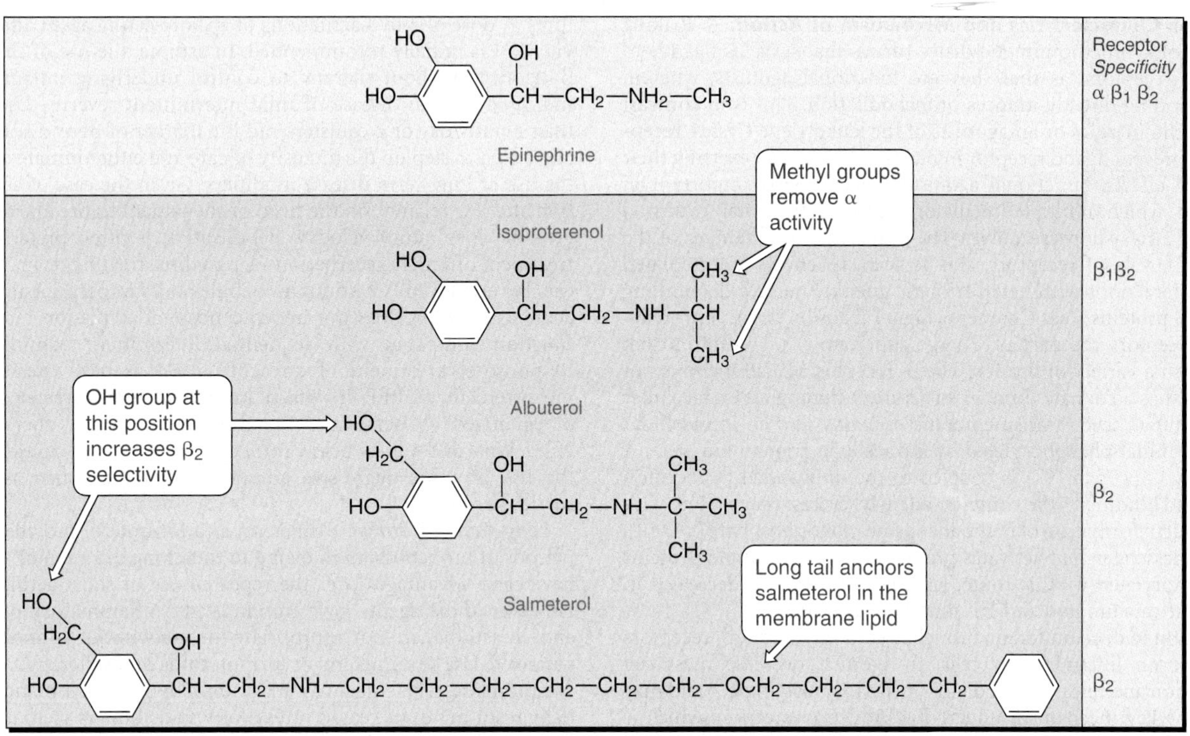

FIGURE 28-2 • Structural functional relationship of sympathomimetic amines.

TABLE 28-3 COMMONLY USED β_2-SPECIFIC AGONISTS

Chemical Name	Trade Name	Dosing Interval (hr)	Onset of Action (min)	Peak Activity (hr)	Duration of Action (hr)	Dosage Range	Comments
SHORT-ACTING*							
Albuterol (salbutamol) *MDI or nebulization*	Proventil; Ventolin; others	4-6	5	1-2	4-6	MDI: 180-720 mcg (2-8 inhalations) HFN: 2.5 mg	Most commonly used short-acting β_2-agonist
Albuterol *oral*	Volmax	6-8	30	2-3	6	2-4 mg	30 min onset of action compared with 5 min with inhaled albuterol
Pirbuterol	Maxair	4-6	5	0.5-1	5	MDI: 200-400 mcg (2 inhalations)	Breath-activated actuator device may be easier to use than pressured MDI
Metaproterenol	Alupent	3-4	5	1	2-4	MDI: 1300-1950 mcg (2-3 inhalations) HFN: 0.4% Solution	Oral formulations also available
LONG-ACTING							
Salmeterol	Serevent	12	30-50	2-4	12	Dry powder: 50-100 mcg (2 inhalations)	Clinical meaningful improvement in FEV_1 between 30 and 50 min
Formoterol	Foradil	12	5	1	12	Dry powder: 12 mcg (2 inhalations)	Clinical meaningful improvement in FEV_1 after 5 min
ENANTIOMER							
Levalbuterol	Xopenex	6-8	5	1.5	6	MDI: 90 mcg (2 inhalations) HFN: 0.63-12.5 mg	(R)-enantiomer of albuterol with similar pharmacokinetic and pharmacodynamic properties
Arformoterol	Brovana	12	5	1-3	12	HFN: 15 μg	(R,R)-enantiomer of formoterol

*Suggested dosage for chronic stable disease; increased dose and frequency are recommended in the setting of acute exacerbation FEV_1, forced expiratory volume in 1 min; HFN, high flow nebulization; MDI, metered-dose inhaler.

Receptor Characteristics and Mechanism of Action. A striking advantage of sympathomimetic drugs (drugs that serve as ligands to adrenergic receptors) is that they are functional agonists, wherein receptor binding directly induces bronchodilation. This is in contrast to the anticholinergics or antagonists of the leukotriene CysLt1 receptor, which prevent ligand receptor interactions, indirectly exerting their therapeutic effects. Functional agonism is particularly important in asthma, in which multiple mediators regulate the final common pathway of airway hyperreactivity. The β_2 receptor is a member of the adrenergic family of receptors, and as such, its effects are mediated through interactions with heterotrimeric guanine nucleotide–binding proteins (G proteins) (see Chapter 6, Signal Transduction). G protein–coupled receptors are part of a large superfamily of receptors that interact with a variety of ligands. The β_2 receptor, like all members of this family, has a cognate domain structure including an extracellular amino terminal, seven transmembrane domains, and an intracellular carboxy terminal phosphorylated by intracellular protein kinases.[22] A stimulatory G protein (G_s) is coupled to the unliganded β_2 receptor. Upon ligand binding to the complex, adenylyl cyclase is activated, with the subsequent formation of cyclic adenosine monophosphate (cAMP), a second messenger that activates protein kinase A. Multiple proteins are phosphorylated by this route, leading ultimately to decreases in intracellular calcium and smooth muscle relaxation.

In addition to distribution on bronchial smooth muscle, β_2 receptors are present on inflammatory cells. β_2-Agonists decrease mast cell degranulation and release of mediators, primarily histamine,[23] and may serve as one key mechanism underlying bronchoprotection, which is the prevention of bronchoconstriction prior to exposure to a usual trigger (such as cold air or aeroallergens). Whereas activation of β_2 receptors on eosinophils, T lymphocytes, macrophages, and neutrophils reduces release of inflammatory mediators in vitro, these receptors are rapidly down-regulated, and their contribution to the therapeutic actions of β_2-agonists is probably minimal. Also, β_2 receptors are located in postcapillary venules, and agonists likely reduce edema induced by the inflammatory asthmatic process.[24] However, in aggregate, the effects of β-agonists independent of bronchodilation are modest, and these agents should not be considered anti-inflammatory drugs.

Dose and Response Characteristics. Upon oral administration, albuterol exhibits an initial onset of bronchodilation after approximately 30 minutes and a peak effect at approximately 3 hours, with duration of action up to about 6 hours. In contrast, after inhalational delivery, most of the short-acting agents demonstrate about 70% of maximum bronchodilation within approximately 5 minutes in asthma and generally have a duration of action of approximately 6 hours. Onset of action is slower in COPD. Inhalational delivery of albuterol is associated with improved bronchodilation versus oral or sublingual administration, with significantly less tremor.[25,26] The dose of drug delivered to the lungs depends upon the delivery device and, in the case of a metered-dose inhaler (MDI) or dry powder, the proper administration technique of the patient. The usual dosage for albuterol is 2 to 4 puffs of an MDI every 4 to 6 hours as needed, with increased frequency in acute exacerbations. Evidence supports the use of inhaled albuterol, and by extension, all short-acting agents, on an as-needed rather than a scheduled basis.[27,28] In the setting of acute exacerbations, short-acting agents can be used at more frequent intervals. Albuterol is primarily biotransformed to a sulfate metabolite and requires no dosage adjustment for renal impairment. Albuterol pharmacokinetics have no significant race or sex differences.[29]

The onset of bronchodilation for salmeterol is slower than that for the short-acting agents, occurring 30 to 50 minutes after a dose with a maximum effect 2 to 3 hours after inhalation. Whereas the plasma half-life is approximately 3 to 4 hours, the clinical efficacy lasts for 12 hours. The duration of action for formoterol is similar to that of salmeterol, although the onset of action is more immediate (~5 min). Despite this faster onset of action, and theoretic potential in acute asthma exacerbation, there is not good evidence to support this for routine use.[29a]

Clinical Use

Quick Relief. Short-acting β_2-agonists are the mainstay treatment for immediate relief of both mild and severe obstructive airway symptoms. A dose of 2 to 4 actuations of a short-acting agent administered via MDI is initially recommended. In asthma, the use of short-acting β_2-agonists without therapy to control underlying inflammation is indicated only in disease of mild intermittent severity. Use of more than 2 puffs/day or 2 canisters/mo is a marker of poor disease control and a sign to step up the intensity of care and either initiate or increase the use of long-term disease modifiers. Given the ease of administration and less reliance on the need of the patient to breathe deeply and generate inspiratory velocity, nebulization is often preferred in the treatment of acute exacerbations. Up to three treatments in 20 minutes can be employed. Continuous nebulization is occasionally used in acute asthma but does not improve hospital admission rates or lung function compared with sequential intermittent administration.[30] Response to treatment of an acute attack is best assessed by the measurement of PEF, in which improvement to greater than 80% of predicted or personal-best values is considered therapeutically efficacious, and values below 50% suggest a poor response requiring the use of more aggressive adjunctive therapies, such as systemic corticosteroids.

Long-Acting Control. Salmeterol and formoterol provide extended periods of bronchodilation owing to their long duration of action and have clear advantages over the repeated use of short-acting agents.[31] However, these agents have minimal anti-inflammatory properties[32] and, in asthma, are not appropriate for use without an inhaled corticosteroid. Use of salmeterol or formoterol as monotherapy can provide symptomatic relief that may mask underlying inflammation, potentially resulting in increased rates of severe asthma exacerbation. Consensus guidelines endorse the use of a long-acting β_2-agonist as the preferred add-on agent for patients taking inhaled corticosteroids who need step-up of their asthma care.[33,34] In these patients, addition of a long-acting β_2-agonist demonstrated improved symptom control and lung function compared with the addition of a leukotriene antagonist or with placebo.[35,36] Similarly, the addition of a long-acting β_2-agonist (versus doubling of the dose of inhaled corticosteroids) improved symptoms, lung function, and use of rescue medications in most studies.[37,38] This synergy may, in part, reflect an increase in glucocorticoid receptors[39,40] or enhanced suppression of inflammatory genes.[41] However, no evidence indicates that outcomes in initial treatment of steroid-naïve patients are better with a combination of a long-acting β_2-agonist and an inhaled steroid compared with inhaled steroid alone. Thus, the role of the long-acting β_2-agonists in the treatment of asthma is as first-line adjunctive therapy to inhaled corticosteroids.[42] In COPD patients with poor reversibility of airway obstruction, evidence demonstrates that the long-acting β_2-agonists reduce exacerbations while improving lung function and quality of life.[43] As with asthma, the long-acting agents do not change the natural history of the disease or the rate of decline in FEV_1. In contrast to asthma, the long acting β_2-agonists can be used as monotherapy without inhaled corticosteroids given the reduced responsiveness of the diverse COPD inflammation to these agents.

Safety. The favorable short-term side effect profile of the β_2-agonists stems in part from the decreased density of β_2 receptors in skeletal muscle and the heart relative to the bronchial wall. The most commonly used β_2-agonists, such as albuterol and salmeterol, are partial agonists, with less than 5% of the intrinsic efficacy at the receptor compared with epinephrine. Thus, these drugs have a greater effect in bronchial smooth muscle cells, which exhibit high densities of β_2 receptors, than nontarget cells exhibiting lower densities of those receptors, especially when the drug is delivered by inhalation.[44] In all cases, systemic side effects can be decreased by use of the inhalational route of drug administration.

Tremor. The propensity for tremor varies among individuals, with older patients being more susceptible, although, in general, this effect is well tolerated. The onset of tremor mirrors that of bronchodilation and is delayed in salmeterol compared with albuterol.[45] Tremor is dose-dependent with larger doses used in acute exacerbations, although tachyphylaxis generally develops with chronic dosing.[46] Thus, tremor is primarily seen in acute administration of high doses or in patients with infrequent or intermittent use of β_2-agonists.

Tachyphylaxis. A disadvantage associated with the use of long-acting agents is the induction of tachyphylaxis, specifically, loss of the bronchoprotective effects of β_2-agonism. In contrast, there is clinically insignificant attenuation in the bronchodilatory properties of short-acting β_2-agonists. However, there is a decrement in bronchoprotection against allergic or induced bronchoprovocative challenges (methacholine, histamine) induced by β_2-agonists after chronic exposure to both long- and short-acting agents.[47] Individuals homozygous for arginine at locus 16 of the β_2 receptor are at greater risk for acute exacerbations than other genotypes, a process that may be related to loss of bronchoprotective effects.[48] In aggregate, the clinical significance of the attenuation of bronchoprotection remains unclear because this effect does not appear to be associated with loss of control of asthma, especially when concomitant inhaled corticosteroids are employed.[49]

Cardiovascular Effects. The heart contains a substantial complement of β_2 receptors. The clinical significance of these receptors in the setting of β-agonist use has not been elucidated. In clinical trials, tachycardia or palpitations were observed in 5% of patients receiving oral and 1% of those receiving aerosolized albuterol. Tachycardia is a greater concern in patients with preexisting cardiac disease and hypoxia, especially at higher doses associated with acute exacerbations. Whereas increased cardiovascular events have been suggested in asthma and COPD patients employing β_2-agonists,[50,51] the data are mixed,[52,53] and these agents are generally well tolerated even in patients with underlying cardiac disease. Based upon published data, if any effect exists, it would be of modest size.

The modest prolongation of the QTc interval caused by albuterol is mediated by its β_2-agonist activity and is a class effect.[54] Accordingly, salmeterol and formoterol prolong the QT interval, though only at approximately 10 times the clinically recommended dose. Adding albuterol to the long-acting β_2-agonist salmeterol causes little change in heart rate or QTc interval.[55] Thus, the clinical significance of QT prolongation with standard use is unclear, though at standard doses it is unlikely that β-agonists cause torsades des pointes. With the exception of sinus tachycardia, arrhythmias tend to be uncommon in patients with near-fatal asthma attacks, suggesting that the mechanism of death from a severe exacerbation is not a drug-induced arrhythmia.[56] However, it is prudent to use β_2-agonists sparingly in patients with congenital long QT syndromes.

Hypokalemia. Activation of β_2 receptors induces the movement of potassium from extracellular to intracellular compartments, and indeed, β_2-agonists are used in the acute treatment of hyperkalemia. As with tremor, decreases in potassium are dose dependent,[57] and tolerance to this effect develops with repeated use. Hypokalemia is more of a concern with patients who have underlying cardiac disease as an arrhythmogenic risk, especially those taking non–potassium-sparing diuretics.[58] Albuterol, salmeterol, and formoterol each decrease serum potassium by approximately 0.45 mEq/L. The duration of this effect is about 120 minutes for albuterol.[59]

Mortality. Soon after the widespread introduction of short-acting β_2-agonists, a number of case-control studies implicated these drugs as modestly increasing asthma-related mortality.[60-62] Postulated etiologies associated with prolonged exposure include loss of bronchoprotection, rebound bronchoconstriction, or undertreatment with effective anti-inflammatory agents owing to a masking of asthmatic symptoms. However, these data have often been contradictory and difficult to interpret. Because β_2-agonist use is a marker of disease severity, the effect appeared to be more strongly associated with specific agents or routes of delivery, and much of these data were collected in an era that predated the widespread use of inhaled corticosteroids.[63] More recent data in which long-acting agents were paired with inhaled steroids suggest that lung function and symptoms improve, with mixed data about effects on the rate of exacerbations.[42,64-66] However, the Salmeterol Multicenter Asthma Research Trial (SMART)[67] was halted early after 26,000 patients owing to poor enrollment, and an interim analysis of suggested treatment with salmeterol was associated with a small absolute increased risk of asthma-related deaths in African Americans. This finding is tempered by a decrease in asthma-related deaths in the United States following the introduction and widespread use of salmeterol in the early 1990s. Separate evidence suggests a subset of patients homozygous for arginine at the 16th amino acid position of the β_2-adrenergic receptor (Arg/Arg) may be at higher risk for exacerbations after chronic β_2 exposure, though there is no consensus on how this should be managed in practice.[68,69] In COPD, high-quality controlled trials have not shown increases in mortality with salmeterol monotherapy.[70] In aggregate, the data on mortality effects of long-acting agents in asthma are unclear. Any effect is diminished or even possibly eliminated through the use of inhaled corticosteroids. From a management perspective, this means using short-acting β_2-agonists only on an as-needed basis and, in asthma, using long-acting β2 agonists only when paired with concomitant inhaled steroids.

Anticholinergics

Background. Plants of the *Datura* genus with anticholinergic constituents, such as Jimson weed or thornapple, have been used in the archaic past to treat asthma through the inhalation of their smoke, with more recent clinical administration in the late 19th century in the form of cigarettes or through early types of inhaler devices (see Chapter 9, Autonomic Pharmacology, for a discussion of parasympathetic pharmacology). Systemic anticholinergic adverse effects limited the therapeutic use of this class of agents until the development of the highly polar anticholinergic agent ipratropium. The positive charge of ipratropium's quaternary amine prevents diffusion across cell membranes after inhalation such that the extent of systemic absorption is minimal (Fig. 28-3). Although basal tone of the airways is controlled primarily by the cholinergic system, antagonism of the pulmonary parasympathetic system leads to only modest clinical benefit in asthma. The inferiority of the muscarinic receptor antagonists in bronchodilatory efficacy compared with that of the β-agonists, even at high doses, has led to this drug's place as a second-line bronchodilator in asthma. However, the unique mechanism of action, safety, and additive effects with sympathomimetics make ipratropium a first-line therapy in COPD and a useful adjunct in severe, acute asthmatic attacks. The two currently available inhaled anticholinergics in the United States include the short-acting agent ipratropium and the long-acting tiotropium (Table 28-4).

Receptor Characteristics and Mechanism of Action. Acetylcholine interaction with lung neuromuscular muscarinic receptors causes an increase in cyclic guanosine monophosphate (cGMP), leading to constriction of bronchial smooth muscles. The anticholinergic agents antagonize this vagally mediated reflex. The inhaled anticholinergics are resistant to diffusion across cell membranes, which localizes drug primarily to the lung. Not surprisingly, serum levels of ipratropium and tiotropium do not correlate with bronchodilation, because this response is mediated by drug deposited in the airway rather than in the systemic vascular compartment. Ipratropium has an onset of bronchodilation after 15 minutes in COPD and reaches peak effectiveness after 1 hour. The onset of action in asthma is shorter.[71] Improvements in FEV_1 generally last for 3 to 4 hours, although some patients enjoy clinical benefits up to 8 hours after dosing. The drug does not distrib-

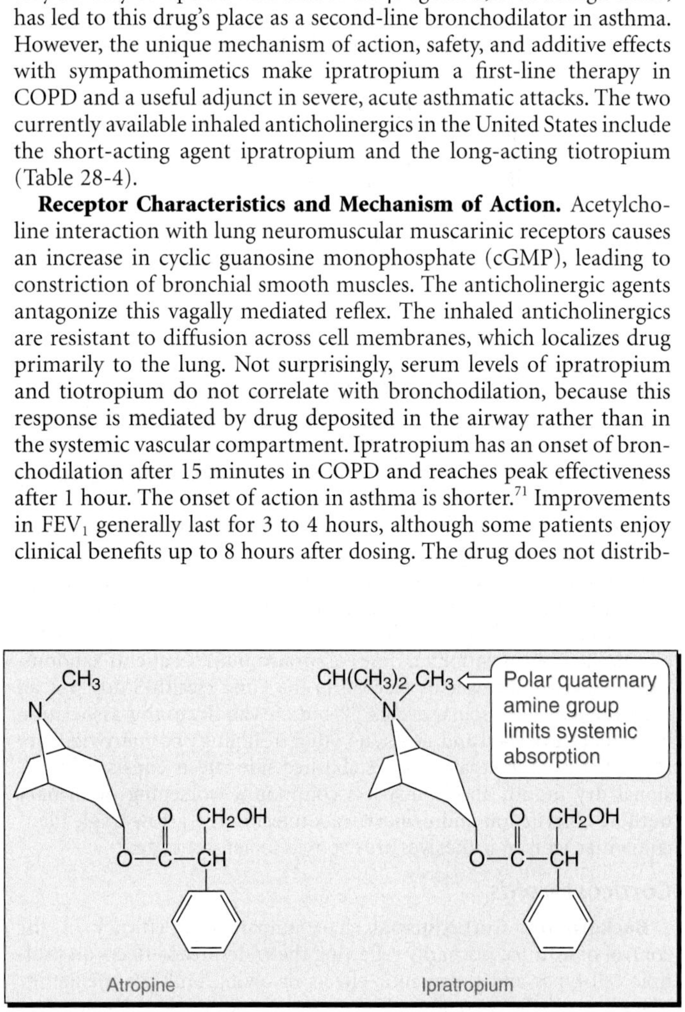

FIGURE 28-3 • Ipratropium and atropine structure.

TABLE 28-4 INHALED ANTICHOLINERGICS

Chemical Name	Trade Name	Dosing Interval (hr)	Onset of Action (min)	Peak Activity (hr)	Duration of Action (hr)	Dosage Range
Ipratropium	Atrovent	6	5-15	1	3-6	MDI: 34 mcg (2 inhalations) HFN: 500 mcg
Tiotropium	Spiriva	12	15	4	36	Dry powder: 18 mcg

HFN, high flow nebulization; MDI, metered-dose inhaler.

ute into the nervous system, minimizing central anticholinergic adverse effects. Because acetylcholine can elicit maximal responses even when only about 50% of receptors are occupied by agonists, systemic anticholinergic effects after inhalation are negligible.[72] Indeed, higher local concentrations of the drug achieved in the bronchial tree after administration by inhalation facilitate full antagonism of muscarinic receptor subtypes M_1, M_2, and M_3. Ipratropium and tiotropium each bind with similar affinity, but tiotropium has a much slower dissociation rate from M_1 and M_3, accounting for a duration of action of more than 24 hours after administration. The relative sparing of M_2 activation is a potential advantage because the M_2 subtype is an autoreceptor on postganglionic cholinergic nerves, which inhibits acetylcholine release.[73]

Clinical Use. Anticholinergics and β_2-agonists are considered first-line bronchodilators for COPD. In acute exacerbations of COPD, short-acting β_2-agonists have a quicker onset of action, but in practice, both agents are administered simultaneously. In stable chronic disease, regular use of inhaled anticholinergics improves symptoms, lung function, exacerbation rates, and health status but does not improve overall or respiratory disease–specific mortality. Ipratropium is administered on a scheduled basis four times a day, whereas tiotropium is inhaled once a day. Tiotropium demonstrates improved clinical outcomes in COPD relative to ipratropium, owing to the relative decrease in M_2 agonism and improved compliance with once-daily administration.[74] Tiotropium as monotherapy has modest superiority over long-acting β_2-agonists,[75] and additive beneficial effects in combination therapy, in more severe COPD. Combination therapy with inhaled corticosteroids is also beneficial (see "Corticosteroids" section).

The anticholinergics in conjunction with β-agonists are beneficial in acute asthma, although this benefit is primarily limited to those patients with the most severe disease.[76] However, given the excellent safety profile and ease of administration with nebulized albuterol, both agents should be given to asthmatics who present to the emergency department with any acute asthma outside of a mild exacerbation. Ipratropium does not appear to provide additional benefit in the long-term management of asthma.[77] The utility of tiotropium in asthma has not been explored. Asthma patients with severe disease or the Arg/Arg genotype may be subsets particularly well suited to the addition of scheduled anticholinergic use though this has not been demonstrated in a systematic fashion.

Safety. Despite potent anticholinergic effects when intravenously administered, inhaled delivery of ipratropium causes remarkably few side effects. Accordingly, no significant cardiovascular or hypokalemic effects occur, even with high doses of ipratropium.[78] Patients randomized to ipratropium versus placebo in the Lung Health Study had an increase in cardiovascular events,[79,80] but the validity of this association has not been verified and, as yet, no other troubling pharmacovigilance signal has been generated.[81-83] Established side effects consist of occasional dry mouth and, much less commonly, worsening of urinary outflow obstruction and urinary tract infections. Narrow-angle glaucoma may worsen if the eyes are exposed to aerosol drug.[84]

Corticosteroids

Background. Corticosteroids have unparalleled efficacy in the control of asthma, primarily reflecting the widespread effects on multiple cell types and therapeutic effects involving multiple mediators. These broad effects are also precisely at the root of the adverse effect profile associated with their use. The efficacy of corticosteroids in asthma was identified not long after these agents were introduced into clinical care. Coupled with the gradual switch to inhaled delivery to minimize systemic adverse effects, this class of drugs has become core elements in the long-term control of anything more severe than mild persistent asthma. Corticosteroids play an important but less of a key role in the treatment of COPD. Parenchymal loss in COPD is not reversed, whereas the inflammatory cells responsible for airway changes are less responsive to the effects of corticosteroids than those in asthma are. A full examination of the cellular effects of corticosteroids is covered in Chapter 41, Adrenal Disorders.

Receptor Characteristics and Mechanism of Action. Corticosteroids are lipophilic and readily cross the membrane bilayer. Glucocorticoid receptors are intracellular and not membrane bound. Two glucocorticoid receptor subtypes exist, with the α form being the functionally active receptor. The β glucocorticoid receptor does not bind corticosteroids, and its role remains unclear. Upon binding of corticosteroid to receptors, a chaperone protein associated with unliganded receptors dissociates, exposing domains that facilitate rapid translocation into the nucleus. In the nucleus, a homodimer of bound receptors forms and binds to specific DNA sequences called *glucocorticoid response elements* (GREs). These GREs reside within promoter regions of steroid-responsive genes, generally increasing transcription of anti-inflammatory mediators. Conversely, inhibition or down-regulation of inflammatory mediators is controlled by inhibition of histone acetyl transferase (HAT). HAT acetylates core histones, altering the charge and unwinding DNA into an open position that allows the transcription of proinflammatory proteins. Glucocorticoids antagonize this function by the recruitment of histone deacetylases (HDACs), which promote the formation of a closed configuration of DNA and decrease transcription of inflammatory genes.[85] There are a number of different HDACs, with varied patterns of expression in cells,[86] which, in part, explains the differential effects of corticosteroids in different tissue types.[87] It is likely that corticosteroids also modulate histone state by other modifications that do not involve acetylation.[88] Other mechanisms of action include increased β_2 receptor expression, decreased mRNA stabilization of inflammatory gene products, and at higher doses, increased transcription of anti-inflammatory genes.

Glucocorticoid receptors are expressed in all cell types in the lung, but the highest density is in the endothelial and epithelial cell types. These structural cells may be of particular importance as major sources of inflammatory mediators and are likely the prime targets responsible for the efficacy of inhaled corticosteroids. Specific cellular effects include decreased cytokine production and eosinophil recruitment and inhibition of inflammatory mediator release.

Dose and Response Characteristics. For acute exacerbations of asthma, oral or intravenous steroids are indicated. Differential efficacy between specific corticosteroids has not been investigated, but prednisone is the most commonly used oral drug and methylprednisolone is the most commonly used parenteral agent. For prednisone, clinical response is seen 3 hours after a dose, with maximal effects noted at 8 to 12 hours. Intravenous methylprednisolone generates a response within 30 minutes, with a maximal effect in 5 hours. Corticosteroids are metabolized, with varying degrees of first-pass hepatic biotransformation depending upon the specific drug.

In chronic asthma, a much more favorable ratio of efficacy to adverse effects is obtained with the use of inhaled, versus systemically administered, corticosteroids. Evidence favors the initial use of a moderate, rather than a high, dose of inhaled steroids.[89] Relative doses for avail-

TABLE 28-5 INHALED CORTICOSTEROID PREPARATIONS IN ADULTS AND CHILDREN (AGES 5-11)

Drug	Trade Name	Low Daily Dose		Medium Daily Dose		High Daily Dose	
		Adult	Child	Adult	Child	Adult	Child
Beclomethasone-HFA	QVAR	80-240	80-160	>240-480	>160-320	>480	>320
Budesonide-DPI	Pulmicort	180-600	180-400	>600-1200	>400-800	>1200	>800
Budesonide inhalation suspension	Pulmicort Respules		0.5 mg		1.0 mg		>1.5 mg
Ciclesonide	Alvesco	80-160	80-160	>160-320	>160-320	>320-1280	>320
Flunisolide HFA	AeroBid	320	160	>320-640	320	>640	>640
Fluticasone HFA/MDI	Flovent HFA	100-250	88-176	250-500	>176-352	>500	>352
Fluticasone DPI	Flovent Diskus	100-300	100-200	>300-500	>200-400	>500	>400
Mometasone	Asmanex	200	100-200	400	>200-400	>400	>400
Triamcinolone	Azmacort	300-750	300-600	>750-1500	>600-900	>1500	>900

Doses are mcg unless otherwise noted.
DPI, dry powder inhaler; HFA, hydrofluoroalkane.
NAEPP #3 and GINA (Global Initiative for Asthma) Global Strategy For Asthma Management And Prevention, update 2007. Available at http://www.ginasthma.com/

able steroid preparations are listed in Table 28-5. Inhaled steroids have a relatively flat dose-response relationship with respect to efficacy, but not safety. Fluticasone has modest dose dependency in terms of beneficial effects (PEF improvement and reduction of oral prednisone dose) and adverse effects, which favors the initial use of a lower dose (200 mcg/day).[90] The choice of dose will also be driven by the severity of the asthma. For example, whereas higher doses of budesonide demonstrate dose-dependent improvements in moderate to severe asthma, lower doses appear to have equal efficacy with moderate and higher doses in mild asthma.[91,92] Similar findings have been obtained with fluticasone[93] and beclomethasone.[94] In adults, the efficacy of high-dose inhaled corticosteroids is similar to that of 5 to 7.5 mg/day of oral prednisone,[95] with fewer systemic adverse events. Clinical trial evidence in COPD has been primarily at moderate to high doses of inhaled corticosteroids.

Because, even at moderate doses, most inhaled corticosteroids are near the maximal effect on their dose-response curves, differences in clinical efficacy between different corticosteroids is difficult to ascertain.[96] Whereas fluticasone may be associated with higher incidence of adrenal suppression,[97,98] most preparations appear to be comparable in terms of efficacy and side effects.[99] Corticosteroids with a higher first-pass metabolism have a theoretical advantage in terms of decreasing systemic absorption after inhaled delivery, however no good evidence exists that these differences are associated with better safety outcomes. Mometasone and budesonide have demonstrated efficacy with once-daily dosing, although only in well-controlled asthma. The optimal dosing time when administered in this fashion is mid to late afternoon.

Clinical Use

Corticosteroids in Chronic Disease. International guidelines universally recommend inhaled corticosteroids as first-line treatment of choice for any disease subtype other than mild persistent asthma.[33,34] High-quality evidence demonstrates improvements in FEV_1, PEF,[100] symptom scores, need for use of short-acting β-agonists, rate of exacerbations,[66] and quality-of-life measures versus placebo. High-quality observational data reveal that regular use of inhaled steroids reduce the risk of asthma deaths and hospitalizations (Fig. 28-4).[101-105] This group of medications has clear efficacy benefits over leukotriene modifiers,[106] long-acting β-agonists, and chromones as monotherapy. For severe asthma, the use of daily oral corticosteroids should be minimized as much as possible owing to toxicity associated with long-term systemic exposure to higher doses. Good evidence indicates that use of one or more second-line agents such as long-acting β_2-agonists[107] can decrease the total dose of corticosteroids while maintaining control of the disease. Unfortunately, inhaled corticosteroids do not appear to prevent asthma in at-risk children,[108] nor is there clear evidence that inhaled steroids change the natural history of asthma or prevent the remodeling of airways seen with long-term disease.

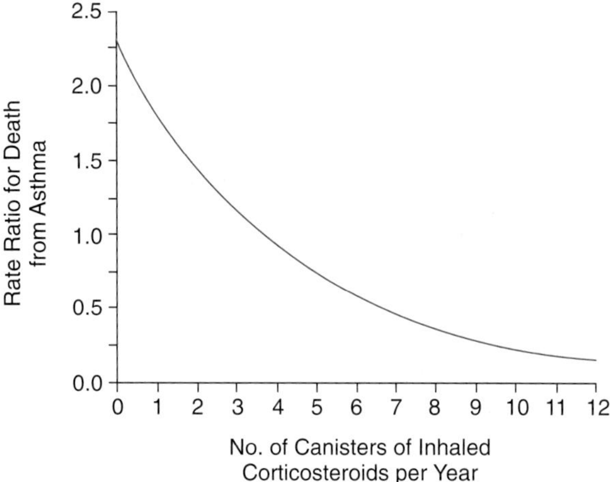

FIGURE 28-4 • Death rate reduction associated with inhaled corticosteroid use. (Adapted from Suissa S, Ernst P, Benayoun S, et al. Low-dose inhaled corticosteroids and the prevention of death from asthma. N Engl J Med 2000;343:332-336.)

International guidelines endorse the use of inhaled corticosteroids in stage 3 (severe) or 4 (very severe) COPD patients with frequent exacerbations. In this patient population, the use of this treatment will decrease exacerbation rate and may provide short-term improvement in FEV_1, though clear evidence demonstrates that inhaled corticosteroids do not change the natural history of COPD or the long-term loss of lung function.[109] Improvements in overall mortality with the use of inhaled corticosteroids in COPD patients, if they exist, are small.[70] The relative merits of the addition of inhaled corticosteroids to long-acting bronchodilators are most compelling in those patients with more advanced disease, because dose-dependent adverse effects are of particular concern in the age group of typical COPD patients. High-quality evidence argues against the use of long-term systemic corticosteroids.

Corticosteroids in Acute Exacerbations. The natural history of asthma and COPD consists of intermittent symptomatic exacerbations driven by flares of inflammation on the cellular level. Appropriate chronic inhaled corticosteroid use will reduce the frequency of, but will not eliminate, asthma exacerbations. Initiation of inhaled corticosteroids, or doubling the dose in those patients already taking them, will generally be sufficient for mild worsening of symptoms. Severe symptoms in both asthmatic and COPD patients require systematic corticosteroids administered orally or parenterally.[110,111] An asthma exacerbation requiring systemic corticosteroids is generally one with less than a 10% improvement in PEF after a dose of an inhaled bronchodilator or a PEF below 70% of predicted after 1 hour of treatment. Exacerbations in COPD are defined primarily by symptomatic changes in dyspnea, cough, or sputum production. Systemic corticosteroids are considered a quick-relief medication. However, given the lag time of a few hours before onset of symptomatic relief, systemic corticosteroids should be started early in any exacerbation. This approach has demonstrated improved outcomes in the emergency department[112] and the office setting. A short course of systemic corticosteroids after an acute exacerbation is associated with decreased relapse rates with minimal adverse effects.[113] Treatment for hospitalized patients generally employs parenteral steroids, although oral formulations have demonstrated good efficacy in acute asthma and are a viable alternative.[114] Evidence supports a dose of 80 mg of methylprednisolone or equivalent for hospitalized acute asthma exacerbation,[115] and a dose of 40 mg is effective in COPD. A typical outpatient asthma exacerbation can be treated with 40 mg of oral prednisone for between 5 and 10 days.[116] This duration of treatment does not require dose tapering. The ideal dose of systemic corticosteroids for COPD exacerbations is not well defined, but a reasonable approach is to use initial doses similar to those cited earlier for asthma, with a rapid taper and treatment for no longer than 2 weeks if treatment response is adequate. Whereas inhaled corticosteroids may provide only modest improvement when added to systemically administered corticosteroids,[117] they should be continued during an acute exacerbation owing to their excellent safety profile and to reinforce the importance of their use to patients.

Safety. The cellular effects of corticosteroids are not limited to the lungs and are the basis for the toxicity observed with corticosteroids. The incidence and severity of adverse effects depends upon both the dose and the duration of therapy. In general, a short burst of oral or parenteral corticosteroids for an acute exacerbation is associated with modest adverse events. In contrast, adverse effects associated with long-term oral administration of corticosteroids are well described and include, but are not limited to, osteoporosis, cataracts, peptic ulcer, accelerated atherosclerosis, and fluid retention. Delivery of corticosteroids to the lungs by the inhaled route increases the therapeutic index by increasing drug deposition at the site of desired action in the lung while reducing total drug dosage and systemic exposure. During inhaled delivery, larger particles are impacted on the oropharynx and swallowed, contributing to adverse effects but not to efficacy. Nonpulmonary corticosteroid systemic exposure for most inhaled agents (i.e., those agents that are extensively metabolized by the liver prior to reaching the systemic circulation) is minimized by first-pass metabolism. Patient techniques to reduce systemic exposure include using a spacer device, which preferentially captures droplets of a nonrespirable size, and rinsing the mouth after inhalation.

Systemic side effects of inhaled corticosteroids are dose dependent, with modest to no effects at mid to lower doses. It has been suggested that the frequency of adverse events with the use of inhaled steroids is not linear and that, at low to moderate doses, some adverse events are of frequencies that make them difficult to differentiate from background.[118] The most rational approach to reduce adverse events associated with inhaled corticosteroids is to use the appropriate dose to control symptoms, with a goal of low to moderate doses, and the adjunctive use of agents with alternate mechanisms of action to control symptoms and minimize the required steroid dose.

Local effects of inhaled corticosteroids are among the most common and consist primarily of dysphonia in as many as 50% of patients and oral candidiasis in fewer than 5%.[119] The use of a spacer device and mouth rinsing after drug administration are particularly effective in reducing these upper airway effects.

Long-term use of inhaled steroids has been associated with cataracts in adults, especially those of the posterior subcapsular type, in a number of case-control studies.[120-122] Inhaled steroid use increases the relative prevalence by up to threefold, although associations have been strongest with long-term use of high doses. Modest increases in intraocular pressure (glaucoma) at high doses has also been observed.[123] The incidence of pneumonia in COPD patients treated with fluticasone may be increased, but this was not a prespecified study end point and the exact relevance of this finding is unclear.[70] Inhaled corticosteroid use, even at moderate doses, is associated with decreased growth velocity in children.[98,124] However, this effect on growth velocity is limited to the first year of drug exposure,[125] and children administered these medications reach normal height in adulthood.[126,127] In adults, osteoporosis is a well-characterized side effect of systemic corticosteroids. The degree to which inhaled corticosteroids cause decreased bone mineral density and increase the risk of fractures at low to moderate doses is not clear,[128-130] in part due to methodological issues of studies that comprise the literature. Those patients treated for extended periods at higher doses have modestly increased risks of fractures.[131] All patients who are maintained on inhaled steroids, especially those on higher doses or those with frequent need for systemic courses of treatment, should be screened and, where indicated, treated for osteoporosis with calcium and bisphosphates, as appropriate.[132] These interventions increase bone mineral density and decrease the rate of fracture in most, but not all, studies.[133]

In aggregate, many studies have demonstrated suppression of the hypothalamic-pituitary-adrenal axis (HPA). HPA function for patients receiving inhaled steroids, though reduced compared with those receiving nonsteroid treatments, was within normal limits. The clinical implications of differences detectable by laboratory evaluation, but otherwise clinically unapparent, is not clear. Case reports of iatrogenic HPA suppression have been noted, specifically with higher doses of inhaled steroids.[134] Low to moderate doses generally have minimal adrenal effects.[135] Overall, inhaled steroids exert a clinically insignificant effect on HPA, although certain patients on higher doses or receiving multiple oral courses may be at risk for insufficiency upon sudden withdrawal of steroid treatment or in the face of a large physiologic stress.[136] Clinicians should be aware of these effects in patients taking large doses over long periods of time, especially in the face of physiologic stressors and concomitant illness. In all cases, the appropriate strategy is to use the minimum amount of corticosteroid that controls the disease, coupled with administration techniques that increase the fraction of drug deposited in the lungs.

Leukotriene Modifiers

Background. The leukotrienes are a class of inflammatory mediators with roles in both early and late responses in asthmatic attacks. Formerly known as "slow-reacting substances of anaphylaxis" owing to their ability to constrict smooth muscle, the name of this class of mediators reflects their initial derivation from leukocytes and a structural formula containing three double bonds in series.[137] The leukotrienes are divided into two groups, the dihydroxy acids, such as leukotriene B_4 (LTB_4), which induce neutrophil chemotaxis, and the cysteinyl leukotrienes, so named because they contain the amino acid cysteine. The cysteinyl leukotrienes C_4, D_4, and E_4 act as potent constrictors on airway smooth muscle, cause eosinophil chemotaxis, mucus hypersecretion, plasma leakage into the interstitium, and proliferation of inflammatory cells in the bone marrow. Leukotrienes are derived from arachidonic acid, a fatty acid component of the plasma membrane phospholipid compartment that serves as the precursor for many eicosanoids[138] (see Chapter 11, Inflammation and Immunomodulation). Free arachidonic acid is liberated from membrane phospholipids by cytosolic phospholipase A_2, which is activated by increases in intracellular calcium induced by immunologic stimuli, including allergen interaction with receptors, or physical stimuli, such as cold air. Following interaction with 5-lipoxygenase–activating protein (FLAP), arachidonic acid is converted by 5-lipoxygenase to leukotriene A_4 (LTA_4). In neutrophils and monocytes, LTA_4 is enzymatically converted to LTB_4. In eosinophils and mast cells, LTA_4 is converted into LTC_4, which, upon secretion, mediates bronchoconstriction, vascular permeability and edema, mucus hypersecretion, smooth muscle hypertrophy, and eosinophil chemotaxis. Cell types that produce leukotrienes include basophils, macrophages, mast cells, lymphocytes, and endothelial cells.[139] Currently available drugs for asthma that target the leukotriene inflammatory cascade either inhibit 5-lipoxygenase, to prevent the generation of LTA_4 (zileuton), or antagonize the cyste-

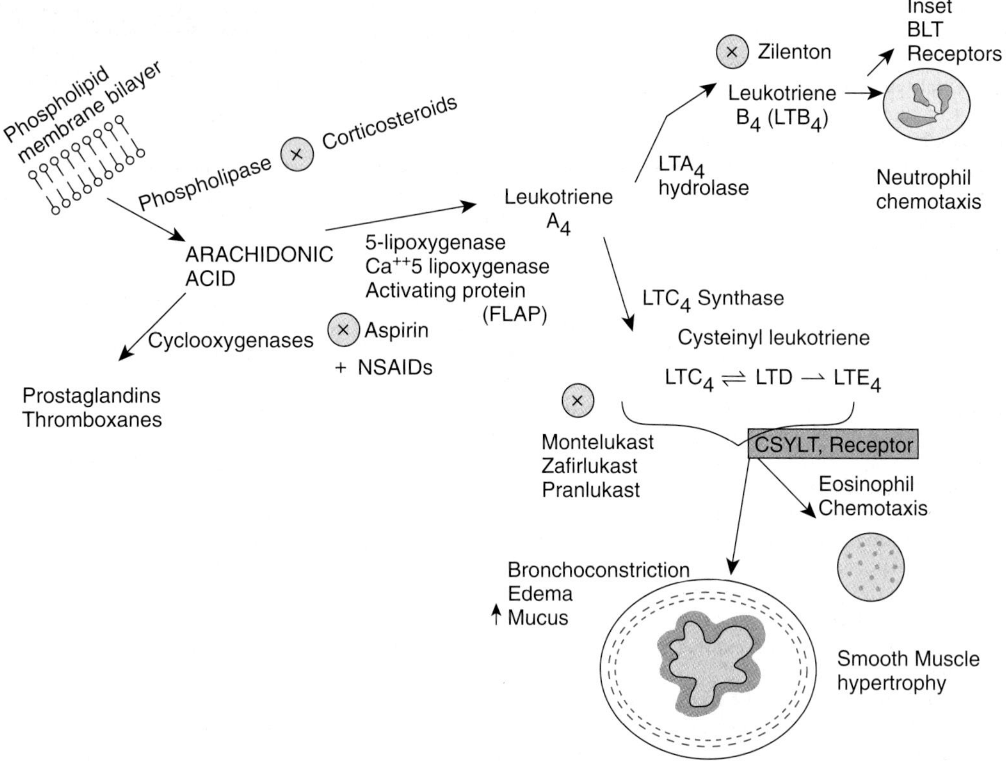

FIGURE 28-5 • Leukotriene pathway. FLAP, 5-lipoxygenase activating protein; NSAIDs, non-steroidal anti-inflammatory drugs.

TABLE 28-6 MODIFIERS OF THE LEUKOTRIENE SYSTEM

Chemical Name	Trade Name	Mechanism of Action	*Typical Dose (mg)* Pediatric	Adult	Dose Interval	Indicated Age Range	Comments
Montelukast	Singulair	CysLT 1 receptor antagonist	4-5	10	qd	>6 mo	Also indicated for use in allergic and perennial rhinitis
Zafirlukast	Accolate	CysLT 1 receptor antagonist	10	20	bid	≥5 yr	Drug interaction with warfarin
Zileuton	Zyflo	5-Lipoxygenase inhibitor	600	600	qid	≥12 yr	Liver enzyme monitoring required due to 2%-5% incidence of hepatitis
	Zyflo CR		1200	1200	bid		Drug interaction with warfarin and theophylline

inyl leukotriene receptor (zafirlukast, montelukast, and pranlukast) (Fig. 28-5).

Receptor Characteristics and Mechanism of Action. The biologic activities of LTB_4 are mediated by binding to the G protein–coupled receptor BLT on leukocytes. Ligand-receptor interaction induces adhesion of leukocytes to the vascular endothelium, followed by migration into the interstitium. Cell types most affected include neutrophils and, to a lesser extent, eosinophils. Specific antagonists to BLT have been developed, although effects on asthma symptoms are modest,[140] suggesting that BLT receptors play only a minor role in the inflammatory cascade in asthma. LTB_4 plays a role in neutrophilic inflammation. Two G protein–coupled receptors, CysLT1 and CysLT2, interact with the cysteinyl leukotrienes LTC_4, LTD_4, and LCE_4.[141] All antagonists in clinical use are specific to the CysLT1 receptor. This receptor is expressed primarily in airway smooth muscle and, to a lesser extent, by eosinophils. This distribution underlies the relative safety of this class of drugs and the utility of systemic, rather than pulmonary, administration. CysLT2 receptors, expressed primarily by lung macrophages and airway smooth muscle cells, are currently not pharmacologic targets in asthma.

Dose and Response Characteristics. All of the agents currently used are administered orally at fixed doses with no dose titration (Table 28-6). Montelukast is well absorbed and dosed daily at 10 mg in adults and 4 or 5 mg in pediatric populations as young as 6 months of age. Zafirlukast is administered twice daily and indicated in children aged 5 and above. Zileuton requires dosing four times a day or twice a day with an extended release preparation.

Clinical response to modifiers of the leukotriene system tends to be variable, with some patients gaining minimal benefit whereas others having a strong clinical response. There is no accurate predictor of a patient's propensity to respond, and assessment of utility in an individual patient is based upon an empirical trial.

Clinical Use. Although inhaled corticosteroids have superior clinical efficacy to the leukotriene antagonists when used as single agents, some elements of asthmatic inflammation, specifically those mediated by neutrophils, do not respond to steroids. Conversely, leukotriene production is unaffected by steroids. These discrete mechanistic differences provide the rationale for combination therapy with leukotriene antagonists and steroids. The leukotriene antagonists have the added benefits of ease of administration by the oral route, excellent safety profile, and added efficacy in allergic rhinitis. Further, use of leukotriene antagonists may be associated with decreased rates of death from asthma.[104] Moreover, leukotriene antagonists have specific efficacy in some subtypes of asthma. Indeed, exercise-induced asthma responds well to leukotriene antagonists, especially in young patients who participate in activities over the course of a day and do not have access to prophylactic β_2-agonists or chromones. The duration of action of leukotriene antagonists provides extended protection in this condition that equals or surpasses that of long-acting β_2-agonists.[142] Similarly, leukotrienes play a key role in the well-described clinical entity of aspirin-induced asthma. In at least some patients, aspirin inhibition of cyclooxygenase potentiates LTB_4 generation by reducing production of the anti-inflammatory prostaglandin E_2, which inhibits LTB_4 synthase and shunts arachidonic acid from the cyclooxygenase to the lipoxygenase pathway.[143,144] All modifiers of the leukotriene pathway exhibit particular clinical efficacy in those patients.[145-147]

The exact role of leukotriene modifiers in acute asthma have not been established, but given the safety and complementary action to standard treatment, their use as an adjunct is advocated.[148,149] Currently available leukotriene modifiers do not have clinical indications in COPD, although scattered reports exist of modest improvement in outcomes with use.[150,151] A much more likely target for COPD treatment within the leukotriene system is antagonism at the BLT_4 receptor, because BLT_4 activation has greater effects on neutrophilic inflammation. However, no BLT_4 antagonists are currently approved for treatment.

Side Effects. Zileuton is associated with elevation in hepatic enzymes in up to 5% of patients, necessitating intermittent laboratory monitoring. Similarly, zafirlukast has been associated with hepatitis, which is generally self limited, but has been linked to hepatic failure. Zafirlukast inhibits cytochrome P-450 2C9 and 3A4, which can serve as a basis for pharmacokinetic adverse drug interactions. Montelukast has an excellent safety profile, with minimal drug interactions. The use of leukotriene antagonists has been associated with Churg-Strauss vasculitis, although this association was observed in severe, steroid-dependent patients and reflects unmasking of the vasculitis by a decrease in steroid dose rather than direct induction by leukotriene antagonists.

Chromones

Background. Cromolyn was first synthesized in Great Britain in 1965 and was identified as a substance that prevented asthmatic response to an allergic challenge.[152] Nedocromil, released in 1993, shares structural homology with cromolyn in their 1,4-benzopyrone moiety. These agents are often called *chromones*, because they share a chromone ring structure.

Receptor Characteristics, Mechanism of Action, and Dose Response. These agents have also been called *mast cell stabilizers*, owing to the observation of inhibition of the degranulation of mast cells in the face of allergens or nonspecific triggers of mediator release. The biologic actions of these agents are mediated by a number of putative mechanisms that work in concert. Inhibition of mediator release is caused by effects on intermediate-conductance chloride channels, the inhibition of which prevents influx of calcium, activation of signaling, and subsequent degranulation.[153] This mechanism appears to prevent mediator release from other inflammatory cells such as eosinophils, neutrophils, monocytes, alveolar macrophages, lymphocytes,[154] and epithelial cells. Effects on sensory nerves may inhibit axonal reflexes or neuropeptide release, reducing airway reactivity and edema. Further, these agents may induce the phosphorylation of a moesin-like protein that inhibits degranulation by direct interactions with the cytoskeleton.[155] In addition, nedocromil appears to prevent the isotype switching of B cells to the IgE phenotype.[156,157] Although all of these effects contribute to a reduction in bronchospasm and prophylactic efficacy, they are not bronchodilators and are ineffective in the setting of acute exacerbation.

Because these agents have no intrinsic antihistamine or bronchodilatory properties, the chromones must be taken at scheduled intervals or before exposure to a known trigger of symptoms. To prevent exposure-induced symptoms, cromolyn or nedocromil should be taken between 10 and 60 minutes prior to exercise. Cromolyn is administered at a dose of 2 puffs four times a day and is available in a nebulized formulation. Nedocromil is administered four times a day until clinical stability is reached, after which the dose can be reduced to twice daily (Table 28-7).

TABLE 28-7 CHROMONES

Chemical Name	Trade Name	Dose	Dosing Interval
Cromolyn sodium	Intal	MDI: 800 mcg/inhalation HFN: 20 mg	qid
Nedocromil	Tilade	MDI: 1.75 mg/inhalation	qid–bid

HFN, high flow nebulization; MDI, metered dose inhaler.

Safety. Side effects of the chromones are generally modest, with occasional dry mouth and hoarseness. Approximately 15% of patients describe dysgeusia associated with nedocromil.

Clinical Use. Cromolyn, and to a lesser extent nedocromil, has a long clinical history as an agent for the long-term control of asthma. Although a Cochrane systematic review[158] examining the issue concluded that efficacy of inhaled cromolyn for asthma in children has not been established and that the body of literature suffers from publication bias, the consensus is that cromolyn and nedocromil are effective in the prophylactic reduction of asthma exacerbations, but with less efficacy than inhaled corticosteroids.[105,125,159]

A useful property of cromolyn and nedocromil is the prophylactic bronchoprotection against an exercise- or allergen-induced challenge. Both cromolyn and nedocromil are equally efficacious in preventing exercise-induced bronchoconstriction,[160] although they are not as effective as the β-agonists for this indication.[161] On the basis of complementary mechanisms of action, the chromones can be paired with a β-agonist for added efficacy prior to an environmental exposure known to induce asthmatic bronchoconstriction.[162] Chromones have no role in the treatment of COPD.

Xanthines

Background. Theophylline is a member of the methylxanthine class of medications, similar in structure to caffeine. Coffee drinking in asthmatics was encouraged by physicians as early as the mid-19th century. The use of theophylline and its water-soluble analogue, aminophylline, dates from the middle of the 20th century. Use of theophylline has been limited primarily by toxicity, although low cost and oral availability have made this a useful adjunct in certain clinical settings.

Receptor Characteristics and Mechanism of Action. Theophylline and aminophylline have been traditionally categorized as bronchodilators. The mechanisms by which these drugs induce clinical effects include the inhibition of phosphodiesterases, prostaglandins, intracellular calcium release, and antagonism of adenosine receptors; and increased IL-10 release, release of catecholamines, and subsequent increases in cyclic nucleotides.[163] The clinical efficacy of theophylline in asthma appears to be greater than that explained by bronchodilation alone. The additional efficacy in asthma is likely due to complementary anti-inflammatory[164] and bronchoprotective[165] effects. Anti-inflammatory effects appear to be mediated, in part, by activation of histone deacetylases. Another putative clinical benefit in COPD is the stimulation of respiratory musculature.

Clinical Use. In asthma guidelines, theophylline is classified as a nonpreferred alternative or adjunct to corticosteroids.[166] This recommendation is based upon the relative inferiority in safety and efficacy of theophylline compared with that of first-line therapies coupled with the availability of alternate oral preparations of long-term controller therapies in the leukotriene modifiers. Methylxanthines should not be used in acute asthma because these agents provide no additional bronchodilation over standard therapy and their use is associated with significant adverse effects.[167]

Theophylline has more utility in COPD than in asthma, although it is still considered inferior to anticholinergics and β-agonists. A Cochrane review concluded that long-acting β-agonists have similar efficacy to that of theophylline but fewer adverse events.[168] Theophylline probably has the greatest role as an adjunct in moderate to severe COPD, particularly in those patients with functional impairment despite maximally optimized therapy with other agents. Despite a prominent side effect profile at therapeutic doses, meta-analysis data confirm clinical observations that many COPD patients have improved symptoms and overall quality of life with the use of theophylline.[169] Theophylline also serves as a viable choice in areas of the world with limited resources for inhaled medications and as an adjunct in those patients unable or unwilling to use inhaled medications.

The therapeutic plasma concentrations of theophylline traditionally have been considered to lie between 10 and 20 mcg/ml. However, anti-inflammatory effects may be achieved at concentrations as low as 5 μg/ml,[170] making a lower dose potentially attractive in asthma. Indeed, the National Asthma Education and Prevention (NAEPP) guidelines suggest that a target range between 5 and 15 μg/ml be used to avoid toxicity in asthma, which is lower than the higher concentrations (15-20 mcg/ml) considered optimal in COPD.[171] The dose required to achieve the desired level varies widely from patient to patient owing to differences in metabolism, reflecting interindividual pharmacogenetic differences and common drug interactions. Because toxicity is associated with peak concentrations, plasma concentrations should be obtained 4 to 6 hours after dosing of a sustained-release product.

Side Effects. The most common side effects of theophylline are nervousness, nausea, vomiting, headache, and anorexia, although no specific symptom predominates[172] and there is no predictable response rate to a given serum concentration. With plasma levels greater than 30 mcg/ml, a risk of cardiac arrhythmias and seizures does exist. These can be fatal and can present without warning signs. Milder side effects are noted even within the therapeutic range for most individuals. Drug interactions with theophylline are common.

INTEGRATED PHARMACOTHERAPEUTIC APPROACH TO THE ASTHMATIC OR COPD PATIENT

The goals of treatment of the obstructive airway diseases are to reduce the cardinal symptoms of obstruction, specifically breathlessness and cough, reduce the rate of acute exacerbations, and improve overall health status. Asthma-specific clinical benchmarks are a reduction in nocturnal awakenings and consumption of short-acting β_2-agonists (Box 28-2). In COPD, maximizing functional status, preventing further disease progression, and improving exercise tolerance are key goals (Box 28-3). Asthma prognosis is generally very good in those patients receiving appropriate, early intervention,[173] although present treatments have done much to reduce the therapeutic nihilism previously accorded COPD.

Treatment outlined in most international guidelines (Box 28-4) involves stepwise pharmacotherapy based on disease severity both at initiation and during the course of treatment. Worsening disease is treated by increasing the dose of a currently used medication or adding a new agent. Similarly, disease severity is assessed periodically to determine whether a step down in treatment intensity is indicated. Since the introduction of consensus guidelines, the prevalence of moderate, but not severe, asthma has been reduced, suggesting some success with present strategies. However, these observations underscore the limits of the present drug armamentarium and the requirement for new drug development and an improved systems approach for the treatment of severe disease.[174]

The keystone of drug therapy in asthma is the use of a long-term controller, supplemented by a short-acting β_2-agonist as a bronchodilator for short-term symptom relief. Inflammation is the key element responsible for asthmatic symptoms, airway hyperreactivity, and probably, airway remodeling. By virtue of their effects on multiple cell types and inflammatory mediators, corticosteroids are the most important

BOX 28-2 GOAL OF THERAPY: CONTROL OF ASTHMA

Reduce Impairment

- Prevent chronic and troublesome symptoms (e.g., coughing or breathlessness in the daytime, in the night, or after exertion).
- Require infrequent use (≤ twice a week) of inhaled SABA for quick relief of symptoms
- Maintain (near) normal pulmonary function.
- Maintain normal activity levels (including exercise and other physical activity and attendance at school or work).
- Meet patients' and families' expectations of and satisfaction with asthma care.

Reduce Risk

- Prevent recurrent exacerbations of asthma and minimize the need for ED visits or hospitalizations.
- Prevent loss of lung function; for children, prevent reduced lung growth.
- Provide optimal pharmacotherapy with minimal or no adverse effects of therapy.

From Expert panel report 3: guidelines for the diagnosis and management of asthma. NIH Publication No. 08-4051. Bethesda, MD: U.S. Department of Health and Human Services; National Institutes of Health; National Heart, Lung, and Blood Institute; National Asthma Education and Prevention Program, 2007.

BOX 28-3 GOALS OF THERAPY: COPD CONTROL

- Relieve symptoms
- Prevent disease progression
- Improve exercise tolerance
- Improve health status
- Prevent and treat complications
- Prevent and treat exacerbations
- Reduce mortality

COPD, chronic obstructive pulmonary disease.
From Global Initiative for Chronic Obstructive Lung Disease, Global Strategy for the Diagnosis, Management, and Prevention of Chronic Obstructive Pulmonary Disease, 2006.

BOX 28-4 INTERNATIONAL CONSENSUS GUIDELINES OF ASTHMA CARE

- National Asthma Education and Prevention Program. Clinical Practice Guidelines Expert Panel Report 3: Guidelines for the Diagnosis and Management of Asthma. DHHS Publication No. NIH 08-4051. Washington, DC: National Institutes of Health National Heart, Lung, and Blood Institute, 2007. Available at http://www.nhlbi.nih.gov
- British guideline on the management of asthma 2007. Available at http://www.sign.ac.uk/guidelines/fulltext/63/index.html
- Global Initiative for Chronic Obstructive Lung Disease 2007. Available at http://www.goldcopd.com/
- National Collaborating Centre for Chronic Conditions, National Institute for Health and Clinical Excellence (NCCCC/NICE). Chronic obstructive pulmonary disease. National clinical guideline on management of chronic obstructive pulmonary disease in adults in primary and secondary care. Thorax 2004;59(Suppl 1):1-232.
- Global Initiative for Asthma 2007 update. Available at http://www.ginasthma.org
- The European Pediatric Asthma Group. Diagnosis and treatment of asthma in childhood: a PRACTALL consensus report. Allergy 2008;63(1):5-34. Available at http://www.blackwell-synergy.com/doi/full/10.1111/j.1398-9995.2007.01586.x

class of drugs used in asthma. Adjunctive long-term controller agents include long-acting β_2-agonists and modifiers of the leukotriene system. Outside of acute exacerbations, instances of step-down in therapy in COPD are generally limited, given the irreversibility of obstruction. Therapy begins with symptom-driven short-acting bronchodilators, followed by add-on therapy with longer-acting bronchodilators; inhaled corticosteroids can be added for more severe disease and in those patients with frequent exacerbations.

In the setting of acute exacerbations, the key elements are the early use of oral prednisone and the aggressive use of inhaled short-acting β_2-agonists. In more severe cases, use of parenteral corticosteroids is well supported by the evidence. In asthma, an inhaled anticholinergic is warranted in severe attacks. Less well supported, but also reasonable in asthma, is the use of nebulized corticosteroids,[175] leukotriene inhibitors,[148] or intravenous magnesium sulfate.[176]

Special Populations

Pregnancy

A primary goal in the treatment of pregnant asthmatic patients is to ensure maternal and fetal health. Although the degree to which non-severe asthma is associated with worse fetal outcomes is not clear, most studies suggest that maternal asthma increases the risks of perinatal mortality, prematurity, low birth weight, and preeclampsia.[177-179] The use of oral steroids during pregnancy is associated with preterm birth, low birth weight, and increased incidence of cleft lip. In contrast, inhaled steroids and β-agonists do not have adverse effects on perinatal or maternal outcomes.[180,181] Most clinical experience with inhaled steroids has been with budesonide, although other inhaled steroid preparations are expected to have similar favorable safety profiles. Similarly, most clinical experience with β-agonists in pregnancy has been with albuterol. The long-acting systemic β-agonists are used as tocolytics in the peripartum period, and the associated neonatal tremor and occasional hypoglycemia are generally managed in a straightforward fashion. Thus, pregnant patients should have their asthma managed with inhaled corticosteroids, with the addition of adjunctive therapies such as long-acting β-agonists and leukotrienes to minimize the need for oral steroids. No human data are available regarding the use of anticholinergics in pregnancy, although minimal systemic absorption and reassuring animal studies with ipratropium suggest a measure of safety.

Pediatrics

Children under the age of 5 are often unable to perform reliable spirometry to confirm the diagnosis of asthma, and children with symptoms suggestive of asthma are treated when alternate diagnoses are excluded. Up to one third of children who wheeze with respiratory infections will develop asthma that persists after age 6.[16] Despite concerns of decreased growth velocity, inhaled corticosteroids remain the primary controller medication. A goal should be to keep doses in the low range, but not at the expense of poor control of asthmatic symptoms. Although inhaled corticosteroids are unmatched for controlling symptoms, they do not prevent asthma or appear to change the natural history of the disease.[108] Inhaled chromones are considered an alternate treatment, but their utility for combination use with inhaled corticosteroids is limited. The leukotriene modifiers montelukast or zafirlukast are acceptable alternatives to corticosteroids as monotherapy in children in whom this therapy is not possible owing to nonadherence to inhaled therapy. These agents also have particular utility in conjunction with inhaled steroids to control symptoms and minimize steroid dose. Long-term controller therapy should be stepped down after 2 to 4 months of good control of symptoms. Another key element of care is the instruction of caregivers in the proper techniques for administration of inhaled therapy.

Alternative Therapies

The binding of circulating IgE by allergen leads to mast cell degranulation and an immediate bronchoconstrictive response. Also, IgE is implicated in up-regulation of the inflammatory response involving other cell types in airways. Exogenous corticosteroids do not influence the rate of IgE production. Omalizumab, a recombinant, humanized monoclonal IgG antibody against circulating IgE, is approved for use in moderate to severe asthmatic patients aged 12 or older who are not controlled with inhaled corticosteroids. Patients must demonstrate a positive skin test or radioallergosorbent test (RAST) to a perennial allergen. The drug is administered by the subcutaneous route every 2 to 4 weeks; the dose is based upon pretreatment serum IgE levels and patient weight. The drug is generally well tolerated, with an anaphylaxis incidence rate of less than 0.1%.

The addition of magnesium sulfate to inhaled β_2-agonists in severe, acute asthma that has not responded to therapy has led to improved lung function and, possibly, rate of hospitalization compared with β_2-agonists used alone.[182] Although histamine is one of the mediators released by the mast cell after degranulation, H_1-antagonists do not improve asthmatic control.[183] Treatment of allergic rhinitis with nasal steroids in patients who also have asthma does appear to improve asthmatic symptoms when coupled with an inhaled corticosteroid.[184] Immunization with influenza and pneumococcal vaccines is safe and effective in both asthmatic and COPD patients. Allergic immunotherapy, usually administered by an allergist, may reduce the dose of medications required and the incidence of exacerbations in asthmatic patients who demonstrate a clear worsening of symptoms in response to specific allergens. However, the therapy does not influence lung function and is associated with a small, but definite, incidence of anaphylaxis. It must be administered over a period of at least 3 to 5 years.[185] Chronic symptomatic or subclinical gastroesophageal reflux is commonly noted in asthma and has been postulated to exacerbate asthma by microaspiration in selected individuals. The use of proton pump inhibitors or histamine antagonists (H_2) has been effective in selected patients. The efficacy of these agents across the spectrum of patients has not been established in clinical trials.[186]

Smoking cessation (see Chapter 56, Nicotine Dependence) is the only therapy proven to reduce the rate of lung function decline and should be fully pursued in all COPD patients. Good evidence supports mortality benefit in the use of oxygen for patients with severe COPD. Benefit is limited to those with hypoxia, defined as oxygen saturation of 60 mm Hg or lower. Hereditary α_1-antitrypsin deficiency can cause an accelerated form of COPD. Replacement therapy is available but reserved only for young patients with documented severe deficiency. The role of antitussives, mucolytics, antioxidants, narcotics,[187] or vasodilators in obstructive airways disease is limited. Long-term antibiotic use is not of benefit, but short courses of antibiotics have been demonstrated to have modest benefit in exacerbations of COPD when increased dyspnea, sputum volume, and sputum purulence are present or in patients with severe exacerbations requiring mechanical ventilation. Antibiotic classes commonly used include β-lactams, cephalosporins, tetracyclines, macrolides, and fluoroquinolones.

In patients with "corticosteroid-resistant" asthma, alternate therapies including intravenous immune globulin (IVIG), colchicine, methotrexate, cyclosporine, and gold have been used. Evidence to support their use is limited, and these agents should remain the purview of subspecialists dedicated to the treatment of severe, treatment-resistant asthma in which adequacy of use of established therapies has been ensured.

Novel Targets

Research into the pathophysiology of asthma has identified a large number of mediators and cell types that could be potential therapeutic targets (Table 28-8). To date, modifiers of the leukotriene system and anti-IgE antibodies are the only therapies targeted at a single mediator that have proved efficacious. Therapies targeting specific cytokines such as IL-12, IL-5, or platelet-activating factor have been unsuccessful,[188-190] reflecting the redundancy of the immunologic system in both health and disease. However, the area remains one of active research, and approaches that combine a number of targets may prove most fruitful. Therapies to influence the long-term decline in

TABLE 28-8 SELECTED POTENTIAL TARGETS FOR NOVEL THERAPEUTICS

Class	Examples
Prostanoids receptors	TXA_2, PGD2
Histamine H_4 antagonists	JNJ 7777120
Phosphodiesterase inhibitors type 4	Cilomilast, roflumilast
Inhibitors of TNF	Infliximab, etanercept
Th2 cytokine inhibitors	Suplatast tosilate
Nicotinic receptor antagonists	1,1-Dimethyl-4-phenylpiperazinium
Inhibitors of adhesion molecules	Efalizumab
lligodeoxynucleotides	CpG ODN conjugated Amb a 1
IKK-2 inhibitors	ML120B, PS-1145
Matrix metalloprotease inhibitors	AZ11557272
α_1 Proteinase inhibitor	Recombinant human
Neutrophil elastase inhibitors	ONO-6818, EPI-hNE4 (DX890)
Leukotriene BLT 1 antagonists	LY29311, SB225002
IL-1 receptor antagonists	Anakinra

IKK, I kappa B kinase; IL-1, interleukin-1; PGD_2, prostaglandin D_2; Th2, T helper lymphocytes; TNF, tumor necrosis factor; TXA_2, thromboxane A_2; Data from references 193-200.

lung function in asthma and to reverse or prevent airway remodeling have been elusive, but remain goals for the future.[191,192]

REFERENCES

1. Bel EH. Clinical phenotypes of asthma. Curr Opin Pulm Med 2004;10:44-50.
2. Caulfield MP, Birdsall NJ. International Union of Pharmacology. XVII. Classification of muscarinic acetylcholine receptors. Pharmacol Rev 1998;50:279-290.
3. Mak JC, Barnes PJ. Autoradiographic visualization of muscarinic receptor subtypes in human and guinea pig lung. Am Rev Respir Dis 1990;141:1559-1568.
4. Watson N, Magnussen H, Rabe KF. Pharmacological characterization of the muscarinic receptor subtype mediating contraction of human peripheral airways. J Pharmacol Exp Ther 1995;274:1293-1297.
5. Wessler I, Kirkpatrick CJ, Racke K. Non-neuronal acetylcholine, a locally acting molecule, widely distributed in biological systems: expression and function in humans. Pharmacol Ther 1998;77:59-79.
6. Barnes PJ. Distribution of receptor targets in the lung. Proc Am Thorac Soc 2004;1:345-351.
7. Fryer AD, Jacoby DB. Muscarinic receptors and control of airway smooth muscle. Am J Respir Crit Care Med 1998;158:154S-160S.
8. Carstairs JR, Nimmo AJ, Barnes PJ. Autoradiographic visualization of beta-adrenoceptor subtypes in human lung. Am Rev Respir Dis 1985;132:541-547.
9. James A. Airway remodeling in asthma. Curr Opin Pulm Med 2005;11:1-6.
10. Ordonez CL, Shaughnessy TE, Matthay MA, Fahy JV. Increased neutrophil numbers and IL-8 levels in airway secretions in acute severe asthma: clinical and biologic significance. Am J Respir Crit Care Med 2000;161:1185-1190.
11. Lemiere C, Pelissier S, Tremblay C, et al. Leukotrienes and isocyanate-induced asthma: a pilot study. Clin Exp Allergy 2004;34:1684-1689.
12. Busse W, Kraft M. Cysteinyl leukotrienes in allergic inflammation: strategic target for therapy. Chest 2005;127:1312-1326.
13. Walker C, Bode E, Boer L, et al. Allergic and nonallergic asthmatics have distinct patterns of T-cell activation and cytokine production in peripheral blood and bronchoalveolar lavage. Am Rev Respir Dis 1992;146:109-115.
14. Humbert M, Menz G, Ying S, et al. The immunopathology of extrinsic (atopic) and intrinsic (non-atopic) asthma: more similarities than differences. Immunol Today 1999;20:528-533.
15. Barnes PJ, Chung KF, Page CP. Inflammatory mediators of asthma: an update. Pharmacol Rev 1998;50:515-596.
16. Williams SG, Schmidt DK, Redd SC, Storms W, and the National Asthma Education and Prevention Program. Key clinical activities for quality asthma care. Recommendations of the National Asthma Education and Prevention Program. MMWR Recomm Rep 2003;52:1-8.
17. Dolovich MB, Ahrens RC, Hess DR, et al. Device selection and outcomes of aerosol therapy: evidence-based guidelines: American College of Chest Physicians/American College of Asthma, Allergy, and Immunology. Chest 2005;127:335-371.
18. Blumenthal M. Herbal Medicine: Expanded Commission E Monographs. Newton MA: Integrative Medicine Communications, 2000.
19. Bullowa JGM, Kaplan DM. On the hypodermic use of adrenalin chloride in the treatment of asthmatic attacks. Med News 1903;83:787-790.
20. Cullum VA, Farmer JB, Jack D, Levy GP. Salbutamol: a new, selective beta-adrenoceptive receptor stimulant. Br J Pharmacol 1969;35:141-151.
21. Persson H, Olsson T. Some pharmacological properties of terbutaline (INN), 1-(3,5-dihydroxyphenyl)-2-(T-butylamino)-ethanol. A new sympathomimetic beta-receptor–stimulating agent. Acta Med Scand Suppl 1970;512:11-19.
22. Insel PA. Seminars in medicine of the Beth Israel Hospital, Boston. Adrenergic receptors—evolving concepts and clinical implications. N Engl J Med 1996;334:580-585.
23. O'Connor BJ, Fuller RW, Barnes PJ. Nonbronchodilator effects of inhaled beta 2 agonists. Greater protection against adenosine monophosphate- than methacholine-induced bronchoconstriction in asthma. Am J Respir Crit Care Med 1994;150:381-387.
24. Baluk P, McDonald DM. The beta 2-adrenergic receptor agonist formoterol reduces microvascular leakage by inhibiting endothelial gap formation. Am J Physiol 1994;266:461-468.
25. Lipworth BJ, Clark RA, Dhillon DP, et al. Pharmacokinetics, efficacy and adverse effects of sublingual salbutamol in patients with asthma. Eur J Clin Pharmacol 1989;37:567-571.
26. Travers A, Jones AP, Kelly K, et al. Intravenous beta2-agonists for acute asthma in the emergency department. Cochrane Database Syst Rev 2001;(2):CD002988.
27. Drazen JM, Israel E, Boushey HA, et al. Comparison of regularly scheduled with as-needed use of albuterol in mild asthma. Asthma Clinical Research Network. N Engl J Med 1996;335:841-847.
28. Dennis SM, Sharp SJ, Vickers MR, et al. Regular inhaled salbutamol and asthma control: the TRUST randomised trial. Therapy Working Group of the National Asthma Task Force and the MRC General Practice Research Framework. Lancet 2000;355:1675-1679.
29. Mohamed MH, Lima JJ, Eberle LV, et al. Effects of gender and race on albuterol pharmacokinetics. Pharmacotherapy 1999;19:157-161.

29a. Lee-Wong M, Chou V, Ogawa Y. Formoterol fumarate inhalation powder vs albuterol nebulizer for the treatment of asthma in the acute care setting. Ann Allergy Asthma Immunol 2008;100:146-152.

30. Rodrigo GJ, Rodrigo C. Continuous vs intermittent beta-agonists in the treatment of acute adult asthma: a systematic review with meta-analysis [Review]. Chest 2002;122:160-165.
31. Walters EH, Walters JA, Gibson PW. Regular treatment with long acting beta agonists versus daily regular treatment with short acting beta agonists in adults and children with stable asthma. Cochrane Database Syst Rev 2002;(4):CD003901.
32. Remington TL, Digiovine B. Long-acting beta-agonists: anti-inflammatory properties and synergy with corticosteroids in asthma. Curr Opin Pulm Med 2005;11:74-78.
33. Expert panel report 3: guidelines for the diagnosis and management of asthma. NIH Publication No. 08-4051. Bethesda, MD: U.S. Department of Health and Human Services; National Institutes of Health; National Heart, Lung, and Blood Institute; National Asthma Education and Prevention Program, 2007.
34. British Thoracic Society, Scottish Intercollegiate Guidelines Network. British guideline on the management of asthma. Thorax 2003;58(suppl 1):i1-i94.
35. Dennis R, Solarte I, Fitzgerald JM. Asthma. Clin Evid 2004;11:1966-1997.
36. Ram FS, Cates CJ, Ducharme FM. Long-acting beta2-agonists versus anti-leukotrienes as add-on therapy to inhaled corticosteroids for chronic asthma. Cochrane Database Syst Rev 2005;(1):CD003137.
37. Pauwels RA, Lofdahl CG, Postma DS, et al. Effect of inhaled formoterol and budesonide on exacerbations of asthma. Formoterol and Corticosteroids Establishing Therapy (FACET) International Study Group [see comment] [erratum appears in N Engl J Med 1998;338:139]. N Engl J Med 1997;337:1405-1411.
38. Shrewsbury S, Pyke S, Britton M. Meta-analysis of increased dose of inhaled steroid or addition of salmeterol in symptomatic asthma (MIASMA). BMJ 2000;320:1368-1373.
39. Eickelberg O, Roth M, Lorx R, et al. Ligand-independent activation of the glucocorticoid receptor by beta2-adrenergic receptor agonists in primary human lung fibroblasts and vascular smooth muscle cells. J Biol Chem 1999;274:1005-1010.
40. Pang L, Knox AJ. Regulation of TNF-alpha–induced eotaxin release from cultured human airway smooth muscle cells by beta2-agonists and corticosteroids. FASEB J 2001;15:261-269.
41. Korn SH, Wouters EF, Wesseling G, et al. Interaction between glucocorticoids and beta2-agonists: alpha and beta glucocorticoid-receptor mRNA expression in human bronchial epithelial cells. Biochem Pharmacol 1998;56:1561-1569.
42. Ni CM, Greenstone I, Ducharme F. Addition of inhaled long-acting beta2-agonists to inhaled steroids as first line therapy for persistent asthma in steroid-naive adults. Cochrane Database Syst Rev 2005;(2):CD005307.
43. Appleton S, Poole P, Smith B, et al. Long-acting beta2-agonists for poorly reversible chronic obstructive pulmonary disease. Cochrane Database Syst Rev 2006;(3):CD001104.
44. Hanania NA, Sharafkhaneh A, Barber R, Dickey BF. Beta-agonist intrinsic efficacy: measurement and clinical significance. Am J Respir Crit Care Med 2002;165:1353-1358.
45. Lotvall J, Lunde H, Svedmyr N. Onset of bronchodilation and finger tremor induced by salmeterol and salbutamol in asthmatic patients. Can Respir J 1998;5:191-194.
46. Lipworth BJ, Struthers AD, McDevitt DG. Tachyphylaxis to systemic but not to airway responses during prolonged therapy with high dose inhaled salbutamol in asthmatics. Am Rev Respir Dis 1989;140:586-592.
47. Salpeter SR, Ormiston TM, Salpeter EE. Meta-analysis: respiratory tolerance to regular beta2-agonist use in patients with asthma. Ann Intern Med 2004;140:802-813.

48. Larj MJ, Bleecker ER. Effects of beta2-agonists on airway tone and bronchial responsiveness. J Allergy Clin Immunol 2002;110:S304-S312.
49. Boulet LP, Cartier A, Milot J, et al. Tolerance to the protective effects of salmeterol on methacholine-induced bronchoconstriction: influence of inhaled corticosteroids. Eur Respir J 1998;11:1091-1097.
50. Salpeter SR, Ormiston TM, Salpeter EE. Cardiovascular effects of beta-agonists in patients with asthma and COPD: a meta-analysis. Chest 2004;125:2309-2321.
51. Au DH, Curtis JR, Every NR, et al. Association between inhaled beta-agonists and the risk of unstable angina and myocardial infarction. Chest 2002;121:846-851.
52. Murray JJ. Cardiovascular risks associated with beta-agonist therapy. Chest 2005;127:2283-2285.
53. Ferguson GT, Funck-Brentano C, Fischer T, et al. Cardiovascular safety of salmeterol in COPD. Chest 2003;123:1817-1824.
54. Crane J, Burgess C, Beasley R. Cardiovascular and hypokalaemic effects of inhaled salbutamol, fenoterol, and isoprenaline. Thorax 1989;44:136-140.
55. Nathan RA, Seltzer JM, Kemp JP, et al. Safety of salmeterol in the maintenance treatment of asthma. Ann Allergy Asthma Immunol 1995;75:243-248.
56. Turner MO, Noertjojo K, Vedal S, et al. Risk factors for near-fatal asthma. A case-control study in hospitalized patients with asthma. Am J Respir Crit Care Med 1998;157:1804-1809.
57. Shrestha M, Bidadi K, Gourlay S, Hayes J. Continuous vs intermittent albuterol, at high and low doses, in the treatment of severe acute asthma in adults. Chest 1996;110:42-47.
58. Lipworth BJ, McDevitt DG, Struthers AD. Prior treatment with diuretic augments the hypokalemic and electrocardiographic effects of inhaled albuterol. Am J Med 1989;86:653-657.
59. Bremner P, Woodman K, Burgess C, et al. A comparison of the cardiovascular and metabolic effects of formoterol, salbutamol and fenoterol. Eur Respir J 1993;6:204-210.
60. Crane J, Pearce N, Flatt A, et al. Prescribed fenoterol and death from asthma in New Zealand, 1981-83: case-control study. Lancet 1989;1:917-922.
61. Spitzer WO, Suissa S, Ernst P, et al. The use of beta-agonists and the risk of death and near death from asthma. N Engl J Med 1992;326:501-506.
62. Pearce N, Grainger J, Atkinson M, et al. Case-control study of prescribed fenoterol and death from asthma in New Zealand, 1977-81. Thorax 1990;45:170-175.
63. Mullen M, Mullen B, Carey M. The association between beta-agonist use and death from asthma. A meta-analytic integration of case-control studies. JAMA 1993;270:1842-1845.
64. Mann M, Chowdhury B, Sullivan E, et al. Serious asthma exacerbations in asthmatics treated with high-dose formoterol. Chest 2003;124:70-74.
65. Ni Chroinin M, Greenstone IR, Danish A, et al. Long-acting beta2-agonists versus placebo in addition to inhaled corticosteroids in children and adults with chronic asthma. Cochrane Database Syst Rev 2005;(4):CD005535.
66. Sin DD, Man J, Sharpe H, et al. Pharmacological management to reduce exacerbations in adults with asthma: a systematic review and meta-analysis. JAMA 2004;292:367-376.
67. Nelson HS, Weiss ST, Bleecker ER, et al, and the SMART Study Group. The Salmeterol Multicenter Asthma Research Trial: a comparison of usual pharmacotherapy for asthma or usual pharmacotherapy plus salmeterol. Chest 2006;129:15-26.
68. Israel E, Chinchilli VM, Ford JG, et al. Use of regularly scheduled albuterol treatment in asthma: genotype-stratified, randomised, placebo-controlled cross-over trial. Lancet 2004;364:1505-1512.
69. Wechsler ME, Lehman E, Lazarus SC, et al. Beta-Adrenergic receptor polymorphisms and response to salmeterol. Am J Respir Crit Care Med 2006;173:519-526.
70. Calverley PM, Anderson JA, Celli B, et al. Salmeterol and fluticasone propionate and survival in chronic obstructive pulmonary disease. N Engl J Med 2007;356:775-789.
71. Ruffin RE, Fitzgerald JD, Rebuck AS. A comparison of the bronchodilator activity of Sch 1000 and salbutamol. J Allergy Clin Immunol 1977;59:136-141.
72. Witek TJ Jr. The fate of inhaled drugs: the pharmacokinetics and pharmacodynamics of drugs administered by aerosol. Respir Care 2000;45:826-830.
73. Barnes PJ. The pharmacological properties of tiotropium. Chest 2000;117:63S-66S.
74. Barr RG, Bourbeau J, Camargo CA, Ram FS. Tiotropium for stable chronic obstructive pulmonary disease: a meta-analysis. Thorax 2006;61:854-862.
75. Rodrigo GJ, Nannini LJ. Tiotropium for the treatment of stable chronic obstructive pulmonary disease: A systematic review with meta-analysis. Pulm Pharmacol Ther 2007;20:495-502.
76. Rodrigo GJ, Rodrigo C. The role of anticholinergics in acute asthma treatment: an evidence-based evaluation. Chest 2002;121:1977-1987.
77. Kerstjens HA, Brand PL, Hughes MD, et al. A comparison of bronchodilator therapy with or without inhaled corticosteroid therapy for obstructive airways disease. Dutch Chronic Non-Specific Lung Disease Study Group. N Engl J Med 1992;327:1413-1419.
78. Dagnone AJ, Parlow JL. Effects of inhaled albuterol and ipratropium bromide on autonomic control of the cardiovascular system. Chest 1997;111:1514-1518.
79. Anthonisen NR, Connett JE, Enright PL, Manfreda J, and the Lung Health Study Research Group. Hospitalizations and mortality in the Lung Health Study. Am J Respir Crit Care Med 2002;166:333-339.
80. Lanes S, Golisch W, Mikl J. Ipratropium and lung health study. Am J Respir Crit Care Med 2003;167:801; author reply 801-802.
81. Sin DD, Tu JV. Lack of association between ipratropium bromide and mortality in elderly patients with chronic obstructive airway disease. Thorax 2000;55:194-197.
82. Gudmundsson G, Gislason T, Lindberg E, et al. Mortality in COPD patients discharged from hospital: the role of treatment and co-morbidity. Respir Res 2006;7:109.
83. Kesten S, Jara M, Wentworth C, Lanes S. Pooled clinical trial analysis of tiotropium safety. Chest 2006;130:1695-1703.
84. Kalra L, Bone MF. The effect of nebulized bronchodilator therapy on intraocular pressures in patients with glaucoma. Chest 1988;93:739-741.
85. Barnes PJ, Adcock IM. How do corticosteroids work in asthma? Ann Intern Med 2003;139:359-370.
86. Gao L, Cueto MA, Asselbergs F, Atadja P. Cloning and functional characterization of HDAC11, a novel member of the human histone deacetylase family. J Biol Chem 2002;277:25748-25755.
87. Peterson CL. HDAC's at work: everyone doing their part. Mol Cell 2002;9:921-922.
88. Berger SL. Histone modifications in transcriptional regulation. Curr Opin Genet Dev 2002;12:142-148.
89. Powell H, Gibson PG. High dose versus low dose inhaled corticosteroid as initial starting dose for asthma in adults and children. Cochrane Database Syst Rev 2004;(2): CD004109.
90. Adams N, Bestall JM, Jones PW. Inhaled fluticasone at different doses for chronic asthma. Cochrane Database Syst Rev 2002;(1):CD003534.
91. Adams N, Bestall J, Jones PW. Budesonide at different doses for chronic asthma. Cochrane Database Syst Rev 2001;(4):CD003271.
92. Masoli M, Holt S, Weatherall M, Beasley R. Dose-response relationship of inhaled budesonide in adult asthma: a meta-analysis. Eur Respir J 2004;23:552-558.
93. Adams N, Bestall J, Lasserson T, Jones P. Inhaled fluticasone versus placebo for chronic asthma in adults and children. Cochrane Database Syst Rev 2005;(2):CD003135.
94. Adams N, Bestall J, Jones P. Inhaled beclomethasone at different doses for long-term asthma. Cochrane Database Syst Rev 2001;(1):CD002879.
95. Mash B, Bheekie A, Jones PW. Inhaled vs oral steroids for adults with chronic asthma. Cochrane Database Syst Rev 2001;(1):CD002160.
96. Beasley R, Sterk PJ, Kerstjens HA, Decramer M. Comparative studies of inhaled corticosteroids in asthma. Eur Respir J 2001;17:579-580.
97. Casale TB, Nelson HS, Stricker WE, et al. Suppression of hypothalamic-pituitary-adrenal axis activity with inhaled flunisolide and fluticasone propionate in adult asthma patients. Ann Allergy Asthma Immunol 2001;87:379-385.
98. Lipworth BJ. Systemic adverse effects of inhaled corticosteroid therapy: a systematic review and meta-analysis. Arch Intern Med 1999;159:941-955.
99. Adams N, Bestall JM, Jones PW. Inhaled beclomethasone versus budesonide for chronic asthma. Cochrane Database Syst Rev 2002;(1):CD003530.
100. Adams NP, Bestall JB, Malouf R, et al. Inhaled beclomethasone versus placebo for chronic asthma. Cochrane Database Syst Rev 2005;(1):CD002738.
101. Suissa S, Ernst P. Inhaled corticosteroids: impact on asthma morbidity and mortality. J Allergy Clin Immunol 2001;107:937-944.
102. Suissa S, Ernst P, Kezouh A. Regular use of inhaled corticosteroids and the long term prevention of hospitalisation for asthma. Thorax 2002;57:880-884.
103. Suissa S, Ernst P, Benayoun S, et al. Low-dose inhaled corticosteroids and the prevention of death from asthma. N Engl J Med 2000;343:332-336.
104. Suissa S, Ernst P. Use of anti-inflammatory therapy and asthma mortality in Japan. Eur Respir J 2003;21:101-104.
105. Donahue JG, Weiss ST, Livingston JM, et al. Inhaled steroids and the risk of hospitalization for asthma. JAMA 1997;277:887-891.
106. Ng D, Salvio F, Hicks G. Anti-leukotriene agents compared to inhaled corticosteroids in the management of recurrent and/or chronic asthma in adults and children. Cochrane Database Syst Rev 2004;(2):CD002314.
107. Gibson PG, Powell H, Ducharme F. Long-acting beta2-agonists as an inhaled corticosteroid-sparing agent for chronic asthma in adults and children. Cochrane Database Syst Rev 2005;(4):CD005076.
108. Guilbert TW, Morgan WJ, Zeiger RS, et al. Long-term inhaled corticosteroids in preschool children at high risk for asthma. N Engl J Med 2006;354:1985-1997.
109. Aaron SD, Vandemheen KL, Fergusson D, et al. Tiotropium in combination with placebo, salmeterol, or fluticasone-salmeterol for treatment of chronic obstructive pulmonary disease: a randomized trial. Ann Intern Med 2007;146:545-555.
110. Smith M, Iqbal S, Elliott TM, et al. Corticosteroids for hospitalised children with acute asthma. Cochrane Database Syst Rev 2003;(2):CD002886.
111. Niewoehner DE, Erbland ML, Deupree RH, et al. Effect of systemic glucocorticoids on exacerbations of chronic obstructive pulmonary disease. Department of Veterans Affairs Cooperative Study Group. N Engl J Med 1999;340:1941-1947.
112. Rowe BH, Spooner C, Ducharme FM, et al. Early emergency department treatment of acute asthma with systemic corticosteroids. Cochrane Database Syst Rev 2001;(1): CD002178.
113. Rowe BH, Spooner CH, Ducharme FM, et al. Corticosteroids for preventing relapse following acute exacerbations of asthma. Cochrane Database Syst Rev 2001;(1): CD000195.
114. Becker JM, Arora A, Scarfone RJ, et al. Oral versus intravenous corticosteroids in children hospitalized with asthma. J Allergy Clin Immunol 1999;103:586-590.
115. Manser R, Reid D, Abramson M. Corticosteroids for acute severe asthma in hospitalised patients. Cochrane Database Syst Rev 2001;(1):CD001740.
116. Jones AM, Munavvar M, Vail A, et al. Prospective, placebo-controlled trial of 5 vs 10 days of oral prednisolone in acute adult asthma. Respir Med 2002;96:950-954.
117. Edmonds ML, Camargo CA Jr, Pollack CV Jr, Rowe BH. The effectiveness of inhaled corticosteroids in the emergency department treatment of acute asthma: a meta-analysis. Ann Emerg Med 2002;40:145-154.
118. Daley-Yates PT, Richards DH. Relationship between systemic corticosteroid exposure and growth velocity: development and validation of a pharmacokinetic/pharmacodynamic model. Clin Ther 2004;26:1905-1919.
119. Roland NJ, Bhalla RK, Earis J. The local side effects of inhaled corticosteroids: current understanding and review of the literature. Chest 2004;126:213-219.
120. Smeeth L, Boulis M, Hubbard R, Fletcher AE. A population based case-control study of cataract and inhaled corticosteroids. Br J Ophthalmol 2003;87:1247-1251.
121. Garbe E, Suissa S, LeLorier J. Association of inhaled corticosteroid use with cataract extraction in elderly patients. JAMA 1998;280:539-543.

122. Cumming RG, Mitchell P, Leeder SR. Use of inhaled corticosteroids and the risk of cataracts. N Engl J Med 1997;337:8-14.
123. Garbe E, LeLorier J, Boivin JF, Suissa S. Inhaled and nasal glucocorticoids and the risks of ocular hypertension or open-angle glaucoma. JAMA 1997;277:722-727.
124. Doull IJ, Freezer NJ, Holgate ST. Growth of prepubertal children with mild asthma treated with inhaled beclomethasone dipropionate. Am J Respir Crit Care Med 1995;151:1715-1719.
125. The Childhood Asthma Management Program Research Group. Long-term effects of budesonide or nedocromil in children with asthma. N Engl J Med 2000;343:1054-1063.
126. Agertoft L, Pedersen S. Effect of long-term treatment with inhaled budesonide on adult height in children with asthma. N Engl J Med 2000;343:1064-1069.
127. Silverstein MD, Yunginger JW, Reed CE, et al. Attained adult height after childhood asthma: effect of glucocorticoid therapy. J Allergy Clin Immunol 1997;99:466-474.
128. Jones A, Fay JK, Burr M, et al. Inhaled corticosteroid effects on bone metabolism in asthma and mild chronic obstructive pulmonary disease. Cochrane Database Syst Rev 2002;(1):CD003537.
129. Johannes CB, Schneider GA, Dube TJ, et al. The risk of nonvertebral fracture related to inhaled corticosteroid exposure among adults with chronic respiratory disease. Chest 2005;127:89-97.
130. Scanlon PD, Connett JE, Wise RA, et al. Loss of bone density with inhaled triamcinolone in Lung Health Study II. Am J Respir Crit Care Med 2004;170:1302-1309.
131. Suissa S, Baltzan M, Kremer R, Ernst P. Inhaled and nasal corticosteroid use and the risk of fracture. Am J Respir Crit Care Med 2004;169:83-88.
132. Gluck O, Colice G. Recognizing and treating glucocorticoid-induced osteoporosis in patients with pulmonary diseases. Chest 2004;125:1859-1876.
133. Campbell IA, Douglas JG, Francis RM, et al, and the Research Committee of the British Thoracic Society. Five year study of etidronate and/or calcium as prevention and treatment for osteoporosis and fractures in patients with asthma receiving long term oral and/or inhaled glucocorticoids. Thorax 2004;59:761-768.
134. Wilson AM, Blumsohn A, Jung RT, Lipworth BJ. Asthma and Cushing's syndrome. Chest 2000;117:593-594.
135. Eichenhorn MS, Wise RA, Madhok TC, et al. Lack of long-term adverse adrenal effects from inhaled triamcinolone: Lung Health Study II. Chest 2003;124:57-62.
136. Martin RJ, Szefler SJ, Chinchilli VM, et al. Systemic effect comparisons of six inhaled corticosteroid preparations. Am J Respir Crit Care Med 2002;165:1377-1383.
137. Drazen JM, Israel E, O'Byrne PM. Treatment of asthma with drugs modifying the leukotriene pathway. N Engl J Med 1999;340:197-206.
138. Braccioni F, Dorman SC, O'Byrne PM, et al. The effect of cysteinyl leukotrienes on growth of eosinophil progenitors from peripheral blood and bone marrow of atopic subjects. J Allergy Clin Immunol 2002;110:96-101.
139. Salvi SS, Krishna MT, Sampson AP, Holgate ST. The anti-inflammatory effects of leukotriene-modifying drugs and their use in asthma. Chest 2001;119:1533-1546.
140. Evans DJ, Barnes PJ, Spaethe SM, et al. Effect of a leukotriene B4 receptor antagonist, LY293111, on allergen induced responses in asthma. Thorax 1996;51:1178-1184.
141. Heise CE, O'Dowd BF, Figueroa DJ, et al. Characterization of the human cysteinyl leukotriene 2 receptor. J Biol Chem 2000;275:30531-30536.
142. Edelman JM, Turpin JA, Bronsky EA, et al. Oral montelukast compared with inhaled salmeterol to prevent exercise-induced bronchoconstriction. A randomized, double-blind trial. Exercise Study Group. Ann Intern Med 2000;132:97-104.
143. Cowburn AS, Sladek K, Soja J, et al. Overexpression of leukotriene C4 synthase in bronchial biopsies from patients with aspirin-intolerant asthma. J Clin Invest 1998;101:834-846.
144. Babu KS, Salvi SS. Aspirin and asthma. Chest 2000;118:1470-1476.
145. Dahlen SE, Malmstrom K, Nizankowska E, et al. Improvement of aspirin-intolerant asthma by montelukast, a leukotriene antagonist: a randomized, double-blind, placebo-controlled trial. Am J Respir Crit Care Med 2002;165:9-14.
146. Lee DK, Haggart K, Robb FM, Lipworth BJ. Montelukast protects against nasal lysine-aspirin challenge in patients with aspirin-induced asthma. Eur Respir J 2004;24:226-230.
147. Nasser SM, Bell GS, Foster S, et al. Effect of the 5-lipoxygenase inhibitor ZD2138 on aspirin-induced asthma. Thorax 1994;49:749-756.
148. Camargo CA Jr, Smithline HA, Malice MP, et al. A randomized controlled trial of intravenous montelukast in acute asthma. Am J Respir Crit Care Med 2003;167:528-533.
149. Silverman RA, Nowak RM, Korenblat PE, et al. Zafirlukast treatment for acute asthma: evaluation in a randomized, double-blind, multicenter trial. Chest 2004;126:1480-1489.
150. Celik P, Sakar A, Havlucu Y, et al. Short-term effects of montelukast in stable patients with moderate to severe COPD. Respir Med 2005;99:444-450.
151. Rubinstein I, Kumar B, Schriever C. Long-term montelukast therapy in moderate to severe COPD—a preliminary observation. Respir Med 2004;98:134-138.
152. Chu EK, Drazen JM. Asthma: one hundred years of treatment and onward. Am J Respir Crit Care Med 2005;171:1202-1208.
153. Alton EW, Norris AA. Chloride transport and the actions of nedocromil sodium and cromolyn sodium in asthma. J Allergy Clin Immunol 1996;98:S102, S105; discussion S105-S106.
154. Storms W, Kaliner MA. Cromolyn sodium: fitting an old friend into current asthma treatment. J Asthma 2005;42:79-89.
155. Theoharides TC, Wang L, Pang X, et al. Cloning and cellular localization of the rat mast cell 78-kDa protein phosphorylated in response to the mast cell "stabilizer" cromolyn. J Pharmacol Exp Ther 2000;294:810-821.
156. Loh RK, Jabara HH, Geha RS. Disodium cromoglycate inhibits S mu–>S epsilon deletional switch recombination and IgE synthesis in human B cells. J Exp Med 1994;180:663-671.
157. Loh RK, Jabara HH, Geha RS. Mechanisms of inhibition of IgE synthesis by nedocromil sodium: nedocromil sodium inhibits deletional switch recombination in human B cells. J Allergy Clin Immunol 1996;97:1141-1150.
158. van der Wouden JC, Tasche MJ, Bernsen RM, et al. Inhaled sodium cromoglycate for asthma in children. Cochrane Database Syst Rev 2003;(3):CD002173.
159. Edwards A, Holgate S, Howell J, et al. Sodium cromoglycate in childhood asthma. Thorax 2001;56:331-332.
160. Kelly K, Spooner CH, Rowe BH. Nedocromil sodium vs. sodium cromoglycate for preventing exercise-induced bronchoconstriction in asthmatics [Review]. Cochrane Database Syst Rev 2000;(4):002731.
161. Spooner CH, Spooner GR, Rowe BH. Mast-cell stabilising agents to prevent exercise-induced bronchoconstriction. Cochrane Database Syst Rev 2003;(4):CD002307.
162. Latimer KM, O'Byrne PM, Morris MM, et al. Bronchoconstriction stimulated by airway cooling. Better protection with combined inhalation of terbutaline sulphate and cromolyn sodium than with either alone. Am Rev Respir Dis 1983;128:440-443.
163. Barnes PJ. Theophylline: new perspectives for an old drug [Review]. Am J Respir Crit Care Med 2003;167:813-888.
164. Kidney J, Dominguez M, Taylor PM, et al. Immunomodulation by theophylline in asthma. Demonstration by withdrawal of therapy. Am J Respir Crit Care Med 1995;151:1907-1914.
165. Magnussen H, Reuss G, Jorres R. Theophylline has a dose-related effect on the airway response to inhaled histamine and methacholine in asthmatics. Am Rev Respir Dis 1987;136:1163-1167.
166. National Asthma Education and Prevention Program. Expert Panel Report: guidelines for the diagnosis and management of asthma—update on selected topics 2002. J Allergy Clin Immunol 2002;110:S141-S219.
167. Siegel D, Sheppard D, Gelb A, Weinberg PF. Aminophylline increases the toxicity but not the efficacy of an inhaled beta-adrenergic agonist in the treatment of acute exacerbations of asthma. Am Rev Respir Dis 1985;132:283-286.
168. Shah L, Wilson AJ, Gibson PG, Coughlan J. Long acting beta-agonists versus theophylline for maintenance treatment of asthma. Cochrane Database Syst Rev 2003;(3):001281.
169. Ram FS, Jardin JR, Atallah A, et al. Efficacy of theophylline in people with stable chronic obstructive pulmonary disease: a systematic review and meta-analysis. Respir Med 2005;99:135-144.
170. Sullivan P, Bekir S, Jaffar Z, et al. Anti-inflammatory effects of low-dose oral theophylline in atopic asthma. Lancet 1994;343:1006-1008.
171. McKay SE, Howie CA, Thomson AH, et al. Value of theophylline treatment in patients handicapped by chronic obstructive lung disease. Thorax 1993;48:227-232.
172. Seddon P, Bara A, Ducharme F, Lasserson T. Oral xanthines as maintenance treatment for asthma in children. Cochrane Database Syst Rev 2006;(1):CD002885.
173. Ernst P, Cai B, Blais L, Suissa S. The early course of newly diagnosed asthma. Am J Med 2002;112:44-48.
174. Bousquet J. Global initiative for asthma (GINA) and its objectives. Clin Exp Allergy 2000;30(suppl 1):2-5.
175. Rodrigo GJ, Rodrigo C. Triple inhaled drug protocol for the treatment of acute severe asthma. Chest 2003;123:1908-1915.
176. Blitz M, Blitz S, Beasely R, et al. Inhaled magnesium sulfate in the treatment of acute asthma. Cochrane Database Syst Rev 2005;(4):CD003898.
177. Bracken MB, Triche EW, Belanger K, et al. Asthma symptoms, severity, and drug therapy: a prospective study of effects on 2205 pregnancies. Obstet Gynecol 2003;102:739-752.
178. Dombrowski MP, Schatz M, Wise R, et al. Asthma during pregnancy. Obstet Gynecol 2004;103:5-12.
179. National Heart, Lung, and Blood Institute, National Asthma Education and Prevention Program Asthma and Pregnancy Working Group. NAEPP Expert Panel Report: managing asthma during pregnancy: recommendations for pharmacologic treatment—2004 update. J Allergy Clin Immunol 2005;115:34-46.
180. Schatz M, Zeiger RS, Hoffman CP, et al. Perinatal outcomes in the pregnancies of asthmatic women: a prospective controlled analysis. Am J Respir Crit Care Med 1995;151:1170-1174.
181. Schatz M, Zeiger RS, Harden KM, et al. The safety of inhaled beta-agonist bronchodilators during pregnancy. J Allergy Clin Immunol 1988;82:686-695.
182. Blitz M, Blitz S, Beasely R, et al. Inhaled magnesium sulfate in the treatment of acute asthma. Cochrane Database Syst Rev 2005;(2):CD003898.
183. Hayashi K, Yanagi M, Wood-Baker R, et al. Oxatomide for stable asthma in adults and children. Cochrane Database Syst Rev 2003;(2):CD002179.
184. Taramarcaz P, Gibson PG. The effectiveness of intranasal corticosteroids in combined allergic rhinitis and asthma syndrome. Clin Exp Allergy 2004;34:1883-1889.
185. Abramson MJ, Puy RM, Weiner JM. Allergen immunotherapy for asthma. Cochrane Database Syst Rev 2003;(4):CD001186.
186. Gibson PG, Henry RL, Coughlan JL. Gastro-oesophageal reflux treatment for asthma in adults and children. Cochrane Database Syst Rev 2003;(2):CD001496.
187. Smith J, Owen E, Earis J, Woodcock A. Effect of codeine on objective measurement of cough in chronic obstructive pulmonary disease. J Allergy Clin Immunol 2006;117:831-835.
188. Leckie MJ, ten Brinke A, Khan J, et al. Effects of an interleukin-5 blocking monoclonal antibody on eosinophils, airway hyper-responsiveness, and the late asthmatic response. Lancet 2000;356:2144-2148.
189. Bryan SA, O'Connor BJ, Matti S, et al. Effects of recombinant human interleukin-12 on eosinophils, airway hyper-responsiveness, and the late asthmatic response. Lancet 2000;356:2149-2153.
190. Spence DP, Johnston SL, Calverley PM, et al. The effect of the orally active platelet-activating factor antagonist WEB 2086 in the treatment of asthma. Am J Respir Crit Care Med 1994;149:1142-1148.

191. Dixon AE, Irvin CG. Early intervention of therapy in asthma. Curr Opin Pulm Med 2005;11:51-55.
192. Pascual RM, Peters SP. Airway remodeling contributes to the progressive loss of lung function in asthma: an overview. J Allergy Clin Immunol 2005;116:477, 486; quiz 487.
193. Leath TM, Singla M, Peters SP. Novel and emerging therapies for asthma. Drug Discov Today 2005;10:1647-1655.
194. Fung-Leung WP, Thurmond RL, Ling P, Karlsson L. Histamine H4 receptor antagonists: the new antihistamines? Curr Opin Investig Drugs 2004;5:1174-1183.
195. Thurmond RL, Desai PJ, Dunford PJ, et al. A potent and selective histamine H4 receptor antagonist with anti-inflammatory properties. J Pharmacol Exp Ther 2004;309:404-413.
196. Gauvreau GM, Becker AB, Boulet LP, et al. The effects of an anti-CD11a mAb, efalizumab, on allergen-induced airway responses and airway inflammation in subjects with atopic asthma. J Allergy Clin Immunol 2003;112:331-338.
197. Catley MC, Sukkar MB, Chung KF, et al. Validation of the anti-inflammatory properties of small-molecule IkappaB Kinase (IKK)-2 inhibitors by comparison with adenoviral-mediated delivery of dominant-negative IKK1 and IKK2 in human airways smooth muscle. Mol Pharmacol 2006;70:697-705.
198. Churg A, Wang R, Wang X, et al. An MMP-9/-12 inhibitor prevents smoke-induced emphysema and small airway remodeling in guinea pigs. Thorax 2007;62:706-713.
199. Karnaukhova E, Ophir Y, Golding B. Recombinant human alpha-1 proteinase inhibitor: towards therapeutic use. Amino Acids 2006;30:317-332.
200. Barnes PJ, Stockley RA. COPD: current therapeutic interventions and future approaches. Eur Respir J 2005;25:1084-1106.

SECTION 7 Renal Therapeutics

29 RENAL INSUFFICIENCY

Kumar Sharma

INTRODUCTION 435
SLOWING THE RATE OF PROGRESSION 435
Pathophysiology 435
Therapeutics 435
Modulators of the Renin-Angiotensin System 435
Investigational Antifibrotic Agents 436
Statins 436
TREATMENT OF THE COMPLICATIONS OF RENAL DYSFUNCTION 437
Volume Overload 437
Hyperkalemia 437
Metabolic Acidosis 437
Hyperphosphatemia 437
Pathophysiology 437
Goals of Therapy 437
Therapeutics 437
Hypocalcemia 437
Pathophysiology 437
Goals of Therapy 438
Therapeutics 438
Renal Osteodystrophy 438
Pathophysiology 438
Goals of Therapy 438
Therapeutics 438
Hypertension 439
Pathophysiology 439
Goals of Therapy 439
Therapeutics 439
Anemia 440
Pathophysiology 440
Goals of Therapy 440
Therapeutics 440
Dyslipidemia 442
Pathophysiology/Goals of Therapy 442
Therapeutics 442
SUMMARY 442

INTRODUCTION

Chronic kidney disease (CKD) is a worldwide public health problem. The incidence and prevalence of renal disease is rising in the United States.[1] In 2002, the National Kidney Foundation (NKF) sponsored the Kidney Disease Outcomes Quality Initiative (K/DOQI) and published guidelines for the evaluation, classification, and management of CKD.[1] The purpose of these guidelines was to create uniform terminology to improve communication among all health care professionals involved in the care of a patient with CKD. CKD is defined as structural abnormalities of the kidney that can lead to decreased kidney function. The K/DOQI Clinical Practice Guidelines for CKD recommend that individuals at high risk, particularly those with diabetes or hypertension or a family history of diabetes, hypertension, or kidney disease, be assessed for CKD.[1] Once the diagnosis is established, CKD should be staged according to the classification proposed by the NKF-K/DOQI Clinical Practice Guidelines for Evaluation, Classification, and Stratification of CKD. This classification, listed in Table 29-1, is based on laboratory evaluation of the severity of kidney disease, as calculated by measuring the glomerular filtration rate (GFR).

The two major outcomes of CKD are (i) loss of kidney function leading to end-stage renal disease (ESRD) and (ii) development of cardiovascular disease (CVD), including coronary artery disease, cerebrovascular disease, peripheral vascular disease, and heart failure. The risk for adverse outcomes is related to the severity of CKD. Increasing evidence indicates that therapeutic interventions at earlier stages of CKD are effective in slowing the progression of CKD and many of its complications.[1] Much of the CKD treatment is targeted at the whole body and is not necessarily kidney specific. An overview of the management of patients with CKD, including (i) the modalities to slow the rate of CKD progression and (ii) the treatment of the complications of CKD, are presented here.

SLOWING THE RATE OF PROGRESSION

Pathophysiology

A variety of diseases, including diabetic nephropathy, hypertensive nephrosclerosis, chronic glomerulonephritis, and polycystic kidney disease, can cause CKD. Diabetes now accounts for 44% of incident cases of ESRD in the United States; the incident rates are similar in Europe and Japan. Studies in animals and humans suggest that progression of CKD may be due to secondary factors that may be unrelated to the activity of the initial disease. These factors include intraglomerular hypertension and glomerular hypertrophy, which lead to glomerular scarring and tubulointerstitial injury.[2] Glomerular injury is mediated by release of cytokines, such as transforming growth factor-β (TGF-β) by the glomerular mesangial cells, which cause an increase in matrix accumulation.[3,4] Tubulointerstitial injury may be caused by angiotensin II (Ang II)–dependent increase in profibrotic factors such as TGF-β, connective tissue growth factor, and other chemokines.[5,6] Data from several large clinical studies confirm that proteinuria and hypertension are independent predictors of the rate of progression of renal dysfunction. If significant injury has already occurred, treatment of the ongoing renal inflammation may not prevent progression of glomerular and tubulointerstitial scarring. Therefore, in addition to treating proteinuria and hypertension, suppressing the development of interstitial fibrosis may retard the progression of CKD.

Therapeutics

Modulators of the Renin-Angiotensin System

Angiotensin-converting enzyme (ACE) inhibitors or Ang II receptor blockers (ARBs) clearly slow the progression of CKD in diabetic nephropathy and nondiabetic CKD. ACE inhibitors and ARBs may have an antifibrotic role in addition to their antihypertensive and antiproteinuric effects.[7]

Mechanisms of Action. Ang II binds to its specific receptors (AT_1 and AT_2) to cause vasoconstriction and arterial wall hypertrophy.[8] Stimulation of the AT_1 receptor has been implicated to mediate Ang II induction of matrix synthesis largely via TGF-β. Inhibition of Ang II formation with an ACE inhibitor diminishes the activity of both receptor subtypes, whereas the ARBs diminish only AT_1 activity.

ACE Inhibitors. ACE inhibitors generally reduce protein excretion by 35% to 45%, which is consistent with a fall in intraglomerular

TABLE 29-1 STAGES OF CHRONIC KIDNEY DISEASE

Stage	Description	GFR (ml/min/1.73 m²)
1	Kidney damage with normal or ↑ GFR	≥90
2	Kidney damage with mild ↓ GFR	60-89
3	Moderate ↓ GFR	30-59
4	Severe ↓ GFR	15-29
5	Kidney failure	<15 (or dialysis)

GFR, glomerular filtration rate.
Adapted from National Kidney Foundation. K/DOQI clinical practice guidelines. Available at http://www.kidney.org/professionals/KDOQI/guidelines.cfm (accessed October 22, 2006).

pressure.[9] The three main trials to date that addressed the potential preferential benefits of ACE inhibitors in patients with CKD of various etiologies were the benazepril trial (comparing benazepril with placebo),[10] the REIN trial (comparing ramipril with placebo),[11,12] and the AASK trial (comparing ramipril with amlodipine and metoprolol).[13,14] All of these trials essentially revealed a decrease in proteinuria, a lower rate of decline in GFR, and a lower number of patients who progressed to ESRD in the ACE inhibitor–treated group. Additional analyses of these trials found that renoprotective benefits were most prominent in patients with current protein excretion of 1 g/day to 2 g/day and a systolic pressure between 110 mm Hg and 129 mm Hg.[15] In comparison, a systolic pressure of less than 110 mm Hg was associated with a higher risk of renal progression and all-cause mortality. The benefit of ACE inhibitors was also demonstrated in patients with type 1 diabetes who already had overt nephropathy.[16] After 4 years, patients treated with captopril had a slower rate of increase in the plasma creatinine concentration and a lesser likelihood of progressing to ESRD or death.[17]

ARBs. Studies in humans have found that Ang II receptor antagonists are as effective as ACE inhibitors in reducing protein excretion in patients with CKD.[18,19] Among patients with immunoglobulin A (IgA) nephropathy, for example, enalapril and irbesartan had similar effects on proteinuria.[20] Two major trials demonstrated a clear benefit in terms of renoprotection with ARBs in patients with nephropathy due to type 2 diabetes. In the Irbesartan Diabetic Nephropathy Trial,[21,22] 1715 hypertensive patients with nephropathy due to type 2 diabetes were randomly assigned to irbesartan (300 mg/day), amlodipine (10 mg/day), or placebo. At 2.6 years, irbesartan was associated with a 20% lower risk of renal disease progression than was amlodipine. In the RENAAL trial,[23] 1513 patients with type 2 diabetes and nephropathy were randomly assigned to losartan (50 mg titrating up to 100 mg once daily) or placebo. In a 3.4-year follow-up, losartan reduced the incidence of a doubling of the plasma creatinine by 25% and of ESRD by 28% versus placebo. As with ACE inhibition, there appears to be a dose effect, with greater reduction of proteinuria at higher doses in both diabetic and nondiabetic patients.[24,25]

Potentially, combination therapy may be more effective that monotherapy because ACE inhibitors block only the formation of Ang II mediated by ACE, but alternative enzymatic pathways exist for the production of Ang II.[26,27] Benefit of an ACE inhibitor/ARB combination was demonstrated in the COOPERATE trial[28] in which 263 Japanese patients with nondiabetic renal failure were randomly assigned to losartan (100 mg/day), trandolapril (3 mg/day), or both agents at equivalent doses. The largest decrease in proteinuria, the slowest time to doubling of the serum creatinine, and the least amount of ESRD were observed with combination therapy. The protective effect had the greatest impact when treatment was initiated early in the course of CKD, usually before the GFR fell below 60 ml/min/1.73 m².

ACE inhibitors and ARBs can cause a decline in renal function and a rise in plasma potassium, both of which typically occur soon after the onset of therapy. As a result, a repeat plasma creatinine and potassium should be measured within 3 to 5 days of treatment initiation. Although many physicians are hesitant to continue ACE inhibitors and/or ARBs with progressive decline in renal function, a recent study indicated that renoprotective benefit remains in patients with advanced renal failure.[29]

K/DOQI Clinical Practice Guidelines recommend a reduction in blood pressure to less than 130/80 mm Hg and a reduction in urinary protein excretion to less than 500 mg/day to 1000 mg/day. As discussed later, in most patients, these aggressive goals will require therapy with multiple drugs.

Investigational Antifibrotic Agents

Pirfenidone down-regulates expression of cytokines and other mediators involved in the development of fibrosis. It has been beneficial in diseases involving scar formation, such as pulmonary fibrosis and focal segmental glomerulosclerosis. Pirfenidone therapy reduced collagen accumulation and increased renal function recovery in rat models with renal interstitial fibrosis. These benefits may be due to reversal of accumulation of extracellular fibrosis by suppression of TGF-β.[30] Currently, an ongoing study is attempting to determine whether pirfenidone can slow the progression of kidney disease in patients with diabetes.[31]

The chemokine receptor CCR-1 is likely to be involved in a variety of proinflammatory diseases. Blockade of CCR-1 with BX471 substantially reduces renal fibrosis in mice with unilateral ureteral obstruction[32] and lupus nephritis.[33] Therefore CCR-1 blockade may represent a new therapeutic strategy for reducing renal fibrosis, a major factor in the progression of CKD to ESRD.

TGF-β blockade with antibodies has been demonstrated to have beneficial effects to protect the kidney in models of type 1 diabetes as well as type 2 diabetes.[34,35] Anti–TGF-β antibodies also reduce fibrosis in rodent models of glomerulonephritis. The antifibrotic effect may be magnified when used in combination with angiotensin inhibition.[36,37] Connective tissue growth factor (CTGF), a downstream mediator of the chronic fibrosis, is activated by TGF-β. It induces fibroblasts to become myofibroblasts that deposit layers of collagen and help form a scar. Studies have demonstrated that the levels of CTGF correlate with the severity of fibrosis in many diseases including diabetic nephropathy, glomerulosclerosis, and IgA nephropathy. Fibrosis has been successfully treated with antibodies such as FG-3019 (a fully human monoclonal antibody) that block CTGF activity in animal models of kidney fibrosis.[38] Bone morphogenetic protein-7 (BMP7) is expressed in adult kidney and inhibits TGF-β–driven fibrogenesis, primarily by preventing the TGF-β–dependent down-regulation of matrix degradation and up-regulation of plasminogen activator inhibitor-1 (PAI-1). BMP7 reduces renal fibrogenesis when given exogenously to rodents with experimental chronic nephropathies.[39] In fact, experimental diabetic nephropathy models have demonstrated decreased levels of renal tubular BMP7 and some of its receptors. Thus, exogenous repletion of these agents may reduce renal fibrogenesis.[40]

Hepatocyte growth factor is a protein that has antifibrogenic activity. It reduces fibrosis via several mechanisms, including inhibition of TGF-β and alpha-smooth muscle actin. It also reduces the tubular expression of proinflammatory chemokines, such as macrophage chemoattractant protein-1 and RANTES.[41-44] Therefore, supplemental therapy with hepatocyte growth factor may be another novel option for prevention and treatment of CKD.

Statins

3-Hydroxy-3-methylglutaryl coenzyme A (HMG CoA) reductase inhibitors (statins), in addition to lowering plasma lipid levels, may directly hinder the progression of renal disease. Hyperlipidemia is common in patients with CKD. Experimental models reveal that hyperlipidemia can cause mesangial cell proliferation and increased production of fibronectin and reactive oxygen species.[45-47] All of these alterations could lead to the glomerular injury. HMG CoA reductase inhibitors inhibit mesangial cell proliferation and production of macrophage chemotactic factors, thereby slowing down renal disease progression.[48] The effect of statins to reduce proteinuria has been quite variable in smaller studies; however, larger studies are under way.[49] Potential benefits of statins will need to be offset against uncommon muscle injury.[50-54]

TREATMENT OF THE COMPLICATIONS OF RENAL DYSFUNCTION

A wide range of disorders may develop as a consequence of loss of renal function. These include disorders of fluid and electrolyte balance (such as volume overload, hyperkalemia, metabolic acidosis, hyperphosphatemia, and hypocalcemia) and hormonal/systemic dysfunctions such as bone disease, hypertension, anemia, and dyslipidemia.

Volume Overload

Patients with CKD and volume overload usually respond to dietary sodium restriction and diuretic therapy. Some studies have shown that limiting sodium intake will also slow the progression of CKD, possibly by lowering the intraglomerular pressure.[55]

Thiazide diuretics in general lower blood pressure more effectively than loop diuretics in patients with hypertension and preserved renal function. However, as the GFR falls below 30 ml/min (stage 4 CKD), thiazide diuretics become less effective, and loop diuretics are more effective antihypertensive agents. The standard treatment includes a loop diuretic given twice daily.[56,57]

The aldosterone antagonists spironolactone and eplerenone can also be used for hypertensive management[58,59] and may have additive antifibrotic effects. A recent study in CKD patients with persistent proteinuria despite conventional management demonstrated that the addition of spironolactone did produce beneficial effects on reducing urinary protein excretion, especially in patients with diabetes.[60] However, benefits on blood pressure control, fibrosis, and proteinuria need to be weighed against the potential for inducing or exacerbating hyperkalemia in CKD patients.[61,62]

Hyperkalemia

Hyperkalemia usually occurs in oliguric patients who have an additional problem, such as a high-potassium diet, increased tissue breakdown, or hypoaldosteronism. Patients who have a serum potassium concentration in the high-normal range (>5 mEq/L) prior to therapy are more likely to develop hyperkalemia with an ACE inhibitor, an ARB, or an aldosterone antagonist. Starting a low-potassium diet or initiating therapy with a thiazide or loop diuretic will decrease the propensity for hyperkalemia. Low-dose sodium polystyrene sulfonate (Kayexalate; 5 g with each meal) can be used to lower the serum potassium concentration without the gastrointestinal side effects seen with larger doses. Patients are also instructed to avoid using medications, such as nonsteroidal anti-inflammatory drugs, that may raise serum potassium.[63] Nonselective β-blockers may cause postprandial rise in the serum potassium concentration but do not produce persistent hyperkalemia.

Metabolic Acidosis

Patients with CKD retain hydrogen ions, which lead to a progressive metabolic acidosis.[64-66] The serum bicarbonate concentration usually stabilizes between 12 mEq/L and 20 mEq/L.[65,67] Two major reasons to treat acidemia in patients with CKD are (i) the worsening bone disease with acidemia because excess hydrogen ions cause release of calcium and phosphate from bone and (ii) increased skeletal muscle breakdown and diminished albumin in uremic acidosis. Alkali therapy is recommended to maintain the serum bicarbonate concentration above 22 mEq/L.[68] Sodium bicarbonate in a daily dose of 0.5 mEq/L to 1 mEq/kg per day is the agent of choice. Because sodium citrate does not produce the bloating linked with bicarbonate therapy, it may be used in some patients who are not able to tolerate sodium bicarbonate.[69]

Hyperphosphatemia

Pathophysiology

Phosphate retention begins early in CKD because its filtration by the kidney is reduced. Hyperphosphatemia leads to elevated blood levels of parathyroid hormone (PTH) and secondary hyperparathyroidism by (i) lowering the levels of ionized calcium, (ii) interfering with the production of $1,25(OH)_2D_3$, and (iii) directly increasing PTH secretion.[70] Because hyperphosphatemia is associated with increased morbidity and mortality in CKD patients, the maintenance of normal serum levels of phosphorus in this population is critical. Therefore, the K/DOQI Clinical Practice Guidelines support intensive control of serum phosphorus in patients with CKD.

Goals of Therapy

Current recommendations in CKD stages 3 and 4 patients state that the serum level of phosphorus should be maintained between 2.7 mg/dL and 4.6 mg/dL. In CKD stage 5 patients and in those on hemodialysis or peritoneal dialysis, the serum levels of phosphorus should be maintained between 3.5 mg/dl and 5.5 mg/dl. The increased intake of calcium may enhance coronary arterial calcification in this setting; therefore, the serum calcium-phosphorus product should also be maintained at below 55 mg^2/dl^2.[70]

Therapeutics

In patients with CKD in whom phosphorus levels cannot be decreased to the target range with dietary phosphorus restriction, phosphate binders should be prescribed. Calcium-based phosphate binders are recommended for use as the initial binder therapy in patients with CKD stages 3 and 4. In patients with CKD stage 5, both calcium-based phosphate binders and noncalcium-based phosphate binders are effective and either may be used as the primary therapy. In dialysis patients who remain hyperphosphatemic (serum phosphorus >5.5 mg/dl), a combination of both calcium-based phosphate binders and noncalcium-containing phosphate-binding agents may be used. The K/DOQI Clinical Practice Guidelines suggest that the total dose of elemental calcium provided by the calcium-based phosphate binders should not exceed 1500 mg/day and the total intake of elemental calcium (including dietary calcium) should not exceed 2000 mg/day. In patients with serum phosphorus levels above 7.0 mg/dl, aluminum-based phosphate binders may be used as a short-term therapy (4 wk), for one course only.[70] Table 29-2 provides the characteristics of various phosphate-binding agents.

Sevelamer hydrochloride, a noncalcium-containing phosphate-binding agent, may also lower total and low-density lipoprotein (LDL) cholesterol in CKD patients.[71] However, the possible induction of metabolic acidosis is a problem associated with this agent.

Lanthanum carbonate (Fosrenol) is a noncalcium-based phosphate binder. Usual doses are 750 mg/dl to 3000 mg/day divided and chewed with meals. No significant clinical adverse effects with lanthanum have yet been reported in studies for up to 2 years.[72,73] The long-term safety of lanthanum use, particularly its possible effect on bone, remains unclear.[74]

Phosphate binders are most effective when taken with meals to bind dietary phosphate. Unfortunately, all of the phosphate binders have a limited phosphorous-binding capacity. Thus, in order to maximize their efficacy in lowering serum phosphorus levels, dietary phosphorus also should be restricted.

Hypocalcemia

Pathophysiology

As chronically reduced levels of calcium cause secondary hyperparathyroidism, have adverse effects on bone mineralization, and may be associated with increased mortality, it is important that CKD patients have normal serum levels of corrected total calcium. Although calcium supplementation may be required in CKD patients to maintain normal calcium levels, high calcium intake should be avoided because it may result in hypercalcemia and soft tissue calcification. During therapy

TABLE 29-2 PHOSPHATE-BINDING COMPOUNDS

Compound	Common Product Name	Estimate of Potential Binding Power	Advantages	Potential Side Effects
Calcium carbonate	TUMS, Oscal, Caltrate, Calci-Mix	Approximately 39 mg phosphorus bound/1 g	Inexpensive, wide availability	Hypercalcemia, extraskeletal calcification, GI side effects
Calcium acetate	PhosLo	Approximately 45 mg phosphorus bound/1 g	Less calcium absorption than calcium acetate	Hypercalcemia, extraskeletal calcification, GI side effects
Aluminum hydroxide	AlternaGEL, Anphojel	Mean binding 22.3 mg phosphorus/5 ml	Noncalcium	Bone mineralization defects, aluminum toxicity, GI distress
Sevelamer HCl	Renagel	Unknown	Noncalcium, nonaluminum	Metabolic acidosis, GI side effects
Lanthanum carbonate	Fosrenol	Unknown	Noncalcium, nonaluminum	Long-term safety unknown

GI, gastrointestinal.
Adapted from National Kidney Foundation. K/DOQI clinical practice guidelines. Available at http://www.kidney.org/professionals/KDOQI/guidelines.cfm (accessed October 22, 2006).

with calcium-based phosphate binders and active vitamin D sterols, hypercalcemia can occur frequently in CKD patients.

Goals of Therapy

The K/DOQI Clinical Practice Guidelines recommend maintaining a corrected total calcium level within the normal range of 8.4 mg/dl to 9.5 mg/dl. If the corrected total serum calcium level exceeds 10.2 mg/dl, therapies that cause an increase in the serum calcium level should be adjusted or avoided. Patients whose serum levels of corrected total calcium are below the recommended minimum (<8.4 mg/dl) should receive therapy to increase serum calcium levels if (i) there are clinical symptoms of hypocalcemia such as paresthesia, Chvostek's and Trousseau's signs, bronchospasm, laryngospasm, tetany, and seizures or (ii) the plasma intact PTH level is above the target range for the particular CKD stage (see later).

Therapeutics

Therapy for hypocalcemia should include calcium salts such as calcium carbonate and oral vitamin D sterols (discussed later). Calcium supplementation is most effective when taken between meals because this maximizes calcium absorption.

Renal Osteodystrophy

Pathophysiology

Changes in mineral metabolism and bone structure are a universal finding in patients with CKD.[75] Osteitis fibrosa, the principal type of renal bone disease, results from secondary hyperparathyroidism. The onset of the disorder is detectable when about 50% of kidney function is lost. Because renal osteodystrophy can be prevented, patients with CKD should be monitored for imbalances in calcium and phosphate homeostasis. They should also be monitored for secondary hyperparathyroidism by measuring the serum calcium, phosphorus, and intact PTH levels. The K/DOQI Clinical Practice Guidelines recommend the use of PTH in the diagnosis and management of osteodystrophy in patients with CKD and a GFR below 60 ml/min/1.73 m^2. The target range of plasma levels of intact PTH in the various stages of CKD are presented in Table 29-3.

Goals of Therapy

Prevention and treatment of osteitis fibrosis in predialysis CKD patients include dietary phosphate restriction, administration of oral phosphate binders, and the administration of vitamin D analogues to directly suppress the secretion of PTH. Patients with CKD are more likely to have lower levels of 25(OH)D than those with no kidney disease. Therefore, in stages 3 and 4 CKD patients, if the serum level of 25(OH)D is less than 30 ng/ml, supplementation with vitamin D_2 (ergocalciferol) should be initiated.[68]

TABLE 29-3 TARGET RANGE OF INTACT PLASMA PTH BY CKD STAGE

CKD Stage	GFR Range (ml/min/1.73 m^2)	Target "Intact" PTH (pg/ml)
3	30-59	35-70
4	15-29	70-110
5	<15 or dialysis	150-300

CKD, chronic kidney disease; GFR, glomerular filtration rate; PTH, parathyropid hormone.
Adapted from National Kidney Foundation. K/DOQI clinical practice guidelines. Available at http://www.kidney.org/professionals/KDOQI/guidelines.cfm (accessed October 22, 2006).

Even though CKD patients with GFR less than 60 ml/min/1.73 m^2 usually have secondary hyperparathyroidism with elevated serum levels of intact PTH, their plasma levels of $1,25(OH)_2D_3$ may be normal.[76] Normal $1,25(OH)_2D_3$ levels in the setting of the high PTH levels are inappropriate, and bone biopsies in such patients are consistent with hyperparathyroid bone disease. Therefore, in patients with CKD stages 3 and 4, therapy with an active (1-hydroxylated) oral vitamin D analogue is indicated when serum levels of 25(OH)D are greater than 30 ng/ml and plasma levels of intact PTH are above the target range for the particular CKD stage. Dose adjustment should be made to keep PTH, phosphorus, and calcium levels within the target ranges for the specific CKD stage (Table 29-3).

Patients with CKD on dialysis usually have low plasma levels of $1,25(OH)_2D_3$. This leads to reduced intestinal calcium absorption (thus contributing to hypocalcemia) and impaired suppression of PTH synthesis. The result is secondary hyperparathyroidism that often progresses. Treatment with an active vitamin D analogue reduces PTH secretion, thus improving hyperparathyroid bone disease and musculoskeletal symptoms. Therefore, patients with CKD stage 5 on hemodialysis or peritoneal dialysis with serum levels of intact PTH greater than 300 pg/ml should receive an active vitamin D analogue to reduce the serum levels of PTH to a target range of 150 pg/ml to 300 pg/ml.[70]

Therapeutics

Vitamin D Analogues. Table 29-4 reviews the recommendations for supplementation. Once patients are replete with vitamin D, supplementation with a vitamin-D–containing multivitamin should be continued and annual reassessment of serum 25(OH)D levels should be performed.

Active Vitamin D Analogues. Three active vitamin D analogues are currently available in the United States: calcitriol, paricalcitol, and doxercalciferol.

TABLE 29-4 RECOMMENDED SUPPLEMENTATION FOR VITAMIN D DEFICIENCY IN PATIENTS WITH CKD STAGES 3 AND 4

Serum 25(OH)D (ng/ml)	Definition	Ergocalciferol Dose (Vitamin D_2)	Duration (mo)
<5	Severe vitamin D deficiency	50,000 IU/wk PO x 12 wk then monthly OR 500,000 IU as a single IM dose	6
5-15	Mild vitamin D deficiency	50,000 IU/wk PO × 4 wk then monthly	6
16-30	Vitamin D deficiency	50,000 IU/mo PO	6

CKD, chronic kidney disease; IM, intramuscular; PO, per os (orally).
Adapted from National Kidney Foundation. K/DOQI clinical practice guidelines. Available at http://www.kidney.org/professionals/KDOQI/guidelines.cfm (accessed October 22, 2006).

Calcitriol: Controversies exist regarding the route (oral vs. intravenous), the dose, and the frequency (intermittent higher "pulse" therapy vs. lower daily therapy) of calcitriol therapy in patients with CKD. Most studies have shown that both routes of administration suppress the PTH equally. The maximum tolerated dose of intermittent calcitriol is usually about 7 mcg/wk to 8 mcg/wk, similar to the normal physiologic production of calcitriol (1 mcg/day).[77] Intravenous therapy is not practical in patients on peritoneal dialysis, and studies in these patients show that pulse oral and daily oral calcitriol therapy are equally effective in suppressing plasma PTH levels.[78]

Paricalcitol: Paricalcitol (Zemplar) has been demonstrated to have less calcemic and phosphatemic effects than calcitriol while retaining the ability to suppress PTH secretion.[79-82] Prospective randomized trials are still needed to further assess the relative effect on mortality of paricalcitol versus calcitriol on hemodialysis patients. Initial starting doses are 1 mcg/day orally or 10 mcg intravenously three times a week at hemodialysis.

Doxercalciferol: Studies show that oral or intravenous doxercalciferol given three times a week during hemodialysis is well tolerated and lowers plasma PTH.[83] An oral formulation, Hectorol, has also been approved for use in the United States. Initial starting doses are 5 mcg/day orally or 2 mcg intravenously three times a week at hemodialysis.

Serum levels of calcium and phosphorus should be monitored at least every 2 weeks for 1 month and then monthly afterward when initiating treatment with active vitamin D sterols or adjusting its dose. The plasma PTH should be checked monthly for at least 3 months and then every 3 months once target levels are achieved. Changes in serum calcium, serum phosphorus, and plasma PTH together should determine the management of active vitamin D analogues in CKD patients.

Calcimimetics. A novel method to decrease PTH secretion while minimizing hypercalcemia is to use a calcimimetic agent that binds to the calcium-sensing receptor (CaSR) in the parathyroid gland thereby increasing its sensitivity to calcium. Numerous studies in mild to severe hyperparathyroid patients on maintenance hemodialysis found that the administration of cinacalcet (Sensipar, AMG 073) or R-568 (norcalcin), a CaSR agonist, resulted in a dose-dependent reduction in the plasma PTH concentration.[84-86] In general, cinacalcet causes a decrease in the PTH, calcium, phosphate, and the Ca x P product. Cinacalcet can be used in combination with vitamin D treatment, phosphate binders, and calcium supplementation to reach the target PTH, phosphorus, and calcium ranges.[87,88] The usual starting dose of cinacalcet is 30 mg/day, with a maximum recommended dose of 180 mg/day. Although cinacalcet is generally safe and well tolerated, low serum calcium levels can occur. The hypocalcemia is usually asymptomatic and can be managed by adjustments in calcium-based phosphate binders or vitamin D sterols or by reductions in cinacalcet dose. However, caution should be used in patients with history of seizure disorder.

Hypertension

Pathophysiology

High blood pressure is both a cause and a complication of CKD. As a complication, hypertension may develop early during the course of CKD in approximately 80% to 85% of patients.[89] It is associated with adverse outcomes including faster loss of kidney function and development of CVD.

Goals of Therapy

The optimal blood pressure in hypertensive patients with CKD is uncertain. Some experts recommend a blood pressure goal of less than 130/80 mm Hg, which is consistent with JNC 7 and the K/DOQI Clinical Practice Guidelines on hypertension and antihypertensive agents in CKD.[90] However, evidence from the Modification of Diet in Renal Disease (MDRD) study, the AASK trial, and a meta-analysis from the ACE Inhibition and Progressive Renal Disease (AIPRD) study group suggests that an even lower blood pressure (<125/75 mm Hg) may be more effective in slowing progressive renal disease in patients with a urinary protein excretion greater than 1000 mg/day.[91] Systolic blood pressure should not be lowered below 110 mm Hg to 120 mm Hg because mortality may increase with systolic pressures below this range.

An integral part of therapy for hypertension in patients with CKD is treating proteinuria. The K/DOQI Clinical Practice Guidelines[90] recommend reduction of urinary protein excretion to less than 500 mg/day to 1000 mg/day. Because this goal can be difficult to achieve, some experts recommend a minimum reduction of at least 60% of baseline urinary protein excretion values.[90]

Therapeutics

All antihypertensive agents can be used to lower blood pressure in patients with CKD. For each patient, a specific agent based on the type of CKD, coexisting CVD, and other comorbid conditions may be used. Figure 29-1 is a sample algorithm included in the K/DOQI Clinical Practice Guidelines for selection of antihypertensive agents in CKD patients.

The target blood pressure can often be safely achieved with combined therapy that usually begins with an ACE inhibitor or an ARB and a diuretic.[92] ACE inhibitors and ARBs, as noted previously, can also slow disease progression, especially in patients with diabetic kidney disease. Because volume expansion contributes to the elevation of blood pressure in CKD, loop diuretics are recommended for the treatment of hypertension, particularly in patients with edema. The thiazide diuretics in conventional dosages become less effective as monotherapy when the GFR falls below 30 ml/min. Thiazide diuretics do have an additive effect when given with a loop diuretic for refractory edema.

The nondihydropyridine calcium channel blockers may have beneficial effects on CKD and CVD. However, a recent study found that verapamil was not as effective as ACE inhibitors to prevent the onset of microalbuminuria in patients with type 2 diabetes.[93] The dihydropyridine calcium channel blockers are usually considered to have a more potent antihypertensive effect than the nondihydropyridine calcium channel blockers; however, they consistently increase proteinuria. Nevertheless, dihydropyridine calcium channel blockers may be very effective in attaining goal blood pressure when used in combination with ACE inhibitors and diuretics.[94,95] These agents should be used with caution in patients with severe left ventricular dysfunction, and the nondihydropyridine calcium channel blockers should be avoided

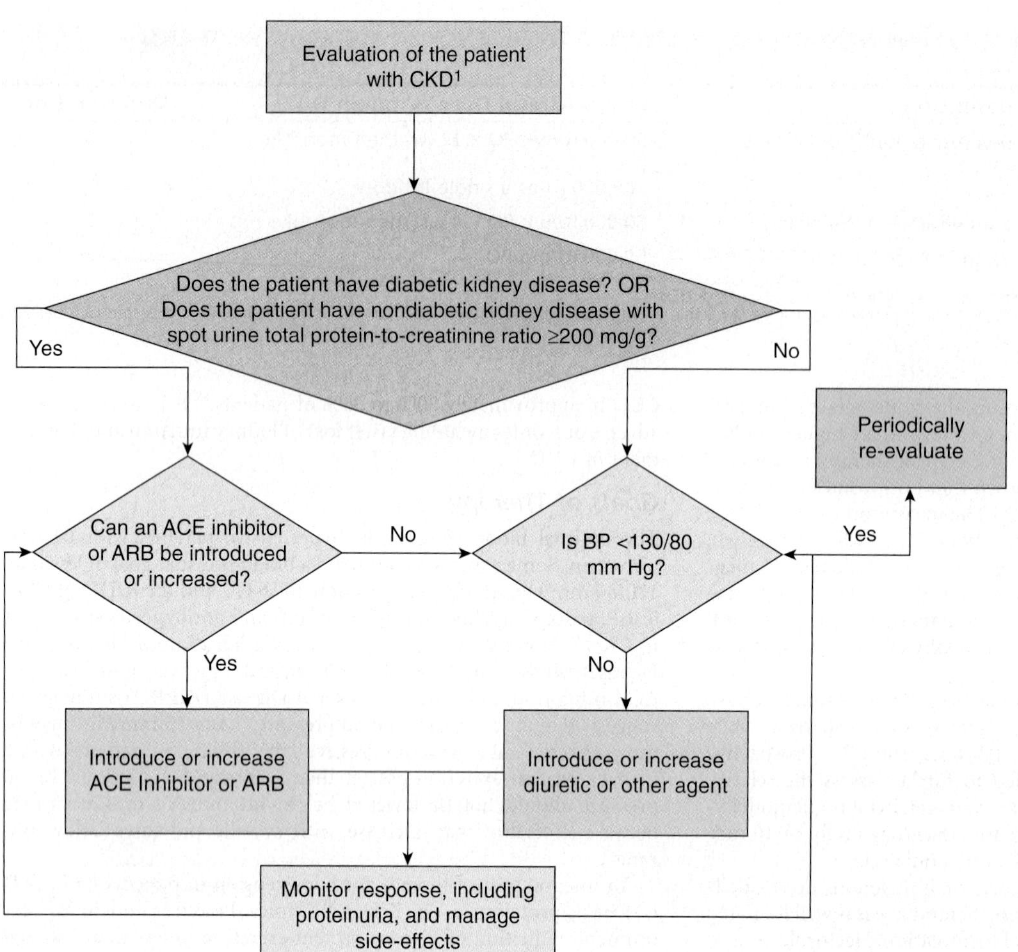

FIGURE 29-1 • Selection of antihypertensive agents in chronic kidney disease patients. (Adapted from National Kidney Foundation. K/DOQI clinical practice guidelines. Available at http://www.kidney.org/professionals/KDOQI/guidelines.cfm [accessed October 22, 2006].)

in patients with sick sinus syndrome or second- or third-degree heart block.

As discussed previously, recent data show that aldosterone receptor antagonists like spironolactone may effectively reduce proteinuria in patients with CKD.[96] However, these patients have an increased risk for hyperkalemia.

Anemia

Pathophysiology

Anemia related to CKD in most patients is primarily due to decreased production of erythropoietin (EPO) by the kidney because of a reduction in functioning renal mass and to shortened red cell survival. Anemia of CKD is normocytic and normochromic. It becomes a common feature in CKD patients as the GFR declines below 60 ml/min per 1.73 m^2.[97,98] The 2006 K/DOQI Clinical Practice Guidelines[99] state that the evaluation of anemia in patients with CKD should begin when the hemoglobin (Hgb) level is less than 12 g/dl in females, and less than 13.5 g/dl in males. The initial evaluation of anemic patients with CKD is the same as the workup for anemic patients without CKD and should include red blood cell indices, absolute reticulocyte count, serum iron, total iron-binding capacity, percent transferrin saturation, serum ferritin, white blood cell count and differential, platelet count, and testing for blood in stool. This assessment should be performed prior to administering erythropoiesis-stimulating agent (ESA) treatment.

Goals of Therapy

Correction of anemia in CKD patients has benefits beyond improving cardiac status, such as (i) improved sense of well-being, quality of life, neurocognitive function, and work capacity; (ii) reduced need for packed red blood cell transfusion; (iii) reduced allosensitization prior to renal transplantation; and (iv) reduced hospitalizations.[99,100] Optimal target Hgb levels have not been determined, but current recommendations are to maintain the level between 11 g/dl and 12 g/dl (hematocrit (Hct) levels between 33% and 36%). In certain circumstances, as in CKD patients with ischemic heart disease, left ventricular hypertrophy, or chronic obstructive lung disease, it may be medically justifiable to maintain the Hgb level above 12 g/dl.[99] According to the K/DOQI Clinical Practice Guidelines,[99] current evidence is insufficient to recommend routinely maintaining Hgb levels at 13.0 g/dl or greater in patients treated with ESA. A recent large study found no benefit to raising Hgb values above 12 g/dl.[100]

Two large prospective trials are ongoing at this time to further evaluate this issue. The Cardiovascular Risk Reduction by Early Anemia Treatment with Epoetin Beta (CREATE) study is designed to evaluate the effects of early intervention to correct Hgb levels to target of 13 g/dl to 15 g/dl versus 10.5 g/dl to 11.5 g/dl on cardiovascular outcomes including left ventricular myocardial infarction and the first cardiovascular event in patients with CKD who are not on dialysis. The Trial to Reduce Cardiovascular Events with Aranesp Therapy (TREAT)[101] is a randomized, placebo-controlled study designed to evaluate the effects of anemia correction (goal Hgb of 13 g/dl) on cardiovascular events in patients with diabetes and CKD who are not on dialysis.

Therapeutics

Two ESAs are currently available in the United States for correcting anemia in CKD.

Erythropoietin alfa: Recombinant human erythropoietin alfa (rHuEpo), the first exogenous erythropoietic protein to be developed, has been in clinical use for well over a decade. Subcutaneous injection is the preferred route of rHuEpo administration in CKD patients. Self-administration is easy to learn and well tolerated by most patients. The recommended starting dose of rHuEpo is 80 units/kg to 120 units/kg per week in one to two doses per week. A reasonable starting dose for most patients is 10,000 units subcutaneously once weekly. If the initial administration of rHuEpo is intravenous for hemodialysis patients, the dose should be 120 units/kg to 180 units/kg per week given in three divided doses.[99] Suggested safe rates of Hgb correction range from 1 g/dl/mo to 2 g/dl/mo and should be less than 2.0 g/dl/mo to 3.0 g/dl/mo.

Darbepoetin alfa: Darbepoetin alfa is a newer erythropoietic protein that differs structurally from rHuEpo. It has a higher sialic acid–containing carbohydrate content, an important determinant of the serum half-life of this molecule. The safety profile of this long-acting erythropoietic agent is similar to that of rHuEpo. Given its threefold longer half-life and greater biologic activity, compared with rHuEpo, darbepoetin alfa is able to maintain target Hgb levels with less frequent dosing. It can be given by either an intravenous or a subcutaneous injection once every other week to successfully correct anemia. The starting dose is 0.45 mcg/kg, and most patients will require a dose of 40 mcg or 60 mcg every other week.[102,103]

PEG-EPO: A PEGylated version of EPO has been developed and should require fewer injections than the non-PEGylated EPO. An added benefit of PEGylation is that less protein than with the unmodified EPO can be administered to patients to achieve the desired therapeutic effect, which may lead to lower patient costs. PEG-EPO is not currently licensed for use in the United States, but the manufacturers are completing the initial clinical trials.[104]

Iron Repletion. An adequate response to ESAs requires the maintenance of sufficient iron stores. Several studies on maintenance iron therapy in patients on EPO found a 33% to 75% reduction in the EPO dose of patients on maintenance iron regimens.[105] The 2006 K/DOQI Clinical Practice Guidelines[99] suggested giving sufficient iron to maintain the percent transferring saturation higher than 20% and the serum ferritin level greater than 200 in CKD patients on hemodialysis and a level greater than 100 in CKD patients on peritoneal dialysis and in CKD patients not yet on renal replacement therapy.[99]

Oral Iron. K/DOQI Clinical Practice Guidelines recommend that when oral iron is used in adults, 200 mg of elemental iron should be administered daily in two to three divided doses. A variety of available oral iron drugs are listed in Table 29-5.

The efficacy of oral iron in CKD patients can be maximized by (i) providing a dose of at least 200 mg of elemental iron per day, (ii) administrating iron between meals and at least 1 hour apart from the ingestion of phosphate binders to maximize iron absorption, and (iii) avoiding delayed-release iron supplements because iron is absorbed in the proximal gastrointestinal tract. All the iron agents can cause gastrointestinal side effects, and little evidence differentiates between them on the basis of efficacy or tolerability.

Intravenous Iron. Even though in patients with CKD not on renal replacement therapy and in those on peritoneal dialysis the route of iron administration can be either intravenous or oral, the preferred route in patients on hemodialyis is intravenous.[99] Intravenous iron is given to maintain appropriate ion indices, but the K/DOQI Clinical Practice Guidelines state that not enough evidence exists to recommend administration of intravenous iron if the serum ferritin level is greater than 500 ng/ml.

The strategy for administering intravenous iron is to anticipate iron deficiency by giving small weekly doses to maintain stable iron stores. Weekly doses of 12.5 mg to 100 mg of intravenous iron may improve responsiveness to rHuEPO. The potential advantage of such an approach lies in linking iron replacement with ongoing iron losses.[106]

Three forms of intravenous iron are most commonly used: iron dextran, iron sucrose, and ferric gluconate.

Iron dextran: Iron dextran has been used for several decades. It is composed of a dense core of iron oxyhydroxide surrounded by a stabilizing shell composed of dextran chains. Although iron dextran is clearly effective, its safety profile remains an issue. It has been estimated that 31 deaths from iron dextran–related anaphylaxis occurred in the United States between 1976 and 1996. Anaphylactic reactions are believed to be related to the drug's dextran component.[107]

Ferric gluconate/iron sucrose: Ferric gluconate and iron sucrose are newer forms of intravenous iron that were approved by the U.S. Food and Drug Administration in 1999 and 2000, respectively. Rather than possessing a dense core of iron hydroxide, as iron dextran does, these agents have polynuclear iron centers. The cores are surrounded by the carbohydrates gluconate and sucrose in ferric gluconate and iron sucrose, respectively. Because these agents do not contain a dextran moiety, they appear to have a far lower risk of anaphylaxis than that of iron dextran.[108] A controlled prospective study of over 2500 hemodialysis patients demonstrated that after single-dose exposure to ferric gluconate, no statistically significant difference could be found in the rate of serious adverse reactions versus placebo.[109] Another large-scale study of hemodialysis patients, including those who had experienced previous intolerance to other intravenous iron preparations, concluded that iron sucrose is safe when given as treatment for iron deficiency or for maintenance of iron stores.[110]

Both iron sucrose and ferric gluconate can be administered by a slow intravenous push without the need for a test dose. Too few studies have directly compared these two agents to be able to reach any conclusions regarding their relative safety and efficacy. At present, it is reasonable to conclude that both are probably as effective as iron dextran and have a much lower risk for immediate, severe reactions.

EPO Resistance. The most frequently encountered source of an inadequate response to ESA is iron deficiency.[111] Other causes include secondary hyperparathyroidism, infection or inflammation, folate or vitamin B_{12} deficiency, occult malignancy, hemoglobinopathies, hemolysis, ACE inhibitors, and malnutrition. An inadequate response to EPO therapy is defined as a failure to achieve target Hgb/Hct levels in the presence of adequate iron store at an intravenous dose of 450 units/kg/wk intravenously or a subcutaneous dose of 300 units/kg/wk within 4 to 6 months or failure to subsequently maintain target Hgb/Hct at that dose.[111] Although the K/DOQI Clinical Practice Guidelines do not support their use, the following therapies have increased erythropoiesis in some EPO-resistant dialysis patients.

Vitamin C: Vitamin C increases the release of iron from ferritin and the reticuloendothelial system, enhances iron utilization during heme synthesis, and has antioxidant properties.[112] Supplementation of 150 mg to 200 mg of oral vitamin C daily has been reported to normalize vitamin C levels in hemodialysis patients. Therapy with long-term intravenous vitamin C in hemodialysis patients has been shown to cause secondary oxalosis.[113] If initiated, therapy with vitamin C should be limited to a 2- to 6-month course of 300 mg to 500 mg intravenously at each hemodialysis session.[111]

L-Carnitine: Use of intravenous L-carnitine in selected patients with CKD and EPO-resistant anemia was recommended in a National Kidney Foundation Carnitine Consensus Conference.[114,115] Therapy with intravenous administration of L-carnitine for a period of 4 to 6 months can be started with a typical dose of 1 g (10 mg/kg-20 mg/kg) after each hemodialysis treatment.

TABLE 29-5 ORAL IRON SUPPLEMENTS

Iron Supplement	Tablet Size (mg)	Amount of Elemental Iron (mg)
Ferrous gluconate	325	35
Ferrous sulfate	325	65
Ferrous fumarate	325	108
Polysaccharide-iron complex	150	150

Adapted from National Kidney Foundation. K/DOQI clinical practice guidelines. Available at http://www.kidney.org/professionals/KDOQI/guidelines.cfm (accessed October 22, 2006).

TABLE 29-6 MANAGEMENT OF DYSLIPIDEMIA IN PATIENTS WITH CKD

Dyslipidemia	Goal	Therapy	Alternative
TG ≥ 500 mg/dl	TG < 500 mg/dl	Fibrate or niacin	Fibrate or niacin
LDL 100-129 mg/dl	LDL < 100 mg/dl	Low-dose statin	Bile acid sequestrant or niacin
LDL ≥ 130 mg/dl	LDL < 100 mg/dl	Maximum-dose statin	Bile acid sequestrant or niacin
TG ≥ 200 mg/dl and non-HDL ≥ 130 mg/dl	Non-HDL < 130 mg/dl	Maximum-dose statin	Fibrate or niacin

HDL, high-density lipoprotein; LDL, low-density lipoprotein; TG, triglyceride.
Adapted from National Kidney Foundation. K/DOQI clinical practice guidelines. Available at http://www.kidney.org/professionals/KDOQI/guidelines.cfm (accessed October 22, 2006).

Androgens: Studies have shown a possible role for androgens in combination with EPO therapy in hemodialysis patients. The results demonstrated a statistically significant increase in Hct levels in patients treated with both EPO and androgen therapy.[116,117] However, the role for supplemental androgens is limited, given their side effect profile in most patients.

Pentoxifylline: Pentoxifylline may result in benefits in EPO-resistant anemia because it may have anti-inflammatory properties.[118] However, routine use of pentoxifylline for EPO-resistant anemia cannot be recommended until a controlled trial is performed.

Statins: Statins are believed to have anti-inflammatory and antioxidant properties. Studies have shown a 25% reduction in EPO requirements in statin-treated dialysis patients.[119] Given the benefits of statins and their low side effect profile, further investigations with these drugs will be valuable.

Dyslipidemia

Pathophysiology/Goals of Therapy

Because abnormal lipid metabolism is common in patients with renal disease, all patients with CKD should be assessed for dyslipidemia. Evaluation should include a fasting lipid profile with total cholesterol, LDL, high-density lipoprotein (HDL), and triglyceride levels.[120] The primary finding in CKD patients is a normal total cholesterol level and a high triglyceride level.[121] Given evidence that mild to moderate degrees of renal failure are associated with an adverse cardiovascular prognosis, CKD is considered a coronary heart disease equivalent. Thus, the target LDL cholesterol level in patients with CKD is less than 100 mg/dl, similar to that in patients with coronary heart disease.

Therapeutics

Table 29-6 summarizes the suggested management of dyslipidemia in adults with CKD. In patients with hypercholesterolemia, a statin can effectively and safely lower the plasma cholesterol concentration to acceptable levels. The 4D trial[122] evaluated the efficacy of lipid lowering in patients with ESRD. In this study, 1255 hemodialysis patients with type 2 diabetes and hyperlipidemia received placebo or atorvastatin. The primary outcome measure was the composite of cardiovascular death, nonfatal myocardial infarction, and stroke. At a median follow-up of 4 years, there was no difference in the incidence of the primary outcome between the two groups. A number of explanations, including limitations in the trial itself and issues related to ESRD, have been proposed for the lack of benefit from atorvastatin. ESRD may be associated with atherosclerotic pathogenic pathways that differ from those in patients without renal disease. The results of 4D, however, cannot be extrapolated to patients with mild to moderate CKD. Despite the absence of clear benefit with statin therapy, the current recommendation is the administration of statin therapy to ESRD patients with elevated levels of serum LDL cholesterol.

In patients with hypertriglyceridemia, treatment with a fibrate or nicotinic acid should be considered.[121] As stated previously, limited data in patients with CKD show that statin therapy may have an additional benefit of slowing the rate of progression of the underlying renal disease.[45-49]

SUMMARY

A phenomenon of reverse epidemiology may hold true in CKD patients. It states that obesity, hypercholesterolemia, and hypertension are paradoxically protective features associated with a greater survival among CKD patients. The hypothesis that "malnutrition-inflammation-cachexia syndrome" is the most likely etiology of the reverse epidemiology. In populations with chronic disease states such as CKD, undernutrition is a common risk factor for adverse cardiovascular events and death. Therefore, obese individuals with high total serum cholesterol and high blood pressure who require dialysis may live longer than those dialysis patients who do not have these factors, normally considered a risk.[123]

Thus, early detection of CKD and aggressive interventions to minimize its progression and complications are the current treatments of CKD. However, in this dynamic era of technology and research, new insight into the mechanisms of progressive renal injury and novel strategies for renoprotective interventions will continue to emerge. The ultimate goal will be to achieve remission of progressive renal disease in the majority of the CKD patients. This strategy will, one hopes, also decrease the overall risk of CVD and mortality observed in patients with decrements in renal function.[124]

REFERENCES

1. National Kidney Foundation. K/DOQI clinical practice guidelines for chronic kidney disease: evaluation, classification, and stratification. Available at http://www.kidney.org/professionals/KDOQI/guidelines_ckd/p1_exec.htm (accessed October 9, 2006).
2. Yu HT. Progression of chronic renal failure. Arch Intern Med 2003;163:1417.
3. Sharma K, Ziyadeh FN. Biochemical, metabolic, and cellular events linking glucose metabolism to the development of diabetic nephropathy. Semin Nephrol 1997;17:80-92.
4. Border W, Noble N. Transforming growth factor-beta in tissue fibrosis. N Engl J Med 1994;331:1286-1291.
5. Ruiz-Ortega M, Ruperez M, Esteban V. Angiotensin II: a key factor in the inflammatory and fibrotic response in kidney diseases. Nephrol Dial Transplant 2006;21:16.
6. Aros C, Remuzzi G. The renin-angiotensin system in progression, remission and regression of chronic nephropathies. J Hypertens Suppl 2002;20:S45.
7. Remuzzi A, Gagliardini E, Sangalli F. ACE inhibition reduces glomerulosclerosis and regenerates glomerular tissue in a model of progressive renal disease. Kidney Int 2006;69:1124.
8. Goodfriend TL, Elliot ME, Catt KJ. Angiotensin receptors and their antagonists. N Engl J Med 1996;334:1649.
9. Gansevoort RT, Sluiter WJ, Hemmelder MH. Antiproteinuric effect of blood-pressure–lowering agents: a meta-analysis of comparative trials. Nephrol Dial Transplant 1995;10:1963.
10. Maschio G, Alberti D, Janin G: Effect of the angiotensin-converting-enzyme inhibitor benazepril on the progression of chronic renal insufficiency. N Engl J Med 1996;334:939.
11. The GISEN Group (Gruppo Italiano di Studi Epidemiologici in Nefrologia). Randomised placebo-controlled trial of effect of ramipril on decline in glomerular filtration rate and risk of terminal renal failure in proteinuric, non-diabetic nephropathy. Lancet 1997;349:1857.
12. Ruggenenti P, Perna A, Gherardi G. Renal function and requirement for dialysis in chronic nephropathy patients on long-term ramipril: REIN Follow-up Trial. Lancet 1998;352:1252.
13. Agodoa LY, Appel L, Bakris GL. Effect of ramipril vs amlodipine on renal outcomes in hypertensive nephrosclerosis: a randomized controlled trial. JAMA 2001;285:2719.
14. Wright JT, Bakris G, Greene T. Effect of blood pressure lowering and antihypertensive drug class on progression of hypertensive kidney disease: results from the AASK Trial. JAMA 2002;288:2421.

15. Jafar TH, Stark PC, Schmid CH. Progression of chronic kidney disease: the role of blood pressure control, proteinuria, and angiotensin-converting enzyme inhibition: a patient-level meta-analysis. Ann Intern Med 2003;139:244.
16. Lewis EJ, Hunsicker LG, Bain RP. The effect of angiotensin-converting enzyme inhibition on diabetic nephropathy. N Engl J Med 1993;329:1456.
17. Wilmer WA, Hebert LA, Lewis EJ. Remission of nephrotic syndrome in type 1 diabetes: long-term follow-up of patients in the Captopril Study. Am J Kidney Dis 1999;34:308.
18. Hilgers KF, Mann JF. ACE Inhibitors versus AT(1) receptor antagonists in patients with chronic renal disease. J Am Soc Nephrol 2002;13:1100.
19. Schmieder RE, Klingbeil AU, Fleischmann EH. Additional antiproteinuric effect of ultrahigh dose candesartan: a double-blind, randomized, prospective study. J Am Soc Nephrol 2005;16:3038.
20. Remuzzi A, Perico N, Sangalli F. ACE inhibition and Ang II receptor blockade improve glomerular size-selectivity in IgA nephropathy. Am J Physiol 1999;276:F457.
21. Lewis EJ, Hunsicker LJ, Clarke WR. Renoprotective effect of the angiotensin-receptor antagonist irbesartan in patients with nephropathy due to type 2 diabetes. N Engl J Med 2001;345:851.
22. Atkins RC, Briganti EM, Lewis JB. Proteinuria reduction and progression to renal failure in patients with type 2 diabetes mellitus and overt nephropathy. Am J Kidney Dis 2005;45:281.
23. Brenner BM, Cooper ME, de Zeeuw D. Effects of losartan on renal and cardiovascular outcomes in patients with type 2 diabetes and nephropathy. N Engl J Med 2001;345:861.
24. Rossing K, Schjoedt KJ, Jensen BR. Enhanced renoprotective effects of ultrahigh doses of irbesartan in patients with type 2 diabetes and microalbuminuria. Kidney Int 2005;68:1190.
25. Aranda P, Segura J, Ruilope LM. Long-term renoprotective effects of standard versus high doses of telmisartan in hypertensive nondiabetic nephropathies. Am J Kidney Dis 2005;46:1074.
26. Chandrasekharan UM, Sanker S, Glynias MJ. Angiotensin II–forming activity in a reconstructed ancestral chymase. Science 1996;271:502.
27. Nishimura H, Hoffmann S, Baltatu O. Angiotensin I converting enzyme and chymase in cardiovascular tissues. Kidney Int Suppl 1996;55:S18.
28. Nakao N, Yoshimura A, Morita H. Combination treatment of angiotensin-II receptor blocker and angiotensin-converting-enzyme inhibitor in non-diabetic renal disease (COOPERATE): a randomized controlled trial. Lancet 2003;361:117.
29. Jaber BL, Midias NE. Benazepril for advanced chronic renal insufficiency. N Engl J Med 2006;354:131-140.
30. Shimizu T, Kuroda T, Hata S. Pirfenidone improves renal function and fibrosis in the post-obstructed kidney. Kidney Int 1998;54:99.
31. Pirfenidone to treat kidney disease in patients with diabetes. Available at http://www.clinicaltrials.gov/ct/show/NCT00105391 (accessed October 7, 2006).
32. Anders HJ, Vielhauer V, Frink M. A chemokine receptor CCR-1 antagonist reduces renal fibrosis after unilateral ureter ligation. J Clin Invest 2002;109:251.
33. Anders HJ, Belemezova E, Eis V. Late onset of treatment with a chemokine receptor CCR1 antagonist prevents progression of lupus nephritis in MRL-Fas(lpr) mice. J Am Soc Nephrol 2004;15:1504.
34. Sharma K, Jin Y, Guo J. Neutralization of TGF-beta by anti-TGF-beta antibody attenuates kidney hypertrophy and the enhanced extracellular matrix gene expression in STZ-induced diabetic mice. Diabetes 1996;45:522-530.
35. Sharma K, Ziyadeh FN. Hyperglycemia and diabetic kidney disease. The case for transforming growth factor-beta as a key mediator. Diabetes 1995;44:1139-1146.
36. Yu L, Border WA, Anderson I. Combining TGF-beta inhibition and angiotensin II blockade results in enhanced antifibrotic effect. Kidney Int 2004;66:1774.
37. Omata M, Taniguch H, Koya D. *N*-Acetyl-seryl-aspartyl-lysyl-proline ameliorates the progression of renal dysfunction and fibrosis in WKY rats with established anti-glomerular basement membrane nephritis. J Am Soc Nephrol 2006;17:674.
38. Anti-CTGF monoclonal antibodies. Available at http://www.fibrogen.com/rd/ctgf/fibrosis.html (accessed October 21, 2006).
39. Wang S, Hirschberg R. Bone morphogenetic protein-7 signals opposing transforming growth factor ß in mesangial cells. J Biol Chem 2004;279:23200-23206.
40. Wang S, Hirschberg R. BMP7 antagonizes TGF-ß–dependent fibrogenesis in mesangial cells. Am J Physiol Renal Physiol 2003;284:F1006-F1013.
41. Yang J, Dai C, Liu Y. Hepatocyte growth factor gene therapy and angiotensin II blockade synergistically attenuate renal interstitial fibrosis in mice. J Am Soc Nephrol 2002;13:2464.
42. Gong R, Rifal A, Tolbert EM. Hepatocyte growth factor ameliorates renal interstitial inflammation in rat remnant kidney by modulating tubular expression of macrophage chemoattractant protein-1 and RANTES. J Am Soc Nephrol 2004;15:2868.
43. Esposito C, Parrilla B, De Mauri A. Hepatocyte growth factor (HGF) modulates matrix turnover in human glomeruli. Kidney Int 2005;67:2143.
44. Dworkin LD, Gong R, Tolbert E. Hepatocyte growth factor ameliorates progression of interstitial fibrosis in rats with established renal injury. Kidney Int 2004;65:409.
45. Keane WF. Lipids and the kidney. Kidney Int 1994;46:910.
46. Rovin BH, Tan LC. LDL stimulates mesangial fibronectin production and chemoattractant expression. Kidney Int 1993;43:218.
47. Keane WF, O'Donnell MP, Kasiske BL. Oxidative modification of low-density lipoproteins by mesangial cells. J Am Soc Nephrol 1993;4:187.
48. Kim SY, Guijarro C, O'Donnell MP. Human mesangial cell production of monocyte chemoattractant protein-1: modulation by lovastatin. Kidney Int 1995;48:363.
49. Agarwal R. Effects of statins on renal function. Am J Cardiol 2006;97:748-755.
50. Graham DJ, Staffa JA, Shatin D. Incidence of hospitalized rhabdomyolysis in patients treated with lipid-lowering drugs. JAMA 2004;292:2585.
51. Smith CC, Bernstein LI, Davis RB. Screening for statin-related toxicity: the yield of transaminase and creatine kinase measurements in a primary care setting. Arch Intern Med 2003;163:688.
52. Ballantyne CM, Corsini A, Davidson MH. Risk for myopathy with statin therapy in high-risk patients. Arch Intern Med 2003;163:553.
53. Rosenson RS, Frauenheim WA. Safety of combined pravastatin-gemfibrozil therapy. Am J Cardiol 1994;74:499.
54. Schrama YC, Hene RJ, de Jonge N. Efficacy and muscle safety of fluvastatin in cyclosporine-treated cardiac and renal transplant recipients. Transplantation 1998;66:1175.
55. Weir MR, Fink JC. Salt intake and progression of chronic kidney disease: an overlooked modifiable exposure? A commentary. Am J Kidney Dis 2005;45:176.
56. Dussol B, Moussi-Frances J, Morange S. A randomized trial of furosemide vs hydrochlorothiazide in patients with chronic renal failure and hypertension. Nephrol Dial Transplant 2005;20:349.
57. Brater DC. Pharmacology of diuretics. Am J Med Sci 2000;319:38.
58. White WB, Duprez D, St. Hillaire R. Effects of the selective aldosterone blocker eplerenone versus the calcium antagonist amlodipine in systolic hypertension. Hypertension 2003;41:1021.
59. Mahmud A, Feely J. Aldosterone-to-renin ratio, arterial stiffness, and the response to aldosterone antagonism in essential hypertension. Am J Hypertens 2005;18:50.
60. Sato A, Hayashi K, Saruta T. Antiproteinuric effects of mineralocorticoid receptor blockade in patients with chronic renal disease. Am J Hypertens 2005;18:44-49.
61. Bianchi S, Bigazzi R, Campese VM. Antagonists of aldosterone and proteinuria in patients with CKD: an uncontrolled pilot study. Am J Kidney Dis 2005;46:45-51.
62. Epstein M: Aldosterone blockade: an emerging strategy for abrogating progressive renal disease. Am J Med 2006;119:912-919.
63. Allon M: Hyperkalemia in end-stage renal disease: mechanisms and management. J Am Soc Nephrol 1995;6:1134.
64. Uribarri J, Douton H, Oh MS. A re-evaluation of the urinary parameters of acid production and excretion in patients with chronic renal acidosis. Kidney Int 1995;47:624.
65. Warnock DG. Uremic acidosis. Kidney Int 1988;34:278.
66. Widmer B, Gerhardt RE, Harrington JT. Serum electrolyte and acid-base composition: the influence of graded degrees of chronic renal failure. Arch Intern Med 1979;139:1099.
67. Wallia R, Greenberg AS, Piraino B. Serum electrolyte patterns in end-stage renal disease. Am J Kidney Dis 1986;8:98.
68. National Kidney Foundation. K/DOQI clinical practice guidelines for nutrition in chronic renal failure. Available at http://www.kidney.org/professionals/KDOQI/guidelines_updates/ doqi_nut.html (accessed October 5, 2006).
69. Uribarri J. Acidosis in chronic renal insufficiency. Semin Dial 2000;13:232.
70. National Kidney Foundation. K/DOQI clinical practice guidelines for bone metabolism and disease in chronic kidney disease. Available at: http://www.kidney.org/professionals/KDOQI/guidelines_bone/index.htm (accessed October 2, 2006).
71. Sadek T, Mazouz H, Bahloul H. Sevelamer hydrochloride with or without alphacalcidol or higher dialysate calcium vs. calcium carbonate in dialysis patients: an open-label, randomized study. Nephrol Dial Transplant 2003;18:582.
72. Chiang SS, Chen JB, Yang WC. Lanthanum carbonate (Fosrenol) efficacy and tolerability in the treatment of hyperphosphatemic patients with end-stage renal disease. Clin Nephrol 2005;63:461.
73. Finn WF. Lanthanum carbonate versus standard therapy for the treatment of hyperphosphatemia: safety and efficacy in chronic maintenance hemodialysis patients. Clin Nephrol 2006;65:191.
74. Lacour B, Lucas A, Auchere D. Chronic renal failure is associated with increased tissue deposition of lanthanum after 28-day oral administration. Kidney Int 2005;67:1062.
75. Hruska KA, Teitelbaum SL. Mechanisms of disease: renal osteodystrophy. N Engl J Med 1995;333:166.
76. Martinez I, Saracho R, Montenegro J. A deficit of calcitriol synthesis may not be the initial factor in the pathogenesis of secondary hyperparathyroidism. Nephrol Dial Transplant 1996;11:22-28.
77. Mazess RB, Elangovan L. A review of intravenous versus oral vitamin D hormone therapy in hemodialysis patients. Clin Nephrol 2003;59:319.
78. Gadallah MF, Arora N, Torres C. Pulse oral versus pulse intraperitoneal calcitriol: a comparison of efficacy in the treatment of hyperparathyroidism and renal osteodystrophy in peritoneal dialysis patients. Adv Perit Dial 2000;16:303.
79. Finch JL, Brown AJ, Kubodera N. Differential effects of 1,25-$(OH)_2D_3$ and 22-oxacalcitriol on phosphate and calcium metabolism. Kidney Int 1993;43:561.
80. Slatopolsky E, Cozzolino M, Finch JL. Differential effects of 19-nor-1,25-$(OH)_2D_2$ and 1alpha-hydroxyvitamin D_2 on calcium and phosphorus in normal and uremic rats. Kidney Int 2002;62:1277.
81. Slatopolsky E, Finch J, Brown A. New vitamin D analogs. Kidney Int Suppl 2003;85:S83.
82. Teng M, Wolf M, Lowrie E. Survival of patients undergoing hemodialysis with paricalcitol or calcitriol therapy. N Engl J Med 2003;349:446.
83. Maung HM, Elangovan L, Frazao JM. Efficacy and side effects of intermittent intravenous and oral doxercalciferol (1alpha-hydroxyvitamin D_2) in dialysis patients with secondary hyperparathyroidism: a sequential comparison. Am J Kidney Dis 2001;37:532.
84. Block GA, Martin KJ, de Francisco AL. Cinacalcet for secondary hyperparathyroidism in patients receiving hemodialysis. N Engl J Med 2004;350:1516.
85. Moe SM, Chertow GM, Coburn JW. Achieving NKF-K/DOQI bone metabolism and disease treatment goals with cinacalcet HCL. Kidney Int 2005;67:760.
86. Lindberg JS, Culleton B, Wong G. Cinacalcet HCl, an oral calcimimetic agent for the treatment of secondary hyperparathyroidism in hemodialysis and peritoneal dialysis: a randomized, double-blind, multicenter study. J Am Soc Nephrol 2005;16:800.

87. Cunningham J, Danese M, Olson K. Effects of the calcimimetic cinacalcet HCl on cardiovascular disease, fracture, and health-related quality of life in secondary hyperparathyroidism. Kidney Int 2005;68:1793.
88. Chertow GM, Blumenthal S, Turner S. Cinacalcet hydrochloride (Sensipar) in hemodialysis patients on active vitamin D derivates with controlled PTH and elevated calcium x phosphate. Clin J Am Soc Nephrol 2006;1:305.
89. Hsu CY, McCulloch CE, Curhan GC. Epidemiology of anemia associated with chronic renal insufficiency among adults in the United States: results from the Third National Health and Nutrition Examination Survey. J Am Soc Nephrol 2002;13:504.
90. National Kidney Foundation. K/DOQI clinical practice guidelines on hypertension and antihypertensive agents in chronic kidney disease. Available at http://www.kidney.org/professionals/KDOQI/guidelines_bp/index.htm (accessed October 3, 2006).
91. Jafar TH, Stark PC, Schmid CH. Progression of chronic kidney disease: the role of blood pressure control, proteinuria, and angiotensin-converting enzyme inhibition: a patient-level meta-analysis. Ann Intern Med 2003;139:244.
92. Lazarus JM, Bourgoignie JJ, Buckalew VM. Achievement and safety of a low blood pressure goal in chronic renal disease. The Modification of Diet in Renal Disease Study Group. Hypertension 1997;29:641.
93. Ruggenenti P, Fassi A, Ilieva AP. Preventing microalbuminuria in type 2 diabetes. N Engl J Med 2004;351:1941-1951.
94. Bakris GL, Weir MR, DeQuattro V. Effects of an ACE inhibitor/calcium antagonist combination on proteinuria in diabetic nephropathy. Kidney Int 1998;54:1283-1289.
95. Bakris GL, Copley JB, Vicknair N. Calcium channel blockers versus other antihypertensive therapies on progression of NIDDM associated nephropathy. Kidney Int 1996;50:1641-1650.
96. Epstein M. Aldosterone as a mediator of progressive renal disease: pathogenetic and clinical implications. Am J Kidney Dis 2001;37:677-688.
97. Astor BC, Muntner P, Levin A. Association of kidney function with anemia: the Third National Health and Nutrition Examination Survey (1988-1994). Arch Intern Med 2002;162:1401.
98. Hsu CY, McCulloch CE, Curhan GC. Epidemiology of anemia associated with chronic renal insufficiency among adults in the United States: results from the Third National Health and Nutrition Examination Survey. J Am Soc Nephrol 2002;13:504.
99. National Kidney Foundation. KDOQI clinical practice guidelines and clinical practice recommendations for anemia in chronic kidney disease. Available at http://www.kidney.org/professionals/KDOQI/guidelines_anemia/index.htm (accessed October 3, 2006).
100. Singh AK, Szczech L, Tang KL. Correction of anemia with epoetin alfa in chronic kidney disease. N Engl J Med 2006;355:2083-2098.
101. Spiegel DM. Anemia management in chronic kidney disease: what have we learned after 17 years? Semin Dial 2006;19:269-272.
102. Allon M, Kleinman K, Walczyk M. The pharmacokinetics of novel erythropoiesis stimulating protein (NESP) following intravenous administration is time- and dose-linear. J Am Soc Nephrol 2000;11:A1308.
103. Graf H, Lacombe J-L, Braun J. Novel erythropoiesis stimulating protein (NESP) effectively maintains Hb (Hb) when administered at a reduced dose frequency compared with recombinant human erythropoietin (r-HuEPO) in ESRD patients. J Am Soc Nephrol 2000;11:A1317.
104. Prolong Pharmaceuticals: less medicine, more efficacy. Available at http://www.prolongpharmaceuticals.com/our_products.php (accessed October 6, 2006).
105. Chang CH, Chang CC, Chiang SS. Reduction in erythropoietin doses by the use of chronic intravenous iron supplementation in iron-replete hemodialysis patients. Clin Nephrol 2002;57:136-141.
106. Besarab A, Amin N, Ahsan M. Optimization of epoetin therapy with intravenous iron therapy in hemodialysis patients. J Am Soc Nephrol 2000;11:530-538.
107. Fishbane S, Ungureanu VD, Maeska JK. The safety of intravenous iron dextran in hemodialysis patients. Am J Kidney Dis 1996;28:529.
108. Faich G, Strobos J. Sodium ferric gluconate complex in sucrose: safer intravenous iron therapy than iron dextrans. Am J Kidney Dis 1999;33:464.
109. Michael B, Coyne DW, Fishbane S. Ferrlecit safety study. Kidney Int 2002;61:1830.
110. Aronaff GR, Bennett WM, Blumenthal S. Iron sucrose in hemodialysis patients: safety of replacement and maintenance regimens. Kidney Int 2004;66:1193-1198.
111. Priyadarshi A, Shapiro JI. Erythropoietin resistance in the treatment of the anemia of chronic renal failure. Semin Dial 2006;19:273-278.
112. Deicher R, Ziai F, Habicht A. Vitamin C plasma levels and response to erythropoietin in patients on maintenance haemodialysis. Nephrol Dial Transplant 2004;19:2319-2324.
113. Canavese C, Petrarulo M, Massarenti P. Long-term, low-dose, intravenous vitamin C leads to plasma calcium oxalate supersaturation in hemodialysis patients. Am J Kidney Dis 2005;45:540-549.
114. Eknoyan G, Latos DL, Lindberg J. Practice recommendations for the use of L-carnitine in dialysis-related carnitine disorder. National Kidney Foundation Carnitine Consensus Conference. Am J Kidney Dis 2003;41:868-876.
115. Golper TA, Goral S, Baker BN: L-Carnitine treatment of anemia. Am J Kidney Dis 2003;41:S27-S34.
116. Ballal SH, Domoto DT, Polack DC. Androgen potentiate the effects of erythropoietin in the treatment of anemia of end-stage renal disease. Am J Kidney Dis 1991;17:29-33.
117. Gaughan WJ, Liss KA, Dunn SR. A 6-month study of low-dose recombinant human erythropoietin alone and in combination with androgens for the treatment of anemia in chronic hemodialysis patient. Am J Kidney Dis 1997;30:495-500
118. Cooper A, Mikhail A, Lethbridge MW. Pentoxifylline improves hemoglobin levels in levels in patients with erythropoietin-resistance anemia in renal failure. J Am Soc Nephrol 2004;15:1877-1882.
119. Sirken G, Kung SC, Raja R. Decreased erythropoietin requirements in maintenance hemodialysis patients with statin therapy. ASAIO J 2003;49:422-425.
120. Appel G. Lipid abnormalities in renal disease. Kidney Int 1991;39:169.
121. National Kidney Foundation. K/DOQI clinical practice guidelines for managing dyslipidemias in chronic kidney disease. Available at http://www.kidney.org/professionals/KDOQI/guidelines_lipids/index.htm (accessed October 10, 2006).
122. Wabber C, Krane V, Marz W. Atorvastatin in patients with type 2 diabetes mellitus undergoing hemodialysis. N Engl J Med 2005;353:238-248.
123. Kalantar-Zadeh K, Block G, Humphreys MH. Reverse epidemiology of cardiovascular risk factors in maintenance dialysis patients. Kidney Int 2003;63:793-808.
124. Go AS, Chertow GM, Fan D. Chronic kidney disease and the risks of death, cardiovascular events, and hospitalization. N Engl J Med 2004;351:1296-1305.

30

VOIDING DYSFUNCTION

Alan J. Wein, Rajiv Saini, and David R. Staskin

INTRODUCTION 445
CLINICAL UROPHARMACOLOGY OF THE LOWER URINARY TRACT: SOME USEFUL CONCEPTS 445
THERAPEUTICS AND CLINICAL PHARMACOLOGY 445
Facilitation of Bladder Emptying 445
Increasing Intravesical Pressure or Facilitating Bladder Contraction 445
Decreasing Outlet Resistance 447
Facilitation of Urine Storage 449
Decreasing Bladder Contractility 450
Increasing Bladder Capacity by Decreasing Sensory (Afferent) Input 453
Increasing Outlet Resistance 453
Circumventing the Problem 454
Antidiuretic Hormone-Like Agents 454
Emerging Targets and Therapeutics 454

INTRODUCTION

The lower urinary tract has two basic functions, the storage and emptying of urine. Bladder filling and urine storage require accommodation of increasing volumes of urine at a low intravesical pressure and with appropriate sensation; a bladder outlet that is closed at rest and remains so during increases in intra-abdominal pressure; and absence of involuntary bladder contractions (caused by non-neurogenic or neurogenic detrusor overactivity). Bladder emptying requires a coordinated contraction by the bladder smooth musculature of adequate magnitude and duration; concomitant lowering of resistance at the level of the smooth sphincter (the smooth muscle of the bladder neck and proximal urethra) and of the striated sphincter (the periurethral and intramural urethral striated musculature); and absence of anatomic obstruction.

This simple overview implies that any type of voiding dysfunction (i.e., of storage, emptying, or a combination of these) must result from an abnormality of one or more of the factors listed previously. Likewise, one can easily classify all known treatments for voiding dysfunction under the broad categories of facilitating either filling-storage or emptying, and achieving this by acting primarily on the bladder or components of the bladder outlet.

As a result of advances in the knowledge of the neuropharmacology and neurophysiology of the lower urinary tract, effective pharmacologic therapy now exists for the management of many types of voiding dysfunction. Because of the number of drug therapies available along with the varying quality and quantity of studies performed using them, the International Consultation on Incontinence was launched by the World Health Organization. The goal of the International Consultation on Incontinence is to classify incontinence and critically assess the evidence for the effectiveness of treatment (Table 30-1).

The focus of this chapter is to summarize the treatments available for female voiding dysfunction within this functional classification. Considerations for male urinary incontinence are also reviewed in the section describing facilitation of urine storage.

CLINICAL UROPHARMACOLOGY OF THE LOWER URINARY TRACT: SOME USEFUL CONCEPTS

The targets of pharmacologic intervention in the bladder body, base, or outlet include nerve terminals that alter the release of specific neurotransmitters, receptor subtypes, cellular second-messenger systems, and ion channels.[1] Peripheral nerves and ganglia, the spinal cord, and supraspinal areas are also sites of action of pharmacologic agents. Voiding is controlled largely by the autonomic nervous system. Because autonomic innervation and receptor content are ubiquitous throughout the human body's organ systems, there are no agents in clinical use that are purely selective for action on the lower urinary tract. The majority of side effects attributed to drugs facilitating bladder storage or emptying are collateral effects on organ systems that share some of the same neurophysiologic or neuropharmacologic characteristics as the bladder.[2] A schematic of mediators of bladder tone and musculature is shown in Figure 30-1.

THERAPEUTICS AND CLINICAL PHARMACOLOGY

Facilitation of Bladder Emptying

Absolute or relative failure to empty results from decreased bladder contractility, increased outlet resistance, or both.[3] Failure of adequate bladder contractility may result from temporary or permanent alteration in any one of the neuromuscular mechanisms necessary for initiating and maintaining a normal detrusor contraction. In neurologically normal individuals, inhibition of the micturition reflex may be secondary to painful stimuli—especially stimuli from the pelvic and perineal areas—or it may be psychogenic. Some drug therapies may inhibit bladder contractility through neurologic or myogenic mechanisms. Bladder smooth muscle function may be impaired from overdistention, severe infection, or fibrosis. Increased outlet resistance is generally secondary to anatomic obstruction but may be secondary to a failure of coordination of the smooth or striated sphincter during bladder contraction. Treatment of failure to empty consists of attempts to increase intravesical pressure, to facilitate the micturition reflex, or to decrease outlet resistance—or some combination of these.

Increasing Intravesical Pressure or Facilitating Bladder Contraction

Parasympathomimetic Agents. A major portion of the final common pathway in physiologic bladder contraction is mediated by parasympathetic postganglionic muscarinic cholinergic receptors (see Chapter 9, Autonomic Pharmacology). Ligands for these receptors, such as acetylcholine (ACh), are effective in treating patients who cannot empty because of inadequate bladder contractility. ACh itself cannot be used for therapeutic purposes because of its off-target

TABLE 30-1 ICI CLASSIFICATION OF INCONTINENCE DRUGS AND EVIDENCE OF EFFICACY

Drug	Level*	Grade†	Dose‡
Antimuscarinics			
Tolterodine	1	A	4 mg/day or 2 mg bid
Trospium	1	A	20 mg bid
Darifenacin	1	A	7.5-15 mg/day
Solifenacin	1	A	5-10 mg/day
Propantheline	2	B	15-30 mg qid
Hyoscyamine	3	C	0.375 mg bid
Drugs with Mixed Actions			
Oxybutynin	1	A	2.5-5 mg tid
Propiverine	1	A	15 mg bid–tid
Dicyclomine	3	C	80 mg qid
Flavoxate	2	D	100 mg tid
Antidepressants			
Imipramine	3	C/D§	25 mg qid
Vasopressin Analogues			
Desmopressin	1	A	20-30 mcg nasal spray at bedtime 0.1-0.4 mg 2 hr before bedtime
α-Adrenergic Antagonists	3	C	
Alfuzosin			10 mg/day
Doxazosin			1-8 mg/day
Terazosin			1-10 mg every night
Tamsulosin			0.4 mg/day
β-Adrenergic Receptor Agonists (terbutaline, albuterol)	3	C	N/A
Estrogens	3	D	
Topical cream			0.5-1.0 g/day; bid after 2 wk
Estradiol ring			One ring every 3 mo
Vaginal tablets			25 mcg/day; twice weekly after 2 wk
Others			
Baclofen	3	C	Up to 120 mg/day in three divided doses
Capsaicin	2	C	N/A
Resiniferatoxin	2	C	N/A
Botulinum toxin	2	B	200-300 units by injection
Bethanechol	3	D	25-100 mg qid

*Level of evidence:
1—Systematic reviews, meta-analyses, good-quality randomized, controlled clinical trials
2—Randomized, controlled trials, good-quality prospective cohort studies
3—Case-controlled studies, case series
4—Expert opinion
†Grade:
A—Based on level 1 evidence (highly recommended)
B—Consistent level 2 or 3 evidence (recommended)
C—Level 4 studies or "majority evidence" (optional)
D—Evidence inconsistent/inconclusive (no recommendation possible)
‡Many doses need to be titrated to effect to avoid adverse effects.
§C, urgency incontinence; D, stress incontinence.
bid, twice daily; N/A, optimal doses not defined; qid, four times daily; tid, three times daily.
Adapted from International Consultation on Incontinence assessments of pharmacotherapy for voiding dysfunction, 2005.[117,118]

actions at central and ganglionic levels and because of its rapid hydrolysis by acetylcholinesterase and butyrylcholinesterase. Of existing cholinergic agonists, only bethanechol chloride has a relatively selective action in vitro on the urinary bladder and gut, with little or no nicotinic action. Bethanechol in vitro causes a contraction of smooth muscle from all areas of the bladder.[4,5]

From the middle of the 20th century, bethanechol has been recommended for the treatment of the atonic or hypotonic bladder,[6] and it has been reported to be effective in achieving what was called "rehabilitation" of the chronically atonic or hypotonic detrusor.[7] When so used, it is recommended that the drug initially be administered subcutaneously in a dose of 5 to 10 mg (usually 7.5 mg) every 4 to 6 hours along with an intermittent bladder-decompression regimen. The patient is asked to try to void 20 to 30 minutes after each dose. When the residual urine volume has decreased to an acceptable level, the dose is gradually decreased and ultimately changed to an oral dose of 50 mg four times daily. In cases of partial bladder emptying, a therapeutic trial with an oral dose of 25 to 100 mg four times daily may be utilized in conjunction with attempted voiding every 4 hours. Bethanechol has also been used to stimulate or facilitate the development of reflex bladder contractions in patients with spinal shock secondary to suprasacral spinal cord injury.[8]

Although anecdotal success in using bethanechol in patients with voiding dysfunction is reported, there is little or no evidence to support its success in facilitating bladder emptying in series.[9] Short-term studies have generally failed to demonstrate significant efficacy in terms of flow and residual urine volume data.[10] Although bethanechol is capable of eliciting an increase in bladder smooth muscle tension, as would be expected from studies in vitro, its ability to stimulate or facilitate a coordinated and sustained physiologic bladder contraction in patients with voiding dysfunction has been unimpressive.[5,9] However, due to the paucity of pharmacotherapy to improve bladder emptying, many clinicians continue to use bethanechol as a first-line treatment in hopes of improving emptying as long as the medication is tolerated without adverse effects by the patient or contraindicated.

The potential side effects of cholinomimetic drugs include flushing, nausea, vomiting, diarrhea, gastrointestinal cramps, bronchospasm,

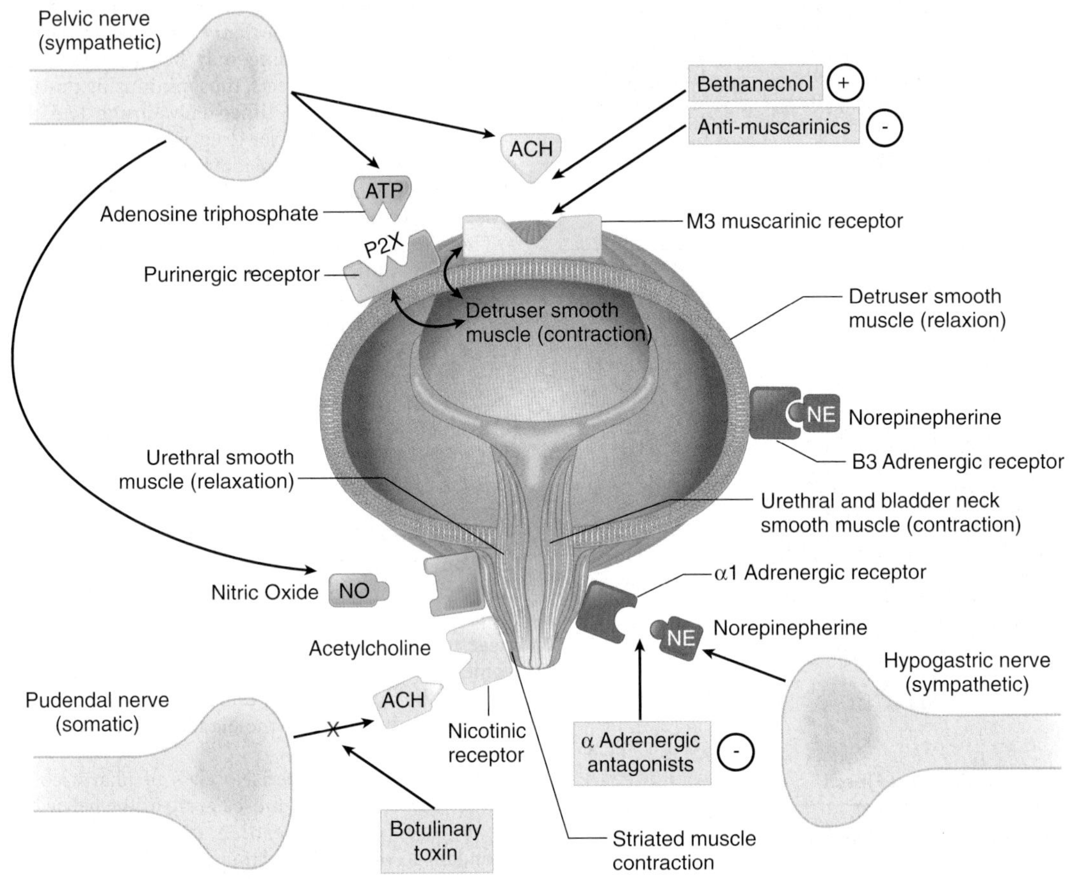

FIGURE 30-1 • **Neurologic innervation and control of bladder musculature.** The lower urinary system has functions of urine storage and elimination. These functions are mediated by autonomic and somatic nerves that innervate smooth muscle in the bladder wall (detrusor) and the smooth and striated muscle of the bladder neck and urethra (external urinary sphincter). Continence is maintained during bladder filling by increased detrusor compliance, coupled with increasing contraction of the external urinary sphincter. During voiding, the external urinary sphincter relaxes and the detrusor contracts to expel urine. Detrusor tone is mediated by the parasympathetic system, primarily through the M_3 muscarinic receptor subtype. M_2 receptors are also present, though their exact role has not been elucidated. Purinergic receptors (P2X) play a minor role in normal physiology, but are important in some cases of overactive bladder. Nitric oxide release causes relaxation of the urethral smooth muscle. Sympathetic modulation is mediated by the hypogastric nerve and involves maintenance of external urinary sphincter pressure by activation of α_1-adrenergic receptors, as well as relaxation of detrusor tone via β_3-adrenergic receptors. Voluntary control of micturition and relaxation of striated musculature of the external urinary sphincter is via the pudendal nerve. Sites of action of drugs commonly used to modulate neuromuscular control of the bladder are listed.

headache, salivation, sweating, and difficulty with visual accommodation. Intramuscular and intravenous use is contraindicated, as it can precipitate acute circulatory failure and cardiac arrest. Other contraindications to the use of this general category of drug include asthma, peptic ulcer, bowel obstruction, recent gastrointestinal surgery, cardiac arrhythmia, hyperthyroidism, and any type of bladder outlet obstruction.

Prostaglandins. The reported use of prostaglandins (PGs) to facilitate emptying is based on the hypothesis that these substances contribute to the maintenance of bladder tone and bladder contractile activity.[11,12] PGE_2 and $PGF_{2\alpha}$ cause bladder contractile responses in vitro and in vivo. PGE_2 causes a net decrease in urethral smooth muscle tone while $PGF_{2\alpha}$ causes an increase.

Prostaglandins have a relatively short half-life, and a mechanistic basis for long-term efficacy based upon limited drug exposure is not clear. Clinical studies with various intravesical preparations have generated a number of conflicting reports, though the quality of most studies has not been high. Potential side effects of PG usage include vomiting, diarrhea, pyrexia, hypertension, and hypotension.

α-Adrenergic Antagonists. Some investigators have suggested that antagonism at the α-adrenergic receptor, in addition to decreasing outlet resistance, may facilitate transmission through pelvic parasympathetic ganglia and thereby enhance bladder contractility. Such an effect may be due solely to an α-adrenergic effect on the outlet, or it may be that α-adrenergic blockade can facilitate the detrusor reflex through either a direct effect on parasympathetic ganglia or an indirect one.[13] An indirect mechanism would be associated with a decrease in urethral resistance.

Opioid Antagonists. It has been hypothesized that endogenous opioids may exert a tonic inhibitory effect on the micturition reflex at various levels,[11,14] and agents such as narcotic antagonists may, therefore, offer possibilities for stimulating reflex bladder activity.

Decreasing Outlet Resistance

The Smooth Sphincter

α-Adrenergic Antagonists. α- and β-Adrenergic receptors populate the bladder and proximal urethral smooth musculature, though the degree of innervation by postganglionic fibers of the sympathetic nervous system is unclear[11,12] (Fig. 30-2). The smooth muscle of the bladder base and proximal urethra contains predominantly α-adrenoceptors. The bladder body contains both types of adrenoceptors, the β type being more common.

α-Receptor antagonists exert their favorable effects on voiding dysfunction primarily by a relaxation effect on the smooth muscle of the bladder neck and proximal urethra. Other mechanisms of action include a decrease in striated sphincter tone and a decrease in bladder contractility. Clinically used agents include alfuzosin, tamsulosin, doxazosin, terazosin, and prazosin.

Prazosin is a short-acting α-receptor antagonist developed initially for hypertension, but has been used in the treatment of voiding dys-

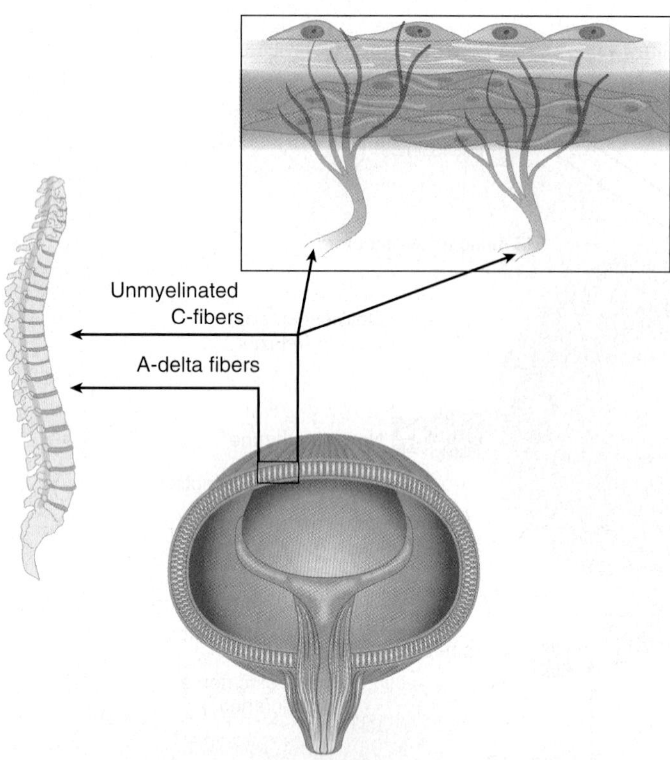

C Sensory Fibers

Receptor	Agonists
Vanilloid	Capsuicia α, anadomide α
Purinergic	ATP
Neurokinin	Substrate P
Endothelin	Endothelin
Cannabiacid	Anadomide

FIGURE 30-2 • **Afferent innervation of the bladder.** Afferent nerves of the bladder travel to sacral and upper lumbar sacral nerve roots. A delta fibers transmit primarily signals in response to bladder distention and contraction of the detrusor. Unmyelinated C fibers innervate detrusor and urinary epithelium. These fibers transmit signals in response to pain and chemical irritation. Aberrant signaling of afferent C fibers may contribute to bladder dysfunction and overactive bladder. Modulation of these receptors may serve as potential therapeutic targets.

function secondary to benign prostatic hyperplasia (BPH). It is used less frequently due to orthostatic hypotension. Terazosin and doxazosin are two relatively selective postsynaptic α_1-blocking drugs. Both are readily absorbed and possess a long plasma half-life, enabling their activity to be maintained over 24 hours following a single dose.[15,16] Efficacy is mediated via interaction with α_1 receptors on the prostatic stroma and capsule. Side effects of orthostatic hypotension and tachycardia are similar to those with prazosin.[17] Retrograde ejaculation due to relaxation of the bladder neck is an adverse effect. Terazosin has the same affinity for α_1 receptors in genitourinary as in vascular tissue and a fourfold greater selectivity for α_1 receptors than doxazosin. Alfuzosin is a selective and competitive antagonist of α_1-mediated contraction of the prostate capsule, bladder base, and proximal urethral smooth muscle, with efficacy similar to that of prazosin.[18] It is more specific for receptors in the genitourinary tract than in the vasculature, raising the possibility that voiding may be facilitated by doses that have minimal vasodilatory effects, thus minimizing postural hypotension.[19] The drug requires three-times-daily dosing (7.5 to 10 mg total). A sustained-release form of the drug, which allows convenient once-daily dosing, is also available.[20] In addition, effects on blood pressure (orthostatic hypotension) were minimal, supporting its selectivity of the lower urinary tract over the vasculature.

There are a number of α_1-receptor subtypes. In the human prostate, the majority of the stromal α_1 receptors are of the α_{1a} subtype.[21] Tamsulosin is an α_1-antagonist that is relatively selective for the α_{1a}- and α_{1d}-receptor subtypes over the α_{1b} subtype.[22] A Cochrane review concluded efficacy similar to that of other α_1-antagonists, with mild but dose-dependent side effects.[23] It is unclear whether highly selective α_{1a}-antagonists will have similar effects in women, as virtually all of the studies reported in the peer-reviewed literature have examined the effects of these agents on benign prostatic obstruction in men. Overall, a systematic review of the published literature has established similar efficacy between different α-receptor antagonists, though alfuzosin and tamsulosin are better tolerated.[24]

Other Potential Nonspecific Therapy. β-Adrenergic stimulation has been shown experimentally to decrease the urethral pressure profile and, by inference, urethral resistance.[25] Progesterone has been suggested as a possible treatment for emptying abnormalities in women via a sphincteric effect.[26] Finally, nitric oxide has been suggested to be a mediator of nonadrenergic, noncholinergic relaxation of the smooth muscle of the bladder outlet that occurs with bladder contraction.[12]

The Striated Sphincter. No class of pharmacologic agents selectively relaxes the striated musculature of the pelvic floor. Three different types of drugs have been used to treat voiding dysfunction secondary to outlet obstruction at the level of the striated sphincter: the benzodiazepines, dantrolene, and baclofen. All are characterized generally as antispasticity drugs. Baclofen and diazepam act predominantly within the central nervous system (CNS), whereas dantrolene acts directly on skeletal muscle. Although these drugs are capable of providing variable relief in specific circumstances, their efficacy is modest, and troublesome muscle weakness, adverse effects on gait, and other side effects limit their overall usefulness. While there are few randomized trials examining use in spinal cord injury–induced spasticity, the weight of clinical experience supports their use.[27]

Benzodiazepines. There are few available published papers that provide valuable data on the use of any of the benzodiazepines for treatment of functional obstruction at the level of the striated sphincter. The rationale for their use is either relaxation of the pelvic floor striated musculature during bladder contraction, or that such relaxation removes an inhibitory stimulus to reflex bladder activity. However, improvement under such circumstances may simply be due to the antianxiety effect of the drug or to the intensive explanation, encouragement, and modified biofeedback therapy that usually accompanies such treatment in these patients. There is a lack of clinical studies showing any advantages of these agents over placebo or aspirin. Typical total daily doses of diazepam, the most widely used agent of this group, range from 4 to 40 mg daily. Side effects of benzodiazepines include nonspecific CNS depression, manifested as sedation, lethargy, drowsiness, slowing of thought processes, and ataxia.[28]

Baclofen. Baclofen depresses monosynaptic and polysynaptic excitation of motor neurons and interneurons in the spinal cord. It was originally thought to function as a γ-aminobutyric acid (GABA) agonist[29]; however, its electrophysiologic and pharmacologic profiles differ radically from those of GABA. Although its effects superficially resemble those of GABA, some specific GABA inhibitors (e.g., bicuculline) do not antagonize the actions of baclofen. Baclofen does not cause depolarization of primary afferent nerve terminals, and there is no evidence that baclofen increases chloride conduction, the most prominent action of GABA. Because both GABA and baclofen can produce some effects that are insensitive to blockade by classic GABA antagonists, two classes of GABA receptors have been proposed: the $GABA_A$

receptor (the classic receptor) and the $GABA_B$ receptor. Baclofen does not bind strongly or specifically to $GABA_A$ receptors but does to $GABA_B$ receptors in brain and spinal membranes. Currently, it is thought that activation of the $GABA_B$ receptors by baclofen causes a decrease in the release of excitatory transmitters onto motor neurons by increasing potassium conductance or by inhibiting calcium influx. The primary site of action of baclofen is in the spinal cord, but it is also reported to be active at more rostral sites in the CNS. Like a $GABA_B$ agonist, baclofen suppresses excitatory neurotransmitter release but also has direct GABAergic activity. Its effect in reducing spasticity is caused primarily by normalizing interneuron activity and decreasing motor neuron activity, perhaps secondary to normalizing interneuron activity.[30]

Baclofen has been found useful for the treatment of skeletal spasticity due to a variety of causes (especially multiple sclerosis and traumatic spinal cord lesions). In regard to its use in treating voiding dysfunction, patients with voiding dysfunction secondary to acute and chronic spinal cord injury respond with lower striated sphincter responses and decreased residual urine volume following baclofen treatment, though response is best with a daily oral dose of approximately 120 mg.[31] Daily intravenous doses of 20 mg are also highly effective.[32]

Intrathecal infusion of baclofen bypasses the blood-brain barrier. Cerebrospinal fluid levels 10 times higher than those reached with oral administration are achieved with infusion amounts 100 times less than those taken orally.[33] Direct administration into the subarachnoid space by an implanted infusion pump has shown promising results, not only for skeletal spasticity but also for striated sphincter dyssynergia and detrusor overactivity. Development of tolerance to intrathecal baclofen with a consequent requirement for increasing doses may prove to be a problem with long-term chronic usage.

Dantrolene. Dantrolene exerts its effects by direct peripheral action on skeletal muscle.[29] While exact molecular mechanisms have not been elucidated, it appears to inhibit the excitation-induced release of calcium ions from the sarcoplasmic reticulum of striated muscle fibers, thereby inhibiting excitation-contraction coupling and diminishing the mechanical force of contraction. Because the blockade of calcium release is not complete, contraction is not completely abolished. Dantrolene reduces reflex more than voluntary contractions, probably because of a preferential action on fast-twitch rather than slow-twitch skeletal muscle fibers. The drug improves voiding function in some patients with classic detrusor striated sphincter dyssynergia. It has been shown to decrease postvoid residuals (33%) and mean urethral closure pressures (49%), thereby allowing improved bladder emptying in patients with urinary retention with detrusor striated sphincter dyssynergia secondary to spinal cord injury.[34] The recommended starting dose is 25 mg daily, which can be gradually increased by increments of 25 mg every 4 to 7 days to a maximum oral dose of 400 mg given in four divided doses. The major side effect of increasing doses is muscle weakness.

Botulinum Toxin. Botulinum toxin (BTX) is a potent inhibitor of ACh release at the neuromuscular junction of striated muscle. It has been used to treat many types of voiding dysfunction. BTX injection into the striated urinary sphincter is used to treat dyssynergia, thereby decreasing bladder outlet resistance. In several small case studies involving hypertonicity of the striated sphincter with poor detrusor contractility, it has demonstrated relaxation of the striated sphincter muscle and facilitate bladder emptying in neurogenic and non-neurogenic causes of urethral sphincter hypertonicity.[35,36] BTX has been used as a intraprostatic injection to decrease outlet resistance in men with BPH in urinary retention.[37] BTX has demonstrated improved voiding parameters, including detrusor pressure at peak flow, peak urinary flow rate, postvoid residual, and prostate volume. The exact mechanism of effect on prostatic tissue in not yet known; however, it may be related to a neurotransmitter pathway that decreases smooth muscle tone in the prostate.[38] Although there are a number of subtypes, BTX-A is the one that has been most studied and is most commonly used and available. There are many protocols involving route of BTX injection and the amount of BTX to be used in total and at each injection site. Currently, the number of patients tested with BTX is small, and more information is needed about criteria for success and side effects.[39]

Facilitation of Urine Storage

The pathophysiology of failure of the lower urinary tract to fill with or to store urine adequately may be secondary to problems related to the bladder, the outlet, or both.[3] Detrusor overactivity can be expressed as discrete involuntary contractions or as reduced compliance with or without phasic contractions. It may manifest itself symptomatically as overactive bladder syndrome, a syndrome of urinary urgency, with or without urgency urinary incontinence, usually with increased micturition frequency during the day and at night (i.e., nocturia). Involuntary bladder contractions are most commonly associated with inflammatory or irritating processes in the bladder wall or with bladder outlet obstruction. They may also be idiopathic. Decreased compliance during filling may be secondary to the sequelae of neurologic injury or disease but may also result from any process that destroys the elastic or viscoelastic properties of the bladder wall. Pure sensory urgency may be idiopathic or result from inflammatory, infectious, neurologic, or psychological factors.

A fixed decrease in outlet resistance may result from degeneration of or damage to innervation of the structural elements of the smooth and/or striated sphincters, neurologic disease or injury, surgical or mechanical trauma, and/or aging. Classic or genuine stress urinary incontinence in women implies a failure of the normal transmission of increases in intra-abdominal pressure to the area of the bladder neck and proximal urethra due to changes in the anatomic position of the vesicourethral junction and proximal urethra during increases in intra-abdominal pressure. As intra-abdominal pressure increases, there is a descent of the bladder neck and urethra due to laxity of the pelvic musculature. This hypermobility prevents normal compression of these structures against the pelvic musculature that would normally prevent stress urinary incontinence. The pathophysiology of stress urinary incontinence may also involve a decrease in reflex striated sphincter contraction, which occurs with a number of maneuvers that increase intra-abdominal pressure. Treatment of abnormalities related to the filling or storage phase of micturition are directed toward inhibiting bladder contractility, increasing bladder capacity, decreasing sensory input during filling, or increasing outlet resistance, either continuously or only during abdominal straining.[1]

In men, detrusor muscle function and innervation is the same as it is in women. Similar to women, male urinary incontinence may be due to detrusor overactivity and overactive bladder. However, a second type of incontinence known as postprostatectomy incontinence may occur following surgical treatments for symptomatic benign prostatic obstruction and surgical and radiation treatment for prostate cancer. The treatment for postprostatectomy incontinence is primarily surgical.

The etiology of overactive bladder in men is often related to bladder outlet obstruction from benign prostatic enlargement or benign prostatic obstruction. Bladder outlet obstruction may result in denervation of bladder smooth muscle, which then allows spontaneous electrical activity to cause small detrusor smooth muscle contractions, giving rise to overactive bladder symptoms. Long-term obstruction can cause bladder smooth muscle decompensation leading to failure to empty the bladder. A parallel theory is that bladder distention results in a more pronounced response to ACh, which causes an increased sense of urgency and other overactive bladder symptoms. Additionally, the aging process may give rise to the development of overactive bladder via a combination of all of these etiologies over time.[40]

Although BPH is a histologic diagnosis, the symptoms of bladder outlet obstruction due to benign prostatic obstruction/benign prostatic enlargement are often referred to as BPH. Patients with clinically significant BPH/benign prostatic enlargement are distinguished by the progressive development of lower urinary tract symptoms. These symptoms are variable and range from nocturia, incomplete emptying, urinary hesitancy, weak stream, frequency, and urgency to the development of acute urinary retention. These symptoms can exist with those of overactive bladder in the same patient.

Treatments focused on treating lower urinary tract symptoms due to BPH can decrease the secondary symptoms of overactive bladder. Pharmacologic treatment for many men with symptomatic BPH has been primarily with α-adrenergic receptor antagonists. These medications work by reducing smooth muscle tone in the prostate and bladder neck. Other medications that may be used include 5α-reductase inhibitors, including finasteride and dutasteride, which have a mechanism of action of reduction of prostate volume by inducing epithelial atrophy. In addition, α-adrenergic receptor antagonists and 5α-reductase inhibitors are often used as combination therapy in men with large prostates.

Confounding the treatment of lower urinary tract symptoms is the often concurrent diagnosis of overactive bladder. The symptom complex of frequency, urgency, and nocturia often overlaps that of lower urinary tract symptoms. Often, these men require combination treatment targeted at decreasing bladder contractility.

Decreasing Bladder Contractility

Anticholinergic/Antimuscarinic Agents. Physiologic bladder contractions are thought to be primarily triggered by ACh-induced stimulation of postganglionic parasympathetic muscarinic cholinergic receptor sites on bladder smooth muscle.[11,12] Atropine, a belladonna alkaloid, and atropine-like agents should depress normal bladder contractions and involuntary bladder contractions of any cause.[41-43] In such patients, the volume to the first involuntary bladder contraction and maximum bladder capacity are generally increased, while the amplitude of the involuntary bladder contraction is decreased. However, although the volume and pressure thresholds at which an involuntary bladder contraction is elicited may increase, urgency incontinence episodes (when present) and the frequency of urgency episodes decrease, but both require an element of behavior modification to achieve optimal levels. Atropine increases both the compliance and the capacity of the neurologically decentralized primate bladder.[44,45] However, this effect in bladders with decreased compliance with normal capacity has not been well studied. In addition, outlet resistance, at least as reflected by urethral pressure measurements, does not seem to be clinically affected by anticholinergic therapy.

Although antimuscarinic agents can produce significant clinical improvement in patients with involuntary bladder contractions and associated symptoms, these agents provide only partial inhibition of vesicular contractions. In many animal models, atropine only partially antagonizes the response of the whole bladder to pelvic nerve stimulation and of bladder strips to field stimulation, although it does completely inhibit the response of bladder smooth muscle to exogenous cholinergic stimulation. Of the theories proposed to explain this phenomenon, termed *atropine resistance*, the most attractive and most commonly cited is the idea that a portion of the neurotransmission involved in the final common pathway of bladder contraction is nonadrenergic, noncholinergic—that is, secondary to release of a transmitter other than ACh or noradrenaline.[11,12,46] Although the existence of atropine resistance in human bladder muscle is by no means agreed upon, this concept is the most common hypothesis invoked to explain clinical difficulty in abolishing involuntary bladder contractions with anticholinergic agents alone, and it is also used to support the rationale of treatment of such types of bladder activity with agents that have different mechanisms of action. Conflicting data regarding atropine resistance has been attributed to marked species-specific responses and, in experimental preparations, also depends on the frequency of nerve stimulation.[47,48] There is little or no atropine resistance in normal human detrusor muscle, though it may exist in morphologically or functionally abnormal bladders.[12]

Messenger RNA has been identified for at least five different muscarinic subtypes in the human bladder (muscarinic receptor genes designated M_1–M_5).[49,50] The nomenclature M_1–M_5 describes the protein products of the M_1–M_5 coding regions (the actual muscarinic receptor subtypes), which are each defined pharmacologically using receptor subtype agonists and antagonists.[12,51,52] Pirenzepine (a selective muscarinic blocker) was originally used to subdivide muscarinic receptors into M_1 and M_2 categories. Using this subclassification, detrusor muscarinic receptors were classified as the M_2 type.[12,53,54] On further analysis of the M_2 receptor population, a small proportion of glandular M_2 receptors were found that could represent the pharmacologic type responsible for muscarinic agonist–induced contractions. This subtype is now called the M_3 receptor.[12,51]

M_2 and M_3 receptors can be found not only on detrusor muscle cells, where M_2 receptors predominate at least 3:1 over M_3 receptors, but also on other bladder structures, which may be of importance for detrusor activation.[49,55] Despite this ratio, in vitro data indicate that most smooth muscle contraction, including that of the urinary bladder, is mediated primarily by the M_3 receptor subtype.[55,56] The exact role of the M_2 receptor is unclear, but it may be important in contributing to bladder contraction in outflow obstruction or denervation.[49]

Muscarinic receptor subtyping becomes important when considering the possibility of pharmacologically selecting (and blocking) those receptors responsible for urinary bladder smooth muscle contraction while minimally affecting other muscarinic receptor sites throughout the body. Ideally, this approach would effectively treat the underlying problem (detrusor overactivity) while eliminating the unpleasant systemic side effects of most nonspecific antimuscarinic agents that, in many cases, are worse than the problem they are treating and result in patient noncompliance.

The clinical utility of available antimuscarinic agents is limited by their lack of selectivity, or "uroselectivity," responsible for the classic peripheral side effects. The potential side effects of all antimuscarinic agents include inhibition of salivary secretion (dry mouth), blockade of the ciliary muscle of the lens to cholinergic stimulation (blurred vision for near objects), tachycardia, drowsiness, decreased cognitive function, and inhibition of gut motility. Those agents that possess some ganglionic blocking activity may also cause orthostatic hypotension and erectile dysfunction at high doses (at which nicotinic activity becomes manifest). Antimuscarinic agents are contraindicated in patients with bladder outlet obstruction because complete urinary retention, gastric retention or other severe conditions with decreased gastrointestinal mobility, and narrow-angle glaucoma may be precipitated. Targeting the M_3 receptor for treatment has the potential to decrease or eliminate some of these side effects; however, the M_3 receptor is present in other anatomic locations in humans.[52] Table 30-2 lists the distribution of muscarinic subtypes in the human body.

The lack of selectivity is a major problem with all antimuscarinic compounds as they tend to affect parasympathetically innervated organs in the same order; generally, larger doses are required to inhibit bladder activity than to affect salivary, bronchial, nasopharyngeal, and sweat secretions. Several receptor antagonists with varying degrees of specificity for the lower urinary tract show some promise in decreasing the side effect profiles of this class of medications without compromising efficacy.

A Cochrane review examined 65 clinical trials employing anticholinergic medications as a class versus placebo for the treatment of overactive bladder syndrome.[57] Anticholinergic medications were associated with a relative risk of 1.39 (95% confidence interval, 1.28 to 1.51) for cure or improvement. Anticholinergic medication use was associated with approximately five fewer trips to the toilet and four fewer leakage episodes every week, with modest improvements in quality of life. Dry mouth was noted in a third of active drug patients, which is about three times that seen with placebo, but withdrawal rates between groups were similar. It should be noted that all products have not been directly compared in head-to-head trials and that outcome measures and patient baseline characteristics differ between trials.

Specific Drugs. Propantheline bromide is the classically described oral agent for producing an antimuscarinic effect in the lower urinary tract. The usual adult oral dose is 15 to 30 mg every 4 to 6 hours, although higher doses are often used. Propantheline is a quaternary ammonium compound that is poorly absorbed after oral administration. No available oral drug has a direct in vitro antimuscarinic binding potential that is closer to that of atropine than propantheline bromide.[58,59] There is a surprising lack of valuable data on the effectiveness of propantheline for the treatment of bladder overactivity.

TABLE 30-2 DISTRIBUTION OF MUSCARINIC RECEPTOR SUBTYPES

	Subtype				
	M_1	M_2	M_3	M_4	M_5
Result of activation	Mobilization of intracellular calcium	Inhibition of adenylyl cyclase activity; activation of nonspecific cation channels, inhibition of K_{ATP} channels	Mobilization of intracellular calcium	Inhibition of adenylyl cyclase activity	Mobilization of intracellular calcium
SITE					
Bladder	Modulates acetylcholine release?	Most numerous (outnumbers M_3 by 3:1); function unclear	Detrusor contraction		
Brain	Abundant in neocortex, hippocampus, neostriatum	Throughout	Low levels throughout	Abundant in neostriatum; present in cortex, hippocampus	Localized to projection neurons of substantia nigra, pars compacta, ventral tegmental area, hippocampus
Salivary glands	High-viscosity lubrication		High- and low-viscosity secretions; saliva volume		
Gastrointestinal tract		Most numerous (outnumbers M_3 by 4:1); contractility?	Gastrointestinal mobility		
Heart	Increases heart rate	Modulates pacemaker activity, atrioventricular conduction, atrial and ventricular contraction	Role unclear		
Eye	7% (ciliary processes, iris sphincter); functional role unclear	5-10%; modulates norepinephrine release?	Predominant: 60-75%; mediates contractility response	5-10%; functional role unclear	5% (iris sphincter only)

Scopolamine, another belladonna alkaloid, is marketed as a soluble salt. It readily enters the CNS due to lipophilicity and has prominent central depressive effects at low doses. It is available as a transdermal patch; however, efficacy has been mixed. The patch provides a continuous delivery of 0.5 mg daily to the circulation for 3 days. Caution should be exercised in the use of the patch in the elderly and young, because of systemic anticholinergic effects and the use of a fixed dose.

Hyoscyamine is reported to have anticholinergic actions and side effects similar to those of other belladonna alkaloids. Methantheline is a quaternary ammonium compound that has similar effects on the lower urinary tract, and some clinicians still prefer it to other anticholinergic agents, though there are few data regarding its efficacy.

Tolterodine and its major metabolite, DD01,[60] show some selectivity for bladder tissue over salivary tissue in vitro and in vivo in the anesthetized cat.[61,62] These tissue-selective effects do not appear to be due to muscarinic receptor subtype selectivity,[60,61] but may be related to differential affinities of the receptors in the salivary gland and detrusor muscle for tolterodine compared with oxybutynin. Although it appears that the binding affinities of tolterodine and oxybutynin to muscarinic receptors in the urinary bladder are similar, the affinity of tolterodine for muscarinic receptors in the parotid gland is eight times lower than that of oxybutynin.[63] Tolterodine is available in two formulations: an immediate-release form (2 mg twice daily) and an extended-release form (2 mg or 4 mg once daily).

The comparative efficacy and safety of tolterodine relative to other agents has been investigated by the Cochrane group in a systemic review of all published studies.[64] Tolterodine and oxybutynin are the drugs that have the best high-quality, comparative clinical investigations, with insufficient studies to make comparative statements with other anticholinergic drugs. Tolterodine has equal efficacy compared to oxybutynin for the end points of patient-perceived improvement and leakage episodes or voids per 24-hour period. Tolterodine is significantly better than oxybutynin with regard to patient withdrawal from treatment due to adverse effects, with dry mouth being the most prominent among them. The side effect profile of tolterodine is dose dependent, with patients taking 2 and 4 mg/day experiencing significantly more adverse effects than those taking 1 mg. Efficacy is not as tightly linked to dose as are adverse events, which supports use of the lowest efficacious dose. The extended-release tolterodine preparation has similar efficacy compared to the immediate-release preparation, though the extended-release preparation is associated with less dry mouth.[65,66]

Darifenacin, a tertiary amine, is a selective muscarinic M_3 receptor antagonist. Its theoretical advantage is its ability to selectively block the M_3 receptor, which is the most important in bladder contraction, thereby decreasing the adverse events related to the blockade of other muscarinic subtypes. It is a substrate for the cytochrome P-450 3A4 isoenzyme system. Several randomized, controlled studies have shown decreases in the frequency and severity of urgency, micturition frequency, and number of incontinent episodes compared to placebo, as well as increases in bladder capacity, with once-daily doses of 7.5 and 15 mg. Efficacy is similar to immediate-release oxybutynin, but with fever episodes of dry mouth or blurred vision. The most common side effects seen were mild to moderate dry mouth and constipation.[67,68]

Solifenacin is a tertiary amine antimuscarinic given at once-daily doses of 5 and 10 mg. It is well absorbed from the gastrointestinal tract and undergoes significant hepatic metabolism by the cytochrome P-450 3A4 isoenzyme. Several large trials have examined the effects of solifenacin, showing a reduction in frequency and in the number of micturition and incontinence episodes over 24 hours, as well as increases in voided volume per micturition. Among patients who were incontinent at baseline, a significant number became continent when compared to placebo. Efficacy is similar to that of tolterodine, though solifenacin has a suggestion of fewer adverse events.[69-71]

Musculotropic Relaxants. Musculotropic relaxants affect smooth muscle directly at a site that is metabolically distal to the cholinergic or other contractile receptor mechanism. Although the agents discussed in this section do relax smooth muscle in vitro by papaverine-like (direct) action, all have also been found to possess variable anticholinergic and local anesthetic properties. There is still some uncertainty about how much of their clinical efficacy is due only to their atropine-like effect. If, in fact, any of these agents does exert a clinically significant inhibitory effect that is independent of antimuscarinic action, a therapeutic rationale exists for combining them with a relatively pure anticholinergic agent.

Oxybutynin chloride is a moderately potent anticholinergic agent that has strong independent musculotropic relaxant activity as well as local anesthetic activity. Efficacy is mediated primarily by antagonism of the muscarinic receptors in the bladder smooth muscle. Immediate-release and extended-release forms of oxybutynin are available. Recommended dosing is 5 mg two to three times daily for immediate release and 5 to 15 mg once daily for extended release. Aside from the ease of once-daily administration, the potential benefit of the extended-release formulation is the stabilization of serum levels throughout the day[72] and decreased incidence of dry mouth.

In an increasing effort to maintain or improve the efficacy of oxybutynin while minimizing its side effects, a 3.9-mg/day oxybutynin transdermal patch has been studied. Although a reduction in dry mouth is often noted, the major side effects for the transdermal form were erythema and pruritus at the application site.[73-75]

Topical application of oxybutynin and other agents to normal or intestinal bladders is another route of administration.[76] This conceptually attractive form of alternative drug administration, delivered by periodic intravesical instillation of either liquid or timed-released pellets, awaits further clinical trials and the development of preparations specifically formulated for this purpose. Several nonrandomized, unblinded and non–placebo-controlled studies have demonstrated the efficacy of this therapy in a variety of patients with neurogenic bladders, showing statistically significant improvements in cystometric capacity, volume at first involuntary bladder contraction, bladder compliance, and overall continence.[77-79] It is not clear whether the anticholinergic effect was due to a local effect or to systemic absorption.[80,81]

Dicyclomine hydrochloride, typically used for gastroenterologic indictions, is also reported to exert a direct relaxant effect on smooth muscle in addition to an antimuscarinic action.[82] Flavoxate hydrochloride has a direct inhibitory action on smooth muscle but very weak anticholinergic properties, and has not demonstrated efficacy in randomized, controlled trials.[43]

Trospium and propiverine are classified as predominantly antispasmodic agents (smooth muscle relaxants) with some anticholinergic effects. Trospium is a quaternary amine and has limited CNS penetration and minimal central cognitive adverse effects.[83-85] It has no selectivity for a muscarinic receptor subtype and is given as 20 mg twice daily. Efficacy is equivalent to extended-release tolterodine or oxybutynin. Propiverine is a musculotropic smooth muscle relaxant that is rapidly absorbed and has a high first-pass metabolism.[86] Propiverine is not available in the United States.

Calcium Antagonists. The role of calcium as a messenger in linking extracellular stimuli to the intracellular environment is well established, including its involvement in excitation-contraction coupling in striated, cardiac, and smooth muscle.[11,12] Interference with calcium inflow or intracellular release is a potent potential mechanism for bladder smooth muscle relaxation.

Nifedipine has been shown to be an effective inhibitor of contraction induced by several mechanisms in human and guinea pig bladder muscle.[43,87] It has also been shown to completely block the noncholinergic portion of the contraction produced by electrical field stimulation in rabbit bladder.

Other calcium antagonist drugs are not widely used in treating voiding dysfunction. A bladder-specific membrane calcium channel is not known to exist, and there is no agent that will specifically block intracellular calcium release only in bladder smooth muscle cells. Available information does not suggest that systemic therapy with calcium antagonists is an effective way to treat detrusor overactivity.[88]

β-Adrenergic Agonists. The presence of β-adrenoceptors in human bladder muscle has prompted attempts to increase bladder capacity with β-adrenergic stimulation. Such stimulation may cause significant increases in the capacity of animal bladders, which contain a moderate density of β-adrenoceptors.[11] Thus far, treatment of overactive bladder/detrusor overactivity with β-agonists has not been successful. The β_3-adrenoceptor is the predominant subtype in the human bladder, and selective treatment with β_3-adrenoceptor agonists may prove to be beneficial.

Tricyclic Antidepressants. Many clinicians have found that tricyclic antidepressants, particularly imipramine hydrochloride, are useful for facilitating urine storage, both by decreasing bladder contractility and by increasing outlet resistance.[5] These agents have been the subject of extensive and highly sophisticated pharmacologic investigation to determine the mechanisms of action responsible for their varied effects.[89] Tricyclic antidepressants possess varying degrees of at least three major pharmacologic actions: (i) they have central and peripheral antimuscarinic effects at some, but not all, sites; (ii) they block the active transport system in the presynaptic nerve ending that is responsible for the reuptake of the released amine neurotransmitters norepinephrine and serotonin; and (iii) they are sedatives, an action that occurs presumably on a central basis but is perhaps related to antihistaminic properties ($\text{histamine}_1 > \text{histamine}_2$). There is also evidence that they desensitize at least some α_2- and β-adrenoceptors.

Imipramine is effective in decreasing bladder contractility and increasing outlet resistance.[90-93] Its mode of action in overactive bladder/detrusor overactivity has not been established. The dose is 25 mg four times a day; however, less frequent dosing is possible due the drug's long half-life. A half-dose can be given in elderly patients, in whom the drug's half-life may be prolonged. The effects of imipramine on the lower urinary tract are often additive to those of anticholinergics. It should be noted that the anticholinergic side effects of the drugs may also be additive.

Doxepin is another tricyclic antidepressant that has been found (using rabbit bladder strips in vitro) to be more potent than other tricyclic compounds with respect to antimuscarinic and musculotropic relaxant activity.[94] When the tricyclic antidepressants are used in the larger doses employed for antidepressant effects, their most frequent side effects are those related to their systemic anticholinergic activity.[89]

Botulinum Toxin. BTX is a presynaptic inhibitor of Ach release and the release of other neurotransmitters. It was previously discussed in regard to its use to facilitate emptying by relaxing the striated sphincter. Similarly, the effects of decreasing muscle contractility can be applied to the bladder by cystoscopic injection of BTX directly into the detrusor muscle. The result is a chemical denervation that is reversible after 6 to 9 months, after which time injections can be repeated to achieve a similar response.

Administration of 200 or 300 units of BTX-A injection into the detrusor muscle of patients with refractory neurogenic detrusor overactivity has, in a small study, demonstrated a decrease in episodes of urinary incontinence by 50%, as well as improvements in maximum detrusor pressure, maximum bladder capacity, and improved quality-of-life score.[95] The results were seen as long as 24 weeks after injection.

Dimethyl Sulfoxide. Dimethyl sulfoxide, a naturally occurring organic compound used as an industrial solvent for many years, has multiple pharmacologic actions (membrane penetration, anti-inflammatory, local analgesic, bacteriostatic, diuretic, cholinesterase inhibitor, collagen solvent, vasodilator) and has been used for the treatment of arthritis and other musculoskeletal disorders. A 50% solution is used for intravesical instillation. Although it has good reported results in interstitial cystitis and has a U.S. Food and Drug Administration (FDA) indication for this condition,[96] it has not been shown to be useful in the treatment of neurogenic and non-neurogenic detrusor overactivity, or in any patient with urgency or frequency without interstitial cystitis.

Polysynaptic Inhibitors. Baclofen has been discussed previously with agents that decrease outlet resistance secondary to striated sphincter dyssynergia. It is also capable of depressing neurogenic detrusor overactivity due to spinal cord injury.[97]

Increasing Bladder Capacity by Decreasing Sensory (Afferent) Input

Vanilloids: Capsaicin and Resiniferatoxin. Decreasing afferent input peripherally is the ideal treatment for both sensory urgency and detrusor overactivity in a bladder with relatively normal elastic or viscoelastic properties in which the sensory afferents constitute the first limb in the abnormal micturition reflex (see Fig. 30-2). Capsaicin produces pain by selectively activating polymodal nociceptive neurons by membrane depolarization and opening a cation-selective ion channel, which can be blocked by ruthenium red. Repeated administration induces desensitization and inactivation of sensory neurons by several mechanisms. Systemic and topical capsaicin produces a reversible antinociceptive and anti-inflammatory action after an initially undesirable analgesic effect. Local or topical application blocks C-fiber conduction and inactivates neuropeptide release from peripheral nerve endings, accounting for local antinociception and reduction of neurogenic inflammation. Resiniferatoxin (RTX) is an analogue of capsaicin, and is approximately 1000 times more potent for desensitization than capsaicin,[98] but only a few hundred times more potent for excitation.[99] Systemic capsaicin produces antinociception by activating specific receptors on afferent nerve terminals in the spinal cord; spinal neurotransmission is subsequently blocked by a prolonged inactivation of sensory neurotransmitter release. With local (intravesical) administration, the potential advantage of capsaicin is a lack of systemic side effects. The actions are highly specific when the drug is applied locally—the compound affects primarily small-diameter nociceptive afferents, leaving the sensations of touch and pressure unchanged, although heat (not cold) perception may be reduced; motor fibers are not affected.[100] The effects are reversible, although it is not known whether initial levels of sensitivity are regained.

An efferent function of capsaicin-sensitive primary afferents is the release of neurotransmitters from the peripheral endings of these sensory neurons, such as tachykinins and calcitonin gene–related peptide.[101] These neurotransmitters can produce events collectively known as neurogenic inflammation, which can include smooth muscle contractions, increased plasma protein extravasation, vasodilation, mast cell degranulation, facilitation of transmitter release from nerve terminals, and recruitment of inflammatory cells. This is another reason why intravesical capsaicin could theoretically be useful in treating the pain and related problems of interstitial cystitis and certain types of bladder overactivity that originate in primary afferents.

The peripheral terminals of capsaicin-sensitive primary afferents form a dense plexus just below the bladder urothelium, and fibers penetrating the urothelium come into contact with the lumen. This location, combined with their peculiar chemosensitivity, permits capsaicin-sensitive primary afferents to detect "backflow" of chemicals across the urothelium, which is thought to occur during conditions leading to breakdown of the "barrier function" of the urothelium.[102] If the barrier theory or "leaky urothelium" theory of the pathogenesis of interstitial cystitis is true, for some or many of the patients with this condition, the capsaicin-sensitive primary afferents may be stimulated by urine constituents leaking back across the urothelium. Under these circumstances, a local release of neuropeptides may well contribute to the production of neurogenic inflammation.

Overall, intravesical capsaicin and RTX treatment may be a promising therapy for detrusor overactivity, and possibly sensory dysfunction of the lower urinary tract; however, many problems exist. Optimal dosage, method and timing of delivery, and delivery vehicle remain unclear. In addition, the patients likely to respond to this therapy are not yet defined.

Increasing Outlet Resistance

α-Adrenergic Agonists. The bladder neck and proximal urethra contain a preponderance of α-adrenergic receptor sites that, when stimulated, produce smooth muscle contraction.[11,12,46] The static infusion urethral pressure profile is altered by such stimulation, producing an increase in mean urethral pressure and maximum urethral closure pressure. Although some clinicians have reported spectacular cure and improvement rates with α-adrenergic agonists and agents that produce an α-adrenergic effect in the outlet of patients with sphincteric urinary incontinence, our own experience coincides with those who report that such treatment often produces satisfactory or some improvement in mild cases but rarely total dryness in patients with severe or even moderate stress incontinence.

α-Adrenergic stimulation generally increases outlet resistance to a variable degree, but these drugs are most often limited by their potential side effects. The FDA has asked manufacturers to voluntarily stop selling α-adrenergic–containing products due to an increase in cerebrovascular incidents noted in women taking the α-adrenergic agent phenylpropanolamine.[49]

β-Adrenergic Antagonists and Agonists. Theoretically, β-adrenergic blocking agents might be expected to "unmask" or potentiate a β-adrenergic effect, thereby increasing urethral resistance. β-Adrenergic stimulation is generally conceded to decrease urethral pressure, but β_2-agonists have been reported to increase the contractility of fast-contracting striated muscle fibers (extensor digitorum longus) from guinea pigs and suppress that of slow-contracting fibers (soleus).[101]

Duloxetine. Duloxetine, a combined serotonin and norepinephrine reuptake inhibitor, increases sphincteric muscle activity during the filling and storage phases of micturition in the model of the irritated feline bladder. This pharmacologic agent has been used clinically as an antidepressant.[104] In a study of its effects on the lower urinary tract in the cat, duloxetine significantly increased bladder capacity[105] (probably through a CNS effect), as well as enhancing external urethral sphincter activity with no effect on sphincter activity during voiding.

A Cochrane systematic review has examined the use of duloxetine for urinary incontinence. The primary benefit has been in the domains of improvement in quality-of-life measures. Objective measures such as 24-hour diaper weight have been less impressive. Side effects, particularly nausea, are common but generally well tolerated.[106] Duloxetine is currently used for treatment of stress urinary incontinence outside the United States, but is not currently FDA approved for this indication.

Estrogens. Although estrogens were recommended for the treatment of female urinary incontinence as early as 1941,[107] there is still controversy over their use and benefit:risk ratio for this purpose. Numerous clinical studies exist; however, there has been little consistency in methodology, many of the studies have been observational, different formulations of estrogens have been tested, and the data can be conflicting.

Estrogens have been considered in the treatment for stress urinary incontinence as the urethra has four estrogen-sensitive layers—the epithelium, vasculature, connective tissue, and musculature—that may play a role in maintaining a positive urethral pressure. Estrogen therapy seems to be capable of facilitating urinary storage in some postmenopausal women. Whether this effect is related just to changes in the autonomic innervation, changes in receptor content or function of the smooth muscle, changes in estrogen binding sites,[108] or changes in the vascular or connective tissue elements of the urethral wall has not been settled. After menopause, urethral pressure parameters normally decrease slightly[109] and, although this change is generally conceded to be related in some way to decreased estrogen levels, it is still largely a matter of speculation whether the actual changes occur in smooth muscle, blood circulation, supporting tissues, or the "mucosal seal mechanism."

Prior meta-analyses have shed some light on the use of estrogen therapy in the treatment of stress urinary incontinence. One suggested a subjective but not objective improvement in stress urinary incontinence.[110] A Cochrane review suggested benefit of estrogen primarily in

TABLE 30-3 EMERGING THERAPEUTICS

Drug	Class	Comments
Fesoterodine[60]	Anticholinergic	Shares the major metabolite DD01 with tolterodine.
Nitric oxide analogues or synthetase stimulators	Nitrate	Involved in relaxation of bladder body smooth muscle.[119]
Prostaglandin synthesis inhibition		Prostaglandins have a potential role in excitatory neurotransmission, development of bladder contractility, emptying contractile response, maintenance of urethral tone during the storage phase of micturition, and release of this tone during the emptying phase.
Dopamine$_1$ receptor agonist	Pergolide	Agonism at receptor inhibits voiding reflex.
Potassium channel openers	Pinacidil	Pinacidil inhibits contractile responses in normal and hypertrophied rat detrusor muscle.[120,121] A preliminary study of this agent was negative.[122]

those with urge incontinence, as well as a potential for worsening of symptoms with the use of estrogen and progestin combination therapy.[111] Both of these studies predated the release of the results of the Woman's Health Initiative,[112] a mega-trial involving 23,296 women whose urinary incontinence symptoms were evaluated. Depending on the presence or absence of a uterus, women were treated with placebo, conjugated equine estrogen (CEE), or a combination of CEE and medroxyprogesterone acetate (MPA). Menopausal hormonal therapy was observed to increase all types of urinary incontinence, with stress urinary incontinence being the most common, after 1 year of use in women who were continent at baseline. For those women with urinary incontinence at baseline, frequency worsened with both CEE alone and the combination of CEE and MPA.

As to the type of estrogen preparation preferred, transdermal seems to be as effective as oral, and subcutaneous implants appear to produce physiologic serum levels. Percutaneous and intramuscular estrogens seem to produce variable serum levels. Vaginal creams produce variable serum levels but physiologic estradiol : estrone ratios.[113]

Circumventing the Problem

Antidiuretic Hormone–Like Agents

The synthetic antidiuretic hormone peptide analogue desmopressin acetate (1-desamino-8-D-arginine vasopressin) has been used for the symptomatic relief of refractory nocturnal enuresis in both children and adults.[114,115] Suggestions have been made that desmopressin might be useful in patients with refractory nocturnal frequency and incontinence who do not belong in the category of primary nocturnal enuresis.[116]

Emerging Targets and Therapeutics

Table 30-3 presents information on several emerging therapeutic options for voiding dysfunction currently under review.

REFERENCES

1. Yoshimura N, Kaiho Y, Miyazato M, et al. Therapeutic receptor targets for lower urinary tract dysfunction. Naunyn Schmiedebergs Arch Pharmacol 2007.
2. Andersson, K-E, Wein AJ. Pharmacology of the lower urinary tract: basis for current and future treatments of urinary incontinence. Pharmacol Rev 2004;56:581-631.
3. Wein AJ. Lower urinary tract dysfunction in neurologic injury and disease. *In* Wein AJ, Kavoussi LR, Novick AC, et al (eds): Campbell-Walsh Urology, 9th ed. Philadelphia: Elsevier Saunders, 2007, pp 2011-2045.
4. Raezer DM, Wein AJ, Jacobowitz DM. Autonomic innervation of canine urinary bladder: cholinergic and adrenergic contributions and interaction of sympathetic and parasympathetic systems in bladder function. Urology 1973;2:211.
5. Barrett DM, Wein AJ. Voiding dysfunction: diagnosis, classification and management. *In* Gillenwater JY, Grayhack JT, Howards ST, Duckett JW (eds): Adult and Pediatric Urology, 2nd ed. St Louis: Mosby–Year Book, 1991, pp 1001-1099.
6. Lee L. The clinical use of urecholine in dysfunctions of the bladder. J Urol 1949;62:300.
7. Sonda L, Gershon C, Diokno A. Further observations on the cystometric and uroflowmetric effects of bethanechol chloride on the human bladder. J Urol 1979;122:775.
8. Perkash I. Intermittent catheterization and bladder rehabilitation in spinal cord injury patients. J Urol 1975;114:230.
9. Barendrecht MM, Oelke M, Laguna MP, Michel MC. Is the use of parasympathomimetics for treating an underactive urinary bladder evidence-based? BJU Int 2007;99:749-752.
10. Sporer A, Leyson J, Martin B. Effects of bethanechol chloride on the external urethral sphincter in spinal cord injury patients. J Urol 1978;120:62.
11. Wein AJ, Levin RM, Barrett DM. Voiding function: relevant anatomy, physiology, and pharmacology. *In* Duckett JW, Howards ST, Grayhack JT, Gillenwater JY (eds): Adult and Pediatric Urology, 2nd ed. St. Louis: Mosby–Year Book, 1991, pp 933-999.
12. Andersson K-E. Pharmacology of lower urinary tract smooth muscles and penile erectile tissues. Pharmacol Rev 1993;45:253.
13. de Groat WC, Booth AM. Autonomic systems to the urinary bladder and sexual organs. *In* Dyck PJ, Thomas PK, Lambert EH (eds): Peripheral Neuropathy. Philadelphia: WB Saunders, 1984, pp 285-299.
14. Steers WD. Physiology of the urinary bladder. *In* Walsh PC, Retik AB, Stamey TA, Vaughan ED (eds): Campbell's Urology, 6th ed. Philadelphia: WB Saunders, 1992, pp 142-169.
15. Taylor SH. Clinical pharmacotherapeutics of doxazosin. Am J Med 1989;87(Suppl 2A):25.
16. Lepor H. Role of long acting selective alpha-1 blockers in the treatment of benign prostatic hyperplasia. Urol Clin North Am 1990;17:651.
17. Wilde M, Fitton A, Sorkin E. Terazosin: a review of its pharmacodynamic and pharmacokinetic properties and therapeutic potential in BPH. Drugs Aging 1993; 3:258.
18. Buzelin JM, Herbert M, Blondin P. Alpha-blocking treatment with alfuzosin in symptomatic benign prostatic hyperplasia: comparative study with prazosin. The PRAZALF Group. Br J Urol 1993;72:922-927.
19. Wilde M, Fitton A, McTavish D. Alfuzosin—a review of its pharmacodynamic and pharmacokinetic properties and its therapeutic potential in BPH. Drugs 1993; 45:410.
20. Buzelin JM, Roth S, Geffriaud-Ricouard C, et al. Efficacy and safety of sustained-release alfuzosin 5 mg in patients with benign prostatic hyperplasia. ALGEBI Study Group. Eur Urol 1997;31:190-198.
21. Lepor H, Tang R, Kobayashi S, et al. Localization of the alpha-1A-adrenoreceptor in the human prostate. J Urol 1995;154:2096-2099.
22. Noble AJ, Williams-Chess R, Couldwell C, et al. The effects of tamsulosin, a high affinity antagonist at functional alpha 1A- and alpha 1D-adrenoceptor subtypes. Br J Pharmacol 1997;120:231-238.
23. Wilt T, MacDonald R, Rutks I. Tamsulosin for benign prostatic hyperplasia. Cochrane Database Syst Rev 2002;(4):CD002081.
24. Djavan B, Marberger M. A meta-analysis on the efficacy and tolerability of alpha1-adrenoceptor antagonists in patients with lower urinary tract symptoms suggestive of benign prostatic obstruction. Eur Urol 1999;36:1-13.
25. Raz S, Caine M. Adrenergic receptors in the female canine urethra. Invest Urol 1971;9:319.
26. Burton G, Dobson C. Progesterone increases flow rates: a new treatment for voiding abnormalities? Neurourol Urodyn 1993;12:398.
27. Taricco M, Adone R, Pagliacci C, Telaro E. Pharmacological interventions for spasticity following spinal cord injury. Cochrane Database Syst Rev 2000;(2):CD001131.
28. Shader RI, Greenblatt DJ. Use of benzodiazepines in anxiety disorders. N Engl J Med 1993;328:1398.
29. Davidoff RA. Antispasticity drugs: mechanisms of action. Ann Neurol 1985; 17:107.
30. Milanov IG. Mechanisms of baclofen action on spasticity. Acta Neurol Scand 1991;85:304.
31. Florante J, Leyson J, Martin B, et al. Baclofen in the treatment of detrusor sphincter dyssynergy in spinal cord injury patients. J Urol 1980;124:82.
32. Hachen H, Krucker V. Clinical and laboratory assessment of the efficacy of baclofen on urethral sphincter spasticity in patients with traumatic paraplegia. Eur Urol 1977;3:327.
33. Penn RD, Savoy SM, Corcos DE. Intrathecal baclofen for severe spinal spasticity. N Engl J Med 1989;320:1517.
34. Hackler RH, Broecker BH, Klein FA, Brady SM. A clinical experience with dantrolene sodium for external urinary sphincter hypertonicity in spinal cord injured patients. J Urol 1980;124:78.
35. Dykstra DD, Sidi AA. Treatment of detrusor-striated sphincter dyssynergia with botulinum A toxin. Arch Phys Med Rehabil 1990;71:24.

36. Leippold T, Reitz A, Schurch B. Botulinum toxin as a new therapy option for voiding disorders: current state of the art. Eur Urol 2003;44:165-174.
37. Kuo HC. Prostate botulinum A toxin injection—an alternative treatment for benign prostatic obstruction in poor surgical candidates. Urology 2005;65:670-674.
38. Wein AJ. Prostate botulinum A toxin injection—an alternative treatment for benign prostatic obstruciton in poor surgical candidates. J Urol 2005;174:1903.
39. Duthie J, Wilson DI, Herbison GP, Wilson D. Botulinum toxin injections for adults with overactive bladder syndrome. Cochrane Database Syst Rev 2007;(3):CD005493.
40. Ng CK, Gonzalez RR, Te AE. Refractory overactive bladder in men: update on novel therapies. Curr Urol Rep 2006;7:456.
41. Jensen D Jr. Pharmacological studies of the uninhibited neurogenic bladder. Acta Neurol Scand 1981;64:145-174.
42. Blaivas J, Labib K, Michalik S, et al. Cystometric response to propantheline in detrusor hyperreflexia: therapeutic implications. J Urol 1980;124:259.
43. Andersson K-E. Current concepts in the treatment of disorders of micturition. Drugs 1988;35:477.
44. McGuire E, Savastano J. Effect of alpha adrenergic blockade and anticholinergic agents on the decentralized primate bladder. Neurourol Urodyn 1985;4:139.
45. Andersson K-E, Ek A, Hedlund H. Effects of prazosin in isolated human urethra and in patients with lower neuron lesions. Invest Urol 1981;19:39.
46. Wein AJ, Van Arsdalen KN, Levin RM. Pharmacologic therapy. *In* Krane RJ, Siroky MB (eds): Clinical Neuro-Urology. Boston: Little Brown, 1991, pp 523-558.
47. Brading A. Physiology of bladder smooth muscle. *In* Torrens M, Morrison JFB (eds): The Physiology of the Lower Urinary Tract. New York: Springer Verlag, 1987, pp 161-192.
48. Brading AF. Physiology of the urinary tract smooth muscle. *In* Webster G, Kirby R, King L, Goldwasser B (eds): Reconstructive Urology. Boston: Blackwell Scientific, 1987, pp 15-26.
49. Abrams P, Andersson KE, Buccafusco JJ, et al. Muscarinic receptors: their distribution and function in body systems, and the implications for treating overactive bladder. Br J Pharmacol 2006;148:565-578.
50. Bonner TI. The molecular basis of muscarinic receptor diversity. Trends Neurosci 1989;12:148.
51. Poli E, Monica B, Zappia L, et al. Antimuscarinic activity of telemyepine on isolated human urinary bladder: no role for M-1 receptors. Gen Pharmacol 1992;23:659.
52. Eglen RM, Watson N. Selective muscarinic receptor agonists and antagonists. Pharmacol Toxicol 1996;78:59-68.
53. Levin RM, Ruggieri MR, Wein AJ. Identification of receptor subtypes in the rabbit and human urinary bladder by selective radio-ligand binding. J Urol 1988;139:844.
54. Levin RM, Ruggieri MR, Lee W, et al. Effect of chronic atropine administration on the rat urinary bladder. J Urol 1988;139:1347.
55. Nilvebrant L, Andersson K-E, Gillberg PG, et al. Tolterodine—a new bladder-selective antimuscarinic agent. Eur J Pharmacol 1997;327:195-207.
56. Tobin G, Sjögren C. In vivo and in vitro effects of muscarinic receptor antagonists on contractions and release of [^{3}H] acetylcholine release in the rabbit urinary bladder. Eur J Pharmacol 1995;281:1-8.
57. Nabi G, Cody JD, Ellis G, et al. Anticholinergic drugs versus placebo for overactive bladder syndrome in adults. Cochrane Database Syst Rev 2006;(4):CD003781.
58. Levin RM, Staskin D, Wein AJ. The muscarinic cholinergic binding kinetics of the human urinary bladder. Neurourol Urodyn 1982;1:221.
59. Peterson JS, Patton AJ, Noronha-Blob L. Mini-pig urinary bladder function: comparisons of in vitro anticholinergic responses and in vivo cystometry with drugs indicated for urinary incontinence. J Auton Pharmacol 1990;10:65-73.
60. Wefer J, Truss MC, Jonas U. Tolterodine: an overview. World J Urol 2001;19:312-318.
61. Nilvebrant L, Hallen B, Larsson G. A new bladder selective muscarinic receptor antagonist: preclinical pharmacological and clinical data. Life Sci 1997;60:1129-1136.
62. Nilvebrant L, Sundquist S, Gillberg PG. Tolterodine is not subtype (m1-m5) selective but exhibits functional bladder selectivity in vivo. Neurourol Urodyn 1996;15:310-311.
63. Nilvebrant L, Glas G, Jonsson A, et al. The in vitro pharmacological profile of tolterodine—a new agent for the treatment of urinary urge incontinence. Neurourol Urodyn 1994;13:433-435.
64. Hay-Smith J, Herbison P, Ellis G, Morris A. Which anticholinergic drug for overactive bladder symptoms in adults? Cochrane Database Syst Rev 2005;(3):CD005429.
65. Diokno AC, Appell RA, Sand PK, et al. OPERA Study Group. Prospective, randomized double-blind study of the efficacy and tolerability of the extended-release formulations of oxybutynin and tolterodine for overactive bladder: results of the OPERA trial. Mayo Clin Proc 2003;78:687.
66. Sussman D, Garely A. Treatment of overactive bladder with once-daily extended-release tolterodine or oxybutynin: the Antimuscarinic Clinical Effectiveness Trial (ACET). Curr Med Res Opin 2002;18:177.
67. Haab F, Stewart L, Dwyer P. Darifenacin, an M3 selective receptor antagonist, is an effective and well-tolerated once-daily treatment for overactive bladder. Eur Urol 2004;45:420.
68. Zinner N, Tuttle J, Marks L. Efficacy and tolerability of darifenacin, a muscarinic M3 selective receptor antagonist (M3 SRA), compared with oxybutynin in the treatment of patients with overactive bladder. World J Urol 2005;23:248-252.
69. Chapple CR, Techberger T, Al-Shukri S, et al. Randomized, double-blind, placebo- and tolterodine-controlled trial of the once-daily antimuscarinic agent solifenacin in patients with symptomatic overactive bladder. BJU Int 2004;93:303.
70. Cardozo L. Solifenacin succinate improves symptoms of an overactive bladder. Int Urogynecol J Pelvic Floor Dysfunct 2003;14(Suppl):S64.
71. Gittleman MC, Kaufman J. Solifenacin succinate 10 mg once daily signficantly improved symptoms of overactive bladder. Int J Gynecol Obstet 2003;83(Suppl 3).
72. Gupta SK, Sathyan G. Pharmacokinetics of an oral once-a-day controlled-release oxybutynin formulation compared with immediate-release oxybutynin. J Clin Pharmacol 1999;39:289-296.
73. Dmochowski RR, Davila GW, Zinner NR, et al. Efficacy and safety of transdermal oxybutynin in patients with urge and mixed urinary incontinence. J Urol 2002;168:580.
74. Davila GW, Daugherty CA, Sanders SW. A short-term, multi-center, randomized double-blind dose titration study of the efficacy and anticholinergic side effects of transdermal compared to immediate release oral oxybutynin treatment of patients with urge urinary incontinence. J Urol 2001;166:140.
75. Dmochowski RR, Sand PK, Zinner NR, et al. Comparative efficacy and safety of transdermal oxybutynin and oral tolterodine versus placebo in previously treated patients with urge and mixed urinary incontinence. Urology 2003;62: 237.
76. Kato K, Kitada S, Chun A, et al. In vitro intravesical instillation of anticholinergic, antispasmodic and calcium blocking agents (rabbit whole bladder model). J Urol 1989;141:1471-1475.
77. Mizunaga M, Miyata M, Kaneko S, et al. Intravesical instillation of oxybutynin hydrochloride therapy for patients with a neuropathic bladder. Paraplegia 1994;32:25-29.
78. Connor JP, Betrus G, Fleming P, et al. Early cystometrograms can predict the response to intravesical instillation of oxybutynin chloride in myelomeningocele patients. J Urol 1994;151:1045-1047.
79. Szollar SM, Lee SM. Intravesical oxybutynin for spinal cord injury patients. Spinal Cord 1996;34:284-287.
80. Madersbacher H, Jilg G. Control of detrusor hyperreflexia by the intravesical instillation of oxybutynin hydrochloride. Paraplegia 1991;19:84.
81. Madersbacher H, Knoll M. Intravesical application of oxybutynin: mode of action in controlling detrusor hyperreflexia. Eur Urol 1995;28:340-344.
82. Downie J, Twiddy D, Awad SA. Antimuscarininc and non-competitive antagonist properties of dicyclomine hydrochloride in isolated human and rabbit bladder muscle. J Pharmacol Exp Ther 1977;201:662.
83. Fusgen I, Hauri D. Trospium chloride: an effective option for medical treatment of bladder overactivity. Int J Clin Pharmacol Ther 2000;38:223.
84. Todorova A, Vonderheid-Guth B, Dimpfel W. Effects of tolterodine, trospium chloride, and oxybutynin on the central nervous system. J Clin Pharmacol 2001; 41:636.
85. Wiedemann A, Fusgen I, Hauri D. New aspects of therapy with trospium chloride for urge incontinence. Eur J Geriatrics 2002;3:41.
86. Madersbacher H, Murz G. Efficacy, tolerability and safety profile of propiverine in the treatment of the overactive bladder (non-neurogenic and neurogenic). World J Urol 2001;19:324.
87. Forman A, Andersson K, Henriksson L, et al. Effects of nifedipine on the smooth muscle of the human urinary tract in vitro and in vivo. Acta Pharmacol Toxicol 1978;43:111-118.
88. Roxburgh C, Cook J, Dublin N. Anticholinergic drugs versus other medications for overactive bladder syndrome in adults. Cochrane Database Syst Rev 2007;(3): CD003190.
89. Hollister LE. Current antidepressants. Annu Rev Pharmacol Toxicol 1986;26:23.
90. Cole A, Fried F. Favorable experiences with imipramine in the treatment of neurogenic bladder. J Urol 1972;107:44.
91. Raezer DM, Benson GS, Wein AJ. The functional approach to the management of the pediatric neuropathic bladder: a clinical study. J Urol 1977;117:649.
92. Tulloch AGS, Creed KE. A comparison between propantheline and imipramine on bladder and salivary gland function. Br J Urol 1981;125:218.
93. Castleden CM, George CF, Renwick AG, et al. Imipramine—a possible alternative to current therapy for urinary incontinence in elderly. J Urol 1981;125:218.
94. Bigger J, Giardino E, Perel JE. Cardiac antiarrhythmic effect of imipramine hydrochloride. N Engl J Med 1977;296:206.
95. Schurch B, Schulte-Baukloh H. Botulinum toxin in the treatment of neurogenic bladder in adults and children. Eur Urol (Suppl) 2006;5:679-684.
96. Sant GR. Intravesical 50% dimethyl sulfoxide (Rimso-50) in treatment of interstitial cystitis. Urology 1987;4(Suppl):17.
97. Kiesswetter H, Schober W. Lioresal in the treatment of neurogenic bladder dysfunction. Urol Int 1975;30:63.
98. Ishizuka O, Mattiasson V, Andersson K-E. Urodynamic effects of intravesical resiniferatoxin and capsaicin in conscious rats with and without outflow obstruction. J Urol 1995;154:611.
99. Szallazi A, Blumgerg PM. Vanilloid receptors: new insights enhance potential as a therapeutic target. Pain 1996;68:195.
100. Craft RM, Porreca F. Treatment parameters of desensitization to capsaicin. Life Sci 1992;51:1767.
101. Maggi CA, Barbanti G, Santicioli P, et al. Cystometric evidence that capsaicin-sensitive nerves modulate the afferent branch of micturition reflex in humans. J Urol 1989;142:150-154.
102. Maggi CA. Therapeutic potential of capsaicin-like molecules—studies in animals and humans. Life Sci 1992;51:1777-1781.
103. Fellenius E, Hedberg R, Holmberg E, et al. Functional and metabolic effects of terbutaline and propranolol in fast and slow contracting skeletal muscle in vitro. Acta Physiol Scand 1980;109:89.
104. Berk M, du Plessis AD, Birkett M, et al. An open-label study of duloxetine hydrochloride, a mixed serotonin and noradrenaline reuptake inhibitor, in patients with DSM-III-R major depressive disorder. Int Clin Psychopharmacol 1997;12:137-140.
105. Thor KB, Katofiasc MA. Effects of duloxetine, a combined serotonin and norepinephrine reuptake inhibitor, on central neural control of lower urinary tract function

in the chloralose-anesthetized female cat. J Pharmacol Exp Ther 1995;274:1014-1024.
106. Mariappan P, Ballantyne Z, N'Dow JMO, Alhasso AA. Serotonin and noradrenaline reuptake inhibitors (SNRI) for stress urinary incontinence in adults. Cochrane Database Syst Rev 2005;(3):CD004742.
107. Donker P, Van Der Sluis C. Action of beta adrenergic blocking agents on the urethral pressure profile. Urol Int 1976;31:6.
108. Batra SC, Iosif CS. Female urethra: a target for oestrogen action. J Urol 1983;129:418.
109. Rud T. Urethral pressure profile in continent women from childhood to old age. Acta Obstet Gynecol Scand 1980;59:331.
110. Fantl JA, Cardozo L, McClish DK. Estrogen therapy in the management of urinary incontinence in postmenopausal women: a meta-analysis. First report of the Hormones and Urogenital Therapy Committee. Obstet Gynecol 1994;83:12.
111. Moehrer B, Hextall A, Jackson S. Oestrogens for urinary incontinence in women. Cochrane Database Syst Rev 2003;(2):CD001405.
112. Hendrix SL, Cochrane BB, Nygaard IE, et al. Effects of estrogen with and without progestin on urinary incontinence. JAMA 2005;293:935.
113. Session DR, Kelly AC, Jewelewicz R. Current concepts in oestrogen replacement therapy in the menopause. Fertil Steril 1993;59:277.
114. Murray K. Medical and surgical management of female voiding difficulty. *In* Drife JO, Hilton P, Stanton SL (eds): Micturition. London: Springer-Verlag, 1990, p 179.
115. Norgaard JP, Rillig S, Djurhuus JC. Nocturnal enuresis: an approach to treatment based on pathogenesis. J Pediatr 1989;114:705.
116. Kinn AC, Larsson PO. Desmopressin: a new principle for symptomatic treatment of urgency and incontinence in patients with multiple sclerosis. Scand J Urol Nephrol 1990;24:109.
117. International Continence Society. Third International Consultation on Incontinence, Monte Carlo, Monaco, June 26-29, 2004.
118. Cardozo L. Pharmacotherapy in stress and mixed incontinence. Eur Urol Suppl 2006;5:854.
119. Taylor MC, Bates CP. A double-blind crossover trial of baclofen: a new treatment for the unstable bladder syndrome. Br J Urol 1979;51:505.
120. Malmgren A, Andersson K, Andersson PO, et al. Effects of cromakalim (BRL 34915) and pinacidil on normal and hypertrophied rat detrusor in vitro. J Urol 1990;143:828.
121. Fovaeus M, Andersson K-E, Hedlund H. The action of pinacidil in isolated human bladder. J Urol 1989;141:637.
122. Hedlund H, Mattiasson A, Andersson K-E. Lack of effect of pinacidil on detrusor instability in men with bladder outlet obstruction. J Urol 1990;143:369A.

31

ACID REFLUX AND ULCER DISEASE

Alex Mejia and Walter K. Kraft

INTRODUCTION 457
PHYSIOLOGY AND PATHOPHYSIOLOGY 457
Regulation of Acid Secretion 457
Central Regulation 457
Peripheral and Cellular Regulation 458
H^+,K^+-ATPase: The Proton Pump 460
Acid-Related Diseases 461
Gastroesophageal Reflux Disease 461
Peptic Ulcer Disease 461
NSAID-Induced Ulcers 462
Stress-Related Ulceration 462
THERAPEUTICS AND CLINICAL PHARMACOLOGY 462
Therapeutics by Class 462
Inhibitors of Gastric Acid 462
Mucosal Protective Agents 467
Therapeutic Strategies for Acid Peptic Disorders 467
Gastroesophageal Reflux Disease 467
Peptic Ulcer Disease 469
NSAID-Induced Ulcers 470
Emerging Targets and Therapeutics 471

INTRODUCTION

The term *peptic* is derived from the Greek *peptos*, which means cooked or digested. Peptic ulcer diseases include a number of conditions primarily affecting the gastrointestinal (GI) tract. Gastroesophageal reflux disease, peptic ulcer secondary to *Helicobacter pylori* infection, and gastric injury caused by nonsteroidal anti-inflammatory drugs are responsible for significant costs to health care and impact the quality of life of afflicted patients. Gastric hydrochloric acid secretion is the resultant of a tight physiological control between mechanisms that protect the epithelial lining and a series of neuronal and hormonal stimulations of receptors on the basolateral membranes that lead to the activation of enzymes located on the surface of the parietal cells. The development of potent, safe drugs based on physiologic targets is an impressive success in modern therapeutics. An example of this success has been the control of gastric acid, and the enhancement of the body's cytoprotective mechanisms.

Acid peptic disorders result from distinctive but overlapping pathogenic mechanisms leading to either excessive acid secretion or diminished mucosal defense. Goals of therapy for these disorders include the relief of symptoms, enhancement of ulcer healing in the affected mucosa (esophagus, stomach, duodenum), and prevention of recurrence milestones in the treatment of these diseases include the discovery of the histamine H_2 receptor and development of functional H_2-receptor antagonists (H_2RAs), the discovery of H^+,K^+-adenosine triphosphatase (H^+,K^+-pumps) and the development of proton pump inhibitors (Fig. 31-1), and the discovery of *H. pylori* and the development of effective eradication regimens.

PHYSIOLOGY AND PATHOPHYSIOLOGY

The stomach has multiple functions, including emptying ingested food in a regulated fashion. The role of acid in normal physiology is to aid in the digestion of proteins, absorption of iron and vitamin B_{12}. The entry of food into the stomach activates acid secretion by a series of balanced but complex pathways that require hormonal, neuronal, and paracrinal signaling. The end result is intracellular calcium accumulation and receptor activation, which promotes the insertion of the gastric H^+,K^+-ATPase proton pumps into the apical surface of the parietal cells. The result is secretion of acid into the parietal cell canaliculus. Activation of any or all of these pathways causes the parietal cell to secrete concentrated acid with a pH at or close to 1.

Several cell types participate in gastric secretion. The most important are the parietal cell and those cells that regulate the output of the parietal cells. The epithelium of the stomach forms deep pits and glands (oxyntic glands). Gastric exocrine cells will originate from stem cells located in the "neck" or midregion of these glands. From there, they migrate upward or downward, maturing into more specialized cells. The parietal cells, which secrete hydrochloric acid and intrinsic factor, are mostly limited to the fundic region of the stomach and are located in the lower two thirds of the oxyntic glands. Chief or peptic cells, responsible for secreting pepsinogen, are also located at the base of the oxyntic glands. Columnar cells and mucus cells line the gastric surface and outer portions of the gastric glands. At least six endocrine cells regulate the activity of the parietal cell: G cells, D cells, enterochromaffin-like (ECL) cells, A-like cells, D1/P cells, and enterochromaffin cells.[1] The final secreted product from the parietal cells will in turn combine with enzymes secreted from chief cells, these pass out of the oxyntic glands up through the mucus gel layer that covers the surface of the stomach (Fig. 31-2 and Table 31-1).

Regulation of Acid Secretion

Acid secretion is initiated by a variety of factors related to food ingestion and can be regulated by a set of mechanisms acting at the central, peripheral, and cellular levels.

Central Regulation

The thought, smell, taste, and swallowing of food can stimulate acid secretion; however, it is underappreciated that the strongest central stimulus is hypoglycemia.[3] The dorsal motor nucleus in the medulla, the hypothalamus, and the nucleus tractus solitarius play key roles in the integration of afferent and efferent information. Most vagal fibers supplying the stomach are afferent,[4] relaying information to the brain about mechanical and chemical changes in the stomach; however, the dorsal motor nucleus supplies its stimulatory fibers to the stomach via the same nerves. The hypothalamus appears to have both stimulatory and inhibitory influences on acid secretion. The nucleus tractus solitarius receives its inputs from taste fibers and plays a role in initiating acid secretion due to the taste of food. In addition, it has also been found to respond with a strong stimulation of acid secretion in response to glucose deprivation. Peptides produced peripherally in the gut can signal the brain directly or by activating afferent neurons that terminate in the spinal cord or brainstem. These include leptin, ghrelin,

TABLE 31-1 OXINTIC GLAND, CELL TYPES AND PRODUCTS

Oxintic Gland Region	Cell Type	Products	% of Gland Cells	Region of Stomach
Isthmus of gland	Mucous cells	Mucus gel layer, mucin PG II	40-46%	Cardiac, pyloric
Neck of gland	Parietal (oxyntic) cells	Gastric acid and intrinsic factor	12-13%	Fundus and body
Base of gland	Chief (zymogenic) cells	Pepsinogen, renin, PG I and leptin(2)	40-44%	Fundic
Base of gland	Enteroendocrine (APUD) cells	Hormones gastrin, histamine, endorphins, serotonin, cholecystokinin and somatostatin	5-6%	Fundic, cardiac, pyloric

PG, prostaglandin.
From Sobhani I, Bado A, Vissuzaine C, et al. Leptin secretion and leptin receptor in the human stomach. Gut 2000;47:178-183.

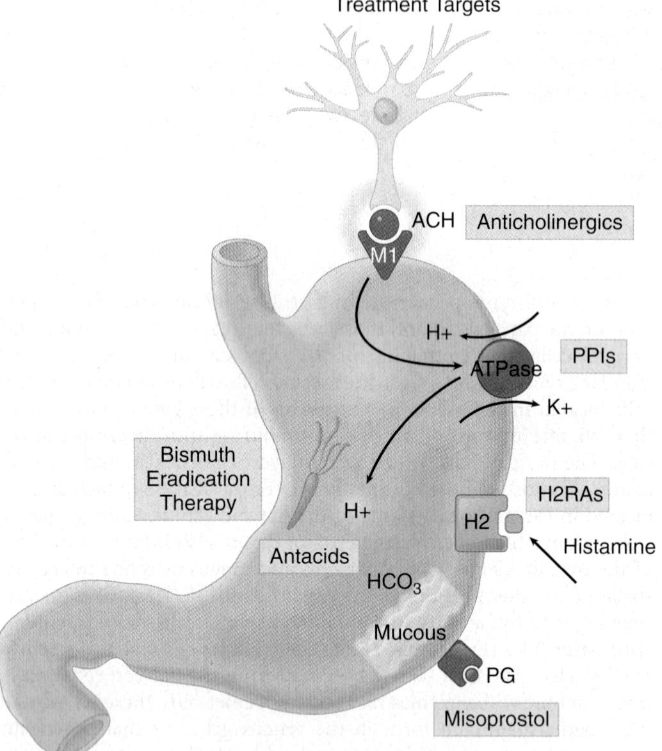

FIGURE 31-1 • Treatment targets.

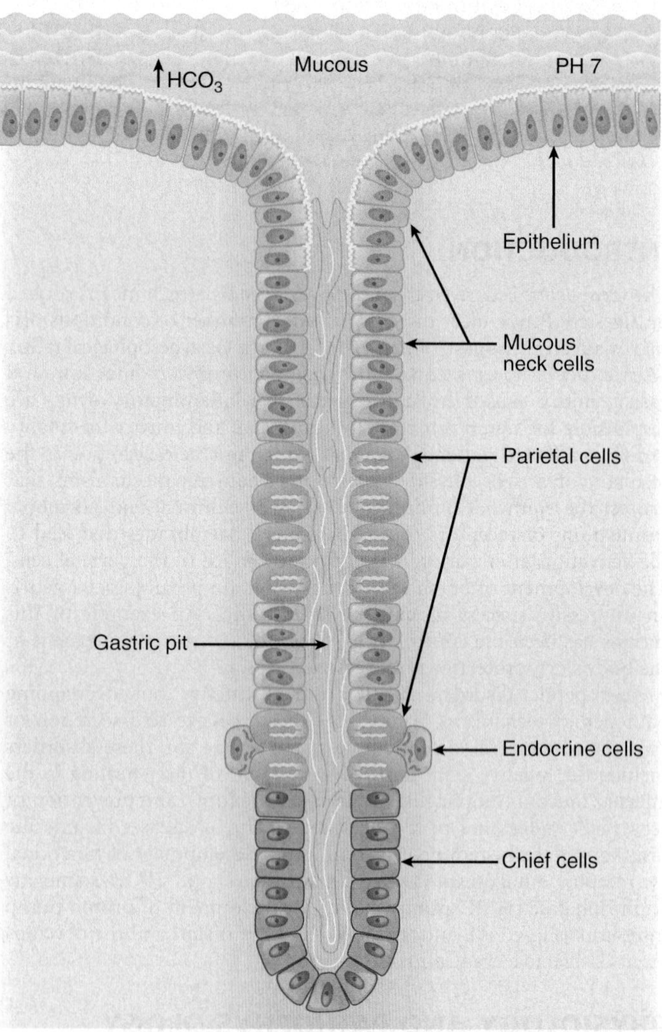

FIGURE 31-2 • Cell locations in the oxyntic gland.

adrenomedullin, orexin A, and neuropeptide Y.[5] Sympathetic receptors of the stomach consist of unmyelinated nerve endings located within the smooth muscle layer detect chemical stimuli and to a lesser degree mechanical stimulation. They play a role in conveying pain sensation associated with inflammatory states such as gastritis. Vagal afferent fibers are located in the smooth muscle layer and the mucosa. They respond to the stretch induced by a full stomach with vasovagal secretory reflexes.[6]

Peripheral and Cellular Regulation

Peripheral regulation of acid secretion includes paracrine, autocrine, neural, and hormonal elements and involves stimulatory and inhibitory modulation. The interaction among three principal gastric endocrine cells (ECL, G, and D cells) and the signals carried by acetylcholine, histamine, and gastrin serve to achieve the common goal of regulating histamine secretion and acid secretion.

Acetylcholine. Local secretion of acetylcholine by parasympathetic vagal efferents is a key modulator of acid secretion. All of the cell bodies of enteric neurons are located within two plexuses, the myenteric (Auerbach's plexus) and the submucosal (Meissner's plexus). Acetylcholine released from postganglionic neurons of the enteric nervous system directly stimulates acid secretion by binding to M3 muscarinic acetylcholine receptors on parietal cells. The M3 receptor is a G protein–coupled receptor consisting of seven connected transmembrane helical domains that activates phospholipase, generating inositol triphosphate (IP3) and releasing intracellular calcium from the endoplasmic reticulum (see Chapter 7, Cell Cycle Pharmacology, Antiproliferation, and Apoptosis). Acetylcholine also directly stimulates histamine release from ECL cells in the fundus. In the antrum, acetylcholine stimulates the release of gastrin from the G cells, which subsequently induces the ECLs to release histamine. Acetylcholine also inhibits the release of somatostatin, which in turn releases a tonic inhibition of gastrin secretion. The importance of acetylcholine in the peptic ulcer diseases has made it a target of anticholinergic drugs. However, the doses usually required to suppress acid secretion are commonly associated with the development of undesirable side effects such as dry mouth, blurred vision, and urinary retention.

Gastrin. Gastrin is found in the G cells of the gastric antrum and duodenum. Gastrin is synthesized in antral-duodenal G cells by post-translational processing of pre-progastrin into acid-stimulatory peptides, of which gastrin-17 and gastrin-34 are the most abundant, and N-terminal fragments, among which progastrin 1-35 and progastrin 1-19 dominate.[7] Although the N-terminal fragments may be the dominant form released into the circulation, their function remains to be determined. Gastrin is the most potent endogenous stimulant for gastric acid secretion, primarily by favoring synthesis and release of histamine from ECL cells. Gastrin also has a trophic effect on the oxyntic mucosa, particularly on ECL cells, which are stimulated to replicate via gastrin/cholecystokinin (CCK)–2 receptors and can induce hyperplasia, hypertrophia, and carcinoids in rat cells.[1] A number of neoplasms are gastrin sensitive, including gastric carcinoids as well as cancers of the stomach, colon, pancreas, and lung,[8] however, long-term drug-induced hypergastrinemia in humans does not appear to be associated with increased incidence of cancer.[9]

The major stimulant for G cell activation in pyloric and duodenal glands is luminal amino acids derived from protein intake. Gastrin and the gastric hormone cholecystokinin (CCK) possess a similar pentapeptide sequence. Two main classes of gastrin/CCK receptors have been characterized: CCK-1 (formerly CCK-A) and CCK-2 (formerly CCK-B).[5] The CCK-1 receptor binds CCK with a 1000-fold greater affinity than gastrin. In the stomach, gastrin mediates its effects primarily through the CCK-2 receptor. The stimulatory pathways for gastrin release are central neural activation, distention of the antrum, and specific chemical components in the food. Neural pathways to the G cells are both inhibitory and stimulatory. Antral vagal influence mediates secretion in response to feeding and hypoglycemia. Paradoxically, selective fundic vagotomy leads to an enhanced release of gastrin, suggesting a vagal-initiated (cholinergic-muscarinic) inhibitory action by the fundus. Despite the fact that cholinergic neurons inhibit pyloric D cells and may enhance gastrin release, bilateral truncal vagotomy leads to sustained elevation of serum gastrin, suggesting that the major central influence involves inhibition while peripheral mechanisms are primarily stimulatory. The peripheral pathways to the G cells are initiated by the presence of food in the stomach, as signaled by mechanical distention, pH, and the presence of specific amino acids. When the pH of the gastric lumen falls below 3, gastrin release is inhibited by a negative feedback. Luminal pH also activates sensory nerve cells, enhancing somatostatin release from antral D cells and suppressing G cells. Somatostatin acts as a paracrine agent to suppress gastrin secretion, with release stimulated by β-adrenergic agonists, CCK, acidification of the antral lumen, and gastrin itself, whereas acetylcholine, through muscarinic receptors, inhibits release.

Histamine. Histamine is the major paracrine stimulator of acid secretion. It is localized both in mucosal mast cells and in endocrine cells, the latter called ECL cells. The ECL cells are localized to the acid-secreting oxyntic or body mucosa, in direct proximity to the parietal cell but not in direct contact with the gastric lumen. Gastrin-stimulated histamine release by the ECL cells has a central role in the regulation of acid secretion. ECL cells also can divide under the influence of gastrin. Conditions in which hypertrophy and hyperplasia of ECL cells become pathologic are those associated with carcinoids and pernicious anemia.

Histamine is produced in ECL cells by decarboxylation of L-histidine by histidine decarboxylase (HDC). HDC promoter activity is upregulated by gastrin, *H. pylori*, and pituitary adenylate cyclase–activating polypeptide. It is inhibited by Krupel-like factor 4 and Yin Yang 1.[10] Histamine is then stored in cytoplasmic vesicles and released in response to gastrin stimulation to the ECL cell via the receptor CCK-B (CCK-2). Targeted gene disruption of HDC and the H_2 receptor demonstrates the key role of histamine in gastrin-stimulated acid secretion. HDC knockout mice produce little or no histamine, resulting in impaired acid secretion and a failure to respond to gastrin.[11]

Of the histamine receptors (H_1, H_2, H_3, and H_4), the constitutively active H_2 receptor has a direct action in the parietal cell. Functional antagonism of the H_2 receptor only partially inhibits the acid secretion stimulated by cholinergic agents and gastrin, suggesting that part of their induced secretion is mediated by histamine. H_2 receptors have an extracellular glycosylation site linked to their amino terminal and an intracellular carboxyl terminal site, making them structurally and functionally different from the H_1 receptor type. Binding of histamine to its receptor leads to activation of stimulatory G protein, which activates a membrane-bound adenylate cyclase favoring the formation of intracellular cyclic AMP (cAMP); this increase is also accompanied by an increase in intracellular calcium. In addition to parietal cell membranes, H_2 receptors have also been found in smooth muscle cells and cardiac myocytes, this may be the reason why certain cardiac arrhythmias have been observed with rapid infusion of intravenous H_2 antagonists. H_3 agonists have been reported to stimulate acid secretion in vitro and inhibit acid secretion in vivo.[12] There are no approved drugs using this target (Fig. 31-3).

Somatostatin. Somatostatin is a physiologic inhibitor of acid secretion. It is released from D cells present in the gastric fundic and antral mucosa. Somatostatin has inhibitory effects on parietal cells, but its major effects are accomplished by the inhibition of histamine release and of gastrin release. The secretion of somatostatin is increased by gastric acid and by gastrin. Somatostatin secretion is also affected by neural inputs. It is suppressed by cholinergic activation and increased by vasoactive intestinal peptide activation. The actions of somatostatin are mediated via five G protein–coupled receptor subtypes, designated SSTR1 to SSTR5. All somatostatin receptors involved in acid secretion are of the SSTR2 subtype. Somatostatin, which is present in D cells, inhibits acid secretion directly by acting on parietal cells and, more importantly, by indirectly inhibiting histamine secretion from ECL cells and gastrin secretion from G cells. The somatostatin analogue octreotide has a theoretical potential in the treatment of acute ulcer bleeding, but has limited actual utilization.[13,14]

Other Mediators. A variety of agents have been reported to stimulate or inhibit acid secretion by direct or indirect actions on the parietal cell. The parietal cell appears to contain receptors in the basolateral membrane for prostaglandins and epidermal growth factor (EGF), and the binding of their ligands appears to inhibit HCl secretion. EGF exerts divergent effects on acid secretion. Acute administration inhibits acid secretion, presumably by activating protein kinase C, whereas prolonged administration increases acid secretion, presumably by inducing both the expression and transcription of the H^+,K^+-ATPase alpha subunit.[15] Nitric oxide (NO) has been reported to either stimulate or inhibit acid secretion.[16] In isolated mouse stomach, low doses of the nitric oxide donor nitroprusside stimulated, whereas higher doses (100 μM to 1 mM) inhibited, acid secretion. The stimulatory effect was blocked by the H_2RA famotidine, suggesting that NO is capable of releasing histamine, presumably from ECL cells.

Ghrelin in the stomach is present in neuroendocrine cells of both the oxyntic and pyloric mucosa, possibly in A-like cells. Fasting and vagotomy increase gastric ghrelin expression and secretion, whereas both feeding and growth hormone treatment decrease them. Peripheral or central administration of ghrelin stimulates gastrin and acid secretion in rats. In humans, intravenous ghrelin enhanced gastric acid secretion, as measured by a wireless pH capsule attached to the gastric mucosa.[17] The pathway appears to involve the vagus nerve and histamine release since the gastric acid stimulatory effect of intravenous ghrelin, in rats, is associated with an increase in HDC messenger RNA and is abolished by vagotomy.[18] However, Levin et al.[19] reported that intravenous infusion of ghrelin has no effect on basal acid secretion and significantly decreases pentagastrin-stimulated acid secretion in awake rats equipped with a gastric fistula.

Leptin, a hormone secreted by adipocytes and thought to function as a satiety signal, is also present in gastric chief and parietal cells. Gastric leptin is released on stimulation by gastrin, CCK, secretin, food

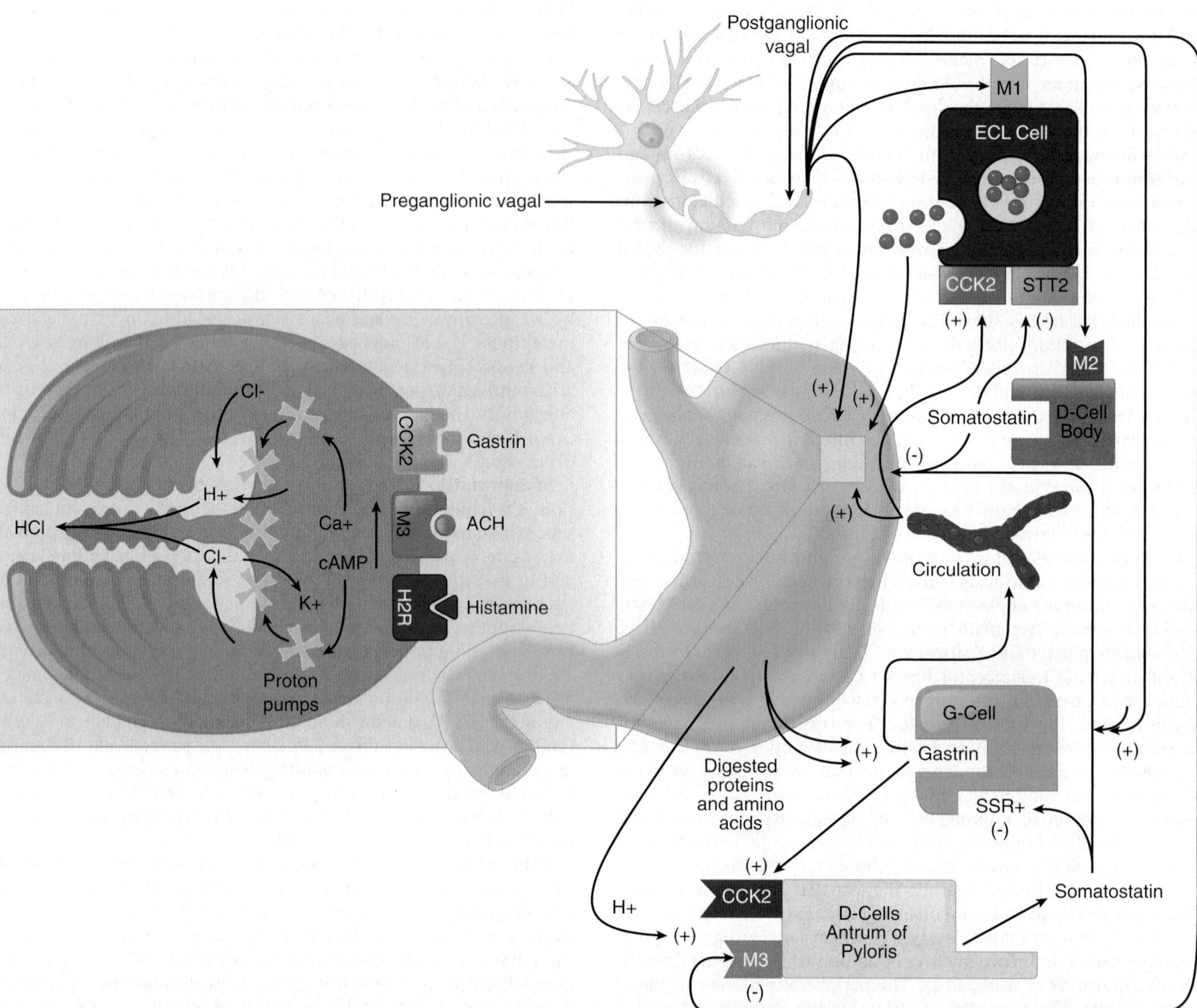

FIGURE 31-3 • Regulation.

ingestion, and vagal nerve activation. In patients infected with *H. pylori*, gastric leptin expression is increased. In humans, insulin-induced hypoglycemia stimulates leptin secretion in men without, but not in those with, highly selective vagotomy, suggesting that leptin can be released by the cephalic phase of gastric secretion. Although the precise physiologic role for gastric leptin remains to be determined, leptin inhibits basal acid and gastrin secretion in vivo in rat and peptone-stimulated acid secretion in humans, suggesting a role for this peptide in the regulation of acid secretion.[5,13,20]

Other neurotransmitters have been associated with acid secretion. The neuropeptide gastrin-releasing peptide (GRP) has been linked with meal-stimulated acid secretion by gastrin release and may also be an important neurotransmitter in the vagal-cholinergic pathway, as demonstrated by the GRP antagonist BIM26226, which blocks vagally mediated acid secretion in humans in ways similar to atropine.[21]

H^+,K^+-ATPase: The Proton Pump

H^+,K^+-ATPase is a magnesium-dependent enzyme found only on secretory membranes of parietal cells, and represents the last step in the secretion of gastric acid. Canaliculi in the apical plasma membrane invaginate into the parietal cell. In the cytoplasmic space, there are abundant membranous structures rich in H^+,K^+-ATPase in the form of microtubules,[22] vesicles, and cisternal sacs called H^+,K^+-ATPase–rich tubulovesicles. When gastric HCl secretion is stimulated, parietal cells undergo a profound morphologic transformation resulting in a 6- to 10-fold increase in apical membrane and a rise in the intracellular levels of cAMP, IP3, diacylglycerol, and Ca^{2+}. This sequence of events induces the tubulovesicles to fuse into the apical plasma membrane, allowing H^+,K^+-ATPase to secrete protons directly into the lumen of the gastric gland.

Acid secretion by parietal cells is an energy-dependent process; the parietal cells have extensive mitochondria to supply this demand. Pumps are phosphorylated and dephosphorylated sequentially during ATP hydrolysis in presence of Mg^{2+}, secreting protons (H^+) from the extracellular fluid compartment to the gastric lumen in exchange for K^+ against a concentration gradient. Chloride ions accompanying hydrogen ions are also secreted against both a parietal cell–to-lumen concentration gradient and an electrical gradient. The availability of protons Mg^{2+} and ATPases makes them less likely to be the rate-limiting factors for proton transport, leaving K^+ as the major factor that controls proton transport.[3] The secretory membrane acquires potassium conductance dependent on the activity of phosphatidylinositol 4,5-bisphosphate or phosphatidylinositol 4,5,6-trisphosphate.[21] Different candidate potassium channels have been identified in the apical membrane of parietal cells: the pH-sensitive KCNQ1channel/KCNE2, the replenisher channels $K_{ir}5.1$ and $K_{ir}4.2$, and the CLIC6 channel K.[22]

Acid is generated in the parietal cell by the enzyme carbonic anhydrase from the hydration of CO_2 to form H^+ and HCO_3^-. The H^+ that is formed in this reaction is secreted by the proton pump in exchange for K^+. The HCO_3^- ions formed during H^+ secretion are exchanged for Cl^- ions at the basolateral membrane of the parietal cell. As a result of HCO_3^-/Cl^- exchange, the pH in the parietal cell remains only slightly alkaline during H^+ secretion. Rapid entry of HCO_3^- from parietal cells into blood has been referred to as the "alkaline tide." Cl^- that entered the parietal cell from the blood in exchange for HCO_3^- is transported into the secretory canaliculus of the stimulated cell via a conductance pathway associated with a K^+ conductance and with H^+,K^+-ATPase.

Structure of the Pump. The proton pump is a dimeric heterodimer P-type pump[22] and carries out the exchange of protons for potassium ions through ATP hydrolysis. It is composed of two subunits: an alpha subunit and a glycosylated beta subunit. The alpha subunit crosses the apical membrane of the parietal cell 10 times, whereas the beta subunit crosses it only once. Complete deletion of either the alpha subunit or the beta subunit in mice was shown to have profound effects on parietal cell structure and function, making them achlorhydric.[23] The alpha subunit reacts with ATP and appears to mediate all of the transport functions of the pump, defines cation binding properties, hydrolyzes ATP, and is the site for binding of proton pump inhibitors (PPIs).[24] The smaller, glycosylated beta subunit contains oligosaccharides, six cysteine residues as oxidized disulfide bonds, and intrinsic protein foldings that are essential for the structural and functional stability of H^+,K^+-ATPase.[13] It appears to play a key role in targeting of the pump to the apical membrane, in the development of the oxyntic mucosa, and in recycling the pump from the "active" secretory canaliculi back to the tubulovesicular membranes when the cell reverts to a "resting" state.

Numerous other proteins play roles in the activation of the parietal cell, proteins involved in trafficking and membrane recycling, regulatory kinases such as protein kinase A and protein kinase C, and cytoskeletal proteins such as actin, ezrin, and others play key yet incompletely understood roles and are potential future targets as pharmacologic inhibitors of H^+ secretion.[23]

Acid-Related Diseases

The term *acid-related diseases* involves a wide variety of disorders that can affect the esophagus, stomach, and duodenum, in some cases involving hydrochloric acid as the principal pathogenic cause and in others involving diminished mucosal defense mechanisms or increase in gastric acid secretion. The concept of acid reflux disorders includes not only the effects of gastroesophageal reflux on the esophageal mucosa but also the role of acid reflux in laryngeal and pulmonary symptoms. Gastritis is defined by endoscopic and histologic criteria and can be classified by the anatomic area, the cellular type that predominates in its inflammatory stage, and the presence or absence of malignant clues. A peptic ulcer is a mucosal defect that extends to or beyond the muscularis mucosa and, in relation to its anatomic location, can be proximal or distal. Other peptic ulcers can occur at areas distant from the stomach, such as in cases of metaplastic gastric mucosa in Meckel's diverticulum or Barrett's esophagus.

Gastroesophageal Reflux Disease

Gastroesophageal reflux disease (GERD) is a common GI disorder. The Montreal Consensus defines GERD as a disease that is associated with troublesome symptoms and/or complications on account of reflux of stomach contents into the esophagus, with complaints divided into esophageal and extraesophageal.[25] Laryngitis, cough, asthma, and dental erosions are recognized as possible extraesophageal manifestations of GERD. GERD is one the most common GI disorders, affecting more that 60 million Americans, with up to 20% of the population having symptoms at least twice a week.[26] Patients with GERD usually complain of heartburn and acid regurgitation as the classic symptoms; however, the frequency and severity of heartburn does not predict the degree of esophageal damage.[27] Chest pain, cough, and other symptoms such as dysphagia and odynophagia are other possible presentations of GERD, but their diagnostic yield is uncertain. Complications such as strictures, Barrett's esophagus, and eventually adenocarcinoma may arise on a long-term basis.

Pathogenesis. GERD results from esophageal mucosa exposure to gastric acidic contents, pepsin, and bile acids. Anatomic and functional interactions involving the stomach, gastroesophageal junction, lower esophageal sphincter (LES), and nervous system lead to altered clearance and protective mechanisms of the esophagus. Hydrochloric acid damages the esophageal lining by disruption of intracellular junctions. Acidic conditions ($pH > 2$) alone will not lead to tissue disruptions or symptoms, but acid in combination with proteolytic enzymes, such as pepsin and trypsin, will disrupt epithelial structures.[28] Pancreatic secretions and bile from duodenal reflux alter the integrity of the esophageal mucosa through a detergent effect on cell membranes. Moreover, in vitro studies provide evidence that bile acids in combination with low pH induce oxidative stress in Barrett's esophagus, which may cause oxidative damage and contribute to the development of esophageal adenocarcinoma.[29] Mechanical factors that contribute to reflux of gastric contents include prolonged esophageal transit times, as well as shorter length and decreased resting pressure of the LES. Acid exposure occurs during transient lower esophageal relaxations. These are thought to be the resultant of a neurally mediated vagal reflex triggered by activation of the stomach stretch receptors. Protective secretions such as bicarbonate, prostaglandin E_2, mucin, and EGF play minor roles in mucosal protection.[30]

Peptic Ulcer Disease

Peptic ulcer disease (PUD) is a relatively common disorder affecting several million people in the United States every year. The anatomic prevalence of ulcer seems to be different among populations. Duodenal ulcers are more prevalent in Western populations, whereas gastric ulcers are more frequent in Asia. The predominant age at which duodenal ulcers occurs is between 20 and 50 years of age, while gastric ulcers predominate in those above 40 years old. The prevalence of gastric ulcer in the United States has shifted in the past 2 decades, from a disease predominantly affecting males to one that is equally present in both sexes. The incidence of PUD has been declining as a result of increasing application of eradication therapy against *H. pylori*, the availability of antisecretory medications, and possibly reduction in smoking rates.[31]

Pathophysiology. Previous concepts of PUD focused on abnormalities in the balance between secretion of gastric acid and pepsin, the defensive factors of the GI tract, and the suppression of acid as a treatment strategy. Duodenal ulcer patients are frequently hypersecretors of acid. In contrast, gastric ulcer patients more commonly have defective mechanisms for protecting the mucosal lining and generally have gastric acid secretion equivalent to that of control subjects. The revolution in PUD human biology occurred in 1983 with reports by Warren and Brown on *H. pylori* as an infectious cause in simultaneous letters to *The Lancet*.[32] Indeed, 90% of ulcers are caused primarily by *H. pylori* infection and/or the use of NSAIDs[31,33] (Tables 31-2 and 31-3).

Helicobacter Pylori. Although chronic gastritis will develop in nearly all individuals who are persistently colonized with *H. pylori*, 80% to 90% will never experience symptoms or develop clinical

TABLE 31-2 RISK FACTORS FOR PEPTIC ULCER DISEASE

Risk Factors	Possibly associated:
• NSAID use	• Corticosteroids (high dose and/or prolonged therapy)
• Smoking cigarettes	• Blood group O
• Family history of ulcers	• HLA-B12, B5, Bw35 phenotypes
• Zollinger-Ellison syndrome (gastrinoma)	• Stress
	• Poverty

NSAID, nonsteroidal anti-inflammatory drug.

TABLE 31-3 ETIOLOGIC FACTORS AND CONDITIONS LEADING TO PEPTIC ULCER DISEASE

Etiology	Associated Conditions with Ulcer Disease
• *H. pylori* infection: 90% of duodenal ulcers and 70%-90% of gastric ulcers • Multifactorial • Ulcerogenic drugs (e.g., NSAIDs) • Hypersecretory syndromes (e.g., Zollinger-Ellison syndrome) Less common: • HSV or CMV infection • Crohn's disease • Vascular insufficiency • Radiation therapy, cancer chemotherapy	• Systemic mastocytosis • Multiple endocrine neoplasia type 1 • Chronic obstructive pulmonary disease • Chronic renal failure • Cirrhosis • Organ transplantation • Hyperparathyroidism • Carcinoid syndrome • Polycythemia rubra vera • Basophilic leukemia • Porphyria cutanea tarda

CMV, cytomegalovirus; HSV, herpes simplex virus; NSAID, nonsteroidal anti-inflammatory drug.

disease. It has not been clearly established as to how the presence of *H. pylori* leads to gastric and duodenal ulcers, but disruption of gastric and duodenal mucosal integrity seems to involve a complex interaction between the host and pathogen.[33] *Helicobacter pylori* is adapted to the gastric environment, it lives within or beneath the gastric mucus layer and induces several mechanisms that lead to the formation of peptic ulcers. After being ingested, the bacteria evade the bactericidal activity of the gastric contents and enter the mucus layer. Urease production and motility are essential for this first step of infection. Urease hydrolyzes urea into carbon dioxide and ammonia, thereby permitting *H. pylori* to survive in an acidic environment.[34]

Helicobacter pylori affects a number of aspects of intestinal biology, having a profound impact on the gastric mucosa and to a lesser extent on gastric physiology (gastrin, somatostatin, and acid secretion). Mucosal defense mechanisms are imbalanced by a decrease in mucosal blood flow and a reduced mucus gel layer. Persistent infection with *H. pylori* can also increase gastric acid secretion, likely mediated through elevated basal and stimulated concentrations of serum gastrin and down-regulation of somatostatin, with inflammatory mediators and the production of virulence factors leading to gastritis, increases in parietal cell mass, and development of ulcers.[31,33]

The presence of *H. pylori* stimulates an inflammatory and immune response triggered by the attachment of bacteria to epithelial cells; mediators such as interleukin (IL)–8, tumor necrosis factor-α, IL-1, and IL-6 lead to persistent gastric mucosal damage as neutrophils, lymphocytes, and plasma cells are recruited to perpetuate the inflammatory state. Further changes to epithelial cells depend on bacterial proteins encoded in the cag-PAI gene and on the translocation of CagA protein into gastric epithelial cells, where it interferes with cell signaling, disrupts apical cell junctions, and induces phenotypic changes in gastric epithelial cells.[31,33] Chronic inflammation also increases epithelial-cell turnover and apoptosis. Proinflammatory polymorphisms of the interleukin-1 gene favor the development of gastritis in the body of the stomach that is associated with hypochlorhydria, gastric atrophy, and gastric adenocarcinoma. In the absence of these proinflammatory polymorphisms, *H. pylori*–mediated gastritis develops predominantly in the antrum in association with a normal to high level of acid secretion.[34]

NSAID-Induced Ulcers

Gastric ulcers in Western countries are most commonly associated with NSAID ingestion, although *H. pylori* may also be present. Up to 25% of patients chronically taking NSAIDs experience upper GI adverse effects. Epidemiologic data on the risk of clinically symptomatic, but uncomplicated, peptic ulcers associated with NSAID intake are quite limited. According to the MUCOSA study,[35] the estimated annualized incidence of NSAID-related ulcer complications was 0.8% for patients without risk factors, 2% with one risk factor, 7.6% to 8.6% with three risk factors, and 18% with four risk factors. A recent population-based cohort study from the United Kingdom reported that the incidence rate of symptomatic uncomplicated peptic ulcer is about one case per 1000 person-years, and that aspirin and nonaspirin NSAIDs multiply this.[36] These findings, together with prior endoscopic evidence, suggest that NSAIDs might not only complicate preexisting peptic ulcers but also cause clinically relevant ones de novo. The risk of developing ulcer is higher in older patients, in those taking high doses of NSAIDs or with concomitant use of corticosteroids, and in those with comorbid conditions. Patients taking aspirin for cardiovascular protective reasons are also at increased risk.[31]

The pathogenesis of symptomatic PUD caused by exposure to NSAIDs is a consequence of systemic inhibition of GI mucosal cyclooxygenase 1 (COX-1) activity and inhibition of thromboxane A_2. There is a decreased production of protective mucosal prostaglandins. Gastric injury by NSAIDs also seems to involve mediators besides prostaglandins, NO as well as various growth factors, such as transforming growth factor (TGF)–β and TGF-α, appear to participate in this process.[37] The role of *H. pylori* infection in NSAID-induced gastritis or ulcer formation is complex, and its role in ulcer risk in patients taking NSAIDs remains undetermined.

Stress-Related Ulceration

Stress ulcers are mucosal erosions that occur in critically ill patients in the stomach and, less frequently, in the duodenum or distal esophagus. They represent a significant cause of morbidity and mortality in critically ill patients in the intensive care unit as they tend to cause oozing of blood from superficial capillary beds, while deeper lesions can erode into the submucosa, causing massive hemorrhage. When occult bleeding (defined as guaiac-positive stools or nasogastric aspirates) is used as an end point, the prevalence ranges from 15% to 50%.[38] The pathophysiology is believed to be multifactorial and is not completely understood.[39] Shock, sepsis and trauma can lead to impaired mucosal healing. Splanchnic hypoperfusion and activation of stress-related responses damage the integrity of the gastric mucosa by reducing GI blood flow, oxygen delivery, and bicarbonate secretion. Gastrointestinal motility is also decreased, delaying the removal of acidic material and other irritants from the stomach. Uremic toxins and reflux of bile salts can also impair the integrity of the mucosal barrier. The most important risk factors for stress-related bleeding are prolonged mechanical ventilation and coagulopathy[38] (Box 31-1).

THERAPEUTICS AND CLINICAL PHARMACOLOGY

Therapeutics by Class

Inhibitors of Gastric Acid

Antacids and Anticholinergic Drugs

Background. Calcium carbonate, in the readily available forms of coral or limestone, has been used to treat dyspepsia for over 2000 years.[40] The use of antacid in the form of bicarbonate of potash for treatment of peptic ulcer was described by William Brinton in 1856 in London.[41] Bertram Sippy's investigations using antacids, often at high doses, in treatment of gastric and duodenal ulcers greatly influenced their use in the United States.[42] In the modern era, the H_2RAs and PPIs

BOX 31-1 RISK FACTORS FOR STRESS ULCERS

- Prolonged mechanical ventilation
- Coagulopathy
- Shock
- Central nervous system injury/surgery
- Multiple trauma
- Prior history of peptic ulcer disease or upper gastrointestinal bleeding
- Multiple organ failure
- Severe sepsis
- Renal failure
- Hepatic failure
- Status post organ transplant
- Burns over 35% of total body surface

have replaced antacids as primary treatment for most acid-related gastric mucosal disorders. However, antacids are inexpensive, readily available, and safe in most populations, and accordingly remain commonly used in the symptom-driven treatment of mild reflux disease and dyspepsia.

Mechanism of Action and Dose-Response Characteristics. Neutralization of stomach pH is the primary mechanism of action of the antacids. These agents often provide prompt and effective pain relief in acid-remediable diseases. The primary effect of antacids on the stomach is due to partial neutralization of gastric hydrochloric acid and inhibition of the proteolytic enzyme pepsin.[43] Symptom relief does not require the gastric contents to become alkaline or neutral in pH. As the pH scale is logarithmic, a 99% reduction in stomach acid translates to increase in gastric pH from 1.3 to 3.5, a level at which symptomatic relief and ulcer healing occur. Other purported mechanisms are acid independent and include delivery of growth factors to injured mucosa, promotion of angiogenesis in injured mucosa, binding of bile acids, and suppression, but not eradication, of *H. pylori.*

Sodium bicarbonate found initial common use as an antacid and is still employed occasionally as a self-prescribed regimen of "baking soda" mixed in water, or in combination products containing aspirin. The fully soluble nature of sodium bicarbonate has made it less desirable. Larger doses can lead to systemic alkalosis, and repeated doses deliver a sizable sodium load, which can be problematic to patients with systolic cardiac dysfunction or renal insufficiency. Most commonly used antacids contain less soluble agents, given alone or in combination. For example, calcium carbonate is sparingly soluble. Reaction with HCl generates soluble calcium chloride, which is converted back to calcium carbonate in the alkaline conditions of the small intestine. This precipitates out into the stool, decreasing absorption. Other commonly used agents are the insoluble antacids aluminum hydroxide and magnesium hydroxide. Aluminum- and calcium-containing products can cause constipation. To counteract this, these agents are often combined with magnesium hydroxide, which when administered alone can cause diarrhea and loose stools.

The potency of an antacid is typically determined by the milliequivalents of hydrochloric acid neutralized under standard conditions. Such ex vivo testing may not reflect actual extent or duration of acid neutralization within the gut lumen. The effective time for antacids to reduce stomach acidity is relatively short on an empty stomach, but can be prolonged to 1 to 3 hours if taken with food. As most agents are insoluble, particle size and solid versus liquid suspension formulation will determine how much of the theoretic acid-neutralizing ability is achieved.

Clinical Use. Antacids have modest efficacy in healing peptic ulcers. However, compliance is limited by the need for frequent dosing and a poor correlation between symptomatic relief and ulcer healing.[44] Accordingly, antacids are not currently used for the treatment of PUD. Meta-analysis data demonstrate antacids not to have a significant effectiveness in trials of nonulcer dyspepsia.[45] This is not surprising in light of the limited number of studies and the weak link between acidity and symptoms in nonulcer dyspepsia.[46] In contrast, antacids do have a modest (10%) improvement in GERD symptoms compared to placebo.[47] Though also effective for stress ulcer prophylaxis in critically ill patients, the present role for these agents is in the treatment of mild symptomatic reflux and dyspepsia.[48] For the clinician, assessing the amount of patient-reported antacid use can help to noninvasively gauge severity of symptoms.

Safety. Adverse events associated with antacids are dose related and were noted more frequently previously, when these agents were used more extensively in the treatment of PUD. Large doses of calcium-containing antacids can cause the milk-alkali syndrome, which consists of hypercalcemia, renal insufficiency, and metabolic alkalosis. Though seen much less commonly since the development of the PPIs, it remains a not-uncommon cause of hypercalcemia.[49,50] Magnesium-containing antacids can cause diarrhea if given alone. Hypermagnesemia can occur in patients with renal insufficiency. Aluminum-containing antacids can cause encephalology and osteomalacia in end-stage renal patients, so calcium carbonate is the preferred antacid in this population.[51] Aluminum does not accumulate to toxic levels in those with normal renal function.[52] All antacids can produce drug interactions by changing gastric or urinary pH; altering rates of absorption, bioavailability, renal elimination, and/or drug dissolution; or reducing gastric acid hydrolysis of drugs. Most antacids, except sodium bicarbonate, may decrease drug absorption by adsorption or chelation of other drugs.[43] Physicians are not always aware of the extent of antacid use by patients, while both patients and physicians are often unaware of specific drug interactions.

H2-Receptor Antagonists

Background. In 1966, Ash and Schild characterized the H_2 receptor, which localized to the gut and was not responsive to classical antihistamines.[53] Antagonists to the H_2 receptor were described in 1972.[54] This class of agents revolutionized the treatment of PUD and have been supplemented only by the development of the PPIs. The improved efficacy of H_2RAs over existing therapies was explained not only by inhibition of histamine-induced acid secretion, but also by partial suppression induced by gastrin or acetylcholine.

Mechanism of Action. The H_2 receptor is a member of the G protein–coupled receptor family. The H_2 receptor is constitutively active, with a tonic production of cAMP. Histamine interaction with the H_2 receptor on parietal cells leads to accumulation of cAMP, which stimulates the production of gastric acid. The class of drugs commonly known as H_2RAs are a group of reversible structural analogues of histamine. These drugs cause the receptor to favor a state of decreased cAMP and ultimately decreased acid production. These agents are inverse agonists with a functional antagonism of histamine activity.[55,56] Specifically, they decrease the tonic activation rate of the receptor, decreasing adenylate cyclase activity and generation of cAMP, and ultimately inhibiting basal acid output as well as meal-stimulated acid secretion. H_2RAs are only partially effective in reducing acid secretion induced by gastrin, the mediator that is released by the gustatory and stomach distention stimuli. Indeed, acid release is not fully suppressed by H_2RAs following food intake.[57] Histamine, in contrast, mediates the basal rate of acid release during nonfeeding periods. This is of particular importance during the nocturnal periods of fasting, which is the rationale for the use of H_2RA dosing at the time of sleep. Models based upon 24-hour pH monitoring and clinical trial data have demonstrated that ulcer healing depends upon the amount of acid suppression, as well as the duration of the portion of the 24-hour cycle with reduced acidity of pH greater than 3 for duodenal ulcer and pH greater than 4 in the esophageal lumen for GERD.[58,59]

The four widely available H_2RAs are cimetidine, ranitidine, famotidine, and nizatidine (Table 31-4). In the United States, all are readily available alone or combined with an antacid in over-the-counter preparations. Roxatidine and ebrotidine are H_2RAs available outside of the United States. Like histamine, cimetidine, ranitidine, famotidine, and nizatidine contain a heterocyclic ring and otherwise have generally similar structural and pharmacokinetic characteristics. H_2RAs are absorbed after oral dosing, achieving peak concentrations within 1 to 3 hours. This rate may be influenced by concomitant use of antacid

TABLE 31-4 PHARMACOLOGIC PROPERTIES OF HISTAMINE$_2$ RECEPTOR ANTAGONISTS

	Cimetidine	Ranitidine	Famotidine	Nizatidine
Trade name	*Tagamet*	*Zantac*	*Pepcid*	*Axid*
Standard daily dose (mg)	400 bid or 800 hs	150 bid or 300 hs	20 bid or 40 hs	150 bid or 300 hs
Onset of action in hr (oral)	1-3	1	1-3	1
Time to peak level (hr)	1-3	2-3	1-3	0.5-3
Half-life (hr)	2.5-3.5	2.5-3	2.5-3.5	1-2
Duration of action (hr)	10-12	13	10-12	12
Bioavailability (%)	50	50	40-60	>70
Labeled pediatric age range (yr)	—	>1 mo	<1 yr	—
IV formulation	+	+	+	–

bid, twice a day; hs, bedtime; IV, intravenous.

therapy but rarely by food ingestion. They are eliminated primarily by renal mechanisms, with between 30% and 60% of drug being excreted unchanged into the urine. Accordingly, dosage adjustments are needed for patients with renal impairment, but not for those with liver disease. The pharmacokinetics of these agents are linear, which assists in dose adjustment.

Dose-Response Characteristics. The therapeutic index of H_2RAs is large, with a few common dose-dependent adverse events. In light of this, and the role histamine plays particularly in nocturnal basal acid secretion, the H_2RAs are often administered once a day just prior to bed. It is not clear if there is added benefit of the addition of a nighttime H_2RA to an existing PPI regimen, even in individuals with known nocturnal acid breakthrough.[60] Effects on acid secretion tend to decline with time, a phenomenon that probably represents an exaggerated first-dose response rather than typical tolerance.[61] Unfortunately, this tachyphylaxis is most pronounced with higher and prolonged doses. Exposure of the H_2 receptor to an H_2RA causes decreased receptor degradation,[62] which may clinically manifest rebound acid secretion upon drug cessation. These characteristics, coupled with the rapid onset of action relative to the PPIs, have made the H_2RAs better suited to a symptom-driven demand use. There is good evidence that demand use relieves heartburn symptoms, though it is not effective in controlling erosive esophagitis.[63]

For over-the-counter use, labeled H_2RA doses (75 mg ranitidine, 10 mg famotidine) are less than those listed in the prescription product insert. At these doses, the over-the-counter drugs are effective in reducing overnight gastric acidity for 12 hours,[64] as well in the face of food-stimulated gastric response.[65,66] Meta-analysis data suggest these doses are also effective in the treatment of symptomatic GERD.[47]

Clinical Use. There is sizeable evidence available regarding the effectiveness of H_2RAs and a number of conclusions can be drawn with a good degree of certainty. H_2RAs have modest efficacy in nonulcer dyspepsia,[45] but are not as effective as PPIs as initial therapy.[67] H_2RA are superior to placebo, but inferior to PPIs in the treatment of esophageal reflux disease.[68-70] Similarly, PPIs are superior to H_2RAs in the prevention of rebleeding of an acute peptic ulcer,[71] on the improvement in ulcer symptoms and in the promotion of healing.[72,73] In the prevention of NSAID-induced injury, standard doses of H_2RAs were effective at reducing the risk of duodenal but not gastric ulcers, while double-dose H_2RAs were effective at reducing the risk of endoscopically visualized duodenal and gastric ulcers.[74] In aggregate, the H_2RAs are less effective than PPIs, though they have a quicker onset of action better suited to rapid symptom control.

Safety. Despite the presence of H_2 receptors outside of the gut, functional antagonism of the H_2 receptor has limited systemic effects. This contributes to the safety of the H_2RAs, as does limited central nervous system (CNS) penetration. In general, the H_2RAs have an excellent safety profile. Cimetidine has a mild antiandrogenic effect, which has been the cause of gynecomastia and impotence, though these are dose dependent and seen usually with prolonged administration. Idiosyncratic cases of myelosuppression, thrombocytopenia, anemia, and neutropenia have been reported with all H_2RA agents. CNS symptoms include confusion, restlessness, headaches, and mental status changes. These seemed to appear more common in elderly patients in the intensive care unit who have hepatic and renal complications. Rarely, cardiac effects are seen following rapid intravenous administration or high-dose therapy, particularly in patients with limited physiologic reserve. Currently there is no clear evidence of teratogenicity when used in gestating patients.[75] There are potential drug interactions with cimetidine due to inhibition of cytochrome P-450 (CYP) isoenzymes, particularly CYP3A4 and 2D6. Cimetidine also inhibits the tubular secretion of some drugs, and it is by this mechanism that the drug also can modestly increase serum creatinine. There is limited potential for drug interactions with other H_2RAs.[76] As there is no differential efficacy benefit, H_2RAs other than cimetidine should be used where feasible.

Proton Pump Inhibitors

Background. In the early 1970s, a screening program using a canine gastric fistula model identified efficacy of an analogue of the antimycobacterial ethionamide. Toxicity and potency issues led to the development of other compounds, ultimately leading to success with omeprazole.[77] At the same time, gastric H^+,K^+-ATPase was identified as the common pathway for acid production, a finding confirmed by correlation of the rate of acid secretion to amount of omeprazole inhibition of the ATPase.[78] This potent inhibition of the final step in the gastric acid production pathway, combined with an excellent safety profile, gives these drugs singular utility that has revolutionized the treatment of diseases of the enteral tract.

Mechanism of Action. The PPIs decrease acid secretion by inhibition of H^+,K^+-ATPase pumps on the parietal cell membrane. This enzyme is the molecular engine of gastric acid secretion and is solely responsible for the release of hydrogen ions into the lumen of the gastric glands and stomach. Acid suppression after a single dose is limited as PPIs are only active on pumps in the secretory canaliculus of parietal cells that are actively secreting acid. Additionally, when plasma levels of drug drop below inhibitory concentrations, newly generated H^+,K^+-ATPase will be fully active. Multiple doses overcome both of these limitations. The effectiveness of PPIs is also enhanced by the irreversible nature of inhibition of H^+,K^+-ATPase by most agents, resulting in a duration of action that exceeds their plasma half-life, as well as an inhibitory mechanism that is independent of histamine, acetylcholine, or gastrin stimulus for acid secretion.[24] In contrast to H_2RAs, the PPIs also decrease pepsin secretion.[79] As pepsin in an acidic environment contributes to mucosal damage, this effect adds to PPI efficacy.

The five widely used PPIs are omeprazole, esomeprazole, lansoprazole, pantoprazole, and rabeprazole (Table 31-5 and Fig. 31-4). These compounds share a common structure consisting of substituted pyri-

TABLE 31-5 PHARMACOLOGIC PROPERTIES OF THE PROTON PUMP INHIBITORS

	Rabeprazole	Pantoprazole	Lansoprazole	Esomeprazole	Omeprazole	Omeprazole IR–Sodium Bicarbonate
Trade name	*AcipHex*	*Protonix*	*Prevacid*	*Nexium*	*Prilosec*	*Zegerid*
Dose for active and maintenance therapy of duodenal ulcers and GERD (mg)	20	40	15	20	20	20
Dose for gastric ulcer and erosive esophagitis (mg)	20-40	40-80	30	40	20-40	20-40
Time to peak plasma concentration (hr)	2-5	1-3	1.7	1.5	0.5-3.5	0.5
Elimination half-life (hr)	1-2	1-2	1.3-1.7	1-1.5	0.5-1	0.4-3.2
Bioavailability (%)	52	77	80	64*	58-70	30-40
Primary route of metabolism	Nonenzymatic	CYP 2C19 and sulfotransferase	CYP 3A4	CYP 2C19	CYP 2C19	CYP 2C19
Labeled pediatric age range (yr)	—	—	>1	>12	>2	—
IV formulations	–	+	+	+	+[†]	–
Controlled release formulation	+	+	+	+	+	N/A
Oral suspension or ability to mix in food	–	+	+	+	+	+

*Increased with repeat dosing.
[†]Available outside of the United States.
CYP, cytochrome P-450; GERD, gastroesophageal reflux disease; IR, immediate release; IV, intravenous.

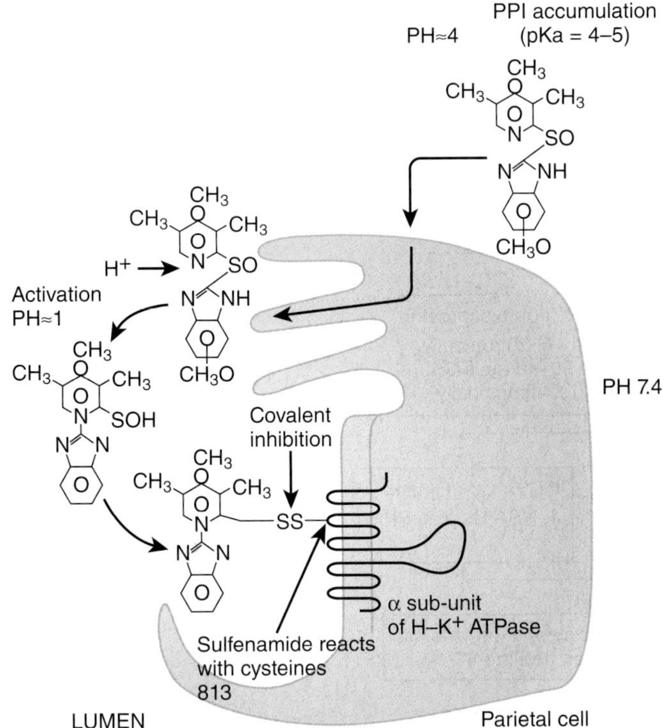

FIGURE 31-4 • Activation and binding of PPIs. PPIs accumulate in the secretory canaliculus of the parietal cell. In this acidic environment, the PPI becomes protonated and converted into the sulfenamide form and binds to the H^+,K^+-ATPase pumps.

dylmethylsulfinyl benzimidazoles and vary in terms of the substitutions on either the pyridine or the benzimidazole ring.[61] PPIs are weak bases that act as prodrugs and need an acidic environment in order to inhibit H^+,K^+-ATPase.[22] They accumulate in the secretory canaliculus of the parietal cell, achieving higher concentrations here when compared to plasma. In this acidic environment, the PPI becomes protonated and converted into the active sulfenamide species, which forms disulfide bonds with cysteine residues in the alpha subunit of H^+,K^+-ATPase. In contrast to the other PPIs, rabeprazole forms a partially reversible bond with the proton pump and is activated at a broader range of gastric pH.

PPIs are well absorbed after oral administration, and despite a short elimination half-life of 1 to 2 hours, they provide prolonged acid inhibition due to covalent binding with the H^+,K^+-ATPase pump. They are more effective if taken immediately before a meal and have to be given with acid-protective coating or with sodium bicarbonate in a combination product to prevent conversion to the active principle in the lumen of the stomach. Agents with a higher bioavailability have a more rapid onset of acid suppression. Dose administration before eating also improves efficacy, due to recruitment of more active H^+,K^+-ATPase to which the drugs can bind. The effects of the PPIs increase with repeat administration, and generally by the third day, a steady state occurs in which the fraction of pumps that remains inhibited over 2 hours reaches about 70% of the pump population. Three days after the cessation of daily dosing, gastric acidity returns to baseline. Accordingly, the occasional use of a PPI taken on an "as-needed" basis does not reliably provide adequate acid inhibition and does not produce a consistent or satisfactory clinical response.[80]

All PPIs undergo some degree of metabolism via hepatic CYP2C19. There is a pharmacogenetic basis for differential metabolism of some of the PPIs. Poor metabolizers make up 2% to 6% of white and 15% to 20% of Asian populations. Poor metabolizers have higher plasma drug levels, more profound acid inhibition, and higher healing rates in PPI-containing *H. pylori* regimens. Differences are largest for omeprazole/esomeprazole, followed by pantoprazole and lansoprazole. Rabeprazole is metabolized by CYP2C19, but the primary biotransformation is nonenzymatic. Improved outcomes using individualized pharmacogenetic guided dosing regimens have been demonstrated in small studies,[81] but the cost-effectiveness and scalable feasibility of such an approach have not been established.

Dose-Response Characteristics. In contrast to the H_2RAs, in which optimal dosing is at night, morning dosing of PPIs is associated with significantly improved acid suppression.[82,83] Although there is no universal definition of PPI failure, only 58% of GERD patients are fully satisfied with their antireflux medications.[84] Several factors have been reported to be associated with PPI failure, though compliance is foremost among them. The degree of acid suppression with PPIs is dose dependent, which lends support for the standard approach of double-dose PPIs for treatment failure. In these patients, better control of acidity is obtained using twice-daily rather than once-a-day dosing.[85] There is not good evidence to support the addition of a nocturnal H_2RA to a twice-daily PPI.[60,86,87] Patients with good control on twice-a-day dosing respond well to step-down therapy to once-a-day treatment.[88] The dose dependency extends down to the over-the-counter 10-mg dose of omeprazole, which provides greater efficacy than placebo, though with less efficacy and more interpatient variability than standard doses.

Intravenous formulations of pantoprazole, lansoprazole, and esomeprazole are available in the United States, while intravenous omeprazole is used in other countries. These agents provide dense temporal inhibition of acid secretion and are particularly useful in the treatment of acute upper gastroenterologic bleeding or for those patients temporarily without enteral intake.

Clinical Use. On the basis of excellent safety and efficacy profiles, the PPIs are the preferred treatment for acid-remediable diseases. This includes erosive esophagitis of all grades.[70] As with the H_2RAs, intermittent or on-demand PPI use does not maintain control in these patients.[63] Symptomatic treatment of heartburn will respond to on-demand PPI use, but the more rapid onset of action makes the H_2RAs a better choice for mild reflux.

PPIs are the primary pharmacologic therapy for acute[89] and chronic treatment of peptic ulcer. Peptic ulcer is uncommon in the absence of *H. pylori* infection or NSAID use.[90] PPIs are a part of all recommended *H. pylori* treatment regimens. Good evidence supports testing and treatment for *H. pylori* in peptic ulcer patients compared to PPI treatment alone.[91] PPIs are also effective in the treatment of nonulcer dyspepsia, though because this heterogeneous population contains patients with symptoms not directly related to acidity, effect size is much less than that with the treatment of GERD or ulcer disease.[92,93] An empirical trial of a PPI with or without *H. pylori* testing is a reasonable approach in patients less than 55 years of age and free of alarm symptoms, particularly if there are associated reflux symptoms.[94]

PPIs are effective in the prophylaxis of endoscopically visualized NSAID-induced mucosal injury[74,95] (Fig. 31-5). Increased use of prophylactic agents in NSAID-using arthritis patients also appears to be associated with fewer peptic ulcers.[96] Efficacy of PPIs is greater than that seen with H_2RAs, but inferior to that of the prostaglandin agent misoprostol. Though the PPI-directed approach may be more cost-effective and associated with fewer side effects than misoprostol,[97] adherence to gastroprotection therapy by any method remains low.[98]

All available PPIs generally have similar efficacy. Esomeprazole may have a modest advantage, particularly over omeprazole, in terms of ulcer healing[99] and reflux symptom relief. However, precise comparable doses between agents have not been established, the magnitude of the

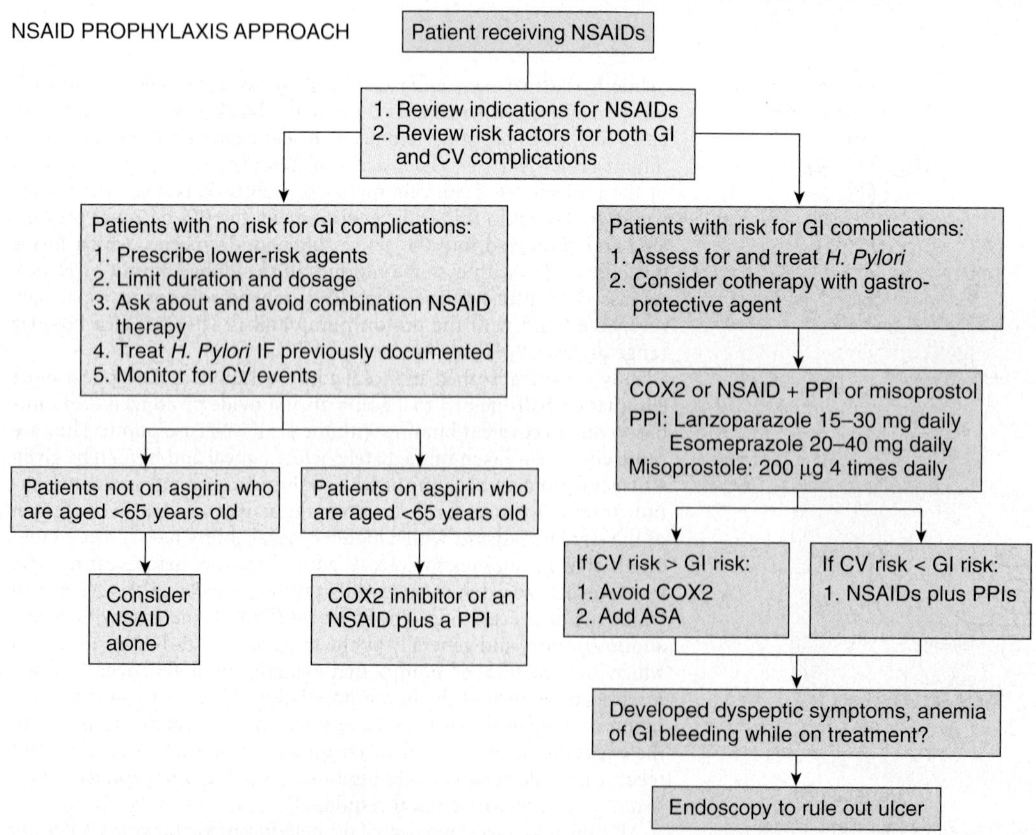

NSAID choice should be done based on an assessment of an individual's cardiovascular (CV) and gastrointestinal (GI) risk factors. For those with competing CV and GI risks, the tradeoffs between reducing adverse GI events (COX-2 inhibitor instead of a nonselective NSAID) must be weighed against concerns about cardiovascular side effects. Gastro protection, although significantly beneficial, does not eliminate risk, particularly among patients at high risk for GI complications.
PPI: proton pump inhibitor, NSAID: nonsteroidal anti-inflammatory drugs, COX2: cyclooxygenase 2 inhibitors

FIGURE 31-5 • NSAID prophylaxis approach.

observed differences is small, and it is not clear if this difference at 8 weeks translates to longer term relative improvement in maintenance.[100,101]

Safety. All PPIs have an excellent safety profile in both clinical trials and postmarketing pharmacovigilance.[102] This includes long-term safety data available for omeprazole, the first marketed PPI. The three main concerns regarding the long-term safety of the class include the effects of prolonged hypergastrinemia, the possible association of PPIs with gastric atrophy, and the effects of chronic hypochlorhydria. Gastrin is a proliferative hormone with a theoretical potential to promote cancer. The original package insert for PPIs contained a black box warning about this potential. This warning was removed as it became clear that the drugs do not appear to be mutagenic, nor are they associated with increased rates of colon cancer or gastric carcinoid.[10] Possible associations with hip fractures,[103] renal complications,[104] and community-acquired pneumonia have also been suggested. Systematic review suggests increased enteric infections (including *Clostridium difficile*) associated with acid suppression.[105] While there is biologic plausibility to such an observation, the data are heterogeneous and a direct causal relationship has not been established. In most cases, the PPIs have favorable risk:benefit ratios for index conditions treated.

As potent inhibitors of acid production, all PPIs can decrease the bioavailability of drugs with acid-dependent absorption. These include the human immunodeficiency virus protease inhibitor atazanavir, as well as ampicillin, iron, and digoxin. Omeprazole is an inhibitor of CYP2C19, which can increase the levels of substrates such as diazepam and phenytoin. Omeprazole has been noted to decrease the platelet inhibitory effect of clopidogrel, but outcomes data of this pharmacodynamic interaction are lacking.[106] PPIs should not be given concomitantly with H_2RAs, prostaglandins, or other antisecretory agents because of the marked reduction in their acid-inhibitory effects when administered simultaneously; however, sufficient time interval between administration of the H_2RA and the PPI is recommended when there is a need of concomitant therapies.

Mucosal Protective Agents

Sucralfate. Sucralfate is a nonabsorbable aluminum salt of sulfated sucrose and aluminum hydroxide. Most of its use is based on the prevention of chemically induced mucosal damage and for the healing of chronic ulcers. In the presence of low intragastric pH, the aluminum hydroxide dissociates; however, this moiety has little impact as an antacid. The sulfate ions then bind to proteins in the damaged gastric tissue of ulcer craters, and this is postulated to stimulate angiogenesis, the delivery of growth factors, and formation of granulation tissue.[107] This binding is favored by a low pH and is the rationale for use 30 to 60 minutes before meals. The drug is excreted in feces, and only a minor increase in serum and urinary aluminum has been reported with its use. Because of this concern, sucralfate is best avoided in patients with kidney failure.

Sucralfate suppresses *H. pylori* and inhibits acid secretion in patients with duodenal ulcers, leading to healing of the ulcer when used in doses of 4 g/day. However, the need for multiple daily doses, as well as the superior efficacy of the PPIs and H_2RAs, have limited its use for this indication. The primary utility is in the prophylaxis of stress ulceration in critically ill patients. There is not a large body of high-quality evidence to compare sucralfate with other modalities. In the best performed study, ranitidine was associated with less GI bleeding.[108] Though initial hopes were that sucralfate would be associated with less ventilator-associated pneumonia than H_2RAs on the basis of the sterilizing effects of an acidic stomach, there is not good clinical evidence to support this.[109,110] There is limited evidence of efficacy in nonulcer dyspepsia,[45] oral mucositis,[111] and radiation-induced proctitis.[112]

Bismuth. Bismuth is a metal with atomic number of 83, and bismuth salts have been used at least since the 18th century. The commonly used salt of salicylic acid, bismuth salicylate, displays anti-inflammatory action and also acts as an antacid and mild antibiotic. It is the active ingredient in a number of over-the-counter preparations. Bismuth suppresses *H. pylori* and has been approved by the U.S. Food and Drug Administration (FDA) for use in combination with other agents for its eradication. Other actions that may promote ulcer healing include inhibition of pepsin activity, and increase in mucosal prostaglandin production and mucus and bicarbonate secretion. It is largely unabsorbed and is excreted in feces. In the colon, it reacts with hydrogen sulfide and forms bismuth sulfide, which blackens the stool. It has modest efficacy in nonulcer dyspepsia,[45] and is presently used in *H. pylori* regimens. Common over-the-counter use is as an antidiarrheal. The safety profile of presently used preparations is excellent.

Prostaglandin Analogues

Mechanism of Action and Clinical Use. In addition to *H. pylori*, NSAID ingestion is a primary cause of PUD. The primary mechanisms of NSAID-induced injury are a reduction in the gastric mucus/bicarbonate protective cap as well as an increase in gastric acid production. The theoretical basis for prostaglandin therapy is to counteract the systemic effects of NSAIDs and enhance epithelial cell growth and repair.[113] Early work led to the development of misoprostol, arbaprostil, enoprostil, and risoprostil. Of these, misoprostol is the only prostaglandin E_2 analogue approved by the FDA for the prevention of NSAID-induced ulcers. It is usually given by mouth, with a good absorption, achieving a peak plasma concentration in 30 minutes, and a half-life of 1.5 hours. The drug has no effect in the CYP system, and its metabolites are excreted in the urine. It enhances mucosal defense mechanisms and inhibits gastric acid secretion in a dose-dependent manner through inhibition of histamine-stimulated cAMP production, reducing nocturnal, basal, and meal-stimulated acid secretion. It is not clear which mechanism predominates, though a combination is most likely. Misoprostol is the only agent that has been shown to reduce serious gastroenterologic complications from NSAID therapy.[95] Misoprostol is uterotropic and is commonly used in an off-label fashion for cervical ripening and the induction of labor.

Safety. Misoprostol also induces uterine contractions and has abortifacient properties, making it contraindicated in women of childbearing potential who do not use contraception. The most common side effects are dose-dependent abdominal cramps and diarrhea. Diarrhea is usually self-limited and will resolve, but it commonly causes discontinuation of therapy and, along with the need for multiple daily doses, limits compliance with therapy and overall use of misoprostol.

Therapeutic Strategies for Acid Peptic Disorders

Gastroesophageal Reflux Disease

The treatment of patients with GERD resides in controlling the symptoms of heartburn and/or acid regurgitation. GERD is a chronic entity that can result in esophageal mucosal injury, usually erosive esophagitis, if left untreated. It is estimated that 50% to 70% of GERD patients never develop esophagitis, and such patients are referred as having nonerosive gastroesophageal reflux disease (NERD). More than 80% of GERD patients need acid-suppressive medications to control their symptoms. Relapse of symptoms occurs in up to 70% to 80% of both esophagitis and NERD patients after they finish an initial course of therapy. Consequently, maintenance treatment is often required for symptom control, resulting in high medication costs for GERD patients.

Therapy for GERD can be approached in two different ways: by means of correction of the mechanisms involved in transient lower esophageal relaxations and an improvement in the esophageal exposure to the acidic gastric content. Consensus opinion suggests that the initial GERD treatment needs a symptom-based approach rather than a pathogenesis-based approach.[114] The primary end points of GERD therapy involve healing and maintenance of healing of moderate to severe lesions and the relief of symptoms for the majority of patients.[84]

A stepwise approach starting with lifestyle and dietary modifications of meals that would otherwise induce symptoms may benefit many patients with GERD. Despite the fact that these strategies have not been evaluated in large clinical trials, the importance of these changes

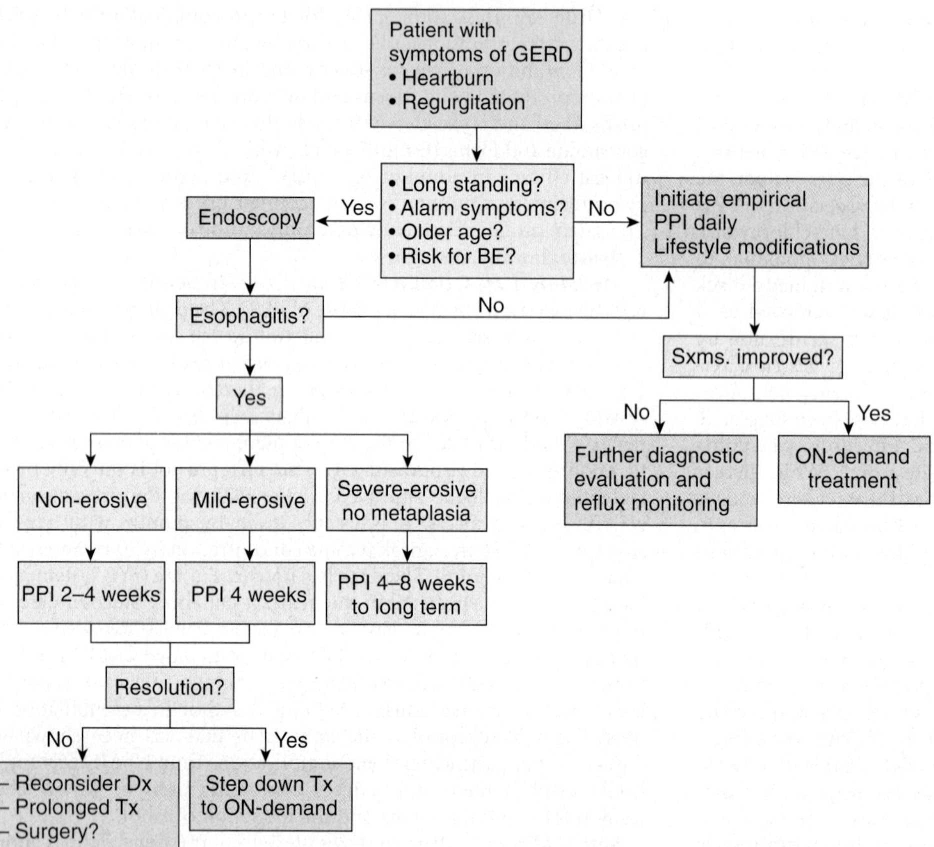

FIGURE 31-6 • GERD therapeutic strategy.

should be encouraged to patients throughout the treatment of this disease.

Most patients with suspected GERD are initially treated empirically, leading to substantial variability in the choice of initial therapy[69] (Fig. 31-6). Guidelines for the medical management of GERD suggest that, when symptoms persist or alarm signs develop, the patient should have further evaluation and treatment.[115,116] Early endoscopy is indicated for those with alarm features (i.e., dysphagia, weight loss), for those having atypical symptoms, or in those patients with long-standing symptoms.

Choice of Agent. Acid suppression represents the mainstay of therapy. Antacids are useful in the treatment of milder forms of GERD, providing rapid but short-lived relief of heartburn. They have been shown to be more effective than placebo in the relief of symptoms induced by a heartburn-promoting meal[115]; however, no trials have demonstrated antacids to be effective in healing esophagitis. Currently their use is focused on the management of mild episodic heartburn, pursuing immediate symptomatic relief in uncomplicated GERD patients with infrequent symptoms. They are usually used concurrently with a more potent antisecretory medication. Moreover, the dosage recommendations for these agents are not clearly established, leading to fluctuations in interval of administration and dosing amount. For these reasons and due to known antacid-drug interactions and the potential of side effects, they are rarely prescribed as a single therapy. The form of a combination therapy may be more beneficial than acid-suppressive therapy alone.[114]

The four H_2RAs are equally effective when used in proper doses, usually twice a day before meals. All four of the H_2RAs are available as over-the-counter formulations, which provides an inexpensive initial management. Given their pharmacokinetics, they are superior for rapid relief of symptoms; nevertheless, their effectiveness deteriorates with time, making the PPIs a better choice for long-term use.[69] There are some differences in potency, duration, and onset of action among the available H_2RAs, but in general the four H_2RAs are equally effective when used in proper doses, usually twice a day before meals, in patients with nonerosive disease. In those patients not responding to twice-daily dosing, or in patients with erosive disease, higher doses or a more frequent interval of administration may be useful.

Symptomatic relief can be expected in up to 60% of patients, and healing rates can be achieved in 50% of patients treated with H_2RAs, whereas corresponding rates for PPIs are 83% and 78%, making PPIs more effective for the empirical treatment of heartburn.[69,115] PPIs are highly effective therapeutic agents for symptom relief, healing, and maintenance of remission in patients with GERD.[117] Guidelines suggest that PPI therapy results in the best medical management for GERD, and with the availability of over-the-counter formulations, the cost of therapy may be reduced.[115]

Because of the wide clinical spectrum associated with GERD, the therapeutic approach is best tailored to the level of severity in the individual patient and several methods have been postulated, among which the step-down or step-up regimens are the most used. Patients should be placed on at least once-daily PPI therapy for 8 weeks, and if symptoms improve, patients can be maintained on continuous therapy or have their therapy titrated downward. Patients whose symptoms do not respond to an 8-week trial of a PPI should be reassessed for compliance with medications and lifestyle modifications. If they are compliant and symptoms remain present, the diagnosis should be reconsidered and confirmatory testing should be performed.[118] Howden et al. divided patients with heartburn into four groups and treated them for 20 weeks with a PPI followed by H_2RA (step-down therapy), an H_2RA followed by PPI (step-up therapy), a continuous PPI, or a continuous H_2RA regimen. They found that treatment with a continuous PPI regimen was the most effective. Therefore, no-step therapy is another good option in treating GERD patients in addition to the step-down or step-up therapies.[119]

Long-term PPI use has been demonstrated to be safe and effective in a number of high-quality studies, indicating that it is likely that different forms of PPI administration will become more acceptable, such as on-demand and intermittent therapy, which also appear to be effective in a significant proportion of patients with NERD.[63] However, to date there are no studies that have determined whether intermittent or on-demand therapy can prevent the long-term sequelae of GERD, such as stricture, Barrett's esophagus, and esophageal adenocarcinoma. Well-controlled studies are limited, and long-term efficacy trials investigating the success of these strategies are needed.[117,120]

Nocturnal Acid Breakthrough. Occasionally PPIs given twice daily do not suppress gastric acid secretion sufficiently overnight. This event, known as nocturnal gastric acid breakthrough (NAB), is arbitrarily defined as intragastric pH less than 4 for more than 1 continuous hour overnight, and occurs in about 70% of both patients with gastroesophageal reflux and normal volunteers. Esophageal acid exposure occurs in 30% to 50% of patients during the NAB period and might be sufficient to produce nocturnal symptoms and mucosal injury in patients with severe erosive esophagitis, Barrett's esophagus, and extraesophageal manifestations of GERD.[121] This NAB and accompanying gastroesophageal reflux may explain why some GERD patients fail to respond to twice-daily PPI treatment.

While some studies have found that adding H_2RAs at bedtime to a high-dose PPI can enhance nocturnal gastric pH control, decrease NAB, and decrease the duration of esophageal acid reflux associated with NAB, overall evidence to support the approach is not high,[60,86,87] and early response may be due to the known exaggerated first-dose phenomenon.[115]

Extraesophageal Syndromes. Extraesophageal manifestations of GERD refer to patients with symptoms not typical of this disease. These include symptoms such as hoarseness, sore throat, asthma, chronic cough, or noncardiac chest pain. Whether PPIs are effective or not in extraesophageal manifestations of GERD remains an important area of controversy and uncertainty.

Clinical suspicion is a critical component in the diagnosis of GERD-induced asthma. An empirical trial of 20 mg of omeprazole twice daily (or equivalent) for several months is a reasonable diagnostic strategy. Esophageal pH monitoring may be useful in patients with asthma with GERD symptoms who do not respond to an empirical trial of PPIs and in patients in whom "silent GERD" may be playing a role in difficult-to-control asthma.[122]

GERD is estimated to be the cause of chronic cough in 10% to 40% of patients and lifestyle modification should be recommended to all patients in whom GERD is suspected to be playing a role in chronic cough. Some authors endorse empirical trials with a high-dose PPI in patients with symptomatic GERD and chronic cough. However the diagnosis of GERD-induced cough is made, no clear guidelines exist regarding medical therapy.[122]

***Helicobacter pylori* in GERD.** The relationship between *H. pylori* and GERD remains unclear, and study results are conflicting.[33] Studies suggest that eradication of *H. pylori* has no influence on relapse of GERD or esophageal acid exposure and that, in patients with pan-gastritis, this may be associated with mild worsening of GERD symptoms, whereas patients with antral-predominant gastritis show improvement of symptoms.[123-125] To date, testing for and eradication of *H. pylori* has not been shown to be advantageous for patients with GERD.[33]

Refractory GERD. In the event of persistence of typical or atypical symptoms of GERD despite adequate medical therapy, the diagnosis of GERD should be reconsidered.[115] The use of higher doses of drug therapy or twice-daily dosing are strategies that may take place prior to other therapeutic approaches such as surgery or novel endoscopic techniques.

Peptic Ulcer Disease

The management of PUD involves an integration of the specific clinical situation, the etiology, and the expected natural history of the disease. Making a firm diagnosis of an etiologic cause is usually the first step in the management of this disease. Testing for *H. pylori* may be influenced by concomitant use of antibiotics, PPIs, or bismuth leading to false-negative results and, when PUD is clinically suspected, a negative test should be confirmed with a different one. Surreptitious NSAID use is common, especially with complicated or refractory ulcers, and it is essential for the physician to rule out NSAID or aspirin use.

Antisecretory therapy is the goal of therapy in patients with no documentation of *H. pylori*, and a number of treatment options are available for the healing of peptic ulcers. These include antacids (rarely used), H_2RAs, and the more effective PPIs. Potential mucosa-offending agents such as NSAIDs, cigarettes, and excess alcohol should be avoided. No firm dietary restrictions are necessary; however, patients should avoid foods that precipitate symptoms.

All four H_2RAs—cimetidine, ranitidine, famotidine, and nizatidine—induce healing rates of 70% to 80% for duodenal ulcer after 4 weeks, and 87% to 94% after 8 weeks, of therapy.[126] Though H_2RAs are effective in the treatment of PUD, PPIs are now the preferred agents because of their ease of use and superior efficacy. Studies of PPIs in patients with PUD have demonstrated superior healing rates, shorter healing time, and faster symptom relief than those obtained with other antisecretory therapies, including H_2RAs. PPIs have been shown to heal peptic ulcers that may be refractory to high-dose H_2RAs, and they also exhibit antimicrobial activity against *H. pylori* in vitro. PPIs only suppress *H. pylori* in vivo without eradicating it, and a combination of adequate acid suppression and antibiotic therapy is necessary for the successful eradication of *H. pylori*. Omeprazole and lansoprazole inhibit gastric acid secretion for many hours, and their effect is probably related to their ability to increase intragastric pH, which optimizes the antimicrobial action of concurrently administered drugs such as amoxicillin. PPI-based triple therapies for PUD result in a markedly reduced ulcer recurrence rate of 12% to 14% assessed from 2 weeks onward.[31]

Eradication of *H. pylori* Infection. Eradication of *H. pylori* infection has revolutionized the approach to treatment of PUD and it is now the mainstay of treatment for this disease, resulting in high ulcer healing rates and decreased recurrence rates, especially for individuals with a duodenal ulcer. In a meta-analysis of 34 studies of patients with duodenal ulcers, *H. pylori* eradication plus antisecretory therapy was superior to an antisecretory drug alone for healing of the ulcer (number needed to treat = 14).[127] *Helicobacter pylori* remains an important factor also linked to the development of gastric malignancy and dyspeptic symptoms[128]; thus eradication of *H. pylori* infection makes sense in view of these risks.

Arriving at a definitive diagnosis of the presence of *H. pylori* is usually the first step in providing care for patients with this disease. Decisions regarding treatment should be based upon patient characteristics, presenting symptoms, and pretest probability of the diagnostic methods employed. Testing for *H. pylori* infection is indicated in patients with active PUD, a past history of documented peptic ulcer, or gastric mucosa–associated lymphoid tissue (MALT) lymphoma.[128]

There is now a worldwide consensus that first-line treatment is based on a combination of PPI-clarithromycin-amoxicillin/metronidazole as a first-choice treatment in populations with less than 15% to 20% clarithromycin resistance prevalence (Table 31-6). In populations with less than 40% metronidazole resistance prevalence, PPI-clarithromycin-metronidazole is preferable.[128,129] Consensus from the European Helicobacter Study Group[129] recommends eradication of *H. pylori* in patients with gastroduodenal diseases, MALT lymphoma, and atrophic gastritis, as well as first-degree relatives of patients with gastric cancer, patients with unexplained iron deficiency anemia, and patients with chronic idiopathic thrombocytopenic purpura. However, there is still no consensus on the optimal duration of treatment (7, 10, or 14 days). Randomized, controlled trials investigating the efficacy of different durations of triple therapy have given similar results,[130-132] showing the potential benefits of shorter regimens, such as better compliance, fewer adverse effects, and lower costs. However, 14 days of therapy provides a moderate eradication rate that is significantly higher than that provided by 7-day therapy. Treatment with PPIs twice daily is superior to treatment once daily. Successful eradication with first-line treatments varies from 70%-95%, and 10-day and 14-day treatments are generally 7-9% more effective than the most commonly used 7-day regimens.[31] Taking into consideration results of several different meta-analyses, the American College of Gastroenterology recommends a 14-day course

TABLE 31-6 TREATMENT REGIMENS FOR *Helicobacter pylori*

Treatment Regimens	Duration of Treatment (Days)	ACG Recommended	European *Helicobacter* Study Group Recommended	FDA Approved	Eradication Rate (%)	Comments
PPI bid + Amoxicillin 1 g bid + Clarithromycin 500 mg bid	14	Yes	Yes	Yes	70-85	Preferred when prevalence of clarithromycin resistance is less than 15%–20%
PPI bid + Amoxicillin 1 g bid + Metronidazole 500 mg bid	10-14	Yes	Yes	No	70-85	Preferred in populations with less than 40% metronidazole resistance
PPI qd–bid **or** H_2RA bid + Bismuth subsalicylate 525 mg qid + Metronidazole 250 mg qid + Tetracycline 500 mg qid	10-14	Yes	Yes	Yes	70-95	Can be used as a salvage or rescue regimen in patients with persistence of infection. Best for PCN allergy cases, but complexity causes decreased compliance
PPI bid + Amoxicillin 1 g bid **Followed by** PPI bid + Clarithromycin 500 mg + Tinidazole 500 mg bid	5 and 5	No	No	No	90	Not associated with increased side effects when compared with other regimens
PPI bid + Amoxicillin 1 g bid + Levofloxacin 500 mg qd	10	No	No	No	87	Treatment should be based on susceptibility
PPI bid + Amoxicillin 1-1.5 g bid + Rifabutin 150 mg qd	12	No	No	No	91	Potential of myelo- and ocular toxicity due to rifabutin; and drug interactions due to rifabutin-induced metabolic enzyme induction

ACG, American College of Gastroenterology; bid, twice a day; FDA, Food and Drug Administration; H_2RA, histamine$_2$ receptor antagonist; PCN, penicillin; PPI, proton pump inhibitor; qd, once a day; qid, four times a day.

of clarithromycin triple therapy, particularly in the United States, where eradication rates have typically been 80% or less with shorter durations of therapy.[128]

Studies indicate that eradication of infection sufficiently heals duodenal ulcers in *H. pylori*–infected individuals and reduces the ulcer recurrence rate.[133] Some studies suggest that maintenance therapy with a PPI after eradication can significantly reduce ulcer recurrence and ulcer complications. Maintenance treatment should be continued with a PPI, following *H. pylori* eradication, in all patients who present with ulcer complications.[31]

NSAID-Induced Ulcers

A relationship between the use of NSAIDs and the development of gastroduodenal injury has been well established.[134] This is considered the major limitation to their use.[135] Guidelines recommend, based on individual risk assessment, a careful selection of the right NSAID for the right patient and to target the management of these patients on preventive measures and treatment of established ulcers.[134] Factors associated with an increased risk of developing GI complications include age greater than 60, prior history of GI event, high dose of NSAIDs, use of steroids, and use of anticoagulation therapy.[134]

The best ulcer-preventive strategy for patients who need to continue NSAID use is still debated.[31] Current prevention strategies to reduce serious NSAID-associated GI events are only cost-effective in patients with risk factors. No strategy shows superiority, but using a selective COX-2 inhibitor would be more cost-effective if it were associated with a reduction of events of the lower GI tract.[136] When faced with a patient in need of ongoing NSAID use, physicians should always consider the patient's underlying cardiovascular and GI risk factors, starting at the lowest effective doses for the shortest period possible and, in order to reduce the risk of gastroduodenal damage, using misoprostol or a PPI together with the NSAID or a selective COX-2 inhibitor with or without a PPI. However, the choice of COX-2 inhibitors is decreasing due to concerns regarding increased cardiovascular side effects.

Misoprostol reduces the risk of endoscopic ulcer and ulcer complications at doses of 800 mcg/day; however, at this dose range, the development of adverse events, specifically diarrhea, is also increased.[74] It is for this reason that this agent is less favored by prescribing physicians when recommending a prophylactic approach. Although commonly used with NSAIDs, single doses of H_2RAs have not been shown to prevent gastric ulcer, the most common NSAID-related lesion,[134] but do prevent duodenal ulcer when used in double doses.[74,137]

Oral PPIs given as single daily doses are effective in the prevention of NSAID-induced gastric and duodenal ulcers. PPIs may be preferred in NSAID users who require a PPI for another condition (e.g., GERD, low-dose aspirin use), those with cardiovascular risk factors, and those with dyspepsia.[138] Oral PPIs have been shown to be superior to H_2RAs in terms of acid suppression,[139] and do not demonstrate tachyphylaxis. They are superior to H_2RAs and misoprostol in reducing ulcers and NSAID-associated dyspepsia,[140] but fail to achieve similar success in prevention of gastric ulcers when compared to misoprostol. Among high-risk patients taking NSAIDs, omeprazole significantly reduced the total number of NSAID-related ulcers when compared with placebo and ranitidine use at standard doses.[134] Systematic reviews also show that omeprazole achieves better results in preventing duodenal but not gastric ulcers when compared to misoprostol.[74]

Once an established ulcer is documented in a patient using NSAIDs, the treatment would imply medications similar to those for non-NSAID ulcers. Discontinuation of the NSAID in use will be a principal therapeutic strategy but one that not always can be reached. Studies show that good healing rates could be obtained at both 4 and 8 weeks with either PPIs at a single daily dose or H_2RAs twice daily and demonstrated that satisfactory healing still occurred with prolonged therapy when it was necessary to continue NSAID treatment.[134]

Users of NSAIDs or aspirin may benefit from routine *H. pylori* testing, specially those patients presenting with ulcer risk factors. A "test and treat" strategy for *H. pylori* infection is not recommended for those already on long-term NSAID therapy and who have a low or absent risk of peptic ulcer, but current guidelines recommend that *H. pylori* infection should be eradicated in anyone in whom it is detected.[31,129] Expert opinion is that *H. pylori*–positive patients with a past or current history of ulcer requiring NSAID therapy should be treated for the infection, as it cannot be determined whether the prior ulcer was due to NSAID therapy or to *H. pylori* infection.[134]

Emerging Targets and Therapeutics

Tenatoprazole (benatoprazole), which is a novel compound with an imidazopyridine backbone in place of the typical substituted benzimidazole, has a prolonged plasma half-life and is under development.[141] Potassium-competitive acid blockers represent a new class of drugs acting through a reversible binding mechanism different from the classical (irreversible) PPIs. Once bound to the enzyme, they induce a conformational change in the structure of the enzyme that inhibits access of K^+ ions to their binding sites, thus preventing the exchange for H^+. Early clinical studies have shown a fast onset of action as they are active in the absence of stimulated acid secretion, achieving a maximum effect after the first dose, whereas classical PPIs need several days to reach their steady state effect.[142] Other neuropeptides being investigated for a possible role in acid secretion include calcitonin gene–related peptide and pituitary adenylate cyclase–activating polypeptide, a member of the secretin-glucagon–vasoactive intestinal polypeptide family, which has also been localized to gastric mucosal neurons and may participate in vagally mediated acid secretion.[21] Potential pharmacologic treatments that reduce the occurrence of transient lower esophageal relaxations in GERD are targeting the neurotransmitters involved using anticholinergics, morphine, and γ-aminobutyric acid agonists.[28]

REFERENCES

1. Cui G, Waldum HL. Physiological and clinical significance of enterochromaffin-like cell activation in the regulation of gastric acid secretion. World J Gastroenterol 2007;13:493-496.
2. Sobhani I, Bado A, Vissuzaine C, et al. Leptin secretion and leptin receptor in the human stomach. Gut 2000;47:178-183.
3. Hersey SJ, Sachs G. Gastric acid secretion. Physiol Rev 1995;75:155-189.
4. Cervero F. Sensory innervation of the viscera: peripheral basis of visceral pain. Physiol Rev 1994;74:95-138.
5. Schubert ML. Gastric secretion. Curr Opin Gastroenterol 2007;23:595-601.
6. Hirschowitz BI, Keeling D, Lewin M, et al. Pharmacological aspects of acid secretion. Dig Dis Sci 1995;40(2 Suppl):3S-23S.
7. Hou W, Schubert ML. Gastric secretion. Curr Opin Gastroenterol 2006;22:593-598.
8. Malfertheiner P, Fass R, Quigley EM, et al. From gastrin to gastro-oesophageal reflux disease—a century of acid suppression. Aliment Pharmacol Ther 2006;23:683-690.
9. Orlando LA, Lenard L, Orlando RC. Chronic hypergastrinemia: causes and consequences. Dig Dis Sci 2007;52:2482-2489.
10. Ai W, Liu Y, Wang TC. Yin Yang 1 (YY1) represses histidine decarboxylase gene expression with SREBP-1a in part through an upstream Sp1 site. Am J Physiol Gastrointest Liver Physiol 2006;290:G1096-G1104.
11. Chen D, Aihara T, Zhao CM, et al. Differentiation of the gastric mucosa. I. Role of histamine in control of function and integrity of oxyntic mucosa: understanding gastric physiology through disruption of targeted genes. Am J Physiol Gastrointest Liver Physiol 2006;291:G539-G544.
12. Schubert ML. Gastric secretion. Curr Opin Gastroenterol 2003;19:519-525.
13. Nikolopoulou VN, Thomopoulos KC, Katsakoulis EC, et al. The effect of octreotide as an adjunct treatment in active nonvariceal upper gastrointestinal bleeding. J Clin Gastroenterol 2004;38:243-247.
14. Leontiadis GI, Howden CW. Pharmacologic treatment of peptic ulcer bleeding. Curr Treat Options Gastroenterol 2007;10:134-142.
15. Kusayanagi S, Takeuchi Y, Todisco A, Mitamura K. Extracellular signal-regulated protein kinases mediate H^+,K^+-ATPase alpha-subunit gene expression. Biochem Biophys Res Commun 2002;290:1289-1294.
16. Hasebe K, Horie S, Komasaka M, et al. Stimulatory effects of nitric oxide donors on gastric acid secretion in isolated mouse stomach. Eur J Pharmacol 2001;420:159-164.
17. Mori M, Suzuki H, Masaoka T, et al. Intravenous ghrelin administration enhances gastric acid secretion—evaluation using wireless pH capsule. Aliment Pharmacol Ther 2006;24(Suppl 4):96-103.
18. Yakabi K, Ro S, Onouhi T, et al. Histamine mediates the stimulatory action of ghrelin on acid secretion in rat stomach. Dig Dis Sci 2006;51:1313-1321.
19. Levin F, Edholm T, Ehrstrom M, et al. Effect of peripherally administered ghrelin on gastric emptying and acid secretion in the rat. Regul Pept 2005;131:59-65.
20. Schubert ML. Gastric secretion. Curr Opin Gastroenterol 2002;18:639-649.
21. Hildebrand P, Lehmann FS, Ketterer S, et al. Regulation of gastric function by endogenous gastrin releasing peptide in humans: studies with a specific gastrin releasing peptide receptor antagonist. Gut 2001;49:23-28.
22. Sachs G, Shin JM, Vagin O, et al. The gastric H,K ATPase as a drug target: past, present, and future. J Clin Gastroenterol 2007;41(6 Suppl 2):S226-S242.
23. Yao X, Forte JG. Cell biology of acid secretion by the parietal cell. Annu Rev Physiol 2003;65:103-131.
24. Caplan MJ. The future of the pump. J Clin Gastroenterol 2007;41(6 Suppl 2):S217-S222.
25. Vakil N, van Zanten SV, Kahrilas P, et al, for the Globale Konsensusgruppe. The Montreal definition and classification of gastroesophageal reflux disease: a global, evidence-based consensus paper. Z Gastroenterol 2007;45:1125-1140.
26. Sifrim D, Mittal R, Fass R, et al. Acidity and volume of the refluxate in the genesis of gastro-oesophageal reflux disease symptoms. Aliment Pharmacol Ther 2007;25:1003-1017.
27. Richter JE. Gastrooesophageal reflux disease. Best Pract Res Clin Gastroenterol 2007;21:609-631.
28. Boeckxstaens GE. The pathophysiology of gastro-oesophageal reflux disease [Review]. Aliment Pharmacol Ther 2007;26:149-160.
29. Dvorak K, Payne CM, Chavarria M, et al. Bile acids in combination with low pH induce oxidative stress and oxidative DNA damage: relevance to the pathogenesis of Barrett's oesophagus. Gut 2007;56:763-771.
30. Moayyedi P, Talley NJ. Gastro-oesophageal reflux disease. Lancet 2006;367:2086-2100.
31. Yuan Y, Padol IT, Hunt RH. Peptic ulcer disease today. Nat Clin Pract Gastroenterol Hepatol 2006;3:80-89.
32. Unidentified curved bacilli on gastric epithelium in active chronic gastritis. Lancet 1983;1:1273-1275.
33. Makola D, Peura DA, Crowe SE. *Helicobacter pylori* infection and related gastrointestinal diseases. J Clin Gastroenterol 2007;41:548-558.
34. Suerbaum S, Michetti P. *Helicobacter pylori* infection. N Engl J Med 2002;347:1175-1186.
35. Silverstein FE, Graham DY, Senior JR, et al. Misoprostol reduces serious gastrointestinal complications in patients with rheumatoid arthritis receiving nonsteroidal anti-inflammatory drugs: a randomized, double-blind, placebo-controlled trial. Ann Intern Med 1995;123:241-249.
36. Garcia Rodriguez LA, Hernandez-Diaz S. Risk of uncomplicated peptic ulcer among users of aspirin and nonaspirin nonsteroidal antiinflammatory drugs. Am J Epidemiol 2004;159:23-31.
37. Chan FK, Graham DY. Prevention of non-steroidal anti-inflammatory drug gastrointestinal complications—review and recommendations based on risk assessment. Aliment Pharmacol Ther 2004;19:1051-1061.
38. Duerksen DR. Stress-related mucosal disease in critically ill patients. Best Pract Res Clin Gastroenterol 2003;17:327-344.
39. Sesler JM. Stress-related mucosal disease in the intensive care unit: an update on prophylaxis. AACN Adv Crit Care 2007;18:119-126.
40. Washington N. Antacids and Anti-Reflux Agents. Boca Raton, FL: CRC Press, 1991.
41. Lam SK, Koo J. New approach with old medicine: antacids and bismuth. *In* Pfeiffer CJ (ed): Therapetutic Agents for Peptic Ulcer. Boca Raton, FL: CRC Press, 1982, p 159.
42. Sippy B. Gastric and duodenal ulcers, medical cure by an efficient removal of gastric juice corrosion. J Am Med Assoc 1915;64:1625.
43. Maton PN, Burton ME. Antacids revisited: a review of their clinical pharmacology and recommended therapeutic use. Drugs 1999;57:855-870.
44. Dunn JP, Etter LE. Inadequacy of the medical history in the diagnosis of duodenal ulcer. N Engl J Med 1962;266:68-72.
45. Moayyedi P, Soo S, Deeks J, et al. Pharmacological interventions for non-ulcer dyspepsia. Cochrane Database Syst Rev 2006;(4):CD001960.

46. Nyren O. Secretory abnormalities in functional dyspepsia. Scand J Gastroenterol Suppl 1991;182:25-28.
47. Tran T, Lowry AM, El-Serag HB. Meta-analysis: the efficacy of over-the-counter gastro-oesophageal reflux disease therapies. Aliment Pharmacol Ther 2007;25:143-153.
48. Aihara T, Nakamura E, Amagase K, et al. Pharmacological control of gastric acid secretion for the treatment of acid-related peptic disease: past, present, and future. Pharmacol Ther 2003;98:109-127.
49. Picolos MK, Orlander PR. Calcium carbonate toxicity: the updated milk-alkali syndrome; report of 3 cases and review of the literature. Endocr Pract 2005;11:272-280.
50. Picolos MK, Lavis VR, Orlander PR. Milk-alkali syndrome is a major cause of hypercalcaemia among non-end-stage renal disease (non-ESRD) inpatients. Clin Endocrinol (Oxf) 2005;63:566-576.
51. National Kidney Foundation. K/DOQI clinical practice guidelines for bone metabolism and disease in chronic kidney disease. Am J Kidney Dis 2003;42(4 Suppl 3): S1-S201.
52. Kaehny WD, Hegg AP, Alfrey AC. Gastrointestinal absorption of aluminum from aluminum-containing antacids. N Engl J Med 1977;296:1389-1390.
53. Ash AS, Schild HO. Receptors mediating some actions of histamine. Br J Pharmacol Chemother 1966;27:427-439.
54. Black JW, Duncan WA, Durant CJ, et al. Definition and antagonism of histamine H_2-receptors. Nature 1972;236:385-390.
55. Parsons ME, Ganellin CR. Histamine and its receptors. Br J Pharmacol 2006;147(Suppl 1):S127-S135.
56. Smit MJ, Leurs R, Alewijnse AE, et al. Inverse agonism of histamine H_2 antagonist accounts for upregulation of spontaneously active histamine H_2 receptors. Proc Natl Acad Sci U S A 1996;93:6802-6807.
57. Merki HS, Halter F, Wilder-Smith C, et al. Effect of food on H_2-receptor blockade in normal subjects and duodenal ulcer patients. Gut 1990;31:148-150.
58. Howden CW, Burget DW, Hunt RH. Appropriate acid suppression for optimal healing of duodenal ulcer and gastro-oesophageal reflux disease. Scand J Gastroenterol Suppl 1994;201:79-82.
59. Burget DW, Chiverton SG, Hunt RH. Is there an optimal degree of acid suppression for healing of duodenal ulcers? A model of the relationship between ulcer healing and acid suppression. Gastroenterology 1990;99:345-351.
60. Pan T, Wang YP, Liu FC, Yang JL. Additional bedtime H_2-receptor antagonist for the control of nocturnal gastric acid breakthrough: a Cochrane systematic review. Chin J Dig Dis 2006;7:141-148.
61. Huang JQ, Hunt RH. Pharmacological and pharmacodynamic essentials of H_2-receptor antagonists and proton pump inhibitors for the practising physician. Best Pract Res Clin Gastroenterol 2001;15:355-370.
62. Osawa S, Kajimura M, Yamamoto S, et al. Alteration of intracellular histamine H_2 receptor cycling precedes antagonist-induced upregulation. Am J Physiol Gastrointest Liver Physiol 2005;289:G880-G889.
63. Zacny J, Zamakhshary M, Sketris I, Veldhuyzen van Zanten S. Systematic review: the efficacy of intermittent and on-demand therapy with histamine H_2-receptor antagonists or proton pump inhibitors for gastro-oesophageal reflux disease patients. Aliment Pharmacol Ther 2005;21:1299-1312.
64. Grimley CE, Cottrell J, Mann SG, et al. Nocturnal intragastric acidity after over-the-counter doses of famotidine, ranitidine or placebo. Aliment Pharmacol Ther 1997;11:881-885.
65. Reilly TG, Singh S, Cottrell J, et al. Low-dose famotidine and ranitidine as single post-prandial doses: a three-period placebo-controlled comparative trial. Aliment Pharmacol Ther 1996;10:749-755.
66. Grimley CE, West JM, Loft DE, et al. Early and late effects of low-dose famotidine, ranitidine or placebo on pentagastrin-stimulated gastric acid secretion in man. Aliment Pharmacol Ther 1996;10:743-747.
67. Delaney B, Ford AC, Forman D, et al. Initial management strategies for dyspepsia. Cochrane Database Syst Rev 2005;(4):CD001961.
68. Khan M, Santana J, Donnellan C, et al. Medical treatments in the short term management of reflux oesophagitis. Cochrane Database Syst Rev 2007;(2): CD003244.
69. van Pinxteren B, Numans ME, Bonis PA, Lau J. Short-term treatment with proton pump inhibitors, H_2-receptor antagonists and prokinetics for gastro-oesophageal reflux disease-like symptoms and endoscopy negative reflux disease. Cochrane Database Syst Rev 2006;(3):CD002095.
70. Wang WH, Huang JQ, Zheng GF, et al. Head-to-head comparison of H_2-receptor antagonists and proton pump inhibitors in the treatment of erosive esophagitis: a meta-analysis. World J Gastroenterol 2005;11:4067-4077.
71. Leontiadis GI, Sharma VK, Howden CW. Proton pump inhibitor treatment for acute peptic ulcer bleeding. Cochrane Database Syst Rev 2006;(1):CD002094.
72. Poynard T, Lemaire M, Agostini H. Meta-analysis of randomized clinical trials comparing lansoprazole with ranitidine or famotidine in the treatment of acute duodenal ulcer. Eur J Gastroenterol Hepatol 1995;7:661-665.
73. Walan A, Bader JP, Classen M, et al. Effect of omeprazole and ranitidine on ulcer healing and relapse rates in patients with benign gastric ulcer. N Engl J Med 1989;320:69-75.
74. Rostom A, Dube C, Wells G, et al. Prevention of NSAID-induced gastroduodenal ulcers. Cochrane Database Syst Rev 2002;(4):CD002296.
75. Garbis H, Elefant E, Diav-Citrin O, et al. Pregnancy outcome after exposure to ranitidine and other H_2-blockers: a collaborative study of the European Network of Teratology Information Services. Reprod Toxicol 2005;19:453-458.
76. Zhou Q, Yan XF, Zhang ZM, et al. Rational prescription of drugs within similar therapeutic or structural class for gastrointestinal disease treatment: drug metabolism and its related interactions. World J Gastroenterol 2007;13:5618-5628.
77. Sjostrand SE, Oble L, Fellenus E. The discovery and development of the proton pump inhibitor. *In* Oble L (ed): The Proton Pump Inhibitors. Basel: Birkhäuser, 1999, p 3.
78. Sachs G, Wallmark B. The gastric H,K-ATPase. *In* Oble L (ed): The Proton Pump Inhibitors. Basel: Birkhäuser, 1999, p 23.
79. Brunner G, Hell M, Hengels KJ, et al. Influence of lansoprazole on intragastric 24-hour pH, meal-stimulated gastric acid secretion, and concentrations of gastrointestinal hormones and enzymes in serum and gastric juice in healthy volunteers. Digestion 1995;56:137-144.
80. Wolfe MM, Sachs G. Acid suppression: optimizing therapy for gastroduodenal ulcer healing, gastroesophageal reflux disease, and stress-related erosive syndrome. Gastroenterology 2000;118(2 Suppl 1):S9-S31.
81. Furuta T, Shirai N, Kodaira M, et al. Pharmacogenomics-based tailored versus standard therapeutic regimen for eradication of *H. pylori*. Clin Pharmacol Ther 2007;81:521-528.
82. Chiverton SG, Howden CW, Burget DW, Hunt RH. Omeprazole (20 mg) daily given in the morning or evening: a comparison of effects on gastric acidity, and plasma gastrin and omeprazole concentration. Aliment Pharmacol Ther 1992;6:103-111.
83. Mussig S, Witzel L, Luhmann R, Schneider A. Morning and evening administration of pantoprazole: a study to compare the effect on 24-hour intragastric pH. Eur J Gastroenterol Hepatol 1997;9:599-602.
84. Coron E, Hatlebakk JG, Galmiche JP. Medical therapy of gastroesophageal reflux disease. Curr Opin Gastroenterol 2007;23:434-439.
85. Timmer W, Ripke H, Kleist P, et al. Effect of four lansoprazole dose levels and one dosage regimen of omeprazole on 24-hour intragastric pH in healthy subjects. Methods Find Exp Clin Pharmacol 1995;17:489-495.
86. Cross LB, Justice LN. Combination drug therapy for gastroesophageal reflux disease. Ann Pharmacother 2002;36:912-916.
87. Vakil N, Guda N, Partington S. The effect of over-the-counter ranitidine 75 mg on night-time heartburn in patients with erosive oesophagitis on daily proton pump inhibitor maintenance therapy. Aliment Pharmacol Ther 2006;23:649-653.
88. Inadomi JM, McIntyre L, Bernard L, Fendrick AM. Step-down from multiple- to single-dose proton pump inhibitors (PPIs): a prospective study of patients with heartburn or acid regurgitation completely relieved with PPIs. Am J Gastroenterol 2003;98:1940-1944.
89. Leontiadis GI, Sreedharan A, Dorward S, et al. Systematic reviews of the clinical effectiveness and cost-effectiveness of proton pump inhibitors in acute upper gastrointestinal bleeding. Health Technol Assess 2007;11(51):iii-iv, 1-164.
90. Huang JQ, Sridhar S, Hunt RH. Role of *Helicobacter pylori* infection and non-steroidal anti-inflammatory drugs in peptic-ulcer disease: a meta-analysis. Lancet 2002;359:14-22.
91. Gisbert JP, Khorrami S, Carballo F, et al. *H. pylori* eradication therapy vs. antisecretory non-eradication therapy (with or without long-term maintenance antisecretory therapy) for the prevention of recurrent bleeding from peptic ulcer. Cochrane Database Syst Rev 2003;(4):CD004062.
92. Moayyedi P, Soo S, Deeks J, et al. Eradication of *Helicobacter pylori* for non-ulcer dyspepsia. Cochrane Database Syst Rev 2006;(2):CD002096.
93. Wang WH, Huang JQ, Zheng GF, et al. Effects of proton-pump inhibitors on functional dyspepsia: a meta-analysis of randomized placebo-controlled trials. Clin Gastroenterol Hepatol 2007;5:178-185.
94. Talley NJ, Vakil NB, Moayyedi P. American Gastroenterological Association technical review on the evaluation of dyspepsia. Gastroenterology 2005;129:1756-1780.
95. Hooper L, Brown TJ, Elliott R, et al. The effectiveness of five strategies for the prevention of gastrointestinal toxicity induced by non-steroidal anti-inflammatory drugs: systematic review. BMJ 2004;329:948.
96. Steen KS, Nurmohamed MT, Visman I, et al. Decreasing incidence of symptomatic gastrointestinal ulcers and ulcer complications in patients with rheumatoid arthritis. Ann Rheum Dis 2008;67:256-259.
97. Brown TJ, Hooper L, Elliott RA, et al. A comparison of the cost-effectiveness of five strategies for the prevention of non-steroidal anti-inflammatory drug-induced gastrointestinal toxicity: a systematic review with economic modelling. Health Technol Assess 2006;10(38):iii-iv, xi-xiii, 1-183.
98. Moore RA, Derry S, Phillips CJ, McQuay HJ. Nonsteroidal anti-inflammatory drugs (NSAIDs), cyxlooxygenase-2 selective inhibitors (coxibs) and gastrointestinal harm: review of clinical trials and clinical practice. BMC Musculoskelet Disord 2006;7:79.
99. Edwards SJ, Lind T, Lundell L. Systematic review: proton pump inhibitors (PPIs) for the healing of reflux oesophagitis—a comparison of esomeprazole with other PPIs. Aliment Pharmacol Ther 2006;24:743-750.
100. Ip S, Bonis P, Tatsoni A, et al. Comparative Effectiveness of Management Strategies for Gastroesophageal Reflux Disease. Comparative Effectiveness Review No. 1. (Prepared by Tufts-New England Medical Center Evidence-based Practice Center under Contract No. 290-02-0022.) December 2005.
101. Vakil N, Fennerty MB. Direct comparative trials of the efficacy of proton pump inhibitors in the management of gastro-oesophageal reflux disease and peptic ulcer disease. Aliment Pharmacol Ther 2003;18:559-568.
102. Salgueiro E, Rubio T, Hidalgo A, Manso G. Safety profile of proton pump inhibitors according to the spontaneous reports of suspected adverse reactions. Int J Clin Pharmacol Ther 2006;44:548-556.
103. Yang YX, Lewis JD, Epstein S, Metz DC. Long-term proton pump inhibitor therapy and risk of hip fracture. JAMA 2006;296:2947-2953.
104. Geevasinga N, Coleman PL, Webster AC, Roger SD. Proton pump inhibitors and acute interstitial nephritis. Clin Gastroenterol Hepatol 2006;4:597-604.
105. Leonard J, Marshall JK, Moayyedi P. Systematic review of the risk of enteric infection in patients taking acid suppression. Am J Gastroenterol 2007;102:2047-2056.
106. Gilard M, Arnaud B, Cornily JC, et al. Influence of omeprazole on the antiplatelet action of clopidogrel associated with aspirin: the randomized, double-blind OCLA (Omeprazole CLopidogrel Aspirin) study. J Am Coll Cardiol 2008;51:256-260.

107. Tarnawski A, Tanoue K, Santos AM, Sarfeh IJ. Cellular and molecular mechanisms of gastric ulcer healing: is the quality of mucosal scar affected by treatment? Scand J Gastroenterol Suppl 1995;210:9-14.
108. Cook D, Guyatt G, Marshall J, et al. A comparison of sucralfate and ranitidine for the prevention of upper gastrointestinal bleeding in patients requiring mechanical ventilation. Canadian Critical Care Trials Group. N Engl J Med 1998;338:791-797.
109. Dodek P, Keenan S, Cook D, et al. Evidence-based clinical practice guideline for the prevention of ventilator-associated pneumonia. Ann Intern Med 2004;141:305-313.
110. Bornstain C, Azoulay E, De Lassence A, et al. Sedation, sucralfate, and antibiotic use are potential means for protection against early-onset ventilator-associated pneumonia. Clin Infect Dis 2004;38:1401-1408.
111. Worthington HV, Clarkson JE, Eden OB. Interventions for preventing oral mucositis for patients with cancer receiving treatment. Cochrane Database Syst Rev 2006;(2): CD000978.
112. Hovdenak N, Sorbye H, Dahl O. Sucralfate does not ameliorate acute radiation proctitis: randomised study and meta-analysis. Clin Oncol (R Coll Radiol) 2005;17:485-491.
113. Duerksen DR. Stress-related mucosal disease in critically ill patients. Best Pract Res Clin Gastroenterol 2003;17:327-344.
114. Tytgat GN, McColl K, Tack J, et al. New algorithm for the treatment of gastro-oesophageal reflux disease. Aliment Pharmacol Ther 2008;27:249-256.
115. DeVault KR, Castell DO, for the American College of Gastroenterology. Updated guidelines for the diagnosis and treatment of gastroesophageal reflux disease. Am J Gastroenterol 2005;100:190-200.
116. Guideline at-a-glance. ACG-revised GERD guidelines focus on proper use of drugs. Geriatrics 2005;60:18.
117. Fennerty MB. Alternative approaches to the long-term management of GERD. Aliment Pharmacol Ther 2005;22(Suppl 3):39-44.
118. Ferguson DD, DeVault KR. Medical management of gastroesophageal reflux disease. Expert Opin Pharmacother 2007;8:39-47.
119. Howden CW, Henning JM, Huang B, et al. Management of heartburn in a large, randomized, community-based study: comparison of four therapeutic strategies. Am J Gastroenterol 2001;96:1704-1710.
120. Inadomi JM, Fendrick AM. PPI use in the OTC era: who to treat, with what, and for how long? Clin Gastroenterol Hepatol 2005;3:208-215.
121. Katz PO, Anderson C, Khoury R, Castell DO. Gastro-oesophageal reflux associated with nocturnal gastric acid breakthrough on proton pump inhibitors. Aliment Pharmacol Ther 1998;12:1231-1234.
122. Napierkowski J, Wong RK. Extraesophageal manifestations of GERD. Am J Med Sci 2003;326:285-299.
123. Moayyedi P, Bardhan C, Young L, et al. *Helicobacter pylori* eradication does not exacerbate reflux symptoms in gastroesophageal reflux disease. Gastroenterology 2001;121:1120-1126.
124. Schwizer W, Thumshirn M, Dent J, et al. *Helicobacter pylori* and symptomatic relapse of gastro-oesophageal reflux disease: a randomised controlled trial. Lancet 2001;357:1738-1742.
125. Tefera S, Hatlebakk JG, Berstad A. The effect of *Helicobacter pylori* eradication on gastro-oesophageal reflux. Aliment Pharmacol Ther 1999;13:915-920.
126. Burget DW, Chiverton SG, Hunt RH. Is there an optimal degree of acid suppression for healing of duodenal ulcers? A model of the relationship between ulcer healing and acid suppression. Gastroenterology 1990;99:345-351.
127. Ables AZ, Simon I, Melton ER. Update on *Helicobacter pylori* treatment. Am Fam Physician 2007;75:351-358.
128. Chey WD, Wong BC, for the Practice Parameters Committee of the American College of Gastroenterology. American College of Gastroenterology guideline on the management of *Helicobacter pylori* infection. Am J Gastroenterol 2007;102:1808-1825.
129. Malfertheiner P, Megraud F, O'Morain C, et al. Current concepts in the management of *Helicobacter pylori* infection: the Maastricht III Consensus Report. Gut 2007;56:772-781.
130. Fuccio L, Minardi ME, Zagari RM, et al. Meta-analysis: duration of first-line proton-pump inhibitor based triple therapy for *Helicobacter pylori* eradication. Ann Intern Med 2007;147:553-562.
131. Lara LF, Cisneros G, Gurney M, et al. One-day quadruple therapy compared with 7-day triple therapy for *Helicobacter pylori* infection. Arch Intern Med 2003;163:2079-2084.
132. Treiber G, Wittig J, Ammon S, et al. Clinical outcome and influencing factors of a new short-term quadruple therapy for *Helicobacter pylori* eradication: a randomized controlled trial (MACLOR study). Arch Intern Med 2002;162:153-160.
133. Ford AC, Delaney BC, Forman D, Moayyedi P. Eradication therapy for peptic ulcer disease in *Helicobacter pylori* positive patients. Cochrane Database Syst Rev 2006;(2):CD003840.
134. Lanza FL. A guideline for the treatment and prevention of NSAID-induced ulcers. Members of the Ad Hoc Committee on Practice Parameters of the American College of Gastroenterology. Am J Gastroenterol 1998;93:2037-2046.
135. Wallace JL. Nonsteroidal anti-inflammatory drugs and gastroenteropathy: the second hundred years. Gastroenterology 1997;112:1000-1016.
136. Lanas A. Economic analysis of strategies in the prevention of non-steroidal anti-inflammatory drug-induced complications in the gastrointestinal tract. Aliment Pharmacol Ther 2004;20:321-331.
137. Taha AS, Hudson N, Hawkey CJ, et al. Famotidine for the prevention of gastric and duodenal ulcers caused by nonsteroidal antiinflammatory drugs. N Engl J Med 1996;334:1435-1439.
138. Laine L. GI risk and risk factors of NSAIDs. J Cardiovasc Pharmacol 2006;47(Suppl 1):S60-S66.
139. Scheiman JM, Yeomans ND, Talley NJ, et al. Prevention of ulcers by esomeprazole in at-risk patients using non-selective NSAIDs and COX-2 inhibitors. Am J Gastroenterol 2006;101:701-710.
140. Scheiman JM. Prevention of NSAID-induced ulcers. Curr Treat Options Gastroenterol 2008;11:125-134.
141. Galmiche JP, Sacher-Huvelin S, Bruley des Varannes S, et al. A comparative study of the early effects of tenatoprazole 40 mg and esomeprazole 40 mg on intragastric pH in healthy volunteers. Aliment Pharmacol Ther 2005;21:575-582.
142. Simon WA, Herrmann M, Klein T, et al. Soraprazan: setting new standards in inhibition of gastric acid secretion. J Pharmacol Exp Ther 2007;321:866-874.

32

MOTILITY DISORDERS

Michael Camilleri and Viola Andresen

INTRODUCTION 475
PATHOPHYSIOLOGY 475
Physiology of Gastrointestinal Motility 475
Basic Control Mechanisms 475
Applied Physiology 476
Motility Disorders 476
Gastroparesis and Chronic Intestinal Pseudo-obstruction 476
Dumping Syndrome and Accelerated Gastric Emptying 477
Slow and Fast Colonic Transit 477
Postoperative Ileus 477
THERAPEUTICS AND CLINICAL PHARMACOLOGY 478
Goals of Therapy 478
Therapeutics by Class 478
Fiber 478
Laxatives 478
Cholinergic Agents 478
Serotonergic Agents 481
Dopamine Antagonists 482
Motilin Agonists 482
Opioid Agents 482
Somatostatin Analogue 483
Chloride Channel Agonist 483
Emerging Targets and Therapeutics 483
Ghrelin 483
Phosphodiesterase Inhibition 483
Guanylate Cyclase-C Agonist 484
Recombinant Human Neurotrophin-3 484
Device-Based Therapies 484

INTRODUCTION

Motility disorders result from impaired control of the neuromuscular apparatus of the gut. Associated symptoms include recurrent or chronic nausea, vomiting, bloating, and abdominal discomfort, constipation, or diarrhea, which occur in the absence of mechanical intestinal obstruction. This chapter briefly reviews the physiology of gastrointestinal motility and describes the neuroenteric mechanisms involved in its regulation.

Motility disorders differ in the degree of morbidity: from occasional dyspeptic symptoms in patients with gastric emptying disturbances to severe abdominal pain, ileus, and cachexia in patients with chronic intestinal pseudo-obstruction. The pathogenesis of most of these disorders is still not completely understood, and usually there are no identifiable causative mechanisms or curative therapies. However, extensive research and increasing knowledge of brain-gut physiology, mechanisms, and neurotransmitters and receptors involved in gastrointestinal motor and sensory functions enable the ongoing development of new therapeutic approaches.

Since there is such a wide range of motility disorders from the esophagus to the anus, it would be impossible to cover all syndromes with sufficient depth. We therefore focus this chapter on the most debilitating disorders, such as gastroparesis, dumping syndrome, and chronic intestinal pseudo-obstruction, and the very common dysfunctions of slow and fast colonic transit and postoperative ileus, for which there has been much progress in pharmacologic treatment. The main pathophysiologic targets and therapeutic approaches of these disorders are presented.

PATHOPHYSIOLOGY

Physiology of Gastrointestinal Motility

Basic Control Mechanisms

Motor function of the gastrointestinal tract depends on the contraction of smooth muscle cells and their integration and modulation by enteric and extrinsic nerves. Disturbances of the mechanisms that regulate gastrointestinal motor function may lead to altered gut motility.[1] Neurogenic modulators of gastrointestinal motility include the central nervous system (CNS), the autonomic nerves, and the enteric nervous system (ENS) (Fig. 32-1).[2] Extrinsic neural control of gastrointestinal motor function consists of the cranial and sacral parasympathetic outflow (excitatory to nonsphincteric muscle) and the thoracolumbar sympathetic supply (excitatory to sphincters, inhibitory to nonsphincteric muscle). The cranial outflow is predominantly through the vagus nerve, which innervates the gastrointestinal tract from the stomach to the right colon and consists of preganglionic cholinergic fibers that synapse with the ENS. The supply of sympathetic fibers to the stomach and small bowel arises from levels T5 to T10 of the intermediolateral column of the spinal cord. The prevertebral ganglia have an important role in the integration of afferent impulses between the gut and the CNS and reflex control of abdominal viscera.

The ENS is an independent nervous system consisting of approximately 100 million neurons organized in ganglionated plexuses.[3] The larger myenteric (or Auerbach's) plexus is situated between the longitudinal and circular muscle layers of the muscularis externa and contains neurons responsible for gastrointestinal motility. The submucosal (or Meissner's) plexus controls absorption, secretion, and mucosal blood flow. The ENS is also important in visceral afferent function, mediating intrinsic neuromuscular or secretory reflexes and extrinsic transmission of visceral sensation via the vagal nerve or the spinal afferents.[4,5]

The main intrinsic reflex serving propulsion of the gut content is the peristaltic reflex[6] (Fig. 32-2). Activation of intrinsic primary afferent neurons follows the release of transmitters such as serotonin (5-hydroxytryptamine [5-HT]) from the enteroendocrine cells in the epithelial layer; these cells serve as both chemical and mechanical transducers. The sensory arm of the peristaltic reflex involves activation of intrinsic primary afferent neurons, which release transmitters including calcitonin gene–related peptide and 5-HT to activate the ascending contractile and descending relaxatory arms of the reflex. The excitatory components of the reflex that result in orad contraction are acetylcholine and tachykinins (substances P and K); descending inhibition in the aborad region is mediated predominantly by vasoactive intestinal polypeptide (VIP) and nitric oxide. Other mediators in the peristaltic reflex include opiates, γ-aminobutyric acid, and somatostatin, involved in the descending relaxation phase of the reflex.

Myogenic factors regulate the electrical activity generated by gastrointestinal smooth muscle cells. The interstitial cells of Cajal (ICCs), some of which are located at the interface of the circular and longitudinal muscle layers, form a non-neural pacemaker system and function as intermediaries between the ENS and muscle cells, with which they

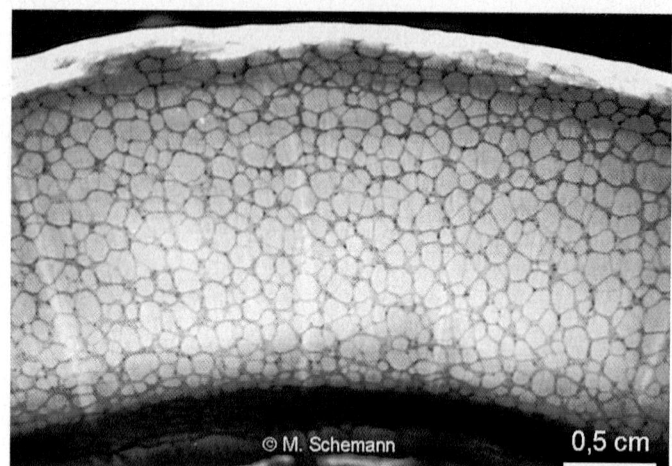

FIGURE 32-1 • Enteric plexus in a whole-mount preparation from the small intestine. (Courtesy of Dr. Michael Schemann, Munich, Germany.)

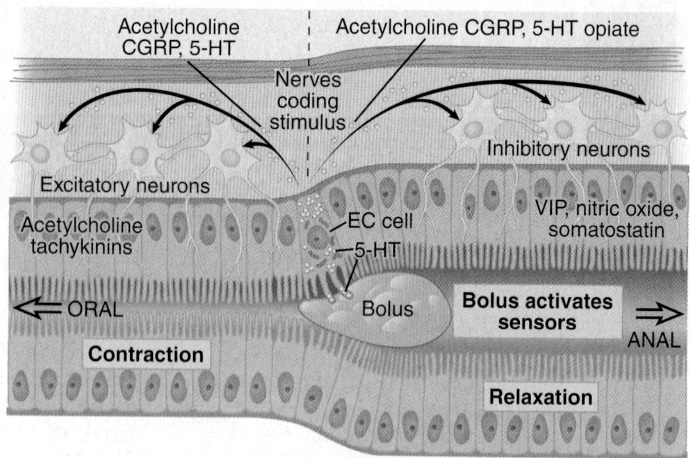

FIGURE 32-2 • Enteric nervous system circuits involved in motility. The peristaltic reflex is the unit of motor function that involves sensing a bolus, ascending contraction, and descending relaxation.

are in proximity.[7,8] Electrical control activity spreads through the contiguous segments of the gut through neurochemical activation by excitatory (e.g., acetylcholine, substance P) and inhibitory (e.g., nitric oxide, somatostatin, VIP) transmitters.[9]

Applied Physiology

Gastric and Small Bowel Motility. The motor functions of the stomach and small intestine are characterized by distinct patterns of activity in the fasting and postprandial periods. The fasting (or interdigestive) period is characterized by a cyclic motor phenomenon called the "interdigestive migrating motor complex" (MMC). In healthy persons, one cycle of the MMC is completed every 60 to 90 minutes.[10,11] The MMC has three phases: a period of quiescence (phase I), a period of intermittent pressure activity (phase II), and an activity front (phase III) during which the stomach and small intestine contract at highest frequency (3 contractions per minute in the stomach and 12 per minute in the upper small intestine). Another characteristic interdigestive motor pattern in the distal small intestine is the "giant migrating complex", or power contraction; it serves to empty residue from the ileum into the colon in bolus transfers.

In the postprandial period, the MMC is replaced in the regions in contact with food by an irregular pressure pattern of variable amplitude and frequency, which enables mixing of food and digestive enzymes. The maximal frequency of contractions is lower than that noted during phase III of the interdigestive MMC. The duration of the postprandial motor activity is proportional to the number of calories consumed during the meal: approximately 1 hour for every 200 kcal ingested. Segments of the small intestine that are not in contact with food continue to display interdigestive motor patterns.

The proximal stomach accommodates food through a decrease in its tone, facilitating the ingestion of food without an increase in pressure. This reflex is mediated by the vagus nerve and involves an intrinsic nitrergic neuron. Liquids empty from the stomach in an exponential manner (Fig. 32-3).[11] The half-emptying time for non-nutrient liquids in healthy persons is usually less than 20 minutes. Solids are selectively retained in the stomach until particles have been triturated to less than 2 mm in diameter. Therefore, gastric emptying of solids is characterized by an initial lag period followed by a linear postlag emptying phase (see Fig. 32-3).

Colonic Motility. The colon serves to provide a site for irregular mixing, absorption, and aboral transit. There are specialized regional functions in the colon.[12] The ascending and transverse regions serve as reservoirs retaining content while fluid and electrolytes are reabsorbed; the descending colon is characterized by relatively rapid transit (conduit); and the sigmoid and rectum constitute a volitional reservoir where stool can be stored until it is socially convenient to pass a bowel

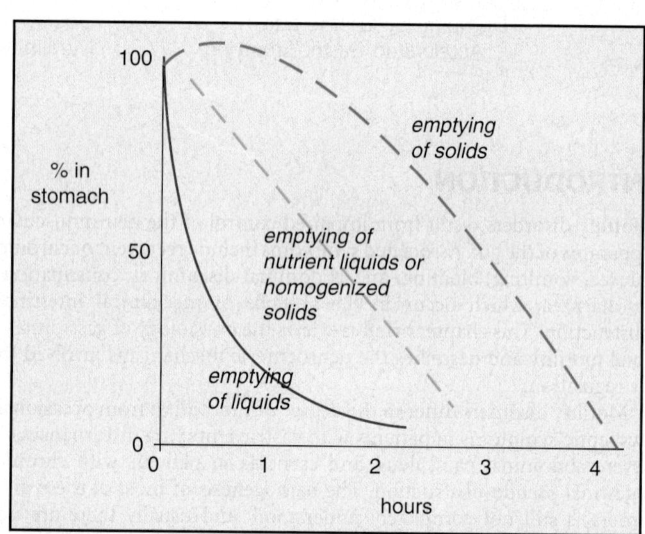

FIGURE 32-3 • Gastric emptying for nutrients of different physical consistencies. Liquids empty exponentially; homogenized solids and nutrient liquids empty in a linear fashion; and solids are initially retained (lag period) for trituration, followed by a generally linear postlag emptying phase.

movement. The colonic contractility consists of a tonic and a phasic component.[13] Bolus transport through the colon occurs through the peristaltic reflex, and mass movements are associated with high-amplitude propagated contractions.

Motility Disorders

Gastroparesis and Chronic Intestinal Pseudo-obstruction

Gastrointestinal motility disturbances result from disorders of the extrinsic nervous system, the ENS, the ICCs (or intestinal pacemakers), or smooth muscle.[1,14] Disorders affecting more than one mechanism occur in systemic sclerosis, amyloidosis, and mitochondrial cytopathy and can present initially with neuropathic patterns; after disease progression, they display myopathic characteristics. Motility disorders can be congenital (affecting the development of the motility apparatus) or acquired.

Gastroparesis is a form of gastric paralysis; chronic symptoms may result from abnormal gastric motility associated with delayed gastric emptying (Fig. 32-4) in the absence of mechanical outlet obstruction, causing significant morbidity.[15] Symptoms are variable and include

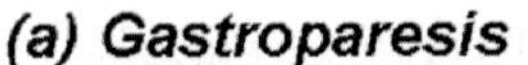

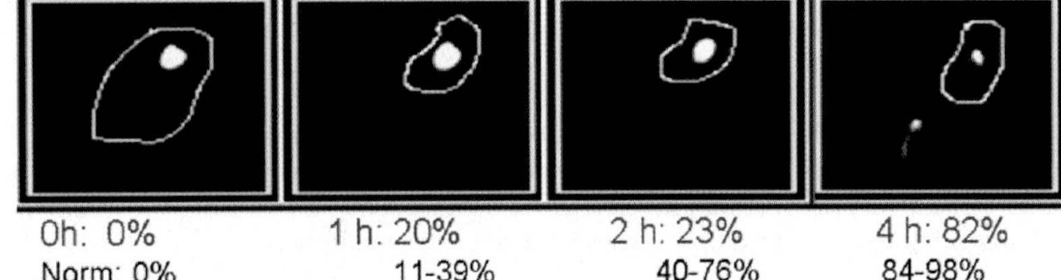

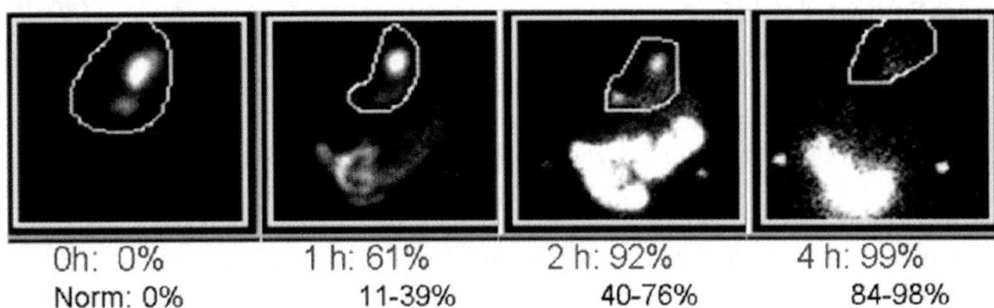

FIGURE 32-4 • Scintigraphic evaluation of gastric emptying by assessing proportion emptied from stomach at hourly intervals. Note delayed gastric emptying, especially at 2 and 4 hours, and accelerated emptying, especially at 1 hour. (From Camilleri M. Clinical Practice: Diabetic gastroparesis. N Engl J Med 2007;356:820-829. Copyright © 1990 Massachusetts Medical Society. All rights reserved.)

early satiety, nausea, vomiting, bloating, and upper abdominal discomfort. Virtually any disease that can induce neuromuscular dysfunction of the gastrointestinal tract may cause gastroparesis. The three most common etiologies are diabetes, idiopathic, and postsurgical. Drugs may be another relevant cause for delayed gastric emptying and gastroparesis. For example, new drugs being developed to restore postprandial normoglycemia may delay gastric emptying. These include analogues of amylin (an enterogastrone produced by pancreatic acinar cells) called pramlintide, and of GLP-1 (an incretin produced by small intestinal enteroendocrine cells) called exenatide. Both retard gastric emptying[16] by inhibition of vagal function, and should be used with caution in gastroparetics. Among diabetics treated with exenatide, 55% of patients developed nausea, and 17% developed vomiting.[17]

Chronic intestinal pseudo-obstruction is an uncommon syndrome characterized by relapsing episodes suggesting intestinal obstruction with no mechanical causes for symptoms.[18,19] Among the variety of etiologies are intrinsic or extrinsic neuropathies, gastrointestinal smooth muscle myopathies, and endocrine, metabolic, and autoimmune diseases. The most common symptoms are nausea, vomiting, abdominal distention, abdominal pain, constipation or diarrhea, and weight loss. These symptoms often present many years before chronic intestinal pseudo-obstruction is diagnosed and are often aggravated by an accompanying intestinal bacterial overgrowth, particularly in myopathic diseases. Malnutrition can cause substantial morbidity and increased mortality.

Dumping Syndrome and Accelerated Gastric Emptying

Dumping syndrome and accelerated gastric emptying (see Fig. 32-4) typically occur after truncal vagotomy and gastric drainage procedures. With the introduction of highly selective vagotomy and the advent of effective antacid secretory therapy, the prevalence of these problems is decreasing.

Rapid gastric emptying is thought to result from impaired gastric accommodation after the ingestion of a meal and the presence of the drainage procedure. A high caloric (usually carbohydrate) content of the liquid phase of the meal evokes a rapid insulin response, with secondary hypoglycemia. These patients also may have impaired antral contractility and gastric stasis of solids, which paradoxically may result in the clinical features of both gastroparesis (for solids) and dumping (for liquids). The most useful investigation is a solid and liquid radioisotopic gastric emptying test.

Slow and Fast Colonic Transit

The two main disturbances in colonic motility are slow colonic transit, resulting in constipation, and fast colonic transit, resulting in diarrhea. Consistency of the stool, which depends on water and electrolyte absorption or secretion, also influences the transit time since more liquid, and hence higher volume stools, are transported through the colon at a faster pace. This is important because pharmacologic methods of influencing colonic transit may be achieved by targeting receptors and neurotransmitters involved in gut motility, and by targeting mechanisms influencing water absorption or secretion.

The cause of abnormal colonic transit in constipation is still incompletely understood. Over the last 2 decades, histologic studies have suggested that there may be quantitative differences in the number of substance P (excitatory nerves reduced) and VIP or nitrergic (inhibitory nerves increased) neurons in the myenteric plexus of resected specimens of colons from patients with severe constipation. More recently, there has been further study of the role of the ICCs in congenital and acquired diseases associated with constipation.

The ICCs are considered the intestinal pacemaker cells. They are typically surrounded by collagen fibers and form close contact with smooth muscle cells, forming gap junctions to transmit the pacemaking activity that reflects the spontaneous oscillation in resting membrane potentials, unaffected by the effects of 10^{-6} M verapamil, an L-type calcium channel blocker. A relative deficiency of tyrosine kinase (c-kit)–positive cells has been reported in Hirschsprung's disease and chronic intestinal pseudo-obstruction. Delayed maturation or maldevelopment of the ICCs may result in neonatal colonic pseudo-obstruction that may be reversible with further maturation of these cells in the myenteric plexus. Megacolon in adults has also been associated with abnormal morphology and ultrastructure of the ICCs.

In patients with acquired slow transit constipation, unassociated with colonic dilation, the number of ICCs in the colon is lower compared to controls (in resection specimens for other indications, typically nonobstructing cancer). Confocal images showed that the ICCs have irregular surface markings and a paucity of branches, and showed reduced numbers of ICCs or of their tyrosine kinase content.

Chronic constipation can also be caused by defecatory disorders due to dysfunction of the pelvic floor or anal sphincter, which may reflexly induce slow colonic transit. A differential diagnosis is important because, in these patients, treatment of the defecatory disorder (e.g., by biofeedback therapy), would be the primary therapy, because restoration of normal defecation would also restore colonic transit in most of these patients. Hence, the diagnostic workup for chronic constipation includes investigation of evacuation disorders by clinical rectal examination, anorectal manometry, and balloon expulsion test.

Postoperative Ileus

Postoperative ileus is a common complication after major abdominal surgery and is characterized by transient intestinal and colonic reduction of motility, or even paralysis.[20,21] The pathophysiology is most likely multifactorial and includes physical manipulation of the bowel, surgical stress, inflammatory mediators (including endogenous opioids), and changes in water and electrolyte balance. It might also be caused or aggravated by the use of opioids in the peri- and postoperative analgesia. The management of postoperative ileus involves a multimodal approach including nasogastric decompression, parenteral nutrition, correction of fluid and electrolyte balance, and substituting nonsteroidal anti-inflammatory drugs for opioids in analgesia.[21,22]

THERAPEUTICS AND CLINICAL PHARMACOLOGY

Goals of Therapy

Drug treatment is only one component of patient management, which should be selected for each patient depending on the regions affected, the severity of the transit abnormality, the presence of dilation (a predictor of bacterial overgrowth), and the nutritional state. The principal methods of management include correction of hydration and nutritional deficiencies, use of prokinetic and antiemetic medications for disorders associated with slow transit, use of agents that retard transit for dumping syndrome, suppression of bacterial overgrowth, decompression, and surgical treatment.[15]

At the mechanistic level, the main targets of current therapy are illustrated in Figure 32-2: acetylcholine, serotonin, somatostatin, and opiates. However, secretory mechanisms at the level of surface epithelial cells (e.g., chloride channels and guanylate cyclase-C) are also targeted to increase fluid secretion and have been shown to accelerate small bowel or colonic transit.

Therapies for fast or slow colonic transit target receptors and neurotransmitters involved in gut motility or mechanisms influencing water absorption or secretion. Novel drugs that modify colonic transit have been specifically evaluated in patients with irritable bowel syndrome (IBS), a highly prevalent functional disorder in which altered bowel habits such as constipation or diarrhea are associated with unexplained abdominal pain, discomfort, and bloating.

Therapeutics by Class

Tables 32-1 and 32-2 summarize the classes of pharmacologic agents used in gastroparesis (Table 32-1) and chronic constipation (Table 32-2). Figure 32-5 also provides a summary of the practical application of pharmacologic and other therapies in gastroparesis based on the severity of gastric emptying delay and nutritional compromise.

Fiber

Increased intake of fluid and fiber increases stool volume and may thereby improve peristalsis and transit. Fiber may be helpful in patients with mild to moderate constipation. However, its use is often limited by the side effects, such as flatulence and bloating. A dose of 12 g is the minimum supplemental dose needed to relieve constipation.

Laxatives

Laxatives may actively or passively (by osmotic gradient) enhance colonic water secretion and stimulate colonic peristalsis. Table 32-2 shows some of the different types of laxatives and their modes of action. Current scientific evidence does not indicate that long-term treatment of laxatives, when used with appropriate care, are harmful. It may be necessary to monitor electrolyte balance in patients who take osmotic laxatives daily or have cardiac or renal insufficiency.

Cholinergic Agents

The gastrointestinal effects of acetylcholine are mediated by nicotinic receptors in the myenteric plexus, and by muscarinic receptor subtypes M_{1-3}, in the myenteric plexus as well as the neuromuscular junction.[23,24] Acetylcholine is the main excitatory neurotransmitter in the gastrointestinal tract.

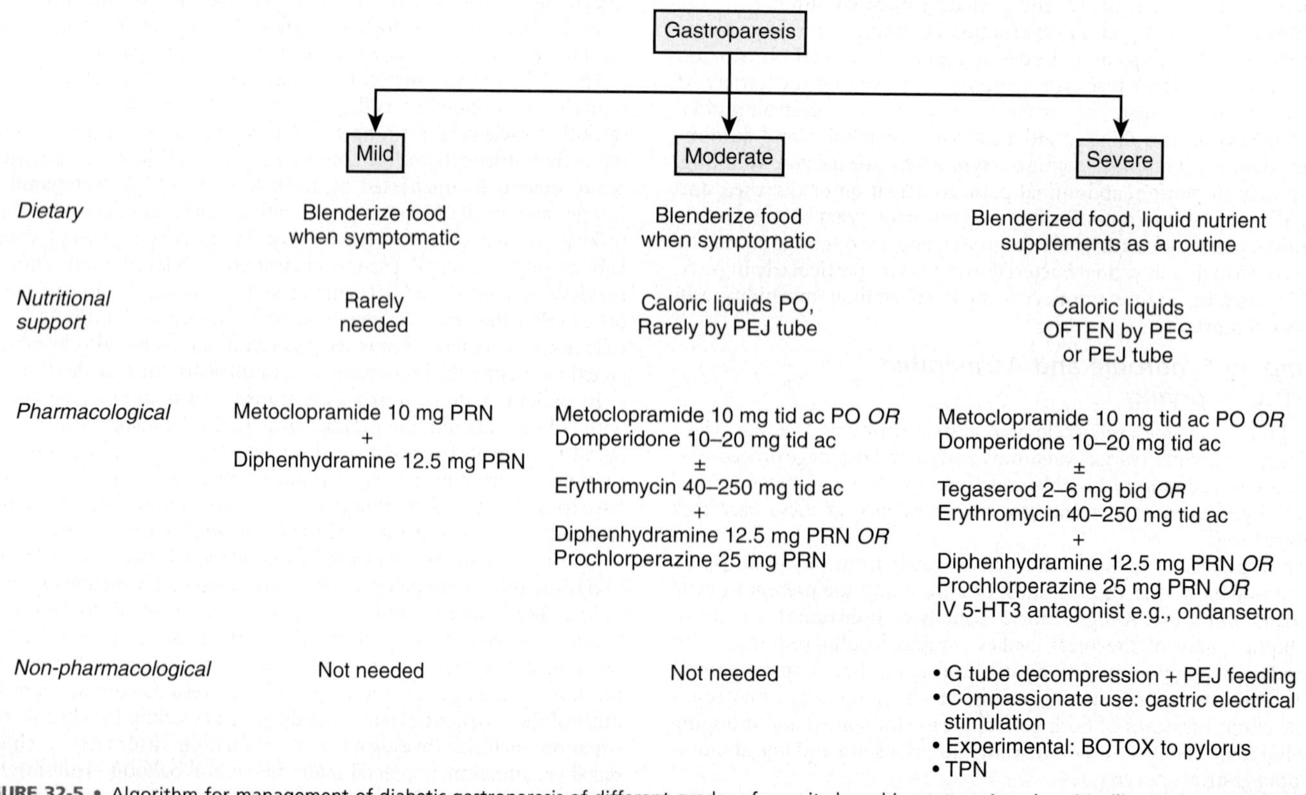

FIGURE 32-5 • Algorithm for management of diabetic gastroparesis of different grades of severity based in part on American Motility Society guidelines[125] and on clinical experience. The degree of gastric retention of solid food at 4 hours provides some guidance, but, generally, progression from left to right and top down is determined by the patient's response to treatment. bid, twice daily; BOTOX, botulinum toxin (40 units × 4 quadrants) injected into pylorus; G tube, gastrostomy tube; IV, intravenous; PEJ, percutaneous endoscopic jejunostomy; PRN, as needed; tid, three times daily. (Adapted from Camilleri M. Clinical Practice: Diabetic gastroparesis. N Engl J Med 2007;356:820-829. Copyright © 1990 Massachusetts Medical Society. All rights reserved.)

TABLE 32-1 PROKINETIC AND ANTIEMETIC MEDICATIONS PROPOSED IN CONSENSUS GUIDELINES* FOR USE IN THE TREATMENT OF GASTROPARESIS

Class of Agent	Examples	Usual Dose (PO Unless Otherwise Stated)	Main Side Effects and Contraindications	Comment
PROKINETICS†				
Dopamine D_2 receptor antagonists, I	Metoclopramide,‡ domperidone§	Start: 5 mg tid Usual dose: 10-20 mg tid, 15 min before meals	Anxiety, depression, extrapyramidal symptoms, rare tardive dyskinesia, galactorrhea	Antiemetic action also provides symptom relief. Metoclopramide (10 mg) also available IM, IV, subQ
Motilin receptor agonists, II	Erythromycin Clarithromycin Azithromycin	40-250 mg tid, 15 min before meals 125-250 mg daily 250 mg daily	Abdominal cramping, appetite loss. Erythromycin contraindicated when drug interactions are anticipated (CYP3A4 metabolism): grapefruit juice, antifungals, cisapride, anticancer drugs (e.g., tamoxifen), antidepressants (e.g., fluoxetine and midazolam), anti-HIV agents (e.g., ritonavir), and antihypertensives (e.g.,verapamil)	Rapid tolerance. Erythromycin useful for acute gastroparesis by IV 3-mg/kg infusion q8h; clarithromycin and azithromycin not formally tested in diabetic gastroparesis.
5-HT_4 receptor agonists, III	Tegaserod Cisapride	2-6 mg bid, 15 min before meals 10-20 mg tid, 15 min before meals	Diarrhea, abdominal pain. Potential for cardiac dysrhythmia with cisapride, cardiovascular events with tegaserod. Cisapride contraindicated when drug interactions anticipated (CYP3A4 metabolism, as above, and erythromycin)	Tegaserod efficacy unclear. Cisapride and tegaserod only available on compassionate use/limited-access program, when other drugs fail.
Muscarinic receptor agonists, III	Bethanechol	10-20 mg tid before meals	Cholinergic side effects (e.g., sweating, bladder dysfunction)	Stimulates gastric emptying; side effects dose limiting; symptom efficacy unclear
Anticholinesterase agents	Physostigmine Neostigmine	30 mg qid 0.5-1 mg IM	Cholinergic side effects (e.g., sweating, bladder dysfunction)	Unclear efficacy
ANTIEMETICS				
Dopamine D_2 receptor antagonists, I	Prochlorperazine Trimethobenzamide	5-10 mg PO, tid, or 5-25 mg PRN q12h rectal suppository 300 mg tid PRN	Extrapyramidal effects, rare jaundice	
Serotonin 5-HT_3 receptor antagonists, III	Ondansetron Granisetron Dolasetron Tropisetron	4-8 mg tid PRN 1 mg bid 50-100 mg PRN Only IV 2-5 mg	Constipation with regular use	Unclear efficacy compared to D_2 antagonists; also available IV
Muscarinic M_1 receptor antagonists, III	Scopolamine patch	1 mg per 3 days	Drowsiness, headache, dry mouth; may be worse on withdrawal Contraindicated with glaucoma, bladder emptying problems	Unclear efficacy for nausea or vomiting of gastroparesis
Histamine H_1 receptor antagonists, II	Dimenhydrinate Meclizine Promethazine	50 mg tid PRN 12.5-25 mg tid PRN 12.5-25 mg IM PRN	Drowsiness, blurred vision, headache, or dry mouth. Contraindicated with glaucoma, bladder emptying problems.	Also available as suppository
Benzodiazepines, III	Lorazepam	0.5-1 mg PRN	Sedation	Unclear efficacy for gastroparesis
Neurokinin NK_1 receptor antagonist, III	Aprepitant	125 mg	Weakness, bowel dysfunction, reduced efficacy of birth control pill. Contraindicated with astemizole, cisapride, pimozide, terfenadine.	Unclear efficacy for gastroparesis

*Guidelines published in Abell et al.[125] and Parkman et al.[126] Two other drug classes, antidepressants and cannabinoid agonists, are included in the list of drugs considered in the consensus guideline published in Abell et al.[125] However, they may both retard gastric emptying and are of unclear efficacy for gastroparesis, and cannabinoids may cause problems with memory and learning, distorted perception, anxiety, or panic attacks.

†Roman numerals refer to line of therapy based on efficacy, cost, ease of administration, and adverse effects.

‡Metoclopramide is the only medication approved by the U.S. Food and Drug Administration (FDA) for this indication.

§Domperidone can be obtained through an FDA investigational new drug application with local Institutional Review Board approval.

bid, twice daily; CYP3A4, cytochrome P-450 isozyme 3A4; IM, intramuscular; IV, intravenous; PRN, as needed; qid, four times daily; subQ, subcutaneous; tid, three times daily.

Adapted from Camilleri M. Clinical Practice: Diabetic gastroparesis. N Engl J Med 2007;356:820-829.

TABLE 32-2 LAXATIVES AND STOOL SOFTENERS FOR THE TREATMENT OF SLOW COLONIC TRANSIT/CONSTIPATION

	Generic Name(s)	Dosage	Comments
Bulk Laxatives			Increase colonic residue, stimulating peristalsis.
	Psyllium	Titrate up to ~20 g	Natural fiber; should be taken with plenty of water to avoid intestinal obstruction. Bacterial degradation may contribute to bloating and flatus. Allergic reactions such as anaphylaxis and asthma are rare.
	Methylcellulose	Titrate up to ~20 g	Semisynthetic cellulose fiber relatively resistant to colonic bacterial degradation.
	Polycarbophil	Titrate up to ~20 g	Synthetic fiber of polymer of acrylic acid, resistant to bacterial degradation.
Osmotic Laxatives			Draw water into the intestines along osmotic gradient
Saline Laxatives			
Magnesium	Magnesium hydroxide Magnesium citrate	15-30 ml daily–bid 150-300 ml PRN	A small percentage of magnesium is actively absorbed in the small intestines. Hypermagnesemia can occur in patients with renal failure and in children.
Phosphate	Sodium phosphate	10-25 ml with 12 oz of water PRN	Hyperphosphatemia in patients with renal insufficiency. Commonly used for bowel preparation prior to colonoscopy.
Poorly Absorbed Sugars			
Disaccharides	Lactulose	15-30 ml daily–bid	Synthetic disaccharide consisting of galactose and fructose linked by bond resistant to disaccharidases; not absorbed by small intestine. Undergoes bacterial fermentation in the colon with formation of short-chain fatty acids. Gas and bloating are common.
Sugar alcohols	Sorbitol or mannitol	15-30 ml daily–bid	Poorly absorbed by human intestine; undergo bacterial fermentation.
Polyethylene glycol	Polyethylene glycol–electrolyte Polyethylene glycol-3350	17-36 g daily–bid 17-36 g daily–bid	Organic polymers, poorly absorbed and not metabolized by colonic bacteria, hence less bloating and cramps.[127] Can be mixed with noncarbonated beverages. Polyethylene glycol-3350 does not include electrolytes and is packaged for regular daily use.
Stimulant Laxatives			Stimulate intestinal motility or secretion
Anthraquinones			Converted by colonic bacteria to their active form
	Cascara sagrada Senna	325 mg (or 5 ml) at bedtime 187 mg daily	May cause pseudo-melanosis coli, a benign condition that is usually reversible within 12 months of cessation. No definitive association between anthraquinones and colon cancer or myenteric nerve damage has been established.
Ricinoleic acid	Castor oil	15-30 ml at bedtime	Hydrolyzed by lipase in the small intestine to ricinoleic acid, which inhibits intestinal water absorption, increases mucosal permeability, and stimulates motor function due to release of neurotransmitters from damage to mucosal enterochromaffin cells. Cramping and severe diarrhea are common.
Diphenylmethane derivatives	Bisacodyl	5-10 mg at bedtime	Hydrolyzed by endogenous esterases and stimulates secretion and motility of small intestine and colon.
	Sodium picosulfate	5-15 mg at bedtime	Hydrolyzed to its active form by colonic bacterial enzymes; affects only the colon.
Stool Softeners	Docusate sodium	100 mg bid	Ionic detergents soften stool by allowing water to interact more effectively with solid stool; modest fluid secretion. Efficacy in constipation is not well established.
Emollient	Mineral oil	5-15 ml PO at bedtime	Emulsified into the stool mass, providing lubrication for the passage of stool. Long-term use can cause malabsorption of fat-soluble vitamins, anal seepage. Lipoid pneumonia may occur in patients predisposed to aspiration of liquids.
Rectal Enemas/ Suppositories	Phosphate enema Mineral oil retention enema Tap water enema Soap suds enema Glycerin Bisacodyl suppositories	120 ml PRN 100 ml PRN 500 ml PRN 1500 ml PRN 10 mg PRN 10 mg PRN	Initiate evacuation by distending the rectum, softening hard stool, and topically stimulating the colonic muscle to contract.[128] Hyperphosphatemia and other electrolyte abnormalities can occur if the enema is retained.

bid, twice daily; PRN, as needed.
Adapted from Lembo A, Camilleri M. Chronic constipation. N Engl J Med 2003;349:1360-1368.

Cholinergics. Neostigmine is a cholinesterase inhibitor that enhances the amount of acetylcholine in the synaptic cleft. In severe cases of acute colonic pseudo-obstruction, intravenous neostigmine was shown to be effective in decompressing the colon.[25,26] Systemic cholinergic side effects would limit its potential use to severe cases of constipation.

Anticholinergics. Nonselective anticholinergics or specific antimuscarinic anticholinergics reduce bowel motility and associated pain. They are often considered with the group of smooth muscle relaxant drugs that act directly on the smooth muscle (e.g., by blocking smooth muscle Ca^{2+} channels). Several compounds (mebeverine, otilinium, pinaverium, and cimetropium) used in Europe as standard treatment of IBS have never been approved in the United States.

Newer anticholinergic agents are being developed to specifically target the muscarinic type 3 receptor (M_3) in the intestinal smooth muscle in order to decrease the nonspecific anticholinergic side effects (dry mouth or increased heart rate). Several agents have shown promising gastrointestinal effects in animal models.[27] The M_3-selective antagonist darifenacin is used to treat overactive bladder, and is associated with increased constipation.[28] Another M_3-selective antagonist, zamifenacin, significantly reduced colonic motility without significant nonspecific anticholinergic effects in a study of 36 IBS patients.[29]

Serotonergic Agents

Serotonin (5-hydroxytryptamine [5-HT]) is found primarily within the gastrointestinal tract (80% of body 5-HT stores), where it is stored in gut enteroendocrine cells (95%) and in enteric neurons (5%). 5-HT plays a pivotal role in the modulation of multiple gut functions such as motility, peristaltic reflex, sensation, blood flow, and secretion. 5-HT also acts as a neurotransmitter in the CNS and the brain-gut axis. Released from enteroendocrine cells in response to luminal mechanical or chemical stimulation, 5-HT acts via a variety of 5-HT receptors either directly (on muscle or enterocytes) or indirectly (through intrinsic neurons) to modulate gastrointestinal function. Serotonergic receptors also occur on vagal and visceral afferent cell bodies.[30] The main receptors involved in the gastrointestinal serotonin functions are the 5-HT_3 and 5-HT_4 receptors.[31,32] The 5-HT_4 receptor appears to play a key role in the peristaltic reflex. 5-HT_3 receptors are involved in visceral, spinal, vagal, brainstem, and limbic sensory mechanisms.

5-HT activity is regulated in part by the 5-HT reuptake transporter protein (SERT). Coates et al. have found that the colonic mucosa of patients with IBS had reduced expression of SERT (messenger RNA and immunohistochemistry).[33] This has not been confirmed in a study from a different laboratory.[34]

Thus, serotonergic mechanisms play a key role in the neurohumoral brain-gut axis in health and disease and are important targets for gut motility disorders.

5-HT_4 Agonists

Established. Cisapride is a 5-HT_4 agonist that facilitates release of acetylcholine from myenteric cholinergic nerves throughout the gut. It was one of the more effective prokinetics; it stimulates antral and duodenal contractions, improves antroduodenal coordination, and accelerates gastric emptying[35,36] and small bowel transit in chronic intestinal dysmotility. Cisapride accelerates gastric emptying and decreases symptoms in patients with gastroparesis for 1 year.[36,37] However, it has been withdrawn from use as it prolongs the QT interval in a dose-dependent manner and was associated with potentially fatal cardiac arrhythmias.[38]

Tegaserod is a selective 5-HT_4 receptor agonist that plays a key role in the peristaltic reflex and has been used in many countries for the treatment of constipation-predominant IBS (C-IBS) and chronic constipation. While several clinical studies demonstrated prokinetic action of tegaserod in the small intestine and the colon,[39,40] data regarding accelerating gastric emptying in humans is less consistent. While animal models of diabetic gastroparesis suggest improvement of gastric emptying, results in healthy humans are contradictory.[41-43]

Tegaserod is also a potent 5-HT_{2B} receptor antagonist, but it is currently unclear whether this contributes to the clinical efficacy profile

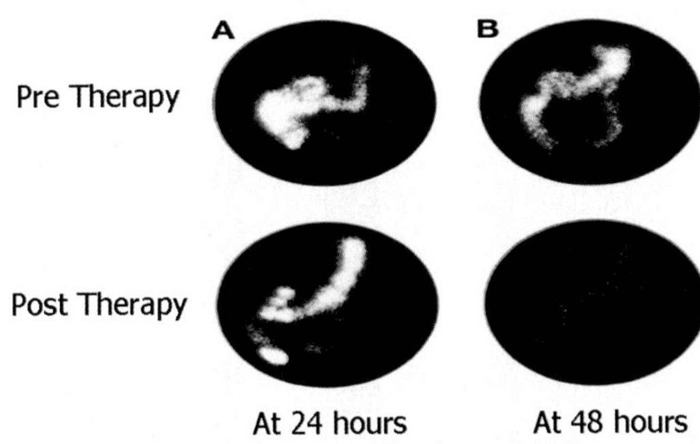

FIGURE 32-6 • Effects of the 5-HT_4 agonist tegaserod on colonic transit time (assessed by scintigraphy) in patients with constipation-predominant irritable bowel syndrome. (From Prather CM, Camilleri M, Zinsmeister AR, et al. Tegaserod accelerates orocecal transit in patients with constipation-predominant irritable bowel syndrome. Gastroenterology 2000;118:463-468.)

of the drug.[44] In pharmacodynamic studies, tegaserod accelerated small bowel transit (2 mg twice daily) and colonic transit (6 mg twice daily) in patients with IBS and constipation[39,40] (Fig. 32-6). A Cochrane meta-analysis[45] reviewed eight randomized, controlled trials in nearly 3000 mostly female patients with C-IBS. The studies showed significant improvement of the subject's overall assessment of relief as the primary end point and of abdominal pain, bowel movement frequency, and consistency as secondary end points. The only relevant adverse effect was transient diarrhea in about 10% of recipients. Other studies supported the efficacy of tegaserod in patients with C-IBS with both repeated[46,47] and long-term treatment.[48] Tegaserod also proved efficacious in the treatment of chronic constipation.[49,50]

Tegaserod was withdrawn by the U.S. Food and Drug Administration (FDA) in March 2007 because of a reported numerical imbalance in the number of patients with cardiovascular adverse events in trials for patients who received tegaserod compared to those on placebo.

Experimental. ATI-7505[51] is a novel, potent agonist of the 5-HT_4 receptor and is chemically related to cisapride. It has been chemically designed to eliminate cardiac liabilities (e.g., QT prolongation, tachycardia) and cytochrome P-450 isozyme 3A4–dependent metabolism at therapeutically relevant concentrations. Available human safety data indicate no cardiac side effects. Recent pharmacodynamic data in healthy human volunteers[52] indicate prokinetic effects with acceleration of gastric emptying (20 mg three times daily) and colonic transit (10 mg three times daily) (Fig. 32-7).

5-HT_3 Receptor Antagonists. 5-HT_3 receptors are located on extrinsic sensory afferents. Antagonism of the 5-HT_3 receptor has been shown to delay gastrointestinal transit, reduce secretion, and increase colonic compliance in response to distention. 5-HT_3 antagonists reduce abdominal pain in diarrhea-prdominant IBS (D-IBS) in clinical trials. This may result from effects on 5-HT_3 receptors of the brain.[53]

Established. Alosetron was the first 5-HT_3 antagonist to be developed for the treatment of D-IBS. At least 10 large, multicenter, randomized, controlled clinical trials reviewed in a meta-analysis[54] have demonstrated alosetron to be effective in improving abdominal pain and discomfort and global IBS symptoms, reducing stool frequency and urgency, and increasing stool consistency in patients with D-IBS or nonconstipated IBS. The estimated relative risk (with 95% confidence intervals [CIs]) for alosetron versus comparators were 1.55 (1.4, 1.72) for global improvement of IBS symptoms, and 1.24 (1.16, 1.34) for relief of abdominal pain and discomfort.

The most important adverse effect of alosetron is constipation, reported in 20% to 30% of patients in trials. Rare cases of ischemic colitis have been attributed to alosetron, with an estimated incidence of approximately 0.1%. The medication can be prescribed for patients with severe D-IBS.

Experimental. Cilansetron is another 5-HT_3 antagonist that is being developed for the treatment of both men and women with D-IBS.

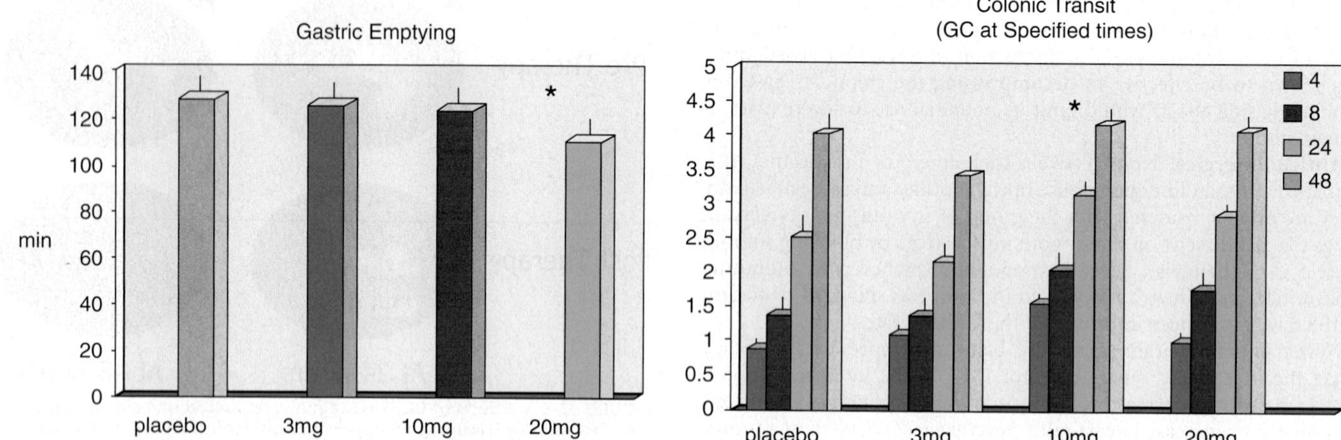

FIGURE 32-7 • Effect of ATI-7570, a novel 5-HT$_4$ agonist, on gastric and colonic transit. (From Camilleri M, Vazquez-Roque MI, Burton D, et al. Pharmacodynamic effects of a novel prokinetic 5-HT$_4$ receptor agonist, ATI-7505, in humans. Neurogastroenterol Motil 2007;19:30-38.)

Efficacy was tested in over 4000 patients and appears to be similar to that of alosetron.[55,56] Cilansetron was also associated with constipation and rare cases of ischemic colitis. It has not been approved for marketing.[57]

The relationship between 5-HT$_3$ antagonists and ischemic colitis is still unclear. It has been reported that IBS itself might be associated with an increased incidence of ischemic colitis.[58] It is conceivable that, in some cases, the initial diagnosis of IBS might have been incorrect due to overlap of nonspecific symptoms. Further research is warranted to identify potential risk factors for ischemic colitis in IBS and potential interactions with 5-HT$_3$ antagonists, to provide these female and male patients with the opportunity to be treated with a class of drugs that is particularly effective for diarrhea, urgency, and pain in IBS.[59,60]

Mixed 5-HT$_4$ Agonist/5-HT$_3$ Antagonist/5-HT$_{2B}$ Antagonist. Another serotonergic agent developed for the treatment of constipation and C-IBS is renzapride, a full agonist of the 5-HT$_4$ receptor and also an antagonist of the 5-HT$_3$ and the 5-HT$_{2B}$ receptors. In a placebo-controlled pharmacodynamic Phase II study,[61] three doses of renzapride (1, 2, and 4 mg) were tested versus placebo in 48 mostly female patients with C-IBS. A statistically significant linear dose response to renzapride was detected for colonic transit and ascending colonic emptying time, but not for gastric emptying or small bowel transit time. The acceleration of colonic transit time was significantly associated with improvement of bowel function scores.[61] No significant adverse clinical, laboratory, or electrocardiogram effects were observed. Phase IIb clinical trials also show efficacy in the relief of symptoms.[62,63] These studies indicate that renzapride may have beneficial effects in patients with constipation and C-IBS.

Dopamine Antagonists

Established. Metoclopramide has both prokinetic actions in the proximal gut and central antiemetic activity. The antiemetic effect results from dopamine (D$_2$) and serotonin (5-HT$_3$) receptor antagonism on vagal and brainstem pathways and on the vomiting center.[64] Prokinetic effects are related to the facilitation of acetylcholine release from enteric cholinergic neurons (5-HT$_4$ receptors), or dopamine D$_2$ receptor antagonism in the myenteric plexus, and to direct smooth muscle contraction via muscarinic receptor sensitization.[65] Metoclopramide is effective for the short-term treatment of gastroparesis for up to several weeks.[66,67] Dopamine D$_2$ receptor antagonism may also result in high prolactin levels and gynecomastia. The long-term utility of metoclopramide has not been proven.[68] Metoclopramide can be administered parenterally (intravenously, intramuscularly, or subcutaneously) when symptoms are severe, but its use is limited by CNS side effects in up to 40% of patients.[68] Restricting the total daily dose to 40 mg per day and using the liquid formula to improve the pharmacokinetics of the drug tend to reduce the central side effects while providing improved efficacy. Efficacy of metoclopramide has been demonstrated mostly in small, often single-center studies rather than in large Phase III trials.

Domperidone is another dopamine D$_2$ receptor antagonist with evidence of efficacy as an antiemetic and prokinetic (at doses up to 20 mg four times daily) in the published literature.[69,70] It is available in the United States through an FDA-approved investigational drug process.

Experimental. Itopride is a novel prokinetic compound with dopamine D$_2$ receptor antagonism and acetylcholinesterase inhibitory actions. While the drug has not yet been evaluated in gastroparesis, a fairly large clinical trial in patients with functional dyspepsia suggested beneficial effects in the treatment of dyspeptic symptoms.[71] A recent pharmacodynamic study could not identify significant effects of the drug on gastric accommodation or emptying in healthy human subjects.[72] A preliminary report of two large Phase III, randomized, controlled trials showed no benefit of itopride over placebo in the treatment of functional dyspepsia.[73]

Motilin Agonists

Established. Erythromycin is most effective when used intravenously (e.g., erythromycin lactobionate, 3 mg/kg every 8 hours by infusion in 100 ml saline over 45 minutes). It stimulates motilin and cholinergic receptors,[74] and induces dumping of food and nondigestible material from the stomach. There is some evidence of efficacy in long-term use of the oral preparation[75] and even in a 4-week trial of patients with scleroderma. Atilmotin, another novel intravenous motilide, also showed promising prokinetic effects on gastric emptying.[76]

Experimental. A novel motilide, mitemcinal (also called GM-611),[77,78] is an acid-resistant macrolide with minimal antibiotic activity, having direct action on muscle motilin receptors. It showed great promise by increasing gastric emptying, and its effects on symptoms of gastroparesis are being evaluated.

Opioid Agents

The three major opioid receptors, μ, δ, and κ, are distributed in the peripheral and central nervous systems. Activation of μ-receptors modulates visceral nociception and slows down gastrointestinal transit.[79-81]

Peripheral μ-Opioid Agonists. The effects of μ-agonists on colonic motility are utilized for the treatment of diarrhea. The classic agents, loperamide and diphenoxylate, do not pass the blood-brain barrier and do not exhibit central effects such as pain relief, sedation, or central addiction. These agents have widely been shown to be effective in the treatment of acute and chronic diarrhea.[82-85]

Experimental Peripheral μ-Opioid Antagonists. Classic pain medications such as codeine or morphine are μ-agonists with both

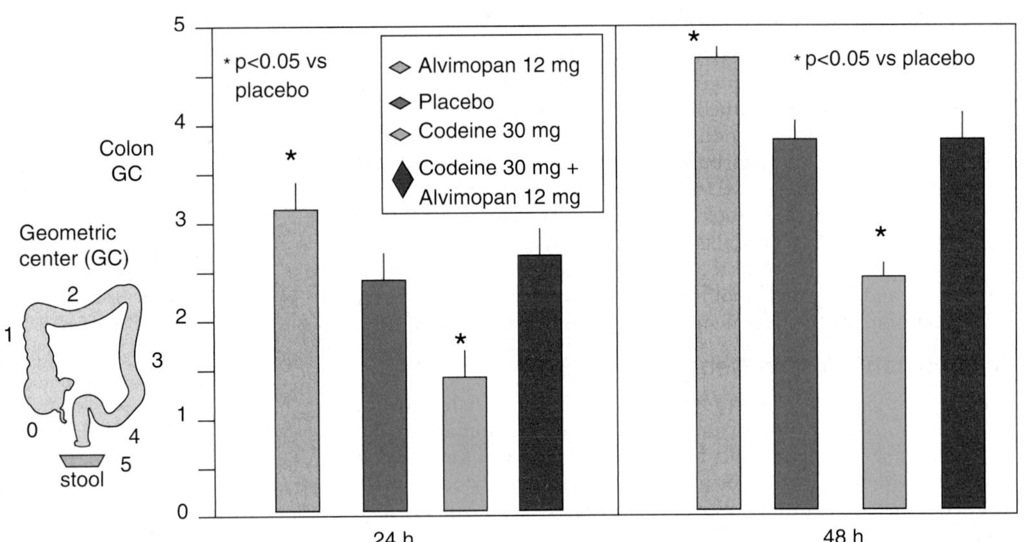

FIGURE 32-8 • Effect of alvimopam, a periplural μ-opioid antagonist on colonic transit, and reversal of effects of codeine. (From Gonenne J, Camilleri M, Ferber I, et al. Effect of alvimopan and codeine on gastrointestinal transit: a randomized controlled study. Clin Gastroenterol Hepatol 2005;3:784-791.)

central and peripheral action, with constipation as a common side effect. Peripherally restricted μ-opioid receptor antagonists may offer new treatment strategies for opioid-induced or slow colonic transit constipation.

Alvimopan, a novel, peripherally restricted μ-opioid antagonist, is effective in the treatment of opioid-induced constipation and postoperative ileus.[86-88] It reverses the peripheral effects of narcotics without influencing the pain relief desired by concomitant opioid administration. A pharmacodynamic study in healthy volunteers[89] confirmed that alvimopan (12 mg twice daily) reversed the colonic transit delay induced by coadministered codeine. Interestingly, alvimopan alone accelerated colonic transit, suggesting that the μ-opiate mechanisms participate in the physiologic control of colonic transit (Fig. 32-8). Future trials to test the effects of alvimopan in patients with constipation, C-IBS, and opiate-induced constipation and to explore dose-related effects are warranted.

Alvimopan reverses the peripheral effects of narcotics without influencing the pain relief desired by concomitant opioid administration. A recent meta-analysis evaluated five clinical trials including more than 2000 patients randomized to alvimopan or placebo for the treatment of postoperative ileus.[90] In this analysis, alvimopan was significantly superior to placebo in restoring gastrointestinal function (cumulative estimated hazard ratio 1.30 [95% CIs: 1.16, 1.45] for the composite end point passage of flatus, stool, and tolerance of solid food) and in reducing time to discharge (cumulative estimated hazard ratio 1.26 [95% CIs: 1.13, 1.40]). Analgesic effects of postoperative opioid therapy remained unchanged by alvimopan, and side effects were similar between alvimopan and placebo.

Methylnaltrexone is another peripherally restricted opioid antagonist that is also being developed for the treatment of opioid-induced side effects, including constipation and postoperative bowel dysfunctions.[91-93]

Somatostatin Analogue

The somatostatin analogue octreotide activates predominantly somatostatin type 2 receptors, reduces gastrointestinal secretion, retards gastrointestinal transit, and has antinociceptive properties. The management of dumping syndrome includes dietary maneuvers (avoidance of high-nutrient liquid drinks and, possibly, addition of guar gum or pectin to retard gastric emptying of liquids). Pharmacologic treatment with octreotide (50 to 100 mcg subcutaneously before meals) may be needed.[94,95] It retards gastrointestinal transit and inhibits the hormonal responses that lead to hypoglycemia.

Subcutaneous octreotide has been shown to reduce carcinoid-associated diarrhea, flush symptoms, and even tumor growth and is therefore widely used in the treatment of carcinoid syndrome.[96] Beneficial effects of octreotide in other disorders associated with chronic diarrhea were demonstrated, for example, in cancer patients with chronic loperamide-refractory diarrhea not related to cancer treatment[97] and in patients with D-IBS.[98,99]

Chlorine Channel Agonist

Volume-regulated chloride channels such as type 2 (ClC_2) and type 3 are found in most mammalian and nonmammalian cell types, including those in the gastrointestinal tract and liver.[100,101] These channels contribute to several cellular functions, including cell volume regulation and epithelial Cl^- transport and fluid secretion. Intestinal Cl^- secretion is critical for intestinal fluid and electrolyte transport. In the gastrointestinal tract, ClC_2 has been found in gastric parietal cells, and small intestinal and colonic epithelia.

Lubiprostone is a prostone that acts as a selective ClC_2 activator and increases intestinal water secretion.[102] Several clinical trials have demonstrated that lubiprostone has positive effects on stool consistency, frequency, and straining, and that it is safe and effective for treating constipation.[103-105] In a pharmacodynamic study, lubiprostone was shown to accelerate small bowel and colonic transit time in healthy volunteers.[106] Side effects of lubiprostone include diarrhea and nausea that is usually mild and transient and not associated with alteration of gastric function.[106] Lubiprostone is approved for the treatment of chronic "idiopathic" constipation.

Emerging Targets and Therapeutics

Ghrelin

Ghrelin has been shown to accelerate gastric emptying in studies in patients with diabetic gastroparesis or idiopathic gastroparesis.[107] These actions require pharmacologic doses far in excess of the doses required to stimulate growth hormone release.[108-110] To date, efficacy in symptom relief appears low. Synthetic ghrelin agonists are being tested.

Phosphodiesterase Inhibition

Phosphodiesterase-5 inhibition with sildenafil restores gastric emptying of liquids in an animal model of diabetes,[111] suggesting sildenafil has potential as a new therapeutic agent for diabetic gastroparesis. Sildenafil also reduced the dysrhythmia of the stomach induced experimentally by hyperglycemia in humans.[112] On the other hand, a thorough study of the effects of sildenafil on human gastric sensorimotor functions showed that the drug significantly increases postprandial gastric volume and slows liquid (though not solid) emptying rate.[113] Sildenafil also inhibits interdigestive motor activity of the antrum and duodenum. Clinical trials are clearly needed before this medication can be considered for the treatment of gastroparesis.

Guanylate Cyclase-C Agonist

Linaclotide (MD-1100 acetate) is a novel, first-in-class compound acting as an agonist of human guanylate cyclase-C, a transmembrane protein located in the gut epithelium. Activation of guanylate cyclase-C induces secretion of fluid, sodium, and bicarbonate in the intestinal lumen and inhibits fluid absorption in the colon.[114-117] In animal and early human safety studies, MD-1100 has been observed to increase stool frequency, decrease stool consistency, and decrease visceral pain.[118] In a recent Phase II trial in patients with IBS and constipation, linaclotide significantly accelerated colonic transit and decreased stool consistency, and increased stool frequency. Therefore, the drug seems to be promising for the treatment of chronic constipation and C-IBS.

Recombinant Human Neurotrophin-3

Neurotrophin-3 (NT-3) is a neurotrophic factor involved in the growth, development, and function of the nervous system. In studies for the treatment of several neurologic disorders, this factor was found to be associated with increased stool frequency and softened stool consistency, which led to investigation of the effects of subcutaneously injected NT-3 on gastrointestinal transit and bowel functions in healthy subjects and patients with functional constipation.

In a pharmacodynamic study,[119] NT-3 accelerated overall colonic transit in health and constipation and gastric and small bowel transit in health. This was associated with an increased stool frequency in healthy and constipated subjects and a decreased stool consistency in constipated patients. A subsequent dose-ranging study in 107 patients with functional constipation[120] confirmed these effects by showing an increased stool frequency, a dose-related softening of stool, and an improved ease of passage. Overall, the most common adverse effects were injection site reactions, mild paresthesia, and decreases in temperature and diastolic blood pressure. High costs related to the recombinant production of human NT-3 may limit its further development for broad indications such as chronic constipation or C-IBS.

Device-Based Therapies

Gastric electrical stimulation may improve symptoms in patients with severe gastroparesis.[121-123] In humans, gastric pacing has not been able to entrain gastric slow waves to normalize gastric dysrhythmias or to accelerate gastric emptying. Gastric electrical stimulation is an approved treatment as a humanitarian use device; further controlled clinical trials are needed to assess the long-term benefits, complications, and optimal selection of patients for this treatment. Electrical stimulation is also an experimental therapy for severe chronic constipation.[124]

REFERENCES

1. Camilleri M. Diagnosis and treatment of enteric neuromuscular diseases. Clin Auton Res 2003;13:10-15.
2. Gershon MD. The enteric nervous system: a second brain. Hosp Pract (Minneap) 1999;34:31-32, 35-38, 41-42 passim.
3. Grundy D, Schemann M. Enteric nervous system. Curr Opin Gastroenterol 2006;22:102-110.
4. Kellow JE, Azpiroz F, Delvaux M, et al. Applied principles of neurogastroenterology: physiology/motility sensation. Gastroenterology 2006;130:1412-1420.
5. Grundy D, Al-Chaer ED, Aziz Q, et al. Fundamentals of neurogastroenterology: basic science. Gastroenterology 2006;130:1391-1411.
6. De Ponti F, Cosentino M, Lecchini S, et al. Physiopharmacology of the peristaltic reflex: an update. Ital J Gastroenterol 1991;23:264-269.
7. Huizinga JD. Physiology and pathophysiology of the interstitial cell of Cajal: from bench to bedside. II. Gastric motility: lessons from mutant mice on slow waves and innervation. Am J Physiol Gastrointest Liver Physiol 2001;281:G1129-G1134.
8. Barajas-Lopez C, Berezin I, Daniel EE, Huizinga JD. Pacemaker activity recorded in interstitial cells of Cajal of the gastrointestinal tract. Am J Physiol Cell Physiol 1989;257:C830-C835.
9. Huizinga JD. Gastrointestinal peristalsis: joint action of enteric nerves, smooth muscle, and interstitial cells of Cajal. Microsc Res Tech 1999;47:239-247.
10. Phillips SF, Camilleri M. Antroduodenal manometry. Dig Dis Sci 1992;37:1305-1308.
11. Camilleri M, Hasler WL, Parkman HP, et al. Measurement of gastrointestinal motility in the GI laboratory. Gastroenterology 1998;115:747-762.
12. Ford MJ, Camilleri M, Wiste JA, Hanson RB. Differences in colonic tone and phasic response to a meal in the transverse and sigmoid human colon. Gut 1995;37:264-269.
13. O'Brien MD, Camilleri M, von der Ohe MR, et al. Motility and tone of the left colon in constipation: a role in clinical practice? Am J Gastroenterol 1996;91:2532-2538.
14. De Giorgio R, Camilleri M. Human enteric neuropathies: morphology and molecular pathology. Neurogastroenterol Motil 2004;16:515-531.
15. Park MI, Camilleri M. Gastroparesis: clinical update. Am J Gastroenterol 2006;101:1129-1139.
16. Edwards CM, Stanley SA, Davis R, et al. Exendin-4 reduces fasting and postprandial glucose and decreases energy intake in healthy volunteers. Am J Physiol Endocrinol Metab 2001;281:E155-E161.
17. Calara F, Taylor K, Han J, et al. A randomized, open-label, crossover study examining the effect of injection site on bioavailability of exenatide (synthetic exendin-4). Clin Ther 2005;27:210-215.
18. Sutton DH, Harrell SP, Wo JM. Diagnosis and management of adult patients with chronic intestinal pseudoobstruction. Nutr Clin Pract 2006;21:16-22.
19. Delgado-Aros S, Camilleri M. [Clinical management of acute colonic pseudo-obstruction in patients: a systematic review of the literature]. Gastroenterol Hepatol 2003;26:646-655.
20. Kehlet H, Holte K. Review of postoperative ileus. Am J Surg 2001;182:3S-10S.
21. Person B, Wexner SD. The management of postoperative ileus. Curr Probl Surg 2006;43:6-65.
22. Holte K, Kehlet H. Postoperative ileus: progress towards effective management. Drugs 2002;62:2603-2615.
23. Goyal RK. Muscarinic receptor subtypes: physiology and clinical implications. N Engl J Med 1989;321:1022-1029.
24. Eglen RM. Muscarinic receptors and gastrointestinal tract smooth muscle function. Life Sci 2001;68:2573-2578.
25. Saunders MD. Acute colonic pseudoobstruction. Curr Gastroenterol Rep 2004;6:410-416.
26. Loftus CG, Harewood GC, Baron TH. Assessment of predictors of response to neostigmine for acute colonic pseudo-obstruction. Am J Gastroenterol 2002;97:3118-3122.
27. Kobayashi S, Ikeda K, Suzuki M, et al. Effects of YM905, a novel muscarinic M3-receptor antagonist, on experimental models of bowel dysfunction in vivo. Jpn J Pharmacol 2001;86:281-288.
28. Foote J, Glavind K, Kralidis G, Wyndaele JJ. Treatment of overactive bladder in the older patient: pooled analysis of three Phase III studies of darifenacin, an M3 selective receptor antagonist. Eur Urol 2005;48:471-477.
29. Houghton LA, Rogers J, Whorwell PJ, et al. Zamifenacin (UK-76,654) a potent gut M3 selective muscarinic antagonist, reduces colonic motor activity in patients with irritable bowel syndrome. Aliment Pharmacol Ther 1997;11:561-568.
30. Hicks GA, Coldwell JR, Schindler M, et al. Excitation of rat colonic afferent fibres by 5-HT_3 receptors. J Physiol (Lond) 2002;544:861-869.
31. Gershon MD. Review article: roles played by 5-hydroxytryptamine in the physiology of the bowel. Aliment Pharmacol Ther 1999;13(Suppl 2):15-30.
32. Gershon MD. Review article: serotonin receptors and transporters—roles in normal and abnormal gastrointestinal motility. Aliment Pharmacol Ther 2004;20(Suppl 7):3-14.
33. Coates MD, Mahoney CR, Linden DR, et al. Molecular defects in mucosal serotonin content and decreased serotonin reuptake transporter in ulcerative colitis and irritable bowel syndrome. Gastroenterology 2004;126:1657-1664.
34. Camilleri M, Andrews CN, Bharucha AE, et al. Alterations in expression of p11 and SERT in mucosal biopsies of patients with irritable bowel syndrome. Gastroenterology 2007;132:17-25.
35. Fraser R, Horowitz M, Maddox A, Dent J. Dual effects of cisapride on gastric emptying and antropyloroduodenal motility. Am J Physiol Gastrointest Liver Physiol 1993;264:G195-G201.
36. Braden B, Enghofer M, Schaub M, et al. Long-term cisapride treatment improves diabetic gastroparesis but not glycaemic control. Aliment Pharmacol Ther 2002;16:1341-1346.
37. Abell TL, Camilleri M, DiMagno EP, et al. Long-term efficacy of oral cisapride in symptomatic upper gut dysmotility. Dig Dis Sci 1991;36:616-620.
38. Wang SH, Lin CY, Huang TY, et al. QT interval effects of cisapride in the clinical setting. Int J Cardiol 2001;80:179-183.
39. Prather CM, Camilleri M, Zinsmeister AR, et al. Tegaserod accelerates orocecal transit in patients with constipation-predominant irritable bowel syndrome. Gastroenterology 2000;118:463-468.
40. Foxx-Orenstein A, Camilleri M, Szarka LA, et al. Non-selective opioid antagonist does not increase small intestine or colon transit effect of tegaserod in subjects with constipation predominant-IBS. Neurogastroenterol Motil 2005;17(Suppl 2):A-43.
41. Talley NJ, Camilleri M, Burton D, et al. Double-blind, randomized, placebo-controlled study to evaluate the effects of tegaserod on gastric motor, sensory and myoelectric function in healthy volunteers. Aliment Pharmacol Ther 2006;24:859-867.
42. Degen L, Petrig C, Studer D, et al. Effect of tegaserod on gut transit in male and female subjects. Neurogastroenterol Motil 2005;17:821-826.
43. Degen L, Matzinger D, Merz M, et al. Tegaserod, a 5-HT4 receptor partial agonist, accelerates gastric emptying and gastrointestinal transit in healthy male subjects. Aliment Pharmacol Ther 2001;15:1745-1751.
44. Beattie DT, Smith JA, Marquess D, et al. The 5-HT4 receptor agonist, tegaserod, is a potent 5-HT2B receptor antagonist in vitro and in vivo. Br J Pharmacol 2004;143:549-560.
45. Evans BW, Clark WK, Moore DJ, Whorwell PJ. Tegaserod for the treatment of irritable bowel syndrome. Cochrane Database Syst Rev 2004(0):CD003960.

46. Muller-Lissner S, Holtmann G, Rueegg P, et al. Tegaserod is effective in the initial and retreatment of irritable bowel syndrome with constipation. Aliment Pharmacol Ther 2005;21:11-20.
47. Tack J, Muller-Lissner S, Bytzer P, et al. A randomised controlled trial assessing the efficacy and safety of repeated tegaserod therapy in women with irritable bowel syndrome with constipation. Gut 2005;54:1707-1713.
48. Layer P, Keller J, Mueller-Lissner S, et al. Tegaserod: long-term treatment for irritable bowel syndrome patients with constipation in primary care. Digestion 2005;71:238-244.
49. Kamm MA, Muller-Lissner S, Talley NJ, et al. Tegaserod for the treatment of chronic constipation: a randomized, double-blind, placebo-controlled multinational study. Am J Gastroenterol 2005;100:362-372.
50. Johanson JF, Wald A, Tougas G, et al. Effect of tegaserod in chronic constipation: a randomized, double-blind, controlled trial. Clin Gastroenterol Hepatol 2004;2:796-805.
51. Dennis D, Palme M, Irwin I, et al. AT-7505 is a novel, selective 5-HT4 receptor agonist that causes gastrointestinal prokinetic activity in dogs. Gastroenterology 2004;126: A-641.
52. Camilleri M, Vazquez-Roque MI, Burton D, et al. Pharmacodynamic effects of a novel prokinetic 5-HT_4 receptor agonist, ATI-7505, in humans. Neurogastroenterol Motil 2007;19:30-38.
53. Mayer EA, Berman S, Derbyshire SW, et al. The effect of the 5-HT3 receptor antagonist, alosetron, on brain responses to visceral stimulation in irritable bowel syndrome patients. Aliment Pharmacol Ther 2002;16:1357-1366.
54. Andresen V, Keller J, Montori V, et al. Effects of 5-HT3 antagonists on symptom relief and constipation in irritable bowel syndrome: a systematic review and meta-analysis of large, multicenter, randomized trials. Neurogastroenterol Motil 2006;18: 687-688.
55. Miner P, Stanton DB, Carter F, et al. Cilansetron in irritable bowel syndrome with diarrhea predominance (IBS-D): efficacy and safety on a 3 month US study. Am J Gastroenterol 2004;99:S277.
56. Bradette M, Monnikes H, Carter F, et al. Cilansetron in irritable bowel syndrome with diarrhea predominance (IBS-D): efficacy and safety in a 6 month global study. Gastroenterology 2004;126:A-42.
57. Cilansetron: KC 9946. Drugs R D 2005;6:169-173.
58. Walker AM, Bohn RL, Cali C, et al. Risk factors for colon ischemia. Am J Gastroenterol 2004;99:1333-1337.
59. Cremonini F, Delgado-Aros S, Camilleri M. Efficacy of alosetron in irritable bowel syndrome: a meta-analysis of randomized controlled trials. Neurogastroenterol Motil 2003;15:79-86.
60. Chang L, Ameen VZ, Dukes GE, et al. A dose-ranging, Phase II study of the efficacy and safety of alosetron in men with diarrhea-predominant IBS. Am J Gastroenterol 2005;100:115-123.
61. Camilleri M, McKinzie S, Fox J, et al. Effect of renzapride on transit in constipation-predominant irritable bowel syndrome. Clin Gastroenterol Hepatol 2004;2:895-904.
62. Meyers NL, Tack J, Middleton S, et al. Efficacy and safety of renzapride in patients with constipation predominant irritable bowel syndrome. Gut 2002;51:A-10.
63. George A, Meyers NL, Palmer RMJ. Efficacy and safety of renzapride in patients with constipation predominant IBS: a Phase-IIb study in the UK primary healthcare setting. Gut 2003;52:A-91.
64. Ramsbottom N, Hunt JN. Studies of the effect of metoclopramide and apomorphine on gastric emptying and secretion in man. Gut 1970;11:989-993.
65. Eisner M. Effect of metoclopramide on gastrointestinal motility in man: a manometric study. Am J Dig Dis 1971;16:409-419.
66. Perkel MS, Hersh T, Moore C, Davidson ED. Metoclopramide therapy in fifty-five patients with delayed gastric emptying. Am J Gastroenterol 1980;74:231-236.
67. Perkel MS, Moore C, Hersh T, Davidson ED. Metoclopramide therapy in patients with delayed gastric emptying: a randomized, double-blind study. Dig Dis Sci 1979;24:662-666.
68. Lata PF, Pigarelli DL. Chronic metoclopramide therapy for diabetic gastroparesis. Ann Pharmacother 2003;37:122-126.
69. Silvers D, Kipnes M, Broadstone V, et al. Domperidone in the management of symptoms of diabetic gastroparesis: efficacy, tolerability, and quality-of-life outcomes in a multicenter controlled trial. DOM-USA-5 Study Group. Clin Ther 1998;20:438-453.
70. Patterson D, Abell T, Rothstein R, et al. A double-blind multicenter comparison of domperidone and metoclopramide in the treatment of diabetic patients with symptoms of gastroparesis. Am J Gastroenterol 1999;94:1230-1234.
71. Holtmann G, Talley NJ, Liebregts T, et al. A placebo-controlled trial of itopride in functional dyspepsia. N Engl J Med 2006;354:832-840.
72. Choung RS, Talley NJ, Peterson JA, et al. A double-blind, randomized, placebo-controlled trial of itopride (100 mg and 200 mg, three times daily) on gastric motor and sensory function in healthy volunteers. Neurogastroenterol Motil 2007;19:180-187.
73. Talley NJ, Tack J, Ptak T, et al. Efficacy and safety of itopride in functional dyspepsia: results of two Phase III, multicentre, randomized, double-blind, placebo-controlled trials. Gastroenterology 2007;132:A93
74. Coulie B, Tack J, Peeters T, Janssens J. Involvement of two different pathways in the motor effects of erythromycin on the gastric antrum in humans. Gut 1998;43:395-400.
75. Richards RD, Davenport K, McCallum RW. The treatment of idiopathic and diabetic gastroparesis with acute intravenous and chronic oral erythromycin. Am J Gastroenterol 1993;88:203-207.
76. Park MI, Ferber I, Camilleri M, et al. Effect of atilmotin on gastrointestinal transit in healthy subjects: a randomized, placebo-controlled study. Neurogastroenterol Motil 2006;18:28-36.
77. McCallum RW, Fogel R, Fang JC, et al. Mitemcinal fumarate (GM-611) provided symptomatic relief of diabetic gastroparesis, especially in type I diabetes: results of a 12-week, multi-center, double-blind, placebo-controlled, randomized Phase 2b study (gm-611-05). Gastroenterology 2005;128:A467.
78. Fang J, McCallum R, DiBase J, et al. Effect of mitemcinal fumarate (GM-611) on gastric emptying in patients with idiopathic or diabetic gastroparesis. Gastroenterology 2004;126:A483.
79. Borody TJ, Quigley EM, Phillips SF, et al. Effects of morphine and atropine on motility and transit in the human ileum. Gastroenterology 1985;89:562-570.
80. Steadman CJ, Phillips SF, Camilleri M, et al. Control of muscle tone in the human colon. Gut 1992;33:541-546.
81. Lembo T, Naliboff BD, Matin K, et al. Irritable bowel syndrome patients show altered sensitivity to exogenous opioids. Pain 2000;87:137-147.
82. Pelemans W, Vantrappen F. A double blind crossover comparison of loperamide with diphenoxylate in the symptomatic treatment of chronic diarrhea. Gastroenterology 1976;70:1030-1034.
83. Mainguet P, Fiasse R, Turine JB. Long-term survey of the treatment of diarrhoea with loperamide. Digestion 1977;16:69-76.
84. Galambos JT, Hersh T, Schroder S, Wenger J. Loperamide: a new antidiarrheal agent in the treatment of chronic diarrhea. Gastroenterology 1976;70:1026-1029.
85. Camilleri M. Management of the irritable bowel syndrome. Gastroenterology 2001;120:652-668.
86. Wolff BG, Michelassi F, Gerkin TM, et al. Alvimopan, a novel, peripherally acting mu opioid antagonist: results of a multicenter, randomized, double-blind, placebo-controlled, Phase III trial of major abdominal surgery and postoperative ileus. Ann Surg 2004;240:728-734; discussion 734-735.
87. Taguchi A, Sharma N, Saleem RM, et al. Selective postoperative inhibition of gastrointestinal opioid receptors. N Engl J Med 2001;345:935-940.
88. Delaney CP, Weese JL, Hyman NH, et al. Phase III trial of alvimopan, a novel, peripherally acting, mu opioid antagonist, for postoperative ileus after major abdominal surgery. Dis Colon Rectum 2005;48:1114-1125; discussion 1125-1126; author reply 1127-1129.
89. Gonenne J, Camilleri M, Ferber I, et al. Effect of alvimopan and codeine on gastrointestinal transit: a randomized controlled study. Clin Gastroenterol Hepatol 2005;3:784-791.
90. Tan EK, Cornish J, Darzi AW, Tekkis PP. Meta-analysis: alvimopan vs. placebo in the treatment of post-operative ileus. Aliment Pharmacol Ther 2007;25:47-57.
91. Methylnaltrexone: MNTX. Drugs R D 2006;7:374-378.
92. Yuan CS. Clinical status of methylnaltrexone, a new agent to prevent and manage opioid-induced side effects. J Support Oncol 2004;2:111-117; discussion 119-122.
93. Yuan CS, Foss JF, O'Connor M, et al. Effects of enteric-coated methylnaltrexone in preventing opioid-induced delay in oral-cecal transit time. Clin Pharmacol Ther 2000;67:398-404.
94. Gray JL, Debas HT, Mulvihill SJ. Control of dumping symptoms by somatostatin analogue in patients after gastric surgery. Arch Surg 1991;126:1231-1235; discussion 1235-1236.
95. Primrose JN. Octreotide in the treatment of the dumping syndrome. Digestion 1990;45(Suppl 1):49-58; discussion 58-59.
96. Saslow SB, O'Brien MD, Camilleri M, et al. Octreotide inhibition of flushing and colonic motor dysfunction in carcinoid syndrome. Am J Gastroenterol 1997;92:2250-2256.
97. Mystakidou K, Katsouda E, Tsilika E, et al. Octreotide long-acting formulation (LAR) in chronic loperamide-refractory diarrhea not related to cancer treatment. Anticancer Res 2006;26:2325-2328.
98. O'Donnell LJ, Watson AJ, Cameron D, Farthing MJ. Effect of octreotide on mouth-to-caecum transit time in healthy subjects and in the irritable bowel syndrome. Aliment Pharmacol Ther 1990;4:177-181.
99. von der Ohe MR, Camilleri M, Thomforde GM, Klee GG. Differential regional effects of octreotide on human gastrointestinal motor function. Gut 1995;36:743-748.
100. Cid LP, Montrose-Rafizadeh C, Smith DI, et al. Cloning of a putative human voltage-gated chloride channel (ClC-2) cDNA widely expressed in human tissues. Hum Mol Genet 1995;4:407-413.
101. Catalan M, Cornejo I, Figueroa CD, et al. ClC-2 in guinea pig colon: mRNA, immunolabeling, and functional evidence for surface epithelium localization. Am J Physiol Gastrointest Liver Physiol 2002;283:G1004-G1013.
102. Lubiprostone: RU 0211, SPI 0211. Drugs R D 2005;6:245-248.
103. Johanson JF, Gargano AM, Holland PC, et al. Phase III, efficacy and safety of RU-0211, a novel chloride channel activator, for the treatment of constipation. Gastroenterology 2003;124:A-48.
104. Johanson JF, Gargano MA, Holland PC, et al. Phase III, randomized withdrawal study of RU-0211, a novel chloride channel activator for the treatment of constipation. Gastroenterology 2004;126:A-100.
105. Johanson JF, Gargano M, Patchen M, Ueno R. Efficacy and safety of a novel compound, RU-0211, for the treatment of constipation. Gastroenterology 2002;122:A-315.
106. Camilleri M, Bharucha AE, Ueno R, et al. Effect of a selective chloride channel activator, lubiprostone, on gastrointestinal transit, gastric sensory and motor functions in healthy volunteers. Am J Physiol Gastrointest Liver Physiol 2006;290:G942-G947.
107. Murray CD, Martin NM, Patterson M, et al. Ghrelin enhances gastric emptying in diabetic gastroparesis: a double blind, placebo controlled, crossover study. Gut 2005;54:1693-1698.
108. Tack J, Depoortere I, Bisschops R, et al. Influence of ghrelin on gastric emptying and meal-related symptoms in idiopathic gastroparesis. Aliment Pharmacol Ther 2005;22:847-853.

109. Tack J, Depoortere I, Bisschops R, et al. Influence of ghrelin on interdigestive gastrointestinal motility in humans. Gut 2006;55:327-333.
110. Cremonini F, Camilleri M, Vazquez Roque M, et al. Obesity does not increase effects of synthetic ghrelin on human gastric motor functions. Gastroenterology 2006;131:1431-1439.
111. Watkins CC, Sawa A, Jaffrey S, et al. Insulin restores neuronal nitric oxide synthase expression and function that is lost in diabetic gastropathy. J Clin Invest 2000;106:373-384.
112. Coleski R, Gonlachanvit S, Owyang C, Hasler WL. Selective reversal of hyperglycemia-evoked gastric myoelectric dysrhythmias by nitrergic stimulation in healthy humans. J Pharmacol Exp Ther 2005;312:103-111.
113. Sarnelli G, Sifrim D, Janssens J, Tack J. Influence of sildenafil on gastric sensorimotor function in humans. Am J Physiol Gastrointest Liver Physiol 2004;287:G988-G992.
114. Currie MG, Fok KF, Kato J, et al. Guanylin: an endogenous activator of intestinal guanylate cyclase. Proc Natl Acad Sci U S A 1992;89:947-951.
115. Hamra FK, Forte LR, Eber SL, et al. Uroguanylin: structure and activity of a second endogenous peptide that stimulates intestinal guanylate cyclase. Proc Natl Acad Sci U S A 1993;90:10464-10468.
116. Giannella RA. *Escherichia coli* heat-stable enterotoxins, guanylins, and their receptors: what are they and what do they do? J Lab Clin Med 1995;125:173-181.
117. Forte LR. Guanylin regulatory peptides: structures, biological activities mediated by cyclic GMP and pathobiology. Regul Pept 1999;81:25-39.
118. Currie MG, Kurtz C, Mahajan-Miklos S, et al. Effects of single dose administration of MD-1100 on safety, tolerability, exposure, and stool consistency in healthy subjects. Am J Gastroenterol 2005;100:S328.
119. Coulie B, Szarka LA, Camilleri M, et al. Recombinant human neurotrophic factors accelerate colonic transit and relieve constipation in humans. Gastroenterology 2000;119:41-50.
120. Parkman HP, Rao SS, Reynolds JC, et al. Neurotrophin-3 improves functional constipation. Am J Gastroenterol 2003;98:1338-1347.
121. Familoni BO, Abell TL, Voeller G, et al. Electrical stimulation at a frequency higher than basal rate in human stomach. Dig Dis Sci 1997;42:885-891.
122. Abell T, McCallum R, Hocking M, et al. Gastric electrical stimulation for medically refractory gastroparesis. Gastroenterology 2003;125:421-428.
123. Abell TL, Van Cutsem E, Abrahamsson H, et al. Gastric electrical stimulation in intractable symptomatic gastroparesis. Digestion 2002;66:204-212.
124. Kamm MA, Dudding TC, Melenhorst J, et al. Sacral nerve stimulation for constipation: an international multi-centre study. Gastroenterology 2007;132:A-40.
125. Abell TL, Bernstein RK, Cutts T, et al. Treatment of gastroparesis: a multidisciplinary clinical review. Neurogastroenterol Motil 2006;18:263-283.
126. Parkman HP, Hasler WL, Fisher RS. American Gastroenterological Association technical review on the diagnosis and treatment of gastroparesis. Gastroenterology 2004;127:1592-1622.
127. Corazziari E, Badiali D, Habib FI, et al. Small volume isosmotic polyethylene glycol electrolyte balanced solution (PMF-100) in treatment of chronic nonorganic constipation. Dig Dis Sci 1996;41:1636-1642.
128. Flig E, Hermann TW, Zabel M. Is bisacodyl absorbed at all from suppositories in man? Int J Pharm 2000;196:11-20.

33

INFLAMMATORY BOWEL DISEASES

Laurence J. Egan and Christian Maaser

OVERVIEW 487
INTRODUCTION 487
Clinical Features 487
Natural History 488
PATHOPHYSIOLOGY OF INFLAMMATORY BOWEL DISEASES 488
Genetics 489
Environmental Factors 489
Importance of the Intestinal Flora 489
Immune Dysregulation 490
THERAPEUTICS AND CLINICAL PHARMACOLOGY OF INFLAMMATORY BOWEL DISEASES 490
Goals of Therapy 490
Induction of Remission 490
Maintenance of Remission 490
Quality-of-Life Improvement 490
Avoidance of Surgery 490
Prevention of Complications 490
Therapeutics by Class 490
Anti-inflammatory Drugs 490
Immunosuppresants 493
Biologics 495
Therapeutic Approach 496
General Considerations 496
Crohn's Disease 496
Ulcerative Colitis 498
Pouchitis 499
Emerging Targets and Therapeutics 499
Anti–Tumor Necrosis Factor-α Alternatives 499
Anticytokines 499
Cytokines and Growth Factors 499
Selective Adhesion Molecule Inhibitor 499
Intracellular Signal Transduction Inhibitors 499
Microbiota 499

OVERVIEW

The purpose of this chapter is to explain what we currently know about the pathogenesis of inflammatory bowel diseases and how this understanding relates to the pharmacologic therapy of those diseases. Early therapeutic efforts in inflammatory bowel disease were based on empirical observations of benefit when certain drugs, notably cortisone and sulfasalazine, when administered for other diseases, improved digestive symptoms in patients who also suffered from inflammatory bowel disease. However, with the tremendous advances of the past 2 decades in our understanding of the pathogenesis and etiology of inflammatory bowel diseases, new therapeutics for these diseases are designed to rationally target key mechanisms of intestinal inflammation.

In this chapter, we first provide an account of current concepts of inflammatory bowel disease pathogenesis. Our current state of knowledge about the causation of inflammatory bowel diseases implicates a genetic disposition to dysregulation of the mucosal immune system that is driven by the normal flora of the gastrointestinal tract, leading to a state of chronic overactivity of cellular and humoral mechanisms of immunity. Next, we provide a detailed account of the pharmacology of the drugs in use to treat inflammatory bowel diseases, with an emphasis on examining how those drugs interrupt pathogenic mechanisms. Many drugs used in inflammatory bowel disease treatment are also used in other immunologic conditions such as autoimmune diseases, and act to modulate or inhibit activity of the immune system. Finally, an approach based on common clinical scenarios is used to synthesize clinical and pharmacologic information into useful therapeutic strategies.

INTRODUCTION

Inflammatory bowel diseases comprise a group of related disorders that are characterized by chronic inflammation of the intestine that results in marked dysfunction of the digestive tract. The two most important and prevalent types of inflammatory bowel disease are Crohn's disease and ulcerative colitis. An additional entity, termed *microscopic colitis*, has also been described but is much less common than Crohn's disease or ulcerative colitis. The cause of any of these related conditions is not known. Crohn's disease and ulcerative colitis were both first described as clinical entities in the early part of the 20th century. The incidence and prevalence of both conditions appeared to rise throughout the 20th century, reaching a plateau in the 1980s or 1990s in most countries.[1,2]

Clinical Features

The clinical manifestations of inflammatory bowel diseases arise as a result of chronic inflammation affecting portions of the digestive tract. Chronic inflammation of any section of this tract can cause edema, bleeding, ulceration, and loss of integrity of the mucosal lining, which impairs an important mechanism of innate immunity. When inflammation extends across the full thickness of the intestinal wall, as occurs in Crohn's disease, fibrotic strictures and penetrating complications such as abscess and fistula can develop. Together, these abnormalities result in symptoms of diarrhea, rectal bleeding, abdominal pain, weight loss, anorexia, and vomiting.

Most patients with inflammatory bowel disease can be categorized on the basis of clinical features as having Crohn's disease or ulcerative colitis (Fig. 33-1). Crohn's disease, also described as regional enteritis, affects any portion of the alimentary tract from mouth to anus, whereas ulcerative colitis remains confined to the large intestine. Inflammation in Crohn's disease can extend through the full thickness of the intestinal wall, whereas in ulcerative colitis the inflammation is more superficial in the mucosa of the colon. Both diseases are characterized histologically by a marked infiltration of the lamina propria of the intestine by acute and chronic inflammatory cells that often extends into the crypts of Lieberkühn, producing crypt abscesses. Noncrotizing granulomata are characteristic of Crohn's disease. Consistent with the transmural extent of inflammation in Crohn's disease, some patients develop complications of abscess or fistula. Abscesses in Crohn's disease can develop in the abdominal cavity, usually in association with a markedly diseased segment of intestine, or in the perineum. Crohn's disease patients are also susceptible to fistulas, which can develop between the intestine and other abdominal or pelvic organs such as other segments of intestine, the bladder, and the vagina.

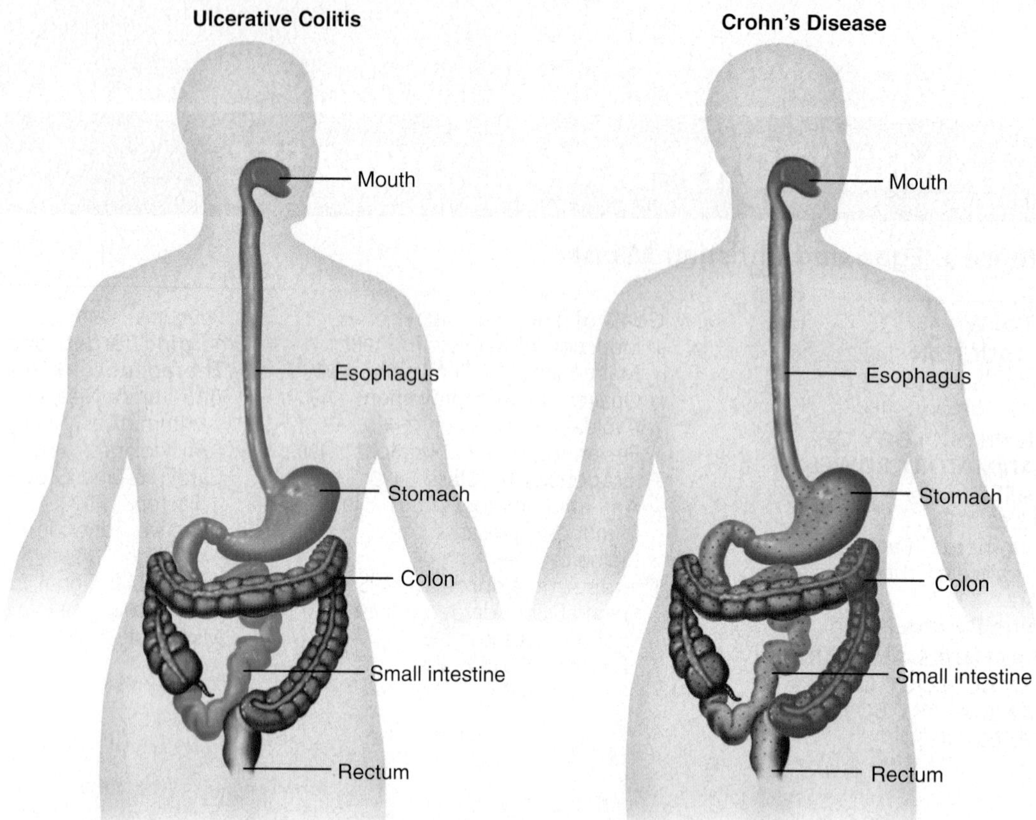

FIGURE 33-1 • Clinical features of ulcerative colitis and Crohn's disease. Commonly affected portions of the intestinal tract are illustrated.

TABLE 33-1 EXTRAINTESTINAL MANIFESTATIONS OF INFLAMMATORY BOWEL DISEASES AND THEIR TREATMENT OPTIONS

Manifestation	Treatment
Arthritis	Sulfasalazine, methotrexate, infliximab
Pyoderma gangrenosum	Cyclosporine, infliximab
Erythema nodosum	Nonsteroidal anti-inflammatory drugs
Primary sclerosing cholangitis	Liver transplantation
Uveitis	Topical corticosteroids

Perianal fistulas connecting the rectum and perineal skin are also common.

Both ulcerative colitis and Crohn's disease can be complicated by extraintestinal manifestations. Treatment of underlying inflammatory bowel disease can sometimes result in resolution of the extraintestinal problems, but this is not always the case. In some situations—for example, the idiopathic bile duct disease primary sclerosing cholangitis—even proctocolectomy does not seem to affect the course of the disease. Table 33-1 lists some of the treatments that have been advocated for certain extraintestinal manifestations of inflammatory bowel disease. Controlled data to support those recommendations are largely lacking, however.

Natural History

Inflammatory bowel disease can develop at any age, but the third decade of life is the period of highest incidence. The severity of disease and consequent morbidity and costs of care vary greatly within populations of patients. Natural history studies indicate that many inflammatory bowel disease patients lead quite normal lives, but others with more severe disease suffer from chronic ill health, and additional morbidity associated with the adverse effects of treatment, both medical and surgical.[3] Many patients experience a relapsing-remitting course of disease. Remissions can occur spontaneously or be induced by medical or surgical intervention, and can be lengthened by medical therapy in some patients. The relapsing-remitting course of inflammatory bowel disease has led to the practice of evaluating the efficacy of drug therapy in the clinical settings of active disease, in which drugs are tested for their ability to induce remission, and in quiescent disease, in which drugs are tested for their ability to maintain remission.

When medical therapy of inflammatory bowel disease fails, surgery is often conducted. In Crohn's disease patients, surgery typically consists of segmental resections of diseased intestine and complications such as abscess and fistula. Primary reanastomosis is often possible, but some patients require temporary or permanent stomas. In ulcerative colitis that requires surgery, proctocolectomy is usually performed, with formation of a permanent ileostomy or ileal pouch–anal anastomosis.

Both Crohn's disease and ulcerative colitis can result in death due to complications of disease, such as cancer and malnutrition, or complications of therapy, such as opportunistic infections or postoperative problems. However, population-based studies have failed to demonstrate any significant shortening of average life expectancy in patients with inflammatory bowel disease.[2,4,5]

PATHOPHYSIOLOGY OF INFLAMMATORY BOWEL DISEASES

A complex and poorly understood interplay between inherited factors, environment, and immune dysregulation in the intestinal mucosal immune system underlies the development of inflammatory bowel diseases (Fig. 33-2).

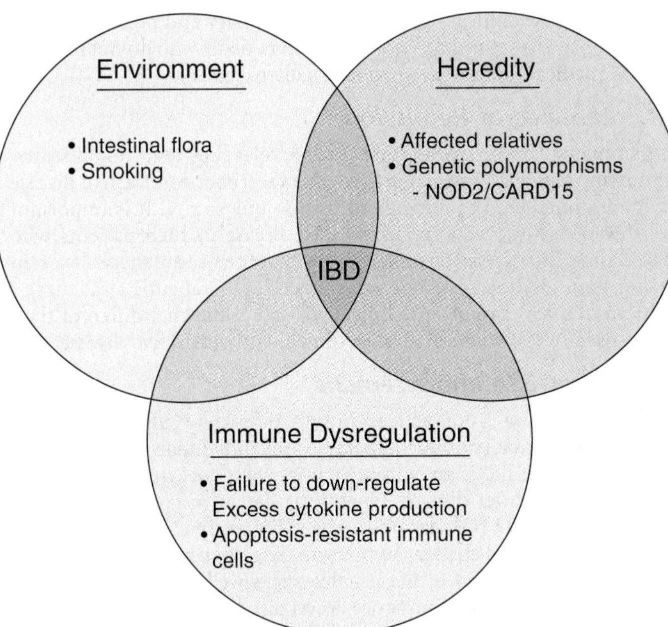

FIGURE 33-2 • Pathophysiology of inflammatory bowel diseases. Environment, heredity, and immune dysregulation combine to cause disease.

Genetics

It has long been recognized that inflammatory bowel diseases run in families. Thus, the relative risk of inflammatory bowel disease is increased in first-degree relatives of an affected patient approximately 10-fold compared to the general population. Moreover, concordance for disease in monozygotic twins, approaching 50%, is considerably higher than that observed in fraternal twins. Recent studies have also emphasized that, within families multiply affected by inflammatory bowel disease, there is a concordance for the phenotypic expression of the disease.[6,7] For example, relatives of a patient with distal ileal Crohn's disease are more likely than nonrelatives to have disease at that location. Despite this epidemiologic evidence supporting a genetic cause for inflammatory bowel disease, it is equally clear that this disease trait is not inherited in a classic monogenetic manner. It is likely that individuals with inflammatory bowel diseases are predisposed to those conditions by the complex interplay of multiple genetic factors.

Significant progress has been made in understanding the genetic contribution to inflammatory bowel diseases through linkage studies of multiply affected families. Numerous genome-wide association studies have been conducted in which an association was sought between genetic markers and occurrence of disease. Through these linkage studies, more than 12 genetic loci associated with inflammatory bowel disease have been identified (reviewed by Schreiber et al.[8]). So far, the most important of these loci is the *IBD1* locus on chromosome 16. The susceptibility gene responsible for linkage of this locus with Crohn's disease has been identified as *NOD2*, also known as *CARD15*.[9] This susceptibility gene was also identified through a candidate gene approach.[10] Three common genetic variants of *CARD15* exist: Arg702Trp, Gly908Arg, and Leu1007fsinsC. The prevalence of any one of those polymorphisms in the general population is around 4%. The possession of one of these variant alleles confers a relative risk for Crohn's disease of approximately 3%. However, individuals with two variant alleles of this gene have a dramatically elevated risk of Crohn's disease, approximately 40-fold that of individuals with two wild-type *CARD15* alleles. Polymorphisms of *CARD15* are not associated with ulcerative colitis. The association of *CARD15* polymorphisms with Crohn's disease has been verified in numerous populations around the world[11] but, interestingly, is not significantly associated with Crohn's disease in Japanese populations.

CARD15 encodes a protein that acts as an intracellular pattern recognition receptor. This protein contains two N-terminal CARD domains that are important for activation of the proinflammatory transcription factor NF-κB. There is a centrally located nuclear binding domain that is important for oligomerization of the protein. There is a C-terminal leucine-rich repeat region that is the site of recognition of bacterial cell wall products. Recent studies have confirmed that CARD15 is a receptor for muramyl dipeptide, a component of the outer wall of certain bacteria. Intensive research is currently underway to elucidate the mechanism by which apparently loss-of-function variants of CARD15, which is required for activation of the innate immune system through NF-κB, can be linked to a chronic inflammatory disease. One leading possibility is that defective function of CARD15 in patients results in a subtle immune deficiency state that hinders the ability of the mucosal immune system to protect against infection by normally harmless microbes.[12]

Apart from *CARD15*, the contribution of other genetic loci to inflammatory bowel disease causation is much less clear. One recent discovery implicates variant alleles of interleukin-23 receptor in protection against inflammatory bowel disease.[13] Ongoing genetic epidemiology research will undoubtedly identify additional inflammatory bowel disease susceptibility genes.

Environmental Factors

Because of the obscure etiology of inflammatory bowel disease and the fact that there is an obvious overactivation of the immune system in affected tissues, many investigators have placed emphasis on trying to establish if these diseases are caused by an infectious agent. One of the most intensively studied microbes has been *Mycobacterium paratuberculosis*. This mycobacterium is a fastidious organism that is quite prevalent in the environment. Many dairy herds, for example, are infected with it. *Mycobacterium paratuberculosis* has been identified in Crohn's disease tissues using a number of methodologies, including polymerase chain reaction and immunohistochemistry.[14] However, efforts to establish Koch's postulates for *M. paratuberculosis* as the causative agent of Crohn's disease have universally failed. Most authorities do not regard this agent as a biologically plausible factor in the causation of inflammatory bowel diseases.

Measles virus has also received considerable attention as a potential cause of Crohn's disease. Epidemiologic studies have demonstrated a coincidence in the rise of the incidence of measles virus infection and Crohn's disease during the 20th century.[15] Measles virus infection can cause a small-vessel vasculitis, and this virus has been identified in small blood vessels of affected Crohn's disease tissues. However, this virus has also been described in vessels of healthy individuals, and despite the low prevalence of measles virus infection in developed countries at present, Crohn's disease remains a relatively common disorder. Little current research focuses on measles virus as a causative agent in Crohn's disease.

Apart from infectious ideologies, epidemiologic studies have also turned up a number of important observations about the pathophysiology of inflammatory bowel diseases. Perhaps the most intriguing of these is the fact that Crohn's disease appears to be positively associated with smoking, whereas ulcerative colitis is negatively associated with smoking.[16,17] This observation has been replicated in many cohorts of patients, and it is clear that, compared to nonsmokers, individuals who smoke cigarettes are more likely to develop Crohn's disease but are less likely to develop ulcerative colitis. The pathophysiologic mechanism underlying this observation has never been elucidated. However, one possibility is that nicotine, which is a weakly effective therapy for ulcerative colitis, might simply be masking subclinical ulcerative colitis in individuals who smoke. It is also possible that the vascular effects of cigarette smoke might contribute to Crohn's disease.

Importance of the Intestinal Flora

The normal fecal stream is an essential factor in the causation of inflammatory bowel diseases. Numerous lines of evidence point toward the fact that the contents of the alimentary canal drive chronic inflammation in patients suffering from inflammatory bowel diseases. For example, surgical diversion of the fecal stream away from involved segments is associated with dramatic resolution of inflammation. Reinstallation of fecal contents in distal bypassed intestine causes disease recurrence.[18] Thus, it appears likely that the microbial flora of the intestinal lumen drives the chronic inflammation in inflammatory bowel disease. This idea is supported by the fact that, in most animal models of inflammatory bowel diseases, when those animals are raised in a germ-free environment, the disease does not manifest.[19] Moreover, antibiotics are at least partially effective in controlling inflammation in rodent models of inflammatory bowel disease and in some patients.[20] Current lines of research indicate that normal intestinal homeostasis depends on active communication between the immune system of gastrointestinal mucosa and the normal intestinal microbial flora.[21,22] Somehow, in inflammatory bowel diseases, this normal communication appears to be disturbed.

Immune Dysregulation

Although it is clear that hereditary and environment play important roles in the causation of inflammatory bowel diseases, it is not known precisely how those factors are translated into the expression of clinical disease. However, a significant body of experimental data has pointed toward imbalances or abnormal regulation of some components of the mucosal immune system in inflammatory bowel disease.[23] For example, the immune system in patients with Crohn's disease appears to become biased toward the response dominated by a particular pattern of cytokine production that is termed *Th1 polarization*. In such patients, there is excessive production of interferon-γ, tumor necrosis factor-α, and interleukin-12.[24] These cytokines are predominantly proinflammatory, stimulating activation of the immune system by promoting the extravasation of leukocytes at the sites of disease and the activation of those cells. In patients with ulcerative colitis, there also is a polarization of cytokine responses in the inflamed tissues that is somewhat different from that seen in Crohn's disease. In ulcerative colitis, the predominant cytokines include interleukin-4 and interleukin-5, which are Th2-polarized cytokines. However, elevated concentrations of interferon-γ and tumor necrosis factor-α are also present, which indicates that ulcerative colitis is not a pure Th2-polarized disease. Many research laboratories are currently working to understanding the cause and effects of dysregulation of the mucosal immune system in inflammatory bowel disease patients.

THERAPEUTICS AND CLINICAL PHARMACOLOGY OF INFLAMMATORY BOWEL DISEASES

Goals of Therapy (Box 33-1)

Induction of Remission

The most important therapeutic goal in patients with active inflammatory bowel disease is to bring about a symptomatic resolution of diarrhea, rectal bleeding, and abdominal pain. This can often be achieved with currently available medications. However, some patients improve with drug therapy, but symptoms do not fully abate. Such patients are said to have achieved a response, but not entered remission. In clinical trials of active inflammatory bowel diseases, it is common to use clinical remission as the primary end point and clinical response as a secondary end point.[25] In patients who do not respond well to medical therapy, surgery is usually necessary.

BOX 33-1 GOALS OF INFLAMMATORY BOWEL DISEASE THERAPY

Induction of clinical remission
Maintenance of clinical remission
Improvement in quality of life
Avoidance of surgery
Prevention of complications

Maintenance of Remission

Inflammatory bowel diseases are chronic relapsing-remitting diseases, and many patients experience flares or exacerbations of active disease that are punctuated by periods of disease quiescence. It is important to prevent symptomatic recurrence of disease in such patients who have come into symptomatic remission, either spontaneously or in response to medical or surgical therapy. The therapeutic strategies to achieve this very important clinical goal are somewhat different than those used to induce remission in the patient with active disease.

Quality-of-Life Improvement

Patients suffering from active Crohn's disease or ulcerative colitis report a lower quality of life than do healthy individuals. Improvement in the quality of life is an extremely important goal in the therapy of inflammatory bowel disease. Quality of life in inflammatory bowel disease patients can be measured using a disease-specific scale, the IBD questionnaire,[26] and changes in this score are often recorded in clinical trials. Although quality of life usually tracks well with measurements of disease activity in inflammatory bowel diseases, drug-associated side effects can have a significant negative impact on quality of life.

Avoidance of Surgery

Many patients with inflammatory bowel diseases have surgery at some point during the disease course. Indeed, in many patients surgery can be life saving. However, the need for surgery can be viewed as a failure of medical therapy. Although surgery is often effective at inducing remission that can be long lasting in some patients, surgery itself can be associated with significant morbidities, especially when it must be repeated.

Prevention of Complications

Complications of inflammatory bowel diseases are common, and when they occur can contribute significantly to the morbidity or even mortality of these diseases. Therefore, the ideal therapeutic approach should encompass attempts to prevent disease complications.

Therapeutics by Class

Anti-inflammatory Drugs

Aminosalicylates. Aminosalicylates are a cornerstone of inflammatory bowel disease therapy. Sulfasalazine is the prototype drug in this class, and was originally developed for the treatment of inflammatory arthritis. This drug was empirically observed to induce benefit in patients who also suffered from inflammatory bowel disease. Sulfasalazine is a conjugate of sulfapyridine and 5-aminosalicylate linked by an azo bond. 5-Aminosalicylate is responsible for the anti-inflammatory effect in inflammatory bowel disease treatment.[27] Because many of the side effects of sulfasalazine are attributed to the sulfapyridine moiety, which has no apparent therapeutic benefit in controlling intestinal inflammation, 5-aminosalicylate has been developed for use free of sulfapyridine. Figure 33-3 shows the chemical structures of several important aminosalicylates. Table 33-2 lists several of the widely used formulations of aminosalicylate, along with dosing and concentrations of active drug.

Pharmacokinetics and Metabolism. A principle of the use of aminosalicylates is that these drugs work best when high concentrations are achieved at the site of disease, usually the distal ileum and colon.[28] In sulfasalazine, the azo bond linking 5-aminosalicylate to sulfapyridine limits absorption of the drug. During its passage through the small bowel, about 10% of an orally administered dose of sulfasalazine is absorbed. Once reaching the colon, the conjugate is separated into sulfapyridine and 5-aminosalicylate by the action of bacterial azoreductases. The majority of sulfapyridine (90%) is absorbed and metabolized in the liver, and the inactive metabolites are then renally excreted. In contrast, less 5-aminosalicylate is absorbed and the major-

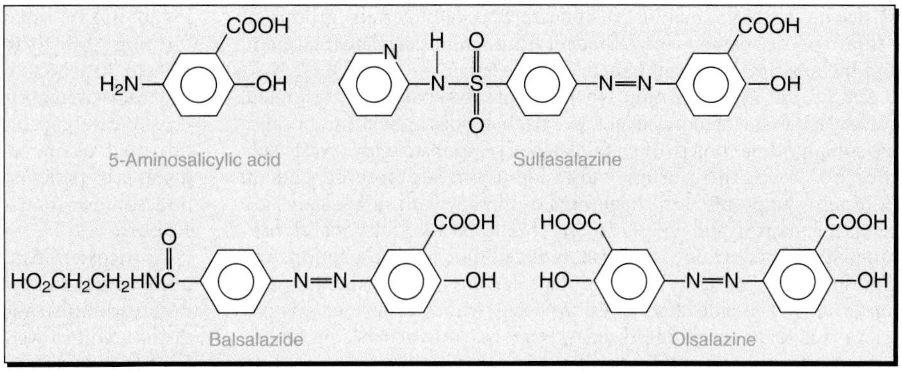

FIGURE 33-3 • Chemical structures of aminosalicylates. Sulfasalazine, balsalazide, and olsalazine are azo-conjugated forms of 5-aminosalicylic acid.

TABLE 33-2 AMINOSALICYLATE PREPARATIONS

Approved Name	Proprietary Name	5-ASA Delivery Mechanism	Sites of Delivery	Luminal 5-ASA Concentration	Absorption	Daily Dose Range
Mesalamine	Rowasa, Salofalk	Enema suspension	Left colon and rectum		13%[193]	1-4 g
Mesalamine	Canasa	Suppository	Rectum		24%	0.5-1.5 g
Mesalamine	Asacol	Eudragit-S–coated tablets (release at pH > 7)	Terminal ileum, colon	Colon: 23 mM[194]	23%[195] 24%[196] 31%[194]	1.6-4.8 g
Mesalamine	Salofalk, Mesasal Claversal	Mesalamine in sodium/glycerine buffer coated with Eudragit-L (release at pH > 6)	Distal jejunum, proximal ileum	Colon: 15 mM[194] Small bowel: 0.3 mM	40%[197] 54%[194]	1.5-4 g
Mesalamine	Pentasa	Ethylcellulose-coated microgranules (time- and pH-dependent release)	Entire small bowel, colon	Small bowel: 0.3 mM Colon: 13 mM[194]	30%[198] 36%[194]	2-4 g
Sulfasalazine	Azulfidine	5-ASA azo-bound to sulfapyridine	Colon	Colonic lumen: 7 mM[199]	11%[195]	1-4 g
Olsalazine	Dipentum	5-ASA dimer, linked by azo bond	Colon	Colonic lumen: 14-23 mM[199] Colon: 24 mM[194]	10%[195] 17%[196] 22%[194]	1-3 g
Balsalazide	Colazide, Colazal	5-ASA azo-bound to inert carrier	Colon			2-6.75 g

5-ASA, 5-aminosalicylic acid.

ity can be recovered in the stool. Similar to sulfasalazine, two other forms of azo-conjugated aminosalicylate have been developed. Balsalazide consists of 5-aminosalicylate conjugated to an inert carrier, and olsalazine consists of a conjugate of two molecules of 5-aminosalicylate.

5-Aminosalicylate is rapidly absorbed from the small intestine when administered orally, so sustained-release preparations have been developed to permit delivery of most of the drug to the more distal bowel, the usual site of inflammatory bowel disease. Sustained-release formulations of 5-aminosalicylate have the approved name mesalazine (North America) or mesalamine (Europe). Sustained-release formulations, which are cellulose-based microcapsulates, show a constant release from the duodenum to the rectum, whereas pH-dependent Eudragit-containing capsules do not release the substance until reaching the distal ileum. Less than one third of the mesalazine is absorbed and reaches the systemic circulation, where it is acetylated in the liver. In contrast to sulfasalazine, the systemic concentration never reaches saturation as long as therapeutic doses are not exceeded, and therefore the rate of elimination is independent from the acetylating phenotype. The systemic half-life of mesalazine is 1 hour, and the inactive metabolite is excreted via the renal route. As a result of oral sustained-release formulations or azo-conjugation, aminosalicylate preparations in clinical use achieve concentrations of 5-aminosalicylate in stool or colonic mucosa in the high micromolar to low millimolar range (see Table 33-2). In addition to the oral sustained-release formulations, mesalazine is also prepared for rectal administration as suppositories and suspension enemas. Despite the variety of formulations of mesalazine, comparative pharmacokinetics studies have revealed that there is little difference among them.[29,30]

5-Aminosalicylate is metabolized in the liver and in intestinal epithelial cells by *N*-acetyltransferase to an inactive metabolite. *N*-acetyltransferase activity is polymorphically expressed, and individuals who inherit one or two low-activity variant alleles of the gene encoding this enzyme have higher levels of active drug. However, a study that explored the possibility that this pharmacogenetic trait might be clinically meaningful did not demonstrate any association between variant alleles of *N*-acetyltransferase 1 and clinical responses to aminosalicylates.[31]

Pharmacodynamics. Many mechanisms of action have been attributed to aminosalicylates that may underlie the therapeutic benefit of these drugs in inflammatory bowel disease. However, the precise action that is relevant is not completely understood. Potentially important mechanisms include inhibition of NF-κB activation,[32] reduced prostaglandin and leukotriene synthesis, and a reduction of reactive oxygen radicals.[33]

Evidence-Based Medicine Clinical Trials. Multiple studies have proven the efficacy of oral aminosalicylates for the treatment of mild to moderately active and quiescent ulcerative colitis,[34-38] as well as for rectal application in proctitis and left-sided colitis.[39,40] In contrast, the role of aminosalicylates for treatment of Crohn's disease is still a matter of debate. In meta-analysis, it appears that only certain groups of Crohn's disease patients might benefit from aminosalicylate treatment, and the magnitude of that benefit is quite small.[41]

Safety/Side Effects. Aminosalicylates are generally well tolerated. Sulfasalazine causes more adverse events than does mesalazine, because the sulfapyridine moiety of sulfasalazine is responsible for several side effects.[42,43] With these drugs, most side effects are dose dependent. Common symptoms at the beginning of therapy with sulfasalazine are headache, nausea, and emesis (about 15% to 20%). Additional significant side effects include skin rash, reduced folic acid absorption, and oligospermia. The latter reduces male fertility during therapy and, importantly, this side effect does not occur with mesalazine. Less frequent side effects include myalgias, bone marrow depression, hemolytic anemia, photosensitivity, interstitial nephritis,[44] pleuropericarditis, and pancreatitis. Allergic reactions presenting as rash and fever can also occur with aminosalicylates.

Pregnancy and Nursing. So far there are few indications of an embryotoxic or teratogenic effect in humans. Sulfasalzine can be detected in breast milk, but harmful effects on breast-fed babies have not been reported.

Interactions. 5-Aminosalicylate elevates the concentrations of the active metabolites of azathioprine and 6-mercaptopurine.[45] Through their effects on intestinal flora, antibiotics can reduce the availability of the active moiety due to less deconjugation of the azo bond. Medications that lower the intestinal pH, such as lactulose, can lower the release of mesalazine from pH-dependent release formulations.

Corticosteroids. Cortisone was the first drug proven efficacious in patients with active ulcerative colitis.[46,47] This drug, along with the development of surgical techniques for proctocolectomy, was probably responsible for reducing the mortality of severe attacks of ulcerative colitis. The most popular corticosteroids in use for inflammatory bowel diseases today are oral prednisone and prednisolone, oral controlled-ileal-release budesonide, and intravenous methylprednisolone or hydrocortisone. These drugs are highly effective and are a key pillar in the management of active ulcerative colitis and Crohn's disease.

Pharmacokinetics and Metabolism. Orally administered corticosteroids such as prednisone and prednisolone are rapidly and almost completely absorbed in the small intestine. Prednisone is a prodrug requiring metabolic activation to prednisolone in the liver. Corticosteroids vary in their relative actions as agonists of glucocorticoid receptors, which mediate their therapeutic benefit, and mineralocorticoid receptors, which may be responsible for their unwanted effects on salt and water homeostasis. This provides a theoretical advantage to the use of corticosteroids with high glucocorticoid and low mineralocorticoid actions, such as methylprednisolone. The plasma elimination half-life of most corticosteroids ranges between 2 and 3 hours, but the efficacy of a single dose lasts up to 18 to 36 hours because of the profound effects of these drugs on gene expression and cellular metabolism. In Table 33-3, the relative potencies of corticosteroids commonly used in inflammatory bowel disease are compared.

Budesonide is an important corticosteroid in the management of Crohn's disease. Due to a high first-pass metabolism by cytochrome P-450 (CYP) isozyme 3A in small intestinal epithelium and liver, forming 6β-hydroxybudesonide and 16α-hydroxyprednisolone, only 10% to 20% of an orally administered dose of budesonide reaches the systemic circulation. This drug has been formulated in controlled-ileal-release capsules that deliver the drug to the distal ileum and proximal colon, the site of disease in many patients with Crohn's disease. In patients with reduced liver function, systemic exposure to budesonide can increase. The median plasma half-life is approximately 4 hours.

Corticosteroids can also be delivered by enema to the rectum and distal colon, an approach that is effective in patients with distal colitis. Rectal administration allows delivery of the drug directly to the site of disease, with lower systemic absorption. However, 10% to 20% of a rectally administered dose of corticosteroid does reach the plasma, and significant side effects can result.

Pharmacodynamics. Corticosteroids exert many effects that contribute to their action as powerful inhibitors of inflammation. All of the known anti-inflammatory effects of corticosteroids are mediated through activation of glucocorticoid receptors (Table 33-4). When a glucocorticoid receptor is activated by binding of the corticosteroid ligand, it translocates into the nucleus and acts as a sequence-specific transcription factor, controlling the expression of numerous genes. Genes that are affected by glucocorticoid receptor binding contain specific sequences in their promoter regions, termed *glucocorticoid response elements*, that mediate receptor binding. This results in multiple effects on different cell types at an inflamed site. For example, corticosteroids lead to inhibition of prostaglandin and leukotriene synthesis via induction of lipocortin and inhibition of phospholipase A_2. Part of the immunosuppressive effect is due to a reduced expression and secretion of proinflammatory cytokines such as tumor necrosis factor-α, interleukin-1, and others. This causes an inhibition of antigen recognition by macrophages as well as blockade of activation of T lymphocytes. Expression of cell adhesion molecules on vascular endothelium, a key event in the recruitment of leukocytes to sites of inflammation, is decreased. Furthermore, these drugs appear to induce apoptosis in monocytes and potentially other cell types important in immune responses.[48] The many side effects of corticosteroids are also mediated by glucocorticoid receptor activation. Therefore, it is currently not possible to uncouple the beneficial anti-inflammatory effects of corticosteroids from harmful adverse effects.

Evidence-Based Medicine Clinical Trials. The efficacy of cortisone in severe attacks of ulcerative colitis was established with one of the first ever randomized, placebo-controlled trials to be conducted.[46] Two large placebo-controlled studies, one in North America[49] and the other in Europe,[50] established the efficacy of prednisolone in active, but not quiescent, Crohn's disease. The data from these controlled trials have been supported by many other smaller studies.[51-56] A controlled clinical trial found a positive effect of budesonide for the treatment of mild to moderate active Crohn's disease in the ileum and the ascending colon. This benefit was somewhat less than observed with conventional corticosteroids, but importantly, fewer adverse effects were observed in budesonide-treated patients.[57] Moreover, compared to placebo,

TABLE 33-3 WIDELY USED CORTICOSTEROIDS IN INFLAMMATORY BOWEL DISEASE

Compound	Glucocorticoid Potency	Mineralocorticoid Potency	Clinical Indication	Dosage
Betamethasone	25-30	0	Topical therapy, UC/CD	5 mg/day, rectal
Hydrocortisone	1	1	Topical therapy, UC/CD	100-200 mg/day, rectal Starting dose 400 mg/day, intravenous
Budesonide	*	*	Crohn's ileitis Left-sided colitis	3-9 mg/day, oral 2 mg/day, rectal
Prednisone	4	0.6	Acute UC/CD	Starting dose 1 mg/kg/day, oral
Prednisolone	4	0.6	Acute UC/CD	Starting dose 1 mg/kg/day, oral
Methylprednisolone	5	0	Acute UC/CD	Starting dose 0.8 mg/kg/day, intravenous

*Data not available.
CD, Crohn's disease; UC, ulcerative colitis.

TABLE 33-4 GENE TARGETS OF GLUCOCORTICOIDS THAT ARE IMPORTANT IN MEDIATING THEIR ANTI-INFLAMMATORY ACTIONS

Target Substance	Effect of Glucocorticoid	Target Cell	Mechanism	Result
IL-1, TNF-α, IL-8	Decrease	Many	Inhibition of NF-κB[200]	Decreasing inflammatory signaling
IL-2	Decrease	Lymphocytes	Inhibition of AP-1[201]	Decreased lymphocyte activation
Inducible nitric oxide synthase	Decrease	Epithelial, endothelial	Inhibition of NF-κB[200]	Decreased vascular permeability
Phospholipase A_2	Decrease	Many	Inhibition of NF-κB, induction of lipocortin gene expression[202]	Decreased eicosanoid production
Cyclooxygenase-2	Decrease	Many	Inhibition of NF-κB[200]	Decreased prostaglandin production
IL-1 receptor type II	Increase	Many	Direct induction of gene expression[203]	Decreased availability of IL-1 for biologic activity
E-selectin	Decrease	Endothelial	Inhibition of NF-κB[204]	Decreased leukocyte extravasation
Intracellular adhesion molecule-1	Decrease	Epithelial, monocytic	Inhibition of NF-κB[205]	Decreased leukocyte migration

IL, interleukin; NF-κB, nuclear factor-κB; TNF, tumor necrosis factor.

budesonide was found to prolong the duration of remission in patients with Crohn's disease.[58] Regarding the treatment of active, distal ulcerative colitis and proctitis, controlled clinical trials have proven budesonide to be both effective and safe.[59-62] Budesonide enemas have been proposed as an alternative treatment for active pouchitis with similar efficacy but better tolerability than oral metronidazole.[63]

Safety/Side Effects. The side effects of corticosteroids are well known and numerous. Typical side effects of long-term corticosteroid therapy include an increased risk of infections, myopathy, osteoporosis, diabetes, and cataract. Fluid retention and hypertension can result from mineralocorticoid effects. Further common side effects at higher dosages are psychosis, increased appetite, and sleep disorder. Long-term use in children can lead to growth retardation. An important but less common side effect is aseptic necrosis of the head of the femur.

Pregnancy and Lactation. Corticosteroids do not have significant known adverse effects on embryonic development and are the class of drugs that can be used with most confidence in inflammatory bowel disease patients during pregnancy. If higher doses of corticosteroids are used until delivery, the newborn should be closely monitored for steroid withdrawal syndrome within the first few days of life.

Immunosuppressants

Azathioprine and 6-Mercaptopurine. Azathioprine is a purine analogue antimetabolite drug that was developed originally as an anticancer drug. It is a prodrug of 6-mercaptopurine, and was developed by Elion and Hitchings as a more long-lived agent that might have a longer duration of action than 6-mercatopurine.[64] Both drugs are important immunomodulators that have been accepted in widespread use for their immune-suppressing properties.

Pharmacokinetics and Metabolism. Azathioprine is almost completely absorbed from the intestinal tract and quickly converted to 6-mercaptopurine by a nonenzymatic reaction after exposure to nucleophiles such as glutathione. 6-Mercatopurine has a number of potential metabolic fates[65] (Fig. 33-4). It can be metabolized by thiopurine methyltransferase to 6-methylmercaptopurine or by xanthine oxidase to 6-thiouric acid. Alternatively, 6-mercaptopurine can be further metabolized to 6-thioguanine nucleotides, the active metabolites, via a multistep enzymatic pathway beginning with hypoxanthine phosphoribosyltransferase followed by inosine triphosphate pyrophosphatase and guanosine monophosphate synthetase. While the plasma half-life of azathioprine and 6-mercatopurine are 1.7 and 1.2 hours, respectively, 6-thioguanine nucleotides are intracellularly stored and are slowly eliminated.

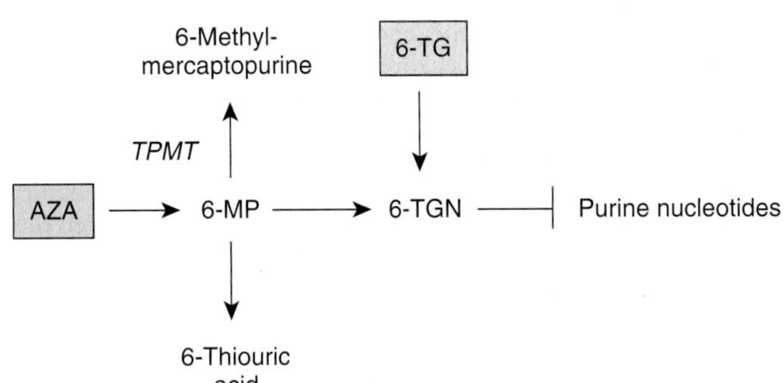

FIGURE 33-4 • **Thiopurine metabolism.** 6-Thioguanine nucleotides (TGN) are the putative active metabolites of azathioprine (AZA) and 6-mercaptopurine (MP). TPMT, a polymorphically expressed enzyme, inactivates 6-mercaptopurine. *Arrows* indicate a pathway of metabolism and the *bar* indicates inhibition of purine production.

The enzyme activities of thiopurine methyltransferase and inosine triphosphate pyrophosphatase are affected by genetic polymorphisms, and the clinical relevance of those genetic polymorphisms is under intense investigation.[65] The gene encoding thiopurine methyltransferase has over 20 known polymorphisms that are distributed heterogeneously among different ethnic groups.[66] Enzyme produced off variant alleles of the thiopurine methyltransferase gene is degraded more quickly than wild-type enzyme, resulting in lower rates of enzyme activity.[67] The population genetics of thiopurine methyltransferase reveal a trimodal distribution of enzyme activity, which correlates with individuals having inherited none, one, or two wild-type alleles. Those with extremely low levels of thiopurine methyltransferase activity are highly susceptible to bone marrow suppression, whereas those with intermediate or high (normal) levels of activity are less likely to develop this complication of therapy with standard doses of azathioprine or 6-mercaptopurine. Some physicians routinely check thiopurine methyltransferase activity in all inflammatory bowel disease patients beginning azathioprine or 6-mercaptopurine therapy, to identify the approximately 1 in 10 patients with intermediate low activity, in whom we prescribe 50% of the normal dose, and the 1 in 300 patients with absent activity, in whom we do not use these drugs.[68]

6-Thioguanine has also been used in patients with inflammatory bowel disease. However, this drug appeared to induce liver disease in children,[69] so its use has been discontinued.

Pharmacodynamics. The major therapeutic mechanism of action of azathioprine and 6-mercaptopurine is the inhibition of purine nucleotide biosynthesis based on a random incorporation of 6-thioguanine nucleotides into DNA, leading to a general inhibition of nucleic acid synthesis.[70] However, this dogma has been questioned recently as more specific, less random mechanisms have been discovered. Recently it was shown that azathioprine-generated 6-thio-guanosine triphosphate prevents T cell-antigen–presenting cell conjugation and the subsequent development of an effective immune response via blockade of Vav activity on Rac proteins.[71] Also, it has been noted that thiopurines appear to block the release of a number of inflammatory genes.[72] Whatever the precise biochemical mechanism of azathioprine or 6-mercaptopurine, it has been shown that these drugs induce apoptosis of activated T lymphocytes, which probably explains their immunomodulating properties.

Evidence-Based Medicine Clinical Trials. There are two positive controlled trials regarding the use of azathioprine for treatment of chronically active ulcerative colitis.[73,74] The effect of 6-mercaptopurine has only been studied in retrospective analysis.[75,76] A steroid-sparing effect for both substances has been well documented. The efficacy of azathioprine and 6-mercaptopurine in inducing and maintaining remission in Crohn's disease with an optimal dose of 2.5 mg/kg and 1.5 mg/kg, respectively, has also been proven in clinical trials.[77-79]

Safety/Side Effects. Dose-independent side effects of azathioprine and 6-mercaptopurine include exanthema, arthralgias, myalgias, and pancreatitis. Dose-dependent effects include nausea, bone marrow suppression, cholestatic hepatitis, and stomatitis. Monitoring is recommended for the detection of leukopenia and hepatitis during therapy. Opportunistic infections occur more commonly in inflammatory bowel disease patients taking azathioprine or 6-mercaptopurine than not, and this can occur even in the absence of overt leukopenia. Several lymphomas have been reported to have occurred in inflammatory bowel disease patients taking these agents. Although not a proven risk factor for lymphoma, many authorities believe that azathioprine and 6-mercaptopurine do confer a small increase in the risk of lymphoma, which may be Epstein-Barr virus associated.[80,81]

Pregnancy and Lactation. No evidence conclusively demonstrates a link between teratogenicity and azathioprine or 6-mercaptopurine treatment in any disease, including inflammatory bowel disease.[82] However, because of the theoretical risk of harm to the fetus due to the antimetabolite effects of these drugs, their continuation in women contemplating conception should be discussed and weighed against the risk of inflammatory bowel disease reactivation.

Interactions. Allopurinol, a drug commonly used in gout, inhibits xanthine oxidase, an enzyme that converts 6-mercaptopurine into inactive metabolites. When coadministered with allopurinol, azathioprine and 6-mercaptopurine are preferentially metabolized into active 6-thioguanine metabolites. This greatly increases the risk of bone marrow suppression. Therefore, this combination should be avoided whenever possible, or the dose of azathioprine or 6-mercaptopurine has to be reduced to 25% of the usual therapeutic dosage. Recently, it has been proposed that the addition of allopurinol to low doses of azathioprine or 6-mercaptopurine can boost the production of active 6-thioguanine metabolites, with potential therapeutic benefits.[83]

Methotrexate. Methotrexate is an analogue of folic acid and, like azathioprine and 6-mercaptopurine, was originally developed as a treatment of leukemia. However, it too was later observed to have significant immunomodulating effects that have been useful in several chronic inflammatory diseases, including inflammatory bowel disease.[84]

Pharmacokinetics and Metabolism. Methotrexate is variably absorbed from the small intestine, with lower bioavailability reported at oral doses above 15 mg. For this reason, and because of significant interindividual variability in absorption, methotrexate is usually administered by subcutaneous or intramuscular injection in inflammatory bowel disease patients.[85] Although its plasma half-life is short (average: 7 hours), methotrexate can last as polyglutamate conjugates in the intracellular space for months, providing a long-lived store of drug.[86] This fact allows for weekly administration of methotrexate, and intracellular stores of methotrexate can be observed to gradually rise over the initial 6 to 8 weeks of therapy (Fig. 33-5).[85] The majority of methotrexate (about 80%) is eliminated unchanged in the kidneys.[86] Due to the renal elimination route, the dosage needs to be reduced in case of renal dysfunction.

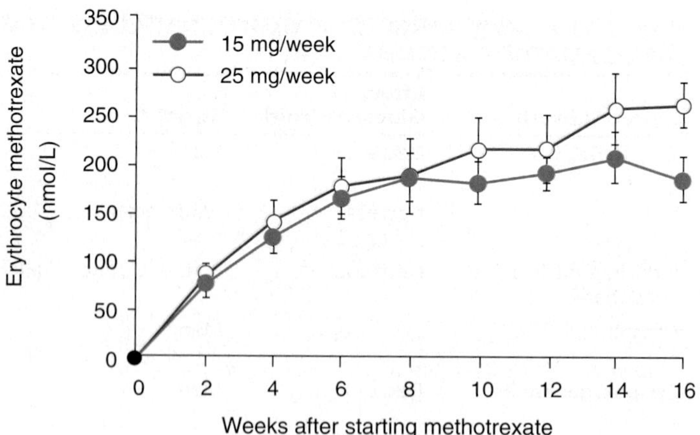

FIGURE 33-5 • Methotrexate accumulates in intracellular stores. Shown are mean erythrocyte methotrexate concentrations in inflammatory bowel disease patients receiving the indicated weekly doses of methotrexate. (From Egan LJ, Sandborn WJ, Tremaine WJ, et al. A randomized dose-response and pharmacokinetic study of methotrexate for refractory inflammatory Crohn's disease and ulcerative colitis. Aliment Pharmacol Ther 1999;13:1597-1604.)

Pharmacodynamics. The classic biochemical mechanism of action of methotrexate is competitive inhibition of dihydrofolate reductase with respect to dihydrofolate as substrate. This inhibits formation of fully reduced folate cofactors that are necessary in one-carbon transfer reactions. The lack of such cofactors impairs de novo synthesis of purine nucleotides and thymidylate. As a result, DNA and RNA synthesis are inhibited. Rapidly cycling cells are most sensitive to the effects of methotrexate, wherein the net result of its depletion of purine nucleotides and thymidylate is often manifest as apoptosis. When used to modulate immune responses, methotrexate has been shown to induce apoptosis of activated but not resting T lymphocytes.[87] This effect is likely to underlie its therapeutic effectiveness in chronic inflammatory diseases. An alternative mechanism was proposed for methotrexate whereby the concentration of the endogenous autocoid adenosine was elevated, which inhibited neutrophil function.[88] However, the importance of this mechanism has not been established in vivo.[89]

Evidence-Based Medicine Based Trials. Methotrexate has been proven in clinical trials to be effective for the induction of remission in chronically active Crohn's disease and for maintenance therapy at a lower dose.[90,91] No controlled trials have examined dose-response rates for treatment of chronically active Crohn's disease, nor have comparisons of oral and parenteral administration been conducted. The use of methotrexate for induction of remission in refractory Crohn's disease was reviewed in a Cochrane analysis.[92] The only controlled trial of the use of methotrexate for treatment of ulcerative colitis was negative, although this may have been due to underdosage.[93]

Safety/Side Effects. The most common side effects are stomatitis, dyspepsia, nausea, emesis, diarrhea, exanthema, and headache. The intake of 5 mg folic acid the day after methotrexate dosing helps to reduce mucosal toxicity by 80% without loss of effectiveness. Quite frequently an elevation of the serum concentration of liver enzymes is detected, which, if transient and not increased more than two- to threefold of normal values, can be tolerated.[94] However, when liver enzyme concentrations are persistently elevated more than two- to threefold, there exists a risk of the development of liver fibrosis and cirrhosis. For this reason, methotrexate should not be used in patients with any preexisting liver disease or risk factors for such diseases, especially alcoholism or nonalcoholic fatty liver disease. For early detection of side effects, it is recommended to check bilirubin, liver enzymes, albumin, and renal parameters before initiation, at weeks 1, 2, 4, 8, and 12 after initiation, and every 12 weeks thereafter. In addition, some guidelines recommend that hepatitis B and C be excluded before treatment. Less common side effects in patients who receive low dosages of methotrexate include myelotoxicity, pneumonitis, and renal toxicity.

Pregnancy and Lactation. Due to teratogenic effects, contraception is essential during methotrexate therapy in women. Some also recommend that male patients taking methotrexate should not conceive, although the risks to offspring in this situation are not known.

Interactions. Coadministration of trimethoprim, another inhibitor of dihydrofolate reductase, can lead to toxicity. Organic acids such as probenicid, sulfonamide, or penicillin can increase the methotrexate concentration due to inhibition of renal elimination.

Cyclosporine. Cyclosporine, the drug that launched organ transplantation, can be beneficial in very carefully selected patients with severely active inflammatory bowel disease.

Pharmacokinetics and Metabolism. The bioavailability of orally administered cyclosporine suspension is highly variable, averaging only about 30%. An emulsion formulation of the drug achieves higher (closer to 50%) and more consistent bioavailability. Cyclosporine is metabolized by CYP3A4, producing inactive metabolites that are cleared only via the biliary route. Cyclosporine can also be administered intravenously. The plasma elimination half-time is about 10 to 15 hours and is increased in the elderly as well as in patients with liver dysfunction. Due to inconsistent absorption, regular measurements of cyclosporine blood levels are required.

Pharmacodynamics. Cyclosporine is a water-insoluble cyclic peptide consisting of 11 amino acids, which is produced by the fungus *Tolypocladium inflatum*. At the molecular level, cyclosporine binds to cyclophilin and inhibits the cytoplasmic phosphatase calcineurin, which is essential for the T-cell receptor–triggered activation of the pivotal transcription factor, nuclear factor of activated T cells.[95] The immunosuppressive effect of cyclosporine is caused by a failure to induce secretion of interleukin-2, a key growth factor that drives T-lymphocyte multiplication during an immune response.

Evidence-Based Medicine Clinical Trials. The efficacy of intravenous cyclosporine for the treatment of steroid-refractory ulcerative colitis has been established in three controlled trials.[96-98] The common response time in the cyclosporine trials was between 7 and 10 days, and the initial remission rate between 63% and 91%. A Cochrane review concluded that the relatively quick response makes the short-term use of cyclosporine attractive, but the uncertain long-term outcomes weigh against the usefulness of this drug.[99] After induction of remission, azathioprine or 6-mercaptopurine should be added for maintenance therapy.[100-102] Intravenous cyclosporine has also been reported to induce clinical responses in patients with highly active Crohn's disease,[103] but when administered orally, this drug was not efficacious at nontoxic doses.[104]

Safety/Side Effects. Dose-related side effects significantly limit the utility of cyclosporine in inflammatory bowel disease. The most common as well as severe side effects are renal toxicity, hypertension, and cholestasis. Less severe side effects include nausea, emesis, diarrhea, headache, tremor, paresthesias, hypertrichosis, gingival hyperplasia, reversible amenorrhea or dysmenorrhea, and hyperuricemia. Allergic reactions, myelotoxic effects, electrolyte imbalance, hyperglycemia, and seizures can also be seen. For monitoring of side effects, it is suggested to check the blood count, bilirubin, uric acid, magnesium, potassium, and liver enzymes as well as renal parameters before therapy, and every 14 days during the first 3 months of therapy. Blood pressure must also be monitored. Seizures on cyclosporine are more common in patients with hypomagnesemia or hypocholesteremia.[105,106]

Interactions. Cyclosporine reduces the elimination of colchicine, digoxin, and prednisolone. Coadministration of cyclosporine with hydroxymethylglutaryl-coenzyme A reductase inhibitors increases the risk of myopathy and rhabdomyolysis caused by those drugs.[107] Substances that inhibit CYP3A4, such as grapefruit juice and ketoconazole, increase the cyclosporine circulating concentration and can cause toxicity.[108]

Tacrolimus. Tacrolimus, also known as FK506, has immunosuppressive actions very similar to those of cyclosporine. Tacrolimus is a macrolide antibiotic and is structurally unrelated to cyclosporine.

Pharmacokinetics and Metabolism. The bioavailability of orally administered tacrolimus ranges from 14% to 32%, but is less variable than cyclosporine. Via CYP3A4, it is processed within the liver to less active metabolites and excreted with bile acids. The usual plasma elimination half-time of 10 hours is increased in patients with liver dysfunction.[109]

Pharmacodynamics. Tacrolimus is extracted from cultures of *Streptomyces tsukubaensis*. Similar to cyclosporine, tacrolimus inhibits the activation of T cells by blocking nuclear factor of activated T cells–induced interleukin-2 production.

Evidence-Based Medicine Clinical Trials. Tacrolimus has been shown to be effective for reducing the number of draining fistulas in patients with perianal Crohn's disease.[110] However, tacrolimus is not efficacious for the induction of fistula remission. There are no other well-controlled trials of tacrolimus in inflammatory bowel disease, although some small studies have suggested benefit in the treatment of chronically active ulcerative colitis.[111-114]

Safety/Side Effects. Some of the more common side effects include tremor, headache, sleeplessness, paresthesia, depression, difficulties with coordination, nervousness, dizziness, and changes in eyesight. Further potential side effects are electrolyte disturbances (hyper- and hypokalemia, hypomagnesemia, hypercalcemia), renal impairment, diabetes, hypertension, anemia, and allergic and anaphylactic reactions.

Interactions. Similar to cyclosporine, important interactions include elevated risk of nephrotoxicity when coadministered with other nephrotoxic drugs and competition with other substrates for CYP3A4, resulting in decreased clearance.

Biologics

Infliximab. The advent of infliximab has revolutionized the management of moderate to severely active inflammatory bowel disease. This agent was developed to neutralize the activity of tumor necrosis factor-α, a pivotal proinflammatory cytokine that was believed to be a major pathogenic factor in septic shock. However, controlled trials revealed a harmful effect of infliximab in such patients. Only later was the beneficial effect of infliximab in Crohn's disease first witnessed.[115]

Pharmacokinetics and Metabolism. Infliximab is administered intravenously, and its dose-concentration relationship follows a linear kinetic over clinically used doses. The degradation of infliximab is not well understood, but most likely it is through the reticuloendothelial system of the liver and spleen. The terminal plasma elimination half-time is about 9 days, and the drug is typically administered once every 8 weeks. Many patients treated with infliximab develop so-called human antichimeric antibodies. These antibodies are associated with shortened plasma half-life and blunted therapeutic effectiveness of infliximab.[116] Infusion reactions are also more common in patients who developed these antibodies. Some reports suggest that the development of human antichimeric antibodies can be minimized by continuous rather than intermittent therapy, pretreatment with intravenous corticosteroid,[117] and concomitant immunomodulation with azathioprine, 6-mercaptopurine, or methotrexate.[118]

Pharmacodynamics. Infliximab is a mouse-human chimeric neutralizing monoclonal antibody against tumor necrosis factor-α. Infliximab binds to soluble and membrane-associated tumor necrosis factor-α. Patients with inflammatory bowel disease have markedly elevated production of this cytokine at sites of disease, predominantly by activated monocytes. The neutralizing effect of this antibody on tumor necrosis factor-α was initially thought to be the main mechanism of action. However, since other tumor necrosis factor-α–neutralizing drugs such as etanercept and onercept did not show significant therapeutic effects for treatment of active Crohn's disease in controlled trials,[119,120] it was suggested that further mechanisms are responsible for the infliximab effect. More recent work suggests that infliximab induces the apoptosis of activated monocytes and lymphocytes that express membrane-associated tumor necrosis factor-α.[121,122] This effect appears to occur through a previously unrecognized signaling pathway from membrane-associated tumor necrosis factor-α directly leading to caspase activation.

Evidence-Based Medicine Clinical Trials. The clinical benefit of infliximab for induction of remission and maintenance therapy for Crohn's disease as well as closure of fistulas has been proven in double-blind, placebo-controlled multicenter trials.[123-126] Furthermore, infliximab has been proven to be effective for induction and maintenance therapy for ulcerative colitis.[127]

Safety/Side Effects. The most significant side effects of infliximab treatment are serious opportunistic infections. Several deaths due to infections have been reported in inflammatory bowel disease patients who were treated with infliximab.[128] The most important opportunistic infection is a reactivation of latent tuberculosis.[129] It is essential to exclude patients with latent tuberculosis from receiving this or any other tumor necrosis factor-α–blocking drugs. For this reason, screening for latent tuberculosis is mandatory in patients in whom infliximab use is planned. Of so-far unknown significance is the increased detection rate of antinuclear and double-stranded DNA antibodies during treatment with infliximab.[130] Due to a potential risk of worsening a preexisting cardiac insufficiency, patients with moderate to severe congestive heart failure should not receive infliximab therapy. Cases of demyelinating disease similar to multiple sclerosis have also been reported after infliximab.[131]

Interactions. No relevant interactions with other medications have been described so far.

Adalimumab

Pharmacokinetics and Metabolism. Adalimumab is an almost fully humanized anti-tumor necrosis factor-α IgG1 antibody, with a half-life of about 12–14 days. It is administered subcutaneously with a usual dosing interval of every 2 weeks. Antibodies against adalimumab have been detected in patients receiving this drug, but their clinical significance is currently not known.

Pharmacodynamics. Adalimumab binds to tumor necrosis factor-α with high affinity and effectively neutralizes its biological activities. Like infliximab, adalimumab appears to be able to induce apoptosis of activated monocytes that express membrane-associated tumor necrosis factor-α.

Evidence-Based Medicine Clinical Trials. Having been a standard medical treatment option in rheumatoid arthritis for several years,[132] it has now also been shown in controlled clinical trials to be efficacious for acute flares of Crohn's disease,[133] as well as maintenance therapy.[134]

Safety/Side Effects. Adalimumab is generally well-tolerated. Some patients have reported injection site reactions that can be managed with antihistamines. The risks of reaction of tuberculosis, other opportunistic infections, and central nervous system demyelination are similar to those encountered with infliximab.

Interactions. No clinically significant drug interactions have been reported with adalimumab.

Natalizumab. Natalizumab, a humanized monoclonal antibody against α4 integrins, is the first inhibitor of leukocyte trafficking to be licensed. Initially, this drug was proven efficacious for the treatment of active multiple sclerosis and Crohn's disease. However, clinical development and licensing were delayed because of fears about the development of a fatal brain disease, progressive multifocal leukoencephalopathy, in patients who received the drug. Eventually in January 2008, natalizumab was approved for use in Crohn's disease by the US Food and Drug Administration, but not by the European Medicines Agency.

Pharmacokinetics and Metabolism. Natalizumab is administered intravenously, with a usual dosing interval of 4 weeks. The average half-life of elimination is about 11 days. Antibodies against natalizumab have been detected in less then 10% of treated patients and their clinical significance is not known.

Pharmacodynamics. Natalizumab blocks the interactions between α4 integrins expressed on the surface of activated lymphocytes and monocytes, and their ligand, vascular cell adhesion molecule-1, expressed on the surface of activated endothelial cells. This decreases the adhesion and subsequent diapedesis of those lymphocytes and monocytes through the capillary wall and migration into inflamed tissues. This blockade of leukocyte extravasation is evident in a sudden rise in circulating white blood cell count after administration of a dose of natalizumab.

Evidence-Based Medicine Clinical Trials. Treatment of flares of Crohn's disease with natalizumab in a double-blind placebo controlled trial did not increase clinical response over placebo.[135] However, patients with initial clinical responses to natalizumab maintained response better when continued on the drug than when switched to placebo.[136] Recently, natalizumab was shown to be superior to placebo for induction of remission in active Crohn's disease.[137]

Safety/Side Effects. In the initial clinical trials of natalizumab for multiple sclerosis and Crohn's disease, 3 out of approximately 2000 patients developed progressive multifocal leukoencephalopathy.[138] All of these patients were receiving additional immunosuppressive drugs. Apart from this very serious adverse reaction, minor infections have been reported to be slightly more common in natalizumab-treated patients than in control patients.

Interactions. No clinically significant drug interactions with natalizumab have been reported yet.

Therapeutic Approach

General Considerations

When approaching a patient with symptomatic inflammatory bowel disease, the physician must consider the following factors:

- Is there evidence of active inflammation?
- What is the location and extent of the disease?
- Is there any evidence of disease complications such as stricture formation or intestinal penetration?
- Are there any extraintestinal manifestations?
- What is the age of the patient?
- Does the patient plan pregnancy?
- Are any comorbidities present?

All of these factors are important in the individual patient because they will dictate the optimum therapeutic approach. It is of the utmost importance when considering medical therapy of inflammatory bowel diseases to establish with as much certainty as possible that the patient's symptoms are caused by active inflamed segments of the intestine and not by complications such as stricture formation or associated comorbidities such as irritable bowel syndrome. This can usually be established with standard clinical investigations including endoscopy, radiology, and laboratory tests. Many inflammatory bowel disease drug therapies require monitoring before and/or during therapy, to detect contraindications to therapy with that drug, or the development of toxicity during therapy with that drug. An outline of appropriate testing is provided in Table 33-5.

Crohn's Disease

Most physicians advocate a stepwise approach to the treatment of Crohn's disease. In this therapeutic approach, Crohn's disease is assessed as mildly, moderately, or severely active. Little consensus exists on the optimum means of assessing Crohn's disease activity, but physicians often consider the anatomic extent of disease, number and size of ulcerations, severity of histologic inflammation and tissue destruction, general condition of the patient, and presence of complications as important factors. This assessment then informs the risk-benefit analysis that guides choice of the initial or next drug. In this therapeutic approach, failure or intolerance of one drug usually prompts a move up the ladder.

Active Inflammatory Crohn's Disease. A stepwise approach to the drug treatment of active inflammatory Crohn's disease is presented in Figure 33-6. Corticosteroids, such as prednisolone at a starting daily dose of 40 mg/day or controlled-ileal-release budesonide 3 mg three times a day, are efficacious for the induction of remission in mildly to moderately active ileal or ileocolonic Crohn's disease.[49-51,53,139,140] Because of significantly less adrenal suppression, controlled-ileal-release budesonide is preferable to conventional corticosteroids in patients with ileal and right colon disease. The dose of conventional corticosteroids such as prednisolone is usually lowered gradually over several weeks after a clinical response has been obtained. One popular approach is to reduce the daily dose of prednisolone by 5 mg every week. Sulfasalazine is another option for left colon disease.[49,50]

Some patients experience adverse effects of corticosteroids (steroid-intolerant patients), some do not improve (steroid-resistant patients), and some flare up when corticosteroids are tapered or stopped (steroid-dependent patients). In such patients, infliximab and adalimumab are very useful. Infliximab, administered as a single infusion of 5 mg/kg, induced remission in 33% of patients and clinical response in 81% of patients, a large benefit compared to placebo.[124] Adalimumab, another anti–tumor necrosis factor-α antibody, was also reported to be efficacious in active Crohn's disease, when administered subcutaneously at a dose of 160 mg initially, followed by 80 mg or 40 mg every other week.[133]

Methotrexate is a useful adjunct to corticosteroids in patients who have persistent disease activity. This drug was found to be efficacious at a weekly dose of 25 mg in such patients.[90] Methotrexate can be administered orally or by injection, and we find the subcutaneous route to be effective and well tolerated by patients.

6-Mercaptopurine or azathioprine are beneficial in patients with active Crohn's disease.[141,142] Best results are obtained when 6-mercaptopurine or azathioprine are initially combined with faster acting drugs such as corticosteroids, infliximab or adalimumab because beneficial effects may take up to 2 or 3 months to develop when 6-mercaptopurine or azathioprine is administered alone. A study of the early use of 6-mercaptopurine in children with Crohn's disease showed that this drug improved long-term outcomes and lowered corticosteroid use.[143] These results provide a rationale for the early introduction of immunomodulators in Crohn's disease, but additional safety data regarding these agents in inflammatory bowel disease is needed.

In patients with moderate to severe active inflammatory Crohn's disease who do not respond fully to the agents discussed above, or who cannot tolerate those agents, natalizumab 300 mg by intravenous infusion may be tried. It is important to carefully weigh the expectation of benefit against the risk of adverse effects in such patients, and to ensure adequate time to allow wash-out of previously administered immunosuppressives.

In summary, patients with active Crohn's disease who do not fully respond to corticosteroids should be treated with 6-mercaptopurine (1.5 mg/kg per day) or azathioprine (2.0 to 2.5 mg/kg per day), subcutaneous methotrexate (25 mg once per week), and infusions of infliximab (5 mg/kg) or injections of adalimumab (160 mg followed by 80 mg or 40 mg every other week). Clinical experience indicates that, among these options, the anti–tumor necrosis factor-α agents will produce the fastest response. Where this therapeutic approach fails or is not tolerated, natalizumab is a good option.

Crohn's Disease in Remission. Most patients with active Crohn's disease can be effectively brought into symptomatic remission with medical therapy or surgery. Prevention of relapses of active disease is a major challenge in the management of this disease.

6-Mercaptopurine and azathioprine, administered at the same doses that are used in active disease, have been extensively studied and are effective in many patients for preventing relapses.[125,141,143,144] In patients who enter durable remission with one of these drugs, studies suggest that the drug should be continued indefinitely.[145] Although clearly beneficial, some patients do not fully respond to azathioprine or 6-mercaptopurine, and these drugs have significant potential for serious toxicity, and require regular toxicity monitoring.

Aminosalicylates are widely used for the maintenance of Crohn's disease remission, yet a critical reading of the literature provides little support for this practice. Although some studies suggested a modest benefit of mesalazine over placebo,[146-148] many studies were negative.[149-155] Meta-analysis showed no significant benefit over placebo in medically induced remission, or a marginal benefit in surgically induced remission.[156] Similarly, sulfasalazine[49,50,157] and olsalazine[158] were found to be not superior to placebo for remission maintenance. For these reasons, we do not recommend the use of aminosalicylates in Crohn's disease patients in remission.

Conventional corticosteroids are not effective for maintaining Crohn's disease remission when used at nontoxic doses. Controlled-ileal-release budesonide 6 mg/day can delay relapse and is an option in some patients who do not tolerate immunomodulators.[159-161]

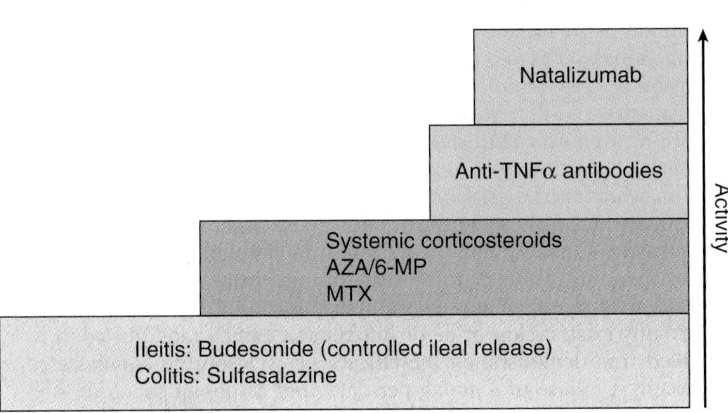

FIGURE 33-6 • Stepwise approach to drug therapy of active inflammatory Crohn's disease. As disease activity increases, the drugs used for therapy are indicated at that step. AZA, azathioprine; MP, mercaptopurine; MTX, methotrexate; TNF, tumor necrosis factor.

TABLE 33-5 TESTING FOR CONTRAINDICATIONS TO AND TOXICITY OF DRUGS USED TO TREAT INFLAMMATORY BOWEL DISEASE

Drug	Before Starting Therapy	During Therapy, Frequency
Aminosalicylates	Serum creatinine	Serum creatinine, every 6 mo
Corticosteroids	None	Not applicable*
Methotrexate	Serum liver enzyme activity Full blood count	Serum liver enzyme activity, every 4 wk Full blood count, every 4 wk
Azathioprine/6-mercaptopurine	Serum liver enzyme activity Full blood count Thiopurine methyltransferase†	Serum liver enzyme activity, every 4 wk Full blood count, every 4 wk
Cyclosporine, intravenous	Cholesterol Creatinine and electrolytes Blood pressure	Creatinine and electrolytes, daily Blood cyclosporine, daily Blood pressure, daily
Anti–tumor necrosis factor-α agents	Chest radiograph and tuberculin skin test	

*Prolonged therapy not recommended.
†Activity or genotype.

Methotrexate maintenance therapy, 15 mg once per week, is effective in preventing clinical relapse in patients who entered remission on this drug.[91]

In patients who enter remission on infliximab, this drug is effective for maintaining remission when continued every 8 weeks at a dose of 5 mg/kg.[126] We usually continue this agent in patients who enter remission after the initial three doses. In patients who flare during maintenance infliximab, the dose can be increased to 10 mg/kg, or the interval between doses can be shortened. Adalimumab, at a dose of 40 mg, is also useful when continued every week or every other week in patients who respond to initial doses.[134] In patients who initially respond to natalizumab, this agent may be continued as a monthly infusion.[162]

In summary, azathioprine or 6-mercaptopurine, methotrexate, infliximab and adalimumab can all be used to prevent relapse in quiescent Crohn's disease. Most patients will relapse without maintenance therapy, so usually one of these drugs should be prescribed. It makes sense to continue the drug that was used successfully to induce remission in an individual patient as the remission maintaining agent. An important exception to this strategy is the patient who has resection of a short segment of distal ileum, entering a surgically induced remission. Many such patients remain asymptomatic for decades, and medical therapy would not be likely to offer much advantage. We commonly stratify such patients for remission-maintaining therapy based on the absence or presence of endoscopic evidence of recurrent disease in the ileum 6 to 12 months postresection.

Perianal Crohn's Disease. Optimal management of perianal Crohn's disease requires accurate definition of the anatomy of fistulas and abscesses and their control using surgery and drainage.[163-165] Medical therapy is commonly undertaken with an antibiotic such as metronidazole, although no controlled evidence supports this practice. Infliximab (5 mg/kg) administered at weeks 0, 2, and 6 and azathioprine (2 to 2.5 mg/kg) or 6-mercaptopurine (1.5 mg/kg) are the drugs with the best established roles for the medical treatment of active fistulizing disease.[125,142] Tacrolimus is an alternative to infliximab and azathioprine, but does not appear to be as effective.[110]

For the maintenance of fistula closure, continuous infliximab infusions every 8 weeks is the optimum strategy.[166] It is not clear if the coadministration of azathioprine or 6-mercaptopurine improves the effectiveness of infliximab in this setting, but these drugs are commonly coadministered in such patients.

Ulcerative Colitis

Similar to Crohn's disease, most physicians advocate a stepwise approach to therapy in ulcerative colitis patients. In this approach, the safest but least active drugs are initially used in patients with mild disease, while more active but potentially toxic drugs are reserved for those patients with more severe disease and those who cannot be well controlled with the less active agents.

Active Ulcerative Colitis. A stepwise approach to drug therapy of active ulcerative colitis is provided in Figure 33-7. Drugs proven effective in the treatment of active ulcerative colitis include the aminosalicylates, corticosteroids, azathioprine, 6-mercaptopurine, cyclosporine, nicotine, and infliximab. The choice of which of these agents to use in an individual patient depends upon the extent and severity of the disease, the responsiveness to and occurrence of toxicities with previous medications, and the presence of any disease complications.

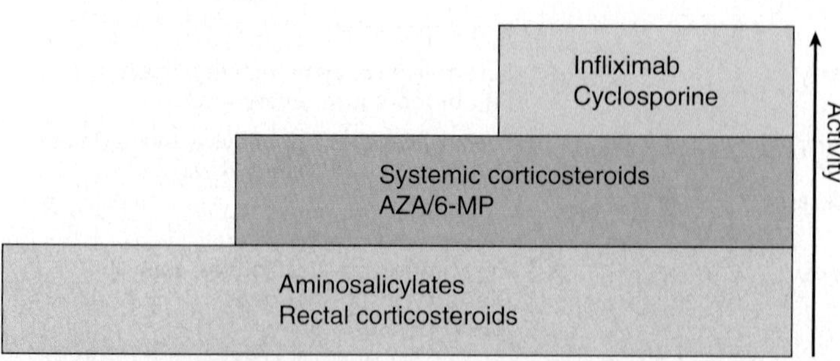

FIGURE 33-7 • Stepwise approach to drug therapy of active ulcerative colitis. As disease activity increases, the drugs used for therapy are indicated at that step. AZA, azathioprine; MP, mercaptopurine.

In patients with mildly to moderately active colitis, an aminosalicylate is usually a good first choice.[34] Clinical responses are typically seen with doses ranging from 1.2 g in divided doses per day, up to a maximum daily dose of 4.8 g. Several reports have suggested that higher doses produce better clinical responses than lower doses.[28] Patients with disease confined to the rectum can usually be treated with suppositories of an aminosalicylate such as mesalazine. In patients with disease extending up to the region of the splenic flexure, enema preparations of mesalazine are quite effective. When the disease extends proximal to the splenic flexure, then oral therapy is usually needed, although it can still be significantly augmented by coadministration of drugs rectally.[167] Most patients prefer to take oral rather than rectal drugs, so even in patients with proctitis, mesalazine tablets can be used successfully. It is important to recognize that some patients do not respond to aminosalicylates, or even experience an exacerbation of symptoms after starting one of these agents.[168] Cessation of mesalazine in such patients is recommended.

In patients with more severe disease activity, or in those who do not respond fully to optimal doses of an aminosalicylate, corticosteroids are indicated. In the outpatient setting, a typical starting dose would be prednisolone 40 mg/day. Usually, a clinical response will begin within a few days, and once the patient has improved considerably (e.g., after about 2 weeks), the dose of prednisolone can be tapered.

Based on observations of ulcerative colitis flares after smoking cessation, nicotine transdermal patches have been evaluated for treatment of mildly active ulcerative colitis. Results show a modest clinical benefit of nicotine over placebo,[169] but side effects including nausea and hypotension severely limit the utility of this therapy.

Patients who do not respond to oral corticosteroids can be treated with intravenous corticosteroids in the hospital.[170] It is critical in this patient population to be alert to the possibility of toxic dilation of the colon, which carries a risk of perforation. Methylprednisolone at a dose of 60 mg once daily is typical, but other corticosteroids are likely to be as effective. If no response occurs within 5 days of intravenous therapy, a decision must be made to proceed to surgery, or move on to another intravenous therapy.[97] If medical therapy is chosen, two viable options currently exist: cyclosporine or infliximab. A small randomized, controlled trial demonstrated the efficacy of cyclosporine administered initially at a dose of 4 mg/kg per day,[96] but a subsequent study suggested that this drug is as effective at the safer intravenous dose of 2 mg/kg per day.[98] Monitoring of cyclosporine blood levels is essential during intravenous therapy. Recent large randomized, controlled trials have established the efficacy of infliximab 5 mg/kg in ulcerative colitis patients with moderate, but not severe, disease activity.[127] Small studies have suggested that infliximab is also effective in the sicker steroid-resistant population.[171] The management of such patients is complex and should ideally involve a team consisting of gastroenterologists and surgeons experienced in the care of sick inflammatory bowel disease patients.

Maintenance of Ulcerative Colitis Remission. Many patients who respond to initial medical therapies for ulcerative colitis will at some point later in the disease experience a flare-up. If flare-ups are very rare and are easily controlled with medications such as aminosalicylates, there is little indication for maintenance therapy. However, in many patients, flares of ulcerative colitis occur soon after stopping medication prescribed to induce remission, and sometimes the flares are severe. In such patients, maintenance therapy is indicated. Drugs proven effective to maintain remission in ulcerative colitis include aminosalicylates, azathioprine, 6-mercaptopurine, and infliximab.

Patients with mild disease usually do well with aminosalicylates such as mesalazine. Effective daily doses range from 1.2 to 2.8 g/day.[172] However, in some patients, aminosalicylates lack efficacy in preventing flares. Those patients should be started on azathioprine at a daily dose of 2 to 2.5 mg/kg per day or 6-mercaptopurine 1.5 mg/kg per day.[74]

Azathioprine and 6-mercaptopurine are slow-acting drugs that may take up to 2 or 3 months to induce a clinical benefit. For this reason, patients must be brought into remission, usually with a further course of corticosteroids or infliximab at the same time that azathioprine or 6-mercaptopurine is started.

Patients who respond to remission induction therapy with infliximab can be treated with maintenance infusions of infliximab with or without coadministration of azathioprine or 6-mercaptopurine.[127] Current data suggest that coadministration of an immunomodulator along with infliximab may prevent development of human antichimeric antibodies, but the results of further studies are needed to establish whether combination therapy is superior to infliximab alone or azathioprine/6-mercaptopurine alone in this clinical setting.

Pouchitis

Patients with ulcerative colitis who have ileal pouch–anal anastomosis surgery can develop inflammatory bowel disease of the pouch, which is termed *pouchitis*. This occurs in more than 50% of patients. Acute flares of pouchitis, which manifest clinically as diarrhea, tenesmus, and bleeding, can usually be managed well with a short course of antibiotics such as metronidazole or ciprofloxacin.[173] If episodes of symptomatic pouchitis occur frequently, short courses of these antibiotics can be used on an ongoing basis, as needed. However, in the minority of patients in whom pouchitis fails to respond fully to antibiotics or who experience flares soon after discontinuing antibiotics, maintenance therapy with an immunomodulator such as azathioprine or 6-mercaptopurine is usually warranted. Small case series also support the use of infliximab in patients with more severe pouchitis.[174]

Emerging Targets and Therapeutics

Anti–Tumor Necrosis Factor-α Alternatives

The effectiveness of infliximab and adalimumab for treatment of certain patients with Crohn's disease and ulcerative colitis is well established. However, one of the main problems of long-term therapy with these antibodies is the development of human antichimeric or antihuman antibodies in a significant percentage of treated patients, leading to a loss of efficacy and/or allergic reactions.[116] A new anti–tumor necrosis factor-α agent, certolizumab has been designed that, in first trials, appear to cause less antibody development and therefore give the hope of a longer efficacy.

Certolizumab Pegol. Certolizumab pegol (CDP870) is a humanized polyethylene glycol (PEG)ylated Fab fragment of an anti–tumor necrosis factor-α monoclonal antibody. In contrast to infliximab and adalimumab, it consists only of a single Fab fragment with no Fc portion. It is engineered for production in *Escherichia coli*. It is linked to 2 × 20 kDa PEG due to which the antibodies' half-life is extended.[175] Furthermore, certolizumab is compatible with subcutaneous administration.

Certolizumab pegol has been shown in two large, controlled trials to be effective for induction of improvement but not symptomatic remission in the treatment of acute flares of Crohn's disease as well as for maintenance therapy. Certolizumab pegol may be licensed for Crohn's disease in the future.[176]

Anticytokines

In addition to targeting tumor necrosis factor-α, further proinflammatory cytokines are the targets of future treatment options for inflammatory bowel disease.

Anti–Interleukin-12. Interleukin-12 is a key cytokine that initiates Th1-mediated inflammatory responses. A human antibody against interleukin-12 was tested for treatment of active Crohn's disease. In the first double-blind trial, anti–interleukin-12 appeared to be able to induce response and remission rates greater than placebo.[177] These initial findings require confirmation in a larger trial.

Anti–Interferon-γ. Another therapeutic aim is to antagonize interferon-γ. Blockade of this Th1 effector cytokine using the humanized antibody fontolizumab showed a beneficial effect for treatment of active Crohn's disease in a placebo-controlled trial. This effect was significant only in a subgroup of patients with elevated levels of C-reactive protein.[178,179]

Anti–Interleukin-6. Interleukin-6 takes part in T- and B-lymphocyte development and differentiation as well as the stimulation of the innate immune system. In several mouse models, administration of a neutralizing interleukin-6 antibody showed promising results such as abolishment of apoptosis resistance of lamina propria T cells.[180] In a first pilot randomized trial of a human anti–interleukin-6 receptor antibody (atlizumab), 80% of treated Crohn's disease patients experienced a response and 20% reached remission at week 12.[181]

Cytokines and Growth Factors

Interleukin-10. Interleukin-10 is a Th2 cytokine that suppresses the expression of the proinflammatory cytokines interleukin-2 and interferon-γ, as well as inhibiting the synthesis of interleukin-12. While initial pilot studies showed a positive effect of intravenously administered interleukin-10 for treatment of Crohn's disease, this effect could not be reproduced in a larger Phase III trial.[182] One group of investigators has cloned interleukin-10 into a nonpathogenic *Lactococcus* strain that temporarily colonizes the gastrointestinal tract, where it locally produces the cytokine. The safety of these genetically modified bacteria has been assessed in a Phase I trial,[183] and the analysis of its efficacy for treatment of inflammatory bowel disease in a large placebo-controlled trial is awaited.

Sargramostim. The hematopoietic growth factor sargramostim, also known as granulocyte-monocyte colony-stimulating factor, has been tested for use in inflammatory bowel disease. This factor stimulates the innate immune system and appears to enhance the disturbed intestinal barrier function in inflammatory bowel disease. Though the primary end point was not reached in a large controlled trial for Crohn's disease, the secondary end point was significant, making sargramostim an interesting potential future alternative approach for treatment of inflammatory bowel disease.[184]

Selective Adhesion Molecule Inhibitor

As the integrin $\alpha_4\beta_7$ recruits leukocytes mainly in the gastrointestinal tract, an antibody against this specific integrin has been developed and tested in a multicenter, double-blind, placebo-controlled trial for treatment of active ulcerative colitis. Initial results with this antibody, MLN02, were positive,[185] and further testing is ongoing.

Intracellular Signal Transduction Inhibitors

Another current focus of clinical research is the modulation of intracellular proinflammatory signal transduction pathways. One example are the mitogen-activated protein (MAP) kinase inhibitors BIRB-769 and RDP58, for which clinical inflammatory bowel disease trials could not show any or showed only minor therapeutic effects, respectively.[186,187] While a pilot study with the MAP kinase inhibitor CNI-1493 showed promising effects in treating acute flares of Crohn's disease,[188] the final results of a follow-up study have not been published.

Microbiota

An interesting alternative new therapeutic approach for inflammatory bowel disease is the administration of the ova of the parasite *Trichiuris suis*. The rationale for this therapy is that countries with a high prevalence of worm infestations have low incidence of inflammatory bowel disease, and the fact that these worms promote Th2 polarization of cytokine responses in the digestive tract. A placebo-controlled trial for treatment of ulcerative colitis showed a moderate effect (response 43% compared to 16% in the placebo group). The results of an uncontrolled trial for treatment of Crohn's disease had a response rate of 79% and remission rate of 72%.[189] Though these results look promising, confirmation in larger multicenter trials is needed.

Probiotics are live nonpathogenic bacteria that exert beneficial effects on health. The mechanisms underlying the benefits of probiotics are not completely understood, but include competition with pathogenic microbes, immunomodulatory effects on cells of the mucosal immune system, and increased mucosal barrier integrity.

Various versions of probiotic bacteria have been thought to serve as treatment options for inflammatory bowel disease. So far, *Escherichia coli* Nissle 1917 has been shown in a controlled trial to be equivalent to mesalazine in maintaining remission in patients with ulcerative colitis.[190] In some countries, *Escherichia coli* Nissle 1917 has therefore been approved for maintenance therapy in those patients intolerant to mesalazine. Furthermore, the probiotic combination VSL#3, containing four strains of lactobacillus, three strains of bifidobacteria, and one streptococcus strain, has shown promising results for treatment of ulcerative colitis in an open-label trial.[191] This needs to be confirmed in placebo-controlled trials. In addition, VSL#3 appears to exert clinically significant anti-inflammatory effects in postoperative pouchitis.[192]

REFERENCES

1. Loftus EV Jr, Silverstein MD, Sandborn WJ, et al. Crohn's disease in Olmsted County, Minnesota, 1940-1993: incidence, prevalence, and survival. Gastroenterology 1998;114:1161-1168.
2. Loftus EV Jr, Silverstein MD, Sandborn WJ, et al. Ulcerative colitis in Olmsted County, Minnesota, 1940-1993: incidence, prevalence, and survival. Gut 2000;46:336-343.
3. Loftus EV Jr, Schoenfeld P, Sandborn WJ. The epidemiology and natural history of Crohn's disease in population-based patient cohorts from North America: a systematic review. Aliment Pharmacol Ther 2002;16:51-60.
4. Winther KV, Jess T, Langholz E, et al. Survival and cause-specific mortality in ulcerative colitis: follow-up of a population-based cohort in Copenhagen County. Gastroenterology 2003;125:1576-1582.
5. Jess T, Loftus EV Jr, Harmsen WS, et al. Survival and cause specific mortality in patients with inflammatory bowel disease: a long term outcome study in Olmsted County, Minnesota, 1940-2004. Gut 2006;55:1248-1254.
6. Colombel JF, Grandbastien B, Gower-Rousseau C, et al. Clinical characteristics of Crohn's disease in 72 families. Gastroenterology 1996;111:604-607.
7. Bayless TM, Tokayer AZ, Polito JM 2nd, et al. Crohn's disease: concordance for site and clinical type in affected family members—potential hereditary influences. Gastroenterology 1996;111:573-579.
8. Schreiber S, Rosenstiel P, Albrecht M, et al. Genetics of Crohn disease, an archetypal inflammatory barrier disease. Nat Rev Genet 2005;6:376-388.
9. Hugot JP, Chamaillard M, Zouali H, et al. Association of NOD2 leucine-rich repeat variants with susceptibility to Crohn's disease. Nature 2001;411:599-603.
10. Ogura Y, Bonen DK, Inohara N, et al. A frameshift mutation in *NOD2* associated with susceptibility to Crohn's disease. Nature 2001;411:603-606.
11. Chamaillard M, Iacob R, Desreumaux P, Colombel JF. Advances and perspectives in the genetics of inflammatory bowel diseases. Clin Gastroenterol Hepatol 2006;4:143-151.
12. Eckmann L, Karin M. NOD2 and Crohn's disease: loss or gain of function? Immunity 2005;22:661-667.
13. Duerr RH, Taylor KD, Brant SR, et al. A genome-wide association study identifies *IL23R* as an inflammatory bowel disease gene. Science 2006;314:1461-1463.
14. McFadden JJ, Butcher PD, Chiodini R, Hermon-Taylor J. Crohn's disease-isolated mycobacteria are identical to *Mycobacterium paratuberculosis*, as determined by DNA probes that distinguish between mycobacterial species. J Clin Microbiol 1987;25:796-801.
15. Daszak P, Purcell M, Lewin J, et al. Detection and comparative analysis of persistent measles virus infection in Crohn's disease by immunogold electron microscopy. J Clin Pathol 1997;50:299-304.
16. Harries AD, Baird A, Rhodes J. Non-smoking: a feature of ulcerative colitis. Br Med J (Clin Res Ed) 1982;284:706.
17. Timmer A, Sutherland LR, Martin F. Oral contraceptive use and smoking are risk factors for relapse in Crohn's disease. The Canadian Mesalamine for Remission of Crohn's Disease Study Group. Gastroenterology 1998;114:1143-1150.
18. D'Haens GR, Geboes K, Peeters M, et al. Early lesions of recurrent Crohn's disease caused by infusion of intestinal contents in excluded ileum. Gastroenterology 1998;114:262-267.
19. Sartor RB. Targeting enteric bacteria in treatment of inflammatory bowel diseases: why, how, and when. Curr Opin Gastroenterol 2003;19:358-365.
20. Isaacs KL, Sartor RB. Treatment of inflammatory bowel disease with antibiotics. Gastroenterol Clin North Am 2004;33:335-345.
21. Rakoff-Nahoum S, Paglino J, Eslami-Varzaneh F, et al. Recognition of commensal microflora by toll-like receptors is required for intestinal homeostasis. Cell 2004;118:229-241.
22. Fukata M, Michelsen KS, Eri R, et al. Toll-like receptor-4 is required for intestinal response to epithelial injury and limiting bacterial translocation in a murine model of acute colitis. Am J Physiol Gastrointest Liver Physiol 2005;288:G1055-G1065.
23. Targan SR, Karp LC. Defects in mucosal immunity leading to ulcerative colitis. Immunol Rev 2005;206:296-305.
24. Cobrin GM, Abreu MT. Defects in mucosal immunity leading to Crohn's disease. Immunol Rev 2005;206:277-295.
25. Sandborn WJ, Feagan BG, Hanauer SB, et al. A review of activity indices and efficacy endpoints for clinical trials of medical therapy in adults with Crohn's disease. Gastroenterology 2002;122:512-530.
26. Maunder RG, Cohen Z, McLeod RS, Greenberg GR. Effect of intervention in inflammatory bowel disease on health-related quality of life: a critical review. Dis Colon Rectum 1995;38:1147-1161.
27. Azad Khan AK, Piris J, Truelove SC. An experiment to determine the active therapeutic moiety of sulphasalazine. Lancet 1977;2:892-895.
28. Hanauer SB. Review article: high-dose aminosalicylates to induce and maintain remissions in ulcerative colitis. Aliment Pharmacol Ther 2006;24(Suppl 3):37-40.
29. Sandborn WJ, Hanauer SB, Buch A. Comparative pharmacokinetics of equimolar doses of 5-aminosalicylate administered as oral mesalamine (Asacol) and balsalazide: a randomized, single-dose, crossover study in healthy volunteers. Aliment Pharmacol Ther 2004;19:1089-1098.
30. Sandborn WJ, Hanauer SB. Systematic review: the pharmacokinetic profiles of oral mesalazine formulations and mesalazine pro-drugs used in the management of ulcerative colitis. Aliment Pharmacol Ther 2003;17:29-42.
31. Ricart E, Taylor WR, Loftus EV, et al. *N*-acetyltransferase 1 and 2 genotypes do not predict response or toxicity to treatment with mesalamine and sulfasalazine in patients with ulcerative colitis. Am J Gastroenterol 2002;97:1763-1768.
32. Egan LJ, Mays DC, Huntoon CJ, et al. Inhibition of interleukin-1-stimulated NF-kappaB RelA/p65 phosphorylation by mesalamine is accompanied by decreased transcriptional activity. J Biol Chem 1999;274:26448-26453.
33. Lauritsen K, Laursen LS, Bukhave K, Rask-Madsen J. Effects of topical 5-aminosalicylic acid and prednisolone on prostaglandin E2 and leukotriene B4 levels determined by equilibrium in vivo dialysis of rectum in relapsing ulcerative colitis. Gastroenterology 1986;91:837-844.
34. Schroeder KW, Tremaine WJ, Ilstrup DM. Coated oral 5-aminosalicylic acid therapy for mildly to moderately active ulcerative colitis: a randomized study. N Engl J Med 1987;317:1625-1629.
35. Hanauer S, Schwartz J, Robinson M, et al. Mesalamine capsules for treatment of active ulcerative colitis: results of a controlled trial. Pentasa Study Group. Am J Gastroenterol 1993;88:1188-1197.
36. Sninsky CA, Cort DH, Shanahan F, et al. Oral mesalamine (Asacol) for mildly to moderately active ulcerative colitis: a multicenter study. Ann Intern Med 1991;115:350-355.
37. Meyers S, Sachar DB, Present DH, Janowitz HD. Olsalazine sodium in the treatment of ulcerative colitis among patients intolerant of sulfasalazine: a prospective, randomized, placebo-controlled, double-blind, dose-ranging clinical trial. Gastroenterology 1987;93:1255-1262.
38. Feurle GE, Theuer D, Velasco S, et al. Olsalazine versus placebo in the treatment of mild to moderate ulcerative colitis: a randomised double blind trial. Gut 1989;30:1354-1361.
39. Gionchetti P, Rizzello F, Venturi A, et al. Comparison of oral with rectal mesalazine in the treatment of ulcerative proctitis. Dis Colon Rectum 1998;41:93-97.
40. Marshall JK, Irvine EJ. Rectal aminosalicylate therapy for distal ulcerative colitis: a meta-analysis. Aliment Pharmacol Ther 1995;9:293-300.
41. Hanauer SB. Review article: aminosalicylates in inflammatory bowel disease. Aliment Pharmacol Ther 2004;20(Suppl 4):60-65.
42. Sutherland LR, May GR, Shaffer EA. Sulfasalazine revisited: a meta-analysis of 5-aminosalicylic acid in the treatment of ulcerative colitis. Ann Intern Med 1993;118:540-549.
43. Singleton JW, Law DH, Kelley ML Jr, et al. National Cooperative Crohn's Disease Study: adverse reactions to study drugs. Gastroenterology 1979;77:870-882.
44. Van Staa TP, Travis S, Leufkens HG, Logan RF. 5-Aminosalicylic acids and the risk of renal disease: a large British epidemiologic study. Gastroenterology 2004;126:1733-1739.
45. Lowry PW, Franklin CL, Weaver AL, et al. Leucopenia resulting from a drug interaction between azathioprine or 6-mercaptopurine and mesalamine, sulphasalazine, or balsalazide. Gut 2001;49:656-664.
46. Truelove SC, Witts LJ. Cortisone in ulcerative colitis; preliminary report on a therapeutic trial. Br Med J 1954;2:375-378.
47. Truelove SC, Witts LJ. Cortisone in ulcerative colitis; final report on a therapeutic trial. Br Med J 1955;2:1041-1048.
48. Schmidt M, Pauels HG, Lugering N, et al. Glucocorticoids induce apoptosis in human monocytes: potential role of IL-1 beta. J Immunol 1999;163:3484-3490.
49. Summers RW, Switz DM, Sessions JT Jr, et al. National Cooperative Crohn's Disease Study: results of drug treatment. Gastroenterology 1979;77:847-869.
50. Malchow H, Ewe K, Brandes JW, et al. European Cooperative Crohn's Disease Study (ECCDS): results of drug treatment. Gastroenterology 1984;86:249-266.
51. Campieri M, Ferguson A, Doe W, et al. Oral budesonide is as effective as oral prednisolone in active Crohn's disease. The Global Budesonide Study Group. Gut 1997;41:209-214.
52. Gross V, Andus T, Caesar I, et al. Oral pH-modified release budesonide versus 6-methylprednisolone in active Crohn's disease. German/Austrian Budesonide Study Group. Eur J Gastroenterol Hepatol 1996;8:905-909.
53. Rutgeerts P, Lofberg R, Malchow H, et al. A comparison of budesonide with prednisolone for active Crohn's disease. N Engl J Med 1994;331:842-845.
54. Brignola C, De Simone G, Belloli C, et al. Steroid treatment in active Crohn's disease: a comparison between two regimens of different duration. Aliment Pharmacol Ther 1994;8:465-468.
55. Chun A, Chadi RM, Korelitz BI, et al. Intravenous corticotrophin vs. hydrocortisone in the treatment of hospitalized patients with Crohn's disease: a randomized double-blind study and follow-up. Inflamm Bowel Dis 1998;4:177-181.
56. Baron JH, Connell AM, Kanaghinis TG, et al. Out-patient treatment of ulcerative colitis: comparison between three doses of oral prednisone. Br Med J 1962;2:441-443.
57. Otley A, Steinhart AH. Budesonide for induction of remission in Crohn's disease. Cochrane Database Syst Rev 2005;4:CD000296.

58. Sandborn WJ, Lofberg R, Feagan BG, et al. Budesonide for maintenance of remission in patients with Crohn's disease in medically induced remission: a predetermined pooled analysis of four randomized, double-blind, placebo-controlled trials. Am J Gastroenterol 2005;100:1780-1787.
59. Hanauer SB, Robinson M, Pruitt R, et al. Budesonide enema for the treatment of active, distal ulcerative colitis and proctitis: a dose-ranging study. U.S. Budesonide Enema Study Group. Gastroenterology 1998;115:525-532.
60. Danielsson A, Hellers G, Lyrenas E, et al. A controlled randomized trial of budesonide versus prednisolone retention enemas in active distal ulcerative colitis. Scand J Gastroenterol 1987;22:987-992.
61. Danielsson A, Lofberg R, Persson T, et al. A steroid enema, budesonide, lacking systemic effects for the treatment of distal ulcerative colitis or proctitis. Scand J Gastroenterol 1992;27:9-12.
62. Lofberg R, Ostergaard Thomsen O, Langholz E, et al. Budesonide versus prednisolone retention enemas in active distal ulcerative colitis. Aliment Pharmacol Ther 1994;8:623-629.
63. Sambuelli A, Boerr L, Negreira S, et al. Budesonide enema in pouchitis—a double-blind, double-dummy, controlled trial. Aliment Pharmacol Ther 2002;16:27-34.
64. Elion GB. The George Hitchings and Gertrude Elion Lecture. The pharmacology of azathioprine. Ann N Y Acad Sci 1993;685:400-407.
65. Egan LJ, Derijks LJ, Hommes DW. Pharmacogenomics in inflammatory bowel disease. Clin Gastroenterol Hepatol 2006;4:21-28.
66. Wang L, Weinshilboum R. Thiopurine S-methyltransferase pharmacogenetics: insights, challenges and future directions. Oncogene 2006;25:1629-1638.
67. Wang L, Sullivan W, Toft D, Weinshilboum R. Thiopurine S-methyltransferase pharmacogenetics: chaperone protein association and allozyme degradation. Pharmacogenetics 2003;13:555-564.
68. Dubinsky MC. Azathioprine, 6-mercaptopurine in inflammatory bowel disease: pharmacology, efficacy, and safety. Clin Gastroenterol Hepatol 2004;2:731-743.
69. Dubinsky MC, Vasiliauskas EA, Singh H, et al. 6-Thioguanine can cause serious liver injury in inflammatory bowel disease patients. Gastroenterology 2003;125:298-303.
70. Lennard L. The clinical pharmacology of 6-mercaptopurine. Eur J Clin Pharmacol 1992;43:329-339.
71. Poppe D, Tiede I, Fritz G, et al. Azathioprine suppresses ezrin-radixin-moesin-dependent T cell-APC conjugation through inhibition of Vav guanosine exchange activity on Rac proteins. J Immunol 2006;176:640-651.
72. Thomas CW, Myhre GM, Tschumper R, et al. Selective inhibition of inflammatory gene expression in activated T lymphocytes: a mechanism of immune suppression by thiopurines. J Pharmacol Exp Ther 2005;312:537-545.
73. Kirk AP, Lennard-Jones JE. Controlled trial of azathioprine in chronic ulcerative colitis. Br Med J (Clin Res Ed) 1982;284:1291-1292.
74. Hawthorne AB, Logan RF, Hawkey CJ, et al. Randomised controlled trial of azathioprine withdrawal in ulcerative colitis. BMJ 1992;305:20-22.
75. Adler DJ, Korelitz BI. The therapeutic efficacy of 6-mercaptopurine in refractory ulcerative colitis. Am J Gastroenterol 1990;85:717-722.
76. George J, Present DH, Pou R, et al. The long-term outcome of ulcerative colitis treated with 6-mercaptopurine. Am J Gastroenterol 1996;91:1711-1714.
77. Pearson DC, May GR, Fick G, Sutherland LR. Azathioprine for maintaining remission of Crohn's disease. Cochrane Database Syst Rev 2000;2:CD000067.
78. Sandborn W, Sutherland L, Pearson D, et al. Azathioprine or 6-mercaptopurine for inducing remission of Crohn's disease. Cochrane Database Syst Rev 2000;2: CD000545.
79. Fraser AG, Orchard TR, Jewell DP. The efficacy of azathioprine for the treatment of inflammatory bowel disease: a 30 year review. Gut 2002;50:485-489.
80. Kandiel A, Fraser AG, Korelitz BI, et al. Increased risk of lymphoma among inflammatory bowel disease patients treated with azathioprine and 6-mercaptopurine. Gut 2005;54:1121-1125.
81. Ang YS, Farrell RJ. Risk of lymphoma: inflammatory bowel disease and immunomodulators. Gut 2006;55:580-581.
82. Ramsey-Goldman R, Mientus JM, Kutzer JE, et al. Pregnancy outcome in women with systemic lupus erythematosus treated with immunosuppressive drugs. J Rheumatol 1993;20:1152-1157.
83. Sparrow MP, Hande SA, Friedman S, et al. Allopurinol safely and effectively optimizes tioguanine metabolites in inflammatory bowel disease patients not responding to azathioprine and mercaptopurine. Aliment Pharmacol Ther 2005; 22:441-446.
84. Egan LJ, Sandborn WJ. Methotrexate for inflammatory bowel disease: pharmacology and preliminary results. Mayo Clin Proc 1996;71:69-80.
85. Egan LJ, Sandborn WJ, Tremaine WJ, et al. A randomized dose-response and pharmacokinetic study of methotrexate for refractory inflammatory Crohn's disease and ulcerative colitis. Aliment Pharmacol Ther 1999;13:1597-1604.
86. Egan LJ, Sandborn WJ, Mays DC, et al. Systemic and intestinal pharmacokinetics of methotrexate in patients with inflammatory bowel disease. Clin Pharmacol Ther 1999;65:29-39.
87. Genestier L, Paillot R, Fournel S, et al. Immunosuppressive properties of methotrexate: apoptosis and clonal deletion of activated peripheral T cells. J Clin Invest 1998;102:322-328.
88. Cronstein BN, Eberle MA, Gruber HE, Levin RI. Methotrexate inhibits neutrophil function by stimulating adenosine release from connective tissue cells. Proc Natl Acad Sci U S A 1991;88:2441-2445.
89. Egan LJ, Sandborn WJ, Mays DC, et al. Plasma and rectal adenosine in inflammatory bowel disease: effect of methotrexate. Inflamm Bowel Dis 1999;5:167-173.
90. Feagan BG, Rochon J, Fedorak RN, et al. Methotrexate for the treatment of Crohn's disease. The North American Crohn's Study Group Investigators. N Engl J Med 1995;332:292-297.
91. Feagan BG, Fedorak RN, Irvine EJ, et al. A comparison of methotrexate with placebo for the maintenance of remission in Crohn's disease. North American Crohn's Study Group Investigators. N Engl J Med 2000;342:1627-1632.
92. Alfadhli AA, McDonald JW, Feagan BG. Methotrexate for induction of remission in refractory Crohn's disease. Cochrane Database Syst Rev 2005;1:CD003459.
93. Oren R, Arber N, Odes S, et al. Methotrexate in chronic active ulcerative colitis: a double-blind, randomized, Israeli multicenter trial. Gastroenterology 1996;110:1416-1421.
94. Te HS, Schiano TD, Kuan SF, et al. Hepatic effects of long-term methotrexate use in the treatment of inflammatory bowel disease. Am J Gastroenterol 2000;95:3150-3156.
95. Liu J, Farmer JD Jr, Lane WS, et al. Calcineurin is a common target of cyclophilin-cyclosporin A and FKBP-FK506 complexes. Cell 1991;66:807-815.
96. Lichtiger S, Present DH, Kornbluth A, et al. Cyclosporine in severe ulcerative colitis refractory to steroid therapy. N Engl J Med 1994;330:1841-1845.
97. D'Haens G, Lemmens L, Geboes K, et al. Intravenous cyclosporine versus intravenous corticosteroids as single therapy for severe attacks of ulcerative colitis. Gastroenterology 2001;120:1323-1329.
98. Van Assche G, D'Haens G, Noman M, et al. Randomized, double-blind comparison of 4 mg/kg versus 2 mg/kg intravenous cyclosporine in severe ulcerative colitis. Gastroenterology 2003;125:1025-1031.
99. Shibolet O, Regushevskaya E, Brezis M, Soares-Weiser K. Cyclosporine A for induction of remission in severe ulcerative colitis. Cochrane Database Syst Rev 2005;1: CD004277.
100. Fernandez-Banares F, Bertran X, Esteve-Comas M, et al. Azathioprine is useful in maintaining long-term remission induced by intravenous cyclosporine in steroid-refractory severe ulcerative colitis. Am J Gastroenterol 1996;91:2498-2499.
101. Domenech E, Garcia-Planella E, Bernal I, et al. Azathioprine without oral ciclosporin in the long-term maintenance of remission induced by intravenous ciclosporin in severe, steroid-refractory ulcerative colitis. Aliment Pharmacol Ther 2002;16:2061-2065.
102. Actis GC, Bresso F, Astegiano M, et al. Safety and efficacy of azathioprine in the maintenance of ciclosporin-induced remission of ulcerative colitis. Aliment Pharmacol Ther 2001;15:1307-1311.
103. Egan LJ, Sandborn WJ, Tremaine WJ. Clinical outcome following treatment of refractory inflammatory and fistulizing Crohn's disease with intravenous cyclosporine. Am J Gastroenterol 1998;93:442-448.
104. Feagan BG, McDonald JW, Rochon J, et al. Low-dose cyclosporine for the treatment of Crohn's disease. The Canadian Crohn's Relapse Prevention Trial Investigators. N Engl J Med 1994;330:1846-1851.
105. de Groen PC, Aksamit AJ, Rakela J, et al. Central nervous system toxicity after liver transplantation: the role of cyclosporine and cholesterol. N Engl J Med 1987;317:861-866.
106. Gijtenbeek JM, van den Bent MJ, Vecht CJ. Cyclosporine neurotoxicity: a review. J Neurol 1999;246:339-346.
107. Corpier CL, Jones PH, Suki WN, et al. Rhabdomyolysis and renal injury with lovastatin use: report of two cases in cardiac transplant recipients. JAMA 1988;260:239-241.
108. Ducharme MP, Provenzano R, Dehoorne-Smith M, Edwards DJ. Trough concentrations of cyclosporine in blood following administration with grapefruit juice. Br J Clin Pharmacol 1993;36:457-459.
109. Venkataramanan R, Jain A, Cadoff E, et al. Pharmacokinetics of FK 506: preclinical and clinical studies. Transplant Proc 1990;22:52-56.
110. Sandborn WJ, Present DH, Isaacs KL, et al. Tacrolimus for the treatment of fistulas in patients with Crohn's disease: a randomized, placebo-controlled trial. Gastroenterology 2003;125:380-388.
111. Fellermann K, Ludwig D, Stahl M, et al. Steroid-unresponsive acute attacks of inflammatory bowel disease: immunomodulation by tacrolimus (FK506). Am J Gastroenterol 1998;93:1860-1866.
112. Baumgart DC, Pintoffl JP, Sturm A, et al. Tacrolimus is safe and effective in patients with severe steroid-refractory or steroid-dependent inflammatory bowel disease—a long-term follow-up. Am J Gastroenterol 2006;101:1048-1056.
113. Fellermann K, Tanko Z, Herrlinger KR, et al. Response of refractory colitis to intravenous or oral tacrolimus (FK506). Inflamm Bowel Dis 2002;8:317-324.
114. Bousvaros A, Kirschner BS, Werlin SL, et al. Oral tacrolimus treatment of severe colitis in children. J Pediatr 2000;137:794-799.
115. D'Haens G, Van Deventer S, Van Hogezand R, et al. Endoscopic and histological healing with infliximab anti-tumor necrosis factor antibodies in Crohn's disease: a European multicenter trial. Gastroenterology 1999;116:1029-1034.
116. Baert F, Noman M, Vermeire S, et al. Influence of immunogenicity on the long-term efficacy of infliximab in Crohn's disease. N Engl J Med 2003;348:601-608.
117. Farrell RJ, Alsahli M, Jeen YT, et al. Intravenous hydrocortisone premedication reduces antibodies to infliximab in Crohn's disease: a randomized controlled trial. Gastroenterology 2003;124:917-924.
118. Sandborn WJ. Preventing antibodies to infliximab in patients with Crohn's disease: optimize not immunize. Gastroenterology 2003;124:1140-1145.
119. Rutgeerts P, Sandborn WJ, Fedorak RN, et al. Onercept for moderate-to-severe Crohn's disease: a randomized, double-blind, placebo-controlled trial. Clin Gastroenterol Hepatol 2006;4:888-893.
120. Sandborn WJ, Hanauer SB, Katz S, et al. Etanercept for active Crohn's disease: a randomized, double-blind, placebo-controlled trial. Gastroenterology 2001;121:1088-1094.
121. Lugering A, Schmidt M, Lugering N, et al. Infliximab induces apoptosis in monocytes from patients with chronic active Crohn's disease by using a caspase-dependent pathway. Gastroenterology 2001;121:1145-1157.

122. Van den Brande JM, Braat H, van den Brink GR, et al. Infliximab but not etanercept induces apoptosis in lamina propria T-lymphocytes from patients with Crohn's disease. Gastroenterology 2003;124:1774-1785.
123. Sands BE, Anderson FH, Bernstein CN, et al. Infliximab maintenance therapy for fistulizing Crohn's disease. N Engl J Med 2004;350:876-885.
124. Targan SR, Hanauer SB, van Deventer SJ, et al. A short-term study of chimeric monoclonal antibody cA2 to tumor necrosis factor alpha for Crohn's disease. Crohn's Disease cA2 Study Group. N Engl J Med 1997;337:1029-1035.
125. Present DH, Rutgeerts P, Targan S, et al. Infliximab for the treatment of fistulas in patients with Crohn's disease. N Engl J Med 1999;340:1398-1405.
126. Hanauer SB, Feagan BG, Lichtenstein GR, et al. Maintenance infliximab for Crohn's disease: the ACCENT I randomised trial. Lancet 2002;359:1541-1549.
127. Rutgeerts P, Sandborn WJ, Feagan BG, et al. Infliximab for induction and maintenance therapy for ulcerative colitis. N Engl J Med 2005;353:2462-2476.
128. Colombel JF, Loftus EV Jr, Tremaine WJ, et al. The safety profile of infliximab in patients with Crohn's disease: the Mayo Clinic experience in 500 patients. Gastroenterology 2004;126:19-31.
129. Keane J, Gershon S, Wise RP, et al. Tuberculosis associated with infliximab, a tumor necrosis factor alpha-neutralizing agent. N Engl J Med 2001;345:1098-1104.
130. Nancey S, Blanvillain E, Parmentier B, et al. Infliximab treatment does not induce organ-specific or nonorgan-specific autoantibodies other than antinuclear and anti-double-stranded DNA autoantibodies in Crohn's disease. Inflamm Bowel Dis 2005;11:986-991.
131. Thomas CW Jr, Weinshenker BG, Sandborn WJ. Demyelination during anti-tumor necrosis factor alpha therapy with infliximab for Crohn's disease. Inflamm Bowel Dis 2004;10:28-31.
132. Navarro-Sarabia F, Ariza-Ariza R, Hernandez-Cruz B, Villanueva I. Adalimumab for treating rheumatoid arthritis. J Rheumatol 2006;33:1075-1081.
133. Hanauer SB, Sandborn WJ, Rutgeerts P, et al. Human anti-tumor necrosis factor monoclonal antibody (adalimumab) in Crohn's disease: the CLASSIC-I trial. Gastroenterology 2006;130:323-333.
134. Colombel JF, Sandborn WJ, Rutgeerts P, et al. Adalimumab for maintenance of clinical response and remission in patients with Crohn's disease: The CHARM Trial. Gastroenterology 2007;132:52-65.
135. Ghosh S, Goldin E, Gordon FH, et al. Natalizumab for active Crohn's disease. N Engl J Med 2003;348:24-32.
136. Sandborn WJ, Colombel JF, Enns R, et al. Natalizumab induction and maintenance therapy for Crohn's disease. N Engl J Med 2005;353:1912-1925.
137. Targan SR, Feagan BG, Fedorak RN, et al. Natalizumab for the treatment of active Crohn's disease: results of the ENCORE Trial. Gastroenterology 2007;132:1672-1683.
138. Van Assche G, Van Ranst M, Sciot R, et al. Progressive multifocal leukoencephalopathy after natalizumab therapy for Crohn's disease. N Engl J Med 2005;353:362-368.
139. Greenberg GR, Feagan BG, Martin F, et al. Oral budesonide for active Crohn's disease. Canadian Inflammatory Bowel Disease Study Group. N Engl J Med 1994;331:836-841.
140. Thomsen OO, Cortot A, Jewell D, et al. A comparison of budesonide and mesalamine for active Crohn's disease. International Budesonide-Mesalamine Study Group. N Engl J Med 1998;339:370-374.
141. Candy S, Wright J, Gerber M, et al. A controlled double blind study of azathioprine in the management of Crohn's disease. Gut 1995;37:674-678.
142. Present DH, Korelitz BI, Wisch N, et al. Treatment of Crohn's disease with 6-mercaptopurine: a long-term, randomized, double-blind study. N Engl J Med 1980;302:981-987.
143. Markowitz J, Grancher K, Kohn N, et al. A multicenter trial of 6-mercaptopurine and prednisone in children with newly diagnosed Crohn's disease. Gastroenterology 2000;119:895-902.
144. Korelitz BI, Hanauer S, Rutgeerts P, et al. Post-operative prophylaxis with 6-MP, 5-ASA or placebo in Crohn's disease: a 2 year multicenter trial. Gastroenterology 1998;114:A1011.
145. Lemann M, Bouhnik Y, Colombel JF, et al. Randomized double blind placebo-controlled multicenter azathioprine withdrawal trial in Crohn's disease. Gastroenterology 2002;122:A174.
146. Arber N, Odes HS, Fireman Z, et al. A controlled double blind multicenter study of the effectiveness of 5-aminosalicylic acid in patients with Crohn's disease in remission. J Clin Gastroenterol 1995;20:203-206.
147. Gendre JP, Mary JY, Florent C, et al. Oral mesalamine (Pentasa) as maintenance treatment in Crohn's disease: a multicenter placebo-controlled study. The Groupe d'Etudes Therapeutiques des Affections Inflammatoires Digestives (GETAID). Gastroenterology 1993;104:435-439.
148. Prantera C, Pallone F, Brunetti G, et al. Oral 5-aminosalicylic acid (Asacol) in the maintenance treatment of Crohn's disease. The Italian IBD Study Group. Gastroenterology 1992;103:363-368.
149. Modigliani R, Colombel JF, Dupas JL, et al. Mesalamine in Crohn's disease with steroid-induced remission: effect on steroid withdrawal and remission maintenance. Groupe d'Etudes Therapeutiques des Affections Inflammatoires Digestives. Gastroenterology 1996;110:688-693.
150. Brignola C, Iannone P, Pasquali S, et al. Placebo-controlled trial of oral 5-ASA in relapse prevention of Crohn's disease. Dig Dis Sci 1992;37:29-32.
151. Sutherland LR, Martin F, Bailey RJ, et al. A randomized, placebo-controlled, double-blind trial of mesalamine in the maintenance of remission of Crohn's disease. The Canadian Mesalamine for Remission of Crohn's Disease Study Group. Gastroenterology 1997;112:1069-1077.
152. Coated oral 5-aminosalicylic acid versus placebo in maintaining remission of inactive Crohn's disease. International Mesalazine Study Group. Aliment Pharmacol Ther 1990;4:55-64.
153. Thomson AB, Wright JP, Vatn M, et al. Mesalazine (Mesasal/Claversal) 1.5 g b.d. vs. placebo in the maintenance of remission of patients with Crohn's disease. Aliment Pharmacol Ther 1995;9:673-683.
154. de Franchis R, Omodei P, Ranzi T, et al. Controlled trial of oral 5-aminosalicylic acid for the prevention of early relapse in Crohn's disease. Aliment Pharmacol Ther 1997;11:845-852.
155. Lochs H, Mayer M, Fleig WE, et al. Prophylaxis of postoperative relapse in Crohn's disease with mesalamine: European Cooperative Crohn's Disease Study VI. Gastroenterology 2000;118:264-273.
156. Akobeng AK, Gardener E. Oral 5-aminosalicylic acid for maintenance of medically-induced remission in Crohn's disease. Cochrane Database Syst Rev 2005;1:CD003715.
157. Lennard-Jones JE. Sulphasalazine in asymptomatic Crohn's disease: a multicentre trial. Gut 1977;18:69-72.
158. Mahmud N, Kamm MA, Dupas JL, et al. Olsalazine is not superior to placebo in maintaining remission of inactive Crohn's colitis and ileocolitis: a double blind, parallel, randomised, multicentre study. Gut 2001;49:552-556.
159. Greenberg GR, Feagan BG, Martin F, et al. Oral budesonide as maintenance treatment for Crohn's disease: a placebo-controlled, dose-ranging study. Canadian Inflammatory Bowel Disease Study Group. Gastroenterology 1996;110:45-51.
160. Lofberg R, Rutgeerts P, Malchow H, et al. Budesonide prolongs time to relapse in ileal and ileocaecal Crohn's disease: a placebo controlled one year study. Gut 1996;39:82-86.
161. Ferguson A, Campieri M, Doe W, et al. Oral budesonide as maintenance therapy in Crohn's disease—results of a 12-month study. Global Budesonide Study Group. Aliment Pharmacol Ther 1998;12:175-183.
162. Schreiber S, Khaliq-Kareemi M, Lawrance IC, et al. Maintenance therapy with certolizumab pegol for Crohn's disease. N Engl J Med 2007;357:239-250.
163. Schwartz DA, Loftus EV Jr, Tremaine WJ, et al. The natural history of fistulizing Crohn's disease in Olmsted County, Minnesota. Gastroenterology 2002;122:875-880.
164. Schwartz DA, Pemberton JH, Sandborn WJ. Diagnosis and treatment of perianal fistulas in Crohn disease. Ann Intern Med 2001;135:906-918.
165. Schwartz DA, Wiersema MJ, Dudiak KM, et al. A comparison of endoscopic ultrasound, magnetic resonance imaging, and exam under anesthesia for evaluation of Crohn's perianal fistulas. Gastroenterology 2001;121:1064-1072.
166. Sands BE, Van Deventer S, Bernstein CN, et al. Long-term treatment of fistulizing Crohn's disease: response to infliximab in the ACCENT II trial through 54 weeks. Gastroenterology 2002;122:A671.
167. Marteau P, Probert CS, Lindgren S, et al. Combined oral and enema treatment with Pentasa (mesalazine) is superior to oral therapy alone in patients with extensive mild/moderate active ulcerative colitis: a randomised, double blind, placebo controlled study. Gut 2005;54:960-965.
168. Sturgeon JB, Bhatia P, Hermens D, Miner PB Jr. Exacerbation of chronic ulcerative colitis with mesalamine. Gastroenterology 1995;108:1889-1893.
169. Sandborn WJ, Tremaine WJ, Offord KP, et al. Transdermal nicotine for mildly to moderately active ulcerative colitis: a randomized, double-blind, placebo-controlled trial. Ann Intern Med 1997;126:364-371.
170. Truelove SC, Jewell DP. Intensive intravenous regimen for severe attacks of ulcerative colitis. Lancet 1974;1:1067-1070.
171. Jarnerot G, Hertervig E, Friis-Liby I, et al. Infliximab as rescue therapy in severe to moderately severe ulcerative colitis: a randomized, placebo-controlled study. Gastroenterology 2005;128:1805-1811.
172. Sutherland L, Macdonald JK. Oral 5-aminosalicylic acid for maintenance of remission in ulcerative colitis. Cochrane Database Syst Rev 2006;2:CD000544.
173. Shen B, Achkar JP, Lashner BA, et al. A randomized clinical trial of ciprofloxacin and metronidazole to treat acute pouchitis. Inflamm Bowel Dis 2001;7:301-305.
174. Colombel JF, Ricart E, Loftus EV Jr, et al. Management of Crohn's disease of the ileoanal pouch with infliximab. Am J Gastroenterol 2003;98:2239-2244.
175. Chapman AP, Antoniw P, Spitali M, et al. Therapeutic antibody fragments with prolonged in vivo half-lives. Nat Biotechnol 1999;17:780-783.
176. Sandborn WJ, Feagan BG, Stoinov S, et al. Certolizumab pegol for the treatment of Crohn's disease. N Engl J Med 2007;357:228-238.
177. Mannon PJ, Fuss IJ, Mayer L, et al. Anti-interleukin-12 antibody for active Crohn's disease. N Engl J Med 2004;351:2069-2079.
178. Reinisch W, Hommes DW, Van Assche G, et al. A dose escalating, placebo controlled, double blind, single dose and multidose, safety and tolerability study of fontolizumab, a humanised anti-interferon gamma antibody, in patients with moderate to severe Crohn's disease. Gut 2006;55:1138-1144.
179. Hommes DW, Mikhajlova TL, Stoinov S, et al. Fontolizumab, a humanised anti-interferon gamma antibody, demonstrates safety and clinical activity in patients with moderate to severe Crohn's disease. Gut 2006;55:1131-1137.
180. Atreya R, Mudter J, Finotto S, et al. Blockade of interleukin 6 trans signaling suppresses T-cell resistance against apoptosis in chronic intestinal inflammation: evidence in Crohn disease and experimental colitis in vivo. Nat Med 2000;6:583-588.
181. Ito H, Takazoe M, Fukuda Y, et al. A pilot randomized trial of a human anti-interleukin-6 receptor monoclonal antibody in active Crohn's disease. Gastroenterology 2004;126:989-996; discussion 947.
182. Fedorak RN, Gangl A, Elson CO, et al. Recombinant human interleukin 10 in the treatment of patients with mild to moderately active Crohn's disease. The Interleukin 10 Inflammatory Bowel Disease Cooperative Study Group. Gastroenterology 2000;119:1473-1482.
183. Braat H, Rottiers P, Hommes DW, et al. A Phase I trial with transgenic bacteria expressing interleukin-10 in Crohn's disease. Clin Gastroenterol Hepatol 2006;4:754-759.
184. Korzenik JR, Dieckgraefe BK, Valentine JF, et al. Sargramostim for active Crohn's disease. N Engl J Med 2005;352:2193-2201.

185. Feagan BG, Greenberg GR, Wild G, et al. Treatment of ulcerative colitis with a humanized antibody to the alpha4beta7 integrin. N Engl J Med 2005;352:2499-2507.
186. Schreiber S, Feagan B, D'Haens G, et al. Oral p38 mitogen-activated protein kinase inhibition with BIRB 796 for active Crohn's disease: a randomized, double-blind, placebo-controlled trial. Clin Gastroenterol Hepatol 2006;4:325-334.
187. Travis S, Yap LM, Hawkey C, et al. RDP58 is a novel and potentially effective oral therapy for ulcerative colitis. Inflamm Bowel Dis 2005;11:713-719.
188. Hommes D, van den Blink B, Plasse T, et al. Inhibition of stress-activated MAP kinases induces clinical improvement in moderate to severe Crohn's disease. Gastroenterology 2002;122:7-14.
189. Summers RW, Elliott DE, Urban JF Jr, et al. *Trichuris suis* therapy in Crohn's disease. Gut 2005;54:87-90.
190. Kruis W, Fric P, Pokrotnieks J, et al. Maintaining remission of ulcerative colitis with the probiotic *Escherichia coli* Nissle 1917 is as effective as with standard mesalazine. Gut 2004;53:1617-1623.
191. Bibiloni R, Fedorak RN, Tannock GW, et al. VSL#3 probiotic-mixture induces remission in patients with active ulcerative colitis. Am J Gastroenterol 2005;100:1539-1546.
192. Mimura T, Rizzello F, Helwig U, et al. Once daily high dose probiotic therapy (VSL#3) for maintaining remission in recurrent or refractory pouchitis. Gut 2004;53:108-114.
193. Almer S, Norlander B, Strom M, Osterwald H. Steady-state pharmacokinetics of a new 4-gram 5-aminosalicylic acid retention enema in patients with ulcerative colitis in remission. Scand J Gastroenterol 1991;26:327-335.
194. Staerk Laursen L, Stokholm M, Bukhave K, et al. Disposition of 5-aminosalicylic acid by olsalazine and three mesalazine preparations in patients with ulcerative colitis: comparison of intraluminal colonic concentrations, serum values, and urinary excretion. Gut 1990;31:1271-1276.
195. Stretch GL, Campbell BJ, Dwarakanath AD, et al. 5-Amino salicylic acid absorption and metabolism in ulcerative colitis patients receiving maintenance sulphasalazine, olsalazine or mesalazine. Aliment Pharmacol Ther 1996;10:941-947.
196. Gionchetti P, Campieri M, Venturi A, et al. Systemic availability of 5-aminosalicylic acid: comparison of delayed release and an azo-bond preparation. Aliment Pharmacol Ther 1996;10:601-605.
197. Norlander B, Gotthard R, Strom M. Pharmacokinetics of a 5-aminosalicylic acid enteric-coated tablet in patients with Crohn's disease or ulcerative colitis and in healthy volunteers. Aliment Pharmacol Ther 1990;4:497-505.
198. Yu DK, Morrill B, Eichmeier LS, et al. Pharmacokinetics of 5-aminosalicylic acid from controlled-release capsules in man. Eur J Clin Pharmacol 1995;48:273-277.
199. Lauritsen K, Staerk Laursen L, Bukhave K, Rask-Madsen J. Longterm olsalazine treatment: pharmacokinetics, tolerance and effects on local eicosanoid formation in ulcerative colitis and Crohn's colitis. Gut 1988;29:974-982.
200. Barnes PJ, Karin M. Nuclear factor-kappaB: a pivotal transcription factor in chronic inflammatory diseases. N Engl J Med 1997;336:1066-1071.
201. Paliogianni F, Raptis A, Ahuja SS, et al. Negative transcriptional regulation of human interleukin 2 (IL-2) gene by glucocorticoids through interference with nuclear transcription factors AP-1 and NF-AT. J Clin Invest 1993;91:1481-1489.
202. Flower RJ, Rothwell NJ. Lipocortin-1: cellular mechanisms and clinical relevance. Trends Pharmacol Sci 1994;15:71-76.
203. Colotta F, Re F, Muzio M, et al. Interleukin-1 type II receptor: a decoy target for IL-1 that is regulated by IL-4. Science 1993;261:472-475.
204. Brostjan C, Anrather J, Csizmadia V, et al. Glucocorticoids inhibit E-selectin expression by targeting NF-kappaB and not ATF/c-Jun. J Immunol 1997;158:3836-3844.
205. Wissink S, van Heerde EC, vand der Burg B, van der Saag PT. A dual mechanism mediates repression of NF-kappaB activity by glucocorticoids. Mol Endocrinol 1998;12:355-363.

34

HEPATIC CIRRHOSIS

Victor J. Navarro, Simona Rossi, and Steven K. Herrine

INTRODUCTION 505
PATHOPHYSIOLOGY 505
The Normal Liver 505
The Diseased Liver 506
Clinical Manifestations of Cirrhosis 506
Models to Predict the Severity of Cirrhosis 507
Parenchymal Failure 507
Portal Hypertension 507
THERAPEUTICS AND CLINICAL PHARMACOLOGY 508
Manifestations of Portal Hypertension and Goals of Therapy 508
Hepatic Vein Pressure Gradient 508
Gastroesophageal Varices 509
Ascites 509
Spontaneous Bacterial Peritonitis 509
Hepatorenal Syndrome 510
Hepatic Encephalopathy 511
Pulmonary Complications of Portal Hypertension 511
Therapeutics by Class 511
Vasoconstrictors 511
Vasodilators 514
Diuretics 514
Disaccharides 515
Antibiotics for Hepatic Encephalopathy 515
Therapeutic Approach 516
Variceal Hemorrhage 516
Ascites 518
Spontaneous Bacterial Peritonitis 518
Hepatorenal Syndrome 519
Hepatic Encephalopathy 520
Pulmonary Complications of Portal Hypertension 520
Emerging Targets and Therapeutics 521
Aquaretics 521
Liver-Specific Nitric Oxide Donors 521
Endothelin Antagonists 521

INTRODUCTION

In the United States, non–alcohol-induced fatty liver disease, seen most frequently in patients with insulin resistance, obesity, and hyperlipidemia, is the most common cause for chronic liver injury, manifested as persistent liver test abnormalities. A significant proportion of patients with this disorder can develop cirrhosis. Viral hepatitis C, affecting 1.8% of the population, is the most common cause for cirrhosis, which develops in approximately 20% of those infected. Viral hepatitis B, alcoholic liver disease, autoimmune diseases, and inherited and metabolic diseases are a few other causes of cirrhosis. Several etiologies of cirrhosis can be treated with targeted therapies; however, a detailed discussion of each cause of cirrhosis and therapies targeted to these underlying causes is beyond the scope of this chapter.

It has been estimated that approximately 5.5 million Americans have cirrhosis.[1] Arguably, the development of portal hypertension is the most important event resulting from cirrhosis. It is responsible for the majority of life-threatening events that occur in cirrhotics. These events can be mitigated or prevented by a carefully measured pharmacologic approach. Thus, the focus of this chapter is to review the current approach to the pharmacotherapy of the manifestations and complications of portal hypertension.

PATHOPHYSIOLOGY

The Normal Liver

The hepatic parenchyma is organized into a repetitive functional unit termed the *acinus* or lobule. Each lobule consists of a central terminal hepatic venule surrounded by as many as four to six terminal portal triads. Hepatocytes are the dominant cell type within the liver, and comprise 80% of its volume.[2] The hepatocyte plays a significant role in the distribution and storage of nutrients, the synthesis of proteins, fatty acids, and lipids, and the formation of bile. Each hepatocyte is in communication with neighboring hepatocytes via gap junctions; in addition, neighboring hepatocytes form bile canaliculi. Hepatocytes are also in communication with endothelial-lined sinusoidal channels via the space of Disse, into which multiple microvilli extend and are involved in active transport.[3]

The hepatocytes, arranged as linear plates one cell thick, extend from the terminal hepatic venule to the portal triads. The sinusoids are filled with blood that flows from the portal triads toward the hepatic vein. Bile flows in the opposite direction, from the hepatocyte, where it is secreted, and empties into bile canaliculi that form between the hepatocytes. These canaliculi coalesce into bile ducts that ultimately drain into the portal triads.[3]

Each acinus is further subdivided into functional zones, which extend from the portal triad to the terminal venule. The zones closer to the portal triad are richer in nutrients and oxygen-filled blood.[3] In addition, the cellular components of each zone have their own unique metabolic and enzymatic responsibility. For instance, the hepatocytes in zone 1 carry large mitochondria and are geared to activities such as fatty acid oxidation, gluconeogenesis, and cholesterol synthesis as well as bile formation, whereas the hepatocytes located in zone 3 are more responsible for the detoxification of drugs as well as their metabolism.[4] Normal hepatic anatomy is depicted in Figure 34-1.

The arrangement of hepatocytes and sinusoids, separated by the space of Disse, allows for movement of products of metabolism freely between the hepatocyte and the vascular space. This system is fed by the liver's vascular supply, comprising the portal vein and the hepatic arteries. The portal vein, which is formed by the confluence of the splenic and superior mesenteric veins, supplies the liver parenchyma with 70% of the blood supply, and although it is rich in nutrients from having passed through the capillary bed of the alimentary tract, it is poor in oxygen. The hepatic artery arises from the celiac artery directly off of the aorta and is responsible for providing the liver with oxygen-rich blood. Both the hepatic artery and the portal vein enter the liver at the hilum and subdivide into progressively smaller branches that terminate in the portal triad. However, significant anatomic variability exists with regard to the hepatic arterial anatomy. Blood exits the liver via the hepatic vein, which forms by the union of the left, middle, and right hepatic veins to drain into the vena cava. In the healthy liver, the sinusoids are a low-pressure and low-resistance system of 2 to 3 mm Hg.[3,5,6]

Among the liver's functions are carbohydrate and amino acid metabolism, lipid and protein metabolism, detoxification of drugs, and the formation of bile. To some extent, the complex metabolic activity can be assessed by biochemical parameters, and injury to the liver can be reflected by abnormalities of these parameters. The aminotransferases, aspartate and alanine aminotransferase, transfer amino groups during gluconeogenesis. An elevation in either enzyme is indicative of hepatocellular damage or injury. Alkaline phosphatase is located at the canalicular membrane of the hepatocyte and the bile duct walls, and is released in greater than usual amounts when there is an impairment to bile flow, termed *cholestasis.* The greater the impairment to bile flow, the greater the accumulation of bilirubin, the breakdown product of hemoglobin metabolism and a major component of bile. Bilirubin is present in conjugated and unconjugated forms, with the former being water soluble and excreted through the kidneys. Unconjugated bilirubin is lipid soluble and not excreted by the kidneys. Whereas an elevation of primarily unconjugated hyperbilirubinemia is seen in extrahepatic disorders such as hemolysis or genetic defects of hepatic conjugation, direct hyperbilirubinemia often results from hepatic disease and/or obstruction.[3,4]

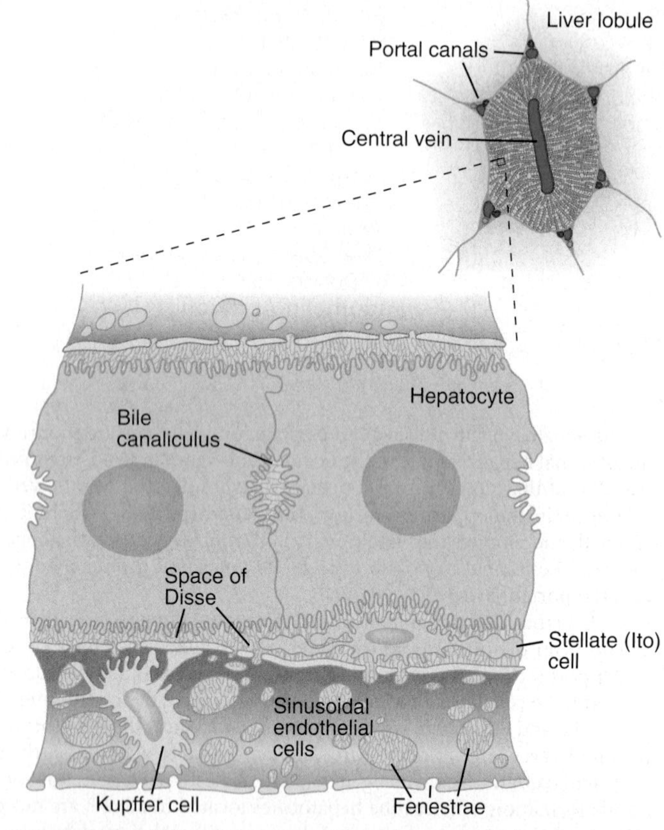

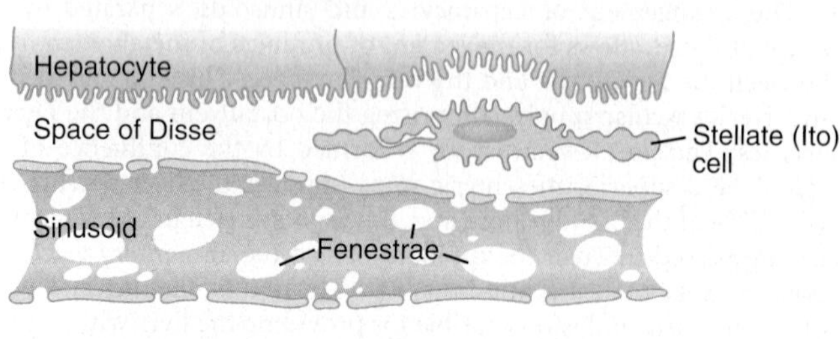

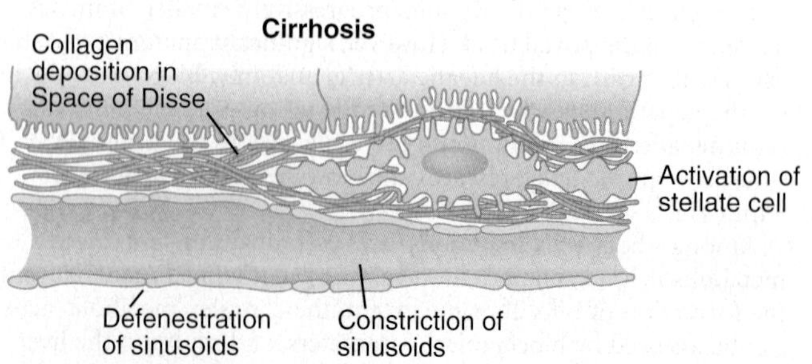

FIGURE 34-1 • Normal anatomy of the main cellular component of the liver, the hepatocyte. Neighboring hepatocytes are in direct communication via gap junctions. Bile canaliculi also pass between hepatocytes and ultimately form larger bile ducts. The exchange of nutrients and metabolic products with the portal circulation occurs at the level of the sinusoid, which communicates with the hepatocyte via the space of Disse. Hepatocytes are arranged in a linear fashion, one cell thick, and extend between the portal triad and the central vein. Each central vein and its linearly arranged hepatocytes extending to the portal triads make up an acinus. Each acinus of the liver is further divided into functional zones depending on their anatomic proximity to the hepatic vein as shown.The lower half of the figure depicts the characteristic changes that occur during the development of cirrhosis. The sinusoidal endothelium undergoes "capillarisation," which is characterized by the loss of normal sinusoidal endothelial fenestrations and thickening of the endothelial lining due to accumulating fibrosis. (Adapted from Wanless IR. Anatomy, histology, embryology, and developmental anomalies of the liver. In Feldman M, Friedman LS, Brandt LJ [eds]: Sleisenger and Fordtran's Gastrointestinal and Liver Disease: Pathophysiology/Diagnosis/Management, 8th ed. Philadelphia: Elsevier Saunders, 2006, pp 1543-1550.)

The Diseased Liver

The normal liver architecture optimizes contact between portal blood, enriched with those substances arriving from the intestine, and sinusoidal endothelium, which interfaces with the systemic circulation. However, several changes occur in the diseased liver that may alter this normal relationship. Most notably, there are changes in blood flow patterns within and around the liver, changes in the behavior of hepatic cells, alteration in the barriers that normally separate and regulate exchange of substances between the vascular space and the subendothelial compartment, and changes in the blood concentration of proteins.

When injured, the liver experiences an influx of inflammatory cells, polymorphonuclear and mononuclear cells, and macrophages. Their activity not infrequently incites hepatocyte inflammation that, in and of itself, may impair hepatic functioning. Hepatic injury is not necessarily accompanied by an impairment in liver function. Chronic liver injury results from a sustained inflammatory assault on the liver due to a variety of causes. By convention, the presence of this injury for more than 6 months is accepted as chronic liver disease. The result of this protracted inflammatory condition is the accumulation of fibrosis. Eventually, the unmitigated production of fibrosis alters the normal hepatic architecture and leads to the formation of cirrhosis.

Cirrhosis, as shown in Figure 34-2, can be defined by the accumulation of fibrosis throughout the substance of the liver, resulting in a subdividing of the hepatic parenchyma into nodules by micro- and macroscopic fibrous septa. These septa contain blood vessels that allow a significant proportion of the portal inflow to escape the usual route of entering the sinuosoid.[7] Also, the sinusoidal endothelium undergoes a process referred to as "capillarization," which is characterized by the loss of normal sinusoidal endothelial fenestrations and thickening of the endothelial lining due to accumulating fibrosis.[8-10] The obvious consequence of this is that substrates in the portal circulation either have limited access to or are excluded from the space of Disse, and thus have limited or no contact with the hepatocytes.

Clinical Manifestations of Cirrhosis

The diagnosis of cirrhosis can be made by clinical, pathologic, and radiologic means. Clinically, the diagnosis is suspected based on a history of an exposure such as a remote blood transfusion that serves as a means of acquisition for hepatitis C, as discussed in Chapter 35 (Infectious Hepatitis), coupled with clinical signs and events consistent

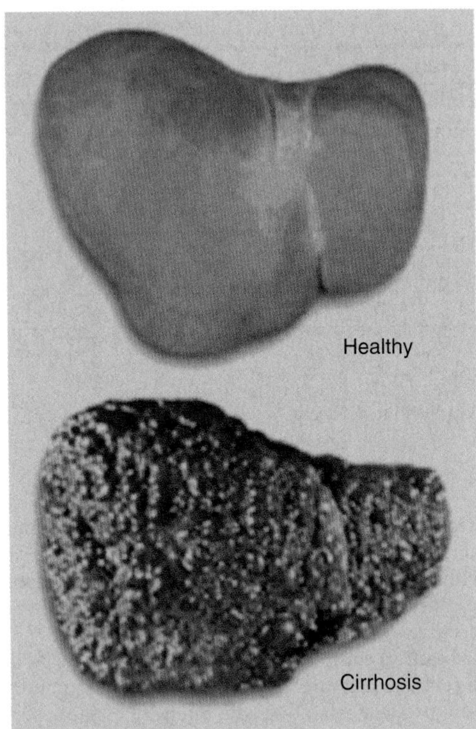

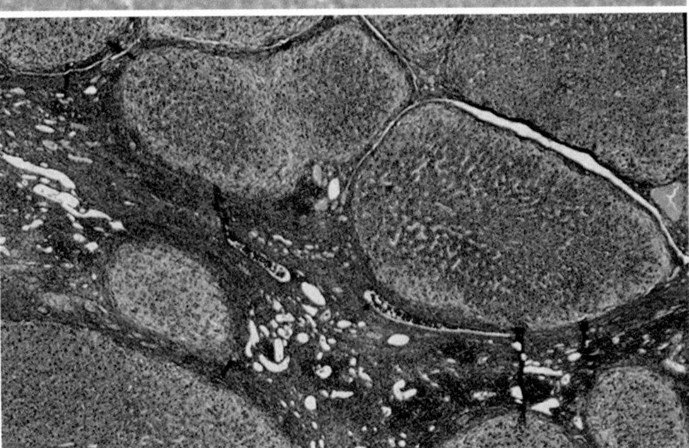

FIGURE 34-2 • Appearance of normal liver. The normal liver has a smooth contour compared to a diseased liver with morphologic evidence of cirrhosis, in which the smooth liver contour takes on a "lumpy" irregular appearance caused by extensive fibrosis throughout the hepatic parenchyma. The lower half of the figure shows normal liver on a histological level. Noted is the development of extensive fibrosis, which is seen as blue fibrous tissue using the trichrome stain. These fibrous septae extend between portal tracts, forming parenchymal nodules that are characteristic of cirrhosis.[7]

with the diagnosis, as discussed later. Often, the clinician's suspicion is confirmed by pathologic or radiologic means. A liver biopsy can be performed during laparotomy or laparoscopy, percutaneously, or through the hepatic veins during a catheterization procedure. The demonstration of fibrous septa and regenerating nodules confirms the suspicion. Also, radiographic studies may be used to identify the surface nodularity and vascular collateralization that support the diagnosis of cirrhosis to a sufficient level of confidence that a biopsy is not needed.

Once a diagnosis of cirrhosis is made, by whatever means, the clinician must assess the extent of functional hepatic impairment, that is, the presence of parenchymal dysfunction or portal hypertension. The presence of cirrhosis does not, in and of itself, imply liver failure. In fact, the enormous resiliency of the liver may allow it to perform normally, despite the presence of extensive fibrosis; the patient may appear well, and have no biochemical evidence of liver dysfunction. Cirrhotic patients with such normal parameters are said to be "compensated." Conversely, patients who develop any complication attributable to cirrhosis, such as ascites, varices, or encephalopathy, as discussed later, are said to be "decompensated." In general, patients with compensated cirrhosis have a longer survival than those with decompensated liver disease, more than 12 and approximately 2 years, respectively.[11]

Models to Predict the Severity of Cirrhosis

The modified Child-Pugh score is a widely used tool to assess the severity and prognosis of cirrhosis.[12] Table 34-1 provides further details about the Child-Pugh score. More recently, the Model for End Stage Liver Disease (MELD) score was developed to predict survival following the transjugular intrahepatic portal-systemic shunt (TIPSS) procedure, and subsequently validated to predict mortality in patients awaiting liver transplantation (Table 34-2).[13] Despite the latter employing more objective parameters, the Child-Pugh score has better predictive accuracy for prognosis.[14]

Parenchymal Failure

In advanced cases of cirrhosis, fibrosis may replace normal hepatocytes to such a degree that normal hepatic functions are compromised. Impaired hepatic function is reflected in abnormalities of those parameters that reflect the liver's synthetic dysfunction, which is characterized by depressed serum albumin and prolonged prothrombin time. Excretory dysfunction is characterized by hyperbilirubinemia and jaundice, indicating an inability of the liver to conjugate bile normally or excrete bile.

Portal Hypertension

Portal hypertension represents the process resulting from cirrhosis that is responsible for most of its life-threatening complications. There have been significant advances in the understanding of portal hypertension.[15] Certainly, portal hypertension results from more than just a simple mechanical obstruction to the inflow of portal blood that may result from scarring of the liver. Rather, a complex sequence of vascular, mechanical, and neurohumoral events occur in cirrhosis that lead to the manifestations of portal hypertension.[16]

The initial event in the development of portal hypertension is an increase in the vascular resistance within the liver. The anatomic changes at the level of the sinusoids have been well characterized.[17] In addition, however, sinusoidal endothelium retains contractile function, which may further contribute to the increased resistance to portal blood inflow.[18] Activated stellate cells contribute to this vascular reactivity.[19,20] Hepatic stellate cells are a heterogeneous and versatile population of cells capable of modulating vascular resistance and, when activated, generating fibrosis.[21,22] Stellate cells are present in the subendothelial space, between the hepatocytes and sinusoidal endothelium. The hepatic stellate cell is the primary source of extracellular matrix in the liver. When activated, typically by an influx of inflammatory

TABLE 34-1 CHILD-PUGH CLASSIFICATION SCHEME*

Parameter	1 Point Each	2 Points Each	3 Points Each
Ascites	None	Slight, diuretic controlled	Moderate or more
Bilirubin (mg/dl)	<2.0	2.0-3.0	>3.0
Albumin (g/dl)	>3.5	2.8-3.5	<2.8
Encephalopathy	None	Stage 1 or 2	Stage 3 or 4
Prolongation of prothrombin time (sec)	<4	4-6	>6
INR	<1.7	1.7-2.3	>2.3
Child's Class	**A**	**B**	**C**
Score	5-6	7-9	≥10
Survival (1 yr)	95%	80%	45%

*The Child-Pugh classification scheme, although originally developed to determine risk for emergent surgery to treat variceal hemorrhage, has been used more broadly to assess the severity of cirrhosis.[11]

TABLE 34-2 MODEL FOR END-STAGE LIVER DISEASE (MELD)*

MELD Score	3-Month Death Rates
≤9	8%
10-19	26%
20-29	56%
30-39	66%
≥40	100%

*The Model for End-Stage Liver Disease (MELD) score was first developed to assess survival following insertion of a transjugular intrahepatic portosystemic shunt (TIPSS) in patients with portal hypertension. This was subsequently validated as a model to assess survival in patients with chronic liver disease not undergoing TIPSS. The MELD score has become the standard by which patients awaiting liver transplantation are allocated an organ. The score is calculated using the serum creatinine, total bilirubin, and international normalized ratio (INR), using the following equation: $3.8\log_e(\text{bilirubin [mg/dl]}) + 11.2\log_e(\text{INR}) + 9.6\log_e(\text{creatinine [mg/dl]}) + 6.4$. This table present a historical data set (used to minimize the impact of liver transplantation, and thus maximize an assessment of the general applicability of the MELD score) of patients with chronic liver disease.[13]

cells, stellate cells transform into a fibrogenic cell. This process is a central event in the development of hepatic fibrosis,[23] but the enhanced vascular tone that occurs within the liver is also modulated by an overexpression of vasoconstrictors and a relative underexpression of vasodilatory substances.[24] The relationship between these substances within the liver is important; principally, a reduction in intrahepatic production of nitric oxide (NO, an important vasodilatory agent)[25-27] and of prostaglandins[28,29] occurs. The end result is an increase in the intrahepatic vascular resistance.

A secondary event that occurs in the pathogenesis of portal hypertension is the development of splanchnic arteriolar vasodilation and a hyperdynamic circulation, resulting from an overexpression of vasodilatory substances, most importantly NO,[30] but also calcitonin gene–related peptide, substance P, and endogenous cannabinoids.[24,27,31-35] The pivotal role that NO plays in portal hypertension is evidenced by several key findings. First, NO appears to be responsible for decreased response to vasoconstrictors that is seen in cirrhosis.[36,37] Second, inhibition of nitric oxide synthase (NOS) mitigates the hyperdynamic circulation.[38,39]

Nitric oxide is an endothelial-derived relaxation factor with a short half-life of only a few seconds and is rapidly reabsorbed.[40] It is synthesized by a family of three isoforms: endothelial nitric oxide synthase (eNOS) and neuronal nitric oxide synthase, which are constitutively expressed, and inducible nitric oxide synthase.[41-44] Each isoform leads to the formation of NO as a by-product of the conversion of arginine to citrulline.[43] In portal hypertension, eNOS appears to be responsible for most of the excess NO in the splanchnic circulation.[45,46] The evidence that supports the complex behavior of NO and its isoforms in portal hypertension has been reviewed elsewhere.[47,48]

The increased flow of blood through the splanchnic circulation leads to more blood flowing into the portal vein, further aggravating the pressure within. Splanchnic arteriolar vasodilation is accompanied by a fall in the systemic vascular resistance, and concurrent hyperdynamic circulation, characterized by an increased cardiac output.[49] This hyperdynamic circulation compensates for the arteriolar vasodilation, thus maintaining arterial pressure. However, as liver disease, and thus portal hypertension, progresses, so does the intensity of the vasodilation. In time, the increase in cardiac output is insufficient to support a normal blood pressure and systemic arterial hypotension develops, in turn leading to appropriate physiologic responses—increased stimulation of the renin-angiotensin and sympathetic nervous systems, and retention of salt and water,[50] as discussed later.

An important dimension of portal hypertension that accounts for many of its clinical manifestations includes the development of portal systemic shunts. These shunts open once a critical threshold pressure has been reached within the portal vein.[51] They permit the portal blood, and its contents, to circumvent the liver and enter into the systemic circulation. The clinical consequences of this shunting include esophageal varices with bleeding, ascites, portal systemic encephalopathy, renal dysfunction, and the pulmonary complications of portal hypertension. These presentations have been termed the *portal hypertensive syndrome.*[52] The sequence of pathophysiologic events that occur in portal hypertension is depicted in Figure 34-3.

THERAPEUTICS AND CLINICAL PHARMACOLOGY

Manifestations of Portal Hypertension and Goals of Therapy

Hepatic Vein Pressure Gradient

In considering the goals of pharmacotherapy for the complications of cirrhosis, one must understand the benefit of measuring, either directly or indirectly, the portal pressure. Direct measurements of the portal vein pressure can be accomplished by direct puncture either percutaneously, at laparotomy, or through transhepatic puncture from the hepatic vein, accessed via the vena cava. Indirect measurement of the portal vein pressures was first introduced in 1951[53] and now is employed routinely. In this procedure, as depicted in Figure 34-4, patients undergo catheterization of the right internal jugular vein or right femoral vein. A catheter is advanced into a terminal hepatic vein, with measurements taken while in the hepatic vein, and again while advanced to the extent of the venule (wedged position). It is now the conventional approach for a balloon-tipped catheter to be used for the wedged measurement. The premise of this procedure is that the wedged pressure reflects the sinusoidal pressure. Arguably, the most important measurement from the catheterization procedure is the hepatic vein pressure gradient (HVPG), which is derived to be the difference between the free hepatic vein pressure, reflecting the pressure within

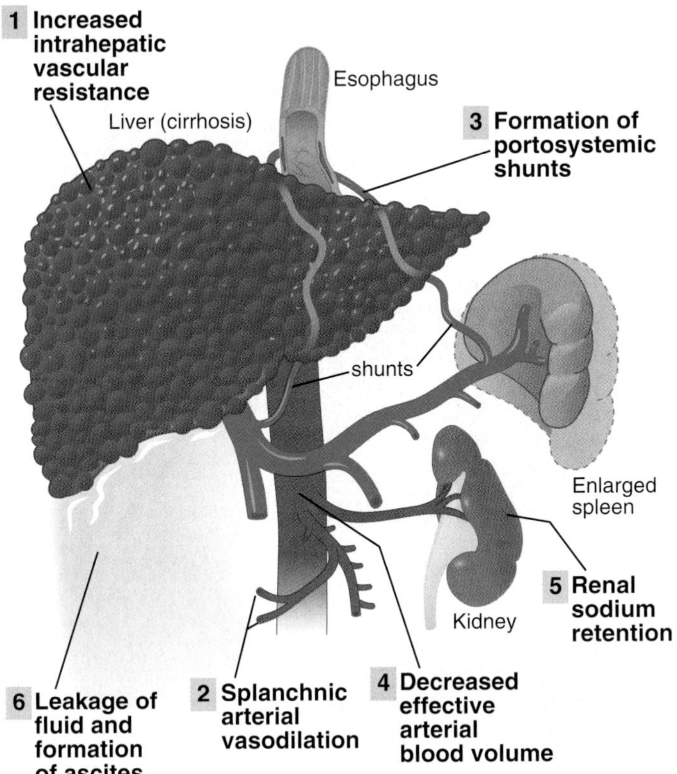

FIGURE 34-3 • **Events leading to clinical manifestations of portal hypertension.** In portal hypertension, a sequence of events occurs leading to its clinical manifestations. This sequence begins with (1) the development of increased intrahepatic vascular resistance, followed by (2) splanchnic arterial vasodilation, (3) the formation of portosystemic shunts (varices), and (4) a decrease in the effective arterial blood volume. These events set the stage for (5) renal sodium retention and volume overload followed, eventually, by (6) the leakage of fluid and formation of ascites.

the postsinusoidal systemic vascular space, and the wedged hepatic vein pressure, reflecting the pressure within the portal vein (presinusoidal space).[54]

The HVPG has become a useful research and clinical tool, particularly in situations in which an assessment of the degree of portal hypertension is required. In fact, the severity of liver disease is accurately reflected by the HVPG; a gradient of greater than or equal to 10 mm Hg is associated with an increased risk of portal hypertensive complications,[55] and a pressure gradient of 12 mm Hg or more identifies varices at risk for rupture.[51] In a recent meta-analysis examining prognostic indicators of survival in cirrhosis, the HVPG proved to be an independent predictor of survival.[11] Moreover, it has been found that a decrease in the baseline of HVPG by 20% translates into protection from variceal bleeding,[56] emphasizing its value as a relevant tool for titration of pharmacotherapeutic interventions. Further, it has been shown that pharmacologic reduction in the HVPG may reduce the risk of other complications of portal hypertension, such as ascites and renal failure.[57]

Gastroesophageal Varices

As described, portosystemic shunts arise as the result of portal hypertension. These shunts, or varices, occur in precarious anatomic locations that predispose them to rupture. Most notably, varices occurring in the esophagus and stomach (gastroesophageal varices) are most prone to bleeding. Gastroesophageal varices have a prevalence of 50% in cirrhotics; they are more likely to occur among patients with more advanced cirrhosis.[58] Patients with large varices have a 30% risk of bleeding.[59,60] The mortality attributable to uncontrolled bleeding is approximately 8%, and the expected mortality at 6 weeks is approximately 20%, despite current therapy.[61] Bleeding stops spontaneously in about 40% of cases.[59] Bacterial infection is associated with failure to control bleeding, and thus with an increased mortality from a bleeding episode.[62]

The goals in treatment of varices can be conceptualized in stages. These include prophylactic therapy, to prevent varices from bleeding; treatment of active bleeding; and finally prevention of rebleeding. Pharmacologic treatments comprise the cornerstone in each stage. As is discussed subsequently, the judicious use of these pharmacotherapies has been advocated and adopted into treatment recommendations.[61]

Ascites

The formation of ascites is typically the earliest manifestation of portal hypertension.[63] Ascites, in and of itself, may lead to additional complications, most importantly spontaneous bacterial peritonitis. Ascites in a cirrhotic patient is an indication of reduced survival; the expected 1-year survival after the formation of ascites is between 45% and 82%.[64]

Sodium retention precedes the formation of ascites, as evidenced by subtle but demonstrable abnormalities in renal sodium handling in cirrhotic patients in the pre-ascitic stage. For example, persistent sodium retention following several days of mineralocorticoid administration, without compensatory renal excretion to regain sodium balance, in some cirrhotics without ascites is indicative of this abnormality. It is speculated that these abnormalities are in response to the splanchnic arterial vasodilation commonly seen in cirrhotics.[65]

The process of ascites formation is one that has been debated. However, the current theory states that portal hypertension initiates arterial vasodilation, which, in turn, leads to a reduction in the effective arterial blood volume (EABV). The reduction in the EABV triggers arterial receptors, then leading to a homeostatic activation of the sympathetic nervous system and the renin-angiotensin-aldosterone system, causing hypersecretion of antidiuretic hormone. The consequence of these events is renal sodium and water retention. As liver disease progresses and arterial vasodilation intensifies, leakage of fluid from the splanchnic circulation into the peritoneal cavity and tissue spaces occurs and ascites develops.[65]

The goal of therapy in cirrhotic patients with ascites is to eliminate the ascites through a combination of dietary salt restriction and diuretics. The absence of ascites leads to an improved nutritional status and a reduction in the risk of spontaneous bacterial peritonitis. Assessing sodium excretion in clinical practice is a useful tool for identifying the response to diuretic therapy. This is done under controlled circumstances, with the patient consuming a low-sodium diet (80 mEq/day, or about 2000 mg/day) and taking no diuretics for at least 5 days prior to a 24-hour urine collection. This method of determining sodium excretion has been described elsewhere.[65] Generally speaking, however, the more impaired the sodium excretion, the higher the doses of diuretics that will be required.

The degree of ascites is highly variable among cirrhotic patients, and within any given patient at any given time. Moreover, the pattern of ascites presentation has an important impact on pharmacotherapy and thus deserves mention. *Uncomplicated ascites* refers to the presence of ascites without renal dysfunction (as discussed later) or infection. Uncomplicated ascites that is detectable only by ultrasound is termed *grade 1*, or mild. *Grade 2* ascites refers to moderate ascites that is detectable as a symmetric distention of the abdomen. Finally, *grade 3* refers to severe ascites with massive distention of the abdomen. *Refractory ascites* is that which cannot be mobilized with dietary sodium restriction and pharmacotherapy; this is further characterized as either *diuretic-resistant ascites* or *diuretic-intractable ascites.* The former refers to ascites that cannot be mobilized or that recurs early after treatment due to a lack of responsiveness to diuretics coupled with dietary sodium restriction; the latter refers to that which cannot be mobilized or that recurs early after treatment due to the development of diuretic-induced complications.[66,67]

Spontaneous Bacterial Peritonitis

Spontaneous bacterial peritonitis (SBP) is, as the name implies, the sudden and unprovoked development of peritoneal fluid infection in a cirrhotic patient. It is defined as the occurrence of greater than 250

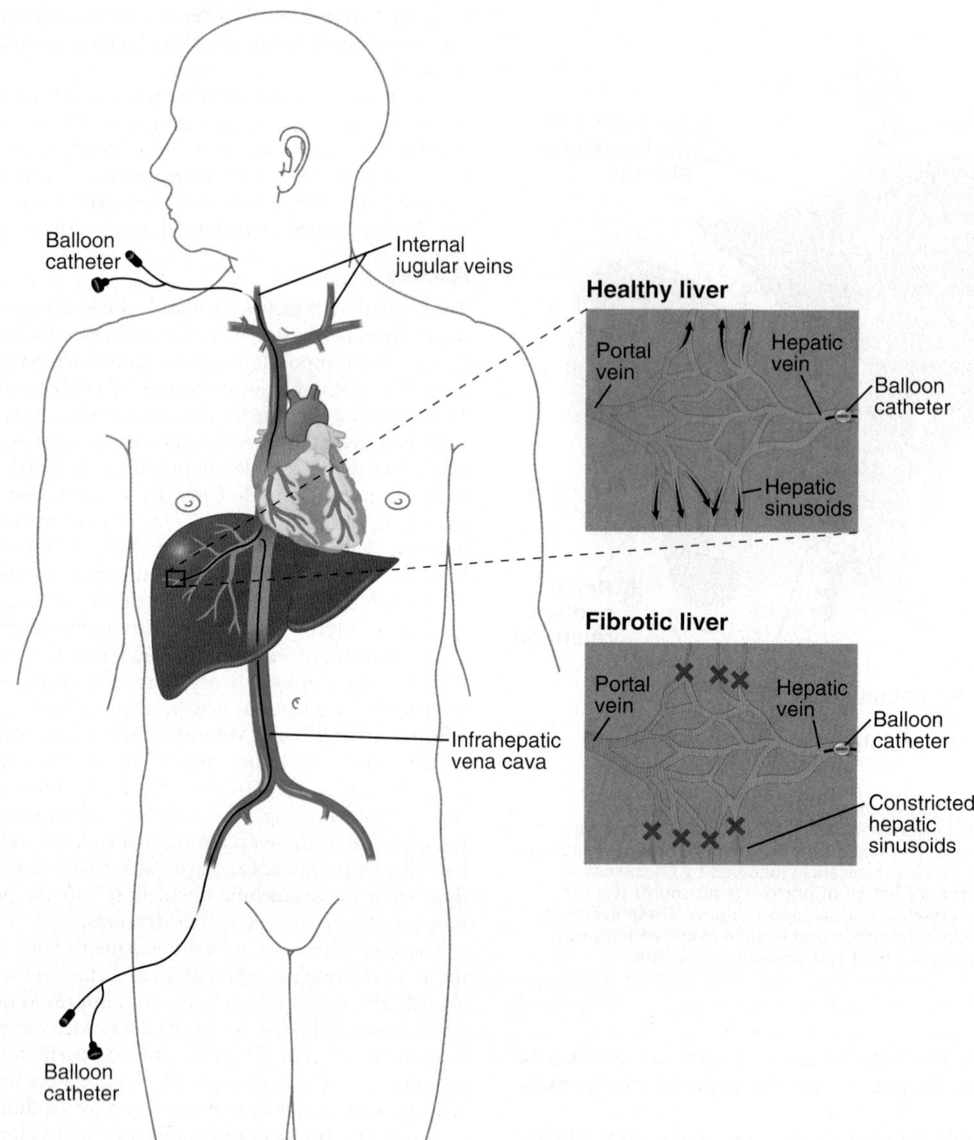

FIGURE 34-4 • Measurement of hepatic vein pressure gradient. Measurement of the hepatic vein pressure gradient (HVPG) is a useful clinical and research intervention. The contemporary technique entails catheterization of the hepatic vein via the internal jugular or infrahepatic vena cava. A balloon tipped pressure transducer catheter is advanced into a terminal hepatic vein, and pressures are measured in the inflated (wedged hepatic vein pressure) and non-inflated (free hepatic vein pressure) positions. The difference between these two values is the HVPG. In the healthy liver, the wedged pressure reflects a normal portal pressure; however, in the fibrotic liver, intrahepatic portal venules are constricted and cannot transmit back pressure as readily. (Adapted from Bosch J: Measurement of portal pressure and its role in the management of chronic liver disease. Semin Liv Dis 2006;26:348-362.)

polymorphonuclear (PMN) leukocytes per cubic milliliter with a positive ascites fluid culture, although approximately 40% of cases over this PMN threshold are culture negative. The most common organisms responsible for this syndrome include gram-negative bacilli followed by gram-positive cocci, in particular, *Streptococcus pneumoniae*.[68] Predisposing factors for development of SBP include advanced stage of liver disease, gastrointestinal bleeding, low ascites fluid protein content (<1 g/dl), urinary tract infection, intestinal bacterial overgrowth, and previous SBP.[68] The most likely pathogenesis for SBP, although speculative, is the translocation of bacteria from the intestinal lumen into the systemic circulation, with subsequent seeding of ascites fluid.[68]

The prevalence of SBP among hospitalized cirrhotic patients with ascites ranges between 7% and 31%.[69] Although patients typically present with symptoms to indicate the presence of infection, such as fever, leukocytosis, or abdominal pain, as many as one third of patients present without localizing symptoms.[68] The prognosis of SBP is poor, overall; the 1-year probability of survival following an episode of SBP has been reported to be as low as 20%.[70]

As is discussed later, the timely institution of pharmacotherapy comprises cornerstone therapy for SBP. In addition, pharmacotherapy is important for the prevention of recurrent episodes of SBP. Drug therapy for SBP is complemented by the infusion of albumin, which mitigates the complications of SBP, such as renal dysfunction.[71]

Hepatorenal Syndrome

In portal hypertension, splanchnic arterial vasodilation leads to the homeostatic activation of the renal volume receptors and baroreceptors, triggering compensatory neural, autonomic, and humoral responses. In particular, splanchnic and peripheral arterial vasodilation and hypotension lead to vigorous stimulation of the renin-angiotensin and sympathetic nervous systems, and eventually antidiuretic hormone.[72] The vasoconstrictive action of these substances are made even more intense by a reduced local synthesis of vasodilators[72,73] and hyporesponsiveness to the action of locally produced vasodilators.[36,37] These events culminate in renal sodium and water retention and expansion of plasma volume with the formation of ascites, as discussed previously. As the hypotension persists, unmitigated vasoconstrictor activity of the renin-angiotensin system occurs at the expense of renal perfusion, thus leading to renal failure. In this clinical situation, the term *hepatorenal syndrome* (HRS) is applied. Cardiac output falls as the severity of arterial vasodilation increases and as HRS develops.[74] A cardiomyopathy has been described in patients with advanced cirrhosis.[75]

HRS occurs in patients with cirrhosis with an incidence of approximately 8% per year.[76] Criteria for the diagnosis of HRS have been established,[66] and two clinical subtypes have been described. HRS type 1 refers to rapidly progressive renal failure, as indicated by a doubling of the creatinine, exceeding 2.5 mg/dl in less than 2 weeks. Type 1 HRS usually results from a precipitating event, such as bleeding or infection, and occurs most often in patients with more advanced cirrhosis and signs of severe circulatory dysfunction. Type 1 HRS portends a very poor prognosis, with only a 2-week median survival time.[76] Type 2 HRS is characterized by a less rapid course, often with moderate reduction or fluctuation in renal function. Circulatory dysfunction is present, but to a lesser degree than in patients with type 1 HRS. Patients with type 2 HRS also have better survival than type 1 HRS, albeit still poor; median survival of 6 months can be expected.

An understanding of the pathogenetic mechanisms involved in HRS and a stratification of its clinical presentation have led to the development of targeted therapies.[77] Namely, current treatments are intended to reverse the splanchnic vasodilation. In addition, restitution of the effective arterial blood volume is another important therapeutic maneuver, with the consummate goal being improvement in renal function. In general, however, the definitive treatment for HRS is liver transplantation, which causes the renal function, in most cases, to return to normal. That notwithstanding, patients with HRS who undergo liver transplantation have a higher mortality than those without renal dysfunction.[77]

Hepatic Encephalopathy

Patients with cirrhosis may experience an alteration in mentation and a decline in cognitive agility. Nomenclature for hepatic encephalopathy (HE) has been established in the context of a consensus conference.[78] In general, there are three types of HE: type A, encephalopathy associated with acute liver failure; type B, encephalopathy associated with portal systemic bypass without intrinsic liver disease; and type C, encephalopathy with cirrhosis and portal hypertension, or portal-systemic shunts.[78]

It is accepted that substances derived from the gut fail to be cleared by the liver, owing to blood that escapes via portosystemic shunts, and act as toxins to the brain. This toxicity is proposed to occur by three mechanisms: an elevation in ammonia, inflammatory responses, and changes in cerebral hemodynamics.[79] Perhaps the most important of these, and one to which most conventional pharmacotherapies are directed, is hyperammonemia.[80,81]

Glutamine taken up in the intestine forms the substrate for the enzyme glutaminase. The action of this enzyme leads to the formation of ammonia and glutamate. In addition, normal flora in the intestine that produce urea also lead to the liberation of ammonia. In the normal situation, the liver converts ammonia and glutamate arriving from the gut via the portal vein into urea and glutamine, respectively. However, as a result of portosystemic shunting, or due to loss of hepatocyte mass due to disease, systemic levels of these substances rise. Ammonia has been shown to be directly toxic to the brain, leading to increased permeability of the blood-brain barrier and astrocyte swelling.[79,82,83]

The pivotal role of the gut for uptake of the substrate for ammonia has made it an obvious target for therapy. In fact, most conventional therapies are targeted at reduction of the substrate for ammonia. These include purgatives and antibiotics, as discussed later.

Pulmonary Complications of Portal Hypertension

Portopulmonary hypertension (PPHTN) is an important complication of portal hypertension for which pharmacotherapy has been employed. In the context of all pulmonary complications associated with cirrhosis and portal hypertension, it is not the most common, however. Hepatopulmonary syndrome (HPS) is the more common pulmonary complication associated with portal hypertension.

HPS is characterized by the presence of intrapulmonary vascular dilatation and hypoxemia, occurring in the setting of chronic liver disease. Patients present with shortness of breath; platypnea (increased shortness of breath with changing from the supine to upright position) and orthodeoxia (a fall in arterial partial pressure of oxygen by 5% or more, or a rise by 4 mm Hg or more, with changing from supine to upright) are typical findings, but not necessary for the diagnosis.[84] Reliable diagnosis depends upon demonstration of arterial hypoxemia and, through the use of contrast-enhanced transthoracic echocardiography, intrapulmonary vascular abnormalities.[85,86] It is hypothesized that the intrapulmonary vascular dilations result from overproduction of NO within the pulmonary vascular bed, as determined by detection of exhaled NO.[87-89] The prevalence of HPS has been reported to be 18% in liver transplantation candidates,[90] but up to 28% in patients with hepatic venous thrombosis (Budd-Chiari syndrome).[91] Pharmacotherapy has little role in the current treatment of patients with HPS, although several agents have been tried in small trials. Definitive therapy of HPS comprises liver transplantation, which leads to reversal of the syndrome in the majority of cases.[92]

Unlike HPS, pharmacotherapy plays an important role in the management of PPHTN, which is defined by the presence of pulmonary arterial hypertension in association with portal hypertension.[84] Specific diagnostic criteria include a mean pulmonary arterial pressure (PAP) of greater than 25 mm Hg at rest or greater than 30 mm Hg during exercise, with a concomitant normal mean pulmonary artery wedge pressure (i.e., <15 mm Hg).[84,93] PPHTN is an infrequent complication of portal hypertension, with an estimated prevalence of up to 2% in patients with cirrhosis and portal hypertension.[94,95] The diagnosis of PPHTN portends a poor prognosis; in one center's experience, 58% of patients died within a year.[94] Five-year survival of 30% has been reported in untreated patients.[96]

The precise etiology of PPHTN is not known, but has been speculated upon and summarized elsewhere.[84] However, salient features of the proposed etiology deserve mention, as they are pertinent to a discussion of the current therapeutic approach. It has been proposed that excess vasoactive substances arrive in the lungs as a consequence of portosystemic shunts.[93,97] The result is a vasoproliferative process, with a histologic appearance indistinguishable from primary pulmonary hypertension. This includes intimal proliferation, smooth muscle hypertrophy, and fibrosis. Neurohumoral factors, such as serotonin and endothelin-1, may lead to pulmonary arterial vasoconstriction and pulmonary hypertension.[98,99] Serotonin uptake has been shown to be reduced in portal hypertension.[100] Endothelin-1, produced by the pulmonary endothelium, binds to receptors on smooth muscle, triggering vasoconstriction.[101,102] Additional factors that may play a role in PPHTN include increased inflammatory activity within the lung vasculature, owing to blood that escapes the liver via portal-systemic shunts. An increase in pulmonary phagocytosis in cirrhotics is evidence, albeit indirect, of increased inflammatory activity.[103]

The goal of pharmacotherapy of PPHTN is to provide relief of symptoms associated with pulmonary hypertension, namely chest pain, dyspnea, and syncope.[104] In addition, a reduction in PAP and in attributable mortality, and an increase in the performance of successful liver transplantation, for which PPHTN is an important contraindication, remain important therapeutic goals. The predicted perioperative mortality for patients undergoing liver transplantation with mean PAP of over 35 mm Hg is more than 50%.[105]

Therapeutics by Class

Vasoconstrictors

Nonselective β-Adrenergic Blockers. These agents reduce portal pressure and flow into the portal vein.[106] Specifically, they produce blockade of the β receptors. As a result, unmitigated α-receptor stimulation occurs. The resulting vasoconstriction yields a reduction in splanchnic vasodilation and reduction in portal inflow. Further, β-

TABLE 34-3 NONSELECTIVE β-BLOCKERS FOR PROPHYLAXIS OF BLEEDING AND PREVENTION OF REBLEEDING FROM GASTROESOPHAGEAL VARICES

Generic Name	Trade Name	Mechanism of Elimination	Half-Life	Dose Range	Dose Interval	Indications in Cirrhosis	Side Effects and Toxicities
Propranolol	Inderal Inderal LA	Renal <1%	PO/IV: 4 hr (IR) PO: 10 hr (SR)	40-320 mg/day (IR) 60-160 mg (SR)	bid–qid (IR) qd (SR)	Prevention of variceal bleeding or rebleeding	Bradycardia Bronchospasm Impedes recognition of hypoglycemia Hyperkalemia CNS (sleep disturbance) Hyperlipidemia
Nadolol	Corgard	Renal Fecal	20 hr	40-320 mg IV: 0.01-0.05 mg/kg Max: 10 mg/day	qd	Prevention of variceal bleeding or rebleeding	Increased in renal failure Less CNS effects than propranolol
Timolol	Blocadren	Renal	4 hr	10-60 mg/day	qd-bid	Prevention of variceal bleeding or rebleeding	Bradyarrhythmia Angina Heart failure Hypotension Dermatologic N/V/D Confusion HA Depression Cough Bronchospasm

bid, twice daily; CNS, central nervous system; HA, headache; IR, immediate-release; IV, intravenous; N/V/D, nausea, vomiting, and diarrheas; PO, oral; qid, four times daily; qd, daily; SR, sustained-release.

adrenergic blockers reduce cardiac output. The combined effect is to reduce portal blood inflow.

The β-adrenergic blockers have no proven value in the prevention of the formation of varices. This was demonstrated in a randomized controlled trial of timolol versus placebo, for the prevention of variceal development. The investigators found no significant difference between the treatment and active groups.[55] In comparison, in patients with moderate to large varices and no history of bleeding, β-adrenergic blockers have been shown to be of significant value in the prevention of an initial bleed. Since the seminal study in 1981,[107] several additional studies have been published that have established the efficacy of these agents for bleeding from esophageal varices in cirrhotics (Table 34-3). Subsequently, a meta-analysis reviewed the 11 randomized controlled trials examining the efficacy of β-adrenergic blockers in the prevention of an initial variceal bleed. These studies comprised 1189 patients with varices; treated patients had an incidence of variceal bleeding of 15%, compared with 24% in the placebo group.[59] Although a statistically significant survival benefit could not be identified, these studies establish the use of β-adrenergic blockers as standard therapy for patients with cirrhosis and moderate or larger varices. The value of nonselective β-adrenergic blockers in patients with very advanced cirrhosis or with very small varices has not yet been established, as such patients were underrepresented in these trials.

There are important considerations when treating cirrhotic patients with β-adrenergic blockers. Namely, there is great variability with regard to the efficacy of the drug, which is determined most precisely by a reduction of the HVPG. In fact, more than half of patients treated do not achieve the targeted reduction in HVPG.[108] Moreover, these drugs are associated with significant side effects that may limit their use. These include hypotension, bradycardia, and bronchospasm. Up to 20% of patients who may benefit from these drugs have contraindications to their use; 15% of patients treated with β-adrenergic blockers develop side effects.[59]

Vasopressin. Endogenous vasopressin is a potent vasoconstrictor that leads to a reduction in the flow of blood through the splanchnic circulation (Table 34-4). As a result of this vasoconstriction, less blood flows into the portal vein and collaterals, and pressure falls.[109,110] The efficacy of vasopressin for reducing the HVPG has been shown.[110] However, its widespread use has been tempered by the frequent and often severe side effects resulting from the intense vasoconstriction. These include cardiac and peripheral vascular ischemia, and hyponatremia and fluid retention reflecting its antidiuretic hormone properties. The use of short- and long-acting nitrates has been advocated to mitigate its side effects.[111] Studies investigating the effect of nitrates on the efficacy of vasopressin in the setting of acute variceal bleeding have been done.[112,113] The evidence supporting its efficacy notwithstanding, the severity of complications associated with its use has made vasopressin an infrequently used drug, yet an important prototype nonetheless.

Terlipressin. An analogue of vasopressin, terlipressin also acts by causing vasoconstriction of the splanchnic vasculature. However, its pharmacokinetic and side effect profiles differ. Specifically, terlipressin has a comparatively longer half-life and few side effects (see Table 34-4). A significant reduction in the HVPG has been shown with an accompanying reduction in collateral blood flow. Its use is associated with reduced mortality and lower rebleeding rates.[114-116] This agent is not yet available in the United States.

Somatostatin. Endogenous somatostatin inhibits the secretion of vasodilatory peptides in the gastrointestinal tract. Perhaps the most important of these enzymes is glucagon, which has been shown to contribute to portal hypertension.[34] Antagonism of the effect of somatostatin by re-introduction of glucagon in an experimental model is further evidence of its important role in portal hypertension.[117] Inhibition of glucagon's effect by somatostatin serves to mitigate the flow of blood into the portal vein, thus reducing pressure and forming the rationale for its use in the treatment of variceal bleeding (Table 34-5).

Somatostatin's clinical use is limited by its short half-life of 1 to 3 minutes,[118] and thus it requires continuous infusion. The standard intravenous dose of somatostatin is 250 mcg followed by a continuous infusion of 250 mcg/hr.[119] Bolus dosing leads to a 50% reduction in portal pressure and collateral flow.[120] Repeated higher bolus dosing (500 mcg) is associated with increased survival in the setting of portal hypertensive bleeding.[121] However, somatostatin is associated with significant gastrointestinal side effects and also potentially deleterious effects on renal function, namely a reduction in renal plasma flow and sodium excretion.[122] As a pharmacotherapeutic for the treatment of esophageal variceal bleeding, somatostatin serves as an important prototype for analogue compounds.

TABLE 34-4 VASOCONSTRICTORS FOR THE TREATMENT OF PORTAL HYPERTENSIVE COMPLICATIONS (VARICEAL BLEEDING AND HEPATORENAL SYNDROME)

Generic Name	Trade Name	Mechanism of Elimination	Half-Life	Dose Range	Dose Interval	Indications in Cirrhosis	Side Effects and Toxicities
Vasopressin	Pitressin	Renal	17-35 min	IV: 0.2 units/min titrated to 1-2 units/min Bolus: 15 units in 15 min	Infusion via central line	Vasoconstriction of splanchnic arterial flow Variceal and other GI bleeding	Facial pallor GI cramping, nausea Coronary constriction Arrythmias Peripheral vasoconstriction Allergic reaction Anaphylaxis Use with nitroglycerin
Terlipressin	Glypressin	Renal	50 min	IV: 2-4 mg, then 1 mg 120 mcg/kg/day	Bolus: q4-6h max	Vasoconstriction of splanchnic arterial flow Variceal and other GI bleeding Hepatorenal syndrome	Hypertension Bradycardia Hypokalemia Bronchoconstriction Urinary retention
Midodrine	Proamatine Orvaten	Renal Fecal	3-4 hr	30 mg/day IV: 5 mg/day	tid IV: qd	Hepatorenal syndrome	Supine hypertension Piloerection Mild GI symptoms

GI, gastrointestinal; IV, intravenous; qd, daily; tid, three times daily.

TABLE 34-5 SOMATOSTATIN AND ITS ANALOGUES, AS VASOCONSTRICTORS, FOR THE TREATMENT OF PORTAL HYPERTENSION AND ITS COMPLICATIONS

Generic Name	Trade Name	Mechanism of Elimination	Half-Life	Dose Range	Dose Interval	Indications in Cirrhosis	Side Effects and Toxicities
Somatostatin			2-3 min	Bolus: 250 mcg Then 250-500 mcg/hr	Infusion	Variceal and nonvariceal bleeding	Reduces hepatic and renal blood flow Can cause malabsorption, cholelithiasis, and diarrhea Glucose intolerance
Octreotide	Sandostatin	Renal	90 min	25-50 mcg/hr Bolus: 50 mcg	Infusion (IV)	Variceal bleeding	Suppresses GI motility and secretion Diarrhea Loose stools Malabsorption Nausea Transient hyperglycemia QT prolongation Bradyarrythmia Hypertension Alopecia Flushing Hypothyroidism Cholelithiasis
Lanreotide	Somatuline	Fecal	90 min 5 days (depot)	IM: 30 mg IM: 60-120 mg 750 mcg subQ	10-14 days 28 days 8 hr	Decreases postprandial portal blood flow	Transient glucose intolerance Cholelithiasis Diarrhea Abdominal pain Hypersensitivity
Vapreotide	Sanvar		164 min	50 mcg Bolus: 50 mcg/hr			HA Fatigue Diarrhea Nausea

GI, gastrointestinal; HA, headache; IM, intramuscular; IV intravenous; subQ, subcutaneous.

The clinical efficacy of somatostatin in the treatment of acute variceal bleeding has been studied in several randomized controlled trials, in comparison to other pharmacologic treatments for portal hypertension or placebo.[59] It has been shown to be superior to placebo, in combination with endoscopic interventions, for achieving control of acute variceal hemorrhage.[123] When compared with other vasoconstrictors, namely vasopressin and terlipressin, studies demonstrate equal efficacy for achieving bleeding cessation; however, somatostatin had a better safety profile than vasopressin.[59]

Somatostatin Analogues

Octreotide. The short half-life and side effect profile of somatostatin led to the search for analogues with more favorable pharmacokinetic and side effect profiles. Octreotide, a cyclic octapeptide, is the most widely used somatostatin analogue. This and other somatostatin analogues, such as lanreotide and vapreotide, demonstrate selective binding to somatostatin receptors, thus having different pharmacodynamic properties[124] (see Table 34-5). Specifically, octreotide is thought to act by inhibiting the secretion of glucagon, an endogenous vasodilatory agent; however, its precise mechanism of action in portal hypertension has not been elucidated.

Pharmacologically, octreotide has a half-life of 2 hours after subcutaneous injection[124] and thus is best given as continuous infusion. Standard dosing of octreotide comprises a 50-mcg intravenous bolus followed by 50 mcg/hr.[119] However, there appears to be rapid desensitization with regard to its portal pressure–lowering effect.[125] Subcutaneous octreotide can be administered, but is of limited clinical use at the present time, due to the lack of evidence for its benefit in the treatment of portal hypertensive complications.[111]

The short-term side effects of octreotide mirror those of somatostatin, including nausea and abdominal cramping; longer term treatment may predispose patients to the formation of cholesterol gallstones owing to gallbladder hypomotility. As a class, however, somatostatin and its analogues also have been associated with ileus, pulmonary edema, and rebound gallbladder hypermotility upon withdrawal.[126]

Randomized controlled trials comparing octreotide to other vasoconstrictors demonstrated it to be more effective than vasopressin, and to have equal efficacy to terlipressin, in controlling variceal bleeding, but with fewer side effects than vasopressin. No difference in terms of survival could be demonstrated among these pharmacologic interventions.[59] A more recent meta-analysis confirmed that octreotide does not improve survival from variceal bleeding.[127] The most consistently reported effect of octreotide is to mitigate the rise in portal pressure that occurs following a meal.[128]

Vasodilators

Nitrates. Nitroglycerin is an NO donor and vasodilator, thus forming the rationale for the use of nitrates in portal hypertension. The hemodynamic response to sublingual administration has been studied in humans.[129] The hemodynamic and clinical effect of a long-acting oral preparation, isosorbide 5-mononitrate, also has been studied.[130,131] Used in combination with nonselective β-blockers, the fall in portal pressure is augmented compared with nonselective β-blockers alone.[132,133] In the largest randomized controlled trial of the use of these agents in combination with nonselective β-blockers for the prevention of variceal bleeding, no clear benefit in the reduction in the risk of bleeding or survival could be attributed to combination therapy.[134] Therefore, the use of nitrates in combination with nonselective β-blockers has not been adopted as part of routine practice.[61]

As the effects of nitrates are not limited to the vascular and splanchnic circulation, their side effects are predictable in patients with cirrhosis (Table 34-6). Most importantly, they may exacerbate the systemic vasodilation already present as a result of the portal hypertensive syndrome. This, in turn, may lead to an exacerbation of sodium and water retention, as well as renal dysfunction.

Epoprostenol. Prostacyclin I_2 (epoprostenol) has a role in the treatment of PPHTN (see Table 34-6). Specifically, its proposed benefit is mitigation of pulmonary arterial vasoconstriction. Epoprostenol is a potent vasodilator and inhibitor of platelet aggregation that is given by continuous intravenous infusion, owing to its short half-life (3 to 5 minutes).[84,135] Side effects of epoprostenol include jaw pain, headache, leg pain, and gastrointestinal distress.[84]

Diuretics

The pharmacology of these agents has been reviewed elsewhere.[65] It is important to emphasize, however, that diuretics are a mainstay in the treatment of patients with cirrhosis, portal hypertension, and fluid overload.

Potassium-Sparing Diuretics. Given the current understanding of the renin-angiotensin-aldosterone system in the development of sodium retention and the formation of ascites, agents that specifically block the action of aldosterone seem to be a rational treatment approach. The agents within this class include spironolactone and amiloride (Table 34-7). The most commonly used agent is spironolactone, which is begun at a dose of 50 to 100 mg/day and titrated to a maximum of 400 mg/day. The peak effect of spironolactone is achieved after 48 hours.[136] Common side effects of spironolactone include painful gynecomastia and hyperkalemia. Amiloride blocks sodium reabsorption at the distal collecting tubule. This is begun at a dose of 5 mg/day and can be titrated up to 30 mg/day. It has more rapid onset of diuretic effect, but is less potent.[137]

Loop Diuretics. Loop diuretics inhibit the apical sodium transporter at the ascending loop of Henle, leading to increased delivery of sodium to the distal tubule. These agents are potent and fast acting, but of limited value as a sole agent in treating cirrhotic patients with ascites, as has been shown in a randomized comparative study.[138] This is due to the hyperaldosterone state induced in portal hypertension, which leads to sodium reabsorption in the distal tuble.[138] However, loop diuretics serve as excellent adjuncts to treatment with aldosterone antagonists, as the latter will block the sodium reabsorption, allowing

TABLE 34-6 VASODILATORS FOR THE TREATMENT OF PORTAL HYPERTENSION AND ITS COMPLICATIONS

Generic Name	Trade Name	Mechanism of Elimination	Half-Life	Dose Range	Dose Interval	Indications in Cirrhosis	Side Effects and Toxicities
Nitroglyerin, sublingual	Nitrostat Nitroquick	Hepatic metabolism	1-3 min	0.3-0.6 mg	5 min	Use in combination with vasopressin to reduce cardiotoxicity of vasopressin	Headache Dizziness Weakness Postural hypotension Tachyphylaxis Cardiac dysrhythmia
Isosorbide mononitrate	Imdur Imdur ER Ismo Monoket	Inactive form by kidney Feces	5 hr	10-20 mg 30-120 mg	q7h qd (ER)	Used in combination with nonselective β-blocker for added portal pressure reduction	Orthostasis N/V/D Dizziness HA Restlessness Arrythmia Heart failure
Epoprostenol (prostacyclin)	Flolan	Mainly urine Less feces	2-3 min[217]	2 ng/kg/min Titrate to 9 ng/kg/min	Continuous infusion	Pulmonary hypertension	Rebound hypertension on withdrawal
Bosentan	Tracleer	Minimal urine Mainly bile	5 hr[218]	PO: 62.5 mg bid Increase to 125 mg bid	bid	Pulmonary hypertension	Edema Flushing Hepatotoxicity Blood dyscrasia Teratogenic

bid, twice daily; ER, extended-release; HA, headache; N/V/D, nausea, vomiting, and diarrheas; PO, oral; qd, daily.

TABLE 34-7 POTASSIUM-SPARING DIURETICS COMMONLY USED FOR THE TREATMENT OF VOLUME OVERLOAD ASSOCIATED WITH PORTAL HYPERTENSION

Generic Name	Trade Name	Mechanism of Elimination	Half-Life	Dose Range	Dose Interval	Indications in Cirrhosis	Side Effects and Toxicities
Spironolactone	Aldactone	Renal Bile	1.4 hr	50-400 mg	q12h	Volume overload and ascites	Hyperkalemia Metabolic acidosis Gynecomastia Impotence Loss of libido Hirsutism Menstrual irregularities PUD/gastritis CNS
Amiloride	Midamor	Renal	6-9 hr	5-30 mg	qd	Volume overload and ascites	CNS GI Musculoskeletal Skin abnormalities Heme dyscrasias N/V/D HA

CNS, central nervous system; GI, gastrointestinal; HA, headache; N/V/D, nausea, vomiting, and diarrheas; PUD, peptic ulcer disease; qd, daily.

TABLE 34-8 LOOP DIURETICS COMMONLY USED FOR THE TREATMENT OF VOLUME OVERLOAD ASSOCIATED WITH PORTAL HYPERTENSION

Generic Name	Trade Name	Mechanism of Elimination	Half-Life	Dose Range	Dose Interval	Indications in Cirrhosis	Side Effects and Toxicities
Furosemide	Lasix	60% Kidney 40% Liver	3.4 hr	40-160 mg	qd	Ascites and edema	Hyponatremia Hypokalemia Hypomagnesemia HLD PSE Hyperglycemia Ototoxicity Hyperuricemia Bone marrow suppression GI disturbance
Bumetanide	Bumex	Metabolized by liver Excreted by kidney, bile, and feces	1-1.5 hr	PO: 0.5-2 mg IV/IM: 0.5-1 mg Max: 10 mg/day	PO: q4-5h IV/IM: q2-3h	Ascites and edema	Hyponatremia Hypokalemia Hypomagnesemia HLD PSE Hyperglycemia Ototoxicity Hyperuricemia Bone marrow suppression GI disturbance
Ethacrynic acid	Edecrin	Renal	1-4 hr	50-200 mg	qd	Ascites and edema	Highest risk for ototoxicity Rash Hyperuricemia Gout Confusion Pancreatitis Heme dyscrasias

HLD, hyperlipidemia; IM, intramuscular; IV, intravenous; PO, oral; PSE, portosystemic encephalopathy; qd, daily.

the natriuresis to take place. Furosemide is the most commonly used loop diuretic and usually is begun, in cirrhotic patients, at a dose of 40 mg/day and titrated to a maximum dose of 160 mg/day (Table 34-8). Its diuretic effect appears rapidly, usually within 30 minutes, and reaches it peak within 2 hours. Common side effects of loop diuretics include hypokalemia, hyponatremia, azotemia, and precipitation of HE. Importantly, cirrhotic patients undergoing aggressive diuresis without preexisting edema may be at particular risk for side effects.[139]

Disaccharides

Lactulose and Lactitol. Nonabsorbable disaccharides are commonly used for the treatment of HE (Table 34-9). The rationale for the use of these agents stems from the goal to reduce the substrate for ammonia. This is, in theory, achieved by a reduction in the pH of the colonic lumen, leaving an environment that is suboptimal for growth of urease-producing bacteria.[140] Although safe, lactulose may be unpalatable due to its sweet taste. Lactitol is a disaccharide analogue of lactulose that is less sweet than lactulose.

Antibiotics for Hepatic Encephalopathy

The rationale behind the use of antibiotics in patients with HE is to reduce the population of urease-producing bacteria that reside in the intestine that liberate ammonia. Neomycin has long been used in cirrhotics with encephalopathy[141] (Table 34-10). An important drawback, however, is that some of this aminoglycoside antibiotic may be absorbed from the small bowel, leading to systemic toxicity.[142]

Currently in the United States, rifaximin is indicated for the treatment of acute self-limited traveler's diarrhea. Rifaximin is an orally

TABLE 34-9 NONABSORBABLE DISACCHARIDES FOR THE MANAGEMENT OF HEPATIC ENCEPHALOPATHY

Generic Name	Trade Name	Mechanism of Elimination	Half-Life	Dose Range	Dose Interval	Indications in Cirrhosis	Side Effects and Toxicities
Lactulose	Cephulac	Minor renal Bile Fecal		20-30 g	tid–qid	Encephalopathy	Flatulance Cramps Abdominal pain Dehydration Hyponatremia Hypokalemia
Lactitol	Neda-lactitol	2% Renal 6.5% Fecal		0.25-0.5 mg/kg/day 20% enema	tid tid	Encephalopathy	Flatulance Cramping Electrolyte disturbances

tid, three times daily; qid, four times daily.

TABLE 34-10 ORAL ANTIBIOTICS FOR THE TREATMENT OF HEPATIC ENCEPHALOPATHY

Generic Name	Trade Name	Mechanism of Elimination	Half-Life	Dose Range	Dose Interval	Indications in Cirrhosis	Side Effects and Toxicities
Neomycin	Neofradin	Fecal Renal	2-3 hr	4-12 g/day	bid Max 2 wk	Encephalopathy	N/V/D Neurologic Ototoxicity Nephrotoxicity Neuromuscular blockade
Rifaximin	Xifaxan	Fecal Renal	5.85 hr	200-400 mg	tid	Encephalopathy	Constipation Vomiting Headache
Metronidazole	Flagyl	Fecal Renal	8 hr	250-500 mg	tid	Encephalopathy	Abdominal discomfort HA Peripheral neuropathy Disulfiram-like reaction with EtOH

bid, twice daily; HA, headache; N/V/D, nausea, vomiting, and diarrheas; qd, daily; tid, three times daily.

administered antibiotic that has gained significant momentum in the United States for the treatment of hepatic encephalopathy. Rifaximin is a synthetic antibiotic with activity against both gram-positive and gram-negative bacteria.[143,144] Less than 0.4% of an oral dose is absorbed systemically. In the few small studies in which it could be assessed, tolerability was better for rifaximin than lactulose.[145] Although uncommon, reported side effects include flatulence, abdominal pain, and weight loss. Metronidazole has also been used to treat HE, although it may cause significant gastrointestinal and neurologic side effects.

Therapeutic Approach

Variceal Hemorrhage

The approach to diagnosis and treatment of the bleeding complications of portal hypertension was the topic of a consensus workshop that provides clinicians with a rational therapeutic approach to varices.[61] This treatment approach is depicted in Figure 34-5.

Prophylactic Therapy. Unfortunately, there are no noninvasive clinical or laboratory parameters that are highly reliable for the prediction of the presence of varices.[146] Rather, it is advised that patients with cirrhosis undergo esophagogastroduodenoscopy to ascertain their presence.[61] Patients with moderate to large varices, judged as being over 5 mm in diameter, are candidates for treatments to prevent bleeding.[59] It is advised that patients who have small varices undergo repeated endoscopic screening on a yearly basis, to assess for growth in variceal size. Those with no varices should undergo endoscopic screening every 2 to 3 years.[147] These intervals are based upon the predicted development and growth of varices, which amounts to a 7% incidence of forming varices, and a more rapid rate of growth in patients with advanced cirrhosis.[148] At present, there is no role for the institution of pharmacologic therapy to prevent the development of varices.[55]

In patients with moderate to large varices, evidence weighs in favor of instituting treatment with nonselective β-blocker therapy for the prevention of bleeding.[59] Although no effect on mortality was determined in a meta-analysis of eight studies comprising 811 patients, the mean weighted bleeding rate at 2 years decreased from 30% to 14%, comparing placebo to treated patients.[59]

Endoscopic variceal band ligation (EVBL) has been demonstrated to be superior to no treatment in prevention of an initial variceal bleed in a meta-analysis.[149] In the same examination of the evidence, including four trials comprising 283 patients who received either EVBL or nonselective β-blocker therapy, EVBL remained superior in the prevention of an initial bleed, but with no significant effect on mortality.[149] A more recent meta-analysis confirmed the findings that EVBL is better than nonselective β-blocker therapy for the prevention of a first variceal bleed, but with no mortality reduction.[150]

Current conventional practice is to treat patients with medium or larger varices with nonselective β-blocker therapy. For those who are intolerant or who have contraindications, EVBL should be used.

Treatment of Active Bleeding. The treatment of patients who present with variceal bleeding depends upon an accurate diagnosis, usually suspected based upon the history provided by the patient or family. Hematemesis, hematochezia, or melena occurring in a patient with known cirrhosis, or with physical findings indicative of advanced liver disease, should raise the suspicion of variceal bleeding. Volume resuscitation, airway management, and cardiopulmonary support are given immediately. Pharmacotherapy is instituted concomitantly. Endoscopic assessment and treatment are performed upon stabilization of the patient.

Institution of vasocontrictors is appropriate, even before diagnostic and therapeutic endoscopy. However, in a meta-analysis of eight trials comprising 939 patients, a combined approach with pharmacotherapy and endoscopic treatment improved rates of initial bleeding control

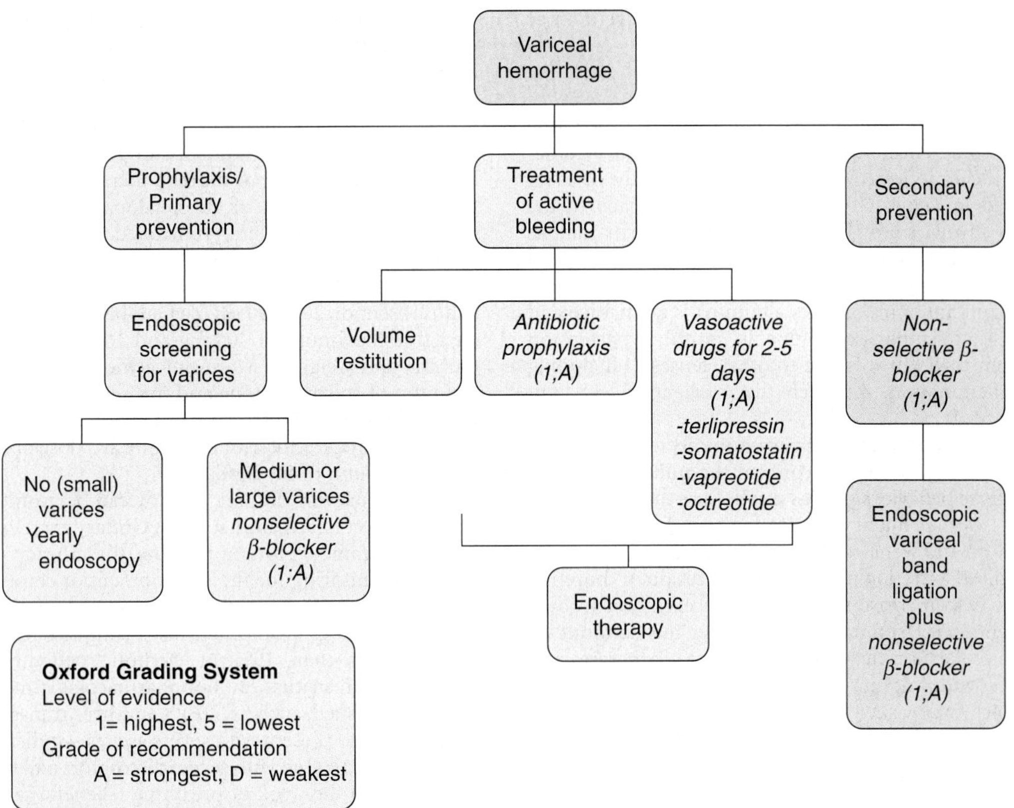

FIGURE 34-5 • Treatment approach to the three important clinical scenarios related to variceal bleeding. These include the prevention of bleeding from varices, the treatment of active bleeding, and the prevention of re-bleeding. The strength of the evidence supporting the therapeutic interventions is given.[61]

and 5-day hemostasis, but with no significant effect on mortality.[151] Agents included somatostatin, octreotide, and vasopressin. This analysis confirms that a combined approach of pharmacologic and endoscopic therapy is the most appropriate approach in the setting of acute variceal hemorrhage.

The efficacy data for the various intravenous vasoconstrictors has been reviewed elsewhere in this chapter. The data most strongly support the use of terlipressin, as it is the only agent associated with a survival benefit.[114] Unfortunately, this agent is not yet available in the United States. Therefore, a somatostatin analogue, such as octreotide, is used most often in combination with endoscopic therapy.

The role of antibiotics in the setting of acute variceal bleeding is strongly supported by the available data. The rationale for their use stems from the higher risk for occurrence of infections in this setting, and the deleterious effect of such infections on the outcome.[62] Infectious complications and mortality are reduced by the early institution of antibiotics, as has been shown in meta-analyses of randomized controlled trials.[152-155] The best regimen for antibiotic prophylaxis also has been investigated in a randomized controlled trial[156] studying norfloxacin 400 mg orally every 12 hours versus ceftriaxone 1 g intravenously every day, for 7 days. The rationale for this study was to identify the optimal prophylactic regimen, given the concern for resistance to quinolones. In fact, the probability of developing infections was higher among those treated with norfloxacin compared with ceftriaxone (33% and 11%, respectively). Therefore, the accepted approach is the institution of ceftriaxone, or another similar third-generation cephalosporin, in patients with acute variceal bleeding.

Prevention of Rebleeding. Patients who have experienced a variceal bleed are at increased risk of another; the risk is greatest within the first few days following the initial bleed. However, the risk remains as high as 60% during the first year, with a 20% mortality rate with each rebleeding episode.[157] Therefore, it is incumbent upon the clinician to pursue some means of prevention of recurrent variceal bleeding.

An early meta-analysis of the available evidence showed that EVBL is an effective way to prevent rebleeding from esophageal varices.[158] Subsequently, a non–placebo-controlled randomized study showed that the combination of nonselective β-blockers and EVBL is superior to EVBL alone in the prevention of rebleeding (14% vs. 38%, respectively, at 16 months).[159] Previously, another non–placebo-controlled randomized trial also demonstrated the benefit of the addition of a nonselective β-blocker (with sucralfate) to EBVL for the prevention of rebleeding.[160] Notwithstanding the limitations to the design of these studies, combination therapy with EBVL and a nonselective β-blocker may be the most effective way to prevent rebleeding.

The benefit of a nonselective β-blocker, alone, for the prevention of rebleeding from varices has been shown. In a meta-analysis of 12 studies that examined the role of these agents for the prevention of rebleeding, these agents not only were associated with an increase in the mean percentage of patients free of rebleeding, but also in survival at 2 years.[161] Pharmacologic therapy is as effective as endoscopic treatment in the prevention of variceal rebleeding.[157] Importantly, there have been no comparisons of pharmacotherapy alone, versus endoscopic therapy alone, for the prevention of variceal rebleeding.

The most effective way to ensure that a patient with cirrhosis will not rebleed is to lower the HVPG adequately.[56] However, measurement of the HVPG is not employed widely, given the perceived risk of catheterization and the necessary expertise in performance of the procedure and interpretation of the data. Given this, the use of pharmacotherapy for the treatment of portal hypertension is often empirical, targeting a 25% reduction in the baseline heart rate. However, given this empirical approach and the understanding that the heart rate may not reflect the portal pressure accurately, some patients may not reach a target portal pressure reduction, and thus fail therapy (i.e., experience recurrent variceal bleeding). Therefore, based on the augmentation of portal pressure reduction with the addition of isosorbide 5-mononitrate to a nonselective β-blocker,[132] it has been suggested to use these agents in combination for the pharmacologic prevention of rebleeding.[157]

Ascites

The management of patients with cirrhosis and ascites has been the focus of a consensus conference[67] as well as the topic of practice guidelines published by the American Association for the Study of Liver Disease and depicted in Figure 34-6.[162] The initial approach to the patient with ascites involves sampling the fluid to confirm that its protein composition is consistent with portal hypertensive ascites, and to exclude infection. In regard to the former, the serum ascites albumin gradient (SAAG: serum albumin – ascites albumin) is a sensitive and specific test for distinguishing ascites due to portal hypertension (SAAG >11 g/L) from that which is due to other causes,[163] including malignancy and inflammation, in which the gradient is less than 11 g/L.

Once the diagnosis of portal hypertensive noninfected ascites has been made, the general approach is to confirm the underlying cause for cirrhosis, to mitigate behaviors such as alcohol use or institute any other specific therapies that might alleviate the portal hypertension, and to institute sodium and water restriction. It is useful to measure a patient's urinary sodium excretion prior to the institution of diuretics. A goal of treatment is to increase urinary sodium excretion to over 78 mmol/day; patients who spontaneously excrete this amount of sodium in a 24-hour collection may not require diuretic therapy, and can mobilize ascites with sodium restriction alone.[162] Targeting a sodium-restricted diet comprising 1.5 to 2.0 g/day will facilitate the elimination of ascites. Fluid restriction of 1 L/day should be instituted in fluid-overloaded patients with hyponatremia (serum Na^+ <125 mmol/L).[162,164] As shown in a randomized controlled trial, the combination of diuretic therapy and sodium restriction is successful in controlling ascites in over 90% of patients.[165] Another goal of therapy is to achieve weight loss, with a loss of 0.5 kg/day being a reasonable target.[139,162] Treatment should be stopped upon the development of any apparent complication of diuretic therapy, such as azotemia, hyponatremia (<120 mmol/L), or encephalopathy.

As reviewed elsewhere, controlled and uncontrolled trials have shown the benefit of spironolactone for the initial treatment of ascites.[67] However, to effectively treat ascites, spironolactone 50 to 100 mg/day and furosemide 20 to 40 mg/day are begun and increased every 3 to 5 days to a maximum of 400 mg and 160 mg, respectively, if adequate diuresis and weight loss are not achieved. Importantly, maintaining this ratio of spironolactone and furosemide tends to avoid hyperkalemia.[162] Patients who experience tender gynecomastia can substitute amiloride for spironolactone, starting at a dose of 5 mg/day and reaching a maximum of 30 mg/day.

The adequacy of diuretic therapy can be monitored by weight loss and reduction in abdominal girth. Urinary excretion of sodium also is a useful parameter for monitoring the efficacy of diuretic therapy. Regular monitoring for the development of complications of diuresis is also necessary. An inadequate response to diuretic therapy, or complications arising from their use, comprise criteria for refractory ascites.[66] Less than 10% of cirrhotic patients develop refractory ascites.[165] In this situation, nonpharmacologic means of ascites treatment are pursued, such as TIPPS and liver transplantation.

Patients who present with severe ascites—indicated by a tense, fluid-filled abdomen, often with severe discomfort and not infrequently with an increase in the work of breathing—benefit from therapeutic paracentesis as an initial maneuver. This is concomitant with the institution of diuretic therapy. In a prospective study, a single large-volume paracentesis of up to 5 L was well tolerated in such patients.[166] The removal of larger amounts of fluid should be accompanied by replacement with intravenous albumin (8 g/L of fluid removed).[167] Massive fluid removal or repeated paracentesis without colloid replacement may predispose patients to renal impairment and hyponatremia.[168] However, a survival advantage to albumin replacement with large-volume paracentesis has not been demonstrated.[162]

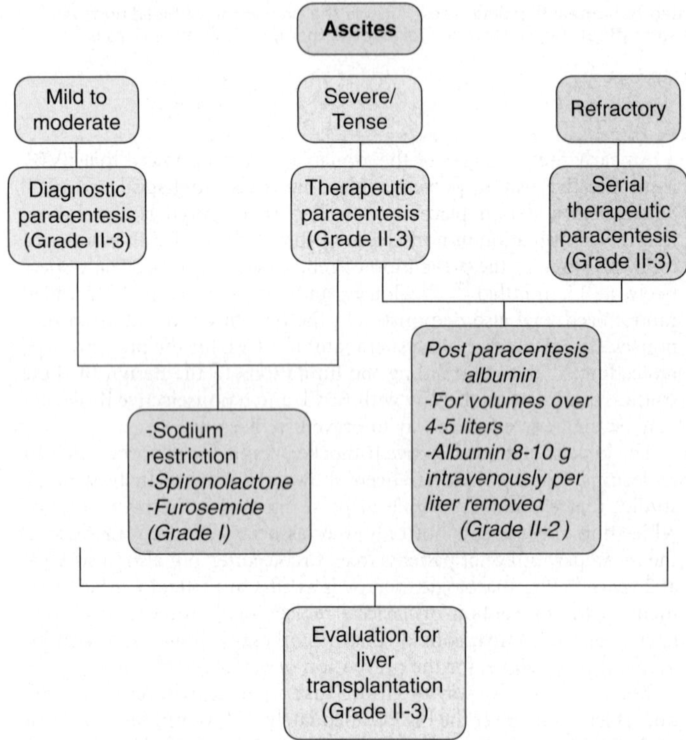

Grade	Definition
I	Randomized controlled trials
II-1	Controlled trials without randomization
II-2	Cohort or case-control analytic studies
II-3	Multiple time series, dramatic uncontrolled experiments
III	Opinions of respected authorities; descriptive epidemiology

FIGURE 34-6 • Treatment approach to the management of ascites. The treatment of ascites, as described in published guidelines,[162] is to a great extent dictated by its severity.

Spontaneous Bacterial Peritonitis

The clinical features and importance of SBP, as well as criteria for diagnosis, have been discussed previously. Diagnostic paracentesis at the time of presentation, or hospitalization, is necessary. Treatment is considered as empirical, active, and preventative.

Empirical therapy is instituted in the setting of a clinical syndrome compatible with infection (fever, leukocytosis, abdominal pain) with a PMN leukocyte count of over 250 cells/mm^3. A positive culture is not necessary to initiate treatment. Clinically, such patients are labeled as having culture-negative neutrocytic ascites, with outcomes no different than those with positive cultures.[169] Thus, treatment of such patients is warranted.[162] Some patients will have a positive ascites culture, but a PMN count less than 250 cells/mm^3; such a scenario is labeled as monomicrobial non-neutrocytic bacterascites.[170] Although this situation may resolve spontaneously in two thirds of patients,[170] those with concurrent clinical signs that are suggestive of infection should be treated empirically.[162]

Several trials have investigated the optimal regimen for treatment of SBP.[71,171-173] Given the organisms most commonly responsible for SBP, an agent with a broad spectrum of action is required. Cefotaxime has been shown to be superior to other therapies and is currently the agent of choice for SBP.[162,171] A dose of 2 g given intravenously every 8 hours leads to high concentration in the ascites fluid.[174] In a randomized trial, a 5-day regimen of therapy and a 10-day regimen were equally effective, making the shorter duration standard practice.[172]

An oral regimen for SBP treatment has also been investigated in a randomized controlled trial.[173] As a cautionary note, however, such therapy has been studied in a highly selected population of patients with SBP, without shock, vomiting, or renal dysfunction.[162,173]

An important study demonstrated, in a randomized controlled format, that the infusion of albumin (1.5 g/kg within 6 hours and then 1.0 g/kg on day 3) in conjunction with cefotaxime yielded decreased mortality (10% compared with those who did not receive albumin).[71] Although this has become conventional practice for treatment of patients with SBP, this study awaits confirmation.

Most patients with SBP respond to the above-outlined therapy. However, the persistence of symptoms or other signs suggesting ongoing or worsening infection merits further investigation by the clinician. A repeat paracentesis is advisable to rule out the possibility of peritonitis from another cause, for which surgical treatment might be needed.[175] Moreover, repeated sampling of fluid, when clinically indicated, may identify an organism resistant to therapy, thus leading to a modification of drug treatment. The current treatment approach to SBP is shown in Figure 34-7.

Patients with ascites and certain risk factors are at increased risk for SBP. These risks include a prior history of SBP, ascites fluid protein less than 1 g/dL, and variceal hemorrhage. Several randomized controlled trials have been conducted to study the optimal regimen for the prevention of SBP.[176-181] Among the scenarios that deserve special attention include prevention of SBP in the setting of gastrointestinal bleeding, for which intravenous ofloxacin (400 mg/day) has been shown to be effective.[180] For those patients who are able to take oral medications, norfloxacin 400 mg for 7 days has been shown to be effective.[179] In a meta-analysis, antibiotic therapy in this setting has shown a survival advantage, compared with untreated patients.[153] Recurrent SBP can effectively be prevented using norfloxacin 400 mg/day.[178] Peritonitis can be prevented in patients with ascites protein less than 1 g/dL using the same regimen.[176] Trimethoprim-sulfamethoxazole is an alternative prophylactic agent; however, there are limited data on its efficacy.[181] The strategy for prevention of SBP is depicted in Figure 34-8.

Indefinite antibiotic therapy for the prevention of SBP necessarily raises the concern for the emergence of resistant organisms.[182] This was investigated in a review of bacterial infections in cirrhotics over a 2-year period. It was found that, among patients on norfloxacin prophylaxis, 50% of all culture-positive cases of SBP were caused by norfloxacin-resistant organisms.[182]

Hepatorenal Syndrome

In determining the approach to the patient with HRS, the distinction between type I and type II HRS is important. Survival without liver transplantation in patients with type I HRS is very short; hence, hemodialysis is of questionable benefit to the patient for whom liver transplantation is not an option. For those patients with type I HRS who are candidates for liver transplantation, renal replacement therapy is used. Continuous venovenous hemofiltration may be better tolerated due to preexisting hypotension. In addition, various pharmacologic preparations have become available for use in patients with type I HRS. However, treatment with vasopressors may be associated with significant ischemic complications.[183]

The combination of octreotide and midodrine has been studied in patients with type I HRS.[184] This combination was shown to improve renal plasma flow, glomerular filtration rate, and urinary sodium excretion; there was a concomitant fall in plasma renin, vasopressin, and glucagon activity.[184] The doses included octreotide up to 200 mg three times a day, subcutaneously, combined with midodrine titrated to achieve a mean increase in blood pressure of 15 mm Hg, up to a maximum oral dose of 12.5 mg three times per day.[184] Although confirmatory studies are needed, midodrine in combination with octreotide is used in many facilities for patients with type I HRS. A randomized, double-blind, placebo-controlled crossover study has shown that octreotide, as a sole pharmaceutical agent, in combination with albumin, is of no benefit in patients with HRS.[185] Although not yet available in the United States, terlipressin alone or in combination

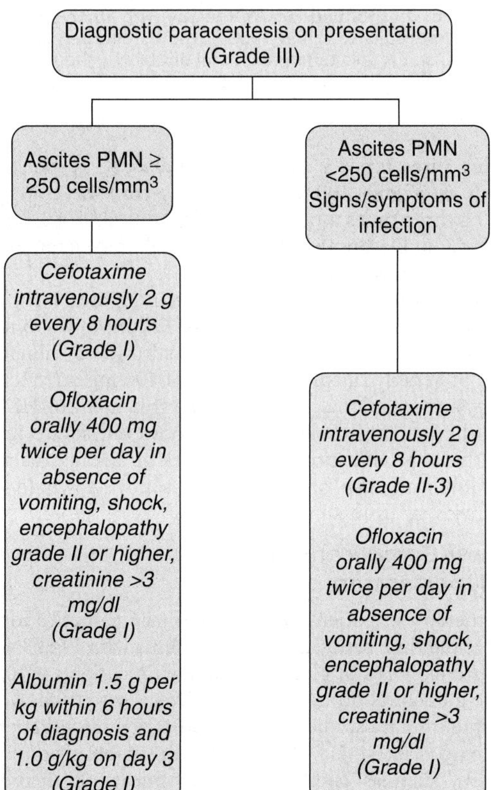

Grade	Definition
I	Randomized controlled trials
II-1	Controlled trials without randomization
II-2	Cohort or case-control analytic studies
II-3	Multiple time series, dramatic uncontrolled experiments
III	Opinions of respected authorities; descriptive epidemiology

FIGURE 34-7 • Current treatment approach to the treatment of spontaneous bacterial peritonitis (SBP). A diagnosis is established by diagnostic paracentesis; those patients with SBP (>250 PMN/mm³) or in whom a strong suspicion of infection exists, despite a lower PMN count, are treated empirically, without awaiting culture evidence. A combination of intravenous antibiotics and albumin comprise the standard approach.[162]

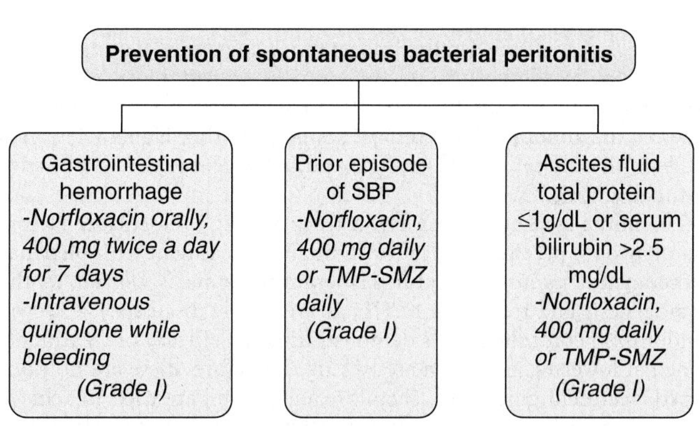

Grade	Definition
I	Randomized controlled trials
II-1	Controlled trials without randomization
II-2	Cohort or case-control analytic studies
II-3	Multiple time series, dramatic uncontrolled experiments
III	Opinions of respected authorities; descriptive epidemiology

FIGURE 34-8 • Current approach to the prevention of SBP. Prophylaxis benefits patients with a prior history of SBP, those with acute gastrointestinal hemorrhage, and with ascites fluid total protein <1 g/dL or serum bilirubin >2.5 mg/dL.[162]

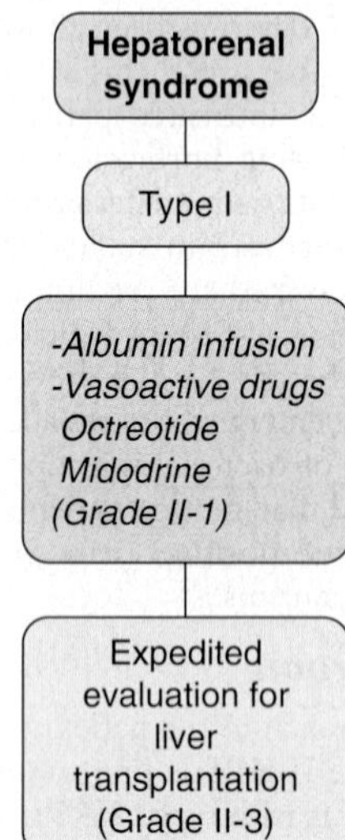

Grade	Definition
I	Randomized controlled trials
II-1	Controlled trials without randomization
II-2	Cohort or case-control analytic studies
II-3	Multiple time series, dramatic uncontrolled experiments
III	Opinions of respected authorities; descriptive epidemiology

FIGURE 34-9 • Management of hepatorenal syndrome (HRS). The evidence is most strong for the treatment of HRS type I, using albumin infusion and vasoactive drugs.[162]

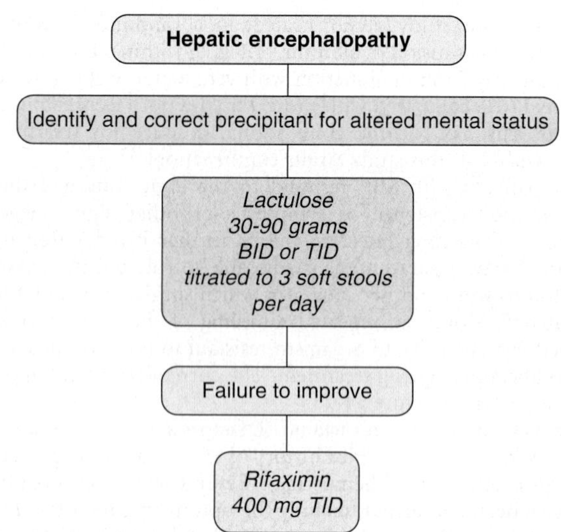

FIGURE 34-10 • At present, there are no consensus guidelines on the management of hepatic encephalopathy (HE). However, a rational approach can be crafted from the literature and clinical experience. The most important initial maneuver is to identify those factors which may contribute to altered mental status in patients with cirrhosis. This includes anatomical neurological abnormalities (such as intracranial bleeding), metabolic disturbances, volume contraction, and sedatives. Concomitant with correction of contributing factors, therapy with a non-absorbable disaccharide is instituted, to achieve about 3 soft stools per day. If the patient's mental status fails to improve, oral antibiotics should be started.

with albumin appears to have some benefit for HRS.[186-189] However, confirmatory studies are awaited. The current approach to the treatment of HRS is depicted in Figure 34-9.

Hepatic Encephalopathy

In diagnosing and thus initiating therapy for HE, it is incumbent upon the clinician to take a circumspect approach to the evaluation of the cirrhotic patient who presents with an altered mental status. A careful history, physical examination, and laboratory and imaging evaluation must be conducted to investigate the causes of altered mentation and possible triggers for HE. This evaluation must include assessment for vascular and anatomic brain abnormalities, metabolic derangements, psychiatric disorders, and infectious processes. Ammonia, as a diagnostic test, is an imperfect tool. That is to say, there is a poor correlation between the ammonia level and the severity of HE.[79] Nonetheless, it is used commonly in clinical practice and, when elevated, is supportive of the diagnosis.

The initial step in treating HE is to correct any remediable factors that may have precipitated it. Concomitantly, treatment with pharmacotherapeutic agents is begun. Hyperammonemia is central to the pathogenesis and treatment of HE, as previously discussed. However, randomized controlled trials demonstrating the efficacy of treatments aimed at lowering ammonia are lacking. Therefore, there are no published treatment guidelines. Lactulose and lactitol are used to achieve three soft bowel movements per day. A typical oral dose to achieve this target catharsis is between 45 and 90 g/day.[79]

A recent meta-analysis reviewed 22 trials of varying quality comparing disaccharides to no treatment, placebo, or antibiotics. A clear benefit of disaccharides could not be demonstrated. This same analysis identified nonabsorbable antibiotics to be superior to disaccharides for the treatment of HE.[190]

Clinical trials of oral antibiotics for the treatment of HE were recently reviewed.[145] The end points assessed in these trials included neurologic signs of encephalopathy and ammonia level. Rifaximin was at least as effective as nonabsorbable disaccharides and other orally administered antibiotics for the treatment of HE. A dose of 1200 mg/day (400 mg three times a day) was found to be optimal.[191] In one recent study, rifaximin (400 mg three time a day) was compared with lactitol (20 g three times a day) in patients with HE in a randomized double-blind, double-dummy, controlled trial; in general, these therapies were similar in efficacy.[192]

A rational treatment approach, as shown in Figure 34-10, is to initiate oral dissacharides to achieve catharsis. Failure to respond with an improvement in mental status warrants institution of nonabsorbable antibiotics, preferably rifaximin at a dose of 400 mg three times a day. Historically, a conventional practice in the treatment of HE has been to restrict the patient's dietary protein; however, severe restrictions may exacerbate the nutritional deficiencies of already malnourished patients. Moreover, such an approach has not shown to have any benefit in recovery from an episode of HE.[193]

Pulmonary Complications of Portal Hypertension

Pharmacotherapy in patients with pulmonary complications of cirrhosis is, for the time being, limited to patients with PPHTN. As there are no controlled trials of pharmacotherapy in patients with PPHTN, therapeutic guidelines do not exist. However, current knowledge and data from preliminary studies can be synthesized into a rational treatment approach (Fig. 34-11).[194] Patients with symptoms of pulmonary hypertension, such as chest pain or dyspnea, and hemodynamic parameters indicative of PPHTN, are candidates for treatment.

In general, patients with portal hypertension are prone to fluid overload, as a result of sodium retention. Like many other complications of cirrhosis, PPHTN may benefit from treatment with diuretics to reduce intravascular volume and right ventricular preload.[194] However, care must be exercised in that overly vigorous diuresis may impede cardiac output.[195] Oxygen supplementation is prudent in patients with PPHTN and arterial hypoxemia.[84]

Given the proposed pathogenesis of PPHTN, vasodilator therapy has become a conventional approach. The acute and chronic effects of continuous infusion of epoprostenol on PPHTN have been reported in small uncontrolled trials and a case series.[196-198] In the largest of these studies, the acute hemodynamic effects of epoprostenol included a reduction in the pulmonary vascular resistance, mean PAP, and cardiac

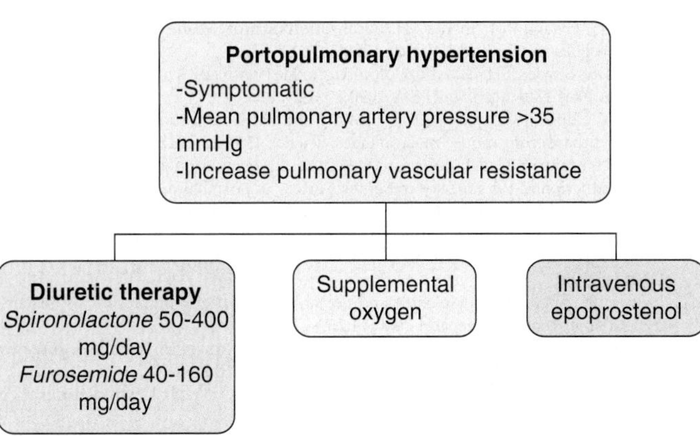

FIGURE 34-11 • Pulmonary complications of portal hypertension. The pulmonary complications of portal hypertension include hepatopulmonary syndrome and portopulmonary hypertension (PPHTN); however, pharmacological interventions have an important role only in the latter. Patients with portal hypertension who are symptomatic (dyspnea, chest pain) and have hemodynamic evidence of pulmonary hypertension (mean Pulmonary Artery Pressure >35 mmHg and an increased Pulmonary Vascular Resistance) are candidates for therapy. At present, there are no consensus guidelines governing the management of patients with PPHTN. However, preliminary evidence supports the use of intravenous epoprostenol. Patients are also treated with supplemental oxygen, when hypoxemic, and diuretics, when volume overload is present.

output. Extended administration produced further reduction in the pulmonary vascular resistance.[197]

Bosentan is a dual endothelin receptor antagonist approved for the treatment of pulmonary artery hypertension. Enthusiasm for its use in the portal hypertensive population has been mitigated by its potential effect on liver enzymes. Notwithstanding this concern, early experience with this drug in patients with PPHTN suggested that it was safe and well tolerated, after one year of therapy, and produced improved symptoms and exercise tolerance.[199] Randomized controlled trials to study the efficacy of bosentan in patients with PPHTN are needed.

Sildenafil (Revatio) was approved in 2005 for the treatment of pulmonary hypertension. Mechanistically, sildenafil is a phosphodiesterase-5 inhibitor that, by impeding the degradation of NO, prolongs its vasodilatory effect. It is an orally active, generally safe compound.[200] In the largest study, 14 patients were administered sildenafil in an uncontrolled format. Walk distance and pulmonary hemodynamics improved after 3 months in most patients.[201] Further studies are needed to determine the efficacy of this drug in PPHTN.

Emerging Targets and Therapeutics

As has been highlighted throughout this chapter, the optimal therapies for various complications of portal hypertension remain unclear. However, new therapies are under investigation.

Aquaretics

Aquaretics selectively increase renal free water excretion and thus may be useful in the management of patients with cirrhosis and hyponatremia,[202] particularly since the progressive decline in sodium portends a poor survival[203] and may be associated with serious side effects. Moreover, severe hyponatremia limits the maximal implementation of diuretic therapy.

In cirrhosis, free water retention is driven, to a great extent, by a homeostatic increase in the secretion of arginine vasopressin (AVP) in response to a reduction in effective arterial blood volume. The antidiuretic effect of vasopressin is mediated through the V2 receptor located on the glomerular collecting ducts. The sequence of events leading to water retention has been reviewed elsewhere.[202] An understanding of this mechanism, however, has led to the development of vasopressin V2 receptor antagonists as a new class of agents to enhance free water excretion.

The pharmacokinetic and pharmacodynamic effects of the AVP antagonist VPA-985 (Lixivaptan) have been studied in a single-dose format in cirrhotic patients with ascites.[204] Dose levels ranged from 25 to 300 mg. This study demonstrated a dose-related increase in urine output and decrease in urine osmolality, as well as significant increase in serum osmolality and serum sodium and vasopressin levels. Peak serum concentrations of VPA-985 were reached at 1 hour, and the elimination half-life ranged from 9 to 22.6 hours.[204]

Phase II clinical trials assessing the safety and efficacy of AVP antagonists have been reviewed recently.[205] Patients with cirrhosis and hyponatremia were included in two trials using VPA-985.[206,207] In these randomized, placebo-controlled trials, dosing over 7 days ranged from 100 mg/day to 250 mg twice daily. Both studies showed a dose-dependent increase in the serum sodium and free water clearance in the treated groups. At the highest dose, however, 50% of patients needed to have dosing withheld on several occasions due to thirst, dehydration, and rapid rises in sodium.[206] Overall, therapy was well tolerated, but side effects included infrequent HE[206] and a dose-dependent increase in thirst.[207]

Liver-Specific Nitric Oxide Donors

The pivotal, and complex, role that NO plays in the generation and perpetuation of portal hypertension has been reviewed here and elsewhere. The differential effect of NO on the liver (vasoconstriction) compared with the splanchnic circulation (vasodilation) raises the possibility of creating a target for pharmacologic manipulation.[208] In theory, supplementation of NO could mitigate the vasoconstriction that gives rise to increased intrahepatic vascular resistance. Systemic delivery of nitrates, or L-arginine as a substrate for NO,[209] has been studied. Only the former, in combination with nonselective β-blockers, has a clinical role. However, targeted delivery of NO to the liver is another strategy that merits attention.[208] The chemical entity 2-(acetyloxy)benzoic acid 3-(nitrooxymethyl)phenyl ester (NCX-1000) was formulated by adding an NO-releasing moiety to the liver-specific bile salt ursodeoxycholic acid. When given to rats with portal hypertension induced by treatment with carbon tetrachloride, a reduction in intrahepatic resistance and reduction in ascites were achieved.[210] Although preliminary, this research gives hope that targeted therapies may be a viable treatment option in the future.

Liver-specific gene transfer of NOSs has also been proposed as a means to raise intrahepatic NO levels.[208] A recombinant adenoviral vector carrying complementary DNA encoding eNOS was injected into the portal circulation of cirrhotic rats, leading to a reduction in portal pressure with no effects on systemic hemodynamics.[211] Such studies in humans have not been reported.

Endothelin Antagonists

Endothelin is a vasoconstrictive substance that regulates hepatic stellate cell function and is thus involved in portal hypertension.[212,213] Specifically, endothelin receptor subtype B is upregulated in animal models[214] and humans.[215] Several lines of evidence, as reviewed elsewhere,[208] suggest that antagonists to endothelin receptors would serve as the most feasible pharmacologic target. Bosentan is an example of a nonselective endothelin receptor antagonist that has found usefulness in the treatment of portal pulmonary hypertension.[199] Experimental evidence exists to suggest that specific receptor blockade may have a more pronounced effect on portal pressure reduction.[216]

REFERENCES

1. Sandler RS, Everhart JE, Donowitz M, et al. The burden of the selected digestive diseases in the United States. Gastroenterology 2002;122:1500-1511.
2. Wanless IR. Physioanatomic considerations. *In* Schiff ER, Sorrell MF, Maddrey WC (eds): Schiff's Diseases of the Liver, 8th ed. Philadelphia: Lippincott–Raven, 1999, pp 3-37.
3. Wanless IR. Anatomy, histology, embryology, and developmental anomalies of the liver. *In* Feldman M, Friedman LS, Brandt LJ (eds): Sleisenger and Fordtran's Gastrointestinal and Liver Disease: Pathophysiology/Diagnosis/Management, 8th ed. Philadelphia: Elsevier Saunders, 2006, pp 1543-1550.
4. Kuntz E, Kuntz H-D. Morphology of the liver. *In* Hepatology: Principles and Practice. New York: Springer-Verlag, 2002, pp 11-24.

5. Jones AL. Anatomy of the liver. *In* Zakim D, Boyer TD (eds): Hepatology: A Textbook of Liver Disease, 3rd ed. Philadelphia: WB Saunders, 1996, pp 3-32.
6. Skandalakis JE, Skandalakis LL, Skandalakis PN, et al. Hepatic surgical anatomy. Surg Clin North Am 2004;84:413-435.
7. Huet PM, Villeneuve JP, Pomier-Layrargues G, et al. Hepatic circulation in cirrhosis. Clin Gastroenterol 1985;14:155-168.
8. Schaffner R, Popper J. Capillarization of hepatic sinusoids in man. Gastroenterology 1963;44:239-242.
9. Fraser R, Dobbs BR, Rogers GW. Lipoproteins and the liver sieve: the role of fenestrated sinusoidal endothelium in lipoprotein metabolism, atherosclerosis, and cirrhosis. Hepatology 1995;21:863-874.
10. Mori T, Okanoue T, Sawa T, et al. Defenestration of the sinusoidal endothelial cell in a rat model of cirrhosis. Hepatology 1993;17:891-897.
11. D'Amico G, Garcia-Tsao G, Pagliaro L. Natural history and prognostic indicators of survival in cirrhosis: a systematic review of 118 studies. J Hepatol 2006;44:217-231.
12. Pugh RWH, Murray-Lyon IM, Dawson JL, et al. Transection of the oesophagus for bleeding oesophageal varices. Br J Surg 1983;60:646-649.
13. Kamath PS, Wiesner RH, Malinchoc M, et al. A model to predict survival in patients with end-stage liver disease. Hepatology 2001;33:464-470.
14. Durand F, Valla D. Assessment of the prognosis of cirrhosis: Child-Pugh versus MELD. J Hepatol 2005;42:S100-S107.
15. Bosch J, Garcia-Pagan JC. Complications of cirrhosis. I. Portal hypertension. J Hepatol 2000;32:141-156.
16. Rockey D. The cellular pathogenesis of portal hypertension: stellate cells contractility, endothelin and nitric oxide. Hepatology 1997;25:2-5.
17. Popper H, Paronetto F, Schaffner F, Perez V. Studies on hepatic fibrosis. Lab Invest 1961;10:265-290.
18. Bhatal PS, Grossman HJ. Reduction of the increased portal vascular resistance of the isolated cirrhotic perfused rat liver by vasodilators. J Hepatol 1985;1:325-329.
19. Bauer M, Zhang JX, Bauer I, et al. ET-1 induced alterations of hepatic microcirculation: sinusoidal and extrasinusoidal sites of action. Am J Physiol 1994;267:G143-G149.
20. Iredale JP. Cirrhosis: new research provides a basis for rational and targeted treatments. BMJ 2003;327:143-147.
21. Sims D. Recent advances in pericyte biology and implications for health and disease. Can J Cardiol 1991;7:431-443.
22. Geerts A. History and heterogeneity of stellate cells, and role in normal liver function. Semin Liver Dis 2001;21:311-336.
23. Friedman SL. Mechanisms of hepatic fibrogenesis. *In* Portal Hypertension in the 21st Century. Dordrecht: Kluwer Academic Publishers, 2004, pp 27-35.
24. Wiest R, Groszmann RJ. The paradox of nitric oxide in cirrhosis and portal hypertension: too much, not enough. Hepatology 2002;35:478-491.
25. Rockey DC. Vascular mediators in the injured liver. Hepatology 2003;37:4-12.
26. Sarela AI, Mihaimeed FM, Batten JJ, et al. Hepatic and splanchnic nitric oxide activity in patients with cirrhosis. Gut 1999;44:749-753.
27. Wiest R, Groszmann RJ. Nitric oxide and portal hypertension: its role in the regulation of intrahepatic and splanchnic vascular resistance. Semin Liver Dis 1999;19:411-426.
28. Graupera M, García-Pagán JC, Titos E, et al. 5-Lipoxygenase inhibition reduces intrahepatic vascular resistance of cirrhotic rat livers: a possible role of cysteinyl-leukotrienes. Gastroenterology 2002;122:387-393.
29. Yokoyama Y, Xu H, Kresge N, et al. Role of thromboxane A1 in early BDL-induced portal hypertension. Am J Physiol Gastrointest Liver Physiol 2003;284:G453-G460.
30. Vallance P, Moncada S. Hyperdynamic circulation in cirrhosis: a role for nitric oxide? Lancet 1991;337:776-778.
31. Vorobioff J, Bredfeldt J, Groszmann RJ. Hyperdynamic circulation in a portal hypertensive rat model: a primary factor for maintenance of chronic portal hypertension. Am J Physiol 1983;244:G52-G56.
32. Pizcueta MP, Pique JM, Bosch J, et al. Effects of inhibiting nitric oxide biosynthesis on the systemic and splanchnic circulation of rats with portal hypertension. Br J Pharmcol 1992;105:105-184.
33. Pizcueta P, Pique JM, Fernandez M, et al. Modulation of the hyperdynamic circulation of cirrhotic rats by nitric oxide inhibition. Gastroenterology 1992;103:1909-1915.
34. Benoit JN, Barrowman JA, Harper SL, et al. Role of humoral factors in the intestinal hyperemia associated with chronic portal hypertension. Am J Physiol 1984;247:G486-G493.
35. Moller S, Bendtsen F, Schifter S, et al. Relation of calcitonin gene-related peptide to systemic vasodilation and central hypovolaemia in cirrhosis. Scand J Gastroenterol 1996;31:928-933.
36. Lee FY, Albillos A, Colombato LA, et al. The role of nitric oxide in the vascular hyporesponsiveness to methoxamine in portal hypertensive rats. Hepatology 1992;16:1043-1048.
37. Sieber C, Lopez-Talavera JC, Groszmann RJ. The role of nitric oxide in the in vitro splanchnic vascular hyporeactivity in ascitic cirrhotic rats. Gastroenterology 1993;104:1750-1754.
38. Niederberger M, Maurtin PY, Gines P, et al. Normalization of nitric oxide production corrects arterial vasodilation and hyperdynamic circulation in cirrhotic rats. Gastroenterology 1995;109:1624-1630.
39. Forrest EH, Jones AL, Dillon JE, et al. The effect of nitric oxide synthase inhibition on portal pressure and azygos blood flow in patients with cirrhosis. J Hepatol 1995;23:254-258.
40. Ignarro LJ. Endothelium-derived nitric oxide: actions and properties. FASEB J 1989;3:31-36.
41. Furchgott RF, Zawadzki JV. The obligatory role of endothelial cells in the relaxation of arterial smooth muscle by acetylcholine. Nature 1980;288:373-376.
42. Bredt DS, Hwang PM, Snyder SH. Localization of nitric oxide synthase indicating a neural role for nitric oxide. Nature 1990;347:768-770.
43. Bredt DS, Snyder SH. Isolation of nitric oxide synthase, a calmodulin-requiring enzyme. Proc Natl Acad Sci U S A 1990;87:682-685.
44. Xie QW, Cho HJ, Calaycay J, et al. Cloning and characterization of inducible nitric oxide synthase from mouse macrophages. Science 1992;256:225-228.
45. Tsai MH, Iwakiri Y, Cadelina G, et al. Mesenteric vasoconstriction triggers nitric oxide overproduction in the superior mesenteric artery of portal hypertensive rats. Gastroenterology 2003;125:1452-1461.
46. Wiest R, Shah V, Sessa WC, et al. NO overproduction by eNOS precedes hyperdynamic splanchnic circulation in portal hypertensive rats. Am J Physiol 1999;276:G1043-G1051.
47. Langer DA, Shah VH. Nitric oxide and portal hypertension: interface of vasoreactivity and angiogenesis. J Hepatol 2006;44:209-216.
48. Iwakiri Y, Groszmann RJ. The hyperdynamic circulation of chronic liver diseases: from the patient to the molecule. Hepatology 2006;43:S121-S131.
49. Abraldes JG, Angermayr B, Bosch J. The management of portal hypertension. Clin Liver Dis 2005;9:685-713.
50. Schrier RW, Arroyo V, Bernardi M, et al. Peripheral arterial vasodilation hypothesis: a proposal for the initiation of renal sodium and water retention in cirrhosis. Hepatology 1988;8:1151-1157.
51. Garcia-Tsao G, Groszmann RJ, Fisher RL, et al. Portal pressure, presence of gastroesophageal varices and variceal bleeding. Hepatology 1985;5:419-424.
52. Blei AT. Portal hypertensive syndrome: its importance and complications. *In* Portal Hypertension in the 21st Century. Dordrecht: Kluwer Academic Publishers, 2004, pp 3-12.
53. Myers JD, Taylor WJ. An estimation of portal venous pressure by occlusive catheterization of an hepatic venule. J Clin Invest 1951;30:662-663.
54. Groszmann R, Wongcharatrawee S. The hepatic venous pressure gradient: anything worth doing should be done right. Hepatology 2004;39:280-282.
55. Groszmann RJ, Garcia-Tsao G, Bosch J, et al. Beta-blockers to prevent gastroesophageal varices in patients with cirrhosis. N Engl J Med 2005;353:2254-2261.
56. Feu F, Garcia-Pagan JC, Bosch J, et al. Relation between portal pressure response to pharmacotherapy and risk of recurrent variceal haemorrhage in patients with cirrhosis. Lancet 1995;346:1056-1059.
57. Abraldes JG, Tarantino I, Turnes J, et al. Hemodynamic response to pharmacological treatment of portal hypertension and long-term prognosis of cirrhosis. Hepatology 2003;37:902-908.
58. Madhotra R, Mulcahy HE, Willner I, et al. Prediction of esophageal varices in patients with cirrhosis. J Clin Gastroenterol 2002;34:81-85.
59. D'Amico G, Pagliaro L, Bosch J. Pharmacological treatment of portal hypertension: an evidence-based approach. Semin Liver Dis 1999;19:475-505.
60. Cales P, Desmorat H, Vinel JP, et al. Incidence of large oesophageal varices in patients with cirrhosis: application to prophylaxis of first bleeding. Gut 1990;31:1298-1302.
61. de Franchis R. Evolving consensus in portal hypertension: report of the Baveno IV Consensus Workshop on methodology of diagnosis and therapy in portal hypertension. J Hepatol 2005;43:167-176.
62. Goulis J, Armonis A, Patch D, et al. Bacterial infection is independently associated with failure to control bleeding in cirrhotic patients with gastrointestinal hemorrhage. Hepatology 1998;27:1207-1212.
63. D'Amico G, Morabito A, Pagliaro L, et al. Survival and prognostic indicators in compensated and decompensated cirrhosis. Dig Dis Sci 1986;31:468-475.
64. Guevara M, Cardenas A, Uriz J, Gines P. Prognosis of patients with cirrhosis and ascites. *In* Gines P, Arroyo V, Rodes J, Schrier RW (eds): Ascites and Renal Dysfunction in Liver Disease, 2nd ed. Malden, MA: Blackwell, 2005, pp 260-270.
65. Fernandez-Llama P, Gines P, Schrier RW. Pathogenesis of sodium retention in cirrhosis: the arterial vasodilation hypothesis of ascites formation. *In* Gines P, Arroyo V, Rodes J, Schrier RW (eds): Ascites and Renal Dysfunction in Liver Disease, 2nd ed. Malden, MA: Blackwell, 2005, pp 201-214.
66. Arroyo V, Gines P, Gerbes AL, et al. Definition and diagnostic criteria of refractory ascites and hepatorenal syndrome in cirrhosis. International Ascites Club. Hepatology 1996;23:164-176.
67. Moore KP, Wong F, Gines P, et al. The management of ascites in cirrhosis: report on the consensus conference of the International Ascites Club. Hepatology 2003;38:258-266.
68. Such J, Guarner C, Runyon B. Pathogenesis and clinical features of spontaneous bacterial peritonitis. *In* Gines P, Arroyo V, Rodes J, Schrier RW (eds): Ascites and Renal Dysfunction in Liver Disease, 2nd ed. Malden, MA: Blackwell, 2005, pp 422-433.
69. Caly WR, Strauss E. A prospective study of bacterial infections in patients with cirrhosis. J Hepatol 1993;18:353-358.
70. Silvain C, Besson I, Ingrand P, et al. Prognosis and long-term recurrence of spontaneous bacterial peritonitis in cirrhosis. J Hepatol 1993;19:188-189.
71. Sort P, Navasa M, Arroyo V, et al. Effect of intravenous albumin on renal impairment and mortality in patients with cirrhosis and spontaneous bacterial peritonitis. N Engl J Med 1999;5:403-409.
72. Arroyo V, Terra C, Torre A, Gines P. Hepatorenal syndrome in cirrhosis: clinical features, diagnosis, and management. *In* Gines P, Arroyo V, Rodes J, Schrier RW (eds): Ascites and Renal Dysfunction in Liver Disease, 2nd ed. Malden, MA: Blackwell, 2005, pp 341-359.
73. Arroyo V, Planas R, Gaya J, et al. Sympathetic nervous activity, renin-angiotensin system and renal excretion of prostaglandin E2 in cirrhosis: relationship to functional renal failure and sodium and water excretion. Eur J Clin Invest 1983;13:271-278.
74. Ruiz-del-Arbol L, Monescillo A, Arocena C, et al. Circulatory function and hepatorenal syndrome in cirrhosis. Hepatology 2005;42:439-447.
75. Ma Z, Lee SS. Cirrhotic cardiomyopathy: getting to the heart of the matter. Hepatology 1996;24:451-459.

76. Gines A, Escorsell A, Gines P, et al. Incidence, predictive factors, and prognosis of hepatorenal syndrome in cirrhosis. Gastroenterology 1993;105:229-236.
77. Arroyo V, Colmenero J. Ascites and hepatorenal syndrome in cirrhosis: pathophysiological basis of therapy and current management. J Hepatol 2003;38:S69-S89.
78. Ferenci P, Lockwood A, Mullen K, et al. Hepatic encephalopathy—definition, n omenclature, diagnosis, and quantification: final report of the working party at the 11th World Congresses of Gastroenterology, Vienna, 1998. Hepatology 2002;35:716-721.
79. Wright G, Jalan R. Management of hepatic encephalopathy in patients with cirrhosis. Best Pract Res Clin Gastroenterol 2007;21:95-110.
80. Butterworth RF. The neurobiology of hepatic encephalopathy. Semin Liver Dis 1996;16:235-244.
81. Norenberg MD. Astrocytic-ammonia interactions in hepatic encephalopathy. Semin Liver Dis 1996;16:245-253.
82. Haussinger D, Kircheis G, Fischer R, et al. Hepatic encephalopathy in chronic liver disease: a clinical manifestation of astrocyte swelling and low-grade cerebral edema? J Hepatol 2000;32:1035-1038.
83. Lockwood AH, Yap EW, Wong WH. Cerebral ammonia metabolism in patients with severe liver disease and minimal hepatic encephalopathy. J Cereb Blood Flow Metab 1991;11:337-341.
84. Rodriguez-Roisin R, Krowka MJ, Herve PH, et al. Pulmonary-hepatic vascular disorders. Eur Respir J 2004;24:861-880.
85. Krowka MJ. Hepatopulmonary syndrome and portopulmonary hypertension: distinctions and dilemmas. Hepatology 1997;25:1282-1284.
86. Lange PA, Stoller JK. The hepatopulmonary syndrome. Ann Intern Med 1995;122:521-529.
87. Rolla G, Brussino L, Colagrande P, et al. Exhaled nitric oxide and impaired oxygenation in cirrhotic patients before and after liver transplantation. Ann Intern Med 1998;129:375-378.
88. Rolla G, Brussino L, Colagrande P, et al. Exhaled nitric oxide and oxygenation abnormalities in hepatic cirrhosis. Hepatology 1997;26:842-847.
89. Cremona G, Higenbottam TW, Mayoral V, et al. Elevated exhaled nitric oxide in patients with hepatopulmonary syndrome. Eur Respir J 1995;8:1883-1885.
90. Martinez GP, Barbera JA, Visa J, et al. Hepatopulmonary syndrome in candidates for liver transplantation. J Hepatol 2001;34:651-657.
91. De BK, Sen S, Biswas PK, et al. Occurrence of hepatopulmonary syndrome in Budd-Chiari syndrome and the role of venous decompression. Gastroenterology 2002;122:897-903.
92. Krowka MJ. Hepatopulmonary syndrome: recent literature (1997-1999) and implications for liver transplantation. Liver Transpl 2000;6(Suppl 1):S31-S35.
93. Krowka MJ. Portopulmonary hypertension: diagnostic advances and caveats. Liver Transpl 2003;9:1336-1337.
94. Hadengue A, Benhayoun MK, Lebrec D, et al. Pulmonary hypertension complicating portal hypertension: prevalence and relation to splanchnic hemodynamics. Gastroenterology 1991;100:520-528.
95. Naeiji R, Melot C, Hallemans R, et al. Pulmonary hemodynamics in liver cirrhosis. Semin Respir Med 1985;7:164-170.
96. Swanson KL, McGoon MD, Krowka MJ. Survival in portopulmonary hypertension [Abstract]. Am J Respir Crit Care Med 2003;167:A683.
97. Herve P, Lebrec D, Brenot F, et al. Pulmonary vascular disorders in portal hypertension. Eur Respir J 1998;11:1153-1166.
98. Kereveu A, Callebert J, Humbert M. High plasma serotonin levels in primary pulmonary hypertension. Arterioscler Thromb Vasc Biol 2000;20:2233-2239.
99. Stewart DJ, Levy RD, Cernacek P, et al. Increased plasma endothelin-1 in pulmonary hypertension. Ann Intern Med 1991;114:464-469.
100. Ahtee L, Briley M, Raisman R, et al. Reduced uptake of serotonin but unchanged ^{3}H-imipiramine binding in the platelets from cirrhotic patients. Life Sci 1981;29:2323-2329.
101. Gerbes AL, Moller S, Gulberg V, et al. Endothelin-1 and -3 plasma concentrations in patients with cirrhosis: role of splanchnic and renal passage and liver function. Hepatology 1995;21:735-739.
102. Bernardi M, Gulberg V, Colantoni A, et al. Plasma endothelin-1 and -3 in cirrhosis: relationship with systemic hemodynamics, renal function, and neurohumoral systems. J Hepatol 1996;24:161-168.
103. Keyes JW, Wilson GA, Quinonest JD. An evaluation of lung uptake of colloid during liver imaging. J Nucl Med 1973;14:687-691.
104. Krowka MJ. Evolving dilemmas and management of portopulmonary hypertension. Semin Liver Dis 2006;26:265-272.
105. Herve P, Le Pavec J, Sztrymf B, et al. Pulmonary vascular abnormalities in cirrhosis. Best Pract Res Clin Gastroenterol 2007;21:141-159.
106. Garcia-Pagan JC, Escorsell A, Moitinho E, et al. Influence of pharmacological agents on portal hemodynamics: basis for its use in the treatment of portal hypertension. Semin Liver Dis 1999;19:427-438.
107. Lebrec D, Poynard T, Hillon P, et al. Propranolol for prevention of recurrent gastrointestinal bleeding in patients with cirrhosis: a controlled study. N Engl J Med 1981;305:1371-1374.
108. Garcia-Tsao G, Grace ND, Groszmann RJ, et al. Short-term effects of propranolol on portal venous pressure. Hepatology 1986;6:101-106.
109. Bosch J, Mastai R, Kravetz D, et al. Measurement of azygous blood flow in the evaluation of portal hypertension in patients with cirrhosis: clinical and hemodynamic correlation in 100 patients. J Hepatol 1985;1:125-129.
110. Bosch J, Bordas JM, Mastai R, et al. Effects of vasopressin on the intravariceal pressure in patients with cirrhosis: comparison with the effects on portal pressure. Hepatology 1988;8:861-865.
111. Minor MA, Grace ND. Pharmacologic therapy of portal hypertension. Clin Liver Dis 2006;10:563-581.
112. Bosch J, Groszmann RJ, Garcia-Pagan JC, et al. Association of transdermal nitroglycerin to vasopression infusion in the treatment of variceal hemorrhage: a placebo-controlled clinical trial. Hepatology 1989;10:962-968.
113. Groszmann RJ, Kravetz D, Bosch J, et al. Nitroglycerin improves the hemodynamic response to vasopressin in portal hypertension. Hepatology 1982;2:757-762.
114. Soderlund C, Manusson I, Torngren S, et al. Terlipressin (triglycyl-lysine vasopressin) controls acute bleeding oesophageal varices: a double-blind, randomized, placebo-controlled trial. Scand J Gastroenterol 1990;25:622-630.
115. Levacher S, Letoumelin P, Paterson D, et al. Early administration of terlipressin plus glyceryl trinitrate to control active upper gastrointestinal bleeding in cirrrhotic patients. Lancet 1995;346:865-868.
116. D'Amico G, Traina M, Vizzini G, et al. Terlipressin or vasopressin plus transdermal nitroglycerin in a treatment strategy for digestive bleeding in cirrhosis: a randomized clinical trial. Liver Study Group of V. Cervello Hospital. J Hepatol 1994;20:206-212.
117. Pizcueta MP, Garcia-Pagan JC, Fernandez M, et al. Glucagon hinders the effects of somatostatin on portal hypertension: a study in rats with partial portal vein ligation. Gastroenterology 1991;101:1710-1715.
118. Sheppard M, Shapiro B, Pimstone B, et al. Metabolic clearance and plasma half-disappearance time of exogenous somatostatin in man. J Clin Endocrinol Metab 1979;48:50-53.
119. Reynaert H, Geerts A. Review article: pharmacological rationale for the use of somatostatin ADN analogues in portal hypertension. Aliment Pharmacol Ther 2003;18:375-386.
120. Cirera I, Feu F, Luca A, et al. Effects of bolus injections and continuous infusions of somatostatin and placebo in patients with cirrhosis: a double-blind hemodynamic investigation. Hepatology 1995;22:106-111.
121. Moitinho E, Planas R, Banares R, et al. Multicenter randomized placebo controlled trial comparing different schedules of somatostatin in the treatment of acute variceal bleeding. J Hepatol 2001;35:712-718.
122. Gines A, Salmeron JM, Gines P, et al. Effects of somatostatin on renal function in cirrhosis. Gastroenterology 1992;103:1868-1874.
123. Avgerinos A, Nevens F, Raptis S, et al. Early administration of somatostatin and efficacy of sclerotherapy in acute oesophageal variceal bleeds: the European Acute Bleeding Oesophageal Variceal Episodes (ABOVE) randomized trial. Lancet 1997;350:1495-1499.
124. Lamberts SW, van der Lely AJ, de Herder WW, et al. Octreotide. N Engl J Med 1996;334:246-254.
125. Escorsell A, Bandi JC, Andreau V, et al. Desensitization to the effects of intravenous octreotide in cirrhotic patients with portal hypertension. Gastroenterology 2001;120:161-169.
126. Abraldes JG, Bosch J. Somatostatin AD analogues in portal hypertension. Hepatology 2002;35:1305-1312.
127. Corley DA, Cello JP, Adkisson W, et al. Octreotide for acute esophageal variceal bleeding: a meta-analysis. Gastroenterology 2001;120:946-954.
128. McCormick PA, Biagino MR, Dick R, et al. Octreotide inhibits the meal-induced increases in portal venous pressure in cirrhotic patients with portal hypertension: a double blind placebo-controlled study. Hepatology 1992;16:1180-1186.
129. Garcia-Tsao G, Groszmann RJ. Portal hemodynamics during nitroglycerin administration in cirrhotic patients. Hepatology 1987;7:805-809.
130. Navasa M, Chesta J, Bosch J, et al. Reduction of portal pressure by isosorbide-5-mononitrate in patients with cirrhosis: effects on splanchnic and systemic hemodynamics and liver function. Gastroentereology 1989;96:1110-1118.
131. Escorsell A, Feu F, Bordad JM, et al. Effects of isosorbide-5-mononitrate on variceal pressure and systemic and splanchnic haemodynamics in patients with cirrhosis. J Hepatol 1996;24:423-429.
132. Garcia-Pagan JC, Feu F, Bosch J, et al. Propranolol compared with propranolol plus isosorbide-5-mononitrate for portal hypertension in cirrhosis: a randomized controlled study. Ann Intern Med 1991;114:869-873.
133. Merkel C, Sacerdoti D, Bolognesi M, et al. Hemodynamic evaluation of the addition of isosorbide-5-mononitrate to nadolol in cirrhotic patients with insufficient response to the beta-blocker alone. Hepatology 1997;26:34-39.
134. Garcia-Pagan JC, Morillas R, Banares R, et al. Propranolol plus placebo versus propranolol plus isosorbide-5-mononitrate in the prevention of a first variceal bleed: a double blind RCT. Hepatology 2003;37:1260-1266.
135. Krowka MJ. Pulmonary hypertension. Mayo Clin Proc 2000;75:625-630.
136. Fogel MR, Sawhney VK, Neal EA, et al. Diuresis in the ascitic patient: a randomized controlled trial of three regimens. J Clin Gastroenterol 1981;3(Suppl 1):73-80.
137. Angeli P, Dalla PM, De Bei F, et al. Randomized clinical study of the efficacy of amiloride and potassium canrenoate in nonazotemic cirrhotic patients with ascites. Hepatology 1994;19:72-79.
138. Perez-Ayuso RM, Arroyo V, Planas R, et al. Randomized comparative study of efficacy of furosemide versus spironolactone in nonazotemic cirrhosis with ascites: relationship between the diuretic response and the activity of the renin-aldosterone system. Gastroenterology 1983;84:961-968.
139. Pockros PJ, Reynolds TB. Rapid diuresis in patients with ascites from chronic liver disease: the importance of peripheral edema. Gastroenterology 1986;90:1827-1833.
140. Riordan SM, Williams R. Treatment of hepatic encephalopathy. N Engl J Med 1997;337:473-479.
141. Conn HO, Leevy CM, Vlahcevic ZR, et al. Comparison of lactulose and neomycin in the treatment of chronic portal-systemic encephalopathy: a double-blind controlled trial. Gastroenterology 1977;72:573-583.
142. Kunin CM, Chalmers TC, Leevy CM, et al. Absorption of orally administered neomycin and kanamycin. N Engl J Med 1960;262:380-385.
143. Hoover WW, Gerlach EH, Hoban DJ, et al. Antimicrobial activity and spetrum of rifaximin, a new topical rifamycin derivative. Diagn Microbiol Infect Dis 1993;16:111-118.

144. Gillis JC, Brogden RN. Rifaximin: a review of its antibacterial activity, pharmacokinetic properties and therapeutic potential in conditions mediated by gastrointestinal bacteria. Drugs 1995;49:467-484.
145. Williams R, Bass N. Rifaximin, a nonabsorbed oral antibiotic, in the treatment of hepatic encephalopathy: antimicrobial activity, efficacy, and safety. Rev Gastroenterol Disord 2005;5(Suppl 1):S10-S18.
146. D'Amico G, Morabito A. Noninvasive markers of esophageal varices: another round, not the last. Hepatology 2004;39:30-34.
147. De Franchis R. Updating consensus in portal hypertension: report of the Baveno III Consensus Workshop on definitions, methodology and therapeutic strategies in portal hypertension. J Hepatol 2000;33:846-852.
148. Merli M, Nicolini G, Angeloni S, et al. Incidence and natural history of small esophageal varices in cirrhotic patients. J Hepatol 2003;38:266-272.
149. Imperiale TF, Chalasani N. A meta-analysis of endoscopic variceal ligation for primary prophylaxis of esophageal variceal bleeding. Hepatology 2001;33:802-807.
150. Khuroo MS, Khuroo NS, Farahat KL, et al. Meta-analysis: endoscopic variceal ligation for primary prophylaxis of oesophageal variceal bleeding. Aliment Pharmacol Ther 2005;21:347-361.
151. Banares R, Albillos A, Rincon D, et al. Endoscopic treatment versus endoscopic plus pharmacologic treatment for acute variceal bleeding: a meta-analysis. Hepatology 2002;35:609-615.
152. Bernard B, Cadranel JF, Valla D, et al. Prognostic significance of bacterial infection in bleeding cirrhotic patients: a prospective study. Gastroenterology 1995;108:1828-1834.
153. Bernard B, Grange JD, Khac EN, et al. Antibiotic prophylaxis for the prevention of bacterial infections in cirrhotic patients with gastrointestinal bleeding: a meta-analysis. Hepatology 1999;29:1655-1661.
154. Soares-Weiser K, Brezis M, Tur-Kaspa R, et al. Antibiotic prophylaxis of bacterial infections in cirrhotic inpatients: a meta-analysis of randomized controlled trials. Scand J Gastroenterol 2003;38:193-200.
155. Carbonell N, Pauwels A, Serfaty L, et al. Improved survival after variceal bleeding in patients with cirrhosis over the past two decades. Hepatology 2004;40:652-659.
156. Fernandez J, Ruiz del Arbol L, Gomez C. Norfloxacin vs ceftriaxone in the prophylaxis of infections in patients with advanced cirrhosis and hemorrhage. Gastroenterology 2006;131:1049-1056.
157. Bosch J, Garcia-Pagan JC. Prevention of variceal rebleeding. Lancet 2003;361:952-954.
158. Laine L, Cook D. Endoscopic ligation compared with sclerotherapy for treatment of esophageal variceal bleeding: a meta-analysis. Ann Intern Med 1995;123:280-287.
159. de la Pena J, Brullet E, Sanchez-Hernandez E, et al. Variceal ligation plus nadolol compared with ligation for prophylaxis of variceal rebleeding: a multicenter trial. Hepatology 2005;41:572-578.
160. Lo GH, Lai KH, Cheng JS, et al. Endoscopic variceal ligation plus nadolol and sucralfate compared with ligation alone for the prevention of variceal rebleeding: a prospective, randomized trial. Hepatology 2000;32:461-465.
161. Bernard B, Lebrec D, Mathurin P, et al. Beta-adrenergic antagonists in the prevention of gastrointestinal rebleeding in patients with cirrhosis: a meta-analysis. Hepatology 1997;25:63-70.
162. Runyon B. Management of adult patients with ascites due to cirrhosis. Hepatology 2004;39:1-16.
163. Runyon BA, Montano AA, Akriviadis EA, et al. The serum-ascites albumin gradient is superior to the exudate-transudate concept in the differential diagnosis of ascites. Ann Intern Med 1992;117:215-220.
164. Gines P, Berl T, Bernardi M, et al. Hyponatremia in cirrhosis: from pathogenesis to treatment. Hepatology 1998;28:851-864.
165. Stanley MM, Ochi S, Lee KK, et al. Peritoneovenous shunting as compared with medical treatment in patients with alcoholic cirrhosis and massive ascites. N Engl J Med 1989;321:1632-1638.
166. Peltekian KM, Wong F, Liu PP, et al. Cardiovascular, renal and neurohumoral responses to single large-volume paracentesis in cirrhotic patients with diuretic-resistant ascites. Am J Gastroenterol 1997;92:394-399.
167. Tito L, Gines P, Arroyo V, et al. Total paracentesis associated with intravenous albumin management of patient with cirrhosis and ascites. Gastroenterology 1990;98:146-151.
168. Gines P, Tito L, Arroyo V, et al. Randomized comparative study of therapeutic paracentesis with and without intravenous albumin in cirrhosis. Gastroenterology 1988;94:1493-1502.
169. Runyon BA, Hoefs JC. Culture-negative neutrocytic ascites: a variant of spontaneous bacterial peritonitis. Hepatology 1984;4:1209-1211.
170. Runyon BA. Monomicrobial nonneutrocytic bacterascites: a variant of spontaneous bacterial peritonitis. Hepatology 1990;12:710-715.
171. Felisart J, Rimola A, Arroyo V, et al. Randomized comparative study of efficacy and nephrotoxicity of ampicillin plus tobramycin versus cefotaxime in cirrhotics with severe infections. Hepatology 1985;5:457-462.
172. Runyon BA, McHutchison JG, Antillon MR, et al. Short-course vs long-course antibiotic treatment of spontaneous bacterial peritonitis: a randomized controlled trial of 100 patients. Gastroenterology 1991;100:1737-1742.
173. Navasa M, Follo A, Llovet JM, et al. Randomized, comparative study of oral ofloxacin versus intravenous cefotaximin in spontaneous bacterial peritonitis. Gastroenterology 1996;111:1011-1017.
174. Runyon BA, Akriviadis EA, Sattler FR, et al. Ascitic fluid and serum cefotaxime and desacetyl cefotaxime levels in patients treated for bacterial peritonitis. Dig Dis Sci 1991;36:1782-1786.
175. Akriviadis EA, Runyon BA. The value of an algorithm in differentiating spontaneous from secondary bacterial peritonitis. Gastroenterology 1990;98:127-133.
176. Runyon BA. Low-protein-concentration ascitic fluid is predisposed to spontaneous bacterial peritonitis. Gastroenterology 1986;91:1343-1346.
177. Soriano G, Teixedo M, Guarner C, et al. Selective intestinal decomtamination prevents spontaneous bacterial peritonitis. Gastroenterology 1991;100:477-481.
178. Gines P, Rimola A, Planas R, et al. Norfloxacin prevents spontaneous bacterial peritonitis recurrence in cirrhosis: results of a double-blind, placebo-controlled trial. Hepatology 1990;12:716-724.
179. Soriano G, Guarner C, Tomas A, et al. Norfloxacin prevents bacterial infection in cirrhotics with gastrointestinal hemorrhage. Gastroenterology 1992;103:1267-1272.
180. Blaise M, Paterson D, Trinchet JC, et al. Systemic antibiotic therapy prevents bacterial infection in cirrhotic patients with gastrointestinal hemorrhage. Hepatology 1994;20:34-38.
181. Singh N, Gayowski T, Yu VL, et al. Trimethoprim-sulfamethoxazole for the prevention of spontaneous bacterial peritonitis in cirrhosis: a randomized trial. Ann Intern Med 1995;122:595-598.
182. Fernandez J, Navasa M, Gomez J, et al. Bacterial infections in cirrhosis: epidemiological changes with invasive procedures and norfloxacin prophylaxis. Hepatology 2002;35:140-148.
183. Guevara M, Gines P, Fernandez-Esparrach G, et al. Reversibility of hepatorenal syndrome by prolonged adminstration of ornipressin and plasma volume expansion. Hepatology 1998;27:35-41.
184. Angeli P, Volpin R, Gerunda G, et al. Reversal of type I hepatorenal syndrome with the administration of midodrine and octreotide. Hepatology 1999;29:1690-1697.
185. Pomier-Layrargues G, Paquin SC, Hassoun Z, et al. Octreotide in hepatorenal syndrome: a randomized, double-blind, placebo-controlled, crossover study. Hepatology 2003;38:238-243.
186. Uriz J, Gines P, Cardenas A, et al. Terlipressin plus albumin infusion: an effective and safe therapy of hepatorenal syndrome. J Hepatol 2000;33:43-48.
187. Ortega R, Gines P, Uriz J, et al. Terlipressin therapy with and without albumin for patients with hepatorenal syndrome: results of a prospective, nonrandomized study. Hepatology 2002;36:941-948.
188. Halimi C, Bonnard P, Bernard B, et al. Effect of terlipressin (Glypressin®) on hepatorenal syndrome in cirrhotic patients: results of a multicentre pilot study. Eur J Gastroenterol Hepatol 2002;14:153-158.
189. Prashant S, Chawla A, Garg R, et al. Beneficial effects of terlipressin in hepatorenal syndrome: a prospective, randomized placebo controlled clinical trial. J Gastroenterol Hepatol 2003;18:152-156.
190. Als-Nielsen B, Gluud LL, Gluud C. Non-absorbable disaccharides for hepatic encephalopathy: systematic review of randomised trials. BMJ 2004;328:1046-1051.
191. Williams R, James OF, Warnes TW, et al. Evaluation of the efficacy and safety of rifaximin in the treatment of hepatic encephalopathy: a double-blind, randomized, dose-finding multi-centre study. Eur J Gastroenterol Hepatol 2000;12:203-208.
192. Mas A, Rodes J, Sunyer L, et al. Comparison of rifaximin and lactitol in the treatment of acute hepatic encephalopathy: results of a randomized, double-blind, double-dummy, controlled clinical trial. J Hepatol 2003;38:51-58.
193. Cordoba J, Lopez-Hellin J, Planas M, et al. Normal protein diet for episodic hepatic encephalopathy: results of a randomized study. J Hepatol 2004;41:38-43.
194. Golbin JM, Krowka MJ. Portopulmonary hypertension. Clin Chest Med 2007;28:203-218.
195. Bosch J, D'Amico G, Garcia-Pagan JC. Portal hypertension. *In* Schiff ER, Dorrell MF, Maddrey WC (eds): Schiff's Diseases of the Liver, 9th ed. Philadelphia: Lippincott Williams & Wilkins, 2003, pp 429-486.
196. Kuo PC, Johnson LB, Plotkin JS, et al. Continuous intravenous infusion of epoprostenol for the treatment of portopulmonary hypertension. Transplantation 1997;63:604-606.
197. Krowka MJ, Frantz RP, McGoon MD, et al. Improvement in pulmonary hemodynamics during intravenous epoprostenol (prostacyclin): a study of 15 patients with moderate to severe portopulmonary hypertension. Hepatology 1999;30:641-648.
198. McLaughlin VV, Genthner DE, Panella MM, et al. Compassionate use of continuous prostacyclin in the management of secondary pulmonary hypertension: a case series. Ann Intern Med 1999;130:740-743.
199. Hoeper MM, Halank M, Marx C, et al. Bosentan therapy for portopulmonary hypertension. Eur Respir J 2005;25:502-508.
200. Galie N, Ghofrani HA, Torbicki A, et al. Sildenafil citrate therapy for pulmonary arterial hypertension. N Engl J Med 2005;353:2148-2157.
201. Reichenberger F, Voswinckel R, Steveling E, et al. Sildenafil treatment for portopulmonary hypertension. Eur Respir J 2006;28:563-567.
202. Gines P, Jimenez W. Aquaretic agents: a new potential treatment of dilutional hyponatremia in cirrhosis. J Hepatol 1996;24:506-512.
203. Arroyo V, Rodes J, Gutierrez-Lizarraga MA, et al. Prognostic value of spontaneous hyponatremia in cirrhosis with ascites. Am J Dig Dis 1976;21:249-256.
204. Guyader D, Patat A, Ellis-Grosse EJ, Orczyk GP. Pharmacodynamic effects of a nonpeptide antidiuretic hormone V2 antagonist in cirrhotic patients with ascites. Hepatology 2002;36:1197-1205.
205. Verbalis JG. AVP receptor antagonists as aquaretics: review and assessment of clinical data. Cleveland Clin J Med 2006;73:S24-S33.
206. Wong F, Blei AT, Blendis LM, Thuluvath PJ. A vasopressin receptor antagonist (VPA-985) improves serum sodium concentration in patients with hyponatremia: a multicenter randomized, placebo-controlled trial. Hepatology 2003;37:182-191.
207. Gerbes AL, Gulberg V, Gines P, et al. Therapy of hyponatremia in cirrhosis with a vasopressin receptor antagonist: a randomized double-blind multicenter trial. Gastroenterology 2003;124:933-939.
208. Reichen J, Lebrec D. The future treatment of portal hypertension. Best Pract Res Clin Gastroenterol 2007;21:191-202.

209. Kakumitsu S, Shijo H, Yokoyama M, et al. Effects of L-arginine on the systemic, mesenteric, and hepatic circulation in patients with cirrhosis. Hepatology 1998;27:377-382.
210. Fiorucci S, Antonelli E, Morelli O, et al. NCX-1000, a NO-releasing derivative of ursodeoxycholic acid, selectively delivers NO to the liver and protects against development of portal hypertension. Proc Natl Acad Sci U S A 2001;98:8897-8902.
211. Van de Casteele M, Omasta A, Janssens S, et al. In vivo gene transfer of endothelial nitric oxide synthase decreases portal pressure in anaesthetised carbon tetrachloride cirrhotic rats. Gut 2002;51:440-445.
212. Pinzani M, Milani S, De Franco R, et al. Endothelin I is overexpressed in human cirrhotic liver and exerts multiple effects on activated hepatic stellate cells. Gastroenterology 1996;110:534-548.
213. Rockey DC, Weisiger RA. Endothelin induced contractility of stellate cells from normal and cirrhotic rat liver: implications for regulation of portal pressure and resistance. Hepatology 1996;24:233-240.
214. Kojima H, Sakurai S, Kuriyama S, et al. Endothelin-1 plays a major role in portal hypertension of biliary cirrhotic rats through endothelin receptor subtype B together with subtype A in vivo. J Hepatol 2001;34:805-811.
215. Yokomori H, Oda M, Yasogawa Y, et al. Enhanced expression of endothelin B receptor at protein and gene levels in human cirrhotic liver. Am J Pathol 2001;159:1353-1362.
216. Cahill PA, Hou MC, Hendrickson R, et al. Increased expression of endothelin receptors in the vasculature of portal hypertensive rats: role in splanchnic hemodynamics. Hepatology 1998;28:396-403.
217. Gomberg-Maitland M, Tapson VF, Benza RL, et al. Transition from intravenous epoprostenol to intravenous treprostinil in pulmonary hypertension. Am J Respir Crit Care Med 2005;172:1586-1589.
218. Kenyon KW, Nappi JM. Bosentan for the treatment of pulmonary arterial hypertension. Ann Pharmacother 2003;37:1055-1062.

35

INFECTIOUS HEPATITIS

Steven K. Herrine, Simona Rossi, and Victor J. Navarro

INTRODUCTION 527
GLOBAL SCOPE OF VIRAL HEPATITIS 527
PATHOPHYSIOLOGY 527
Hepatitis A Virus 527
Epidemiology 527
Pathogenesis 528
Clinical Presentation 528
Hepatitis B/Hepatitis D Viruses 528
Epidemiology 528
Pathogenesis 529
Clinical Presentation 529
Hepatitis C Virus 530
Epidemiology 530
Pathogenesis 531
Clinical Presentation 532
Hepatitis E Virus 533
Epidemiology 533
Pathogenesis 534
Clinical Presentation 534
THERAPEUTICS AND CLINICAL PHARMACOLOGY 534
Hepatitis A 534
Prevention 534
Prophylaxis 534
Hepatitis B/Hepatitis D 534
Prevention 534
Prophylaxis 535
Current HBV Vaccination Recommendations 535
Treatment of HBV Infection 535
Pharmacologic Approach to Treatment of HBV 537
Hepatitis C 539
Prevention 539
Prophylaxis 539
Treatment of HCV Infection 540
Hepatitis E 542
Prevention 542
Prophylaxis 542
Treatment of Acute HEV Infection 542

INTRODUCTION

Hepatotropic virus infection is a disease state that appears to be as old as civilization itself. Numerous ancient texts refer to epidemic jaundice; the relationship between icterus and the liver was also understood. Knowledge of hepatic anatomy appears to be quite ancient, a likely result of the importance of animal liver in divination. Greek medicine was able to identify specific liver disorders, including abscess, inflammation, cirrhosis, hepatomegaly, and ductal abnormalities.[1] The epidemic nature of jaundice seen among soldiers implied an infectious cause to some clinicians. European epidemics in the 17th and 18th centuries added to the credence of this theory. The parenteral etiology of some forms of infectious hepatitis was hinted at by post–smallpox vaccination outbreaks in 1883. Parenteral infections during the subsequent period were described in the setting of mercurial therapy for syphilis, laboratory testing in diabetics, outbreaks in laboratory workers, and yellow fever vaccination. That blood products could transmit the agent of infectious hepatitis was discovered around World War II, when pooled plasma and whole blood infusions were used with increasing frequency. By 1944, two filterable agents had been identified, causing infectious "type A" and serum "type B" hepatitis.

In 1965, Blumberg and colleagues developed a serologic marker for type B hepatitis.[2] Detected in the serum of an Australian aborigine, the serum reactant was coined the Australian antigen. Eponymously named Dane particles, representing intact hepatitis B virions, were identified by electron microscopy in 1970.[3] By the end of the 1970s, hepatitis B serologic measures had become recognizable in a form still used today.

Hepatitis A virus (HAV) was seen in feces of patients by electron microscopy by 1973 and was propagated in vitro by 1979.[4,5] Despite these advances, investigators still knew of at least one other infectious agent that caused posttransfusion hepatitis. This virus was termed non-A, non-B hepatitis until 1989, when in a molecular biologic tour de force, hepatitis C virus (HCV) was identified.[6]

GLOBAL SCOPE OF VIRAL HEPATITIS

Hepatitis B virus (HBV) infection is an enormous global health burden. Current estimates put the prevalence of HBV infection at around 2 billion persons globally, with some 350 million chronically infected. Hepatitis B infection is the 10th leading cause of global mortality. Hepatocellular carcinoma, much of which is related to chronic HBV infection, accounts for over 300,000 deaths annually and is the third leading cause of global cancer mortality. HBV vaccine, available since 1982, has led to dramatic decreases in these grim statistics in countries where inoculation programs have been adopted. Nonetheless, in the absence of large-scale vaccination programs, HBV morbidity and mortality promise to grow in the coming decades.[7,8]

Hepatitis C is highly endemic in many disparate parts of the globe. The Centers for Disease Control and Prevention (CDC) estimates that there are currently some 170 million carriers of the virus worldwide with approximately 3 to 4 million new infections per year. The highest endemicity has been reported in northern and central Africa, the eastern Mediterranean, and the Ukraine, citing figures that are probably conservative due to underreporting. In the United States, current data suggest a prevalence of 1.8%, but the limitation of the National Health and Nutrition Examination Survey (NHANES) reporting system may also render this estimate conservative. Although the incidence of HCV infection in the United States has been on the decline since the 1980s, the prevalence of chronic infection is expected to rise well into the first 2 decades of the 21st century. Total economic burden of HCV in the United States has been estimated at over $1 billion per annum.[9]

PATHOPHYSIOLOGY

Hepatitis A Virus

Epidemiology

HAV is seen with varying levels of endemicity across the globe. The epidemiology of infection similarly varies, based on the prevalence of symptoms in different age groups and the incidence of naturally occurring neutralizing antibodies in these populations. In some parts of the world—for example Africa, Asia, and parts of Central and South America—HAV infection is highly endemic, with most exposures occurring in infancy or childhood. These infections are largely asymptomatic and well tolerated, leading to a high prevalence of HAV immunity in the adult population. In areas of low endemicity of HAV, infection later in life is the common scenario. HAV infection in adults can be a serious disease, with the majority of such cases leading to symptoms and an appreciable case fatality rate. The prevalence of HAV in any given country is roughly inversely proportional to the socioeconomic status of the region. As development and improved sanitation are seen, a shift of cases from the younger to the older age group is seen.

In the United States, a region of relatively low HAV endemicity, a significant number of acute HAV infections continue to be reported. It has been estimated that HAV infection is among the most common vaccine-preventable infections seen in the United States today. HAV infection tends to come in clusters, largely due to community outbreaks, such as in households or extended families. Outbreaks associated with contaminated food are also reported. Regional variations of HAV incidence have helped to predict locations of outbreaks and to focus vaccine programs.[10]

Pathogenesis

HAV was first isolated from human volunteers and visualized by electron microscopy in 1973.[11] The virus was cloned in the ensuing years, allowing development of a vaccine by 1990. The virus is classified within the Picornaviridae family, defining a new genus, *Hepatovirus*. HAV is a positive-strand RNA virus lacking a lipid envelope. Similar to the best known picornavirus, poliovirus, the RNA genome is packaged within icosahedral protein capsids. Unlike poliovirus, HAV does not appear to require nonstructural proteins for replication.[12] The actual structure of the HAV virus is an area of ongoing investigation, but recent studies suggest significant differences from other known members of the Picornaviridae family.[13]

Hepatitis A is generally transmitted via the oral-fecal route, explaining the higher prevalence of disease in regions with poorer sanitation facilities. The virus is stable at low temperatures and in acidic environments and is resistant to detergents. After infection, HAV appears to replicate in the liver and to be excreted via the bile into the intestinal lumen. Large amounts of virus are shed in the feces within 1 to 4 weeks of infection. Maximal fecal shedding and hence greatest infectivity are seen immediately prior to the onset of hepatocellular injury. Long-term fecal shedding of virus does not appear to occur.[12] Hepatocellular injury resulting from hepatitis A infection appears to be immune mediated. Human leukocyte antigen–restricted, virus-specific, cytotoxic, $CD8^+$ T cells have been recovered from infected humans.[14,15] Interferon gamma in response to HAV infection has been isolated from this cell type.[16] Anti-HAV, first as immunoglobulin M (IgM) followed shortly thereafter by immunoglobulin G (IgG), is detectable in infected individuals within weeks of infection, indicative of the robust immune response generated against this infection. Immunity is conferred for life. Reexposure to HAV will increase levels of HAV IgG, but does not lead to recurrent liver disease[17] (Fig. 35-1).

Clinical Presentation

HAV infection is the most common cause of acute viral hepatitis in the United States. After exposure, the clinical presentation can range from essentially asymptomatic to the dramatic picture of fulminant hepatic failure. In general, the severity of acute HAV infection–related symptoms is inversely proportional to age. In the adult population, acute infection often has its onset with a viral prodrome including myalgia, fever, lassitude, fatigue, and varying degrees of right upper quadrant abdominal discomfort. In mild cases, physical examination is nonspecific and may be entirely unremarkable. In more severe cases, tender hepatomegaly, icterus, and even peripheral edema and ascites may be seen on presentation. In the setting of profound immune-mediated hepatocellular necrosis, the diagnosis of fulminant hepatic failure may be encountered, usually defined as the onset of liver failure within 6 weeks of the recognition of liver disease. From a pragmatic point of view, this almost always means varying degrees of encephalopathy and even coma following the onset of jaundice. Laboratory assessment is characterized by elevation of serum aminotransferase, with alanine aminotransferase (ALT) predominant. On occasion, aminotransferase elevation can be dramatic, even exceeding 10,000 U/L. The presence of increased prothrombin time is indicative of severe

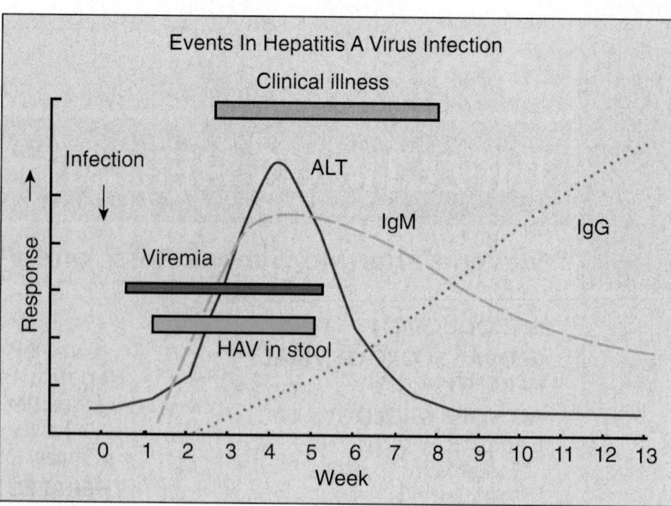

FIGURE 35-1 • Clinical events following hepatitis A infection. Large amounts of virus are shed in the feces within 1 to 4 weeks of infection. Maximal fecal shedding and hence greatest infectivity are seen immediately prior to the onset of hepatocellular injury. Anti-HAV, first as IgM followed shortly thereafter by IgG, is detectable in infected individuals within weeks of infection. (Figure from CDC. http://www.cdc.gov/NCIDOD/Diseases/Hepatitis/slideset/index.htm)

hepatocellular dysfunction and risk of acute liver failure: such a presentation should lead to prompt admission to the hospital and consideration of transfer to a center offering liver transplantation.

The recognition of an index case of acute hepatitis A should prompt the identification of other persons at risk for infection. Intimate and household contacts should be offered both passive and active immunoprophylaxis with immunoglobulin and HAV vaccination, respectively. In institutional settings, large-scale use of immunoglobulin can decrease the risk of an epidemic. The lack of symptoms in exposed contacts should not dissuade the use of immunoprophylaxis, since the virus is transmitted during the prodromic phase.

Unlike the other major hepatotropic viruses, hepatitis A does not lead to chronic infection, the development of cirrhosis, or increased risk for the development of hepatocellular carcinoma. Rarely, acute HAV infection can present with prolonged cholestasis. The use of corticosteroids in this setting has been anecdotally reported to lessen the duration of symptoms and laboratory abnormalities. A relapsing form of HAV has also been described, although this presentation is unusual and carries no additional risk of long-term sequelae.

Hepatitis B/Hepatitis D Viruses

Epidemiology

Hepatitis B is widely prevalent throughout the world. There are geographic significant differences, however, in the endemicity of the virus. The CDC has divided the globe into areas of high endemicity (≥8%), moderate endemicity (2% to 7%) and low endemicity (<2%) (Fig. 35-2). Transmission patterns vary greatly by endemicity, with vertical transmission predominant in areas of high endemicity and horizontal transmission predominant in areas of lower endemicity.[18] The virus is often present in very high concentrations in infected persons. Most transmission is by percutaneous or mucosal exposure to infected blood or other bodily fluids. The major mode of transmission is person to person, but because the virus tends to be stable and infectious for up to a week on surfaces, infection can take place via these fomites.[19] Vertical transmission, that is, from mother to infant, is the most common global mode of transmission. Most of these infections take place at the time of parturition, although a smaller percentage take place in utero. Infectivity appears to be directly proportional to viral burden of the mother and the presence of hepatitis B e antigen (HBeAg, a marker of viral replication). Horizontal transmission is most often seen in the setting of sexual transmission. Sexual acquisition of HBV is significantly more frequent in those with multiple heterosexual part-

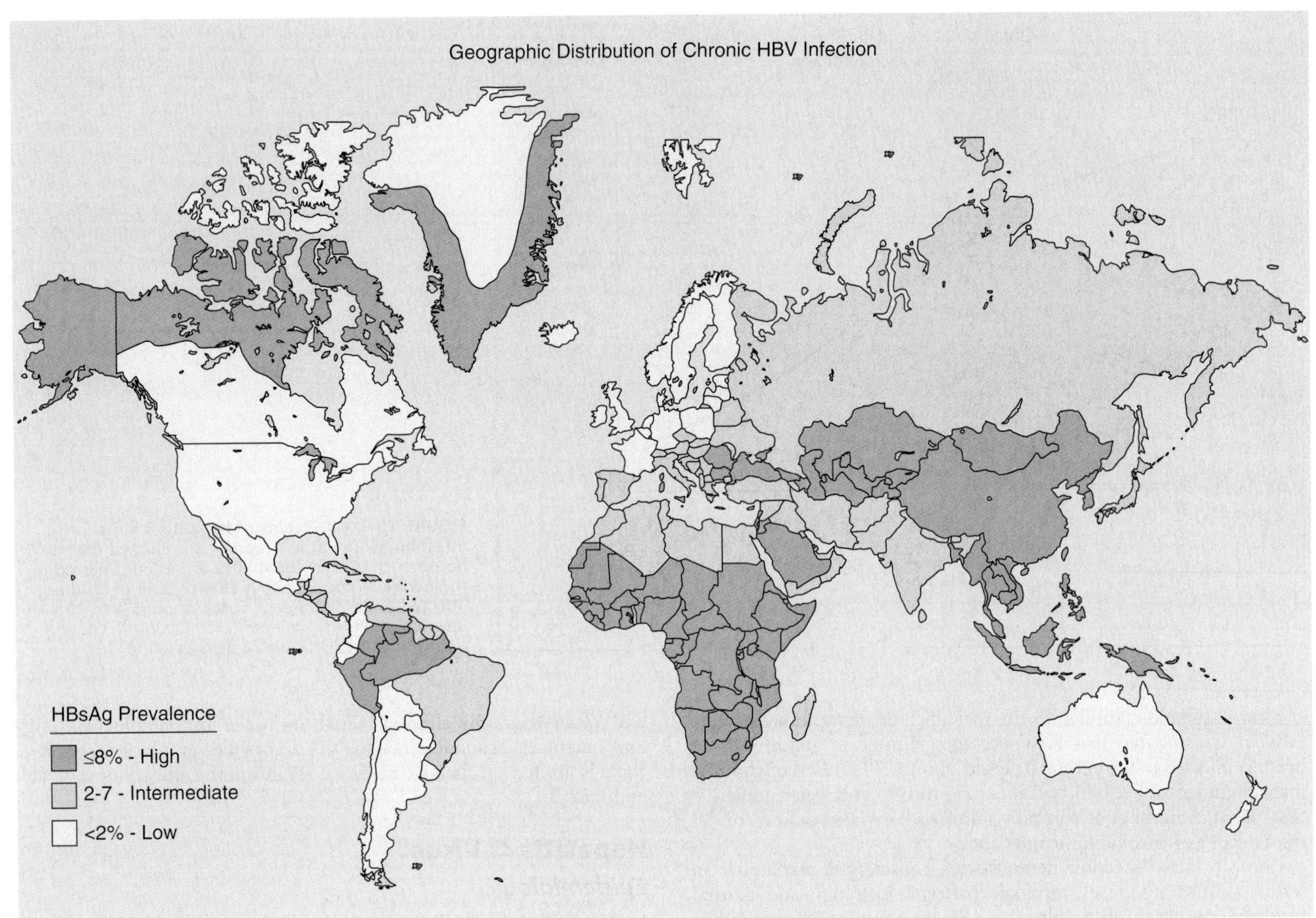

FIGURE 35-2 • Geographic distribution of chronic hepatitis B infection. The CDC has divided the globe into areas of high endemicity (≥8%), moderate endemicity (2% to 7%), and low endemicity (<2%). (Figure from CDC. http://www.cdc.gov/NCIDOD/Diseases/Hepatitis/slideset/index.htm)

ners and in men who have sex with men.[20-22] Intravenous drug use is known to be a risk factor for HBV infection. The prevalence of new intravenous drug use–related HBV infections has been on the decline for about a decade, largely due to increased awareness of the need for changes in practice among drug users.

HBV transmission by unsafe medical injection practices is of particular importance in the developing world, where reusable syringes are frequently encountered. Such contaminated injections have been reported to be responsible for over 20% of new HBV cases worldwide.[23] In the developed nations, HBV infection in the setting of health care delivery has similarly been reported through a variety of devices. Hemodialysis, formerly an important risk factor for new HBV acquisition, has significantly diminished in importance as a mode of HBV transmission.[24] The incidence of such events is overshadowed by other modes of transmission, however.[25,26]

Pathogenesis

HBV is a partially double-stranded DNA virus classified in the family Hepadnaviridae. Virions are 42 to 47 nm in size and enter the bloodstream through the parenteral route. Replication takes place only in the liver. The HBV genome contains four major overlapping open reading frames encoding the envelope, nucleocapsid, polymerase, and X proteins.[27,28] HBV is unique among DNA viruses in that it employs a reverse transcriptase during replication, a fact that has significant therapeutic implications, as is discussed later. HBV replication, which can exceed 10^{11} virions per day, lacks proofreading ability, resulting in a high mutation rate.[29] The most important clinical mutations involve the precore and core-promoter regions, again resulting in significant implications for therapy. Although many mutant strains of HBV have been identified, the most clinically significant strains include the precore and core-promoter variants and the surface and polymerase mutants. A number of HBV genotypes have been detected. Denoted HBV genotypes A through G, there are distinct patterns of geographic predominance but, to date, no clear clinical applicability regarding natural history or pharmacologic responsiveness.[30]

Clinical Presentation

Acute HBV Infection. Like HAV, HBV infection can present across the clinical spectrum from subclinical infection through a self-limiting icteric illness to the dramatic presentation of fulminant hepatic failure. The severity of illness is generally inversely proportional to the age of virus acquisition. Specifically, greater than 90% of perinatal infections are asymptomatic, compared to 5% to 15% of infections in children less than the age of 5 and 33% to 50% in older children and adults.[31] Symptomatic infection can be characterized by a combination of nonspecific symptoms such as fatigue, myalgia, and low-grade fever and also includes more specific findings such as jaundice, right upper quadrant abdominal pain, acholic stool, dark urine, and nausea and vomiting.

Chronic HBV Infection. Chronic HBV infection is defined as the persistent presence of circulating hepatitis B surface antigen (HBsAg) for at least 6 months following exposure to the virus. HBsAg is also seen in acute HBV, so the clinical context must be taken into account. IgM antibody against the hepatitis B core antigen will be present in acute cases and can be used to differentiate acute from chronic hepatitis B if the distinction is not clinically apparent. HBV infection becomes chronic with an incidence inversely proportional to the age

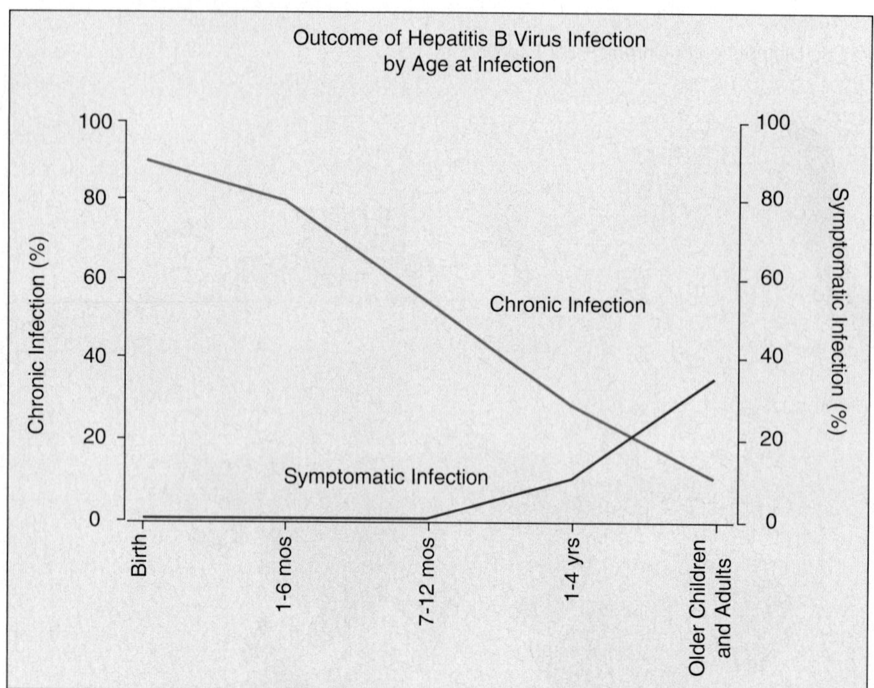

FIGURE 35-3 • Outcome of hepatitis B virus infection by age at infection. It is estimated that HBV becomes chronic in about 90% of persons infected in the perinatal period, about 25% to 50% of children infected under the age of 5, and about 5% to 10% of infected adults. (Figure from CDC. http://www.cdc.gov/NCIDOD/Diseases/Hepatitis/slideset/index.htm)

at viral acquisition, similar to the incidence of asymptomatic acute HBV. It is estimated that HBV becomes chronic in about 90% of persons infected in the perinatal period, about 25% to 50% of children infected under the age of 5, and about 5% to 10% of infected adults[30-32] (Fig. 35-3). A number of clinical syndromes have been defined under the category of chronic HBV infection.

Chronic HBV infection demonstrates considerable variability in serum aminotransferases, serologic patterns, histology, and natural history. Typically chronic replicative HBV infection is characterized by elevated aminotransferases, high HBV DNA, positivity of HBeAg, and evidence of histologic inflammation. It is increasingly recognized that a subset of patients with HBeAg-positive serologic status and high HBV DNA have normal transaminases and minimal histologic activity, a state that is referred to as "immune tolerant." This pattern is more common in younger HBV patients and appears to connote a benign prognosis, although more evidence regarding natural history is sought.[33] Chronic replicative HBV infection can lead to cirrhosis in some individuals, but others undergo a seroconversion with loss of HBeAg, development of anti-HBe, and diminution of HBV DNA. Conversion to this state, referred to as "inactive carrier state," can be associated with a flare in aminotransferases. Inactive carrier state HBV generally follows a benign course, but can be complicated by reactivation of viremia, sometimes in the setting of immune suppression. Others will undergo reactivation of HBV replication, but without reappearance of HBeAg.[35,36]

Recommendations for treatment of chronic hepatitis B based on these categories is in an active state of flux, but currently available guidelines are presented later. Although many individuals with chronic HBV infection are minimally affected and will die from nonhepatic diseases, it is estimated that some 15% to 25% of chronically infected individuals will eventually die as a direct result of hepatic disease or HBV-induced hepatocellular carcinoma.[37,38]

A number of extrahepatic manifestations of chronic HBV infection have been described. Among the most commonly seen and clinically significant are cryoglobulinemia, polyarteritis nodosa, leukocytoclastic vasculitis, membranous glomerulonephritis, and membranoproliferative glomerulonephritis.

Because HBV is a leading risk factor for the development of hepatocellular carcinoma, many authorities have recommended screening programs for this malignancy in high-risk populations. Common approaches include biannual measurements of serum α-fetoprotein and ultrasonography, although serial computed tomography scanning and magnetic resonance imaging are sometimes employed. To date, there is limited prospective evidence regarding the efficacy of such an approach.[33,39]

Hepatitis C Virus

Epidemiology

HCV infection is a leading cause of hepatic morbidity and mortality around the world. Although the prevalence of chronic HCV infection varies geographically, it has recently been estimated that global prevalence is about 2%, or some 123 million persons.[40] The existence of and quality of seroprevalence data vary widely across the globe. It is generally agreed that the infection is most prevalent in Africa and Asia, with lower seroprevalence rates in the industrialized countries such as those of the Americas, Europe, and Australia. Some of the highest reported seroprevalence rates are from Egypt (22%), Pakistan (4%), and China (3.2%). The lowest reported rates are from Germany (0.6%), India (0.9%), Australia (1.1%), and France (1.1%). Somewhat higher rates are reported in the United States (1.8%), Japan (1.5% to 2.3%), and Italy (2.2%)[41] (Fig. 35-4). Peak incidence of HCV infections appears to have taken place during the decade of the 1980s, with significantly lower incidence in subsequent years. This decreased incidence is thought to be a result of lower transmission rates among those persons injecting drugs, rather than screening of the blood supply. Because of the prolonged latency of HCV infectious complications, prevalence and impact of chronic infection are expected to increase over the next 2 decades.[42,43]

The leading modes of transmission of HCV infection, like prevalence rates, vary globally, but the majority can be attributed to intravenous drug use, blood transfusion, and unsafe therapeutic injection practices. Other parenteral exposure risks, such as medical procedures, tattooing, body piercing, scarification practices, and sexual transmission, are less important modes of transmission. In the United States, Europe, and Australia, intravenous drug use has been the leading mode of HCV transmission since the discovery of the virus. Rates of such transmission are clearly diminishing due in large part to safer injection practices. In the developing world, unsafe therapeutic injection has emerged as a major source of new HCV infections, accounting for an estimated 2 million new HCV infections in 2000.[23] An important example of this set of risk factors is Egypt's schistosomiasis eradication

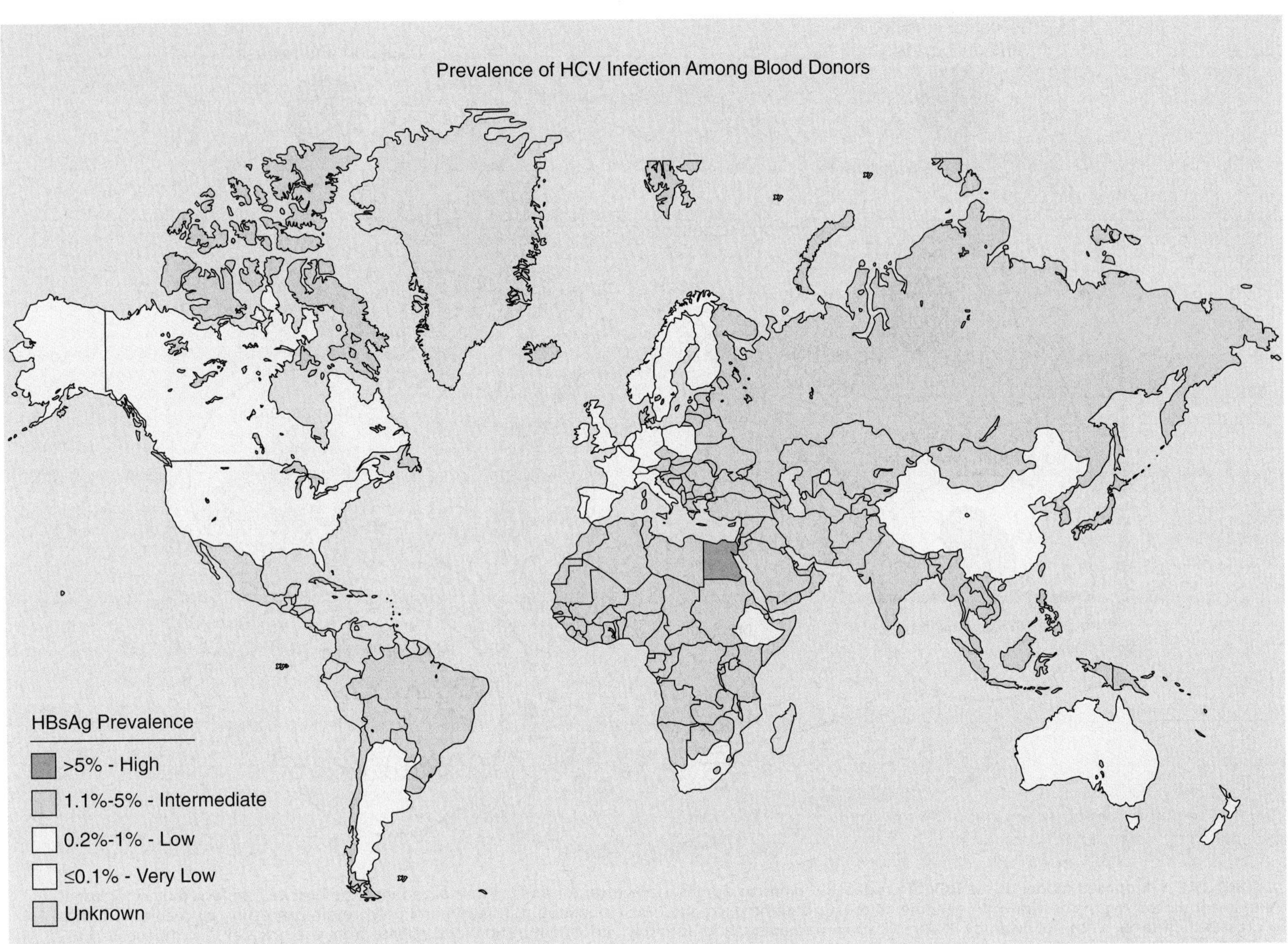

FIGURE 35-4 • Prevalence of HCV infection among blood donors. HCV infection is a leading cause of hepatic morbidity and mortality around the world. Although the prevalence of chronic HCV infection varies geographically, it has recently been estimated that global prevalence is about 2%, or some 123 million persons. (Figure from CDC. http://www.cdc.gov/NCIDOD/Diseases/Hepatitis/slideset/index.htm)

campaign, which resulted in the world's highest seroprevalance of HCV from reusable glass syringes.[44] Other significant data regarding this transmission mode are available from Pakistan[45] and Taiwan.[46]

Despite the rarity of blood transfusion–related HCV transmission in the industrialized nations, such transfusion is likely to contribute significantly to HCV incidence in the developing world. Transfusion-related infection has virtually disappeared from the United States, Europe, and Australia, largely to the adoption of all-volunteer donation systems but further aided by blood product screening for ALT, anti-HCV antibody, and HCV RNA.[47] Many countries around the world continue to use paid blood donors.[48,49] Furthermore, the World Health Organization estimated than only some 42% of blood products are screened for infectious agents.[50] Sexual transmission is thought to exist as a risk factor for HCV acquisition, but is considered to be inefficient and relatively unimportant from a public health standpoint.[51,52] The CDC recommends no change in sexual practices for monogamous couples in which one is chronically infected with HCV. Vertical transmission rates have been estimated at between 2.7% and 8.4% and appear to be increased in mothers co-infected with HCV and human immunodeficiency virus (HIV).[53,54]

Pathogenesis

The discovery of HCV as the major cause of non-A, non-B hepatitis in 1989 was accomplished through incisive use of the modern tools of molecular biology.[6] Since that time, progress on understanding the pathophysiology of HCV has been hampered by the lack of suitable laboratory models. The HCV replicon system has been the standard tool used to investigate HCV replication and inhibition.[55,56] HCV functional pseudoparticles and other modeling systems have added to the investigative armamentarium.[57,58] HCV has been classified as a flavivirus of the *Hepacivirus* genus. Similar viruses include yellow fever virus, dengue virus, and bovine diarrhea virus. Molecularly, HCV contains a 9.6-kb plus-strand RNA genome composed of a 5′ noncoding region, a long open reading frame encoding a polyprotein precursor of about 3000 amino acids, and a 3′ noncoding region. The structural proteins include the core protein, thought to represent the viral nucleocapsid, and the envelope glycoproteins E1 and E2. The envelope proteins form a noncovalent complex, the function of which is not fully understood.

The life cycle of HCV, as is implied by the previous discussion, is incompletely understood, but the following model has been proposed: HCV binding to a cell surface receptor; internalization into the host cell; cytoplasmic release and uncoating of the viral RNA genome; internal ribosome entry site–mediated translation and polyprotein processing by cellular and viral proteases; RNA replication, packaging, and assembly; and virion maturation and release from the host cell[59] (Fig. 35-5). Although a number of receptor candidates for HCV infection are being investigated, the details of this process are not understood.[60] A number of nonstructural proteins have been identified and characterized, providing potential strategies for therapeutic intervention. For example, the NS3 serine protease[61] and the NS5B RNA–dependent RNA polymerase[62] have emerged as potential targets for antiviral therapies.

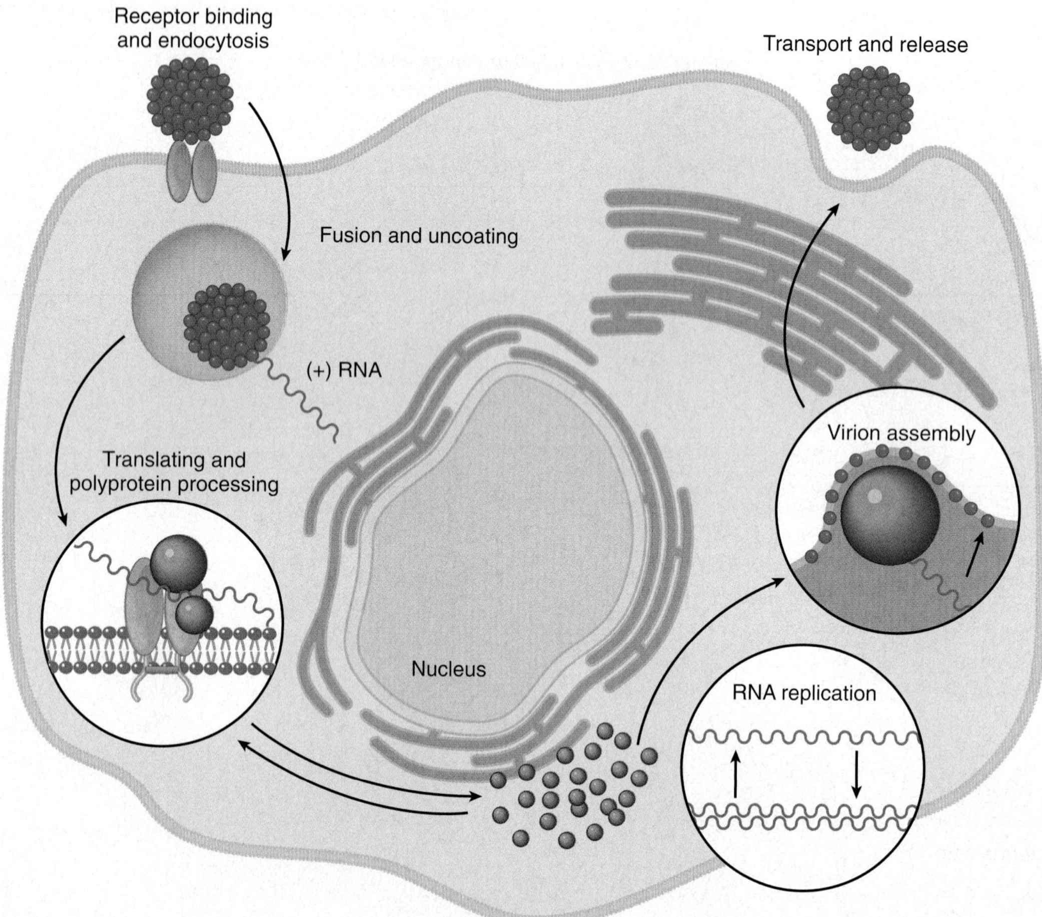

FIGURE 35-5 • Proposed model of the HCV life cycle. HCV binds to a cell surface receptor and is internalized into the host cell, followed by cytoplasmic release and uncoating of the viral RNA genome. Internal ribosome entry site (IRES)-mediated translation and polyprotein processing by cellular and viral proteases then takes place, followed by RNA replication, packaging, and assembly; virion maturation; and release from the host cell. (From Lindenbach BD, Rice CM. Unravelling hepatitis C virus replication from genome to function. Nature 2005;436:933-938.)

Clinical Presentation

Acute HCV Infection. The overwhelming majority of HCV infections that are seen clinically are chronic in nature. It should be noted, however, that there is a growing recognition of acute HCV infection, especially in the context of needle stick injury and intravenous drug use. The realization that acute infection, when treated early, has a very high therapeutic response rate has led to increased vigilance and surveillance for such infections. Acute hepatitis C presents in a fashion similar to the other hepatotropic viruses. Many infections will be subclinical, and others may present with classic symptoms such as nausea, vomiting, right upper quadrant pain, and malaise. A smaller percentage of cases will present with jaundice. There have been very few reported cases of HCV presenting with fulminant hepatic failure. The acute symptoms are self-limited, but the duration and severity of symptoms give no indication of the probability of chronicity. The significant spontaneous clearance rate of acute HCV infection has led to specific treatment delay recommendations when taking a clinical approach to such patients.

Chronic HCV Infection. Chronic HCV is the most common hepatotropic virus infection in the industrialized nations. The frequency with which the infection becomes chronic is in the range of 85% of exposed persons, explaining the high prevalence of chronic infection. Many cases of chronic HCV infection are asymptomatic or associated only with mild, nonspecific symptoms such as fatigue. Such nonspecific symptoms can be disruptive or even disabling, with consistently lower quality-of-life scores in HCV patients compared to matched controls. The most common presentation of chronic HCV is the incidental finding of mildly elevated serum aminotransferases. In such patients with a positive anti-HCV antibody, viremia can be detected in about 85%, denoting chronic infection. In those patients with detectable anti-HCV antibody but repeatedly undetectable virus, the difference between false-positive antibody test and resolved infection can be delineated by the recombinant immunoblot assay. Up to 30% of chronically infected patients will have persistently normal aminotransferases, so a high index of suspicion for potential infectious risk factors is necessary.[63] Natural history studies have shown that some 20% of chronically infected patients will develop hepatic cirrhosis over a period estimated to range from 20 to 30 years (Fig. 35-6). Although clinical evidence of cirrhosis may be suggested in some patients by physical examination, laboratory assessment, or radiographic studies, most patients, even those with significant liver fibrosis, will not demonstrate such findings. Therapeutic decisions regarding antiviral therapy must incorporate the estimated rate of progression.[64] Fibrotic progression is higher in male patients, those who drink larger amounts of alcohol, those with HIV co-infection, and those who have evidence of fibrosis on a liver biopsy. Most hepatologists prefer to include an examination of liver histology in the management of patients with chronic HCV infection.[65,66]

The quantification of HCV RNA has become an important part of the therapy for patients with chronic HCV infection; however, it is important to note that there is no correlation between viral load and disease severity.[67] The quantitative HCV polymerase chain reaction (PCR) provides information on treatment success and duration but not about natural history of disease. HCV has six major genotypes and more than 50 subtypes. Although HCV genotype does not correlate with disease severity, response rates to interferon-based regimens are substantially higher in patients infected with genotype 2 or 3.[68] Types 1, 2, and 3 are most common in Western Europe, North America,

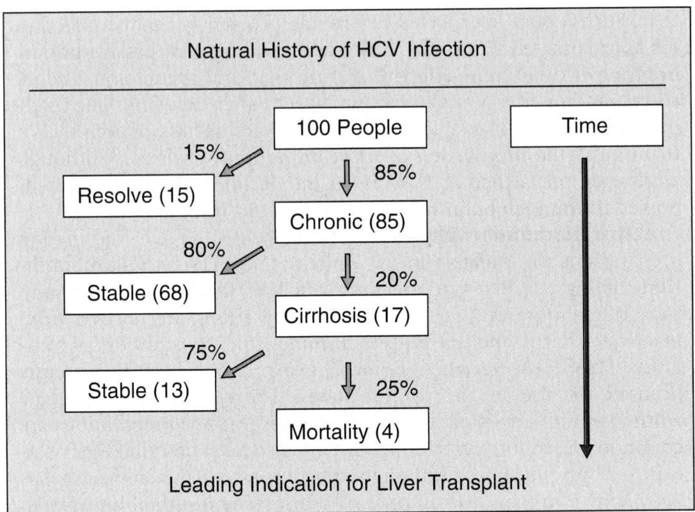

FIGURE 35-6 • Natural history of HCV infection. The frequency with which HCV infection becomes chronic is in the range of 85% of exposed persons, explaining the high prevalence of chronic infection. Natural history studies have shown that some 20% of chronically infected patients will develop hepatic cirrhosis over a period estimated at 20 to 30 years.

Australia, and the Far East.[69] Among U.S. patients with HCV infection, approximately 70% have genotype 1, 15% have genotype 2, and 10% have genotype 3.[70] Type 4, which has been reported to respond poorly to interferon-based therapies, is found especially in the Middle East and in central and northern Africa.[71] Genotype 5 is predominately found in South Africa, while genotype 6 is found almost exclusively in Southeast Asia.

Hepatitis E Virus

Epidemiology

Hepatitis E virus (HEV) is an enterically transmitted hepatotropic viral infection that was recognized and cloned in 1980 and sequenced shortly thereafter. It appears that this infection is relatively recent in humans, and it currently appears to be restricted to certain geographic areas characterized by poor environmental sanitation. Infection is frequently water borne, with outbreaks associated with flooding and contamination of the drinking supply.[72] HEV infection has been seen especially in epidemics, rather than sporadically. Affected areas of the globe include the Indian subcontinent, eastern Asia, Central Asia, and to a lesser extent Mexico, Africa, and the Middle East (Fig. 35-7). Besides large outbreaks such as the one seen in China in 1986-1988, sporadic cases can be seen in endemic areas.[73] Sporadic cases in other parts of the world appear to be restricted to recent travelers to endemic areas. The most affected population is 15- to 40-year-olds, with a slight

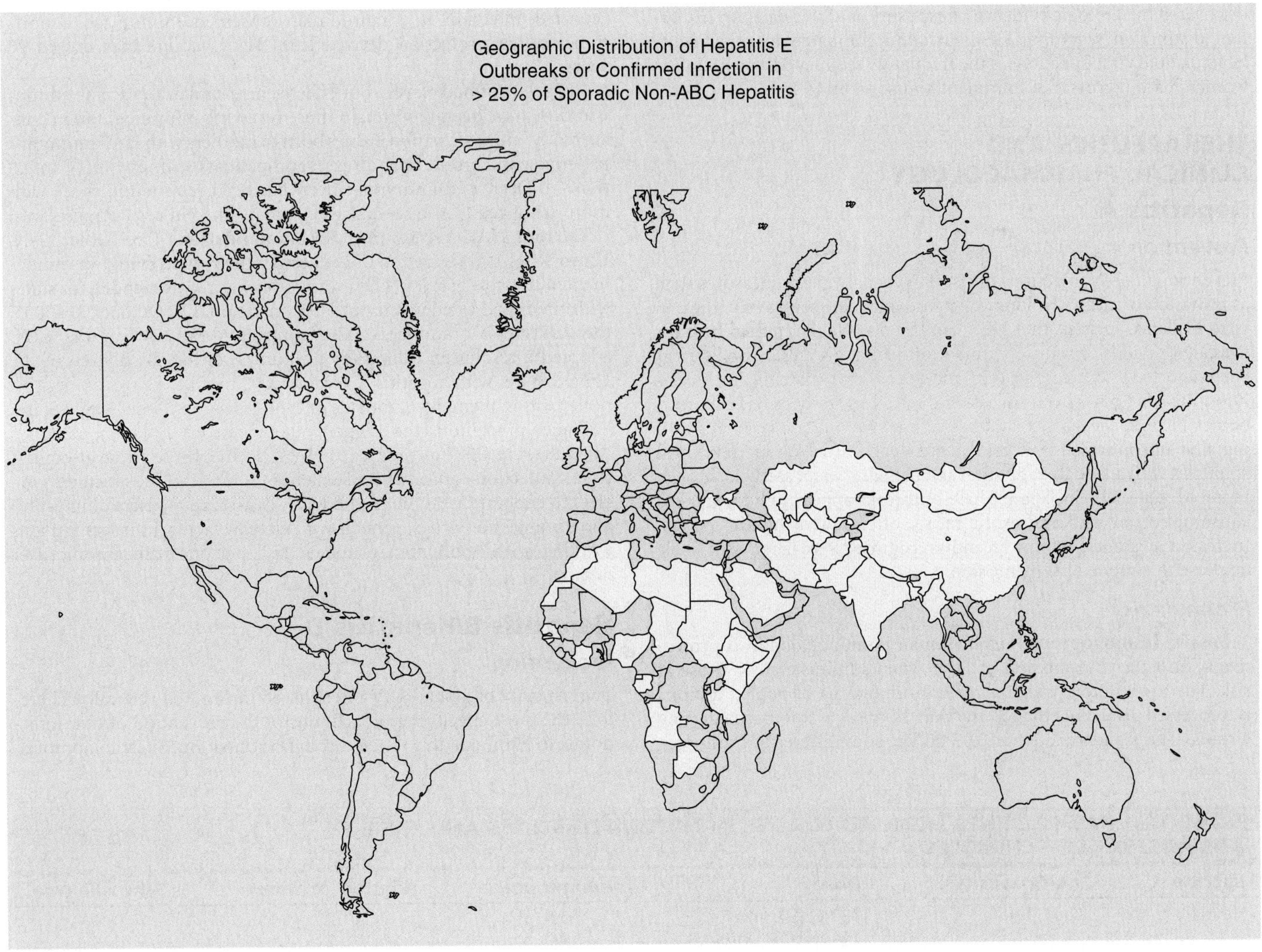

Geographic Distribution of Hepatitis E
Outbreaks or Confirmed Infection in
> 25% of Sporadic Non-ABC Hepatitis

FIGURE 35-7 • Geographic distribution of hepatitis E. HEV infection has been seen especially in epidemics, rather than sporadically. Affected areas of the globe include the Indian subcontinent, eastern Asia, central Asia, and to a lesser extent Mexico, Africa, and the Middle East. (Figure from CDC. http://www.cdc.gov/NCIDOD/Diseases/Hepatitis/slideset/index.htm)

male predominance. The very young have been noted to be relatively spared. For reasons that are not understood, HEV infection in pregnant women, especially in the third trimester, carries a high rate (15% to 25%) of fulminant hepatitis and death.[74-76]

Pathogenesis

HEV is a small, nonenveloped, 32- to 34-nm diameter virus provisionally classified in the family Caliciviridae, genus *Calicivirus*.[77] The HEV genome of 7.5 kb contains three overlapping open reading frames that are thought to code for structural and nonstructural proteins. Similar to the study of HCV, details of viral entry and replication are poorly delineated due to the lack of a reliable tissue culture system.[78,79] Several strains of the virus have been isolated, the two primary types being delineated the Burmese and the Mexican types. Other strains with a significant lack of genetic homology to the Burmese and Mexican strains have also been isolated.[80,81]

Clinical Presentation

Acute HEV Infection. Acute infection with HEV presents with symptoms similar to any acute hepatitis. The incubation period of 2 to 10 weeks can be associated with a viral prodrome, including symptoms of lassitude, myalgias, headache, and arthralgias; this prodrome often predates the onset of more severe symptoms, should the latter occur at all.[78] The majority of reported cases present in the icteric phase, often with right upper quadrant abdominal pain, nausea, and vomiting. Pruritis has been reported in up to 50% of cases.[82] Like other forms of viral hepatitis, HEV infection can be asymptomatic, only discovered by serologic evidence of exposure at a later date. An important distinction regarding HEV infection compared to other acute hepatotropic viral infections is the frequently seen severity in pregnant women, with reports of a fulminant course in up to 25%.[76]

THERAPEUTICS AND CLINICAL PHARMACOLOGY

Hepatitis A

Prevention

Prevention of HAV infection consists largely of hygienic measures such as provision of clean drinking water and adequate sewage facilities. In vitro evidence suggests that HEV can live outside the human host for extended periods of time. Treatment of drinking water by boiling has been reported to decrease severity and duration of epidemic outbreaks. Zoonotic spread has been suggested due to the presence of HAV antibodies in pigs, sheep, rats, and cattle, but this mode of transmission remains unconfirmed.[83] Recently, outbreaks of HAV in developed countries with adequate sanitation and drinking water safety have been reported, especially in Japan. These outbreaks appear to be related to consumption of wild and exotic meats, often raw or lightly cooked. Increased awareness of this recently recognized risk factor will likely decrease this mode of transmission.

Prophylaxis

Passive Immunoprophylaxis. Human immunoglobulin is protective against the transmission of HAV when administered to those at risk. The preparation, which is made from plasma of pooled donors, is processed by cold ethanol fractionation so as to inactivate any viruses. The standard dose is 0.02 ml/kg, administered intramuscularly. Such a dose is expected to provide protection against infection for approximately 3 months.[84] The administration of passive immunoprophylaxis is most effective during the viral incubation period, corresponding to a period of about 2 weeks after exposure. The coadministration of immunoglobulin and HAV vaccine has not been shown to diminish the effectiveness of active immunoprophylaxis.[85] Although worldwide prevalence of HAV is on the decline, the effectiveness of pooled immunoglobulin has not been thought to be attenuated.[86]

Active Immunoprophylaxis. Currently, two HAV vaccination preparations are available in the United States: Havrix (GlaxoSmithKline Biologicals, Rixensart, Belgium) and VAQTA (Merck & Company, Inc., Whitehouse Station, NJ). Both preparations are derived from inactivated virus and are highly immunogenic. In addition, a combined HAV/HBV vaccine (Twinrix; GlaxoSmithKline) is currently licensed for use in the United States. The schedules for vaccine administration are listed in Table 35-1. HAV vaccine preparations are commonly used for prevention, but have also been described for postexposure prophylaxis.[87] Although effectiveness of this approach has been shown in a limited number of trials, some health authorities in Canada and Europe have recommended vaccine rather than immunoglobulin for postexposure immunoprophylaxis.[88]

The chief use of HAV vaccine is preexposure prophylaxis in children. Studies have confirmed the immunogenicity and effectiveness of both U.S.-licensed preparations, with immunity rates in this setting of 94% to 100%.[89,90] Several lines of evidence have suggested that protection after the recommended vaccination series is quite long lasting. High protective antibody levels, kinetics models, and the lack of reported infection in longitudinally observed immunized cohorts indicate that protection derived from HAV vaccine may exceed 20 years.[91-93]

Reduced antibody levels, but effectiveness similar to vaccine administration, have been reported in those receiving immunoglobulin concurrently with vaccination, babies born to mothers with HAV immunity, patients with chronic liver disease, and patients with early HIV infection.[94-96] Decreased immunogenicity has been reported in those with more advanced HIV disease and recipients of solid organ transplants.

Current HAV Vaccination Recommendations (see Table 35-1). Universal HAV vaccination of children in the United States was implemented in two steps: in 1999, vaccination was recommended for states with the highest endemicity of HAV infection. On October 27, 2005, the Advisory Committee on Immunization Practices of the CDC adopted a resolution calling for immunization of all children in the United States with hepatitis A vaccine at 12 months of age.[97] Since this policy was implemented, the rate of HAV infection in the United States has fallen precipitously to 1.9 per 100,000 persons in the population.[98] In adults, the CDC recommends HAV vaccination to those at highest risk of infection and/or its consequences. Specific groups include travelers to endemic areas, men who have sex with men, users of injection and noninjection drugs, persons with clotting factor disorders, persons working with nonhuman primates, and persons with chronic liver disease.[99]

Hepatitis B/Hepatitis D

Prevention

The majority of global HBV infection is transmitted vertically. Therefore, the most effective approach toward the prevention of new infection is to eliminate this mode through vaccination. Such an approach

TABLE 35-1 HAV VACCINES LICENSED FOR USE IN THE UNITED STATES AND THEIR ADMINISTRATION SCHEDULES

Vaccine	Age Groups (yr)	Dose	Volume (ml)	Number of Doses	Schedule (mo)
Havrix	1-18	720 ELISA units	0.5	2	0, 6-12
	≥19	1440 ELISA units	1.0	2	0, 6-12
VAQTA	1-18	25 units	0.5	2	0, 6-12
	≥19	50 units	1.0	2	0, 6-12
Twinrix	≥18	720/20 ELISA units	1.0	3	0, 1, 6

is clearly effective in providing long-lasting immunity to large populations.[100] HBV vaccination was first routinely recommended in Chinese infants in 1992. With support from the World Health Organization, timely vaccination (within 24 hours of birth) has increased from 29.1% to 75.8% in the period from 1997 to 2003.[101] It is reasonable to assume, based on reports from smaller vaccination cohorts, that these interventions will dramatically reduce the burden of HBV-related disease in the coming decades.[102] In the United States, HBV remains a sexually transmitted disease, in addition to being transmitted through parenteral and vertical exposure. Therefore, prevention techniques, besides widespread use of the vaccine, must include education of high-risk groups. Because hepatitis D virus (HDV) can only affect those persons with chronic HBV infection, the strategy to prevent HDV infection is identical to efforts regarding HBV.

Prophylaxis

Postexposure HBV prophylaxis is indicated in a number of specific circumstances. Because standard immunoglobulin preparations do not contain adequate concentrations of anti-HBs to provide effective passive immunoprophylaxis, concentrated preparations are necessary. Hepatitis B immunoglobulin is derived from pooled blood donors and has found use in the setting of prevention of neonatal HBV infection and the prevention of reinfection of transplanted hepatic allografts.[103,104] Reactivation of HBV infection in previously exposed persons undergoing immunosuppression, especially cytotoxic chemotherapy, has led to the recommendation of lamivudine prophylaxis for certain high-risk groups.[105] It is likely that alternative antivirals or combination therapy will be required in this setting due to the development of lamivudine-resistant strains.[106,107]

Current HBV Vaccination Recommendations

Three hepatitis B vaccination products are currently available in the United States (Table 35-2). The CDC recommends the following HBV strategy[108]:

- Universal vaccination of infants beginning at birth
- Prevention of perinatal HBV infection through (i) routine screening of all pregnant women for HBeAg and (ii) immunoprophylaxis of infants born to HBeAg-positive women or to women with unknown HBeAg status
- Routine vaccination of previously unvaccinated children and adolescents
- Vaccination of previously unvaccinated adults at risk for HBV infection

Treatment of HBV Infection

Interferon

Mechanism of Action. Interferons are naturally occurring cytokines that have important innate antiviral effects in vivo. Type 1 interferons, the type used in the therapy of hepatitis B and C, include interferons α, β, γ, and ω. All of these types of interferons are thought to have innate antiviral, antiproliferative, and immunomodulatory properties. To date, it is the α interferons that have yielded the most results as pharmaceutical agents. The human interferon alfa family consists of at least 15 subtypes, ranging in molecular size from 17.5 to 23 kDa, each containing 165 or 166 amino acids. There is approximately 80% sequence homology between members of the group of proteins.[109] The mechanism of action of interferon alfa is not precisely known, but much has been elucidated about its action. Interferon, which is currently only parenterally administered, binds to and leads to dimerization of interferon cell surface receptor subunits. The next step involves activation of the receptor-associated Janus-activated kinase 1 and tyrosine kinase 2.[110] Transcription proteins 1 and 2 (STAT 1 and STAT 2) are in turn activated by these activated kinases. The activated STAT1/2 complex then migrates to the cell nucleus, forming a complex with interferon regulatory factor 9, where interaction with cellular DNA leads to expression of interferon-stimulated genes. A wide variety of gene products are expressed, many involved in antiviral activity.[111-115]

Pharmacokinetics. Oral absorption of interferons is low due to proteolysis of the protein in the digestive tract. To date, the only effective delivery of interferon is via the parenteral route. Intramuscular and submucosally administered interferon alfa is about 70% to 80% absorbed. Peak plasma concentrations are reached within 1 to 8 hours, and interferon can be measured in the serum for up to 24 hours following a single injection. Intravenous administration results in lower peak concentrations and shorter duration of serum levels.[109,116,117]

Following parenteral administration, interferon alfa concentrations decline in a biexponential pattern. Terminal elimination half-life has been measured at between 4 to 16 hours. Volume of distribution of interferon has been variously measured at 12 to 40 L/kg, corresponding to 20% to 60% of body weight. Interferon does not appear to cross the blood-brain barrier, but does cross the human placenta.[118,119]

Much of the research in interferon metabolism has been performed in animals. Alfa interferons are filtered through the kidney by luminal endocytosis, followed by proximal tubular reabsorption and lysosomal proteolysis, so that little interferon is found in the urine. The liver appears to play little role in the catabolism and elimination of interferon, which is not found in the bile. Estimated clearance of interferons is in the range of 5 to 32 L/hr.[109,116]

Interferon administration leads to a variety of physical side effects that vary widely among individuals. Acute side effects include influenza-like symptoms such as myalgias, arthralgias, pyrexia, headache, and lassitude. These side effects tend to subside with clearance of the drug from the system. Later and more persistent side effects with repeated administration include fatigue, weight loss, anorexia, and an assortment of neuropsychiatric side effects ranging from mild attention deficits through emotional lability to anger and depression. Suicide resulting from interferon-related depression has been described.[120] Serotonin reuptake inhibitors and other antidepressants have been used with success in ameliorating interferon-induced neuropsychiatric side effects.[121] Interferon also causes myelosuppressive effects, predominantly leukopenia and thrombocytopenia, although suppression of erythropoiesis is also encountered.[122] Interferon has been reported to reduce levels of microsomal cytochrome P-450 and thus affect levels of other drugs dependent on this pathway for clearance. It is unclear that this effect has clinical significance in humans.[109]

Peginterferon. Pegylation, the process of molecularly affixing a polyethylene glycol (PEG) moiety to a protein, was first described by Davis et al. in 1978.[68] This process allows for prolongation of the half-life of biologically active proteins by decreasing renal clearance and proteolytic degradation. Pegylated interferon was first designed using a 5-kDa PEG chain. Efficacy of the compound was unacceptable, leading to the development of peginterferons with larger PEG moieties.[123] Currently, two peginterferons are available for clinical use: peginterferon alfa-2a (Pegasys; Roche Laboratories, Nutley, NJ) and peginterferon alfa-2b (PEG-Intron; Schering-Plough, Kenilworth, NJ). Peginterferon alfa-2a utilizes two monomethoxy PEG chains, each with molecular weight of 20 kDa, linked to lysine residues in the interferon protein chain. Peginterferon alfa-2b utilizes a linear 12-kDa PEG moiety bound primarily to histidine residues. Given the difference in drug design, it is not surprising that the two molecules have differing pharmacokinetic characteristics.

Peginterferon alfa-2a, with a molecular weight of 40 kDa, when administered to healthy volunteers in the recommended 180-mcg subcutaneous dose, leads to detectable plasma concentration within 3 to 8 hours, with peak plasma levels between 72 and 96 hours. Absorption half-life is in the range of 60 hours. Mean elimination half-life is approximately 80 hours. Peginterferon alfa-2a appears to be restricted

TABLE 35-2 HBV VACCINES LICENSED FOR ADULT USE IN THE UNITED STATES AND THEIR ADMINISTRATION SCHEDULES

Vaccine	Dose	Volume (ml)	Number of Doses	Schedule (mo)
Recombivax	10 mcg	1.0	3	0, 1, 6
Engerix-B	20 mcg	1.0	3	0, 1, 6
Twinrix	20 mcg	1.0	3	0, 1, 6

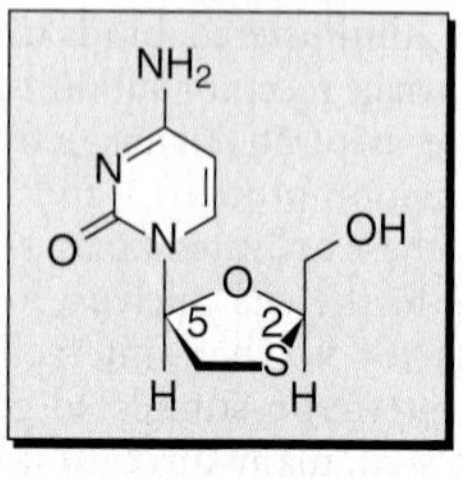

FIGURE 35-8 • Molecular structure of lamivudine.

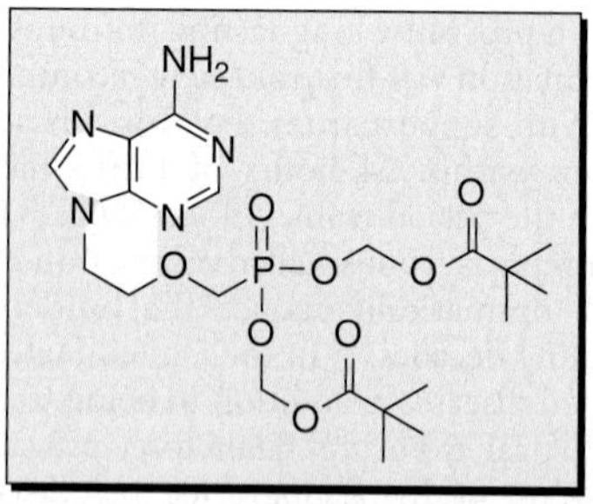

FIGURE 35-9 • Molecular structure of adefovir dipivoxil.

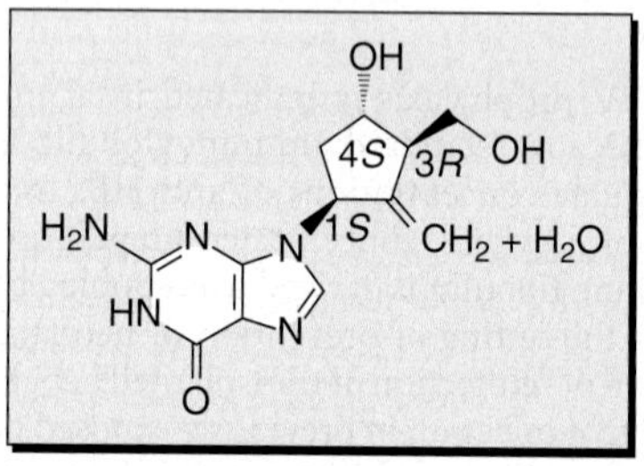

FIGURE 35-10 • Molecular structure of entecavir.

primarily to the intravascular compartment, with a volume of distribution of 4 to 16 L/kg, which corresponds to some four times less than unmodified interferon alfa. As a result, peginterferon alfa-2a is administered in a fixed dose regardless of body weight.

Peginterferon alfa-2b, with a molecular weight of 12 kDa, has an absorption half-life of 4.6 hours, with peak serum concentrations being reached by 15 to 44 hours. The volume of distribution of peginterferon alfa-2b, about 1.0 L/kg, is closer to that of unmodified interferon due to the smaller PEG moiety. As a result, this drug is dosed according to body weight. The currently licensed dose is 1.5 mcg/kg per week, although unconfirmed data suggest that 1.0 mcg/kg per week may have similar efficacy in certain circumstances.[124] The longer serum half-life of peginterferon alfa-2b is in large part due to the decreased elimination half-life of the drug, which is approximately 40 hours, some seven times greater than unmodified interferon.[123]

Lamivudine

Mechanism of Action. Lamivudine is a cytosine nucleoside analogue, which acts as a reverse transcriptase inhibitor. Lamivudine is the negative enantiomer of 2′-deoxy-3′-thiacytidine, which makes it less toxic than the positive enantiomer and more resistant to molecular degradation through deamination and the cleavage of 3′-5′ exonucleases[125] (Fig. 35-8). Its action as an L-nucleoside inhibits HBV DNA synthesis by disrupting DNA chain formation.

Pharmacokinetics. Lamivudine is readily and rapidly absorbed via the oral route, with peak concentrations reached approximately 30 to 90 minutes following administration.[126,127] Bioavailability is above 80% in adults, but some 10% lower in children.[125] Timing of meals does not affect lamivudine absorption.[128] Lamivudine exhibits linear pharmacokinetics with area under the curve (AUC) values corresponding to the magnitude of the dose, with parameters that are not affected by gender or race.[125]

The volume of distribution of lamivudine is approximately 1.3 L/kg when given intravenously.[126] The drug readily crosses the placenta and is present in breast milk.[129] Lamivudine crosses the blood-brain barrier, with cerebrospinal fluid concentrations of 4% to 8% and serum concentrations of 9% to 17% in adults and children, respectively.[129,130]

Lamivudine is primarily eliminated via the renal route, with some 70% of the unchanged drug found in urine.[131] Therefore, lamivudine dosing needs to be altered for patients with renal insufficiency, but not reduced in patients with hepatic dysfunction.[125,131] The elimination half-life of lamivudine approximates 5 to 7 hours, with an active 5′-triphosphate metabolite having a prolonged half-life of 10.5 to 15.5 hours.[125]

No interaction between lamivudine and cytochrome P-450 3A isozymes has been demonstrated. Other than a reduced extraction ratio of the drug seen with trimethoprim, no important drug interactions have been described.[125] Lamivudine is remarkably well tolerated, with a side effect profile similar to that of placebo in registration trials for treatment of HBV.[132]

Adefovir Dipivoxil

Mechanism of Action. Adefovir dipivoxil is the diester prodrug of adefovir, which is an acyclic deoxyadenosine monophosphate analogue (Fig. 35-9). Adefovir exerts its influence on HBV replication in the diphosphate form, which incorporates into HBV DNA during replication, inhibiting HBV reverse transcriptase.[133]

Pharmacokinetics. Phamacokinetic parameters for intravenous adefovir are independent of dose. Adefovir has poor oral bioavailability, although the dipivoxil modification significantly improves such bioavailability, to some 59%. Absorption is increased in the presence of food.[134] Peak concentrations in humans with chronic HBV infection occur around 1.75 hours following the dose.

The steady state volume of distribution of adefovir is 352 to 392 ml/kg. The drug is not significantly protein bound in humans.[133] In preclinical studies, it was found that the drug is distributed widely, but has especially high concentrations in the kidney, which may account for some of the clinically observed dose-limiting renal toxicity.[135]

Adefovir undergoes biexponential decline in the serum following intravenous administration.[133] Terminal elimination half-life ranges from 0.1 to 7 hours for the intravenous form. The oral dipivoxil form demonstrates a terminal elimination half-life of about 7.5 hours.[136] About 45% of the total adefovir dose is eliminated in the urine as unchanged drug.

Adefovir dipivoxil is a well-tolerated drug, with a side effect profile similar to that of placebo during registration trials.[137] Asthenia and diarrhea were among the most common reported adverse effects in the 10-mg daily dose, while pharnygitis and anorexia were seen with higher than placebo incidence in the 30-mg daily dose. Dose-dependent nephrotoxicity is the most significant adverse effect of the drug, with median increase in serum creatinine of 0.2 mg/dl in the 30-mg daily dosing groups. Exacerbation of HBV viremia and significant elevations of serum aminotransferases have been seen with discontinuation of adefovir therapy.

Entecavir

Mechanism of Action. Entecavir is a carbocyclic analogue of 2-deoxyguanosine (Fig. 35-10). It has very potent activity against HBV. Compared to adefovir and lamivudine, it shows greater than 100 times the potency against wild-type virus.[138] It inhibits viral replication by inhibiting priming, reverse transcription, and DNA elongation.

Pharmacokinetics. Entecavir is rapidly absorbed in a dose-dependent manner when administered orally, with peak plasma concentration occuring at approximately 0.6 to 1.0 hour. Steady state plasma concentrations of entecavir are reached at approximately day 6 to 10.[139,140] Mean AUC at steady state is dose dependent. Entecavir absorption is decreased when administered with food.[140]

Entecavir is widely distributed into tissues, with protein binding estimated at 13%. It has a mean terminal half-life ranging from 128 to 149 hours. Elimination is predominantly through the renal route, with 62% to 73% of the unchanged drug found in the urine.[139] Renal insuf-

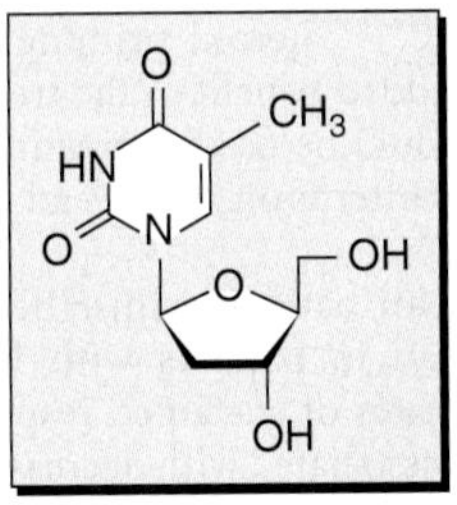

FIGURE 35-11 • Molecular structure of telbivudine.

ficiency causes accumulation of entecavir, but pharmacokinetic measures are not significantly affected by hepatic impairment.[140]

The side effect profile of entecavir, like that of the other HBV nucleoside and nucleotide analogues, is excellent. Percentages of adverse events were not significantly different than those reported by placebo arms in the registration trials. The most common adverse effects (reported in >10% of patients) were headache, upper respiratory tract infection, cough, nasopharyngitis, upper abdominal pain, fatigue, and fever.

Telbivudine

Mechanism of Action. Telbivudine (β-L-2′-deoxythymidine) is an L-enantiomer of thymidine (Fig. 35-11). Telbivudine demonstrates potent anti-HBV activity through the dual inhibition of reverse transcriptase and DNA polymerase. Activity requires biotransformation to the triphosphate form, which competes with thymidine triphosphate during DNA elongation.[141]

Pharmacokinetics. Telbivudine is well absorbed via the oral route, with an estimated bioavailability of 68%. The time to peak serum concentration is 0.8 to 2.8 hours, with AUC ranging from 1.1 to 47.5 mcg/ml per hour.[142] At steady state, the maximum concentration and AUC values are higher than with a single dose, indicating drug accumulation.[142]

Telbivudine is primarily excreted in a monophasic manner via the renal route, without the development of active metabolites. Maximum telbivudine exposure and concentration do not significantly differ in patients with renal or hepatic insufficiency, but increased elimination half-life in subjects with renal impairment has led to recommended dose reduction in such persons. Coadministration with food does not appear to affect the pharmacokinetics of telbivudine.[143]

Like the other HBV oral antivirals, telbivudine is well tolerated in clinical trials, with reports of adverse reactions not exceeding that reported by recipients in control groups. Although no significant drug-drug interactions have been described with telbivudine, caution with coadministration of allopurinol and probencid, which are inhibitors of nucleoside elimination, should be exercised.[141]

Other Agents

Tenofovir. Tenofovir is an acyclic adenine nucleotide, which is approved for use in HIV infection. Tenofovir has been shown to be efficacious in the treatment of patients co-infected with HIV/HBV who are resistant to lamivudine and/or interferon.[144] It also appears that tenofovir may be more potent than adefovir in non-HIV patients with known lamivudine-resistant infection, with a greater capability of inducing complete viral suppression.[145]

Emtricitabine. Emtricitabine, or 5-fluorocytidine, is a compound structurally similar to lamivudine. It is not yet approved for the treatment of HBV. The antiviral efficacy of the compound is good, rivaling other drugs in the class. Like lamivudine, emtricitabine is limited by the high development of HBV resistance after prolonged use, especially in patients with HBeAg-positive infection.[146]

Clevudine. Clevudine, a pyrimidine nucleoside analogue, has potent activity in vitro and in HBV-infected patients. Viral reductions appear to be sustained once the drug is discontinued, and drug-resistant viral strains have not yet been reported.[102,147]

Pharmacologic Approach to Treatment of HBV

Acute HBV Infection. In adults, the majority of acute HBV cases are self-limited and result in full recovery, with the subsequent development of neutralizing anti-HBs antibodies. However, it is known that a small proportion of acute HBV-infected persons can progress to acute liver failure, with the resulting need for liver transplantation, or death.[148] A number of case reports suggest the effectiveness of antiviral agents, especially lamivudine, in the setting of acute HBV infection, but a randomized trial failed to show improved outcomes, despite significant reductions in viremia in the treated groups.[149-151]

TABLE 35-3 THERAPEUTIC APPROACH FOR CHRONIC HEPATITIS B INFECTION

HBV DNA	ALT	Recommendation
HBeAg-Positive HBV		
<20,000	Normal	• No treatment. • Monitor every 6-12 mo. • Consider therapy in patients with known histologic disease even if low-level replication.

≥20,000	Normal	• Consider liver biopsy, especially if older than 35-40 yr.
		• Treat if significant histologic disease.
		  • Peginterferon
		  • Adefovir
		  • Entecavir
		• In absence of treatment, monitor every 6-12 mo.

≥20,000	Elevated	• Treatment recommended.
		  • Peginterferon
		  • Adefovir
		  • Entecavir
		• If "high" HBV DNA, oral agents preferred over peginterferon.

HBeAg-Negative HBV		
HBV DNA	**ALT**	**Recommendation**
<20,000	Normal	• No treatment. • Monitor every 6-12 mo. • Consider therapy in patients with known histologic disease even if low-level replication.

≥20,000	Normal	• Consider liver biopsy, especially if older than 35-40 yr.
		• Treat if significant histologic disease.
		  • Peginterferon
		  • Adefovir
		  • Entecavir
		• In absence of treatment, monitor every 6-12 mo.

≥20,000	Elevated	• Treatment recommended.
		  • Peginterferon
		  • Adefovir
		  • Entecavir
		• Long-term therapy required for oral agents.

Adapted from Keeffe EB, Dieterich DT, Han SH, et al. A treatment algorithm for the management of chronic hepatitis B virus infection in the United States: an update. Clin Gastroenterol Hepatol 2006;4:936-962.

Chronic HBV Infection (Table 35-3). Given the high morbidity of chronic HBV, even in the absence of established cirrhosis, treatment is aimed at suppressing viral replication to prevent progression of liver disease and diminish the development of cirrhosis, decompensated liver disease, or hepatocellular cancer. In patients with HBeAg-positive disease, the goal is to achieve seroconversion to HBeAg-negative disease. However, in patients with HBeAg-negative disease and persistent viral replication—that is, those with the precore mutant variety of chronic hepatitis B, which does not express HBeAg—the goal is persistent viral suppression. This goal often requires ongoing long-term treatment.[152]

In order to understand and compare efficacy of different treatments in clinical trials, similar definitions of response to treatment should be used and specific end points should be reported. Response can be defined in three categories: biochemical response refers to normalization of ALT, virologic response is defined as undetectable HBV DNA levels and seroconversion to HBeAg-negative status, and histologic response is a decrease in histologic activity by at least 2 points in the absence of advancing fibrosis. A complete response is defined by achieving all three of these end points. Failure to decrease HBV DNA to less than 2 $\log_{10}$ IU/ml on oral treatment is called "primary nonresponse," while increase in HBV DNA of greater than 1 $\log_{10}$ IU/ml upon discontinuation of treatment is referred to as "virologic relapse." Treatment success is further defined as response maintained while on treatment, at the end of treatment, sustained at 6 months, and sustained at 12 months.[38,39,152]

Determining whom to treat is important in the management of HBV. Many patients have chronic inactive infection or normal histologic findings that do not warrant treatment. This is especially true with the development of oral therapies, where the limits of potential viral resistance must be balanced against the potential for progressive liver disease or hepatic decompensation.[152] In general, treatment should be reserved for patients who have high viral loads, abnormal liver tests, and/or evidence of histologically progressive disease. As HBeAg-negative patients tend to have lower viral loads even in the presence of significant inflammatory disease, a lower threshold of HBV DNA should be used in considering initiation of treatment in this group of patients.[38,39]

Interferon. Interferon exerts its affect on HBV through both antiviral and antiproliferative means. In addition, it has been shown to stimulate natural killer cells, which play a role in HBV clearance.[153] Numerous trials have evaluated the efficacy of interferon in HBV treatment. One of the key factors affecting this drug's ability is the presence of HBeAg, which implies replication and the lack of resistance-inducing viral mutations. A meta-analysis of the effect of interferon in HBeAg-positive patients treated with interferon ranging from 7 to 30 MU/wk for 3 to 6 months showed 33% sustained eradication of viral replication, 37% loss of HBeAg, and 7.8% loss of HBsAg.[154] Higher doses of interferon are associated with higher rates of response. HIV co-infection, Asian origin, and lower pretreatment ALT are associated with lower response to interferon.[155] Other factors that have been associated with higher interferon response in the treatment of chronic HBV include chronic active hepatitis on liver biopsy, low hepatitis HBV DNA, high aspartate aminotransferase pretreatment levels, and shorter duration of HBV infection.[156] HBV genotype, which has not yet seen wide clinical use, may also play a role in predicting response to interferon.[157] The lack of consistently reported paired liver biopsies makes conclusions on histologic response inaccurate. Response to interferon in HBeAg-positive HBV infection appears to be long lasting, with persistent loss of viremia in the majority of responders. One trial reported loss of HBeAg in 65% of such responders, with no evidence of clinical progression of disease.[158] Survival data based on interferon treatment response have yielded mixed results, but most investigators describe improved outcomes, particularly in patients with pretreatment hepatic cirrhosis.[159-163] Steroid priming followed by interferon treatment provides no added benefit in the treatment of chronic HBV infection.[164] Caution should be used in treating patients with decompensated cirrhosis as interferon can lead to worsening clinical status.[165]

Interferon treatment for patients with HBeAg-negative disease has been less successful than in patients with HBeAg-positive disease, mainly due to the low rates of sustained response.[166] However, interferon treatment may be associated with decrease in fibrosis progression in those patients who do achieve a sustained virologic response.[167] Re-treatment or prolonged treatment in patients who do not initially respond to interferon may offer biochemical and histologic benefits.[168,169]

Peginterferon. The easier administration, higher serum interferon levels, and prolonged half-life of peginterferon make the agent an attractive choice in the treatment of HBV. In HBeAg-positive patients, 48 weeks of peginterferon alfa-2b yielded HBeAg seroconversion in 32%, HBV DNA levels below 100,000 copies/ml in 32%, and HBsAg seroconversion in 3.8% after 24 weeks of follow-up.[170] Successful peginterferon therapy is significantly associated with younger age, female gender, high baseline ALT, low baseline HBV DNA, and HBV genotype other than type D.[171] The use of smaller doses or shorter treatment duration is under further study.[172] Peginterferon is more efficacious than lamivudine monotherapy in HBeAg-positive disease. Combination treatment with peginterferon and lamivudine appears to add no benefit over the use of peginterferon alone.[170,173]

Unlike the experience with unmodified interferon, peginterferon has been used successfully in the treatment of HBeAg-negative chronic HBV. Treatment with 48 weeks of peginterferon alfa-2a resulted in HBV DNA levels less than 20,000 copies/ml in 59%, sustained HBV DNA less than 400 copies/ml in 19%, and loss of HBsAg in 3.4% of patients after 24 weeks of follow-up.[174] Based on these studies, peginterferon-alpha 2a was approved for the treatment of hepatitis B in the United States in May of 2005.

Nucleoside and Nucleotide Analogues (Table 35-4). It has become clear that HBV treatment paradigms now take two major forms: time-limited treatment regimens, in which e-antigen seroconversion and persistent loss of HBV replication following therapy is the goal; and suppressive regimens, in which the expectation of longer, even indefinite pharmacologic therapy provides ongoing viral suppression. The nucleotide and nucleoside analogues, although initially evaluated as drugs that could provide sustained response, have evolved into agents for which long-term use is standard, especially in e-antigen–negative chronic HBV infection.

Lamivudine was the first nucleoside analogue to enter the HBV armamentarium. Registration trials showed histologic response in 52% of patients, loss of HBeAg in 32%, sustained suppression of HBV DNA in 44%, sustained normalization of serum ALT in 41%, and "triple seroconversion," defined as the loss of HBeAg, undetectable levels of serum HBV DNA, and the appearance of antibodies against HBeAg, in 17% after 52 weeks of lamivudine 100 mg daily.[175] The drug showed similar effectiveness in Asian patients and is well tolerated.[176] Longer

TABLE 35-4 DRUGS APPROVED FOR HBV THERAPY: RESULTS OF VARIOUS PARAMETERS AFTER 1 YEAR OF THERAPY

		Peg %	Lam %	Emt %	Tel %	Ent %	Ade %	Pla %
eAg⁺	Loss of HBsAg	3	<1	<1	<1	1.7	<1	<1
	Loss of HBeAg	30	22	14	26	22	24	12
	Lack of DNA	25	39	39	60	67	21	1
	ALT normal	39	66	65	77	68	48	21
	Improved histology	38	59	62	65	72	53	25
eAg⁻	Loss of HBsAg	4	<1	<1	<1	<1	<1	<1
	Lack of DNA	63	72	79	88	90	51	2
	ALT normal	38	74	65	74	78	72	24
	Improved histology	48	63	59	66	70	64	28

Ade, adefovir; ALT, alanine aminotransferase; Emt, emtricitabine; Ent, entecavir; HBeAg, hepatitis B e antigen; HBsAg, hepatitis B surface antigen; Lam, lamivudine; Tel, telbivudine; Peg, peginterferon; Pla, placebo.

Adapted from Hoofnagle JH, Doo E, Liang TJ, et al. Management of hepatitis B: summary of a clinical research workshop. Hepatology 2007;45:1056-1075.

duration of therapy has been associated with improved outcomes in those who respond, but are associated with significant incidences of viral mutation and drug resistance.[132,177] Lamivudine resistance, which can be estimated at a rate of 15% to 20% per year on therapy, has resulted in resistance rates of up to 80% of patients at 5 years of treatment. Viral breakthrough associated with the emergence of mutation can be associated with flares in serum transaminases and worsening clinical outcomes. Even in the absence of such events, there is no benefit to continued lamivudine treatment after the development of HBV mutation.[178] The concern about the emergence of treatment-resistant viral mutants has resulted in many treatment algorithms not including lamivudine as first-line therapy.[179]

Adefovir dipivoxil, the prodrug of adefovir, was the second oral agent approved for use for the treatment of chronic HBV in the United States. The agent is not as potent an antiviral as lamivudine, but histologic responses are similar and the drug has been associated with considerably lower rates of viral mutation and drug resistance.[35] In e-antigen–positive patients, adefovir for 48 weeks at the best tolerated dose, 10 mg daily, was associated with histologic improvement in 53%, reduction of HBV DNA to less than 400 copies/ml in 21%, normalization of ALT in 48%, and HBeAg seroconversion in 12%.[137] In e-antigen–negative patients, 48 weeks of adefovir 10 mg daily resulted in histologic improvement in 77%, reduction of HBV DNA to less than 400 copies/ml in 51%, and normalization of ALT in 72%.[180] Discontinuation of adefovir in e-antigen–negative patients resulted in loss of benefit, while continuation of therapy for up to 144 weeks was well tolerated and associated with a viral resistance rate of 5.9%.[181] Adefovir has significant activity against strains of HBV with lamivudine resistance, although resistance has been reported to adefovir/lamivudine combination therapy.[182]

Entecavir, which was approved for use in the United States by the U.S. Food and Drug Administration (FDA) in 2005, is an acyclic adenine nucleotide with significant anti-HBV activity. Compared to adefovir and lamivudine, entecavir has greater than 100 times the potency against wild-type virus. In HBV e-antigen–positive patients, entacavir 0.5 mg daily for 52 weeks was associated with histologic improvement in 72%, reduction of HBV DNA to levels undetectable by PCR in 67%, normalization of ALT in 68%, and HBeAg seroconversion in 21%.[183] In HBV e-antigen–negative patients, entacavir 0.5 mg daily for 52 weeks was associated with histologic improvement in 70%, reduction of HBV DNA to levels undetectable by PCR in 90%, and normalization of ALT in 78%.[184] Viral resistance was very low in the registration trials and has remained at low rates in subsequent follow-up.[185,186] Entecavir is approved for the treatment of lamivudine-resistant HBV, but a daily dose of 1.0 mg needs to be employed, and such strains are prone to the development of entecavir resistance.[187] Entecavir-resistant HBV strains appear to be sensitive to adefovir therapy.

Telbivudine, or β-L-2′-deoxythymidine, is a nucleoside analogue with greater potency than, but a resistance profile similar to, lamivudine. In a study of 921 HBeAg-positive and 446 HBeAg-negative chronic hepatitis B patients, telbivudine resulted in significantly superior viral suppression and ALT normalization than in those patients treated with lamivudine. HBeAg loss and seroconversion were statistically more likely in the telbivudine group if the pretreatment ALT was greater than two times the upper limit of normal. For HBeAg-negative disease, telbivudine was statistically superior to lamivudine with regard to HBV DNA suppression but identical to lamivudine with regard to ALT normalization. Like lamivudine, telbivudine has a significant resistance profile. At the end of 2 years of treatment, patients on telbivudine experienced 21.6% genotypic resistance for HBeAg-positive disease and 8.6% genotypic resistance for HBeAg-negative disease. The resistance pattern overlapped that of lamivudine, thus limiting the use of telbivudine in lamivudine-exposed patients.[188]

Emtricitabine, or 5-fluorocytidine, is a compound structurally similar to lamivudine. As of this writing, the drug is not yet FDA approved for the treatment of HBV. Like lamivudine, emtricitabine is limited by its high development of resistance to HBV after prolonged use, especially in patients with HBeAg-positive infection. In terms of efficacy, emtricitabine is similar to lamivudine. A recent study comparing 52 weeks of emtricitabine 200 mg daily versus placebo for both HBeAg-positive and HBeAg-negative disease showed viral response rates of 39% and 79%, respectively.[146]

Emerging Therapies for HBV Infection. Many new HBV therapies are nucleoside or nucleotide analogues that target HBV reverse transcriptase. In addition to the currently available compounds (see Table 35-4), nucleoside analogues under development include tenofovir, clevudine, elvucitabine, valtoricitabine, amdoxovir, and racivir as well as several other compounds in preclinical or early clinical phases. A promising target for HBV drug development is agents that block encapsidation and HBV core antigen translation. Heteroaryldihydropyrimidines inhibit HBV replication by binding and degrading HBV core protein, preventing formation of the HBV nucleocapsid. Phenylpropenamides are agents that appear to directly prevent nucleocapsid formation, although these agents have not entered clinical trials. Glucosidase inhibitors block capsid assembly by blocking glycosylation of HBV envelope proteins. Immunomodulatory agents designed to activate HBV-specific $CD4^+$ T helper (Th) and $CD8^+$ cytotoxic T lymphocytes are also under development. Therapeutic vaccination has been under investigation for some years as a method to stimulate humoral or cellular immunity in persons chronically infected with HBV. A variety of other approaches to HBV infection are in early phases of development, including TLR ligands, cytotoxic T lymphocyte–based immunotherapy, cytokine manipulation, and gene therapy.[189,190]

Hepatitis C

Prevention

Transmission of HCV now only rarely takes place in the setting of blood product infusion due to the recognition of the virus, its antibody, and widespread screening of the blood supply by serologic and molecular methods. In the developed nations, the most common mode of transmission remains the use of intravenous drugs. Since this recognition, the incidence of HCV has declined steadily, most likely due to changes in behavior of intravenous drug users. Other measures that have contributed to a decreased incidence of HCV include more careful infection control measures in health care settings, particularly hemodialysis units (Fig. 35-12). Ongoing reports of nosocomial infection indicate the need for continued surveillance, education, and regulatory attention.

Prophylaxis

Because antibodies produced in response to HCV infection classically do not provide protective immunity, infusion of such antibodies is not expected to provide preexposure or postexposure prophylaxis. Recent

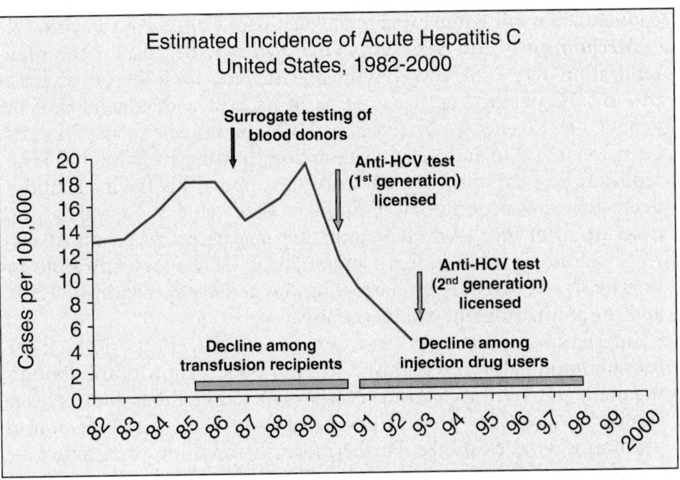

FIGURE 35-12 • Estimated incidence of acute HCV infection. The incidence of HCV has declined steadily since discovery of the virus, most likely due to changes in behavior of intravenous drug users. Other measures that have contributed to decreased incidence of HCV include more careful infection control measures in health care settings, particularly hemodialysis units.

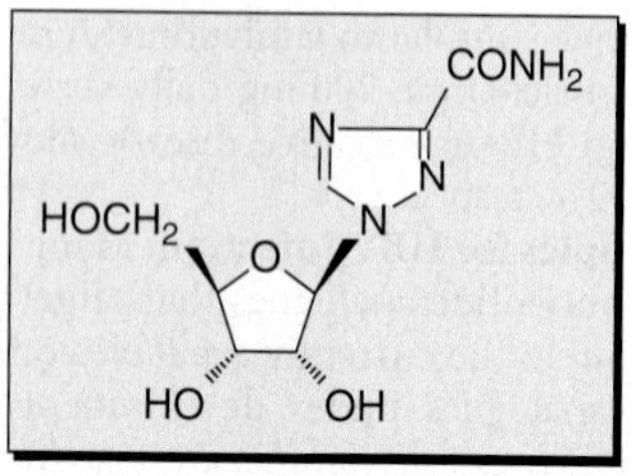

FIGURE 35-13 • Molecular structure of ribavirin.

work has focused on the production of monoclonal antibodies against the E2 envelope protein of HCV, which has been demonstrated to interfere with HCV infection in a murine model. Early human use is targeted for prevention of reinfection of liver allografts following transplantation.[191] In the clinical setting of acute exposure to HCV, early detection of seroconversion with prompt interferon-based treatment has yielded excellent clearance rates.

Treatment of HCV Infection

Interferon. The mechanism of action and pharmacokinetics of interferon in the treatment of HCV infection are the same as those for HBV infection (see Hepatitis B/Hepatitis D earlier).

Ribavirin

Mechanism of Action. Ribavirin is a guanosine analogue that has been used as an antiviral in a number of applications since its synthesis in 1972[192] (Fig. 35-13). Early use of ribavirin included oral administration for treatment of Lassa fever, measles, and hepatitis A.[193-195] In the United States its use, until recently, had been largely in the form of an aerosol for the treatment of respiratory syncytial virus in infants and influenza in young adults.[196-198] Although the mechanism of action is incompletely understood, several mechanisms have been proposed: direct inhibition of HCV replication, inhibition of inosine monophosphate dehydrogenase (IMPDH), promotion of viral mutagenesis, immunomodulation, and intracellular synergy with interferon.[199]

Intracellular phosphorylation of ribavirin forms a monophosphate, a diphosphate, and a triphosphate. Incorporation of ribavirin triphosphate by RNA polymerases appears to cause early chain termination.[115] The concentrations of ribavirin able to cause this effect in experimental models are clinically untenable, thus this mechanism cannot account for the demonstrated clinical efficacy. Another of the products of ribavirin metabolism, ribavirin monophosphate, is a competitive inhibitor of IMPDH. IMPDH leads to depletion of the GTP necessary for viral RNA synthesis. This effect is only partially reversible by addition of GTP to the HCV replicon system. Again, this effect is thought to contribute to, but not entire explain, the therapeutic effects of ribavirin.[115]

Mechanism of Interferon/Ribavirin Synergy. Because of the high replication rate of HCV, combined with lack of RNA polymerase proofreading ability, the virus exists in its host with a great deal of genetic heterogeneity, referred to as HCV quasispecies. Ribavirin has been theorized to induce viral mutation, leading to failure of viral replication.[200] Experimental evidence to support this theory includes decreased transfection of HCV in the replicon system[201] as well as the description of increased HCV mutation in patients receiving ribavirin.[202] Thus, ribavirin-induced mutation of HCV may contribute to interferon effectiveness by narrowing the genetic spectrum of HCV and preventing mutant escape variants.

Interferon is understood to exert its antiviral effects through an immunomodulatory mechanism. Immunomodulation is also among the many putative mechanisms of ribavirin action. Ribavirin has been shown to favor the production of Thl over Th2 $CD4^+$ response, promoting viral clearance. Furthermore, the addition of ribavirin to interferon results in more potent HCV-specific T-cell responses and increased sustained virologic response.[203,204] That ribavirin can synergize the intracellular action of interferon has been demonstrated by the favorable up- and down-regulation of cytokines that have been implicated in interferon-based antiviral effects.[205]

Pharmacokinetics. Ribavirin is rapidly and efficiently (85%) absorbed from the gastrointestinal tract, with bioavailability of approximately 50%. Mean time to maximal serum concentration is about 1.5 hours, with half-life of the distribution phase of about 3.7 hours.[206,207] Food increases plasma levels significantly.[206] With multiple dosing, ribavirin accumulates in plasma, with maximal concentration being achieved in about 4 weeks. Maximal concentration with multiple-dose administration is nearly five times that of mean maximal concentration with a single dose.[207]

The volume of distribution of ribavirin is estimated at about 10 L/kg, largely due to extensive cellular uptake of the drug. Ribavirin does not bind to plasma proteins, but rather appears to be absorbed into various cellular compartments due to the ubiquity of nucleoside transporter molecules.[208] Ribavirin is phosphorylated by adenosine kinase into ribavirin monophosphate, which is dephosphorylated in nucleated cells but accumulates in anucleate cells such as the erythrocyte.

Ribavirin pharmocokinetics are characterized by a rapid absorption and distribution phase, but prolonged elimination phase. Single-dose elimination half-life is about 79 hours, with a terminal elimination phase of about 100 hours.[199] Ribavirin is about 5% to 15% renally cleared, with the major route of elimination being metabolic. The similar elimination behavior of the drug in subjects with normal versus diseased livers is taken as evidence of the lack of significant hepatic metabolism. Elimination from erythrocytes is slow, with a half-life estimated at around 40 days, likely due to splenic hemolysis. Ribavirin clearance is significantly slowed in individuals with renal insufficiency.[199]

The major dose-limiting side effect of ribavirin is hemolytic anemia. In early registration trials, anemia led to dose reductions in up to 40% of subjects and discontinuation of ribavirin therapy in up to 20%.[124,209] Ribavirin is a known teratogen; effective contraception for women of childbearing potential and their partners is required.[210]

Clinical Use of Interferon, Ribavirin, Peginterferon, and Combination Therapy

Treatment Definitions. Clinical trials of HCV antivirals involve specific outcome measures to assess efficacy. Biochemical response is defined as normalization of serum aminotransferases, especially ALT. Such a response can be maintained during treatment, at the end of treatment, or sustained at a given time length after cessation of treatment. Biochemical response is now considered of limited significance when compared to virologic response, which is defined as lack of detectible circulating virus during, at the completion of, or following antiviral therapy. The most important treatment landmarks are the end-of-treatment virologic response (ETVR) and the sustained virologic response (SVR), the latter usually defined as 6 months following completion of therapy. The difference between ETVR and SVR can be taken as the relapse rate.

Treatment of Acute Hepatitis. Natural history studies suggest that at least 15% of those individuals exposed to HCV will resolve their infection spontaneously. Therefore, prophylactic treatment of exposed individuals, even with evidence of seroconversion and viremia, is not recommended.[211] Because antiviral therapy of acute HCV is associated with considerably higher response rates than treatment of chronic infection, early treatment is tempting to both the clinician and the exposed individual. Careful consideration is required in choosing candidates for and the timing of treatment of acute infection. Heterogeneity of early studies led to difficulty in determining the optimal form of interferon, need for ribavirin combination therapy, appropriate delay in commencement of therapy, and duration of treatment.[212,213] A number of prospective randomized trials have now made more evidence-based recommendations possible.

Regarding acceptable delay prior to initiation of treatment, a U.S. group compared treatment initiations of 8 weeks, 12 weeks, and 20 weeks following infection, noting sustained virologic response rates of 95%, 92%, and 76%, respectively, with overall SVR of 87%.[214] Regarding duration of antiviral therapy, the same investigators compared treatment durations of 8 weeks, 12 weeks, and 24 weeks with peginterferon alfa-2b, noting sustained virologic response rates of 67%, 82%, and 91%, respectively. All responses were durable 48 weeks following cessation of antiviral therapy.[215] A European investigative group

TABLE 35-5 DRUGS APPROVED FOR HCV THERAPY

Generic Name	Trade Name	Dosing	SVR	SVR G1	SVR G2/G3	Reference
Interferon alfa	Intron A Referon Infergen	3 MU tiw 3 MU tiw 9-15 mcg tiw	8% 11% 12%	N/A N/A N/A	N/A N/A N/A	218 225 248
Interferon + ribavirin	Rebetron	IFN: 3 MU tiw RBV: 1000-1200 mg daily divided bid	38%	28%	66%	70
Peginterferon alfa-2a	Pegasys	180 mcg subQ weekly	39%	28%	N/A	226
Peginterferon alfa-2b	PEG-Intron	1.5 mcg/kg subQ weekly	23%	14%	49%	227
Peginterferon alfa-2a + ribavirin	—	IFN: 180 mcg subQ weekly RBV: 1000-1200 mg daily divided bid	56%	46%	76%	209
Peginterferon alfa-2b + ribavirin	—	IFN: 1.5 mcg/kg subQ weekly RBV: 400 mg PO bid	54%	42%	82%	124

bid, twice daily; G1, HCV genotype 1; G2, HCV genotype 2; G3, HCV genotype 3; IFN, interferon; MU, million units; N/A, information not available; PO, orally; RBV, ribavirin; subQ, subcutaneously; SVR, sustained virologic response; tiw, three times weekly.

reported slightly less efficacy, with ETVR in 82% and SVR in 71% of those treated with peginterferon alfa-2b for 24 weeks. When the group adhering to 80% or more of the recommended dose for 80% or more of the recommended treatment duration was subjected to subanalysis, the ETVR was 94% and the SVR 89%.[216] Based upon extent data, it seems reasonable to recommend a treatment delay of no longer than 12 weeks, followed by at least 24 weeks of peginterferon. The role of longer treatment durations and the addition of ribavirin remain unproven.

Treatment of Chronic Hepatitis (Table 35-5). Interferon alfa monotherapy was approved for use in the treatment of HCV in 1991. Response was initially defined by sustained normalization of serum aminotransferases, which was seen in approximately 25% of treated persons.[217] Meta-analysis has estimated end-of-treatment ALT normalization levels in 45% to 51% of treated patients, and sustained ALT normalization 3 to 6 months after cessation of therapy in 21% to 22% of subjects.[122,163] With development of accurate and readily available molecular assays, it became clear that ALT response overestimated actual viral response. Furthermore, a significant proportion of persons chronically infected with HCV have persistently normal serum aminotransferases. In a meta-analysis performed after virologic testing became widely available, ETVR was observed in 29% of treated patients, with 6-month SVR in 8% of treated patients. Increasing the duration of therapy to 12 months increased the frequency of SVR to nearly 20%. Dose and frequency escalations were not associated with more favorable rates of SVR.[218,219]

Ribavirin, an orally administered nucleoside analogue, although not as effective as monotherapy,[220] was found in pilot studies[221,222] to have significant synergy with interferon alfa. Combination of interferon with ribavirin yielded notable improvement in efficacy, with SVR rates of 38% to 43% in registration trials. During these trials, evidence emerged that SVR was associated with lower viral loads, less fibrosis on liver biopsy, and especially viral genotypes other than genotype 1.[70,223]

By the late 1990s, pegylated forms of interferon alfa became available for general use. These compounds, which use various forms of PEG to prolong drug half-life, resulted in enhanced rates of SVR.[224] Peginterferon alfa-2a, which employs a 40-kDa PEG moiety, was shown in registration trials to result in SVRs of 28% to 39%.[225,226] Of note, the SVR rate was only modestly diminished in patients with advanced fibrosis or cirrhosis, in stark contradistinction to response rates with unmodified interferon.[153] When combined with ribavirin, peginterferon yields SVRs as high as 56%.[209] Peginterferon alfa-2b, which employs a PEG moiety of 12 kDa in size, has been shown to provide an SVR of 25% to 28% as monotherapy[227] and of 54% when combined with oral ribavirin.[124] Of note, when used as monotherapy, peginterferon alfa-2b had similar efficacy in both standard and reduced doses. Retrospective analysis of registration trials suggested that shorter duration and lower dose of therapy in those patients infected with HCV genotypes 2 and 3 resulted in SVR rates similar to those with standard dosing.[228] Retrospective analysis also led to the insight, ultimately confirmed in prospectively designed trials, that significant reduction of circulating virus at time points early in therapy is predictive of ultimate sustained virologic response, or lack thereof. Currently, eradication of virus or viral reduction of 2 logs at 12 weeks of therapy is termed "early virologic response," while the same condition met at 4 weeks of therapy is termed "rapid virologic response."[229,230]

TABLE 35-6 DRUGS UNDER DEVELOPMENT FOR THE TREATMENT OF HEPATITIS C

Compound	Mechanism of Action	Phase of Development
ISIS 14803	Antisense oligonucleotide	II
BILN 2061	Protease inhibitor	Suspended
VX-950	Protease inhibitor	II
SCH503034	Protease inhibitor	II
ITMN B	Protease inhibitor	I
NM-283	Polymerase inhibitor	II
R1626	Polymerase inhibitor	II
HCV-796	Polymerase inhibitor	II
MX-3256	α-Glucosidase inhibitor	II
CPG10101	Toll-like receptor 9 agonist	II
IDN-6556	Caspase inhibitor	II

Other HCV Agents (Tables 35-6 and 35-7). Development of novel agents for use in the treatment of acute and chronic hepatitis C infection is an active area of research.[231] Current approaches focus on identifying steps in the viral life cycle amenable to pharmacologic interference (Fig. 35-14). Given the prodigious replicative ability of HCV virus, coupled with the slower turnover of infected hepatocytes, it is vital not only to cease infection of hepatocytes, but also to suppress viral replication in previously infected hepatocytes.[232] Candidate drugs under development can be categorized by the various aspects of the viral life cycle against which they are targeted. Agents designed to stop viral attachment to the cell include neutralizing antibodies delivered by infusion (passive) or induction (vaccination).[233,234] Mimicry of the CD81 receptor has also been targeted in order to inhibit viral cell attachment and entry.[235] After viral entry, uncoating and release of viral RNA allows for translation of viral proteins via the action of the HCV internal ribosome entry site (IRES). Antisense oligonucleotides aimed against highly conserved portions of the IRES have theoretical applicability in the treatment of HCV, but such approaches have met with difficulty in clinical applicability.[236]

After translation of viral proteins, posttranslational processing of the viral polyprotein takes place, yielding multiple viral peptides.

TABLE 35-7 THERAPEUTIC APPROACH FOR CHRONIC HEPATITIS C INFECTION

	Evidence Level*
SCREENING	
Universal screening is not recommended.	I
Screening is recommended in high risk groups: persons who • received transfusion prior to 1992 • received clotting factors prior to 1988 • have frequent percutaneous exposures • have biochemical or clinical evidence of chronic liver disease • are spouses of persons with chronic HCV infection	III
PREVENTION	
Persons with chronic HCV are candidates for hepatitis A and hepatitis B vaccinations.	III
DIAGNOSIS AND PRETREATMENT EVALUATION	
Persons with HCV viremia and evidence of chronic hepatitis with compensated liver disease are candidates for antiviral therapy.	I
Abnormal aminotransferases are not a requirement for therapy.	I
Histologic examination of the liver is indicated, especially in persons infected with HCV genotype 1.	I
TREATMENT	
The current standard of care for treatment of chronic HCV is combination peginterferon alfa and ribavirin.	I
There is no significant difference in efficacy between the two available peginterferons.	I
Ribavirin should be administered in a dose of 1000-1200 mg daily, divided twice daily for maximum efficacy.	I
Genotype 1 HCV should be treated for 48 weeks.	I
Genotypes 2 and 3 HCV should be treated for 24 weeks with a lower dose of ribavirin.	I
Failure to eliminate or reduce viral load by 2 log at 12 weeks of treatment should prompt early cessation of therapy.	I
ACUTE HEPATITIS C	
Treatment delay should be no longer that 3 months.	II-2b
Peginterferon monotherapy for 24 weeks is recommended.	II-2b

*Levels of evidence: I, well-designed randomized, controlled trials; II-2b, well-designed cohort (prospective) study with historical controls; III, large differences from comparisons between times and/or places with and without intervention (in some circumstances these may be equivalent to level II or I).

Structural proteins are produced in great excess for unclear reasons. Nonstructural proteins, especially the NS3-NS4a serine protease, have emerged as leading targets for drug development. The initial protease inhibitor, BILN 2061 (Boehringer Ingelheim; Ingelheim, Germany), showed rapid diminution of circulating virus in human trials, but development was stopped with emergence of animal cardiac toxicity. Two newer protease inhibitors, VX-950 (Telaprevir, Vertex Pharmaceuticals, Cambridge, MA) and SCH503034 (Boceprevir, Schering Plough, Kenilworth, NJ), are currently in Phase III clinical trials. Both agents appear well tolerated, potent, and possibly synergistic with interferon.[237-240]

HCV RNA transcription is reliant upon HCV RNA–dependent RNA polymerase. Nucleoside and non-nucleoside inhibitors of RNA polymerase are under development. NM-283 (valopicitabine; Idenix Pharmaceutical, Cambridge, MA) showed early promise in large scale human trials, but development has been suspended due to gastrointestinal toxicity. Two other polymerase inhibitors, R1626 (Roche Pharmaceuticals, Nutley, NJ) and HCV-796 (Viropharma Inc., Exton, PA), are in earlier phases of clinical development.[232] Other newer approaches to HCV pharmacotherapy include α-glucosidase inhibitors to inhibit viral assembly, toll-like receptor 9 agonists to function as a non-interferon immune modulator, and caspase inhibitors to increase apoptosis of infected hepatocytes.

Hepatitis E

Prevention

The primary mode of prevention of HEV is attention to hygienic practices. Outbreaks have been reported in Asia, Africa, and the Middle East, all associated with overcrowded situations amenable to contamination of water. HEV does not appear to be transmitted from human to human, thus eradication of water-borne reservoirs of the virus by boiling or chemical treatment should greatly diminish the frequency and severity of outbreaks.[241] The realization that HEV may also be transmitted as a zoonotic virus can allow preventive measures to reduce this less common form of transmission. Because most of the HEV seen in nontropical and developed countries appears linked to travel, preventive measures aimed at this population are advisable.[242]

Prophylaxis

The standard-preparation immunoglobulin for HEV postexposure prophylaxis appears to be relatively inefficient.[243,244] Prophylactic efforts have focused on the development of a safe and effective HEV vaccine. HEV exists as four genotypes, of which genotype 1 is by far the most prominent. The presence of a single HEV serotype has facilitated the development of a vaccine that should have global applicability.[245] The development of a recombinant genotype 1 HEV vaccine has recently led to a large randomized trial in the Nepalese Army.[246] In this group of young men who were at substantial risk of HEV infection, vaccine effectiveness was in excess of 95% with an excellent safety profile.[247] Given the high burden of HEV infection in large areas of the world, further studies and more extensive use of the vaccine are expected.

Treatment of Acute HEV Infection

Treatment of acute HEV infection is supportive. Because viral shedding takes place during the incubation period, careful attention to hygiene and proper disposal of sewage is vital to avoid epidemic outbreaks. Particular vigilance for the development of liver failure, manifested by coagulopathy and encephalopathy, should be given to pregnant women.

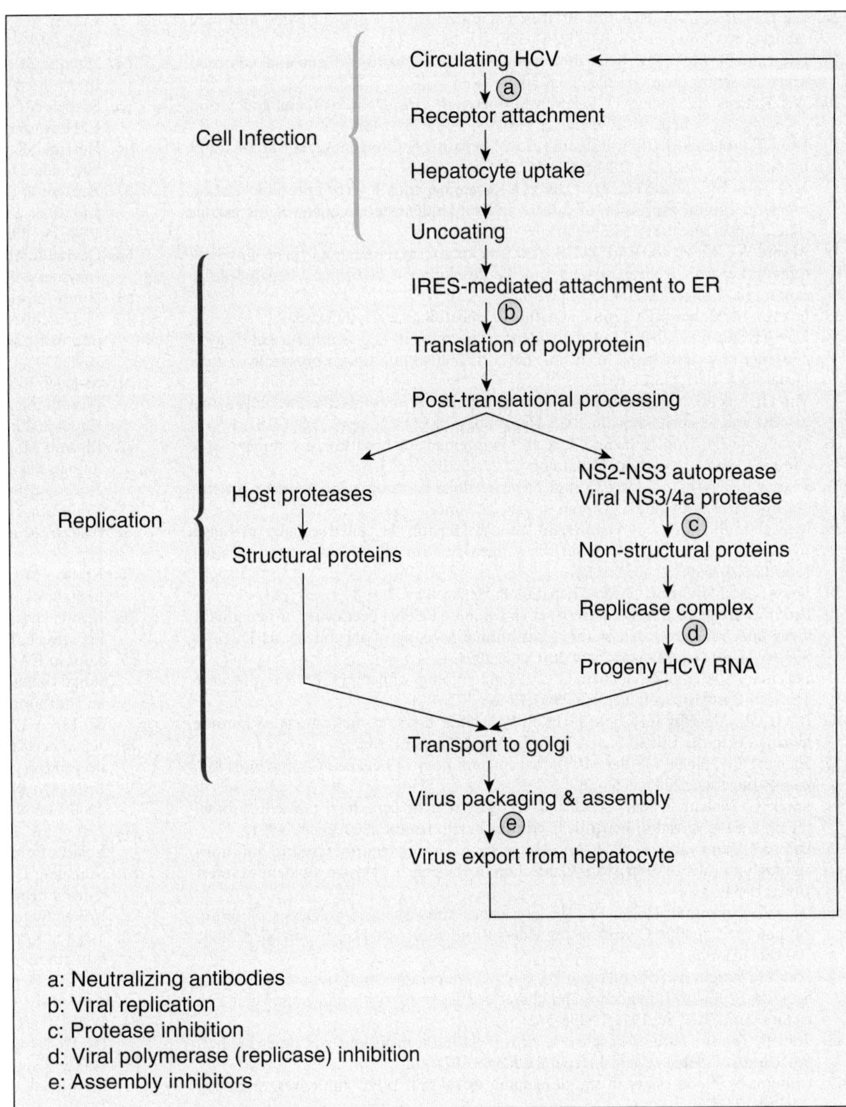

FIGURE 35-14 • Mechanism of HCV therapies in the context of the viral life cycle.

REFERENCES

1. Chen TS, Chen PS. Understanding the Liver. Westport, CT: Greenwood Press, 1984.
2. Blumberg BS. Polymorphisms of serum proteins and the development of isoprecipitins in transfused patients. Bull N Y Acad Med 1964;40:377-386.
3. Dane DS, Cameron CH, Briggs M. Virus-like particles in serum of patients with Australia-antigen-associated hepatitis. Lancet 1970;1:695-698.
4. Dienstag JL, Feinstone SM, Kapikian AZ, Purcell RH. Faecal shedding of hepatitis-A antigen. Lancet 1975;1:765-767.
5. Frosner GG, Deinhardt F, Scheid R, et al. Propagation of human hepatitis A virus in a hepatoma cell line. Infection 1979;7:303-305.
6. Choo QL, Kuo G, Weiner AJ, et al. Isolation of a cDNA clone derived from a blood-borne non-A, non-B viral hepatitis genome. Science 1989;244:359-362.
7. World Health Organization. The World Health Report. Geneva: World Health Organization, 1997.
8. World Health Organization. Hepatitis B: World Health Organization Fact Sheet 204 (Revised October 2000). Available at *http://who.int/inf-fs/en/fact204.html*
9. Brown RS, Gaglio PJ. Scope of worldwide hepatitis C problem. Liver Transpl 2003;9:S10-S13.
10. Bell BP. Global epidemiology of hepatitis A: implications for control strategies. Presented at the 10th International Symposium on Viral Hepatitis and Liver Disease, Atlanta, April 9-13, 2000. Antivir Ther 2000;5(Suppl 1):13-18.
11. Feinstone SM, Kapikian AZ, Purcell RH. Hepatitis A: detection by immune electron microscopy of a virus like antigen associated with acute illness. Science 1973;182:1026-1028.
12. Martin A, Lemon SM. The molecular biology of hepatitis A virus. In Ou J-H (ed): Hepatitis Viruses. Norwell, MA: Kluwer Academic Publishers, 2002, pp 23-50.
13. Martin A, Lemon SM. Hepatitis A virus: From discovery to vaccines. Hepatology 2006;43:S164-S172.
14. Fleischer B, Fleischer S, Maier K, et al. Clonal analysis of infiltrating T lymphocytes in liver tissue in viral hepatitis A. Immunology 1990;69:14-19.
15. Vallbracht A, Gabriel P, Maier K, et al. Cell-mediated cytotoxicity in hepatitis A virus infection. Hepatology 1986;6:1308-1314.
16. Maier K, Gabriel P, Koscielniak E, et al. Human gamma interferon production by cytotoxic T lymphocytes sensitized during hepatitis A virus infection. J Virol 1988;62:3756-3763.
17. Stapleton JT, Lange DK, LeDuc JW, et al. The role of secretory immunity in hepatitis A virus infection. J Infect Dis 1991;163:7-11.
18. Shepard CW, Simard EP, Finelli L, et al. Hepatitis B virus infection: epidemiology and vaccination. Epidemiol Rev 2006;28:112-125.
19. Bond WW, Petersen NJ, Favero MS. Viral hepatitis B: aspects of environmental control. Health Lab Sci 1977;14:235-252.
20. Alter MJ, Margolis HS. The emergence of hepatitis B as a sexually transmitted disease. Med Clin North Am 1990;74:1529-1541.
21. Alter MJ, Ahtone J, Weisfuse I, et al. Hepatitis B transmission between heterosexuals. JAMA 1986;256:1307-1310.
22. Dietzman DE, Harnisch JP, Ray CG, et al. Hepatitis B surface antigen (HBsAg) and antibody to HBsAg: prevalence in homosexual and heterosexual men. JAMA 1977; 238:2625-2626.
23. Hauri AM, Armstrong GL, Hutin YJF. The global burden of disease attributable to contaminated injections given in health care settings. Int J STD AIDS 2004;15:7-16.
24. Centers for Disease Control and Prevention. Recommendations for preventing transmission of infections among chronic hemodialysis patients. MMWR Recomm Rep. 2001;50(RR-5):1-43.
25. Williams IT, Perz JF, Bell BP. Viral hepatitis in ambulatory care settings. Clin Infect Dis 2004;38:1592-1598.
26. Samandari T, Malakmadze N, Balter S, et al. A large outbreak of hepatitis B virus infections associated with frequent injections at a physician's office. Infect Control Hosp Epidemiol 2005;26:745-750.

27. Lee JY, Locarnini S. Hepatitis B virus: pathogenesis, viral intermediates, and viral replication. Clin Liver Dis 2004;8:301-320.
28. Locarnini S, McMillan J, Bartholomeusz A. The hepatitis B virus and common mutants. Semin Liver Dis 2003;23:5-20.
29. Wei Y, Tavis JE, Ganem D. Relationship between viral DNA synthesis and virion envelopment in hepatitis B viruses. J Virol 1996;70:6455-6458.
30. Wai CT, Fontana RJ. Clinical significance of hepatitis B virus genotypes, variants, and mutants. Clin Liver Dis 2004;8:321-352.
31. McMahon BJ, Alward WL, Hall DB, et al. Acute hepatitis B virus infection: relation of age to clinical expression of disease and subsequent development of the carrier state. J Infect Dis 1985;151:599-603.
32. Alward WL, McMahon BJ, Hall DB, et al. The long-term serological course of asymptomatic hepatitis B virus carriers and the development of primary hepatocellular carcinoma. J Infect Dis 1985;151:604-609.
33. Lok AS, McMahon BJ. Chronic hepatitis B. Hepatology 2007;45:507-539.
34. Liaw YF, Sheen IS, Chen TJ, et al. Incidence, determinants and significance of delayed clearance of serum HBsAg in chronic hepatitis B virus infection: a prospective study. Hepatology 1991;13:627-631.
35. Yim HJ, Lok AS. Natural history of chronic hepatitis B virus infection: what we knew in 1981 and what we know in 2005. Hepatology 2006;43(2 Suppl 1):S173-S181.
36. Hoofnagle JH, Doo E, Liang TJ, et al. Management of hepatitis B: summary of a clinical research workshop. Hepatology 2007;45:1056-1075.
37. Beasley RP, Hwang LY, Lin CC, et al. Hepatocellular carcinoma and hepatitis B virus: a prospective study of 22,707 men in Taiwan. Lancet 1981;2:1129-1133.
38. McMahon BJ, Alberts SR, Wainwright RB, et al. Hepatitis B-related sequelae: prospective study of 1400 hepatitis B surface antigen-positive Alaska Native carriers. Arch Intern Med 1990;150:1051-1054.
39. Lok AS, McMahon BJ. Chronic hepatitis B. Hepatology 2001;34:1225-1241.
40. Perz JF, Farrington LA, Pecoraro C, et al. Estimated global prevalence of hepatitis C virus infection. Presented at the 42nd Annual Meeting of the Infectious Diseases Society of America, Boston, Sept 30-Oct 3, 2004.
41. Bellentani S, Miglioli L, Bedogni G, et al. Epidemiology of hepatitis C virus infection. Minerva Gastroenterol Dietol 2005;51:15-29.
42. Davis GL, Albright JE, Cook SF, et al. Projecting future complications of chronic hepatitis C in the United States. Liver Transpl 2003;9:331-338.
43. Shepard CW, Finelli L, Alter MJ. Global epidemiology of hepatitis C virus infection. Lancet Infect Dis 2005;5:558-567.
44. Frank C, Mohamed MK, Strickland GT. The role of parenteral antischistosomal therapy in the spread of hepatitis C virus in Egypt. Lancet 2000;355:887-891.
45. Luby SP, Qamruddin K, Shah AA. The relationship between therapeutic injections and high prevalence of hepatitis C infection in Hafizabad, Pakistan. Epidemiol Infect 1997;119:349-356.
46. Lin CC, Hwang SJ, Chiou ST. The prevalence and risk factors analysis of serum antibody to hepatitis C virus in the elders in northeast Taiwan. J Chin Med Assoc 2003;66:103-108.
47. Seeff LB, Wright EC, Zimmerman HJ, et al. VA cooperative study of post-transfusion hepatitis, 1969-1974: incidence and characteristics of hepatitis and responsible risk factors. Am J Med Sci 1975;27:355-362.
48. Prati D. Transmission of hepatitis C virus by blood transfusions and other medical procedures: a global review. J Hepatol 2006;45:607-616.
49. Dhingra N. Blood safety in the developing world and WHO initiatives. Vox Sang 2002;83:173-177.
50. World Health Organization. Global database on blood safety 2001-2002. Available at *http://www.who.int/bloodsafety/GDBS_Report_2001-2002.pdf* (accessed May 28, 2007).
51. Terrault NA. Sexual activity as a risk factor for hepatitis C. Hepatology 2002;36:S99-S105.
52. Vandelli C, Renzo F, Romano L. Lack of evidence of sexual transmission of hepatitis C among monogamous couples: results of a 10-year prospective follow-up study. Am J Gastroenterol 2004;99:855-859.
53. Yeung LTF, King SM, Roberts EA. Mother-to-infant transmission of hepatitis C virus. Hepatology 2001;34:223-229.
54. Ferrero S, Lungaro P, Bruzzone BM, et al. Prospective study of mother-to-infant transmission of hepatitis C virus: a 10-year survey (1990-2000). Acta Obstet Gynecol Scand 2003;82:229-234.
55. Lohmann V, Korner F, Koch J, et al. Replication of subgenomic hepatitis C virus RNAs in a hepatoma cell line. Science 1999;285:110-113.
56. Blight KJ, Kolykhalov AA, Rice CM. Efficient initiation of HCV RNA replication in cell culture. Science 2000;290:1972-1974.
57. Bartosch B, Dubuisson J, Cosset FL. Infectious hepatitis C virus pseudo-particles containing functional E1-E2 envelope protein complexes. J Exp Med 2003;197:633-642.
58. Hsu M, Zhang J, Flint M, et al. Hepatitis C virus glycoproteins mediate pH-dependent cell entry of pseudotyped retroviral particles. Proc Natl Acad Sci U S A 2003;100:7271-7276.
59. Moradpour D, Blum HE. A primer on the molecular virology of hepatitis C. Liver Int 2004;24:519-525.
60. Barth H, Liang TJ, Baumert TF. Hepatitis C virus entry: molecular biology and clinical implications. Hepatology 2006;44:527-535.
61. Lamarre D, Anderson PC, Bailey M, et al. An NS3 protease inhibitor with antiviral effects in humans infected with hepatitis C virus. Nature 2003;426:186-189.
62. Lesburg CA, Cable MB, Ferrari E, et al. Crystal structure of the RNA-dependent RNA polymerase from hepatitis C virus reveals a fully encircled active site. Nat Struct Biol 1999;6:937-943.
63. Piton A, Poynard T, Imbert-Bismut F, et al. Factors associated with serum alanine transaminase activity in healthy subjects: consequences for the definition of normal values, for selection of blood donors, and for patients with chronic hepatitis C. Hepatology 1998;27:1213-1219.
64. Herrine SK. Approach to the patient with chronic hepatitis C virus infection. Ann Intern Med 2002;136:747-757.
65. Saadeh S, Cammell G, Carey WD, et al. The role of liver biopsy in chronic hepatitis C. Hepatology 2001;33:196-200.
66. Herrine SK, Friedman LS. Divining the role of liver biopsy in hepatitis C. J Hepatol 2005;43:374-376.
67. Zeuzem S, Franke A, Lee JH, et al. Phylogenetic analysis of hepatitis C virus isolates and their correlation to viremia, liver function tests, and histology. Hepatology 1996;24:1003-1009.
68. Davis FF, Abuchowski A, Van Es T. Enzyme-polyethylene glycol adducts: modified enzymes with unique properties. Enzyme Eng 1978;4:169-173.
69. Simmonds P. Variability of hepatitis C virus. Hepatology 1995;21:570-583.
70. McHutchison JG, Gordon SC, Schiff ER, et al. Interferon alfa-2b alone or in combination with ribavirin as initial treatment for chronic hepatitis C. N Engl J Med 1998;339:1485-1492.
71. Al-Faleh FZ, Aljumah A, Rezeig M, et al. Treatment of chronic hepatitis C genotype IV with interferon-ribavirin combination in Saudi Arabia: a multicentre study. J Viral Hepat 2000;7:287-291.
72. Khuroo MS. Study of an epidemic of non-A, non-B hepatitis: possibility of another human hepatitis virus distinct from post-transfusion non-A, non-B type. Am J Med 1980;68:818-823.
73. Krawczynski K. Hepatitis E. Hepatology 1993;17:932-941.
74. Balayan MS. Epidemiology of hepatitis E virus infection. J Viral Hepat 1997;4:155-165.
75. Khuroo MS, Teli MR, Skidmore S, et al. Incidence and severity of viral hepatitis in pregnancy. Am J Med 1981;70:252-255.
76. Krawczynski K, Kamili S, Aggarwal R. Global epidemiology and medical aspects of hepatitis E. Forum (Genova) 2001;11:166-179.
77. Koonin EV, Gorbalenya AE, Purdy MA, et al. Computer-assisted assignment of functional domains in the nonstructural polyprotein of hepatitis E virus: delineation of an additional group of positive-strand RNA plant and animal viruses. Proc Natl Acad Sci U S A 1992;89:8259-8263.
78. Acharya SK, Panda SK. Hepatitis E virus: epidemiology, diagnosis, pathology and prevention. Trop Gastroenterol 2006;27:63-68.
79. Krawczynski K, Aggarwal R, Kamili S. Hepatitis E. Infect Dis Clin North Am 2000;14:669-687.
80. Tsarev SA, Binn LN, Gomatos PJ, et al. Phylogenetic analysis of hepatitis E virus isolates from Egypt. J Med Virol 1999;57:68-74.
81. Schlauder GG, Dawson GJ, Erker JC, et al. The sequence and phylogenetic analysis of a novel hepatitis E virus isolated from a patient with acute hepatitis reported in the United States. J Gen Virol 1998;79:447-456.
82. Tsega E, Krawczynski K, Hansson BG, et al. Outbreak of acute hepatitis E virus infection among military personnel in northern Ethiopia. J Med Virol 1991;34:232-236.
83. Teo CG. Hepatitis E indigenous to economically developed countries: to what extent a zoonosis? Curr Opin Infect Dis 2006;19:460-466.
84. Winokur PL, Stapleton JT. Immunoglobulin prophylaxis for hepatitis A. Clin Infect Dis 1992;14:580-586.
85. Walter EB, Hornick RB, Poland GA, et al. Concurrent administration of inactivated hepatitis A vaccine with immune globulin in healthy adults. Vaccine 1999;17:1468-1473.
86. Bianco E, De Masi S, Mele A, et al. Effectiveness of immune globulins in preventing infectious hepatitis and hepatitis A: a systematic review. Dig Liver Dis 2004;36:834-842.
87. Sagliocca L, Amoroso P, Stroffolini T, et al. Efficacy of hepatitis A vaccine in prevention of secondary hepatitis A infection: a randomised trial. Lancet 1999;353:1136-1139.
88. Wasley A, Fiore A, Bell BP. Hepatitis A in the era of vaccination. Epidemiol Rev 2006;28:101-111.
89. Innis BL, Snitbhan R, Kunasol P, et al. Protection against hepatitis A by an inactivated vaccine. JAMA 1994;271:1328-1334.
90. Werzberger A, Mensch B, Kuter B, et al. A controlled trial of a formalin-inactivated hepatitis A vaccine in healthy children. N Engl J Med 1992;327:453-457.
91. Werzberger A, Mensch B, Nalin DR, et al. Effectiveness of hepatitis A vaccine in a former frequently affected community: 9 years' followup after the Monroe field trial of VAQTA. Vaccine 2002;20:1699-1701.
92. Van Herck K, Van Damme P, Lievens M, et al. Hepatitis A vaccine: indirect evidence of immune memory 12 years after the primary course. J Med Virol 2004;72:194-196.
93. Van Damme P, Banatvala J, Fay O, et al. Hepatitis A booster vaccination: is there a need? Lancet 2003;362:1065-1071.
94. Letson GW, Shapiro CN, Kuehn D, et al. Effect of maternal antibody on immunogenicity of hepatitis A vaccine in infants. J Pediatr 2004;144:327-332.
95. Majda-Stanislawa E, Bednarek M, Kuydowicz J. Immunogenicity of inactivated hepatitis A vaccine in children with chronic liver disease. Pediatr Infect Dis J 2004;23:571-573.
96. Stark K, Gunther M, Neuhaus R, et al. Immunogenicity and safety of hepatitis A vaccine in liver and renal transplant recipients. J Infect Dis 1999;180:2014-2017.
97. Karayiannis P, Main J, Thomas HC. Hepatitis vaccines. Br Med Bull 2004;70:29-49.
98. Wasley A, Samandari T, Bell BP. Incidence of hepatitis A in the United States in the era of vaccination. JAMA 2005;294:194-201.
99. Fiore AE, Wasley A, Bell BP. Prevention of hepatitis A through active or passive immunization: recommendations of the Advisory Committee on Immunization Practices (ACIP). MMWR Recomm Rep 2006;55(RR-7):1-23.

100. Ni YH, Huang LM, Chang MH, et al. Two decades of universal hepatitis B vaccination in Taiwan: impact and implication for future strategies. Gastroenterology 2007;132:1287-1293.
101. Centers for Disease Control and Prevention. Progress in hepatitis B prevention through universal infant vaccination—China, 1997-2006. MMWR Morb Mortal Wkly Rep 2007;56:441-445.
102. Chang TT, Jia JD, Omata M, et al. New therapies for chronic hepatitis B infection. Liver Int 2006;26(Suppl 2):30-37.
103. McGory RW, Ishitani MB, Oliveira WM, et al. Improved outcome of orthotopic liver transplantation for chronic hepatitis B cirrhosis with aggressive passive immunization. Transplantation 1996;61:1358-1364.
104. Young BW, Lee SS, Lim WL, et al. The long-term efficacy of plasma-derived hepatitis B vaccine in babies born to carrier mothers. J Viral Hepat 2003;10:23-30.
105. Yeo W, Chan PK, Zhong S, et al. Frequency of hepatitis B virus reactivation in cancer patients undergoing cytotoxic chemotherapy: a prospective study of 626 patients with identification of risk factors. J Med Virol 2000;62:299-307.
106. Coiffier B. Hepatitis B virus reactivation in patients receiving chemotherapy for cancer treatment: role of lamivudine prophylaxis. Cancer Invest 2006;24:548-552.
107. Schnepf N, Sellier P, Bendenoun M, et al. Reactivation of lamivudine-resistant occult hepatitis B in an HIV-infected patient undergoing cytotoxic chemotherapy. J Clin Virol 2007;39:48-50.
108. Mast EE, Weinbaum CM, Fiore AE, et al. A comprehensive immunization strategy to eliminate transmission of hepatitis B virus infection in the United States: recommendations of the Advisory Committee on Immunization Practices (ACIP). Part II: immunization of adults. MMWR Recomm Rep 2006;55(RR-16):1-33.
109. Wills RJ. Clinical pharmacology of interferons. Clin Pharmacokinet 1990;19:390-399.
110. Gale M Jr. Effector genes of interferon action against hepatitis C virus. Hepatology 2003;37:975-978.
111. de Veer MJ, Holko M, Frevel M, et al. Functional classification of interferon-stimulated genes identified using microarrays. J Leukocyte Biol 2001;69:912-920.
112. Feld JJ, Hoofnagle JH. Mechanism of action of interferon and ribavirin in treatment of hepatitis C. Nature 2005;436:967-972.
113. Sen GC. Viruses and interferons. Annu Rev Microbiol 2001;55:255-281.
114. Bekisz J, Schmeisser H, Hernandez J, et al. Human interferons alpha, beta and omega. Growth Factors 2004;22:243-251.
115. Tilg H. New insights into the mechanisms of interferon: an immunoregulatory and anti-inflammatory cytokine. Gastroenterology 1997;112:1017-1021.
116. Haria M, Benfield P. Interferon-alfa-2a: a review of its pharmacological properties and therapeutic use in the management of viral hepatitis. Drugs 1995;50:873-896.
117. Wills RJ, Dennis S, Spiegel HE, et al. Interferon kinetics and adverse reactions after intravenous, intramuscular, and subcutaneous injection. Clin Pharmacol Ther 1984;35:722-727.
118. Smith RA, Norris F, Palmer D, et al. Distribution of alpha interferon in serum and cerebrospinal fluid after systemic administration. Clin Pharmacol Ther 1985;37:85-88.
119. Waysbort A, Giroux M, Mansat V, et al. Experimental study of transplacental passage of alpha interferon by two assay techniques. Antimicrob Agents Chemother 1993;37:1232-1237.
120. Janssen HL, Brouwer JT, van der Mast RC, et al. Suicide associated with alfa-interferon therapy for chronic viral hepatitis. J Hepatol 1994;21:241-243.
121. Schaefer M, Schwaiger M, Garkisch AS, et al. Prevention of interferon-alpha associated depression in psychiatric risk patients with chronic hepatitis C. J Hepatol 2005;42:793-798.
122. Poynard T, Leroy V, Cohard M, et al. Meta-analysis of interferon randomized trials in the treatment of viral hepatitis C: effects of dose and duration. Hepatology 1996;24:778-789.
123. Reddy KR. Development and pharmacokinetics and pharmacodynamics of pegylated interferon alfa-2a (40 kD). Semin Liver Dis 2004;24(Suppl 2):33-38.
124. Manns MP, McHutchison JG, Gordon SC, et al. Peginterferon alfa-2b plus ribavirin compared with interferon alfa-2b plus ribavirin for initial treatment of chronic hepatitis C: a randomised trial. Lancet 2001;358:958-965.
125. Johnson MA, Moore KH, Yuen GJ, et al. Clinical pharmacokinetics of lamivudine. Clin Pharmacokinet 1999;36:41-66.
126. van Leeuwen R, Lange JM, Hussey EK, et al. The safety and pharmacokinetics of a reverse transcriptase inhibitor, 3TC, in patients with HIV infection: a Phase I study. AIDS 1992;6:1471-1475.
127. Yuen GJ, Morris DM, Mydlow PK, et al. Pharmacokinetics, absolute bioavailability, and absorption characteristics of lamivudine. J Clin Pharmacol 1995;35:1174-1180.
128. Angel JB, Hussey EK, Hall ST, et al. Pharmacokinetics of 3TC (GR109714X) administered with and without food to HIV infected patients. Drug Invest 1993;6:70-74.
129. Blaney SM, Daniel MJ, Harker AJ, et al. Pharmacokinetics of lamivudine and BCH-189 in plasma and cerebrospinal fluid of nonhuman primates. Antimicrob Agents Chemother 1995;39:2779-2782.
130. Lewis LL, Venzon D, Church J, et al. Lamivudine in children with human immunodeficiency virus infection: a Phase I/II study. The National Cancer Institute Pediatric Branch–Human Immunodeficiency Virus Working Group. J Infect Dis 1996;174:16-25.
131. Heald AE, Hsyu PH, Yuen GJ, et al. Pharmacokinetics of lamivudine in human immunodeficiency virus-infected patients with renal dysfunction. Antimicrob Agents Chemother 1996;40:1514-1519.
132. Lau DT, Khokhar MF, Doo E, et al. Long-term therapy of chronic hepatitis B with lamivudine. Hepatology 2000;32:828-834.
133. Cundy KC, Barditch-Crovo P, Walker RE, et al. Clinical pharmacokinetics of adefovir in human immunodeficiency virus type 1-infected patients. Antimicrob Agents Chemother 1995;39:2401-2405.
134. Barditch-Crovo P, Toole J, Hendrix CW, et al. Anti-human immunodeficiency virus (HIV) activity, safety, and pharmacokinetics of adefovir dipivoxil (9-[2-(bis-pivaloyloxymethyl)-phosphonylmethoxyethyl]adenine) in HIV-infected patients. J Infect Dis 1997;176:406-413.
135. Cundy KC. Clinical pharmacokinetics of the antiviral nucleotide analogues cidofovir and adefovir. Clin Pharmacokinet 1999;36:127-143.
136. Rivkin AM. Adefovir dipivoxil in the treatment of chronic hepatitis B. Ann Pharmacother 2004;38:625-633.
137. Marcellin P, Chang TT, Lim SG, et al. Adefovir dipivoxil for the treatment of hepatitis B e antigen-positive chronic hepatitis B. N Engl J Med 2003;348:808-816.
138. Chang TT, Gish RG, Hadziyannis SJ, et al. A dose-ranging study of the efficacy and tolerability of entecavir in lamivudine-refractory chronic hepatitis B patients. Gastroenterology 2005;129:1198-1209.
139. Yan JH, Bifano M, Olsen S, et al. Entecavir pharmacokinetics, safety, and tolerability after multiple ascending doses in healthy subjects. J Clin Pharmacol 2006;46:1250-1258.
140. Robinson DM, Scott LJ, Plosker GL. Entecavir: a review of its use in chronic hepatitis B. Drugs 2006;66:1605-1622.
141. Kim JW, Park SH, Louie SG. Telbivudine: a novel nucleoside analog for chronic hepatitis B. Ann Pharmacother 2006;40:472-478.
142. Zhou XJ, Lim SG, Lloyd DM, et al. Pharmacokinetics of telbivudine following oral administration of escalating single and multiple doses in patients with chronic hepatitis B virus infection: pharmacodynamic implications. Antimicrob Agents Chemother 2006;50:874-879.
143. Zhou XJ, Fielman BA, Lloyd DM, et al. Pharmacokinetics of telbivudine in healthy subjects and absence of drug interaction with lamivudine or adefovir dipivoxil. Antimicrob Agents Chemother 2006;50:2309-2315.
144. Ristig MB, Crippin J, Aberg JA, et al. Tenofovir disoproxil fumarate therapy for chronic hepatitis B in human immunodeficiency virus/hepatitis B virus-coinfected individuals for whom interferon-alpha and lamivudine therapy have failed. J Infect Dis 2002;186:1844-1847.
145. van Bommel F, Wunsche T, Mauss S, et al. Comparison of adefovir and tenofovir in the treatment of lamivudine-resistant hepatitis B virus infection. Hepatology 2004;40:1421-1425.
146. Lim SG, Ng TM, Kung N, et al. A double-blind placebo-controlled study of emtricitabine in chronic hepatitis B. Arch Intern Med 2006;166:49-56.
147. Yoo BC, Kim JH, Chung YH, et al. Twenty-four-week clevudine therapy showed potent and sustained antiviral activity in HBeAg-positive chronic hepatitis B. Hepatology 2007;45:1172-1178.
148. Yuki N, Nagaoka T, Yamashiro M, et al. Long-term histologic and virologic outcomes of acute self-limited hepatitis B. Hepatology 2003;37:1172-1179.
149. Reshef R, Sbait W, Tur-Kaspa R. Lamivudine in the treatment of acute hepatitis B. N Engl J Med 2000;343:1123-1124.
150. Schmilovitz-Weiss H, Ben-Ari Z, Sikuler E, et al. Lamivudine treatment for acute severe hepatitis B: a pilot study. Liver Int 2004;24:547-551.
151. Kumar M, Satapathy S, Monga R, et al. A randomized controlled trial of lamivudine to treat acute hepatitis B. Hepatology 2007;45:97-101.
152. Tillmann HL. Antiviral therapy and resistance with hepatitis B virus infection. World J Gastroenterol 2007;13:125-140.
153. Heathcote EJ, Shiffman ML, Cooksley WG, et al. Peginterferon alfa-2a in patients with chronic hepatitis C and cirrhosis. N Engl J Med 2000;343:1673-1680.
154. Wong DK, Cheung AM, O'Rourke K, et al. Effect of alpha-interferon treatment in patients with hepatitis B e antigen-positive chronic hepatitis B: a meta-analysis. Ann Intern Med 1993;119:312-323.
155. Lok AS, Lai CL, Wu PC, et al. Long-term follow-up in a randomised controlled trial of recombinant alpha 2-interferon in Chinese patients with chronic hepatitis B infection. Lancet 1988;2:298-302.
156. Brook MG, Karayiannis P, Thomas HC. Which patients with chronic hepatitis B virus infection will respond to alpha-interferon therapy? A statistical analysis of predictive factors. Hepatology 1989;10:761-763.
157. Chu CJ, Keeffe EB, Han SH. Hepatitis B virus genotypes in the United States: results of a nationwide study. Gastroenterology 2003;125:444-451.
158. Korenman J, Baker B, Waggoner J, et al. Long-term remission of chronic hepatitis B after alpha-interferon therapy. Ann Intern Med 1991;114:629-634.
159. Lin SM, Sheen IS, Chien RN, et al. Long-term beneficial effect of interferon therapy in patients with chronic hepatitis B virus infection. Hepatology 1999;29:971-975.
160. Yuen MF, Hui CK, Cheng CC, et al. Long-term follow-up of interferon alfa treatment in Chinese patients with chronic hepatitis B infection: the effect on hepatitis B e antigen seroconversion and the development of cirrhosis-related complications. Hepatology 2001;34:139-145.
161. Lau DT, Everhart J, Kleiner DE, et al. Long-term follow-up of patients with chronic hepatitis B treated with interferon alfa. Gastroenterology 1997;113:1660-1667.
162. Fattovich G, Giustina G, Realdi G, et al. Long-term outcome of hepatitis B e antigen-positive patients with compensated cirrhosis treated with interferon alfa. European Concerted Action on Viral Hepatitis (EUROHEP). Hepatology 1997;26:1338-1342.
163. Niederau C, Heintges T, Haussinger D. Treatment of chronic hepatitis C with α-interferon: an analysis of the literature. Hepatogastroenterology 1996;43:1544-1556.
164. Perrillo RP, Schiff ER, Davis GL, et al. A randomized, controlled trial of interferon alfa-2b alone and after prednisone withdrawal for the treatment of chronic hepatitis B. The Hepatitis Interventional Therapy Group. N Engl J Med 1990;323:295-301.

165. Hoofnagle JH, Di Bisceglie AM, Waggoner JG, et al. Interferon alfa for patients with clinically apparent cirrhosis due to chronic hepatitis B. Gastroenterology 1993;104:1116-1121.
166. Brunetto MR, Oliveri F, Demartini A, et al. Treatment with interferon of chronic hepatitis B associated with antibody to hepatitis B e antigen. J Hepatol 1991;13:S8-S11.
167. Papatheodoridis GV, Petraki K, Cholongitas E, et al. Impact of interferon-alpha therapy on liver fibrosis progression in patients with HBeAg-negative chronic hepatitis B. J Viral Hepat 2005;12:199-206.
168. Lampertico P, Del Ninno E, Vigano M, et al. Long-term suppression of hepatitis B e antigen-negative chronic hepatitis B by 24-month interferon therapy. Hepatology 2003;37:756-763.
169. Manesis EK, Hadziyannis SJ. Interferon alpha treatment and retreatment of hepatitis B e antigen-negative chronic hepatitis B. Gastroenterology 2001;121:101-109.
170. Lau GK, Piratvisuth T, Luo KX, et al. Peginterferon alfa-2a, lamivudine, and the combination for HBeAg-positive chronic hepatitis B. N Engl J Med 2005;352:2682-2695.
171. Bonino F, Marcellin P, Lau GK, et al. Predicting response to peginterferon alpha-2a, lamivudine and the two combined for HBeAg-negative chronic hepatitis B. Gut 2007;56:699-705.
172. Cooksley WG, Piratvisuth T, Lee SD, et al. Peginterferon alpha-2a (40 kDa): an advance in the treatment of hepatitis B e antigen-positive chronic hepatitis B. J Viral Hepat 2003;10:298-305.
173. Chan HL, Leung NW, Hui AY, et al. A randomized, controlled trial of combination therapy for chronic hepatitis B: comparing pegylated interferon-alpha2b and lamivudine with lamivudine alone. Ann Intern Med 2005;142:240-250.
174. Marcellin P, Lau GK, Bonino F, et al. Peginterferon alfa-2a alone, lamivudine alone, and the two in combination in patients with HBeAg-negative chronic hepatitis B. N Engl J Med 2004;351:1206-1217.
175. Dienstag JL, Schiff ER, Wright TL, et al. Lamivudine as initial treatment for chronic hepatitis B in the United States. N Engl J Med 1999;341:1256-1263.
176. Lai CL, Chien RN, Leung NW, et al. A one-year trial of lamivudine for chronic hepatitis B. Asia Hepatitis Lamivudine Study Group. N Engl J Med 1998;339:61-68.
177. Liaw YF, Leung NW, Chang TT, et al. Effects of extended lamivudine therapy in Asian patients with chronic hepatitis B. Asia Hepatitis Lamivudine Study Group. Gastroenterology 2000;119:172-180.
178. Liaw YF, Chien RN, Yeh CT. No benefit to continue lamivudine therapy after emergence of YMDD mutations. Antivir Ther 2004;9:257-262.
179. Keeffe EB, Dieterich DT, Han SH, et al. A treatment algorithm for the management of chronic hepatitis B virus infection in the United States: an update. Clin Gastroenterol Hepatol 2006;4:936-962.
180. Hadziyannis SJ, Tassopoulos NC, Heathcote EJ, et al. Adefovir dipivoxil for the treatment of hepatitis B e antigen-negative chronic hepatitis B. N Engl J Med 2003;348:800-807.
181. Hadziyannis SJ, Tassopoulos NC, Heathcote EJ, et al. Long-term therapy with adefovir dipivoxil for HBeAg-negative chronic hepatitis B. N Engl J Med 2005;352:2673-2681.
182. Brunelle MN, Jacquard AC, Pichoud C, et al. Susceptibility to antivirals of a human HBV strain with mutations conferring resistance to both lamivudine and adefovir. Hepatology 2005;41:1391-1398.
183. Chang TT, Gish RG, de Man R, et al. A comparison of entecavir and lamivudine for HBeAg-positive chronic hepatitis B. N Engl J Med 2006;354:1001-1010.
184. Lai CL, Shouval D, Lok AS, et al. Entecavir versus lamivudine for patients with HBeAg-negative chronic hepatitis B. N Engl J Med 2006;354:1011-1020.
185. Sherman M, Yurdaydin C, Sollano J, et al. Entecavir for treatment of lamivudine-refractory, HBeAg-positive chronic hepatitis B. Gastroenterology 2006;130:2039-2049.
186. Colonno R, Rose R, Levine S, et al. Entecavir two year resistance update: no resistance observed in nucleoside naïve patients and low frequency resistance emergence in lamivudine refractory patients. Hepatology 2005;42(Suppl 1):573A.
187. Tenney DJ, Levine SM, Rose RE, et al. Clinical emergence of entecavir-resistant hepatitis B virus requires additional substitutions in virus already resistant to lamivudine. Antimicrob Agents Chemother 2004;48:3498-3507.
188. Lai CL, Lim SG, Brown NA, et al. A dose-finding study of once-daily oral telbivudine in HBeAg-positive patients with chronic hepatitis B virus infection. Hepatology 2004;40:719-726.
189. Wu GY, Chen HS. Novel approaches towards conquering hepatitis B virus infection. World J Gastroenterol 2007;13:830-836.
190. Yerly D, Di Giammarino L, Bihl F, Cerny A. Targets of emerging therapies for viral hepatitis B and C. Expert Opin Ther Targets 2006;10:833-850.
191. Eren R, Landstein D, Terkieltaub D, et al. Preclinical evaluation of two neutralizing human monoclonal antibodies against hepatitis C virus (HCV): a potential treatment to prevent HCV reinfection in liver transplant patients. J Virol 2006;80:2654-2664.
192. Gilbert BE, Knight V. Biochemistry and clinical applications of ribavirin. Antimicrob Agents Chemother 1986;30:201-205.
193. McCormick JB, King IJ, Webb PA, et al. Lassa fever: effective therapy with ribavirin. N Engl J Med 1984;314:20-26.
194. Banks G, Fernandez H. Clinical use of ribavirin in measles: a summarized review. In Smith RA, Knight V, Smith JAD (eds): Clinical Applications of Ribavirin. New York: Academic Press, 1984, pp 203-209.
195. Sanchez FA, Sosa IRG, Vargas GM, et al. Treatment of type A hepatitis with ribavirin. In Smith RA, Knight V, Smith JAD (eds): Clinical Applications of Ribavirin. New York: Academic Press, 1984, pp 193-201.
196. Gilbert BE, Wilson SZ, Knight V, et al. Ribavirin small-particle aerosol treatment of infections caused by influenza virus strains A/Victoria/7/83 (H1N1) and B/Texas/1/84. Antimicrob Agents Chemother 1985;27:309-313.
197. Hall CB, McBride JT, Gala CL, et al. Ribavirin treatment of respiratory syncytial virus infection in infants with underlying cardiopulmonary disease. JAMA 1985;254:3047-3051.
198. Taber LH, Knight V, Gilbert BE, et al. Ribavirin aerosol treatment of bronchiolitis associated with respiratory syncytial virus infection in infants. Pediatrics 1983;72:613-618.
199. Dixit NM, Perelson AS. The metabolism, pharmacokinetics and mechanisms of antiviral activity of ribavirin against hepatitis C virus. Cell Mol Life Sci 2006;6:832-842.
200. Crotty S, Maag D, Arnold JJ, et al. The broad-spectrum antiviral ribonucleoside ribavirin is an RNA virus mutagen. Nature Med 2000;6:1375-1379.
201. Zhou S, Liu R, Baroudy BM, et al. The effect of ribavirin and IMPDH inhibitors on hepatitis C virus subgenomic replicon RNA. Virology 2003;310:333-342.
202. Young KC, Lindsay KL, Lee KJ, et al. Identification of a ribavirin-resistant NS5B mutation of hepatitis C virus during ribavirin monotherapy. Hepatology 2003;38:869-878.
203. Tam RC, Pai B, Bard J, et al. Ribavirin polarizes human T cell responses towards a type 1 cytokine profile. J Hepatol 1999;30:376-382.
204. Cramp ME, Rossol S, Chokshi S, et al. Hepatitis C virus-specific T-cell reactivity during interferon and ribavirin treatment in chronic hepatitis C. Gastroenterology 2000;118:346-355.
205. Zhang Y, Jamaluddin M, Wang S, et al. Ribavirin treatment up-regulates antiviral gene expression via the interferon-stimulated response element in respiratory syncytial virus-infected epithelial cells. J Virol 2003;77:5933-5947.
206. Glue P. The clinical pharmacology of ribavirin. Semin Liv Dis 1999;19:17-24.
207. Khakoo S, Glue P, Grellier L, et al. Ribavirin and interferon alfa-2b in chronic hepatitis C: assessment of possible pharmacokinetic and pharmacodynamic interactions. Br J Clin Pharmacol 1998;46:563-570.
208. Jarvis SJ, Thorn JA, Glue P. Ribavirin uptake by human erythrocytes and the involvement of nitrobenzylthioinosine-sensitive (es)-nucleoside transporters. Br J Clin Pharmacol 1998;123:1587-1592.
209. Fried MW, Shiffman ML, Reddy KR, et al. Peginterferon alfa-2a plus ribavirin for chronic hepatitis C virus infection. N Engl J Med 2002;347:975-982.
210. Cusson JR. Ribavirin: a word of caution. CMAJ 1987;136:563.
211. Hofer H, Watkins-Riedel T, Janata O, et al. Spontaneous viral clearance in patients with acute hepatitis C can be predicted by repeated measurements of serum viral load. Hepatology 2003;37:60-64.
212. Heller T, Rehermann B. Acute hepatitis C: a multifaceted disease. Semin Liver Dis 2005;25:7-17.
213. Poynard T, Regimbeau C, Myers RP, et al. Interferon for acute hepatitis C. Cochrane Database Syst Rev 2002;(1):CD000369.
214. Kamal SM, Fouly AE, Kamel RR, et al. Peginterferon alfa-2b therapy in acute hepatitis C: impact of onset of therapy on sustained virologic response. Gastroenterology 2006;130:632-638.
215. Kamal SM, Moustafa KN, Chen J, et al. Duration of peginterferon therapy in acute hepatitis C: a randomized trial. Hepatology 2006;43:923-931.
216. Wiegand J, Buggisch P, Boecher W, et al. Early monotherapy with pegylated interferon alpha-2b for acute hepatitis C infection: the HEP-NET acute-HCV-II study. Hepatology 2006;43:250-256.
217. Hoofnagle JH, Mullen KD, Jones DB, et al. Treatment of chronic non-A, non-B hepatitis with recombinant human alpha interferon: a preliminary report. N Engl J Med 1986;315:1575-1578.
218. Carithers RLJ, Emerson SS. Therapy of hepatitis C: meta-analysis of interferon alfa-2b trials. Hepatology 1997;26(Suppl 1):83S-88S.
219. Myers RP, Regimbeau C, Thevenot T, et al. Interferon for interferon naïve patients with chronic hepatitis C. Cochrane Database Syst Rev 2002;(2):CD000370.
220. Di Bisceglie AM, Conjeevaram HS, Fried MW, et al. Ribavirin as therapy for chronic hepatitis C: a randomized, double-blind, placebo-controlled trial. Ann Intern Med 1995;123:897-903.
221. Schalm SW, Hansen BE, Chemello L, et al. Ribavirin enhances the efficacy but not the adverse effects of interferon in chronic hepatitis C: meta-analysis of individual patient data from European centers. J Hepatol 1997;26:961-966.
222. Schvarcz R, Yun ZB, Sonnerborg A, et al. Combined treatment with interferon alpha-2b and ribavirin for chronic hepatitis C in patients with a previous non-response or non-sustained response to interferon alone. J Med Virol 1995;46:43-47.
223. Poynard T, Marcellin P, Lee SS, et al. Randomised trial of interferon 2b plus ribavirin for 48 weeks or for 24 weeks versus interferon 2b plus placebo for 48 weeks for treatment of chronic infection with hepatitis C virus. Lancet 1998;352:1426-1432.
224. Glue P, Fang JW, Rouzier-Panis R, et al. Pegylated interferon-alpha2b: pharmacokinetics, pharmacodynamics, and preliminary efficacy data. Clin Pharmacol Ther 2000;68:556-567.
225. Pockros PJ, Carithers R, Desmond P, et al. Efficacy and safety of two-dose regimens of peginterferon alpha-2a compared with interferon alpha-2a in chronic hepatitis C: a multicenter, randomized controlled trial. Am J Gastroenterol 2004;99:1298-1305.
226. Zeuzem S, Feinman SV, Rasenack J, et al. Peginterferon alfa-2a in patients with chronic hepatitis C. N Engl J Med 2000;343:1666-1672.
227. Lindsay KL, Trepo C, Heintges T, et al. A randomized, double-blind trial comparing pegylated interferon alfa-2b to interferon alfa-2b as initial treatment for chronic hepatitis C. Hepatology 2001;34:395-403.
228. Hadziyannis SJ, Sette H Jr, Morgan TR, et al. Peginterferon alfa-2a and ribavirin combination therapy in chronic hepatitis C: randomized study of treatment duration and ribavirin dose. Ann Intern Med 2004;140:346-355.
229. Dienstag JL, McHutchison JG. American Gastroenterological Association technical review on the management of hepatitis C. Gastroenterology 2006;130:231-264.
230. Hoofnagle JH, Seeff LB. Peginterferon and ribavirin for chronic hepatitis C. N Engl J Med 2006;355:2444-2451.

231. Stauber RE, Stadlbauer V. Novel approaches for therapy of chronic hepatitis C. J Clin Virol 2006;36:87-94.
232. Davis GL. New therapies: oral inhibitors and immune modulators. Clin Liver Dis 2006;10:867-880.
233. Krawczynski K, Alter MJ, Tankersley DL, et al. Effect of immune globulin on the prevention of experimental hepatitis C virus infection. J Infect Dis 1996;173:822-828.
234. Di Bisceglie AM, Frey S, Gorse GJ, et al. A Phase I safety and immunogenicity trial of a novel E1E2/MF59C.1 hepatitis C vaccine candidate in healthy HCV-negative adults. Hepatology 2005;42:750A.
235. Petracca R, Falugi F, Galli G, et al. Structure-function analysis of hepatitis C virus envelope-CD81 binding. J Virol 2000;74:4824-4830.
236. Gordon SC, Bacon BR, Jacobson IM, et al. A Phase II, 12-week study of ISIS 14803, an antisense inhibitor of HCV for the treatment of chronic hepatitis C. Hepatology 2002;36:362A.
237. Summa V. VX-950 (Vertex/Mitsubishi). Curr Opin Investig Drugs 2005;6:831-837.
238. Lin C, Kwong AD, Perni RB. Discovery and development of VX-950, a novel, covalent, and reversible inhibitor of hepatitis C virus NS3.4A serine protease. Infect Disord Drug Targets 2006;6:3-16.
239. Sarrazin C, Rouzier R, Wagner F, et al. SCH 503034, a novel hepatitis C virus protease inhibitor, plus pegylated interferon alpha-2b for genotype 1 nonresponders. Gastroenterology 2007;132:1270-1278.
240. Reesink HW, Zeuzem S, Weegink CJ, et al. Initial results of a 14-day study of the hepatitis C virus inhibitor VX-950, in combination with peginterferon-alfa 2a. J Hepatol 2006;44(Suppl 2):S272.
241. Emerson SU, Purcell RH. Hepatitis E virus. Rev Med Virol 2003;13:145-154.
242. Arankalle VA. Hepatitis A vaccine strategies and relevance in the present scenario. Indian J Med Res 2004;119:iii-vi.
243. Arankalle VA, Chadha MS, Dama BM, et al. Role of immune serum globulins in pregnant women during an epidemic of hepatitis E. J Viral Hepat 1998;5:199-214.
244. Khuroo MS, Dar MY. Hepatitis E: Evidence for person-to-person transmission and inability of low dose immune serum globulin from an Indian source to prevent it. Indian J Gastroenterol 1992;11:113-116.
245. Worm HC, Wirnsberger G. Hepatitis E vaccines: progress and prospects. Drugs 2004;64:1517-1531.
246. Tsarev SA, Tsareva TS, Emerson SU, et al. Successful passive and active immunization of cynomolgus monkeys against hepatitis E. Proc Natl Acad Sci U S A 1994;91:10198-10202.
247. Shrestha MP, Scott RM, Joshi DM, et al. Safety and efficacy of a recombinant hepatitis E vaccine. N Engl J Med 2007;356:895-903.
248. Melian EB, Plosker GL. Interferon alfacon-1: a review of its pharmacology and therapeutic efficacy in the treatment of chronic hepatitis C. Drugs 2001;61:1661-1691.

36

OBESITY AND NUTRITION

Robert F. Kushner

INTRODUCTION 549
PATHOPHYSIOLOGY 549
THERAPEUTICS AND CLINICAL PHARMACOLOGY 550
Goals of Therapy 550
Therapeutics by Class 550
Amphetamine-Derived Centrally Acting Anorexiants 550
Nonamphetamine Centrally Acting Anorexiants 551
Lipase Inhibitors 552
Cannabinoid-1 Receptor Blocker 552
Therapeutic Approach 553
Diet Therapy 553
Exercise Therapy 553
Pharmacotherapy 553
Emerging Targets and Therapeutics 554

INTRODUCTION

Obesity in adults is clinically defined as a body mass index (BMI; weight in kg/[height in meters]^2) ≥ 30 kg/m^2, where the healthy range is 18.5 to 24.9 kg/m^2, overweight is 25 to 29.9 kg/m^2, class 1 obesity is 30 to 34.9 kg/m^2, class 2 obesity is 35 to 39.9 kg/m^2, and class 3 obesity is 40 kg/m^2. The older terminology of "morbid obesity," empirically defined as more than 100 pounds or 100% over ideal body weight, has been replaced with newer descriptive terms, including "class 3 obesity," "extreme obesity," or "clinically severe obesity." The term *morbid obesity*, however, is still listed in the International Classification of Diseases, Ninth Revision, Clinical Modification (ICD-9-CM), where it is used for coding, and is also used by the National Library of Medicine and in journals and texts.

The prevalence of obesity continues to rise each year, with a disproportionate increase in class 3 obesity and among minority women. According to the 2001-2002 National Health and Nutrition Examination Survey (NHANES), 65% of the U.S. adult population has a BMI of ≥25 kg/m^2 and an estimated 30% are categorized as obese.[1] Obesity is associated with increased morbidity and mortality affecting nine organ systems that involve at least 40 medical conditions, including type 2 diabetes, hypertension, dyslipidemia, heart disease, nonalcoholic fatty liver disease, and some forms of cancer, among many others. Despite the medical, social, and economic impact of obesity, few pharmacologic agents are currently available. This is due, in part, to the complexities of the biologic systems that govern appetite regulation and energy expenditure as well as the multifactorial etiology of the disorder.

PATHOPHYSIOLOGY

The etiology of obesity is multifaceted, brought about by an interaction between predisposing genetic and metabolic factors and a rapidly changing "modern" environment. Based on over a million years of genetic evolution, homo sapiens are physiologically engineered for survival amidst an environment where there is ample physical activity balanced by a marginal or near-sufficient energy supply. Thus, there is a strong selection bias in favor of regulatory systems that vigorously defend against deficits in body weight.[2] The metabolic regulatory system includes feedback loops between the central and autonomic nervous systems, the endocrine glands, and adipose tissue that operate to adjust hunger, satiety, and energy expenditure. Physiologically, weight maintenance is now considered to be governed by a combination of short-term mechanisms originating in the gastrointestinal tract, and longer term processes that monitor total adipose mass involving feedback to the central nervous system. However, over the past century, we have experienced a rapid and unprecedented technological advancement in the availability of food coupled with a reduced need for daily physical activity. These social, economic, and behavioral influences have resulted in an unintended disturbance in energy balance, where "energy in" exceeds "energy out." Thus, the societal pressures that expose individuals to high-calorie, large-portion convenience foods along with technical advances that promote sedentary behavior are at odds with our genetically derived physiology.

Insights into the metabolic and genetic control systems that govern regulation of body weight have been broadened over the past several decades with the identification of gut-derived hormones and the discovery of the *ob* gene and its protein product called leptin (from the Greek work *leptos*, meaning "thin"). Short-term regulation of appetite (hunger and satiety) is influenced by release of the gut hormones cholecystokinin, ghrelin, peptide $YY_{3\text{-}36}$, and glucagon-like peptide-1 (GLP-1), along with signals originating from the vagus afferent neurons within the gastrointestinal tract that respond to mechanical deformation, macronutrients, pH, tonicity, and hormones.[3,4] Whereas ghrelin stimulates food intake, cholecystokinin, peptide $YY_{3\text{-}36}$, and GLP-1 enhance satiety. Gut-derived hunger and satiety signals are shown in Figure 36-1.[4]

For longer term energy regulation, neural and humoral signals derived from the periphery are integrated in specific regions of the hypothalamus and brainstem. Energy homeostasis is maintained by a balance between pathways that stimulate food intake and promote weight gain (anabolic or orexigenic) and pathways that promote reduced food intake and depletion of body fat (catabolic or anorexigenic). Leptin has emerged as the long-sought adipose-derived "satiety hormone." Leptin is secreted from fat cells in response to an increase in fat mass and acts over hours. The hormone's site of action is the arcuate nucleus of the hypothalamus, where it appears to have a dual action: (i) inhibiting neurons that coexpress the orexigenic hormones neuropeptide Y and agouti-related protein; and (ii) stimulating neurons that coexpress the anorexigenic hormones α-melanocyte-stimulating hormone (α-MSH), a cleavage product of pro-opiomelanocortin and cocaine- and amphetamine-regulated transcript (CART). Alpha-MSH subsequently binds to its receptor, MC4R, resulting in downstream appetite control and energy balance.[5,6] A tonic inhibition of the melanocortin cells predominates whenever the neuropeptide Y/agouti-related protein neurons are active.[7] Hypothalamic integration of these neuropeptides is shown in Figure 36-2.[8] This orexigenic dominance in the hypothalamus promotes hunger over satiety, leading to a positive energy balance. Thus far, no successful strategies have emerged that target this system for the treatment of obesity.

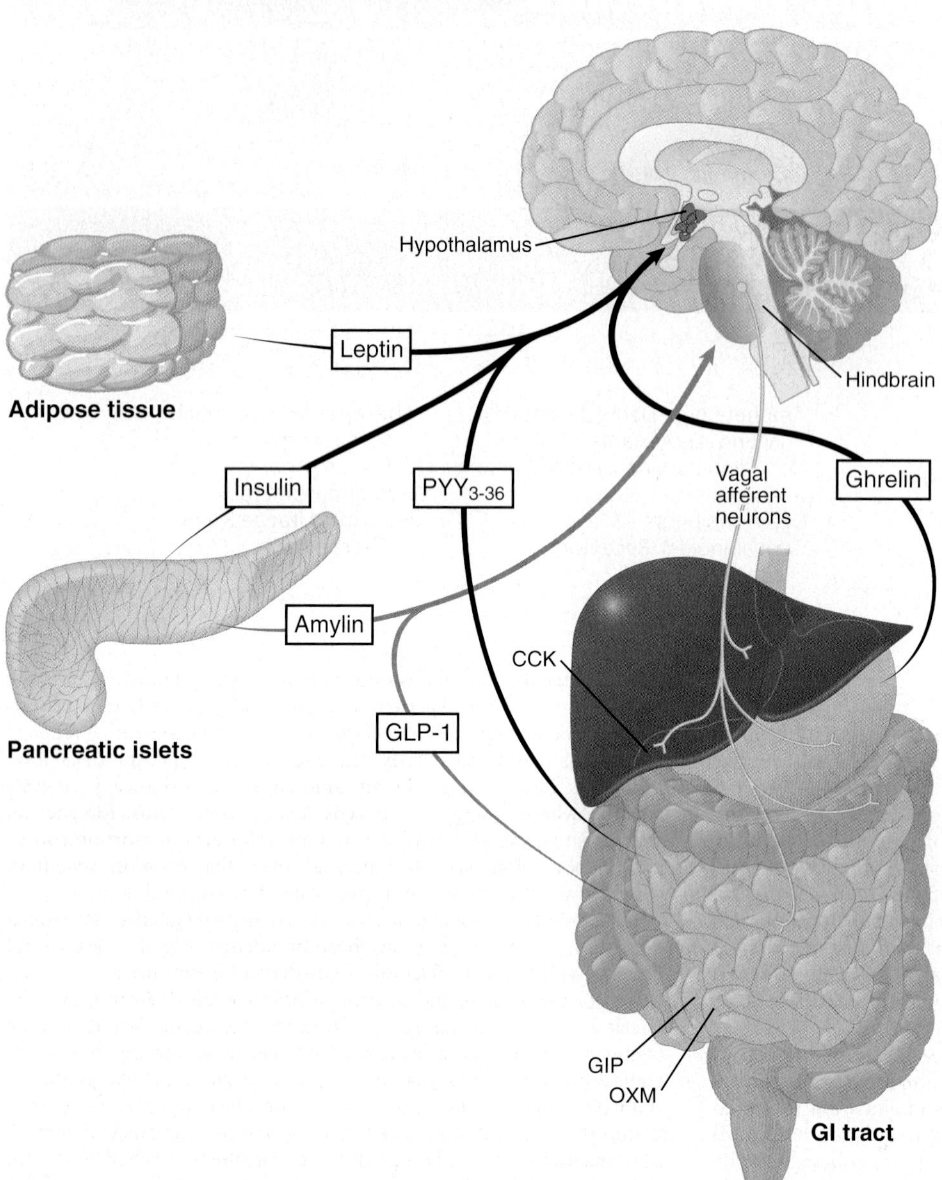

FIGURE 36-1 • Representation of gut peptides and the hypothalamus. Hormones released by the gut have incretin-, hunger-, and satiety-stimulating actions. CCK, cholecystokinin; GIP, glucose-dependent insulinotropic polypeptide; GLP-1, glucagon-like peptide-1; OXM, oxyntomodulin; PYY_{3-36}, peptide YY_{3-36}. (From Badman MK, Flier JS. The gut and energy balance: visceral allies in the obesity wars. Science 2005;307:1909-1914. Reprinted with permission of AAAS.)

THERAPEUTICS AND CLINICAL PHARMACOLOGY

Goals of Therapy

The goals of obesity treatment are to (i) stop weight gain, (ii) reduce body weight, (iii) maintain a lower body weight over the long term, and (iv) improve obesity-related comorbid conditions and reduce the risk of future illness. The choice of treatment modalities is determined by the patient's risk status, his or her abilities and desires, and available resources. The initial target goal of weight loss is to decrease body weight by about 10% of baseline weight over 6 months of therapy.[9] Lifestyle management is used throughout the treatment continuum, while pharmacotherapy and surgery are used as adjunctive modalities in accordance with increasing BMI level and risk level.

Therapeutics by Class

Since appetite, energy expenditure, and body weight are regulated by multiple complex pathways, it has been difficult to identify effective and safe medications for the treatment of obesity. Historically, safety concerns have outweighed benefit for many weight loss drugs. Since 1997, five drugs have been removed from markets around the world due to lack of safety: fenfluramine hydrochloride, dexfenfluramine hydrochloride, and phenylpropanolamine hydrochloride worldwide and diethylpropion hydrochloride and phentermine hydrochloride in Europe. Thereafter, only three drugs have been introduced into the marketplace: sibutramine hydrochloride, orlistat, and rimonabant. In this section, only medications currently available in the United States or Europe are reviewed.

Amphetamine-Derived Centrally Acting Anorexiants

Appetite suppressing drugs, or anorexiants, effect *satiation* (the processes involved in the termination of a meal), *satiety* (the absence of hunger after eating), and *hunger* (a biologic sensation that initiates eating). By increasing satiation and satiety and decreasing hunger, these agents help patients reduce caloric intake while providing a greater sense of control without deprivation. In the 1930s, amphetamines were first introduced as anorexiants. However, amphetamine was addictive and had euphoric side effects. By modifying the side chain of amphetamine's α-phenylethylamine structure, the anorectic effect of the parent compound was retained while reducing the stimulatory properties and potential for addiction. These amphetamine congeners produced a wide range of pharmacologic responses that influence dopaminergic and noradrenergic neurotransmission. Among the centrally acting adrenergic agents that have been marketed for the treatment of obesity, four compounds—phentermine, benzphetamine, phendimetrazine, and diethylpropion—increase the release of norepinephrine from the nerve terminals into the interneuronal cleft and inhibit its reuptake, thus increasing the amount of norepinephrine interacting with postganglionic neuronal α_2-adrenergic receptors. The fifth compound, mazindol, is structurally related to the tricyclic antidepressants and functions by blocking norepinephrine reuptake.[10,11] By 1960, all five of the sympathomimetic amines were approved as adjuncts in the management of obesity. Due to their addictive potential, they are all scheduled by the U.S. Drug Enforcement Agency as Schedule III or IV drugs.

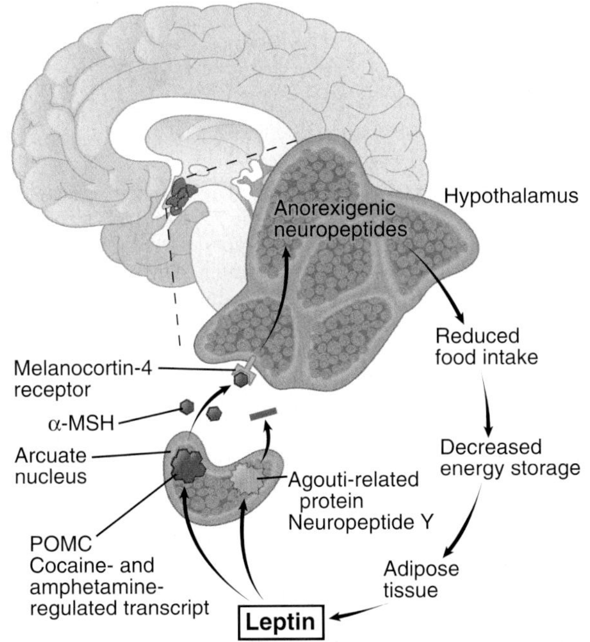

FIGURE 36-2 • Representation of hypothalamic control of appetite regulation and energy balance. Leptin stimulates neurons in the arcuate nucleus of the hypothalamus that coexpress the anorexigenic hormones α-melanocyte-stimulating hormone (α-MSH, a cleavage product of pro-opiomelanocortin [POMC]) and cocaine- and amphetamine-related transcript. Leptin also inhibits the orexigenic hormones agouti-related protein and neuropeptide Y. (Adapted from List JF, Habener JF. Defective melanocortin 4 receptors in hyperphagia and morbid obesity. N Engl J Med 2003;348:1160-1163. Copyright © 1990 Massachusetts Medical Society. All rights reserved.)

Among the anorectics, phentermine is the most commonly prescribed agent.[12] Approved for the treatment of obesity as a resin complex in 1959 and in hydrochloride form in 1973, phentermine is currently approved by the U.S. Food and Drug Administration (FDA) for short-term use only (8 to 12 weeks) in conjunction with a low-calorie diet and exercise. Current treatment strategy, however, dictates long-term administration of this medication. There are limited long-term data on the effectiveness of phentermine. A 2002 review of six randomized, controlled trials using phentermine for weight control found that patients lost 0.6 to 6.0 additional kg of weight compared to placebo over 2 to 24 weeks of treatment.[13] Treatment is typically started with a 15-mg daily dose administered $^1/_2$ hour before or 1 to 2 hours after a meal, with the dose titrated up to a maximum of 37.5 mg/day. The most common side effects of the amphetamine-derived anorexiants are restlessness, insomnia, dry mouth, constipation, and increased blood pressure and heart rate. Phentermine is primarily excreted by the kidneys and should be used with caution in patients with abnormal renal function.

Nonamphetamine Centrally Acting Anorexiants

Sibutramine is the first of a new class of compounds that have dual serotonin and norepinephrine reuptake inhibition that primarily affects satiation. The drug undergoes rapid and extensive metabolism in the liver to produce two demethylated primary and secondary amine metabolites that have greater pharmacologic activity than the parent compound.[14] These metabolites have long elimination half-lives of 14 to 16 hours, allowing once-daily dosing. Unlike the sympathomimetic amines, sibutramine is not pharmacologically related to amphetamine and has no addictive potential. Sibutramine was approved by the FDA in 1997 for weight loss and weight maintenance in conjunction with a reduced-calorie diet at 5-, 10-, and 15-mg doses. The pharmacologic properties of the drug are summarized in Table 36-1.[15]

In clinical trials, weight loss is apparent at 4 weeks and is at near maximum at approximately 24 weeks. A meta-analysis on sibutramine efficacy reported a mean difference in weight loss (compared to placebo) of 3.43 kg at 6 months and 4.45 kg at 12 months.[16] Categorically, adults taking sibutramine for 1 year are 19% to 34% more likely to achieve 5% weight loss and 12% to 31% more likely to achieve 10% weight loss than those taking placebo.[17] One trial evaluated the utility of sibutramine for weight maintenance.[18] By using the Last Observation Carried Forward (LOCF) method, participants receiving sibutramine versus those receiving placebo maintained 4.0 kg more weight

TABLE 36-1 PHARMACOLOGIC PROPERTIES OF SIBUTRAMINE, ORLISTAT, AND RIMONABANT

	Sibutramine	Orlistat	Rimonabant
Mechanism of action	Monoamine reuptake inhibitor (primarily norepinephrine and serotonin)	Gastric and pancreatic lipase inhibitor	Endocannabinoid (CB_1) receptor blocker
Typical dose	10-15 mg once daily	120 mg twice daily with meals*	20 mg daily
Absorption	77%	Minimal	Not known
Plasma protein binding	94%	99%	99.9%
Time to peak concentration	1-2 hr (2.5-3.6 hr for metabolites)	8 hr	2 hr
Metabolism	Primarily via hepatic cytochrome P-450 3A4 isozyme to active M1 and M2 metabolites	Some metabolism within gastrointestinal wall to inactive metabolites	Hepatic cytochrome P-450 3A4 isozyme and aminohydrolase pathways to inactive metabolites
Elimination	Primarily urine (77%)	Feces (over 96% of total drug ingested; 83% unchanged)	Biliary excretion and fecal elimination (86%)
Elimination half-life	1-2 hr (M1 metabolite, 14 hr; M2 metabolite, 16 hr)	14-19 hr	6-9 days (16 days in obese patients)

*Over-the-counter dose is 60 mg.
From Padawal RS, Majumdar SR. Drug treatments for obesity: orlistat, sibutramine, and rimonabant. Lancet 2007;369:71-77.

TABLE 36-2 SUMMARY OF WEIGHT LOSS OUTCOMES AND ADVERSE EFFECTS FOR SIBUTRAMINE, ORLISTAT, AND RIMONABANT

	Sibutramine	Orlistat	Rimonabant
Mean % weight loss (95% CI)*	4.6 (3.8-5.4)	2.9 (2.3-3.4)	4.6 (4.3-5.0)†
5% weight loss (% patients to reach threshold)‡	34 (28-40)	21 (19-24)	33 (29-39)
10% weight loss (% patients to reach threshold)	15 (4-27)	12 (8-16)	21 (17-25)
Common adverse effects	Insomnia, dry mouth, headache, constipation, increased blood pressure and heart rate	Fatty stool, urgency, oily spotting, fecal incontinence	Nausea, dizziness, insomnia, depression, anxiety

*Placebo-subtracted percent weight loss; CI, confidence interval.
†20-mg rimonabant group.
‡Categorical responses; percent of patients reaching 5% and 10% placebo-subtracted weight loss thresholds: mean % of patients (95% CI).
Adapted from Padawal RS, Majumdar SR. Drug treatments for obesity: orlistat, sibutramine, and rimonabant. Lancet 2007;369:71-77.

loss at 2 years. Efficacy and safety beyond 2 years of treatment are unknown. A meta-analysis of eight studies in diabetic patients receiving sibutramine showed a mean weight loss of 5.53 ± 2.2 kg for those treated with sibutramine and 0.90 ± 0.17 kg for the placebo-treated patients.[19]

The most commonly reported adverse events of sibutramine are headache, dry mouth, insomnia, and constipation (Table 36-2). These are generally mild and well tolerated. The principal concern is a dose-related increase in blood pressure and heart rate that may require discontinuation of the medication. A dose of 10 to 15 mg/day causes an average increase in systolic and diastolic blood pressure of 2 to 4 mm Hg and an increase in heart rate of 4 to 6 beats/min. For this reason, all patients should be monitored closely and seen back in the office within 1 month after initiating therapy. The risk of adverse effects on blood pressure is no greater in patients with controlled hypertension than in those who do not have hypertension, and the drug does not appear to cause cardiac valve dysfunction. Contraindications to sibutramine use include uncontrolled hypertension, congestive heart failure, symptomatic coronary artery disease, arrhythmias, or history of stroke. Similar to other antiobesity medications, weight reduction is enhanced when the drug is used along with behavior therapy, and body weight increases once the medication is discontinued.

Lipase Inhibitors

Orlistat was approved by the FDA in 1999 as the first lipase inhibitor for obesity management, including weight loss and weight maintenance, when used in conjunction with a reduced-calorie diet. Based on its safety profile, the medication was approved as an over-the-counter medication in the United States in 2007 at half the prescription dose. The drug is a synthetic hydrogenated derivative of a naturally occurring lipase inhibitor, lipostatin, produced by the mold *Streptomyces toxytricini.* Orlistat is a potent, slowly reversible inhibitor of pancreatic, gastric, and carboxylester lipases and phospholipase A_2, which are required for the hydrolysis of dietary fat in the gastrointestinal tract into fatty acids and monoacylglycerols.[20] The drug's activity takes place in the lumen of the stomach and small intestine by forming a covalent bond with the active serine residue site of these lipases, rendering the inactivated enzymes unable to hydrolyze dietary fat. Orlistat is minimally (<1%) absorbed from the gastrointestinal tract and primarily eliminated in the feces. When taken as directed (120-mg capsule three times per day with meals or up to 1 hour after a meal), the drug blocks the digestion and absorption of approximately 30% of dietary fat. Thus, if taken with a 30-g fat meal, 10 g or 90 calories of fat will be malabsorbed. Higher doses do not increase weight loss. On discontinuation of the drug, fecal fat usually returns to normal concentrations within 48 to 72 hours.

Multiple randomized, double-blind, placebo-controlled studies have shown that, after 1 to 2 years, mean weight loss in orlistat-treated patients averages approximately 2.7 to 3.19 kg greater than that in placebo-treated patients.[21-23] Total weight lost in the orlistat-treated patients (diet and drug) is approximately 7.1 to 8.1 kg. Categorically, more subjects randomized to orlistat compared to placebo lose greater than 5% (average 55% vs. 33%) and greater than 10% (average 34% vs. 16%) of body weight. In the longest published follow-up study, mean weight loss after 4 years for the orlistat-treated patients was 5.8 kg compared to 3.0 kg with placebo.[24]

Since orlistat is minimally absorbed from the gastrointestinal tract, it has no systemic side effects. Tolerability to the drug is related to the malabsorption of dietary fat and subsequent passage of fat in the feces. Six gastrointestinal tract adverse effects have been reported to occur in at least 10% of orlistat-treated patients: oily spotting, flatus with discharge, fecal urgency, fatty/oily stool, oily evacuation, and increased defecation. The events are generally experienced early, diminish as patients control their dietary fat intake, and infrequently cause patients to withdraw from clinical trials. Psyllium mucilloid is helpful in controlling the orlistat-induced gastrointestinal side effects when taken concomitantly with the medication. Serum concentrations of the fat-soluble vitamins D and E and β-carotene have been found to be significantly lower in some of the trials, although generally remaining within normal ranges. The manufacturer's package insert for orlistat recommends that patients take a vitamin supplement along with the drug to prevent potential deficiencies. Since the medication decreases absorption of fat and cholesterol, improvement in serum total cholesterol, low-density lipoprotein cholesterol, and high-density lipoprotein (HDL) cholesterol has been observed independent of weight loss.[25]

Orlistat is contraindicated in patients with cholestasis and malabsorptive syndromes and in women who are pregnant or breast-feeding. Orlistat can affect blood levels of cyclosporine and amiodarone, so patients on these medications should be closely monitored. International normalized ratio values should be followed closely in patients on warfarin during the first month of treatment with orlistat, as it can decrease vitamin K levels.

Cannabinoid-1 Receptor Blocker

Rimonabant, a first-in-class cannabinoid-1 receptor blocker, was approved by the European Agency for the Evaluation of Medicinal Products in 2006 as an adjunct to diet and exercise for the treatment of obese or overweight patients with associated risk factors. The company withdrew its application to the FDA in June 2007 due to safety considerations. Cannabinoid receptors and their endogenous ligands have been implicated in a variety of physiologic functions, including feeding, modulation of pain, emotional behavior, and peripheral lipid metabolism. The cannabinoid receptors, the endocannabinoids, and the enzymes catalyzing their biosynthesis and degradation constitute the endocannabinoid system.[26] Cannabis and its main ingredient, Δ^9-tetrahydrocannabinol (THC), are exogenous cannabinoid compounds. Two endocannabinoids have been identified, anandamide and 2-arachidonyl glyceride. Two cannabinoid receptors have been cloned: CB_1 (abundant in the brain) and CB_2 (present in immune cells). The brain endocannabinoid system is thought to control food intake through reinforcing motivation to find and consume foods with high incentive value and regulate actions of other mediators of appetite.[27] The primary function of the CB_1 receptors is thought to be inhibition of neurotransmitter release, specifically γ-aminobutyric acid (GABA) or glutamate.[28] The first selective cannabinoid CB_1 receptor antagonist, called rimonabant, was discovered in 1994. The medication is effective in antagonizing the orexigenic effect of THC and suppressing appetite when given alone in animal models.

Thus far, four large prospective, randomized, controlled clinical trials designated the RIO studies (*R*imonabant *I*n *O*besity) have been published that compare rimonabant 5 mg and 20 mg with placebo. RIO-Lipids and RIO-Diabetes[29,30] were 1-year trials; RIO-Europe and RIO-North America were 2-year trials.[31,32] Mean placebo-subtracted 1-year weight loss for the 20-mg dose ranged from 3.9 kg (RIO-Diabetes) to 5.4 kg (RIO-Lipids). Concomitant improvements were seen in waist circumference (−3.3 to −4.7 cm), serum triglycerides (−13.2% to −16.4%), HDL cholesterol (7.2% to 8.9%), and glucose control (hemoglobin A_{1c} −0.7% relative to placebo). Although nausea is the most frequent adverse effect of the drug, psychiatric events are the most common reason for early discontinuation from the clinical trials. Specifically, depressed mood disorders and anxiety were reported more frequently among the medication group. The psychiatric side effects pose the greatest safety concern for this drug.

Therapeutic Approach

To provide guidance to the primary care practitioner and evidence for the effects of treatment, the National Heart, Lung, and Blood Institute (NHLBI) published the "Clinical Guidelines on the Identification, Evaluation, and Treatment of Overweight and Obesity in Adults" in 1998.[9] The "Practical Guide to the Identification, Evaluation, and Treatment of Overweight and Obesity in Adults" was subsequently developed cooperatively by the NHLBI and North American Association for the Study of Obesity and published in 2000.[33] In 2003, as part of their Roadmaps for Clinical Practice series, the American Medical Association published "Assessment and Management of Adult Obesity: A Primer for Physicians."[34] These guidelines recommend proactive obesity care in the primary care setting, beginning with identification, classification, and categorization of risk.

Therapy for obesity always begins with lifestyle management and may include pharmacotherapy or surgery. Lifestyle management incorporates the three essential components of obesity care: dietary therapy, physical activity, and behavior therapy. Lifestyle management has been shown to result in a modest (typically 3 to 5 kg) weight loss compared to no treatment or usual care.[35]

Diet Therapy

The primary focus of diet therapy is on reducing overall consumption of calories. The NHLBI Guidelines[9] recommend initiating treatment with a diet producing a calorie deficit of 500 to 1000 kcal/day. In general, this translates into prescribing diets containing 1000 to 1200 kcal/day for most women and between 1200 and 1600 kcal/day for men. The macronutrient composition of the diet will vary depending on the patient's preference and medical condition. The revised Dietary Reference Intakes for Macronutrients released by the Institute of Medicine recommend an adult diet that has 45% to 65% of calories from carbohydrates, 20% to 35% from fat, and 10% to 35% from protein.[36] The guidelines also recommend daily fiber intake of 38 g (men) and 25 g (women) for persons over 50 and 30 g (men) and 21 g (women) for those under 50 years of age. The 2005 U.S. Department of Agriculture (USDA) *Dietary Guidelines for Americans*, which focus on health promotion and risk reduction, can be applied to treatment of the overweight and obese patient.[37] The dietary recommendations include maintaining a diet rich in whole grains, fruits, vegetables, and dietary fiber, consuming two servings (8 oz) of fish high in ω-3 fatty acids per week, decreasing sodium to less than 2300 mg/day, consuming 3 cups of milk (or equivalent low-fat or fat-free dairy products) per day, limiting cholesterol to less than 300 mg/day, and keeping total fat between 20% and 35% of daily calories and saturated fats to less than 10% of daily calories. Application of these guidelines to specific calorie goals can be found on the USDA web site at *www.mypyramid.gov*.

A current area of controversy is the use of low-carbohydrate, high-protein diets for weight loss. In recent years, several randomized, controlled trials have demonstrated greater weight loss at 6 months with improvement in coronary artery disease risk factors, including an increase in HDL cholesterol and a decrease in triglyceride levels. However, weight loss between groups did not remain statistically significant at 1 year.[38] Low-carbohydrate diets appear to be at least as effective as low-fat diets in inducing weight loss for up to 1 year. Another dietary approach to consider is the concept of energy density. Dietary studies have demonstrated that people tend to ingest a constant volume of food, regardless of caloric or macronutrient content. The energy density approach to weight loss comes from this observation. Energy density refers to the number of calories (energy) a food contains per unit of weight. This value is affected by the water, macronutrient (fat, carbohydrate, and protein), and fiber content of the food. The theory holds that a smaller number of calories can be consumed for a given weight of food if the food is low in energy density. Adding water or fiber to a food decreases its energy density by increasing weight without affecting caloric content. Examples of foods with low energy density include soups, fruits, vegetables, oatmeal, and lean meats. Dry foods and high-fat foods such as pretzels, cheese, egg yolks, potato chips, and red meat have a high energy density. Studies on the topic suggest that diets containing low energy density foods control hunger and result in decreased caloric intake and weight loss.

Exercise Therapy

Although exercise alone is only moderately effective for weight loss, the combination of dietary modification and exercise is the most effective behavioral approach for treatment of obesity. Additionally, physical activity is beneficial for improved cardiorespiratory fitness, cardiovascular disease and cancer risk reduction, and improved mood and self-esteem. Currently, the *minimum* public health recommendation for physical activity is 30 minutes of moderate-intensity physical activity on most, preferably all, days of the week.[39] Studies have demonstrated that lifestyle activities are as effective as structured exercise programs in improving cardiorespiratory fitness and weight loss.

The most important role of exercise appears to be in the maintenance of weight loss, for which exercise at a higher level than generally recommended for public health is necessary. The American College of Sports Medicine (ACSM) recommends that overweight and obese individuals progressively increase to a minimum of 150 minutes of moderate-intensity physical activity per week as a first goal.[40] However, for long-term weight loss, higher amounts of exercise (e.g., 200 to 300 minutes per week or ≥2000 kcal/wk) are needed. The *Dietary Guidelines for Americans* published in 2005 found compelling evidence that at least 60 to 90 minutes of daily moderate-intensity physical activity (420 to 630 minutes per week) is needed to sustain weight loss.[37] The ACSM also recommends that resistance exercise supplement the endurance exercise program. Many patients would benefit from consultation with an exercise physiologist or personal trainer.

Pharmacotherapy

Adjuvant pharmacologic treatments should be considered for patients with a BMI greater than 30 kg/m^2, or those with a BMI greater than 27 kg/m^2 who also have concomitant obesity-related risk factors or diseases and for whom dietary and physical activity therapy has not been successful. Whether the medication acts centrally to suppress appetite or peripherally to block the absorption of fat, patients must deliberately and consciously alter their behavior for weight loss to occur. In other words, for all antiobesity drugs, the pharmacologic action must be *translated* into behavior change. For anorexiants, a reduced sense of hunger and/or increased satiety must be translated into choosing smaller, healthier meals and reduced snacking. Failure to sense and act upon these inhibitory internal signals will result in modest or no weight loss. Similarly, if a patient takes an intestinal fat-blocking agent and does not limit the consumption of dietary fat to 30% or less, he or she will discontinue the medication due to intolerable side effects. Moreover, failure to incorporate physical activity as part of the lifestyle change will seriously hinder maintenance of the initial weight loss. Thus, there is a bidirectional, mutually beneficial relationship between antiobesity drugs and lifestyle management, with each therapy enhancing the efficacy of the other.

In a randomized trial by Wadden et al.[41] evaluating the benefits of lifestyle modification in the pharmacologic treatment of obesity, investigators showed that the efficacy of sibutramine-induced mean weight loss at 1 year was significantly enhanced when subjects also attended a lifestyle support group (−10.8%) or attended a lifestyle support group plus maintained a portion-controlled diet (−16.5%) versus sibutramine alone (−4.1%). The importance of combining pharmacotherapy with lifestyle modification was confirmed in a subsequent study by the same group.[42] Thus, when prescribed an antiobesity medication, patients must be actively engaged in a lifestyle program that provides the strategies and skills needed to effectively use the drug.

Emerging Targets and Therapeutics

An emerging theme in pharmacotherapy for obesity is to target several points in the regulatory pathways that control body weight. Although this is considered common practice in the treatment of other chronic diseases such as diabetes, hypertension, and asthma, it has not been embraced in the development of antiobesity therapies until recently.[43] Several combination drug therapies are entering or currently in Phase III trials. Bupropion and naltrexone (Contrave), a dopamine and norepinephrine reuptake inhibitor and an opioid receptor antagonist, respectively, both enhance the release of the anorexiant neuropeptides α-MSH and CART in the hypothalamus. Excalia (bupropion and zonisamide, an anticonvulsant that has serotonergic and dopaminergic activity) similarly enhances the release of α-MSH and CART. Qnexa—phentermine and topiramate, a catecholamine releaser and an anticonvulsant, respectively—is due to enter Phase III trials. Topiramate's action on body weight is thought to be mediated through its modulation of GABA receptors to reduce food intake. At doses of 96 mg and 192 mg, topiramate resulted in a mean loss of 15.4% and 16.5% of baseline body weight, respectively, versus 8.9% for placebo-treated patients.[44] Although effective, the associated adverse events of cognitive impairment and paresthesias caused the sponsor to terminate development of the drug as an antiobesity agent. Other drugs in development include locaserin, a selective 5-hydroxytryptamine$_{2c}$ receptor agonist that causes hypophagia,[45] and compounds that target the melanocortin system—melanin-concentrating hormone receptor antagonists.[46]

Another emerging area is drugs that act peripherally to affect appetite. Two gut-derived peptides, GLP-1 and amylin, have both been exploited for the treatment of type 2 diabetes since they act as insulin sensitizers. They also significantly enhance satiety when administered exogenously. Exenatide, a GLP-1 analogue produced in the salivary gland of the Gila monster lizard, has been shown to decrease food intake by 19%[47] and result in moderate weight loss in patients enrolled in clinical trials for type 2 diabetes. Pramlintide, a human analogue of amylin, has also been shown to significantly reduce food intake after single injections[48] and cause modest weight loss in patients with type 2 diabetes. Clinical trials of these agents for patients with obesity are pending.

REFERENCES

1. Ogden CL, Carroll MD, Curtin LR, et al. Prevalence of overweight and obesity in the United States, 1999-2004. JAMA 2006;295:1549-1555.
2. Schwartz MW, Woods SC, Seeley RJ, et al. Is the energy homeostasis system inherently biased toward weight gain? Diabetes 2003;52:232-238.
3. Druce MR, Small CJ, Bloom SR. Minireview: Gut peptides regulating satiety. Endocrinology 2004;145:2660-2665.
4. Badman MK, Flier JS. The gut and energy balance: visceral allies in the obesity wars. Science 2005;307:1909-1914.
5. Schwartz MW, Woods SC, Porte D, et al. Central nervous system control of food intake. Nature 2000;404:661-671.
6. Korner J, Aronne LJ. The emerging science of body weight regulation and its impact on obesity treatment. J Clin Invest 2003;111:565-570.
7. Horvath TL. The hardship of obesity: a soft-wired hypothalamus. Nat Neurosci 2005;8:561-565.
8. List JF, Habener JF. Defective melanocortin 4 receptors in hyperphagia and morbid obesity. N Engl J Med 2003;348:1160-1163.
9. National Heart, Lung, and Blood Institute (NHLBI) and National Institute for Diabetes and Digestive and Kidney Diseases (NIDDKD). Clinical guidelines on the identification, evaluation, and treatment of overweight and obesity in adults: the evidence report. Obes Res. 1998;6(Suppl 2):51S-210S.
10. Bray GA, Greenway FL. Current and potential drugs for treatment of obesity. Endocrine Rev 1999;20:805-875.
11. Kordik CP, Reitz AB. Pharmacological treatment of obesity: therapeutic strategies. J Med Chem 1999;42:181-201.
12. Stafford RS, Radley DC. National trends in antiobesity medication use. Arch Intern Med 2003;163:1046-1050.
13. Haddock CK, Poston WSC, Dill PL, et al. Pharmacotherapy for obesity: a quantitative analysis of four decades of published randomized clinical trials. Int J Obes 2002;26:262-273.
14. McNeely W, Goa KL. Sibutramine: a review of its contribution to the management of obesity. Drugs 1998;56:1093-1124.
15. Padawal RS, Majumdar SR. Drug treatments for obesity: orlistat, sibutramine, and rimonabant. Lancet 2007;369:71-77.
16. Shekelle PG, Morton SC, Maglione M, et al. Pharmacological and Surgical Treatment of Obesity: Summary Evidence Report/Technology Assessment No. 103 (AHRQ publication no. 04-E028-1). Rockville, MD: Agency for Healthcare Research and Quality, 2004.
17. Arterburn DE, Crane PK, Veenstra DL. The efficacy and safety of sibutramine for weight loss: a systematic review. Arch Intern Med 2004;164:994-1003.
18. James WP, Astrup A, Finer N, et al. Effect of sibutramine on weight maintenance after weight loss: a randomized trial. STORM Study Group. Sibutramine Trial of Obesity Reduction and Maintenance. Lancet 2000;356:2119-2125.
19. Vettor R, Serra R, Pagano C, Federspil G. Effect of sibutramine on weight management and metabolic control in type 2 diabetes: a meta-analysis of clinical studies. Diabetes Care 2005;28:942-949.
20. Lucas KH, Kaplan-Machlis B. Orlistat—a novel weight loss therapy. Ann Pharmacother 2001;35:314-328.
21. Padawal R, Li SK, Lau DCW. Long-term pharmacotherapy for overweight and obesity: a systematic review and meta-analysis of randomized controlled trials. Int J Obes 2003;27:1437-1446.
22. Li Z, Maglione M, Tu W, et al. Meta-analysis: pharmacologic treatment of obesity. Ann Intern Med 2005;142:532-546.
23. O'Meara SO, Riemsma R, Shirran L, et al. A systematic review of the clinical effectiveness of orlistat used for the management of obesity. Obes Rev 2004;5:51-68.
24. Torgerson JS, Hauptman J, Boldrin MN, Sjostrom L. XENical in the prevention of diabetes in Obese Subjects (XENDOS) Study. Diabetes Care 2004;27:155-161.
25. Hutton B, Fergusson D. Changes in body weight and serum lipid profile in obese patients treated with orlistat in addition to a hypocaloric diet: a systematic review of randomized clinical trials. Am J Clin Nutr 2004;80:1461-1468.
26. Di Marzo V, Bifulco M, De Petrocellis L. The endocannabinoid system and its therapeutic exploitation. Nat Rev Drug Discov 2004;3:771-784.
27. Pagotto U, Marsicano G, Cota D, et al. The emerging role of the endocannabinoid system in endocrine regulation and energy balance. Endocrine Rev 2006;27:73-100.
28. Mackie K. Mechanisms of CB_1 receptor signaling: endocannabinoid modulation of synaptic strength. Int J Obes 2006;30(Suppl 1):S19-S23.
29. Despres JP, Golay A, Sjostrom L. Effects of rimonabant on metabolic risk factors in overweight patients with dyslipidemia. N Engl J Med 2005;353:2121-2134.
30. Scheen AJ, Finer N, Hollander P, et al. Efficacy and tolerability of rimonabant in overweight or obese patients with type 2 diabetes: a randomized controlled study. Lancet 2006;368:1660-1672.
31. Van Gaal LF, Rissanen AM, Scheen AJ, et al. Effects of the cannabinoid-1 receptor blocker rimonabant on weight reduction and cardiovascular risk factors in overweight patients: 1-year experience from the RIO-Europe study. Lancet 2005;365:1389-1397.
32. Pi-Sunyer FX, Aronne LJ, Heshmati HM, et al. Effect of rimonabant, a cannabinoid-1 receptor blocker, on weight and cardiometabolic risk factors in overweight or obese patients. RIO-North America: a randomized controlled trial. JAMA 2006;295:761-775.
33. National Heart, Lung, and Blood Institute (NHLBI) and North American Association for the Study of Obesity (NAASO). Practical Guide on the Identification, Evaluation, and Treatment of Overweight and Obesity in Adults (NIH publication no. 00-4084). Bethesda, MD: National Institutes of Health, 2000.
34. Kushner RF. Roadmaps for Clinical Practice: Case Studies in Disease Prevention and Health Promotion—Assessment and Management of Adult Obesity: A Primer for Physicians. Chicago: American Medical Association, 2003. Available at *www.ama-assn.org/ama/pub/category/10931.html*
35. U.S. Preventive Services Task Force. Screening for obesity in adults: recommendations and rationale. Ann Intern Med 2003;139:930-932.
36. Institute of Medicine (IOM). Institute of Medicine of the National Academies: Dietary Reference Intakes for Energy, Carbohydrate, Fiber, Fat, Fatty Acids, Cholesterol, Protein, and Amino Acids (Macronutrients). A report of the Panel on Macronutrients, Subcommittees on Upper Reference Levels of Nutrients and Interpretation and Uses of Dietary Reference Intakes, and the Standing Committee on the Scientific Evaluation of Dietary Reference Intakes. Washington, DC: Institute of Medicine, 2002.
37. U. S. Department of Agriculture and U.S. Department of Health and Human Services. Nutrition and Your Health: Dietary Guidelines for Americans, 5th ed (Home and

Garden Bulletin No. 232). Washington, DC: U.S. Department of Health and Human Services, 2005.
38. Noble CA, Kushner RF. An update on low-carbohydrate, high-protein diets. Curr Opin Gastroenterol 2006;22;153-159.
39. Pate RR, Pratt M, Blair SN, et al. Physical activity and public health: a recommendation from the Centers for Disease Control and Prevention and the American College of Sports Medicine. JAMA 1995;273:402-407.
40. Jakacic JM, Clark K, Coleman E, et al. Appropriate intervention strategies for weight loss and prevention of weight regain for adults. Med Sci Sports Exerc 2001;33:2145-2156.
41. Wadden TA, Berkowitz RI, Sarwer DB, et al. Benefits of lifestyle modification in the pharmacologic treatment of obesity: a randomized trial. Arch Intern Med 2001;161:218-227.
42. Wadden TA, Berkowitz RI, Womble LG, et al. Randomized trial of lifestyle modification and pharmacotherapy for obesity. N Engl J Med 2005;353:2111-2120.
43. Aronne LJ, Thornton-Jones ZD. New targets for obesity pharmacotherapy. Clin Pharmacol Ther 2007;81:748-752.
44. Astrup A, Caterson I, Zelissen P, et al. Topiramate: long-term maintenance of weight loss induced by a low-calorie diet in obese subjects. Obes Res 2004;12:1658-1669.
45. Halford JC, Harrold JA, Boyland EJ, et al. Serotonergic drugs: effects on appetite expression and use for the treatment of obesity. Drugs 2007;67:27-55.
46. Hervieu G. Further insights into the neurobiology of melanin-concentrating hormone in energy and mood balances. Expert Opin Ther Targets 2006;10:211-229.
47. Edwards CM, Stanley SA, Davis R, et al. Exendin-4 reduces fasting and postprandial glucose and decreases energy intake in healthy volunteers. Am J Physiol Endocrinol Metab 2001;281:E155-E161.
48. Chapman I, Parker B, Doran S, et al. Low-dose pramlintide reduced food intake and meal duration in healthy, normal-weight subjects. Obesity 2007;15:1179-1186.

37

DIABETES MELLITUS

Robert A. Rizza and Adrian Vella

INTRODUCTION 557
PATHOPHYSIOLOGY 557
THERAPEUTICS AND CLINICAL PHARMACOLOGY 558
Goals of Therapy 558
Therapeutics by Class 559
α-Glucosidase Inhibitors 559
Pramlintide 559
Incretin-Based Therapy 560
Meglitinides 561
Biguanides 561
Sulfonylureas 562
Thiazolindinediones 562
Insulin 562
Therapeutic Approach 566
Emerging Targets and Therapeutics 568
Prevention of Type 2 Diabetes and Early Intervention in Prediabetes 568
MODY and Implications of Therapy 568
Combination PPAR Agonists 568

INTRODUCTION

Diabetes comprises a heterogeneous group of conditions characterized by hyperglycemia caused by a relative or absolute deficiency of insulin. Most patients with diabetes fall into two broad categories: type 1 or "immune-mediated" diabetes, which is characterized by infiltration and destruction of the pancreatic islets by autoreactive T cells, and type 2 or "non–immune-mediated" diabetes, which is often associated with obesity and a sedentary lifestyle (Fig. 37-1). Although the distinction between the two broad categories is relatively straightforward for the majority of patients with diabetes, a substantial minority tend to be more difficult to classify.[1]

This distinction may be more than academic given that patients with severe insulin deficiency are unlikely to achieve glycemic control without insulin replacement and are at risk of unrestrained gluconeogenesis, ketogenesis, and diabetic ketoacidosis. In addition, immune-mediated diabetes could theoretically be amenable to immune modulation to prevent islet destruction and insulin dependency. At the present time, treatment has focused on the use of exogenous insulin to replace endogenous secretion of this hormone. Therefore, detailed discussion of the therapeutic agents in this chapter focuses mainly on their use in people with type 2 diabetes.

PATHOPHYSIOLOGY

Diabetes arises out of a complex interaction between genes and the environment. Type 1 and type 2 diabetes have a distinct genetic predisposition that is conferred by multiple genes with weak to moderate effect on disease development.[2,3] Maturity-onset diabetes of the young (MODY) is a distinct subset of diabetes that is inherited in an autosomal dominant fashion—a fact that may have therapeutic relevance.[4]

In nondiabetic humans, glucose concentrations average 4.5 to 5.5 mmol/L following a 6- to 12-hour overnight fast (Fig. 37-2). At this time, the rate of entry of glucose into the circulation (glucose production) approximates the rate of removal (glucose utilization). Within 5 to 6 hours after a meal, essentially all glucose entering the circulation comes from the liver and is derived from glycogenolysis and gluconeogenesis. Gluconeogenesis is responsible for approximately 50% to 60% of endogenous glucose production following an overnight fast, with the proportion increasing with increasing duration of the fast. Gluconeogenesis utilizes three-carbon precursors to synthesize glucose molecules. These substrates include lactate, alanine, and glycerol.[5]

Increases in plasma glucose (which occur within 5 to 10 minutes after eating) stimulate insulin secretion and suppress glucagon secretion. The reciprocal changes in hepatic sinusoidal insulin and glucagon concentrations, in concert with the elevated glucose concentrations, enhance peripheral and hepatic glucose uptake and suppress hepatic glucose production. These coordinated changes in hepatic and extrahepatic glucose metabolism generally limit the postprandial rise in glucose to 7 to 8 mmol/L.

In people with diabetes, fasting glucose concentrations are elevated and there is an accompanying excessive glycemic excursion following carbohydrate ingestion. Insulin secretion is typically decreased and delayed following food ingestion, and this abnormality is observed early in the evolution of diabetes. In addition to defects in insulin secretion, people with diabetes commonly exhibit defects in insulin action. Numerous studies have shown that insulin-induced stimulation of glucose uptake in muscle and adipose tissues as well as insulin-induced suppression of glucose production are impaired in diabetics.[6-8]

The more significant the defects in insulin secretion and action, the higher glucose concentrations have to rise to balance glucose appearance and disappearance. Glucose appearance is elevated due to failure to suppress hepatic glucose production since the systemic rate of appearance of ingested glucose does not differ from that observed in nondiabetic individuals. Defects in insulin secretion and action both contribute to postprandial hyperglycemia. A delay in the early rise in insulin concentrations causes a delay in suppression of glucose production, which in turn results in an excessive glycemic excursion. In contrast, a decrease in insulin action results in sustained hyperglycemia but has minimal effect on peak glucose concentrations. Whereas an isolated alteration in either hepatic or extrahepatic insulin action impairs glucose tolerance, a defect in both results in severe hyperglycemia.[6]

Glucose also is an important regulator of its own metabolism. In the presence of basal insulin concentrations, an increase in plasma glucose stimulates glucose uptake and suppresses glucose production. The ability of glucose to regulate its own metabolism is impaired in diabetes. This is commonly referred to as a defect in "glucose effectiveness."[7] Inhibition of glucagon secretion lowers both fasting glucose and postprandial glucose concentrations. However, failure to appropriately suppress glucagon secretion has minimal effect on glucose production and glucose tolerance when insulin secretion is intact.[9] In contrast, it causes marked hyperglycemia when insulin secretion is decreased and delayed, as is typical of diabetes.[9,10] Therefore the ideal therapy for diabetes would be an agent that simultaneously improves insulin secretion, insulin action, and glucose effectiveness as well as glucagon secretion.

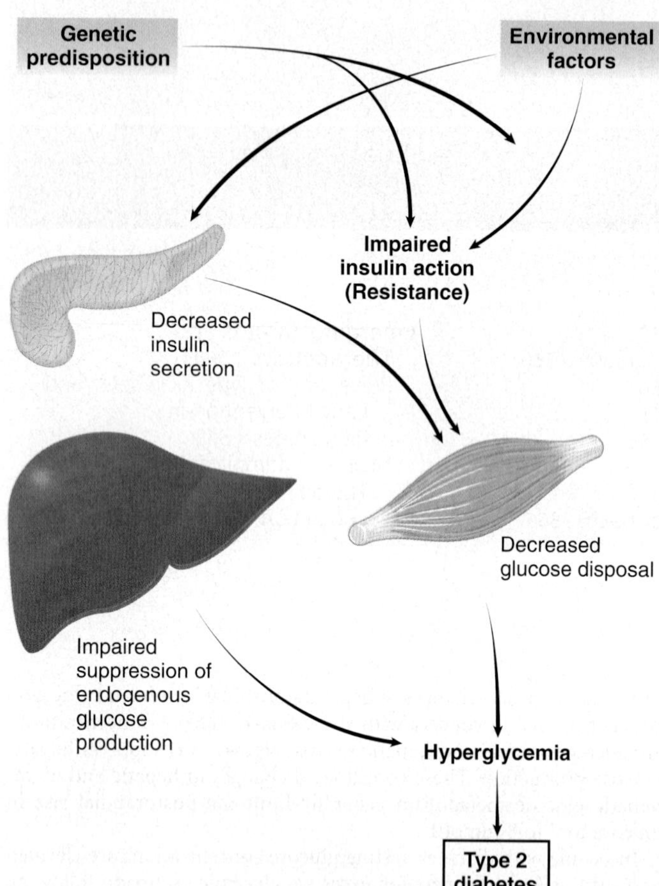

FIGURE 37-1 • **Pathogenesis of type 2 diabetes mellitus.** (Adapted from Porth CM. Pathophysiology: Concepts of Altered Health States, 7th ed. Philadelphia: Lippincott Williams & Wilkins, 2005.)

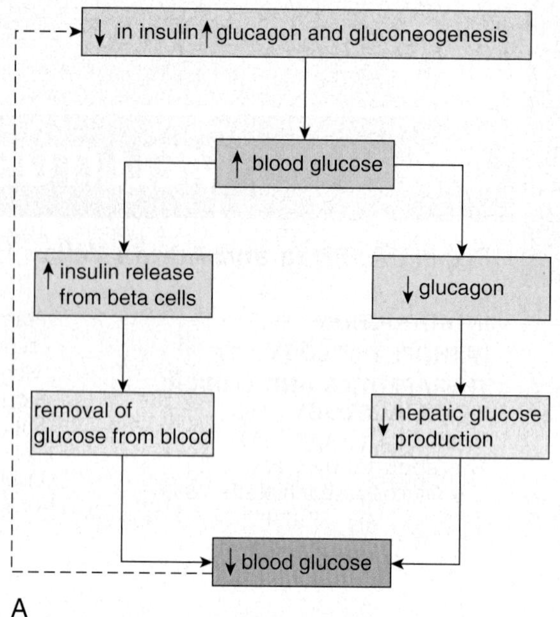

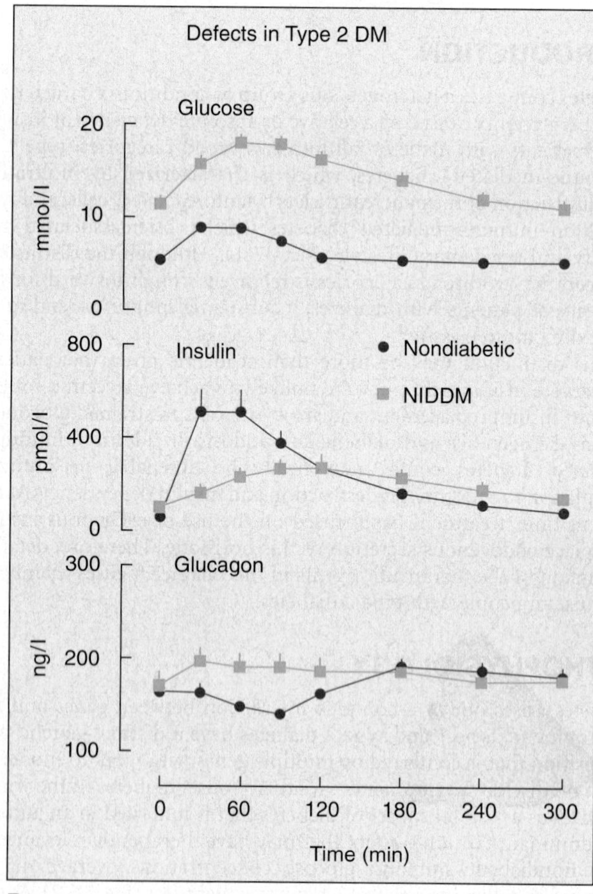

FIGURE 37-2 • **A,** Hormonal and hepatic regulation of blood glucose. **B,** The defects present in type 2 diabetes. Compared to healthy controls, people with diabetes have higher fasting and postprandial glucose concentrations. This is due in part to the delayed and blunted insulin secretion and the impaired suppression of glucagon secretion in response to meal ingestion. (Adapted from Porth CM. Pathophysiology: Concepts of Altered Health States, 7th ed. Philadelphia: Lippincott Williams & Wilkins, 2005.)

THERAPEUTICS AND CLINICAL PHARMACOLOGY

Goals of Therapy

Chronic hyperglycemia leads to the micro- and macrovascular complications that frequently accompany diabetes. The Diabetes Control and Complications Trial was able to show that "tight" glucose control (i.e., glucose concentrations closer to the normal physiologic range as measured by hemoglobin A_{1c} [HbA_{1c}]) compared to "conventional" control prevented or delayed retinopathy and nephropathy in people with type 1 diabetes.[11] Similar findings have been reported by the United Kingdom Prospective Diabetes Study (UKPDS) group for type 2 diabetes.[12,13] Since hypoglycemia can also produce acute and chronic, potentially catastrophic, complications, the goal of diabetes therapy has been to safely achieve glucose concentrations as close to the normal physiologic range as possible while avoiding hypoglycemia.

In addition, because diabetes is associated with adverse cardiovascular risk and with other cardiovascular risk factors, improving cardiovascular risk has also been a goal of therapy. Some agents may affect cardiovascular risk beyond their ability to lower glucose concentrations and may also affect progression of complications or beta cell failure. This is discussed later in the relevant sections.

Antihypertensive therapy and therapy of dyslipidemia is covered in other chapters (see Chapter 27, Pulmonary Arterial Hypertension; and Chapter 23, Dyslipidemias). Exercise, weight loss and appropriate diet are important foundations on which therapy for diabetes is based, and addressing these issues may allow simpler regimens to be used or enhance the successful achievement of glycemic control. Pharmacotherapy for obesity is discussed in another chapter (see Chapter 36, Obesity and Nutrition).

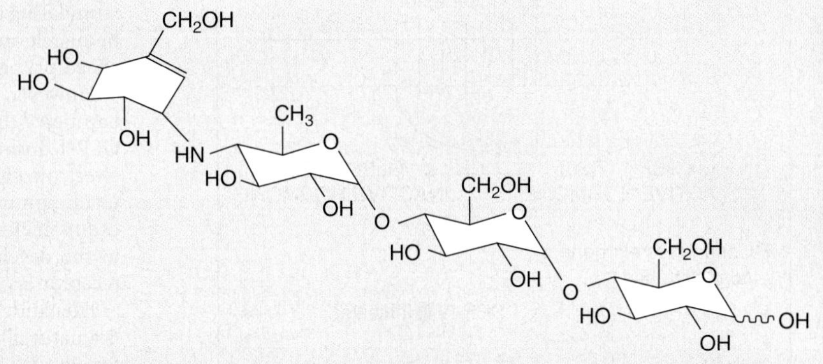

FIGURE 37-3 • Acarbose.

TABLE 37-1 α-GLUCOSIDASE INHIBITORS

Drug	Dose	Duration of Action	Excretion
Acarbose	25-100 mg with each meal	Inactivated by intestinal bacteria. Peak effect ~1 hr after ingestion	Poor absorption, but what is absorbed is excreted unchanged in the urine
Miglitol	25-100 mg with each meal	Half-life of 2 hr. Duration extended in renal impairment.	Excreted unchanged in the urine.

Therapeutics by Class

α-Glucosidase Inhibitors

α-Glucosidase enzymes are present at the intestinal brush border and hydrolyze nonabsorbable oligosaccharides and polysaccharides into absorbable monosaccharides. Inhibition of these enzymes leads to decreased postprandial glucose excursions and improved glycemic control.[14]

The prototype molecule, acarbose (Fig. 37-3), is a pseudotetrasaccharide that has a high affinity for the carbohydrate-binding site of the α-glucosidase enzymes that cleave maltose, isomaltose, and sucrose. It acts as a competitive inhibitor since it cannot be cleaved by these enzymes. It is active throughout the small intestine and is minimally absorbed from the gastrointestinal tract. Acarbose is subsequently metabolized by the colonic flora.

Inhibition of the α-glucosidase enzymes retards entry of glucose into the systemic circulation, thereby better matching systemic appearance of ingested glucose with the blunted and delayed insulin secretion seen in people with diabetes. It has been suggested that a greater delivery of nutrients to the distal small intestine results in increased secretion of incretin hormones compared to that seen in the absence of acarbose and other α-glucosidase inhibitors.[15] However this is uncertain.[16]

The usual starting dose is 25 mg with meals, and dosage is titrated up to maximum doses of 75 to 100 mg three times daily (Table 37-1). Since the drug must be present in the small intestine at the time of meal absorption, it must be administered prior to or with the meal. In clinical trials, acarbose has been shown to decrease fasting glucose values by 25 to 30 mg/dl and HbA_{1c} values by 0.7% to 1.0%. A greater decrease in peak postprandial glucose concentrations has been observed (~50 mg/dl) commensurate with its expected mode of action.[17] Although triglyceride concentrations may be decreased by acarbose, high-density and low-density lipoprotein concentrations are unaffected. Body weight is not significantly altered by acarbose therapy.[17]

The side effects of acarbose are mostly gastrointestinal in nature and include bloating, flatulence, and diarrhea. Occasional patients complain of fecal incontinence, but these symptoms are usually transient and diminish with continued drug use. Patients taking these medications often recognize foods that are especially likely to cause side effects and change their dietary behavior accordingly. Reversible increases in liver transaminase concentrations have been observed with high doses of acarbose. The drug is contraindicated in patients with malabsorption or inflammatory bowel disease and in the presence of significant renal impairment (creatinine > 2.0 mg/dl). Although the drug is contraindicated in cirrhosis, a randomized, placebo-controlled, double-blind crossover study recently demonstrated that acarbose was superior to lactulose in preventing hepatic encephalopathy in patients with type 2 diabetes and cirrhosis.[18]

Since acarbose does not directly interfere with insulin secretion, hypoglycemia does not occur in diabetic patients using this medication as monotherapy. However, if hypoglycemia (due to another medication such as a sulfonylurea) does occur, pure glucose should be used to treat this, as absorption of disaccharides or more complex carbohydrates will be retarded.[19]

Pramlintide

Pramlintide is an analogue of a gut-derived hormone that has therapeutic utility in diabetes. Symlin (pramlintide acetate) was approved by the U.S. Food and Drug Administration (FDA) for use in people with type 1 or type 2 diabetes receiving insulin. It is an analogue of amylin, a neuroendocrine hormone synthesized by pancreatic beta cells and co-secreted with insulin. Amylin delays gastric emptying through a vagally mediated mechanism and may contribute to glycemic control in the postprandial period.[20,21] In addition, amylin decreases glucagon secretion and therefore contributes to the suppression of endogenous glucose production after a meal.[22] Pramlintide differs from amylin in that proline replaces an alanine and two serines at positions 25, 28, and 29, respectively. This change to the native sequence improves the stability and solubility of the native hormone in water.[23]

Pramlintide is administered by subcutaneous injection prior to meal ingestion (three times daily) in a dose ranging from 30 to 120 mcg. It is metabolized by the kidneys and has a half-life of 45 to 60 minutes. However, the primary metabolite, which has a similar half-life, is also bioactive. Studies in patients with moderate to severe renal impairment (creatinine clearance > 20 to 50 ml/min) did not show toxicity or adverse events.

Pramlintide is indicated for the prevention and treatment of postprandial hyperglycemia, as an adjunct to mealtime insulin, and is also associated with a short-term decrease in caloric intake. It has been associated with some minimal weight loss in clinical studies.[24] Since type 1 diabetes is an amylin-deficient state, whereas type 2 diabetes is a state of relative amylin excess, the dosage requirements vary according to diabetes type. This may also be the reason why nausea and vomiting in association with pramlintide therapy is more commonly

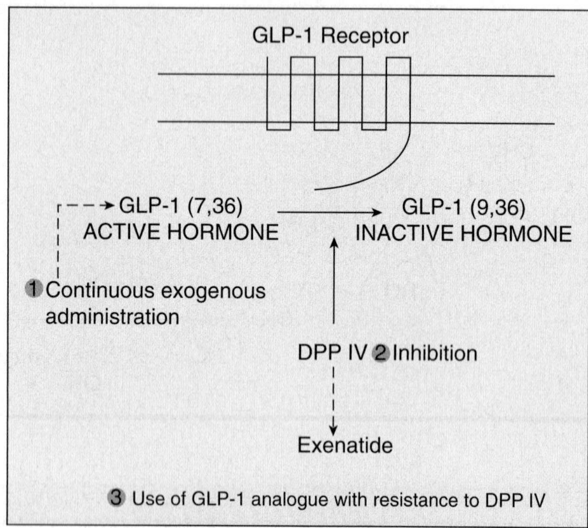

FIGURE 37-4 • GLP-1 based therapy.

encountered in people with type 1 diabetes than those with type 2 diabetes. It has been recommended that pramlintide be administered as a starting dose of 60 mcg, increasing to 120 mcg, as opposed to 30 mcg, increasing by 15-mcg increments to 60 mcg, in people with type 2 diabetes. Pramlintide is supplied in liquid form.

Since pramlintide delays gastric emptying reduction in meal-associated insulin dosing is recommended to avoid hypoglycemia. Pramlintide cannot be mixed with insulin, so people with type 1 diabetes who are receiving multiple daily injections of insulin will need to take an additional injection of pramlintide with each meal. Occasional patients with type 2 diabetes who are receiving basal insulin alone and experiencing large postprandial glycemic excursions may benefit from the addition of pramlintide before meals. Glucose lowering associated with the addition of pramlintide therapy leads to reductions in HbA_{1c} of approximately 0.5%.

Incretin-Based Therapy

Physiologists have long recognized that administration of glucose via the gut produced greater insulin secretion than when an equivalent amount of glucose is administered intravenously. This was hypothesized to be due to "incretins"—hormones released by the gut in response to nutrient ingestion that aid in the postabsorptive assimilation of these nutrients.[25] Glucagon-like peptide-1 (GLP-1) is one such hormone (Fig. 37-4). It arises from posttranscriptional processing of proglucagon in intestinal L cells by the prohormone convertase-1, which leads to the formation of GLP-1 and GLP-2. The latter peptide hormone acts as a growth factor for intestinal epithelium. Although it has a short half-life in the circulation secondary to its rapid inactivation by dipeptidyl peptidase 4 (DPP-4, an enzyme that is widely distributed and cleaves all peptides whose second N-terminal amino acid is a proline or alanine), it is a potent insulin secretagogue; it inhibits glucagon secretion and also delays gastric emptying. Unlike other secretagogues, GLP-1 stimulates insulin secretion in a glucose-dependent fashion. That is, insulin secretion is stimulated only in the presence of physiologic hyperglycemia, therefore minimizing the risk of hypoglycemia. When combined with the ability to delay gastric emptying, GLP-1–based therapy seems an ideal remedy for postprandial hyperglycemia.[26]

Short-term GLP-1 administration has been shown to restore insulin secretion in patients with type 2 diabetes who have experienced failure of oral hypoglycemic agents. Activation of GLP-1 receptor signaling leads to enhanced expression of messenger RNA transcripts for insulin in beta cell lines. Subsequently, evidence has accumulated to suggest that GLP-1 inhibits cytokine-induced B-cell apoptosis, as well as that induced by the administration of streptozotocin. In partially pancreatectomized mice, GLP-1 administration expanded B-cell mass by stimulating neogenesis and proliferation. All of these observations may be of relevance in individuals with type 2 diabetes who have experienced primary or secondary failure of oral agents.[27]

However, the short half-life of active GLP-1 in the circulation has hampered the use of GLP-1 as a therapeutic agent. Bolus subcutaneous GLP-1 dosing leads to delayed gastric emptying but little long-lasting effect on glycemic control. Continuous infusion of GLP-1 using an insulin pump has been utilized in clinical studies, but this is of limited utility in clinical practice. Consequently, GLP-1–based therapy has led to the development of various compounds that either act as GLP-1 receptor agonists or inhibit GLP-1 breakdown by DPP-4.

Exenatide is the first GLP-1–based therapy to gain FDA approval. It is a naturally occurring analogue of GLP-1 that acts as a GLP-1 receptor agonist. It is found in the saliva of large reptiles such as *Heloderma horridum* and, since its second amino acid is a glycine, it is resistant to degradation by DPP-4. It has a half-life of approximately 2 hours as opposed to the 2 to 5 minutes of native GLP-1. Detectable concentrations are present for up to 10 hours after administration. It is thought to regulate satiety in *Heloderma horridum* and other related species. Various trials in humans have demonstrated that this compound is a powerful insulin secretagogue, suppresses glucagon secretion, and delays gastric emptying. There is often accompanying weight loss in patients treated with exenatide.[28]

Treatment is recommended as adjunctive therapy for patients with type 2 diabetes mellitus who have failed to achieve adequate glycemic control with metformin and/or a sulfonylurea. It is administered by subcutaneous injection 30 to 60 minutes prior to the morning and evening meals. The initial recommended starting dose is 5 mcg given by subcutaneous injection twice daily. This can be increased to 10 mcg depending on effect and how well the initial dose is tolerated.

Adverse events are related to its effects on gastrointestinal motility, with symptoms such as early satiety, epigastric fullness, reflux, nausea, and vomiting. Most of these symptoms are mild and resolve over time, but this is not always the case. Patients with delayed gastric emptying may be more likely to develop these symptoms, and patients with known gastroparesis should not be treated with this compound. Drug interactions could theoretically arise out of the delayed absorption secondary to prolonged gastric emptying that this drug engenders. However, in clinical trials, although the absorption of statins or antihypertensive medications was delayed, no net effect on lipid profiles or blood pressure was observed.

Exenatide per se does not cause hypoglycemia because of the glucose-dependent nature of its effect on insulin secretion. However, when used as an adjunct to sulfonylurea treatment, the incidence of hypoglycemia increases significantly. A recently published trial noted an approximately 30% incidence of self-reported hypoglycemia in patients receiving 10 mcg of exenatide.[29] This is in contrast to the incidence of hypoglycemia when exenatide was added to an insulin sensitizer (metformin); the incidence did not differ from that observed in patients receiving placebo.[28]

Exenatide is an important new addition to the therapeutic armamentarium for the treatment of type 2 diabetes; however, its place in the armamentarium is still being debated. Should exenatide be used early in the treatment of obese patients who have developed diabetes? Should it be added to metformin alone or in combination with a sulfonylurea? Does it have a role in patients receiving insulin who exhibit poor postprandial glucose control and/or are gaining weight? The additional glucose-lowering effect of this medication translates into a lowering of HbA_{1c} by about 1%.

Various inhibitors of DPP-4 are being developed, although at the time of writing only one, sitagliptin, has been approved for clinical use. This class of agents inhibits the breakdown of endogenous incretin hormones, and other hormones such as insulin-like growth factor-1 and GLP-2, and therefore raises incretin concentrations after meal ingestion. In clinical trials, these compounds have no effect on weight but also have not been associated with nausea, vomiting, or other gastrointestinal symptoms.[30] This is probably related to the magnitude of elevation in active GLP-1 concentrations (as well as the duration of that elevation) seen when DPP-4 is inhibited. The rise in active GLP-1 seen with DPP-4 inhibition is transient and does not reach the concentrations encountered during continuous GLP-1 infusions that delay gastric emptying.[31] Glucose lowering is accompanied by suppression of glucagon concentrations and minimal effect, if any, on insulin concentrations, leading some authors to mistakenly conclude that DPP-4 inhibitors do not increase insulin secretion. In fact, mathematical modeling has shown that indeed insulin secretion is higher for a given glucose concentration in the presence of DPP-4 inhibitors.[32]

Meglitinides

Repaglinide and nateglinide (Fig. 37-5) are short-acting nonsulfonylurea insulin secretagogues collectively known as meglitinides (Table 37-2). Both compounds are rapidly absorbed and rapidly cleared from the circulation so that administration results in a rapid, but brief, rise in insulin secretion. This necessitates dosing prior to each meal. The corollary of this is that hypoglycemia is unlikely to occur, but these drugs are chiefly effective at decreasing postprandial glucose concentrations with less apparent effect on fasting glucose concentrations.

Like the sulfonylureas, repaglinide acts by stimulating release of insulin from beta cells by inhibiting ATP-sensitive K^+ channels, thereby activating the Ca^{2+} channels, leading to an increase in intracellular calcium and subsequent insulin release. However, repaglinide acts on a distinct binding site in addition to that with which conventional sulfonylureas bind.[33] Repaglinide is not effective in the absence of functioning beta cells.

Nateglinide is a derivative of phenylalanine, while repaglinide is a derivative of benzoic acid. Repaglinide is completely metabolized by oxidative biotransformation and direct conjugation with glucuronate. None of its metabolites contribute to its glucose-lowering effect. It has a half-life of approximately 1 hour. Nateglinide, in contrast, has metabolites that exhibit some glucose-lowering activity, and this may explain why its effective half-life is approximately 90 minutes. Although dosing should be carefully titrated upward in patients with hepatic impairment, mild to moderate renal impairment does not contraindicate their use.

Although clearly less effective than conventional sulfonylureas and metformin, this class of agents may be useful in people with renal impairment and/or hepatic impairment in whom therapy with conventional agents is contraindicated. They may be used to treat patients with isolated impairment of glucose tolerance and occasionally in conjunction with basal insulin therapy. Given the low likelihood of hypoglycemia associated with these agents, they may be used in elderly patients who are vulnerable to hypoglycemia secondary to comorbidity, metabolic impairment, or social circumstances.

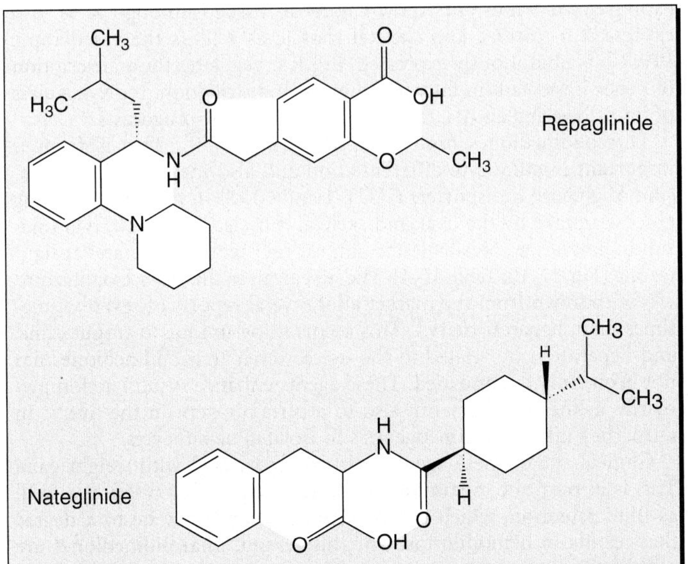

FIGURE 37-5 • Repaglinide and nateglinide.

Biguanides

Metformin is the only biguanide approved for use in the United States. Phenformin was previously approved but was withdrawn because it caused lactic acidosis. Unlike phenformin, metformin has low lipid solubility and rarely causes lactic acidosis in diabetic patients with normal renal function.

Metformin seems to improve insulin action in hepatic and extrahepatic tissues (Fig. 37-6). It may decrease endogenous glucose production by inhibiting glycogenolysis and gluconeogenesis. In muscle, it increases insulin receptor tyrosine kinase activity, and increases the number and activity of GLUT-4 transporters, all of which enhances glucose disposal.[34] However, the receptor(s) through which metformin mediates these actions are as yet unknown. As would be anticipated from its known efficacy of improving insulin action in patients with type 2 diabetes, fasting and postprandial insulin secretion falls with metformin therapy. This is secondary to the normal compensatory response of the pancreas to the improved insulin action and lower glucose concentrations prevailing while on therapy with metformin.

Gastrointestinal side effects such as nausea, dyspepsia, abdominal discomfort, and diarrhea are the most common symptoms reported. In most cases these can be minimized or avoided by slow titration. Hypoglycemia in patients treated with metformin monotherapy is unlikely and should prompt a search for other causes of hypoglycemia. Studies have demonstrated that, when used in therapeutic doses and in the absence of hepatic, renal, or cardiorespiratory insufficiency, metformin does not interfere with lactate metabolism or raise plasma lactate concentrations.[13] Indeed, the absence of lactic acidosis in most studies utilizing long-term metformin raises the possibility that lactic acidosis is due to the severity of the underlying medical disorder and not metformin therapy.

Metformin should not be used in patients with renal disease because the drug is excreted by the kidneys. Serum creatinine concentration has been used as a guideline to determine if metformin can be safely used in patients. However, serum creatinine is not a reliable indicator of renal function in elderly patients with reduced muscle mass; in these situations, creatinine clearance estimation should be undertaken prior to using the drug. In terms of efficacy, metformin is effective therapy when used alone or in combination with other oral medications or insulin for the treatment of type 2 diabetes. Its use has sometimes been advocated in people with type 1 diabetes because of its beneficial effects on weight and lipid concentrations.[35] Most studies show that weight gain does not occur in patients with type 2 diabetes treated with metformin alone or in combination. Indeed modest weight loss may be experienced during the first months of therapy.[36]

TABLE 37-2 THE MEGLITINIDES

Drug	Dose	Duration of Action	Excretion
Repaglinide	0.5-2 mg with each meal	Peak plasma concentrations 1 hr after ingestion. Half-life of 1 hr.	Oxidation and glucuronidation
Nateglinide	60-240 mg with each meal	Peak plasma concentrations 1 hr after ingestion. Half-life of 1.5 hr.	Hydroxylation followed by glucuronidation

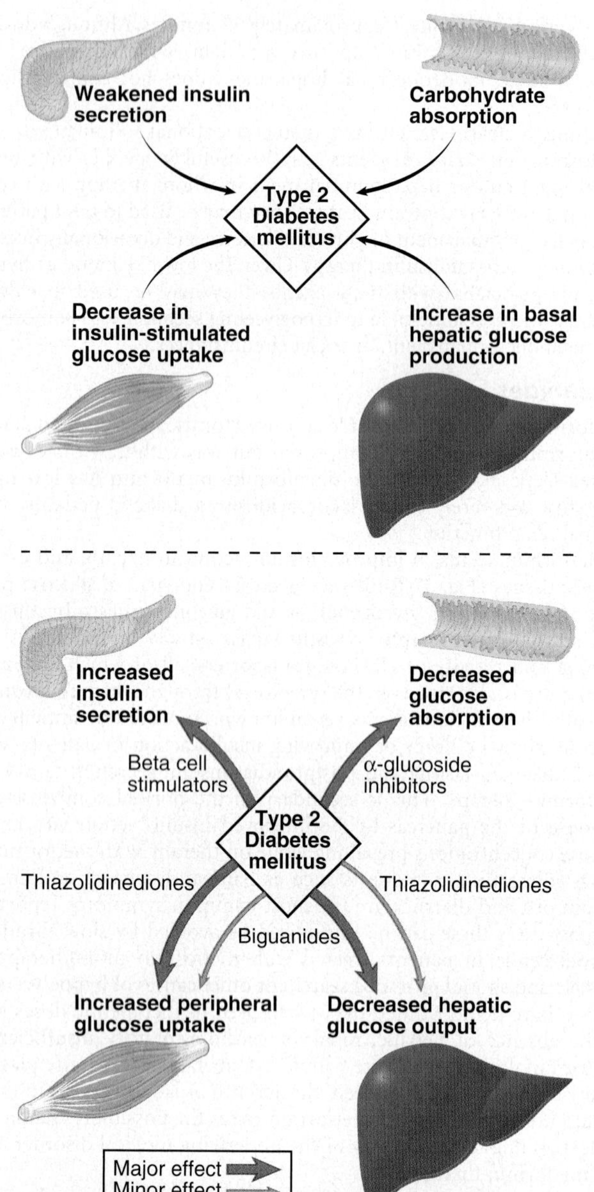

FIGURE 37-6 • (Top) Mechanisms of elevated blood glucose in type 2 diabetes. **(Bottom)** Action sites of oral hypoglycemic agents and mechanisms of lowering blood glucose in type 2 diabetes. (Adapted from Porth CM. Pathophysiology: Concepts of Altered Health States, 7th ed. Philadelphia: Lippincott Williams & Wilkins, 2005.)

Sulfonylureas

Sulfonylureas were the first class of oral agents used to treat type 2 diabetes (Fig. 37-7; Table 37-4). The sulfonylurea receptor on pancreatic beta cells is part of a potassium channel complex that regulates potassium influx into the cell. Binding to the sulfonylurea complex leads to decreased potassium influx, depolarization of the beta cell membrane, and a subsequent increase of calcium flux into the cell (Fig. 37-8). This results in activation of the secretory machinery of the cell, culminating in the exocytosis of insulin from secretory granules that are translocated to the cell surface by the cytoskeleton.[37]

The resulting insulin secretion suppresses endogenous glucose production and stimulates glucose disappearance. This results in lowering of fasting as well as postprandial blood glucose levels. However, and unlike incretin-based therapy, this effect is not glucose dependent, and all patients treated with sulfonylureas are theoretically at risk of hypoglycemia. In practice, patients with blood sugars close to the normal range, variable dietary and exercise habits, and impaired clearance mechanisms are most at risk of sulfonylurea-induced hypoglycemia. Sulfonylurea-induced hypoglycemia can be distinguished from other causes of hypoglycemia by the evidence of inappropriate endogenous insulin secretion (inappropriate C-peptide concentrations for the prevailing glucose concentrations) and detectable sulfonylurea at the time of hypoglycemia.[38] Chronic hyperglycemia will impair insulin secretion and action—a phenomenon referred to as glucose toxicity, which can be reversed by improved glycemic control. Most investigators believe that the improvement in insulin action associated with sulfonylurea therapy is due to reversal of glucose toxicity.[19]

As expected, the integrity of islet insulin secretion determines response to sulfonylureas. Patients with evidence of severely impaired secretion (fasting glucose > 15 mmol/L, low fasting C-peptide concentrations) or evidence of islet autoimmunity are unlikely to respond adequately to therapy. Good initial response to therapy followed by subsequent failure is often referred to as "secondary failure." This may be due to patient-related factors (poor compliance with therapy or lifestyle modification, comorbidities that preclude sulfonylurea use) as well as disease progression. It has been commonly believed that sulfonylureas may predispose to or directly contribute to beta cell failure, but a similar rate of secondary failure with metformin has been observed in the UKPDS.[39]

Thiazolidinediones

The peroxisome proliferator activated receptor (PPAR) is activated by fatty acids and fatty acid–derived eicosanoids. It exists in three isoforms with different tissue specificity. Activation of PPAR leads to the formation of heterodimers with retinoid-X receptors, which bind to DNA-sequences that act as PPAR response elements, which act as transcriptional regulators of PPAR-regulated genes. The PPAR-α isoform is expressed in tissues where active fatty acid catabolism occurs—most notably the liver, heart, and brown fat. PPAR-γ is mainly expressed in white and brown adipose tissue, although it is also expressed in cardiac and skeletal muscle as well as the vasculature. PPAR-δ is ubiquitously expressed. PPAR-α regulates the transcription of genes important in fatty acid uptake and oxidation. Indeed, a class of lipid-lowering agents, the fibrates, act as PPAR-α agonists.[40]

Thiazolidinediones bind to PPAR-γ (Fig. 37-9). This isoform is important in adipocyte differentiation and also mediates the expression of glucose transporters GLUT-1 and GLUT-4, thereby increasing glucose uptake by the liver and skeletal muscle. At present, two thiazolidinediones are available for clinical use: pioglitazone and rosiglitazone (Fig. 37-10; Table 37-4). The first agent in this class, troglitazone, was withdrawn from the market after several reports of severe, sometimes fatal, hepatotoxicity.[41] This seems to be unique to troglitazone, and hepatotoxicity related to the use of other thiazolidinediones has not been truly documented. These agents enhance insulin action primarily in the periphery but also to a certain extent in the liver.[42] In vitro, they inhibit gluconeogenesis in isolated hepatocytes.

Clinical use of these agents has been associated with weight gain. This is in part due to stimulation of adipocyte differentiation as well as fluid retention, which can be significant and may be to a degree that results in hemodilution. For this reason, thiazolidinediones are contraindicated in situations in which fluid retention is a problem (e.g., congestive heart failure).[43] PPAR-γ agonists promote uptake of free fatty acids in subcutaneous adipose tissue rather than in visceral adipose. This may be the reason for the paradoxical improvement in insulin action despite the weight gain observed in clinical studies.

Insulin

The discovery of insulin (Fig. 37-11) and the ability to extract active insulin from animal sources marked a turning point in the therapy of diabetes. Bovine and porcine insulin was utilized until the advent of recombinant DNA technology made it feasible to synthesize human insulin in quantities sufficient to meet clinical demand. This had the advantage of being less immunogenic and less likely to cause atrophy

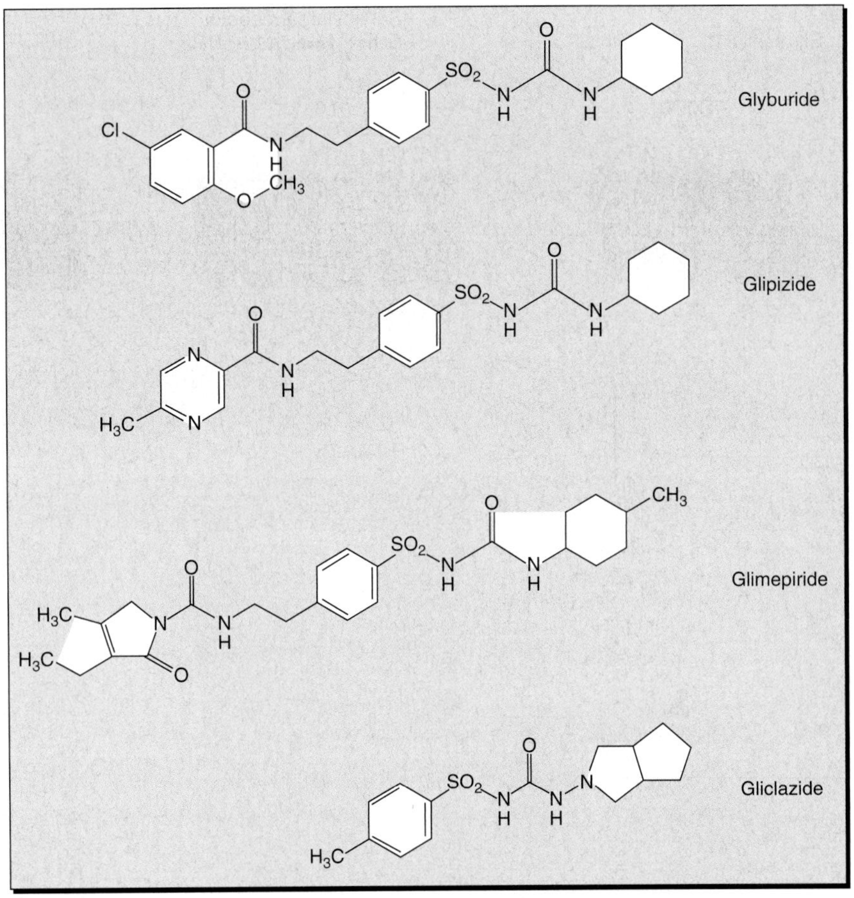

FIGURE 37-7 • **Glyburide, glipizide, glimepiride, and gliclazide.**

TABLE 37-3 SULFONYLUREAS

Drug	Dose	Duration of Action	Excretion
Tolbutamide	100-1000 mg	Half-life of 4-6 hr. Duration of action is 6-12 hr.	Hepatic metabolism and renal excretion of inactive metabolites.
Acetohexamide	250-1000 mg	High protein binding. Active metabolite has a half-life of 6 hr. Duration of action is 8-24 hr.	Hepatic metabolism, but 70% of the active metabolite is excreted by the kidneys.
Chlorpropamide	100-500 mg	Interferes with water excretion—may cause hyponatremia. Half-life of 36 hr. Duration of action is 60-72 hr.	Biotransformed in the liver but active and inactive metabolites renally excreted.
Tolazamide	100-250 mg	Half-life of 7 hr. Duration of action is 10-20 hr.	Hepatic metabolism and renal excretion of inactive metabolites.
Glyburide	1.5-12 mg	Half-life of 10 hr. Duration of action is 12-24 hr.	50% renal excretion and 50% biliary excretion.
Glipizide	5-40 mg	Half-life of 2-4 hr. Duration of action is 12-24 hr.	Renal excretion of inactive metabolites. Less than 10% excreted unchanged.
Glimepiride	1-8 mg	Half-life of 5-9 hr. Duration of action is 16-24 hr.	60% of inactive metabolite renally excreted.
Gliclazide	80-320 mg	Half-life of 10 hr. Duration of action is 24 hr.	Biotransformed in the liver but excreted by the kidneys.

TABLE 37-4 THE THIAZOLIDINEDIONE DRUGS

Drug	Dose	Duration of Action	Excretion
Pioglitazone	15-45 mg	Half-life of 16-24 hr. For onset and offset of action, see Troglitazone.	Hydroxylation and oxidation; the metabolites are glucuronidated or sulfated.
Rosiglitazone	2-8 mg as single or divided dose	Half-life of 3-5 hr. For onset and offset of action, see Troglitazone.	Demethylation and hydroxylation followed by sulfation and glucuronidation.
Troglitazone*	200-600 mg	Initial response 2-4 wk after initiation of dosing. Peak response achieved by 12-14 wk of dosing. Elimination half-life of 24 hr.	Three metabolites: a sulfate conjugate, a quinone metabolite, and a glucuronide conjugate.

*Withdrawn.

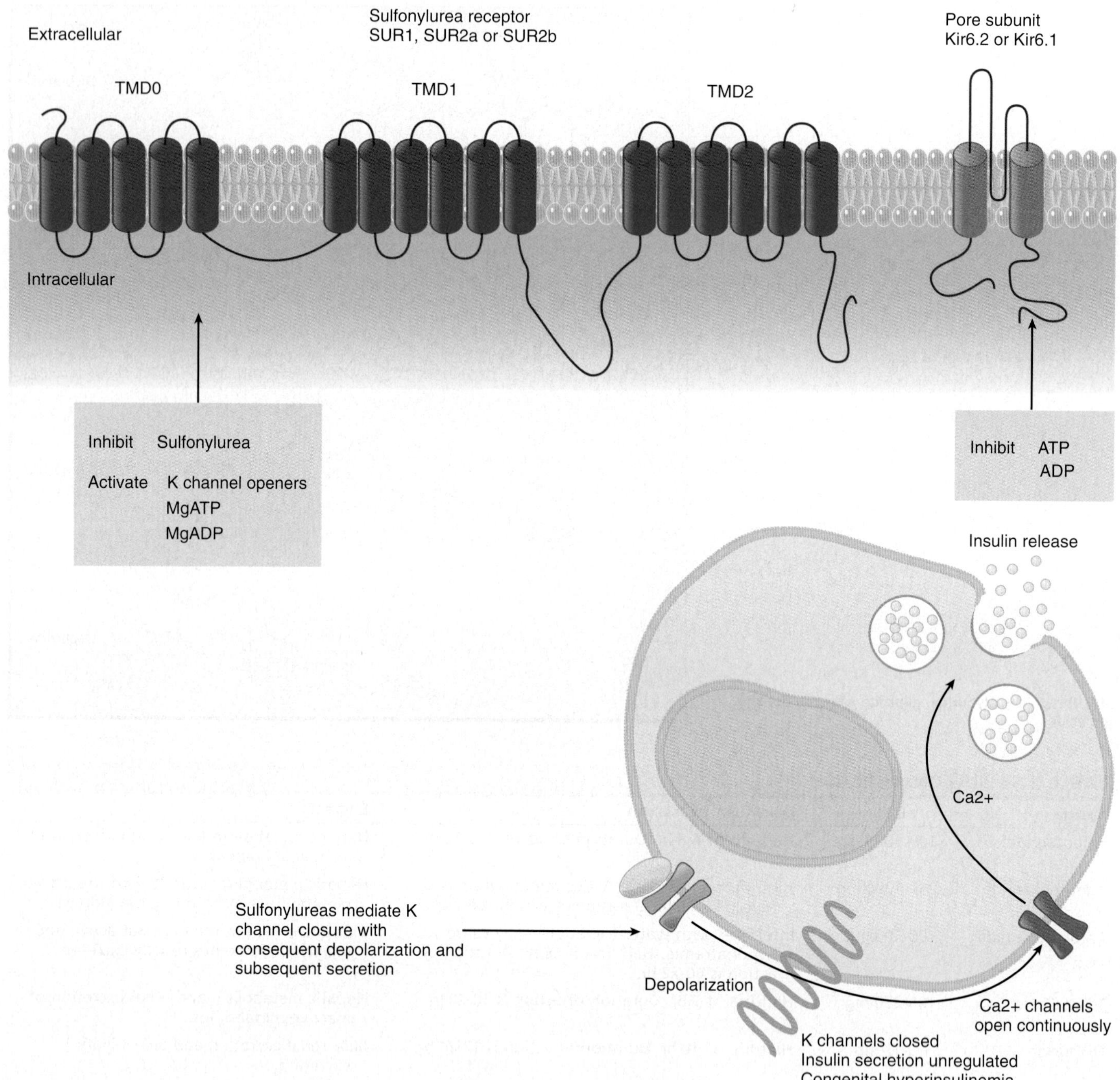

FIGURE 37-8 • Sulfonylureas mediate potassium channel closure with consequent depolarization and subsequent secretion. (Modified from Ashcroft FM. ATP-sensitive potassium channelopathies: focus on insulin secretion. J Clin Invest 2005;115:2047-2058. With permission of the American Society for Clinical Investigation.)

of subcutaneous fat (lipoatrophy) at the site of injection. The development of insulin antibodies in response to injection of animal insulin often led to binding of exogenous insulin by antibody in a fashion that altered the pharmacokinetics of the injectable preparation. In addition to making therapy with human insulin a feasible proposition, the ability to synthesize insulin using recombinant DNA led to the possibility of modifications to the native insulin sequence so as to alter the rate of onset and offset of its action.

Insulin is secreted continuously by the pancreas, with the rate increasing in response to meal ingestion and then subsiding to lower secretory rates encountered during fasting. The hormone is secreted directly into the hepatic portal vein, and approximately 60% of insulin is extracted by the liver in the first pass. Therefore, there is a portal-peripheral gradient of insulin concentration that is lost when insulin is injected subcutaneously. The significance of this is unclear.

Insulin regimens over the years have attempted to match this secretory pattern by using combinations of "basal" long-acting preparations and "bolus" short-acting preparations (Fig. 37-12). Since the hormone is injected subcutaneously, retarding uptake from the injection site could alter characteristics of absorption and therefore lead to a longer acting preparation. When injected subcutaneously, *regular insulin* reaches peak onset of action around 2 hours after injection, and its actions last for 4 to 6 hours. This is in part due to the properties of insulin to dimerize and self-aggregate. In fact, dissociation from these

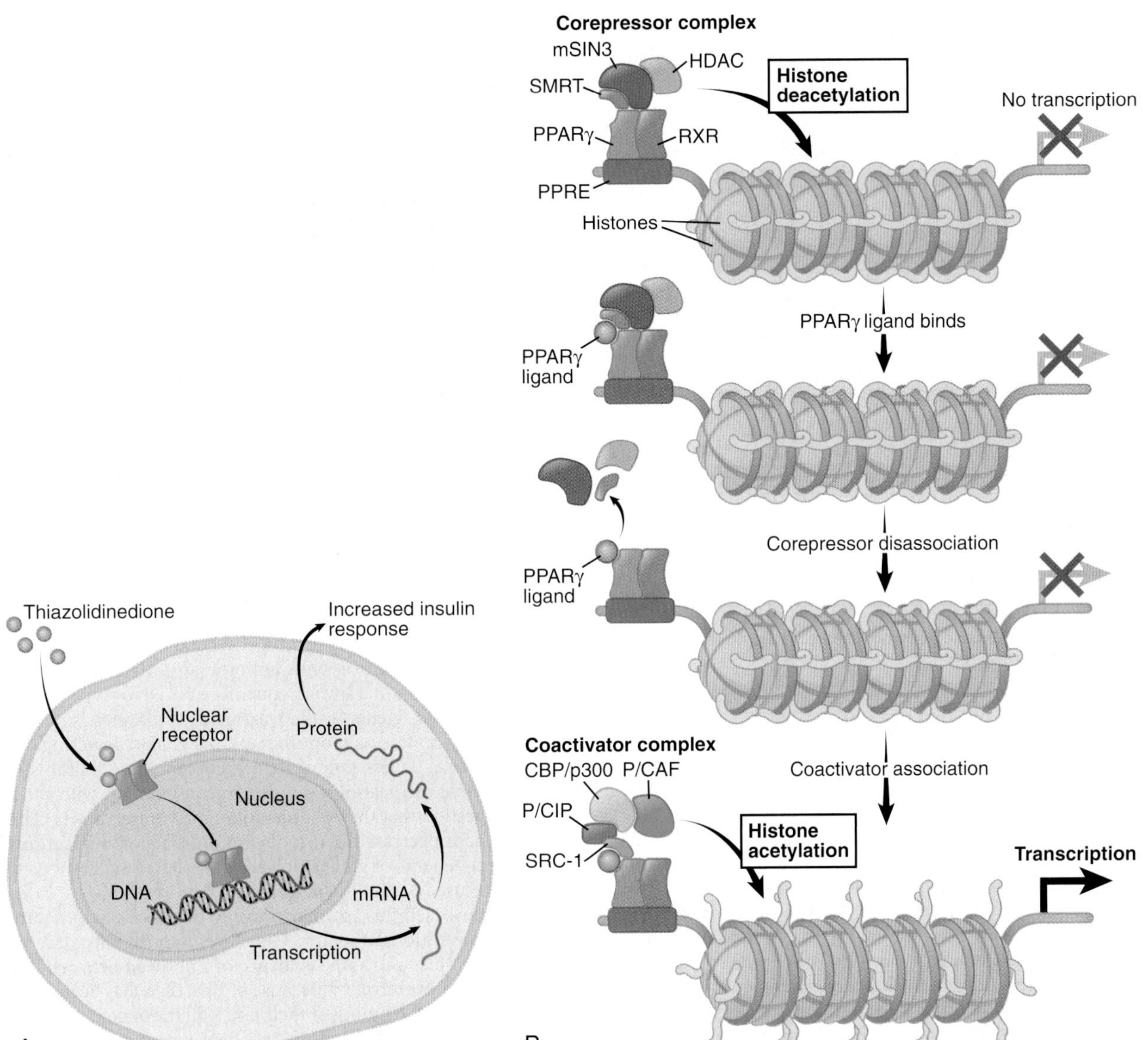

FIGURE 37-9 • **A,** Action of the thiazolidinediones on activation of the PPAR-γ receptor that regulates gene transcription of proteins that regulate glucose uptake and reduce fatty acid release. (Adapted from Porth CM. Pathophysiology: Concepts of Altered Health States, 7th ed. Philadelphia: Lippincott Williams & Wilkins, 2005.) **B,** In the absence of a TZD, the PPAR-γ receptor exists as a heterodimer with the retinoid-X receptor (RXR) nuclear receptor; the heterodimer is located on a PPAR response element (PPRE) of a target gene. This receptor heterodimer complex is associated with a multicomponent co-repressor complex, which physically interacts with the PPAR-γ receptor. The co-repressor complex contains histone deacetylase activity, and the deacetylated state of histone inhibits transcription. After PPAR-γ ligand binding, the co-repressor complex is dismissed and a coactivator complex is recruited to the heterodimer PPAR-γ receptor (bottom). The coactivator complex contains histone acetylase activity, leading to chromatin remodeling, facilitating active transcription. (Adapted from Glass CK, Rosenfeld MG. The coregulator exchange in transcriptional functions of nuclear receptors. Genes Dev 2000;14:121-141.)

self-aggregates is the rate-limiting step for absorption from the subcutaneous injection site. Indeed, if regular insulin is to be used to prevent postprandial hyperglycemia, it is recommended that injection take place 30 minutes prior to meal ingestion.

The dimerization of insulin occurs because of the flexibility at the C-terminal region of the insulin B-chain (residues B24-B26), which allows it to bind to the equivalent region of a second monomer in an antiparallel β-sheet structure. Site-directed mutagenesis affecting the adjacent region (residues B26-B30) alters the self-association properties of insulin. Sequence reversal of the proline and lysine at positions B28 and B29, respectively, led to the creation of *lispro insulin*, which has an onset of action of approximately 15 minutes after injection and peak activity within 1 hour (Fig. 37-13). It is cleared within 4 hours of injection. Similarly, the substitution of the proline at B28 with aspartate also reduces the self-aggregation of insulin. This insulin analogue—*aspart insulin*—has pharmacodynamics similar to lispro insulin. *Insulin glulisine* differs from human insulin in that the amino acid asparagine at position B3 is replaced by lysine and the lysine in position B29 is replaced by glutamic acid. Again, its pharmacokinetics are similar to the other rapid-acting insulin analogues.[44]

Conversely, promoting aggregation has been used to produce long-acting insulin. For example, protamine, a highly basic polypeptide, complexes with insulin, which is acidic. This forms a microcrystalline precipitate when it comes into contact with the neutral tissue fluid and is the basis of the intermediate-acting insulin *neutral protamine Hagedorn (NPH) insulin*. It reaches peak activity in 6 to 8 hours and has a duration of action of 14 to 20 hours. Zinc ions stabilize insulin hexamers, consisting of three insulin dimers and zinc together with protamine, that confer properties on *lente insulin* that are similar to NPH

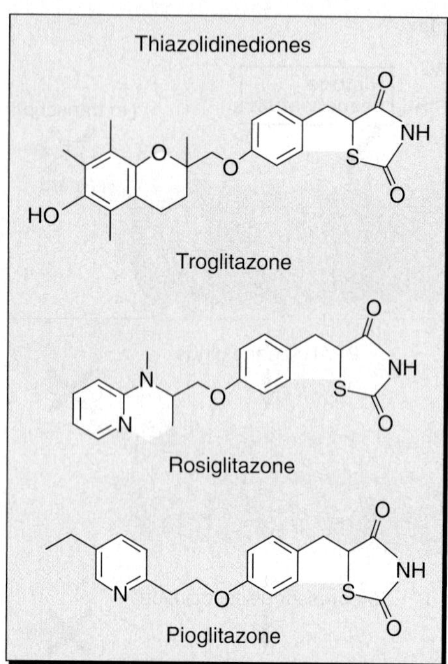

FIGURE 37-10 • Thiazolidinediones: troglitazone, rosiglitazone, and pioglitazone.

insulin. *Ultralente insulin*, now withdrawn from the market, contained a still higher percentage of zinc to produce even greater duration of action.

Insulin glargine is a long-acting insulin analogue (see Fig. 37-13). It is the result of the addition of two arginine residues to the C-terminus of the insulin B-chain. This changes the isoelectric point of insulin from a pH of 5.4 to 6.7 so that it precipitates in the neutral environment of the subcutaneous tissues. In addition, the asparagine at A21 is substituted with glycine, which may also contribute to the stability of the formulation. Insulin glargine has a relatively rapid onset (1 to 2 hours) but a long duration of action (24 hours).

Insulin detemir differs from human insulin in that the amino acid threonine at position B30 has been omitted, and a C14 fatty acid chain has been attached to the amino acid B29. It is a long-acting insulin that is administered by single or twice-daily dosing. Onset of action is usually between 2 and 4 hours, with offset about 12 to 14 hours after administration.

Recently inhaled insulin has been approved for clinical use in humans. *Exubera* is a rapid-acting insulin in powder form. This product contains insulin particles (<7.5 μm) combined with a dry powder carrier. The preparation is supplied as a blister pack, and a specialized inhaler is used to deliver the drug to the lungs by generating a pulse of compressed air, thus mobilizing the dry powder insulin into a cloud that can be inhaled. One milligram of the dry powder is equivalent to 3 units of insulin. The bioavailability of this product is approximately 10%, compared with regular human insulin administered by subcutaneous injection. Its onset of action is similar to rapid-acting insulin analogues. However, it can cause bronchospasm and has been associated with changes in lung diffusing capacity. Its efficacy and safety in smokers or people with chronic obstructive lung disease or asthma is unknown.

Therapeutic Approach

Optimal therapy for diabetes has been the subject of much opinion and controversy with respect to tailoring the optimal approach for each individual patient. Traditionally most physicians treating patients with diabetes have favored a stepwise approach with sequential addition of therapy intended to achieve and maintain glycemic goals. It is important to realize that the time of presentation in the course of the disease is extremely variable and may influence initial therapy.

In type 1 diabetes, patients usually present emergently with acute hyperglycemia and occasionally frank diabetic ketoacidosis, which requires insulin therapy together with intravenous rehydration and replacement of electrolytes. A few patients with type 1 diabetes present with mild asymptomatic elevations of fasting blood glucose and/or HbA_{1c} discovered incidentally. Islet autoimmunity may be documented at that time. Others are treated with oral agents but experience early treatment failure. Some have advocated using fasting C-peptide values together with the secretory response to glucagon to determine whether such patients require insulin therapy.[45]

In type 2 diabetes (Fig. 37-14), lifestyle modification forms the basis of all successful pharmacotherapy and, depending on the preceding habits of the individual as well as the degree of hyperglycemia at presentation, may be advocated as the sole intervention at presentation. This is reasonable provided close follow-up is maintained. Often metformin therapy is initiated as first-line therapy. Various rationales support this prescribing habit—it is unlikely to cause hypoglycemia, may benefit the cardiovascular risk profile of the individual, and may cause weight loss or at least prevent the weight gain associated with improved glycemic control.

Sulfonylureas are a reasonable first choice for monotherapy if hypoglycemia and/or weight loss are not significant clinical issues (see Fig. 37-14). However, like metformin, a substantial proportion of patients will not achieve control with monotherapy. Metformin and sulfonylurea combination therapy is frequently utilized for type 2 diabetes. The place for newer agents in the treatment of diabetes is still uncertain. When they are used as monotherapy, the glucose lowering of the thiazolidinediones is less potent than metformin and sulfonylureas, and usually these medications are used in combination with other agents. The suggestion that thiazolidinediones may preserve beta cell function and perhaps decrease the risk of cardiovascular complications beyond the direct benefits of glucose lowering has led to suggestions that these agents be used earlier in combination therapy.[46]

Incretin-based therapy may prove to be a useful adjunct to patients failing conventional therapy. GLP-1 receptor agonists are associated with weight loss and some evidence of improved beta cell function, at least in the short term.[28,29] Because of this, there has been some discussion regarding the timing of their use. Will the benefit be greatest when used at the time of diagnosis in obese patients with diabetes as an adjunct to aggressive lifestyle modification? Should therapy be reserved for patients in whom oral medications are failing, or is it reasonable to use these agents in combination with insulin? The necessity of administering these medications by subcutaneous injection has limited their use to a subset of the patient population. In theory, DPP-4 inhibitors offer many of the same benefits of the GLP-1 receptor agonists. However, they have not been associated with weight loss and have less marked effects on glycemic control.[47] Their role in the therapy of type 2 diabetes is yet to be ascertained. The theoretical benefits of GLP-1–based therapy on beta cell function have not been truly demonstrated in clinical practice.

Insulin therapy in diabetes can occur in a variety of ways. Multiple daily injections of insulin attempt to replicate fasting and prandial insulin secretion through a combination of a premeal bolus insulin and a basal insulin. An increasingly popular alternative is continuous subcutaneous insulin infusion by means of a portable pump. This can be programmed to provide a premeal bolus as well as basal insulin, at varying rates, throughout the rest of the day. Such complex patterns of insulin administration are usually reserved for patients with type 1 diabetes.[48]

The insulin regimens used in type 2 diabetes tend to be simpler and are sometimes combined with oral medications. Bedtime insulin–daily sulfonylurea is one such combination. More commonly, insulin is used in conjunction with an insulin sensitizer. Such combinations may be useful in certain situations, but their appropriateness and the risks and benefits involved should be evaluated for the individual patient. A combination of metformin and insulin therapy usually results in

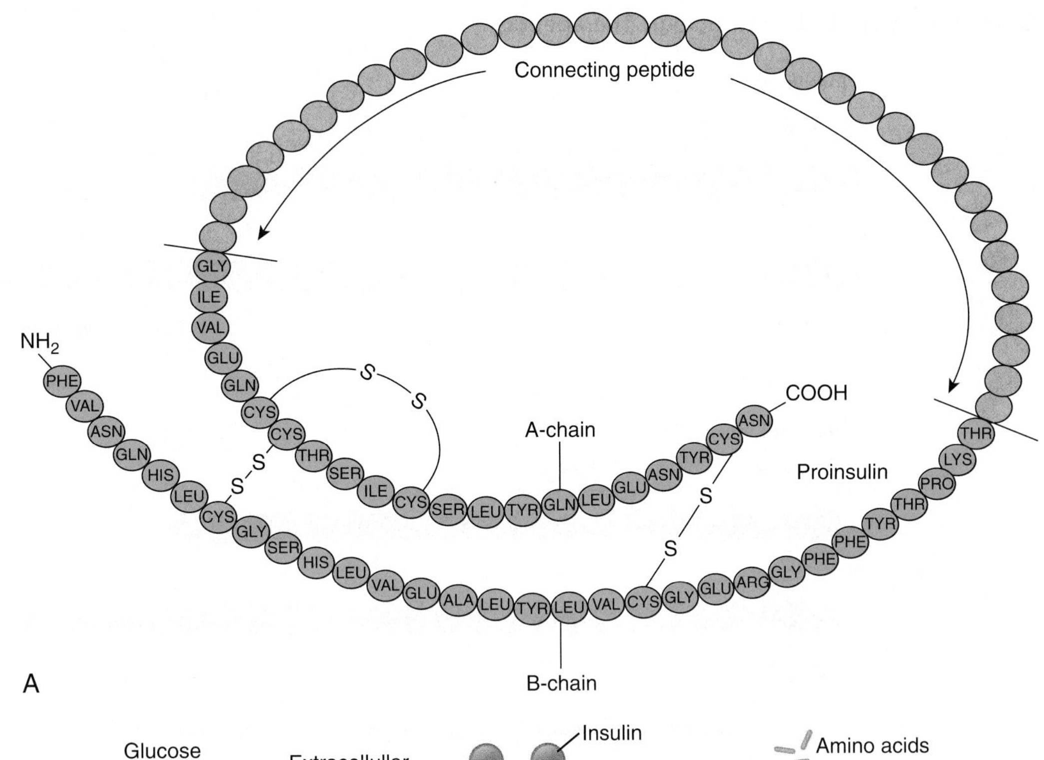

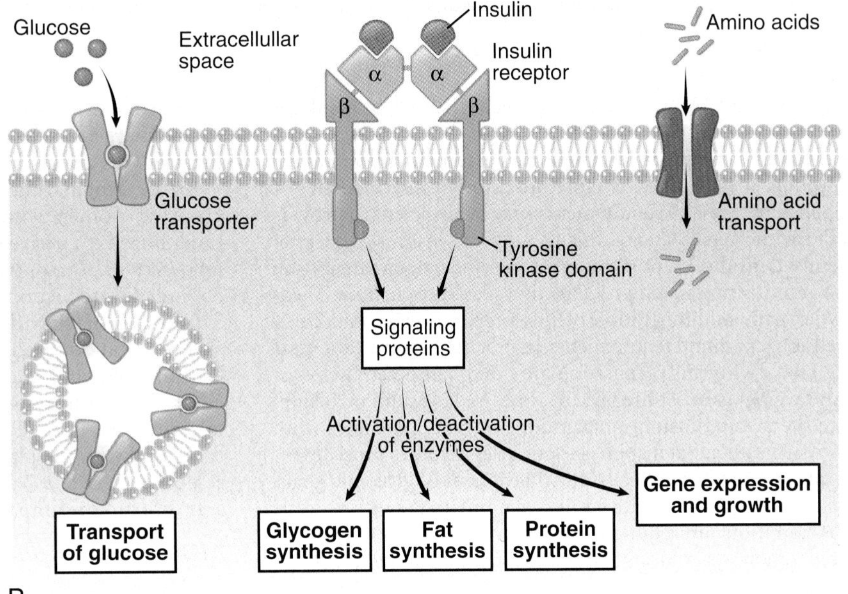

FIGURE 37-11 • Structure of proinsulin and insulin receptor. A, With removal of the connecting peptide (C-peptide), proinsulin is converted to insulin. **B,** Insulin binds to the alpha subunits of the insulin receptor, which increases glucose transport and causes autophosphorylation of the beta subunit of the receptor, which induces tyrosine kinase activity. Tyrosine phosphorylation, in turn, activates a cascade of intracellular signaling proteins that mediate the effects of insulin on glucose, fat, and protein metabolism. (Adapted from Porth CM. Pathophysiology: Concepts of Altered Health States, 7th ed. Philadelphia: Lippincott Williams & Wilkins, 2005.)

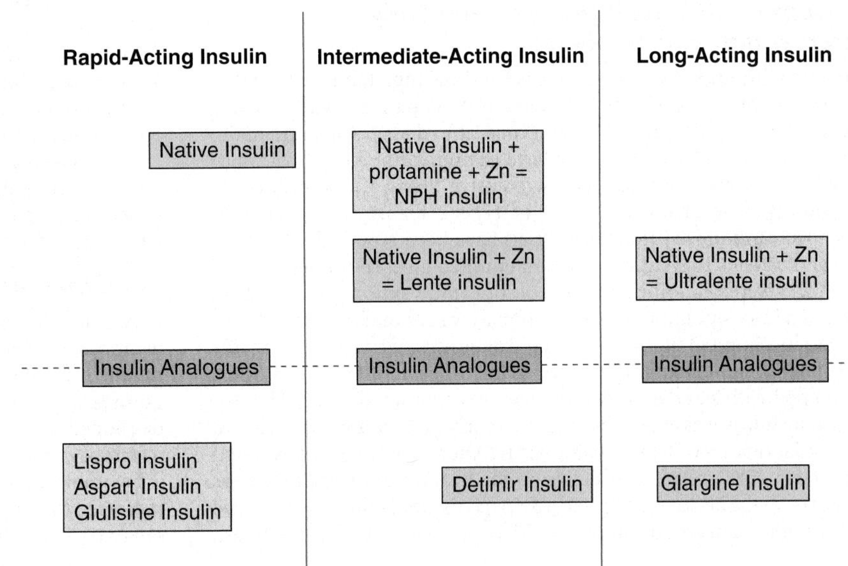

FIGURE 37-12 • A classification of insulin and insulin analogue preparations that are used clinically.

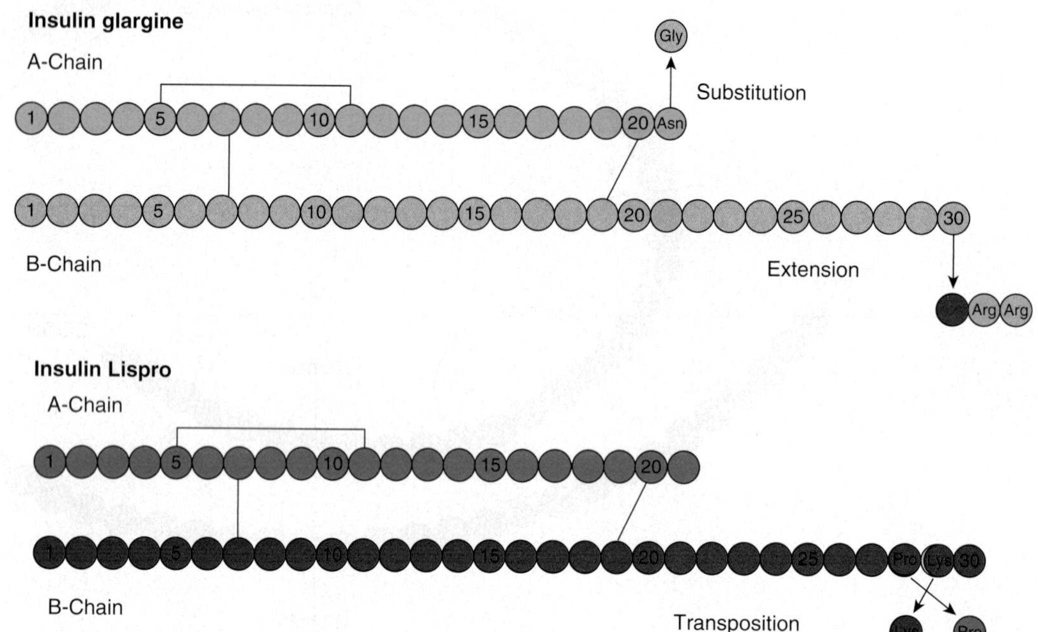

FIGURE 37-13 • Two examples of insulin analogues outlining the changes to the native insulin sequence that result in the altered pharmacokinetics of the analogues.

improved glycemic control with less weight gain than when insulin is used alone.

In type 2 diabetes, simple insulin regimens assume that the patient is able to produce insulin, and therefore provision of intermediate- or long-acting insulin for basal requirements may be sufficient to provide a "scaffold" for the pancreas on which to secrete insulin (e.g., after meals). Premixed insulin is a preparation of intermediate-acting insulin mixed with rapid-acting insulin (70/30) in a fixed proportion. Theoretically, twice-daily administration of this preparation should cover meals as well as background requirements. In practice however, attempts at lowering HbA_{1c} with this preparation are often hampered by hypoglycemia and weight gain. At the present time, NPH insulin or insulin glargine are the favored insulin preparations in type 2 diabetes, with some studies suggesting that insulin glargine is less likely to cause hypoglycemia and is more likely to facilitate achievement of glycemic goals. However, single daily dosing with insulin glargine may not be a realistic proposition if insulin requirements are greater than 50 units/day, and this preparation is significantly more expensive than NPH insulin.

Emerging Targets and Therapeutics

Prevention of Type 2 Diabetes and Early Intervention in Prediabetes

Patients with impaired fasting glucose and/or impaired glucose tolerance are at high risk of type 2 diabetes. Indeed, patients with a fasting glucose between 100 and 125 mg/dl convert to diabetes at a rate of 5% to 10% per year. Various studies have examined the benefit of pharmacologic intervention as well as intensive lifestyle modification in preventing or delaying the onset of type 2 diabetes. Several well-designed randomized, controlled trials have been reported.

The Diabetes Prevention Program enrolled glucose-intolerant subjects who were randomized to one of four intervention groups, which included intensive lifestyle modification as well as medication (administered in a blinded fashion) in three groups: the metformin group, the troglitazone group, or the placebo group. These interventions were combined with standard diet and exercise recommendations. The troglitazone intervention was discontinued early in the study secondary to the initial reports of fatal hepatotoxicity. After an average follow-up of 2.8 years, a 58% relative reduction in the progression to diabetes was observed in the lifestyle group and a 31% relative reduction was observed in the metformin group compared with control subjects.[49] Interestingly, in the troglitazone arm of the Diabetes Prevention Program, troglitazone markedly reduced the incidence of diabetes during the period the drug was given—an effect that has been sustained.[50]

In the Troglitazone in Prevention of Diabetes (TRIPOD) study, Hispanic women with previous gestational diabetes mellitus were randomized to receive either placebo or troglitazone. After a median follow-up of 30 months, troglitazone treatment was associated with a 56% relative reduction in progression to diabetes.[51]

In the STOP-IDDM trial, participants with impaired glucose tolerance were randomized in a double-blind fashion to receive either acarbose or a placebo. After a mean follow-up of 3.3 years, a 25% relative risk reduction in progression to diabetes, based on one oral glucose tolerance test (OGTT), was observed in the acarbose-treated group compared with the placebo group. If this diagnosis was confirmed by a second OGTT, a 36% relative risk reduction was observed in the acarbose group compared with the placebo group.[52,53]

MODY and Implications of Therapy

MODY is a heterogeneous group of disorders in which diabetes is inherited as an autosomal dominant trait. It manifests in young (typically before age 25) individuals, but absolute insulin dependence is not usually a feature at least initially.[4] Patients with mutations in glucokinase or *HNF1α* as well as mutations in *KCNJ11* respond to insulin secretagogues but not to insulin sensitizers.[54] In contrast, patients with mutations in *HNF1β* do not respond to sulfonylureas and rapidly require treatment with exogenous insulin.[55]

Such observations provide important insights into the pathophysiology of monogenic forms of diabetes, and more importantly how genetics can influence response to pharmacotherapy. This continues to be an area of active investigation.

Combination PPAR Agonists

Given the clinical benefits of therapy with PPAR-α ligands such as gemfibrozil, which lower triglyceride concentrations, and the improvements in insulin action associated with PPAR-γ ligands, several compounds that act as agonists of both PPAR subtypes have been developed.[56] Clinical trials utilizing one of these compounds, muraglitazar, have shown their ability to lower HbA_{1c} together with inducing a favorable lipid profile.[57] Despite this, it seems that muraglitazar increased the risk of death, myocardial infarction, and stroke.[58] Further safety trials will be needed for this and related compounds.

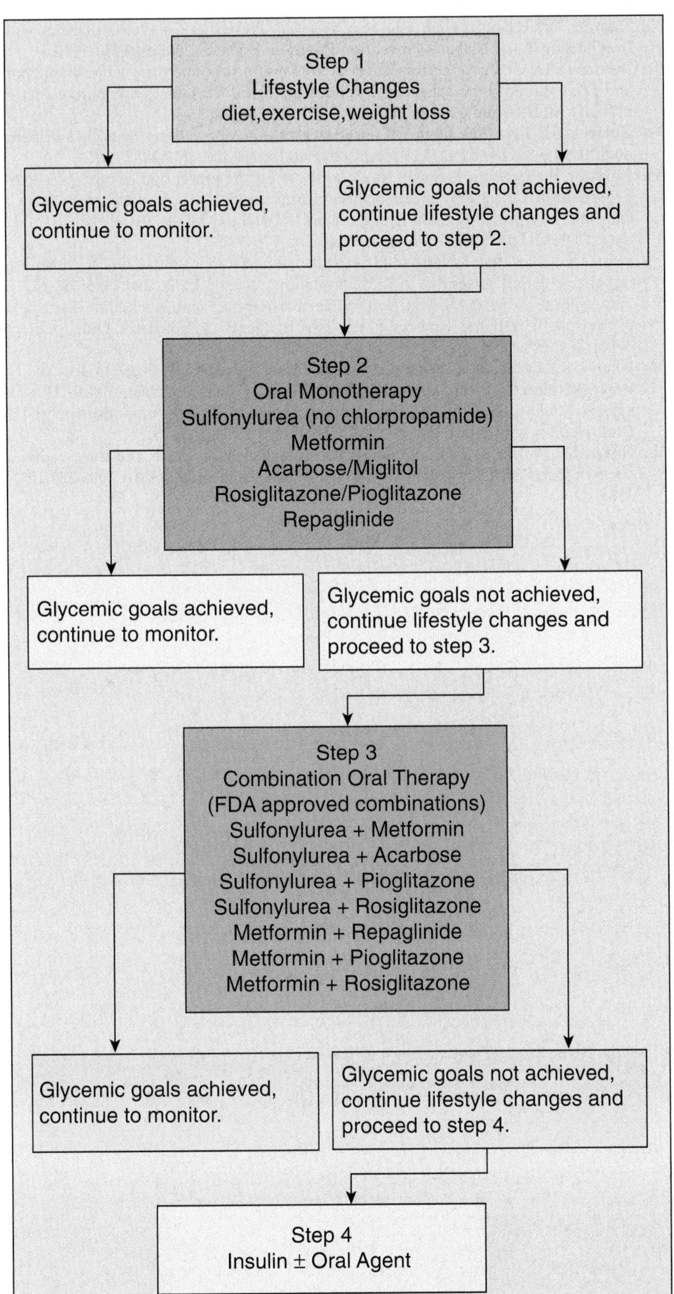

FIGURE 37-14 • Treatment of diabetes mellitus.

REFERENCES

1. Report of the Expert Committee on the Diagnosis and Classification of Diabetes Mellitus. Diabetes Care 1997;20:1183-1197.
2. Florez JC, Hirschhorn J, Altshuler D. The inherited basis of diabetes mellitus: implications for the genetic analysis of complex traits. Annu Rev Genomics Hum Genet 2003;4:257-291.
3. Todd JA. Genetics of type 1 diabetes. Pathol Biol (Paris) 1997;45:219-227.
4. Hattersley AT. Molecular genetics goes to the diabetes clinic. Clin Med 2005;5:476-481.
5. Dinneen S, Gerich J, Rizza R. Carbohydrate metabolism in non-insulin-dependent diabetes mellitus. N Engl J Med 1992;327:707-713.
6. Basu A, Alzaid A, Dinneen S, et al. Effects of a change in the pattern of insulin delivery on carbohydrate tolerance in diabetic and nondiabetic humans in the presence of differing degrees of insulin resistance. J Clin Invest 1996;97:2351-2361.
7. Basu A, Caumo A, Bettini F, et al. Impaired basal glucose effectiveness in NIDDM: contribution of defects in glucose disappearance and production, measured using an optimized minimal model independent protocol. Diabetes 1997;46:421-432.
8. Vella A, Camilleri M, Rizza RA. The gastrointestinal tract and glucose tolerance. Curr Opin Clin Nutr Metab Care 2004;7:479-484.
9. Shah P, Basu A, Basu R, Rizza R. Impact of lack of suppression of glucagon on glucose tolerance in humans. Am J Physiol Endocrinol Metab 1999;277(2 Pt 1):E283-E290.
10. Shah P, Vella A, Basu A, et al. Lack of suppression of glucagon contributes to postprandial hyperglycemia in subjects with type 2 diabetes mellitus. J Clin Endocrinol Metab 2000;85:4053-4059.
11. The effect of intensive treatment of diabetes on the development and progression of long-term complications in insulin-dependent diabetes mellitus. The Diabetes Control and Complications Trial Research Group. N Engl J Med 1993;329:977-986.
12. Intensive blood-glucose control with sulphonylureas or insulin compared with conventional treatment and risk of complications in patients with type 2 diabetes (UKPDS 33). UK Prospective Diabetes Study (UKPDS) Group. Lancet 1998;352:837-853.
13. Effect of intensive blood-glucose control with metformin on complications in overweight patients with type 2 diabetes (UKPDS 34). UK Prospective Diabetes Study (UKPDS) Group. Lancet 1998;352:854-865.
14. Lebovitz HE. α-Glucosidase inhibitors. Endocrinol Metab Clin North Am 1997;26:539-551.
15. Enc FY, Imeryuz N, Akin L, et al. Inhibition of gastric emptying by acarbose is correlated with GLP-1 response and accompanied by CCK release. Am J Physiol Gastrointest Liver Physiol 2001;281:G752-G763.
16. Hucking K, Kostic Z, Pox C, et al. α-Glucosidase inhibition (acarbose) fails to enhance secretion of glucagon-like peptide 1 (7-36 amide) and to delay gastric emptying in type 2 diabetic patients. Diabet Med 2005;22:470-476.
17. Chiasson JL, Josse RG, Hunt JA, et al. The efficacy of acarbose in the treatment of patients with non-insulin-dependent diabetes mellitus: a multicenter controlled clinical trial. Ann Intern Med 1994;121:928-935.
18. Gentile S, Guarino G, Romano M, et al. A randomized controlled trial of acarbose in hepatic encephalopathy. Clin Gastroenterol Hepatol 2005;3:184-191.
19. DeFronzo RA. Pharmacologic therapy for type 2 diabetes mellitus. Ann Intern Med 1999;131:281-303.
20. Samsom M, Szarka LA, Camilleri M, et al. Pramlintide, an amylin analog, selectively delays gastric emptying: potential role of vagal inhibition. Am J Physiol Gastrointest Liver Physiol 2000;278:G946-G951.
21. Vella A, Lee JS, Camilleri M, et al. Effects of pramlintide, an amylin analogue, on gastric emptying in type 1 and 2 diabetes mellitus. Neurogastroenterol Motil 2002;14:123-131.
22. Young A, Pittner R, Gedulin B, et al. Amylin regulation of carbohydrate metabolism. Biochem Soc Trans 1995;23:325-331.
23. Rink TJ, Beaumont K, Koda J, Young A. Structure and biology of amylin. Trends Pharmacol Sci 1993;14:113-118.
24. Ryan GJ, Jobe LJ, Martin R. Pramlintide in the treatment of type 1 and type 2 diabetes mellitus. Clin Ther 2005;27:1500-1512.
25. Kieffer TJ, Habener JF. The glucagon-like peptides. Endocr Rev 1999;20:876-913.
26. Drucker DJ. Development of glucagon-like peptide-1-based pharmaceuticals as therapeutic agents for the treatment of diabetes. Curr Pharm Des 2001;7:1399-1412.
27. Drucker DJ. Glucagon-like peptides: regulators of cell proliferation, differentiation, and apoptosis. Mol Endocrinol 2003;17:161-171.
28. DeFronzo RA, Ratner RE, Han J, et al. Effects of exenatide (exendin-4) on glycemic control and weight over 30 weeks in metformin-treated patients with type 2 diabetes. Diabetes Care 2005;28:1092-1100.
29. Kendall DM, Riddle MC, Rosenstock J, et al. Effects of exenatide (exendin-4) on glycemic control over 30 weeks in patients with type 2 diabetes treated with metformin and a sulfonylurea. Diabetes Care 2005;28:1083-1091.
30. Ristic S, Byiers S, Foley J, Holmes D. Improved glycaemic control with dipeptidyl peptidase-4 inhibition in patients with type 2 diabetes: vildagliptin (LAF237) dose response. Diabetes Obes Metab 2005;7:692-698.
31. Meier JJ, Gallwitz B, Salmen S, et al. Normalization of glucose concentrations and deceleration of gastric emptying after solid meals during intravenous glucagon-like peptide 1 in patients with type 2 diabetes. J Clin Endocrinol Metab 2003;88:2719-2725.
32. Mari A, Sallas WM, He YL, et al. Vildagliptin, a dipeptidyl peptidase-IV inhibitor, improves model-assessed beta-cell function in patients with type 2 diabetes. J Clin Endocrinol Metab 2005;90:4888-4894.
33. Fuhlendorff J, Rorsman P, Kofod H, et al. Stimulation of insulin release by repaglinide and glibenclamide involves both common and distinct processes. Diabetes 1998;47:345-351.
34. Klip A, Leiter LA. Cellular mechanism of action of metformin. Diabetes Care 1990;13:696-704.
35. Urakami T, Morimoto S, Owada M, Harada K. Usefulness of the addition of metformin to insulin in pediatric patients with type 1 diabetes mellitus. Pediatr Int 2005;47:430-433.
36. Campbell IW, Howlett HC. Worldwide experience of metformin as an effective glucose-lowering agent: a meta-analysis. Diabetes Metab Rev 1995;11(Suppl 1):S57-S62.
37. Siconolfi-Baez L, Banerji MA, Lebovitz HE. Characterization and significance of sulfonylurea receptors. Diabetes Care 1990;13(Suppl 3):2-8.
38. Service FJ. Hypoglycemia. Endocrinol Metab Clin North Am 1997;26:937-955.
39. United Kingdom Prospective Diabetes Study 24: a 6-year, randomized, controlled trial comparing sulfonylurea, insulin, and metformin therapy in patients with newly diagnosed type 2 diabetes that could not be controlled with diet therapy. United Kingdom Prospective Diabetes Study Group. Ann Intern Med 1998;128:165-175.
40. Staels B, Fruchart JC. Therapeutic roles of peroxisome proliferator-activated receptor agonists. Diabetes 2005;54:2460-2470.
41. Vella A, de Groen PC, Dinneen SF. Fatal hepatotoxicity associated with troglitazone. Ann Intern Med 1998;129:1080.
42. Inzucchi SE, Maggs DG, Spollett GR, et al. Efficacy and metabolic effects of metformin and troglitazone in type II diabetes mellitus. N Engl J Med 1998;338:867-872.

43. Nesto RW, Bell D, Bonow RO, et al. Thiazolidinedione use, fluid retention, and congestive heart failure: a consensus statement from the American Heart Association and American Diabetes Association. Diabetes Care 2004;27:256-263.
44. Bhatnagar S, Srivastava D, Jayadev MS, Dubey AK. Molecular variants and derivatives of insulin for improved glycemic control in diabetes. Prog Biophys Mol Biol 2006;91:199-228.
45. Service FJ, Rizza RA, Zimmerman BR, et al. The classification of diabetes by clinical and C-peptide criteria: a prospective population-based study. Diabetes Care 1997;20:198-201.
46. Dormandy JA, Charbonnel B, Eckland DJ, et al. Secondary prevention of macrovascular events in patients with type 2 diabetes in the PROactive Study (PROspective pioglitAzone Clinical Trial In macroVascular Events): a randomised controlled trial. Lancet 2005;366:1279-1289.
47. Ahren B, Landin-Olsson M, Jansson PA, et al. Inhibition of dipeptidyl peptidase-4 reduces glycemia, sustains insulin levels, and reduces glucagon levels in type 2 diabetes. J Clin Endocrinol Metab 2004;89:2078-2084.
48. Rizza RA, Gerich JE, Haymond MW, et al. Control of blood sugar in insulin-dependent diabetes: comparison of an artificial endocrine pancreas, continuous subcutaneous insulin infusion, and intensified conventional insulin therapy. N Engl J Med 1980;303:1313-1318.
49. Knowler WC, Barrett-Connor E, Fowler SE, et al. Reduction in the incidence of type 2 diabetes with lifestyle intervention or metformin. N Engl J Med 2002;346:393-403.
50. Knowler WC, Hamman RF, Edelstein SL, et al. Prevention of type 2 diabetes with troglitazone in the Diabetes Prevention Program. Diabetes 2005;54:1150-1156.
51. Buchanan TA, Xiang AH, Peters RK, et al. Preservation of pancreatic beta-cell function and prevention of type 2 diabetes by pharmacological treatment of insulin resistance in high-risk Hispanic women. Diabetes 2002;51:2796-2803.
52. Chiasson JL, Josse RG, Gomis R, et al. Acarbose for prevention of type 2 diabetes mellitus: the STOP-NIDDM randomised trial. Lancet 2002;359:2072-2077.
53. Chiasson JL, Josse RG, Gomis R, et al. Acarbose for the prevention of type 2 diabetes, hypertension and cardiovascular disease in subjects with impaired glucose tolerance: facts and interpretations concerning the critical analysis of the STOP-NIDDM Trial data. Diabetologia 2004;47:969-975; discussion 976-977.
54. Pearson ER, Flechtner I, Njolstad PR, et al. Switching from insulin to oral sulfonylureas in patients with diabetes due to Kir6.2 mutations. N Engl J Med 2006;355:467-477.
55. Hattersley AT, Pearson ER. Minireview: Pharmacogenetics and beyond: the interaction of therapeutic response, beta-cell physiology, and genetics in diabetes. Endocrinology 2006;147:2657-2663.
56. Lebovitz H. Diabetes: assessing the pipeline. Atheroscler Suppl 2006;7:43-49.
57. Buse JB, Rubin CJ, Frederich R, et al. Muraglitazar, a dual (alpha/gamma) PPAR activator: a randomized, double-blind, placebo-controlled, 24-week monotherapy trial in adult patients with type 2 diabetes. Clin Ther 2005;27:1181-1195.
58. Nissen SE, Wolski K, Topol EJ. Effect of muraglitazar on death and major adverse cardiovascular events in patients with type 2 diabetes mellitus. JAMA 2005;294:2581-2586.

38

DISORDERS OF THE THYROID

Helen L. Baron and Peter A. Singer

HYPOTHYROIDISM 571
Introduction 571
Pathophysiology 571
Clinical and Metabolic Features 572
Cardiovascular 572
Respiratory 573
Gastrointestinal 573
Hematologic 573
Neuromuscular 574
Reproductive 574
Dermatologic 574
Weight Gain 574
Laboratory Diagnosis 574
Therapeutics and Clinical Pharmacology 574
Levothyroxine 574
Other Thyroid Hormone Preparations 575
Special Therapeutic Circumstances 576
Subclinical Hypothyroidism 576
Coronary Heart Disease 576
Pregnancy 576
Secondary Hypothyroidism 576
Surgical Patients 576
Myxedema Coma 576
HYPERTHYROIDISM 576
Introduction 576
Pathophysiology 577
Clinical and Metabolic Features 577
Cardiovascular 577
Respiratory 577
Gastrointestinal 578
Hematologic 578
Neuromuscular 578
Skeletal 578
Renal 578
Reproductive 578
Dermatologic 578
Ocular 579
Metabolic Abnormalities 579
Laboratory Diagnosis 579
Therapeutics and Clinical Pharmacology 580
β-Adrenergic Blockade 580
Thionamides 580
Radioactive Iodine Therapy 581
Surgery 581
Toxic Nodular Goiter 581
Special Therapeutic Circumstances 581
Subclinical Hyperthyroidism 581
Pregnancy 582
Apathetic Hyperthyroidism 582
Thyroid Storm 582

HYPOTHYROIDISM

Introduction

Hypothyroidism is likely the most common thyroid disorder encountered in clinical practice. According to the U.S. National Health and Nutrition Examination Survey (NHANES III), hypothyroidism was found in 4.6% (0.3% overt and 4.3% subclinical) of 13,344 persons without previously known thyroid dysfunction.[1]

Hypothyroidism is approximately nine times more common in women than in men, and increases with age in both sexes. By age 75 years, hypothyroidism affects approximately 20% of women and approximately 15% of men.[2] African Americans are affected less frequently than whites, Hispanics, and Asians.[1,3,4] Hypothyroidism typically has an insidious onset and, because of the subtlety of many of the symptoms and signs, may not be readily recognized either by the affected persons or by their physicians. Fortunately, both the biochemical diagnosis and the treatment of hypothyroidism are relatively straightforward.

Pathophysiology

Hypothyroidism may arise from a defect anywhere along the hypothalamic-pituitary-thyroid axis (Fig. 38-1). The vast majority of hypothyroidism is due to thyroid gland dysfunction, and is termed *primary hypothyroidism* (Fig. 38-2). Hypothyroidism is infrequently due to insufficient secretion of thyroid-stimulating hormone (TSH; thyrotropin) from the pituitary or thyrotropin-releasing hormone (TRH) from the hypothalamus, which is termed *secondary hypothyroidism.*[5]

Primary hypothyroidism may be present in one of two forms: subclinical hypothyroidism or overt hypothyroidism. Subclinical hypothyroidism is defined as having normal serum levels of the thyroid hormones thyroxine (T_4) and triiodothyronine (T_3), in conjunction with an elevated serum TSH level.[6] Few if any symptoms of hypothyroidism are present. Overt hypothyroidism is defined as having low thyroid hormone levels with an elevation in the serum TSH concentration. The majority of these patients will present with the signs and symptoms of hypothyroidism.

There are multiple etiologies of primary hypothyroidism, and they include such divergent causes as autoimmune disease, surgical removal of the thyroid gland, radioablation, inflammation, pharmacologic agents, infiltrative disorders, and congenital hypothyroidism (Box 38-1). Worldwide, the most common etiology of hypothyroidism is iodine deficiency, a disorder virtually eliminated from the industrialized world.

The most common form of primary hypothyroidism in iodine-sufficient areas of the world is chronic autoimmune (Hashimoto's) thyroiditis. This disorder is caused by both cellular and antibody-mediated destruction of the thyroid gland.[7] Hypothyroidism secondary to Hashimoto's thyroiditis is generally permanent, so that once the diagnosis of hypothyroidism is established, thyroid hormone replacement therapy is lifelong. The other most common causes of hypothyroidism include thyroidectomy (usually for treatment of thyroid cancer, symptomatic goiter, and thyrotoxicosis), and radioiodine ablation, generally for thyrotoxic Graves' disease.

Primary hypothyroidism may also occasionally be transient, either due to inflammation or due to the effects of certain pharmacologic agents, including the antiarrhythmic amiodarone, lithium, interferon alfa, and interleukin-2.[8] Amiodarone, a unique pharmacologic agent that is a commonly used antiarrhythmic, may cause hypothyroidism either by causing inflammation of the thyroid gland or from the inhibitory effects of excess iodides.[9,10] High doses of exogenous iodides decrease the organification of iodide within the thyroid gland, resulting in a decrease in thyroid hormone synthesis (Wolff-Chaikoff effect).[11,12] This results in hypothyroidism, and occurs almost exclusively in individuals with underlying Hashimoto's thyroiditis. It is estimated that a 200-mg dose of amiodarone releases 6 mg/day of iodine into circulation, compared to the 0.3 mg/day of iodine in the typical diet in the United States.[13] Exogenous iodides also act by directly inhibiting thyroid hormone release, an effect also observed with the antidepressant lithium carbonate. Lithium's effects on thyroid function also

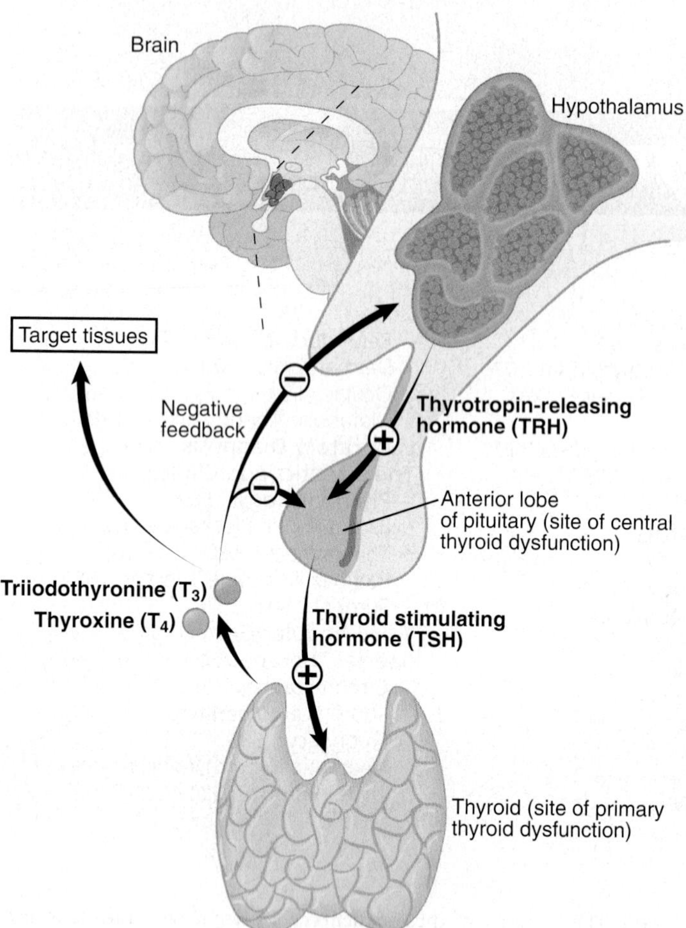

FIGURE 38-1 • The hypothalamic-pituitary-thyroidal axis.

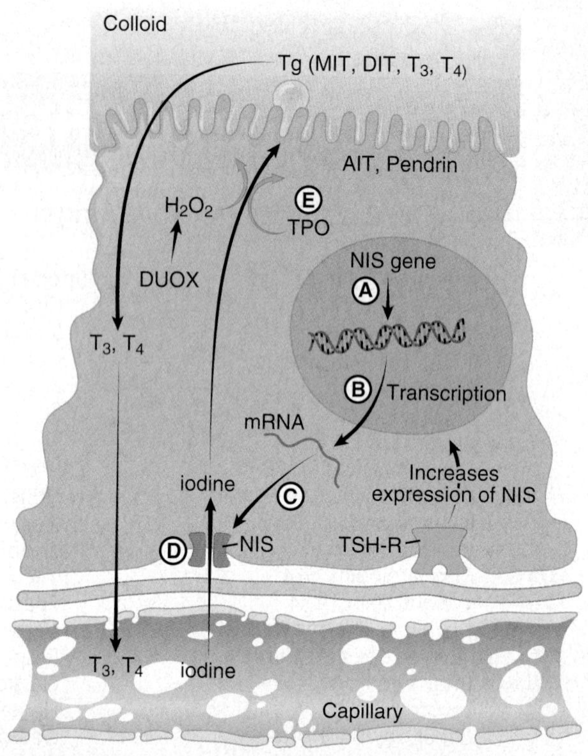

FIGURE 38-2 • Iodine metabolism in normal thyroid cells. TSH signaling via the TSH receptor (which is shown at the bottom of the thyrocyte on the left) controls thyroid hormone synthesis, and it can increase expression of NIS in the basolateral membrane of thyrocytes. As shown in the thyrocyte on the right, NIS takes up iodide from the blood. The proteins involved in efflux of iodide at the apical membrane are not known, and the roles of AIT and pendrin are unclear. As shown in the left-hand thyrocyte, iodide is organified in the tyrosyl residues of Tg in a reaction catalyzed by TPO, in the presence of H_2O_2, which is produced by DUOX. Tg contains MIT, DIT, T_3, and T_4 and is stored in colloid until T_3 and T_4 need to be released into the blood. Among potential defects of iodide metabolism in thyroid cancer cells, decreased iodide uptake may be related to the following features: **(A)** an NIS gene abnormality (not yet found); **(B)** decreased NIS gene expression; **(C)** abnormal NIS protein maturation (glycosylation); or **(D)** abnormal NIS protein targeting to the plasma membrane. **(E)** Decreased iodide organification may be related to decreased TPO expression and to posttranslational abnormalities. (AIT, apical iodine transporter; DIT, diiodotyrosine; DUOX, dual oxidase; MIT, monoiodotyrosine; mRNA, messenger RNA; NIS, sodium iodide symporter; T_3, triiodothyronine; T_4, thyroxine; Tg, thyroglobulin; TPO, thyroid peroxidase; TSH-R, thyroid-stimulating hormone receptor.)

appear to occur mainly in patients with underlying Hashimoto's thyroiditis, and may be seen in up to 20% of individuals treated with lithium.[14-16]

Congenital hypothyroidism occurs in approximately 1 of every 3500 live births in the United States.[17] The most common causes of congenital hypothyroidism include agenesis and dysgenesis of the thyroid, although worldwide, iodine deficiency is the most common cause of congenital hypothyroidism.[18] Because of the severity of developmental and neurologic defects associated with congenital hypothyroidism, there is mandatory neonatal screening of thyroid function in virtually all developed countries.

Hypothyroidism due to insufficient secretion of TSH from the pituitary or TRH from the hypothalamus commonly occurs as a result of a mass lesion in the area of the sella turcica, generally a pituitary tumor or a craniopharyngioma, but may also be due to hemorrhage, external radiation, or infiltrative disorders.[19]

Clinical and Metabolic Features

Thyroid hormone has a critical role in normal growth and development in infancy and childhood, as well as in the metabolic activity of adults. Thyroid hormone affects the function of nearly every human organ system, through a canonical signaling mechanism (Fig. 38-3), and its deficiency results in a typical constellation of signs, symptoms, and metabolic alterations. Physical examination of the thyroid gland generally reveals a firm, diffusely enlarged gland, although it may be nodular and, in some cases, atrophied and nonpalpable. Noteworthy is that virtually all of the clinical features attributable to hypothyroidism are reversible with appropriate thyroid hormone replacement (Box 38-2).

Cardiovascular

The hypothyroid state reduces the need for oxygen and substrate utilization by all major organ systems in the body. This decrease in metabolic demand results in a reduction in cardiac output, due to decreases in cardiac contractility, decreases in heart rate, and increases in peripheral vascular resistance.[20,21] Increases in systemic vascular resistance also result in diastolic hypertension, which occurs in approximately 20% to 40% of hypothyroid patients.[21] Pericardial effusion may be noted as well, although only in the context of severe, long-standing hypothyroidism, and is rarely hemodynamically significant.

Hyperlipidemia is common, and is due to decreases in circulating lipid clearance. The predominant pattern includes high total cholesterol and low-density lipoprotein cholesterol concentrations, and there is a direct relationship between the degree of hypothyroidism and the degree of cholesterol elevation.[3,22,23] Elevations in very-low-density lipoprotein cholesterol concentrations and isolated hypertriglyceridemia are not as commonly noted. High-density lipoprotein cholesterol concentrations are not affected.[3] Hyperhomocystinemia is also prevalent, due to decreases in metabolic clearance.[24,25]

BOX 38-1 ETIOLOGIES OF HYPOTHYROIDISM

Primary Hypothyroidism

Permanent Hypothyroidism

- Chronic autoimmune (Hashimoto's) thyroiditis (most common cause in industrialized countries)
- Thyroid ablation (radioactive iodine therapy or thyroidectomy)
- External radiotherapy (for head and neck cancer, lymphoma)
- Congenital (~1 in 3500 live births in the United States; due to thyroid agenesis)
- Infiltrative disorders (hemochromatosis, amyloidosis, Riedel's thyroiditis, cystinosis, scleroderma, leukemia)
- Iodine deficiency (principally in Africa and in some areas of Latin America)
- Iodine excess (from iodine-containing medications, such as amiodarone or saturated solution of potassium iodide; this process occurs in patients with underlying autoimmune thyroid disease)

Transient Hypothyroidism

- Subacute painful (viral) thyroiditis
- Subacute painless thyroiditis (frequently seen postpartum)
- Drug-induced thyroiditis
  - Interferon alfa, interleukin-2, amiodarone (these drugs induce a thyroiditis-like response)
  - Exogenous iodides, including amiodarone (euthyroidism returns after drug withdrawal)
  - Methimazole, propylthiouracil (resolves after medication withdrawal)
  - Lithium carbonate (resolves after medication withdrawal; occurs only in patients with underlying autoimmune thyroid disease)

Secondary (Central) Hypothyroidism

- Pituitary adenoma, craniopharyngioma
- Pituitary apoplexy, Sheehan's syndrome
- Lymphocytic hypophysitis
- Pituitary irradiation
- Cranial irradiation
- Pituitary stalk section, other major head trauma
- Congenital hypopituitarism
- Infiltrative disorders: Langerhans cell histiocytosis, hemochromatosis
- Granulomatous disorders: sarcoidosis

Adapted from Singer PA. Hypothyroidism. *In* Rakel RE, Bope ET (eds): Conn's Current Therapy. Philadelphia: Elsevier Saunders, 2006, pp 802-806.

Respiratory

Hypothyroidism may cause respiratory muscle weakness, with resultant alveolar hypoventilation and a reduction in hypoxic respiratory drive.[26,27] In addition, there may be a decrease in hypercapnic ventilatory drive, particularly with profound hypothyroidism, such as myxedema coma.[28] Obstructive sleep apnea may be seen in hypothyroid patients; possible mechanisms for this include depression in ventilatory drive and myxedematous changes of the tongue, pharynx, and larynx.[29,30] Respiratory muscle weakness results from a diffuse skeletal muscle myopathy, which may also be clinically evident in patients with significant hypothyroidism.[26,31]

Gastrointestinal

Decreases in gut motility are commonly seen in hypothyroidism and frequently lead to constipation. This is one of the most common complaints of patients with hypothyroidism. In severe cases of hypothyroidism, intestinal slowing may even progress to ileus.

Hematologic

The predominant hematologic abnormality seen in hypothyroidism is a normochromic, normocytic, hypoproliferative anemia, due to a

BOX 38-2 SYMPTOMS AND SIGNS OF HYPOTHYROIDISM

Common Symptoms

- Fatigue
- Increased need for sleep
- Cold intolerance
- Dry skin and hair
- Weight gain (mild)
- Constipation
- Intellectual slowing

Common Signs

- Relative bradycardia
- Slowed speech
- Dry, flaky skin
- Pallor (with overt hypothyroidism)
- Goiter
- Periorbital edema
- Distant heart tones (with marked hypothyroidism)
- Delayed deep tendon reflexes

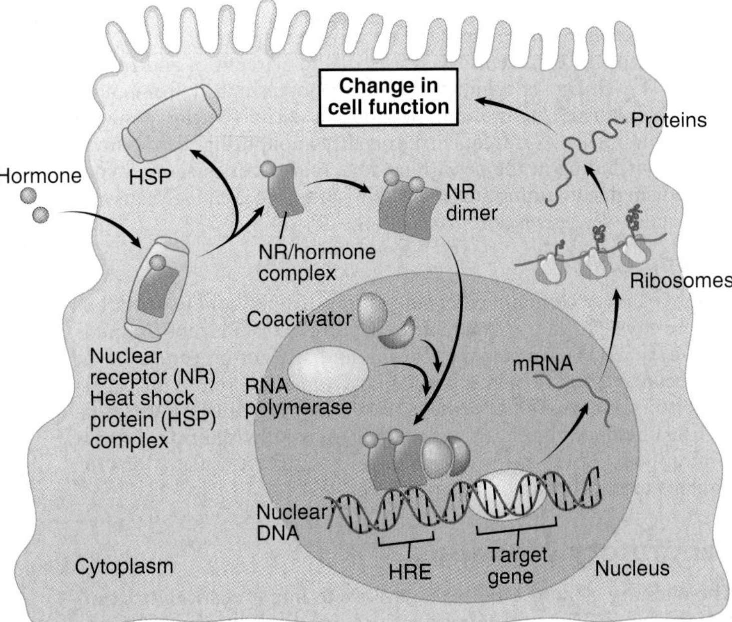

FIGURE 38-3 • Thyroid hormone signaling. The mechanism of thyroid hormone receptor, a class I nuclear receptor (NR), which, in the absence of ligand, is located in the cytosol. Hormone binding triggers dissociation of heat shock proteins (HSP), dimerization, and translocation to the nucleus, where it binds to a specific sequence of DNA known as a hormone response element (HRE). The nuclear receptor DNA complex in turn recruits other proteins that are responsible for transcription of downstream DNA into messenger RNA (mRNA), which is eventually translated into protein, which results in a change in cell function.

decrease in serum erythropoietin concentrations leading to a decrease in erythropoiesis.[32] Menstruating women may present with iron deficiency anemia secondary to the increased menstrual losses frequently noted with hypothyroidism.[33] Mild problems with coagulation, manifested by bleeding and easy bruisability, may be seen with hypothyroidism due to a decrease in factor VIII concentrations and a prolonged partial thromboplastin time.[34] Pernicious anemia may also be seen in autoimmune hypothyroidism due to the presence of antiparietal antibodies. Pernicious anemia may be seen in up to 10% of patients with Hashimoto's hypothyroidism.[34,35]

Neuromuscular

Hypothyroidism results in a generalized slowing of the neurologic processes. Common symptoms include generalized muscle weakness (more frequently seen in the proximal muscles), stiffness, fatigue, excessive sleepiness, and slowing of thought processes. Delayed deep tendon reflexes are a common sign in hypothyroidism. Impairment of short-term memory may also be observed.[36] Carpal tunnel syndrome may also be present, due to mechanical compression of the median nerve as it passes through the volar aspect of the wrist. This is a local effect resulting from the hypothyroid patient's generalized edema.[37,38] Frank psychosis ("myxedema madness") or even coma may be seen in patients with decompensated hypothyroidism.[39] Common signs of myxedema madness include typical clinical features seen in hypothyroidism, in addition to altered mentation and slow, slurred speech.

Reproductive

Menstrual irregularities are frequently seen in women with hypothyroidism, and may range from oligomenorrhea or anovulatory amenorrhea to hypermenorrhea and menorrhagia. Such menstrual changes may result in decreased fertility due to impaired ovulation.[40,41] If a hypothyroid woman becomes pregnant, her risk for a first-trimester abortion is increased.[40,41] Hypothyroid men may experience decreases in seminal volume, and motility abnormalities with their sperm may also be noted. Sperm count and sperm morphology do not typically change in hypothyroid men.[42]

Dermatologic

Dermatologic complaints are common with hypothyroidism, and indeed may be the initial complaints of patients. Patients complain of dry flaky skin, decreased sweating, coarse and thinning hair, and brittle nails. In addition, the skin may be pale due to concurrent anemia and surface vessel vasoconstriction. Moreover, the skin may have a yellow-orange cast, due to hypercarotenemia associated with the decreased clearance of carotene.[43] Thinning or absence of the lateral third of the eyebrows may also be observed in patients with significant hypothyroidism. Autoimmune vitiligo may be periorbital ("raccoon eyes"), or it may occur on the extensor surfaces of the extremities and on the trunk. The vitiligo is symmetric, thus distinguishing it from other forms of vitiligo.[44,45] Autoimmune alopecia areata (patchy alopecia) may occur but is very infrequent. Generalized nonpitting edema (myxedema), including in the periorbital area, may occur in severe hypothyroidism due to infiltration of the skin with glycosaminoglycans and subsequent water retention[46] (Fig. 38-4).

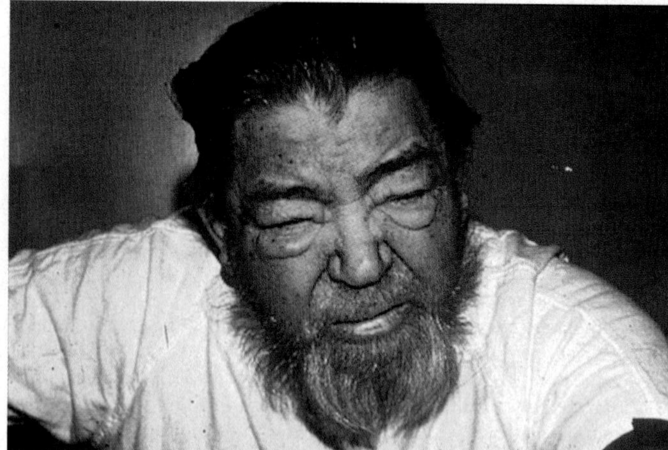

FIGURE 38-4 • Severe hypothyroidism in an adult male. Note the marked periorbital puffiness. (From Singer PA. Thyroid dysfunction of the elderly. In Korenman SG [ed]: Atlas of Clinical Endocrinology. Philadelphia: Blackwell Science, 1999, pp 147-159.)

Weight Gain

Weight gain is a common complaint among hypothyroid patients, but the direct weight gain attributable to hypothyroidism is modest and is due to generalized metabolic slowing and the accumulation of an extracellular fluid rich in glycosaminoglycans that results in classic nonpitting edema. The appetite is usually decreased in hypothyroidism, so obesity, when present, is not due to hypothyroidism.[46] From a clinical perspective, this is one of the most difficult explanations for patients to understand or, indeed, accept.

Laboratory Diagnosis

The pituitary gland is exquisitely sensitive to minor changes in serum free thyroxine (FT_4) concentrations, such that small changes in FT_4 are reflected by amplified reciprocal changes in TSH.[47] TSH is thus the most sensitive marker for alterations in thyroid hormone secretion. An elevation in serum TSH, then, indicates a diagnosis of primary hypothyroidism, and the degree of hypothyroidism should lead to the evaluation of FT_4. A low FT_4 level confirms the diagnosis of overt hypothyroidism, while mild elevations of TSH—generally between 5 and 20 mU/L (normal 0.5 to 5 mU/L)—with normal FT_4 indicate the presence of subclinical hypothyroidism.

In the patient with suspected hypothyroidism, a low or normal serum TSH, coupled with a low FT_4 level, would suggest central hypothyroidism, and further investigation for hypothalamic-pituitary dysfunction should ensue. Nevertheless, central hypothyroidism is by far the exception, and the serum TSH is the single best test to screen for thyroid dysfunction.[48,49]

TSH levels must be interpreted with caution in hospitalized patients, since ill individuals may have alterations of serum TSH ranging from high to low values depending on the degree of illness, even in the face of normal FT_4 levels.[50,51] Medications utilized in the intensive care unit, such as dopamine and high doses of glucocorticoids, may inhibit TSH secretion.[52,53]

Antithyroid antibodies are usually present in the sera of patients with primary hypothyroidism, specifically in chronic autoimmune (Hashimoto's) thyroiditis. The most commonly encountered antibodies are directed against thyroid peroxidase (TPO), and thyroglobulin. The vast majority of patients with Hashimoto's hypothyroidism will have detectable thyroid antibodies, with TPO antibodies seen in more than 90% of affected individuals and thyroglobulin antibodies detectable in 80% to 90% of these patients.[54] As anti-TPO concentrations are typically higher and more frequently seen with Hashimoto's thyroiditis, antithyroglobulin antibodies do not need to be routinely tested. Antithyroglobulin antibodies may be measured in those patients with a high index of suspicion for autoimmune hypothyroidism in whom anti-TPO antibodies are negative[54,55] (Fig. 38-5).

Therapeutics and Clinical Pharmacology

Levothyroxine

The optimal treatment for hypothyroidism is replacement with levothyroxine sodium (L-T4). A number of formulations of L-T4 exist, both as branded and as generic preparations. It is the position of the American Thyroid Association, the Endocrine Society, and the American Association of Clinical Endocrinologists that branded prepara-

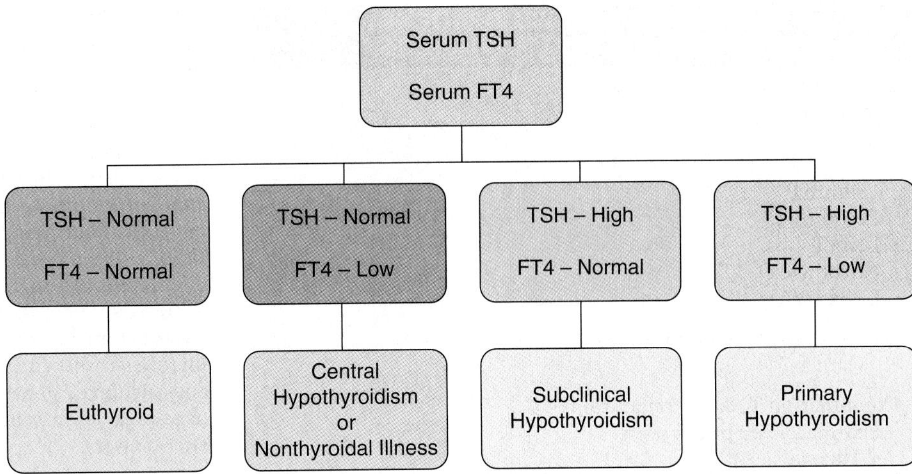

FIGURE 38-5 • Suggested schema for the evaluation of suspected hypothyroidism.

tions should be employed, because of inconsistent bioavailability of some generic preparations.[56,57] If a patient's L-T4 brand is changed, or if a generic form is substituted, then serum TSH should be checked 6 weeks later to determine if re-titration of the thyroid hormone dose is needed.[57]

Typical daily oral replacement doses of L-T4 average 1.6 mcg/kg but may vary. Approximately 80% of oral L-T4 is absorbed, and L-T4 should be taken on an empty stomach, about 1 hour before eating, in order to maximize absorption. Care should be given to avoid taking calcium and iron supplements at the same time as L-T4, since they appear to inhibit L-T4 absorption, albeit to a minor degree.[58-60] As such, ingestion of these supplements should be separated from the L-T4 dose by at least 4 hours.

Young, otherwise healthy hypothyroid individuals may be started on full replacement L-T4 doses, but individuals older than 50 years of age are generally started on lower doses of L-T4, between 25 and 50 mcg/day, and the dose is titrated upward by 25 mcg until euthyroidism is achieved. Adjustments in L-T4 dosing should be no more frequent than every 6 to 8 weeks, since it takes up to 6 to 8 weeks for TSH to equilibrate.[61]

The goal of thyroid hormone replacement therapy is to achieve a normal TSH level, preferably 0.5 to 2 mU/L.[1] Once the TSH has normalized, and a maintenance dose of L-T4 has been determined, serum TSH may be measured once yearly or more often if a change in the patient's clinical status occurs.

There are a number of clinical conditions, as well as various pharmacologic agents, that may alter L-T4 requirements (Box 38-3). L-T4 requirements may be influenced to varying degrees by thyroid-binding globulin (TBG) concentrations, gastrointestinal absorption, and medications that may alter the metabolism of thyroid hormone. Pharmacologic agents that increase TBG concentrations, and thus increase L-T4 requirements, include estrogen (including oral contraceptives and pregnancy) and selective estrogen receptor modulators.[62,63] Androgens and glucocorticoids lower TBG concentrations, resulting in minor decreases in L-T4 requirements.[61] Impaired gastrointestinal absorption of L-T4 is seen with celiac disease, inflammatory bowel disease, and ingestion of iron and calcium carbonate supplements, and in individuals who consume large amounts of fiber, bran, or soy protein.[59,60,64-67] In cases of impaired gastrointestinal absorption, L-T4 doses may need to be increased. L-T4 should be taken at least 4 hours apart from the ingestion of iron or calcium carbonate supplements.[61] Drugs that induce hepatic microsomal enzymes, such as rifampin and commonly prescribed anticonvulsants such as phenytoin and carbamazepine, increase the rate of L-T4 metabolism, resulting in increased L-T4 requirements.[68] Significant weight gain increases L-T4 requirements, while significant weight loss decreases L-T4 requirements. Patients older than 75 or 80 years of age may experience decreased L-T4 requirements.[69]

BOX 38-3 FACTORS AFFECTING LEVOTHYROXINE (L-T4) DOSE

Increased L-T4 Dose Requirements

- Increases in thyroxine-binding globulin (TBG)
  - Pregnancy
  - Oral estrogen therapy
  - Selective estrogen receptor modulators
- Impairment in gastrointestinal absorption of L-T4
  - Inflammatory bowel disease, celiac disease
  - Vitamins and supplements containing iron or calcium carbonate
  - Aluminum hydroxide gels
  - Sucralfate
  - Bile acid–binding sequestrants (cholestyramine, cholestipol)
  - Diet very high in soy protein or fiber
- Drugs increasing L-T4 metabolism
  - Phenytoin
  - Carbamazepine
  - Phenobarbital
  - Rifampin
- Unknown mechanism
  - Sertraline
  - Lovastatin
- Significant weight gain

Decreased L-T4 Dose Requirement

- Decreases in TBG
  - Androgen therapy
  - Nephrotic syndrome
  - Congenital TBG deficiency
- Aging (old age)
- Significant weight loss

Adapted from Singer PA. Hypothyroidism. *In* Rakel RE, Bope ET (eds): Conn's Current Therapy. Philadelphia: Elsevier Saunders, 2006, pp 802-806.

Other Thyroid Hormone Preparations

Other thyroid hormone preparations include liothyronine sodium (L-T3; Cytomel), and combinations of L-T4 and L-T3, such as desiccated thyroid (Box 38-4). Most endocrinologists believe that these agents should not be used as first-line replacement therapy for hypothyroidism. Combination preparations may vary in bioavailability, and are used infrequently. In addition, patients treated with L-T3 may experience wide variations in serum T_3 concentrations due to its rapid gastrointestinal absorption and short half-life of 1 day. Individuals with underlying heart disease may experience an increase in anginal

BOX 38-4 THYROID HORMONE PREPARATIONS COMMONLY AVAILABLE IN THE UNITED STATES

Levothyroxine (T_4) Preparations
- Synthroid
- Levoxyl
- Thyro-Tab
- Unithroid
- Levothroid
- Levo-T
- Novothyrox
- L-thyroxine

Liothyronine (T_3) Preparations
- Cytomel

Combination T_4 & T_3 Preparations
- Pharmacologic preparation
  - Thyrolar
- Dessicated thyroid extract
  - Thyroid USP
  - Armour Thyroid

symptoms and/or arrhythmias because of supraphysiologic levels of T_3.[70]

Studies have been published advocating the addition of L-T3 to an L-T4 treatment regimen, in order to more effectively treat patients' hypothyroid symptoms and to improve their general well-being. The majority of studies have failed to demonstrate superiority of T_4-T_3 combination therapy to L-T4 monotherapy for the management of hypothyroid symptoms.[71-76] In particular, a recent systematic review of nine randomized trials revealed that only one study reported beneficial effects of combination T_4-T_3 therapy on mood, quality of life, and psychometric performance when compared to L-T4 therapy alone.[77]

Special Therapeutic Circumstances

Subclinical Hypothyroidism

Vague, nonspecific constitutional symptoms may be seen in patients with subclinical hypothyroidism, but are poorly correlated with serum TSH values. In addition, there is ongoing debate as to whether or not the disorder is associated with significant clinical consequences, although most endocrinologists believe that it is.[78] One indisputable fact is that patients with subclinical hypothyroidism with positive TPO antibodies progress to overt hypothyroidism, at a rate of approximately 3% to 5% per year, which suggests that, if treatment with L-T4 is not initiated, then careful surveillance is indicated.[4] Evidence suggests that there is an increase in the prevalence and progression of coronary artery disease, as well as all-cause mortality, in patients with subclinical hypothyroidism.[79-82] In view of this, most thyroid specialists agree that patients with serum TSH concentrations greater than 10 mU/L should be treated with L-T4.[78] At issue is whether or not patients with TSH levels below 10 mU/L should be treated, and the consensus appears to be that clinical judgment should be considered in such cases.[78,83]

Coronary Heart Disease

Hypothyroid individuals with known coronary artery disease or significant cardiovascular factors such as diabetes mellitus, hypertension, dyslipidemia, or metabolic syndrome should have their thyroid hormone replaced cautiously. Thyroid hormone replacement increases myocardial oxygen demand, and thus may be associated with a risk of inducing anginal symptoms, cardiac arrhythmias, and myocardial infarction. These patients should be started on L-T4 at a dose of 25 mcg/day and the dose should be increased by 25 mcg/day every 6 to 8 weeks until serum TSH has normalized.[84] Hypothyroid patients may safely undergo angioplasty or coronary bypass surgery before or soon after L-T4 therapy has been initiated.[85]

Pregnancy

Thyroid hormone requirements increase during pregnancy because of increased T_4 clearance, transfer of maternal T_4 to the fetus, and an estrogen-mediated increase in TBG concentration.[86-89] It is essential for the pregnant woman to be euthyroid throughout her pregnancy, as thyroid hormone is essential for normal fetal growth and intellectual development. The increase in maternal T_4 requirements begins at approximately 8 weeks of gestation, and plateaus by about 16 weeks of gestation.[89] On average, hypothyroid pregnant patients require approximately 40% more L-T4 to maintain normal TSH levels.[90] Some endocrinologists recommend empirically increasing the L-T4 dose by 30% to 40% once pregnancy is confirmed, while others monitor serum TSH levels before adjusting the L-T4 dose.[70] Pregnant women with hypothyroidism should take their prenatal vitamins (which contain iron and calcium carbonate) several hours apart from their L-T4 dose.[91] The dose of L-T4 may be reduced to the prepregnant level immediately after delivery.

Secondary Hypothyroidism

Unlike treatment for primary hypothyroidism, TSH is of no use in assessing adequacy of L-T4 replacement, because of impairment of TSH secretion. Therefore, treatment is monitored by serum T_4 levels, with the goal of therapy being an FT_4 level in the upper half of the normal range.

Surgical Patients

Adverse effects may be encountered in hypothyroid patients who undergo surgery. The most common complications noted are perioperative ileus, hyponatremia, slower wound healing, and greater difficulty in extubating patients. Hypothyroid patients also manifest less fever in response to serious infections, and may have more prolonged effects of anesthesia and opioids than euthyroid patients.[92,93] If possible, then, elective surgical procedures in hypothyroid patients should be postponed until euthyroidism is achieved with L-T4. Urgent surgical procedures may proceed, however, with patients being managed expectantly for postoperative complications. L-T4 therapy may even be administered parenterally if hypothyroidism is severe.

Myxedema Coma

Myxedema coma is an endocrine emergency characterized by severe hypothyroidism, hypothermia, and altered mental status.[94] There is usually a precipitating cause, such as an infection, myocardial infarction, stroke, or cold exposure. The mortality rate of untreated myxedema coma can be as high as 30% to 40%.[95,96] Treatment includes aggressive replacement of thyroid hormone, usually intravenous L-T4, although L-T3 has been advocated as well.[94] Supportive measures are essential to the treatment of myxedema coma and include intravenous fluids, passive rewarming, mechanical ventilation if needed, and empirical broad-spectrum antibiotics until cultures are proven negative. Investigation for the precipitating cause of myxedema coma is crucial to its treatment.[97]

HYPERTHYROIDISM

Introduction

The term *hyperthyroidism* refers to a group of heterogeneous disorders, all of which are characterized by elevations in serum thyroid hormone concentrations, but that are distinguished by their diverse etiologies and clinical presentations. The term *hyperthyroidism* is also often used interchangeably with the term *thyrotoxicosis,* and will be for the purposes of this discussion as well. Graves' disease is the most common thyrotoxic disorder encountered in the United States.[98] It primarily affects women of childbearing age, and has a female:male ratio of approximately 5:1.[98] The overall prevalence of Graves' disease is approximately 0.5%, although the lifetime probability of a woman developing Graves' disease is approximately 2%.[1-3,99] Regardless of etiology, all forms of hyperthyroidism share two common features. These include the catabolic tissue effects of excessive circulating thyroid hormone, and a β-adrenergic–mediated symptom complex that varies in severity according to the degree of hyperthyroidism present. The treatment of hyperthyroidism depends on establishing the cause of the excessive production of thyroid hormone.

Pathophysiology

The etiologies of hyperthyroidism may be classified into two major groups: those that increase thyroidal radioiodine uptake, and those in which iodine uptake is decreased (Box 38-5). Causes of hyperthyroidism that have a high radioiodine uptake include Graves' disease, toxic thyroid nodules (either solitary or multiple), the hyperthyroid phase of chronic autoimmune disease ("hashitoxicosis"), and rarely, TSH-producing pituitary tumors and choriocarcinomas.

The causes of hyperthyroidism with low radioiodine uptake include excess thyroid hormone ingestion; various forms of inflammatory diseases that destroy thyroid tissue, including subacute granulomatous thyroiditis, painless lymphocytic thyroiditis, and thyroiditis due to therapeutic cytokines (interferon alfa, interleukin-2); the antiarrhythmic amiodarone; and, rarely, lithium carbonate. In addition, rare causes of low thyroidal radioiodine uptake hyperthyroidism include struma ovarii and metastatic functioning follicular thyroid cancer.[100]

Graves' disease is the most common cause of hyperthyroidism, accounting for approximately 70% to 75% of patients with thyrotoxicosis.[4] Graves' disease is an autoimmune condition, and the resultant thyrotoxicosis is mediated via the stimulation of the thyroid gland by TSH receptor antibodies. TSH receptor antibodies are secreted by B lymphocytes that have been stimulated by helper T lymphocytes.[101,102] T cells are activated via thyroid autoantigen presentation by human leukocyte antigen (HLA) class II expression on thyroid cells. HLA class II expression, as part of the major histocompatibility complex (MHC) class II molecules, has been demonstrated on thyroid cells in patients with Graves' disease, but not on thyroid cells from normal individuals.[103] The presence of MHC class II molecules on thyroid cells allows for continued activation of thyroid-specific autoreactive T cells, and thus furthers the development of autoimmune disease.[104]

BOX 38-5 ETIOLOGIES OF HYPERTHYROIDISM

Hyperthyroidism with Elevated RAIU*
- Graves' disease
- Toxic multinodular goiter
- Toxic adenoma
- TSH-secreting pituitary tumor
- Hydatidiform mole
- Choriocarcinoma
- Pituitary resistance to thyroid hormone

Hyperthyroidism with Low RAIU*
- Factitious
- Subacute granulomatous thyroiditis
- Subacute lymphocytic thyroiditis
  - Postpartum
  - Sporadic
- Drug-induced thyroiditis
  - Amiodarone
  - Interleukin-2†
  - Interferon alfa†
  - Iodine-induced hyperthyroidism
  - Radiation-induced thyroiditis
  - Metastatic functioning follicular tumor
  - Struma ovarii

*In probable decreasing order of frequency.
†Immune-modulating agents.
RAIU, radioactive iodine uptake; TSH, thyroid-stimulating hormone.
Adapted from Bruman KD. Hypothyroidism. *In* Rakel RE, Bope ET (eds): Conn's Current Therapy. Philadelphia: Elsevier Saunders, 2006, pp 806-811.

Clinical and Metabolic Features

All causes of hyperthyroidism share two common features: the catabolic tissue effects of excessive circulating thyroid hormone and the β-adrenergic–mediated symptom complex. The signs and symptoms of hyperthyroidism, as well as its metabolic effects, vary according to both the severity and the duration of the disorder (Box 38-6). Typical symptoms include nervousness, heat intolerance, irritability, palpitations, and increases in bowel motility, with increases in frequency of bowel movements. Common physical finding include an enlarged thyroid, tachycardia, and weight loss (Figs. 38-6 and 38-7). Many of these symptoms are β-adrenergic mediated, in particular, the symptoms of nervousness, tachycardia, palpitations, and impaired sleep habits. Other symptoms, such as increases in appetite, weight loss, muscle weakness, and fatigue, are the results of the catabolic effects of thyrotoxicosis. Excessive thyroid hormone adversely affects all tissues.

Cardiovascular

The most common cardiovascular symptoms of hyperthyroidism include tachycardia, palpitations, and dyspnea on exertion. Frequent physical findings include systolic hypertension and a widening of the pulse pressure. The hyperthyroid state results in an increase in cardiac output, an increase in cardiac contractility, and a decrease in peripheral resistance. Because of an increase in metabolic demand, the heart may not be able to withstand the increases in oxygen demand. A reversible cardiomyopathy, or even congestive heart failure, may ensue due to the increases in metabolic requirements.[105]

Atrial fibrillation may occur in 10% to 20% of individuals with hyperthyroidism, and is more commonly seen in elderly individuals, especially in older men. While most patients revert to normal sinus rhythm once euthyroidism is achieved, anticoagulation for atrial fibrillation is indicated, especially if atrial enlargement is present.[21,84,106,107]

Respiratory

The shortness of breath commonly seen in thyrotoxicosis occurs more with exertion than at rest. The etiology of this dyspnea on exertion is not clearly understood, and is probably multifactorial. Possible explanations include respiratory muscle weakness (as part of the generalized muscle weakness experienced by some thyrotoxic patients), high-output heart failure, increases in ventilatory drive, increases in airway resistance, and decreases in lung compliance.[108] In the case of significant obstructive thyromegaly, tracheal compression may also be seen. Thyrotoxicosis increases oxygen consumption and carbon dioxide production. This leads to increases in minute ventilation and tachypnea.[108] A thyrotoxic individual with normal lung function should be able to tolerate these metabolic demands, but patients with underlying

BOX 38-6 SYMPTOMS AND SIGNS OF HYPERTHYROIDISM

Common Symptoms
- Nervousness
- Palpitations
- Easy fatigability
- Insomnia
- Heat intolerance
- Excessive perspiration
- Weight loss
- Hyperdefecation

Common Signs
- Thyroid enlargement (goiter)
- Infiltrative eye signs (in Graves' disease)
- Tachycardia
- Fine tremor
- Smooth, moist skin
- Hyperkinesis
- Brisk deep tendon reflexes

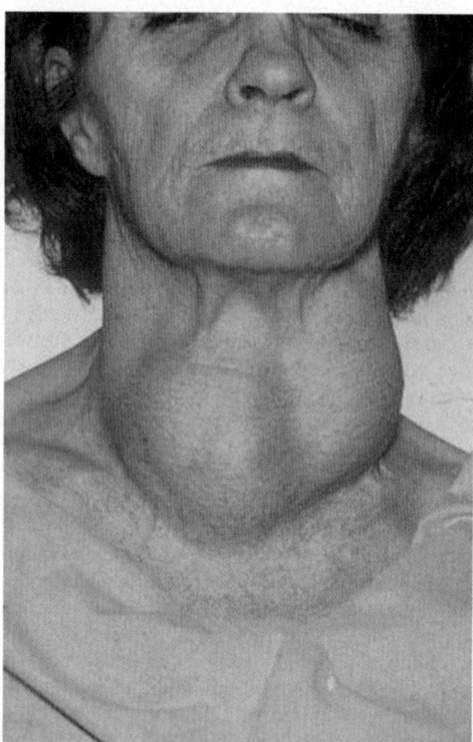

FIGURE 38-6 • Patient with huge toxic multinodular goiter. (From Singer PA. Thyroid dysfunction of the elderly. In Korenman SG [ed]: Atlas of Clinical Endocrinology. Philadelphia: Blackwell Science, 1999, pp 147-159.)

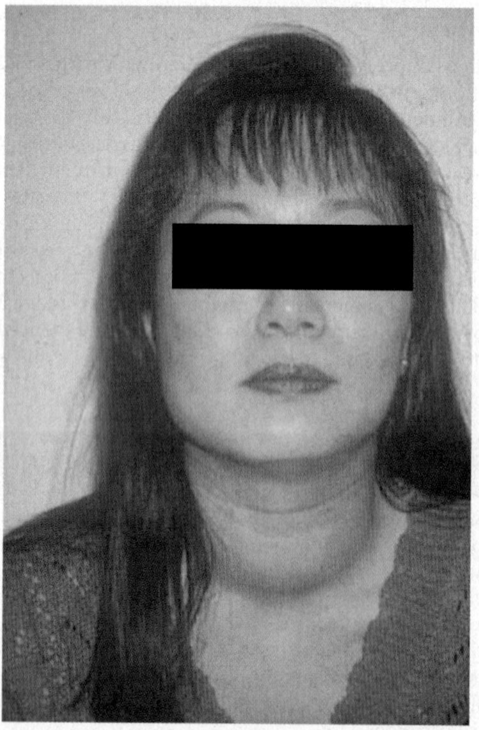

FIGURE 38-7 • Patient with Graves' disease and diffuse goiter.

pulmonary pathology may not be able to compensate, and thus might experience decreases in exercise tolerance and dyspnea with exertion, and possibly at rest.[109,110]

Gastrointestinal

Calorigenesis increases in hyperthyroidism, and in an effort to mitigate tissue breakdown, appetite increases. Despite this increase in food intake, however, weight loss is usual. This is contributed to by increases in gut motility, hyperdefecation, and malabsorption. Celiac disease has a higher prevalence in individuals with hyperthyroidism than in the general population, and this may exacerbate the malabsorption already seen in hyperthyroidism.[111] Anorexia and significant weight loss may also be seen in the elderly population.[112]

Hematologic

The plasma volume increases in hyperthyroidism, resulting in a dilutional normochromic, normocytic anemia even though the red blood cell mass also increases. Graves' disease may be associated with other autoimmune conditions, such as pernicious anemia, which occurs in 1% to 3% of patients with thyrotoxicosis.[32,113-115] Other hematologic conditions occasionally seen in thyrotoxicosis include idiopathic thrombocytopenic purpura and granulocytopenia. Although the cause of the granulocytopenia is unknown, antineutrophil antibodies have been detected in up to 50% of patients with Graves' disease.[116] The level of contribution of these antibodies to the observed granulocytopenia is uncertain.[116]

Neuromuscular

Nervousness, anxiety, emotional lability, and difficulty sleeping are common symptoms seen with hyperthyroidism.[117] Hyperthyroidism is associated with a generalized increase in neuromuscular activity, hyperkinesis, tremor, and brisk deep tendon reflexes.[117,118] Proximal muscle weakness, particularly of the shoulder girdle, hip flexors, and thigh muscles, is commonly seen in hyperthyroidism, as is a generalized decrease in lean muscle mass.[118-120] Myasthenia gravis may be seen in 3% to 10% of patients with Graves' disease.[117,121] Hypokalemic thyrotoxic periodic paralysis may occur with thyrotoxicosis, and it has a predilection for Asian men. These bouts of paralysis are typically provoked by high-carbohydrate meals and/or excessive alcohol intake.[122]

Skeletal

Bone reabsorption increases with hyperthyroidism. Cortical bone is lost to a greater degree than is trabecular bone.[123] With severe and long-standing hyperthyroidism, markers of bone turnover, such as serum alkaline phosphatase and osteocalcin, may increase. Rarely, serum calcium concentrations may increase.[123]

Renal

Thyrotoxicosis increases heart rate and cardiac output, decreases peripheral resistance, and increases blood flow to all organs, including the kidneys. Glomerular filtration rate thus increases.[124] In addition, renal tubular transport of sodium increases due to increased ATPase activity.[124] Occasional patients with thyrotoxicosis experience both polyuria and polydipsia. In thyrotoxic patients, the thirst response is initiated at a lower serum osmolality than in the euthyroid patient.[125] This increase in thirst response leads to polydipsia, which results in polyuria. The thirst response returns to normal after successful treatment of thyrotoxicosis, with the subsequent resolution of both the polydipsia and polyuria.[124,125]

Reproductive

Increases in sex hormone–binding globulin levels are seen in both men and women with hyperthyroidism. This leads to increases in total sex hormones, but may not alter the concentration of free sex hormones.[126] In women, decreases in luteinizing hormone concentrations lead to reduced midcycle luteinizing hormone surges, which may then result in oligomenorrhea, if not frank amenorrhea, with resultant difficulty with fertility.[126,127]

Dermatologic

In hyperthyroidism, the skin is warm due to increases in blood flow, and is also smooth, due to decreases in the keratin layer.[43] Sweating increases due to the increased β-adrenergic state, and is usually accompanied by the complaint of heat intolerance. Notable signs include onycholysis and softening of the nails, and thinning of the hair. Other cutaneous manifestations include vitiligo, alopecia areata (rare), and infiltrative dermopathy (pretibial myxedema).[43]

Ocular

Stare and lid lag may be present, regardless of the cause of hyperthyroidism, due to stimulation of β-adrenergic receptors on the levator palpebrae muscles, but among thyrotoxic disorders, infiltrative ophthalmopathy is seen only in patients with Graves' disease.[128] Graves' ophthalmopathy may result in exophthalmos, secondary to the lymphocytic infiltration of extraocular muscles and retro-orbital fat.[129]

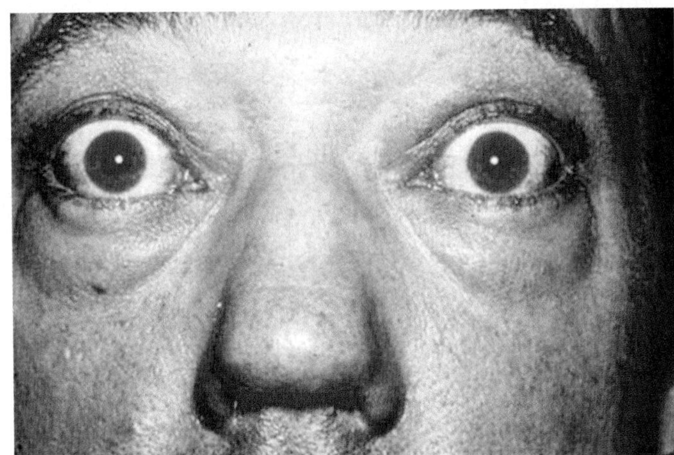

FIGURE 38-8 • Ocular findings in an adult with Graves' disease. Note the stare, proptosis, and infraorbital edema.

Restriction of extraocular movements causes diplopia, and is the result of fibrosis of the ocular muscles.[128] Commonly noted ocular symptoms in addition to diplopia include grittiness, eye irritation, and photophobia. Periorbital edema and injected conjunctivae may also be noted in Graves' ophthalmopathy (Fig. 38-8). Corneal ulceration may occur as a result of proptosis with lid retraction and corneal exposure, and severe proptosis may cause optic neuropathy and even blindness.[129-131]

Metabolic Abnormalities

Thyroid hormone antagonizes the peripheral actions of insulin, thus leading to increases in insulin resistance and impairments in glucose tolerance. Thus, hyperglycemia may be seen in hyperthyroidism, despite β-receptor–mediated stimulation of insulin secretion.[132] Diabetic individuals who become hyperthyroid may have worsening glycemic control until euthyroidism is reestablished.[133]

Laboratory Diagnosis

The diagnosis of hyperthyroidism is established by confirmation of elevated serum T_4 and/or T_3 levels, and a suppressed serum TSH concentration. Once the diagnosis of hyperthyroidism has been made, a radioiodine uptake and scan may be performed to help determine the etiology. If the radioiodine uptake is elevated and a diffuse goiter is present, the diagnosis is Graves' disease. Antiperoxidase antibodies may be obtained, as they are found to be positive in approximately 80% of patients with Graves' disease.[134] Some specialists, especially in countries other than the United Sates, also obtain levels of thyroid-stimulating immunoglobulins (TSIs, or TSH receptor antibodies) in order to confirm the diagnosis of Graves' disease. It is not recommended to routinely check these antibodies, unless the diagnosis of Graves' disease is in doubt[135] (Fig. 38-9).

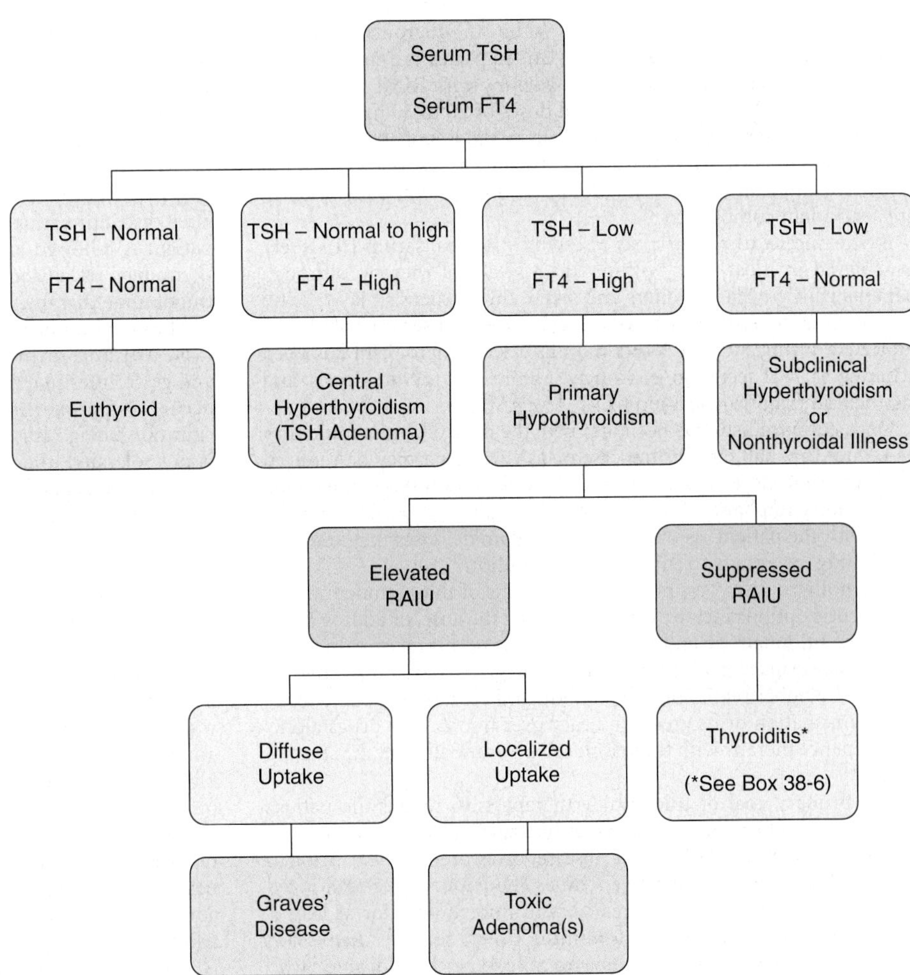

FIGURE 38-9 • Schema for the evaluation of suspected hyperthyroidism.

Therapeutics and Clinical Pharmacology

The treatment of hyperthyroidism is directed toward the relief of symptoms, the reduction of thyroid hormone concentrations, and in certain circumstances—specifically Graves' disease and toxic nodular goiter—the specific cause of thyrotoxicosis. Since Graves' disease is the most common thyrotoxic disorder, most of the following discussion of the treatment of hyperthyroidism pertains to this condition.

β-Adrenergic Blockade

β-Adrenergic blocking agents quickly ameliorate the hyperadrenergic symptoms of hyperthyroidism, including tremulousness, nervousness, anxiety, tachycardia, palpitations, and heat intolerance. Propranolol is a nonselective β-blocker, and is frequently used in the treatment of hyperthyroidism. The typical starting dose of propranolol ranges between 20 and 40 mg every 6 hours, with the goal of therapy being the resolution of hyperadrenergic symptoms and a heart rate of about 80 beats per minute. Propranolol must be given every 6 hours due to its very short half-life. This fact actually makes propranolol the preferred β-blocker for the amelioration of thyrotoxic symptoms, since patients may learn to titrate their own medication, depending on their symptoms. As patients improve during the course of their definitive therapy of hyperthyroidism, they may be able to omit more doses of propranolol. Other longer acting β-blockers, such as atenolol, nadolol, and metoprolol, may also be employed. Atenolol offers the additional convenience of once-daily dosing, and may be started at 50 to 100 mg daily. These long-acting β-blockers are cardioselective, and so are not contraindicated in individuals with asthma, as is propranolol.[136-138]

Thionamides

Thionamide drugs normalize thyroid hormone levels pharmacologically. These medications inhibit the synthesis of thyroid hormone by blocking the organification of iodine within the thyroid.[138] The two thionamides available for use in the United States are methimazole (MMI), and propylthiouracil (PTU). Therapy with MMI is generally given two to three times daily, in total doses of 20 to 30 mg/day. PTU is usually given three to four times daily in total doses of 300 to 400 mg/day. MMI is often preferred over PTU because of its longer duration of action, thus allowing for less frequent dosing and, consequently, greater patient compliance.[139]

Biochemical euthyroidism, as assessed by normal serum FT_4 levels, is achieved in most cases within 6 to 8 weeks of therapy, although patients with very large goiters and severe thyrotoxicosis may take up to 3 months to become euthyroid. Measurement of serum TSH is not indicated during the first 3 to 4 months after euthyroidism has been achieved as TSH secretion is strongly inhibited by thyrotoxicosis, and lags behind the normalization of FT_4 levels.[138]

Once euthyroidism has been attained, the dose of thionamide may be reduced by half, and in the case of MMI, dosing may be reduced from multiple doses a day to once-daily dosing, further enhancing medication compliance. Compliance with medication must be emphasized with the patient, as omission of thionamide doses may result in continuing, or even worsening, hyperthyroidism.[138]

If hypothyroidism occurs during the course of thionamide therapy, therapeutic options include further reducing the dose, or adding L-T4. Combined thionamide and L-T4 therapy has been preferred by some thyroid specialists, and some studies suggested that this therapy resulted in higher remission rates, although there has not been consistent confirmation of its greater efficacy over thionamide drugs alone. Maintenance therapy with thionamide drugs is usually half the starting dose.[140,141]

The primary goal of thionamide therapy is to render the patient euthyroid. This form of treatment may be used in an attempt to achieve a long-term remission of Graves' disease, or as pretreatment prior to ablative therapy with radioactive iodine. The frequency of prolonged remission in Graves' patients treated with thionamides for at least 1 year is approximately 20% to 30% in the United States.[142] Remission rates tend to be higher in patients with mild hyperthyroidism or who have a small goiter, in those older than 40 years of age, and in those with a negative family history of Graves' disease.[143,144] Rapid correction of thyrotoxicosis and shrinkage of the thyroid gland with thionamide therapy are also favorable indicators of a long-term remission. Patients with continued suppression of serum TSH after 6 months of therapy with thionamides are unlikely to go into remission, and a decision about the wisdom of continued therapy with thionamides should be made.[143-145]

After completion of a course of treatment with either MMI or PTU, the drug is discontinued, and the patient is followed for signs of recurrent hyperthyroidism. Patients are typically monitored about 6 weeks after discontinuation of therapy, and if biochemically euthyroid, the patient is followed at increasingly longer intervals. Recurrent hyperthyroidism usually occurs within the first year after discontinuation of thionamide therapy.[145]

Thionamides have several potential side effects, including pruritis, rash, urticaria, arthralgias, arthritis, fever, abnormal taste sensation, and gastrointestinal discomfort. One or more of these side effects may occur in approximately 10% of patients on thionamides, the most common being rash and arthralgias[146] (Box 38-7). If one thionamide is not tolerated, then another may be substituted, but up to 50% of patients will experience cross-sensitivity.[138] Most side effects, although bothersome, are not particularly serious. More serious and potentially life-threatening adverse reactions due to thionamides include agranulocytosis and hepatotoxicity.[138]

Agranulocytosis is a rare, but potentially fatal complication of thionamide therapy, occurring in 0.2% to 0.5% of patients.[147] This side effect is more commonly seen in the elderly population, and in individuals taking higher doses of thionamides.[148] Presenting symptoms include fever and signs of infection, especially a sore throat. Patients with these complaints should be instructed to discontinue their thionamide immediately, and contact their treating physician so that a white blood cell count with a differential count may be obtained. Spontaneous recovery of the white blood cell count occurs within several days after discontinuation of the thionamide. In addition to prompt discontinuation of the thionamide, these patients should be hospitalized with neutropenic precautions, and broad-spectrum antibiotics should be administered. Granulocyte colony-stimulating factor has been used as adjunctive therapy in severe cases of agranulocytosis, but its efficacy is uncertain.[149,150] Usually agranulocytosis develops so suddenly that

BOX 38-7 SIDE EFFECTS OF THIONAMIDE DRUGS

Most Common (1% to 5%)
- Pruritis
- Arthralgias
- Fever

Uncommon (<1%)
- Gastrointestinal complaints
- Abnormalities of taste and smell
- Arthritis

Rare (<0.5%)
- Agranulocytosis
- Aplastic anemia
- Thrombocytopenia
- Hepatic dysfunction
  - Toxic hepatitis with PTU
  - Cholestatic hepatitis with MMI
- Vasculitis
- Systemic lupus–like syndrome
- Hypoprothrombinemia with PTU
- Hypoglycemia (due to anti-insulin antibodies) with MMI

MMI, methimazole; PTU, propylthiouracil.
Adapted from Cooper DS. Treatment of thyrotoxicosis. *In* Braverman LE, Utiger RD (eds): Werner & Ingbar's The Thyroid: A Fundamental and Clinical Text, 9th ed. Philadelphia: Lippincott Williams & Wilkins, 2005, p 671.

routine monitoring of the leukocyte count during thionamide therapy is thought to be of little value.[151]

Hepatotoxicity is a rare but serious complication of thionamide therapy. Liver transaminases increase slightly in up to one third of patients taking PTU, but these changes are not typically predictive of hepatotoxicity.[152] Baseline liver function tests are not predictive of this change, as they are usually mildly elevated in hyperthyroid patients. The elevations in liver transaminases typically resolve with discontinuation of PTU.[152] Rarely, PTU has been associated with fulminant hepatic necrosis.[152,153] MMI has been associated infrequently with cholestatic jaundice.[154] Patients should be warned of these possible adverse reactions, and should be counseled to discontinue their thionamide drug and inform their physician if they develop malaise, jaundice, or dark urine.[153,154]

Antineutrophil cytoplasmic antibody–positive vasculitis has been reported in association with thionamides, especially PTU.[155,156] Another rare but serious complication associated with thionamide use is the development of a lupus-like syndrome, which is characterized by typical skin involvement, glomerulonephritis, and arthralgias seen with lupus.[155,156]

Radioactive Iodine Therapy

Radioactive iodine therapy, in the form of sodium ^{131}I, is widely used in the treatment of Graves' hyperthyroidism and is the preferred treatment for Graves' disease among physicians in the United States. This is in sharp contrast to thyroid experts in both Europe and Japan, where the majority of physicians favor thionamide drugs as the primary form of therapy.[157] After oral administration, ^{131}I is rapidly concentrated in the thyroid gland, but its maximum effect may take up to 3 months. The goal of radioactive iodine therapy is complete ablation of the thyroid gland, since remission cannot be achieved with its use.

Prior to radioactive iodine administration, patients may be rendered biochemically euthyroid with thionamides. In these cases, the thionamide is discontinued 3 to 5 days prior to radioiodine administration, although some physicians prefer to administer radioactive iodine without thionamide pretreatment.[139]

Radioactive iodine is contraindicated during pregnancy, and women of childbearing age must have a negative pregnancy test before its administration. In women inadvertently given radioactive iodine after the first trimester, after the fetal thyroid has developed, fetal hypothyroidism may occur.[158] Radioiodine treatment is effective and predictable and appears to be free of side effects other than the predicted development of hypothyroidism.

Careful follow-up, after more than 50 years of radioiodine use, has failed to demonstrate a statistically increased rate of malignancy in treated individuals, or of genetic defects in offspring of ^{131}I-treated patients. Of note, however, one recent study involving over 7000 radioiodine-treated patients revealed a slight increase in small bowel cancers, but an overall decrease in cancer incidence.[138,159,160]

The goal of radioactive iodine therapy is thyroid ablation. After radioactive iodine administration, patients should be evaluated clinically and biochemically at 4- to 6-week intervals, and when hypothyroidism develops, L-T4 therapy is initiated. Patients who continue to be thyrotoxic 6 months after ^{131}I will require additional therapy with radioactive iodine. Up to 10% of patients may fail their first dose of radioactive iodine treatment, and thus require additional doses. Such patients typically have severe hypothyroidism, or very large goiters.[161]

Of note, patients who receive radioactive iodine will emit radiation for some time after dosing. If they intend to travel or pass through security checkpoints during this time, they may be identified by law enforcement personnel as emitting radiation. These patients should be forewarned of this possibility, and should be provided with a letter from their treating physician documenting that they have recently ingested therapeutic radioactive iodine.[162]

Surgery

Surgery is infrequently employed in the treatment of hyperthyroidism in the United States and is generally reserved for patients with very large goiters (especially if obstructive symptoms are present), pregnant patients, children and teenagers, and those individuals who refuse radioiodine therapy, are allergic to thionamides, or are unable to comply with their medication. Patients with a coexisting thyroid nodule that is worrisome for malignancy may also elect to proceed with surgery.[163,164]

Prior to surgery, the patient should preferably be rendered euthyroid via the use of thionamide drugs. Exogenous iodides, in the form of saturated solution of potassium iodide (SSKI), 5 drops a day in water, are also administered for 10 days prior to surgery in order to decrease the vascularity of the thyroid gland.[165]

Subtotal thyroidectomy is the preferred operation, and is rapidly curative of hyperthyroidism. Postoperative hypothyroidism is usual, and L-T4 replacement is required. Hyperthyroidism may recur due to regrowth of tissue, however, if insufficient thyroid tissue was removed. Surgery is not without its associated risks; injury to the recurrent laryngeal nerve and permanent hypoparathyroidism may occur in 1% to 3% of all cases.[166,167]

Toxic Nodular Goiter

Toxic adenomas and toxic multinodular goiters are second in prevalence to Graves' disease, with toxic multinodular goiter more common than toxic adenoma.[168] The typical presentation of an individual with a toxic adenoma is that of a hyperthyroid patient with a single, palpable nodule, usually greater than 3 centimeters in size, that on thyroid scanning demonstrates focal increased uptake of radioactive iodine, with suppression of radioiodine uptake in the remainder of the thyroid. An individual with a toxic multinodular goiter will have a radioiodine uptake that reveals multiple focal areas of increased uptake. Toxic multinodular goiter is more frequently seen in older individuals from iodine-deficient areas of the world; in the United States, it is most often encountered in individuals who emigrated from areas of iodine deficiency.[168,169]

Treatment of hyperthyroidism due to toxic nodular goiter is similar to the treatment of Graves' disease in that a dual approach is required to both relieve β-adrenergic–mediated symptoms via β blockade, and to reduce thyroid hormone production with the use of thionamide drugs. In contrast to Graves' disease, however, toxic adenomas and toxic multinodular goiter do not remit with prolonged thionamide therapy. Thionamides are therefore only used to achieve euthyroidism in preparation for radioiodine ablation or surgery.[170]

Radioiodine is the preferred treatment method for older individuals with toxic nodular goiter, and in contrast to Graves' disease, euthyroidism is usual due to the fact that the radioiodine preferentially accumulates in the hyperfunctioning nodules and spares the remaining thyroid tissue. Approximately 10% to 20% of patients with toxic nodular goiter may fail to become euthyroid after one dose of radioiodine, usually if the uptake of radioiodine is relatively low.[171]

Subtotal thyroidectomy is indicated for patients with very large goiters with obstructive symptoms. It is also preferred for individuals younger than 40 years of age with a solitary toxic adenoma. In such patients, hemithyroidectomy would be the treatment option of choice.[172]

Special Therapeutic Circumstances

Subclinical Hyperthyroidism

Subclinical hyperthyroidism is characterized by low serum TSH concentrations and normal serum T_4 and T_3 concentrations. Since patients do not manifest typical signs and symptoms of hyperthyroidism, the diagnosis is usually made during routine screening of thyroid function. The most common causes of subclinical hyperthyroidism in the United States include overzealous thyroid hormone replacement for individuals with hypothyroidism, and the treatment of patients in whom TSH suppression is the goal, such as patients with differentiated thyroid cancer. Subclinical hyperthyroidism may also be seen in individuals with other thyroid disorders[173] (Box 38-8).

The skeleton and the cardiovascular system are the major organ systems adversely affected by subclinical hyperthyroidism. Thyroid

BOX 38-8 ETIOLOGIES OF SUBCLINICAL HYPERTHYROIDISM

- Overzealous thyroid hormone replacement therapy
- Thyroid hormone suppressive therapy (treatment of thyroid cancer)
- Autonomously functioning thyroid adenoma(s)
- Concurrent treatment for Graves' disease
  - Remission after thionamide therapy
- After treatment of thyrotoxicosis, before recovery of the hypothalamic-pituitary-thyroidal axis
- After radioiodine ablative therapy
- Severe nonthyroidal illness

Adapted from Ross DS. Subclinical thyrotoxicosis. *In* Braverman LE, Utiger RD (eds): Werner & Ingbar's The Thyroid: A Fundamental and Clinical Text, 9th ed. Philadelphia: Lippincott Williams & Wilkins, 2005, p 1080.

hormone has a direct resorptive effect on bone, and overt thyrotoxicosis is known to be associated with increased bone resorption and increases in fracture rate.[123,174] Studies have shown that reductions in bone mineral density, primarily at cortical bone sites, occur in postmenopausal women with subclinical hyperthyroidism.[175-179] Data regarding fracture risk for patients with subclinical hyperthyroidism (including postmenopausal women), however, are still inconclusive.[180]

The frequency of atrial fibrillation is increased in thyrotoxic individuals, and studies have demonstrated that there is a threefold increased risk of developing atrial fibrillation among individuals with subclinical hyperthyroidism who are 60 years of age or older and who have a low serum TSH (≤0.1 mU/L).[181] Atrial fibrillation in older patients is associated with increased cardiovascular and cerebrovascular mortality, primarily due to thromboembolic events.[182-184] In addition, other effects on cardiac function due to subclinical hyperthyroidism include increases in heart rate and premature atrial beats, increases in cardiac contractility, reduced exercise tolerance, aggravation of anginal symptoms, and congestive heart failure.[181-186]

Thus, since subclinical hyperthyroidism appears to have adverse effects on both the cardiovascular and skeletal systems in older individuals, it should be avoided where possible. Careful attention should be paid to dosing with L-T4, and when subclinical hyperthyroidism is endogenous, it should be treated appropriately.[181-187]

Pregnancy

Hyperthyroidism during pregnancy presents several potential complications for both the mother and fetus. Maternal risk factors include increased rates of spontaneous abortion, premature labor, preeclampsia, and heart failure. Fetal aspects of hyperthyroidism include fetal goiter, growth retardation, increased rates of stillbirth, and low birth weight. Any form of hyperthyroidism may complicate pregnancy, but Graves' disease is the most common cause.[188]

Treatment options for pregnant hyperthyroid women include symptomatic treatment with β-adrenergic blocking agents, thionamides, and surgery. Radioiodine is contraindicated during pregnancy. β-Blockers may be given to pregnant women for the first few weeks of treatment in order to ameliorate the symptoms of hyperthyroidism.[188] Their use should be minimized during pregnancy, however, so as to lessen the potential fetal risks of neonatal growth restriction, hypoglycemia, respiratory depression, and bradycardia.[189]

Thionamides are used to treat hyperthyroidism during pregnancy. PTU is usually preferred over MMI, primarily due to very rare fetal malformations attributed to MMI use, namely aplasia cutis, tracheo-esophageal fistulas, and choanal atresia.[190,191] The goal of thionamide therapy is to give the lowest dose needed to maintain maternal thyroid hormone levels in the upper half of the normal range. This will minimize fetal exposure to thionamides, thereby reducing the potential for fetal goiter and fetal hypothyroidism. Hyperthyroid pregnant patients should be examined at least every 4 to 6 weeks with assessment of maternal thyroid status. Fetal thyroid status may be monitored by the obstetrician by checking fetal heart rate and by serial ultrasonography to assess fetal growth. Thyroidectomy during pregnancy may be necessary for women who are intolerant of or allergic to thionamides. Surgery should be performed in the second trimester, as surgery during the first trimester carries an increased risk of spontaneous abortion, and surgery in the third trimester carries an increased risk of preterm labor.[188,192-194]

Both PTU and MMI are secreted in human breast milk, but only in small concentrations, especially if the maternal doses of thionamides are minimized (<20 mg/day MMI, or <150 mg/day PTU).[195,196] The total daily dose of thionamides may be given in divided doses during the day, following breast-feedings.[196] This way, the risk to nursing infants of developing hypothyroidism from mothers taking thionamides is practically negligible.[195,196]

Neonatal hyperthyroidism is a potential complication of hyperthyroid pregnancies. Neonatal hyperthyroidism is considered to be uncommon, occurring in approximately 1% of pregnancies in patients with Graves' disease in North America.[197] The risk of neonatal hyperthyroidism is highest in women with poorly controlled thyrotoxicosis, and in women with very elevated TSH receptor antibody titers.[197] Fetal hyperthyroidism is caused by the transfer of maternal TSIs to the fetus.[188] When present in high concentrations in the mother, they may cross the placental barrier, stimulate the fetal thyroid, and cause fetal and neonatal hyperthyroidism. When the pregnant woman receives thionamides, the thionamide crosses the placenta, and so protects the fetus against fetal hyperthyroidism. After delivery, maternal TSI antibodies may temporarily persist, but the benefit of antithyroid medications (via placental passage) is lost. Thus, neonatal hyperthyroidism may develop within a few days after birth.[188] Signs of neonatal hyperthyroidism include congestive heart failure, goiter, proptosis, jaundice, hyperirritability, failure to thrive, and tachycardia. The diagnosis is confirmed by suppressed neonatal TSH concentrations and elevated FT_4 concentrations. Neonatal hyperthyroidism is usually transient, and so medical therapy (which may include β blockade and/or thionamides) is supportive.[188]

Apathetic Hyperthyroidism

Hyperthyroidism in the geriatric population may not present with the classical clinical features (large goiter, typical eye findings) of Graves' hyperthyroidism (Fig. 38-10). These individuals may instead present with fatigue, apathy, anorexia, and weight loss, often out of proportion to the degree of thyrotoxicosis. Indeed, some patients may even be initially evaluated for a suspected malignancy due to the degree of unintentional weight loss, weakness, and a paucity of overt signs of hyperthyroidism. Supraventricular tachycardias are commonly seen, and atrial fibrillation may be a presenting sign of hyperthyroidism in apathetic hyperthyroidism. Patients with apathetic hyperthyroidism should be treated with radioactive iodine, following pretreatment with thionamide therapy to reduce the risk of exacerbation of thyrotoxicosis after radioactive iodine is administered.[181-186,198] The goal of ablative therapy is to quickly resolve thyrotoxicosis, and to minimize the chance for recurrence.[49]

Thyroid Storm

Thyroid storm (also known as thyrotoxic crisis) is a severe and potentially life-threatening form of thyrotoxicosis characterized by exaggerated manifestations of hyperthyroidism, fever, and altered mental status.[199] Often a precipitating event such as an infection, trauma, or surgery causes this decompensation in individuals with long-standing, poorly controlled hyperthyroidism. Prompt recognition and appropriate treatment of this condition are essential to minimizing morbidity and mortality.[199]

The treatment of the thyrotoxicosis associated with thyroid storm (Table 38-1) involves the use of β-blockers and thionamides, but these medications are given in higher doses than in typical Graves' disease.[200] In addition to thionamide drugs, exogenous iodides such as SSKI should be administered. Exogenous iodides acutely inhibit thyroid hormone release from the thyroid gland, and serve as a potent inhibi-

TABLE 38-1 TREATMENT OF THYROID STORM

Drug	Typical Adult Dose	Action
ANTITHYROID AGENTS		
Propylthiouracil (also called PTU)	1200-1500 mg/day, given in 200- to 250-mg increments PO or via gastric tube	Prevents production of more T_4 and T_3 in the thyroid, and blocks conversion of T_4 to T_3 outside the thyroid
Methimazole (Tapazole)	120 mg given in 20-mg increments PO or via gastric tube	Prevents production of more thyroid hormone
IODIDES		
Lugol's solution Saturated solution of potassium iodide (Pima, SSKI)	10 drops twice a day PO or via gastric tube 8 drops every 6 hr PO or via gastric tube	Block release of stored thyroid hormone from thyroid gland
GLUCOCORTICOIDS		
Dexamethasone (Decadron) Hydrocortisone	2 mg every 6 hr, PO or IV 100 mg every 8 hr	Block conversion of T_4 to T_3
β-BLOCKERS		
Propranolol (Inderal) Esmolol (Brevibloc Injection)	1 mg/min IV as required, then 60-80 mg every 4 hr PO or via gastric tube 500 mcg/kg/min for 1 min, then 50-100 mcg/kg/min for 4 min	Reduce symptoms (tachycardia, tremor, restlessness) caused by heightened response to catecholamines; block conversion of T_4 to T_3

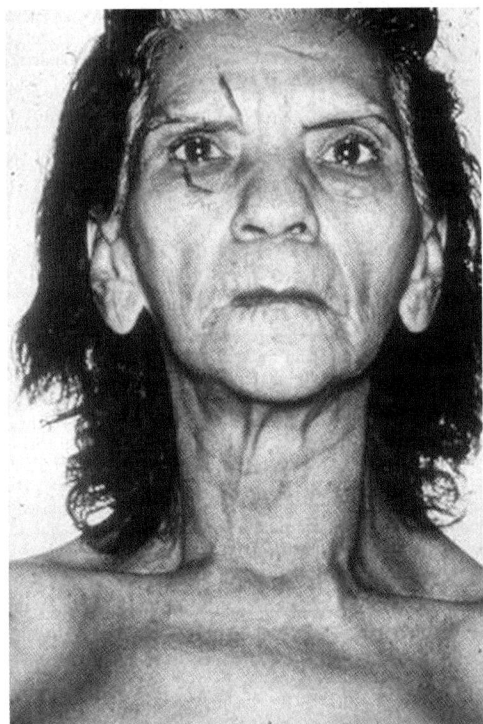

FIGURE 38-10 • **Patient with apathetic hyperthyroidism.** Note the absence of a visible goiter, or the eye findings commonly seen with Graves' disease. (From Singer PA. Thyroid dysfunction of the elderly. In Korenman SG [ed]: Atlas of Clinical Endocrinology. Philadelphia: Blackwell Science, 1999, pp 147-159.)

tor of peripheral T_4-to-T_3 conversion.[11,12,201] SSKI may be administered as 10 drops in water three times daily, or sodium iodide, 500 mg intravenously, may be administered if the patient is unable to take oral medications. Iodides should be administered at least 1 hour after the first dose of a thionamide has been administered, so that the iodine will not serve as a substrate for further thyroid hormone synthesis. Some clinicians also use pharmacologic doses of glucocorticoids in an attempt to further reduce peripheral T_4-to-T_3 conversion (although their clinical efficacy has not been reliably demonstrated).[200]

In addition to these specific treatments directed toward restoring a euthyroid state, supportive measures are essential in the management of thyroid storm. These patients should be managed in the intensive care unit, with careful attention to identification and management of the precipitating or intercurrent illness. Acetaminophen is preferred over aspirin for treating fever, as aspirin may increase FT_4 and T_3 concentrations by interfering with their protein binding to albumin.[200]

REFERENCES

1. Hollowell JG, Staehling NW, Flanders W, et al. Serum TSH, T_4, and thyroid antibodies in the United States population (1988 to 1994): National Health and Nutrition Examination Survey (NHANES III). J Clin Endocrinol Metab 2002;87:489-499.
2. Vanderpump MP. The epidemiology of thyroid diseases. *In* Braverman LE, Utiger RD (eds): Werner & Ingbar's The Thyroid: A Fundamental and Clinical Text, 9th ed. Philadelphia: Lippincott Williams & Wilkins, 2005, pp 398-406.
3. Canaris GJ, Manowitz NR, Mayor G, et al. The Colorado Thyroid Disease Prevalence Study. Arch Intern Med 2000;160:526-534.
4. Vanderpump MP, Tunbridge WM, French JM, et al. The incidence of thyroid disorders in the community: a twenty-year follow up of the Whickham survey. Clin Endocrinol (Oxf) 1995;43:55-68.
5. Braverman L, Utiger R. Introduction to hypothyroidism. *In* Braverman LE, Utiger RD (eds): Werner & Ingbar's The Thyroid: A Fundamental and Clinical Text, 9th ed. Philadelphia: Lippincott Williams & Wilkins, 2005, pp 697-699.
6. Ross DS. Subclinical hypothyroidism. *In* Braverman LE, Utiger RD (eds): Werner & Ingbar's The Thyroid: A Fundamental and Clinical Text, 9th ed. Philadelphia: Lippincott Williams & Wilkins, 2005, pp 1070-1078.
7. Weetman AP. Chronic autoimmune thyroiditis. *In* Braverman LE, Utiger RD (eds): Werner & Ingbar's The Thyroid: A Fundamental and Clinical Text, 9th ed. Philadelphia: Lippincott Williams & Wilkins, 2005, pp 701-713.
8. Singer PA. Primary hypothyroidism due to other causes. *In* Braverman LE, Utiger RD (eds): Werner & Ingbar's The Thyroid: A Fundamental and Clinical Text, 9th ed. Philadelphia: Lippincott Williams & Wilkins, 2005, pp 745-753.
9. Harjai KJ, Licata AA. Effects of amiodarone on thyroid function. Ann Intern Med 1997;126:63-73.
10. Trip MD, Wiersinga W, Plomp TA, et al. Incidence, predictability, and pathogenesis of amiodarone-induced thyrotoxicosis and hypothyroidism. Am J Med 1991;91:507-511.
11. Wolff J, Chaikoff IL. Plasma inorganic iodide as a homeostatic regulator of thyroid function. J Biol Chem 1948;174:555-564.
12. Wolff J, Chaikoff IL, et al. The temporary nature of the inhibitory action of excess iodine on organic iodine synthesis in the normal thyroid. Endocrinology 1949;45:504-513.
13. Roti E, Vagenakis AG. Effect of excess iodide: clinical aspects. *In* Braverman LE, Utiger RD (eds): Werner & Ingbar's The Thyroid: A Fundamental and Clinical Text, 9th ed. Philadelphia: Lippincott Williams & Wilkins, 2005, pp 288-305.
14. Berens SC, Berstein RS, Robbins J, et al. Antithyroid effects of lithium. J Clin Invest 1970;49:1357-1367.
15. Spaulding SW, Burrow GN, Bermudez F, et al. The inhibitory effect of lithium on thyroid hormone release in both euthyroid and thyrotoxic patients. J Clin Endocrinol Metab 1972;35:905-911.

16. Emerson CH, Dyson WL, Utiger RD, et al. Serum thyrotropin and thyroxine concentrations in patients receiving lithium carbonate. J Clin Endocrinol Metab 1973;36:338-346.
17. Devos H, Rodd C, Gagne N, et al. A search for the possible molecular mechanisms of thyroid dysgenesis: sex ratios and associated malformations. J Clin Endocrinol Metab 1999;84:2502-2506.
18. Andersson M, Takkouche B, Egli I, et al. Current global iodine status and progress over the last decade towards the elimination of iodine deficiency. Bull World Health Organ 2005;83:518-525.
19. Samuels MH, Ridgway EC. Central hypothyroidism. Endocrinol Metab Clin North Am 1992;21:903-919.
20. Woeber KA. Thyrotoxicosis and the heart. N Engl J Med 1992;327:94-98.
21. Klein I, Ojamaa K. Cardiovascular manifestations of endocrine disease. J Clin Endocrinol Metab 1992;75:339-342.
22. O'Brien T, Dinneen SF, O'Brien PC, et al. Hyperlipidemia in patients with primary and secondary hypothyroidism. Mayo Clin Proc 1993;68:860-866.
23. Diekman T, Lansberg PJ, Kastelein JP, et al. Prevalence and correction of hypothyroidism in a large cohort of patients referred for dyslipidemia. Arch Intern Med 1995;155:1490-1495.
24. Catargi B, Parrot-Roulaud F, Cochet C, et al. Homocysteine, hypothyroidism, and effect of thyroid hormone replacement. Thyroid 1999;9:1163-1166.
25. Hussein WI, Green R, Jacobsen DW, et al. Normalization of hyperhomocysteinemia with L-thyroxine in hypothyroidism. Ann Intern Med 1999;131:348-351.
26. Siafakas NM, Salesiotou V, Filaditaki V. Respiratory muscle strength in hypothyroidism. Chest 1992;102:189-194.
27. Ladenson PW, Goldenheim PD, Ridgway EC. Prediction and reversal of blunted ventilatory responsiveness in patients with hypothyroidism. Am J Med 1988;83:877-883.
28. Zwillich CW, Pierson DJ, Hofeldt FD, et al. Ventilatory control in myxedema and hypothyroidism. N Engl J Med 1975;292:662-665.
29. Rajagopal KR, Abbrecht PH, Derderian SS, et al. Obstructive sleep apnea in hypothyroidism. Ann Intern Med 1984;101:491-494.
30. Lin CC, Tsan KW, Chen PJ. The relationship between sleep apnea syndrome and hypothyroidism. Chest 1992;102:1663-1667.
31. Khalleli AA, Griffith DG, Edwards RH. The clinical presentation of hypothyroid myopathy and its relationship to abnormalities in structure and function in skeletal muscle. Clin Endocrinol 1987;19:365-376.
32. Das KC, Mukherjee, Sarkar TK, et al. Erythropoiesis and erythropoietin in hypo- and hyperthyroidism. J Clin Endocrinol Metab 1975;40:211-220.
33. Krassas GE, Pontikides N, Kaltsas T, et al. Disturbances of menstruation in hypothyroidism. Clin Endocrinol (Oxf) 1999;50:655-659.
34. Marqusee E, Mandel SJ. The blood in hypothyroidism. *In* Braverman LE, Utiger RD (eds): Werner & Ingbar's The Thyroid: A Fundamental and Clinical Text, 9th ed. Philadelphia: Lippincott Williams & Wilkins, 2005, pp 803-805.
35. Tudhope GR, Wilson GM. Deficiency of vitamin B_{12} in hypothyroidism. Lancet 1962;1:703-706.
36. Burmeister LA, Ganguli M, Dodge HH, et al. Hypothyroidism and cognition: preliminary evidence for a specific defect in memory. Thyroid 2001;11:1177-1185.
37. Laureno R. Neurologic manifestations of thyroid disease. Endocrinologist 1996;6:467-472.
38. Purnell DC, Daly D, Lipscomb PR. Carpal tunnel syndrome associated with myxedema. Arch Intern Med 1961;108:751-756.
39. Watanakunakorn G, Hodges RE, Evans TC. Myxedema: a study of 400 cases. Arch Intern Med 1965;116:183-190.
40. Thomas R, Reid RL. Thyroid disease and reproductive dysfunction: a review. Obstet Gynecol 1987;70:789-798.
41. Davis LE, Leveno KJ, Cunningham FG. Hypothyroidism complicating pregnancy. Obstet Gynecol 1988;72:108-112.
42. Corrales Hernandez JJ, Miralles Garcia JM, Garcia Diez LC. Primary hypothyroidism and human spermatogenesis. Arch Androl 1990;25:21-27.
43. Heymann WR. Cutaneous manifestations of thyroid disease. J Am Acad Dermatol 1992;26:885-902.
44. Diven DG, Gwinup G, Newton RC. The thyroid. Dermatol Clin 1989;7:547-557.
45. Ai J, Leonhardt JM, Heymann WR. Autoimmune thyroid diseases: etiology, pathogenesis, and dermatologic manifestations. J Am Acad Dermatol 2003;48:641-659.
46. Smith TJ, Bahn RS, Gorman CA. Connective tissue, glycosaminoglycans and diseases of the thyroid. Endocr Rev 1989;10:266-391.
47. Spencer CA, LoPresti JS, Patel A, et al. Applications of a new chemiluminometric thyrotropin assay to subnormal measurement. J Clin Endocrinol Metab 1990;70:453-460.
48. Caldwell G, Kellett HA, Gow SM, et al. A new strategy for thyroid function testing. Lancet 1985;1:1117-1119.
49. Nicoloff JT, Spencer CA. The use and misuse of the sensitive thyrotropin assays. J Clin Endocrinol Metab 1990;71:553-558.
50. Chopra IJ. Euthyroid sick syndrome: is it a misnomer? J Clin Endocrinol Metab 1997;82:329-334.
51. Utiger RD. Altered thyroid function in nonthyroidal illness and surgery: to treat or not to treat? N Engl J Med 1995;333:1562-1563.
52. Kakucska I, Qi Y, Lechan RM. Changes in adrenal status affect hypothalamic thyrotropin-releasing hormone gene expression in parallel with corticotrophin-releasing hormone. Endocrinology 1995;136:2795-2802.
53. Scanlon MF, Weightman DR, Shale DJ, et al. Dopamine is a physiological regulator of thyrotropin (TSH) secretion in normal man. Clin Endocrinol (Oxf) 1979;10:7-15.
54. Marcocci C, Marino M. Thyroid-directed antibodies. *In* Braverman LE, Utiger RD (eds): Werner & Ingbar's The Thyroid: A Fundamental and Clinical Text, 9th ed. Philadelphia: Lippincott Williams & Wilkins, 2005, pp 361-372.
55. Spencer CA. Thyroglobulin. *In* Braverman LE, Utiger RD (eds): Werner & Ingbar's The Thyroid: A Fundamental and Clinical Text, 9th ed. Philadelphia: Lippincott Williams & Wilkins, 2005, pp 345-359.
56. Blakesley V, Awni W, Locke C, et al. Are bioequivalence studies of levothyroxine sodium formulations in euthyroid volunteers reliable? Thyroid 2004;14:191-200.
57. Joint statement on the U.S. Food and Drug Administration's decision regarding bioequivalence of levothyroxine sodium. Thyroid 2004;14:486.
58. Fish LH, Schwartz HL, Cavanaugh J, et al. Replacement dose, metabolism, and bioavailability of levothyroxine in the treatment of hypothyroidism: role of triiodothyronine in pituitary feedback in humans. N Engl J Med 1987;316:764-770.
59. Campbell NRC, Hasinoff BB, Stalts H, et al. Ferrous sulfate reduces thyroxine efficacy in patients with hypothyroidism. Ann Intern Med 1992;117:1010-1013.
60. Singh N, Singh PN, Hershman JM. Effect of calcium carbonate on the absorption of levothyroxine. JAMA 2000;283:2822-2825.
61. Woeber KA. Treatment of hypothyroidism. *In* Braverman LE, Utiger RD (eds): Werner & Ingbar's The Thyroid: A Fundamental and Clinical Text, 9th ed. Philadelphia: Lippincott Williams & Wilkins, 2005, pp 864-869.
62. Arafah BM. Increased need for thyroxine in women with hypothyroidism during estrogen therapy. N Engl J Med 2001;344:1743-1749.
63. Kostoglou-Athanassiou I, Ntalles K, Markopoulos C, et al. Thyroid function in postmenopausal women with breast cancer on tamoxifen. Eur J Gynaecol Oncol 1998;19:150-154.
64. D'Esteve-Bonetti L, Bennet AP, Malet D, et al. Gluten-induced enteropathy (celiac disease) revealed by resistance to treatment with levothyroxine and alfacalcidol in a sixty-eight-year-old patient: a case report. Thyroid 2002;12:633-636.
65. Liel Y, Harman-Boehm I, Shany S. Evidence for a clinically important adverse effect of fiber-enriched diet on the bioavailability of levothyroxine in adult hypothyroid patients. J Clin Endocrinol Metab 1996;80:857-859.
66. Bell DSH, Ovalle F. Use of soy protein supplement and resultant need for increased dose of levothyroxine. Endocr Pract 2001;7:193-194.
67. Curran PG, DeGroot LJ. The effect of hepatic enzyme-inducing drugs on thyroid hormones and the thyroid gland. Endocr Rev 1991;12:135-150.
68. Isojarvi JI, Turrka J, Pakarinen AJ, et al. Thyroid function in men taking carbamazepine, oxcarbazepine, or valproate for epilepsy. Epilepsia 2001;42:930-934.
69. Sawin CT, Herman T, Molitch ME, et al. Aging and the thyroid: decreased requirements for thyroid hormone in older hypothyroid patients. Am J Med 1983;75:206-209.
70. Singer PA. Hypothyroidism. *In* Rakel RE, Bope ET (eds): Conn's Current Therapy 2006. Philadelphia: Elsevier Saunders, 2006; pp 802-806.
71. Walsh JP, Shiels L, Lim EM, et al. Combined thyroxine/liothyronine treatment does not improve well-being, quality of life, or cognitive function compared to thyroxine alone: a randomized controlled trial in patients with primary hypothyroidism. J Clin Endocrinol Metab 2003;88:4543-4550.
72. Sawka AM, Gerstein HC, Marriott MJ, et al. Does a combination regimen of thyroxine (T_4) and 3,5,3′-triiodothyronine improve depressive symptoms better than T_4 alone in patients with hypothyroidism? Results of a double-blind, randomized, controlled trial. J Clin Endocrinol Metab 2003;88:4551-4555.
73. Siegmund W, Spieker K, Weike AI, et al. Replacement therapy with levothyroxine plus triiodothyronine (bioavailable molar ratio 14:1) is not superior to thyroxine alone to improve well-being and cognitive performance in hypothyroidism. Clin Endocrinol (Oxf) 2004;60:750-757.
74. Escobar-Morreale HF, Botella-Carretero JI, Gomez-Bueno M, et al. Thyroid hormone replacement therapy in primary hypothyroidism: a randomized trial comparing L-thyroxine plus liothyronine with L-thyroxine alone. Ann Intern Med 2005;142:412-424.
75. Saravanan P, Simmons DJ, Greenwood R, et al. Partial substitution of thyroxine (T_4) with triiodothyronine in patients on T_4 replacement therapy: results of a large community-based randomized controlled trial. J Clin Endocrinol Metab 2005;90:805-812.
76. Appelhof BC, Fliers E, Wekking EM, et al. Combined therapy with levothyroxine and liothyronine in two ratios, compared with levothyroxine monotherapy in primary hypothyroidism: a double-blind, randomized, controlled clinical trial. J Clin Endocrinol Metab 2005;90:2666-2674.
77. Escobar-Morreale HF, Botella-Carretero JI, Escobar del Rey F, et al. Treatment of hypothyroidism with combinations of levothyroxine plus liothyronine [Review]. J Clin Endocrinol Metab 2005;90:4946-4954.
78. Gharib H, Tuttle M, Baskin HJ, et al. Consensus statement. Subclinical thyroid dysfunction: a joint statement on management from the American Association of Clinical Endocrinologists, the American Thyroid Association, and the Endocrine Society. J Clin Endocrinol Metab 2005;90:581-585.
79. Hak AE, Pols HA, Visser TJ, et al. Subclinical hypothyroidism is an independent risk factor for atherosclerosis and myocardial infarction in elderly women: the Rotterdam Study. Ann Intern Med 2000;132:270-278.
80. Lindeman RD, Romero LJ, Schade DS, et al. Impact of subclinical hypothyroidism on serum total homocysteine concentrations, the prevalence of coronary heart disease (CHD), and CHD risk factors in the New Mexico Elder Health Survey. Thyroid 2003;13:595-600.
81. Imaizumi M, Akahoshi M, Ichimaru S, et al. Risk for ischemic heart disease and all-cause mortality in subclinical hypothyroidism. J Clin Endocrinol Metab 2004;89:3365-3370.
82. Rodondi N, Aujesky D, Vittinghoff E. Subclinical hypothyroidism and the risk of coronary heart disease: a meta-analysis. Am J Med 2006;119:541-551.
83. Surks MI, Ortiz E, Daniels GH, et al. Subclinical thyroid disease: scientific review and guidelines for diagnosis and management. JAMA 2004;291:228-238.
84. Klein I, Ojamaa K. Thyroid hormone and the cardiovascular system. N Engl J Med 2001;344:501-509.

85. Klein IL. The cardiovascular system in hypothyroidism. *In* Braverman LE, Utiger RD (eds): Werner & Ingbar's The Thyroid: A Fundamental and Clinical Text, 9th ed. Philadelphia: Lippincott Williams & Wilkins, 2005, pp 774-780.
86. Ain K, Mori Y, Refetoff S. Reduced clearance rate of thyroxine binding globulin (TBG) with increased sialylation: a mechanism for estrogen-induced elevation of serum TBG concentration. J Clin Endocrinol Metab 1987;65:689-696.
87. Ballabio M, Posyyachinda M, Ekins RP. Pregnancy-induced changes in thyroid function: role of human chorionic gonadotropin as a putative regulator of maternal thyroid. J Clin Endocrinol Metab 1991;73:824-831.
88. Burrow GN, Fisher DA, Larsen PR. Maternal and fetal thyroid function. N Engl J Med 1994;331:1072-1078.
89. Mestman JH, Goodwin M, Montoro MM. Thyroid disorders of pregnancy. Endocrinol Metab Clin North Am 1995;24:41-71.
90. Alexander EK, Marqusee E, Lawrence J, et al. Timing and magnitude of increase in levothyroxine requirements during pregnancy in women with hypothyroidism. N Engl J Med 2004;351:241-249.
91. Chopra IJ, Baber K. Treatment of primary hyperthyroidism during pregnancy: is there an increase in thyroxine dose requirement in pregnancy? Metabolism 2003;52:122-128.
92. Weinberg AD, Brennan MD, Gorman CA, et al. Outcome of anesthesia and surgery in hypothyroid patients. Arch Intern Med 1983;143:893-897.
93. Ladenson PW, Levin AA, Ridgway EC, et al. Complications of surgery in hypothyroid patients. Am J Med 1984;77:261-266.
94. Wartofsky L. Myxedema coma. *In* Braverman LE, Utiger RD (eds): Werner & Ingbar's The Thyroid: A Fundamental and Clinical Text, 9th ed. Philadelphia: Lippincott Williams & Wilkins, 2005, pp 850-855.
95. Hylander B, Rosenqvist U. Treatment of myxoedema coma: factors associated with fatal outcome. Acta Endocrinol 1985;108:65.
96. Yamamoto T, Fukuyama J, Fujiyoshi A. Factors associated with mortality of myxedema coma: report of eight cases and literature survey. Thyroid 1999;9:1167-1174.
97. Nicoloff JT, LoPresti JS. Myxedema coma: a form of decompensated hypothyroidism. Endocrinol Metab Clin North Am 1993;22:279-290.
98. Tunbridge WMG, Vanderpump MPJ. Population screening for autoimmune thyroid disease. Endocrinol Metab Clin North Am 2000;29:239-253.
99. Tunbridge WMG, Evered DC, Hall R, et al. The spectrum of thyroid disease in the community: the Whickham Survey. Clin Endocrinol (Oxf) 1977;7:481-491.
100. Braverman LE, Utiger RD. Introduction to thyrotoxicosis. *In* Braverman LE, Utiger RD (eds): Werner & Ingbar's The Thyroid: A Fundamental and Clinical Text, 9th ed. Philadelphia: Lippincott Williams & Wilkins, 2005, pp 453-455.
101. McLachlan SM, Pegg CA, Atherton MC, et al. TSH receptor antibody synthesis by thyroid lymphocytes. Clin Endocrinol (Oxf) 1986;24:223-230.
102. Rees Smith B, McLachlan SM, Furmaniak J. Autoantibodies to the thyrotropin receptor. Endocr Rev 1988;9:106-121.
103. Hanafusa T, Pujol Borrell R, Chiovato L, et al. Aberrant expression of HLA-DR antigen on thyrocytes in Graves' disease: relevance for autoimmunity. Lancet 1983;2:1111-1115.
104. Davies TF. The pathogenesis of Graves' disease. *In* Braverman LE, Utiger RD (eds): Werner & Ingbar's The Thyroid: A Fundamental and Clinical Text, 9th ed. Philadelphia: Lippincott Williams & Wilkins, 2005, pp 457-473.
105. Biondi B, Palmieri A, Lombardi G, et al. Effects of thyroid hormone on cardiac function: the relative importance of heart rate, loading conditions, and myocardial contractility in the regulation of cardiac performance in human hyperthyroidism. J Clin Endocrinol Metab 2002;87:968-974.
106. Osman F, Gammage MD, Franklyn JA. Hyperthyroidism and cardiovascular morbidity and mortality. Thyroid 2002;12:483-487.
107. Osman F, Gammage MD, Sheppard MC, et al. Cardiac dysrhythmias and thyroid dysfunction: the hidden menace? J Clin Endocrinol Metab 2002;87:963-967.
108. Ingbar DH. The pulmonary system in thyrotoxicosis. *In* Braverman LE, Utiger RD (eds): Werner & Ingbar's The Thyroid: A Fundamental and Clinical Text, 9th ed. Philadelphia: Lippincott Williams & Wilkins, 2005, pp 569-581.
109. Ayres J, Rees J, Clark TJH, et al. Thyrotoxicosis and dyspnea. Clin Endocrinol 1982;16:65-71.
110. Kahaly G, Hellermann J, Mohr-Kahaly S, et al. Impaired cardiopulmonary exercise capacity in patients with hyperthyroidism. Chest 1996;109:57-61.
111. Ch'ng CL, Biswas M, Benton A, et al. Prospective screening for celiac disease in patients with Graves' hyperthyroidism using anti-gliadin and tissue tranglutaminase antibodies. Clin Endocrinol (Oxf) 2005;62:303-306.
112. Nordyke RA, Gilbert FI Jr, Harada AS. Graves' disease: influence of age on clinical findings. Arch Intern Med 1988;148:626-631.
113. Fein HG, Rivlin RS. Anemia in thyroid disease. Med Clin North Am 1975;59:1133-1145.
114. Alperin JB, Haggard ME, Haynie TP. A study of vitamin B_{12} requirements in a patient with pernicious anemia and thyrotoxicosis: evidence of an increased need for vitamin B_{12} in the presence of hyperthyroidism. Blood 1970;36:632-641.
115. Perros P, Singh RK, Ludlam CA, et al. Prevalence of pernicious anemia in patients with type I diabetes mellitus and autoimmune thyroid disease. Diabetic Med 2000;17:749-751.
116. Weitzman SA, Stossel TP, Harmon DC, et al. Antineutrophil autoantibodies in Graves' disease. J Clin Invest 1985;75:119-123.
117. Gardner DF. The neuromuscular system and brain in thyrotoxicosis. *In* Braverman LE, Utiger RD (eds): Werner & Ingbar's The Thyroid: A Fundamental and Clinical Text, 9th ed. Philadelphia: Lippincott Williams & Wilkins, 2005, pp 637-643.
118. Duyff RF, Van den Bosch J, Laman DM, et al. Neuromuscular findings in thyroid dysfunction: a prospective clinical and electrodiagnostic study. J Neurol Neurosurg Psychiatry 2000;68:750-755.
119. Zurcher RM, Horber FF, Grunig BE, et al. Effect of thyroid dysfunction on thigh muscle efficiency. J Clin Endocrinol Metab 1989;69:1082-1086.
120. Norrelund H, Hove KY, Brems-Dalgaard E, et al. Muscle mass and function in thyrotoxic patients before and during medical treatment. Clin Endocrinol (Oxf) 1999;51:693-699.
121. Marino M, Ricciardi R, Pinchera A, et al. Mild clinical expression of myasthenia gravis associated with autoimmune thyroid diseases. J Clin Endocrinol Metab 1997;82:438-443.
122. Gharib H. Thyrotoxic periodic paralysis. Endocr Pract 1998;4:178-179.
123. Ross DS. Hyperthyroidism, thyroid hormone and bone. Thyroid 1994;4:319-326.
124. Kaptein EM. The kidneys and electrolyte metabolism in thyrotoxicosis. *In* Braverman LE, Utiger RD (eds): Werner & Ingbar's The Thyroid: A Fundamental and Clinical Text, 9th ed. Philadelphia: Lippincott Williams & Wilkins, 2005, pp 582-588.
125. Evered DC, Hayter CJ, Surveyor I. Primary polydipsia in thyrotoxicosis. Metabolism 1972;21:393-404.
126. Ridgway EC, Maloof F, Longcope C. Androgens and estrogen dynamic in hyperthyroidism. J Endocrinol 1982;95:105-115.
127. Koutras DA. Disturbances of menstruation in thyroid disease. Ann N Y Acad Sci 1997;816:280-284.
128. Perros P, Dickinson AJ. Ophthalmopathy. *In* Braverman LE, Utiger RD (eds): Werner & Ingbar's The Thyroid: A Fundamental and Clinical Text, 9th ed. Philadelphia: Lippincott Williams & Wilkins, 2005, pp 474-487.
129. Burch HB, Wartofsky L. Graves' ophthalmopathy: current concepts regarding pathogenesis and management. Endocr Rev 1993;14:747-793.
130. Bilezekian JP, Loeb JN. The influence of hyperthyroidism and hypothyroidism on alpha- and beta-adrenergic receptor systems and adrenergic responsiveness. Endocr Rev 1983;4:378-388.
131. Bahn RS, Heufelder AE. Pathogenesis of Graves' ophthalmopathy. N Engl J Med 1993;329:1468-1475.
132. Silva EJ. Thermogenesis and the sympathoadrenal system in thyrotoxicosis. *In* Braverman LE, Utiger RD (eds): Werner & Ingbar's The Thyroid: A Fundamental and Clinical Text, 9th ed. Philadelphia: Lippincott Williams & Wilkins, 2005, pp 607-620.
133. Andersen OO, Friis T, Ottesen B. Glucose tolerance and insulin secretion in hyperthyroidism. Acta Endocrinol 1977;84:576-587.
134. McIver B, Morris JC. The pathogenesis of Graves' disease. Endocrinol Metab Clin North Am 1998;27:73-89.
135. Surks MI, Chopra I, Mariash C, et al. American Thyroid Association guidelines for use of laboratory tests in thyroid disorders. JAMA 1990;263:1529-1532.
136. Singer PA, Cooper D, Levy E, et al. Treatment guidelines for patients with hyperthyroidism and hypothyroidism. JAMA 1995;273:808-812.
137. Franklyn JA. The management of hyperthyroidism. N Engl J Med 1994;130:1731-1738.
138. Cooper DS. Treatment in thyrotoxicosis. *In* Braverman LE, Utiger RD (eds): Werner & Ingbar's The Thyroid: A Fundamental and Clinical Text, 9th ed. Philadelphia: Lippincott Williams & Wilkins, 2005, pp 665-694.
139. Singer PA. Hyperthyroidism. *In* Rakel RE, Bope ET (eds): Conn's Current Therapy 2008. Philadelphia: Elsevier Saunders, 2008; pp 650-655.
140. Rittmaster RS, Zwicker H, Abbott EC, et al. Effect of methimazole with or without exogenous L-thyroxine on serum concentrations of thyrotropin (TSH) receptor antibodies in patients with Graves' disease. J Clin Endocrinol Metab 1996;81:3283-3288.
141. Tamai H, Hayaki I, Kawai K, et al. Lack of effect of thyroxine administration on elevated thyroid stimulating hormone receptor antibody levels in treated Graves' disease patients. J Clin Endocrinol Metab 1995;80:1481-1484.
142. Cooper DS. Antithyroid drugs. N Engl J Med 2005;352:905-917.
143. Vitti P, Rayo T, Chiovato L, et al. Clinical features of patients with Graves' disease undergoing remission after antithyroid drug treatment. Thyroid 1997;7:369-375.
144. Allahabadia A, Daykin J, Holder RL, et al. Age and gender predict the outcome of treatment for Graves' hyperthyroidism. J Clin Endocrinol Metab 2000;85:1038-1042.
145. Allannic H, Fauchet R, Orgiazzi J, et al. Antithyroid drugs and Graves' disease: a prospective randomized evaluation of the efficacy of treatment duration. J Clin Endocrinol Metab 1990;70:675-679.
146. Werner MC, Romaldini JH, Bromberg N, et al. Adverse effects related to thionamide drugs and their dose regimen. Am J Med Sci 1989;297:216-219.
147. van Staa TP, Boulton F, Cooper C, et al. Neutropenia and agranulocytosis in England and Wales: incidence and risk factors. Am J Hematol 2003;72:248-254.
148. Cooper DS, Goldminz D, Levin A, et al. Agranulocytosis associated with antithyroid drugs: effects of patient age and drug dose. Ann Intern Med 1983;98:26-29.
149. Balkin MS, Buchholtz M, Ortiz J, et al. Propylthiouracil (PTU)-induced agranulocytosis treated with recombinant human granulocyte colony-stimulating factor (G-CSF). Thyroid 1993;3:305-309.
150. Fukata S, Kuma K, Sugawara M. Granulocyte colony stimulating factor (GCSF) does not improve recovery from antithyroid drug-induced agranulocytosis: a prospective study. Thyroid 1999;9:29-31.
151. Tajiri J, Noguchi S, Murakami T, et al. Antithyroid drug-induced agranulocytosis: the usefulness of routine white blood cell count monitoring. Arch Intern Med 1990;150:621-624.
152. Liaw Y-F, Huang M-J, Fan K-D, et al. Hepatic injury during propylthiouracil therapy in patients with hyperthyroidism. Ann Intern Med 1993;118:424-428.
153. Williams KV, Nayak S, Becker D, et al. Fifty years of experience with propylthiouracil-associated hepatotoxicity: what have we learned? J Clin Endocrinol Metab 1997;82:1727-1733.

154. Arab DM, Malatjalian DA, Rittmaster RS. Severe cholestatic jaundice in uncomplicated hyperthyroidism treated with methimazole. J Clin Endocrinol Metab 1995; 80:1083-1085.
155. Gunton JE, Stiel J, Caterson RJ, et al. Anti-thyroid drugs and antineutrophil cytoplasmic antibody positive vasculitis: a case report and review of the literature. J Clin Endocrinol Metab 1999;84:13-16.
156. Harper L, Chin L, Daykin J, et al. Propylthiouracil and carbimazole associated-antineutrophil cytoplasmic antibodies (ANCA) in patients with Graves' disease. Clin Endocrinol (Oxf) 2004;60:671-675.
157. Wartofsky L, Glinoer D, Solomon B, et al. Differences and similarities in the diagnosis and treatment of Graves' disease in Europe, Japan, and the United States. Thyroid 1991;1:129-135.
158. Stoffer SS, Hamburger JI. Inadvertent ^{131}I therapy for hyperthyroidism in the first trimester of pregnancy. J Nucl Med 1976;17:146-149.
159. Safa AM, Schumacher OP, Rodriguez-Antunez A. Long-term follow-up results in children and adolescents treated with radioactive iodine (^{131}I) for hyperthyroidism. N Engl J Med 1975;292:167-171.
160. Franklyn JA, Maisonneuve P, Sheppard M, et al. Cancer incidence and mortality after radioiodine treatment for hyperthyroidism: a population-based cohort study. Lancet 1999;353:2111-2115.
161. Holm LE, Lundell G, Dahlqvist I, et al. Cure rate after ^{131}I therapy for hyperthyroidism. Acta Radiol 1981;20:161-166.
162. Buettner C, Surks MI. Police detainment of a patient following treatment with radioactive iodine [Letter]. JAMA 2002;288:2687.
163. Patwardhan NA, Moront M, Rao S, et al. Surgery still has a role in Graves' hyperthyroidism. Surgery 1993;114:1108-1112.
164. Winsa B, Rastad J, Larsson E, et al. Total thyroidectomy in therapy-resistant Graves' disease. Surgery 1994;116:1068-1074.
165. Chang DCS, Wheeler MH, Woodcock JP, et al. The effect of preoperative Lugol's iodine on thyroid blood flow in patients with Graves' hyperthyroidism. Surgery 1987;102:1055-1061.
166. Palit TK, Miller CC III, Miltenburg DM. The efficacy of thyroidectomy for Graves' disease: a meta-analysis. J Surg Res 2000;90:161-165.
167. Sosa JA, Bowman HM, Tielsch JM, et al. The importance of surgeon experience for clinical and economic outcomes from thyroidectomy. Ann Surg 1998;228:320-330.
168. Laurberg P, Pedersen KM, Vestergaard H, et al. High incidence of multinodular goiter in the elderly population in a low iodine intake area vs. high incidence of Graves' disease in the young in a high iodine intake area: comparative surveys of thyrotoxicosis epidemiology in East-Jutland Denmark and Iceland. J Intern Med 1991;229:415-420.
169. Delange F, de Benoist B, Pretell E, et al. Iodine deficiency in the world: where do we stand at the turn of the century? Thyroid 2001;11:437-447.
170. Hegedus L, Bonnema SJ, Bennedbaek FN. Management of simple nodular goiter: current status and future perspectives. Endocr Rev 2003;24:102-132.
171. Nygaard B, Hegedus L, Nielsen KG, et al. Long-term effect of radioactive iodine on thyroid function and size in patients with solitary autonomously functioning toxic thyroid nodules. Clin Endocrinol (Oxf) 1999;50:197-202.
172. Thomusch O, Machens A, Sekulla C, et al. Multivariate analysis of risk factors for postoperative complications in benign goiter surgery: prospective multicenter study in Germany. World J Surg 2000;24:1335-1341.
173. Charkes ND. The many causes of subclinical hyperthyroidism. Thyroid 1996;5:391-396.
174. Solomon BL, Wartofsky L, Burman KD. Prevalence of fractures in postmenopausal women with thyroid disease. Thyroid 1993;3:17-23.
175. Foldes J, Tarjan G, Szathmari M, et al. Bone mineral density in patients with endogenous subclinical thyrotoxicosis: is this thyroid status a risk factor for osteoporosis? Clin Endocrinol (Oxf) 1993;39:521-527.
176. Gurlek A, Gedik O. Effect of endogenous subclinical hyperthyroidism on bone metabolism and bone mineral density in premenopausal women. Thyroid 1999;9:539-543.
177. Baldini M, Gallazzi M, Orsati A, et al. Treatment of benign nodular goiter with mildly suppressive doses of L-thyroxine: effects on bone mineral density and on nodule size. J Intern Med 2002;251:407-414.
178. Mikosch M, Obermayer-Pietsch B, Jost R, et al. Bone metabolism in patients with differentiated thyroid carcinoma receiving suppressive levothyroxine treatment. Thyroid 2003;13:347-356.
179. Kumeda Y, Inaba M, Tahara H, et al. Persistent increase in bone turnover in Graves' patients with subclinical thyrotoxicosis. J Clin Endocrinol Metab 2000;85:4157-4161.
180. Ross DS. Subclinical thyrotoxicosis. *In* Braverman LE, Utiger RD (eds): Werner & Ingbar's The Thyroid: A Fundamental and Clinical Text, 9th ed. Philadelphia: Lippincott Williams & Wilkins, 2005, pp 1079-1085.
181. Sawin CT, Geller A, Wolf PA, et al. Low serum thyrotropin concentrations as a risk factor for atrial fibrillation in older persons. N Engl J Med 1994;331:1249-1252.
182. Osman F, Gammage MD, Franklyn JA. Hyperthyroidism and cardiovascular morbidity and mortality. Thyroid 2002;12:483-487.
183. Parle JV, Maisonneuve P, Sheppard MC, et al. Prediction of all-cause and cardiovascular mortality in elderly people from one low serum thyrotropin result: a 10-year cohort study. Lancet 2001;358:861-865.
184. Boelaert K, Franklyn JA. Thyroid hormone in health and disease. J Endocrinol 2005;187:1-15.
185. Auer J, Scheibner P, Mische T, et al. Subclinical hyperthyroidism as a risk factor for atrial fibrillation. Am Heart J 2001;142:838-842.
186. Cappola AR, Fried LP, Arnold AM, et al. Thyroid status, cardiovascular risk, and mortality in older adults. JAMA 2006;295:1033-1041.
187. Biondi B, Palmieri EA, Fazio S, et al. Endogenous subclinical thyrotoxicosis affects quality of life and cardiac morphology and function in young and middle-aged patients. J Clin Endocrinol Metab 2000;85:4701-4705.
188. Mestman JH. Hyperthyroidism and pregnancy. Best Pract Res Clin Endocrinol Metab 2004;18:267-288.
189. Rubin PC. Beta-blockers in pregnancy. N Engl J Med 1981;305:1323-1326.
190. Milham S Jr. Scalp defects in infants of mothers treated for hyperthyroidism with methimazole or carbimazole during pregnancy. Teratology 1985;32:321.
191. Wilson LC, Kerr BA, Wilkinson R, et al. Choanal atresia and hypothelia following methimazole exposure in utero: a second report. Am J Med Genet 1998;75:220-222.
192. Mortimer RH, Cannell GR, Addison RS, et al. Methimazole and propylthiouracil equally cross the perfused human term placental lobule. J Clin Endocrinol Metab 1997;82:3099-3102.
193. Momotani N, Noh J, Oyanagi H, et al. Antithyroid drug therapy for Graves' disease during pregnancy: optimal regimen for fetal thyroid status. N Engl J Med 1986;315:24-28.
194. Bankowski BJ, Hearne AE, Lambrou NC, et al. Surgical disease and trauma in pregnancy. *In* Johns Hopkins Manual of Gynecology & Obstetrics, 2nd ed. Philadelphia: Lippincott Williams & Wilkins, 2002, p 232.
195. Azizi F, Khoshniat M, Bahrainian M, et al. Thyroid function and intellectual development of infants nursed by mothers taking methimazole. J Clin Endocrinol Metab 2000;85:3233-3238.
196. Momotani N, Yamashita R, Makino F, et al. Thyroid function in wholly breast-feeding infants whose mothers take high doses of propylthiouracil. Clin Endocrinol (Oxf) 2000;53:177-181.
197. Glinoer D. Thyroid disease during pregnancy. *In* Braverman LE, Utiger RD (eds): Werner & Ingbar's The Thyroid: A Fundamental and Clinical Text, 9th ed. Philadelphia: Lippincott Williams & Wilkins, 2005, pp 1086-1108.
198. Solomon B, Glinoer D, Lagasse R, et al. Current trends in the management of Graves' disease. J Clin Endocrinol Metab 1990;70:1518-1524.
199. Burch HB, Wartofsky L. Life-threatening thyrotoxicosis: thyroid storm. Endocrinol Metab Clin North Am 1993;22:263-277.
200. Wartofsky L. Thyrotoxic storm. *In* Braverman LE, Utiger RD (eds): Werner & Ingbar's The Thyroid: A Fundamental and Clinical Text, 9th ed. Philadelphia: Lippincott Williams & Wilkins, 2005, pp 651-657.
201. Wartofsky L, Ransil BJ, Ingbar SH. Inhibition by iodine of the release of thyroxine from the thyroid glands of patients with thyrotoxicosis. J Clin Invest 1970;49:78-86.

39

DISORDERS OF CALCIUM METABOLISM AND BONE MINERALIZATION

Bart L. Clarke and Sundeep Khosla

OVERVIEW 587
PATHOPHYSIOLOGY 587
Calcium Metabolism 587
Hypercalcemia 588
Hypocalcemia 589
Regulation of Calcium and Phosphate Metabolism 589
Parathyroid Hormone 589
Vitamin D 590
Bone Physiology 593
Osteoporosis 594
Paget's Disease of Bone 595
Renal Osteodystrophy 595
THERAPEUTICS AND CLINICAL PHARMACOLOGY 595
Goals of Therapy 595
Therapeutics by Class 595
Calcium 595
Vitamin D 596
Vitamin D Analogues 596
Therapeutic Uses of Vitamin D 597
Calcimimetics 598
Calcilytics 598
Anticatabolic Agents 598
Anabolic Agents 603
Therapeutic Approach 604
Emerging Targets and Therapeutics 605
Non–FDA-Approved Anticatabolic Agents 605
Non–FDA-Approved Anabolic Agents 605
Non–FDA-Approved Mixed Agents 605

OVERVIEW

This chapter describes the pharmacology and addresses the therapeutics of disorders of calcium metabolism and bone mineralization. The first part of the chapter reviews current concepts regarding normal calcium metabolism and bone physiology, and then briefly reviews the major disorders affecting calcium metabolism and the skeleton. The second half of the chapter discusses the pharmacology of calcium, vitamin D, vitamin D analogues, and drugs used to treat disorders of calcium metabolism and bone mineralization.

New drugs that interact with the calcium-sensing receptor (CaSR), including the first calcimimetic, cinacalcet, and the category of calcilytics, are reviewed. Drugs used to treat disorders of bone mineralization are then discussed, including anticatabolic agents that prevent bone loss, including U.S. Food and Drug Administration (FDA)–approved agents such as oral and intravenous bisphosphonates, hormone therapy, the selective estrogen receptor modulator (SERM) raloxifene, calcitonin, and the only bone anabolic agent currently approved by the FDA, teriparatide (PTH 1-34). A variety of non–FDA-approved agents currently being investigated are briefly discussed, including several oral and intravenous bisphosphonates, other SERMs, tibolone, denosumab, parathyroid hormone (PTH)–related peptide, cathepsin K inhibitors, and PTH 1-84, a non–FDA-approved anabolic agent. Other medications not yet approved by the FDA to treat disorders of bone mineralization are agents that do not meet criteria for pure anticatabolic or anabolic action. These drugs, including strontium ranelate and nandrolone decanoate, are reviewed briefly to conclude the chapter.

PATHOPHYSIOLOGY

Calcium Metabolism

Extracellular ionized calcium in the millimolar range is physiologically important for maintenance of skeletal metabolism, nerve and muscle function, and cell activity. Intracellular ionized calcium in the micromolar range functions as a cytoplasmic second messenger. Basal cytoplasmic intracellular ionized calcium is maintained normally at around 0.1 μM, due to active intracellular calcium extrusion by Ca^{2+}-ATPases and by Na^+/Ca^{2+} exchange across the plasma membrane, and by intracellular uptake into mitochondria and the endoplasmic reticulum.

Serum calcium normally ranges from 8.5 to 10.5 mg/dl. Circulating serum calcium is bound to proteins (40%), primarily albumin (90%) but also β-globulin, α_2-globulin, α_1-globlin, and γ-globulin, as well as anions such as phosphate, citrate, or sulfate (10%). The balance of serum calcium is found in free ionized form (50%). Only free ionized calcium is physiologically active, with a normal range of 4.25 to 5.25 mg/dl. Diffusible calcium includes serum ionized calcium plus a proportion of protein- and anion-complexed calcium. Only diffusable calcium can cross cell membranes via calcium channels or calcium transporters. Men typically have total body calcium content of about 1300 g, and women about 1000 g. More than 99% of total body calcium is sequestered in the bones and teeth.

Several factors affect measurement of serum total or ionized calcium. Alterations in serum albumin alter serum calcium without affecting ionized calcium. Decreases in serum albumin below 4.0 mg/dl decrease serum total calcium by 0.8 mg/dl for each 1.0-mg/dl decrease in serum albumin, whereas increases above 4.0 mg/dl increase serum total calcium by 0.8 mg/dl for each 1.0-mg/dl increase in serum albumin. Dehydration increases serum total calcium due to hemoconcentration. Acid-base disturbances affect serum ionized calcium without affecting total calcium. Acidemia increases serum ionized calcium, and alkalemia decreases ionized calcium. Serum ionized calcium is usually measured in complex clinical situations associated with changes in serum albumin levels and/or acid-base balance, but under normal circumstances, serum total calcium measurement is adequate.

Extracellular calcium is tightly regulated by hormones that affect absorption of calcium from the intestine, excretion of calcium from the kidney, and absorption or release of calcium from the skeleton. The serum calcium concentration reflects the balance between calcium influx into extracellular fluid from intestinal absorption, skeletal resorption, and renal resorption and calcium efflux from extracellular fluid through intestinal secretion, skeletal uptake, and renal excretion.

Other factors indirectly affect the serum calcium concentration. Increased PTH or parathyroid hormone–related peptide (PTHrp) directly stimulates renal tubular reabsorption of filtered calcium, thereby limiting renal calcium excretion. Hypercalcemia interferes with antidiuretic hormone–stimulated free water reabsorption in the distal renal tubule, and thereby may induce nephrogenic diabetes insipidus. Nausea and vomiting caused by hypercalcemia may cause further hemoconcentration. Severe volume depletion may reduce renal calcium clearance. Immobilization, especially in younger individuals, patients with Paget's disease of bone, or astronauts in a microgravity environment, may directly increase bone resorption.

The G protein–coupled extracellular CaSR plays a major role in regulation of extracellular calcium.[1] This receptor is found on parathyroid cells, renal tubular cells, osteoblasts, intestinal mucosal cells, and adipocytes, as well as a variety of other cells in other tissues. The CaSR regulates secretion of PTH by parathyroid cells and renal tubular cell reabsorption of calcium from the urine, and may regulate bone turnover or intestinal calcium absorption as well. This receptor is a seven-transmembrane segment receptor, with a large extracellular portion that binds ionized calcium and a shorter intracellular portion that interacts with a variety of G proteins and signal transduction pathways. It may be part of a larger family of calcium- or cation-binding receptors.

Skeletal calcium is contained in a crystalline form complexed with phosphorus and hydroxyl groups known as hydroxyapatite $[Ca_{10}(PO_4)_6(OH)_2]$. The hydroxyapatite crystalline lattice also contains small amounts of sodium, potassium, magnesium, and fluoride. A small portion of skeletal calcium is available in an easily mobilized labile pool that exchanges with interstitial fluid. Exchange of skeletal calcium with interstitial fluid is regulated by sex steroids, PTH, vitamin D, various medications, and other factors that regulate bone turnover and interstitial fluid calcium.

Figure 39-1 illustrates the various components of daily whole body calcium turnover based on metabolic balance studies. Calcium is absorbed from the intestine primarily by facilitated diffusion. Vitamin D–dependent calcium absorption occurs mainly in the proximal duodenum, whereas facilitated diffusion occurs throughout the small intestine. The intestine obligatorily excretes 150 mg of calcium each day due to losses from mucosal and biliary secretions and intestinal cell death. Intestinal fractional absorption of calcium depends on total body calcium stores and dietary calcium intake. Consumption of a low-calcium diet leads to increased fractional calcium absorption due in part to increased renal synthesis of 1,25-dihydroxyvitamin D. The efficiency of this adaptive mechanism is decreased in older adults. Intestinal calcium absorption is decreased in patients with malabsorption or rapid intestinal transit, or in patients taking glucocorticoids or phenytoin.

Urinary calcium excretion represents the difference between the renal daily filtered calcium load and the amount reabsorbed by the kidneys. The kidneys filter about 9000 mg of calcium each day, with the proximal renal tubules reabsorbing about 98% (8800 mg). Tubular reabsorption of calcium is regulated mainly by the circulating PTH level, but also by the filtered sodium load, presence of non-reabsorbed urinary anions, and diuretic use (see Chapter 22, Hypertension; and Chapter 26, Heart Failure). High sodium intake increases urinary calcium excretion, and low sodium intake may decrease urinary calcium excretion. Loop diuretics such as furosemide act on the ascending limb of the loop of Henle to increase calcium excretion, whereas thiazide diuretics uncouple sodium and calcium excretion, leading to increased sodium excretion and decreased calcium excretion. Increased dietary protein intake increases urinary calcium excretion, presumably through the effect of sulfur-containing amino acids on renal tubular function.

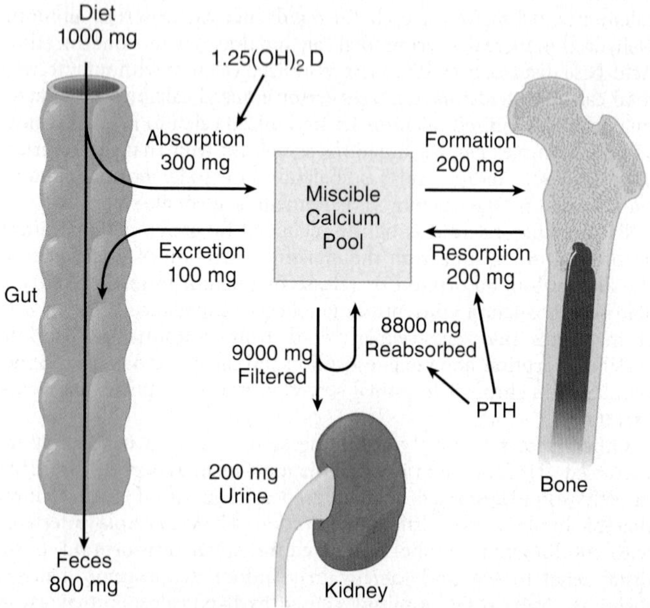

FIGURE 39-1 • Whole body daily calcium turnover.

Hypercalcemia

Hypercalcemia usually results from increased skeletal resorption or intestinal absorption in combination with normal or decreased renal excretion, but may also result from normal calcium influx in association with decreased renal excretion or skeletal mineralization. Increased skeletal resorption typically is due to accelerated osteoclast recruitment and activation, most often under the influence of PTH, PTHrp, or 1,25-dihydroxyvitamin D. Cytokines that may stimulate osteoclast recruitment or function include interleukin (IL)-1α, IL-1β, IL-6, tumor necrosis factor-α, lymphotoxin, or transforming growth factor-β. Increased intestinal absorption of calcium is a less common cause of hypercalcemia than increased skeletal resorption, but may occur with increased production of 1,25-dihydroxyvitamin D or absorptive hypercalciuria. Regardless of the cause of increased calcium influx into extracellular fluid, serum calcium levels do not typically increase unless the kidneys fail to compensate with increased urinary calcium excretion.

Mild increases in serum calcium to the 10.5- to 12-mg/dl range often do not cause symptoms. Moderate increases to the 12- to 15-mg/dl range may cause few if any symptoms if they develop slowly or are long standing, but an acute rise in serum calcium to this range usually causes fatigue, weakness, loss of appetite, depression, and constipation. Ingestion of large amounts of calcium rarely causes hypercalcemia except in the setting of hyperthyroidism[2] or milk-alkali syndrome,[3] in which intake of large amounts of milk or other dairy products and antacids cause decreased renal excretion of calcium.

The most common cause of hypercalcemia in healthy adults in the outpatient setting is primary hyperparathyroidism, due to oversecretion of PTH.[4] Secondary hyperparathyroidism most often results from chronic kidney disease, and is usually associated with a normal or decreased serum calcium level. Tertiary hyperparathyroidism, in which the parathyroid glands become autonomously functioning due to long-standing chronic stimulation from secondary hyperparathyroidism, is associated with hypercalcemia. Signs and symptoms of primary hyperparathyroidism are more than those associated with hypercalcemia, and include fatigue, weakness, thirst, frequent urination, calcium-containing kidney stones, hematuria, bone loss or osteoporosis, joint or bone pain, loss of appetite, heartburn or reflux, peptic ulcer disease, constipation, difficulty concentrating, decreased memory, and depression. Most individuals diagnosed with primary hyperparathyroidism are asymptomatic or vaguely symptomatic, and do not develop kidney stones or bone disease such as osteitis fibrosa cystica.[5] Patients with primary hyperparathyroidism usually have low-normal or mildly decreased serum phosphate levels and high-normal to increased serum PTH. Serum PTH levels assessed by current "full-length" immunoradiometric assays measure PTH 1-84, whereas "intact" PTH assays measure both PTH 1-84 and the major fragment, PTH 7-84.[6]

Familial benign hypercalcemia, also known as familial hypocalciuric hypercalcemia (FHH), is an autosomal dominant inherited disorder associated with mild hypercalcemia, low-normal or mildly decreased serum phosphate, increased serum PTH, and 24-hour urine calcium excretion inappropriately low for the level of serum calcium.[7,8] This disorder is caused by heterozygous mutations in the CaSR,[9] but the biochemical findings mimic primary hyperparathyroidism and may be mistaken for primary hyperparathyroidism, leading to unnecessary neck surgery to remove abnormal parathyroid glands. FHH is not associated with the long-term complications seen with primary hyperparathyroidism, and surgical removal of parathyroid glands does not cure the condition. Infants with homozygous CaSR mutations have severe hypercalcemia that requires life-saving emergent parathyroidectomy shortly after birth.

The most common cause of hypercalcemia in hospitalized adult patients is cancer.[10] Malignancy may cause hypercalcemia due to oversecretion of PTHrp[11] or other cytokines or prostaglandins, or due to bone destruction caused by metastasis. PTHrp is most often oversecreted by squamous cell or epithelial cancers, but may be overproduced by myeloma cells also. PTHrp interacts with the PTH/PTHrp-1 receptor to cause increased bone resorption leading to hypercalcemia. Some patients with lymphomas or granulomatous disorders, such as sarcoidosis or tuberculosis, may overproduce 1,25-dihydroxyvitamin D due to 1α-hydroxylase expression in tumor cells or macrophages, respectively, which then causes increased intestinal absorption of calcium.[12,13] Patients with hypercalcemia of malignancy may have more severe hypercalcemia, often in the 15- to 20-mg/dl range or higher, with marked fatigue, malaise, somnolence, nausea, vomiting, thirst, and frequent urination.

Increased exogenous vitamin D intake may cause increased serum 25-hydroxyvitamin D levels, leading to increased intestinal calcium absorption, usually with associated decreased serum PTH and 1,25-dihydroxyvitamin D levels. Individuals with hyperthyroidism may develop hypercalcemia due to increased skeletal resorption caused by increased thyroid hormone levels. Hypercalcemia may be associated with volume depletion or dehydration of any cause, and is associated with adrenocortical insufficiency and oversecretion of vasoactive intestinal peptide. Pheochromocytomas may cause hypercalcemia due to increased secretion of PTHrp in the setting of multiple endocrine neoplasia syndrome type IIA.

Hypocalcemia

Mild hypocalemia in the range of 8.0 to 8.5 mg/dl is usually asymptomatic, but lower levels of serum total or ionized calcium usually cause tingling paresthesias, cramps, increased neuromuscular excitability, tetany, laryngospasm, bronchospasm, or tonic-clonic seizures.[14] Low serum calcium due to chronic hypoparathyroidism may be associated with total body hair loss (alopecia totalis) developing in infancy or childhood, grooved fingernails, dental enamel hypoplasia, cataracts, brain basal ganglia calcifications, and depression, anxiety, or delusions.

Vitamin D deficiency and/or low calcium intake, as occurs with poor nutrition, starvation, or malabsorptive disorders, commonly causes hypocalcemia. Malabsorption may also be associated with hypophosphatemia, hypoalbuminemia, hypoproteinemia, hypomagnesemia, or edema. Magnesium deficiency may potentiate hypocalcemia by decreasing the secretion and/or action of PTH. Long-standing severe nutritional calcium deficiency may rarely lead to rickets in infants or children.[15]

Hypocalcemia due to hypoparathyroidism in adults most commonly develops after thyroid or other neck surgery or neck radiation therapy. In children it may result from genetic disorders such as DiGeorge syndrome, which causes parathyroid aplasia. Adults may develop hypoparathyroidism due to autoimmune disease[16] or iron or copper overload syndromes. Hypoparathyroidism is usually associated with hyperphosphatemia, resulting from decreased PTH effects on renal tubular phosphate transport.

Pseudohypoparathyroidism causes hypocalcemia and hyperphosphatemia due to tissue resistance to PTH action. PTH resistance in this disorder is not due to mutations in the PTH/PTHrp-1 receptor, but rather mutations in the G_sa (*GNAS1*) protein linked to the PTH/PTHrp-1 receptor, which mediates PTH-induced adenylate cyclase activation.[17] Variable phenotypic expression of pseudohypoparathyroidism results from differential genomic imprinting of the maternal and paternal G_sa alleles.[18] Some patients with *GNAS1* mutations also have resistance to other hormones such as thyroid-stimulating hormone, luteinizing hormone, follicle-stimulating hormone, glucagon, calcitonin, or growth hormone–releasing hormone.

Hypocalcemia may develop and persist for several days to weeks after removal of overactive parathyroid glands, such as after removal of a parathyroid adenoma causing primary hyperparathyroidism. This results from suppression of the remaining normal parathyroid glands by the previous hypercalcemia, and rapid uptake of calcium by the skeleton. Rapid uptake of calcium by the skeleton after removal of a parathyroid adenoma, known as "hungry bones syndrome," may require treatment with significant amounts of oral and/or intravenous calcium and vitamin D for several days to weeks after surgical cure of primary hyperparathyroidism.

Infants may develop tetany shortly after birth if their mothers had hyperparathyroidism during pregnancy, due to suppression of the baby's parathyroid glands by transplacental transfer of the mother's high circulating level of calcium. These infants usually recover from tetany as soon as their serum calcium levels begin to rise, as their parathyroid glands recover the ability to produce adequate PTH. Hypocalcemia may occur in patients with chronic kidney disease due to hyperphosphatemia and metabolic acidosis, but most patients with renal insufficiency or failure do not develop symptoms from hypocalcemia unless treatment of their acid-base disturbance causes lowering of their serum ionized calcium. Hyperphosphatemia inhibits renal 1α-hydroxylase activity in this setting, decreasing synthesis of serum 1,25-dihydroxyvitamin D and thereby limiting intestinal calcium absorption. Transfusion of large amounts of citrated blood may chelate sufficient serum calcium to cause hypocalcemia.

Regulation of Calcium and Phosphate Metabolism

PTH and 1,25-dihydroxyvitamin D (calcitriol) regulate calcium and phosphate homeostasis through their effects on the kidneys, intestine, and parathyroid glands. PTH is a peptide hormone that simulates the kidneys to reabsorb calcium and excrete phosphorus, and stimulates renal 1α-hydroxylase synthesis of 1,25-dihydroxyvitamin D from circulating 25-hydroxyvitamin D. PTH indirectly stimulates the intestine to absorb calcium via its stimulation of renal synthesis of 1,25-dihydroxyvitamin D. 1,25-Dihydroxyvitamin D is the only biologically active metabolite of vitamin D, while 25-hydroxyvitamin D is biologically inert, and stored in body fat as a reservoir hormone. Figure 39-2 illustrates the regulation of calcium and phosphate metabolism by PTH and 1,25-dihydroxyvitamin D.

Parathyroid Hormone

The parathyroid glands were first identified by Sir Richard Owen, curator of the British Museum of Natural History, as he was dissecting a rhinoceros that had died in the London Zoo. Human parathyroid glands were first identified by Sandstrom in 1890.[19] In 1891, von Recklinghausen described the parathyroid-associated bone disease "osteitis fibrosa cystica" for the first time, and Ashkenazy reported this condition in a patient with a parathyroid adenoma for the first time in 1904. Gley described the physiologic consequences of complete thyroparathyroidectomy in animals in 1914. Vassale and Generali reported seizures and death after complete parathyroidectomy in animals unless calcium was given postoperatively. MacCallum and Voegtlin documented that complete parathyroidectomy in animals caused decreased serum calcium, and several investigators subsequently demonstrated that parathyroid gland extracts prevented or treated hypocalcemic tetany in parathyroidectomized animals and caused increased serum calcium levels.

Human, bovine, and porcine PTH are 84–amino acid peptides with molecular weights of about 9500 Da. Biologic activity resides in the amino-terminal end of the PTH molecule, which binds to PTH receptors. PTH is initially synthesized as pre-proparathyroid hormone, with 115 amino acids, and converted to proparathyroid hormone by removal of the proximal 25 amino-terminal residues while in the endoplasmic reticulum. Proparathyroid hormone subsequently moves to the Golgi complex and is converted to PTH 1-84 by removal of an additional six

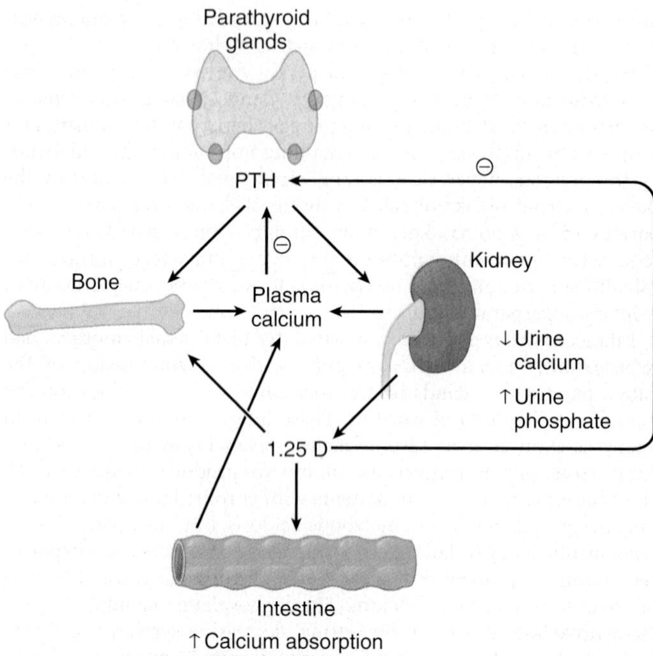

FIGURE 39-2 • Regulation of calcium metabolism by parathyroid hormone (PTH) and 1,25-dihydroxyvitamin D.

amino acids. PTH 1-84 is sequestered within cytoplasmic secretory granules until released into the circulation. Neither pre-proparathyroid hormone nor proparathyroid hormone is normally released into the circulation.[20]

PTH 1-84 is proteolytically hydrolyzed into several major and minor fragments within the parathyroid cell before release, and subsequently further metabolized in various tissues after release. PTH 7-84 and other amino-truncated fragments accumulate during chronic kidney disease because they are normally removed from the circulation by the kidneys, as well as by the liver and other tissues. PTH 7-84 interacts with PTH receptors on specific target cells and may cause them to undergo internalization from the cell surface.[21] During acute hypocalcemia, more intact PTH 1-84 is secreted by the parathyroid cell, and less is hydrolyzed to PTH 7-84 intracellularly. During prolonged hypocalcemia, the parathyroid glands synthesize increased amounts of PTH and eventually undergo hypertrophy and subsequently hyperplasia.

PTH 1-84 has a half-life of 2 to 5 minutes in the circulation, and is removed from the circulation largely by metabolism in the liver and kidneys. Measurement of intact PTH 1-84 by immunoradiometric assays is complicated by multiple circulating fragments of PTH. Previous two-site monoclonal antibody assays directed against the amino- and mid-terminal regions of the PTH 1-84 molecule have recently been shown to cross-react with PTH 7-84. More recent second-generation PTH assays have been developed that are capable of differentiating between PTH 1-84 and PTH 7-84.[22]

PTH 1-84 increases extracellular fluid calcium into the normal range by stimulating renal calcium reabsorption and bone release of calcium. PTH 1-84 also binds to PTH receptors in cartilage, vascular smooth muscle, placenta, liver, pancreatic islets, brain, dermis, and lymphocytes, where its function is less certain.[23] PTH actions in all target tissues are mediated by at least two PTH receptors. The PTH/PTHrp-1 receptor binds both PTH 1-84 and PTHrp, and is found mainly in the bone and kidneys. The PTH-2 receptor binds PTH 1-84 only, and is found in blood vessels, testis, brain, pancreas, and placenta. The natural ligand for the PTH-2 receptor was recently reported to be hypothalamic tuberoinfundibular peptide of 39 residues (TIP39).[24] The PTH/PTHrp-1 and PTH-2 receptors are linked to the phospholipase C and protein kinase A signaling pathways via G_s and G_q in specific cells. The phospholipase D signaling pathway is activated via a $G_{12/13}$-RhoA pathway in some cells.[25] Initial evidence suggests that at least one PTH carboxyl-terminal fragment receptor, called the C-PTH receptor, exists in some tissues and binds to certain C-terminal fragments.[26]

PTH secretion is rapidly and tightly regulated by serum ionized calcium. As serum ionized calcium decreases, PTH secretion increases rapidly, and as serum ionized calcium increases, PTH secretion decreases rapidly. Prolonged hypocalcemia leads eventually to parathyroid cell hypertrophy with associated increased uptake of amino acids and nucleic acids and cytoplasmic enlargement. Serum ionized calcium appears to regulate PTH synthesis and secretion, as well as parathyroid cell growth. Ionized calcium regulates PTH synthesis and secretion through binding to the plasma membrane–bound CaSR,[27] which is linked to the G_q–phospholipase C signaling pathway and G_i. Binding of ionized calcium to the CaSR inhibits PTH secretion, whereas decreased binding of ionized calcium to the CaSR increases PTH secretion. Hypercalcemia causes decreased cyclic AMP (cAMP) generation and inhibition of protein kinase C (PKC) activity, whereas hypocalcemia leads to increased cAMP generation and PKC activity. Other compounds that increase PKC activity, such as β-adrenergic receptor agonists and dopamine, also increase PTH secretion to a small degree, but physiologic regulation of PTH secretion is mainly by ionized calcium. 1,25-Dihydroxyvitamin D directly suppresses PTH gene transcription, thereby decreasing PTH secretion. Serum phosphate does not regulate PTH secretion directly, except via indirect effects on serum calcium. Hypomagnesemia commonly decreases PTH secretion, but hypermagnesemia may also decrease PTH secretion.

Chronically increased PTH levels classically stimulate bone resorption via interaction with osteoblast PTH receptors,[20] which subsequently cause osteoclast activation and release of ionized calcium into extracellular fluid. Chronically increased PTH levels generally inhibit osteoblast function, but acutely increased PTH levels may stimulate osteoblast function. The mechanism(s) behind the radically different effects of chronically increased PTH versus intermittently increased PTH on bone remain the subject of ongoing investigation.[28]

PTH stimulates PTH/PTHrp-1 receptors on the apical border of proximal renal tubular cells, resulting in increased tubular reabsorption of calcium, decreased tubular reabsorption of phosphorus, and increased 1α-hydroxylase activity.[29] These effects reduce urinary calcium excretion, increase urinary phosphorus excretion, and increase renal 1,25-dihydroxyvitamin D production, which causes increased intestinal calcium absorption. Chronically increased PTH levels may increase the renal filtered calcium load enough to overwhelm the ability of the kidneys to reabsorb calcium, and hypercalciuria may develop.

PTH decreases renal tubular reabsorption of phosphorus by down-regulating proximal renal tubular cell luminal membrane Na^+-P_i cotransport protein expression, rather than inhibiting its activity. The effects of PTH on phosphorus reabsorption are mediated by cAMP expression, and a portion of cAMP synthesized in the renal cortex in response to PTH, called nephrogenous cAMP, is normally excreted in the urine. Urinary cAMP may be measured as a marker of PTH action in the kidney.

PTH also increases renal tubular reabsorption of magnesium, resulting in decreased urinary magnesium and increased serum magnesium. PTH increases renal excretion of water, amino acids, citrate, sodium, chloride, and sulfate, while it decreases excretion of hydrogen ions.

PTH rapidly and significantly stimulates proximal renal tubular cell 1α-hydroxylase activity, leading to increased serum 1,25-hydroxyvitamin D synthesis and release. Low serum phosphorus and calcium also directly stimulate renal tubular cell 1α-hydroxylase activity. Serum 1,25-dihydroxyvitamin D increases intestinal calcium absorption and bone release of calcium.

Vitamin D

Renally synthesized serum 1,25-dihydroxyvitamin D primarily acts indirectly via intestinal calcium absorption to increase serum calcium and extend PTH action.[30] More recently, 1,25-dihydroxyvitamin D has been found to interact with cells and tissues unrelated to bone or mineral metabolism. Vitamin D receptors have been found on hematopoietic cells, lymphocytes, epidermal cells, myocytes, and neurons, and 1,25-dihydroxyvitamin D promotes maturation and differentiation of mononuclear cells involved with cytokine production and immune function, differentiation of malignant cells, and differentiation of epidermal cells.[31]

Figure 39-3 illustrates the pathways of vitamin D production and metabolism. Vitamin D is available as both animal-derived cholecalciferol (vitamin D_3) and plant-derived ergocalciferol (vitamin D_2). Vitamin D_2 and vitamin D_3 are fat soluble. Prior to discovery of vitamin D, children in temperate zone urban centers frequently developed rickets. Rickets was initially thought to be due to lack of fresh air, although dietary deficiency was thought responsible by some investigators. Mellanby and Huldschinsky showed that cod liver oil supplementation or sunshine prevented or cured rickets in children. Animal chow irradiation was discovered to be as efficacious as whole animal irradiation in treating rachitic animals in 1924. These observations eventually led to the isolation and purification of cholecalciferol and ergocalciferol. DeLuca and Shnoes[32] and Mason et al.[33] showed that vitamin D requires metabolism in the liver and kidneys to become physiologically active.

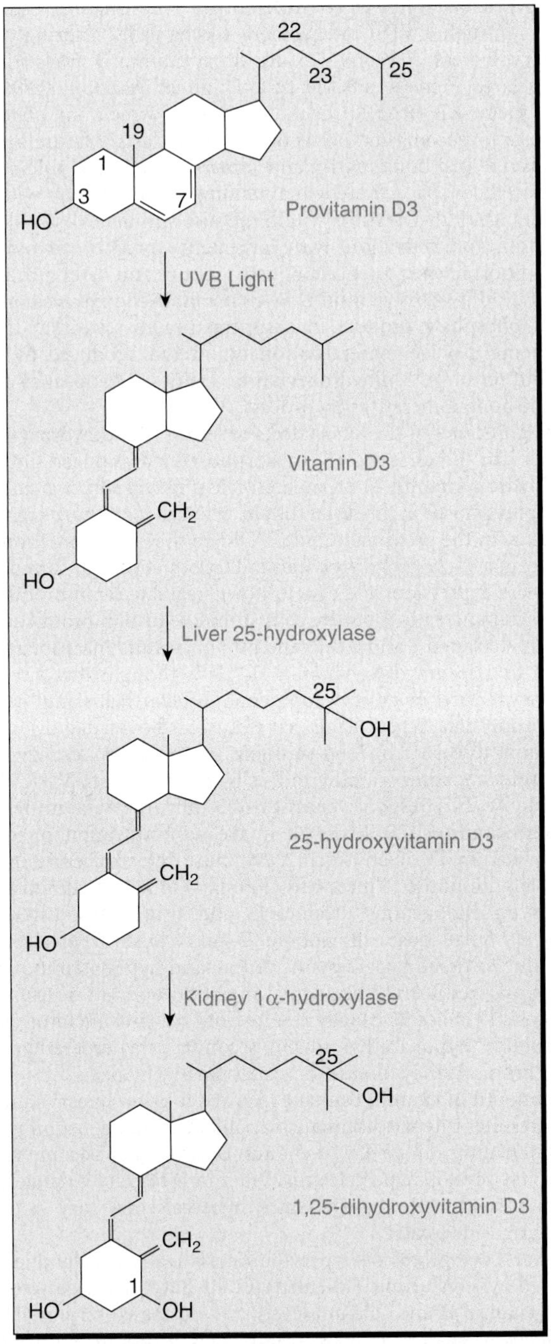

FIGURE 39-3 • **Pathways of vitamin D production and metabolism.**

Ultraviolet B light (290 to 315 nm) irradiation of 7-dehydrocholesterol in the skin of animals increases production of cholecalciferol (vitamin D_3). Ergocalciferol (vitamin D_2) is synthesized from ergosterol in plants. The main structural difference between vitamin D_2 and vitamin D_3 is that vitamin D_2 has a double bond between C22 and C23, and a methyl group at C24, whereas D_3 has neither. Vitamin D_2 is commonly found in commercially available vitamins or supplements, and in irradiated bread or milk. Dietary and supplemental sources of vitamin D_3 may be derived from oily fish such as salmon and mackerel, as well as fish liver oils such as cod liver oil. Clinical experience has shown that vitamins D_2 and D_3 are equally efficacious for treatment of rickets, although vitamin D_3 was recently demonstrated to have greater bioavailability in serum.

Adequate sunlight exposure may stimulate production of sufficient 25-hydroxyvitamin D levels in many humans, but recent studies have shown that low serum 25-hydroxyvitamin D levels are more common in the United States than previously recognized, with re-emergence of nutritional vitamin D–deficiency rickets in some populations.[34,35] Possible explanations for the increased prevalence of vitamin D deficiency include decreased intake of vitamin D–fortified foods due to efforts to reduce dietary fat intake, reduced intake of vitamin D–supplemented calcium-rich foods such as milk in adolescents or young women having children, increased use of sunscreens and protective coverings, and decreased sunlight exposure to reduce risk of skin cancer and premature aging of skin.

Vitamins D_2 and D_3 are absorbed from the small intestine via passive absorption with assistance from bile (see Chapter 34, Hepatic Cirrhosis). Both forms of vitamin D are transferred to chylomicrons initially, and then absorbed via the lymphatics. Both forms are excreted in bile through the intestine, with a small amount excreted in the urine.

Absorbed vitamin D circulates bound to the α-globulin vitamin D–binding protein with a plasma half-life of 19 to 25 hours. Vitamin D is usually stored in body fat for months. For vitamin D to become physiologically active, it must be activated sequentially by the liver and kidney. Liver cytochrome P-450 (CYP) 25-hydroxylase enzyme (CYP27A1) 25-hydroxylates circulating cholecalciferol or ergocalciferol to 25-hydroxyvitamin D_3 or D_2, respectively, which have a plasma half-life of 19 days. Serum 25-hydroxyvitamin D levels optimally range between 25 and 80 ng/ml, with vitamin D deficiency currently defined as less than 10 ng/ml. Vitamin D toxicity, associated with hypercalcemia, typically occurs with serum 25-hydroxyvitamin D levels above 120 ng/ml.

Renal CYP 1α-hydroxylase (CYP27B1) is stimulated by decreased serum calcium[36] or phosphorus,[37] increased PTH, or vitamin D deficiency to produce increased serum 1,25-dihydroxyvitamin D. Figure 39-4 shows the physiologic regulation of renal 1α-hydroxylase activity. Renal 1α-hydroxylase is localized in mitochondria in proximal renal tubules. PTH rapidly stimulates 1-hydroxylase via a cAMP-dependent signaling pathway. 1α-Hydroxylase is also found at low levels in macrophages, osteoblasts, keratinocytes, and cells in the prostate, colon, breast, and placenta, but these cells are not thought to contribute significantly to serum 1,25-dihydroxyvitamin D production under normal circumstances.[31] Serum prolactin and estrogen may also increase renal 1α-hydroxylase activity. Serum 1,25-dihydroxyvitamin D has a plasma half-life of 3 to 5 days in humans. Increased serum calcium, phosphorus, and 1,25-dihydroxyvitamin D levels suppress renal 1-hydroxylase activity. Increased serum calcium upregulates renal CYP 24-hydroxylase enzyme (CYP24), which causes increased production of biologically inactive 1,24,25-trihydroxyvitamin D and 24,25-hydroxyvitamin D. Serum 1,25-dihydroxyvitamin D is also metabolized by side chain hydroxylations, resulting in cleavage between carbons 23 and 24, which produces water-soluble calcitroic acid. Although more than 50 different metabolites of vitamin D have been

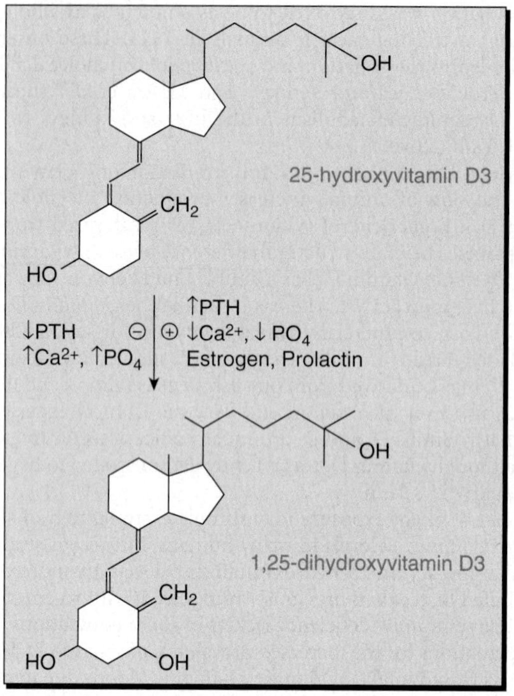

25-hydroxyvitamin D3

↓PTH ↑Ca^{2+}, ↑PO_4 ⊖ | ⊕ ↑PTH ↓Ca^{2+}, ↓ PO_4 Estrogen, Prolactin

1,25-dihydroxyvitamin D3

FIGURE 39-4 • Regulation of 1α-hydroxylase activity.

identified, 1,25-dihydroxyvitamin D is the only biologically active form of vitamin D necessary for intestinal absorption of calcium and phosphate, and for recruitment of bone marrow monocytic cells to become mature osteoclasts that mobilize bone calcium for release into the circulation.[38]

Although the most well-known function of 1,25-dihydroxyvitamin D is to stimulate absorption and retention of calcium and phosphorus, it is recognized that 1,25-dihydroxyvitamin D has multiple other functions independent of its effect on calcium metabolism or bone mineralization. The vitamin D receptor (VDR) is found in brain, prostate, breast, gonads, colon, pancreas, monocytes, and activated T and B lymphocytes.[31] Serum 1,25-dihydroxyvitamin D enters target cells by passive diffusion, and binds to a single form of VDR associated with heat-shock protein chaperones. The VDR belongs to the steroid and thyroid hormone receptor superfamily. The VDR binds 1,25-dihydroxyvitamin D with 1000-fold higher affinity than 25-hydroxyvitamin D or other dihydroxylated forms of vitamin D. The 1,25-dihydroxyvitamin D–VDR complex dissociates from associated heat-shock proteins and undergoes heterodimer formation with retinoid-X receptors in the nucleus after nuclear translocation to bind to vitamin D response elements of genes regulated by vitamin D. Vitamin D also has nongenomic actions that appear to require functional membrane-bound VDR.[39] VDR polymorphisms have been linked to bone loss or osteoporosis in some studies, but not others.[40]

1,25-Dihydroxyvitamin D maximally stimulates intestinal calcium absorption in the duodenum, with less effect in the jejunum or ileum.[41] The colon also absorbs calcium to a lesser degree. Serum 1,25-dihydroxyvitamin D increases duodenal enterocyte transcellular calcium absorption by upregulating expression of the luminal border calcium channel TRPV6[42] and other calcium transporters, cytoplasmic calbindin-D_{9K}, and serosal surface plasma membrane Ca^{2+}-ATPase. Upregulation of these various genes leads to increased transfer of calcium from the lumen of the intestine into the brush border cell, diffusion of calcium through the cell, and energy-dependent extrusion of calcium into the circulation at the serosal surface plasma membrane.[41] The proximal small intestine absorbs calcium inefficiently in the absence of 1,25-dihydroxyvitamin D through thermodynamically passive mass action, mostly through the paracellular pathway, in which calcium is absorbed across gap junctions between the enterocytes via the lateral intercellular spaces. With vitamin D deficiency, no more than 10% to 15% of dietary calcium, and no more than 60% of dietary phosphorus, is absorbed. With vitamin D sufficiency, about 30% of dietary calcium and 70% to 80% of dietary phosphorus is absorbed. Calcium absorption may increase to as much as 50% to 80% of dietary intake during pregnancy, lactation, or growth spurts due to increased serum 1,25-dihydroxyvitamin D levels.[31]

There is little evidence to suggest that vitamin D directly affects bone mineralization. Most of the effect of vitamin D on bone mineralization appears to be mediated by intestinal calcium absorption.[38] The low bone density seen in VDR knockout mice is completely reversed by a high-calcium diet, and patients with rickets due to VDR mutations may be treated successfully with intravenous calcium infusion. Physiologic vitamin D supplementation increases calcium mobilization from bone by recruitment of osteoclasts, and pharmacologic doses increase bone turnover by multiple mechanisms. Mature osteoclasts do not express VDR, however. Osteoclast precursors are stimulated by 1,25-dihydroxyvitamin D to differentiate into mature osteoclasts possibly through a VDR-independent mechanism.[43] During calcium deficiency, increased serum 1,25-dihydroxyvitamin D levels stimulate osteoblasts to increase surface production of receptor activator of nuclear factor-κB (RANK) ligand (RANKL), which stimulates pre-osteoclasts to become mature activated osteoclasts. Mature activated osteoclasts resorb bone matrix and mineral and release calcium into the extracellular space, thereby maintaining serum calcium within the normal range. 1,25-Dihydroxyvitamin D also stimulates osteoblast differentiation and activation, with increased expression of osteoblast alkaline phosphatase, osteocalcin, osteopontin, and several cytokines. Serum 1,25-dihydroxyvitamin D helps maintain the extracellular fluid calcium phosphate product in a supersaturated state that leads to spontaneous passive mineralization of osteoid produced by osteoblasts, but serum 1,25-dihydroxyvitamin D does not appear to directly affect the bone mineralization process.

The significance of the renal effects of serum 1,25-dihydroxyvitamin D on calcium and phosphorus reabsorption remains uncertain. Serum 1,25-dihydroxyvitamin D stimulates calcium reabsorption independent of phosphorus in the distal tubule, whereas phosphorus reabsorption occurs in the proximal tubule. VDRs in the kidney are thought to down-regulate 1,25-dihydroxyvitamin D production and stimulate 24-hydroxylase expression, and also to down-regulate renin production.

VDRs in pancreatic islet beta cells stimulate insulin production and secretion. Activated T and B cells and monocytes and macrophages also respond to 1,25-dihydroxyvitamin D.[44] It is thought that vitamin D sufficiency reduces risk of development of osteoarthritis, multiple sclerosis, fibromyalgia, type 1 diabetes mellitus, cardiovascular disease, and periodontal disease.[31] In long-standing secondary or tertiary hyperparathyroidism, some parathyroid cells down-regulate VDR expression and lose their responsiveness to 1,25-dihydroxyvitamin D.[43]

Hypervitaminosis D. Excessive intake, administration, or production of vitamin D of any form may cause hypercalcemia in some individuals. Response to increased vitamin D intake or administration depends on endogenous production and tissue responsiveness to vitamin D. Small doses of vitamin D may cause hypercalcemia in infants due to tissue hyperresponsiveness, and hypervitaminosis D in children may result from accidental ingestion of adult doses. Hypervitaminosis D in adults usually results from overtreatment of vitamin D deficiency, hypoparathyroidism, secondary hyperparathyroidism due to chronic kidney disease, or excess dietary intake.

The amount of vitamin D intake required to cause hypervitaminosis D with resultant hypercalcemia is variable. Patients consuming more than 50,000 units once a day of vitamin D_2 or D_3 may become vitamin D toxic and develop hypercalcemia. Vitamin D toxicity is dangerous in patients treated with digoxin since hypercalcemia may potentiate cardiac glycoside toxicity.

Signs and symptoms of hypervitaminosis D are usually due to the associated hypercalcemia. Patients typically have increased serum 25-hydroxyvitamin D and calcium levels, and decreased serum PTH and 1,25-dihydroxyvitamin D levels. Moderately severe hypercalcemia in children may cause growth arrest lasting for 6 months or longer, and hypervitaminosis D in pregnant women may cause fetal development of supravalvular aortic stenosis.

Hypovitaminosis D. Low serum vitamin D levels result in hypocalcemia and hypophosphatemia, with resultant secondary hyperparathyroidism. Children with hypovitaminosis D accumulate unmineralized newly formed bone and cartilage, leading to development of rickets characterized by irregular, frayed epiphyses on radiographs and bowing of the bones when children start to walk or bear weight.

Hypovitaminosis D in adults leads to osteomalacia, in which unmineralized newly formed bone accumulates throughout the skeleton without associated epiphyseal abnormalities. Since growth and maturation of the skeleton is complete, the bones typically do not bow and growth plates are normal on radiographs. Patients with mild osteomalacia may be asymptomatic, but those with moderate or severe osteomalacia may describe diffuse, aching bone pain away from their joints, especially with weight bearing, and have significant proximal or other muscle weakness. Bone deformity, pseudofractures, or fractures may occur with severe or long-standing hypovitaminosis D. A serum 25-hydroxyvitamin D level of less than 10 ng/ml is predictive of osteomalacia.

Rickets and Osteomalacia. Rickets and osteomalacia are caused by deficiency of or resistance to vitamin D synthesis or action. Hypophosphatemic vitamin D–resistant rickets is usually an X-linked disorder characterized by hypophosphatemia and an inappropriately low-normal or decreased serum 1,25-dihydroxyvitamin D level. Patients typically heal their osteomalacia when treated with large doses of inorganic phosphorus and vitamin D. Serum 1,25-dihydroxyvitamin D levels may remain inappropriately low-normal or decreased with treatment. X-linked hypophosphatemic rickets is due to mutations in *PHEX* (*P*hosphate-regulating gene with *H*omologies to *E*ndopeptidases on the *X* chromosome), which produces a neutral endopeptidase that normally cleaves fibroblast growth factor-23 (FGF-23) and other peptides that stimulate proximal renal tubular phosphate loss.[45] Loss of activity of this neutral endopeptidase results in increased serum FGF-23 and other phosphaturic factor levels, which result in proximal renal tubular phosphate wasting. Autosomal dominant hypophosphatemic rickets is caused by mutations in the FGF-23 gene that prevent serum FGF-23 degradation by neutral endopeptidase.[46,47] Hereditary hypophosphatemic rickets with hypercalciuria is due to mutations in the renal tubular sodium-phosphate cotransporter NaPi-Lc.

Pseudovitamin D–deficiency rickets (previously known as vitamin D–dependent rickets type I) is an autosomal recessive disorder characterized by inactivating mutations in the renal 1α-hydroxylase gene (*CYP27B1*).[48,49] In this disorder, serum calcium, phosphorus, and 1,25-dihydroxyvitamin D levels are low, whereas serum 25-hydroxyvitamin D is normal and serum PTH increased. Treatment with physiologic doses of 1,25-dihydroxyvitamin D is effective.[50]

Hereditary vitamin D–resistant rickets (previously known as vitamin D–dependent rickets type II) is an autosomal recessive disorder characterized by VDR inactivating mutations.[51] Mutations have been reported in the VDR zinc finger domain, ligand-binding domain, domain required for heterodimerization with the retinoid-X receptor, and transactivation domain. These mutations cause low serum calcium and phosphorus, increased serum 1,25-dihydroxyvitamin D and PTH, and normal serum 25-hydroxyvitamin D. Affected individuals variably develop hair loss beginning in the first year of life, which may progress to alopecia totalis (total body hair loss). Chronic treatment with pharmacologic doses of vitamin D or 1,25-dihydroxyvitamin D is effective in about half of these patients who have residual VDR function, whereas chronic intravenous calcium is required for those who lack VDR function.[50]

Renal osteodystrophy is caused by chronic kidney disease and characterized by decreased renal 1α-hydroxylase activity and decreased serum 1,25-dihydroxyvitamin D levels. Lack of renal clearance of serum phosphate causes hyperphosphatemia, with resultant hypocalcemia and secondary hyperparathyroidism. Low serum 1,25-dihydroxyvitamin D levels cause decreased intestinal calcium absorption and decreased mobilization of calcium from bone. Aluminum deposition previously played a role in renal osteodystrophy when patients with chronic kidney disease were treated with aluminum-containing phosphate binders to lower serum phosphate, and when aluminum-containing fluids were used for dialysis in end-stage renal failure patients.

Bone Physiology

The skeleton contains 213 bones that function to support bodily structures, provide a framework for muscle attachment to allow mobility, protect vital internal organs, and provide for hematopoiesis. The skeleton is composed largely of mineralized matrix, with a small component of metabolically active bone cells. Endochondral bone is formed in the long bones by gradual mineralization of previously synthesized unmineralized matrix, and membranous bone is formed in flat bones by gradual mineralization of membranous bone.

The skeleton is composed of the axial skeleton, including the central bones of the skull, spine, ribs, and pelvis, and the appendicular skeleton, including the peripheral bones of the arms and legs. The appendicular skeleton contains 80% of total skeletal mass, and is predominantly composed of cortical bone. The axial skeleton contains the remaining 20% of skeletal mass, and is composed of a large amount of trabecular bone surrounded by a thin shell of cortical bone. Trabecular bone is composed of highly connected bony plates forming a meshwork within which bone marrow and fat are found. Bone turnover, reflecting both new bone formation and old bone resorption, is greater in the axial skeleton than the appendicular skeleton, largely due to the greater surface area in trabecular bone and the intimate connection between bone cell precursors in the bone marrow and adjacent bone surfaces.

Peak bone mass normally occurs in the third decade of life for both men and women. Bone acquisition occurs during normal growth and development in infancy and childhood, and accelerates significantly around the time of puberty. About 60% of final adult bone mass is acquired within 2 years before and 2 years after puberty, during the period of greatest skeletal growth velocity. Near-maximum bone mass is achieved by age 17 in women and age 20 in men, with further slower acquisition occurring over the next decade. Peak adult bone mass is determined largely by genetic inheritance, but also affected by circulating sex steroid levels, physical activity level, calcium intake, and diseases affecting skeletal bone mass acquisition.

Bone mineral density (BMD) and fracture risk are determined by bone mass, factors affecting eventual or previous peak BMD at skeletal maturity in the third decade, and rate of bone loss after achievement of skeletal maturity in the third decade. Previous studies using dual-energy x-ray absorptiometry (DXA) showed that BMD remained relatively stable in women from the third decade until the early 50s, when rapid bone loss began in women starting their transition through menopause. Rapid bone loss continued for 5 to 8 years, before slowing and continuing at a slower rate until the end of life. DXA studies in men showed that men lost bone density at a relatively constant rate from their 50s until the end of life. Recent studies using quantitative computed tomography scanning have shown that trabecular bone loss begins in adult men and women in the mid-20s, and that cortical bone loss begins in the mid-50s.[52,53]

Skeletal growth occurs longitudinally throughout childhood and adolescence, and formed bone adapts to biomechanical stresses in a process known as modeling.[54] Previously formed endochondral bone is continuously reworked throughout life by a process of sequential bone resorption and formation known as bone remodeling.[54] Remodeling is carried out by millions of bone remodeling units active throughout the skeleton at any one time, affecting about 10% of total bone area at a given time. About 90% of bone surfaces are inactive at any one time, and covered by a thin layer of lining cells.

Figure 39-5 illustrates the bone remodeling cycle. In response to local microtrauma[55] and other as-yet unknown signals, bone marrow monocytic precursors are recruited to specific sites on the bone surface to fuse and form multinucleated osteoclasts, which resorb a given packet of bone by secreting hydrogen ions and a variety of enzymes that digest bone mineral and matrix proteins. Osteoclast formation and activation are regulated by a variety of cytokines such as IL-1 and

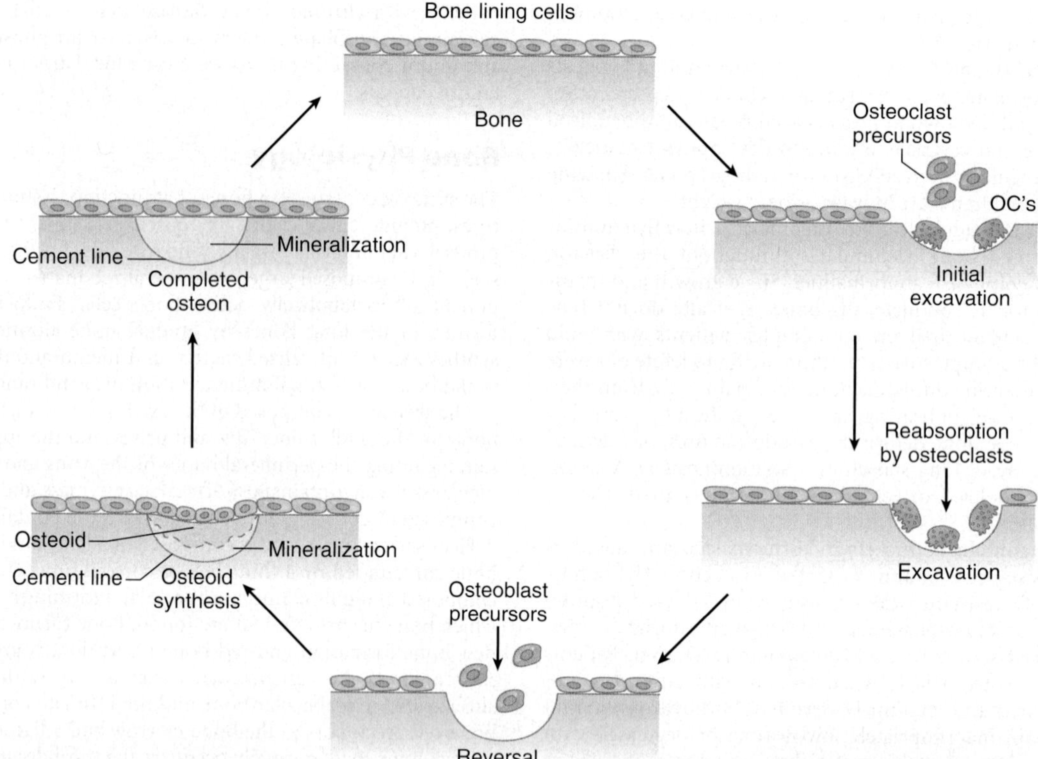

FIGURE 39-5 • Bone remodeling cycle.

IL-6 produced by osteoblasts, but primarily through osteoblast precursor production of RANKL.[56,57] Figure 39-6 illustrates how RANKL regulates osteoclast formation and activation. RANKL stimulates RANK expressed by osteoclasts, and causes osteoclast activation and osteoclast precursor differentiation. Osteoblasts also produce membrane-bound and soluble osteoprotegerin (OPG), which functions as a decoy receptor for RANKL. Increased production of OPG may lead to decreased osteoclast activity, which leads to decreased bone resorption. Decreased production of OPG, as occurs in postmenopausal estrogen deficiency or glucocorticoid therapy, may lead to increased osteoclast activity, which leads to increased bone resorption.

After osteoclasts in a bone remodeling unit complete bone resorption over 2 to 4 weeks, the unit undergoes a reversal phase in which osteoclasts disappear and osteoblast precursors migrate from the marrow stromal space. Osteoblast precursors differentiate into osteoblasts and begin to form proteinaceous matrix known as osteoid,

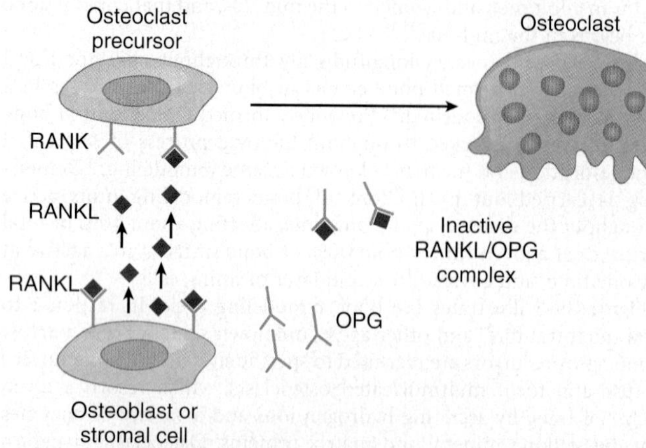

FIGURE 39-6 • RANK ligand and osteoclast formation.

which contains predominantly type I collagen, but also osteocalcin and a variety of other noncollagenous proteins. Once the newly formed osteoid seam reaches about 20 μm in thickness, unmineralized osteoid begins to mineralize. The bone formation phase, including mineralization, typically lasts about 4 to 6 months.

If the amounts of bone removed by bone resorption and new bone formed by bone formation are equal, bone mass will remain the same. In order to gain bone, the balance between bone formation and resorption must favor formation. To lose bone mass, bone resorption must exceed formation. Age-related bone loss occurs due to the accumulation of small deficits in each remodeling cycle since skeletal maturity. Alterations in factors affecting bone metabolism may increase or decrease the number of bone remodeling units active at any time, as well as influence activity levels of osteoblasts or osteoclasts. For example, hyperthyroidism increases the number and activity of bone remodeling units throughout the skeleton, whereas glucocorticoid therapy decreases osteoblast function.[58]

At any given time, millions of bone resorption spaces are present throughout the skeleton. The sum of these spaces represents a transient bone deficit called the remodeling space. This space may expand or contract, depending on the number and activity of bone remodeling units and therapies given to patients.

Osteoporosis

Osteoporosis is a disorder characterized by low bone mass and decreased bone quality, both of which predispose to fractures with minimal or no trauma. Decreased bone quality is attributed to abnormalities in bone microarchitecture, increased bone turnover, microdamage accumulation, and mineralization abnormalities. Osteoporosis is a public health problem in developed countries. In the United States, about 50% of 50-year-old white women and 17% of 50-year-old white men will sustain a clinical fracture during their remaining lifetime. Fractures most commonly affect the vertebrae, distal radius, proximal femur, and other bones, but the entire skeleton is vulnerable. Fracture risk increases exponentially with age, and is associated with decreased survival after any type of fracture.[59]

Osteoporosis is usually classified as primary or secondary. Albright and Reifenstein attributed primary osteoporosis to both menopausal estrogen loss and the effects of normal aging in 1947.[60] Secondary osteoporosis is due to systemic illness or medications that cause bone loss. It was previously thought that type I osteoporosis was primarily due to trabecular bone loss due to estrogen deficiency and led to Colles' fractures, whereas type II osteoporosis caused both cortical and trabecular bone loss due to age-related changes in bone remodeling, decreased dietary calcium and vitamin D intake, and increased PTH secretion, and led to vertebral and hip fractures. It is now understood that these two types of osteoporosis are not entirely distinct, and that they overlap during much of postmenopausal life. Regardless of the type of osteoporosis, this disorder responds to treatment of underlying secondary causes and therapies to decrease bone loss or stimulate bone formation.

Paget's Disease of Bone

Paget's disease of bone is characterized by disordered remodeling in one or more bones of the skeleton, and it is currently hypothesized that paramyxoviral infection of giant multinucleated osteoclasts may play a role in its pathogenesis.[61] Paget's disease is estimated to affect 2% to 3% of the population in North America, Europe, and Australia, and to be less common in other parts of the world. Paget's disease has decreased in prevalence over the last several decades in the United Kingdom[62] and New Zealand.[63] Paget's disease is due to increased bone resorption by abnormal osteoclasts, coupled to increased bone formation by normal osteoblasts, with the result that abnormal disorganized woven bone is formed in place of normal lamellar bone during the remodeling process. Pagetic bone is structurally weaker than normal, and subject to bowing, stress fractures, or fractures. Joints adjacent to pagetic bone may develop osteoarthritis due to adjacent inflammation. Deafness, spinal cord compression, high-output cardiac failure, and rare malignant transformation to osteogenic sarcoma are recognized complications of Paget's disease of bone.

Renal Osteodystrophy

Renal osteodystrophy is composed of a spectrum of metabolic bone disease associated with chronic kidney disease and its treatment. High-turnover renal osteodystrophy is characterized by osteitis fibrosa cystica due to hyperparathyroidism, caused by hypocalcemia, hyperphosphatemia, low serum 1,25-dihydroxyvitamin D, and skeletal resistance to PTH. Low-turnover renal osteodystrophy may be associated with adynamic bone disease with very low bone formation rates, in some cases with associated osteomalacia due to low serum 1,25-dihydroxyvitamin D and mineralization defects. Osteomalacia in the setting of chronic kidney disease may have been due primarily to aluminum deposition at the mineralization front in the past, when aluminum-containing phosphate binders were used and dialysate fluid contained aluminum. Low-turnover bone disease is attributed mainly to relative hypoparathyroidism due to oversuppression of PTH with calcium and vitamin D supplementation.

THERAPEUTICS AND CLINICAL PHARMACOLOGY

Goals of Therapy

The goals of therapy for disorders of calcium metabolism and bone mineralization are to cure or improve abnormalities associated with disease, and to ameliorate pain and other symptoms. These goals may often be successfully achieved with an increasing armamentarium of treatment options that beneficially affect calcium metabolism and bone mineralization.

Therapeutics by Class

Calcium

The current U.S. Dietary Reference Intake for elemental calcium is 1000 mg/day in healthy men or women of age less than 50 years, 1200 mg/day in healthy men and women over age 50 years, and 1300 mg/day in healthy adolescents.[64] About three fourths of this intake is achieved through dairy products in the United States, but calcium-supplemented soy milk, fish, and certain vegetables such as broccoli and spinach are also good sources of dietary calcium. Based on National Health and Nutrition Examination Survey III data, the current estimated average calcium intake in men is 600 to 700 mg/day, whereas women have an estimated intake of 500 to 600 mg/day.

Hypercalcemia. Hypercalcemia is most often mild, but may be moderate or severe. Large amounts of oral or intravenous normal saline help reverse dehydration and improve renal clearance of calcium in almost all settings, and should be considered first-line therapy for all patients except those with congestive heart failure or fluid overload states. Patients may require as much as 3 to 6 L of fluid per day for 1 to 3 days to decrease serum calcium levels toward normal. After patients are adequately hydrated, loop diuretics such as furosemide or torsemide will further improve renal clearance of serum calcium (see Chapter 22, Hypertension; and Chapter 26, Heart Failure). Loop diuretics should not be given until patients have been adequately rehydrated to avoid worsening hypercalcemia due to further volume depletion and hemoconcentration.

Intravenous bisphosphonates are very effective in management of hypercalcemia because they decrease skeletal calcium release into the circulation by potently inhibiting osteoclast-mediated bone resorption. Oral bisphosphonates may be helpful for treating hypercalcemia, but are less potent and less rapidly effective than intravenous bisphosphonates. Pamidronate (Aredia) is usually given as 60 to 90 mg intravenously over 2 to 24 hours.[65] Zoledronic acid (Zometa) is usually given as 4 mg intravenously over 15 minutes.[66] Serum calcium typically reaches its postinfusion nadir within 5 to 7 days after pamidronate infusion, and the therapeutic effect usually persists for several weeks to months. Serum calcium typically reaches its nadir within 3 to 5 days after a zoledronic acid infusion, with the effect persisting for several months to as long as a year.

Hypercalcemia due to endogenous overproduction of 1,25-dihydroxyvitamin D may occur in sarcoidosis, tuberculosis, Crohn's disease, other granulomatous diseases, or lymphoma. This situation responds well to high-dose glucocorticoids. Prednisone is usually given as 40 to 80 mg/day initially for several weeks, followed by a slow tapering course over the next several months. Hydrocortisone may be given as 200 to 300 mg/day intravenously for 3 to 5 days. Glucocorticoids typically take several weeks to maximally lower serum calcium.

Injectable salmon calcitonin (Calcimar) rapidly lowers serum calcium, but is less potent than bisphosphonates or glucocorticoids for this purpose. The major advantage of calcitonin is its rapid onset of action, typically within 2 to 6 hours. Calcitonin is usually given initially as 4 units/kg body weight by subcutaneous injection every 12 hours, with an increase to 8 units/kg every 12 hours after 1 to 2 days if the response is slower than desired. Calcitonin may be further increased to a maximum of 8 units/kg every 6 hours after an additional 2 days without adequate response.

Plicamycin (Mithracin) is a cytotoxic antibiotic that blocks osteoclast messenger RNA synthesis. This may sometimes be used to decrease serum calcium by blocking bone resorption. The usual dose given is relatively low at 15 to 25 mcg/kg body weight to minimize bone marrow, renal, or hepatic toxicity. The hypocalcemic effect of plicamycin occurs within 24 to 48 hours of starting therapy.

Gallium nitrate is approved for treatment of hypercalcemia, but not used widely due to less potent effects than bisphosphonates and calcitonin. Gallium has nephrotoxic effects and is contraindicated in renal failure.

Oral sodium phosphate was used in the past to lower serum calcium, but this is no longer recommended due to the availability of more effective medications, and the possibility that this treatment may cause soft tissue calcium phosphate deposition.

Once acute hypercalcemia is controlled, the underlying cause of the hypercalcemia must still be addressed. If hypercalcemia is due to symptomatic primary hyperparathyroidism, parathyroidectomy remains the only cure. Patients with symptomatic primary hyperparathyroidism should undergo surgery to prevent recognized complications such as osteoporosis, fractures, kidney stones, renal dysfunction, esophageal reflux, peptic ulcer disease, or neuropsychiatric complaints. U.S. national consensus guidelines recommend surgery in patients with asymptomatic primary hyperparathyroidism who have persistent hypercalcemia greater than 1.0 mg/dl above the normal range, hypercalciuria greater than 400 mg/day, renal function decreased by more than 30% below age- and sex-matched controls, osteoporosis defined as T-score below −2.5 at any skeletal site, or age younger than 50 years.[67] Primary hyperparathyroidism is due to a single adenoma in about 80% to 85% of cases, parathyroid hyperplasia in about 15% to 20% of cases, and parathyroid carcinoma in less than 0.5% of cases. In patients who undergo surgery, primary hyperparathyroidism is cured by experienced surgeons in 95% to 98% of cases. Complications of parathyroidectomy include postoperative hypocalcemia due to hungry bones syndrome, hypocalcemia due to permanent hypoparathyroidism, or hoarseness due to recurrent laryngeal nerve injury during surgery.

Cinacalcet is a calcimimetic compound that decreases PTH secretion by activating the parathyroid cell CaSR.[68,69] This medication appears able to control hypercalcemia in patients with primary hyperparathyroidism who refuse or cannot tolerate surgery, but is currently approved for treatment of parathyroid carcinoma or tertiary hyperparathyroidism due to chronic kidney disease.[70]

Hypercalcemia of malignancy responds best to treatment of the underlying cancer. Intravenous bisphosphonates typically work well if the tumor is not able to be controlled by surgery, chemotherapy, or radiation.[65]

Hypocalcemia. A variety of calcium salts are available to treat acute hypocalcemia. Calcium gluconate is typically given intravenously for severe symptomatic hypocalcemia as a 10% solution containing 9.3 mg Ca^{2+}/ml, for a total dose of 10 to 15 mg/kg body weight over 4 to 6 hours. Patients may benefit from more rapid infusion of 10 ml of 10% solution diluted in 50 ml of 5% dextrose in water (D_5W) or 0.9% sodium chloride given by slow injection over more than 5 minutes, with repeat doses as needed to control symptoms. Calcium gluconate should not be given intramuscularly because it may cause abscess formation at the injection site.

Hypocalcemic tetany or laryngospasm may be treated with intravenous calcium chloride. Calcium chloride infusion may cause peripheral vasodilation and result in a cutaneous burning sensation at the infusion site. Extravasation of calcium chloride during infusion causes soft tissue inflammation and necrosis, leading to sloughing of tissue, so many centers now require intravenous calcium chloride to be given through a central venous line. Calcium chloride is usually given as a 10% solution containing 1.36 mEq Ca^{2+}/ml, at a rate of not greater than 1 ml/min to prevent cardiac arrhythmias due to resultant hypercalcemia. Calcium chloride infusion may cause a moderate decrease in blood pressure due to associated vasodilation.

Calcium gluceptate may be given as a 22% solution containing 18 mg Ca^{2+}/ml in a volume of 5 to 20 ml intravenously for severe hypocalcemic tetany. Rapid intravenous infusion may cause pain or tingling in the vein used for infusion. Gluteal intramuscular injections of calcium gluceptate may be given at up to 5 ml if intravenous infusion is not an option.

Oral calcium supplementation is usually sufficient to control milder or more chronic hypocalcemic symptoms, typically with vitamin D supplementation. Hypocalcemia due to hypoparathyroidism is usually treated with high-dose oral calcium and vitamin D supplementation. Calcium salts stimulate gastric acid secretion, and patients may find that calcium supplementation worsens hyperacidity or reflux. Oral calcium is available as calcium carbonate, calcium citrate, calcium phosphate, calcium lactate, or calcium gluconate. Calcium carbonate is widely used since it is commonly available and inexpensive, but it requires adequate stomach acid to digest the tablet before calcium can be absorbed. Calcium citrate does not require stomach acid digestion prior to absorption. Hypocalcemic patients are usually treated with 1 to 2 g of elemental calcium per day, but may require as much as 3 to 5 g/day for adequate control in more severe cases.

Calcium carbonate or acetate may be used to decrease intestinal phosphorus absorption in patients with chronic kidney disease, or oxalate absorption in inflammatory bowel disease. Intravenous calcium gluconate may be infused to prevent cardiorespiratory arrest in patients with serum K^+ greater than 7.0 mmol/l. Calcium in this situation reverses the cardiac effects of hyperkalemia, which may allow time to reduce serum potassium by other means. Intravenous calcium is approved for treatment of black widow spider bites and magnesium toxicity.

Vitamin D

Vitamin D preparations are used for a variety of purposes in disorders of bone and mineral metabolism. Vitamin D is commonly used to prevent or treat nutritional rickets. Vitamin D is also used to treat other types of rickets or osteomalacia, particularly osteomalacia in patients with chronic kidney disease. Vitamin D is helpful in treating hypoparathyroidism, and recommended for treatment of most forms of osteoporosis.

The optimal intake of vitamin D remains controversial. The current recommended daily allowance of vitamin D for infants and children is 400 international units (IU) (10 mcg), based on the historical observation that 1 teaspoon of cod liver oil each day, which contains 400 IU of vitamin D, was safe and effective in curing rickets in children.[71] The current recommended daily allowance of vitamin D for adults less than 50 years is arbitrarily set at 200 IU, based on the fact that adults require less vitamin D than children.

The Food and Nutrition Board of the U.S. Institute of Medicine published Dietary Reference Intakes for vitamin D in 1997.[72] Vitamin D intake of 200 IU/day was recommended for healthy adults through age 50 years, 400 IU/day for adults from age 50 to 70 years, and 600 IU/day for adults over 70 years. Pregnant or lactating women may require as much as 1000 IU/day to maintain optimal serum 25-hydroxyvitamin D levels of greater than 30 ng/ml (75 nmol/L). Doses of vitamin D as high as 10,000 IU/day do not typically cause vitamin D toxicity. Vitamin D toxicity is usually associated with serum 25-hydroxyvitamin D levels greater than 120 ng/ml.

Vitamin D is available in a variety of oral or intravenous preparations. Vitamin D_2 (ergocalciferol) or vitamin D_3 (cholecalciferol) may be given orally to prevent vitamin D deficiency and to treat familial hypophosphatemia, hypoparathyroidism, and hereditary vitamin D–resistant rickets (previously known as vitamin D–dependent rickets type II), at doses of 25,000 to 100,000 IU from once each day to three times each week.

Calcitriol (Rocaltrol, Calcijex) is water soluble and may be given orally or intravenously. Calcitriol-induced hypercalcemia resolves quickly once it is stopped, which helps prevent persistent hypercalcemia that may last for months in patients toxic from fat-soluble forms of vitamin D.

Vitamin D Analogues

Figure 39-7 shows the structures of several available vitamin D analogues. Doxercalciferol (1α-hydroxyvitamin D_2; Hectorol) is activated by liver 25-hydroxylase to form 1,25-dihydroxyvitamin D_2, and approved for oral or intravenous treatment of secondary hyperparathyroidism. Doxercalciferol is available as 0.5- and 2.5-mcg capsules and a solution containing 2 mcg/ml for infusion, and usually given orally or intravenously at 10 to 20 mcg three times a week.

Dihydrotachysterol (DHT) is a reduced form of vitamin D_2 that is converted in the liver to the active form of 25-hydroxytachysterol. DHT has less than 1% the activity of calcitriol in stimulating intestinal calcium absorption, but significantly more effect in stimulation of skeletal release of calcium at high doses, so is often used to treat refractory rickets, hypoparathyroidism, or renal osteodystrophy. Oral DHT increases serum calcium maximally after 2 weeks of daily treatment, and is available as 0.125-, 0.2-, and 0.4-mg capsules. It is typically given as 0.2 to 1.0 mg/day. The hypercalcemic effect of this water-soluble vitamin D analogue wears off 2 to 4 weeks after it is stopped.

1α-Hydroxycholecalciferol (alphacalcidol) is a synthetic analogue of 1,25-dihydroxyvitamin D_3 approved for use in Europe and elsewhere, but not in the United States. Alfacalcidol is 25-hydroxylated in the liver

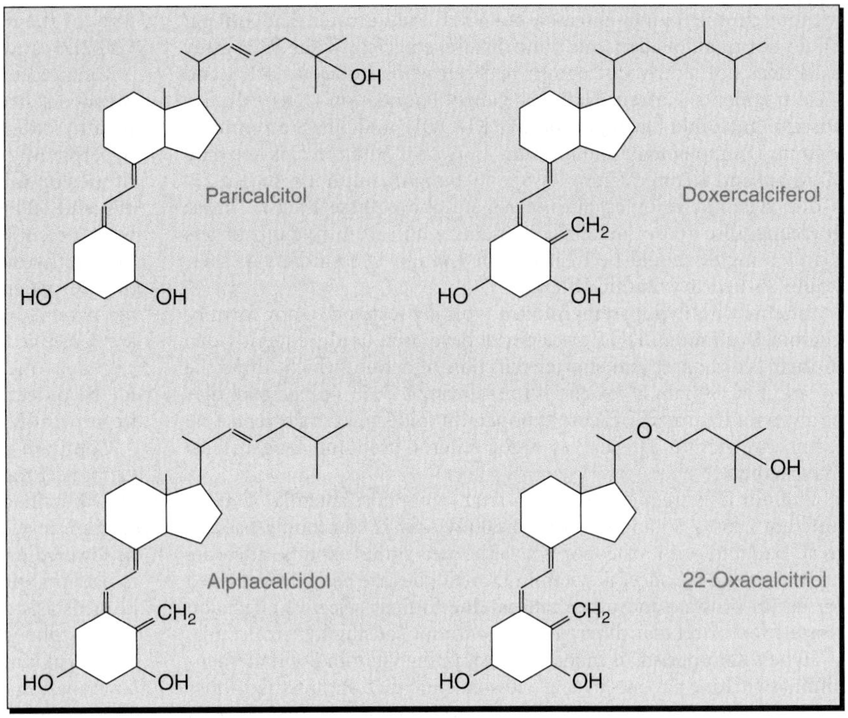

FIGURE 39-7 • Vitamin D analogues.

to form 1,25-dihydroxyvitamin D_3, and is equally effective as 1,25-dihydroxyvitamin D_3 in stimulating intestinal calcium absorption and promoting bone mineralization. It has the advantage of not requiring renal 1α-hydroxylation, so may be used to treat renal osteodystrophy.

Calcipotriol (calcipotriene) is a synthetic calcitriol analogue with a modified side chain containing a C22-C23 double bond, 24(S)-hydroxyl group, and cyclopropane ring containing C25-C27. Calcipotriol binds to the VDR with equal affinity as calcitriol, but stimulates intestinal calcium absorption with less than 1% of the effect of calcitriol. It is approved for treatment of psoriasis (see Chapter 71, Psoriasis), and is available as a topical preparation (Dovonex) for this purpose. It appears to be slightly more effective than glucocorticoids in treating psoriasis.

Paricalcitol (Zemplar) is a synthetic calcitriol analogue lacking the exocyclic C19, and containing the D2 rather than the D3 side chain. It binds to the PTH gene vitamin D response element and directly suppresses PTH transcription without stimulating intestinal calcium or phosphorus absorption.[73] Paricalcitol is available as 1-, 2-, and 4-mcg capsules and a 5-mcg/ml solution for intravenous infusion, and is usually given as 2 to 4 mcg orally three times each week, or started at 0.04 to 0.1 mcg/kg intravenously every other day and titrated up to 0.24 mcg/kg every other day as needed. Paricalcitol is approved to treat secondary hyperparathyroidism.

22-Oxacalcitriol (maxicalcitol; Oxarol) is a synthetic calcitriol analogue with an oxygen atom substituted for C22, with low affinity for vitamin D–binding protein and more rapid metabolism than calcitriol. 22-Oxacalcitriol potently suppresses PTH transcription and has limited intestinal or bone effects. It is available orally, but not yet approved to treat secondary hyperparathyroidism.

Therapeutic Uses of Vitamin D

Nutritional rickets develops due to inadequate sunlight exposure or lack of adequate intake of vitamin D in the diet. This condition was once thought to be rare in the United States and other developed countries where vitamin D has been added to various foods, but is now increasing in prevalence again.[31,34,35] Infants fed breast milk or formula without vitamin D supplementation are advised to take vitamin D supplementation of 400 IU/day. Vitamins D and A are often given in combination due to the availability of preparations containing both vitamins. Since the fetal skeleton acquires more than 85% of its calcium content during the third trimester, premature infants are at risk of rickets and may benefit from vitamin D supplementation. Treatment of developed rickets requires larger doses of vitamin D than required for prevention. Treatment of patients with rickets with vitamin D 1000 IU/day normalizes serum calcium and phosphorus levels within about 10 days, and usually heals radiographic evidence of rickets after about 3 weeks. Larger doses of vitamin D, such as 3000 to 4000 IU/day, may be given to promote more rapid healing of rickets, especially if associated with respiratory compromise due to rickets affecting the rib cage. Oral or intravenous vitamin D preparations may be given to prevent or treat vitamin D deficiency associated with intestinal malabsorption, such as occurs with gastric bypass surgery, pancreatic insufficiency, or celiac disease.

Osteomalacia associated with renal osteodystrophy may benefit from treatment with vitamin D. Osteomalacia is characterized by excessive accumulation of unmineralized bone matrix (osteoid) throughout the skeleton. It most often is due to vitamin D or phosphorus deficiency. Replacement with vitamin D and adequate phosphorus typically allows osteomalacia to heal over several weeks to months.

Renal osteodystrophy is the term used to describe the spectrum of bone disease in patients with chronic kidney disease, which ranges from high-turnover hyperparathyroidism to low-turnover adynamic bone disease. The approach to treatment of renal osteodystrophy depends on the predominant form of bone disease present. High-turnover bone disease with low bone density due to hyperparathyroidism and 1,25-dihydroxyvitamin D deficiency benefits from dietary phosphate restriction, non–aluminum-containing phosphate binders, and calcitriol in some cases. Overuse of calcium-containing phosphate binders and calcitriol may lead to suppression of PTH into the normal range for patients without chronic kidney disease, which may lead to adynamic bone disease due to skeletal resistance to PTH action. Sevelamer hydrochloride (RenaGel) is a nonabsorbable phosphate-binding polymer composed of cross-linked poly[allylamine hydrochloride], which is approved for lowering serum phosphorus levels in patients on dialysis treatment.[74] Sevelamer may cause nausea, vomiting, diarrhea, or dyspepsia, but does not affect absorption of commonly used medications such as digoxin or warfarin. Adynamic bone disease is more likely to be present when serum PTH levels are less than 100 pg/ml (with a normal range of 10 to 65 pg/ml in patients without chronic kidney disease), but PTH levels greater than 100 pg/ml do not rule out adynamic bone disease, especially if the PTH assay used does not clearly distinguish between whole-molecule PTH and PTH fragments. Current National Kidney Foundation (NKF) Kidney Disease Outcomes Quality Initiative (KDOQI) guidelines recommend vitamin D supplementation if serum 25-hydroxyvitamin D is less than 30 ng/ml and serum calcium less than 9.5 mg/dl, but not if serum 25-hydroxyvitamin D or calcium levels are above these levels.[75] These guidelines also recommend that patients with serum calcium of less than 9.5 mg/dl should be treated with vitamin D regardless of their serum 25-hydroxyvitamin D level.

Patients with hypoparathyroidism typically respond to any form of vitamin D, although DHT or calcitriol have been used frequently due to their faster onset and shorter duration of action, which limits the duration of vitamin D toxicity if this develops. DHT or calcitriol may be given for treatment of acute hypoparathyroidism, with slower acting forms of vitamin D such as ergocalciferol used for longer term management.

Vitamin D is frequently used to treat hypophosphatemia of many different causes. Vitamin D 400 to 800 IU/day is commonly used to treat patients with osteoporosis, although some experts advocate higher doses. Noncalcemic vitamin D analogues are being investigated for use in prostate and other cancers due to their selective effects on stimulation of cellular differentiation without causing hypercalcemia.

Hypervitaminosis D is managed by stopping vitamin D supplementation, switching patients over to a low-calcium diet, starting high-dose glucocorticoids to block calcium absorption and stimulate renal calcium excretion, and increasing oral fluid intake or starting intravenous fluids. With treatment, serum calcium gradually improves toward normal, soft tissue calcium deposits are mobilized, and renal dysfunction improves toward normal.

Calcimimetics

Calcimimetics are CaSR agonists that act like calcium, thereby inhibiting PTH secretion by the parathyroid glands.[76] These agents increase the sensitivity of the CaSR to extracellular calcium, leading to lowering of the extracellular calcium level at which PTH secretion is suppressed. Type II calcimimetics are longer acting phenylalkylamine analogues of the shorter acting type I calcimimetics such as NPS R-568, which was designed based on the structure of fendiline and other agents that block voltage-sensitive calcium channels.[77]

Cinacalcet (Sensipar) is approved for treatment of secondary hyperparathyroidism due to chronic kidney disease[78] and control of hypercalcemia in parathyroid carcinoma.[79] Figure 39-8 shows the structure of cinacalcet. Cinacalcet also lowers serum calcium and PTH levels in patients with normal renal function, and doses of 20 to 100 mg/day lower PTH levels in a dose-dependent manner. Cinacalcet has been shown to normalize PTH levels in primary hyperparathyroidism for up to 3 years.[69] Resistance to cinacalcet has not yet been reported. It has not yet been established that cinacalcet reduces long-term outcomes of chronic kidney disease, such as increased mortality, cardiovascular disease, or hyperparathyroidism-induced bone disease.

Cinacalcet is synthesized as a racemic mixture of optical isomers. The (*R*-) enantiomer is 10- to 100-fold more potent in humans than the (*S*-) enantiomer. Cinacalcet exhibits first-order absorption kinetics with oral dosing, with peak serum levels achieved 2 to 6 hours after administration, and maximum PTH suppression within 2 to 4 hours. The plasma half-life of cinacalcet is between 30 and 40 hours, with 85% of the drug absorbed cleared by the kidneys. Hepatic CYP3A4, CYP2D5, and CYP1A2 enzymes metabolize cinacalcet.

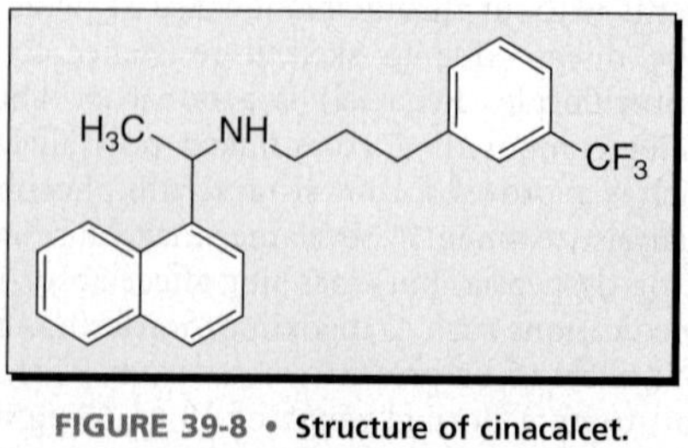

FIGURE 39-8 • Structure of cinacalcet.

Cinacalcet is available as 30-, 60-, and 90-mg tablets, with the recommended starting dose of 30 mg/day in patients with secondary hyperparathyroidism, and 30 mg twice daily in patients with primary hyperparathyroidism or parathyroid carcinoma. The initial dose is titrated upward every 2 to 4 weeks to achieve serum PTH levels between 150 and 300 pg/ml in secondary hyperparathyroidism in accordance with current NKF KDOQI guidelines, and to normalize serum calcium in parathyroid carcinoma. The maximum dose for chronic kidney disease patients on dialysis is 180 mg/day, and the maximum dose for patients with parathyroid carcinoma 360 mg/day. Some patients are sensitive to low-dose cinacalcet and develop symptomatic hypocalcemia on low daily doses, and 30 mg every other day appears to be effective for some patients with primary or secondary hyperparathyroidism.

Common side effects of cinacalcet are hypocalcemia and nausea. Cinacalcet should not be used if serum calcium is less than 8.4 mg/dl, and the cinacalcet dose should be lowered or stopped if the serum calcium level is lower than the normal range. Cinacalcet should also be lowered or stopped if serum PTH decreases to less than 150 pg/ml in patients with chronic kidney disease. Medications that affect calcium homeostasis or hinder cinacalcet absorption, such as vitamin D analogues, phosphate binders, bisphosphonates, calcitonin, glucocorticoids, gallium nitrate, or cisplatin, should be used with caution in combination with cinacalcet. Medications metabolized by CYP3A4, CYP2D5, or CYP1A2 enzymes may affect cinacalcet levels.

Calcilytics

Calcilytic compounds have the opposite effect of calcimimetic compounds on the CaSR, and cause allosteric inhibition of the CaSR, which leads to increased PTH secretion.[77] These CaSR antagonists potentially could be used as anabolic agents to treat osteoporosis, or to stimulate PTH secretion in patients with hypoparathyroidism. Calcilytics are also synthesized as racemic mixtures of optical isomers, with the (*R*-) enantiomer being more potent in humans. Calcilytic compounds derived from NPS 2143 stimulate PTH secretion under normal calcium concentrations, but are not active under very low or very high calcium concentrations. Human clinical trials have not yet been conducted with calcilytic agents, and they are not further discussed here.

Anticatabolic Agents

Bisphosphonates. Bisphosphonates are pyrophosphate analogues with a central phosphorus-carbon-phosphorus bond resistant to biologic degradation.[80] The geminal carbon atom in these compounds binds to R1 and R2 moieties. Figure 39-9 shows the structures of available bisphosphonates. The R1 moiety in second- and third-generation bisphosphonates typically is a hydroxyl group, to increase avidity of binding to hydroxyapatite, and the R2 moiety an amino-containing side chain, which increases drug potency. When bisphosphonates are added to solutions or suspensions of calcium phosphate, hydroxyapatite crystal formation slows and previously formed crystals dissolve. These compounds bind avidly to hydroxyapatite while potently inhibiting bone resorption, and therefore remain in the skeleton for several years.

Bisphosphonates are highly negatively charged membrane-impermeable compounds, so only a very small percentage of the administered dose (<1% of an alendronate or risedronate dose, and <6% of an etidronate or tiludronate dose) is absorbed. Oral bisphosphonates in clinical use are recommended to be taken with a full 8-ounce glass of water on an empty stomach, at least 30 minutes before other food or medication, with advice to remain upright for at least 30 minutes after a dose. Absorbed bisphosphonate concentrates in skeletal remodeling sites, and is incorporated into the bone matrix by fluid-phase endocytosis,[81] where it remains until the bone matrix is remodeled. During resorption, bisphosphonates incorporated in bone matrix are released into the resorption lacunae beneath osteoclasts, from where they are taken up by osteoclasts to inhibit osteoclast activity and/or cause osteoclast apoptosis.

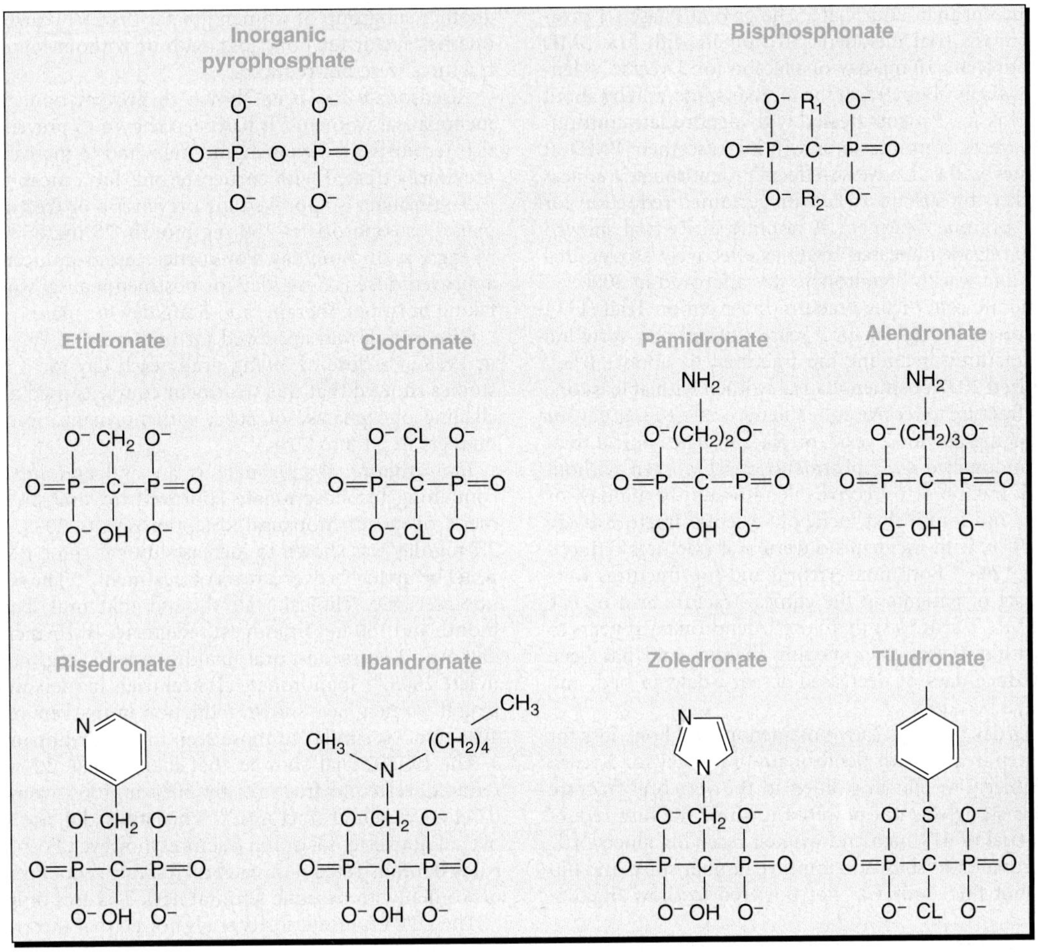

Inorganic pyrophosphate

Bisphosphonate

Etidronate

Clodronate

Pamidronate

Alendronate

Risedronate

Ibandronate

Zoledronate

Tiludronate

FIGURE 39-9 • Bisphosphonate structures.

Etidronate was the first bisphosphonate developed for clinical use, and this was designed specifically to inhibit mineralization in patients with ectopic mineralization in soft tissues. Other first-generation bisphosphonates, including clodronate and tiludronate, have modest anticatabolic effect. Later second- and third-generation bisphosphonates were designed to minimize inhibition of mineralization and to maximally inhibit osteoclast bone resorption. Second-generation bisphosphonates, such as alendronate and pamidronate, have a nitrogen-containing R2 side chain, and are 10 to 100 times more potent than etidronate at inhibiting osteoclasts. Third-generation bisphosphonates have their R2-side chain nitrogen contained within a heterocyclic ring, and are up to 10,000 times more potent than etidronate.

Nitrogen-containing bisphosphonates inhibit farnesyl pyrophosphate synthase in the hydroxymethylglutaryl coenzyme A reductase pathway, which leads to decreased posttranslational prenylation of small membrane-bound GTP-binding proteins such as ras, rab, and rho.[80] Reduced prenylation of these proteins causes reduced osteoclast bone resorption and accelerated osteoclast apoptosis. These actions do not require osteoclast apoptosis.[82] Non–nitrogen-containing bisphosphonates produce toxic analogues of ATP that lead to osteoclast apoptosis.[83]

Bisphosphonates are excreted mainly by the kidneys. Dose adjustment guidelines for renal insufficiency have been advised for multiple myeloma patients receiving zoledronic acid. Alendronate should not be given if the creatinine clearance is less than 35 ml/min; all other approved oral and intravenous bisphosphonates should not be used if creatinine clearance is less than 30 ml/min.

The major side effect of oral bisphosphonates is upper gastrointestinal irritation, which occurred in as many as 30% of patients during clinical trials. Gastrointestinal symptoms may be treated successfully with proton pump inhibitors or histamine$_2$-receptor blockers in some cases. Other side effects may include esophageal or stomach ulcers or diarrhea. Intravenous bisphosphonates may cause a self-limited tumor necrosis factor-α–associated systemic inflammatory response associated with low-grade fever, myalgias, and arthralgias starting within several hours of the first dose in 10% to 15% of patients that typically resolves spontaneously within 48 hours after the dose. Premedication with prednisone or aspirin may help prevent this reaction in some patients. Intravenous zoledronic acid may cause renal dysfunction in some patients when given rapidly over less than 15 minutes. Osteonecrosis of the jaw is reported in 1% to 10% of cancer patients receiving monthly intravenous bisphosphonates, typically over 2 to 3 years, for multiple myeloma or skeletal breast or prostate cancer metastases, but appears to be very rare in patients taking oral bisphosphonates for postmenopausal osteoporosis.

Bisphosphonates prevent bone loss caused by normal aging, estrogen deficiency, and glucocorticoid therapy, and prevent fractures in patients with postmenopausal osteoporosis and women and men with glucocorticoid-induced osteoporosis. Oral alendronate, risedronate, and ibandronate are currently approved by the FDA for prevention and treatment of osteoporosis. Intravenous zoledronic acid and pamidronate are approved for treatment or prevention of multiple myeloma and skeletal metastases from breast or prostate cancer. Intravenous etidronate, pamidronate, and zoledronic acid are approved for treatment of hypercalcemia of malignancy. Oral alendronate, risedronate, and tiludronate, and intravenous pamidronate, are approved for treatment of Paget's disease of bone.

Alendronate. Alendronate is an oral nitrogen-containing bisphosphonate, and was the first bisphosphonate approved for prevention and treatment of postmenopausal osteoporosis in 1995. Alendronate is 700 times more potent than etidronate. The pivotal Phase III postmenopausal osteoporosis trial included 530 women with low BMD randomized to alendronate 10 mg/day or placebo for 3 years.[84] Alendronate increased BMD by about 9% at the lumbar spine, and by about 6% at the hip over 3 years. Patients treated with alendronate continuously for up to 10 years continue to slowly increase their BMD at different skeletal sites without adverse effect.[85] Alendronate reduces bone turnover markers by 50% to 70%, with sustained reduction for as long as patients continue treatment. A noninferiority trial showed that alendronate 70 mg/wk increased BMD as effectively as alendronate 10 mg/day,[86,87] and weekly alendronate was approved in 2000.

The vertebral fracture arm of the Fracture Intervention Trial (FIT) showed that alendronate 10 mg/day for 3 years reduced new vertebral and nonvertebral fractures, including hip fractures, by about 50%.[88] This study randomized 2027 postmenopausal women with at least one prevalent vertebral fracture to receive either alendronate 10 mg/day for 1 year, alendronate 5 mg/day for 2 years, or placebo. The clinical fracture arm of FIT randomized 4432 postmenopausal women without prevalent vertebral fractures to receive alendronate 10 mg/day or placebo for 3 years, and found that incident vertebral fractures were reduced by about 50%, with incident nonvertebral fractures reduced by a nonsignificant 12%.[89] Both nonvertebral and hip fractures were reduced in the subset of patients in the clinical fracture arm of FIT with baseline hip BMD T-score less than –2.5. Alendronate appears to reduce fractures within 1 year after starting therapy, and has been demonstrated to reduce days of decreased activity, days in bed, and utilization of hospital bed days.

Alendronate 5 mg/day prevents early postmenopausal bone loss for up to 5 years.[90] In men treated with alendronate 10 mg/day for 2 years, BMD increased similarly to that in women in the vertebral fracture arm of FIT, but this study was not powered to show fracture reduction.[91] In a clinical trial of 477 men and women receiving glucocorticoid therapy, alendronate was shown to improve lumbar spine and hip BMD over 1 year, but this study was not powered to show fracture reduction.[92]

Alendronate is approved for treatment of postmenopausal osteoporosis at 70 mg/wk or 10 mg/day, and for prevention of postmenopausal osteoporosis at 35 mg/wk or 5 mg/day. For glucocorticoid-induced osteoporosis, the approved dose is 10 mg/day for postmenopausal women not on estrogen, and 5 mg/day for postmenopausal women on estrogen and for men.

Alendronate was approved for treatment of Paget's disease of bone in the fall of 1995 at a dose of 40 mg/day orally for 6 months, based on a study of 89 patients with moderate to severe Paget's disease who were randomized to receive alendronate 40 mg/day or etidronate 400 mg/day for 6 months.[93] Alendronate normalized serum alkaline phosphatase in more than 63%, compared to 17% for etidronate. Alendronate decreased serum alkaline phosphatase by 79%, compared to 44% for etidronate. A 6-month course of alendronate may induce a remission of Paget's disease lasting 12 to 18 months.

Risedronate. Risedronate is an oral nitrogen-containing bisphosphonate approved for prevention and treatment of postmenopausal osteoporosis in 1998. Risedronate is 1000 times more potent than etidronate. Risedronate 5 mg/day for 3 years increased lumbar spine BMD by 5%, and hip BMD by up to 4% in postmenopausal women, and decreased markers of bone turnover by 40% to 60% for as long as treatment was given.[94] Risedronate 35 mg/wk was shown to be equivalent to 5 mg/day in a noninferiority study, and approved in 2003.[95]

Risedronate was shown to reduce vertebral fractures by about 50% in two 3-year clinical trials involving a total of 3600 postmenopausal women with at least one baseline prevalent vertebral fracture.[94,96] Vertebral fracture reduction was evident by 1 year of therapy. One of these studies showed nonvertebral fracture reduction by 39%.[94] The Hip Intervention Program clinical trial randomized 9331 women over age 70 to risedronate 2.5 mg/day or 5 mg/day, or placebo, and found that hip fractures were reduced by 30% overall in the combined treatment arms compared to placebo.[97] In a subgroup of women ages 70 to 79 years with baseline hip BMD T-scores of less than –3.0, with at least one risk factor for bone loss, hip fractures were reduced by 40%. In another subgroup of women greater than 80 years of age with at least one risk factor for bone loss, with or without low baseline hip BMD, fractures were not reduced.

Risedronate has been shown to prevent bone loss in early postmenopausal women.[98] It has been shown to prevent bone loss in corticosteroid-treated women and men, and to increase BMD in patients previously treated with corticosteroids for a mean of 5 years.[99]

Risedronate is approved for prevention or treatment of postmenopausal osteoporosis at 150 mg/month, 75 mg/day for 2 days/month, 35 mg/wk, or 5 mg/day. For corticosteroid-induced osteoporosis, the approved dose is 5 mg/day for postmenopausal women taking or not taking hormone therapy, and 5 mg/day for men.

Risedronate was approved for treatment of Paget's disease of bone in 1998 at a dose of 30 mg orally each day for 2 months.[100] Clinical studies showed that this treatment course caused a decrease in serum alkaline phosphatase of 80%, with normalization of bone turnover markers in 50% to 70%.

Ibandronate. Ibandronate is an oral and intravenous nitrogen-containing bisphosphonate approved for oral prevention and treatment of postmenopausal osteoporosis in 2003. Oral ibandronate 2.5 mg/day was shown to increase lumbar spine BMD by 5% and hip BMD by up to 4% over 3 years of treatment.[101] The subsequent MOBILE noninferiority clinical trial showed that oral ibandronate 100 mg/month and 150 mg/month caused greater BMD increases than 2.5 mg/day over 2 years, and oral ibandronate 150 mg/month was approved in late 2005.[102] Ibandronate clinical trials in men and early postmenopausal women have shown reduction in markers of bone turnover of 40% to 60%, similar to those seen in postmenopausal women.

The BONE trial showed that ibandronate 2.5 mg/day for 3 years reduced vertebral fractures by 50% in 1964 women with prevalent baseline vertebral fractures.[101] This study did not show reduction in overall nonvertebral or hip fractures, however. Post-hoc analysis of this study demonstrated nonvertebral fracture reduction of 69% in a subset of women with baseline femoral neck T-scores of less than –3.0.

The DIVA noninferiority trial showed that intravenous ibandronate 3 mg over 15 to 30 seconds every 3 months for 2 years was more effective at preventing bone loss than oral ibandronate 2.5 mg/day.[103] Markers of bone turnover were suppressed by intravenous ibandronate for up to 3 months. This trial was not powered to show fracture reduction. A previous study of intravenous ibandronate 1 mg every 3 months demonstrated an increase of lumbar spine BMD of 2.9%, but did not show fracture reduction, perhaps because markers of bone turnover did not remain completely suppressed between doses.[104]

Oral ibandronate is approved for prevention and treatment of postmenopausal osteoporosis at 2.5 mg/day or 150 mg/month, and intravenous ibandronate at 3 mg over 15 to 30 seconds every 3 months.

Etidronate. Etidronate was the first oral bisphosphonate approved for treating patients with metabolic bone disease in the United States in 1983, and is the least potent bisphosphonate currently available in the United States. It is available as 200- and 400-mg tablets. Because higher doses of 20 mg/kg per day may cause inhibition of mineralization, it was investigated for use in postmenopausal osteoporosis in a cyclical intermittent regimen of 400 mg/day (5 mg/kg per day) orally for 2 weeks every 3 months.[105,106] Clinical studies demonstrated improved BMD, but were not powered to show fracture reduction. Cyclical intermittent etidronate has been shown to prevent bone loss in early postmenopausal women[107] and patients with glucocorticoid-induced osteoporosis.[108] One small open study showed improved BMD in men.

Etidronate is approved for treatment of Paget's disease of bone[109,110] and hypercalcemia of malignancy, but not osteoporosis. Etidronate is given to patients with Paget's disease at a daily dose of 400 mg (5 mg/kg per day) for 6 months, with the subsequent 6 months off therapy. This regimen causes a reduction in markers of bone turnover of about 50%. Higher doses may cause inhibition of mineralization. Etidronate is contraindicated in Paget's disease patients with advancing lytic lesions in weight-bearing bones.

Tiludronate. Tiludronate is about 10 times more potent than etidronate, but does not cause a mineralization defect at the clinically approved dose. Tiludronate is not approved for treatment of osteoporosis because fracture reduction was not demonstrated in Phase III clinical trials, perhaps because the dose used was too small. Tiludronate was approved for treatment of Paget's disease in 1997, and is available in 200-mg tablets. Two tablets are given once a day for 3 months, with a posttreatment drug-free interval of 3 months. Clinical trials with tiludronate showed that serum total alkaline phosphatase normalized in 24% to 35% of patients with moderately active Paget's disease.[111,112] The duration of effect is estimated to be 3 to 4 months. Tiludronate appears to have efficacy similar to etidronate, but without causing a mineralization defect.

Pamidronate. Pamidronate is not approved for treatment of osteoporosis, but is approved for treatment of hypercalcemia of malignancy and Paget's disease of bone. Intravenous pamidronate increases BMD or prevents bone loss in postmenopausal osteoporosis,[113] in early menopausal women, and in patients with corticosteroid-induced osteoporosis.[114] Pamidronate is usually given off-label to women with postmenopausal osteoporosis not able to tolerate other therapies as 60 to 90 mg intravenously over 2 to 4 hours. Pamidronate 30 mg may be given intravenously over 2 hours.[115] Oral pamidronate is available in Europe and other countries, but not in the United States.

Pamidronate is about 100 times as potent as etidronate, and was approved in 1995 for intravenous treatment of Paget's disease and hypercalcemia of malignancy. It is commonly given to patients with mild to moderate Paget's disease as 30 to 90 mg intravenously in 300 to 500 ml normal saline or D_5W over 2 to 4 hours every 3 months.[116,117] The FDA-approved dose is 30 mg intravenously in 300 to 500 ml normal saline or D_5W over 4 hours each day for 3 days sequentially, but this regimen is impractical for many patients. Patients with moderate to severe Paget's disease may require multiple infusions of 60 to 90 mg over 2 hours each week for several weeks. Markers of bone turnover are typically suppressed within several days of an infusion, but serum alkaline phosphatase may take as long as 2 to 3 weeks to reach its nadir. A successful course of therapy may normalize markers of bone turnover and suppress disease activity for up to 1 year. Side effects include low-grade fever, myalgias, arthralgias, and flulike symptoms within the first 48 hours of infusion. Subsequent doses are less likely to cause flulike symptoms. Pamidronate may cause mild and transient hypocalcemia, hypophosphatemia, and lymphopenia, so patients should be calcium and vitamin D replete before each infusion. Patients may develop resistance to pamidronate over time.

Zoledronic Acid. Zoledronic acid is the most potent intravenous bisphosphonate currently available. It is approved for treatment of hypercalcemia of malignancy, and prevention or treatment of skeletal metastases. A Phase II study showed that zoledronic acid 4 mg once a year increased bone density and reduced bone turnover for at least 12 months.[118] Phase III clinical trials in postmenopausal osteoporosis and Paget's disease were recently completed. The Phase III fracture reduction trial involving over 7700 postmenopausal women randomized to zoledronic acid 5 mg intravenously once a year or placebo for 3 years demonstrated 70% reduction in vertebral fractures and 40% reduction in hip fractures.[119] Markers of bone turnover were suppressed as expected. Side effects included low-grade fever and flulike symptoms in 15% of patients with the first infusion, with 1% to 3% of patients having symptoms with their second or third infusions.

A Phase III clinical trial in Paget's disease of bone in which 357 patients were randomized to zoledronic acid 5 mg over 15 minutes once a year or risedronate 30 mg/day orally for 2 months showed that 89% of patients treated with zoledronic acid, and 58% of patients with risedronate, had normal serum alkaline phosphatase levels within 6 months.[120] The main side effect was low-grade fever and flulike symptoms in about 10% of patients, and bone pain in 5% of patients within the first 48 hours of treatment.

The FDA approved zoledronic acid 5 mg intravenously over 15 minutes once a year for treatment of postmenopausal osteoporosis, and 5 mg intravenously over 15 minutes intermittently as needed for treatment of Paget's disease.

Estrogen or Hormone Therapy. Estrogen therapy has a variety of benefits for calcium metabolism and bone mineralization, among its many effects on many tissues, and aspects pertinent to bone and mineral metabolism are reviewed here. Estrogen therapy was first demonstrated to prevent calcium loss in postmenopausal women with osteoporotic fractures by Fuller Albright in 1947.[60,121] Since the 1970s, controlled clinical trials have convincingly shown that estrogen therapy prevents bone loss in estrogen-deficient women. Estrogen, or estrogen plus progestin, has historically been given as conjugated equine estrogen at 0.625 mg/day or the equivalent with the goal of decreasing bone remodeling to premenopausal levels.

Three small controlled studies have shown that estrogen therapy reduces fracture risk. The first demonstrated that transdermal estrogen reduced vertebral fracture risk by 50% over 2 years of therapy.[122] The other two studies showed that oral estrogen over 9 to 10 years reduced radiologic vertebral fractures and clinical fractures.[123,124] During the time these studies were conducted, multiple large epidemiologic studies suggested that estrogen treatment reduced clinical fracture risk, including hip and nonvertebral fracture risk, in postmenopausal women.[125-128] Some concern was raised that the results of these studies were influenced by the fact that women taking hormone therapy are generally healthier and exhibit more health-seeking behaviors than those who do not.[129]

Two larger European clinical trials showed that estrogen and progestin therapy prevented Colles' and clinical nonvertebral fractures in early postmenopausal women.[130,131] Two subsequent National Institutes of Health–funded studies in the United States, the Postmenopausal Estrogen/Progestin Intervention (PEPI) study and the Women's Health Initiative (WHI) study, were designed to determine the effects of estrogen with or without progestin on bone density[132] and clinical fractures in women, respectively.[133-135] The PEPI study showed that conjugated equine estrogen 0.625 mg/day for 3 years in 800 early postmenopausal women prevented bone loss, and that addition of medroxyprogesterone acetate or microionized progesterone had no effect on BMD.[132] More than 90% of postmenopausal women receiving estrogen in this study did not lose BMD, and stopping estrogen caused bone loss to recur. The Heart and Estrogen/Progestin Replacement Study (HERS) was published after the PEPI study, and showed that estrogen therapy in postmenopausal women with established cardiovascular disease failed to prevent either fractures or adverse cardiovascular events. The HERS study remains the only large randomized controlled trial of estrogen that did not demonstrate fracture reduction.[136]

The WHI clinical trial evaluated the effects of conjugated equine estrogens or conjugated equine estrogens plus medroxyprogesterone acetate on fractures in postmenopausal women with a mean age of 62 years, and demonstrated fracture reduction as expected from previous observational and randomized controlled trials. The first WHI cohort of 16,000 postmenopausal women was treated with conjugated equine estrogens 0.625 mg/day and medroxyprogesterone acetate 2.5 mg/day for 8 years,[133,134] and the second cohort of 10,000 hysterectomized women was treated with conjugated equine estrogens alone at 0.625 mg/day for 8 years.[135] The combination estrogen plus progestin study was stopped at 5.2 years due to increased global risk due to combination therapy. The estrogen-alone study was stopped at 6.2 years due to increased stroke risk, but interpretation of this study is complicated by the fact that more than 50% of trial participants discontinued the study or were lost to follow-up by the time the study was halted. Overall fracture risk was reduced by 24% in both cohorts, even though subjects were not recruited based on baseline bone density or previous fractures. Despite the fact that bone density was measured in only 10% of subjects in the combination therapy study, and only 9% were found to have osteoporosis, hip and clinical vertebral fractures decreased by 30%. Vertebral morphometric fractures were not assessed by spine films in the WHI study. Combination hormone therapy was associated with increased risk of myocardial infarction, stroke, deep venous thrombosis, pulmonary embolism, and breast cancer, and decreased risk of colon cancer.[133,134] Estrogen therapy alone was associated with increased risk of deep venous thrombosis, pulmonary embolism, and stroke.[135]

Because of concerns regarding the adverse outcomes seen in the WHI studies, low-dose hormone therapy has been advocated for patients with vasomotor instability. Two studies done in the early 1980s with conjugated equine estrogen did not show prevention of bone loss sufficient to reduce fractures, and it was presumed that low-dose hormone therapy would have no skeletal benefit.[137,138] More recent studies with low-dose estrogen have suggested that there may be some benefit. A large population-based study showed that postmenopausal women with serum estradiol levels of 10 to 15 pg/ml had higher bone density levels than postmenopausal women with serum estradiol levels of less than 5 pg/ml, and that women with the lowest serum estradiol levels had the highest risk of vertebral and hip fractures.[139]

Low-dose estrogen therapy has been shown to reduce bone remodeling at all doses of conjugated equine estrogens used, regardless of whether a progestin is added or not. One study showed that markers of bone turnover were only slightly less suppressed with 0.3 mg/day compared to 0.625 mg/day, and that bone density increased at all doses, with more than 90% of subjects responding to treatment by either maintaining or gaining bone density at the lumbar spine and hip.[140] Another study with ultra-low-dose transdermal estrogen of 0.014 mg/day showed reduction in markers of bone turnover and prevention of bone loss.[141]

Stopping postmenopausal hormone therapy causes bone loss to begin immediately, but it is not yet clear that the rate of bone loss occurring after discontinuation of hormone therapy is as high as it is after ovariectomy.[142-144] Some studies have found that fracture risk increases immediately after stopping postmenopausal estrogen or hormone therapy, whereas other studies have demonstrated a more prolonged reduction in fracture risk after therapy is stopped.[145,146]

Since the WHI study findings were published, treatment guidelines have recommended that estrogen or hormone therapy be given only to early postmenopausal women with intolerable hot flashes or other vasomotor symptoms, and then only at the lowest dose tolerated for as short a time as possible. Early postmenopausal women of age less than 55 years may have less risk of adverse outcomes than seen in the WHI. The benefits and risks of other hormone preparations may be quite different than for conjugated equine estrogens and medroxyprogesterone acetate, but these have not been investigated in detail.

SERMs. Selective estrogen receptor modulators are estrogen-like compounds that bind to estrogen receptors with tissue-specific actions. These agents may cause benefits of estrogen action in certain tissues, and minimize the risk of estrogen action in other tissues.[147] Raloxifene is a polyhydroxylated nonsteroidal compound with a benzothiophene core that has high affinity for both estrogen receptor (ER)α and ERβ.[148] Raloxifene is approved for prevention and treatment of osteoporosis.

Raloxifene acts as a partial estrogen agonist in bone, and therefore causes an anticatabolic effect on bone resorption. Raloxifene 60 mg/day increases lumbar spine BMD by 2% and reduces vertebral fractures by 30%, whereas raloxifene 120 mg/day reduces vertebral fractures by 50%, in postmenopausal women.[149,150] Raloxifene modestly lowers serum total and low-density lipoprotein cholesterol, but does not increase high-density lipoprotein cholesterol or normalize increased serum plasminogen activator inhibitor-1 in postmenopausal women.[150] Raloxifene does not appear to cause proliferation or thickening of the endometrium. Raloxifene reduces the risk of ER-positive breast cancers, but not ER-negative cancers, in postmenopausal women at high risk,[151] and does not increase cardiovascular risks in this population. Adverse effects include hot flashes, a threefold increased risk of blood clots, and lower extremity cramps.

Raloxifene binds to the ligand-binding pocket of both ERα and ERβ and competitively inhibits binding of 17β-estradiol. ERα and ERβ are held in tissue-specific conformations prior to ligand binding by association with different co-repressors and coactivators in different target tissues. The ER conformation, and associated co-repressors and coactivators, change depending on the ligand bound, which is thought to explain the tissue-specific actions of different ER ligands.[147]

Raloxifene is absorbed rapidly after oral dosing. It has an absolute bioavailability of about 2%. The half-life of raloxifene is about 28 hours, with metabolism by hepatic glucuronidation, followed by excretion in the bile and stool being the major route of elimination. Raloxifene is not significantly metabolized by the liver CYP system.

Calcitonin. Calcitonin is a peptide hormone that causes lowering of serum calcium in rodents and dogs, but not in humans. It was discovered and named by Copp in 1962, after he demonstrated that perfusion of dog parathyroid and thyroid glands with hypercalcemic blood caused a more rapid and temporary decrease in serum calcium than had been seen in parathyroidectomized animals.[152] Copp interpreted his findings as demonstrating that the parathyroid or thyroid glands produce a calcium-lowering hormone he named calcitonin in response to hypercalcemia, thereby normalizing serum calcium levels. Munson et al. noted that rats parathyroidectomized by cautery developed more severe hypocalcemia than rats undergoing thyroparathyroidectomy, and hypothesized that the thyroid gland in these animals produced a hypocalcemic product. These investigators subsequently demonstrated that thyroid extracts could cause hypocalcemia in rats, and named the putative product thyrocalcitonin. Subsequent studies confirmed that calcitonin and thyrocalcitonin are identical, and that calcitonin is produced by the parafollicular C cells of the thyroid gland, which are derived from neural crest ectoderm. Nonmammalian vertebrates produce calcitonin in their ultimobranchial bodies, which are anatomically distinct from the thyroid gland. Human C cells are distributed in the thyroid, parathyroid, and thymus glands.

Calcitonin is a 32–amino acid single-chain peptide, composed of 8 conserved amino acids including a C-terminal prolinamide and disulfide bridge between cysteines at positions 1 and 7. Both the prolinamide and disulfide bridge are necessary for calcitonin to exert biologic activity. Mid-peptide amino acids are less constant, and contribute to the potency and duration of action of the peptide. Salmon and eel calcitonins are more potent than mammalian calcitonins in mammals, even though they differ from human calcitonin by 13 and 16 amino acids, respectively. Salmon calcitonin is about 20 times more potent that human calcitonin in humans, apparently because it is cleared from the human circulation more slowly than human calcitonin.

The 135–amino acid calcitonin propeptide is synthesized from the 6-exon calcitonin gene on chromosome 11p. C-cell calcitonin messenger RNA is differentially spliced so that mature calcitonin contains portions of exons 1 to 4. Figure 39-10 shows the alternative splicing of calcitonin gene messenger RNA to produce calcitonin (CT), katacalcin (Kc), and calcitonin gene–related peptide (CGRP). Neural tissue calcitonin messenger RNA is processed such that exon 4 is excluded, and exons 1 to 3, 5, and 6 included to form CGRP. CGRP is a 37–amino acid product that interacts with CGRP receptors. Thyroid C cells normally produce little if any CGRP. CGRP and its receptors are widely distributed in the central nervous system, where CGRP serves as a neurotransmitter. CGRP is found in bipolar neurons in sensory ganglia, and causes vasodilation.

Multiple forms of calcitonin are released into the circulation, including higher molecular-weight aggregates and cross-linked complexes. The complexity of the circulating forms of calcitonin delayed development of calcitonin assays. Serum calcium regulates calcitonin synthesis and secretion by thyroid C cells in humans. Increased serum calcium increases release of calcitonin, whereas decreased serum calcium decreases serum calcitonin secretion. Women have a greater calcitonin response to calcium or pentagastrin. Secretion of calcitonin is stimulated by catecholamines, glucagon, gastrin, and cholecystokinin, but these do not play a physiologic role in regulation of calcitonin secretion. Circulating calcitonin has a half-life of about 10 minutes, with circulating concentrations less than 15 pg/ml in men and less than 10 pg/ml in women.

Unlike in rodents or dogs, the physiologic role of calcitonin in humans remains unknown. Calcitonin deficiency in humans does not cause hypercalcemia or other detectable effects on calcium metabolism. Calcitonin excess in humans with thyroid C-cell hyperplasia or medullary thyroid carcinoma does not cause hypocalcemia or other detectable effects on calcium metabolism. Medullary thyroid carcinoma associated with multiple endocrine neoplasia type II is transmitted in an autosomal dominant manner, so family members of patients are advised to be screened for causative *RET* proto-oncogene mutations.

Calcitonin directly inhibits osteoclast bone resorption by binding to calcitonin receptors on osteoclasts. Six calcitonin receptor subtypes

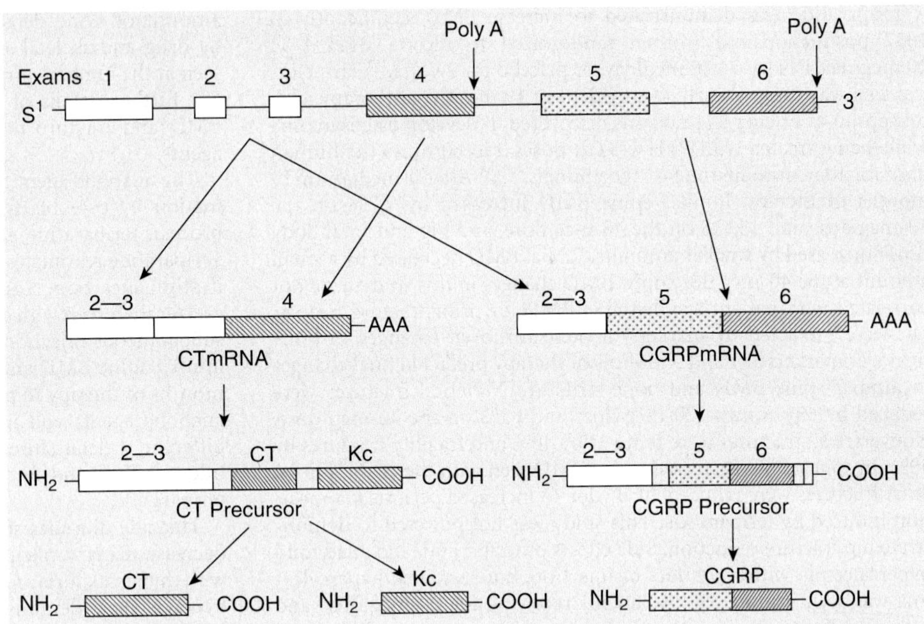

FIGURE 39-10 • Alternative splicing of calcitonin/calcitonin gene–related peptide (CGRP).

have been identified, synthesized through alternative splicing of coding and noncoding exons. Osteoclasts exposed to calcitonin lose their ruffled borders and withdraw from sites of active bone resorption.[153] Osteoclasts may escape the inhibitory effects of calcitonin after long-term exposure due to development of anticalcitonin antibodies or down-regulation of calcitonin receptors.[154,155]

Injectable calcitonin decreases serum calcium and phosphate levels in patients with hypercalcemia, with the effect of a single dose lasting for 6 to 10 hours. Patients typically become unresponsive to injected calcitonin after a few days, likely due to down-regulation of calcitonin receptors. In postmenopausal women, nasal spray calcitonin 200 IU each day increases lumbar spine trabecular bone density by 1% to 2% over 2 years, but has no significant effect on cortical bone density. Nasal spray calcitonin at this dose has no effect on trabecular or cortical bone density in men, but may reduce bone loss in patients receiving glucocorticoid therapy. In a large multicenter trial involving 1255 women postmenopausal for at least 5 years, with lumbar spine T-scores less than −2.0 and prevalent vertebral fractures in 78%, nasal spray calcitonin 200 IU/day for 5 years reduced vertebral fractures by 36%, but had no effect on hip fractures.[156] Lumbar spine BMD increased by about 1.5% over the 5 years of the study, but no BMD changes were seen at other skeletal sites. The significant reduction in vertebral fracture risk despite minimal changes in bone density suggests that calcitonin reduces fractures primarily by decreasing bone turnover or improving bone quality in as-yet undefined ways.

Injected calcitonin is approved for treatment of symptomatic Paget's disease of bone. Calcitonin has been shown to be effective in patients with moderate to severe Paget's disease with increased serum alkaline phosphatase and urinary markers of bone resorption. In these patients, injected calcitonin reduces markers of bone turnover by about 30%, with corresponding reductions in pain. Nasal spray calcitonin has not been shown to be effective in treatment of Paget's disease. Oral salmon calcitonin has been shown to provide cartilage protection in osteoarthritis. Injectable or nasal spray calcitonin may reduce pain after vertebral fracture in some patients, and is unique among all osteoporosis therapies in this regard, and may reduce bone pain in patients with Paget's disease of bone and metastatic disease.[157]

Salmon calcitonin is approved in the United States for treatment of postmenopausal osteoporosis in women at least 5 years after menopause. Nasal spray salmon calcitonin is given as 200 IU in alternating nostrils each day, whereas injectable salmon calcitonin is given initially as 100 IU each day, with subsequent decreases to 50 IU every day and then every other day. Nasal spray calcitonin causes nasal irritation in about 12% of postmenopausal women, whereas injectable calcitonin typically causes nausea, hives, facial flushing, or intestinal cramping (rarely). Treatment with calcitonin is often reserved for postmenopausal patients with osteoporosis on multiple medications who are not able to tolerate other anticatabolic therapies, or with acute back pain related to recent vertebral fracture.

Anabolic Agents

Anabolic agents for treatment of osteoporosis reduce fracture risk by increasing bone density and improving bone quality via stimulation of new bone formation. By contrast, anticatabolic agents primarily function to decrease bone loss.

Teriparatide (PTH 1-34). Teriparatide (recombinant human PTH 1-34) is the only currently approved anabolic agent available in the United States for treatment of postmenopausal women or men with severe osteoporosis, high risk of fracture, or failure on or intolerance of other therapies.[158] Teriparatide causes larger increases in BMD, particularly in the spine, than anticatabolic agents. Teriparatide initially stimulates bone formation directly, followed by stimulation of both bone resorption and formation, while maintaining a positive bone balance throughout both phases of the response.[159] Bone histomorphometry studies show that teriparatide stimulates new bone formation by causing restoration of bone microarchitecture, increased trabecular connectivity, and increased cortical thickness.[160] Teriparatide also stimulates periosteal new bone formation, leading to increased bone diameter, which results in greater biomechanical strength of bone.[161] The anabolic effect of PTH was first described in rodents in the 1930s by Hans Selye, but these findings were overlooked until the 1970s, when clinical trials of PTH resumed.

Teriparatide is approved for use at a dose of 20 mcg/day by subcutaneous injection for up to 2 years in the United States, and up to 18 months in Europe. Maximum serum PTH 1-34 concentrations are achieved 30 minutes after injection, and these decrease to undetectable within 3 hours, whereas maximum serum calcium concentrations occur 4 to 6 hours after a dose. Teriparatide is 95% bioavailable, and cleared by the liver and other tissues. The serum half-life of teriparatide is 1 hour when given subcutaneously and 5 minutes when given intravenously. Teriparatide is contraindicated in patients less than 18 years old with open epiphyses, as well as patients with Paget's disease of bone, history of skeletal radiation therapy, unexplained increased serum alkaline phosphatase, metastatic bone cancer, multiple myeloma, hyperparathyroidism, or hypercalcemia.

Teriparatide was demonstrated to increase BMD significantly in 1637 postmenopausal women randomized to receive PTH 1-34 20 mcg/day, PTH 1-34 40 mcg/day, or placebo for 2 years.[162] This clinical trial was stopped early at a median of 19 months of therapy after one group of Fischer 344 rats was discovered to develop osteosarcoma while being treated with PTH 1-34 at doses 3 to 60 times the human dose for the entire lifetime of the animals.[163,164] After a median of 19 months of therapy, lumbar spine BMD increased by 9.7% on the 20-mcg dose and 13.7% on the 40-mcg dose, and hip and total body BMD increased by smaller amounts. Radial BMD decreased by a small amount at the 40-mcg dose only. BMD changes in this study were not correlated with patient age, baseline BMD, or prior fracture history, but were predicted by markers of bone turnover. Changes in bone turnover markers at 1 and 3 months of therapy predicted final changes in lumbar spine BMD and bone structure. Vertebral fractures were reduced by 65% on the 20-mcg dose and 69% on the 40-mcg dose. Nonvertebral fractures were reduced by 40% and fragility fractures by 50%. In spite of the decreased radial BMD seen with the 40-mcg dose, wrist fractures were reduced, likely due to increased periosteal apposition induced by teriparatide. This study was not powered to demonstrate hip fracture reduction. Side effects of teriparatide included mild hypercalcemia within 6 hours of injection, but sustained hypercalcemia was seen in only 3% of patients receiving the 20-mcg dose and 11% of patients receiving the 40-mcg dose. There were no differences between the teriparatide and placebo groups in regard to deaths, hospitalizations, cardiovascular disorders, kidney stones, or gout, despite an average increase in 24-hour urine calcium of 40 mg and an average increase in serum uric acid of 25%. No subjects developed osteosarcoma during the human clinical trial, and no patients have developed osteosarcoma to date despite over 250,000 patients having received treatment worldwide. The main side effects in the clinical trial were dizziness, leg cramps, and irritation at the injection sites. Nausea, arthralgias, myalgias, fatigue, and weakness were reported by some patients.

Therapeutic Approach

Regular weight-bearing moderate physical activity, adequate calcium and vitamin D intake, and positive lifestyle changes will decrease or prevent bone loss and reduce fractures in many patients. For individuals younger than their mid-30s, moderate physical activity, adequate calcium and vitamin D intake, avoidance of lifestyle choices that adversely affect BMD, and preservation of normal gonadal steroid secretion will help them achieve their genetically determined potential peak bone mass. Use of postmenopausal hormone therapy has been significantly reduced in recent years as a result of the WHI, which confirmed that estrogen alone and estrogen plus progesterone prevent fractures, but also that estrogen alone causes increased risk of stroke, and that estrogen plus progesterone causes increased risk of stroke, myocardial infarction, deep venous thrombosis, and breast cancer.[133-135] Hormone therapy is now reserved for postmenopausal women with intolerable hot flashes or other vasomotor instability symptoms, but only at as low a dose as tolerated, for as short a time as possible.

A variety of anticatabolic agents and a single anabolic agent have been approved in the United States for prevention and treatment of postmenopausal osteoporosis. Anticatabolic agents primarily act by decreasing the rate of bone resorption by osteoclasts, and therefore prevent future bone loss. A relatively small increase in BMD occurs as the remodeling space open at the beginning of anticatabolic therapy fills in over the next several years, until a new steady state level is achieved, over which time bone density slowly increases to a new plateau. Because bone remodeling is a coupled process, anticatabolic agents also decrease the rate of bone formation, which further limits the increase in BMD possible with these agents. Retrospective evaluation of the major clinical trials with anticatabolic agents has determined that only 3% to 30% of the fracture reduction benefit seen with these agents results from the increase in bone density seen, and that 70% to 97% of the fracture reduction benefit results from decreased bone turnover and stabilization of bone microarchitecture.[165-167] The amount of bone density increase seen with different agents varies by drug and skeletal site, but a maximum increase of about 10% is seen at the lumbar spine after 3 years of therapy with oral alendronate. For further details of the effects of specific anticatabolic agents on BMD and fracture reduction, see the previous discussion of these agents.

The anabolic agent teriparatide primarily stimulates new bone formation by osteoblasts, but because bone remodeling is a coupled process, teriparatide also stimulates bone resorption by osteoclasts. Teriparatide stimulates bone formation sooner and more rapidly than it stimulates bone resorption, so increases in BMD are somewhat greater than seen with anticatabolic agents. Teriparatide 20 mcg/day by subcutaneous injection causes a maximum increase of about 15% in lumbar spine BMD and 3% increase in total hip bone density over 18 months of therapy in postmenopausal women.[162] It is likely that other anabolic agents will increase bone density by different amounts at different skeletal sites. For further details of the effects of teriparatide on BMD and fracture reduction, see the previous discussion of teriparatide.

Thiazide diuretics such as hydrochlorothiazide and chlorthalidone decrease urinary calcium excretion and reduce bone loss in patients with hypercalciuria. Clinical trials of thiazides in patients without hypercalciuria demonstrated relatively small increases in BMD over several years, and several studies suggest that thiazides may reduce hip fractures.[168] For a more detailed discussion of thiazide diuretics, see Chapter 22, Hypertension; and Chapter 26, Heart Failure.

Adequate calcium intake likely improves bone health throughout life. Recommended intakes for children and adolescents help the skeleton increase bone mineral content during growth and development,[169] but it is not yet proven that calcium intake in youth or adolescence increases peak BMD. Increased calcium intake during young adulthood increases BMD during the last phase of skeletal mineral acquisition.[170] Early postmenopausal bone loss due to estrogen deficiency may be limited by calcium intake, but calcium alone is usually not sufficient to stabilize BMD. Calcium supplementation has little effect on trabecular bone loss in early postmenopausal years, but may help prevent cortical bone loss. Calcium intake has been shown to decrease bone turnover, increase BMD, and reduce fractures in elderly individuals.[171]

Most adults taking 1000 mg supplemental elemental calcium in addition to their dietary intake of 500 to 600 mg elemental calcium achieve the recommended 1200 to 1500 mg elemental calcium intake for postmenopausal women and elderly men. Elemental calcium intake of more than 2500 mg/day may cause hypercalciuria. Intake of more than 2000 mg/day may cause constipation. Calcium carbonate supplements are most often recommended to be taken between meals in younger individuals with adequate gastric acid secretion, and with meals in older individuals in whom gastric acid secretion may be decreased. Calcium citrate absorption does not depend on stomach acid production.

Vitamin D supplementation of 400 IU/day is recommended for women and men over age 50 years in the belief that it increases calcium absorption at a time in life where intestinal calcium absorption is normally decreasing. At least half the individuals in the United States on therapy for postmenopausal osteoporosis were found to be vitamin D insufficient or deficient in a recent study.[35] It is still controversial whether vitamin D supplementation alone, or vitamin D in combination with calcium intake, can reduce osteoporotic fractures. The WHI calcium and vitamin D trial showed that elemental calcium 1000 mg/day plus vitamin D 400 IU/day did not reduce fractures at any skeletal site in a very large study population. Of the 18,000 individuals taking calcium plus vitamin D, 41% were noncompliant with therapy, making it difficult to interpret the intention-to-treat analysis.[172] Per-protocol analysis of this study with the 59% of patients who were compliant with therapy showed that calcium plus vitamin D reduced hip fractures by 29%, but not fractures at other sites. Calcitriol and alfacalcidol are used in some countries to prevent bone loss and reduce fractures in postmenopausal women who are not vitamin D deficient or insufficient, on the assumption that suppression of PTH secretion by calcitriol will reduce bone loss. Clinical trials with calcitriol in the United

States have not consistently demonstrated benefit, and have caused hypercalcemia and hypercalciuria.

Raloxifene is the only SERM approved in the United States for prevention and treatment of osteoporosis. Other SERMs, such as clomiphene, tamoxifen, or toremifene, are approved for other clinical indications. Raloxifene is an estrogen agonist in bone and liver, estrogen antagonist in the breast, and inactive in the uterus. Raloxifene modestly increases bone density and decreases vertebral fractures, but not hip or other nonvertebral fractures.[150] Raloxifene was recently demonstrated to be as effective as tamoxifen in reducing breast cancer risk in postmenopausal women at high risk,[173] and to not increase their cardiovascular risk.[174] Raloxifene should not be used for premenopausal women since it causes bone loss at this stage of life.[175]

Nasal spray calcitonin has been shown to stabilize BMD and reduce vertebral fracture risk by 36% in postmenopausal women, but not nonvertebral fractures.[156] The benefits of calcitonin may be greatest in women with the highest rates of bone turnover.

Because individual anticatabolic therapies are relatively potent, combination therapy with two anticatabolic agents is not generally recommended. Clinical trials of combination therapy with alendronate plus estrogen showed a slightly greater increase in BMD and minimal difference in fracture reduction compared to monotherapy.[176] Combination therapy with an anabolic agent plus an anticatabolic agent appears reasonable, given how these medications are believed to work, but clinical trials with alendronate plus PTH 1-84 in postmenopausal women and men showed blunting of the expected increase in bone density due to teriparatide.[177,178] Another trial with raloxifene plus PTH 1-84 showed potentiation of the expected increase in bone density due to teriparatide, suggesting that the potency of the anticatabolic agent influences the bone density response seen with combination anabolic plus anticatabolic therapy.[179] None of the available clinical trials with combination anabolic plus anticatabolic therapy has been powered to show fracture reduction. Sequential therapy with PTH 1-84 followed by alendronate in postmenopausal women caused a greater increase in bone density than alendronate or estrogen alone.[180]

Most patients with Paget's disease of bone are asymptomatic and do not require therapy. A small percentage of patients develop pain, progressive bone deformity, stress fractures, pathologic fractures, compression of cranial or peripheral nerves, hypercalcemia, or high-output congestive heart failure, and require treatment. Several oral and intravenous bisphosphonates and injectable calcitonin are approved for treatment of Paget's disease.[93,100,109,116,117,120] The bisphosphonates typically reduce bone turnover, as assessed by increased serum alkaline phosphatase and urinary NTx-telopeptide, or other markers of bone turnover, within several weeks to months. Bone pain and other symptoms typically improve over the same time course. A single treatment course with any of these agents will usually induce a remission lasting several months to years. If and when symptoms recur, another course of the same or a different agent may be tried. Oral etidronate at higher doses of 20 mg/kg per day for longer than 6 months has been shown to cause osteomalacia, and lower doses of 5 mg/kg per day have been reported to cause occasional focal osteomalacia. None of the other oral or intravenous bisphosphonates or calcitonin has been shown to cause abnormalities in skeletal mineralization. Most patients with Paget's disease of bone requiring therapy use oral or intravenous bisphosphonates due to their greater potency, more rapid and longer lasting effects, lower cost, and fewer side effects. Most patients using injectable calcitonin eventually develop resistance to calcitonin. Mithramycin (plicamycin) may be used in patients not responding to, or unable to tolerate, bisphosphonates or calcitonin, but hematologic and other toxicities limit its use.

Emerging Targets and Therapeutics

Given the relatively small number of choices and limitations on use of the various medications available, a variety of medications are under active investigation for use in disorders of calcium metabolism and bone mineralization. These therapies are all based on new molecular targets, and several of these are briefly described here.

Non–FDA-Approved Anticatabolic Agents

Bisphosphonates. Clodronate, neridronate, olpadronate, and other bisphosphonates are being investigated for use in management of postmenopausal osteoporosis, hypercalcemia of malignancy, osteogenesis imperfecta, and skeletal metastases.[181] Clodronate is currently approved in Europe and Canada to treat hypercalcemia of malignancy.[182]

SERMs. Arzoxifene,[183] lasofoxifene,[184] and several other SERMs are or have been undergoing long-term clinical investigation for use in treatment of postmenopausal osteoporosis. Most of these agents are still in early-stage clinical trials or beginning Phase III clinical trials.

Tibolone. Tibolone is a hormonal therapy with combined estrogenic, androgenic, and progestogenic properties.[185,186] Use of tibolone has been advocated for multiple purposes, but future use in the United States will likely be limited due to blood clotting effects seen in one osteoporosis clinical trial.

Denosumab. Denosumab is a monoclonal antibody to RANKL being investigated for use in postmenopausal osteoporosis and rheumatoid arthritis.[187,188] This antibody is given by subcutaneous injection twice a year. The Phase II osteoporosis clinical trial showed that a denosumab injection is able to reduce bone turnover markers for 6 months.

Sclerostin Monoclonal Antibody. Sclerostin is a small molecule secreted by osteocytes within bone that diffuses through the canalicular network to the surface of bone, where it inhibits osteoblast function via antagonism of various bone morphogenetic proteins. A monoclonal antibody to sclerostin is being developed to disinhibit osteoblasts, with the anticipation that this will have an anabolic effect on bone.[189,190]

PTH-Related Peptide. Full-length and amino-terminal PTH-related peptide have been or are being investigated for use in treatment of postmenopausal osteoporosis.[191,192]

Cathepsin K Inhibitors. Cathepsin K inhibitors are small-molecule inhibitors of cathepsin K, one of the major lysosomal enzymes produced by activated osteoclasts to resorb bone matrix. Cathepsin K inhibitors have been shown to decrease bone resorption in ovariectomized rodents.[193,194]

Non–FDA-Approved Anabolic Agents

PTH 1-84. Injectable full-length PTH 1-84 is currently being investigated for treatment of postmenopausal osteoporosis. A Phase II clinical trial randomized 217 postmenopausal women of mean age 64.5 years to receive PTH 1-84 at 50, 75, or 100 mcg/day by subcutaneous injection, or placebo, for 2 years. Lumbar spine BMD demonstrated a dose-dependent increase in this study, but hip and total body BMD did not.[195]

The Treatment of Osteoporosis trial randomized 2532 postmenopausal osteoporotic women of mean age 64 years to receive PTH 1-84 100 mcg/day or placebo.[196] Nineteen percent of study subjects had prevalent vertebral fractures. Lumbar spine BMD increased by 7.9%, compared to placebo. Per-protocol analysis showed that PTH 1-84 reduced incident vertebral fractures by 66%, regardless of whether prevalent vertebral fractures were present. No data have been published regarding nonvertebral fracture reduction in this trial. Hypercalcemia occurred in 28.3% of women receiving PTH 1-84 and 4.7% of women receiving placebo.[197]

Non–FDA-Approved Mixed Agents

Strontium Ranelate. Strontium ranelate has been approved for treatment of osteoporosis in Europe, Australia, and several other countries. Strontium ranelate is supplied as a powder in a sachet packet, and taken by drinking the dissolved 2-g contents of one packet in an 8-ounce glass of water each day. This agent has been shown to reduce the risk of both vertebral and hip fractures, similar to teriparatide.[198-201] Strontium is incorporated into the skeleton, and part of the increase in bone density seen during therapy is due to its higher atomic weight. Although the magnitude of its effects on bone density and fracture reduction are similar to teriparatide, strontium is classified as a mixed category agent because it simultaneously stimulates markers of bone formation and suppresses markers of bone resorption.[202] Side effects include nausea, cramps, and intestinal upset.

Nandrolone Decanoate. Nandrolone decanoate is an androgenic anabolic steroid that has been investigated in small clinical trials for several years in an effort to stimulate bone formation.[203,204] This compound has not proven to be very useful for increasing bone density or preventing fractures.

REFERENCES

1. Tfelt-Hansen J, Brown EM. The calcium-sensing receptor in normal physiology and pathophysiology: a review. Crit Rev Clin Lab Sci 2005;42:35-70.
2. Benker G, Breuer N, Windeck R, et al. Calcium metabolism in thyroid disease. J Endocrinol Invest 1988;11:61-69.
3. Beall DP, Scofield RH. Milk-alkali syndrome associated with calcium carbonate consumption. Medicine 1995;74:89-96.
4. al Zahrani A, Levine MA. Primary hyperparathyroidism. Lancet 1997;349:1233-1238.
5. Silverberg SJ, Bilezikian JP. The diagnosis and management of asymptomatic primary hyperparathyroidism. Nat Clin Pract Endocrinol Metab 2006;2:494-503.
6. Gao P, Scheibel S, D'Amour P, et al. Development of a novel immunoradiometric assay exclusively for biologically active whole parathyroid hormone 1-84: implications for improvement of accurate assessment of parathyroid function. J Bone Miner Res 2001;16:605-614.
7. Law WM Jr, Heath H III. Familial benign hypercalcemia (hypocalciuric hypercalcemia): clinical and pathogenetic studies in 21 families. Ann Intern Med 1985;102: 511-519.
8. Marx SJ, Attie MF, Levine MA, et al. The hypocalciuric or benign variant of familial hypercalcemia: clinical and biochemical features in fifteen kindreds. Medicine 1981;60:397-412.
9. Thakker RV. Diseases associated with the extracellular calcium-sensing receptor. Cell Calcium 2004;35:275-282.
10. Stewart AF. Clinical Practice. Hypercalcemia associated with cancer. N Engl J Med 2005;352:373-379.
11. Strewler GJ. The physiology of parathyroid hormone-related protein. N Engl J Med 2000;342:177-185.
12. Adams JS, Singer FR, Gacad MA, et al. Isolation and structural identification of 1,25-dihydroxyvitamin D3 produced by cultured alveolar macrophages in sarcoidosis. J Clin Endocrinol 1985;60:960-966.
13. Adams JS, Fernandez M, Gacad MA, et al. Vitamin D metabolite-mediated hypercalcemia and hypercalciuria in patients with AIDS- and non-AIDS-associated lymphoma. Blood 1989;73:235-239.
14. Thakker RV. Hypocalcemia: pathogenesis, differential diagnosis, and management. *In* Favus MJ (ed): Primer on the Metabolic Bone Diseases and Disorders of Mineral Metabolism, 6th ed. Washington, DC: American Society for Bone and Mineral Research, 2006, pp 213-215.
15. Kooh SW, Fraser D, Reilly BJ, et al. Rickets due to calcium deficiency. N Engl J Med 1977;297:1264-1266.
16. Eisenbarth GS, Gottlieb PA. Autoimmune polyendocrine syndromes. N Engl J Med 2004;350:2068-2079.
17. Yu D, Yu S, Schuster V, et al. Identification of two novel deletion mutations with the $G_s\alpha$ gene (*GNAS1*) in Albright hereditary osteodystrophy. J Clin Endocrinol Metab 1999;84:3254-3259.
18. Levine MA, Germain-Lee E, Jan de Beur S. Genetic basis for resistance to parathyroid hormone. Horm Res 2003;60(Suppl 3):87-95.
19. Carney JA. The glandulae parathyroideae of Ivar Sandstrom: contributions from two continents. Am J Surg Pathol 1996;20:1123-1144.
20. Brown EM, Jüeppner H. Parathyroid hormone: synthesis, secretion, and action. *In* Favus MJ (ed): Primer on the Metabolic Bone Diseases and Disorders of Mineral Metabolism, 6th ed. Washington, DC: American Society for Bone and Mineral Research, 2006, pp 90-99.
21. Sneddon WB, Syme CA, Bisello A, et al. Activation-independent parathyroid hormone receptor internalization is regulated by NHERF1 (EBP50). J Biol Chem 2003:278: 43787-43796.
22. Monier-Faugere MC, Geng Z, Mawad H, et al. Improved assessment of bone turnover by the PTH (1-84)/large C-PTH fragments ratio in ESRD patients. Kidney Int 2001;60:1460-1468.
23. Tian J, Smogorzewski M, Kede L, et al. Parathyroid hormone-parathyroid hormone-related protein receptor messenger RNA is present in many tissues besides the kidney. Am J Nephrol 1993;13:210-213.
24. Usdin TB, Hoare SRJ, Wang T, et al. A new neuropeptide and PTH2-receptor agonist from hypothalamus. Nat Neurosci 1999;2:941-943.
25. Singh A, Gilchrist A, Voyno-Yasenetskaya T, et al. $G_{\alpha 12}$ and $G_{\alpha 13}$ subunits of heterotrimeric G proteins mediate parathyroid hormone activation of phospholipase D in UMR-106 osteoblastic cells. Endocrinology 2005;146:2171-2175.
26. Murray TM, Rao LG, Divieti P, et al. Parathyroid hormone secretion and action: evidence for discrete receptors for the carboxyl-terminal region and related biological actions of carboxyl-terminal ligands. Endocr Rev 2005;26:78-113.
27. Brown EM, MacLeod RJ. Extracellular calcium sensing and extracellular calcium signaling. Physiol Rev 2001;81:239-297.
28. Dempster DW, Cosman F, Parisien M, et al. Anabolic actions of parathyroid hormone on bone. Endocr Rev 1993;14:690-709.
29. Friedman PA. Calcium transport in the kidney. Curr Opin Nephrol Hypertens 1999;8:589-595.
30. Raisz LG. Pathogenesis of osteoporosis: concepts, conflicts, and prospects. J Clin Invest 2005;115:3318-3325.
31. Holick MF. High prevalence of vitamin D inadequacy and implications for health. Mayo Clin Proc 2006;81:353-373.
32. DeLuca HF, Shnoes HK. Metabolism and mechanism of action of vitamin D. Annu Rev Biochem 1976;45:631-666.
33. Mason JB, Hay RW, Leresche J, et al. The story of vitamin D: from vitamin to hormone. Lancet 1974;1:325-329.
34. Gaugris S, Heaney RP, Boonen S, et al. Vitamin D inadequacy among post-menopausal women: a systematic review. Q J Med 2005;98:667-676.
35. Holick MF, Siris ES, Binkley N, et al. Prevalence of vitamin D inadequacy among postmenopausal North American women receiving osteoporosis therapy. J Clin Endocrinol Metab 2005;90:3215-3224.
36. Bland R, Walker EA, Hughes SV, et al. Constitutive expression of 25-hydroxyvitamin D_3-1α-hydroxylase in a transformed human proximal tubule cell line: evidence for direct regulation of vitamin D metabolism by calcium. Endocrinology 1999;140: 2027-2034.
37. Yoshida T, Yoshida N, Monkawa T, et al. Dietary phosphorus deprivation induces 25-hydroxyvitamin D_3 1α-hydroxylase gene expression. Endocrinology 2001;142: 1720-1726.
38. Suda T, Ueno Y, Fujii K, et al. Vitamin D and bone. J Cell Biochem 2003;88:259-266.
39. Zanello LP, Norman AW. Rapid modulation of osteoblast ion channel responses by 1α,25$(OH)_2$-vitamin D_3 requires the presence of a functional vitamin D nuclear receptor. Proc Natl Acad Sci U S A 2004;101:1589-1594.
40. Macdonald HM, McGuigan FE, Stewart A, et al. Large-scale population-based study shows no evidence of association between common polymorphism of the VDR gene and BMD in British women. J Bone Miner Res 2006;21:151-162.
41. Bronner F. Mechanisms of intestinal calcium absorption. J Cell Biochem 2003;88:387-393.
42. Barley NF, Howard A, O'Callaghan D, et al. Epithelial calcium transporter expression in human duodenum. Am J Physiol Gastrointest Liver Physiol 2001;280:G285-G290.
43. Hendy GN, Hruska KA, Mathew S, et al. New insights into mineral and skeletal regulation by active forms of vitamin D. Kidney Int 2006;69:218-223.
44. Hayes CE, Nashold FE, Spach KM, et al. The immunological functions of the vitamin D endocrine system. Cell Mol Biol 2003;49:277-300.
45. HYP Consortium. A gene (*PEX*) with homologies to endopeptidases is mutated in patients with X-linked hypophosphatemic rickets. Nat Genet 1995;11:130-136.
46. Econs MJ, McEnery PT, Lennon F, et al. Autosomal dominant hypophosphatemic rickets is linked to chromosome 12 p13. J Clin Invest 1997;100:2653-2657.
47. White KE, Jonsson KB, Carn G, et al. The autosomal dominant hypophosphatemic rickets (ADHR) gene is a secreted polypeptide overexpressed by tumors that cause phosphate wasting. J Clin Endocrinol 2001;86:497-500.
48. Fraser D, Kooh SW, Kind KP, et al. Pathogenesis of hereditary vitamin D-dependent rickets: an inborn error of vitamin D metabolism involving defective conversion of 25-hydroxyvitamin D to 1α-25-dihydroxyvitamin D. N Engl J Med 1973;289:817-822.
49. Drezner MK, Feinglos MN. Osteomalacia due to 1α,25-dihydroxycholecalciferol deficiency. J Clin Invest 1977;60:1046-1053.
50. Demay MB. Rickets caused by impaired vitamin D activation and hormone resistance: pseudovitamin D deficiency rickets and hereditary vitamin D-resistant rickets. *In* Favus MJ (ed): Primer on the Metabolic Bone Diseases and Disorders of Mineral Metabolism, 6th ed. Washington, DC: American Society for Bone and Mineral Research, 2006, pp 338-341.
51. Brooks MH, Bell NH, Love L, et al. Vitamin D-dependent rickets type II: resistance of target organs to 1,25-dihydroxyvitamin D_3. N Engl J Med 1978;298:996-999.
52. Khosla S, Riggs BL, Atkinson EJ, et al. Effects of sex and age on bone microstructure at the ultradistal radius: a population-based noninvasive in vivo assessment. J Bone Miner Res 2006;21:124-131.
53. Khosla S, Melton LJ 3rd, Achenbach SJ, et al. Hormonal and biochemical determinants of trabecular microstructure at the ultradistal radius in women and men. J Clin Endocrinol Metab 2006;91:885-891.
54. Dempster DW. Anatomy and functions of the adult skeleton. *In* Favus MJ (ed): Primer on the Metabolic Bone Diseases and Disorders of Mineral Metabolism, 6th ed. Washington, DC: American Society for Bone and Mineral Research, 2006, pp 7-11.
55. Burr DB, Forwood MR, Fyhrie DP, et al. Perspective: bone microdamage and skeletal fragility in osteoporotic and stress fractures. J Bone Miner Res 1997;12:6-15.
56. Boyle WJ, Simonet WS, Lacey DL. Osteoclast differentiation and activation. Nature 2003;423:337-342.
57. Suda T, Takahashi N, Udagawa N, et al. Modulation of osteoclast differentiation and function by the new members of the tumor necrosis factor receptor and ligand families. Endocr Rev 1999;20:345-357.
58. Weinstein RS, Jilka RL, Parfit AF, et al. Inhibition of osteoblastogenesis and promotion of apoptosis of osteoblasts and osteocytes by glucocorticoids. J Clin Invest 1998; 102:272-282.
59. Center JR, Nguyen TV, Schneider D, et al. Mortality after all major types of osteoporotic fracture in men and women: an observational study. Lancet 1999;353: 878-882.
60. Albright F. The effect of hormones on osteoporosis in man. Rec Prog Horm Res 1947;1:293-353.
61. Kurihara N, Reddy SV, Menaa C, et al. Osteoclasts expressing the measles virus nucleocapsid gene display a pagetic phenotype. J Clin Invest 2000;105:607-614.
62. Cooper C, Schafheutle K, Dennison E, et al. The epidemiology of Paget's disease in Britain: is the prevalence decreasing? J Bone Miner Res 1999;14:192-197.

63. Cundy T, McAnulty K, Wattie D, et al. Evidence for secular changes in Paget's disease. Bone 1997;20:69-71.
64. Food and Nutrition Board. Dietary Reference Intakes: Calcium Phosphorus, Magnesium, Vitamin D, and Fluoride. Washington, DC: National Academy Press, 1997.
65. Stewart AF. Hypercalcemia associated with cancer. N Engl J Med 2005;352:373-379.
66. Major P, Lortholay A, Hon J, et al. Zoledronic acid is superior to pamidronate in the treatment of hypercalcemia of malignancy: a pooled analysis of two randomized, controlled clinical trials. J Clin Oncol 2001;19:558-567.
67. Bilezikian JP, Potts JT, El Hajj-Fuleihan G, et al. Summary statement from a workshop on asymptomatic primary hyperparathyroidism: a perspective for the 21st century. J Bone Miner Res 2002;17(Suppl 2):N2-N11.
68. Shoback DM, Bilezikian JP, Turner SA, et al. The calcimimetic cinacalcet normalizes serum calcium in patients with primary hyperparathyroidism. J Clin Endocrinol Metab 2003;88:5644-5649.
69. Peacock M, Bilezikian JP, Klassen P, et al. Cinacalcet HCl maintains long-term normocalcemia in patients with primary hyperparathyroidism. J Clin Endocrinol Metab 2005;90:135-141.
70. Moe SM, Chertow GM, Coburn JW, et al. Achieving the NKF-K/DOQI bone metabolism and disease treatment goals with cinacalcet HCl. Kidney Int 2005;67:760-771.
71. Vieth R. Vitamin D supplementation, 25-hydroxyvitamin D concentrations, and safety. Am J Clin Nutr 1999;69:842-856.
72. Institute of Medicine Subcommittee on Interpretation and Uses of Dietary Reference Intakes, Standing Committee on the Scientific Evaluation of Dietary Reference Intakes. Dietary Reference Intakes: Application in Dietary Planning. Washington, DC: National Academy Press, 2003, p 237.
73. Martin KJ, Gonzalez EA, Gellens M, et al. 10-Nor-1-α-25-dihydroxyvitamin D_2 (paricalcitol) safely and effectively reduces the levels of intact parathyroid hormone in patients on hemodialysis. J Am Soc Nephrol 1998;9:1427-1432.
74. Chertow GM, Burke SK, Lazarus JM, et al. Poly[allylamine hydrochloride] (RenaGel): a noncalcemic phosphate binder for the treatment of hyperphosphatemia in chronic renal failure. Am J Kidney Dis 1997;29:66-71.
75. Eknoyan G, Levin A, Levin NW. Bone metabolism and disease in chronic kidney disease. Am J Kidney Dis 2003;42(Suppl 3):1-201.
76. Hebert SC. Therapeutic use of calcimimetics. Annu Rev Med 2006;57:349-364.
77. Nemeth EF. Calcimimetic and calcilytic drugs: just for parathyroid cells? Cell Calcium 2004;35:283-289.
78. Block GA, Martin KJ, de Francisco AL, et al. Cinacalcet for secondary hyperparathyroidism in patients receiving hemodialysis. N Engl J Med 2004;350:1516-1525.
79. Barman Balfour J, Scott L. Cinacalcet hydrochloride. Drugs 2005;65:271-281.
80. Russell RG. Bisphosphonates: from bench to bedside. Ann N Y Acad Sci 2006;1068:367-401.
81. Stenbeck G, Horton MA. A new specialized cell-matrix interaction in actively resorbing osteoclasts. J Cell Sci 2000;113:1577-1587.
82. Halasy-Nagy MR, Rodan GA, Reszka AA. Inhibition of bone resorption by alendronate and risedronate does not require osteoclast apoptosis. Bone 2001;29:553-559.
83. Frith JC, Monkkonen J, Blackburn GM, et al. Clodronate and liposome-encapsulated clodronate are metabolized to a toxic ATP analog, adenosine 5′-(beta,gamma-dichloromethylene) triphosphate, by mammalian cells in vitro. J Bone Miner Res 1997;12:1358-1367.
84. Liberman UA, Weiss SR, Broll J, et al. Effect of oral alendronate on bone mineral density and the incidence of fractures in postmenopausal osteoporosis. N Engl J Med 1995;333:1437-1443.
85. Bone HG, Hosking D, Devogelaer JP, et al, for the Alendronate Phase III Osteoporosis Treatment Study Group. Ten years' experience with alendronate for osteoporosis in postmenopausal women. N Engl J Med 2004;350:1189-1199.
86. Schnitzer T, Bone HG, Crepaldi G, et al. Therapeutic equivalence of alendronate 70 mg once-weekly and alendronate 10 mg daily in the treatment of osteoporosis. Alendronate Once-Weekly Study Group. Aging Clin Exp Res 2000;12:1-12.
87. Rizzoli R, Greenspan SL, Bone G 3rd, et al, for the Alendronate Once-Weekly Study Group. Two-year results of once-weekly administration of alendronate 70 mg for the treatment of postmenopausal osteoporosis. J Bone Miner Res 2002;17:1988-1996.
88. Black DM, Cummings SR, Karpf DB, et al. Randomised trial of effect of alendronate on risk of fracture in women with existing vertebral fractures. Lancet 1996;348:1535-1541.
89. Cummings SR, Black DM, Thompson DE, et al. Effect of alendronate on risk of fracture in women with low bone density but without vertebral fractures: results from the Fracture Intervention Trial. JAMA 1998;280:2077-2082.
90. Ravn P, Weiss SR, Rodriguez-Portales JA, et al. Alendronate in early postmenopausal women: effects on bone mass during long-term treatment and after withdrawal. Alendronate Osteoporosis Prevention Study Group. J Clin Endocrinol Metab 2000;85:1492-1497.
91. Orwoll E, Ettinger M, Weiss S, et al. Alendronate for the treatment of osteoporosis in men. N Engl J Med 2000;343:604-610.
92. Saag KG, Emkey R, Schnitzer TJ, et al. Alendronate for the prevention and treatment of glucocorticoid-induced osteoporosis. Glucocorticoid-Induced Osteoporosis Intervention Study Group. N Engl J Med 1998;339:292-299.
93. Siris E, Weinstein RS, Altman R, et al. Comparative study of alendronate vs. etidronate for the treatment of Paget's disease of bone. J Clin Endocrinol Metab 1996;81:961-967.
94. Harris ST, Watts NB, Genant HK, et al. Effects of risedronate treatment on vertebral and nonvertebral fractures in women with postmenopausal osteoporosis: a randomized controlled trial. Vertebral Efficacy with Risedronate Therapy (VERT) Study Group. JAMA 1999;282:1344-1352.
95. Brown JP, Kendler DL, McClung MR, et al. The efficacy and tolerability of risedronate once a week for the treatment of postmenopausal osteoporosis. Calcif Tiss Int 2002;71:103-111.
96. Reginster J, Minne HW, Sorenson OH, et al, for the Vertebral Efficacy with Risedronate Therapy Study Group. Randomized trial of the effects of risedronate on vertebral fractures in women with established postmenopausal osteoporosis. Osteoporos Int 2000;11:83-91.
97. McClung MR, Geusens P, Miller PD, et al. Effect of risedronate on the risk of hip fracture in elderly women. N Engl J Med 2001;344:333-340.
98. Fogelman I, Ribot C, Smith R, et al. Risedronate reverses bone loss in postmenopausal women with low bone mass: results from a multinational, double-blind, placebo-controlled trial. BMD-MN Study Group. J Clin Endocrinol Metab 2000;85:1895-1900.
99. Cohen S, Levy RM, Keller M, et al. Risedronate therapy prevents corticosteroid-induced bone loss: a twelve-month, multicenter, randomized, double blind, placebo-controlled, parallel-group study. Arthritis Rheum 1999;42:2309-2318.
100. Miller PD, Adachi JD, Brown JP, et al. Risedronate vs. etidronate: duration of remission of Paget's disease with only 2 months of 30 mg risedronate. J Bone Miner Res 1997;12:S269.
101. Chestnut CH III, Skag A, Christiansen C, et al. Oral Ibandronate Osteoporosis Vertebral Fracture Trial in North America and Europe (BONE): effects of oral ibandronate administered daily or intermittently on fracture risk in postmenopausal osteoporosis. J Bone Miner Res 2004;19:1241-1249.
102. Miller PD, McClung MR, Macovei L, et al. Monthly oral ibandronate therapy in postmenopausal osteoporosis: 1-year results from the MOBILE study. J Bone Miner Res 2005;20:1315-1322.
103. Delmas PD, Adami S, Strugala C, et al. Intravenous ibandronate injections in postmenopausal women with osteoporosis: one-year results from the dosing intravenous administration study. Arthritis Rheum 2006;54:1838-1846.
104. Recker R, Stakkestad JA, Chesnut CH 3rd, et al. Insufficiently dosed intravenous ibandronate injections are associated with suboptimal antifracture efficacy in postmenopausal osteoporosis. Bone 2004;34:890-899.
105. Storm T, Thamsborg G, Steiniche T, et al. Effect of intermittent cyclical etidronate therapy on bone mass and fracture rate in women with postmenopausal osteoporosis. N Engl J Med 1990;322:1265-1271.
106. Watts NB, Harris ST, Genant HK, et al. Intermittent cyclical etidronate treatment of postmenopausal osteoporosis. N Engl J Med 1990;323:73-79.
107. Herd RJ, Balena R, Blake GM, et al. The prevention of early postmenopausal bone loss by cyclical etidronate therapy: a 2-year, double-blind, placebo-controlled study. Am J Med 1997;103:92-99.
108. Adachi JD, Bensen WG, Brown J, et al. Intermittent etidronate therapy to prevent corticosteroid-induced osteoporosis. N Engl J Med 1997;337:382-387.
109. Altman RD, Johnston CC, Khairi MRA, et al. Influence of disodium etidronate on clinical and laboratory manifestations of Paget's disease of bone (osteitis deformans). N Engl J Med 1973;289:1379-1384.
110. Canfield R, Rosner W, Skinner J, et al. Diphosphonate therapy of Paget's disease of bone. J Clin Endocrinol Metab 1977;44:96-106.
111. Roux C, Gennari C, Farrerons J, et al. Comparative prospective, double-blind, multicenter study of the efficacy of tiludronate and etidronate in treatment of Paget's disease of bone. Arthritis Rheum 1995;38:851-858.
112. McClung MR, Tou CPK, Goldstein NH, et al. Tiludronate therapy for Paget's disease of bone. Bone 1995;17:493S-496S.
113. Peretz A, Body JJ, Dumon JC, et al. Cyclical pamidronate infusions in postmenopausal osteoporosis. Maturitas 1996;25:69-75.
114. Boutsen Y, Jamart J, Esselinckx W, et al. Primary prevention of glucocorticoid-induced osteoporosis with intravenous pamidronate and calcium: a prospective controlled 1-year study comparing a single infusion, an infusion given once every 3 months, and calcium alone. J Bone Miner Res 2001;16:104-122.
115. Tyrrell CJ, Collinson M, Madsen EL, et al. Intravenous pamidronate: infusion rate and safety. Ann Oncol 1994;5(Suppl 7):S27-S29.
116. Siris ES. Perspectives: a practical guide to the use of pamidronate in the treatment of Paget's disease. J Bone Miner Res 1994;9:303-304.
117. Harinck HI, Papapoulos SE, Blanksma HJ, et al. Paget's disease of bone: early and late responses to three different modes of treatment with aminohydroxypropylidene bisphosphonate (APD). Br Med J (Clin Res Ed) 1987;295:1301-1305.
118. Reid IR, Brown JP, Burckhardt P, et al. Intravenous zoledronic acid in postmenopausal women with low bone mineral density. N Engl J Med 2002;346:653-661.
119. Black DM, Delmas PD, Eastell R, et al. Once-yearly zoledronic acid for treatment of postmenopausal osteoporosis. N Engl J Med 2007;356:1809-1822.
120. Reid IR, Miller P, Lyles K, et al. A single infusion of zoledronic acid improves remission rates in Paget's disease: a randomized controlled comparison with risedronate. N Engl J Med 2005;353:898-908.
121. Albright F, Bloomberg E, Smith PH. Postmenopausal osteoporosis. Trans Assoc Am Physicians 1940;55:298-305.
122. Lufkin EG, Wahner HW, O'Fallon WM, et al. Treatment of postmenopausal osteoporosis with transdermal estrogen. Ann Intern Med 1992;117:1-9.
123. Lindsay R, Hart DM, Forrest C, Baird C. Prevention of spinal osteoporosis in oophorectomized women. Lancet 1980;2:1151-1153.
124. Nachtigall LE, Nachtigall RH, Nachtigall RD, et al. Estrogen replacement therapy I: a 10-year prospective study in the relationship to osteoporosis. Obstet Gynecol 1979;53:277-281.
125. Cauley JA, Seeley DG, Ensrud K, et al. Estrogen replacement therapy and fractures in older women. Ann Intern Med 1995;122:9-16.
126. Kiel DP, Felson DT, Anderson JJ, et al. Hip fracture and the use of estrogens in postmenopausal women. The Framingham Study. N Engl J Med 1987;317:1169-1174.
127. Ettinger B, Genant HK, Cann CE. Long-term estrogen replacement therapy prevents bone loss and fractures. Ann Intern Med 1985;102:319-324.
128. Michaëlsson K, Baron JA, Farahmand BY, et al. Hormone replacement therapy and risk of hip fracture: population based case-control study. BMJ 1998;316:1858-1863.

129. Barrett-Connor E. Postmenopausal estrogen and prevention bias. Ann Intern Med 1991;115:455-456.
130. Komulainen MH, Kroger H, Tuppurainen MT, et al. HRT and vitamin D in prevention of non-vertebral fractures in postmenopausal women: a 5 year randomized trial. Maturitas 1998;31:45-54.
131. Mosekilde L, Beck-Nielsen H, Sorenson OH, et al. Hormonal replacement therapy reduces forearm fracture incidence in recent postmenopausal women: results of the Danish Osteoporosis Prevention Study. Maturitas 2000;36:181-193.
132. PEPI Writing Group. Effects of hormone therapy on bone mineral density: results from the Postmenopausal Estrogen/Progesterone Interventions (PEPI) trial. JAMA 1996;276:1389-1396.
133. Rossouw JE, Anderson GL, Prentice RL, et al. Risks and benefits of estrogen plus progestin in healthy postmenopausal women: principal results from the Women's Health Initiative randomized controlled trial. JAMA 2002;288:321-333.
134. Cauley JA, Robbins J, Chen Z, et al, for the Women's Health Initiative Investigators. Effects of estrogen plus progestin on risk of fracture and bone mineral density. The Women's Health Initiative randomized trial. JAMA 2003;290:1729-1738.
135. Anderson GL, Limacher M, Assaf AR, et al, for the Women's Health Initiative Steering Committee. Effects of conjugated equine estrogen in postmenopausal women with hysterectomy. The Women's Health Initiative randomized controlled trial. JAMA 2004;291:1701-1712.
136. Cauley JA, Black DM, Barrett-Connor E, et al. Effects of hormone replacement therapy on clinical fractures and height loss. The Heart and Estrogen/Progestin Replacement Study (HERS). Am J Med 2001;110:442-450.
137. Genant HK, Cann CE, Ettinger B, et al. Quantitative computed tomography of vertebral spongiosa: a sensitive method for diagnosing early bone loss after oophorectomy. Ann Intern Med 1982;97:699-705.
138. Lindsay R, Hart DM, Clarie AC. The minimum effective dose of estrogen for prevention of postmenopausal bone loss. Obstet Gynecol 1986;63:759-763.
139. Cummings SR, Browne WS, Bauer D, et al. Endogenous hormones and the risk of hip and vertebral fractures. N Engl J Med 1998;339:733-738.
140. Lindsay R, Gallagher JC, Kleerekoper M, et al. Effect of lower doses of conjugated equine estrogens with and without medroxyprogesterone acetate on bone in early postmenopausal women. JAMA 2002;287:2668-2676.
141. Cummings SR, Yankov V, Ensrud K, et al. Ultra low dose estradiol increases BMD and decreases bone turnover in older women, particularly those with undetectable estradiol. The Ultra Trial. J Bone Miner Res 2003;18(Suppl 2):1207.
142. Greendale GA, Espeland ME, Slone S, et al. Bone mass response to discontinuation or long-term use of hormone replacement therapy: results from the Postmenopausal Estrogen/Progestin Interventions (PEPI) Safety Follow-Up Study. Arch Intern Med 2002;162:665-672.
143. Lindsay R, Hart DM, MacLean A, et al. Bone response to termination of oestrogen treatment. Lancet 1978;1:1325-1327.
144. Christiansen C, Christiansen MS, Transbol I, et al. Bone mass in postmenopausal women after withdrawal of estrogen/gestagen replacement therapy. Lancet 1981;1:459-461.
145. Felson DT, Zhang Y, Hannan MT, et al. The effect of postmenopausal estrogen therapy on bone density in elderly women. N Engl J Med 1993;329:1141-1146.
146. Yates J, Barrett-Connor E, Barias S, et al. Rapid loss of hip fracture protection after estrogen cessation: evidence from National Osteoporosis Risk Assessment. Obstet Gynecol 2002;103:440-446.
147. Smith CL, O'Malley BW. Coregulator function: a key to understanding tissue specificity of selective receptor modulators. Endocr Rev 2004;25:45-71.
148. Kuiper GG, Carlsson B, Grandien K, et al. Comparison of the ligand binding specificity and transcript tissue distribution of estrogen receptors ERα and β. Endocrinology 1997;138:863-870.
149. Delmas PD, Bjarnason NH, Mitlak BH, et al. Effects of raloxifene on bone mineral density, serum cholesterol concentrations, and uterine endometrium in postmenopausal women. N Engl J Med 1997;337:1641-1647.
150. Ettinger B, Black DM, Mitlak BH, et al. Reduction of vertebral fracture risk in postmenopausal women with osteoporosis treated with raloxifene: results from a 3-year randomized clinical trial. Multiple Outcomes of Raloxifene Evaluation (MORE) Investigators. JAMA 1999;282:637-645.
151. Cummings SR, Eckert S, Krueger KA, et al. The effect of raloxifene on risk of breast cancer in postmenopausal women: results from the MORE randomized trial. Multiple Outcomes of Raloxifene Evaluation. JAMA 1999;281:2189-2197.
152. Azria M, Copp SH, Zanelli JM. 25 years of salmon calcitonin: from synthesis to therapeutic use. Calcif Tiss Int 1995;57:405-408.
153. Chambers TJ, Moore A. The sensitivity of isolated osteoclasts to morphological transformation by calcitonin. J Clin Endocrinol Metab 1983;57:819-824.
154. Singer FR, Aldred JP, Neer RM, et al. An evaluation of antibodies and clinical resistance to salmon calcitonin. J Clin Invest 1972;51:2331-2338.
155. Takahashi S, Goldring S, Katz M, et al. Downregulation of calcitonin receptor mRNA expression by calcitonin during human osteoclast-like cell differentiation. J Clin Invest 1995;95:167-171.
156. Chestnut CH, Silverman S, Andriano K, et al. A randomized trial of nasal spray calcitonin in postmenopausal women with established osteoporosis. The Prevent Recurrence of Osteoporotic Fractures Study. Am J Med 2000;109:267-276.
157. Silverman SL, Azria M. The analgesic effect of calcitonin following osteoporotic fracture. Osteoporos Int 2002;13:858-867.
158. Hodsman AB, Bauer DC, Dempster DM, et al. Parathyroid hormone and teriparatide for the treatment of osteoporosis: a review of the evidence and suggested guidelines for its use. Endocr Rev 2005;26:688-703.
159. Arlot M, Meunier PM, Boivin G, et al. Differential effects of teriparatide and alendronate on bone remodeling in postmenopausal women assessed by histomorphometric parameters. J Bone Miner Res 2005;20:1244-1253.
160. Dempster DW, Cosman F, Kurland ES, et al. Effects of daily treatment with parathyroid hormone on bone microarchitecture and turnover in patients with osteoporosis: a paired biopsy study. J Bone Miner Res 2001;16:1846-1853.
161. Parfitt AM. PTH and periosteal bone expansion. J Bone Miner Res 2002;17:1741-1743.
162. Neer RM, Arnaud CD, Zanchetta JR, et al. Effect of parathyroid hormone (1-34) on fractures and bone mineral density in postmenopausal women with osteoporosis. N Engl J Med 2001;344:1434-1441.
163. Vahle JL, Sato M, Long GG, et al. Skeletal changes in rats given daily subcutaneous injections of rhPTH(1-34) for 2 years and relevance to human safety. Toxicol Pathol 2002;30:312-321.
164. Vahle JL, Long GG, Sandusky G, et al. Bone neoplasms in F344 rats given teriparatide [rhPTH(1-34)] are dependent on duration of treatment and dose. Toxicol Pathol 2004;32:426-438.
165. Cummings SR, Karpf DB, Harris F, et al. Improvement in spine bone density and reduction in risk of vertebral fractures during treatment with antiresorptive drugs. Am J Med 2002;112:281-289.
166. Sarkar S, Mitlak B, Wong M, et al. Relationships between bone mineral density and incident vertebral fracture risk with raloxifene therapy. J Bone Miner Res 2002;17:1-10.
167. Li Z, Meredith MP, Hoseyni MS. A method to assess the proportion of treatment effect explained by a surrogate endpoint. Stat Med 2001;20:3175-3188.
168. Schoofs MW, van der Klift M, Hofman A, et al. Thiazide diuretics and the risk for hip fracture. Ann Intern Med 2003;139:476-482.
169. Johnston CC Jr, Miller JZ, Slemenda CW, et al. Calcium supplementation and increases in bone mineral density in children. N Engl J Med 1992;327:882-887.
170. Recker RR, Davies KM, Hinders SM, et al. Bone gain in young adult women. JAMA 1992;268:2403-2408.
171. Dawson-Hughes B, Harris SS, Krall EA, et al. Effect of calcium and vitamin D supplementation on bone density in men and women 65 years of age or older. N Engl J Med 1997;337:670-676.
172. Jackson RD, LaCroix AZ, Gass M, et al. Calcium plus vitamin D supplementation and the risk of fractures. N Engl J Med 2006;354:669-683.
173. Vogel VG, Costantino JP, Wickerham DL, et al. Effects of tamoxifen vs raloxifene on the risk of developing invasive breast cancer and other disease outcomes. The NSABP Study of Tamoxifen and Raloxifene (STAR) P-2 trial. JAMA 2006;295:2727-2741.
174. Barrett-Connor E, Mosca L, Collins P, et al. Effects of raloxifene on cardiovascular events and breast cancer in postmenopausal women. N Engl J Med 2006;355:125-137.
175. Powles TJ, Hickish T, Kanis JA, et al. Effect of tamoxifen on bone mineral density measured by dual-energy x-ray absorptiometry in healthy premenopausal and postmenopausal women. J Clin Oncol 1996;14:78-84.
176. Greenspan SL, Emkey RD, Bone HG, et al. Significant differential effects of alendronate, estrogen, or combination therapy on the rate of bone loss after discontinuation of treatment of postmenopausal osteoporosis: a randomized, double-blind, placebo-controlled trial. Ann Intern Med 2002;137:875-883.
177. Black DM, Greenspan SL, Ensrud K, et al. The effects of parathyroid hormone and alendronate alone or in combination in postmenopausal women. N Engl J Med 2003;349:1207-1215.
178. Finkelstein JS, Hayes A, Hunzelman JL, et al. The effects of parathyroid hormone, alendronate, or both in men with osteoporosis. N Engl J Med 2003;349:1216-1226.
179. Deal C, Omizo M, Schwartz EN, et al. Combination teriparatide and raloxifene therapy for postmenopausal osteoporosis: results from a 6-month double-blind placebo-controlled trial. J Bone Miner Res 2005;20:1905-1911.
180. Black DM, Bilezikian JP, Ensrud KE, et al. One year of alendronate after one year of parathyroid hormone (1-84) for osteoporosis. N Engl J Med 2005;353:555-565.
181. Michaelson MD, Smith MR. Bisphosphonates for treatment and prevention of bone metastases. J Clin Oncol 2005;23:8219-8224.
182. Dando TM, Wiseman LR. Clodronate: a review of its use in the prevention of bone metastases and the management of skeletal complications associated with bone metastases in patients with breast cancer. Drugs Aging 2004;21:949-962.
183. Munster PN. Arzoxifene: the development and clinical outcome of an ideal SERM. Expert Opin Investig Drugs 2006;15:317-326.
184. Epstein S. Update of current therapeutic options for the treatment of postmenopausal osteoporosis. Clin Ther 2006;28:151-173.
185. Kloosterboer HJ. Tissue-selectivity: the mechanism of action of tibolone. Maturitas 2004;48(Suppl 1):S30-S40.
186. Devogelaer JP. A review of the effects of tibolone on the skeleton. Expert Opin Pharmacother 2004;5:941-949.
187. McClung MR, Lewiecki EM, Cohen SB et al, for the AMG 162 Bone Loss Study Group. Denosumab in postmenopausal women with low bone mineral density. N Engl J Med 2006;354:821-831.
188. Bekker PJ, Holloway DL, Rasmussen AS, et al. A single-dose placebo-controlled study of AMG 162, a fully human monoclonal antibody to RANKL, in postmenopausal women. J Bone Miner Res 2005;20:2275-2282.
189. Van Bezooijen RL, ten Dijke P, Papapoulos SE, et al. SOST/sclerostin, an osteocyte-derived negative regulator of bone formation. Cytokine Growth Factor Rev 2005;16:319-327.
190. Poole KE, van Bezooijen RL, Loveridge N, et al. Sclerostin is a delayed secreted product of osteocytes that inhibits bone formation. FASEB J 2005;19:1842-1844.
191. Kronenberg HM. PTHrP and skeletal development. Ann N Y Acad Sci 2006;1068:1-13.
192. Horwitz MJ, Tedesco MB, Sereika SM, et al. Continuous PTH and PTHrP infusion causes suppression of bone formation and discordant effects on 1,25$(OH)_2$ vitamin D. J Bone Miner Res 2005;20:1792-1803.

193. Kim MK, Kim HD, Park JH, et al. An orally active cathepsin K inhibitor, furan-2-carboxylic acid, 1-{1-[4-fluoro-2-(2-oxo-pyrrolidin-1-yl)-phenyl]-3-oxo-piperidin-4-ylcarbamoyl}-cyclohexyl)-amide (OST-4077), inhibits osteoclast activity in vitro and bone loss in ovariectomized rats. J Pharmacol Exp Ther 2006;318:555-562.
194. Lark MW, Stroup GB, James IE, et al. A potent small molecule, nonpeptide inhibitor of cathepsin K (SB 331750) prevents bone matrix resorption in the ovariectomized rat. Bone 2002;30:746-753.
195. Hodsman AB, Hanley DA, Ettinger MP, et al. Efficacy and safety of human parathyroid hormone (1-84) in increasing bone mineral density in postmenopausal osteoporosis. J Clin Endocrinol Metab 2003;88:5212-5220.
196. Ettinger MP, Greenspan SL, Marriott TB, et al. PTH(1-84) prevents first vertebral fracture in postmenopausal women with osteoporosis: results from the TOP study. Arthritis Rheum 2004;50:3060.
197. Greenspan SL, Bone HG, Marriott TB, et al. Preventing the first vertebral fracture in postmenopausal women with low bone mass using PTH(1-84): results from the TOP study [Abstract]. J Bone Miner Res 2005;20(Suppl 1):S56.
198. Seeman E, Vellas B, Benhamou C, et al. Strontium ranelate reduces the risk of vertebral and nonvertebral fractures in women eighty years of age and older. J Bone Miner Res 2006;21:1113-1120.
199. Roux C, Reginster JY, Fechtenbaum J, et al. Vertebral fracture risk reduction with strontium ranelate in women with postmenopausal osteoporosis is independent of baseline risk factors. J Bone Miner Res 2006;21:536-542.
200. Reginster JY, Seeman E, De Vernejoul MC, et al. Strontium ranelate reduces the risk of nonvertebral fractures in postmenopausal women with osteoporosis. Treatment of Peripheral Osteoporosis (TROPOS) study. J Clin Endocrinol Metab 2005;90:2816-2822.
201. Meunier PJ, Roux C, Seeman E, et al. The effects of strontium ranelate on the risk of vertebral fracture in women with postmenopausal osteoporosis. N Engl J Med 2004;350:459-468.
202. Riggs BL, Parfitt AM. Drugs used to treat osteoporosis: the critical need for a uniform nomenclature based on their action on bone remodeling. J Bone Miner Res 2005;20:177-184.
203. Frisoli A Jr, Chaves PH, Pinheiro MM, et al. The effect of nandrolone decanoate on bone mineral density, muscle mass, and hemoglobin levels in elderly women with osteoporosis: a double-blind, randomized, placebo-controlled clinical trial. J Gerontol A Biol Sci Med Sci 2005;60:648-653.
204. Flicker L, Hopper JL, Larkins RG, et al. Nandrolone decanoate and intranasal calcitonin as therapy in established osteoporosis. Osteoporos Int 1997;7:29-35.

40

DISORDERS OF THE HYPOTHALAMIC-PITUITARY AXIS

Run Yu and Glenn D. Braunstein

INTRODUCTION 611
DISEASES OF ABNORMAL LEVELS OF ARGININE VASOPRESSIN 611
Central Diabetes Insipidus 611
Pathophysiology 611
Goals of Therapy 612
Syndrome of Inappropriate Secretion of Antidiuretic Hormone 613
Pathophysiology 613
Goals of Therapy 613
FUNCTIONAL HYPOTHALAMIC AMENORRHEA 614
PITUITARY HORMONE DEFICIENCY 614
Growth Hormone Deficiency 614
Pathophysiology 614
Goals of Therapy 615
PITUITARY TUMORS 616
Prolactinoma 616
Pathophysiology 616
Goals of Therapy 616
Growth Hormone–Secreting Tumors 617
Pathophysiology 617
Goals of Therapy 618
Cushing's Disease 619
Other Pituitary Tumors 619
RECOMBINANT HUMAN THYROID-STIMULATING HORMONE 619
EMERGING TARGETS AND THERAPEUTICS 620

INTRODUCTION

The neuroendocrine portion of the hypothalamus and pituitary are anatomically and functionally closely connected and can be considered as a functional unit. The hypothalamus is a complex organ and has multiple functions, including regulating biorhythms, autonomic nervous system activity, and pituitary hormone secretion (Fig. 40-1). The hypothalamus receives neural inputs from various part of the brain and senses humoral factors and physiochemical parameters from the circulation. The hypothalamus integrates this multitude of signals and elaborates hormones that either regulate functions of the pituitary or directly act on peripheral targets. The pituitary gland anatomically and functionally divides into the posterior and anterior pituitary. The posterior pituitary is composed of axons of hypothalamic neurons and, thus, is an extension of the hypothalamus. The anterior pituitary is a true endocrine organ and receives hypothalamic hormonal inputs through the hypothalamohypophyseal portal vein system, which collects venous blood from the hypothalamus and drains it to the pituitary. The pituitary hormones stimulate peripheral endocrine organs to produce their respective hormones, which negatively or positively feed back on the hypothalamus and pituitary to achieve physiologic hormonal balance. Table 40-1 summarizes the hormones secreted by the hypothalamus and pituitary and their peripheral endocrine organs.

Hypothalamic diseases are rare. Tumors, hamartomas, inflammatory disorders, metabolic derangements, and developmental abnormalities are among the most common hypothalamic disorders. They present with distinct hypothalamic syndromes affecting water metabolism, body temperature regulation, food intake, puberty onset, mood, behavior, and pituitary hormone secretion. Treatment for most hypothalamic diseases is symptomatic or part of systemic treatment; currently there are only a few specific therapies for hypothalamic diseases. Disorders affecting arginine vasopressin (AVP) production and secretion and hypothalamic amenorrhea are reviewed in this chapter.

Pituitary diseases are more common. Acquired pituitary diseases include tumors, trauma, infiltrative diseases, and vascular diseases, while congenital pituitary diseases include abnormal pituitary development and birth trauma. Clinical presentations of pituitary diseases involve pituitary hormone excess or deficiency and space-occupying effects on vital structures such as the optic chiasm, hypothalamus, and cavernous sinuses in the vicinity of the pituitary. Therapies are available for growth hormone (GH) deficiency and for prolactin- and GH-secreting tumors, and they are covered in this chapter. Recombinant thyroid-stimulating hormone (TSH) is discussed as it is increasingly being used as part of the treatment regimen for patients with thyroid disorders. Therapies for adrenocorticotropin (ACTH) deficiency or excess, hypothyroidism from TSH deficiency, and gonadotropin abnormalities are covered in Chapter 38 (Disorders of the Thyroid), Chapter 41 (Adrenal Disorders), and Chapter 42 (Reproductive Health).

DISEASES OF ABNORMAL LEVELS OF ARGININE VASOPRESSIN

AVP (also called antidiuretic hormone [ADH]) is a peptide hormone containing 9 amino acid residues produced by neurons in the supraoptic nuclei (SON) and paraventricular nuclei (PVN) in the hypothalamus (Fig. 40-2).[1,2] These neurons send axons through the pituitary stalk to the posterior pituitary, where the secretory vesicles accumulate. While AVP secretion is stimulated by profoundly low intravascular pressure, AVP secretion is primarily regulated physiologically by plasma osmolality. The neuron bodies in SON and PVN sense the plasma osmolality, and AVP secretion from the posterior pituitary is increased when plasma osmolality rises above the normal 285 mOsm/kg. AVP acts on its renal V2 receptor in the distal nephron to redistribute water channels (aquaporins) to the interstitial side of cell membranes to enhance water reabsorption.

Central Diabetes Insipidus

Pathophysiology

Central diabetes insipidus (CDI), also called hypothalamic diabetes insipidus, is characterized by excessive renal excretion of water due to partial or complete AVP deficiency.[1] Any hereditary or acquired pathologic processes that alter the AVP gene or damage the neurons in SON and PVN in the hypothalamus, the pituitary stalk, or the posterior pituitary will result in partial or complete AVP deficiency. Insufficient AVP secretion causes continuous water loss even in the face of increased plasma osmolality, leading to dehydration, altered mental status, and even death. Some pregnant women develop CDI due to the placental production of vasopressinase (cysteine aminopeptidase), which exces-

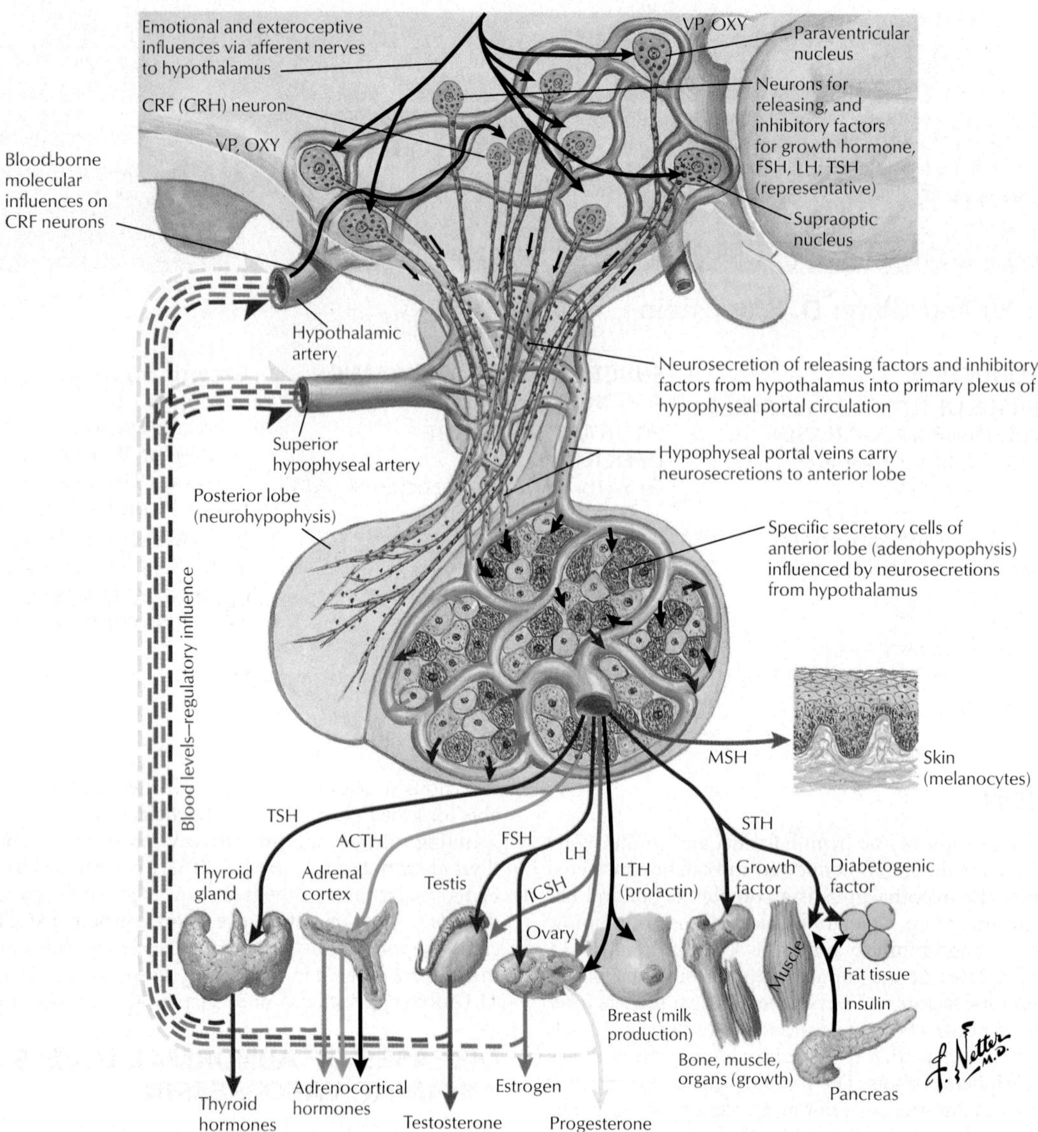

FIGURE 40-1 • The hypothalamus and pituitary control a complex neuroendocrine system that governs metabolism, growth, and reproduction. The hypothalamus produces both inhibitory and releasing neuropeptides and hormones, which reach the pituitary via a hypophysial portal system. Hypothalamic hormones trigger release of anterior pituitary hormones, which are sent to target organs where they induce hormone synthesis. Most of these endocrine-organ systems function via negative feedback—e.g., hypothalamic CRH stimulates pituitary ACTH-secretion, which stimulates adrenal cortisol secretion, which in turn inhibits CRH and ACTH secretion. Hypothalamic and pituitary hormones are used as tools in stimulation tests to diagnose hypofunctioning or hyperfunctioning endocrine states. For example, ACTH and CRH, which target the adrenal cortex, aid adrenal insufficiency diagnosis. Pituitary hormones are also used as replacement therapy for deficiencies such as hypopituitarism. (Reprinted from Netter Anatomy Illustration Collection,)

sively destroys the circulating AVP.[3] Common clinical CDI syndromes include miscellaneous hereditary conditions; any tumors that involve the hypothalamus, pituitary stalk, or posterior pituitary; neurosurgical complications; brain trauma; and infiltrative diseases, such as sarcoidosis or Langerhans cell histiocytosis.

Goals of Therapy

The underlying pathologic processes that cause CDI are usually irreversible except in some cases of transient CDI, such as those occurring during pregnancy or immediately following pituitary surgery. AVP deficiency by itself does not cause harm so long as the patient has intact thirst sense and is able to drink large amounts of water. Treatment is needed, however, in order to reduce the disruption of the patient's life caused by the frequent need to drink and urinate. The goal of treatment is to conveniently provide a sufficient amount of exogenous AVP or AVP analogue to normalize fluid intake and urine production.[1] Modern treatment involves only one medication, desmopressin, a synthetic AVP analogue that is resistant to vasopressinase.[4] Exogenous AVP itself has the untoward action of increasing blood pressure and has a short half-life; therefore, its use has largely been replaced by desmopressin.

AVP is a 9–amino acid peptide. Desmopressin was synthesized in 1967 by deamination of the first amino acid residue and replacing L-arginine at the eighth residue with D-arginine. Desmopressin's antidiuretic-to-vasopressive activity ratio is 3000-fold higher than that of AVP. Numerous clinical trials and more than 30 years of successful clinical experience demonstrate that desmopressin is the first-line treatment for CDI in both children and adults.[1,4] Desmopressin is a selective agonist of the V2 AVP receptor in the distal nephron of the kidney, simulating the natural AVP effects on water retention by the kidney. Desmopressin is given either nasally, intravenously, subcutaneously, or orally.[5] The most commonly used is the nasal route, and one spray delivers a dose of 10 μg. Individual variability exists, and the total daily requirement is usually 10 to 40 μg given in two divided doses. The plasma half-life has two components, a distributive half-life of 6.5 to 9 minutes and a terminal elimination half-life of 30 to 117 minutes.

TABLE 40-1 HYPOTHALAMUS AND PITUITARY HORMONES AND THEIR PERIPHERAL TARGETS*

Hypothalamus Hormones	Pituitary Hormones	Peripheral Hormone (organ)
PITUITARY HORMONE–RELEASING HORMONES		
Thyrotropin-releasing hormone (TRH)	↑ Thyroid-stimulating hormone (TSH)	↑ Thyroxine (thyroid)
Corticotropin-releasing hormone (CRH)	↑ Adrenocorticotropic hormone (ACTH)	↑ Cortisol (adrenal cortex)
Gonadotropin-releasing hormone (GnRH)	↑ Luteinizing hormone (LH) ↑ Follicle-stimulating hormone (FSH)	↑ Sex steroids (gonads) ↑ Inhibin (gonads)
Growth hormone–releasing hormone (GHRH)	↑ Growth hormone (GH)	↑ Insulin-like growth factor-I (IGF-I) (liver)
PITUITARY HORMONE–INHIBITING HORMONES		
Somatostatin	↓ GH, ↓ TSH	
Dopamine	↓ Prolactin	
HORMONES ACTING DIRECTLY ON THE PERIPHERY		
Arginine vasopressin		
Oxytocin		

*Functionally, the hypothalamus secretes three types of hormones. The pituitary hormone–releasing hormones stimulate the synthesis and secretion of pituitary hormones, which then stimulate peripheral endocrine organs to produce their respective hormones. For example, TRH stimulates the pituitary to secrete TSH and TSH stimulates the thyroid to secrete thyroxine. The pituitary hormone–inhibiting hormones inhibit the synthesis and secretion of pituitary hormones. For example, dopamine inhibits prolactin secretion. Vasopressin and oxytocin act directly on peripheral organs.

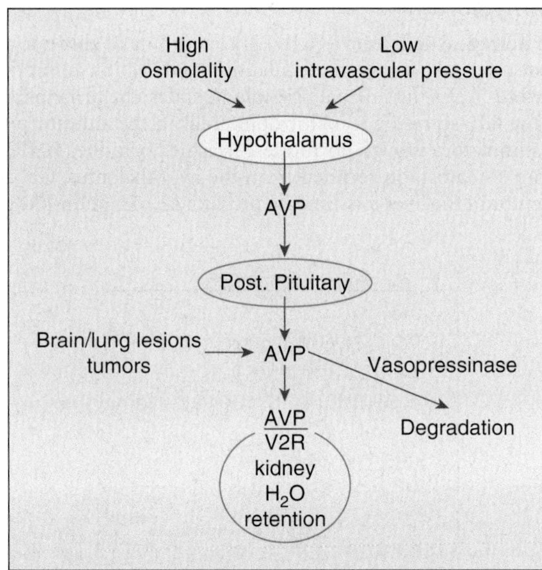

FIGURE 40-2 • Arginine vasopressin actions. Arginine vasopressin (AVP) secretion by the hypothalamus is regulated by both osmolality (under a physiologic state) and intravascular pressure (during hypotension). AVP is produced in the hypothalamus and transported to the posterior pituitary. High-plasma osmolality stimulates AVP release. AVP activates the V2 AVP receptor in the kidney, which then retains water. Brain and lung lesions and various tumors autonomously secrete AVP. AVP is degraded by placental vasopressinase in some pregnancies.

Elimination is mostly by renal excretion. After one nasal spray, the antidiuretic effect lasts 6 to 20 hours. If the patient has severe allergic rhinitis or still has nasal packing after transsphenoidal pituitary surgery, the subcutaneous or intravenous route can be used. Oral desmopressin is an attractive alternative for routine use, although the necessary dose is much higher due to trypsin digestion in the digestive tract.[5,6] The typical oral desmopressin dose is 100 to 400 μg every 8 hours. Oral desmopressin is particularly useful in patients with chronic rhinitis, those allergic to components of nasal formulations, or those with visual impairment.

The most common significant adverse effect of desmopressin is water intoxication, which is related to overdosing; the lowest dose of desmopressin should be used to maintain normal water balance.[4,7] Clinical and laboratory monitoring and dosing adjustment are needed in patients with heart failure, acute renal failure, and severe hypovolemic hypernatremia. Rarely allergic reactions develop.

Treatment of CDI is straightforward without much controversy. Desmopressin should be started once CDI is diagnosed and should continue if the CDI is permanent. The dose should be tapered or discontinued in cases of transient CDI. There are no official guidelines regarding CDI therapy.

Syndrome of Inappropriate Secretion of Antidiuretic Hormone

Pathophysiology

Syndrome of inappropriate secretion of ADH (SIADH) is a syndrome with multiple causes, but the central feature is absolute or relative excessive AVP secretion even when plasma osmolality is lower than normal.[8,9] Clinically, euvolemic hyponatremia and relatively concentrated urine are the main manifestations of SIADH. Common clinical scenarios involving SIADH are brain or lung diseases, medications, and tumors. Pathophysiologically, there are four types of SIADH. In the first type, various tumors (such as small-cell lung cancers) autonomously secrete AVP ectopically, and AVP levels are consistently high with random variations and do not respond to plasma osmolality. In the second type, basal AVP levels are higher than normal but additional AVP secretion is regulated appropriately by plasma osmolality. The third type is a reset of the hypothalamic osmostat after prolonged hypo-osmolality or hyponatremia. AVP levels are very low in the fourth type despite typical SIADH presentations. Except for the first type, most types of SIADH have multiple causes. For example, the fourth type of SIADH can be caused by renal V2 AVP receptor activation by medications or endogenous substances, or the V2 receptor can harbor mutations that render it constitutively active.[10,11] Conversely, the underlying disease for SIADH can cause multiple types of SIADH in a patient.

Goals of Therapy

Goals of therapy are to relieve symptoms, restore sodium levels, and normalize osmolality. The clinical presentation depends upon the underlying cause and the rapidity of fall of the serum sodium. Mild transient SIADH often does not require specific treatment, and clinical and laboratory monitoring is sufficient. Severe SIADH requires treatment, and attention should be paid to the speed of SIADH development and hyponatremia correction due to the concern of central pontine myelinolysis by too-rapid changes in serum osmolality. Treatment of SIADH should be aimed at correcting hyponatremia and addressing causes of SIADH; clinical judgment dictates where the emphasis should be. If no underlying causes are found or they are not correctable and symptoms are mild, water and fluid restriction is the first step in treatment. Fluid restriction should be tailored to urine output and not cause volume depletion. It may take several days for sodium levels to rise. Severe symptoms from a very low osmolality or due to a rapid fall in serum sodium may require an infusion of hypertonic (3%) saline and the administration of a loop diuretic, such as furosemide, to increase free water clearance.[12]

Pharmacologic treatments are available for SIADH. Demeclocycline is an antibiotic that causes nephrogenic diabetes insipidus; thus the kidney cannot produce hypertonic urine.[13] It is used at 600 to 1200 mg/day orally in divided doses. Its renal toxicity seriously limits demeclocycline's use except in severe SIADH.[14]

AVP receptor antagonists are a category of drugs that can be used in treating SIADH.[15] As inappropriately high levels of AVP are a common pathophysiologic mechanism in all diseases presenting SIADH, AVP receptors are a rational target for designing pharmaceuticals that antagonize AVP. Early attempts in the 1970s to 1980s to design peptide AVP receptor antagonists failed due to their low efficacy. Nonpeptide AVP receptor antagonists were found through screening numerous chemical compounds. Conivaptan, one such antagonist, is approved for use in SIADH. Conivaptan is a benzodiazepine derivative and an antagonist to both the V1a (in vascular smooth muscle and myocardium) and V2 AVP receptors.[15,16] In a placebo-controlled randomized trial, serum sodium concentrations in patients treated with intravenous conivaptan infusion (40 to 80 mg/day) for 2 days were 6 mEq/L higher than those treated with placebo.[15] Conivaptan-treated patients achieved a net water clearance of 900 ml in 4 days compared with patients treated with placebo. It is approved for intravenous infusion only at present. Conivaptan is metabolized by and potently inhibits its cytochrome P-450 (CYP) isoenzyme 3A4, a major liver isoenzyme for drug metabolism. The most common adverse effects are infusion site reactions for intravenous infusion. Conivaptan should not be used with other CYP 3A4–inhibiting medications such as ketoconazole, itraconazole, clarithromycin, ritonavir, and indinavir, and caution should be taken to avoid overdosing of drugs that are metabolized by CYP 3A4. Conivaptan also raises digoxin concentrations; thus, digoxin levels should be carefully monitored to avoid toxicity. As there has been limited clinical experience in using this drug and the effects on hyponatremia appear modest, it is still not clear what the best indications are for conivaptan. As absolute high AVP levels are present in tumor-induced SIADH, this type of SIADH may benefit most from AVP receptor antagonists.

The potential benefits of inhibiting the V1a receptor by conivaptan in heart failure are being investigated.[15,17] Several other oral nonpeptide V2 AVP receptor antagonists are in various stages of development and show efficacy in SIADH, congestive heart failure, cirrhosis, polycystic kidney disease, and certain forms of congenital nephrogenic diabetes insipidus (V2 antagonists translocate cytoplasmically stranded V2 receptors to the plasma membrane).[18,19]

SIADH is a clinical syndrome, and treatment for SIADH should be individualized according to the severity of hyponatremia and likely causes of the syndrome. Fluid and free water restriction is sufficient in most mild cases. AVP receptor antagonists may probably be reserved for the subtype of SIADH in which AVP levels are elevated. There are no official guidelines regarding SIADH therapy.

FUNCTIONAL HYPOTHALAMIC AMENORRHEA

Functional hypothalamic amenorrhea is often seen in underweight young women experiencing physical or emotional stresses.[20] There are no anatomic abnormalities in the brain as demonstrated by brain imaging. Levels of gonadotropin-releasing hormone (GnRH), luteinizing hormone (LH), follicle-stimulating hormone (FSH), and estradiol are all lower than those in normal women in the same age. It is not clear what mechanisms decrease GnRH, but as hypothalamic amenorrhea is often associated with energy deficits and low levels of leptin, leptin deficiency may play a primary role.

PITUITARY HORMONE DEFICIENCY

Hypopituitarism refers to decreased secretion of one or more hormones from the anterior pituitary.[21,22] Hypopituitarism can be either due to diseases that damage the pituicytes or due to hypothalamic diseases that result in decreased secretion of hypothalamic releasing hormones. Hypopituitarism can be either acquired or congenital. Tumors, trauma, infiltrative diseases, and vascular accidents are among the most common causes of acquired hypopituitarism, while mutations of genes critical for pituitary development and birth trauma are the most common causes of congenital hypopituitarism.[23] Therapeutic goals for hypopituitarism are to optimally replace the normal hormonal milieu.

Prolactin is not replaced, and lactation may proceed without prolactin.[24] Hormonal treatment of GH deficiency is discussed here. Although hormonal replacement is a great achievement in medicine and reaches satisfactory clinical and biochemical end points in most patients, the current replacement therapy still does not completely mimic normal physiologic hormone secretion.[25]

Growth Hormone Deficiency

Pathophysiology

Growth hormone deficiency (GHD) is a syndrome of absolute or relative inadequate GH secretion. Regulation of GH action is summarized in Figure 40-3. During normal physiologic states, the principal regulators of the GH-secreting somatotrophic cells in the anterior pituitary are the stimulatory growth hormone–releasing hormone (GHRH) and inhibitory somatostatin secreted from the hypothalamus. GH acts on GH receptor in the liver to stimulate production of insulin-like growth

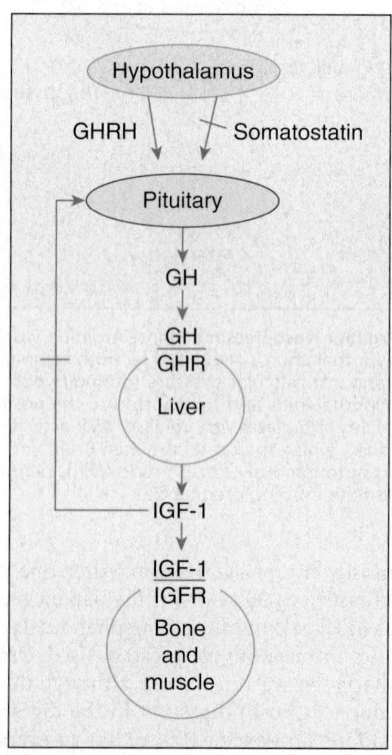

FIGURE 40-3 • Regulation of growth hormone actions. Growth hormone (GH) secretion is stimulated by growth hormone–releasing hormone (GHRH) and inhibited by somatostatin from the hypothalamus. GH activates GH receptor in the liver, which then secretes insulin-like growth factor-I (IGF-I). IGF-I acts on its own receptor on bone and muscle and promotes growth. IGF-I also negatively feeds back on the pituitary to inhibit GH secretion. (Modified from Herman-Bonert V, Melmed S. Growth hormone. In Melmed S [ed]: The Pituitary, 2nd ed. Malden, MA: Blackwell, 2002, pp 79-118.)

factor-I (IGF-I) and IGF binding protein 3 (IGFBP3). IGF-I and GH then activate their respective receptors on bone and muscle to promote growth in children or preserve muscle mass and bone mass in adults. Abnormal functioning of any steps in this chain of action results in GHD. Inadequate GHRH secretion can be idiopathic, as in idiopathic isolated GHD in children, or secondary to tumors involving the hypothalamus, as in craniopharyngioma. Neonatal injury to the pituitary stalk cuts off GHRH stimulation and invariably causes GHD. Mutations in homeobox genes such as *PROP1* and *Pit1* disrupt pituitary organogenesis and cause a decrease in somatotroph numbers, resulting in GHD and other pituitary hormone deficiencies. Pituitary tumors and surgical and radiation therapy for pituitary tumors or other intracranial neoplasms can damage the somatotrophs as well. Mutations in the genes for GH receptor, postreceptor signaling molecules, and IGF-I can all contribute to resistance to GH (Laron syndrome).[26] Rarely, IGF-I resistance occurs in patients with abnormal IGF binding proteins. Clinically, GHD is mostly idiopathic in children, but due to acquired pituitary or hypothalamic diseases in adults.

Goals of Therapy

GHD in children needs to be treated. The goals of treatment should be to restore normal growth as much as possible while avoiding GH excess and a long delay in puberty for several years.[27-29] Although treatment of adult GHD offers some measurable benefits, the goals of treatment are less clearly defined.[29,30] As its pathophysiology indicates, GHRH, GH, and IGF-I are each used in GHD treatment; among them, GH is by far the most important agent.

Growth Hormone. The rationale of using GH to treat GHD in children is straightforward as GH is the hormone that is lacking in most patients with GHD. Since recombinant human GH (rhGH) made in genetically modified *Escherichia coli* strains was approved for treatment of childhood GHD in 1985, it has become the mainstay for GHD treatment. Several brands are available in the U.S. market.[29] rhGH is a 22-kDa, single-chain polypeptide with 191 amino acid residues, similar to the native human pituitary GH.[31] Numerous clinical trials and extensive clinical experience have convincingly demonstrated that rhGH is an effective and safe treatment for most forms of GHD.[27-31] Data from National Cooperative Growth Study on more than 12,000 U.S. children demonstrated that rhGH therapy started at an average (±SD) age of 9.2 ± 4.1 years increased growth velocity from 4.4 ± 2.8 cm/yr before treatment to 10.0 ± 3.1 cm/yr 1 year after treatment, and improved the low height standard deviation scores from −2.6 ± 1.1 to −0.5 ± 1.1 after 7 years of treatment.[32]

After one subcutaneous injection of rhGH, plasma rhGH levels peak in 2 to 6 hours, and IGF-I levels peak in about 20 hours after injection.[27-31] The plasma half-life of rhGH is 20 to 30 minutes, and it is metabolized by the liver, kidney, and other organs. For GHD in children, rhGH is administered subcutaneously every day in the evening for 6 to 7 days a week. For younger children, 1 day without injection per week constitutes a "rest" and may improve compliance. The starting dose is 0.3 mg/kg of body weight per week divided evenly into 6 or 7 daily injections. rhGH therapy should continue until final height or epiphyseal closure is reached. Dose titration is based on the growth curve and serum IGF-I and IGFBP3 levels and targeted to achieve sufficient catch-up linear growth and normalize IGF-I and IGFBP3 in order to avoid overdosing. Higher doses can be used if GHD is diagnosed in late childhood to maximize growth within the therapeutic window.

During the transition period from late adolescence to adulthood, GH function should be re-evaluated in those patients with childhood GHD.[33,34] Patients with idiopathic or isolated childhood GHD tend to develop normal GH secretion, while those with GHD and multiple pituitary hormone deficiencies, genetic abnormalities, and structural damage to the hypothalamus or pituitary usually remain GH deficient. All those with clear GHD during the transition and afterward would benefit from GH therapy. Patients with irreversible causes of GHD should continue GH therapy, but rhGH doses should be continuously titrated down to avoid overdosing and to maintain normal GH status. When restarting GH therapy, it is suggested to begin with 0.4 to 0.8 mg/day and to increase the dose by 0.2 to 0.4 mg/day every 4 to 6 weeks until a maintenance dose of 1.2 to 2.0 mg/day is achieved.[29] The maintenance dose may need to be titrated down periodically to avoid adverse effects.

Adverse effects of rhGH are related to overdosing.[27-31] Children may develop coarse facial features. Rare allergic reactions may occur. Due to the concern that rhGH may promote tumor growth, rhGH treatment in tumor survivors should be coordinated with a pediatric oncologist or neurosurgeon in order to monitor for tumor relapse. Current data do not indicate that rhGH causes such a relapse, although the risk of secondary neoplasms appears to increase.[35]

rhGH therapy is also approved for treating other childhood diseases characterized by short stature or relative GHD. These diseases are Turner's syndrome, chronic renal failure, small for gestational age, Prader-Willi syndrome, and severe idiopathic short stature. rhGH treatment in these diseases varies, and readers should refer to published guidelines.[29]

The decision to treat GHD in adults should be made on an individual basis, and rhGH treatment probably most benefits those with clear structural pituitary diseases, with demonstrated laboratory abnormalities in GH secretion following provocative testing, and low IGF-I levels.[29-31,36] In these patients, rhGH therapy increases lean body mass and decreases fat mass, increases bone mineral density, lowers LDL and total cholesterol levels, and improves the quality of life. rhGH is injected subcutaneously daily, and dosing should be titrated up from a conservative starting dose, which is usually 0.3 mg/day. A body weight–based regimen commonly causes overdosing and should not be used in adults. Dosing is increased by 0.1 to 0.2 mg/day every 1 to 2 months, targeting the clinical response (such as improvements in energy levels and muscle mass) and keeping IGF-I levels in the upper half of normal range. The optimal duration of rhGH treatment is not clear, but treatment perhaps can continue indefinitely if rhGH produces expected benefits. Although there is only weak and controversial evidence suggesting that rhGH treatment for adult GHD may facilitate tumor growth, current guidelines suggest that rhGH treatment is contraindicated in patients with concurrent malignancies; clinicians should make a balanced decision regarding rhGH usage with concurrent malignancy.

Several studies show that administration of exogenous GH to healthy elderly without GHD modestly increases lean body mass and decreases fat mass.[37-40] The increase in muscle mass, however, does not translate into increase in muscle strength or functioning levels. If the healthy elderly undergo muscle strength training, GH does not give any additional benefits. In addition, some individuals treated with GH develop carpal tunnel syndrome, gynecomastia, or hyperglycemia. Malignancy associated with GH therapy is also a theoretical concern. Due to these issues, GH should not be used as an antiaging agent, and prescribing GH for "antiaging" purposes is unwise (and illegal) in the United States. The limited benefits extra GH can confer to a healthy elderly adult can be easily achieved with exercise.[41,42] rhGH is also used for treating lipodystrophy in adult and pediatric patients infected with human immunodeficiency virus.[43,44]

Insulin-like Growth Factor-I. As IGF-I is the major hormonal mediator of GH actions, IGF-I therapy is a rational treatment of patients with GH resistance.[45-48] Recombinant human IGF-I (rhIGF-I) and recombinant human IGF-I/IGFBP3 complex (rhIGF-I/rhIGFBP3) were both approved for treatment of primary IGF-I deficiency. rhIGF-I is produced in genetically modified *E. coli* strains and is a 7.6-kDa single-chain polypeptide of 70 amino acid residues. The amino acid sequence of rhIGF-I is identical to that of natural human IGF-I. rhIGF-I binds to IGF-I receptor and stimulates skeletal growth. Five clinical trials including a total of 71 children (chronological age 6.7 years at time of starting treatment) with primary IGF-I deficiency treated with rhIGF-I for 1 to 8 years demonstrated that rhIGF-I accelerates height velocity from 2.8 cm/yr before treatment to 8.0 cm/year in the first year of treatment. In the 13 patients who completed 8 years of rhIGF-I treatment, standard deviation score went from −6.7 to −5.2. Bioavailability of rhIGF-I after one subcutaneous injection is close to 100% in normal volunteers. rhIGF-I binds to endogenous IGFBP3 in the plasma. Plasma rhIGF-I concentration peaks in 2 hours after injection, and half-time for elimination is 5.8 hours. rhIGF-I is metabolized by the liver and kidney. rhIGF-I dosing should be individualized. The starting dose is 40 to 80 μg/kg of body weight twice a day injected subcutaneously. The dose can be increased by 40 μg/kg per dose, to a maximum of 120 μg/kg given twice a day. Mild to moderate hypoglycemia occurs in 42% of patients, consistent with the structural homology between rhIGF-I and insulin. Other adverse events include lipohypertrophy at injection sites and rarely benign intracranial hypertension.

The adverse effects of rhIGF-I may be related to high free IGF-I levels. To avoid these adverse effects, rhIGF-I has been mixed at a 1 : 1 molar ratio with rhIGFBP3.[49] The rhIGF-I/rhIGFBP3 complex has a longer plasma half-life than free IGF-I, which is more rapidly eliminated from the circulation. Produced also in *E. coli*, rhIGFBP3 is a 29-kDa single-chain polypeptide of 264 amino acid residues. The amino acid sequence of rhIGFBP3 is identical to that of natural human IGFBP3. The efficacy of rhIGF-I/IGFBP3 has been established in a prospective, open-label clinical trial of 36 children (chronological age 8.7 years at time of starting treatment) with IGF-I deficiency. rhIGF-I/IGFBP3 accelerates height velocity from 2 to 3 cm/yr before treatment to 7 to 9 cm/year in the first 6 months of treatment. Standard deviation score improved by 0.4. Plasma rhIGF-I and IGFBP3 concentrations peak in 11 to 19 hours after injection, and half-time for elimination is 13.4 hours for IGF-I and 54 hours for IGFBP3. rhIGF-I dosing should also be individualized. The starting dose is 0.5 mg/kg of body weight subcutaneously once a day. The dose can be increased to a maximal of 1 to 2 mg/kg daily. Adverse effects are fewer and less severe than those caused by rhIGF-I alone.

There has been limited experience with rhIGF-I and rhIGF-I/rhIGFBP3 in the treatment of primary IGF-I deficiency. Generally their efficacy is less impressive compared with that of rhGH for common GHD, suggesting that GH has IGF-I–independent growth benefits. These agents, however, are valuable as rhGH does not work well in the treatment of primary IGF-I deficiency.[45-48]

Growth Hormone–Releasing Hormone. GHRH is used for both diagnosis and treatment of GHD.[50-52] GHRH cannot be used alone in the diagnosis of GHD as responses to GHRH are variable between individual subjects. GHD is credibly diagnosed by applying both GHRH and arginine. For this test, recombinant analogue GHRH (1-29) 1 μg/kg of body weight is injected intravenously at time 0 and arginine hydrochloride 0.5 g/kg of body weight is infused intravenously during the first 30 minutes, and GH levels are measured every 15 minutes for 90 minutes. Insufficient elevation of GH levels after stimulation is diagnostic of GHD.

Therapeutically, GHRH is used to treat GHD in children. Synthetic GHRH (Sermorelin) was approved in 1998 for GHD treatment, but the manufacturer (Serono) withdrew it from the U.S. market in 2002, so no U.S. Food and Drug Administration (FDA)–approved GHRH is available for routine use now. A synthetic GHRH analogue, CJC-1295, with a longer in vivo half-life has been tested in normal subjects and proven to increase GH and IGF-I.[53]

The GH Research Society (2000) and the Lawson Wilkins Pediatric Endocrinology Society (2003) have published guidelines on treatment of GHD in children.[27,28] The American Association of Clinical Endocrinologists (AACE) has a 2003 guideline on rhGH use for GHD in adults and children.[29] The Endocrine Society has a 2006 guideline on treatment of GHD in adults.[30] Several authoritative reviews also give advice on GH use.[31,33,41] We synthesize a summary here incorporating all agents. In children with GHD, rhGH should be started once the diagnosis is made and terminated when the target height is reached. rhGH should be restarted in the late teenage years or young adulthood if GHD proves to be permanent on repeat testing or with a low IGF-I level in the presence of a structural lesion. rhIGF-I can be used for children with GH resistance. It is not practical in most cases to use GHRH as it is not commercially available in the United States. Whichever agent is to be used, dosing should be individualized and clinical and laboratory responses monitored. rhGH therapy should be used in definitive adult GHD.

PITUITARY TUMORS

Pituitary tumors comprise 10% of intracranial tumors.[54] Clinically, most pituitary tumors are benign adenomas from the anterior pituitary. These adenomas either do not secrete functioning hormones (thus called nonfunctioning) or secrete autonomously one or more hormones that cause endocrine disturbances. The adenoma itself may also cause mass effect by growth and invasion of surrounding organs, including the pituitary stalk, optic chiasm, and hypothalamus. The goals of managing all pituitary adenomas are normalizing the levels of the hormone(s) the adenoma secretes and reducing the tumor size. Surgical, medical, and radiation therapies are all employed.

Prolactinoma

Pathophysiology

Prolactinoma is an adenoma of the anterior pituitary lactotrophic cells.[55-57] It secretes excess amounts of prolactin and damages the pituitary and surrounding structures through mass effects. Prolactin receptors are present in the mammary glands, hypothalamus, pituitary, and many other organs.[58] Physiologic prolactin secretion is important in the development of mammary glands and lactation; inhibition of gonadal function during lactation has evolutionary value in hindering ovulation and pregnancy during lactation. Abnormally high levels of prolactin outside the context of pregnancy and normal lactation cause galactorrhea by stimulating milk production, and central hypogonadism by suppressing secretion of hypothalamic GnRH and pituitary LH and FSH. Prolactin secretion from prolactinomas is still under negative control by dopamine via the D_2 receptor and positive control by estrogen via the estrogen receptor; both receptors are present in normal lactotrophs and in prolactinoma cells. By virtue of a space-occupying lesion, prolactinoma can cause headache, hypopituitarism, visual field defects, and blindness.

Goals of Therapy

Goals of therapy should be normalization of prolactin levels and tumor shrinkage in most cases.[55,56,59,60] For small prolactinomas (microadenomas) with low levels of prolactin in women, symptomatic management with estrogen with or without progesterone or watchful observation is also reasonable. Except in a few selected cases in which surgical resection is optional, medical treatment with dopamine agonists is the best approach.

Bromocriptine. Bromocriptine is a semisynthetic ergot derivative first synthesized in the late 1960s and found to have dopamine activity, to lower prolactin levels, and to shrink prolactinomas.[52,61,62] Bromocriptine was first FDA-approved for hyperprolactinemia in 1978 and later for the specific treatment of prolactinomas in 1985. It is an agonist of the D_2 dopaminergic receptor, which couples to the inhibitory G protein (G_i).[63] Bromocriptine lowers intracellular cyclic AMP levels in normal lactotrophs and in prolactinoma cells, and decreases prolactin production and secretion. Bromocriptine also causes prolactinoma cell shrinkage and inhibits prolactinoma cell division. Bromocriptine thus is an ideal medical treatment for prolactinoma, leading to both a decrease in prolactin levels and tumor shrinkage. These changes are somewhat irreversible after long-term bromocriptine treatment. The efficacy of bromocriptine has been attested by numerous clinical trials and more than 20 years of clinical experience.[55,56,59,60] Bromocriptine normalized prolactin levels in 70% to 80% of patients, but some patients resumed normal menses even with slightly elevated prolactin levels. Tumor shrinkage of more than 50% is achieved in 40% of patients, shrinkage of 25% to 50% in 29% of patients, and shrinkage of less than 25% in 13% of patients. Only about 20% of patients have no change in tumor size.

The bioavailability of bromocriptine after an oral dose is 28%.[55,56,59,60] After absorption from the gastrointestinal tract into the circulation, bromocriptine sustains extensive first-pass biotransformation by the liver. After an oral dose, plasma levels peak in 1 to 3 hours and prolactin-lowering effects start in 1 to 2 hours, and the effects last 12 hours. Bromocriptine is metabolized and excreted by the liver and has two components in the elimination half-life. The second component of half-life is about 15 hours.

Bromocriptine therapy should be started with a low dose and titrated up gradually.[55,56,59,60] It is recommended to start with a dose of 0.625 mg taken orally daily at bedtime with a snack for a week. A morning dose of 1.25 mg is then added. The dose is increased by 1.25 mg every week until the full dose of 5.0 mg is reached. Dose can be further increased if prolactin levels are not normalized. Optimal effects can be achieved with a twice-daily regimen (e.g., 2.5 mg twice daily).

The most common adverse effects are nausea and vomiting.[55,56,59,60] Orthostatic hypotension, digital vasospasm, nasal congestion, and depression are less common. Bromocriptine is safe during pregnancy.

Bromocriptine was approved for Parkinson's disease in 1978, although it is now a second-line agent for this condition. Bromocriptine was also approved for acromegaly in 1984 (this use is to be discussed under GH-secreting tumor). Bromocriptine should not be used for the purpose of lactation suppression in postpartum women.[64] It was approved for such use in 1980, but the manufacturer withdrew the drug from such use in 1994 due to variable efficacy and rare vascular complications.

Cabergoline. Cabergoline was first synthesized in the early 1980s as an ergot derivative and approved for treatment for hyperprolactinemic disorders in the United States in 1996.[55,56,59,60] Due to better patient compliance and greater tumor size reduction, cabergoline is preferable over bromocriptine in the routine treatment of prolactinoma. Compared with bromocriptine, cabergoline acts similarly on the D_2 dopaminergic receptor, but its actions are longer lasting and its side effects are more tolerable. Clinical trials and extensive experience both demonstrate that cabergoline's effects on prolactin level normalization are similar to those of bromocriptine, but tumor shrinkage by cabergoline is more evident than that by bromocriptine. Cabergoline's prolonged action is due to its long half-life in the pituitary and high affinity for the D_2 receptor, as well as enterohepatic circulation. After one oral dose, plasma levels peak in 2 to 3 hours and the elimination half-life is over 60 hours. The prolactin-lowering effect starts at 3 hours after ingestion and remains active for as long as 120 hours. Cabergoline therapy also starts with a low dose and is titrated up gradually until the prolactin concentration is normalized. The starting dose is 0.25 mg taken orally twice a week. The dose is increased by 0.25 mg twice weekly every month up to 1 mg twice weekly. The usual therapeutic dose is 0.25 to 0.5 mg twice weekly. Cabergoline has adverse effects similar to those of bromocriptine, but they are less severe and less frequent. At doses approximately 30-fold higher than that used for prolactinoma, cabergoline is associated with structural and functional heart valve defects during treatment for Parkinson's disease. There are no data on whether the low-dose treatment of cabergoline for prolactinoma is associated with similar complications. We advise using bromocriptine and avoiding cabergoline in patients with prolactinoma and heart murmurs or history of valvular heart diseases before the risks of low-dose cabergoline on heart valve damage are ascertained.[64a,64b]

Pergolide and quinagolide are two other D_2 receptor agonists used for prolactinoma in Europe and Canada, but they are not approved for such use in the United States.[59,60]

Special Issues During Dopamine Agonist Therapy. A minority of prolactinomas are resistant to dopamine agonists. The exact definition of resistance has been variable.[59,60,65] An authoritative review defined dopamine agonist resistance as failure to normalize prolactin levels or failure to shrink prolactin tumor size by more than 50%. Resistance is usually due to low expression levels of D_2 receptors and the inhibitory G protein in the adenoma. Strategies for managing resistance include switching to another dopamine agonist and cautiously increasing the dose of the better drug. If the second dopamine agonist also meets resistance, surgery and radiation therapies are reasonable.

For most women desiring pregnancy, either bromocriptine or cabergoline can be used to treat the prolactinoma, although the former has a longer and more reliable safety record.[59,60,66] Once pregnancy is established, the dopamine agonist should be discontinued. If the tumor grows during pregnancy, bromocriptine can be used. Dopamine agonists should not be used by nursing women but should be resumed in women who do not breast-feed.

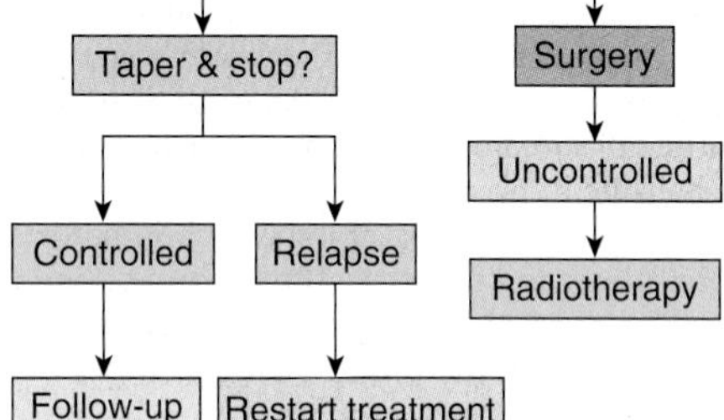

FIGURE 40-4 • Guideline for managing prolactinoma. Medical treatment with a dopamine agonist (DA) is first-line therapy. The choice of agent depends on availability, cost, and physician experience. Cabergoline is usually the first choice in the United States. In select patients with microprolactinoma, surgical resection is an alternative. After medical treatment, if patients have normalized prolactin and tumors are undetectable on magnetic resonance imaging for 2 years, tapering or withdrawal from medical treatment can be attempted with careful monitoring. (From Casanueva FF, Molitch ME, Schlechte JA, et al. Guidelines of the Pituitary Society for the diagnosis and management of prolactinomas. Clin Endocrinol 2006;65:265-273.)

Chronic visual changes associated with macroprolactinoma are not surgical emergencies and are treated with dopamine agonists,[56] while acute visual impairment in a patient with a macroadenoma may represent enlargement from hemorrhage into the tumor ("pituitary apoplexy"), which is a neurosurgical emergency.[67]

The duration of medical treatment is under active investigation.[60,68] In some patients, treatment may be lifelong. Large trials of withdrawal from bromocriptine are lacking, whereas a trial provides some practical guidance for cabergoline withdrawal. It is recommended that, for patients who have been on cabergoline treatment for at least 2 years with normalization of prolactin levels and no residual tumors on magnetic resonance imaging, cabergoline withdrawal can be attempted; the remission rate is as high as 70% at 8 years after withdrawal. Menopause is another opportunity to discontinue medical treatment. A small study shows that 45% of patients normalize prolactin after menopause while off medication.[69]

The Pituitary Society has a 2006 guideline on diagnosis and management of prolactinoma.[70] Several authoritative reviews are also available.[56,59,60] The Pituitary Society guideline is shown in Figure 40-4 with our comments in the legend.

Growth Hormone–Secreting Tumors

Pathophysiology

GH-secreting tumors are adenomas of the pituitary somatotrophic cells.[71] These tumors autonomously secrete large amounts of GH and, like prolactinomas, can also expand to damage the pituitary and invade surrounding organs and tissues. GH secretion from GH-secreting tumors is still under negative control by somatostatin and IGF-I. The high levels of GH act on the normal GH signaling pathway and cause exaggerated biologic effects. In children, these tumors cause gigantism; in adults, they cause acromegaly and organomegaly, as well as other abnormalities including diabetes, hypertension, sleep apnea, osteoarthritis, skin tags, cardiovascular diseases, and possibly malignancy.

Goals of Therapy

Goals of therapy should be normalization of GH and IGF-I levels and reduction in tumor size in most cases.[71,72] Unlike prolactinoma, for which medical treatment is first line, GH secreting tumors demand a more individualized treatment plan. In most cases, surgical resection is a reasonable first option, especially for patients with microadenomas (<1 cm), but surgery achieves biochemical cure in less than 50% of patients with macroadenomas (>1 cm). Somatostatin analogues as primary medical therapy is more appropriate in patients with low likelihood of surgical cure, high operative risks, or without sellar compression, or in patients who decline surgery.[72,73] A comparison of primary surgical and primary medical treatments is shown in Table 40-2. The role of radiation therapy is less defined and rather controversial.

Somatostatin Analogues. GH secretion by adenomas is negatively regulated by somatostatin, but somatostatin is unsuitable for therapeutic use due to its short half-life in plasma (2 to 3 minutes) and nonselective actions on all somatostatin receptor subtypes.[74-76] Somatostatin analogues with longer half-lives and selective affinity for sst2 and sst5 somatostatin receptor subtypes are the mainstay of medical treatment for GH-secreting adenomas. Two somatostatin analogues, octreotide and lanreotide, are used to treat GH-secreting tumors.

Octreotide is a synthetic octapeptide that was first synthesized as a somatostatin analogue in the early 1980s and was soon found to inhibit GH secretion in patients with acromegaly.[77-82] Octreotide also lowers IGF-I levels and reduces pituitary tumor size. The beneficial effects of octreotide on acromegaly are produced by multiple mechanisms. Octreotide directly inhibits GH secretion for GH-secreting adenomas and causes adenoma cell apoptosis and subsequent tumor shrinkage.[83,84] Octreotide also reduces GHRH secretion from the hypothalamus. In addition, octreotide inhibits GH binding to its receptors and reduces IGF-I production in the liver. At the molecular level, octreotide binds to sst2 and sst5 receptor subtypes, which are coupled to G_i. Inhibition of GHRH and GH secretion is mediated by lowering cyclic AMP and cytoplasmic calcium levels in the hypothalamic and pituitary somatotrophic cells.

The efficacy of octreotide as primary medical treatment for acromegaly is well established. A critical analysis of six clinical trials published before 2004 demonstrates that 43% to 79% of patients normalize GH levels (measured by GH suppression during a glucose tolerance test), and 53% to 68% of patients normalize IGF-I after octreotide (regular or long-acting release [LAR]) treatment for 1 to 5 years.[72] The degree of biochemical control is comparable to that from surgery. When used preoperatively on macroadenomas, octreotide also increased the cure rate of surgery; octreotide is unlikely to further increase the already high surgical cure rate of microadenomas.[96] Octreotide is similarly effective in patients who have undergone surgery and in those for whom octreotide is primary treatment. Surgical debulking of large tumors may enhance octreotide efficacy.[85]

Two preparations of octreotide are available: regular octreotide and octreotide LAR. Regular octreotide was approved for acromegaly in 1994. In acromegalic patients, plasma levels peak at 40 minutes after one subcutaneous injection and the biologic action of one subcutaneous dose is up to 12 hours. The elimination half-time is 1.7 to 1.9 hours. Most octreotide is degraded in the liver, but 30% is excreted into the urine. Dosing should be adjusted in patients with renal failure. Octreotide therapy usually starts at 50 μg injected subcutaneously three times a day. The dose is titrated up every 2 weeks based on IGF-I levels; the usual dose is 100 μg three times a day, but higher doses may be needed in some patients. As medical treatment may be lifelong and the frequent injections negatively affect patient compliance, octreotide LAR was invented and was approved for acromegaly in 1998. It is composed of biodegradable microspheres to which octreotide is attached and gradually released after intramuscular injection. Once octreotide is released into the circulation, it behaves as regular octreotide and has the same pharmacokinetics. Following one intramuscular injection, plasma octreotide levels have two peaks. The first peak appears within 1 hour, and plasma levels gradually drop and the trough is reached at 3 to 5 days. Plasma levels gradually increase, and the second peak appears at 3 weeks. After multiple injections every 4 weeks, steady state octreotide plasma levels are reached. The manufacturer (Novartis) and experts recommend starting octreotide LAR after an initial trial of regular octreotide in order to determine the efficacy in lowering GH and IGF-I and patient tolerance.[73] This recommendation is reasonable as one injection of octreotide LAR results in therapeutic octreotide plasma levels for up to 60 days. A trial with 34 patients, however, showed that the efficacy and tolerability of octreotide LAR are satisfactory when it is used as initial therapy without previous regular octreotide.[86] Octreotide LAR is started at 20 mg every 4 weeks, and the dose is adjusted every 3 months according to GH and IGF-I levels.

As octreotide is an analogue of somatostatin, a hormone with numerous physiologic functions, octreotide tends to have multiple adverse effects, although most of them are subclinical.[72,73] The most common are injection site pain and gastrointestinal distress, including diarrhea, abdominal cramps, and fatty stools. Most patients tolerate these well. More than half of the patients develop gallbladder sludge or gallstones that are usually asymptomatic. A minority of patients develop bradycardia, hypo- or hyperglycemia, or hypothyroidism. Patients with pre-existing heart disease, diabetes, or thyroid disorders need to be monitored carefully during octreotide treatment for exacerbation of the coexisting condition.

TABLE 40-2 DECIDING THE IDEAL PRIMARY THERAPY FOR PATIENTS HARBORING GH-SECRETING ADENOMAS: FACTORS TO CONSIDER WHEN CHOOSING BETWEEN SURGERY AND SOMATOSTATIN ANALOGUES

	Transphenoidal Surgery	Long-Acting Somatostatin Analogues
Cost	One-time cost (when cure achieved)	Lifelong therapy
Recurrence rate	Up to 10%	No tachyphylaxis reported
Side effects	<10% morbidity (DI, CSF leak, meningitis, severe sinusitis, hypopituitarism); mortality <1%	Transient GI symptoms 25%, asymptomatic gallstones 15%
Reversal of compressive effects	Tumor excision leads to immediate relief of optic tract pressure and is mandatory for progressive deterioration of visual fields.	Some degree of tumor shrinkage occurs in most patients; a decrease in volume >25% and >50% occurs in ~50% and ~25% of patients, respectively.
Biochemical control	70%-90% of microadenomas <50% of macroadenomas	50%-80% overall
Anesthetic/surgical risk	Avoid surgery if high risk	
Patient preference	Weigh informed risks versus benefits	Weigh informed risks versus benefits

CSF, cerebrospinal fluid; DI, diabetes insipidus; GI, gastrointestinal.
From Donangelo I, Melmed S. Treatment of acromegaly: future. Endocrine 2005;28:123-128.

Another long-acting somatostatin analog, lanreotide acetate, was approved for medical treatment of acromegaly in 2007. Lanreotide acetate had been used in Europe for several years. Its indications, efficacy, and adverse effects are comparable to those of octreotide LAR. Lanreotide acetate is given as a deep subcutaneous injection monthly. The starting dose is 90 mg/month and the dose is titrated every three months according to GH and IGF-1 levels.[73,86a,86b]

Dopamine Agonists. The dopamine agonist bromocriptine has limited efficacy in acromegaly, but cabergoline has substantial benefits on the condition.[72,87] At doses usually higher than used for prolactinoma, cabergoline alone normalized IGF-I levels in 35% of patients. Cabergoline is used as an adjunct therapy in partially octreotide-resistant acromegaly and in tumors secreting both GH and prolactin.[88,89]

Growth Hormone Receptor Antagonist. Molecular biology has allowed rational design of a GH antagonist, pegvisomant, which was approved for acromegaly in 2003. Normal GH binds to two GH receptors and induces GH receptor dimerization, a critical step for GH signaling.[90] Pegvisomant is a recombinant mutant GH molecule with four to six polyethylene glycol (PEG) polymers covalently linked to lysine or phenylalanine residues.[91-93] The mutant GH harbors 9 amino acid residue substitutions that result in increased affinity to one GH receptor but much decreased affinity to another, preventing GH receptor dimerization. The PEG polymers attached to the mutant GH increase its molecular weight from 22 kDa to 42, 47, or 52 kDa, thus decreasing renal clearance but without jeopardizing affinity to GH receptor. Pegvisomant has been subjected to several clinical trials that demonstrated that up to 18 months of therapy decreases IGF-I levels in every patient, normalizes IGF-I levels in 97% of patients, and alleviates many symptoms of acromegaly.[94-96] In patients who are resistant to octreotide, replacement with or addition of pegvisomant normalizes IGF-I levels.[96,97] After one subcutaneous injection, pegvisomant plasma levels peak at 33 to 77 hours, and half-time for elimination is about 6 days, primarily through renal clearance. Pegvisomant therapy starts with a dose of subcutaneous injections of 10 mg daily, and the dose is titrated up every 4 to 6 weeks based on IGF-I levels; the maximum dose can be as high as 80 mg/day.[98] The goals of therapy are normalization of IGF-I levels and alleviation of symptoms and signs of acromegaly.

There is limited clinical experience on using pegvisomant for acromegaly treatment. The most common side effects are injection site reactions and headache.[94-96] GH levels increase twofold in most patients partly due to removal of IGF-I negative feedback, and partly due to cross reaction of pegvisomant with GH. Serious adverse effects include GH-secreting tumor enlargement and elevation of liver enzymes in a few patients. Overtreatment is a potential issue, and there is no satisfactory marker of optimal dosage as IGF-I may be normal in adult patients with GHD.[72]

The Acromegaly Treatment Workshop, participated in by neuroendocrinologists and neurosurgeons, established by consensus a guideline on acromegaly management in 2000 that was amended in 2003.[99,100] The AACE has a 2004 guideline for acromegaly treatment.[101] Several authoritative reviews are also available.[71-73] The amended algorithm by the Acromegaly Treatment Workshop is shown in Figure 40-5 with our comments in the legend.

Cushing's Disease

Cushing's disease is caused by an ACTH-secreting pituitary adenoma.[102] Autonomous ACTH secretion stimulates overproduction of cortisol with resultant multisystem abnormalities such as obesity, fat accumulation in the face and trunk, muscle wasting, collagen thinning, hypertension, diabetes mellitus, and hirsutism. Primary treatment is surgical resection of the disease-causing pituitary tumor.

Corticotropin-releasing hormone (CRH) is clinically used in a CRH stimulation test and in petrosal sinus venous sampling for the diagnosis of Cushing's disease.[103,104] Chemically synthesized ovine or human CRH is injected intravenously at a dose of 1 μg/kg of body weight or 100 μg to stimulate ACTH release. The half-life of ovine CRH is longer than that of human CRH, and therefore ovine CRH has longer stimulation on ACTH production.

Other Pituitary Tumors

Pituitary tumors of the nonfunctioning, gonadotrophic, and thyrotropin-secreting types are primarily treated surgically and therefore not discussed in this chapter.

RECOMBINANT HUMAN THYROID-STIMULATING HORMONE

TSH deficiency alone or with deficiency of other pituitary hormones causes central hypothyroidism, and treatment is with thyroxine replacement (see Chapter 38, Disorders of the Thyroid). Although recombinant human TSH (rhTSH) is not used for treatment of hypothalamic or pituitary diseases, rhTSH is now widely used for diagnos-

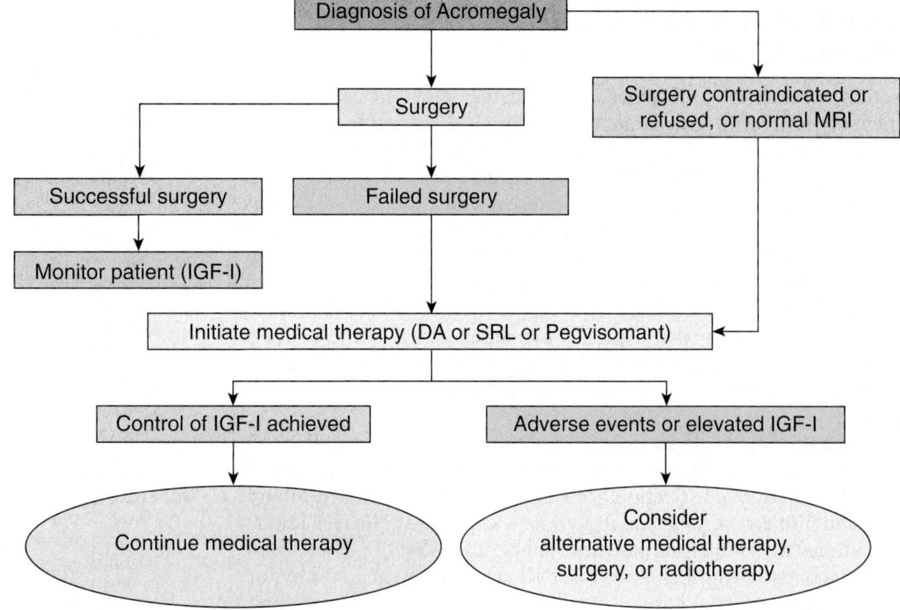

FIGURE 40-5 • Guideline for managing acromegaly. First-line therapy is surgical resection. Primary medical therapy is appropriate in patients with low likelihood of surgical cure, high operative risks, and without sellar compression, and in patients who decline surgery. The choice of agent depends on availability, cost, and physician experience. In the United States, octreotide is usually the first choice. Cabergoline is useful for tumors secreting both GH and prolactin. Addition of pegvisomant or cabergoline to patients resistant to octreotide is reasonable. DA, dopamine agonist. (From Clemmons DR, Chihara K, Freda PU, et al. Optimizing control of acromegaly: integrating a growth hormone receptor antagonist into the treatment algorithm. J Clin Endocrinol Metab 2003;88:4759-4767.)

tic purposes and for the treatment of thyroid cancer and goiter based on the fact that TSH stimulates uptake of radiolabeled iodine into normal or cancerous thyroid tissue.[105] Due to the ease of protocol and better patient quality of life, rhTSH administration has partly replaced the thyroxine withdrawal method, which stimulates endogenous TSH elevation in thyroid cancer patients treated with an initial dose of radioactive iodine for ablation of residual thyroid tissue following total thyroidectomy. rhTSH is a glycoprotein comprising two noncovalently linked subunits.[106,107] The alpha subunit has 92 amino acids and two N-linked glucosylation sites, while the beta subunit has 112 amino acids and one N-linked glucosylation site. Both subunits are identical to those of natural human TSH in amino acid sequence. rhTSH is produced by a Chinese hamster ovary cell clone that is stably transfected with plasmids encoding the complimentary DNA for the two subuits. rhTSH is secreted into the cell culture medium and purified biochemically.

Like natural TSH, rhTSH binds to and activates the G_s-coupled TSH receptor and increases intracellular cyclic AMP levels.[105-107] The signaling cascade eventually leads to increased production and secretion of thyroxine, triiodothyronine, and thyroglobulin, and increased uptake of radioiodine and glucose in both normal thyroid follicular cells and thyroid cancer cells in vitro and in vivo. rhTSH can be assayed with the same method used for natural TSH. After an intramuscular injection of 0.9 mg of rhTSH, peak serum concentration is reached in an average of 10 hours and the serum rhTSH plateau lasts for about 20 hours. The volume of distribution is 69 L. The half-time for rhTSH elimination is about 22 hours, and rhTSH is possibly metabolized by the liver and kidney.

Clinical use of rhTSH is based on the fact that rhTSH stimulates radioactive iodine and glucose uptake and thyroglobulin production and secretion.[105] rhTSH is used diagnostically for monitoring remnant and metastatic thyroid cancer by whole body radioactive iodine scan, positron emission tomography, and thyroglobulin levels. Therapeutically, rhTSH facilitates radioactive iodine treatment of thyroid cancer and multinodular goiter. rhTSH 0.9 mg is given intramuscularly on two consecutive days, and on the third day, radioactive iodine is given for diagnosis or treatment. Positron emission tomography is also performed on the third day if intended. Diagnostic whole body radioactive iodine scan and thyroglobulin measurements take place on the fifth day.

The common rhTSH side effects are nausea and headache.[105] Severe side effects are related to the increase in thyroid cancer or goiter volume induced by rhTSH, which can lead to neurologic deterioration in patients with thyroid cancer brain metastasis, or to respiratory distress in those with large goiters.

EMERGING TARGETS AND THERAPEUTICS

Leptin, a hormone secreted by adipose tissue, has been used experimentally to treat hypothalamic amenorrhea.[108] (The leptin effects on obesity are discussed in Chapter 36, Obesity and Nutrition, and Chapter 37, Diabetes Mellitus). Human leptin is a 16-kDs polypeptide comprising 146 amino acids.[109] Leptin receptors are found in the hypothalamus and other brain areas. A recombinant methionyl human leptin (r-metHuLeptin) is given subcutaneously daily at 0.08 mg/kg of body weight in divided doses for 2 to 3 months. This regimen improves LH levels and LH pulsatility, as well as estradiol levels, and induces ovulation in women with hypothalamic amenorrhea. Some patients resumed ovulatory menstruation. Leptin's role for functional hypothalamic amenorrhea is only experimental, and further studies are needed.

A somatostatin analogue, SOM230, has much higher affinity for sst5 somatostatin receptors and slightly lower affinity for sst2 receptors.[110] SOM230 inhibits GH secretion from cultured human normal pituitary cells and pituitary tumors and in acromegalic patients. The GH-lowering efficacy in acromegalic patients is higher than that of octreotide in some patients.[111] Another series of novel agents have dual affinity for sst2 somatostatin receptor and D_2 dopamine receptor.[112] They inhibit secretion of both GH and prolactin from human tumor cells. Clinical trials of these novel compounds are under way and will determine if the compounds are useful clinically.

RELATED TOPICS IN OTHER CHAPTERS

- For information on rimonibant, see Chapter 37 (Diabetes Mellitus).
- For medications used in appetite control, see Chapter 36 (Obesity and Nutrition) and Chapter 37 (Diabetes Mellitus).
- For information on diagnostic use of ACTH in adrenal insuffciency, see Chapter 41 (Adrenal Disorders).
- For information on therapeutic use of LH, FSH, clomiphene, and leuprolide (Lupron), see Chapter 42 (Reproductive Health).

REFERENCES

1. Robertson GL. Diabetes insipidus. Endocrinol Metab Clin North Am 1995;24:549-572.
2. Birnbaumer M. Vasopressin receptors. Trends Endocrinol Metab 2000;11:406-410.
3. Durr JA, Hoggard JG, Hunt JM, et al. Diabetes insipidus in pregnancy associated with abnormally high circulating vasopressinase activity. N Engl J Med 1987;316:1070-1074.
4. Kim RJ, Malattia C, Allen M, et al. Vasopressin and desmopressin in central diabetes insipidus: adverse effects and clinical considerations. Pediatr Endocrinol Rev 2004;2(Suppl 1):115-123.
5. Lam KS, Wat MS, Choi K, et al. Pharmacokinetics, pharmacodynamics, long-term efficacy and safety of oral 1-deamino-8-D-arginine vasopressin in adult patients with central diabetes insipidus. Br J Clin Pharmacol 1996;42:379-485.
6. Fukuda I, Hizuka N, Takano K. Oral DDAVP is a good alternative therapy for patients with central diabetes insipidus: experience of five-year treatment. Endocr J 2003;50:437-443.
7. Thumfart J, Roehr CC, Kapelari K, et al. Desmopressin associated symptomatic hyponatremic hypervolemia in children: are there predictive factors? J Urol 2005;174:294-298.
8. Robertson GL. Regulation of arginine vasopressin in the syndrome of inappropriate antidiuresis. Am J Med 2006;119:S36-S42.
9. Miller M. Hyponatremia and arginine vasopressin dysregulation: mechanisms, clinical consequences, and management. J Am Geriatr Soc 2006;54:345-353.
10. Chan TY. Drug-induced syndrome of inappropriate antidiuretic hormone secretion: causes, diagnosis and management. Drugs Aging 1997;11:27-44.
11. Feldman BJ, Rosenthal SM, Vargas GA, et al. Nephrogenic syndrome of inappropriate antidiuresis. N Engl J Med 2005;352:1884-1890.
12. Gross P, Wehrle R, Bussemaker E. Hyponatremia: pathophysiology, differential diagnosis and new aspects of treatment. Clin Nephrol 1996;46:273-276.
13. Forrest JN Jr, Cox M, Hong C, et al. Superiority of demeclocycline over lithium in the treatment of chronic syndrome of inappropriate secretion of antidiuretic hormone. N Engl J Med 1978;298:173-177.
14. Janicic N, Verbalis JG. Evaluation and management of hypo-osmolality in hospitalized patients. Endocrinol Metab Clin North Am 2003;32:459-481.
15. Greenberg A, Verbalis JG. Vasopressin receptor antagonists. Kidney Int 2006;69:2124-2130.
16. Verbalis JG, Bisaha JG, Smith N. Novel vasopressin V1A and V2 antagonist (conivaptan) increased serum sodium concentration and effective water clearance in patients with hyponatremia. Circulation 2004;110(Suppl 3):III-723.
17. Abraham WT, Shamshirsaz AA, McFann K, et al. Aquaretic effect of lixivaptan, an oral, non-peptide, selective V2 receptor vasopressin antagonist, in New York Heart Association functional class II and III chronic heart failure patients. J Am Coll Cardiol 2006;47:1615-1621.
18. Gerbes AL, Gulberg V, Gines P, et al. Therapy of hyponatremia in cirrhosis with a vasopressin receptor antagonist: a randomized double-blind multicenter trial. Gastroenterology 2003;124:933-939.
19. Wang X, Gattone V 2nd, Harris PC, et al. Effectiveness of vasopressin V2 receptor antagonists OPC-31260 and OPC-41061 on polycystic kidney disease development in the PCK rat. J Am Soc Nephrol 2005;16:846-851.
20. Ahima RS. Body fat, leptin, and hypothalamic amenorrhea. N Engl J Med 2004;351:959-962.
21. Vance ML. Hypopituitarism. N Engl J Med 1994;330:1651-1662.
22. Lamberts SW, de Herder WW, van der Lely AJ. Pituitary insufficiency. Lancet 1998;352:127-134.
23. Zhu X, Lin CR, Prefontaine GG, et al. Genetic control of pituitary development and hypopituitarism. Curr Opin Genet Dev 2005;15:332-340.
24. De Coopman J. Breastfeeding after pituitary resection: support for a theory of autocrine control of milk supply? J Hum Lact 1993;9:35-40.
25. Romijn JA, Smit JW, Lamberts SW. Intrinsic imperfections of endocrine replacement therapy. Eur J Endocrinol 2003;149:91-97.
26. Laron Z. Laron syndrome (primary growth hormone resistance or insensitivity): the personal experience 1958-2003. J Clin Endocrinol Metab 2004;89:1031-1044.
27. Growth Hormone Research Society. Consensus guidelines for the diagnosis and treatment of growth hormone (GH) deficiency in childhood and adolescence: summary statement of the GH Research Society. J Clin Endocrinol Metab 2000; 85:3990-3993.

28. Wilson TA, Rose SR, Cohen P, et al. Update of guidelines for the use of growth hormone in children: the Lawson Wilkins Pediatric Endocrinology Society Drug and Therapeutics Committee. J Pediatr 2003;143:415-421.
29. Gharib H, Cook DM, Saenger PH, et al. American Association of Clinical Endocrinologists medical guidelines for clinical practice for growth hormone use in adults and children—2003 update. Endocr Pract 2003;9:64-76.
30. Molitch ME, Clemmons DR, Malozowski S, et al. Evaluation and treatment of adult growth hormone deficiency: an Endocrine Society Clinical Practice Guideline. J Clin Endocrinol Metab 2006;91:1621-1634.
31. Vance ML, Mauras N. Growth hormone therapy in adults and children. N Engl J Med 1999;341:1206-1216.
32. Wyatt D. Lessons from the National Cooperative Growth Study. Eur J Endocrinol 2004;151(Suppl 1):S55-S59.
33. Allen DB. Issues in the transition from childhood to adult growth hormone therapy. Pediatrics 1999;104:1004-1010.
34. Shalet S. Stepping into adulthood: the transition period. Horm Res 2004;62(Suppl 4):15-22.
35. Ergun-Longmire B, Mertens AC, Mitby P, et al. Growth hormone treatment and risk of second neoplasms in the childhood cancer survivor. J Clin Endocrinol Metab 2006;91:3494-3498.
36. Hoffman AR. Treatment of the adult growth hormone deficiency syndrome: directions for future research. Growth Horm IGF Res 2005;15(Suppl A):48-52.
37. Rudman D, Feller AG, Nagraj HS, et al. Effects of human growth hormone in men over 60 years old. N Engl J Med 1990;323:1-6.
38. Taaffe DR, Pruitt L, Reim J, et al. Effect of recombinant human growth hormone on the muscle strength response to resistance exercise in elderly men. J Clin Endocrinol Metab 1994;79:1361-1366.
39. Papadakis MA, Grady D, Black D, et al. Growth hormone replacement in healthy older men improves body composition but not functional ability. Ann Intern Med 1996;124:708-716.
40. Blackman MR, Sorkin JD, Munzer T, et al. Growth hormone and sex steroid administration in healthy aged women and men: a randomized controlled trial. JAMA 2002;288:2282-2292.
41. Vance ML. Can growth hormone prevent aging? N Engl J Med 2003;348:779-780.
42. Perls TT, Reisman NR, Olshansky SJ. Provision or distribution of growth hormone for "antiaging": clinical and legal issues. JAMA 2005;294:2086-2090.
43. Burgess E, Wanke C. Use of recombinant human growth hormone in HIV-associated lipodystrophy. Curr Opin Infect Dis 2005;18:17-24.
44. Krause JC, Toye MP, Stechenberg BW, et al. HIV-associated lipodystrophy in children. Pediatr Endocrinol Rev 2005;3:45-51.
45. Walker JL, Van Wyk JJ, Underwood LE. Stimulation of statural growth by recombinant insulin-like growth factor I in a child with growth hormone insensitivity syndrome. J Pediatr 1992;121:641-646.
46. Laron Z, Anin S, Klipper-Aurbach Y, et al. Effects of insulin-like growth factor on linear growth, head circumference and body fat in patients with Laron-type dwarfism. Lancet 1992;339:1258-1261.
47. Laron Z. Insulin-like growth factor-I (IGF-I): safety and efficacy. Pediatr Endocrinol Rev 2004;2(Suppl 1):78-85.
48. Backeljauw PF, Underwood LE. Growth hormone insensitivity syndrome. Therapy for 6.5-7.5 years with recombinant insulin-like growth factor I in children with growth hormone insensitivity syndrome: a clinical research center study. J Clin Endocrinol Metab 2001;86:1504-1510.
49. Camacho-Hubner C, Rose S, Preece MA, et al. Pharmacokinetic studies of recombinant human insulin-like growth factor I (rhIGF-I)/rhIGF-binding protein-3 complex administered to patients with growth hormone insensitivity syndrome. J Clin Endocrinol Metab 2006;91:1246-1253.
50. Ghigo E, Aimaretti G, Arvat E, et al. Growth hormone-releasing hormone combined with arginine or growth hormone secretagogues for the diagnosis of growth hormone deficiency in adults. Endocrine 2001;15:29-38.
51. Thorner MO, Reschke J, Chitwood J, et al. Acceleration of growth in two children treated with human growth hormone-releasing factor. N Engl J Med 1995;312:4-9.
52. Thorner M, Rochiccioli P, Colle M, et al. Once daily subcutaneous growth hormone-releasing hormone therapy accelerates growth in growth hormone-deficient children during the first year of therapy. Geref International Study Group. J Clin Endocrinol Metab 1996;81:1189-1196.
53. Teichman SL, Neale A, Lawrence B, et al. Prolonged stimulation of growth hormone (GH) and insulin-like growth factor I secretion by CJC-1295, a long-acting analog of GH-releasing hormone, in healthy adults. J Clin Endocrinol Metab 2006;91:799-805.
54. Melmed S. Mechanisms for pituitary tumorigenesis: the plastic pituitary. J Clin Invest 2003;112:1603-1618.
55. Molitch ME. Prolactinoma. In Melmed S (ed): The Pituitary, 2nd ed. Malden, MA: Blackwell, 2002, pp 455-495.
56. Schlechte JA. Prolactinoma. N Engl J Med 2003;349:2035-2041.
57. Spada A, Mantovani G, Lania A. Pathogenesis of prolactinomas. Pituitary 2005;8:7-15.
58. Davis JR. Prolactin and reproductive medicine. Curr Opin Obstet Gynecol 2004;16:331-337.
59. Molitch ME. Medical management of prolactin-secreting pituitary adenomas. Pituitary 2002;5:55-65.
60. Mary PG, Molitch ME, Lombardi G, et al. Advances in the treatment of prolactinomas. Endocr Rev 2006;27:485-534.
61. Besser GM, Parke L, Edwards CR, et al. Galactorrhoea: successful treatment with reduction of plasma prolactin levels by brom-ergocryptine. Br Med J 1972;3:669-672.
62. Sobrinho LG, Nunes MC, Santos MA, et al. Radiological evidence for regression of prolactinoma after treatment with bromocriptine. Lancet 1978;2:257-258.
63. Missale C, Nash SR, Robinson SW, et al. Dopamine receptors: from structure to function. Physiol Rev 1998;78:189-225.
64. Spitz AM, Lee NC, Peterson HB. Treatment for lactation suppression: little progress in one hundred years. Am J Obstet Gynecol 1998;179:1485-1490.
64a. Schade R, Andersohn F, Suissa S, et al. Dopamine agonists and the risk of cardiac-valve regurgitation. N Engl J Med 2007;356:29-38.
65b. Zanettini R, Antonini A, Gatto G, et al. Valvular heart disease and the use of dopamine agonists for Parkinson's disease. N Engl J Med 2007;356:39-46.
65. Molitch ME. Pharmacologic resistance in prolactinoma patients. Pituitary 2005;8:43-52.
66. Bronstein MD. Prolactinomas and pregnancy. Pituitary 2005;8:31-38.
67. Randeva HS, Schoebel J, Byrne J. Classical pituitary apoplexy: clinical features, management and outcome. Clin Endocrinol 1999;51:181-188.
68. Colao A, Di Sarno A, Cappabianca P, et al. Withdrawal of long-term cabergoline therapy for tumoral and nontumoral hyperprolactinemia. N Engl J Med 2003;349:2023-2033.
69. Karunakaran S, Page RC, Wass JA. The effect of the menopause on prolactin levels in patients with hyperprolactinaemia. Clin Endocrinol 2001;54:295-300.
70. Casanueva FF, Molitch ME, Schlechte JA, et al. Guidelines of the Pituitary Society for the diagnosis and management of prolactinomas. Clin Endocrinol 2006;65: 265-273.
71. Ben-Shlomo A, Melmed S. Acromegaly. Endocrinol Metab Clin North Am 2001; 30:565-583.
72. Donangelo I, Melmed S. Treatment of acromegaly: future. Endocrine 2005;28:123-128.
73. Vance ML, Laws ER Jr. Role of medical therapy in the management of acromegaly. Neurosurgery 2005;56:877-885.
74. Lamberts SW, van der Lely AJ, de Herder WW, et al. Octreotide. N Engl J Med 1996;334:246-254.
75. Olias G, Viollet C, Kusserow H, et al. Regulation and function of somatostatin receptors. J Neurochem 2004;89:1057-1091.
76. Lahlou H, Guillermet J, Hortala M, et al. Molecular signaling of somatostatin receptors. Ann N Y Acad Sci 2004;1014:121-131.
77. Yen SS, Siler TM, DeVane GW. Effect of somatostatin in patients with acromegaly: suppression of growth hormone, prolactin, insulin and glucose levels. N Engl J Med 1974;290:935-938.
78. Lamberts SW, Oosterom R, Neufeld M, et al. The somatostatin analog SMS 201-995 induces long-acting inhibition of growth hormone secretion without rebound hypersecretion in acromegalic patients. J Clin Endocrinol Metab 1985;60:1161-1165.
79. Lamberts SW, Uitterlinden P, del Pozo E. SMS 201-995 induces a continuous decline in circulating growth hormone and somatomedin-C levels during therapy of acromegalic patients for over two years. J Clin Endocrinol Metab 1987;65:703-710.
80. Barkan AL, Lloyd RV, Chandler WF, et al. Preoperative treatment of acromegaly with long-acting somatostatin analog SMS 201-995: shrinkage of invasive pituitary macroadenomas and improved surgical remission rate. J Clin Endocrinol Metab 1988;67:1040-1048.
81. Moller DE, Moses AC, Jones K, et al. Octreotide suppresses both growth hormone (GH) and GH-releasing hormone (GHRH) in acromegaly due to ectopic GHRH secretion. J Clin Endocrinol Metab 1989;68:499-504.
82. Ho KY, Weissberger AJ, Marbach P, et al. Therapeutic efficacy of the somatostatin analog SMS 201-995 (octreotide) in acromegaly: effects of dose and frequency and long-term safety. Ann Intern Med 1990;112:173-181.
83. Murray RD, Kim K, Ren SG, et al. Central and peripheral actions of somatostatin on the growth hormone-IGF-I axis. J Clin Invest 2004;114:349-356.
84. Wasko R, Jankowska A, Kotwicka M, et al. Effects of treatment with somatostatin analogues on the occurrence of apoptosis in somatotropinomas. Neuroendocrinol Lett 2003;24:334-338.
85. Ben-Shlomo A, Melmed S. Clinical Review 154: The role of pharmacotherapy in perioperative management of patients with acromegaly. J Clin Endocrinol Metab 2003:88:963-968.
86. Colao A, Pivonello R, Rosato F, et al. First-line octreotide-LAR therapy induces tumour shrinkage and controls hormone excess in patients with acromegaly: results from an open, prospective, multicentre trial. Clin Endocrinol 2006;64:342-351.
86a. Ciccarelli A, Daly A, Beckers A. Lanreotide Autogel for acromegaly: a new addition to the treatment armamentarium. Treatments Endocrinol 2004;3:77-81.
86b. Tolis G, Angelopoulos NG, Katounda E, et al. Medical treatment of acromegaly: comorbidities and their reversibility by somatostatin analogs. Neuroendocrinology 2006;83:249-257.
87. Abs R, Verhelst J, Maiter D, et al. Cabergoline in the treatment of acromegaly: a study in 64 patients. J Clin Endocrinol Metab 1998;83:374-378.
88. Cozzi R, Attanasio R, Lodrini S, et al. Cabergoline addition to depot somatostatin analogues in resistant acromegalic patients: efficacy and lack of predictive value of prolactin status. Clin Endocrinol 2004;61:209-215.
89. Freda PU, Reyes CM, Nuruzzaman AT, et al. Cabergoline therapy of growth hormone & growth hormone/prolactin secreting pituitary tumors. Pituitary 2004;7:21-30.
90. Herrington J, Carter-Su C. Signaling pathways activated by the growth hormone receptor. Trends Endocrinol Metab 2001;12:252-257.
91. Chen WY, Wight DC, Wagner TE, et al. Expression of a mutated bovine growth hormone gene suppresses growth of transgenic mice. Proc Natl Acad Sci U S A 1990;87:5061-5065.
92. Fuh G, Cunningham BC, Fukunaga R, et al. Rational design of potent antagonists to the human growth hormone receptor. Science 1992;256:1677-1680.
93. Clark R, Olson K, Fuh G, et al. Long-acting growth hormones produced by conjugation with polyethylene glycol. J Biol Chem 1996;271:21969-21977.
94. Trainer PJ, Drake WM, Katznelson L, et al. Treatment of acromegaly with the growth hormone-receptor antagonist pegvisomant. N Engl J Med 2000;342:1171-1177.

95. van der Lely AJ, Hutson RK, Trainer PJ, et al. Long-term treatment of acromegaly with pegvisomant, a growth hormone receptor antagonist. Lancet 2001;358:1754-1759.
96. Herman-Bonert VS, Zib K, Scarlett JA, et al. Growth hormone receptor antagonist therapy in acromegalic patients resistant to somatostatin analogs. J Clin Endocrinol Metab 2000;85:2958-2961.
97. Gola M, Bonadonna S, Mazziotti G, et al. Resistance to somatostatin analogs in acromegaly: an evolving concept? J Endocrinol Invest 2006;29:86-93.
98. Feenstra J, de Herder WW, ten Have SM, et al. Combined therapy with somatostatin analogues and weekly pegvisomant in active acromegaly. Lancet 2005;365:1644-1646.
99. Melmed S, Casanueva FF, Cavagnini F, et al. Guidelines for acromegaly management. J Clin Endocrinol Metab 2002;87:4054-4058.
100. Clemmons DR, Chihara K, Freda PU, et al. Optimizing control of acromegaly: integrating a growth hormone receptor antagonist into the treatment algorithm. J Clin Endocrinol Metab 2003;88:4759-4767.
101. AACE Acromegaly Guidelines Task Force. AACE Medical Guidelines for Clinical Practice for the diagnosis and treatment of acromegaly. Endocr Pract 2004;10:213-225.
102. Newell-Price J, Bertagna X, Grossman AB, et al. Cushing's syndrome. Lancet 2006;367:1605-1617.
103. Nieman LK. Diagnostic tests for Cushing's syndrome. Ann N Y Acad Sci 2002;970:112-118.
104. Nieman LK, Loriaux DL. Corticotropin-releasing hormone: clinical applications. Annu Rev Med 1989;40:331-339.
105. Woodmansee WW, Haugen BR. Uses for recombinant human TSH in patients with thyroid cancer and nodular goiter. Clin Endocrinol 2004;61:163-173.
106. Cole ES, Lee K, Lauziere K, et al. Recombinant human thyroid stimulating hormone: development of a biotechnology product for detection of metastatic lesions of thyroid carcinoma. Bio/Technology 1993;11:1014-1024.
107. Weintraub BD, Szkudlinski MW. Development and in vitro characterization of human recombinant thyrotropin. Thyroid 1999;9:447-450.
108. Welt CK, Chan JL, Bullen J, et al. Recombinant human leptin in women with hypothalamic amenorrhea. N Engl J Med 2004;351:987-997.
109. Mantzoros CS. The role of leptin in human obesity and disease: a review of current evidence. Ann Intern Med 1999;130:671-680.
110. Murray RD, Kim K, Ren SG, et al. The novel somatostatin ligand (SOM230) regulates human and rat anterior pituitary hormone secretion. J Clin Endocrinol Metab 2004;89:3027-3032.
111. van der Hoek J, de Herder WW, Feelders RA, et al. A single-dose comparison of the acute effects between the new somatostatin analog SOM230 and octreotide in acromegalic patients. J Clin Endocrinol Metab 2004;89:638-645.
112. Ren SG, Kim S, Taylor J, et al. Suppression of rat and human growth hormone and prolactin secretion by a novel somatostatin/dopaminergic chimeric ligand. J Clin Endocrinol Metab 2003;88:5414-5421.

41

ADRENAL DISORDERS

Lisa Hamaker and Serge Jabbour

INTRODUCTION 623
GLUCOCORTICOID EXCESS: CUSHING'S SYNDROME 623
Pathophysiology 623
Therapeutics and Clinical Pharmacology 623
Goals of Therapy 623
Therapeutics by Class 624
Therapeutic Approach 625
Emerging Targets and Therapeutics 625
GLUCOCORTICOID AND MINERALOCORTICOID DEFICIENCIES: ADRENAL INSUFFICIENCY 626
Pathophysiology 626
Therapeutics and Clinical Pharmacology 626
Goals of Therapy 626
Therapeutics by Class 626
Therapeutic Approach 627
Emerging Targets and Therapeutics 627
CATECHOLAMINE EXCESS: PHEOCHROMOCYTOMAS 627
Pathophysiology 627
Therapeutics and Clinical Pharmacology 628
Goals of Therapy 628
Therapeutics by Class 628
Therapeutic Approach 628
MINERALOCORTICOID EXCESS: PRIMARY HYPERALDOSTERONISM 629
Pathophysiology 629
Therapeutics and Clinical Pharmacology 629
Goals of Therapy 629
Therapeutics by Class 629
Therapeutic Approach 629

INTRODUCTION

The adrenal glands are endocrine organs located above the kidneys that play an integral role in human physiology. The adrenal cortex or outer layer consists of three distinct zones: the zona glomerulosa, the zona fasciculata, and the zona reticularis, which secrete mineralocorticoids, glucocorticoids, and sex steroids, respectively. The adrenal medulla is responsible for catecholamine synthesis.

The hypothalamic-pituitary-adrenal (HPA) axis is responsible for glucocorticoid production by the adrenal glands, and dysfunction at any level can lead to either overproduction (Cushing's disease) or underproduction (adrenal insufficiency) of glucocorticoids. Thus, although the chapter is entitled "Adrenal Disorders," physiology and selected pathology of the entire HPA axis will be reviewed. Production of aldosterone is regulated by the renin-angiotensin-aldosterone system, and primary adrenal insufficiency can result in a deficiency of this hormone by destruction of the zona glomerulosa. Overproduction of catecholamines by the adrenal medulla is caused by a pheochromocytoma. The chapter will focus on pathophysiology and treatment of the above conditions with the emphasis on drug therapeutics.

GLUCOCORTICOID EXCESS: CUSHING'S SYNDROME

Pathophysiology

In normal subjects, corticotropin-releasing hormone (CRH) is released from the hypothalamus into the hypophysial portal blood and stimulates the anterior pituitary to synthesize and release corticotropin (adrenocorticotropic hormone; ACTH) and other pro-opiomelanocortin–derived peptides. ACTH in turn stimulates adrenal cortisol secretion. ACTH secretion is pulsatile in nature, with the highest concentrations in the morning and the lowest in the evening and early morning hours. Cortisol inhibits further hypothalamic CRH synthesis and secretion, blocks the effects of CRH in the pituitary, and inhibits the synthesis and release of ACTH (Fig. 41-1). CRH secretion is tightly regulated by this negative feedback as well as by inputs from higher brain centers, the circadian pacemaker, and stress.

The biochemical pathways involved in adrenal steroidogenesis are shown in Figure 41-2. The initial rate-limiting step is the transport of cholesterol from the outer to the inner mitochondrial membrane for conversion to pregnenolone by cytochrome P-450_{scc}. Steroidogenic acute regulatory protein (StAR) is essential in mediating its effect. Steroidogenesis is the result of concerted action of several enzymes. Cortisol exists in two forms in serum: free and bound to corticosteroid-binding globulin. Its secretion normally reflects that of ACTH and is also pulsatile.

In 1912, Harvey Cushing described a patient with obesity, hirsutism, and amenorrhea who he postulated had a primary pituitary abnormality causing adrenal hyperplasia. The term *Cushing's disease* is thus reserved for pituitary lesions causing ACTH production and resultant glucocorticoid excess. *Cushing's syndrome* is used to describe all causes of excess glucocorticoid production, whether endogenous or exogenous in nature.

Cushing's syndrome may be either ACTH-dependent or ACTH-independent. Causes of ACTH-dependent Cushing's syndrome result in adrenocortical hyperplasia and include Cushing's disease, ectopic secretion of ACTH by nonpituitary tumors, ectopic CRH production, and iatrogenic or factitious Cushing's syndrome due to administration of exogenous ACTH. ACTH-dependent causes are responsible for approximately 85% of cases of endogenous Cushing's syndrome in adults.[1]

ACTH-independent causes are responsible for the remainder of cases of Cushing's syndrome in adults.[1] The most common cause of ACTH-independent Cushing's disease by far is iatrogenic, resulting from exogenous administration of glucocorticoids, generally for their anti-inflammatory effects. The remainder of ACTH-independent causes are adrenal in nature. In adults, most cases of adrenal Cushing's syndrome are caused by adenomas, but carcinomas and nodular adrenal hyperplasia also occur. In Cushing's syndrome due to primary adrenocortical disease, increased cortisol secretion suppresses both CRH and ACTH secretion and causes the pituitary corticotrophs and the normal adrenal tissue to atrophy. This can result in adrenal insufficiency when the underlying pathology is resected.

Therapeutics and Clinical Pharmacology

Goals of Therapy

Therapy of choice for Cushing's disease is transsphenoidal surgery. Pituitary irradiation is also used, most commonly in patients who are

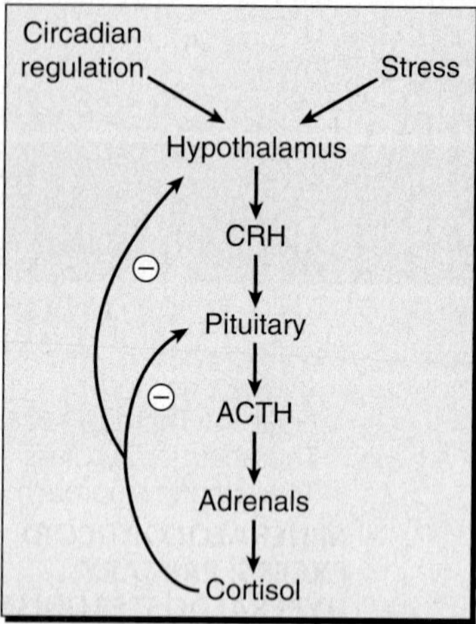

FIGURE 41-1 • The hypothalamic-pituitary-adrenal axis. Adrenocorticotropic hormone (ACTH) is secreted from the anterior pituitary under the influence of corticotropin-releasing hormone (CRH). CRH secretion is regulated by circadian rhythm and stressors operating through the hypothalamus. Secretion of CRH and ACTH is inhibited by cortisol.

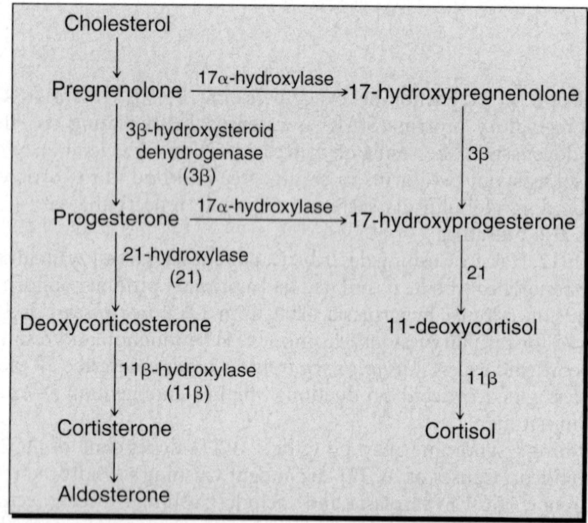

FIGURE 41-2 • Adrenal steroidogenesis. Aldosterone and cortisol are synthesized through the coordinated action of a series of steroidogenic enzymes in a zone-specific fashion.

poor surgical candidates or refuse surgery and in those patients who fail surgery. It may be considered as initial therapy in children because it is as likely to cure them as transsphenoidal surgery. Patients who fail transsphenoidal surgery and/or irradiation are candidates for adrenalectomy, which can be achieved either surgically or medically. A complication of this approach, especially in patients who have not had pituitary irradiation, is Nelson's syndrome, in which an enlarging tumor is associated with progressive hyperpigmentation due to very high ACTH concentrations. It occurs in 20% to 25% of adults with Cushing's disease who undergo total adrenalectomy without prior irradiation, but it is less common with medical adrenalectomy.[2] Cortisol release can also be diminished by the administration of drugs that inhibit enzymes involved in cortisol synthesis.

In patients with ectopic ACTH or CRH production, surgical removal of the malignancy is clearly the most important approach. However, in patients with nonresectable cancers, chemotherapy is the principal therapy. In these cases, cortisol hypersecretion can be medically treated by adrenal enzyme inhibitors or, in indolent malignancies, with surgical or medical adrenalectomy.

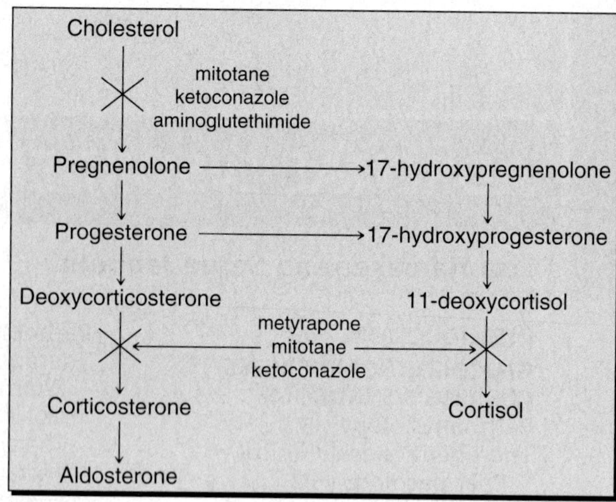

FIGURE 41-3 • Sites of action of mitotane, metyrapone, ketoconazole, and aminoglutethimide.

In Cushing's syndrome due to primary adrenocortical disease, surgical removal of the adenoma or carcinoma is the primary therapy. Patients with nonresectable or recurrent adrenal carcinoma are usually treated with mitotane.

Some of the adrenal enzyme inhibitors may also be used in the management of Cushing's syndrome during pregnancy.

Therapeutics by Class

Mitotane. Mitotane, also known as 1,1-dichlorodiphenildichloroethane (o,p′-DDD), was discovered as the active component of the insecticide dichlorodiphenyltrichloroethane (DDT). It acts on the mitochondria of adrenocortical cells, both normal and neoplastic, to inhibit the 11β-hydroxylase and cholesterol side-chain cleavage enzymes (Fig. 41-3). Its metabolite causes mitochondrial destruction and necrosis of adrenocortical cells; thus, it can be given to produce a "medical" adrenalectomy. It is most commonly used in patients with adrenal carcinoma but can also be used in cases of Cushing's disease in which patients are not cured by pituitary irradiation or surgery and in patients with ectopic ACTH or CRH syndromes.

Therapy should be started at 0.5 g once daily and increased weekly by 0.5 g as the patient tolerates to reach a final dose of 2 to 3 g/day. One half of the dose should be taken at bedtime to reduce nausea. Doses of 2 to 3 g/day generally result in therapeutically effective but safe mitotane concentrations (14 to 25 μg/ml) in 3 to 5 months.[3] After this time period, concentrations can usually be maintained by doses of 1 to 2 g/day. The usual duration of mitotane therapy in patients with Cushing's disease is 6 to 9 months. If patients cannot tolerate 1 g/day, surgical adrenalectomy should be performed.

Mitotane is expensive and has many side effects that are mainly dose related. Major side effects are nausea, vomiting, and anorexia, but rash, diarrhea, ataxia, confusion, gynecomastia, and leukopenia can also occur. Hypercholesterolemia, hypouricemia, and hepatotoxicity are also known side effects. Some side effects may be due to glucocorticoid deficiency. A trial of increased glucocorticoid dosage may mitigate symptoms. Monitoring plasma levels is useful in decreasing major toxicity as major neurologic toxicity is generally present only in patients with levels greater than 20 mg/dl.[4]

It is difficult to predict when a patient will develop cortisol deficiency after beginning treatment with mitotane. It may be safest to begin replacement glucocorticoids when mitotane treatment is begun. Mitotane increases the metabolism of dexamethasone and fludrocortisone, so normal physiologic glucocorticoid replacement with dexamethasone (0.5 mg daily) will not be adequate.[5] It may be necessary to increase the dose of dexamethasone (and fludrocortisone if mineralocorticoid replacement is necessary) to three to seven times the usual dose. Dosage should be adjusted based on symptoms. Mitotane does not alter metabolism of cortisol and prednisolone, so the dose of

TABLE 41-1 INHIBITORS OF GLUCOCORTICOID SYNTHESIS

Agent	Effective Dosage	Mechanism of Action	Side Effects
Mitotane	2-3 g/day	Inhibits 11β-hydroxylase and cholesterol side-chain cleavage enzymes; metabolite causes necrosis of adrenal cortex	Nausea/vomiting, anorexia, rash, diarrhea, ataxia, gynecomastia, leukopenia
Metyrapone	Primary therapy: 4 g/day Adjunctive therapy: 500-750 mg tid–qid	Inhibits 11β-hydroxylase	Hypertension, acne, hirsutism
Aminoglutethimide	250 mg bid–tid	Blocks conversion of cholesterol to pregnenolone	Excessive somnolence at doses of >1 g/day, transient pruritic rash, bone marrow suppression, goiter, hypothyroidism, cholestasis, headache
Ketoconazole	200-400 mg bid–tid	Blocks conversion of cholesterol to pregnenolone; inhibits 11β-hydroxylase	Headache, sedation, amenorrhea in women, gynecomastia and impotence in men, reversible hepatotoxicity

prednisone does not need to be adjusted (usually 5 mg daily).[5] Since mitotane is taken up by fatty tissues and thus remains active for several weeks to months following discontinuation, the dose of glucocorticoid may have to be tapered to the usual replacement dosage over some time following completion of treatment with mitotane.

Mitotane tends to spare the zona glomerulosa, so there is a good possibility that patients will retain normal aldosterone secretion. This puts the patient at lower risk of developing adrenal crisis. This is an advantage over surgical adrenalectomy.

Adrenal Enzyme Inhibitors. Metyrapone, aminoglutethimide, ketoconazole, and etomidate all inhibit one or more of the enzymes involved in cortisol synthesis and can be used in treatment of Cushing's disease (Table 41-1). These agents are most commonly used in patients who are not cured by transsphenoidal surgery, who do not have a complete response with or cannot tolerate mitotane, or who cannot be treated by adrenalectomy. However, pharmacologic blockade is often incomplete and the increase in ACTH secretion overcomes the blockade, resulting in continued cortisol overproduction.

Metyrapone is an inhibitor of 11β-hydroxylase, which regulates the final step of cortisol biosynthesis (see Fig. 41-3). 11β-Hydroxylase also inhibits aldosterone secretion, but its effect on electrolyte balance is mitigated by increased production of 11-deoxycorticosterone, which has mineralocorticoid activity. Metyrapone may also inhibit ACTH secretion directly in high doses.[6] Metyrapone at doses of 4 g/day decreases cortisol secretion in untreated patients with Cushing's disease, but it does not return the levels to normal and can result in greatly increased side effects, including hypertension, hirsutism, and acne, due to increased production of mineralocorticoids and androgens. It is useful as adjunctive therapy in doses of 500 to 750 mg three to four times daily in patients with mild disease or after pituitary irradiation.[7]

Aminoglutethimide is an anticonvulsant drug that blocks the first step in cholesterol synthesis: conversion of cholesterol to pregnenolone (see Fig. 41-3). The synthesis of mineralocorticoids can also be reduced due to the early site of action of the drug. Renin increases but not to levels high enough to overcome the blockade, so aldosterone remains low. Fludrocortisone replacement may be required. Dosage is 250 mg two to three times daily. The drug can be increased to 2 g/day, but doses of 1 g/day or higher are associated with excessive somnolence in adults. A transient, pruritic rash can occur on medication initiation and can be treated symptomatically with an antihistamine without stopping the medication. Other side effects include rare bone marrow suppression and cholestasis, and headache, goiter, and hypothyroidism. Aminoglutethimide is less expensive than the other adrenal enzyme inhibitors but is also less effective. If patients taking aminoglutethimide need glucocorticoid replacement, prednisone may be the replacement glucocorticoid of choice since it is unaffected by aminoglutethimide. Aminoglutethimide increases the metabolism of dexamethasone.[8]

Ketoconazole inhibits the first step of cortisol biosynthesis and to a lesser extent the final step, conversion of 11-deoxycortisol to cortisol (see Fig. 41-3). It may be more effective in treatment of Cushing's syndrome than metyrapone and aminoglutethimide because it also inhibits ACTH secretion at therapeutic doses by impairing corticotroph adenylate cyclase activity.[9] Therapeutic doses are usually 200 to 400 mg two or three times daily. Side effects include headache, sedation, and amenorrhea in premenopausal women, and gynecomastia and impotence in men secondary to testosterone deficiency. Ketoconazole is also a rare cause of reversible hepatotoxicity, so liver function tests should be followed. In elderly patients with Cushing's disease, ketoconazole has been used as definitive long-term therapy.[10]

Therapeutic Approach

As stated earlier, medical adrenalectomy with mitotane is used in Cushing's disease patients who fail transsphenoidal surgery and/or irradiation. It can also be used to treat patients with ectopic ACTH or CRH production and nonresectable, indolent malignancies and in patients with nonresectable or recurrent adrenal carcinoma. The use of mitotane as adjuvant therapy after surgery for adrenal carcinoma is somewhat controversial, but recent evidence of its efficacy at doses of 1.5 to 2 g/day is encouraging.[11]

Adrenal enzyme inhibitors are used most commonly in the management of Cushing's disease during pregnancy (with the exception of ketoconazole, which is teratogenic), in patients with nonresectable ACTH- or CRH-producing tumors, and in those with nonresectable or recurrent adrenal carcinoma. They may also be used in patients with Cushing's disease who do not respond to and/or refuse pituitary irradiation or surgical or medical adrenalectomy.

Treatment with adrenal enzyme inhibitors usually begins with ketoconazole. Since it acts quickly, its effect can be assessed within 24 hours by measuring serum cortisol or 24-hour urine cortisol excretion. The starting dose of ketoconazole is usually 200 mg three times daily. If increasing doses of ketoconazole do not control cortisol secretion, another enzyme inhibitor should be added, most likely metyrapone. If maximum doses of ketoconazole and metyrapone are ineffective, then aminoglutethimide should be added at its maximum dosage. Using the medications in combination commonly allows one to obtain the maximum therapeutic benefit with the lowest incidence of side effects. Adrenal insufficiency can be avoided by starting dexamethasone as soon as cortisol secretion approaches the normal range.

Emerging Targets and Therapeutics

Mifepristone, an antiprogestational drug, is a competitive inhibitor of glucocorticoids at their receptor and has been used acutely in several patients with Cushing's disease.[12] It appears to be effective, although cortisol secretion increases. It also blocks the effects of exogenous glucocorticoids, making it difficult to treat the glucocorticoid deficiency it may induce. Further study is necessary to clarify efficacy of this agent in treatment of Cushing's syndrome.

GLUCOCORTICOID AND MINERALOCORTICOID DEFICIENCIES: ADRENAL INSUFFICIENCY

Pathophysiology

The HPA axis is responsible for production of glucocorticoids in the zona fasciculata of the adrenal cortex. The hypothalamus produces CRH, which stimulates the pituitary to synthesize ACTH, which further stimulates the adrenal gland to produce cortisol, the main endogenous glucocorticoid. Cellular receptors for cortisol are abundant in cell cytoplasm, reflecting the life-sustaining role glucocorticoids play. Cortisol feeds back negatively on the hypothalamus and pituitary gland. For further discussion of the HPA axis, please see the section on glucocorticoid excess.

Recent estimates of glucocorticoid secretion are approximately 5 to 10 mg/m^2 per day of cortisol.[13] Glucocorticoid levels have diurnal variation, with the peak level between 4:00 and 8:00 AM and minimal production of cortisol during the evening. Synthesis of cortisol can be increased by a factor of 10 under conditions of severe stress.[14]

The zona glomerulosa of the adrenal cortex is responsible for production of aldosterone, which plays an essential role in sodium and potassium homeostasis. Cortisol at high concentrations can bind to and activate the aldosterone receptor in the collecting tubules of the kidney. However, cortisol does not act as a major mineralocorticoid because collecting tubule cells contain enzymes, such as 11β-hydroxysteroid dehydrogenase, that convert cortisol to cortisone and other inactive metabolites.[15] Thus aldosterone is the physiologically active agonist of the receptor.

Aldosterone secretion is controlled by the renin-angiotensin-aldosterone system (Fig. 41-4). In brief, renal hypoperfusion, produced by volume depletion or hypotension, results in production of renin by the juxtaglomerular cells of the kidney. Renin causes conversion of angiotensinogen to angiotensin, which is further converted to angiotensin II by angiotensin-converting enzyme (ACE). Angiotensin II stimulates the zona glomerulosa cells of the adrenal cortex to produce aldosterone. An additional stimulus for aldosterone release is potassium level. Secretion increases linearly as the plasma potassium concentration rises above 3.5 mEq/L. Aldosterone acts primarily in the distal nephron to increase the reabsorption of sodium and the secretion of potassium and to maintain intravascular volume.

When Thomas Addison first described adrenal insufficiency in 1855, the most common cause of primary adrenal insufficiency, as well as adrenal insufficiency in general, was bilateral adrenal destruction by tuberculosis. Now tuberculosis is responsible for only 7% to 20% of cases of Addison's disease (which includes all causes of primary adrenal insufficiency). The most common cause is autoimmune disease, accounting for 70% to 90% of cases.[16] Other causes include other infectious diseases, such as disseminated fungal infections, human immunodeficiency virus infection, and syphilis; replacement by metastatic cancer or hemorrhage; and drugs. Disseminated tuberculosis and fungal infections are still a major cause of adrenal insufficiency in countries in which there is a high incidence of these diseases. Primary adrenal insufficiency develops in patients who have greater than 90% destruction or replacement of the adrenal glands.[16]

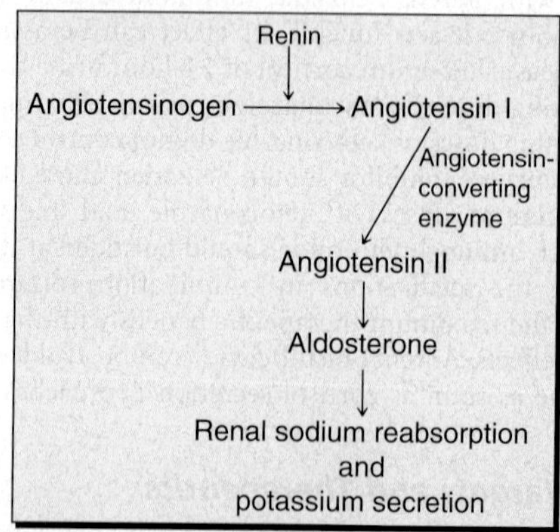

FIGURE 41-4 • The renin-angiotensin-aldosterone regulatory system. Renin is secreted by the kidney and converts angiotensin, which is produced by the liver, to angiotensin I. Angiotensin I is converted into biologically active angiotensin II by angiotensin-converting enzyme, mainly in the lung. Angiotensin II stimulates aldosterone secretion by the adrenal glands.

Since destruction of the adrenal gland is not limited to the zona fasciculata, cortisol is not the only hormone deficient in primary adrenal insufficiency. With primary adrenal insufficiency, mineralocorticoids (e.g., aldosterone) are also deficient.

Secondary adrenal insufficiency is caused by pituitary dysfunction or destruction with resultant insufficient ACTH production. Destruction can be caused by pituitary tumors or craniopharyngiomas, radiation, head trauma, infiltrative diseases, infectious diseases, or lymphocytic hypophysitis. Other causes include pituitary infarction, which can occur with childbirth if hypotension occurs (Sheehan's syndrome) or with hemorrhage into a pituitary tumor (pituitary apoplexy).

The most common causes of tertiary adrenal insufficiency are cessation of chronic glucocorticoid therapy and cure of Cushing's syndrome. High doses of glucocorticoids decrease CRH secretion, which results in decreased secretion of ACTH by the pituitary corticotrophs, which decrease in size and number. In the absence of ACTH stimulation, the zona fasciculata and zona reticularis of the adrenal medulla atrophy. Aldosterone deficiency does not occur in patients with secondary or tertiary adrenal insufficiency because this function depends mostly on the renin-angiotensin system. Any process that involves the hypothalamus, such as tumors, infiltrative diseases, and radiation, can result in tertiary adrenal insufficiency as well.

Therapeutics and Clinical Pharmacology

Goals of Therapy

The goal of therapy in adrenal insufficiency is to correct the glucocorticoid and/or mineralocorticoid deficiency. In general, one should strive for the lowest dose of glucocorticoid that relieves symptoms of deficiency, which include fatigue, weakness, dizziness, nausea, and vomiting, and decreases hyperpigmentation without inducing symptoms or signs of Cushing's syndrome. Mineralocorticoid replacement is required in all patients with primary adrenal insufficiency to prevent sodium loss, intravascular volume depletion, and hyperkalemia.

Therapeutics by Class

Glucocorticoids. The average daily secretion of cortisol in normal subjects is 10 to 20 mg/day,[17] but replacement doses range somewhat secondary to variability in steroid metabolism and absorption. Patients with adrenal insufficiency are usually treated with the longer-acting glucocorticoids such as dexamethasone or prednisone. It is only necessary to take these medications once daily, and they avoid the marked changes in concentrations that occur when hydrocortisone or cortisone acetate is given in two or three daily doses. Usual replacement dosages for prednisone and dexamethasone are 5 mg and 0.5 mg daily, respectively. Obese patients may require higher doses and thin patients may require less. The dose of glucocorticoid also may need to be increased in patients taking drugs that accelerate hepatic steroid metabolism, such as phenytoin, mitotane, and aminoglutethimide.[18]

Traditionally, shorter-acting glucocorticoids such as cortisone acetate (25 to 37.5 mg/day) or hydrocortisone (20 to 30 mg/day) were given, in two or three divided doses. Typical regimens consisted of taking two thirds of the daily dose upon arising in the morning and one third in the afternoon or evening. The goal was to simulate normal circardian rhythm of cortisol, but this does not occur since normal subjects secrete little cortisol from 6:00 PM to 3:00 AM. In addition, serum cortisol concentrations rise rapidly following ingestion of cortisone or hydrocortisone, exceeding the binding capacity of corticosteroid-binding globulin, and thus reaching higher concentrations than normal. The free cortisol is then rapidly filtered into the urine, resulting in a rapid decline in cortisol levels.[19] Short-acting corticosteroid preparations also do not simulate endogenous cortisol production in that endogenous cortisol already reaches a peak before the patient takes the morning cortisol dose. This may be responsible for symptoms of transient early-morning adrenal insufficiency, manifesting in symptoms of fatigue, nausea, and headache that resolve following the morning dose of hydrocortisone. Due to periods of relative adrenal insufficiency with the traditional regimen, there is inadequate regulation of ACTH secretion. Of note, these preparations have some mineralocorticoid activity so, if they are used, fludrocortisone should be decreased appropriately.

Mineralocorticoids. Mineralocorticoid replacement is required in all patients with primary adrenal insufficiency to prevent sodium loss and dehydration. The endogenous mineralocorticoids, aldosterone and deoxycorticosterone, are not used because of rapid hepatic degradation and the high cost of aldosterone. Fludrocortisone (9-α-fluorohydrocortisone) is a potent synthetic mineralocorticoid that can be given orally in a usual dose of 0.1 mg/day. Some patients may require doses of up to 0.2 mg/day in order to bring their plasma renin activity into the upper-normal range.[20] Patients on hydrocortisone or cortisone may be able to be maintained on lower doses (such as 0.05 mg/day).

Therapeutic Approach

Patients with adrenal insufficiency may present in acute adrenal crisis or with more subtle symptoms of chronic glucocorticoid and/or mineralocorticoid deficiency. Adrenal crisis is a life-threatening emergency that requires immediate treatment. When the diagnosis is suspected, therapy should not be delayed to obtain confirmatory results. The initial goal of therapy is restoration of intravascular volume and correction of electrolyte abnormalities. Large volumes of isotonic saline and intravenous glucocorticoids should be infused as quickly as possible. Dexamethasone (4 mg) or hydrocortisone (100 mg) are the most commonly used glucocorticoids. Dexamethasone is preferred as it is long acting and does not interfere with measurement of serum cortisol in subsequent ACTH stimulation tests. If hydrocortisone is used, 100 mg should be given every 6 to 8 hours. Mineralocorticoid replacement is not useful in the acute setting as its effects may take several days and sodium replacement can occur with saline.

Unless there is a complicating illness, high-dose parenteral therapy can be tapered over 1 to 2 days and changed to oral maintenance therapy. Patients are generally started on 5 mg of prednisone or 0.5 mg of dexamethasone once daily. Since endogenous ACTH secretion begins to increase at 3:00 to 4:00 AM, this would be the ideal time to administer the prednisone or dexamethasone. As this is not convenient, the next best time to administer the medication is at bedtime. This will lower the morning plasma ACTH concentrations into the normal range.

The goal of corticosteroid replacement should be to use the smallest dose that relieves the patient's symptoms, decreases hyperpigmentation, and lowers the early-morning plasma ACTH concentration into the normal range. If the patient continues to have symptoms at the standard maintenance dosages, the dosage should be increased. However, if increasing the dosage does not promptly relieve symptoms, the steroid dosage should be decreased back to baseline.

Patients may feel better on larger doses of steroids, but may develop long- and short-term complications of cortisol excess, including symptoms or signs of Cushing's syndrome such as weight gain. A concern of excessive long-term glucocorticoid therapy is the risk of osteoporosis.[21] Although elevated risk is not universally confirmed in the literature,[22] the possible increased risk does highlight the importance of avoiding excessive glucocorticoid doses.

The starting dose for mineralocorticoid replacement is typically 0.1 mg/day of fludrocortisone. The adequacy of treatment can be assessed by asking about symptoms of postural hypotension as well as monitoring blood pressure, serum sodium and potassium, and plasma renin activity. Plasma renin activity should be kept in the upper-normal range.[23] Some experts recommend measuring plasma renin activity in newly diagnosed and treated patients and routinely once yearly, as well as in patients with symptoms consistent with mineralocorticoid deficiency, such as nausea and salt craving.[24]

The dose of mineralocorticoid may need to be increased in summer when a greater amount of salt loss occurs in sweat. Salt intake in patients with adrenal insufficiency should generally be liberal. Signs of excess mineralocorticoid replacement are hypertension, edema, and hypokalemia. In these instances, caution should be taken in lowering the plasma renin level to normal. Hypertension in patients with adrenal insufficiency can be treated by lower doses of fludrocortisone and decreased salt intake.

Patients with adrenal insufficiency require supplemental glucocorticoid therapy in addition to their normal corticosteroids when they have an acute illness or undergo a stressful procedure. Given large variation in cortisol production in healthy patients undergoing stress, it is difficult to exactly predict the needs of patients, and some controversy exists about the amount of additional glucocorticoid that is needed. There is no universal consensus regarding treatment, but in general, the more invasive the procedure or severe the illness, the higher the dose of corticosteroid used. For critically ill patients or those undergoing major surgery, such as heart surgery, a typical regimen is hydrocortisone 100 mg every 8 hours with a taper to maintenance regimen as clinical condition improves.

Emerging Targets and Therapeutics

Corticosteroid insufficiency can occur during the course of a severe acute illness in individuals without obvious structural defects in the HPA axis. This deficiency has been termed *functional adrenal insufficiency* and is usually transient. It is thought to be due to many factors occurring during severe illness, including the inhibition of adrenal cortisol synthesis by high levels of inflammatory cytokines in patients with sepsis.[25] Diagnosis and treatment of "functional adrenal insufficiency" is still somewhat controversial and demands more research. In general, patients in whom corticosteroid therapy is started should be treated with intravenous or intramuscular hydrocortisone at 50 mg every 6 hours and, as the acute illness resolves, steroids should be tapered.[25]

In women, the adrenal cortex is the primary source of androgen in the form of dehydroepiandrosterone (DHEA) and dehydroepiandrosterone sulfate (DHEA-S). The physiologic role of these androgens is not known, and replacement has not generally been performed in patients with adrenal insufficiency. Treatment may result in improved sense of well-being and sexuality, but trials have been limited by short treatment–phase durations.[26,27] In addition, safety data for DHEA therapy is lacking. Further study is needed.

CATECHOLAMINE EXCESS: PHEOCHROMOCYTOMAS

Pathophysiology

Pheochromocytomas are tumors that arise from neuroectodermal chromaffin cells in the sympathetic nervous system and can release epinephrine, norepinephrine, dopamine, and/or a wide variety of active peptides. Tumors that arise from chromaffin cells of the adrenal medulla are referred to as pheochromocytomas and those in paraganglia (neural crest cells that have migrated) are referred to as paragangliomas or extra-adrenal pheochromocytomas.

Epinephrine is synthesized in the adrenal medulla and released into the systemic circulation. Norepinephrine is synthesized and stored at the peripheral nerve endings. Dopamine acts primarily as a neurotransmitter in the central nervous system. Specific catecholamine receptors (α_1, α_2, β_1, β_2) mediate their activity.

Catecholamines are formed from the amino acid tyrosine in neuroendocrine tissues (Fig. 41-5). L-Norepinephrine is converted to L-epinephrine by phenylethanolamine-*N*-methyltransferase, whose expression is regulated by the presence of glucocorticoids, which are

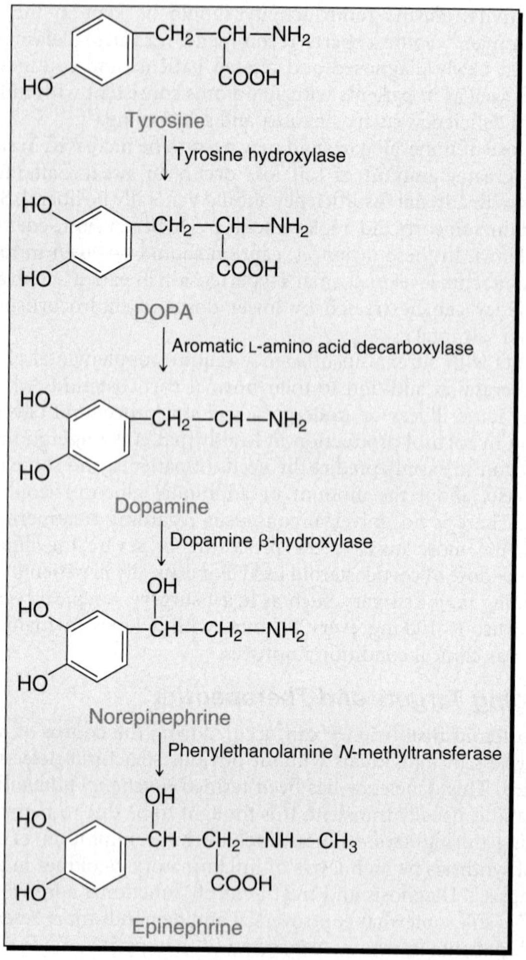

Tyrosine

↓ Tyrosine hydroxylase

DOPA

↓ Aromatic L-amino acid decarboxylase

Dopamine

↓ Dopamine β-hydroxylase

Norepinephrine

↓ Phenylethanolamine *N*-methyltransferase

Epinephrine

FIGURE 41-5 • Catecholamine synthesis.

in high concentration in the medulla through the corticomedullary system. In normal adrenal medullary tissue, approximately 80% of the catecholamines released are epinephrine. Small adrenal pheochromocytomas tend to secrete predominately epinephrine, whereas larger tumors often secrete predominately norepinephrine, probably due to less exposure of tumor cells to cortisol.

Metabolism of catecholamines occurs through two enzyme pathways with the end products of normetanephrine, vanillylmandelic acid, and metanephrine. The diagnosis of pheochromocytoma is made with demonstration of an elevation of these metabolites or catecholamines, either circulating or urinary.

Therapeutics and Clinical Pharmacology

Goals of Therapy

Surgical removal of the tumor is the treatment of choice, with the exception of patients with widely metastatic disease or in those with serious medical comorbidities making surgery too dangerous to perform. All patients require preoperative medical therapy with the goal of controlling hypertension (including a hypertensive crisis during surgery) and volume expansion. Patients with undiagnosed pheochromocytomas who undergo surgery for another reason (and thus have not had preoperative medical therapy) have high surgical mortality rates due to hypertensive crises and organ failure.[28]

Therapeutics by Class

α-Adrenergic Blockers. α-Blockers block adrenergic effects of catecholamines on vascular smooth muscle α receptors, causing a lowering of peripheral vascular resistance and blood pressure, and thus attenuating catecholamine-induced vasoconstriction. They may be reversible or irreversible in their receptor interaction and may be selective or nonselective.

Phenoxybenzamine is the α-adrenergic blocking agent of choice for patients with pheochromocytoma undergoing surgery. It binds covalently to α receptors, causing an irreversible blockade of long duration (14 to 48 hours or longer) and is nonselective (binds to both α_1 and α_2 receptors). Initial dosage is 10 mg once or twice daily, and the dose is increased every 2 days as needed to reduce blood pressure to normal levels. The final dosage of phenoxybenzamine is typically between 20 and 100 mg daily. Side effects derive from its α receptor–blocking actions, including orthostasis and tachycardia. It may also cause nonspecific symptoms of fatigue, sedation, and nausea.

Selective α_1-adrenergic blocking agents (prazosin, terazosin, or doxazosin) are not used routinely preoperatively because of incomplete α-adrenergic blockade. However, with their more favorable side effect profiles, they may be used in cases in which long-term pharmacologic treatment is needed, as in cases of metastatic pheochromocytoma.

β-Adrenergic Blockers. β-Adrenergic blockers are useful in pheochromocytoma once adequate α-adrenergic blockade has been achieved. Blockade of vasodilatory peripheral β receptors without α blockade can lead to unopposed α receptor stimulation and further elevations in blood pressure. No specific agents have been studied. Caution should be used in patients with coexisting lung disease or congestive heart failure. Chronic catecholamine excess in pheochromocytoma patients can lead to undetected cardiomyopathy, so caution should be taken with medication administration.

Calcium Channel Blockers. Although there is less experience with calcium channel blockers than with α- or β-blockers in perioperative treatment of pheochromocytoma, they may be as effective when used as the primary mode of therapy.[29] Nicardipine is the most commonly used calcium channel blocker in this setting. The starting dose is 30 mg twice daily of the sustained preparation preoperatively, and it is given as an intravenous infusion intraoperatively. Its sole use does not prevent all hemodynamic changes, but its use is associated with a low morbidity and mortality.[30] Currently the main role for this class is to supplement the combined α and β blockade when blood pressure control is inadequate or when patients have intolerable side effects.

Metyrosine. Metyrosine (α-methyl-*para*-tyrosine) can be used to treat pheochromocytoma as well. Metyrosine is a competitive inhibitor of tyrosine hydroxylase, which converts tyrosine to dopa, and is the rate-limiting step in catecholamine synthesis (see Fig. 41-5). In doses of 1 to 4 g/day, metyrosine decreases the amounts of norepinephrine and epinephrine secreted by the tumor.

Side effects can be disabling, with sedation, diarrhea, depression, and anxiety among the most common. Crystalluria can occur, so patients are instructed to increase their fluid intake to avoid crystal formation. For these reasons, metyrosine is generally used in patients when other agents have been ineffective, in those with inoperable pheochromocytoma, or in those in whom tumor manipulation or destruction will be marked (e.g., radiofrequency ablation of hepatic metastases). However, some use metyrosine in addition to α blockade preoperatively. In one study, patients given metyrosine as well as α blockade had better blood pressure control and a smoother perioperative course than those who had α blockade alone.[31]

Therapeutic Approach

There is no universally accepted method of surgical preparation of pheochromocytoma patients. One approach is to start an α-blocker preoperatively until normal blood pressure levels are reached and blood volume expansion is achieved. Close blood pressure monitoring on an outpatient basis should be performed. Target blood pressure is less than 120/80 mm Hg seated, with systolic blood pressure greater than 90 mm Hg while standing. On the second or third day of α blockade, patients should start a diet high in sodium content to avoid orthostatic hypotension. The degree of volume expansion needs to be adjusted for patients with congestive heart failure or renal insufficiency.

β-Blockers should be started only once adequate α blockade has been achieved and are usually reserved for patients with recurrent arrhythmias or persistent tachycardia. They should be used cautiously and at a low dose.

The roles of calcium channel blockers and metyrosine in perioperative management remain undetermined and, at present, these drugs are mostly used in cases in which α- and β-blockers cause intolerable side effects.

MINERALOCORTICOID EXCESS: PRIMARY HYPERALDOSTERONISM

Pathophysiology

Primary hyperaldosteronism is caused by increased aldosterone secretion from the adrenals, which results primarily from two major subtypes[32]: (i) unilateral aldosterone-producing adenoma (APA) or Conn's syndrome (50% to 60% of cases) and (ii) idiopathic hyperaldosteronism (IHA) or bilateral adrenal hyperplasia (40% to 50% of cases).

A rare subtype is renin-responsive adenoma, which morphologically and in response to adrenalectomy appears as APA, but it responds to physiologic maneuvers, as do hyperplastic glands of IHA. Another rare subtype is primary adrenal hyperplasia, in which a hyperplastic adrenal gland morphologically resembles that in IHA but mimics the APA response to physiologic maneuvers and unilateral adrenalectomy. The last rare subtype is glucocorticoid-remediable aldosteronism (GRA), which is autosomal dominant in inheritance and is associated with variable degrees of hyperaldosteronism that are suppressible with exogenous glucocorticoids. Rarely, aldosterone can be secreted by adrenocortical carcinomas and ovarian tumors.

The autonomous secretion of aldosterone leads to suppression of renin activity, as opposed to secondary hyperaldosteronism (such as renal artery stenosis), in which the high renin leads to high aldosterone (see "Pathophysiology" in the section on glucocorticoid and mineralocorticoid deficiencies).

Routine laboratory studies can show hypernatremia, hypokalemia, and metabolic alkalosis resulting from the action of aldosterone on the distal tubule of the kidney (i.e., enhancing sodium reabsorption and potassium and hydrogen ion excretion). Almost 20% of patients have impaired glucose tolerance resulting from the inhibitory affect of hypokalemia on insulin action and secretion; however, diabetes mellitus is rare. Normokalemia does not exclude primary hyperaldosteronism. Several studies have shown that 7% to 38% of patients with primary hyperaldosteronism have baseline serum levels of potassium that are in the reference range. The hypokalemia becomes evident with liberalization of dietary sodium intake. Screening[33] is performed by obtaining a morning sample for plasma aldosterone (PA) and plasma renin activity (PRA). A PA/PRA ratio of 20 (with a PA = 15 ng/dl) provides a sensitivity of 100% and a specificity of 80%, indicating the need for further study to confirm primary hyperaldosteronism. The most commonly used confirmatory test is a 24-hour urine aldosterone level obtained after 3 days of salt loading. The patient can be instructed to maintain a sodium intake of at least 200 mEq/day (1 teaspoon of salt three times daily) for 3 days. Care must be taken to ensure that potassium stores are replete and the patient is normokalemic at the time of testing because hypokalemia can inhibit aldosterone release and salt loading can exacerbate hypokalemia. A 24-hour aldosterone excretion rate of greater than 14 μg (with a concomitant 24-hour urine sodium >200 mEq) is diagnostic of primary hyperaldosteronism.

Therapeutics and Clinical Pharmacology

Goals of Therapy

In patients with primary hyperaldosteronism, the goal of treatment is to prevent the morbidity and mortality associated with hypertension and hypokalemia. The appropriate treatment depends on the cause (Conn's syndrome vs. IHA).[34] Although hypertension is frequently cured after unilateral adrenalectomy in patients with Conn's syndrome, the mean cure rate is only 19% after unilateral or bilateral adrenalectomy in patients with IHA, in whom treatment mainly is medical. In the case of APA, medical therapy is used preoperatively to control blood pressure and correct hypokalemia, thus decreasing surgical risk. Medical therapy is administered to patients with persistent hypertension postoperatively, poor surgical candidates, those who refuse surgery, and patients with IHA. It consists of a low-sodium diet and spironolactone or eplerenone (first-line agents). Additional antihypertensives can be used to control blood pressure.

Therapeutics by Class

Spironolactone. Spironolactone competes with aldosterone for receptor sites in distal renal tubules, increasing water excretion while retaining potassium and hydrogen ions. It may block the effects of aldosterone on arteriolar smooth muscles. The usual dose is 100 mg daily, which can be increased to 400 mg/day for control of blood pressure.

As side effects, spironolactone blocks testosterone biosynthesis and peripheral androgen action, causing impotence, decreased libido, and gynecomastia in men. In women, it may cause menstrual irregularities. High doses increase the half-life of digoxin (digoxin dose must be adjusted), and concomitant therapy with ACE inhibitors or indomethacin has been associated with severe hyperkalemia.

Eplerenone. Eplerenone selectively blocks aldosterone at mineralocorticoid receptors in epithelial (e.g., kidney) and nonepithelial (e.g., heart, blood vessels, brain) tissues; thus, it decreases blood pressure and sodium reabsorption. The usual dose is 50 mg daily; it can be increased after 4 weeks to 100 mg/day. As side effects, it may cause hyperkalemia, hypertriglyceridemia, headache, and dizziness.

Therapeutic Approach

Surgery[34-36] is the main therapy for Conn's syndrome. A laparoscopic adrenalectomy is favored, when possible. In patients with Conn's syndrome, the blood pressure response to spironolactone preoperatively is a predictor of the blood pressure response to unilateral adrenalectomy. Surgical risk can be decreased by correcting the hypokalemia and controlling the blood pressure by administering spironolactone for at least 1 to 2 weeks, preferably 6 weeks, before surgery. Hypertension typically does not resolve immediately postoperatively but, rather, over 3 to 6 months; however, almost all patients have improved control of blood pressure after surgery. Long-term cure rates with unilateral adrenalectomy for Conn's syndrome average 69%. Persistent hypertension may be related to resetting of baroreceptors, established hemodynamic changes, structural changes in the blood vessels, or coincidental essential hypertension.

Medical therapy[34-36] is administered to patients with persistent hypertension postoperatively, poor surgical candidates, those who refuse surgery, and patients with IHA:

- A sodium-restricted diet (<80 mEq or <2 g of sodium per day), maintenance of ideal body weight, and regular aerobic exercise contribute substantially to the success of pharmacologic treatment.
- Frequently, hypertension and hypokalemia can be controlled with a potassium-sparing agent such as spironolactone or a selective aldosterone blocker such as eplerenone. Hypokalemia is promptly corrected, but hypertension may take as long as 4 to 8 weeks to correct. Potassium supplementation should not be routinely administered with spironolactone because of the potential for the development of hyperkalemia. If hypertension persists despite titration, a second-step agent is added to the treatment.
- Second-step agents include thiazide diuretics, ACE inhibitors, calcium channel antagonists, and angiotensin II blockers.
- GRA is treated with physiologic doses of glucocorticoid, which correct the hypertension and hypokalemia.

REFERENCES

1. Newell-Price J, Trainer P, Besser M, et al. The diagnosis and differential diagnosis of Cushing's syndrome and pseudo-Cushing's states. Endocr Rev 1998;19:647-672.
2. Periera MA, Halpern A, Salgado LR, et al. A study of patients with Nelson's syndrome. Clin Endocrinol (Osf) 1998;49:533-539.
3. Terzolo M, Pia A, Berruti A, et al. Low-dose monitored mitotane treatment achieves the therapeutic range with manageable side effects in patients with adrenocortical cancer. J Clin Endocrinol Metab 2000;85:2234-2238.
4. Baudin E, Pellegriti G, Bonnay M, et al. Impact of monitoring plasma 1,1-dichlorodiphenildichloroethane (o,p′DDD) levels on the treatment of patients with adrenocortical carcinoma. Cancer 2001;92:1385-1392.
5. Robinson BG, Hales IB, Henniker AJ, et al. The effect of o,p′-DDD on adrenal steroid replacement therapy requirements. Clin Endocrinol 1987;27:437-444.
6. Takamatsu J, Kitazawa A, Nakata K, et al. Does mitotane reduce endogenous ACTH secretion? [Letter]. N Engl J Med 1981;305:957.
7. Verhelst JA, Trainer PJ, Howlett TA, et al. Short and long-term responses to metyrapone in the medical management of 91 patients with Cushing's syndrome. Clin Endocrinol 1991;35:169-178.
8. Santen RJ, Wells SA, Runic S, et al. Adrenal suppression with aminoglutethimide. I. Differential effects of aminoglutethimide on glucocorticoid metabolism as a rationale for use of hydrocortisone. J Clin Endocrinol Metab 1977;45:469-479.
9. Stalla GK, Stalla J, Huber M, et al. Ketoconazole inhibits corticotropic cell function in vitro. Endocrinology 1988;122:618-623.
10. Berwaerts JJ, Verhelst JA, Verheart GC, et al. Corticotropin-dependent Cushing's syndrome in older people: presentation of five cases and therapeutical use of ketoconazole. J Am Geriatr Soc 1998;46:880-884.
11. Dickstein G, Shechner C, Arad E, et al. Is there a role for low doses of mitotane (o′p-DDD) as adjuvant therapy in adrenocortical carcinoma? J Clin Endocrinol Metab 1998;83:3100-3103.
12. Bertagna X, Bertagna C, Laudat MH, et al. Pituitary-adrenal response to the antiglucocorticoid action of RU 486 in Cushing's syndrome. J Clin Endocrinol Metab 1986;63:639-643.
13. Estaban NV, Loughlin T, Yergey A, et al. Daily cortisol production in man determined by stable isotope dilution/mass spectrometry. J Clin Endocrinol Metab 1991;72:39-45.
14. Lamberts SWJ, Bruining HA, DeJong FJ. Corticosteroid therapy in severe illness. N Engl J Med 1997;337:1285-1292.
15. Kenouch S, Coutry N, Farman N, Bonvalet J-P. Multiple patterns of 11β-hydroxysteroid dehydrogenase catalytic activity along the mammalian nephron. Kidney Int 1992;42:56-60.
16. Coursin DB, Wood KI. Corticosteroid supplementation for adrenal insufficiency. JAMA 2002;287:236-240.
17. Kraan GP, Dullaart RP, Pratt JJ, et al. The daily cortisol production reinvestigated in healthy men: the serum and urinary cortisol production rates are not significantly different. J Clin Endocrinol Metab 1998;83:1247-1252.
18. Elias AN, Gwinup G. Effects of some clinically encountered drugs on steroid synthesis and degradation. Metabolism 1980;29:582-595.
19. Groschl M, Rauh M, Dorr HG. Cortisol and 17-hydroxyprogesterone kinetics in saliva after oral administration of hydrocortisone in children and young adolescents with congenital adrenal hyperplasia due to 21-hydroxylase deficiency. J Clin Endocrinol Metab 2002;87:1200-1204.
20. Oelkers W. Adrenal insufficiency. N Engl J Med 1996;335:1206-1212.
21. Peacey SR, Guo CY, Robinson AM, et al. Glucocorticoid replacement therapy: are patients overtreated and does it matter? Clin Endocrinol 1997;46:255-261.
22. Valero MA, Leon M, Ruiz Valdepenas MP, et al. Bone density and turnover in Addison's disease: effect of glucocorticoid treatment. Bone Miner 1994;26:9-17.
23. Oelkers W, Diederich S, Bahr V. Diagnosis and therapy surveillance in Addison's disease: rapid adrenocorticotropin (ACTH) test and measurement of plasma ACTH, renin activity, and aldosterone. J Clin Endocrinol Metab 1992;75:259-264.
24. Nieman LK. Treatment of adrenal insufficiency. In: Rose BD (ed): UpToDate. Wellesley, MA, 2006. Available at *http://www.uptodate.com.*
25. Cooper MS, Stewart PM. Corticosteroid insufficiency in acutely ill patients. N Engl J Med 2003;348:727-734.
26. Hunt PJ, Gurnell EM, Huppert FA, et al. Improvement in mood and fatigue after dehydroepiandrosterone replacement in Addison's disease in a randomized, double-blind trial. J Clin Endocinol Metab 2000;85:4650-4656.
27. Panjari, M, Davis SR. DHEA therapy for women: effect on sexual function and wellbeing. Hum Reprod Update 2007;13:239-248.
28. Lo CY, Lam KY, Wat MS. Adrenal pheochromocytoma remains a frequently overlooked diagnosis. Am J Surg 2000;179:212-215.
29. Ulchaker JC, Goldfarb DA, Bravo EL. Successful outcomes in pheochromocytoma surgery in the modern era. J Urol 1999;161:764-767.
30. Lebuffe G, Dosseh ED, Tek G. The effect of calcium channel blockers on outcome following the surgical treatment of phaeochromocytomas and paragangliomas. Anaesthesia 2005;60:439-444.
31. Steinsapir J, Carr AA, Prisant LM. Metyrosine and pheochromocytoma. Arch Intern Med 1997;157:901-906.
32. Jabbour SA, De Papp AE. Pitfalls in the diagnosis and management of primary hyperaldosteronism. Endocrinologist 1999;9:395-398.
33. Young WF Jr. Clinical practice: the incidentally discovered adrenal mass. N Engl J Med 2007;356:601-610.
34. Young WF Jr, Hogan MJ, Klee GG, van Heerden JA. Primary aldosteronism: diagnosis and treatment. Mayo Clin Proc 1990;65:96-110.
35. Gill JR. Primary aldosteronism: strategies for diagnosis and treatment. Endocrinologist 1991;1:365-369.
36. Bravo EL. Primary aldosteronism: new approaches to diagnosis and management. Cleveland Clin J Med 1993;60:379-386.

42

REPRODUCTIVE HEALTH

Dale W. Stovall and Jerome F. Strauss, III

OVERVIEW 631
INTRODUCTION TO THE HYPOTHALAMIC-PITUITARY-GONADAL AXIS 631
GONADOTROPIN-RELEASING HORMONE ANALOGUES AND GONADOTROPINS 631
Gonadotropin-Releasing Hormone 631
Biochemistry 631
Available Products 632
Clinical Utility 632
Side Effects 632
Gonadotropins 632
Biochemistry 632
Available Products and Clinical Utility 633
Side Effects 633
Conclusions and Evidence-Based Recommendations 633
GnRH Analogues and Endometriosis 633
GnRH Analogues and Uterine Leiomyoma 633
Gonadotropins and Infertility 633
ESTROGENS AND PROGESTERONE 633
Estrogens 634
Biochemistry 634
Mechanism of Action 634
Pharmacokinetics and Administration 634
Progesterone 635
Biochemistry 635
Mechanism of Action 635
Pharmacokinetics and Administration 635
Selective Estrogen Receptor Modulators, Estrogen Antagonists, and Aromatase Inhibitors 636
Selective Estrogen Receptor Modulators 636
Estrogen Antagonists 636
Aromatase Inhibitors 636
Clinical Uses 636
Contraception 636
Fertility Therapy 639
Menopause 639

OVERVIEW

The protein and steroidal hormones of the hypothalamic-pituitary-gonadal axis have numerous physiologic actions. The primary roles of these hormones are related to reproduction. Agonists and antagonists of the reproductive system have been used for assisted reproduction, contraception, and the treatment of menopausal symptoms and various gynecologic diseases. This chapter reviews the regulation of the hormones of the hypothalamic-pituitary-gonadal axis and builds upon these concepts to provide the rationale for the clinical utility and side effects of both agonists and antagonists derived from this axis.

INTRODUCTION TO THE HYPOTHALAMIC-PITUITARY-GONADAL AXIS

A neuroendocrine cascade with integrated feedback regulation involving the hypothalamus, pituitary, and gonads controls the reproductive systems in men and women (Fig. 42-1). The cascade begins with a neuronal oscillator in the mediobasal hypothalamus, primarily in the arcuate nucleus, which fires at intervals that coincide with bursts of a hypothalamic releasing factor, gonadotropin-releasing hormone (GnRH). GnRH is then released into the hypothalamic-pituitary portal vasculature and interacts with its receptor on the pituitary gonadotropes that make up approximately 20% of the hormone-secreting cells in the anterior pituitary gland. The intermittent release of GnRH is associated with an increase in the synthesis of gonadotropin subunits and a pulsatile secretion of the gonadotropins luteinizing hormone (LH) and follicle-stimulating hormone (FSH). In men, LH acts on testicular Leydig cells to stimulate the synthesis of testosterone and FSH acts on Sertoli cells to stimulate the production of proteins required for sperm maturation. In women, FSH stimulates the growth of developing ovarian follicles and induces the expression of LH receptors on theca and granulosa cells. FSH also regulates the activity of aromatase in granulosa cells, stimulating the production of estradiol. LH acts on the theca cells to stimulate the production of androstenedione, the major precursor to estradiol production by the ovary. LH is also required for the signaling of ovulation of the dominant follicle. The gonadal steroids, primarily estradiol and progesterone, regulate the frequency of GnRH release and the amplitude of gonadotropin secretion.[1,2] In the follicular phase, estradiol feedback effects are inhibitory and gradually reduce gonadotropin levels. At midcycle, serum estradiol levels rise above a threshold of 150 to 200 pg/ml for approximately 36 hours, producing a brief positive feedback on the pituitary that triggers the preovulatory surge of LH and FSH. In the luteal phase, progesterone, acting on the hypothalamus, decreases the firing rate of the pulse generator. Acting on the pituitary, progesterone increases the amplitude of LH pulses. When the ovaries are removed or cease to function at menopause, there is an overproduction of FSH and LH.

In addition to steroid hormones, the ovaries and testes secrete protein hormones that modulate gonadotropin secretion through actions on the pituitary under normal gonadal function. Included are inhibin A and inhibin B. After menopause, hormone replacement therapy does not reduce serum FSH and LH levels to premenopausal levels because of the loss of inhibin production by the ovaries.

GONADOTROPIN-RELEASING HORMONE ANALOGUES AND GONADOTROPINS

Gonadotropin-Releasing Hormone

Biochemistry

GnRH is a decapeptide that is derived by proteolytic cleavage of a 92–amino acid precursor. GnRH signals through a specific G protein–coupled receptor on gonadotropes that stimulates the phospholipase C–inositol-1,4,5-triphosphate–Ca^{2+} pathway. The half-life of GnRH is only 2 to 4 minutes. The fact that intermittent secretion of GnRH results in the synthesis and release of FSH and LH was first demonstrated by Knobil.[3] It was also Knobil who noted that, while pulsatile GnRH secretion is essential for the maintenance of normal ovulatory menstrual cycles, continuous GnRH infusion results in a cessation of gonadotropin release and ovarian steroid production. The cessation of FSH and LH production is the result of down-regulation (internalization) and desensitization (uncoupling) of GnRH receptors. It is this

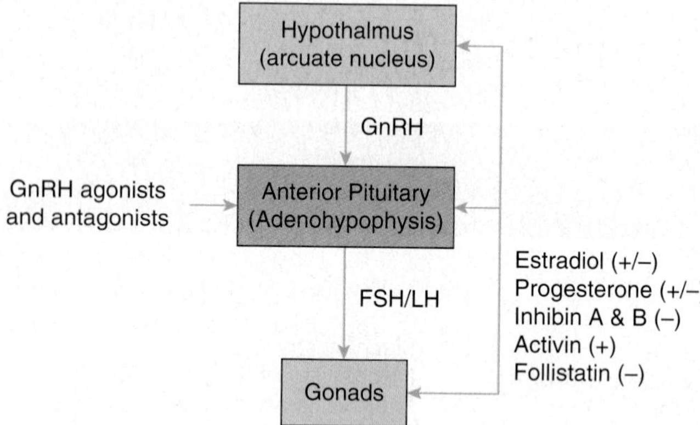

FIGURE 42-1 • The hypothalamic-pituitary-gonadal axis. The figure illustrates the sites of production and release of hormones, their feedback mechanisms, and the site of action of GnRH agonists and antagonists.

TABLE 42-1 AVAILABLE GNRH AGONISTS AND ANTAGONISTS

Generic Name (Trade Names)	Routes of Administration
AGONISTS	
GnRH (Factrel, Lutrepulse)	IV, subQ
Leuprolide (Lupron, Eligard, Viadur)	IM, subQ, depot
Buserelin (Suprefact)	subQ, IN
Nafarelin (Synarel)	IN
Deslorelin	subQ, IM, depot
Histrelin (Supprelin)	subQ
Triptorelin (Trelstar)	IM, depot
Goserelin (Zoladex)	subQ implant
ANTAGONISTS	
Cetrorelix (Cetrotide)	subQ implant
Ganirelix (Antagon)	subQ
Abarelix (Plenaxis)	subQ depot

GnRH, gonadotropin-releasing hormone; IV, intravenous: IM, intramuscular; IN, intranasal; subQ, subcutaneous.

concept that is utilized in the therapeutic role of GnRH agonists. GnRH receptors are also found in the ovary and testis, but their physiologic significance is yet to be determined.

Available Products

A number of U.S. Food and Drug Administration (FDA)–approved GnRH agonists and antagonists are currently available (Table 42-1). GnRH (gonadorelin) is available under the trade names Factrel and Lutrepulse. The GnRH analogues contain substitutions of the amino acid glycine at position 6, which protects against proteolysis. Substitutions at the C-terminus end improve receptor affinity. These analogues exhibit enhanced potency and a prolonged duration of action compared to native GnRH. When a GnRH agonist is administered, there is an initial release of gonadotropins and sex steroids that persists for a few days. In contrast, when a GnRH antagonist is administered, there is no initial increase in gonadotropin release. The first antagonists synthesized caused local and systemic release of histamine and severe flushing. The currently available antagonists elicit fewer of these undesired effects.

Clinical Utility

Synthetic GnRH (gonadorelin hydrochloride [Factrel]) is marketed for diagnostic purposes to differentiate between pituitary and hypothalamic defects in patients with delayed puberty and hypogonadotropic hypogonadism. After a baseline serum LH is drawn, a single 100-mcg dose of GnRH is administered either subcutaneously or intravenously. An increase in serum LH of greater than 10 mIU/ml is considered a positive response. Synthetic GnRH (gonadorelin acetate [Lutrepulse]) is marketed for the treatment of infertile women who are anovulatory and have GnRH deficiency. In this protocol, GnRH is administered in pulses by a pump to promote a physiologic cycle. Because of the complexity of administration, this treatment modality was rarely used and this product is no longer available in the United States.

As GnRH agonists and antagonists significantly inhibit gonadotropin secretion and decrease the production of gonadal steroids, they are useful in disorders that respond to hypogonadism. The current FDA-approved indications for these therapies include gonadotropin-dependent precocious puberty, palliative therapy for prostate cancer, and endometriosis. Depot preparations of goserelin (Zoladex), leuprolide (Lupron Depot, Elegard) or triptorelin (Trelstar LA), which can be administered subcutaneously or intramuscularly as infrequently as every 3 months, can be very useful for long-term treatment. In the case of precocious puberty, the cessation of gonadotropin release halts pubertal progression. The GnRH agonist is continued until the chronologic and bone ages of the individual match. With discontinuation of GnRH therapy, pubertal development is reinitiated. For endometriosis, a 6-month interval of therapy has been approved. In patients with endometriosis, dysmenorrhea is common and, as GnRH agonist therapy results in amenorrhea, reduction in pelvic pain is common. Furthermore, the hypoestrogenemia that is obtained with long-term GnRH administration results in regression of endometriosis implants; however, the implants do not tend to permanently regress and there is return of symptoms in up to 50% of patients within a year. GnRH analogues have also been prescribed for the treatment of uterine leiomyomas and for patients with blood dyscrasias in whom long-term amenorrhea and compliance are paramount.

Both GnRH agonists and antagonists have been used to suppress the LH surge and thus prevent ovulation prior to oocyte retrieval in assisted reproduction cycles such as in vitro fertilization (IVF). If a GnRH agonist is used, it can be initiated either in the midluteal phase or in the early follicular phase in conjunction with gonadotropins. Therapy is continued until human chorionic gonadotropin (hCG) is administered. GnRH antagonists can also be used to suppress the LH surge in IVF cycles. Their advantage in this regard is that they can be initiated a few days after gonadotropin therapy is begun, as they do not cause an initial release of endogenous gonadotropins. To date, most studies have demonstrated that slightly higher doses of gonadotropins are required for ovarian stimulation when GnRH antagonists are used in IVF cycles as compared to the use of GnRH agonists. Down-regulation of gonadotropins with GnRH agonists can cause luteal phase insufficiency; therefore, all patients are given luteal phase support following oocyte retrieval.

Side Effects

As administration of GnRH agonists and antagonists results in cessation of estrogen production and hypoestrogenemia, side effects include hot flashes, vaginal dryness, and, over time, bone loss. The average amount of bone loss in a premenopausal woman on a GnRH analogue is approximately 1% per month. Because of these side effects, therapy for non–life-threatening diseases such as endometriosis has been limited to 6 months. However, the addition of a progestin, such as norethindrone 2.5 mg orally per day, or a combination of estrogen and a progestin, known as "add-back" therapy, can reduce hot flashes and prevent bone loss (see later sections).

Gonadotropins

Biochemistry

The gonadotropins (LH, FSH, and hCG), together with thyroid-stimulating hormone, constitute the glycoprotein family of pituitary hormones. Each hormone is a glycosylated heterodimer containing a common alpha subunit and a distinct beta subunit that confers specificity of action. Among the beta subunits of this family, that of hCG is the most unique because it contains a carboxyl-terminal extension of 30 amino acids and extra carbohydrate residues. The carbohydrate residues on the gonadotropins play a role in signal transduction at the gonadotropin receptors and also influence the rates of clearance of the gonadotropins from the circulation and thus their serum half-lives. The hCG beta subunit gene is also expressed in trophoblast-derived hydatidiform moles and in choriocarcinomas. The oligosaccharides found on the hCG molecule produced by trophoblasts from normal pregnancies are identical to those found on the hCG molecule produced by benign hydatidiform moles. However, the oligosaccharides found on the hCG molecule from choriocarcinoma-derived hCG are different from those found in normal pregnancies or hydatidiform moles.[4]

The actions of both LH and hCG are mediated through the same receptor, the LH receptor. FSH binds to its unique receptor. Both the LH and FSH receptors are coupled to a G protein and have large, glycosylated extracellular domains that contribute to their affinity and specificity for their ligands. The FSH and LH receptors couple to G_s to activate the adenyl cyclase–cyclic AMP pathway. However, not all actions are mediated by cyclic AMP. At higher ligand concentrations, the agonist-occupied gonadotropin receptors also activate protein kinase C and Ca^{2+} signaling pathways through G_q-mediated effects on phospholipase Cβ.

Available Products and Clinical Utility

The gonadotropins are almost exclusively used for assisted reproduction purposes.[5] In general, FSH and LH are used to promote follicular development and hCG is used to trigger ovulation. Unlike GnRH, there are no LH, FSH, or hCG antagonists or long-acting agonists available. However, the currently marketed gonadotropin products do come from various sources. Menotropins (e.g., Pergonal, Repronex) that contain essentially equal amounts of FSH and LH are products from the urine of postmenopausal women. Because they contain other urinary proteins, they can cause hypersensitivity reactions. Urofollitropin (uFSH; Bravelle) is a highly purified FSH prepared by immunoconcentration with monoclonal antibodies and does not cause the same hypersensitivity problems as the menotropins. FSH and LH are also available as recombinant DNA preparations. Recombinant FSH is prepared by expressing complementary DNAs encoding the alpha and beta subunits of FSH in a mammalian cell line, yielding products whose glycosylation patterns mimic that of FSH produced by gonadotropes. The three recombinant FSH preparations available (Gonal-F, Puregon, and Follistim) are known as follitropins and differ slightly in their carbohydrate structures. Recombinant forms of LH (Luveris, Lhadi) are also available and are currently under investigation. The purported advantages of the purified FSH products, including reduced dosing and improved efficacy, have not been borne out in clinical trials. Furthermore, the recombinant products are more expensive as compared to the naturally derived hormones. Ovulation induction with FSH with or without LH requires monitoring with serial ultrasound imaging and serum estradiol levels and should only be performed by physicians experienced in assisted reproduction technologies.

Like FSH and LH, hCG is available as both a urine-derived product and a recombinant preparation. The urine-derived hCGs (e.g., Pregnyl, Novarel, Profasi) and recombinant hCG (choriogonadotropin alfa [Ovidrel]) mimic the action of LH. These compounds are given as opposed to LH to trigger ovulation either after administration of clomiphene citrate in women who do not produce an LH surge, or in women who are undergoing induction of ovulation with FSH. In this regard, hCG is administered when ultrasound imaging reveals one or more dominant follicles. Ovulation begins approximately 36 hours after the administration of hCG.

Side Effects

The primary risks of the use of gonadotropins for ovulation induction are the increased risk of multiple gestations and the risk of ovarian hyperstimulation syndrome (OHSS). Twin pregnancies occur in approximately 1.2% of births in women who are not taking fertility medications. In women undergoing induction of ovulation with gonadotropins, the rate of twin pregnancies is approximately 20% to 25% and the rate of more than twins is approximately 5%.

OHSS is believed to result from increased ovarian secretion of substances that increase vascular permeability and is characterized by rapid accumulation of fluid in the peritoneal cavity, the thorax, and, in rare cases, the pericardium. Signs and symptoms include abdominal pain and/or distention, nausea and vomiting, diarrhea, marked ovarian enlargement, dyspnea, and oliguria. OHSS can lead to hypovolemia, electrolyte abnormalities, ascites, pleural effusions, acute respiratory distress syndrome, thromboembolic events, and hepatic dysfunction. OHSS usually does not occur if hCG is not administered; therefore, in cases in which estrogen levels are excessively high or a large number of follicles are obtained with administration of FSH, hCG can be withheld.

Conclusions and Evidence-Based Recommendations

GnRH Analogues and Endometriosis

Endometriosis is rarely seen in women after menopause, so medications that induce a menopause-like state should be effective in treating endometriosis. GnRH analogues do appear to be an effective treatment for endometriosis-associated pelvic pain. However, there are no data to suggest that GnRH analogues are effective in the treatment of endometriosis-associated infertility or that GnRH analogues are more effective than other medical therapies such as danazol or gestrinone in the treatment of endometriosis-associated pelvic pain. GnRH analogues do differ from other medical therapies in regard to their side effects.[6]

GnRH Analogues and Uterine Leiomyoma

Uterine leiomyomas are the most common benign gynecologic tumors. Leiomyomas can cause heavy and/or irregular uterine bleeding and pelvic pain. Therefore, leiomyomas are a common indication for hysterectomy. Like endometriosis implants, leiomyomas possess estrogen receptors and tend to regress after menopause. Treatment with GnRH analogues has been shown to reduce the size of leiomyomas up to 50% after 3 months of therapy. Treatment with GnRH analogues for leiomyomas is most appropriate in the perimenopause to hasten the onset of the hypoestrogenic state, and as a preoperative therapy to stop bleeding and increase the patient's blood count and/or allow for a vaginal hysterectomy.

Gonadotropins and Infertility

The use of gonadotropins for induction of ovulation in women who fail to ovulate or conceive after induction of ovulation from clomiphene citrate, tamoxifen, or an aromatase inhibitor is appropriate. It is not considered first-line therapy for simple ovulation induction, especially in the young, reproductive-age female. The expense of gonadotropin therapy may be inhibitory for many individuals.

ESTROGENS AND PROGESTERONE

By 1900, ovarian control of the female reproductive system via hormonal production was established by Kramer, who demonstrated that symptoms from gonadectomy were relieved through the transplant of ovarian tissue. In 1923, Allen and Doisy devised a bioassay for ovarian extracts base on a vaginal smear in rats. In 1933, Corner and Allen isolated a hormone called progestin from the corpora lutea of sows; a few years later, the name was changed to progesterone. Russel Marker was the first to synthesize progesterone from the plant product diosgenin in the 1940s. Then in the early 1950s, Carl Djerassi synthesized the first orally active progestin, a 19-nortestosterone compound called norethindrone. By 1960, Jensen and colleagues had demonstrated the presence of intracellular receptors for estrogen, now known as estrogen receptor α (ERα), in target organs. A second estrogen receptor was identified in 1996 and termed estrogen receptor β (ERβ). The progesterone receptor was found to be present in two isoforms, A and B,

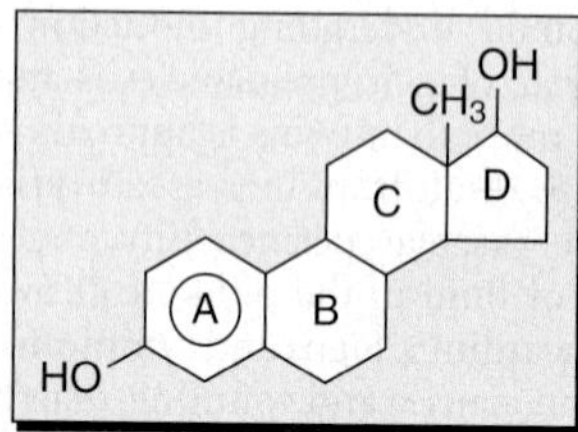

FIGURE 42-2 • **Estradiol.** The figure also depicts the basic structure of an estrogen with 18 carbons and A, B, C, and D rings. The D ring is a benzene ring.

which arise from a single gene by transcription initiated from different promoters.

Estrogens

Biochemistry

Estrogens are endogenous hormones that produce a multitude of physiologic actions. The principal actions of endogenous estrogens are pubertal development in girls and preparation of the female reproductive tract for implantation of the fertilized ovum. However, many nonreproductive tissues, including liver, bone, central nervous system (CNS), heart, and vascular endothelium, express low levels of both estrogen receptors. The most potent naturally occurring estrogen in humans is 17β-estradiol, followed by estrone and estriol. Each of these estrogens is an 18-carbon compound with an A, B, C, and D ring (Fig. 42-2). Steroidal estrogens arise from one of two precursors, androstenedione or testosterone, through aromatization of the A ring. The machinery necessary for this aromatization process is contained in the ovarian granulosa cell, testicular Sertoli and Leydig cells, adipose stroma, the placental syncytiotrophoblast, preimplantation blastocysts, bone, and various regions in the brain.[7] In premenopausal women, the ovaries are the principal source of circulating estrogen, where the production of testosterone from androstenedione and estradiol from estrone is favored. In postmenopausal women, the principal source of circulating estrogen is adipose tissue stroma, where estrone is synthesized from dehydroepiandrosterone secreted by the adrenals.

Many steroidal and nonsteroidal compounds that possess estrogenic or antiestrogenic activity occur in plants and fungi. Included are flavones, isoflavones, and coumestan derivatives. Synthetic agents, including pesticides, plasticizers, and a variety of other industrial chemicals, also have hormonal or antihormonal activity.

Mechanism of Action

Estrogens exert their effects primarily through interactions with the ERα or ERβ receptors. Both ERs are ligand-activated transcription factors that have different tissue distributions and transcriptional regulatory effects on a wide number of target genes.[8] The ER has numerous functional domains, including the ligand-binding domain, DNA-binding domain, and transcription activation domain. There are significant differences between the two receptor isoforms in the ligand-binding and transactivation domains, and the receptors appear to have different biologic functions and respond differently to various estrogenic compounds.[9] ERα is expressed most abundantly in the female reproductive tract, but is also expressed in the mammary gland, hypothalamus, endothelial cells, and vascular smooth muscle. ERβ is expressed most abundantly in the prostate and ovaries, but is also expressed in lung, brain, bone, and vasculature. Many cells express both ERs.

The concept of ligand-mediated changes in ER confirmation is central to understanding the mechanism of action of estrogen agonists and antagonists. After estrogen enters the cell via passive diffusion through the cell membrane, it binds to an ER in the nucleus. Upon binding to estrogen, the ER undergoes a conformational change that causes receptor dimerization, which increases the affinity and rate of receptor binding to the DNA.[10] Both ERα and ERβ homodimers and ERα/ERβ heterodimers can be produced depending on the receptor complement in a given cell. The ER dimer binds to estrogen response elements located in the promoter region of target genes. The ER-DNA complex recruits a cascade of coactivators and other proteins to the promoter region to form a transcription apparatus. In contrast, interactions of ERs with antagonists also promote dimerization and DNA binding. However, an antagonist produces a different confirmation change in the ER as compared to the agonist-occupied receptor.[11] The antagonist-induced conformation facilitates binding of co-repressors and other proteins that together reduce the ability of the transcription apparatus to form initiation complexes.

Other estrogen-associated signaling systems are present in humans. Several studies have suggested that some ERs are located on the plasma membrane of cells. It appears that the same gene that encodes ERα also encodes this form of ER, but it is transported to the plasma membrane.[12] Still other signaling systems may activate the nuclear ER by ligand-independent mechanisms. Finally, estrogen is known to initiate cell activities through nongenomic actions.

Pharmacokinetics and Administration

Estradiol, ethinyl estradiol, and other estrogens are extensively bound to plasma proteins. Estradiol is primarily bound to sex hormone binding globulin (SHBG) and to a lesser degree to serum albumin. Ethinyl estradiol, in contrast, is bound extensively to serum albumin but not SHBG. Unbound estrogens are rapidly distributed, and estradiol undergoes rapid hepatic biotransformation and has a plasma half-life of only a few minutes.

Estrogens also undergo enterohepatic recirculation through sulfate and glucuronide conjugation in the liver, biliary secretion of the conjugates in the intestine, and hydrolysis in the gut followed by reabsorption. Ethinyl estradiol is cleared much more slowly than estradiol due to decreased hepatic metabolism, and its elimination phase half-life ranges from 13 to 27 hours. As discussed next, a variety of estrogen preparations are available for oral, transdermal, parenteral, and topical administration (Table 42-2).

Oral. Because estrogen is lipophilic, it is generally well absorbed. Micronized estradiol (e.g., Estrace) is available for administration, as is ethinyl estradiol, which contains an ethinyl group at C17. Micronization yields a large surface for rapid absorption, but because of the first-pass effect, high doses of micronized estradiol must be given to maintain a significant bioavailability (e.g., 1 to 2 mg). Substitution of an ethinyl group at C17 inhibits first-pass hepatic metabolism, allowing for a lower dose to be used (e.g., 20 to 35 mcg). Conjugated equine estrogens (e.g., Premarin) that primarily contain the sulfate esters of estrone have been available for many decades, and a mixture of conjugated estrogens prepared from plant sources (e.g., Cenestin) has been made available more recently. For these conjugated estrogens to be absorbed across the intestinal epithelium, enzymes present in the lower gut must hydrolyze them to remove the charged sulfate groups. Another preparation, estropipate (e.g., Ortho-est and Ogen), contains estrone sulfate that is stabilized with piperazine. Plant-derived products, primarily from soy, are available as nonprescription items. These products may contain flavonoids such as genistein that demonstrate estrogenic activity in laboratory tests but are much less potent than estradiol. To date, their relevant doses and efficacy have not been established in clinical trials[13] (see Chapter 90, Complementary and Alternative Medicine, Nutraceuticals, and Dietary Supplements).

Transdermal. Estradiol is available for transdermal administration through patches and topical creams. Unlike oral administration, transdermal administration does not provide high levels of drug into the liver via the hepatic portal circulation; therefore, the hepatic effects of estrogen should be reduced. Furthermore, transdermal patches (e.g., Estraderm, Vivelle, Alora, Climara) provide a slow, constant release of estradiol with more constant serum levels as compared to oral administration. Topical creams (e.g., Estrasorb) that are applied to the upper thigh and calf and gels (e.g., Estrogel) that are applied to the arm are available. Estrogen cream preparations can also be used for vaginal administration. Vaginal estrogen creams must not be used in patients in whom estrogen in contraindicated, as vaginally administrated estrogen is systemically absorbed. Other vaginal estrogen preparations

TABLE 42-2 AVAILABLE ESTROGEN AND PROGESTOGEN PREPARATIONS

Product	Type of Estrogen/ Progestogen	Formulation
ESTROGEN (ORAL)		
Cenestin	Synthetic conjugated estrogens	Tablets
Enjuvia	Synthetic conjugated estrogens	Tablets
Estrace	Estradiol (micronized)	Tablets
Femtrace	Estradiol	Tablets
Menest	Esterified estrogens	Tablets
Ogen	Estropipate	Tablets
Ortho-Est	Estropipate	Tablets
Premarin	Conjugated equine estrogens	Tablets
ESTROGEN (TRANSDERMAL)		
Alora	Estradiol	Patch (matrix)
Climara	Estradiol	Patch (matrix)
Esclim	Estradiol	Patch (matrix)
Estraderm	Estradiol	Patch (reservoir)
Estrasorb	Estradiol	Emulsion (topical)
Estrogel	Estradiol	Gel (topical)
Menostar	Estradiol	Patch (matrix)
Vivelle	Estradiol	Patch (matrix)
Vivelle-Dot	Estradiol	Patch (matrix)
ESTROGEN (VAGINAL)		
Estrace	Estradiol	Cream
Estring	Estradiol	Ring
Femring	Estradiol	Ring
Premarin	Conjugated estrogens	Cream
Vagifem	Estradiol	Vaginal tablets
PROGESTOGEN (ORAL)		
Aygestin	Norethindrone acetate	Tablets
Prometrium	Progesterone (micronized)	Capsules
Provera	Medroxyprogesterone acetate	Tablets

include a 3-month vaginal ring (e.g., Estring, Femring) and a vaginal tablet (Vagifem).

Parenteral. When dissolved in oil and injected, esters of estradiol are well absorbed. The aryl and alkyl esters of estradiol become less polar as the size of the substitutes increases; therefore, the rate of absorption of oily preparations is progressively slowed and the duration of action can be prolonged. A single dose of compounds such as estradiol valerate (Delestrogen) or estradiol cypionate (Depo-estradiol) may be absorbed over several weeks following a single intramuscular injection. Suspensions containing estrone or a combination of esters also may be given via intramuscular injection.

Progesterone

Biochemistry

Progestins, like estrogens, are endogenous hormones. Unlike estrogens, which contain three naturally occurring compounds in humans, the only naturally occurring progestin in humans is progesterone, a 21-carbon compound. The principal actions of progesterone are development of the mammary gland, preparation of the endometrium for embryo implantation, maintenance of early gestation, thickening of the cervical mucus, and inhibition of milk production before parturition. Progesterone also may have depressant and hypnotic effects in the CNS, possibly accounting for the reports of drowsiness after administration. Metabolic actions of progesterone include increasing basal insulin levels and a rise in insulin levels after carbohydrate ingestion, but it does not normally alter glucose tolerance. Medroxyprogesterone acetate (MPA) has been shown to increase low-density lipoprotein cholesterol and decrease high-density lipoprotein cholesterol levels.[14] Other physiologic effects of progesterone include decreasing the frequency of GnRH pulses, which is the major mechanism of action of progestin-containing contraceptives. Progestins also act as natural antiestrogenic compounds by reducing the replenishment of estrogen receptors. Progesterone is secreted by the ovary, primarily from the corpus luteum during the second half of the menstrual cycle. Between 7 and 10 weeks of gestation, the synthesis of progesterone shifts from the corpus luteum to the placenta.

Numerous synthetic progestins are available. There are the pregnanes such as MPA (Provera) and megestrol acetate (Megace), the 19-nortestosterone derivatives or estranes (e.g., norethindrone, norethynodrel), and the gonanes (e.g., norgestrel, norgestimate, desogestrel, trimegestone). The most recent generation of gonanes have been engineered to have fewer androgenic effects. These 19-nor compounds are known to display limited binding to glucocorticoid, androgen, and mineralocorticoid receptors, a property that accounts for their non-progestational activities. A spironolactone derivative, drospirenone, acts both as a progestin and as a mineralocorticoid receptor antagonist.

Mechanism of Action

A single gene encodes for two isoforms of the progesterone receptor (PR): PR-A and PR-B. The ratios of the individual isoforms vary in reproductive tissues as a consequence of the tissue type, developmental status, and hormone levels. The ligand-binding domains of the two PR isoforms are identical. Like the ERs, after ligand binding, the ligand-receptor complexes form both homo- and heterodimers and then bind to the progesterone response elements located on the target genes.[15] Similar to the estrogen mechanisms, the PR-DNA complex recruits a cascade of coactivators and other proteins to the promoter region to form a transcription apparatus. Progesterone, like estrogen, causes up-regulation of its own receptors. Progesterone antagonists, like estrogen antagonists, recruit co-repressor proteins that render a target promoter inaccessible to the transcription apparatus. Two progesterone antagonists are RU486 and asoprisnil. RU486 has been used to inhibit implantation. Asoprisnil has been studied in the treatment of leiomyomas, but both agents could theoretically be effective in the treatment of dysfunctional uterine bleeding and endometriosis. RU486 has androgenic and corticosteroid activity.

Pharmacokinetics and Administration

In the plasma, progesterone is bound by albumin and corticosteroid binding globulin, but is not appreciably bound to SHBG. The 19-nor compounds bind to SHBG and albumin, and esters such as MPA bind primarily to albumin. The elimination half-life of progesterone is approximately 5 minutes, and, like estrogen, it is metabolized primarily in the liver to hydroxylated metabolites and their sulfate and glucuronide conjugates, which are eliminated in the urine. The synthetic progestins have much longer half-lives: norethindrone, approximately 7 hours; gestodene, approximately 12 hours; and MPA, approximately 24 hours.

A variety of progestin preparations are available. Progesterone undergoes rapid first-pass metabolism, and therefore high doses of progesterone must be given to obtain even a low bioavailability. Oral micronized progesterone (e.g., Prometrium) is available and is administered in doses of 100 to 200 mg/day. Both MPA and megestrol acetate (Megace) can be administered orally due to decreased hepatic metabolism. The 19-nor compounds have good oral activity because they contain an ethinyl substitute at the C17 position. Progesterone is also available as a vaginal gel (e.g., Crinone, Prochieve) and is contained within an intrauterine device (e.g., Progestasert). Finally, progesterone is available in oil solution for injection, and esters such as hydroxyprogesterone caproate (e.g., Hyalutin) and MPA (Depo-Provera) are available as intramuscular injections. 17α-Hydroxyprogesterone caproate has been shown in a large, randomized, multicenter trial to reduce the rate of preterm birth. Progestin-containing implants are also available (see Table 42-2).

Selective Estrogen Receptor Modulators, Estrogen Antagonists, and Aromatase Inhibitors

Currently, the primary use of estrogen and progesterone receptor antagonists is in the treatment and prevention of breast cancer and infertility. Many estrogen and progesterone antagonists are currently under investigation for these and other indications, including leiomyomas, osteoporosis, and endometriosis. Ligands that discriminate between ERα and ERβ have been developed but are not yet in clinical use.

Selective Estrogen Receptor Modulators

Selective estrogen receptor modulators (SERMs) are compounds with tissue-selective actions. The pharmacologic goal of these drugs is to produce beneficial estrogenic actions in certain tissues (e.g., bone, brain), but antagonistic activity in tissues such as breast and endometrium, where estrogen actions might be deleterious. Currently approved drugs in the United States in this class are tamoxifen citrate (e.g., Nolvadex), raloxifene hydrochloride (Evista), and toremifene (Fareston), which is chemically related to and has actions similar to tamoxifen. Tamoxifen and toremifene are approved for treatment of breast cancer, and raloxifene is currently approved for the prevention and treatment of osteoporosis.

Tamoxifen is a triphenylethylene with the same stilbene nucleus as diethylstilbestrol; it is given orally, and peak plasma levels are reached in 4 to 6 hours. It displays two elimination phases with half-lives of 7 to 14 hours and 4 to 11 days. Tamoxifen has an antiresorptive effect in bone and stimulates proliferation of endometrial cells. It causes a two- to threefold increase in deep venous thrombosis and pulmonary embolism and a twofold increase in endometrial cancer.[16] Tamoxifen also produces hot flashes, cataracts, and nausea. It has been shown to induce ovulation and to be similarly effective as compared to clomiphene citrate (see later).

Raloxifene is a polyhydroxylated nonsteroidal compound with a benzothiophene core. It is absorbed rapidly after oral administration and has an absolute bioavailability of about 2%. The drug has a half-life of about 28 hours. Raloxifene is an estrogen agonist in bone, where it exerts an antiresorptive effect. The drug does not cause endometrial stimulation and significantly reduces the risk of ER-positive breast cancer. Adverse effects include hot flashes and leg cramps.

Estrogen Antagonists

Antiestrogens are distinguished from the SERMs in that they are pure antagonists in all tissues studied. Clomiphene citrate (e.g., Clomid, Serophene) is approved for the treatment of infertility in anovulatory women, and fulvestrant (Faslodex) is used for the treatment of breast cancer in women with disease progression after tamoxifen.

Clomiphene citrate is a triphenylethylene with two isomers, *cis*-clomiphene and *trans*-clomiphene, that are a weak estrogen agonist and a potent antagonist, respectively. Clomiphene is well absorbed following oral administration, and has a long plasma half-life of 5 to 7 days. It increases gonadotropin secretion and stimulates ovulation. It increases the amplitude of LH and FSH pulses without changing the pulse frequency.[17] The drug is administered in the early follicular phase, most commonly for 5 days. It does increase the risk for multiple gestations, with the risk for twins being approximately 5% to 10%. It commonly causes hot flashes and less frequently causes ovarian cysts. There are rare reports of visual disturbances with clomiphene citrate.

Aromatase Inhibitors

The recognition that circulating estrogens may play a significant role in breast cancer has greatly stimulated interest in the use of aromatase inhibitors to selectively block production of estrogens. Both steroidal (e.g., formestane and exemestane [Aromasin]) and nonsteroidal agents (e.g., anastrozole [Arimidex] and letrozole [Femara]) are available. Steroidal, or type I, agents are substrate analogues that act as suicide inhibitors to irreversibly inactivate aromatase, while the nonsteroidal, or type II, agents interact reversibly with the heme groups of cytochrome P-450 enzymes.[18] Currently, the agents in this class are approved for the treatment of breast cancer. However, letrozole has been shown to induce ovulation by reducing the negative feedback of estradiol to the hypothalamic-pituitary axis and thereby increasing endogenous FSH and LH, which promotes folliculogenesis. One potential advantage of ovulation induction with letrozole as compared to clomiphene citrate is a lack of estrogen antagonism in the endometrium and uterine cervix. Caution must be used when prescribing aromatase inhibitors to women who are or may become pregnant because of the potential risk for developmental defects. Another agent that has been successfully used to induce ovulation in women with polycystic ovary disease is metformin. Metformin is an oral hypoglycemic that is purported to induce ovulation by reducing insulin levels, which in turn leads to a reduction in ovarian stroma–driven androgen production that inhibits folliculogenesis.

Clinical Uses

The therapeutic uses of estrogens and progestins primarily reflect their physiologic activities. The most common uses of these agents are contraception and menopausal hormone therapy in women. Progestins are also used in the treatment of patients with endometriosis, primary dysmenorrhea, and dysfunctional uterine bleeding. Continuous progestin therapy leads to an endometrium that is secretory, yet atrophic. One common side effect of continuous progestin therapy is irregular uterine bleeding. When estrogen and progestins are used in combination, irregular bleeding is less common.

Contraception (Table 42-3)

Combination Estrogen and Progestin Oral Contraceptives. Combination oral contraceptives act by preventing ovulation. They have been in use for 45 years. Over that time period, much has been learned about their risks and benefits. The consequences of not providing effective contraception for women is well illustrated by the experience in many countries, where inadequate family planning services have resulted in high rates of induced, and in some cases unsafe, abortion. When used properly, the effectiveness rate of combination oral contraceptives is approximately 99.9%. However, in practice, failure rates are as high as 8%.[19]

The first question to answer with any method of contraception is what screening needs to be performed prior to its use. Screening is supported only if evidence indicates that the early detection of a condition affects its natural history, the test is cost effective and acceptable to women screened and service providers, and adequate treatment exists. Current scientific evidence suggests only two prerequisites for the safe provision of combination oral contraceptives: a careful personal and family medical history with particular attention to cardiovascular risk factors, and an accurate blood pressure measurement. Only a small minority of women will require any further assessment. A personal history of myocardial infarction, stroke, or venous thromboembolism (VTE) contraindicates combination oral contraceptive use.[20] Women with a substantial and sustained increase in blood pressure should be advised to consider changing to other methods of contraception. Caution is also necessary when prescribing combination oral contraceptives to women who are over 35 and smoke, and perhaps to women who are obese. A current Papanicolaou (Pap) smear is not a reason not to prescribe any method of contraception, but rather should be considered a separate important medical issue.[21]

For decades, combination oral contraceptives have been administered in a 28-day package that contains 3 weeks of hormone-containing pills followed by 1 week of placebo pills. The rationale behind the 28-day package of pills is for patients to have a menstrual period every month. One of the problems with oral contraceptives is their side

TABLE 42-3 AVAILABLE ORAL CONTRACEPTIVES

Type Progestin/Estrogen	Product	Progestin (mg)	Estrogen (mcg)
COMBINATION EXTENDED CYCLE			
Levonorgestrel/EE	Seasonale	0.15	30
COMBINATION MONOPHASIC			
Norethindrone/EE or norethindrone acetate*/EE	Brevicon	0.5	35
	Junel 21 1/20	1*	20
	Junel Fe 1/20	1*	20
	Junel 21 1.5/30	1.5*	30
	Junel Fe 1.5/30	1.5*	30
	Loestrin 1/20	1*	20
	Loestrin Fe 1/20	1*	20
	Loestrin 24 Fe	1.5	20
	Loestrin 1.5/30	1.5*	30
	Norinyl 1 + 35	1	35
	Nortrel 0.5/35	0.5	35
	Nortrel 1/35	1	35
	Ortho-Novum 1/35	1	35
	Ovcon-35	0.4	35
	Ovcon-35 chewable	0.4	35
	Ovcon-50	1	50
Levonorgestrel/EE	Alesse	0.1	20
	Aviane	0.1	20
	Lessina	0.1	20
	Levlite	0.1	20
	Levlen	0.15	30
	Nordette	0.15	30
	Portia	0.15	30
Norgestrel/EE	Cryselle	0.3	30
	Lo/Ovral	0.3	30
	Ovral	0.5	50
Ethynodiol diacetete/EE	Demulen 1/35	1	35
	Demulen 1/50	1	50
	Kelnor 1/35	1	35
Norethindrone/mestranol	Norinyl 1 + 50	1	50
	Ortho-Novum 1/50	1	50
Desogestrel/EE	Apri	0.15	30
	Desogen	0.15	30
	Ortho-Cept	0.15	30
Drospirenone/EE	Yasmin	3	30
	Yaz	3	30
Norgestimate/EE	Ortho-Cyclen	0.25	35
	Sprintec	0.25	35
COMBINATION BIPHASIC			
Norethindrone/EE	Ortho-Novum 10/11	0.15 1	35 35
Desogestrel/EE	Kariva	0.15 —	20 10
	Mircette	0.15 —	20 10
COMBINATION TRIPHASIC			
Desogestrel/EE	Cyclessa	0.1 0.125 0.15	25 25 25
	Velivet	0.1 0.125 0.15	25 25 25
Norethindrone/EE	Aranelle	0.5 1 0.5	35 35 35
	Nortrel 7/7/7	0.5 0.75 1	35 35 35
	Ortho-Novum 7/7/7	0.5 0.75 1	35 35 35
	Tri-Nprinyl	0.5 1 0.5	35 35 35

Continued

TABLE 42-3 AVAILABLE ORAL CONTRACEPTIVES—cont'd

Type Progestin/Estrogen	Product	Progestin (mg)	Estrogen (mcg)
Norgestimate/EE	Ortho Tri-Cyclen Lo	0.18	25
		0.215	25
		0.25	25
	Ortho Tri-Cyclen	0.18	35
		0.215	35
		0.25	35
	Tri-Sprintec	0.18	35
		0.215	35
		0.25	35
Levonorgestrel/EE	Enpresse	0.05	30
		0.075	40
		0.125	30
	Tri-Levlen	0.05	30
		0.075	40
		0.125	30
	Triphasil	0.05	30
		0.075	40
		0.125	30
COMBINATION ESTROPHASIC			
Norethindrone acetate/EE	Estrostep Fe	1	20
		1	30
		1	35
Progestin-only	Camila	0.35	None
	Errin	0.35	None
	Micronor	0.35	None
	Nor-QD	0.35	None
Norgestrel	Ovrette	0.075	None

EE, ethinyl estradiol.

effects, which include irregular menstrual bleeding, amenorrhea, headaches, bloating, and fatigue. In an effort to improve the side effect profile of oral contraceptives, pharmaceutical companies have developed oral contraceptives with lower doses of hormone, new progestins, and new schedules of administration. The last few decades have seen a change from first- to second- and finally to third-generation progestins used in oral contraceptives. During this same time, new modes of administration of the progestins within oral contraceptives have been developed, including biphasic and triphasic pills that provide different amounts of hormone over a 3-week period. More recently, a pill package containing 3 months of hormone-containing pills followed by 1 week of placebo pills has been added to the market (Seasonale). The rationale behind this extended pill package is for the patient to have a menstrual period less often, only once every 3 months in this case. Finally, there has been some concern that third-generation progestins increase the risk for VTEs. Most of the data regarding this issue reveal a slight but significant increase in venous thrombosis with the use of third-generation progestins.

Progestin-Only Contraceptives. Several agents are available for progestin-only contraception. They are only slightly less efficacious than combination oral contraceptives, with reports of theoretical efficacy of 99%. Specific preparations include the "minipill": low doses of progestins (e.g., 350 mcg of norethindrone [Nor-QD, Micronor] or 75 mcg of norgestrel [Ovrette]) taken daily without interruption. Their primary side effects are irregular menstrual bleeding and spotting. Their primary advantage is that they can be used when estrogen is contraindicated and a pill is desired.

Long-Term Reversible Contraception. Although oral contraceptives may be administered throughout the reproductive years, and therefore are an acceptable long-term method of contraception, there are also contraceptive methods that provide protection from pregnancy for more than 3 months with a single administration. The options currently available in the United States include depot MPA (DMPA-IM 150), the levonorgestrel-releasing intrauterine system (LNG-IUS), the Copper T intrauterine device (IUD), and a single-rod progestin implant (Implanon) that was recently approved for use by the FDA. DMPA prevents pregnancy for 3 months, the single-rod progestin implant provides contraception for 3 years, LNG-IUS provides protection for up to 5 years, and the IUD can be used for up to 10 years. The primary advantage of long-term reversible contraception is the low first-year failure rates: 3.0% (DMPA), 0.1% (LNG-IUS), and 0.8% (Copper T). Further, as these methods do not contain estrogen, they can be used when estrogen is contraindicated, such as in patients with a personal history of myocardial infarction, stroke, or VTE.

The long-term reversible contraceptive methods do have their disadvantages. The primary disadvantages of DMPA are its adverse effect on menstrual bleeding patterns, characterized by persistent spotting and unpredictable bleeding, and its adverse effects on bone mineral density (BMD). Because DMPA suppresses estradiol production, it may decrease BMD. The most recent data suggest a decrease in BMD of only 4% per year with DMPA.[22] Currently, however, DMPA has a "black box" warning stating that the agent should not be used for more than 2 years unless other contraceptive methods are inadequate.

The primary disadvantages of the LNG-IUS and the IUD include their initial costs, which may be an obstacle for some patients. Pain and cramping may be experienced during insertion. There is also a small risk of uterine perforation with insertion, and expulsion of these devices occurs in about 2% to 3% of parous women. Therefore, a follow-up visit should be scheduled after the next menses. The risk of pelvic inflammatory disease (PID) with IUDs appears to be concentrated in the first 20 days following insertion. Thereafter, the risk falls to a low level (1 infection per 1000 person-years of experience) and remains low for a period of 8 years.[23] As this and other data have demonstrated a low risk of PID with IUD use, the new package insert for the Copper T IUD now permits its use in women with a history of PID.

Emergency Contraception. Emergency contraception, also called the "morning-after pill" and postcoital contraception, is therapy used to prevent pregnancy after an unprotected or inadequately protected act of sexual intercourse. Currently, the only FDA-approved methods of emergency contraception are the administration of progestin-only or combination estrogen-progestin oral contraceptive pills. The progestin-only regimen consists of a total dose of 1.5 mg levonorgestrel

(Plan B). The package insert recommends patients take one 0.75-mg pill as soon as possible after unprotected intercourse and take a second 0.75-mg pill 12 hours after the first dose. However, randomized trials have shown that taking both pills at the same time or 24 hours apart is equally effective and does not increase the risk of side effects.[24] Therapy should be initiated as soon as possible. Although many package inserts recommend their use only within 72 hours of intercourse, some studies have shown that emergency contraception is still moderately effective when the first dose is taken up to 120 hours after intercourse. Recently, the FDA has approved the use of Plan B as an over-the-counter method of emergency contraception in women 18 and over. For women under age 18, it is available by prescription.

The levonorgestrel-only regimen is associated with significantly lower incidences of nausea and vomiting than the combined regimen. Nausea and vomiting occurs in approximately 18% and 4%, respectively, of women who take the levonorgestrel-only regimen as compared to 43% and 16%, respectively, of women who take the combined regimen. Other side effects include breast tenderness, abdominal pain, dizziness, headache, and fatigue.

Conclusions and Evidence-Based Recommendations

Biphasic or Triphasic Versus Monophasic Oral Contraceptives. There are no data to support the hypothesis that either biphasic or triphasic oral contraceptives significantly reduce the irregular menstrual bleeding associated with monophasic oral contraceptives.[25,26]

Estrogen Pills: 20 mcg Versus >20 mcg. Because combination oral contraceptives that contain 20 mcg of ethinyl estradiol contain a low dose of estrogen, they are theoretically safer. However, when compared to combination oral contraceptives that contain greater than 20 mcg of ethinyl estradiol, 20-mcg pills caused an increase in the rate of bleeding pattern disruptions and resulted in higher discontinuation rates. Therefore, it is recommended to start patients on a monophasic pill that contains 30 or 35 mcg of ethinyl estradiol.

Contraceptive Pills and Patches and Weight Gain. The fear of weight gain may prevent women from using contraception. There is no evidence that either contraceptive pills or patches cause weight gain, or that weight gain has been a significant cause for stopping the use of these contraceptives in clinical trials.

Combination Oral Contraceptives Versus Progestin-Only Contraceptives and Lactation. Some studies have suggested differences between combination and progestin-only oral contraceptives in the quality or quantity of breast milk. Based upon the data to date, it is unclear whether the quality or quantity of breast milk is significantly affected by either combination oral contraceptives or progestin-only contraceptives. However, none of the trials to date has shown a significant difference in infant growth or weight due to hormonal contraceptives taken during lactation.

Comparison of Various Progestins in Combination Contraceptives. Company-sponsored randomized trials have demonstrated that second- and third-generation progestins are preferred over first-generation progestins with regard to breakthrough bleeding, spotting, and amenorrhea. However, data from independently conducted, well-designed clinical trials to compare second- and third-generation progestins are needed.

Contraceptives and Ectopic Pregnancy. Both oral contraceptives and IUDs reduce the rate of ectopic pregnancy.[27]

Contraindications to Hormone-Containing Contraceptives. Women with uncontrolled hypertension are not candidates for estrogen-containing oral contraceptives because of an increased risk for stroke. Furthermore, women with thrombogenic mutations such as factor V Leiden, protein C, and protein S deficiency should not be given estrogen-containing oral contraceptives. Varicose veins are not a contraindication to oral contraceptive use. Women who are over age 35 and who smoke should not be given oral contraceptives.

Fertility Therapy

Both clomiphene citrate and tamoxifen are effective in inducing ovulation and increasing pregnancy rates, and no differences have been demonstrated between these two therapies in regard to these outcomes. They are both inexpensive and, unlike FSH, require less extensive monitoring of ovulation induction. Preliminary data regarding the use of aromatase inhibitors such as letrozole and anastrozole in induction of ovulation are promising but inconsistent. It is still too early to recommend aromatase inhibitors as first-line therapy for ovulation induction.

Menopause

Estrogen Alone. Data from the Women's Health Initiative (WHI) demonstrate that, after an average of 6.8 years of therapy, estrogen therapy alone revealed no significant increased risk for coronary artery disease (relative risk [RR] = 0.91), pulmonary embolism (RR = 1.34), breast cancer (RR = 0.77), colorectal cancer (RR = 1.08), or total mortality (RR = 1.04). However, the risk for stroke was significantly increased (39%) and the risk for hip fracture was reduced (39%).[28]

Combination Estrogen and Progestins. Data from both the WHI and observational studies agree that estrogen and progestin therapy in menopausal women increases the risk of stroke (RR = 1.5), pulmonary embolism (RR = 2.0), and breast cancer (RR = 1.25) and decreases the risk of hip fractures (RR = 0.3) and colon cancer (RR = 0.4).[29] Although it is still unclear, there is speculation that the timing of initiation of hormone therapy in relation to stage of atherosclerosis may be important. According to this theory, initiation of hormone therapy in the first few years after menopause may be cardioprotective.[30] However, this theory has yet to be substantiated by a randomized trial.

Conclusions and Evidence-Based Recommendations

Vasomotor Symptoms. Estrogen with or without a progestin is effective and FDA approved for the treatment of vasomotor symptoms such as hot flashes and night sweats that are associated with menopause. The lowest effective dose should be used for the shortest period of time. Any therapy that is under investigation for the treatment of vasomotor symptoms must be assessed in masked trials against a placebo because of the large placebo effect seen in most randomized trials.

Symptoms of Vaginal Atrophy. Estrogen administration is effective and is FDA approved for the treatment of symptoms of vaginal atrophy, including vaginal dryness and itching. Estrogen administration via creams, pessaries, tablets, and the estrogen vaginal ring appears to be equally effective in treating these symptoms. Although estrogen is effective in the treatment of vaginal atrophy, it is not effective for the treatment of urinary incontinence.

Osteoporosis and Colon Cancer. Estrogen therapy significantly increases BMD and is FDA approved for the prevention of osteoporosis. Estrogen therapy alone or continuous combined estrogen and progestin therapy (after 4 years) significantly reduced the risk of osteoporosis-associated fractures and colon cancer.

Uterine Bleeding and Endometrial Hyperplasia. Unopposed estrogen therapy is associated with an increased risk of endometrial hyperplasia, irregular bleeding, and noncompliance. The addition of oral progestins to oral estrogen therapy is associated with a reduced risk of hyperplasia and improved compliance. Irregular bleeding is more common in the first year of therapy with continuous progestin and estrogen as compared to cyclic, once-per-month, progestin and continuous estrogen. The risk of endometrial hyperplasia is higher when progestins are administered every 3 months as compared to every month.

Cardiovascular Disease, Breast Cancer, and Other Risks of Therapy. Although short-term use of estrogen and progestins appears safe in healthy, younger menopausal-age women, long-term therapy for treatment and prevention of chronic diseases in menopause-age women is not indicated. In healthy women, combined continuous hormone therapy significantly increases the risk of venous thromboembolism, coronary event (after 1 year's use), stroke (after 3 years), breast cancer (after 5 years), gallbladder disease, and dementia (in women over 65 years). The highest risk for coronary events occurs in the first year of therapy. Therefore, combined estrogen and progestin hormone therapy should not be initiated or continued in postmenopausal women for the prevention of cardiovascular disease.

Weight Gain. Weight is normally gained during the menopausal years. There is no evidence that estrogen therapy alone or in combination with a progestin causes an increase or decrease in weight gain or body mass index during the menopause. There is also no evidence that estrogen therapy has any effect on the waist-hip ratio or redistribution of body fat.

REFERENCES

1. Hewitt SC, Korach KS. Oestrogen receptor knockout mice: roles for oestrogen receptors α and β in reproductive tissues. Reproduction 2003;125:269-277.
2. Conneely OM, Mulac-Jericevic B, DeMayo F, et al. Reproductive functions of progesterone receptors. Recent Prog Horm Res 2002;57:339-355.
3. Knobil E. Patterns of hypophysiotropic signals and gonadotropin secretion in the rhesus monkey. Biol Reprod 1981;24:44-49.
4. Kobata A. Structures, function, and transformational changes of the sugar chains of glycohormones. J Cell Biochem 1988;37:79-90.
5. Huirne JAF, Lambalk CB, Van Loenen AC, et al. Contemporary pharmacological manipulation in assisted reproduction. Drugs 2004;64:297-322.
6. Prentice A, Deary AJ, Goldbeck-Wood S, et al. Gonadotrophin-releasing hormone analogues for pain associated with endometriosis. Cochrane Database of Systemic Reviews 1999,(2):CD000346.
7. Simpson ER, Clyne C, Rubin G, et al. Aromatase—a brief overview. Annu Rev Physiol 2002;64:93-127.
8. Hanstein B, Djahansouzi S, Dall P, et al. Insights into the molecular biology of the estrogen receptor define novel therapeutic targets for breast cancer. Eur J Endocrinol 2004;150:243-255.
9. Kuiper GG, Carlsson B, Grandien K, et al. Comparison of the ligand binding specificity and transcript tissue distribution of estrogen receptors ER α and β. Endocrinology 1997;138:863-870.
10. Cheskis BJ, Karathanasis S, Lyttle CR. Estrogen receptor ligands modulate its interaction with DNA. J Biol Chem 1997;272:11384-11391.
11. Smith CL, O'Malley BW. Coregulator function: a key to understanding tissue specificity of selective receptor modulators. Endocr Rev 2004;25:45-71.
12. Zhu W, Smart EJ. Caveolae, estrogen and nitric oxide. Trends Endocrinol Metab 2003;14:114-117.
13. Fitzpatrick LA. Soy isoflavones: hope or hype? Maturitas 2003;44(Suppl 1):S21-S29.
14. Writing Group for the PEPI Trial. Effects of estrogen or estrogen/progestin regimens on heart disease risk factors in postmenopausal women. The Postmenopausal Estrogen/Progestin Interventions (PEPI) Trial. JAMA 1995;273:199-208.
15. Giangrande PH, McDonnell DP. The A and B isoforms of the human progesterone receptor: two functionally different transcription factors encoded by a single gene. Recent Prog Horm Res 1999;54:291-313.
16. Smith RE. A review of selective estrogen receptor modulators and National Surgical Adjuvant Breast and Bowel Project clinical trials. Semin Oncol 2003;30(Suppl 16):4-13.
17. Kettel LM, Roseff SJ, Berga SL, et al. Hypothalamic-pituitary-ovarian response to clomiphene citrate in women with polycystic ovary syndrome. Fertil Steril 1993;59:532-538.
18. Haynes BP, Dowsett M, Miller WR, et al. The pharmacology of letrozole. J Steroid Biochem Mol Biol 2003;87:35-45.
19. Trussell J. Contraceptive failure in the United States. Contraception 2004;70:89-96.
20. Hannaford PC, Webb AM. Evidence-guided prescribing of combined oral contraceptives: consensus statement. Contraception 1996;54:125-129.
21. Stewart FH, Harper CC, Ellertson CE, et al. Clinical breast and pelvic examination requirements for hormonal contraception: current practice versus evidence. JAMA 2001;285:2232-2239.
22. Clark MK, Sowers MR, Nichols S, Levy B. Bone mineral density changes over two years in first-time users of depot medroxyprogesterone acetate. Fertil Steril 2004;82:1580-1586.
23. Farley TMM, Rosenberg MJ, Rowe PJ, et al. Intrauterine devices and pelvic inflammatory disease: an international perspective. Lancet 1992;339:785-788.
24. von Hertzen H, Piaggio G, Ding J, et al. Low dose mifepristone and two regimens of levonorgestrel for emergency contraception: a WHO multicentre randomized trial. WHO Research Group on Post-Ovulatory Methods of Fertility Regulation. Lancet 2002;360:1803-1810.
25. Percival-Smith RK, Yuzpe AA, Desrosiers JA, et al. Cycle control on low-dose oral contraceptives: a comparative trial. Contraception 1990;42:253-262.
26. Larranaga A, Sartoretto JN, Winterhalter M, Navas Filho F. Clinical evaluation of two biphasic and one triphasic norgestrel/ethinyl estradiol regimens. Int J Fertil 1978;23:193-199.
27. Franks AL, Beral V, Cates W Jr, Hogue CJ. Contraception and ectopic pregnancy risk. Am J Obstet Gynecol 1990;163(4 Pt I):1120-1123.
28. Anderson GL, Limacher M, Assaf AR, et al. Effects of conjugated equine estrogen in postmenopausal women with hysterectomy: the Women's Health Initiative randomized controlled trial. JAMA 2004;291:1701-1712.
29. Michels KB, Manson JE. Postmenopausal hormone therapy: a reversal of fortune. Circulation 2003;107:1830-1833.
30. Manson JE, Bassuk SS, Harman SM, et al. Postmenopausal hormone therapy: new questions and the case for new clinical trials. Menopause 2006;13:139-147.

43

ALZHEIMER'S DISEASE AND DEMENTIAS

Wael N. Haidar and Ronald C. Petersen

INTRODUCTION 641
PATHOPHYSIOLOGY 641
Mild Cognitive Impairment 641
Alzheimer's Disease 641
Other Dementias 643
THERAPEUTICS AND CLINICAL PHARMACOLOGY 643
Therapeutics by Class 643
Symptomatic 643
Disease-Modifying Agents 645
Vitamin E 645
Emerging Targets and Therapeutics 645
Anti-inflammatory Drugs 645
Estrogen Replacement Therapy 646
Investigational Drugs 646
Herbal/Alternative Therapies 646
Treatment of Noncognitive Symptoms 646
Motor Symptoms 646
Behavioral Management/ Psychosis 647
Apathy/Depression 647
Sleep Disorders 647

INTRODUCTION

Over the past 50 years, most industrialized nations have been witnessing an aging of their population resulting in an increased awareness of geriatric syndromes and diseases of the elderly. Among the most prominent, and with devastating consequences for the patient and the family, are the cognitive disorders. In the year 2000, there were an estimated 4.5 million Americans with Alzheimer's disease (AD), with an expected increase to 8.5 million by the year 2030.[1]

While a significant amount of research to evaluate cognition and aging has been conducted, identifying the changes that may constitute "normal aging" remains difficult and controversial. Several investigators developed and published normative data for specific neuropsychological tests.[2] However, other investigators have argued that data may have been contaminated with subjects with incipient cognitive impairment.[3] Furthermore, the overlapping nature of the different constructs and different stages of dementia makes cutoffs somewhat arbitrary (Fig. 43-1).

PATHOPHYSIOLOGY

Mild Cognitive Impairment

The concept of mild cognitive impairment (MCI) arose with the need to frame the group of patients who had some evidence of cognitive decline but were not demented. While there are no consensus criteria, the following were initially described: cognitive decline compared to his or her baseline, cognitive deficit based on age and education, global cognition preserved, functionally near normal, and not demented.[4,5] The only domain affected in MCI is usually memory.

MCI can further be characterized based on the number of domains affected and if any of those include memory. Amnestic MCI (memory impairment), particularly if there is evidence of neuron degeneration, is likely to evolve into AD. Work is underway to clarify the relationship between other subtypes and conversion to dementia. Evaluation of patients with MCI is similar to that of patients with clinically probable AD.

The American Academy of Neurology's (AAN's) most recently released practice parameter paper recommends a close follow-up of patients diagnosed with MCI because they have a higher risk of converting to AD compared to the general population.[6] While no treatment has been found to be effective in slowing or preventing conversion, it remains a hot area in research, and many potential therapies are currently being investigated. More recently, a broader framework has been proposed by an international forum of experts.[7]

Alzheimer's Disease

AD is by far the most common dementia. Its hallmark is initial memory involvement and a slowly progressive dementia.[8] Eventually, other cognitive domains may be involved. As mentioned earlier, age remains the most important risk factor. The incidence and prevalence of AD double every 5 years after age 65. AD prevalence in women is higher than in men, likely reflecting their longer life expectancy.[9-11]

Definite AD is a pathologic diagnosis, the classical pathology being neuritic plaques and neurofibrillary tangles.[12] Currently, abnormal processing or deposition of amyloid is thought to have a central role in the pathogenesis of AD resulting in neuritic plaques. Amyloid precursor protein (APP) is usually cleaved by α-secretase enzyme, leading to the formation of a p3 fragment (β-amyloid $[A\beta]_{17-42}$), which is soluble (Fig. 43-2). However, when APP is cleaved by β- and γ-secretases, it results in the formation of $A\beta_{1-40}$ and $A\beta_{1-42}$, which are subsequently deposited in the brain. The insoluble deposits produce an inflammatory response eventually leading to cell death (Fig. 43-3). Similarly, neurofibrillary tangles are formed by the abnormal processing of tau. However, its exact role in AD pathogenesis remains unclear. An understanding of both pathways to AD is paramount to the development of a variety of potential drug therapy targets that may prevent or stop the progression of the disease.

Clinically, we are able to diagnose possible and probable AD. Several published criteria exist for the diagnosis. In its practice parameters paper, the AAN believed the criteria in the *Diagnostic and Statistical Manual of Mental Disorders, Fourth Edition* (DSM-IV) were reliable.[13] These are summarized in Box 43-1. The diagnosed patient should have a memory impairment associated with other cognitive deficits. The deficits should impact the patient's functional status and the course of the disease (slow and progressive). Finally, the symptoms should not be explained by another neurologic disorder.[14]

Patient history remains essential for obtaining the information and establishing the diagnosis of dementia. The clinician should interview the patient and preferably a caregiver or close family member to assess

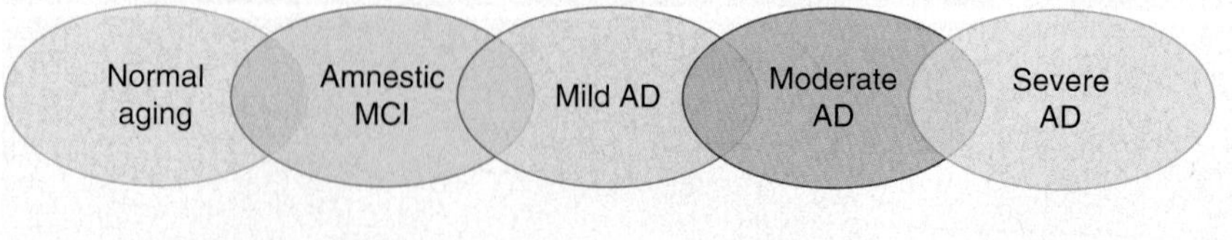

FIGURE 43-1 • Spectrum of progression of cognition from normal aging to severe Alzheimer's disease.

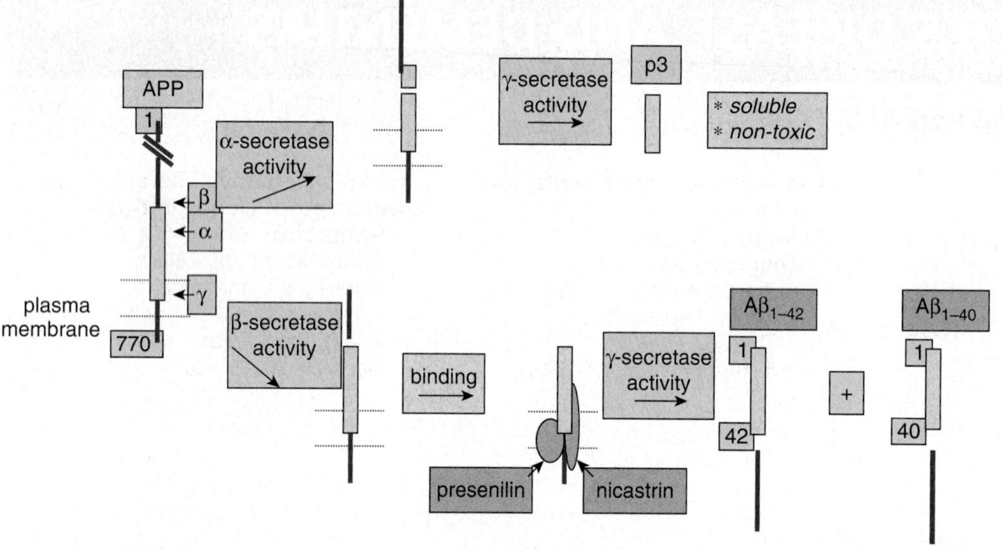

FIGURE 43-2 • Amyloid precursor protein processing by secretases.

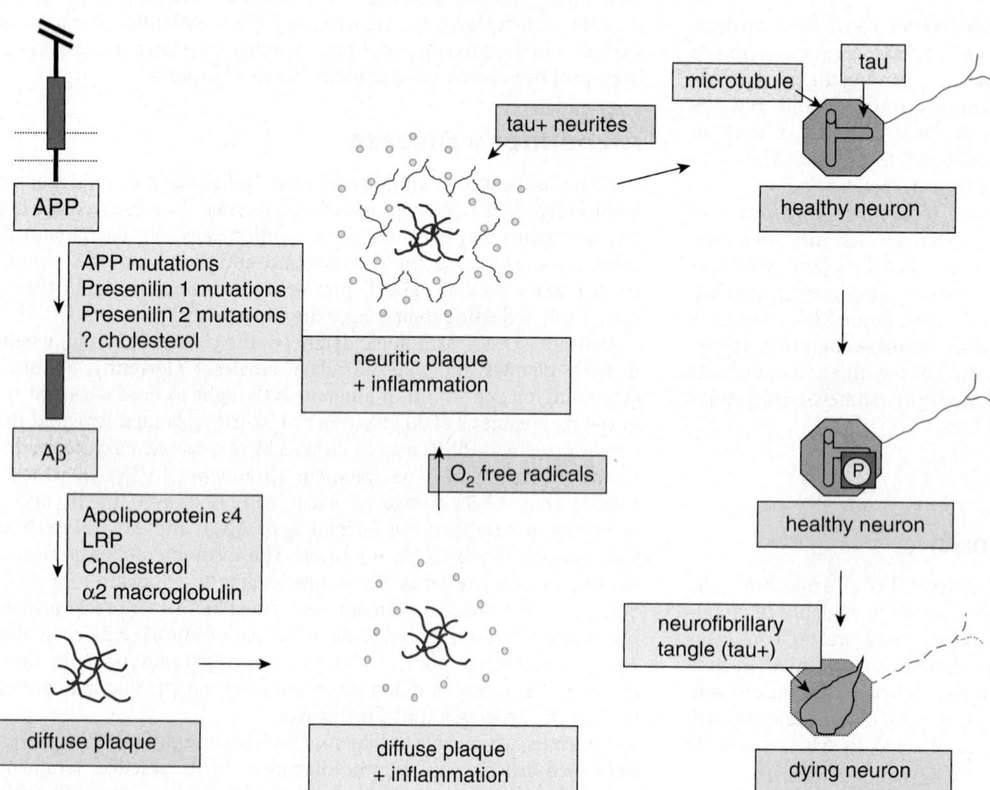

FIGURE 43-3 • Amyloid hypothesis and the pathogenesis of Alzheimer's disease.

the cognitive complaints, change compared to baseline, functional status, and effects of cognitive symptoms on the patient's ability to carry out his or her usual daily activities. The clinician should also assess the patient's cognition using a standardized instrument such as the Mini-Mental State Examination (MMSE) or the Kokmen Short Test of Mental Status.[15,16] Neuropsychological testing may have several important contributions to the diagnosis and long-term follow-up of patients with dementia. It helps assess the cognitive function of the patient as compared to other individuals of similar age, gender, and education. In addition, the testing profile might help differentiate the dementias based on the domain involvement. Another important use of neuropsychological testing is to establish a baseline assessment. This is particularly useful when the symptoms are subtle or unclear and a follow-up is planned.

BOX 43-1 ADAPTED DSM-IV CRITERIA FOR THE DIAGNOSIS OF DEMENTIA

1. Impairment in more than one cognitive domain, usually memory (learning or recall) plus an additional cognitive domain.
2. Cognitive deficits of sufficient severity to affect social or occupational functioning, and this represents a change from previous level.
3. Clinical course is gradual onset and progressive decline.
4. Not due to delirium.
5. No other central nervous system explanation (e.g., cerebrovascular disease, Parkinson's disease).

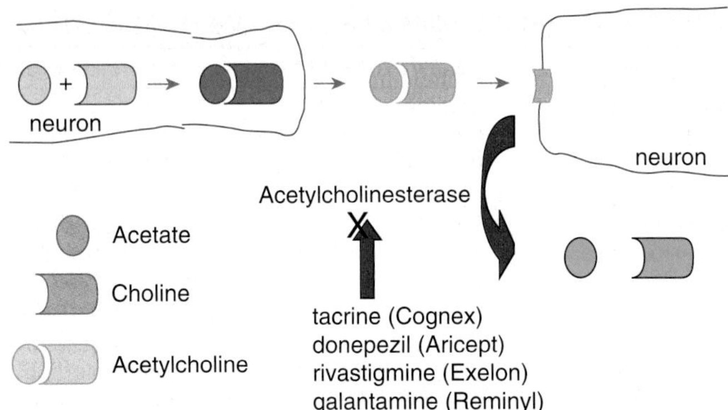

FIGURE 43-4 • **Mechanism of action of cholinesterase inhibitors in the synaptic cleft.**

Neurologic examination may play a supporting role in confirming the diagnosis of AD since it is usually normal early on in the disease and might help determine the etiology of the patient's symptoms. For example, parkinsonism may suggest dementia with Lewy bodies (DLB) and lateralizing signs may suggest a cerebrovascular accident. A general medical examination may help rule out systemic etiologies. The most useful laboratory tests to diagnose AD, according to the AAN practice parameter paper, are thyroid function tests and serum vitamin B_{12} levels.[13] While it is common to obtain more laboratory testing, it is important to note that there is no evidence to support routine screening. Scanning and imaging technologies also play a role in the diagnosis of AD. A computed tomography scan or magnetic resonance imaging of the head will help rule out potential causes for the cognitive symptoms and help assess the presence and degree of neuron degeneration. Other modalities have limited clinical usefulness.

Several genetic mutations have been associated with AD. Mutations have been identified on chromosome 1, 14, and 21.[17] However, genetic testing is reserved for individuals with very early onset and where a strong family history is present. Appropriate genetic counseling prior to testing is essential. With regard to late-onset AD, a growing body of literature suggests an increased risk in individuals with a specific apolipoprotein E (apo E) polymorphism.[18,19] Testing for apo E4 may help augment the clinician's diagnostic acumen.[20] However, routine testing for symptomatic individuals is not recommended.

A final area of great interest in AD diagnosis is biomarkers in the blood and cerebrospinal fluid. Patients with AD were found to have reduced spinal fluid levels of $A\beta_{1\text{-}42}$ and elevated levels of tau relative to controls.[21] However, the use of these biomarkers in a clinical setting has not been investigated, and it is unclear what role if any they may have in the diagnostic strategy.[22] In its practice parameters paper, the AAN does not recommend the use of biomarkers, functional imaging, or genetic testing based on the current evidence.[13]

Other Dementias

DLB is thought to be the second most common form of dementia, with an estimated prevalence of 15% to 25%. The main difference from AD is in the relative sparing of memory with involvement of other cognitive domains, particularly attention/concentration and visuospatial abilities.[23,24] DLB has strong association with parkinsonism and rapid-eye-movement (REM) sleep behavior disorder.[25] Fluctuation in cognitive status and visual hallucinations are common, and neuroleptic sensitivity is an important feature that may have treatment implications.[26]

In vascular dementia, cognitive deficits are thought to be secondary to vascular injury. However, the contribution of white matter ischemic disease to the cognitive deficits is unclear. Evaluation of vascular dementia is similar to that of AD. Neuroimaging modalities have a particular importance given the nature of brain injury.

Frontotemporal lobar degeneration encompasses a wide variety of clinical syndromes characterized by behavioral and/or language dysfunction. Diverse findings are also present on pathology. Clinical diagnosis often relies on history, with confirmation made only at autopsy. There are no disease-modifying treatments as of now; there is a lot of interest and research at the moment, and there are several plausible targets for therapy. For the management of symptoms, the clinician may follow recommendations for other dementias.

THERAPEUTICS AND CLINICAL PHARMACOLOGY

Therapeutics by Class

Management of the patient with dementia may require several different classes of pharmacologic agents. Treatment should address not only the dementia but also the associated syndromes. Among the former, treatment is mostly symptomatic, though a few disease-modifying agents have been explored.

Symptomatic

Currently five drugs have been approved by the U.S. Food and Drug Administration (FDA) for the treatment of clinically probable AD. Cholinesterase inhibitors (ChEIs) have been the mainstay of AD therapy for the past 10 years. In 2004, an *N*-methyl-D-aspartate (NMDA) receptor antagonist was introduced to clinical practice. Table 43-1 summarizes the main characteristics of the FDA-approved drugs.

Cholinesterase Inhibitors. Several studies evaluating the pathophysiology of AD have suggested that patients with AD have a cholinergic deficit.[27] Autopsy-based neurochemical studies in the late 1970s demonstrated deficits in the enzymes responsible for synthesis of acetylcholine in patients with AD. Subsequent work demonstrated marked cell loss of the cholinergic projection neurons lateral and anterior to the hypothalamus in AD.[28-32]

Cholinesterase is an enzyme that is present in the synaptic cleft. It functions mainly as a catalyst for the hydrolysis of the acetylcholine into choline and acetate, effectively allowing the cholinergic neuron to return to its resting state. ChEIs bind to the active site of the enzyme, enhancing and prolonging the stimulation of the postsynaptic neuron (Fig. 43-4). There are several inhibitors that have a wide variety of uses. In the setting of AD, there are currently four active agents. All four bind to the enzyme in a reversible fashion.

The most common side effects for this class are gastrointestinal (GI) in nature, and they are usually mild and self-limited. Rarely, they can have an effect on cardiac rate and rhythm. Though uncommon, the patient with underlying conduction abnormalities may be at risk. Routine electrocardiography prior to initiating therapy is not recommended but may be considered in high-risk patients such as those over 70 years of age or those with known heart disease. ChEIs can also affect respiratory function and should be used judiciously in patients known to have asthma or severe chronic obstructive pulmonary disease. Their use may interfere with administration of general anesthesia. Some patients may experience vivid dreams while on these drugs, particularly when taken at night.

TABLE 43-1 DRUGS APPROVED FOR MANAGEMENT OF ALZHEIMER'S DISEASE

Drug Name	Mechanism of Action	Pharmacologic Properties	Side Effects	Typical Dosing
Tacrine (Cognex)	Reversible acetylcholinesterase inhibitor	Oral bioavailability: 36% Protein binding: 55% Half-life: 2-4 hr Hepatic metabolism	Elevated transaminases, nausea, vomiting, diarrhea, dyspepsia, myalgia, anorexia, ataxia	Available in 10-, 20-, 30-, and 40-mg tablets. Dosing 4 times daily.
Donepezil (Aricept)	Reversible acetylcholinesterase inhibitor	Oral bioavailability: 100% Protein binding: 96% Half-life: 70 hr Hepatic metabolism	Nausea, diarrhea, insomnia, vomiting, muscle cramp, fatigue, anorexia	Available in 5- and 10-mg tablets. Dosing once daily.
Rivastigmine (Exelon)	Inhibits both butyrylcholinesterase and acetylcholinesterase	Oral bioavailability: 36% Protein binding: 40% Half-life: 1.5 hr Hepatic metabolism	Nausea, vomiting, weight loss, loss of appetite, dizziness	Available in 3- and 6-mg tablets. Dosing 2 times daily.
Galantamine (Reminyl, Razadyne)	Reversible acetylcholinesterase inhibitor	Oral bioavailability: 90% Protein binding: 18% Half-life: 7 hr Hepatic metabolism–partial	Nausea, vomiting, diarrhea, anorexia, weight loss	Available in 4-, 8-, and 12-mg tablets. Dosing 2 times daily.
Memantine (Namenda, Ebixa)	*N*-methyl-D-aspartate receptor antagonist	Oral bioavailability: 100% Protein binding: 45% Half-life: 60-80 hr Hepatic metabolism–partial	Fatigue, hypertension, dizziness, headache, constipation, vomiting, back pain, confusion, somnolence, hallucination, cough, dyspnea	Available in 10- and 20-mg tablets. Dosing 2 times daily.

Tacrine (Cognex). Tacrine, also known as tetrahydroaminoacridine, was the first ChEI to be commercially available for the treatment of probable AD. It was approved by the FDA in 1993. Its use was limited by the toxicity profile and its dosing regimen. The agent had to be administered four times daily, and it was associated with liver toxicity, which necessitated monitoring of liver functions regularly. It was rarely used in clinical practice.

Donepezil (Aricept). Donepezil was first approved in 1996 for mild to moderate AD, and in December 2006 for severe AD. It has 100% bioavailability with a half-life of 70 hours, thus allowing for a once-daily regimen. It requires no laboratory monitoring. The starting dose is 5 mg/day, and if that is tolerated well, in 4 to 6 weeks the dose is increased to 10 mg/day. The most common side effects are an increase in bowel frequency, nausea, and vomiting, which appear to be dose related.

Studies have showed modest improvement in cognitive function as measured by scales such as the Alzheimer's Disease Assessment Scale–Cognitive Subscale (ADAS-Cog) and the Clinician's Interview-Based Impression of Change. Effects have been studied up to 52 weeks. Rapid deterioration back to baseline can occur when stopping the medication.[33] Two recent clinical trials in nursing home patients from Sweden and Japan evaluated initiation of donepezil in severe AD patients.[34,35] Primary outcomes were improvements on neuropsychological testing. They both showed a statistically significant improvement in some tests at 6 months.

Donepezil has been studied in patients with MCI in a large, multicenter, randomized controlled trial (RCT). The trial showed a reduced risk of developing the clinical diagnosis of AD for 12 months. The differences were statistically significant, but the two groups were similar at 36 months. Subgroup analysis suggested that patients who were apo E4 positive may have a more persistent benefit such that this subgroup had a reduced risk of developing AD for 24 months.[36] However, routine genetic testing for apo E4 status is not recommended. No therapy is currently FDA approved for the treatment of MCI.

Rivastigmine (Exelon). Rivastigmine was approved in 1997 for mild to moderate AD.[37] In 2006, it became the only agent approved for mild to moderate Parkinson's disease–associated dementia.[38] It has 96% bioavailability and a half-life of 1.5 hours. It requires twice-daily dosing and is usually started at 1.5 mg twice a day and increased in increments of 1.5 mg per dose to a maximum of 6 mg twice daily.

Some of the unique features of rivastigmine include a slow dissociation from acetylcholinesterase, and inhibition of butyrylcholinesterase. The significance of the latter remains unknown. Rivastigmine has a greater cholinesterase inhibition at the highest dose but may also be prone to an increased frequency of side effects. The side effects profile is similar to that of donepezil, with a higher incidence of GI symptoms.

The therapeutic effect size of rivastigmine on neuropsychological testing is approximately the same as that of donepezil.[37,39] Recently, the FDA approved a patch form for the administration of the drug.

Galantamine (Reminyl, Razadyne). Galantamine is an alkaloid that acts as a reversible inhibitor of cholinesterase. It has also been shown to have some nicotinic receptor activity, which may give it an additional benefit over the other cholinesterase inhibitors. It has 80% to 100% bioavailability and a half-life of 7 hours. The initial dose is 4 mg twice daily, which is then increased to 8 mg twice daily and ultimately to 12 mg twice daily if tolerated. The side effects profile is similar to those of the other cholinesterase inhibitors with potential GI, cardiac, and pulmonary concerns. In clinical trials, the therapeutic effect size of galantamine was similar to donepezil and rivastigmine.[40] In a recent study, galantamine had an effect on activities of daily living and behavior. One of the latest studies with galantamine looked at potential use in MCI. However, there was an increased risk of sudden cardiac death in the treatment group. The FDA has cautioned against the use of galantamine in this setting.[41]

ChEIs and DLB. Neuronal loss in DLB appears to be less severe than in other dementias; however, the cholinergic depletion in the basal forebrain may be more profound.[42,43] Many case studies and open-label studies have looked at potential treatment with ChEIs with modest results.[44-47] Autopsy reports of patients with AD treated with ChEIs suggested that those who responded well were more likely to have DLB pathology.[48,49] Two RCTs with rivastigmine have been performed[50,51]; the largest had 120 patients. The treatment group had significant improvement in psychiatric symptoms (apathy, hallucinations) and had better performance on neuropsychological testing.[50] The side effect profile of ChEIs in patients with DLB is similar to that in patients with AD.

N-Methyl-D-Aspartate (NMDA) Receptor Antagonist. Research over the past 10 years has suggested an important role for the glutaminergic system in the symptomatology of AD.[52] It has been shown that abnormal stimulation of the glutaminergic system may lead to neuronal excitotoxicity and may contribute to neurodegeneration in the setting of dementia. A potential target for therapy consideration was the NMDA receptor[52] (Fig. 43-5).

Memantine (Namenda, Ebixa) is the only drug in this class that is currently approved by the FDA (in 2004) for the treatment of moderate to severe AD. It is thought to have a low to moderate affinity for the NMDA receptor and to act as an noncompetitive antagonist, reducing calcium influx to the cytoplasm.[52] It has been shown to have no activity on cholinesterase inhibition and thus can be used as a stand-alone therapy or in combination with ChEIs.[53] Memantine also acts as an noncompetitive antagonist at the 5-hydroxytryptamine$_3$ receptor, the significance of which in AD remains unknown.[54] It has 100% bioavailability with an extended half-life (60 to 80 hours). Common side effects include fatigue, dizziness, headache, nausea, and vomiting. There has been a slight increase in blood pressure with its use. Common psychiatric manifestations include agitation and visual hallucinations. Its therapeutic effect size has not been consistent, with a wide variability in reported results. When used as a stand-alone therapy, it has been shown to reduce nursing care, delay nursing home admission, and increase quality of life in moderate to severe AD.

There have been two main trials with memantine, one in Europe and another in the United States[55,56]; both included patients with moderate to severe AD and vascular dementia. They were both placebo controlled and showed improvement in the clinician-based Clinical Global Impression of Change and functional improvement on the Behavioral Rating Scale for Geriatric Patients.[55,56] Another randomized trial in patients with moderate to severe AD on a stable dose of donepezil showed improvement in memory, language, and praxis in post-hoc analysis.[57,58] There was also functional improvement; item analysis showed better function in grooming, toileting, conversing, watching television, and being left alone.[57,58] Memantine was also studied in mild to moderate AD in a placebo-controlled RCT for 24 weeks. The data showed a significant difference between the two groups at 24 months on neuropsychological testing and activities of daily living.[59] A small RCT in China comparing memantine to donepezil in mild to moderate possible or probable AD showed no significant difference between the two groups, with both showing significant improvement compared to baseline.[60]

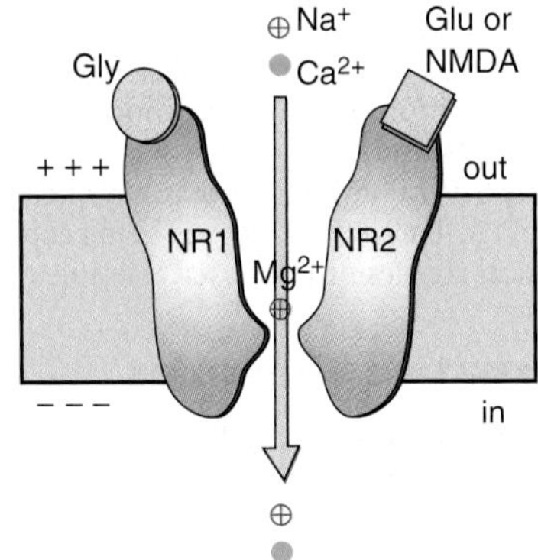

FIGURE 43-5 • Structure of N-methyl-D-aspartate receptor.

Disease-Modifying Agents

Vitamin E

Data from large epidemiologic studies have suggested a lower prevalence of AD in patients receiving antioxidants, including vitamins C and E.[61] Other studies suggested enhanced memory performance in the old and very old.[62] This has led to a large RCT with vitamin E and selegiline on clinical disease progression in moderate AD patients.[63] The study was interpreted positively for vitamin E; however, vitamin E therapy is not FDA approved for this indication. Selegiline results were considered to be less robust with higher side effects, and selegiline has not been recommended or used clinically. The AAN practice parameter paper considered treatment with vitamin E 1000 IU twice a day to slow progression of disease to be an acceptable attempt.[64] However, a recent meta-analysis, released after the AAN practice parameter paper, evaluating patients taking vitamin E (not only those with dementia) suggested an increased risk of mortality when the daily dose exceeds 200 IU.[65] Consequently, high-dose vitamin E (400 IU or greater) is generally not recommended.

Emerging Targets and Therapeutics

Table 43-2 presents a summary of selected therapies currently in Phase II or III clinical trials. Table 43-3 summarizes some of the main studies that were halted.

Anti-inflammatory Drugs

Steroids/Nonsteroidal Anti-inflammatory Drugs. Data from observational studies have suggested a protective effect of nonsteroidal anti-inflammatory drugs (NSAIDs) on prevalence of AD. Epidemiologic studies showed lower prevalence of AD in patients using NSAIDs regularly.[66,67] Patients with rheumatoid arthritis were found to die from AD 5 times less often than the general population.[68] Some clinical

TABLE 43-2 SELECTED DRUG THERAPIES FOR ALZHEIMER'S DISEASE UNDER INVESTIGATION

Drug Name	Company	Status	Mechanism of Action
AAC-001	Wyeth and Elan	Phase II	Active immunization
Alzhemed (tramiprosate)	Neurochem	Phase III	Prevents fibrillation and accumulation of Aβ
Bapineuzumab	Wyeth and Elan	Phase II	Monoclonal antibody to Aβ
LY2062430	Eli Lilly	Phase II	May influence β-amyloid production
LY450139	Eli Lilly	Phase II	γ-Secretase inhibitor
Flurizan (MPC-7869)	Myriad	Phase III	Modulates the action of γ-secretase and reduces selectively $A\beta_{42}$
PBT-2	Prana Biotechnology	Phase II	Decreases levels of Aβ protein
TTP488	TransTech Pharma	Phase II	Reduces amyloid burden

TABLE 43-3 SELECTED INVESTIGATIONAL THERAPIES THAT HAVE BEEN HALTED

Drug Name	Company	Results	Mechanism of Action
AN1792	Elan/Wyeth	Halted Phase II	$A\beta_{1-42}$ vaccination; halted secondary to meningoencephalitis.
Clioquionol	Prana Biotech	Halted Phase II	
Phenserine	Axonyx	Halted Phase III	Cholinesterase inhibitor; lowers $A\beta_{42}$ peptide. Study failed to show any significant difference in primary outcomes.

studies with anti-inflammatory drugs had limitations; others showed no effect.[69,70] Traditional NSAID trials had high dropout rates. A small diclofenac trial had more than a 50% dropout rate in the treatment group.[71] A trial with low-dose prednisone for 1 year showed no difference on the ADAS-Cog, and the treatment group showed worsening of behavioral symptoms.[72] One of the larger trials, the ADAPT trial, started in 2001, aimed at evaluating potential effects of naproxen and celecoxib on primary prevention of AD. However, the study had to be halted over concern of increased cardiovascular events. Cyclooxygenase-2 inhibitors are better tolerated, but studies thus far have been negative for dementia or MCI. In addition, in view of the increased cardiac mortality that has been suggested recently, it is unlikely that any further trials will be attempted in the near future.

Statins. Epidemiologic studies in 2000 suggested a protective effect, with reduced prevalence of probable AD, among the cohort using hydroxymethylglutaryl-coenzyme A reductase inhibitors. Animal and in vitro studies showed that cholesterol and statins modulate APP processing.[73] In vitro studies with simvastatin showed that treatment reduced levels of $A\beta_{42}$ and $A\beta_{40}$ in hippocampal cell structures. Treatment of guinea pigs resulted in reduced Aβ levels in cerebrospinal fluid (CSF).[73] Several studies suggested that plasma levels of amyloid protein were not different between those individuals taking statins and those who were not.[74] However, these findings remain controversial as other investigators have shown a reduction in the serum levels among statins users. An RCT with simvastatin for 26 weeks in patients with AD showed no significant reduction in CSF amyloid in the treatment group.[75]

Currently, investigators believe that reduction in brain inflammation may play a more important role in the prevention of AD, rather than a direct effect on amyloidogenic proteins. At the time of writing this chapter, two large primary prevention trials were underway: a Phase III clinical trial with simvastatin and a Phase II clinical trial with atorvastatin.

Estrogen Replacement Therapy

Similar to anti-inflammatory drugs, the earliest indication of potential beneficial effects of estrogens came from large epidemiologic studies. They have suggested a potential protective effect for estrogen on cognition and reduced risk of dementia.[76-78] However, two RCTs have produced negative results. The larger of the two involved 120 patients with mild to moderate AD who were treated with placebo or estrogen over a period of 1 year. There was no effect on ADAS-Cog or global change measures.[79,80] Certain researchers suggested a role for estrogen as a prophylactic therapy, yet recent data from the Women's Health Initiative suggested that long-term use of estrogen replacement therapy may increase risk of breast cancer and stroke.[81] Estrogen and progestin therapy increased the risk of dementia. In the same study, women were not protected by the treatment from developing MCI.[82] Current recommendations for therapy do not include any role for estrogen replacement.

Investigational Drugs

Amyloid Treatments. Amyloid-based therapy remains the most promising disease-modifying strategy for the treatment of AD. There has been a surge in interest and research work in the field, and most major pharmaceutical companies have at least one drug in clinical trials. Table 43-2 summarizes selected ongoing Phase II/III trials for some of those.

Immunotherapy. Several research teams have been working on active and passive immunotherapy strategies. The largest active immunization trial was a multicenter RCT of $A\beta_{1\text{-}42}$ immunization (AN1792) in patients with mild to moderate AD. The study was stopped early when some of the immunized patients developed encephalitis (6%). Data analysis showed that 19.7% achieved the predetermined antibody response. There were no differences on ADAS-Cog, Disability Assessment for Dementia, Clinical Dementia Rating, MMSE, or Clinical Global Impression of Change scores. Further analysis of z scores on the Neuropsychological Test Battery showed differences in favor of the immunized group.[83,84] Postmortem analysis of brain tissue from a few patients suggested resolution of amyloid plaque with focal absence of amyloid deposit. However, vascular amyloid was preserved or even slightly increased.[85] Other active immunization agents are currently in Phase II trials.

Passive vaccination trials using monoclonal or polyclonal antibodies are being pursued. Bapineuzumab (AAB-001) is a monoclonal antibody that binds circulating Aβ and increases its clearance. Other planned studies include using polyclonal intravenous immune globulins.

Aβ-Acting Agents. Several agents in this group are currently being investigated; results from two of the most promising agents should be available during 2007-2008.

Tramiprozate (Alzhemed) is a small molecule that easily crosses the blood-brain barrier. It is thought to prevent fibrillation and reduce amyloid accumulation by interfering in the interaction of Aβ with glycosaminoglycans. It may also play a role in binding circulating Aβ. Recent data have suggested protection of nerve cells from neurotoxicity of $A\beta_{42}$. The drug is currently in Phase III clinical trial. A Phase II trial consisted of 58 patients randomly assigned to receive placebo or the active drug for 3 months. It was followed by an open-label extension for 17 months. At 3 months, mild AD patients had 33% decrease of CSF $A\beta_{42}$ concentrations and moderate AD patients had a 14% decrease in $A\beta_{42}$ concentrations. However, there were no significant differences in cognitive measures at 3 months.[86]

Flurizan (MPC-7869), a selective amyloid-lowering agent, has been shown to reduce levels of $A\beta_{42}$ in cultured human cells and in animal models. Primary action is through modulation of γ-secretase. A Phase II clinical trial has been completed. Patients who took 800 mg of the active drug daily had a statistically significantly lower rate of deterioration in activities of daily living and global function; they also had slower decline in cognition, but this did not reach significance.[87] A Phase III clinical trial is underway.

Tau Treatments. Several animal models have been established and some experimental tau-based therapies are being explored. There have been no large clinical studies of tau-based therapies.

Herbal/Alternative Therapies

There has been a large amount of public interest and research involving herbal medicines for memory. The description of all reported herbal therapies is beyond the scope of this chapter. We will cover some of the better studied remedies. A recent systematic review identified two herbs and two herbal formulations that were associated with cognitive improvement in AD: *Salvia officinalis* (Yi-Gan San) and *Melissa* (Ba Wei Di Huang Wan).[88] In a separate meta-analysis, *Gingko biloba* had shown mild effectiveness in cognition in patient with mild symptoms.[89] A 24-week RCT comparing gingko extract EGb 761, donepezil, and placebo showed no difference between both treatment groups.[90] However, the study was of relatively short duration and the donepezil dose used was only 5 mg. The Ginkgo Evaluation of Memory study is underway to further qualify potential therapeutic benefit of gingko treatment. Huperazine A, an extract of the Chinese herb *Huperzia serrata* that acts as a ChEI, is currently in clinical trials.

Treatment of Noncognitive Symptoms

Noncognitive symptoms are often as difficult for the patient and family as the cognitive symptoms. The frequency varies significantly between individuals and type of dementia. Box 43-2 summarizes the most frequent behavioral and psychiatric manifestations associated with AD.[91]

Motor Symptoms (see Chapter 44, Parkinson's Disease)

Parkinsonism may be particularly prevalent in DLB but may also occur in AD and frontotemporal lobal degeneration. Treatment with levodopa may be considered. Dopamine agonists, and to a lesser extent levodopa, can have significant effects on cognition, and their use should be closely monitored.

BOX 43-2 BEHAVIORAL AND PSYCHIATRIC SYMPTOMS IN ALZHEIMER'S DISEASE

Agitation: 50%-70%
Anxiety: 30%-50%
Depression: 25%-50%
Disinhibition: 20%-35%
Delusions: 15%-50%
Hallucinations: 10%-25%
Aggression: 25%
Sexual disinhibition: 5%-10%

TABLE 43-4 TREATMENT RECOMMENDATIONS FOR BEHAVIORAL MANIFESTATIONS OF ALZHEIMER'S DISEASE

Symptom	Medication	Usual Daily Dose (Range)
Delusions	Risperidone (Risperdal)	1 mg (0.05-2 mg)
	Olanzapine (Zyprexa)	5 mg (5-10 mg)
	Quetiapine (Seroquel)	400 mg (50-400 mg)
	Haloperidol (Haldol)	1 mg (0.5-3 mg)
Agitation/ aggression	Risperidone (Risperdal)	1 mg (0.05-2 mg)
	Olanzapine (Zyprexa)	5 mg (5-10 mg)
	Quetiapine (Seroquel)	400 mg (50-400 mg)
	Haloperidol (Haldol)	1 mg (0.5-3 mg)
	Trazodone (Desyrel)	100 mg (100-400 mg)
	Buspirone (Buspar)	15 mg (15-30 mg)
	Propranolol (Inderal)	120 mg (80-240 mg)
	Carbamazepine (Tegretol)	400 mg (200-1200 mg)
	Divalproex (Depakote)	500 mg (250-2000 mg)
	Lorazepam (Ativan)	1 mg (0.5-6 mg)

Behavioral Management/Psychosis

Agitation is common in the setting of all dementias, particularly with a more advanced stage of the disease.[92] The clinician should pay careful attention at the evaluation stage as agitation may reflect an acute medical illness. Assessment of the environment is essential; changes in nursing staff, family visits, and absence of familiar objects may all play a role in increasing psychosis. Delusions are common in certain dementias; most commonly they involve paranoia, and misidentification syndromes (Capgras and Fregoli delusions) are sometime seen. Hallucinations can also be seen; visual hallucinations may be more frequent in DLB. Typically, medication therapy (Table 43-4) involves the use of neuroleptics. Neuroleptics (often referred to as antipsychotics) target mainly the D_2 dopamine receptor in the brain. They are further classified into two groups: typical antipsychotics block the D_2 receptors in several dopamine pathways in the brain, thus increasing their side effects profile. Atypical antipsychotics, in contrast, are more selective for the mesolimbic pathway (which is thought to mediate their sedating effects). They have some activity against serotonin receptors.

The safety profile of atypical antipsychotics makes them a better alternative for the demented population. Several studies have showed reduced psychosis and improved behavioral control with olanzapine, risperidone, and quetiapine.[93-96] However, the cost of these newer agents is considerable compared to the traditional antipsychotics. A recent study suggested increased mortality with the use of atypical antipsychotics in some psychiatric conditions. Their use was associated with increased cardiovascular abnormalities and stroke. Subsequently, the FDA has issued a "black box" warning with regard to the use of this class of medications in elderly demented patients. These drugs remain useful in clinical practice but should be used with caution.

Apathy/Depression (see Chapter 53, Depression and Bipolar Disorders)

Apathy is the most common noncognitive symptom associated with AD. It may improve with treatment with ChEIs, stimulants (methylphenidate), dopamine agonists, or antidepressants. Depression is another common psychiatric comorbidity with dementia. Selective serotonin reuptake inhibitors have been used successfully. Tricyclic antidepressants should be avoided because of their anticholinergic properties. All antidepressants may worsen cognitive function.

Sleep Disorders (see Chapter 57, Insomnia (Narcolepsy)-Related Disorders)

Many sleep disorders may coexist with the diagnosis of dementia; treatment should be considered as it may help improve cognitive abilities and functional capacity. REM sleep behavior disorder is highly associated with DLB; in a small study involving seven patients, melatonin improved symptoms in five of them. A sleep medicine consultation is recommended, because confirmation of the diagnosis often requires a polysomnogram.

REFERENCES

1. Brookmeyer R, Gray S, Kawas C. Projections of Alzheimer's disease in the United States and the public health impact of delaying disease onset. Am J Public Health 1998;88:1337-1342.
2. Ivnik RJ, Smith GE, Lucas JA, et al. Testing normal older people three or four times at 1- to 2-year intervals: Defining normal variance. Neuropsychology 1999;13:121-127.
3. Sliwinski M, Lipton RB, Buschke H, Stewart W. The effects of preclinical dementia on estimates of normal cognitive functioning in aging. J Gerontol B Psychol Sci Soc Sci 1996;51:217-225.
4. Petersen RC (ed). Mild Cognitive Impairment: Aging to Alzheimer's Disease. New York: Oxford University Press, 2003.
5. Petersen RC. Aging, mild cognitive impairment, and Alzheimer's disease. Neurol Clin 2000;18:789-805.
6. Petersen RC, Stevens JC, Ganguli M, et al. Practice Parameter: Early detection of dementia: mild cognitive impairment (an evidence-based review). Report of the Quality Standards Subcommittee of the American Academy of Neurology. Neurology 2001;56:1133-1142.
7. Petersen RC. Mild cognitive impairment as a diagnostic entity. J Intern Med 2004;256:183-194.
8. Fleming K, Adams A, Petersen R. Dementia: diagnosis and evaluation. Mayo Clin Proc 1995;70:1093-1107.
9. Kukull WA, Ganguli M. Epidemiology of dementia: concepts and overview. Neurol Clin 2000;18:923-949.
10. Evans DA, Funkenstein HH, Albert MS, et al. Prevalence of Alzheimer's disease in a community population of older persons: higher than previously reported. JAMA 1989;262:2551-2556.
11. Kokmen E, Beard CM, Offord K, Kurland LT. Prevalence of medically diagnosed dementia in a defined United States population: Rochester, Minnesota, January 1, 1975. Neurology 1989;39:773-776.
12. The National Institute on Aging and Reagan Institute Working Group on Diagnostic Criteria for the Neuropathological Assessment of Alzheimer's Disease. Consensus recommendations for the postmortem diagnosis of Alzheimer's disease. Neurobiol Aging 1997;18(4 Suppl):S1-S2.
13. Knopman DS, DeKosky ST, Cummings JL, et al. Practice Parameter: Diagnosis of dementia (an evidence-based review). Report of the Quality Standards Subcommittee of the American Academy of Neurology. Neurology 2001;56:1143-1153.
14. American Psychiatric Association. Diagnostic and Statistical Manual of Mental Disorders, 4th ed. Washington, DC: American Psychiatric Association, 1994.
15. Folstein MF, Folstein SE, McHugh PR. "Mini-Mental State": a practical method for grading the cognitive state of patients for the clinician. J Psychiatr Res 1975;12:189-198.
16. Kokmen E, Smith GE, Petersen RC, et al. The Short Test of Mental Status: correlations with standardized psychometric testing. Arch Neurol 1991;48:725-728.
17. Hardy J, Gwinn-Hardy K. Genetic classification of primary neurodegenerative disease. Science 1998;282:1075-1079.
18. Roses AD. Apolipoprotein E and Alzheimer's disease. In Rosenberg RN, Prusiner SB, DiMauro S, Barchi RL (eds): The Molecular and Genetic Basis of Neurological Disease, Vol. 2. Boston: Butterworth-Heinemann, 1997, pp 000-000.
19. Farrer LA, Cupples LA, Haines JL, et al. Effects of age, sex, and ethnicity on the association between apolipoprotein E genotype and Alzheimer disease: a meta-analysis. APOE and Alzheimer Disease Meta Analysis Consortium. JAMA 1997;278:1349-1356.
20. Mayeux R, Saunders AM, Shea S, et al. Utility of the apolipoprotein E genotype in the diagnosis of Alzheimer's disease. Alzheimer's Disease Centers Consortium on Apolipoprotein E and Alzheimer's Disease. N Engl J Med 1998;338:506-511.
21. Galasko D, Chang L, Motter R, et al. High cerebrospinal fluid tau and low amyloid beta42 levels in the clinical diagnosis of Alzheimer disease and relation to apolipoprotein E genotype. Arch Neurol 1998;55:937-945.
22. Hulstaert F, Blennow K, Ivanoiu A, et al. Improved discrimination of AD patients using beta-amyloid(1-42) and tau levels in CSF. Neurology 1999;52:1555-1562.
23. Ferman TJ, Boeve BF, Smith GE, et al. REM sleep behavior disorder and dementia: cognitive differences when compared with AD. Neurology 1999;52:951-957.
24. Ferman TJ, Smith GE, Boeve BF, et al. Neuropsychological differentiation of dementia with Lewy bodies from normal aging and Alzheimer's disease. Clin Neuropsychol 2006;20:623-636.

25. Boeve B, Silber M, Ferman T. REM sleep behavior disorder in Parkinson's disease and dementia with Lewy bodies. J Geriatr Psychiatry Neurol 2004;17:146-157.
26. McKeith IG, Perry EK, Perry RH. Report of the Second Dementia with Lewy Body International Workshop: diagnosis and treatment. Consortium on Dementia with Lewy Bodies. Neurology 1999;53:902-905.
27. Whitehouse PJ, Price DL, Clark AW, et al. Alzheimer disease: evidence for selective loss of cholinergic neurons in the nucleus basalis. Ann Neurol 1981;10:122-126.
28. Bowen DM, Smith CB, White P, et al. Neurotransmitter-related enzymes and indices of hypoxia in senile dementia and other abiotrophies. Brain 1976;99:459-496.
29. Davies P, Maloney AJ. Selective loss of central cholinergic neurons in Alzheimer's disease. Lancet 1976;2:1403.
30. Perry EK, Tomlinson BE, Blessed G, et al. Correlation of cholinergic abnormalities with senile plaques and mental test scores in senile dementia. BMJ 1978;2:1457-1459.
31. Rasool CG. Neurofibrillary degeneration of cholinergic and noncholinergic neurons of the basal forebrain in Alzheimer's disease. Ann Neurol 1986;20:482-488.
32. Whitehouse PJ, Price DL, Struble RG, et al. Alzheimer's disease and senile dementia: loss of neurons in the basal forebrain. Science 1982;215:1237-1239.
33. AD 2000 Collaborative Group. Long-term donepezil treatment in 565 patients with Alzheimer's disease (AD2000): randomized double-blind trial. Lancet 2004;363:2105-2115.
34. Winblad B, Kilander L, Eriksson S, et al., for the Severe Alzheimer's Disease Study Group. Donepezil in patients with severe Alzheimer's disease: double-blind, parallel-group, placebo-controlled study. Lancet 2006;9516:1057-1065.
35. Data presented at the 10th International Conference on Alzheimer's Disease (ICAD) and Related Disorders in Madrid, Spain, July 15-20, 2006.
36. Petersen RC, Thomas RG, Grundman M, et al., for the Alzheimer's Disease Cooperative Study Group. Vitamin E and donepezil for the treatment of mild cognitive impairment. N Engl J Med 2005;352:2379-2388.
37. Rosler M, Anand R, Cicin-Sain A, et al. Efficacy and safety of rivastigmine in patients with Alzheimer's disease: international randomized controlled trial. BMJ 1999;318:633-638.
38. Emre M, Aarsland D, Albanese A, et al. Rivastigmine for dementia associated with Parkinson's disease. N Engl J Med 2004;351:2509-2518.
39. Rosler M, Retz W, Retz-Junginger P, Dennler HJ. Effects of two-year treatment with the cholinesterase inhibitor rivastigmine on behavioral symptoms in Alzheimer's disease. Behav Neurol 1998;11:211-216.
40. Tariot PN, Solomon PR, Morris JC, et al. A 5-month, randomized, placebo-controlled trial of galantamine in AD. Neurology 2000;54:2269-2276.
41. Center for Drug Evaluation and Research. Alert for healthcare professionals on galantamine hydrochloride (marketed as Razadyne, formerly Reminyl). U.S. Food and Drug Administration web site, updated August 9, 2006. Available at *http://www.fda.gov/cder/drug/InfoSheets/HCP/galantamineHCP.htm* (accessed February 28, 2007).
42. Dickson D. Dementia with Lewy bodies: neuropathology. J Geriatr Psychiatr Neurol 2002;15:210-216.
43. Dickson DW, Crystal H, Mattiace LA, et al. Diffuse Lewy body disease: light and electron microscopic immunocytochemistry of senile plaques. Acta Neuropathol 1989;78:572-584.
44. Querfurth HW, Allam GJ, Geffroy MA, et al. Acetylcholinesterase inhibition in dementia with Lewy bodies: results of a prospective pilot trial. Dement Geriatr Cogn Disord 2000;11:314-321.
45. Lanctot KL, Herrmann N. Donepezil for behavioural disorders associated with Lewy bodies: a case series. Int J Geriatr Psychiatry 2000;15:338-345.
46. Samuel W, Caligiuri M, Galasko D, et al. Better cognitive and psychopathologic response to donepezil in patients prospectively diagnosed as dementia with Lewy bodies: a preliminary study. Int J Geriatr Psychiatry 2000;15:794-802.
47. Edwards KR, Hershey L, Wray L, et al. Efficacy and safety of galantamine in patients with dementia with Lewy bodies: a 12-week interim analysis. Dement Geriatr Cogn Disord 2004;17(Suppl 1):40-48.
48. Levy R, Eagger S, Griffiths M, et al. Lewy bodies and response to tacrine in Alzheimer's disease. Lancet 1994;343:176.
49. Liberini P, Memo M, Spano PF. Lewy body pathology and heterogeneity in Alzheimer's disease. JAMA 1995;274:1199.
50. McKeith IG, Del Ser T, Spano PF, et al. Efficacy of rivastigmine on dementia with Lewy bodies: a randomized, double blind, placebo-controlled international study. Lancet 2000;356:2031-2036.
51. Grace J, Daniel S, Stevens T, et al. Long-term use of rivastigmine in patients with dementia with Lewy bodies: an open-label trial. Int Psychogeriatr 2001;13:199-205.
52. Cacabelos R, Takeda M, Winblad B. The glutamatergic system and neurodegeneration in dementia: preventive strategies in Alzheimer's disease. Int J Geriatr Psychiatry 1999;14:3-47.
53. Wenk GL, Quack G, Moebius HJ, Danysz W. No interaction of memantine with acetylcholinesterase inhibitors approved for clinical use. Life Sci 2000;66:1079-1083.
54. Rammes G, Rupprecht R, Ferrari U, et al. The N-methyl-D-aspartate receptor channel blockers memantine, MRZ 2/579 and other amino-alkyl-cyclohexanes antagonise 5-HT 3 receptor currents in cultured HEK-293 and N1E-115 cell systems in a non-competitive manner. Neurosci Lett 2001;306:81-84.
55. Winblad B, Poritis N. Memantine in severe dementia: results of the 9M-Best Study Benefit and efficacy in severely demented patients during treatment with memantine. Int J Geriatr Psychiatry 1999;14:135-146.
56. Reisberg B, Doody R, Stoffler A, et al., for the Memantine Study Group. Memantine in moderate-to-severe Alzheimer's disease. N Engl J Med 2003;348:1333-1341.
57. Feldman HH, Schmitt FA, Olin JT for the Memantine MEM-MD-02 Study Group. Cognitive response to memantine in moderate to severe Alzheimer disease patients already receiving donepezil: an exploratory reanalysis. Alzheimer Dis Assoc Disord 2006;20:255-262.
58. Feldman HH, Schmitt FA, Olin JT for the Memantine MEM-MD-02 Study Group. Activities of daily living in moderate-to-severe Alzheimer disease: an analysis of the treatment effects of memantine in patients receiving stable donepezil treatment. Alzheimer Dis Assoc Disord 2006;20:263-268.
59. Peskind ER, Potkin SG, Pomara N, et al. Memantine treatment in mild to moderate Alzheimer disease: a 24-week randomized, controlled trial. Am J Geriatr Psychiatry 2006;14:704-715.
60. Hu HT, Zhang ZX, Yao JL, et al. Clinical efficacy and safety of akatinol memantine in treatment of mild to moderate Alzheimer disease: a donepezil-controlled, randomized trial. Zhonghua Nei Ke Za Zhi 2006;45:277-280.
61. Morris MC, Beckett LA, Scherr PA, et al. Vitamin E and vitamin C supplements use and risk of incident Alzheimer disease. Alzheimer Dis Assoc Disord 1998;12:121-126.
62. Perrig WJ, Perrig P, Stahelin HB. The relation between antioxidants and memory performance in the old and very old. J Am Geriatr Soc 1997;45:718-724.
63. Sano M, Ernesto C, Thomas R, et al. A controlled trial of selegiline, alpha-tocopherol, or both as treatment for Alzheimer's disease: The Alzheimer's Disease Cooperative Study. N Engl J Med 1997;336:1216-1222.
64. Doody RS, Stevens JC, Beck C, et al. Practice Parameter: Management of dementia (an evidence-based review). Report of the Quality Standards Subcommittee of the American Academy of Neurology. Neurology 2001;56:1154-1166.
65. Miller ER 3rd, Pastor-Barriuso R, Dalal D, et al. Meta-analysis: high-dosage vitamin E supplementation may increase all-cause mortality. Ann Intern Med 2005;142:37-46.
66. Breitner JCS, Gau BA, Welsh KA, et al. Inverse association of anti-inflammatory treatments and Alzheimer's disease: initial results of a co-twin control study. Neurology 1994;44:227-232.
67. Andersen K, Launer LJ, Ott A, et al. Do nonsteroidal anti-inflammatory drugs decrease the risk for Alzheimer's disease? The Rotterdam Study. Neurology 1995;45:1441-1445.
68. Myllykangas-Luosujarvi R, Isomaki H. Alzheimer's disease and rheumatoid arthritis. Br J Rheumatol 1994;33:501-502.
69. McGeer PL, Rogers J. Anti-inflammatory agents as a therapeutic approach to Alzheimer's disease. Neurology 1992;42:447-449.
70. Rogers J, Kirby LC, Hempelman SR, et al. Clinical trial of indomethacin in Alzheimer's disease. Neurology 1993;43:1609-1611.
71. Scharf S, Mander A, Ugoni A, et al. A double-blind, placebo-controlled trial of diclofenac/misoprostol in Alzheimer's disease. Neurology 1999;53:197-201.
72. Aisen PS, Davis KL, Berg JD, et al. A randomized controlled trial of prednisone in Alzheimer's disease: Alzheimer's Disease Cooperative Study. Neurology 2000;54:588-593.
73. Fassbender K, Simons M, Bergmann C, et al. Simvastatin strongly reduces levels of Alzheimer's disease beta-amyloid peptides Abeta 42 and Abeta 40 in vitro and in vivo. Proc Natl Acad Sci U S A 2001;98:5856-5861.
74. Hoglund K, Syversen S, Lewczuk P, et al. Statin treatment and a disease-specific pattern of beta-amyloid peptides in Alzheimer's disease. Exp Brain Res 2005;164:205-214.
75. Simons M, Schwarzler F, Lutjohann D, et al. Treatment with simvastatin in normocholesterolemic patients with Alzheimer's disease: a 26-week randomized, placebo-controlled, double-blind trial. Ann Neurol 2002;52:346-350.
76. Henderson VW, Paganini-Hill A, Emanuel CK, et al. Estrogen replacement therapy in older women: comparisons between Alzheimer's disease cases and nondemented control subjects. Arch Neurol 1994;51:896-900.
77. Kawas C, Resnick S, Morrison A, et al. A prospective study of estrogen replacement therapy and the risk of developing Alzheimer's disease: the Baltimore Longitudinal Study of Aging. Neurology 1997;48:1517-1521.
78. Tang MX, Jacobs D, Stern Y, et al. Effect of estrogen during menopause on risk and age at onset of Alzheimer's disease. Lancet 1996;348:429-432.
79. Mulnard RA, Cotman CW, Kawas C, et al. Estrogen replacement therapy for treatment of mild to moderate Alzheimer disease: a randomized controlled trial. Alzheimer's Disease Cooperative Study. JAMA 2000;283:1007-1015.
80. Henderson VW, Paganini-Hill A, Miller BL, et al. Estrogen for Alzheimer's disease in women: randomized, double-blind, placebo-controlled trial. Neurology 2000;54:295-301.
81. Writing Group for the Women's Health Initiative Investigators. Risks and benefits of estrogen plus progestin in healthy postmenopausal women: principal results from the Women's Health Initiative randomized controlled trial. JAMA 2002;288:321-333.
82. Shumaker SA, Legault C, Rapp SR, et al. Estrogen plus progestin and the incidence of dementia and mild cognitive impairment in postmenopausal women. JAMA 2003;289:2651-2662.
83. Orgogozo JM, Gilman S, Dartigues JF, et al. Subacute meningoencephalitis in a subset of patients with AD after Abeta42 immunization. Neurology 2003;61:46-54.
84. Rovira MB, Forette F, Orgogozo JM for the AN1792 (QS-21)-201 Study Team. Clinical effects of Abeta immunization (AN1792) in patients with AD in an interrupted trial. Neurology 2005;64:1553-1562.
85. Ferrer I, Boada Rovira M, Sanchez Guerra ML, et al. Neuropathology and pathogenesis of encephalitis following amyloid-beta immunization in Alzheimer's disease. Brain Pathol 2004;14:11-20.
86. Aisen PS, Saumier D, Briand R, et al. A Phase II study targeting amyloid-beta with 3APS in mild-to-moderate Alzheimer disease. Neurology 2006;67:1757-1763.
87. Data presented at the 10th International Conference on Alzheimer's Disease (ICAD) and Related Disorders in Madrid, Spain, July 15-20, 2006.
88. Dos Santos-Neto LL, de Vilhena Toledo MA, Medeiros-Souza P, de Souza GA. The use of herbal medicine in Alzheimer's disease—a systematic review. Evid Based Complement Alternat Med 2006;3:441-445.
89. Kurz A, Van Baelen B. Ginkgo biloba compared with cholinesterase inhibitors in the treatment of dementia: a review based on meta-analyses by the Cochrane Collaboration. Dement Geriatr Cogn Disord 2004;18:217-226.

90. van Dongen MC, van Rossum E, Kessels AG, et al. The efficacy of ginkgo for elderly people with dementia and age-associated memory impairment: new results of a randomized clinical trial. J Am Geriatr Soc 2000;48:1183-1194.
91. Reisberg B, Borenstein J, Salob SP, et al. Behavioral symptoms in Alzheimer's disease: phenomenology and treatment. J Clin Psychiatry 1987;48(Suppl):9-15.
92. Deutsch LH, Bylsma FW, Rovner BW, et al. Psychosis and physical aggression in probable Alzheimer's disease. Am J Psychiatry 1991;148:1159-1163.
93. Sultzer DL, Gray KF, Gunay I, et al. A double-blind comparison of trazodone and haloperidol for treatment of agitation in patients with dementia. Am J Geriatr Psychiatry 1997;5:60-69.
94. Katz IR, Jeste DV, Mintzer JE, et al. Comparison of risperidone and placebo for psychosis and behavioral disturbances associated with dementia: a randomized, double-blind trial. Risperidone Study Group. J Clin Psychiatry 1999;60:107-115.
95. McManus DQ, Arvanitis LA, Kowalcyk BB. Quetiapine, a novel antipsychotic: experience in elderly patients with psychotic disorders. Seroquel Trial 48 Study Group. J Clin Psychiatry 1999;60:292-298.
96. Street J, Clark WS, Gannon KS, et al. Olanzapine treatment of psychotic and behavioral symptoms in patients with Alzheimer's disease in nursing care facilities. Arch Gen Psychiatry 2000;57:968-976.

44

PARKINSON'S DISEASE

Ludy Shih and Daniel Tarsy

OVERVIEW 651
INTRODUCTION 651
PATHOPHYSIOLOGY 651
THERAPEUTICS AND CLINICAL PHARMACOLOGY 653
Goals of Therapy 653
Therapeutics by Class 654
Symptomatic 654
Therapeutic Approach 660
Emerging Targets and Therapeutics 660
CONCLUSIONS 660

OVERVIEW

Pharmacologic treatment of Parkinson's disease (PD) has been enabled by critical observations on the pathophysiologic and biochemical properties of the disease. From early findings of dopamine deficiency to current investigations into the pharmacologic mechanisms responsible for both motor and nonmotor complications in the advanced stages, PD patients are enjoying a multitude of treatment options that enhance their quality of life and delay significant disability that would otherwise occur without the existing treatments.

In this chapter, we review the underpinnings of disease symptomatology, targets for pharmacologic intervention, the evidence for their clinical effectiveness, and practical considerations regarding their use. Also, we identify areas for future research and possible targets for new therapies to be developed.

INTRODUCTION

PD is a neurodegenerative disease characterized by rigidity, tremor, and slowness or paucity of movements (termed *bradykinesia*). After Alzheimer's disease, PD is the most common neurodegenerative disorder, affecting approximately 0.3% of the entire population of industrialized countries and 1% of all persons over the age of 60.[1] The annual cost of PD has been estimated at anywhere from $8000 to $10,000 for costs directly related to patient care and treatment and $25,000 per patient in indirect costs, including loss of productivity and uncompensated caregiving, suggesting an estimated loss of $25 to $35 billion annually within the United States alone.[2-4] Though the disease has a slowly progressive course compared to other neurodegenerative diseases such as amyotrophic lateral sclerosis and Huntington's disease, which progress more rapidly, it causes morbidity, decline in ability to carry out activities of daily living, and reduced life expectancy compared to age-matched controls.[5]

PD was recognized as a clinical entity in the early 19th century and was brought to attention by James Parkinson's "An Essay on the Shaking Palsy."[6] The first attempts at treating PD were reported in the 1860s with the use of anticholinergic drugs such as hyoscine; thereafter, synthetic anticholinergics became the mainstay of treatment.[7] However, beginning in the early 20th century, findings in the brains of PD patients described striking pallor and neuronal loss in the substantia nigra.[8-10] This observation, coupled with the discovery of profound deficiency of the monoamine neurotransmitter dopamine,[11] led to efforts to replete dopamine in PD patients. Levodopa was the first antiparkinsonian drug discovered for this disease based on this mechanism, and subsequently much of pharmacologic therapy has been focused upon enhancing dopamine action or replacing the low levels of dopamine within the nigrostriatal system. However, other sites in the brainstem, cortex, and autonomic ganglia are affected as well, resulting in noradrenergic, serotonergic, and cholinergic loss with corresponding nonmotor symptoms such as autonomic dysfunction, depression, and dementia; the predominance of the latter resulted in the recognition of a related disorder called dementia with Lewy bodies (DLB) (Fig. 44-1).[12] Therefore, various new strategies are emerging to treat nonmotor symptoms of PD in addition to identifying neuroprotective agents that slow down the progression of the disease.

PATHOPHYSIOLOGY

The motor symptoms and signs of PD arise from dysfunction in the basal ganglia, which include the subthalamic nucleus, caudate, putamen, globus pallidus, and substantia nigra pars compacta and pars reticulata. Collectively, this group of structures is thought to be responsible for the automatic execution of learned motor plans.[13] The striatum, consisting of the caudate and putamen, receives major input from two areas, the cortex and the substantia nigra. The effect of dopaminergic release from the axon terminals of substantia nigra pars compacta neurons chiefly depends upon two populations of medium spiny neurons in the striatum, those whose cell bodies and dendrites contain D_1-like dopamine receptors (including D_1 and D_5 receptors), mediated through increased adenylate cyclase activity and cyclic adenosine monophosphate (AMP), and those containing D_2-like receptors (including D_2, D_3, and D_4 receptors), mediated through decreased adenylate cyclase activity and cyclic AMP. The outflow from the striatum into the globus pallidus, subthalamus, and thalamus, and ultimately back to the cortex, has been divided into indirect and direct pathways. The direct pathway is facilitated by dopaminergic activation of striatal neurons, which contain D_1 receptors. From the striatum, γ-aminobutyric acidergic (GABAergic) neurons send inhibitory projections to the internal globus pallidus, which in turn projects GABA-mediated inhibitory projections to the ventral anterior and ventrolateral thalamic nuclei, which serve to stimulate the cortex through excitatory glutamatergic pathways. The internal globus pallidus is akin to a "brake" on the facilitation of movements. The overall effect of dopamine is thus a facilitation of movement via excitation of neurons that inhibit the internal globus pallidus, thereby allowing for facilitation of activity in the thalamocortical system.

The indirect pathway arises from D_2 receptor–containing striatal neurons whose activity is inhibited by dopamine. GABAergic neurons project from the striatum to the external globus pallidus, which in turns sends inhibitory GABAergic projections to the subthalamic nucleus. The subthalamic nucleus sends excitatory glutamatergic projections to the internal globus pallidus, which in turn sends inhibitory GABAergic projections to the thalamus. It has been suggested that, when dopaminergic projections from the substantia nigra to the striatum are reduced as in PD, the indirect pathway is disinhibited and the direct pathway is facilitated, both thereby leading to enhanced pallidal-thalamic inhibition followed by reduced thalamocortical facilitation. The net functional effect of this is inhibition of motor function.[14,15]

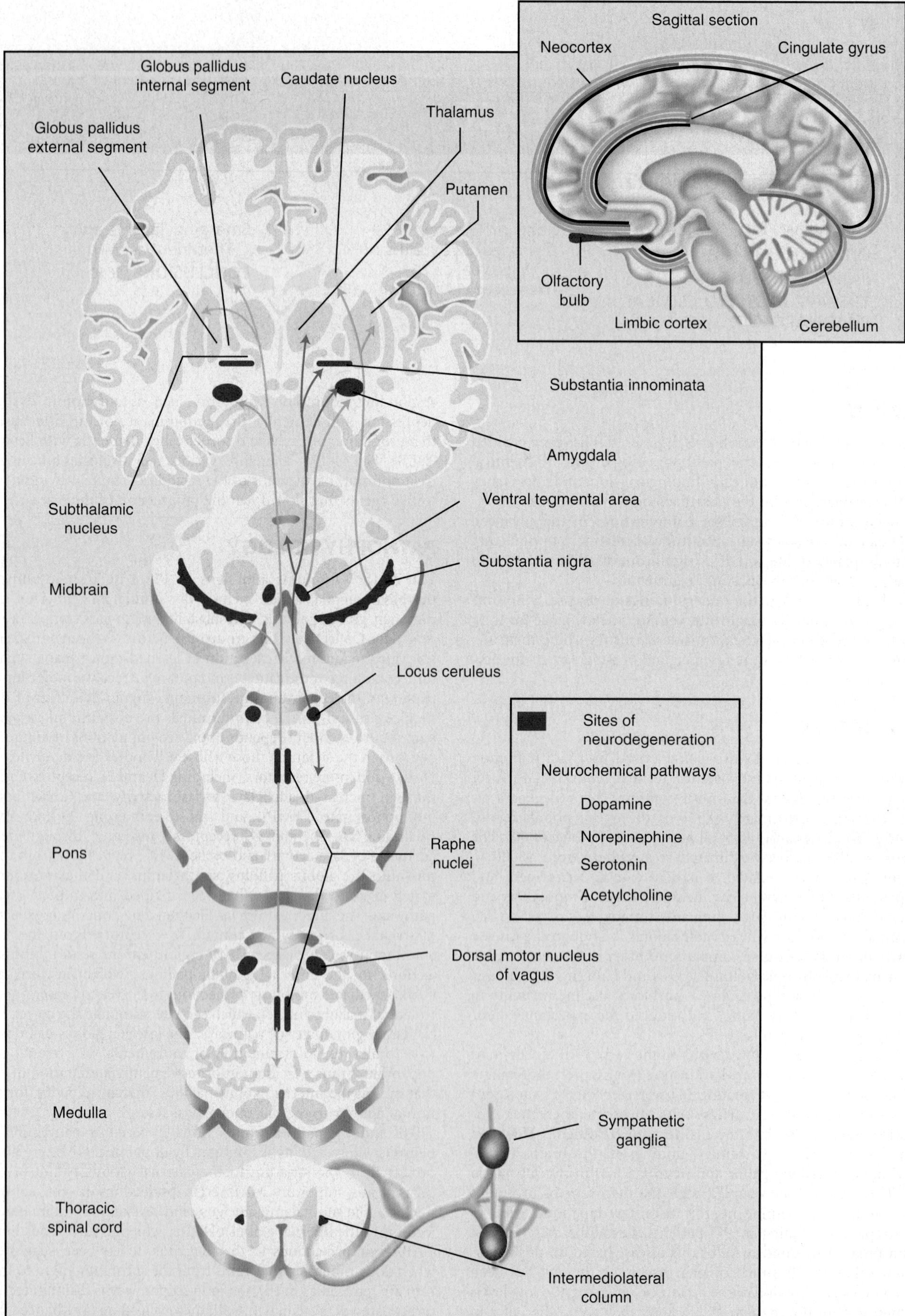

FIGURE 44-1 • Neurotransmitter pathways and sites involved in Parkinson's disease. (Adapted from Lang AE, Lozano AM. Medical progress: Parkinson's disease—first of two parts. N Engl J Med 1998;339:1044-1053. Copyright © 1990 Massachusetts Medical Society. All rights reserved.)

There is evidence, however, that this model of basal ganglia physiology is oversimplified and also fails to explain several important clinical observations. One of these is the relief of dyskinesias and dystonia by pallidal ablation or deep brain stimulation (DBS), which, according to the simple model described previously, should increase rather than decrease hyperkinetic disorders by removing pallidal inhibition of thalamocortical activity.[16] A more likely explanation for the benefit of pallidal ablation or DBS is elimination of the effect of abnormal patterns of pallidal neuronal firing on thalamocortical activity.[17]

The hallmark pathologic finding in PD is pallor and gliosis of the ventral tier of the substantia nigra, pars compacta. Eosinophilic intracytoplasmic inclusions called Lewy bodies are found in surviving neurons of this region and are characteristic of idiopathic PD, although not restricted to this region. Lewy bodies and neuronal degeneration are often found in other nuclei containing pigmented catecholaminergic neurons, such as the locus ceruleus, dorsal motor nucleus of the vagus, hypothalamus, Edinger-Westphal nucleus, dorsal raphe nuclei, olfactory bulb, autonomic ganglia, and nucleus basalis of Meynert, which contains predominantly cholinergic neurons.[18] Within Lewy bodies are protein aggregates, chief among which is an insoluble complex of α-synuclein and other proteins that have been implicated as being neurotoxic. Evidence for a possibly important role for α-synuclein in PD came from study of a large Greek-Italian family with autosomal dominant levodopa-responsive parkinsonism in whom mutations in the gene encoding for α-synuclein, *PARK1*, were found.[19] α-Synuclein is thought to play a role in synaptic vesicle formation and neurotransmitter release. When α-synuclein mutates, it accumulates, perhaps due to faulty degradation, thereby leading to protein aggregation and cell death. Further evidence for the role of protein degradation in this disease was found when mutations in a gene encoding for parkin, a ubiquitin E3 ligase that prepares substrates for protein degradation mediated through the ubiquitin proteasome system, were found in an autosomal recessive juvenile form of parkinsonism.[20,21] Parkin gene knockout animal models have implicated mitochondrial dysfunction, perhaps mediated through its protective effects against mitochondrial-mediated apoptosis.[22] Investigation is currently in progress to determine whether animals exposed to proteasomal inhibitors can accurately model human PD.[23]

Other theories advanced regarding contributing factors to nigrostriatal neuronal death include environmental neurotoxins, mitochondrial dysfunction, and oxidative stress. The discovery of subacute and acute parkinsonism in human adults induced by the ingestion of 1-methyl-4-phenyl-1,2,3,6-tetrahydropyridine (MPTP), a byproduct of synthesized meperidine, led to observations that MPTP may cause parkinsonism by inducing mitochondrial dysfunction.[24] MPTP is oxidized by monoamine oxidase B to 1-methyl-4-phenypyridinium (MPP+), and MPP+ inhibits mitochondrial complex I activity as well as mitochondrial respiration. In addition, MPP+ may also induce apoptosis.[25] There is also concern that dopamine itself may lead to increased oxidative stress and increased formation of free radicals and quinones, which can lead to DNA damage.[26] A recent clinical trial comparing the use of levodopa early versus late in PD did not appear to show a more rapid progression of disease in early users.[27]

Regardless of the etiology of nigrostriatal neuronal loss, the observation that dopamine deficiency is present in the central nervous systems of PD patients has been the most critical discovery for management of disease symptoms. Early observations by Carlsson and colleagues in 1957 revealed that levodopa administration could reverse the akinesia of catecholamine-depleted animals and led to the hypothesis that dopamine deficiency was the basis for akinesia in PD.[28] Subsequent demonstrations of striatal dopamine deficiency in brains of PD patients as well as in urine by Hornykiewicz and Barbeau led to clinical trials of levodopa in PD patients.[11,29-31] Since the 1960s, levodopa repletion or enhancement of dopamine action has been the mainstay of pharmacologic therapy for PD.[25] As a result of well-elaborated observa-tions on the physiology and pharmacology of dopamine, drug therapy has been targeted at several different steps in its production and metabolism.

Accordingly, drugs that block dopamine receptors or deplete dopamine are well known to cause parkinsonism. Examples of presynaptic dopamine depleters include reserpine or tetrabenazine, which is used in Canada and Europe to treat choreiform movements. A major class of dopamine receptor blockers are the antipsychotic drugs, also known as neuroleptics, used for treatment of schizophrenia and other acute psychoses. Some atypical antipsychotics, such as quetiapine and clozaril, are postulated to have less D_2-blocking activity compared to the typical antipsychotics and are thought to carry a lower risk of drug-induced parkinsonism.[32] Certain antiemetics, such as prochlorperazine and metoclopramide, also contain D_2 receptor–blocking activity and are known to cause parkinsonism as well as chorea and dystonia.

Dopamine is synthesized in the brain from tyrosine via a two-step process. The first step is rate limiting and requires the enzyme tyrosine hydroxylase, which converts tyrosine to the intermediate product L-3,4-dihydroxyphenylalanine, also known as L-dopa or levodopa. L-Dopa is converted by amino acid decarboxylase (AADC) to dopamine. It is worth noting that L-AAAD is found in the gastric mucosa as well as the central nervous system, leading to peripheral synthesis of dopamine when levodopa is administered orally. Dopamine is normally then taken up and stored into synaptic vesicles via the vesicular monoamine transporter, which is the site of action of reserpine, the catecholamine-depleting agent used by Carlsson and colleagues in their seminal studies of the effects of dopamine depletion on motor behavior.[28] The capacity for dopamine storage is critical for proper regulation of dopamine release. Putamenal dopamine storage capacity is greatly reduced in PD,[33] and motor fluctuations alternating between akinesia and hyperkinesias may more directly reflect the amount of dopamine in the synapse. Termination of dopamine action occurs either by presynaptic neuronal reuptake via the dopamine transporter or by enzymatic inactivation. Two enzymes are responsible for the breakdown of dopamine: monoamine oxidase (MAO) and catechol *O*-methyltransferase (COMT). MAO exists in two forms, type A, which has higher affinity for norepinephrine and 5-hydroxytryptophan, and type B, which has higher affinity for *o*-phenylethylamines such as dopamine (Fig. 44-2). Subsequently, drugs targeting these enzymes have also been useful in the treatment of PD.

In advanced PD, with continued exposure to dopaminergic agents and continued degeneration of dopaminergic neurons, involuntary movements of the head, neck, and limbs called dyskinesia develop. This has been attributed to up-regulation of dopamine receptors due to decreased endogenous synaptic dopamine, which, combined with intermittent stimulation of receptors by dopamine or dopamine agonists, leads to oversensitization of striatal dopamine receptors.[34] Other neurotransmitter receptors may be involved as well, including adenosine type A2A, glutamate *N*-methyl-D-aspartate (NMDA)- and α-amino-3-hydroxy-5-methyl-4-isoxazolepropionate (AMPA)-type receptors, and serotonin.[34] Because dyskinesia sometimes represents a major disability in advanced treated PD, therapeutic targets are being identified to suppress these movements (Fig. 44-3).

THERAPEUTICS AND CLINICAL PHARMACOLOGY

Goals of Therapy

Symptom management remains the mainstay of antiparkinsonian treatments. Controlling rest tremor, rigidity, and bradykinesia improves quality of life. Early in the disease, agents enhancing dopaminergic transmission generally improve rigidity and bradykinesia and, to a variable extent, tremor. These symptoms and signs are most often formally assessed by clinical rating scales, the most widely used being the Unified Parkinson Disease Rating Scale (UPDRS). This scale includes subscales for assessments of mood/cognition, motor function, activities of daily living, and complications of therapy, with higher values representing more severe clinical signs. As the disease advances, fluctuations in the patient's response to medications often occurs, characterized by predictable wearing off of dopamine effects requiring more frequent dosing intervals, prolonged delays to onset of clinical effect, medication failures with individual doses, sudden and unpredictable wearing off, dyskinesias, and painful dystonias.

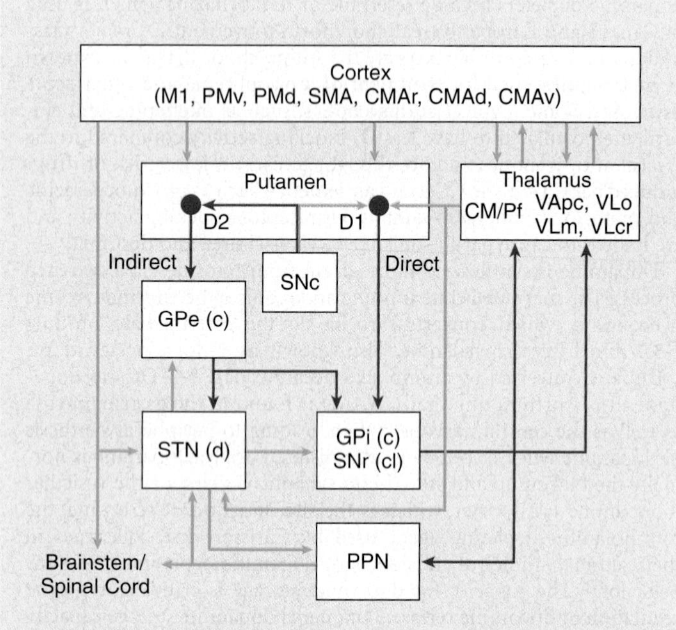

FIGURE 44-2 • Intrinsic circuit anatomy of the motor circuit. The cortical motor areas give rise to a specific motor subcircuit. *Red arrows* indicate inhibitory (γ-aminobutyric acid [GABA]-ergic) connections; *green arrows* indicate excitatory (glutamatergic) connections. c, caudal; cl, caudolateral; CM, centromedian nucleus of thalamus; CMAd, dorsal portion of cingulate motor area; CMAr, rostral portion of cingulate motor area; CMAv, ventral portion of cingulate motor area; d, dorsal; GPe, external segment of the globus pallidus; GPi, internal segment of the globus pallidus; M1, primary motor cortex; Pf, parafascicular nucleus of the thalamus; PMd, dorsal premotor cortex; PMv, ventral premotor cortex; PPN, pedunculopontine nucleus; SMA, supplementary motor area; SNc, substantia nigra pars compacta; SNr, substantia nigra pars reticulata; STN, subthalamic nucleus; VApc, ventral anterior nucleus of thalamus pars parvocellularis; VLcr, ventrolateral nucleus of thalamus rostral pars caudalis; VLm, ventrolateral nucleus of thalamus pars medialis; VLo, ventrolateral nucleus of thalamus pars oralis. (Adapted from DeLong ME, Wichmann T. Circuits and circuit disorders of the basal ganglia. Arch Neurol 2007;64:20-24. With permission of the American Medical Association.)

Management of nonmotor symptoms is increasingly recognized as important for improving quality of life for patients with PD.[35] Estimates of prevalence of depression vary widely from 7% to 76% depending upon definitions of depression and methods of sampling.[36] Efforts at estimating prevalence of anxiety are hampered by similar methodologic difficulties. Dementia has been increasingly recognized as a comorbidity. A recent review of prevalence estimates of dementia in PD patients suggests that 24% to 31% of PD patients suffer from dementia.[37] With growing recognition of these symptoms, there has been increased interest in identifying and managing them, which is addressed below. In addition, PD patients often experience sleep disorders and autonomic dysfunction such as orthostatic hypotension, bladder and bowel dysfunction, and sexual dysfunction. Because of the lack of controlled clinical trials, the treatment of these symptoms will not be reviewed here.

Therapeutics by Class

Symptomatic

Dopamine Agonists (Table 44-1). Currently, dopamine agonists are widely used as monotherapy for initiation of treatment in PD. This is largely due to the observation that dopamine agonists have a lower risk of resulting in motor complications in comparison to levodopa.[38-40] Another common use for dopamine agonists is as adjunct therapy to levodopa in order to lower the levodopa dose to reduce levodopa-induced dyskinesias and to provide more sustained antiparkinsonian effect to alleviate wearing-off effects. Three ergot-derived agents, bromocriptine, pergolide, and cabergoline, and three non–ergot-derived dopamine agonists, pramipexole, ropinirole, and rotigotine are available for use in PD.

Bromocriptine, a tetracyclic ergoline derivative, was the first dopamine agonist introduced for use in PD and was initially marketed as an adjunct to levodopa. It acts primarily as a D_2 agonist with mixed D_1 agonist/antagonist activity. It has agonist activity at lower concentrations and antagonist activity at higher ones. Like all ergotamine-derived dopamine agonists, it is extensively metabolized in the liver. It was shown to be effective in reducing UPDRS scores in placebo-controlled trials as well as reducing levodopa doses required by patients.[41,42] In addition, several studies found that, as an alternative therapy to levodopa, it was effective in reducing motor complications related to levodopa.[42] Currently bromocriptine is less commonly used in PD than the more modern dopamine agonists. Cabergoline, also a tetracyclic ergoline derivative, has selective D_2 receptor affinity, while pergolide mesylate has activity at both D_1 and D_2 receptors. Both were shown to be effective in reducing off-time and increasing on-time and, like bromocriptine, delayed motor complications in comparison to levodopa.[43-47] Both cabergoline and pergolide have been associated with cardiac valvulopathy.[48,49] However, the relationship between dose, duration, and which ergot-derived dopamine agonists are more likely to cause valvulopathy has yet to be evaluated with prospective screening studies. Additionally, because of dopaminergic inhibition of prolactin secretion, pergolide, bromocriptine, and cabergoline are also indicated for hyperprolactinemia. Therefore, they are expected to suppress lactation. Dopamine also exerts some regulatory control over growth hormone, and bromocriptine is therefore indicated for acromegaly as well.

Treatment with ergot-derived dopamine agonists has decreased in favor of non–ergot-derived dopamine agonists such as pramipexole and ropinirole because of risk of pleuropulmonary fibrosis and valvulopathy.[50,51] Pramipexole is a nonergot dopamine agonist with high relative in vitro specificity and full intrinsic activity at the D_2 subfamily of dopamine receptors, binding with higher affinity to D_3 than to D_2 or D_4 receptor subtypes. Ropinirole differs only in that it has full activity at the D_3 receptor subtypes as well as D_2 receptors.[52] These drugs also effectively treat motor symptoms of PD compared to placebo[53-58] and can be used to reduce motor fluctuations when given as adjunct therapy to levodopa.[39,59-63] They have also both been shown to delay the development of motor complications such as mild dyskinesia and wearing-off effects compared to levodopa.[38,58,64] Ropinirole and pramipexole have different methods of metabolism. Ropinirole is metabolized by cytochrome P-450 isozyme 1A2, and its clearance may be reduced when concomitantly taken with various drugs, including ciprofloxacin and estrogen. Pramipexole is excreted renally and should be used with caution and at modified doses in patients with renal failure.

Other side effects common to this class of medication include symptoms related to peripheral dopaminergic activity in the gastrointestinal and vascular systems. Nausea occurs in 40% to 60% of patients and orthostatic hypotension in about 10% to 12%.[55,56] Leg edema has also been reported in about 8% of patients taking pramipexole[56] and also occurs with ropinirole. Sleepiness and even "sleep attacks" have been reported with the use of both pramipexole and ropinirole.[65] Other symptoms particularly common in the elderly are visual hallucinations, paranoia, and confusion, likely due to dopamine actions in the central nervous system. Another notable side effect currently under active investigation is the development of impulsive and compulsive behaviors such as gambling, shopping, eating, and sexual behaviors.[66,67] The frequency of these behaviors is currently uncertain. Dopaminergic medications may influence the underlying physiologic role of dopamine in reward processing, particularly in PD patients in whom the ventral tegmental area, a site central to reward-based learning, is also affected by dopaminergic neuronal degeneration. The risk of compulsive behaviors appears to be increased with concurrent use of any of the dopamine agonists and a prior history of impulse control disorder.[66,67]

Ropinirole is generally taken at a starting dose of 0.25 mg three times daily to a maximum of 24 mg daily. Pramipexole is taken at a

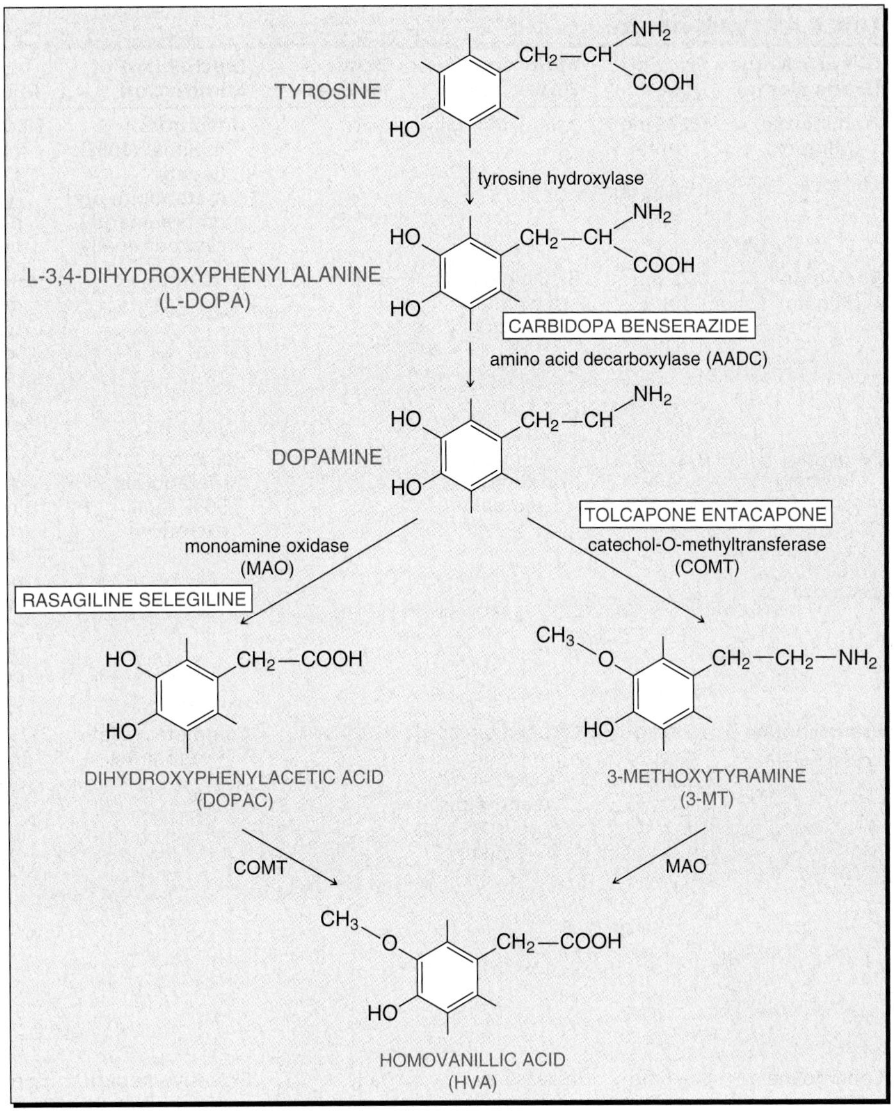

TYROSINE

tyrosine hydroxylase

L-3,4-DIHYDROXYPHENYLALANINE (L-DOPA)

CARBIDOPA BENSERAZIDE

amino acid decarboxylase (AADC)

DOPAMINE

monoamine oxidase (MAO)

RASAGILINE SELEGILINE

TOLCAPONE ENTACAPONE

catechol-O-methyltransferase (COMT)

DIHYDROXYPHENYLACETIC ACID (DOPAC)

3-METHOXYTYRAMINE (3-MT)

COMT

MAO

HOMOVANILLIC ACID (HVA)

FIGURE 44-3 • Synthesis and metabolism of dopamine and targets of pharmacotherapy. (Adapted from Micheli F, Cersosimo MG, Wooten GF. Neurochemistry and neuropharmacology of Parkinson's disease. In Watts RL, Koller WC (eds): Movement Disorders: Principles and Practice, 2nd ed. New York: McGraw-Hill, 2004, p. 199.)

starting dose of 0.125 mg three times daily to a maximum of 4.5 mg daily, although there is no evidence that 4.5 mg daily is more effective than 1.5 mg daily.

Apomorphine is another dopamine agonist that is given parenterally and is finding use in "rescue therapy" of PD patients in a severely bradykinetic and rigid off state.[68] It can be effective within 20 minutes but, given the significant risk of nausea, vomiting, increased dyskinesia, and orthostatic hypotension, its use should be reserved for treating unpredictable and severe off states that occur despite optimal medical therapy. Because of concern for syncope, it is recommended that initial test doses should be administered under clinician supervision with monitoring of supine and standing blood pressure at baseline and 20, 40, and 60 minutes after the dose. Patients who experience significant orthostatic hypotension should not be offered further treatment. In addition, at least at the start, apomorphine should not be given with a non–5-hydroxytryptamine$_3$ (5-HT$_3$) antagonist antiemetic because of the risk of profound hypotension when given concomitantly with 5-HT$_3$ antagonists such as ondansetron and dolasetron. Lisuride is a dopamine agonist available in Europe that is available parenterally and used in similar circumstances.[69] Domperidone, a selective D$_2$ receptor blocker that is not available in the United States, may also be given to limit side effects of nausea. Rotigotine was recently approved as the first transdermal dopamine agonist in the treatment of early stage PD. It has activity at D1, D2 and D3 receptors. Premarketing clinical trials demonstrated mild reduction in UPDRS scores but further studies are currently underway to determine whether this mode of administration is helpful for motor fluctuations or more severe motor symptoms in advanced PD.

Dopamine Precursors (Table 44-2). Levodopa, also known as L-dopa or L-3,4-dihydroxyphenylalanine, has remained the "gold standard" of PD treatment in part due to the existence of class I and II evidence that reduction of motor symptoms is more robust with levodopa than with dopamine agonists.[58,64] Dopamine does not cross the blood-brain barrier, therefore requiring the use of its precursor. In the oral form, it is absorbed by the gastrointestinal system and then rapidly distributed systemically. The elimination half-life is approximately 60 to 90 minutes, and carbidopa/levodopa is excreted renally. Its uptake into the central nervous system depends upon a large neutral amino acid transporter. The gastric mucosa contains large amounts of AADC and COMT, which convert levodopa into dopamine and O-methyldopa before it crosses the blood-brain barrier. For this reason, AADC inhibitors, such as carbidopa and benserazide, are coadministered to increase bioavailability to the nervous system and to reduce side effects due to conversion to dopamine in the periphery, such as nausea, vomiting, and hypotension.

Carbidopa/levodopa is usually started at 12.5/50 or 25/100 mg three times daily and is gradually increased according to response and as the patient's motor symptoms progress. With disease progression, levodopa continues to remain effective for most motor symptoms but gradually produces shorter duration of benefit following each dose. This is

TABLE 44-1 DOPAMINE AGONISTS

Generic Name (Trade Name)	Starting Dose	Maintenance Dose	Dose Interval	Mechanism of Elimination	Toxicity	Special Considerations
Pramipexole (Mirapex)	0.125 mg three times daily	1.5-4.5 mg daily	8 hr	Undergoes minimal (10%) hepatic metabolism and predominantly cleared renally	Nausea, vomiting, orthostatic hypotension, sleep attacks, visual hallucinations, psychosis, compulsive behaviors	Clearance reduced by cimetidine
Ropinirole (Requip)	0.25 mg three times daily	8-16 mg/daily; maximum 24 mg daily	8 hr	Hepatic	Nausea, vomiting, orthostatic hypotension, syncope, sleep attack, somnolence, visual hallucinations, psychosis, compulsive behaviors	Metabolized by cytochrome P-450 isozyme 1A2; clearance may be reduced by ciprofloxacin or estrogens
Pergolide (Permax)	0.05 mg daily	1.5-3 mg daily; maximum 5 mg daily	8 hr	Hepatic metabolism, 50% renal excretion	Constipation, diarrhea, dyspepsia, nausea, insomnia, somnolence, rhinitis, ergot-related side effects: Raynaud's phenomenon, erythromelalgia, retroperitoneal or pulmonary fibrosis, peripheral vasospasm, cardiac valvulopathy	Contraindicated with hypersensitivity to pergolide or other ergot derivatives
Bromocriptine (Parlodel)	1.25 mg twice daily	Can be increased by 2.5 mg every 2-4 weeks. Typical dose is 20-40 mg daily.	12-24 hr	Complete hepatic metabolism	Hypotension, vasoconstriction, constipation, nausea, vomiting, dizziness, headache, fatigue, ergot-related side effects	Contraindicated during postpartum period in women with history of coronary artery disease or other severe cardiovascular conditions, hypersensitivity to bromocriptine products, or sensitivity to ergot alkaloids, and in uncontrolled hypertension
Cabergoline (Dostinex)	0.5-1 mg daily in morning	Increase by 0.5 mg in weekly intervals or longer; maximum 10 mg daily	Daily	Extensive hepatic metabolism; elimination half-life 63-69 hr	Constipation, nausea, dizziness, headache, somnolence, depression, fatigue, orthostatic hypotension, ergot-related side effects	
Apomorphine (Apokyn)	2 mg (0.2 ml) as a test dose	Can be increased by 1 mg as needed; maximum 5 mg	As needed for rescue of severe "off" episodes	Unknown; blood levels are increased in hepatic and renal impairment; elimination half-life 30-60 min	Nausea, vomiting, syncope, hypotension, hallucinations, injection site reactions	Should be administered with an antiemetic but not with the 5-HT_3 antagonist class due to reports of profound hypotension and loss of consciousness
Rotigotine (Neupro)	2 mg/24 hr patch daily	Increase by 2 mg/24 hr weekly to 6 mg/24 hr patch	Daily	Renally excreted; elimination half-life after removal of patch is 5–7 hr	Nausea, application site reaction, somnolence, dizziness, headache, vomiting, insomnia	Patch application site should be rotated daily over 14 days to minimize risk of site reaction

5-HT_3, 5-hydroxytryptamine$_3$.

believed to be due to the progressively reduced dopamine storage capability in remaining nigral neurons. It is therefore not unusual for patients with advanced disease with motor fluctuations to take up to 1200 to 1500 mg of levodopa daily in divided doses given as often as every 2 hours. By contrast, midline motor symptoms such as gait disturbance, postural instability, voice impairment, and dysphagia become more apparent with disease progression and are usually less responsive to levodopa. In higher doses, nausea, vomiting, hallucinations, and orthostatic hypotension can ensue, and troublesome dyskinesias, usually related to peak systemic levels, can necessitate reductions in dosing. Diphasic dyskinesias are much less common but can occur. These correlate with the rise and fall of plasma levels and are usually

TABLE 44-2 DOPAMINE PRECURSORS

Generic Name (Trade Name)	Starting Dose	Maintenance Dose	Dosing Interval	Mechanism of Elimination	Toxicity	Special Considerations
Carbidopa/levodopa (Sinemet), available in 10/100-, 25/100-, and 25/250-mg tablets	25/100 mg three times daily	Some patients may require up to 1200 mg daily or more. Maximum dose is determined by side effects.	2-8 hr	Broken down in the CNS to various metabolites when given with carbidopa; 70%-80% renally excreted; elimination half-life 60-90 min	Nausea, vomiting, dyskinesia, hypotension, visual hallucinations, psychosis, confusion	Carbidopa/levodopa should be taken at least 30 min before or 60 min after meals because of competition with other amino acids for gastrointestinal absorption.
Carbidopa/levodopa sustained release (Sinemet CR), available in 25/100- and 50/200-mg tablets	50/200 mg twice daily	In combination with regular Sinemet	6-12 hr	Metabolized in CNS when given with carbidopa; 70%-80% renally excreted	Nausea, vomiting, dyskinesia, hypotension, visual hallucinations, psychosis, confusion	Increase by 30% to adjust for less bioavailability in this formulation.
Levodopa/carbidopa disintegrating tablet (Parcopa)	25/100 mg three times daily	Same as levodopa/ carbidopa	2-8 hr		Nausea, vomiting, dyskinesia, hypotension	Does not reach systemic circulation faster than regular oral tablets; best used for patients with swallowing dysfunction.

CNS, central nervous system.

TABLE 44-3 CATECHOL O-METHYLTRANSFERASE INHIBITORS

Generic Name (Trade Name)	Starting Dose	Maintenance Dose	Dosing Interval	Mechanism of Elimination	Toxicity	Special Considerations
Tolcapone (Tasmar)	100 mg three times daily	Up to 200 mg three times daily	8 hr	99% hepatic metabolism, 60% renal excretion	Dyskinesia, nausea, diarrhea, loss of appetite, dream disorder, sleep disorder, fulminant hepatic failure (rare)	Baseline liver function tests, followed by every 2-4 weeks for 6 months. Reduction of levodopa dose by 25% is often necessary.
Entacapone (Comtan)	200 mg with each levodopa/ carbidopa dose	Maximum recommended dose is 1600 mg daily	2-8 hr	100% hepatic metabolism, 90% biliary excretion, 10% renal excretion	Dyskinesia, nausea, diarrhea, abdominal pain, constipation, discolored urine	Reduction of levodopa dose is sometimes necessary.

very problematic. Dopamine agonists and COMT inhibitors are often used to reduce these side effects by reducing the need for levodopa. When the therapeutic window for levodopa becomes so narrow that the same dose required to produce symptomatic relief also produces severe dyskinesia, and when levodopa and adjunctive medications are taken at high frequency and in large amounts, patients are often considered for DBS surgery targeted at the subthalamic nucleus (STN), which has been shown to reduce motor fluctuations and also reduce dyskinesias, mostly by virtue of reducing levodopa and levodopa equivalent medication doses used for treatment of PD.[70]

Catechol *O*-Methyltransferase Inhibitors (Table 44-3). Tolcapone was the first drug of this class available for use in the United States. Like entacapone, it is a reversible inhibitor of COMT that converts levodopa to 3-*O*-methyldopa. COMT is located in the gut, liver, and blood. Both tolcapone and entacapone are extensively metabolized in the liver and have half-lives of approximately 1.5 hours. Both drugs have been shown to reduce off-time and increase on-time in patients already receiving levodopa treatment. The effect amounts to approximately 1 to 2 hours more on-time during a 24-hour period and may also allow the reduction of the daily levodopa dose by about 100 mg.[71,72] Tolcapone is taken in a dose of 100 to 200 mg three times daily. Entacapone 200 mg is taken with each dose of levodopa, up to a maximum of eight doses daily.

Side effects of COMT inhibitors are related to enhanced dopaminergic action, which may cause worsening of dyskinesias, hallucinations, and nausea. These can generally be managed by reducing the dose of levodopa. Diarrhea occurs in 14% to 20% of patients taking either entacapone or tolcapone. Only 2% to 5% of patients were forced to discontinue entacapone because of adverse effects during clinical trials, whereas 7% to 22% of patients discontinued tolcapone due to adverse effects.[71-74] Urine discoloration with entacapone developed in approximately 10% of patients during clinical trials.

There were three fatal cases of fulminant liver failure following treatment with tolcapone over the course of 40,000 patient-years in the period shortly following its introduction.[75] All three cases occurred within the first 6 months of treatment. Surveillance of tolcapone effects since that time has shown a very small incidence of reversible hepatotoxicity and no additional deaths. Based on recently amended U.S. Food and Drug Administration (FDA) recommendations, the manufacturer recommends checking baseline alanine aminotranferase (ALT) and aspartate aminotransferase (AST) values and then checking values periodically (i.e., every 2 to 4 weeks) for the first 6 months of therapy. After the first 6 months, periodic monitoring is recommended at intervals deemed clinically relevant. No specific monitoring frequency is recommended, although more frequent monitoring increases the chances of early detection. Enzymes should be checked

TABLE 44-4 MONOAMINE OXIDASE INHIBITORS

Generic Name (Trade Name)	Starting Dose	Maintenance Dose	Dosing Interval	Mechanism of Elimination	Toxicity	Special Considerations
Selegiline (Eldepryl)	5 mg daily	5 mg two times daily	12 h	Metabolized by several cytochrome P-450 enzymes	Confusion, headache, insomnia, hypotension, diarrhea	Contraindicated for use with meperidine. Serotonin syndrome with concomitant use of SSRI thought to be uncommon.
Selegiline (Zelapar)	1.25 mg daily	2.5 mg daily if no benefit after 6 weeks on starting dose	Daily	Metabolized by several cytochrome P450 enzymes	Dizziness, nausea, pain headache, insomnia, dyskinesia	Contraindicated for use with meperidine. Should not be used with tramadol, methadone, propoxyphene, dextromethorphan or other MAO inhibitors.
Rasagiline (Azilect)	As adjunctive therapy, 0.5 mg daily; as monotherapy, 1 mg daily	1 mg daily	Daily	Extensively metabolized in the liver via the cytochrome P-450 isozyme 1A2	Headache, flulike syndrome, malaise	Contraindicated for use with meperidine, sympathomimetic amines such as pseudoephedrine; theoretical concerns with concomitant use with SSRI or the tyramine "cheese effect."

SSRI, selective serotonin reuptake inhibitor.

before any increase in dose and thereafter every 2 to 4 weeks for the next 6 months of therapy. If ALT and AST values rise to greater than two times the upper limit of normal, tolcapone should be discontinued.[76]

Monoamine Oxidase Inhibitors (Table 44-4). Selegiline, also known as deprenyl, is a selective, irreversible inhibitor of MAO-B. In contrast to MAO-A, which metabolizes serotonin and norepinephrine, MAO-B deaminates dopamine, which results in the formation of dihydroxyphenylacetaldehyde,[77] which is then converted to dihydroxyphenylacetic acid. This in turn is metabolized by COMT to become homovanillic acid, the principal metabolite of dopamine. MAO inhibitors are believed to enhance dopaminergic transmission by increasing the half-life of dopamine in the synapse. Selegiline has an elimination half-life of 1.2 hours and is predominantly metabolized by hepatic cytochrome P-450 enzymes.[78] Selegiline is metabolized to *N*-desmethylselegiline, L-amphetamine, and L-methamphetamine,[79] which are thought to be less potent than their D-isoforms. Amphetamine is believed to enhance dopaminergic action by inducing vesicular release of dopamine.

Clinical trials with selegiline showed only modest improvement in the UPDRS score, and therefore selegiline is often used in early PD when only mild motor improvements are required. The magnitude of motor improvement is on the order of 1 to 2 points on the UPDRS motor subscale.[80] It can also be used as adjunctive therapy with levodopa. Two clinical trials have shown that off-time is decreased and on-time is increased.[81,82]

Selegiline has also been examined in a large clinical trial for the possibility of neuroprotective effect. After it was suggested that selegiline protected dopaminergic neurons from MPTP-induced toxicity in animals, it was tested in a large, randomized, controlled clinical trial called the DATATOP study, which involved 800 patients with PD duration of less than 5 years.[80,83] This study showed that, after a mean follow-up period of 14 months, the time until levodopa therapy was added was a median of 9 months later than in patients receiving placebo. The authors concluded that this was due to a neuroprotective effect, but this conclusion was confounded by the fact that selegiline also produces mild symptomatic benefit, thereby casting doubt on this conclusion. In follow-up studies on patients who did not reach the end point of requiring levodopa within the study time frame, all 310 of these patients were given 10 mg selegiline daily regardless of their initial assignment. This group of subjects was monitored for the next 18 months. Those who were placed on selegiline initially reached disability earlier than those not given selegiline, suggesting that whatever initial symptomatic benefits selegiline offered were not sustained over the longer term.[84] Meta-analyses on the subject as well as practice guidelines developed by the American Academy of Neurology (AAN) have concluded that there is insufficient evidence to support a neuroprotective effect for selegiline on progression of PD.[85,86]

Rasagiline is a newly available selective irreversible MAO-B inhibitor that produces fewer amphetamine-like metabolites than selegiline. Its symptomatic clinical effect is similar to that of selegiline in de novo PD patients, producing an improvement in UPDRS scores on the order of 3 to 4 points compared to those taking placebo.[87] It has also been shown to be modestly beneficial in decreasing off-time by 0.9 hours beyond that caused by placebo, an effect which is probably similar to that of entacapone.[88,89] Finally, like selegiline, a possible neuroprotective benefit has been proposed for rasagiline. A delayed start protocol with rasagiline showed a 2.3-point smaller increase in mean total UPDRS score in patients treated for 12 months compared with those treated with placebo for 6 months followed by rasagiline, 2 mg/day, for 6 months.[90] However, larger and more prolonged studies are necessary and are currently in progress to determine whether rasagiline slows the rate of decline in UPDRS scores.

Selegiline is started at 5 mg daily and can be taken twice daily, although evidence is lacking that 10 mg is more effective than 5 mg daily. Rasagiline is started at 0.5 mg daily if used as adjunctive therapy and at 1 mg daily if used as monotherapy. It is recommended that neither medication be taken with sympathomimetic medications such as pseudoephedrine, because of concern of developing hypertensive crisis, and meperidine and tricyclic antidepressants, which can produce autonomic instability, coma, hyperpyrexia, and convulsions. The concomitant use of selective serotonin reuptake inhibitors (SSRIs) is also not recommended due to case reports of serotonin syndrome (hyperthermia, rigidity, myoclonus, autonomic instability with rapid vital sign fluctuations, and mental status changes progressing to extreme agitation, delirium, and coma) in patients receiving SSRIs and selegiline. However, in Phase III clinical trials, amitriptyline, trazodone, citalopram, sertraline, and paroxetine were not excluded and serotonin syndrome did not occur. Finally, ingestion of foods containing tyramine is also cautioned against out of concern of developing hypertensive crisis. Tyramine, which is present in certain foods, is normally metabolized by MAO. When taken concomitantly with MAO inhibitors, tyramine is able to induce release of norepinephrine through peripheral adrenergic terminals.[91] Although it is recommended that patients be educated about which foods contain tyramine (red wine, fermented cheeses, aged meats, etc.), clinical experience has not borne out a significant incidence of these symptoms.

TABLE 44-5 ANTICHOLINERGICS

Generic Name (Trade Name)	Starting Dose	Maintenance Dose	Dosing Interval	Mechanism of Elimination	Toxicity	Special Considerations
Trihexyphenidyl (Artane)	1 mg twice daily	2 mg twice to three times daily	8-12 hr	Excreted renally	Nausea, xerostomia, constipation, blurred vision, dizziness, angle-closure glaucoma, disorientation	Contraindicated in narrow-angle glaucoma
Benztropine (Cogentin)	0.5 mg twice daily, increase by 0.5 mg every 5-6 days	2 mg twice daily	12 hr	Excreted renally	Tachyarrhythmia, constipation, nausea, xerostomia, hyperpyrexia, confusion	

Anticholinergics (Table 44-5). Anticholinergic medications were among the first medications used for the treatment of PD. It is not known exactly why anticholinergics have a beneficial impact on dopamine neurotransmission, but several observations have been made regarding the muscarinic-mediated blocking of dopamine reuptake; the coexpression of muscarinic receptors on striatal neurons and cholinergic interneurons containing D_1 and D_2 receptors, allowing for disinhibition of cholinergic effects in a setting of dopamine insufficiency; and the enhancement of D_1-mediated locomotor activity in muscarinic receptor knockout mice.[92-95]

Current indications for anticholinergic drugs are for patients under the age of 65, without dementia and with predominant symptoms of tremor and rigidity rather than akinesia. Randomized, controlled clinical trials have been conducted on benzhexol, also known as trihexyphenidyl, benztropine, and forms more commonly used outside the United States, such as orphenadrine and bornaprine. A recent review of these trials suggested that anticholinergics were better than placebo in treating some features of PD. However, the quality of studies was generally low, sample sizes were quite small, and all were done prior to 1986.[96]

Trihexyphenidyl and benztropine are excreted renally and can be taken twice to three times daily. A typical starting dose for trihexyphenidyl is 1 mg twice daily, titrated to a maximum daily dose of 6 to 8 mg. Benztropine is started at 0.5 mg twice daily and may be titrated to a total daily dose of 4 mg. A number of significant side effects can occur, especially in PD patients, who may already have cognitive or autonomic symptoms. These include memory impairment, confusion, psychosis, mood changes, visual hallucinations, dry mouth, blurred vision, constipation, nausea, urinary retention, impaired sweating, tachycardia, and precipitation of narrow-angle glaucoma.[97]

Glutamate Antagonists. Amantadine is an anti-influenza agent that was serendipitously observed by Schwab and colleagues in 1969 to have mild antiparkinsonian effects.[98] It exerts antagonist activity at the NMDA glutamate receptor and may also exert anticholinergic effects. Since its introduction, many uncontrolled trials have provided evidence for symptomatic benefit in PD as monotherapy or adjunct therapy, but a recent meta-analysis of randomized, controlled trials found insufficient evidence that it provides symptomatic benefit over placebo.[99] Amantadine has also been used to reduce levodopa-induced dyskinesias. Several randomized, controlled crossover studies have examined its use in this regard. These trials, reviewed in a recent meta-analysis, demonstrated a 24% to 60% reduction in dyskinesias, but owing to a lack of a washout period, data from these trials were weak in supporting a true antidyskinetic effect.[100-103]

Treatment with amantadine is 200 to 300 mg daily divided in two or three doses. It is renally excreted. Neuropsychiatric adverse effects, including confusion, hallucinations, and nightmares, have been documented in large trials and occurred as frequently as 10% of the time in an elderly population.[104] Therefore, caution is recommended when using it in elderly patients. Other notable side effects include livedo reticularis and ankle edema.

Antidepressants. Several randomized controlled clinical trials have investigated the use of antidepressants for depression in patients with PD. Citalopram, sertraline, fluoxetine, amitriptyline, and nortriptyline have been among those tested.[105-109] Somewhat surprisingly, no significant benefit was found for any of these agents except for amitriptyline. However, because of its anticholinergic side effects and occasional adverse effects on gait and balance, this may not be a suitable first-line agent for treatment of depression in this population. A recent practice parameter put forth by the AAN suggested that none of the previously mentioned studies had sufficient power to exclude or confirm efficacy and that larger scale randomized, placebo-controlled trials are needed to resolve this issue.[110]

Neuroleptics. Psychosis in PD patients ranges from benign visual hallucinations with preserved insight to more frightening visual hallucinations associated with paranoid delusions. Neuroleptics have been used with caution in PD patients since the mechanism of action for most neuroleptics involves blockade of dopamine receptors, which can worsen parkinsonism. A recent concern with prescribing atypical antipsychotic drugs for psychosis related to dementia is the increased mortality seen in elderly patients taking these medications.[111]

Olanzapine, clozapine, and quetiapine have been evaluated in randomized controlled studies for treatment of psychosis in PD patients. A class I study of clozapine, which has a relative high affinity for D_4 subtype receptors, showed improved psychosis using a clinical global impression scale (CGIS) and Brief Psychiatric Rating Scale (BPRS).[112] Another study involving clozapine and quetiapine, which has D_2 and 5-hydroxytryptamine$_2$ antagonist activity, showed similar improvements in CGIS and BPRS scores.[113] Two studies involving olanzapine showed that it worsened motor symptoms and did not improve psychosis.[114,115] Clozapine's disadvantage is the need for frequent monitoring that is required because of the 1.3% incidence of agranulocytosis. Monitoring of blood counts is required weekly for the first 6 months of therapy and every 2 weeks for the next 6 months, and thereafter maintained at every 4 weeks. Other disadvantages of clozapine are its potential side effects of confusion, weight gain, and drooling.

Cholinesterase Inhibitors. Recent focus on the cognitive deficits associated with PD has stimulated interest in cholinesterase inhibitors, which are used to treat memory deficit symptoms in Alzheimer's disease. To date, only rivastigmine has been FDA approved for dementia associated with PD. In a double-blind, randomized, placebo-controlled study involving 410 patients, there was a mean improvement of 2.1 points in the 70-point cognitive subscale of the Alzheimer's Disease Assessment Scale from a baseline score of 23.8, as compared with a 0.7-point worsening in the placebo group, from a baseline score of 24.3 ($P < 0.001$). Clinically meaningful improvements in the scores for the AD Cooperative Study–Clinical Global Impression of Change were observed in 19.8% of patients in the rivastigmine group and 14.5% of those in the placebo group, while clinically meaningful worsening was observed in 13.0% and 23.1%, respectively.[116] Similar to other cholinesterase inhibitors, rivastigmine was associated with nausea, vomiting, and tremor, which likely relate to its cholinergic enhancing properties. Trials involving donepezil have shown mild improvement in neuropsychological testing as well as clinician impressions of improvement, but sample sizes were small and therefore no definitive conclusions can be drawn regarding the efficacy of donepezil. However, the similar magnitude of effect demonstrated in these trials suggests that a class effect probably exists.[117-119] Although theoretical concerns of worsening parkinsonism by enhancing cholinergic action are well founded, these have not been reported as an adverse effect in the larger clinical trials.

Rivastigmine is started at 1.5 mg twice daily and subsequently increased to a maximum of 6 mg twice daily. Nausea, vomiting, and diarrhea occurred in 29%, 17%, and 7%, respectively, compared with 11%, 3%, and 4%, respectively, in the placebo group. Worsening of PD is a theoretical concern given the balance of dopamine-acetylcholine regulation and was observed in 3% versus 1% of patients taking placebo (Exelon package label).

Therapeutic Approach

The AAN has developed Practice Guidelines regarding pharmacologic management on several topics in Parkinson's disease, including the initiation of treatment for PD, management of motor fluctuations, management of depression and psychosis, and neuroprotective strategies.[86,110,120,121]

For initiating treatment for PD, the following conclusions were made (Box 44-1):

1. Selegiline has very mild symptomatic benefit (level A, class II evidence) with no evidence for neuroprotective benefit (level U, class II evidence).
2. For PD patients requiring initiation of symptomatic therapy, either levodopa or a dopamine agonist can be used. However, levodopa provides superior motor benefit but is associated with a higher risk of dyskinesia (level A, class I, and class II evidence).
3. No evidence was found that initiating treatment with sustained-release levodopa provides an advantage over immediate-release levodopa (level B, class II evidence).

BOX 44-1 RATINGS AND DEFINITIONS FOR STUDIES

Ratings for the Quality of the Evidence

Class I—Prospective, randomized, controlled clinical trial with masked outcome assessment, in a representative population. The following are required: (a) primary outcome(s) is/are clearly defined; (b) exclusion/inclusion criteria are defined; (c) adequate accounting for dropouts and crossovers with numbers sufficiently low to have minimal potential for bias; and (d) relevant baseline characteristics are presented and substantially equivalent among treatment groups or there is appropriate statistical adjustment for differences.

Class II—Prospective matched group cohort study in a representative population with masked outcome assessment that meets criteria a through d above *or* a randomized controlled trial in a representative population that lacks one of criteria a through d.

Class III—All other controlled trials (including well-defined natural history controls or patients serving as own controls) in a representative population, where outcome assessment is independent of patient treatment.

Class IV—Evidence from uncontrolled studies, case series, case reports, or expert opinion.

Definitions for the Strength of the Recommendations

A—Established as effective, ineffective, or harmful for the given condition in the specified population. Level A rating requires at least one convincing class I study or at least two consistent, convincing class II studies.

B—Probably effective, ineffective, or harmful for the given condition in the specified population. Level B rating requires at least one convincing class II study or at least three consistent class III studies.

C—Possibly effective, ineffective, or harmful for the given condition in the specified population. Level C rating requires at least two convincing and consistent class III studies.

U—Data inadequate or conflicting; given current knowledge, treatment is unproven.

For treating motor complications related to PD, the following conclusions were made:

1. Entacapone and rasagiline should be offered to reduce off-time (Level A).
2. Pergolide, pramipexole, ropinirole, and tolcapone should be considered to reduce off-time (Level B).
3. Apomorphine, cabergoline, and selegiline may be considered to reduce off-time (Level C).
4. The available evidence does not establish superiority of one medicine over another in reducing off-time (Level B).
5. Sustained-release carbidopa/levodopa and bromocriptine may be disregarded to reduce off-time (Level C).
6. Amantadine may be considered to reduce dyskinesia (Level C).
7. STN DBS may be considered to improve motor function and reduce off-time, dyskinesia, and medication usage (Level C).
8. Preoperative response to levodopa predicts better outcome after DBS of the STN (Level B).

For treating depression, dementia, and psychosis in PD, the following conclusions were drawn:

1. Amitriptyline may be considered to treat depression in PD without dementia (Level C).
2. For psychosis in PD, clozapine should be considered (Level B), quetiapine may be considered (Level C), but olanzapine should not be considered (Level B).
3. Donepezil or rivastigmine should be considered for dementia in PD (Level B) and rivastigmine should be considered for DLB (Level B).

Emerging Targets and Therapeutics

Development of new pharmacotherapies for PD lies chiefly in identifying neuroprotective or disease-modifying strategies as well as in reducing motor fluctuations in advanced PD. Currently, DBS is a neurosurgical technique that applies high-frequency electric current to various nuclei within the basal ganglia. The most commonly used target in PD is the STN. DBS has been demonstrated to reduce off-time, motor fluctuations, and dyskinesias as well as the total daily dose of levodopa or levodopa equivalent doses in a randomized best medical therapy–controlled trial.[70] However, not all advanced PD patients are good candidates for surgery due to medical comorbidities or the presence of dementia. Therefore, efforts are aimed at discovering drugs that can be delivered in a continuous fashion, nondopaminergic agents that may ameliorate motor complications,[122] and potential neuroprotective agents. Several candidates for neuroprotective effects include newer MAO-B inhibitors; mitochondrial enhancers, including creatine[123] and coenzyme Q10[124]; NMDA antagonists; anti-inflammatory agents; antiapoptotic agents; and various neurotrophic factors.[125] Of drugs that can be delivered to provide continuous enhancement of dopamine effect in the central nervous system, intraduodenal levodopa and transdermally administered rotigotine[126-128] are used in Europe and are undergoing clinical trials in the US. Small open-label studies of transdermal lisuride and apomorphine have also been carried out.[129,130] New dopamine agonists have been developed in hopes of developing agents effective against dyskinesias. In addition, because of evidence that glutamate (NMDA and AMPA), adenosine A_{2A}, α-adrenergic, 5-hydroxytryptamine$_{1A}$ and 5-hydroxytryptamine$_{2A}$, cannabinoid, and neuropeptide receptors are potentially involved in the development of dyskinesias, agents that target these receptors are also being developed.[122]

CONCLUSIONS

PD is a neurodegenerative illness that continues to cause progressive morbidity and disability despite the availability of effective symptomatic treatments. The hallmark pathophysiologic finding of PD related to motor deficits is that of degenerating nigrostriatal neurons containing dopamine. Current treatments are aimed at enhancing dopamine neurotransmission, targeting dopamine receptors, blocking enzymes responsible for the breakdown of dopamine, or blocking acetylcholine-mediated influences on dopamine action. A number of other medications are being investigated for management of comorbid nonmotor aspects of PD, such as depression, dementia, and psychosis. As investigations elaborate on other neuropharmacologic mechanisms that operate in the basal ganglia, new drugs are being developed for both symptomatic and neuroprotective effects.

REFERENCES

1. de Lau LM, Breteler MM. Epidemiology of Parkinson's disease. Lancet Neurol 2006;5:525-535.
2. Huse DM, Schulman K, Orsini L, et al. Burden of illness in Parkinson's disease. Mov Disord 2005;20:1449-1454.
3. Noyes K, Liu H, Li Y, et al. Economic burden associated with Parkinson's disease on elderly Medicare beneficiaries. Mov Disord 2006;21:362-372.
4. Whetten-Goldstein K, Sloan F, Kulas E, et al. The burden of Parkinson's disease on society, family, and the individual. J Am Geriatr Soc 1997;45:844-849.
5. Morens DM, Davis JW, Grandinetti A, et al. Epidemiologic observations on Parkinson's disease: incidence and mortality in a prospective study of middle-aged men. Neurology 1996;46:1044-1050.
6. Parkinson J. An Essay on the Shaking Palsy. London: Sherwood, Neely and Jones; 1817.
7. Charcot JM. Leçons sur les Maladies du Système Nerveux faites a La Salpétrière. Paris: A. Delahaye, 1872.
8. Foix C, Nicolesco J. Anatomie cérebrale: les noyaux gris centraux et la région mesenchephalo-soux-optique. *En* Series Anatomie cérebrale. Paris: Masson, 1925.
9. Hassler R. Zur Pathologie der Paralysis agitans und des postenzephalitischen Parkinsonismus. J Psychol Neurol 1938;48:387-476.
10. Tretiakoff C. Contributions a l'étude de l'anatomie pathologique du locus niger de Soemmering avec quelques déductions relatives à la pathogènie des troubles de tonus musculaire et de la maladie de Parkinson. Thesis, Paris, 1919.
11. Birkmayer W, Hornykiewicz O. [The L-3,4-dioxyphenylalanine (DOPA)-effect in Parkinson-akinesia.]. Wien Klin Wochenschr 1961;73:787-788.
12. Braak H, Muller CM, Rub U, et al. Pathology associated with sporadic Parkinson's disease—where does it end? J Neural Transm Suppl 2006;89-97.
13. Kopell BH, Rezai AR, Chang JW, et al. Anatomy and physiology of the basal ganglia: implications for deep brain stimulation for Parkinson's disease. Mov Disord 2006;21(Suppl 14):S238-S246.
14. Albin RL, Young AB, Penney JB. The functional anatomy of basal ganglia disorders. Trends Neurosci 1989;12:366-375.
15. Alexander GE, Crutcher MD, DeLong MR. Basal ganglia-thalamocortical circuits: parallel substrates for motor, oculomotor, "prefrontal" and "limbic" functions. Prog Brain Res 1990;85:119-146.
16. Lang AE, Lozano AM. Parkinson's disease: second of two parts. N Engl J Med 1998;339:1130-1143.
17. Anderson ME, Postupna N, Ruffo M. Effects of high-frequency stimulation in the internal globus pallidus on the activity of thalamic neurons in the awake monkey. J Neurophysiol 2003;89:1150-1160.
18. Gearing M, Mirra S. Neuropathology of movement disorders: an overview. *In* Watts R, Koller W (eds): Movement Disorders: Neurologic Principles and Practice, 2nd ed. New York: McGraw-Hill, 2004, pp 143-158.
19. Polymeropoulos MH, Lavedan C, Leroy E, et al. Mutation in the alpha-synuclein gene identified in families with Parkinson's disease. Science 1997;276:2045-2047.
20. Kitada T, Asakawa S, Hattori N, et al. Mutations in the *parkin* gene cause autosomal recessive juvenile parkinsonism. Nature 1998;392:605-608.
21. Eriksen JL, Wszolek Z, Petrucelli L. Molecular pathogenesis of Parkinson disease. Arch Neurol 2005;62:353-357.
22. Shen J, Cookson MR. Mitochondria and dopamine: new insights into recessive parkinsonism. Neuron 2004;43:301-304.
23. Beal F, Lang A. The proteasomal inhibition model of Parkinson's disease: "boon or bust"? Ann Neurol 2006;60:158-161.
24. Langston JW, Ballard P, Tetrud JW, et al. Chronic parkinsonism in humans due to a product of meperidine-analog synthesis. Science 1983;219:979-980.
25. Mizuno Y, Hattori N, Mochizuki H. Etiology of Parkinson's disease. *In* Watts R, Koller W (eds): Movement Disorders: Neurologic Principles and Practice, 2nd ed. New York: McGraw-Hill, 2004, pp 209-231.
26. Ogawa N, Asanuma M, Miyazaki I, et al. L-DOPA treatment from the viewpoint of neuroprotection: possible mechanism of specific and progressive dopaminergic neuronal death in Parkinson's disease. J Neurol 2005;252(Suppl IV):IV23-IV31.
27. Fahn S. Does levodopa slow or hasten the rate of progression of Parkinson's disease? J Neurol 2005;252(Suppl IV):IV37-IV42.
28. Carlsson A, Lindqvist M, Magnusson T. 3,4-Dihydroxyphenylalanine and 5-hydroxytryptophan as reserpine antagonists. Nature 1957;180:1200.
29. Barbeau A, Sourkes TL, Murphy CF. Les catecholamine dans la maladie de Parkinson. In de Ajuriguerra J (ed): Monoamines et Systeme Nerveaux Central. Geneva: George, 1962, pp 247-262.
30. Barbeau A, Murphy GF, Sourkes TL. Excretion of dopamine in diseases of basal ganglia. Science 1961;133:1706-1707.
31. Cotzias GC, Van Woert MH, Schiffer LM. Aromatic amino acids and modification of parkinsonism. N Engl J Med 1967;276:374-379.
32. Tarsy D, Baldessarini RJ, Tarazi FI. Effects of newer antipsychotics on extrapyramidal function. CNS Drugs 2002;16:23-45.
33. Piccini P, Pavese N, Brooks DJ. Endogenous dopamine release after pharmacological challenges in Parkinson's disease. Ann Neurol 2003;53:647-653.
34. Brotchie JM, Lee J, Venderova K. Levodopa-induced dyskinesia in Parkinson's disease. J Neural Transm 2005;112:359-391.
35. Pfeiffer R, Bodis-Wollner I (eds). Parkinson's Disease and Nonmotor Dysfunction. Totowa, NJ: Humana Press, 2005.
36. Veazey C, Aki SO, Cook KF, et al. Prevalence and treatment of depression in Parkinson's disease. J Neuropsychiatry Clin Neurosci 2005;17:310-323.
37. Aarsland D, Zaccai J, Brayne C. A systematic review of prevalence studies of dementia in Parkinson's disease. Mov Disord 2005;20:1255-1263.
38. Dopamine transporter brain imaging to assess the effects of pramipexole vs levodopa on Parkinson disease progression. JAMA 2002;287:1653-1661.
39. Lieberman A, Olanow CW, Sethi K, et al. A multicenter trial of ropinirole as adjunct treatment for Parkinson's disease. Ropinirole Study Group. Neurology 1998;51:1057-1062.
40. Whone AL, Watts RL, Stoessl AJ, et al. Slower progression of Parkinson's disease with ropinirole versus levodopa: the REAL-PET study. Ann Neurol 2003;54:93-101.
41. Staal-Schreinemachers AL, Wesseling H, Kamphuis DJ, et al. Low-dose bromocriptine therapy in Parkinson's disease: double-blind, placebo-controlled study. Neurology 1986;36:291-293.
42. Comparisons of therapeutic effects of levodopa, levodopa and selegiline, and bromocriptine in patients with early, mild Parkinson's disease: three year interim report. Parkinson's Disease Research Group in the United Kingdom. BMJ 1993;307:469-472.
43. Hutton JT, Koller WC, Ahlskog JE, et al. Multicenter, placebo-controlled trial of cabergoline taken once daily in the treatment of Parkinson's disease. Neurology 1996;46:1062-1065.
44. Olanow CW, Myllyla VV, Sotaniemi KA, et al. Effect of selegiline on mortality in patients with Parkinson's disease: a meta-analysis. Neurology 1998;51:825-830.
45. Pezzoli G, Martignoni E, Pacchetti C, et al. A crossover, controlled study comparing pergolide with bromocriptine as an adjunct to levodopa for the treatment of Parkinson's disease. Neurology 1995;45:S22-S27.
46. Rinne UK, Bracco F, Chouza C, et al. Cabergoline in the treatment of early Parkinson's disease: results of the first year of treatment in a double-blind comparison of cabergoline and levodopa. The PKDS009 Collaborative Study Group. Neurology 1997;48:363-368.
47. Inzelberg R, Nisipeanu P, Rabey JM, et al. Double-blind comparison of cabergoline and bromocriptine in Parkinson's disease patients with motor fluctuations. Neurology 1996;47:785-788.
48. Peralta C, Wolf E, Alber H, et al. Valvular heart disease in Parkinson's disease vs. controls: an echocardiographic study. Mov Disord 2006;21:1109-1113.
49. Yamamoto M, Uesugi T, Nakayama T. Dopamine agonists and cardiac valvulopathy in Parkinson disease: a case-control study. Neurology 2006;67:1225-1229.
50. Bhatt MH, Keenan SP, Fleetham JA, et al. Pleuropulmonary disease associated with dopamine agonist therapy. Ann Neurol 1991;30:613-616.
51. Frans E, Dom R, Demedts M. Pleuropulmonary changes during treatment of Parkinson's disease with a long-acting ergot derivative, cabergoline. Eur Respir J 1992;5:263-265.
52. Reavill C, Boyfield I, Coldwell M, et al. Comparative pharmacological study of ropinirole (SKF-101468) and its metabolites in rats. J Pharm Pharmacol 2000;52:1129-1135.
53. Brooks DJ, Abbott RJ, Lees AJ, et al. A placebo-controlled evaluation of ropinirole, a novel D2 agonist, as sole dopaminergic therapy in Parkinson's disease. Clin Neuropharmacol 1998;21:101-107.
54. Hubble JP, Koller WC, Cutler NR, et al. Pramipexole in patients with early Parkinson's disease. Clin Neuropharmacol 1995;18:338-347.
55. Adler CH, Sethi KD, Hauser RA, et al. Ropinirole for the treatment of early Parkinson's disease. The Ropinirole Study Group. Neurology 1997;49:393-399.
56. Shannon KM, Bennett JP Jr, Friedman JH. Efficacy of pramipexole, a novel dopamine agonist, as monotherapy in mild to moderate Parkinson's disease. The Pramipexole Study Group. Neurology 1997;49:724-728.
57. Safety and efficacy of pramipexole in early Parkinson disease: a randomized dose-ranging study. Parkinson Study Group. JAMA 1997;278:125-130.
58. Pramipexole vs. levodopa as initial treatment for Parkinson disease: A randomized controlled trial. Parkinson Study Group. JAMA 2000;284:1931-1938.
59. Rascol O, Lees AJ, Senard JM, et al. Ropinirole in the treatment of levodopa-induced motor fluctuations in patients with Parkinson's disease. Clin Neuropharmacol 1996;19:234-245.
60. Lieberman A, Ranhosky A, Korts D. Clinical evaluation of pramipexole in advanced Parkinson's disease: results of a double-blind, placebo-controlled, parallel-group study. Neurology 1997;49:162-168.
61. Guttman M. Double-blind comparison of pramipexole and bromocriptine treatment with placebo in advanced Parkinson's disease. International Pramipexole-Bromocriptine Study Group. Neurology 1997;49:1060-1065.
62. Wermuth L. A double-blind, placebo-controlled, randomized, multi-center study of pramipexole in advanced Parkinson's disease. Eur J Neurol 1998;5:235-242.
63. Pinter MM, Pogarell O, Oertel WH. Efficacy, safety, and tolerance of the non-ergoline dopamine agonist pramipexole in the treatment of advanced Parkinson's disease: a double blind, placebo controlled, randomised, multicentre study. J Neurol Neurosurg Psychiatry 1999;66:436-441.
64. Rascol O, Brooks DJ, Korczyn AD, et al. A five-year study of the incidence of dyskinesia in patients with early Parkinson's disease who were treated with ropinirole or levodopa. 056 Study Group. N Engl J Med 2000;342:1484-1491.
65. Frucht S, Rogers JD, Greene PE, et al. Falling asleep at the wheel: motor vehicle mishaps in persons taking pramipexole and ropinirole. Neurology 1999;52:1908-1910.
66. Voon V, Hassan K, Zurowski M, et al. Prospective prevalence of pathologic gambling and medication association in Parkinson disease. Neurology 2006;66:1750-1752.

67. Weintraub D, Siderowf AD, Potenza MN, et al. Association of dopamine agonist use with impulse control disorders in Parkinson disease. Arch Neurol 2006;63:969-973.
68. Dewey RB Jr, Hutton JT, LeWitt PA, et al. A randomized, double-blind, placebo-controlled trial of subcutaneously injected apomorphine for parkinsonian off-state events. Arch Neurol 2001;58:1385-1392.
69. Stocchi F, Ruggieri S, Vacca L, et al. Prospective randomized trial of lisuride infusion versus oral levodopa in patients with Parkinson's disease. Brain 2002;125:2058-2066.
70. Deuschl G, Schade-Brittinger C, Krack P, et al. A randomized trial of deep-brain stimulation for Parkinson's disease. N Engl J Med 2006;355:896-908.
71. Baas H, Beiske AG, Ghika J, et al. Catechol-O-methyltransferase inhibition with tolcapone reduces the "wearing off" phenomenon and levodopa requirements in fluctuating parkinsonian patients. J Neurol Neurosurg Psychiatry 1997;63:421-428.
72. Rinne UK, Larsen JP, Siden A, et al. Entacapone enhances the response to levodopa in parkinsonian patients with motor fluctuations. Nomecomt Study Group. Neurology 1998;51:1309-1314.
73. Rajput AH, Martin W, Saint-Hilaire MH, et al. Tolcapone improves motor function in parkinsonian patients with the "wearing-off" phenomenon: a double-blind, placebo-controlled, multicenter trial. Neurology 1997;49:1066-1071.
74. Merello M, Lees AJ, Webster R, et al. Effect of entacapone, a peripherally acting catechol-O-methyltransferase inhibitor, on the motor response to acute treatment with levodopa in patients with Parkinson's disease. J Neurol Neurosurg Psychiatry 1994;57:186-189.
75. Borges N. Tolcapone-related liver dysfunction: implications for use in Parkinson's disease therapy. Drug Saf 2003;26:743-747.
76. Olanow CW. Tolcapone and hepatotoxic effects. Tasmar Advisory Panel. Arch Neurol 2000;57:263-267.
77. Burke WJ, Li SW, Chung HD, et al. Neurotoxicity of MAO metabolites of catecholamine neurotransmitters: role in neurodegenerative diseases. Neurotoxicology 2004;25:101-115.
78. Mahmood I. Is 10 milligrams selegiline essential as an adjunct therapy for the symptomatic treatment of Parkinson's disease? Ther Drug Monit 1998;20:717-721.
79. Heinonen EH, Anttila MI, Lammintausta RA. Pharmacokinetic aspects of l-deprenyl (selegiline) and its metabolites. Clin Pharmacol Ther 1994;56:742-749.
80. Effects of tocopherol and deprenyl on the progression of disability in early Parkinson's disease. The Parkinson Study Group. N Engl J Med 1993;328:176-183.
81. Golbe LI, Lieberman AN, Muenter MD, et al. Deprenyl in the treatment of symptom fluctuations in advanced Parkinson's disease. Clin Neuropharmacol 1988;11:45-55.
82. Waters CH, Sethi KD, Hauser RA, et al. Zydis selegiline reduces off time in Parkinson's disease patients with motor fluctuations: a 3-month, randomized, placebo-controlled study. Mov Disord 2004;19:426-432.
83. Mytilineou C, Cohen G. Deprenyl protects dopamine neurons from the neurotoxic effect of 1-methyl-4-phenylpyridinium ion. J Neurochem 1985;45:1951-1953.
84. Impact of deprenyl and tocopherol treatment on Parkinson's disease in DATATOP subjects not requiring levodopa. Parkinson Study Group. Ann Neurol 1996;39:29-36.
85. Macleod AD, Counsell CE, Ives N, Stowe R. Monoamine oxidase B inhibitors for early Parkinson's disease. Cochrane Database Syst Rev 2005;(3):CD004898.
86. Miyasaki JM, Martin W, Suchowersky O, et al. Practice parameter: Initiation of treatment for Parkinson's disease (an evidence-based review). Report of the Quality Standards Subcommittee of the American Academy of Neurology. Neurology 2002;58:11-17.
87. A controlled trial of rasagiline in early Parkinson disease: the TEMPO Study. Arch Neurol 2002;59:1937-1943.
88. Rascol O, Brooks DJ, Melamed E, et al. Rasagiline as an adjunct to levodopa in patients with Parkinson's disease and motor fluctuations (LARGO, Lasting effect in Adjunct therapy with Rasagiline Given Once daily, study): a randomised, double-blind, parallel-group trial. Lancet 2005;365:947-954.
89. A randomized placebo-controlled trial of rasagiline in levodopa-treated patients with Parkinson disease and motor fluctuations: the PRESTO study. Arch Neurol 2005;62:241-248.
90. A controlled, randomized, delayed-start study of rasagiline in early Parkinson disease. Arch Neurol 2004;61:561-566.
91. Youdim MBH, Riederer PF. A review of the mechanisms and role of monoamine oxidase inhibitors in Parkinson's disease. Neurology 2004;63:S32-S35.
92. Gomeza J, Zhang L, Kostenis E, et al. Enhancement of D1 dopamine receptor-mediated locomotor stimulation in M_4 muscarinic acetylcholine receptor knockout mice. Proc Natl Acad Sci U S A 1999;96:10483-10488.
93. Weiner DM, Levey AI, Brann MR. Expression of muscarinic acetylcholine and dopamine receptor mRNAs in rat basal ganglia. Proc Natl Acad Sci U S A 1990;87:7050-7054.
94. Coyle JT, Snyder SH. Antiparkinsonian drugs: inhibition of dopamine uptake in the corpus striatum as a possible mechanism of action. Science 1969;166:899-901.
95. Ding J, Guzman JN, Tkatch T, et al. RGS4-dependent attenuation of M4 autoreceptor function in striatal cholinergic interneurons following dopamine depletion. Nat Neurosci 2006;9:832-842.
96. Katzenschlager R, Sampaio C, Costa J, Lees A. Anticholinergics for symptomatic management of Parkinson's disease. Cochrane Database Syst Rev 2003;(3): CD003735.
97. Tarsy D. Initial treatment of Parkinson's disease. Curr Treat Options Neurol 2006;8:224-35.
98. Schwab RS, England AC Jr, Poskanzer DC, et al. Amantadine in the treatment of Parkinson's disease. JAMA 1969;208:1168-1170.
99. Crosby N, Deane KHO, Clarke CE. Amantadine in Parkinson's disease. Cochrane Database Syst Rev 2003;(1):CD003468.
100. Luginger E, Wenning GK, Bosch S, et al. Beneficial effects of amantadine on L-dopa-induced dyskinesias in Parkinson's disease. Mov Disord 2000;15:873-878.
101. Snow BJ, Macdonald L, McAuley D, et al. The effect of amantadine on levodopa-induced dyskinesias in Parkinson's disease: a double-blind, placebo-controlled study. Clin Neuropharmacol 2000;23:82-85.
102. Verhagen Metman L, Del Dotto P, van den Munckhof P, et al. Amantadine as treatment for dyskinesias and motor fluctuations in Parkinson's disease. Neurology 1998;50:1323-1326.
103. Crosby NJ, Deane KHO, Clarke CE. Amantadine for dyskinesia in Parkinson's disease. Cochrane Database Syst Rev 2003;(2):CD003467.
104. Keyser LA, Karl M, Nafziger AN, et al. Comparison of central nervous system adverse effects of amantadine and rimantadine used as sequential prophylaxis of influenza A in elderly nursing home patients. Arch Intern Med 2000;160:1485-1488.
105. Wermuth L SP, Timm B, Utzon NP, et al. Depression in idiopathic Parkinson's disease treated with citalopram—a placebo-controlled trial. Nordic J Psychiatry 1998;52:163-169.
106. Andersen J, Aabro E, Gulmann N, et al. Anti-depressive treatment in Parkinson's disease: a controlled trial of the effect of nortriptyline in patients with Parkinson's disease treated with L-DOPA. Acta Neurol Scand 1980;62:210-219.
107. Avila A, Cardona X, Martin-Baranera M, et al. Does nefazodone improve both depression and Parkinson disease? A pilot randomized trial. J Clin Psychopharmacol 2003;23:509-513.
108. Leentjens AF, Vreeling FW, Luijckx GJ, et al. SSRIs in the treatment of depression in Parkinson's disease. Int J Geriatr Psychiatry 2003;18:552-554.
109. Serrano-Duenas M. [A comparison between low doses of amitriptyline and low doses of fluoxetin used in the control of depression in patients suffering from Parkinson's disease]. Rev Neurol 2002;35:1010-1014.
110. Miyasaki JM, Shannon K, Voon V, et al. Practice parameter: Evaluation and treatment of depression, psychosis, and dementia in Parkinson disease (an evidence-based review). Report of the Quality Standards Subcommittee of the American Academy of Neurology. Neurology 2006;66:996-1002.
111. Schneider LS, Dagerman KS, Insel P. Risk of death with atypical antipsychotic drug treatment for dementia: meta-analysis of randomized placebo-controlled trials. JAMA 2005;294:1934-1943.
112. Low-dose clozapine for the treatment of drug-induced psychosis in Parkinson's disease. The Parkinson Study Group. N Engl J Med 1999;340:757-763.
113. Morgante L, Epifanio A, Spina E, et al. Quetiapine versus clozapine: a preliminary report of comparative effects on dopaminergic psychosis in patients with Parkinson's disease. Neurol Sci 2002;23(Suppl 2):S89-S90.
114. Ondo WG, Levy JK, Vuong KD, et al. Olanzapine treatment for dopaminergic-induced hallucinations. Mov Disord 2002;17:1031-1035.
115. Breier A, Sutton VK, Feldman PD, et al. Olanzapine in the treatment of dopamimetic-induced psychosis in patients with Parkinson's disease. Biol Psychiatry 2002;52:438-445.
116. Emre M, Aarsland D, Albanese A, et al. Rivastigmine for dementia associated with Parkinson's disease. N Engl J Med 2004;351:2509-2518.
117. Aarsland D, Laake K, Larsen JP, et al. Donepezil for cognitive impairment in Parkinson's disease: a randomised controlled study. J Neurol Neurosurg Psychiatry 2002;72:708-712.
118. Leroi I, Brandt J, Reich SG, et al. Randomized placebo-controlled trial of donepezil in cognitive impairment in Parkinson's disease. Int J Geriatr Psychiatry 2004;19: 1-8.
119. Ravina B, Putt M, Siderowf A, et al. Donepezil for dementia in Parkinson's disease: a randomised, double blind, placebo controlled, crossover study. J Neurol Neurosurg Psychiatry 2005;76:934-939.
120. Pahwa R, Factor SA, Lyons KE, et al. Practice parameter: Treatment of Parkinson disease with motor fluctuations and dyskinesia (an evidence-based review). Report of the Quality Standards Subcommittee of the American Academy of Neurology. Neurology 2006;66:983-995.
121. Suchowersky O, Gronseth G, Perlmutter J, et al. Practice parameter: Neuroprotective strategies and alternative therapies for Parkinson disease (an evidence-based review). Report of the Quality Standards Subcommittee of the American Academy of Neurology. Neurology 2006;66:976-982.
122. Bonuccelli U, Del Dotto P. New pharmacologic horizons in the treatment of Parkinson disease. Neurology 2006;67:S30-S38.
123. Bender A, Koch W, Elstner M, et al. Creatine supplementation in Parkinson disease: a placebo-controlled randomized pilot trial. Neurology 2006;67:1262-1264.
124. Shults CW, Oakes D, Kieburtz K, et al. Effects of coenzyme Q10 in early Parkinson disease: evidence of slowing of the functional decline. Arch Neurol 2002;59:1541-1550.
125. Tilley BC, Palesch YY, Kieburtz K, et al. Optimizing the ongoing search for new treatments for Parkinson disease: using futility designs. Neurology 2006;66:628-633.
126. Morgan JC, Sethi KD. Rotigotine for the treatment of Parkinson's disease. Expert Rev Neurother 2006;6:1275-1282.
127. Poewe W, Luessi F. Clinical studies with transdermal rotigotine in early Parkinson's disease. Neurology 2005;65:S11-S14.
128. Nyholm D. Enteral levodopa/carbidopa gel infusion for the treatment of motor fluctuations and dyskinesias in advanced Parkinson's disease. Expert Rev Neurother 2006;6:1403-1411.
129. Priano L, Albani G, Brioschi A, et al. Transdermal apomorphine permeation from microemulsions: a new treatment in Parkinson's disease. Mov Disord 2004;19:937-942.
130. Woitalla D, Müller T, Benz S, et al. Transdermal lisuride delivery in the treatment of Parkinson's disease. J Neural Transm Suppl 2004;(68):89-95.

45

SEIZURE DISORDERS

Scott Mintzer

OVERVIEW 663
PATHOPHYSIOLOGY OF DISEASE 663
THERAPEUTICS AND CLINICAL PHARMACOLOGY 665
Goals of Therapy 665
Therapeutics by Class 666
Barbiturates and Primidone 666
Phenytoin 667
Benzodiazepines 669
Succinimides 670
Carbamazepine and Oxcarbazepine 670
Valproate 672
Felbamate 673
Gabapentin and Pregabalin 673
Lamotrigine 674
Topiramate 674
Tiagabine 675
Zonisamide 675
Levetiracetam 676
Vigabatrin 676
Therapeutic Approach 677
Emerging Targets and Therapeutics 679

OVERVIEW

The story of drug treatment for seizures is virtually a history of drug treatment itself, as this area includes some of the oldest agents still in common use in the modern formulary, alongside the steady stream of new compounds that have been brought to market in the last 15 years—and continue to appear. As the pathophysiology of seizures remains almost wholly obscure, the methods of development have remained largely unchanged since the discovery of phenytoin's anticonvulsant effects by Merritt and Putnam in 1938.[1] This may have much to do with the fact that the new generation of antiepileptic drugs (AEDs), while bringing welcome improvements in safety and side effect profiles, has unfortunately done little to reduce the burden of drug-resistant epilepsy, which afflicts one third of seizure patients.[2] Thus, one may view the current state of epilepsy treatment as a great triumph of empiricism and a simultaneous demonstration of empiricism's limits.

Epilepsy (a disease for which the term *seizure disorder* is essentially a euphemism) afflicts an estimated 0.5% to 1% of the population in both developed and developing countries[3]—a sizable market from the pharmaceutical companies' perspective, but not one that justifies the large number of unique agents currently available and in development. The continued activity in this sphere is almost certainly a consequence of the expansion of this class of agents for uses other than seizures, including migraine (valproate, topiramate), pain (gabapentin, pregabalin), and psychiatric conditions such as bipolar disorder (lamotrigine). All of this makes it even more worthwhile for the clinician or pharmacology student to learn about this class of drugs. But if this is your first foray into the area, be forewarned: rather than a profusion of "me too" drugs that sort themselves into easy classes, the epilepsy field features a host of unique agents with considerable variation in pharmacologic properties, side effect profiles, and spectrum of action. What follows is an attempt to make more digestible an area that is inherently challenging even to those who use these drugs on a regular basis.

PATHOPHYSIOLOGY OF DISEASE

Since epilepsy can be defined as a predisposition to spontaneous seizures, it is helpful to understand the different types of seizures and of epilepsy syndromes. A *seizure* is a paroxysmal, rhythmic change in cortical electrical activity that is almost always accompanied by a change in behavior. This change may be purely subjective (i.e., sensory symptoms that are not apparent to an outside observer), and on occasion such electrical activity produces no symptoms at all—a so-called *subclinical* or *electrographic* seizure. A *focal* or *partial* seizure is one that originates in one hemisphere; the generator may be a small area, or a large multilobar network within a hemisphere, and the discharge may subsequently spread to involve both hemispheres diffusely. A *generalized* seizure originates from both hemispheres simultaneously. There are several different types of generalized seizures, the most common of which is the *tonic-clonic* ("grand mal") type in which loss of consciousness with tonic stiffening is followed by gradually increasing clonic (back-and-forth) muscle activity, all lasting about a minute. There are also isolated *clonic* seizures and isolated *tonic* seizures, each featuring the respective form of motor activity without the other kind, as well as the dreaded *atonic* seizures, in which the patient abruptly loses all muscle tone and collapses to the ground, frequently producing self-injury. Commonly seen in children are *absence* ("petit mal") seizures, episodes of loss of awareness and behavioral arrest for a few seconds, sometimes accompanied by eye fluttering, with the patient immediately returning to his or her previous activities as if nothing had happened (and usually unaware that anything has happened). Finally, *myoclonic* seizures—sudden, split-second, lightning-like contraction of a muscle or group of muscles, accompanied by a diffuse change on electroencephalography (EEG)—are often not mentioned by the patient and usually have little effect themselves on the patient's well-being but can provide very important clues to properly categorizing the patient's epilepsy syndrome.

This latter point bears some elaboration: it is important to recognize that the aforementioned seizure types are not haphazardly distributed among patients, but instead occur in discrete syndromes. For example, in the syndrome of juvenile myoclonic epilepsy, myoclonic seizures occur preferentially upon awakening in the morning, sometimes leading to a generalized tonic-clonic seizure, and with 10% to 30% of patients also experiencing absence seizures. A full discussion of epilepsy syndromes can be important for the proper use of AEDs in some patients but is far beyond the purview of this chapter; the reader is referred to a comprehensive textbook in the field for more information about this.[4] For our purposes here, it is enough to understand two principles: first, that the epilepsies are classified as *generalized* or *focal* (*partial*), depending on whether the patient is predisposed to generalized or focal seizures, respectively; and second, that the generalized epilepsies are further subdivided into *idiopathic* (*primary*) and *symptomatic* (*secondary*), with the former patients having normal intelligence and brain function, and the latter having generalized seizures secondary to some diffuse brain disease (e.g., congenital hypoxia, tuberous sclerosis) that has also produced mental retardation.

If you would like to learn more about the pathophysiology of epilepsy, then by all means join the rest of us—epilepsy is one of the few diseases in medicine for which our ability to treat far exceeds our understanding of the pathogenic mechanisms. It is widely believed that the primary generalized epilepsies are genetic in nature, and there are numerous specific genes that have been associated with various generalized epilepsy syndromes, only some of which have clearly identified functions. The inheritance and penetrance patterns appear to be complex, however, and the genes thus far discovered account for only a small percentage of patients with primary generalized epilepsy.[5]

The best understood of the seizure types from a pathophysiologic standpoint is the absence seizure. In this condition, brief lapses of consciousness are accompanied by generalized sharp-appearing discharges on EEG at a rate of three per second. Strong evidence suggests that these 3-Hz discharges are the product of reverberating circuits that link thalamic relay neurons with virtually the entire cerebral cortex in a diffuse fashion (Fig. 45-1). Neurons in the reticular nucleus of the thalamus act as intermediaries in this circuit, providing GABAergic inhibition (via $GABA_B$ receptors) to other thalamic neurons. This inhibition activates a slow depolarizing current, which in turn activates fast depolarizing calcium spikes via the low-threshhold, transient, "T-type" calcium current. After the calcium spikes, the cell becomes transiently hyperpolarized, and the cycle repeats itself. This circuit functions in the generation of normal oscillatory sleep activity, but appears to be appropriated for the generation of the generalized discharges.[6] The importance of the aforementioned circuit is reinforced by the fact that most anti-absence drugs block T-type calcium currents, while drugs that enhance stimulation of $GABA_B$ receptors (e.g., the γ-aminobutyric acid [GABA] uptake inhibitor tiagabine) may make these seizures worse, as does direct thalamic infusion of $GABA_B$ agonists in rat models.[7] The precise neurophysiologic alteration that permits this appropriation in afflicted patients remains unclear, however.

Focal epilepsy, at the "macro" level, may be caused by a host of focal lesions occurring anywhere in the cerebral cortex, including cortical dysplasias, neoplasms, heterotopias and hamartomas, congenital malformations, infarctions, hemorrhages, vascular malformations, traumatic injuries, and central nervous system infections of various kinds. The most well-studied cause of focal epilepsy is hippocampal sclerosis, a condition with a very particular pattern of neuronal cell loss and gliosis that differs from what is seen with anoxic damage, Alzheimer's disease, or other hippocampal pathologies.[8] Hippocampal sclerosis is often associated with a neurologic "hit" in childhood (e.g., a prolonged febrile seizure, meningitis), and it is likely the most common cause of drug-resistant focal epilepsy, often requiring resective surgery (discussed later in the chapter). Despite extensive study, and the striking success of hippocampal resection for this condition, it remains entirely unclear what it is about this condition that generates the seizures at a systems level.

At the "micro" level, seizures have been conceptualized as being due to excessive neuronal excitation, inadequate inhibition, or both. Focal

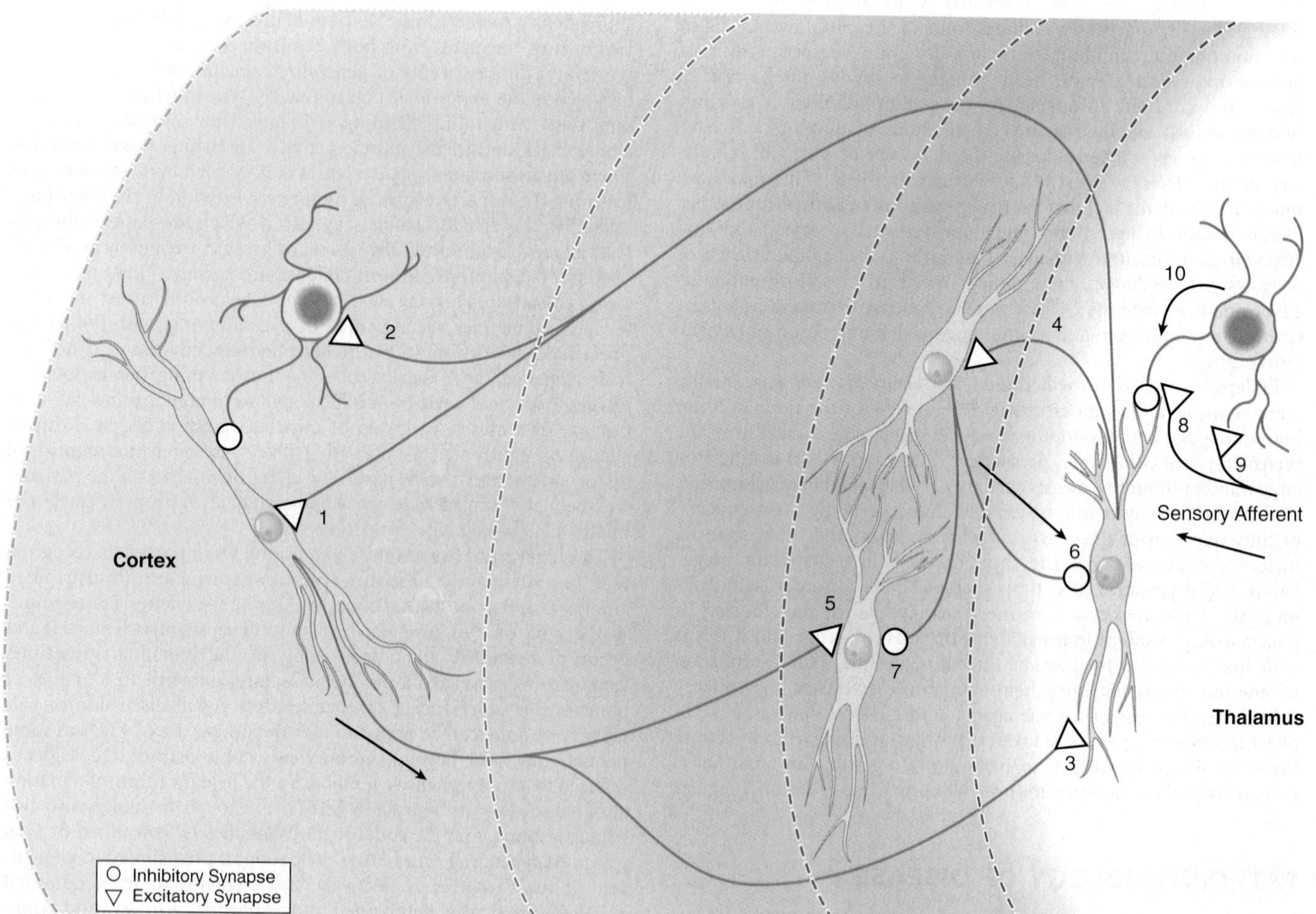

FIGURE 45-1A • The basic thalamocortical circuit. Thalamic neurons in primary sensory relay nuclei project to layers III/IV and V/VI of the cerebral cortex. This projection terminates both on pyramidal neurons (synapse 1) and on the inhibitory interneurons (synapse 2) in the cortex. Layer VI pyramidal neurons reciprocally innervate the same area as the thalamus from which an ascending afferent is received (synapse 3). Both the thalamocortical and corticothalamic projections send an axon collateral to the nucleus reticularis thalami (NRT; synapse 4 and 5). The NRT provides inhibitory GABAergic innervations to the thalamus (synapse 6) and to other NRT neurons (synapse 7). The major sensory afferents of the thalamus synapse onto the dendrites of both thalamic relay neurons (synapse 8) and inhibitory interneurons (synapse 9). The dendrites of inhibitory interneurons can function as both pre- and postsynaptic elements and can provide inhibitory innervation of thalamic relay neuron dendrites (synapse 10), as well as conventional axonal synaptic connections (synapse 10).

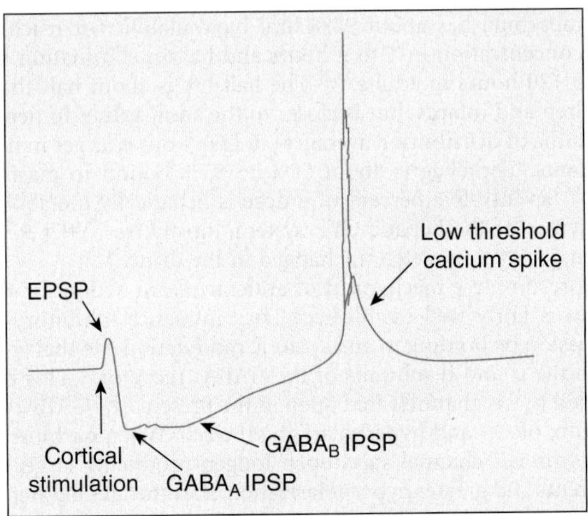

FIGURE 45-1B • Response of a thalamic neuron to stimulation of the corticothalamic afferents. Note that the stimulation triggers an excitatory postsynaptic potential/inhibitory postsynaptic potential (EPSP/IPSP) sequence, followed by a rebound low-threshold calcium spike. The EPSP is mediated by the corticothalamic afferent, and the IPSP is mediated by corticothalamic activation of the nucleus reticularis thalami (NRT), which, in turn, provides inhibitory innervation of the thalamus. Also note that the IPSP has two components, mediated by activation of GABA$_A$ and GABA$_B$ receptors. The IPSP-elicited hyperpolarization de-inactivates the T current in the thalamic neuron, which then triggers a rebound burst as the IPSP decays.

seizures are a product of groups of electrically hyperexcitable neurons that fire synchronously, producing a rhythmic, evolving electrical discharge. In between seizures, most such groups of neurons produce much briefer synchronous depolarizations; in electrical field recordings such as EEGs these manifest as sharp-appearing waves (*interictal epileptiform activity*, also called *spikes* or *sharp waves*). These waves—and presumably the seizures that arise from the same neurons—result from the summation of many *paroxysmal depolarizing shifts* in postsynaptic neurons, which have been presumed to be due to excitatory postsynaptic potentials resulting from neurotransmitter release by presynaptic neurons.[9,10] While recent evidence suggests that the excitatory neurotransmitters underlying many paroxysmal depolarizing shifts may come from astrocytes rather than neurons,[11] it is clear regardless that glutamate and its ionotropic receptors play a role in the generation of epileptiform activity. Some anticonvulsant drugs may work through glutamate, at least in part (e.g., *N*-methyl-D-aspartate [NMDA] receptor antagonism), while others may work by reducing fast-frequency neuronal firing so that less glutamate is released at the synapses. In an analogous fashion, GABA, the predominant inhibitory neurotransmitter in the central nervous system, can clearly impede the development of epileptiform activity and reduce seizures, and several anticonvulsant drugs (e.g., barbiturates, benzodiazepines, tiagabine) appear to exert their anticonvulsant properties by increasing synaptic GABA or potentiating its effects. It is worth noting that, in some circumstances (e.g., in absence seizures, as described previously), neuronal hypersynchrony may be produced by excessive, rather than inadequate, inhibition, depending on the epileptogenic circuitry.

One near-universal feature of seizures is that individual events terminate within a few minutes, or even seconds. If the pathophysiologic underpinnings of seizure onset are largely unknown, those underlying seizure termination remain even more obscure. Occasionally a seizure fails to terminate, resulting in an ongoing, rhythmic cortical discharge, usually with a profound clinical correlate, referred to as *status epilepticus.* It is presumed that the occurrence of a seizure engages inherent ictal termination mechanisms within the brain, and that status epilepticus results from failure of these termination mechanisms. Status epilepticus is a medical emergency under most circumstances, so that while the pharmacologic mechanisms engaged in combating it are similar to those employed for recurrent single seizures, the mode of delivery is generally more aggressive (e.g., intravenous [IV], rectal, etc.).

THERAPEUTICS AND CLINICAL PHARMACOLOGY

Goals of Therapy

It might seem intuitively evident that the fundamental goal of treatment in epilepsy is the complete prevention of seizures, yet this obvious conclusion is belied by the actual clinical practices of too many physicians, who consider patients "stable" if their seizure frequency is unchanging and opt to simply refill prescriptions rather than make aggressive attempts to eliminate seizures. Others pursue repeated medication trials far beyond the point of diminishing returns instead of pursuing nonpharmacologic options. These efforts are in part a product of the plethora of options for the treatment of epilepsy, and in part a product of fundamental misunderstandings about the challenges faced by seizure patients.

First and foremost, patients with active seizures suffer from a profound lack of independence, not only from the helplessness that must be endured with every seizure but also from the brute fact of being unable to legally drive a car. Both the pervasive sense of fear (of having a seizure at work, or in a social situation) and the driver's license revocation persist until the patient has been completely seizure-free for a period of time. Driving laws vary widely by state, but in many a seizure-free period of 6 months is required to legally drive, so that as few as two seizures per year are sufficient to completely curtail driving indefinitely. The psychosocial consequences of this lack of independence are often profound.

Beyond this, both declining cognitive function and increased mortality are important but often overlooked issues in patients with epilepsy. Mounting evidence suggests that recurrent seizures over many years are associated with structural damage to the brain[12] and declines in performance on cognitive tests.[13] This is particularly well established in patients with seizures arising from the mesial temporal lobes (e.g., those with hippocampal sclerosis), and the most prominent declines are seen in memory function, but the physical and functional changes extend well beyond these areas.[12,13] Mortality is also considerably elevated in patients with uncontrolled seizures, with standardized mortality ratios three times higher than those in the general population.[14] This relates to a host of causes, including sudden unexplained death in epilepsy. The latter appears not to occur when seizures are completely eliminated, but it can occur even when seizures are infrequent.[15]

It should not be surprising, then, that quality of life in patients with epilepsy is not significantly improved by treatment measures unless seizure freedom is obtained,[16] so complete seizure freedom should be aggressively sought in the majority of patients. There are some exceptions. Many patients with exclusively nocturnal seizures, or those who suffer only simple partial seizures (focal seizures without any impairment of awareness) can keep their driver's licenses and thus may feel far less burdened by their disease. A significant percentage of patients with symptomatic generalized epilepsy simply cannot be made seizure free by any means, but the vast majority of such patients are severely mentally retarded and thus do not drive, hold jobs, date, or the like. In these patients, the typical palliative goal of care is to reduce or eliminate seizures that are productive of self-injury, particularly atonic seizures. It is also worth noting that, in patients with simple partial seizures, it is not clear that mortality is elevated or that cognitive function is at risk; evidence addressing these issues is greatly needed. In addition, patients with idiopathic epilepsies appear to have mortality rates that are only modestly higher than the general population,[17] and may not experience cognitive decline, though all the other aforementioned difficulties of epilepsy apply, making seizure freedom the appropriate goal for such patients anyway.

Aside from seizure freedom, two other important factors are highly relevant to therapy goals. The first is depression, which is rampant among patients with epilepsy and makes a very strong—some might say overwhelming[18]—contribution to quality of life.[19] Depression should be assiduously sought in this population, and aggressively treated—without fear of antidepressants lowering the seizure threshold, which appears to be more myth than reality.[20] The treatment of comorbid depression in epilepsy is largely similar to that employed in the general population, which is covered in more detail in Chapter 53 (Depression and Bipolar Disorders).

The second factor, particularly relevant to this chapter, is that of medication side effects. The vast majority of patients who suffer seizures take medications for prolonged periods of time—at least 2 years, and often lifelong. Thus, any medication side effects that amount to more than a minor nuisance can become a significant and persistent problem. Paradoxically, the most obvious side effects are often the ones least likely to affect quality of life: a patient who becomes severely dizzy, or nauseated, or sleepy, will almost certainly register a complaint, with a resultant change of medication (or, failing an appropriate response, a change of physician). But many of the side effects of anticonvulsants can be insidious, or not obviously connected to the drug in the patient's or physician's mind, thereby remaining "under the radar" and possibly producing a prolonged negative impact: cognitive impairment with topiramate, weight gain with valproate, irritability with levetiracetam, or lamotrigine-induced insomnia are all examples of the latter.

Just as patients are often implicitly "told" by their physicians that they must live with seizures (rather than pursuing other forms of aggressive treatment), so too are patients often implicitly given the message that they must live with medication side effects as an unavoidable concomitant to their epilepsy treatment. As an illustration of this, the author once received a panicked call from a generally stoic patient who insisted that her phenytoin blood level must have dropped because she felt "too good." (She was right!) In truth, anticonvulsant side effects are rarely, if ever, unavoidable, particularly in light of the number of drug options currently available (see the section on Therapeutic Approach later). In fact, detailed efforts to uncover and ameliorate medication side effects result in improved quality of life in the majority of patients with epilepsy, even those who were being seen in tertiary epilepsy centers.[21] It should also be noted that, even when patients tolerate medications well, there may be detrimental metabolic effects that can cause significant difficulty; thus, valproate is frequently associated with the development of symptoms of polycystic ovary syndrome, particularly in women with primary generalized epilepsy,[22] while drugs that induce the cytochrome P-450 (CYP) enzyme system may produce bone loss,[23-25] sexual dysfunction,[26] or abnormalities in serum lipids and other serologic indices of vascular risk.[27]

In status epilepticus, the goal of treatment simply becomes complete cessation of seizures as quickly as possible. In resistant cases, or when there is serious comorbid medical illness, it may be tricky to accomplish this without undue suppression of blood pressure or respiration from the high doses of IV agents required.

Therapeutics by Class

The agents in common use against seizures are presented in this section in chronologic order of their entry (or the entry of the first drug of the class) into the U.S. market. Note that, where not specifically cited, pharmacokinetics and usage data have been obtained from the manufacturer's package insert. Drugs that are only occasionally used as anticonvulsants under specific circumstances (e.g., acetazolamide, adrenocorticotropic hormone, propofol) are not discussed.

Barbiturates and Primidone

While the first truly effective antiepileptic agents were the bromides, barbiturates are the oldest anticonvulsants still in clinical use. These are derivatives of barbituric acid, and the most prominent member of this class by far is phenobarbital, which was first developed for human use as a sedative-hypnotic agent in 1912 and inadvertantly found to be an effective anticonvulsant. Mephobarbital, which is metabolized into phenobarbital but also has independent anticonvulsant properties, is virtually unused at present.

Phenobarbital has about 95% oral bioavailability. It reaches peak serum concentration in 1 to 3 hours and has an elimination half-life of 90 to 120 hours in adults.[28,29] The half-life is about half that value in children and infants, but is closer to the adult values in neonates.[30] The volume of distribution averages 0.6 L/kg[28] but is larger in neonates and infants. The drug is about 50% to 55% bound to plasma proteins.[31,32] Seventy-five percent of a dose is hepatically metabolized by the enzymes of the hepatic CYP system, mostly by CYP2C9.[33,34] The remaining 25% is excreted unchanged in the urine.[34]

The presumptive mechanism of anticonvulsant action for the barbiturates is fairly well established. They influence inhibitory neurotransmission by binding to an allosteric modulation site that is present on both the α and β subunits of the $GABA_A$ receptor.[35] This receptor is coupled to Cl^- channels that open in the presence of GABA, permitting influx of Cl^- and hyperpolarizing the cell. When barbiturates are present, the Cl^- channel stays open longer, producing larger inward Cl^- currents and greater hyperpolarization. Barbiturates neither change the frequency of channel opening nor increase its conductance.[36]

Phenobarbital is clearly effective for both focal seizures and generalized tonic-clonic seizures,[37] though the evidence is imperfect owing to the "grandfathered" status of the compound. It is clearly ineffective for absence seizures, and there is little evidence concerning its effect on myoclonic seizures. The drug is used in all age groups, though it is not considered a first-line drug, particularly in adults,[38] owing to widespread concerns about its side effects. While there is strong clinical experience informing these concerns, the evidentiary basis for this is mixed.[39] Nonetheless it certainly has a place, particularly for economic reasons: it costs mere pennies per tablet, thus making it an option for patients in developing countries, or for those in the United States who lack the means to obtain other drugs. In addition, it remains the drug of choice for neonatal seizures, as intravenous phenytoin can be particularly difficult to use in neonates owing to the nonlinear pharmacokinetics, and more recently introduced IV agents have not been studied.

In adults, phenobarbital may be prescribed once per day at a dose of 1 to 3 mg/kg per day, more commonly at the low end of this range. Dosing in children is similar, while neonates and infants are given doses at the upper end of this range. Phenobarbital is also available in an IV form that is used for rapid loading of the drug or for status epilepticus. In this context, it is typically given in doses of 15 to 20 mg/kg at a rate of no more than 100 mg/min. The typical target serum level for therapy is 15 to 40 mg/dl; for patients in status epilepticus, especially neonates, even higher doses may be sought.

The most common and notorious side effects of phenobarbital are sedation, depression of mood, and cognitive impairment.[40] Behavioral side effects, particularly hyperactivity, are also common in children. Rash, hepatotoxicity, and bone marrow suppression are uncommon but potentially serious risks. Baseline and periodic monitoring of blood counts and liver function is often performed. In addition, barbiturates are very potent inducers of the CYP system,[41] thereby increasing the hepatic metabolism of a host of compounds. This itself may lead to significant metabolic side effects, including megaloblastic anemia and osteopenia (both presumably due to effects on serum vitamin levels)[42,43] and elevated cholesterol.[44,45] These effects are elaborated in more detail in the later section on phenytoin. CYP induction also leads to a very large number of drug interactions, particularly reductions in the serum levels of other agents, including other AEDs; most of the drugs mentioned in the phenytoin and carbamazepine sections of this chapter are likely also affected by barbiturates. As a practical matter, it is probably wise to assume that any other drug the patient is taking that is hepatically metabolized might have a reduced circulating level in the presence of phenobarbital. Conversely, other drugs that induce or inhibit CYP2C19 may reduce or increase, respectively, the serum level of phenobarbital. Thus, its level is reduced in the presence of phenytoin, and increased when given concurrently with valproate.[46,47]

Pentobarbital is an IV barbiturate that is employed regularly as a treatment for refractory status epilepticus or to induce coma in patients with severe brain injury. In this setting, it is given intravenously at doses of 1 to 5 mg/kg per hour after a load of 5 to 15 mg/kg. It is heavily sedating and produces marked respiratory suppression, so that its use requires intubation and mechanical ventilation. For this reason, it is held in abeyance until other drugs have failed to break the seizures. Pentobarbital is hepatically metabolized and has a half-life of 18 to 48 hours,[48] so if a pentobarbital-treated critically ill patient is oversedated, expect to wait 1 to 2 days before dose reduction has any clinical effect.

Primidone, developed in 1952, is very similar to phenobarbital in structure, but with a single carbonyl group replaced. It has two major metabolites, one of which is phenobarbital itself; studies have estimated that roughly 20% to 25% of a dose of primidone is metabolized into phenobarbital.[49,50] The other metabolite is phenylethylmalonamide (PEMA), the potency of whose anticonvulsant properties remains uncertain but is probably low.[51] Because of the complexity of its metabolism, it has been difficult to parse out the effects of the parent compound proper, which has very low protein binding, excellent distribution across the blood-brain barrier, a volume of distribution similar to that of phenobarbital, and a half-life of 10 to 15 hours.[52-54] Primidone is clearly more than just a phenobarbital prodrug, however, as demonstrated by its well-established therapeutic effect in essential tremor, for which it is a drug of first choice; neither phenobarbital nor PEMA has any efficacy in this regard.[55,56] In fact, primidone is probably used far more for essential tremor than for epilepsy in contemporary neurologic practice. This is reinforced by the results of a large, randomized trial demonstrating that primidone was clearly less well tolerated than other equally efficacious anticonvulsants (as was phenobarbital).[37] Nonetheless, the drug is effective for focal and secondarily generalized seizures, and it is also effective for primary generalized tonic-clonic seizures. All the aforementioned side effects of phenobarbital apply to primidone. In addition, the drug seems to produce a syndrome of acute toxicity in some patients, with drowsiness, dizziness, ataxia, and nausea occurring after a single dose, so it is extremely important to start the drug very gradually—125 mg once daily, increasing every several days to a target dose of 10 to 20 mg/kg per day. This is traditionally divided into three daily doses because of the short half-life of the parent compound in some patients. However, the utility of measuring primidone levels is unclear, and phenobarbital levels are generally used to target therapy. Like phenobarbital, primidone is not considered a first-line AED at present.[38]

Phenytoin

Phenytoin remains the veritable "granddaddy" of AEDs, at least in the United States, where it is probably the most commonly prescribed anticonvulsant. Any discussion of the drug must begin with its unusual pharmacokinetics. Phenytoin is one of the only drugs in the modern formulary for which the appropriate metabolizing enzymes—in this case, CYP2C9 and CYP2C19—saturate around doses that are typically used in clinical practice. The precise saturation point varies among patients, but the net effect of this property is that, when increasing a patient's phenytoin dose, the increase in serum level may not be proportional: if the metabolizing enzymes have been saturated, then all additional drug remains active in the serum, increasing the concentration by far more than the relative dose increase. Thus, a graph of dose versus concentration will not be a straight line (Fig. 45-2)—a phenomenon referred to as *nonlinear kinetics* (which inevitably makes its way into exam questions). This can make dose adjustment difficult (see later). It also makes the elimination half-life dependent upon the serum concentration. To understand why, consider that half-life is equal to

$$0.693 * V_d * (K_m + C)/V_{max}$$

where V_d is the volume of distribution, C is the serum concentration of the drug, V_{max} is the maximum velocity of the relevant enzyme(s), and K_m is the concentration at which the enzyme system attains half of maximum velocity—or, to put it colloquially, a measure of how much the enzyme system can handle (see Chapter 13, Pharmacokinetics, for more detailed discussion of these parameters). All of these are essentially constant for a given drug except for C, of course, which will vary according to the administered dose. For almost all drugs, C is considerably lower than K_m, so it contributes little to the equation. But for phenytoin, typical therapeutic serum concentrations—ranging from 10 to 20 mcg/ml—are about two to four times larger than the typical K_m, so that C affects the equation considerably, making elimination half-life directly proportional to concentration.[57] In the vast majority of adult patients, elimination half-life is over 12 hours even at subtherapeutic concentrations, and over 24 hours once therapeutic levels are reached. V_{max} is about 50% greater in children, reducing the half-life,[58] but nearly all children had a half-life of 12 hours or more at therapeutic serum concentrations.[59]

The vast majority of a dose of phenytoin is hepatically metabolized by the aforementioned CYP isoenzymes into inactive metabolites, which are then glucuronidated.[57] Bioavailability of the original brand-name drug (Dilantin), a sustained-release capsule, is approximately 86%, but bioavailability may be different with other formulations. Complicating matters further is the fact that 30-mg and 100-mg cap-

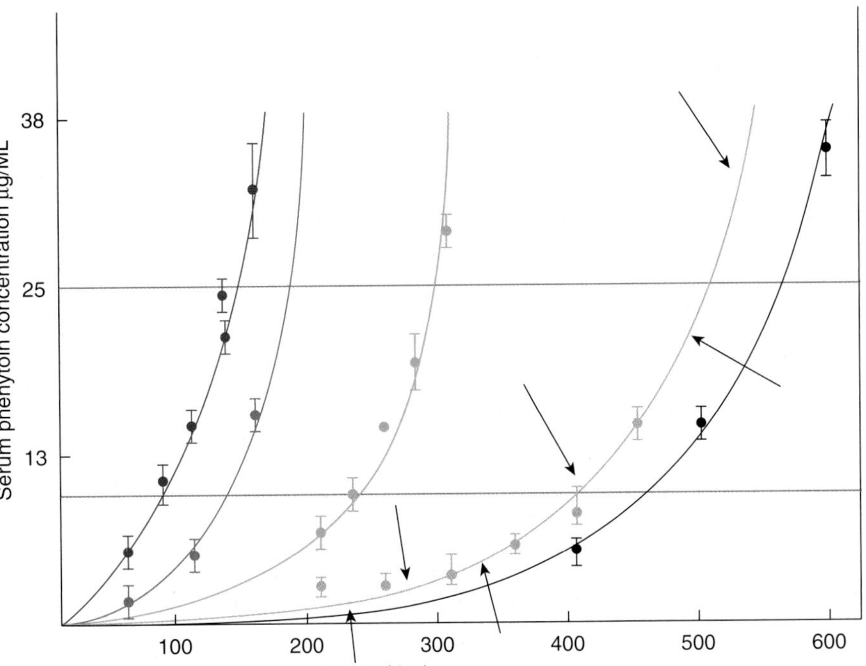

FIGURE 45-2A • Relationship between serum phenytoin concentration and daily dose in five patients. Each point represents the mean (± standard deviation) of three to eight measurements of serum phenytoin concentration at steady state. The curves were fitted by computer using the Michaelis-Menton equation.

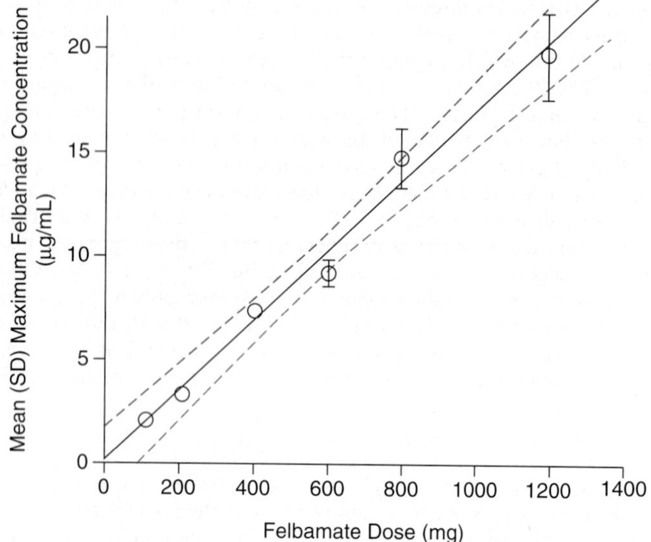

FIGURE 45-2B • Felbamate concentration versus dose.

sules are made using the sodium salt, while 50-mg immediate-release chewable tablets are made using the acid, which contains 8.5% more phenytoin on a milligram-for-milligram basis. For most drugs, the significance of these variances would be dubious, but for phenytoin, in light of the nonlinear kinetics, they may be significant, so it is wise to use one preparation rather than "mixing and matching" and to avoid changing it unless it is necessary.

Phenytoin appears to exert its anticonvulsant properties via neuronal Na^+ channels, but it is not a simple Na^+ channel blocker. Instead it appears to bind to the channels in their inactive state and increase the time it takes for them to recover to the active state. The result of this action is that neurons fire action potentials of normal amplitude and duration, but the prolonged recovery time limits high-frequency firing.[60] This limitation of high-frequency firing is also voltage dependent, being less prominent when the cell is hyperpolarized and more prominent when the cell is depolarized; this property should reduce the tendency of neurons to fire rapid, repetitive action potentials in the setting of a paroxysmal depolarizing shift.

Phenytoin is quite effective for focal seizures with and without secondary generalization. It is also sometimes effective for primary generalized tonic-clonic seizures, but less so than valproate[61] and possibly less so than the other "broad-spectrum" anticonvulsants (lamotrigine, topiramate, zonisamide, levetiracetam). In addition, it helps little for atonic seizures, has no effect on absence seizures, and is more likely to worsen patients with myoclonic seizures than to improve them.[62,63] As a consequence, phenytoin is of little use in patients with generalized epilepsies and is not considered a first choice for such patients.[38] Phenytoin is also manufactured in an IV preparation formulated with a mixture of solvents, including propylene glycol and alcohol in an extremely basic solution (pH 12); this form of phenytoin is generally considered first-line treatment for focal or generalized convulsive status epilepticus.

The saturable hepatic metabolism, the bioavailability variations, the extensive (90%) protein binding, and the fact that phenytoin (like the barbiturates) is a potent inducer of CYP isoenzymes combine to make phenytoin one of the most difficult drugs in the entire modern pharmacopeia to use properly. It is ironic, then, that widespread use of the drug in America continues to be perpetuated by non-neurologists who tend to be unfamiliar with its complexities. For example, the traditional knee-jerk practice of acutely loading an adult patient with 1000 mg of IV phenytoin, followed by chronic outpatient therapy at 100 mg orally three times daily, is wrong on both counts. When there is a need to get the drug on board in an effective dose quickly, loading doses of 15 to 20 mg/kg are used; this can be IV (given at a rate no faster than 50 mg/min) or oral (usually divided into two oral doses several hours apart), but a dose of 1 g will likely be inadequate for all but petite women. Outpatient therapy in adults is initiated at 4 to 7 mg/kg per day, generally once daily, so that the 300-mg daily dose is likely to undershoot for all but small-sized adults, and the thrice-daily dosing will encourage noncompliance in a disease state in which compliance is crucial. In children 10 years or older, initial dosing should be twice daily at the high end of the adult range (6 to 8 mg/kg per day), and in younger children it should be even higher (8 to 10 mg/kg per day).[64]

When phenytoin is loaded, serum levels may be checked within hours. Subsequent dose adjustments must be made carefully, as it is hard to know when enzyme saturation will occur. A good rule of thumb is to increase the dose by 100 mg daily if the level is below the traditional therapeutic range of 10 to 20 mcg/ml, but to increase by only 30 to 50 mg daily if the level is within that range. Be prepared to wait several weeks to reliably assess the results of the change, particularly with higher levels, because the time to reach steady state is increased as serum concentration increases due to the nonlinear kinetics.[57] In the acute hospital setting, when higher levels are needed, take the level you want (say, 20 mcg/ml), subtract the level you have (say, 11 mcg/ml), and divide this by the V_d of phenytoin, which is about 0.8 L/kg in non-neonates, to arrive at the additional loading dose needed (in this example, $9/0.8 \cong 11$ mg/kg). Maintenance doses—but not loading doses—should be lower in patients with hepatic failure. Renal failure should theoretically have no effect upon phenytoin dosing, but in practice patients with renal failure are often hypoalbuminemic, resulting in a larger free fraction of phenytoin than would be expected and necessitating lower daily doses. Phenytoin is not significantly dialyzed,[65,66] but dialysis may increase the protein binding of phenytoin by opening up binding sites, resulting in lower free fractions even when total serum phenytoin is unchanged.[67] In fact, since only nonbound phenytoin is pharmacologically active, measurements of free phenytoin (generally 10% of total, or 1.0 to 2.0 mcg/ml as a therapeutic target) are a more accurate gauge of effective drug level in all patients. As a practical matter, these levels are more expensive and take much longer to obtain, however, and the free fraction remains constant in a given patient unless there are systemic changes that affect protein binding, so one strategy is to obtain both total and free serum levels simultaneously on one occasion, determine the free fraction for that patient, and then follow total levels thereafter.

With regard to adverse effects, yet another myth concerning phenytoin—and other AEDs—is that serum levels above 20 mcg/ml are somehow "toxic" and necessitate immediate dose decrease. This is often done even when the level has been obtained in the emergency room after presentation for a recurrent seizure—precisely when an acute reduction in drug dose is the least helpful course of action. In point of fact, while many patients will complain of acute side effects at such levels, there is nothing inherently "toxic" or dangerous about phenytoin levels in the 20s, or even in the 30s (stratospheric levels of 40 mcg/ml or more may lead to paradoxical seizure exacerbation, however), and patients with elevated levels who have no complaints should be left alone. The acute dose-related side effects of phenytoin include sedation, dizziness, cognitive impairment, nausea, ataxia, and nystagmus. Choreiform and other extrapyramidal movement disorders occasionally occur but are reversible.[68] Medically dangerous side effects include rash (which can assume the very severe forms of Stevens-Johnson syndrome or toxic epidermal necrolysis), and hepatic toxicity; the latter may be more common in African Americans, generally occurs within 6 weeks of exposure to the drug, and virtually always occurs in association with a rash, suggesting that it is a hypersensitivity-mediated reaction.[69] Phenytoin can also cause declines in neutrophils, red cells, platelets, or all three, and rarely even full-blown aplastic anemia. Periodic monitoring of both blood counts and liver function is traditionally performed, at least in the early stages of treatment, though it is of uncertain benefit. Acute IV administration of phenytoin can cause hypotension and cardiac arrhythmia (in fact, phenytoin is considered a class Ib antiarrythmic and was for many years the treatment of choice for digitalis toxicity). This limits its IV infusion rate to

50 mg/min. The IV preparation is toxic to tissue—possibly due to the propylene glycol vehicle, or the strongly basic pH of the solution—and can cause phlebitis or, with extravasation, tissue necrosis. More rare is the "purple glove syndrome," in which edema, purplish discoloration, and pain occur in the limb in which an IV phenytoin infusion has been given. This can occasionally be severe, even causing ulcerations and necessitating skin grafts,[70] but a prospective study found the incidence to be only 1.7%, with all cases being mild.[71] Intravenous phenytoin precipitates in dextrose and so must never be mixed in a dextrose solution.

Many other side effects of phenytoin are more insidious. Among the most common are cosmetic effects, which include gingival hyperplasia (the scorn of dentists, seen in perhaps 50% of phenytoin-treated patients), hirsutism, and coarsening of facial features with long-standing use. These changes may be particularly problematic in women, causing some to forswear its use. Chronic neurologic toxicity may include peripheral neuropathy and atrophy of the cerebellum, though the association of phenytoin with the former is not fully established, while the latter, strangely, is never symptomatic. Perhaps most importantly, phenytoin can produce a host of chronic metabolic effects, likely owing to its potent induction of hepatic CYP isoenzymes and other enzymes. Folate deficiency is reported to be common and may contribute to elevated homocysteine or, more rarely, megaloblastic anemia.[72,73] The decades-long suspicion that phenytoin is bad for bone mass has had recent confirmation, with one large community-based study showing clear acceleration of osteopenia among phenytoin-treated elderly women[23] and other studies demonstrating hypocalcemia and evidence of elevated bone turnover.[74] Men on phenytoin have significant decreases in circulating serum testosterone and significantly lower sexual function scores than those treated with nothing or with a noninducing drug.[26] The author's own work,[27] together with some work already published,[75] suggests that phenytoin may also have significant adverse effects upon serum lipids and other vascular risk factors.

Finally, phenytoin is involved in a host of drug interactions. Some of these are a product of its extensive protein binding, with competition for available binding sites on albumin, but most are a result of its extensive enzyme-inducing properties, which cause levels of other hepatically metabolized drugs to be reduced. The list of drugs that may interact with phenytoin is so extensive as to be beyond the scope of this chapter, but a few of these are particularly noteworthy. Phenytoin reduces the levels of oral contraceptive hormones to the point where their efficacy may be reduced[76]; while some advocate higher dose hormone preparations to combat this, there is no evidence establishing the utility of this approach, and the author's policy is to have the patient choose either a new anticonvulsant or a new method of contraception. Certain drugs with narrow therapeutic indices, such as warfarin and digoxin, may have their levels reduced to an extent that jeopardizes their therapeutic benefit. Antineoplastic agents may also fall into this category; in fact, a recent study in glioblastoma patients found that those treated with phenytoin had a shorter life expectancy than those treated with noninducing AEDs, presumably because of reduction of the effect of the chemotherapeutic agent.[77] Both cyclosporine and corticosteroids are significantly reduced with phenytoin co-medication; this, combined with its other pharmacokinetic and metabolic complexities, suggests that phenytoin is poorly suited for use in the transplant population. As with phenobarbital, it is probably best to assume that any heptically metabolized drug might be reduced in effectiveness or require higher doses when phenytoin is used.

Fos-phenytoin is an intravenous phenytoin prodrug consisting of a phenytoin molecule esterified to a monophosphate moiety. The latter is rapidly cleaved by nonspecific phosphorylases in the circulation and in local tissues, yielding phenytoin; this reaction has a half-life of approximately 10 minutes. Fos-phenytoin is mixed in a simple aqueous solution, which makes it nonirritating to vascular and dermal tissues. It also does not precipitate in dextrose. It can be administered at rates up to 150 mg/min, three times faster than phenytoin, though the additional time necessary for the phosphate group to be cleaved prevents the drug from reaching a therapeutic concentration much faster. It can also be administered intramuscularly, which is occasionally beneficial in circumstances in which rapid onset of action is needed but IV access is limited. Because of the additional phosphate group, fos-phenytoin weighs more than phenytoin, such that the former is equivalent to the latter in a 3:2 ratio. To avoid confusion, fos-phenytoin is dosed in "phenytoin equivalents," or PEs, so that if a patient requires a dose of 1200 mg of phenytoin, you may order 1200 mg *PE* of fos-phenytoin instead. In comparison to IV phenytoin, fos-phenytoin produces less local venous irritation, is less injurious with extravasation, does not produce the purple glove syndrome, and may produce less hypotension[78]; it is not clear that the incidence of cardiac arrhythmia is different. Whether or not this justifies the marked price difference between the two is a matter of considerable debate within hospital formulary committees.

Benzodiazepines

Available since the marketing of chlordiazepoxide in 1957, benzodiazepines retain a unique and prominent place as drugs of first choice for the acute treatment of seizures. The ones primarily used in this capacity in the United States are diazepam and lorazepam; midazolam, a very short-acting agent, is also used for the treatment of refractory status epilepticus. The utility of benzodiazepines as chronic anticonvulsants is severely limited by tolerance to their effects; the only one used commonly for this indication in the United States is clonazepam (occasionally clorazepate is also used this way). Nitrazepam and clobazam are used in other countries for long-term daily treatment but are not available in the United States at present and are not discussed further.

Benzodiazepines exert their effects via $GABA_A$ receptors, though not as direct agonists. Instead, they bind to an allosteric modulation site on the $GABA_A$ receptor that is distinct from the one to which barbiturates bind. The $GABA_A$ receptor is linked to a Cl^- channel that, when opened, causes Cl^- influx and hyperpolarization of the neuron. When both GABA and benzodiazepines are bound to the receptor, there is much more frequent channel opening than there is in the presence of GABA alone.[79] The duration of individual channel opening is the same, however. This contrasts with the actions of barbiturates, which cause the Cl^- channel to open at the same frequency but stay open longer.[36]

Clonazepam has about 90% bioavailability, a time to peak concentration (T_{max}) of 1 to 4 hours, and a V_d of 1.5 to 4.4 L/kg; is 86% bound to plasma proteins; and is hepatically metabolized by CYP3A4 to inactive metabolites. The elimination half-life is 17 to 56 hours.[80] It is predominantly used to treat myoclonic seizures, as well as the atypical absence seizures of the Lennox-Gastaut syndrome; its chronic effectiveness for other seizure types, such as absence, is limited by tolerance to its anticonvulsant effects.[81] In adults, therapy may be initiated at 0.5 mg twice daily and increased by a similar amount every 3 days up to 1 to 2 mg twice daily; in children start with 0.01 to 0.03 mg/kg divided twice daily and increase by 0.25 to 0.5 mg every 3 days to a target of 0.2 mg/kg. Sedation, depression, and incoordination are the predominant side effects.

Diazepam is available in oral, IV, and rectal formulations. The oral and IV forms have essentially complete bioavailability, and the rectal is about 90% bioavailable. T_{max} is 30 to 90 minutes orally[82] and 30 to 60 minutes rectally.[83] The drug is over 95% protein bound, and concentrations in the cerebrospinal fluid (CSF) are equal to the unbound plasma fraction.[84] The volume of distribution is approximately 1 L/kg. The drug is almost completely metabolized by CYP isoenzymes 2C19 and 3A4 into desmethyldiazepam, oxazepam, and temazepam, which are highly active metabolites.[85] Thus, while diazepam has a typical half-life of 40 hours, this can be much longer in patients with less activity of 2C19; furthermore, even this is misleading regarding the duration of its activity, because desmethyldiazepam reaches concentrations higher than that of diazepam itself and has an elimination half-life of 3 days or more. Despite this, the drug's clinical utility is limited by its two-stage distribution process, with initial rapid distribution across the blood-brain barrier followed by rapid redistribution out of the brain into adipose and other peripheral tissues, resulting in an initial-phase brain half-life of only 30 minutes.[86] The half-life is halved in children and adolescents.[87] For acute indications, the IV dose is 10 to 20 mg in adults or 0.25 to 0.5 mg/kg in children, given at a rate of 1 to 5 mg/min, while the rectal dose is similar (0.5 mg/kg in young children, 0.3 mg/kg in school-age children, 0.2 mg/kg in adolescents or adults). For short-term oral use, doses of 5 to 10 mg up to twice daily are used in adults.

Lorazepam, available in oral and IV formulations, is often considered the drug of choice for status epilepticus. Oral bioavailability is over 94%, with a T_{max} of 1 to 2 hours and a V_d of 0.85 to 1.5 L/kg.[88] It is 93% bound to plasma proteins,[89] and CSF concentrations are 10% to 15% of those in plasma.[90] The large majority of a dose is hepatically glucuronidated into an active metabolite.[91] The elimination half-life of the drug in patients over the age of 7 years ranges from 17 to 56 hours[88,92]; it is much longer in neonates, and likely longer than adults in children under age 3. Acute IV dosing for status epilepticus is up to 0.1 mg/kg in children and adults (in adults this may be given in rapid, serial 2-mg increments until seizures are controlled in an effort to avoid respiratory suppression and mechanical ventilation).

Midazolam, a short-acting IV agent, is used only in cases of refractory status epilepticus, typically after both phenytoin and phenobarbital have failed to control seizures. It is very highly protein bound, produces maximal effects within a few minutes, and is completely metabolized by CYP3A4, with a half-life of 1.5 to 4 hours, into much less active metabolites.[93] Because of its short duration of effect, it is given as an IV bolus of 0.2 mg/kg followed by a continuous IV infusion at 0.1 to 0.5 mg/kg per hour.

Side effects of all benzodiazepines are similar, and include sedation, depression, and incoordination with oral use, and sedation and respiratory suppression with parental administration. With the exception of myoclonic seizures, tolerance to the anticonvulsant effects of benzodiazepines develop within weeks to months (reviewed extensively by Löscher and Schmidt[94]), so that chronic oral use is unlikely to be beneficial; in fact, because of the tendency of the drugs to produce withdrawal seizures upon discontinuation, chronic use is more likely to be problematic than beneficial. While oral benzodiazepines do not cause significant respiratory suppression by themselves, they may do so in the presence of other sedative agents. Intravenous use of more than modest doses of these agents is likely to necessitate mechanical ventilation.

Succinimides

This class consists of two drugs in current clinical use: Ethosuximide, the original member of the class, was developed in 1958 and remains a mainstay of treatment for absence seizures, while methsuximide has a broader spectrum of action but more side effects and is used rarely. Ethosuximide was the first drug to ever demonstrate effectiveness against absence seizures. It has a T_{max} of 3 to 5 hours[95] with near-complete bioavailability. V_d is 0.7 L/kg. It is completely unbound by plasma proteins, and CSF concentrations are comparable to those in blood.[96] About 80% of a dose of ethosuximide is metabolized hepatically, almost all by CYP3A4,[97] with the remaining 20% excreted unchanged in urine. The elimination half-life of the drug is quite long, averaging 50 hours in adults[95] and 35 hours in children.[98]

Ethosuximide appears to exert its actions via blockade of voltage-dependent T-type Ca^{2+} channels in the thalamus,[99] which have been strongly implicated in the pathogenesis of absence seizures (see discussion earlier in the chapter). It has no relevant effects on voltage-gated Na^+ channels, or on the release of excitatory or inhibitory neurotransmitters, consistent with its status as the "one-trick pony" of epilepsy therapeutics: It is ineffective for virtually all seizure types besides absence. For that purpose, children generally require doses of 20 to 40 mg/kg per day, but therapy should be initiated at one third to one half that dose and gradually increased over 1 to 2 weeks. In adults or older children, initiation is at 250 mg once daily, with increases of 250 to 500 mg/week up to a target of 750 to 2000 mg/day. While the half-life of the drug should permit once-daily dosing, it is usually given two or three times daily to minimize gastrointestinal upset, which is a common problem. Dosing may be guided by plasma levels, with the generally accepted therapeutic range for ethosuximide being 40 to 100 mcg/ml. Serum levels, and repeated EEGs with hyperventilation, may be particularly useful and important in treating absence epilepsy, a condition in which patients are frequently unaware of their seizures.

The use of ethosuximide is limited by the fact that many patients with absence seizures also suffer from generalized tonic-clonic or myoclonic seizures for which ethosuximide will be ineffective; in these patients, another "broad-spectrum" drug such as lamotrigine or valproate is generally preferable. Another drawback of ethosuximide is the common occurrence of side effects. Gastrointestinal complaints are very common, sometimes requiring dose reduction or dosing with meals. More typical AED side effects, including sedation, dizziness, and fatigue, are also fairly common. Another category of side effects from ethosuximide is that of behavioral changes, ranging from irritability and aggression to depression to frank psychosis. Headaches are reported in a fair number of children on ethosuximide. Extrapyramidal reactions, including dystonia, akathisia, and parkinsonism, have been reported with chronic use. Dose-related granulocytopenia can be seen and improves when the dose is lowered, but more significant hematologic reactions, including pancytopenia and full-blown aplastic anemia, which may be fatal, may very rarely be seen.[100] Allergic skin reactions, occasionally severe, may also be seen.

Methsuximide is approved for use against absence seizures (though it may be less effective than ethosuximide), but it is also effective against partial seizures and all other types of generalized seizures, including myoclonic seizures.[101] Its mechanisms of action are unknown, though based on its structural similarity to ethosuximide, one might infer that it shares a similar anti-absence mechanism. It is absorbed completely, has a T_{max} of 1 to 4 hours, does not bind to plasma proteins, and is rapidly (half-life ~ 2 hours) converted to an active metabolite, *N*-desmethylmethsuximide, which is itself hepatically metabolized with a mean half-life of 40 hours and is 45% to 60% protein bound.[102] The acute toxic side effects are similar to those of ethosuximide but more common, and rash can occur, but severe hepatic or hematologic toxicity has not been documented. Therapy is initiated at 300 mg/day (or half that in children) and titrated by that amount every 1 to 2 weeks to a target of 10 mg/kg, divided two to three times daily, like ethosuximide, to minimize side effects. Tolerability has limited the use of methsuximide, though it can occasionally be a helpful adjunct, particularly in patients with refractory primary generalized epilepsy, in whom options are limited.

Carbamazepine and Oxcarbazepine

Carbamazepine, a compound related to the tricyclic antidepressants, was first marketed in the United States in 1974. It rapidly became a preferred treatment option for patients with focal epilepsy, primarily because it demonstrated efficacy equal to phenytoin but without any of the latter's cosmetic side effects.[37] Even today, carbamazepine is still generally considered the "gold standard" of therapy for partial seizures and is the drug most often used as a head-to-head comparitor with other drugs. Whether it should remain the first choice for therapy in the face of so many new competitors is a matter of considerable debate.[38,103]

Carbamazepine is thought to have incomplete bioavailability,[104] though one study comparing an IV solution with an oral syrup found the latter to be fully bioavailable, with a V_d of about 1 L/kg.[105] T_{max} varies considerably depending on the preparation, with the suspension peaking at 1.5 hours, the immediate-release tablet around 4.5 hours, the extended-release capsules at 6 hours, and another brand of extended-release tablets peaking in a range between 3 and 12 hours. Note that these values apply to chronic administration of the drug; initial T_{max} times are longer (see later). Carbamazepine is about 75% bound to plasma proteins; concentrations in CSF are about equal to the unbound fraction. Carbamazepine is 97% hepatically metabolized, with CYP3A4 being predominantly responsible for the formation of the major metabolite, carbamazepine epoxide, and CYP2C8 and CYP1A2 playing smaller roles in carbamazepine biotransformation. Carbamazepine epoxide appears to be a highly active metabolite with effects very similar to the parent compound,[106] and its serum level may be measured when carbamazepine levels are measured both for assessment of potential efficacy and for toxicity. Carbamazepine epoxide is itself metabolized by a hepatic microsomal enzyme into a dihydroxylated compound. Amazingly, little information is available about the effects of renal or hepatic insufficiency on carbamazepine usage, though one would expect that dosing should be reduced in the former setting, and case reports indicate that carbamazepine is dialyzable.[107]

Carbamazepine has the property of potently inducing its own metabolism, a process referred to as *autoinduction.* Put in real terms, initial doses of carbamazepine have an elimination half-life of anywhere between 25 and 65 hours, but after 3 to 5 weeks of daily dosing, the half-life declines to 12 to 17 hours and remains stable thereafter. The half-life is shorter in children. Autoinduction also affects the T_{max} of the drug, which is much longer with initial doses than after chronic treatment.

The mechanism of carbamazepine's anticonvulsant effects is well described. It produces a frequency- and voltage-dependent blockade of Na^+ channels, likely by binding to them in the inactive state and delaying their recovery to the active state, thereby limiting sustained high-frequency neuronal firing of action potentials in a manner very similar to that of phenytoin.[106,108] It must have additional physiologic or chemical actions, however, because the spectrum of action of carbamazepine extends to trigeminal neuralgia and acute mania, conditions for which it is a first-line treatment and for which phenytoin is ineffective (see Chapter 48, Headache, and Chapter 53, Depression and Bipolar Disorders, for more on these indications). Carbamazepine has also been shown to block currents through the NMDA subtype of glutamate receptors,[109] but whether this has any bearing upon its anticonvulsant or other clinical actions remains unknown.

As an anticonvulsant, carbamazepine is formally indicated for the treatment of both partial seizures and generalized tonic-clonic seizures. It has little or no effect on absence, atypical absence, myoclonic, or atonic seizures, and in fact it is far more likely to make such patients worse than better.[63,110] It is unclear whether carbamazepine is as efficacious for primary generalized tonic-clonic seizures as it is for focal seizures with secondary generalization, but the drug clearly should not be a first-line choice in patients with generalized epilepsies. In adults, carbamazepine may be initiated at 200 mg twice daily and increased by 200 mg/week to a typical target dose of around 10 mg/kg per day (usually 600 to 1000 mg daily) divided thrice daily (standard preparations) or twice daily (extended-release preparations). Doses up to 1600 mg daily may be used if necessary and tolerated. In school-age children, this titration schedule may be halved, but young children metabolize the drug more rapidly, so initiation of therapy is at 10 mg/kg per day with titration to a maximum of 35 mg/kg per day. It is crucial that carbamazepine not be started at full dose in patients naive to the drug, as the reduced initial metabolism virtually guarantees that they will become acutely toxic and transfer their care to another practitioner. Therapy may be targeted by checking serum levels, with the traditionally accepted therapeutic range for carbamazepine being 4 to 12 mcg/ml. While the overall utility of "therapeutic ranges" is much debated, the author finds the range for carbamazepine to be particularly accurate, as the large majority of patients develop signs of toxicity at levels around 12 mcg/ml.

While carbamazepine lacks the cosmetic side effects of phenytoin, it has many other side effects that are similar. The acute toxic side effects include dizziness, somnolence, ataxia, nystagmus, nausea, and diplopia; the latter is rarely seen with phenytoin but is common with carbamazepine toxicity, which appears to be more toxic to the vestibular pathways. Hyponatremia is commonly seen in carbamazepine-treated patients but is rarely clinically relevant; the author ignores Na^+ values of more than 125 mmol/L. A more medically important side effect is skin rash, which is fairly common and, in rare cases, dangerous (e.g., Stevens-Johnson syndrome). Hematologic toxicity is also seen with carbamazepine, most commonly in the form of leukopenia that may be transient or persistent. The clinical relevance of these self-limited reductions in neutrophil count remains uncertain. The greatest concern with carbamazepine use is that of more serious hematologic toxicity, including agranulocytosis or aplastic anemia; in fact, the appearance of several such cases early on led to a delay in the drug's development and marketing. It was subsequently determined that the risk of these had been exaggerated, and current estimates place the incidence at 8 in 1 million. Hepatic toxicity can occur with carbamazepine, but it is far less frequent than with phenytoin; nonetheless, baseline and "periodic" evaluations of liver function are officially recommended.

Like phenytoin and the barbiturates, carbamazepine is a very potent inducer of the hepatic CYP system. This property appears to lead to a host of adverse metabolic effects on various systems, among them male sexual function,[26] thyroid function,[111] and serum lipids.[27,112] Loss of bone mass has not been conclusively demonstrated with carbamazepine as it has with phenytoin, but carbamazepine clearly reduces circulating vitamin D levels and increases bone turnover, both of which would be expected to lead to loss of bone mass over time.[25] The CYP induction properties of carbamazepine (and its own metabolism by the CYP system) also lead to a very large number of drug-drug interactions, many of which are similar to those of phenytoin. As with the latter, it is probably wise to assume that any hepatically metabolized drug a patient may be taking could be significantly reduced in concentration when carbamazepine is given concurrently, and there is specific evidence for carbamazepine-induced metabolism of tricyclic antidepressants, atypical antipsychotics, oral contraceptives (see Phenytoin section earlier), corticosteroids, cyclosporine, warfarin, dihydropyridine calcium channel blockers, and almost every anticonvulsant discussed in this chapter (excepting gabapentin, pregabalin, and levetiracetam, which are not metabolized). This list is incomplete, and the reader is referred to a detailed text for further information.[113] In addition to these effects of carbamazepine on other drugs, carbamazepine is itself affected by the many drugs that inhibit CYP3A4, including erythromycin, propoxyphene, and ketoconazole. Carbamazepine metabolism may also be induced by other inducing AEDs.

Carbamazepine's very close cousin oxcarbazepine was developed with the rationale of avoiding the unstable epoxide metabolite, which was considered possibly to be responsible for some of the adverse effects of carbamazepine. Oxcarbazepine is completely absorbed, whereupon over 80% of a dose is metabolized into its monohydroxy derivative (MHD); oxcarbazepine itself has an elimination half-life of only 2 hours, and most of its anticonvulsant effects are believed to occur via the actions of the MHD. The MHD has a T_{max} of 4.5 hours and a very high apparent V_d of 49 L. It is 40% bound to plasma proteins. About one third of the MHD is excreted unchanged in urine, with most of the remainder undergoing glucuronidation.[114] The elimination half-life of the MHD is 9 hours; in renal failure, the half-life is doubled, while children under 8 have an area under the concentration-time curve (AUC) 30% to 40% lower than adults. Both oxcarbazepine and the MHD appear to act by mechanisms very similar to those of carbamazepine,[115] though the MHD has the additional property of blocking N-type Ca^{2+} channels, which carbamazepine does not share.[116]

Oxcarbazepine is indicated as monotherapy or add-on therapy in patients age 4 years and older with focal epilepsy. In adults, the drug is started at 150 to 300 mg twice daily and increased by a similar amount weekly to a target of 600 mg twice daily; doses up to 2400 mg daily may be used. In children, begin with 8 to 10 mg/kg per day and titrate by a similar amount weekly to a target of 900 to 1200 mg/day. Oxcarbazepine has been found to be therapeutically equivalent to carbamazepine at a ratio of approximately 3:2—for example, in a comparative study of the two, the mean dose of oxcarbazepine was almost precisely 50% greater than the mean dose of carbamazepine.[117] The latter study also demonstrated that oxcarbazepine was equally efficacious but better tolerated than carbamazepine. The most common side effect of oxcarbazepine is dizziness, with the other acute side effects of carbamazepine also seen. Rash, both mild and severe, is less common with oxcarbazepine, and neither hepatic nor hematologic toxicity has been reported. Another advantage is that oxcarbazepine is not an inducer of the CYP system, and as a consequence it is devoid of almost all of carbamazepine's drug interactions; it does appear to induce the metabolism of oral contraceptives, however. Oxcarbazepine may also avoid most of the metabolic effects of carbamazepine on lipids[118] and sex hormones,[119] but unfortunately it appears to have similar effects on bone metabolism.[25] The biggest drawback of oxcarbazepine is an increased frequency of hyponatremia; Na^+ values under 125 mmol/L, a level low enough to potentially exacerbate seizures, are seen in 2.5% of patients. This may occur more commonly in the elderly[120] and in patients taking diuretics. On balance, in view of the improved tolerability, greater safety, obviation of periodic phlebotomy, and avoidance of drug interactions, it may be appropriate to consider oxcarbazepine a modest but significant improvement over carbamazepine. Many have debated whether these benefits are worth the additional cost, but such arguments will soon become moot in the United States with the recent expiration of oxcarbazepine's patent protection.

Valproate

Valproate was the first of the so-called broad-spectrum anticonvulsants, and as such represented a real advance in therapy when it was brought to market in 1978. Up until that time, any patient with a primary generalized epilepsy who suffered from multiple seizure types might, for example, have been obliged to take phenytoin for tonic-clonic seizures, ethosuximide for absences, and a benzodiazepine for myoclonic events. Valproate's simultaneous effectiveness for all of these seizure types, and all other kinds of generalized seizures, allowed for "one-stop shopping," greatly simplifying therapy. It is also quite effective for focal seizures,[121] though the company did not obtain a formal U.S. Food and Drug Administration (FDA) indication for this until relatively recently. In addition, as befits a broad-spectrum AED, the spectrum of effectiveness extends to conditions beyond epilepsy; valproate is considered a drug of first choice for mania (see Chapter 53, Depression and Bipolar Disorders), and it is also quite effective as a preventive agent for migraine headaches (see Chapter 48, Headache).

Valproate is available in several different chemical forms. The original pill formulation was of valproic acid, and this is still available, but it has largely been supplanted by an enteric-coated version of divalproex, a 1:1 chemical complex of the acid and the sodium salt, which is thought to reduce gastrointestinal upset. Divalproex was more recently introduced in an extended-release formulation. The sodium valproate salt itself is also available in an oral syrup and in an IV formulation for acute therapy. The oral formulations have virtually complete bioavailability except for the extended-release preparation, which is about 85% bioavailable. T_{max} varies from about 1 to 4 hours depending on the preparation, but the extended-release pill has a much longer T_{max} of over 19 hours.[122] T_{max} is greater when given with food. Valproate is largely bound to plasma proteins, but the binding appears to saturate and is thus concentration dependent, ranging from 92% at low therapeutic serum levels to around 80% at high levels. V_d is around 0.17 L/kg. CSF concentrations are equal to the unbound fraction. Over 97% of a dose of valproate is hepatically metabolized via a mixture of mitochondrial β-oxidation, CYP-mediated processes, and glucuronidation. The elimination half-life is 13 to 15 hours in young or elderly adults,[123,124] 9 to 12 hours in children,[125,126] and 26 to 40 hours in neonates.[127] This is lessened by about 40% in the presence of enzyme inducers. Overall AUC is equivalent for all dosage formulations with the exception once again of the extended-release tablet, which yields an AUC about 11% less and thus requires a dose roughly that much higher for equivalence with other preparations.[122]

Despite 30 years of widespread use, valproate's mechanisms of action remain largely obscure. The drug clearly produces increases in synaptic GABA, apparently through a combination of increased synthesis and decreased degradation.[128,129] It appears to reduce sustained rapid firing of neurons, consistent with a frequency-dependent effect on voltage-gated Na^+ channels, though its effects are somewhat different from those of phenytoin.[108,128] Valproate has also been shown to reduce excitation mediated by NMDA-type glutamate receptors.[128,130] The relative contribution of any or all of these mechanisms to clinical anticonvulsant activity remains entirely unclear, however. Valproate has been found to block voltage-dependent T-type Ca^{2+} channels in a peripheral ganglion preparation,[131] which may relate to its anti-absence activity, though this has not been verified in thalamic neurons.

Valproate is indicated as monotherapy or add-on therapy for patients with partial seizures and those with absence or atypical absence seizures. As mentioned, it is clearly effective for all other seizure types too, including primary generalized tonic-clonic seizures and atonic seizures. Therapy is begun at 10 to 15 mg/kg per day in two or three divided doses (the extended-release form may be given as a single daily dose) and may be titrated upward by 5 to 7 mg/kg per week to a maximum of 50 to 60 mg/kg per day (though doses of 15 to 30 mg/kg per day are more typical). The traditional therapeutic range of serum concentrations is 50 to 100 mcg/ml, though higher levels are sometimes sought. The IV formulation is used in exactly the same manner; in addition, some practitioners have begun to use larger initial IV doses, run in very rapidly, for treatment of acute seizures or status epilepticus.[132]

Valproate is most commonly used in the treatment of generalized epilepsies. Comparative data have been lacking until very recently,[133] but many practitioners consider valproate the most effective drug for generalized epilepsy syndromes. Unfortunately, valproate's efficaciousness in this population comes at the cost of many potential problematic side effects. Gastrointestinal upset may be the most common and can occasionally preclude its use altogether. Valproate can also produce the typical acute side effects seen in most AEDs—sedation, cognitive impairment, dizziness, and ataxia—along with its own trio of unique and frustrating chronic side effects: weight gain, hair loss, and tremor. The latter condition is usually not a true impediment to the patient (though it can be, particularly with higher doses), and hair loss, while it can be profuse and concerning, is rarely cosmetically consequential. Weight gain, on the other hand, is probably the single biggest problem with the use of the drug. It affects a significant number of patients and can be substantial (even 15 kg or more). In children, on the other hand, anorexia and weight loss are sometimes seen. Peripheral edema may be seen with chronic use, particularly in the mentally retarded population, though without any evidence of cardiac or renal disease.

Other side effects may be even more consequential. Valproate can be hepatotoxic, with effects ranging from mild elevations of hepatic enzyme levels to fulminant hepatic failure; the latter is rare, but children under age 2—particularly those with mental retardation or metabolic disorders or who are taking multiple AEDs—are at higher risk. Baseline and periodic assessments of liver function are typically performed. Acute pancreatitis is also a rare but dangerous complication. Severe hematologic reactions (e.g., pancytopenia) are extremely rare with valproate, but reductions in platelet count and platelet function are fairly common; thrombocytopenia occurs exclusively at higher doses and is exquisitely dose dependent, but a mild bleeding diathesis may be present even when platelet count is normal. Acute encephalopathy or even coma can be seen in valproate-treated patients, associated with elevated blood ammonia levels; once identified, this responds rapidly to drug discontinuation.

A significant endocrinologic issue occurring with valproate use is that many women, particularly those with primary generalized epilepsy syndromes, develop a constellation of symptoms that strongly resembles polycystic ovary syndrome (PCOS).[22,134] While the association of PCOS and valproate use is still debated by some,[135] the author finds the evidence overwhelming.[136-138] Another very important reproductive issue pertaining to valproate is its teratogenicity. It is the single AED most clearly associated with birth defects, including a 2.5% incidence of neural tube defects.[139-141] Several recent studies have also shown reduced cognitive abilities in children who were exposed to valproate in utero.[142,143] Because of the potential for weight gain, PCOS, and teratogenicity, some epileptologists (including the author) have a significant disinclination to use this drug in the reproductive-age female population unless other options have been exhausted.

Last but not least, valproate is a potent inhibitor of the hepatic CYP system, and that, along with its extensive and competitive protein binding, leads to a fair number of drug-drug interactions. Among the most prominent are its interactions with other AEDs, particularly lamotrigine, barbiturates, and ethosuximide, in which the other drug's levels are increased by the hepatic inhibition. Valproate tends to displace phenytoin from binding sites on serum albumin, leading to higher free phenytoin levels even as total phenytoin is unchanged (or decreased). When used with carbamazepine, valproate can lead to inhibition of metabolism of the carbamazepine-epoxide metabolite, causing toxicity even in the setting of unchanged carbamazepine levels. Reciprocally, phenytoin and the other inducing AEDs will increase the metabolism of valproate and reduce valproate levels; the combination of each drug's effect on the other can be very complex and may require frequent monitoring of both total and free serum levels as any adjustments are made.

Felbamate

Upon its release in 1993, felbamate was the first new anticonvulsant introduced to the U.S. market in over 15 years and generated considerable excitement, particularly because of its seeming efficacy in patients with refractory generalized epilepsies such as Lennox-Gastaut syndrome, among whom it drastically reduced devastating atonic seizures in about half of patients who had previously been untreatable.[144] The joy was short lived, however, as cases of aplastic anemia and liver failure, many fatal, emerged during the first postmarketing year without warning. By the time the dust had settled, the vast majority of patients had been taken off the drug, though it was allowed to remain on the market (albeit with limited use recommendations). It took the introduction of several more new AEDs, and several years, to convince many neurologists that it was safe to start using new therapies again.

Felbamate is highly absorbed, with a T_{max} of 1.5 to 2 hours[145] and a V_d around 0.75 L/kg, averaging 51 L.[146] It is roughly 25% bound to plasma proteins. It is approximately 55% metabolized (to a minor extent by CYP3A4), with the remainder excreted unchanged in urine, with an overall elimination half-life of around 19 hours.[147] It has several putative mechanisms of action, including blockade of voltage-sensitive Na^+ channels, protection against seizures induced by non-NMDA glutamate receptor antagonists,[148] and blockade of glycine binding to its receptor.[149] It is approved for use as monotherapy or add-on therapy in patients 14 years and older with focal seizures, in whom it is begun at 400 mg three times daily and titrated by 600 mg every 2 weeks to a target of 800 mg three times daily. It is also approved for use in children with Lennox-Gastaut syndrome, in whom it is started at 15 mg/kg per day and increased by a similar amount weekly up to 45 mg/kg per day in three divided doses. Common side effects include nausea and vomiting, headache, dizziness, somnolence, and insomnia—the latter due to its sometime stimulating properties. Weight loss is also common, and allergic rash can be seen. The incidence of aplastic anemia has been estimated at approximately 1 in 4000, and fatal liver failure has been estimated to occur at a rate of roughly 1 in 30,000.[150] It has been postulated that a specific atropaldehyde metabolite of felbamate could be responsible for these severe reactions,[151] but this hypothesis has been impossible to test because of the low number of new exposures to the drug. At least one case of toxic epidermal necrolysis has been reported.[152] As a consequence of these risks, it is recommended that written informed consent be obtained prior to the use of felbamate. Finally, felbamate has been found to simultaneously *induce* CYP3A4 and *inhibit* CYP2C19, leading to a complicated panel of interactions with other AEDs.[147]

Gabapentin and Pregabalin

A stupendous example of serendipity in drug design, gabapentin was specifically designed to reduce seizures by acting as an agonist at the GABA receptor—which it has been clearly found *not* to do.[153] That did not stop it from demonstrating true anticonvulsant efficacy via other mechanisms, nor did it stop the drug from finding a cozy and wholly unanticipated home in the neurologic armamentarium as a reliever of neuropathic and other chronic pain conditions; in fact, the latter are said to account for 90% of prescriptions for this agent in the United States. As a consequence, we probably have gabapentin to thank for the continued interest in finding new indications for anticonvulsant drugs—and by extension, for most of the recent and current pipeline of AEDs.

The pharmacology of gabapentin is complicated by issues pertaining to gastric absorption; bioavailability of the drug varies inversely with the dose administered, topping out at around 1200 mg total. This may be mediated by the neutral amino acid transporter in the gastrointestinal tract and its saturation by gabapentin administration.[154] T_{max} is 2 to 3 hours. Binding to plasma proteins is negligible. Concentrations in CSF are about 20% of those in plasma. Gabapentin undergoes no metabolism at all and is excreted unchanged in the urine with a half-life of 5 to 7 hours. The half-life increases as creatinine clearance decreases, ultimately resulting in an effective half-life of 132 hours in dialysis-dependent patients on nondialysis days (reduced to 4 hours on dialysis days). Pharmacokinetics are similar in children and adults, although children under 5 years of age had a higher clearance, resulting in an AUC about 30% less than older subjects, and should therefore require higher doses.

Early studies regarding gabapentin's mechanism of action largely focused on ways in which it *failed* to affect the GABAergic neurotransmitter system. More recently, the drug was found to bind avidly and specifically with the $\alpha 2\delta$ subunit of the presynaptic voltage-dependent calcium channel on neurons, resulting in reduction in synaptic release of a number of neurotransmitters, including glutamate, acetycholine, and noradrenaline.[155] This action is believed to be plausibly responsible for both the anticonvulsant and analgesic properties of the drug; in fact, this makes more sense than any GABAergic hypothesis ever did, since no drug that acts on the GABA system had ever before demonstrated any pain-relieving properties. With regard to the latter, of particular interest is the finding that one of the neurotransmitter systems most affected by gabapentin is the substance P/calcitonin gene–related peptide system, in which gabapentin causes reduction of transmitter release by 60% to 70%.[156]

Gabapentin is approved in the United States for add-on treatment of focal seizures in patients 3 years of age and older. It appears effective as initial monotherapy as well,[157,158] though one recent large comparative trial found it significantly less effective than carbamazepine or lamotrigine.[103] Aside from focal seizures that secondarily generalize, it is not likely to be effective for any other seizure types. It is also approved for the treatment of postherpetic neuralgia and is very commonly used in a host of different chronic pain conditions (covered in more detail in Chapter 61, Treatment of Pain). In adults with epilepsy, therapy is typically initiated at 300 to 400 mg three times daily and titrated upward weekly in a similar amount up to a target dose of 600 to 1200 mg three times daily. Individual doses of greater than 1200 mg are unlikely to be of benefit due to the aforementioned absorption limits; the dosing interval may be increased to four times daily to allow higher daily doses, but this is rarely done. In children 12 years and under, dosing is initiated at 10 to 15 mg/kg per day and titrated up to 25 to 50 mg/kg per day.

One of gabapentin's greatest assets is its side effect profile. Typically this may include sedation, ataxia, or dizziness, but these occur in only a minority of patients (and, in the author's experience, at low doses rather than during dose escalation). The one side effect that appears more problematic at higher doses is weight gain, never extreme but commonly in the range of 5% to 10% of body weight.[159] Essentially no medically dangerous side effects have been reported, and the drug is not known to have any drug interactions of any kind.

Pregabalin was brought to market in an effort to overcome the limits of gabapentin's effectiveness imposed by the ceiling on absorption. It is freely absorbed, with a bioavailability of over 90% regardless of the dose administered. Peak serum levels are reached in 1.5 hours (but delayed to hours when given with food). Otherwise it shares most of the pharmacologic properties of gabapentin, as well as its apparent mechanism of action, and its indications are similar (though it does not have approval for pediatric use as of this writing). Adult treatment is initiated at 150 mg/day in two or three divided doses; studies have shown this to be an effective dose, but it may be titrated upward to a maximum of 600 mg/day. Steady state levels occur in 24 to 48 hours. The side effects are similar to those of gabapentin, including weight gain. Peripheral edema, not related to renal or cardiac function, also seems to occur in some patients (this can also occur with gabapentin on occasion). Whether pregabalin has any real advantages over gabapentin remains to be seen, but the ability to start treatment at an effective dose and to use a twice-daily rather than thrice-daily regimen may be useful.

Lamotrigine

Lamotrigine was developed out of a program to design antineoplastic agents; since many of the previously existing AEDs lowered folate levels, it was thought (erroneously) that this property might relate to their anticonvulsant effects. Ironically, lamotrigine actually has no antifolate effects[160]—and even more ironically, it is now considered by many epileptologists to be the AED of choice in pregnancy (see later).

Lamotrigine has virtually complete absorption and bioavailability, with a T_{max} of about 2 hours. It is 55% bound to plasma proteins, with CSF concentrations roughly 50% to 60% of that found in serum.[161] V_d ranges from 0.9 to 1.3 L/kg. The large majority (~81%) of a dose is glucuronidated by hepatic enzymes, with an elimination half-life that averages 25 hours but can be as low as 12 hours; the half-life is increased two- to threefold when valproate is used concurrently or when there is moderately severe hepatic insufficiency, and halved in the presence of one of the enzyme-inducing AEDs (phenytoin, carbamazepine, barbiturates). Only 20% of a dose is disposed of during a 4-hour hemodialysis session.

Lamotrigine appears to exert its actions via blockade of voltage-dependent Na^+ channels, leading to decreased glutamate release.[162,163] In this regard, its physiologic effects may be similar to those of phenytoin and carbamazepine.[163] However, this clearly does not fully explain the relevant effects of lamotrigine in view of the differences in its spectrum of action and side effect profile from the former drugs. Lamotrigine has also been found to block influx through voltage-dependent Ca^{2+} channels[164] and to enhance hyperpolarizing K^+ currents.[165] Both of these effects would be expected to reduce neuronal depolarization and prevent seizures, but their clinical relevance remains to be determined.

Lamotrigine is indicated for add-on therapy for focal seizures, for primary generalized tonic-clonic seizures, and for the generalized seizures of the Lennox-Gastaut syndrome in patients 2 years and older. It also carries the curious indication of monotherapy conversion in adults taking one of the older generation AEDs. In reality, lamotrigine is clearly effective against all seizure types, including absence,[166,167] and is frequently used as initial monotherapy despite the lack of an indication for this. One therapeutic oddity of lamotrigine is that it is effective in the majority of patients with myoclonic seizures, but in a significant minority the myoclonic seizures are made worse[168]; this likely points to the genetic heterogeneity of (otherwise clinically similar) myoclonic epilepsies. The near absence of sedative or cognitive side effects[169-171] makes it unique among available AEDs; in fact, the drug clearly has some mood-elevating and stimulating properties,[172,173] and insomnia is one of the most common dose-related side effects. The antidepressant properties have led to a formal FDA indication for bipolar depression, for which many consider it the drug of first choice (see Chapter 53, Depression and Bipolar Disorders, for more on this). Other dose-related side effects include dizziness and ataxia, though these occur much less frequently than with the older Na^+ channel–blocking drugs. Worsening of migraine headaches is sometimes seen, as is tremor, particularly at higher doses or with concurrent use of valproate. Lamotrigine has no hepatic or hematologic effects, but its one potentially dangerous side effect is rash. The overall incidence of rashes with the drug ranges from 2% to 10%, but almost all of these are nonserious, and many are likely not even drug related. Very serious cutaneous reactions, including toxic epidermal necrolysis or Stevens-Johnson syndrome, occur with an incidence of 0.1% to 0.3% in the adult population and 0.8% in the pediatric population, with rare deaths reported. It is believed that the risk of rash may be higher in patients already on valproate, and when the initial titration is too rapid. Thus, the rash risk, which is the drug's main drawback, leads directly to its second major drawback: a slow and complex titration schedule, with a consequent delay of 6 to 8 weeks until the drug reaches steady therapeutic serum concentrations. This makes the drug unsuitable for circumstances in which seizure prevention is urgently needed. Some practitioners exhibit a reluctance to use the drug at all because of the rash risks, a practice that is not entirely rational, since many of these same people instead prescribe "tried and true" carbamazepine, which appears to have a similar risk of skin eruptions.[174-176] The author strongly advises that any patient started on lamotrigine who complains of rash be seen in the office as soon as possible for a direct assessment, as the large majority of such complaints yield skin findings that are not drug-related. In addition, virtually all lamotrigine-related rashes occur within the first 2 to 3 months of treatment, so the risk is not chronic.

In adults, when there are no other inducing or inhibiting AEDs being used concurrently, lamotrigine is started at 25 mg/day and doubled every 2 weeks up to a typical target dose of 100 to 200 mg twice daily; further increases of 100 mg weekly may then be made if needed. It is crucial that, in the presence of valproate co-medication, the drug be started at 25 mg every *other* day for 2 weeks, after which the aforementioned schedule may be followed; valproate effectively doubles the lamotrigine level, so the target should be lower as well. When lamotrigine is being used with an inducing AED, take the aforementioned schedule and double it, including the target dose. In children, start at 0.6 mg/kg per day, double it in 2 weeks and again at 4 weeks, and then increase by 1.2 mg/kg per day up to an initial target dose of 5 mg/kg per day. Again, this schedule should be halved in patients on valproate and doubled in patients on inducers. Note that lamotrigine and carbamazepine appear to have a pharmacodynamic interaction that leads to a greater frequency of typical carbamazepine side effects (dizziness, ataxia) without any change in circulating drug levels; it responds to a decrease in the dosage of either drug, but the use of this combination is probably not worth the trouble, and the author generally tapers carbamazepine as lamotrigine is raised.

One important area of use for lamotrigine is that of planned pregnancy, a common occurrence in a disease that affects many young patients. While data on anticonvulsant use in pregnancy are far from adequate, there is nonetheless a fair body of literature suggesting that the prospectively determined rate of birth defects in infants exposed to lamotrigine in utero is around 3%,[177,178] a number little different from the rate seen in women with epilepsy who are unmedicated. This, and the relative paucity of data on other drugs, has led to the widespread use of lamotrigine in the pregnant population. A recent report suggesting an increased incidence of cleft palate with lamotrigine exposure has put a bit of a damper on this, but other pregnancy registries have failed to confirm the finding, making its significance uncertain. More pregnancy data are clearly necessary for this and all other AEDs.

Topiramate

Topiramate was released to the U.S. market in 1996. Structurally it consists of a fructose ring with a sulfamate group substitution. The drug is 80% bioavailable and reaches a peak concentration in about 2 hours. It binds only modestly (15% to 30%) to plasma proteins. It crosses the blood-brain barrier very readily, reaching unbound CSF concentrations nearly identical to those in plasma. About 70% of a dose is excreted unchanged in the urine, with the remainder being processed by the liver into a half-dozen minor metabolites. The half-life of the drug is 21 hours. Reabsorption of the drug from the proximal renal tubule may play a role in its persistence in the serum. Since clearance is reduced by about half in patients with renal failure, the dose should be halved in this population as well. During hemodialysis, the drug is cleared at a rate four to six times faster than it is cleared in patients with normally functioning kidneys, so dosage after dialysis is probably warranted.

There are multiple putative mechanisms of action for topiramate, a reliable sign that its true mechanism of action remains uncertain. It may have some effect on Na^+ channels, but this effect is fairly modest overall and differs significantly from neuron to neuron, which is quite unlike the effects of phenytoin, carbamazepine, or lamotrigine.[179] Topiramate has been shown to block currents induced by kainate at its specific subtype of glutamate receptor while having no effect on currents evoked at the NMDA subtype of glutamate receptor.[180] It has also been shown to enhance $GABA_A$ receptor–mediated inhibitory currents in some neurons, and to do so in a manner that is clearly distinct from the benzodiazepines.[181] Finally, the drug inhibits carbonic anhydrase, though whether this relates to its anticonvulsant activity is highly debatable, and in any case the inhibition of carbonic anhydrase produced by topiramate is only 1% to 10% of that seen with acetazolamide, the prototype of the class.[182]

Topiramate is clearly a "broad-spectrum" anticonvulsant in that it demonstrates efficacy against partial seizures and many types of primary generalized seizures. It is indicated for both add-on therapy (ages 2 years and up) and initial monotherapy (ages 10 and up) for both partial seizures and primary generalized tonic-clonic seizures, and as add-on therapy for children or adults with the Lennox-Gastaut syndrome of mental retardation and multiple generalized seizure types. Clinical experience suggests that it can be effective for tonic, atonic, and myoclonic seizures, but it is usually ineffective for absence seizures.[183] In the adult population, initial dosing is 25 mg once daily, increasing weekly up to 50 to 100 mg twice daily. Doses of 200 mg twice daily or higher may be used, but are more likely to produce side effects than clinical benefit; in fact, in the initial monotherapy population, strong randomized double-blind data indicate that 50 mg twice daily yields the same seizure-free rate as 100 mg twice daily.[184] In children, therapy is initiated at 1 to 3 mg/kg per day, increasing by a similar amount weekly to a target of 5 to 9 mg/kg per day in two divided doses. Starting topiramate at full dose is virtually guaranteed to provoke side effects, but in refractory nonconvulsive status epilepticus, when this is not a concern, it can be done and may be successful at terminating seizures.[185,186]

Topiramate stands out from other AEDs because of two potentially beneficial side effects. The first is reduction in frequency of migraine headaches, an effect so prominent that it was formally studied and approved for this indication. (This is discussed further in Chapter 48, Headache.) This is particularly noteworthy in light of the fact that a large number of patients with epilepsy suffer from comorbid migraines. The second beneficial side effect is weight loss, which is seen in a large fraction of patients and can sometimes be considerable. The mechanism for weight loss is unclear. Useful as these effects are, they can be counterbalanced by adverse effects, the most troublesome of which is cognitive impairment. This can take the form of poor concentration, impaired processing abilities, or—most uniquely—word-finding difficulty. These effects may resolve spontaneously after several weeks, and occur more frequently when topiramate is used in conjunction with other drugs, and when patients have partial seizures emanating from the dominant hemisphere.[187] Other common side effects include sedation; behavioral symptoms such as aggression, psychosis, or depression[188]; peripheral paresthesias; and nephrolithiasis (1.5% incidence). The latter two effects are presumably due to the carbonic anhydrase activity. This activity is also responsible for the occurrence of metabolic acidosis, which is rarely clinically relevant. Two other very rare but serious side effects are secondary angle-closure glaucoma and the oligohydrosis/hyperthermia reaction first described with zonisamide (see later); both are reversible with discontinuation of the drug.

Tiagabine

Like gabapentin, tiagabine was an attempt to leverage the GABA pathway for anticonvulsant effects, but a more accurate one; the drug clearly acts by inhibition of GABA reuptake, increasing its concentration at the synapse. Tiagabine is almost fully absorbed and has a total bioavailability of 90%. T_{max} is 0.75 hours, but much longer (2.5 hours) when given with a fatty meal. V_d is a little less than 1 L/kg and is dependent upon height in a nonlinear fashion.[189] It is 96% bound to plasma proteins. Tiagabine undergoes metabolism almost completely, with most of it done by hepatic CYP3A4. The elimination half-life averages 6 to 8 hours at typical therapeutic dose ranges[190] but is considerably shorter in patients taking enzyme-inducing AEDs concurrently. The drug is unaffected by renal failure or hemodialysis, but hepatic insufficiency reduces clearance by 60%, necessitating a lower total daily dose.

Tiagabine is indicated as add-on therapy for partial seizures in patients over the age of 12. The drug has also demonstrated at least some efficacy in monotherapy conversion in partial epilepsy patients using a low-dose versus high-dose design,[191] but in one initial monotherapy comparison study, published in abstract form only, tiagabine appeared to be inferior to carbamazepine. Low doses of both drugs were used in the latter study, which may limit its general applicability.[192] Tiagabine is contraindicated in generalized epilepsies as it has no demonstrated efficacy in this group, and it can worsen generalized spike-and-wave abnormalities on EEG, leading to an increase in seizures or even nonconvulsive status epilepticus.[193,194] The involvement of GABAergic neurons in the generation of generalized spike-wave discharges (see earlier discussion) may be responsible for this. For this reason, if the type of epilepsy (focal vs. generalized) is unclear, then tiagabine is best avoided. Initiation of therapy is at 4 mg/day, with subsequent increases of 4 mg/week to a target dose of 16 mg/day in patients not on inducing drugs, or 30 to 32 mg/day when there is concurrent inducing AED use. Side effects commonly include sedation, fatigue, dizziness, and difficulty with memory or concentration. In addition, a host of reports suggest that tiagabine can produce nonconvulsive status epilepticus in patients with focal epilepsy[195,196] or even in patients who do not have epilepsy at all.[197-199] As is apparent, essentially all known adverse reactions to tiagabine are central nervous system related, and no systemic side effects have been described. Fairly or unfairly, the drug remains something of a "poor stepchild" among the new generation of AEDs and is not commonly used.

Zonisamide

Zonisamide was first synthesized in Japan and introduced there in 1989, with subsequent introduction to the U.S. market 11 years later after a long hiatus in its development due to concerns about its propensity to produce renal stones. As a consequence, unlike many of the newer AEDs, clinical use in America has been informed by over 15 years of use in Japan and South Korea. Zonisamide is a sulfonamide compound, chemically unrelated to other AEDs. Its gastrointestinal absorption is complete and unaffected by food, and bioavailability is assumed to be 100% but has never formally been reported. T_{max} occurs in 2 to 6 hours (on the later end if given with food), and V_d is 1.45 L/kg. Zonisamide is 40% bound to plasma proteins, but it also has the property—unique among AEDs—of binding extensively to red blood cells, owing to the drug's affinity for carbonic anhydrase within erythrocytes. This binding is rapidly saturable at low concentrations, however, so it is of little clinical relevance. Concentrations in CSF approximate the free fraction in plasma.[200] About one third of a dose of zonisamide is excreted unchanged in the urine, and another one half is reduced by CYP3A4, with the remainder undergoing acetylation. The elimination half-life of the drug is 63 hours. This is reduced by about half in patients taking inducing AEDs. There is no change with concomitant valproate therapy.[201] Marked renal insufficiency increases AUC by 35%; the effects of hepatic insufficiency on zonisamide have not been studied.

Zonisamide has multiple neurophysiologic and neurochemical effects, two of which are most relevant to its clinical actions. First, it reduces current through voltage-dependent Na^+ channels, likely by binding to them in the inactive state and delaying their recovery to the active state. This impairs high-frequency firing of action potentials.[202] Second, zonisamide blocks T-type Ca^{2+} channel currents.[203] These actions are similar to those of several of the older anticonvulsants and likely explain the drug's broad spectrum of action, which encompasses partial seizures, generalized tonic-clonic seizures, and absence seizures. Zonisamide has also been shown to facilitate dopaminergic and serotonergic neurotransmission by increasing synthesis of these monoamines, though it is unclear that this has anything to do with its anticonvulsant actions. Finally, zonisamide is well established to inhibit carbonic anydrase, but at low potency. Its carbonic anhydrase activity does not appear to be correlated with its anticonvulsant actions.[204]

In the United States, zonisamide is indicated only as add-on therapy for partial epilepsy in adults, but its indications in Japan and Korea, along with clinical experience, make it clear that its spectrum of action extends to all types of generalized seizures, to the pediatric population, and to monotherapy use.[205,206] Zonisamide is even effective in a significant subset of patients with infantile spasms, an uncommon but devastating form of epilepsy that can be extremely difficult to treat.[207,208] In adults, therapy is initiated at 100 mg/day and increased every 2 weeks (the drug takes that long to reach steady state) to a target dose of 200 to 400 mg once daily. In children, a starting dose of 2 to 4 mg/kg per day may be doubled in 2 weeks to reach the target dose.

The author finds the once-daily dosing of zonisamide to be a significant therapeutic advantage for some patients, particularly those unaccustomed to taking daily medications or those more interested in their social lives than their health (e.g., adolescents and 20-somethings). Maximizing compliance is particularly crucial for a condition in which one or two missed doses could theoretically put the patient at risk. While there are other once-daily AEDs (phenytoin, phenobarbital, valproate extended release), all have the drawbacks of drug interactions, tolerability issues, and adverse metabolic effects. Nonetheless, while zonisamide is overall well tolerated, it is certainly not free of adverse effects itself. Typical dose-related AED effects on the central nervous system, including dizziness, fatigue, somnolence, cognitive impairment, and ataxia, can be seen (though probably less frequently than with the older AEDs). Behavioral or psychiatric side effects, including irritability, depression, and occasionally even psychosis, can be seen with zonisamide. Peripheral paresthesias are common, and symptomatic nephrolithiasis occurs at a rate of about 1.2%—both of these effects are also seen with topiramate, and for the same reason (carbonic anhydrase inhibition). Nephrolithiasis likely has a pharmacogenetic component, as the incidence of zonisamide-related renal stones in the Japanese population is far lower.[209] Weight loss is also sometimes seen with zonisamide, though it seems less potent than topiramate in this regard.

With respect to dangerous side effects, the oligohydrosis/hyperthermia reaction, which can also be seen with topiramate, was first reported in children taking zonisamide. In this situation, normal heat-related perspiration becomes severely impaired, which can lead to a clinical picture resembling heat stroke when patients are exposed to hot weather. All cases have resolved after discontinuation, and it has not been reported in adults to date. Rash can occur with zonisamide just as it does with sulfonamide antibiotics, and in fact zonisamide is contraindicated in patients with a sulfa allergy. The rash can rarely manifest as a dangerous condition such as Stevens-Johnson syndrome or toxic epidermal necrolysis, and seven rash-related deaths were documented during the first 11 years of marketing in Japan. A handful of cases of pancytopenia and aplastic anemia have been reported, but they are rare enough that any association with the drug is unclear.

Levetiracetam

Levetiracetam caused something of a stir within the epilepsy pharmacology community upon its initial release in 2000 because it failed to demonstrate efficacy in one of the two standard animal screening models for anticonvulsants, a profile that would typically have consigned a candidate compound to the scrap heap. The company persisted in further testing nonetheless, yielding a drug that not only is effective, but appears to work via mechanisms completely different from those known for all other anticonvulsant drugs. One cannot help but wonder how many other similarly effective compounds may have been abandoned based upon animal models which are clearly less than ideal.

Levetiracetam is a pyrrolidine derivative with virtually complete absorption, distribution into all body water ($V_d = 0.5$ to 0.7 L/kg), and a T_{max} of about 1 hour. It is not bound to plasma proteins to any relevant degree. About two thirds of a dose is excreted unchanged in the urine, while one quarter is minimally metabolized by hydrolysis in a manner independent of hepatic enzyme systems. The elimination half-life is approximately 7 hours, but despite this the drug is clearly effective with twice-daily dosing. It has no known interactions with other drugs. As would be expected of a renally cleared compound, the dose should be reduced by roughly 50% in patients with renal impairment. About half of a dose is cleared with hemodialysis, so supplemental dosing of a similar amount immediately after a dialysis session is warranted.

The mechanism of action of levetiracetam appears to be unique among currently available AEDs, as the drug has been shown to have no effect on Na^+ channels or T-type Ca^{2+} channels, and no direct effects on GABA or glutamate neurotransmission. It has been shown to increase brain concentrations of taurine,[210] and to selectively block N-type Ca^{2+} channels in the hippocampus.[211] A specific, saturable binding site for the drug in the brain was subsequently identified, and more recently its identity has been revealed as the synaptic vesicle protein SV2A.[212] The latter investigators demonstrated that the correlation between a given compound's SV2A binding affinity and its anticonvulsant properties is very high, strongly suggesting that this is the true underlying mechanism of the drug's action. Further elaboration remains, however, since the precise function of SV2A is not itself clear, though it probably functions in presynaptic vesicle fusion.[212]

Like all the newer AEDs, levetiracetam was approved by the FDA for add-on therapy in adult patients with focal seizures, and like all other drugs its true utility in this regard is modest at best.[213] Again, like many of the others, levetiracetam is widely used by clinicians in monotherapy for patients with partial epilepsy, for which purpose it appears quite effective despite the lack of a formal indication.[214] In addition, the drug was found to have efficacy for myoclonic seizures, and was recently given FDA approval for this seizure type. It also appears to be effective for the primary generalized tonic-clonic seizures that are almost invariably a concomitant of myoclonic seizures.[215] Adoption of the drug has undoubtedly been abetted by its great ease of use and rapid onset of action; the drug may be started at a full therapeutic dose of 500 mg twice daily, which demonstrates anticonvulsant efficacy within 24 to 48 hours.[216] This property represents a significant advantage over the majority of newer generation AEDs. Some clinicians prefer to start at 250 mg twice daily and then increase to 500 mg twice daily within a week. The dose may be increased up to 1500 mg twice daily, or even higher, but there is little improvement in efficacy.[217] In children, for whom there is no formal FDA indication, the drug is started at 20 mg/kg per day in two divided doses, and may be increased up to 40 mg/kg per day as needed.

Levetiracetam has an excellent safety record, with essentially no medically dangerous side effects having been reported to date. The two most common side effects by far are fatigue and irritability; the author recommends specifically inquiring about the latter both with the patient and family members, since some patients may not be aware of the change themselves, and family members may attribute this to the patient's reaction to the disease. Other psychiatric side effects are also occasionally seen, including psychosis (incidence of 1% to 1.5%) and depression. As is fitting for a drug with a mechanism of action different from its peers, the drug has yet to demonstrate any utility in treating migraine, neuropathic pain, or psychiatric conditions.

The excellent water solubility of levetiracetam permitted the creation of an IV formulation, which was recently released to the U.S. market. Infusion of a full dose (1500 mg or more) can be done in 15 minutes, with somnolence and fatigue being the predominant adverse reactions. Its approved indication is as an alternative for add-on use in patients with focal epilepsy when oral treatment may not be feasible. The utility of the drug for more urgent indications, such as status epilepticus, has not yet been studied.

Vigabatrin

This drug is not available in the United States as of this writing, but is briefly discussed here because of a few noteworthy scientific and clinical properties. Vigabatrin was specifically (and successfully) designed to selectively inhibit GABA transaminase, the major enzyme responsible for the metabolism of GABA, in yet another attempt to leverage the GABAergic system for anticonvulsant effects. Vigabatrin is excreted in the urine in unchanged form with a half-life of roughly 5 hours,[218] but the drug binds irreversibly to GABA transaminase, leading to biologic effects that persist for days, including increases in central nervous system GABA on the order of two- to threefold.[219] It is indicated worldwide for partial seizures (though it may be less effective than carbamazepine[220]), but, more uniquely, it is also clearly effective for infantile spasms, a devastating and treatment-resistant form of epilepsy that often leaves its young victims permanently handicapped.[221] Infantile spasms may be cryptogenic or associated with a diffuse neurologic condition, most commonly tuberous sclerosis, and while vigabatrin can reduce infantile spasms from any cause, it appears to be a veritable "magic bullet" for infantile spasms due to tuberous sclerosis.[222] Such is its effectiveness that parents of affected infants in the United States are frequently counseled to cross the nearest border (Canadian or Mexican) to obtain it. The drug remains unavailable in this country nonetheless because it has been found to produce significant restrictions of peripheral visual fields in up to 40% of patients; the field loss is asymptomatic in the vast majority of cases, but unfortunately it is also usually irreversible.[223] It is presumed that vigabatrin-induced impairment of GABAergic cells in the retina may be responsible, though neither tiagabine nor any other GABAergic drug has ever been found to affect peripheral vision. While the FDA has not approved vigabatrin for this reason, many hope that the drug might at least be approved for use in children with infantile spasms, for whom visual field constriction would be the least of concerns.

Therapeutic Approach

First, decide whether treatment is appropriate for a given patient; a good rule of thumb is that a first seizure is typically not treated while a second seizure usually is,[224] but there are many exceptions that are beyond the scope of this chapter, and the reader is referred to an epilepsy text for further discussion of this fundamental question.[4] Once the decision to treat has been made, the next step—a crucial one that is often overlooked—is to determine what type of epilepsy the patient has. Often a specific syndromic diagnosis cannot be made, but at the very least an understanding of whether the patient has focal epilepsy or generalized epilepsy is necessary to establish appropriate treatment options. This can almost always be done simply by taking a careful and detailed history, but when there is doubt, then sleep-deprived EEG, magnetic resonance imaging of the brain, or inpatient video-EEG monitoring can be used to sort out the diagnosis. (N.B.: The occurrence of generalized tonic-clonic seizures does *not* necessarily mean that the patient has generalized epilepsy, as they may be secondarily generalized from a focal area.)

Once the type of epilepsy is known, then consider your options. For a patient with focal epilepsy, every drug marketed in the United States—with the exception of ethosuximide—is efficacious. For patients with generalized epilepsy, only the broad-spectrum AEDs (valproate, lamotrigine, zonisamide, and sometimes topiramate and levetiracetam) are likely to be of benefit. If you cannot be sure what kind of epilepsy you are dealing with, it pays to hedge your bet by choosing one of these agents. For patients with generalized epilepsy, diagnosis of specific seizure types may be helpful in choosing optimal therapy; for example, if the patient has absence seizures, then subtract topiramate and levetiracetam from your list, but ethosuximide may be a consideration.

Now comes the hard part. In choosing an AED, there are many guidelines, but no clear algorithms. One set of guidelines is that produced jointly by the American Academy of Neurology and the American Epilepsy Society,[225] whose panel members evaluated data on the newer AEDs in new-onset epilepsy patients, emphasizing prospective, blinded, randomized controlled trials. These authors found that there was evidence of efficacy for oxcarbazepine and topiramate for partial and generalized tonic-clonic seizures, lamotrigine for these types and for absence seizures, and gabapentin for partial seizures. From there, they stated, "Choice of AED will depend on individual patient characteristics."

Using considerably more rigorous criteria, a subcommittee of the International League Against Epilepsy assessed randomized monotherapy studies in both the older and newer AEDs, with an emphasis on trials of long (≥48 weeks) duration having adequate power to detect 20% differences between treatment arms.[226] Their results were sobering: High-level evidence was available only for focal seizures, not for any of the generalized seizure types and syndromes, and this evidence favored only a few drugs for each population: carbamazepine, phenytoin, and valproate in adults; gabapentin and lamotrigine in the elderly; and oxcarbazepine in children. They commented: "There is an especially alarming lack of well-designed, properly conducted randomized controlled trials for patient with generalized seizures/epilepsies and for children in general."

Take these two major guidelines together and you get quite a paradox: using moderately stringent criteria, there was evidence that a number of newer AEDs were effective in monotherapy (while the older ones, as "standard" treatments, were presumed effective); yet using highly stringent criteria, only a few AEDs were demonstrated effective, and for limited patient populations. Furthermore, since the vast majority of epilepsy trials are sponsored by the pharmaceutical companies, these evidence-based guidelines are, in effect, largely held hostage to the sponsors' motivations, which have more to do with marketing than science. This means that other drugs for which good monotherapy trials have not yet been pursued (e.g., zonisamide) might very well be just as effective—and, in fact, are commonly used as monotherapy. In the end, both of these guidelines tell us the same thing: we need better trials, possibly by more disinterested sponsors, in order to choose among the many options for treatment.

One other set of "guidelines" is not strictly a guideline, nor even evidence based: A large panel of experts was asked to rank treatment options for various hypothetical patient scenarios, and the results were quantitatively analyzed.[38] This "Expert Consensus" sits at the opposite end of the spectrum from the aforementioned guidelines: largely unscientific, yet potentially just as useful to the practitioner precisely by virtue of being more akin to the real world and less beholden to the artificial milieu of clinical trial design. The full results of this process are too extensive to detail here, but in summary, for new-onset treatment in adolescents and adults, the consensus top choices were carbamazepine, oxcarbazepine, and lamotrigine for focal epilepsy, and valproate for most of the generalized seizure types. An analogous survey done regarding treatment in children yielded fairly similar recommendations.[227]

One final method for choosing an AED might be called the "concrete differences" method: certain drugs have concrete benefits over others that either (i) have been demonstrated in trials, or (ii) are so clear cut that no one would dispute them. These might include treatment of comorbid conditions such as migraine (topiramate, valproate) or obesity (topiramate); rapid titration and onset of action (levetiracetam, oxcarbazepine); once-daily dosing (zonisamide, valproate); or low cost (phenytoin, carbamazepine, phenobarbital) (Fig. 45-3).

The author is of the opinion that—aside from the financially disadvantaged—it is getting harder and harder to justify use of the older enzyme-inducing drugs in light of the mounting evidence of their adverse metabolic effects, their requirement for blood monitoring, and their profuse drug-drug interactions. In addition, valproate is associated with enough reproductive and endocrine difficulties that the author believes it should not be used in reproductive-age women unless other options have been extensively explored.

As discussed earlier, complete freedom from disabling seizures (i.e., those involving loss of awareness or disruption of activities) is the goal. So if your patient has one or more recurrent seizures on a reasonable dose of an AED, what next? It used to be standard teaching that one should maximize the dose of the current AED—that is, continue to increase until the first side effects, then come down to the maximum tolerated dose to demonstrate conclusively whether or not that drug will be effective for that patient. Yet the available evidence does not support this practice. Kwan and Brodie[228] found that 91% to 94% of patients who became seizure free on their first AED did so at very modest doses: ≤800 mg/day of carbamazepine, ≤300 mg/day of lamotrigine, or ≤1500 mg/day of valproate. Another study involving topiramate clearly demonstrated that seizure-free rates are the same whether using 50 mg or 100 mg twice daily; the higher dose yielded nothing but a higher rate of side effects.[184] Thus, while a drug should be increased at least to a moderate dose if tolerated, increases beyond this appear to yield very little in terms of incremental seizure freedom.

So should you change to another drug? Absolutely—but don't get your hopes up. In a landmark study, Kwan and Brodie[2] prospectively treated and followed a large cohort of patients with untreated epilepsy to assess their long-term response to therapy. They found that 36% of patients could not be made seizure free, and the response to the first

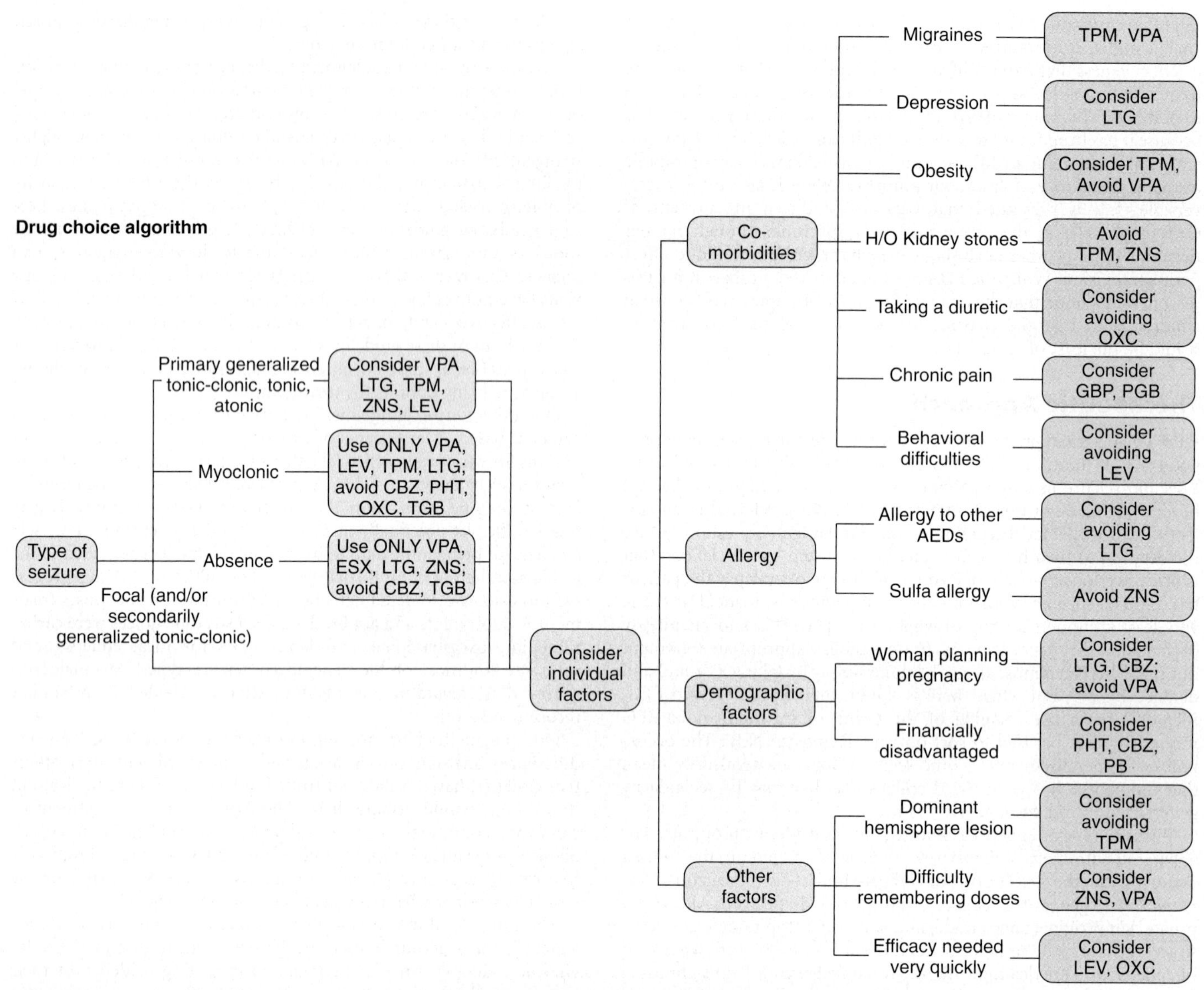

FIGURE 45-3 • Drug choice algorithm.

drug was telling: *only 11% of those who failed the first drug due to lack of efficacy ever became seizure free.* The authors concluded that refractory epilepsy could be identified very early in its course. Two recent studies suggest that this prognosis may be a bit overly pessimistic[229,230] but do not alter the greater conclusion that sequential drug trials reach a point of diminishing returns fairly rapidly.

So what then? Consistent evidence indicates that patients with focal epilepsy who cannot be made free from disabling seizures using drugs should be considered for focal surgical resection. The process of assessing candidacy for epilepsy surgery involves an extensive evaluation that is described elsewhere.[4] Resection is most commonly performed for seizures arising from the temporal lobes, a population in which a randomized trial has demonstrated the overwhelming superiority of surgery over continued medical therapy.[231] The results are long lasting, with over 60% of patients remaining seizure free even when followed out for 5 years.[232] Nonetheless, patients with seizures arising from other regions, such as the frontal lobes, can also achieve very good results with surgery in some cases.[233] Achieving seizure freedom not only benefits quality of life[234] but also significantly improves mortality.[15] There is a broad consensus in the field that patients with focal epilepsy who have not been rendered seizure free after two or three trials of different AEDs should be referred to a specialized epilepsy center so that surgery may be considered.

Whether surgery is being considered or not, referral to an epilepsy center is important after two or three failed medication trials simply so the diagnosis of epilepsy can be verified. This is a crucial step to avoid long-term inappropriate AED treatment in patients who do not have epilepsy. The most common mimicker of epilepsy is psychogenic seizures, but occasionally cardiac arrhythmia, migraine variants, and paroxysmal basal ganglia or neuromuscular disorders are mistaken for epilepsy as well. Careful history taking by a specialist and long-term video-EEG monitoring usually establish the appropriate diagnosis. The fundamental algorithm for the treatment of presumed epileptic seizures is outlined in Figure 45-4.

Not all patients are amenable to resective surgery, including those whose epileptic foci cannot be localized, those whose foci are in unresectable regions, and those with multifocal epilepsy. Patients with refractory generalized epilepsy are also not amenable to resection; furthermore, in this group of patients, there are very few data on the comparative efficacy of different AEDs, so that—in contrast to focal epilepsy—essaying various drugs and drug combinations to find the "magic bullet" for a given patient cannot be dismissed as a treatment strategy. Future studies will hopefully shed light on this. Nonpharmacologic treatment options for this group, and for the refractory focal epilepsy patients who are not candidates for resection, include vagus nerve stimulation,[235] corpus callosotomy,[236] or the ketogenic diet.[237] All

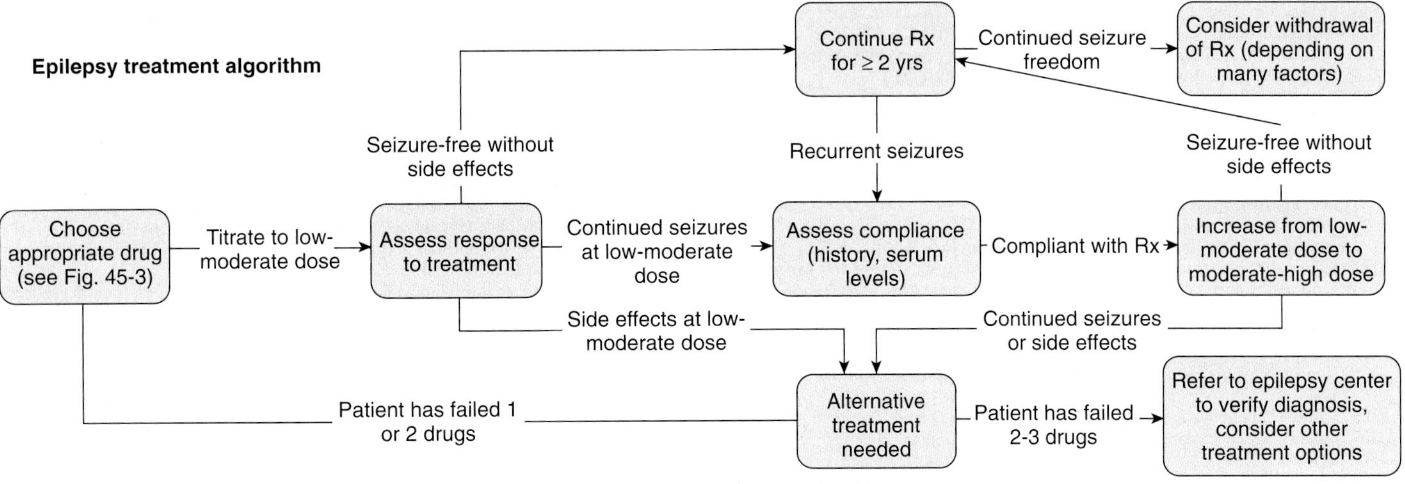

FIGURE 45-4 • Epilepsy treatment algorithm.

of these produce seizure freedom only rarely, however, so they should be viewed as palliative treatment options for those who cannot be "cured" by surgical resection.

Emergency treatment for status epilepticus is fairly well standardized. Two randomized trials[238,239] demonstrated that lorazepam and diazepam are equally effective, though the former drug is used more often owing to diazepam's short brain half-life, which requires the use of IV phenytoin in tandem. Phenytoin should be used in either case if seizures continue despite multiple doses of the benzodiazepine, and should be pushed aggressively if needed. Should status persist despite high (≥25 to 30 mcg/ml) concentrations of phenytoin, then IV phenobarbital is traditionally used. If seizures still persist despite high therapeutic serum phenobarbital levels, then the patient is intubated and a continuous IV anesthetic drip is used; pentobarbital, midazolam, or propofol are the most common choices. The role of the newer IV AEDs, valproate and levetiracetam, in the treatment of status epilepticus has yet to be determined.

Emerging Targets and Therapeutics

In spite of the crowded market, much activity continues in the area of AED development, with a bevy of compounds in various stages of the pipeline; an incomplete list of these follows.

Seletracetam is related to levetiracetam but far more potent, having a higher affinity for binding at synaptic vesicle protein SV2A.[240] *Brivaracetam*, another in the same class, not only has 10 times the binding affinity for SV2A, but also appears to have some Na^+ channel blocking properties.[241] *Carisbamate* (formerly known as RWJ-333369) is structurally related to felbamate but does not form an atropaldehyde metabolite.[242] *Rufinamide* is structurally unrelated to other AEDs and functions as an inactivator of voltage-gated Na^+ channels,[243] but appears to have a much better therapeutic index than the older AEDs. *Lacosamide* (formerly known as harkoseride), related to the amino acid serine, has two potentially relevant biochemical properties: selective enhancement of the slow inactivation of voltage-dependent Na^+ channels[244] and modulation of collapsin response mediator protein 2, resulting in retardation of axon growth.[245] *Ganaxolone* is a neuroactive steroid that is closely related to the progesterone metabolite allopregnanolone, and like that molecule, it acts as an allosteric modulator of the $GABA_A$ receptor.[246] *Retigabine* has a broad spectrum of anticonvulsant activity and a completely novel mechanism of action: enhancement of M-current through neuronal K^+ channels.[247] *Talampanel* is structurally related to the benzodiazepines but acts instead as a noncompetitive antagonist at the AMPA subtype of glutamate receptor.[248] *Stiripentol*, discovered over 20 years ago, is still in development but is licensed as an orphan drug in France to treat severe myoclonic epilepsy of infancy, another devastating and difficult-to-treat condition for which it appears to have considerable efficacy. It increases synaptic GABA via several mechanisms, including blockade of GABA transaminase; development has been hampered by its impressive tendency to interact with other AEDs.[249]

In addition to the many novel AEDs in the development pipeline, many organizations have been pursuing truly novel treatment modalities for refractory epilepsy. Several trials underway involve continuous or intermittent electrical stimulation of brain structures, either in the cortex or in subcortical structures such as the thalamus or basal ganglia. Continuous stimulation would mimic the implantable neurostimulators currently in use for patients with Parkinson's disease and other movement disorders, while intermittent stimulation would ideally be combined with some manner of computerized prosthetic device that was capable of recording the patient's EEG activity and determining that a seizure was occurring—or, even better, that one was about to occur. This could then allow the delivery of electrical stimulation or a rapid-acting drug to terminate the process. While treatment modalities of this nature are many years away, there is enough active work on the various pieces of this science fiction–like scenario to permit hope that it may eventually come to fruition.

REFERENCES

1. Merritt HH, Putnam TJ. Landmark article Sept 17, 1938: Sodium diphenyl hydantoinate in the treatment of convulsive disorders. JAMA 1984;251:1062-1067.
2. Kwan P, Brodie MJ. Early identification of refractory epilepsy. N Engl J Med 2000;342:314-319.
3. Hauser WA, Hesdorffer DH. Epilepsy: Frequency, Causes and Consequences. New York: Demos Press, 1990.
4. Engel J Jr, Pedley TA. Epilepsy: A Comprehensive Textbook. Philadelphia: Lippincott–Raven, 1998.
5. Berkovic SF. Genetics of epilepsy syndromes. *In* Engel J, Pedley T (eds): Epilepsy: A Comprehensive Textbook. Philadelphia: Lippincott–Raven, 1997.
6. Steriade M, Contreras D. Relations between cortical and thalamic cellular events during transition from sleep patterns to paroxysmal activity. J Neurosci 1995;15:623-642.
7. Hosford DA, Clark S, Cao Z, et al. The role of $GABA_B$ receptor activation in absence seizures of lethargic (*lh/lh*) mice. Science 1992;257:398-401.
8. Mathern GW, Babb TL, Leite JP, et al. The pathogenic and progressive features of chronic human hippocampal epilepsy. Epilepsy Res 1996;26:151-161.
9. Prince DA, Futamachi KJ. Intracellular recordings in chronic focal epilepsy. Brain Res 1968;11:681-684.
10. Dichter M, Spencer WA. Penicillin-induced interictal discharges from the cat hippocampus. I. Characteristics and topographical features. J Neurophysiol 1969;32:649-662.
11. Tian GF, Azmi H, Takano T, et al. An astrocytic basis of epilepsy. Nat Med 2005;11:973-981.
12. Seidenberg M, Kelly KG, Parrish J, et al. Ipsilateral and contralateral MRI volumetric abnormalities in chronic unilateral temporal lobe epilepsy and their clinical correlates. Epilepsia 2005;46:420-430.
13. Hermann BP, Seidenberg M, Dow C, et al. Cognitive prognosis in chronic temporal lobe epilepsy. Ann Neurol 2006;60:80-87.
14. Nilsson L, Tomson T, Farahmand BY, et al. Cause-specific mortality in epilepsy: a cohort study of more than 9,000 patients once hospitalized for epilepsy. Epilepsia 1997;38:1062-1068.
15. Sperling MR, Feldman H, Kinman J, et al. Seizure control and mortality in epilepsy. Ann Neurol 1999;46:45-50.

16. Birbeck GL, Hays RD, Cui X, Vickrey BG. Seizure reduction and quality of life improvements in people with epilepsy. Epilepsia 2002;43:535-538.
17. Cockerell OC, Johnson AL, Sander JW, et al. Mortality from epilepsy: results from a prospective population-based study. Lancet 1994;344:918-921.
18. Tracy JI, Dechant V, Sperling MR, et al. The association of mood with quality of life ratings in epilepsy. Neurology 2007;68:1101-1107.
19. Gilliam FG. Diagnosis and treatment of mood disorders in persons with epilepsy. Curr Opin Neurol 2005;18:129-133.
20. Kanner AM, Kozak AM, Frey M. The use of sertraline in patients with epilepsy: is it safe? Epilepsy Behav 2000;1:100-105.
21. Gilliam FG, Fessler AJ, Baker G, et al. Systematic screening allows reduction of adverse antiepileptic drug effects: a randomized trial. Neurology 2004;62:23-27.
22. Isojarvi JI, Laatikainen TJ, Pakarinen AJ, et al. Polycystic ovaries and hyperandrogenism in women taking valproate for epilepsy. N Engl J Med 1993;329:1383-1388.
23. Ensrud KE, Walczak TS, Blackwell T, et al. Antiepileptic drug use increases rates of bone loss in older women: a prospective study. Neurology 2004;62:2051-2057.
24. Pack AM, Olarte LS, Morrell MJ, et al. Bone mineral density in an outpatient population receiving enzyme-inducing antiepileptic drugs. Epilepsy Behav 2003;4:169-174.
25. Mintzer S, Boppana P, Toguri J, DeSantis A. Vitamin D levels and bone turnover in epilepsy patients taking carbamazepine or oxcarbazepine. Epilepsia 2006;47:510-515.
26. Herzog AG, Drislane FW, Schomer DL, et al. Differential effects of antiepileptic drugs on sexual function and hormones in men with epilepsy. Neurology 2005;65:1016-1020.
27. Mintzer S, Skidmore C, Abidin C, et al. The effects of antiepileptic drugs on serum lipids, homocysteine, and C-reactive protein. Epilepsia 2007;48(Suppl 6):404.
28. Nelson E, Powell JR, Conrad K, et al. Phenobarbital pharmacokinetics and bioavailability in adults. J Clin Pharmacol 1982;22:141-148.
29. Viswanathan CT, Booker HE, Welling PG. Bioavailability of oral and intramuscular phenobarbital. J Clin Pharmacol 1978;18:100-105.
30. Vining EP. Use of barbiturates and benzodiazepines in treatment of epilepsy. Neurol Clin 1986;4:617-632.
31. Ehrnebo M, Agurell S, Jalling B, Boreus LO. Age differences in drug binding by plasma proteins: studies on human foetuses, neonates and adults. Eur J Clin Pharmacol 1971;3:189-193.
32. Nishihara K, Uchino K, Saitoh Y, et al. Estimation of plasma unbound phenobarbital concentration by using mixed saliva. Epilepsia 1979;20:37-45.
33. Goto S, Seo T, Murata T, et al. Population estimation of the effects of cytochrome P450 2C9 and 2C19 polymorphisms on phenobarbital clearance in Japanese. Ther Drug Monit 2007;29:118-121.
34. Bernus I, Dickinson RG, Hooper WD, Eadie MJ. Urinary excretion of phenobarbitone and its metabolites in chronically treated patients. Eur J Clin Pharmacol 1994;46:473-475.
35. Verdoorn TA, Draguhn A, Ymer S, et al. Functional properties of recombinant rat $GABA_A$ receptors depend upon subunit composition. Neuron 1990;4:919-928.
36. MacDonald RL, Rogers CJ, Twyman RE. Barbiturate regulation of kinetic properties of the $GABA_A$ receptor channel of mouse spinal neurones in culture. J Physiol (Lond) 1989;417:483-500.
37. Mattson RH, Cramer JA, Collins JF, et al. Comparison of carbamazepine, phenobarbital, phenytoin, and primidone in partial and secondarily generalized tonic-clonic seizures. N Engl J Med 1985;313:145-151.
38. Karceski S, Morrell MJ, Carpenter D. Treatment of epilepsy in adults: expert opinion, 2005. Epilepsy Behav 2005;7(Suppl 1):S1-64; quiz S65-S67.
39. Kwan P, Brodie MJ. Phenobarbital for the treatment of epilepsy in the 21st century: a critical review. Epilepsia 2004;45:1141-1149.
40. Meador KJ, Loring DW, Moore EE, et al. Comparative cognitive effects of phenobarbital, phenytoin, and valproate in healthy adults. Neurology 1995;45:1494-1499.
41. Waxman DJ, Azaroff L. Phenobarbital induction of cytochrome P-450 gene expression. Biochem J 1992;281(Pt 3):577-592.
42. Hosseinpour F, Ellfolk M, Norlin M, Wikvall K. Phenobarbital suppresses vitamin D3 25-hydroxylase expression: a potential new mechanism for drug-induced osteomalacia. Biochem Biophys Res Commun 2007;357:603-607.
43. Formiggini G, Bovina C, Marchi-Marchetti M, Marchetti M. Effect of phenobarbitone on folic acid metabolism in the rat. Pharmacol Res Commun 1984;16:467-478.
44. Sonmez FM, Demir E, Orem A, et al. Effect of antiepileptic drugs on plasma lipids, lipoprotein (a), and liver enzymes. J Child Neurol 2006;21:70-74.
45. Verrotti A, Basciani F, Domizio S, et al. Serum lipids and lipoproteins in patients treated with antiepileptic drugs. Pediatr Neurol 1998;19:364-367.
46. Morselli PL, Rizzo M, Garattini S. Interaction between phenobarbital and diphenylhydantoin in animals and in epileptic patients. Ann N Y Acad Sci 1971;179:88-107.
47. Wilder BJ, Willmore LJ, Bruni J, Villarreal HJ. Valproic acid: interaction with other anticonvulsant drugs. Neurology 1978;28:892-896.
48. Reidenberg MM, Lowenthal DT, Briggs W, Gasparo M. Pentobarbital elimination in patients with poor renal function. Clin Pharmacol Ther 1976;20:67-71.
49. Bogan J, Smith H. The relation between primidone and phenobarbitone blood levels. J Pharm Pharmacol 1968;20:64-67.
50. Olesen OV, Dam M. The metabolic conversion of primidone (Mysoline) to phenobarbitone in patients under long-term treatment: an attempt to estimate the independent effect of primidone. Acta Neurol Scand 1967;43:348-356.
51. Bourgeois BF, Dodson WE, Ferrendelli JA. Primidone, phenobarbital, and PEMA: I. Seizure protection, neurotoxicity, and therapeutic index of individual compounds in mice. Neurology 1983;33:283-290.
52. Houghton GW, Richens A, Toseland PA, et al. Brain concentrations of phenytoin, phenobarbitone and primidone in epileptic patients. Eur J Clin Pharmacol 1975;9:73-78.
53. Kauffman RE, Habersang R, Lansky L. Kinetics of primidone metabolism and excretion in children. Clin Pharmacol Ther 1977;22:200-205.
54. Cloyd JC, Miller KW, Leppik IE. Primidone kinetics: effects of concurrent drugs and duration of therapy. Clin Pharmacol Ther 1981;29:402-407.
55. Sasso E, Perucca E, Calzetti S. Double-blind comparison of primidone and phenobarbital in essential tremor. Neurology 1988;38:808-810.
56. Calzetti S, Findley LJ, Pisani F, Richens A. Phenylethylmalonamide in essential tremor: a double-blind controlled study. J Neurol Neurosurg Psychiatry 1981;44:932-934.
57. Browne TR, Leduc B. Phenytoin and other hydantoins: chemistry and biotransformation. *In* Levy RH, Mattson RH, Meldrum BS, Perucca E (eds): Antiepileptic Drugs, 5th ed. Philadelphia: Lippincott Williams & Wilkins, 2002, pp 565-580.
58. Eadie MJ, Tyrer JH, Bochner F, Hooper WD. The elimination of phenytoin in man. Clin Exp Pharmacol Physiol 1976;3:217-224.
59. Dodson WE. Phenytoin elimination in childhood: effect of concentration-dependent kinetics. Neurology 1980;30:196-199.
60. McLean MJ, Macdonald RL. Multiple actions of phenytoin on mouse spinal cord neurons in cell culture. J Pharmacol Exp Ther 1983;227:779-789.
61. Wilder BJ, Ramsay RE, Murphy JV, et al. Comparison of valproic acid and phenytoin in newly diagnosed tonic-clonic seizures. Neurology 1983;33:1474-1476.
62. Eldridge R, Iivanainen M, Stern R, et al. "Baltic" myoclonus epilepsy: hereditary disorder of childhood made worse by phenytoin. Lancet 1983;2:838-842.
63. Genton P, Gelisse P, Thomas P, Dravet C. Do carbamazepine and phenytoin aggravate juvenile myoclonic epilepsy? Neurology 2000;55:1106-1109.
64. O'Mara NB, Jones PR, Anglin DL, et al. Pharmacokinetics of phenytoin in children with acute neurotrauma. Crit Care Med 1995;23:1418-1424.
65. Hays DP, Primack WA, Abroms IF. Phenytoin clearance by continuous ambulatory peritoneal dialysis. Drug Intell Clin Pharm 1985;19:429-431.
66. Martin E, Gambertoglio JG, Adler DS, et al. Removal of phenytoin by hemodialysis in uremic patients. JAMA 1977;238:1750-1753.
67. Dasgupta A, Abu-Alfa A. Increased free phenytoin concentrations in predialysis serum compared to postdialysis serum in patients with uremia treated with hemodialysis: role of uremic compounds. Am J Clin Pathol 1992;98:19-25.
68. Chadwick D, Reynolds EH, Marsden CD. Anticonvulsant-induced dyskinesias: a comparison with dyskinesias induced by neuroleptics. J Neurol Neurosurg Psychiatry 1976;39:1210-1218.
69. Parker WA, Shearer CA. Phenytoin hepatotoxicity: a case report and review. Neurology 1979;29:175-178.
70. O'Brien TJ, Cascino GD, So EL, Hanna DR. Incidence and clinical consequence of the purple glove syndrome in patients receiving intravenous phenytoin. Neurology 1998;51:1034-1039.
71. Burneo JG, Anandan JV, Barkley GL. A prospective study of the incidence of the purple glove syndrome. Epilepsia 2001;42:1156-1159.
72. Scott JM, Weir DG. Drug-induced megaloblastic change. Clin Haematol 1980;9:587-606.
73. Sener U, Zorlu Y, Karaguzel O, et al. Effects of common anti-epileptic drug monotherapy on serum levels of homocysteine, vitamin B12, folic acid and vitamin B6. Seizure 2006;15:79-85.
74. Pack AM, Morrell MJ, Marcus R, et al. Bone mass and turnover in women with epilepsy on antiepileptic drug monotherapy. Ann Neurol 2005;57:252-257.
75. Nikolaos T, Stylianos G, Chryssoula N, et al. The effect of long-term antiepileptic treatment on serum cholesterol (TC, HDL, LDL) and triglyceride levels in adult epileptic patients on monotherapy. Med Sci Monit 2004;10:MT50-MT52.
76. O'Brien MD, Guillebaud J. Contraception for women with epilepsy. Epilepsia 2006;47:1419-1422.
77. Oberndorfer S, Piribauer M, Marosi C, et al. P450 enzyme inducing and non-enzyme inducing antiepileptics in glioblastoma patients treated with standard chemotherapy. J Neurooncol 2005;72:255-260.
78. Browne TR. Fosphenytoin (Cerebyx). Clin Neuropharmacol 1997;20:1-12.
79. Rogers CJ, Twyman RE, Macdonald RL. Benzodiazepine and beta-carboline regulation of single $GABA_A$ receptor channels of mouse spinal neurones in culture. J Physiol (Lond) 1994;475:69-82.
80. Kaplan SA, Alexander K, Jack ML, et al. Pharmacokinetic profiles of clonazepam in dog and humans and of flunitrazepam in dog. J Pharm Sci 1974;63:527-532.
81. Sato T. The prognosis of epileptic seizures—review of the literatures. Folia Psychiatr Neurol Jpn 1977;31:279-289.
82. Kaplan SA, Jack ML, Alexander K, Weinfeld RE. Pharmacokinetic profile of diazepam in man following single intravenous and oral and chronic oral administrations. J Pharm Sci 1973;62:1789-1796.
83. Cloyd JC, Lalonde RL, Beniak TE, Novack GD. A single-blind, crossover comparison of the pharmacokinetics and cognitive effects of a new diazepam rectal gel with intravenous diazepam. Epilepsia 1998;39:520-526.
84. Kanto J, Kangas L, Siirtola T. Cerebrospinal-fluid concentration of diazepam and its metabolites in man. Acta Pharmacol Toxicol (Copenh) 1975;36:328-334.
85. Kanto J, Sellman R, Haataja M, Hurme P. Plasma and urine concentrations of diazepam and its metabolites in children, adults and in diazepam-intoxicated patients. Int J Clin Pharmacol Biopharm 1978;16:258-264.
86. Celesia GG, Booker HE, Sato S. Brain and serum concentrations of diazepam in experimental epilepsy. Epilepsia 1974;15:417-425.
87. Anderson GD, Miller JW. Benzodiazepines: chemistry, biotransformation, and pharmacokinetics. *In* Levy RH, Mattson RH, Meldrum BS, Perucca E (eds): Antiepileptic Drugs, 5th ed. Philadelphia: Lippincott Williams & Wilkins, 2002.
88. Greenblatt DJ, Shader RI, Franke K, et al. Pharmacokinetics and bioavailability of intravenous, intramuscular, and oral lorazepam in humans. J Pharm Sci 1979;68:57-63.
89. Moschitto LJ, Greenblatt DJ. Concentration-independent plasma protein binding of benzodiazepines. J Pharm Pharmacol 1983;35:179-180.

90. Ochs HR, Busse J, Greenblatt DJ, Allen MD. Entry of lorazepam into cerebrospinal fluid. Br J Clin Pharmacol 1980;10:405-406.
91. Elliott HW. Metabolism of lorazepam. Br J Anaesth 1976;48:1017-1023.
92. Kearns GL, Mallory GB Jr, Crom WR, Evans WE. Enhanced hepatic drug clearance in patients with cystic fibrosis. J Pediatr 1990;117:972-979.
93. Smith MT, Eadie MJ, Brophy TO. The pharmacokinetics of midazolam in man. Eur J Clin Pharmacol 1981;19:271-278.
94. Löscher W, Schmidt D. Experimental and clinical evidence for loss of effect (tolerance) during prolonged treatment with antiepileptic drugs. Epilepsia 2006;47:1253-1284.
95. Eadie MJ, Tyrer JH, Smith GA, McKauge L. Pharmacokinetics of drugs used for petit mal "absence" epilepsy. Clin Exp Neurol 1977;14:172-183.
96. Loscher W, Frey HH. Kinetics of penetration of common antiepileptic drugs into cerebrospinal fluid. Epilepsia 1984;25:346-352.
97. Bachmann K, He Y, Sarver JG, Peng N. Characterization of the cytochrome P450 enzymes involved in the in vitro metabolism of ethosuximide by human hepatic microsomal enzymes. Xenobiotica 2003;33:265-276.
98. Buchanan RA, Fernandez L, Kinkel AW. Absorption and elimination of ethosuximide in children. J Clin Pharmacol J New Drugs 1969;9:393-398.
99. Coulter DA, Huguenard JR, Prince DA. Characterization of ethosuximide reduction of low-threshold calcium current in thalamic neurons. Ann Neurol 1989;25:582-593.
100. Massey GV, Dunn NL, Heckel JL, et al. Aplastic anemia following therapy for absence seizures with ethosuximide. Pediatr Neurol 1994;11:59-61.
101. Hurst DL. Methsuximide therapy of juvenile myoclonic epilepsy. Seizure 1996;5:47-50.
102. Wad N, Bourgeois B, Kramer G. Serum protein binding of desmethyl-methsuximide. Clin Neuropharmacol 1999;22:239-240.
103. Marson AG, Al-Kharusi AM, Alwaidh M, et al. The SANAD study of effectiveness of carbamazepine, gabapentin, lamotrigine, oxcarbazepine, or topiramate for treatment of partial epilepsy: an unblinded randomised controlled trial. Lancet 2007;369:1000-1015.
104. Cotter LM, Smith G, Hooper WD, et al. The bioavailability of carbamazepine. Proc Aust Assoc Neurol 1975;12:123-128.
105. Gerardin A, Dubois JP, Moppert J, Geller L. Absolute bioavailability of carbamazepine after oral administration of a 2% syrup. Epilepsia 1990;31:334-338.
106. McLean MJ, Macdonald RL. Carbamazepine and 10,11-epoxycarbamazepine produce use- and voltage-dependent limitation of rapidly firing action potentials of mouse central neurons in cell culture. J Pharmacol Exp Ther 1986;238:727-738.
107. Tapolyai M, Campbell M, Dailey K, Udvari-Nagy S. Hemodialysis is as effective as hemoperfusion for drug removal in carbamazepine poisoning. Nephron 2002;90:213-215.
108. Vreugdenhil M, Wadman WJ. Modulation of sodium currents in rat CA1 neurons by carbamazepine and valproate after kindling epileptogenesis. Epilepsia 1999;40:1512-1522.
109. Lampe H, Bigalke H. Carbamazepine blocks NMDA-activated currents in cultured spinal cord neurons. Neuroreport 1990;1:26-28.
110. Thomas P, Valton L, Genton P. Absence and myoclonic status epilepticus precipitated by antiepileptic drugs in idiopathic generalized epilepsy. Brain 2006;129:1281-1292.
111. Isojarvi JI, Pakarinen AJ, Ylipalosaari PJ, Myllyla VV. Serum hormones in male epileptic patients receiving anticonvulsant medication. Arch Neurol 1990;47:670-676.
112. Bramswig S, Sudhop T, Luers C, et al. Lipoprotein(a) concentration increases during treatment with carbamazepine. Epilepsia 2003;44:457-460.
113. Wurden CJ, Levy RH. Carbamazepine: interactions with other drugs. *In* Levy RH, Mattson RH, Meldrum BS, Perucca E (eds): Antiepileptic Drugs, 5th ed. Philadelphia: Lippincott Williams & Wilkins, 2002, pp 247-261.
114. Schutz H, Feldmann KF, Faigle JW, et al. The metabolism of ^{14}C-oxcarbazepine in man. Xenobiotica 1986;16:769-778.
115. McLean MJ, Schmutz M, Wamil AW, et al. Oxcarbazepine: mechanisms of action. Epilepsia 1994;35(Suppl 3):S5-S9.
116. Stefani A, Pisani A, De Murtas M, et al. Action of GP 47779, the active metabolite of oxcarbazepine, on the corticostriatal system. II. Modulation of high-voltage-activated calcium currents. Epilepsia 1995;36:997-1002.
117. Dam M, Ekberg R, Loyning Y, et al. A double-blind study comparing oxcarbazepine and carbamazepine in patients with newly diagnosed, previously untreated epilepsy. Epilepsy Res 1989;3:70-76.
118. Isojarvi JI, Pakarinen AJ, Rautio A, et al. Liver enzyme induction and serum lipid levels after replacement of carbamazepine with oxcarbazepine. Epilepsia 1994;35:1217-1220.
119. Isojarvi JI, Pakarinen AJ, Rautio A, et al. Serum sex hormone levels after replacing carbamazepine with oxcarbazepine. Eur J Clin Pharmacol 1995;47:461-464.
120. Dong X, Leppik IE, White J, Rarick J. Hyponatremia from oxcarbazepine and carbamazepine. Neurology 2005;65:1976-1978.
121. Beydoun A, Sackellares JC, Shu V. Safety and efficacy of divalproex sodium monotherapy in partial epilepsy: a double-blind, concentration-response design clinical trial. Depakote Monotherapy for Partial Seizures Study Group. Neurology 1997;48:182-188.
122. Dutta S, Reed RC. Distinct absorption characteristics of oral formulations of valproic acid/divalproex available in the United States. Epilepsy Res 2007;73:275-283.
123. Bowdle AT, Patel IH, Levy RH, Wilensky AJ. Valproic acid dosage and plasma protein binding and clearance. Clin Pharmacol Ther 1980;28:486-492.
124. Perucca E, Grimaldi R, Gatti G, et al. Pharmacokinetics of valproic acid in the elderly. Br J Clin Pharmacol 1984;17:665-669.
125. Chiba K, Suganuma T, Ishizaki T, et al. Comparison of steady-state pharmacokinetics of valproic acid in children between monotherapy and multiple antiepileptic drug treatment. J Pediatr 1985;106:653-658.
126. Cloyd JC, Fischer JH, Kriel RL, Kraus DM. Valproic acid pharmacokinetics in children. IV. Effects of age and antiepileptic drugs on protein binding and intrinsic clearance. Clin Pharmacol Ther 1993;53:22-29.
127. Gal P, Oles KS, Gilman JT, Weaver R. Valproic acid efficacy, toxicity, and pharmacokinetics in neonates with intractable seizures. Neurology 1988;38:467-471.
128. Loscher W. Valproate: a reappraisal of its pharmacodynamic properties and mechanisms of action. Prog Neurobiol 1999;58:31-59.
129. Larsson OM, Gram L, Schousboe I, Schousboe A. Differential effect of gamma-vinyl GABA and valproate on GABA-transaminase from cultured neurones and astrocytes. Neuropharmacology 1986;25:617-625.
130. Zeise ML, Kasparow S, Zieglgansberger W. Valproate suppresses N-methyl-D-aspartate-evoked, transient depolarizations in the rat neocortex in vitro. Brain Res 1991;544:345-348.
131. Kelly KM, Gross RA, Macdonald RL. Valproic acid selectively reduces the low-threshold (T) calcium current in rat nodose neurons. Neurosci Lett 1990;116:233-238.
132. Misra UK, Kalita J, Patel R. Sodium valproate vs phenytoin in status epilepticus: a pilot study. Neurology 2006;67:340-342.
133. Marson AG, Al-Kharusi AM, Alwaidh M, et al. The SANAD study of effectiveness of valproate, lamotrigine, or topiramate for generalised and unclassifiable epilepsy: an unblinded randomised controlled trial. Lancet 2007;369:1016-1026.
134. Morrell MJ, Giudice L, Flynn KL, et al. Predictors of ovulatory failure in women with epilepsy. Ann Neurol 2002;52:704-711.
135. Genton P, Bauer J, Duncan S, et al. On the association between valproate and polycystic ovary syndrome. Epilepsia 2001;42:295-304.
136. Isojarvi JI, Rattya J, Myllyla VV, et al. Valproate, lamotrigine, and insulin-mediated risks in women with epilepsy. Ann Neurol 1998;43:446-451.
137. Herzog AG, Schachter SC. Valproate and the polycystic ovarian syndrome: final thoughts. Epilepsia 2001;42:311-315.
138. Isojarvi JI, Tauboll E, Tapanainen JS, et al. On the association between valproate and polycystic ovary syndrome: a response and an alternative view. Epilepsia 2001;42:305-310.
139. Lindhout D, Schmidt D. In-utero exposure to valproate and neural tube defects. Lancet 1986;1:1392-1393.
140. Vajda FJ, Hitchcock A, Graham J, et al. Foetal malformations and seizure control: 52 months data of the Australian Pregnancy Registry. Eur J Neurol 2006;13:645-654.
141. Meador KJ, Baker GA, Finnell RH, et al. In utero antiepileptic drug exposure: fetal death and malformations. Neurology 2006;67:407-412.
142. Adab N, Kini U, Vinten J, et al. The longer term outcome of children born to mothers with epilepsy. J Neurol Neurosurg Psychiatry 2004;75:1575-1583.
143. Vinten J, Adab N, Kini U, et al. Neuropsychological effects of exposure to anticonvulsant medication in utero. Neurology 2005;64:949-954.
144. Efficacy of felbamate in childhood epileptic encephalopathy (Lennox-Gastaut syndrome). The Felbamate Study Group in Lennox-Gastaut Syndrome. N Engl J Med 1993;328:29-33.
145. Sachdeo R, Narang-Sachdeo SK, Shumaker RC, et al. Tolerability and pharmacokinetics of monotherapy felbamate doses of 1,200-6,000 mg/day in subjects with epilepsy. Epilepsia 1997;38:887-892.
146. Graves NM, Ludden TM, Holmes GB, et al. Pharmacokinetics of felbamate, a novel antiepileptic drug: application of mixed-effect modeling to clinical trials. Pharmacotherapy 1989;9:372-376.
147. Pellock JM, Perhach JL, Sofia RD. Felbamate. *In* Levy RH, Mattson RM, Meldrum BS, Perucca E (eds): Antiepileptic Drugs, 5th ed. Philadelphia: Lippincott Williams & Wilkins, 2002, pp 301-318.
148. White HS, Wolf HH, Swinyard EA, et al. A neuropharmacological evaluation of felbamate as a novel anticonvulsant. Epilepsia 1992;33:564-572.
149. McCabe RT, Wasterlain CG, Kucharczyk N, et al. Evidence for anticonvulsant and neuroprotectant action of felbamate mediated by strychnine-insensitive glycine receptors. J Pharmacol Exp Ther 1993;264:1248-1252.
150. French J, Smith M, Faught E, Brown L. Practice Advisory: The use of felbamate in the treatment of patients with intractable epilepsy: report of the Quality Standards Subcommittee of the American Academy of Neurology and the American Epilepsy Society. Neurology 1999;52:1540-1545.
151. Thompson CD, Gulden PH, Macdonald TL. Identification of modified atropaldehyde mercapturic acids in rat and human urine after felbamate administration. Chem Res Toxicol 1997;10:457-462.
152. Travaglini MT, Morrison RC, Ackerman BH, et al. Toxic epidermal necrolysis after initiation of felbamate therapy. Pharmacotherapy 1995;15:260-264.
153. Lanneau C, Green A, Hirst WD, et al. Gabapentin is not a $GABA_B$ receptor agonist. Neuropharmacology 2001;41:965-975.
154. Stewart BH, Kugler AR, Thompson PR, Bockbrader HN. A saturable transport mechanism in the intestinal absorption of gabapentin is the underlying cause of the lack of proportionality between increasing dose and drug levels in plasma. Pharm Res 1993;10:276-281.
155. Taylor CP, Angelotti T, Fauman E. Pharmacology and mechanism of action of pregabalin: the calcium channel alpha2-delta (alpha2-delta) subunit as a target for antiepileptic drug discovery. Epilepsy Res 2007;73:137-150.
156. Fehrenbacher JC, Taylor CP, Vasko MR. Pregabalin and gabapentin reduce release of substance P and CGRP from rat spinal tissues only after inflammation or activation of protein kinase C. Pain 2003;105:133-141.
157. Beydoun A. Monotherapy trials with gabapentin for partial epilepsy. Epilepsia 1999;40(Suppl 6):S13-S16; discussion S73-S74.
158. Brodie MJ, Chadwick DW, Anhut H, et al. Gabapentin versus lamotrigine monotherapy: a double-blind comparison in newly diagnosed epilepsy. Epilepsia 2002;43:993-1000.
159. DeToledo JC, Toledo C, DeCerce J, Ramsay RE. Changes in body weight with chronic, high-dose gabapentin therapy. Ther Drug Monit 1997;19:394-396.

160. Gidal BE, Tamura T, Hammer A, Vuong A. Blood homocysteine, folate and vitamin B-12 concentrations in patients with epilepsy receiving lamotrigine or sodium valproate for initial monotherapy. Epilepsy Res 2005;64:161-166.
161. Rambeck B, Jurgens UH, May TW, et al. Comparison of brain extracellular fluid, brain tissue, cerebrospinal fluid, and serum concentrations of antiepileptic drugs measured intraoperatively in patients with intractable epilepsy. Epilepsia 2006;47:681-694.
162. Lees G, Leach MJ. Studies on the mechanism of action of the novel anticonvulsant lamotrigine (Lamictal) using primary neurological cultures from rat cortex. Brain Res 1993;612:190-199.
163. Sitges M, Chiu LM, Guarneros A, Nekrassov V. Effects of carbamazepine, phenytoin, lamotrigine, oxcarbazepine, topiramate and vinpocetine on Na^+ channel-mediated release of [^{3}H]glutamate in hippocampal nerve endings. Neuropharmacology 2007;52:598-605.
164. Wang SJ, Sihra TS, Gean PW. Lamotrigine inhibition of glutamate release from isolated cerebrocortical nerve terminals (synaptosomes) by suppression of voltage-activated calcium channel activity. Neuroreport 2001;12:2255-2258.
165. Zona C, Tancredi V, Longone P, et al. Neocortical potassium currents are enhanced by the antiepileptic drug lamotrigine. Epilepsia 2002;43:685-690.
166. Beran RG, Berkovic SF, Dunagan FM, et al. Double-blind, placebo-controlled, crossover study of lamotrigine in treatment-resistant generalised epilepsy. Epilepsia 1998;39:1329-1333.
167. Frank LM, Enlow T, Holmes GL, et al. Lamictal (lamotrigine) monotherapy for typical absence seizures in children. Epilepsia 1999;40:973-979.
168. Biraben A, Allain H, Scarabin JM, et al. Exacerbation of juvenile myoclonic epilepsy with lamotrigine. Neurology 2000;55:1758.
169. Meador KJ, Loring DW, Ray PG, et al. Differential cognitive and behavioral effects of carbamazepine and lamotrigine. Neurology 2001;56:1177-1182.
170. Meador KJ, Loring DW, Vahle VJ, et al. Cognitive and behavioral effects of lamotrigine and topiramate in healthy volunteers. Neurology 2005;64:2108-2114.
171. Gilliam F, Vazquez B, Sackellares JC, et al. An active-control trial of lamotrigine monotherapy for partial seizures. Neurology 1998;51:1018-1025.
172. Cramer JA, Hammer AE, Kustra RP. Improved mood states with lamotrigine in patients with epilepsy. Epilepsy Behav 2004;5:702-707.
173. Ettinger AB, Kustra RP, Hammer AE. Effect of lamotrigine on depressive symptoms in adult patients with epilepsy. Epilepsy Behav 2007;10:148-154.
174. Brodie MJ, Overstall PW, Giorgi L. Multicentre, double-blind, randomised comparison between lamotrigine and carbamazepine in elderly patients with newly diagnosed epilepsy. The UK Lamotrigine Elderly Study Group. Epilepsy Res 1999; 37:81-87.
175. Brodie MJ, Richens A, Yuen AW. Double-blind comparison of lamotrigine and carbamazepine in newly diagnosed epilepsy. UK Lamotrigine/Carbamazepine Monotherapy Trial Group. Lancet 1995;345:476-479.
176. Steiner TJ, Dellaportas CI, Findley LJ, et al. Lamotrigine monotherapy in newly diagnosed untreated epilepsy: a double-blind comparison with phenytoin. Epilepsia 1999;40:601-607.
177. Cunnington M, Ferber S, Quartey G. Effect of dose on the frequency of major birth defects following fetal exposure to lamotrigine monotherapy in an international observational study. Epilepsia 2007;48:1207-1210.
178. Morrow J, Russell A, Guthrie E, et al. Malformation risks of antiepileptic drugs in pregnancy: a prospective study from the UK Epilepsy and Pregnancy Register. J Neurol Neurosurg Psychiatry 2006;77:193-198.
179. McLean MJ, Bukhari AA, Wamil AW. Effects of topiramate on sodium-dependent action-potential firing by mouse spinal cord neurons in cell culture. Epilepsia 2000;41(Suppl 1):S21-S24.
180. Gibbs JW 3rd, Sombati S, DeLorenzo RJ, Coulter DA. Cellular actions of topiramate: blockade of kainate-evoked inward currents in cultured hippocampal neurons. Epilepsia 2000;41(Suppl 1):S10-S16.
181. White HS, Brown SD, Woodhead JH, et al. Topiramate modulates GABA-evoked currents in murine cortical neurons by a nonbenzodiazepine mechanism. Epilepsia 2000;41(Suppl 1):S17-S20.
182. Dodgson SJ, Shank RP, Maryanoff BE. Topiramate as an inhibitor of carbonic anhydrase isoenzymes. Epilepsia 2000;41(Suppl 1):S35-S39.
183. Cross JH. Topiramate monotherapy for childhood absence seizures: an open label pilot study. Seizure 2002;11:406-410.
184. Privitera MD, Brodie MJ, Mattson RH, et al. Topiramate, carbamazepine and valproate monotherapy: double-blind comparison in newly diagnosed epilepsy. Acta Neurol Scand 2003;107:165-175.
185. Kahriman M, Minecan D, Kutluay E, et al. Efficacy of topiramate in children with refractory status epilepticus. Epilepsia 2003;44:1353-1356.
186. Towne AR, Garnett LK, Waterhouse EJ, et al. The use of topiramate in refractory status epilepticus. Neurology 2003;60:332-334.
187. Mula M, Trimble MR, Thompson P, Sander JW. Topiramate and word-finding difficulties in patients with epilepsy. Neurology 2003;60:1104-1107.
188. Mula M, Trimble MR, Lhatoo SD, Sander JW. Topiramate and psychiatric adverse events in patients with epilepsy. Epilepsia 2003;44:659-663.
189. Ingwersen SH, Pedersen PC, Groes L, et al. Population pharmacokinetics of tiagabine in epileptic patients on monotherapy. Eur J Pharm Sci 2000;11:247-254.
190. Gustavson LE, Mengel HB. Pharmacokinetics of tiagabine, a gamma-aminobutyric acid-uptake inhibitor, in healthy subjects after single and multiple doses. Epilepsia 1995;36:605-611.
191. Schachter SC. Tiagabine monotherapy in the treatment of partial epilepsy. Epilepsia 1995;36(Suppl 6):S2-S6.
192. Kälviäinen R. Tiagabine: clinical efficacy and use in epilepsy. *In* Levy RH, Mattson RH, Meldrum BS, Perucca E (eds): Antiepileptic Drugs, 5th ed. Philadelphia: Lippincott Williams & Wilkins, 2002, pp 698-704.
193. Genton P. When antiepileptic drugs aggravate epilepsy. Brain Dev 2000;22:75-80.
194. Knake S, Hamer HM, Schomburg U, et al. Tiagabine-induced absence status in idiopathic generalized epilepsy. Seizure 1999;8:314-317.
195. Koepp MJ, Edwards M, Collins J, et al. Status epilepticus and tiagabine therapy revisited. Epilepsia 2005;46:1625-1632.
196. Vinton A, Kornberg AJ, Cowley M, et al. Tiagabine-induced generalised non convulsive status epilepticus in patients with lesional focal epilepsy. J Clin Neurosci 2005;12:128-133.
197. Jette N, Cappell J, VanPassel L, Akman CI. Tiagabine-induced nonconvulsive status epilepticus in an adolescent without epilepsy. Neurology 2006;67:1514-1515.
198. Vollmar C, Noachtar S. Tiagabine-induced myoclonic status epilepticus in a nonepileptic patient. Neurology 2007;68:310.
199. Zhu Y, Vaughn BV. Non-convulsive status epilepticus induced by tiagabine in a patient with pseudoseizure. Seizure 2002;11:57-59.
200. Kumagai N, Seki T, Yamada T, et al. Concentrations of zonisamide in serum, free fraction, mixed saliva and cerebrospinal fluid in epileptic children treated with monotherapy. Jpn J Psychiatry Neurol 1993;47:291-292.
201. Ragueneau-Majlessi I, Levy RH, Brodie M, et al. Lack of pharmacokinetic interactions between steady-state zonisamide and valproic acid in patients with epilepsy. Clin Pharmacokinet 2005;44:517-523.
202. Rock DM, Macdonald RL, Taylor CP. Blockade of sustained repetitive action potentials in cultured spinal cord neurons by zonisamide (AD 810, CI 912), a novel anticonvulsant. Epilepsy Res 1989;3:138-143.
203. Suzuki S, Kawakami K, Nishimura S, et al. Zonisamide blocks T-type calcium channel in cultured neurons of rat cerebral cortex. Epilepsy Res 1992;12:21-27.
204. Masuda Y, Noguchi H, Karasawa T. Evidence against a significant implication of carbonic anhydrase inhibitory activity of zonisamide in its anticonvulsive effects. Arzneimittelforschung 1994;44:267-269.
205. Kothare SV, Kaleyias J, Mostofi N, et al. Efficacy and safety of zonisamide monotherapy in a cohort of children with epilepsy. Pediatr Neurol 2006;34:351-354.
206. Tosches WA, Tisdell J. Long-term efficacy and safety of monotherapy and adjunctive therapy with zonisamide. Epilepsy Behav 2006;8:522-526.
207. Suzuki Y, Nagai T, Ono J, et al. Zonisamide monotherapy in newly diagnosed infantile spasms. Epilepsia 1997;38:1035-1038.
208. Yanai S, Hanai T, Narazaki O. Treatment of infantile spasms with zonisamide. Brain Dev 1999;21:157-161.
209. Yagi K, Seino M. Methodological requirements for clinical trials in refractory epilepsies—our experience with zonisamide. Prog Neuropsychopharmacol Biol Psychiatry 1992;16:79-85.
210. Tong X, Patsalos PN. A microdialysis study of the novel antiepileptic drug levetiracetam: extracellular pharmacokinetics and effect on taurine in rat brain. Br J Pharmacol 2001;133:867-874.
211. Lukyanetz EA, Shkryl VM, Kostyuk PG. Selective blockade of N-type calcium channels by levetiracetam. Epilepsia 2002;43:9-18.
212. Lynch BA, Lambeng N, Nocka K, et al. The synaptic vesicle protein SV2A is the binding site for the antiepileptic drug levetiracetam. Proc Natl Acad Sci U S A 2004;101:9861-9866.
213. Grant R, Shorvon SD. Efficacy and tolerability of 1000-4000 mg per day of levetiracetam as add-on therapy in patients with refractory epilepsy. Epilepsy Res 2000;42: 89-95.
214. Brodie MJ, Perucca E, Ryvlin P, et al. Comparison of levetiracetam and controlled-release carbamazepine in newly diagnosed epilepsy. Neurology 2007;68:402-408.
215. Berkovic SF, Knowlton RC, Leroy RF, et al. Placebo-controlled study of levetiracetam in idiopathic generalized epilepsy. Neurology 2007.
216. French J, Arrigo C. Rapid onset of action of levetiracetam in refractory epilepsy patients. Epilepsia 2005;46:324-326.
217. Cereghino JJ, Biton V, Abou-Khalil B, et al. Levetiracetam for partial seizures: results of a double-blind, randomized clinical trial. Neurology 2000;55:236-242.
218. Ben-Menachem E, Persson LI, Mumford J, et al. Effect of long-term vigabatrin therapy on selected neurotransmitter concentrations in cerebrospinal fluid. J Child Neurol 1991;Suppl 2:S11-S16.
219. Ben-Menachem E, Hamberger A, Mumford J. Effect of long-term vigabatrin therapy on GABA and other amino acid concentrations in the central nervous system—a case study. Epilepsy Res 1993;16:241-243.
220. Chadwick D. Safety and efficacy of vigabatrin and carbamazepine in newly diagnosed epilepsy: a multicentre randomised double-blind study. Vigabatrin European Monotherapy Study Group. Lancet 1999;354:13-19.
221. Appleton RE, Peters AC, Mumford JP, Shaw DE. Randomised, placebo-controlled study of vigabatrin as first-line treatment of infantile spasms. Epilepsia 1999;40:1627-1633.
222. Aicardi J, Mumford JP, Dumas C, Wood S. Vigabatrin as initial therapy for infantile spasms: a European retrospective survey. Sabril IS Investigator and Peer Review Groups. Epilepsia 1996;37:638-642.
223. Kalviainen R, Nousiainen I, Mantyjarvi M, et al. Vigabatrin, a GABAergic antiepileptic drug, causes concentric visual field defects. Neurology 1999;53:922-926.
224. Hauser WA, Rich SS, Lee JR, et al. Risk of recurrent seizures after two unprovoked seizures. N Engl J Med 1998;338:429-434.
225. French JA, Kanner AM, Bautista J, et al. Efficacy and tolerability of the new antiepileptic drugs I: treatment of new onset epilepsy. Report of the Therapeutics and Technology Assessment Subcommittee and Quality Standards Subcommittee of the American Academy of Neurology and the American Epilepsy Society. Neurology 2004;62:1252-1260.
226. Glauser T, Ben-Menachem E, Bourgeois B, et al. ILAE treatment guidelines: evidence-based analysis of antiepileptic drug efficacy and effectiveness as initial monotherapy for epileptic seizures and syndromes. Epilepsia 2006;47:1094-1120.

227. Wheless JW, Clarke DF, Carpenter D. Treatment of pediatric epilepsy: expert opinion, 2005. J Child Neurol 2005;20(Suppl 1):S1-S56; quiz S59-S60.
228. Kwan P, Brodie MJ. Effectiveness of first antiepileptic drug. Epilepsia 2001;42:1255-1260.
229. Callaghan BC, Anand K, Hesdorffer D, et al. Likelihood of seizure remission in an adult population with refractory epilepsy. Ann Neurol 2007;62:382-389.
230. Luciano AL, Shorvon SD. Results of treatment changes in patients with apparently drug-resistant chronic epilepsy. Ann Neurol 2007;62:375-381.
231. Wiebe S, Blume WT, Girvin JP, Eliasziw M. A randomized, controlled trial of surgery for temporal-lobe epilepsy. N Engl J Med 2001;345:311-318.
232. Sperling MR, O'Connor MJ, Saykin AJ, Plummer C. Temporal lobectomy for refractory epilepsy. JAMA 1996;276:470-475.
233. Jobst BC, Siegel AM, Thadani VM, et al. Intractable seizures of frontal lobe origin: clinical characteristics, localizing signs, and results of surgery. Epilepsia 2000;41:1139-1152.
234. McLachlan RS, Rose KJ, Derry PA, et al. Health-related quality of life and seizure control in temporal lobe epilepsy. Ann Neurol 1997;41:482-489.
235. A randomized controlled trial of chronic vagus nerve stimulation for treatment of medically intractable seizures. The Vagus Nerve Stimulation Study Group. Neurology 1995;45:224-230.
236. Nei M, O'Connor M, Liporace J, Sperling MR. Refractory generalized seizures: response to corpus callosotomy and vagal nerve stimulation. Epilepsia 2006;47:115-122.
237. Kinsman SL, Vining EP, Quaskey SA, et al. Efficacy of the ketogenic diet for intractable seizure disorders: review of 58 cases. Epilepsia 1992;33:1132-1136.
238. Leppik IE, Derivan AT, Homan RW, et al. Double-blind study of lorazepam and diazepam in status epilepticus. JAMA 1983;249:1452-1454.
239. Treiman DM, Meyers PD, Walton NY, et al. A comparison of four treatments for generalized convulsive status epilepticus. Veterans Affairs Status Epilepticus Cooperative Study Group. N Engl J Med 1998;339:792-798.
240. Bennett B, Matagne A, Michel P, et al. Seletracetam (UCB 44212). Neurotherapeutics 2007;4:117-122.
241. von Rosenstiel P. Brivaracetam (UCB 34714). Neurotherapeutics 2007;4:84-87.
242. Yao C, Doose DR, Novak G, Bialer M. Pharmacokinetics of the new antiepileptic and CNS drug RWJ-333369 following single and multiple dosing to humans. Epilepsia 2006;47:1822-1829.
243. Arroyo S. Rufinamide. Neurotherapeutics 2007;4:155-162.
244. Errington AC, Coyne L, Stohr T, et al. Seeking a mechanism of action for the novel anticonvulsant lacosamide. Neuropharmacology 2006;50:1016-1029.
245. Doty P, Rudd GD, Stoehr T, Thomas D. Lacosamide. Neurotherapeutics 2007;4:145-148.
246. Nohria V, Giller E. Ganaxolone. Neurotherapeutics 2007;4:102-105.
247. Porter RJ, Nohria V, Rundfeldt C. Retigabine. Neurotherapeutics 2007;4:149-154.
248. Howes JF, Bell C. Talampanel. Neurotherapeutics 2007;4:126-129.
249. Chiron C. Stiripentol. Expert Opin Investig Drugs 2005;14:905-911.

46

MULTIPLE SCLEROSIS

Benjamin M. Greenberg, John N. Ratchford, and Peter A. Calabresi

OVERVIEW 685
INTRODUCTION 685
Epidemiology 685
Genetics 685
Clinical Features 685
Diagnosis 686
PATHOPHYSIOLOGY 687
THERAPEUTICS AND CLINICAL PHARMACOLOGY 689
Goals of Therapy 689
Therapeutics by Class 689
Immunomodulators 689
Immunosuppressants 691
Therapeutic Approach 692
Treatment with DMT: Patient Selection and Initiation 692
First-Line Treatment for RRMS 693
Treatments Helpful in SPMS 694
Treatments Helpful in PPMS 695
Definition of Treatment Failure 695
Management of Breakthrough Disease Activity 695
Management of Acute Relapses 695
Treatments Helpful for Common MS-Related Symptoms 696
Treatment Considerations Related to Pregnancy 697
Treating the Pediatric MS Patient 697
Emerging Targets and Therapeutics 698

OVERVIEW

Multiple sclerosis (MS) is a complex disease of the central nervous system (CNS) with the potential to cause significant physical and emotional disability. Approximately 350,000 Americans are currently diagnosed with MS, and the direct and indirect costs associated with the disease are about $14 billion per year.[1] MS is the most common nontraumatic cause of neurologic disability in early to middle adulthood. There is an inherent variability from patient to patient with regard to disease course and severity. Some patients experience frequent exacerbations with escalating disability while others have a relatively benign course. Most commonly the disease begins with episodic relapses that are separated by periods of remission. In the later stages of the disease, many patients will develop slowly progressive neurologic disability. Most evidence points to an immune-mediated pathophysiology involving B and T lymphocytes, macrophages, and microglia. According to this hypothesis, an autoimmune response against CNS myelin is initiated, leading to demyelination and axonal injury. To date, the most effective therapies have been immunosuppressant and immunomodulatory drugs. While none of the approaches can be described as curative, the presently approved drugs have led to significant reductions in relapse rates and disability.

INTRODUCTION

Epidemiology

The typical age of onset for MS is between 20 and 40. The disease is unusual before adolescence, but onset has been described as young as age 2 and as old as age 74. The ratio of affected women to men is between 1.7:1 and 2.5:1, although the ratio is more even at older ages of onset. Several important epidemiologic observations have been made about the geographic distribution of MS. In both the northern and southern hemispheres, the prevalence of the disease increases with increasing distance from the equator. There is also a difference in risk for different ethnic groups, independent of latitude. For example, England and Japan are at the same latitude, but the prevalence of MS differs significantly in the two countries (85 per 100,000 for England versus 1.4 per 100,000 in Japan). Caucasians tend to have the highest risk, while lower risk is seen in people of African or Asian descent. The highest prevalence is seen in the northern United States, southern Canada, northern Europe, and southern Australia. The southern United States and southern Europe have a moderate prevalence. The lowest prevalence is seen in Japan, China, Latin America, and equatorial Africa. Migration studies have also added to our understanding of the relationship between geography and risk of MS. Children born to parents who migrated from a low- to a high-risk area had an increase in their risk of developing MS, and vice versa.[2] By analyzing the ages of migrants, it was suggested that one's environmental risk was determined by about age 15.[2] This has led to hypotheses that the risk of MS is partly determined by viral exposures during childhood. Recent data suggest that the incidence of MS may be increasing, especially in women, although issues regarding ascertainment and diagnosis make these studies challenging.

Genetics

In addition to environmental factors, genetics influences the risk of developing MS. Family clusters are known to occur. Twin studies have found that the monozygotic twin of an MS patient has about a 30% chance of developing MS. Dizygotic twins have a risk that is similar to that of any sibling of an MS patient, about 2% to 5%. The risk in children of MS patients is slightly lower than for siblings. Second- and third-degree relatives of an MS patient also carry some elevated risk. Genetic studies have found the strongest association with the major histocompatibility complex (MHC), particularly the HLA-DRB1 locus. More recently, two additional genes were identified in genome-wide scans,[3] the interleukin-2 receptor alpha gene and the interleukin-7 receptor alpha gene. The fact that all three genes are part of the immune system serves as an important confirmation of the autoimmune nature of this disease.

Clinical Features

MS has classically been separated into four different subtypes: relapsing-remitting, secondary progressive, primary progressive, and progressive relapsing MS (Fig. 46-1). Relapsing-remitting MS (RRMS) is the most common clinical subtype, representing about 85% of patients at diagnosis. It is marked by intermittent exacerbations that may partly or completely resolve over weeks to months. These relapses are separated by periods of clinical stability. However, patients may continue to experience symptoms from prior relapses that healed incompletely. After a variable period of time, a majority of RRMS patients will enter a secondary progressive phase of the disease (SPMS). SPMS patients experience a slowly progressive worsening of disability that may or may not have superimposed relapses. About 10% to 15% of patients will have a primary progressive course (PPMS), marked by slowly progressive worsening from the outset without relapses. A small number of patients are labeled as having progressive relapsing MS. These patients begin with a progressive course but develop one or more relapses. Patients who have had a single demyelinating event, but do not yet meet criteria for MS, are referred to as having a clinically isolated syndrome.

MS can present with a large number of symptoms possibly referable to the CNS. The symptoms may be transient and often difficult to describe. Classic MS symptoms include unilateral blurred vision with brow pain on lateral eye movement, weakness, numbness, paresthesias, pain, imbalance, double vision, bladder and bowel dysfunction, impaired coordination, fatigue, depression, cognitive impairment, heat intolerance, and sexual dysfunction. On exam, common signs include visual impairment, brainstem dysfunction, nystagmus, dysarthria, spasticity, hyperreflexia, weakness, sensory loss, and ataxia. Several paroxysmal phenomena can be associated with MS, including tonic spasms, trigeminal neuralgia, and myokymia. New clinical symptoms are thought to result from new areas of inflammation and demyelination, while the acquisition of long-term disability is more related to axonal damage.[4,5]

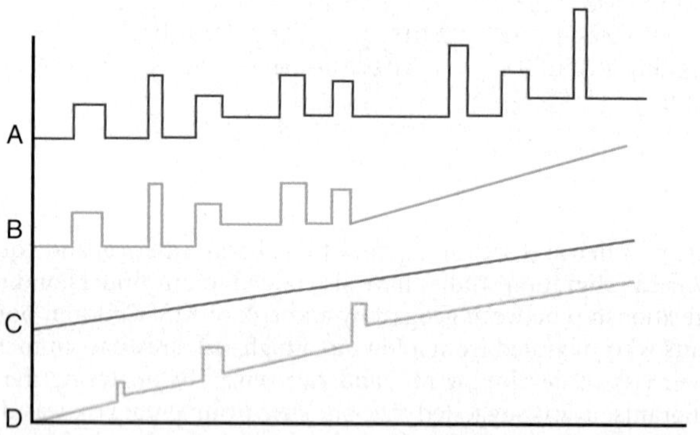

FIGURE 46-1 • A diagrammatic representation of disability by time for different subtypes of MS. A, Relapsing-remitting MS. **B,** Secondary progressive MS. **C,** Primary progressive MS. **D,** Progressive relapsing MS.

Diagnosis

The diagnosis of MS can be challenging as there is no single test with adequate sensitivity or specificity and there are several potential mimics. MS was classically diagnosed by the identification of lesions attributable to the CNS white matter that were separated in time and space with objective findings on neurologic exam and no better explanation.[6] However, the advent of magnetic resonance imaging (MRI) has significantly changed how the diagnosis is made. Currently, the most widely used diagnostic criteria are the McDonald criteria, which were last revised in 2005 (Table 46-1).[7] These criteria endorsed the use of MRI as a surrogate marker for defining separation in time and space.

Brain MRI in MS classically shows lesions that are hyperintense on T2-weighted sequences (Fig. 46-2). Lesions are frequently in the periventricular white matter, often extending perpendicular to the ventricle. Lesions of the corpus callosum are common in MS, as are lesions in the subcortical white matter, cerebellum, brainstem, and spinal cord. Newer imaging techniques are also identifying an increased number of lesions in the cortex. Acute lesions will often enhance with gadolinium, indicating active inflammation with blood-brain barrier (BBB) breakdown. Areas of hypointensity on T1 sequences are also seen. T1 hypointensity is observed transiently in acute lesions. However, when it is present chronically, it likely represents an area of significant axonal damage. Disability correlates more strongly with the T1 hypointensity volume than the volume of T2 hyperintensities. With time, the accumulating axonal damage will often manifest as global cerebral atrophy. Only about 5% to 10% of lesions seen on MRI are associated with clinical symptoms. Gray matter lesions are also common in MS, but are not well seen on conventional MRI.

TABLE 46-1 REVISED MCDONALD CRITERIA

Clinical Presentation	Additional Data Needed for MS Diagnosis
2 or more attacks; objective clinical evidence of 2 or more lesions	• None
2 or more attacks; objective clinical evidence of 1 lesion	• Dissemination in space, demonstrated by: →MRI *or* →2 or more MRI-detected lesions consistent with MS plus positive CSF *or* →Await further clinical attack implicating a different site
1 attack; objective clinical evidence of 2 or more lesions	• Dissemination in time, demonstrated by: →MRI *or* →Second clinical attack
1 attack; objective clinical evidence of 1 lesion (monosymptomatic presentation; clinically isolated syndrome)	• Dissemination in space, demonstrated by: →MRI *or* →2 or more MRI-detected lesions consistent with MS plus positive CSF *and* • Dissemination in time, demonstrated by: →MRI *or* →Second clinical attack
Insidious neurologic progression suggestive of MS	• One year of disease progression (retrospectively or prospectively determined) *and* • Two out of three of the following: a. Positive brain MRI (9 T2 lesions or 4 or more T2 lesions with positive visual evoked potentials) b. Positive spinal cord MRI (2 or more focal T2 lesions) c. Positive CSF

CSF, cerebrospinal fluid; MRI, magnetic resonance imaging; MS, multiple sclerosis.
From Polman CH, Reingold SC, Edan G, et al. Diagnostic criteria for multiple sclerosis: 2005 revisions to the "McDonald Criteria." Ann Neurol 2005;58:840-846.

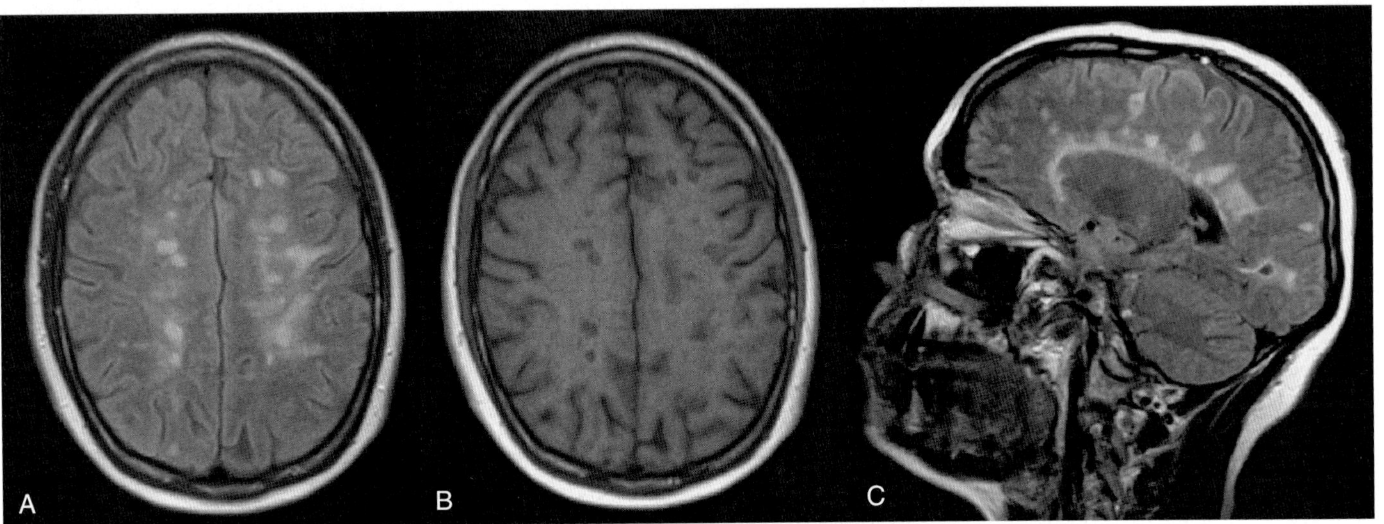

FIGURE 46-2 • **Brain MRI of a patient with MS. A,** Axial fluid-attenuated inversion recovery (FLAIR) image showing multiple hyperintensities. **B,** Axial T1-weighted image at the same level. Some of the areas of FLAIR hyperintensity are also hypointense on T1-weighted images. **C,** Sagittal FLAIR image showing periventricular hyperintensities.

In the past, a cerebrospinal fluid (CSF) exam was a common part of the MS diagnosis. The presence of an elevated protein, oligoclonal bands, or an elevated immunoglobulin G index is supportive of the diagnosis. Although CSF analysis is still important in some cases to rule out other diagnoses such as infections, it is often unnecessary in routine cases. Evoked potentials of the visual, auditory, or somatosensory pathways can be helpful in some cases to detect subclinical lesions that cannot be seen on MRI.

PATHOPHYSIOLOGY

Classically, MS has been described as an immune-mediated demyelinating disease affecting the brain, spinal cord, and optic nerves.[8] Recent research has reemphasized the concomitant presence of both gray matter pathology and extensive axonal damage in the brains of patients diagnosed with MS.[9,10] The exact cause(s) of MS have not been determined, but a combination of genetic and environmental factors coalesces in some people to lead to demyelination and axonal damage. One theory is that certain viruses may share sequence homology with myelin proteins and, through molecular mimicry, mediate aberrant activation of cross-reactive T cells. Viruses may also cause bystander activation through release of cytokines or stimulation of antigen-presenting cells. It is possible that MS is actually a syndrome of various related diseases that cause episodic demyelination and neuronal damage. Four pathologic subtypes of MS have been described, as discussed later, confirming a variety of immunopathogenetic mechanisms involved in different types of MS. While most of these types have an immune-mediated component, there are some aspects of MS that may be independent of the immune system. For example, the degeneration of chronically demyelinated axons that occurs in the secondary progressive phase of the disease appears to be noninflammatory. To date, the only successful treatment strategies for MS have involved immunomodulatory or immunosuppressive approaches, supporting the role that the immune system plays. Moreover, these therapies generally are effective only during the relapsing-remitting phase, the most inflammatory phase of the disease.

Pathologic examination of the CNS in patients with MS typically identifies an inflammatory response involving cellular and humoral immune systems. Whether or not the immune system begins by recognizing a foreign antigen and then strays against self or begins by recognizing self-antigens is unknown. Fundamental to the classic description of MS pathogenesis is the inappropriate disruption of the BBB. Normally, the BBB is composed of specialized endothelial cells with an intricate network of tight junctions. Functionally, the BBB significantly restricts the diffusion of molecules from the periphery into the CNS. Disruption of the BBB by immune cells in MS is responsible for gadolinium-enhancing lesions on MRI and "attacks" in MS patients. Lymphocytes are able to migrate across the BBB via a series of adhesion molecule interactions. Critical to this process is a connection between very late antigen-4 (VLA-4) on lymphocytes and monocytes and its ligands vascular cell adhesion molecule-1 (VCAM-1) on endothelial cells and fibronectin in the basement membrane.[11] Presumably, once effector cells from the immune system have gained access to the CNS, they secrete a cascade of cytokines that lead to demyelination and ultimately axonal damage (Fig. 46-3).

Numerous studies have analyzed the relative role that $CD4^+$ and $CD8^+$ T cells play in disease pathogenesis. Epidemiologic studies and mouse models have linked MS to MHC class II genes, which present antigens to $CD4^+$ T cells.[12-14] Thus, $CD4^+$ T cells have been of interest for years. The production of tumor necrosis factor (TNF) from $CD4^+$ T cells correlates with the number of T2-hyperintense lesions on MRI.[15] While autoreactive T cells have been identified in patients with MS and in healthy volunteers, the $CD4^+$ T cells are functionally different in patients with MS. Specifically, they tend to be more differentiated and have a higher level of T helper cell type 1 (Th1) phenotypes in patients with MS compared to controls.[16] Yet, therapy directed against $CD4^+$ T cells made only a small difference in patients treated in clinical trials.[17,18] Therapy that depleted both $CD4^+$ and $CD8^+$ T cells, however, led to a reduction in disease activity.[19-21] The role of T helper type 17 (Th17) cells in MS is less clear. This newly described subset of T cells has been implicated in an animal model of MS, experimental autoimmune encephalomyelitis, and interleukin (IL)-17 expression can be seen in MS brain-infiltrating cells.

Several studies have identified the potential role of $CD8^+$ T cells in MS. Genetic studies have implicated various MHC class I genes as being associated with increased risk of MS while some MHC class I genes are protective.[22,23] Persistence of autoreactive $CD8^+$ T cells in the CSF of patients with MS has been described.[24] In mouse studies, $CD8^+$ T cells have been shown to potentiate immune-mediated demyelinating disease.[25] Yet, there are also data that suggest a possible neuroprotective role for self-reactive $CD8^+$ T cells.[26] While $CD4^+$ T cell production of TNF-α has correlated with the number of T2-hyperintense lesions on MRI, certain $CD8^+$ T cell populations have been negatively correlated with T1-hypointense lesions.[15,27]

In one study, a systematic review of biopsies and autopsy specimens from MS patients identified four distinct pathologic patterns.[28] Two patterns were noteworthy for T-cell infiltrates and preservation of oligodendrocytes, with one pattern additionally having deposition of

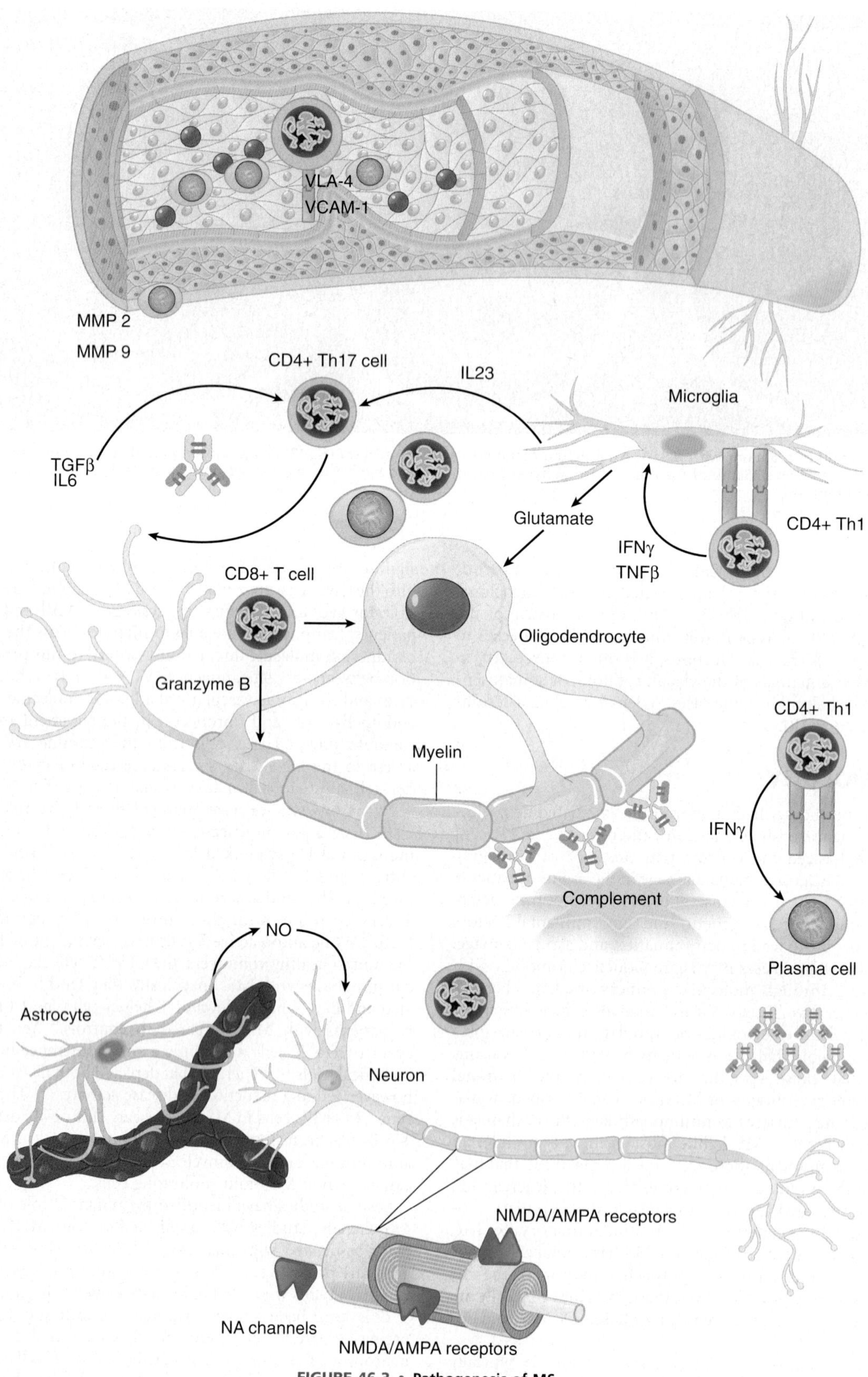

FIGURE 46-3 • Pathogenesis of MS.

antibodies and complement. A third pattern was notable for a T-cell infiltrate without antibody deposition, but there was a loss of myelin-associated glycoprotein in tissues and oligodendrocyte apoptosis with preserved myelin around veins and venules. Finally, the fourth pattern was notable for T-cell inflammation, but also oligodendrocyte cell death. This research identified heterogeneous pathology between patients with MS, but the findings within each individual patient were homogeneous. Presumably, these patterns represent various forms of MS, but only one form is occurring in any given patient at one time. However, the selection bias that is inherent in this study (patients presenting for biopsy or autopsy) could account for some of the homogeneity, and other groups have not confirmed these patterns in their MS brain tissue examinations.

Clinically, patients may experience new symptoms in the setting of new inflammation and demyelination affecting clinically eloquent parts of the CNS. Often the inflammation resolves partly, and there can be partial remyelination with varying degrees of gliotic scarring and axonal damage. Much of the disease accumulates in a silent manner and is not evident until compensatory mechanisms begin to break down, years into the disease process. Thus, progression of disability occurs slowly with time but becomes most noticeable after years of accumulated axonal damage.[4] Therapeutic possibilities include immunomodulatory, immunosuppressive, neuroprotective, and neuroreparative strategies.

THERAPEUTICS AND CLINICAL PHARMACOLOGY

Goals of Therapy

There are two types of therapies for MS: disease-modifying therapies (DMTs) and symptomatic treatments. All of the DMTs currently approved by the U.S. Food and Drug Administration (FDA) for MS act by immunomodulation or immunosuppression. These treatments are effective at reducing the frequency of disease relapses and decreasing the number of new lesions seen on MRI in RRMS. Some have also been shown to delay the accumulation of disability. While these immunomodulatory treatments are beneficial in relapsing-remitting patients, they have not been proven effective in SPMS or PPMS. Immunomodulation is probably ineffective in progressive MS because the nerve damage in these groups is less dependent on inflammation. Consequently, there is a major need for treatments for progressive MS patients.

While the DMTs decrease the incidence of new relapses, they are not helpful in repairing damage that has already occurred. Prior relapses often leave patients with residual symptoms. A number of medications are available to help these MS-related symptoms. Alleviating pain, spasticity, bladder dysfunction, depression, and anxiety makes up a significant portion of the care offered to patients with MS.

Therapeutics by Class

Immunomodulators

Interferons. The first drug specifically approved for use in relapsing MS was interferon beta-1b (Betaseron in North America/Betaferon in Europe). Subsequent to that, two different preparations of interferon beta-1a were released (Avonex and Rebif). While the interferon beta-1a preparations are identical to human interferon-β in terms of amino acid sequence and glycosylation, interferon beta-1b is produced in bacterial cells, has a few amino acid changes, and is not glycosylated. All of the interferons are FDA approved for RRMS and are therefore not recommended for PPMS or SPMS without relapses.

Mechanism of Action. A variety of mechanisms of action have been proposed for beta interferons. First, immunologically, there is a down-regulation of CD80$^+$ B cells in patients treated with interferon beta.[29] This protein is responsible for co-stimulation of T cells and leads to Th1-type cytokine secretion. Interferon beta also suppresses the expression of interferon-γ–induced MHC class II antigens on antigen-presenting cells.[30,31] Several studies have demonstrated a direct effect on T cells, including suppression of matrix metalloproteinases (MMPs) and promotion of the production of anti-inflammatory cytokines such as IL-4 and IL-10.[32-34] These processes complement each other and lead to an overall shift in T-cell cytokine profiles, favoring a T helper cell type 2 (Th2) response over Th1.[33]

A complementary immunomodulatory effect of interferon beta is that it alters the permeability of the BBB, making it more difficult for autoreactive T cells to enter the parenchyma.[35,36] Clinically, patients on interferon beta have markedly fewer gadolinium-enhancing lesions.[37-40] Reducing the ability of reactive immune cells to enter the CNS would lower the number of new demyelinating lesions and axonal damage. The mechanisms underlying this effect likely relate both to direct immune effects on T cells (decreased MMP production and T-cell activation) and direct effects on endothelial cells. This includes shedding of VCAM-1 into a soluble circulating form that may saturate T-cell ligands and decrease cell migration across the BBB.[41]

Interferon beta also has potential neuroprotective qualities. T cells from patients treated with interferon beta stimulate human brain endothelial cells to secrete nerve growth factor. This protein may play a role in protecting axons from inflammation-mediated damage.[42]

Dosing. The three preparations of interferon beta vary in their dose and route of administration. Interferon beta-1b (Betaseron/Betaferon) is administered every other day via a subcutaneous injection at a dose of 250 mcg. One version of interferon beta-1a (Avonex) is administered intramuscularly once a week at a dose of 30 mcg. The other version of interferon beta-1a (Rebif) is administered subcutaneously three times a week at a dose of either 22 or 44 mcg per injection. Dose titration is recommended for the subcutaneous formulations to decrease the chance of side effects at the onset of therapy. There have been a series of large-scale, double-blind, placebo-controlled trials of these medications in RRMS.

The specific biologic activity is not readily comparable between the different interferon beta preparations. A variety of bioassays are used to quantify interferon beta activity.[43] One strategy utilizes a series of biomarkers that quantify the antiviral effects of interferon beta. Markers such as MXA protein, neopterin, and 2′,5′-oligoadenylate synthetase can be measured in vitro and in vivo and used to compare the relative biologic activity of the three interferons.

Clinical Efficacy. Pivotal studies have found that interferon beta reduces relapse rates by approximately a third and the appearance of new lesions on MRI by approximately 50% to 70%.[40,44-46] Two head-to-head trials have compared low-dose (Avonex) and high-dose (Betaseron/Betaferon or Rebif) interferons to determine whether or not there is a dose-dependent effect. These trials identified a more robust effect of higher dose interferon, especially early on in therapy.[47,48] There is evidence to indicate that interferon can lose its clinical efficacy if a patient develops persistently high titers of neutralizing antibodies.[49,50] This may explain why the higher efficacy of high-dose interferons wanes over time when compared to low-dose interferon.

Adverse Effects. Clinically, patients taking interferon injections may experience a variety of potential side effects. The most common are flulike symptoms including fever, chills, muscle aches, and fatigue. These symptoms are usually self-limited and diminish with successive doses. They can be managed with the use of prophylactic acetaminophen and/or ibuprofen or naproxen taken 1 hour before an injection and are a rare cause of discontinuing medication. Taking the medicine at bedtime can also be useful so that the patient is asleep during the peak period of side effects. Patients utilizing a subcutaneous route of administration have an increased potential for developing site reactions in the skin when compared to the intramuscular injection route. Injection site necrosis can be seen in patients using subcutaneous interferon beta[51] but is rare now with proper injection technique. Some data have linked the use of interferon to an increased rate of depression.[52,53] Drops in peripheral blood counts in all cell lines have been seen, and interferons have rarely caused severe hepatic injury. Consequently, it is advised that patients have their complete blood count with differential, platelet count, blood chemistries, and liver function tests checked periodically. Patients taking Rebif or Betaseron are advised to have these tests at 1, 3, and 6 months after initiation of therapy and periodically thereafter. Avonex patients are advised to have monitoring at least every 6 months. Thyroid function should also be monitored every 6 months, and a pregnancy test should be sent before starting therapy in women of childbearing age. Other rare adverse effects observed with interferon beta are seizures, cardiomyopathy, menstrual irregularities, and autoimmune disorders (especially thyroid dysfunction).

Glatiramer Acetate. Glatiramer acetate (Copaxone) is a collection of peptides randomly formed from four amino acids (alanine, glutamate, lysine, and tyrosine) combined in a molar ratio of 4.2 : 1.4 : 3.4 : 1.0. The peptides have lengths ranging between 40 and 100 residues. This compound has sequence homology with myelin basic protein and was originally tested as an agent for inducing demyelination in mice. Instead, the compound offered protection for mice with experimental autoimmune encephalitis. Glatiramer acetate is FDA approved for reducing the frequency of relapses in RRMS.

Mechanism of Action. After injection, glatiramer acetate binds MHC class II molecules and is presented to T lymphocytes. Glatiramer acetate biases T cells toward a Th2 $CD4^+$ T-cell profile.[32,54,55] In mice these glatiramer acetate–reactive T cells can be isolated from the CNS and may both ameliorate inflammation and promote neuroprotection and repair via the release of growth factors such as brain-derived neurotrophic factor (BDNF).[32,56-58] Further evidence implicates a shift in peripheral immune system–derived T cells, including upregulation of $CCR7^+$ T central memory $CD4^+$ cells and of $CD8^+$ T cells in response to glatiramer acetate therapy[59,60] (Fig. 46-4).

Beyond effects on T cells, there is in vitro and in vivo evidence that glatiramer acetate exerts an effect on antigen-presenting cells. Monocytes alter their cytokine expression in response to glatiramer acetate, increasing IL-10 levels and decreasing IL-12 levels.[61] Thus, glatiramer acetate–treated monocytes promote a Th2 type T-cell response. Furthermore, there is evidence to indicate the monocyte activity is inhibited by glatiramer acetate, as evidenced by diminished CD25, CD69, and TNF-α expression.[62] These effects may play a direct role in the drug's clinical activity.

Finally, more recent evidence supports a possible role for glatiramer acetate in promoting neuroprotection. The T cells generated by treatment produce BDNF, which promotes neuronal survival.[57,63,64] While this feature is not unique to glatiramer acetate–treated T cells, animal models suggest that these T cells are uniquely primed to migrate to sites of injury within the CNS and promote repair.[65,66]

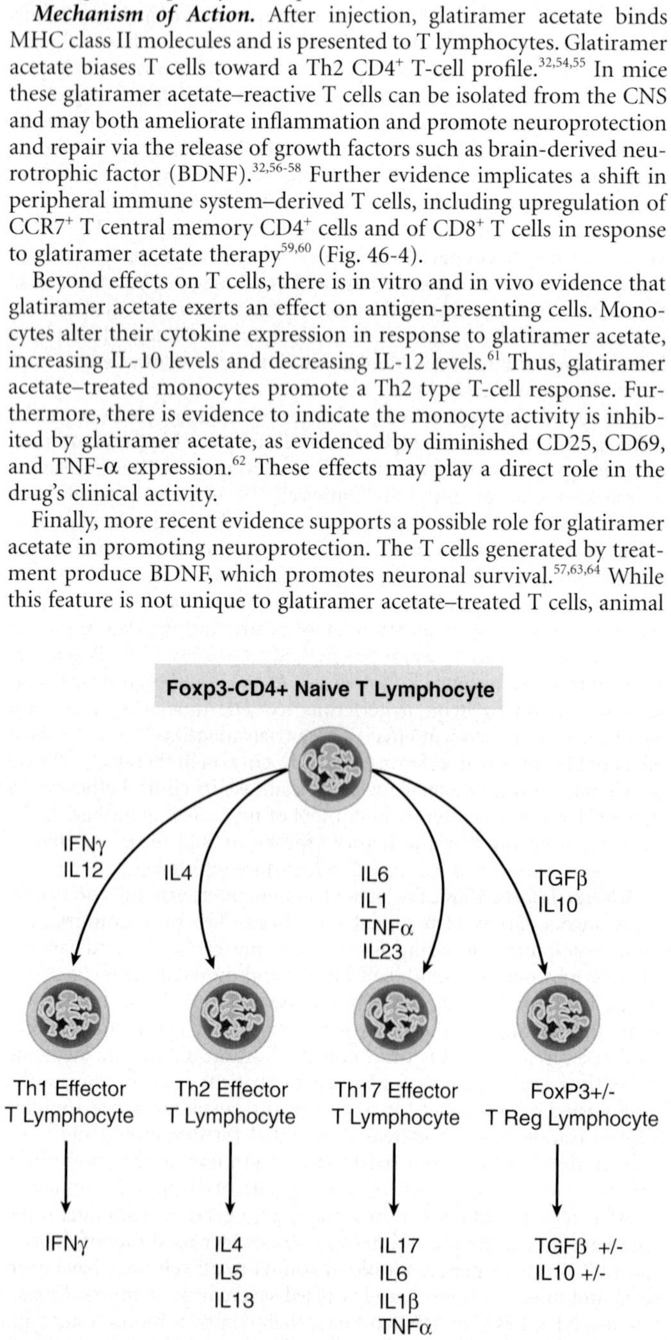

Dosing. Glatiramer acetate is administered as a daily subcutaneous injection of 20 mg. Dose titration is not needed. The available data on pharmacokinetics are very limited.

Clinical Efficacy. The clinical benefit of glatiramer acetate was proven in a double-blind, placebo-controlled trial where the outcomes were relapse rate and disability progression.[67] Further studies also identified a benefit as measured by MRI parameters (a reduction in the number of enhancing lesions and T2-hyperintense lesions).[68] Currently, the combination of interferon and glatiramer acetate is being studied to determine whether the efficacy of each would be additive.[69] There have been no convincing data indicating that the development of antibodies against glatiramer acetate are clinically relevant.[70]

Adverse Events. Tolerability of daily glatiramer acetate injections is quite good. Unlike interferon, there are no flulike side effects, but, because of the subcutaneous nature of the injection, site reactions are common. Patients may experience lipoatrophy at injection sites, causing dimpling of skin.[71] About 10% of patients experience an idiosyncratic reaction shortly after injection of the drug, characterized by chest tightness, shortness of breath, palpitations, and flushing. It is a self-limited event that does not require intervention.[72] It does not represent an allergic reaction, and patients are able to take their next dose with little risk of recurrence. Some study patients experienced this once while others had several episodes. Occasional transient chest pain without the other associated symptoms has also been observed, but it does not appear to have any important clinical sequelae. Routine blood monitoring is not needed, but, as with all of the DMTs, women of childbearing age should have a pregnancy test before beginning therapy.

Natalizumab. Natalizumab (Tysabri) is a humanized monoclonal antibody that was FDA approved for use in MS in November 2004.[73] Subsequent to its release, two patients who had been enrolled in the combination natalizumab and interferon beta-1a (Avonex) trial developed progressive multifocal leukoencephalopathy (PML), a serious viral brain infection, and one died. Subsequently, a third patient with PML was discovered postmortem. That patient had been exposed to four doses of natalizumab and several other chronic immunosuppressive medications for Crohn's disease. This prompted the voluntary withdrawal of natalizumab from the market while a safety analysis could be completed. Natalizumab was re-released for use as monotherapy in the summer of 2006 under a monitoring program designed to identify potential PML cases early. The FDA has approved natalizumab for use in relapsing forms of MS to delay the accumulation of physical disability and reduce the frequency of clinical exacerbations. It is recommended for patients who have had an inadequate response to, or are unable to tolerate, alternate MS therapies.

Mechanism of Action. Natalizumab is a humanized monoclonal antibody that binds to the α4 chain of the VLA-4 integrin dimer on the cell surface of all leukocytes except neutrophils. Normally, VLA-4 binds to targets such as VCAM-1 on the surface of activated vascular endothelium. Natalizumab interferes with this interaction and thereby prevents migration of leukocytes across the BBB to sites of inflammation. This is believed to lead to decreased CNS inflammation and demyelination.

Dosing. Natalizumab is administered as a 300-mg intravenous (IV) infusion every 4 weeks. Steady state levels are reached approximately 24 weeks after monthly dosing, and the mean half-life of the drug is 11 days. Dosing in renal or hepatic insufficiency has not been studied.

Clinical Efficacy. Two large, randomized, double-blind, placebo-controlled studies of natalizumab have been published.[73,74] One was a study of natalizumab monotherapy (AFFIRM) and the other was a study of natalizumab in combination with interferon beta-1a (SENTINEL). The AFFIRM trial found a 42% reduction in the risk of sustained disability progression after 2 years in the natalizumab group compared to placebo.[73] In the natalizumab group, the annualized relapse rate was reduced by 68% and the number of new or enlarging T2 hyperintensities was reduced by 83%.[73] The mean number of

FIGURE 46-4 • The differentiation of $CD4^+$ T lymphocytes. (Adapted from Weaver CT, Harrington LE, Mangan PR, et al. Th17: an effector CD4 T cell lineage with regulatory T cell ties. Immunity 2006;24:677-688.)

gadolinium-enhancing lesions was also reduced significantly with natalizumab (92% reduction).

Adverse Events. The greatest concern about the use of natalizumab is the risk of developing PML. In the Phase III studies, the risk was found to be approximately 1 in 1000 patients. However, the three patients that developed PML were all treated with other immunomodulating drugs, so the risk of PML in monotherapy may be lower. The two MS patients who were diagnosed with PML developed it after 2 years of treatment. The patient with Crohn's disease who developed PML received 8 months of treatment. It is not known whether early detection of PML and discontinuation of the medication will help new cases. Unfortunately, the mortality rate for PML is high and there are no effective treatments. The real rate of PML with natalizumab in clinical practice will not be known for several years. As required by the FDA-mandated safety program, patients receiving natalizumab who develop new neurologic symptoms or signs need to be evaluated by a neurologist and have a brain MRI performed to help rule out PML.

Complications of natalizumab therapy go beyond possible PML. Patients can have immediate infusion-related reactions (2%), which are common to almost all therapeutic monoclonal antibodies. These include chest tightness, shortness of breath, urticaria, and rarely anaphylaxis. Patients on natalizumab had a higher rate of headaches and urinary tract infections when compared to placebo.[73,75] Persistent antibodies to natalizumab were seen in 6% of patients treated in trials and were associated with decreased efficacy of the drug.[76] Periodic monitoring of liver function is recommended with this treatment. Natalizumab remains a very potent and well-tolerated therapeutic option for MS. However, due to a still unknown risk of PML, it is prudent to limit natalizumab use to patients with more aggressive forms of relapsing MS who do not respond to first-line treatments.

Immunosuppressants

Mitoxantrone. Mitoxantrone (Novantrone) is a synthetic intercalating chemotherapeutic agent that is used in the treatment of MS. It has shown efficacy in RRMS and subsets of SPMS.[77-79] It is FDA approved for reducing neurologic disability and/or frequency of clinical relapses in SPMS, progressive relapsing, and worsening RRMS. Of note, it is the only FDA-approved treatment for SPMS. Mitoxantrone is also approved for use in the treatment of acute nonlymphocytic leukemia and for pain related to advanced hormone-refractory prostate cancer. This drug has significant potential toxicities, including cardiotoxicity, myelosuppression, and risk of leukemia. Consequently, it is reserved for use in patients with aggressive disease.

Mechanism of Action. Mitoxantrone readily crosses the BBB and inhibits DNA replication and RNA synthesis in leukocytes.[80] It also inhibits topoisomerase II, interfering with DNA repair.[81] The effect in MS, beyond a global immunosuppressive effect, might be related to its demonstrated specificity for antigen-specific T cells.[82] Mitoxantrone may also have effects on monocytes, inhibiting their ability to migrate across the BBB.[83] Finally, there are also data indicating that mitoxantrone interferes with antigen-presenting cell function.[84]

Dosing. The FDA-approved dose for mitoxantrone is 12 mg/m^2 IV every 3 months. However, one clinical trial also used a mitoxantrone dose of 20 mg IV monthly combined with a monthly dose of methylprednisolone.[85] The drug is eliminated in a three-compartment model with half-lives of 6 to 12 minutes, 1.1 to 3.1 hours, and an elimination half-life of 23 to 215 hours.[86] It is 78% bound to plasma proteins and is excreted in urine and feces either as unchanged drug or as inactive metabolites. Mitoxantrone should not be used in MS patients with hepatic impairment because its clearance is significantly reduced in these patients. It is also contraindicated in patients with a left ventricular ejection fraction (LVEF) less than 50% or patients whose cumulative lifetime dose is greater than 140 mg/m^2.

Clinical Effects. In a pivotal study, mitoxantrone was tested on patients who had a measurable worsening of disability in the prior 18 months. This was either a stepwise worsening in RRMS patients or a gradual progression of disability in patients with SPMS (with or without superimposed relapses). When dosed at 12 mg/m^2 every 3 months for 24 months, mitoxantrone decreased the number of relapses and decreased the chance of having disability progression compared to placebo.[87] A second trial gave mitoxantrone 20 mg IV and methylprednisolone 1 g IV monthly or methylprednisolone alone for 6 months to patients with very active disease based on clinical and MRI criteria.[88] The group receiving monthly mitoxantrone and methylprednisolone had fewer new enhancing lesions on MRI compared to the methylprednisolone-alone group. Relapse rate and mean disability scores also improved in the mitoxantrone group.

Adverse Effects. There are two major potential complications of mitoxantrone therapy: cardiomyopathy and leukemia. Congestive heart failure (CHF) can occur during therapy or months to years after discontinuation of mitoxantrone. In cancer patients receiving up to 140 mg/m^2, the risk of CHF was estimated at 2.6%.[86] The risk of an asymptomatic decrease in LVEF is likely higher. It is recommended that all MS patients receiving mitoxantrone have evaluation of their ejection fraction by echocardiogram or multigated radionuclide angiography at baseline and before each dose of mitoxantrone. MS patients with a clinically significant drop in LVEF or an LVEF below 50% should not receive mitoxantrone. Contraindications to use include prior history of cardiovascular disease, history of mediastinal radiotherapy, previous use of anthracyclines or anthracenediones, and concomitant use of cardiotoxic drugs. The cardiac toxicity is dose related, prompting the mandated lifetime maximum dose of 140 mg/m^2.

The other major concern is a risk of secondary acute myelogenous leukemia, which has been seen in 0.25% of MS patients treated with mitoxantrone.[86] Myelosuppression is seen with this treatment, typically beginning 8 to 14 days after a single large dose and persisting for 4 to 10 days. Other potential side effects include nausea, alopecia, changes in menstrual cycle, amenorrhea, urinary tract infections, and transaminitis. Prior to each dose, a complete blood count, platelet count, and liver function tests should be checked. The medication should not be administered to patients with an absolute neutrophil count less than 1500 cells/mm^3 or a platelet count less than 100,000/mm^3. Due to potential teratogenic effects of mitoxantrone, women of childbearing age should have a pregnancy test prior to each dose of mitoxantrone. The potential complications and relatively limited clinical benefit have diminished the use of mitoxantrone under this protocol. Yet, there are several ongoing studies examining the usefulness of mitoxantrone as an inducing agent in regimens for RRMS.[89] These studies are determining whether a lower dose of mitoxantrone prior to starting an injectable DMT will improve clinical outcomes.

Corticosteroids. Corticosteroids dampen the inflammatory cellular response and cytokine cascade through a variety of mechanisms that are incompletely understood. Cytokines are proteins released by inflammatory cells that can amplify the immune response as well as mediate direct damage to the nervous system.[90,91] Corticosteroids suppress gene expression and secretion of many of the proinflammatory cytokines implicated in MS.[92,93] Second, corticosteroids stop T cells and B cells from activating by interfering with cell signaling.[94] Third, corticosteroids decrease the extravasation of immune cells into the CNS by suppressing MMPs and adhesion molecules.[95] Finally, corticosteroids actually have proapoptotic effects on activated immune cells.[96] The effects of corticosteroids are not limited to peripheral immune cells. Corticosteroids may decrease BBB permeability by suppressing adhesion molecule expression on endothelial cells, and suppressing effector functions of glial cells in the CNS. Both pro- and antiapoptotic effects of corticosteroids on neurons have been reported.[97]

Clinical indications for using corticosteroids in MS are controversial. There is compelling evidence from large trials that a pulse of high-dose IV corticosteroids can accelerate the recovery from a relapse.[98] The most widely cited study of corticosteroids in demyelinating disease is the Optic Neuritis Treatment Trial.[99] This study was a double-blind, placebo-controlled trial that enrolled patients with a first episode of isolated optic neuritis. The three groups were (i) IV corticosteroids (methylprednisolone 250 mg IV every 6 hours for 3 days) followed by an oral prednisone taper, (ii) an oral prednisone taper in isolation, and (iii) oral placebo. Over 450 patients were followed prospectively to track visual recovery and risk of other episodes of demyelination. While the long-term outcomes for all three groups were similar, patients receiving IV corticosteroids had a faster recovery. Another observation from this study was that patients who received only oral corticosteroids had the highest rate of recurrent optic neuritis. Thus, when relapses of demyelinating disease occur, the usual course of treatment involves a pulse dose of IV corticosteroids with or without an oral taper. Only small clinical studies have been performed analyzing the potential role of corticosteroids in long-term disease management.[100] While some data have supported the use of quarterly pulses of corticosteroids, longer term, controlled studies will be required to validate these findings. Potential adverse effects of acute treatment with corticosteroids include elevated blood pressure, hyperglycemia, insomnia, mania or psychosis, and weight gain. Additional adverse effects of long-term treatment include risk of peptic ulcers, infections, and osteoporosis.

Cyclophosphamide. Cyclophosphamide (Cytoxan) is an alkylating agent that is used to treat malignancies and some autoimmune conditions. Cyclophosphamide has also been used to treat MS, although it is not FDA approved for this indication. A 1983 study randomized patients with severe, progressive MS to IV cyclophosphamide plus adrenocorticotrophic hormone (ACTH), ACTH alone, or plasma exchange with ACTH and oral cyclophosphamide.[101] The study was neither blinded nor placebo controlled. It found that 80% of patients treated with IV cyclophosphamide plus ACTH had stabilized at 1 year compared to 20% in the group treated with ACTH alone. Other studies of cyclophosphamide in progressive MS have been negative.[102,103] Subgroup analyses determined that younger patients with a shorter duration of progressive disease and an inflammatory component to their disease as evidenced by MRI or clinical activity may be more likely to respond to cyclophosphamide.[104] Several small, open-label studies have also used monthly pulses of cyclophosphamide in RRMS patients with continued disease activity while on interferon beta or glatiramer acetate.[105-108] At doses varying from 500 to 1500 mg/m^2 IV monthly, these studies have shown benefits on both MRI and clinical outcomes.

Possible adverse effects seen with cyclophosphamide include infertility, amenorrhea, alopecia, cardiotoxicity, infections, and secondary malignancies. Hemorrhagic cystitis is more commonly associated with long-term oral cyclophosphamide treatment; however, patients receiving cyclophosphamide should be adequately hydrated. A complete blood count and urinalysis should be performed periodically to monitor the white blood cell count and to rule out hematuria. A pregnancy test should be sent prior to initiation of therapy.

Azathioprine. Azathioprine (Imuran) is a purine analogue that is used for posttransplantation immunosuppression, rheumatoid arthritis, and other autoimmune conditions. It is not FDA approved for MS, but it is used commonly in Europe in MS patients, partly because it is relatively inexpensive. An evidence-based review concluded that azathioprine was helpful in patients who experience frequent relapses.[109] An open-label clinical trial studied the effect of adding azathioprine to interferon beta-1b in patients experiencing an exacerbation or disease progression while on interferon beta.[110] Patients were maintained on interferon beta-1b and titrated up to a goal dose of 3 mg/kg of azathioprine as tolerated. However, only 1 of the 15 patients was able to tolerate the full dose of azathioprine. MRI scans on the combination therapy had 65% fewer gadolinium-enhancing lesions when compared to baseline scans in the same patients when they were on interferon beta monotherapy. The authors found that a total white blood count less than 4800 was the best predictor of MRI response.

Possible adverse effects with azathioprine include myelosuppression, gastrointestinal side effects, infections, elevated transaminases, and secondary malignancies. At the onset of therapy, patients should have a complete blood count and pregnancy test. The blood count should then be monitored weekly for the first month, twice monthly for the second and third months, and then monthly. About 0.3% of the population is homozygous for a nonfunctional form of the TPMT enzyme, which metabolizes azathioprine.[111] These patients are at risk for life-threatening myelosuppression if given azathioprine. Heterozygotes may also be at an elevated risk of myelosuppression. These patients can be identified by genotyping or by testing enzyme activity levels prior to the initiation of azathioprine treatment.

Methotrexate. Methotrexate is a folate analogue used to treat some malignancies, rheumatoid arthritis, and other autoimmune conditions. It has been used for a number of years in MS, but it is not FDA approved for this diagnosis. The Avonex Combination Trial randomized patients with continued disease activity on Avonex to receive Avonex plus either methotrexate, pulse dose corticosteroids, or methotrexate and pulse dose corticosteroids. Although trends favored the combination group, there was not a statistically significant difference among the treatment groups.[112] The full results of this trial have not yet been published. In an open-label study of 15 patients, weekly oral methotrexate (20 mg) and interferon beta-1a were given to patients who had breakthrough disease on interferon beta.[113] MRI scans on the combination therapy showed 44% fewer gadolinium-enhancing lesions when compared to baseline scans in the same patients when they were on interferon beta monotherapy.

Adverse events associated with methotrexate include gastrointestinal toxicity, myelosuppression, hepatotoxicity, secondary lymphomas, infections, fetal death or congenital anomalies, lung disease, skin reactions, and encephalopathy. At baseline, patients should be screened with a complete blood count including platelet count, liver function tests, renal function tests, chest radiograph, and pregnancy test, as applicable. Hematologic monitoring is recommended at least monthly, and renal and liver function should be checked every 1 to 2 months. Patients should be counseled that pregnancy should be avoided if either partner is receiving methotrexate.

Mycophenolate Mofetil. Mycophenolate mofetil (Cellcept) blocks purine metabolism and is used for posttransplantation immunosuppression. Although not FDA approved for MS, several uncontrolled studies have reported benefits using this treatment.[114-116] Further studies are needed to better establish the utility of this treatment in MS. Potential adverse effects include infections, leukopenia, gastrointestinal bleeding, diarrhea, and secondary malignancies. Complete blood counts are needed weekly during the first month, twice monthly for the second and third months, and monthly through the first year. Women of childbearing age should be tested for pregnancy and advised that the use of mycophenolate during pregnancy increases the risk of fetal loss and congenital malformations.

Intravenous Immune Globulin. Intravenous immune globulin (IVIG) is used to treat a number of autoimmune neurologic diseases such as myasthenia gravis and acute inflammatory demyelinating polyneuropathy. Several trials have tested IVIG in MS. A randomized trial of monthly 0.15- to 0.2-g/kg IVIG or placebo found a 59% reduction of the annual relapse rate in the IVIG group relative to placebo.[117] A more recent placebo-controlled trial of two doses of IVIG did not find a difference in its primary outcome of the proportion of relapse-free patients, although the full results have not yet been published.[118] The role of IVIG in MS remains unclear. One interesting use of IVIG has been to reduce the risk of relapses in the postpartum period, but its role in this situation is unclear (see "Treatment Considerations Related to Pregnancy" section later). IVIG can cause allergic reactions, headache, fluid overload, aseptic meningitis, encephalopathy, renal failure, and thrombosis/hyperviscosity syndromes.

Therapeutic Approach

Several important issues regarding treatment of patients with MS remain unresolved. In some instances, high-quality evidence is available to guide our decisions, but in many instances these data are lacking and treatment decisions must be based on uncontrolled trials, expert opinion, or personal experience. Several key treatment issues and the available evidence are reviewed in this section.

Treatment with DMT: Patient Selection and Initiation

The initial trials of the first DMTs, interferon beta and glatiramer acetate, were on patients with clinically definite RRMS with relatively high relapse rates. All these agents were shown to reduce relapse rate in RRMS. For interferons, the rate of relapse reductions ranged from 18% to 32% depending on the study.[44,119,120] The reduction in relapse rate was 29% in the pivotal study of glatiramer acetate.[121] All interferon formulations and glatiramer have also shown a beneficial effect on MRI measures of disease activity. Based upon these data, the FDA has approved glatiramer acetate and three formulations of interferon beta for use in relapsing forms of MS. Demonstration of an effect on disability was more variable in these trials.

After interferon beta was proven to benefit RRMS patients, questions arose about whether it might also help patients who have had a single clinical episode of CNS inflammation and are deemed to be at high risk of developing MS. Diagnostic criteria for MS require two episodes of CNS inflammation that are disseminated in time and space. Patients who have had a single attack are referred to as having a "clinically isolated syndrome" (CIS). Criteria for MS can be fulfilled by waiting for a second attack or, in some cases, by using paraclinical evidence of MS such as the development of new lesions on an MRI. When evaluating patients with CIS, it is important to consider their risk of having further events that would qualify them for the diagnosis of MS. The best tool to stratify risk of developing MS is brain MRI. The Optic Neuritis Treatment Trial enrolled patients with new optic neuritis and followed them prospectively. It found that patients with one or more lesions typical of MS on brain MRI had a 56% chance of developing MS (defined as a second clinical attack) after 10 years versus a 22% risk for those with a normal brain MRI.[122] Therefore, a study was undertaken in which patients with an initial clinical demyelinating event and subclinical demyelination on MRI were randomized to weekly intramuscular interferon beta-1a or placebo.[123] Patients receiving interferon beta-1a had a 44% lower chance of progressing to clinically definite MS during the follow-up period, and there were fewer new lesions on MRI. Similar findings were seen in studies using the other formulations of interferon beta.[124,125] A trial using glatiramer acetate in CIS showed that this drug reduced the risk of developing MS and delayed the development of MS in individuals with CIS.[126]

The American Academy of Neurology (AAN) published guidelines on the treatment of MS in 2002 (reaffirmed in 2003).[127] The guidelines concluded that, on the basis of several class I studies (see Table 46-2 for a summary of levels of evidence), interferon beta and glatiramer acetate have been demonstrated to reduce the attack rate in patients with MS (level A recommendation). Interferon beta also reduces the attack rate in patients with CIS who are at high risk for developing MS (level A). Consequently, the guidelines concluded that it is appropriate to consider interferon beta treatment for any patient who is at high risk for developing MS or who already has RRMS or SPMS and is still experiencing relapses (level A). Glatiramer acetate is appropriate to consider for treatment of any patient with RRMS (level A). It was concluded that there were insufficient data to recommend interferon beta or glatiramer for SPMS without relapses (level U recommendation). They also thought that there was insufficient evidence to determine whether certain populations of MS patients (e.g., those with more attacks or at earlier disease stages) are better candidates for therapy than others (level U recommendation). Most MS experts believe that early treatment of MS with a DMT offers patients the best chance of minimizing relapses and preventing or delaying disability.

First-Line Treatment for RRMS

Opinions differ regarding what is the optimal first-line RRMS therapy. Since the three interferon beta formulations and glatiramer acetate all have similar efficacy in reducing relapse rates, the choice of therapy is often best guided by the characteristics and preferences of the individual patient. These treatments do differ in the type of injection, frequency of injection, side effects, and frequency and significance of neutralizing antibody formation.

The three formulations of interferon beta have several differences. Betaseron (or Betaferon in Europe) is subcutaneous interferon beta-1b 250 mcg every other day, Avonex is intramuscular interferon beta-1a 30 mcg weekly, and Rebif is subcutaneous interferon beta-1a 44 mcg three times per week. Avonex is considered to be a "low-dose" interferon, while Rebif and Betaseron are considered "high-dose." The AAN treatment guidelines note that evidence indicates that it is "probable that there is a dose-response curve associated with the use of interferon beta" (level B recommendation); that is, a higher dose or higher frequency of administration probably improves efficacy.[127]

Avonex has the lowest frequency of shots (once per week), while the others are about three times per week and glatiramer acetate is daily. This makes Avonex advantageous for patients who are particularly averse to injections. However, Avonex requires a deeper, intramuscular

TABLE 46-2 SUMMARY OF EVIDENCE GRADES

Rating of Recommendation	Translation of Evidence to Recommendations	Rating of Therapeutic Articles
A = Established as effective, ineffective, or harmful for the given condition in the specified population	Level A rating requires at least one convincing class I study or at least two consistent convincing class II studies	**Class I:** Prospective, randomized, controlled clinical trial with masked outcome assessment, in a representative population. The following are required: a) primary outcome(s) is/are clearly defined b) exclusion/inclusion criteria are clearly defined c) adequate accounting for dropouts and crossovers with numbers sufficiently low to have minimal potential for bias d) relevant baseline characteristics are presented and substantially equivalent among treatment groups or there is appropriate statistical adjustment for differences
B = Probably effective, ineffective, or harmful for the given condition in the specified population	Level B rating requires at least one convincing class II study or at least three consistent class III studies	**Class II:** Prospective matched group cohort study in a representative population with masked outcome assessment that meets a–d above *or* an RCT in a representative population that lacks one of criteria a–d
C = Possibly effective, ineffective, or harmful in the specified population	Level C rating requires at least two convincing and consistent class III studies	**Class III:** All other controlled trials (including well-defined natural history controls or patients serving as own controls) in a representative population, where outcome assessment is independent of patient treatment
U = Data inadequate or conflicting. Given current knowledge, treatment is unproven.		**Class IV:** Evidence from uncontrolled studies, case series, case reports, or expert opinion

injection with a needle that is larger than what is used for the subcutaneous injections for the other medications.

The interferon beta preparations also differ in their frequency of inducing neutralizing antibodies (NAbs). NAbs are antibodies that bind to the interferon molecule and potentially can decrease its clinical efficacy. Estimates of the frequency of NAbs have differed significantly depending on the type of study and the definition of NAb positivity. Betaseron is associated with the highest rate of NAb formation, which was 38% in the Phase III study.[44] For Rebif, NAb positivity was seen in 14% of patients in the Phase III study.[120] The manufacturers of Rebif are testing a new formulation that may decrease the development of NAbs. The Phase III trial of Avonex had a 22% rate of NAb positivity[119]; however, using a newly formulated product, most studies have found NAb formation to be less than 7%.[128] Therefore, Avonex appears to have the lowest rate of NAb formation, while Betaseron has the highest. The clinical significance of NAbs has been debated. To address this question, the AAN published a practice guideline on NAbs in 2007.[129] The authors concluded that "it is probable that the presence of NAbs, especially in persistently high titers, is associated with a reduction in the radiographic and clinical effectiveness of interferon beta treatment (level B recommendation)."[128] They also concluded that the rate of NAb formation is probably less with interferon beta-1a compared to interferon beta-1b (level B) and the rate of NAb formation probably depends on the formulation, dose, route of administration, or frequency of administration (level B). NAbs to glatiramer acetate have not been found.[129]

The side effect profile differs significantly between interferon beta and glatiramer acetate. Interferon beta causes flulike symptoms, including fever, myalgia, headache, and fatigue, in up to 75% of patients at initiation of therapy.[130] Interferon beta can cause a transient worsening of preexisting MS symptoms, especially spasticity.[131,132] This often accompanies flulike symptoms in the first 12 weeks. These effects resemble the worsening seen in MS patients with stress, heat, or inflammation. Interferon beta treatment requires blood monitoring for leukopenia or elevated transaminases; glatiramer acetate does not require any blood monitoring. Depression is a common comorbidity in MS. Data have been conflicting on the role of interferon beta in exacerbating depression; however, it appears that this treatment can induce or exacerbate depression in some patients. Other side effects of interferon beta include menstrual disorders and exacerbation of migraine headaches. Glatiramer acetate is associated with a rare immediate post-injection reaction. This reaction is benign but can be frightening for the patient. The reaction occurs within minutes of the injection and can include flushing, chest tightness or pain, dyspnea, palpitations, and anxiety that can last from seconds up to 30 minutes. This reaction is considered benign and not associated with cardiac dysfunction. It is relatively uncommon, occurring from one to seven times during the 30-month Phase III trial in 15% of patients.[121] Anaphylaxis has been reported as a rare event with both glatiramer and interferon beta.[133,134]

Some direct comparisons have been made between different interferon beta formulations. The EVIDENCE trial randomized patients with RRMS to receive either Rebif or Avonex.[135] Due to different routes and frequencies of administration, the patients and treating physicians were not blinded, but relapses and disability were evaluated by a second physician who was blinded. The study found a 17% reduction in annualized relapse rate in the Rebif group compared to the Avonex group. The number of patients needed to treat with Rebif compared to Avonex for one additional patient to remain relapse-free is 12. The INCOMIN study randomized patients with RRMS to Betaseron or Avonex and followed them for 2 years.[136] Patients and physicians were unblinded in this study, but the MRI assessments were blinded. They found a 31% relative risk reduction of annualized relapse rate in the Betaseron group relative to the Avonex group. The Betaseron group also had a higher proportion of patients remaining relapse-free, and MRI measures favored Betaseron. However, interpretation of the results must take into account the lack of blinding regarding clinical outcomes.

Randomized trials comparing interferon beta and glatiramer acetate have also been performed. The REGARD trial randomized patients with RRMS to Rebif or glatiramer acetate.[137] There was no significant difference in the primary end point of time to first relapse. In a prespecified subgroup analysis, the subgroup of patients with lower baseline disability had a greater time to first relapse in the Rebif group relative to the glatiramer group. The authors noted that patients in this trial had much lower relapse rates than had been predicted based on prior studies. The BECOME trial is an MRI study that randomized patients to glatiramer or Betaseron and followed them for up to 2 years with monthly MRI scans.[138] The primary outcome of the number of new MRI lesions was not significantly different in the two treatment groups. Taken together, these two studies support the conclusion that the efficacy of glatiramer and high-dose interferon are similar.

Based on the data discussed here, a few suggestions can be made regarding initial choice of therapy in RRMS. Glatiramer acetate has the best side effect profile and is a good choice for patients who want to avoid flulike symptoms and do not mind daily injections. Patients who are very averse to injections may prefer the weekly injection of Avonex. For patients with particularly active disease, the additional efficacy of high-dose interferon (Rebif or Betaseron) may be preferred over a low-dose interferon. The lower risk of NAb formation with Avonex may be an advantage over high-dose formulations for some patients. Also, between high-dose formulations, the lower frequency of NAb formation in Rebif may make it preferable to Betaseron. The presence of a history of depression or migraine headache favors use of glatiramer over interferon beta.

Treatments Helpful in SPMS

The results of treatment trials in SPMS have been mixed, and this stage of the disease is more difficult to treat than RRMS. Mitoxantrone is the only FDA-approved treatment for SPMS. As discussed earlier, mitoxantrone was given to patients with worsening RRMS or SPMS who had experienced an increase in disability over the prior 18 months.[87] The effective dose used in this double-blind, randomized, placebo-controlled study was 12 mg/m^2 IV every 3 months for 2 years. Relapse rate and disability measures were better in the group receiving mitoxantrone.

Use of mitoxantrone is a reasonable strategy in patients with very active RRMS or rapidly progressive SPMS. For SPMS patients, it is probably most useful in patients who still have a significant inflammatory component to their disease, such as patients in a transitional phase between RRMS and SPMS. Patients with later stages of SPMS are less likely to benefit. The major limitation of this treatment strategy is the adverse effect profile of mitoxantrone. As discussed previously, mitoxantrone is associated with cardiomyopathy, myelosuppression, secondary leukemias, and other side effects. The AAN published guidelines on the use of mitoxantrone in MS in 2003.[139] The authors concluded that "it appears that mitoxantrone may have a beneficial effect on disease progression in patients with MS whose clinical condition is deteriorating" (level B recommendation). However, they cautioned that "this agent is of limited use and of potentially great toxicity. Therefore, it should be reserved for patients with rapidly advancing disease who have failed other therapies."

Although it is not FDA approved for this indication, several trials have shown positive results with cyclophosphamide in SPMS. A 1983 study randomized patients with severe, progressive MS to IV cyclophosphamide plus ACTH, ACTH alone, or plasma exchange with ACTH and oral cyclophosphamide.[101] Although the study was neither blinded nor placebo controlled, it found that 80% of patients treated with cyclophosphamide had stabilized at 1 year compared to 20% in the group treated with ACTH alone. Other studies of cyclophosphamide in progressive MS have been negative.[103,104] Post-hoc analyses of these studies have identified subgroups that are most likely to respond to cyclophosphamide—specifically, younger patients with a shorter duration of progressive disease with an inflammatory component to their disease as evidenced by MRI or clinical activity.[105] Based on this evidence, the AAN treatment guidelines concluded that pulse cyclophosphamide treatment does not seem to alter the course of progressive MS (level B recommendation), but that it is possible that younger patients with progressive MS might derive some benefit from pulse plus booster cyclophosphamide treatment (level U recommendation).[127]

The utility of interferons in SPMS has been an area of controversy. A European study randomized SPMS patients to subcutaneous interferon beta-1b or placebo.[140] SPMS was defined as a period of deterioration independent of relapses sustained for 6 months, and patients needed to have a history of two or more relapses or an increase in disability in the prior 2 years. This study was terminated early due to a benefit in the interferon beta-1b group for the primary outcome of time to confirmed disability progression. Based on these data, the European Union approved interferon beta-1b for use in SPMS. In contrast, a North American study of interferon beta-1b in SPMS had completely different results.[141] This study enrolled patients with MS for at least 2 years who had had at least one relapse and a progressive course for at least 6 months. Patients also had to have an increase in disability in the preceding 2 years. This study found no benefit of interferon beta for the primary outcome of time to progression. In fact, the study was stopped early due to futility. However, the interferon beta group did show benefit on some secondary outcome measures, including a reduction in relapse rate and number of new MRI lesions. A post-hoc combined analysis of the two trials was performed.[142] The patients in the European study were more likely to be at an earlier phase of SPMS and had more inflammatory activity as evidenced by relapse rate and MRI activity. The authors concluded that SPMS patients with pronounced disability progression and continuing relapse activity are more likely to respond to interferon beta. AAN treatment guidelines state that it is appropriate to consider interferon beta for treatment of SPMS patients who are still experiencing relapses (level A recommendation); however, the effectiveness of interferon beta in patients with SPMS without relapses is uncertain (level U recommendation).[127]

Treatments Helpful in PPMS

Unlike RRMS, attempts to find treatments for PPMS have been disappointing. There are currently no FDA-approved treatments for PPMS; this is a major unmet medical need. With the exception of natalizumab, the approved therapies for RRMS have been tested in PPMS. The PROMiSe trial randomized PPMS patients to receive glatiramer acetate or placebo and followed them for 3 years.[88] The primary end point was time to sustained progression of disability. The study found no significant treatment effect. Interferon beta-1b has been tested in a randomized, placebo-controlled trial of patients with PPMS or transitional MS, defined as progressive disease with a history of a single relapse prior to, at the onset of, or during the progressive phase.[143] Preliminary results were reported, but the full results have not yet been published. There was no difference in the groups with respect to the outcome of confirmed 6-month progression. However, the interferon group had better Multiple Sclerosis Functional Composite scores and better results on some MRI measures. A double-blind, placebo-controlled trial of mitoxantrone in PPMS has been completed. The preliminary analysis indicated that there was no benefit on clinical outcomes, but the results have not yet been published.[144] A trial of rituximab in PPMS was reported to be negative in a company press release.

Definition of Treatment Failure

Many physicians struggle with how to define treatment failure in MS. Although no universal definition of treatment failure exists, most people would agree that more than two relapses per year, an evolving MRI, or development of new disability should prompt consideration of a change in therapy. However, we know from clinical trials that first-line therapies such as interferon beta and glatiramer acetate only decrease the relapse rate by about one third. Consequently, it may be unrealistic to expect complete quiescence with these medications. If one knows the pretreatment relapse rate or the frequency at which new MRI lesion developed, then this can be used as a comparison. Unfortunately, decisions must usually be made without these data.

The most challenging situation is the patient with about one relapse per year or no relapses but continued development of new MRI lesions. The management of this patient often depends on several questions: Are they true relapses (as opposed to heat- or infection-related "pseudorelapses")? How severe are they? How well does the patient recover? Are there prognostic factors that portend a worse disease course? Does the patient want to change treatments? What other treatments are available, and what are their risk: benefit ratios? An important consideration when faced with breakthrough disease activity is the patient's compliance. As with any disease, a treatment only works if a patient takes it. Another consideration in patients on interferon beta is the possible presence of NAbs. Although the clinical importance of NAbs remains controversial, an AAN guideline concluded that it is probable that the presence of NAbs, especially in persistently high titers, is associated with a reduction in the radiographic and clinical effectiveness of interferon beta treatment (level B recommendation).[128] The presence of high-titer NAbs in the context of breakthrough disease activity should prompt consideration of changing to a non-interferon treatment. Antibodies to natalizumab have also been observed.[76] Persistent antibodies were seen in 6% of trial patients and were associated with decreased efficacy of the drug. Testing for antibodies to interferon beta and natalizumab is commercially available. The presence of other non-MS pathologies should also be a consideration in breakthrough disease (e.g., PML in a patient receiving natalizumab).

Management of Breakthrough Disease Activity

Breakthrough disease activity remains a common problem with our current armamentarium of treatments. As discussed previously, assessment of treatment compliance and consideration of the presence of NAbs to interferon beta or natalizumab should be considered. If it is decided that the degree of disease activity is not acceptable, then several strategies are available. Opinions on how to manage ongoing disease activity differ significantly, and there are limited data to guide decision making. Some clinicians will change a patient from a low-dose to high-dose interferon, although there are no data to support this. Switching from interferon beta to glatiramer acetate or vice versa is another strategy. The combination of interferon beta and glatiramer was found to be safe in a pilot trial,[145] and a large National Institutes of Health–sponsored trial is underway to test the effectiveness of this regimen.[69]

Another approach for managing breakthrough disease activity is to switch to a more potent agent. Two FDA-approved treatments that can be used in this circumstance are natalizumab and mitoxantrone. Clinical trials with natalizumab showed robust effects on relapse rate and MRI measures in relapsing MS. However, due to the risk of PML, a potentially fatal viral infection of the brain, natalizumab should only be used as monotherapy in patients with relapsing forms of MS who have had an inadequate response to alternate MS therapies. As described earlier, mitoxantrone is indicated for treatment of SPMS or worsening RRMS. Although not FDA approved for this indication, IV cyclophosphamide has often been used for MS patients with relatively aggressive disease. One trial randomized RRMS patients who continued to have very active disease on interferon beta to receive 6 months of pulse corticosteroids or pulse corticosteroids plus IV cyclophosphamide (800 mg/m^2) in addition to interferon beta.[107] In the 18-month follow-up, there were a lower relapse rate and fewer new gadolinium-enhancing lesions in the group receiving IV cyclophosphamide, pulse corticosteroids, and interferon beta.

Other non–FDA-approved therapies are commonly used in breakthrough MS. Some clinicians will add pulse dose corticosteroids, azathioprine, methotrexate, mycophenolate mofetil, cladribine, cyclosporine, or IVIG to the patient's regimen. The data for use of these agents are often limited. The AAN treatment guidelines concluded that regular pulse corticosteroids may be useful in the long-term management of RRMS (level C recommendation),[127] azathioprine may reduce relapse rate in MS (level C), cladribine does not appear to favorably affect the disease course (level C), cyclosporine may possibly have some benefit in MS (level C), and IVIG could possibly affect relapse rate (level C).

Management of Acute Relapses

The treatment of an acute MS relapse largely depends on its severity. Early in the disease, most relapses are followed by significant recovery even in the absence of treatment. Studies have shown that high-dose IV corticosteroids can speed up the recovery from a relapse (level A recommendation).[127] However, there does not appear to be any long-term benefit to a brief use of corticosteroids in an acute relapse (level B recommendation). Therefore, many clinicians will use high-dose IV steroids for any relapse that causes functional impairment (e.g., weakness, notable visual impairment). For milder symptoms not causing functional impairment (e.g., a mild sensory disturbance), corticosteroids are often withheld. A typical regimen is methylprednisolone 1000 mg IV daily for 3 to 7 days. Some clinicians will follow this with a 10- to 14-day oral prednisone taper, although many do not. The Optic Neuritis Treatment Trial found that optic neuritis patients treated with a moderate dose of oral corticosteroids (prednisone 1 mg/kg) had a higher risk of developing a new optic neuritis than the groups treated with placebo or high-dose IV methylprednisolone.[99] Therefore, moderate-dose oral corticosteroids are not recommended. High-dose oral and IV corticosteroid regimens have been compared in small randomized trials.[146,147] They have found no difference in efficacy, suggesting that high-dose oral regimens may be a more convenient and less expensive option to IV methylprednisolone. The AAN treatment guidelines found that there is no compelling evidence to indicate that the route, type, or dosage of corticosteroid affects the clinical benefit that is observed, at least at the dosages that have been studied (level C recommendation).

For patients with a severe relapse that does not respond to high-dose corticosteroids, one option is plasma exchange. In one trial patients with severe deficits that did not respond to high-dose corticosteroids were randomized to seven courses of plasma exchange or sham treatment.[148] The group receiving plasma exchange was significantly more likely to experience at least moderate neurologic recovery. This treatment was given a level C recommendation in the AAN treatment guidelines.[127]

Treatments Helpful for Common MS-Related Symptoms

Besides disease-modifying agents, physicians will often need to prescribe medication for symptomatic therapy. Patients with MS suffer from a variety of secondary symptoms including spasticity, incontinence, fatigue, pain, and depression. Successful management of those symptoms is a significant part of improving patients' quality of life. Table 46-3 lists various therapeutic options for common secondary symptoms and their potential side effects. At times, a side effect profile can be used to the patient's advantage. For example, if a patient presents with insomnia, depression, neuropathic pain, and incontinence, he or she may not need four prescriptions. Using amitriptyline as an antidepressant may treat all four symptoms based on its anticholinergic properties (causing drowsiness in the evenings and decreased urination) as well as its ability to treat neuropathic pain.[149-151] It is critical to determine the root cause of various symptoms before prescribing a medication. An MS patient with fatigue may be suffering from sleep apnea rather than MS-related fatigue. Successful treatment of these symptoms will only occur if all potential causes have been considered.

Spasticity is a velocity-dependent increase in muscle tone that results from lesions of the descending corticospinal tract. Commonly, patients will complain of stiffness of gait, loss of dexterity, or painful muscle spasms. Physical therapy can be helpful in improving spasticity and preventing contractures. Baclofen (Lioresal) is a γ-aminobutyric acid B receptor agonist that is used to treat spasticity. Patients should begin at a dose of 5 mg three times per day and be titrated up as tolerated. The dose-limiting side effect is usually sedation. In addition, decreased muscle tone can sometimes make it more difficult for patients to walk. Patients should be cautioned not to stop the medicine abruptly due to risk of withdrawal seizures. Tizanidine (Zanaflex) is another centrally acting antispasmodic agent. It is an agonist of α_2-adrenergic receptors. Sedation is the most common side effect encountered with tizanidine. Botulinum toxin injections can be used to relieve localized adductor spasms. However, these large muscles often require a high dose to be effective. Other treatments used to relieve spasticity include benzodiazepines, dantrolene, dronabinol, and an intrathecal baclofen pump.

TABLE 46-3 COMMONLY USED SYMPTOMATIC THERAPIES

	Potential Side Effects
SPASTICITY	
Baclofen	Drowsiness, headache, insomnia, nausea, confusion, seizures
Dantrolene	Drowsiness, dizziness, diarrhea, constipation, headache, palpitations, hepatotoxicity
Diazepam	Drowsiness, dizziness, fatigue, constipation, headache, blurred vision, confusion, ataxia
Dronabinol	Dizziness, insomnia, mood changes, ataxia, anxiety, paranoia, unusual thoughts, increased appetite
Tizanidine	Drowsiness, fatigue, dry mouth, dizziness
NEUROPATHIC PAIN	
Amitriptyline	Drowsiness, dizziness, dry mouth, headache, urinary retention, weight gain
Carbamazepine	Ataxia, clumsiness, dizziness, drowsiness, nausea
Gabapentin	Drowsiness, dizziness, fatigue, irregular eye movements
Lamotrigine	Rash, headache, fatigue, dizziness, blurred vision, ataxia
Paroxetine	Drowsiness, nausea, diarrhea, insomnia, dry mouth, tremor, decreased libido, sexual dysfunction
Topiramate	Paresthesias, weight loss, dizziness, cognitive difficulties, ataxia, somnolence
Tramadol	Nausea, constipation, dizziness, lowered seizure threshold
FATIGUE	
Amantadine	Nausea, drowsiness, headache, constipation, rash
Modafinil	Headache, anxiety, insomnia

Bladder dysfunction is a very common complaint among MS patients. Furthermore, bladder and kidney stones, renal dysfunction, and urosepsis can be major sources of morbidity in MS. When patients present with a new urinary complaint, it is important to perform a urine culture to evaluate for an infection. There are three general types of urinary problems in MS. It is often difficult to distinguish them based on history, and urodynamic studies can be helpful in some cases. First is the atonic bladder, which presents with difficulty voiding and overflow incontinence. Urinary tract infections are common. Cholinergic medications such as bethanecol can sometimes assist with bladder emptying. However, many patients will need to perform clean intermittent bladder catheterization. Patients with frequent urinary tract infections may benefit from the use of urine acidifiers such as cranberry juice or vitamin C. The second type of bladder problem is the spastic bladder. Patients are unable to store urine well, resulting in urinary urgency and incontinence. Anticholinergics such as oxybutynin (Ditropan) and tolterodine (Detrol) can alleviate some of these symptoms. The third bladder problem is detrusor-sphincter dyssynergia. This occurs when the detrusor muscle and external urinary sphincter contract simultaneously, leading to high pressures in the bladder. This is also best treated with clean intermittent catheterization, but α-blockers such as terazosin (Hytrin) can be helpful. Constipation can be treated with dietary changes and stool softeners. Bowel incontinence is less common, but more distressing. Use of a bulk fiber agent such as psyllium (Metamucil) can be suggested.

Fatigue is the most commonly reported symptom of MS, with an estimated frequency between 76% and 92%.[152] The first step in managing fatigue is to evaluate for a cause other than MS. Hypothyroidism, anemia, depression, sleep apnea, or medication effects all can contribute to fatigue. The patient's sleep habits should be explored, including the frequency of awakenings due to nocturia. Regular exercise can improve endurance and should be recommended. If this is insufficient, several pharmacologic interventions can be tried. About 30% of patients will respond well to amantadine (Symmetrel) 100 mg in the morning and 100 mg in the early afternoon. Patients may experience livedo reticularis or anticholinergic effects with this treatment. Modafinil (Provigil) is a medication that promotes wakefulness and is used in narcolepsy. The evidence for its utility in MS fatigue is mixed. Although benefits were seen in an open-label study of MS fatigue, a randomized, double-blind, placebo-controlled trial failed to show a benefit.[153] Nonetheless, many experts believe that a subset of patients will respond favorably to Modafinil. CNS stimulants such as methylphenidate (Ritalin) are an option for patients with severe fatigue that has not responded to other treatments. One double-blind, placebo-controlled, crossover study of aspirin 1300 mg daily showed a benefit on fatigue scores in MS.[154] Although not FDA approved in the United States, 4-aminopyridine has been used for many years for management of MS symptoms. It is thought that it may improve conduction in demyelinated nerves through blocking currents in the $K_v1.4$ potassium channels on axons. Its use has been limited by an increased seizure risk, but a longer acting formulation (fampridine) is being tested in clinical trials.

MS patients can experience both musculoskeletal pain and centrally mediated dysesthesias. For neuropathic pain, commonly used treatments include gabapentin (Neurontin), tricyclic antidepressants such as amitriptyline or nortriptyline, tramadol (Ultram), pregabalin (Lyrica), duloxetine (Cymbalta), topiramate (Topamax), baclofen (Lioresal), carbamazepine (Tegretol), and lamotrigine (Lamictal). In MS, trigeminal neuralgia can result from a demyelinating plaque at the dorsal root entry zone of the trigeminal nerve. Carbamazepine, gabapentin, and phenytoin (Dilantin) are frequently used for this condition, although some patients may require gamma knife or neurosurgical intervention. Musculoskeletal pain can be treated with nonsteroidal anti-inflammatory medications.

Several other symptoms are commonly encountered in MS patients. Patients can experience cognitive dysfunction, particularly with regard to sustained attention, working memory, and speed of information processing. It is hoped that use of DMTs will decrease the development of cognitive impairment. Studies of acetylcholinesterase inhibitors for cognitive impairment in MS have generally been negative, although subsets of patients may benefit from this approach.[155] Cognitive rehabilitation can be tried. Depression and bipolar disorder are seen at a higher frequency in MS patients. Treatment of these conditions is the same as for non-MS patients with these conditions. Sexual dysfunction is also identified commonly in MS patients. Since many patients will not spontaneously report this problem, it is often useful to question patients about it. As with other symptoms, a contribution of depression, other medical conditions, or medication effects should be ruled out. Men may experience erectile dysfunction, which can be treated with phosphodiesterase-5 inhibitors such as sildenafil (Viagra). Women may report decreased libido, decreased vaginal lubrication, or decreased perineal sensation. Water-soluble lubricants can assist with vaginal dryness, but pharmacologic options are not available for other causes of sexual dysfunction.

Treatment Considerations Related to Pregnancy

Given that MS is most commonly diagnosed in women between 20 and 40, clinicians are frequently faced with questions relating to pregnancy. Many women with MS have successful deliveries, and there is no evidence that MS has any adverse effects on the health of the baby. Epidemiologic studies of pregnant patients have found that the MS relapse rate is lower during pregnancy, especially during the third trimester.[156] However, the risk of relapses is increased in the 3-month period following delivery. After that 3-month period, the relapse rate returns to the prepregnancy level, indicating that pregnancy does not accelerate the disease process. Taken together, the relapse rate for the 1-year period including the pregnancy is the same as the rate in non-pregnant patients. In addition, neither epidural analgesia nor breast-feeding is associated with an increased relapse rate or disease progression.[156]

None of the DMTs has been proven to be safe in pregnancy or breast-feeding. Glatiramer acetate is in FDA Pregnancy Category B (animal reproduction studies have not demonstrated a fetal risk, but there are no controlled studies in pregnant women, or animal reproduction studies have shown an adverse effect [other than a decrease in fertility] that was not confirmed in controlled studies in women in the first trimester [and there is no evidence of a risk in later trimesters]). Interferon beta and natalizumab are Category C (either studies in animals have revealed adverse effects on the fetus and there are no controlled studies in women, or studies in women and animals are not available). Mitoxantrone is Category D (there is positive evidence of human fetal risk, but the benefits from its use in pregnant women may be acceptable despite the risk). For women who want to get pregnant, the first step is to discuss what is known about pregnancy and MS. For women on interferon, it should be discontinued 1 to 2 months before the woman wants to start trying to get pregnant because of the known abortifacient potential of this class. As for any woman, the use of prenatal vitamins and folic acid supplementation is recommended prior to and during pregnancy. If a pregnancy is discovered while the woman is on a DMT, the treatment should be stopped immediately. The potential effects of using these therapies while breast-feeding are unknown. Consequently, it should be recommended that they not be used while breast-feeding.

Management of the postpartum patient can be challenging. However, 72% of women will not have a relapse in the 3 months after pregnancy.[157] In the Pregnancy in Multiple Sclerosis study, the best predictors of which patients were most likely to experience a postpartum relapse were the prepregnancy relapse rate, relapse rate during pregnancy, and a higher disability score.[157] In other words, those with active disease before and during pregnancy were most likely to have a postpartum relapse. The decision about whether to forego breast-feeding in order to resume a DMT after delivery should depend on the clinician's estimate of the likelihood of a postpartum relapse, the severity of prior relapses, and the patient's preferences.

One strategy that has been employed to try to decrease postpartum relapses is the use of IVIG. In a retrospective analysis of patients treated with different IVIG regimens during and/or after pregnancy, one group found a lower relapse rate compared to untreated patients.[158] A prospective randomized trial of postpartum IVIG was performed for the purpose of identifying an optimal dose.[159] The first group received one dose of 150 mg/kg IVIG and the second group received 450, 300, and 150 mg/kg on days 1, 2, and 3 after delivery, respectively. Both groups then received 150 mg/kg of IVIG every 4 weeks for five treatments. The treatment regimens did not differ with respect to the outcome of the number of patients remaining relapse-free in the first 3 months postpartum. The postpartum relapse rate was not significantly higher than the relapse rate before pregnancy, leading the authors to conclude that IVIG appears to decrease the postpartum relapse rate.

Treating the Pediatric MS Patient

Although MS classically has its onset in early adulthood, approximately 3% to 10% of cases will have onset before age 18.[160] In some instances it can initially be difficult to differentiate pediatric MS from conditions such as acute disseminated encephalomyelitis (ADEM). To assist with this, Krupp et al. have published proposed diagnostic criteria for pediatric MS and related conditions.[161] None of the therapies used in MS are FDA approved for use in children. However, based on the same rationale for use in adults, glatiramer acetate and all three forms of interferon beta have been assessed in clinical trials in children.[160] These studies have generally found that the side effect profile in children is similar to that of adults,[162] although children under 10 may be more likely to develop abnormal liver function tests with interferon beta.[162,163] Although these smaller studies were not generally designed to look for treatment effects, most studies have found a lower relapse rate in the treated group.[162] Data on long-term safety and efficacy are not available.

A recent review by the International Pediatric MS Study Group recommended that immunomodulatory therapy should be started in children with active relapsing-remitting disease.[162] The authors defined this as more than one exacerbation in a period of 1 to 2 years and new T2-hyperintense lesions or gadolinium-enhancing lesions on repeat brain MRI scans over the same time frame. They cautioned that, in patients whose initial episode includes encephalopathy, the use of DMTs should be delayed until a second or third attack with more typical MS features has occurred to avoid giving inappropriate treatment to a child with ADEM. Interferon beta or glatiramer acetate is an appropriate first-line therapy. The choice should be made based on a discussion with the child and parents. IVIG can be considered as an alternative, especially for children under 6 years, in whom there is limited knowledge about the tolerability of these medications.[162] Azathioprine is an option for patients who cannot tolerate injections.[162] Dose adjustment for interferon beta may be necessary for children younger than 10 years or those with a low body weight, especially at the initiation of therapy.[162]

Emerging Targets and Therapeutics

As the pathogenesis of MS has been further elucidated, a variety of novel therapeutic targets have been identified. There are currently over a dozen clinical trials of new therapies and new combinations of therapies for MS. Some treatments aim to modify or suppress the immune system. Other drugs are being tested as putative neuroprotectants. These agents are meant to protect neurons from damage regardless of inflammation-mediated demyelination. Beyond the mechanisms of action, the other area of change is in the route of administration—the newer agents include a number of oral and infusible drugs.

FTY720 (fingolimod) is an agonist to sphingosine-1 phosphate (S1P) receptors on the surface of lymphocytes (specifically the S1P1 receptor). Binding of this receptor results in its internalization, which then prevents normal lymphocyte egress from the secondary lymph organs. This reduces the number of circulating lymphocytes available to mount an autoimmune attack in the CNS. This agent, derived from the fungus *Isaria sinclairii,* has been studied in MS and kidney transplantation patients.[164,165] A Phase II double-blind, placebo-controlled trial randomized 281 patients with RRMS to 1.25 mg or 5 mg of FTY720 or placebo. Patients were followed for 6 months, after which most patients participated in an extension study.[166] There was a significant reduction in relapses and new MRI lesions. Side effects included an increased risk of nasopharyngitis, influenza, headache, and diarrhea. Two Phase III trials are underway.

BG-12 is an oral fumarate that is currently in Phase III clinical trials for RRMS. While the exact mechanism of action is unknown, there is some evidence for an anti-inflammatory effect that ameliorates immune-mediated CNS damage.[167] A promising Phase II trial analyzed three doses of BG-12 (120, 360, and 720 mg) versus placebo and reported a reduction in relapse rate and MRI benefits. The most common adverse events were flushing, gastrointestinal disorders, headache, and nasopharyngitis.

Laquinimod is a synthetic compound with excellent oral bioavailability that is structurally related to linomide. In Phase II and III studies, linomide was effective at preventing new lesions on MRI, but was discontinued due to side effects including myocardial infarction and serositis.[168] A Phase II double-blind, placebo-controlled trial of laquinimod (0.1 and 0.3 mg/day) versus placebo reported a reduction in the appearance of new MRI lesions.[169] Phase III trials will be conducted in order to confirm these results and further evaluate the safety profile in a larger cohort of patients.

Teriflunomide is another oral immunomodulatory agent that inhibits pyrimidine synthesis in T cells.[170,171] After showing promising results in animal models of MS, Phase I and II studies were conducted.[172] A 36-week, double-blind, placebo-controlled trial compared two doses of teriflunomide (7 and 14 mg/day) to placebo. Patients receiving the higher dose of teriflunomide had fewer relapses, fewer new MRI lesions, and less accrual of disability (albeit over a short period).[172] A Phase III trial is currently underway.

Cladribine (Leustatin) is an immunosuppressant that is cytotoxic for resting and proliferating lymphocytes. T lymphocytes are preferentially depleted compared to B cells.[173] Injectable versions of this drug have shown efficacy in RRMS.[174,175] Studies attempting to identify a beneficial effect on progressive forms of MS failed to achieve clinically significant outcomes.[176,177] The major toxicity of this agent has been myelosuppression.[178] Currently, a Phase III trial of oral cladribine in RRMS is underway.

In addition to oral agents, a variety of monoclonal antibodies have shown significant potential in MS. Rituximab (Rituxan) is a chimeric monoclonal antibody that binds to CD20, a molecule on the surface of all B cells except plasma cells. Originally used to treat B-cell lymphoma, this agent has become an attractive therapy for several autoimmune disorders. Indeed, rituximab has been FDA approved for use in certain regimens for rheumatoid arthritis.[179] This treatment causes death of B cells via complement-mediated cytotoxicity, antibody-dependent cell-mediated cytotoxicity, and apoptosis.[180] Given that B cells are a source of IL-6 and TNF-α, depleting the B-cell population with rituximab would also reduce these proinflammatory cytokines. When patients with MS were treated with rituximab, CSF analysis revealed a decrease in the number of B and T cells.[181] Small Phase I and II trials have found a reduction in relapses and new MRI lesion formation.[182,183] Whether this clinical outcome implicates antibodies in the pathogenesis of MS or indicates the importance of B cells as antigen-presenting cells is unclear.

Daclizumab (Zenapax) is a humanized monoclonal antibody that recognizes CD25, the alpha subunit of the IL-2 receptor on T cells. This antibody interferes with IL-2 signaling pathways in T cells, but does not cause apoptosis or cell death.[184] While T-cell function is altered with daclizumab, the number of $CD56^+$ natural killer cells increases. The effect of this cell population on the pathogenesis of MS is unknown, but they may have protective capabilities.[185] Two small open-label studies of daclizumab for patients with RRMS have indicated that the drug is well tolerated and there is a significant improvement in both MRI and clinical end points.[186,187]

Alemtuzumab (Campath) is a monoclonal antibody that recognizes CD52, a molecule found on mature lymphocytes. While the mechanism of action has not been elucidated in vivo, some studies have shown that alemtuzumab can induce apoptosis in lymphocytes.[188,189] It has been approved by the FDA for treatment-refractory chronic lymphocytic leukemia.[190] Multiple open-label studies of alemtuzumab in RRMS and SPMS have shown promising clinical results.[19,21,191] While larger studies are currently underway, some concerning side effects have been identified. Specifically, many patients develop autoimmune hyperthyroidism and infusion reactions.[192,193] Also, there is an increased risk of opportunistic infections with agents such as cytomegalovirus. In data presented at the 59th AAN meeting, the CAMMS223 study comparing alemtuzumab to interferon beta showed a significant reduction in relapses and progression to disability. Adverse events included a significant increase in autoimmune thyroid disease and several unexpected cases of idiopathic thrombocytopenic purpura (ITP).[193,194] Unfortunately, one case of ITP resulted in a fatal intracerebral hemorrhage. The side effect profile may significantly limit this drug's clinical utility.

Various drugs that are currently indicated for the treatment of other conditions have shown promise in MS. In animal studies and small human trials, drugs such as minocycline, statins, and estriol have shown promise as MS therapies.[195-201] Experimental data suggest that minocycline could function as an MMP inhibitor, thereby reducing the migration of lymphocytes into the parenchyma.[202] Statins are thought to have both neuroprotective effects and a capability to alter the permeability of the BBB.[203-205] The sex hormone estriol has been shown to alter chemokine expression and T-cell migration.[206,207] Thus, each of these drugs, as well as many others, is being investigated in clinical trials.

While the majority of therapeutics studied to date suppress or modulate the immune system, more recent strategies have targeted neuroprotection. Multiple studies have identified axonal loss early in the course of MS, and axonal loss is predictive of the development of disability.[4,208-210] Moreover, in progressive forms of MS, axonal damage appears to be at least partly independent of inflammation, and immunosuppression is usually ineffective. Therapeutically, it would be advantageous to have neuroprotective therapies that could lessen or prevent axonal damage and disability accrual. Several agents have shown promise in early clinical trials. One theory of the cause of neuronal damage is glutamate-mediated excitotoxicity. Riluzole (Rilutek), a glutamate/N-methyl-D-aspartate pathway blocker, was tested in a small group of patients with PPMS. Results suggested a slowing of neuronal loss.[211,212] Use of erythropoietin (Epogen, Procrit) is another potential neuroprotective strategy. When examined in preclinical studies, results suggested that erythropoietin may help maintain neuronal integrity despite intense inflammation.[213] A third neuroprotective strategy is based on the observation that certain sodium channels are implicated in axonal damage.[214] Agents that block sodium channels have shown a benefit in animal models of MS and are progressing to clinical trials.[215-217] These are just a few of the potential strategies that are being investigated from a neuroprotection perspective.

Both immunomodulatory and neuroprotective strategies, however, achieve clinical efficacy by preventing future damage in patients with MS. There are no approved therapies that are targeted at promoting or inducing repair of the damaged nervous system. Restorative therapies currently under investigation include drugs that will promote remyelination and cell-based therapies (e.g., stem cells) that are meant to re-create normal CNS circuitry. There are natural inhibitors of axonal regeneration, such as the Nogo pathway. The Nogo receptor utilizes a series of proteins, such as LINGO-1, to transduce its signal.[218] Strategies that interfere with this signaling pathway may promote regeneration within the CNS after inflammation. Likewise, a multitude of researchers are pursuing cell-based therapies as a way to induce repair within a damaged CNS. Glial-restricted precursor cells have the potential to repair CNS damage from inflammatory processes.[219] These approaches require significant preclinical data before human trials will commence.

REFERENCES

1. Kobelt G, Berg J, Atherly D, Hadjimichael O. Costs and quality of life in multiple sclerosis: a cross-sectional study in the United States. Neurology 2006;66:1696-1702.
2. Kurtzke JF. The epidemiology of multiple sclerosis. *In* Raine CS, McFarland H, Tourtellotte WW (eds): Multiple Sclerosis: Clinical and Pathogenetic Basis. London: Chapman & Hall, 1997, pp 91-139.
3. The International Multiple Sclerosis Genetics Consortium. Risk alleles for multiple sclerosis identified by a genomewide study. N Engl J Med 2007;357:851-862.
4. De Stefano N, Narayanan S, Francis GS, et al. Evidence of axonal damage in the early stages of multiple sclerosis and its relevance to disability. Arch Neurol 2001;58:65-70.
5. van Waesberghe JH, Kamphorst W, De Groot CJ, et al. Axonal loss in multiple sclerosis lesions: magnetic resonance imaging insights into substrates of disability. Ann Neurol 1999;46:747-754.
6. Schumacher GA. Multiple sclerosis. Arch Neurol 1966;14:571-573.
7. Polman CH, Reingold SC, Edan G, et al. Diagnostic criteria for multiple sclerosis: 2005 revisions to the "McDonald Criteria." Ann Neurol 2005;58:840-846.
8. Ikuta F, Zimmerman HM. Distribution of plaques in seventy autopsy cases of multiple sclerosis in the United States. Neurology 1976;26(6 Pt 2):26-28.
9. Filippi M, Bozzali M, Rovaris M, et al. Evidence for widespread axonal damage at the earliest clinical stage of multiple sclerosis. Brain 2003;126(Pt 2):433-437.
10. Miller DH, Thompson AJ, Filippi M. Magnetic resonance studies of abnormalities in the normal appearing white matter and grey matter in multiple sclerosis. J Neurol 2003;250:1407-1419.
11. Hartung HP, Archelos JJ, Zielasek J, et al. Circulating adhesion molecules and inflammatory mediators in demyelination: a review. Neurology 1995;45(6 Suppl 6):S22-S32.
12. Yeo TW, De Jager PL, Gregory SG, et al. A second major histocompatibility complex susceptibility locus for multiple sclerosis. Ann Neurol 2007;61:228-236.
13. Brassat D, Salemi G, Barcellos LF, et al. The HLA locus and multiple sclerosis in Sicily. Neurology 2005;64:361-363.
14. Khare M, Mangalam A, Rodriguez M, David CS. HLA DR and DQ interaction in myelin oligodendrocyte glycoprotein-induced experimental autoimmune encephalomyelitis in HLA class II transgenic mice. J Neuroimmunol 2005;169:1-12.
15. Killestein J, Kalkers NF, Meilof JF, et al. TNFalpha production by CD4+ T cells predicts long-term increase in lesion load on MRI in MS. Neurology 2001;57:1129-1131.
16. Crawford MP, Yan SX, Ortega SB, et al. High prevalence of autoreactive, neuroantigen-specific CD8+ T cells in multiple sclerosis revealed by novel flow cytometric assay. Blood 2004;103:4222-4231.
17. Lindsey JW, Hodgkinson S, Mehta R, et al. Repeated treatment with chimeric anti-CD4 antibody in multiple sclerosis. Ann Neurol 1994;36:183-189.
18. van Oosten BW, Lai M, Hodgkinson S, et al. Treatment of multiple sclerosis with the monoclonal anti-CD4 antibody cM-T412: results of a randomized, double-blind, placebo-controlled, MR-monitored Phase II trial. Neurology 1997;49:351-357.
19. Coles A, Deans J, Compston A. Campath-1H treatment of multiple sclerosis: lessons from the bedside for the bench. Clin Neurol Neurosurg 2004;106:270-274.
20. Coles AJ, Wing MG, Molyneux P, et al. Monoclonal antibody treatment exposes three mechanisms underlying the clinical course of multiple sclerosis. Ann Neurol 1999;46:296-304.
21. Paolillo A, Coles AJ, Molyneux PD, et al. Quantitative MRI in patients with secondary progressive MS treated with monoclonal antibody Campath 1H. Neurology 1999; 53:751-757.
22. Harbo HF, Lie BA, Sawcer S, et al. Genes in the HLA class I region may contribute to the HLA class II-associated genetic susceptibility to multiple sclerosis. Tissue Antigens 2004;63:237-247.
23. Fogdell-Hahn A, Ligers A, Gronning M, et al. Multiple sclerosis: a modifying influence of HLA class I genes in an HLA class II associated autoimmune disease. Tissue Antigens 2000;55:140-148.
24. Skulina C, Schmidt S, Dornmair K, et al. Multiple sclerosis: brain-infiltrating CD8+ T cells persist as clonal expansions in the cerebrospinal fluid and blood. Proc Natl Acad Sci U S A 2004;101:2428-2433.
25. Huseby ES, Liggitt D, Brabb T, et al. A pathogenic role for myelin-specific CD8+ T cells in a model for multiple sclerosis. J Exp Med 2001;194:669-676.
26. Schwartz M, Kipnis J. Protective autoimmunity and neuroprotection in inflammatory and noninflammatory neurodegenerative diseases. J Neurol Sci 2005;233:163-166.
27. Killestein J, Eikelenboom MJ, Izeboud T, et al. Cytokine producing CD8+ T cells are correlated to MRI features of tissue destruction in MS. J Neuroimmunol 2003;142:141-148.
28. Lucchinetti C, Bruck W, Parisi J, et al. Heterogeneity of multiple sclerosis lesions: implications for the pathogenesis of demyelination. Ann Neurol 2000;47:707-717.
29. Genc K, Dona DL, Reder AT. Increased CD80+ B cells in active multiple sclerosis and reversal by interferon beta-1b therapy. J Clin Invest 1997;99:2664-2671.
30. Jiang H, Milo R, Swoveland P, et al. Interferon beta-1b reduces interferon gamma-induced antigen-presenting capacity of human glial and B cells. J Neuroimmunol 1995;61:17-25.
31. Joseph J, Knobler RL, D'Imperio C, Lublin FD. Down-regulation of interferon-gamma-induced class II expression on human glioma cells by recombinant interferon-beta: effects of dosage treatment schedule. J Neuroimmunol 1988;20:39-44.
32. Aharoni R, Teitelbaum D, Sela M, Arnon R. Copolymer 1 induces T cells of the T helper type 2 that crossreact with myelin basic protein and suppress experimental autoimmune encephalomyelitis. Proc Natl Acad Sci U S A 1997;94:10821-10826.
33. Kozovska ME, Hong J, Zang YC, et al. Interferon beta induces T-helper 2 immune deviation in MS. Neurology 1999;53:1692-1697.
34. Ma Z, Qin H, Benveniste EN. Transcriptional suppression of matrix metalloproteinase-9 gene expression by IFN-gamma and IFN-beta: critical role of STAT-1alpha. J Immunol 2001;167:5150-5159.
35. Floris S, Ruuls SR, Wierinckx A, et al. Interferon-beta directly influences monocyte infiltration into the central nervous system. J Neuroimmunol 2002;127:69-79.
36. Kraus J, Oschmann P. The impact of interferon-beta treatment on the blood-brain barrier. Drug Discov Today 2006;11:755-762.
37. Stone LA, Frank JA, Albert PS, et al. Characterization of MRI response to treatment with interferon beta-1b: contrast-enhancing MRI lesion frequency as a primary outcome measure. Neurology 1997;49:862-869.
38. Barbero P, Bergui M, Versino E, et al. Every-other-day interferon beta-1b versus once-weekly interferon beta-1a for multiple sclerosis (INCOMIN Trial) II: analysis of MRI responses to treatment and correlation with Nab. Mult Scler 2006;12:72-76.
39. Pozzilli C, Bastianello S, Koudriavtseva T, et al. Magnetic resonance imaging changes with recombinant human interferon-beta-1a: a short term study in relapsing-remitting multiple sclerosis. J Neurol Neurosurg Psychiatry 1996;61:251-258.
40. Fieschi C, Pozzilli C, Bastianello S, et al. Human recombinant interferon beta in the treatment of relapsing-remitting multiple sclerosis: preliminary observations. Mult Scler 1995;1(Suppl 1):S28-S31.
41. Calabresi PA, Prat A, Biernacki K, et al. T lymphocytes conditioned with interferon beta induce membrane and soluble VCAM on human brain endothelial cells. J Neuroimmunol 2001;115:161-167.
42. Biernacki K, Antel JP, Blain M, et al. Interferon beta promotes nerve growth factor secretion early in the course of multiple sclerosis. Arch Neurol 2005;62:563-568.
43. Antonetti F, Finocchiaro O, Mascia M, et al. A comparison of the biologic activity of two recombinant IFN-beta preparations used in the treatment of relapsing-remitting multiple sclerosis. J Interferon Cytokine Res 2002;22:1181-1184.
44. Interferon beta-1b is effective in relapsing-remitting multiple sclerosis. I. Clinical results of a multicenter, randomized, double-blind, placebo-controlled trial. The IFNB Multiple Sclerosis Study Group. Neurology 1993;43:655-661.
45. Evidence of interferon beta-1a dose response in relapsing-remitting MS: the OWIMS Study. The Once Weekly Interferon for MS Study Group. Neurology 1999;53:679-686.
46. Liu C, Blumhardt LD. Randomised, double blind, placebo controlled study of interferon beta-1a in relapsing-remitting multiple sclerosis analysed by area under disability/time curves. J Neurol Neurosurg Psychiatry 1999;67:451-456.
47. Panitch H, Goodin DS, Francis G, et al. Randomized, comparative study of interferon beta-1a treatment regimens in MS. The EVIDENCE Trial. Neurology 2002;59:1496-1506.

48. Durelli L, Verdun E, Barbero P, et al. Every-other-day interferon beta-1b versus once-weekly interferon beta-1a for multiple sclerosis: results of a 2-year prospective randomised multicentre study (INCOMIN). Lancet 2002;359:1453-1460.
49. Bertolotto A, Gilli F, Sala A, et al. Persistent neutralizing antibodies abolish the interferon beta bioavailability in MS patients. Neurology 2003;60:634-639.
50. Tomassini V, Paolillo A, Russo P, et al. Predictors of long-term clinical response to interferon beta therapy in relapsing multiple sclerosis. J Neurol 2006;253:287-293.
51. Betaseron® Prescribing Information. Emeryville, CA: Chiron, 2003.
52. Loftis JM, Hauser P. The phenomenology and treatment of interferon-induced depression. J Affect Disord 2004;82:175-190.
53. Patten SB, Francis G, Metz LM, et al. The relationship between depression and interferon beta-1a therapy in patients with multiple sclerosis. Mult Scler 2005;11:175-181.
54. Chen M, Gran B, Costello K, et al. Glatiramer acetate induces a Th2-biased response and crossreactivity with myelin basic protein in patients with MS. Mult Scler 2001;7:209-219.
55. Duda PW, Schmied MC, Cook SL, et al. Glatiramer acetate (Copaxone) induces degenerate, Th2-polarized immune responses in patients with multiple sclerosis. J Clin Invest 2000;105:967-976.
56. Aharoni R, Kayhan B, Eilam R, et al. Glatiramer acetate-specific T cells in the brain express T helper 2/3 cytokines and brain-derived neurotrophic factor in situ. Proc Natl Acad Sci U S A 2003;100:14157-14162.
57. Ziemssen T, Kumpfel T, Klinkert WE, et al. Glatiramer acetate-specific T-helper 1- and 2-type cell lines produce BDNF: implications for multiple sclerosis therapy. Brain-derived neurotrophic factor. Brain 2002;125(Pt 11):2381-2391.
58. Ziemssen T, Kumpfel T, Schneider H, et al. Secretion of brain-derived neurotrophic factor by glatiramer acetate-reactive T-helper cell lines: implications for multiple sclerosis therapy. J Neurol Sci 2005;233:109-112.
59. Allie R, Hu L, Mullen KM, et al. Bystander modulation of chemokine receptor expression on peripheral blood T lymphocytes mediated by glatiramer therapy. Arch Neurol 2005;62:889-894.
60. Karandikar NJ, Crawford MP, Yan X, et al. Glatiramer acetate (Copaxone) therapy induces CD8$^+$ T cell responses in patients with multiple sclerosis. J Clin Invest 2002;109:641-649.
61. Kim HJ, Ifergan I, Antel JP, et al. Type 2 monocyte and microglia differentiation mediated by glatiramer acetate therapy in patients with multiple sclerosis. J Immunol 2004;172:7144-7153.
62. Weber MS, Starck M, Wagenpfeil S, et al. Multiple sclerosis: glatiramer acetate inhibits monocyte reactivity in vitro and in vivo. Brain 2004;127(Pt 6):1370-1378.
63. Chen M, Valenzuela RM, Dhib-Jalbut S. Glatiramer acetate-reactive T cells produce brain-derived neurotrophic factor. J Neurol Sci 2003;215:37-44.
64. Ziemssen T. Neuroprotection and glatiramer acetate: the possible role in the treatment of multiple sclerosis. Adv Exp Med Biol 2004;541:111-134.
65. Kipnis J, Yoles E, Porat Z, et al. T cell immunity to copolymer 1 confers neuroprotection on the damaged optic nerve: possible therapy for optic neuropathies. Proc Natl Acad Sci U S A 2000;97:7446-7451.
66. Gilgun-Sherki Y, Panet H, Holdengreber V, et al. Axonal damage is reduced following glatiramer acetate treatment in C57/bl mice with chronic-induced experimental autoimmune encephalomyelitis. Neurosci Res 2003;47:201-207.
67. Johnson KP, Brooks BR, Cohen JA, et al. Extended use of glatiramer acetate (Copaxone) is well tolerated and maintains its clinical effect on multiple sclerosis relapse rate and degree of disability. Copolymer 1 Multiple Sclerosis Study Group. Neurology 1998;50:701-708.
68. Comi G, Filippi M, Wolinsky JS. European/Canadian multicenter, double-blind, randomized, placebo-controlled study of the effects of glatiramer acetate on magnetic resonance imaging—measured disease activity and burden in patients with relapsing multiple sclerosis. European/Canadian Glatiramer Acetate Study Group. Ann Neurol 2001;49:290-297.
69. National Institutes of Health. Combination therapy in patients with relapsing-remitting multiple sclerosis. 2005. Available at *http://www.clinicaltrials.gov*.
70. Vartanian TK, Zamvil SS, Fox E, Sorensen PS. Neutralizing antibodies to disease-modifying agents in the treatment of multiple sclerosis. Neurology 2004;63(11 Suppl 5):S42-S49.
71. Edgar CM, Brunet DG, Fenton P, et al. Lipoatrophy in patients with multiple sclerosis on glatiramer acetate. Can J Neurol Sci 2004;31:58-63.
72. Galetta SL, Markowitz C. US FDA-approved disease-modifying treatments for multiple sclerosis: review of adverse effect profiles. CNS Drugs 2005;19:239-252.
73. Polman CH, O'Connor PW, Havrdova E, et al. A randomized, placebo-controlled trial of natalizumab for relapsing multiple sclerosis. N Engl J Med 2006;354:899-910.
74. Rudick RA, Stuart WH, Calabresi PA, et al. Natalizumab plus interferon beta-1a for relapsing multiple sclerosis. N Engl J Med 2006;354:911-923.
75. Sheremata WA, Vollmer TL, Stone LA, et al. A safety and pharmacokinetic study of intravenous natalizumab in patients with MS. Neurology 1999;52:1072-1074.
76. Calabresi PA, Giovannoni G, Confavreux C, et al. The incidence and significance of anti-natalizumab antibodies: results from AFFIRM and SENTINEL. Neurology 2007;69:1391-1403.
77. Noseworthy JH, Hopkins MB, Vandervoort MK, et al. An open-trial evaluation of mitoxantrone in the treatment of progressive MS. Neurology 1993;43:1401-1406.
78. Jain KK. Evaluation of mitoxantrone for the treatment of multiple sclerosis. Expert Opin Investig Drugs 2000;9:1139-1149.
79. Mauch E, Kornhuber HH. [Immunosuppressive therapy of multiple sclerosis with mitoxantrone]. Fortschr Neurol Psychiatr 1993;61:410-417.
80. Fox EJ. Mechanism of action of mitoxantrone. Neurology 2004;63(12 Suppl 6):S15-S18.
81. Thielmann HW, Popanda O, Gersbach H, Gilberg F. Various inhibitors of DNA topoisomerases diminish repair-specific DNA incision in UV-irradiated human fibroblasts. Carcinogenesis 1993;14:2341-2351.
82. Neuhaus O, Wiendl H, Kieseier BC, et al. Multiple sclerosis: mitoxantrone promotes differential effects on immunocompetent cells in vitro. J Neuroimmunol 2005;168:128-137.
83. Kopadze T, Dehmel T, Hartung HP, et al. Inhibition by mitoxantrone of in vitro migration of immunocompetent cells: a possible mechanism for therapeutic efficacy in the treatment of multiple sclerosis. Arch Neurol 2006;63:1572-1578.
84. Neuhaus O, Kieseier BC, Hartung HP. Mechanisms of mitoxantrone in multiple sclerosis—what is known? J Neurol Sci 2004;223:25-27.
85. Edan G, Miller D, Clanet M, et al. Therapeutic effect of mitoxantrone combined with methylprednisolone in multiple sclerosis: a randomised multicentre study of active disease using MRI and clinical criteria. J Neurol Neurosurg Psychiatry 1997;62:112-118.
86. Novantrone® prescribing information. Rockland, MA: Serono Inc., 2006.
87. Hartung HP, Gonsette R, Konig N, et al. Mitoxantrone in progressive multiple sclerosis: a placebo-controlled, double-blind, randomised, multicentre trial. Lancet 2002;360:2018-2025.
88. Wolinsky JS, Narayana PA, O'Connor P, et al. Glatiramer acetate in primary progressive multiple sclerosis: results of a multinational, multicenter, double-blind, placebo-controlled trial. Ann Neurol 2007;61:14-24.
89. Ramtahal J, Jacob A, Das K, Boggild M. Sequential maintenance treatment with glatiramer acetate after mitoxantrone is safe and can limit exposure to immunosuppression in very active, relapsing remitting multiple sclerosis. J Neurol 2006;253:1160-1164.
90. Dorr J, Roth K, Zurbuchen U, et al. Tumor-necrosis-factor-related apoptosis-inducing-ligand (TRAIL)-mediated death of neurons in living human brain tissue is inhibited by flupirtine-maleate. J Neuroimmunol 2005;167:204-209.
91. Kaplin AI, Deshpande DM, Scott E, et al. IL-6 induces regionally selective spinal cord injury in patients with the neuroinflammatory disorder transverse myelitis. J Clin Invest 2005;115:2731-2741.
92. Bartosik-Psujek H, Magrys A, Montewka-Koziol M, Stelmasiak Z. [Change of interleukin-4 and interleukin-12 levels after therapy of multiple sclerosis relapse with methylprednisolone.]. Neurol Neurochir Pol 2005;39:207-212.
93. Dinkel K, MacPherson A, Sapolsky RM. Novel glucocorticoid effects on acute inflammation in the CNS. J Neurochem 2003;84:705-716.
94. Sloka JS, Stefanelli M. The mechanism of action of methylprednisolone in the treatment of multiple sclerosis. Mult Scler 2005;11:425-432.
95. Harkness KA, Adamson P, Sussman JD, et al. Dexamethasone regulation of matrix metalloproteinase expression in CNS vascular endothelium. Brain 2000;123(Pt 4):698-709.
96. Leussink VI, Jung S, Merschdorf U, et al. High-dose methylprednisolone therapy in multiple sclerosis induces apoptosis in peripheral blood leukocytes. Arch Neurol 2001;58:91-97.
97. Diem R, Hobom M, Maier K, et al. Methylprednisolone increases neuronal apoptosis during autoimmune CNS inflammation by inhibition of an endogenous neuroprotective pathway. J Neurosci 2003;23:6993-7000.
98. Brusaferri F, Candelise L. Steroids for multiple sclerosis and optic neuritis: a meta-analysis of randomized controlled clinical trials. J Neurol 2000;247:435-442.
99. Beck RW, Cleary PA, Trobe JD, et al. The effect of corticosteroids for acute optic neuritis on the subsequent development of multiple sclerosis. N Engl J Med 1993;329:1764-1769.
100. Zivadinov R, Rudick RA, De Masi R, et al. Effects of IV methylprednisolone on brain atrophy in relapsing-remitting MS. Neurology 2001;57:1239-1247.
101. Hauser SL, Dawson DM, Lehrich JR, et al. Intensive immunosuppression in progressive multiple sclerosis: a randomized, three-arm study of high-dose intravenous cyclophosphamide, plasma exchange, and ACTH. N Engl J Med 1983;308:173-180.
102. Canadian Cooperative Multiple Sclerosis Study Group. The Canadian cooperative trial of cyclophosphamide and plasma exchange in progressive multiple sclerosis. Lancet 1991;337:441-446.
103. Likosky W, Fireman B, Elmore R, et al. Intense immunosuppression in chronic progressive multiple sclerosis: the Kaiser study. J Neurol Neurosurg Psychiatry 1991;54:1055-1060.
104. Gauthier SA, Weiner HL. Use of cyclophosphamide and other immunosuppressants to treat multiple sclerosis. *In* Cohen JA, Rudick RA (eds): Multiple Sclerosis Therapeutics, 3rd ed. Oxon, UK: Informa Healthcare, 2007.
105. Gobbini MI, Smith ME, Richert ND, et al. Effect of open label pulse cyclophosphamide therapy on MRI measures of disease activity in five patients with refractory relapsing-remitting multiple sclerosis. J Neuroimmunol 1999;9:142-149.
106. Patti F, Cataldi M, Nicoletti F. Combination of cyclophosphamide and interferon-beta halts progression in patients with rapidly transitional multiple sclerosis. J Neurol Neurosurg Psychiatry 2001;71:404-407.
107. Smith DR, Weinstock-Guttman B, Cohen JA, et al. A randomized blinded trial of combination therapy with cyclophosphamide in patients with active multiple sclerosis on interferon beta. Mult Scler 2005;11:573-582.
108. Reggio E, Nicoletti A, Fiorilla T, et al. The combination of cyclophosphamide plus interferon beta as rescue therapy could be used to treat relapsing-remitting multiple sclerosis patients: twenty-four months follow-up. J Neurol 2005;252:1255-1261.
109. Casetta I, Iuliano G, Filippini G. Azathioprine for multiple sclerosis. Cochrane Database Syst Rev 2007;(4):CD003987.
110. Pulicken M, Bash CN, Costello K, et al. Optimization of the safety and efficacy of interferon beta 1b and azathioprine combination therapy in multiple sclerosis. Mult Scler 2005;11:169-174.
111. Imuran® Prescribing Information. San Diego: Prometheus Laboratories, Inc., 2002.
112. Cohen J, Calabresi P, Eickenhorst T, et al. Results of the Avonex Combination Trial [Abstract]. Neurology 2007;68(Suppl 1):A100.

113. Calabresi PA, Wilterdink JL, Roqq JM, et al. An open-label trial of combination therapy with interferon beta-1a and oral methotrexate in MS. Neurology 2002;58:314-317.
114. Ahrens N, Salama A, Haas J. Mycophenolate mofetil in the treatment of refractory multiple sclerosis. J Neurol 2001;248:713-714.
115. Frohman EM, Brannon K, Racke MK, Hawker K. Mycophenolate mofetil in multiple sclerosis. Clin Neuropharmacol 204;27:80-83.
116. Vermersch P, Waucquier N, Michelin E, et al. Combination of IFN beta-1a (Avonex) and mycophenolate mofetil (Cellcept) in multiple sclerosis. Eur J Neurol 2007;14:85-89.
117. Fazekas F, Deisenhammer F, Strasser-Fuchs S, et al. Randomised placebo-controlled trial of monthly intravenous immunoglobulin therapy in relapsing-remitting multiple sclerosis. Austrian Immunoglobulin in Multiple Sclerosis Study Group. Lancet 1997;349:589-593.
118. Fazekas F, Freedman MS, Hartung HP, et al. Prevention or relapse with intravenous immunoglobulin study: initial results of a dose-finding trial in relapsing-remitting multiple sclerosis. J Neurol 2006;253(Suppl 2):101.
119. Jacobs LD, Cookfair DL, Rudick RA, et al. Intramuscular interferon beta 1a for disease progression in relapsing multiple sclerosis. Ann Neurol 1996;39:285-294.
120. The PRISMS Study Group. Randomised double-blind placebo-controlled study of interferon beta-1a in relapsing-remitting multiple sclerosis. Lancet 1998;352:1498-1504.
121. Johnson KP, Brooks BR, Cohen JA, et al. Copolymer 1 reduces relapse rate and improves disability in relapsing-remitting multiple sclerosis: results of a Phase III multicenter, double blind placebo-controlled trial. Neurology 1995;45:1268-1276.
122. Beck RW, Trobe JD, Moke PS, et al. High- and low-risk profiles for the development of multiple sclerosis within 10 years after optic neuritis: experience of the Optic Neuritis Treatment Trial. Arch Ophthalmol 2003;121:944-949.
123. Jacobs LD, Beck RW, Simon JH, et al. Intramuscular interferon beta-1a therapy initiated during a first demyelinating event in multiple sclerosis. N Engl J Med 2000;343:898-904.
124. Comi G, Filippi M, Barkhof F, et al. Effect of early interferon treatment on conversion to definite multiple sclerosis: a randomized study. Lancet 2001;357:1576-1582.
125. Kappos L, Polman CH, Freedman MS, et al. Treatment with interferon beta-1b delays conversion to clinically definite and McDonald MS in patients with clinically isolated syndromes. Neurology 2006;67:1242-1249.
126. Comi GC, et al. Treatment with glatiramer acetate delays conversion to clinically definite multiple sclerosis (CDMS) in patients with clinically isolated syndromes (CIS) [Abstract]. Presented at the American Academy of Neurology meeting, 2008.
127. Goodin DS, Frohman EM, Garmany GP, et al. Disease modifying therapies in multiple sclerosis: Subcommittee of the American Academy of Neurology and the MS Council for Clinical Practice Guidelines. Neurology 2002;58:169-178.
128. Goodin DS, Frohman EM, Hurwitz B, et al. Neutralizing antibodies to interferon beta: assessment of their clinical and radiographic impact. An evidence report. Report of the Therapeutics and Technology Assessment Subcommittee of the American Academy of Neurology. Neurology 2007;68:977-984.
129. Johnson KP, Teitelbaum D, Arnon R, Sela M. Antibodies to copolymer 1 do not interfere with its clinical effect. Neurology 1995;38:973.
130. Walther EU, Hohlfeld R. Multiple sclerosis: side effects of interferon beta therapy and their management. Neurology 1999;53:1622-1627.
131. European Study Group in Interferon β-1b in Secondary Progressive MS. Placebo-controlled multicentre randomized trial of interferon β-1b in treatment of secondary progressive multiple sclerosis. Lancet 1998;352:1491-1497.
132. Lublin FD, Whitaker JN, Eidelman BH, et al. Management of patients receiving interferon beta-1b for multiple sclerosis: report of a consensus conference. Neurology 1996;46:12-18.
133. Rauschka H, Farina C, Sator P, et al. Severe anaphylactic reaction to glatiramer acetate with specific IgE. Neurology 2005;64:1481-1482.
134. Corona T, Leon C, Ostrosky-Zeichner L. Severe anaphylaxis with recombinant interferon beta. Neurology 1999;52:425.
135. Panitch H, Goodin D, Francis G, et al. Benefits of high-dose, high-frequency interferon beta-1a in relapsing-remitting multiple sclerosis are sustained to 16 months: final comparative results of the EVIDENCE trial. J Neurol Sci 2005;239:67-74.
136. Durelli L, Verdun E, Barbero P, et al. Every-other-day interferon beta-1b versus once-weekly interferon beta-1a for multiple sclerosis: results of a 2-year prospective randomized multicentre study (INCOMIN). Lancet 2002;359:1453-1460.
137. Mikol DD, Barkhof F, Chang P, et al. The REGARD trial: a randomized assessor-blinded trial comparing interferon beta-1a and glatiramer acetate in relapsing-remitting multiple sclerosis [Abstract]. Presented at the European Committee for Treatment and Research in Multiple Sclerosis meeting, 2007.
138. Wolansky L, Cook S, Skurnick J, et al. Betaseron vs. copaxone in MS with triple-dose gadolinium and 3-T MRI endpoints (BECOME): Announcement of final primary study outcome [Abstract]. Multiple Sclerosis 2007;13(Suppl 2):S58.
139. Goodin DS, Arnason BG, Coyle PK, et al. The use of mitoxantrone (Novantrone) for the treatment of multiple sclerosis: report of the Therapeutics and Technology Assessment Subcommittee of the American Academy of Neurology. Neurology 2003;61:1332-1338.
140. Kappos L, Polman C, Pozzilli C, et al. Final analysis of the European multicenter trial on IFNbeta-1b in secondary-progressive MS. Neurology 2001;57:1969-1975.
141. Panitch H, Miller A, Paty D, Weinshenker B, for the North American Study Group on Interferon beta-1b in Secondary Progressive MS. Interferon beta-1b in secondary progressive MS: results from a 3-year controlled study. Neurology 2004;63:1788-1795.
142. Kappos L, Weinshenker B, Pozzilli C, et al. Interferon beta-1b in secondary progressive MS: a combined analysis of the two trials. Neurology 2004;63:1779-1787.
143. Montalban X. Overview of European pilot study of interferon β-1b in primary progressive multiple sclerosis. Mult Scler 2004;10:S62-S64.
144. Kita M, Cohen JA, Fox RJ, et al. A Phase II trial of mitoxantrone in patients with primary progressive multiple sclerosis [Abstract]. Neurology 2004;62(Suppl 5):A99.
145. Lublin F, Cutter G, Elfont R, et al. A trial to assess the safety of combining therapy with interferon beta-1a and glatiramer acetate in patients with relapsing MS [Abstract]. Neurology 2001;56(Suppl 3):A148.
146. Barnes D, Hughes RA, Morris RW, et al. Randomised trial of oral and intravenous methylprednisolone in acute relapses of multiple sclerosis. Lancet 1997;349:902-906.
147. Alam SM, Kyriakides T, Lawden M, Newman PK. Methylprednisolone in multiple sclerosis: a comparison of oral with intravenous therapy at equivalent high doses. J Neurol Neurosurg Psychiatry 1993;56:1219-1220.
148. Weinshenker BG, O'Brien PC, Petterson TM, et al. A randomized trial of plasma exchange in acute central nervous system inflammatory demyelinating disease. Ann Neurol 1999;46:878-886.
149. McCarson KE, Ralya A, Reisman SA, Enna SJ. Amitriptyline prevents thermal hyperalgesia and modifications in rat spinal cord $GABA_B$ receptor expression and function in an animal model of neuropathic pain. Biochem Pharmacol 2005;71:196-202.
150. Saarto T, Wiffen PJ. Antidepressants for neuropathic pain. Cochrane Database Syst Rev 2005;(3):CD005454.
151. Vu TN. Current pharmacologic approaches to treating neuropathic pain. Curr Pain Headache Rep 2004;8:15 18.
152. UK Multiple Sclerosis Society. MS Symptom Management Survey. London: UK Multiple Sclerosis Society, 1997.
153. Stankoff B, Waubant E, Confavreux C, et al. Modafinil for fatigue in MS: a randomized placebo-controlled double-blind study. Neurology 2005;64:1139-1143.
154. Wingerchuk DM, Benarroch EE, O'Brien PC, et al. A randomized controlled cross-over trial of aspirin for fatigue in multiple sclerosis. Neurology 2005;64:1267-1269.
155. Krupp LB, Christodoulou C, Melville P, et al. Donepezil improved memory in multiple sclerosis in a randomized clinical trial. Neurology 2004;63:1579-1585.
156. Confavreux C, Hutchinson M, Hours MM, et al. Rate of pregnancy-related relapse in multiple sclerosis. Pregnancy in Multiple Sclerosis Group. N Engl J Med 1998;329:285-291.
157. Vukusic S, Hutchinson M, Hours M, et al. Pregnancy and multiple sclerosis (the PRIMS study): clinical predictors of post-partum relapse. Brain 2004;127:1353-1360.
158. Achiron A, Kishner I, Dolev M, et al. Effect of intravenous immunoglobulin treatment on pregnancy and postpartum-related relapses in multiple sclerosis. J Neurol 2004;258:1133-1137.
159. Haas J, Hommes OR. A dose comparison study of IVIG in postpartum relapsing-remitting multiple sclerosis. Mult Scler 2007;13:900-908.
160. Banwell B, Ghezzi A, Bar-Or A, et al. Multiple sclerosis in children: clinical diagnosis, therapeutic strategies, and future directions. Lancet Neurol 2007;6:887-902.
161. Krupp LB, Banwell B, Tenembaum S, for the International Pediatric MS Study Group. Consensus definitions proposed for pediatric multiple sclerosis and related disorders. Neurology 2007;68:S7-S12.
162. Pohl D, Waubant E, Banwell B, et al. Treatment of pediatric multiple sclerosis and variants. Neurology 2007;68:S54-S65.
163. Banwell B, Reder AT, Krupp L, et al. Safety and tolerability of interferon beta-1b in pediatric multiple sclerosis. Neurology 2006;66:472-476.
164. Budde K, Schutz M, Glander P, et al. FTY720 (fingolimod) in renal transplantation. Clin Transpl 2006;20(Suppl 17):17-24.
165. Segoloni GP, Quaglia M. New immunosuppressive drugs for prevention and treatment of rejection in renal transplant. J Nephrol 2006;19:578-586.
166. Kappos L, Antel J, Comi G, et al. Oral fingolimod (FTY720) for relapsing multiple sclerosis. N Engl J Med 2006;355:1124-1140.
167. Schilling S, Goelz S, Linker R, et al. Fumaric acid esters are effective in chronic experimental autoimmune encephalomyelitis and suppress macrophage infiltration. Clin Exp Immunol 2006;145:101-107.
168. Tan IL, Lycklama a Nijeholt GJ, Polman CH, et al. Linomide in the treatment of multiple sclerosis: MRI results from prematurely terminated Phase-III trials. Mult Scler 2000;6:99-104.
169. Polman C, Barkhof F, Sandberg-Wollheim M, et al. Treatment with laquinimod reduces development of active MRI lesions in relapsing MS. Neurology 2005;64:987-991.
170. Cherwinski HM, Byars N, Ballaron SJ, et al. Leflunomide interferes with pyrimidine nucleotide biosynthesis. Inflamm Res 1995;44:317-322.
171. Cherwinski HM, Cohn RG, Cheung P, et al. The immunosuppressant leflunomide inhibits lymphocyte proliferation by inhibiting pyrimidine biosynthesis. J Pharmacol Exp Ther 1995;275:1043-1049.
172. O'Connor PW, Li D, Freedman MS, et al. A Phase II study of the safety and efficacy of teriflunomide in multiple sclerosis with relapses. Neurology 2006;66:894-900.
173. Selby R, Brandwein J, O'Connor P. Safety and tolerability of subcutaneous cladribine therapy in progressive multiple sclerosis. Can J Neurol Sci 1998;25:295-299.
174. Grieb P, Ryba M, Stelmasiak Z, et al. Cladribine treatment of multiple sclerosis. Lancet 1994;344:538.
175. Stelmasiak Z, Bartosik-Psujek H, Belniak-Legiec E, Mitosek-Szewczyk K. The effect of cladribine on some parameters of blood and cerebrospinal fluid in patients with relapsing-remitting multiple sclerosis (RR-MS). Ann Univ Mariae Curie Sklodowska [Med] 2000;55:221-225.
176. Goodin DS. The cladribine trial in secondary progressive MS: response. Neuroepidemiology 2000;19:53-54.
177. Rice GP, Filippi M, Comi G. Cladribine and progressive MS: clinical and MRI outcomes of a multicenter controlled trial. Cladribine MRI Study Group. Neurology 2000;54:1145-1155.

178. Beutler E, Koziol JA, McMillan R, et al. Marrow suppression produced by repeated doses of cladribine. Acta Haematol 1994;91:10-15.
179. Edwards JC, Szczepanski L, Szechinski J, et al. Efficacy of B-cell-targeted therapy with rituximab in patients with rheumatoid arthritis. N Engl J Med 2004;350:2572-2581.
180. Cerny T, Borisch B, Introna M, et al. Mechanism of action of rituximab. Anticancer Drugs 2002;13(Suppl 2):S3-S10.
181. Cross AH, Stark JL, Lauber J, et al. Rituximab reduces B cells and T cells in cerebrospinal fluid of multiple sclerosis patients. J Neuroimmunol 2006;180:63-70.
182. Bar-Or A, Calabresi PA, Arnold DL, et al. A Phase I, open-label, multicenter study to evaluate the safety and activity of rituximab in adults with relapsing-remitting multiple sclerosis (RRMS) [Abstract]. Neurology 2007;68(Suppl 1):S02.001.
183. Hauser S, Waubant E, Arnold DL, et al. A Phase II randomized, placebo-controlled, multicenter trial of rituximab in adults with relapsing-remitting multiple sclerosis (RRMS) [Abstract]. Neurology 2007;68(Suppl 1):S12.003.
184. Goebel J, Stevens E, Forrest K, Roszman TL. Daclizumab (Zenapax) inhibits early interleukin-2 receptor signal transduction events. Transpl Immunol 2000;8:153-159.
185. Bielekova B, Catalfamo M, Reichert-Scrivner S, et al. Regulatory CD56(bright) natural killer cells mediate immunomodulatory effects of IL-2Ralpha-targeted therapy (daclizumab) in multiple sclerosis. Proc Natl Acad Sci U S A 2006;103:5941-5946.
186. Bielekova B, Richert N, Howard T, et al. Humanized anti-CD25 (daclizumab) inhibits disease activity in multiple sclerosis patients failing to respond to interferon beta. Proc Natl Acad Sci U S A 2004;101:8705-8708.
187. Rose JW, Watt HE, White AT, Carlson NG. Treatment of multiple sclerosis with an anti-interleukin-2 receptor monoclonal antibody. Ann Neurol 2004;56:864-867.
188. Mone AP, Cheney C, Banks AL, et al. Alemtuzumab induces caspase-independent cell death in human chronic lymphocytic leukemia cells through a lipid raft-dependent mechanism. Leukemia 2006;20:272-279.
189. Stanglmaier M, Reis S, Hallek M. Rituximab and alemtuzumab induce a nonclassic, caspase-independent apoptotic pathway in B-lymphoid cell lines and in chronic lymphocytic leukemia cells. Ann Hematol 2004;83:634-645.
190. Alinari L, Lapalombella R, Andritsos L, et al. Alemtuzumab (Campath-1H) in the treatment of chronic lymphocytic leukemia. Oncogene 2007;26:3644-3653.
191. Coles AJ, Wing M, Smith S, et al. Pulsed monoclonal antibody treatment and autoimmune thyroid disease in multiple sclerosis. Lancet 1999;354:1691-1695.
192. Keating MJ, Flinn I, Jain V, et al. Therapeutic role of alemtuzumab (Campath-1H) in patients who have failed fludarabine: results of a large international study. Blood 2002;99:3554-3561.
193. Sullivan H. ITP following the treatment of multiple sclerosis patients with alemtuzumab in CAMMS233: case reports and risk management plan implementation [Abstract]. Neurology 2007;68(Suppl 1):S32.004.
194. Coles A. Efficacy of alemtuzumab in treatment-naive relapsing remitting multiple sclerosis [Abstract]. Neurology 2007;68(Suppl 1):S12.004.
195. Giuliani F, Fu SA, Metz LM, Yong VW. Effective combination of minocycline and interferon-beta in a model of multiple sclerosis. J Neuroimmunol 2005;165:83-91.
196. Zabad RK, Metz LM, Todoruk TR, et al. The clinical response to minocycline in multiple sclerosis is accompanied by beneficial immune changes: a pilot study. Mult Scler 2007;13:517-526.
197. Davignon J, Leiter LA. Ongoing clinical trials of the pleiotropic effects of statins. Vasc Health Risk Manag 2005;1:29-40.
198. Neuhaus O, Hartung HP. Evaluation of atorvastatin and simvastatin for treatment of multiple sclerosis. Expert Rev Neurother 2007;7:547-556.
199. Sena A, Pedrosa R, Morais MG. Beneficial effect of statins in multiple sclerosis: is it dose-dependent? Atherosclerosis 2007;191:462.
200. Kim S, Liva SM, Dalal MA, et al. Estriol ameliorates autoimmune demyelinating disease: implications for multiple sclerosis. Neurology 1999;52:1230-1238.
201. Palaszynski KM, Liu H, Loo KK, Voskuhl RR. Estriol treatment ameliorates disease in males with experimental autoimmune encephalomyelitis: implications for multiple sclerosis. J Neuroimmunol 2004;149:84-89.
202. Yong VW, Zabad RK, Agrawal S, et al. Elevation of matrix metalloproteinases (MMPs) in multiple sclerosis and impact of immunomodulators. J Neurol Sci 2007;259:79-84.
203. Ifergan I, Wosik K, Cayrol R, et al. Statins reduce human blood-brain barrier permeability and restrict leukocyte migration: relevance to multiple sclerosis. Ann Neurol 2006;60:45-55.
204. Stepien K, Tomaszewski M, Czuczwar SJ. Neuroprotective properties of statins. Pharmacol Rep 2005;57:561-569.
205. Stuve O. Statins and the blood-brain barrier: plugging the holes. Ann Neurol 2006;60:1-2.
206. Pelfrey CM, Moldovan IR, Cotleur AC, et al. Effects of sex hormones on costimulatory molecule expression in multiple sclerosis. J Neuroimmunol 2005;167:190-203.
207. Zang YC, Halder JB, Hong J, et al. Regulatory effects of estriol on T cell migration and cytokine profile: inhibition of transcription factor NF-kappa B. J Neuroimmunol 2002;124:106-114.
208. Brettschneider J, Petzold A, Junker A, Tumani H. Axonal damage markers in the cerebrospinal fluid of patients with clinically isolated syndrome improve predicting conversion to definite multiple sclerosis. Mult Scler 2006;12:143-148.
209. Bruck W. Inflammatory demyelination is not central to the pathogenesis of multiple sclerosis. J Neurol 2005;252(Suppl 5):v10-v15.
210. Pirko I, Lucchinetti CF, Sriram S, Bakshi R. Gray matter involvement in multiple sclerosis. Neurology 2007;68:634-642.
211. Gilgun-Sherki Y, Panet H, Melamed E, Offen D. Riluzole suppresses experimental autoimmune encephalomyelitis: implications for the treatment of multiple sclerosis. Brain Res 2003;989:196-204.
212. Killestein J, Kalkers NF, Polman CH. Glutamate inhibition in MS: the neuroprotective properties of riluzole. J Neurol Sci 2005;233:113-115.
213. Sattler MB, Merkler D, Maier K, et al. Neuroprotective effects and intracellular signaling pathways of erythropoietin in a rat model of multiple sclerosis. Cell Death Differ 2004;11(Suppl 2):S181-S192.
214. Smith KJ. Sodium channels and multiple sclerosis: roles in symptom production, damage and therapy. Brain Pathol 2007;17:230-242.
215. Bechtold DA, Yue X, Evans RM, et al. Axonal protection in experimental autoimmune neuritis by the sodium channel blocking agent flecainide. Brain 2005;128(Pt 1):18-28.
216. Black JA, Liu S, Hains BC, et al. Long-term protection of central axons with phenytoin in monophasic and chronic-relapsing EAE. Brain 2006;129(Pt 12):3196-3208.
217. Hains BC, Saab CY, Lo AC, Waxman SG. Sodium channel blockade with phenytoin protects spinal cord axons, enhances axonal conduction, and improves functional motor recovery after contusion SCI. Exp Neurol 2004;188:365-377.
218. Satoh J, Tabunoki H, Yamamura T, et al. TROY and LINGO-1 expression in astrocytes and macrophages/microglia in multiple sclerosis lesions. Neuropathol Appl Neurobiol 2007;33:99-107.
219. Cao Q, Xu XM, Devries WH, et al. Functional recovery in traumatic spinal cord injury after transplantation of multineurotrophin-expressing glial-restricted precursor cells. J Neurosci 2005;25:6947-6957.

47

DYSAUTONOMIAS

Kyoko Sato, André Diedrich, and David Robertson

INTRODUCTION 703
PATHOPHYSIOLOGY OF AUTONOMIC DISORDERS 703
Neurally Mediated Syncope 703
Postural Tachycardia Syndrome (Orthostatic Intolerance) 705
Pure Autonomic Failure 707
Multiple System Atrophy 708
Dopamine β-Hydroxylase Deficiency 708
Baroreflex Failure 709
THERAPEUTICS AND CLINICAL PHARMACOLOGY 710
Medications 710
Fludrocortisone 710
Midodrine 711
Indomethacin 711
Clonidine 712
Droxidopa (L-DOPS) 712
Yohimbine 712
Erythropoietin 712
Therapeutic Approach 713
Management of Autonomic Failure 713
Management of Orthostatic Intolerance 715
Management of Neurally Mediated Syncope 715
Management of Baroreflex Failure 715
SUMMARY 716

INTRODUCTION

If the discipline of clinical pharmacology can claim academic ownership of any of the human organ systems, it is probably the autonomic nervous system. It would be difficult to identify an area in which the role of pharmacology has been so pivotal from the earliest days of elucidation of neurotransmitters and their receptors 100 years ago to the current era. The autonomic nervous system has a large role in the practice of medicine also. About 10% of prescriptions written in the United States are for agents that act through effects on the autonomic nervous system, and another 25% of drugs have consequential toxicity or overdose effects that are autonomic in nature.

The autonomic nervous system exerts widespread control over homeostasis.[1-3] Almost every organ system receives regulatory information from the central nervous system (CNS) through the autonomic efferents (Fig. 47-1), and increasingly we recognize that afferent input into the central autonomic network regulates not only the output of the autonomic system, but much CNS function not generally considered to be autonomic in nature. The emerging concept is one of far more pervasive integration of autonomic activities with the brain and the body than previously thought. Furthermore, we continue to find new and more widespread reach of autonomic control, most recently to bone and adipose tissue.[4]

The afferent inputs to autonomic regulation are likewise protean, but understanding them is crucial for all that follows. Baroreceptors in the carotid sinus sense stretch and convey information about distention of the vessel wall to the brainstem via the glossopharyngeal nerve (cranial nerve IX). Other baroreceptors in the aortic arch and the great vessels of the thorax transmit similar information by the vagus nerve (cranial nerve X) to the same brainstem nuclei. In addition, blood volume in the thorax is sensed by low-pressure receptors linked by the vagus nerve to the brainstem. The brainstem structure receiving this information is the *nucleus tractus solitarii*, which lies in the dorsal medulla at the level of the fourth ventricle. Neurotransmitters and neuromodulators such as glutamate and nitric oxide released in the nucleus tractus solitarii lead to cardiovascular effects. The caudal ventrolateral medulla and the rostral ventrolateral medulla are crucial brainstem structures involved in the modulation of sympathetic outflow. Afferent nerve traffic from the thorax and abdomen also provides input to central cardiovascular centers after traveling with sympathetic nerves back to the spinal cord, and sometimes on to medullary cardiovascular control centers. The precise role of these "sympathetic afferents" is currently an area of active investigation. Table 47-1 provides instructive examples of how biochemical tests may be combined to make diagnostic discoveries.

Evidence-based approaches in discussion of disorders and their management are ideal in disciplines in which a critical mass of carefully controlled studies exists. In uncommon disorders, there is rarely an adequate basis for such an approach. In the autonomic disorders, for example, there are probably fewer than five double-blind studies of chronic drug efficacy in homogeneous dysautonomic populations. Reasons for this include limited numbers of clinical investigators with an interest in these diseases, poorly characterized pathophysiologic mechanisms of many entities, and a high likelihood that many autonomic disorders are heterogeneous in etiology, which may require individualized therapy. With increasing interest in autonomic disorders, improved therapy based on optimally designed trials can be anticipated. In the section that follows, the six dysautonomias most likely to be encountered by clinical pharmacologists are outlined and the rationale for therapeutic approaches described.

PATHOPHYSIOLOGY OF AUTONOMIC DISORDERS (Table 47-2)

Neurally Mediated Syncope

Perhaps 30% of people faint at least once in their lives.[5,6] Syncope accounts for 3% of emergency room visits to American teaching hospitals annually.[7] Although isolated episodes are common, 3% of patients will experience recurrent episodes.[5,6] A majority of these patients faint for reasons poorly understood but considered to be benign, and are considered to have neurally mediated syncope (NMS), in the absence of structural heart disease.[8,9] Frequent NMS is associated with a poor quality of life that improves when the frequency of syncope is reduced.[10,11] Unfortunately, the pathophysiology of NMS is likely to be heterogeneous, and is still poorly understood.[12]

NMS most commonly occurs during standing, but it can also occur in the seated and occasionally even in the lying posture during sleep.[13] It can occur with exercise (at initiation or at peak exercise) or with emotional/psychological triggers such as phlebotomy. Standing upright elicits marked hemodynamic changes. Upon standing, about 750 ml of blood is pooled in the capacitance vessels of the lower abdomen, buttocks, and legs, and plasma moves from the blood into the interstitium (~14% of the plasma volume over 30 minutes).[14,15] There is consequentially a decrease in venous return, stroke volume, and cardiac output.[14] Baroreceptor afferent nerves detect reduced stretch,[16] and convey this

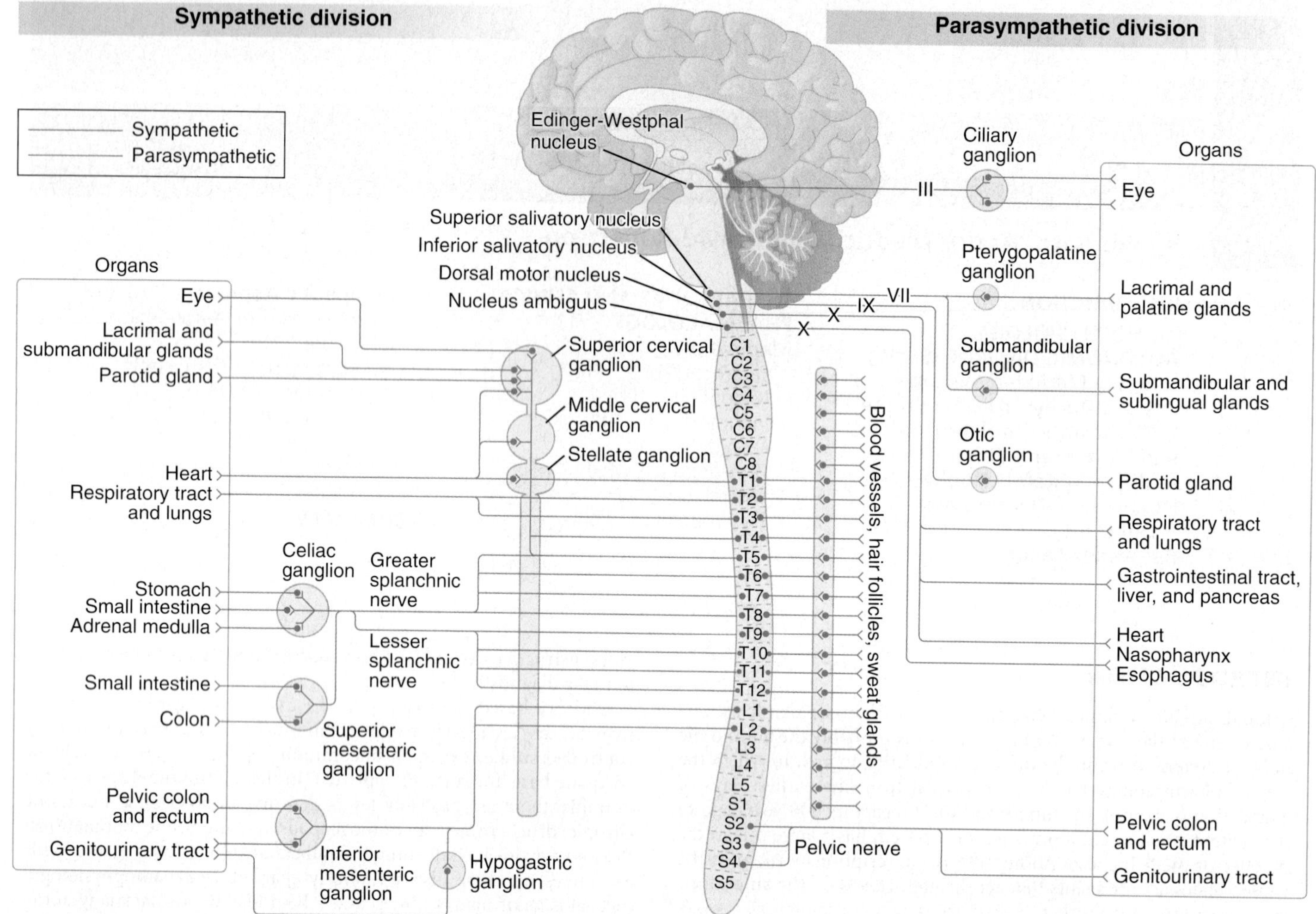

FIGURE 47-1 • Schematic diagram of the sympathetic and parasympathetic divisions of the peripheral autonomic nervous system. The paravertebral chain of the sympathetic division is illustrated on both sides of the spinal outflow to demonstrate the full range of target structures innervated. Although the innervation pattern is diagrammatically illustrated to be direct connections between preganglionic outflow and postganglionic neurons, there is overlap of innervation such that more than one spinal segment provides innervation to neurons within the ganglia. (Modified from Hamill RW, et al. In Robertson D [ed]: Primer on the Autonomic Nervous System, 2nd ed. Boston: Elsevier Academic Press, 2004, pp 20-33.)

information to the nucleus tractus solitarii, setting in motion a decrease in parasympathetic tone and an increase in sympathetic activity, with release of norepinephrine and a rise in peripheral resistance.[17] Low-pressure baroreflexes may also activate sympathetic tone, vasopressin, and the secretion of renin when thoracic blood volume is decreased while standing. This could partly explain why standing diastolic blood pressure is often higher than supine blood pressure. In patients with NMS, some aspect of this important integrative function fails on occasion.

A ventricular theory of NMS[18] is an organizing principle in most efforts to understand syncope. This theory suggests that, when the baroreceptor detects a decrease of blood pressure, a reflex increase in efferent sympathetic activity develops. The increase in sympathetic tone attempts to enhance total peripheral resistance and produces positive chronotropic and inotropic effects in the heart. The presence of increased cardiac sympathetic stimulation in a setting of ventricular hypovolemia is believed to result in large pressure transients evoked by contraction of the ventricular muscle on an empty chamber. This strong contraction of the hypovolemic ventricle is thought to stimulate vagal afferents in the left ventricle. Activation of these afferents might trigger an inhibitory response similar to that of the Bezold-Jarisch reflex,[19] resulting in hypotension and bradycardia. However, several observations are inconsistent with this hypothesis. First, given the critical role of hypovolemia in the model, one might think that patients susceptible to NMS would be more hypovolemic than controls. Total blood volume, however, is not different between syncope patients and control subjects,[20] nor does it predict response to head-up tilt.[21] Second, direct recordings of ventricular afferent fibers found that only a very small percentage fired in response to a hemorrhagic hypovolemia in an animal model.[22] Third, patients with denervated hearts (after cardiac transplantation) can nevertheless have NMS with sympathetic withdrawal.[23-26]

Investigations of autonomic nervous system function over the last 25 years have revealed a seeming paradox. On the one hand, peroneal sympathetic nerve activity decreases precipitously, and may entirely disappear, immediately prior to syncope.[27,28] This disappearance of sympathetic nerve activity occurs at a time when circulating epinephrine levels are greatly elevated. The rise in plasma epinephrine definitely precedes the actual syncope. Does the epinephrine release contribute to the production of the syncope, or does it prepare the fainting subject for a subsequent recovery of hemodynamic functional integrity? This is an important area for further investigation. One reason it has received little attention relates to the logistics of sampling and the fact that the venous epinephrine level hovers around the limit of detection using the high-performance liquid chromatography assay, even as arterial levels of epinephrine rise noticeably. For this reason, it has been challenging for us to appreciate the role of epinephrine.

The physical examination should focus on ruling out structural heart disease and focal neurologic lesions. One useful maneuver is carotid sinus massage, performed by massage of the carotid sinus for

TABLE 47-1 TESTS OF NEUROTRANSMITTER RECEPTOR RESPONSIVENESS

Name	Administration	Receptor	Response
AGONISTS			
Phenylephrine	IV, eye	α_1	Pressor; pupillary dilation
Clonidine	Oral	α_2, I	Depressor (central); MSNA
Isoproterenol	IV IV local	β_1 β_2	Increased HR Depressor; vascular resistance
Acetylcholine	IV local	Muscarinic	Decreased vascular resistance
Methacholine	Eye	Muscarinic	Pupillary constriction
Nicotine	IV	Nicotinic	Increased HR
ANTAGONISTS			
Phentolamine	IV	α_1, α_2	Depressor
Yohimbine	IV	α_2	Increased BP, plasma NE
Propranolol	IV IV local	β_1 β_2	Reduced HR Increased vascular resistance
Atropine	IV	Muscarinic	Increased HR
Trimethaphan	IV	Nicotinic	Depressor; MSNA
NEUROTRANSMITTER-RELEASING AGENTS			
Tyramine	IV	α, β	Increased BP, plasma NE
Hydroxyamphetamine	Eye	α_1	Pupillary dilation
PHEOCHROMOCYTOMA-PROVOKING AGENTS			
Histamine	IV	α_1, β	Increased BP, plasma NE
Glucagon	IV	α_1, β	Increased BP, plasma NE

BP, blood pressure; HR, heart rate; I, imidazoline; IV, intravenous; MSNA, muscle sympathetic nerve activity; NE, norepinephrine.
Modified from Hamill RW, et al. In Robertson D (ed): Primer on the Autonomic Nervous System, 2nd ed. Boston: Elsevier Academic Press, 2004, pp 213-216.

10 seconds in both the supine and upright postures, with a positive result requiring a drop in blood pressure or heart rate with an associated reproduction of presenting symptoms. This procedure must be approached with care, however, as it has been associated in rare cases with neurologic complications.

Tilt-table testing has been widely used in evaluating syncope since the late 1980s, though there are increasing indications that its clinical utility has been overestimated. The patient is subjected to head-up tilt at angles of 60 to 80 degrees, aiming to induce either syncope or intense presyncope, with reproduction of presenting symptoms. Passive tilt tests simply use upright tilt for up to 45 minutes to induce vasovagal syncope (sensitivity ~40%, specificity ~90%). Provocative tilt tests use a simultaneous combination of orthostatic stress and drugs such as isoproterenol, nitroglycerin, or adenosine to provoke syncope with a slightly higher sensitivity, but reduced specificity. There is little agreement about the best protocol. Many physicians are more comfortable treating patients if a diagnosis can be established with a tilt-table test. Unfortunately, it is very uncommon for a tilt study to actually provide a reliable diagnosis. Recent studies with implantable loop recorders (heart rate and rhythm recording and playback device that continuously monitor the heart rate for up to 14 months) have called the value of tilt testing into question. The International Study on Syncope of Uncertain Etiology (ISSUE) investigators reported that, in the absence of significant structural heart disease, patients with tilt-positive syncope and tilt-negative syncope have similar patterns of recurrence (34% in each group over a follow-up of 3 to 15 months), with electrocardiographic recording during episodes consistent with NMS.[29] Despite these data, tilt-table testing has not yet disappeared from the diagnostic armamentarium. Tilt tests are no longer a central feature of our evaluation of NMS. The test is contraindicated if aortic stenosis or serious coronary artery disease is suspected.

Most patients with NMS have a favorable outlook, with only about a 25% likelihood of syncope recurrence after tilt testing in patients who receive neither drugs nor a device. The cause for this apparently great reduction in syncope frequency may be due to spontaneous remission, reassurance, or advice about the pathophysiology of syncope, and postural maneuvers to prevent syncope. However, patients with a high frequency of syncopal spells are more likely to faint in follow-up. The time to the first recurrence of syncope after tilt testing is a simple and individualized measure of eventual syncope frequency, as those patients who faint early after a tilt test tend to continue to faint more frequently.

Postural Tachycardia Syndrome (Orthostatic Intolerance)

Postural tachycardia syndrome (POTS) is defined by an increase in heart rate of 30 bpm or more on standing associated with symptoms of sympathetic activation. Orthostatic symptoms include lightheadedness, palpitations, tremulousness, visual changes, discomfort or throbbing of the head, poor concentration, tiredness, weakness, and occasionally fainting. There is usually little or no fall in blood pressure on standing. Additional criteria sometimes used for the diagnosis of POTS include a plasma norepinephrine of at least 600 pg/ml on standing. Standing plasma norepinephrine levels greater than 2000 pg/ml have been encountered, and such patients much be carefully studied to rule out pheochromocytoma. Many POTS patients also have a bluish-red discoloration of the skin in the lower extremities on standing. POTS patients often present with a reduced plasma volume of about 500 ml.[30]

POTS affects an estimated 250,000 to 500,000 Americans and causes a wide range of disabilities. There is a 4 : 1 female preponderance, typically in the 15- to 45-year age group. Symptom severity is sometimes catamenial. Possible reasons for these cyclical changes include an estrogen-dependent change of plasma volume or a direct estrogen receptor–mediated modulation of vascular reactivity. Other than essential hypertension and NMS, POTS is the most common chronic disorder of blood pressure regulation. It is also the most frequently encountered dysautonomia, accounting for almost half of patients referred to centers specializing in autonomic disorders.

TABLE 47-2 PATHOPHYSIOLOGY OF AUTONOMIC DISORDERS

Disorder	Presentation	Diagnosis	Prognosis
Neurally mediated syncope (NMS)	Syncope characterized by hypotension and/or bradycardia without other structural cardiac or neurologic diseases.	Exclude other organic cardiac or neural diseases. Passive tilt-table testing for up to 45 min has been widely used, but is not often definitive. Its sensitivity is ~40% while specificity is ~90%.	*Usually* favorable even without receiving any specific treatment. About 25% of NMS patients experience recurrent symptoms.
Postural tachycardia syndrome (POTS) (orthostatic intolerance)	Symptoms of inadequate cerebral perfusion on upright posture, usually in the absence of a significant fall (sometimes even an increase) in blood pressure.	Heart rate increase of 30 bpm or more on standing associated with symptoms (e.g., light-headedness, palpitations, tremulousness, visual changes, weakness, occasionally fainting). Additional criteria: • Plasma norepinephrine of at least 600 pg/ml on standing • A bluish-red discoloration of skin in the lower extremities on standing • A reduced plasma volume of about 500 ml	Most POTS patients benefit from low dose propranolol, and often require no therapy after 5 years
Pure autonomic failure (PAF)	Autonomic failure (e.g., urinary incontinence, male erectile dysfunction, loss of sweating) with orthostatic hypotension. Often supine hypertension. Mild anemia.	Often supine plasma norepinephrine is below 100 pg/ml. Absence of another cause of autonomic failure. Lewy bodies in autonomic tissue.	Generally good. Many patients live for 20 years or more after the onset of their disease.
Multiple system atrophy (MSA)	Autonomic failure, especially orthostatic hypotension and genitourinary abnormalities. Extrapyramidal symptoms and cerebellar dysfunction in any combination.	Autonomic plus extrapyramidal or cerebellar problems. Often near-normal supine blood norepinephrine. Cardiac [^{123}I]-MIBG or ^{18}F-dopa PET might help the differential diagnosis from Parkinson's disease or PAF. The only definitive diagnosis is presence of glial cytoplasmic inclusions at autopsy.	Poor. Common causes of death are pneumonia and pulmonary embolus.
Dopamine β-hydroxylase (DBH) deficiency	Lifelong severe orthostatic hypotension. Renal function abnormalities.	Absent or extremely low levels of norepinephrine and its metabolites in a setting of excessive levels of dopamine and its metabolites.	Near normal.
Baroreflex failure	Wide excursions of blood pressure and heart rate. Labile or episodic hypertension.	Detailed clinical history taking; trauma from injury, tumor, radiation, surgical intervention, brainstem stroke, genetic disorder, or family history. Work up to exclude pheochromocytoma. Absence of bradycardic response to the pressor effect of phenylephrine or the tachycardic response to a depressor agent.	Dependent on underlying pathophysiology.

MIBG, metaiodobenzylguanide; PET, positron emission tomography.

The cause of POTS in most individuals still eludes us. However, recently it has become clear that most such individuals have more than mere deconditioning. The onset of POTS often occurs in the wake of a viral infection, pregnancy, or a major surgical procedure, encouraging consideration of an autoimmune etiology. It is important to view POTS not as a disease but as a syndrome, a final common pathway by which many different pathophysiologies may present. Potential pathophysiologic mechanisms include a partial autonomic neuropathy, excessive venous pooling, a gravity-dependent fluid shift, diminished plasma volume or red cell mass, and a centrally mediated hyperadrenergic state. Some of these are shown in Figure 47-2. Figure 47-2B shows a schematic of neuropathic POTS. Patchy denervation of the sympathetic innervation of the blood vessels is shown in the extremities (especially the legs) and the kidneys, with subsequent hypovolemia and increased orthostatic venous pooling, in neuropathic POTS. This feeds back to the brain to increase sympathetic nervous system outflow in a compensatory effort that is sensed most in the heart, where there is no denervation. In central hyperadrenergic POTS (Fig. 47-2C), there is increased central sympathetic outflow to multiple structures, without peripheral denervation. This excessive sympathetic nervous outflow from the brain affects the blood vessels, kidneys, and heart. This form of POTS is often associated with orthostatic hypertension. Central hyperadrenergic POTS patients might benefit from peripheral β-adrenergic blockage. Also, central sympatholytics such as clonidine or methyldopa can be used for hyperadrenergic POTS. Genetic etiologies of POTS are beginning to emerge. The clearest example is the illustrative but quite rare form of POTS due to norepinephrine transporter (NET) deficiency. This derives from a unique A453P mutation yielding loss of gene function.[31] Since the NET clears norepinephrine from the synaptic cleft, in its functional absence, plasma norepinephrine rises and sympathetic hyperactivity emerges. Other polymorphisms in the NET gene may have related but distinct phenotypes.[32]

Mastocytosis is a disorder that may underlie POTS in some individuals.[33] It is due to increased numbers or increased responsiveness of mast cells. Release of histamine and prostaglandin D_2 into the circulation dominates the clinical picture. Characteristic chronic skin changes (erythematous acneiform papular lesions) are seen in only a minority of patients, but red flushing and urticaria are common during attacks. Palpitations, with or without chest pain, headaches, nausea, vomiting, diarrhea, and dyspnea, may occur. Perhaps 25% of cases are

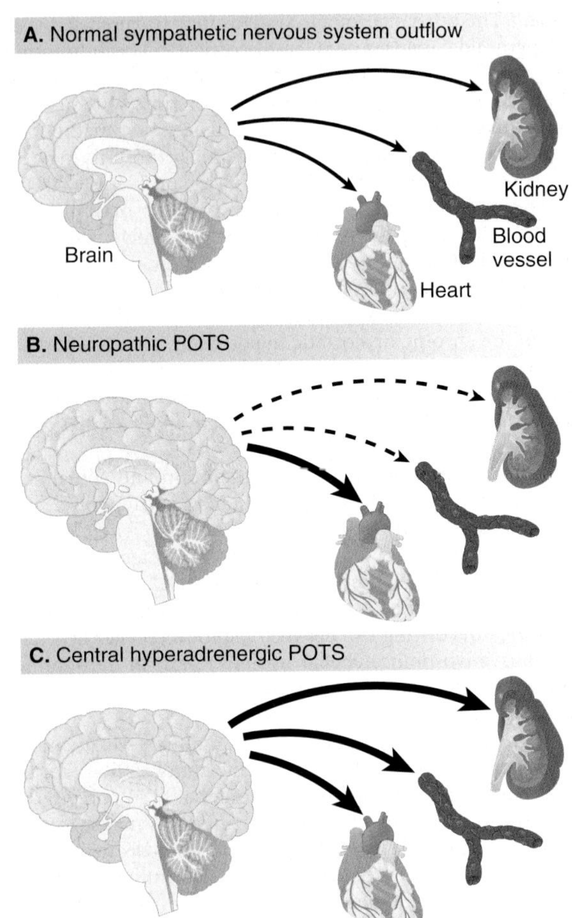

FIGURE 47-2 • Pathophysiologic schema for two of the most clearly established etiologies of POTS. A, A basal situation with a normal amount of sympathetic nervous system outflow from the brain that activates receptors in the blood vessels (vascular tone and venous return), heart (heart rate and contractility), and kidney (blood volume regulation through renin). **B,** In neuropathic POTS, patchy denervation of the sympathetic innervation of the blood vessels is shown in the extremities and the kidney. This feeds back to the brain to increase sympathetic nervous system outflow in a compensatory effort that is sensed most in the heart, where there is no denervation. **C,** A schematic of central hyperadrenergic POTS, with increased central sympathetic outflow to multiple structures without peripheral denervation. (Modified from Raj SR. The Postural Tachycardia Syndrome [POTS]: pathophysiology, diagnosis & management. Indian Pacing Electrophysiol J 2006;6:84-99.)

familial (autosomal dominant). Many patients respond well to treatment with histamine H_1- and H_2-receptor antagonists, but some have severe attacks with hypotension that must be treated by epinephrine infusion. Increases in blood pressure have also been seen. During severe attacks, disturbances in mental status may seem out of proportion to the hypotension. Patients may also seem to be unconscious for 5 to 20 minutes after syncope, but may indicate after recovery that they heard what was said to them in the minutes after syncope but were unable to reply to questions. Along with histamine and prostaglandin D_2, substantial quantities of heparin are present in mast cells, and, during attacks, sometimes enough heparin is released to raise the partial thromboplastin time.

It is well known that orthostatic symptoms similar to POTS occur in up to 64% of returning astronauts.[34] The underlying mechanisms remain unclear. The reduction in stroke volume[34] consistent with their reduced red blood cell masses[35] and hypovolemia[36] may contribute to the development of postflight orthostatic intolerance as well as the increased baseline sympathetic neural outflow and exaggerated sympathetic response to lower body negative pressure.[37]

We need to know more about the interrelationships of POTS and physical deconditioning. Both share many clinical features, and their separation can prove challenging. Perhaps more challenging is the fact that many patients with POTS respond to their illness by reducing their physical activity. When they present to physicians, they therefore present with both POTS and deconditioning.

The majority of patients with POTS have a relatively mild disorder that improves over succeeding weeks and months. Most patients will eventually be free of symptoms. However, in some patients, the symptoms are more severe, the duration of the illness may be longer, and the expected recovery may not occur. Overall, most POTS patients improve sufficiently to require no therapy after 5 years.

Pure Autonomic Failure

Pure autonomic failure (PAF) is a neurodegenerative disorder of the autonomic nervous system presenting in mid to late life. The disorder is confined to the sympathetic and parasympathetic nervous systems. PAF patients have autonomic failure resulting in peripheral but not central involvement.[38]

PAF involves sympathetic fibers preferentially. The adrenal medulla is relatively spared. The initial feature in men is male erectile dysfunction, but the symptom that usually brings patients to the physician is orthostatic hypotension. The orthostatic hypotension may be described as unsteadiness or faintness upon standing. It is worst in the morning, and improves as the day goes on. Supine hypertension may be marked during the night. Orthostatic hypotension is made more severe by meals, exercise, fever, or environmental heat. Sometimes if the orthostatic hypotension is not severe enough to induce syncope, patients complain of orthostatic pain in the neck, shoulders, or occiput, relieved by lying down. While orthostatic hypotension is defined as a decline in systolic blood pressure of 20/10 mm Hg after at least 1 minute of standing, most PAF patients have a decrease in systolic blood pressure of 50 mm Hg or greater. A diagnosis of PAF cannot be excluded on the basis of a single measurement of upright blood pressure that does not meet these criteria. Many patients who carry the diagnosis of PAF may actually have an autonomic neuropathy instead. Several measurements of orthostatic blood pressure should be made. About 5% of PAF patients have what appears to be angina pectoris, usually in the absence of significant angiographically demonstrable coronary atherosclerosis. PAF patients tolerate high altitude very poorly, perhaps because they hyperventilate in this situation, and hyperventilation induces a substantial fall in blood pressure in dysautonomia. Even with severe supine hypertension, cardiac function can be well preserved and contractility may even be raised.

A reduced basal metabolic rate is typical. There is usually hypohidrosis or at least an asymmetric distribution of sweating. Nocturia is an invariable accompaniment of PAF, and may cause the patient to get up as many as five times per night to pass substantial amounts of urine. Urinary hesitancy, urgency, dribbling, and occasional incontinence may also occur. Some patients develop urinary retention and may have repeated urinary tract infections in consequence. It is noteworthy that patients with PAF do not usually have fevers as high as healthy subjects; nevertheless, any fever will significantly lower their blood pressure and consequently decrease their functional capacity of daily activity. A sudden decline in functional mobility in a patient with PAF is suggestive of a surreptitious infection, usually of the urinary tract.

The pathology of PAF is characterized by Lewy bodies, a loss of cells in the intermediolateral column of the spinal cord, and a loss of catecholamine uptake and catecholamine fluorescence in sympathetic postganglionic neurons. PAF must be distinguished from multiple system atrophy (MSA) and Parkinson's disease with autonomic failure. PAF is less disabling than these other syndromes. In PAF, there should be no indication from the history or physical examination of cerebellar, striatal, pyramidal, or extrapyramidal dysfunction.

PAF patients have greatly reduced levels of catecholamines. Plasma and urinary norepinephrine levels are usually greatly reduced, sometimes to 10% of normal. Plasma norepinephrine is virtually always under 200 pg/ml and often under 100 pg/ml. Plasma levels of epinephrine are also reduced but usually to a lesser extent than norepinephrine.

Dopamine levels in urine are usually about 50% of normal values. There is marked hypersensitivity to all pressor and depressor stimuli.

Patients with PAF have a generally good outlook; many live for 20 years or more after the onset of their disease. However, they need to learn to live within the limitations imposed by their symptoms. The most common cause of death in these patients is pulmonary embolus or intercurrent infection. The incidence of both myocardial infarction and stroke appears to be significantly reduced in PAF.

Multiple System Atrophy

MSA (Shy-Drager syndrome) is a progressive neurodegenerative disorder encompassing autonomic, extrapyramidal, cerebellar, and pyramidal features. Extrapyramidal involvement is about threefold more common than cerebellar involvement. The pathologic hallmark of MSA is neuronal loss and gliosis within multiple sites in the brain, intermediolateral columns, and Onuf's nucleus in the spinal cord, with characteristic glial cytoplasmic inclusions (GCIs) containing α-synuclein and ubiquitin. These inclusions are quite distinct from Lewy bodies, which also contain ubiquitin. The GCIs tend to be irregular in outline, in contrast to the target-shaped concentric circular Lewy bodies of Parkinson's disease.

Onset of MSA averages 53 years, and there is no confirmed case under age 30. Onset beyond age 70 is rare. There is no gender predilection. It is estimated that 25,000 to 75,000 Americans suffer from MSA. In some patients the disease presents as orthostatic hypotension or urinary tract symptoms, but in other cases, extrapyramidal symptoms or cerebellar symptoms predominate in the early stages. When orthostatic hypotension antedates other neurologic involvement, differentiation from autonomic neuropathy or PAF may be difficult.[39,40]

The broad range of symptoms in MSA include male erectile dysfunction, micrographia, slurred speech, sleep apnea, difficulty with urination, urinary tract infections, headache, neck pain, dimming of vision, and leg discomfort. Orthostatic hypotension is common, even though blood pressure while lying down may be very high. There are several unusual features of MSA that are often missed, but may be important in making this diagnosis. Patients frequently note emotional lability, with short (sometimes only 1- or 2-minute) episodes of crying due to happiness or sadness in response to a relatively minor environmental stimulus, such as a song or an event in a television program or movie. This is usually self-limited, but may be a harbinger of depression, and should be treated with a selective serotonin reuptake inhibitor. Patients sometimes have periodic gasping respirations punctuating the medical interview. They only last 1 or 2 seconds, but seem labored. Finally, many patients will discontinue the use of nicotine-containing products at the onset of their disease. It sometimes appears that they no longer enjoy the nicotine. Ultimately, nicotine may provoke worsened tremor in some of these patients. A final symptom that occurs in occasional patients is diplopia.

In contrast to patients with PAF, the supine plasma and urinary concentrations of norepinephrine are often near normal in patients with MSA, but they do not rise appropriately on assumption of the upright posture.[41] Such patients have a constitutive release of peripheral autonomic neurotransmitters in the absence of normal central control. Noteworthy is the biochemical evidence of central abnormalities in the dopamine, acetylcholine, and serotonin systems. Other diagnostic tests include brain magnetic resonance imaging or urodynamic testing. There is much current enthusiasm for diagnostic ^{123}I-metaiodobenzylguanide (MIBG) scanning; the rationale for this is that uptake of this compound, a congener of norepinephrine, into the noradrenergic-rich tissues such as the heart will be impaired in conditions such as PAF and Parkinson's disease, whereas in MSA, [^{123}I]-MIBG uptake will be comparatively normal.[42] Also, ^{18}F-fluorodopamine (^{18}F-dopa) positron emission tomography could demonstrate cardiac sympathetic denervation in PAF and Parkinson's disease in contrast to relatively preserved cardiac sympathetic innervation in MSA.[42]

Autonomic failure in MSA is widespread and is associated with impairment in other neurologic systems. When autonomic failure dominates the disease presentation, it is sometimes called Shy-Drager syndrome.[43] The other neurologic systems may be cerebellar, extrapyramidal, pyramidal, neuromuscular, or cortical.[44] The autonomic dysfunction in MSA can be viewed as a predominantly CNS defect with an inability to engage the postganglionic autonomic system. The result is a constitutive, poorly organized, postganglionic sympathetic release of norepinephrine.[45] In these patients, chronic orthostatic hypotension may be a presenting symptom; in other cases, problems with balance due to extrapyramidal or cerebellar involvement may predominate early in the course. In patients with cerebellar involvement, tremor is worsened by nicotine, and MSA patients often spontaneously discontinue smoking at the onset of their disease. A significant minority of patients will also experience a painful neuropathy in the lower extremities. When the chronic orthostatic hypotension antedates other neurologic involvement, it may be very difficult to differentiate the MSA from the more benign PAF. Clinical symptoms of autonomic failure discussed earlier with respect to PAF often apply to patients with MSA.

Pathologically, multiple sites within the brain and spinal cord are involved. Sympathetic and parasympathetic postganglionic neurons, however, appear relatively spared in most patients. Characteristic GCIs that are quite distinct from the Lewy bodies encountered in Parkinson's disease occur in oligodendroglia and neurons.[46] Very likely, MSA will ultimately be found to represent several distinct clinical entities. Some investigators distinguish between a spinocerebellar degeneration (spontaneous olivospinocerebellar atrophy) and an autonomic dysfunction associated with extrapyramidal involvement (striatonigral degeneration).

The prognosis is more guarded in MSA than in PAF. It is rare for a patient to survive 12 years. The autonomic abnormalities are seldom the direct cause of death. A significant number of MSA patients develop laryngeal stridor and difficulty in swallowing. This may lead to recurrent episodes of pneumonia, a frequent cause of death. In addition, many patients with MSA experience sleep apnea. Pulmonary hypertension may occur during apnea. In spite of the frequency of these two problems, however, one of the most common causes of death in patients with MSA is pulmonary embolus.

There is no known cure for MSA, so management involves treating patients symptomatically.[47,48] This includes treatment of the depression, tremor and gait disturbances, and orthostatic hypotension, and possible self-catheterization when urinary retention is severe.

Dopamine β-Hydroxylase Deficiency

Dopamine β-hydroxylase (DBH) deficiency is due to selective absence of norepinephrine and all its metabolites.[49] It has only been described in a few patients but has a disproportionate importance because it illuminates human noradrenergic function. Affected patients have absent sympathetic noradrenergic function but normal parasympathetic and sympathetic cholinergic function. DBH-deficient patients exhibit profound orthostatic hypotension. Although present from birth, the disorder is often unrecognized until adulthood. In the perinatal period, DBH deficiency has been complicated by vomiting, dehydration, hypotension, hypothermia, and profound hypoglycemia requiring repeated hospitalization; children have reduced exercise capacity. By early adulthood, individuals have profound orthostatic hypotension, greatly reduced exercise tolerance, ptosis of the eyelids, and supine nasal stuffiness. Presyncopal symptoms include dizziness, blurred vision, dyspnea, nuchal discomfort, and chest pain. Neuropsychiatric symptoms are surprisingly mild, and most patients are not considered to have CNS abnormalities prior to diagnosis driven by their orthostatic hypotension. During adult life, some DBH-deficient patients develop renal function abnormalities, including raised creatinine. Life expectancy is not known with certainty but appears to be near normal.

The diagnosis of DBH deficiency is based on clinical findings, including orthostatic hypotension, intact sweating, ptosis of the eyelids, and arched palate. Biochemical features include minimal or undetectable plasma, cerebrospinal, and urinary norepinephrine and epinephrine, and a 5- to 10-fold elevation of plasma dopamine, a finding pathognomonic of DBH deficiency. Patients lack urinary normetanephrine, metanephrine, and vanillylmandelic acid. DBH molecular genetic testing is available on a research basis only.

A disorder with biochemical similarities to DBH deficiency is Menkes' syndrome. DBH is a copper-containing enzyme, and congenital disorders of impaired copper may present with certain features similar to DBH deficiency. Male infants with Menkes' syndrome present with stubby, tangled, sparse hair (often white or gray in color), pudgy cheeks, spasticity, seizures, hypothermia, retarded growth, and decreased visual function. Subdural hematoma, jaundice, and osteoporosis are also seen. The abnormality in copper handling leads to defective DBH functional efficiency. The incidence is between 1 : 50,000 and 1 : 100,000.

DBH deficiency is the first neurotransmitter defect for which a uniquely efficacious replacement strategy has been developed. Administration of droxidopa (L-threo-3,4-dihydroxyphenylserine [L-DOPS]) alleviates the orthostatic hypotension and other symptoms. Individuals do not respond well to standard therapeutic approaches for autonomic failure. Surgery can correct ptosis. Renal function is assessed every 5 years, or more often if loss of function emerges.

Baroreflex Failure

Human baroreflexes buffer blood pressure against excessive rise or fall. It is well known the impairment of baroreflex plays a significant role in several cardiovascular diseases.[50-52] Baroreflex failure itself is perhaps the most dramatic neurologic disorder of blood pressure regulation.[53] Acute baroreflex failure can be associated with stress-induced systolic blood pressure surges to over 300 mm Hg, and provides evidence of the great capacity of the human CNS to barogenerate cardiovascular excitation. It is quite distinct from autonomic failure, resembling the clinical pattern of pheochromocytoma more than it does a typical dysautonomia. Baroreflex failure occurs when afferent baroreceptive input via the vagus or glossopharyngeal nerves or their central connections becomes impaired. This results in wide excursions of blood pressure and heart rate. Such excursions may derive from endogenous factors such as anger or drowsiness, which result in high and low pressures, respectively. They may also derive from exogenous factors such as environmental stressors like excessive cold or bright light.

Acute baroreflex impairment may produce hypertensive crisis. Over succeeding days to weeks, or in the absence of an acute event, volatile hypertension with periods of hypotension occurs. In some individuals, after months to years there is ultimately orthostatic hypotension. Usually bilateral destruction of baroreflex afferent function results in concomitant destruction of much efferent vagal function. Loss of vagal parasympathetic tone to the heart prevents bradycardia during stimuli that would ordinarily elicit parasympathetic activation (e.g., sedation or sleep). However, if the baroreflex failure occurs with relative sparing of the parasympathetic efferent vagal fibers, sleep or sedation may lead to malignant vagotonia with severe bradycardia and hypotension and episodes of sinus arrest[45] (Jordan syndrome) (Fig. 47-3). Along with the hypertensive episodes encountered in the other forms of baroreflex failure, patients with this form may have episodes of hypotension with a systolic pressure below 50 mm Hg. Accompanying symptoms include fatigue and dizziness, with possible progression to frank syncope. The most severe episodes tend to occur during early morning sleep, and periods of asystole longer than 20 seconds have been observed. Episodes have also occurred following intravenous nitroprusside and sublingual nitroglycerin.

Impairment in the vascular baroreceptors, the glossopharyngeal or vagal nerves, or their brainstem connections can all potentially lead to baroreflex failure. Trauma from injury, tumor, radiation, surgical intervention, or brainstem stroke may cause baroreflex failure. Demyelination of the afferents in Guillain-Barré syndrome also causes baroreflex disorder.[54] It occurs in familial paraganglioma syndrome owing to bilateral local tumor growth invading structures at or near the glossopharyngeal and vagal nerves. Radiation therapy of throat carcinoma may incur collateral damage to cranial nerves, and this damage tends to occur after an interval of months or, in some cases, years following

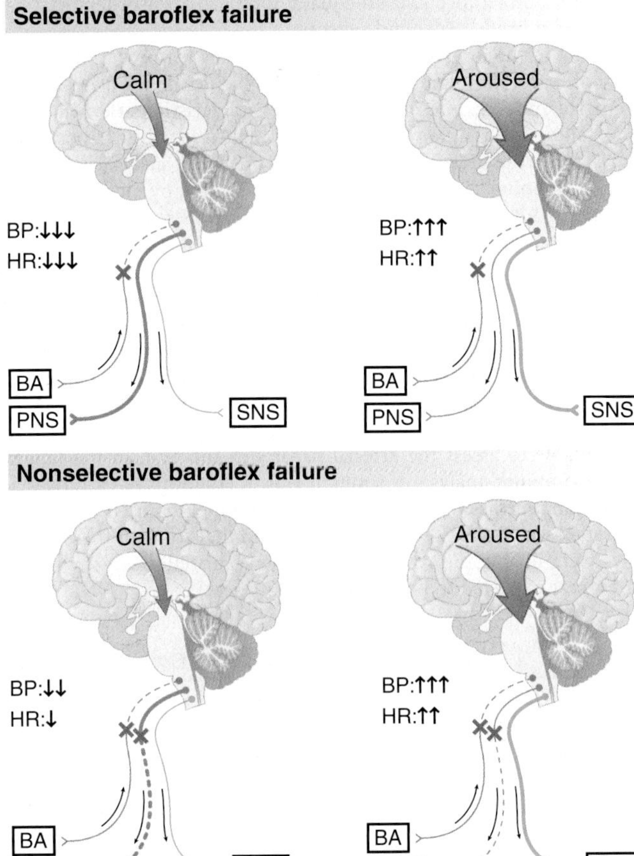

FIGURE 47-3 • Selective baroreflex failure (top) contrasted with nonselective baroreflex failure (bottom). Baroreflex afferents (BA) are damaged in patients with selective and nonselective baroreflex failure. The efferent sympathetic (SNS) and parasympathetic (PNS) nerves are intact in selective baroreflex failure. In nonselective baroreflex failure, efferent parasympathetic nerves are at least in part damaged. BP, blood pressure; HR, heart rate. (Modified from Jordan J, Shannon JR, Black BK, et al. Malignant vagotonia due to selective baroreflex failure. Hypertension 1997;30:1072-1077.)

the irradiation, perhaps reflecting local fibrosis as the pathophysiology whereby the nerves are damaged. Also, patients who have received radiotherapy for head and neck cancer may present with lightheadedness or syncope due to baroreceptor damage. A baroreflex failure patient with impaired function of the nucleus tractus solitarii but no history of radiation, tumor, or trauma was ultimately found to have Leigh's syndrome. Some genetic disorders that appear to entail baroreflex dysfunction have been described: the Groll-Hirschowitz syndrome, in which carotid sinus nerve dysfunction, sensory neuropathy, and duodenal diverticula occur, and the syndrome of autosomal dominant hypertension and brachydactyly with loss of baroreflex buffering. Abnormal elastic fiber assembly at the arterial level in Williams syndrome may alter baroreceptor discharges and cause their reduced baroreflex sensitivity.[55] The *PHOX2B* mutation associated with congenital central hypoventilation syndrome (Ondine's curse) also causes baroreflex failure because the impaired ontogeny of the visceral reflexes includes the baroreceptive pathway, mainly its vagal component.[56]

Because of the protean manifestations of baroreflex failure, the differential diagnosis can be extensive. The most important consideration is usually pheochromocytoma. The diagnosis of baroreflex failure often emerges following a negative workup for pheochromocytoma. Other entities from which it must be distinguished include generalized anxiety disorder, migraine, PAF, hyperthyroidism, alcohol withdrawal, and drug use (e.g., amphetamine, cocaine). Renovascular hypertension frequently presents with volatility and brittleness, and may sometimes mimic baroreflex failure. There is a long list of entities that can produce orthostatic intolerance and an equally long list of disorders that can present with bradycardia and syncope.

In spite of the long differential diagnosis, key features in the evaluation of baroreflex failure make it possible to definitively address whether or not it is present. The most characteristic pattern in baroreflex failure is baseline pressures in the high-normal or hypertensive range, but with pressor surges accompanied by tachycardia lasting minutes to hours. These pressor surges are elicited by mental or physical stress, during which sympathetic outflow is increased, and are characterized by palpitations and often severe headaches. Continuous blood pressure recordings clearly differentiate autonomic neuropathy from baroreflex failure. The great variability of baroreflex failure might be shown.[57] The best test is to document normal or excess excursions of heart rate during normal daily activities (confirming autonomic control of heart rate), and then document an absence of bradycardic response of the heart rate to the pressor effect of phenylephrine or the tachycardic heart rate response to a depressor agent. Several methods are available to assess the arterial baroreflex function in the laboratory.[58] Computer analysis of spontaneous fluctuations of cardiovascular variables recorded with noninvasive equipment is used to estimate baroreflex sensitivity.[59] Recent study showed that some of these procedures were unable to provide results when baroreflex sensitivity estimates were expected to be very low in data sets.[60]

There is profuse sweating during many of these attacks. Tremulousness, anxiety, and irritability are typical of these episodes, sometimes acting as the triggering event for the surge. Mild and transient elevations in plasma glucose have also occasionally been seen, as well as a positive correlation between blood pressure and intraocular pressure. During such pressor surges, plasma norepinephrine levels reach values not much less than those seen in pheochromocytoma. Norepinephrine levels of 1000 pg/ml in the supine posture during a pressor surge would be typical, and values above 2000 pg/ml are occasionally seen. These pressor surges can also be punctuated by hypotensive valleys, especially during periods of quiet, sedation, or sleep, when sympathetic outflow is diminished. In practice, the history of prior trauma exposure is usually the most important consideration in suspecting the diagnosis of baroreflex failure.

THERAPEUTICS AND CLINICAL PHARMACOLOGY

Medications (Table 47-3)

Fludrocortisone

For all disorders associated with chronic orthostatic hypotension, fludrocortisone is the treatment of choice when nonpharmacologic

TABLE 47-3 MEDICATIONS USED TO TREAT DYSAUTONOMIAS

Medication	Mechanism of Action	Efficacy	Adverse Effects and Disadvantages	Dose
Fludrocortisone	Mineralocorticoid. Initial increase in plasma volume due to sodium retention that develops over several days.	Orthostatic hypotension Hypovolemic orthostatic intolerance	Hypokalemia (50%), hypomagnesemia (5%) Drug should not be used in patients who are unable to tolerate an increased fluid load (e.g., congestive heart failure patients) A common adverse effect of fludrocortisone is headache	0.1 mg (usually up to 0.4 mg) once or twice a day, orally
Midodrine	α-Adrenoreceptor agonist. Constriction of arterioles and veins.	Orthostatic hypotension	Urinary retention Supine hypertension	2.5-10 mg every 3-4 hr (in daytime)
Indomethacin (NSAIDs)	Probably prostanoid synthesis inhibition.	Orthostatic hypotension	Gastrointestinal: abdominal pain, constipation, diarrhea Central nervous system: dizziness, headache, somnolence	25-30 mg three times a day Maximum 200 mg/day
Clonidine	α_2-Receptor agonist. Central sympathetic inhibition. Peripheral vascular smooth muscle contraction (high doses only).	May occasionally increase blood pressure in complete sympathetically denervated patients, but these are very rare.	Hypotension (may be severe) CNS effects (e.g., sedation, hallucinations)	0.4-0.8 mg/day
Droxidopa (L-DOPS)	Analogue of norepinephrine. Converted directly into norepinephrine.	Orthostatic hypotension of DBH deficiency. Pressor agent in MSA, PAF, and other autonomic neuropathies.	Hypertension at high doses	200-600 mg two or three times a day
Yohimbine	Central and peripheral α_2-adrenergic receptor antagonist. Increase efferent sympathetic activity.	Orthostatic hypotension	CNS effect (anxiety, nervousness) Diarrhea	2.5-5.4 mg three times a day
Erythropoietin	Recombinant human erythropoietin. Increases erythrocytes and perhaps intravascular volume. Direct vasopressor effect.	Orthostatic hypotension	Cost and inconvenience of this treatment Supine hypertension Unknown long-term safety	25-75 U/kg three times weekly intravenously or subcutaneously. Treat until hematocrit is in the normal gender-based range.

CNS, central nervous system; DBH, dopamine β-hydroxylase; MSA, multiple system atrophy; PAF, pure autonomic failure.

measures no longer suffice. The value of fludrocortisone for raising blood pressure in a patient with autonomic failure was first demonstrated by Grant W. Liddle on December 18, 1956, and fludrocortisone subsequently became the treatment of choice for this purpose.[61]

Certain special features of fludrocortisone complicate its successful use. First, most of its blood pressure raising effect is due to sodium retention, which develops over several days; therefore, the full pressor action of fludrocortisone is seen in 1 to 2 weeks, rather than on the day it is first administered. Doses should be altered no more often than weekly, commencing with a dose of 0.1 mg once a day, orally. Since patients usually expect a drug to work the first day, it is wise to discuss this delayed action so they are not disappointed by the lack of immediate salutary effect. They should also be aware that they may need to gain 5 to 8 pounds in order for fludrocortisone to have its maximal favorable effect to raise their blood pressure. Sleeping with 6 to 8 inches of head upright tilt will prevent excessive nocturnal volume loss, and consequently increase the efficacy of fludrocortisone.

There are occasional complications of fludrocortisone therapy. Almost 50% of patients will develop hypokalemia within 2 weeks, and about 5% will also develop hypomagnesemia. The former can be treated with potassium supplementation and the latter with small doses of magnesium sulfate.

Since fluid retention is critical to fludrocortisone's beneficial effect, the drug should not be used in patients who are unable to tolerate an increased fluid load (e.g., congestive heart failure patients). In point of fact, patients with congestive heart failure usually have increased (rather than reduced) orthostatic tolerance, and we have seen patients with mild autonomic failure experience a lessening of their orthostatic hypotension when they develop congestive heart failure. We have never encountered a case of pulmonary edema in a patient with autonomic failure that did not respond immediately to assumption of the seated or upright posture. It seems prudent, however, to avoid weight gains greater than 10 pounds.

A common adverse effect of fludrocortisone is headache. This appears to be a greater problem in younger and healthier persons than in elderly or sick persons. Headache has limited the use of fludrocortisone in astronauts, who experience a very high incidence of orthostatic intolerance on return from space. Few patients with severe autonomic failure complain of headache. In patients who need fludrocortisone most of all, the headache is usually not noticed.

Recently, there have been a number of improvements in our understanding of fludrocortisone actions. Whereas it was initially thought that mineralocorticoid receptors acted within the nucleus of the cell to alter gene transcription, it is becoming evident that some actions of mineralocorticoids are due to cell surface receptors that act through second messengers without requiring engagement of the DNA. Such mechanisms might be activated more rapidly than those requiring involvement of cellular transcription machinery. For this reason, a better understanding of the pharmacokinetic profile of fludrocortisone has been important. Fludrocortisone is rapidly and nearly completely absorbed following oral administration and declines with a half-life of 2 to 3 hours. Because of this relatively short half-life, it may be more efficacious to give the drug in a twice-daily regimen rather than the once-daily regimen more commonly used. However, many patients have clearly received benefit even with a once-daily regimen.

The recommended dosage in the published literature of fludrocortisone in autonomic failure varies over a wide range (0.05 to 2.00 mg daily, orally). It is unusual to have any benefit from a dosage smaller than 0.05 mg daily. In practice, 0.1 mg/day is usually the starting dose. That dose can be increased by 0.1-mg oral increments at 1- to 2-week intervals. Few patients will require more than 0.4 mg orally daily. There appears to be little if any glucocorticoid effect at low (0.1- to 0.2-mg) daily doses of fludrocortisone, but adrenocorticotropic hormone suppression as manifested by reduced cortisol level can be seen following one oral dose of 2.0 mg fludrocortisone. In using fludrocortisone or any other pressor agent, it is important to be guided by relief of unacceptable symptoms (syncope), rather than any a priori level of upright blood pressure.

Midodrine

Midodrine is a prodrug that, following absorption, is metabolized to desglymidodrine, an α_1-adrenoreceptor agonist that differs from methoxamine only in lacking a methyl group on the side chain.[62] There is a long history of successful clinical use of the α_1-adrenoreceptor agonist class of drugs. A theoretical advantage of midodrine is that it is absorbed as the prodrug with limited direct effect to constrict the vasculature of the gastrointestinal tract; it is metabolized to desglymidodrine, which has an order of magnitude greater potency to raise blood pressure in the peripheral circulation. It is more than 90% absorbed following oral administration. The peak concentration in plasma occurs in 20 to 30 minutes, with a half-life of 30 minutes. The plasma concentration of desglymidodrine peaks at 1 hour, with a half-life of approximately 3 hours. The metabolites are predominantly excreted through the urinary tract.

Oral midodrine results in all the typical effects of an α_1-adrenoreceptor agonist. Such drugs lead to arterial and venous constriction with attendant increased peripheral vascular resistance and central redistribution of blood volume. The trigone and sphincter of the urinary bladder are stimulated. There is contraction of the radial muscle of the iris leading to pupillary dilation. Pilomotor muscles are stimulated, leading to a sensation of hair standing on end (piloerection or horripilation). Noradrenergic sweating may occur transiently.

Midodrine directly raises blood pressure by constriction of arterioles and veins. It is best used to raise blood pressure during the daytime, especially in the morning, so that the maximum effect occurs at a time when the patient wants to be upright. In the supine posture (e.g., during the night), blood pressure is always sufficiently high in autonomic failure, and raising it further at that time with this or some other agent is counterproductive. For all these reasons, administration of midodrine early in the day is the means to achieve the greatest benefit.

The initial dose of midodrine typically needs to be increased after a day or so to maintain the same effect because desensitization of the α_1-receptor–mediated responses may occur initially. This desensitization does not continue, however, after the first week. Usually midodrine is begun with 2.5 mg at breakfast and lunch, but the dose is escalated at 2.5-mg increments daily until a satisfactory response occurs or a dosage of 30 mg daily is achieved. Many patients will benefit from 5 or 10 mg on arising, a similar dose mid-morning, and a third dose in the early afternoon. Only by individualization of the use of this drug can its therapeutic benefit be maximized. It is also important that the functional capacity, as assessed by standing time in severely affected patients and by systolic blood pressure in more mildly affected patients, be the ultimate guide in structuring the regimen. Through personal observation, patients may develop considerable facility in the use of agents such as midodrine, and input from knowledgeable and medically sophisticated patients can greatly enhance the efficacy of this agent, particularly in regard to dosage scheduling.

The adverse effects of midodrine are mechanism based. Almost all patients receiving effective doses will experience the sensation of gooseflesh (piloerection), paresthesia of the scalp, or pruritus. All three of these symptoms probably relate to effects of muscle contraction on integumentary hairs. In many patients, these symptoms are very mild. In some cases, these symptoms may become a welcome sign that the blood pressure is about to rise. Occasional patients, however, are severely bothered by these sensations. Sometimes it is sufficiently bothersome that they will request discontinuation of the medication. The most serious complication of administration of midodrine is hypertension, particularly in the supine posture, that may be of considerable concern.

Indomethacin

Indomethacin (25 to 50 mg) will raise blood pressure about 20 mm Hg in most but not all severely affected patients with autonomic failure. The response is more dramatic in the postprandial period than at other times of the day. Since patients may have troubling gastrointestinal or

CNS adverse effects with indomethacin, other nonsteroidal anti-inflammatory drugs (NSAIDs), such as ibuprofen, have also been successfully employed, although their relative efficacies and toxicities have not been compared. The precise mechanism of the pressor action of NSAIDs in autonomic failure is not established.

Clonidine

The use of α-adrenergic receptor agonists and antagonists has been extensively studied.[63-66] In the vasomotor center, α_2-adrenergic receptor stimulation inhibits sympathetic outflow; however, centrally active α_2-receptor agonists also have direct activity on muscular α_2 receptors in the periphery. In the rare patient in whom sympathetic denervation is complete (plasma norepinephrine levels <25 pg/ml), clonidine does not decrease blood pressure, and the direct effects of clonidine on vascular smooth muscle α-adrenergic receptors promote smooth muscle contraction. This can result in a dramatic elevation in blood pressure, particularly with oral dosages of 0.4 to 0.8 mg.[67] However, the major limitation of clonidine is its depressor effect, observed when this agent is administered to a patient with partial autonomic failure. Sometimes patients with partial autonomic impairment may develop quite severe orthostatic hypotension in response to clonidine. In such patients, although only a low level of sympathetic activity remains, it may be pivotal in the maintenance of blood pressure, and the administration of clonidine, particularly at low doses, may result in incapacitating hypotension. This is especially likely to occur in patients with baroreflex failure. Finally, some patients given clonidine for the management of low blood pressure have marked CNS effects, such as sedation or hallucinations. For all these reasons, clonidine should only rarely and cautiously be used in the management of orthostatic hypotension.

Droxidopa (L-DOPS)

Droxidopa (L-DOPS) is an analogue of norepinephrine to which a carboxyl group has been attached. This agent is uniquely beneficial in patients with DBH deficiency.[66] The advantage of this agent in this disorder is that L-DOPS is already β-hydroxylated and can be converted directly into norepinephrine by the enzyme dopa decarboxylase, which lacks substrate specificity (Fig. 47-4).

Although this agent has occasionally been used in other forms of autonomic impairment,[68,69] it is of greatest benefit in DBH deficiency, where it circumvents the enzymatic defect. Dosages of 200 to 600 mg two or three times daily have a dramatic pressor effect in patients with DBH deficiency. In general, the drug has been well tolerated. Orthostatic tolerance is greatly enhanced during therapy with this agent, and plasma norepinephrine concentrations, previously undetectable, usually rise into the normal range. A concomitant fall in plasma concentrations of dopamine usually occurs, perhaps because the rate-limiting tyrosine hydroxylase activity is decreased by the newly synthesized feedback inhibition actions of norepinephrine now present in the patient's sympathomimetic neurons. Studies in patients with autonomic neuropathy, PAF, and MSA are currently underway in order to bring droxidopa to the American market.

Yohimbine

The α_2-adrenergic receptor antagonist yohimbine is sometimes useful in patients with autonomic failure.[64,66,70] Yohimbine increases sympathetic nervous system efferent output by antagonizing central or presynaptic α_2-adrenergic receptors, or both. Although it might seem paradoxical that both α_2-adrenergic receptor agonists, such as clonidine, and α_2-adrenergic receptor antagonists, such as yohimbine, would be employed in treating low blood pressure, they are useful in different subgroups of patients. While clonidine should be restricted to patients who have no sympathetic function remaining, yohimbine may be useful in proportion to the amount of sympathetic activity the patient still possesses. In a sense, yohimbine may be a particularly physiologic approach in that it enhances the patient's own sympathetic nervous system activation, whereas most other drugs merely supplement or compensate for it. Adverse effects with yohimbine are predominantly anxiety, nervousness, and diarrhea.

Erythropoietin

Recombinant human erythropoietin is available in a preparation with a 165–amino acid sequence "backbone" identical to that of erythropoietin. The recombinant erythropoietin available for clinical use has been given the generic name epoetin alfa. It can be given intravenously or subcutaneously, and has the same physiologic actions as endogenous erythropoietin. Patients with severe autonomic failure often have mild anemia (hematocrit 32 to 38), usually in proportion to the degree to which the plasma norepinephrine level is subnormal.[71] This anemia typically elicits an inadequate endogenous erythropoietin response. The anemia is dramatically responsive to epoetin alfa.[72] The pressor effect of erythropoietin was probably due to the red cell mass, although erythropoietin may have direct vascular effects as well.[73] For this reason, when simpler measures are insufficient, a trial of epoetin alfa may be undertaken. The greatest disadvantage of this agent is that it must be administered parenterally.

Epoetin alfa usually is administered in doses of 25 to 75 U/kg three times weekly. An increase in the reticulocyte count usually is detected within 10 days, and an increase in hematocrit is detectable in 2 to 6 weeks. The goal of using epoetin alfa for patients with autonomic failure is to achieve a hematocrit in the normal gender-based range. This is a somewhat higher target than is usually sought in other diseases for which epoetin alfa has been recommended. It should be recognized that, because epoetin alfa has still been used in only a few hundred patients with autonomic failure, there may be refinements in our use of it in the future. Recently, darbepoetin alfa (Aranesp), a

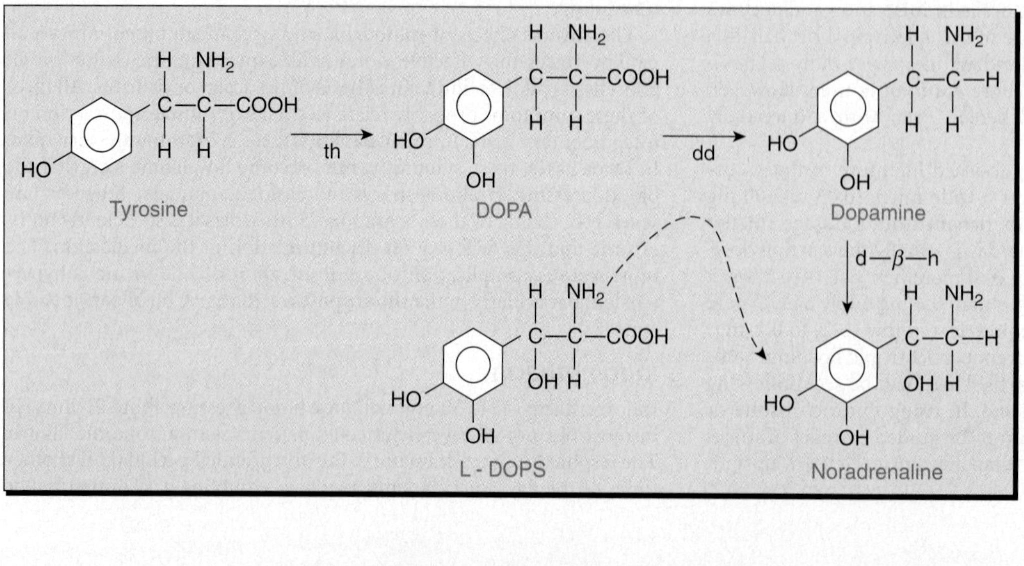

FIGURE 47-4 • Primary biosynthetic pathway of catecholamines (*solid arrows*) and alternative formation of norepinephrine (*dotted arrow*) from DOPS. d-β-h, dopamine β-hydroxylase; dd, dopa decarboxylase; th, tyrosine hydroxylase. (Modified from Biaggioni I, Robertson D. Endogenous restoration of noradrenaline by precursor therapy in dopamine-beta-hydroxylase deficiency. Lancet 1987;2:1170-1172.)

synthetic form of erythropoietin, has become available, and has the convenience of once-weekly administration.

In addition to the increase in red blood cell count that occurs with epoetin alfa, blood pressure often rises slightly. The mechanism by which this occurs is not entirely clear. It does not appear to be entirely explained by viscosity changes in the blood. The possibility that epoetin alfa might possess an effect on the vasculature heretofore not recognized must remain open.

Occasional patients with autonomic failure experience an acute increase in blood pressure with the first dose, which does not necessarily occur with subsequent doses. The mechanism of this increase remains unclear. During the period when the hematocrit is increasing, iron deficiency is particularly prone to develop. This should be anticipated in patients with marginal iron levels. Supplementation may be required during the first 2 months of therapy, and, in some cases, for an indefinite period thereafter.

Many patients are able, once they have reached their target hematocrit, to reduce the dosage of epoetin alfa. Some patients are able to be maintained long term on doses as low as 25 U/kg three times weekly. It is not uncommon for patients to experience a greatly increased sense of well-being and improved appetite on this regimen. Conversely, because erythropoietin is a growth factor, the outcome of long-term use on susceptibility to hematologic and other malignancies is being watched carefully.

Therapeutic Approach

For many individuals with dysautonomias, management of orthostatic symptoms is key to maintaining an active and productive lifestyle. The purpose of therapeutic interventions is to increase the patient's functional capacity rather than to achieve any particular level of blood pressure. Factors such as prior ingestion of food and drugs as well as the rate of ventilation should be taken into account when assessing the patient's standing time or blood pressure. Hyperventilation lowers[74] and hypoventilation raises blood pressure. Strenuous exercise may markedly lower blood pressure in these patients, but an appropriate exercise program may have long-term benefits.

Patient education is the cornerstone of treating individuals with postural hypotension. Many patients discover for themselves that they are less able to carry out vigorous activities following meals. This association may not have been made by other patients, who should be advised to utilize the period before meals for most of their activities and to limit their activities in the hour or so following a large meal.

Management of Autonomic Failure (Box 47-1)

Orthostatic Hypotension. Orthostatic hypotension is a dominant symptom in autonomic failure patients. However, it is a highly variable phenomenon. In many patients, it is completely absent at certain times of the day. In other patients, it may be present in the morning but not later in the day, after a large breakfast but not before breakfast, or after climbing a flight of stairs but not before.[75] In other individuals, orthostatic hypotension may be present at all times, while its degree remains variable. Other major determinants of the degree of hypotension include hyperventilation,[76] fever, and environmental temperature. In the most severely affected patients, admittedly a small subgroup of all patients with orthostatic symptoms, the upright blood pressure can be as low as 60/40 mm Hg. At this cuff estimate of blood pressure, the oscillatory (automatic) sphygmomanometer is inadequate to assess true intra-arterial blood pressure. For this reason, in severely affected patients, it is useful to monitor the severity of disease and its response to therapy by the standing time. The standing time is primarily of value in monitoring individuals who are unable to stand motionless for as long as 3 minutes. The importance of the standing time is that many individuals who have an increase in standing time from 30 to 120 seconds may have a substantial increase in functional capacity, even though they may have no change in their level of upright blood pressure as assessed by the sphygmomanometer. A patient with a standing time under 30 seconds usually cannot live alone, while a patient with a standing time greater than 60 seconds generally can. Thus, the standing time determination greatly facilitates the management of the most severely affected patients with orthostatic hypotension.

BOX 47-1 SUMMARY OF TREATMENTS FOR AUTONOMIC FAILURE

Aim to enable patients to stand for at least for 3 minutes.

Pharmacologic Treatments

Orthostatic Hypotension

- Fludrocortisone 0.1-0.2 mg once or twice a day orally, with increased salt intake
- Short-acting pressor agents, as needed, twice to three times in daytime
  - Midodrine 5-10 mg
  - Yohimbine 5.4 mg
  - Indomethacin 50 mg
  - Pyridostigmine 60 mg
- Recombinant erythropoietin if necessary

Supine Hypertension

- Transdermal nitroglycerin 0.1-0.2 mg/hr at night, remove in the morning
- Short-acting calcium blocker (nifedipine 30 mg) at bedtime

Nonpharmacologic Treatments

- Eliminate all prescription medications that may cause orthostatic hypotension.
- Increase fluid intake (drink 16 oz tap water).
- Avoid low-sodium diet.
- Avoid excessive activity in the 2-hour period after meals.
- A snack or a glass of wine can be exploited to treat supine hypertension at night.
- Elevate the head of the bed to 5-20 degrees during nighttime.
- Avoid standing quickly or standing motionless.
- Wear waist-high pressure stockings with abdominal binder.
- Avoid supine position during the daytime.
- Avoid hot environment.
- Avoid activities that involve straining.

Maximizing circulating blood volume is extremely important in treating orthostatic hypotension in severely affected patients with autonomic failure. Even healthy young people pool 350 ml of blood in their legs on standing, and this pooling is, of course, much more marked in patients with autonomic failure. There is a reduction in central blood volume, and most patients have a reduced total blood volume as well. Low-normal values of central venous pressure, right atrial pressure, and pulmonary wedge pressure are frequently seen in severely affected patients with autonomic failure even in the supine position. Liver blood flow is reduced considerably by upright posture, and drug metabolism (e.g., lidocaine) may thus be altered.[77] Fludrocortisone is commonly used to increase central volume because it increases plasma volume. Fludrocortisone can induce or worsen supine hypertension, which might have a relationship with its long-term safety. Erythropoietin therapy for anemia also increases intravascular volume. However, the degree of symptomatic improvement is not sufficient to justify the cost and inconvenience of this treatment in some patients.

All prescription medications should be carefully screened for their potential effects on blood pressure. In particular, antihypertensive medicines prescribed for supine hypertension and drugs such as tricyclic antidepressants can greatly reduce blood pressure. Patients with autonomic failure are extremely sensitive to vasodilating agents. They have increased sensitivity to the effects of sympathomimetic amines and have an exaggerated sensitivity to β_2-agonist stimulation compared with α_1-agonist stimulation.[78] Consequently, β-agonists may exert a marked vasodepressor effect in these patients. The dramatic vasoactive effects of many classes of drugs make use of anesthetics especially difficult in these patients.[79]

Patients should avoid certain nonprescription medications such as diet pills containing phenylpropanolamine or nasal sprays containing phenylephrine or oxymetazoline (a congener of clonidine). Although acutely pressor, these agents, when ingested in excess over time, can lead to significant orthostatic hypotension.

Finally, short-acting pressor agents (e.g., midodrine, yohimbine) may contribute to normalize activity of patients. We recommend using them as needed, 30 to 45 minutes before the activity.

Supine Hypertension. Supine hypertension and its attendant diuresis can be minimized by elevating the head of the bed on blocks to approximately 5 to 20 degrees.[80] In addition to attenuating nocturnal diuresis, this will reduce the notable worsening of symptoms in the morning. Six to eight degrees of head-up tilt at night also may minimize nocturnal shifts of interstitial fluid from the legs into the circulation. Interstitial fluid in the legs on standing may exert greater support and oppose the tendency of blood to pool. Supine blood pressure usually is highest just after a person goes to bed at night. Most treatment modalities raise supine as well as upright blood pressure. Thus, head-up tilt can minimize the effect of pressor drugs during the night, a time when pressor actions are no longer necessary and may in fact be harmful. Tilt-table conditioning has led to improved functional capacity in some patients with autonomic failure.[81] Also, patients should avoid pressor agents and fluid intake at bedtime. Patients may need pharmacologic treatment if these approaches are not sufficient to control supine hypertension. Transdermal nitroglycerin (0.1 to 0.2 mg/hr) and short-acting nifedipine (30 mg) at bedtime decrease supine blood pressure in autonomic failure patients.[82] Other vasodilators such as hydralazine may be useful in some cases. Patients who are prescribed these regimens should be warned about potential risks of falls if they get up during the night.

Sodium and Food Management. Patients with autonomic failure have inadequately conserved sodium during low salt intake.[83] This may be due to decreased noradrenergic activity in the kidney, to relatively enhanced dopamine actions, or to other effects. In addition, renin responses to a low-salt diet and upright posture are reduced or absent during autonomic failure.[84] Almost all of these patients have elevated supine systemic vascular resistance that does not increase with upright posture. This elevated supine pressure probably also contributes to the failure of the kidney to conserve salt and water. At night, when supine, these patients inappropriately waste sodium in the urine, leading to relative hypovolemia and a degree of orthostatic hypotension that is worse in the morning and improves during the day. It is interesting that angiotensin-converting enzyme inhibitors can sometimes reduce blood pressure in spite of the very low plasma renin activity levels present in these patients, raising the possibility of the involvement of a kallikrein mechanism. For this reason, sodium intake should be liberalized in all patients except those few with coexisting congestive heart failure.[85] Slight pedal edema is well tolerated and implies higher intravascular volume as well as increased interstitial hydrostatic pressure in the legs.

Food exerts a dramatic depressor effect in patients with chronic orthostatic hypotension.[86-88] In normal subjects, there is a slight tachycardia with little or no fall in blood pressure after eating. However, patients with autonomic failure, the elderly, and those taking sympatholytic agents may exhibit large postprandial falls in blood pressure. Digestion shifts blood flow to the hepatic and splanchnic beds, and, as already noted, these patients are exquisitely sensitive to changes in circulating blood volume. In addition, several vasoactive substances such as histamine and adenosine, and a variety of vasodilatory gastrointestinal hormones, may be released into the circulation during a meal. Although their precise role in altering blood pressure is uncertain, these substances, acting either as local vasodilators or systemic hormones, can contribute to the hypotensive response. For example, simple measures such as a cup of coffee with meals may attenuate the postprandial hypotensive response, perhaps because of the ability of caffeine to block adenosine receptors. Presser agents should be administered in such a way that peak effects occur in the postprandial period when they are needed most. The depressor effect of meals can also be exploited in these patients. Those who have supine hypertension benefit from a small meal or snack at bedtime in order to lower their nocturnal blood pressure. This is especially important in those who have been receiving pressor agents during the day. Alcohol tends to lower blood pressure in these patients and can worsen symptoms. However, alcohol can be exploited in order to treat supine hypertension at night. We often advise our patients to have a glass of wine before retiring, as it elicits a fall of 10 to 20 mm Hg in blood pressure.

Patients should avoid excessive activity in the 2-hour period after meals, since at these times, especially after breakfast, they are most likely to have symptomatic orthostatic hypotension. Patients should also eat smaller meals and limit confections to minimize this effect. In diabetic patients, alterations in insulin levels and the consequences of hypoglycemia may dramatically affect blood pressure and autonomic function.[89] As strange as it may seem, the ingestion of tap water elicits a profound pressor response in most patients with autonomic failure. This effect of 16 oz of water is evident within several minutes, peaks at about 30 minutes, and is sustained for about 1 hour.[45]

Physical and Environmental Management. When autonomic reflexes fail, many physical maneuvers and life habits have a much greater effect on blood pressure than they have in normal subjects. This can be used to advantage in patient management. Wouter Wieling and his collaborators have introduced a range of simple physical maneuvers such as leg crossing or squatting that can improve the patient's ability to stand upright.[90-92]

A support garment that exerts graded pressure on the legs and abdomen, and increases interstitial hydrostatic pressure, is often helpful. When the patient stands, this hydrostatic pressure will tend to keep blood from pooling in the legs. However, patients must be cautioned not to wear these stockings at night or when supine, since they will increase central blood volume, contribute to diuresis, and decrease interstitial fluid in the legs. Support stockings are not of much help unless they go at least to the waist. In fact, an abdominal binder in association with elastic stockings is even more useful. This augments venous return from the splanchnic bed, a major source of venous pooling. Antigravity suits and shock trousers have been used in the past with some success, but can be awkward.

Increased abdominal and intrathoracic pressure significantly compromises venous return and can precipitate hypotension. Lifting heavy objects, reaching up, coughing, and straining at stool or with voiding can bring on hypotension. Working with one's arms above shoulder level (e.g., shaving) can lower pressure dramatically, because this maneuver and lifting are often accompanied by an unconscious Valsalva-like increase in thoracic pressure. Ambulation or shifting weight from leg to leg, as opposed to standing motionless, takes advantage of muscular pumping on the veins. A slightly stooped walking posture may be helpful to the most severely affected patients. Patients may hang their legs over the side of the bed before standing. This minimizes hemodynamic stress, since assumption of the upright posture is broken down into two movements: assumption of the seated posture and standing from the seated posture.

Some mechanical aids may allow patients to carry on activities of daily living more easily. For instance, a "derby chair" (a cane when folded, and a small seat when unfolded) can be used by severely affected patients to extend their walking range. Patients may use the cane for support while walking, and when symptoms ensue, they can unfold the chair and sit until they are ready to walk again. Recliner chairs are used so that patients can rest during the day without lying flat. This is especially important when pressor drugs are administered during the day, conferring added risk for supine hypertension.

Although exhaustive isometric exercise in normal subjects raises blood pressure via sympathetic activation, it can precipitate hypotension in patients with autonomic failure. A graded program of isotonic exercise such as walking may be beneficial.[93] More vigorous exercise such as jogging is rarely tolerated because of marked decreases in blood pressure that may occur. Climbing stairs is a common hypotensive stimulus. Exercise, even while a patient is supine, may cause hypotension.

The ideal exercise for patients with autonomic failure is swimming. While the patient is submerged in water, his or her tolerance of upright

BOX 47-2 SUMMARY OF TREATMENT FOR ORTHOSTATIC INTOLERANCE

Pharmacologic Treatments
- Fludrocortisone 0.05-0.1 mg once or twice a day orally, plus salt
- Low-dose propranolol 10-20 mg twice to four times a day orally
- Midodrine 2.5-10 mg three times a day orally
- Clonidine 0.05-0.1 mg twice a day orally
- Methyldopa 125-250 mg three times a day orally
- Recombinant erythropoietin, if necessary

Nonpharmacologic Treatments
- Mild exercise
- Consumption of 16 oz of water as prophylaxis against symptoms in the upright posture (lasts about 60-120 minutes)
- Acute 1-L intravenous saline infusion

posture is almost unlimited. In this situation, hydrostatic pressure prevents blood pooling in the legs and abdomen, and blood pressure is well maintained. We recommend that our patients undertake a graded program of swimming. Leaving the swimming pool, however, may pose difficulty. Furthermore, patients with Shy-Drager syndrome may find swimming more of a challenge if the extrapyramidal disease restricts their mobility.

Periods of inactivity and prolonged bed rest should be avoided, since they will worsen tolerance to standing. Prolonged bed rest, even in normal subjects, may cause mild orthostatic hypotension. Astronauts who are very physically fit experience orthostatic hypotension on return to Earth after the weightlessness of outer space. Even well-trained and healthy young pilots, during the positive G accelerations of aerial maneuvers, may experience quite severe hypotension leading to unconsciousness and seizures. Small wonder that, in severely affected patients with autonomic failure, quite mild acceleration, such as that encountered in an ordinary elevator, can bring on symptoms.

Other environmental stresses can also worsen orthostatic hypotension. Symptoms are more pronounced in hot weather. This is not so much due to volume loss from sweating (which is usually reduced) as to vasodilation and increased blood flow to the skin. In addition, fever in patients with autonomic failure may contribute markedly to orthostatic hypotension. Patients are also especially at risk in the shower or arising from a hot bath.

New Therapeutic Methods and Future Possibilities. While atrial tachypacing has been advocated in the management of autonomic failure, our results have been poor. This approach may be used with caution in the face of significant persistent bradycardia. Recently a novel therapeutic strategy, a bionic baroreflex system, has been proposed and its efficacy demonstrated in a model of sudden hypotension during surgery.[94] The bionic baroreflex system consisted of a computer-controlled negative feedback circuit that sensed arterial pressure and automatically computed the frequency of a pulse train required to stimulate sympathetic nerves via an epidural catheter placed at the level of the lower thoracic spinal cord. However, further clinical trials and evaluations are needed.

Management of Orthostatic Intolerance (Box 47-2)

Because orthostatic intolerance is such a heterogeneous disease and because its various pathophysiologies are still incompletely understood, it has been difficult to develop therapeutic regimens genuinely effective for everyone. The most commonly used agents are low-dose propranolol, fludrocortisone plus salt, midodrine, low-dose clonidine or methyldopa, and, where anemia is present, erythropoietin. The rationale for some of these drugs is to increase blood volume or vascular tone, while for others it is to attenuate the increased sympathetic tone. Acute intravenous saline infusion (1 L over 1 hour) is effective at acute heart rate control and improving symptoms.[95] In order to ensure adequate hydration, we recommend patients ingest 16 oz of water prophylactically to lower their heart rates.[96] Results are often disappointing with each of these therapies. Controlled trials conducted over a long period of time are needed to fully evaluate these and other approaches (e.g., phenobarbital, pyridostigmine, acetazolamide, hydralazine). Finally some patients benefit from an exercise program. This must be approached cautiously beginning in the most severely affected patients with no more than "orthostatic exercise," standing against a wall for incrementally increasing periods each day (see next section). More vigorous exercise programs are currently being studied.

BOX 47-3 SUMMARY OF TREATMENTS FOR NEURALLY MEDIATED SYNCOPE

Pharmacologic Treatments
- No drug proven effective yet.
- Selective serotonin reuptake inhibitors suggested to be helpful in some cases.

Nonpharmacologic Treatments
- Increase salt intake.
- Institute orthostatic training 30-40 minutes, one or two times per day.
- Cardiac pacemaker implantation is controversial.

Management of Neurally Mediated Syncope (Box 47-3)

Unlike most conditions discussed in this chapter, NMS is episodic. Most patients should simply be reassured about the usual benign course of NMS and instructed to avoid those situations that precipitate fainting. The use of increased salt intake may be helpful. They should be taught to recognize an impending faint and urged to lie down (or sit down if that is not possible) quickly. This will not be enough for some patients, and other treatment options may be necessary.

No drug has been proven to be of benefit in this disorder, but a number are sometimes used. Although salt replenishment and fludrocortisone have not been rigorously studied, they are both commonly used because of their low side effect profile and possible efficacy. A study is currently underway that will determine if fludrocortisone is of benefit. Although commonly used, there is only poor evidence for the effectiveness of β-blockers. The α_1-agonist midodrine has been reported to decrease the rate of recurrent syncope among frequent fainters, whereas another α_1-agonist, etilefrine, was not found to be useful. Orthostatic (standing) training has been suggested as an effective nonpharmacologic therapy for patients with recurrent NMS. This treatment involves having patients lean upright against a wall for 30 to 40 minutes one or two times per day. While the initial results from this therapy are quite promising, it has not yet been subjected to a proper trial.

Permanent dual-chamber pacemakers may reduce recurrent syncope among highly symptomatic patients with NMS, but their value remains controversial. This therapy is both expensive and invasive. At this time, permanent pacemaker implantation can rarely be recommended in therapy for NMS.[97]

Because bradycardia often occurs in association with syncopal attacks, agents that increase heart rate by reducing parasympathetic tone (disopyramide and other muscarinic antagonists) have been employed with varying degrees of success. In a carefully conducted study in a small number of subjects, Mosqueda-Garcia et al.[98] noted attenuated sympathetic activity on tilt and reasoned that enhancing sympathetic tone with a centrally acting α_2-adrenoreceptor antagonist might be beneficial. They showed significant improvement in orthostatic tolerance in patients with neurally mediated syncope in response to oral yohimbine.[98] A larger and more prolonged trial of this agent is needed.

Management of Baroreflex Failure (Box 47-4)

Treatment of baroreflex failure aims to reduce the frequency and magnitude of life-threatening surges in blood pressure and heart rate. A secondary goal of therapy is to attenuate symptomatic hypotensive

BOX 47-4 SUMMARY OF TREATMENTS FOR BAROREFLEX FAILURE

Pharmacologic Treatments

- Clonidine 0.6-2.5 mg a day orally (transdermal also effective)
- Propranolol LA 80 mg twice a day
- Benzodiazepine
- Low-dose fludrocortisone (0.05 mg once or twice a day orally) plus salt for hypotensive episode

Nonpharmacologic Treatments

- Calming self-controlling method, such as biofeedback
- Cardiac pacemaker implantation for severe bradycardia (<40 bpm)

episodes. The pharmacologic treatment of choice for blood pressure surges is clonidine. This is a physiologic approach to treatment because this agent acts centrally and peripherally to attenuate sympathetic activation, and limit the extent to which pressor surges can occur. Also, clonidine may increase the baroreflex sensitivity.[99] The nonspecific α-adrenoreceptor blocker phenoxybenzamine has been relatively unsuccessful in reducing the frequency of pressor surges, though the magnitude of surges (but not tachycardia) is controlled. The sedative effects of the α_2-adrenoreceptor agonists such as clonidine may assist patients in preventing hypertensive episodes. The initial sustained hypertension phase requires hospitalization in an intensive care unit and control with nitroprusside and sympatholytic agents. In the first 2 or 3 days, apneic spells occasionally occur when powerful pain medications are employed, so monitoring is necessary. Once the chronic labile phase is reached, clonidine, either orally or in the form of a clonidine patch, is extremely effective, but quite high doses (0.6 to 2.5 mg daily in divided doses) are sometimes initially required. While commencement with 0.1 mg three times daily is usual, escalation every other day may be required until blood pressure surges are brought under control. Such agents may make hypotensive episodes worse in some patients.

A practical point in the management of patients in the first few weeks after baroreflex failure develops is recognition of the relationship between emotional upset and pressor crises. Patients may over time learn to control the onset of the pressor crises (usually recognized by flushing or headache) by exerting calming self-control. Thus, in some cases, the patient may develop a spontaneous biofeedback treatment of his or her disorder that may result in a reduction in both the number and severity of attacks. Over long periods of time, most patients may be graduated from clonidine to benzodiazepine with continued adequate control.

The patient with selective baroreflex failure may have the additional problem of episodic malignant vagotonia, especially severe bradycardia (<40 bpm). In such patients, therapy may have to begin with placement of a pacemaker to prevent cardiac arrest.

Until its withdrawal from the American market owing to declining use, the sympathoplegic agent guanethidine was the treatment of choice for baroreflex failure with excessive hypertension. Some compounding pharmacies may still provide it. However, in some patients, prevention of hypotension is also required. This is quite difficult, as the hypotensive episodes are usually short lived and most agents have a longer half-life than the hypotensive spell duration. In spite of all its difficulties, fludrocortisone may still be the best way to treat this problem. Since some patients with baroreflex failure have reduced plasma volume as well, fludrocortisone along with high salt intake might have beneficial effects on this variable. Generally, low doses (0.05 mg twice a day) are all that is required. Noteworthy, though, is that fludrocortisone requires a week or two for its full effect to be realized.

SUMMARY

Patients with disorders of the autonomic nerve system are often referred to clinical pharmacologists for evaluation and therapy. The evaluation of such patients entails the application of a combination of physiologic, pharmacologic, and biochemical tests at the bedside. Subsequent tailoring of the optimal therapeutic regimen is driven by these clinical pharmacologic interventions. Few medical conditions in the 21st century are as dependent on bedside clinical acumen and application of pharmacologic probes as disorders of the autonomic nervous system.

REFERENCES

1. Mathias CJ, Bannister R. Autonomic Failure: A Textbook of Clinical Disorders of the Autonomic Nervous System. Oxford, UK: Oxford University Press, 2002.
2. Goldstein DS. The Autonomic Nervous System in Health and Disease. New York: Marcel Dekker, 2001.
3. Robertson D, Biaggioni I, Burnstock G, Low PA. Primer on the Autonomic Nervous Sustem, 2nd ed. Amsterdam: Elsevier, 2004.
4. Elefteriou F, Ahn JD, Takeda S, et al. Leptin regulation of bone resorption by the sympathetic nervous system and CART. Nature 2005;434:514-520.
5. Savage DD, Corwin L, McGee DL, et al. Epidemiologic features of isolated syncope: the Framingham Study. Stroke 1985;16:626-629.
6. Chen LY, Shen WK, Mahoney DW, et al. Prevalence of self-reported syncope: an epidemiologic study from Olmsted County, MN. J Am Coll Cardiol 2002;39:114A-115A.
7. Day SC, Cook EF, Funkenstein H, Goldman L. Evaluation and outcome of emergency room patients with transient loss of consciousness. Am J Med 1982;73:15-23.
8. Strickberger SA, Benson DW, Biaggioni I, et al. AHA/ACCF Scientific Statement on the evaluation of syncope: from the American Heart Association Councils on Clinical Cardiology, Cardiovascular Nursing, Cardiovascular Disease in the Young, and Stroke, and the Quality of Care and Outcomes Research Interdisciplinary Working Group, and the American College of Cardiology Foundation, in collaboration with the Heart Rhythm Society; endorsed by the American Autonomic Society 74. Circulation 2006;113:316-327.
9. Sheldon R, Rose S, Koshman ML. Comparison of patients with syncope of unknown cause having negative or positive tilt-table tests. Am J Cardiol 1997;80:581-585.
10. Rose MS, Koshman ML, Spreng S, Sheldon R. The relationship between health-related quality of life and frequency of spells in patients with syncope. J Clin Epidemiol 2000;53:1209-1216.
11. Sheldon R, Koshman ML, Wilson W, et al. Effect of dual-chamber pacing with automatic rate-drop sensing on recurrent neurally mediated syncope. Am J Cardiol 1998;81:158-162.
12. Raj SR, Sheldon RS. Syncope: investigation and treatment. Curr Cardiol Rep 2002;4:363-370.
13. Jardine DL, Krediet CT, Cortelli P, Wieling W. Fainting in your sleep? Clin Auton Res 2006;16:76-78.
14. Jacob G, Ertl AC, Shannon JR, et al. Effect of standing on neurohumoral responses and plasma volume in healthy subjects. J Appl Physiol 1998;84:914-921.
15. Jacob G, Raj SK, Ketch T, et al. Postural pseudoanemia: posture-dependent change in hematocrit. Mayo Clin Proc 2005;80:611-614.
16. Landgren S. On the excitation mechanism of the carotid baroceptors. Acta Physiol Scand 1952;26:1-34.
17. Spyer KM. The central nervous organization of reflex circulatory control. In Loewy AD, Spyer KM (eds): Central Regulation of Autonomic Function. New York: Oxford University Press, 1990, pp 168-188.
18. Sharpey-Schafer EP. Syncope. Br Med J 1956;1:506-509.
19. Mark AL. The Bezold-Jarisch reflex revisited: clinical implications of inhibitory reflexes originating in the heart. J Am Coll Cardiol 1983;1:90-102.
20. Tarazi RC, Dustan HP, Frohlich ED, et al. Plasma volume and chronic hypertension. Relationship to arterial pressure levels in different hypertensive diseases. Arch Intern Med 1970;125:835-842.
21. Jaeger FJ, Maloney JD, Castle LW, Fouad-Tarazi FM. Is absolute hypovolemia a risk factor for vasovagal response to head-up tilt? Pacing Clin Electrophysiol 1993;16(4 Pt 1):743-750.
22. Oberg B, Thoren P. Increased activity in left ventricular receptors during hemorrhage or occlusion of caval veins in the cat: a possible cause of the vaso-vagal reaction. Acta Physiol Scand 1972;85:164-173.
23. Fitzpatrick AP, Banner N, Cheng A, et al. Vasovagal reactions may occur after orthotopic heart transplantation. J Am Coll Cardiol 1993;21:1132-1137.
24. Lightfoot JT, Rowe SA, Fortney SM. Occurrence of presyncope in subjects without ventricular innervation. Clin Sci (Lond) 1993;85:695-700.
25. Morgan-Hughes NJ, Kenny RA, Scott CD, et al. Vasodepressor reactions after orthotopic cardiac transplantation: relationship to reinnervation status. Clin Auton Res 1994;4:125-129.
26. Scherrer U, Vissing S, Morgan BJ, et al. Vasovagal syncope after infusion of a vasodilator in a heart-transplant recipient. N Engl J Med 1990;322:602-604.
27. Wallin BG, Sundlof G. Sympathetic outflow to muscles during vasovagal syncope. J Auton Nerv Syst 1982;6:287-291.
28. Ziegler MG, Echon C, Wilner KD, et al. Sympathetic nervous withdrawal in the vasodepressor (vasovagal) reaction. J Auton Nerv Syst 1986;17:273-278.
29. The Steering Committee of the ISSUE. International Study on Syncope of Uncertain Etiology 2: the management of patients with suspected or certain neurally mediated syncope after the initial evaluation. Rationale and study design. Europace 2003;5:317-321.
30. Raj SR, Biaggioni I, Yamhure PC, et al. Renin-aldosterone paradox and perturbed blood volume regulation underlying postural tachycardia syndrome. Circulation 2005;111:1574-1582.

31. Shannon JR, Flattem NL, Jordan J, et al. Orthostatic intolerance and tachycardia associated with norepinephrine-transporter deficiency. N Engl J Med 2000;342:541-549.
32. Kim CH, Hahn MK, Joung Y, et al. A polymorphism in the norepinephrine transporter gene alters promoter activity and is associated with attention-deficit hyperactivity disorder. Proc Natl Acad Sci U S A 2006;103:19164-19169.
33. Shibao C, Arzubiaga C, Roberts LJ, et al. Hyperadrenergic postural tachycardia syndrome in mast cell activation disorders. Hypertension 2005;45:385-390.
34. Buckey JC Jr, Lane LD, Levine BD, et al. Orthostatic intolerance after spaceflight. J Appl Physiol 1996;81:7-18.
35. Alfrey CP, Udden MM, Leach-Huntoon C, et al. Control of red blood cell mass in spaceflight. J Appl Physiol 1996;81:98-104.
36. Johnson PC, Driscokk TB, Leblanc AC. Blood volume changes. In Johnston RS, Dietlein LE (eds): Biomedical Results from Skylab. Washington, DC: National Aeronautics and Space Administration, 1997, pp 235-241.
37. Ertl AC, Diedrich A, Biaggioni I, et al. Human muscle sympathetic nerve activity and plasma noradrenaline kinetics in space. J Physiol (Lond) 2002;538(Pt 1):321-329.
38. Mabuchi N, Hirayama M, Koike Y, et al. Progression and prognosis in pure autonomic failure (PAF): comparison with multiple system atrophy. J Neurol Neurosurg Psychiatry 2005;76:947-952.
39. Seppi K, Schocke MF, Wenning GK, Poewe W. How to diagnose MSA early: the role of magnetic resonance imaging. J Neural Transm 2005;111:1574-1582.
40. Geser F, Wenning GK, Poewe W, McKeith I. How to diagnose dementia with Lewy bodies: state of the art. Mov Disord 2005;20(Suppl 12):S11-S20.
41. Ziegler MG, Lake CR, Kopin IJ. The sympathetic-nervous-system defect in primary orthostatic hypotension. N Engl J Med 1977;296:293-297.
42. Goldstein DS, Holmes C, Cannon RO, et al. Sympathetic cardioneuropathy in dysautonomias. N Engl J Med 1997;336:696-702.
43. Consensus Committee of the American Autonomic Society and American Academy of Neurology. Consensus statement on the definition of orthostatic hypotension, pure autonomic failure, and multiple system atrophy. Neurology 1996;46:1470.
44. Wenning GK, Tison F, Ben SY, et al. Multiple system atrophy: a review of 203 pathologically proven cases. Mov Disord 1997;12:133-147.
45. Jordan J, Shannon JR, Black BK, et al. Malignant vagotonia due to selective baroreflex failure. Hypertension 1997;30:1072-1077.
46. Papp MI, Lantos PL. Accumulation of tubular structures in oligodendroglial and neuronal cells as the basic alteration in multiple system atrophy. J Neurol Sci 1992;107:172-182.
47. Wenning GK, Geser F, Poewe W. Therapeutic strategies in multiple system atrophy. Mov Disord 2005;20(Suppl 12):S67-S76.
48. Freeman R. Treatment of orthostatic hypotension. Semin Neurol 2003;23:435-442.
49. Robertson D, Garland EM. Dopamine beta hydroxylase deficiency. GeneClinics 2005; (3). Available at: *http://www.geneclinics.org/servlet/access?db=geneclinics&id=8888891&key=YFQfVXIfQFoXz&gry=&fcn=y&fw=1017&filename=/profiles/dbh/index.html*
50. Bristow JD, Honour AJ, Pickering GW, et al. Diminished baroreflex sensitivity in high blood pressure. Circulation 1969;39:48-54.
51. Osculati G, Grassi G, Giannattasio C, et al. Early alterations of the baroreceptor control of heart rate in patients with acute myocardial infarction. Circulation 1990;81:939-948.
52. La Rovere MT, Bigger JT Jr, Marcus FI, et al. Baroreflex sensitivity and heart-rate variability in prediction of total cardiac mortality after myocardial infarction. ATRAMI (Autonomic Tone and Reflexes After Myocardial Infarction) Investigators. Lancet 1998;351:478-484.
53. Timmers HJ, Wieling W, Karemaker JM, Lenders JW. Denervation of carotid baro- and chemoreceptors in humans. J Physiol (Lond) 2003;553(Pt 1):3-11.
54. Annane D, Baudrie V, Blanc AS, et al. Short-term variability of blood pressure and heart rate in Guillain-Barre syndrome without respiratory failure. Clin Sci (Lond) 1999;96:613-621.
55. Girard A, Sidi D, Aggoun Y, et al. Elastin mutation is associated with a reduced gain of the baroreceptor–heart rate reflex in patients with Williams syndrome. Clin Auton Res 2002;12:72-77.
56. Trang H, Girard A, Laude D, Elghozi JL. Short-term blood pressure and heart rate variability in congenital central hypoventilation syndrome (Ondine's curse). Clin Sci (Lond) 2005;108:225-230.
57. Elghozi JL, Girard A, Ribstein J. Baroreflex failure syndrome: an uncommon case of an extreme blood pressure variability. Rev Med Interne 2001;22:1261-1268.
58. Parati G, Di Rienzo M, Mancia G. How to measure baroreflex sensitivity: from the cardiovascular laboratory to daily life. J Hypertens 2000;18:7-19.
59. Di Rienzo M, Castiglioni P, Mancia G, et al. Advancements in estimating baroreflex function. IEEE Eng Med Biol Mag 2001;20(2):25-32.
60. Laude D, Elghozi JL, Girard A, et al. Comparison of various techniques used to estimate spontaneous baroreflex sensitivity (the EuroBaVar study). Am J Physiol Regul Integr Comp Physiol 2004;286:R226-R231.
61. Chobanian AV, Volicer L, Tifft CP, et al. Mineralocorticoid-induced hypertension in patients with orthostatic hypotension. N Engl J Med 1979;301:68-73.
62. McTavish D, Goa KL. Midodrine: a review of its pharmacological properties and therapeutic use in orthostatic hypotension and secondary hypotensive disorders. Drugs 1989;38:757-777.
63. Goldberg MR, Robertson D. Yohimbine: a pharmacological probe for study of the alpha 2-adrenoreceptor. Pharmacol Rev 1983;35:143-180.
64. Onrot J, Goldberg MR, Biaggioni I, et al. Oral yohimbine in human autonomic failure. Neurology 1987;37:215-220.
65. Onrot J, Goldberg MR, Hollister AS, et al. Management of chronic orthostatic hypotension. Am J Med 1986;80:454-464.
66. Freeman R, Young J, Landsberg L, Lipsitz L. The treatment of postprandial hypotension in autonomic failure with 3,4-DL-threo-dihydroxyphenylserine. Neurology 1996;47:1414-1420.
67. Robertson D, Goldberg MR, Hollister AS, et al. Clonidine raises blood pressure in severe idiopathic orthostatic hypotension. Am J Med 1983;74:193-200.
68. Biaggioni I, Robertson RM, Robertson D. Manipulation of norepinephrine metabolism with yohimbine in the treatment of autonomic failure. J Clin Pharmacol 1994;34:418-423.
69. Kaufmann H. Could treatment with DOPS do for autonomic failure what DOPA did for Parkinson's disease? Neurology 1996;47:1370-1371.
70. Seibyl JP, Krystal JH, Price LH, Charney DS. Use of yohimbine to counteract nortriptyline-induced orthostatic hypotension. J Clin Psychopharmacol 1989;9:67-68.
71. Biaggioni I, Robertson D, Krantz S, et al. The anemia of primary autonomic failure and its reversal with recombinant erythropoietin. Ann Intern Med 1994;121:181-186.
72. Hoeldtke RD, Streeten DH. Treatment of orthostatic hypotension with erythropoietin. N Engl J Med 1993;329:611-615.
73. Heidenreich S, Rahn KH, Zidek W. Direct vasopressor effect of recombinant human erythropoietin on renal resistance vessels. Kidney Int 1991;39:259-265.
74. Onrot J, Bernard GR, Biaggioni I, et al. Direct vasodilator effect of hyperventilation-induced hypocarbia in autonomic failure patients. Am J Med Sci 1991;301:305-309.
75. Robertson D, Wade D, Robertson RM. Postprandial alterations in cardiovascular hemodynamics in autonomic dysfunction states. Am J Cardiol 1981;48:1048-1052.
76. Burnum JF, Hickam JB, Stead EA. Hyperventilation in postural hypotension. Circulation 1954;10:362-365.
77. Feely J, Wade D, McAllister CB, et al. Effect of hypotension on liver blood flow and lidocaine disposition. N Engl J Med 1982;307:866-869.
78. Kronenberg MW, Forman MB, Onrot J, Robertson D. Enhanced left ventricular contractility in autonomic failure: assessment using pressure-volume relations. J Am Coll Cardiol 1990;15:1334-1342.
79. Parris WCV, Goldberg MR, Hollister AS, Robertson D. The anesthetic management of autonomic dysfunction. Anesthesiol Rev 1984;11:17-23.
80. MacLean AR, Allen EV, Magath TB. Orthostatic tachycardia and orthostatic hypotension: defects in the return of venous blood to the heart. Am Heart J 1944;27:145-163.
81. Hoeldtke RD, Cavanaugh ST, Hughes JD. Treatment of orthostatic hypotension: interaction of pressor drugs and tilt table conditioning. Arch Phys Med Rehabil 1988;69:895-898.
82. Jordan J, Shannon JR, Pohar B, et al. Contrasting effects of vasodilators on blood pressure and sodium balance in the hypertension of autonomic failure. J Am Soc Nephrol 1999;10:35-42.
83. Bachman D, Youmans WB. Effects of posture on renal excretion of sodium and chloride in orthostatic hypotension. Circulation 1953;7:413-421.
84. Gordon RD, Kuchel O, Liddle GW, Island DP. Role of the sympathetic nervous system in regulating renin and aldosterone production in man. J Clin Invest 1967;46:599-605.
85. Wilcox CS, Puritz R, Lightman SL, et al. Plasma volume regulation in patients with progressive autonomic failure during changes in salt intake or posture. J Lab Clin Med 1984;104:331-339.
86. Sanders AO. Postural hypotension with tachycardia: a case report. Am Heart J 1932;7:808-813.
87. Robertson RM, Robertson D. The Bezold-Jarisch reflex: possible role in limiting myocardial ischemia. Clin Cardiol 1981;4:75-79.
88. Jansen RW, Lipsitz LA. Postprandial hypotension: epidemiology, pathophysiology, and clinical management. Ann Intern Med 1995;122:286-295.
89. Davis SN, Shavers C, Davis B, Costa F. Prevention of an increase in plasma cortisol during hypoglycemia preserves subsequent counterregulatory responses. J Clin Invest 1997;100:429-438.
90. Wieling W, Colman N, Krediet CT, Freeman R. Nonpharmacological treatment of reflex syncope. Clin Auton Res 2004;14(Suppl 1):62-70.
91. Krediet CT, de Bruin IG, Ganzeboom KS, et al. Leg crossing, muscle tensing, squatting, and the crash position are effective against vasovagal reactions solely through increases in cardiac output. J Appl Physiol 2005;99:1697-1703.
92. van Dijk N, Quartieri F, Blanc JJ, et al. Effectiveness of physical counterpressure maneuvers in preventing vasovagal syncope: the Physical Counterpressure Manoeuvres Trial (PC-Trial). J Am Coll Cardiol 2006;48:1652-1657.
93. Youmans JB, Akeroyd JH, Frank H. Changes in the blood and circulation with changes in posture: the effect of exercise and vasodilatation. J Clin Invest 1935;14:739-753.
94. Yamasaki F, Ushida T, Yokoyama T, et al. Artificial baroreflex: clinical application of a bionic baroreflex system. Circulation 2006;113:634-639.
95. Jacob G, Shannon JR, Black B, et al. Effects of volume loading and pressor agents in idiopathic orthostatic tachycardia. Circulation 1997;96:575-580.
96. Shannon JR, Diedrich A, Biaggioni I, et al. Water drinking as a treatment for orthostatic syndromes. Am J Med 2002;112:355-360.
97. Mosqueda-Garcia R, Furlan R, Tank J, Fernandez-Violante R. The elusive pathophysiology of neurally mediated syncope. Circulation 2000;102:2898-2906.
98. Mosqueda-Garcia R, Fernandez-Violante R, Tank J, et al. Yohimbine in neurally mediated syncope: pathophysiological implications. J Clin Invest 1998;102:1824-1830.
99. Tank J, Jordan J, Diedrich A, et al. Clonidine improves spontaneous baroreflex sensitivity in conscious mice through parasympathetic activation. Hypertension 2004;43:1042-1047.

48

HEADACHE

Alfredo Bianchi

OVERVIEW 719
INTRODUCTION 719
General Concepts 719
Historical Notes 719
PATHOPHYSIOLOGY 720
Theories of Primary Headache Pathogenesis 724
THERAPEUTICS AND CLINICAL PHARMACOLOGY 725
Goals of Therapy and Therapeutic Approach 725
Therapeutics by Class 726
Acute Abortive Therapy of Headache Attacks 726
Prophylactic or Preventive Therapy 734
Adjuvant Pharmacotherapeutic Strategies 736
Emerging Targets and Therapeutics 737

OVERVIEW

Headache, or cephalalgia—a disturbance consisting in a painful state located in one or more parts of the head, as well as in the back of the neck—may have many different causes. In accordance with the 2004 classification of the International Headache Society,[1] headache is categorized in three different groups: (i) primary or direct headaches (headache as a disease: no other causative disorders); (ii) secondary headaches (headache as a symptom: caused by or attributed to another disorder); and (iii) cranial neuralgias, central and primary facial pain, and other headaches. In the first group are included, with their respective subtypes: (a) migraine with and without aura, (b) tension-type headache, (c) cluster headache and other trigeminal autonomic cephalalgias (TACs), and (d) other primary headaches. The second group encompasses headaches secondary to (a) head or neck traumas; (b) cranial or cervical vascular disorders; (c) intracranial nonvascular disorders; (d) drug usage or withdrawal; (e) infections; (f) homeostatic disorders; (g) disorders of facial or cranial structures; and (h) psychiatric disorders. The third group comprises headache-like syndromes or headaches of uncertain origin and nature.

This chapter deals mostly with primary headaches and the fourth subgroup of secondary headaches, those connected to drug abuse, which are frequently associated with primary headaches. In consideration of the multiple possible pathogeneses of headaches, which are not yet clearly defined for primary headaches, their therapy involves a broad variety of drugs, either symptomatic or prophylactic. Patients with secondary headaches and headaches of the third group must be evaluated for the differential diagnosis necessary for correct pharmacologic therapy.

Triptans and fast-acting nonsteroidal anti-inflammatory drugs (NSAIDs) are employed in the preventive treatment of painful headache attacks. Among the various prophylactic or preventive drugs, also directed to counteract trigger factors, antidepressants and antiepileptics, β-blockers, and calcium antagonists have a prominent role. Vitamins, coenzymes, minerals, and nutriceuticals in general represent valuable adjuvant pharmacotherapeutic strategies. Psychotherapy and other extrapharmacologic therapies may be useful adjuncts to pharmacotherapy, as may be an accurate evaluation of precipitating factors (see Box 48-2 later) and the adoption of measures able to avoid or limit their influence on disease onset and severity.

INTRODUCTION

General Concepts

Primary headaches occur in populations all over the world (>12% for migraine and tension-type headache). Their main sign is a nociceptive pain generated in the trigeminal-vascular complex related to the meningeal dural territory. These headaches may be preceded, in the forms defined as "with aura," by focal neurologic phenomena, mostly visual but also sensory or motor, lasting between 5 and 60 minutes. The intensity of painful attacks can be moderate to very strong and their frequency often gradually increases; their duration, long lasting for migraine and tension-type-headache, is short or variable in other forms. Because of these characteristics and associated signs, among which the most recurrent are intolerance to light, noise, odors, and movement, primary headaches may markedly impair the quality of life.

Among secondary headaches, according to their etiology, are grouped a large number of syndromes, having different natures, clinical evolution, and prognoses ranging from quite severe to very mild and quickly reversible.

Historical Notes

Headaches were well known in remote antiquity—migraine is clearly mentioned in the Ebers papyrus, written more than 1550 years ago but probably based on older documents. On stone tablets at the Epidaurus temple, of the prehippocratic period, is recorded the history of Agestratos, a young man suffering fom headache who dreamed of being cured by Asclepius and then recovered so well that shortly afterward he won the Nemean games of wrestling. At the time of Hippocrates (460-370 BC), there was the first description of visual symptoms associated with migraine and of some secondary forms of headache. Remarkable progress was made in the Roman age by Cornelius Celsus, Areteus of Cappodocia, and especially Galen, the author of the term *hemicrania*, later known as "migraine" in French and English, for which he gave the first precise definition.

In middle ages, the famous Salerno Medical School, the Arabian physicians Abucalsis and Avicenna, Hildegard of Bingen, Maimonides, and the authors of the *Codex Vindobonensis* were advancing the work of the Greeks and Romans. In the following centuries, Le Pois and Tissot from France, Wepfer from Switzerland, Willis and Liveing from England, Ramazzini from Italy, and others added new important pillars in the knowledge of headaches. However, the treatment of headaches, apart from a few exceptions such as caffeine and feverfew (still included in the modern therapeutic armamentarium), remained archaic and scarcely efficacious until a few decades ago, thus justifying the famous comment of George Bernard Shaw, who, after recovering from a devastating headache attack, asked the Arctic explorer Nansen whether he had discovered a cure for this disease. When Nansen, amazed, denied that he had, Shaw replied: "Well, it is most astonishing that you have spent your life in trying to discover the North Pole, which nobody on earth cares two pence about and you have never attempted to discover a cure for the headache, which every living person is crying aloud for."

The first specific treatment for headache was ergotamine tartrate, which was introduced before and consolidated after the report of Graham and Wolff[2] and the subsequent studies of Wolff.[3,4] Since the discovery of triptans, the therapy of headaches has progressed. Recently, a number of molecules possessing symptomatic or preventive activity have been discovered, and new targets are arising every day. It is difficult to forecast what developments will occur in this field over the next 10 years.

PATHOPHYSIOLOGY

The pain sensation, contributing to the preservation of homeostatic balance, is elicited by the activation of specific receptors situated in peripheral nerve fibers, at the level of cutaneous and visceral structures (see Chapter 61, Treatment of Pain; and Chapter 87, Over-the-Counter Medications). Following physical and chemical stimuli, they produce action potentials able to carry painful afferent messages along primary sensory neurons of the spinal dorsal roots and, thereafter, along second-order sensory neurons, reaching thalamocortical centers. The conduction of these messages shows significant variability, according to the dimension and myelinization of the nociceptive fibers. A delta fibers—myelinated, of small diameter (2 to 3 μm), and slow conducting (5 to 25/msec)—as well as C fibers—unmyelinated, of very small diameter (0.3 to 1.3 μm), and very slow conducting (0.1 to 2.0/msec)—both of which are largely distributed in meninges, are involved in migraine and other primary headaches pain (Fig. 48-1 and Table 48-1).[5,6] Their electrical stimulation, in animal experimental models, provokes the release of endogenous neuropeptides such as calcitonin gene–related peptide (CGRP), neurokinin A (NKA), and substance P (SP), all of which play fundamental roles in the induction of migraine.

Nociceptors are sensitized by noxious agents produced in inflammatory or traumatic events and acting as endogenous triggers (Table 48-2).[7] Hydrogen (H^+) or potassium (K^+) ions, bradykinin, histamine, and serotonin, liberated by inflamed tissues, activate nociceptors with different mechanisms. Following the stimulation of serotonin receptors, specific ionic channels are open. Through its B2 receptors, bradykinin induces the synthesis, mediated by the enzyme phospholipase C,

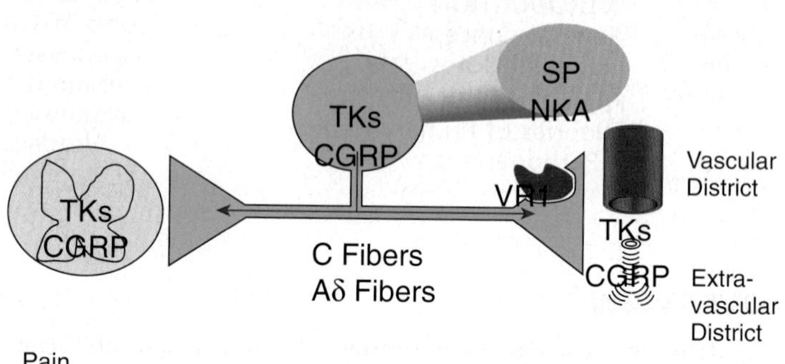

FIGURE 48-1 • Main characteristics of primary sensitive neurons. TKs, tachykinins.

TABLE 48-1 SUSCEPTIBILITY OF VARIOUS TYPES OF NERVE FIBERS TO BLOCKADE

Conduction Biophysical Classification	Anatomic Location	Myelin	Diameter (μm)	Conduction Velocity (m/sec)	Function
A fibers					
A alpha, A beta	Afferent to and efferent from muscles and joints	Yes	6-22	10-85	Motor and proprioception
A gamma	Efferent to muscle spindles	Yes	3-6	15-35	Muscle tone
A delta	Sensory roots and afferent peripheral nerves	Yes	1-4	5-25	Pain, temperature, touch
B fibers	Preganglionic sympathetic	Yes	<3	3-15	Vasomotor, visceromotor, sudomotor, pilomotor
C fibers					
Sympathetic	Postganglionic sympathetic	No	0.3-1.3	0.7-1.3	Vasomotor, visceromotor, sudomotor, pilomotor
Dorsal root	Sensory roots and afferent peripheral nerves	No	0.4-1.2	0.1-2.0	Pain, temperature, touch

Adapted from Carpenter RL, Mackey DC. Local anesthetics. In Barash PG, Cullen BF, Stoelting RK (eds): Clinical Anesthesia. Philadelphia: Lippincott, 1992, pp 509-541.

TABLE 48-2 SUBSTANCES RELEASED DURING INFLAMMATION ABLE TO ACTIVATE OR SENSITIZE NOCICEPTORS

Substance	Source	Activity on Primary Afferent Fibers
K^+ or H^+	Injured cells	Activation
Serotonin	Platelets	Activation
Bradykinin	Plasmatic kyninogen	Activation
Histamine	Mast cells	Activation
Prostaglandins	Injured cells, macrophages	Sensitization
Substance P, neurokinin A, calcitonin gene–related peptide	Primary afferent fibers	Sensitization

Data from Bianchi A, Caraci F, Salomone S. The pain in primary headache. In Capasso A (ed): Recent Developments in Pain Research. Trivandrum, India: Research Signpost, 2005, pp 343-357.

of the intracellular second messenger inositol triphosphate and of diacylglycerol (DG). Protein kinase C, activated by diacylglycerol, raises the conductance for Na^+ and Ca^{2+}, thereby eliciting, through an action potential, the release of CGRP, SP, and NKA, which are able to induce vasodilation and increase vascular permeability.

Peripheral endings of sensory nociceptive neurons can also exert efferent functions. A subgroup of them are sensitive to the excitatory and desensitizing activities of capsaicin, which is able to mediate the synthesis of neuropeptides in their cell bodies. At the peripheral nerve endings, a low pH present in inflamed tissues because of the high content of protons may induce antidromic reflexes and release of vasoactive neuropeptides, as well as passage in the interstitial spaces of kininogen, the precursor of bradykinin. The subsequent synthesis of bradykinin further amplifies this vicious circle, stimulating the synthesis and release of histamine, serotonin, and prostaglandins, especially prostaglandin E_2 (PGE_2). While the first two substances directly excite polymodal nociceptors, PGE_2, produced by the enzymatic activity of cyclooxygenase (COX) on its substrate arachidonic acid in mast cells, macrophages, and other inflammatory cells, provokes hyperalgesia at the level of injured tissues, mostly through a nociceptor sensitization. Allodynia, which is a consequence, becomes evident and therefore could be defined as the "marker" of the sensitization (see Box 48-4 later). Actually, these events decrease the action potential threshold, facilitating the activation of nociceptive fibers. As a result of this sequence, afferent endings of sensory capsaicin-sensitive neurons are stimulated, with increase of intracellular cyclic AMP levels and consequent activation of protein kinase A, phosphorylating both voltage-dependent Ca^{2+} channels and tetrodotoxin-resistant Na^+ channels. All these phenomena are thought to happen in connection with neuronal stimulations in a syndrome known as neurogenic inflammation.[8] The mechanism of action of aspirin and other NSAIDs, employed in the therapy of migraine pain and related symptoms, is based on the reduction of prostaglandins synthesis (see Chapter 11, Inflammation and Immunomodulation), subsequent to the inhibition of COX-1 and COX-2.

At the level of the sensory neurons are located several receptors able to modulate pain generation and propagation (Table 48-3). Afferent fibers of nociceptive primary neurons, ending in the superficial part of the ipsilateral spinal horn, form synaptic connections with second-order excitatory glutamatergic neurons. Glutamate activates different types of receptors (ionotropic and metabotropic) at central and peripheral sites. α-Amino-3-hydroxy-5-methyl-4-isoxazolepropionic acid (AMPA) and kainate receptors (ionotropic) provoke excitatory postsynaptic potentials (EPSPs), with a rapid onset and a short duration (a few milliseconds). *N*-methyl-D-aspartate (NMDA) receptors, also ionotropic, induce slower EPSPs, lasting about 100 msec. Metabotropic glutamate receptors (mGluR) play an important modulating role in the hyperalgesic response, some positive (mGluR4 and mGluR6-8) and others negative (mGluR1 and mGluR5). Through G proteins, these receptors activate intracellular metabolic pathways. The phosphorylation of intracellular substrates, such as ionic channels, is able to modulate different phases of synaptic transmission, and the activation of mGluR5 can also increase the sensitivity of ionotropic receptors for glutamate itself. All glutamate receptors seem to be involved in the phenomenon of central sensitization and consequent hyperalgesia.[9,10]

Cortical spreading depression (CSD) is characterized by a massive failure of ion homeostasis associated with a transient cessation of neuronal function and believed to be involved in migraine pathogenesis. It requires the release of glutamate and NMDA receptors, which play a crucial role in the propagation of this process.[9,10] Electrical stimulation in the presence of ifenprodil, a selective NMDA receptor antagonist, of murine brain entorhinal cortex slices containing the NMDA receptor-mediated component of extracellularly recorded field EPSPs, is nearly unable to reproduce CSD.[11]

In anesthetized cats, by recording the trigeminal-cervical complex function evoked by the electrical stimulation of the superior sagittal sinus and activated by L-glutamate, it has been shown that CGRP receptor antagonists α-CGRP and BIBN4096BS, given by microiontophoresis onto neurons of the trigeminal-vascular complex or intravenously, significantly inhibit the evoked activity. These data suggest that there are non-presynaptic CGRP receptors in the trigeminal-cervical complex that can be inhibited by CGRP receptor blockade, and therefore that a CGRP receptor antagonist could be effective in the acute treatment of migraine and cluster headache.[12] An in vitro study in human embryonic kidney has shown that a selective and noncompetitive Glu-K5 antagonist is able to inhibit L-glutamate and domoate-evoked currents, blocking the kainate subtype of glutamatergic receptors.[13] Nociceptive spinal neurons present a high degree of plasticity, revealed by the increased intensity and duration of neuronal discharges after repeated injuries and prolonged activation of C fibers. Windup and long-term potentiation processes could be jointly responsible for the chronic pain manifestations that are at the basis of chronic migraine. Windup and long-term potentiation are fundamental in NMDA receptor activation,[14] which induces an increase in intracellular Ca^{2+} concentration, thereby stimulating nitric oxide synthase (NOS), a Ca^{2+}/calmodulin-dependent enzyme, able to increase the formation of nitric oxide (NO). This last compound is active at the location where it is produced as well as in the extracellular space (reached by diffusion), where it stimulates the guanylate cyclases of adjacent neuronal endings. This provokes a further release of glutamate,[9,15,16] with the involvement of inhibitory transmitters such as opioids, adenosine, and γ-aminobutyric acid (GABA), which have a balancing role in inflammatory conditions. This phenomenon does not happen in neuropathic states because of the nerve damage. The transmission of nociceptive messages from afferent primary fibers as well as the activity of spinal nociceptive neurons are modulated by presynaptic and postsynaptic mechanisms, through GABAergic, glycinergic, purinergic, and enkephalinergic spinal interneurons.[14] The repeated and intense stimulation of NMDA receptors occurring during migraine attacks and the

TABLE 48-3 RECEPTORS PRESENT AT THE LEVEL OF SENSORY PRIMARY NEURONS AND POSSIBLE EFFECTS ON THE RELEASE OF NEUROPEPTIDES INVOLVED IN NEUROGENIC INFLAMMATION AND MIGRAINE PAIN

Receptors	Ligands	Activity on the Sensory Primary Neuron
5-HT_{1D}	Serotonin	Decreased release of CGRP and SP
$GABA_A$	GABA	Decreased release of CGRP and SP
CB-1	Anandamide*	Decreased release of CGRP and SP
Ionotropic and metabotropic	Glutamate	Increased release of vasoactive peptides
VR-1	Capsaicin or anandamide†	Increased release of CGRP and SP
PAR-2	Peptidic chains SLIGRL and SLIGKV	Increased release of CGRP and SP

*At nanomolar concentrations.
†At micromolar concentrations.
CB, cannabinoid; CGRP, calcitonin gene–related peptide; GABA, γ-aminobutyric acid; 5-HT, 5-hydroxytryptamine; PAR, protease-activated receptor; SP, substance P; VR, vanilloid receptor.
Data from Bianchi A, Caraci F, Salomone S. The pain in primary headache. In Capasso A (ed): Recent Developments in Pain Research. Trivandrum, India: Research Signpost, 2005, pp 343-357.

consequent onset of sensitization could explain the progressive evolution from a form of headache with many free intervals to the daily chronic headache, inducing the patient to assume daily doses of analgesics with the risk of abuse.[17,18]

Gelatinous substance, located in the spinal posterior horn gray matter, is the first control station for painful afferent impulses. Gelatinous substance is rich in opioid peptides (enkephalins and dynorphins) and, of course, in opioid receptors μ and κ, as well as their interneurons, which are able to selectively inhibit the neurotransmitters release from A delta and C fibers, thus creating an access gate to painful afferent pathways. Opioid peptides exert a prevalent inhibition on neuronal activity due to the opening of K^+ membrane channels, operated by μ and δ receptors, or to the closing of Ca^{2+} channels, induced by κ-opioid receptors. Spinal nociceptive circuits and especially enkephalinergic neurons are under the control of neuronal systems descending from the brainstem, able to exert facilitating or inhibiting effects and therefore playing an important role in the regulation of nociceptive reflexes and pain perception.[17-19]

The periaqueductal grey (PAG), the nucleus raphe magnus, and the nucleus reticularis paragigantocellularis and magnocellularis, as well as the locus ceruleus, together form the inhibitory descending system. PAG neurons project onto the nucleus raphe magnus, where descending serotoninergic fibers arise, and onto the nucleus reticularis paragigantocellularis and magnocellularis; in the locus ceruleus are stored the vesicular monoamine transporters and the C-terminus of neuropeptide Y. These structures form the so-called migraine generator region of the human brainstem (see Fig. 48-5 later), and from them noradrenergic and serotoninergic descending fibers, directed to the spinal cord, take origin. Serotoninergic and noradrenergic pathways activate spinal enkephalinergic interneurons, negatively modulating (through a presynaptic inhibition) the transmission of nociceptive messages. In this way opioid agonists such as morphine, fentanyl, pentazocine, and buprenorphine exert their analgesic effect.[18,19]

Though the opioid system has not received major consideration in the study of migraine pathogenesis, its involvement can be postulated. As far as morphine is concerned, according to several observations, it seems that this drug could worsen rather than attenuate the migraine pain. In the United States, since 1992 a nasal spray formulation of butorphanol has been employed in the therapy of severe migraine attacks, showing a rapid onset of action with a pain relief lasting from 3 to 5 hours. Interactions between butorphanol and sumatriptan were not observed when the drugs were administered close together,[20] but widespread reports of abuse and dependence have induced its manufacturer to voluntarily request the FDA to reschedule butorphanol as a narcotic.[21]

Opioid analgesics also appear to be generally not indicated in the management of chronic daily headache. The study of pathophysiologic models of opioidergic pathways for migraine and chronic daily headache, as well as of neural plasticity in the context of neuropathic pain states, has contributed to promote the concept of chronic daily headache as a neuropathic pain syndrome.[22,23]

The brain is not provided with pain-sensitive endings, while meninges are rich in nociceptors. The ophthalmic branch of the trigeminal nerve reaches extracerebral vessels at the level of the meninges (dura mater, arachnoid, and pia mater), which receive peripheral fibers coming from pseudo-unipolar neurons present in the trigeminal ganglion. All these fibers form the neuroanatomic circuit known as the trigeminal-vascular system, forwarding stimuli received from afferent peripheral endings to the trigeminal nucleus caudalis and to other brainstem nuclei, such as the superior salivatory nucleus. According to Edvinsson and Goadsby,[24] through these pathways an afferent cholinergic pathway of the VIIth cranial nerve could be activated, with the release at the meningeal level of vasoactive intestinal polypeptide, able to provoke further vasodilation and hyperactivation of trigeminal fibers. An important role is attributed to parasympathetic pathways in primary headache pathogenesis, especially with respect to explaining symptoms such as tearing, conjunctival blood injection, and rhinorrhea, often observed primarily in patients suffering from cluster headache. The trigeminal-vascular system, with its different components,

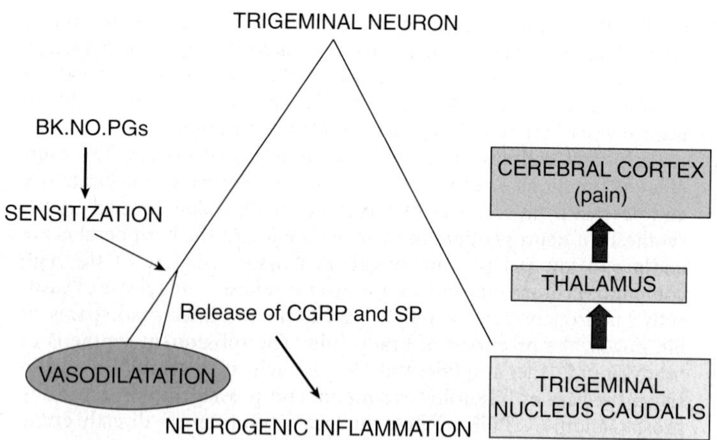

FIGURE 48-2 • Role of the trigeminal neuron in a migraine attack. Attack-eliciting factors at the subcortical level provoke the dilation of cranial vessels with activation of trigeminal sensory afferent endings and a consequent neurogenic inflammation process, due to the release of CGRP and SP or NKA. BK, bradykinin; CGRP, calcitonin gene–related peptide; NKA, neurokinin A; NO, nitric oxide; SP, substance P. (From Bianchi A, Caraci F, Salomone S. The pain in primary headache. In Capasso A [ed]: Recent Developments in Pain Research. Trivandrum, India: Research Signpost, 2005, pp 343-357.)

therefore represents the most important anatomic and functional area for the study of headache pathophysiology.

The characterization of 5-hydroxytryptamine (5-HT) receptors within trigeminal sensory neurons has vastly improved our knowledge regarding the pathogenesis and treatment of migraine. The stimulation of subtypes B and D of 5-HT_1 receptors inhibits the release of vasoactive and pain-transmitter peptides such as CGRP, SP, and NKA,[25] which are involved in dural plasma extravasation following neurogenic inflammation. In experimental animal models, this involvement was found to be due to the depolarization provoked by the electric stimulation of peripheral trigeminal fibers. The release of CGRP caused by the activation of trigeminal fibers leads to dilation of meningeal vessels and plasma extravasation, which, in turn, bring about the hyperactivation of central and peripheral trigeminal endings responsible for pain (Fig. 48-2). These pathophysiologic mechanisms, from which arises the trigeminal-vascular theory of Moskowitz,[8-10] as demonstrated in the rat, could be at the root of migraine pain. However, this hypothesis has been not yet definitively validated in humans, though it has received strong support from the significant therapeutic activity exerted by triptans toward the primary headache pain. Another indirect proof of the possible application of Moskowitz's theory to humans seems to reside in some observations made by Goadsby et al.[26]; according to them, CGRP levels increase in the external jugular vein blood during migraine attacks. Edvinsson has shown the correlation between the decrease of blood CGRP levels and the therapeutic efficacy of triptans.[15]

Among receptors with a prevalent inhibitory activity, an important role is played by GABA receptors located in trigeminal sensory neurons. It has been proven in the rat, by means of immunoreactivity, that neurons projecting to the thalamus from the caudal trigeminal spinal tract nucleus receive GABAergic input via $GABA_A$ receptors containing $gamma_1$ and $gamma_2$ subunits, while many neurons expressing AMPA-type receptors do not project to the thalamus.[27] In another experimental model, the inhibition of trigeminal nociceptive neurons exerted by bicuculline injected into rat PAG was maintained in the presence of PAG P/Q-type calcium channels blocked by ν-toxin. These findings suggest that, in disorders such as migraine, involving the PAG and/or P/Q-type calcium channels, the two systems could be separately modulated and thus require preventive treatments by two different approaches.[28] Valproate, as are the other anticonvulsants, seems to be provided with several mechanisms of action, being able to inhibit GABA transaminase, which causes GABA degradation, and, at the same time, activate glutamic acid decarboxylase and succinic semialdehyde dehydrogenase, which induce GABA synthesis, stimulating GABA transporter-3 (GAT-3) and prolonging the inactivation of voltage-activated sodium channels. Therefore, following its administration, GABA extracellular concentrations in the proximity of GABAergic endings are increased[29-31] (see Chapter 45, Seizure Disorders).

Valproate, currently used in the preventive treatment of migraine, in animal experimental models was found to block dural plasmatic extravasation induced by neurogenic inflammation, due to either the electrical stimulation of trigeminal fibers or the intravenous administration of SP.[32] Experimental fundamental data in laboratory animals were obtained after clinical evidence, at which time the use of valproate in migraine therapy was already consolidated, providing strong support to the hypothesis that the activation of trigeminal sensory neurons is an initial step in the neurogenic inflammation process and in the pathogenesis of CSD and primary headaches.[9,32-34]

Cannabinoid receptors, vanilloid receptors, and protease-activated receptors (PARs) are also present at the level of peripheral and central endings of primary sensory neurons. These receptors, characterized only a few years ago (see Table 48-3), seem to play an important role in headache pain pathophysiology. Like eicosanoids and platelet-activating factor, the endocannabinoids anandamide and 2-acylglycerol, having a lipidic structure, derive from membrane phospholipids, and their pharmacodynamic profile is similar to that of the principle active ingredient of *Cannabis*, Δ^9-tetrahydrocannabinol, and other natural and synthetic cannabinoids. The synthesis of anandamide is regulated by phospholipase D, while another intracellular enzyme, fatty acid amide hydrolase, is responsible for its degradation, followed by the taking back of its constituents in phospholipids.[35] Unlike neurotransmitters and neuropeptides, which are continuously synthesized and then stored in special depot sites, from which they are released following the excitation of nerve endings, endogenous cannabinoids are produced from endothelial cells, macrophages, and peripheral cells only when their holocrine-paracrine function is expressed, that is, during the inflammation process and in all conditions of cellular injury.[36,37]

Once released into the extracellular space, anandamide activates, at nanomolar concentrations, its own cannabinergic receptors (CB), generally distinguished as CB-1 and CB-2, while, at micromolar concentrations, it stimulates vanilloid receptors (e.g., VR-1), inducing CGRP release and vasodilation.[38] CB receptors of both types are coupled, through G protein, with adenylate cyclase. CB-1 receptors mediate analgesic effects of anandamide either peripherally or centrally; CB-2 receptors, present in B lymphocytes and natural killer cells, seem able to produce an anti-inflammatory action when activated.[39] Thus, anandamide, at nanomolar concentrations, exerts an inhibitory effect on pain either centrally or peripherally, due to the contemporaneous activation of encephalic (as in the PAG, in relation to the activation of group III mGlu receptors) and spinal (10th lamina) CB-1 receptors,[40,41] as well as CB-1 receptors in peripheral sensory neurons, such as at the level of peptidergic capsaicin-sensitive endings, where anandamide is able to reduce the release of CGRP and SP.[39,41-43] Hohmann and Herkenham[44] have demonstrated, by means of histochemical techniques, the presence of CB-1 in peripheral nerve endings.

In conclusion, endocannabinoids such as anandamide activate CB and VR-1 receptors (at nanomolar concentrations) or transient receptor potential vanilloid-1 (TRPV-1) receptors (at micromolar concentrations). The latter are capsaicin sensitive,[38] with opposite effects on pain, on which they exert a dual activity—inhibitory or stimulatory, analgesic or algogenic. Thus they assume a balancing role, either peripherally or centrally, sustained by the opposite modifications of Ca^{2+} intracellular content they can promote.[39]

The capsaicin receptor is a nonselective receptor channel of 838 amino acids, discovered in 1977, that can be activated by protons as well as by capsaicin and capsaicin-like substances (Figs. 48-3 and 48-4), semi-lipidic structures with a vanilloid group.[45,46] Capsaicin-sensitive fibers have a small diameter (A delta and C fibers) and are peptidergic, causing the release of the inflammation mediators CGR, SP, and NKA[47,48] with pain. This polymodal receptor, when activated by capsaicin and other agonists, is able to induce the inflow of extracellular Ca^{2+} and Na^+ in response to the loss of extracellular Ca^{2+}, transducing physical (heat from 42° to 53° C), physicochemical (pH 5-6), and various chemical stimuli in nociceptive sensations, through a Ca^{2+}-dependent mechanism, not only at the peripheral level but also centrally, in spinal endings of primary sensory neurons.[49] *N*-acyl-dopamine has agonistic activity on the VR-1 receptor, thus interacting, like all other agonists and antagonists listed in Box 48-1, with anandamide and other pain

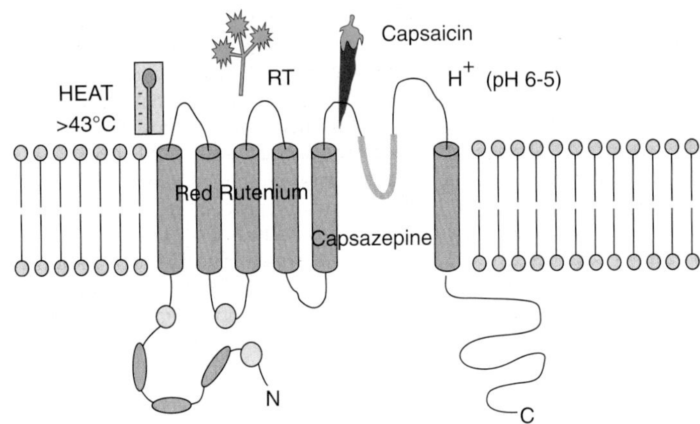

FIGURE 48-3 • General structure of vanilloid receptor VR-1 with main agonists and antagonists. RT, resinoferotoxin.

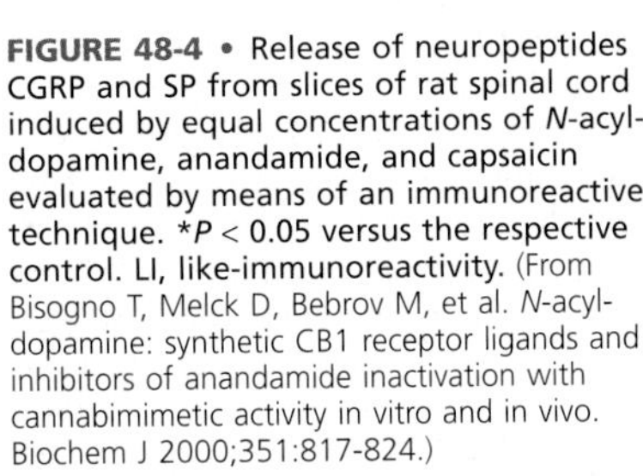
FIGURE 48-4 • Release of neuropeptides CGRP and SP from slices of rat spinal cord induced by equal concentrations of *N*-acyl-dopamine, anandamide, and capsaicin evaluated by means of an immunoreactive technique. *$P < 0.05$ versus the respective control. LI, like-immunoreactivity. (From Bisogno T, Melck D, Bebrov M, et al. *N*-acyl-dopamine: synthetic CB1 receptor ligands and inhibitors of anandamide inactivation with cannabimimetic activity in vitro and in vivo. Biochem J 2000;351:817-824.)

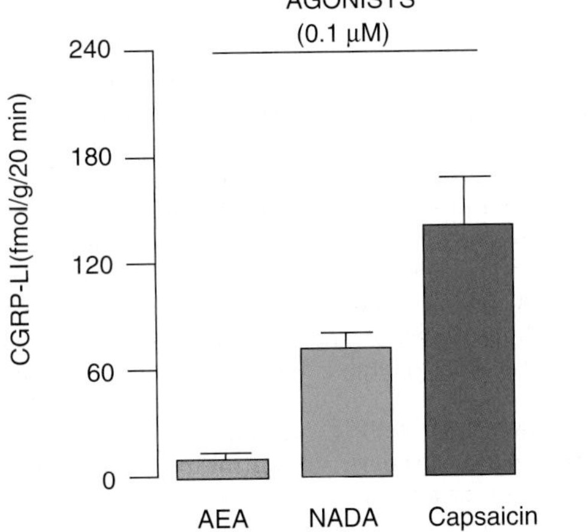

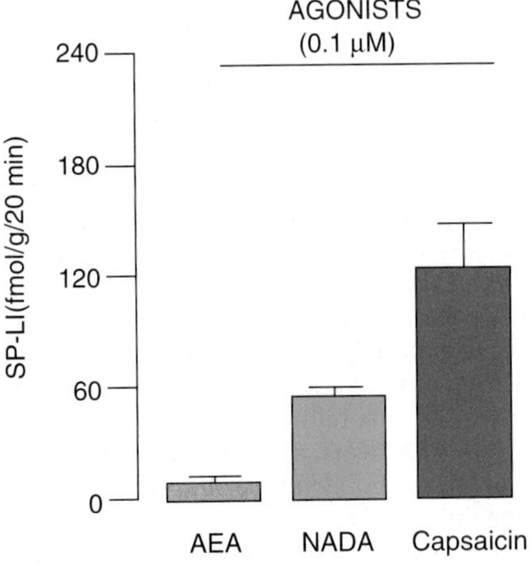

BOX 48-1 VANILLOID RECEPTOR 1 (VR-1) RECEPTOR AGONISTS AND ANTAGONISTS

Agonists
Capsaicin
Resiniferotoxin
Arvanil
Olvanil
Anandamide
NADA*
Ethanol
Leukotrienes
Protons (pH < 6)
Temperature > 43° C

Antagonists
Capsazepine
Ruthenium red†
L-Resiniferotoxin
SB-366791

*N-acyl-dopamine.
†Noncompetitive and calcium antagonist.
From Caterina MJ, Schumacher MA, Tominaga M, et al. The capsaicin receptor: a heat activated ion channel in the pain pathway. Nature 1997;389:816-824.

TABLE 48-4 HUMAN AND ANIMAL CORRELATES OF CORTICAL SPREADING DEPRESSION

Human Observations	Animal Studies
Slow evolution of migraine aura	Slow spread of neuronal activity in animals
Spreading oligemia on imaging studies during migraine	Waves of reduced apparent diffusion coefficient, below ischemic levels
Magnetoencephalographic DC shifts in migraine	DC shifts in animal experiments of CSD
CGRP is released during migraine	Pial dilation following CSD is partially mediated by CGRP

CGRP, calcitonin gene–related peptide; CSD, cortical spreading depression; DC, direct current.
Adapted from Buchanan TM, Ramadan NM, Aurora S. Future pharmacologic targets for acute and preventive treatments of migraine. Expert Rev Neurother 2004;4:391-430.

mediators.[50] At the first application, capsaicin produces an intense painful effect, desensitizing the afferent fibers, so that subsequent applications provoke a clear-cut analgesic response.[49] Ethanol also potentiates the VR-1 nociceptive response.[51]

Another class of receptors, the PARs (generally distinguished as PAR-1 and PAR-2), has been isolated in the rat, by means of immunohistochemical techniques,[52] in capsaicin-sensitive primary sensory neurons, at the level of trigeminal and spinal dorsal root ganglia. Here PAR-2 receptors are co-located with VR-1 receptors, probably involved also being in primary headache pathogenetic mechanisms. The PAR-2 receptor[52] is selectively activated by the SLIGRL and SLIGKV peptides trypsin and tryptase, proteases abundantly contained in mast cells and released by them during the inflammatory process; in many tissues, mast cells are in close contact with the endings of capsaicin-sensitive primary sensory neurons containing neuropeptides. The activation of PAR-2 provokes Ca^{2+} mobilization and release of both CGRP and SP in slices of rat isolated neurons and in vascular intracranial structures cultured in vitro, while in vivo CGRP-induced swelling of the rat paw is observed. Cannabimimetic and vanilloid mechanisms seem to be involved in the neurogenic inflammation process and in CSD, validating Moskowitz's theory.[8,9,53] Also, traditional medicine of the 19th century was using cannabis in the treatment of headache.[54] Therefore, CB, VR, and PAR receptors, with their ligands, seem worthy of attention in the study of pain pathophysiology and therapeutic problems related to primary headaches.[52-55]

Theories of Primary Headache Pathogenesis

The complexity of the interactions taking place in the sensory neuronal network, with the mediation of all the different neurotransmitters involved, gives the measure of the extreme difficulty connected with the study of the pathogenesis of primary headaches, and in particular of their cardinal sign, the pain. This is the case in spite of the very significant scientific contributions of these last years, from which the issue has received enormous broadening and enlightenment. Many theories have been formulated in the past 60 years about the pathogenesis of migraine and other forms of primary headache, but it is still far from being fully clarified.

The first theory, originally conceived in 1938 by Graham and Wolff[2] and later elaborated by Wolff,[3] is built upon a vascular basis, considering three main aspects: (i) during the migraine attack, extracranial vessels are dilated and throbbing in a large percentage of patients; (ii) the stimulation of intracranial vessels provokes an ipsilateral headache; and (iii) vasoconstrictor drugs, such as ergot derivatives, exert a curative effect, while vasodilators, such as nitrates, may induce an attack. With the support of these observations, Wolff hypothesized that intracranial vasoconstriction could be responsible for the migraine aura and the following hyperemic reaction associated with local vasodilation, with the consequent stimulation of perivascular nociceptive endings generating the headache attack. Heyck[56] completed the theory with the concept that, during the attack, arteriovenous anastomoses are closed, thus explaining the decreased oxygen extraction observed on the symptomatic side. Successive theories underlined the importance of vasoactive and neuroactive substances (such as plasmatic kinins, endorphins, serotonin, histamine, endocannabinoids, adenosine, prostaglandins, NO, and endothelin-1), released in perivascular areas, which could be directly and/or indirectly involved in the neurogenic inflammation and its symptoms.[57-66] In the previously mentioned theory of Moskowitz,[8-10] based on the presence of neurogenic inflammation in the trigeminal-vascular area and the integration of painful messages in the cerebral cortex, can be seen the confluence of all the theories reported up to the present.

Another attractive possibility to interpret headache pathogenesis, related to the previously mentioned CSD, is the depression of electrical cerebrocortical activity. This depression, observed in animal experimental models by Leão long ago,[67] consists in the suppression of cortical hyperexcitation produced by electrical stimuli, progressing by contiguity within the cerebral structures in a posterior-anterior direction at a speed of 2 to 5 mm/min and associated with vasodilation.[68,69] Animal studies indicate that CSD activates the trigeminal system via unmyelinated A delta and C fibers, and similarities have been seen between experimental CSD in the rat and human migraine visual aura and perhaps other migraine auras (Table 48-4). According to Moskowitz,[70] experimental and clinical studies are giving a strong support to the hypothesis that CSD, due to physical or chemical stimuli, can induce at the trigeminal-vascular level the activation of trigeminal afferents innervating meninges, which, traveling to the brainstem, trigger parasympathetic efferents, thereby inducing a sustained reflex vasodilation in the dura mater.

CSD also causes the activation of a class of enzymes called matrix metalloproteinases, constituents of an inflammatory cascade triggered by the intracerebral generation of reactive oxygen species (e.g., NO), which provides indirect evidence for the up-regulation of a proinflammatory state in the brain and its connective tissue coverings. CSD can be considered the pathophysiologic substrate of migraine, taking part in the generation of pain through the previously mentioned mechanisms. Genetic and environmental factors may modulate individual susceptibility to CSD, lowering its threshold through genes able to control the translocation of Ca^{2+}, Na^{+}, and K^{+} ions, as can happen in the pathophysiology of different migraine subtypes. Recently, mice carrying a human familial hemiplegic migraine-1 mutation were found to exhibit a very low CSD threshold associated with enhanced neurotransmitter release. CSD causes a transient propagated increase in cortical blood flow, with a drastic decrease in the middle meningeal artery; therefore, the migraine pain could arise from the dural ischemia induced by CSD.[71] CSD regulates genes that are intrinsic to its propagation, that identify accompanying vascular responses as a potential source of pain, and that protect against its potential pathologic consequences. These include genes related to vasoactive peptides and to the vasodilator atrial natriuretic peptide, which are induced by CSD, or related to the vasoconstrictor neuropeptide Y, which is conversely down-regulated, as happens also for L-type calcium channel messenger RNA (mRNA); other genes specifically regulated by CSD are those involved in oxidative stress responses.[72] In xenon-133 studies, decreased cerebral blood perfusion lasting about 1 hour, especially in the occipital area, has been observed as a consequence of CSD. These data have been validated by means of magnetoelectroencephalography, single-photon emission computed tomography, magnetic resonance imaging, and positron emission tomography studies,[73-76] especially for migraine with aura and at least partially for migraine without aura. Mitochondrial alterations and a decrease in Mg^{2+} blood levels have also been associated with migraine in neuroimaging investigations.[77-80]

Lance,[60] Diener and May,[81] and Welch et al.[82] have proposed consideration of the participation of frontal, occipital, and limbic cortical areas, subcortical nuclei, and brainstem structures specialized in sensory controlling mechanisms in migraine pathogenesis. These structures interact with several neurotransmitters such as noradrenaline, serotonin, dopamine, and others, and are considered "migraine generators," participating in CSD. They can be modified in the presence of calcium channel genetic mutations (Fig. 48-5).

In relation to episodic and chronic tension-type headache, it is not clear whether their pathogenesis is similar or different, and to what extent, with respect to that of migraine.[83] New concepts emphasize the role of peripheral pain mechanisms in episodic tension-type headache and central nociceptive pathway sensitization involving the NO system and *N*-methyl-D-aspartate receptors in chronic tension-type headache; the influence of stress and of protracted muscular contraction have also been investigated in both conditions.[84] With respect to cluster headache, among other theories, the immunologic theory seems worthy of interest. This theory deals mostly with interleukin and cytokine receptors and involves the complex relationship between neuropsychic, endocrine, and immunologic systems,[85] as demonstrated by the reduced response of cortisol to *meta*-chlorophenylpiperazine.[86] During the attack, there is activation of the hypothalamic gray area ipsilateral to the affected side.[87] Recent findings suggest the possibility of a link between *HCRTR1* and *HCRTR2*, encoding for the hypocretin/orexin receptors OX1 and OX2, and cluster headache and migraine; if so, the hypocretin/orexin system, influencing a wide range of physiologic and behavioral processes, among which are also pain threshold and nociceptive transmission, has been involved in the pathogenesis of primary headache. In the rat, the orexin-1 receptor antagonist SB-334867 has been found to be able to counteract the neurogenic dural vasodilation induced by local electrical stimulation, inhibiting CGRP prejunctional release from trigeminal neurons.[88,89]

Finally, it is necessary to assess again the importance of genetic factors and mitochondrial abnormalities[77-80,89-92] in the pathogenesis of migraine, tension-type headache, and cluster headache.The knowledge of headache pathophysiology, as already stressed, has improved remarkably in recent years because of the advances realized by molecular and clinical pharmacology, which presage further progress in the near future.

THERAPEUTICS AND CLINICAL PHARMACOLOGY

Goals of Therapy and Therapeutic Approach

The main goals to be reached with a pharmacologic therapy applied to headache patients are essentially two: abortion of the head pain at the attack onset, implying the early administration of an appropriate analgesic, and the prevention of cephalalgic episodes through the daily use for some months, in repeatable cycles, of prophylactic drugs able to correct neurovascular disorders at the basis of the disturbance. At the same time, the impact of trigger factors (Box 48-2) must be avoided or limited. Headaches actually are the expression—the primary forms directly and the secondary ones indirectly—of a pathologic state of the sensory nervous system, while vascular-related structures have in general a concurrent but not causative role. Causes and mechanisms of primary forms have not yet been well elucidated, although they appear identifiable for secondary forms of headache.

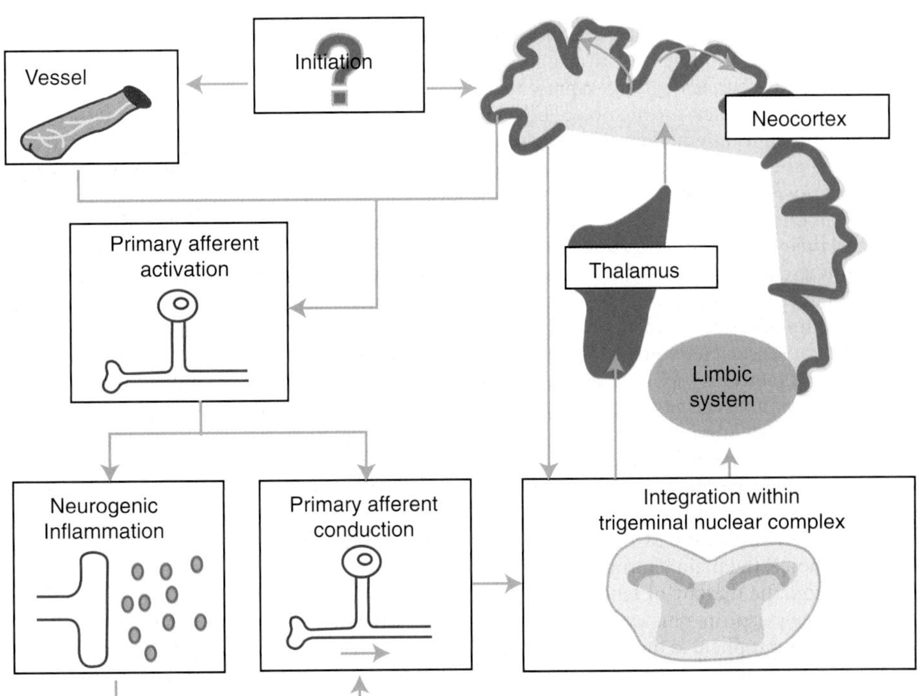

FIGURE 48-5 • A schematic representation of pathways involved in the generation of migraine attacks.

BOX 48-2 HEADACHE TRIGGERS OR AGGRAVATING/ PRECIPITATING FACTORS

Migraine With and Without Aura, Tension Type
Stress
Hunger
Alcohol
Anxiety
Schedule change
Menstruation
Menopause
Ovulation
Smoke
Intense light
Exposure to sun
Altitude
Indoor and outdoor air abnormalities
Weather changes
Relaxation after stress
Noise
Sleep disorders
Postural disorders
Head trauma
Sex
Foods
Additives
Drugs
Odors

Cluster and Other TACS
Alcohol, especially during the cluster remission phase
Sexual activity
Lying down

Trigeminal Neuralgia
Trigger point stimulation: speaking, eating, drinking, facial muscular activity, local temperature changes, air conditioning

It has already been determined that migraine and other primary headaches have an important genetic component, located on chromosome 19p13 and chromosome 1 in familial hemiplegic migraine, and genetic investigations on the causes of migraine are demonstrating the existence of inheritable impairments of ionic Ca^{2+}, Na^+, and K^+ channels. Thus, the development of drugs able to correct these dysfunctions, known as channelopathies, represents an important strategy in the search for new therapeutic tools. The beneficial effects of magnesium depend on its interactions with calcium and glutamate. Migraine attacks are the result of a complex and multifactorial disorder of central sensory control systems on which many local and general regulatory parameters, specially of endocrine, thalamic, or cortical nature, can exert their influence, generating the characteristic pain in intracranial neurovascular structures of trigeminal origin, present around large endocranial vessels and in meninges. On these bases, primary cephalalgic manifestations fundamentally imply a pronounced sensitivity of extracerebral sensory nervous structures, with a reduced resistance to all stressing conditions such as a decreased blood flow and also simple mechanical stimuli such as that caused by the vascular stretching associated with vasodilation. Pharmacologic means directed to counteract in different ways this neurovascular vulnerability, in which nervous components play the prevalent role, can represent valuable prophylactic approaches to primary headache therapy.[93]

In the abortive therapy of migraine acute attacks, triptans are the drugs of choice, the main alternative drugs being NSAIDs and ergots. The symptomatic therapy of tension-type headache is based on acetaminophen or aspirin plus caffeine or anti–COX-2, other NSAIDs (naproxen, ibuprophen, ketorolac, etc.), and, when there is an intense muscular involvement, muscle relaxants. For acute treatment of cluster headaches and TACs, subcutaneous sumatriptan is used first, while normobaric or hyperbaric oxygen inhalation (7 to 9 L/min every 15 minutes) also seems able to produce good results. In chronic daily headache attacks, it is very difficult to achieve symptomatic therapy because, in the presence of a syndrome of abuse, it is necessary to avoid the medication responsible. In cases of triptan abuse, these drugs cannot be utilized and, in the case of de novo CDH, it is advisable that their use be practiced in a moderate way.

For migraines, prophylactic or preventive therapy is based mainly on the following classes of pharmacologic agents: beta-adrenergic blockers, antiepileptics, calcium channel blockers antidepressants, botulinum toxin A, short-term prophylaxis (NSAIDs, triptans, muscle relaxants), serotonin antagonists and ergots, angiotensin antagonists and angiotensin-converting enzyme (ACE) inhibitors, and other agents (hormones, histamine H_3 agonists, neuroleptics, feverfew, Petasites); antiemetic, antinausea, and gastroprotective drugs are often used as adjuncts. For the preventive therapy of tension headache, the following therapies are used: antidepressants, botulinum toxin A, and short-term treatment with NSAIDs and muscle relaxants when muscular contraction is present. The preventive therapy of cluster headache and other TACs includes verapamil, corticosteroids, lithium, topiramate, and civamide by the intranasal route.

Supportive therapy consists of minerals, coenzymes, vitamins, and nutraceuticals in general, (i.e., naturally occurring substances or formulations of these substances). Most of the latter are dietary supplements.

With regard to secondary headaches, treatment is primarily focused on dealing with the disease from which they have origin and/or to which they are related. The risk that a drug, when abused or misused, could be the cause of such a disturbance is in direct relation to its blood concentration and toxicodynamic potential, as well as to the duration and frequency of the exposure. Headaches induced by drug abuse are, in a high percentage of cases, complications of primary headaches, specially migraine. In reality, all drugs used for the abortive therapy of attacks may generate a syndrome of abuse, especially when they are taken with great frequency and/or elevated dosages.

Many chemical agents present in drugs or in foods may induce or trigger headaches, relative to the blood levels they reach. Foods that induce headaches are numerous; chocolate in particular is notorious, but worthy of mention are also yeasts and some additives and preservatives (Box 48-3). In these cases a specific therapy is indicated, associated with a detoxification strategy (Table 48-5). Narcotics in general may induce headache, either with acute or chronic administrations or following their withdrawal in addicted subjects, because of abstinence phenomena they can generate (see Box 48-3). The risk of chronic daily headache, with the possibility of addiction, is high in migraineurs ingesting analgesics, especially barbiturates; the abuse of butalbital is emblematic.

Therapeutics by Class

Acute Abortive Therapy of Headache Attacks

The acute therapy of headache is directed against pain and other symptoms characteristic of headache attacks, while preventive or prophylactic therapy has the scope to avoid the repetition or worsening of acute episodes. Adjuvant extrapharmacologic therapeutic strategies (psychotherapy, physiotherapy, biofeedback and acupuncture, trigger control, and dietary habits), can be usefully integrated with prophylactic or preventive therapies.

Triptans. It has long been observed that 5-HT_1 serotonin receptors are strongly involved in the pathogenesis of primary headaches, and the precursors of serotonin, L-5-hydroxytryptophan and L-tryptophan, are effective in migraine therapy.[94] Triptans (indole derivatives substituted in positions 3 and 5), also known as 5-HT_1 receptor agonists (Fig. 48-6), are very active against acute attacks in the majority of primary headaches.

They represent the first choice of specific drugs in the symptomatic treatment of migraine and cluster headache. It is well known that triptans inhibit CGRP gene transcription in trigeminal sensory neurons, but it has not yet been clarified whether this action is medi-

BOX 48-3 CHEMICAL AGENTS WHOSE USE (A, B, D) OR WITHDRAWAL (C) MAY INDUCE HEADACHE

A. Acute Exposure
1. Nitric oxide (NO) donors, such as nitrates and nitrites, in drugs, food (hot dog), siloed fodders, and gunpowder
2. Foods: histamine releasers (oligantigenic substances) or those containing vasotropic compounds—tyramine and phenylethylamines (chocolate; seasoned, fermented, or lipid-rich foods or drinks)
3. Additives (aspartame) or preservatives (monosodium glutamate: Chinese restaurant headache)
4. Calcitonin gene–related peptide
5. Phosphodiesterase inhibitors (sildenafil, tadalafil, vardenafil, etc.)
6. Carbon monoxide (CO) (natural calamities, fires, work or domestic accidents)
7. Ethyl alcohol (with or without hangover)
8. Cocaine
9. Cannabis
10. Volatile substances (sniffing)
11. Various drugs: atropine, cardiac glycosides, insulin and oral hypoglycemic agents, hydralazine, disulfiram, imipramine, nicotine, nifedipine, nimodipine, tolazoline, etc.
12. Inorganic compounds: arsenic, bromine, chlorine, copper, lead, lithium, and mercury derivatives
13. Organic compounds: long-chain alcohols, aniline, balsams, camphor, carbon disulfide, EDTA, sulfhydric acid, kerosene, methyl alcohol, halogenated methyl esters, naphthalenes, organophosphates

B. Chronic Exposure and Abuse
14. Ergotamine and ergot derivatives
15. Non-narcotic analgesics (NSAIDs), simple or compound
16. Narcotic analgesics (barbiturates, opiates)
17. Triptans
18. Tobacco
19. Hydroxymethylglutaryl-coenzyme A antagonists (statins, etc.)
20. Antihypertensive drugs (clonidine, methyldopa, dipyridamole, etc.)
21. Monoamine oxidase inhibitors
22. Tricyclic antidepressants
23. Corticosteroids
24. Estrogens

C. Withdrawal in the Course of Abuse With or Without Dependence
25. Ergotamine annd ergot derivatives
26. Caffeine
27. Nicotine (tobacco)
28. Opiates and other narcotics

D. With Unknown and Complex Mechanisms
29. Estrogens, progestins, and hormonal contraceptives
30. Antiandrogens

Adapted from Headache Classification Subcommittee of the International Headache Society. The International Classification of Headache Disorders, 2nd ed. Cephalalgia 2004;24(Suppl 1):9-160.

TABLE 48-5 THERAPEUTIC MEASURES TO BE ADOPTED IN DRUG ABUSE SYNDROMES

Drug Abused	Symptoms	Pharmacologic Treatment	Other Therapeutic Measures
Triptans	Rebound headache paresthesia, pain in the chest, dizziness Serotonin syndrome in cases of interactions	Withdrawal Cyproheptadine (5-HT_{2A} antagonists) Benzodiazepines Ziprasidone Prophylactic therapy	Administration of intravenous fluids Control of vital functions Control of agitation and autonomic instability
NSAIDs (nonselective COX inhibitors)	Gastroduodenal ulcerations Alterations in renal function	Withdrawal Other analgesics Proton pump inhibitors Leukotriene receptor antagonists	Prophylactic agents Inhibitors of 5-lipoxygenase Riboflavin
Butalbital	Psychological and physical dependence Withdrawal syndrome Rebound headache	Phenobarbital + caffeine Dihydroergotamine Propranolol	Propranolol Dihydroergotamine Metoclopramide Selective serotonin reuptake inhibitors
Ergots	Rebound headache Nausea and vomiting Ergotism	Withdrawal Anticoagulants Low-molecular-weight dextran	Vasodilators Sodium nitroprusside Phenothiazines

ated, as far as the presynaptic level is concerned, only by the activation of 5-HT_{1D} and 5-HT_{1F} or also of 5-HT_{1B} receptors, this last subtype having been isolated, as mRNA, only in human trigeminal ganglial neurons. A histochemical demonstration is still lacking of the B subtype of 5-HT_1 receptors at both central and peripheral endings, as for 5-HT_{1D} and 5-HT_{1F}.[25,95,96] Centrally, for example, at the level of the nuclei tractus solitarii, which is an important site of action for triptan antimigraine drugs, trigeminal-vascular activation triggers nausea and vomit, frequently associated with pain in a migraine attack.[97] Numerous trigeminal afferent fibers arrive at this site, which is involved in the pathogenesis of migraine symptoms connected with the autonomous nervous system. Therefore, the therapeutic activity of triptans on the previously mentioned symptoms, associated with their analgesic effect, could be exerted either directly in situ or indirectly, as a consequence of the inhibition of the trigeminal nociceptive system.

Thus, through their agonist activity on 5-$HT_{1D\text{-}F}$ receptors, and perhaps also 5-HT_{1B} receptors, triptans could inhibit, at the presynaptic level, the release of neuropeptides able to provoke either the intracranial vasodilation or pain characteristic of migraine and related to the stimulation of primary trigeminal nociceptive neurons, which is the first step in pain generation and transmission. These neurons in turn activate, through their central endings, second-order nociceptive neurons at the level of the brainstem and nucleus caudalis. 5-HT_{1F} and 5-HT_{1D} receptors have been found there, as well as at peripheral endings of trigeminal ganglion neurons, in which they could have a function analogous to that of 5-HT_{1D} receptors.[95,98,99] The activation produced by the electrical stimulation of this nucleus and of dura mater in anesthetized rats is selectively inhibited by agonists of 5-HT_{1F}, such as LY 3334370 and LY344864, which inhibit glutamate release and block pain transmission to central areas of

Practice: Neuropharmacologic Therapeutics

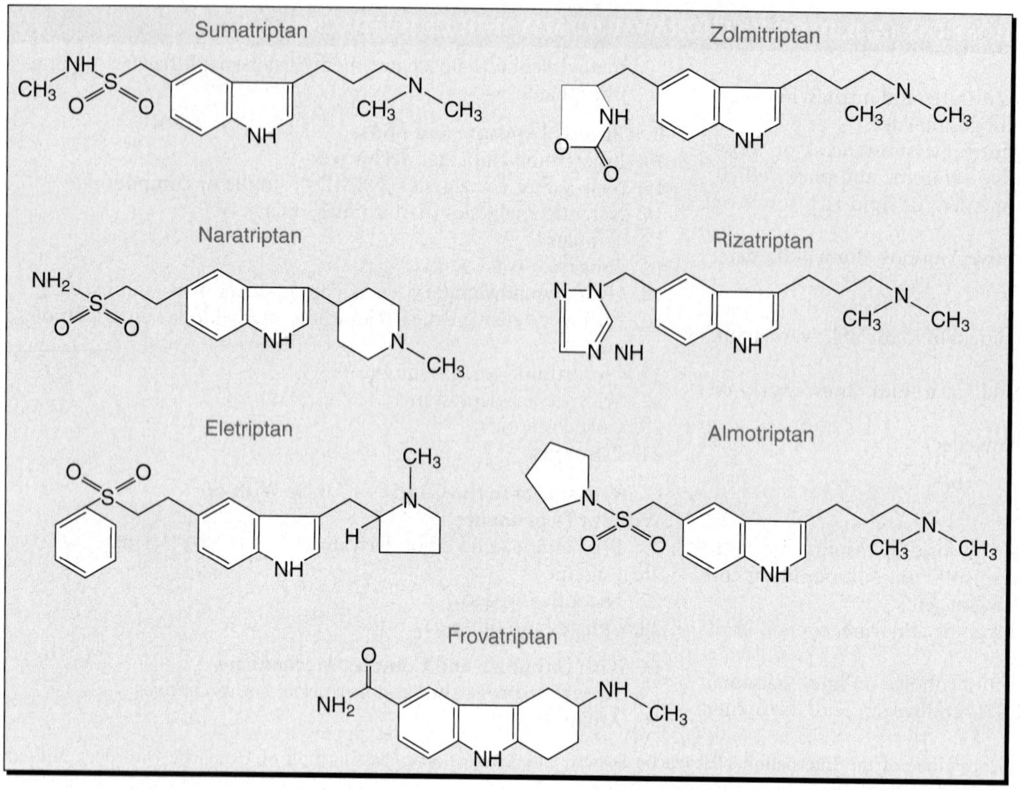

FIGURE 48-6 • Chemical structures of triptans.

nociceptive inputs through the trigeminal ganglion and nucleus caudalis.[98-100]

According to Levy et al.,[101] the analgesic action of triptans is exerted through presynaptic 5-$HT_{1B\text{-}D}$ receptors in the dorsal horn by blocking the synaptic transmission from axon terminals of the trigeminal-vascular neurons to cell bodies of their central counterparts. On this basis, the analgesic action of triptans could be specifically obtained mostly in the absence of a central sensitization. Therefore, early treatment with triptans provides a powerful means of prevention of the central sensitization triggered by chemical stimulation of meningeal nociceptors.[102]

Preclinical investigations in rats have shown that triptan compounds exert their effect not only by blocking the release of neuropeptide transmitters from sensory nerve terminals and directly constricting blood vessel smooth muscles, but also by modulating the release of glutamate and NO.[98,103] Actually, the majority of 5-HT_{1B}, 5-HT_{1D}, and 5-HT_{1F} receptors are co-located with glutamate receptors, as demonstrated by means of immunohistochemical staining techniques.[104]

Sumatriptan succinate, synthetized in 1984 and available for clinical use since 1992 in the United States, is the prototype of this group of migraine-aborting drugs, able to activate presynaptic and postjunctional 5-HT_{1B}, 5-HT_{1D}, and 5-HT_{1F} receptors located in the trigeminal-vascular system. The results of several studies suggest that the stimulation of 5-HT_{1B} receptors produces constriction of dural, pial, and intracranial vessels, but the presence of these receptors in other vascular walls, such as saphenous vein and basilar and coronary arteries, contraindicates the use of triptans in patients with cardiovascular disease. The contemporary activation of 5-HT_{1B}, 5-HT_{1D}, and/or 5-HT_{1F} receptors blocks the neurogenic inflammation, characterized by the plasma protein extravasation, caused by the release from trigeminal neurons of neurogenic vasoactive peptides SP, NKA, and endothelin 3. The first two of these peptides stimulate tachykinin receptor 1, with subsequent vasodilation and increase in dural vascular permeability, and the third activates endothelin receptor B, with vasoconstriction followed by vasodilation, secondary to NO release. CGRP, which is also released from trigeminal neurons in neurogenic inflammation, also causes vasodilation. In conclusion, all three subtypes of 5-HT_1 receptors, being able to inhibit trigeminal neurons in the brainstem and upper spinal cord, participate in the central blockade of pain transmission. Because of sensitization phenomena hindering the activity of triptans, their potency of action is inversely proportional to the pain intensity and to the lag time between the onset of the attack and their administration. Consequently, the migraine becomes more difficult to treat, for the same pain intensity, with passing time.[9,64,105,106] Triptans have to be ingested immediately after the appearance of the headache pain[107] in order to act on initiating neuronal mechanisms of the migraine cycle (Fig. 48-7), before sensitization is achieved and allodynia may appear (Box 48-4). If the pain persists, the same dose can be repeated 2 hours later (4 hours later for naratriptan), but no more can be taken in the following 24 hours.

Sumatriptan plasma concentrations attain their peak in about 12 minutes after subcutaneous administration, and between 1 and 2 hours later when administered by the oral route. The bioavailability for subcutaneous and oral or nasal spray administrations is, respectively, 97%, 14%, and 17%. The metabolism of triptans occurs mainly by means of monoamine oxidase (MAO) A and cytochrome P-450 isoenzymes; relative metabolites are excreted with the urine. Thus, their use is not suitable when renal and/or hepatic function is impaired, or in association with inhibitors of enzymes involved in their metabolism (ketoconazole, itoconazole) or with proteases used in the treatment of acquired immunodeficiency syndrome. Plasma protein binding of triptans ranges between 14% (rizatriptan, sumatriptan) and 30% (naratriptan).

Tables 48-6, 48-7, and 48-8 summarize the main pharmacokinetic properties and receptor affinities of the triptans available in the clinical practice,[96,108,109] and dosages at which they are used for different administration routes. Although triptans are the most specific drugs known to date for the treatment of migraine and other primary headache attack, 25% to 35% of patients are reported to be nonresponsive to them; the reasons for this refractoriness has only barely been investigated. A poor response to rizatriptan seems to be related to a lesser degree of trigeminal and autonomic activation, as confirmed by the presence of reduced levels of specific markers.[110,111]

Following sumatriptan administration by subcutaneous, nasal spray, or oral routes, many patients report transient mild pain at the site of

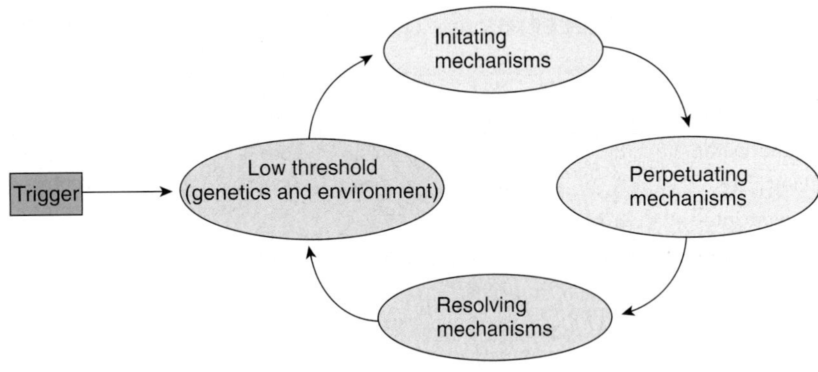

FIGURE 48-7 • Model of a migraine cycle. (From Buchanan TM, Ramadan NM, Aurora S. Future pharmacologic targets for acute and preventive treatments of migraine. Expert Rev Neurother 2004;4:391-430.)

TABLE 48-6 MAIN PHARMACOKINETIC CHARACTERISTICS OF TRIPTANS

Substance and Oral Doses (mg)	T_{max} (hr) and C_{max} (ng/ml)	$T_{1/2}$ (hr)/ AUC (mg/L)	Metabolism and Renal Elimination % (RE)	Bioavailability (%)	Lipophilia Log D pH 7.4
Almotriptan 12.5-25	T_{max}: 1.5-3 C_{max}: 3-103	3.5/80-558	CYP 3A4-2D6, MAO-A, sulfonamide group; RE 50	70	+0.35
Eletriptan 40-80	T_{max}: 1.0-3 C_{max}: 82-246	4/670-1660	CYP 3A4, sulfonamide group; RE 9	50	+0.5
Frovatriptan 2.5-40	T_{max}: 2.3-3.5 C_{max}: 7-53.4	26/94-881	CYP 1A2, sulfonamide group; RE 33	30	
Naratriptan 2.5 5 10	T_{max}: 2-4 C_{max}: 12.6 23.9 46.1	6/98 200 387	CYP 1A2, sulfonamide group; RE 70	74	−0.2
Rizatriptan 5-10	T_{max}: 1-1.5 C_{max}: 7.8-19.8	2/17.4-50	CYP 2D6-1A2, MAO-A; RE 30	42	−0.7
Sumatriptan 50-100	T_{max}: 2-2.5 C_{max}: 31-54	2/118-158	MAO-A, sulfonamide group; RE 20	15	−1.3
Zolmitriptan 2.5	T_{max}: 2-2.5 C_{max}: 3	3/17	CYP 1A2, MAO-A; RE 10	40	−0.7

AUC, area under the curve; C_{max}, maximum concentration; CYP, cytochrome P-450; MAO-A, monoamine oxidase A; $T_{1/2}$, half-life; T_{max}, time of maximum concentration.
From Lanteri-Minet M. Utilisation clinique des triptans dans la prise en charge de la migraine. CNS Drugs 2006;20(Spec Issue 1):12-23.

BOX 48-4 ALLODYNIA IN MIGRAINE

Definition

Pain triggered by stimuli not normally painful and that may occur in locations other than the area stimulated. *Ipsilateral cutaneous allodynia* is a common sign of migraine, especially with aura, and is due to the sensitization of central trigeminal-vascular neurons receiving sensory inputs from the scalp and facial skin.

Types of Stimuli and Testing Methods

Brush allodynia (BA): tested by cutaneous stimulation with a gauze pad

Pressure allodynia (PA): tested by cutaneous stimulation with Frey's hairs (camel hairs of different thickness mounted inside a thin tube)

Localization and Clinical Meaning

- Allodynia is located in the periorbital and temporal skin areas.
- Allodynia may occur during the attack in response to activities such as combing, shaving, taking a shower, or wearing glasses or earrings.
- Analgesic medication with triptans is not efficacious.

administration and elsewhere, in addition to bitter taste, nausea, and sweating, which are the most recurrent side effects. Coronary vasospasm is sometimes observed following triptan administration, which may be associated, in cardiopathic or hypertensive patients, with myocardial ischemia or infarction, or atrial or ventricular arrhythmias. For this reason, triptans are contraindicated in hypertensive and cardiopathic patients. In the absence of sufficient data on the tolerability of triptans in embryonic and fetal life and in children and adolescents, as well as in the elderly, their use should be avoided in pregnant or lactating women and practiced with caution in patients younger than 18 and older than 65 years. Only sumatriptan per nasal spray is allowed between 12 and 18 years.

Dangerous interactions between drugs used in symptomatic and/or prophylactic headache therapy may occur (Table 48-9), the most severe event being the serotonin syndrome,[112-116] a potentially life-threatening condition involving rhabdomyolysis, disseminated intravascular coagulation, and acute respiratory distress. Serotonin syndrome is caused by a drug-induced increase of intrasynaptic 5-HT concentration due to an increase in serotonin production or release (tryptophan, amphetamines, cocaine), an excessive concentration of serotoninergic (triptans) or dopaminergic (bromocriptine, levodopa) agonists, intensive nonselective (selegiline) or reversible (moclobemide) MAO inhibition, or greatly reduced monoamine reuptake (tricyclic antidepressants, selective serotonin reuptake inhibitors [SSRIs], venlafaxine, trazodone, meperidine, lithium). The occurrence of severe serotonin syndrome (Fig. 48-8) in patients misusing triptans is rare because of the high dosages of the mentioned drugs required to initiate it. In genetically

TABLE 48-7 5-HT RECEPTOR AFFINITY OF TRIPTANS

Substance	Pk1 5-HT_{1B}	Pk1 5-HT_{1D}	Pk1 5-HT_{1F}	Other Affinities
Almotriptan	8	8	7.7	5-HT_7
Eletriptan	8	8.94	7.99	5-HT_{1E}
Frovatriptan	8.23	8.52	7.2	
Naratriptan	8.09	8.09	8.18	5-HT_{1E}
Rizatriptan	6.89	7.04	6.81	
Sumatriptan	7.37	8.04	7.88	
Zolmitriptan	7.69	8.88	7.54	5-HT_{1E}, 5-HT_7

5-HT, 5-hydroxytryptamine.
Data from Lanteri-Minet M. Utilisation clinique des triptans dans la prise en charge de la migraine. CNS Drugs 2006;20(Spec Issue 1):12-23.

TABLE 48-8 DOSES OF TRIPTANS (IN MG) FOR DIFFERENT ROUTES OF ADMINISTRATION

	Route of Administration			
Substance	Oral	Subcutaneous	Rectal	Nasal Spray
Almotriptan	12.5			
Eletriptan	20, 40			
Frovatriptan	2.5			
Naratriptan	1-2.5			
Rizatriptan	5-10			
Sumatriptan	50-100	6	25	10-20
Zolmitriptan	2.5			

predisposed subjects, however, the syndrome may have a significant incidence, so it is advisable to apply all the measures suggested by pharmacogenomic studies in order to avoid or limit its severe consequences by means of a combination of medical education and technological advances.[115-117]

Long-term treatment with triptans in rats did not attenuate 5-HT_1 receptor–dependent functions, though it was able to alter the mRNA receptor expression in several tissues relevant to migraine pathophysiology.[118] In the development or maintenance of chronic daily headache, clinical investigations of Bigal et al. have demonstrated that the overuse of triptans is less frequent than that of other drugs (butalbital, acetaminophen, other NSAIDs, opioids) utilized symptomatically for the headache attack.[119] Among 456 patients with transformed migraine and acute medication overuse, seen in a tertiary headache center from 2000 to 2004, they found the following overused substances: butalbital combination products, 48%; acetaminophen, 46.2%; other NSAIDs, 40.8%; opioids, 33.3%; triptans, 17.8%; and ergotamine tartrate, 11.8%. The majority of patients observed with chronic daily headache from drug abuse (69.7%) were able to undergo detoxification without returning to medication overuse within 1 year of follow-up, while the remaining patients under observation (30.3%) did not discontinue medication overuse. The comparison between the two groups showed, in detoxified patients, a decrease in headache frequency of 73.3% versus 17.2% in the continuing-use group and equivalent outcomes with respect to headache duration and score. On the basis of these results, these authors concluded that successful detoxification may ensure a significant improvement of the headache status in patients overusing, in a large percent of the cases, more than one type of medication.[119]

Box 48-5 presents a clinical evaluation of the triptans. The improvement of pharmacokinetic properties, included lipophilicity, which is necessary for crossing the blood-brain barrier, has been the objective for the development of second-generation triptans (almotriptan, eletriptan, frovatriptan, naratriptan, rizatriptan, zolmitriptan, donitriptan, IS-159), together with greater clinical efficacy and reduced incidence and intensity of adverse reactions, especially at the cardiovascular level. However, the newer triptans, in spite of better

TABLE 48-9 POSSIBLE INTERACTIONS BETWEEN DRUGS USED IN HEADACHE THERAPY

Drug A	Drug B	Effect	Onset	Mechanism of Action
Triptans	Triptans	Sustained vasoconstriction	Fast	Synergic activity
Triptans	MAO inhibitors	Serotonin syndrome	Fast	5-HT receptor activation
Triptans (high doses)	SSRIs, TCAs, venlafaxine, trazodone, meperidine, lithium	Serotonin syndrome	Fast	5-HT receptor activation
Triptans	Ergotamine	Sustained vasoconstriction	Fast	Potentiated vasoconstriction
Triptans	Methysergide	Long-lasting vasoconstriction	Fast	Potentiated vasoconstriction
Rizatriptan	Propranolol	Increase of rizatriptan plasma concentration	Fast	Inhibition of rizatriptan metabolism
Aspirin	Diclofenac	Gastroenteric lesions	Fast	Gastric mucosa irritation
Aspirin	Indomethacin	Gastroenteric lesions	Delayed	Gastric mucosa irritation
Aspirin	COX-2 inhibitors	Increased risk of gastroenteric hemorrhage	Delayed	Gastric mucosa irritation
NSAIDs	NSAIDs	Gastroenteric lesions	Fast	Gastric mucosa irritation
SSRIs	MAO inhibitors	Serotonin syndrome	Fast	5-HT receptor activation
TCAs	Sertraline	Serotonin syndrome	Fast	5-HT receptor activation
Valproate	Amitriptyline	Serotonin syndrome	Delayed	Inhibition of amitryptiline metabolism
β-Blockers	Verapamil	Hypotension, bradycardia	Fast	Potentiation of cardiovascular effects and reduced metabolism of β-blockers

COX, cyclooxygenase; 5-HT, 5-hydroxytryptamine; MAO, monoamine oxidase; NSAIDs, nonsteroidal anti-inflammatory drugs; SSRIs, selective serotonin reuptake inhibitors; TCAs, tricyclic antidepressants.

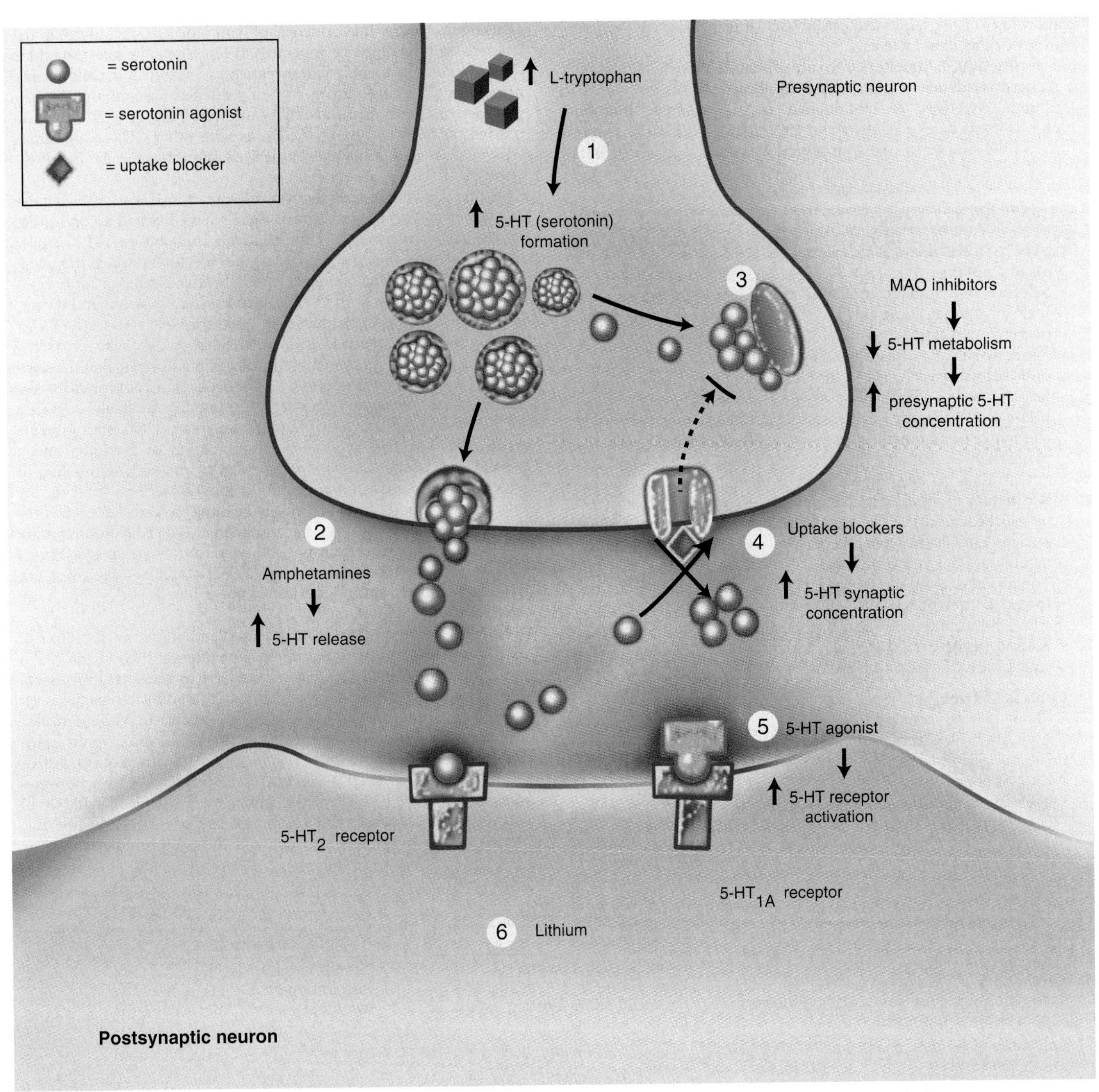

FIGURE 48-8 • Mechanisms of serotonin syndrome. *1*, Increased doses of L-tryptophan will proportionally increase serotonin (5-HT) formation. *2*, Amphetamines and other drugs increase the release of stored 5-HT. *3*, Inhibition of serotonin metabolism by monoamine oxidase (MAO) inhibitors will increase presynaptic 5-HT concentration. *4*, Impairment of 5-HT transport into the presynaptic neuron by uptake blockers (e.g., selective serotonin reuptake inhibitors, tricyclic antidepressants such as amitriptyline) increases synaptic 5-HT concentration. *5*, Direct serotonin agonists can stimulate postsynaptic 5-HT receptors. *6*, Lithium increases postsynaptic 5-H receptor responses. (Adapted from Mills KC. Serotonin syndrome: a clinical update. Crit Care Clin 1997;13:763-783.)

pharmacokinetic and pharmacodynamic profiles in preclinical investigations, did not exhibit more favorable profiles than sumatriptan in clinical practice.[109] The gap can be explained by the difficulty of constructing reliable experimental models of primary headaches in laboratory animals.[15,120,121] Thus, new, different pharmacologic approaches are necessary in order to find compounds providing these features and begin the post-triptan era in the pharmacotherapy of headache.

Nonsteroidal Anti-Inflammatory Drugs (Simple or Compound). NSAIDs, extensively discussed in Chapter 11 (Inflammation and Immunomodulation), are a class of drugs very widely used in the symptomatic therapy of headache. Their therapeutic effects derive mainly from their inhibitory activity on both isoforms of cyclooxygenase (COX-1, or constitutive, and COX-2, or inducible), microsomal enzymes playing a fundamental role in prostaglandin synthesis. Aspirin, which is the acetyl ester of sodium salicylate, and all traditional NSAIDs, or nonselective COX inhibitors, have three characteristic effects: analgesic, antipyretic, and anti-inflammatory; an exception is acetaminophen, for which the third effect is practically lacking. Aspirin, especially in a highly buffered effervescent preparation, is largely used with good results in the treatment of acute migraine attacks.[122] Moreover, its "cardioprotective" activity may be beneficial in conditions of comorbidity of migraine with cardiovascular disorders (see Section 5, Cardiovascular Therapeutics).

Selective COX-2 inhibitors or coxibs, discovered much later, present a reduced incidence of gastrointestinal adverse effects compared to traditional NSAIDs. Acetaminophen or paracetamol, inhibiting both cyclooxygenases, each by about 50%, shows a clinical pharmacologic profile similar to coxibs in several aspects and therefore is not contraindicated in the presence of pathologic states affecting the stomach and the digestive apparatus. It represents the safest migraine symptomatic treatment in elderly patients,[123] as well as in children and pregnant or lactating women.[124,125] In particular, acetaminophen analgesic activity depends on its ability to block PGE_2 generation within the central nervous system (CNS), as with other COX-1 inhibitors, while it fails to inhibit platelet-derived thromboxane A_2 and PGE_2 synthesis.[126]

BOX 48-5 CLINICAL PHARMACOLOGY OF TRIPTANS: ESSENTIAL POINTS

Pros of Triptans

- Selective symptomatic drugs for migraine attacks, triptans are ineffective in tension-type headache, the only primary headache in which they fail.
- Sumatriptan, at a dose of 6 mg by the subcutaneous route, is the only really active therapy in the cluster headache attack.
- Triptans have shown to be active in the acute and short-term prophylactic therapy of orgasmic headache, being a valuable alternative to indomethacin, which is not well tolerated by many patients.[134]
- Sumatriptan has been shown to be effective also in the symptomatic therapy of severe secondary headaches in which the pain may be blocked at the level of transmission from the trigeminal nucleus caudalis to second-order neurons, and therefore in any meningeal nociceptive process.[196,197]
- Triptans have a rapid onset of action.
- In case of lack of response, the administration can be repeated after 2 hours and once more in the following 24 hours.
- Abuse syndrome is less frequent and more manageable than with ergots, barbiturates, and NSAIDs.

Contras of Triptans

- About 25% nonresponders
- Contraindicated in patients with cardiovascular disturbances
- Use not permitted during pregnancy and lactation
- Use not permitted in children
- Use with caution in elderly and adolescents
- Possibility of negative interactions (see Table 48-9)

Although acting differently from triptans, NSAIDs are still effective in migraineurs when nociceptive signals have reached second-order trigeminal-vascular neurons and allodynia is established. The adjunct use of triptans with NSAIDs could be the basis for a rational treatment in patients developing allodynia, specially after 1 hour or more from the onset of the attack.[127,128] Clinical studies have shown that the combination of a fast-acting triptan such as rizatriptan with selective COX-2 inhibitors is effective in migraineurs. The lower headache recurrence observed in the group treated with rofecoxib and rizatriptan in comparison with the group receiving only rizatriptan could indicate the possibility of a synergic response[129]; dexamethasone might be useful for a limited population of migraine patients still presenting recurrence after a treatment with the combination of a triptan and a NSAID.[129] Recent investigations have led to the conclusion that, in patients at cardiovascular risk, COX-2 inhibitors could facilitate the onset of thrombotic events[130]; for this reason rofecoxib has been withdrawn from the market by its manufacturer. Nevertheless, according to several authors, a certain possibility of cardiovascular side effects would exist also for the traditional NSAIDs and nonselective COX inhibitors, except aspirin, and not only for new NSAIDs, which are selective COX-2 inhibitors.[131]

NSAIDs are among the most overused and abused medications in migraine patients.[119] Indomethacin is a member of this class to which some forms of primary headaches resistant to other treatments are responsive; these include some trigeminal-autonomic cephalgias, such as paroxysmal and continuous hemicrania, Valsalva-induced headache, primary stabbing headache, orgasmic headache, and hypnic headache.[132-134] The use of indomethacin is associated with frequent gastrointestinal and CNS adverse effects and the risk of overuse syndromes when it is combined with prochlorperazine and caffeine.[135] Table 48-10 lists the NSAIDs, simple and combined, largely used in the abortive therapy of headache, their dosages, and their contraindications. Box

TABLE 48-10 NSAID PHARMACOTHERAPEUTIC CHARACTERISTICS

Drug	Dosages (mg)	Contraindications[105]
Acetaminophen tablet Acetaminophen + codeine tablet Acetaminophen + aspirin + caffeine tablet Acetaminophen suppository	Oral: 325-650 Oral: 325 + 30 Oral: 250 + 250 + 65 Rectal: 120-600	Do not exceed 4 g/day Risk in hepatic disease patients Insomnia
Aspirin tablet (enteric coated) Aspirin suppository	Oral: 325-650 every 4-6 hr Rectal: 120, 300, and 600 mg	Risk in active peptic ulcer patients
Diclofenac tablet or sachet	Oral: 50 (3/day)	Risk in active peptic ulcer patients Interacts with tacrolimus and methotrexate
Ibuprofen tablet	Oral: 200-800	Do not exceed 3200 mg/day
Ketoprofen capsule Ketoprofen parenteral injection Ketoprofen suppository	Oral: 50-150 Intramuscular: 75 Rectal: 100	Risk in active peptic ulcer, renal impairment, obstetric patients Incomplete hemostasis
Ketorolac coated tablet or drops Ketorolac parenteral injection	Oral: 10-40 Intramuscular: 30-60	Do not exceed 90 mg/day Risk in active peptic ulcer, renal impairment, obstetric patients Incomplete hemostasis Interacts with lithium
Naproxen tablet	Oral: 275-550	Risk in active peptic ulcer patients
Piroxicam capsule	Oral: 10-20	Risk in active peptic ulcer patients
Nimesulide tablet	Oral: 100	Cardiovascular diseases
Coxibs: celecoxib (C), valdecoxib (V), parecoxib (P), etoricoxib (E), lumiracoxib (L)	Oral: C 200; V 10-20; E 60-120; L 200 Parenteral: P 20-40	Risk in cardiovascular disease and atherosclerosis patients

BOX 48-6 CLINICAL EVALUATION OF NSAIDs AND OTHER NONTRIPTAN DRUGS USED IN HEADACHE ABORTIVE THERAPY

- Headache abortive therapy is today based first of all on triptans, but NSAIDs, if correctly used, are still very important in non-triptan responders and in primary headaches in which triptans are ineffective.
- The combination of triptans with NSAIDs is efficacious in migraineurs with allodynia,[127-129] and the triple combination of triptans, NSAIDs, and dexamethasone significantly decreases migraine recurrence.[129]
- All the medications used to abort an attack must be taken as soon as possible after the headache onset (see Table 48-6).
- Mild migraine should have a trial of NSAIDs, eventually in combination with an antiemetic and/or caffeine; moderate to severe migraine should be treated with either dihydroergotamine or triptans.
- The leading choice treatment for tension-type headache[198] is ibuprofen (800 mg), because of its good gastrointestinal tolerance, followed by naproxen sodium (825 mg).
- Ergots, in spite of their side effects, can represent a useful alternative. In general, triptans are considered to be safer than ergots and dihydroergotamine better tolerated than ergotamine; however, either drug carries a consistent risk in patients with coronary pathology.
- Triptans cannot be used within 24 hours of dihydroergotamine treatment, and dihydroergotamine cannot be used before 6 hours after triptan administration.
- It is necessary to remember that the symptomatic approach to migraine and other cephalgias should have a temporary duration—just the time necessary to reduce, with a calibrated and individually tailored preventive cure, the intensity and frequency of attacks, thus avoiding the later need of other acute pharmacologic strategies.
- Options for the emergency management of severe headaches include triptans (see Box 48-5), NSAIDs (specially ketorolac IV), sodium valproate IV (start with 10-15 mg/kg per day, divided into 6-hour intervals, while monitoring liver function), ergots, and neuroleptics.
- Over-the-counter products such as isometheptene (a sympathomimetic drug), alone or in combination with dichoralfenazone (a chloral hydrate derivative), and acetaminophen,[93] on the market in the United States as lysine clonixinate, or NSAIDs[199] and dipyrone,[200] used, respectively, in Latin America and in Europe, may be also helpful options.
- Antinauseants (metoclopramide), myorelaxants, antiemetics (neuroleptics), and gastroprotective medications (domperidone, acid-suppressive drugs) are combined, when indicated, especially with NSAIDs and ergots.
- The role of COX-2 inhibitors is not clearly defined, since their pharmacodynamic profile is still under investigation. They may offer some interesting perspectives in cancer prevention.[201]

48-6 reports a comparative clinical evaluation of NSAIDs and other drugs in the acute therapy of primary headaches.

Ergots. This group of drugs comprises natural alkaloids of *Claviceps purpurea*, a fungus that grows on rye and other grains, and their semisynthetic derivatives, all having origin from the tetracyclic compound 6-methylergoline (see Chapter 8, Neurotransmitters). They possess a complex pharmacodynamic profile, behaving as partial agonists or antagonists of α-adrenergic, dopaminergic, and serotoninergic receptors (Table 48-11). Ergots, the first specific antimigraine therapy available, have been used in the past also as prophylactic agents in the therapy of migraine, but at present they have almost been abandoned for this indication because of their tendency to produce dependence manifestations. For either symptomatic or preventive indications, ergots expose the user to the risk of abuse, with resultant chronic daily headache, which begins after a longer term of treatment than with triptans but with more severe adverse effects,[119] especially for ergotamine; in this respect, dihydroergotamine is better tolerated.[136,137] In randomized clinical trials, oral, sublingual, and intranasal ergot preparations were found to have inferior antimigraine efficacy than triptans, while the contrary was resulting for the rectal route.[138] Table 48-12 lists the available preparations and doses, adverse effects, and contraindications of ergots.

TABLE 48-11 RECEPTOR TYPES AND SUBCLASSES AFFECTED BY ERGOTAMINE AND DIHYDROERGOTAMINE (AND OTHER ERGOT ALKALOIDS AND THEIR DERIVATIVES)

Serotonin Receptors	Adrenergic Receptors	Dopamine Receptors
$5\text{-}HT_{1A}$	α_1	DA_1
$5\text{-}HT_{1B}$	α_2	DA_2
$5\text{-}HT_{1B/2A/2C}$	α_1, $\alpha_2 > \beta$	$DA_2 > DA_1$

Data from Silberstein[139] and Saper and Silberstein.[140]

TABLE 48-12 PHARMACOTHERAPY OF ERGOTS

Preparations	Route of Administration and Doses
Ergotamine tartrate (1-mg tablets; 2-mg suppositories) + caffeine 100 mg	Oral: 2 mg every 30 min (6 mg/24 hr; 10 mg/wk)
Dihydroergotamine mesylate	
Ampules (1 mg/ml)	IV: 0.75 mg; can be repeated after 1 hr; 2 mg/24 hr; 6 mg/wk IM or subQ: 1 mg; can be repeated after 1 hr; 3 mg/24 hr; 6 mg/wk
Nasal spray (4 mg/ml)	0.5 (one spray) in each nostril; may be repeated in 15 min, for a total dose of 2-3 mg (4-6 sprays) in 24 hr and 4 mg (8 sprays) in 1 wk
Ergostine	Oral: 2 mg
α-Dihydroergocryptine	Oral: 10 mg twice a day

IM, intramuscular; IV, intravenous; subQ, subcutaneous.

Ergots are contraindicated in pregnant or lactating women and in patients with cardiovascular diseases, septic states, and hepatic or renal impairment. The concomitant use of caffeine 200 mg may improve the absorption of ergotamine and ergostine administered by the oral route.

Other Drugs

Barbiturates and Opioids. Butalbital, simple or compound, at the oral dose of 50 mg, has been widely used in the acute therapy of migraine, but this drug is associated with a high risk of addiction, with the onset of a chronic daily headache that is quite difficult to treat. The same is true for butorphanol and other opioids, the only exceptions being, in certain instances, tramadol 100 mg by the intramuscular route.[139]

Valproate Sodium. Valproate sodium, by the intravenous route, is used in the therapy of very severe migraine attacks (see Box 48-6).

Muscle Relaxants. These medications are applied more frequently in prophylactic therapy than in symptomatic therapy of tension-type headache associated with pericranial tenderness.

Oxygen. For the acute treatment of cluster headache attacks, 100% O_2, at a flow of at least 7 L/min over 15 minutes, as an alternative to sumatriptan, is considered a drug of first choice.[140]

Others. Other options for the abortive or symptomatic therapy of primary headaches are lidocaine 4% to 6% nasal drops and intranasal capsaicin or its *z*-isomer civamide.[141,142]

Prophylactic or Preventive Therapy

The objectives of prophylactic therapy, based on the previously mentioned classes of agents, are to reduce the intensity, frequency, and duration of attacks and to make them more responsive to acute treatments, thereby improving the quality of life of headache sufferers. Prophylaxis is also indicated when acute medications produce adverse effects, are inefficacious, or are contraindicated, as can happen in the presence of comorbid conditions.[143] According to Silberstein and Goadsby,[144] prophylactic agents raise the threshold of activation of migraine and other primary headaches, enhancing antinociception, inhibiting CSD, and, when administered chronically to experimental animals,[70,106] blocking peripheral and central sensitization and neurogenic inflammation and modulating sympathetic, parasympathetic, and 5-HT tone. Table 48-13 lists drugs currently used in primary headache preventive therapy.

β-Adrenergic-Blockers (see Chapter 8, Neurotransmitters). Propranolol, timolol, and metoprolol, as well as, with less support from clinical data, other β-blocking drugs (nadolol, pindolol, atenolol), are first-line pharmacologic agents for migraine prevention,[143,145] and they can also be used in chronic daily headaches,[146] being particularly useful in the presence of comorbidity with hypertension. The mechanism of action hypothesized for the prophylactic effect of propranolol and other compounds of the same group, which are devoid of adrenergic intrinsic activity and known to modulate vascular tone, is the normalization of abnormal catecholamine response in migraine patients, produced by blocking an endothelial β-adrenergic receptor activating NOS or by blocking an endothelial 5-HT receptor, also coupled to NOS.[147] β-Blockers also have anxiolytic effects and, as with other drugs acting on adrenergic receptors tried in the prophylactic therapy of primary headache, such as the α_2-selective adrenergic agonists clonidine and tizanidine,[148,149] could exert their activity also on the locus

TABLE 48-13 AGENTS USED IN THE PROPHYLACTIC THERAPY OF PRIMARY HEADACHES AND TRIGEMINAL NEURALGIA

Pharmacologic Class	Drugs	Mean Daily Dose (mg/ml)	Main Indications
β-Adrenergic receptor antagonists	Propranolol Timolol Metoprolol Nadolol Pindolol Atenolol	40-160 10-20 50-200 40-240 5-20 50-200	Migraine, chronic daily headache, headache associated with hypertension
Anticonvulsants	Valproate	500-1500 (10-15 IV/die*)	Migraine, emergency migraine,* chronic migraine, hemicrania continua, cluster headache, SUNCT
	Topiramate	50-200	Migraine, cluster headache, chronic daily headache, pediatric migraine, SUNCT
	Gabapentin	600-2000	Migraine, chronic daily headache, SUNCT, cluster headache
	Tiagabine	30-50	Migraine, anxiety
	Lamotrigine	25-100	Migraine with aura, SUNCT, paroxysmal hemicrania
	Zonisamide	100-400	Refractory pediatric migraine, chronic daily headache, paroxysmal hemicrania
	Levetiracetam	500-1000	Migraine with aura
	Carbamazepine	200-800	Trigeminal neuralgia
	Oxcarbazepine	300-600	SUNCT
	Pregabalin	150-600	Trigeminal neuropathic pain
Calcium channel blockers	Verapamil	240-320	Cluster headache
	Flunarizine	5-10	Migraine without aura, pediatric migraine
	Cinnarizine	5-75	Migraine without aura, pediatric migraine
Antidepressants	Amitryptiline	10-150	Tension-type headache, migraine
	Venlafaxine	75-150	Tension-type headache, migraine
	SSRIs	20-40	Migraine with mood disorders
Muscle relaxants	Tizanidine	Start with max. 2 tid, increase gradually in order to reach 8 tid (10-12 wk); 10 tid for 10-12 wk	Tension-type headache with pericranial tenderness, chronic daily headache, neuralgias (topical application)
	Baclofen		Migraine, cluster headache
Short-term prophylaxis	Methylprednisolone or equivalent corticosteroids	100 up to 500 per day (IV same dose), over 5 days, then tapering down in 3-4 days to	Cluster headache
	Lithium carbonate	150-300 2-3 times per day for 10-15 days, monitoring blood levels	
Serotonin antagonists and ergots	Cyproheptadine	Syrup: 0.25 kg/day, divided into 3 doses	Pediatric migraine
	Dihydroergocryptine	Start with 5 bid; increase of 5 every 3-4 days, to reach 20 bid	Migraine
Angiotensin modulators	Lisinopril Candesartan	20 16	Migraine

ceruleus and other structures participating in the "migraine generator" (see Fig. 48-5). Furthermore, according to Shields and Goadsby,[150] they may exert some of their effects in migraine through β_1-adrenoceptor antagonist actions in the thalamus. This hypothesis seems attractive considering the complex and widespread nature of the sensory disturbance in migraine, defined by Sicuteri[57]—a pathology affecting at the same time the nociceptive function, the autonomic nervous system, and the affective sphere.

In clinical practice, propranolol is given by the oral route, at a mean daily dose of 40 to 120 mg for 3-month cycles of therapy. This treatment, in the absence of contraindications, is generally well tolerated and induces a significant decrease of migraine index, with appreciable anxiolytic activity. The side effects of β-blockers, in general rather rare and mild at the doses currently utilized in clinical practice, are orthostatic hypotension, fatigue, depression, and sexual dysfunction. These drugs are contraindicated in patients having as comorbid conditions asthma and Raynaud's disease, and must not be given to pregnant or lactating women. The combination of propranolol with rizatriptan or calcium channel blockers may produce pharmacokinetic and pharmacodynamic interactions, such as elevation of rizatriptan concentrations[151] or reduction of β-blocker metabolism and synergism of cardiac effects (see Table 48-9).

Antiepileptics (see Chapter 45, Seizure Disorders). In this class of pharmacologic agents there is a remarkable array of new drugs in the course of development,[31] and several of the currently marketed agents show clear-cut activity in the therapy of primary headaches.

Valproate is an anticonvulsant drug currently used in the preventive treatment of migraine, and also assayed as a second-order analgesic in the therapy of cluster headache.[29,33,34,152] Its mechanism of action, not yet clearly elucidated, involves GABAergic transmission, which is increased, with suppression of migraine-related events in the cortex, perivascular parasympathetic endings, and trigeminal nucleus caudalis. It reduces the release of excitatory amino acids and/or blocks their effects, blocks voltage-gated sodium channels, and modulates dopaminergic and serotoninergic tone. Valproic acid is about 90% bound to plasma proteins and metabolized by microsomal glucuronide conjugation, mitochondrial beta oxidation and cytochrome P-450–dependent omega-1,2 oxidation. The elimination half-life is between 9 and 18 hours, becoming shorter when enzyme-inducing agents are coadministered. Valproic acid is able to inhibit the metabolic transformation of other drugs, such as lamotrigine and certain drugs used in the treatment of human immunodeficiency virus. Reported adverse effects include gastrointestinal disturbances, weight gain, and, at high serum concentrations, tremor, platelet disorders, pancreatitis, and liver toxicity. It is therefore advisable to monitor the serum levels of valproate during long-term prophylactic medication. The drug is not to be used in infants below 2 years of age and in pregnant or lactating women, and the risk of teratogenicity is high.[152-155]

Good results have also been obtained in the treatment of primary headaches with more recent anticonvulsants such as topiramate, gabapentin, lamotrigine, tiagabine, zonisamide, and levetiracetam. Topiramate has recently received approval for migraine prevention in the United States and in other countries. Based on cellular phosphorylation, it blocks voltage-dependent sodium channels and potentiates GABA receptor activity, inhibiting AMPA/kainate receptors and L-type and N-type calcium channels. Side effects are fatigue, paresthesia, and weight loss, and contraindications include hepatopathies, glaucoma, and nephrolithiasis. Gabapentin acts on $GABA_A$ and $GABA_B$ receptors, modulating the nonpore alpha$_2$-delta subunit of P/Q type calcium channels and reducing neuronal excitability as a consequence of decreased release of glutamate/aspartate and inhibition of AMPA receptors activity on noradrenergic tone. It may induce somnolence and dizziness. All antiepileptics possess a teratogenic potential, especially valproate. Comparative evaluations of data relating to clinical effectiveness, safety, and tolerability of these drugs did not show significant differences between them.[106,141,144,146,156-163] Their clinical applications in the prophylaxis of primary headaches are listed in Table 48-13.

Calcium Channel Blockers (see Chapter 8, Neurotransmitters; Chapter 24, Coronary Artery Disease; and Chapter 25, Rhythm Disorders). Calcium channel blockers produce a reduction of Ca^{2+} flux through voltage-dependent calcium channels of L, N, and P/Q types located in presynaptic terminals of trigeminal-vascular structures, by binding to alpha$_1$ subunits, which are modulated by alpha$_2$, delta, and beta subunits. With this mechanism, they modify the release of neurotransmitters and vasoactive neuropeptides, especially CGRP,[164] dural blood vessel dilation, and headache attack.[165] Verapamil also exerts other activities, such as the inhibition of neuronal NOS, the blockade of hyperalgesia, and the potentiation of analgesia from opioids and acetaminophen. Flunarizine and cinnarizine (lomerizine[166]) have been tried in Japan, and new agents of this group are in development. They are well tolerated also in the pediatric age range, and their side effects are constipation, sedation, and weight gain.[106]

Antidepressants (see Chapter 53, Depression and Bipolar Disorders). A large percentage of migraine and other primary headache sufferers present with mood disorders, anxiety, and reactive depression. For this reason, and because neurotransmitters involved in the pathophysiology of depression also have a prevalent role in central sensitization mechanisms of primary headaches, especially in tension-type headache and chronic daily headache, amitriptyline, the prototype of the tricyclic antidepressants, has been tried as a preventive agent, alone or in combination with tizanidine.[149] The main pharmacodynamic properties of this drug are (i) blockade of sodium channels, causing the inhibition of peripheral sensitization; (ii) activation of adenosine A_1 receptors, with enhancement of descending modulation of the rostro-ventral-medial nucleus; (iii) 5-HT_2 down-regulation; and (iv) increase of GABA-mediated inhibition due to a positive modulation of $GABA_A$, and reduced function of GABA transporters GAT-1 and GAT-3. In an attempt to find among the antidepressants of the same group (selective norepinephrine reuptake inhibitors) or of other groups, such as the SSRIs, a drug providing a larger therapeutic index in comparison with amitriptyline, other antidepressants have been clinically assayed, but none has been demonstrated to exert equal activity. The only ones found to be effective and rather well tolerated are venlafaxine and duloxetine, selective for the 5-HT transporter at low doses, the norepinephrine transporter at medium doses, and the dopamine transporter at high doses. Amitriptyline and other tricyclic antidepressants, being provided with antimuscarinic effects, are contraindicated in glaucoma and may cause several side effects, such as sedation, weight gain, dry mouth, sour taste, epigastric distress, urinary retention, blurred vision, dizziness, tachycardia, orthostatic hypotension, weakness, and fatigue. SSRIs, devoid of anticholinergic effects, may be useful in conditions of comorbidity with anxiety and mood disorders, but it is advisable to consider the relative risk (see Table 48-9) connected to their adjunct use with triptans.[106,143]

Botulinum Toxin A. Botulinum toxin A, a neurotoxin produced by the anaerobic bacterium *Clostridium botulinum*, is a locally acting protein that inhibits the release of acetylcholine from presynaptic nerve endings. It belongs to the muscle relaxant agent class, acting as an antispastic in the CNS at higher centers and on the spinal cord. Furthermore, botulinum toxin, which has as its receptor the synaptic vesicle protein SV2 (isoforms A, B, and C), may exert an analgesic action in the prophylactic treatment of chronic forms of migraine and tension-type headache and in chronic daily headache that seems to be based on the inhibition of peripheral release of excitatory amino acids and proinflammatory and nociceptive neuropeptides.[146,148,167] Botulinum is injected into the pericranial muscles, such as the glabellar, frontalis, temporalis, and others (see Table 48-13). The treatment is tolerated rather well, the noxious side effects being moderate and transient. They include muscular weakness, muscle pain at the injection site, blepharoptosis, dysphagia, and asthenia. There are still conflicting opinions on the efficacy of botulinum toxin, and further study is necessary. Another problem is the cost of the treatment.

Short-Term Prophylaxis. NSAIDs, especially naproxen, ketoprofen, and tolfenamic acid, may be effective as prophylactic agents for primary headaches; aspirin, 500 mg daily or three times a week, is also effective for relatively long-term treatment. Triptans have also been used for short-term prophylaxis (e.g., naratriptan and sumatriptan in perimenstrual migraine).[168] Muscle relaxants acting on the CNS have seen clinical application in the short-term prophylactic treatment of tension-type headache, as well as in symptomatic treatment; these include tizanidine,[148] often combined with amitriptyline[149]; baclofen, a $GABA_B$ receptor agonist; and benzodiazepines.[169] $GABA_B$ receptors also have been implicated in migraine pathogenetic mechanisms. The coupling between GABA and $GABA_B$ receptors induces the activation of a specific G protein, exerting an inhibitory effect on the enzyme adenylate cyclase, with the reduction of intracellular cyclic AMP levels and a decreased phosphorylation rate. Consequently, GABA agonists produce a functional block of voltage-dependent Ca^{2+} channels involved in neurotransmitter release, inhibiting the release of many neurotransmitters, GABA included. Baclofen in fact has been shown to inhibit the activation of the trigeminal-vascular system at the level of the spinal trigeminal caudate nucleus, thereby exerting significant antinociceptive activity, as observed in many clinical trials on patients suffering from migraine or cluster headache.[29,30,170,171] Corticosteroids and lithium are used for short periods in the preventive therapy of cluster headache, with continuous monitoring of the patient's clinical condition because of the low tolerability of these pharmacologic agents.[141]

Serotonin Antagonists and Ergots. Agents of this group are cyproheptadine, pizotifen, and the ergots α-dihydroergocryptine and methysergide ($5\text{-}HT_{2B}$ and $5\text{-}HT_{2C}$ receptor antagonists), and lisuride, an isoergolenyl derivative found effective in migraine prevention. Cyproheptadine, an antihistamine$_1$ agent and a weak anticholinergic, is used in migraine prevention in children, being well tolerated; pizotifen and α-dihydrocryptine, not available in the United States, are other efficacious migraine preventive agents, generally with poor tolerability for the high incidence of tiredness and/or drowsiness and weight gain. Methysergide is able to exert a potent beneficial effect in primary headache prevention, but because of the serious adverse events it can produce, among which are retroperitoneal, pleuropulmonary, coronary, and endocardial fibrosis, for prolonged treatment, its usage should remain under the supervision of a specialist and be reserved for severe cases in which other preventive drugs are not effective.[144,172] Lisuride also provides central dopaminergic activity.[173] For information on ergotamine tartrate and dihydroergotamine mesylate, used much less today in the preventive therapy of migraine, see Table 48-12.

Angiotensin Antagonists and ACE Inhibitors. Candesartan, an angiotensin II AT1-receptor inhibitor, and lisinopril, an ACE inhibitor, were found effective in migraine prophylaxis in patients not responsive to triptans or in hypertensive patients, in whom triptans are not indicated. While the mechanism of action is unknown for candesartan, for ACE inhibitors the antimigraine activity is thought to be due to modifications of vasoreactivity and sympathetic tone induced by these medications and also to their influence on the turnover of proinflammatory peptides, such as SP, enkephalins, and bradykinin.[107,145]

Other Agents. The complex and multifactorial pathogenesis of primary headaches involves practically the entire hormonal constellation. Therefore, many hormones have been proposed in the preventive therapy of different primary headaches, but the only ones thus far recognized to have a precise role and a certain effectiveness are corticosteroids in cluster headache (see Table 48-13). Testosterone replacement therapy was effective in episodic and chronic cluster headache in male patients showing low levels of the hormone. In female patients suffering from the same type of headache, a combination testosterone/estrogen was given with good results.[174] Recent neuroendocrine and sleep studies suggest consideration of melatonin and other hormones that could interact at the hypothalamic level for cluster headache and all autonomic trigeminal headaches, as well as for migraine. In contrast, short-term perimenstrual hormonal therapy, using combined oral contraceptives or progestins alone, has been tried in severe menstrual migraine and in menopausal migraine, with equivocal results.[174-176]

Millan-Guerrero et al.[66] have demonstrated, in a double-blind, placebo-controlled clinical study, that the histamine catabolite *N*-α-methylhistamine, a selective histamine$_3$ (H_3) receptor agonist, given subcutaneously at doses of 1 to 3 ng twice a week to 60 patients with migraine, induced a significant reduction, compared to placebo, in headache intensity, frequency, and duration and analgesic intake. They concluded that H_3 agonists may specifically inhibit the neurogenic edema response involved in migraine physiopathology.[66] Intranasal preparations of capsaicin and its *z*-isomer civamide have been used for the treatment of migraine, and cluster headache studies are still in progress.[141,142] According to Slow et al., there is widespread evidence supporting the use of neuroleptics in headache treatment.[177]

In a recent multicenter clinical study, the officinal herb feverfew (*Tanacetum parthenium*) was shown to be effective at 6.25 mg three times daily and very well tolerated in migraine preventive therapy; the mechanism of action of parthenolides, its active principles, is thought to be the blockade of nuclear factor-κB activation, resulting in attenuation of inducible NOS and inhibition of the proinflammatory cascade.[106] The root of *Petasites hybridus*, a perennial shrub used in popular medicine for hundreds of years for many pathologic conditions, is sold as butterbur root over the counter for migraine therapy in Germany. Recently it has been demonstrated that, at its optimal effective daily dose of 75 mg twice daily, it is able to produce a mean decrease in migraine frequency of 48% versus 26% with placebo. The drug may exert vasodilatory effects from direct antagonism on the activity of L-type calcium channels in vascular smooth muscle as well as anti-inflammatory effects due to leukotriene inhibition.[106]

Adjuvant Pharmacotherapeutic Strategies

The complexity of primary headache pathogenesis, with the involvement of many receptor functions and related metabolic pathways, and with frequent comorbidities, has resulted in the use of a large number of drugs in prophylactic therapy. In recent years, increasing value has been seen in the adjuvant use of naturally occurring products, such as minerals, coenzymes, and vitamins, in order to obtain favorable synergistic activity with other therapeutic agents.

Minerals. The mineral most studied for adjuvant use in headache prophylaxis is magnesium, which counteracts vasospasm, inhibits platelet aggregation, and stabilizes cell membranes.[80] As a result of these activities, magnesium is able to modulate serotonin receptors and other related receptors and neurotransmitters, NO synthesis and release, and inflammatory mediators, reducing eicosanoid and vasoactive neuropeptide formation. Current evidence suggests that, during an acute attack, migraine patients with and without aura have lowered levels of ionized magnesium in blood plasma and red cells. In light of its potential deficiency in migraine and other primary headaches, as well as its ability to inhibit platelet aggregation and interact in neurotransmitter turnover and receptor activity (clinically documented in several studies together with good tolerability), the use of magnesium pidolate (300 to 600 mg) is indicated in the prevention therapy of primary headaches.[178,179]

Coenzymes. Mitochondrial dysfunction with impaired oxygen metabolism has been suggested for migraine pathogenesis. Coenzyme Q_{10} (ubiquinone or ubidecarenone), an endogenous enzyme cofactor produced in all living cells in humans, functions to promote the proton-electron translocation in mitochondria, transferring electrons from complexes I and II to cytochrome *c*. At the same time, it protects mitochondria from free radical damage and plays a role in the permeability transition of the inner mitochondrial membrane. Coenzyme Q_{10} is a useful therapeutic agent in conditions associated with increased oxidative stress and in patients suffering from mitochondrial encephalomyopathies, being able to improve exercise tolerance, muscle weakness, and brain energy metabolism. Exogenous coenzyme Q_{10}, which can be administered either orally or parenterally, decreases serum pyruvate and lactate levels. On the basis of this evidence, Rozen et al.[180] in an open study investigated the efficacy of ubidecarenone as a preventive medication for migraine headaches, at a daily oral dosage of 150 mg for 3 months. A greater than 50% reduction in number of days with migraine headache was observed in 61.3% of the patients. The average number of days with migraine during the baseline period was 7.34, and this decreased to 2.95, which was a statistically significant response; the mean migraine attack frequency was reduced by 55.3% after 3 months of treatment. No side effects were noted. Coenzyme Q_{10}

was equally effective in migraine without aura and in migraine with aura. Doses greater than 150 mg/day can be used in children also, considering its safety profile.

Vitamins. Riboflavin, or vitamin B_2, an essential constituent and precursor of riboflavin 5′-phosphate, also known as flavin mononucleotide or flavin adenine dinucleotide, is required for the activity of flavoenzymes involved in the electron transport chain. Altered mitochondrial energy metabolism may play a role in migraine pathogenesis, and patients with migraine demonstrate a reduction in mitochondrial phosphorylation potential in between attacks. Riboflavin may work by increasing mitochondrial energy efficiency. In a study by Schoenen et al.,[181] an oral daily dose of 400 mg given for 3 months to patients suffering from migraine with and without aura induced a significant reduction in both attack frequency and headache days, with a mean global improvement of 68.2%. Amitriptyline increases the renal excretion of riboflavin.

Cobalamins (methylcobalamin, adenosylcobalamin, and hydroxycobalamin) are involved in several important pathways, among which is a scavenging action against NO by hydroxycobalamin; NO plays a definite role in the pathogenesis of migraine. The chronic use of NSAIDs, specially anti–COX-1, induces gastric damage that favors the development of *Helicobacter pylori*, with a decrease of intrinsic factor production and consequent reduction of vitamin B_{12} absorption, which ultimately affects the important metabolic functions regulated by this vitamin. Migraine intensity, duration, and frequency can be significantly reduced by a therapy with vitamin B_{12}. A few studies have examined the relationship between dysfunction of the vitamin B_{12} pathway and headache pathogenesis.

Hyperhomocysteinemia is an independent risk factor for coronary artery disease, and can be associated with cerebrovascular disorders. Low serum levels of vitamin B_{12} and folate correlate with high levels of homocystinemia, and plasma levels of homocysteine can be lowered by supplementation of folic acid. Multiple genetic and environmental factors can lead to hyperhomocysteinemia. In particular, a polymorphism in the 5,10-methylenetetrahydofolate reductase gene (*MTHFR*) has been observed, and individuals homozygous for the mutation C677T exhibit reduced enzymatic activity and elevated homocysteine concentration, especially in cases of folate deprivation. The prevalence of *MTHFR* mutations and other polymorphisms of the enzyme has been demonstrated in migraine and tension-type headache patients, in whom a reduction of vitamin B_{12} and folate serum concentrations has also been observed. Moreover, basal levels of homocystinemia were increased in these patients, indicating that this compound is a reliable marker of vitamin B_{12} deficiency and that hyperhomocysteinemia is often associated with migraine. Homocysteic acid acts physiologically as an endogenous agonist of NMDA receptors, playing a significant role in the initiation, propagation, and duration of CSD. Elevated homocysteic acid levels, secondary to hyperhomocysteinemia, could sensitize the dura mater and cerebral arteries and/or promote the activation of the trigeminal-vascular system, thus predisposing patients to migraine attacks or increasing the disease's severity (Fig. 48-9).

Vitamin B_{12} seems to exert a prominent role in migraine therapy for its scavenging and neurotrophic properties, as well as for its other physiologic and pharmacodynamic roles, such as hepatoprotection and antianemic activity. An intriguing and interesting relationship is that existing between vitamin B_{12} and homocysteine, often based on an inverse order of concentration in biologic means. The meaning of this relationship is not yet clarified, but it offers many attractive options for fundamental and clinical research, as well as in the field of primary headache pathogenesis and therapy.[179]

Emerging Targets and Therapeutics

The number of prospective potential targets in the pharmacotherapy of headaches is very large,[9,15,33,71,105,106,120,182,183] considering the multifaceted pathogenesis of these headaches and the plurality of nervous structures involved (Fig. 48-10 and Box 48-7). As always happens in scientific progress, a number of attempts, often supported by convincing precedents, have led to unpredictable flops (Table 48-14). In addition, there are contrasting opinions about some drugs, such as lamotrigine.

A rational perspective for the future includes modulators of ionotropic or metabotropic glutamate receptors. Such agents should result in efficacious treatment of chronic daily headaches, since the glutamatergic system is implicated in CSD, neurogenic inflammation, and sensitization pathways generating allodynia, as demonstrated by experimental research and confirmed by clinical studies.[17,18,183-185] New compounds such as LY-293558,[186] a novel AMPA/GluR5 antagonist, provided there is good tolerability, will probably be designed and developed shortly.

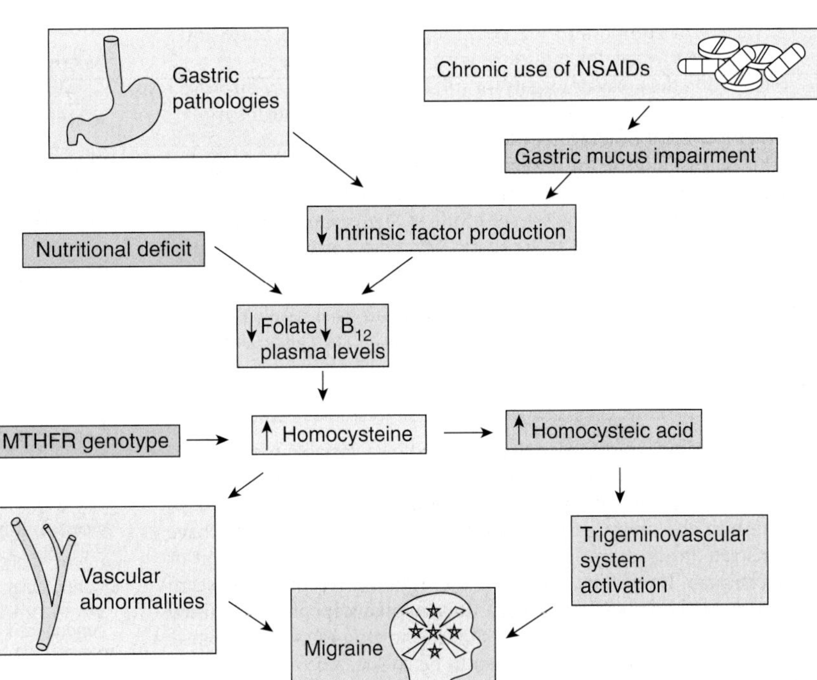

FIGURE 48-9 • Role of vitamin B_{12} in migraine pathogenesis. Gastric pathologies and/or chronic use of nonselective NSAIDs in migraine patients impair the production of intrinsic factor, with a reduction in vitamin B_{12} absorption. Nutritional deficits may also contribute to vitamin B_{12} deficit. Low plasma levels of B_{12} and/or mutation in the methylenetetrahydrofolate reductase (*MTHFR*) gene can lead to the elevation of the homocystinemia. The increase in homocysteic acid levels, secondary to hyperhomocysteinemia, could activate the trigeminal-vascular system, thus favoring the onset of migraine attacks. (From Bianchi A, Salomone S, Caraci F, et al. Role of magnesium, coenzyme Q10, riboflavin, and vitamin B12 in migraine prophylaxis. Vitam Horm 2004;69:297-312.)

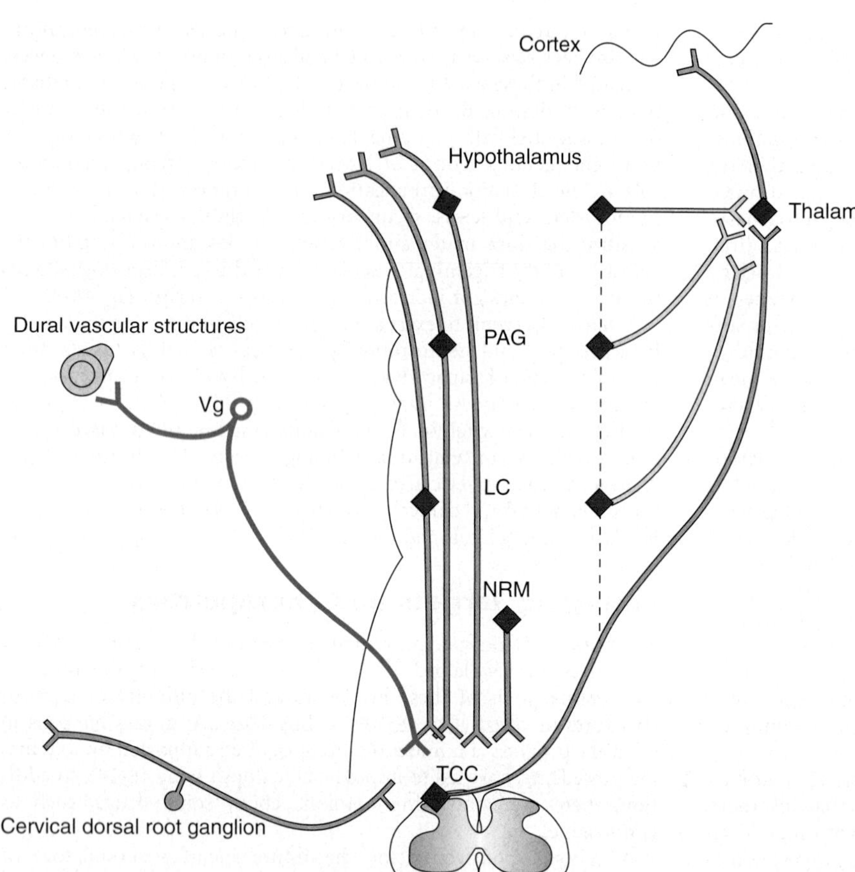

FIGURE 48-10 • Selected pathways and modulatory centers associated with migraine. Inputs from dural vascular structures are projected by the ophthalmic division of the trigeminal nerve, with cell bodies in the trigeminal ganglion (Vg) project, along with branches of the upper cervical nerve roots, onto second-order neurons in the trigeminal nucleus caudalis and dorsal horns of C1 and C2; together, these are known as the trigeminocervical complex (TCC). These neurons, in turn, project largely into the contralateral thalamus and cortex. Modulatory projections from the hypothalamus, periaqueductal grey (PAG) matter, locus ceruleus (LC), and medullary nucleus raphe magnus (NRM) can modulate activity in the TCC, and, for many of these structures, also modulate thalamic activity (as shown). Migraine is probably caused by dysfunction of the modulatory sensory matrix that controls afferent inputs. Therefore, suitable drug development targets either can be located in the primary pathways (such as the TCC) or are those altering the behavior of modulatory centers (such as the PAG). (From Goadsby PJ. Can we develop neurally acting drugs for the treatment of migraine? Nature Rev Drug Discov 2005;4:741-750.)

BOX 48-7 KEY ISSUES FOR NEW TARGETS IN THE PHARMACOTHERAPY OF HEADACHE

- Advances in the understanding of migraine pathophysiology have allowed selective targeting of key steps in the migraine cascade; however, we are still far from the ideal acute and preventive therapy for migraine.
- Selective targets may lead to the development of future therapies with greater effectiveness and fewer adverse effects.
- A variety of compounds are being reviewed for both acute and preventive therapy for migraine, with a range of targets.
- Expanding the array of targets for migraine therapy may improve the success rate for pharmacotherapy and allow physicians more precise control of treatment for their patients.
- Although many of the investigative therapies will not become standard treatment, target-based drug design confirmed with randomized clinical trials may result in increasing success as a result of advances in technology, genomics, proteomics, and metabonomics.

From Buchanan TM, Ramadan NM, Aurora S. Future pharmacologic targets for acute and preventive treatments of migraine. Expert Rev Neurother 2004;4:391-430.

Since migraine is a disorder characterized by a variable pain threshold and many clinical expressions, linked to different genes, investigations on the polymorphous opioid receptors could also contribute to reduction of the migraine pain threshold, though many studies have demonstrated the adverse effects of opiates[20-23] in the management of headache pain. Interesting aspects of the opioid receptor family seem to be presented by nociceptin/orphanin, a heptadecapeptide identified as the endogenous ligand for the nociceptin opioid receptor like-1 (ORL-1). Nociceptin has been shown to be co-located with CGRP, SP, NOS, and pituitary adenylate cyclase–activating peptide, which implies

TABLE 48-14 EXAMPLES OF FAILED DRUGS IN ACUTE AND PREVENTIVE MIGRAINE THERAPY

Drug Tested in RCT	Mechanism of Action	Reason(s) for Failure
Zatosetron	5-HT_3 antagonist	Negative RCT (acute)
PNU-142633	5-HT_{1D} agonist	Negative RCT (acute) Weak 5-HT_{1D}
LY-334370	5-HT_{1F} agonist	Animal toxicity (acute)
Avitriptan (BMS-180048)	5-$HT_{1B/D}$ agonist	Animal toxicity (acute)
Alniditan (R91214)	5-$HT_{1B/D}$ agonist	Withdrawn
CP-122, 228	PPE inhibitor	Failed RCT (acute), dosing?
4991W93	PPE inhibitor	Failed RCT (acute), dosing?
Bosentan	$ET_{A/B}$ blocker	Failed RCT (acute)
Lanepitant	NK-1 antagonist	Failed RCT (acute, prevention)
GR205171	NK-1 antagonist	Negative RCT (acute)
L-758298	NK-1 antagonist	Negative RCT (acute)
Ganaxolone	$GABA_A$ modulator	Negative RCT (acute)
Lamotrigine	Sodium channel blocker	Negative RCT (prevention)
Montelukast	LD_4 antagonist	Negative RCT (prevention), dosing?

ET, endothelin; GABA, γ-aminobutyric acid; 5-HT, 5-hydroxytryptamine (serotonin); LD, leukotriene; NK, neurokinin; PPE, plasma protein extravasation; RCT, randomized controlled trial.

Adapted from Buchanan TM, Ramadan NM, Aurora S. Future pharmacologic targets for acute and preventive treatments of migraine. Expert Rev Neurother 2004;4:391-430.

a role in trigeminal sensory transmission and vascular regulation,[182] with inhibition of neurogenic dural vasodilation. The ORL-1 receptor offers a new research objective in antimigraine therapy.

Calignano et al.[187] have observed that CB-1 agonists, such as WIN552122, when applied on the skin, are able to reduce the nociceptive activity of formalin. After a protracted and intense noxious stimulation, sufficient to provoke an inflammatory reaction, central and peripheral neuronal excitability can be significantly increased, with the possibility of inducing the onset of pain and hyperalgesia by normally innocuous events (allodynia). Cannabinoids, in animal experimental models, antagonize either hyperalgesia or allodynia.[41-44,188,189] In contrast, CB-1 antagonists, such as SR141716A, decrease the activation threshold, raising the response to mechanic and thermic stimuli. Therefore, it may be that, after repeated or long-lasting injury, as after trauma or in the course of inflammation, endocannibanoid levels appear significantly augmented either in sensory terminals or in CNS structures (e.g., in the PAG), while a sensitization of CB-1 receptors can be observed. Experimental data seem to demonstrate the fundamental role of endocannabinoids in pain pathways, disclosing a possible interaction of these new targets in the treatment of various clinical forms of pain, headache included. A study conducted by Chichewitz[190] in experimental models has demonstrated the existence of an intimate connection between cannabinoid and opioid signaling pathways in the modulation of pain perception, which indicates that the analgesic effect of Δ^9-tetrahydrocannabinol, the major psychoactive constituent of marijuana, could be mediated, at least in part, through the activation of CB-1 receptors associated with δ- and κ-opioid receptors. This study suggests the development of a novel analgesic regimen based on the use of low-dose cannabinoids and opioids to effectively treat the acute and chronic pain of headache.

On the basis of the results obtained by Amenta et al.[54] in an epidemiologic study conducted on marijuana smokers, cannabis seems to produce a statistically significant analgesic effect on migraineurs, as shown in Figure 48-11. This observation supports the view of Russo,[53] who has hypothesized that migraine and other painful conditions alleviated by cannabis, such as fibromyalgia, irritable bowel syndrome, and related conditions often displaying associated clinical, biochemical, and pathophysiologic patterns, could be the expression of a state of endocannabinoid deficiency. Further studies on the role of endocannabinoids and CB, VR, and PAR receptors will establish whether, how, and to what extent they participate in the pathogenetic mechanisms of headache, and may open interesting therapeutic possibilities. In conclusion, CB, as well as VR and PAR receptors with their ligands, seem worthy of attention in the study of pain pathophysiology and therapeutic problems related to primary headaches.[39,41-46,49-55,187-190]

The development of agents able to inhibit second-order neurons from the trigeminal nucleus caudalis, such as adenosine A1 receptor agonists GR79236 and GR190178, without concomitant vasoconstriction, suggests their utilization for the treatment of migraine.[63,182] Hypothalamic peptides and orexin A can be also taken in consideration; they determine, through protein kinase C, the phosphorylation of voltage-activated channels, with the production of analgesic effects having a mechanism not yet elucidated.[71,89,182] In addition, the research on new antiepileptics,[31] GABA agonists,[29,30] calcium channel blockers[106,107] such as dotarizine and alfa-eudesmol,[106,189] $5\text{-HT}_{1D\text{-}F}$ nontriptans and/or nonvasoactive 5-HT_1 agonists, 5-HT_2 antagonists, NOS inhibitors, and SP antagonists[47,106,107,182,183] will keep scientists in the field of primary headaches pharmacotherapy busy for the coming years.

Since drugs used in primary headache prophylaxis, when administered chronically in experimental animals, are able to suppress dose-dependent CSD, research is focused on the development of more effective migraine prophylactic agents directed to target specific cellular and molecular mechanisms underlying the important role of CSD and related modifications in migraine pathogenesis.[70]

Clinical trials performed for testing whether selective neurokinin-1 receptor antagonists are effective in migraine therapy have produced negative results. For this reason, the role of plasma protein extravasation mediated by neurokinin-1 receptor activation (SP/NKA operated) has been questioned in migraine. Conversely, high-affinity nonpeptide antagonists of human CGRP were found effective in reducing both headache and associated phenomena of migraine attacks, without affecting cardiovascular parameters.[191-193]

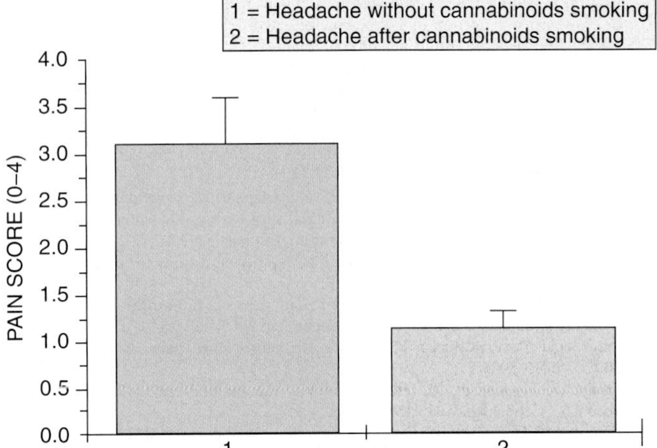

FIGURE 48-11 • Pain variations induced by cannabinoids in 25 headache sufferers, after smoking marijuana. (From Amenta V, Pitari GM, Caff M, et al. An epidemiological study on the activity of cannabis in idiopathic headache. In Olesen J, Edvinsson L [eds]: Frontiers in Headache Research Series, Vol 7: Headache Pathogenesis: Monoamines, Purines and Nitric Oxide. Philadelphia: Lippincott–Raven, 1997, pp 107-109.)

Continuing pharmacogenomic investigations are expected to give new insights about qualitative and quantitative differences in the genetic expression of 5-HT receptors and related carriers and enzymatic functions. This research should provide a significant contribution to the improvement of therapeutic possibilities related to the dysfunction, by mutation, of Ca^{2+} channels, especially P/Q type, and of other ionic channels involved in primary headaches, with respect to their role in 5-HT release and in CSD, estimated to be the basis of migraine aura,[194] pain mechanisms, and their control.[195]

REFERENCES

1. Headache Classification Subcommittee of the International Headache Society. The International Classification of Headache Disorders, 2nd ed. Cephalalgia 2004;24(Suppl 1):9-160.
2. Graham JR, Wolff HG. Mechanism of migraine headache and action of ergotamine tartrate. Arch Neurol Psychiatr 1938;39:737-763.
3. Wolff HG. Headache and Other Head Pain. New York: Oxford University Press, 1963.
4. Lance JW, Goadsby PJ. Mechanism and Management of Headache, 6th ed. Oxford: Butterworth, 1998, pp xv, 1-8.
5. Hardman JG, Limbard LE, Goodman Gilman A (eds). Goodman & Gilman's the Pharmacological Basis of Therapeutics, 10th ed. New York: McGraw-Hill, 2001, p 372.
6. Carpenter RL, Mackey DC. Local anesthetics. In Barash PG, Cullen BF, Stoelting RK (eds): Clinical Anesthesia. Philadelphia: Lippincott, 1992, pp 509-541.
7. Bianchi A, Caraci F, Salomone S. The pain in primary headache. In Capasso A (ed): Recent Developments in Pain Research. Trivandrum, India: Research Signpost, 2005, pp 343-357.
8. Moskowitz MA. Neurogenic versus vascular mechanisms of sumatriptan and ergot alkaloids in migraine. Trends Pharmacol Sci 1992;13:307-311.
9. Waeber C, Moskowitz MA. Therapeutic implications of central and peripheral neurologic mechanisms in migraine. Neurology 2003;61(8 Suppl 4):S9-S20.
10. Waeber C, Moskowitz MA. Migraine as an inflammatory disorder. Neurology 2005;64(10 Suppl 2):S9-S15.
11. Faria LC, Mody I. Protective effect of ifenprodil against spreading depression in the mouse enthorinal cortex. J Neurophysiol 2004;92:2610-2614.
12. Storer RJ, Akerman S, Goadsby PJ. Calcitonin gene-related peptide (CGRP) modulates nociceptive transmission in the cat. Br J Pharmacol 2004;142:1171-1181.
13. Christensen JK, Varming T, Ahring PK, et al. In vitro characterization of 5-carboxyl-2,4-di-benzamidobenzoic acid (NS3769), a noncompetitive antagonist of GLUK 5 receptors. J Pharmacol Exp Ther 2004;309:1003-1010.
14. Dickenson AH, Chapman V, Green GM. The pharmacology of excitatory and inhibitory aminoacid-mediated events in the transmission and modulation of pain in the spinal cord. Gen Pharmacol 1997;28;633-638.
15. Edvinsson L. Neuronal signal substances as biomarkers of migraine. Headache 2006;46:1088-1094.

16. Kowara R, Moraleja KL, Chakravarthy B. Involvement of nitric oxide synthase and ROS-mediated activation of L-type voltage gated Ca^{2+} channels in NMDA-induced DPYSL3 degradation. Brain Res 2006;1119:40-49.
17. Gallai V, Alberti A, Gallai B, et al. Glutamate and nitric oxide pathway in chronic daily headache: evidence from cerebrospinal fluid. Cephalalgia 2003;23:166-174.
18. Tajti J, Uddman R, Edvinsson L. Neuropeptide localization in the "migraine generator" region of the human brainstem. Cephalalgia 2001;21:96-101.
19. Staud R, Rodriguez ME. Mechanisms of disease: pain in fibromyalgia syndrome. Nat Clin Pract Rheumatol 2006;2:90-98.
20. Vachharajani NN, Shyu WC, Nichola PS, et al. A pharmacokinetic interaction study between butorphanol and sumatriptan nasal sprays in healthy subjects: importance of the timing of butorphanol administration. Cephalalgia 2002;22:283-287.
21. Loder E. Post-marketing experience with an opioid nasal spray for migraine: lessons for the future. Cephalalgia 2006;26:89-97.
22. Biondi DM. Opioid resistance in chronic daily headache: a synthesis of ideas from the bench and bedside. Curr Pain Headache Rep 2003;7:67-75.
23. Przewlocki R, Prezwlocka B. Opioids in neuropathic pain. Curr Pharm Des 2005;11:3013-3025.
24. Edvinsson L, Goadsby PJ. Neuropeptides in the cerebral circulation: relevance to headache. Cephalalgia 1995;15:272-276.
25. Longmore J, Shaw D, Smith D, et al. Differential distribution of 5HT1D- and 5HT1B-receptor immunoreactivity within the human trigemino-cerebrovascular system: implications for the discovery of new antimigraine drugs. Cephalalgia 1997;17:833-842.
26. Goadsby PJ, Edvinsson L, Ekman R. Vasoactive peptide release in the extracerebral circulation of humans during migraine headache. Ann Neurol 1990;28:183-187.
27. Kondo E, Kiyama H, Yamano M, et al. Expression of glutamate (AMPA type) and gamma-aminobutyric acid (GABA)A receptors in the rat caudal trigeminal spinal nucleus. Neurosci Lett 1995;186:169-172.
28. Knight YE, Bartsch T, Goadsby PJ. Trigeminal antinoception induced by bicuculline in the periaqueductal gray (PAG) is not affected by PAG P/Q-type calcium channel blockade in rat. Neurosci Lett 2003;336:113-116.
29. Johannessen CU. Mechanisms of action of valproate: a commentatory. Neurochem Int 2000;37:103-110.
30. GaoY, Lei LS, Wu SG. Changes in GAT-3 and GABA-T mRNA expression of C6 glioma cells in response to a 2-week treatment with sodium valproate and withdrawal. Di Yi Jun Yi Da Xue Xue Bao 2003;23:885-887.
31. Rogawski MA. Diverse mechanisms of antiepileptic drugs in the development pipeline. Epilepsy Res 2006;69:273-294.
32. Lee WS, Limmroth V, Ayata C, et al. Peripheral GABA-A receptor-mediated effects of sodium valproate on dural plasma protein extravasation to substance P and trigeminal stimulation. Br J Pharmacol 1995;116:1661-1667.
33. Parsons AA. Cortical spreading depression: its role in migraine pathogenesis and possible therapeutic intervention strategies. Curr Pain Headache Rep 2004;8:410-416.
34. Ayata C, Jin H, Kudo C, et al. Suppression of cortical spreading depression in migraine prophylaxis. Ann Neurol 2006;59:652-661.
35. Piomelli D, Beltramo M, Giuffrida A, et al. Endogenous cannabinoid signaling. Neurobiol Dis 1998;5:462-473.
36. Wagner JA, Varga K, Ellis EF, et al. Activation of peripheral CB1 cannabinoid receptors in haemorrhagic shock. Nature 1997;390:518-521.
37. Varga K, Wagner JA, Bridgen DT, et al. Platelet- and macrophage-derived endogenous cannabinoids are involved in endotoxin-induced hypotension. FASEB J 1998;12:1035-1044.
38. Zygmunt PM, Petersson J, Andersson DA, et al. Vanilloid receptors on sensory nerves mediate the vasodilator action of anandamide. Nature 1999;400:452-457.
39. Pertwee RG. Pharmacological actions of cannabinoids. Handb Exp Pharmacol 2005;(168):1-51.
40. Maione S, Oliva P, Marabese I, et al. Periaqueductal gray matter metabotropic glutamate receptors modulate formalin-induced nociception. Pain 2000;85:183-189.
41. Martin WJ, Coffin PO, Attias E, et al. Anatomical basis for cannabinoid-induced antinociception as revealed by intracerebral microinjections. Brain Res 1999;822:237-242.
42. Ahluwalia J, Urban L, Capogna M, et al. Cannabinoid 1 receptors are expressed in nociceptive primary sensory neurons. Neuroscience 2000;100:685-688.
43. Johanek LM, Simone DA. Cannabinoid agonist, CP 55,940, prevents capsaicin-induced sensitization of spinal cord dorsal horn neurons. J Neurophysiol 2005;93:989-997.
44. Hohmann AG, Herkenham M. Cannabinoid receptors undergo axonal flow in sensory nerves. Neuroscience 1999;92:1171-1175.
45. Szallasi A, Blumberg PM. Vanilloid receptors: new insights enhance potential as a therapeutic target. Pain 1996;68:195-208.
46. Caterina MJ, Schumacher MA, Tominaga M, et al. The capsaicin receptor: a heat activated ion channel in the pain pathway. Nature 1997;389:816-824.
47. Regoli D, Boudon A, Fauchère JL. Receptors and antagonists for substance P and related peptides. Pharmacol Rev 1994;46:551-599.
48. Tsuchiya M, Sakakibara A, Yamamoto M. A tachykinin NK1 receptor antagonist attenuates the 4 beta-phorbol-12-myristate-13-acetate-induced nociceptive behaviour in the rat. Eur J Pharmacol 2005;507:29-34.
49. Tognetto M, Amadesi S, Harrison S, et al. Anandamide excites central terminals of dorsal root ganglion neurons via vanilloid receptor-1 activation. J Neurosci 2001;21:1104-1109.
50. Bisogno T, Melck D, Bebrov M, et al. *N*-acyl-dopamine: synthetic CB1 receptor ligands and inhibitors of anandamide inactivation with cannabimimetic activity in vitro and in vivo. Biochem J 2000;351:817-824.
51. Trevisani M, Smart D, Gunthorpe MJ, et al. Ethanol elicits and potentiates nociceptor responses via the vanilloid receptor-1. Nat Neurosci 2002;5:546-551.
52. Dai Y, Moriyama T, Higashi T, et al. Proteinase-activated receptor 2-mediated potentiation of transient receptor potential vanilloid subfamily 1 activity reveals a mechanism for proteinase-induced inflammatory pain. J Neurosci 2004;24:4293-4299.
53. Russo EB. Clinical endocannabinoid deficiency (CECD): can this concept explain therapeutic benefits of cannabis in migraine, fibromyalgia, irritable bowel syndrome and other treatment-resistant conditions? Neuro Endocrinol Lett 2004;25:31-39.
54. Amenta V, Pitari GM, Caff M, et al. An epidemiological study on the activity of cannabis in idiopathic headache. In Olesen J, Edvinsson L (eds): Frontiers in Headache Research Series, Vol 7: Headache Pathogenesis: Monoamines, Purines and Nitric Oxide. Philadelphia: Lippincott–Raven, 1997, pp 107-109.
55. Steinhoff M, Buddenkotte J, Shpacovitch V, et al. Proteinase-activated receptors: transducers of proteinase-mediated signalling in inflammation and immune response. Endocr Rev 2005;26:1-43.
56. Heyck H. Neue Beiträge für Klinik un Pathogenese der Migräne. Stuttgart, Thieme, 1956.
57. Sicuteri F. Hypothesis: migraine, a central biochemical dysnociception. Headache 1976;16:145-159.
58. Sicuteri F. Dopamine, the second putative protagonist in headache. Headache 1977;17:129-131.
59. Sicuteri F. Endorphins, opiate receptors and migraine headache. Headache 1978;17:253-257.
60. Lance JW. The pathophysiology of migraine: a tentative synthesis. Pathol Biol 1992;40;355-360.
61. Hoskin KL, Bulmer DC, Goadsby JP. Fos expression in the trigeminovascular complex of the cat after stimulation of the superior sagittal sinus is reduced by L-NAME. Neurosci Lett 1999;266:173-176.
62. Sarchielli P, Alberti A, Codini M, et al. Nitric oxide metabolites, prostaglandins and trigeminal vasoactive peptides in internal jugular vein blood during spontaneous migraine attacks. Cephalalgia 2000;20:907-918.
63. Giffin NJ, Kowacs F, Libri V, et al. Effect of the adenosine A1 receptor agonist GR79236 on trigeminal nociception with blink reflex recordings in healthy human subjects. Cephalalgia 2003;23:287-292.
64. Peroutka SJ. Neurogenic inflammation and migraine: implications for the therapeutics. Mol Interv 2005;5:304-311.
65. Cupini LM, Bari M, Battista N, et al. Biochemical changes in endocannabinoid are expressed in platelets of female but not male migraineurs. Cephalalgia 2006;26:277-281.
66. Milan-Guerrero RO, Isais-Millan R, Benjamin TH, et al. *N*-alpha-methylhistamine safety and efficacy in migraine prophylaxis: Phase III study. Can J Neurol Sci 2006;33:195-199.
67. Leão AAP. Spreading depression of activity in the cerebral cortex. J Neurophysiol 1944;7:359-390.
68. Lauritzen M. Pathophysiology of the migraine aura: the spreading depression theory. Brain 1994;117:199-210.
69. Lauritzen M. Cortical spreading depression in migraine. Cephalalgia 2001;21:757-760.
70. Moskowitz MA. Migraine headache: from models to mechanism. J Headache Pain 2006;7:243-244.
71. Lambert GA, Michalicek J. Cortical spreading depression reduces dural blood flow—a possible mechanism for migraine pain? Cephalalgia 1994;14:430-436.
72. Choudhuri R, Cui L, Yong C, et al. Cortical spreading depression and gene regulation: relevance to migraine. Ann Neurol 2005;51:499-506.
73. Gilkey SJ, Ramadan NM, Aurora TK, et al. Cerebral blood flow in chronic posttraumatic headache. Headache 1997;37:583-587.
74. Koroleva VI, Davydov VI, Roschchina GY. Suppression of EEG gamma activity—an informative measure of spreading depression waves in the neocortex of the conscious rabbit. Neurosci Behav Physiol 2006;36:625-630.
75. May A. A review of diagnostic and functional imaging in headache. J Headache Pain 2006;7:174-184.
76. Cohen AS, Goadsby JP. Functional neuroimaging of primary headache disorders. Expert Rev Neurother 2006;6:1159-1171.
77. Peroutka SJ. Genetic basis of migraine. Clin Neurosci 1998;5:34-37.
78. Rozen T, Shanske S, Otaegui D, et al. Study of mitochondrial DNA mutations in patients with migraine with prolonged aura. Headache 2004;44:674-677.
79. Koga Y, Nataliya P. Migraine headache and mitochondrial DNA abnormality. Nippon Rinsho 2005;63:1720-1726.
80. Lodi R, Iotti S, Cortelli P, et al. Deficient energy metabolism is associated with low free magnesium in the brains of patients with migraine and cluster headache. Brain Res Bull 2001;54:437-441.
81. Diener HC, May A. New aspects of migraine physiopathology: lessons learned from positron emission tomography. Curr Opin Neurol 1996;9:199-201.
82. Welch KM, Cao Y, Aurora S, et al. MRI of the occipital cortex, red nucleus, and substantia nigra during visual aura of migraine. Neurology 1998;51:1465-1469.
83. Turkdogan D, Cagirici S, Soylemez D, et al. Characteristic and overlapping features of migraine and tension type headache. Headache 2006;46:461-468.
84. Mathew NT. Tension-type headache. Curr Neurol Neurosci Rep 2006;6:100-105.
85. Giacovazzo M, Martelletti P, Valeri M, et al. A new immunological aspect of cluster headache: the increase of monocyte and NK cell populations. Headache 1986;26:134-136.
86. Leone M, Attanasio A, Croci D, et al. The *m*-chlorophenylpiperazine test in cluster headache: a study on central serotoninergic activity. Cephalalgia 1997;17:662-672.
87. Leone M. Deep brain stimulation in headache. Lancet Neurol 2006;5:873-877.
88. Holland PR, Akerman S, Goadsby PJ. Orexin 1 receptor activation attenuates neurogenic dural vasodilatation in an animal model of trigeminovascular nociception. J Pharmacol Exp Ther 2005;315:1380-1385.

89. Schurks M, Kurth T, Geissler I. Cluster headache is associated with the G1246A polymorphism in the hypocretin receptor 2 gene. Neurology 2006;66:1917-1919.
90. Gardner KL. Genetics of migraine: an update. Headache 2006;46(Suppl 1):19-24.
91. Russell MB, Saltyte-Benth J, Levi N. Are infrequent episodic, frequent episodic and chronic tension-type headache inherited? A population-based study of 11,199 twin pairs. J Headache Pain 2006;7:119-126.
92. Baumber L, Sjostrand C, Leone M, et al. A genome-wide scan and *HCRTR2* candidate gene analysis in a European cluster headache cohort. Neurology 2006;66:1888-1893.
93. Silberstein SD, Lipton RG, Goadsby PJ, et al. Headache in Primary Care: 5. The Pathophysiology of Primary Headache. Oxford: Isis Medical Media, 1999, pp 39-49.
94. Sicuteri F. The ingestion of serotonin precursors (L-5-hydroxytryptophan and L-tryptophan) improves migraine headache. Headache 1973;13:19-22.
95. Bouchelet I, Cohen Z, Case B, et al. Differential expression of sumatriptan sensitive 5-hydroxytryptamine receptors in human trigeminal ganglia and cerebral blood vessels. Mol Pharmacol 1996;50:219-232.
96. Lanteri-Minet M. Utilisation clinique des triptans dans la prise en charge de la migraine. CNS Drugs 2006;20(Spec Issue 1):12-23.
97. Hoskin KL, Lambert GA, Donaldson C, et al. The 5-hydroxytryptamine 1B/1D/1F receptor agonists eletriptan and naratriptan inhibit trigeminovascular input to the nucleus tractus solitarius in the cat. Brain Res 2004;998:91-99.
98. Ramadan NM, Skljarevski V, Phebus LA, et al. 5-HT1F receptor agonists in acute migraine treatment: a hypothesis. Cephalalgia 2003;23:776-785.
99. Shepheard S, Edvinsson L, Cumberbatch M, et al. Possible antimigraine mechanisms of action of the 5HT1F receptor agonist LY 334370. Cephalalgia 1999;19:851-858.
100. Goldstein DJ, Roon KI, Offen WW, et al. Selective serotonin 1F ($5HT_{1F}$) receptor agonist LY 334370 for acute migraine: a randomized controlled trial. Lancet 2001;358:1230-1234.
101. Levy D, Jakubowski M, Burstein R. Disruption of communication between peripheral and central trigeminovascular neurons mediates the antimigraine action of 5HT1B/1D receptor agonists. Proc Natl Acad Sci U S A 2004;101:4274-4279.
102. Burstein R, Jakubowski M. Unitary hypothesis for multiple triggers of the pain and strain of migraine. J Comp Neurol 2005;493:9-14.
103. Lambert GA, Hoskin KL, Zagami AS. Nitrergic and glutamatergic neuronal merchanisms at the trigeminovascular first-order synapse. Neuropharmacology 2004;47:92-105.
104. Ma QP. Co-localization of 5-HT (1B/1D/1F) receptors and glutamate in trigeminal ganglia in rats. Neuroreport 2001;12:1589-1591.
105. Arulmozhi DK, Veeranjaneyulu A, Bodhankar SL. Migraine: current therapeutic targets and future avenues. Curr Vasc Pharmacol 2006;4:117-128.
106. Ramadan NM, Buchanan TM. New and future migraine therapy. Pharmacol Ther 2006;112:199-212.
107. Buchanan TM, Ramadan NM, Aurora S. Future pharmacologic targets for acute and preventive treatments of migraine. Expert Rev Neurother 2004;4:391-430.
108. Pini LA, Cicero AFG. Triptans: the experience of a clinical pharmacologist in clinical practice. J Headache Pain 2001;2:S103-S106.
109. Ferrari MD, Goadsby PJ, Roon KI, et al. Triptans (serotonin, 5-HT1B/1D agonists) in migraine: detailed results and methods of a meta-analysis of 53 trials. Cephalalgia 2002;22:833-658.
110. Barbanti P, Fabbrini G, Vanacore N, et al. Sumatriptan in migraine with unilateral cranial autonomic symptoms: an open study. Headache 2003;43:400-403.
111. Sarchielli P, Pini LA, Zanchin G, et al. Clinical-biochemical correlates of migraine attacks in rizatriptan responders and non responders. Cephalalgia 2006;26:257-265.
112. Lejoyeux M, Rouillon F, Leon A, et al. The serotonin syndrome: review of the literature and description of an original study. Encephale 1995;21:537-543.
113. Guzelcan Y, Kleinpenning AS. Life-threatening serotonin syndrome following a single dose of a serotonin reuptake inhibitor during maintenance therapy with a monoamine oxidase inhibitor. Ned Tijdschr Geneeskd 2006;50:1081-1084.
114. Birmes P, Coppin D, Schmitt L, et al. Serotonin syndrome: a brief review. CMAJ 2003;168:1439-1442.
115. Boyer EW, Shannon M. The serotonin syndrome. N Engl J Med 2005;352:1112-1120.
116. Wooltorton E. Triptan migraine treatments and antidepressants: risk of serotonin syndrome. CMAJ 2006;175:874-876.
117. Mills KC. Serotonin syndrome: a clinical update. Crit Care Clin 1997;13:763-783.
118. Reuter U, Salomone S, Ickenstein GW, et al. Effects of chronic sumatriptan and zolmitriptan treatment on 5-HT1 receptor expression and function in rats. Cephalalgia 2003;23:398-407.
119. Bigal ME, Rapoport AM, Sheftell FD, et al. Transformed migraine and medication overuse in a tertiary headache centre—clinical characteristics and treatment outcomes. Cephalalgia 2004;24:483-490.
120. Akerman S, Goadsby PJ. The role of dopamine in a model of trigeminovascular nociception. J Pharmacol Exp Ther 2005;314:162-169.
121. Arulmani U, Gupta S, Van Den Brink AM, et al. Experimental migraine models and their relevance in migraine therapy. Cephalalgia 2006;26:642-659.
122. Diener HC, Lampl C, Reimnitz P, et al. Aspirin in the treatment of acute migraine attacks. Expert Rev Neurother 2006;6:563-573.
123. Sarchielli P, Mancini ML, Calabresi P. Practical considerations for the treatment of elderly patients with migraine. Drugs Aging 2006;23:461-489.
124. Hamailanen ML. Migraine in children and adolescents: a guide to drug treatment. CNS Drugs 2006;20:813-820.
125. Silberstein SD. Headaches in pregnancy. Neurol Clin 2004;22:727-756.
126. Aronoff DM, Oates JA, Boutaud O. New insights into the mechanism of action of acetaminophen: its clinical pharmacologic characteristics reflect its inhibition of the two prostaglandin H2 synthases. Clin Pharmacol Ther 2006;79:9-19.
127. Buzzi MG. Allodynia and early treatment of migraine attacks with triptans. J Headache Pain 2006;7:265-266.
128. Loder E. Fixed drug combination for the acute treatment of migraine: place in therapy. CNS Drugs 2006;19:769-784.
129. Krymchantowski AV, Barbosa JS. Dexamethasone decreases recurrence observed after treatment with a triptan combined with a nonsteroidal anti-inflammatory drug. Arq Neuropsiquiatr 2001;59:708-711.
130. Kroetz F, Schiele TM, Klauss V, et al. Selective COX-2 inhibitors and risk of myocardial infarction. J Vasc Res 2005;42:312-324.
131. Valat JP, Deray G, Heloire F. Are there any differences in the cardiovascular tolerance between classical NSAIDs and coxibs? Presse Med 2006;35:1525-1534.
132. Dodick DW. Indomethacin-responsive headache syndromes. Curr Pain Headache Rep 2004;8:19-26.
133. Giammarco R. The nurse with jabbing headaches. In Purdy RA, Rapoport AM, Sheftel FD, et al (eds): Advanced Therapy of Headache, 2nd ed. Hamilton, Ontario: BC Decker, 2005, pp 125-128.
134. Frese A, Gantenbein A, Marziiak M, et al. Triptans in orgasmic headache. Cephalalgia 2006;26:1458-1461.
135. Ferrari A, Savino G, Gallesi D, et al. Effect of the antimigraine combination of indomethacin, prochlorperazine and caffeine (IPC) on the disposition of its components in chronic headache patients. Pharmacol Res 2006;54:142-149.
136. Silberstein SD. The pharmacology of ergotamine and dihydroergotamine. Headache 1997;37(Suppl 1):S15-S25.
137. Saper JR, Silberstein SD. Pharmacology of dihydroergotamine and evidence for efficacy and safety in migraine. Headache 2006;46(Suppl 4):S171-S181.
138. Bigal ME, Tepper SJ. Ergotamine and dihydroergotamine: a review. Curr Pain Headache Rep 2003;7:55-62.
139. Engindeniz Z, Demircan C, Karli, et al. Intramuscular tramadol for the acute treatment of acute migraine attacks in emergency department: a prospective, randomized, double-blind study. J Headache Pain 2005;6:143-148.
140. Rapoport AM. Acute treatment of headache. J Headache Pain 2006;7:355-359.
141. May A, Leone M, Afra J, et al. EFNS guidelines on the treatment of cluster headache and other trigeminal-autonomic cephalalgias. Eur J Neurol 2006;13:1066-1077.
142. Rapoport AM, Bigal ME, Tepper SJ, et al. Intranasal medications for the treatment of migraine and cluster headache. CNS Drugs 2004;18:671-685.
143. Buchanan TM, Ramadan NM. Prophylactic pharmacotherapy for migraine headaches. Semin Neurol 2006;26:188-198.
144. Silberstein SD, Goadsby PJ. Migraine: preventive treatment. Cephalalgia 2002;22:491-512.
145. Modi S, Lowder DM. Medication for migraine prophylaxis. Am Fam Physician 2006;73:72-78.
146. Mathew NT. Views and Perspectives. The prophylactic treatment of chronic daily headache. Headache 2006;46:1552-1564.
147. Tvedskov JF, Thomsen LL, Thomsen LL, et al. The effect of propranolol on glyceryltrinitrate-induced headache and arterial response. Cephalalgia 2004;24:1076-1087.
148. Freitag G. Preventative treatment for migraine and tension-type headaches: do drugs having effects on muscle spasm and tone have a role? CNS Drugs 2003;17:373-381.
149. Bettucci D, Testa L, Calzoni S, et al. Combination of tizanidine and amitriptyline in the prophylaxis of chronic tension-type headache: evaluation of efficacy and impact on quality of life. J Headache Pain 2006;7:34-36.
150. Shields KG, Goadsby PJ. Propranolol modulates trigeminovascular responses in thalamic ventroposteromedial nucleus: a role in migraine? Brain 2005;128:86-97.
151. Goldberg MR, Sciberras D, De Smet M, et al. Influence of beta-adrenoceptor antagonists on the pharmacokinetics of rizatriptan, a 5-HT1B/1D agonist: differential effects of propranolol, nadolol and metoprolol. Br J Clin Pharmacol 2001;52:69-76.
152. Gallagher RM, Mueller LL, Freitag FG. Divalproex sodium in the treatment of migraine and cluster headache. J Am Ostheopath Assoc 2002;102:92-94.
153. Cutrer FM, Limmroth V, Moskowitz MA. Possible mechanisms of valproate in migraine prophylaxis. Cephalalgia 1997;17:93-100.
154. Freitag FG, Collins SD, Carlson HA, et al. A randomized trial of divalproex sodium extended-release tablets in migraine prophylaxis. Neurology 2002;58:1652-1659.
155. Perucca E. Pharmacological and therapeutic properties of valproate: a summary after 35 years of clinical experience. CNS Drugs 2002;16:695-714.
156. Mathew NT. Antiepileptic drugs in migraine prevention. Headache 2001;41(Suppl 1): S18-S24.
157. Matharu MS, Bradbury P, Swash M. Clinical Correspondence. Hemicrania continua: side alternation and response to topiramate. Cephalalgia 2006;26:341-344.
158. Pakalnis A, Kring D. Zonisamide prophylaxis in refractory pediatric headache. Headache 2006;46:804-807.
159. Ashkenazi A, Benlifer A, Korenblit J, et al. Zonisamide for migraine prophylaxis in refractory patients. Cephalalgia 2006;26:1199-1202.
160. Anzai Y, Ayashi M, Ohia T. Zonisamide eradicated paroxysmal headache with EEG abnormalities triggered by hypertensive encephalopathy due to purpura nephritic syndrome. Brain Dev 2006;28:610-613.
161. Brighina F, Palermo A, Aloisio A, et al. Levetiracetam in the prophylaxis of migraine with aura: a 6-month open-label study. Clin Neuropharm 2006;29:338-342.
162. Wilby J, Kainth A, Hawkins N, et al. Clinical effectiveness, tolerability and cost-effectiveness of newer drugs for epilepsy in adults: a systematic review and economic evaluation. Health Technol Assess 2005;9:1-157.
163. Perucca E, Meador KJ. Adverse effects of antiepileptic drugs. Acta Neurol Scand Suppl 2005;181:30-35.
164. Greenberg DA. Calcium channels in neurological disease. Ann Neurol 1997;42:275-282.
165. Akerman S, Williamson DJ, Goadsby PJ. Voltage-dependent calcium channels are involved in neurogenic dural vasodilatation via a presynaptic transmitter release mechanism. Br J Pharmacol 2003;140:558-566.
166. Hara H, Shimazava M, Hashimoto M, et al. Anti-migraine effects of lomerizine. Nippon Yakurigaku Zasshi 1998;112(Suppl 1):138P-142P.
167. Dong M, Yeh F, Tepp WH, et al. SV2 is the protein receptor for botulinum neurotoxin A. Science 2006;312:540-541.

168. Silberstein SD. Headache and female hormones: what you need to know. Headache 2001;14:323-333.
169. D'Amico D, Grazzi L, Leone M, et al. A review of the treatment of primary headaches. Part II: Tension-type headache. Ital J Neurol Sci 2005;19:2-9.
170. Hering-Hanit R. Baclofen for prevention of migraine. Cephalalgia 1999;19:589-591.
171. Hering-Hanit R, Gadoth N. Baclofen in cluster headache. Headache 2000;40:48-51.
172. Bussone G, Cerbo R, Martucci N, et al. Alpha-dihydroergocryptine in the prophylaxis of migraine: a multicenter double-blind study versus flunarizine. Headache 1999;39:426-431.
173. Soyka D, Frieling B. Lisuride for the prevention of migraine: results of a multicenter study. Fortschr Med 1989;107:763-766.
174. Stillman MJ. Testosterone replacement therapy for treatment of refractory cluster headache. Headache 2006;46:925-933.
175. Gupta S, Mehrotra S, Villalon CM, et al. Potential role of female sex hormones in the pathophysiology of migraine. Pharmacol Ther 2007;113:321-340.
176. Silberstein SD, Saper JR, Freitag FG. Migraine: diagnosis and treatment. In Silberstein SD, Lipton RB, Dalessio DJ (eds): Wolff's Headache and Other Head Pain, 7th ed. Oxford: Oxford University Press, 2001, pp 8-237.
177. Slow HC, Young WB, Silberstein SD. Neuroleptics in headache. Headache 2005;45:358-371.
178. Aloisi P, Marrelli A, Porto C, et al. Visual evoked potentials and serum magnesium levels in juvenile migraine patients. Headache 1997;37:383-385.
179. Bianchi A, Salomone S, Caraci F, et al. Role of magnesium, coenzyme Q10, riboflavin, and vitamin B12 in migraine prophylaxis. Vitam Horm 2004;69:297-312.
180. Rozen TD, Oshinsky ML, Gebeline CA, et al. Open label trial of coenzyme Q10 as a migraine preventive. Cephalalgia 2002;22:137-141.
181. Schoenen J, Jacquy J, Lenaerts M. Effectiveness of high dose riboflavin in migraine prophylaxis: a randomized controlled trial. Neurology 1998;50:466-470.
182. Goadsby PJ. Can we develop neurally acting drugs for the treatment of migraine? Nature Rev Drug Discov 2005;4:741-750.
183. Stam AH, Haan J, Frants RR, et al. Migraine: new treatment options from molecular biology. Expert Rev Neurother 2005;5:563-661.
184. Nicolodi M, Sicuteri F. Negative modulators of excitatory amino acids in episodic and chronic migraine: preventing and reverting chronic migraine. Int J Clin Pharmacol Res 1998;18:93-100.
185. Kaube H, Herzog J, Kaufer T, et al. Aura in some patients with familial hemiplegic migraine can be stopped by intranasal ketamine. Neurology 2000;55:139-141.
186. Sang CN, Ramadan NM, Wallihan RG, et al. LY-293558, a novel AMPA/GluR5 antagonist, is efficacious and well tolerated in acute migraine. Cephalalgia 2004;24:596-602.
187. Calignano A, La Rana G, Giuffrida A, Piomelli D. Control of pain initiation by endogenous cannabinoids. Nature 1998;394:277-281.
188. Li J, Daughters RS, Bullis C, et al. The cannabinoid receptor agonist WIN 55,212-2 mesylate blocks the development of hyperalgesia produced by capsaicin in rats. Pain 1999;81:25-33.
189. Martin WJ, Loo CM, Basbaum AI. Spinal cannabinoids are anti-allodynic in rats with persistent inflammation. Pain 1999;82:199-205.
190. Chichewitz DL. Synergistic interactions between cannabinoid and opioid analgesic. Life Sci 2004;74:1317-1324.
191. Olesen J, Diener HC, Husstedt IW, et al. Calcitonin gene related peptide receptor antagonist BIBN 4096 2BS for the acute treatment of migraine. N Engl J Med 2004;350:1104-1110.
192. Geppetti P, Trevisani M, Nicoletti P, et al. Novel therapeutic targets. Neurol Sci 2006;27(Suppl 2):S111-S114.
193. Strassman AM, Levy D. Response properties of dural nociceptors in relation to headache. J Neurophysiol 2006;95:1298-1306.
194. Nyholt DR, Morley KI, Ferreira MA, et al. Genomewide significant linkage to migrainous headache on chromosome 5q21. Am J Hum Genet 2005;77:500-512.
195. Craven A, Olesen J, Parsons A. From migraine and other headaches to neurovascular regulation and basic mechanisms of head pain. J Neurol Neurosurg Psychiatry 2006;77(Suppl 1):134-135.
196. Manfredi PL, Shenoy S, Payne R. Sumatriptan for headache caused by head and neck cancer. Headache 2000;40:758-760.
197. Rosenberg JH, Silberstein SD. The headache of SAH responds to sumatriptan. Headache 2005;45:597-598.
198. Fumal A, Schoenen J. Tension-type headache. Rev Neurol (Paris) 2005;161:720-722.
199. Krymchantowski AV, Peixoto P, Higashi P, et al. Lysine clonixinate vs naproxen sodium for the acute treatment of migraine: a double-blind, randomized, crossover study. MedGenMed 2005;7:69.
200. Tulunay FC, Ergun H, Gulmez SE, et al. The efficacy and safety of dypirone (Novalgin) tablets in the treatment of acute migraine attacks: a double-blind, crossover, randomized, placebo-controlled, multi-centre study. Funct Neurol 2004;19:197-202.
201. Cha YI, Dubois RN. NSAIDs and cancer prevention: targets downstream of COX-2. Annu Rev Med 2007;58:239-252.

49

STROKE

Rodney Bell, Kiwon Lee, Carissa Pineda, and David Brock

EPIDEMIOLOGY 743
PATHOPHYSIOLOGY 743
THERAPEUTICS AND CLINICAL PHARMACOLOGY 743
Acute Reperfusion Therapy for Ischemic Stroke 743
Alteplase 743
Pro-urokinase 744
Stroke Prevention 744
Primary Stroke Prevention 746
Secondary Stroke Prevention 746
Lifestyle Modification 746
Clinical Risk Factors 748

EPIDEMIOLOGY

Stroke is a major public health care issue. Worldwide, it is estimated that 5.5 million people die from a stroke each year, making stroke the second leading cause of death, while 15.5 million are left with a significant disability. In the United States, stroke remains the third leading cause of death. The annual incidence of stroke is approximately 700,000 cases in America, with a prevalence of 4.7 million. Stroke is the leading cause of adult disability. The cost of stroke to the U.S. economy is estimated to be about $57 billion. In patients with stroke, there is often an overlap with other systemic vascular diseases such as coronary artery disease (56%) and peripheral vascular disease (28%). The mortality after the first stroke is approximately 22% and doubles (41%) with the second stroke. The risk of having the second stroke is about 12% in the first year and falls to about 5% per year in subsequent years.[1]

Stroke results from brain injury that can be classified into two major categories: ischemic or hemorrhagic. Of all strokes in the United States, 88% are ischemic in nature, and 9% are due to intracerebral hemorrhage and 3% to subarachnoid hemorrhage. The incidence and prevalence of stroke are anticipated to increase as a result of the aging of the population and changes in racial demographics, and with increased prevalence of atrial fibrillation, hypertension, diabetes mellitus, and cardiovascular diseases. The risk of stroke increases with increasing age, the majority occurring after 65 years of age.[2] Therefore, the incidence and rate of stroke are expected to increase over the next several decades.

PATHOPHYSIOLOGY

Ischemic stroke occurs when a blood vessel is occluded, causing interruption of blood flow to a region of the brain. Hemorrhagic stroke, in contrast, occurs when a blood vessel ruptures. Ischemic stroke can be embolic (i.e., from a source outside of the brain) or can result from the occlusion of a blood vessel generally from in situ thrombosis within an atherosclerotic blood vessel or an enhanced tendency for the blood to clot. An embolus can originate from the heart, such as a thrombus in the left atrium in patients with atrial fibrillation or the ventricles after a heart attack, from a myxoma, or from atheroemboli from the aortic arch, the carotid artery, or intrinsic arteries of the brain. Atherothrombosis can occur in any portion of the arterial tree. Abnormalities of coagulation proteins due to elevated levels or function resulting from disease conditions (e.g., cancer, connective tissue diseases) or inherited disorders (mutation or polymorphisms) causing a hypercoagulable state also increase predisposition to the formation of arterial clots (Box 49-1).[3-5]

Ischemic stroke occurs following occlusion of an artery or severe narrowing that reduces blood flow below a critical threshold. This threshold varies between white and gray matter and between different areas of the brain. Certain areas of the brain, such as the hippocampus, are highly vulnerable to hypoxia or decreased flow. This selective vulnerability predicts to some degree the areas of brain damage and resulting functional deficits. Within minutes after the cessation of blood flow, irreversible damage to the brain tissue may result, which is surrounded by areas that are viable but not functional. This has been referred to as the ischemic penumbra. Within this penumbral region, biochemical events proceed in a cascade that can be potentially targeted for pharmacologic intervention.[6] Numerous clinical trials have been conducted to modulate this ischemic cascade and salvage the ischemic penumbra from ultimate cellular death. These attempts to salvage the penumbra and thereby limit the ischemic infarct have thus far been unsuccessful, and have included the use of GM_1 gangliosides, calcium channel blockers, anticoagulants, free radical scavengers, glutamate receptor antagonists, neurotrophic factors and the like.[7-9]

THERAPEUTICS AND CLINICAL PHARMACOLOGY

Acute Reperfusion Therapy for Ischemic Stroke

Restoration of blood flow to the brain (reperfusion) acutely after a blood vessel is occluded has been the only successful strategy in improving functional outcomes. Intravenous (IV) recombinant tissue-type plasminogen activator (rt-PA) within 3 hours of stroke symptom onset is the only U.S. Food and Drug Administration (FDA)–approved therapy for acute ischemic stroke. The National Institute of Neurological Disorders and Stroke acute stroke trial proved the efficacy of rt-PA (Alteplase) when given at a 0.9-mg/kg dose, with 10% administered as an initial IV bolus followed by a continuous IV infusion for 1 hour (up to a maximum dose of 90 mg).[10] The clinical criteria recommended by the American Heart Association for administering rt-PA are listed in Box 49-2.

Alteplase

Alteplase (the only FDA-approved therapy) is a tissue plasminogen activator produced by recombinant DNA technology. It is a sterile, purified glycoprotein of 527 amino acids. It is synthesized using the complementary DNA for natural human tissue-type plasminogen activator obtained from a human melanoma cell line. It is available as a sterile, white to off-white, lyophilized powder for IV administration after reconstitution with sterile water.

Alteplase is a serine protease, which has the property of fibrin-enhanced conversion of plasminogen to plasmin (hence the term *plasminogen activator*). It produces limited conversion of plasminogen in the absence of fibrin. When introduced into the systemic circulation at pharmacologic concentration, alteplase binds to fibrin within a thrombus and converts the entrapped plasminogen to plasmin. This initiates local fibrinolysis with limited systemic proteolysis. Following administration of 100 mg alteplase, there is a decrease (16% to 36%) in circulating fibrinogen.[11,12] The initial volume of distribution of alteplase approximates plasma volume. It is rapidly cleared from the plasma with an initial half-life of less than 5 minutes and a plasma clearance rate of 380 to 570 ml/min,[11,12] mediated primarily by the liver.

Pro-urokinase

Pro-urokinase, another thrombolytic agent, given intra-arterially directly into the middle cerebral artery, was also shown to be beneficial, but has not been approved by the FDA.[13] Despite this, many centers use intra-arterial thrombolysis (IAT) for proximal middle cerebral or basilar artery thrombosis. There is now a renewed interest in the use of IAT, following IV rt-PA, because of the low rate of recanalization (10%) after IV rt-PA for major vessel occlusion.[14]

Direct mechanical disruption or removal of the arterial clot is an alternative strategy to restore blood flow to the ischemic brain, and a clot removal device (MERCI device) has been approved by the FDA.[15]

Stroke Prevention

The only approved treatment for acute ischemic stroke is alteplase (rt-PA); however, its use is limited due to the strict inclusion and exclusion criteria (summarized in Box 49-2) to ensure its safety, and only 3% to 5% of stroke patients actually receive rt-PA. Since a neuroprotective compound affecting the ischemic penumbra has yet to be identified and proven efficacious in clinical trials, primary and secondary prevention become increasingly important to reduce mortality, up to 22% after the first stroke and as high as 40% with the second stroke.[1] The risk factors associated with stroke, underlying pathogenesis, and therapeutic targets for prevention of stroke are summarized in Table 49-1.

The most important risk factor that increases predisposition to ischemic stroke is the presence of atherosclerotic vascular disease, which also increases the risk for coronary artery and peripheral vascular

BOX 49-1 HEMOSTATIC RISK FACTORS FOR STROKE

- Hyperhomocysteinemia
- Elevated C-reactive protein
- Antiphospholipid antibodies
- Elevated fibrinogen
- Factor VII
- Factor V Leiden
- Prothrombin G20210A mutations
- Elevated cardiolipin immunoglobulin G antibodies
- Lupus anticoagulant
- Plasminogen activator inhibitor-1
- Hereditary thrombophilias
- Platelet hyperreactivity

BOX 49-2 CRITERIA FOR THROMBOLYTIC THERAPY

- Diagnosis of ischemic stroke causing measurable neurologic deficit
- The neurologic signs should not be clearing spontaneously
- The neurologic signs should not be minor and isolated
- Caution should be exercised in treating a patient with major deficits
- The symptoms of stroke should not be suggestive of subarachnoid hemorrhage
- Onset of symptoms less than 3 hours before beginning treatment
- No head trauma or prior stroke in the previous 3 months
- No myocardial infarction in the previous 3 months
- No gastrointestinal or urinary tract hemorrhage in the previous 21 days
- No major surgery in the previous 14 days
- No arterial puncture at a noncompressible site in the previous 7 days
- No history of previous intracranial hemorrhage
- Blood pressure not elevated (systolic <185 mm Hg and diastolic <110 mm Hg)
- No evidence of active bleeding or acute trauma (fracture) on examination
- Not taking an oral anticoagulant or, if anticoagulant being taken, international normalized ratio 1.7
- If receiving heparin in previous 48 hours, activated partial thromboplastin time must be in normal range
- Platelet count 100,000 mm^3
- Blood glucose concentration 50 mg/dl (2.7 mmol/L)
- No seizure with postictal residual neurologic impairments
- Computed tomography does not show a multilobar infarction (hypodensity >$^1/_3$ cerebral hemisphere)
- The patient or family understand the potential risks and benefits from treatment

Adapted from American Heart Association guidelines.

TABLE 49-1 RISK FACTORS, UNDERLYING MECHANISMS, AND STRATEGIES TO REDUCE RISK OF STROKE

Risk Factors	Mechanism	Treatments
NONMODIFIABLE		
Age	Atherosclerosis	Treat risk factors BP and lipid control
Gender	Unclear	Avoid hormone replacement therapy
Race/ethnicity	Unclear	Treat risk factors
Heredity	Familial lipid abnormalities	Lower lipids
MODIFIABLE		
Hypertension	Endothelial dysfunction ↑ Angiotensin II ↑ Cholesterol synthesis ↑ Oxidized LDL ↑ Smooth muscle proliferation ↑ Monocyte activation ↑ Oxidative stress ↑ Platelet aggregation ↑ Insulin resistance ↑ Apoptosis	BP control ACE inhibitors ARB Ca channel blocker Diuretic

TABLE 49-1 RISK FACTORS, UNDERLYING MECHANISMS, AND STRATEGIES TO REDUCE RISK OF STROKE—cont'd

Risk Factors	Mechanism	Treatments
Cigarette smoking	↑ Leukocytes ↑ CRP ↑ Endothelial superoxide ↑ Cytokines (IL-6, interleukin beta, TNF) ↑ Platelet-derived growth factor expression ↑ Monocyte adhesion Metalloproteinase activation	Stop smoking; baseline in about 5 yr
Diabetes	↑ Inflammation ↑ Microvascular disease	Strict glucose control for microvascular disease
Prior stroke or TIA	Generalized atherosclerosis or cardiac arrhythmia (atrial fibrillation or flutter)	Reduction in risk factors for atherosclerosis Statins Antiplatelet agents Anticoagulation
Dyslipidemia	↑ Progression of atherosclerosis, endothelial dysfunction, and activation of platelet and coagulation proteins and inflammation	Statins Diet modification
Obesity/metabolic syndrome	Progressive atherosclerosis ↑ Insulin resistance ↑ Triglycerides and LDL ↓ HDL ↑ Hypertension ↑ PAI-1 ↑ CRP ↑ Renin, angiotensin, ACE ↑ Protein S, von Willebrand factor	Weight loss Exercise Control of BP and glucose
Excessive alcohol	↓ Platelets, abnormal platelet function Hypertension	↓ Alcohol consumption
Physical inactivity	↑ Inflammation ↓ HDL ↑ CRP ↑ IL-6 ↑ TNF-α	Exercise and diet
Carotid artery disease	Embolic and hemodynamic	Surgery or stents Antiplatelet agents Statins
Atrial fibrillation	Embolic	Anticoagulation
Heart disease: CHF, MI, cardiomyopathy	Embolic	Anticoagulation or antiplatelet agents
Patent foramen ovale (PFO)	Embolic	Anticoagulation or closure of PFO
Polycythemia	Vascular obstruction, hemorrhage	Normalize hematocrit
Sickle cell anemia	Vascular obstruction	Exchange transfusion
Elevated homocysteine level	Promotes atherosclerosis	Unclear if lowering makes a difference (folate, B_{12}, B_6)
Cocaine and other substance abuse	↑ BP ↑ Inflammation	Abstinence
Obstructive sleep apnea	↑ BP Same as for obesity	Weight loss CPAP
EMERGING RISK FACTORS		
Inflammatory markers: ICAM, hs-CRP	CRP may play an independent role in addition to an inflammatory marker ↑ Endothelial activation and dysfunction ↑ Adhesion molecule expression	
Infectious agents: CMV, *Chlamydia pneumoniae, Helicobacter pylori*	Infections associated with generalized inflamation	
Renin-angiotensin	See above	ACE ARB
Lipoproteins: LP(a), LDL, small dense LDL	Oxidized LDL	Statins

ACE, angiotensin-converting enzyme; ARB, angiotensin II receptor blocker; BP, blood pressure; Ca, calcium; CHF, congestive heart failure; CMV, cytomegalovirus; CPAP, continuous positive airway pressure; CRP, C-reactive protein; HDL, high-density lipoprotein; ICAM, intracellular adhesion molecule; IL, interleukin; LP(a), lipoprotein (a); LDL, low-density lipoprotein; MI, myocardial infarction; PAI-1, plasminogen activator inhibitor-1; TIA, transient ischemic attack; TNF, tumor necrosis factor.

disease. Therefore, factors that increases atherosclerosis are the primary targets for the primary and seconary prophylaxis for stroke (see Table 49-1). Atherosclerosis is a progressive chronic disease characterized by the response of the blood vessel wall to a multifactorial injury that produces atheromatous or fibrous plaques. The plaques are asymmetric focal thickenings of the intima of the blood vessel wall and consist of cells, connective tissue elements, lipids, debris, blood-borne immune and inflammatory cells, and vascular endothelial and smooth muscle cells. The earliest manifestation of atheroma formation is the fatty streak, which contains macrophages and T cells underneath the endothelium. This leads to endothelial dysfunction and damage that increases predisposition to leukocyte and platelet adhesion and release of inflammatory mediators (cytokines) that in turn potentiate vascular smooth muscle proliferation and accumulation of peroxidized lipids. The center of the plaque consists of foam cells and extracellular lipid droplets surrounded by a cap of smooth muscle cells and a collagen-rich matrix. Thrombosis occurs when an activated plaque ruptures, exposing the core of phospholipids, tissue factors, and platelet adhesive matrix molecules to the circulating blood, which induces clot formation. Matrix metalloproteinases and cysteine proteases have been implicated in plaque activation and subsequent rupture.[16,17]

Key to the initiation of atherosclerosis is abnormality of endothelium, a metabolically active tissue involved in the regulation of vasomotor tone, hemostasis, and vascular permeability, protecting against oxidative stress and inhibiting cell adhesion and migration. The endothelium releases two classes of vasoactive substances with opposing effects, endothelium-derived relaxing factors (EDRFs) and endothelium-derived contracting factors (EDCFs). EDRFs, such as nitric oxide (NO), protect the vessels from atherogenic insults, while EDCFs contribute to the progression of vascular disease. Endothelial dysfunction can be thought of as a reduction in the bioavailability of EDRFs. This is characterized by increased permeability of the plasma membrane and decreased NO synthesis and release, with overexpression of mediators that attract inflammatory cells (chemoattractants) and molecules that adhere to the endothelial surface. This causes a state of "endothelial activation" characterized by a proinflammatory, proliferative, procoagulatory milieu that favors progression of atherosclerosis and activation of atherosclerotic plaque that ruptures, exposing prothrombotic material such as tissue factor, platelet adhesion molecules, and phospholipids to the blood.[18,19]

Atherosclerotic plaque initiation is aggravated by various cardiovascular risk factors and characterized by an accumulation of lipids and lipoproteins. These factors include shear forces at the bifurcation of the arterial tree, hypertension, hypercholesterolemia, diabetes, chemicals such as tobacco, vasoactive amines such as norepinephrine and angiotensin II, and perhaps infectious agents (see Table 49-1). These changes promote recruitment and internalization of inflammatory cells within the intimal layer of the vascular wall, with subsequent proliferation of vascular smooth muscle cells and progression of atherosclerosis.

These changes in the vascular wall can be thought of as occurring in stages (Fig. 49-1). In stage one, there is deposition and accumulation of low-density lipoprotein (LDL) that is then oxidized in the intima. The oxidized LDL in areas of high oscillatory shear stress (bifurcations of arteries) causes increased expression of adhesion molecules and inflammatory genes by the endothelial cells. Oxidized LDL is also toxic to endothelial and smooth muscle cells. This promotes a proinflammatory state by inhibiting the secretion of tissue plasminogen activator and stimulating the secretion of plasminogen activator inhibitor-1 (PAI-1). This creates an inflammatory response in the artery that can be considered the second stage, with the recruitment of inflammatory cells (leukocytes, monocytes, and T lymphocytes). The inflammatory cells are attracted to the endothelium by the adhesion molecules vascular cell adhesion molecule-1 (VCAM-1) and intracellular adhesion molecule-1 (ICAM-1). Chemokines that are produced in the intima stimulate these cells to migrate through the interendothelial junctions into the subendothelial space. In the third stage, monocytes are recruited and evolve into macrophages that express scavenger receptors that bind oxidized LDL. The oxidized LDL is engulfed by the macrophages, which forms foam cells within the fatty streak. In the fourth stage of plaque formation, there is migration of smooth muscle cells from the media into the intimal layers of the arterial wall, which is facilitated by platelet-derived growth factor (PDGF) secreted by the macrophages. Likewise, smooth muscle cells divide, contributing to the growth of the plaque. These cells seem to undergo apoptosis or programmed cell death in response to inflammatory cytokines. Extracellular matrix macromolecules such as proteoglycans, collagen, and elastin are secreted by the smooth muscle cells, marking the fourth stage. These molecules that hold the plaque together are in a state of formation and destruction. The destruction is catalyzed by metalloproteinases and cysteine proteases. The breakdown of these molecules allows outward growth of the plaque into the arterial lumen. When the rate of breakdown exceeds the rate of formation, the fibrous cap becomes weakened and may disrupt. Activated macrophages, T cells, and mast cells produce matrix metalloproteinases, cysteine proteases, free radicals, inflammatory cytokines, and vasoactive molecules that destabilize the plaque. In the fifth stage, the plaque is disrupted, releasing the thrombogenic core of collagen and lipids with its high concentration of tissue factor. The exposure of tissue factor to the blood containing circulating coagulation factors (VIIa and Xa) causes the cleavage of prothrombin to thrombin, triggering coagulation, fibrin deposition, and platelet activation, leading to thrombus formation. Platelet adhesion and activation result in the release of thromboxane A_2, serotonin, adenosine diphosphate, platelet-activating factor, thrombin, and tissue factor, which stimulate further platelet recruitment and narrowing of the artery.[20,21]

Systemic inflammation plays an important role in atherosclerosis and plaque rupture, manifest by elevation of inflammatory markers such as C-reactive protein (CRP), fibrinogen, interleukin (IL)–7, IL-8, soluble CD40 ligand, and the CRP-related protein pentraxin 3. CRP, in addition to being a marker for inflammation, also participates in the inflammatory process itself.[22-26] Structural heart disease, including severe valvular disease with cardiac enlargement, contractile dysfunction, and atrial fibrillation, also increases the risk for thromboembolism and stroke. Targeting of these risk factors thus becomes an important part of primary and secondary stroke prevention strategies to prevent or slow progression of atherosclerosis and thromboembolism.

Primary Stroke Prevention

Primary stroke prevention, prevention before an event occurs, deals with risk factors for first stroke. These risk factors are similar to those for secondary stroke prevention, and since most studies deal with secondary prevention (i.e., prevention of recurrence of a cerebrovascular event after a stroke or transient ischemic attack [TIA]), these factors are addressed together. Lifestyle changes, control of blood pressure, blood glucose, and lipids, regular exercise, smoking cessation, and moderation of alcohol intake are all important in stroke prevention. Warfarin, statins, and aspirin are useful drugs for primary prevention of stroke. Warfarin use with an International Normalized Ratio of 2 to 3 is used for the primary prevention of stroke in patients with atrial fibrillation. Use of statins has also been shown to reduce the risk for stroke.[27] Aspirin has been shown to be useful in the primary prevention of stroke in women, but not men. The Women's Health Study randomized 39,876 women to receive 100 mg of aspirin or placebo every other day. Women who received aspirin had significantly fewer ischemic strokes ($P = 0.009$).[28]

Secondary Stroke Prevention

Lifestyle Modification

Smoking Cessation. Smoking is one of the most modifiable of the lifestyle risk factors. In the year 2000, smoking caused an estimated 1.69 million cardiovascular deaths in the 1 billion smokers in the world. Smoking is associated with approximately 30% of strokes and 12% to 14% of stroke deaths.[29] Smoking contributes to the risk of stroke by multiple mechanisms, including accelerated atherosclerosis

Stage 0 Normal

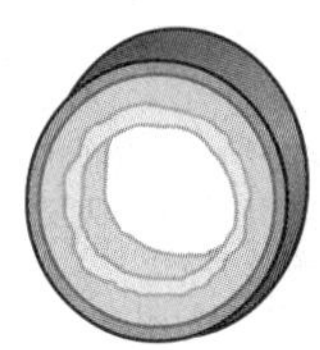

Risk factors
Age
Hypertension
Smoking
Diabetes
Lack of exercise
Hyperlipidemia
Excessive alcohol

Stage 1 Endothelial dysfunction

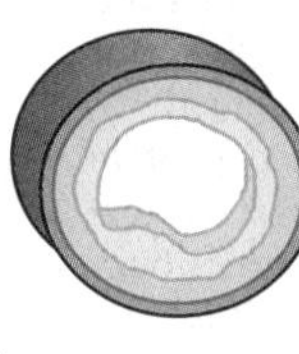

Endothelial dysfunction

Activation of adhesion molecules and inflammatory genes

Deposition of LDL and subsequent oxidation

Stage 0 Normal Risk factors	Stage 1 Endothelial Dysfunction	Stage 2 Inflammatory Response	Stage 3 Monocytes to Macrophages	Stage 4 Migration of smooth muscle cells and plaque growth	Stage 5 Plaque rupture and clot formation
Age	Endothelial dysfunction from risk factors	Leukocytes	Monocytes converted to macrophages	Migration of smooth muscle cells from media to intima	Plaque rupture releasing thrombogenic core of collegen and lipids with a high concentration of tissue factor
Hypertension	Activation of adhesion molecules and inflammatory genes	Monocytes	Macrophages ingest oxidized LDL producing fatty streak	Smooth muscle cells devide	Triggers coagulation cascade
Smoking	Deposition of LDL and subsequent oxidation	T lymphocytes		Smooth muscle cells secrete extracellular matrix molecules	Activates platelets
Diabetes		Migration into the subendothelial space		Plaque growth and destruction	Clot fromation
Lack of exercise				Break down activates the plaque	
Hyperlipidemia					
Excessive Alcohol					

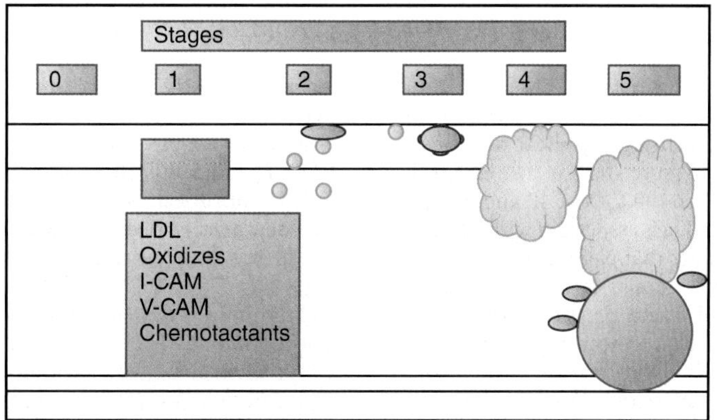

FIGURE 49-1 • Vascular wall changes by stage.

and inflammation with increase in circulating leukocytes, CRP, IL-6, IL-1β, tumor necrosis factor (TNF), and soluble adhesion molecule type 1. Cigarette smoking also increases endothelial superoxide production, activates metalloproteinases in mast cells and T lymphocytes, increases PDGF expression from platelets, and promotes monocyte adhesion to endothelial cells.[30] Cessation of smoking decreases the risk of stroke to the level of risk in the general nonsmoking population by 5 years.

Moderation of Alcohol Consumption. Excessive alcohol consumption is associated with increased risk of stroke. Low to moderate alcohol intake is associated with a decrease in the incidence of stroke, thus giving the J-shaped curve in which modest intake of alcohol is protective, whereas excessive alcohol is deleterious.[31]

The mechanisms by which alcohol reduces the risk for stroke are multifactorial. Regular alcohol consumption increases the protective high-density lipoprotein (HDL) cholesterol levels. Statistically, the higher HDL cholesterol levels in moderate drinkers account for about half of their lower cardiovascular risk. Moderate alcohol also decreases the inflammatory markers CRP, ICAM-1, VCAM-1, E-selectin, and fibrinogen, which are known to play a role in inflammation and atherosclerosis.[32] The type of beverage may make a difference. Polyphenolic compounds such as flavonids and resveratrol found in plants and red wine have antioxidant and anti-inflammatory properties. Resveratrol has been shown in animal studies to increase insulin sensitivity, reduce insulin-like growth factor-1, increase AMP-activated protein kinases and peroxisome proliferator-activated receptor-γ coactivator-1α, increase mitochondrial number, and improve motor function.[33] Whether resveratrol or other compounds in wine can be purified and used to reduce cardiovascular events without deleterious effects of excessive alcohol is being investigated.

Metabolic Syndrome and Obesity. The metabolic syndrome, defined by the presence of abdominal obesity, hypertension, insulin resistance with impaired glucose tolerance, and low HDL cholesterol and high triglyceride and LDL cholesterol concentrations, increases the risk of cardiovascular events and stroke.[34] This syndrome is associated with increased concentrations of PAI-1, CRP, and other markers of inflammation.[35] The adipocytes are metabolically active cells producing molecules involved in the regulation of blood pressure (renin, angiotensin), lipid metabolism (retinol-binding protein-1 and cholesteryl-ester transfer protein), and the coagulation and fibrinolytic pathways. Urokinase-type plasminogen activator, protein S, and von Willebrand factor are all upregulated in obesity.[36] Appropriate diet (e.g., the Mediterranean diet and increased fish consumption) is associated with lower levels of inflammatory markers, including CRP, IL-6, fibrinogen, and white blood cell counts. Exercise and weight loss decrease CRP and, in some individuals, IL-6 and TNF-α. Rimonabant, a cannabinoid receptor blocker that produces weight loss, decreases triglycerides, and increases HDL cholesterol, is being investigated for treatment of the metabolic syndrome and associated risk of cardiovascular events.[37]

Clinical Risk Factors

Diabetes. Diabetes is present in 15% to 33% of patients with ischemic stroke. Consequently, patients with diabetes require particularly rigorous control of blood pressure and blood lipids to reduce the risk of cerebrovascular events.[29] Tight glycemic control has been shown to reduce microvascular disease and other end points, such as diabetic neuropathy.[38] Current recommendations from the American Heart Association (AHA) and the American Stroke Association (ASA) suggest more rigorous control of blood pressure with angiotensin-converting enzyme (ACE) inhibitors or angiotensin receptor blockers (ARBs) (class I, level of evidence A), control of lipids, and tight glycemic control to reduce microvascular complications (class IIB, level of evidence B).[29]

Hypertension. Hypertension is the most modifiable risk factor for stroke protection. There appears to be a strong log-linear relationship between stroke mortality and blood pressure starting at 115 mm Hg systolic and 75 mm Hg diastolic. Between the ages of 40 and 69 years, an increase in blood pressure by 20 mm Hg is associated with a twofold increase in stroke mortality.[39] This implies that patients who are in the normotensive range of blood pressure are also at risk and that risk increases further with the elevation of blood pressure levels for any decade of life, especially if accompanied by other risk factors such as diabetes mellitus, hyperlipidemia, or target end-organ damage.[40] Overall, a 30% reduction in the risk of stroke can be achieved by effectively controlling hypertension.[41]

Several classes of antihypertensives, including diuretics, β-blockers, calcium channel blockers (CCBs), α-adrenergic blockers, and modulators of the renin-angiotensin-aldosterone system (RAAS), have been studied for stroke prevention. The thiazide diuretics act by inhibiting tubular resorption of sodium and chloride in the ascending loop of Henle and early distal tubule, resulting in excretion of water, sodium, and chloride producing a net effect of decreasing peripheral vascular resistance. Thiazide diuretic use has been demonstrated to reduce the risk of stroke in the Post-stroke Antihypertensive Treatment Study (PATS), which showed a 29% relative risk reduction (RRR) for stroke at 3 years,[42] and the PROGRESS trial, in which combination therapy with perindopril reduced the risk for recurrent stroke.[43]

β-Adrenergic receptor blockers antagonize the effect of catecholamine in the myocardium and vasculature. Joint National Committee guidelines consider congestive heart failure and secondary cardioprotection in the hypertensive patient an indication for the use of β-blockers. However, their utility in controlling blood pressure and the risk of stroke has been recently questioned and appears to be less than other antihypertensives, including modulators of the RAAS. The Losartan Intervention For Endpoint reduction (LIFE) study recruited more than 9000 patients with hypertension and left ventricular hypertrophy. In this study, despite comparable lowering of blood pressure, a losartan-based regimen produced a significant 25% reduction in the incidence of fatal and nonfatal stroke when compared to the β-blocker atenolol.[44]

CCBs decrease blood pressure by reducing entry of calcium ions into vascular smooth muscle cells by inhibiting the voltage-gated L-type calcium channels. In the Systolic Hypertension in Europe (Syst-Eur) study, hypertensive patients age 60 or older were randomized to nitrendipine or placebo. The nitrendipine-treated group had a decreased incidence of stroke (relative risk [RR], 36%).[45]

α-Adrenergic receptor blockers act by antagonizing central nervous system α_2-adrenergic or peripheral α-adrenergic receptors. Treatment with an α-blocker (doxazosin) in the Antihypertensive and Lipid-Lowering to prevent Heart Attack Trial (ALLHAT) was associated with an increase in cardiovascular events.[46]

The modulators of the RAAS, ACE inhibitors and ARBs, are antihypertensive medications that have been demonstrated to effectively reduce blood pressure in hypertensive patients and decrease the risk of cardiovascular events. Angiotensin II is involved in remodeling of the arterial blood vessel wall in both hypertension and atherogenesis. It appears to play a role in mediation of the early stage 1 of vascular endothelial dysfunction and inflammation that lead to the formation and growth of the atherosclerotic plaque. Specifically, angiotensin II promotes insulin resistance[47] and modifies LDL molecules, promoting deposition of oxidized LDL and reactive oxygen species production, increasing smooth muscle cell proliferation and monocyte activation, and facilitating adhesion of monocytes and leukocytes to endothelial cells.[48] Angiotensin II also promotes a state of oxidative stress by the activation of NADP/NADP oxidase, production of superoxide radicals, and degradation of NO.[49] In addition, angiotensin II is prothrombogenic, and stimulates the synthesis of PAI-1 in both normal and hypertensive individuals and enhances collagen- and epinephrine-induced platelet aggregation in normotensive subjects.

While it is clear that lowering the blood pressure reduces the risk for stroke, it is not clear which is the best antihypertensive agent. Data from the ALLHAT study in which 33,357 patients with a history of hypertension and at least one other cardiovascular risk factor were randomly assigned to receive a thiazide diuretic (chlorthalidone 12.5 mg daily), a CCB (amlodipine 2.5 to 5 mg daily), an ACE inhibitor (lisinopril 10 to 40 mg daily), or an α-adrenergic blocker (doxazosin) demonstred a differential effect of these antihypertensive agents on cardiovascular events. Patients in this study were an average of 67 years old, 47% female, and 32% black. The α-adrenergic blocker arm was terminated because of the excess of end points when compared to chlorthalidone. There was a 15% excess of stroke in the doxazosin versus the chlorthalidone group. In blacks, there was a 40% excess of stroke in those assigned lisinopril compared with chlorthalidone. The finding of an increased incidence of stroke in those patients treated with ACE inhibitors compared to diuretics are controversial as it is at odds with the results of other clinical trials.[46]

The Heart Outcomes Prevention Evaluation (HOPE) trial enrolled 9297 patients with risk factors for coronary artery disease, stroke, peripheral vascular disease, or diabetes, plus one or more cardiovascular risk factors. The subjects were randomized to receive either ramipril (ACE inhibitor) or placebo. Despite only a modest blood pressure–lowering effect (by 3 to 4 mm Hg), ramipril reduced the rate of the composite end point of cardiovascular mortality by 22% when compared to placebo.[50] Similarly, in the Anglo-Scandinavian Cardiac Outcomes Trial–Blood Pressure Lowering Arm (ASCOT-BPLA), which enrolled 19,257 patients with hypertension randomized to amlodipine (5 to 10 mg/day) adding perindopril (4 to 8 mg/day) as required versus atenolol (50 to 100 mg/day) adding bendroflumethiazide (1.25 to

2.5 mg/day) as needed, indicated a difference in effectiveness of these antihypertensives in reducing the risk of stroke. Fewer individuals on the amlodipine regimen had fatal and nonfatal stroke (23%) compared to the β-blocker/thiazide combination, despite almost identical lowering of blood pressure. The incidence of new-onset diabetes was also higher in the atenolol/thiazide group.[51]

In the Morbidity and Mortality After Stroke, Eprosartan Compared with Nitrendipine for Secondary Prevention (MOSES) trial, 1405 patients treated with eprosartan (an ARB) or nitrendipine (a CCB) after a stroke were followed for a mean of 2.5 years. Despite virtually identical blood pressure control, the risk of all-cause mortality, cerebrovascular events, or cardiovascular events was lower in the eprosartan than the nitrendipine group.[52]

Thus, control of hypertension appears to be a major mechanism that helps reduce the risk for stroke (class I, level of evidence A). ACE inhibitors and ARBs seem to be particularly effective. Differences between most studies with ACE inhibitors and ALLHAT may result from relative poor blood pressure control in the ALLHAT study, which enrolled a larger population of African American patients who respond less well to ACE inhibitors and ARBs due to their low-renin hypertension. The choice of specific drugs therefore should be individualized on the basis of population and specific patient characteristics (class IIb, level of evidence C).[29]

Control of Hyperlipidemia. Before the development of the statins, attempts to reduce total blood cholesterol, either by diet or by fibric acid–based therapy, were ineffective in significantly reducing the incidence of stroke.[53] Over the past decade, however, numerous large-scale trials for lowering cholesterol with statins have demonstrated a reduction in vascular events, including stroke, documenting their use in primary prevention of stroke. The statins are lipid-lowering agents that act by inhibition of 3-hydroxy-3-methylglutaryl coenzyme A (HMG-CoA) reductase. This enzyme is responsible for the conversion of HMG-CoA to mevalonate. Products of mevalonate metabolism are critical for several cellular processes, and inhibition of the mevalonate pathway by statins has pleiotropic effects. It has been reported that statins inhibit the migration and proliferation of vascular smooth muscle cells; reduce IL-6 expression; upregulate NO synthetase, increasing NO and improve endothelium-dependent vasodilation; and inhibit the expression of PAI-1 and matrix metalloproteinases in endothelial cells.[54-56] These effects of statins are independent of plasma cholesterol level, and can be antagonized by exogenous mevalonate and some isoprenoids. These findings suggest that statins exert direct anti-atherosclerotic effects on the vascular wall beyond their effects on plasma lipids. Numerous lipid-lowering trials have shown that treatment with statins is associated with a significant decrease in the risk of stroke and TIA in patients with multiple risk factors for atherosclerosis. Statins can retard or reverse the progression of carotid atherosclerosis as measured by serial ultrasound.[57]

The Heart Protection Study (20,536 patients randomized to simvastatin or placebo) provided evidence for the efficacy of statins as secondary prevention in cerebral ischemia patients. This included 3,280 patients with a history of stroke or TIA. Major vascular event rates were significantly reduced from 29.8% to 24.7% ($P < 0.001$), and stroke from 5.7% to 4.3% ($P < 0.0001$). These benefits occurred regardless of the entry level of cholesterol (minimum entry level 135 mg/dl).[58] These results formed the basis for FDA approval of simvastatin for secondary stroke prevention.

Reduction in stroke risk has also been demonstrated for atorvastatin in the lipid-lowering limb of the ASCOT trial that enrolled hypertensive patients. In this study, atorvastatin was added to the treatment regimen of 2532 patients with type 2 diabetes. There was a significant reduction in the number of fatal and nonfatal strokes ($P < 0.024$).[59] This benefit was additive to the lowering of the blood pressure by antihypertensive agents. Similarly, in the SPARCL trial, which randomized 4731 patients with recent stroke or TIA and without coronary artery disease to atorvastatin (80 mg/day) or placebo, the risk of stroke and cardiovascular events was significantly reduced ($P = 0.03$).[60]

In patients with ischemic stroke or TIA with elevated cholesterol and evidence of atherosclerotic disease, statin agents are recommended

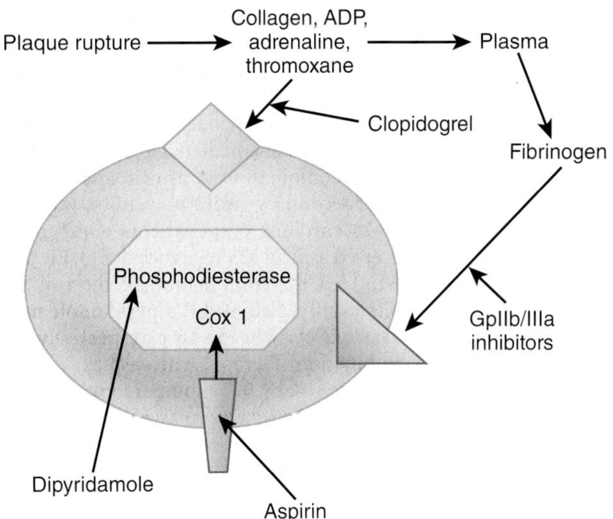

FIGURE 49-2 • Mechanism of anti-platelet agents.

with the goal of achieving an LDL cholesterol level less than 100 mg/dl, or less than 70 mg/dl for persons with multiple risk factors (class I, level of evidence A). Patients with ischemic stroke or TIA presumed to be due to an atherosclerotic origin but with no preexisting indications for statins (normal cholesterol, no coronary artery disease) are reasonable candidates for treatment with a statin to reduce the risk of vascular events (class IIa, level of evidence B).[29]

Platelet Inhibition. Platelets are essential for thrombus formation (Fig. 49-2). Therefore, inhibition of platelet activity has become a mainstay of secondary stroke prevention. Currently, three classes of antiplatelet compounds are in clinical use: the cyclooxygenase (COX) inhibitors (e.g., aspirin), the phosphodiesterase inhibitors (e.g., dipyridamole), and the adenosine diphosphate (ADP) inhibitors (e.g., clopidogrel).[61]

Aspirin. Aspirin's actions are mediated by irreversibly acetylating the enzyme COX. COX has two isoforms: COX-1 and COX-2. Aspirin selectively inhibits COX-1 over COX-2 by 166-fold. The antithrombotic action of aspirin is mainly due to inhibition of platelet COX-1, which prevents the synthesis of thromboxane A_2. COX-2 is induced by inflammatory stimuli and results in the production of prostaglandins that contribute to the inflammatory response. COX-2 inhibition is responsible for the analgesic and anti-inflammatory effect of aspirin and other nonsteroidal anti-inflammatory agents. COX-2 suppresses the formation of prostacyclin (prostaglandin I_2 [PGI_2]), leaving the production of thromboxane A_2 (TXA_2) unaltered. PGI_2 is a key COX product in the endothelium that inhibits platelet aggregation, causes vasodilation, and prevents proliferation of vascular smooth muscle cells. In contrast to PGI_2, the COX-1–derived prostanoid TXA_2 causes platelet aggregation, vasoconstriction, and vascular proliferation, and therefore its inhibition helps reduce the risk of thrombosis.[62]

A meta-analysis of 11 randomized, placebo-controlled studies showed that aspirin reduces the incidence of stroke recurrence by 15% (RR 0.85; 95% confidence interval [CI], 0.77 to 0.94) and that efficacy seems consistent across doses from 50 to 1500 mg/day.[63,64] Aspirin doses of 75 mg/day and less have been suggested to be more desirable because they "spare" prostacyclin, a platelet antiaggregant and potent vasodilator, and are safer because they are associated with less gastrotoxicity.[64] The incidence of total bleeding, particularly gastrointestinal bleeding, is related to dosage used, with the incidence around 3.6% for a 100-mg/day dose compared to 9.1% for 100 to 325 mg/day.[64] Major bleeding incidence has not been well correlated to aspirin dose; however, studies may have been underpowered to detect this difference. For primary stroke prevention, aspirin has been shown to be more effective in women than men.[28]

The early use of aspirin in patients treated within 48 hours of an acute stroke onset has been shown in the Chinese Acute Stroke Trial and the International Stroke Trial to reduce both stroke recurrence risk and mortality.[65,66]

Dipyridamole. Dipyridamole is an antiplatelet agent that inhibits phosphodiesterase, increases cyclic AMP levels, stimulate prostacyclin production, and reduce cellular uptake of adenosine. Dipyridamole may also directly enhance prostacyclin-mediated platelet inhibition and inhibit thromboxane. The combination of aspirin and extended-release (ER) dipyridamole for secondary stroke prevention was evaluated in a large trial (ESPS-2) enrolling 6602 patients with previous stroke or TIA.[67] Patients received aspirin (25 mg twice daily), ER dipyridamole (200 mg twice daily), or the combination of the two twice daily. During the 2-year follow-up, aspirin or ER dipyridamole monotherapy reduced the risk of stroke by 18% and 16%, respectively, compared with placebo. Combination therapy with aspirin plus ER dipyridamole reduced the stroke risk by 37% compared with placebo. Thus in the secondary prevention of stroke, combination therapy with aspirin plus ER dipyridamole was twice as effective as either agent alone, with an absolute risk reduction of 3% after 2 years. The risk of bleeding with the combination therapy was not higher compared to aspirin monotherapy. The most common adverse event experienced in patients receiving dipyridamole was headache.[68] A post-hoc analysis of patients with coronary disease or history of myocardial infarction at the time of enrollment in ESPS-2 mitigated fears that dipyridamole may increase the number of cardiac events by causing cardiac "steal" and showed that it was safe and beneficial in this population.[69] A second post-hoc analysis stratified efficacy data by risk subgroup and found that patients at highest risk accrued the greatest benefit from the combination of aspirin and ER dipyridamole therapy.[70]

The European/Australian Stroke Prevention in Reversible Ischemia Trial (ESPRIT) included 2739 patients with history of stroke of arterial origin who received aspirin 30 to 325 mg/day (median, 75 mg/day) with or without dipyridamole 200 mg twice daily; ER dipyridamole was used by 83% (n = 1131) of patients taking the combination regimen.[71] The primary composite cardiovascular end point of death, stroke, or myocardial infarction occurred in 13% of patients taking combination therapy and 16% of patients taking aspirin monotherapy, demonstrating a benefit with the combination (hazard ratio 0.80; 95% CI, 0.66 to 0.98). Addition of these data to the meta-analysis of previous trials resulted in an overall risk ratio for the composite of vascular-related death, stroke, or myocardial infarction of 0.82 (95% CI, 0.74 to 0.91). There was no significant difference in the incidence of bleeding between groups; however, more patients did discontinue therapy in the combination group, mainly due to headache.[71] ESPS-2 and ESPRIT results are consistent and provide evidence that the combination of aspirin and ER dipyridamole improves secondary stroke prevention and prevention of other vascular events following stroke or TIA compared with aspirin monotherapy, without increasing bleeding risk.

Current guidelines by the American College of Chest Physicians (ACCP) and the AHA and ASA recommend the combination of aspirin 25 mg and ER dipyridamole 200 mg twice daily for initial therapy for patients with noncardioembolic stroke or TIA. They also suggest use of this combination over aspirin monotherapy (grade 2A [ACCP] and class IIa, level of evidence A [ASA/AHA]).[29]

Platelet Receptor Antagonists. The ADP receptor antagonists clopidogrel and ticlodipine inhibit ADP activity by preventing its binding to the platelet receptor. ADP stimulates expression of the glycoprotein (GP) IIb/IIIa receptor and may mediate release of other aggregation agonists and enhance platelet binding of von Willebrand factor. Hence, the end result of ADP inhibition is impairment of platelet aggregation and fibrinogen-mediated platelet cross-linking. The GP IIb/IIIa receptor antagonists block the final common pathway in platelet activation. The intravenous GP IIb/IIIa receptor antagonists are effective in the management of ischemic events related to percutaneous interventions and in patients hospitalized for unstable angina and non–ST-segment elevation myocardial infarction.[72]

The Clopidogrel versus Aspirin in Patients at Risk of Ischaemic Events (CAPRIE) trial compared aspirin 325 mg/day with clopidogrel 75 mg/day in 19,185 patients with atherosclerotic vascular disease. The results showed a significant RRR of 8.7% with clopidogrel in the composite end point of ischemic stroke, myocardial infarction, or vascular death. However, these results were primarily driven by the results of the peripheral vascular disease cohort, whereas in the ischemic stroke cohort, there was only a nonsignificant trend toward benefit with clopidogrel. Safety of clopidogrel appeared similar to that of aspirin therapy.[73] Current ACCP and ASA/AHA guidelines indicate that clopidogrel should be used in patients with hypersensitivity to aspirin (grade 1C+ [ACCP] and class IIa, level of evidence B [ASA/AHA]) and should be considered instead of aspirin therapy (grade 2B [ACCP] and class IIa, level of evidence B [ASA/AHA]).[29]

Two trials, Management of Atherothrombosis With Clopidogrel in High-Risk Patients (MATCH)[74] and Clopidogrel for High Atherothrombotic Risk and Ischemic Stabilization, Management, and Avoidance (CHARISMA),[75] were designed to evaluate whether dual antiplatelet therapy with aspirin and clopidogrel was superior to monotherapy with either drug. The MATCH study evaluated 7599 high-risk patients specifically for secondary stroke prevention. Patients received the combination of aspirin 75 mg/day plus clopidogrel 75 mg/day or clopidogrel monotherapy. No significant benefit of dual antiplatelet treatment was observed for the primary composite cardiovascular end point (RRR 6.4%; 95% CI, −4.6 to 16.3; P = 0.244) or reduction in ischemic stroke (RRR 7.1%; 95% CI, −8.5 to 20.4; P = 0.353), while the risk of life-threatening bleeding was significantly increased (RR 1.26; 95% CI, 0.64 to 1.88; $P < 0.0001$).[74] The CHARISMA trial examined 15,603 patients with clinically evident cardiovascular disease or multiple risk factors who were receiving the combination of aspirin (75 to 162 mg/day) and clopidogrel or aspirin monotherapy. There was no significant difference between groups in the primary composite end point of myocardial infarction, stroke, or cardiovascular death. There was a suggestion of benefit for dual antiplatelet therapy in patients with evidence of cardiovascular disease, although the results were only marginally significant (RR 0.88; 95% CI, 0.77 to 0.998; P = 0.046). There was a trend toward greater incidence of major bleeding (RR 1.25; 95% CI, 0.97 to 1.61; P = 0.09) and a statistically significant increase in moderate bleeding (requiring transfusion) with the combination group (RR 1.62; 95% CI, 1.27 to 2.08; $P < 0.001$).[75]

Taken together, the results of MATCH and CHARISMA indicate that clinicians should exercise great caution when considering the use of the combination of aspirin and clopidogrel therapy for secondary stroke prevention, owing to lack of demonstrated superior efficacy, increased risk of serious bleeding complications, and increased cost compared with low-dose monotherapy with either agent. The ASA/AHA guidelines state that the addition of aspirin to clopidogrel increases the risk of hemorrhage and is not routinely recommended for patients with ischemic stroke or TIA (class III, level of evidence A).[29]

The Profess Study randomized 20,232 patients with stroke age greater than 55 within 90 days or 50-54 years of age within 90-120 days following a stroke and that had two other vascular risk factors. Patients were randomized to clopidogrel 75 mg plus telmisartan 80 mg, clopidogrel plus placebo, extended released dipyridamole 200 mg plus 25 mg ASA (ER-DP 200 mg + ASA 25 mg bid) plus telmisartan, or ER-DP 200 mg + ASA 25 mg bid plus placebo. The primary endpoint was stroke. There was no difference in the primary outcome ER-DP 200 mg + ASA 25 mg bid vs. Clopidogrel 75 mg (9.0% vs. 8.8%; HR 1.01 (0.92-1.11), p = 0.783) (unpublished data).

Intracerebral Hemorrhage. Intracerebral hemorrhage (ICH) accounts for approximately 9% of strokes, which is approximately 37,000 to 52,400 patients per year. Uncontrolled hypertension and the use of anticoagulation with warfarin increase the ICH risk 7- to 10-fold. ICH is also more common in certain ethnic populations, including African Americans, Hispanics, and Japanese. Heavy alcohol consumption also increases the risk of ICH, and evidence suggests that cigarette smokers may be at increased risk. Among young men and women, independent risk factors for ICH include current cigarette smoking and consumption of ≥2 alcohol drinks daily.[76]

ICH has been traditionally associated with dismal mortality and morbidity rates and high costs. In some reports, the 6-month mortality rate is 30% to 50%.[2-4] Only 20% of patients regain functional independence at 6 months. The most consistent predictors of outcome across studies are the hematoma volume, neurologic status (e.g., Glasgow Coma Scale score), and the presence and volume of the intraventricular hemorrhage. The most powerful individual predictor appears to be the volume of ICH measured on initial computed tomography scan.[77] Since hematoma volume is a critical predictor of outcome, removal of the clot or limiting its expansion seems reasonable. However, surgical removal of the hematoma is not more effective than medical therapy.[78] The FAST trial randomized 399 patients with ICH diagnosed by computed tomography within 3 hours after onset to receive placebo or doses of 40, 80, or 160 mcg/kg of recombinant activated factor VII (rFVIIa). Hematoma expansion and 90-day mortality were less in the treated group.[79] However, subsequent results of the Phase III FAST trial indicate that the rFVIIa did not improve the long-term outcome compared to placebo.[80]

REFERENCES

1. Sanossian N, Ovbiagele B. Multimodality stroke prevention. Neurologist 2006; 12:14-31.
2. Rosamond W, Flegal K, Friday G, et al. Heart disease and stroke statistics—2007 updated: a report from the American Heart Association Statistics Committee and Stroke Statistics Subcommittee. Circulation 2007;115:69-171.
3. Voetsch B, Loscalzo J. Genetic determinants of arterial thrombosis. Thromb Vasc Biol 2004;24:216-229.
4. Crowther M, Kelton J. Congenital thrombophilic states associated with venous thrombosis: a qualitative overview and proposed classification system. Ann Intern Med 2003;138:128-134.
5. Feinbloom D, Bauer K. Assessment of hemostatic risk factors in predicting arterial thrombotic events. Arterioscler Thromb Vasc Biol 2005;25:2043-2053.
6. Bandera E, Botteri M, Minelli C, et al. Cerebral blood flow threshold of ischemic penumbra and infarct core in acute ischemic stroke. Stroke 2006;37:1334-1339.
7. Kidwell C, Liebeskind D, Starkman S, et al. Trends in acute ischemic stroke trials through the 20th century. Stroke 2001;32:1349-1359.
8. Fischer M. Recommendations for advancing development of acute stroke therapies. Stroke Therapy Academic Industry Roundtable 3. Stroke 2003;34:1539-1546.
9. Schouten J. Neuroprotection in traumatic brain injury: a complex struggle against the biology of nature. Curr Opin Crit Care 2007;13:134-142.
10. NINDS rt-PA Stroke Study Group. Tissue plasminogen activator for acute ischemic stroke. N Engl J Med 1995;333:1581-1587.
11. Seifried E, Tanswell P, Ellbrück D, et al. Pharmacokinetics and haemostatic status during consecutive infusions of recombinant tissue-type plasminogen activator in patients with acute myocardial infarction. Thromb Haemost 1989;61:497-501.
12. Tanswell P, Tebbe U, Neuhaus K-L, et al. Pharmacokinetics and fibrin specificity of alteplase during accelerated infusions in acute myocardial infarction. J Am Coll Cardiol 1992;19:1071-1075.
13. Furlan A, Higashida R, Wechsler L, et al. Intra-arterial prourokinase for acute ischemic stroke. JAMA 1999;282:2003-2011.
14. Shaltoni H, Albright K, Gonzales N, et al. Is intra-arterial thrombolysis safe after full-dose intravenous recombinant tissue plasminogen activator for acute ischemic stroke? Stroke 2007;38:80-84.
15. Smith W, Sung G, Starkman S, et al, for the MERCI Trial Investigators. Safety and efficacy of mechanical embolectomy in acute ischemic stroke. Stroke 2005;36:1432-1438.
16. Inoue T, Node K. Vascular failure: a new clinical entity for vascular disease. J Hypertens 2006;24:2121-2130.
17. Koenig W, Kuseyinova N. Biomarkers of arterosclerotic plaque instability. Arterioscler Thromb Vasc Biol 2007;27:15-26.
18. Szmitko P, Wang C, Weisel R, et al. New markers of inflammation and endothelial activation. Circulation 2003;108:1917-1923.
19. Deanfield J, Donald A, Ferri C, et al. Endothelial function and dysfunction. Part 1. Methodological issues for assessment in the different vascular beds: a statement by the Working Group on Endothelin and Endothelial Factors of the European Society of Hypertension. J Hypertens 2005;23:7-17.
20. Munger M, Hawkins D. Atherothrombosis: epidemiology, pathophysiology, and prevention. J Am Pharm Assoc 2004;44(2 Suppl 1):S5-S13.
21. Faxon DP, Fuster V, Libby P, et al. Atherosclerotic Vascular Disease Conference: Writing Group III: Pathophysiology. Circulation 2004;109:2617-2625.
22. Jialal I, Devaraj S, Venugopal S. C-reactive protein: risk marker or mediator in atherothrombosis. Hypertension 2004;44:6-11.
23. Stoll G, Bendsus M. Inflamation and atherosclerosis: novel insights into plaque formation and destabilization. Stroke 2006;37:1923-1932.
24. Paoletti R, Gotto A, Hajjar D. Inflammation in atherosclerosis and implications for therapy. Circulation 2004;109:20-26.
25. Libby P, Ridker P, Maseri A. Inflammation and atherosclerosis. Circulation 2002; 105:1135-1143.
26. Hansson G. Inflammation, atherosclerosis and coronary artery disease. N Engl J Med 2005;352:1685-1695.
27. Goldstein L, Adams R, Alberts M, et al. Primary prevention of stroke: a guideline from the American Heart Association/American Stroke Association Stroke Council. Stroke 2006;37:1583-1633.
28. Ridker P, Cook N, Lee I, et al. A randomized trial of low-dose aspirin in the primary prevention of cardiovascular disease in women. N Engl J Med 2005;352:1293-1304.
29. Sacco R, Adams R, Albers G, et al. Guidelines for prevention of stroke in patients with ischemic stroke or transient ischemic attack: a statement for healthcare professionals from the American Heart Association/American Stroke Association Council on Stroke. Stroke 2006;37:577-617.
30. Perlstein T, Lee R. Smoking, metalloproteinases, and vascular disease. Arterioscler Throb Vasc Biol 2006;26:250-256.
31. Sacco R, Elkind M, Boden-Albala B, et al. The protective effect of moderate alcohol consumption on ischemic stroke. JAMA 1999;281:53-60.
32. Li J, Mukamal K. An update on alcohol and atherosclerosis. Curr Opin Lipidol 2004;15:673-680.
33. Baur J, Pearson K, Price N, et al. Resveratrol improves health and survival of mice on a high calorie diet. Nature 2006;444:337-342.
34. Suk S, Sacco R, Boden-Albala B, et al. Abdominal obesity and the risk of ischemic stroke: the Northern Manhattan Stroke Study. Stroke 2003;34:1586-1592.
35. Dandona P, Aljada A, Chaudhuri A, et al. Metabolic syndrome: a comprehensive perspective based on interactions between obesity, diabetes and inflammation. Circulation 2005;111:1448-1454.
36. Lee Y, Pratley R. Abdominal obesity and cardiovascular disease risk: the emerging role of the adipocyte. J Cardiopulm Rehabil Prev 2007;27:2-10.
37. Rosenstock J, Iranmanesh A, Hollander PL. Serenade: rimonibant monotherapy for treatment of multiple cardiometabolic risk factors in treatment-naïve patients with type 2 diabetes. Diabet Med 2007;24(Suppl 1):1-29.
38. American Diabetes Association. Standards of care for patients with diabetes mellitus. Diabetes Care 2003;26(Suppl):S33-S50.
39. Rodgers A, MacMahon S, Gamble G, et al. Blood pressure and risk of stroke in patients with cerebrovascular disease: the United Kingdom Transient Ischaemic Attack Collaborative Group. BMJ 1996;313;147.
40. Lawes C, Bennett D, Feigin V, et al. Blood pressure and stroke: an overview of published reviews. Stroke 2004;35:776-785.
41. Chalmers J, Todd A, Chapman N, et al. International Society of Hypertension (ISH): statement on blood pressure lowering and stroke prevention. J Hypertens 2003;21:651-663.
42. Post-stroke Antihypertensive Treatment Study: a preliminary result. PATS Collaborating Group. Chin Med J (Engl) 1995;108:710-717.
43. PROGRESS Collaborative Group. Randomized trial of a perindopril-based blood-pressure-lowering regimen among 6105 individuals with previous stroke or transient ischemic attack. Lancet 2001;358:1033-1041.
44. Dahlof B, Devereux R, Kjeldsen S, et al. Cardiovascular morbidity and mortality in the Losartan Intervention For Endpoint reduction hypertension study (LIFE): a randomized trial against atenolol. Lancet 2002;359:1003.
45. Staessen J, Fagard R, Thijs L, et al. Randomized double-blind comparison of placebo and active treatment for older patients with isolated systolic hypertension Lancet 1997;350:757-764.
46. Major outcomes in high-risk hypertensive patients randomized to angiotensin-converting enzyme inhibitor or calcium channel blocker vs. diuretic: the Antihypertensive and Lipid-Lowering Treatment to Prevent Heart Attack Trial (ALLHAT). JAMA 2002;288:2981-2997.
47. Karin A, Jandeleit-Dahm, Tikellis C, et al. Why blockade of the renin-angiotensin system reduces the incidence of new-onset diabetes. J Hypertens 2005;23:463-473.
48. Carlos F, Richmond R, Smith R, et al. Renin-angiotensin system as a therapeutic target in managing atherosclerosis. Am J Ther 2004;11:44-53.
49. Thone-Reineke C, Steckelings U, Unger T. Angiotensin receptor blockers and cerebral protection. J Hypertens 2006:24(Suppl):S115-S121.
50. Heart Outcomes Prevention Evaluation (HOPE) Study Investigators. Effect of ramipril on cardiovascular and microvascular outcome in patients with diabetes mellitus: results of the HOPE and MICRO-HOPE substudy. Lancet 2000;355:253-259.
51. Dahlof B, Server P, Poulter N, et al. Prevention of cardiovascular events with an antihypertensive regimen of amlodipine adding perindopril as required versus atenolol adding bendroflumethiazide as required, in the Anglo-Scandinavian Cardiac Outcomes Trial Blood Pressure Lowering Arm (ACCOT-BPLA): a multicenter randomized controlled trial. Lancet 2005;366:895-906.
52. Schrader J, Luders S, Lulschewski A, et al. Morbidity and mortality after Stroke, Eprosartan compared with nitrendipine for Secondary prevention: principal results of a prospective randomized controlled study (MOSES). MOSES Study Group. Stroke 2005;36:1218-1226.
53. Corvol J, Bouzamondo A, Sirol M, et al. Differential effects of lipid-lowering therapies on stroke prevention: a meta-analysis of randomized trials. Arch Intern Med 2003;163:669-676.
54. Stancu C, Sima A. Statins: mechanism of action and effects. J Cell Mol Med 2001;5:378-387.
55. Aikawa M. Effects of statin therapy on vascular dysfunction. Coron Artery Dis 2004;15:227-233.
56. Walter D, Zeiher A, Dimmeler S. Effects of statins on endothelium and their contribution to neovascularization by mobilization of endothelial progenitor cells. Coron Artery Dis 2004;15:235-242.
57. Furberg C, Adams H, Applegate W, et al. Effect of lovastatin on early carotid atherosclerosis and cardiovascular events. Asymptomatic Carotid Artery Progression Study (ACAPS) research group. Circulation 1994;90:1679-1687.
58. Heart Protection Study Collaborative Group. MRC/BHF heart protection study of cholesterol lowering with simvastatin in 20 536 high-risk individuals: a randomised placebo-controlled trial. Lancet 2002;360:7-22.

59. Sever P, Poulter N, Dahlof B, et al. Reduction in cardiovascular events with atorvastatin in 2,532 patients with type 2 diabetes. Anglo-Scandinavian Cardiac Outcomes Trial-Lipid Lowering Arm (ASCOT-LLA). Diabetes Care 2005;28:1151-1157.
60. The Stroke Prevention by Aggressive Reduction in Cholesterol Levels (SPARCL) Investigators. High-dose atorvastatin after stroke or transient ischemic attack. N Engl J Med 2006;355:549-559.
61. Billett H. Antiplatelet agents and arterial thrombosis. Clin Geriatr Med 2006;22:57-74.
62. Iadecola C, Gorelick P. The Janus face of cyclooxygenase-2 in ischemic stroke: shifting toward downstream targets. Stroke 2005;36:182-185.
63. Yadav JS, Wholey MH, Kuntz RE, et al, for the Stenting and Angioplasty with Protection in Patients at High Risk for Endarterectomy Investigators. Protected carotid-artery stenting versus endarterectomy in high-risk patients. N Engl J Med 2004;351:1493-1501.
64. Antithrombotic Trialists' Collaboration. Collaborative meta-analysis of randomized trials of antiplatelet therapy for prevention of death, myocardial infarction, and stroke in high-risk patients. BMJ 2002;321:71-87.
65. Serebruany VL, Malinin AI, Eisert RM, et al. Risk of bleeding complications with antiplatelet agents: meta-analysis of 338,191 patients enrolled in 50 randomized trials. Am J Hematol 2004;75:40-47.
66. International Stroke Trial Collaborative Group. The International Stroke Trial (IST): a randomized trial of aspirin, subcutaneous heparin, both, or neither among 19,435 patients with acute ischemic stroke. Lancet 1997;349:1569-1581.
67. CAST (Chinese Acute Stroke Trial) Collaborative Group. CAST: randomized placebo-controlled trial of early aspirin use in 20,000 patients with acute ischemic stroke. Lancet 1997;349:1641-1649.
68. Diener H-C, Cunha L, Forbes C, et al. European Stroke Prevention Study. 2. Dipyridamole and acetylsalicylic acid in the secondary prevention of stroke. J Neurol Sci 1996;143:1-13.
69. Diener H, Darius H, Bertrand-Hardy J, et al. Cardiac safety in the European Stroke Prevention Study 2 (ESPS2). Int J Clin Pract 2001;55:162-163.
70. Sacco RL, Sivenius J, Diener H-C. Efficacy of aspirin plus extended-release dipyridamole in preventing recurrent stroke in high risk populations. Arch Neurol 2005;62:403-408.
71. ESPRIT Study Group. Aspirin plus dipyridamole versus aspirin alone after cerebral ischaemia of arterial origin (ESPRIT): randomised controlled trial. Lancet 2006;367: 1665-1673.
72. The Clopidogrel in Unstable Angina to Prevent Recurrent Events Trial Investigators. Effects of clopidogrel in addition to aspirin in patients with acute coronary syndromes with ST-segment elevation. N Engl J Med 2001;345:495-502.
73. CAPRIE Steering Committee. A randomised, blinded trial of clopidogrel versus aspirin in patients at risk of ischaemic events (CAPRIE). Lancet 1996;348:1329-1339.
74. Diener H-C, Bogousslavsky J, Brass LM, et al. Aspirin and clopidogrel compared with clopidogrel alone after recent ischaemic stroke or transient ischaemic attack in high-risk patients (MATCH): randomized, double-blind, placebo-controlled trial. Lancet 2004;364:331-337.
75. Bhatt DL, Fox KAA, Hacke W, et al. Clopidogrel and aspirin versus aspirin alone for the prevention of atherothrombotic events. N Engl J Med 2006;354:1706-1717.
76. Broderick J, Adams H, Barsan W, et al. Guidelines for the management of spontaneous intracerebral hemorrhage: a statement for healthcare professionals from a special writing group of the Stroke Council, American Heart Association. Stroke 1999;30:905-915.
77. Qureshi A, Tuhrim S, Broderick J, et al. Spontaneous intracerebral hemorrhage. N Engl J Med 2001;344:1450-1460.
78. Mendelow A, Gregson B, Fernandes H, et al. Early versus initial conservative treatment in patients with spontaneous supratentorial intracerebral hematoma in the International Surgical Trial in Intracerebral Haemorrhage (STICH): a randomized trial. Lancet 2005;365:387-397.
79. Mayer S, Brun N, Begtrup K, et al. Recombinant activated factor VII for acute intracerebral hemorrhage. N Engl J Med 2005;352:777-785.
80. Mayer S, Brun N, Begtrup K, et al. Efficacy and safety of recombinant factor VII for acute intracerebral hemorrhage. N Engl J Med 2008;358:2127-2137.

50

OBSESSIVE-COMPULSIVE DISORDERS

Darin D. Dougherty and Michael A. Jenike

OVERVIEW 753
INTRODUCTION 753
PATHOPHYSIOLOGY 754
THERAPEUTICS AND CLINICAL PHARMACOLOGY 754
Goals of Therapy 754
Behavior Therapy 754
Therapeutics by Class 755
Serotonin Reuptake Inhibitors 755
Alternative Monotherapies 755
SRI Augmentation 756
Emerging Targets and Therapeutics 756
Ablative Limbic System Surgery 756
Device-Based Approaches 757
Combined Neurosurgical/Device-Based Approaches 757

OVERVIEW

Obsessive-compulsive disorder (OCD) is a relatively common anxiety disorder that is manifested by obsessions and compulsions (described later). First-line pharmacotherapy for OCD is serotonin reuptake inhibitors (SRIs). In addition to SRIs, behavior therapy is also considered a first-line therapy. The available data suggest that behavior therapy is at least as effective as medication and may be superior in regard to risks, costs, and enduring benefits. Second-line pharmacotherapy for OCD includes alternative monotherapies and augmentation of SRIs with dopamine antagonists. Emerging therapeutics for OCD include surgical and/or device-related interventions.

INTRODUCTION

OCD is a relatively common condition, with lifetime prevalence estimates of approximately 2% to 3% in the United States and comparable lifetime prevalence rates worldwide.[1-3] The defining signs and symptoms of OCD include intrusive unwanted thoughts (i.e., obsessions) and repetitive behaviors (i.e., compulsions)[4] (Box 50-1). Obsessions are thoughts, images, or impulses that occur over and over again and that feel out of control. The individual does not want to have these obsessive thoughts, and they are usually experienced as disturbing and intrusive. Most OCD sufferers recognize that the obsessive thoughts do not make sense. Common obsessions include contamination fears (of germs, chemicals, bodily fluids, etc.), pathologic doubting (e.g., imagining having harmed someone, having said the wrong thing, having not locked doors or turned off appliances), intrusive violent or sexual thoughts or urges, concerns with symmetry or ordering (i.e., a need to have things "just so"), and religious scrupulosity. Compulsions are acts that the person performs over and over again, often according to certain "rules." Individuals with OCD perform these compulsions in response to and in order to minimize their obsessions. Of course, afterward the obsessions return and the OCD sufferer becomes trapped in a cycle of obsessions and compulsions. Common compulsions include repeated washing, cleaning, checking, touching, counting, and arranging behaviors. Most OCD sufferers have multiple obsessions and multiple compulsions.[3]

Everyone experiences occasional unwanted thoughts, performs occasional repetitive or ritualistic behaviors, and has occasional transient feelings of anxiety. In order to meet the criteria for OCD, the obsessions and compulsions must be sufficiently intense or frequent to cause marked distress or impair functioning. Many people with OCD are severely impaired by the symptoms of their disease, performing rituals for hours each day, and may become housebound due to avoidance. Most people with OCD recognize that their thoughts and behaviors are extreme or nonsensical (i.e., they have insight into their symptoms), and are often embarrassed or ashamed of their condition and frightened that they may be "going crazy." In a small percentage (~10%) of cases of OCD, sufferers have poor insight as obsessions progress to overvalued ideas, prompting the special diagnostic designation of "OCD with poor insight."[4]

The differential diagnosis of OCD includes other psychiatric disorders that are characterized by repetitive thoughts or behaviors (Box 50-2). For instance, the obsessions of OCD must be distinguished from ruminations of major depression, the racing thoughts associated with mania, the delusional thoughts of psychosis, and the preoccupation with food and body image associated with eating disorders. Likewise, the compulsions of OCD must be distinguished from the tics of Tourette's syndrome (TS), the ritualized self-injurious behaviors of borderline personality disorder, the rhythmic movements that can present in autism or mental retardation, and the stereotypies of complex partial seizures. By definition, the diagnosis of OCD should not be made if the symptoms can be attributed to another disorder or are the consequence of substance use.[4]

Although the current diagnostic scheme classifies OCD as an anxiety disorder, a variety of disorders from other categories within the *Diagnostic and Statistical Manual of Mental Disorders, Fourth Edition* (DSM-IV)[4] are also characterized by repetitive thoughts and/or behaviors.[5-7] The term *obsessive-compulsive spectrum disorders* (OCSDs) has been introduced that includes similar disorders that share common phenomenologic, etiologic, and perhaps pathophysiologic characteristics. Such OCSDs include TS (characterized by intrusive sensations and urges, as well as a drive to perform motor and vocal tics), trichotillomania (characterized by compulsive hair pulling), and body dysmorphic disorder (characterized by a preoccupation with certain aspects of one's own appearance). It remains to be seen whether the concept of OCSDs will prove clinically useful or neurobiologically valid, as well as which disorders can be meaningfully grouped together and by what criteria. Lastly, comorbidity with OCD is common. OCSDs are much more prevalent in patients with OCD than in the general population. Therefore, it is important to screen for OCSDs in any patient with OCD and vice versa.[2,3] The prevalence of major depression is much higher in patients with OCD than in the general population. Studies suggest that the point prevalence of major depression in patients with OCD is approximately one third, while the lifetime prevalence of major

BOX 50-1 DSM-IV CRITERIA FOR OBSESSIVE-COMPULSIVE DISORDER

A. Either obsessions or compulsions:
Obsessions as defined by (1), (2), (3), and (4):
1. recurrent and persistent thoughts, impulses, or images that are experienced, at some time during the disturbance, as intrusive and inappropriate and that cause marked anxiety or distress
2. the thoughts, impulses, or images are not simply excessive worries about real-life problems
3. the person attempts to ignore or suppress such thoughts, impulses, or images, or to neutralize them with some other thought or action
4. the person recognizes that the obsessional thoughts, impulses, or images are a product of his or her own mind (not imposed from without as in thought insertion)

Compulsions as defined by (1) and (2):
1. repetitive behaviors (e.g., hand washing, ordering, checking) or mental acts (e.g., praying, counting, repeating words silently) that the person feels driven to perform in response to an obsession, or according to rules that must be applied rigidly
2. the behaviors or mental acts are aimed at preventing or reducing distress or preventing some dreaded event or situation; however, these behaviors or mental acts either are not connected in a realistic way with what they are designed to neutralize or prevent or are clearly excessive

B. At some point during the course of the disorder, the person has recognized that the obsessions or compulsions are excessive or unreasonable. **Note:** This does not apply to children.
C. The obsessions or compulsions cause marked distress, are time consuming (take more than 1 hour a day), or significantly interfere with the person's normal routine, occupational (or academic) functioning, or usual social activities or relationships.
D. If another Axis I disorder is present, the content of the obsessions or compulsions is not restricted to it (e.g., preoccupation with food in the presence of an Eating Disorder; hair pulling in the presence of Trichotillomania; concern with appearance in the presence of Body Dysmorphic Disorder; preoccupation with drugs in the presence of a Substance Use Disorder; preoccupation with having a serious illness in the presence of Hypochondriasis; preoccupation with sexual urges or fantasies in the presence of a Paraphilia; or guilty ruminations in the presence of Major Depressive Disorder).
E. The disturbance is not due to the direct physiological effects of a substance (e.g., a drug of abuse, a medication) or a general medical condition.

From American Psychiatric Association. Diagnostic and Statistical Manual of Mental Disorders, 4th ed. Washington, DC: American Psychiatric Press, 1994, pp 422-423.

BOX 50-2 DIFFERENTIAL DIAGNOSIS OF OCD

- Ruminations of major depression
- Racing thoughts of mania
- Delusional thoughts of psychosis
- Preoccupation with food and body image associated with eating disorders
- Tics of Tourette's syndrome
- Ritualized self-injurious behaviors
- Rhythmic movements that may be present in autism or mental retardation
- Stereotypies of complex partial seizures

depression in patients with OCD may be as high as two thirds. Other anxiety disorders and substance use disorders are highly comorbid with OCD as well.

PATHOPHYSIOLOGY

Genetic studies suggest that there may be multiple etiologic subtypes of OCD.[8,9] One issue that confounds genetic studies is that in some cases OCD seems to arise sporadically, whereas in others there exists an apparent familial relationship. Reviews of twin studies find concordance rates of 50% to 60% in monozygotic twins and only 10% in dizygotic twins.[10,11] In addition, heritabilities of 44% for obsessive-compulsive traits and 47% for obsessive-compulsive symptoms have been reported.[12] Although the pathophysiology of OCD is incompletely understood, contemporary neurobiologic models implicate dysfunction in a segregated corticostriatal-thalamic circuit that includes the caudate nucleus, thalamus, orbitofrontal cortex (OFC), and anterior cingulate cortex (ACC) (Fig. 50-1).[13-18] Supporting evidence for this model includes subtle structural abnormalities in the caudate nucleus in OCD patients, as well as functional dysregulation of neural circuits comprising the OFC, ACC, thalamus, and caudate both at rest and during symptom provocation. Interestingly, following successful treatment of OCD symptoms, these abnormalities attenuate.[18] Autoimmune processes, precipitated by β-hemolytic streptococcal infection, may cause damage to striatal neurons in rare sporadic childhood-onset cases of OCD.[19-22] While these cases are rare, they provide further evidence of the central role of the striatum in the pathophysiology of OCD. Neurochemically, both serotonergic and dopaminergic systems have been implicated in the pathophysiology of OCD.[17,23,24] This is because there are prominent serotonergic and dopaminergic projections to and from the striatum and because serotonergic and dopaminergic medications are effective for the treatment of OCD.[25-29]

THERAPEUTICS AND CLINICAL PHARMACOLOGY

Goals of Therapy

The single most important factor in successfully treating OCD is correctly diagnosing OCD. While a thorough clinical evaluation should result in the correct diagnosis the majority of the time, it is important to consider the differential diagnosis (as described earlier). Comorbid diagnoses are the rule rather than the exception in patients with OCD (as described earlier), and adequate treatment of these comorbid conditions is essential. If treatment of comorbid conditions is suboptimal, the symptoms associated with these comorbid conditions may interfere with the treatment of the OCD symptoms. Fortunately, SRIs are the first-line treatment both for OCD and for many of these comorbid diagnoses.

It is also important that both the treatment provider and the patient understand what is considered to be response to treatment for OCD. While the goal of treatment of major depression, for example, is remission, remission is rare in OCD. The "gold standard" for assessing the severity of OCD symptoms is the Yale-Brown Obsessive Compulsive Scale (Y-BOCS),[30,31] a clinician-administered scale that assesses the frequency, interference, distress, resistance, and control of both obsessions and compulsions. The majority of pharmacotherapy trials for OCD have used a reduction of 25% to 35% in Y-BOCS score from baseline as the definition of response. Therefore, it is important to recognize that many patients who are characterized as responders will often still have significant residual symptoms.

Behavior Therapy

The specific type of behavior therapy used to treat OCD is exposure and response prevention (ERP). ERP involves exposing the patient to provocative stimuli (e.g., touching a "contaminated" object) and then preventing his or her usual response or compulsion (e.g., refraining from hand washing).[32-34] Virtually all controlled trials of ERP behavior

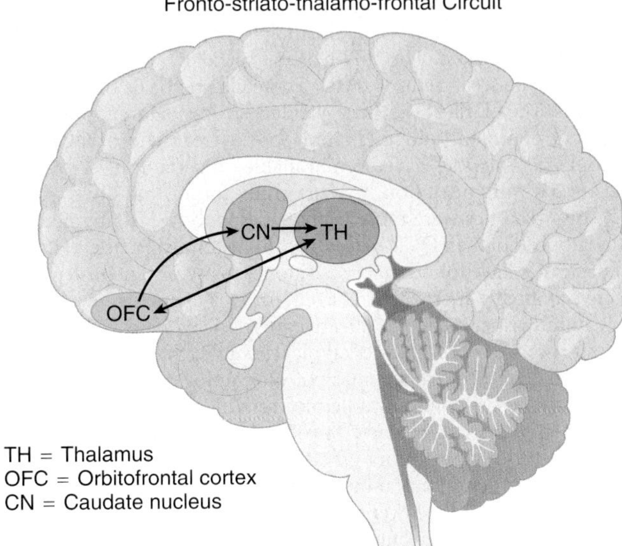

FIGURE 50-1 • The segregated corticostriatal-thalamic circuit (CSTC) associated with the pathophysiology of OCD.

therapy have demonstrated antiobsessional efficacy,[35-41] with dropout rates for these studies averaging approximately 20%.[42] Response to ERP appears to be sustained for up to 1 to 5 years after discontinuation of active treatment, although some studies were confounded by occasional "booster" sessions.[35,39,43,44] A meta-analysis[45,46] based on data from 38 studies between 1961 and 1984 found comparable effect sizes for medication treatment with clomipramine (1.7) and behavior therapy (1.8) at the end of treatment; the benefits from exposure and response prevention persisted at a mean 80-week follow-up (effect size = 1.7), whereas no such follow-up data were available for clomipramine. Thus, behavior therapy may produce the highest mean effect size and the most enduring gains following discontinuation of active treatment.

Some studies directly comparing behavior therapy versus medication have been conducted. One study found that clomipramine was more effective for reducing obsessional doubt, whereas behavior therapy was more effective for reducing compulsive rituals.[47] Nonetheless, medication and behavior therapy are routinely used in concert, as a subset of patients do respond better to the combination of medication and behavioral therapy when compared to either treatment used alone.[48,49] Four studies[50-53] have demonstrated that the combination of behavior therapy and medication is more effective than either treatment alone, whereas three studies[54-56] found that the addition of SRIs to patients being treated with either cognitive or behavior therapy was not superior to either cognitive or behavior therapy alone.

Therapeutics by Class

Serotonin Reuptake Inhibitors

The first-line pharmacotherapy treatment for OCD is the SRIs. These include all of the selective SRIs—fluoxetine (Prozac), sertraline (Zoloft), paroxetine (Paxil), fluvoxamine (Luvox), citalopram (Celexa), and escitalopram (Lexapro)—as well as clomipramine (Anafranil), a tricyclic antidepressant with a mechanism of action that primarily involves serotonin reuptake inhibition. The efficacy of the SRIs for the treatment of OCD was first demonstrated with clomipramine and then by a subsequent large number of randomized, double-blind, placebo-controlled trials.[25,27,57-60] A meta-analysis of these trials found that, in most studies, 40% to 60% of patients respond to the SRIs with a 20% to 40% mean decrease in OCD symptoms.[61] While fewer controlled head-to-head trials of one SRI compared to another SRI for the treatment of OCD have been conducted, it does not appear that any SRI is more efficacious than another SRI for the treatment of OCD.[62] However, it is important for clinicians to note that controlled head-to-head trials

TABLE 50-1 STANDARD RECOMMENDED DOSES OF THE SRIS FOR THE TREATMENT OF OCD

Medication	Dose (mg/day)	Length of Treatment (wk)
Clomipramine (Anafranil)	Up to 250	12
Fluoxetine (Prozac)	Up to 80	12
Sertraline (Zoloft)	Up to 200	12
Fluvoxamine (Luvox)	Up to 300	12
Paroxetine (Paxil)	Up to 60	12
Citalopram (Celexa)	Up to 60	12
Escitalopram (Lexapro)	Up to 20-30	12

of SRIs and tricyclic antidepressants in the treatment of OCD have demonstrated that SRIs are more efficacious than tricyclic antidepressants (other than clomipramine) and that tricyclic antidepressants are no more efficacious than placebo.[63] Therefore, tricyclic antidepressants other than clomipramine are not recommended for the treatment of OCD.

There are major differences in how the SRIs are used for the treatment of OCD when compared to how SRIs are used to treat other psychiatric illnesses. First, studies have shown that higher doses of SRIs than are typically used to treat other disorders, such as major depression, are usually required to achieve response in OCD. Standard recommended doses of the SRIs for the treatment of OCD (Table 50-1) are 80 mg/day of fluoxetine, 200 mg/day of sertraline, 60 mg/day of paroxetine, 300 mg/day of fluvoxamine, 60 mg/day of citalopram, 20 to 30 mg/day of escitalopram, and 250 mg/day of clomipramine. Some patients will respond to lower SRI doses; however, the clinician cannot identify these patients initially, and studies show that a higher percentage of patients will respond to the higher doses of the SRIs rather than lower doses. Therefore, when treating patients with OCD, it is most advantageous to treat all patients with high doses of the SRIs (if tolerated). Second, while patients with major depression treated with SRIs usually respond within 2 to 6 weeks, response may not occur in OCD patients for 10 to 12 weeks. Most clincians escalate the dose of SRIs relatively quickly so that the required 10- to 12-week trial period may begin because a 10- to 12-week trial following each dose escalation (e.g., fluoxetine 20 mg/day, 40 mg/day, 60 mg/day, and, finally, 80 mg/day) could take as long as a year. However, if a lower dose is desired (e.g., due to side effects) after response has been achieved, the dose can be lowered to determine whether the side effects dissipate and response is maintained.

Little is known about the recommended length of treatment with SRIs; few medication discontinuation trials have been conducted in OCD patients. Most of this small number of medication discontinuation trials found clinically significant relapse rates following SRI discontinuation.[63-68] Therefore, it is important for clinicians and patients to understand that OCD is a chronic condition that may require chronic treatment. Rather than medication discontinuation, another strategy may be to use a lower SRI dose for maintenance treatment. While a small number of studies have suggested that lower SRI doses can be used for maintenance treatment,[69,70] further research is needed. At this time there is not enough evidence to support lower SRI dose maintenance treatment. Lastly, many experts believe that the combination of ERP and medication lessens the chance for relapse following medication discontinuation.

Alternative Monotherapies

Because it is believed that the serotonergic and dopaminergic systems are involved in the pathophysiology of OCD, it might be expected that other agents that influence the serotonergic and dopaminergic systems may be useful in the treatment of OCD. However, data from clinical trials of such alternative monotherapies for the treatment of OCD have not convincingly demonstrated that any of these potential alternative monotherapies are efficacious. The results of these trials are summarized in this section.

Other Antidepressants. Because venlafaxine is a dual serotonergic and noradrenergic reuptake inhibitor, it has been studied for the treatment of OCD. Initial evidence supporting the efficacy of venlafaxine for the treatment of OCD includes small open-label studies and case reports. While one double-blind, head-to-head study comparing venlafaxine to paroxetine found that the two agents were equally efficacious, with response rates of approximately 40% for each treatment group,[71] another found that venlafaxine was no more effective than placebo.[72] Monoamine oxidase inhibitors (MAOIs) block the degradation of monoamines such as serotonin and dopamine by, as the name suggests, inhibiting the enzyme monoamine oxidase. Because this block of degradation would be expected to increase levels of serotonin in the brain, MAOIs have been the focus of numerous controlled trials for the treatment of OCD.[73-76] Unfortunately, three of the four published trials of the MAOIs for the treatment of OCD failed to demonstrate efficacy.[73-75] In summary, at this point it does not appear that antidepressants other than SRIs are effective for treating OCD. However, further trials with existing antidepressants are still warranted.

Anxiolytics. Because OCD is an anxiety disorder and because anxiolytics are often used as supplementary therapy for the anxiety associated with OCD, some investigators have studied anxiolytics as monotherapy for OCD. There have been three controlled trials of anxiolytics for the treatment of OCD. Two of these three studies involved clonazepam, and the results were mixed, with one study finding that clonazepam demonstrated efficacy comparable to clomipramine (and both superior to placebo)[71] and another failing to demonstrate a difference between clonazepam and placebo.[77] Lastly, one controlled trial of buspirone, a 5-hydroxytryptamine$_{1A}$ partial agonist, versus clomipramine found them equally efficacious for the treatment of OCD.[78] These results conflict, however, with results of two controlled trials of buspirone augmentation of SRIs for the treatment of OCD that did not demonstrate efficacy.[79,80] Therefore, at this point there is not enough evidence to support monotherapy for OCD with anxiolytics. Anxiolytics are often effective as supplemental treatment of the nonspecific anxiety associated with OCD.

Other Experimental Agents. There is not enough evidence to support the use of other experimental agents for the treatment of OCD at this juncture. It should be noted, though, that there have been mixed results of trials of agents such as inositol, antiandrogens, glutamatergic agents, and opioids as monotherapy for OCD. Further trials of these agents may inform future treatment of OCD.

SRI Augmentation

Neuroleptics. As described previously, the striatum and the dopaminergic system are implicated in the pathophysiology of OCD. Neuroleptics, or dopamine antagonists, block dopamine transmission, especially in the striatum where the majority of dopamine receptors in the brain are located. For this reason, neuroleptics have long been studied for the treatment of OCD. These clinical trials of neuroleptic augmentation of the SRIs have yielded strong data supporting the efficacy of neuroleptic augmentation for the treatment of OCD. Conventional neuroleptics have been available longer and have long been used for SRI augmentation.[81,82] One study found that OCD patients with comorbid tics were more likely to respond to SRI augmentation with haloperidol than OCD patients without comorbid tics.[82] However, recent studies have found that risperidone, an atypical neuroleptic, was effective as an SRI augmentation agent for OCD patients,[28,83,84] and one study found risperidone was effective for OCD patients both with and without comorbid tics.[28] Newer atypical neuroleptics have been studied as well, with one controlled study of olanzapine augmentation demonstrating efficacy,[85] one controlled study of olanazapine augmentation failing to demonstrate efficacy,[86] two controlled studies of quetiapine augmentation demonstrating efficacy,[29,87] and one controlled trial of quetiapine augmentation failing to demonstrate efficacy.[88]

Typically doses at the lower end of those recommended for the treatment of psychosis are adequate for SRI augmentation in OCD patients. For example, the controlled study by McDougle et al.[28] used doses of 1 to 4 mg/day of risperidone for SRI augmentation. An advantage of SRI augmentation with neuroleptics over initiating a trial with another monotherapeutic agent is that only a 4-week trial is needed for augmentation while another 10- to 12-week trial would be necessary for the monotherapy trial. Lastly, it is important to note that atypical neuroleptics may be a useful treatment strategy when employed in combination with SRIs, but there are numerous reports of atypical neuroleptics inducing or worsening obsessive-compulsive symptoms when used without an SRI.[89]

Emerging Targets and Therapeutics

Ablative Limbic System Surgery

For patients with intractable OCD (i.e., those who have failed to respond to medications and behavior therapy), neurosurgery may be a viable option. Ablative limbic system procedures have been used for decades for treatment-refractory OCD and include anterior cingulotomy, limbic leukotomy, and anterior capsulotomy. Anterior cingulotomy and limbic leukotomy procedures always require a craniotomy. An anterior cingulotomy involves ablation of a small amount of bilateral dorsal ACC (Fig. 50-2). A limbic leukotomy includes both an anterior cinguolotomy and a subcaudate tractotomy, where white matter tracts connecting the striatum and ventral prefrontal cortex are

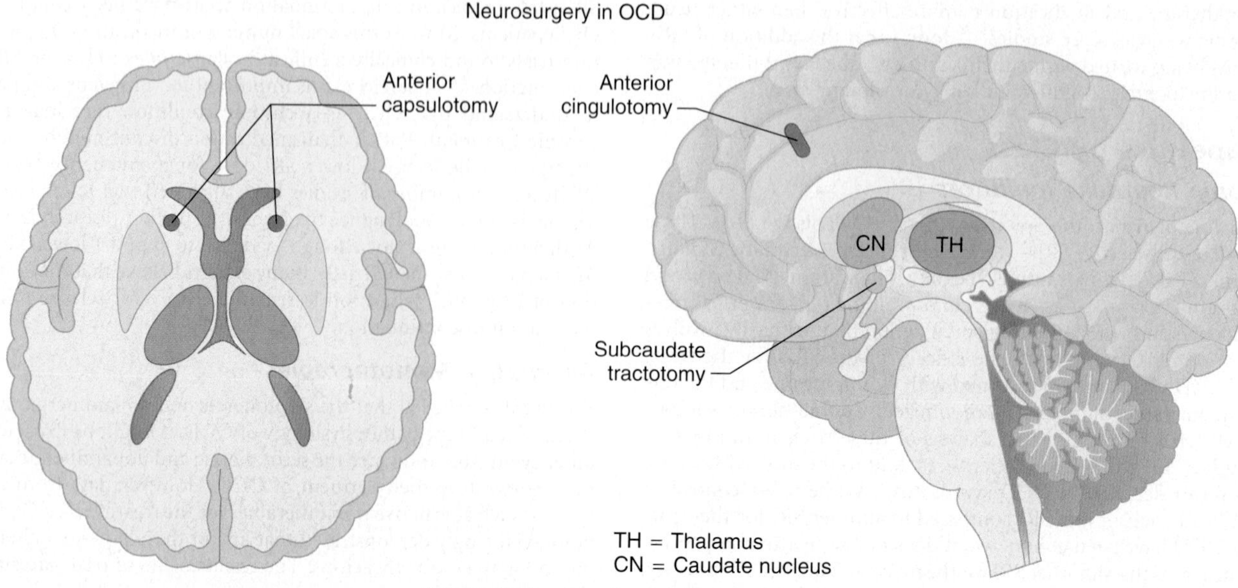

FIGURE 50-2 • Anterior cingulotomy lesion.

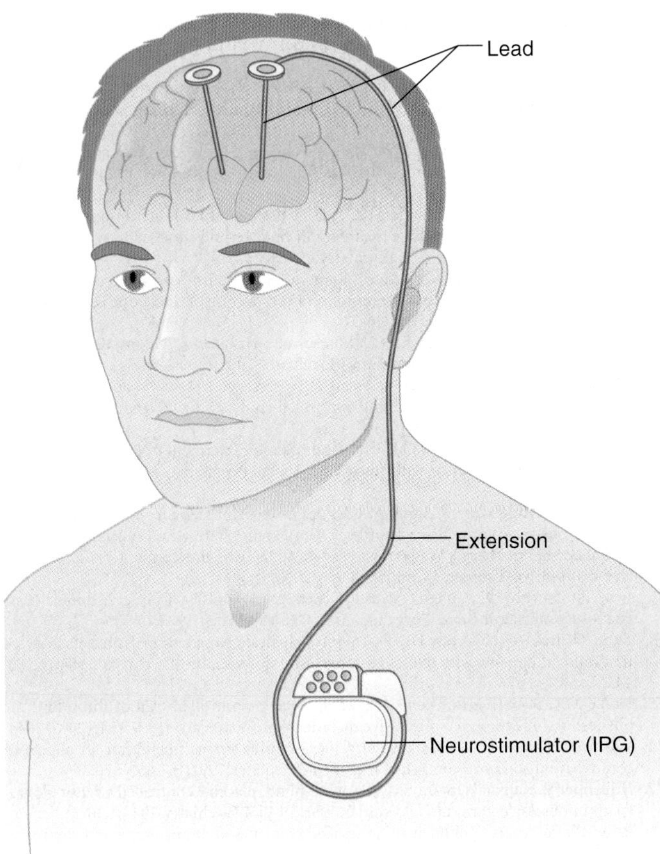

FIGURE 50-3 • **Deep brain stimulation.**

partially ablated. An anterior capsulotomy can be performed via craniotomy or noninvasively using a gamma knife. As the name suggests, an anterior capsulotomy involves bilateral ablation of the anterior limb of the internal capsule. Anterior cingulotomy and limbic leukotomy cannot be performed using a gamma knife because the volume of tissue ablated during these procedures is too large.

The mechanism of action of these procedures is unknown, but it is hypothesized that the lesions disrupt dysfunctional circuitry associated with OCD. Prospective trials of anterior cingulotomy and anterior capsulotomy have demonstrated response rates as high as 45%.[58,90,91] Because patients had to have failed most or all other available treatments to be eligible for these procedures, these response rates are quite clinically significant. If these patients were followed naturalistically without surgical intervention, the response rates would almost certainly be near zero.

Device-Based Approaches

There are no controlled data regarding the efficacy of electroconvulsive therapy (ECT) for OCD. Although utilizing ECT to treat comorbid affective illness may be warranted, there is little evidence to support the use of ECT for obsessive-compulsive symptoms. Transcranial magnetic stimulation (TMS) is another device currently being studied primarily for the treatment of affective disorders. This technology uses a magnetic field to alter neurotransmission in focal areas of cortex. A small amount of preliminary data suggest that TMS, administered to lateral prefrontal regions, may be an effective treatment for OCD.[92] Further studies are certainly needed before TMS could be considered as a possible treatment for OCD.

Combined Neurosurgical/Device-Based Approaches

Deep brain stimulation (DBS) utilizes electrodes implanted in specific targets within the brain and then turned on to either chronically stimulate or inhibit surrounding brain tissue (Fig. 50-3). DBS has been widely used to treat neurologic illnesses such as Parkinson's disease. Some preliminary studies of DBS for treatment-refractory OCD have been encouraging.[93,94] While the DBS leads are placed in the striatum for Parkinson's disease, the initial studies of DBS for OCD have involved DBS lead placement at the same site as would be ablated during an anterior capsulotomy (i.e., the anterior limb of the internal capsule). Further studies of DBS for the treatment of OCD are needed as well.

REFERENCES

1. Angst J. The epidemiology of obsessive compulsive disorder. *In* Hollander E, Zohar J, Marazziti D, et al (eds): Current Insights in Obsessive Compulsive Disorder. Chichester, UK: Wiley, 1994, pp 93-104.
2. Karno M, Golding JM, Sorenson SB, et al. The epidemiology of obsessive-compulsive disorder in five US communities. Arch Gen Psychiatry 1988;45:1094-1099.
3. Rasmussen SA, Eisen JL. The epidemiology and differential diagnosis of obsessive compulsive disorder. J Clin Psychiatry 1994;55:5-14.
4. American Psychiatric Association. Diagnostic and Statistical Manual of Mental Disorders, 4th ed. Washington, DC: American Psychiatric Press, 1994.
5. Hollander E. Obsessive compulsive spectrum disorders. Psychiatr Ann 1993;23:355-407.
6. Hollander E, Kwon JH, Stein DJ, et al. Obsessive-compulsive and spectrum disorders: overview and quality of life issues. J Clin Psychiatry 1996;57(Suppl 8):306.
7. McElroy SL, Phillips KA, Keck PE. Obsessive compulsive spectrum disorder. J Clin Psychiatry 1994;55(Suppl):15-32.
8. Pauls DL, Leckman JF. The inheritance of Gilles de Tourette's syndrome and associated behaviors: evidence for autosomal dominant transmission. N Engl J Med 1986;315:993-997.
9. Pauls DL, Alsobrook JP, Goodman WK, et al. A family study of obsessive-compulsive disorder. Am J Psychiatry 1995;152:76-84.
10. Carey G, Gottesman II. Twin and family studies of anxiety phobic and obsessive disorders. *In* Klein DF, Rabkin J (eds): Anxiety: New Research and Changing Concepts. New York: Raven Press, 1981, pp 117-136.
11. Rasmussen SA, Tsuang MT. Clinical characteristics and family history in DSM III obsessive-compulsive disorder. Am J Psychiatry 1986;143:317-322.
12. Clifford CA, Murray RM, Fulker DW. Genetic and environmental influences on obsessional traits and symptoms. Psychol Med 1984;14:791-800.
13. Baxter LR, Schwartz JM, Guze BH, et al. Neuroimaging in obsessive-compulsive disorder: seeking the mediating neuroanatomy. *In* Jenike MA, Baer L, Minichiello WE (eds): Obsessive Compulsive Disorder: Theory and Management, 2nd ed. Chicago: Year Book Medical Publishers, 1990, pp 167-188.
14. Insel TR. Toward a neuroanatomy of obsessive-compulsive disorder. Arch Gen Psychiatry 1992;49:739-744.
15. Rapoport JL, Wise SP. Obsessive-compulsive disorder: evidence for basal ganglia dysfunction. Psychopharmacol Bull 1988;24:380-384.
16. Rauch SL, Jenike MA. Neurobiological models of obsessive-compulsive disorder. Psychosomatics 1993;34:20-32.
17. Rauch SL, Whalen PJ, Dougherty D, et al. Neurobiologic models of obsessive-compulsive disorder. *In* Jenike MA, Baer L, Minichiello WE (eds): Obsessive-Compulsive Disorders: Practical Management, 3rd ed. St. Louis: Mosby–Year Book, 1998, pp 222-253.
18. Deckersbach T, Dougherty DD, Rauch SL. Functional imaging of mood and anxiety disorders. J Neuroimaging 2006;16:1-10.
19. Allen AJ, Leonard HL, Swedo SE. Case study: A new infection-triggered, autoimmune subtype of pediatric OCD and Tourette's syndrome. J Am Acad Child Adolesc Psychiatry 1995;34:307-311.
20. Swedo SE. Sydenham's chorea: a model for childhood autoimmune neuropsychiatric disorders. JAMA 1994;272:1788-1791.
21. Swedo SE, Leonard HL, Kiessling LS. Speculations on antineuronal antibody-mediated neuropsychiatric disorders of childhood. Pediatrics 1994;93:323-326.
22. Swedo SE, Leonard HL, Garvey M, et al. Pediatric autoimmune neuropsychiatric disorders associated with streptococcal infections: clinical description of the first 50 cases. Am J Psychiatry 1998;155:264-271.
23. Denys D, Zohar J, Westenberg HG. The role of dopamine in obsessive-compulsive disorder: preclinical and clinical evidence. J Clin Psychiatry 2004;65:11-17.
24. Denys D, van der Wee N, Janssen J, et al. Low level of dopaminergic D_2 receptor binding in obsessive-compulsive disorder. Biol Psychiatry 2004;55:1041-1045.
25. Dougherty DD, Rauch SL. Serotonin-reuptake inhibitors in the treatment of OCD. *In* Hollander E, Stein DJ (eds): Obsessive-Compulsive Disorders: Diagnosis–Etiology–Treatment. New York: Marcel Dekker, 1997, pp 145-160.
26. Dougherty DD, Rauch SL, Jenike MA. Pharmacological treatments for obsessive-compulsive disorder. *In* Nathan PE, Gorman JM (eds): A Guide to Treatments That Work, 2nd ed. New York: Oxford University Press, 2002, pp 387-410.
27. Dougherty DD, Rauch SL, Jenike MA. Pharmacotherapy for obsessive-compulsive disorder. J Clin Psychol 2004;60:1195-1202.
28. McDougle CJ, Epperson CN, Pelton GH, et al. A double-blind, placebo-controlled study of risperidone addition in serotonin reuptake inhibitor-refractory obsessive-compulsive disorder. Arch Gen Psychiatry 2000;57:794-801.
29. Denys D, de Geus F, van Megen HJ, et al. A double-blind, placebo-controlled trial of quetiapine addition in patients with obsessive-compulsive disorder refractory to serotonin reuptake inhibitors. J Clin Psychiatry 2004;65:1040-1048.
30. Goodman WK, Price LH, Rasmussen SA, et al. Efficacy of fluvoxamine in obsessive-compulsive disorder: a double-blind comparison with placebo. Arch Gen Psychiatry 1989;46:36-44.

31. Goodman WK, Price LH, Rasmussen SA, et al. The Yale-Brown Obsessive Compulsive Scale (Y-BOCS), Part I: development, use, and reliability. Arch Gen Psychiatry 1989;46:1006-1011.
32. Emmelkamp PMG, de Lange I. Spouse involvement in the treatment of obsessive-compulsive patients. Behav Res Ther 1983;21:341-346.
33. Emmelkamp PMG, Kraanen J. Therapist-controlled exposure in vivo versus self-controlled exposure in vivo: a comparison with obsessive-compulsive patients. Behav Res Ther 1977;15:491-495.
34. Emmelkamp PMG, Van Der Helm M, Van Zanten BL, et al. Treatment of obsessive-compulsive patients: the contribution of self-instructional training to the effectiveness of exposure. Behav Res Ther 1980;18:61-66.
35. Boulougouris JC. Variables affecting the behavior modification of obsessive-compulsive patients treated by flooding. *In* Boulougouris JC, Rabavilas AD (eds): The Treatment of Phobic and Obsessive Compulsive Disorders. Oxford, UK: Pergamon Press, 1977, pp 73-84.
36. Fals-Stewart W, Marks AP, Schafer J. A comparison of behavioral group therapy and individual behavior therapy in treating obsessive-compulsive disorder. J Nerv Ment Dis 1993;181:189-193.
37. Foa EB, Steketee G, Grayson JB, et al. Deliberate exposure and blocking of obsessive-compulsive rituals: immediate and long-term effects. Behav Ther 1984;15:450-472.
38. Lindsay M, Crino R, Andrews G. Controlled trial of exposure and response prevention in obsessive-compulsive disorder. Br J Psychiatry 1997;171:135-139.
39. Marks IM, Hodgson R, Rachman S. Treatment of chronic obsessive-compulsive neurosis by in-vivo exposure: a two-year follow-up and issues in treatment. Br J Psychiatry 1975;127:349-364.
40. Rachman S, Hodgson R, Marks IM. The treatment of chronic obsessive-compulsive neurosis. Behav Res Ther 1971;9:237-247.
41. Rachman S, Marks IM, Hodgson R. The treatment of obsessive-compulsive neurotics by modeling and flooding in vivo. Behav Res Ther 1973;11:463-471.
42. Rachman SJ, Hodgson RJ. Obsessions and Compulsions. Englewood Cliffs, NJ: Prentice-Hall, 1980.
43. Marks IM. Review of behavioral psychotherapy: I. Obsessive-compulsive disorders. Am J Psychiatry 1981;138:584-592.
44. Mawson D, Marks IM, Ramm L. Clomipramine and exposure for chronic obsessive-compulsive rituals: III. Two year follow-up and further findings. Br J Psychiatry 1982;140:11-18.
45. Christensen H, Hadzi-Pavlovic D, Andrews G, et al. Behavior therapy and tricyclic medication in the treatment of obsessive-compulsive disorder: a quantitative review. J Consult Clin Psychol 1987;55:701-711.
46. Quality Assurance Project. Treatment outlines for the management of obsessive-compulsive disorders. Aust N Z J Psychiatry 1985;19:240-253.
47. Solyom L, Sookman D. A comparison of clomipramine hydrochloride (Anafranil) and behaviour therapy in the treatment of obsessive neurosis. J Int Med Res 1977;5(Suppl 5):49-106.
48. Baer L, Minichiello WE. Behavior therapy for obsessive-compulsive disorder. *In* Jenike MA, Baer L, Minichiello WE (eds): Obsessive-Compulsive Disorders: Practical Management, 3rd ed. St. Louis: Mosby–Year Book, 1998, pp 337-367.
49. Rauch SL, Jenike MA. Management of treatment resistant obsessive-compulsive disorder: concepts and strategies. *In* Berend B, Hollander E, Marazitti D, et al (eds): Current Insights in Obsessive-Compulsive Disorder. Chichester, UK: Wiley, 1994, pp 227-244.
50. Honagen F, Winkelman G, Rasche-Rauchle H, et al. Combination of behaviour therapy with fluvoxamine in comparison with behaviour therapy and placebo. Br J Psychiatry 1998;173(Suppl 35):71-78.
51. Marks IM, Stern RS, Mawson D, et al. Clomipramine and exposure for obsessive-compulsive rituals. Br J Psychiatry 1980;136:1-25.
52. Marks IM, Lelliott P, Basoglu M, et al. Clomipramine, self-exposure and therapist-aided exposure for obsessive-compulsive rituals. Br J Psychiatry 1988;152:522-534.
53. O'Connor K, Todorov C, Robillard S, et al. Cognitive-behaviour therapy and medication in the treatment of obsessive-compulsive disorder: a controlled study. Can J Psychiatry 1999;44:64-71.
54. Foa EB, Liebowitz MR, Kozak MJ, et al. Randomized, placebo-controlled trial of exposure and ritual prevention, clomipramine, and their combination in the treatment of obsessive-compulsive disorder. Am J Psychiatry 2005;162:151-161.
55. van Balkom AJ, de Haan E, van Oppen P, et al. Cognitive and behavioral therapies alone versus in combination with fluvoxamine in the treatment of obsessive-compulsive disorder. J Nerv Ment Dis 1998;186:492-499.
56. Rachman S, Cobb J, Grey S, et al. The behavioural treatment of obsessional-compulsive disorders, with and without clomipramine. Behav Res Ther 1979;17:467-478.
57. Cartwright C, Hollander E. SSRIs in the treatment of obsessive-compulsive disorder. Depress Anxiety 1998;8:105-113.
58. Dougherty DD, Baer L, Cosgrove GR, et al. Prospective long-term follow-up of 44 patients who received cingulotomy for treatment-refractory obsessive-compulsive disorder. Am J Psychiatry 2002;159:269-275.
59. Greist JH, Chouinard G, DuBoff E, et al. Double-blind comparison of three doses of sertraline and placebo in the treatment of outpàtients with obsessive compulsive disorder. Arch Gen Psychiatry 1995;52:289-295.
60. Jenike MA. Drug treatment of obsessive-compulsive disorders. *In* Jenike MA, Baer L, Minichiello WE (eds): Obsessive-Compulsive Disorders: Practical Management, 3rd ed. St. Louis: Mosby–Year Book, 1998, pp 469-532.
61. Griest JH, Jefferson JW, Kobak KA, et al. Efficacy and tolerability of serotonin transport inhibitors in obsessive-compulsive disorder: a meta-analysis. Arch Gen Psychiatry 1995;52:53-60.
62. Pigott TA, Seay SM. A review of the efficacy of selective serotonin reuptake inhibitors in obsessive-compulsive disorders. J Clin Psychiatry 1999;60:101-106.
63. Thoren P, Asberg M, Cronholm B, et al. Clomipramine treatment of obsessive compulsive disorder: I. A controlled clinical trial. Arch Gen Psychiatry 1980;37:1281-1285.
64. Pato MT, Zohar-Kaduch R, Zohar J, et al. Return of symptoms after discontinuation of clomipramine in patients with obsessive compulsive disorder. Am J Psychiatry 1988;145:1521-1525.
65. Hollander E, Allen A, Steiner M, et al. Acute and long-term treatment and prevention of relapse of obsessive-compulsive disorder with paroxetine. J Clin Psychiatry 2003;64:1113-1121.
66. Leonard HL, Swedo SE, Lenane MC, et al. A double-blind desipramine substitution during long-term clomipramine treatment in children and adolescents with obsessive-compulsive disorder. Arch Gen Psychiatry 1991;48:922-927.
67. Romano S, Goodman W, Tamura R, et al. Long-term treatment of obsessive-compulsive disorder after an acute response: a comparison of fluoxetine versus placebo. J Clin Psychopharmacol 2001;21:46-52.
68. Koran LM, Hackett E, Rubin A, et al. Efficacy of sertraline in the long-term treatment of obsessive-compulsive disorder. Am J Psychiatry 2002;159:88-95.
69. Mundo E, Bareggi SR, Pirola R, et al. Long-term pharmacotherapy of obsessive-compulsive disorder: a double-blind controlled study. J Clin Psychopharmacol 1997; 17:4-10.
70. Tollefson GD, Birkett M, Koran L, et al. Continuation treatment of OCD: double-blind and open-label experience with fluoxetine. J Clin Psychiatry 1994;55(Suppl 10):69-76.
71. Hewlett W, Vinogradov S, Agras W. Clomipramine, clonazepam, and clonidine treatment of obsessive compulsive disorder. J Clin Psychopharmacol 1992;12:420-430.
72. Hollander E, Friedberg J, Wasserman S, et al. Venlafaxine in treatment-resistant obsessive-compulsive disorder. J Clin Psychiatry 2003;64:546-550.
73. Insel TR, Murphy DL, Cohen RM, et al. Obsessive-compulsive disorder: a double-blind trial of clomipramine and clorgyline. Arch Gen Psychiatry 1983;40:605-612.
74. Zahn TP, Insel TR, Murphy DL. Psychophysiological changes during pharmacological treatment of patients with obsessive-compulsive disorder. Br J Psychiatry 1984;145:39-44.
75. Jenike MA, Baer L, Minichiello WE, et al. Placebo-controlled trial of fluoxetine and phenelzine for obsessive-compulsive disorder. Am J Psychiatry 1997;154:1261-1264.
76. Vallejo J, Olivares J, Marcos T, et al. Clomipramine versus phenelzine in obsessive-compulsive disorder: a controlled trial. Br J Psychiatry 1992;161:665-670.
77. Hollander E, Kaplan A, Stahl SM. A double-blind, placebo-controlled trial of clonazepam in obsessive-compulsive disorder. World J Biol Psychiatry 2003;4:30-34.
78. Pato MT, Pigott TA, Hill JL, et al. Controlled comparison of buspirone and clomopramine in obsessive-compulsive disorder. Am J Psychiatry 1991;148:127-129.
79. Pigott TA, L'Heureux F, Hill JL, et al. A double-blind study of adjuvant buspirone hydrochloride in clomipramine-treated patients. J Clin Psychopharmacol 1982;12:11-18.
80. Grady TA, Pigott TA, L'Heureux F, et al. A double-blind study of adjuvant buspirone hydrochloride in fluoxetine treated patients with obsessive compulsive disorder. Am J Psychiatry 1993;150:819-821.
81. McDougle CJ, Goodman WK, Price LH, et al. Neuroleptic addition in fluvoxamine refractory obsessive compulsive disorder. Am J Psychiatry 1990;147:652-654.
82. McDougle CJ, Goodman WK, Leckman JF, et al. Haloperidol addition in fluvoxamine-refractory obsessive-compulsive disorder: a double-blind, placebo-controlled study in patients with and without tics. Arch Gen Psychiatry 1994;51:302-308.
83. Hollander E, Baldini Rossi N, Sood E, et al. Risperidone augmentation in treatment-resistant obsessive-compulsive disorder: a double-blind, placebo-controlled study. Int J Neuropsychopharmacol 2003;6:397-401.
84. Li X, May RS, Tolbert LC, et al. Risperidone and haloperidol augmentation of serotonin reuptake inhibitors in refractory obsessive-compulsive disorder: a crossover study. J Clin Psychiatry 2005;66:736-743.
85. Bystritsky A, Ackerman SL, Rosen RM, et al. Augmentation of serotonin reuptake inhibitors in refractory obsessive-compulsive disorder using adjunctive olanzapine: a placebo-controlled trial. J Clin Psychiatry 2004;65:565-568.
86. Shapira NA, Ward HE, Mandoki M, et al. A double-blind, placebo-controlled trial of olanzapine addition in fluoxetine-refractory obsessive-compulsive disorder. Biol Psychiatry 2004;55:553-555.
87. Atmaca M, Kuloglu M, Tezcan E, et al. Quetiapine augmentation in patients with treatment resistant obsessive-compulsive disorder: a single-blind, placebo-controlled study. Int Clin Psychopharmacol 2002;17:115-119.
88. Carey PD, Vythilingum B, Seedat S, et al. Quetiapine augmentation of SRIs in treatment refractory obsessive-compulsive disorder: a double-blind, randomized, placebo-controlled study. BMC Psychiatry 2005;5:5.
89. Lykouras L, Alevizos B, Michalopoulou P, et al. Obsessive-compulsive symptoms induced by atypical antipsychotics: a review of the reported cases. Prog Neuropsychopharmacol Biol Psychiatry 2003;27:333-346.
90. Cosgrove GR, Rauch SL. Stereotactic cingulotomy. Neurosurg Clin N Am 2003;14:225-235.
91. Greenberg BD, Price LH, Rauch SL, et al. Neurosurgery for intractable obsessive-compulsive disorder and depression: critical issues. Neurosurg Clin N Am 2003;14:199-212.
92. Greenberg BD, George MS, Dearing J, et al. Effect of prefrontal repetitive transcranial magnetic stimulation (rTMS) in obsessive compulsive disorder: a preliminary study. Am J Psychiatry 1997;154:867-869.
93. Gabriels L, Cosyns P, Nuttin B, et al. Deep brain stimulation for treatment-refractory obsessive-compulsive disorder: psychopathological and neuropsychological outcome in three cases. Acta Psychiatr Scand 2003;107:241-243.
94. Greenberg BD, Malone DA, Friehs GM, et al. Three-year outcomes in deep brain stimulation for highly resistant obsessive-compulsive disorder. Neuropsychopharmacology 2006;31:2384-2393.

51

ATTENTION-DEFICIT/HYPERACTIVITY DISORDER

David A. Mrazek and Kathryn M. Schak

INTRODUCTION 759
ADHD IN CHILDHOOD AND ADOLESCENCE 759
Components of Assessment 759
THERAPEUTICS AND CLINICAL PHARMACOLOGY 759
Psychostimulants 759
Amphetamines 760
Methylphenidates 762
Psychostimulant Side Effects 765
Nonstimulant Medications 765
Atomoxetine 765
Tricyclic Antidepressants 766
Bupropion 766
α-Agonists 766
Pemoline 766
Pharmacogenomics 767
Dopamine Transporter Gene (SLC6A3) 767
Dopamine D_4 Receptor Gene (DRD4) 767
Synaptosomal-Associated Protein 25 Gene (SNAP25) 767
ADHD IN ADULTS 767
CONCLUSIONS 767

INTRODUCTION

Attention-deficit/hyperactivity disorder (ADHD) is a neurobehavioral condition that is characterized by features of inattention, hyperactivity, and impulsivity. The precise prevalence of ADHD in school-age children has been difficult to establish, but rates as high as 9% have been reported.[1] In 1937, Dr. Bradley first documented the use of *d,l*-amphetamine to improve inattention and behavior problems in hospitalized children.[2] At the time, *d,l*-amphetamine sulfate was available as Benzedrine.[3] A variety of names for ADHD have been used to diagnostically label hyperactive children. Early diagnostic classifications included "minimal brain dysfunction" and "hyperkinetic reaction of childhood." In 1980, these children were labeled as having "attention deficit disorder with or without hyperactivity." In 1994, the current diagnostic label of "attention-deficit/hyperactivity disorder" was adopted.

ADHD IN CHILDHOOD AND ADOLESCENCE

Eighteen symptoms that are currently used to make the diagnosis of ADHD in children and adolescents are listed in Box 51-1. These symptoms must occur for at least 6 months, be maladaptive, and be inconsistent with the developmental level of the child. Impairment from symptoms must occur in at least two settings, and the onset of symptoms must occur before 7 years of age. There are three subtypes of ADHD: the combined type, the predominantly inattentive type, and the predominantly hyperactive-impulsive type. The most common subtype in children is the combined type, which requires six or more inattention symptoms and six or more hyperactivity or impulsivity symptoms. For the predominantly inattentive or predominantly hyperactive-impulsive types, at least six symptoms are respectively required in the labeled category with less than six symptoms occurring in the other category.

To make the diagnosis of ADHD in children and adolescents, symptom reports from both the parent(s) and teacher should be documented. Direct contact with the teacher of the child in order to accurately document school day behavior is optimal. However, it is common practice to review behavioral checklists such as the Conners Teacher Rating Scale that are completed by the teacher of the child. The Conners Parent Rating Scale is also available to systematically document parental observations.

Components of Assessment

A detailed psychiatric history should be conducted that includes systematic documentation of the symptoms of ADHD, previous medication trials, comorbid psychiatric conditions, a family psychiatric history, and a review of cardiac symptoms. Baseline blood pressure, heart rate, height, and weight should be documented and subsequently monitored (Box 51-2).

THERAPEUTICS AND CLINICAL PHARMACOLOGY

Psychostimulants

The psychostimulants are the first-line medications for the treatment of ADHD symptoms in children and adults. The psychostimulants are divided into two classes: amphetamines and methylphenidates.

The psychostimulants are structurally similar to the dopamine and norepinephrine molecules. The effects of psychostimulants on neurochemical functions have been identified at both the presynaptic and postsynaptic neurons. Psychostimulants are believed to displace norepinephrine and dopamine from presynaptic stores in the synaptic space and block the reuptake of dopamine by the dopamine transporter (DAT) (Fig. 51-1). Psychostimulants also appear to be direct adrenergic agonists of the postsynaptic neuron (see Fig. 51-1). Dextroamphetamine (Dexedrine) was the first drug approved for the treatment of ADHD by the U.S. Food and Drug Administration (FDA). Methylphenidate (Ritalin) was subsequently approved by the FDA in 1961. The FDA approval of Adderall in 1996 for treatment of ADHD has been followed by an increase in development and availability of psychostimulants, particularly the methylphenidates. Currently, there are over 15 available psychostimulants that vary by duration of action (short acting, intermediate acting, long acting) and administration route (tablet, sprinkles, liquid, chewable tablet, and dermal patch) (Table 51-1).

Psychostimulants provide an immediate and often dramatic improvement in the target symptoms of ADHD. However, a response to stimulant treatment is not diagnostic of ADHD as normal children and adults have similar cognitive and behavioral responses to psychostimulants.[4] Despite its less intense psychostimulant properties, caffeine has also been shown to improve ADHD symptoms in children.[5]

Many controlled studies support the efficacy of psychostimulants in treating childhood ADHD.[6] However, two large placebo-controlled trials, supported by the National Institute for Mental Health (NIMH), have been widely recognized as supporting the use of psychostimulant treatment for ADHD.

The NIMH Multimodal Treatment Study of ADHD (MTA)[7] was a multisite clinical trial of school-age children with ADHD that compared psychostimulant treatment to psychosocial treatments designed to reduce ADHD symptoms. The MTA study participants were divided

BOX 51-1 DSM-IV CRITERIA FOR ATTENTION-DEFICIT/HYPERACTIVITY DISORDER

Either six of the inattention symptoms or six of the hyperactivity-impulsivity symptoms have persisted for at least 6 months to a degree that is maladaptive and inconsistent with developmental level.

- If six symptoms from each of the inattention and hyperactivity-impulsivity criteria are met then the diagnosis is combined type.
- If only six inattentive symptoms, then the diagnosis is predominantly inattentive type.
- If only six symptoms of hyperactivity-impulsivity, then the diagnosis is predominantly hyperactive-impulsive type.

Inattention

1. Often fails to give close attention to details or makes careless mistakes in schoolwork, work, or other activities
2. Often has difficulty sustaining attention in tasks or play activities
3. Often does not seem to listen when spoken to directly
4. Often does not follow through on instructions and fails to finish schoolwork, chores, or duties in the workplace (not due to oppositional behavior or failure to understand instructions)
5. Often has difficulty organizing tasks and activities
6. Often avoids, dislikes, or is reluctant to engage in task that require sustained mental effort (such as schoolwork or homework)
7. Often loses things necessary for tasks or activities (e.g., toys, school assignments, pencils, books, or tools)
8. Is often easily distracted by extraneous stimuli
9. Is often forgetful in daily activities

Hyperactivity-Impulsivity

Hyperactivity

1. Often fidgety with hands or feet or squirms in seat
2. Often leaves seat in classroom or in other situations in which remaining seated is expected
3. Often runs about or climbs excessively in situations in which it is inappropriate (in adolescents or adults, may be limited to subjective feelings of restlessness)
4. Often has difficulty playing or engaging in leisure activities quietly
5. Is often "on the go" or often acts as if "driven by a motor"
6. Often talks excessively

Impulsivity

1. Often blurts out answers before questions have been completed
2. Often has difficulty awaiting turn
3. Often interrupts or intrudes on others (e.g., butts into conversations or games)

Additionally, the following criteria must be met:

- Some hyperactive-impulsive or inattentive symptoms that caused impairment were present before age 7 years.
- Some impairment from the symptoms present in two or more settings.
- There must be clear evidence of clinically significant impairment in social, academic, or occupational functioning.

Adapted from American Psychiatric Association. Diagnostic and Statistical Manual of Mental Disorders, Fourth Edition. Washington, DC: American Psychiatric Association, 1994.

BOX 51-2 CLINICAL DATA NECESSARY PRIOR TO INITIATING PSYCHOSTIMULANT TREATMENT

Key Elements of History

- Current ADHD symptoms
- Comorbid Axis I conditions, including mood, anxiety, and psychotic symptoms
- Comorbid medical conditions, including tic disorder, cardiac conditions, and seizure disorders
- If a previous history of ADHD is detected, clarification of the longitudinal course and treatment

Baseline Data

- Blood pressure
- Heart rate
- Height
- Weight
- ADHD symptoms

BOX 51-3 GENERAL RECOMMENDATIONS FOR PSYCHOSTIMULANT DOSING

1. Use the recommended starting dose of each stimulant.
2. Increase in weekly increments of 5 to 10 mg/dose for methylphenidate or 2.5 to 5 mg for amphetamines.
3. Effective dosing has not been correlated with age, body mass, or gender.
4. Slow titration of dose should be monitored until optimal efficacy is achieved with minimal tolerable side effects.

into four study groups: (i) medication alone, (ii) intensive behavioral treatment, (iii) combined medication and behavioral treatment, and (iv) standard community care. The study included 579 children between the ages of 7 and 10 years with combined-type ADHD. Subjects were followed for 14 months. The MTA study demonstrated that children receiving psychostimulant medication alone or medication in combination with behavioral treatment showed significantly greater improvement in ADHD symptoms than children receiving either behavioral treatment alone or standard community care.[7]

The NIMH Preschool ADHD Treatment Study (PATS)[8] was the first controlled multisite study that examined the safety and efficacy of psychostimulant treatment in younger children. The PATS study included 303 children with combined or predominantly hyperactive ADHD who were treated with methylphenidate. These children were between 3 and 5.5 years of age. Preschoolers in the PATS study responded to a mean daily dose of 14.2 mg.[8]

The American Academy of Child and Adolescent Psychiatry practice parameters recommend initial treatment with either an amphetamine or methylphenidate. If an initial trial is unsuccessful, subsequent treatment with the alternative class of stimulant medication or treatment with a nonstimulant is recommended. Approximately 70% of children with ADHD have been demonstrated to respond to stimulant treatment.[6] Initial dosing for most methylphenidates is 5 to 10 mg/dose, and amphetamines 2.5 to 5 mg/dose. The dose can be gradually increased until symptom control is achieved or until side effects become a problem. Once a maintenance dose is established, targeted ADHD symptoms and side effects should be monitored as well as blood pressure, heart rate, height, and weight.

The duration of action can be regulated by the selection of the formulations used. In younger children, the administration route is also an issue. Long-acting psychostimulant formulations are more convenient, while shorter acting formulations allow minimization of side effects (Box 51-3).

Amphetamines

Short-Acting Amphetamines

Dextroamphetamine Sulfate. Dextroamphetamine sulfate is the dextro isomer of the compound *d,l*-amphetamine sulfate and is available as Dexedrine and Dextrostat (Fig. 51-2). These immediate release formulations begin to have an effect within 30 minutes to 1 hour after administration and have duration of action of 4 to 6 hours. Dextroamphetamine was the first amphetamine formulation to be approved by the FDA for use in children older than 2 years of age for

TABLE 51-1 CURRENTLY AVAILABLE STIMULANT MEDICATIONS

Effect Duration	Administration Form	Methylphenidates	Amphetamines
Short acting (bid or tid)	Tablet only	Ritalin Methylin Focalin	Adderall Dexedrine Dextrostat Desoxyn
	Chewable tablet	Methylin	None
	Liquid	Ritalin Methylin	Dextrostat
Intermediate acting (one q A.M. or bid)	Tablet only	Ritalin SR Methylin ER Metadate ER	None
Long acting (one q A.M.)	Tablet only Tablet that may be sprinkles	Concerta Metadate CD Ritalin LA Focalin XR	Dexedrine Spansule Adderall XR Vyvanse
	Skin patch	Daytrana	None

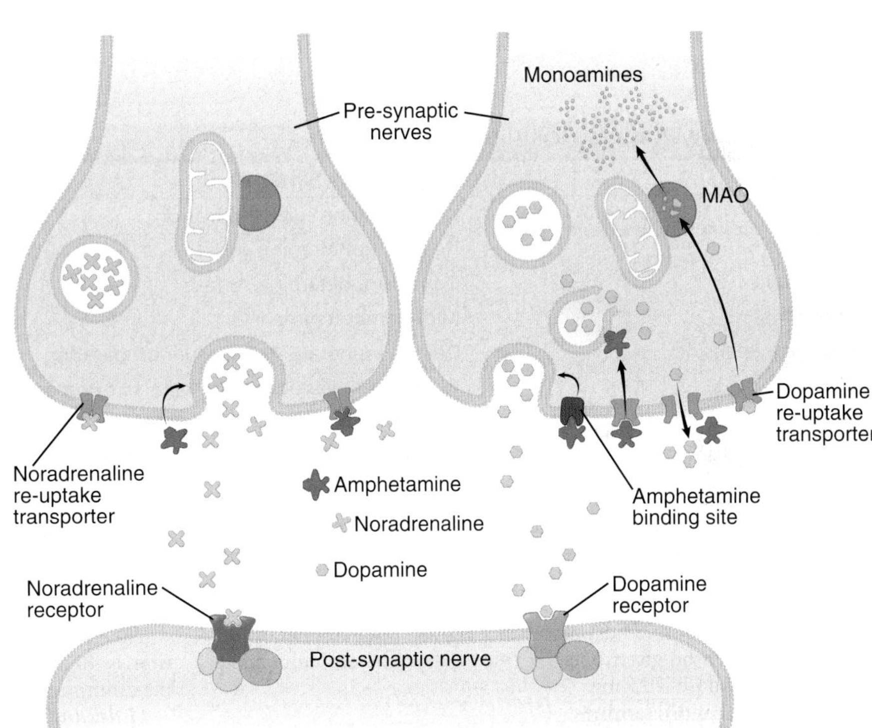

FIGURE 51-1 • The mechanism of action of psychostimulants such as amphetamine. Low-dose amphetamine can modify the action of dopamine and noradrenaline in the brain. Amphetamine increases the concentration of dopamine in the synaptic cleft in three ways. *1,* It can bind to the presynaptic membrane of dopaminergic neurons and induce the release of dopamine from the nerve terminal. *2,* Amphetamine can interact with dopamine-containing synaptic vesicles, releasing free dopamine into the nerve terminal. *3,* Amphetamine can bind to the dopamine reuptake transporter, causing it to act in reverse and transport free dopamine out of the nerve terminal. Amphetamine can also cause an increased release of noradrenaline into the synaptic cleft.

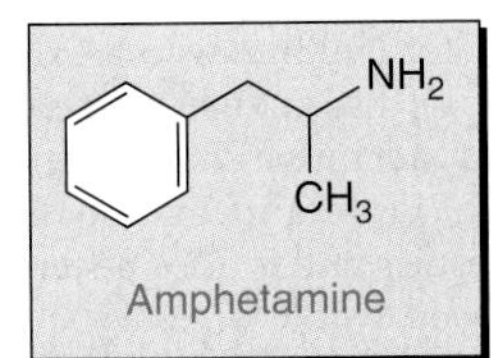

FIGURE 51-2 • Amphetamine.

treatment of ADHD. Dexedrine is available in scored 5-mg tablets (Table 51-2). Dextrostat is available in scored 5- and 10-mg tablets as well as a liquid with a concentration of 5 mg/ml.

The initial recommended dose for dextroamphetamine sulfate in children who are 3 to 5 years of age is 2.5 mg once a day, with dose adjustments of 2.5 mg/wk. The maximum recommended daily dose in this age group is 40 mg. The initial recommended dose for children who are older than 5 years of age is 5 mg, with dose adjustments of 5 mg/wk. The maximum recommended daily dose for children in this age group is also 40 mg. Two to three doses a day may be required with the first dose in the morning and additional doses at 4- to 6-hour intervals.

Amphetamine Salt Preparation. An amphetamine salt combination of the neutral sulfate salts of dextroamphetamine and amphetamine is available as Adderall. This compound is composed of the dextro isomer of amphetamine saccharate and *d,l*-amphetamine aspartate monohydrate. This salt preparation was approved in 1996 for use in children older than 2 years of age and is an immediate-release medication with clinical effects occurring within 45 minutes of administration, a peak effect at 1 to 2 hours, and a duration of action between 4 and 6 hours. This preparation is available in 5-, 7.5-, 10-, 12.5-, 15-, 20-, and 30-mg tablets (Table 51-3).

The initial recommended dose for this salt preparation in children 3 to 5 years of age is 2.5 mg once daily, with dose adjustments of 2.5 mg/wk. This preparation can be given once or twice a day; the maximum recommended daily dose is 40 mg. The initial dose in children who are older than 5 years of age is 5 mg daily, with dose adjustments of 5 mg/wk. This preparation can be given once or twice a day. The maximum recommended daily dose is also 40 mg in this age group.

Methamphetamine Hydrochloride. Methamphetamine hydrochloride is a short-acting formulation that is available as Desoxyn. Meth-

TABLE 51-2 SUMMARY OF PRESCRIBING INFORMATION FOR CURRENTLY AVAILABLE AMPHETAMINES

Trade Name	Doses (mg)	Approved Use for Ages 3-5 Yr	Form	Initial Dose (mg)	Maximum Daily Dose (mg)	Daily Doses	Peak Effect (hr)	Duration of Effect (hr)
SHORT ACTING								
Adderall	5, 7.5, 10, 12.5, 15, 20, 30	Yes	Tablet	3-5 yr: 2.5 6 yr & older: 5	40	1-2	3	4-6
Dexedrine	5 5 mg/1 ml	Yes	Tablet Liquid	3-5 yr: 2.5 6 yr & older: 5	40	1-2	2-3	4-6
Dextrostat	5, 10		Tablet	3-5 yr: 2.5 6 yr & older: 5	40	1-2	2-3	4-6
Desoxyn	5	No	Tablet	5	25	1-2	2-3	4-5
LONG ACTING								
Dexedrine Spansule	5, 10, 15	Yes	Capsule	5	40	1	8	8-10
Adderall XR	5, 10, 15, 20, 25, 30	No	Tablet (XR)	5	30	1	7	10-12
Vyvanse	30, 50, 70	No	Capsule	30	70	1		

XR, extended release.

TABLE 51-3 AVAILABLE DOSE OF AMPHETAMINES

Trade Name	Preparation Type	Available Doses (mg)
Adderall	Amphetamine salt preparation	5, 7.5, 10, 12.5, 15, 20, 30
Dexedrine	Dextroamphetamine sulfate	5
Dextrostat	Dextroamphetamine sulfate	5, 10
Desoxyn	Methamphetamine HCl	5
Dexedrine Spansule	Dextroamphetamine spansule preparation	5, 10, 15
Adderall XR	Extended-release amphetamine salt preparation	5, 10, 15, 20, 25, 30
Vyvanse	Lisdexamfetamine dimesylate	30, 50, 70

amphetamine hydrochloride has a peak effect within 2 to 3 hours of administration and a duration of action 4 to 5 hours. It is approved for use in children who are older than 5 years of age. Methamphetamine hydrochloride is available in 5-mg tablets.

The initial recommended dose for methamphetamine hydrochloride is 5 mg, with dose adjustments of 5 mg/wk. Methamphetamine hydrochloride can be given once or twice a day. The recommended maximum daily dose is 25 mg.

Long-Acting Amphetamines

Dextroamphetamine Spansule Preparations. Dextroamphetamine spansule capsules are an extended-release formulation of dextroamphetamine that is administered once a day and is available as Dexedrin Spansules. This spansule preparation contains both immediate-release and extended-release dextroamphetamine. The peak effect of these spansules occurs at 8 hours. The duration of action may extend to 10 hours. The spansule preparation is approved for use in children older than 2 years of age. The spansule preparation is available in 5- and 10-mg capsules. These capsules must be swallowed intact and cannot be divided, crushed, or chewed.

The initial recommended dose for the spansule preparation is 5 mg/day, with dose adjustments of 5 mg/wk. The maximum recommended daily dose is 40 mg. If a patient is taking dextroamphetamine, he or she may change to the spansules preparation by taking the total daily dose in the morning.

Extended Amphetamine Salt Preparation. An extended-release amphetamine salt preparation is available as Adderall XR. This preparation is given once a day and contains 50% short-acting amphetamine and 50% delayed-release amphetamine. The extended-release salt preparation was designed to replace the twice-daily dosing that is often required when taking the short-acting salt preparation. Initial effects occur within 1.5 hours, the peak effect occurs at 7 hours, and the duration of action can last up to 12 hours. The extended-release salt preparation was approved by the FDA for use in children who are older than 5 years of age. It is available in 5-, 10-, 15-, 20-, 25-, and 30-mg capsules. The capsules may be swallowed as whole capsules or alternatively may be administered by sprinkling the capsule contents on a small amount of food such as applesauce.

The initial recommended dose of the extended-release salt preparation is 10 mg daily, with dose adjustments of 5 to 10 mg/wk. The maximum recommended daily dose is 30 mg.

Lisdexamfetamine Dimesylate. Lisdexamfetamine dimesylate is a prodrug that is metabolized to dextroamphetamine and is available as Vyvanse. It was designed to reduce abuse potential because dextroamphetamine is released only after the removal of *l*-lysine. This prodrug preparation is approved for children who are older than 5 years of age. The peak concentration of lisdexamfetamine occurs in 1 hour, while the maximum dextroamphetamine concentration does not occur until 3.5 hours after ingestion. Lisdexamfetamine dimesylate is available in 30-, 50-, and 70-mg capsules and is administered in the morning. The capsule may be swallowed whole or may be dissolved in a glass of water.

The initial recommended dose of lisdexamfetamine dimesylate is 30 mg/day, with dose adjustments of 20 mg/wk. The maximum recommended dose of lisdexamfetamine is 70 mg.

Methylphenidates

Short-Acting Methylphenidate Formulations

Methylphenidate Hydrochloride. Methylphenidate hydrochloride (*d,l*-methylphenidate; Fig. 51-3) is available as Ritalin and Methylin. The effects of methylphenidate begin at 30 to 60 minutes after administration. Peak effects occur within 1 to 2 hours, and the duration of action is usually about 4 hours. Methylphenidate has been approved for treatment of ADHD symptoms in children who are older than 5 years of age.

Methylphenidate is available in 5-, 10-, and 20-mg tablets as well as 2.5-, 5-, and 10-mg grape-flavored chewable tablets (Table 51-4). It is also available in a grape-flavored oral solution in two concentrations (5 mg/5 ml and 10 mg/5 ml).

The initial dosing recommendation for short-acting methylphenidate formulations in school-age children is 5 mg once or twice daily. Dose adjustments of 5 to 10 mg are recommended on a weekly basis, with a maximum daily dose of 60 mg.

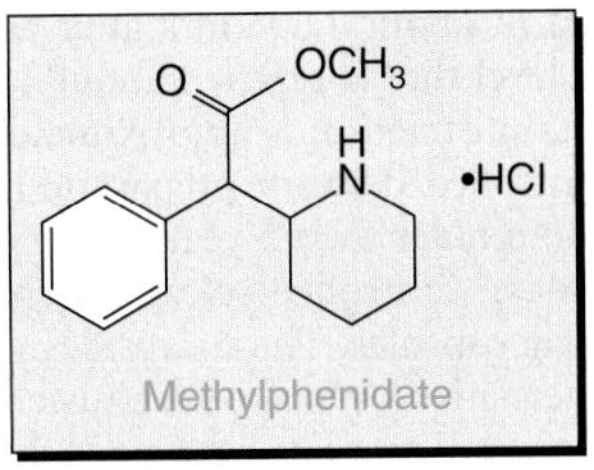

FIGURE 51-3 • Methylphenidate.

Dexmethylphenidate Hydrochloride. Dexmethylphenidate hydrochloride (*d*-methylphenidate) is the *d*-isomer of the racemic mixture of *d,l*-methylphenidate and is available as Focalin. Given that the *d*-isomer is the only active isomer of methylphenidate, the *d*-isomer preparation is twice as potent as the racemic preparation. The FDA approved dexmethylphenidate for children older than 5 years of age in 2001. Peak effects occur in 1 to 1.5 hours, and the duration of action is approximately 4 hours. Dexmethylphenidate hydrochloride is available in 2.5-, 5-, and 10-mg tablets (Table 51-5).

The initial recommended dose is 2.5 mg once or twice daily, which is often given before or after breakfast and lunch. Dose adjustments of 2.5 to 5 mg/wk are recommended. The maximum daily dose is 20 mg, which is typically given in two 10-mg doses. When changing from the racemic methylphenidate preparation to the *d*-isomer preparation, the methylphenidate dose should be decreased by half.

Intermediate-Acting Methylphenidate Formulations

Sustained-Release Formulations of Methylphenidate. Methylphenidate hydrochloride sustained-release formulations are available as Ritalin SR, Methylin ER, and Metadate ER. The first sustained-release

TABLE 51-4 SUMMARY OF PRESCRIBING INFORMATION FOR CURRENTLY AVAILABLE METHYLPHENIDATE PREPARATIONS

Trade Name	Doses (mg)	Form	Initial Dose (mg)	Maximum Daily Dose (mg)	Daily Doses	Peak Effect (hr)	Duration of Effect (hr)
SHORT ACTING							
Ritalin	5, 10, 20	Tablet	5	60	2-3	1-2	2-4
Methylin	2.5, 5, 10 5 mg/5 ml, 10 mg/5 ml	Tablet and chewable tablet Liquid	5	60			
Focalin	2.5, 5, 10	Tablet	2.5	20	2-3	1-1.5	2-5
INTERMEDIATE ACTING							
Ritalin SR	20	Tablet (SR)	20	60	1	3-5	6-8
Methylin ER	10, 20	Tablet (XR)	10	60	1		
Metadate ER	10, 20	Tablet (XR)	10	60	1		
LONG ACTING							
Metadate CD	10, 20, 30, 40, 50, 60	Capsule* (XR)	20	60	1	1.5 & 4.5	8-9
Ritalin LA	10, 20, 30, 40	Capsule* (XR)	10	60	1	2 & 6.5	8-10
Concerta	18, 27, 36, 54	Tablet (XR)	18	6-12 yr: 54 13-17 yr: 72	1	6-8	10-12
Focalin XR	5, 10, 20	Capsule* (XR)	5	20	1	1.5 & 6.5	12
Daytrana	10, 15, 20, 30	Dermal patch	10	30	1	7-9	12

*Indicates form may be sprinkled.
SR, sustained release; XR, extended release.

TABLE 51-5 AVAILABLE DOSES OF METHYLPHENIDATES

Trade Name	Preparation Type	Available Doses (mg)
Ritalin	Methylphenidate HCl	5, 10, 20
Methylin	Methylphenidate HCl	2.5, 5, 10
Focalin	Dexmethylphenidate HCl	2.5, 5, 10
Ritalin SR	Sustained-release methylphenidate HCl	20
Methylin ER	Sustained-release methylphenidate HCl	10, 20
Metadate ER	Sustained-release methylphenidate HCl	10, 20
Metadate CD	Methylphenidate controlled-delivery preparation	10, 20, 30, 40, 50, 60
Ritalin LA	Extended-release methylphenidate HCl	10, 20, 30, 40
Concerta	Methylphenidate OROS	18, 27, 36, 54
Focalin XR	Extended-release dexmethylphenidate HCl	5, 10, 20
Daytrana	Methylphenidate transdermal patch	10, 15, 20, 30

methylphenidate formulation was approved by the FDA in 1984. These sustained-release methylphenidate formulations have varying durations of effect that range from 3 to 5 hours. The durations of action range between 6 and 8 hours. All three sustained-release formulations have been approved by the FDA in children older than 5 years of age. Ritalin SR is available in 20-mg tablets. Methylin ER and Metadate ER are each available in 10- and 20-mg tablets. Each of these sustained-release tablets must be swallowed whole and cannot be sprinkled, divided, crushed, or chewed.

The initial recommended dose of the sustained-release methylphenidate formulations is 10 to 20 mg once to twice daily, with dose adjustments of 10 mg weekly. The maximum daily recommended dose is 60 mg. Patients may be initiated on a short-acting methylphenidate formulation with dosing equivalently converted to a sustained-release formulation. For example, a patient receiving methylphenidate 10 mg twice daily may be alternatively given 20 mg of a sustained-release methylphenidate each morning.

Long-Acting Methylphenidate Formulations. There are five extended-release methylphenidate formulations that provide both immediate and long-acting benefits: Concerta, Metadate CD, Ritalin LA, Focalin XR, and Daytrana. Each is used as the initial treatment for ADHD or used after the initiation of treatment with shorter acting methylphenidate formulations. Extended-release methylphenidate formulations may reduce breakthrough symptoms in the middle of the day and improve adherence by eliminating a midday dose that often must be administered at school. Extended-release psychostimulants are also less subject to abuse and diversion. Metadate CD and Ritalin LA have a duration of action of about 8 hours and are designed for the treatment of ADHD symptoms during the school day. These two formulations are less likely to result in persistent loss of appetite or insomnia than Concerta or Focalin XR.

Methylphenidate OROS. Methylphenidate OROS is an extended-release methylphenidate formulation that is available as Concerta. Methylphenidate OROS was the first 12-hour extended-release methylphenidate formulation approved by the FDA and was designed to replace short-acting methylphenidate formulations that required two or three doses per day. The OROS preparation is composed of three layers. The short-acting component of the tablet begins to work in the first hour, followed by the controlled release of longer acting core layers over a period of 6 to 8 hours. The duration of action of this preparation is 10 to 12 hours. The OROS preparation is approved for use in children who are older than 5 years of age. It is available in 18-, 27-, 36-, or 54-mg tablets. These tablets must be swallowed whole and cannot be divided, crushed, or chewed.

The initial recommended dose of the OROS preparation is 18 mg in the morning. The maximum daily dose for children who are 6 to 12 years of age is 54 mg. The maximum daily dose for children who are 13 to 17 years of age is 72 mg. However, the total daily dose should not exceed 2 mg/kg per day. To convert from shorter acting methylphenidate preparations, the recommendation is to use the OROS preparation that contains slightly less of the immediate-release dose in the outer layer. For example, if the patient is currently receiving methylphenidate 10 mg twice daily, the recommended OROS preparation dose would be the 36-mg tablet, which contains 8 mg of the immediate-release form in the outer layer (Table 51-6).

TABLE 51-6 RECOMMENDED DOSE CONVERSION: METHYLPHENIDATE TO OROS PREPARATION

Original Methylphenidate Dose (Either bid or tid)	Total OROS Preparation Dose	Amount of OROS Preparation Dose Released Immediately
5 mg	18 mg	4 mg
10 mg	36 mg	8 mg
15 mg	54 mg	12 mg

Methylphenidate Controlled-Delivery Preparation. Methylphenidate "controlled delivery" is an extended-release methylphenidate formulation that is available as Metadate CD. The controlled-delivery preparation was the second extended-release methylphenidate formulation that was approved for treatment of ADHD in 2001. It is designed to replace the twice-daily dosing of short-acting methylphenidate and provide symptom control over the duration of the school day. Metadate CD contains 30% short-acting beads. The pharmacokinetic profile for this controlled-delivery preparation includes a first peak plasma level that is achieved in about 1.5 hours after administration and a second peak plasma level that is reached about 4.5 hours after taking the tablet. The duration of action is approximately 8 to 9 hours. The methylphenidate controlled-delivery preparation is approved by the FDA for use in children older than 5 years of age.

The methylphenidate controlled-release preparation is available in 10-, 20-, and 30-mg capsules. These capsules may be swallowed as whole capsules or alternatively may be administered by sprinkling the capsule contents on a small amount of food such as applesauce.

The initial recommended dose for the methylphenidate controlled-delivery preparation is 20 mg each morning, with dose adjustments of 10 to 20 mg/wk. The maximum recommended daily dose is 60 mg daily.

Methylphenidate Hydrochloride Extended Release. Methylphenidate hydrochloride extended release is available as Ritalin LA. This preparation consists of a capsule containing 50% short-acting beads and 50% extended-release beads. The methylphenidate extended-release capsule is designed to replace taking two daily doses of short-acting methylphenidate, and it has a duration of action of 8 hours. Its pharmacokinetic profile includes a first peak effect at 2 hours followed by a second peak effect at 6.5 hours. The extended-release formulation is approved for children older than 5 years of age.

The methylphenidate extended-release preparation is available in 10-, 20-, 30-, and 40-mg capsules. These capsules may be swallowed as whole capsules or alternatively may be administered by sprinkling the capsule contents on a small amount of food such as applesauce.

The initial recommended dose of the extended-release preparation is 20 mg each morning, with dose adjustments of 10 mg at weekly intervals. The maximum recommended daily dose is 60 mg. A single capsule of the extended-release preparation provides the equivalent total amount of two tablets of immediate-release methylphenidate. Consequently, a patient receiving methylphenidate 10 mg twice daily would receive a single extended-release dose of 20 mg.

Dexmethylphenidate Hydrochloride Extended Release. Dexmethylphenidate hydrochloride extended-release formulation is available as Focalin XR and contains 50% short-acting beads and 50% enteric-coated, delayed-release beads. Dexmethylphenidate hydrochloride extended release has a first peak effect at 1.5 hours and a second peak effect at 6.5 hours. The duration of action is approximately 12 hours. The dexmethylphenidate hydrochloride extended-release preparation is approved for children older than 5 years of age.

Dexmethylphenidate hydrochloride extended release is available in 5-, 10-, and 20-mg capsules. Dexmethylphenidate hydrochloride extended-release capsules may be swallowed as whole capsules or alternatively may be administered by sprinkling the capsule contents on a small amount of food such as applesauce.

The initial recommended dose of dexmethylphenidate hydrochloride extended release is 5 mg each morning, with dose adjustments of 5 mg/wk. The maximum recommended daily dose is 20 mg. Dexmethylphenidate hydrochloride extended-release capsules are designed to provide a single dose of medication that is equivalent to two doses of dexmethylphenidate hydrochloride. Dexmethylphenidate hydrochloride extended release is twice as potent as extended-release methylphenidate hydrochloride. Consequently, a patient receiving extended-release methylphenidate hydrochloride 40 mg would require only 20 mg of dexmethylphenidate hydrochloride extended release.

Methylphenidate Transdermal Patch. The methylphenidate transdermal patch is available as Daytrana and is the only psychostimulant transdermal patch that has been approved for the treatment of ADHD. The pharmacokinetic profile for this transdermal patch includes a first effect at 1.5 hours and a second peak effect at 6.5 hours. The duration

TABLE 51-7 MANAGEMENT OF COMMON PSYCHOSTIMULANT SIDE EFFECTS

Side Effect	Action
Delayed sleep onset	Lower or discontinue last dose. If using long-acting formulation, consider changing to shorter acting formulation. Consider adjunctive treatment with sedative agent at bedtime, such as clonidine.
Decreased appetite	Administer psychostimulant with meals or shortly after meals.
Weight loss	Administer psychostimulant after meals. Hold psychostimulant on weekends and vacations from school.
Rebound hyperactivity	Use longer acting preparations such as once-daily dosing formulation, or a combination of sustained release with immediate release. Change timing of medications with overlapping coverage to avoid medication troughs. Concomitant use of a nonstimulant such as clonidine.
Irritability	Rule out rebound hyperactivity. Rule out comorbid conditions. Decrease dose. Switch to longer acting formulation. Trial with a non-psychostimulant.
Slowed height growth	Hold psychostimulant on weekends and vacations from school. Trial with an alternate psychostimulant. Trial with a non-psychostimulant.
Tics	Decrease or discontinue psychostimulant. Trial with a non-psychostimulant. Attempt trial with alternate psychostimulant class. Concomitant use of psychostimulant with clonidine.

of action is approximately 12 hours. The patch is approved for children older than 5 years of age. Side effects specific to the patch include contact dermatitis at the site of the patch administration. Patients who develop a contact sensitization to transdermal methylphenidate may not be able to tolerate methylphenidate in any form. The transdermal patch is available in 10-mg (12.5 cm^2), 15-mg (18.75 cm^2), 20-mg (25 cm^2), and 30-mg (37.5 cm^2) patches that are designed to be worn for approximately 9 hours.

The initial recommended dose for the transdermal patch is 10 mg, with dose adjustments of 5 or 10 mg each week. The maximum recommended daily dose is 30 mg (see Table 51-6).

Psychostimulant Side Effects

No differences have been found in side effect profiles between the methylphenidate formulations and the amphetamines. The more common psychostimulant side effects are delayed sleep onset, loss of appetite, weight loss, and rebound hyperactivity (Table 51-7). Other side effects include irritability, slowed height growth, and tics. Side effects usually resolve when the dose is decreased. If a side effect occurs when taking one psychostimulant, the alternate class of stimulant or a non-psychostimulant medication may be used.

Delay in the onset of sleep is often managed by decreasing or discontinuing the last dose of the day. Alternatively, a change from a long-acting preparation to a shorter acting preparation may be helpful. Decrease in appetite can be managed by taking doses during or immediately after meals. If weight loss occurs, the total dose can be decreased or a drug holiday initiated.

Rebound hyperactivity includes the symptoms of irritability, motor hyperactivity, agitation, excitability, and oppositional behavior that occur at times when the medication serum level is dropping. This problem is often managed by changing to a longer acting psychostimulant formulation or by adding a small dose of short-acting medication in the afternoon.

Psychostimulant treatment has also been associated with increased aggression. If persistent aggressive behavior occurs, discontinuation of these medications may be required.

Psychostimulants may slow the growth of some children.[8,9] However, it is not clear if the use of psychostimulants is associated with a decrease in the ultimate height of patients, and one study did not demonstrate a significant negative impact on growth.[10] An increase in growth has been demonstrated during periods of psychostimulant discontinuation.[11,12] Consequently, discontinuation of psychostimulants on weekends or during summer breaks from school may result in more consistent growth, although the reoccurrence of ADHD symptoms during these periods may have a negative impact on social interactions. Yet another consideration is that children with ADHD may have a more prolonged growth trajectory than other children that is independent of their treatment.[13]

Psychostimulants may precipitate tics or exacerbate a preexisting tic disorder. If tics occur, ADHD symptoms may be treated using other medications.[14] An alternative treatment strategy is to continue to treat the patient with stimulants, but initiate concomitant treatment with an α-agonist to decrease the occurrence of tics.

The precipitation of psychotic symptoms is a relatively infrequent side effect of psychostimulants. Reported psychotic symptoms included tactile hallucinations, visual hallucinations, and delusions. Euphoria can be precipitated by psychostimulants. In patients who experience either psychotic symptoms or euphoria, psychostimulants should usually be discontinued.

An increase in cardiac symptoms has been associated with psychostimulant use. Twenty-one fatal cases have been documented. Patients with congenital cardiac conditions, including structural cardiovascular defects and cardiomyopathies, should be carefully monitored if prescribed psychostimulants.

Psychostimulants are designated by the Drug Enforcement Agency as Schedule II drugs with established abuse potential. Concern of possible abuse has risen due to the increase in production and prescribing rates of methylphenidate. Ironically, it has been suggested that early treatment with psychostimulants may actually provide protection against the development of substance abuse.[15] Furthermore, adolescents with ADHD who are treated with psychostimulants appear to have lower rates of substance use than those untreated adolescents with ADHD.[16] The use of the extended-release preparations of the psychostimulants may minimize this risk.

Nonstimulant Medications

Atomoxetine

Atomoxetine is a selective norepinephrine reuptake inhibitor (see Fig. 51-1) that was approved by the FDA in 2003 for children who are older than 5 years of age. Atomoxetine (Strattera) is available in 10-, 18-, 25-, 40-, 60-, 80-, and 100-mg capsules (Table 51-8). Atomoxetine has

TABLE 51-8 SUMMARY OF PRESCRIBING INFORMATION FOR NONSTIMULANT MEDICATIONS USED TO TREAT ADHD

Medication	Doses (mg)	Form	Initial Dose	Maximum Daily Dose (mg)	Daily Doses	Side Effects
Atomoxetine	10, 18, 25, 40, 60, 80, 100	Capsule	70 kg & under: 0.5 mg/kg/day Over 70 kg: 40 mg	70 kg & under: 1.4 mg/kg/day or 100 mg Over 70 kg: 100 mg	1-2	Decreased appetite, GI upset, sedation
Bupropion	75, 100	Tablet	75	300	1-3	Irritability, decreased appetite, insomnia; lowers seizure threshold, may exacerbate tics
Bupropion SR	100, 150, 200	Tablet	100	300	1-2	
Bupropion XL	150, 300	Tablet	150	300	1	
Clonidine	0.1, 0.2, 0.3	Tablet	0.05 qhs	0.5	1-4	Sedation, depression, dry mouth, hypotension, rebound hypertension with abrupt discontinuation
Guanfacine	1, 2	Tablet	0.5 qhs	5	1-3	

GI, gastrointestinal.

an overall effect size for the treatment of ADHD of 0.6 to 0.7[17,18] as compared to an effect size for psychostimulants that exceeds 0.8.[19] (The calculation of effect sizes allows for direct comparison of efficacy between different compounds. Values close to zero reflect small effect sizes while values closer to 1.0 are very large effect sizes.)

The initial recommended dose of atomoxetine is determined by body weight in children. For children up to 70 kg, a starting dose of 0.5 mg/kg per day is recommended, with an increase after a minimum of 3 days to a target dose of 1.2 mg/kg per day. The maximum dose is 1.4 mg/kg per day or 100 mg. For children over 70 kg and adults, a starting dose of 40 mg daily with increases after a minimum of 3 days to a target dose of 80 mg daily is recommended. A maximum dose of 100 mg a day may be utilized after 2 to 4 additional weeks in patients who have not achieved an adequate clinical response on lower doses.

The effects of atomoxetine may be seen within a few days to 1 week. However, the full benefit may not be evident for a month. Atomoxetine is typically given in the morning, but may be given at night if the patient experiences sedation.

Side effects in children include decreased appetite, gastrointestinal discomfort, and sedation. Side effects in adults include insomnia, sexual side effects, and increased blood pressure. Given that atomoxetine is a selective norepinephrine reuptake inhibitor, there is a black box warning of potential increased thoughts of suicidal ideation and suicidal behavior in children and young adults.

Atomoxetine is metabolized by the cytochrome P-450 (CYP) 2D6 enzyme. Caution should be used with concomitant use of medications that inhibit CYP2D6 as a decrease in the rate of metabolism of atomoxetine may require a decrease in the dose. Genetically determined poor metabolizers of the CYP2D6 enzyme have two inactive copies of the 2D6 gene. These poor CYP2D6 metabolizers have been found to have up to 500% higher plasma levels compared to extensive metabolizers following atomoxetine ingestion.[20] Despite reports suggesting that poor CYP2D6 metabolizers can tolerate atomoxetine at doses up to 1.8 mg/kg per day,[21] clinical 2D6 genotyping prior to prescription can be used to identify poor metabolizers and minimize side effects.

Tricyclic Antidepressants

The tricyclic antidepressants have historically been used to treat ADHD and have demonstrated efficacy and safety.[6] However, tricyclic antidepressants are no longer first-line agents for the treatment of ADHD. One factor that is associated with this change has been the sudden death of at least eight children who had been taking either desipramine or imipramine. Desipramine is primarily metabolized by the CYP2D6 enzyme, and poor metabolizers of CYP2D6 substrates are more likely to have increased serum levels. Consequently, 2D6 genotyping has been recommended before using desipramine in children.[22]

The use of tricyclics may be indicated in treating patients with ADHD and comorbid depression and tic disorders. Tricyclic antidepressant side effects include irritability, insomnia, gastrointestinal symptoms, headaches, potential withdrawal symptoms, and blood pressure changes. However, the use of tricyclic antidepressants requires serum level and electrocardiographic monitoring. Like all antidepressant medications, there is a black box warning that use in children and young adults may be associated with suicidal thoughts and behavior.

Bupropion

Bupropion is approved by the FDA for use as an antidepressant that inhibits the reuptake of dopamine, serotonin, and norepinephrine (see Fig. 51-1) and is available as Wellbutrin. While bupropion is not approved by the FDA for treatment of ADHD, it has been used for this purpose. Dosing recommendations vary depending on the formulation (immediate-, sustained-, and extended-release forms). Common side effects include irritability, decreased appetite, and insomnia. Bupropion may lower seizure threshold and exacerbate tics. Furthermore, use of bupropion may be associated with an increase in suicidal ideation and suicidal behavior.

α-Agonists

α-Agonists have been used as a second line to treat ADHD. Specifically, clonidine (Catapres) and guanfacine (Tenex) have been used as a monotherapy for children who do not tolerate psychostimulants. An α-agonist may specifically target hyperactivity, impulsivity, and aggression in children. α-Agonists have also been used concomitantly with psychostimulants to target sleeplessness and rebound hyperactivity.

Clonidine is an α-agonist with a primary clinical indication for use in the treatment of adult hypertension. Clonidine is available in 0.1-, 0.2-, and 0.3-mg tablets. Clonidine has an onset of action in 30 to 60 minutes, with duration of action of 3 to 6 hours. Initial dosing is 0.05 mg at bedtime, with dosing increase in increments of 0.05 mg to a maximum daily dose of 0.2 to 0.6 mg (0.5 mg/kg per day), which is typically given in three divided doses.

Guanfacine is a more selective α-agonist and is available in 1- and 2-mg tablets. Guanfacine does have less incidence of rebound hypertension secondary to its longer half-life. Guanfacine has an onset of action of 1 to 4 hours with duration of action of 6 to 8 hours. Initial dosing is 0.5 at bedtime, with dosing increases to 3 times daily, with a maximum daily dose of 5 mg divided into two or three doses daily.

α-Agonist side effects include sedation, depression, dry mouth, hypotension, and possible rebound hypertension with abrupt discontinuation. There have been reports of death in children who were receiving both clonidine and psychostimulants.

Pemoline

Pemoline was previously a commonly used medication for the treatment of ADHD symptoms that required a single daily dose. Pemoline is still available as Cylert. However, pemoline has been documented to cause severe hepatic failure in 15 patients, of whom 12 died or required transplantation within 4 weeks of liver failure (see *http://www.fda.*

gov/medWatch/safety/1999/cylert.htm). As a result of this hepatic toxicity, blood monitoring of liver function every 2 weeks is required when prescribing pemoline. While pemoline continues to be FDA approved, with the black box warning, for the treatment of ADHD in children less than 6 years of age, it is rarely used.

Pharmacogenomics

The ability to identify genes associated with ADHD may help in both making the diagnosis of ADHD and selecting appropriate treatment options. The primary current benefit of pharamacogenetic testing is the avoidance of toxic reactions and adverse events.[23]

ADHD is a highly heritable condition[24,25] with an estimated heritability in the range of 70% to 80%.[26] A number of candidate genes have been studied that may be involved in increasing susceptibility to developing ADHD (Box 51-4).[27] Many of these genes have been studied because they code for proteins that influence neurotransmission, and variation in these genes could modify the effects of stimulants.

Dopamine Transporter Gene (SLC6A3)

The dopamine transporter gene *SLC6A3* contains a segment that is composed of a variable number of tandem repeats located within the 3′ untranslated region.[28] There are at least 10 variations based on the number of tandem repeats in this unit. The 10-repeat allele is believed to be one of the more active common variants, and it has been reported to be associated with an increased risk for ADHD in some studies. Pooled study results suggest that there is a significant association between this variant of *SLC6A3* and ADHD.[24,27]

The association between the *SLC6A3* gene and methylphenidate response is being investigated. In some studies of white populations, patients with ADHD who have two copies of the 10-repeat dopamine transporter allele have been found to have an enhanced response to methylphenidate.[29,30] A positive study between the homozygous 10-repeat *SLC6A3* variants and methylphenidate response has also been shown in a sample of Korean children.[31] However, other studies have shown a decreased response to methylphenidate in African American children who are homozygous for the 10-repeat variant.[32] A decreased response has also been reported in Brazilian children with the homozygous 10-repeat allele.[33] More support for the 10-repeat allele being associated with a positive response to methylphenidate has recently been reported in a French Canadian population.[34] Further pharmacogenomic research is clearly needed to clarify the relationship of *SLC6A3* variation and response to psychostimulant treatment.

Dopamine D_4 Receptor Gene (DRD4)

The *DRD4* gene has been associated with differential responses to methylphenidate. An association with the 7-repeat allele of the VNTR polymorphism was associated with a greater dose requirement of methylphenidate in a predominantly African American sample.[35] A complementary finding of a better response to methylphenidate in Korean children who had the homozygous *4-repeat allele has recently been reported.[36]

Synaptosomal-Associated Protein 25 Gene (SNAP25)

The *SNAP25* gene has been associated with an increased risk of developing ADHD. Two linked single-nucleotide polymorphisms have been described, T1069C and T1065G. Pooled analyses of these variations in the SNAP gene have confirmed that there is an association with ADHD.[24] A genotype-dose interaction has suggested that the G allele is associated with a better response to psychostimulants. Patients with two copies of the T allele have been reported to have an improved psychostimulant response and less sleep disturbance than carriers of the G allele.[37]

BOX 51-4 GENES ASSOCIATED WITH ADHD

- Dopamine 4 receptor gene (*DRD4*)
- Dopamine 5 receptor gene (*DRD5*)
- Dopamine β-hydroxylase gene (*DBH*)
- Dopamine transporter gene (*DAT1*)
- Serotonin HTR1B receptor gene (*HTR1B*)
- Serotonin transporter gene (*5HTT*)
- Synaptosomal-associated protein 25 gene (*SNAP25*)

ADHD IN ADULTS

Studies have found that up to 60% of the pediatric population diagnosed with ADHD will continue to experience impairing symptoms into their third decade of life.[38] Furthermore, 4% of children with ADHD may continue to meet full criteria for ADHD into adulthood.[39] These estimates vary widely based on whether one disabling symptom continues into adulthood or whether full criteria for ADHD are met in adulthood.

The prevalence of ADHD in adults has been estimated to be 4.4%.[1] Currently, the diagnostic criteria developed for the diagnosis of ADHD in children are being used to make the diagnosis of ADHD in adults. This approach to making the diagnosis is clearly problematic.

Psychostimulants, norepinephrine reuptake inhibitors, and antidepressants have been reported to be helpful in adult ADHD. A recent literature review of pharmacologic therapies for adult ADHD identified 15 studies using psychostimulants and 27 studies using nonstimulant medications.[40] The response rate for the treatment of adult ADHD has varied from 25% to 78% in randomized control studies.[41,42] Longer acting psychostimulants have been studied in adult ADHD in two placebo-controlled trials. The first used methylphenidate OROS, which had a beneficial effect.[43] The second used extended-release mixed amphetamine salts and also reported an improvement.[44] These data suggest that adults with ADHD symptoms may benefit from treatment with psychostimulants, but this literature has a number of limitations and further research is needed.

The first medication approved specifically for use in adults with ADHD was atomoxetine. There are two randomized, placebo-controlled atomoxetine studies reporting a 56% response rate in treating adult ADHD.[45] Bupropion has also been demonstrated to reduce ADHD symptoms in adults in controlled trials, with response rates of 53% to 76%.[46,47] A double-blind, placebo-controlled study of the use of desipramine in treating adults with ADHD demonstrated a response rate of 68%, which is similar to the response rate of children with ADHD treated with desipramine.[48]

CONCLUSIONS

The use of psychostimulants has been extensively studied in children and adolescents and found to improve attentional symptoms. Many stimulant preparations are currently available. Atomoxetine, tricyclic antidepressants, buproprion, and α-agonists are alternative medications that have been successfully used to treat ADHD.

While pharmacogenomics research is advancing, there are no available clinical tests that identify children who will more consistently respond to currently available medications used to treat ADHD. More pharmacogenomics research is clearly needed but promises to greatly improve the effectiveness of treatment of ADHD.

ADHD in adults is believed to also respond to medication. However, additional research is needed to more accurately diagnose ADHD in adults. Once better diagnostic criteria become available, additional well-designed clinical trials are clearly needed to establish both efficacy and effectiveness.

REFERENCES

1. Kessler RC, Adler L, Barkley R, et al. The prevalence and correlates of adult ADHD in the United States: results from the National Comorbidity Survey Replication. Am J Psychiatry 2006;163:716-723.
2. Bradley C. The behavior of children receiving benzedrine. Am J Psychiatry 1937;94:577-585.
3. Iversen L. Speed, Ecstacy, Ritalin: The Science of Amphetamines. New York: Oxford University Press, 2006.

4. Rapoport JL, Berg CJ, Ismond DR, et al. Dextroamphetamine: its cognitive and behavioral effects in normal and hyperactive boys and normal men. Arch Gen Psychiatry 1980;37:933-943.
5. Schnackenberg RC. Caffeine as a substitute for Schedule II stimulants in hyperkinetic children. Am J Psychiatry 1973;130:796-798.
6. Spencer T, Biederman J, Wilens T, et al. Pharmacotherapy of attention-deficit hyperactivity disorder across the life cycle [Comment]. J Am Acad Child Adolesc Psychiatry 1996;35:409-432.
7. A 14-month randomized clinical trial of treatment strategies for attention-deficit/hyperactivity disorder. The MTA Cooperative Group. Multimodal Treatment Study of Children with ADHD [Comment]. Arch Gen Psychiatry 1999;56:1073-1086.
8. Greenhill L, Kollins S, Abikoff H, et al. Efficacy and safety of immediate-release methylphenidate treatment for preschoolers with ADHD. J Am Acad Child Adolesc Psychiatry 2006;45:1284-1293.
9. Charach A, Figueroa M, Chen S, et al. Stimulant treatment over 5 years: effects on growth. J Am Acad Child Adolesc Psychiatry 2006;45:415-421.
10. Biederman J, Faraone SV, Monuteaux MC, et al. Growth deficits and attention-deficit/hyperactivity disorder revisited: impact of gender, development, and treatment. Pediatrics 2003;111(5 Pt 1):1010-1016.
11. Safer DJ, Allen RP, Barr E. Growth rebound after termination of stimulant drugs. J Pediatr 1975;86:113-116.
12. Klein RG, Landa B, Mattes JA, et al. Methylphenidate and growth in hyperactive children: a controlled withdrawal study. Arch Gen Psychiatry 1988;45:1121-1130.
13. Spencer T, Biederman J, Wilens T. Growth deficits in children with attention deficit hyperactivity disorder. Pediatrics 1998;102(2 Pt 3):501-506.
14. Law SF, Schachar RJ. Do typical clinical doses of methylphenidate cause tics in children treated for attention-deficit hyperactivity disorder? J Am Acad Child Adolescent Psychiatry 1999;38:944-951.
15. Biederman J. Pharmacotherapy for attention-deficit/hyperactivity disorder (ADHD) decreases the risk for substance abuse: findings from a longitudinal follow-up of youths with and without ADHD. J Clin Psychiatry 2003;64(Suppl 11):3-8.
16. Wilens TE, Biederman J, Millstein RB, et al. Risk for substance use disorders in youths with child- and adolescent-onset bipolar disorder. J Am Acad Child Adolesc Psychiatry 1999;38:680-685.
17. Michelson D, Faries D, Wernicke J, et al. Atomoxetine in the treatment of children and adolescents with attention-deficit/hyperactivity disorder: a randomized, placebo-controlled, dose-response study. Pediatrics 2001;108:E83.
18. Michelson D, Allen A, Busner J, et al. Once-daily atomoxetine treatment for children and adolescents with attention deficit hyperactivity disorder: a randomized, placebo-controlled study. Am J Psychiatry 2002;159:1896-1901.
19. Spencer T, Biederman J, Wilens T. Pharmacotherapy of attention deficit hyperactivity disorder. Child Adolesc Psychiatr Clin N Am 2000;9:77-97.
20. Farid NA, Bergstrom RF, Ziege EA, et al. Single-dose and steady-state pharmacokinetics of tomoxetine in normal subjects. J Clin Pharmacol 1985;25:296-301.
21. Michelson D, Read HA, Ruff DD, et al. CYP2D6 and clinical response to atomoxetine in children and adolescents with ADHD. J Am Acad Child Adolesc Psychiatry 2007;46:242-251.
22. Bhagia J, Westergren M, Mrazek D. Tricyclic antidepressant fatality in children: consideration of 2D6 genotype. *In* Finding R (ed): Proceedings of the 51st Annual Meeting of the American Academy of Child & Adolescent Psychiatry. Washington, DC: American Academy of Child & Adolescent Psychiatry, 2004, p 150.
23. Sallee FR, DeVane CL, Ferrell RE. Fluoxetine-related death in a child with cytochrome P-450 2D6 genetic deficiency. J Child Adolesc Psychopharmacol 2000;10:27-34.
24. Faraone SV, Perlis RH, Doyle AE, et al. Molecular genetics of attention-deficit/hyperactivity disorder. Biol Psychiatry 2005;57:1313-1323.
25. McGough JJ, Smalley SL, McCracken JT, et al. Psychiatric comorbidity in adult attention deficit hyperactivity disorder: findings from multiplex families. Am J Psychiatry 2005;162:1621-1627.
26. Faraone SV, Doyle AE. The nature and heritability of attention-deficit/hyperactivity disorder. Child Adolesc Psychiatr Clin N Am 2001;10:299-316.
27. Faraone SV, Khan SA. Candidate gene studies of attention-deficit/hyperactivity disorder. J Clin Psychiatry 2006;67(Suppl 8):13-20.
28. Sano A, Kondoh K, Kakimoto Y, et al. A 40-nucleotide repeat polymorphism in the human dopamine transporter gene. Hum Genet 1993;91:405-406.
29. Kirley A, Lowe N, Hawi Z, et al. Association of the 480 bp dat1 allele with methylphenidate response in a sample of Irish children with ADHD. Am J Med Genet Part B Neuropsychiatr Genet 2003;121B:50-54.
30. Stein MA, Waldman ID, Sarampote CS, et al. Dopamine transporter genotype and methylphenidate dose response in children with ADHD. Neuropsychopharmacology 2005;30:1374-1382.
31. Cheon KA, Ryu YH, Kim JW, et al. The homozygosity for 10-repeat allele at dopamine transporter gene and dopamine transporter density in Korean children with attention deficit hyperactivity disorder: relating to treatment response to methylphenidate. Eur Neuropsychopharmacol 2005;15:95-101.
32. Winsberg BG, Comings DE. Association of the dopamine transporter gene (*DAT1*) with poor methylphenidate response [Comment]. J Am Acad Child Adolesc Psychiatry 1999;38:1474-1477.
33. Roman T, Szobot C, Martins S, et al. Dopamine transporter gene and response to methylphenidate in attention-deficit/hyperactivity disorder. Pharmacogenetics 2002;12:497-499.
34. Joober R, Grizenko N, Sengupta S, et al. Dopamine transporter 3′-UTR VNTR genotype and ADHD: a pharmaco-behavioural genetic study with methylphenidate. Neuropsychopharmacology 2007;32:1370-1376.
35. Hammarman S, Fossella J, Ulger C, et al. Dopamine receptor 4 (drd4) 7-repeat allele predict methylphenidate dose response in children with attention deficit hyperactivity disorder: A pharmacogenetic study. J Child Adolesc Psychopharm 2004;14:564-574.
36. Cheon K-A, Kim B-N, Cho S-C. Association of 4-repeat allele of the dopamine D4 receptor gene exon III polymorphism and response to methylphenidate treatment in Korean ADHD children. Neuropsychopharmacology 2007;32:1377-1383.
37. McGough J, McCracken J, Swanson J, et al. Pharmacogenetics of methylphenidate response in preschoolers with ADHD. J Am Acad Child Adolesc Psychiatry 2006;45:1314-1322.
38. Weiss G, Hechtman L, Milroy T, et al. Psychiatric status of hyperactives as adults: a controlled prospective 15-year follow-up of 63 hyperactive children. J Am Acad Child Psychiatry 1985;24:211-220.
39. Mannuzza S, Klein RG, Bessler A, et al. Adult psychiatric status of hyperactive boys grown up. Am J Psychiatry 1998;155:493-498.
40. Wilens TE. Drug therapy for adults with attention-deficit hyperactivity disorder. Drugs 2003;63:2395-2411.
41. Mattes JA, Boswell L, Oliver H. Methylphenidate effects on symptoms of attention deficit disorder in adults. Arch Gen Psychiatry 1984;41:1059-1063.
42. Spencer T, Biederman J, Wilens T, et al. A large, double-blind, randomized clinical trial of methylphenidate in the treatment of adults with attention-deficit/hyperactivity disorder. Biol Psychiatry 2005;57:456-463.
43. Biederman J, Spencer TJ, Wilens TE, et al. Treatment of ADHD with stimulant medications: Response to Nissen perspective in the *New England Journal of Medicine*. J Am Acad Child Adolesc Psychiatry 2006;45:1147-1150.
44. Weisler RH, Biederman J, Spencer TJ, et al. Mixed amphetamine salts extended-release in the treatment of adult ADHD: a randomized, controlled trial. CNS Spectrums 2006;11:625-639.
45. Michelson D, Adler L, Spencer T, et al. Atomoxetine in adults with ADHD: two randomized, placebo-controlled studies. Biol Psychiatry 2003;53:112-120.
46. Wilens TE, Spencer TJ, Biederman J, et al. A controlled clinical trial of bupropion for attention deficit hyperactivity disorder in adults. Am J Psychiatry 2001;158:282-288.
47. Wilens TE, Haight BR, Horrigan JP, et al. Bupropion XL in adults with attention-deficit/hyperactivity disorder: a randomized, placebo-controlled study. Biol Psychiatry 2005;57:793-801.
48. Wilens T, Biederman J, Jefferson P, et al. Six-week, double-blind, placebo-controlled study of desipramine for adult attention deficit hyperactivity disorder. Am J Psychiatry 1996;153:1147-1153.

52

ANXIETY

Chi-Un Pae and Ashwin A. Patkar

INTRODUCTION 769
PATHOPHYSIOLOGY 769
Basic Neurocircuit of Anxiety 769
Neurobiologic Findings of Specific Anxiety Disorders 769
Panic Disorder 769
Generalized Anxiety Disorder 770
Obsessive-Compulsive Disorder 770
Posttraumatic Stress Disorder 770
Social Anxiety Disorder 771
Diagnostic Classification of Anxiety Disorders 771
Clinical Features of Anxiety Disorders 772
THERAPEUTICS AND CLINICAL PHARMACOLOGY 772
Goals of Therapy 772
General Guidelines for Pharmacotherapy 772
Therapeutics for Individual Anxiety Disorders 772
Treatment of Panic Disorder 772
Treatment of Generalized Anxiety Disorder 775
Treatment of Obsessive-Compulsive Disorder 776
Treatment of Posttraumatic Stress Disorder 777
Treatment of Social Anxiety Disorder 778
Role of Behavioral Interventions in Anxiety Disorders 780
Panic Disorder 780
Generalized Anxiety Disorder 780
Obsessive-Compulsive Disorder 780
Posttraumatic Stress Disorder 780
Social Anxiety Disorder 780
SUMMARY AND CONCLUSIONS 780

"A crust eaten in peace is better than a banquet partaken in anxiety."

Aesop

INTRODUCTION

Anxiety is a state of fear or a subjective feeling of apprehension, foreboding, or dread that may be experienced with or without specific causes. It is often accompanied by other psychological symptoms such as insomnia and by several somatic symptoms such as tremulousness, excessive sweating, and palpitation that are associated with hyperarousal of the autonomic nervous system.[1] Animal models have implicated the reticular activating system, the amygdala and its connections with the hippocampus, and the medial frontal cortex as the principal neurocircuits underlying the pathophysiology of anxiety.[2,3]

Serotonergic and noradrenergic neurons are the primary neurotransmitter systems that modulate anxiety by reciprocal interaction with other neuronal pathways in the central nervous system.[2-7] Other possible biologic mechanisms include disturbances of γ-aminobutyric acid (GABA),[8,9] disruption of corticosteroids,[10-12] alteration in neuropeptides,[13] and genetic susceptibilities.[14,15] The environmental influences mediating anxiety include stress, personality, and coping styles.[16,17]

Therefore, a better understanding of neural mechanisms related to anxiety disorders may lead to the development of more specific treatment agents for anxiety disorders.

PATHOPHYSIOLOGY

Basic Neurocircuit of Anxiety

The amygdala plays a critical role in anxiety by linking external stimuli to defense responses (Fig. 52-1). It registers the emotional significance of the stimuli and also plays a role in the development of emotional memories.[18-22] The lateral nucleus of the amygdala receives sensory information from the thalamus and cortex[23] and consolidates the development of conditioned emotional memories.[23] The output pathway nuclei of the amygdala, in particular the central nucleus, receives convergent information from multiple amygdala regions and coordinates behavioral responses that reflects a final summation of neural activities.[20,22,24,25] The amygdala gives multiple projections to specific nuclei in the hypothalamus, midbrain, medulla, and other brain regions that eventually account for the clinical manifestations as anxiety.[22,24-26]

The amygdala, hippocampus, and prefrontal cortex comprise the pivotal neurocircuit for the development of anxiety.[20,21,24,26-29] Overall, the common pathway for the pathophysiology in anxiety disorders is exaggerated output through the central nucleus of the amygdala to different regions of the brain.[24,30] For example, in panic disorder (PD), the core fear is impending death; in social anxiety disorder (SAD), it is imminent embarrassment; in posttraumatic stress disorder (PTSD), it is the emotional memory of trauma or threatened events; in obsessive-compulsive disorder (OCD), it is intrusive obsessive ideas; and in generalized anxiety disorder (GAD), it is free-floating anxiety.[24]

Neurobiologic Findings of Specific Anxiety Disorders

Panic Disorder

Most symptoms of panic attacks reflect somatic discomforts from autonomic arousal. Norepinephrine has long been the main neurotransmitter implicated in the pathophysiology of PD. Provocation studies with yohimbine (an α_2-adrenoreceptor antagonist) have found increases of norepinephrine in the locus ceruleus.[31,32] Other findings have supported alterations in the function or sensitivity of the α_2-adrenoreceptor and β-adrenoreceptor in PD.[33,34]

Disturbances in the serotonin (5-hydroxytryptamine [5-HT]) system also appear to contribute to PD. Pharmacologic manipulations of the 5-HT system employing fenfluramine, tryptophan depletion, and *meta*-chlorophenylpiperazine (mCPP) have implicated alteration in 5-HT receptor activity in the PD.[35] For example, provocation tests with fenfluramine showed greater increases in anxiety, plasma prolactin, and cortisol in PD subjects compared with controls.[36] Studies have also found a significant decrease in serotonin transporter (5-HTT) binding in the midbrain, temporal lobes, and thalamus in patients with PD compared to controls.[37] The sensitivity of PD patients to the panicogenic effects of agents such as cholecystokinin (CCK)-4, flumazenil, and carbon dioxide (CO_2) has been reported to be reduced by selective serotonin reuptake inhibitors (SSRIs).[35] SSRIs may exert their thera-

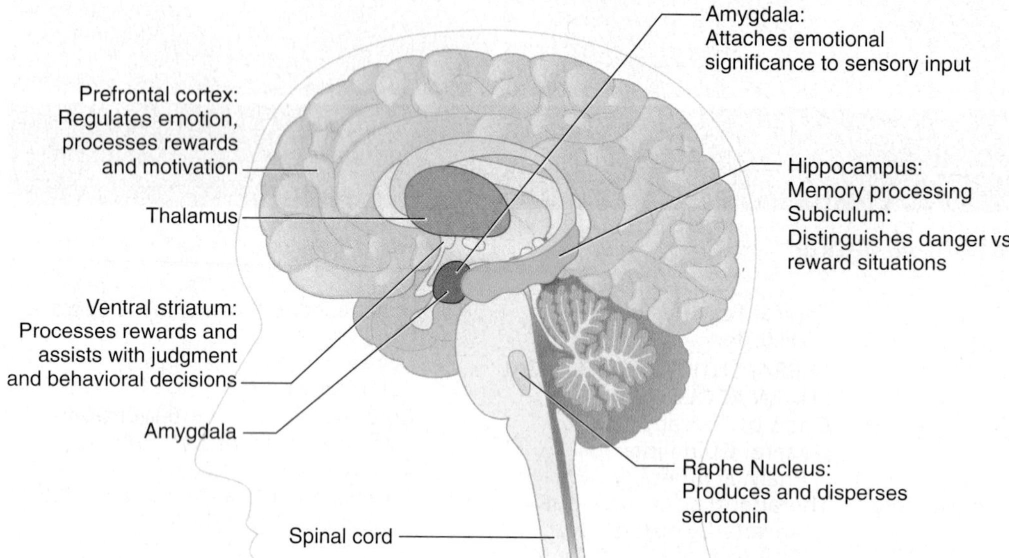

FIGURE 52-1 • **The bipolar brain.**

peutic effects in PD by increasing the synaptic availability of 5-HT,[38] which is supported by subsequent studies showing that tryptophan depletion reversed the antipanic effect of chronic SSRIs treatment in PD patients.[39]

A considerable body of evidence suggests that activation of the hypothalamic-pituitary-adrenal (HPA) axis leading to an increased release of corticotropin-releasing hormone,[40] adrenocorticotropic hormone,[41] and cortisol[42] may mediate the development of PD. Reductions in GABA and CCK have also been documented in PD subjects, but the evidence is still sparse. There is no consistent evidence that enhanced dopamine release in the prefrontal cortex following anxiogenic challenge directly mediates anxiety-like behavioral responses.[43-47]

It has been suggested that patients with PD have CO_2 hypersensitivity, which can be caused by a deranged suffocation alarm monitor. This finding substantiates the false suffocation alarm theory proposed for PD, and it is physiologically specific for PD.[48]

Genetic variability may have a distinctive influence on PD. The lifetime prevalence of panic was 10.7% among relatives of panic probands compared to 1.4% among relatives of controls, yielding a relative risk of 6.8.[49] Accumulating evidence also suggest that vulnerability to panic attacks and PD may be related to several genes such as those for 5-HTT (*5HTTLPR*),[50] the 5-HTR_{2A} receptor, the dopamine D1 receptor, and CCK[51] (Fig. 52-2).

Generalized Anxiety Disorder

Compared to the data in PD, the findings are less consistent regarding the role of norepinephrine in GAD. Increases, decreases, or no changes in levels of plasma 3-methoxy-4-hydroxyphenylglycol (MHPG),[52] no alteration of resting plasma norepinephrine levels,[53] a blunted growth hormone (GH) response to clonidine,[54] and normal responses to yohimbine[52] have all been reported in GAD patients.

A considerable amount of attention has been currently focused on the role of 5-HT in GAD. Findings include reduced cerebrospinal fluid (CSF) 5-HT levels, exaggerated response to mCPP,[55] and decreased [^{3}H]paroxetine binding.[56]

There is increasing evidence to show that the GABA system is involved in GAD (Fig. 52-3). Studies have shown a consistent decrease in peripheral benzodiazepine receptors (pBZrs)[57] and increased density of pBZrs.[58] The $GABA_A$ receptor complex has also been suggested to be implicated in the pathogenesis of GAD, with the development of new anxiolytics based on its neurobiologic role.[59] Many neurosteroids function as positive or negative allosteric modulators at the $GABA_A$ receptor complex; however, there is no direct evidence of neurosteroid involvement in the development of GAD.[59]

Obsessive-Compulsive Disorder

A functional abnormality in the circuitry of the basal-thalamic-orbitofrontal-cortical circuit has been consistently implicated in the pathophysiology of OCD. Increased "resting" cerebral blood flow and glucose metabolism in the orbital cortex, putamen, thalamus, and caudate nucleus has been replicated in OCD patients.[36]

The most prevalent hypothesis for OCD is that an aberration in the 5-HT system, in particular the 5-HT_{1D} receptor, may contribute to the pathophysiologic process of OCD. A number of studies demonstrated that sumatriptan (5-HT_{1D} agonist) and mCPP (5-HT_{1A}, 5-HT_{1B}, and 5-HT_{1D} agonist; 5-HT_3 partial agonist) can provoke or worsen OCD symptoms. 6-Chloro-2-(1-piperazinyl)pyrazine (MK-212; a 5-HT_{1A}, 5-HT_{1B}, and 5-HT_{2C} agonist) and ipsapirone (5-HT_{1A} agonist) were not associated with OCD, which support a primary role of the 5-HT_{1D} receptor and a partial role of the 5-HT_{2C} receptor.[60] Decreased [^{3}H]paroxetine and serotonin reuptake sites in platelets have been also reported in OCD patients. A family-based association study complemented the 5-HT_{1D} receptor hypothesis by showing that the 5-HT_{1D} receptor gene is transmitted to patients with OCD.[61] Other family-based association studies supported the possible contribution of the "*l*" allele of *5HTTLPR* to the development of OCD.[62] Recent linkage studies have shown that chromosomes 3q27-28, 6q, 7p, 1q, and 15q may be possible loci containing candidate genes for OCD.[63]

To date, several neurobiologic studies have suggested that dopamine or noradrenergic neurons are less likely to play a critical role in the development of OCD.[64] However, indirect evidence such as potential benefits from atypical antipsychotic augmentation and an alteration of the $dopamine_2$ receptor and dopamine transporter densities in neuroimaging studies indicate that further investigation of the dopamine system may be necessary.[60]

Posttraumatic Stress Disorder

Considerable evidence indicates that noradrenergic, serotonergic, and GABA function is abnormal in PTSD patients. Norepinephrine disturbances include increased heart and blood pressure rates, and increased levels of plasma MHPG after a yohimbine challenge and increased sensitivity of platelet α_2-adrenoreceptors.[36] In addition, elevated urinary levels of epinephrine and norepinephrine have been found in PTSD patients compared to the controls.[65] Geracioti and colleagues reported that CSF norepinephrine concentrations were significantly higher in the PTSD patients than in the controls and were positively correlated with the severity of PTSD symptoms.[66]

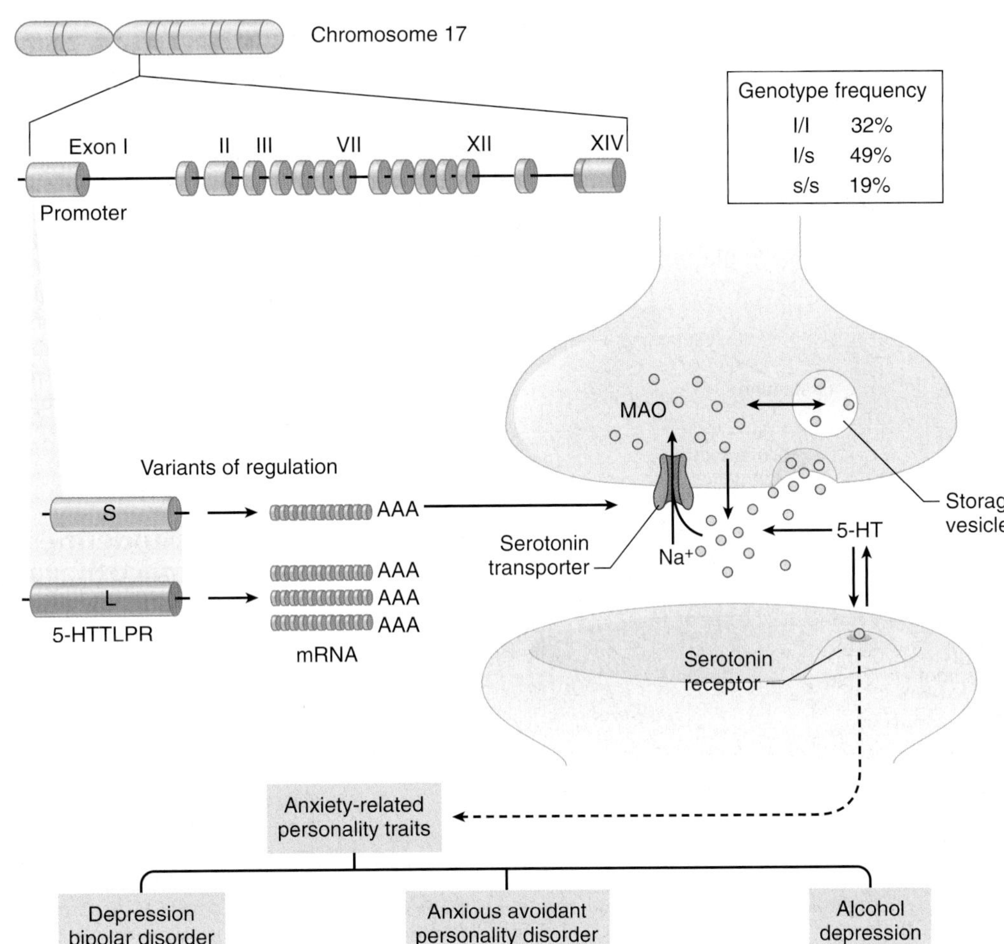

FIGURE 52-2 • Allelic variation of serotonin transporter function in anxiety-related disorders. LPR, linked polymorphic region; MAO, monoamine oxidase.

Evidence also supports the involvement of the 5-HT system in PTSD. Decreased [^{3}H]paroxetine and 5-HT reuptake site in platelets have been reported in PTSD patients. In addition, mCPP challenges have aggravated the core symptoms of PTSD.[67]

Reduction of pBZrs in PTSD patients suggests the possible involvement of the GABA system in PTSD. Increased glucocorticoid receptors, elevated corticotropin releasing factor in the CSF, and hypersuppression with the dexamethasone suppression test have also been reported, pointing to an alteration of the HPA axis in PTSD. There is some evidence of opioid peptide and thyroid function abnormalities in PTSD as well.[1,36]

Social Anxiety Disorder

Neuroanatomic areas implicated in SAD include the amygdala, prefrontal cortex, hippocampus, and striatum. Increased neural activity in the left postcentral gyrus and the lenticulate, right inferior frontal, and middle temporal gyri have been reported in SAD patients.[68]

Since autonomic hyperarousal (manifested by flushing, tachycardia, and tremulousness) is a common symptom of SAD patients, understanding autonomic nervous system function in these patients might shed light on the dysfunctional circuitry involved in SAD.[69] Patients with SAD appear to produce higher levels of norepinephrine in response to postural changes than those with PD.[70] Increased plasma concentration of MHPG has been found, and yohimbine aggravates the social anxiety symptoms in SAD patients.[71] A reduced GH response to clonidine (α_2-adrenergic agonist) has been also reported in SAD patients.[72]

Serotonergic pathways may also play a major role in SAD, as shown by the clinical effectiveness of SSRIs and other related findings. Platelet 5HT$_2$ receptor density was positively correlated with symptom severity in SAD patients. An augmented cortisol response to fenfluramine[73] and increased anxiety responses to mCPP[74] in SAD patients have been also reported compared to controls.

Low striatal dopamine$_2$ receptor binding or low dopamine transporter density in SAD patients has been reported, although there is a paucity of consistent data concerning the involvement of dopaminergic system alteration in SAD.[75] A hyperactivation of the HPA axis in response to psychological stress has been observed.[76]

Several challenge tests with lactate, caffeine, or flumazenil have been used to reproduce phobic anxiety, and show that patients with SAD carry less sensitivity to these substances than those with PD, and are more sensitive to CO$_2$ than patients with PD.[77]

Molecular genetic studies have identified candidate genes for the several neurotransmitter systems implicated in SAD, for example, 5-HT$_{2A}$T102C polymorphism[78] and *5HTTLPR*.[79] Moreover, reduction in SAD symptoms during SSRI treatment was significantly associated with the *5HTTLPR* genotype.[80]

Diagnostic Classification of Anxiety Disorders

Anxiety disorders represent a group of syndromes with a symptom cluster of excessive worrying, intense fears, hypervigilance, or multiple somatic symptoms, in the absence of a real threatening situation, that is associated with socio-occupational impairment. The *Diagnostic and Statistical Manual of Mental Disorders, Fourth Edition* provides a phenomenologic classification of anxiety disorders with specific symptomatology[1] (Table 52-1). Early and accurate diagnosis is the cornerstone of optimal treatment. A suggested diagnostic approach toward a patient with suspected anxiety disorder has been developed by the Canadian Psychiatric Association.[81]

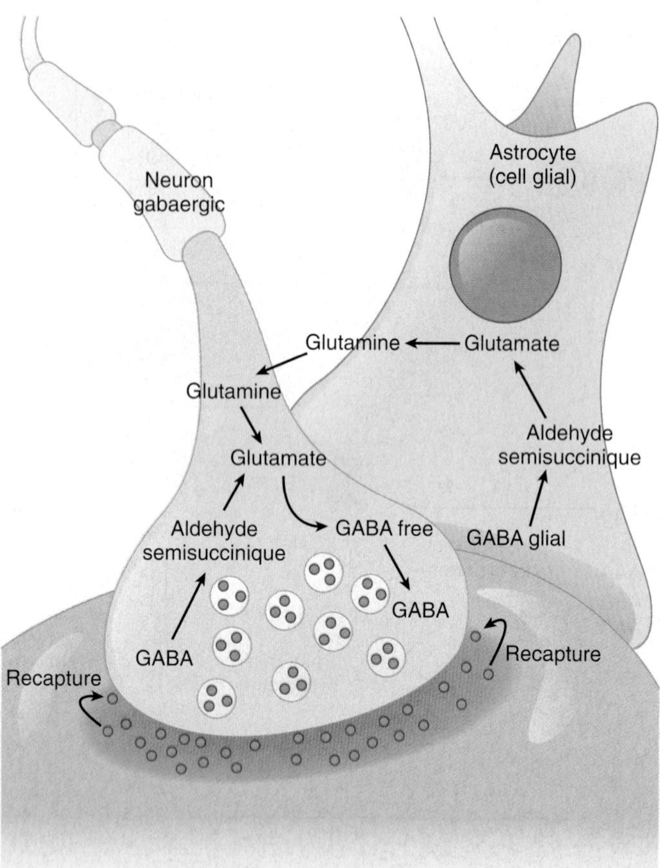

FIGURE 52-3 • GABA neuronal circuitry. There are receptors in the brain that receive the neurotransmitter γ-aminobutyric acid (GABA). When GABA is transmitted to the receptor, there is a reduction in neuronal electrical activity. Generalized anxiety disorder occurs either due to impeded GABA interactions with existing receptors or due to reduced/aberrant expression of those receptors. Without GABA signaling, neurons are disinhibited, leading to improper electrical activity, ultimately precipitating manifestation of anxiety traits.

Clinical Features of Anxiety Disorders

The lifetime prevalence of anxiety disorders is estimated to be 28.8% and 21% in the general population in the United States and Europe, respectively.[82] Data from the National Comorbidity Survey suggest that the higher ratio of 12-month to lifetime prevalence indicates that anxiety disorders are more chronic than earlier suspected.[83,84]

The most common anxiety disorder is SAD, with a lifetime prevalence 12.1%, followed by PTSD (6.8%) and GAD (5.7%).[1,84] GAD is the most common mental disorder diagnosed in the primary care setting. Among patients with major depression, 85% have symptoms of anxiety and 58% have a diagnosis of an anxiety disorder during their lifetime.[85] The common comorbid conditions of anxiety disorders include major depression, substance abuse, and another concurrent anxiety disorder. Anxiety disorders with comorbid conditions are related to more severe symptomatologies, a higher rate of suicide attempts, more hospitalizations, a less favorable response, and poor compliance with treatment.[86] Anxiety disorders have a waxing and waning course, which results in repeated remission and relapse over the patient's lifetime.[85]

Anxiety disorders are commonly related to underlying medical conditions as well, such as thyroid diseases, pheochromocytoma, or even coronary artery disease. The majority of patients with anxiety disorder (83%) present to their physician with somatic symptoms.[87-89] Studies have shown that physicians are less likely to recognize psychiatric illness, in particular anxiety disorders, if presented with physical symptoms alone.[89]

THERAPEUTICS AND CLINICAL PHARMACOLOGY

Goals of Therapy

Pharmacotherapy alone or in combination with psychotherapy is generally considered the standard for treatment of most anxiety disorders.[90] Most patients with anxiety disorders can benefit from behavioral treatment to improve functional impairment. Appropriate treatment starts with managing stressful symptoms and individualizing treatment strategies.[91] A clinically meaningful improvement in overall symptoms should be the initial target of treatment.[92] A full remission of anxiety symptoms and functional recovery should be the overall goal.[92-94] Coexisting psychiatric disorders are common in patients with anxiety disorders, and appropriate treatment for comorbid conditions should be a part of treatment.[95] Finally, successful long-term maintenance—that is, prevention of relapse and recurrence—should be a long-term strategy.[92]

General Guidelines for Pharmacotherapy

Antidepressants, benzodiazepines, and other anxiolytics are currently available for the treatment of anxiety disorders. Treatments with these agents also include combining different drug classes to augment response or switching from one class to an alternative class in case of resistance to the first-line agent.[88,89,96]

The selection of a particular drug class (and of a specific drug within that class) should be determined principally by the evidence-based data supporting its use, and also by whether the patient had previous treatment experience with that compound.[89] SSRIs are broadly effective and are generally accepted as the first-line treatment agents for most anxiety disorders.[87,88,96,97] The use of other drugs such as tricyclic antidepressants (TCAs), monoamine oxidase inhibitors (MAOIs), buspirone, antipsychotics, β-blockers, and anticonvulsants needs to be considered in the context of the supportive evidence for specific conditions and their individual risks and benefits.

Patients with anxiety disorders are particularly sensitive to medication side effects, so a gradual titration of dosage and tapering of medication is desirable when antidepressants are selected as the first-line agents.[88,96,98] Concomitant use of benzodiazepines with antidepressants is often helpful to manage acute anxiety symptoms.[87,88,96] When an adequate first-line treatment has failed, a switch to a drug from a different class or augmentation with other efficacious agents should be considered.[99] It is important to confirm an accurate diagnosis prior to considering treatment failure. When initiating combination or augmentation therapy, drug-to-drug interactions should be considered, especially if MAOIs are selected.[89] An adequate trial period in the acute phase is 4 to 6 weeks. Maintenance treatment is recommended for at least 6 to 12 months.[87-89,96,98] A mounting body of evidence suggests that most anxiety disorders have a chronic course, low rates of remission, and high rates of relapse, which indicates the need for frequent clinical evaluation.[88,100] For example, in the case of PD, controlled studies have indicated that the relapse rate with 12-month treatment was 3% to 13%.[96,101]

Therapeutics for Individual Anxiety Disorders

Treatment of Panic Disorder

A summary of evidence-based recommended pharmacologic agents for PD is presented in Table 52-2.

SSRIs. Several SSRIs (e.g., paroxetine, fluoxetine, sertraline) have been approved for the treatment of PD by the U.S. Food and Drug Administration (FDA).

A number of double-blind, placebo-controlled randomized clinical trials (RCTs) have demonstrated the efficacy and safety of paroxetine (Paxil) for the treatment of PD in short-term (up to 12-week) or long-

TABLE 52-1 ANXIETY DISORDERS ACCORDING TO DIAGNOSTIC AND STATISTICAL MANUAL (DSM-IV) CLASSIFICATION*

Classification	Characteristic Symptoms
Generalized Anxiety Disorder	Chronic anxiety, exaggerated worry and tension, even when there is little or nothing to provoke it; lasts at least 6 mo
Panic Disorder (with/without agoraphobia)	Unexpected and repeated episodes of panic attack accompanied by physical symptoms that may include chest pain, heart palpitations, shortness of breath, dizziness, or abdominal distress; usually lasts more than 10 min
Obsessive-Compulsive Disorder	Recurrent, unwanted thoughts (obsessions) and/or repetitive behaviors (compulsions)
Posttraumatic Stress Disorder	Exposure to a variety of traumatic incidents; reexperience, avoidance, and increased arousal; usually begins within 3 mo of the incident
Social Phobia	Experience of fear, apprehension, or worry regarding social situations and being evaluated by others
Agoraphobia (with/without panic attack)	Severe and pervasive anxiety about being in situations from which escape might be difficult or avoidance of situations such as being alone outside of the home; traveling in a car, bus, or airplane; or being in a crowded area
Substance-Induced Anxiety Disorder	Persistent anxiety symptoms, including panic attacks, originating from a substance
Specific Phobia	Fear caused by a specific object or situation
Adjustment Disorder	Development of emotional or behavioral symptoms in response to an identifiable stressor(s) occurring within 3 mo of the onset of the stressor(s)
Acute Stress Disorder	Exposure to a traumatic event or distressing events: subjective sense of numbing, detachment, or absence of emotional responsiveness; reduction in awareness of surroundings; derealization; depersonalization; dissociative amnesia
Anxiety Disorder due to General Medical Condition	Persistent anxiety symptoms, including panic attacks, originating from a general medical condition
Anxiety Disorder Not Otherwise Specified	Prominent anxiety or phobic avoidance that does not meet criteria for any specific anxiety disorder, adjustment disorder with anxiety, or adjustment disorder with mixed anxiety and depressed mood

*All *Diagnostic and Statistical Manual of Mental Disorders, Fourth Edition* (DSM-IV) anxiety disorder diagnoses include a criterion of severity. The anxiety must be severe enough to interfere significantly with the patient's occupational or educational functioning, social activities or close relationships, and other customary activities.
Adapted from American Psychiatric Association. Diagnostic and Statistical Manual of Mental Disorders, Fourth Edition. Washington, DC: American Psychiatric Press, 1994.

term (36-week) treatment periods.[99,102-105] A controlled-release (CR) formulation of paroxetine has also proven to be efficacious for the treatment of PD in a recent large multicenter RCT (mean dose 50 mg/day in completers).[106] Paroxetine has a side effect profile comparable to other SSRIs, but the potential for discontinuation syndrome, sexual dysfunction, and weight gain appears to be slightly higher.[107-110] Paroxetine has been currently categorized as an FDA Pregnancy Category D drug for its use in pregnancy. The effective dose is 40 mg/day.[99,104,111] The dose of paroxetine should be started at 10 mg/day, with dose increases in 10-mg/day increments at intervals of at least 1 week up to 60 mg/day. The initial dose of paroxetine CR should be 12.5 mg/day; dose changes should occur in 12.5-mg/day increments and at intervals of at least 1 week. The maximum dosage should not exceed 75 mg/day.

The efficacy and safety of fluoxetine (Prozac) and weekly fluoxetine have been demonstrated for the treatment of PD in short-term and long-term RCTs (12 to 24 weeks).[101,112,113] The common side effects include nausea and insomnia; a relatively low incidence of discontinuation symptoms have been reported due to its long half-life.[112,113] Treatment should be initiated with 10 mg/day, with a dose increase after 1 week based on tolerability. The target dose should be 20 mg/day. A further dose increase may be considered after several weeks if no clinical improvement is observed. Fluoxetine doses above 60 mg/day have not been systematically evaluated in PD patients.

Both short-term (10-12 weeks) and long-term (28-week) RCTs have shown that sertraline (Zoloft) is efficacious and safe for the treatment of PD.[114-118] No efficacy differences were found for the fixed-dose studies comparing 50, 100, and 200 mg/day of sertraline.[116,117] Common side effects include ejaculation failure, dry mouth, and dizziness.[116,117] Treatment should be initiated with a dose of 25 mg/day. Titration should be in 50-mg/day increment at intervals of at least 1 week. Patients not responding to a 50-mg/day dose may benefit from dose increases up to a maximum of 200 mg/day.

Several RCTs of fluvoxamine (Luvox) have been conducted yielding mixed results.[119-122] A dose of 100 to 300 mg/day may be effective for the treatment of PD.[87,88] The long-term efficacy of fluvoxaime for the treatment in PD has not been systemically established.

Citalopram (Celexa) has no indication for treatment of anxiety disorders, although some RCTs showed superior efficacy for citalopram (10 to 60 mg/day) compared to placebo and similar efficacy compared to TCAs in short-term and long-term studies.[123,124] The effective dose of citalopram for PD is 20 to 30 mg/day.[125] Common side effects in the studies were nausea, insomnia, and dizziness. Escitalopram (Lexapro) also has been studied for the treatment of PD and showed modest efficacy compared to placebo.[126] Escitalopram has not been approved for treatment of PD in the United States, but has an approval in Europe. The long-term efficacy of escitalopram for the treatment of PD has not been systemically investigated.

Newer Antidepressants. Venlafaxine (Effexor) has not been FDA approved for treatment of anxiety disorders. In one 8-week RCT, venlafaxine demonstrated superior efficacy compared to placebo (mean dose 150 mg/day).[127] Recently, several adequately powered, 10-week RCTs provided evidence that venlafaxine extended release (XR) (75 to 225 mg/day) has efficacy in the treatment of PD,[128] and the drug has been approved for PD. In short-term comparative studies with paroxetine and placebo, it was as efficacious as paroxetine and superior to placebo at a dose of 225 mg/day.[111,129,130] The long-term efficacy of venlafaxine XR has not yet been proven. Common side effects were similar to those of SSRIs, but dose-related hypertension has been reported, in particular at the upper end of the therapeutic dosage (225 mg/day).[88] The recommended initial dose of venlafaxine XR is 37.5 mg/day for 7 days. Dose increments should be weekly increases of 75 mg/day to a maximum dose of 225 mg/day.

Other antidepressants also show promise for the treatment of PD, but are not FDA approved for this indication. Mirtazapine (Remeron)

TABLE 52-2 SUMMARY OF EVIDENCE-BASED PHARMACOLOGIC AGENTS FOR PANIC DISORDER*

Therapeutic Agents	Starting Dose (mg/day)	Therapeutic Dose (mg/day)	STE	LTE
SSRIs				
Paroxetine†,1	10	20-50	+	+
Paroxetine CR†,1	12.5	25-75	+	+
Citalopram1	10	20-60	+	+
Escitalopram1	10	20-60	+	+
Fluoxetine†,1	10	20-60	+	+
Fluvoxamine1	50	100-300	+	–
Sertraline†,1	25	50-200	+	+
NEWER ANTIDEPRESSANTS				
Venlafaxine2	75	75-225	+	–
Venlafaxine XR†,1	75	75-225	+	–
Mirtazapine‡,2	15	15-45	+	–
TCAs				
Imipramine2	25	75-250	+	+
Clomipramine2	25	75-250	+	+
MAOIs				
Phenelzine	15	45-90	+	–
BENZODIAZEPINES				
Alprazolam†,2	0.25 or 0.5	1-10	+	+
Clonazepam†,2	0.5	1-4	+	–
Lorazepam2	0.5	2-8	+	–
Diazepam2	2-10 mg	5-20	+	–

*This table has been created based on cited references, individual drugs' prescribing information, and published treatment guidelines for anxiety disorders. Studies included proven efficacy for panic disorder in one or more randomized, double-blind, placebo-controlled study.
†Approved by the U.S. Food and Drug Administration (FDA).
‡Randomized, double-blind, comparative study only.
1First-line agent.
2Second-line agent.
CR, controlled release; LTE, long-term efficacy; MAOIs, monoamine oxidase inhibitors; SSRIs, selective serotonin reuptake inhibitors; STE, short-term efficacy; TCAs, tricyclic antidepressants; XR, extended release.

in 15- to 45-mg/day doses showed an efficacy comparable to paroxetine (24 weeks) or fluoxetine (6 weeks) in two randomized comparative studies.[131,132] To date there are insufficient data from RCTs to support the use of bupropion (Wellbutrin) and duloxetine (Cymbalta) in PD.[133]

TCAs. Before the availability of SSRIs, TCAs such as imipramine (Tofranil) and amitriptyline (Elavil) were first-line agents for PD, although they lacked FDA approval. Imipramine (100 to 225 mg/day) has consistently shown superior efficacy compared to placebo in short-term RCTs (8 to 12 weeks).[134] The imipramine dose should be titrated from 25 mg/day to a target dose of 100 mg/day, maintaining the same dose for at least 4 weeks to determine the therapeutic response (maximum dose 300 mg/day).[88] Long-term trials (3 to 12 months) have shown imipramine to be effective to prevent relapse of PD.[135-137] Long-term trials with other TCAs have been found to be equivocal.[87] Clomipramine (Anafranil) has also been found to be effective for the treatment of PD in RCTs at doses of 50 to 100 mg for 6 to 12 weeks.[134,138] Currently, TCAs are not commonly prescribed for the treatment of PD because of tolerability concerns, in particular anticholinergic and cardiac effects, cognitive disturbances, and safety concerns with overdose.[87-89]

MAOIs. There are no FDA-approved MAOIs for the treatment of PD. However, some agents such as phenelzine (Nardil) showed efficacy comparable to TCAs such as imipramine or clomipramine in short-term RCTs (8 to 10 weeks).[139]

Benzodiazepines. Alprazolam (Xanax) and clonazepam (Klonopin) have been approved by the FDA for the treatment of PD and have been the most extensively studied agents among the benzodiazepines. Alprazolam was found to be superior to placebo in the treatment of panic attacks in both short-term (8-week) and long-term (24-week) RCTs.[140,141] The effective dose range was 3 to 6 mg/day. A sustained-release formulation of alprazolam is also effective in the acute treatment of PD at doses comparable to those of standard alprazolam (mean dose 4.7 mg/day).[142] RCTs of diazepam (Valium) (5 to 20 mg/day),[143] lorazepam (Ativan) (2 to 8 mg/day),[144] and clonazepam (1 to 4 mg/day)[145] suggest efficacy similar to alprazolam or the TCAs at doses equipotent with alprazolam. Common side effects of benzodiazepines include sedation, ataxia, memory impairment, and withdrawal symptoms.[88] Alprazolam in particular has potential for abuse and physical dependence. In an RCT, 35% of the alprazolam-treated group suffered from discontinuation syndrome, compared to 0% of the placebo-treated group.[146] It is generally advised to taper benzodiazepines over a sufficiently prolonged period (at least 8 weeks), especially where high doses are employed.[146] Clinically, benzodiazepines have the advantage of rapid response, and a combination of a benzodiazepine and an antidepressant may potentiate early response compared with antidepressant monotherapy, although clinicians should be alert for possible additive side effects.

Other Agents. The use of buspirone (BuSpar), a 5-HT_{1A} receptor partial agonist, in the treatment of PD is not encouraging. Buspirone at a dose of 60 mg/day was not superior to placebo on any of the outcome measures of PD in a 8-week RCT.[147]

There are no consistent data supporting the use of anticonvulsants such as carbamazepine (Epitol, Tegretol) and valproate (Depakote) in PD.[148,149] Novel anticonvulsants such as tiagabine (Gabitril)[150] and gabapentin (Neurontin)[151] have been tested for PD in RCTs, and the results need to be replicated in subsequent independent studies.

β-Blockers have not been proposed as first-line agents for the treatment of PD. Some limited number of RCTs and open-label trials (OLTs) of β-blockers, including propranolol (Inderal) and pindolol (Visken), have been conducted with inconsistent results.[152,153]

There are no robust data supporting the efficacy of atypical antipsychotics such as olanzapine (Zyprexa)[154] and quetiapine (Seroquel),[155] clonidine (Catapres) (α_2-adrenergic agonist),[156] trazodone (Desyrel),[157] nefazodone (Serzone),[158] and inositol[159] in PD. In general, studies using these agents were small uncontrolled trials that investigated mainly the drugs' effectiveness as an augmentation therapy for PD. More data will be necessary to evaluate the efficacy of these agents.

Summary. The evidence and practice guidelines indicate that SSRIs should be considered first-line pharmacologic agents for PD. Escitalopram, citalopram, and venlafaxine XR may be switched if first-line agents fail. Benzodiazepines may be preferred as the first choice when there is a history of poor response or adverse effects with SSRIs. Benzodiazepines may be combined with SSRIs to potentiate early or partial response to SSRIs for patients not at risk for substance abuse. Other antidepressants such as venlafaxine, mirtazapine, TCAs, and MAOIs should be considered as second-line agents. The therapy should be continued for at least 6 months, and the drugs should be slowly tapered.

Treatment of Generalized Anxiety Disorder

A summary of evidence-based recommended pharmacologic agents for GAD is presented in Table 52-3.

SSRIs. Currently paroxetine and escitalopram have been approved for the treatment of GAD by the FDA. Paroxetine has been found to be efficacious and safe for the treatment of GAD in short-term (8-week)[160,161] and long-term (24- to 32-week)[108,162] RCTs. The recommended starting and target dose is 20 mg/day. There is not sufficient evidence to suggest a greater benefit to doses higher than 20 mg/day. Paroxetine CR 12.5, 25, and 37.5 mg/day has been tested for GAD with inconsistent results.[163]

The efficacy and safety of sertraline (50 to 150 mg/day) have been proven in a series of short-term RCTs (10 to 12 weeks).[164,165] There are no long-term RCT data. Sertraline (50 to 200 mg/day) was also found to be efficacious for retractable GAD in a recent 12-week RCT.[166] Finally, a small RCT suggested that sertraline at 50 mg/day may be efficacious for the treatment of GAD in children and adolescents.[167]

The efficacy of fluoxetine, citalopram, and fluvoxamine for GAD has not been established in RCTs.[168] Both short-term (8-week)[169] and long-term (24-week)[108,170] RCTs have shown escitalopram to be efficacious and safe for GAD. One long-term study found that escitalopram would be more tolerable compared to paroxetine, based on early dropout rates due to adverse events (6.6% vs. 22.6%; $P = 0.02$).[108] The effective dose of escitalopram in short-term and long-term trials was 20 mg/day. The recommended starting dose is 10 mg/day.

Newer Antidepressants. Venlafaxine has not been approved for treatment of GAD in the United States, although a recent RCT suggested that 75 mg/day of venlafaxine may be efficacious for GAD.[171] However, venlafaxine has received an indication for GAD in Europe at the dose of 75 mg/day.[171] Venlafaxine XR (75, 150, and 225 mg/day) has been approved for GAD based on the results from short-term (8-week) RCTs.[172,173] The long-term (24-week) efficacy of velafaxine XR (75, 150, and 225 mg/day) has also been established.[174] The dose-response relationship shows that 150 and 225 mg/day are more advantageous than 75 mg/day, although all three doses were efficacious for GAD.[172] Several comparative studies showed that venlafaxine XR (75 to 225 mg/day) was superior to fluoxetine (20 to 60 mg/day) in major depressive disorder patients with comorbid GAD[175] and superior to buspirone (30 mg/day) for acute treatment of GAD.[173] The recommended starting and maximum doses of venlafaxine XR are 75 mg/day and 225 mg/day, respectively. Dose increases should be in increments of up to 75 mg/day with intervals of at least 1 week.

TABLE 52-3 SUMMARY OF EVIDENCE-BASED PHARMACOLOGIC AGENTS FOR GENERALIZED ANXIETY DISORDER*

Therapeutic Agents	Starting Dose (mg/day)	Therapeutic Dose (mg/day)	STE	LTE
SSRIs				
Paroxetine[†,1]	10	20-50	+	+
Escitalopram[†,1]	10	20-60	+	+
Sertraline[1]	25	50-200	+	–
NEWER ANTIDEPRESSANTS				
Venlafaxine XR[†,1]	75	75-225	+	+
TCAs				
Imipramine[2]	25	75-200	+	–
BENZODIAZEPINES				
Alprazolam[†,2]	0.25 or 0.5	2-10	+	–
Diazepam[2]	2-10 mg	5-15	+	–
OTHER AGENTS				
Buspirone[†,2]	15	15-60	+	–
Hydroxyzine	10	37.5-75	+	–
Pregabalin[2]	150	150-600	+	–
Trifluoperazine	2	2-6	+	–
Risperidone[‡]	0.5	0.5-1.5	+	–
Olanzapine[‡]	2.5	2.5-10	+	–

*This table has been created based on cited references, individual drugs' prescribing information, and published treatment guidelines for anxiety disorders. Studies included proven efficacy for generalized anxiety disorder in one or more randomized, double-blind, placebo-controlled study.

†Approved by the U.S. Food and Drug Administration (FDA).

‡Placebo-controlled augmentation study.

1First-line agent.

2Second-line agent.

LTE, long-term efficacy; SSRIs, selective serotonin reuptake inhibitors; STE, short-term efficacy; TCAs, tricyclic antidepressants; XR, extended release.

Mirtazapine (30 mg/day) was effective for GAD in an OLT for 12 weeks. However, the efficacy and safety of mirtazapine for GAD should be supported by RCT data.[176] There is no published evidence from an RCT to support the efficacy of duloxetine, mirtazapine, or bupropion for GAD.

TCAs. In a short-term RCT, imipramine (150 mg/day) was efficacious for GAD.[177] In addition, it may be effective in reduction of benzodiazepine discontinuation symptoms among GAD patients who have been on long-term benzodiazepine use (average duration of use, 8.5 years).[178]

MAOIs. The efficacy and safety of MAOIs have not been established in treatment of GAD.

Benzodiazepines. Alprazolam (2 mg/day)[179] and diazepam (15 mg/day)[180] were superior to placebo in short-term (4-week) RCTs in GAD.

Other Agents. Buspirone (BuSpar) was efficacious for GAD in three short-term RCTs (4 to 14 weeks).[173,181,182] Buspirone was particularly useful for benzodiazepine-naive patients. In comparative studies, buspirone was equally efficacious compared to benzodiazepines but less effective than velafaxine XR.[173,181] The recommended initial dose is 15 mg/day, and the dosage may be increased by 5 mg/day with intervals of 2 to 3 days. The effective dose is 30 mg/day and could be titrated up to 60 mg/day if clinically indicated.

A small number of RCTs support the augmenting efficacy of atypical antipsychotics such as risperidone (0.5 to 1.5 mg/day, 5 weeks)[183] and olanzapine (mean dose 9.0 mg/day, 6 weeks)[184] for GAD. Trifluoperazine (Stelazine), a typical antipsychotic agent (2 to 6 mg/day, 4 weeks) has also shown superior efficacy over placebo for GAD.[185]

Two short-term (4- to 6-week) RCTs have demonstrated pregabalin (300 to 600 mg/day) to be superior to placebo and equal to lorazepam (6 mg/day), alprazolam (1.5 mg/day), and venlafaxine (75 mg/day) in treatment of GAD.[171,186] Long-term controlled trial data are not available.

Hydroxyzine (Atarax) (50 mg/day) was found to be superior to placebo in 4-week and 12-week RCTs. The most common side effect with hydroxyzine is transient sleepiness.[187,188] A 3-week RCT failed to find efficacy and safety of propranolol for GAD.[189]

Summary. Evidence indicates that paroxetine, escitalopram, sertraline, and venlafaxine XR are recommended as first-line agents for GAD. Buspirone, imipramine, and pregabalin should be considered second-line treatments due to limited data.[190] The optimal duration of treatment has not been fully established yet, but it seems reasonable to continue pharmacologic treatment for at least 6 months.

Treatment of Obsessive-Compulsive Disorder

A summary of evidence-based recommended pharmacologic agents for OCD is presented in Table 52-4.

SSRIs. Among the currently available SSRIs, paroxetine, fluoxetine, sertraline, and fluvoxamine have been approved for the treatment of OCD.

The efficacy and safety of paroxetine (40 to 60 mg/day) in OCD has been demonstrated in short-term (12-week)[191] and long-term (24-week)[192] RCTs. A dose-response relationship has been established in those studies, where paroxetine 40 to 60 mg/day was effective in OCD but paroxetine 20 mg/day failed to demonstrate benefit.[192,193] In a 12-week RCT,[191] paroxetine (20 to 60 mg/day) was as effective as clomip-

TABLE 52-4 SUMMARY OF EVIDENCE-BASED PHARMACOLOGIC AGENTS FOR OBSESSIVE-COMPULSIVE DISORDER*

Therapeutic Agents	Starting Dose (mg/day)	Therapeutic Dose (mg/day)	STE	LTE
SSRIs				
Paroxetine[†,1]	20	20-60	+	+
Fluoxetine[†,1]	20	40-80	+	+
Sertraline[†,1]	50	50-200	+	+
Fluvoxamine[†,1]	50	100-300	+	–
Citalopram[2]	20	20-60	+	–
NEWER ANTIDEPRESSANTS				
Venlafaxine XR[‡,2]	75	150-300	+	–
Mirtazapine[‡,2]	15	15-30	+	–
TCAs				
Clomipramine[†,2]	50	75-300	+	+
MAOIs				
Phenelzine[§]	15	75	+	–
BENZODIAZEPINES				
Clonazepam	0.5	5	+	–
OTHER AGENTS				
Buspirone[§]	15	60	+	–
Haloperidol[§]	1	1-3.0	+	–
Pindolol[§]	5	7.5	+	–
Quetiapine[§]	50	100-300	+	–
Risperidone[§]	0.5	0.5-3.0	+	–
Olanzapine[§]	5	5-15	+	–

*This table has been created based on cited references, individual drugs' prescribing information, and published treatment guidelines for anxiety disorders. Studies included proven efficacy for obsessive-compulsive disorder in one or more randomized, double-blind, placebo-controlled study.
[†]Approved by the U.S. Food and Drug Administration (FDA).
[‡]Randomized, double-blind comparative study.
[§]Randomized, placebo-controlled augmentation study.
[1]First-line agent.
[2]Second-line agent.
LTE, long-term efficacy; MAOIs, monoamine oxidase inhibitors; SSRIs, selective serotonin reuptake inhibitors; STE, short-term efficacy; TCAs, tricyclic antidepressants; XR, extended release.

ramine (50 to 250 mg/day) in the treatment of OCD. The efficacy of paroxetine (10 to 50 mg/day) was also evaluated in children (7 to 11 years of age) and adolescents (12 to 17 years of age) in a 10-week RCT. In these studies, paroxetine was superior to placebo and was well tolerated among younger OCD patients.[194] However, SSRIs have not been FDA approved for treatment of OCD in pediatric populations. Patients should be started on 20 mg/day, and the dose can be increased in 10-mg/day increments at intervals of at least 1 week. The maximum dosage should not exceed 60 mg/day. Paroxetine CR has not been systemically evaluated for the treatment of OCD.

A series of RCTs (20 to 60 mg/day for 13 weeks) supported the acute efficacy of fluoxetine for the treatment of OCD.[193] The long-term efficacy of fluoxetine has also been established in a 52-week RCT.[195,196] Forty milligrams per day of fluoxetine is considered an effective dose for OCD.[197] Fluoxetine (20 to 60 mg/day) was also efficacious in child and adolescent populations in a 13-week RCT.[198] A dose range of 20 to 60 mg/day is recommended; however, doses of up to 80 mg/day have been well tolerated in open studies of OCD.[196] The maximum dose should not exceed 80 mg/day. The full therapeutic effect may be delayed until 5 weeks of treatment or longer.

The efficacy and safety of fluvoxamine and fluvoxamine CR (100 to 300 mg/day) for OCD have been demonstrated in RCTs (10 to 12 weeks).[199-202] The effective dose of fluvoxamine ranged from 100 to 300 mg/day.[201] The efficacy and safety of fluvoxamine (50 to 200 mg/day, 10 weeks) was also demonstrated in children and adolescents in an RCT.[203] The recommended starting dose for fluvoxamine is 50 mg/day. The dose should be increased in 50-mg/day increments every 4 to 7 days, and the maximum dose is 300 mg/day.

Short-term (10- to 12-week)[204,205] and long-term[206] RCTs have shown sertraline (50 to 200 mg/day) to be efficacious and safe in OCD. The efficacy and safety of sertraline (50 to 200 mg/day) was also comparable to that of clomipramine (50 to 200 mg/day).[207] Sertraline should be initiated with a dose of 50 mg/day. The dose should be increased in 50-mg/day increments every week up to maximum of 200 mg/day.

The efficacy of citalopram (20, 40, and 60 mg/day) for OCD has been shown in a short-term RCT (12 weeks).[208] Another small OLT has shown intravenous citalopram (20 to 80 mg/day, 3 weeks) to be effective and safe for treatment-resistant OCD.[209] Escitalopram has no published data derived from an RCT in OCD.

Newer Antidepressants. There is a single small RCT of venlafaxine for OCD that did not demonstrate a significant benefit.[210] Double-blind, crossover (12-week)[211] or comparative (12-week)[212,213] studies have shown efficacy of venlafaxine XR (75 to 300 mg/day; 300 mg/day) similar or comparable to paroxetine (15 to 60 mg/day; 60 mg/day) or clomipramine (150 to 225 mg/day). Mirtazapine augmentation (15 to 30 mg/day) of an SSRI (citalopram, 20 to 80 mg/day) was efficacious in a small RCT.[214] Bupropion did not demonstrate efficacy in a small OLT.[215] Published data supporting the utility of bupropion and duloxetine in OCD are not available.

TCAs. Clomipramine has been the gold standard for the treatment of OCD since the early 1980s. A large number of short- and long-term RCTs have established the efficacy of clomipramine for OCD. In addition, comparative studies found clomipramine to have efficacy comparable to SSRIs in OCD.[216,217] In short-term RCTs, the effective dose of clomipramine was 200 to 300 mg/day.[218] The long-term efficacy of clomipramine for OCD (52 weeks) has also been established, but tolerability was an issue, with nearly 25% of subjects dropping out due to adverse events.[219] A small 12-week double-blind study found clomipramine to be superior to imipramine in OCD.[220] Clomipramine should be initiated at 25 mg/day and increased to 100 mg/day during the first 2 weeks. The dosage may be increased gradually over the next several weeks, in 2-week increments, up to a maximum of 300 mg/day.

MAOIs. In a double-blind comparative study (12 weeks), phenelzine (75 mg/day) was as effective as clomipramine (225 mg/day),[221] although a subsequent small 10-week RCT failed to demonstrate the efficacy of phenelzine (60 mg/day) in OCD.[222]

Benzodiazepines. Although one small RCT found clonazepam to be effective for OCD,[223] there is insufficient evidence to support the efficacy of clonazepam for OCD.[224,225]

Other Agents. Buspirone (60 mg/day) was efficacious as an augmentation therapy in the treatment of patients who failed to respond to SSRIs in a short-term RCT for OCD.[226] Pindolol augmentation (7.5 mg/day) of an SSRI has proven to be effective in treatment-resistant OCD.[227] Combination of haloperidol (3 mg/day),[228] risperidone (2.0 mg/day),[229] olanzapine (5 to 15 mg/day),[230] and quetiapine (200 to 300 mg/day)[231] with SSRIs was also efficacious for OCD. A recent meta-analysis confirmed the efficacy of augmentation of SSRIs with antipsychotics in the treatment of OCD.[232]

Summary. Paroxetine, fluoxetine, fluvoxamine, and sertraline should be considered first-line agents for both acute and longer term treatment of OCD. Lack of head-to-head comparative studies between first-line agents suggests that clinicians should choose individualized treatment agents based on the patient's previous response history and the tolerability profile of the medications. The treatment response is usually gradual and partial, and many patients (40% to 60%) fail to respond adequately to first-line treatment. Pharmacologic options for nonresponders or partial responders to first-line therapy include switching from SSRIs to clomipramine or venlafaxine XR, combining SSRIs with other antidepressants, or augmenting SSRIs with antipsychotic agents.[218]

Treatment of Posttraumatic Stress Disorder

A summary of evidence-based recommended pharmacologic agents for PTSD is presented in Table 52-5.

SSRIs. Currently two SSRIs, paroxetine and sertraline, have been approved for the treatment of PTSD by the FDA. The efficacy and safety of paroxetine (20 to 40 mg/day) has been demonstrated for core PTSD symptoms (reexperiencing, avoidance/numbness, and hyperarousal), depressive symptoms, and functional outcomes in several 12-week RCTs with a fixed-dose (20 or 40 mg/day) or a flexible-dose (20 to 50 mg/day) design.[233,234] No dose-response relationship has been observed.[233] There are no long-term RCT data on paroxetine for PTSD, although paroxetine was effective for relapse prevention at doses of 20 to 40 mg/day in an unpublished, open-label, 52-week maintenance study.[235] The recommended starting dose for paroxetine is 20 mg/day, and dose changes should occur in 10-mg/day increments at intervals of at least 1 week to reach a target dose of 20 to 40 mg/day.

Short-term (10- to 12-week), flexible-dose RCTs have shown that 50 to 200 mg/day of sertraline was efficacious and safe in PTSD.[236-238] Sertraline (50 to 200 mg/day, mean dose 137 mg/day) was also effective for relapse prevention of PTSD in a 28-week RCT.[237] The starting dose of sertraline should be 25 mg/day, and the dose increments should be 50 mg/day at at least 1-week intervals. The maximum dose of sertraline in PTSD is 200 mg/day.

Although fluoxetine has not been approved by the FDA, its efficacy and safety in PTSD have been observed in short-term (20 to 80 mg/day for 12 weeks)[239-241] and long-term (65 mg/day for 24 weeks)[240,242] RCTs.

The efficacy of fluvoxamine for PTSD has not been studied in RCTs. A small, 14-week OLT showed that fluvoxamine was effective for PTSD at mean dose of 150 mg/day.[243]

Citalopram was not associated with significant improvement in PTSD symptoms compared with placebo in an RCT,[238] although citalopram (20 to 40 mg/day) demonstrated efficacy in PTSD in small OLTs (8 weeks).[244,245] Data are not yet available on escitalopram in PTSD.

Newer Antidepressants. In a 12-week RCT,[246] venlafaxine XR (37.5 to 300 mg/day; mean dose 164.4 mg/day) demonstrated superiority to placebo and efficacy comparable to sertraline (25 to 200 mg/day, mean dose 110.2 mg/day) in PTSD. The long-term efficacy of venlafaxine XR in PTSD has not been investigated. There are no published data for venlafaxine or duloxetine in PTSD. Mirtazapine (15 to 45 mg/day) showed efficacy in PTSD in a small 8-week RCT.[247] Bupropion sustained-release (150 to 300 mg/day) failed to show efficacy in PTSD in a 12-week RCT.[248]

TCAs. Amitriptyline (mean dose 170 mg/day)[249] and imipramine (mean dose 225 mg/day)[250] demonstrated efficacy for PTSD in short-term RCTs. Desipramine (Norpramin) (mean dose 165 mg/day) failed to show efficacy for PTSD in a small 4-week RCT.[251]

TABLE 52-5 SUMMARY OF EVIDENCE-BASED PHARMACOLOGIC AGENTS FOR POSTTRAUMATIC STRESS DISORDER*

Therapeutic Agents	Starting Dose (mg/day)	Therapeutic Dose (mg/day)	STE	LTE
SSRIs				
Paroxetine[†,1]	20	20-50	+	–
Sertraline[†,1]	25	50-200	+	+
Fluoxetine[1]	20	20-80	+	+
NEWER ANTIDEPRESSANTS				
Venlafaxine XR[1]	75	100-375	+	+
Mirtazapine[2]	15	15-45	+	–
TCAs				
Imipramine[2]	75	75-200	+	–
Amitriptyline[2]	75	75-200	+	–
MAOIs				
Phenelzine[2]	15	45-90	+	–
OTHER AGENTS				
Risperidone[‡]	0.5	1-3	+	
Olanzapine[‡]	10	10-20	+	
Lamotrigine	25	25-500	+	–
Propranolol	15	40	+	–

*This table has been created based on cited references, individual drugs' prescribing information, and published treatment guidelines for anxiety disorders. Studies included proven efficacy for posttraumatic stress disorder in one or more randomized, double-blind, placebo-controlled study.
†Approved by the U.S. Food and Drug Administration (FDA).
‡Randomized, placebo-controlled augmentation study.
1First-line agent.
2Second-line agent.
LTE, long-term efficacy; MAOIs, monoamine oxidase inhibitors; SSRIs, selective serotonin reuptake inhibitors; STE, short-term efficacy; TCAs, tricyclic antidepressants; XR, extended release.

MAOIs. Two 8-week RCTs supported superior efficacy of phenelzine (mean dose 70 mg/day) over imipramine and placebo for PTSD.[250] Moclobemide, a reversible inhibitor of monoamine oxidase, was proven not to be efficacious for PTSD.[252]

Benzodiazepines. Alprazolam[253] and clonazepam[254] failed to show significant benefits over placebo for PTSD. Severe discontinuation syndrome with alprazolam, even with a gradual tapering of medication, has been reported, which limits the use of this medication for treating PTSD.[255] Benzodiazepines are not recommended as a monotherapy for PTSD patients, despite widespread use in clinical practice.[88]

Other Agents. Lamotrigine (25 to 500 mg/day, mean dose 230 mg/day) demonstrated efficacy in the treatment of PTSD in a small 12-week RCT.[256] Other anticonvulsants such as gabapentin, tiagabine, valproate, and carbamazepine, and lithium may be considered as augmentation treatment.[257-260] Risperidone (1 to 3 mg/day, 16 weeks)[261] and olanzapine (10 to 20 mg/day, 12 weeks)[262] have shown encouraging results as adjuncts with first-line agents for PTSD in short-term RCTs. A small RCT supported the efficacy of propranolol (40 mg/day) for prevention of subsequent PTSD symptoms immediately after traumatic events.[263]

Summary. Currently available data suggest that paroxetine, sertraline, fluoxetine, and venlafaxine XR should be the first-line agents in PTSD. Mirtazapine and TCAs can be considered second-line agents. An appropriate duration of trial should be at least 8 to 12 weeks. For partial or nonresponders, augmentation by lamotrigine or atypical antipsychotics may be considered. The findings of maintenance trials support the value of long-term treatment in increasing the efficacy of medication and preventing relapse.[264]

Treatment of Social Anxiety Disorder

A summary of evidence-based recommended pharmacologic agents for SAD is presented in Table 52-6.

SSRIs. Currently three SSRIs—paroxetine, paroxetine CR, and sertraline—have been approved for the treatment of SAD by the FDA. Escitalopram, fluvoxamine, and fluvoxamine CR have also shown efficacy for SAD, although they have not been FDA approved for SAD.

Paroxetine (20 to 60 mg/day) has demonstrated efficacy for SAD in a number of short-term (12-week)[265-267] and long-term (24-week)[268] RCTs. There does not appear to be any additional benefit with doses above 20 mg/day. Paroxetine CR (12.5 to 37.5 mg/day) was also found to have efficacy for SAD.[269] The mean daily dose of paroxetine CR at the end of the study was 32.3 mg/day.[269] There have been no long-term RCTs of paroxetine CR for SAD. The recommended dosage of paroxetine in SAD is 20 to 60 mg/day. Paroxetine CR should be started at 12.5 mg/day. Dose increases of paroxetine CR should occur at intervals of at least 1 week, in increments of 12.5 mg/day, up to a maximum of 37.5 mg/day.

Fluoxetine have shown mixed results for the treatment of SAD in RCTs.[270,271] However, a large 14-week RCT demonstrated efficacy of fluoxetine for SAD (10 to 60 mg/day, mean dose 43.6 mg/day). In another study, fluoxetine was as efficacious as cognitive behavioral therapy (CBT) and superior to placebo.[272] The long-term efficacy of fluoxetine has not yet been studied.

The efficacy and safety of sertraline (50 to 200 mg/day) in SAD has been established in short-term (10- to 12-week)[166,273] and long-term (20- to 24-week)[274,275] RCTs. In both short-term and long-term RCTs, the mean dose of sertraline was 150 mg/day. The starting dose of sertraline in SAD is 25 mg/day, and the dose increments should be 50 mg/day at an interval of at least 1 week. The maximum dose is 200 mg/day.

Fluvoxamine (150 mg/day) was efficacious in SAD in a short-term (12-week) RCT.[276] In another large 12-week RCT, fluvoxamine (mean dose 202 mg/day) demonstrated efficacy for SAD.[277] A large 24-week RCT also confirmed the long-term benefit of fluvoxamine CR (100 to 300 mg/day) in SAD.[278,279]

In a small short-term (6-week) RCT,[280] citalopram (40 mg/day) was shown to be efficacious for SAD. There are no published long-term treatment data for citalopram. Escitalopram (5, 10, and 20 mg/day)

TABLE 52-6 SUMMARY OF EVIDENCE-BASED PHARMACOLOGIC AGENTS FOR SOCIAL ANXIETY DISORDER*

Therapeutic Agents	Starting Dose (mg/day)	Therapeutic Dose (mg/day)	STE	LTE
SSRIs				
Paroxetine[†,1]	20	20-60	+	+
Paroxetine CR[†,1]	12.5	12.5-37.5	+	–
Sertraline[†,1]	50	50-200	+	+
Fluoxetine	10	10-60	+	–
Fluvoxamine[1]	50	100-300	+	–
Fluvoxamine CR[1]	50	100-300	+	+
Citalopram[2]	20	40	+	–
Escitalopram[1]	5	5-20	+	+
NEWER ANTIDEPRESSANTS				
Venlafaxine XR[†,1]	75	75-225	+	+
MAOIs				
Phenelzine[2]	15	45-90	+	+
RIMA				
Moclobemide[2]	300	300-600	+	+
BENZODIAZEPINES				
Clonazepam[2]	0.5	0.5-3	+	–
Alprazolam[2]	0.5	2-6.5	+	–
OTHER AGENTS				
Olanzapine	5	5-20	+	–
Pregabalin[2]	150	600	+	–
Gabapentin[2]	300	900-3600	+	–

*This table has been created based on cited references, individual drugs' prescribing information, and published treatment guidelines for anxiety disorders. Studies included proven efficacy for social anxiety disorder in one or more randomized, double-blind, placebo-controlled study.
†Approved by the U.S. Food and Drug Administration (FDA).
[1]First-line agent.
[2]Second-line agent.
CR, controlled release; LTE, long-term efficacy; MAOIs, monoamine oxidase inhibitors; RIMA, reversible inhibitor of monoamine oxidase; SSRIs, selective serotonin reuptake inhibitors; STE, short-term efficacy; XR, extended release.

demonstrated efficacy for SAD in a short-term (12-week) and long-term (24-week) RCT.[281] In a 24-week RCT, escitalopram (10 and 20 mg/day) was also effective in relapse prevention.[282]

Newer Antidepressants. There are no published RCTs of venlafaxine in SAD. In a 12-week RCT, venlafaxine XR (75 to 225 mg/day) was as efficacious as paroxetine (20 to 50 mg/day).[283,284] Two dose ranges of venlafaxine XR (75 mg/day and 150 to 225 mg/day) were tested for long-term treatment (28 weeks) and both doses were equally effective.[285] Recently, venlafaxine XR has been approved for SAD. Dose increment should be the same as with PD and GAD treatment. Although OLTs have shown promise for bupropion and mirtazapine, there are no data from RCTs to support their use in SAD. Duloxetine has no evidence to support its use in SAD.

TCAs. Although clomipramine has been proven to be effective for SAD in a large OLT,[286] there are no published RCTs of TCAs in SAD.

MAOIs. The efficacy of phenelzine (45 to 90 mg/day) in SAD has been established in short-term (8- to 16-week)[287-290] and long-term (24-week)[291] RCTs. The mean doses in these controlled trials ranged from 55 to 75.7 mg/day. Phenelzine should be started at 7.5 to 15 mg/day and increased at a minimum of 2-week intervals to reach 60 mg/day. The maximum dose is 90 mg/day. Selegiline was found to be effective in a small OLT.[292] A recently introduced novel formulation of selegiline, the selegiline transdermal system (EMSAM), does not require any dietary modifications for the 6 mg/24 hr patch that was found to be effective in major depression. It is possible that transdermal selegiline may have a role in SAD, although RCTs have not been performed.[293] The reversible MAOI moclobemide has mixed efficacy results for SAD in a number of RCTs.[289,294-296]

Benzodiazepines. Alprazolam (2.1 to 6.3 mg/day, mean dose 4.2 mg/day, 12 weeks)[288] and clonazepam (0.5 to 3 mg/day, mean dose 2.4 mg/day, 10 weeks)[297] have shown benefit for SAD in OLTs. However, there are no published RCT data for long-term efficacy of benzodiazepines.

Other Agents. Gabapentin (900 to 3600 mg/day for 14 weeks)[298] and pregabalin (150 and 600 mg/day for 10 weeks)[299] have shown positive results in RCTs for SAD. Buspirone (15 to 30 mg/day),[300] propranolol,[301] and atenolol (25 to 100 mg/day)[287,302] have failed to demonstrate significant benefit for SAD in RCTs. A small 8-week RCT has shown olanzapine monotherapy (5 to 20 mg/day, mean dose 9 mg/day) to be efficacious for SAD.[303] However, it would be preferable for olanzapine to be considered as an augmentation with first-line agents based on its tolerability issues.[303]

Summary. SSRIs should be considered first-line agents for SAD. Although several of the SSRIs have been found to be efficacious, to date paroxetine, paroxetine CR, sertraline, and venlafaxine XR have FDA approval in SAD. MAOIs such as phenelzine have substantial evidence in SAD, although safety concerns about food and drug interactions have limited their use. Long-term treatment (12 to 24 months) is necessary to optimize medication response and prevent relapse and recurrence. It is preferable to wait for at least 10 weeks before deciding that a patient is a nonresponder and switching to another agent. There are no data to support the use of benzodiazepines as monotherapy, but they may be considered as adjuncts to antidepressants for selected cases. Other agents such as gabapentin, pregabalin, and olanzapine have limited evidence to support their use as monotherapy in SAD.[304]

Role of Behavioral Interventions in Anxiety Disorders

Although pharmacologic treatment is beneficial for anxiety disorders, there is substantial evidence to demonstrate that behavioral interventions, in particular CBT, are also effective and may be comparable to medications in terms of efficacy.[89] While there are few head-to-head comparisons of pharmacologic plus behavioral treatments versus either intervention alone, it has been considered that a combination of medication and CBT may be superior to medication alone, especially for relapse prevention.[305]

The choice of pharmacologic or behavioral treatment depends on several factors. Patient motivation and preference are the most important factors. Other factors are prior treatment history, accessibility to and reimbursement for behavioral interventions, clinician's experience, and presence of comorbid medical or psychiatric disorders. Combination of medication and behavioral treatments is especially recommended for patients who do not respond fully to medications or who have recurrence of symptoms after being stable on medications.[81,89,305]

Panic Disorder

Short-term RCTs have demonstrated CBT to be efficacious in PD and equally effective as SSRIs,[306] MAOIs,[307] and TCAs.[306] A recent large meta-analysis including 124 studies also supported that CBT is as efficacious as pharmacologic treatment for PD[308] and may have more efficacy in preventing relapse (1 to 5 years) than pharmacologic treatment.[309,310] Evidence for the efficacy of CBT for medication nonresponders has been also reported.[311] It appears that CBT is as effective as pharmacologic treatment, but there is no solid evidence supporting routine combination of CBT and pharmacologic treatment in PD.

Generalized Anxiety Disorder

A number of RCTs have shown that CBT is efficacious, with comparable magnitude of efficacy, compared to pharmacologic treatment for GAD in short-term and long-term treatment periods.[312,313] However, there is little evidence to support the routine combination of CBT and pharmacologic treatment for GAD.[313]

Obsessive-Compulsive Disorder

CBT alone has clearly shown efficacy for OCD in short-term and long-term trials.[81] Several well-designed RCTs evaluated the comparative efficacy of pharmacologic treatment alone, CBT alone, or combination treatment without finding any clear evidence of the benefit of combination treatment.[200,314-316] A recent stringent meta-analysis also failed to find a clear advantage for combination of pharmacologic agents and CBT over CBT alone, which is similar to experts' recommendation that CBT alone may be the first-line treatment for OCD as well as pharmacologic treatment.[317]

Posttraumatic Stress Disorder

CBT has demonstrated short-term and long-term efficacy for PTSD in several RCTs regardless of the CBT model employed.[318] However, there is no strong evidence to conclude whether CBT is comparable to pharmacologic treatment in PTSD.[81] Current evidence shows that either CBT or pharmacologic treatment alone is efficacious for PTSD.

Social Anxiety Disorder

An increasing number of RCTs have demonstrated CBT alone to be efficacious for SAD.[319,320] Long-term CBT (1 year) may also reduce risk of relapse.[270] However, there is little evidence that combined treatment is superior to either monotherapy in patients with SAD.[270,319,320]

SUMMARY AND CONCLUSIONS

Since the introduction of distinct anxiety disorders in the *Diagnostic and Statistical Manual of Mental Disorders, Third Edition*, there has been a growing interest in these conditions, leading to a wealth of pharmacotherapy trials and several medications receiving FDA approval. SSRIs remain the drugs of choice for treatment of anxiety disorders. Within the SSRI class, some agents have more evidence to support their use in a particular subtype of anxiety disorder, and it is preferable for clinicians to utilize FDA-approved agents as drugs of first choice. There is growing evidence that some of the newer antidepressants, such as the serotonin-norepinephrine reuptake inhibitor venlafaxine, are effective in certain types of anxiety disorders. Benzodiazepines may be preferred when rapid relief of symptoms is a priority or if patients do not tolerate SSRIs, and can be used in combination with antidepressants for augmentation of response. While TCAs and MAOIs have evidence of efficacy in anxiety disorders, tolerability concerns limit their use to patients who have failed SSRIs.

Evidence-based guidelines and algorithms for the treatment of anxiety disorders have been developed on the basis of systematic reviews of the literature and expert consensus in areas where data are lacking. Pharmacotherapy algorithms have the potential advantage of being concise and evidence based. However, such algorithms run the risk of oversimplifying complex clinical realities, and are only as good as the data on which they rest. Dugan and Cohen[321] suggested that "before physicians view guidelines as precise tools to use in the construction of optimal patient care, they must be convinced that guidelines contain clear, evidence-based recommendations, and that there is a distinct advantage to them in changing practice styles to follow guidelines." Unfortunately there is a large gap between recommended pharmacologic treatment guidelines and actual delivery of care for the treatment of anxiety disorders. For example, despite the American Psychiatric Association guidelines recommending SSRIs as the first-line treatment for PD, a large longitudinal study found that treatment patterns of practitioners did not change significantly and benzodiazepines remained the most commonly used medication for PD.[322] These findings also highlight the need for increased effectiveness research to examine the factors associated with promoting and inhibiting the implementation of treatment guidelines for anxiety disorder in real-world settings. These factors may help improve and modify existing treatment guidelines and thus help minimize the gap between clinical research and actual delivery of care. Finally, anxiety disorders are often chronic and are associated with significant functional impairment and reduced quality of life.

A systematic approach to treatment of anxiety disorders should include comprehensive assessment, patient education, use of empirically proven pharmacologic treatments that may need to be combined with behavioral treatments, and appropriate monitoring and duration of treatment.

REFERENCES

1. American Psychiatric Association. Diagnostic and Statistical Manual of Mental Disorders, Fourth Edition. Washington, DC: American Psychiatric Press, 1994.
2. Balaban CD. Neural substrates linking balance control and anxiety. Physiol Behav 2002;77:469-475.
3. Perry B. Neurophysiological aspects of anxiety disorders in children. *In* Coffey CE, Brumback RA (eds): Textbook of Pediatric Neuropsychiatry. Washington, DC: American Psychiatric Press, 1998.
4. Moore RY, Bloom FE. Central catecholamine neuron systems: anatomy and physiology of the norepinephrine and epinephrine systems. Annu Rev Neurosci 1979;2:113-168.
5. Moore RY, Bloom FE. Central catecholamine neuron systems: anatomy and physiology of the dopamine systems. Annu Rev Neurosci 1978;1:129-169.
6. Shephard RA. Neurotransmitters, anxiety and benzodiazepines: a behavioral review. Neurosci Biobehav Rev 1986;10:449-461.
7. Ressler KJ, Nemeroff CB. Role of serotonergic and noradrenergic systems in the pathophysiology of depression and anxiety disorders. Depress Anxiety 2000;12(Suppl 1):2-19.
8. Roy-Byrne PP. The gaba-benzodiazepine receptor complex: structure, function, and role in anxiety. J Clin Psychiatry 2005;66(Suppl 2):14-20.
9. Nutt DJ, Malizia AL. New insights into the role of the $GABA_A$-benzodiazepine receptor in psychiatric disorder. Br J Psychiatry 2001;179:390-396.
10. De Kloet ER, Vreugdenhil E, Oitzl MS, et al. Brain corticosteroid receptor balance in health and disease. Endocr Rev 1998;19:269-301.
11. Korte SM. Corticosteroids in relation to fear, anxiety and psychopathology. Neurosci Biobehav Rev 2001;25:117-142.
12. Le Melledo JM, Baker G. Role of progesterone and other neuroactive steroids in anxiety disorders. Expert Rev Neurother 2004;4:851-860.
13. Sajdyk TJ, Fitz SD, Shekhar A. The role of neuropeptide Y in the amygdala on corticotropin-releasing factor receptor-mediated behavioral stress responses in the rat. Stress 2006;9:21-28.

14. Beidel DC, Turner SM. At risk for anxiety: I. Psychopathology in the offspring of anxious parents. J Am Acad Child Adolesc Psychiatry 1997;36:918-924.
15. Turner SM, Beidel DC, Costello A. Psychopathology in the offspring of anxiety disorders patients. J Consult Clin Psychol 1987;55:229-235.
16. Bienvenu OJ, Samuels JF, Costa PT, et al. Anxiety and depressive disorders and the five-factor model of personality: a higher- and lower-order personality trait investigation in a community sample. Depress Anxiety 2004;20:92-97.
17. Hettema JM, Neale MC, Myers JM, et al. A population-based twin study of the relationship between neuroticism and internalizing disorders. Am J Psychiatry 2006;163:857-864.
18. Linke R, Braune G, Schwegler H. Differential projection of the posterior paralaminar thalamic nuclei to the amygdaloid complex in the rat. Exp Brain Res 2000;134:520-532.
19. LeDoux JE, Cicchetti P, Xagoraris A, et al. The lateral amygdaloid nucleus: sensory interface of the amygdala in fear conditioning. J Neurosci 1990;10:1062-1069.
20. LeDoux J. The emotional brain, fear, and the amygdala. Cell Mol Neurobiol 2003;23:727-738.
21. LeDoux J. Fear and the brain: where have we been, and where are we going? Biol Psychiatry 1998;44:1229-1238.
22. Ninan PT. The functional anatomy, neurochemistry, and pharmacology of anxiety. J Clin Psychiatry 1999;60(Suppl 22):12-17.
23. Sigurdsson T, Doyère V, Cain CK, LeDoux JE. Long-term potentiation in the amygdala: a cellular mechanism of fear learning and memory. Neuropharmacology 2007;52:215-227.
24. Ninan PT, Dunlop BW. Neurobiology and etiology of panic disorder. J Clin Psychiatry 2005;66(Suppl 4):3-7.
25. Kaplan H, Sadock B. Kaplan and Sadock's Synopsis of Psychiatry: Behavioral Sciences/Clinical Psychiatry, 9th ed. Philadelphia: Lippincott Williams & Wilkins, 2002.
26. Davis M. The role of the amygdala in fear-potentiated startle: implications for animal models of anxiety. Trends Pharmacol Sci 1992;13:35-41.
27. Quirk GJ, Likhtik E, Pelletier JG, et al. Stimulation of medial prefrontal cortex decreases the responsiveness of central amygdala output neurons. J Neurosci 2003;23:8800-8807.
28. Grace AA, Rosenkranz JA. Regulation of conditioned responses of basolateral amygdala neurons. Physiol Behav 2002;77:489-493.
29. Tamminga CA. The anatomy of fear extinction. Am J Psychiatry 2006;163:961.
30. LeDoux JE, Iwata J, Cicchetti P, et al. Different projections of the central amygdaloid nucleus mediate autonomic and behavioral correlates of conditioned fear. J Neurosci 1988;8:2517-2529.
31. Redmond DE Jr, Huang YH. Current concepts. II. New evidence for a locus coeruleus-norepinephrine connection with anxiety. Life Sci 1979;25:2149-2162.
32. Bremner JD, Krystal JH, Southwick SM, et al. Noradrenergic mechanisms in stress and anxiety: I. Preclinical studies. Synapse 1996;23:28-38.
33. Stein D. The neurobiology of panic disorder: toward an integrated model. CNS Spectr 2005;9(Suppl 12):12-24.
34. Gurguis GN, Blakeley JE, Antai-Otong D, et al. Adrenergic receptor function in panic disorder. Neutrophil beta 2 receptors: G_s protein coupling, effects of imipramine treatment and relationship to treatment outcome. J Psychiatr Res 1999;33:309-322.
35. Maron E, Shlik J. Serotonin function in panic disorder: important, but why? Neuropsychopharmacology 2006;31:1-11.
36. Charney DS, Drevets WC. Neurobiological basis of anxiety disorders. *In* Neuropsychopharmacology: The Fifth Generation of Progress. Nashville, TN: American College of Neuropsychopharmacology, 2005, pp 901-930.
37. Maron E, Kuikka JT, Shlik J, et al. Reduced brain serotonin transporter binding in patients with panic disorder. Psychiatry Res 2004;132:173-181.
38. Nutt DJ, Forshall S, Bell C, et al. Mechanisms of action of selective serotonin reuptake inhibitors in the treatment of psychiatric disorders. Eur Neuropsychopharmacol 1999;9(Suppl 3):S81-S86.
39. Bell C, Forshall S, Adrover M, et al. Does 5-HT restrain panic? A tryptophan depletion study in panic disorder patients recovered on paroxetine. J Psychopharmacol 2002;16:5-14.
40. Gold PW, Pigott TA, Kling MA, et al. Basic and clinical studies with corticotropin-releasing hormone: implications for a possible role in panic disorder. Psychiatr Clin North Am 1988;11:327-334.
41. Strohle A, Holsboer F, Rupprecht R. Increased ACTH concentrations associated with cholecystokinin tetrapeptide-induced panic attacks in patients with panic disorder. Neuropsychopharmacology 2000;22:251-256.
42. Belgorodsky A, Knyazhansky L, Loewenthal U, et al. Effects of the cortisol synthesis inhibitor metyrapone on the response to carbon dioxide challenge in panic disorder. Depress Anxiety 2005;21:143-148.
43. Wall PM, Blanchard RJ, Yang M, et al. Infralimbic D2 receptor influences on anxiety-like behavior and active memory/attention in CD-1 mice. Prog Neuropsychopharmacol Biol Psychiatry 2003;27:395-410.
44. Abercrombie ED, Keefe KA, DiFrischia DS, et al. Differential effect of stress on in vivo dopamine release in striatum, nucleus accumbens, and medial frontal cortex. J Neurochem 1989;52:1655-1658.
45. Goddard AW, Mason GF, Almai A, et al. Reductions in occipital cortex GABA levels in panic disorder detected with ^{1}H-magnetic resonance spectroscopy. Arch Gen Psychiatry 2001;58:556-561.
46. Goddard AW, Mason GF, Appel M, et al. Impaired GABA neuronal response to acute benzodiazepine administration in panic disorder. Am J Psychiatry 2004;161:2186-2193.
47. Koszycki D, Torres S, Swain JE, et al. Central cholecystokinin activity in irritable bowel syndrome, panic disorder, and healthy controls. Psychosom Med 2005;67:590-595.
48. Klein DF. False suffocation alarms, spontaneous panics, and related conditions: an integrative hypothesis. Arch Gen Psychiatry 1993;50:306-317.
49. Gorwood P, Feingold J, Ades J. Genetic epidemiology and psychiatry: scope and limitations of familial studies. Case of panic disorder. Encephale 1999;25:21-29.
50. Maron E, Lang A, Tasa G, et al. Associations between serotonin-related gene polymorphisms and panic disorder. Int J Neuropsychopharmacol 2005;8:261-266.
51. Maron E, Nikopensius T, Koks S, et al. Association study of 90 candidate gene polymorphisms in panic disorder. Psychiatr Genet 2005;15:17-24.
52. Charney DS, Woods SW, Heninger GR. Noradrenergic function in generalized anxiety disorder: effects of yohimbine in healthy subjects and patients with generalized anxiety disorder. Psychiatry Res 1989;27:173-182.
53. Gerra G, Zaimovic A, Zambelli U, et al. Neuroendocrine responses to psychological stress in adolescents with anxiety disorder. Neuropsychobiology 2000;42:82-92.
54. Abelson JL, Glitz D, Cameron OG, et al. Blunted growth hormone response to clonidine in patients with generalized anxiety disorder. Arch Gen Psychiatry 1991;48:157-162.
55. Goddard AW, Woods SW, Money R, et al. Effects of the CCK_B antagonist CI-988 on responses to mCPP in generalized anxiety disorder. Psychiatry Res 1999;85:225-240.
56. Iny LJ, Pecknold J, Suranyi-Cadotte BE, et al. Studies of a neurochemical link between depression, anxiety, and stress from [^{3}H]imipramine and [^{3}H]paroxetine binding on human platelets. Biol Psychiatry 1994;36:281-291.
57. Rocca P, Beoni AM, Eva C, et al. Peripheral benzodiazepine receptor messenger RNA is decreased in lymphocytes of generalized anxiety disorder patients. Biol Psychiatry 1998;43:767-773.
58. Chiu S, Singh AN, Chiu P, et al. Inverse agonist binding of peripheral benzodiazepine receptors in anxiety disorder. Eur Arch Psychiatry Clin Neurosci 2001;251:136-140.
59. Strous RD, Maayan R, Weizman A. The relevance of neurosteroids to clinical psychiatry: from the laboratory to the bedside. Eur Neuropsychopharmacology 2006;16:155-169.
60. Zohar J, Kennedy JL, Hollander E, et al. Serotonin-1D hypothesis of obsessive-compulsive disorder: an update. J Clin Psychiatry 2004;65(Suppl 14):18-21.
61. Mundo E, Richter MA, Zai G, et al. 5HT1D beta receptor gene implicated in the pathogenesis of obsessive-compulsive disorder: further evidence from a family-based association study. Mol Psychiatry 2002;7:805-809.
62. McDougle CJ, Epperson CN, Price LH, et al. Evidence for linkage disequilibrium between serotonin transporter protein gene (SLC6A4) and obsessive compulsive disorder. Mol Psychiatry 1998;3:270-273.
63. Shugart YY, Samuels J, Willour VL, et al. Genome wide linkage scan for obsessive-compulsive disorder: evidence for susceptibility loci on chromosomes 3q, 7p, 1q, 15q, and 6q. Mol Psychiatry 2006;11:763-770.
64. Azzam A, Mathews CA. Meta-analysis of the association between the catecholamine-O-methyl-transferase gene and obsessive-compulsive disorder. Am J Med Genet B Neuropsychiatr Genet 2003;123:64-69.
65. Hawk LW, Dougall AL, Ursano RJ, et al. Urinary catecholamines and cortisol in recent-onset posttraumatic stress disorder after motor vehicle accidents. Psychosom Med 2000;62:423-434.
66. Geracioti TD Jr, Baker DG, Ekhator NN, et al. CSF norepinephrine concentrations in posttraumatic stress disorder. Am J Psychiatry 2001;158:1227-1230.
67. Southwick SM, Krystal JH, Bremner JD, et al. Noradrenergic and serotonergic function in posttraumatic stress disorder. Arch Gen Psychiatry 1997;54:749-758.
68. Kilts CD, Kelsey JE, Knight B, et al. The neural correlates of social anxiety disorder and response to pharmacotherapy. Neuropsychopharmacology 2006;31:2243-2253.
69. Mathew SJ, Coplan JD, Gorman JM. Neurobiological mechanisms of social anxiety disorder. Am J Psychiatry 2001;158:1558-1567.
70. Stein MB, Tancer ME, Uhde TW. Heart rate and plasma norepinephrine responsivity to orthostatic challenge in anxiety disorders: comparison of patients with panic disorder and social phobia and normal control subjects. Arch Gen Psychiatry 1992;49:311-317.
71. Potts NL, Book S, Davidson JR. The neurobiology of social phobia. Int Clin Psychopharmacol 1996;11(Suppl 3):43-48.
72. Tancer ME, Stein MB, Uhde TW. Growth hormone response to intravenous clonidine in social phobia: comparison to patients with panic disorder and healthy volunteers. Biol Psychiatry 1993;34:591-595.
73. Tancer ME, Mailman RB, Stein MB, et al. Neuroendocrine responsivity to monoaminergic system probes in generalized social phobia. Anxiety 1994;1:216-223.
74. Hollander E, Kwon J, Weiller F, et al. Serotonergic function in social phobia: comparison to normal control and obsessive-compulsive disorder subjects. Psychiatry Res 1998;79:213-217.
75. Tiihonen J, Kuikka J, Bergstrom K, et al. Dopamine reuptake site densities in patients with social phobia. Am J Psychiatry 1997;154:239-242.
76. Condren RM, O'Neill A, Ryan MC, et al. HPA axis response to a psychological stressor in generalised social phobia. Psychoneuroendocrinology 2002;27:693-703.
77. Coupland NJ. Social phobia: etiology, neurobiology, and treatment. J Clin Psychiatry 2001;62(Suppl 1):25-35.
78. Lochner C, Hemmings S, Seedat S, et al. Genetics and personality traits in patients with social anxiety disorder: a case-control study in South Africa. Eur Neuropsychopharmacol 2007;17:321-327.
79. Grabe HJ, Lange M, Wolff B, et al. Mental and physical distress is modulated by a polymorphism in the 5-HT transporter gene interacting with social stressors and chronic disease burden. Mol Psychiatry 2005;10:220-224.
80. Stein MB, Seedat S, Gelernter J. Serotonin transporter gene promoter polymorphism predicts SSRI response in generalized social anxiety disorder. Psychopharmacology (Berl) 2006;187:68-72.
81. Canadian Psychiatric Association. Clinical practice guidelines: management of anxiety disorders. Can J Psychiatry 2006;51:9S-91S.

82. Wittchen HU, Jacobi F. Size and burden of mental disorders in Europe—a critical review and appraisal of 27 studies. Eur Neuropsychopharmacol 2005;15:357-376.
83. Kessler RC, McGonagle KA, Zhao S, et al. Lifetime and 12-month prevalence of DSM-III-R psychiatric disorders in the United States: results from the National Comorbidity Survey. Arch Gen Psychiatry 1994;51:8-19.
84. Kessler RC, Berglund P, Demler O, et al. Lifetime prevalence and age-of-onset distributions of DSM-IV disorders in the National Comorbidity Survey replication. Arch Gen Psychiatry 2005;62:593-602.
85. Mulsant BH, Reynolds CF 3rd, Shear MK, et al. Comorbid anxiety disorders in late-life depression. Anxiety 1996;2:242-247.
86. Lecrubier Y. The impact of comorbidity on the treatment of panic disorder. J Clin Psychiatry 1998;59(Suppl 8):11-14; discussion 15-16.
87. Royal Australian and New Zealand College of Psychiatrists Clinical Practice Guidelines Team for Panic Disorder and Agoraphobia. Australian and New Zealand clinical practice guidelines for the treatment of panic disorder and agoraphobia. Aust N Z J Psychiatry 2003;37:641-656.
88. American Psychiatric Association. Practice Guidelines for the Treatment of Psychiatric Disorders: Compendium 2006. Washington, DC: American Psychiatric Press, 2006.
89. Baldwin DS, Anderson IM, Nutt DJ, et al. Evidence-based guidelines for the pharmacological treatment of anxiety disorders: recommendations from the British Association for Psychopharmacology. J Psychopharmacol 2005;19:567-596.
90. Devane CL, Chiao E, Franklin M, et al. Anxiety disorders in the 21st century: status, challenges, opportunities, and comorbidity with depression. Am J Manag Care 2005;11:S344-S353.
91. Roy-Byrne PP, Wagner A. Primary care perspectives on generalized anxiety disorder. J Clin Psychiatry 2004;65(Suppl 13):20-26.
92. Goodman WK. Selecting pharmacotherapy for generalized anxiety disorder. J Clin Psychiatry 2004;65(Suppl 13):8-13.
93. Ballenger JC. Treatment of anxiety disorders to remission. J Clin Psychiatry 2001;62(Suppl 12):5-9.
94. Doyle AC, Pollack MH. Establishment of remission criteria for anxiety disorders. J Clin Psychiatry 2003;64(Suppl 15):40-45.
95. Kessler RC, Chiu WT, Demler O, et al. Prevalence, severity, and comorbidity of 12-month DSM-IV disorders in the National Comorbidity Survey replication. Arch Gen Psychiatry 2005;62:617-627.
96. Bandelow B, Zohar J, Hollander E, et al. World Federation of Societies of Biological Psychiatry (WFSBP) guidelines for the pharmacological treatment of anxiety, obsessive-compulsive and posttraumatic stress disorders. World J Biol Psychiatry 2002;3:171-199.
97. Mitte K, Noack P, Steil R, et al. A meta-analytic review of the efficacy of drug treatment in generalized anxiety disorder. J Clin Psychopharmacol 2005;25:141-150.
98. Ballenger JC, Davidson JR, Lecrubier Y, et al. Consensus statement on panic disorder from the International Consensus Group on Depression and Anxiety. J Clin Psychiatry 1998;59:47-54.
99. Ballenger JC, Wheadon DE, Steiner M, et al. Double-blind, fixed-dose, placebo-controlled study of paroxetine in the treatment of panic disorder. Am J Psychiatry 1998;155:36-42.
100. Bruce SE, Yonkers KA, Otto MW, et al. Influence of psychiatric comorbidity on recovery and recurrence in generalized anxiety disorder, social phobia, and panic disorder: a 12-year prospective study. Am J Psychiatry 2005;162:1179-1187.
101. Michelson D, Pollack M, Lydiard RB, et al. Continuing treatment of panic disorder after acute response: randomised, placebo-controlled trial with fluoxetine. The Fluoxetine Panic Disorder Study Group. Br J Psychiatry 1999;174:213-218.
102. Pollack MH, Doyle AC. Treatment of panic disorder: focus on paroxetine. Psychopharmacol Bull 2003;37(Suppl 1):53-63.
103. Oehrberg S, Christiansen PE, Behnke K, et al. Paroxetine in the treatment of panic disorder: a randomised, double-blind, placebo-controlled study. Br J Psychiatry 1995;167:374-379.
104. Lecrubier Y, Bakker A, Dunbar G, et al. A comparison of paroxetine, clomipramine and placebo in the treatment of panic disorder. Collaborative Paroxetine Panic Study Investigators. Acta Psychiatr Scand 1997;95:145-152.
105. Lecrubier Y, Judge R. Long-term evaluation of paroxetine, clomipramine and placebo in panic disorder. Collaborative Paroxetine Panic Study Investigators. Acta Psychiatr Scand 1997;95:153-160.
106. Sheehan DV, Burnham DB, Iyengar MK, et al. Efficacy and tolerability of controlled-release paroxetine in the treatment of panic disorder. J Clin Psychiatry 2005;66:34-40.
107. Bogetto F, Bellino S, Revello RB, et al. Discontinuation syndrome in dysthymic patients treated with selective serotonin reuptake inhibitors: a clinical investigation. CNS Drugs 2002;16:273-283.
108. Bielski RJ, Bose A, Chang CC. A double-blind comparison of escitalopram and paroxetine in the long-term treatment of generalized anxiety disorder. Ann Clin Psychiatry 2005;17:65-69.
109. Fava M, Judge R, Hoog SL, et al. Fluoxetine versus sertraline and paroxetine in major depressive disorder: changes in weight with long-term treatment. J Clin Psychiatry 2000;61:863-867.
110. Pae CU, Patkar AA. Paroxetine: current status in psychiatry. Expert Rev Neurother 2007;7:107-120.
111. Pollack MH, Lepola U, Koponen H, et al. A double-blind study of the efficacy of venlafaxine extended-release, paroxetine, and placebo in the treatment of panic disorder. Depress Anxiety 2006;24:1-14.
112. Michelson D, Lydiard RB, Pollack MH, et al. Outcome assessment and clinical improvement in panic disorder: evidence from a randomized controlled trial of fluoxetine and placebo. The Fluoxetine Panic Disorder Study Group. Am J Psychiatry 1998;155:1570-1577.
113. Michelson D, Allgulander C, Dantendorfer K, et al. Efficacy of usual antidepressant dosing regimens of fluoxetine in panic disorder: randomised, placebo-controlled trial. Br J Psychiatry 2001;179:514-518.
114. Bandelow B, Behnke K, Lenoir S, et al. Sertraline versus paroxetine in the treatment of panic disorder: an acute, double-blind noninferiority comparison. J Clin Psychiatry 2004;65:405-413.
115. Pohl RB, Wolkow RM, Clary CM. Sertraline in the treatment of panic disorder: a double-blind multicenter trial. Am J Psychiatry 1998;155:1189-1195.
116. Pollack MH, Otto MW, Worthington JJ, et al. Sertraline in the treatment of panic disorder: a flexible-dose multicenter trial. Arch Gen Psychiatry 1998;55:1010-1016.
117. Londborg PD, Wolkow R, Smith WT, et al. Sertraline in the treatment of panic disorder: a multi-site, double-blind, placebo-controlled, fixed-dose investigation. Br J Psychiatry 1998;173:54-60.
118. Rapaport MH, Wolkow R, Rubin A, et al. Sertraline treatment of panic disorder: results of a long-term study. Acta Psychiatr Scand 2001;104:289-298.
119. Bakish D, Hooper CL, Filteau MJ, et al. A double-blind placebo-controlled trial comparing fluvoxamine and imipramine in the treatment of panic disorder with or without agoraphobia. Psychopharmacol Bull 1996;32:135-141.
120. Asnis GM, Hameedi FA, Goddard AW, et al. Fluvoxamine in the treatment of panic disorder: a multi-center, double-blind, placebo-controlled study in outpatients. Psychiatry Res 2001;103:1-14.
121. Sandmann J, Lorch B, Bandelow B, et al. Fluvoxamine or placebo in the treatment of panic disorder and relationship to blood concentrations of fluvoxamine. Pharmacopsychiatry 1998;31:117-121.
122. Nair NP, Bakish D, Saxena B, et al. Comparison of fluvoxamine, imipramine, and placebo in the treatment of outpatients with panic disorder. Anxiety 1996;2:192-198.
123. Leinonen E, Lepola U, Koponen H, et al. Citalopram controls phobic symptoms in patients with panic disorder: randomized controlled trial. J Psychiatry Neurosci 2000;25:24-32.
124. Lepola UM, Wade AG, Leinonen EV, et al. A controlled, prospective, 1-year trial of citalopram in the treatment of panic disorder. J Clin Psychiatry 1998;59:528-534.
125. Perna G, Bertani A, Caldirola D, et al. A comparison of citalopram and paroxetine in the treatment of panic disorder: a randomized, single-blind study. Pharmacopsychiatry 2001;34:85-90.
126. Stahl SM, Gergel I, Li D. Escitalopram in the treatment of panic disorder: a randomized, double-blind, placebo-controlled trial. J Clin Psychiatry 2003;64:1322-1327.
127. Pollack MH, Worthington JJ 3rd, Otto MW, et al. Venlafaxine for panic disorder: results from a double-blind, placebo-controlled study. Psychopharmacol Bull 1996;32:667-670.
128. Bradwejn J, Ahokas A, Stein DJ, et al. Venlafaxine extended-release capsules in panic disorder: flexible-dose, double-blind, placebo-controlled study. Br J Psychiatry 2005;187:352-359.
129. Pollack M, Emilien G, Tzanis E, Whitaker T. Venlafaxine XR and paroxetine in the short-term treatment of panic disorder. Presented at the meeting of the World Federation for the Societies of Biological Psychiatry, Sydney, Australia, 2004.
130. Pollack M, Mangano R, Entsuah R, Tzanis E. Short-term treatment of panic disorder: venlafaxine XR vs paroxetine or placebo. Presented at the 158th Annual Meeting of the American Psychiatric Association, Atlanta, 2005.
131. Wade A, Crawford GM, Angus M, et al. A randomized, double-blind, 24-week study comparing the efficacy and tolerability of mirtazapine and paroxetine in depressed patients in primary care. Int Clin Psychopharmacol 2003;18:133-141.
132. Hong CJ, Hu WH, Chen CC, et al. A double-blind, randomized, group-comparative study of the tolerability and efficacy of 6 weeks' treatment with mirtazapine or fluoxetine in depressed Chinese patients. J Clin Psychiatry 2003;64:921-926.
133. Crippa JA, Zuardi AW. Duloxetine in the treatment of panic disorder. Int J Neuropsychopharmacol 2006;9:633-634.
134. Modigh K, Westberg P, Eriksson E. Superiority of clomipramine over imipramine in the treatment of panic disorder: a placebo-controlled trial. J Clin Psychopharmacol 1992;12:251-261.
135. Mavissakalian MR, Perel JM. Long-term maintenance and discontinuation of imipramine therapy in panic disorder with agoraphobia. Arch Gen Psychiatry 1999;56:821-827.
136. Barlow DH, Gorman JM, Shear MK, et al. Cognitive-behavioral therapy, imipramine, or their combination for panic disorder: a randomized controlled trial. JAMA 2000;283:2529-2536.
137. Mavissakalian M, Perel JM. Protective effects of imipramine maintenance treatment in panic disorder with agoraphobia. Am J Psychiatry 1992;149:1053-1057.
138. McTavish D, Benfield P. Clomipramine: an overview of its pharmacological properties and a review of its therapeutic use in obsessive compulsive disorder and panic disorder. Drugs 1990;39:136-153.
139. Sheehan DV, Ballenger J, Jacobsen G. Treatment of endogenous anxiety with phobic, hysterical, and hypochondriacal symptoms. Arch Gen Psychiatry 1980;37:51-59.
140. Schweizer E, Rickels K, Weiss S, et al. Maintenance drug treatment of panic disorder. I. Results of a prospective, placebo-controlled comparison of alprazolam and imipramine. Arch Gen Psychiatry 1993;50:51-60.
141. Ballenger JC, Burrows GD, DuPont RL Jr, et al. Alprazolam in panic disorder and agoraphobia: results from a multicenter trial. I. Efficacy in short-term treatment. Arch Gen Psychiatry 1988;45:413-422.
142. Schweizer E, Patterson W, Rickels K, et al. Double-blind, placebo-controlled study of a once-a-day, sustained-release preparation of alprazolam for the treatment of panic disorder. Am J Psychiatry 1993;150:1210-1215.
143. Noyes R Jr, Burrows GD, Reich JH, et al. Diazepam versus alprazolam for the treatment of panic disorder. J Clin Psychiatry 1996;57:349-355.
144. Schweizer E, Pohl R, Balon R, et al. Lorazepam vs. alprazolam in the treatment of panic disorder. Pharmacopsychiatry 1990;23:90-93.

145. Beauclair L, Fontaine R, Annable L, et al. Clonazepam in the treatment of panic disorder: a double-blind, placebo-controlled trial investigating the correlation between clonazepam concentrations in plasma and clinical response. J Clin Psychopharmacol 1994;14:111-118.
146. Pecknold JC, Swinson RP, Kuch K, et al. Alprazolam in panic disorder and agoraphobia: results from a multicenter trial. III. Discontinuation effects. Arch Gen Psychiatry 1988;45:429-436.
147. Sheehan DV, Raj AB, Harnett-Sheehan K, et al. The relative efficacy of high-dose buspirone and alprazolam in the treatment of panic disorder: a double-blind placebo-controlled study. Acta Psychiatr Scand 1993;88:1-11.
148. Baetz M, Bowen RC. Efficacy of divalproex sodium in patients with panic disorder and mood instability who have not responded to conventional therapy. Can J Psychiatry 1998;43:73-77.
149. Uhde TW, Stein MB, Post RM. Lack of efficacy of carbamazepine in the treatment of panic disorder. Am J Psychiatry 1988;145:1104-1109.
150. Schwartz TL. The use of tiagabine augmentation for treatment-resistant anxiety disorders: a case series. Psychopharmacol Bull 2002;36:53-57.
151. Pande AC, Pollack MH, Crockatt J, et al. Placebo-controlled study of gabapentin treatment of panic disorder. J Clin Psychopharmacol 2000;20:467-471.
152. Noyes R Jr, Anderson DJ, Clancy J, et al. Diazepam and propranolol in panic disorder and agoraphobia. Arch Gen Psychiatry 1984;41:287-292.
153. Hirschmann S, Dannon PN, Iancu I, et al. Pindolol augmentation in patients with treatment-resistant panic disorder: a double-blind, placebo-controlled trial. J Clin Psychopharmacol 2000;20:556-559.
154. Sepede G, De Berardis D, Gambi F, et al. Olanzapine augmentation in treatment-resistant panic disorder: a 12-week, fixed-dose, open-label trial. J Clin Psychopharmacol 2006;26:45-49.
155. Takahashi H, Sugita T, Yoshida K, et al. Effect of quetiapine in the treatment of panic attacks in patients with schizophrenia: 3 case reports. J Neuropsychiatry Clin Neurosci 2004;16:113-115.
156. Coplan JD, Liebowitz MR, Gorman JM, et al. Noradrenergic function in panic disorder: effects of intravenous clonidine pretreatment on lactate induced panic. Biol Psychiatry 1992;31:135-146.
157. Mavissakalian M, Perel J, Bowler K, et al. Trazodone in the treatment of panic disorder and agoraphobia with panic attacks. Am J Psychiatry 1987;144:785-787.
158. Papp LA, Coplan JD, Martinez JM, et al. Efficacy of open-label nefazodone treatment in patients with panic disorder. J Clin Psychopharmacol 2000;20:544-546.
159. Palatnik A, Frolov K, Fux M, et al. Double-blind, controlled, crossover trial of inositol versus fluvoxamine for the treatment of panic disorder. J Clin Psychopharmacol 2001;21:335-339.
160. Rickels K, Zaninelli R, McCafferty J, et al. Paroxetine treatment of generalized anxiety disorder: a double-blind, placebo-controlled study. Am J Psychiatry 2003;160:749-756.
161. Pollack MH, Zaninelli R, Goddard A, et al. Paroxetine in the treatment of generalized anxiety disorder: results of a placebo-controlled, flexible-dosage trial. J Clin Psychiatry 2001;62:350-357.
162. Stocchi F, Nordera G, Jokinen RH, et al. Efficacy and tolerability of paroxetine for the long-term treatment of generalized anxiety disorder. J Clin Psychiatry 2003;64:250-258.
163. GlaxoSmithKline. Study ID 29060/791: a randomized, double-blind, placebo-controlled, flexible dosage trial to evaluate the efficacy and tolerability of paroxetine CR in patients with generalized anxiety disorder (GAD). Obtained from GSK Clinical Trial Register Website.
164. Allgulander C, Dahl AA, Austin C, et al. Efficacy of sertraline in a 12-week trial for generalized anxiety disorder. Am J Psychiatry 2004;161:1642-1649.
165. Brawman-Mintzer O, Knapp RG, Rynn M, et al. Sertraline treatment for generalized anxiety disorder: a randomized, double-blind, placebo-controlled study. J Clin Psychiatry 2006;67:874-881.
166. Liebowitz MR, DeMartinis NA, Weihs K, et al. Efficacy of sertraline in severe generalized social anxiety disorder: results of a double-blind, placebo-controlled study. J Clin Psychiatry 2003;64:785-792.
167. Rynn MA, Siqueland L, Rickels K. Placebo-controlled trial of sertraline in the treatment of children with generalized anxiety disorder. Am J Psychiatry 2001;158:2008-2014.
168. The Research Unit on Pediatric Psychopharmacology Anxiety Study Group. Fluvoxamine for the treatment of anxiety disorders in children and adolescents. N Engl J Med 2001;344:1279-1285.
169. Goodman WK, Bose A, Wang Q. Treatment of generalized anxiety disorder with escitalopram: pooled results from double-blind, placebo-controlled trials. J Affect Disord 2005;87:161-167.
170. Davidson JR, Bose A, Wang Q. Safety and efficacy of escitalopram in the long-term treatment of generalized anxiety disorder. J Clin Psychiatry 2005;66:1441-1446.
171. Montgomery SA, Tobias K, Zornberg GL, et al. Efficacy and safety of pregabalin in the treatment of generalized anxiety disorder: a 6-week, multicenter, randomized, double-blind, placebo-controlled comparison of pregabalin and venlafaxine. J Clin Psychiatry 2006;67:771-782.
172. Rickels K, Pollack MH, Sheehan DV, et al. Efficacy of extended-release venlafaxine in nondepressed outpatients with generalized anxiety disorder. Am J Psychiatry 2000;157:968-974.
173. Davidson JR, DuPont RL, Hedges D, et al. Efficacy, safety, and tolerability of venlafaxine extended release and buspirone in outpatients with generalized anxiety disorder. J Clin Psychiatry 1999;60:528-535.
174. Katz IR, Reynolds CF 3rd, Alexopoulos GS, et al. Venlafaxine ER as a treatment for generalized anxiety disorder in older adults: pooled analysis of five randomized placebo-controlled clinical trials. J Am Geriatr Soc 2002;50:18-25.
175. Silverstone PH, Ravindran A. Once-daily venlafaxine extended release (XR) compared with fluoxetine in outpatients with depression and anxiety. Venlafaxine XR 360 Study Group. J Clin Psychiatry 1999;60:22-28.
176. Gambi F, De Berardis D, Campanella D, et al. Mirtazapine treatment of generalized anxiety disorder: a fixed dose, open label study. J Psychopharmacol 2005;19:483-487.
177. Rickels K, Downing R, Schweizer E, et al. Antidepressants for the treatment of generalized anxiety disorder: a placebo-controlled comparison of imipramine, trazodone, and diazepam. Arch Gen Psychiatry 1993;50:884-895.
178. Rickels K, DeMartinis N, Garcia-Espana F, et al. Imipramine and buspirone in treatment of patients with generalized anxiety disorder who are discontinuing long-term benzodiazepine therapy. Am J Psychiatry 2000;157:1973-1979.
179. Moller HJ, Volz HP, Reimann IW, et al. Opipramol for the treatment of generalized anxiety disorder: a placebo-controlled trial including an alprazolam-treated group. J Clin Psychopharmacol 2001;21:59-65.
180. Boyer WF, Feighner JP. A placebo-controlled double-blind multicenter trial of two doses of ipsapirone versus diazepam in generalized anxiety disorder. Int Clin Psychopharmacol 1993;8:173-176.
181. Chessick CA, Allen MH, Thase M, et al. Azapirones for generalized anxiety disorder. Cochrane Database Syst Rev 2006;(3):CD006115.
182. Feighner JP, Cohn JB. Analysis of individual symptoms in generalized anxiety—a pooled, multistudy, double-blind evaluation of buspirone. Neuropsychobiology 1989;21:124-130.
183. Brawman-Mintzer O, Knapp RG, Nietert PJ. Adjunctive risperidone in generalized anxiety disorder: a double-blind, placebo-controlled study. J Clin Psychiatry 2005;66:1321-1325.
184. Pollack MH, Simon NM, Zalta AK, et al. Olanzapine augmentation of fluoxetine for refractory generalized anxiety disorder: a placebo controlled study. Biol Psychiatry 2006;59:211-215.
185. Mendels J, Krajewski TF, Huffer V, et al. Effective short-term treatment of generalized anxiety disorder with trifluoperazine. J Clin Psychiatry 1986;47:170-174.
186. Feltner DE, Crockatt JG, Dubovsky SJ, et al. A randomized, double-blind, placebo-controlled, fixed-dose, multicenter study of pregabalin in patients with generalized anxiety disorder. J Clin Psychopharmacol 2003;23:240-249.
187. Ferreri M, Hantouche EG, Billardon M. Value of hydroxyzine in generalized anxiety disorder: controlled double-blind study versus placebo. Encephale 1994;20:785-791.
188. Llorca PM, Spadone C, Sol O, et al. Efficacy and safety of hydroxyzine in the treatment of generalized anxiety disorder: a 3-month double-blind study. J Clin Psychiatry 2002;63:1020-1027.
189. Meibach RC, Dunner D, Wilson LG, et al. Comparative efficacy of propranolol, chlordiazepoxide, and placebo in the treatment of anxiety: a double-blind trial. J Clin Psychiatry 1987;48:355-358.
190. Kapczinski F, Lima MS, Souza JS, et al. Antidepressants for generalized anxiety disorder. Cochrane Database Syst Rev 2003;(2):CD003592.
191. Zohar J, Judge R. Paroxetine versus clomipramine in the treatment of obsessive-compulsive disorder. OCD Paroxetine Study Investigators. Br J Psychiatry 1996;169:468-474.
192. Hollander E, Allen A, Steiner M, et al. Acute and long-term treatment and prevention of relapse of obsessive-compulsive disorder with paroxetine. J Clin Psychiatry 2003;64:1113-1121.
193. Montgomery SA, McIntyre A, Osterheider M, et al. A double-blind, placebo-controlled study of fluoxetine in patients with DSM-III-R obsessive-compulsive disorder. The Lilly European OCD Study Group. Eur Neuropsychopharmacol 1993;3:143-152.
194. Geller DA, Wagner KD, Emslie G, et al. Paroxetine treatment in children and adolescents with obsessive-compulsive disorder: a randomized, multicenter, double-blind, placebo-controlled trial. J Am Acad Child Adolesc Psychiatry 2004;43:1387-1396.
195. Romano S, Goodman W, Tamura R, et al. Long-term treatment of obsessive-compulsive disorder after an acute response: a comparison of fluoxetine versus placebo. J Clin Psychopharmacol 2001;21:46-52.
196. Tollefson GD, Birkett M, Koran L, et al. Continuation treatment of OCD: double-blind and open-label experience with fluoxetine. J Clin Psychiatry 1994;55(Suppl):69-76; discussion 77-78.
197. Lopez-Ibor JJ Jr, Saiz J, Cottraux J, et al. Double-blind comparison of fluoxetine versus clomipramine in the treatment of obsessive compulsive disorder. Eur Neuropsychopharmacol 1996;6:111-118.
198. Geller DA, Hoog SL, Heiligenstein JH, et al. Fluoxetine treatment for obsessive-compulsive disorder in children and adolescents: a placebo-controlled clinical trial. J Am Acad Child Adolesc Psychiatry 2001;40:773-779.
199. Goodman WK, Kozak MJ, Liebowitz M, et al. Treatment of obsessive-compulsive disorder with fluvoxamine: a multicentre, double-blind, placebo-controlled trial. Int Clin Psychopharmacol 1996;11:21-29.
200. Hohagen F, Winkelmann G, Rasche-Ruchle H, et al. Combination of behaviour therapy with fluvoxamine in comparison with behaviour therapy and placebo: results of a multicentre study. Br J Psychiatry Suppl 1998;(35):71-78.
201. Koran LM, McElroy SL, Davidson JR, et al. Fluvoxamine versus clomipramine for obsessive-compulsive disorder: a double-blind comparison. J Clin Psychopharmacol 1996;16:121-129.
202. Hollander E, Koran LM, Goodman WK, et al. A double-blind, placebo-controlled study of the efficacy and safety of controlled-release fluvoxamine in patients with obsessive-compulsive disorder. J Clin Psychiatry 2003;64:640-647.
203. Riddle MA, Reeve EA, Yaryura-Tobias JA, et al. Fluvoxamine for children and adolescents with obsessive-compulsive disorder: a randomized, controlled, multicenter trial. J Am Acad Child Adolesc Psychiatry 2001;40:222-229.

204. Greist J, Chouinard G, DuBoff E, et al. Double-blind parallel comparison of three dosages of sertraline and placebo in outpatients with obsessive-compulsive disorder. Arch Gen Psychiatry 1995;52:289-295.
205. Kronig MH, Apter J, Asnis G, et al. Placebo-controlled, multicenter study of sertraline treatment for obsessive-compulsive disorder. J Clin Psychopharmacol 1999;19:172-176.
206. Greist JH, Jefferson JW, Kobak KA, et al. A 1 year double-blind placebo-controlled fixed dose study of sertraline in the treatment of obsessive-compulsive disorder. Int Clin Psychopharmacol 1995;10:57-65.
207. Bisserbe J, Lane R, Flament M. A double-blind comparison of sertraline and clomipramine in outpatients with obsessive compulsive disorder. Eur Psychiatry 1997;12:37-44.
208. Montgomery SA, Kasper S, Stein DJ, et al. Citalopram 20 mg, 40 mg and 60 mg are all effective and well tolerated compared with placebo in obsessive-compulsive disorder. Int Clin Psychopharmacol 2001;16:75-86.
209. Pallanti S, Quercioli L, Koran LM. Citalopram intravenous infusion in resistant obsessive-compulsive disorder: an open trial. J Clin Psychiatry 2002;63:796-801.
210. Yaryura-Tobias JA, Neziroglu FA. Venlafaxine in obsessive-compulsive disorder. Arch Gen Psychiatry 1996;53:653-654.
211. Denys D, van Megen HJ, van der Wee N, et al. A double-blind switch study of paroxetine and venlafaxine in obsessive-compulsive disorder. J Clin Psychiatry 2004;65:37-43.
212. Denys D, van der Wee N, van Megen HJ, et al. A double blind comparison of venlafaxine and paroxetine in obsessive-compulsive disorder. J Clin Psychopharmacol 2003;23:568-575.
213. Albert U, Aguglia E, Maina G, et al. Venlafaxine versus clomipramine in the treatment of obsessive-compulsive disorder: a preliminary single-blind, 12-week, controlled study. J Clin Psychiatry 2002;63:1004-1009.
214. Pallanti S, Quercioli L, Bruscoli M. Response acceleration with mirtazapine augmentation of citalopram in obsessive-compulsive disorder patients without comorbid depression: a pilot study. J Clin Psychiatry 2004;65:1394-1399.
215. Vulink NC, Denys D, Westenberg HG. Bupropion for patients with obsessive-compulsive disorder: an open-label, fixed-dose study. J Clin Psychiatry 2005;66:228-230.
216. Flament MF, Bisserbe JC. Pharmacologic treatment of obsessive-compulsive disorder: comparative studies. J Clin Psychiatry 1997;58(Suppl 12):18-22.
217. Piccinelli M, Pini S, Bellantuono C, et al. Efficacy of drug treatment in obsessive-compulsive disorder: a meta-analytic review. Br J Psychiatry 1995;166:424-443.
218. Fineberg NA, Gale TM. Evidence-based pharmacotherapy of obsessive-compulsive disorder. Int J Neuropsychopharmacol 2005;8:107-129.
219. Katz RJ, DeVeaugh-Geiss J, Landau P. Clomipramine in obsessive-compulsive disorder. Biol Psychiatry 1990;28:401-414.
220. Volavka J, Neziroglu F, Yaryura-Tobias JA. Clomipramine and imipramine in obsessive-compulsive disorder. Psychiatry Res 1985;14:85-93.
221. Vallejo J, Olivares J, Marcos T, et al. Clomipramine versus phenelzine in obsessive-compulsive disorder: a controlled clinical trial. Br J Psychiatry 1992;161:665-670.
222. Jenike MA, Baer L, Minichiello WE, et al. Placebo-controlled trial of fluoxetine and phenelzine for obsessive-compulsive disorder. Am J Psychiatry 1997;154:1261-1264.
223. Hewlett WA, Vinogradov S, Agras WS. Clomipramine, clonazepam, and clonidine treatment of obsessive-compulsive disorder. J Clin Psychopharmacol 1992;12:420-430.
224. Hollander E, Kaplan A, Stahl SM. A double-blind, placebo-controlled trial of clonazepam in obsessive-compulsive disorder. World J Biol Psychiatry 2003;4:30-34.
225. Crockett BA, Churchill E, Davidson JR. A double-blind combination study of clonazepam with sertraline in obsessive-compulsive disorder. Ann Clin Psychiatry 2004;16:127-132.
226. McDougle CJ, Goodman WK, Leckman JF, et al. Limited therapeutic effect of addition of buspirone in fluvoxamine-refractory obsessive-compulsive disorder. Am J Psychiatry 1993;150:647-649.
227. Dannon PN, Sasson Y, Hirschmann S, et al. Pindolol augmentation in treatment-resistant obsessive compulsive disorder: a double-blind placebo controlled trial. Eur Neuropsychopharmacol 2000;10:165-169.
228. McDougle CJ, Goodman WK, Leckman JF, et al. Haloperidol addition in fluvoxamine-refractory obsessive-compulsive disorder: a double-blind, placebo-controlled study in patients with and without tics. Arch Gen Psychiatry 1994;51:302-308.
229. McDougle CJ, Epperson CN, Pelton GH, et al. A double-blind, placebo-controlled study of risperidone addition in serotonin reuptake inhibitor-refractory obsessive-compulsive disorder. Arch Gen Psychiatry 2000;57:794-801.
230. Bystritsky A, Ackerman DL, Rosen RM, et al. Augmentation of serotonin reuptake inhibitors in refractory obsessive-compulsive disorder using adjunctive olanzapine: a placebo-controlled trial. J Clin Psychiatry 2004;65:565-568.
231. Carey PD, Vythilingum B, Seedat S, et al. Quetiapine augmentation of SRIs in treatment refractory obsessive-compulsive disorder: a double-blind, randomised, placebo-controlled study [ISRCTN83050762]. BMC Psychiatry 2005;5:5.
232. Skapinakis P, Papatheodorou T, Mavreas V. Antipsychotic augmentation of serotonergic antidepressants in treatment-resistant obsessive-compulsive disorder: a meta-analysis of the randomized controlled trials. Eur Neuropsychopharmacol 2007;17:79-93.
233. Marshall RD, Beebe KL, Oldham M, et al. Efficacy and safety of paroxetine treatment for chronic PTSD: a fixed-dose, placebo-controlled study. Am J Psychiatry 2001;158:1982-1988.
234. Tucker P, Zaninelli R, Yehuda R, et al. Paroxetine in the treatment of chronic posttraumatic stress disorder: results of a placebo-controlled, flexible-dosage trial. J Clin Psychiatry 2001;62:860-868.
235. GlaxoSmithKline. Study ID = BRL29060A/799: clinical evaluation of BRL29060A (paroxetine hydrochloride hydrate) in posttraumatic stress disorder (PTSD)—a 52-week, non-comparative, uncontrolled study for the clinical use experience. 2005. Obtained from GSK Clinical Trial Register Website.
236. Brady K, Pearlstein T, Asnis GM, et al. Efficacy and safety of sertraline treatment of posttraumatic stress disorder: a randomized controlled trial. JAMA 2000;283:1837-1844.
237. Davidson JR, Rothbaum BO, van der Kolk BA, et al. Multicenter, double-blind comparison of sertraline and placebo in the treatment of posttraumatic stress disorder. Arch Gen Psychiatry 2001;58:485-492.
238. Tucker P, Potter-Kimball R, Wyatt DB, et al. Can physiologic assessment and side effects tease out differences in PTSD trials? A double-blind comparison of citalopram, sertraline, and placebo. Psychopharmacol Bull 2003;37:135-149.
239. Martenyi F, Brown EB, Zhang H, et al. Fluoxetine versus placebo in posttraumatic stress disorder. J Clin Psychiatry 2002;63:199-206.
240. Martenyi F, Soldatenkova V. Fluoxetine in the acute treatment and relapse prevention of combat-related post-traumatic stress disorder: analysis of the veteran group of a placebo-controlled, randomized clinical trial. Eur Neuropsychopharmacol 2006;16:340-349.
241. van der Kolk BA, Dreyfuss D, Michaels M, et al. Fluoxetine in posttraumatic stress disorder. J Clin Psychiatry 1994;55:517-522.
242. Martenyi F, Brown EB, Zhang H, et al. Fluoxetine v. placebo in prevention of relapse in post-traumatic stress disorder. Br J Psychiatry 2002;181:315-320.
243. Escalona R, Canive JM, Calais LA, et al. Fluvoxamine treatment in veterans with combat-related post-traumatic stress disorder. Depress Anxiety 2002;15:29-33.
244. English BA, Jewell M, Jewell G, et al. Treatment of chronic posttraumatic stress disorder in combat veterans with citalopram: an open trial. J Clin Psychopharmacol 2006;26:84-88.
245. Seedat S, Stein DJ, Emsley RA. Open trial of citalopram in adults with post-traumatic stress disorder. Int J Neuropsychopharmacol 2000;3:135-140.
246. Davidson J, Rothbaum BO, Tucker P, et al. Venlafaxine extended release in posttraumatic stress disorder: a sertraline- and placebo-controlled study. J Clin Psychopharmacol 2006;26:259-267.
247. Davidson JR, Weisler RH, Butterfield MI, et al. Mirtazapine vs. placebo in posttraumatic stress disorder: a pilot trial. Biol Psychiatry 2003;53:188-191.
248. Hertzberg MA, Moore SD, Feldman ME, et al. A preliminary study of bupropion sustained-release for smoking cessation in patients with chronic posttraumatic stress disorder. J Clin Psychopharmacol 2001;21:94-98.
249. Davidson J, Kudler H, Smith R, et al. Treatment of posttraumatic stress disorder with amitriptyline and placebo. Arch Gen Psychiatry 1990;47:259-266.
250. Frank JB, Kosten TR, Giller EL Jr, et al. A randomized clinical trial of phenelzine and imipramine for posttraumatic stress disorder. Am J Psychiatry 1988;145:1289-1291.
251. Reist C, Kauffmann CD, Haier RJ, et al. A controlled trial of desipramine in 18 men with posttraumatic stress disorder. Am J Psychiatry 1989;146:513-516.
252. Neal LA, Shapland W, Fox C. An open trial of moclobemide in the treatment of post-traumatic stress disorder. Int Clin Psychopharmacol 1997;12:231-237.
253. Braun P, Greenberg D, Dasberg H, et al. Core symptoms of posttraumatic stress disorder unimproved by alprazolam treatment. J Clin Psychiatry 1990;51:236-238.
254. Cates ME, Bishop MH, Davis LL, et al. Clonazepam for treatment of sleep disturbances associated with combat-related posttraumatic stress disorder. Ann Pharmacother 2004;38:1395-1399.
255. Risse SC, Whitters A, Burke J, et al. Severe withdrawal symptoms after discontinuation of alprazolam in eight patients with combat-induced posttraumatic stress disorder. J Clin Psychiatry 1990;51:206-209.
256. Hertzberg MA, Butterfield MI, Feldman ME, et al. A preliminary study of lamotrigine for the treatment of posttraumatic stress disorder. Biol Psychiatry 1999;45:1226-1229.
257. Hamner MB, Brodrick PS, Labbate LA. Gabapentin in PTSD: a retrospective, clinical series of adjunctive therapy. Ann Clin Psychiatry 2001;13:141-146.
258. Connor KM, Davidson JR, Weisler RH, et al. Tiagabine for posttraumatic stress disorder: effects of open-label and double-blind discontinuation treatment. Psychopharmacology (Berl) 2006;184:21-25.
259. Fesler FA. Valproate in combat-related posttraumatic stress disorder. J Clin Psychiatry 1991;52:361-364.
260. Sutherland SM, Davidson JR. Pharmacotherapy for post-traumatic stress disorder. Psychiatr Clin North Am 1994;17:409-423.
261. Bartzokis G, Lu PH, Turner J, et al. Adjunctive risperidone in the treatment of chronic combat-related posttraumatic stress disorder. Biol Psychiatry 2005;57:474-479.
262. Stein MB, Kline NA, Matloff JL. Adjunctive olanzapine for SSRI-resistant combat-related PTSD: a double-blind, placebo-controlled study. Am J Psychiatry 2002;159:1777-1779.
263. Pitman RK, Sanders KM, Zusman RM, et al. Pilot study of secondary prevention of posttraumatic stress disorder with propranolol. Biol Psychiatry 2002;51:189-192.
264. Stein DJ, Ipser JC, Seedat S. Pharmacotherapy for post traumatic stress disorder (PTSD). Cochrane Database Syst Rev 2006;(1):CD002795.
265. Stein MB, Liebowitz MR, Lydiard RB, et al. Paroxetine treatment of generalized social phobia (social anxiety disorder): a randomized controlled trial. JAMA 1998;280:708-713.
266. Baldwin D, Bobes J, Stein DJ, et al. Paroxetine in social phobia/social anxiety disorder: randomised, double-blind, placebo-controlled study. Paroxetine Study Group. Br J Psychiatry 1999;175:120-126.
267. Liebowitz MR, Stein MB, Tancer M, et al. A randomized, double-blind, fixed-dose comparison of paroxetine and placebo in the treatment of generalized social anxiety disorder. J Clin Psychiatry 2002;63:66-74.
268. Stein DJ, Versiani M, Hair T, et al. Efficacy of paroxetine for relapse prevention in social anxiety disorder: a 24-week study. Arch Gen Psychiatry 2002;59:1111-1118.
269. Lepola U, Bergtholdt B, St. Lambert J, et al. Controlled-release paroxetine in the treatment of patients with social anxiety disorder. J Clin Psychiatry 2004;65:222-229.

270. Clark DM, Ehlers A, McManus F, et al. Cognitive therapy versus fluoxetine in generalized social phobia: a randomized placebo-controlled trial. J Consult Clin Psychol 2003;71:1058-1067.
271. Kobak KA, Greist JH, Jefferson JW, et al. Fluoxetine in social phobia: a double-blind, placebo-controlled pilot study. J Clin Psychopharmacol 2002;22:257-262.
272. Davidson JR, Foa EB, Huppert JD, et al. Fluoxetine, comprehensive cognitive behavioral therapy, and placebo in generalized social phobia. Arch Gen Psychiatry 2004; 61:1005-1013.
273. Katzelnick DJ, Kobak KA, Greist JH, et al. Sertraline for social phobia: a double-blind, placebo-controlled crossover study. Am J Psychiatry 1995;152:1368-1371.
274. Walker JR, Van Ameringen MA, Swinson R, et al. Prevention of relapse in generalized social phobia: results of a 24-week study in responders to 20 weeks of sertraline treatment. J Clin Psychopharmacol 2000;20:636-644.
275. Van Ameringen MA, Lane RM, Walker JR, et al. Sertraline treatment of generalized social phobia: a 20-week, double-blind, placebo-controlled study. Am J Psychiatry 2001;158:275-281.
276. van Vliet IM, den Boer JA, Westenberg HG. Psychopharmacological treatment of social phobia: a double blind placebo controlled study with fluvoxamine. Psychopharmacology (Berl) 1994;115:128-134.
277. Stein MB, Fyer AJ, Davidson JR, et al. Fluvoxamine treatment of social phobia (social anxiety disorder): a double-blind, placebo-controlled study. Am J Psychiatry 1999;156:756-760.
278. Westenberg HG, Stein DJ, Yang H, et al. A double-blind placebo-controlled study of controlled release fluvoxamine for the treatment of generalized social anxiety disorder. J Clin Psychopharmacol 2004;24:49-55.
279. Stein DJ, Westenberg HG, Yang H, et al. Fluvoxamine CR in the long-term treatment of social anxiety disorder: the 12- to 24-week extension phase of a multicentre, randomized, placebo-controlled trial. Int J Neuropsychopharmacol 2003;6:317-323.
280. Furmark T, Appel L, Michelgard A, et al. Cerebral blood flow changes after treatment of social phobia with the neurokinin-1 antagonist GR205171, citalopram, or placebo. Biol Psychiatry 2005;58:132-142.
281. Lader M, Stender K, Burger V, et al. Efficacy and tolerability of escitalopram in 12- and 24-week treatment of social anxiety disorder: randomised, double-blind, placebo-controlled, fixed-dose study. Depress Anxiety 2004;19:241-248.
282. Montgomery SA, Nil R, Durr-Pal N, et al. A 24-week randomized, double-blind, placebo-controlled study of escitalopram for the prevention of generalized social anxiety disorder. J Clin Psychiatry 2005;66:1270-1278.
283. Allgulander C, Mangano R, Zhang J, et al. Efficacy of venlafaxine ER in patients with social anxiety disorder: a double-blind, placebo-controlled, parallel-group comparison with paroxetine. Hum Psychopharmacol 2004;19:387-396.
284. Liebowitz MR, Gelenberg AJ, Munjack D. Venlafaxine extended release vs placebo and paroxetine in social anxiety disorder. Arch Gen Psychiatry 2005;62:190-198.
285. Stein MB, Pollack MH, Bystritsky A, et al. Efficacy of low and higher dose extended-release venlafaxine in generalized social anxiety disorder: a 6-month randomized controlled trial. Psychopharmacology (Berl) 2005;177:280-288.
286. Beaumont G. A large open multicentre trial of clomipramine (anafranil) in the management of phobic disorders. J Int Med Res 1977;5(Suppl 5):116-123.
287. Liebowitz MR, Schneier F, Campeas R, et al. Phenelzine vs atenolol in social phobia: a placebo-controlled comparison. Arch Gen Psychiatry 1992;49:290-300.
288. Gelernter CS, Uhde TW, Cimbolic P, et al. Cognitive-behavioral and pharmacological treatments of social phobia: a controlled study. Arch Gen Psychiatry 1991;48:938-945.
289. Versiani M, Nardi AE, Mundim FD, et al. Pharmacotherapy of social phobia: a controlled study with moclobemide and phenelzine. Br J Psychiatry 1992;161:353-360.
290. Heimberg RG, Liebowitz MR, Hope DA, et al. Cognitive behavioral group therapy vs phenelzine therapy for social phobia: 12-week outcome. Arch Gen Psychiatry 1998;55:1133-1141.
291. Liebowitz MR, Heimberg RG, Schneier FR, et al. Cognitive-behavioral group therapy versus phenelzine in social phobia: long-term outcome. Depress Anxiety 1999;10:89-98.
292. Simpson HB, Schneier FR, Marshall RD, et al. Low dose selegiline (L-deprenyl) in social phobia. Depress Anxiety 1998;7:126-129.
293. Patkar AA, Pae CU, Masand PS. Transdermal selegiline: the new generation of monoamine oxidase inhibitors. CNS Spectr 2006;11:363-375.
294. Blanco C, Raza MS, Schneier FR, et al. The evidence-based pharmacological treatment of social anxiety disorder. Int J Neuropsychopharmacol 2003;6:427-442.
295. The International Multicenter Clinical Trial Group on Moclobemide in Social Phobia. Moclobemide in social phobia: a double-blind, placebo-controlled clinical study. Eur Arch Psychiatry Clin Neurosci 1997;247:71-80.
296. Stein DJ, Cameron A, Amrein R, et al. Moclobemide is effective and well tolerated in the long-term pharmacotherapy of social anxiety disorder with or without comorbid anxiety disorder. Int Clin Psychopharmacol 2002;17:161-170.
297. Davidson JR, Potts N, Richichi E, et al. Treatment of social phobia with clonazepam and placebo. J Clin Psychopharmacol 1993;13:423-428.
298. Pande AC, Davidson JR, Jefferson JW, et al. Treatment of social phobia with gabapentin: a placebo-controlled study. J Clin Psychopharmacol 1999;19:341-348.
299. Pande AC, Feltner DE, Jefferson JW, et al. Efficacy of the novel anxiolytic pregabalin in social anxiety disorder: a placebo-controlled, multicenter study. J Clin Psychopharmacol 2004;24:141-149.
300. van Vliet IM, den Boer JA, Westenberg HG, et al. Clinical effects of buspirone in social phobia: a double-blind placebo-controlled study. J Clin Psychiatry 1997;58:164-168.
301. Falloon IR, Lloyd GG, Harpin RE. The treatment of social phobia: real-life rehearsal with nonprofessional therapists. J Nerv Ment Dis 1981;169:180-184.
302. Liebowitz MR. Social phobia. Mod Probl Pharmacopsychiatry 1987;22:141-173.
303. Barnett SD, Kramer ML, Casat CD, et al. Efficacy of olanzapine in social anxiety disorder: a pilot study. J Psychopharmacol 2002;16:365-368.
304. Stein DJ, Ipser JC, van Balkom AJ. Pharmacotherapy for social anxiety disorder. Cochrane Database Syst Rev 2000;(4):CD001206.
305. Black DW. Efficacy of combined pharmacotherapy and psychotherapy versus monotherapy in the treatment of anxiety disorders. CNS Spectr 2006;11:29-33.
306. Bakker A, van Dyck R, Spinhoven P, et al. Paroxetine, clomipramine, and cognitive therapy in the treatment of panic disorder. J Clin Psychiatry 1999;60:831-838.
307. Loerch B, Graf-Morgenstern M, Hautzinger M, et al. Randomised placebo-controlled trial of moclobemide, cognitive-behavioural therapy and their combination in panic disorder with agoraphobia. Br J Psychiatry 1999;174:205-212.
308. Mitte K. A meta-analysis of the efficacy of psycho- and pharmacotherapy in panic disorder with and without agoraphobia. J Affect Disord 2005;88:27-45.
309. Bruce TJ, Spiegel DA, Hegel MT. Cognitive-behavioral therapy helps prevent relapse and recurrence of panic disorder following alprazolam discontinuation: a long-term follow-up of the Peoria and Dartmouth studies. J Consult Clin Psychol 1999;67:151-156.
310. Clark DM, Salkovskis PM, Hackmann A, et al. Brief cognitive therapy for panic disorder: a randomized controlled trial. J Consult Clin Psychol 1999;67:583-589.
311. Heldt E, Gus Manfro G, Kipper L, et al. One-year follow-up of pharmacotherapy-resistant patients with panic disorder treated with cognitive-behavior therapy: outcome and predictors of remission. Behav Res Ther 2006;44:657-665.
312. Linden M, Zubraegel D, Baer T, et al. Efficacy of cognitive behaviour therapy in generalized anxiety disorders: results of a controlled clinical trial (Berlin CBT-GAD study). Psychother Psychosom 2005;74:36-42.
313. Power KG, Simpson RJ, Swanson V, et al. Controlled comparison of pharmacological and psychological treatment of generalized anxiety disorder in primary care. Br J Gen Pract 1990;40:289-294.
314. Cottraux J, Mollard E, Bouvard M, et al. A controlled study of fluvoxamine and exposure in obsessive-compulsive disorder. Int Clin Psychopharmacol 1990;5:17-30.
315. van Balkom AJ, de Haan E, van Oppen P, et al. Cognitive and behavioral therapies alone versus in combination with fluvoxamine in the treatment of obsessive compulsive disorder. J Nerv Ment Dis 1998;186:492-499.
316. Foa EB, Liebowitz MR, Kozak MJ, et al. Randomized, placebo-controlled trial of exposure and ritual prevention, clomipramine, and their combination in the treatment of obsessive-compulsive disorder. Am J Psychiatry 2005;162:151-161.
317. Foa EB, Franklin ME, Moser J. Context in the clinic: how well do cognitive-behavioral therapies and medications work in combination? Biol Psychiatry 2002;52:987-997.
318. Bisson J, Andrew M. Psychological treatment of post-traumatic stress disorder (PTSD). Cochrane Database Syst Rev 2007;(3):CD003388.
319. Blomhoff S, Haug TT, Hellstrom K, et al. Randomised controlled general practice trial of sertraline, exposure therapy and combined treatment in generalised social phobia. Br J Psychiatry 2001;179:23-30.
320. Schuurmans J, Comijs H, Emmelkamp PM, et al. A randomized, controlled trial of the effectiveness of cognitive-behavioral therapy and sertraline versus a waitlist control group for anxiety disorders in older adults. Am J Geriatr Psychiatry 2006;14:255-263.
321. Dugan E, Cohen SJ. Improving physicians' implementation of clinical practice guidelines: enhancing primary care practice. *In* Shumaker S, Schron E, Ockene J, McBee W (eds): The Handbook of Health Behavior Change. New York: Springer, 1998, pp 283-304.
322. Bruce SE, Vasile RG, Goisman RM, et al. Are benzodiazepines still the medication of choice for patients with panic disorder with or without agoraphobia? Am J Psychiatry 2003;160:1432-1438.

53

DEPRESSION AND BIPOLAR DISORDERS

Wade Berrettini

INTRODUCTION 787
PATHOPHYSIOLOGY 787
Unipolar Disorder 787
Bipolar Disorder 787
THERAPEUTICS AND CLINICAL PHARMACOLOGY 788
Goals of Therapy 788
Pharmacotherapy of Unipolar Disorder 788
Selective Serotonin Reuptake Inhibitors 790
Serotonin and Norepinephrine Reuptake Inhibitors 791
Bupropion 791
Mirtazepine 791
Tricyclic Antidepressants 791
Monoamine Oxidase Inhibitors 791
Stimulation of Central Nervous System Neurogenesis: A Novel Approach to Antidepressant Activity 792
Summary 792
Pharmacotherapy of Bipolar Disorder 792
Lithium 792
Anticonvulsant Mood Stabilizers 793
Atypical Antipsychotic Mood Stabilizers 794

INTRODUCTION

The main focus of this chapter is the pharmacotherapy of the two major types of mood disorder, unipolar disorder (UP), also known as major depressive disorder and bipolar disorder (BP) also known as manic-depressive illness. It should be emphasized that this chapter does not include any discussion of the various effective psychotherapies for these mood disorders, such as cognitive behavioral therapy, as these topics are beyond the scope of the chapter. However, comprehensive, optimal treatment of these mood disorders should include a psychotherapeutic modality in addition to the pharmacotherapy (for reviews of psychotherapies of mood disorders, see Swartz et al.,[1] Friedman and Thase,[2] and Markowitz[3]).

This chapter reviews agents approved in the United States for the pharmacotherapy of UP and BP. Although there are valuable UP/BP medications not available in the United States, this review is restricted to those agents approved for UP and/or BP in the United States.

There are two main goals for the pharmacotherapy of UP and BP: (i) remission of symptoms for an acute episode of the mood disorder and (ii) prevention of recurrence. Because these disorders are highly recurrent in nature,[4] and because each episode carries with it substantial morbidity and risk for suicide, prevention of recurrence is a key goal in pharmacotherapy of UP and BP.

PATHOPHYSIOLOGY

Unipolar Disorder

UP (Fig. 53-1) is operationally defined in the Diagnostic and Statistical Manual of Mental Disorders, Fourth Edition (DSM-IV).[5] Women are affected more often than men, in a ratio of 3:2. The lifetime risk for UP is a function of its definition, and the range for lifetime risk is approximately 10% to 20%. The age at onset is quite variable, as many individuals suffer a first episode late in life, after the loss of a loved one or a serious medical illness. Typical age at onset is young adulthood; however, prepubertal onset is less common. There is substantial evidence that that age at onset for UP is decreasing, for uncertain reasons. The World Health Organization Global Burden of Disease study found that UP is responsible for more disability than any other condition during the middle years of life.[6]

This group of disorders is recurrent in nature.[4] After two episodes (depending on episode severity and duration, as well as the period of euthymia), many authorities recommend prophylactic (also known as preventative or maintenance) pharmacotherapy, to reduce the risk of recurrence.[7,8] It is impossible to predict the time at which a recurrence will develop. It is also impossible to predict the severity or duration of a recurrence. In retrospect, stressful life events are often identified as "precipitants" of a recurrence. Such stressful life events include job change, retirement, death of a relative or spouse, illness, and certain drugs (e.g., corticosteroids). However, it is impossible to predict whether any stressful life event will precipitate an episode of UP. (For a comprehensive review of the symptoms, epidemiology and course of illness for UP, see Goodwin et al.[9])

Suicide is the outcome for approximately 15% of individuals with UP. Most individuals with UP will have vague suicidal ideation ("I would be better off dead"), and many will have specific plans ("I thought about locking myself in the garage with the car running."). While there are certain characteristics of suicide completers (e.g., family or personal history of suicide attempts, psychotic symptoms, living alone), it is impossible to predict a suicide attempt accurately. A vulnerable period for suicide attempt may occur when a depressed individual is initially responding to antidepressant therapy. UP disorder is often comorbid with drug/alcohol abuse and/or dependence, which increases risk for suicide. Anxiety disorders are also frequently comorbid with UP. (For a review of suicide in UP, see Mann and Currier.[10])

Little is known concerning the origins of UP. It is clear that genetic influences explain a substantial fraction of the risk; this fraction of risk increases when one considers only early-onset recurrent UP. A review of twin studies in recurrent UP disorder estimated heritability at 37%, with a substantial component of unique individual environmental risk, but little shared environmental risk.[11] Many promising candidate genes are under investigation for their putative role in UP (for review, see Berrettini[12]). Several studies have indicated that putative genetic risk factors for UP, such as a functional repeated element in the promoter of the serotonin transporter gene, interact with a life history of "negative environmental events" to produce high risk for UP.[13]

Bipolar Disorder

BP (Fig. 53-2) is defined as the occurrence of one or more manic episodes, usually accompanied by episodes of major depressive disorder. Manic episodes are operationally defined in the DSM-IV.[5] BP is divided into two forms, BP I and BP II, the difference being that individuals with BP II typically have recurrent major depressive episodes plus milder manic syndromes, termed *hypomanias*, for which there is no impairment/incapacitation in an individual's functioning. Individuals with BP I have the full manic syndrome, with impairment or incapacitation in a major life role of the individual. Occasionally, individuals may have "mixed" episodes in which symptoms of major depressive disorder and mania are intermixed. (For a comprehensive review of the symptoms, course of illness, and epidemiology of BP, see Goodwin and Jamieson.[14])

BP affects 2% to 3% of the world population, and is a major public health problem.[15] The typical age at onset (defined as first episode of depression or mania) is in late adolescence. Prepubertal onset is uncommon, as is onset after age 50. Women and men are equally at risk. BP is highly recurrent in nature. Unfortunately, it is impossible to predict the timing of future episodes of BP, or whether they will be severe or mild, or manic or depressive in nature. Because each episode of BP is associated with significant morbidity and mortality, prevention of recurrence is a primary treatment goal, along with resolution of the acute episode. (For a review of the epidemiology of BP, see Goodwin et al.[9])

BP shares with UP a high rate of suicide, approximately 15% across the lifetime.[10] BP is frequently comorbid with anxiety disorders and alcohol/drug abuse and/or dependence.

1. Sad mood for ≥2 weeks
2. Impairment/Incapacitation & at least 5 of the following:

A. Sleep disturbance
B. Appetite change
C. Anhedonia
D. Worthlessness
E. Suicidal ideation
F. Loss of energy
G. Difficulty concentrating
H. Psychomotor retardation or agitation

FIGURE 53-1 • Unipolar disorder.

1. Elevated or irritable mood for ≥1 week
2. Impairment/Incapacitation & at least 4 of the following:

A. Distractibility
B. Racing thoughts
C. Grandiosity
D. Increased activity
E. Increased talking
F. Decreased need for sleep
G. Inappropriate/reckless behaviors

FIGURE 53-2 • Bipolar disorder.

The pathophysiology of BP is largely unknown. BP is a partially genetic disorder, with estimates of heritability from twin studies approaching approximately 80%.[16] Many promising candidate genes are under investigation for BP (see Berrettini[12] for review).

THERAPEUTICS AND CLINICAL PHARMACOLOGY

Goals of Therapy

For both UP and BP pharmacotherapy, the goals of treatment are twofold: (i) remission of symptoms for the acute episode and (ii) prevention of recurrence. Concerning pharmacotherapy of UP, it is important to differentiate antidepressant (AD) *response* (defined as >50% decrease in severity of depression symptoms on a rating scale) from *remission*, the virtual absence of depressive symptoms (Fig. 53-3). The goal of remission is key to optimal long-term patient outcome, because longitudinal research demonstrates that remitted UP patients have a much better long-term outcome than those UP patients who have responded to AD therapy with a decrease in depressive symptoms, but have residual difficulties[17] (Fig. 53-4).

For UP pharmacotherapy, prevention of recurrence most often involves continuation of the same pharmacotherapy regimen beyond the acute and continuation phases of treatment into a maintenance phase. Typically, the full AD dose that was associated with remission of symptoms is used for prevention of recurrence.[7,8]

For BP disorder, prevention of recurrence typically involves treatment with one or more "mood stabilizers," a class of compounds that may be defined as those agents that decrease risk for recurrence of depression and mania in BP patients. It should be noted that mood stabilizers are often (but not always) distinct from those medications used to treat acute episodes of mania and/or depression.

Pharmacotherapy of Unipolar Disorder

ADs can be classified according to presumed mechanism of action and/or by chemical structure as shown in Figure 53-5. *No one AD is superior to another in efficacy or in onset of clinical response.* ADs differ remarkably in side effects, dosing schedules, pharmacodynamics, pharmacokinetics, and therapeutic index. In short-term (6 to 8 weeks) double-blind, placebo-controlled clinical trials of an AD, approximately 60% of UP patients are responders (>50% decrease in depression symptom severity from baseline) and approximately 30% enter

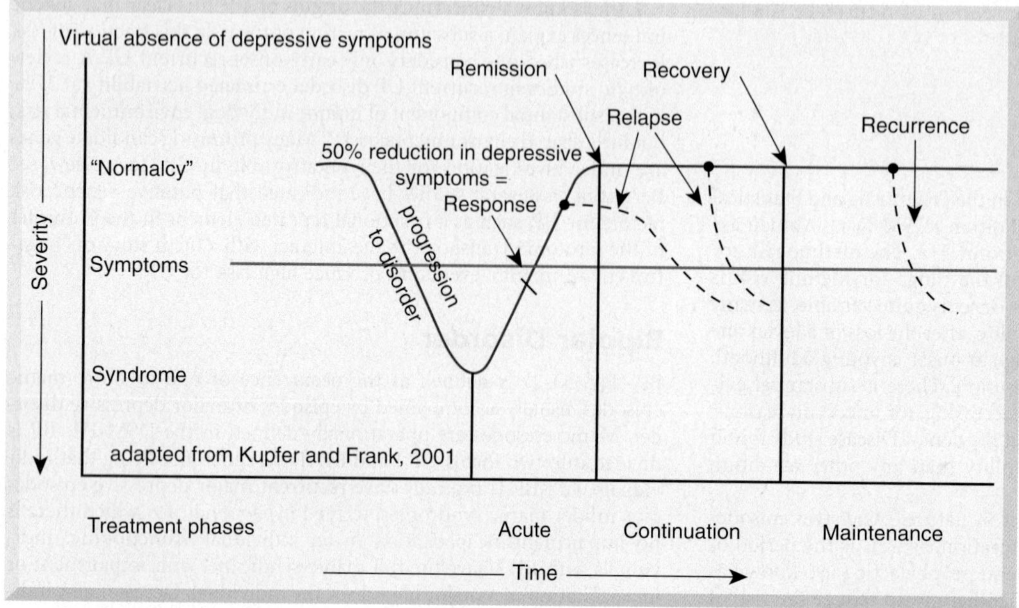

FIGURE 53-3 • Unipolar disorder: response, remission, recovery, relapse, and recurrence.

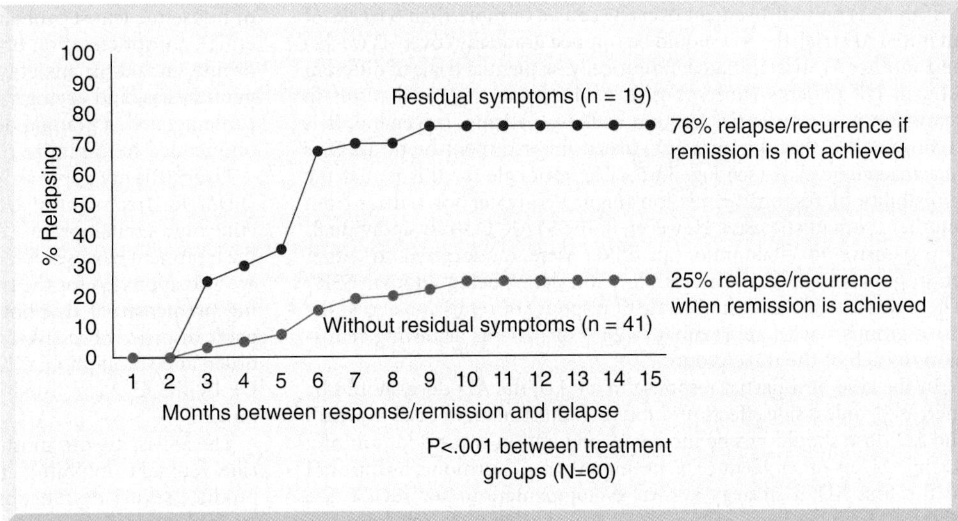

FIGURE 53-4 • Failure to achieve remission increases the risk of relapse.

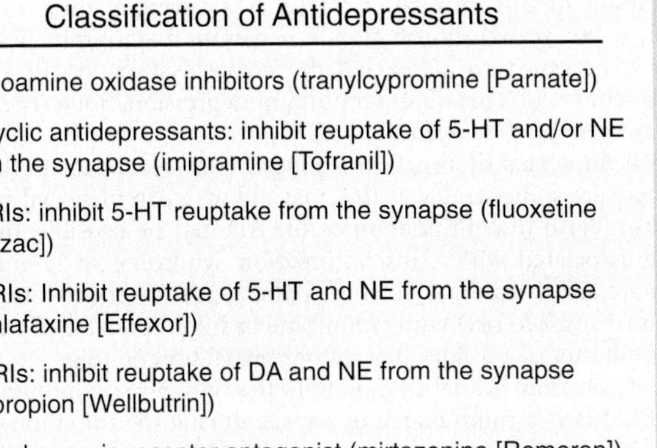

Classification of Antidepressants

- Monoamine oxidase inhibitors (tranylcypromine [Parnate])
- Tricyclic antidepressants: inhibit reuptake of 5-HT and/or NE from the synapse (imipramine [Tofranil])
- SSRIs: inhibit 5-HT reuptake from the synapse (fluoxetine [Prozac])
- SNRIs: Inhibit reuptake of 5-HT and NE from the synapse (venlafaxine [Effexor])
- DNRIs: inhibit reuptake of DA and NE from the synapse (bupropion [Wellbutrin])
- α-2 adrenergic receptor antagonist (mirtazepine [Remeron])

SSRI = selective serotonin reuptake inhibitor
SNRI = selective serotonin/norepinephrine reuptake inhibitor
DNRI = dopamine/norepinephrine reuptake inhibitor

FIGURE 53-5 • Pharmacotherapy of unipolar disorder.

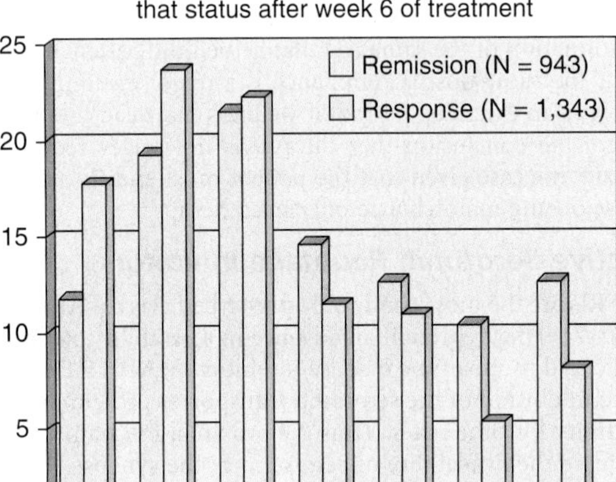

FIGURE 53-6 • Time to response and remission in STAR*D trial.

remission (virtual absence of depressive symptoms). ADs typically require at least 2 weeks for the clinical response to be detectable, and the reason for this delay is not clear.

For the untreated, first-episode UP individual, the selection of an AD should be guided by two main concerns: (i) family history of AD response (i.e., the physician should choose the AD associated with good response in a similarly affected first-degree relative); and (ii) side effect profile (i.e., the patient's medical history should be considered in light of the side effect profile for an AD). Regarding the second point, for example, if a person with UP has a history of epilepsy, the physician should avoid bupropion, as it can elicit a seizure in the susceptible individual.

For the untreated UP individual with a history of good therapeutic response to a given AD, that same AD should be prescribed again. In this instance, long-term maintenance therapy should be given serious consideration.

In general, the selected AD should be prescribed at a lower effective dose for at least 3 weeks. If there is no improvement in symptoms during that time, the dose should be gradually increased, as tolerated, to the maximal recommended dose. If no improvement is observed at the maximal recommended (or tolerated) dose after several weeks, the person with UP should be considered nonresponsive to the medication, as long as noncompliance is not present. If noncompliance is suspected, the physician should ask the patient to bring the medication to each subsequent appointment, so that the physician can determine that the prescription was filled, and that the correct amount of pills are missing from the supply originally dispensed.

What duration of exposure to effective doses of an AD is required for an adequate trial? The answer to this question is not straightforward. Previously, a 6-week trial was thought to be adequate, if it included at least 2 weeks at the maximum recommended (or maximally tolerated) dose. The Sequenced Treatment Alternatives to Relieve Depression (STAR*D) trial was an open-label, flexible-dose (20 to 60 mg daily) trial of citalopram (a selective serotonin reuptake inhibitor [SSRI]) in approximately 4000 individuals with UP[18] for 14 weeks. In this trial, a significant fraction of individuals responded only after more than 6 weeks of citalopram (Fig. 53-6). Thus, a much longer trial of an AD might yield response or remission. In any case, a minimum duration of 6 weeks is necessary before a patient can be judged as a nonresponder.

Several authors have designed UP treatment algorithms[19] as guidelines for the sequential treatment of persons with UP. These algorithms allow for flexible selection of second-, third-, and fourth-tier ADs for the UP patient who has not responded to the initially chosen AD. These algorithms are useful guides to rational pharmacotherapy of UP.

If there is no improvement over the course of more than 6 weeks of an initial AD trial, the AD should be stopped gradually (over ~2 weeks) and another AD trial initiated. Empirically, sequential trials of different ADs in UP patients (unresponsive to the initial AD) will result in remission in a substantial fraction of these patients. In general, it is recommended that the next AD chosen for treatment be of another pharmacologic class (see Fig. 53-5). The rationale for this is that the probability of response/remission might be greater for a drug from another mechanistic class. However, in the STAR*D study, individuals unresponsive to citalopram (an SSRI) were randomized to either bupropion, venlafaxine, or sertraline, the latter being another SSRI. There was no difference in the rate of response or remission across the three groups,[20] with approximately 25% of patients achieving remission in each of the three groups.

In the case of a partial response to an AD, the AD dose should be increased, unless side effects prohibit this adjustment. In cases in which the AD dose should not be increased, one option is the addition of a second AD or other agent (e.g., lithium, thyroid hormone, buspirone) to the first AD, a strategy known as augmentation (for review, see Blier[21]). Much has been written about the decision to switch from one AD to another, versus augmentation of an AD, because a partial response to an AD is very common.

Because a large fraction of UP is recurrent,[4] after two episodes, maintenance therapy may be indicated.[7,8] Maintenance therapy refers to continuation of the same AD that helped the patient achieve remission, at the same dose. Compliance is a major issue in maintenance therapy, as an extended period of wellness may lead the patient to the questionable conclusion that the AD is no longer required. This is especially the case given that the patient must endure side effects and expense during maintenance pharmacotherapy.

Selective Serotonin Reuptake Inhibitors

The SSRIs are the most commonly prescribed class of ADs in use today (Fig. 53-7). They represent an advance in tolerability, *not efficacy,* over tricyclic and monoamine oxidase inhibitor (MAOI) ADs, due to their specific inhibition of the serotonin transporter protein, with relatively low affinity for other sites. Thus the proximal mechanism of action is to increase the availability of serotonin at the synapse. They are relatively safe in overdose, a consideration for any AD. Readily absorbed from the gastrointestinal tract, these agents circulate tightly bound to plasma proteins.

SSRIs are metabolized by microsomal liver enzymes, then conjugated with glucuronide and excreted in the urine. Therefore, hepatic or renal deficits will reduce clearance. The individual cytochrome P-450 (CYP) enzymes involved in metabolism of SSRIs have been delineated.[22] All these agents and/or their active metabolites have relatively long half-lives (>12 hours), so that once-daily dosing is appropriate. Fluoxetine is rapidly converted to the active metabolite norfluoxetine, which has a very long half-life (~7 days). With the possible exception of fluoxetine (most probably because of the long half-life of norfluoxetine), abrupt cessation of an SSRI can lead to a discontinuation syndrome, including anxiety, insomnia, agitation, headache, irritability, paresthesias, and crying.[23] Thus, when discontinuation of an SSRI is contemplated, a gradual decrease in SSRI dosage over 2 weeks is recommended to minimize risk for discontinuation symptoms.

Five SSRIs are approved by the U.S. Food and Drug Administration (FDA) for treatment of UP: fluoxetine, sertraline, citalopram, paroxetine, and escitalopram. (A sixth SSRI, fluvoxamine, is approved for the treatment of obsessive-compulsive disorder.) Several of these drugs are also approved for the treatment of various other disorders, including premenstrual dysphoric disorder, posttraumatic stress disorder, panic disorder, obsessive-compulsive disorder, generalized anxiety disorder, and social phobia. The five SSRIs approved for the treatment of UP by the FDA are listed in Table 53-1 with the recommended dose ranges.

The SSRIs, as with most ADs, including serotonin and norepinephrine reuptake inhibitors (SNRIs), MAOIs, and tricyclic ADs, may produce sexual dysfunctions, including decreased libido, inability to achieve erection, and delayed orgasm. Some form of sexual dysfunction may be present in approximately 50% of individuals taking one of these ADs.[24] (Bupropion and mirtazepine are notable exceptions.) These sexual side effects represent the most common adverse event leading to discontinuation of an AD during maintenance therapy. However, sexual dysfunction is a common symptom in depression. It is necessary to judge that the sexual dysfunction in a recovering patient is not a residual symptom of depression, but a true treatment-emergent adverse event.

If the sexual dysfunction is judged to be secondary to the AD, then there are some strategies that may allow return of sexual functioning. Short-term discontinuation of the AD may be possible, but this may be associated with a discontinuation syndrome or re-emergence of depressive symptoms. In some patients, short-term treatment (1 to 2 hours prior to sex) with yohimbine or inhibitors of cyclic GMP phosphodiesterase epsilon may restore sexual functioning.

Apart from sexual dysfunction, the only other common side effect of SSRIs is a mild degree of nausea during the initiation of therapy. This is rarely severe enough to be accompanied by vomiting, and it does not usually cause the patient to stop treatment. Reassurance and the suggestion to take the medication with food may help.

Recently, it has been suggested that SSRIs might increase risk for suicidal ideation and behavior in adolescents and children,[25] based on analysis of three unpublished studies in which paroxetine did not differentiate from placebo. The FDA has mandated a label warning about increased risk for suicidal ideation with SSRIs in adolescents and children. In a meta-analysis of 40,000 adults participating in 477 randomized, placebo-controlled trials of SSRIs, there were 16 suicides, 172 episodes of nonfatal self-harm, and 177 episodes of suicidal ideation. There was no evidence that SSRIs increased risk for suicide or suicidal

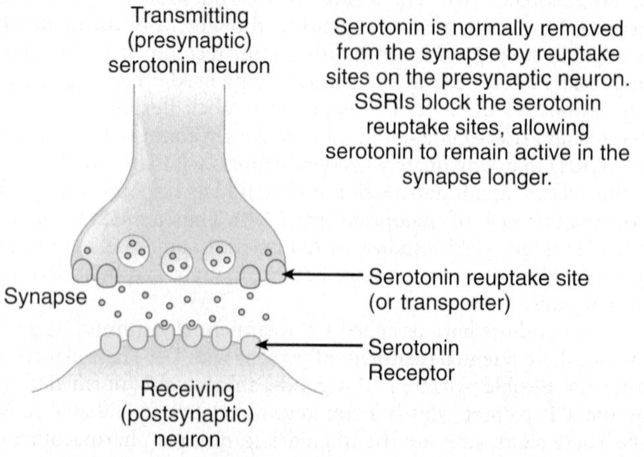

FIGURE 53-7 • Selective serotonin reuptake inhibitors.

TABLE 53-1 SSRIs APPROVED FOR TREATMENT OF UNIPOLAR DISORDER

Medication	FDA-Approved Dose Range (mg)	FDA-Approved Indications
Fluoxetine	20-80	UP, bulimia nervosa, OCD, panic disorder, PDD, PTSD
Paroxetine	20-50	UP, GAD, PDD, social phobia, panic disorder, PTSD
Sertraline	50-200	UP, OCD, panic disorder, PTSD, PDD, social phobia
Citalopram	20-60	UP
Escitalopram	5-40	UP

FDA, U.S. Food and Drug Administration; GAD, generalized anxiety disorder; OCD, obsessive-compulsive disorder; PDD, premenstrual dysphoric disorder; PTSD, posttraumatic stress disorder; UP, unipolar disorder.

ideation in this population.[26] There is some evidence that increased rates of SSRI prescriptions, when analyzed by county, are associated with decreased suicide rates in children and adolescents.[27] At present, there are insufficient data to address the issue of increased risk for suicide among individuals treated with SSRIs. This lack of data underscores the importance of careful evaluation of the UP patient taking any AD, as suicide is the outcome in approximately 15% of individuals with UP.

Serotonin and Norepinephrine Reuptake Inhibitors

Venlafaxine and duloxetine are dual SNRIs approved by the FDA for UP pharmacotherapy. Venlafaxine has also been approved for the treatment of generalized anxiety disorder and social phobia. The venlafaxine dosage range is 75 to 375 mg daily, with some evidence that a minimum effective dose (at which clinically optimal blockade of norepinephrine reuptake sites might occur) is approximately 150 mg/day. Although it has a short half-life, requiring at least twice-daily dosing, there is an extended-release version suitable for once-daily administration. This drug is not tightly bound to plasma proteins, a difference from SSRIs. It is metabolized by the CYP2D6 enzyme and excreted in the urine. Venlafaxine may have a slight propensity to increase blood pressure at the higher end of the dosage range, although clinically significant increases in blood pressure are uncommon. There is some evidence that venlafaxine may increase the rate of remission among UP patients in short-term, placebo-controlled trials when compared with SSRIs, especially in the more severely affected patients.

The duloxetine dosage range is 20 to 60 mg daily. An extended-release form permits once-daily dosing. It is metabolized by CYP2D6 and CYP1A2. It is also approved by the FDA for neuropathic pain. Venlafaxine and duloxetine, as SNRIs, have some of the characteristics of SSRIs, including nausea, sexual dysfunction,[28] and risk for discontinuation syndrome upon abrupt cessation.[29]

Bupropion

Bupropion is a dopamine and norepinephrine reuptake inhibitor. It is FDA approved for UP pharmacotherapy and for smoking cessation (the effective dose being 150 to 300 mg daily for the latter indication). The minimal recommended dose for UP pharmacotherapy is 300 mg daily, with the maximal dose being approximately 450 mg daily. Although it has a short half-life, with active metabolites, there are extended-release preparations suitable for once-daily dosing. The side effect profile is generally benign (anxiety, agitation, insomnia, and palpitations occur uncommonly), with little sexual dysfunction. At higher doses, there is a small risk for seizures in the susceptible individual, such that the medication should not be used in the seizure-prone individual.

Mirtazepine

Mirtazepine is a 5-hydroxytryptamine (5-HT) 5-HT_{2A} receptor antagonist for α_2-adrenergic receptors, approved by the FDA for UP pharmacotherapy. These α_2-adrenergic receptors generally inhibit the release of norepinephrine and serotonin. Thus blockade of these receptors facilitates presynaptic release of norepinephrine and serotonin. Due to histamine receptor blockade, mirtazepine exhibits sedative effects, with benefit to the person with UP troubled by insomnia. Also related to the histamine receptor blockade, mirtazepine may cause increased appetite and weight gain. Due to 5-HT_2 blockade, it has some anxiolytic properties. Although it is metabolized by CYP1A1, CYP2D6, and CYP2C19, it is not an inhibitor of those enzymes.

Tricyclic Antidepressants

Tricyclic ADs are thought to work through blockade of norepinephrine and/or serotonin reuptake (see Fig. 53-7). The first tricyclic AD, imipramine, was initially found to be effective in depression, and this was an impetus to test compounds of similar structure. Other tricyclics were synthesized, tested, and found to have similar efficacy, and the tricyclic ADs became the cornerstone of UP pharmacotherapy for the next 25 years.

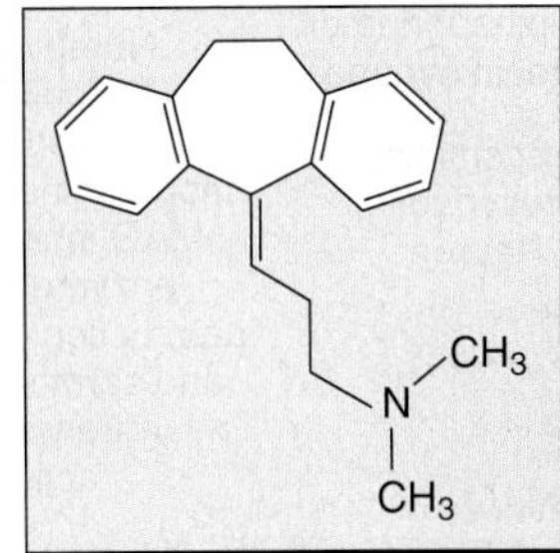

FIGURE 53-8 • Structure of amitriptyline.

These compounds have in common a core of three heterocyclic carbon rings, with a side chain (see the structure of amitriptyline in Fig. 53-8). At times, during the synthesis of a series of tricyclics, medicinal chemists would create a fourth ring from the side chain, giving rise to some closely related tetracyclic compounds (e.g., maprotiline) that also had AD efficacy. It has been found empirically that the tertiary amine (see side chain in amitriptyline structure in Fig. 53-8) conveys more serotonergic reuptake blockade, while the desmethyl metabolite (a secondary amine) has more norepinephrine reuptake blockade. Thus most teriary amine tricylic ADs, such as imipramine and amitriptyline, due to their desmethyl active metabolites, block reuptake of both serotonin and norepinephrine. The secondary amine tricyclics (desipramine, nortriptyline) preferentially block norepinephrine reuptake.

As a class of ADs, the tricyclics are unsurpassed in efficacy for pharmacotherapy of UP. They are also effective in treatment of anxiety disorders.[30] Because they have several difficult side effects due to blockade of α_1, histaminic H_1, and cholinergic receptors (sedation, dry mouth, constipation, orthostatic hypotension), it is best to begin with a small dose (e.g., 25 to 50 mg of imipramine, amitriptyline, desipramine, or nortriptyline) and increase to an effective dose (~150 mg at bedtime) over approximately 1 week. Because of their sedative side effects and long half-lives, tricyclics are best prescribed in once-daily dosing at bedtime. As with other ADs, a 2- to 3-week time lag is seen between starting the medication and clinical improvement. If no response is seen at the end of 3 weeks, gradual increase in dosage (as side effects permit) should be attempted. The maximal recommended dose of many tricyclics is approximately 300 mg daily. Protriptyline is a notable exception, for which the recommended dosing range is 20 to 60 mg daily.

Tricyclic ADs are lethal in overdose, often when a 10-day supply is ingested at once. Tricyclics may be fatal in overdose because of their propensity to induce cardiac arrhythmias. These compounds have a quinidine-like effect on cardiac conduction, slowing conduction.

Tricyclics undergo demethylation and aromatic ring hydroxylation in the liver as a function of CYP enzymes, including CYP2D6. The demethylated compounds are active in blocking norepinephrine reuptake. Because functional polymorphisms of CYP2D6 are common, some patients may require lower doses, for example, individuals of Asian and African background.[31]

Monoamine Oxidase Inhibitors

MAOIs are effective antidepressants that have been in use since the 1950s. The first MAOI, iproniazid, was discovered to improve mood during testing for antibacterial efficacy in patients with tuberculosis. By inhibiting degradation of monoamines (Fig. 53-9), these agents increase the availability of monoamine neurotransmitters for release into the synapse. Because MAOIs also augment the activity of dopamine, these agents may permit therapeutic response in individuals unresponsive to SSRIs, tricyclic ADs, and SNRIs (for review, see Potter et al.[30]). MAOIs may be particularly useful in the treatment of atypical depressive symptoms such as hypersomnia, hyperphagia, anergy, and low energy,[32] as well as anxiety disorders.

Three MAOIs are approved by the FDA for UP pharmacotherapy in the United States: phenelzine (dosage range 45 to 90 mg daily),

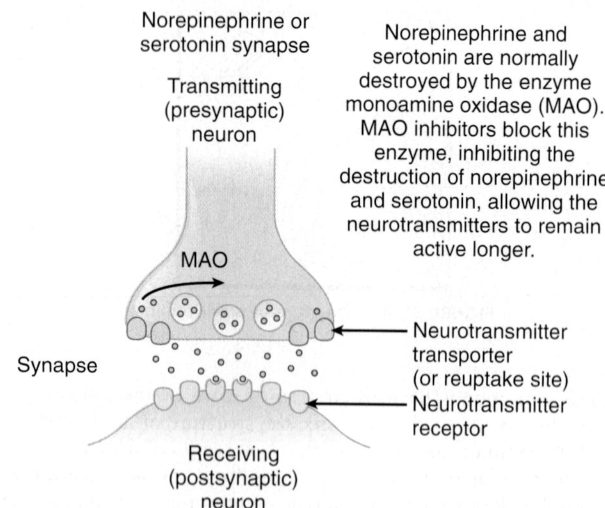

FIGURE 53-9 • Monamine oxidase inhibitors.

Placebo-Controlled Trials in BP

Drug	Bipolar Depression		Mania	
	Acute	Maintenance	Acute	Maintenance
Lithium (Li)	++	++	++	++
Carbamazepine	–	–	++	+
Divalproex	–	+	++	+
Lamotrigine	++	++	–	+
Olanzapine	++*	+	++	++
Risperidone	–	–	++	–
Quetiapine	++	–	++	–
Ziprasidone	–	–	+	–
Aripiprazole	–	+	++	++

*++ in combination with fluoxetine; quality of evidence/effect size: ++ = marked, + = moderate, ± = mild, – = minimal/inadequate evidence

FIGURE 53-10 • Pharmacotherapy of bipolar disorder.

tranylcypromine (dosage range 30 to 60 mg), and isocarboxazid (dosage range 30 to 60 mg). MAOIs have unsurpassed efficacy in the treatment of UP, but they have, as a class, several limitations that constrain their tolerability and safety. Orthostatic hypotension, headache, myoclonic jerks, weakness, peripheral edema, and insomnia are common adverse events (for review, see Potter et al.[30]). Additionally, when combined with sympathomimetics (ephedrine, pseudoephedrine, phenylpropanolamine, amphetamine, etc.), serious (and sometimes fatal) hypertensive crises may result. Thus, many medications, including nonprescription items, must be avoided. Several opioid agonists (e.g., meperidine) can cause a syndrome of coma, hyperpyrexia, and hypertension when given to a patient taking MAOIs. MAOIs must not be combined with SSRIs, or a serotonin syndrome may result. Although MAOIs may be cautiously combined with tricyclics for treatment-resistant depression, there is a risk for hypertensive crisis. It is prudent for the patient taking an MAOI to refrain from eating foods associated with high levels of tyramine and/or other sympathomimetic amines, although the necessity for complete abstinence has been questioned.[33] It is critical to maintain avoidance of interacting drugs for at least 1 week after cessation of an MAOI, because enzymatic inhibition continues for an extended period, until new enzyme is synthesized.

Stimulation of Central Nervous System Neurogenesis: A Novel Approach to Antidepressant Activity

ADs increase the availability of neurotransmitter monoamines (serotonin, norepinephrine, and/or dopamine) at central nervous system (CNS) synapses, either through blockade of reuptake (SSRIs, SNRIs, bupropion) or by inhibition of degradation (MAOIs). Although the inhibition of reuptake of monoamine oxidase is immediate, clinical recovery requires weeks of AD administration. This delay in clinical response has never been explained, suggesting that the monoamine action is a proximal event leading to cascades of CNS change, requiring weeks of adaptation through which the clinically observable AD response occurs.

One promising theory of the CNS adaptation to AD administration is stimulation of neurogenesis through increasing levels of brain-derived neurotrophic factor (BDNF) (see Castrén et al.[34] for review). Multiple different ADs and electroconvulsive therapy increase levels of BDNF in rodent brain after chronic treatment,[35,36] while BDNF has AD-like effects on rodents in models of depression.[37,38] BDNF-deficient mice have depressive behaviors in rodent models of depression, such as the forced swim test.[39] Hippocampal neurogenesis, an effect of BDNF, seems to be required for AD activity in rodents.[40] From clinical studies, acutely depressed UP patients have decreased levels of serum BDNF, which return toward normal after AD treatment.[41,42] Finally, BDNF gene alleles have been associated repeatedly with BP[43-45] and UP,[46] although the UP association is controversial.[47]

Summary

There are multiple classes of AD drugs, but no one drug has superior efficacy over another. No one class of medications has a more rapid onset than another. All these agents require at least 2 to 3 weeks for the onset of clinical symptom reduction. Because they have fewer side effects, the newer agents (SSRIs, SNRIs, bupropion, mirtazepine) are more easily tolerated than the older agents, the tricyclics and MAOIs. Recent developments from the STAR*D study bring into question the issue of duration for an adequate trial for an AD. Previously, a 6- or 8-week trial was assumed to be adequate, but many citalopram-treated patients in the STAR*D study developed a response only after a longer period of treatment.[18]

Pharmacotherapy of Bipolar Disorder

Although algorithms for the treatment of BP have been constructed,[48] such an algorithm is beyond the scope of this chapter. However, a guiding principle of BP pharmacotherapy is that all such patients should be treated continuously with one or more mood-stabilizing agents. A mood-stabilizing agent (Fig. 53-10) may be defined as a medication that lessens the probability of recurrence for both depression and mania. Lithium, anticonvulsants (lamotrigine, carbamazepine, divalproex), and atypical antipsychotics (e.g., olanzapine, aripiprazole) may be considered mood stabilizers. It is useful to consider the various mood stabilizers as exhibiting different capacities to stabilize mood from below (i.e., stabilize mood to a euthymic state from an episode of depression without increasing risk for mania) and from above (stabilize mood to a euthymic state from an episode of mania/hypomania, without increasing risk for depression) (for review, see Muzina and Calabrese[48]).

No one mood-stabilizing agent has been shown to be superior in efficacy to another, so that selection of an agent is less than a straightforward process. Since BP is a chronic recurring illness with onset in adolescence, a lifetime of treatment is envisioned, so that the mood-stabilizing agent(s) must be tolerable and affordable. Most BP patients will not have an optimal response to a single mood stabilizer, and combinations of two or more mood stabilizers may be required to prevent recurrence in most BP patients.

Lithium

For more than 50 years, lithium has been a first-line medication for the treatment of BP (for review, see Keck and McElroy[49]). Lithium has efficacy in the acute treatment of manic[50] and depressive[51] phases of BP and in the prevention of BP recurrence. Although several of the initial trials were done as long as approximately 50 years ago (e.g.,

Schou et al.[50]), more recent double-blind, placebo-controlled trials, in which lithium was an active comparator, continue to prove its efficacy for mania and for prevention of recurrence[52,53] in relation to the newer agents.

The mechanism of action for lithium remains undefined. Perhaps the most prominent theory of its mechanism of action involves the inhibition of inositol monophosphatase and/or inositol polyphosphate phosphatase, key enzymes in the inositol triphosphate (a CNS second messenger) cycle.[54] Such an inhibition would theoretically deplete the CNS of myoinositol. This is an active area of investigation.

Lithium carbonate is given orally in sufficient doses to achieve a therapeutic blood level of 0.8 to 1.3 mEq/L for treatment of acute mania. The response in acute mania requires as long as 2 weeks, although the response time can be shortened by rapid titration (20 mg/kg per day) to a full therapeutic dose.[49] The entire range of manic symptoms responds to lithium monotherapy, including psychotic symptoms (e.g., grandiose delusions). Acute side effects of lithium include increased thirst, increased urination, hand tremor, nausea, diarrhea, cognitive slowing, weight gain, and somnolence. Most side effects are less prominent at lower blood levels. Since lithium is excreted almost entirely by the kidney, reduced doses must be used in individuals with impaired renal function. Lithium has a narrow range of blood levels in which it is effective, and toxicity can develop over time if the recommended dose is exceeded by 20%. Presenting symptoms of lithium toxicity can include nausea, diarrhea, vomiting, unsteady gait, blurred vision, and delirium. Lithium is dangerous in overdose.

Evidence from maintenance therapy trials with lithium has been generated in multiple long-term studies,[49] with the conclusion that lithium prevents the recurrence of both depressive and manic phases of illness. Maintenance lithium therapy generally involves somewhat lower blood levels (~0.6 to 0.9 mEq/L) compared to those recommended to treat acute mania. This is especially important given that side effects are more prominent at higher blood levels. One of the benefits of maintenance lithium therapy is reduction in risk for suicide.[55] In general, BP patients with an optimal response to lithium include those with classic euphoric mania, less psychosis, and fewer mixed states.

Although lithium monotherapy has been a very successful maintenance strategy for many BP patients, only approximately 50% of patients will have an adequate long-term response to lithium monotherapy. In general, when lithium monotherapy is unsuccessful in prevention of recurrence (e.g., when a compliant individual with BP has more than two "breakthrough" episodes), addition of a second mood stabilizer should be considered. If the breakthrough episodes are depressive in nature, addition of lamotrigine should be considered, as this agent may have particular efficacy in preventing recurrence of depressive episodes.[48] If breakthrough episodes are manic, addition of divalproex or an atypical antipsychotic (e.g., aripiprazole) may be considered, as these agents may have particular efficacy in preventing manic recurrence.

Lithium may produce, as a long-term adverse effect, an interstitial nephritis with gradual loss of renal function, as evidenced by decreasing glomerular filtration rate. It is impossible to predict who will develop this adverse effect, and nephrology consultation is indicated. The loss of renal function is permanent, and, in many cases, cessation of lithium therapy may be indicated. Another maintenance therapy issue is the development of subclinical hypothyroidism. Lithium therapy may cause elevated levels of thyroid-stimulating hormone and lower triiodothyronine and thyroxine levels in approximately 5% of patients. This may occur through interference with the thyroid-stimulating hormone signaling system in thyroid gland cells. The thyroid abnormalities can be corrected by addition of synthetic thyroid hormone (levothyroxine). Upon cessation of lithium therapy, the thyroid abnormalities revert to baseline. Because of these renal and thyroid adverse events during chronic pharmacotherapy, lithium-treated individuals should have renal and thyroid blood tests on an annual basis, as a minimum.

Addition of lithium to an AD is an effective "augmentation" strategy when a UP patient has a partial response to an AD. For reasons that are unclear, this combination may allow for a more complete response than the AD alone. Evidence for significant improvement after lithium augmentation has been observed with tricylics, MAOIs, and SSRIs (for review, see Freeman et al.[56]). In general, lithium levels in the maintenance treatment range (0.6 to 0.9 mEq/L) are used for UP AD augmentation. The time course of response is not defined in this augmentation strategy.

Anticonvulsant Mood Stabilizers

Divalproex. Several anticonvulsants have demonstrated efficacy in BP, as noted in Figure 53-10. Divalproex is an enteric-coated version of valproic acid, and was the second agent after lithium to be FDA approved for the treatment of acute manic episodes (for review, see Nasrallah et al.[57]), as well as mixed episodes. There are no double-blind, placebo-controlled trials of divalproex in maintenance therapy of BP that demonstrate efficacy, although the agent is widely used for maintenance on the basis of less rigorous evidence.[53,58,59] Its mechanism of action in BP is unknown. There is limited evidence for efficacy of divalproex in the depressive phase of BP.[60,61]

Divalproex pharmacotherapy is often initiated at low doses (e.g., 250 mg twice daily) with gradual increases, according to tolerability, in two divided doses daily, to achieve a blood level of 50 to 125 mcg/dl. An extended-release version permits once-daily dosing. For the severely manic patient, requiring rapid titration, doses of 20 mg/kg per day can be initiated in the hospitalized patient. Somewhat higher doses (e.g., 1 g twice daily) are used to treat acute mania, compared to doses (e.g., 500 mg twice daily) for maintenance therapy. Prior to the initiation of divalproex therapy, a complete blood count, thyroid function tests, and liver function tests should be obtained. Divalproex is associated with mild increases in liver enzymes, which typically resolve with time. A decrease in platelet count, with a report of easy bruising, can be observed. Elevated thyroid-stimulating hormone is an uncommon adverse event that can be treated with low doses of levothyroxine. These tests should be repeated every 6 months. Somnolence, tremor, dizziness, asthenia, and weight gain are common difficulties (for review, see Nasrallah et al.[57]). In the 1-year maintenance study of divalproex,[53] 21% of divalproex-treated patients gained more than 5% of baseline weight. This degree of weight gain limits the acceptability of divalproex. Rarely, severe pancreatitis or hepatic necrosis has been observed. Increased risk to the fetus for teratogenic events (neural tube defects) indicates that divalproex should not be used in women of childbearing age unless a secure form of birth control is employed.[62] Divalproex also increases risk for polycystic ovarian syndrome, which developed in approximately 10% of 89 women on divalproex compared to 1% of 143 women with BP taking other mood stabilizers.[63] Therefore, the use of divalproex in women who wish to have children must be considered in this light.

Divalproex is also FDA-approved for the treatment of epilepsy and for migraine. The latter indication is significant, as migraine is comorbid with BP.

Lamotrigine. Lamotrigine is an anticonvulsant that is FDA approved for maintenance treatment of BP, on the basis of two placebo-controlled trials.[64,65] Although this medication is efficacious for the treatment of acute BP depression,[66] there is no evidence for efficacy in acute mania. Lamotrigine is believed to have particular efficacy in preventing relapse in BP to the depressive phase. Its mechanism of action in BP is unknown. Its anticonvulsant activity may be due to inhibition of voltage-sensitive sodium channels.

The target dose of lamotrigine in BP is 100 mg twice daily, for treatment of acute BP depression or for maintenance. This target dose should be reached using a very gradual increase from 25 mg twice daily over a 6-week period. This gradual titration schedule is thought to reduce risk for a potentially life-threatening but uncommon (~1 in 5000) side effect, a severe skin rash. Lamotrigine is glucuronated to inactive metabolites and excreted almost entirely by the kidney. The most common side effects are somnolence and nonserious skin rash. Unfortunately, the nonserious skin rash is difficult to differentiate from the severe rash, so immediate discontinuation of the drug is recommended (until expert evaluation is obtained) if a rash develops.

Carbamazepine and Oxcarbamazepine. Carbamazepine (CBZ) is an anticonvulsant that is FDA approved for the treatment of acute mania and mixed episodes, on the basis of two placebo-controlled trials.[67,68] The effective dose range is wide, from 200 to 1600 mg/day, based on these studies,[67,68] which employed a sustained-release preparation allowing for once-daily dosing. Dosing is usually initiated at 100 mg twice daily (or 200 mg daily in an extended-release preparation), with gradual increases based on tolerability. Plasma levels in the range of 8 to 12 mcg/ml have been used to optimize therapy in epilepsy, but their use in BP may not be necessary.[67,68] Although not approved by the FDA for maintenance therapy, evidence from 10 randomized, double-blind studies using lithium as the comparative agent indicated that CBZ was effective for the prophylactic treatment of BP. Response rates to CBZ and lithium were generally similar, with no consistent trends indicating one medication to be superior (for review, see Nasrallah et al.[57]). There are no double-blind, placebo-controlled studies of CBZ in BP depression that are of adequate size to draw conclusions about efficacy.

CBZ is oxidized in the liver by CYP3A4 to the active epoxide metabolite, oxcarbamazepine. After further metabolism and glucuronidation, most of the CBZ derivatives appear in urine. Drugs that inhibit CYP3A4 (e.g., macrolide antibiotics, fluvoxamine, fluoxetine) may lead to CBZ toxicity. The most common side effects of CBZ are dizziness, ataxia, skin rash, somnolence, and diplopia. Because CBZ induces its own metabolism, during the first several weeks of treatment, small increases in dosage may be key to optimal pharmacotherapy. Mild elevations in liver function tests occur in approximately 5% of patients. Mild leukopenia and thrombocytopenia can occur. For these reasons, baseline liver function tests and a complete blood count should be obtained at baseline and at 6-month intervals. While blood levels of CBZ are not essential to BP pharmacotherapy, they can guide dosing and are a useful check on compliance. There is low risk for agranulocytosis and aplastic anemia (~1 in 500,000). Because there is a small increase in risk for spina bifida, the use of CBZ in women of childbearing potential should be limited to those patients using an acceptable form of birth control. CBZ is also FDA approved for the treatment of epilepsy and trigeminal neuralgia.

Oxcarbamazepine, the active metabolite of CBZ, is FDA approved for epilepsy. It may have a milder side effect profile, and it presumably has equal efficacy in BP with its parent compound, although there are no systematic studies that address this.

Atypical Antipsychotic Mood Stabilizers

All typical and atypical antipsychotics have proven to be useful in the treatment of acute manic or mixed episodes, even in the absence of overt psychotic symptoms. Both classes of antipsychotics effectively block D_2 dopamine receptors. The atypicals also block $5\text{-}HT_{2A}$ serotonin receptors. Although there are no studies that address this issue, it is presumed that the same mechanisms of action that explain their antipsychotic action also explain their antimanic action. Several large, well-designed, placebo-controlled trials of some atypicals for maintenance BP pharmacotherapy have been published (for review, see Gitlin[69]). This section reviews evidence for efficacy of these atypicals in maintenance therapy for BP and for acute depression. For dosing, metabolism, mechanisms, side effects, and excretion information, the reader is referred to Chapter 54 (Psychosis and Schizophrenia) regarding treatment of schizophrenia.

Olanzapine (5 to 20 mg/day) and the combination of olanzapine/fluoxetine (6/25 to 12/50 mg/day) proved superior to placebo in the treatment of acute BP depression in a large 8-week randomized, double-blind trial of 833 BP I patients.[70] There was no difference in risk for manic outcome for the three treatment groups. A comparison of divalproex versus olanzapine (5 to 20 mg/day) for acute mania and maintenance in BP I patients over a 47-week trial showed no difference in recurrence of mania for the two groups.[71] Subsequently, a randomized, double-blind trial of olanzapine (5 to 20 mg/day) versus lithium for maintenance therapy of BP I patients[72] demonstrated equivalent efficacy in recurrence risk for the two treatment groups. Thus, for olanzapine, there are substantial well-designed trials indicating its efficacy in treatment of acute mania and acute BP depression, and in prevention of recurrence.

Olanzapine has a common and highly significant side effect of weight gain, which limits its acceptance by many patients. Mean weight gain over 1 year on olanzapine may be approximately 5 kg, with the fraction of patients gaining greater than 7% of body weight approaching 30%.[72] Because obesity is frequently comorbid in BP, olanzapine can worsen a common medical comorbidity. It has considerable sedation as a side effect, making it useful in the agitated manic patient.

Aripiprazole is an atypical antipsychotic with a relatively unique receptor binding profile. It is a partial agonist/antagonist at the D_2 dopamine receptor and an antagonist at $5\text{-}HT_{1A}$ serotonin receptors. It has efficacy in the treatment of acute BP manic and mixed episodes[73] and in maintenance treatment of BP.[74,75] There are no well-designed trials of aripiprazole in BP depression. This medication is weight neutral, and has little sedation.

Quetiapine is an atypical antipsychotic, with D_2 dopamine and $5\text{-}HT_{2A}$ receptor antagonism, that is FDA approved for the treatment of acute mania. Quetiapine was significantly more effective than placebo as monotherapy for BP I or II depression (dosages of 300 or 600 mg/day), beginning at week 1, in a large ($N = 542$), double-blind, placebo-controlled trial. The two quetiapine dosage options did not differ in response rates (58%) compared to 36% for placebo ($P < 0.001$), suggesting that the lower dose is preferred for most patients, to minimize risk for side effects.[76] Quetiapine has significant sedation, making it useful in the agitated manic patient. The sedation is also useful for the insomnia that accompanies BP depression.

In summary, atypical antipsychotics, in particular olanzapine and aripiprazole, may have mood-stabilizing properties that prevent recurrence in BP. While all atypicals probably have efficacy in BP mania, quetiapine and olanzapine are particularly useful in BP depression.

REFERENCES

1. Swartz HA, Frank E, Kupfer DJ. Psychotherapy for bipolar disorder. *In* Stein DJ, Kupfer DJ, Schatzberg AF (eds): Textbook of Mood Disorders. Washington, DC: American Psychiatric Press, 2006, pp 405-420.
2. Friedman ES, Thase ME. Cognitive-behavioral therapy for depression and dysthymia. *In* Stein DJ, Kupfer DJ, Schatzberg AF (eds): Textbook of Mood Disorders. Washington, DC: American Psychiatric Press, 2006, pp 353-372.
3. Markowitz JC. Interpersonal psychotherapy for depression and dysthymic disorder. *In* Stein DJ, Kupfer DJ, Schatzberg AF (eds): Textbook of Mood Disorders. Washington, DC: American Psychiatric Press, 2006, pp 383-388.
4. Angst J, Preisig M. Course of unipolar, bipolar affective and schizoaffective disorders: results of a prospective study from 1959 to 1985. Swiss Arch Neurol Psychiatry 1995;146:5-16.
5. American Psychiatric Association. Diagnostic and Statistical Manual of Mental Disorders, Fourth Edition. Washington, DC: American Psychiatric Association, 1994.
6. Murray CJL, Lopez AD. The Global Burden of Disease: A Comprehensive Assessment of Mortality and Disability from Diseases, Injuries and Risk Factors in 1990 and Projected to 2020. Cambridge, MA: Harvard Univeristy Press, 1996.
7. Geddes JR, Carney SM, Davies C, et al. Relapse prevention with antidepressant drug treatment in depressive disorders: a systematic review. Lancet 2003;361:653-661.
8. Kupfer DJ, Frank E. The interaction of drug and psychotherapy in the long-term treatment of depression. J Affect Disords 2001;62:131-137.
9. Goodwin RF, Jacobi F, Bittner A, Wittchen H-U. Epidemiology of mood disorders. *In* Stein DJ, Kupfer DJ, Schatzberg AF (eds): Textbook of Mood Disorders. Washington, DC: American Psychiatric Press, 2006, pp 33-54.
10. Mann JJ, Currier D. Understanding and preventing suicide. *In* Stein DJ, Kupfer DJ, Schatzberg AF (eds): Textbook of Mood Disorders. Washington, DC: American Psychiatric Press, 2006, pp 485-496.
11. Sullivan PF, Neale MC, Kendler KS. Genetic epidemiology of major depression: review and meta-analysis. Am J Psychiatry 2000;157:1552-1562.
12. Berrettini WH. Genetics of bipolar and unipolar disorders. *In* Stein DJ, Kupfer DJ, Schatzberg AF (eds): Textbook of Mood Disorders. Washington, DC: American Psychiatric Press, 2006, pp 235-250.
13. Caspi A, Sugden K, Moffitt TE, et al. Influence of life stress on depression: moderation by a polymorphism in the 5-HTT gene. Science 2003;301:386-389.
14. Goodwin FK, Jamieson KJ. Manic-Depressive Illness. New York: Oxford University Press, 2003.
15. Kessler RC, Chiu WT, Demler O, et al. Prevalence, severity, and comorbidity of 12-month DSM-IV disorders in the National Comorbidity Survey Replication. Arch Gen Psychiatry 2005;62:617-627.
16. McGuffin P, Rijsdijk S, Andrew M, et al. The heritability of bipolar affective disorder and the genetic relationship to unipolar depression. Arch Gen Psychiatry 2003;60:497-502.
17. Paykel ES, Ramana R, Cooper Z, et al. Residual symptoms after partial remission: an important outcome in depression. Psychol Med 1995;25:1171-1180.

18. Trivedi MH, Rush AJ, Wisniewski SR, et al, for the STAR*D Study Team. Evaluation of outcomes with citalopram for depression using measurement-based care in STAR*D: implications for clinical practice. Am J Psychiatry 2006;163:28-40.
19. Trivedi MH, Rush AJ, Crismon ML, et al. Clinical results for patients with major depressive disorder in the Texas Medication Algorithm Project. Arch Gen Psychiatry 2004;61:669-680.
20. Rush AJ, Trivedi MH, Wisniewski SR, et al, for the STAR*D Study Team. Bupropion-SR, sertraline, or venlafaxine-XR after failure of SSRIs for depression. N Engl J Med 2006;354:1231-1234.
21. Blier P. Medication combination and augmentation strategies in the treatment of major depression. *In* Stein DJ, Kupfer DJ, Schatzberg AF (eds): Textbook of Mood Disorders. Washington, DC: American Psychiatric Press, 2006, pp 509-526.
22. Stein DJ, Kupfer DJ, Schatzberg AF (eds). The American Psychiatric Publishing Textbook of Mood Disorders. Washington, DC: American Psychiatric Publishing, 2005.
23. van Geffen EC, Hugtenburg JG, Heerdink ER, et al. Discontinuation symptoms in users of selective serotonin reuptake inhibitors in clinical practice: tapering versus abrupt discontinuation. Eur J Clin Pharmacol 2005;61:303-307.
24. Ferguson JM. The effects of antidepressants on sexual functioning in depressed patients: a review. J Clin Psychiatry 2001;62(Suppl 3):22-34.
25. Wooltorton E. Paroxetine (Paxil, Seroxat): an increased risk of suicide in pediatric patients. CMAJ 2003;169:446.
26. Gunnell D, Saperia J, Ashby D. Selective serotonin reuptake inhibitors (SSRIs) and suicide in adults: meta-analysis of drug company data from placebo controlled, randomized controlled trials submitted to the MHRA's safety review. BMJ 2005;330:385.
27. Gibbons RD, Hur K, Bhaumik DK, Mann JJ. The relationship between antidepressant prescription rates and rate of early adolescent suicide. Am J Psychiatry 2006;163:1898-1904.
28. Thase ME, Clayton AH, Haight BR, et al. A double-blind comparison between bupropion XL and venlafaxine XR: sexual functioning, antidepressant efficacy, and tolerability. J Clin Psychopharmacol 2006;26:482-488.
29. Perahia DG, Kajdasz DK, Desaiah D, Haddad PM. Symptoms following abrupt discontinuation of duloxetine treatment in patients with major depressive disorder. J Affect Disord 2005;89:207-212.
30. Patil S, Ahmed S, Potter WZ. Advances in treatment and perspectives for new interventions in mood and anxiety disorders. In Soares JC, Gershon S, Soares C (eds): Handbook of Medical Psychiatry. New York: Informa Health Care, 2003, pp 807-826.
31. Gaedigk A, Bradford LD, Marcucci KA, Leeder JS. Unique CYP2D6 activity distribution and genotype-phenotype discordance in black Americans. Clin Pharmacol Ther 2002;72:76-89.
32. Stewart JW, Quitkin FM, Davies C. Atypical depression, dysthymia and cyclothymia. *In* Stein DJ, Kupfer DJ, Schatzberg AF (eds): Textbook of Mood Disorders. Washington, DC: American Psychiatric Press, 2006, pp 547-559.
33. Shulman KI, Walker SE, McKenzie S, Knowles S. Dietary restriction, tyramine and the use of monoamine oxidase inhibitors. J Clin Psychopharmacol 1989;9:397-402.
34. Castrén E, Võikar V, Rantamäki T. Role of neurotrophic factors in depression. Curr Opin Pharmacol 2007;7:18-21.
35. Altar CA, Whitehead RE, Chen R, et al. Effects of electroconvulsive seizures and antidepressant drugs on brain-derived neurotrophic factor protein in rat brain. Biol Psychiatr 2003;54:703-709.
36. Rantamäki T, Hendolin P, Kankaanpää A, et al. Pharmacologically diverse antidepressants rapidly activate brain-derived neurotrophic factor receptor TrkB and induce phospholipase-Cγ signaling pathways in mouse brain. Neuropsychopharmacology 2007;32:2152-2162.
37. Siuciak JA, Lewis DR, Wiegand SJ, Lindsay RM. Antidepressantlike effect of brain-derived neurotrophic factor (BDNF). Pharmacol Biochem Behav 1997;56:131-137.
38. Shirayama Y, Chen AC, Nakagawa S, et al. Brain-derived neurotrophic factor produces antidepressant effects in behavioral models of depression. J Neurosci 2002;22:3251-3261.
39. Monteggia LM, Luikart B, Barrot M, et al. Brain-derived neurotrophic factor conditional knockouts show gender differences in depression-related behaviors. Biol Psychiatry 2007;61:187-197.
40. Santarelli L, Saxe M, Gross C, et al. Requirement of hippocampal neurogenesis for the behavioral effects of antidepressants. Science 2003;301:805-809.
41. Karege F, Perret G, Bondolfi G, et al. Decreased serum brain-derived neurotrophic factor levels in major depressed patients. Psychiatry Res 2002;109:143-148.
42. Shimizu E, Hashimoto K, Okamura N, et al. Alterations of serum levels of brain-derived neurotrophic factor (BDNF) in depressed patients with or without antidepressants. Biol Psychiatry 2003;54:70-75.
43. Lohoff FW, Sander T, Ferraro TN, et al. Confirmation of association between the Val66Met polymorphism in the brain-derived neurotrophic factor (BDNF) gene and bipolar I disorder. Am J Med Genet 2005;139:51-53.
44. Neves-Pereira M, Mundo E, Muglia P, et al. The brain-derived neurotrophic factor gene confers susceptibility to bipolar disorder: evidence from a family-based association study. Am J Hum Genet 2002;71:651-655.
45. Sklar P, Gabriel SB, McInnis MG, et al. Family-based association study of 76 candidate genes in bipolar disorder: BDNF is a potential risk locus. Mol Psychiatry 2002;7:579-593.
46. Schumacher J, Jamra RA, Becker T, et al. Evidence for a relationship between genetic variants at the brain-derived neurotrophic factor (BDNF) locus and major depression. Biol Psychiatry 2005;58:307-314.
47. Surtees PG, Wainwright NW, Willis-Owen SA, et al. No association between the BDNF Val66Met polymorphism and mood status in a non-clinical community sample of 7389 older adults. J Psychiatr Res 2006;41:404-409.
48. Muzina DJ, Calabrese JR. Guidelines for the treatment of bipolar disorder. *In* Stein DJ, Kupfer DJ, Schatzberg AF (eds): Textbook of Mood Disorders. Washington, DC: American Psychiatric Press, 2006, pp 463-483.
49. Keck PE, McElroy SL. Lithium and mood stabilizers. *In* Stein DJ, Kupfer DJ, Schatzberg AF (eds): Textbook of Mood Disorders. Washington, DC: American Psychiatric Press, 2006, pp 281-288.
50. Schou M, Juel-Nelson M, Stromgren E, et al. The treatment of manic psychoses by administration of lithium salts. J Neurol Neurosurg Psychiatry 1954;17:250-260.
51. Zornberg GL, Pope HG. Treatment of depression in bipolar disorder: new directions for research. J Clin Psychopharmacol 1993;13:397-408.
52. Bowden CL, Brugger AM, Swann AC, et al. Efficacy of divalproex versus lithium and placebo in the treatment of mania. JAMA 1994;271:918-924.
53. Bowden CL, Calabrese JR, McElroy SL, et al. Efficacy of divalproex versus lithium and placebo in maintenance treatment of bipolar disorder. Arch Gen Psychiatry 2000;57:481-489.
54. Berridge MJ, Downes CP, Hanley MR. Neural and developmental actions of lithium: a unifying hypothesis. Cell 1989;59:411-419.
55. Goodwin FK, Fireman B, Simon GE, et al. Suicide risk in bipolar disorder during treatment with lithium and divalproex. JAMA 2003;290:1467-1473.
56. Freeman MP, Wiegand C, Gelenbery AJ. Lithium. *In* Schatzberg AF, Nemeroff CB (eds): Textbook of Psychopharmacology, 3rd ed. Washington, DC: American Psychiatric Press, 2004, pp 547-565.
57. Nasrallah HA, Ketter TA, Kalili AH. Carbamazepine and valproate for the treatment of bipolar disorder: a review of the literature. J Affect Dis 2006;95:69-78.
58. Findling RL, McNamara NK, Youngstrom EA, et al. Double-blind 18-month trial of lithium versus divalproex maintenance treatment in pediatric bipolar disorder. J Am Acad Child Adolesc Psychiatry 2005;44:409-417.
59. Calabrese JR, Shelton MD, Rapport DJ, et al. A 20-month, double-blind, maintenance trial of lithium versus divalproex in rapid-cycling bipolar disorder. Am J Psychiatry 2005;162:2152-2161.
60. Gyulai L, Bowden CL, McElroy SL, et al. Maintenance efficacy of divalproex in the prevention of bipolar depression. Neuropsychopharmacology 2003;28:1374-1382.
61. Davis LL, Bartolucci A, Petty F. Divalproex in the treatment of bipolar depression: a placebo-controlled study. J Affect Disord 2005;85:259-266.
62. Meador KJ, Baker GA, Finnell RH, et al, for the NEAD Study Group. In utero antiepileptic drug exposure: fetal death and malformations. Neurology 2006;67:407-412.
63. Joffe H, Cohen L, Suppes T, et al. Valproate is associated with new-onset oligomenorrhea with hyperandrogenism in women with bipolar disorder. Biol Psychiatry 2006;59:1078-1086.
64. Bowden CL, Calabrese JR, Sachs G, et al, for the Lamictal 606 Study Group. A placebo-controlled 18-month trial of lamotrigine and lithium maintenance treatment in recently manic or hypomanic patients with bipolar I disorder. Arch Gen Psychiatry 2003;60:392-400.
65. Calabrese JR, Bowden CL, Sachs G, et al, for the Lamictal 605 Study Group. A placebo-controlled 18-month trial of lamotrigine and lithium maintenance treatment in recently depressed patients with bipolar I disorder. J Clin Psychiatry 2003;64:1013-1024.
66. Calabrese JR, Bowden CL, Sachs G, et al, for the Lamictal 602 Study Group. A double-blind placebo-controlled study of lamotrigine monotherapy in outpatients with bipolar I depression. J Clin Psychiatry 1999;60:79-88.
67. Weisler RH, Kalali AH, Ketter TA, for the SPD417 Study Group. A multicenter, randomized, double-blind, placebo-controlled trial of extended-release carbamazepine capsules as monotherapy for bipolar disorder patients with manic or mixed episodes. J Clin Psychiatry 2004;65:478-484.
68. Weisler RH, Keck PE, Swann AC, et al. Extended-release carbamazepine capsules as monotherapy for acute mania in bipolar disorder: a multicenter, randomized, double-blind, placebo-controlled trial. J Clin Psychiatry 2005;66:323-330.
69. Gitlin M. Treatment-resistant bipolar disorder. Mol Psychiatry 2006;11:227-240.
70. Tohen M, Vieta E, Calabrese J, et al. Efficacy of olanzapine and olanzapine-fluoxetine combination in the treatment of bipolar I depression. Arch Gen Psychiatry 2003;60:1079-1088.
71. Tohen M, Ketter TA, Zarate CA, et al. Olanzapine versus divalproex sodium for the treatment of acute mania and maintenance of remission: a 47-week study. Am J Psychiatry 2003;160:1263-1271.
72. Tohen M, Greil W, Calabrese J, et al. Olanzapine versus lithium in the maintenance treatment of bipolar disorder: a 12-month, randomized, double-blind, controlled clinical trial. Am J Psychiatry 2005;162:1281-1290.
73. Sachs G, Sanchez R, Marcus R, et al, for the Aripiprazole Study Group. Aripiprazole in the treatment of acute manic or mixed episodes in patients with bipolar I disorder: a 3-week placebo-controlled study. J Psychopharmacol 2006;20:536-546.
74. Keck PE Jr, Calabrese JR, McQuade RD, et al, for the Aripiprazole Study Group. A randomized, double-blind, placebo-controlled 26-week trial of aripiprazole in recently manic patients with bipolar I disorder. J Clin Psychiatry 2006;67:627-637.
75. McQuade R, Sanchez R, Marcus R, et al. Aripiprazole for relapse prevention in bipolar disorder: a 26-week placebo controlled study. Int J Neuropsychopharmacol 2004;7(Suppl 2):S161.
76. Calabrese JR, Keck PE, Macfadden W, et al. A randomized, double-blind, placebo-controlled trial of quetiapine in the treatment of bipolar I or II depression. Am J Psychiatry 2005;162:1351-1360.

54

PSYCHOSIS AND SCHIZOPHRENIA

Steven J. Siegel, Mary E. Dankert, and Jennifer M. Phillips

OVERVIEW 797
INTRODUCTION 797
Diagnostic Criteria for Schizophrenia 797
Types of Schizophrenia 798
PATHOPHYSIOLOGY 799
Genetic and Environmental Contributions 799
Genetic Vulnerability 799
Environmental Factors 799
Neuropathology 799
Physical Abnormalities 801
Behavioral Models of Schizophrenia 801
Physiologic Abnormalities 801
Gating of Event-Related Potentials 801
THERAPEUTICS AND CLINICAL PHARMACOLOGY 801
Goals of Therapy 801
Pharmacologic Targets 802
Positive Symptoms 802
Negative Symptoms 802
Cognitive Deficits 803
Motor Manifestations 803
Antipsychotics 804
Historical Development of Antipsychotic Medication 804
Clozapine 804
Therapeutic Approach 805
Emerging Targets and Therapeutics 812
NMDA Agonists 812
Nicotinic Agents 812
Phosphodiesterase Inhibitors 812
erbB Antagonists 812
Nonadherence to Treatment 812
SUMMARY 813

OVERVIEW

Schizophrenia is among the most devastating of all illnesses, affecting approximately 1% to 2% of the world population. Age of onset is generally between 20 and 30 years, with a chronic, unremitting disease course for the duration of the patient's life. Schizophrenia is characterized by two main symptom clusters, termed *positive symptoms* and *negative symptoms*, as well as lasting cognitive and functional disability. Positive symptoms include hallucinations, delusions, and disorganized, often bizarre thoughts and behavior. Negative symptoms include loss of interest and motivation, as well as loss of normal ability to both feel and express emotion. Lasting functional decline is a hallmark of the illness leading to the enormous personal, familial, and societal costs due to disability and lost productivity.

Although there have been effective medications for the positive symptoms of schizophrenia since the mid-1950s, there has been relatively little progress on effective treatments for the negative, cognitive, and functional domains. Recent large-scale multicenter studies and meta-analyses demonstrate that newer, formerly called atypical, medications have had little impact on improved efficacy, tolerability, or compliance with treatment. Additionally, nonadherence to existing medications significantly complicates treatment because the majority of patients do not take medication consistently. Future treatments will focus on both new mechanisms of action and improved delivery systems to target unmet needs in schizophrenia.

INTRODUCTION

This chapter addresses historical and current approaches to the treatment of schizophrenia. Although schizophrenia remains among the most severe and debilitating illnesses known to medicine, its treatment has remained virtually unchanged for over 50 years due to a lack of significant advances in our understanding of pharmacologic targets. This is in part due to a lack of adequate animal models and preclinical screening tools to identify biologic, mechanistic, or molecular therapeutic targets that will address the pathophysiology of negative symptoms and cognitive deficits. Major concepts in this chapter include the use of dopamine receptor type 2 (D_2) antagonists for the treatment of psychosis. Additionally, the limitations of the concept of "typical" versus "atypical" classifications for antipsychotic drugs is reviewed. The final portion of the chapter discusses several promising areas for future therapeutic advances, including improved drug delivery strategies that have the potential to effect rapid and dramatic improvements in schizophrenia outcomes.

Diagnostic Criteria for Schizophrenia

Like all psychiatric diagnoses, schizophrenia remains a behaviorally defined illness. Diagnostic criteria for schizophrenia, according to the Diagnostic and Statistical Manual of Mental Disorders, Fourth Edition, Text Revision (DSM-IV-R), include a constellation of positive and negative symptoms coupled with duration of greater than 6 months, significant disability, and a lack of other, obvious causes[1] (Fig. 54-1).

Positive symptoms are named for the presence of behaviors that should not be present. These include

1. Hallucinations—false sensory experiences that may occur in all modalities
2. Delusions—fixed false beliefs that are inconsistent with the individual's cultural beliefs
3. Disorganization—can include thoughts, speech, and behavior

Negative symptoms are named for the lack of normal behaviors or capabilities. These include

1. Alogia—decreased speech
2. Anhedonia—lack of emotion
3. Asociality—lack of normal social interactions or drive
4. Avolition or amotivation—lack of desire to do things and lack of action
5. Affective flattening—lack of facial expression and normal body language

An individual must have at least two positive symptoms (hallucinations, delusions, disorganization) or one positive symptom and one negative symptom (alogia, anhedonia, asociality, avolition, affective flattening) to meet the so-called A criterion for the illness. There are, however, two symptoms that can fulfill this criterion alone. One is bizarre delusions, defined as beliefs that are not possible (e.g., "an alien is living inside my head directing my behavior") as opposed to thoughts that are unlikely albeit possible (e.g., "the police and CIA are tapping my phone and following me around"). The other symptom that can fulfill Criterion A alone is a running commentary of voices, which typically consists of an auditory hallucination that announces the

Diagnostic Criteria for Schizophrenia

Criteria A - Positive and negative symptoms: At least 2 of the following:

1. Delusions (bizarre delusions alone are sufficient)
2. Disorganization (behavior, speech, or thought process)
3. Hallucinations (a voice commenting or voices conversing is sufficient)
4. Negative symptoms (alogia, anhedonia, asociality, avolition, affective)

Criteria B - Social or Occupational Decline: The person demonstrates a marked decline in function with either loss of previous milestones or failure to progress to expected level. For example, patients may experience dropping out of school, inability to work, or inability to care for home and family despite previously normal development.

Criteria C - Duration: Criteria A and B must be present for at least 6 months. Following treatment, positive symptoms may be diminished or disappear. Negative symptoms and functional decline generally persist during treatment.

FIGURE 54-1 • Criteria for schizophrenia according to the DSM-IV-R.[1]

individual's thoughts and movements in real time or two or more voices conversing with each other.

An important distinction that is often overlooked by clinicians regards the difference between hallucinations and ruminations. Hallucinations are best defined as true sensory experiences, indistinguishable from the sensation from real external stimuli. For example, many patients deny hallucinations, rather stating that they have developed extraordinary hearing that enables them to overhear conversations through walls or over great distances. The sensation can then become positive reinforcement for delusions of superior hearing or mind reading as well as providing content for other delusional beliefs. Alternatively, "hearing thoughts in one's head" that are distinct from true sensory experiences are best regarded as ruminations and should not be ascribed to abnormalities in the perceptual domain.

In addition to the symptomatic criteria, there are requirements for both sufficient duration and disability to justify a diagnosis of schizophrenia. The functional requirement for schizophrenia is designated Criterion B. In order to receive a diagnosis of schizophrenia, a person must display social or occupational decline as evidenced by a marked decline in function with either loss of previous milestones or failure to progress to an expected level. For example, patients may drop out of school or develop inability to work or to care for their home and/or family despite previously normal development. To meet criteria for schizophrenia, the symptoms (Criterion A) and disability (Criterion B) must also be present for a sufficient duration to rule out less severe or temporary conditions. The duration requirement, Criterion C, is operationally defined as a period of at least 6 months. If the individual is successfully treated with medication, positive symptoms may be diminished or disappear during this interval. However, negative symptoms and functional decline generally persist during treatment.

Types of Schizophrenia

Schizophrenia is a heterogeneous illness with a great deal of variation in both the presentation and severity. In recognition of this variability, four categories have been defined by the relative weight of different symptom clusters (paranoid, catatonic, disorganized, and undifferentiated) and a fifth category is defined by late stage of illness (residual). The *paranoid* type is characterized by a relative prominence of delusions and/or severe hallucinations without severe disorganization, catatonia, or negative symptoms. All domains may be present, but the most severe dimensions in this type of schizophrenia are hallucinations and delusions. The paranoid type is thought to have a good outcome relative to other types. This may reflect a more benign form of illness or unique neurobiology and etiology. Alternatively, it likely reflects the fact that current medications are effective for hallucinations and delusions but do little for catatonia or negative symptoms. Thus, paranoid schizophrenia is a form of the illness that is marked by treatable symptoms and thus may appear more benign.

The *catatonic* type is a relatively severe form of schizophrenia that is characterized by catalepsy or immobility with waxy flexibility; echolalia or echopraxia (reflexive repetition of words or motions of another person); purposeless motor activity; negativism or resistance to physical or verbal directions; maintenance of a rigid, inappropriate posture; mutism; stereotopies or repetitive purposeless movements; and grimacing. At least two of these behaviors must be present to meet criteria for catatonic schizophrenia, and the extent to which catatonic symptoms exist is variable across the course of illness. Unlike other symptoms of schizophrenia, catatonia is often responsive to benzodiazepines. However, once the effects of the medication wear off, the catatonia returns until the underlying cause is addressed. Thus it is crucial to recognize that catatonia can be a manifestation of many illnesses. For example, it is difficult to diagnose schizophrenia during the catatonic phase, because catatonia itself can also be a manifestation of depression. If depression is the underlying cause, then electroconvulsive therapy is often required. The diagnosis of schizophrenia must generally be made during a nonmute/noncatatonic period.

The *disorganized* type of schizophrenia is intermediate in severity and prognosis between the relatively benign paranoid type and more severe catatonic type. Disorganized schizophrenia is characterized by prominence of disorganized behavior and speech in the presence of flat or inappropriate affect. The fourth category of schizophrenia is called *undifferentiated* type due to a lack of prominence of any single symptom constellation in the presence of sufficient symptoms to meet the threshold for schizophrenia. The final category, *residual* type, is orthogonal to the previous groups in that it is marked by the absence of prominent positive symptoms, due to treatment or late stage of illness, in the presence of negative symptoms and disability. Thus this form of schizophrenia is in fact defined by the dimensions of schizophrenia that are amenable to current treatment modalities. As noted earlier, most antipsychotic medications diminish positive symptoms such as hallucinations, delusions, and disorganization but are not effective for negative symptoms and thus do little to restore function.[2]

Although not part of the formal DSM-IV-R scheme, there is an additional dimension called deficit syndrome that can be added as a modifier to the aforementioned categories based on prominence of negative symptoms.[3-5] The deficit category is defined as prominent negative symptoms that cannot be attributed to depression or medication side effects.[3] Thus individuals with this constellation of symptoms display relatively isolated lives in the absence of significant motivation, interpersonal contacts, emotional connection, or role functioning. This modifier has been particularly useful in that the presence of the deficit syndrome has both functional and prognostic significance.

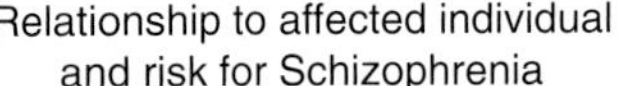

Several studies have suggested that the presence of deficit syndrome is predictive of poor outcome.[2,6,7]

PATHOPHYSIOLOGY

Approximately 1% of people develop schizophrenia. Unlike many psychiatric disorders that are defined by cultural norms, the incidence and expression of schizophrenia is remarkably constant throughout the world and across time. This observation led schizophrenia to be among the first of the psychiatric disorders to be recognized as a neurologic or brain disorder. Although the distinction between a brain disorder and psychological disorder seems antiquated today, most psychiatric disorders were not recognized as having concrete biologic substrates until the last quarter century.

Genetic and Environmental Contributions

Genetic Vulnerability

Approximately 50% of the risk for schizophrenia can be ascribed to genetic factors. This assertion comes from familial and adoption studies that show that the risk for schizophrenia is proportional to an individual's relationship to an affected patient. For example, there is a 1% prevalence for the disorder in the general population. This risk is increased 10-fold if one has a single first-degree relative who is already diagnosed. For example, the risk for developing schizophrenia is 10% if either parent or a sibling is affected. There is no additional risk conferred if that sibling is a dizygotic twin. However, if a monozygotic twin develops the illness, the relative risk is 50, suggesting fully half of the risk is conferred by sharing the same genome. Similarly, there is a 50% risk of developing schizophrenia if both parents are affected, again supporting the idea that receiving 100% of your genetic material from affected individuals results in 50% risk of illness. There is a proportional dilution affect such that nieces, nephews, and grandchildren of affected patients have approximately 2% to 5% risk, again reflecting approximately one quarter to one half of the risk of a first-degree relation[8] (Fig. 54-2).

Despite this consistent evidence that genes contribute to the vulnerability to schizophrenia, identifying specific genes that confer risk has been more elusive. A variety of genes have been linked to increased risk, but few are replicated in independent samples and none accounts for more than a minimal increase in risk relative to other alleles.[9] A review by Prathikanti and Weinberger provides an overview of this topic in more detail.[10] Several candidate genes and pathways have been implicated, but much needs to be done to validate and replicate these findings before definitive statements can be made regarding specific genetic risks.

Environmental Factors

A variety of environmental factors have also been shown to add minimal to modest increased risk for schizophrenia. Among these factors, most have yielded mixed results across studies, again suggesting that no one factor reliably increases risk. For example, several studies have suggested that prenatal infections may increase risk.[11] These studies generally rely on very slight increase in the prevalence of the disease among offspring that were born following an influenza epidemic. However, approximately as many studies fail to find this association.[12-15] Similarly, prenatal stress has been suggested as a risk for schizophrenia. These studies include increased prevalence among people born during war or if there is a death of the father during gestation.[16-19] Prenatal nutrition and length of gestation have also been implicated as risks, as evidenced by isolated findings of increased incidence among children born during famine or with premature births.[20,21] Some of these factors can be traced to an individual (premature birth, death of the father during gestation), but most cannot (famine, influenza epidemic, war). This hinders the ability to link specific cases with identifiable risk exposure. Other environmental factors that increase risk include being born in winter months or in an urban setting.[22]

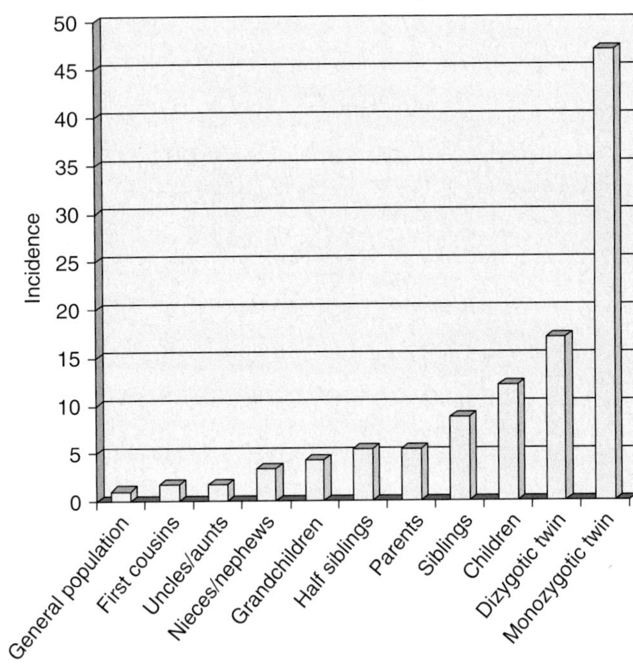

FIGURE 54-2 • The incidence of schizophrenia varies in proportion to the degree of genetic similarity with an affected individual. For example, the relative risk for developing the disorder increases 2-fold for first cousins, uncles, and aunts; 5-fold for grandchildren; 10-fold for siblings and other first-degree relatives; and 50-fold for monozygotic twins.[8]

Neuropathology

"Schizophrenia is the graveyard of neuropathologists."[23]

This quote characterized neuroanatomic studies of schizophrenia for the first half of the 20th century.[23,24] However, this former period of scientific quiescence in psychiatry gave way to the current explosion of biologic research, led in part and perhaps best exemplified by schizophrenia research. Initial neuroanatomic findings were limited to the observation of enlarged ventricles in schizophrenia. Although this remains the most consistent and replicable finding in the field, it lacks specificity. Subsequent studies have elucidated some possible mechanisms of this increased ventricle-to-brain ratio, including smaller neuron size and decreased neuron counts in select brain regions.[23] However, with this explosion of research, the lack of data that characterized the early 20th century has been supplanted by a gross excess of findings without either replication or a coherent sense of how these myriad findings fit together. Thus, the challenge for the early 21st century is no longer to find abnormalities, but to separate the proverbial chaff from the wheat and determine which findings are real, and which will persevere to form a meaningful piece of the puzzle. Several high-quality reviews have attempted to bring order to small subsets of the data. For example, a review by David Lewis and colleagues argues convincingly that there is a selective decrease in a subset of γ-aminobutyric acid (GABA)ergic interneurons that express the calcium binding protein parvalbumin.[25] These cells are notable for sending their axons to the axon initial segment of neocortical pyramidal cells in layer 4, thus having the potential to act as gatekeepers for the cortical output from a specific cortical region or column[26] (Fig. 54-3).

Additionally, this subset of parvalbumin-containing neurons has the highest proportion of *N*-methyl-D-aspartate (NMDA) receptors relative to other GABAergic cell classes as defined by their calcium binding proteins.[27] Thus there has been a convergence of this line of neuroanatomic research with one of the major pharmacologic, neurotransmit-

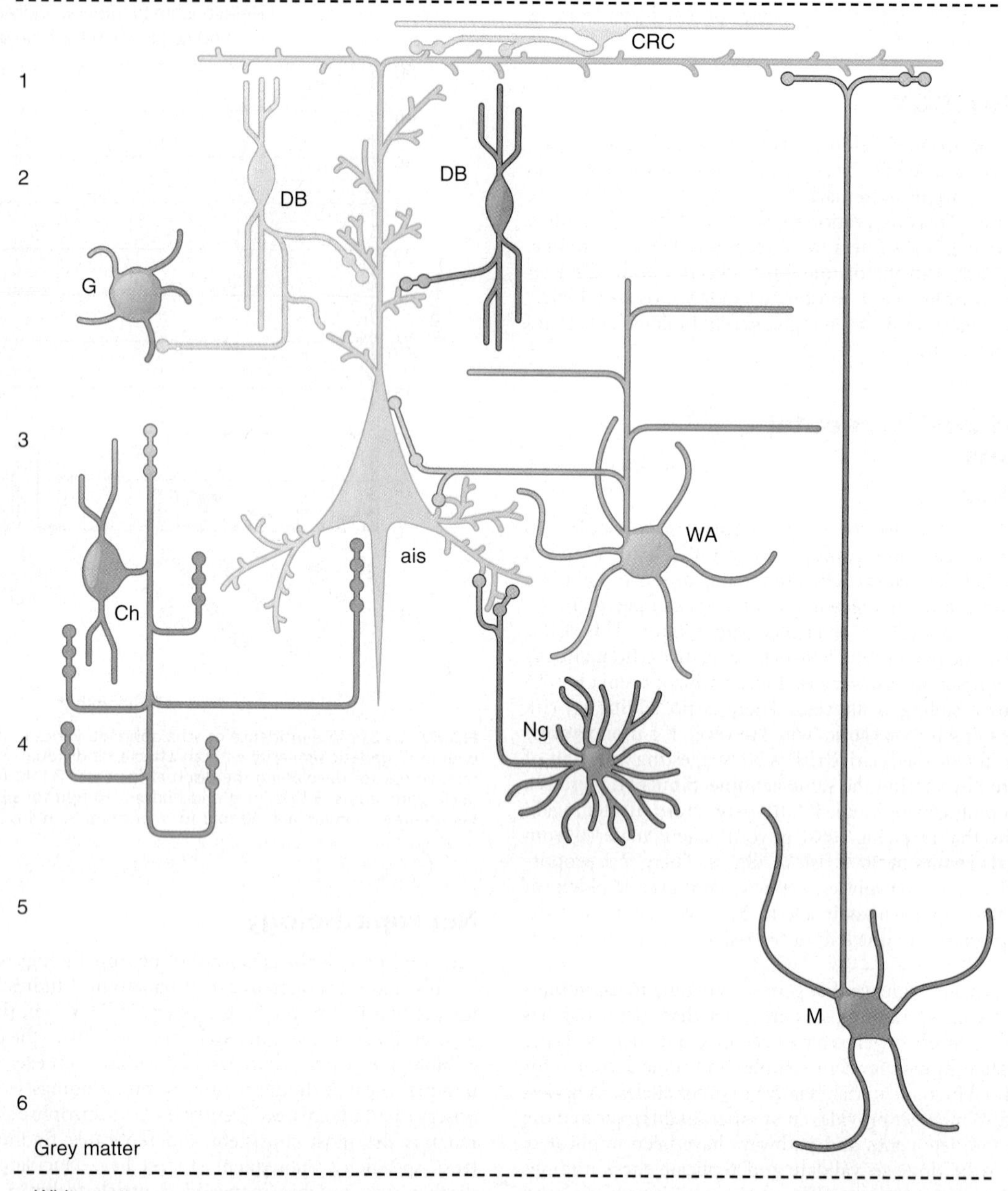

FIGURE 54-3 • Morphologic and biochemical features of subpopulations of cortical GABA neurons in the dorsolateral prefrontal cortex. The diagram illustrates the calcium-binding proteins parvalbumin (*blue*), calbindin (*red*), and calretinin (*yellow*) and the locations of inhibitory synaptic inputs to a pyramidal neuron (*green*) by different morphologic classes of cortical γ-aminobutyric acid (GABA) neurons. The chandelier (Ch) and wide arbor (WA) or basket neurons provide inhibitory input to the axon initial segment (ais) and the cell body proximal dendrites, respectively, of pyramidal neurons. By contrast, the calbindin-expressing double bouquet (red DB), neurogliaform (Ng), and Martinotti (M) neurons tend to provide inhibitory inputs to the distal dendrites of pyramidal neurons. Finally, calretinin-expressing (yellow) DB and Cajal-Retzius cell (CRC) neurons appear to target both pyramidal cell distal dendrites and other GABA (G) neurons. *1-6*, Layers of dorsolateral prefrontal cortex. (Adapted from Lewis DA, Volk DW, Hashimoto T. Selective alterations in prefrontal cortical GABA neurotransmission in schizophrenia: a novel target for the treatment of working memory dysfunction. Psychopharmacology (Berl) 2004;174:143-150.)

ter-based theories of schizophrenia, namely the NMDA receptor hypofunction theory of schizophrenia. This line of studies has postulated that people with schizophrenia have a reduction in NMDA-type glutamate-mediated transmission. These theories were initially based on the observation that NMDA antagonists such as phencyclidine and ketamine result in behavioral, cognitive, and physiologic profiles similar to those seen in schizophrenia. Subsequent studies have extended this line of research with anatomic studies of NMDA receptors in postmortem brains and genetic studies to examine the genes for proteins involved in the NMDA receptor–mediated signal transduction.[28] Among these, the genes for neuregulin-1 and dysbindin have been among the most promising to date.[28,29] However, as noted earlier, genetic studies thus far have only been able to account for a very small amount of the variance for developing schizophrenia, and few have been replicated across populations.[10] In this respect, the dysbindin association is perhaps the most consistent. However, mutations in this gene result in muscular dystrophy rather than schizophrenia-like syndromes, complicating interpretation of the genetic findings. Alternatively, functional studies in postmortem brains show increased neuregulin-1 activity in schizophrenia.[28] Neuregulin-1 is thought to inhibit NMDA receptor–mediated glutamate transmission.[30] Therefore, increased neuregulin-1 activity is among the most promising mechanistic leads for beginning a molecular or mechanistic understanding of schizophrenia.

Physical Abnormalities

Several studies have demonstrated that physical abnormalities in schizophrenia may extend beyond brain anatomy. For example, minor physical anomalies are thought to include facial asymmetry, cleft palate, hair whorls, abnormal palmar crease, furrowed tongue, flat occiput, and primitive shape of ears.[31-34] One study found that 60% of schizophrenia patients and 38% of their siblings, but only 5% of control subjects, had a high rate of minor physical anomalies (i.e., six or more).[35] Several investigators have concluded that minor physical anomalies are an indirect index for early prenatal central nervous system maldevelopment, suggesting that schizophrenia results at least in part from neurodevelopmental damage.[36,37] Furthermore, some studies have suggested that this relationship is most noticeable for males.[38,39]

Behavioral Models of Schizophrenia

Sensorimotor gating is a basic neural process in which a weak sensory stimulus (sound) causes the inhibition of a subsequently elicited motor response. This process has been proposed as a heuristic model for the ability of a person to automatically filter out extraneous sensory information.[40] Reduced sensorimotor gating has been observed in several psychiatric disorders, including but not limited to schizophrenia.[41] Sensorimotor gating deficits are particularly relevant to the study of schizophrenia, however, because the ability of a drug to increase sensorimotor gating in some rodent models predicts the clinical efficacy of medications used to treat positive symptoms.[42] Some investigators have also suggested that symptoms experienced by patients with schizophrenia may result, in part, from the inability to filter sensory information.[43] There is also a high degree of conservation across species for neuronal processes involved in sensorimotor gating.[40,42] Therefore, mouse and rat models have been used to study gating using a task called prepulse inhibition of acoustic startle, in which the presentation of a nonstartling acoustic stimulus (prepulse) inhibits the startle response elicited by a later startling stimulus. The extent to which an animal inhibits the subsequent startle response is thought to reflect the animal's ability to filter or gate sensory information.[42] These studies suggest that several neurotransmitter systems, including dopamine, serotonin, and glutamate, regulate sensorimotor gating, indicating convergence on a common mechanism or pathway.[43]

Physiologic Abnormalities

Several endophenotypic markers of schizophrenia are viewed as potential biologic intermediaries linking the clinical diagnosis to its underlying neurobiologic substrates. Auditory event-related potentials (ERPs) are among the most extensively studied endophenotypic markers of schizophrenia.[44-50] In these studies, an auditory stimulus evokes a series of electroencephalographic (EEG) responses corresponding to progression of brain activity throughout the auditory pathway. Early components (below 10 msec) originate in the cochlea and auditory nuclei of the brainstem, while midlatency components, including a positive deflection at approximately 50 msec in humans (P50), reflect activation of the auditory thalamus and auditory cortex.[48,51,52] Longer latency components, including a negative deflection at approximately 100 msec in humans (N100), have been localized to the primary auditory cortex and cortical association areas.[53] Abnormalities in the P50 and N100 components are postulated to reflect abnormal neuronal architecture related to the generation and modulation of auditory responses, and may be informative about more generalized neurologic impairments in schizophrenia.[54,55]

Gating of Event-Related Potentials

Many ERP studies in schizophrenia have utilized a series of paired clicks to assess brain mechanisms of sensory processing. In these tasks, the amplitude of the EEG response to the first stimulus is larger than the response to the second. Although this approach has been extensively applied to study the P50 component, it should be noted that multiple components, including N100, also decrease in amplitude following the second stimulus.[48,56-59] Several studies indicate that unmedicated schizophrenia patients have reduced amplitude of the P50 component following the first stimulus in a paired click task, with resulting loss in gating of the second stimulus.[46,47] Although this finding has been replicated in some studies of patients treated with antipsychotic medications, other studies indicate that antipsychotic treatment results in an increased amplitude for both the first and second responses, maintaining the loss of gating.[44,46,60] This profile of equal amplitude of response to the first and second stimuli has been conceptualized as impaired gating.[55] Importantly, nicotine has been shown to restore gating among medicated schizophrenia patients. Some studies have attributed this effect to a reduction in the second response, while others indicate that nicotine acts primarily to increase the amplitude of the first[61-63] (Fig. 54-4).

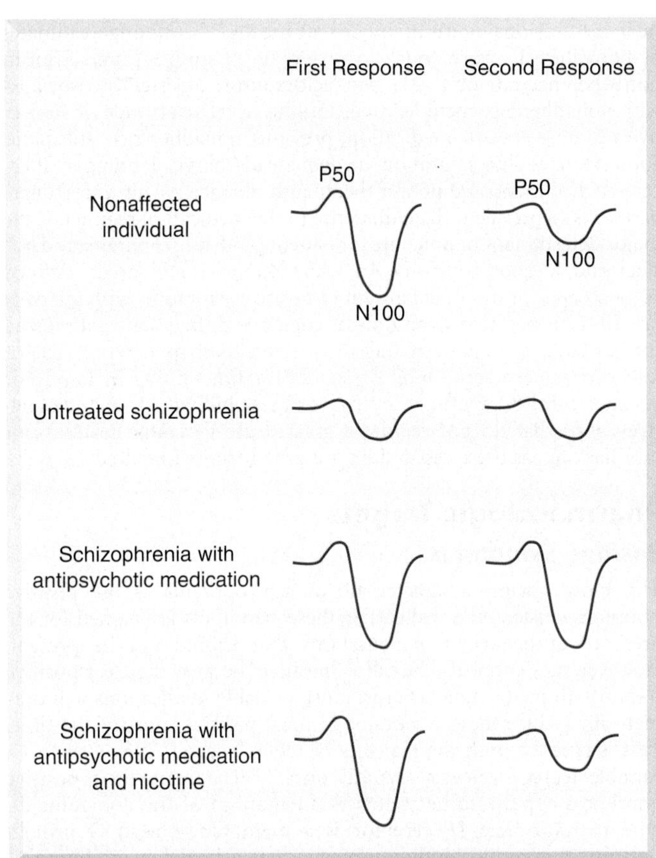

FIGURE 54-4 • Schematic representation of schizophrenia phenotypes for the P50 and N100 responses. A, The normal pattern of P50 and N100 responses in nonaffected individuals. Note that the first response is large and the second is decreased. **B,** In unmedicated schizophrenia, both the first and second responses are diminished for the P50 and N100 components. **C,** Antipsychotic treatment results in increased amplitude of both the first and second responses for the P50 and N100 components among schizophrenia patients, yielding the pattern of normal amplitude with impaired gating often described among medicated patients. **D,** Nicotine reduces the amplitude of the second response among medicated schizophrenia patients.[63]

THERAPEUTICS AND CLINICAL PHARMACOLOGY

Goals of Therapy

The term *therapeutic goal* in schizophrenia must unfortunately be divided into "realistic goals" and "idealized or eventual goals." Using current treatments, therapy for schizophrenia can realistically be expected to reduce positive symptoms in about 70% of patients, most of the time.[64] This will usually be complicated by very low adherence rates in schizophrenia such that up to 70% to 90% of patients take their medications intermittently or erratically.[65-67] Although estimates of nonadherence vary widely, a review of 39 studies found a mean nonadherence rate of 41.2%, and factors most consistently associated with nonadherence included poor insight, negative attitude or subjective response toward medication, previous nonadherence, substance abuse, shorter illness duration, inadequate discharge planning or aftercare environment, and poorer therapeutic alliance.[68] This unfortunate pattern is so prevalent that adherence to the medication regimen is the major determinant of outcome for patients with schizophrenia today.[69] That said, a "good" outcome for schizophrenia is still largely defined as an absence or minimal amount of positive symptoms with virtually no effect on negative symptoms or cognitive difficulties, as discussed further later. A small percentage of patients, perhaps 10% to 15% or less, can achieve some level of significant functioning in family or vocational roles.[70] Optimal settings for these individuals include low-stress jobs that do not require a great deal of mental flexibility or multitasking, as these capabilities are usually quite impaired.

Pharmacologic Targets

Positive Symptoms

The most obvious characteristic of schizophrenia is the positive symptom cluster. As noted earlier, these symptoms are named for the presence of behaviors or sensations that should not be present. However, they could also be called "positive" because there is a positive response to medication. That is, most available medications will dramatically reduce these symptoms in most patients most of the time. This is true for both the majority of older, "typical" agents and to a variable degree for newer "atypical" ones.[71,72] The treatment of positive symptoms appears to be related to antagonism of the dopamine D_2 type receptor. The D_2 receptor is a membrane-bound G protein (guanine nucleotide–binding proteins) that is linked to inhibition of adenylyl cyclase through its alpha subunit. When dopamine binds to this receptor subtype, it leads to a cascade of events that decrease adenylyl cyclase activity, which in turn decreases cyclic adenosine monophosphate (cAMP) formation and reduces activation of protein kinase A (cAMP-dependent protein kinase). This in turn reduces phosphorylation of many intracellular substrates, including ion channels and DNA-binding proteins. Thus, in the presence of a D_2 receptor antagonist, this process is reduced and there is an increase in intracellular cAMP and its downstream effects. There have been some limited efforts to recapitulate this effect using novel receptor-independent mechanisms, including inhibition of the enzymes that degrade cAMP (Fig. 54-5). These are limited thus far to basic science studies using animal models of schizophrenia.[73] However, these efforts have not yielded therapeutic interventions thus far.

Preclinical screening tools for the development of new medications have relied heavily on behaviors and systems that detect D_2 antagonism. These models include blocking the effects of either direct dopamine agonists such as apomorphine or indirect agonists such as amphetamine on locomotor activity, prepulse inhibition of startle response, or ERPs, to name just a few.[42,43,73,74] These models have yielded a high degree of positive predictive validity for identifying compounds that effectively reduce positive symptoms. However, there appears to be little predictive value in these approaches for the treatment of negative symptoms.

Negative Symptoms

Early claims for new antipsychotic medications (those introduced since the early 1990s) included improved efficacy for negative symptoms.[75] However, these claims have not been substantiated over time.[72,76] These newer drugs were formerly called "atypical" antipsychotic medications for a variety of reasons, including proposed efficacy for negative symptoms. However, the use of this definition of atypicality has diminished due to a number of studies that found no difference between older and new medications for negative symptom domains. The term *primary negative symptom* refers to the reduction in normal emotion, motivation, and action that is due to the illness. This is dis-

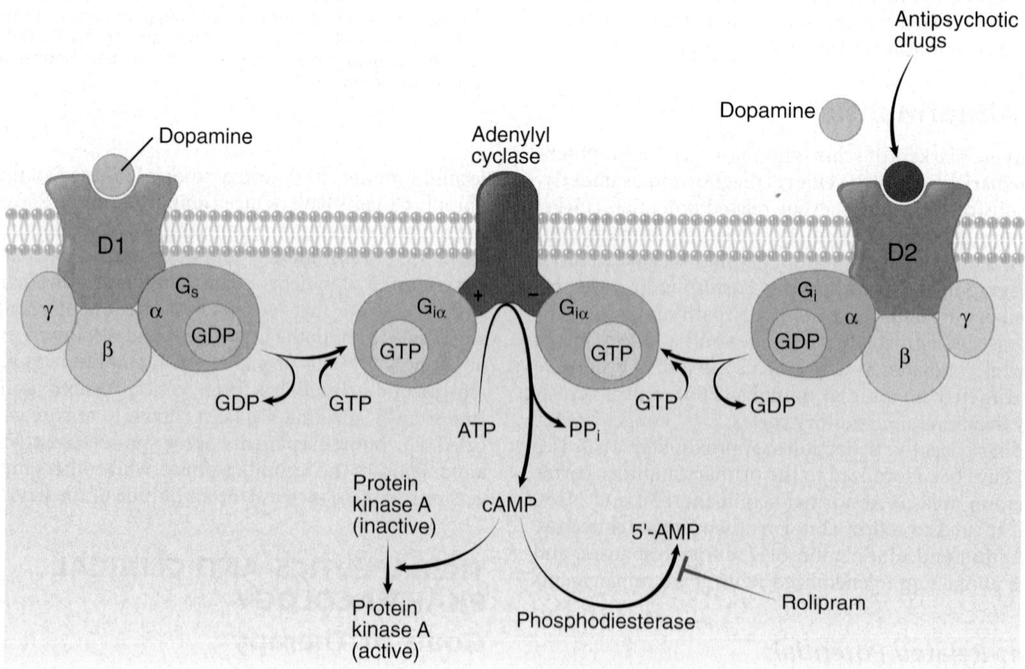

FIGURE 54-5 • All currently available antipsychotic medications act by reducing dopamine signaling at the G_i-coupled dopamine D_2 receptor. When dopamine binds this receptor, it activates an inhibitory G protein alpha subunit, which reduces the baseline activity of adenylyl cyclase with a subsequent reduction in cAMP formation. In the presence of a D_2 antagonist, dopamine is less able to reduce intracellular cAMP, leading to increased cAMP-mediated processes, including activation of protein kinase A (PKA). Recent preclinical studies have examined the idea that phosphodiesterase inhibitors, which block degradation of cAMP, could achieve a similar end point of increasing cAMP concentration and PKA activation. For example, one study demonstrated antipsychotic-like properties of the phosphodiesterase inhibitor rolipram using auditory evoked potentials in mice.[111]

tinguished from secondary, or medication-induced, negative symptoms that have been postulated to result from excessive doses of antipsychotic medication leading to either motor abnormalities (stiffness) or sedation. As doses have been lowered with changing standards of practice over the past 20 years, these difficulties have become less prominent. Since this change in practice style has been coincident with the availability of new medications, it has been difficult to parse the benefits of lower doses from inappropriately ascribing reduced side effects to improved medications.

This lack of efficacy for the negative symptom domain may reflect a loss of brain substrates that are necessary for normal emotional and motivated behaviors by the time the diagnosis is made. Alternatively, preclinical screening tools that have historically isolated D_2 antagonists may simply not be assessing the relevant neurobiologic and pharmacologic targets for negative symptoms. This argument becomes circular as we have no agents that improve negative symptoms in humans and therefore no mechanism to validate positive predictive value for any animal models or targeted therapeutic approach. However, this gap in current preclinical screening tools for therapeutic approaches to social and emotional deficits is starting to be addressed. For example, mouse models for abnormal social behaviors are now being developed and validated to identify drug candidates and genes related to negative symptoms in schizophrenia and other human illnesses[77,78] (Fig. 54-6). Similarly, current medications have little or no effect on other aspects of schizophrenia, such as cognitive deficits, that contribute to the lifelong disability.[70,79]

Cognitive Deficits

The DSM-IV-R definition captures the most obvious manifestations of schizophrenia, but does not address other aspects that have emerged as important therapeutic targets and determinants of outcome. For example, schizophrenia is marked by profound cognitive disabilities that leave patients unable to perform many simple tasks or maintain vocational or role-appropriate function (employment, student, or homemaker).[80,81] This has become an area of intense research and clinical interest in recent years. Despite earlier claims that new medications had superior effect on cognitive outcome, this assertion has not been substantiated.[79] The National Institutes of Health (NIH) and the U.S. Food and Drug Administration have attempted to address this gap in therapeutic development by sponsoring a consensus panel. This panel, entitled Measurement and Treatment Research to Improve Cognition in Schizophrenia (MATRICS), was created to define cognitive domains, tasks, and targets for future drug development.[82-84] The MATRICS initiative is intended to provide a framework to standardize criteria for assessing cognitive function and therefore for demonstrating cognitive improvement.[83] However, there is still no clear consensus that the MATRICS battery will be adopted among pharmaceutical companies that may favor faster, more automated computerized batteries that offer increased reliability, standardization across clinical sites, and ease of use. Such batteries are being rapidly developed in a variety of settings, with some made freely available[80] (Fig. 54-7).

Motor Manifestations

Although antipsychotic medication treatment can cause motor impairments such as stiffness (discussed later), schizophrenia itself can include abnormalities in coordination and movement.[85] These problems can be subtle, requiring a neurologic exam to reveal, or grossly apparent in the form of tardive dyskinesia (TD).[86] TD is a late-onset, age-dependent emergence of abnormal movements.[87] The incidence of TD increases with age, such that approximately 40% of schizophrenia patients will exhibit TD by 60 years of age.[88] One of the greatest misconceptions in psychiatry today is that antipsychotic medications cause TD. However, there is irrefutable evidence that TD is actually part of the illness rather than a manifestation of treatment. This evi-

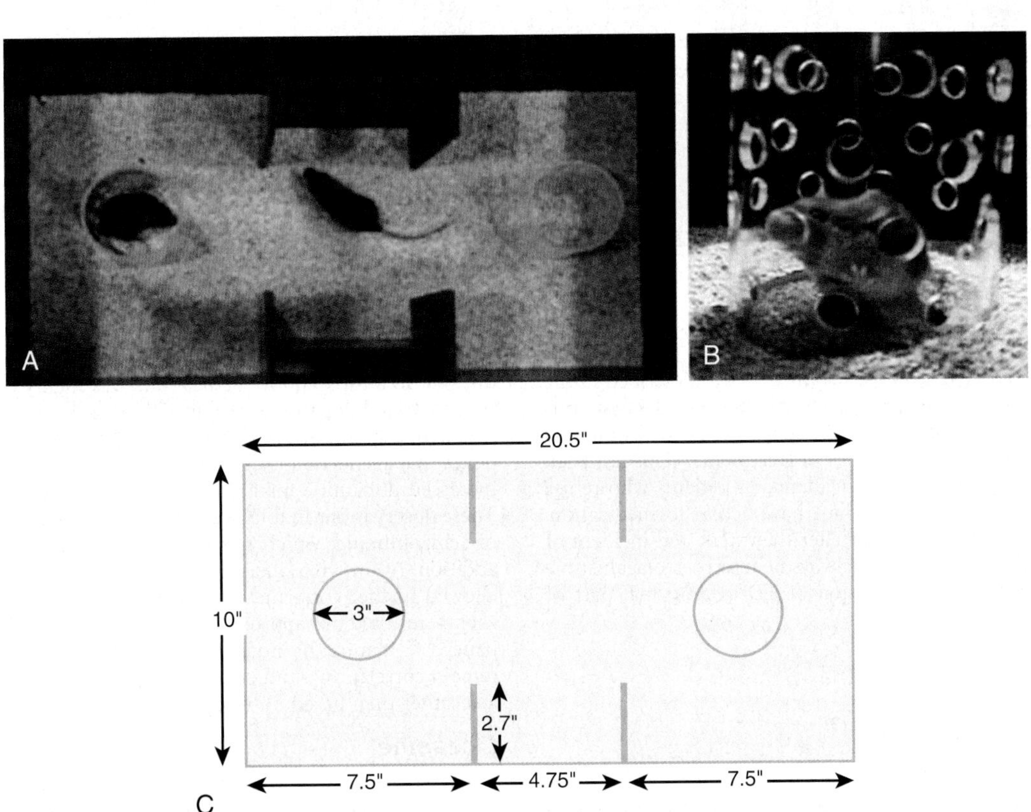

FIGURE 54-6 • Behavioral testing apparatus. A, The social approach-avoidance testing apparatus viewed from above. There is a clear Plexiglass cylinder in each of the two end chambers, and the center chamber is empty. Prior to the start of each test, one of the end chambers was arbitrarily designated the "social side" (the side into which the stimulus mouse would be introduced), and the other end chamber was designated the "nonsocial side." **B,** Multiple small holes are evenly spaced over the entire surface of the cylinders in each end chamber. **C,** Dimensions of the behavioral testing apparatus. (**A** provided by Dr. E. Brodkin.)

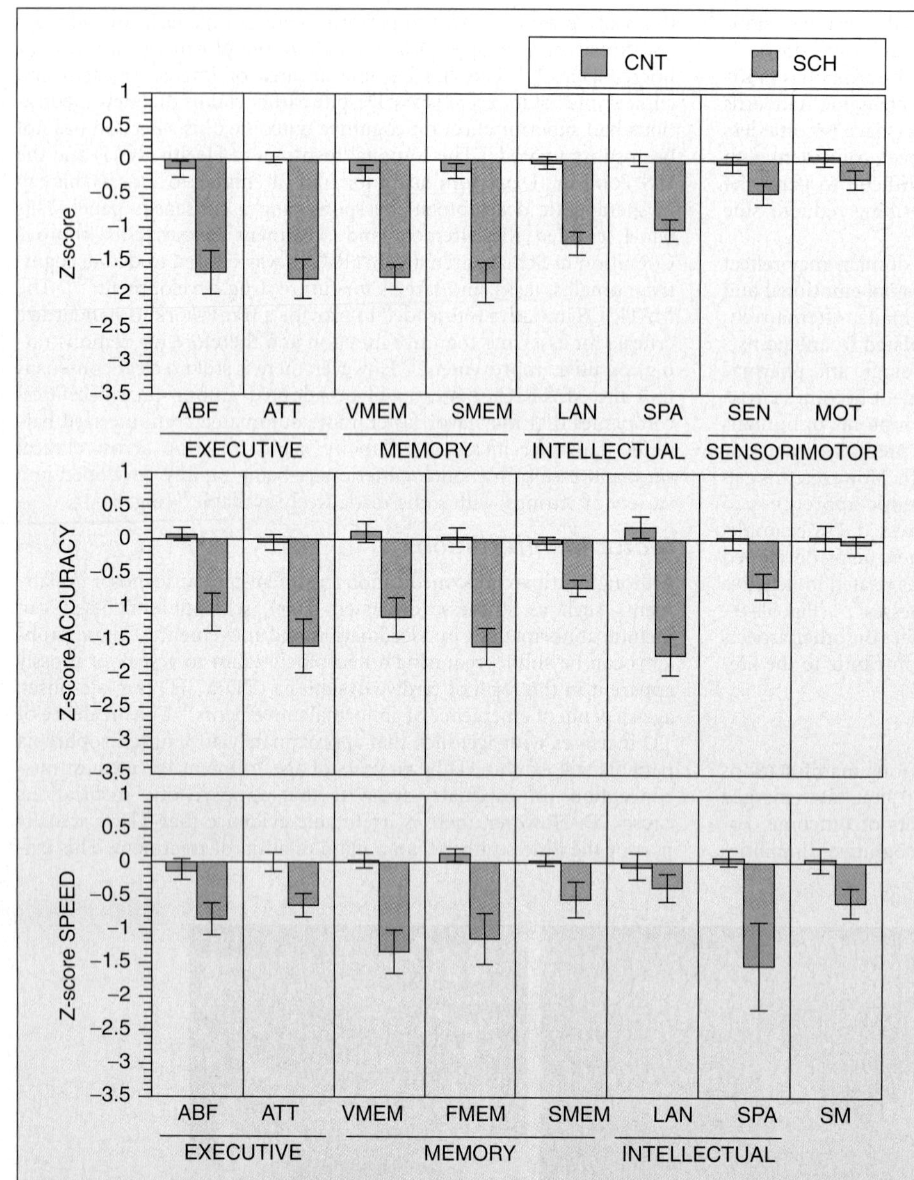

FIGURE 54-7 • The neurocognitive profile of patients with schizophrenia and healthy controls (means ± SEM) on the traditional battery (*top bar*) and the computerized scan accuracy (*middle*) and speed (*bottom*).[80]

dence includes the fact that TD in schizophrenia was described in the late 19th century, over 50 years prior to the discovery of the first antipsychotic medication, and that approximately 40% of schizophrenia patients will develop TD in the absence of treatment.[88] This has been demonstrated both by observing its incidence in patients who refuse treatment and in countries that do not have access to medication. There is evidence that treatment may alter the extent and incident of TD risk; however, these studies must always be interpreted against the background of age-emergent expression of TD as a normal part of schizophrenia.

Antipsychotics

Historical Development of Antipsychotic Medication

The use of medicine for the treatment of schizophrenia dates back to 1952 with the serendipitous observation that chlorpromazine yielded symptomatic improvement when given as a preanesthetic agent.[89-91] This was followed by the empirical discovery of other chemical entities with similar therapeutic effects. Approximately 10 years later, a seminal article by Seeman and colleagues documented that the clinically derived dose of all antipsychotic medications was highly correlated with the IC_{50} at striatal dopamine receptors[92,93] (Fig. 54-8).

A similarly important discovery resulted from complimentary evidence that agents that improved psychosis in schizophrenia resulted in increased dopamine metabolites in brain and cerebrospinal fluid.[94,95] These observations in total were the basis for the dopamine hypothesis of schizophrenia, which remains as valid today as it was then. The addition of in vivo imaging with positron emission tomography allowed further confirmation that therapeutic doses of antipsychotic agents resulted in approximately 70% to 80% D_2 receptor occupancy.[96,97] It must be noted, however, that all of these observations remain correlations, and dose finding for these medications is empirical rather than based on receptor affinity.

Clozapine

The next major advance in the treatment of psychosis resulted from the observation by John Kane and colleagues that clozapine appeared to have superior efficacy as compared with other agents among a population of treatment-resistant patients.[98] One notable feature of this medication was that it also appeared to achieve significant improvement without the typical motor side effects seen with most other agents. This lack of motor side effects at therapeutic doses led to the

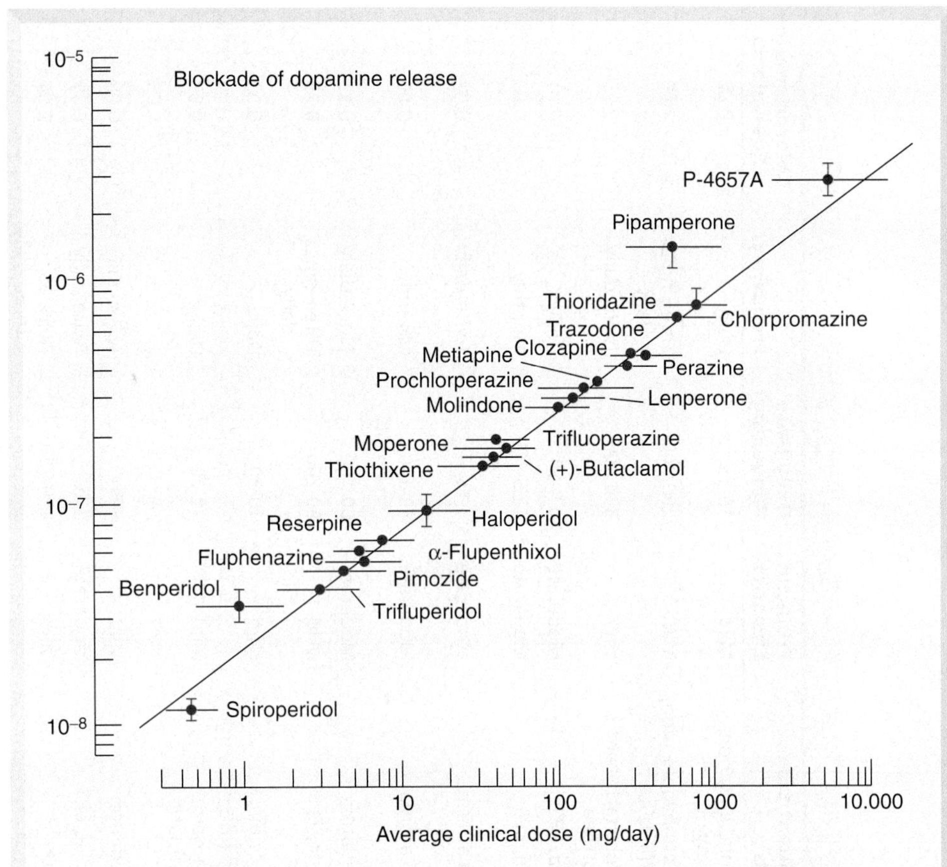

FIGURE 54-8 • The neuroleptic IC_{50} values (the neuroleptic concentrations that inhibited the stimulated release of dopamine by 50%) correlate with the average clinical doses (in milligrams per day) for controlling schizophrenia. The horizontal bars indicate the range of clinical doses. The vertical bars show the 20% variation in the IC_{50} values. The correlation includes such diverse compounds as phenothiazines, butyrophenones, reserpine, pimozide, trazodone, clozapine, and (+)– butaclamol. *Trans*-thiothixene (P-4657A) is of the order of one-hundredth the potency of its *cis*-isomer.[111]

term *atypical antipsychotic* for clozapine. Unfortunately, the term *atypical* medication took on broader meaning as it was applied to newer medications over time. For example, many theories have been put forward to suggest why clozapine displays efficacy without the same degree of dopamine blockade as other drugs. However, a close inspection of the data presented in the landmark Seeman and Lee article[92] clearly shows that clozapine sits squarely on the same correlation line as all other drugs for dopamine blockade and dose. Thus, the observation is more accurately stated that clozapine appears to have a lower degree of motor side effects despite the same level of dopamine blockade as other medications.

Much attention was then placed on decomposing the receptor binding profile for clozapine to discover which receptor binding properties might contribute to the relative lack of motor side effects. This led to the initial hypotheses that the ratio of serotonin type 2 to dopamine type 2 receptor binding was a key feature of atypicality.[99-101] However, this theory has failed to yield any medications that match clozapine in efficacy. Additionally, chlorpromazine (the first antipsychotic medication) actually meets this and many other definitions of "atypicality" since it has significant serotonin type 2 and dopamine type 2 binding at clinical doses.[102] A number of other theories have been put forward in an attempt to retain the idea that newer medications are categorically, mechanistically, or clinically distinguished from older ones. For example, one theory posits that "atypical" agents have less prolactin elevation than typical ones.[103] However, risperidone, which is considered atypical, has among the highest prolactin elevation among all antipsychotic medications, and chlorpromazine, the original agent, has only moderate increases.[104-107]

Similarly, several authors have hypothesized that "atypical" agents might improve cognition.[108] However, several studies have not found cognitive benefits for newer agents over older ones, and a recent large-scale comparison of newer agents versus the "typical" agent perphenazine showed that the older, typical agent showed a slight but significant advantage over newer drugs for cognitive improvement.[79,109,110] Other definitions have similarly failed to distinguish any classlike properties among older (pre-risperidone) and newer (risperidone and newer) agents. Table 54-1 provides a summary of antipsychotic agents available in the United States, and Table 54-2 lists the receptor affinity for a subset of these medications.[111]

Therapeutic Approach

There is little consensus regarding the best approach to choosing antipsychotic medication. Some experts have advocated the use of newer medications based on early reports that these agents had either therapeutic benefit or reduced side effects. However, the purported benefit of these agents in a subset of industry-sponsored clinical trials has been disputed by some clinicians, who fail to see any meaningful distinction based on the nomenclature of "typical" for older off-patent agents and "atypical" for newer on-patent agents. The one caveat to this controversy is the widely held belief that clozaril remains unparalleled in its efficacy. However, it is also unparalleled in side effect burden and logistic difficulty for both the patient and physician. These factors—side effects and logistics—together continue to cause the gross underutilization of clozapine among patients who could benefit from its superior efficacy. Several large meta-analyses and clinical trials have now shown that clozapine remains superior to all other agents, with small advantages for olanzapine and risperidone over older medications for some domains and small advantages for older medication over all newer ones on other domains[71,72,76,110] (Fig. 54-9).

Therefore, the main factor in choosing a medication is generally matching of side effect liability with both patient and physician preferences and risk tolerance. For example, a number of medications that work well for positive symptoms, such as haloperidol and risperidone, have a relatively high risk of causing motor side effects such as stiffness and tremor as well as a feeling of restlessness called akathisia. However,

TABLE 54-1 LIST OF ANTIPSYCHOTIC MEDICATIONS

Medication	Category	Class	Metabolism	Prominent Side Effects	Prolactin Elevation	Daily Dose Range (mg)	Frequency	Chlorpromazine Equivalents
Aripiprazole	Newer	Quinolinone	CYP2D6, 3A4	Insomnia, agitation, anxiety	Mild	10-15	Daily	0.02
Chlorpromazine	Older	Phenothiazine	CYP2D6	Sedation, hypotension, shuffling gait	Mild	200-800	Three times daily	1.00
Clozapine	Older	Dibenzodiazepine	CYP1A2, 2D6, 3A4	Sedation, tachycardia, sialorrhea	Low	300-600	Twice daily	0.75
Fluphenazine	Older	Phenothiazine	CYP2D5	Nausea, EPS	Moderate	0.5-10	Daily	0.01
Fluphenazine decanoate	Long-acting	Phenothiazine with 10-carbon ester linkage	CYP2D6	Nausea, EPS	Moderate	12.5-100 per month	Monthly	0.00
Haloperidol	Older	Butyrophenone	CYP2D6, 3A4; 2D6 inhibitor	EPS, akathisia	Moderate	1-15	Twice daily	0.02
Haloperidol decanoate	Long-acting	Butyrophenone with 10-carbon ester linkage	CYP2D6, 3A4	EPS, akathisia	Moderate	50-100 monthly	Monthly	0.00
Loxapine	Older	Dibenzodiazepine	CYP enzyme unknown	EPS, sedation	Moderate	60-100	Twice daily	0.13
Molindone	Older	Dihydroindolene	CYP enzyme unknown	Sedation, EPS	Mild	50-200	Three times daily	0.25
Olanzapine	Newer	Thienobenzodiazepine	CYP1A2, 2D6, 2C18	Weight gain, constipation	Mild	10-20	Daily	0.03
Olanzapine—rapidly dissolving	Newer	Thienobenzodiazepine	CYP1A2, 2D6, 2C19	Weight gain, constipation	Mild	10-20	Daily	0.03
Perphenazine	Older	Phenothiazine	CYP2D6	EPS, sedation	Mild	8-64	Twice daily	0.08
Pimozide	Older	Diphenylbutylpiperidine	CYP1A2, 3A4	Akathisia, EPS	Moderate	2-10	Twice daily	0.01
Quetiapine	Newer	Dibenzothiazepine	CYP3A4	Sedation	Mild	150-750	Twice to three daily	0.94
Risperidone	Newer	Benzisoxazole	CYP2D6	EPS, hypotension, hyperprolactinema	Severe	1-4	Daily	0.01
Risperidone microspheres	Long-acting	Risperidone in PLGA microspheres	CYP2D6	EPS, hypotension, hyperprolactinema	Severe	25-50 every 2 wk	Bimonthly	0.00
Thioridazine	Older	Phenothiazine	CYP2D6	Sedation, dry mouth, constipation	Mild	200-800	Twice to three daily	1.00
Thiothixene	Older	Thioxanthene	CYP enzyme unknown	Akathisia, EPS	Moderate	4-15	Twice daily	0.02
Trifluoperazine	Older	Phenothiazine	CYP enzyme unknown	Hypotension, EPS	Moderate	4-10	Twice daily	0.01
Ziprasidone	Newer	Benzothiazolylpiperazine	CYP3A4	Sedation, headache	Mild	80-160	Twice daily	0.20

CYP, cytochrome P-450; EPS, extrapyramidal symptoms.

TABLE 54-2 RADIOLIGAND-INDEPENDENT DISSOCIATION CONSTANTS

	D2*	D4*	5-HT$_{2A}$*	D$_2$:5-HT$_{2A}$ Ratio	D$_2$:D$_4$ Ratio
Chlorpromazine	0.66 ± 0.05 (12)	1.15 ± 0.04 (9)	3.5 ± 0.06 (9)	0.19	0.58
Clozapine	44 ± 8 (27)	1.6 ± 0.4 (96)	11 ± 3.5 (9)	4.00	28.00
Fluphenazine	0.32 ± 0.03 (7)	50 ± 10 (11)	80 ± 19 (6)	0.004	0.0064
Haloperidol	0.35 ± 0.05 (18)	0.84 ± 0.05 (54)	25 ± 8 (5)	0.014	0.42
Molindone	6 ± 3 (9)	2400 ± 800 (11)	5800 ± 1300 (6)	0.001	0.0025
Olanzapine	3.7 ± 0.6 (12)	2 ± 0.4 (22)	5.8 ± 0.7 (14)	0.64	1.85
Quetiapine	78 ± 28 (13)	3000 ± 300 (14)	2500 ± 600 (5)	0.03	0.026
Risperidone	0.3 ± 0.1 (19)	0.25 ± 0.1 (17)	0.14 ± 0.1 (5)	2.14	1.2
Thioridazine	0.4 ± 0.12 (12)	1.5 ± 0.5 (16)	60 ± 15 (6)	0.007	0.27
Trifluoperazine	0.96 ± 0.2 (11)	44 ± 6 (11)	135 ± 50 (6)	0.007	0.022

*In nanomoles ± standard error (*n* experiments in duplicate).
From Seeman P, Corbett R, Van Tol HH. Atypical neuroleptics have low affinity for dopamine D2 receptors or are selective for D4 receptors. Neuropsychopharmacology 1997;16:93-110, discussion 111-135.

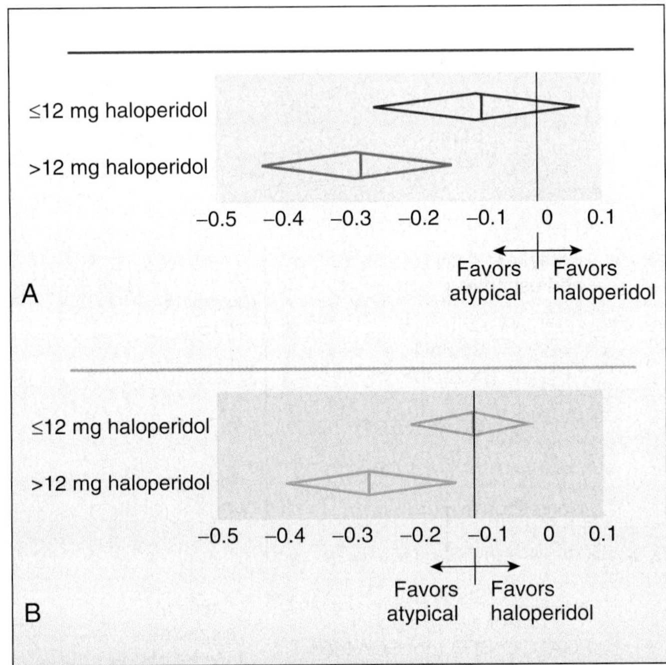

FIGURE 54-9 • **A,** Overall symptom score by dose of comparator drug in trials of patients with schizophrenia or related disorders (standardized weighted mean difference and 95% confidence intervals). **B,** Dropout rates by dose of comparator drug in trials of patients with schizophrenia or related disorders (risk difference and 95% confidence intervals).[72]

these risks can be dramatically reduced by the use of low doses (i.e., 3 to 4 mg/day of risperidone or 4 to 8 mg/day of haloperidol). Additionally, there are countermeasures, including the use of anticholinergic medications such as benztropine that block the manifestation, but not root causes, of motor side effects. There are two distinct approaches to the use of anticholinergic medication based on the physician's risk preferences. One approach favors starting without anticholinergic medication coadministration to minimize unnecessary exposure. In this strategy, one can warn the patient that he or she may experience stiffness or tremor, but that you will be able to give an "antidote" if this should occur.

The counter approach is to start anticholinergic medication immediately as prophylaxis, so as to minimize the chances that the patient will have an unpleasant experience. The latter approach leads to risk of anticholinergic side effects of dry mouth, constipation, and possibly cognitive impairment, which have sometimes then been inappropriately attributed to the antipsychotic medication. It also leads some clinicians to apply the strategy in concert with medications for which it is not indicted. For example, olanzapine has high affinity as an anticholinergic agent, likely accounting for its lower motor side effect risk. Therefore, additional anticholinergic medication is unlikely to be indicated. Conversely, olanzapine's liability is that it causes patients to lose their sense of satiety when eating, yielding increased appetite leading to weight gain, often of 20 pounds or more. Pharmacologic countermeasures for this unfortunate and potentially deleterious side effect include off-label use of appetite suppressants such as topirimate. However, this agent has its own serious side effects, including profound memory disturbances. Therefore the use of topirimate to counter the appetite problems with olanzapine is not recommended. This leaves only behavioral countermeasures such as diet and exercise. Although these measures are completely effective if used, patients with schizophrenia are no more likely to adhere to proper eating and physical activity programs than the general public, which is quite poor at both. Thus physicians still tend to use medications of habit, coupled with loose guidelines to avoid olanzapine in obese patients and avoid risperidone and other high-potency agents in patients with a history of or existing severe motor problems.

There have been few efforts to create an evidenced-based algorithm for initiation and maintenance of medication for schizophrenia. The only clear decision is that all patients need some form of medication all of the time. There has been one major initiative to provide guidelines for treatment. Although the Texas Algorithm was created prior to widespread realization that newer agents held little if any advantage over older ones, it does provide a strategy for treatment.[112] One possible concern with this algorithm is that it does not distinguish among more and less efficacious medications. Rather, this algorithm gives preference to newer medications that many practitioners would argue are actually less effective and have higher side effect liability than many older ones (Fig. 54-10).

To address this potential limitation in the Texas Algorithm, we propose an alternative algorithm based on clinical experience and the literature (Fig. 54-11). This algorithm is based on the following basic principles and hypotheses:

1. Clozapine is the most efficacious agent available, albeit one with many side effects that is difficult for patients to take.
2. There is a slight advantage for either risperidone or olanzapine over haloperidol and other older agents in large meta-analyses.
3. Other new antipsychotic medications do not offer substantial benefit and may actually be worse than older agents in some respects, including both efficacy and side effects.
4. Nonadherence to medication is the major cause of all treatment failures, so injectable long-acting agents should be used early in the therapeutic progression.

Text continued on p. 812.

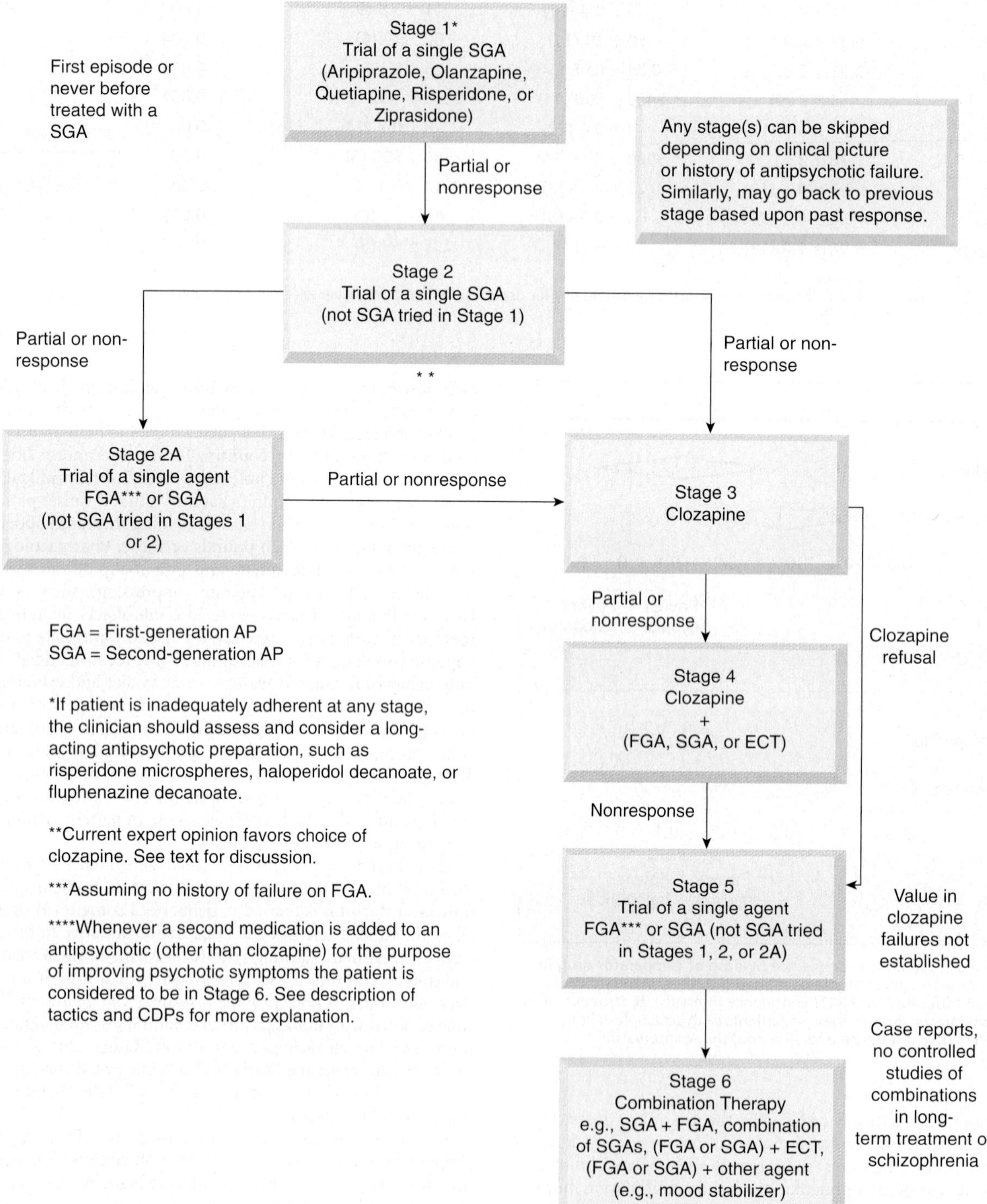

FIGURE 54-10 • Texas Algorithm. The Texas Algorithm has been among the first major efforts to operationalize treatment recommendations based on expert consensus. The major limitation to this approach is that it favors newer agents. The preponderance of data now clearly demonstrate that there is no benefit for efficacy, side effects, or tolerability of functional/cognitive outcome from new agents. Therefore, the tendency to start with more expensive, newer medications is unjustified by evidence-based practice principals.

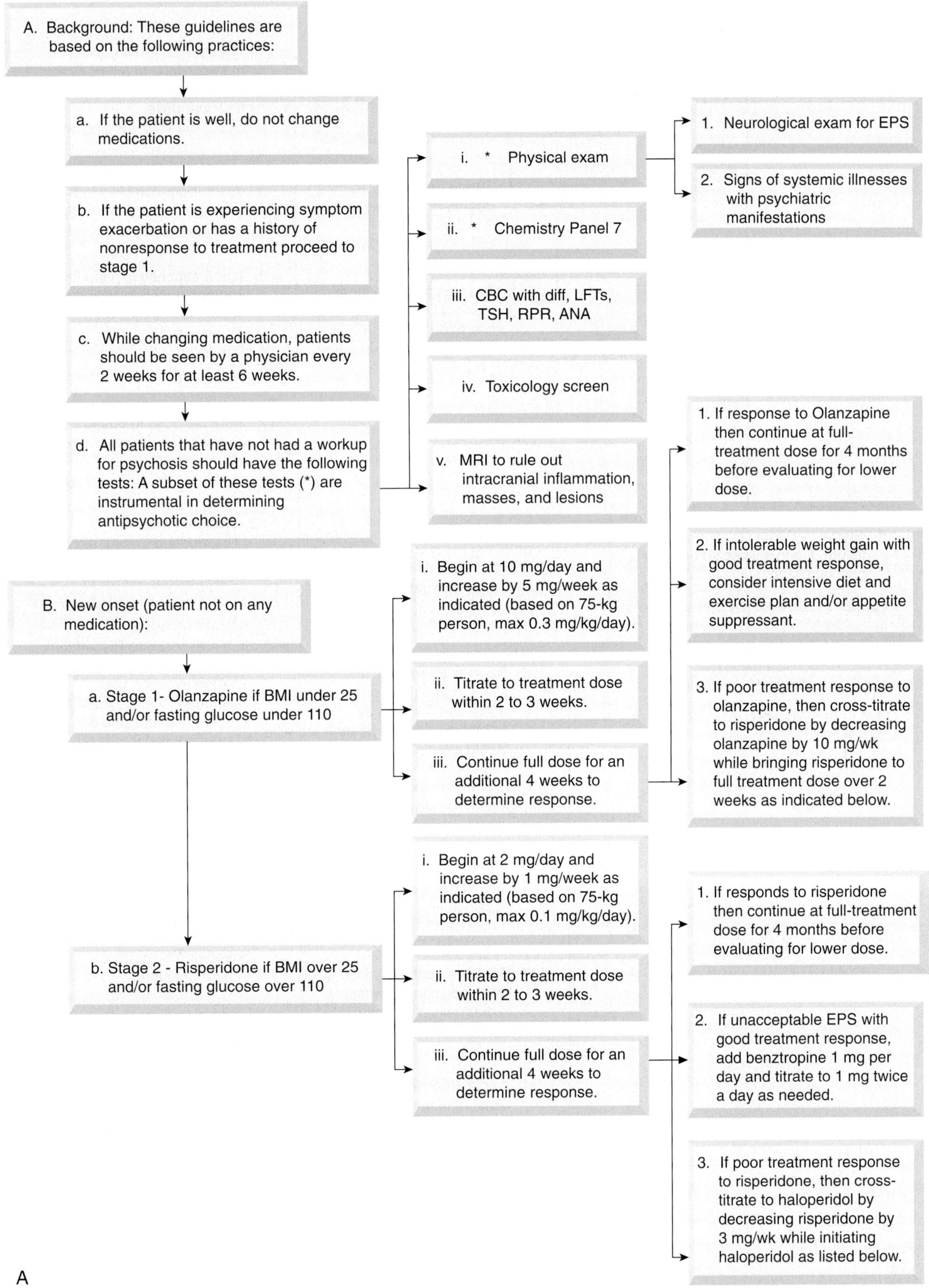

FIGURE 54-11 • Algorithm for antipsychotic treatment. The authors propose an algorithm for treatment that incorporates stage of illness (i.e., new onset or previously treated), prevailing risk factors (e.g., obesity, existing tremor), comorbid medical conditions (e.g., type 1 diabetes, cardiovascular disease), and patient behavior (e.g., compliance) to tailor treatment in a logical progression to achieve lowest risk and highest efficacy.

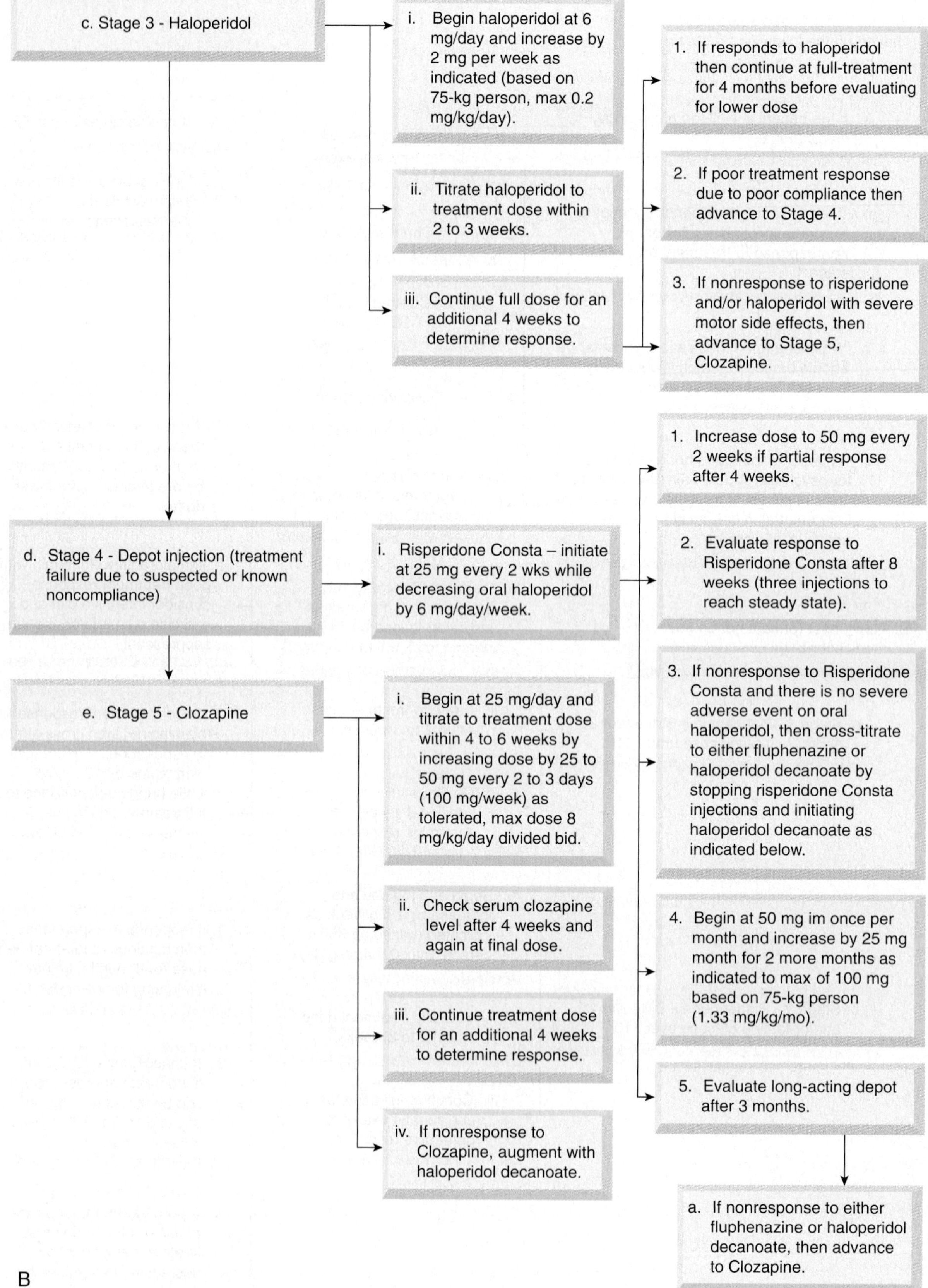

FIGURE 54-11, cont'd

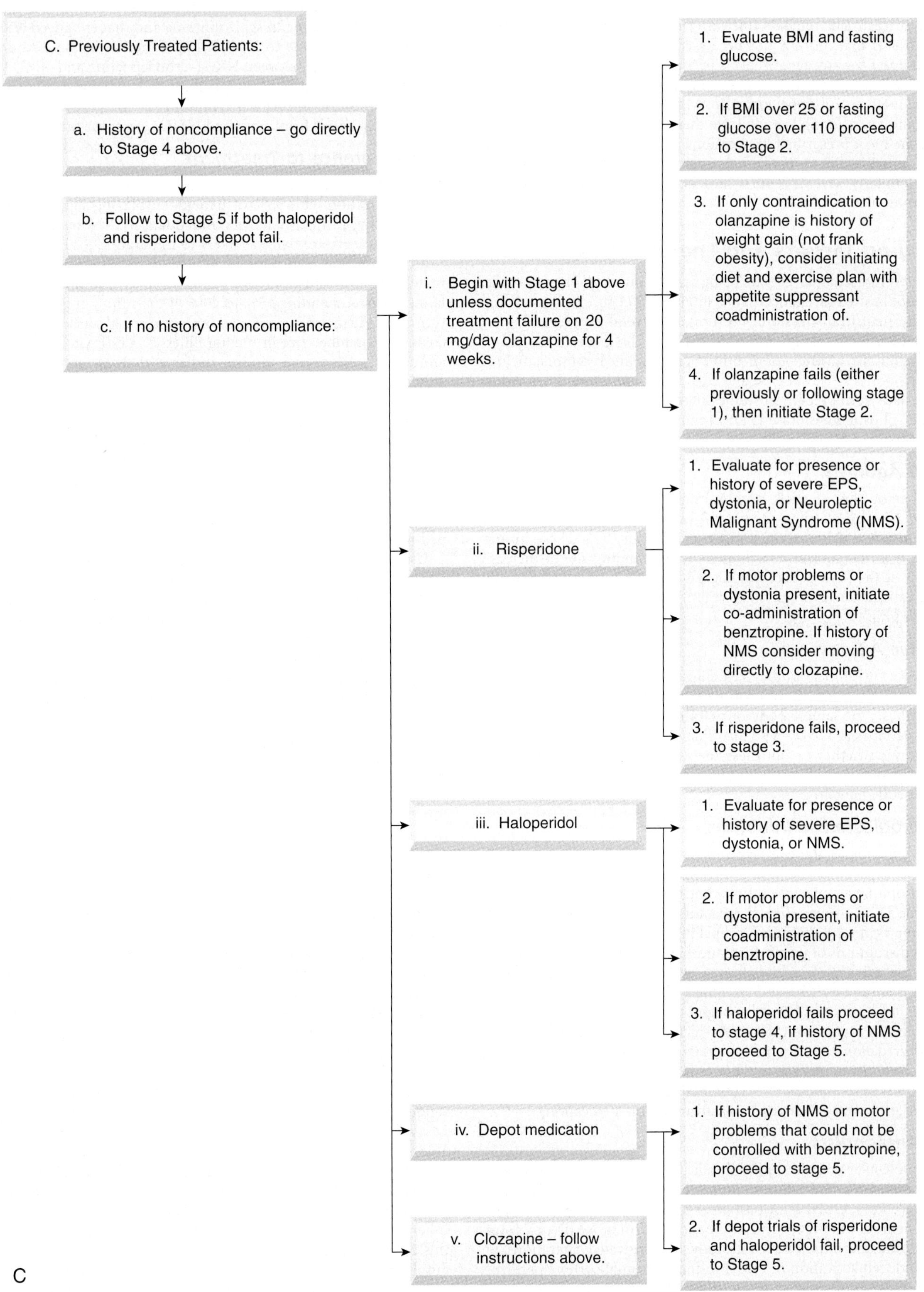

FIGURE 54-11, cont'd

Of note, aripirizole is relatively new at the time of this chapter, so its role in treatment remains unclear. Thus far, one observation that seems clear is that more is not necessarily better beyond the recommended doses for any agent. This is perhaps more true for aripirizole, which takes on characteristics of a full dopamine agonist above about 15 mg in a 60- to 70-kg person. Also, while many clinicians find quetiapine and ziprasidone less effective than other agents, quetiapine is among the most prescribed medications in psychiatry, largely outside of schizophrenia due to its relative paucity of side effects and calming nature. Similarly, several reports have suggested ziprasidone may be useful in bipolar psychosis.

Emerging Targets and Therapeutics

Several new molecular targets are being actively pursued. These include, but are not limited to, agents that facilitate NMDA receptor–mediated glutamate neurotransmission. Additionally, several investigators and pharmaceutical companies are investigating a possible role for full or partial agonists at a variety of nicotinic acetylcholine receptors, including the α_7 homomeric subtype and $\alpha_4\beta_2$ heteromeric receptors. Additionally, data from preclinical studies suggests that there may be a role for either phosphodiesterase (PDE) inhibitors or erbB antagonists in future treatment of schizophrenia.

NMDA Agonists

A number of clinical trials have examined the role for agents that facilitate NMDA receptor–mediated glutamate transmission. These agents include gylcine, serine, and D-cycloserine.[113-117] These amino acids bind to the allosteric facilitator glycine binding site to increase efficiency at the NMDA receptor. Despite being among the first truly novel treatments to emerge in 50 years, some data thus far has been disappointing.[115,118]

Nicotinic Agents

A number of preclinical studies have suggested that people with schizophrenia may have deficits in nicotinic acetylcholine receptor function. Among these, the largest body of literature has examined a possible role for agonists at the α_7-type nicotinic receptor.[119-122] Future studies will examine whether or not these theoretical links, based largely on electrophysiologic studies in animal models and patients, will translate to therapeutic benefit.

Phosphodiesterase Inhibitors

As noted previously, there are convergent lines of evidence suggesting impairments in intracellular cAMP regulation in schizophrenia. The observation that all effective antipsychotic medications antagonize the dopamine D_2 G protein–linked receptor, which itself inhibits cAMP formation, is among the most compelling of these arguments. Additionally, disruptions of cAMP formation in animals recapitulate many phenotypic markers of schizophrenia, including deficits in prepulse inhibition of startle, ERPs, and learning and memory problems.[74,123,124] However, recent studies have also begun to address alternative molecular targets to increase cAMP levels, including those responsible for cAMP degradation. For example, inhibitors of PDE, which degrade cAMP, have been shown to meet several key criteria as antipsychotic agents in preclinical animal models.[73,125] Thus PDE inhibitors may represent a new class of receptor-independent schizophrenia medications.

erbB Antagonists

Recent molecular genetic studies implicate neuregulin-1 (NRG1) and its receptor erbB in the pathophysiology of schizophrenia.[126,127] Among NRG1 receptors, erbB4 is of particular interest because of its crucial roles in neurodevelopment and in the modulation of NMDA receptor signaling. Furthermore, a recent study demonstrated alterations of NRG1-induced activation of erbB4 in the prefrontal cortex in schizophrenia using a postmortem tissue-stimulation approach.[28] This study found that NRG1 stimulation suppresses NMDA receptor activation in the human prefrontal cortex and that NRG1-induced suppression of NMDA receptor activation was more pronounced in schizophrenia subjects than in controls. These data suggest there may be enhanced NRG1-erbB4 signaling in schizophrenia and that enhanced NRG1 signaling may contribute to NMDA hypofunction in the disorder. This mechanistic linkage between NRG1-erbB signaling and NMDA receptor hypofunction further suggests that erbB antagonists may present a novel approach to alleviating symptoms or manifestations of schizophrenia that result from impaired NMDA receptor function.

Nonadherence to Treatment

Medication nonadherence is the major risk factor for relapse and rehospitalization with 55% of patients displaying significant difficulties adhering to treatment recommendations.[69] Nonadherent schizophrenia patients are twice as likely to undergo rehospitalization from relapse, resulting in a poor quality of life.[128] For example, approximately 50% of schizophrenia patients relapse within 1 year of their latest episode, spending 15% to 20% of their time in psychiatric institutions.[129] Furthermore, the economic and social burden of health care costs for nonadherence in mental illnesses is estimated at $2.3 billion annually.[130] Additional studies indicate that an actual medication adherence rate of 23% is in stark contrast to the patient-reported rate of 55%, while others find that as few as 12% of patients achieve 1 year of uninterrupted antipsychotic medication.[131,132] Although many studies report medication adherence rates of 50%, it is increasingly thought that such data may be skewed, as many patients cease medication treatment once outside clinical trials.[133] This was recently demonstrated in the NIH-sponsored Clinical Antipsychotic Trials of Intervention Effectiveness (CATIE), where 74% of patients discontinued their medication despite being in a clinical trial.[76]

Use of Depot Preparations. Previous approaches to improve adherence through parenteral administration were introduced in the mid-1960s and have proven effective.[134-137] Depot injections work well to deliver antipsychotic drugs over several weeks with enhanced efficacy over oral dosing.[138] However, limitations of depot formulations restrict more significant improvements in adherence and efficacy. For example, adverse effects are occasionally manifest and must be endured for the remainder of the treatment interval due to the inability to remove depot formulations. Prolonged pain often persists at repeated injection sites, leading many patients to cease treatment.[139] Decanoate formulations are further limited by chemistry, with many compounds unable to form the ester linkage needed to make prodrug molecules. Recently, PLGA microspheres have been used to administer a biweekly formulation of risperidone that does not require formation of a prodrug (Risperidone Consta; Janssen Pharmaceutica). Although this approach shows promise in controlled studies, injections must be administered biweekly, requiring 24 annual treatment decisions.[140,141] Despite early promise, it is not yet clear what effect such a short delivery interval will have on practical application of this technology since adherence rates in the real world are estimated to be substantially lower than those in well-funded, labor-intensive clinical trials.[142] Thus depot medications may not provide adequate sustained care to many patients.

Indications to Develop Antipsychotic Implants. To address the need for more sustained treatment adherence, new methods of long-term medication delivery have been investigated using implantable systems for the treatment of schizophrenia.[143-145] Implantable systems have the capability to optimize a medication's therapeutic properties, rendering treatments that are more safe, efficacious, and reliable.[146] Less medication is required and side effects can be minimized. Implantable systems can also be removed by a physician in case of adverse side effects, offering a degree of reversibility not available with depot injections. Additionally, mandatory removal at the end of the delivery interval is eliminated with biodegradable systems, cutting in half the inherent invasiveness to the patient.[147] Recent studies by the authors of this chapter also indicate that more than 40% of patients and 75% of family members favor implants as a mechanism to maintain long-term medication adherence and health[148] (M. Dankert, unpublished data). Thus long-term delivery systems that guarantee adherence to medication could offer a solution to the most intractable, yet addressable cause of poor outcomes in schizophrenia.

SUMMARY

Schizophrenia is among the most severe, debilitating, and devastating illnesses across all fields of medicine. It takes hold of an individual during late adolescence or young adulthood and dominates the remainder of his or her life course. Additionally, schizophrenia affects the patient's entire family and social structure due to the pervasive nature of disability and alternating course of remissions and exacerbations. Both genetic and environmental factors contribute to the risk for schizophrenia, although neither specific genes nor behaviors can be definitively linked to disease expression. All current medications treat the positive symptom cluster, including hallucinations, delusions, and disorganization. Unfortunately, none treats the negative or cognitive symptoms. Despite concerted efforts over the last 2 decades to create improved medications, it is now clear that antipsychotic medications have not changed in basic mechanism (dopamine D_2 receptor antagonism) since the invention of chlorpromazine in 1952. Accordingly, the prognosis for schizophrenia remains poor, with the majority of patients unable to fully integrate into either their former social or occupational roles. The future of medication development for schizophrenia remains unclear due to a dearth of well-established, validated targets. However, some efforts are focused on functional NMDA receptor agonists, nicotine receptor agonists, and modulators of intracellular cAMP levels. Additionally, interventions that increase adherence to medication, such as long-term delivery systems, are likely to have the greatest potential impact on improved outcome in schizophrenia in the near future.

REFERENCES

1. American Psychiatric Association. Diagnostic and Statistical Manual of Mental Disorders, Fourth Edition, Text Revision. Washington, DC: American Psychiatric Association, 2000.
2. Arango C, Buchanan RW, Kirkpatrick B, Carpenter WT. The deficit syndrome in schizophrenia: implications for the treatment of negative symptoms. Eur Psychiatry 2004;19:21-26.
3. Carpenter WT Jr, Heinrichs DW, Wagman AM. Deficit and nondeficit forms of schizophrenia: the concept. Am J Psychiatry 1988;145:578-583.
4. Wagman AM, Heinrichs DW, Carpenter WT Jr. Deficit and nondeficit forms of schizophrenia: neuropsychological evaluation. Psychiatry Res 1987;22:319-330.
5. Carpenter WT Jr. The deficit syndrome. Am J Psychiatry 1994;151:327-329.
6. Fenton WS, McGlashan TH. Antecedents, symptom progression, and long-term outcome of the deficit syndrome in schizophrenia. Am J Psychiatry 1994;151:351-356.
7. Mayerhoff DI, Loebel AD, Alvir JM, et al. The deficit state in first-episode schizophrenia. Am J Psychiatry 1994;151:1417-1422.
8. Gottesman I. Schizophrenia Genesis: The Origins of Madness. New York: Freeman, 1991.
9. O'Tuathaigh CM, Babovic D, O'Meara G, et al. Susceptibility genes for schizophrenia: characterisation of mutant mouse models at the level of phenotypic behaviour. Neurosci Biobehav Rev 2007;31:60-78.
10. Prathikanti S, Weinberger DR. Psychiatric genetics—the new era: genetic research and some clinical implications. Br Med Bull 2005;73-74:107-122.
11. Battle YL, Martin BC, Dorfman JH, Miller LS. Seasonality and infectious disease in schizophrenia: the birth hypothesis revisited. J Psychiatr Res 1999;33:501-509.
12. Cooper SJ. Schizophrenia after prenatal exposure to 1957 A2 influenza epidemic. Br J Psychiatry 1992;161:394-396.
13. Crow TJ, Done DJ. Prenatal exposure to influenza does not cause schizophrenia. Br J Psychiatry 1992;161:390-393.
14. Sham PC, O'Callaghan E, Takei N, et al. Schizophrenia following pre-natal exposure to influenza epidemics between 1939 and 1960. Br J Psychiatry 1992;160:461-466.
15. Kendell RE, Kemp IW. Maternal influenza in the etiology of schizophrenia. Arch Gen Psychiatry 1989;46:878-882.
16. van Os J, Selten JP. Prenatal exposure to maternal stress and subsequent schizophrenia: the May 1940 invasion of The Netherlands. Br J Psychiatry 1998;172:324-326.
17. Myhrman A, Rantakallio P, Isohanni M, et al. Unwantedness of a pregnancy and schizophrenia in the child. Br J Psychiatry 1996;169:637-640.
18. Huttunen MO, Niskanen P. Prenatal loss of father and psychiatric disorders. Arch Gen Psychiatry 1978;35:429-431.
19. Yaktin US, Labban S. Traumatic war: stress & schizophrenia. J Psychosoc Nurs Ment Health Serv 1992;30(6):29-33.
20. Smits L, Pedersen C, Mortensen P, van Os J. Association between short birth intervals and schizophrenia in the offspring. Schizophr Res 2004;70:49-56.
21. Boog G. Obstetrical complications and subsequent schizophrenia in adolescent and young adult offsprings: is there a relationship? Eur J Obstet Gynecol Reprod Biol 2004;114:130-136.
22. Freeman H. Schizophrenia and city residence. Br J Psychiatry Suppl 1994;(23):39-50.
23. Harrison PJ. The neuropathology of schizophrenia: a critical review of the data and their interpretation. Brain 1999;122(Pt 4):593-624.
24. Plum F. Prospects for research on schizophrenia. 3. Neurophysiology: neuropathological findings. Neurosci Res Program Bull 1972;10:384-388.
25. Lewis DA, Hashimoto T, Volk DW. Cortical inhibitory neurons and schizophrenia. Nat Rev Neurosci 2005;6:312-324.
26. Lewis DA, Volk DW, Hashimoto T. Selective alterations in prefrontal cortical GABA neurotransmission in schizophrenia: a novel target for the treatment of working memory dysfunction. Psychopharmacology (Berl) 2004;174:143-150.
27. Huntley GW, Vickers JC, Morrison JH. Quantitative localization of NMDAR1 receptor subunit immunoreactivity in inferotemporal and prefrontal association cortices of monkey and human. Brain Res 1997;749:245-262.
28. Hahn CG, Wang HY, Cho DS, et al. Altered neuregulin 1-erbB4 signaling contributes to NMDA receptor hypofunction in schizophrenia. Nat Med 2006;12:824-828.
29. Talbot K, Eidem WL, Tinsley CL, et al. Dysbindin-1 is reduced in intrinsic, glutamatergic terminals of the hippocampal formation in schizophrenia. J Clin Invest 2004;113:1353-1363.
30. Gu Z, Jiang Q, Fu AK, et al. Regulation of NMDA receptors by neuregulin signaling in prefrontal cortex. J Neurosci 2005;25:4974-4984.
31. Gourion D, Goldberger C, Bourdel MC, et al. Minor physical anomalies in patients with schizophrenia and their parents: prevalence and pattern of craniofacial abnormalities. Psychiatry Res 2004;125:21-28.
32. Sivkov ST, Akabaliev VH. Minor physical anomalies in schizophrenic patients and normal controls. Psychiatry 2003;66:222-233.
33. Trixler M, Tenyi T, Csabi G, Szabo R. Minor physical anomalies in schizophrenia and bipolar affective disorder. Schizophr Res 2001;52:195-201.
34. Guy JD, Majorski LV, Wallace CJ, Guy MP. The incidence of minor physical anomalies in adult male schizophrenics. Schizophr Bull 1983;9:571-582.
35. Ismail B, Cantor-Graae E, McNeil TF. Minor physical anomalies in schizophrenic patients and their siblings. Am J Psychiatry 1998;155:1695-1702.
36. Hata K, Iida J, Iwasaka H, et al. Minor physical anomalies in childhood and adolescent onset schizophrenia. Psychiatry Clin Neurosci 2003;57:17-21.
37. Green MF, Satz P, Soper HV, Kharabi F. Relationship between physical anomalies and age at onset of schizophrenia. Am J Psychiatry 1987;144:666-667.
38. Green MF, Satz P, Gaier DJ, et al. Minor physical anomalies in schizophrenia. Schizophr Bull 1989;15:91-99.
39. Firestone P, Peters S. Minor physical anomalies and behavior in children: a review. J Autism Dev Disord 1983;13:411-425.
40. Braff DL, Geyer MA, Light GA, et al. Impact of prepulse characteristics on the detection of sensorimotor gating deficits in schizophrenia. Schizophr Res 2001;49:171-178.
41. Braff DL, Grillon C, Geyer MA. Gating and habituation of the startle reflex in schizophrenic patients. Arch Gen Psychiatry 1992;49:206-215.
42. Swerdlow NR, Braff DL, Geyer MA. Animal models of deficient sensorimotor gating: what we know, what we think we know, and what we hope to know soon. Behav Pharmacol 2000;11:185-204.
43. Geyer MA, Krebs-Thomson K, Braff DL, Swerdlow NR. Pharmacological studies of prepulse inhibition models of sensorimotor gating deficits in schizophrenia: a decade in review. Psychopharmacology (Berl) 2001;156:117-154.
44. Clementz BA, Keil A, Kissler J. Aberrant brain dynamics in schizophrenia: delayed buildup and prolonged decay of the visual steady-state response. Brain Res Cogn Brain Res 2004;18:121-129.
45. Boutros NN, Zouridakis G, Overall J. Replication and extension of P50 findings in schizophrenia. Clin Electroencephalogr 1991;22:40-45.
46. Freedman R, Adler LE, Waldo MC, et al. Neurophysiological evidence for a defect in inhibitory pathways in schizophrenia: comparison of medicated and drug-free patients. Biol Psychiatry 1983;18:537-551.
47. Jin Y, Potkin SG, Patterson JV, et al. Effects of P50 temporal variability on sensory gating in schizophrenia. Psychiatry Res 1997;70:71-81.
48. Erwin RJ, Mawhinney-Hee M, Gur RC, Gur RE. Midlatency auditory evoked responses in schizophrenia. Biol Psychiatry 1991;30:430-442.
49. Siegel C, Waldo M, Mizner G, et al. Deficits in sensory gating in schizophrenic patients and their relatives: evidence obtained with auditory evoked responses. Arch Gen Psychiatry 1984;41:607-612.
50. Umbricht D, Javitt D, Novak G, et al. Effects of clozapine on auditory event-related potentials in schizophrenia. Biol Psychiatry 1998;44:716-725.
51. Picton TW, Hillyard SA. Human auditory evoked potentials. II. Effects of attention. Electroencephalogr Clin Neurophysiol 1974;36:191-199.
52. Picton TW, Hillyard SA, Krausz HI, Galambos R. Human auditory evoked potentials. I. Evaluation of components. Electroencephalogr Clin Neurophysiol 1974;36:179-190.
53. Gallinat J, Mulert C, Bajbouj M, et al. Frontal and temporal dysfunction of auditory stimulus processing in schizophrenia. Neuroimage 2002;17:110-127.
54. Freedman R, Adler LE, Bickford P, et al. Schizophrenia and nicotinic receptors. Harv Rev Psychiatry 1994;2:179-192.
55. Adler LE, Olincy A, Waldo M, et al. Schizophrenia, sensory gating, and nicotinic receptors. Schizophr Bull 1998;24:189-202.
56. Erwin RJ, Shtasel D, Gur RE. Effects of medication history on midlatency auditory evoked responses in schizophrenia. Schizophr Res 1994;11:251-258.
57. Boutros NN, Belger A, Campbell D, et al. Comparison of four components of sensory gating in schizophrenic and normal subjects: a preliminary report. Psychiatry Res 1999;88:119-130.
58. Boutros NN, Korzyukov O, Jansen B, et al. Sensory gating deficits during the midlatency phase of information processing in medicated schizophrenia patients. Psychiatry Res 2004;126:203-215.
59. Rosburg T. Effects of tone repetition on auditory evoked neuromagnetic fields. Clin Neurophysiol 2004;115:898-905.

60. Clementz BA, Geyer MA, Braff DL. Multiple site evaluation of P50 suppression among schizophrenic and normal comparison subjects. Schizophr Res 1998;30:71-80.
61. Crawford HJ, McClain-Furmanski D, Castagnoli N Jr, Castagnoli K. Enhancement of auditory sensory gating and stimulus-bound gamma band (40 Hz) oscillations in heavy tobacco smokers. Neurosci Lett 2002;317:151-155.
62. Adler G, Gattaz WF. Auditory evoked potentials in schizophrenic patients before and during neuroleptic treatment: relationship to psychopathological state. Eur Arch Psychiatry Clin Neurosci 1993;242:357-361.
63. Siegel SJ, Maxwell CR, Majumdar S, et al. Monoamine reuptake inhibition and nicotine receptor antagonism reduce amplitude and gating of auditory evoked potentials. Neuroscience 2005;133:729-738.
64. Dixon LB, Lehman AF, Levine J. Conventional antipsychotic medications for schizophrenia. Schizophr Bull 1995;21:567-577.
65. Adams SG Jr, Howe JT. Predicting medication compliance in a psychotic population. J Nerv Ment Dis 1993;181:558-560.
66. Cramer JA, Rosenheck R. Compliance with medication regimens for mental and physical disorders. Psychiatr Serv 1998;49:196-201.
67. Valenstein M, Copeland LA, Owen R, et al. Adherence assessments and the use of depot antipsychotics in patients with schizophrenia. J Clin Psychiatry 2001;62:545-551.
68. Lacro JP, Dunn LB, Dolder CR, et al. Prevalence of and risk factors for medication nonadherence in patients with schizophrenia: a comprehensive review of recent literature. J Clin Psychiatry 2002;63:892-909.
69. Corriss DJ, Smith TE, Hull JW, et al. Interactive risk factors for treatment adherence in a chronic psychotic disorders population. Psychiatry Res 1999;89:269-274.
70. Rosenheck R, Leslie D, Keefe R, et al. Barriers to employment for people with schizophrenia. Am J Psychiatry 2006;163:411-417.
71. Davis JM, Chen N, Glick ID. A meta-analysis of the efficacy of second-generation antipsychotics. Arch Gen Psychiatry 2003;60:553-564.
72. Geddes J, Freemantle N, Harrison P, Bebbington P. Atypical antipsychotics in the treatment of schizophrenia: systematic overview and meta-regression analysis. BMJ 2000;321:1371-1376.
73. Maxwell CR, Kanes SJ, Abel T, Siegel SJ. Phosphodiesterase inhibitors: a novel mechanism for receptor-independent antipsychotic medications. Neuroscience 2004;129: 101-107.
74. Maxwell CR, Liang Y, Kelly MP, et al. Mice expressing constitutively active $G_s$alpha exhibit stimulus encoding deficits similar to those observed in schizophrenia patients. Neuroscience 2006;141:1257-1264.
75. Remington G. Understanding antipsychotic "atypicality": a clinical and pharmacological moving target. J Psychiatry Neurosci 2003;28:275-284.
76. Lieberman JA, Stroup TS, McEvoy JP, et al. Effectiveness of antipsychotic drugs in patients with chronic schizophrenia. N Engl J Med 2005;353:1209-1223.
77. Brodkin ES. Quantitative trait locus analysis of aggressive behaviours in mice. Novartis Found Symp 2005;268:57-69; discussion 69-77, 96-99.
78. Brodkin ES, Hagemann A, Nemetski SM, Silver LM. Social approach-avoidance behavior of inbred mouse strains towards DBA/2 mice. Brain Res 2004;1002:151-157.
79. Siegel SJ, Irani F, Brensinger CM, et al. Prognostic variables at intake and long-term level of function in schizophrenia. Am J Psychiatry 2006;163:433-441.
80. Gur RC, Ragland JD, Moberg PJ, et al. Computerized neurocognitive scanning: II. The profile of schizophrenia. Neuropsychopharmacology 2001;25:777-788.
81. Green MF, Kern RS, Heaton RK. Longitudinal studies of cognition and functional outcome in schizophrenia: implications for MATRICS. Schizophr Res 2004;72:41-51.
82. Marder SR, Fenton W, Youens K. Schizophrenia, IX: Cognition in schizophrenia—the MATRICS initiative. Am J Psychiatry 2004;161:25.
83. Green MF, Nuechterlein KH. The MATRICS initiative: developing a consensus cognitive battery for clinical trials. Schizophr Res 2004;72:1-3.
84. Geyer MA, Heinssen R. New approaches to measurement and treatment research to improve cognition in schizophrenia. Schizophr Bull 2005;31:806-809.
85. Kopala LC. Spontaneous and drug-induced movement disorders in schizophrenia. Acta Psychiatr Scand Suppl 1996;389:12-17.
86. Fenton WS, Wyatt RJ, McGlashan TH. Risk factors for spontaneous dyskinesia in schizophrenia. Arch Gen Psychiatry 1994;51:643-650.
87. Fenton WS, Blyler CR, Wyatt RJ, McGlashan TH. Prevalence of spontaneous dyskinesia in schizophrenic and non-schizophrenic psychiatric patients. Br J Psychiatry 1997;171:265-268.
88. Fenton WS. Prevalence of spontaneous dyskinesia in schizophrenia. J Clin Psychiatry 2000;61(Suppl 4):10-14.
89. Delay J, Deniker P, Harl JM, Grasset A. [N-dimethylamino-prophylchlorophenothiazine (4560 RP) therapy of confusional states.] Ann Med Psychol (Paris) 1952;110:398-403.
90. Delay J, Deniker P, Harl JM. [Therapeutic use in psychiatry of phenothiazine of central elective action (4560 RP).] Ann Med Psychol (Paris) 1952;110:112-117.
91. Shen WW. A history of antipsychotic drug development. Compr Psychiatry 1999;40:407-414.
92. Seeman P, Lee T. Antipsychotic drugs: direct correlation between clinical potency and presynaptic action on dopamine neurons. Science 1975;188:1217-1219.
93. Seeman P, Chau-Wong M, Tedesco J, Wong K. Brain receptors for antipsychotic drugs and dopamine: direct binding assays. Proc Natl Acad Sci U S A 1975;72:4376-4380.
94. Carlsson A, Lindqvist M. Effect of chlorpromazine or haloperidol on formation of 3-methoxytyramine and normetanephrine in mouse brain. Acta Pharmacol Toxicol (Copenh) 1963;20:140-144.
95. Sedvall G. Relationships among biochemical, clinical, and pharmacokinetic variables in neuroleptic-treated schizophrenic patients. Adv Biochem Psychopharmacol 1980;24:521-528.
96. Farde L, Hall H, Ehrin E, Sedvall G. Quantitative analysis of D2 dopamine receptor binding in the living human brain by PET. Science 1986;231:258-261.
97. Farde L, Wiesel FA, Jansson P, et al. An open label trial of raclopride in acute schizophrenia: confirmation of D2-dopamine receptor occupancy by PET. Psychopharmacology (Berl) 1988;94:1-7.
98. Kane J, Honigfeld G, Singer J, Meltzer H. Clozapine for the treatment-resistant schizophrenic: a double-blind comparison with chlorpromazine. Arch Gen Psychiatry 1988;45:789-796.
99. Ereshefsky L, Watanabe MD, Tran-Johnson TK. Clozapine: an atypical antipsychotic agent. Clin Pharm 1989;8:691-709.
100. Nordstrom AL, Farde L, Halldin C. High 5-HT2 receptor occupancy in clozapine treated patients demonstrated by PET. Psychopharmacology (Berl) 1993;110:365-367.
101. Nordstrom AL, Farde L, Nyberg S, et al. D1, D2, and 5-HT2 receptor occupancy in relation to clozapine serum concentration: a PET study of schizophrenic patients. Am J Psychiatry 1995;152:1444-1449.
102. Trichard C, Paillere-Martinot ML, Attar-Levy D, et al. Binding of antipsychotic drugs to cortical 5-HT2A receptors: a PET study of chlorpromazine, clozapine, and amisulpride in schizophrenic patients. Am J Psychiatry 1998;155:505-508.
103. Rauser L, Savage JE, Meltzer HY, Roth BL. Inverse agonist actions of typical and atypical antipsychotic drugs at the human 5-hydroxytryptamine$_{2C}$ receptor. J Pharmacol Exp Ther 2001;299:83-89.
104. Gruen PH, Sachar EJ, Langer G, et al. Prolactin responses to neuroleptics in normal and schizophrenic subjects. Arch Gen Psychiatry 1978;35:108-116.
105. Langer G, Sachar EJ, Gruen PH, Halpern FS. Human prolactin responses to neuroleptic drugs correlate with antischizophrenic potency. Nature 1977;266:639-640.
106. Cheer SM, Wagstaff AJ. Quetiapine: a review of its use in the management of schizophrenia. CNS Drugs 2004;18:173-199.
107. Kinon BJ, Stauffer VL, McGuire HC, et al. The effects of antipsychotic drug treatment on prolactin concentrations in elderly patients. J Am Med Dir Assoc 2003;4:189-194.
108. Meltzer HY, McGurk SR. The effects of clozapine, risperidone, and olanzapine on cognitive function in schizophrenia. Schizophr Bull 1999;25:233-255.
109. Keefe R, Gu H, Perkins D, et al. A comparison of the effects of olanzapine, quetiapine, and risperidone on neurocognitive function in first-episode psychosis. *In* Proceedings of the 44th Annual Meeting of the American College of Neuropsychopharmacology. Nashville, TN: American College of Neuropsychopharmacology, 2005, p 127.
110. Keefe RS. Neurocognitive effects of antipsychotic medications in patients with chronic schizophrenia in the CATIE Trial. Biol Psychiatry 2006;59(Suppl):965.
111. Seeman P, Corbett R, Van Tol HH. Atypical neuroleptics have low affinity for dopamine D2 receptors or are selective for D4 receptors. Neuropsychopharmacology 1997;16:93-110; discussion 111-135.
112. Miller AL, Hall CS, Buchanan RW, et al. The Texas Medication Algorithm Project antipsychotic algorithm for schizophrenia: 2003 update. J Clin Psychiatry 2004;65:500-508.
113. Javitt DC. Is the glycine site half saturated or half unsaturated? Effects of glutamatergic drugs in schizophrenia patients. Curr Opin Psychiatry 2006;19:151-157.
114. Zylberman I, Javitt DC, Zukin SR. Pharmacological augmentation of NMDA receptor function for treatment of schizophrenia. Ann N Y Acad Sci 1995;757:487-491.
115. van Berckel BN, Evenblij CN, van Loon BJ, et al. D-cycloserine increases positive symptoms in chronic schizophrenic patients when administered in addition to antipsychotics: a double-blind, parallel, placebo-controlled study. Neuropsychopharmacology 1999;21:203-210.
116. Rosse RB, Theut SK, Banay-Schwartz M, et al. Glycine adjuvant therapy to conventional neuroleptic treatment in schizophrenia: an open-label, pilot study. Clin Neuropharmacol 1989;12:416-424.
117. Javitt DC, Zylberman I, Zukin SR, et al. Amelioration of negative symptoms in schizophrenia by glycine. Am J Psychiatry 1994;151:1234-1236.
118. Goff DC, Herz L, Posever T, et al. A six-month, placebo-controlled trial of D-cycloserine co-administered with conventional antipsychotics in schizophrenia patients. Psychopharmacology (Berl) 2005;179:144-150.
119. Freedman R, Leonard S, Waldo M, et al. Characterization of allelic variants at chromosome 15q14 in schizophrenia. Genes Brain Behav 2006;5(Suppl 1):14-22.
120. Freedman R, Olincy A, Ross RG, et al. The genetics of sensory gating deficits in schizophrenia. Curr Psychiatry Rep 2003;5:155-161.
121. Simosky JK, Stevens KE, Kem WR, Freedman R. Intragastric DMXB-A, an alpha7 nicotinic agonist, improves deficient sensory inhibition in DBA/2 mice. Biol Psychiatry 2001;50:493-500.
122. Adler LE, Cawthra EM, Donovan KA, et al. Improved p50 auditory gating with ondansetron in medicated schizophrenia patients. Am J Psychiatry 2005;162:386-388.
123. Gould TJ, Bizily SP, Tokarczyk J, et al. Sensorimotor gating deficits in transgenic mice expressing a constitutively active form of Gs alpha. Neuropsychopharmacology 2004;29:494-501.
124. Kelly MP, Isiegas C, Cheung YF, et al. Constitutive activation of Gαs causes deficits in sensorimotor gating because of PKA-dependent decreases in cAMP. Neuropsychopharmacology 2007;32:577-588.
125. Kanes S, Tokarczyk J, Siegel S, et al. Rolipram: a specific phosphodiesterase 4 inhibitor with potential antipsychotic activity. Neuroscience 2007;144:239-246.
126. Stefansson H, Sigurdsson E, Steinthorsdottir V, et al. Neuregulin 1 and susceptibility to schizophrenia. Am J Hum Genet 2002;71:877-892.
127. Stefansson H, Steinthorsdottir V, Thorgeirsson TE, et al. Neuregulin 1 and schizophrenia. Ann Med 2004;36:62-71.

128. Svarstad BL, Shireman TI, Sweeney JK. Using drug claims data to assess the relationship of medication adherence with hospitalization and costs. Psychiatr Serv 2001;52:805-811.
129. Ayuso-Gutierrez JL, del Rio Vega JM. Factors influencing relapse in the long-term course of schizophrenia. Schizophr Res 1997;28:199-206.
130. Menzin J, Boulanger L, Friedman M, et al. Treatment adherence associated with conventional and atypical antipsychotics in a large state Medicaid program. Psychiatr Serv 2003;54:719-723.
131. McCombs JS, Nichol MB, Stimmel GL, et al. Use patterns for antipsychotic medications in Medicaid patients with schizophrenia. J Clin Psychiatry 1999;60(Suppl 19):5-11; discussion 12-13.
132. Velligan DI, Lam F, Ereshefsky L, Miller AL. Psychopharmacology: perspectives on medication adherence and atypical antipsychotic medications. Psychiatr Serv 2003;54:665-667.
133. Seeman MV. Clinical trials in psychiatry: do results apply to practice? Can J Psychiatry 2001;46:352-355.
134. Blachly PH. Depot fluphenazine enanthate treatment of outpatient schizophrenics. J New Drugs 1965;64:114-116.
135. Laffan RJ, High JP, Burke JC. The prolonged action of fluphenazine enanthate in oil after depot injection. Int J Neuropsychiatry 1965;1:300-306.
136. Moldenhauer B. [Long-term therapy with depot-fluphenazine Dapotum in schizophrenia]. Med Welt 1966;27:1477-1481.
137. McIlrath WA. Experience with a depot phenothiazine in the treatment of schizophrenia. Med J Aust 1967;1:760-762.
138. Adams CE, Fenton MK, Quraishi S, David AS. Systematic meta-review of depot antipsychotic drugs for people with schizophrenia. Br J Psychiatry 2001;179:290-299.
139. Kane JM, Aguglia E, Altamura AC, et al. Guidelines for depot antipsychotic treatment in schizophrenia. European Neuropsychopharmacology Consensus Conference in Siena, Italy. Eur Neuropsychopharmacol 1998;8:55-66.
140. Martin SD, Libretto SE, Pratt DJ, et al. Clinical experience with the long-acting injectable formulation of the atypical antipsychotic, risperidone. Curr Med Res Opin 2003;19:298-305.
141. Harrison TS, Goa KL. Long-acting risperidone: a review of its use in schizophrenia. CNS Drugs 2004;18:113-132.
142. Visco AG, Weidner AC, Cundiff GW, Bump RC. Observed patient compliance with a structured outpatient bladder retraining program. Am J Obstet Gynecol 1999;181:1392-1394.
143. Siegel SJ. Extended release drug delivery strategies in psychiatry: theory to practice. Psychiatry 2005 2005;2:22-31.
144. Hans ML, Dan L, Winey KI, et al. Daily to annual biodegradable drug delivery strategies for psychoactive compounds. *In* Mallapragada SK (ed): Handbook of Biodegradable Polymeric Materials & Applications. Stevenson Ranch, CA: American Scientific Publishers, 2004.
145. Siegel SJ, Winey KI, Gur RE, et al. Surgically implantable long-term antipsychotic delivery systems for the treatment of schizophrenia. Neuropsychopharmacology 2002;26:817-823.
146. Dash AK, Cudworth GC 2nd. Therapeutic applications of implantable drug delivery systems. J Pharmacol Toxicol Methods 1998;40:1-12.
147. Fischel-Ghodsian F, Newton JM. Analysis of drug release kinetics from degradable polymeric devices. J Drug Target 1993;1:51-57.
148. Irani F, Dankert M, Brensinger C, et al. Patient attitudes towards surgically implantable, long-term delivery of psychiatric medicine. Neuropsychopharmacology 2004;29:960-968.

55

DRUG ADDICTION

Doo-Sup Choi, Victor M. Karpyak, Mark A. Frye, Daniel K. Hall-Flavin, and David A. Mrazek

OVERVIEW 817
INTRODUCTION 817
PATHOPHYSIOLOGY 817
The Commonality of Addiction 817
Pathophysiology of Main Drugs of Abuse 818
Genetic Factors Directly Associated with Addiction 818
Alcoholism 818
Opiate Addiction 821
Nicotine Addiction 821
Cocaine Addiction 822
Amphetamine Addiction 823
Marijuana Addiction 823
THERAPEUTICS AND CLINICAL PHARMACOLOGY 823
Goals of Therapy 823
Prevention and Prophylaxis 823
Symptom Management 824
Treatment 825
Therapeutics by Class 825
Pharmacotherapeutics Approved by the FDA 825
Behavioral Treatment Programs 826
Therapeutic Approach 826
Alcoholism 826
Heroin Addiction 829
Nicotine Addiction 831
Emerging Targets and Therapeutics 832
Novel Pharmacotherapies 832
Pharmacogenomics: Individualized Treatment 833

OVERVIEW

In this chapter, we review addiction to alcohol and other drugs, and current approaches to treatment. Drug dependence (used here interchangeably with the term *addiction*) as defined in the *Diagnostic and Statistical Manual of Mental Disorders, Fourth Edition* (DSM-IV) requires the presence of at least three of seven symptoms occurring at any time in the same 12-month period as listed in Box 55-1.[1] Although many categories of drugs could be abused and potentially cause addiction (Table 55-1), we focus on the six most highly addictive substances: alcohol, opiates, nicotine, cocaine, amphetamine, and marijuana.

Recent advances made in molecular neurobiology, behavioral science, and genetic studies have provided the foundation for several well-established treatment methods. Thus, we summarize the current knowledge of pathophysiology of addiction underlying pharmacologic actions of available pharmacotherapies, and the clinical approaches to the patient. We then discuss promising new therapies that are currently under development or in clinical trials.

INTRODUCTION

The impact that drug addiction poses economically and socially is substantial. In the United States alone, annual economic loss due to drug addiction exceeds $300 billion. This figure includes direct liabilities such as costs for detoxification, addiction treatment, and other health care costs associated with comorbid medical and psychiatric conditions. Drug addiction also imposes indirect losses due to unemployment, legal consequences, and criminal behavior.[2] In the United States, more than 11,000 specialized facilities provide addiction rehabilitative services, including counseling, behavior therapies, 12-step programs, and medication initiation and management.

Common features of drug or substance addiction include (i) a compulsion to seek out and take drugs. (ii) loss of control in limiting intake, and (iii) evidence of physiologic dependence marked by a withdrawal syndrome upon cessation of use or when a substantial decline in physiologically significant use is experienced.[3] Addiction represents a complex, multifaceted disorder or set of disorders influenced by genetic predisposition interacting with environmental factors (e.g., stress) and sociocultural determinants (e.g., group attitudes toward availability and use). Current and future treatment interventions must therefore incorporate these considerations in order to achieve an acceptable level of risk and success. This chapter focuses on the neurobiologic vulnerability and the structural and physiologic change that occurs with drug addiction.

Chronic exposure to abusive drugs disrupts the normal brain circuits related to reward and motivation. Consequently, for most addicts, the act of drug use is no longer volitional, and use may continue despite impressive negative consequence, defying obvious rational explanation. Long-term drug exposure is associated with neuronal adaptation to the irresistible stimuli associated with drug use, ultimately causing aberrant behavior in an affected individual. Many of these adaptive patterns in neural circuits of reward are irreversible.[4] Therefore, the goal for treatment is not to change the brain back to a predrug use state, but rather to compensate for those brain changes and normalize any physiologic functions that are disrupted by drug use.

Molecular targets in the brain for treatment interventions are diverse, ranging from neurotransmitter receptors to signaling molecules in the cytoplasm of cells within the dopamine, opioid, glutamate, γ-aminobutyric acid (GABA), adenosine, and serotonin signaling systems. This review focuses on the pharmacologic agents that have been successfully employed in clinical trials that can block withdrawal syndromes, inhibit the drug-seeking desire, and help to maintain prolonged abstinence.

PATHOPHYSIOLOGY

The Commonality of Addiction

Drug addiction is a chronic brain disease and is defined by the enduring vulnerability to relapse to drug use once the addictive state is established. As shown in Figure 55-1, initial exposure to the drug can lead to this state through several steps. In this process, acute reinforcement and tolerance to a drug may be prerequisites for addiction. Interestingly, statistics showed that only a portion of regular drug users (5% to 30%) fall into addiction, and some drugs are associated with higher rates of addiction compared with others. This provides evidence that a subset of the population exposed to a particular drug has a genetic vulnerability to addiction. Once addiction is established, recovery efforts are focused on avoiding relapse after abstinence from use of the drug is achieved.

The most prominent feature of drug addiction is that the reward system is drastically altered by acute and/or chronic exposure to the

BOX 55-1 DSM-IV CRITERIA FOR SUBSTANCE DEPENDENCE AND SUBSTANCE ABUSE

The following are DSM-IV criteria for substance dependence:

A maladaptive pattern of substance use leading to clinically significant impairment of distress, as manifested by three (or more) of the following, occurring at any time in the same 12-month period:

1. Tolerance, as defined by either of the following:
   a. A need for markedly increased amounts of the substance to achieve intoxication or designed effect
   b. Markedly diminished effect with continued use of the same amount of the substance
2. Withdrawal, as manifested by either of the following:
   a. The characteristic withdrawal syndrome for the substance
   b. The same (or a closely related) substance is taken to relieve or avoid withdrawal symptoms
3. The substance is often taken in larger amounts or over a longer period than was intended.
4. There is a persistent desire or unsuccessful efforts to cut down or control substance use.
5. A great deal of time is spent in activities necessary to obtain the substance (e.g., visiting multiple doctors or driving long distances), use the substance (e.g., chain-smoking), or recover from its effects.
6. Important social, occupational, or recreational activities are given up or reduced because of substance use.
7. The substance use is continued despite knowledge of having a persistent or recurrent physical or psychological problem that is likely to have been caused or exacerbated by the substance (e.g., current cocaine use despite recognition of cocaine-induced depression, or continued drinking despite recognition that an ulcer was made worse by alcohol consumption).

The following are DSM-IV criteria for substance abuse:

A. A maladaptive pattern of substance use leading to clinically significant impairment or distress, as manifested by one (or more) of the following, occurring within a 12-month period:
   1. Recurrent substance use resulting in a failure to fulfill major role obligations at work, school, or home (e.g., repeated absences or poor work performance related to substance use; substance-related absences, suspensions or expulsions from school; neglect of children or household)
   2. Recurrent substance use in situations in which it is physically hazardous (e.g., driving an automobile or operating a machine when impaired by substance use)
   3. Recurrent substance-related legal problems (e.g., arrests for substance-related disorderly conduct)
   4. Continued substance use despite having persistent or recurrent social or interpersonal problems caused or exacerbated by the effects of the substance (e.g., arguments with spouse about consequences of intoxication, physical fights)

B. The symptoms have never met the criteria for Substance Dependence for this class of substance.

substance(s) of use, resulting in compulsive drug-seeking behavior in vulnerable individuals. Although acute exposure to various drugs of abuse impacts upon different neurotransmitter signaling pathways in the central and peripheral nervous systems, the mesocorticolimbic circuit (i.e., dopaminergic neurons in the ventral tegmental area [VTA] and glutamatergic neurons in the prefrontal cortex [PFC]) and its targets in the limbic forebrain, especially the nucleus accumbens (NAc), appear to be the common pathway that mediates rewarding and reinforcing properties of the drugs of abuse (Fig. 55-2). In addition, several drugs (e.g., heroin) modify this main reward circuit by interacting with opioid receptors found within the VTA-NAc pathway (see Fig. 55-2). Upon chronic exposure, recruitment of several other brain regions (including the amygdala, hippocampus, and hypothalamus) produces an abnormal synaptic interrelationship within the PFC-VTA-NAc. Repeated use of the drug diminishes the positive reinforcing effect of the drug and requires an increased dose to achieve the same effect previously experienced.

Chronic drug intake is associated with craving, which is considered a central characteristic experienced in the development and maintenance of drug addiction. Craving can be defined as the desire or urge to reexperience the effect of a previously used psychoactive substance.[5] Changes mediated through the mesocorticolimbic circuit have been associated with the subjective experience of craving when the drug of abuse is absent or not available, or when an individual is exposed to cues associated with drug use. Many pharmacotherapies are targeted to reduce craving since it bears a strong causal relationship with involuntary relapse to drug use. Adapted neurocircuits with altered gene expressions in the VTA-NAc pathway contribute to eliciting the nature of the craving (Fig. 55-3). Subsequently, several transcription factor–mediated gene expressions, including delta fosB and CREB, are considered to be crucial in neuroadaptation.[4]

Pathophysiology of Main Drugs of Abuse

Genetic Factors Directly Associated with Addiction

Family and twin epidemiologic studies demonstrate that genetic factors significantly contribute to the vulnerability to drug addiction,[6] with estimates ranging from 30% to 60%. Several genetic variants are commonly associated with most drug addiction. However, many genetic variants are thought to be specific to addiction to a specific drug. Genes involved in a drug's effect at a receptor and its impact on receptor-mediated signaling, and genes involved in the pharmacokinetic profile of a drug in the susceptible individual (due to alteration of ion channel activity and changes in gene expression altering a drug's absorption, distribution, metabolism, and excretion), are responsible for vulnerability to drug addiction.

Studies attempting to identify particular genes responsible for these changes may be broadly categorized into (i) family-based "linkage analysis" that investigates the transmission of genetic markers within specific genomic regions of interest and phenotypic expression in pedigrees, and (ii) "association studies" that examine whether a particular gene allele is more prevalent in study patients compared with control subjects. Recently, the Collaborative Study on the Genetics of Alcoholism, sponsored by the National Institute on Alcohol Abuse and Alcoholism (NIAAA), completed a family-based linkage study across all states in the United States. The group, led by Dr. George Uhl, has developed, validated, and applied a new genetic platform that has allowed them to generate the equivalent of more than 29 million individual genotypes and subsequently analyze 104,268 genetic variations from unrelated alcohol-dependent and control individuals.[7] Association studies are able to detect linked variants (i) if they are within 40,000 to 80,000 nucleotides of the genotyped variant, (ii) if linkage disequilibrium is relatively high, and (iii) if the effect sizes are moderate to high. Table 55-2 shows the currently known genes associated with drug addiction as evidenced by linkage or association studies.[6]

From the vantage point of pharmacotherapy, genetic variations between individuals may determine the nature of the therapeutic response to a specific medication. This is the primary focus of pharmacogenomic research (see Chapter 15, Pharmacogenetics and Pharmacogenomics). A goal of pharmacogenomic studies is to define DNA sequence variability associated with a favorable outcome, which can then be used to guide the selection of appropriate drugs and determine a reasonable dose of a drug that will be effective for an individual patient.[8]

Alcoholism

Alcohol is easily absorbed from the gastrointestinal tract and distributed throughout the body, readily entering most tissues, including the brain. It passes the placental barrier, with the potential to cause defects

TABLE 55-1 COMMONLY ABUSED DRUGS*

Category	Examples of *Commercial* and Street Names	DEA Schedule[†]/How Administered	*Intoxication Effects*/Potential Health Consequences
Cannabinoids			*Euphoria, slowed thinking and reaction time, confusion, impaired balance and coordination*/cough, frequent respiratory infections, impaired memory and learning, increased heart rate, anxiety, panic attacks
Hashish	boom, chronic, ganster, hash, hash oil, hemp	I/swallowed, smoked	
Marijuana	blunt, dope, ganja, grass, herb, joints, Mary Jane, pot, reefer, sinsemilla, skunk, weed	I/swallowed, smoked	
Depressants			*Reduced anxiety, feeling of well-being, lowered inhibition, lowered blood pressure, impaired coordination*/fatigue, confusion, impaired coordination, respiratory depression For barbiturates and benzodiazepines—*sedation, drowsiness*/unusual excitement, fever, slurred speech For flunitrazepam—visual and gastrointestinal disturbances, urinary retention
Alcohol	Beer, wine, hard liquor	NA/ingested	
Barbiturates	*Amytal, Nembutal, Seconal, Phenobarbital*; babs, reds, red birds, phennies, tooies, yellow, yellow jackets	II, III, IV/injected, swallowed	
Benzodiazepines	*Ativan, Halcion, Librium, Valium, Xanax*; CNDU, downers, tranks	IV/swallowed, injected	
Flunitrazepam	*Rohypnol*; forget-me pill, Mexican valium	IV/swallowed, snorted	
GHB	*γ-Hydroxybutyrate*; G, Georgia home boy, liquid ecstasy	I/swallowed	
Hallucinogens			*Altered states of perception and feeling, nausea*/persisting perception disorder (flashbacks) For LSD and mescaline—*increased body temperature, heart rate, blood pressure; loss of appetite, sleeplessness, numbness, weakness, tremors* For psilocybin—*nervousness, paranoia*
LSD	*Lysergic acid diethylamide*; blotter, boomers, cubes	I/swallowed, absorbed through mouth tissues	
Mescaline	buttons, cactus, mesc	I/swallowed, smoked	
Psilocybin	magic mushroom, purple passion, shrooms	I/swallowed	
Opioids and Morphine Derivatives			*Pain relief, euphoria, drowsiness*/nausea, constipation, confusion, sedation, respiratory depression and arrest For codeine—*less analgesia, sedation, and respiratory depression than morphine* For heroin—*staggering gait*
Codeine	*Robitussin A-C*; Captain Cody, schoolboy, pancakes and syrup	II, III, IV/injected, swallowed	
Heroin	*Diacetylmorphine*; brown sugar, dope	I/injected, smoked, snorted	
Morphine	*Roxonal, Duramorph*; Miss Emma, monkey, white stuff	II, III/injected, swallowed, smoked	
Opium	*Laudanum, paregoric*; big O, black stuff, block	II, III, IV/swallowed, smoked	
Stimulants			*Increased heart rate, blood pressure, and metabolism; feelings of exhilaration, energy, increased mental alertness*/rapid or irregular heartbeat, reduced appetite, weight loss, heart failure, nervousness, insomnia For amphetamines—*rapid breathing*/tremor, loss of coordination, irritability, delirium For cocaine—*increased temperature*/chest pain, nausea, abdominal pain For MDMA—*mild hallucinogenic effects, increased tactile sensitivity, empathic feelings*
Nicotine	Tobacco, cigarettes, cigars	NA/smoked, chewed, snorted	
Amphetamines	*Biphetamine, Dexedrin*; bennies, black beauties, crosses, heart	II/injected, swallowed, smoked, snorted	
Cocaine	*Cocaine hydrochloride*; blow, bump, Charlie, coke, crack, flake, rock, snow, toot	II/injected, smoked, snorted	
MDMA	Adam, clarity, ecstasy, Eve, lover's speed	I/swallowed	
Methamphetamine	*Desoxyn*; chalk, crank, crystal, fire, glass, go fast, ice, meth	II/injected, swallowed, smoked, snorted	
Other compounds			
Anabolic steroids	*Anadrol, Oxandrin, Durabolin, Depot-Testosterone, Euipoise*; roids, juice	III/injected, swallowed, applied to skin	*No intoxication effects*/hypertension, blood clotting and cholesterol changes, liver cyst and cancer, hostility and aggression
Inhalants	Solvents (paint thinners, gasoline, glues), gases (butane, propane, aerosol propellants, nitrous oxide)	NA/inhaled	*Stimulation, loss of inhibition, headache, nausea or vomiting, slurred speech, loss of motor coordination*/cramps, weight loss, muscle weakness, depression

*This table represent a summary of the list available from the National Institute on Drug Abuse (*http://www.nida.nih.gov*) that contain more complete names, intoxication effects, and potential health consequences.

[†]Schedule I and II drugs have a high potential for abuse. They require greater storage security and have a quota on manufacturing, among other restrictions. Schedule I drugs are available for research only and have no approved medical use; Schedule II drugs are available only by prescription (unrefillable) and require a form for ordering. Schedule III and IV drugs are available by prescription, may have five refills in 6 months, and may be ordered orally. Most Schedule V drugs are available over the counter.

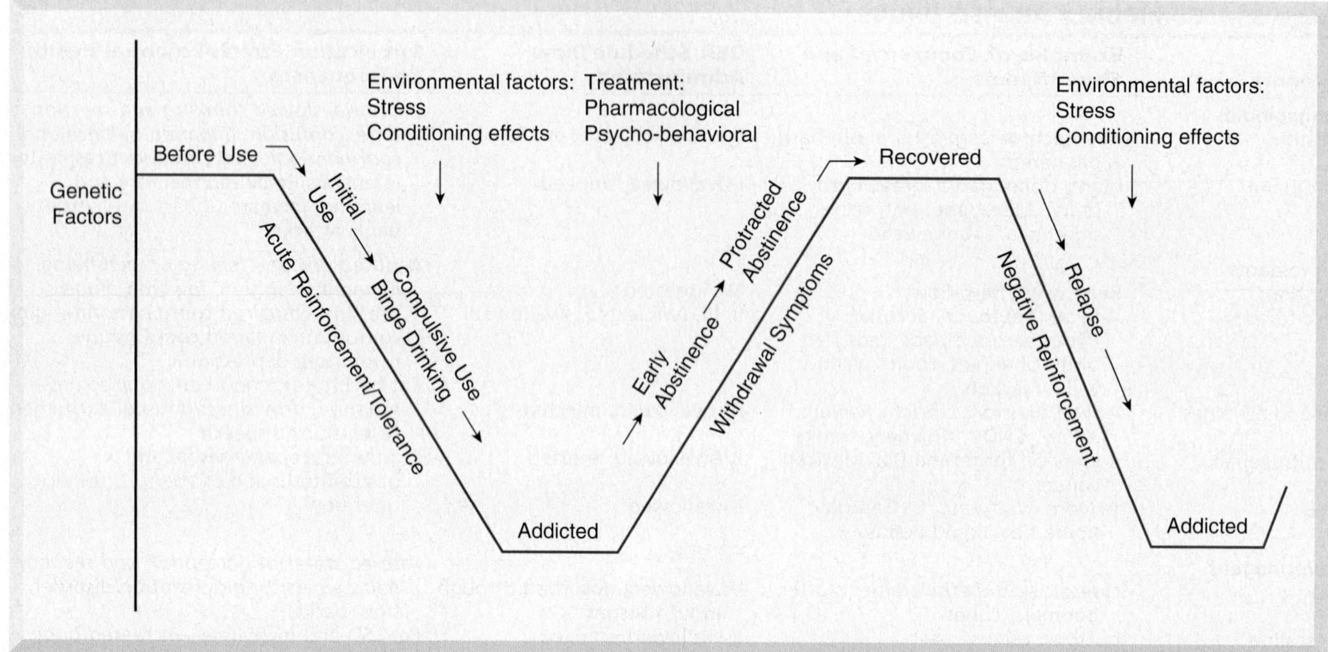

FIGURE 55-1 • Steps and time course of drug addiction. Initial drug use can trigger an individual to compulsive drug taking or binge alcohol consumption. In this process, genetic factors and environmental factors such as stress and conditioning contribute to the vulnerability of entering into a cycle of drug abuse and addiction. Once addicted, most individuals try to abstain from the drug when they experience adverse psychological and physical effects. However, over 80% fall into relapse without the use of medication or systemic treatment. (Modified from Koob and Le Moal[3] and Dahchour and De Witte.[63])

TABLE 55-2 GENES HAVING ONE OR MORE VARIANTS ASSOCIATED WITH DRUG ADDICTION IN HUMANS

System	Gene	Protein	Substance*	Location
Opioid	*OPRM1*	μ-Opioid receptor	Alc, H/O	6q24-25
	OPRK1	κ-Opioid receptor	H/O	8q11.2
	PDYN	Preprodynophin	C/S	20pter-p12.2
Dopaminergic	*TH*	Tyrosine hydroxylase	Alc	11p15.5
	DRD2	Dopamine receptor D_2	Alc	11q23
	DRD3	Dopamine receptor D_3	Alc, C/S	3q13.3
	DRD4	Dopamine receptor D_4	Alc, H/O, C/S	11p15.5
	DBH	Dopamine-β-hydroxylase	C/S	9q34
	DAT	Dopamine transporter	Alc	5p15.3
Serotonergic	*TPH1*	Tryptophan hydroxylase 1	Alc	11p15.3-14
	TPH2	Tryptophan hydroxylase 2	Alc, H/O	12q21.1
	HTR1B	Serotonin receptor 1B	Alc, H/O	6q13
	HTR2A	Serotonin receptor 2A	Alc	13q14-21
	SERT	Serotonin transporter	Alc, H/O	17q11.1-12
Catecholaminergic	*MAOA*	Monoamine oxidase A	Alc	Xp11.23
	COMT	Catechol-*O*-methyltransferase	Alc, H/O	22q11.2
GABAergic	*GABRA1*	GABA receptor subunit $alpha_1$	Alc	5q34-35
	GABRA6	GABA receptor subunit $alpha_6$	Alc	5q31.1-35
	GABRB1	GABA receptor subunit $beta_1$	Alc	4p13-12
Cannabinoid	*CNR1*	Cannabinoid receptor 1	Alc, C/S	6q14-15
	FAAH	Fatty acid amide hydroxylase	Alc	1p35-34
EtOH metabolism	*ADH1B*	Alcohol dehydrogenase 1B	Alc	4q22
	ADH1C	Alcohol dehydrogenase 1C	Alc	4q22
	ALDH2	Aldehyde dehydrogenase 2	Alc	12q24.2
Cholinergic	*CHRM2*	Muscarinic acetylcholine receptor M2	Alc	7q35-36
Neuromodulatory	*NPY*	Neuropeptide Y	Alc	7p15.1
Drug metabolism	*CYP2D6*	Cytochrome P-450	H/O	22q13.1
Signaling	*ANKK1*	Ankyrin repeat and kinase domain–containing 1	Alc	11q23.2

*Alc, alcohol; C/S, cocaine or stimulants; H/O, heroin or opiate.

Modified from Kreek MJ, Nielsen DA, Butelman ER, LaForge KS. Genetic influences on impulsivity, risk taking, stress responsivity and vulnerability to drug abuse and addiction. Nat Neurosci 2005;8:1450-1457.

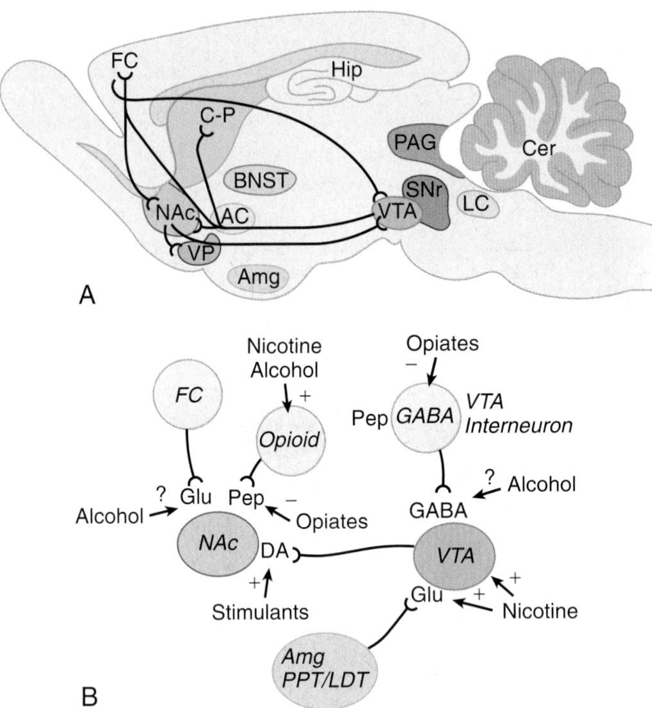

FIGURE 55-2 • Neurocircuits of drug addiction and acute actions of drugs of abuse on the VTA-NAc pathway. A, Sagittal section through a representative rodent brain illustrating the dopamine, glutamate, and γ-aminobutyric acid (GABA) interactions in the mesocorticolimbic region, which is hypothesized to be involved in the neurocircuitry of drug dependence. Approximately 95% of neurons in the dorsal (C-P) and ventral (NAc) striatum are medium-sized spiny neurons, which use GABA as their main neurotransmitter (*green*). These neurons receive glutamatergic projections (*blue*) from the cerebrofrontal cortex (FC), which form well-defined synapses on the heads of dendritic spines, whereas the dopaminergic neurons (*red*) from the VTA interact with stems of dentrites. (Modified from Hyman SE, Malenka RC. Addiction and the brain: the neurobiology of compulsion and its persistence. Nat Rev Neurosci 2001;2:695-703.)

B, Highly simplified scheme of converging acute actions of drugs of abuse on the VTA-NAc pathway. Drugs of abuse, despite diverse initial actions, produce some common effects on the VTA-NAc pathway. Stimulants directly increase dopaminergic transmission in the NAc. Opiates inhibit GABAergic interneurons in the VTA, which disinhibits VTA dopamine neurons. Nicotine seems to activate VTA dopamine neurons directly via stimulation of nicotinic cholinergic receptors on those neurons and indirectly via stimulation of its receptors on glutamatergic nerve terminals that innervate the dopamine cells. Alcohol may inhibit GABAergic terminals in the VTA and hence disinhibit VTA dopamine neurons. It also may inhibit glutamatergic terminals that innervate NAc neurons. (Modified from Nestler EJ. Is there a common molecular pathway for addiction? Nat Neurosci 2005;8:1445-1449.)

AC, anterior commissure; Amg, amygdala; BNST, bed nucleus stria terminalis; Cer, cerebellum; C-P, caudate-putamen; DA, dopamine; FC, cerebrofrontal cortex; Glu, glutamate; Hip, hippocampus; LC, locus ceruleus; NAc, nucleus accumbens; PAG, periaqueductal gray; Pep, opioid peptides; PPT/LDT, peduncular pontine tegmentum/lateral dorsal tegmentum; SNr, substantia nigra pars reticulata; VP, ventral pallidum; VTA, ventral tegmental area.

in the developing infant (fetal alcohol effects, fetal alcohol syndrome). About 90% to 95% of alcohol is metabolized to acetic acid in the liver through a two-step dehydrogenase enzymatic reaction involving alcohol dehydrogenase and acetaldehyde dehydrogenase. About 5% to 10% of alcohol is excreted unchanged in expired air through the lungs. While many factors can impact on the relationship between amount of alcohol ingested and blood alcohol concentration (BAC), in general, 0.04 BAC produces detectable behavioral effects, which requires approximately two drinks (1 drink = 5 oz or 132 cc of 12% wine, 12 oz or 317 cc of 5% beer, or 1.5 oz of distilled spirits) for a 160-pound adult male.

Although there are no alcohol-specific receptors in the central nervous system (CNS), low to moderate doses of alcohol (0.02 to 0.08 BAC) enhance GABA-mediated inhibition by possible direct interaction with $GABA_A$ receptors,[9] increasing endogenous opioids and inhibiting excitatory neurotransmitters signaling such as N-methyl-D-aspartate receptor function and calcium influx through voltage-gated calcium channels.[10] The same dose of alcohol can produce a euphoric effect with a relaxed feeling and a reduced social inhibition, which can render the individual more gregarious, talkative, and friendly, promoting the reward circuitry. This initial positive reinforcing effect of alcohol is accompanied by neuronal adaptation to a higher responsiveness of dopamine release in the mesolimbic brain regions. Repeated alcohol intake requires a higher dose to obtain the same levels of intoxicating effect. Physical tolerance may lead to an individual consuming higher doses of alcohol (>0.1 BAC) and to associated adverse physiologic conditions in the long term, such as brain damage (Wernicke-Korsakoff syndrome and alcoholic dementia) and liver dysfunction (alcoholic hepatitis and cirrhosis).

Withdrawal from repeated heavy drinking produces an intense withdrawal syndrome that develops within a few hours after the drinking stops and may continue for 2 to 4 days or longer.

Opiate Addiction

Morphine and its analogue heroin (converted to morphine in the brain) interact with three distinct opioid receptors: μ, δ, and κ. The numerous natural, semisynthetic, and synthetic narcotics bind to these receptors with different affinities, manifesting distinct effects in the CNS (see Fig. 55-2). Naloxone, a μ-opioid antagonist, quickly reverses the intoxicating effects of opiates, indicating that receptor-mediated signaling is a key action of opiates.

The μ-opioid receptor has a high affinity for morphine and related opiate drugs, and is widely expressed both in the brain and spinal cord.[11] Different brain regions are thought to mediate the diverse function of morphine. Analgesic effects are mediated within the medial thalamus, periaqueductal gray, median raphe, and spinal cord. Reward and positive effects appear to be processed within the nucleus accumbens. The brainstem is responsible for effects upon the cardiovascular and respiratory systems (opioid-induced suppression), coughing, and nausea/vomiting. Sensorimotor integration is localized to the thalamus and striatum.

Expression of δ-receptors, which is similar to that of μ-opioid receptors, appears to be more prevalent in the forebrain regions, including the neocortex, olfactory areas, and striatum. This suggests that δ-opioid receptors modulate cognitive function, olfaction, motor integration, and reinforcement.

The κ-opioid receptor initially was identified as possessing a high affinity for binding to ketocyclazocine, an opiate analogue, causing hallucinations and dysphoria. This receptor is uniquely expressed in the hypothalamus and pituitary glands, where it mediates pain perception, gut mobility, and dysphoria.

Opiates have a dramatic pain-reducing effect but are highly reinforcing, and chronic use leads to tolerance and ultimately to physical dependence. Like other drugs of abuse, dopamine release in the nucleus accumbens is implicated in the reinforcing effects of opiates. In contrast, stimulation of κ-opioid receptors in the NAc reduces dopaminergic neuronal activity and produces aversion, indicating that mesolimbic opioid receptors mediate not only reinforcement of opiates but also the aversive effects of this class of drugs. κ-Opioid receptor agonists decrease heroin, cocaine, and ethanol self-administration, and block heroin and cocaine conditioned place preference in rats. Opiate withdrawal is marked by physical discomfort, musculoskeletal pain, dysphoria, restlessness, fearfulness, and flulike symptoms. The time course of withdrawal is dependent upon its half-life. In the case of morphine, it peaks 36 to 48 hours after the last administration, and disappears within 7 to 10 days. Although several brain regions are implicated in opiate withdrawal, the periaqueductal gray and locus ceruleus are the main regions involved in mediating withdrawal-induced anxiety (see Fig. 55-2).

Nicotine Addiction

Nicotine is an alkaloid found in tobacco leaves and a main addictive ingredient of cigarette smoke. The amount of nicotine absorbed from

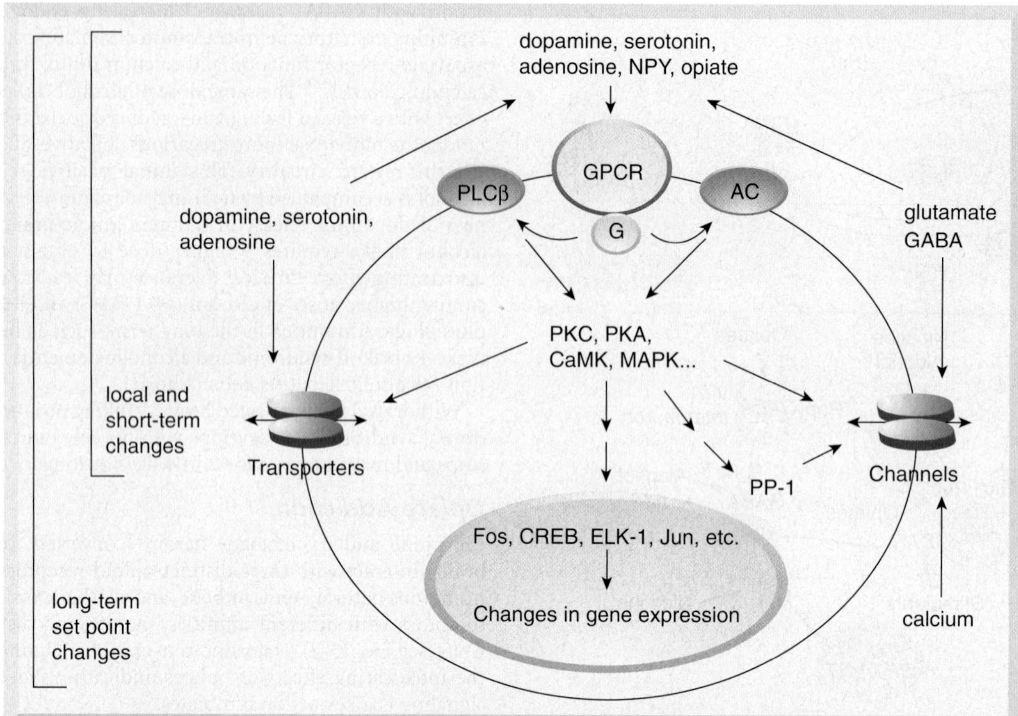

FIGURE 55-3 • Molecular mechanisms of neuroadaptation. Upon acute exposure, drugs of abuse mostly interact with membrane proteins such as G protein–coupled receptors, transporters, and ion channels, which regulate the neuronal firing and subsequent signaling mechanism in the cytoplasm. The receptors modulate levels of the second messengers such as cyclic AMP and Ca^{2+}, which in turn regulate the activity of protein kinases such as PKA, PKC, CaMK, and MAPK. Long-term functional changes, which may happen upon chronic exposure to drugs of abuse, are associated with reprogramming of gene expression. AC, adenylyl cyclase; CaMK, calcium/calmodulin kinases; GPCR, G protein–coupled receptors; MAPK, mitogen activated kinases; PKA, protein kinase A; PKC, protein kinase C; PLCβ, phospholipase Cβ; PP-1, protein phosphatase 1.

a typical smoked cigarette is about 0.8 to 1.5 mg, which causes the plasma nicotine concentration to reach 100 to 200 nmol/L.[12] The nicotine reaches the brain in about 7 seconds, which is approximately twice as fast as when a drug is administered intravenously, causing powerful reinforcing effects on smoking behavior compared to alternative routes of administration. About 70% to 80% of nicotine is converted into cotinine, a principal metabolite, by a specific liver enzyme, cytochrome P-450 2A6. Cotinine and other nicotine metabolites are excreted mainly in the urine.[13]

Nicotine binds to nicotinic acetylcholine receptors (nAChRs) with especially high affinity for the $alpha_4$ and $beta_2$ subunits, found[14] in many parts of the brain including the cerebral cortex, thalamus, striatum, hippocampus, VTA, locus ceruleus, and raphe nuclei. The activation of the nAChRs enables Na^+ influx into the cell and depolarizes the cell membranes, leading to a fast excitatory response. Some nAChRs also allow significant amounts of Ca^{2+} influx, thereby stimulating Ca^{2+}-dependent signaling pathways. Presynaptic nAChRs enhance the neurotransmitter release from the terminal. Nicotine enhances cognitive function in humans[15] and working memory in animals.[16]

The activation of VTA nAChRs directly stimulates dopamine release in the nucleus accumbens (see Fig. 55-2), which establishes the strong reinforcement associated with smoking tobacco. Repeated exposure to nicotine leads to either a tolerance or subsequent sensitization. In the same day, smokers experience a lower level of response toward the end of the day, which is mainly attributed to the desensitization of nAChR-mediated dopamine release in the mesolimbic brain region.[17] This short-sustaining acute tolerance explains the increased sensitization to the first cigarette of the day after an overnight abstinence. Chronic tolerance is evident after long-term exposure to nicotine and is superimposed on the tolerance that occurs with acute use. The subcutaneous injection of a high dose of nicotine elicited an aversive reaction in nonsmokers, whereas no sign of such reactions is observed in smokers, indicating that the initial aversive effects could be overcome by nicotine's reinforcing effects through repeated smoking.[18] Abstinence from smoking causes withdrawal symptoms such as tobacco craving, restlessness, insomnia, hunger, and weight gain. The symptoms last approximately 4 weeks following abstinence. In one study, although nicotine gum effectively prevented almost all of the withdrawal symptoms except for hunger and weight gain, two thirds of the subjects relapsed at a 6-month follow-up test.[13] Animal studies demonstrated that mecamylamine, an nAChR antagonist, precipitated nicotine withdrawal and nicotine-dependent dopamine release in the NAc, suggesting that nAChRs also participate in nicotine withdrawal.[19]

Cocaine Addiction

The plasma concentration of cocaine varies depending on the route of administration.[20] Cocaine is rapidly metabolized and eliminated within 0.5 to 1.5 hours after absorption. However, major metabolites, including benzoylecgonine, can be detected in the urine several days after the last dose.

Cocaine mainly blocks three presynaptic neurotransmitter transporters: dopamine, norepinephrine, and serotonin transporters. It does so with different binding affinities, causing increased neurotransmitter levels in the synapses.[13] Although cocaine binds most strongly to the serotonin transporter, blockade of dopamine reuptake appears to produce the stimulating and reinforcing properties of the compound. Cocaine inhibits voltage-gated sodium channels in nerve axons, blocking nerve conduction. This pharmacologic action of cocaine was applied to the development of two widely used local anesthetics, procaine and lidocaine, which are cocaine derivatives (see Chapter 61, Treatment of Pain).[13]

As a psychomotor stimulant, cocaine has a remarkable ability to augment alertness and heighten arousal, leading to behavioral excitement with feelings of exhilaration and euphoria. Cocaine also activates the sympathetic nervous system, which mediates cocaine's physiologic effects such as increased heart rate, vasoconstriction, hypertension, and hyperthermia. Higher doses of cocaine can be toxic or even fatal, with risk of seizures, heart failure, stroke, or intracranial hemorrhage. Since cocaine has the ability to block dopamine reuptake, it is evident that dopamine plays a central role in reinforcement, leading to addiction similar to that experienced with the chronic use of other psychostimulants. Studies with dopamine transporter (DAT)– and serotonin transporter (SERT)–null mice reveal that DAT and SERT serve complimentary roles in producing conditioned place preference to cocaine.[21,22] Volkow and colleagues found that baseline dopamine activity and the rate of transporter occupancy determine the subjective "high" experienced with cocaine and methylphenidate use.[23,24] Methylphenidate is a stimulant that blocks DAT and is used clinically to treat attention-deficit/hyperactivity disorder (see Chapter 51, Attention Deficit Disorder). Cocaine produces short-lasting acute tolerance that leads to taking a higher dose during a binge administration setting. At the same time, it fosters a longer term sensitization that may be critical for strong reinforcement and craving. Cocaine withdrawal is accompanied by an inability to experience normal pleasure, a lack of energy, and anxiety.

Amphetamine Addiction

Amphetamine and methamphetamine produce a long-lasting "high" compared to cocaine, due to a longer half-life ranging from 7 to 30 hours. Amphetamines inhibit monoamine oxidase–mediated catecholamine metabolism and increase the availability of dopamine in synapses. As a result, these substances exhibit a psychomotor response similar to that observed with cocaine administration.

In animal studies, multiple doses of methamphetamine cause severe neurotoxic effects with reduction in baseline activity of striatal dopamine, tyrosine hydroxylase, and DAT.[25] Recent human studies indicate that dopamine neurotoxicity can increase one's vulnerability to developing Parkinson's disease. In addition, heavy use of amphetamines and methamphetamines can cause a psychotic state similar to that seen in paranoid schizophrenia.

Methylenedioxymethamphetamine (MDMA), an amphetamine analogue, is one of the popular street drugs for young adults, and primarily enhances serotonin levels. This mediates most of the behavioral effects of the drug, including mild euphoria, enhanced sensory perception, and feelings of well-being and self-confidence. MDMA also produces a variety of physiologic responses, including increased heart rate, increased blood pressure, elevated body temperature, and sweating. Repeated exposure to MDMA causes neurotoxicity, as demonstrated by reduced numbers of serotoninergic axon terminals in the cortex and hippocampus.[26]

Marijuana Addiction

A typical marijuana cigarette contains 0.5 to 1 g of cannabis and 20 to 40 mg of Δ^9-tetrahydrocannabinol (THC), the primary active ingredient. About 20% (4 to 8 mg) of THC is absorbed into the lungs by smoking, and rapidly distributed to the bloodstream within 20 minutes. It is then metabolized over the next 2 hours.[27] THC is converted into several metabolites in the liver, and it is excreted primarily in feces (75%) and urine (25%). Although THC levels in the bloodstream decline rapidly, complete elimination takes a much longer time due to lipid-soluble metabolites in fatty tissues, which can be detected more than 2 weeks after a single use in nonchronic users.

THC and other metabolites bind to the CB1 receptor in the CNS, which was first characterized pharmacologically,[28] followed by molecular cloning.[29] The CB1 receptor is a widely distributed G protein–coupled metabotropic receptor that is negatively coupled with adenylyl cyclase activity and decreases cyclic AMP levels. Upon activation, it inhibits a voltage-sensitive Ca^{2+} channel and activates K^+ channels. The CB1 receptor is primarily expressed presynaptically in axon terminals and can inhibit the release of many neurotransmitters, including acetylcholine, dopamine, serotonin, glutamate, and GABA.[30] The endocannabinoids, naturally occurring ligands, are generated from arachidonic acid and pass through membranes rather than being stored in the vesicles. Postsynaptic endocannabinoids can regulate the presynpatic release of neurotransmitters by functioning as a retrograde messenger. For example, retrograde signaling by endocannabinoids reduces GABAergic inhibition of pyramidal neurons in the hippocampus.[13]

Inhibition of the CB1 receptor increases pain sensitivity, suggesting that the release of endocannabinoids decreases certain types of painful stimuli.[31,32] Other research using CB1-knockout mice revealed that endocannabinoids may mediate eating behaviors,[33] and may be implicated in extinction of the fear response.[34] Marijuana produces several physiologic responses, including increased blood flow to the skin and increased hunger. Marijuana has also been associated with pathophysiologic responses such as anxiety, panic, paranoia, and even a state of delirium.

Cannabinoid reinforcement has been shown to depend on both CB1 receptor and μ-opioid receptor activation. Like other drugs of abuse, dopamine release in the NAc is critical to the reinforcement process. Microinjection of the μ-opioid receptor antagonist naloxoenazine into the VTA of rats blocked THC-induced dopamine release.[35] In contrast, in human studies with another opioid antagonist, naltrexone, an increase rather than a decrease in the positive subjective effects of oral THC in regular heavy marijuana smokers was noted.[36] Since the conditioned place aversion produced by a higher THC dose is abolished in κ-opioid–null mice,[37] the balance between the positive reinforcing properties versus the aversive effects determines the net effect of the drug on an individual. Repeated use of cannabinoids causes the development of behavioral and physiologic tolerance, which may be due to down-regulation and desensitization of the brain CB1 receptors. Abstinence from long-term use leads to a withdrawal syndrome with symptoms of irritability, increased anxiety, depressed mood, sleep disturbances, highlighted aggressiveness, and decreased appetite.[38]

THERAPEUTICS AND CLINICAL PHARMACOLOGY

Goals of Therapy

Prevention and Prophylaxis

The best way to prevent drug addiction is to minimize exposure to potential drugs of abuse. Although this is a clinical recommendation, particularly in those with a family history of addictive disorders, it is almost impossible to remove all available psychoactive substances in our current society. In fact, many potential psychoactive substances (alcohol, nicotine, caffeine) are culturally integrated into modern society, with easy access and acceptance. Advances in chemistry during the 19th century made it possible to purify primary active ingredients such as morphine and cocaine, allowing more concentrated forms with higher addictive properties. Initially, current illegal substances were popular medicines before adverse and addictive effects become obvious. Levying higher taxes on alcohol and tobacco and legal interdiction of illegal substances reduced the access and thereby the risk of abuse to some extent. However, it is evident with the widespread use of marijuana and MDMA (ecstasy) that these and other illicit drugs are easily accessible in this society. Nearly all addicted individuals believe in the beginning that they can stop using drugs volitionally, and most try to stop without treatment. The neurobiologic vulnerability of recreational use progressing to addiction and subsequent need of treatment is not fully understood.

As noted previously, drug addictions result from complex gene-gene and gene-environment interactions.[39] Clinical and epidemiologic data indicate specific risk groups based on ancestry (i.e., sons of alcoholic fathers) or on the presence of specific endophenotypes (i.e., low response to alcohol).[40] In addition, ancestral (i.e., East Asian origin), genetic (i.e., the presence of the *ALDH2*2* allele), and phenotypic ("flushing") factors may represent protective factors predicting greater resilience to developing alcohol dependence.[41] As current treatment options related to genotype are presently limited to research, primary and secondary prevention efforts are focused on education, particularly in youth or at-risk populations, and on use in moderation (alcohol) or controlled supervision (prescription stimulants, sedatives, and analgesics). Specific recommendations for what is considered excessive alcohol consumption (Box 55-2) are widely published and supported by robust national and international epidemiologic data.

Symptom Management

Though treatment of substance dependence targeting the etiologic foundations of addiction is not yet available, specific methods for symptom management have been developed (Table 55-3). These are focused on critical physiologic manifestations of substance dependence, including tolerance, withdrawal, craving, and relapse prevention. As presented in this section, the majority of symptom management has focused on alcohol dependence, withdrawal syndrome, craving, and relapse prevention and to a lesser extent on narcotics.

Symptom Management 1: Tolerance. Tolerance (i.e., a need for markedly increased amounts of the substance to achieve intoxication or designed effect or markedly diminished effect with continued use of the same amount of the substance) is the first DSM-IV criterion for establishing a diagnosis of substance dependence (see Box 55-1), and is also the first target symptom for pharmacotherapy.

In 1951, the U.S. Food and Drug Administration (FDA) approved disulfiram (Antabuse) as an adjunctive treatment for alcohol dependence. Twenty years later, the antiprotozoal and antibiotic metronidazole, having an effect on human aldehyde dehydrogenase (ALDH)[42] similar to that of disulfiram, was used "off-label" for the same purpose.[43,44] In contrast to newer agents, both of these agents are viewed as aversive disincentives for use of alcohol because of the toxic effects of acetaldehyde accumulation in cases of alcohol consumption (via accumulation of aldehyde by-products of alcohol metabolism).

In 1984, naltrexone was approved by the FDA for treatment of narcotic dependence. Animal studies indicated that naltrexone can effectively block morphine tolerance and physical dependence.[45] Early studies in humans indicated that chronic use of naltrexone reversed tolerance and supersensitivity to heroin effects on pituitary-gonadal hormones[46] and negatively affected the ability of ex-addicts to tolerate morphine injection, which resulted in a dysphoric rather than euphoric response.[47] Compliance problems resulted in less common use of naltrexone in opioid addicts. Several clinical studies[48-50] led to the approval of oral naltrexone in a lower dosage form (ReVia) for the treatment of alcohol dependence. Recently, an intramuscular sustained-release form of naltrexone (Vivitrol) has been approved for use in alcohol dependence. The injectable form may be more useful for treatment of opioid addiction. Naloxone is also known to inhibit tolerance and dependence to morphine,[51] but was never approved for this purpose. Instead, it has been approved as a component of Suboxone to prevent intravenous abuse of this medication.

Symptom Management 2: Withdrawal. Evidence supports the use of benzodiazepines in the treatment of withdrawal syndrome in alcohol and sedative-hypnotic drug dependence.[52,53] Though no official FDA approval has been issued, practical guidelines highlight the similarity of the clinical presentation and treatment approaches for both conditions, emphasizing more protracted withdrawal in patients abusing sedative-hypnotic drugs. Conversion tables and detailed taper recommendations can be found elsewhere.[53] Evidence-based guidelines for the management of alcohol withdrawal are discussed later in this chapter.

Symptom Management 3: Craving and Relapse Prevention. The chronic relapsing nature of substance dependence is the most important target for treatment efforts. Historically,[54] craving has been considered the main reason for relapse, and medications developed for combating relapse were seen as a new class of "anticraving (antidipsotropic)" medications.[55] In this chapter, we review medications targeting relapse prevention within the same theoretical framework and use the same terminology. It is noted, however, that the effect on craving is not

BOX 55-2 HAZARDOUS LEVELS OF DRINKING (BASED ON NIAAA GUIDELINES)

One standard drink is equivalent to 12 ounces of beer, 5 ounces of wine, or 1.5 ounces of 80-proof spirits.

For healthy **men up to age 65**
- more than **4** drinks in a **day** AND
- more than **14** drinks in a **week**

For healthy **women** (and healthy **men over age 65**)
- more than **3** drinks in a **day** AND
- more than **7** drinks in a **week**

TABLE 55-3 PHARMACOLOGIC APPROACH TO ADDICTION TREATMENT

	Target Symptoms		
	Tolerance/Sensitivity	**Withdrawal**	**Craving/Relapse Prevention**
	Medication Type		
Drug of Abuse	**Aversive**	**Cross-tolerant**	**Antidipsotropic**
Alcohol	Disulfiram* (Antabuse)	Benzodiazepines Chlormetiazole Valproic acid Carbamazepine	Naltrexone tablets* (ReVia) Naltrexone extended-release injectable suspension* (Vivitrol) Acamprosate tablets* (Campral) Ondansetron (Zofran) Baclofen Topiramate (Topamax)
Opiates	Naltrexone* (ReVia) Naloxone	Buprenorphine sublingual tablets* (Subutex) Methadone oral solution* Clonidine	Buprenorphine-naloxone combined tablets* (Suboxone) Methadone oral solution*
Nicotine		Nicotine gum/lozenge* (Nicorette) Nicotine transdermal system* (Nicoderm) Nicotine inhaler* (Nicotrol) Varenicline tablets* (Chantix)	Bupropion sustained-release tablets* (Zyban) Varenicline tablets* (Chantix)
Sedatives		Benzodiazepines Anticonvulsants	
Stimulants	None	None	Dexamphetamine
Cocaine	None	None	Disulfiram
Cannabis	None	None	None

*FDA-approved medications.

TABLE 55-4 OPTIONS AT DIFFERENT STAGES OF RECOVERY

	Detoxification/Withdrawal	Intensive Treatment	Early Recovery	Recovery Maintenance
Duration	Days-4 wk	3-4 wk	1.5-3 mo	Years
Cross-tolerant medications	×	×	×	×
Aversive medications		×	×	×
Antidipsotropics		×	×	×

As a complete cure is not available, special importance in treatment programs is paid to development of the therapeutic environment and a social system supportive of recovery. Description of this component is beyond the scope of this chapter. More information can be found elsewhere.[52]

officially cited by the FDA in their approval statements for naltrexone, acamprosate, or other medications designed to prevent relapse. In part, this is related to the fact that the theoretical construct of "craving" remains undeveloped and there is a lack of consensus on the availability of research tools that allow a reliable measurement of craving.[56,57]

Effective control of each of these symptoms is crucial during specific stages of recovery (Table 55-4) and for overall treatment success. Specifically, successful management of withdrawal allows smooth recovery from intoxication, builds trusting relationships, and minimizes mood fluctuations, which may affect commitment to recovery. Commitment to recovery needs to be solidified during a period of intensive treatment, which provides an individual with general knowledge about chemical dependency and how this can be applied to his or her particular clinical situation. It also allows for the development of effective coping strategies relevant to his or her individual case. The severity of craving, role of the environmental cues, and subject's behavior are reviewed. In this context, the use of antidipsotropics and/or aversive medications is discussed. For example, individuals with a clear, identifiable craving for alcohol often are interested in the use of antidipsotropic medications, which establish a goal of craving suppression in avoiding relapse. Other individuals prefer to use medications with aversive properties (i.e., disulfiram) and avoid drinking because of a fear of the toxicity. Both types of medications continue to be useful in recovery. The flexibility and adjustments to contemporary life circumstances of the patient are paramount. Existing evidence and guidelines for the use of specific drugs of each class are reviewed in the section on Therapeutics by Class.

Treatment

The ultimate goal of addiction therapy is to return individuals to productive functioning in the family, workplace, and community. The overall treatment success rate is similar to those for other chronic diseases such as diabetes, hypertension, and asthma. Several studies demonstrate that treatment interventions reduce drug use by 40% to 60% and significantly decrease criminal activity during and after treatment.[58]

Several different pharmacologic approaches are being used to treat drug addiction. First, using short-term substitution of a cross-tolerant, nonaddictive drug to alleviate withdrawal symptoms is effective. Second, long-term substitutions such as methadone for opiate withdrawal and nicotine patches or chewing gums for nicotine addiction are being used. Third, pharmacologic blocking of the primary drug targets is a direct method to counter drug use. Naltrexone, a μ-opioid receptor antagonist, and mecamylamine, a nicotinic receptor antagonist, sometimes are used to treat opiate and nicotine addiction, respectively. Fourth, aversive medications, such as disulfiram in the treatment of alcohol dependence, are being used. Finally, medications designed to limit craving or other components of relapse are used.

Therapeutics by Class

Pharmacotherapeutics Approved by the FDA

Alcoholism. Disulfiram inhibits ALDH, leading to increased blood acetaldehyde levels following intake of alcohol accompanied by various adverse symptoms such as facial flushing, tachycardia, nausea, and vomiting. This method is used to induce an aversive effect of drugs (see Table 55-3). In 1951, the FDA approved disulfiram (Antabuse) as an adjunctive treatment for alcohol dependence. A recent study shows that disulfiram has limited efficacy secondary to poor treatment adherence,[59] indicating that compliance, perhaps related to its aversive mechanism of action, is a major issue in using disulfiram. Overall, disulfiram may be clinically useful for those who are very determined to avoid alcohol.

Naltrexone was approved by the FDA for treatment of narcotic dependence in 1984 and for the treatment of alcohol dependence in 1995. Naltrexone is an opioid receptor antagonist with relative selectivity for the μ-opioid receptor at lower doses. This positive effect seems logical since ethanol administration increases the release of endogenous opioid peptides and subsequently leads to the release of dopamine in the NAc, with subsequent positive reinforcing effect.[60] Consistently, μ-opioid–null mice do not self-administer ethanol.[61] Numerous clinical trials have shown that naltrexone decreases relapse severity and diminishes craving.[62] Overall, naltrexone is effective during short-term treatment; in combination with behavior therapy, it improves treatment retention rate and efficacy.

Acamprosate is the most recent FDA-approved agent (in 2004) for treatment of alcohol dependence. It is a functional glutamate antagonist whose precise molecular mechanisms of action remain unclear. Acamprosate inhibits the effects of the hyperglutamatergic state that characterizes alcohol withdrawal in rats,[63] indicating that it abolishes the negative reinforcing effect of alcohol. Additional studies showed that acamprosate can normalize the progressive recruitment of elevated extracellular glutamate levels by repeated cycles of intoxication and withdrawal.[64,65] Recently, Spanagel and colleagues demonstrated that a hyperglutamatergic state in clock gene *per2*-mutant mice contributes to excessive alcohol drinking, and that acamprosate normalizes glutamate levels as well as reversing excessive drinking in the mice.[66] Like naltrexone, acamprosate has a modest and significant beneficial effect on treatment retention. In this regard, additional behavioral treatment to enhance the retention rate helps to increase the efficacy of acamprosate use.

Heroin Addiction. Methadone is a full agonist of the μ-opioid receptor. The methadone maintenance program has been in use in both detoxification and treatment for heroin addiction since 1964, and was approved by the FDA in 1973. The active form of methadone has a half-life of approximately 36 hours, while the half-life of the inactive form is around 16 hours.[67] A very well-established evidence base exists to support the notion that it is the cornerstone of opioid addiction treatment. Since methadone can produce a "rush" of euphoria if it is injected intravenously, most programs require a supervised daily administration of oral methadone. It has been demonstrated that progressive tolerance does not develop in patients maintained on doses of methadone ranging from 80 to 150 mg/day for over 35 years.[68]

L-α-acetyl morphine (LAAM) is a synthetic cogener of methadone with a longer duration of action, approved by the FDA for use in 1993. LAAM is metabolized in the gut wall and converted to its active metabolites, nor-LAAM and dinor-LAAM, via demethylation.[67] Because of its longer duration of action, it can be administered less frequently than methadone while maintaining similar or better effects. LAAM is usually dispensed in a specially licensed clinic two to three times per week. Recent findings demonstrated that LAAM can cause prolongation of QT intervals in the electrocardiograms of patients and a potentially life-threatening arrhythmia, which limited the clinical usefulness of LAAM.[67] Because of these side effects, LAAM is no longer being used in clinics.

Buprenorphine possesses partial agonist activity at μ-opioid receptors. Thus, it can attenuate the effects of full agonists such as morphine and heroin. Like LAAM, buprenorphine has a slow onset and a long duration of action. It is well absorbed sublingually. Coadministration with naloxone, an opioid antagonist, is known to be effective in preventing potential diversion of buprenorphine as it is not absorbed well sublingually but would induce withdrawal symptoms if dissolved and injected. Because of this, sublingual administration is commonly used to treat opioid dependence. The FDA approved buprenorphine monotherapy (Subetex) and the buprenorphine-naloxone treatment method (Suboxone) in 2002.

Nicotine Addiction. Nicotine replacement therapies (NRTs) help smoking cessation by providing nicotine indirectly and by lessening nicotine withdrawal symptoms. Currently, there are many forms of nicotine replacement methods available, including nicotine-containing chewing gum, transdermal nicotine patches, nicotine nasal spray, a nicotine inhaler, and nicotine lozenges. Most NRTs are available over the counter except the nasal spray and inhaler, which require a prescription.

Bupropion is a selective catecholamine (norepinephrine and dopamine) reuptake inhibitor. This drug was approved by the FDA in 1985 and marketed as an antidepressant. Despite several label revisions for formulation changes, seizure risk, and most recently a class label change for suicidality, it is a first-line antidepressant for many patients with depression and is the only FDA-approved treatment for seasonal affective disorder. Bupropion has also antagonist activity at the $alpha_3$ $beta_4$ nAChR-like ibogaine, which is known to be effective in reducing severity of nicotine cravings and withdrawal syndromes. The bupropion treatment course lasts between 7 and 12 weeks. Bupropion is metabolized in the liver and eliminated through excretion into the urine. The half-life of bupropion is 20 hours.

Combination treatment is useful in improving treatment outcome if a single agent shows a poor response. In nicotine addiction, a combination of NRTs or of NRTs and bupropion is known to be more effective than monotherapy.[69]

Behavioral Treatment Programs

Self-help groups such as Alcoholics Anonymous (AA), Narcotics Anonymous (NA), and Cocaine Anonymous (CA), which are based on a 12-step model, and other self-help groups such as Smart Recovery, can complement and extend the effects of pharmacotherapies. These groups also emphasize the central role of spirituality in recovery.

Therapeutic Approach

Clinical guidelines for the assessment of alcohol and/or drug use problems and for performance measurement of clinical addiction treatment programs have been published by several major organizations, including the American Psychiatric Association,[70] the Veteran's Administration,[71] the Institute of Medicine,[72] and the Washington Circle.[73] In addition, clinical principles of treatment have been well presented by the National Institute on Drug Abuse (*http://www.nida.nih.gov/*). The American Society of Addiction Medicine has published treatment-matching guidelines for individuals in need of formal therapeutic intervention, as well as evidence-based guidelines for the management of alcohol withdrawal and alcohol withdrawal delirium.[74-76] It is beyond the scope of this chapter to outline each of these guidelines in detail; this review focuses on a synthesis of the primary principles of assessment and intervention that are common to each of these guidelines and that define the standard of care in the field, with particular reference to evidence-based data on the effectiveness of drugs targeting addiction pathophysiology (Table 55-5).

The clinical assessment of alcohol and/or other drug use proceeds through a series of several stages and is predicated on the clinician's diagnostic and therapeutic acumen. The NIAAA[77] has recently published a four-step approach that (modified to include other substances of use) encapsulates the primary principles of assessment and intervention noted earlier, informally known as the "Four As":

1. Asking about alcohol and/or other drug use
2. Assessing for alcohol and/or other drug-related problems
3. Advising appropriate action
4. Assisting the patient in accessing treatment services and monitoring progress toward mutually agreed-upon therapeutic goals appropriately

Often the most prominent hurdle to overcome is inattention to inquiry about use.

While several screening instruments have enjoyed widespread popularity, recent research has supported the use of a single question in identifying "at-risk" drinkers deserving of further screening: "On any single occasion during the past 3 months, have you had more than five drinks containing alcohol?"[78] In addition, the Alcohol Use Disorders Identification Test (AUDIT) developed by the NIAAA is a sensitive and specific screening tool for identifying at-risk drinkers.[79] Individuals who score positively on these screening instruments should be referred to the next level of assessment, which includes measures of quantity and frequency as well as an assessment of patterns and consequences of use. Data exist that correlate quantity-frequency measures and the potential risk for abuse of or dependence upon alcohol.[80] In addition, relative risk data exist estimating the dependence-producing potential of a variety of substances of abuse.[81]

Individuals who do not qualify for a diagnosis of alcohol abuse or dependence (see Box 55-1) are advised either to abstain or to set drinking goals. As denial is a hallmark of addiction,[82] obtaining objective information from reliable sources is critical to the diagnosis of substance use disorders. Referral to a specialist is indicated if there is evidence of impaired control over use of the substance, preoccupation, continued use despite adverse consequence, craving, or evidence of physiologic dependence (changes in tolerance and/or withdrawal symptoms on cessation of use). Abstinence is advised if an individual demonstrates any of the following: (i) evidence of alcohol dependence, (ii) pregnancy or active attempts to conceive, (iii) comorbid psychiatric or medical conditions likely to be negatively impacted by alcohol use, and (iv) the possibility of drug-drug interactions occasioned by the introduction of alcohol.

Assisting patients in establishing drinking goals, accessing treatment if needed, and monitoring progress on an ongoing basis is crucial to an individual's success. It is important to keep in mind that behavior change occurs over time and progresses through several stages, including precontemplation, contemplation, preparation, action, and maintenance.[83] In addition, actual behavior change is more likely to occur if an individual perceives there is a behavior that needs to be changed, that indeed there exists a means of addressing the problem, and that he or she can play an active role in bringing about that change. Engaging the services of a substance abuse professional can be invaluable in matching an individual's clinical needs to the variety of therapeutic approaches available.

Until recently, addiction-specific pharmacologic interventions were limited for the individual with an alcohol or other drug use disorder. Pharmacologic emphasis was placed primarily on treating substance-related withdrawal syndromes, and treatment of psychiatric and/or medical comorbidity. Within the past 10 years, additional agents have been added to the armamentarium available to clinicians in these areas. However, it is likely that we are standing on the verge of a new era of addiction-specific pharmacotherapy targeting the enduring vulnerability to relapse that occurs once an addiction is physiologically established.[84]

Alcoholism

Drugs used to treat alcohol dependence are usually grouped into those that are used to treat alcohol withdrawal, and those used to prevent relapse to alcohol use once an individual has discontinued drinking. While this review primarily is devoted to examining the latter category, a brief mention of evidence-based reviews of agents used to treat alcohol withdrawal is in order.

TABLE 55-5 PHARMACOLOGIC CHARACTERISTICS OF MEDICATIONS USED FOR ADDICTION TREATMENT

Medication	Addiction Substance	Target Symptom	Main Target Protein	Common Side Effects	Contraindications and Warnings
Naltrexone	Alcohol Opioids	Craving Tolerance	Agonist: μ-Opioid receptor	Nausea or vomiting; abdominal pain or discomfort; anxiety; nervousness; fatigue; restlessness, trouble sleeping; headache; joint or muscle pain	• Allergic reaction to naltrexone • Active use of opioid drugs • Hepatic failure • Acute hepatitis • Risk for hepatotoxicity
Acamprosate	Alcohol	Craving	Unknown	Diarrhea; flatulence; asthenia	• Hypersensitivity to acamprosate • Severe renal impairment (creatinine clearance ≤30 ml/min) • Mild increase in suicidal ideation
Ondansetron	Alcohol	Craving	Antagonist: 5-HT_3 receptor	Headache; diarrhea; constipation; malaise/fatigue; dizziness	• Hypersensitivity to ondansetron
Baclofen	Alcohol	Withdrawal	Agonist: $GABA_B$ receptor	Bloody or dark urine; chest pain; fainting; hallucinations; depression or other mood changes; ringing or buzzing in the ears; skin rash or itching	• Hypersensitivity to baclofen (CNS toxicity more likely in elderly who have renal function impairment)
Topiramate	Alcohol	Craving	Agonist: $GABA_A$ receptor Antagonist: voltage-activated Na^+ and Ca^{2+} channels; AMPA and kainate receptors Inhibitor: carbonic anhydrase	Vision problems; uncontrolled eye movements; eye pain; eye redness; increased eye pressure; burning, prickling, or tingling sensations; clumsiness or unsteadiness; confusion; dizziness; drowsiness; generalized slowing of mental and physical activity; memory problems; nervousness; speech or language problems; trouble in concentrating or paying attention; unusual tiredness or weakness; menstrual changes; menstrual pain	• Hypersensitivity to topiramate • Hyperchloremic, non–anion gap, metabolic acidosis may develop • Primary narrow-angle glaucoma has been reported
Buprenorphine	Opioids	Craving	Partial agonist: μ-Opioid receptor Antagonist: κ-Opioid receptor	Dizziness, light-headedness, or feeling faint; drowsiness; nausea or vomiting; unusual tiredness or weakness. Psychotomimetic effects less likely compared to other opioid agonist/antagonist analgesics. Less dependence or abuse liability compared to other potent opioid analgesics.	• Hypersensitivity to buprenorphine • Significant respiratory depression has been associated with intravenous combination with benzodiazepines, alcohol, and other opioids or in patients with compromised respiratory function
Methadone	Opioids	Craving Withdrawal	Agonist: μ-Opioid receptor	Cold, clammy skin; redness or flushing of face; sweating	• Hypersensitivity to methadone? • Overdose may cause dizziness; confusion; drowsiness; low blood pressure; nervousness or restlessness; pinpoint pupils; slow heartbeat; slow or troubled breathing; weakness
Bupropion	Nicotine	Craving	Antagonist: $alpha_3$ $beta_2$ and $alpha_3$ $beta_4$ nAChR subunits Inhibitor: DAT and NET	Dry mouth and insomnia. Bupropion has low abuse potential. Few cases of drug dependence and withdrawal symptoms associated with the immediate-release formulation have been reported.	• Allergic response to bupropion • Seizure disorder • Bulimia or anorexia nervosa • Abrupt discontinuation of alcohol or sedatives • Concurrent administration with monoamine oxidase inhibitor • Worsening of depression and suicide risk in adolescents • Incidence of seizures is dose dependent

Continued

TABLE 55-5 PHARMACOLOGIC CHARACTERISTICS OF MEDICATIONS USED FOR ADDICTION TREATMENT—cont'd

Medication	Addiction Substance	Target Symptom	Main Target Protein	Common Side Effects	Contraindications and Warnings
Varenicline	Nicotine	Craving	Partial agonist: alpha$_4$ beta$_2$ nAChR subunit	Nausea; headache; insomnia and abnormal dreams	• Severe renal impairment may increase varenicline exposure
Nicotine	Nicotine	Withdrawal	Agonist: nAChRs	Vivid dreams or other sleep disturbances; increased heart rate; high blood pressure; local irritation (nasal, skin, etc.)	• Hypersensitivity or allergy to nicotine or to menthol (for inhaler and nasal spray)
Naloxone	Opioids	Tolerance	Antagonist: μ-, δ-, κ-Opioid receptors	Nausea and vomiting	
Disulfiram	Alcohol	Tolerance	Inhibitor: ALDH	Cases of hepatitis, and hepatic failure resulting in transplantation or death, have been reported. Occasional skin eruptions. Psychotic reactions have been noted, attributable in most cases to high dosage, combined toxicity (with metronidazole or isoniazid), or the unmasking of underlying psychoses in patients stressed by the withdrawal of alcohol.	• Hypersensitivity to disulfiram or to other thiuram derivatives used in pesticides and rubber vulcanization • Recent use of metronidazole, paraldehyde, alcohol, or alcohol-containing preparations (e.g., cough syrups, tonics aftershave lotions and back rubs) • Severe myocardial disease or coronary occlusion • Psychoses
Metronidazole	Alcohol	Tolerance	Inhibitor: ALDH	Numbness, tingling, pain, or weakness in hands or feet; seizures (usually with high doses)	• Hypersensitivity to metronidazole • Severe myocardial disease or coronary occlusion • Psychoses
Clonidine	Opioids	Withdrawal	Agonist: α_2-Adrenoreceptor	Constipation; dizziness; drowsiness; dryness of mouth; weakness, fatigue; headache	• Known hypersensitivity to clonidine • Sudden cessation of clonidine treatment may cause agitation, nervousness, headache, and tremor, accompanied or followed by a rapid rise in blood pressure

ALDH, aldehyde dehydrogenase; AMPA, α-amino-3-hydroxy-5-methyl-4-isoxazolepropionate; CNS, central nervous system; DAT, dopamine transporter; GABA, γ-aminobutyric acid; 5-HT, 5-hydroxytryptamine (serotonin); nAChR, nicotinic acetylcholine receptor; NET, norepinephrine transporter.

Two evidence-based practice guidelines have been published dealing with the management of alcohol withdrawal. The first of these, sponsored by the American Society of Addiction Medicine and authored by Mayo-Smith,[75] examined the extant literature to the date of publication utilizing a Level I-V system of assessing evidence (Level I, randomized controlled trial with low false-positive and low false-negative errors, to Level V, case series without controls) and a three-tiered system of recommendations (Grades A through C). The authors concluded that benzodiazepines reduce withdrawal severity and reduce incidence of delirium and seizures, and that individualizing therapy with withdrawal scales resulted in administration of substantially less medication and shorter treatment durations. β-Blockers, clonidine, and carbamazepine reduced withdrawal severity, but evidence was inadequate to determine effect on delirium and seizures. Phenothiazines ameliorated withdrawal seizures but were judged to be less effective than benzodiazepines in reducing delirium or seizures.

Mayo-Smith and colleagues also used a similar system of assessment for levels of evidence and recommendations in an evidence-based practice guideline for the management of alcohol withdrawal delirium.[76] In this study, the authors concluded that control of agitation should be achieved using parenteral rapid-acting sedative-hypnotic agents that are cross-tolerant with alcohol, and that adequate doses, enough to achieve light somnolence, should be used for the duration of the delirium, coupled with comprehensive supportive and medical care. Spies and Rommelspacher have addressed the prevention and treatment of alcohol withdrawal in the special circumstance of the postoperative intensive care unit patient.[85]

Garbutt et al. evaluated the efficacy of the drugs used to treat alcohol addiction into four distinct grades based on the consistency across studies, quality of studies, sample size, and magnitude of effects.[86] The grades are

Good (A): Data are sufficient for evaluating efficacy. The sample size is adequate. The data are consistent and indicate that the key drug is clearly superior to placebo for treating alcohol dependence.

Fair (B): Data are sufficient for evaluating efficacy. The sample size is adequate. The data indicate that there are inconsistencies in the findings between the key therapy and placebo and that the efficacy of the key therapy for treating alcohol dependence is not clearly established.

Poor (C): Data are sufficient for evaluating efficacy. The sample size is adequate. The data show that the key therapy is no more efficacious for treating alcohol dependence than placebo.

Incomplete evidence (I): Data are insufficient for assessing the efficacy of the key therapy for treating alcohol dependence based on limited sample size or poor methodology.

Disulfiram

Oral Disulfiram (Maintenance Dosage: 200 to 250 mg/day, Grade B). After alcohol intake under the influence of disulfiram, the concentration of acetaldehyde in the blood may be 5 to 10 times higher compared to normal alcohol metabolism, resulting in adverse flulike symptoms, including flushing, hypotension, nausea, and weakness. The effects start 5 to 10 minutes after alcohol intake and last 30 minutes to several hours depending on the individual. The five studies with 1207 subjects, including three double-blind, randomized controlled trials, provide modest evidence that disulfiram reduces drinking frequencies without significant improvement of abstinence rates.[87-89] Compliance with the use of disulfiram is critical to its success.

Disulfiram Implants (One-Time Dose: 800 to 1000 mg, Grade B). This method has been developed to ensure compliance and is currently being investigated. The six studies with 282 enrolled subjects revealed diverse outcomes without notable advantages over the tablet maintenance treatment.[86]

Naltrexone (Dose: 50 to 100 mg/day, Grade A). Bouza et al. recently summarized 19 studies addressing naltrexone efficacy; 17 of the 19 studies were single- or double-blind randomized clinical trials. To evaluate the efficacy, the studies were grouped by duration of treatment. For short-term treatment (≤12 weeks), naltrexone produced an effect with respect to the following secondary outcomes: time to relapse, percentage of drinking days, number of drinks per drinking day, days of abstinence, total consumption during treatment, and γ-glutamyl transpeptidase and aspartate aminotransferase levels.[62] However, Anton et al. reported that 14-week follow-up studies after the 12-week naltrexone treatment with 131 subjects does not support the effectiveness of naltrexone.[90] For midterm treatment (6 months), naltrexone has a favorable effect on both abstinence and relapse rates. However, there were no significant differences in amount of alcohol consumption or degree of compliance.[62] Interestingly, intensive behavior therapy increased the efficacy of naltrexone in the midterm treatment paradigm, whereas there was no significant effect of behavior therapy in short-term treatment.[91] This implies that the main benefit of behavioral treatment is to enhance patient compliance with naltrexone treatment. Recently, a depot preparation was shown to increase compliance and efficacy.[86] For long-term treatment (>12 months), available data have demonstrated no differences between naltrexone and placebo in terms of percentage of drinking days or number of drinks per drinking day at 12 months of treatment.[92]

Recently, the large-scale Combined Pharmacotherapies and Behavioral Interventions (COMBINE) studies revealed that all three treatment groups—(i) naltrexone + medical management (n = 302), (ii) a combined behavioral intervention + medical management (n = 305), and (iii) naltrexone + combined behavioral intervention + medical management (n = 309)—had a higher percentage of days abstinent (80.6, 79.2, and 77.1, respectively) compared to the control group (n = 305) assigned to placebo plus medical management (percentage days abstinent, 75.1). Naltrexone also reduced the number of heavy drinking days over time.[93]

Acamprosate (Dose: 1300 to 3000 mg/day, Grade A). Acamprosate has been available in Europe for more than a decade, and during that time there have been 16 published clinical trials that have included over 4500 subjects. In 14 of these 16 studies, acamprosate was shown to lengthen time to relapse, reduce drinking days, or increase complete abstinence among alcohol-dependent patients.[94] The first U.S. study was conducted in 21 outpatient clinics across the United States and published in 2006.[95] Research subjects were given the standard 2-g dose (n = 258), an exploratory 3-g dose (n = 83), or a placebo (n = 260) to evaluate the efficacy of acamprosate in a double-blind, placebo-controlled 6-month trial. The double-blind treatment period was 24 weeks, with research assessments at weeks 1, 2, 4, 8, 12, 16, 20, and 24. A one-time follow-up study was done 8 weeks after the treatment. The percentage of abstinent days was similar among three groups: 54.3% for placebo, 56.1% for 2 g, and 60.7% for 3 g. However, acamprosate significantly increased the percentage of abstinence days for the motivated subgroup having a baseline goal of abstinence (58.1% for placebo, 70% for 2 g, and 72.5% for 3 g; P = 0.02).

Conflicting data have been reported in the recent COMBINE study sponsored by the NIAAA. In this study, the authors concluded in their primary analysis that there is no advantage of acamprosate versus placebo.[93] This study also showed a lack of clinical advantage in combining acamprosate and naltrexone, which had been suggested to increase the bioavailability of acamprosate.[96] A 2006 abstract from the Research Society on Alcoholism meeting reported that acamprosate treatment with extensive behavior therapies was significantly effective for a majority of motivated patients utilizing abstinence as the study reference point and in the Penn Alcohol Craving Scale (PACS) and the Obsessive Compulsive Drinking Scale (OCDS) measures.[97,98] O'Malley noted that a secondary analysis of the COMBINE data is underway to determine what factors may account for the discrepancy between their study results and the substantial majority of the clinical trials currently published citing efficacy of acamprosate.[99] Several authors have noted informally that efficacy in these studies may be determined by degree of severity of alcohol dependence. It is possible that (i) well-managed behavior therapies and patient motivation are essential for the outcome of acamprosate treatment and (ii) pharmacogenomic profiles of individual patients may be important to determine drug efficacy.

Heroin Addiction

The treatment of opioid addiction can be broadly classified into two categories: that utilizing antagonist therapies (e.g., naltrexone) with abstinence as a goal, and that using agonist therapies (e.g., methadone, LAAM, and buprenorphine) with maintenance strategies as the cornerstone of treatment. Prior to the introduction of buprenorphine into the list of agents used to treat opioid addiction, the Veterans Administration (VA) reviewed the efficacy of both agonist and antagonist forms of therapy for heroin and other opioid addiction.[71] In grading the evidence, the rating scheme published by the U.S. Preventive Service Task Force was utilized. References were reviewed for scientific merit, clinical relevance, and applicability to populations served by the VA. Quality of Evidence (QE) Grades I-III were assigned based on experimental design and overall quality. These may be summarized as follows:

Grade I: Evidence obtained from at least one properly randomized controlled trial.

Grade II-1: Evidence obtained from well-designed controlled trials without randomization.

Grade II-2: Evidence obtained from well-designed cohort or case-control analytic studies, preferably from more than one center or research group.

Grade II-3: Evidence obtained from multiple time series with or without the intervention. Dramatic results in uncontrolled experiments could also be regarded as this type of evidence.

Grade III: Opinions of respected authorities based on clinical experience, descriptive studies and case reports, or reports of expert committees.

In addition, a recommendation rating scheme of Grades A-E in descending order of recommended use was developed by the working group, based primarily on the scientific evidence. Grade A represented a strong recommendation of efficacy, while Grade E reflected the opinion that the agent should be excluded from consideration. Recommendations in a treatment algorithm carried both sets of grading in their justifications.

Methadone (Dose: 80 to 120 mg/day; Grade: VA QE Level I; Recommendation Grade: A). For over 40 years since its introduction by Dole and Nyswander,[100] methadone agonist (or maintenance) therapy has been a cornerstone of treatment for opiate dependence. In one of the earliest clinical trials, methadone was administered orally in doses of 20 to 40 mg initially and increased by 10 mg/week to a target range of 80 to 120 mg/day. During this treatment, withdrawal signs and symptoms were abolished and craving was significantly reduced. The patients in the methadone maintaining program with 80 to 120 mg/day for 150 days could not discriminate the difference between heroin, morphine, hydromorphine, and methadone versus saline under controlled, double-blind conditions, suggesting that the long-term methadone exposure led to development of cross-tolerance to other opiates.[100] In the 1970s, a group conducted a clinical study in Hong Kong.[101] In this double-blind study, 100 volunteers with heroin addiction were initially admitted to a hospital for 2 weeks for stabilization on 60 mg of methadone before being assigned at random to one of two groups: one group received methadone (range 30 to 130 mg, average 97 mg/day); those in the other group had their dose of methadone reduced at the rate of 1 mg/day and were then maintained on placebo. All subjects were provided with a broad range of supportive services. After 32 weeks, 10% of the controls were still in treatment, compared with 76% of those receiving methadone. At the end of the 3-year project, only 1 of the original 50 placebo subjects still turned up for treatment (2%), whereas the retention rate (proportion still in treatment) for methadone subjects was 56%. Subjects who had dropped out of the study and were readmitted for methadone treatment under known conditions had the same retention rate as the original treatment group. This study clearly demonstrated that methadone increased treatment retention rate. In the 1990s, a study led by Strain et al. demonstrated that a higher dose group experienced the greatest beneficial effect on relapse compared to a moderate-dose group.[102] In this study, 192 patients were enrolled and divided into two groups depending on methadone doses. One group was treated with 40 to 50 mg/day (n = 97) and the other group was administered 80 to 100 mg/day (n = 95) with concurrent counseling. By intent-to-treat analysis through week 30, the high-dose group had significantly reduced opiate use compared with patients in the moderate-dose group. These differences persisted during withdrawal from methadone.

As of 2002, about 180,000 (~20%) of 898,000 chronic opiate users in the United States were enrolled in methadone treatment programs and another 100,000 were being treated by other methods.[67] Up to 80% of patients remain abstinent for 1 to 3 years during the treatment, and one 6-year follow-up study showed that 40% of former methadone patients were abstinent from opiates.[103]

LAAM (Dose: 75 to 115 mg, 3 times/wk; Grade: VA QE Level I; Recommendation Grade: A). LAAM is a long-acting μ-opioid agonist provided in the context of specialized opioid maintenance treatment programming. It is typically dosed three times weekly. Multicenter double-blind trials have been conducted to compare LAAM and methadone dosing levels. In one study, LAAM was compared with two dosage strengths of methadone with 430 street heroin addicts from 12 VA hospitals. The starting sample consisted of 146 patients receiving low-dose methadone, and 142 patients who were given LAAM. The LAAM patients with the 80-mg dose regimen (three times per week) demonstrated greater reductions in opiate use than those in the low-dose (50-mg) methadone group.[104] Another multicenter trial was performed to evaluate the effects of LAAM.[105] This study compared patients who had continued methadone use with those who transferred from the methadone treatment program to a LAAM treatment program. Subjects were randomly assigned to continued maintenance on methadone (n = 308) or transferred to LAAM (n = 328) for a period of 40 weeks. This study suggested that LAAM is as safe as methadone and, when given three times a week, is an acceptable and effective maintenance drug for many heroin addicts. However, LAAM-transferred patients had a lower retention rate (31%) compared to the methadone group (60%).

The FDA approved LAAM for marketing in 1993, and initially 421 out of an estimated 9000 narcotic treatment programs registered to dispense LAAM to 5100 patients in the United States.[106] To evaluate the clinical efficacy of different doses of LAAM in the treatment of opioid dependence, a randomized, controlled, double-blind, parallel group, 17-week study was conducted.[106] In this study, opioid-dependent volunteers (n = 180) were recruited and thrice-weekly (Monday/Wednesday/Friday) oral LAAM dose regimens of 25/25/35 mg, 50/50/70 mg, and 100/100/140 mg were offered, and voluntary counseling was provided. Results showed that the self-reported heroin use decreased in a dose-related manner. At final assessment, patients in the high-dose condition reported using heroin 2.5 of 30 days as compared with 4.1 or 6.3 days for patients in the medium-dose and low-dose conditions, respectively. Consistently, the urinalysis results were similarly dose related, suggesting that the clinical efficacy of LAAM is positively related to dose. Recently, Johnson et al. compared the efficacy of LAAM (75 to 115 mg), buprenorphine (16 to 32 mg), and high-dose (60 to 100 mg) and low-dose (20 mg) methadone as treatments for opioid dependence in a 17-week randomized study of 220 patients.[107] In this study, LAAM and buprenorphine were administered three times a week while methadone was administered daily. The data suggest that higher dose methadone, LAAM, and buprenorphine reduced illicit opiate use compared to the low-dose methadone group.[107] In 2001, the FDA approved taking LAAM at home without supervision. However, LAAM was removed from the market in 2003 because of severe side effects.

Buprenorphine. Two formulations of buprenorphine from Reckitt Benckiser have been approved in the United States to treat opioid addiction: Subutex (flavorless sublingual, no active additives; in 2- and 8-mg dosages) and Suboxone (orange-flavored sublingual, one part naloxone for every four parts buprenorphine; in 2- and 8-mg dosages). A recent clinical trial led by Ling and colleagues demonstrated the clinical effectiveness of buprenorphine-naloxone (bup-nx) over clonidine for opioid detoxification in inpatient and outpatient community treatment programs.[108] In this study, opioid-dependent individuals seeking short-term treatment were randomly assigned, in a 2 : 1 ratio favoring bup-nx, to a 13-day detoxification using bup-nx or clonidine. Bup-nx combination tablets in dosages of 2 mg buprenorphine/0.5 mg naloxone and/or 8 mg buprenorphine/2.0 mg naloxone were used. A total of 113 inpatients (77 bup-nx, 36 clonidine) and 231 outpatients (157 bup-nx, 74 clonidine) participated. Supportive interventions included appropriate ancillary medications and standard counseling procedures guided by a self-help handbook. The criterion for treatment success was defined as the proportion of participants in each condition who were both retained in the study for the entire duration and provided an opioid-free urine sample on the last day of clinic attendance. Secondary outcome measures included use of ancillary medications, number of side effects reported, and withdrawal and craving ratings. A total of 59 of the 77 inpatients assigned to the bup-nx condition (77%) achieved the treatment success criterion compared to 8 of the 36 assigned to clonidine (22%), whereas 46 of the 157 outpatients assigned to the bup-nx condition (29%) achieved the treatment success criterion, compared to 4 of the 74 assigned to clonidine (5%).

Another recent study with a small number of participants showed that the combination of buprenorphine and carbamazepine leads to a better clinical outcome compared to a combination of methadone and carbamazepine in the detoxification of opioid addicts.[109] In this study, 26 patients with opioid dependence participated and received randomly either a combination of an 11-day low-dose buprenorphine and a 14-day carbamazepine regimen (n = 14) or a combination of an 11-day methadone and a 14-day carbamazepine regimen (n = 12) in a double-blind, randomized 14-day inpatient detoxification treatment. Patients taking buprenorphine and carbamazepine showed a significantly better psychological state after the first and second weeks of treatment. Above all, the buprenorphine-treated patients demonstrated less fatigue, less sensitivity, and less dysphoria as well as more prominent mood elevation during the detoxification process. Consistent with the Ling et al.[108] study, this trial supports the effectiveness of buprenorphine in opioid detoxification.

A study led by Fiellin's group at Yale University investigated the use of counseling and different frequencies of medication dispensing in primary care treatment with buprenorphine-naloxone.[110] They conducted a 24-week randomized, controlled clinical trial with 166 patients assigned to one of three treatments: standard medical management and either once-weekly or thrice-weekly medication dispensing, or enhanced medical management and thrice-weekly medication dispensing. Standard medical management was brief, manual-guided, medically focused counseling; enhanced management was similar, but each session was extended. The primary outcomes were self-reported frequency of illicit opioid use, the percentage of opioid-negative urine specimens, and the maximum number of consecutive weeks of abstinence from illicit opioids. The three treatments had similar efficacies with respect to the mean percentage of opioid-negative urine specimens (standard medical management and once-weekly medication dispensing, 44%; standard medical management and thrice-weekly medication dispensing, 40%; and enhanced medical management and thrice-weekly medication dispensing, 40%; $P = 0.82$) and the maximum number of consecutive weeks during which patients were abstinent from illicit opioids. All three treatments were associated with significant reductions from baseline in the frequency of illicit opioid use, but there were no significant differences among the treatments. The proportion of patients remaining in the study at 24 weeks did not differ significantly among the patients receiving standard medical management and once-weekly medication dispensing (48%) or thrice-weekly medication dispensing (43%) or enhanced medical management and thrice-weekly medication dispensing (39%) ($P = 0.64$). Adherence to buprenorphine-naloxone treatment varied; increased adherence was associated with improved treatment outcomes. This study indicated that, although there were no beneficial effects of extended counseling or thrice-weekly medication dispensing over the relatively limited nurse-administered counseling and once-weekly dispensing, the results support the feasibility of buprenorphine-naloxone maintenance in primary care.

Nicotine Addiction

Nicotine Replacement Therapies. Nicotine gum was approved as a pharmacotherapeutic aid in the treatment of nicotine dependence in 1984 under the trade name "Nicorette," followed by approval of other forms of NRT, including the transdermal nicotine patch. In 1994, a group led by Hurt et al. demonstrated the efficacy of the nicotine patch. In this trial, patients were treated with a 22-mg nicotine patch in a randomized, double-blind, placebo-controlled trial.[111] Subjects were 240 healthy volunteers who were smoking at least 20 cigarettes per day, and were randomly assigned to 8 weeks of a 22-mg nicotine or placebo patch. Main outcome measures were (i) abstinence from smoking, verified by expired air carbon monoxide levels; (ii) withdrawal symptoms, recorded during patch therapy; and (iii) percentage of nicotine replacement, as calculated by dividing serum nicotine and cotinine levels at week 8 of patch therapy by levels obtained while smoking. They found a higher smoking cessation rate in the active nicotine patch group at 8 weeks (46.7% vs. 20%) ($P < 0.001$) and at 1 year (27.5% vs. 14.2%) ($P = 0.011$). Higher smoking cessation rates were also observed in subjects assigned to the active patch who had lower serum levels of nicotine and cotinine at baseline, and withdrawal symptom relief was greater in the active patch group compared with placebo. This study demonstrated that clinically significant smoking cessation can be achieved using nicotine patch therapy combined with physician intervention, nurse counseling, follow-up, and relapse prevention. Smokers with lower baseline nicotine and cotinine levels had improved rates of cessation. This provides indirect evidence that more adequate nicotine replacement was achieved with this fixed dose of transdermal nicotine than in those smokers with higher baseline levels.

In 2002, Silagy et al. reviewed the over 90 randomized trials of NRT then published.[112] Following this, a clinical trial was conducted by the same group: (i) to evaluate the effectiveness of the different forms of NRT (chewing gum, transdermal patches, nasal spray, inhalers, and tablets) in achieving abstinence from cigarettes, or a sustained reduction in amount smoked; (ii) to determine whether the effect is influenced by the clinical setting in which the smoker is recruited and treated, the dosage and form of the NRT used, or the intensity of additional advice and support offered to the smoker; (iii) to determine whether combinations of NRT are more effective than one type alone; and (iv) to determine the effectiveness of NRT compared to other pharmacotherapies.[113] In this study, they measured a main outcome as abstinence from smoking after at least 6 months of follow-up. They identified 123 trials; 103 contributed to the primary comparison between NRT and a placebo or non-NRT control group. The odds ratio (OR) for abstinence with NRT compared to control was 1.77 (95% confidence interval [CI], 1.66 to 1.88). The ORs for the different forms of NRT were 1.66 (95% CI, 1.52 to 1.81) for gum, 1.81 (95% CI, 1.63 to 2.02) for patches, 2.35 (95% CI, 1.63 to 3.38) for nasal spray, 2.14 (95% CI, 1.44 to 3.18) for inhaled nicotine, and 2.05 (95% CI, 1.62 to 2.59) for nicotine sublingual tablet/lozenge. These odds were largely independent of the duration of therapy, the intensity of additional support provided, or the setting in which the NRT was offered. In highly dependent smokers, there was a significant benefit of 4-mg gum compared with 2-mg gum (OR 2.20; 95% CI, 1.85 to 3.25). There was weak evidence that combinations of forms of NRT are more effective. Higher doses of nicotine patch may produce small increases in cessation rates.

Only one study directly compared NRT to another pharmacotherapy. In this study, cessation rates with bupropion were higher than with nicotine patch or placebo. The authors concluded that all of the commercially available forms of NRT (gum, transdermal patch, nasal spray, inhaler, and sublingual tablets/lozenges) are effective as part of a strategy to promote smoking cessation. The effectiveness of NRT appears to be largely independent of the intensity of additional support provided to the smoker.

Bupropion (150 to 300 mg/day). Bupropion sustained-release (SR) was approved for smoking cessation in the United States in 1997. In the same year, Hurt et al. published a double-blind, placebo-controlled trial of a sustained-release form of bupropion for smoking cessation.[114] The 615 subjects were randomly assigned to receive placebo or bupropion at a dose of 100, 150, or 300 mg/day for 7 weeks. At the end of 7 weeks of treatment, the rates of smoking cessation as confirmed by carbon monoxide measurements were 19.0% in the placebo group, 28.8% in the 100-mg group, 38.6% in the 150-mg group, and 44.2% in the 300-mg group ($P < 0.001$). They concluded that a sustained-release form of bupropion was effective for smoking cessation and was accompanied by reduced weight gain and minimal side effects.

In 2003, Ferry and Johnston reviewed the efficacy and safety of bupropion SR for treatment of tobacco dependence based on data from clinical trials and 5 years of postmarketing experience, through June 2001.[115] There were approximately 32 million patient exposures to bupropion (9 million for smoking cessation) in clinical practice, and more than 8000 patients had been studied in clinical trials for tobacco dependence. In clinical trials, bupropion SR was more effective than placebo at improving initial and long-term abstinence rates and preventing relapse. Bupropion SR is generally well tolerated. The most common adverse event in clinical trials or clinical practice is insomnia, which can also be a symptom of nicotine withdrawal. The two main risks of treatment with bupropion SR are major motor seizure and hypersensitivity reaction. Clinical trials data suggest that the incidence of seizure is approximately 0.1%, and that of serious cases of hypersensitivity approximately 0.12%. Benefit-risk assessment, assuming a 30% 1-year cessation rate, demonstrates that, for every 10,000 smokers treated with bupropion SR, 19 lives are saved and 86 cases of smoking-attributed morbidity are averted in a 5-year period, while the risk of experiencing one of the two potentially serious adverse events during treatment is 0.22%. These data further establish both the efficacy and safety of bupropion SR and its use in preventing the adverse health effects of chronic tobacco use.

Varenicline Tartrate. Varenicline tartrate, a selective nAChR partial agonist, represents a novel type of therapy for smoking cessation. It was approved by the FDA in May 2006 as an aid for smoking cessation. Oncken et al.[116] evaluated the efficacy, safety, and tolerability of four varenicline dose regimens, two with progressive dosing over the first week (e.g., titrated) and two with a fixed dosing schedule (e.g., nontitrated), for promoting smoking cessation. They found that, on weeks 9 through 12, continuous quit rates were greater in the 1.0-mg group (49.4%) and the 0.5-mg group (44.0%) versus placebo (11.6%; $P <$ 0.001 vs. both doses). On weeks 9 through 52, abstinence rates were greater in the 1.0-mg group (22.4%; $P < 0.001$) and the 0.5-mg group (18.5%; $P < 0.001$) versus placebo (3.9%). Varenicline was generally well tolerated, with nausea occurring in 16% to 42% of varenicline-treated subjects. Reports of nausea were lower for the titrated versus nontitrated dosing and infrequently led to medication discontinuation. Authors of this study concluded that varenicline tartrate,

0.5 mg and 1.0 mg twice daily, is efficacious for smoking cessation.[116] In a Phase II, multicenter, randomized, double-blind, placebo-controlled study of healthy smokers, the same group of researchers demonstrated both short-term (1 mg twice daily and 1 mg once daily) and long-term (1 mg twice daily) efficacy of varenicline tartrate versus placebo and favorable effects of the 1-mg twice daily dose versus bupropion.[117]

Emerging Targets and Therapeutics

Novel Pharmacotherapies

Given the neuroplastic change that results from chronic drug exposure, receptor antagonist therapies designed to circumvent acute reinforcement, used alone, are unlikely to achieve efficacy or effectiveness in treating addictive behavior. Altered brain circuits persist, and are hardly reversible by blocking a primary site of action. It is not surprising, therefore, that agonists or partial agonists that can compensate for and mitigate the effect of the addictive drug without causing another addiction have shown the most successful treatment effects thus far. Once a person is addicted, the therapeutic focus shifts to those secondary or multiple neurotransmitter systems that mediate craving, withdrawal syndromes, and relapse.

As one of the major precipitants of relapse is associated with drug-specific cues and general stress, drugs that can modify the cue-related cognitive function and relieve the stress-induced priming system represent another therapeutic target for consideration. Also, modifying the pharmacokinetics of drugs and developing sustained-release forms may improve treatment outcome in individuals for whom compliance is an issue. Slowing the kinetics of entry into the brain via the blood-brain barrier (e.g., through the use of vaccines) may hold promise. In this section, several examples of agents with novel therapeutic targets are reviewed.

Alcoholism. Several new medications are currently being developed in addition to three FDA approved drugs.[117a] Ondansetron is a serotonin 5-HT_3 receptor antagonist currently used to treat nausea and vomiting in humans. In 1993, Johnson et al. demonstrated that pretreatment with ondansetron significantly attenuated the positive reinforcing effects of alcohol along with reducing the craving for alcohol.[118] Recently, ondansetron has been shown to be effective in treating early-onset alcoholics compared to placebo, but not for late-onset alcoholics.[119] Ondansetron appears to be safe and well tolerated.

Baclofen is a $GABA_B$ receptor agonist and is used to treat spastic movement at a spinal level. The usefulness of baclofen in treating alcoholism was suggested long ago.[120] However, recently the use of baclofen in alcoholism was more specifically examined in humans,[121,122] showing that baclofen reduced alcohol craving and intake. In rodent experiments, baclofen has been shown to inhibit acquisition of alcohol consumption[123] and to suppress motivation to obtain alcohol.[124] Baclofen may have potential in the treatment of addiction to other drugs such as opiates, cocaine, and nicotine.[125]

Topiramate is an anticonvulsant that has also been effective in the treatment of obesity.[126] Its mechanism of action in the treatment of addiction has not been clearly delineated. Recently, topiramate has been shown to potentiate GABA signaling[127] and to antagonize glutamatergic signaling at kainite receptors.[128] Johnson et al. have demonstrated that topiramate is more efficacious than placebo as an adjunct to standardized medication compliance regimens in the treatment of alcohol dependence.[129,130] Interestingly, topiramate is useful for the treatment of cigarette smoking in alcohol-dependent individuals.[131] There has been a steady interest in the evaluation of mood-stabilizing anticonvulsants as potential treatments for alcohol withdrawal and/or alcohol abuse relapse prevention. This interest is from the standpoint of the similarity of preclinical models of alcoholism to bipolar disorder.[132]

A recently developed LY686017 is a neurokinin 1 (substance P) receptor antagonist. A clinical study demonstrated that LY686017 suppressed spontaneous alcohol cravings, improved overall well being, blunted cravings induced by a challenge procedure, and attenuated concomitant cortisol responses.[132a] Most importantly, the fMRI study showed that this compound suppresses the stress and negative emotions that drive anxious alcoholics to drink.[132a] Further studies with a larger population will warrant the usefulness of LY686017 in the clinics.

Nicotine Addiction. Several nonapproved but clinically available pharmacologic treatments have been used for nicotine addiction.[69] Clonidine, an α_2-adrenoreceptor agonist, was approved originally for the treatment of hypertension. Later this compound was found to be effective in reducing opiate withdrawal symptoms. Combined data from nine double-blind, placebo-controlled trials ($N = 813$), showed a smoking quit rate with clonidine that was significantly greater than placebo. Further analysis suggested that behavior therapy potentiated this effect. Interestingly, it appeared that female smokers benefited more substantially from clonidine than male smokers.[133] However, clonidine shows significant side effects such as sedation, constipation, and orthostatic hypotension, limiting its use, and it is currently considered as a second-line cessation pharmacotherapy.

Mecamylamine is a noncompetitive antagonist for the high-affinity nAChR. Nemeth-Coslett et al.[134] demonstrated that mecamylamine decreased several measures of cigarette smoking, including number of cigarettes, number of puffs per cigarette, and expired air carbon monoxide level, in multiple measures of cigarette smoking during 90-minute test sessions in normal volunteers. Before sessions, subjects received oral doses of mecamylamine (2.5, 5.0, 10, or 20 mg) or placebo. Each dose and placebo was given three times in a randomized block sequence. Currently, several studies of mecamylamine in combination with NRTs are underway.

A nicotine vaccine produces antibodies that bind to nicotine and prevent it from crossing the blood-brain barrier to act on receptors in the brain. Vaccination of animals attenuates nicotine effects[135] and suppresses dopamine release in the nucleus accumbens.[136] These results suggest that a nicotine vaccine could reduce relapse to smoking by attenuating the pharmacologic effects of nicotine during the first few months after quitting.[137] This new approach for improving the success of smoking cessation is currently under clinical trials.[138]

Cocaine Addiction. Since there is no FDA-approved medication available for cocaine and amphetamine addiction, many studies are underway searching for effective pharmacotherapies for cocaine and/or other psychostimulant-related addictions (for details, see the tables in two recent reviews[60,84]). Here we review several clinically promising medications.

Desipramine is a tricyclic antidepressant that inhibits the reuptake of norepinephrine. It is used to treat depression and was later found to be effective in treating neuropathic pain. Oliveto et al. presented data indicating that the desipramine and amantadine groups appeared to have greater increases in opioid- and cocaine-free urines than the fluoxetine group in a double-blind, 12-week trial.[139] A recent clinical study from a randomized, placebo-controlled, 12-week clinical trial in 165 opioid- and cocaine-dependent patients who were treated with desipramine in combination with buprenorphine or methadone showed that the desipramine effect was significant in patients maintained on buprenorphine, but not on methadone.[140]

In rodents, the dopamine$_3$ receptor antagonists SB-277011A and NGB 2904 inhibit cocaine- and/or stress-induced reinstatement of drug-seeking behavior. Interestingly, BP-897 (a mixed dopamine$_3$ receptor agonist/antagonist) produced a 70% inhibition of cue-induced reinstatement at a dose of 3 mg/kg.[141]

Marijuana Addiction. The CB1-selective antagonist SR141716 has been shown to inhibit the acute psychological and physiologic effects of marijuana in human volunteers.[142] In this study, 63 healthy men with a history of marijuana use were randomly assigned to receive oral SR141716 or a placebo in an escalating-dose (1, 3, 10, 30, and 90 mg) design. Each subject smoked an active (2.64% THC) or placebo marijuana cigarette 2 hours later. Single oral doses of SR141716 produced a significant dose-dependent blockade of marijuana-induced subjective intoxication and tachycardia. The 90-mg dose produced 38% to 43% reductions in visual analog scale ratings and produced a 59% reduction in heart rate. SR141716 was well tolerated by all subjects. Therefore, this compound is promising for the future.

Pharmacogenomics: Individualized Treatment

Interestingly, statistics show that only a small portion of regular drug users actually develop an addictive disorder. For example, only 5% to 10% of regular alcohol drinkers and cocaine users, and 25% to 30% of snorting active opiate users, become addicted.[60] Thus, a subset of the population may have genetic susceptibilities or, conversely, genetically related resilience. A recent pharmacogenomic study demonstrated that alcoholic patients who carry at least one allele of Asp40 (A118G) of mu-opioid receptor could have a significantly higher benefit from naltrexone treatment regardless of behavioral treatment whereas Asn40 non-carrier alcoholics have no beneficial effects from naltrexone treatment.[143] This finding opens up the possibility to select subgroups based on genetic predisposition to maximize pharamcotherapies. Therefore, the promise of genomic medicine as applied in this population will be to help identify individuals who have particular susceptibilities that can be effectively matched to specific primary, secondary, or tertiary prevention efforts.

REFERENCES

1. American Psychiatric Association. Diagnostic and Statistical Manual of Mental Disorders, Fourth Edition. Washington, DC: American Psychiatric Press, 2004.
2. Pouletty P. Drug addictions: towards socially accepted and medically treatable diseases. Nat Rev Drug Discov 2002;1:731-736.
3. Koob GF, Le Moal M. Neurobiology of Addiction. San Diego: Elsevier, 2006.
4. Nestler EJ. Is there a common molecular pathway for addiction? Nat Neurosci 2005;8:1445-1449.
5. United Nations International Drug Control Programme and World Health Organization Informal Expert Committee on the Craving Mechanism. Technical Report Series No. V. Geneva: World Health Organization, 1992.
6. Kreek MJ, Nielsen DA, Butelman ER, LaForge KS. Genetic influences on impulsivity, risk taking, stress responsivity and vulnerability to drug abuse and addiction. Nat Neurosci 2005;8:1450-1457.
7. Johnson C, Drgon T, Liu QR, et al. Pooled association genome scanning for alcohol dependence using 104,268 SNPs: validation and use to identify alcoholism vulnerability loci in unrelated individuals from the collaborative study on the genetics of alcoholism. Am J Med Genet B Neuropsychiatr Genet 2006;141:844-853.
8. Weinshilboum R, Wang L. Pharmacogenomics: bench to bedside. Nat Rev Drug Discov 2004;3:739-748.
9. Boehm SL 2nd, Ponomarev I, Jennings AW, et al. γ-Aminobutyric acid A receptor subunit mutant mice: new perspectives on alcohol actions. Biochem Pharmacol 2004;68:1581-1602.
10. Krystal JH, Petrakis IL, Mason G, et al. *N*-methyl-D-aspartate glutamate receptors and alcoholism: reward, dependence, treatment, and vulnerability. Pharmacol Ther 2003;99:79-94.
11. Mansour A, Khachaturian H, Lewis ME, et al. Anatomy of CNS opioid receptors. Trends Neurosci 1988;11:308-314.
12. Rang H, Dale MM, Ritter JM, Moore PK. Pharmacology, 5th ed. Edinburgh: Churchill Livingstone, 2003.
13. Meyer JH, Quenzer LH. Psychopharmacology: Drugs, The Brain, and Behavior. Sunderland, MA: Sinauer Associates, 2005.
14. Cordero-Erausquin M, Marubio LM, Klink R, Changeux JP. Nicotinic receptor function: new perspectives from knockout mice. Trends Pharmacol Sci 2000;21:211-217.
15. Cobb MH, Boulton TG, Robbins DJ. Extracellular signal-regulated kinases: ERKs in progress. Cell Regul 1991;2:965-978.
16. Picciotto MR, Zoli M, Zachariou V, Changeux JP. Contribution of nicotinic acetylcholine receptors containing the beta 2-subunit to the behavioural effects of nicotine. Biochem Soc Trans 1997;25:824-829.
17. Pidoplichko VI, DeBiasi M, Williams JT, Dani JA. Nicotine activates and desensitizes midbrain dopamine neurons. Nature 1997;390:401-404.
18. Foulds J, Stapleton JA, Bell N, et al. Mood and physiological effects of subcutaneous nicotine in smokers and never-smokers. Drug Alcohol Depend 1997;44:105-115.
19. Hildebrand BE, Panagis G, Svensson TH, Nomikos GG. Behavioral and biochemical manifestations of mecamylamine-precipitated nicotine withdrawal in the rat: role of nicotinic receptors in the ventral tegmental area. Neuropsychopharmacology 1999;21:560-574.
20. Jones RT. The pharmacology of cocaine smoking in humans. NIDA Res Monogr 1990;99:30-41.
21. Sora I, Hall FS, Andrews AM, et al. Molecular mechanisms of cocaine reward: combined dopamine and serotonin transporter knockouts eliminate cocaine place preference. Proc Natl Acad Sci U S A 2001;98:5300-5305.
22. Uhl GR, Hall FS, Sora I. Cocaine, reward, movement and monoamine transporters. Mol Psychiatry 2002;7:21-26.
23. Volkow ND, Wang GJ, Fowler JS, et al. Blockade of striatal dopamine transporters by intravenous methylphenidate is not sufficient to induce self-reports of "high." J Pharmacol Exp Ther 1999;288:14-20.
24. Volkow ND, Wang GJ, Fowler JS, et al. Dopamine transporter occupancies in the human brain induced by therapeutic doses of oral methylphenidate. Am J Psychiatry 1998;155:1325-1331.
25. McCann UD, Ricaurte GA. Amphetamine neurotoxicity: accomplishments and remaining challenges. Neurosci Biobehav Rev 2004;27:821-826.
26. Hatzidimitriou G, McCann UD, Ricaurte GA. Altered serotonin innervation patterns in the forebrain of monkeys treated with (±)3,4-methylenedioxymethamphetamine seven years previously: factors influencing abnormal recovery. J Neurosci 1999;19:5096-5107.
27. Agurell S, Halldin M, Lindgren JE, et al. Pharmacokinetics and metabolism of delta 1-tetrahydrocannabinol and other cannabinoids with emphasis on man. Pharmacol Rev 1986;38:21-43.
28. Devane WA, Dysarz FA 3rd, Johnson MR, et al. Determination and characterization of a cannabinoid receptor in rat brain. Mol Pharmacol 1988;34:605-613.
29. Matsuda LA, Lolait SJ, Brownstein MJ, et al. Structure of a cannabinoid receptor and functional expression of the cloned cDNA. Nature 1990;346:561-564.
30. Iversen L. Cannabis and the brain. Brain 2003;126(Pt 6):1252-1270.
31. Calignano A, La Rana G, Giuffrida A, Piomelli D. Control of pain initiation by endogenous cannabinoids. Nature 1998;394:277-281.
32. Richardson JD, Aanonsen L, Hargreaves KM. Hypoactivity of the spinal cannabinoid system results in NMDA-dependent hyperalgesia. J Neurosci 1998;18:451-457.
33. Black SC. Cannabinoid receptor antagonists and obesity. Curr Opin Investig Drugs 2004;5:389-394.
34. Marsicano G, Wotjak CT, Azad SC, et al. The endogenous cannabinoid system controls extinction of aversive memories. Nature 2002;418:530-534.
35. Tanda G, Pontieri FE, Di Chiara G. Cannabinoid and heroin activation of mesolimbic dopamine transmission by a common mu1 opioid receptor mechanism. Science 1997;276:2048-2050.
36. Haney M, Bisaga A, Foltin RW. Interaction between naltrexone and oral THC in heavy marijuana smokers. Psychopharmacology (Berl) 2003;166:77-85.
37. Ghozland S, Matthes HW, Simonin F, et al. Motivational effects of cannabinoids are mediated by mu-opioid and kappa-opioid receptors. J Neurosci 2002;22:1146-1154.
38. Kouri EM, Pope HG Jr. Abstinence symptoms during withdrawal from chronic marijuana use. Exp Clin Psychopharmacol 2000;8:483-492.
39. Goldman D, Oroszi G, Ducci F. The genetics of addictions: uncovering the genes. Nat Rev Genet 2005;6:521-532.
40. Schuckit MA, Smith TL. The relationship of behavioural undercontrol to alcoholism in higher-functioning adults. Drug Alcohol Rev 2006;25:393-402.
41. Luczak SE, Shea SH, Hsueh AC, et al. *ALDH2*2* is associated with a decreased likelihood of alcohol-induced blackouts in Asian American college students. J Stud Alcohol 2006;67:349-353.
42. Edwards JA, Price J. Metronidazole and human alcohol dehydrogenase. Nature 1967;214:190-191.
43. Mottin JL. Drug-induced attenuation of alcohol consumption: a review and evaluation of claimed, potential or current therapies. Q J Stud Alcohol 1973;34:444-472.
44. Wilson CW, O'Brien C, MacAirt JG. The effect of metronidazole on the human taste threshold to alcohol. Br J Addict Alcohol Other Drugs 1973;68:99-110.
45. Bhargava HN, Matwyshyn GA, Gerk PM, et al. Effects of naltrexone pellet implantation on morphine tolerance and physical dependence in the rat. Gen Pharmacol 1994;25:149-155.
46. Mendelson JH, Ellingboe J, Kuehnle JC, Mello NK. Heroin and naltrexone effects on pituitary-gonadal hormones in man: interaction of steroid feedback effects, tolerance and supersensitivity. J Pharmacol Exp Ther 1980;214:503-506.
47. Kleber HD, Kosten TR, Gaspari J, Topazian M. Nontolerance to the opioid antagonism of naltrexone. Biol Psychiatry 1985;20:66-72.
48. Volpicelli JR, Alterman AI, Hayashida M, O'Brien CP. Naltrexone in the treatment of alcohol dependence. Arch Gen Psychiatry 1992;49:876-880.
49. Volpicelli JR, Davis MA, Olgin JE. Naltrexone blocks the post-shock increase of ethanol consumption. Life Sci 1986;38:841-847.
50. O'Malley SS, Jaffe AJ, Chang G, et al. Naltrexone and coping skills therapy for alcohol dependence: a controlled study. Arch Gen Psychiatry 1992;49:881-887.
51. Yano I, Takemori AE. Inhibition by naloxone of tolerance and dependence in mice treated acutely and chronically with morphine. Res Commun Chem Pathol Pharmacol 1977;16:721-734.
52. Berglund M. A better widget? Three lessons for improving addiction treatment from a meta-analytical study. Addiction 2005;100:742-750.
53. Miller NS, Gold MS. Management of withdrawal syndromes and relapse prevention in drug and alcohol dependence. Am Fam Physician 1998;58:139-146.
54. Jellinek EM. Phases of alcohol addiction. Q J Stud Alcohol 1952;13:673-684.
55. O'Brien CP. Anticraving medications for relapse prevention: a possible new class of psychoactive medications. Am J Psychiatry 2005;162:1423-1431.
56. Verheul R, van den Brink W, Geerlings P. A three-pathway psychobiological model of craving for alcohol. Alcohol Alcohol 1999;34:197-222.
57. Ooteman W, Koeter M, Verheul R, et al. Development and validation of the Amsterdam Motives for Drinking Scale (AMDS): an attempt to distinguish relief and reward drinkers. Alcohol Alcohol 2006;41:284-292.
58. National Institute of Drug Abuse. Principles of Drug Addiction Treatment. Bethesda, MD: National Institutes of Health, 1999.
59. Bergland M, Thelander S, Jonsson E (eds). Treating Alcohol and Drug Abuse: An Evidence Based Review. Weinheim, Germany: Wiley, 2003.
60. Kreek MJ, LaForge KS, Butelman E. Pharmacotherapy of addictions. Nat Rev Drug Discov 2002;1:710-726.
61. Roberts AJ, McDonald JS, Heyser CJ, et al. mu-Opioid receptor knockout mice do not self-administer alcohol. J Pharmacol Exp Ther 2000;293:1002-1008.
62. Bouza C, Angeles M, Munoz A, Amate JM. Efficacy and safety of naltrexone and acamprosate in the treatment of alcohol dependence: a systematic review. Addiction 2004;99:811-828.
63. Dahchour A, De Witte P. Ethanol and amino acids in the central nervous system: assessment of the pharmacological actions of acamprosate. Prog Neurobiol 2000;60:343-362.

64. COMBINE Study Research Group. Testing combined pharmacotherapies and behavioral interventions for alcohol dependence (the COMBINE study): a pilot feasibility study. Alcohol Clin Exp Res 2003;27:1123-1131.
65. De Witte P, Pinto E, Ansseau M, Verbanck P. Alcohol and withdrawal: from animal research to clinical issues. Neurosci Biobehav Rev 2003;27:189-197.
66. Spanagel R, Pendyala G, Abarca C, et al. The clock gene *Per2* influences the glutamatergic system and modulates alcohol consumption. Nat Med 2005;11:35-42.
67. Kreek MJ, Vocci FJ. History and current status of opioid maintenance treatments: blending conference session. J Subst Abuse Treat 2002;23:93-105.
68. Davis AM, Inturrisi CE. *d*-Methadone blocks morphine tolerance and *N*-methyl-D-aspartate-induced hyperalgesia. J Pharmacol Exp Ther 1999;289:1048-1053.
69. George TP, O'Malley SS. Current pharmacological treatments for nicotine dependence. Trends Pharmacol Sci 2004;25:42-48.
70. Work Group on Substance Use Disorders (Kleber HD WR, Anton RF, et al); Steering Committee on Practice Guidelines, American Psychiatric Association (McIntyre JS, Charles SC, Anzia DJ, et al). Clinical practice guidelines: Treatment of patients with substance use disorders, second edition. Am J Psychiatry 2006;163(8 Suppl):5-82.
71. Veterans Administration/Department of Defense Evidence-Based Clinical Practice Guideline Working Group, Veterans Health Administration, Department of Veterans Affairs; and Health Affairs, Department of Defense. Management of Substance Use Disorders in Primary and Specialty Care (Office of Quality and Performance Publication 10Q-CPG/SUD-01). Washington, DC: Department of Veterans Affairs, 2001.
72. Institute of Medicine, Committee on Crossing the Quality Chasm. Adaptation to Mental Health and Addictive Disorders: Improving the Quality of Health Care for Mental and Substance-Use Conditions. Washington, DC: National Academies Press, 2006.
73. McCorry F, Garnick D, Bartlett J. Developing performance measures for alcohol and other drug services in managed care plans. Joint Commission J Quality Improvement 2000;26:633-643.
74. American Society of Addiction Medicine. ASAM Patient Placement Criteria for the Treatment of Substance Abuse Disorders, 2nd ed, rev. Chevy Chase, MD: American Society of Addiction Medicine, 2001.
75. Mayo-Smith MF. Pharmacological management of alcohol withdrawal: a meta-analysis and evidence-based practice guideline. JAMA 1997;278:144-151.
76. Mayo-Smith MF, Beecher LH, Fischer TL, et al. Management of alcohol withdrawal delirium: an evidence-based practice guideline. Arch Intern Med 2004;164:1405-1412.
77. National Institute on Alcohol Abuse and Alcoholism. Helping Patients Who Drink Too Much: A Clinician's Guide (NIH Publication 05-3769). Bethesda, MD: National Institutes of Health, 2005.
78. Canagasaby A, Vinson D. Screening for hazardous or harmful drinking using one or two quantity-frequency questions. Alcohol Alcohol 2005;40:208-213.
79. Reinert DF, Allen JP. The Alcohol Use Disorders Identification Test (AUDIT): a review of recent research. Alcohol Clin Exp Res 2002;26:272-279.
80. Dawson DA, Grant BF, Stinson FS, et al. Effectiveness of the derived Alcohol Use Disorders Identification Test (AUDIT-C) in screening for alcohol use disorders and risk drinking in the US general population. Alcohol Clin Exp Res 2005;29:844-854.
81. Anthony JC, Warner LA, Kessler RC. Comparative epidemiology of dependence on tobacco, alcohol, controlled substances, and inhalants: basic findings from the National Comorbidity Survey. Exp Clin Psychopharmacol 1994;2:244-268.
82. Morse RM, Flavin DK. The definition of alcoholism. JAMA 1992;268:1012-1014.
83. Prochaska JO, DiClemente CC. Towards a comprehensive model of change. *In* Miller WR, Heather N (eds): Treating Addictive Behaviors: Processes of Change. New York: Plenum Press, 1986, pp. 3-27.
84. Vocci F, Ling W. Medications development: successes and challenges. Pharmacol Ther 2005;108:94-108.
85. Spies CD, Rommelspacher H. Alcohol withdrawal in the surgical patient: prevention and treatment. Anesth Analg 1999;88:946-954.
86. Garbutt JC, West SL, Carey TS, et al. Pharmacological treatment of alcohol dependence: a review of the evidence. JAMA 1999;281:1318-1325.
87. Fuller R, Roth H, Long S. Compliance with disulfiram treatment of alcoholism. J Chronic Dis 1983;36:161-170.
88. Fuller RK, Branchey L, Brightwell DR, et al. Disulfiram treatment of alcoholism. A Veterans Administration Cooperative Study. JAMA 1986;256:1449-1455.
89. Fuller RK, Roth HP. Disulfiram for the treatment of alcoholism: an evaluation in 128 men. Ann Intern Med 1979;90:901-904.
90. Anton RF, Moak DH, Latham PK, et al. Posttreatment results of combining naltrexone with cognitive-behavior therapy for the treatment of alcoholism. J Clin Psychopharmacol 2001;21:72-77.
91. Volpicelli JR, Rhines KC, Rhines JS, et al. Naltrexone and alcohol dependence: role of subject compliance. Arch Gen Psychiatry 1997;54:737-742.
92. Krystal JH, Cramer JA, Krol WF, et al. Naltrexone in the treatment of alcohol dependence. N Engl J Med 2001;345:1734-1739.
93. Anton RF, O'Malley SS, Ciraulo DA, et al. Combined pharmacotherapies and behavioral interventions for alcohol dependence. The COMBINE study: a randomized controlled trial. JAMA 2006;295:2003-2017.
94. Mason BJ. Acamprosate and naltrexone treatment for alcohol dependence: an evidence-based risk-benefits assessment. Eur Neuropsychopharmacol 2003;13:469-475.
95. Mason BJ, Goodman AM, Chabac S, Lehert P. Effect of oral acamprosate on abstinence in patients with alcohol dependence in a double-blind, placebo-controlled trial: the role of patient motivation. J Psychiatr Res 2006;40:383-393.
96. Johnson BA, O'Malley SS, Ciraulo DA, et al. Dose-ranging kinetics and behavioral pharmacology of naltrexone and acamprosate, both alone and combined, in alcohol-dependent subjects. J Clin Psychopharmacol 2003;23:281-293.
97. Hall-Flavin D, Karpyak V, Vander Weg M, et al. The use of acamprosate in a clinical population: initial Mayo Clinic experience. Alcohol Clin Exp Res 2006;30:106A.
98. Vander Weg M, Karpyak V, Hall-Flavin D, et al. Comparability of the Penn Alcohol Craving Scale and the Obsessive Compulsive Drinking Scale for assessing craving in a clinical sample. Alcohol Clin Exp Res 2006;30:161A.
99. O'Malley S. Public Communication. Presented at the International Society of Addiction Medicine Annual Meeting, Porto, Portugal, September 29, 2006.
100. Dole VP, Nyswander ME, Kreek MJ. Narcotic blockade. Arch Intern Med 1966;118:304-309.
100. Newman RG, Whitehill WB. Double-blind comparison of methadone and placebo maintenance treatments of narcotic addicts in Hong Kong. Lancet 1979;2:485-488.
102. Strain EC, Bigelow GE, Liebson IA, Stitzer ML. Moderate- vs high-dose methadone in the treatment of opioid dependence: a randomized trial. JAMA 1999;281:1000-1005.
103. Bertschy G. Methadone maintenance treatment: an update. Eur Arch Psychiatry Clin Neurosci 1995;245:114-124.
104. Ling W, Charuvastra C, Kaim SC, Klett CJ. Methadyl acetate and methadone as maintenance treatments for heroin addicts. A Veterans Administration Cooperative Study. Arch Gen Psychiatry 1976;33:709-720.
105. Ling W, Klett CJ, Gillis RD. A cooperative clinical study of methadyl acetate. I. Three-times-a-week regimen. Arch Gen Psychiatry 1978;35:345-353.
106. Eissenberg T, Bigelow GE, Strain EC, et al. Dose-related efficacy of levomethadyl acetate for treatment of opioid dependence: a randomized clinical trial. JAMA 1997;277:1945-1951.
107. Johnson RE, Chutuape MA, Strain EC, et al. A comparison of levomethadyl acetate, buprenorphine, and methadone for opioid dependence. N Engl J Med 2000;343:1290-1297.
108. Ling W, Amass L, Shoptaw S, et al. A multi-center randomized trial of buprenorphine-naloxone versus clonidine for opioid detoxification: findings from the National Institute on Drug Abuse Clinical Trials Network. Addiction 2005;100:1090-1100.
109. Seifert J, Metzner C, Paetzold W, et al. Mood and affect during detoxification of opiate addicts: a comparison of buprenorphine versus methadone. Addict Biol 2005;10:157-164.
110. Fiellin DA, Pantalon MV, Chawarski MC, et al. Counseling plus buprenorphine-naloxone maintenance therapy for opioid dependence. N Engl J Med 2006;355:365-374.
111. Hurt RD, Dale LC, Fredrickson PA, et al. Nicotine patch therapy for smoking cessation combined with physician advice and nurse follow-up: one-year outcome and percentage of nicotine replacement. JAMA 1994;271:595-600.
112. Silagy C, Lancaster T, Stead L, et al. Nicotine replacement therapy for smoking cessation. Cochrane Database Syst Rev 2002;(4):CD000146.
113. Silagy C, Lancaster T, Stead L, et al. Nicotine replacement therapy for smoking cessation. Cochrane Database Syst Rev 2004;(3):CD000146.
114. Hurt RD, Sachs DP, Glover ED, et al. A comparison of sustained-release bupropion and placebo for smoking cessation. N Engl J Med 1997;337:1195-1202.
115. Ferry L, Johnston JA. Efficacy and safety of bupropion SR for smoking cessation: data from clinical trials and five years of postmarketing experience. Int J Clin Pract 2003;57:224-230.
116. Oncken C, Gonzales D, Nides M, et al. Efficacy and safety of the novel selective nicotinic acetylcholine receptor partial agonist, varenicline, for smoking cessation. Arch Intern Med 2006;166:1571-1577.
117. Nides M, Oncken C, Gonzales D, et al. Smoking cessation with varenicline, a selective alpha4beta2 nicotinic receptor partial agonist: results from a 7-week, randomized, placebo- and bupropion-controlled trial with 1-year follow-up. Arch Intern Med 2006;166:1561-1568.
117a. Miller G. Psychopharmacology. Tackling alcoholism with drugs. Science 2008;320:168-170.
118. Johnson BA, Campling GM, Griffiths P, Cowen PJ. Attenuation of some alcohol-induced mood changes and the desire to drink by 5-HT3 receptor blockade: a preliminary study in healthy male volunteers. Psychopharmacology (Berl) 1993;112:142-144.
119. Kranzler HR, Pierucci-Lagha A, Feinn R, Hernandez-Avila C. Effects of ondansetron in early- versus late-onset alcoholics: a prospective, open-label study. Alcohol Clin Exp Res 2003;27:1150-1155.
120. Cott J, Carlsson A, Engel J, Lindqvist M. Suppression of ethanol-induced locomotor stimulation by GABA-like drugs. Naunyn Schmiedebergs Arch Pharmacol 1976;295:203-209.
121. Addolorato G, Caputo F, Capristo E, et al. Ability of baclofen in reducing alcohol craving and intake: II—Preliminary clinical evidence. Alcohol Clin Exp Res 2000;24:67-71.
122. Colombo G, Agabio R, Carai MA, et al. Ability of baclofen in reducing alcohol intake and withdrawal severity: I—Preclinical evidence. Alcohol Clin Exp Res 2000;24:58-66.
123. Colombo G, Serra S, Brunetti G, et al. The $GABA_B$ receptor agonists baclofen and CGP 44532 prevent acquisition of alcohol drinking behaviour in alcohol-preferring rats. Alcohol Alcohol 2002;37:499-503.
124. Colombo G, Vacca G, Serra S, et al. Baclofen suppresses motivation to consume alcohol in rats. Psychopharmacology (Berl) 2003;167:221-224.
125. Cousins MS, Roberts DC, de Wit H. $GABA_B$ receptor agonists for the treatment of drug addiction: a review of recent findings. Drug Alcohol Depend 2002;65:209-220.
126. Li Z, Maglione M, Tu W, et al. Meta-analysis: pharmacologic treatment of obesity. Ann Intern Med 2005;142:532-546.
127. White HS, Brown SD, Woodhead JH, et al. Topiramate enhances GABA-mediated chloride flux and GABA-evoked chloride currents in murine brain neurons and increases seizure threshold. Epilepsy Res 1997;28:167-179.

128. Gryder DS, Rogawski MA. Selective antagonism of GluR5 kainate-receptor-mediated synaptic currents by topiramate in rat basolateral amygdala neurons. J Neurosci 2003;23:7069-7074.
129. Johnson BA, Ait-Daoud N, Bowden CL, et al. Oral topiramate for treatment of alcohol dependence: a randomised controlled trial. Lancet 2003;361:1677-1685.
130. Johnson BA, Ait-Daoud N, Akhtar FZ, Ma JZ. Oral topiramate reduces the consequences of drinking and improves the quality of life of alcohol-dependent individuals: a randomized controlled trial. Arch Gen Psychiatry 2004;61:905-912.
131. Johnson BA, Ait-Daoud N, Akhtar FZ, Javors MA. Use of oral topiramate to promote smoking abstinence among alcohol-dependent smokers: a randomized controlled trial. Arch Intern Med 2005;165:1600-1605.
132. Frye MA, Altshuler LL, McElroy SL, et al. Gender differences in prevalence, risk, and clinical correlates of alcoholism comorbidity in bipolar disorder. Am J Psychiatry 2003;160:883-889.
132a. George DT, Gilman J, Hersh J, et al. Neurokinin 1 receptor antagonism as a possible therapy for alcoholism. Science 2008;319:1536-1539.
133. Covey LS, Glassman AH. A meta-analysis of double-blind placebo-controlled trials of clonidine for smoking cessation. Br J Addict 1991;86:991-998.
134. Nemeth-Coslett R, Henningfield JE, O'Keeffe MK, Griffiths RR. Effects of mecamylamine on human cigarette smoking and subjective ratings. Psychopharmacology (Berl) 1986;88:420-425.
135. Pentel P, Malin D. A vaccine for nicotine dependence: targeting the drug rather than the brain. Respiration 2002;69:193-197.
136. de Villiers SH, Lindblom N, Kalayanov G, et al. Active immunization against nicotine suppresses nicotine-induced dopamine release in the rat nucleus accumbens shell. Respiration 2002;69:247-253.
137. Vocci FJ, Chiang CN. Vaccines against nicotine: how effective are they likely to be in preventing smoking? CNS Drugs 2001;15:505-514.
138. Hall WD. Will nicotine genetics and a nicotine vaccine prevent cigarette smoking and smoking-related diseases? PLoS Med 2005;2:e266; quiz e351.
139. Oliveto A, Kosten TR, Schottenfeld R, et al. Desipramine, amantadine, or fluoxetine in buprenorphine-maintained cocaine users. J Subst Abuse Treat 1995;12:423-428.
140. Kosten T, Sofuoglu M, Poling J, et al. Desipramine treatment for cocaine dependence in buprenorphine- or methadone-treated patients: baseline urine results as predictor of response. Am J Addict 2005;14:8-17.
141. Gilbert JG, Newman AH, Gardner EL, et al. Acute administration of SB-277011A, NGB 2904, or BP 897 inhibits cocaine cue-induced reinstatement of drug-seeking behavior in rats: role of dopamine D3 receptors. Synapse 2005;57:17-28.
142. Huestis MA, Gorelick DA, Heishman SJ, et al. Blockade of effects of smoked marijuana by the CB1-selective cannabinoid receptor antagonist SR141716. Arch Gen Psychiatry 2001;58:322-328.
143. Anton RF, Oroszi G, O'Malley S, et al. An evaluation of mu-opioid receptor (OPRM1) as a predictor of naltrexone response in the treatment of alcohol dependence: results from the Combined Pharmacotherapies and Behavioral Interventions for Alcohol Dependence (COMBINE) study. Arch Gen Psychiatry 2008;65:135-144.

56

NICOTINE DEPENDENCE

Neal L. Benowitz

INTRODUCTION 837
Epidemiology of Cigarette Smoking 837
Smoking-Related Disease 837
GENERAL ADDICTION CONCEPTS 837
TARGETS FOR THERAPY OF NICOTINE ADDICTION 837
PATHOPHYSIOLOGY OF NICOTINE DEPENDENCE 837
PHARMACOKINETICS AND METABOLISM 840
PHARMACODYNAMICS 841
DRUG INTERACTIONS WITH NICOTINE AND TOBACCO 841
Drug Metabolism 841
Pharmacodynamic Interactions 843
THERAPEUTICS AND CLINICAL PHARMACOLOGY 843
Goals of Therapy 843
Therapeutics by Class 843
Nicotine-Replacement Therapy 843
Bupropion 845
Varenicline 845
Other Medications for Smoking Cessation 845
Therapeutic Approach 845
Emerging Targets and Therapeutics 846

INTRODUCTION

Cigarette smoking remains a leading cause of premature morbidity and mortality in the United States and in many countries around the world. An average of 435,000 people in the United States die prematurely from tobacco-related disease each year, which includes 1 in 5 overall deaths. A lifelong smoker has about a 1 in 3 chance of dying prematurely from a complication of smoking.

Smoking is relevant to many areas of medicine because it is a major cause of premature atherosclerotic vascular disease, chronic lung disease, cancer, and infectious disease. Smoking also influences responses to various drugs, by both pharmacokinetic and pharmacodynamic mechanisms.

Epidemiology of Cigarette Smoking

Currently, about 45 million individuals (21% of the adult population) in the United States are cigarette smokers, including 23% of men and 18% of women.[1] People who are less well educated and/or have unskilled occupations are more likely to smoke. For example, 35.6% of people with 9 to 11 years of education are smokers, versus 16.5% of those with a college degree. Other forms of tobacco use include pipes and cigars (used by 9% of men and 0.3% of women) and smokeless tobacco (5.5% of men and 1% of women). Smokeless tobacco use in the United States is primarily oral snuff and chewing tobacco.

Smoking-Related Disease

Tobacco use is a major cause of death from cancer, cardiovascular disease, and pulmonary disease (Box 56-1). Cigarette smoking is also a risk factor for respiratory tract and other infections, osteoporosis, reproductive disorders, adverse postoperative events, delayed wound healing, duodenal and gastric ulcers, and the development of diabetes. Smoking is also a major cause of fire-related and trauma-related injuries. The pathophysiology of smoking-induced disease is quite complex and beyond the scope of this chapter. Smoking-related disease is a consequence of exposure to toxins in tobacco smoke; however, the primary cause of smoking-related disease is addiction to nicotine.

GENERAL ADDICTION CONCEPTS (Fig. 56-1)

Drug dependence and addiction are used interchangeably in this chapter. Drug dependence has been defined by the World Health Organization as "a behavioral pattern in which the use of a psychoactive drug is given sharply higher priority over other behaviors which once had significantly higher value." In other words, the drug has come to control behavior to an extent that is considered detrimental to the individual, to society, or to both. The U.S. Surgeon General has developed criteria for drug dependence related to the scientific basis of drug dependence (Box 56-2). The major criteria are highly controlled or compulsive use of a drug that has psychoactive effects and evidence that drug-taking behavior is reinforced by the effects of that drug. A number of additional phenomena commonly occur as part of drug addiction, including the development of tolerance and physical dependence. Physical dependence, as differentiated from drug dependence broadly, refers to a state of physical withdrawal that is caused when a drug that has been taken is abruptly discontinued. The American Psychiatric Association has developed diagnostic criteria for psychoactive substance dependence (Box 56-3). Common to all definitions of drug addiction is the loss of control of drug use.

TARGETS FOR THERAPY OF NICOTINE ADDICTION

This chapter focuses on nicotine dependence and not on the many diseases caused by nicotine dependence. The general goal of treatment is to aid smokers to quit smoking. For reasons described later, smoking is a complex and multifactorial behavioral disorder that requires substantial modification of behavior in order to quit. Medications are aids to smoking cessation, working primarily by reducing withdrawal symptoms after cessation, although some more recently marketed medications may also block the reinforcing effects of nicotine. As is true for all drug addictions, behavioral therapy increases the likelihood of quitting. For cigarette smoking, the effects of behavioral therapy and medications appear to be multiplicative. That is, adding medication appears to approximately double the quit rate that is seen from whatever level of behavioral therapy a person is provided (from 2%-3% without behavioral therapy to 20% or more with intensive behavioral therapy).

PATHOPHYSIOLOGY OF NICOTINE DEPENDENCE

Tobacco contains thousands of chemicals. Nicotine is the chemical responsible for most of the pharmacologic actions of tobacco and for addiction. Tobacco contains primarily *S*-nicotine, which binds to nicotinic cholinergic receptors in autonomic ganglia, the adrenal medulla, neuromuscular junctions, and the brain.

BOX 56-1 TOBACCO USE AS A CAUSE OF DISEASE

Cancer
- Lung
- Urinary tract
- Oral cavity
- Oro- and hypopharynx
- Esophagus
- Larynx
- Pancreas
- Nasal cavity, sinuses, nasopharynx
- Stomach
- Liver
- Kidney
- Uterine cervix
- Myeloid leukemia

Cardiovascular Disease
- Sudden death
- Acute myocardial infarction
- Unstable angina
- Stroke
- Peripheral arterial occlusive disease (including thromboangiitis obliterans)
- Aortic aneurysm

Pulmonary Disease
- Lung cancer
- Chronic bronchitis
- Emphysema
- Asthma
- Increased susceptibility to pneumonia and to pulmonary tuberculosis
- Increased susceptibility to desquamative interstitial pneumonitis
- Increased morbidity from viral respiratory infection

Gastrointestinal Disease
- Peptic ulcer
- Esophageal reflux

Reproductive Disturbances
- Reduced fertility
- Premature birth
- Lower birth weight
- Spontaneous abortion
- Abruptio placentae
- Premature rupture of membranes
- Increased perinatal mortality

Oral Disease (Smokeless Tobacco)
- Oral cancer
- Leukoplakia
- Gingivitis
- Gingival recession
- Tooth staining

Other
- Non–insulin-dependent diabetes mellitus
- Earlier menopause
- Osteoporosis
- Cataract
- Tobacco amblyopia (loss of vision)
- Age-related macular degeneration
- Premature skin wrinkling
- Aggravation of hypothyroidism
- Altered drug metabolism or effects

Infectious Diseases
- Pneumococcal pneumonia
- Legionnaire's disease
- Meningococcal disease
- Periodontal disease
- *Helicobacter pylori*
- Common cold
- Influenza
- HIV infection
- Tuberculosis

HIV, human immunodeficiency virus.

BOX 56-2 SURGEON GENERAL'S CRITERIA FOR DRUG DEPENDENCE

Primary Criteria
- Highly controlled or compulsive use
- Psychoactive effects
- Drug-reinforced behavior

Additional Criteria

Addictive behavior often involves
- Stereotypic patterns of use
- Use despite harmful effects
- Relapse after abstinence
- Recurrent drug cravings

Dependence-producing drugs often produce
- Tolerance
- Physical dependence
- Pleasant (euphoriant) effects

From U.S. Department of Health and Human Services Public Health Service. The Health Consequences of Smoking: Nicotine Addiction. A Report of the Surgeon General. DHHS (CDC) Publication No. 88-8406. Washington DC: Government Printing Office, 1988.

When a person inhales smoke from a cigarette, nicotine is distilled from the tobacco and is carried in smoke particles into the lungs, where it is absorbed rapidly into the pulmonary venous circulation. It then enters the arterial circulation and moves quickly to the brain. Nicotine diffuses readily into brain tissue, where it binds to nicotinic cholinergic receptors (nAChRs), which are ligand-gated ion channels. When a cholinergic agonist binds to the outside of the channel, the channel opens, allowing the entry of cations, including sodium and calcium. These cations further activate voltage-dependent calcium channels, allowing further calcium entry.

The nAChR complex is composed of five subunits. Much diversity is present in nAChRs, with nine α-subunit isoforms, α_2 through α_{10}, and three β-subunit isoforms, β_2 through β_4, identified in brain tissues.[2] The most abundant nAChRs are the α_4- and β_2-containing receptors, accounting for 90% of high-affinity nicotine binding in the rat brain. The presence of the β_2-subunit is critical for dopamine release and for the behavioral effects of nicotine, including self-administration.[3] The α_4-subunit is an important determinant of sensitivity to nicotine.[4] The $\alpha_3\beta_4$-subtype is believed to mediate the cardiovascular effects of nicotine. $\alpha7$ Homomeric receptors are believed to be involved in rapid synaptic transmission and may play a role in learning and sensory gating.

Nicotinic receptor activation works, at least in part and possibly in the main, by facilitating the release of neurotransmitters. Most of this release is believed to occur via modulation by presynaptic nAChRs. Dopamine release is critical to the reinforcing effects of nicotine and other drugs of abuse.[5] Chemically or anatomically lesioning dopamine neurons in the brain prevents nicotine self-administration in rats. Other neurotransmitters, including norepinephrine, acetylcholine, serotonin, γ-aminobutyric acid, glutamate, and endorphins, are released as well, mediating various behaviors of nicotine (Fig. 56-2). Nicotine releases dopamine in the mesolimbic area, the corpus striatum, and the prefrontal cortex. Of particular importance are the dopa-

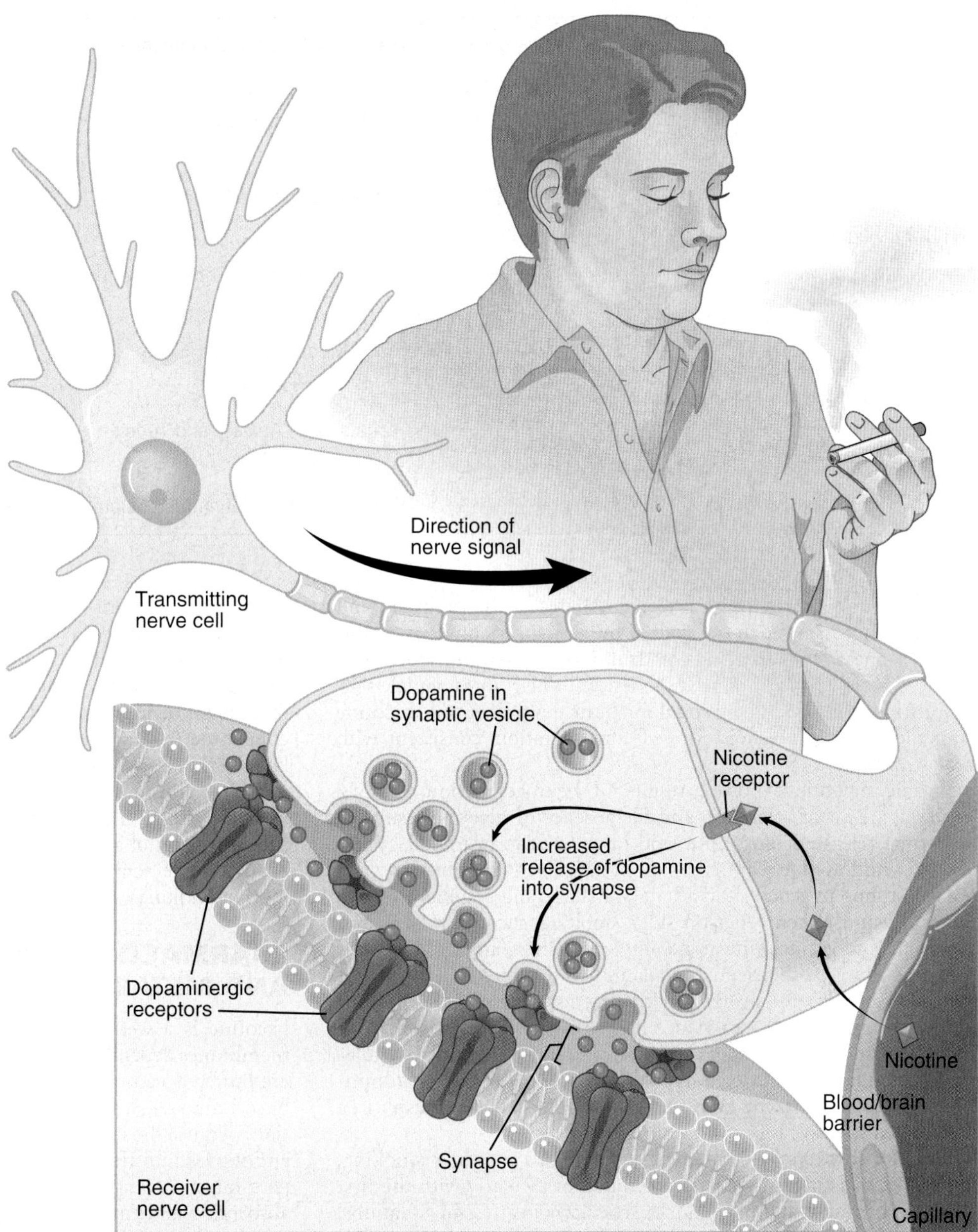

FIGURE 56-1 • General addiction concepts.

BOX 56-3 APA CRITERIA FOR NICOTINE DEPENDENCE

A maladaptive pattern of substance use, leading to clinically significant impairment or distress, as manifested by three or more of the following occurring at any time in the same 12-month period:

1. Tolerance, as defined by either of the following:
   a. Need for markedly increased amounts of the substance to achieve intoxication or desired effect.
   b. Markedly diminished effect with continued use of the same amount of the substance.
2. Withdrawal, as manifested by either of the following:
   a. The characteristic withdrawal syndrome for the substance.
   b. The same (or closely related) substance is taken to relieve or avoid withdrawal symptoms.
3. The substance is often taken in larger amounts or over a longer period than was intended.
4. There is a persistent desire or unsuccessful efforts to cut down or control substance use.
5. A great deal of time is spent in activities necessary to obtain the substance, use the substance, or recover from its effects.
6. Important social, occupational, or recreational activities are given up or reduced because of substance use.
7. The substance use is continued despite knowledge of having had a persistent or recurrent physical or psychological problem that is likely to have been caused or exacerbated by the substance.

APA, American Psychiatric Association.

From American Psychiatric Association. Diagnostic and Statistical Manual of Mental Disorders (DSM-IV), 4th ed. Washington, DC: American Psychiatric Association, 1994.

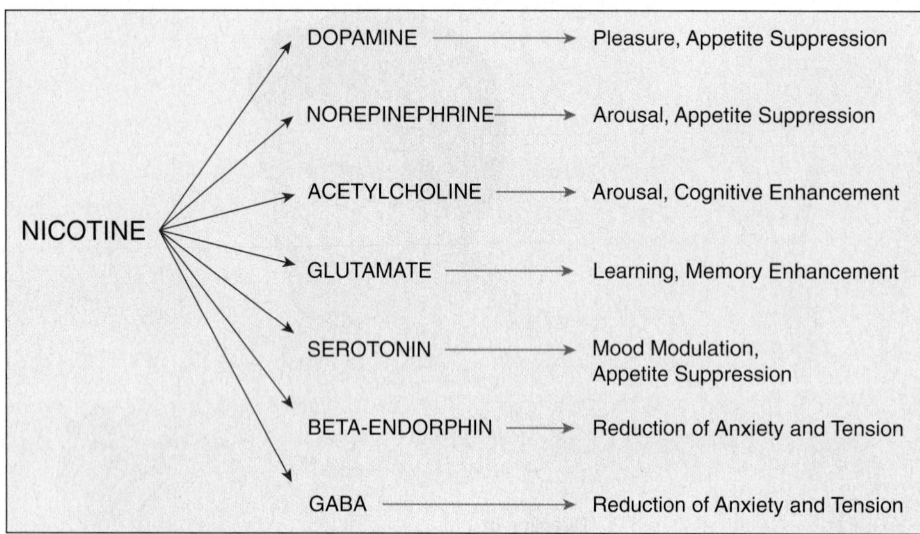

FIGURE 56-2 • Nicotine receptor activation promotes the release of neurotransmitters, which then mediate various behavioral effects of nicotine. (Adapted from Benowitz NL. Nicotine addiction. Prim Care 1999;26:611-613.)

minergic neurons in the ventral tegmental area of the midbrain and the release of dopamine in the shell of the nucleus accumbens, as this pathway appears to be critical for drug-induced reward. Dopamine release signals a pleasurable experience. When intracranial self-administration is used as a model for brain reward in rats, nicotine acutely lowers the threshold for self-administration, consistent with greater reward.[6]

Chronic nicotine exposure results in neuroadaptation, that is, the development of tolerance; and the absence of nicotine results in subnormal release of dopamine and other neurotransmitters. Thus, nicotine withdrawal results in the state of deficient dopamine responses to novel stimuli in general and a state of malaise and inability to experience pleasure. When a person stops smoking, nicotine withdrawal symptoms emerge, including irritability, restlessness, anxiety, problems of getting along with friends and family, difficulties concentrating, increased hunger and eating, and craving for tobacco. The state of malaise and inability to experience pleasure associated with nicotine withdrawal has been termed *hedonic dysregulation*. Hedonic dysregulation may explain craving, and its rapid reversal by nicotine readministration may explain why even a single cigarette can easily result in a return to compulsive tobacco use.

Although smokers give different explanations for their smoking, most agree that smoking produces arousal, particularly with the first cigarette of the day, and relaxation, particularly in stressful situations. Consistent with reports of arousal, electroencephalographic desynchronization with an upward shift in the dominant alpha frequency and a decreased total alpha and theta power follows cigarette smoking or administration of nicotine.

Addiction to tobacco is multifactorial, including a desire for the direct pharmacologic actions of nicotine, relief of withdrawal symptoms, and learned associations. Smokers cite a variety of reasons for smoking, including pleasure, arousal, enhanced vigilance, improved performance, relief of anxiety or depression, reduced hunger, and control of body weight. Environmental cues—such as the smell of a cigarette, observing friends who are smoking, a meal, cup of coffee, talking on the phone, or an alcoholic beverage—often trigger an urge to smoke. Functional imaging studies indicate that exposure to drug-associated cues activates cortical regions of the brain, including the insula. Smoker who acquire damage to the insula (e.g., owing to brain trauma) are more likely to quit smoking soon after the injury, are more likely to remain abstinent, and are less likely to experience conscious urges to smoke compared with smokers with brain injury that does not affect the insula.[7] Smoking and depression are strongly linked. Smokers are more likely than nonsmokers to have a history of major depression. When smokers with a history of depression do quit, depression is more apt to be a prominent withdrawal symptom.

Most tobacco use begins in childhood or adolescence. Risk factors for youth smoking include peer and parental influences; behavioral problems (e.g., poor school performance); personality characteristics such as rebelliousness or risk taking, depression, and anxiety; and genetic influences. Twin studies have provided strong evidence for the presence of a genetic vulnerability for nicotine dependence.[8] Environmental influences such as advertising and smoking in movies also contribute to youth smoking. Although smoking rates among adults have declined since the 1970s, initiation rates for youth have remained relatively constant since the mid 1980s. Approaches to preventing tobacco addiction in youth include educational activities in schools, aggressive antitobacco media campaigns, taxation of tobacco products, changing the social and environmental norms (such as restricting indoor smoking), and deglamorizing smoking.

PHARMACOKINETICS AND METABOLISM

Nicotine is a weak base (pKa = 8.0). Absorption through mucous membranes depends on pH. Chewing tobacco, snuff, and nicotine gum are buffered with an alkaline pH to facilitate absorption through the buccal mucosa. Smoking is a highly efficient form of drug administration, because the drug enters the circulation rapidly through the lungs and moves into the brain within seconds. Inhaled drugs escape first-pass intestinal and hepatic metabolism. The more rapid the rate of absorption and entry of a drug into the brain, the greater is the "rush" and the more reinforcing the drug. Smoking produces high concentrations of a drug in the brain that are comparable with those seen after intravenous administration. It is not surprising that a number of substances of abuse, including marijuana, cocaine, opiates, phencyclidine, and organic solvents, are abused by the inhalational route because access to the brain is so rapid. The smoking process also allows precise dose titration, so a smoker may obtain desired effects.

Nicotine is rapidly and extensively metabolized by the liver, primarily by the liver enzyme cytochrome P-450 (CYP) 2A6, to the chemical cotinine[9] (Fig. 56-3). The metabolite cotinine is widely used as a quantitative marker for exposures to nicotine and is useful as a diagnostic test for the use of tobacco and as a measure of compliance with treatments for smoking cessation. The half-life of nicotine averages about 2 hours. Considerable genetic polymorphism in CYP2A6 activity is associated with wide individual variability and racial differences in the rate of nicotine metabolism.[9] Asians and African Americans metabolize nicotine, on average, more slowly than do whites or Hispanics. Sex hormones also substantially affect CYP2A6 activity. The rate of nicotine metabolism is faster in women than in men.[10] Among women, nicotine metabolism is faster in those taking estrogen-containing oral contraceptives and even faster during pregnancy than in other women.

The peak-to-trough oscillation in blood levels from cigarette to cigarette is considerable. However, consistent with the half-life of 2

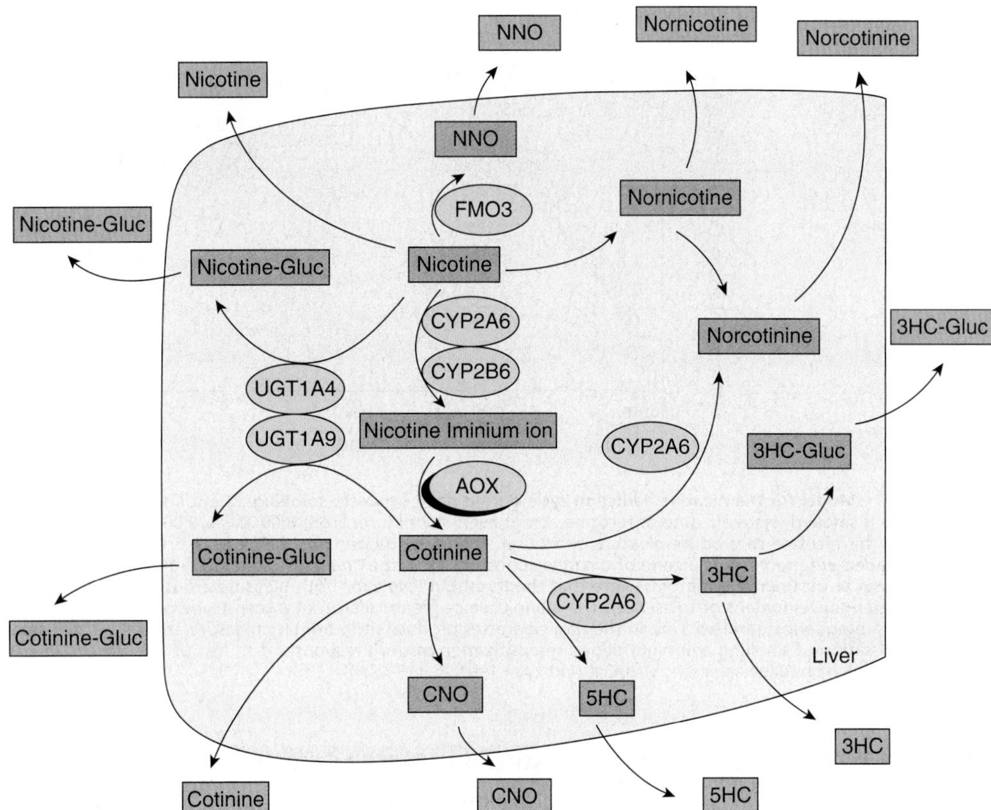

FIGURE 56-3 • Summary of nicotine metabolism in human liver cell.

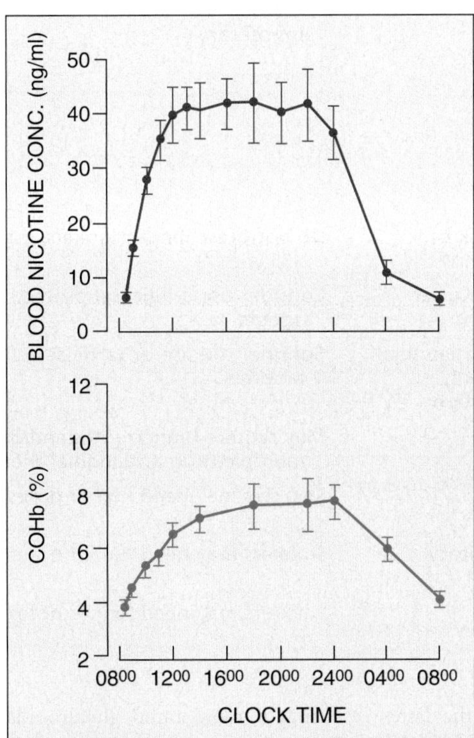

FIGURE 56-4 • Circadian blood nicotine and carboxyhemoglobin concentrations during regular cigarette smoking. Mean (± standard error of the mean [SEM]) blood nicotine and carboxyhemoglobin (COHb) concentrations (conc) in cigarette smokers. Subjects smoked cigarettes every half hour from 8:30 AM to 11:00 PM, for a total of 30 cigarettes a day. (Reprinted with permission from Benowitz NL, Kuyt F, Jacob P 3rd. Circadian blood nicotine concentrations during cigarette smoking. Clin Pharmacol Ther 1982;32:758-764.)

hours, nicotine accumulates in the body over 6 to 9 hours of regular smoking (Fig. 56-4). Thus, smoking results not in intermittent and transient exposure to nicotine but in an exposure that lasts 24 hours a day. Arteriovenous differences in nicotine concentration during cigarette smoking are substantial, with arterial levels exceeding venous levels 6- to 10-fold. The persistence of nicotine in the brain throughout the day and night results in changes in the structure and function of nicotinic receptors and in intracellular processes of neuroadaptation, as mentioned previously.

PHARMACODYNAMICS

Two issues are particularly relevant in understanding the pharmacodynamics of nicotine. First, the nicotine dose-response relationship is complex. Low doses may stimulate neural systems, whereas higher doses depress them. For example, low doses of nicotine produce central or peripheral nervous system stimulation with arousal and an increase in heart rate or blood pressure. At high doses, such as during nicotine intoxication, nicotine produces ganglionic blockade resulting in bradycardia, hypotension, and depressed mental status. A second important pharmacodynamic issue is the development of tolerance. Tolerance develops rapidly to the dysphoria, nausea, and vomiting that often occur when smoking one's first cigarette. Tolerance to subjective effects and to the acceleration of heart rate produced by nicotine develops within the day in many smokers. Thus, within even a single day, because of the development of tolerance, the positive rewards of smoking diminish, and smoking becomes motivated more by relief of withdrawal symptoms (Fig. 56-5).

DRUG INTERACTIONS WITH NICOTINE AND TOBACCO

Drug Metabolism

Cigarette smoking may interact with medications through effects on drug metabolism or pharmacodynamics. Smoking is well known to

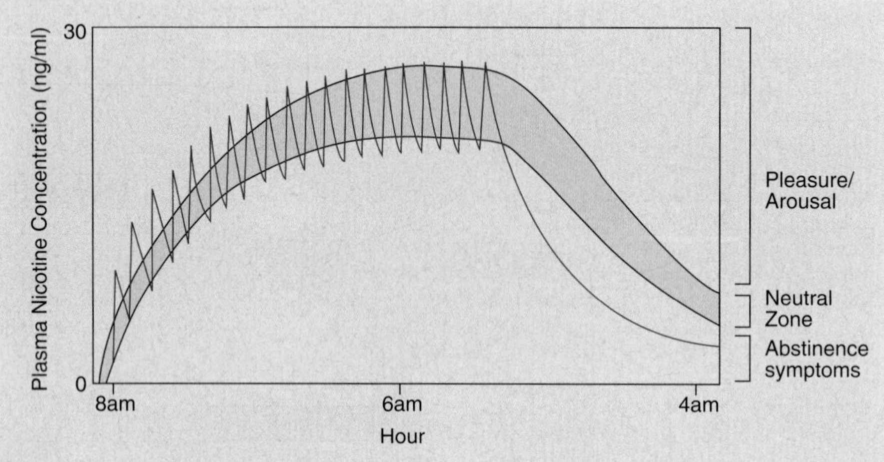

FIGURE 56-5 • Model for the nicotine addiction cycle during daily cigarette smoking. The *solid line* represents venous plasma concentrations of nicotine as a cigarette is smoked (systemic dose of nicotine, 1 mg) every 40 minutes from 8:00 AM to 9:00 PM. The *upper dashed line* indicates the threshold concentration for nicotine to produce pleasure or arousal. The *lower dashed line* indicates the concentrations at which symptoms of abstinence from nicotine occur. The *shaded area* represents a zone of nicotine concentrations (the "neutral" zone) in which the smoker is comfortable without experiencing either pleasure/arousal or abstinence symptoms. Note that the threshold levels for both pleasure/arousal and abstinence rise progressively during smoking owing to neuroadaptation (development of tolerance). The magnitude of pleasure/arousal is seen to be greatest with the first cigarette of the day and becomes less intense with subsequent cigarettes. Late in the day, cigarettes produce little primary pleasure/arousal but are smoked primarily to relieve abstinence symptoms. Cessation of smoking overnight allows resensitization of drug responses (i.e., loss of tolerance). (Reprinted with permission from Benowitz NL. Cigarette smoking and nicotine addiction. Med Clin North Am 1992;76:415-437.)

TABLE 56-1 CIGARETTE SMOKING AND DRUG INTERACTIONS

Drugs		Interaction (Effects Compared with Nonsmokers)	Significance
Antipyrine Caffeine Chlorpromazine Clozapine Desmethyldiazepam Erlotinib Estradiol Estrone Flecainide Fluvoxamine Haloperidol	Imipramine Irinotecan Lidocaine Olanzapine Oxazepam Pentazocine Phenacetin Phenylbutazone Propranolol Tacrine Theophylline	Accelerated metabolism	May require higher doses in smokers, reduced doses after quitting. Reduced toxicity with standard doses (e.g., irinotecan)
Oral contraceptives		Enhanced thrombosis, increased risk of stroke and myocardial infarction	Do not prescribe to smokers, especially if >35 yr
Cimetidine and other H_2 blockers		Lower rate of ulcer healing, higher ulcer recurrence rates	Consider using mucosal protective agents
Propranolol		Less antihypertensive effect, less antianginal efficacy; more effective in reducing mortality after myocardial infarction	Consider the use of cardioselective β blockers
Nifedipine (and probably other calcium blockers)		Less antianginal effect	May require higher doses and/or multiple-drug antianginal therapy
Diazepam, chlordiazepoxide (and possibly other sedative-hypnotics)		Less sedation	Smokers may need higher doses
Chlorpromazine (and possibly other neuroletics)		Less sedation, possibly reduced efficacy	Smokers may need higher doses
Propoxyphene		Reduced analgesia	Smokers may need higher doses

accelerate the metabolism of many drugs, particularly those metabolized by CYP1A2, including caffeine, clozapine, olanzapine, tacrine, theophylline, erlotinib, and others. As an example of the clinical consequences of enzyme induction from smoking, accelerated metabolism of erlotinib most likely explains the poorer response of smokers versus nonsmokers with non–small cell lung cancer.[11] Polycyclic aromatic hydrocarbons appear to be responsible for the induction of CYP1A2. Cigarette smoking also appears to induce drug metabolism by CYP2E1 and by some uridine diphosphate glucuronosyltransferase (UGT) pathways, the latter resulting in more rapid glucuronidation of a number of drugs. Cigarette smoking is associated with a decreased risk of hematologic toxicity of irinotecan, a drug widely used for metastatic colon cancer and other solid tumors.[12] Smoking accelerates the metabolism of irinotecan to its active metabolite SN-38, and further accelerates the glucuronidation of SN-38, explaining the reduced toxicity, but also suggesting that smoking could reduce efficacy.

Drugs whose metabolism is accelerated by cigarette smoking are listed in Table 56-1.

Pharmacodynamic Interactions

Several pharmacodynamic interactions arise from the cardiovascular effects of nicotine and cigarette smoke. The relevant cardiovascular effects include constriction of skin and coronary blood vessels, increase in heart rate and myocardial contractility, induction of a hypercoagulable state, and impaired oxygen release to body tissues (the latter owing to the effects of carbon monoxide in smoke). By reducing the blood flood to the skin and subcutaneous tissue, cigarette smoking slows absorption of insulin from subcutaneous sites. In patients with angina pectoris, the frequency of angina and the duration of exercise before the development of chest pain or electrocardiographic changes are improved less by β blockers or calcium channel blockers in smokers versus nonsmokers. Cigarette smoking and oral contraceptives interact synergistically to increase the risk of stroke and premature myocardial infarction in women owing to induction of a hypercoagulable state. Cigarette smoking enhances the procoagulant effects of estrogens. For this reason, oral contraceptives are relatively contraindicated in women who smoke cigarettes.

Another pharmacodynamic interaction is related to the central nervous system–stimulating effects of nicotine. Cigarette smokers experience less sedation from several drugs that act on the central nervous system than do nonsmokers. These agents include diazepam, chlordiazepoxide, and chlorpromazine. The efficacy of analgesic drugs such as propoxyphene may be reduced in cigarette smokers, even in the absence of pharmacokinetic interactions. Cigarette smoking is also a major risk factor for the development and recurrence of peptic ulcer disease. Smoking adversely affects mucosal protective factors and impairs the therapeutic effects of histamine H_2-receptor antagonists.

THERAPEUTICS AND CLINICAL PHARMACOLOGY

Goals of Therapy

Among smokers, 70% would like to quit, and 46% try to quit each year. The goals of smoking-cessation therapy are to facilitate quitting and to prevent relapse of smoking after quitting. Spontaneous quit rates are approximately 1% per year. Simple physician advice increases the quit rate to 3%. Minimal intervention programs increase quit rates to 5% to 10%, whereas more intensive treatments, including smoking-cessation clinics, can yield quit rates of 25% to 30%. The effects of medication to aid smoking cessation interact with the effects of behavioral therapy. For example, if the odds ratio for quitting is 2.0, which is typical for nicotine-replacement therapy, then nicotine treatment will double whatever the cessation rate is owing to a particular level of behavioral counseling.

The main strategies for cessation are behavioral counseling, pharmacologic intervention, or a combination of the two. Many smokers try over-the-counter smoking-cessation medications prior to discussing smoking with their health care providers. The efficacy of over-the-counter medications may be limited by improper use of the medications and concomitant untreated issues such as depression, alcoholism, or other factors. Assessing stress, exposure to family members or roommates who smoke, and whatever factors are known for an individual to have prompted relapse to smoking in the past is an important part of history taking before undertaking a therapeutic intervention.

Therapeutics by Class (Table 56-2)

Currently, three classes of medications have been approved for smoking cessation: nicotine-replacement products (patch, gum, spray, inhaler, and lozenge), bupropion, and most recently, varenicline. Although not approved by regulatory authorities for smoking cessation, clinical trials have also demonstrated the efficacy of nortriptyline and clonidine, which are considered to be second-line drugs.

Nicotine-Replacement Therapy

Nicotine medications act on nAChRs to mimic or replace the effects of nicotine from tobacco. Nicotine-replacement medications are believed to facilitate smoking cessation in several ways. The principal action is the relief of withdrawal symptoms when a person stops tobacco use. Amelioration of withdrawal symptoms is observed with relatively low blood levels of nicotine. A second mechanism of benefit is positive reinforcement, particularly for the arousal and stress-relieving effects. The degree of positive reinforcement is related to the rapidity of absorption and the peak nicotine level achieved in arterial blood. Positive reinforcement is most relevant with rapid-delivery formulations, such as nicotine nasal spray and, to a lesser extent, nicotine gum, inhaler, and lozenge. The use of these products allows smokers to dose themselves with nicotine when they have the urge to smoke cigarettes. Conversely, nicotine patches deliver nicotine gradually and produce sustained nicotine levels throughout the day, thus, they do not provide much positive reinforcement.

A third possible mechanism of benefit is related to the ability of nicotine medications to desensitize nicotinic receptors. This desensitization results in a reduced effect of nicotine from cigarettes, so that when a person lapses to smoking while on nicotine-replacement therapy, the cigarette is less satisfying and the person is less likely to resume smoking.

The first nicotine-replacement therapy to be marketed was nicotine polacrilex gum. Nicotine gum was developed by Ove Ferno, a Swedish pharmaceutical scientist, in response to learning that submariners in the Swedish navy, who had been smokers but were not allowed to smoke on board submarines, used smokeless tobacco to prevent the discomfort usually experienced when they were unable to smoke. Nicotine is bound to an ion exchange resin (polacrilex) from which it is slowly released when chewed. Because nicotine is a weak base, the gum is buffered to an alkaline pH so as to facilitate absorption across the buccal membranes. Nicotine is absorbed gradually over 30 minutes (Fig. 56-6). The optimal use of nicotine gum includes instructions to chew slowly, to chew 8 to 10 pieces per day, and to continue for an adequate period of time for the smoker to be comfortable without cigarettes, usually 3 months or longer. Because buccal absorption depends on an alkaline pH, smokers should be advised to avoid drinking acidic liquids such as juice or coffee within 15 or 20 minutes of using nicotine gum. Side effects of nicotine gum are primarily local and include jaw fatigue, sore mouth and throat, upset stomach, and hiccups.

Nicotine passes readily through the skin, as it does through other membranes. Tobacco leaf harvesters may experience nicotine intoxication owing to dermal absorption (termed *green tobacco sickness*), and many poisonings have been described owing to cutaneous exposure to nicotine insecticides. Given the relatively short half-life of nicotine (2 hr), it is not surprising that transdermal nicotine preparations have been developed and marketed. Several transdermal nicotine preparations are available as patches; these deliver 21 or 22 mg over a 24-hour period, or 15 mg over a 16-hour period. Some brands offer lower-dose patches for tapering. Patches are applied in the morning and removed either the next morning or at bedtime, depending on the patch and the wishes of the patient. Patches intended for 24-hour use can also be removed at bedtime if the patient is experiencing insomnia or disturbing dreams, which are known side effects of nicotine. Full-dose patches are recommended for most smokers for the first 1 to 3 months, followed by one or two tapering doses for 2 to 4 weeks each period.

Nicotine is also readily absorbed through the nasal mucosa. Nicotine nasal spray, 1 spray into each nostril, delivers about 0.5-mg nicotine systemically and can be used every 30 to 60 minutes. Local irritation of the nose commonly produces burning, sneezing, and watery eyes during the initial treatment, but tolerance to these effects develops in 1 to 2 days. The nicotine inhaler actually delivers nicotine to the throat and upper airway, from which it is absorbed at a rate similar to that of nicotine from gum or lozenge. The nicotine inhaler is marked as a cigarette-like plastic device and can be used *ab libitum*.

Most recently, nicotine lozenges have been marketed over the counter. The lozenges are available at 2- and 4-mg strengths and are placed in the buccal cavity, where they are slowly absorbed over 30 minutes. Smokers are instructed to choose their dose according to how

TABLE 56-2 PHARMACOTHERAPY

Pharmacotherapy	Precautions/ Contraindications	Adverse Effects	Dosage	Duration	Availability
FIRST-LINE					
Sustained-release bupropion hydrochloride	History of seizure History of eating disorders	Insomnia Dry mouth	150 mg every morning for 3 days then 150 mg twice daily (begin treatment 1-2 wk before quitting)	7-12 wk maintenance up to 6 mo	Prescription only
Nicotine gum	Temporomandibular joint disorder	Mouth soreness Dyspepsia	1-24 cigarettes/day; 2 mg gum (≤24 pieces/day) ≥25 cigarettes/day; 4 mg gum (≤24 pieces/day)	Up to 12 wk	OTC only
Nicotine inhaler		Local irritation of mouth and throat	6-16 cartridges/day	≤6 mo	Prescription only
Nicotine nasal spray	Chronic nasal disorders including rhinitis, polyps, and sinusitis	Nasal irritation Throat burning	8-40 doses/day	3-6 mo	Prescription only
Nicotine patch	Skin diseases such as atopic or eczematous dermatitis	Local skin reaction Insomnia	21 mg/24 hr 14 mg/24 hr 7 mg/24 hr 15 mg/16 hr	4 wk then 2 wk then 2 wk 8 wk	Prescription and OTC
Varenicline	Kidney failure	Nausea	0.5 mg/once daily for 3 days 0.5 mg/twice daily for 4 days 1.0 mg/twice daily (begin treatment 7 days before quit date)	12 wk; if not smoking at 12 wk, may continue for an additional 12 wk	Prescription only
SECOND-LINE					
Clonidine	Rebound hypertension	Dry mouth Drowsiness Dizziness Sedation	0.15-0.75 mg/day	3-10 wk	Prescription only (oral formulation) Prescription only (patch)
Nortriptyline	Risk of arrhythmias	Sedation Dry mouth	75-100 mg/day	12 wk	Prescription only

OTC, over the counter.
Adapted from The Tobacco Use and Dependence Clinical Practice Guideline Panel, Staff, and Consortium Representatives. A clinical practice guideline for treating tobacco use and dependence: a U.S. Public Health Service report. JAMA 2000;283:3244-3254.

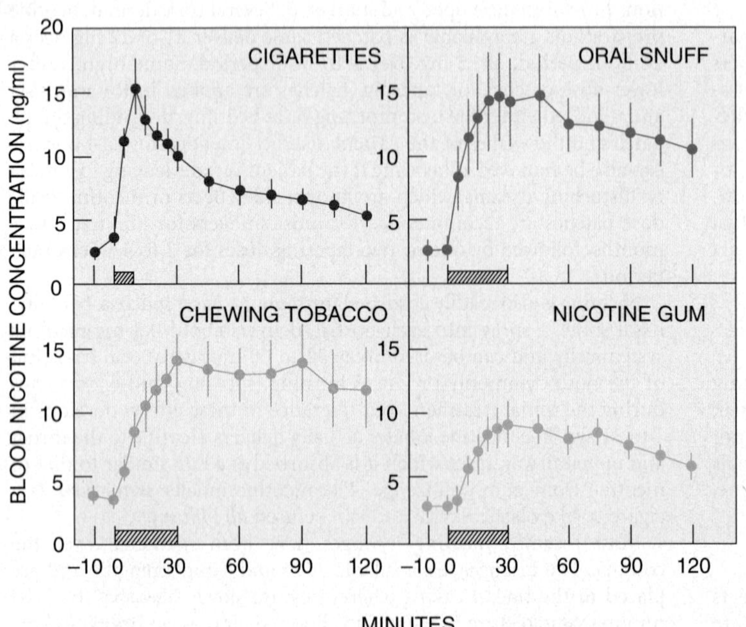

FIGURE 56-6 • Blood nicotine concentrations with use of various forms of tobacco and nicotine medications. Mean (±SEM) blood concentrations of nicotine in 10 subjects who smoked cigarettes for 9 minutes ($1\frac{1}{3}$ cigarettes), used oral snuff (2.5 g), used chewing tobacco (mean, 7.9 g), and chewed nicotine gum (two 2-mg pieces). *Shaded bars* above the time axis indicate the period of exposure to tobacco or nicotine gum. (Reprinted with permission from Benowitz NL, Porchet H, Sheiner L, Jacob P 3rd. Nicotine absorption and cardiovascular effects with smokeless tobacco use: comparison with cigarettes and nicotine gum. Clin Pharmacol Ther 1988;44:23-28.)

long after awakening in the morning they smoke their first cigarette (a measure of level of dependence). Those who smoke within 30 minutes are advised to use a 4-mg lozenge, whereas those who smoke their first cigarette more than 30 minutes after awakening are advised to use the 2-mg lozenges. Use is recommended every 1 to 2 hours.

Nicotine medications appear to be safe for use by patients with cardiovascular diseases and should be offered to cardiovascular patients. Although smoking-cessation medications are recommended by the manufacturer for relatively short-term use (generally 3-6 mo), the use of these medications for 6 months or longer is safe and may be helpful to smokers who fear relapse without medication.

Bupropion

Bupropion is a dopamine and norepinephrine neuronal reuptake inhibitor. Bupropion was marketed as an antidepressant medication before it was marketed for smoking cessation. The serendipitous observation of spontaneous smoking cessation among veterans treated for bupropion for depression led to the exploration of bupropion as a smoking-cessation medication. Bupropion increases brain levels of dopamine and norepinephrine, simulating the effects of nicotine on these neurotransmitters. Bupropion also has some nicotine receptor blocking activity, which could contribute to reduced reinforcement from a cigarette in the case of a lapse.

Bupropion is marketed under different brand names (and with different package inserts) for different indications: Wellbutrin for depression and Zyban for smoking cessation, although generic bupropion is also available. Clinical trials with bupropion for smoking cessation were conducted with bupropion sustained release (SR), dosed twice daily. Bupropion has a half-life of 21 hours and has active metabolites with similarly long half-lives. Bupropion is metabolized primarily by CYP2B6. Bupropion is to be started 7 to 14 days before the target quit date to allow the achievement of steady state levels of bupropion and its metabolites. Typically, smokers start with 150 mg of bupropion SR each morning for 3 days, then increasing to 150 mg SR twice daily for 6 to 12 weeks. Bupropion has stimulant properties and can cause anxiety and insomnia. Bupropion in excessive doses can cause seizures. It should not be used in individuals with a history of seizures or with eating disorders (such as bulimia or anorexia).

Clinical trials have demonstrated that the combination of bupropion and a nicotine patch is safe and may be more effective than bupropion alone. Bupropion has been studied in clinical studies for 1 year and was demonstrated to be safe and significantly better than placebo at promoting cessation. Given its antidepressant properties, bupropion would seem to be a logical choice for depressed smokers. However, bupropion has been shown to have equal efficacy in smokers with and without depression.

Varenicline

Varenicline was synthesized with the goal of developing a specific antagonist for the $\alpha 4\beta 2$ nAChR.[13] Varenicline is an analogue of cytisine, a plant alkaloid reported to have some benefit in smoking cessation, but is believed to have generally poor oral bioavailability. Varenicline was shown in vitro receptor binding studies to have high affinity for the $\alpha 4\beta 2$ nAChR and very little effect on other nAChR subtypes or neurotransmitter receptors. Varenicline is a partial agonist of the $\alpha 4\beta 2$ receptor in vivo, as demonstrated by studies of dopamine release, measured with microdyalisis in the nucleus accumbens of conscious rats. Nicotine, a full agonist, causes substantial dopamine release. Varenicline, a partial agonist, produces less of a response than that of nicotine (about 50%) but, at the same time, blocks the effects of any nicotine added to the system (Fig. 56-7).

Varenicline is excreted primarily unchanged by the kidney, and in humans, almost 90% of an oral dose is recovered in urine as unchanged varenicline. A small percentage of the dose is metabolized. The oral clearance of varenicline in humans averages about 175 ml/min for a person weighing 70 kg. Because this clearance is higher than the glomerular filtration rate, renal clearance involves both filtration and net secretion. Varenicline is a substrate for any organic cation transporter 2, a renal transporter that actively secretes cationic

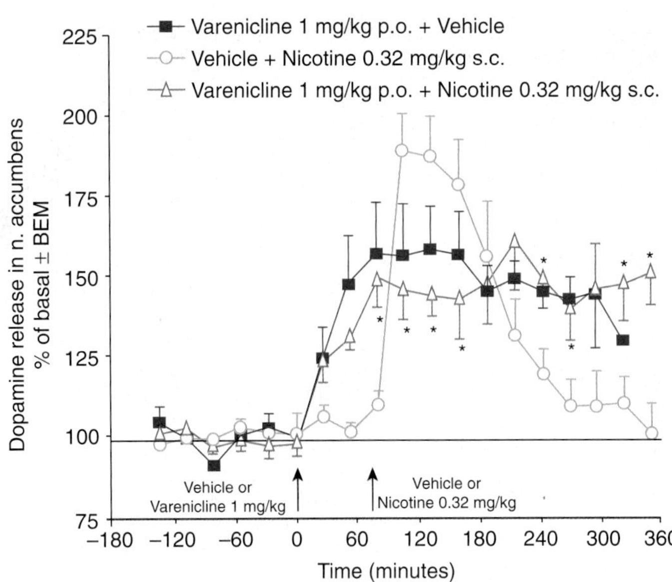

FIGURE 56-7 • Effects of nicotine, varenicline, and nicotine and varenicline in combination on extracellular dopamine levels in the nucleus accumbens of conscious rats. (Reprinted with permission from Coe JW, Brooks PR, Vetelino MG, et al. Varenicline: an alpha4beta2 nicotinic receptor partial agonist for smoking cessation. J Med Chem 2005;48:3474-3477.)

drugs. The half-life of varenicline averages 17 hours, allowing dosing once or twice daily. Because of the minimal extent of varenicline metabolism, the oral bioavailability of varenicline is high and fairly consistent, and there is no concern about metabolic drug interactions. Cimetidine reduces the clearance of varenicline by about 25%, most likely acting as a competitor for transporters in the renal secretion of varenicline.

Varenicline has been studied in several clinical trials, including two that compared it with bupropion.[14] In these trials, abstinence rates averaged 44% for varenicline, 30% for bupropion, and 18% for placebo at the end of treatment. The most common side effect of varenicline is nausea, reported by about 30% of patients. Nausea is usually mild to moderate and rarely results in treatment discontinuation.

Varenicline should be started at least 7 days before the target quit date to allow blood levels to reach steady state. The recommended dose of varenicline is 0.5 mg once daily for 3 days, 0.5 mg twice daily for 4 days, and then 1 mg twice daily for 12 weeks. This gradual escalation is done to minimize the development of nausea. Smokers who have stopped smoking after 12 weeks should be offered an additional 12 weeks of varenicline therapy to help maintain nonsmoking.[15]

Other Medications for Smoking Cessation

Nortriptyline is a norepinephrine reuptake blocker and, as such, simulates the actions of nicotine in the brain. Clonidine is an α_2-adrenergic receptor agonist that acts primarily on the brain to reduce sympathetic neural outflow. Its effects include sedation and anxiolysis as well as, potentially, hypotension, bradycardia, and dry mouth. The mechanism of clonidine's benefit in smoking cessation is believed to be related to its calming and anxiolytic effects. This drug appears to be most useful in smokers who experience a high degree of anxiety when they try to quit smoking. Both nortriptyline and clonidine have been reported to have odds ratios of about 2 compared with placebo in clinical trials.

Therapeutic Approach

Evidence-based guidelines for the treatment of tobacco addiction emphasize identifying all tobacco users in a physician's practice and ascertaining each patient's intent with respect to quitting smoking (see Fig. 56-7). Identification of tobacco use is facilitated by the implementation of an office-based system so that patients are queried about tobacco use at every visit. Tobacco use should be treated as a vital sign

TABLE 56-3 STRATEGIES TO HELP THE PATIENT TO QUIT TOBACCO USE

Strategies for Implementation	Action
Ask—Systematically identify all tobacco users at every visit	Implement an office-wide system that ensures that, for every patient at every clinic visit, tobacco-use status is queried and documented.
Advise—Strongly urge all tobacco users to quit	In a clear, strong, and personalized manner, urge every tobacco user to quit.
Assess—Determine willingness to make a quit attempt	Ask every tobacco user if he/she is willing to make a quit attempt at this time (e.g., within the next 30 days).
Assist—Aid the patient in quitting	Help the patient with a quit plan. Provide practical counseling (problem solving/skills training). Provide intratreatment social support. Help patient obtain extratreatment social support. Recommend the use of approved pharmacotherapy except in special circumstances.
Arrange—Schedule follow-up contact	Schedule follow-up contact, either in person or via telephone.

Adapted from The Tobacco Use and Dependence Clinical Practice Guideline Panel, Staff, and Consortium Representatives. A clinical practice guideline for treating tobacco use and dependence: a U.S. Public Health Service report. JAMA 2000;283:3244-3254.

BOX 56-4 GUIDELINES FOR SMOKING CESSATION

- In general, all smokers trying to quit smoking should be offered pharmacotherapy.
- Six first-line smoking-cessation medications are available—four types of nicotine-replacement therapy, sustained-release bupropion, and varenicline. Data are inadequate to rank these in order of efficacy. The choice of the first-line therapy should be governed by patient preference, familiarity of the clinician with the medication, contraindications in specific patients, and previous experience of the patient with specific pharmacotherapies.
- Second-line therapies include clonidine and nortriptyline. These drugs should be reserved for individuals with contraindications or failure of response to first-line medications.
- Several pharmacotherapies may delay, but not prevent, weight gain after smoking cessation. It is recommended that patients start or increase physical activity, but strict dieting is discouraged because it appears to increase the likelihood of relapse to smoking. Patients should be reassured that weight gain after quitting is self-limited and poses much less of a risk to health than smoking does.
- Transdermal nicotine (patches) and nicotine gum appear to be safe for patients with chronic cardiovascular disease. Other medications are probably much safer than smoking in the presence of medical disease, but need further evaluation.
- In smokers with prolonged withdrawal symptoms or in an individual who is unable not to smoke in the absence of medication, long-term therapy with nicotine-replacement medication or bupropion appears to be safe and reasonable.
- Research suggests that combining bupropion with nicotine patches or combining nicotine patches with ad libitum use of nicotine gum or nicotine nasal spray increases abstinence rates, compared with the rates produced by a single form of therapy.

Adapted from The Tobacco Use and Dependence Clinical Practice Guideline Panel, Staff, and Consortium Representatives. A clinical practice guideline for treating tobacco use and dependence: a U.S. Public Health Service report. JAMA 2000;283:3244-3254.

by using tobacco status stickers on patients' charts, electronic medical records, or computer reminder systems. The practice of routinely recording a patient's tobacco use status increases the odds ratio for quitting twofold.

Brief strategies to help a patient quit (Table 56-3 and Box 56-4) can be implemented in as little as 3 minutes during an office visit and can increase cessation rates significantly. Although brief physician advice increases quit rates by 70%, intensive behavioral treatment produces higher success rates and is cost effective. Clinicians with training in intensive smoking-cessation therapy should be identified as a referral source for smokers who are interested in behavioral counseling. As an alternative, smokers can be referred to telephone quit lines, which also provide smoking-cessation counseling.

The recent U.S. Public Health Service guideline recommends that all smokers trying to quit should be offered pharmacotherapy.[16] There are three classes of smoking-cessation medication, as mentioned previously. The choice of first-line therapy should be governed by patient preference, familiarity of the clinician with the medication, contraindications for specific patients, and prior experience of the patient with specific pharmacotherapies. Second-line therapies, clonidine and nortriptyline, should be reserved for individuals with contraindications to, or failure of, a response to first-line medications. In smokers with prolonged withdrawal symptoms, or in an individual who is unable to quit smoking in the absence of medication, long-term pharmacotherapy appears to be safe and reasonable. Recent research suggests that combining bupropion with nicotine patches or combining nicotine patches with *ab libitum* use of nicotine gum or nicotine nasal spray increases abstinence rates over those of a single form of therapy.

Emerging Targets and Therapeutics

Rimonabant is a cannabinoid (CB-1) receptor antagonist that has been developed for the treatment of obesity and the metabolic syndrome. Clinical studies have also shown rimonabant to be effective as an aid for smoking cessation.[17] Cannabinoid receptors are believed to contribute to the reinforcing effects of nicotine action.

Nicotine vaccines are currently undergoing clinical trials.[18] Acute immunization is performed to develop antibodies to nicotine. The antibody binds nicotine and slows its entry into the brain, thereby reducing the reinforcing effects of cigarette smoking. The nicotine vaccine is a logical approach to preventing relapse, which occurs in a large proportion of smokers after cessation.

Other potential future medications for smoking cessation include monamine oxidase inhibitors (MAO_A and MAO_B), which inhibit the metabolism of dopamine and, therefore, increase dopamine levels in the brain; and dopamine receptor D_3 receptor antagonists and partial agonists, which modulate activity of a receptor involved in drug-seeking behaviors.[19] Inhibitors of CYP2A6 activity have also been proposed as smoking-cessation aids; these work by increasing nicotine levels from tobacco use, thereby reducing urges to smoke. Methoxsalen and tranylcypromine inhibit CYP2A6 activity and slow nicotine metabolism, but both have significant toxicity, making routine clinical use problematic. Finally, selective nAChR agonists and antagonists in addition to varenicline are in early stages of development.

REFERENCES

1. State-specific prevalence of cigarette smoking and quitting among adults—United States, 2004. MMWR Morb Mortal Wkly Rep 2005;54:1124-1127.
2. Dajas-Bailador F, Wonnacott S. Nicotinic acetylcholine receptors and the regulation of neuronal signalling. Trends Pharmacol Sci 2004;25:317-324.
3. Maskos U, Molles BE, Pons S, et al. Nicotine reinforcement and cognition restored by targeted expression of nicotinic receptors. Nature 2005;436:103-107.
4. Tapper AR, McKinney SL, Nashmi R, et al. Nicotine activation of alpha4* receptors: sufficient for reward, tolerance, and sensitization. Science 2004;306:1029-1032.
5. Nestler EJ. Is there a common molecular pathway for addiction? Nat Neurosci 2005;8:1445-1449.

6. Kenny PJ, Markou A. Conditioned nicotine withdrawal profoundly decreases the activity of brain reward systems. J Neurosci 2005;25:6208-6212.
7. Naqvi NH, Rudrauf D, Damasio H, Bechara A. Damage to the insula disrupts addiction to cigarette smoking. Science 2007;315:531-534.
8. Madden PA, Pedersen NL, Kaprio J, et al. The epidemiology and genetics of smoking initiation and persistence: crosscultural comparisons of twin study results. Twin Res 2004;7:82-97.
9. Hukkanen J, Jacob P 3rd, Benowitz NL. Metabolism and disposition kinetics of nicotine. Pharmacol Rev 2005;57:79-115.
10. Benowitz NL, Lessov-Schlaggar CN, Swan GE, Jacob P 3rd. Female sex and oral contraceptive use accelerate nicotine metabolism. Clin Pharmacol Ther 2006;79: 480-488.
11. Hamilton M, Wolf JL, Rusk J, et al. Effects of smoking on the pharmacokinetics of erlotinib. Clin Cancer Res 2006;12:2166-2171.
12. van der Bol JM, Mathijssen RH, Loos WJ, et al. Cigarette smoking and irinotecan treatment: pharmacokinetic interaction and effects on neutropenia. J Clin Oncol 2007;25:2719-2726.
13. Coe JW, Brooks PR, Vetelino MG, et al. Varenicline: an alpha4beta2 nicotinic receptor partial agonist for smoking cessation. J Med Chem 2005;48:3474-3477.
14. Gonzales D, Rennard SI, Nides M, et al. Varenicline, an alpha4beta2 nicotinic acetylcholine receptor partial agonist, vs sustained-release bupropion and placebo for smoking cessation: a randomized controlled trial. JAMA 2006;296:47-55.
15. Tonstad S, Tonnesen P, Hajek P, et al. Effect of maintenance therapy with varenicline on smoking cessation: a randomized controlled trial. JAMA 2006;296:64-71.
16. The Tobacco Use and Dependence Clinical Practice Guideline Panel, Staff, and Consortium Representatives. A clinical practice guideline for treating tobacco use and dependence: a U.S. Public Health Service report. JAMA 2000;283:3244-3254.
17. Tucci SA, Halford JC, Harrold JA, Kirkham TC. Therapeutic potential of targeting the endocannabinoids: implications for the treatment of obesity, metabolic syndrome, drug abuse and smoking cessation. Curr Med Chem 2006;13:2669-2680.
18. Hatsukami DK, Rennard S, Jorenby D, et al. Safety and immunogenicity of a nicotine conjugate vaccine in current smokers. Clin Pharmacol Ther 2005;78:456-467.
19. Siu EC, Tyndale RF. Non-nicotinic therapies for smoking cessation. Annu Rev Pharmacol Toxicol 2007;47:541-564.
20. Benowitz NL. Nicotine addiction. Prim Care 1999;26:611-631.
21. Benowitz NL, Kuyt F, Jacob P 3rd. Circadian blood nicotine concentrations during cigarette smoking. Clin Pharmacol Ther 1982;32:758-764.
22. Benowitz NL. Cigarette smoking and nicotine addiction. Med Clin North Am 1992;76:415-437.
23. Benowitz NL, Porchet H, Sheiner L, Jacob P 3rd. Nicotine absorption and cardiovascular effects with smokeless tobacco use: comparison with cigarettes and nicotine gum. Clin Pharmacol Ther 1988;44:23-28.
24. U.S. Department of Health and Human Services Public Health Service. The Health Consequences of Smoking: Nicotine Addiction. A Report of the Surgeon General. DHHS (CDC) Publication No. 88-8406. Washington DC: Government Printing Office, 1988.
25. American Psychiatric Association. Diagnostic and Statistical Manual of Mental Disorders (DSM-IV), 4th ed. Washington, DC: American Psychiatric Association, 1994.

57

INSOMNIA (NARCOLEPSY)-RELATED DISORDERS

Teofilo Lee-Chiong and James F. Pagel

OVERVIEW 849
INSOMNIA 849
Introduction 849
Pathophysiology 849
Therapeutics and Clinical Pharmacology 849
Goals of Therapy 849
Therapeutics by Class 849
Therapeutic Approach 851
Emerging Targets and Therapeutics 851
HYPERSOMNIA 851
Introduction 851
Pathophysiology 851
Therapeutics and Clinical Pharmacology 851
Goals of Therapy 851
Therapeutics by Class 852
Therapeutic Approach 853
PARASOMNIAS 853
Introduction 853
Pathophysiology 853
Therapeutics and Clinical Pharmacology 853
Goals of Therapy 853
Therapeutics of Specific Parasomnias 853

OVERVIEW

Sleep disorders encompass conditions in which an imbalance between wakefulness and sleep areas in the central nervous system (Fig. 57-1) causes sleeplessness (insomnia), excessive sleepiness (hypersomnia) or inappropriate behavior or movements during sleep (parasomnias). Not surprisingly, sedating medications used to treat insomnia can lead to excessive sleepiness; conversely, adverse effects of psychostimulants indicated for the therapy of excessive sleepiness include the development of insomnia.

INSOMNIA

Introduction

Insomnia is defined as repeated difficulty with either initially falling asleep (sleep onset insomnia) or remaining asleep (sleep maintenance insomnia) despite adequate opportunity, condition, and time for sleep. Insomnia is the most common sleep disorder. About a third of adults report having occasional insomnia, and approximately 10% have chronic insomnia.

Pathophysiology

Insomnia is a symptom with numerous and diverse etiologies. Causes of insomnia include primary sleep disturbances; other sleep disorders; disturbances of the circadian sleep-wake rhythm; medical, neurologic, and psychiatric illnesses; behavior disorders; and medication use or withdrawal.

Therapeutics and Clinical Pharmacology

Goals of Therapy

Therapy of insomnia should address both nighttime sleep disturbance and its daytime consequences. Because insomnia may be due to many causes, the clinician should attempt to identify and manage factors that may precipitate or perpetuate sleep disruption. Many patients with chronic insomnia will benefit from therapy incorporating sleep hygiene education, behavior modification, and administration of hypnotic agents.

Pharmacotherapy is generally effective for transient insomnia arising from acute stressors, jet lag, or shift work, and may be useful in selected patients with more persistent sleep complaints.

Therapeutics by Class

Hypnotic agents that have been used to treat insomnia include benzodiazepines, non-benzodiazepine benzodiazepine receptor agonists (NBBRAs), and sedating antidepressants. Benzodiazepines and the NBBRAs act at the γ-aminobutyric acid (GABA)–benzodiazepine (BZ) receptor complex (Fig. 57-2). The various GABA-BZ receptor subunits (BZ1, BZ2, and BZ3) differ in their action. BZ1 is primarily responsible for the agent's hypnotic and amnesic actions. The BZ2 and BZ3 receptors are involved with its effect on memory and cognitive functioning, muscle relaxation, and antiseizure and antianxiety properties. Nonprescription hypnotic agents such as histamine antagonists, melatonin, and herbal compounds are commonly self-administered by patients with insomnia.

Benzodiazepines. Benzodiazepines bind nonselectively to the different GABA-BZ receptor subunits. They are effective hypnotic agents, anxiolytics, muscle relaxants, and anticonvulsants. As a class, they decrease sleep latency (time it takes to fall asleep), increase total sleep time, and decrease frequency of awakenings. Based on duration of action, benzodiazepines can be classified into short half-life (<3 hours), medium half-life (8 to 24 hours), and long half-life (>24 hours) agents (Box 57-1).

Disadvantages of benzodiazepines include potential lethality during overdose, especially when co-ingested with other central nervous system depressants or alcohol; dependency and abuse liability; development of tolerance; and rebound insomnia (worsening of sleep disturbance compared to baseline sleep quality) and withdrawal symptoms (e.g., agitation, anxiety, confusion, restlessness, tremulousness) after abrupt cessation of chronic use.[1] Short-acting agents are associated with greater withdrawal symptoms and rebound daytime anxiety, whereas long-acting drugs, by virtue of their longer elimination half-lives, may give rise to daytime sleepiness and cognitive impairment.

The use of benzodiazepine should generally be avoided during pregnancy or lactation, and in patients with untreated obstructive sleep apnea and significant obstructive and restrictive ventilatory dysfunction (e.g., emphysema and obesity-hypoventilation syndrome).

Non-benzodiazepine Benzodiazepine Receptor Agonists. NBBRAs selectively bind to the GABA-BZ1 receptor subunit. In contrast to the benzodiazepines, NBBRAs possess no anticonvulsant or muscle relaxant activity. They are also less likely to alter sleep architecture. The hypnosedative action of the NBBRAs is comparable with that of benzodiazepines.[2]

Zolpidem has a quick onset of action and a short half-life of approximately 2.4 hours. Zaleplon has a rapid onset but short duration of

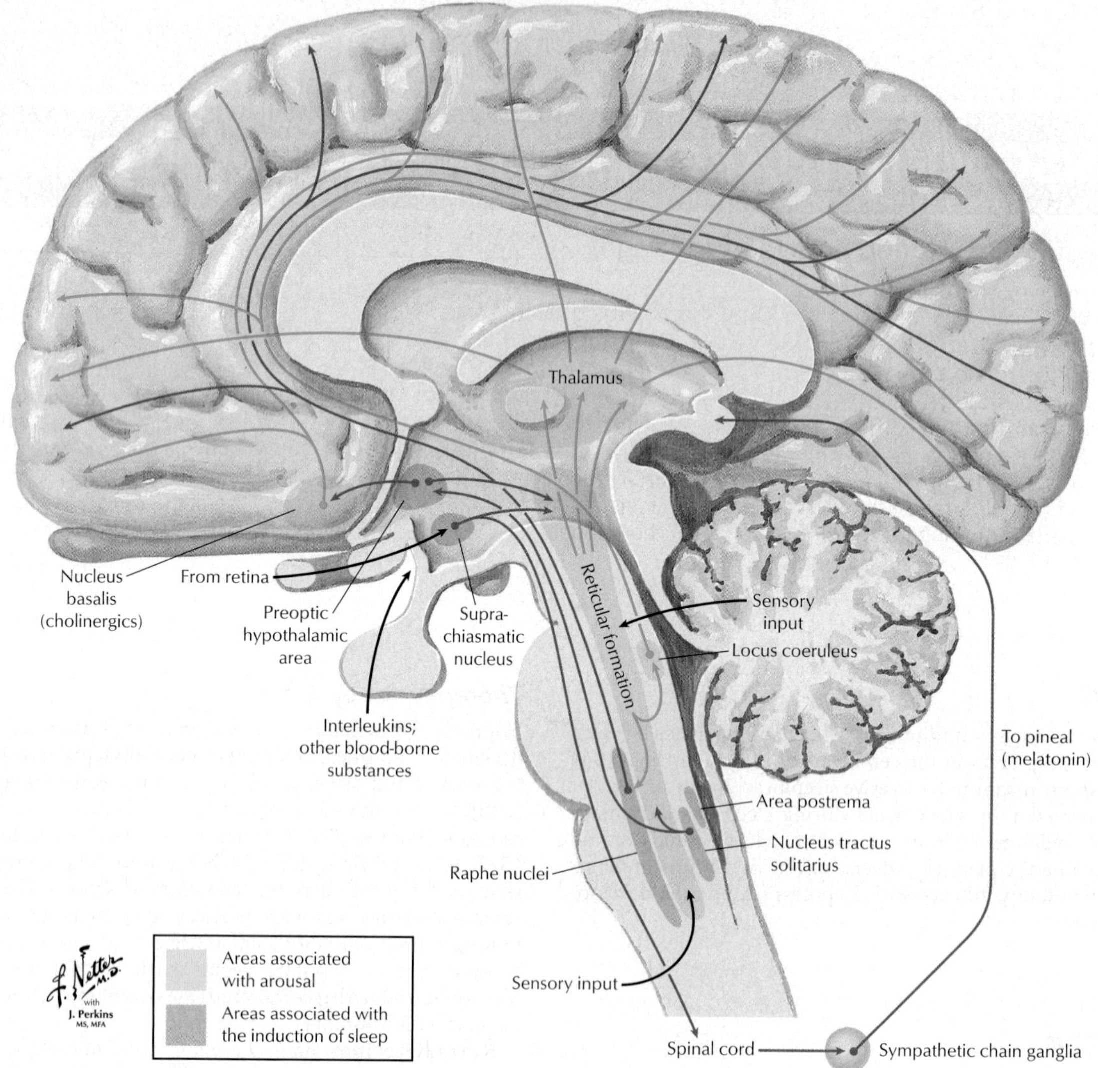

FIGURE 57-1 • Sleep and wakefulness control. Critical areas in the central nervous system are color coded. (Reprinted from Netter Anatomy Illustration Collection, © Elsevier Inc. All rights reserved.)

action, with a half-life of only about 1 hour. It has minimal effects on sleep architecture, and no significant risk of tolerance to its sleep-promoting effects or rebound insomnia after its discontinuation.[3] Eszopiclone has a relatively long duration of action and is approved for chronic treatment of persistent primary insomnia.[4] Compared to conventional benzodiazepines, NBBRAs are less likely to cause significant rebound insomnia or tolerance.[5]

Most published studies on benzodiazepines and NBBRAs lack data regarding long-term follow-up.

Sedating Antidepressants. Although sedating antidepressants (e.g., amitriptyline, doxepin, mirtazapine, trazodone, trimipramine) are widely prescribed to aid sleep in individuals with chronic insomnia, their effectiveness in this population has not been clearly established, particularly in those individuals without mood disorders.

Mirtazapine acts by antagonizing central α_2-adrenergic and 5-hydroxytryptamine $(5\text{-HT})_2$ and 5-HT_3 receptors. When given to patients with major depression and insomnia, it can significantly improve sleep latency, sleep efficiency, and wake after sleep onset.[6]

Trazodone is a 5-HT_2 and α_1 receptor antagonist that possesses both anxiolytic and sedative properties.[7] Adverse effects include cardiac arrhythmias, priapism, and the development of the serotonin syndrome. There is no significant tolerance or dependence potential.

Melatonin Receptor Agonists. Ramelteon, a melatonin receptor agonist, is highly selective for ML1 receptors located mainly in cells of the suprachiasmatic nucleus, and has little affinity for other ML receptor subtypes, such as ML2. Its use may result in a significantly shorter mean latency to persistent sleep and a longer mean total sleep time compared to placebo.[8]

Nonprescription Hypnotic Agents. Patients with insomnia commonly self-administer nonprescription sleep agents, to manage their sleep disturbances.

Histamine Antagonists. Most over-the-counter hypnotic agents are antihistamines. The first-generation histamine_1 antagonists (e.g., diphenhydramine, chlorpheniramine) readily cross the blood-brain barrier and are sedating. In contrast, second-generation agents, such as loratadine and fexofenadine, are less likely to cause sedation. There are only a few published studies on the efficacy of antihistamines as hypnotic agents, and their use for the management of chronic insomnia is not well established. In one study, diphenhydramine improved sleep latency to a significantly greater degree than did placebo.[9] Tolerance to the hypnotic effects of diphenhydramine may develop rapidly.

Melatonin. Secretion of endogenous melatonin by the pineal gland is increased at night (Fig. 57-3). Studies evaluating melatonin's effect on sleep are primarily on insomnia related to circadian rhythm sleep disorders, with more limited data on its use for therapy of primary insomnia.[10]

Herbal Preparations. Patients with insomnia often use nonprescription herbal preparations, such as kava (*Piper methysticum*),

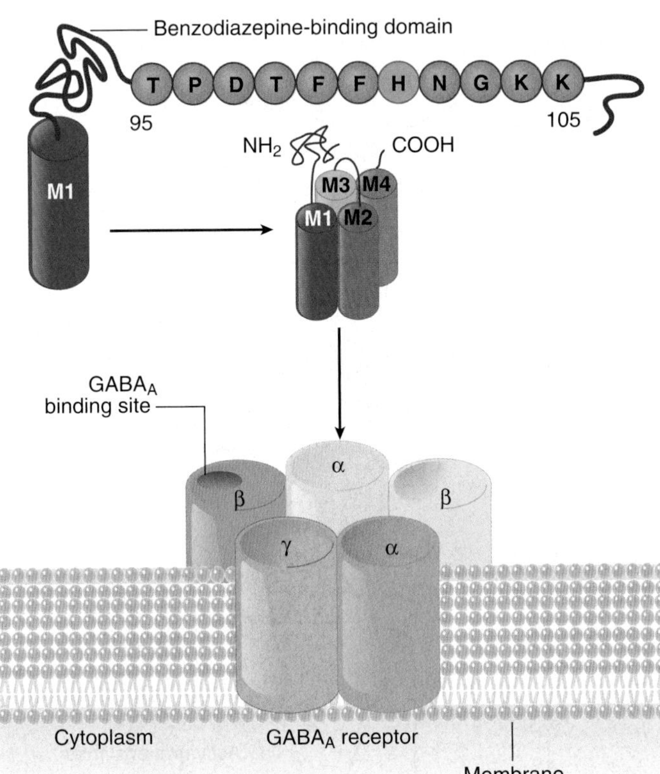

FIGURE 57-2 • The structure of gamma-aminobutyric acid (GABA)-benzodiazepine receptor complex. $GABA_A$ receptors are ligand-gated ion channels. The opening of each ion channel is surrounded by five peptide subunits. Each of the five subunits consists of four membrane-spanning domains (M1, M2, M3, and M4). The benzodiazepine-binding site is located on the extracellular portion of the M1 segment of a subunit. The substitution of one amino acid, arginine, at position 101 for histidine (H) in the N-terminal domain renders the receptor insensitive to benzodiazepines. The binding site for GABA itself is in a different domain of the receptor complex. (Adapted from Weinberger DR: Anxiety at the frontier of molecular medicine. N Engl J Med 2001;344:16.)

BOX 57-1 DURATION OF ACTION OF BENZODIAZEPINES

Short-Acting Agents
Alprazolam (Xanax)
Oxazepam (Serax)
Triazolam (Halcion)

Intermediate-Acting Agents
Estazolam (ProSom)
Temazepam (Restoril)

Long-Acting Agents
Clorazepate (Tranxene)
Diazepam (Valium)
Flurazepam (Dalmane)
Quazepam (Doral)

valerian (*Valeriana officinalis*), passionflower (*Passiflora incarnata*), and skullcap (*Scutellaria laterifolia*).[11] These agents are commonly combined in commercial botanical products. However, few clinical trials of their use in the therapy of insomnia are published in the medical literature, and additional studies are necessary to define their mechanisms of action and their roles in the management of patients with either transient or chronic insomnia.

Therapeutic Approach

Selection among the many available hypnotic agents should take into account the specific characteristics of the patient (age, presence of medical or psychiatric illnesses, pregnancy or lactation, and occupation), pharmacologic profile of the agent (hypnotic efficacy, absorption, elimination, onset and duration of action, effect on sleep stages, risks of tolerance, dependency and withdrawal, abuse potential, and possible drug interactions), and the duration and timing of insomnia. Short-acting agents are appropriate for sleep onset insomnia, while agents with intermediate duration of action are indicated for patients with both sleep onset and maintenance insomnia. Finally, long-acting compounds are useful for those with early morning awakenings and daytime anxiety.

Response to and adverse effects from pharmacotherapy should be closely monitored in every patient, especially in the older adult. Indications for use should be reassessed on a regular basis whenever these agents are used for longer periods.

Emerging Targets and Therapeutics

A number of hypnotic medications are currently under development. One promising drug is indiplon, a non-benzodiazepine $GABA_A$ receptor modulator that has been shown to improve sleep latency and sleep efficiency.[12]

HYPERSOMNIA

Introduction

Persons who are excessive sleepy are unable to consistently achieve and sustain wakefulness and alertness to accomplish the tasks of daily living. Episodes of sleep, therefore, occur unintentionally or at inappropriate times or places.

Pathophysiology

It is important to distinguish excessive sleepiness from fatigue, exhaustion, tiredness, or weakness, which may closely mimic it. Insufficient sleep is the most common cause of excessive sleepiness. *Insufficient sleep syndrome* consists of chronic voluntary failure to obtain sufficient duration of nighttime sleep to achieve and maintain normal alertness while awake. *Narcolepsy* is a neurologic disorder characterized by excessive sleepiness, cataplexy (brief loss or reduction of postural muscle tone occurring during wakefulness that is triggered by intense emotion such as laughter) in a subset of patients, sleep paralysis (transient inability to move occurring at sleep onset or upon awakening), and hallucinations (hallucinatory phenomena that can be visual, auditory, tactile, or kinetic, occurring during wakefulness at sleep onset [hypnagogic] or upon awakening [hypnopompic]). Narcolepsy is believed to be due to abnormalities involving the hypocretin, cholinergic, monoamine, and dopaminergic pathways of the central nervous system. Patients with *idiopathic hypersomnia* report severe and constant sleepiness that occurs despite sufficient or even increased amounts of nighttime sleep and without any identifiable cause. Excessive sleepiness can result from central nervous system trauma; other sleep disorders (obstructive sleep apnea syndrome or Kleine-Levin recurrent hypersomnia syndrome); circadian sleep-wake rhythm disorders; medical, neurologic, and psychiatric conditions; and the use of substances and medications.

Therapeutics and Clinical Pharmacology

Goals of Therapy

Psychostimulants are commonly required to control pathologic sleepiness. These agents improve alertness, cognitive performance, and mood. Commonly used agents include caffeine, amphetamines (e.g., dextroamphetamine, methamphetamine), methylphenidate, and modafinil.[13] They generally increase the availability of norepinephrine and dopamine at the synaptic junctions.

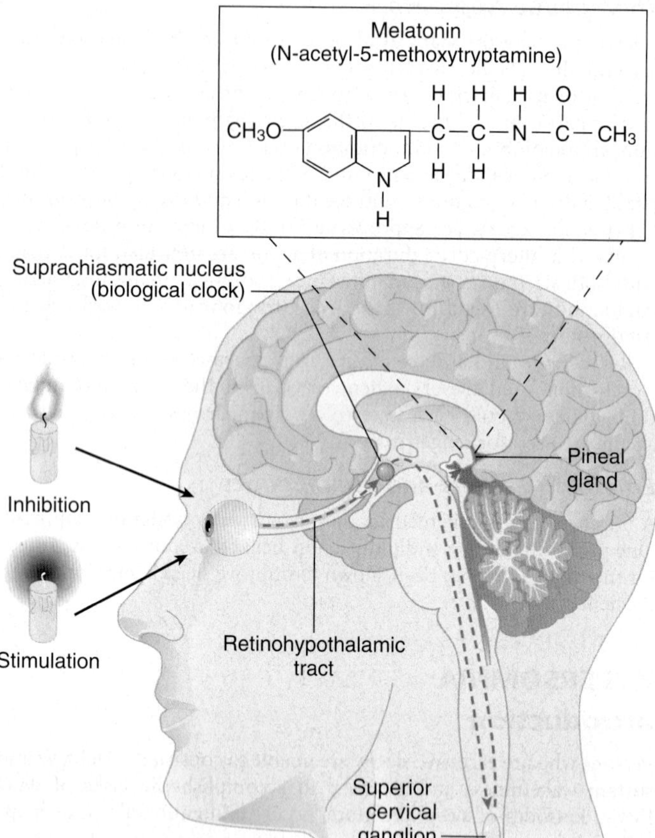

FIGURE 57-3A • Physiology of melatonin secretion. Melatonin (with structure shown in inset) is produced in the pineal gland. The production and secretion of melatonin are mediated largely by postganglionic retinal nerve fibers that pass through the retinohypothalamic tract to the suprachiasmatic nucleus, then to the superior cervical ganglion, and finally to the pineal gland. This neuronal system is activated by darkness and suppressed by light. The activation of α_1- and β_1-adrenergic receptors in the pineal gland raises cyclic AMP and calcium concentrations and activates arylalkylamine *N*-acetyltransferase, initiating the synthesis and release of melatonin. The daily rhythm of melatonin secretion is also controlled by an endogenous, free-running pacemaker located in the suprachiasmatic nucleus. (Adapted from Brzezinski A: Melatonin in humans. N Engl J Med 1997;336:186-195.)

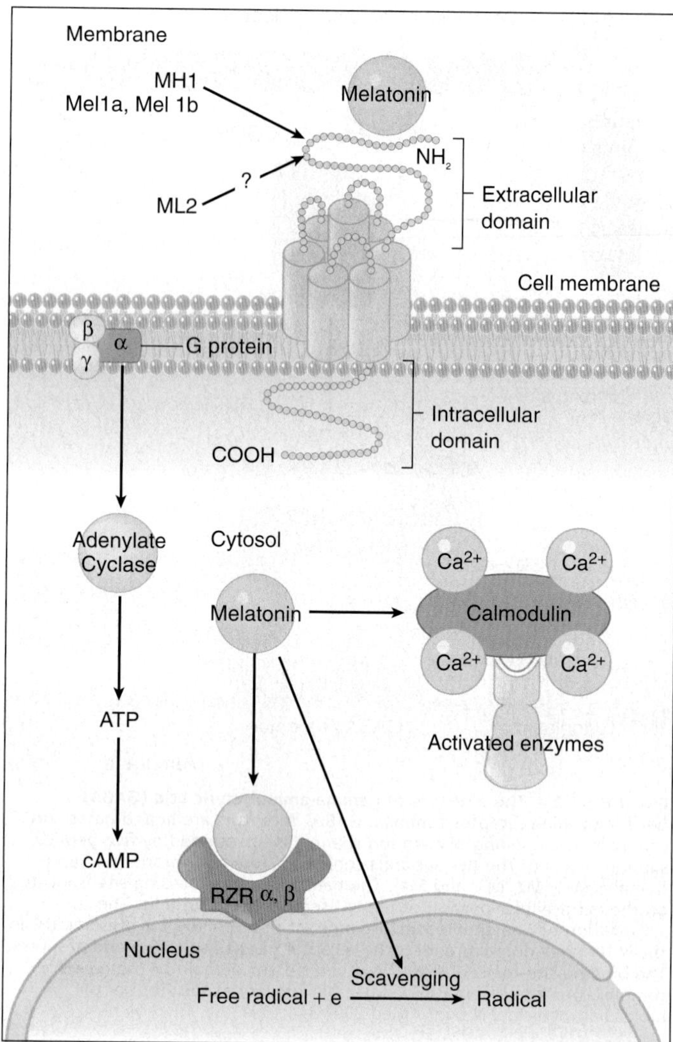

FIGURE 57-3B • Mechanisms of action of melatonin at the cellular level. Two membrane-bound melatonin receptors have been identified: ML1 (a high-affinity receptor) and ML2 (a low-affinity receptor). ML1 has two subtypes, designated Mel1a and Mel1b. By binding to its membrane-bound receptors, melatonin changes the conformation of the α subunit of specific intracellular G proteins, which then bind to adenylate cyclase and activate it. Cytosolic and nuclear binding sites have also been described. On binding to cytosolic calmodulin, melatonin may directly affect calcium signaling by interacting with target enzymes, such as adenylate cyclase and phosphodiesterase, and structural proteins. The nuclear binding sites are retinoid Z receptors (RZR) α and β. Melatonin scavenges oxygen-centered free radicals, especially the highly toxic hydroxyl radical, and neutralizes them by a single electron transfer (e), which results in detoxified radicals. The hormone may therefore protect macromolecules, particularly DNA, from oxidative damage. The question marks indicate mechanisms of action that have not been proved. cAMP denotes cyclic AMP. (Adapted from Brzezinski A: Melatonin in humans. N Engl J Med 1997;336:186-195.)

Therapeutics by Class

Caffeine. Caffeine acts by inhibiting adenosine transmission. Major sources of caffeine include coffee, tea, and caffeinated sodas. It increases both subjective and objective (e.g., Multiple Sleep Latency Test) measures of alertness.[14] Physiologic changes related to its use include increases in metabolic rate, blood pressure, heart rate, and body temperature. Habitual use can give rise to tolerance and withdrawal symptoms. It has a mean half-life of approximately 5 hours.

Amphetamine. Amphetamine (dextroamphetamine and methamphetamine) acts by releasing norepinephrine and dopamine at neuronal terminals. Administration of amphetamines prolongs sleep latency, decreases total sleep time, and enhances alertness, cognitive performance, memory, and mood. Incidence of physiologic effects (tachycardia and hypertension) and adverse effects (insomnia, nervousness, headaches, tremulousness, agitation, palpitations, and arrhythmias) is dose dependent.[14] Amphetamines have a high abuse liability and risk of dependency. Tolerance develops rapidly. Withdrawal symptoms are common after drug discontinuation. Amphetamine is indicated for the therapy of sleepiness secondary to narcolepsy.

Methylphenidate. Methylphenidate acts by blocking dopamine reuptake and enhancing release of dopamine and norepinephrine. It improves alertness and psychomotor performance.[14] Like the amphetamines, methylphenidate administration is associated with increases in heart rate and blood pressure. Methylphenidate appears to have less abuse liability than amphetamines. It is indicated for the treatment of excessive sleepiness related to narcolepsy. Methylphenidate is available in an immediate-release form (elimination half-life of approximately 2.5 to 3.5 hours), an extended-release form (duration of action of 8 to 12 hours), and combinations of both immediate- and extended-release formulations.

Modafinil. The precise mechanism of action for the alerting and wakefulness-promoting properties of modafinil is incompletely understood. It is believed to involve the histaminergic, dopaminergic, noradrenergic, GABA, and hypocretin systems. Administration of the drug to sleep-deprived individuals results in a dose-dependent improvement in alertness, psychomotor performance, and reaction time.

Physiologic effects consist of increases in blood pressure, heart rate, and body temperature, especially at higher doses.[15,16] Modafinil has less abuse liability compared to amphetamine or methylphenidate, and is not associated with tolerance. Adverse effects include the development of nausea and headaches. It is indicated for the treatment of excessive sleepiness due to narcolepsy or shift work sleep disorder. It is also approved for treating persistent sleepiness despite continuous positive airway pressure (CPAP) therapy in patients with obstructive sleep apnea syndrome. The usual starting dose is 100 to 200 mg daily, and the maximum dose is 400 mg daily.

Therapeutic Approach

Therapy of excessive sleepiness generally involves proper sleep hygiene practices, including maintaining a regular sleep-wake schedule and obtaining an adequate amount of sleep each night, and specific management of any underlying medical, neurologic, or psychiatric disorder that can give rise to or contribute to sleepiness. Patients who continue to have significant daytime sleepiness may benefit from judicious use of stimulant agents.

General guidelines regarding the use of psychostimulants include using the lowest possible effective dose, monitoring clinical response as well as adverse effects, and timing drug administration to meet specific individual needs.

PARASOMNIAS

Introduction

Parasomnias are undesirable physical events or experiences that occur during the sleep period. They involve sleep-related movements or behaviors over which the sleeper has no conscious deliberate control.

Pathophysiology

The pathophysiology of most parasomnias remains incompletely understood. It is believed that parasomnias arise from the simultaneous occurrence of, or rapid oscillation between, the various state-determining variables of wakefulness, non–rapid-eye-movement (NREM) sleep, and rapid-eye-movement (REM) sleep, with intrusion of elements of one state into another.

Therapeutics and Clinical Pharmacology

Goals of Therapy

No treatment of parasomnias is necessary beyond proper diagnosis and reassurance, if the parasomnia is not associated with nocturnal injury or adverse effects on waking function. Current treatments of parasomnias are largely anecdotal and based on case reports, with almost no clinical trials utilizing placebo controls.

The more common parasomnias, the NREM disorders of arousal and the REM sleep-associated parasomnias, are sleep stage specific. One facet of medication treatment of parasomnias involves sleep stage manipulation (Box 57-2). Therefore, medications that suppress REM sleep may be useful in the treatment of REM sleep–associated parasomnias, whereas agents that alter or suppress NREM stage 3 and 4 sleep have been proven useful in the treatment of the NREM disorders of arousal (see Box 57-2).

Therapeutics of Specific Parasomnias

Disorders of Arousal. This group of parasomnias consists of confusional arousals, sleepwalking, and sleep terrors. They occur out of NREM sleep, particularly stages 3 and 4 sleep, often during the first third of the night. Disorders of arousal are most prevalent during childhood and become less frequent with increasing age. *Confusional arousals* are characterized by episodes of confusion, disorientation, or inappropriate behavior following spontaneous or forced arousals from sleep. *Sleepwalking*, or somnambulism, refers to ambulation that occurs during sleep, accompanied by diminished arousability, impaired judgment, and inappropriate behavior. *Sleep terrors* (pavor nocturnus) consist of abrupt awakenings with profound fear, inconsolability, misperception of the environment, confusion, amnesia for the episode, and autonomic and behavioral manifestations of intense fear.

BOX 57-2 MEDICATIONS THAT CAN ALTER SLEEP STAGES

Medication Classes Suppressing REM Sleep
- Antidepressants (monoamine oxidase inhibitors, selective serotonin reuptake inhibitors, tricyclic antidepressants)
- Barbituates and barbiturate-like agents
- Benzodiazepines

Medications That Decrease NREM Stages 3 and 4 Sleep
- Amphetamines
- Benzodiazepines
- Selective serotonin reuptake inhibitors
- Tricyclic antidepressants

Medications That Increase NREM Stages 3 and 4 Sleep
- γ-Hydroxybutyrate
- Lithium
- Opiates

Environmental protection of the sleeper and family reassurance are important. Specific therapy may be indicated for cases that are potentially injurious or associated with significant distress to the patient or household members. Benzodiazepines, particularly clonazepam, have been used in the treatment of disorders of arousal.[17] Other medications that have been used successfully to treat sleep terrors or sleepwalking include the selective serotonin reuptake inhibitors (SSRIs; e.g., paroxetine), other benzodiazepines (e.g., alprazolam, diazepam), and imipramine.[18]

Exploding Head Syndrome. Exploding head syndrome is a rare disorder with a characteristic presentation. Persons describe a sensation of an "explosion" or a "sudden loud noise" in their head as they are falling asleep or upon awakening. There are often no complaints of significant pain. Anecdotal treatment success with medication has been obtained with indomethacin, nifedipine, and clomipramine.[19]

Nightmare Disorder. Nightmares are unpleasant and frightening dreams that occur during REM sleep. Once awakened, the person is fully alert and profoundly fearful and anxious, can recall vividly the preceding dream, and has difficulty returning to sleep. Occasional nightmares are not uncommon. Generally, no specific therapy aside from reassurance that the condition is benign is necessary. In some cases, treatment may be desired because of the frequency of events or extremely disturbing nature of the dream content.

Frequent nightmares associated with decreased sleep quality and sleep disruption can occur independently of any psychiatric disorder. Nightmares can occur as a medication side effect (Table 57-1). Nightmares can affect daytime functioning and give rise to psychological distress, and targeted therapy of nightmares can lead to improvements in sleep disturbance, psychological distress, and severity of associated psychiatric conditions.

Frequent nightmares associated with significant physical or psychological trauma are the most common symptom of posttraumatic stress disorder (PTSD). A meta-analysis of the literature on the pharmacotherapy of PTSD concluded that pharmacotherapy is useful in the treatment of PTSD. The SSRI antidepressants are currently the medications of choice for the treatment of PTSD.[20] Other medications that have shown to be effective include antianxiety agents, nonbenzodiazepine hypnotics, antidepressants, mood stabilizers, anticonvulsants, and antipsychotics.[21] The effects on nightmare frequency in PTSD have not been addressed for most of these agents, except for the antidepressants (e.g., trazodone, nefazodone, fluvoxamine), which have been shown to improve both the nightmare frequency and

TABLE 57-1 MEDICATIONS THAT MAY CAUSE NIGHTMARES

Neuroreceptor Affected	Agents
Norepinephrine	β-Blockers (atenolol, bisoprolol, labetalol, oxprenolol, propranolol) Guanethidine
Serotonin	Selective serotonin reuptake inhibitors (escitalopram, fluoxetine, paroxetine)
Serotonin and norepinephrine	Risperidone Venlafaxine
Dopamine	Dopamine agonists (amantadine, levodopa, ropinirole, selegiline) Amphetamine-like agents (bethanidine, fenfluramine, phenmetrazine)
γ-Aminobutyric acid (GABA)	γ-Hydroxybutyrate Triazolam Zopiclone
Miscellaneous agents	Angiotensin-converting enzyme inhibitors (enalapril, losartan, quinapril) Antihistamines (chlorpheniramine) Antimicrobials and immunosuppressants (amantadine, fleroxacin, ganciclovir, gusperimus) Antipsychotics (clozapine) Digoxin Naproxen Verapamil

insomnia associated with chronic PTSD.[20] The acute use of hypnotics after a traumatic event does not prevent the development of PTSD.[22]

It is postulated that some patients with PTSD exhibit abnormalities in noradrenergic function.[23] Antihypertensive agents affect noradrenergic central nervous system receptors, and these drugs have been shown to affect both REM sleep and reports of dreaming. The effects of these agents on both dreams and nightmares are often opposite to the drugs' known pharmacologic effects on REM sleep.[24] A reduction in dream recall occurs with use of both α-agonists (REM suppressants) and β-blockers (NREM suppressants). Prazosin is the α-agonist most commonly used for the treatment of recurrent nightmares in PTSD patients.[25] An agent's effect on REM sleep may or may not be associated with an associated change in reported dreaming. The use of β-blockers depresses REM sleep percentages yet can result in increased reports of dreaming, nightmares, and hallucinations. β-Blockers (e.g., propranolol) have been shown to be effective in treating PTSD.

REM Sleep Behavior Disorder. In REM sleep behavior disorder (RBD), abnormal behavior develops during REM sleep accompanied by loss of REM-related muscle atonia or hypotonia. Affected individuals appear to be "acting out their dreams," with abnormal behaviors ranging from simple motions to highly elaborate activities, such as screaming, punching, or kicking. These dream-enacting behaviors can result in injury to the sleeper or bed partner. Clonazepam is the most commonly utilized medication for the treatment of RBD. It is effective in treating the behavioral and dream-disordered components of RBD with few reports of tolerance or abuse.[26] Positive responses have also been noted for SSRIs, tricylic antidepressants (e.g., impramine, desipramine), other benzodiazepines (e.g., alprazolam, triazolam), and anticonvulsants (e.g., carbamazepine).[27] Anecdotal and case reports suggest beneficial effects from melatonin, tryptophan, monoamine oxidase inhibitors, valproic acid, gabapentin, clonidine, levodopa/carbidopa, and clozapine in specific cases.[28]

Sleep Enuresis. Sleep enuresis is characterized by recurrent involuntary bed-wetting occurring during sleep after 5 years of age. Sleep enuresis is classified as *primary* if a child older than 5 years of age has not been able to consistently stay dry during sleep, or *secondary* if bed-wetting recurs after the child or adult has maintained dryness for at least 6 consecutive months. Patients with nocturnal enuresis may not demonstrate the normal nocturnal increase in antidiuretic hormone. Desmopressin (DDAVP) pills or nasal spray are effective and used commonly for the treatment of nocturnal enuresis. Imipramine has a long history of use in children for the treatment of functional enuresis; however, children are more sensitive than adults to acute overdosage, and electrocardiographic abnormalities have been noted with routine use. The goal of medication therapy for enuresis is the maintenance of dry nights pending the eventual urologic-neurogenic maturity that comes with increasing patient age. Enuresis responds well to behavioral treatments, with success rates in excess of 90% noted for combination therapies that include bed-wetting alarms, rewards, and responsibility training.[29]

Sleep Paralysis. Sleep paralysis can occur either at sleep onset (hypnagogic) or upon awakening (hypnopompic). There is a generalized transient inability to move the head, body, and extremities, with sparing of the ocular and respiratory muscles. Isolated sleep paralysis is generally a benign condition with no known complications. In the absence of other symptoms of narcolepsy such as excessive sleepiness or cataplexy, further evaluation is unwarranted. If indicated, REM suppressant agents, such as SSRIs or tricyclic antidepressants, have been used. However, only anecdotal reports are cited in the literature as to the efficacy of these drugs.[30]

Sleep-Related Dissociative Disorders. Nighttime episodes of dissociative disorder can consist of screaming, running, violent or sexualized behavior, or self-mutilation. The dissociative disorders and their associated psychiatric conditions require long-term therapy of the underlying disorder. Treatment is usually initialized in a specialized inpatient setting. Nocturnal utilization of benzodiazepine agents may aggravate a nocturnal dissociative disorder.

Sleep-Related Eating Disorder. Sleep-related eating disorder (SRED) consists of repetitive arousals from sleep with involuntary eating or drinking. In many individuals, the awakenings appear to be triggered by learned behavior rather than real hunger or thirst. Patients are typically unaware or only partly conscious of the abnormal behavior. Treatment of SRED should be directed toward treating any underlying sleep disorders, such as obstructive sleep apnea. In cases associated with sleepwalking and restless leg syndrome, therapy with dopamine agonists (pramipexole or ropinirole), benzodiazepines (clonazepam), or opiates (codeine) can be effective. Fluoxetine and bupropion can be useful as adjunctive therapies. Psychological and behavioral treatments are usually ineffective.

Sleep-Related Groaning (Catathrenia). Catathrenia consists of expiratory groaning during sleep occurring predominantly or exclusively during REM sleep. The course tends to be chronic with a nightly occurrence. Sleep-related groaning may occur in association with obstructive sleep apnea. Treatments attempted to this point, however, including CPAP and several medications, have not been shown to be effective.[31]

REFERENCES

1. Schweizer E, Rickels K. Benzodiazepine dependence and withdrawal: a review of the syndrome and its clinical management. Acta Psychiatr Scand Suppl 1998;393:95-101.
2. Terzano MG, Rossi M, Palomba V, et al. New drugs for insomnia: comparative tolerability of zopiclone, zolpidem and zaleplon. Drug Saf 2003;26:261-282.
3. Walsh JK, Vogel GW, Scharf M, et al. A five week, polysomnographic assessment of zaleplon 10 mg for the treatment of primary insomnia. Sleep Med 2000;1:41-49.
4. Krystal AD, Walsh JK, Laska E, et al. Sustained efficacy of eszopiclone over 6 months of nightly treatment: results of a randomized, double-blind, placebo-controlled study in adults with chronic insomnia. Sleep 2003;26:793-799.
5. Hajak G, Muller WE, Wittchen HU, et al. Abuse and dependence potential for the non-benzodiazepine hypnotics zolpidem and zopiclone: a review of case reports and epidemiological data. Addiction 2003;98:1371-1378.
6. Winokur A, DeMartinis NA 3rd, McNally DP, et al. Comparative effects of mirtazapine and fluoxetine on sleep physiology measures in patients with major depression and insomnia. J Clin Psychiatry 2003;64:1224-1229.
7. Saletu-Zyhlarz GM, Abu-Bakr MH, Anderer P, et al. Insomnia in depression: differences in objective and subjective sleep and awakening quality to normal controls and acute effects of trazodone. Prog Neuropsychopharmacol Biol Psychiatry 2002;26:249-260.

8. Erman M, Seiden D, Zammit G. Phase II study of the selective ML-1 receptor agonist TAK-375 in subjects with primary chronic insomnia [Abstract]. Sleep 2003;26(Suppl): A298.
9. Rickels K, Morris RJ, Newman H, et al. Diphenhydramine in insomniac family practice patients: a double-blind study. J Clin Pharmacol 1983;23:234-242.
10. Almeida Montes LG, Ontiveros Uribe MP, Cortes Sotres J, et al. Treatment of primary insomnia with melatonin: a double-blind, placebo-controlled, crossover study. J Psychiatry Neurosci 2003;28:191-196.
11. Fugh-Berman A, Jerry M, Cott J. Dietary supplements and natural products as psychotherapeutic agents. Psychosom Med 1999;61:712-728.
12. Walsh JK, Lankford DD, Krystal A, et al. Efficacy and tolerability of four doses of indiplon (NBI-34060) modified-release in elderly patients with sleep maintenance insomnia [Abstract]. Sleep 2003;26(Suppl):A78.
13. Mitler MM, Hajdukovic R. Relative efficacy of drugs for the treatment of sleepiness in narcolepsy. Sleep 1991;14:218-220.
14. Bonnet MH, Balkin TJ, Dinges DF, et al, for the Sleep Deprivation and Stimulant Task Force of the American Academy of Sleep Medicine. The use of stimulants to modify performance during sleep loss: a review by the Sleep Deprivation and Stimulant Task Force of the American Academy of Sleep Medicine. Sleep 2005;28:1163-1187.
15. U.S. Modafinil in Narcolepsy Multicenter Study Group. Randomized trial of modafinil as a treatment for the excessive daytime somnolence of narcolepsy. Neurology 2000;54:1166-1175.
16. Schwartz JR, Hirshkowitz M, Erman MK, et al. Modafinil as adjuct therapy for daytime sleepiness in obstructive sleep apnea: a 12-week, open-label study. Chest 2003;124:2192-2199.
17. Schenck CH, Mahowald MW. Long term nightly benzodiazepine treatment of injurous parasomnias and other disorders with disrupted nocturnal sleep in 170 adults. Am J Med 1996;100:333-337.
18. Lillywhite AR, Wilson SJ, Nutt DJ. Successful treatment of night terrors and somnambulism with paroxetine. Br J Psychiatry 1994;164:551-554.
19. Casucci G, d'Onofrio F, Torelli P. Rare primary headaches: clinical insights. Neurol Sci 2004;25(Suppl 3):S77-S83.
20. Singareddy RK, Balon R. Sleep in posttraumatic stress disorder. Ann Clin Psychiatry 2002;14:183-190.
21. Putnam FW, Hulsmann JE. Pharmacotherapy for survivors of childhood trauma. Semin Clin Neuropsychiatry 2002;7:129-136.
22. Mellman TA, Bustamante V, David D, et al. Hypnotic medication in the aftermath of trauma. J Clin Psychiatry 2002;63:1183-1184.
23. Southwick SM, Krystal JH, Morgan CA, et al. Abnormal noradrenergic function in posttraumatic stress disorder. Arch Gen Psychiatry 1993;50:266-274.
24. Pagel JF, Helfter P. Drug induced nightmares—an etiology based review. Hum Psychopharmacol 2003;18:59-67.
25. Raskind MA, Peskind ER, Kanter ED, et al. Reduction of nightmares and other PTSD symptoms in combat veterans by prazosin: a placebo-controlled study. Am J Psychiatry 2003;160:371-373.
26. Chiu HF, Wing YK. REM sleep behaviour disorder: an overview. Int J Clin Pract 1997;51:451-454.
27. Schenck CH, Boyd JL, Mahowald MW. A parasomnia overlap disorder involving sleepwalking, sleep terrors, and REM sleep behavior disorder in 33 polysomnographically confirmed cases. Sleep 1997;20:972-981.
28. Wills L, Garcia J. Parasomnias: epidemiology and management. CNS Drugs 2002;16:803-810.
29. Challamel MJ, Cochat P. Nocturnal enuresis in children. *In* Lee-Chiong T (ed): Sleep—A Comprehensive Handbook. Hoboken, NJ: John Wiley & Sons, 2006, pp 443-448.
30. Queshi A. Other parasomnias. *In* Lee-Chiong T (ed): Sleep—A Comprehensive Handbook. Hoboken, NJ: John Wiley & Sons, 2006, pp 463-470.
31. Vetrugno R, Provini F, Plazzi G, et al. Catathrenia (nocturnal groaning): a new type of parasomnia. Neurology 2001;56:681-683.

58

DRUGS IN OPHTHALMOLOGY

Douglas J. Rhee and William S. Tasman

INTRODUCTION: OPTICAL PHYSICS AND ANATOMY 857
BASIC CONCEPTS OF OCULAR PHARMACOLOGY 857
Intraocular "Circulation" 857
The Eye as a Separate Bioavailable Site 857
Basic Ocular Pharmacokinetics 857
Intraocular Penetration of Systemic Medications 857
Topical Administration 857
THERAPEUTICS AND CLINICAL PHARMACOLOGY 858
Therapeutics by Class 858
Antibiotics 858
Mydriatics and Cycloplegics 859
Anti-inflammatories 859
Antiglaucoma Agents 860
Antiangiogenesis Agents 861
Lubricants 861

INTRODUCTION: OPTICAL PHYSICS AND ANATOMY

The eye is a sensory organ designed to gather electromagnetic energy (i.e., light). Based on the absorption spectra of the three principle pigments within the red, green, and blue cones of the retina, visible light is between the wavelengths of 380 and 700 nm; light of lower frequency is named ultraviolet, followed by x-rays, while light of higher frequency is called infrared, followed by microwave (Fig. 58-1). Light enters the eye and is focused by the cornea and the lens onto the retina. The photons of light are eventually absorbed by the photosensitive pigments of the rods (rhodopsin; peak absorption 500 nm) and cones (red, green, and blue opsins). This energy is converted into electrochemical signals that are eventually transmitted through the optic nerve to the brain, where the information is mapped and processed. "Vision" is the brain's interpretation of that information.

There are many unique anatomic and physiologic aspects of the eye that make the pharmacokinetics of treating ocular disease different from treating disease of other organs. Since the eyes have approximately 30% of their front surfaces exposed, there is direct access allowing topical and direct intraocular administration.

The outer coat of the eye is the sclera and cornea, which are composed of fibroblasts embedded in an extracellular matrix comprising collagens, elastin, and proteoglycans. The sclera and cornea range in thickness between 0.5 and 1.5 mm. Internally, the eye is divided into the anterior and posterior chambers; these spaces are separated by the crystalline lens. Within the anterior chamber (i.e., front of the eye) is aqueous humor. The posterior chamber is filled with the vitreous humor, which is a clear gel that has a scaffolding ultrastructure with a density approximating jelly.

BASIC CONCEPTS OF OCULAR PHARMACOLOGY

Intraocular "Circulation"

The lens, cornea, and trabecular meshwork (the principle drain of the eye) receive their nutrients and have their metabolic waste eliminated by the flow of aqueous humor since there is no direct blood supply to these tissues. Aqueous is formed in the ciliary processes (pars plicata region of the retina) (Fig. 58-2). The epithelial cells of the inner nonpigmented layer are the principle tissue of aqueous production. Aqueous is produced by a combination of active secretion, ultrafiltration, and diffusion; active secretion is the predominant mechanism. Many of the intraocular pressure–lowering agents used to treat glaucoma work by decreasing aqueous secretion in the ciliary body (Fig. 58-3). Aqueous then flows through the pupil and into the anterior chamber, nourishing the lens, cornea, and iris.

Aqueous drains through the anterior chamber angle, which contains the trabecular meshwork and ciliary body face. Between 80% and 90% of aqueous outflow is through the trabecular meshwork ("conventional pathway"), with the remaining 10% to 20% through the ciliary body face ("uveoscleral" or "alternative pathway"). The trabecular meshwork is thought to be the region where regulation of aqueous humor outflow takes place.

The Eye as a Separate Bioavailable Site

Physiologically and immunologically, the eye is a relatively isolated structure. There are several "barriers." The blood-aqueous barrier[1] is created by tight junctions between the cells of ciliary epithelium. The blood-retina barrier[2] is maintained by tight junctions between cells of retinal capillary endothelium of the retina and iris. These barriers may allow some molecules smaller than 500 Da to pass.

Basic Ocular Pharmacokinetics

Intraocular Penetration of Systemic Medications

Systemically delivered medications penetrate the intraocular cavities very poorly because of the blood-retina and blood-aqueous barriers.[1,2] Fluoroquinolone antibiotics[3] and oral carbonic anhydrase inhibitors[4] are notable exceptions.

Topical Administration

Absorption begins in the conjunctival cul-de-sac with mixing of the drug with the tears to give some unknown concentration.[1,5] The cul-de-sac has a volume of 7 μl, which can expand momentarily and variably up to 30 μl. The typical drop volume dispensed from a commercial drop bottle is 25 to 35 μl. (The practical lower limit of commercial drop bottles is 20 to 25 μl.) The relatively stagnant precorneal tear film layer has a thickness of about 7 to 9 μm. The basal rate of tear flow is approximately 1 μl/min, with a physiologic turnover rate of 10% to 15% per minute (in the nonirritated eye). If instillation causes irritation and stimulates lacrimation, the turnover rate increases to approximately 30%/min. The washout effect of spontaneous tear flow results in almost complete disappearance of the drug from the cul-de-sac within 5 minutes. At least 80% of the drop leaves via lacrimal drainage. Blinking of the eyelids forces part of the instilled volume out through the puncta into the nasolacrimal duct. Each blink eliminates about 2 µl of fluid from the cul-de-sac. Generally, a small fraction of the instilled dose (1% to 10%) reaches the internal structures of the eye. Absorption into the eye takes time (Box 58-1).

The cornea is the most significant barrier to topical drug absorption.[1,5] Making the molecule more lipophilic increases its permeability. Within the cornea, the epithelial cell layer poses the major barrier to absorption, more so for hydrophilic than for lipophilic compounds. The lipid content of the epithelium and endothelium is 100 times greater than the stroma. The stroma is more of a barrier to lipophilic than hydrophilic drugs; the epithelium is more tortuous but less porous than the stroma. Most drugs exhibit similar times to peak concentration in the aqueous humor as the material drains out of the cul-de-sac within the first 5 minutes. For this reason, the time it takes for most drugs to reach their peak concentration in the aqueous falls within 20 to 60 minutes. Normally the turnover of aqueous is rapid (half-life of 52 minutes). After topical administration, the highest concentrations of most drugs, in descending order, are found in the cornea, iris, ciliary body, aqueous humor, sclera, and conjunctiva (Box 58-2). Binding by melanin is also an important factor.

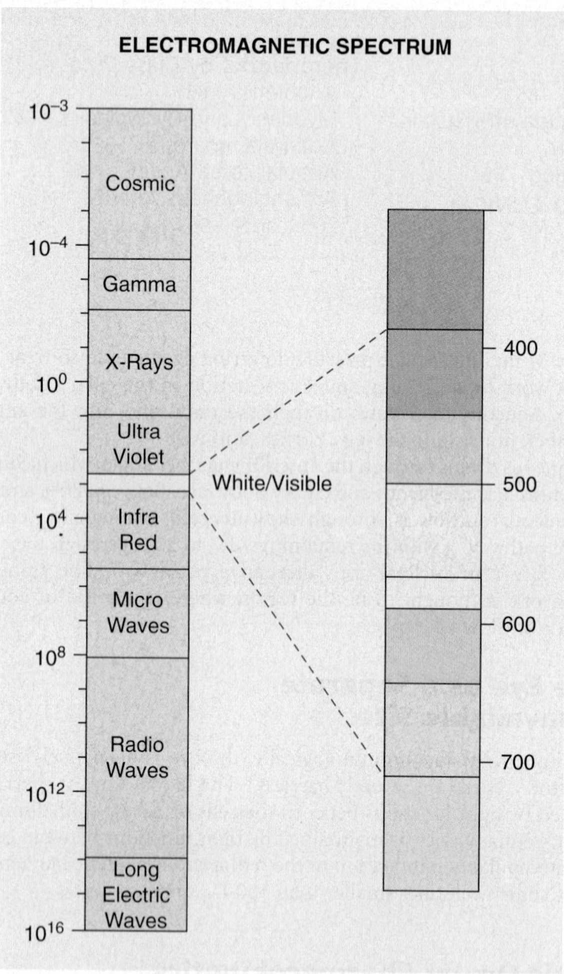

FIGURE 58-1 • Electromagnetic spectrum.

THERAPEUTICS AND CLINICAL PHARMACOLOGY

Therapeutics by Class

Antibiotics

The eye is susceptible to surface infection, abscess formation (e.g., endophthalmitis), and endogenous infections by bacteria, fungi, viruses, and parasites. The most commonly encountered infections in developed nations are bacterial.[6] In underdeveloped nations, parasites such as *Chlamydia trachomatis* (trachoma) and *Onchocera volvulus* (river blindness) are major public health issues as they both are blinding diseases. Exposure results from poor water and sewage handling, and blindness occurs often from delays in treatment or lack of access to health care.

BOX 58-1 SEPARATION OF DOSES TO AVOID WASHOUT

Clinical Pearl: If the patient is prescribed more than one topical medication, instruct him or her to separate the two doses by 5 to 6 minutes. Otherwise, the second drop will wash out the first medication. Specifically:

- 30-second interval: washout with 45% loss of drug effect
- 2-minute interval: 17% loss of effect
- 5-minute interval: no washout

Example: The corneal concentration of 1% prednisolone phosphate followed by a second drop of antibiotic in the rabbit is as follows:

Interval between 2 Drops	Corneal Concentration
Prednisolone alone	8.96 µg/g
30 seconds	3.98 µg/g
60 seconds	5.09 µg/g
120 seconds	6.85 µg/g

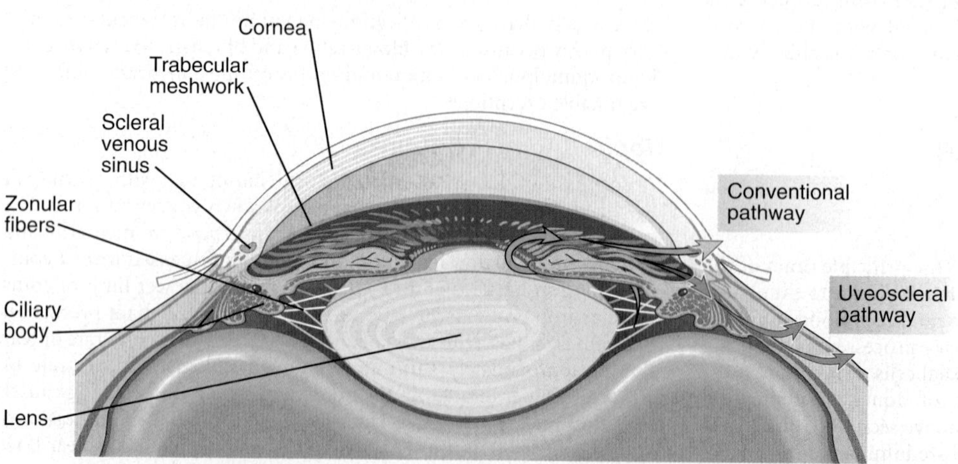

FIGURE 58-2 • Normal anatomy and physiology of aqueous humor flow. Aqueous is produced within the epithelium of the ciliary body processes, and flows from behind the iris, through the pupil, and into the anterior chamber.

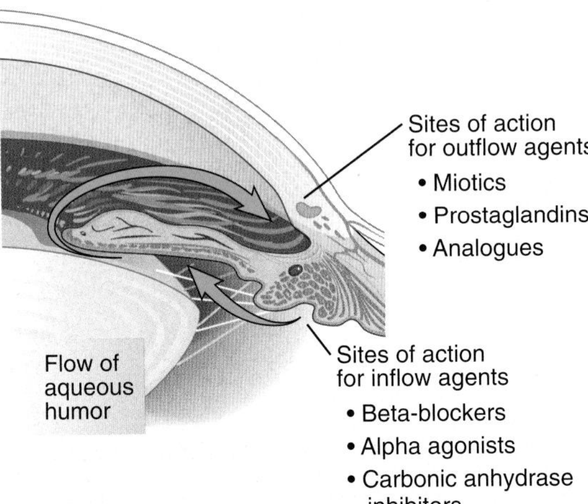

FIGURE 58-3 • Medication sites of action.

BOX 58-2 CLINICAL PEARLS

- Systemic absorption of locally administered medications: some amount certainly gets absorbed primarily through the mucosa of the nasolacrimal system.
- Advantage of local delivery: allows you to achieve higher local concentrations with relatively lower systemic side effects.

With surface infections of the conjunctiva and cornea, topical administration of antibiotics coupled with low systemic absorption allow much higher concentrations to be achieved than with systemically administered medications.[7] The practical implication is that some organisms that might be "resistant" to certain medications delivered within the body are susceptible to those medications when applied topically.

Topically administered medications can be given as liquid drops (solution or suspension) or as an ointment; ointments allow the medication to stay at the ocular surface a little longer than liquid drops, but there is significant blurring of vision with the ointments.

The most commonly utilized topical antibacterials are the fluoroquinolones[8] (Table 58-1). Except for the third- and fourth-generation fluoroquinolones, systemically administered antibiotics achieve poor intraocular penetration. However, certain antibiotics can be directly injected into the vitreous chamber. Some antibiotics are also administered subconjunctivally to provide a depot reservoir of medication allowing slow release over a greater time period than ointments.

For fungal infections, amphotericin B, flucytosine, miconazole, and natamycin can be administered topically. Intravitreal injections of amphotericin B are sometimes used for serious fungal endophthalmitis.

For viral infections of the cornea, a combination of topical antivirals and oral antivirals are typically used. In the case of herpetic keratitis, systemic prophylaxis with oral antiviral medications is maintained indefinitely.[9] Rarely, a viral infection of the retina can occur, which is generally treated with systemic antivirals. Topical antivirals include acyclovir, idoxuridine, trifluridine, and vidarabine.

In the United States, one of the most common parasitic infections encountered in the eye is *Acanthamoeba* infection of the cornea related to contact lens use with poor hygiene; typically a combination of topical and oral medications are used.[10] *Toxoplasma gondii* and *Pneumocystis jiroveci* retinochoroidal infections are also encountered and generally treated with systemic medications.

Mydriatics and Cycloplegics

The iris contains the dilator and constrictor muscles (Fig. 58-4). The sphincter muscle and circular muscle in the ciliary body, controlling accommodation, are innervated by the parasympathetic system. The iris dilator muscle is innervated by the sympathetic system.

TABLE 58-1 TOPICAL ANTIBACTERIALS

Drug	Preparation
Bacitracin	Soln; 10,000 units/ml Oint; 500 units/g
Cefazolin	Soln; 5% Oint; 1%
Ciprofloxacin	Soln; 0.3% Oint; 0.3%
Erythromycin	Oint; 0.5%
Gatifloxacin	Soln; 0.3%
Gentamicin	Soln; 0.3% Oint; 0.3% Soln; 1.5%
Levofloxacin	Soln; 0.5%
Moxifloxacin	Soln; 0.5%
Norfloxacin	Soln; 0.3%
Ofloxacin	Soln; 0.3%
Oxytetracycline/polymyxin B	Oint; 0.5%/10,000 units per ml
Polymyxin B/bacitracin	Oint; 10,000 units per ml/500 units per ml
Polymyxin B/neomycin	Soln; 16,250 units per ml/0.35% Oint; 10,000 units per ml/0.35%
Polymyxin B/neomycin/bacitracin	Oint; 5000 units per ml/0.5%/400 units per ml Oint; 10,000 units per ml/0.35%/400 units per ml
Polymyxin B/neomycin/gramicidin	Soln; 10,000 units per ml/0.35%/0.025%
Polymyxin B/trimethoprim	Soln; 10,000 units per ml/0.1%
Sulfacetamide	Soln; 10% Oint; 10%
Sulfacetamide/phenylephrine	Soln; 15%/0.125%
Sulfisoxazole	Soln; 4% Oint; 4%
Tetracycline	Soln; 1%
Tobramycin	Soln; 0.3% Oint; 0.3% Soln; 1.5%
Vancomycin	Soln; 5%

Oint, ointment; soln, solution.

Anticholinergic agents act by blocking the parasympathetic innervation to the iris sphincter muscle, allowing unopposed action by the dilator muscle. Sympathomimetic agents act by stimulating the sympathetic fibers, activating the dilator muscle.

These agents are used to dilate the pupil for three primary purposes: (i) to allow diagnostic examination of the retina or measurement of refractive error, (ii) for splinting of the iris (i.e., to prevent pupillary movement) during intraocular inflammation, and (iii) for monocular blurring of vision to treat amblyopia. All have the potential for systemic side effects. Additionally, these agents have the potential to incite acute angle-closure glaucoma in susceptible individuals who have narrow anterior chamber angles.

Some commonly used parasympathetic agents include tropicamide, scopolamine, homatropine, cyclopentolate, and atropine. Phenylephrine is the most commonly used sympathomimetic agent for dilation.

Anti-inflammatories

Topical corticosteroids of varying potency and nonsteroidal anti-inflammatory drugs (NSAIDs) are frequently used in ophthalmology. The intraocular potency of the corticosteroids depends not only on

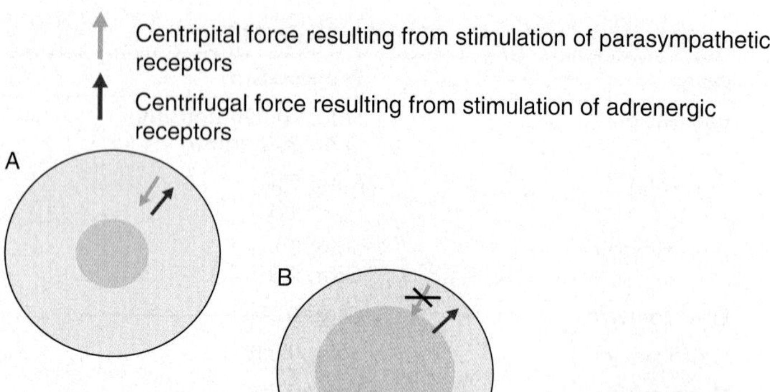

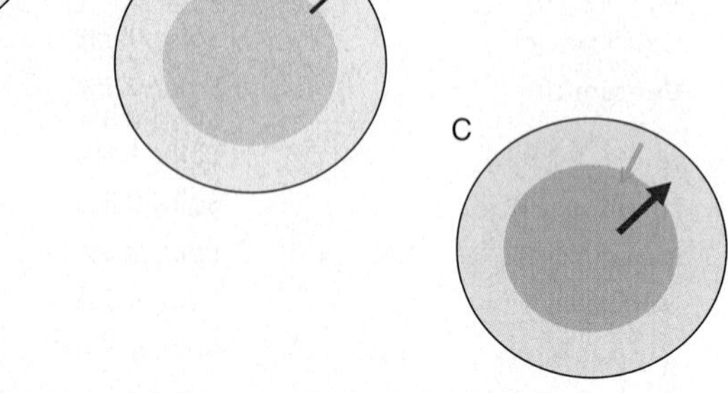

C

FIGURE 58-4 • Schematic of the mechanisms of mydriatic and cycloplegic agents. Frontal view of iris; *black circle* represents pupil size. **A,** Normal tone of the iris, and hence degree of pupil dilation, is a balance of the opposing forces of the iris sphincter (constricts the pupil) and the iris dilator (opens the pupil). **B,** Anticholinergics block the parasympathetic tone, leaving an unopposed dilator muscle. **C,** Adrenergic agents increase the tone of the dilator muscle.

receptor binding, but also on their ability to traverse the cornea to enter the anterior chamber. Acetates are more lipophilic and will penetrate the intact cornea (Table 58-2). Phosphate formulations will not achieve good intraocular concentrations, but will be very potent on the surface. Corticosteroids can also be delivered as depot subtenons and intraocular injections.

Systemic complications are rarely seen with topically administered corticosteroids. However, local complications such as elevated intraocular pressure causing glaucomatous optic nerve damage and cataract formation are common with chronic use.

The topical NSAIDs are primarily used for postoperative pain management for minor procedures, prevention and treatment of macular edema following cataract surgery, mild intraocular inflammation, and ocular involvement of seasonal allergies.[11] Commonly used topical NSAIDs include diclofenac, ketorolac, bromfenac, and flurbiprofen.

TABLE 58-2 TOPICAL CORTICOSTEROIDS

Potency	Drug
Low	Cortisone Hydrocortisone
Mild	Fluorometholone Medrysone
Moderate	Fluorometholone acetate Dexamethasone phosphate Rimexolone
High	Loteprednol etabonate
Highest	Prednisolone phosphate Dexamethasone acetate Prednisolone acetate

Antiglaucoma Agents

Glaucoma is a group of over 30 conditions (the glaucomas) that share a relatively elevated intraocular pressure as well as characteristic optic nerve and visual field (i.e., peripheral vision) changes. All antiglaucoma medications lower intraocular pressure.[12,13] Mechanistically, they work by either decreasing aqueous production or enhancing aqueous drainage (see Fig. 58-2). When systemically absorbed through the nasal mucosa, many of the glaucoma medications have the potential to cause significant generalized side effects.

There are six classes of antiglaucoma medications defined by their mechanism of action. α-Agonists, which include apraclonidine and brimonidine, activate α_2-adrenergic receptors in the ciliary body epithelium and inhibit aqueous secretion; there is weak evidence that brimonidine, a highly selective α_2-adrenergic agent, may also enhance uveoscleral drainage. Potential side effects include local irritation, allergy, mydriasis, dry mouth, dry eye, hypotension, and lethargy. Brimonidine should be avoided in children younger than 2 years of age because it has been associated with apnea in children.

β-Blockers, which include betaxolol, carteolol, levobetaxolol, levobunolol, metipranolol, timolol hemihydrate, and timolol maleate, are antagonists of the β-adrenergic receptors in the ciliary body epithelium and decrease aqueous humor production. Betaxolol is relatively "cardioselective," meaning that it has a greater specificity for β_2-adrenergic receptors. Carteolol has some intrinsic sympthomimetic activity that may decrease the rate of side effects compared with other agents. The other agents are nonselective for the various β-adrenergic receptors. Potential side effects include blurred vision, corneal anesthesia, bradycardia/heart block, bronchospasm, fatigue, mood change, impotence, decreased sensitivity to hypoglycemic symptoms in insulin-dependent diabetics, and worsening of myasthenia gravis. Topical β-blockers should be avoided in patients with asthma, severe chronic obstructive pulmonary disease, bradycardia, heart block, congestive heart failure, and myasthenia gravis.

Carbonic anhydrase inhibitors (CAIs) include acetazolamide, brinzolamide, dorzolamide, and methazolamide. CAIs are kinetic inhibitors of the enzyme carbonic anhydrase and decrease aqueous production by the ciliary body (Fig. 58-5). Potential side effects of topical therapy include bitter taste, diuresis, fatigue, gastrointestinal upset, Stevens-Johnson syndrome, and a theoretical risk of aplastic anemia. Systemic therapy has been associated with hypokalemia/acidosis, renal stones, paresthesias, nausea, cramps, diarrhea, malaise, lethargy, depression, impotence, unpleasant taste, aplastic anemia, and Stevens-Johnson syndrome. CAIs should be avoided in patients with a history of a sulfonamide allergy and used with great caution in patients with hyponatremia/hypokalemia, recent renal stones, and thiazide diuretic and digitalis use.

Hyperosmolar agents, which include isosorbide and mannitol, dehydrate the vitreous and decrease intraocular fluid volume by osmotically drawing fluid into the intravascular space. The agents are given orally or intravenously. Potential side effects include congestive heart failure, urinary retention in men, backache, myocardial infarction, headache, and mental confusion. Hyperosmolar agents should be used with caution in patients with congestive heart failure, diabetic ketoacidosis, subdural or subarachnoid hemorrhage, or preexisting severe dehydration.

Miotic agents include echothiophate iodide, physostigmine, demecarium bromide, acetylcholine, carbachol, and pilocarpine. Pilocarpine and acetylcholine are direct acting agonists of muscarinic

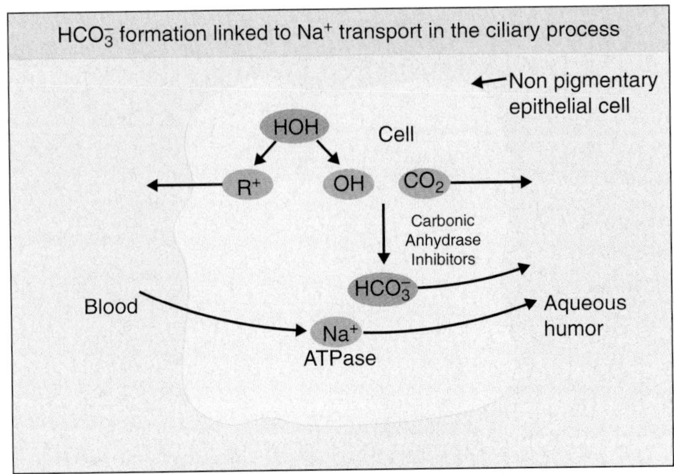

FIGURE 58-5 • Mechanism of carbonic anhydrase inhibitors in the eye to reduce production of aqueous. Aqueous humor is secreted into the posterior chamber by the nonpigmented epithelium of the ciliary process, which is dependent upon the active transport of sodium by the Na^+,K^+-ATPase pump. Aqueous secretion can be decreased by inhibiting the formation of the counter-ion, bicarbonate, by carbonic anhydrase, which catalyzes the hydration of carbon dioxide to bicarbonate.

receptors, while the other agents are indirect cholinergics that inhibit the enzyme acetylcholinesterase. Carbachol may have both direct and indirect activity. Miotics cause pupillary muscle constriction, which is believed to pull open the trabecular meshwork to increase trabecular outflow. Potential side effects of direct cholinergic agents include brow ache, breakdown of the blood-aqueous barrier, angle closure (increases pupillary block and causes the lens/iris diaphragm to move anteriorly), decreased night vision, variable myopia, retinal tear/detachment, and possibly anterior subcapsular cataracts; systemic side effects with topically administered direct-acting agents are rare. Topically applied indirect-acting mitotics can be associated with retinal detachment, cataract, myopia, intense miosis, angle closure, increased postsurgery bleeding, punctal stenosis, and increased formation of posterior synechiae in chronic uveitis. Systemic side effects such as diarrhea, abdominal cramps, enuresis, and increased effects of succinylcholine may also be seen. Direct-acting cholinergic agents should be used with caution in patients with peripheral retinal pathology, central media opacity, and uveitis. Indirect-acting mitotics should be avoided in patients undergoing concurrent succinylcholine administration, who have a predisposition to retinal tear, or with anterior subcapsular cataract, ocular surgery, or uveitis.

Prostaglandin analogues, which include bimatoprost, latanoprost, and travoprost, are analogues of prostaglandin $F_{2\alpha}$ and are agonists of the FP prostamide receptors. They increase uveoscleral outflow by increasing extracellular matrix turnover in the ciliary body face. Potential side effects include an increase in melanin pigmentation in the iris, blurred vision, and eyelid redness; cystoid macular edema and anterior uveitis have also been reported. Systemic side effects are rare and include upper respiratory infection–like symptoms, backache, and myalgia. Prostaglandin analogues should be used with caution during pregnancy or active uveitis.

Antiangiogenesis Agents

Age-related macular degeneration is the leading cause of blindness in the United States.[14] Macular degeneration is a dysfunction of the

TABLE 58-3 ANTIANGIOGENESIS AGENTS

Drug	Preparation
Verteporfin	Solution, 2 mg/ml (supplied as 15 mg of lyophilized powder to be diluted in 7.5 ml of sterile water)
Pegaptanib sodium	0.3 mg intravitreal q 6 wk
Ranibizumab	0.3 mg or 0.5 mg intravitreal q mo
Bevacizumab	1.25 mg intravitreal
Triamcinolone acetate	4.0 mg intravitreal 20 mg intravitreal

retinal pigment epithelial cells causing death of the overlying photoreceptors of the retina. There are two subclassifications: "dry" and "wet." The wet form refers to the development of choroidal neovascularization. Studies are ongoing with anti-inflammatory agents (e.g., triamcinolone) for clinically significant diabetic maculopathy, as are studies of branch retinal vein occlusion with ranbizumab[15] (Table 58-3).

Lubricants

Tear film dysfunction is a common cause of symptomatic discomfort.[16] It is treated by over-the-counter lubricants known as artificial tears; most are varying concentrations of polyvinyl alcohol.[17] One prescription formulation exists (cyclosporine 0.05%) to address the inflammatory aspect of the pathophysiology.

REFERENCES

1. Urtti A. Challenges and obstacles of ocular pharmacokinetics and drug delivery. Adv Drug Deliv Rev 2006;58:1131-1135.
2. Cunha-Vaz JG. The blood-retinal barriers system: basic concepts and clinical evaluation. Exp Eye Res 2004;78:715-721.
3. Thompson AM. Ocular toxicity of fluoroquinolones. Clin Exp Ophthalmol 2007;35:566-577.
4. Costa VP, Harris A, Stefánsson E, et al. The effects of antiglaucoma and systemic medications on ocular blood flow. Prog Retin Eye Res 2003;22:769-805.
5. Ghate D, Edelhauser HF. Ocular drug delivery. Expert Opin Drug Deliv 2006;3:275-287.
6. Donahue SP, Khoury JM, Kowalski RP. Common ocular infections: a prescriber's guide. Drugs 1996;52:526-540.
7. Sheikh A, Hurwitz B. Topical antibiotics for acute bacterial conjunctivitis: Cochrane systematic review and meta-analysis update. Br J Gen Pract 2005;55:962-964.
8. Mah FS. Fourth-generation fluoroquinolones: new topical agents in the war on ocular bacterial infections. Curr Opin Ophthalmol 2004;15:316-320.
9. Guess S, Stone DU, Chodosh J. Evidence-based treatment of herpes simplex virus keratitis: a systematic review. Ocul Surf 2007;5:240-250.
10. Awwad ST, Petroll WM, McCulley JP, Cavanagh HD. Updates in *Acanthamoeba* keratitis. Eye Contact Lens 2007;33:1-8.
11. Schalnus R. Topical nonsteroidal anti-inflammatory therapy in ophthalmology. Ophthalmologica 2003;217:89-98.
12. Alward WL. Medical management of glaucoma. N Engl J Med 1998;339:1298-1307.
13. Whitson JT. Glaucoma: a review of adjunctive therapy and new management strategies. Expert Opin Pharmacother 2007;8:3237-3249.
14. de Jong PT. Age-related macular degeneration. N Engl J Med 2006;355:1474-1485.
15. Brown DM, Regillo CD. Anti-VEGF agents in the treatment of neovascular age-related macular degeneration: applying clinical trial results to the treatment of everyday patients. Am J Ophthalmol 2007;144:627-637.
16. Montes-Mico R. Role of the tear film in the optical quality of the human eye. J Cataract Refract Surg 2007;33:1631-1635.
17. Perry HD, Donnenfeld ED. Dry eye diagnosis and management in 2004. Curr Opin Ophthalmol 2004;15:299-304.

SECTION 13 Anesthesia

59

LOCAL ANESTHESIA

John E. Tetzlaff

INTRODUCTION 863
PHYSIOLOGY 863
Physiologic Basis of Conduction Block 863
Organic Chemistry of Local Anesthetic Molecules 863
Structure 863
Acid-Base Behavior 864
Pharmacokinetics of Conduction Blockade 864
Speed of Onset 864
Potency 864
Duration of Action 864
Toxicity of Local Anesthetics 864
CNS Toxicity 864
Cardiac Toxicity 864
Methemoglobinemia 865
Tissue Toxicity 865
Allergy to Local Anesthetics 865
THERAPEUTICS AND CLINICAL PHARMACOLOGY 865
Goals of Therapeutic Application of Local Anesthetics 865
Therapeutic Actions of Local Anesthetics by Class 865
Esters 866
Amides 867
Emerging Targets 870

INTRODUCTION

The goal of anesthesia is to create an interruption of neural activity in a reversible manner to allow a painful procedure (surgery, fracture reduction, and so forth) to be performed. Local anesthetics (LAs) are the oldest class of drugs known to provide anesthesia. Native tribes in South America have known for centuries of the properties of the coca leaf to create numbness and euphoria.[1] While it was the mood-altering properties that caused cocaine to be brought to Europe, it was the almost coincidental discovery of dense topical anesthesia of the cornea by Koller in 1884 that created regional anesthesia. Within 2 years, topical anesthesia of the eye with cocaine solution had revolutionized ophthalmologic surgery.[2] Topical anesthesia of mucous membranes advanced other surgery as well as the infant science of endoscopy. With the invention of the hypodermic needle, infiltration, plexus block, and even subarachnoid block were possible, although tissue irritation from cocaine was greater than ideal. This led to the creation of procaine and the advent of modern regional anesthesia.

As neuroscience advanced, it became possible to explain the mechanism of the actions of LAs. When the physiology of neural transmission and excitable membranes became clear, it was possible to understand reversible interruption of neural transmission (conduction block) and the organic chemistry of molecules capable of local anesthesia. It was then also possible to define those chemical properties that determine the speed of onset of conduction block, the duration of action, and the density of the block as well as the serious side effects, including tissue injury, seizure activity, and cardiac events.

In the present, mature phase of regional anesthesia, it is possible to select the correct LA to achieve a desired clinical end point among a wide range of options, from topical anesthesia to complete motor/sensory block to analgesia with motor function preserved for labor or postoperative acute pain control. With alteration of existing molecules, it is possible to reduce serious toxic properties (selective cardiac toxicity) while preserving optimum clinical properties (e.g., creation of ropivacaine from bupivacaine).

PHYSIOLOGY

Physiologic Basis of Conduction Block

The role of the nervous system is the rapid conduction of signals from one location to another, sometimes at a considerable distance. The basis of this unique property of the nervous system is the excitable cell (neuron). The excitability property originates from a specialized cell membrane (axon) embedded with ion-specific channels[3] for sodium and potassium. The potassium channels allow free movement of potassium, which creates the electronegativity (about −90 mV) of the intracellular side of the axon. The sodium channel is gated, with sodium movement only allowed when the channel is open (activated). The result is sodium becoming the predominant extracellular cation, balancing potassium dominance on the intracellular side. The origin of a signal is a spontaneous depolarization at one site, triggered by a mechanical distortion or a chemical neurotransmitter; thus depolarization causes adjacent sodium channels at specialized gaps (nodes of Ranvier) of the surface insulation of the axon (myelin) to open and sodium to rush in, creating local depolarization.[4] This in turn causes the sodium channels at the next adjacent node to open. This sequential process results in propagation of the impulse, which is the physiologic basis for neural conduction. After the signal passes, the original electronegativity is restored, initially by passive efflux of potassium and subsequently by active ion transport via sodium-potassium ATPase, rapidly restoring the axon to a state in which impulse conduction could occur again.

The common characteristic of molecules capable of LA action is the ability to reversibly block activation of sodium channels. This is theoretically possible on the intracellular or the extracellular side of the channels. The only known molecules that block the extracellular side do so in a covalent manner, eliminating the reversibility requirement (organophosphates, various snake venoms) for clinical conduction block.[5] Interruption of sodium channel activation is possible by ionic (reversible) bonding at the cytoplasmic opening. Organic chemicals that can be deposited close to a neural structure, cross the axon membrane, and occupy (inactivate) a sodium channel have LA activity.

Although there is considerable diversity among the chemicals with LA action, there are a number of common denominators: structure, acid-base behavior, and properties that determine clinical action.

Organic Chemistry of Local Anesthetic Molecules

Structure (Fig. 59-1)

Clinically useful LAs are all amphipathic molecules, meaning that they contain two chemically different elements. The LA molecule contains

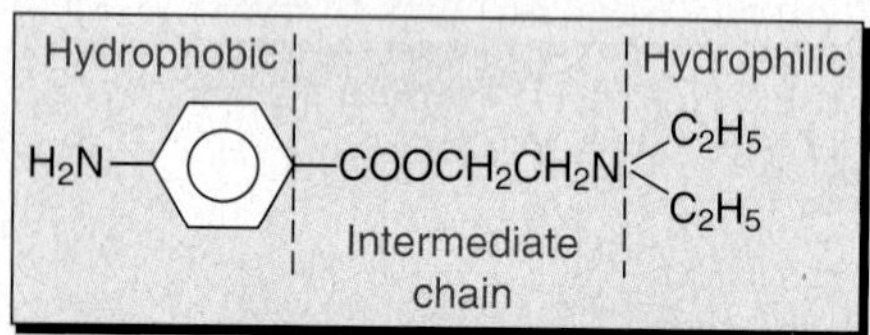

FIGURE 59-1 • Genetic structure of a local anesthetic molecule. (Adapted from Tetzlaff JE: Clinical Pharmacology of Local Anesthetics. Philadelphia: Butterworth-Heinemann, 2000.)

a hydrophilic element and a hydrophobic element separated by a critical interval. The hydrophilic element is a tertiary amine for all the LAs except benzocaine (secondary amine). The tertiary amine is the element of the LA that interacts with the hydrophilic elements of the open sodium channel, preventing sodium ion movement (inactivation). The hydrophobic elements are ringed structures that derive from aniline for the amide LA class or *para*-aminobenzoic acid (PABA) for the ester LA class. The hydrophobic group is the primary determinant of lipid solubility for the molecule and, therefore, the potential to cross the lipoprotein axon membrane. Although both of these key elements must be present, they also must be separated by a critical distance of between 3 and 7 carbon equivalents. When this intermediate chain is either less or more, the LA activity virtually disappears. This critical separation may be related to the opposing chemical properties of the two poles of the molecule causing the alignment of the tertiary amine toward the sodium channel, perhaps while the hydrophobic group is still embedded within the lipoprotein membrane. The final common structural element is the covalent bond within the intermediate chain that separates the amphipathic sides of the molecule. The molecule would have LA action without the bond, but could be difficult to manufacture, and the metabolic half-life would be long enough that the toxicity profile could be problematic. The bonds define the two major chemical classes and evolve from precursor molecules (aniline for amides and PABA for esters).

Acid-Base Behavior

All of the clinically useful LAs are weak bases with a PK_a (pH at which base/cation ratio = 50/50) from 7.6 to 9.3. Because of poor solubility in water of the base form of the tertiary amines, they are prepared commercially as hydrochloride salts (at the tertiary amine) or hydrocarbonate salt (outside the United States) to facilitate maintaining the molecule in solution.[6] The molecules are much more soluble in the cationic form, and as a result the pH of the solution is adjusted to 5.0 to 5.5. One exception is a commercial solution prepared with epinephrine, which is pH adjusted to 2.0 to 2.5 to decrease spontaneous hydrolysis of epinephrine. Another exception is the eutectic mixture of local anesthetics (EMLA). At neutral or higher pH, the base form at high concentrations moves into an emulsion state and an equal mixture of 5% lidocaine and 5% prilocaine base becomes a suspension of 2.5% of both that is suited to topical application.[7]

Pharmacokinetics of Conduction Blockade

The characteristics of conduction blockade that characterize individual LAs are speed of onset, potency, and duration of action.

Speed of Onset

If LAs could be delivered intracellularly without irreversible damage to the axon, the speed of onset would be very rapid. However, intraneural injection is a morbid event, and the clinical practice of regional anesthesia requires delivery close to the neural structure. The latency to onset is from the moment of injection until impulse extinction occurs when a critical mass of sodium channels are inactivated.[8] This requires the LA molecules to cross the neural membrane and the tertiary amine to occupy the cytoplasmic opening of the sodium channel.[9] The LA injected is pH 5.0 to 5.5 with a pK_a greater than 7.6. This means that there is a large majority (100/1 to 1000/1) in the ionic (cation) form. However, the ability to cross the axonal membrane is more than 1000 times greater in the neutral (base) form.[10] An element of latency is the time for the extracellular buffering (predominately the bicarbonate system) of the agent to reach the physiologic range where the concentration of the base becomes significant. Because of the rapid equilibrium, as one base LA crosses the axon membrane, another is instantly created from a cation. This establishes a concentration gradient into the axoplasm. The rate-limiting step is the buffering, which occurs at a rate proportional to the pH. As the pK_a of the LAs increases, the proportion of base to cation is lower and the speed of onset slower. In simple terms, speed of onset is inversely proportional to pK_a.

Potency

Potency is that characteristic of LA molecules that determines how much of the agent gets to the target. The principle barrier is the neural membrane and the property that determines crossing is lipid solubility.[9] The greater the lipid solubility, the greater the potency.[11] Anything that increases the lipid solubility of a given LA will increase the potency.[12] There are several examples among existing agents. For one of the oldest LAs, procaine, adding a four-carbon aliphatic chain to the hydrophobic region of the molecule creates tetracaine, which increases lipid solubility of the molecule and potency of LA action in direct proportion to the lipid solubility. When a two-carbon aliphatic group is added to the intermediate chain of lidocaine, the result is the more potent LA etidocaine. When a four-carbon (butyl) aliphatic group is substituted for the one-carbon (methyl) on the tertiary amine aliphatic group of mepivacaine, the result is the most potent LA, bupivacaine.

Duration of Action

The duration of LA activity is determined by the time that the tertiary amine group remains in contact with the sodium channel. This is related to how long the other element of the molecule remains embedded in the neural membrane. Since this is a lipoprotein membrane and hydrophobic area, the LA characteristics that predict duration of action are lipid solubility and protein binding. As both increase, so does duration of LA action. Clinical examples support this hypothesis. The commercially available LA with the lowest lipid solubility and least capacity for protein binding is chloroprocaine, which has the shortest duration of action. Conversely, bupivacaine has the highest lipid solubility and protein binding and, following the rule, the longest duration of action.

Toxicity of Local Anesthetics

LA use is associated with potential adverse actions, including central nervous system (CNS) toxicity, selective cardiac toxicity, methemoglobinemia, tissue toxicity, and allergy. The mechanisms are different, and are presented separately.

CNS Toxicity

CNS toxicity from LAs is related to the action of the unbound fraction of the agent within the limbic brain.[13] Because of differential sensitivity, inhibitory tracts are blocked prior to excitatory fibers, resulting in selective activity of excitatory tracts.[14,15] If the accumulation of free (unbound) LA is gradual, the initial effects are primitive emotions (fear, anxiety, and so forth) and cranial nerve paresthesia (facial numbness, metallic taste, strong odor, loud tinnitus, and so forth). As the level increases further, uncontrolled motor activity occurs, which evolves toward jacksonian seizure activity. If the rate of rise is rapid or a bolus (intra-arterial injection of the vertebral/carotid artery), the excitement phase is brief and seizure activity is the first manifestation. For the agents with low protein binding, the progression of the promontory signs is more apparent. With a highly protein-bound agent such as bupivacaine, there is very little evidence of CNS LA action until the protein-binding capacity is reached, and additional LA can have a bolus effect with little or no warning.[16]

Cardiac Toxicity

At very high concentrations, all LAs will cause cardiac standstill by massive sodium channel block of the cardiac conducting system.[17] At doses appropriate for clinical use, cardiac toxicity is rare with some notable exceptions. Cocaine is associated with cardiovascular consequences due to systemic action. Plasma levels of cocaine cause a dose-dependent block of the reuptake of catecholamines, which causes generalized vasoconstriction, hypertension, and direct adrenergic effects on the myocardium, including increased heart rate and contractility. This can induce myocardial ischemia based on oxygen supply-demand issues. In a subset of patients, exposure to cocaine can cause coronary artery vasospasm, even in apparently normal coronary arteries.[18] This has caused myocardial infarction in healthy, young adults involved in illicit use of cocaine[19,20] and has caused cardiac events during clinical use of cocaine.[21] With other LAs besides cocaine, an analogous event can occur with intravascular injection of a solution mixed with epinephrine based on the adrenergic bolus.

The highly lipid-soluble agents (bupivacaine, etidocaine) have been determined to have selective cardiac toxicity not found in their less lipid-soluble precursors (mepivacaine, lidocaine). The first reports in the 1970s involved attempted epidural anesthesia with boluses of concentrated bupivacaine (0.75%). These cases had in common cardiac arrest that responded very poorly to resuscitation, resulting in morbidity or mortality in a majority. In those monitored at the time of collapse, the precipitating event was a lethal ventricular arrhythmia (ventricular tachycardia, ventricular fibrillation) that was unresponsive to countershock and antiarrhythmics.[22] Investigation into the cause of these disasters identified a unique pharmacokinetic profile of sodium channel block on the cardiac conducting system with these large, highly lipid-soluble LAs. In contrast to lidocaine, which enters and exits sodium channels at the same rate, bupivacaine exits substantially slower, resulting in accumulation.[23] Since the affinity is much greater in the open position, and the time in the open position increases with heart rate, accumulation increases with tachycardia.[24] When the primary conducting system is fully blocked, reentrant pathways become active and predisposed toward lethal ventricular arrhythmia.[25] This also explains the ineffective response to antiarrhythmics and defibrillation due to the long-duration block of the cardiac conducting system. Further investigation implicated the butyl group as causative for this selective cardiac toxicity and led to the synthesis of ropivacaine (one carbon shorter) to preserve the unique clinical properties of bupivacaine with reduced cardiac toxicity. The manufacture of ropivacaine led to another discovery. The molecule was prepared as the levo-isomer, and the question was raised about whether the isomeric forms were different. With bupivacaine, it was determined that the dextro-isomer was significantly slower in exiting the sodium channels of the cardiac conducting system, and therefore much more cardiotoxic. This led to the creation of the levo-isomeric form of bupivacaine (levobupivacaine).

Methemoglobinemia

Metabolites of prilocaine and, to a lesser extent, benzocaine have a high affinity to oxidize the ferric iron of hemoglobin to the ferrous form, creating methemoglobin.[26] When the level exceeds 10%, cyanosis is evident. The oxygen-carrying capacity of methemoglobin is reduced. Overall oxygen delivery is not significantly reduced,[27] although the clinical appearance of the patient cannot be distinguished from that of desaturation and hypoxemia. Spontaneous reversal occurs with exposure to reductase enzyme activity in red cells, and treatment is rarely necessary.[26] In patients with diminished cardiopulmonary reserves who become symptomatic, treatment can be initiated with methylene blue (a reducing agent) 1 to 2 mg/kg intravenously, and may need to be repeated 12 hours later if continued absorption of the inciting LA occurs.[28]

Tissue Toxicity

At high concentrations, all LAs have a direct cytotoxic effect.[29] This property is proportional to the potency and unique to the tissue type. Axons and nerve cell bodies can demonstrate edema at histologic exam after LA exposure.[30] At supraclinical doses, conduction block is irreversible and related to membrane disruption. Lidocaine may produce some neurotoxicity at clinical doses, although the effect is usually transient. Injection into muscle can cause myonecrosis and/or rhabdomyolysis.[31] The tissue irritant properties of cocaine make injection excessively painful and limit the efficacy of cocaine to topical application. In vitro evidence implicates chloroprocaine in neurotoxic effects in cell culture of respiratory epithelium and fibroblasts.

Various LA additives also have the potential for tissue toxicity, including epinephrine (vasoconstriction), other vasoconstrictors, and the preservatives sodium bisulfite (direct neurotoxicity)[32] and ethylenediaminetetra-acetic acid (EDTA) (calcium derangement in skeletal muscle).[33] In the history of regional anesthesia, contaminants from detergents and bactericidal solutions used to sterilize glass ampules of LA and reusable needles have caused tissue injury.

Allergy to Local Anesthetics

The incidence of true allergy to LAs is fortunately very rare,[34] although the clinical experience with patients "allergic to LAs" is much more common. The LA molecule is too small to be an ideal allergen by itself, although these molecules bind to proteins and, as haptens, can become allergenic. The allergy profile of LAs is determined by the class, with ester agents having a much higher incidence. This is related to the precursor of the ester agents, PABA, having a significant presence in cosmetics and sunscreens.[35] The incidence of allergy to amides is exceedingly rare, with the exception of lidocaine multidose vials, in which the allergen historically was the added preservative methylparaben.[36] When there is true allergy, the cross-reactivity between amides and esters is very low.

The reason for the large difference between the true incidence of LA allergy and the number of patients labeled as such is related to clinical events that occur during LA use. When LA solutions with various additives achieve rapid, high plasma levels, the resulting symptoms can be attributed to allergy. The low protein-bound LAs procaine and chloroprocaine can create an intense prodrome from CNS actions. Rapid plasma levels of an LA with an opioid will create the euphoria/dysphoria related to the opioid. LA solutions with concentrated epinephrine are uniquely suited to the mistaken diagnosis of allergy. When a bolus of epinephrine becomes intravascular rapidly, the resulting adrenergic symptoms are easy to mistake as allergy in an unmonitored setting.[37] The classic example is the injection of an LA with concentrated epinephrine for maxillary dental procedures. Intraosseous injection is common,[38] and the sudden adrenergic response, with increase in heart rate, contractility, and blood pressure creates symptoms of palpitation and flushing that are easily attributable to allergy.[39] A further confusing variable historically was the use of latex barrier devices for dental procedures, since latex is significantly more allergenic than LAs.

The only way to confirm allergy to LAs is by intradermal skin testing. Unfortunately, the sensitivity and specificity of skin testing for LA allergy is low.[40,41] If allergy to an ester is reported, use of an amide agent is a reasonable clinical choice in a monitored setting.

THERAPEUTICS AND CLINICAL PHARMACOLOGY

Goals of Therapeutic Application of Local Anesthetics

The universal goal of LA use is reversible neural blockade. The most common indication is the need to perform painful procedures or to relieve pain caused by surgery or trauma. The versatility of LAs is related to the wide range of different ways they can be used, including topical application to skin and mucous membranes, superficial infiltration, field block, peripheral nerve block, plexus block, intra-articular injection, intracavitary (thorax, peritoneum, bladder) injection, and neuraxial (spinal, epidural, caudal) block. The choice of the agent depends on the target and the intended duration of the block.

Therapeutic Actions of Local Anesthetics by Class

The main classification of LAs with clinical relevance is ester and amide agents. This separation determines clinical activity as well as therapeu-

TABLE 59-1 ESTER LOCAL ANESTHETIC AGENTS

Agents	Trade Name	Molecular Weight	% Protein Binding	PK_a	Partition Coefficient (Lipid Solubility)	Maximum Dose
Procaine	Novocaine	236	6	9.0	1.7	>1000 mg
Chloroprocaine	Nessicaine	271	<1	9.0	9.0	800-1000 mg
Tetracaine	Pontocaine	264	75	8.5	221	120 mg
Benzocaine	None	165	<1	2.5	<1	200-300 mg

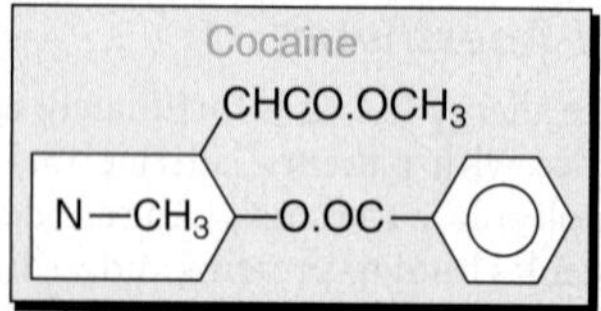

FIGURE 59-2 • **Structure of cocaine.** (Adapted from Tetzlaff JE: Clinical Pharmacology of Local Anesthetics. Philadelphia: Butterworth-Heinemann, 2000.)

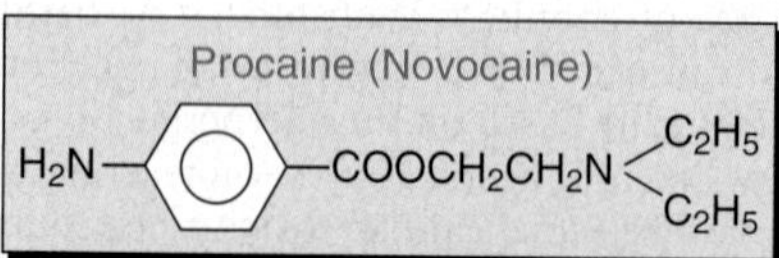

FIGURE 59-3 • **Structure of procaine.** (Adapted from Tetzlaff JE: Clinical Pharmacology of Local Anesthetics. Philadelphia: Butterworth-Heinemann, 2000.)

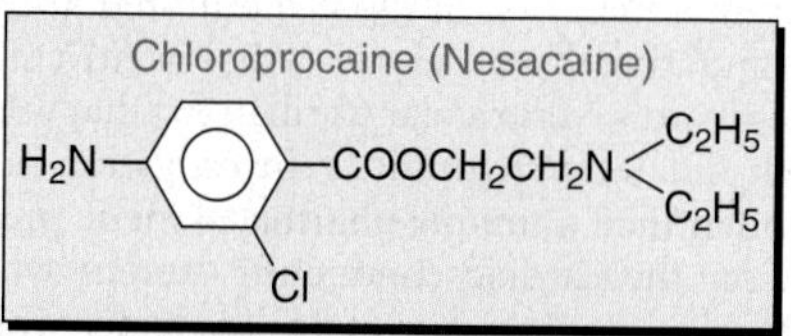

FIGURE 59-4 • **Structure of chloroprocaine.** (Adapted from Tetzlaff JE: Clinical Pharmacology of Local Anesthetics. Philadelphia: Butterworth-Heinemann, 2000.)

tic approach and metabolism. Within the ester class of LAs, the commercially available options are cocaine, procaine, chloroprocaine, tetracaine, and benzocaine. The clinical options within the amide class (not all available in the United States) include lidocaine, mepivacaine, prilocaine, dibucaine, etidocaine, bupivacaine, ropivacaine, and levobupivacaine.

Esters (Table 59-1)

Cocaine (Fig. 59-2). Cocaine is the oldest LA. Use of coca leaves for topical anesthesia and euphoric side effects has been reported in South America for centuries.[42] Experimentation in Peru in the 1860s demonstrated anesthesia after topical application of these leaves to mucous membranes and reactions that were undoubtedly seizures.[43] Confirmation of the therapeutic potential of cocaine was confirmed after export to Europe.[44] In Germany, Koller accidentally discovered that a few drops of a solution made from crystals of cocaine produced rapid, complete anesthesia of the cornea that was reversible and nontoxic to the eye. Lacking the train fare to go to Munich, he arranged for a more affluent colleague to present this finding to the German Society of Ophthalmologists in 1882. Although this denied Koller credit for the discovery, the technique achieved worldwide recognition very rapidly within the field of ophthalmology.[2]

Cocaine is prepared as an alkaloid solution in a 1% to 10% concentration for topical application. The previous crystal and ETOH solutions are no longer manufactured due to the propensity for diversion related to the ease of illicit use. Applied properly to skin and especially mucous membranes, cocaine produces dense anesthesia up to 1 cm in depth and intense vasoconstriction. The double-ring structure of the tertiary amine results in tissue irritation and slow metabolism. Up to 10% is excreted intact in the urine, with the balance eliminated by hydrolysis of one of the two ester bonds. The maximum dose for the average-size adult is 160 mg or about 3 mg/kg.[45] Euphoric effects are related to plasma levels in the CNS, and the hemodynamic effects are related to block of reuptake of catecholamines described previously. Plasma levels occur 30 to 60 minutes after application. Peak levels can be decreased by incremental application.

In addition to topical anesthesia of the cornea (currently uncommon), the combination of dense topical anesthesia and vasoconstriction is well suited to manipulation of mucous membranes. Cocaine was the first LA used for endoscopy, although toxicity has virtually eliminated this use. It remains ideal for intranasal procedures such as rhinoplasty or manipulation of nasal fracture. Historically, cocaine was the first LA used for peripheral nerve and plexus block by Halstead and Crile in the early 20th century. However, tissue irritation and subsequent neuritis made this less than ideal, and this role was rapidly and permanently replaced by procaine and other LAs that followed. Cocaine is used in concentrated solution mixed with tetracaine and epinephrine (adrenaline) as TAC. Although this mixture has some efficiency for topical anesthesia for lacerations, especially in children, there have also been numerous reports of disasters related to toxic uptake of cocaine, causing seizures and death, especially in children.[46,47] With the creation of EMLA, this role for cocaine has virtually disappeared.

Procaine (Fig. 59-3). The recognition that benzoic acid esters besides cocaine had LA properties led to the search for an agent with less tissue irritation than cocaine. This led to the discovery of procaine by Einhorn of Germany in 1904. Procaine rapidly displaced cocaine from every application except topical anesthesia and was the only LA for injection for the first half of the 20th century.

Like all other members of the ester class, procaine is a chemical derivative of PABA and has a pK_a of 8.9. The ester bond is unstable at alkaline pH, and procaine is prepared as a hydrochloride salt at pH less than 6.0. It has limited lipid solubility, low affinity for protein binding, and a relatively high pK_a, resulting in an agent profile of slow onset, low potency, and short duration of action. The toxicity potential is very low because of the rapid hydrolysis of the ester bond by plasma cholinesterase and the high potential for intact renal elimination.[48]

Historically, procaine has been used for every injection technique of regional anesthesia, including infiltration and peripheral nerve, plexus, and neuraxial blocks. Other agents have displaced procaine from most of these roles except for some infiltration techniques (scalp for awake craniotomy) in which high volumes are needed and compounded with other agents for obstetric spinal anesthesia. Although not commonly available, procaine is used as a 1% solution for subarachnoid block, and has been available in the past in a wide range of concentrations up to 4% for dental anesthesia. Although procaine ("novocaine") is virtually synonymous with dental anesthesia, the actual use of this agent for dental anesthesia has almost disappeared, mainly due to the slow onset and short duration.

Chloroprocaine (Fig. 59-4). In the second half of the 20th century, experiments in Sweden focused on chemical alteration of procaine to achieve specific clinical goals. A chloride substitution on the aromatic ring of procaine increases the susceptibility of the ester ring to hydrolysis and even more rapid metabolism in serum. Named 2-chloroprocaine (2-CP) in 1955, the low toxicity allowed use of high total doses to achieve rapid onset of conduction block. This substitution produced

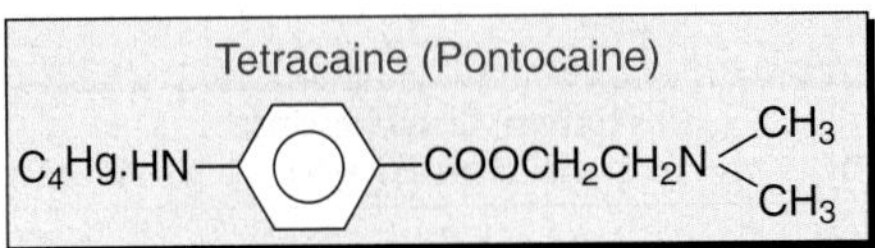

FIGURE 59-5 • Structure of tetracaine. (Adapted from Tetzlaff JE: Clinical Pharmacology of Local Anesthetics. Philadelphia: Butterworth-Heinemann, 2000.)

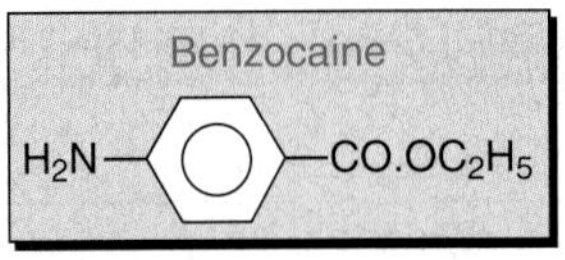

FIGURE 59-6 • Structure of benzocaine. (Adapted from Tetzlaff JE: Clinical Pharmacology of Local Anesthetics. Philadelphia: Butterworth-Heinemann, 2000.)

the most alkaline LA, with a pK_a of 9.0. Like procaine, the ester bond is subject to spontaneous hydrolysis and is manufactured as a hydrochloride salt at pH 2.5 to 4.0. It has very low lipid solubility and very low affinity for protein binding, and, with the high pK_a, the clinical profile for the agent is slow onset, short duration, and low potency. The ability to use a high total dose overcomes both the slow onset and low potency, presenting an agent that can be used for rapid onset of dense conduction block of a short duration. Because of high water solubility, a large fraction (up to 50%) can be excreted intact in the urine. The plasma half-life is 23 seconds, and the ester bond is rapidly cleaved by plasma cholinesterase.[49] Assuming normal plasma cholinesterase levels and activity, doses of 800 to 1000 mg can be used with very low risk of CNS toxicity and no concern for selective cardiotoxicity. In the historical evolution of 2-CP manufacture, two additives have been associated with toxicity. The first commercial preparation was stabilized with sodium metabisulfate, which was determined to be causative for several cases of severe transverse myelitis after accidental intrathecal infection during attempted epidural anesthesia.[50-52] The next formulation included EDTA, which deletes calcium and caused paravertebral muscle spasms after recovery from ambulatory epidural anesthesia.

2-CP can produce short-duration, dense neural block with infiltration and peripheral nerve, plexus, and neuraxial blocks. For peripheral injection, the 2% solution is chosen, producing dense anesthesia and motor block of brief duration (30 to 60 minutes). The single most common use is for epidural anesthesia for cesarean section in a patient with an existing epidural catheter. For analgesia with low motor block, the 2% solution can be diluted. Reinjection is required at 30- to 45-minute intervals. For dense sensory and motor block (e.g., cesarean section), the 3% solution is used. The onset is rapid and the duration brief, requiring redosing at 30 to 45 minutes. Low lipid solubility ensures very low agent transfer to the fetus.[53] Ironically, even though massive intrathecal injection causing transverse myelitis almost caused 2-CP to disappear from use, it is currently being used for outpatient spinal anesthesia in the preservative-free form with some success.[54-56]

Tetracaine (Fig. 59-5). Further experimental work in Sweden led to the association of potency of LAs with lipid solubility. Theoretically, increasing the lipid solubility of procaine would increase its potency and duration of action by increasing protein binding. When the two-carbon branches of the tertiary amine of procaine were reduced by one and a four-carbon group was added to the aromatic ring, the lipid solubility was increased and the resulting molecule was named tetracaine. Although the pK_a (8.6) is lower than procaine, the profile of the agent is slow onset, high potency, and long duration of action. Because of the high lipid solubility, the potential for CNS is also high. Early in the clinical experience with tetracaine, use of high volumes of tetracaine solution for endoscopy in unmonitored settings resulted in disasters related to CNS toxicity, and tetracaine acquired a reputation for being highly toxic.[57,58] However, with appropriate regional anesthesia techniques, tetracaine has had an excellent safety record. Although the increased lipid solubility decreases the susceptibility of the ester bond to hydrolysis, the plasma half-life is still short (120 to 150 seconds), and the potential for toxicity is much lower than its reputation.[59]

With good lipid solubility, tetracaine has an excellent profile for topical anesthesia. It remains the agent of choice for ophthalmic topical anesthesia in a 1% solution. Although it has been used for topical anesthesia of mucous membranes, the enthusiasm for tetracaine to facilitate endoscopy has been tempered by the very long duration and concern about toxicity.[60] The high lipid solubility limits the diffusion through tissues and, combined with slow onset, makes tetracaine an uncommon choice for tissue infiltration or peripheral blocks unless as part of a compounded solution with another LA. In that setting, the tetracaine is used for long duration of action mixed with a short-onset agent. Compounding 0.1% to 0.2% tetracaine with 0.5% to 1.0% lidocaine or mepivacaine is a common choice for peripheral or epidural block involving tetracaine. It can be used in the same compounded solutions for caudal or epidural action with the same rationale. Tetracaine (1.0% solution) is the most common choice for subarachnoid block in the United States, producing a dense block of long duration (120 to 180 minutes or longer with epinephrine added), with a dose range of 5 to 20 mg. It can be used plain in this role or mixed with glucose to produce a hyperbaric solution for gravity distribution.

Benzocaine (Fig. 59-6). Benzocaine is a benzoic acid derivative that as a secondary amine, is the only commercially available LA that is not a tertiary amine. Because of poor solubility in water, it is prepared in a concentrated solution (20%) designed for topical anesthesia by inhalation or metered spray, or in a suspension for direct application to mucous membranes. For any benzocaine that reaches plasma, the ester bond is hydrolyzed at about the same rate as procaine. Because of limited aqueous solubility, very little is excreted intact in the urine. If a significant plasma level occurs, benzocaine has the propensity to oxidize the ferric iron of hemoglobin to ferrous, creating methemoglobin.[61] This would only occur with application to disrupted (trauma, burn) surfaces or application of large amounts to children or infants.[62-64] Even methemoglobin at 30% should not be symptomatic unless cardiopulmonary reserves are reduced, in which case the treatment is methylene blue. The principle clinical role for benzocaine is topical nebulized or aerosol application to the oropharynx for endoscopy. The concentrated (10% to 20%) gel suspensions have been used for analgesia of the external ear canal during painful otitis media. Benzocaine has also been used to decrease the pain and discomfort experienced after episiotomy for childbirth[65] and for topical analgesia for rectal pain.[66]

Amides (Table 59-2)

Lidocaine (Fig. 59-7). The first half-century of regional anesthesia was dominated by ester agents—cocaine and procaine. The search for a more versatile agent led to the discovery of tertiary amine derivatives of aniline that had the chemical properties necessary to act as clinically useful LAs. The discovery in 1948 of lidocaine by Lofgren of Sweden initiated the amino amide era of regional anesthesia, which has been dominant ever since. Although many other amides have been introduced, none is as versatile as lidocaine, the original member of the class.

Lidocaine has a pK_a of 7.8 and is prepared as hydrochloride salt in the United States, with pH adjusted to 5.0 to 5.5 for stability and antimicrobial effect. Lidocaine is also prepared as a hydrocarbonate salt solution in Canada and the United Kingdom, with a lower pH and high level of dissolved carbon dioxide ("carbonation"). The low pK_a, intermediate lipid solubility, and intermediate protein-binding potential of lidocaine presents an agent with rapid onset, dense anesthesia at higher concentrations, and an intermediate duration of action. The amide bond is very resistant to hydrolysis, and very little is excreted intact in the urine. Redistribution is the primary means of termination of LA action. Metabolism is slow in the amide class and starts with biotransformation in the liver followed by hydrolysis of the amide bond and elimination of metabolites in the urine. Maximum doses of 500 to 600 mg (7 to 8 mg/kg) are generally considered safe. Because of the use of lidocaine as a parenteral antiarrhythmic, more is known about the

TABLE 59-2 AMIDE LOCAL ANESTHETIC AGENTS

Agents	Trade Name	Molecular Weight	% Protein Binding	PK_a	Partition Coefficient (Lipid Solubility)	Maximum Dose
Lidocaine	Xylocaine	234	64	7.9	2.4	500 mg
Prilocaine	Citanest	220	55	7.9	25	600 mg
Etidocaine	Duranest	276	94	7.7	800	300 mg
Mepivacaine	Polocaine, Carbocaine	246	77	7.8	21	400-500 mg
Bupivacaine	Sensorcaine, Marcaine	288	96	8.2	346	200-300 mg
Ropivacaine	Intropin	262	95	8.2	115	300 mg
Levobupivacaine	Chirocaine	288	96	8.2	346	300 mg

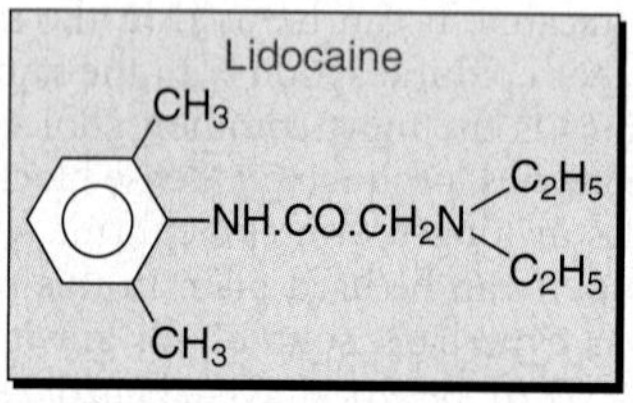

FIGURE 59-7 • Structure of lidocaine. (Adapted from Tetzlaff JE: Clinical Pharmacology of Local Anesthetics. Philadelphia: Butterworth-Heinemann, 2000.)

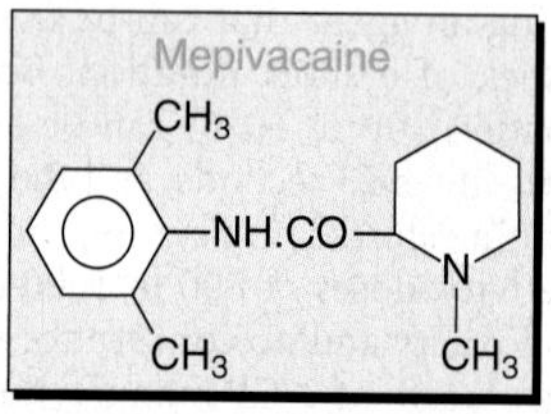

FIGURE 59-8 • Structure of mepivacaine. (Adapted from Tetzlaff JE: Clinical Pharmacology of Local Anesthetics. Philadelphia: Butterworth-Heinemann, 2000.)

relationship between blood levels of lidocaine and toxicity. At plasma levels of 5 μg/dl, lidocaine is rarely toxic, whereas at 10 μg/dl it is rarely asymptomatic. Although sudden massive boluses of lidocaine can cause irreversible cardiac arrest, at clinical levels there is no selective cardiac toxicity. Although millions of spinal anesthetics have been performed with lidocaine, there have been reports of irritation of the cauda equina and/or lumbosacral nerve roots after spinal anesthesia.[67] Because these symptoms resolve rapidly, this phenomenon has become known as transient neurologic symptoms (TNS).[68,69] The presentation of TNS is typically burning dysesthesia in the buttocks and posterior thighs that can be fairly intense and resolves over 3 to 5 days without treatment.[70]

Lidocaine is capable of every clinical use reported for LAs. Parenteral lidocaine can be used as an antiarrhythmic because it suppresses activity in reentrant pathways. It is also used parenterally to diagnosis and treat chronic pain conditions related to abnormal neural activity (e.g., central pain, some chronic regional pain syndromes). Combined lipid and aqueous solubility make lidocaine the most commonly used topical anesthetic, with a shorter duration than tetracaine and much less risk of toxicity for high-volume topical use (e.g., bronchoscopy). It can be used for infiltration, field block, peripheral nerve block, and plexus block as well as neuraxial block. By altering the concentration, a range from analgesia to anesthesia with dense motor block can be achieved, although other amides have a wider separation between motor and sensory block and may be better suited to tasks in which sparing motor block is important. Very high volumes of dilute (0.3% to 0.5%) lidocaine can be injected into fatty subcutaneous tissue under high pressure (tuminescent technique) with very little plasma uptake. Lidocaine is the most common choice in the United States for intravenous regional anesthesia (a.k.a. Bier block). Although lidocaine has become less popular, 2% lidocaine for surgical epidural anesthesia remains a gold standard, as does 1.0% to 1.5% lidocaine for plexus and peripheral nerve blocks.

Mepivacaine (Fig. 59-8). In 1957, Ekenstam combined the advantages of the ring structure of cocaine and the amide family with the introduction of mepivacaine, the first member of the pipecolylxylide subgroup of the amides, which would later include bupivacaine, ropivacaine, and levobupivacaine. Mepivacaine was designed with more lipid solubility and protein-binding potential, with the intent to create an LA with higher potency and longer duration than lidocaine. Although this is the clinical signature of the agent, it is similar enough to lidocaine that it has never achieved the widespread recognition of lidocaine except among those users who recognize the subtle advantages. With a low pK_a and intermediate lipid solubility and protein binding, it has a profile very similar to lidocaine, although, for equivalent applications, it is 20% to 30% more potent and has a longer duration of action. Because of the ring structure, the metabolism is significantly slower in adults. This is especially true of the fetus because of delayed development of the enzyme capable of the first step in biotransformation.[71] Because of the high maternal-fetal transfer (similar to lidocaine) and the delayed fetal metabolism, mepivacaine is not used for high-dose applications in obstetrics (e.g., cesarean section) to avoid "the floppy baby."[72]

Mepivacaine can be used for every application that lidocaine is used for while achieving a duration of action 20% to 30% longer than lidocaine. Ironically, with TNS causing hesitation to use lidocaine for spinal anesthesia, there has been increased interest in mepivacaine spinal anesthesia. Two percent mepivacaine consistently produces the best quality motor block for epidural anesthesia in cases in which dense motor block is important, with a redose interval at 60 to 90 minutes. There is extensive evidence of the efficiency of mepivacaine to produce dense anesthesia and motor block with 1.0% to 1.5% for peripheral nerve or plexus block,[73,74] with a 2-to 3-hour duration that is 50% longer with epinephrine added. Compounded with 0.1% to 0.2% tetracaine ("supercaine"), the result is a fast onset of complete anesthesia with long-duration postoperative analgesia. There are reports of mepivacaine use for intravenous regional anesthesia with no obvious advantage over lidocaine.

Prilocaine (Fig. 59-9). Prilocaine was designed as a member of the amide family with the intent to create a molecule with quicker hydrolysis of the amide bond, but preserving the versatile LA activity of lidocaine. With a pK_a of 7.9% and similar lipid solubility and protein-binding potential, the rapid speed of metabolism is a theoretical advantage over lidocaine. Unfortunately, the propensity to create methemoglobin (previously described) has more than neutralized this advantage.

Prilocaine has an active role in topical anesthesia as one of the constituents of EMLA. Like lidocaine, in the base form, it forms an emulsion when diluted (from 5.0% to 2.5%). For those willing to ignore the risk of methemoglobinemia, prilocaine is an excellent choice for intravenous regional anesthesia[75] or topical anesthesia.[76] Prilocaine has an active application in dental anesthesia, being able to suppress noxious stimuli better than procaine and lidocaine. Intra-articular prilocaine has been found to create excellent conditions for knee arthroscopy and

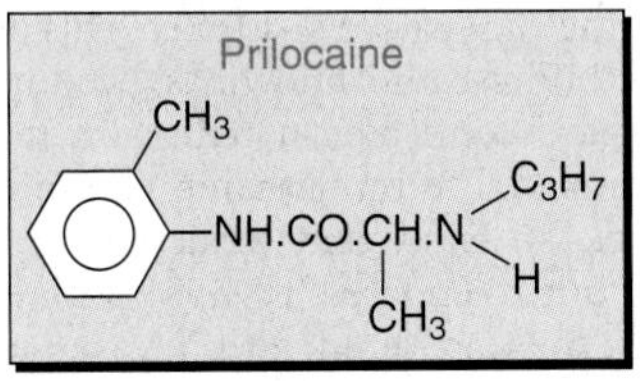

FIGURE 59-9 • Structure of prilocaine. (Adapted from Tetzlaff JE: Clinical Pharmacology of Local Anesthetics. Philadelphia: Butterworth-Heinemann, 2000.)

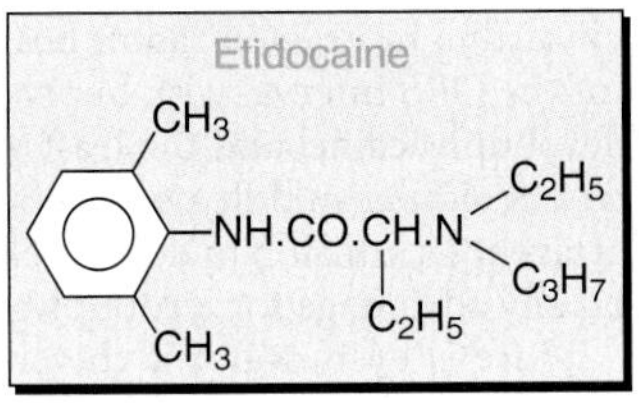

FIGURE 59-10 • Structure of etidocaine. (Adapted from Tetzlaff JE: Clinical Pharmacology of Local Anesthetics. Philadelphia: Butterworth-Heinemann, 2000.)

minor arthroscopic surgery. Although solutions of prilocaine create good topical anesthesia, the high absorbance would be associated with the potential for methemoglobinemia. Peripheral nerve, plexus, and neuraxial anesthesia have all been performed with prilocaine, resulting in anesthesia comparable to lidocaine with shorter duration. This agent is not available in the United States for these applications.

Etidocaine (Fig. 59-10). Etidocaine is a chemical modification of lidocaine designed with the same strategy as the creation of tetracaine from procaine. The alteration that created etidocaine is the addition of an ethyl (two-carbon aliphatic) group to the intermediate chain of lidocaine. The result is an agent with a pK_a of 7.9 and high lipid solubility and protein-binding potential. The resulting profile is an agent with slow onset, high potency, and long duration of action. As previously described, selective cardiotoxicity related to fast-in, slow-out affinity for the cardiac sodium channels makes high plasma levels of this agent problematic. One interesting clinical property of etidocaine is a selectively greater motor compared to sensory block, with very long duration of motor block,[77] exceeding sensory block by up to 25%.[78] This makes etidocaine an ideal choice to salvage a continuous block when the motor block is not complete. On the other hand, as a sole agent it is capable of creating an immobile patient who has retained sensation, a less than ideal characteristic.

Clinical use of etidocaine has concentrated on epidural use.[79] Dense topical anesthesia was described, but the rapid plasma uptake and narrow therapeutic/toxic range makes this less than ideal. It is not optimal for infiltration or peripheral/plexus block because of sensory sparing. Dense motor block with epidural anesthesia for surgery can be achieved at high doses for some cases as long as adequate sensory anesthesia is confirmed.[80] Because of the selective cardiac toxicity and sensory sparing, there is very little use of etidocaine in the United States, and the agent is not commercially available.

Bupivacaine (Fig. 59-11). Bupivacaine was designed as a modification of mepivacaine to achieve a more potent, longer acting agent. The modification is the swap of a one-carbon methyl group on the pipecolyl ring (mepivacaine) to a four-carbon butyl group (bupivacaine). The result is a molecule with high pK_a, high lipid solubility, and high protein-binding potential, creating an LA with slow onset, high potency, and long duration of action. For all three of these characteristics, bupivacaine is the leader. There are unique elements to the conduction block with bupivacaine that are the opposite of the profile of etidocaine. At high concentration, dense sensory block of very long duration[81] can occur while motor function may remain partially intact. At low concentrations, sensory block may create analgesia with little or no motor block, ideal for obstetric analgesia[82] or postoperative pain control during active rehabilitation.[83] The amide bond is the most

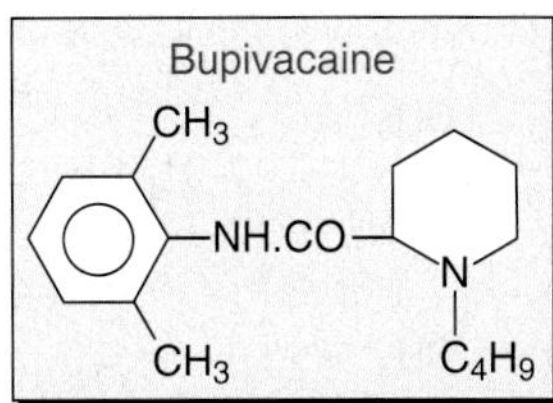

FIGURE 59-11 • Structure of bupivacaine. (Adapted from Tetzlaff JE: Clinical Pharmacology of Local Anesthetics. Philadelphia: Butterworth-Heinemann, 2000.)

resistant to hydrolysis, and metabolism is very slow, requiring at least two steps prior to urinary elimination. Even redistribution is slow due to high protein-binding potential. With potency and toxicity being closely related, there is a narrow range from therapeutic to toxic concentrations. This is complicated further by avid protein-binding affinity, because it is the unbound LA that creates the prodrome during CNS exposure to plasma LA. With bupivacaine, there may be no prodrome at all until moments prior to a serious reaction. Also, the type of reaction can be very different from those with other members of the pipecolylxylide family. With mepivacaine, there will likely be a prodrome (cranial nerve paresthesia) followed by seizure activity. With bupivacaine, the patient may be asymptomatic until moments before seizure or lethal arrhythmia (or both) present suddenly.[84] All of this leads to a relatively conservative safe upper limit of 2 mg/kg of bupivacaine for most applications of regional anesthesia.

Bupivacaine has the potential for any application of regional anesthesia, although many are restricted by concern for toxicity. Bupivacaine creates excellent topical anesthesia of mucous membranes, but the plasma uptake is also rapid so that toxicity would be a concern with more than very limited use. Diluted bupivacaine is used for infiltration and field block because of the long duration,[85] when motor block is not needed or specifically avoided. At lower concentrations (0.25% to 0.5%), an adequate volume can be used to perform high-volume peripheral blocks (e.g., brachial plexus), although motor block may be incomplete.[86,87] At a higher concentration (0.625% or 0.75%), the motor block may be more complete, but the volume required for some regional anesthesia techniques may approach or exceed the toxic range. Bupivacaine has a significant role in all neuraxial blocks. Bupivacaine is selected for postoperative analgesia via pediatric control block with 0.25% and 0.5% concentrations at lower volume to provide motor block for pelvis and lower extremity surgery. Bupivacaine is the second most commonly selected agent for adult spinal anesthesia, either as a hyperbaric solution for a high block[88] or as a plain solution for lower block.[89] For spinal anesthesia, bupivacaine creates nearly equivalent motor and sensory block.

The range of action for bupivacaine is best demonstrated with epidural anesthesia. At 0.75%, long-duration anesthesia with good motor block occurs. At 0.5%, the motor block is not always complete, although the sensory block still creates anesthesia. At 0.25%, the motor block can be very limited and the sensory block is partial, blocking nociceptive signals but sparing some elements of light touch and proprioception. Below 0.1%, there is virtually no motor block and sensation is present simultaneously with analgesia. This makes 0.1% bupivacaine and below an ideal concentration for analgesia for labor, where motor block could prevent active participation in stage 2 of labor. Similarly, analgesia with intact sensation makes 0.1% bupivacaine an ideal choice for postoperative analgesia after lower extremity procedures, since ambulation and active range of motion are possible.[83] Intravenous regional anesthesia has been reported successfully with bupivacaine,[90] but obvious concerns with cardiac toxicity severely restrict this option. There are no parenteral applications for bupivacaine.

Ropivacaine (Fig. 59-12). Ropivacaine was designed as a modification of bupivacaine to address the cardiac toxicity. The idea for the chemical substitution came from a toxicity profile of the two members of the pipecolylxylide family. Bupivacaine has selective cardiac toxicity, whereas mepivacaine does not. Since the unique elements of bupivacaine came from adding three carbons to a methyl

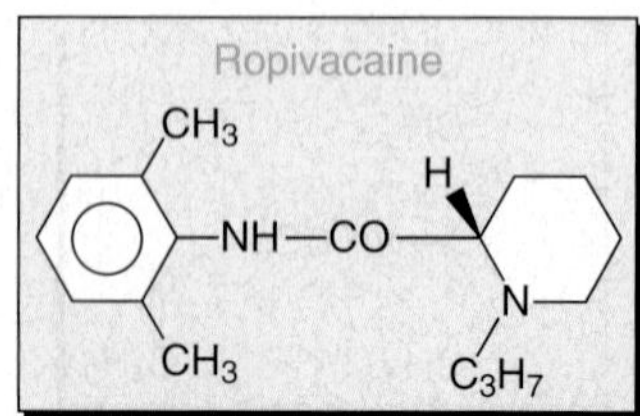

FIGURE 59-12 • Structure of ropivacaine. The chemical formula of ropivacaine resembles that of the amino amides mepivacaine and bupivacaine. (Adapted from Tetzlaff JE: Clinical Pharmacology of Local Anesthetics. Philadelphia: Butterworth-Heinemann, 2000.)

group of mepivacaine, it was logical to reduce one in the hope that the favorable characteristics of bupivacaine would be retained. The substitution of an isopropyl for the butyl group of bupivacaine creates ropivacaine. The result is an agent with a pK_a of 8.1%, high lipid solubility, and high protein-binding potential. The question of cardiac toxicity was investigated with the first trials of ropivacaine. In cell cultures, ropivacaine had less interference with cardiac cell energy handling,[91] and less impact on the arrhythmia threshold with intracoronary injection,[92] compared to bupivacaine. When infused parenterally (human volunteers), ropivacaine had less effect on cardiac contractility[93] compared to bupivacaine. During U.S. Food and Drug Administration trials with ropivacaine, there were no reports of selective cardiac toxicity. There were several reports of inadvertent overdoses or intravascular injection with ropivacaine not associated with cardiac toxicity.[94,95] The toxicity profile was much more like mepivacaine than bupivacaine.

The clinical profile of ropivacaine is remarkably similar to that of bupivacaine. One exception is the discovery that ropivacaine is a weak vasoconstrictor, in comparison to bupivacaine (and all other LAs except cocaine), which vasodilates by a direct action on vascular smooth muscle. This vasoconstriction is not great enough to make ropivacaine a candidate for nasal surgery. It could be a useful choice for infiltration except for skin supplied by end-artery circulation (fingers, toes, earlobes, genitalia), where vasoconstriction is relatively contraindicated. This would also be a theoretical risk with spinal anesthesia,[96] although ropivacaine reduces spinal cord blood flow much less than the doses of epinephrine used routinely with spinal anesthesia. The quality of clinical block with ropivacaine appears to be very similar in onset, duration, and quality to that of bupivacaine,[97] and ropivacaine provides excellent analgesia postoperatively when used for wound infiltration or epidural infusion.[98] At 0.5%, there is a low level of motor block when injected in the epidural space.[99] At lower concentrations, there may be even less motor block than with bupivacaine at comparable analgesia.[100] Analgesia is equivalent between 0.25% and 0.5% ropivacaine for femoral nerve block after total knee replacement, equal to 0.25% bupivacaine, and has increased motor block with 0.5% ropivacaine.[101] When 0.1% and 0.2% ropivacaine are compared to the same concentrations of bupivacaine, the analgesia is equivalent between bupivacaine and ropivacaine, with no improved analgesia at the higher doses.[102] After open shoulder surgery with continuous interscalene block with 0.75% ropivacaine, an infusion of 0.2% ropivacaine provides profound analgesia with no cumulative toxicity for up to 48 hours.[103] Thoracic epidural analgesia with ropivacaine/fentanyl at 0.15% or 0.2% was equivalent to 0.1% bupivacaine with no obvious advantage for the ropivacaine except the theoretical reduced cardiotoxicity.[104]

Levobupivacaine (see Fig. 59-11). All of the members of the mepivacaine family have asymmetric substitutions of a central (chiral) carbon. This means that there are two potential mirror image versions of the molecules, called stereoisomers. Mepivacaine and bupivacaine were first released as mixtures (racemic). Investigation into the causes of cardiac toxicity for bupivacaine revealed that the right-sided (dextro) version had three to four times as much potential for cardiac toxicity due to slower exit from cardiac sodium channels during diastole compared to the left-sided (levo) molecule.[105] For this reason, ropivacaine was prepared from the start as a levo-isomer. This observation also led to the creation of L-bupivacaine, known as levobupivacaine.[106]

Animal studies have confirmed a reduction in cardiac effects of levobupivacaine compared to bupivacaine. In swine, ropivacaine and levobupivacaine have an equivalent reduction in lethal dose during intracoronary injection compared to bupivacaine.[107] An equivalent reduction in lethal dose was found with intravenous levobupivacaine in sheep compared to bupivacaine.[108] Also in sheep, a significant reduction in arrhythmia was noted at nonlethal infusion rates.[109] In human volunteers, less negative inotropy, less conduction delay, and less arrhythmia were found during intravenous infusion of levobupivacaine compared to bupivacaine.[110] In comparing levobupivacaine to ropivacaine and bupivacaine in isolated rabbit heart tissue, there was more prolongation of the QRS interval with bupivacaine, an intermediate amount with levobupivacaine, and the least with ropivacaine in a ratio of 1.0/0.4/0.3.[111] A similar middle position for levobupivacaine was found during intravenous infusion in dogs.[112] Not all of the animal studies demonstrated any advantage for levobupivacaine over bupivacaine, however.[113,114] There is even doubt if the chirality is the most important determinant of toxicity, versus molecular size, supported by evidence that ropivacaine is less cardiotoxic than either bupivacaine or levobupivacaine.[115] Although stereospecificity reduces cardiotoxicity with bupivacaine, there are no advantages in this respect between the possible isomers of ropivacaine, although only the levo version is available for clinical use.[116]

There are no unique clinical properties of levobupivacaine compared to bupivacaine. Apart from the cardiac toxicity and the cost differential, levobupivacaine can be used interchangeably with bupivacaine. Clinical studies reported to date have found no difference in the clinical behavior of levobupivacaine compared to equivalent concentrations of bupivacaine.[117,118] Murdoch et al. evaluated levobupivacaine for postoperative epidural analgesia after orthopedic surgery, looking at 0.0625%, 0.0125%, and 0.25% concentrations, and found the best analgesia with 0.25% with no difference in motor block.[119]

Emerging Targets

Future evolution of LA pharmacology will undoubtedly focus on improvements in the prevention and treatment of pain. Techniques and devices are being investigated to deliver LAs for days after surgery via catheters, pumps, and even home delivery devices (gravity, elastomeric, and so forth). Other strategies focus on longer-acting agents, such as encapsulation of LA molecules so they become a sustained-release compound, such that one injection near the target could provide prolonged analgesia. Additives to LA solutions have also been studied to achieve sustained analgesia by interfering with ascending nociceptive signals. The theoretical epidural "cocktail" of the future could suspend ascending nociceptive signals (complete pain relief) without side effects, depending on how the components were mixed and how they were prepared chemically. Extending this vision further, long-acting LA cocktails may be constructed to silence abnormally active elements within the neuraxis that create and sustain chronic pain states. Eventually, it may be possible to select a very small needle and inject a solu-tion that would either prevent acute pain or treat the chronic pain states originating or sustained within distinct neuraxial (or cranial?) dermatomes.

REFERENCES

1. Cohen S. Cocaine. JAMA 1975;231:74-75.
2. Leonard M. Carl Koller: Mankind's greatest benefactor? The story of local anesthesia. J Dent Res 1998;77:535-538.
3. Smythies JRA, Benington F, Bradley RJ, et al. The molecular structure of the sodium channel. J Theor Biol 1974;43:29-42.
4. Catterall WA. Cellular and molecular biology of voltage-gated sodium channels. Physiol Rev 1992;72:S15-S41.
5. Cahalan MD, Almers W. Interactions between quaternary lidocaine, the sodium channel gates, and tetrodotoxin. Biophys J 1979;27:39-55.
6. Geddes IC. Local anaesthetics. Laval Med 1971;42:787-793.
7. Gajraj NM, Pennant JH, Watcha F. Eutectic mixture of local anesthetics (EMLA) cream. Anesth Analg 1994;78:574-583.

8. Strichartz G. Molecular mechanisms of nerve block by local anesthetics. Anesthesiology 1976;45:421-441.
9. Butterworth JF, Strichartz GR. Molecular mechanisms of local anesthesia: a review. Anesthesiology 1990;72:711-734.
10. Narahashi T, Frazier DT, Yamada M. The site of action and the active form of local anesthetics: theory and pH experiments with tertiary compounds. J Pharmacol Exp Ther 1970;171:32-44.
11. Piccinini F, Chiarra A, Villani F. The active form of local anesthetic drugs. Experientia 1972;28:140-141.
12. Strichartz GR, Sanchez V, Arthur GR, et al. Fundamental properties of local anesthetics II. Measured octanol: buffer partition coefficients and pKa values of clinically used drugs. Anesth Analg 1990;71:58-70.
13. Munson ES, Wagman IH. Action of lidocaine in the central nervous system. Anesthesiology 1969;30:3-4.
14. de Jong RH, Robles R, Corbin RW. Central actions of lidocaine—synaptic transmission. Anesthesiology 1969;30:19-23.
15. Warnick JE, Kee RD, Yim GKW. The effects of lidocaine on inhibition in the cerebral cortex. Anesthesiology 1971;34:327-332.
16. Rosenberg PH, Kalso EA, Tuominen MK, Linden HB. Acute bupivacaine toxicity as a result of venous leakage under the tourniquet cuff during a Bier block. Anesthesiology 1983;58:95-98.
17. Thomas RD, Behbehani MM, Coyle D, Denson DD. Cardiovascular toxicity of local anesthetics: an alternative hypothesis. Anesth Analg 1986;65:444-450.
18. Lange RA, Cigarroa RG, Yancy CW, et al. Cocaine-induced coronary-artery vasospasm. N Engl J Med 1989;321:1557-1562.
19. Chiu YC, Brecht K, DasGupta DS, Mhoon E. Myocardial infarction with topical cocaine anesthesia for nasal surgery. Arch Otolaryngol Head Neck Surg 1986;112:988-990.
20. Lustik SJ, Chibber AK, van Vliet M, Pomerantz RM. Ephedrine-induced coronary vasospasm in a patient with prior cocaine use. Anesth Analg 1997;84:931-933.
21. Minor RL, Scott BD, Brown DD, Winniford MD. Cocaine-induced myocardial infarction in patients with normal coronary arteries. Ann Intern Med 1991;115:797-806.
22. Davis NL, deJong RH. Successful resuscitation following massive bupivacaine overdose. Anesth Analg 1982;61:62-64.
23. Clarkson CW, Hondeghem LM. Mechanism for bupivacaine depression of cardiac conduction: fast block of sodium channels during the action potential with slow recovery from block during diastole. Anesthesiology 1985;62:396-405.
24. Reiz S, Nath S. Cardiotoxicity of local anaesthetic agents. Br J Anaesth 1986;58:736-746.
25. Bruelle P, Lefrant JY, de La Coussaye JE, et al. Comparative electrophysiologic and hemodynamic effects of several amide local anesthetic drugs in anesthetized dogs. Anesth Analg 1996;82:648-656.
26. Bellamy MC, Hopkins PM, Halsall PJ, Ellis FR. A study into the incidence of methemoglobinaemia after "three-in-one" block with prilocaine. Anaesthesia 1992;47:1084-1085.
27. Harris WH, Cole DW, Mital M, Laver MB. Methemoglobin formation and oxygen transport following intravenous regional anesthesia using prilocaine. Anesthesiology 1968;29:65-69.
28. Johnson D. Perioperative methemoglobinemia. Can J Anaesth 2005;52:665-668.
29. Kalichman MW, Moorhouse DF, Powell HC, Myers RR. Relative neural toxicity of local anesthetics. J Neuropathol Exp Neurol 1993;52:234-240.
30. Kalichman MW, Powell HC, Myers RR. Qualitative histologic analysis of local anesthetic-induced injury to rat sciatic nerve. J Pharmacol Exp Ther 1989;250:406-413.
31. Basson MD, Carlson BM. Myotoxicity of single and repeated injections of mepivacaine (Carbocaine) in the rat. Anesth Analg 1980;59:275-282.
32. Moore DC, Bridenbaugh LD, Thompson GE, et al. Factors determining dosages of amide-type local anesthetic drugs. Anesthesiology 1977;47:263-268.
33. Fibuch EF, Opper SE. Back pain following epidurally administered Nesacaine-MPF. Anesth Analg 1989;69:113-115.
34. Bromage PB. Allergy to local anaesthetics. Anaesthesia 1975;30:239.
35. Caro I. Contact allergy/photo allergy to glyceryl PABA and benzocaine. Contact Dermatitis 1978;4:381-382.
36. Glinert RJ, Zachary CB. Local anesthetic allergy: its recognition and avoidance. J Dermatol Surg Oncol 1991;17:491-496.
37. Giovannitti JA, Bennett CR. Assessment of allergy to local anesthetics. J Am Dent Assoc 1979;98:701-706.
38. Bartlett FZ. Clinical observations on the effects of injection of local anesthetics preceded by aspiration. Oral Surg Oral Med Oral Pathol 1972;33:520-523.
39. Johnson WT, DeStigter T. Hypersensitivity to procaine, tetracaine, mepivacaine and methyl paraben: report of a case. J Am Dent Assoc 1983;106:53-56.
40. Adriani J. The clinical pharmacology of local anesthetics. J Clin Pharmacol Exp Ther 1960;1:645.
41. Sindel LJ, deShazo RD. Accidents resulting from local anesthetics: true or false allergy? Clin Rev Allergy 1991;9:379-395.
42. Petersen RC. History of cocaine. NIDA Res Monogr 1977;13:17-34.
43. Grinspoon L, Bakalar JB. Coca and cocaine as medicines: an historical review. J Ethnopharmacol 1981;3:149-159.
44. Siegel RK, Hirschman A. Moreno and the first study on cocaine: a historical note and translation. J Psychoactive Drugs 1983;15:219-220.
45. Grienwald JH, Holtel MR. Absorption of topical cocaine in rhinologic procedures. Laryngoscope 1996;106:1223-1225.
46. Tipton GA, DeWitt G, Eisenstein SJ. Topical TAC (tetracaine, adrenaline, cocaine) solution for local anesthesia in children: prescribing inconsistency and acute toxicity. South Med J 1989;82:1344-1346.
47. Dailey RH. Fatality secondary to misuse of TAC solution. Ann Emerg Med 1988;17:159-160.
48. Gadalla MAF, El-Hak RY. Serum levels of procaine in humans after peri-oral injections. Pharmazie 1985:40:118-120.
49. Kuhnert BR, Kuhnert PM, Philipson EH, et al. The half-life of 2-chloroprocaine. Anesth Analg 1986;65:273-278.
50. Ravindran RS, Bond VK, Tasch MD, et al. Prolonged neural blockade following regional analgesia with 2-chloroprocaine. Anesth Analg 1980;59:447-452.
51. Reisner LS, Hochman BN, Plumer MH. Persistent neurologic deficit and adhesive arachnoiditis following intrathecal 2-chloroprocaine injection. Anesth Analg 1980;59:452-454.
52. Wang BC, Hillman DE, Spielholz NI, Turndorf H. Chronic neurological deficits and nesacaine-CE and effect of the anesthetic, 2-chloroprocaine, or the antioxidant, sodium bisulfite. Anesth Analg 1984;63:445-447.
53. Datta S, Corke BC, Alper MH, et al. Epidural anesthesia for cesarean section: a comparison of bupivacaine, chloroprocaine and etidocaine. Anesthesiology 1980;52:48-51.
54. Kopacz DJ. Spinal 2-chloroprocaine: minimum effective dose. Reg Anesth Pain Med 2005;30:36-42.
55. Casati A, Danelli G, Berti M, et al. Intrathecal 2-chloroprocaine for lower limb outpatient surgery: a prospective, randomized, double-blind, clinical evaluation. Anesth Analg 2006;103:234-238.
56. Yoos JR, Kopacz DJ. Spinal 2-chloroprocaine for surgery: an initial 10-month experience. Anesth Analg 2004;99:553-558.
57. Adriani J, Campbell D. Fatalities following topical application of local anesthetic to mucous membranes. J Am Med Assoc 1956;162:1527-1530.
58. Campbell D, Adriani J. Absorption of local anesthetics. J Am Med Assoc 1958;168:873-877.
59. Porush I, Shiumamura A, Takahashi LT. Determination of tetracaine in blood. J Pharm Sci 1965;54:1809-1810.
60. Stevens JB, Vories PA, Walker SC. Nebulized tetracaine attenuates the hemodynamic response to tracheal intubation. Acta Anaesthesiol Scand 1996;40:757-759.
61. Collins JF. Methemoglobinemia as a complication of 20% benzocaine spray for endoscopy. Gastroenterology 1990;98:211-213.
62. Kellett PB, Copeland CS. Methemoglobinemia associated with benzocaine-containing lubricant. Anesthesiology 1983;59:463-464.
63. Seibert RW, Seibert JJ. Infantile methemoglobinemia induced by a topical anesthetic, cetacaine. Laryngoscope 1984;94:816-817.
64. Sherman JM. Methemoglobinemia owing to rectal-probe lubrication. Am J Dis Child 1979;133:439-440.
65. Goldstein PJ, Lipman M, Luebehusen J. A controlled clinical trial of two local agents in postepisiotomy pain and discomfort. South Med J 1977;70:806-808.
66. Lee E, Boorse R, Marcinczyk M. Methemoglobinemia secondary to benzocaine topical anesthetic. Surg Laparosc Endosc 1996;6:492-493.
67. Strichartz GR. Every problem is an opportunity, or one person's poison is another person's remedy. Reg Anesth Pain Med 1998;23:3-6.
68. Hampl KF, Heinzmann-Wiedmer S, Luginbuehl I, et al. Transient neurologic symptoms after spinal anesthesia. Anesthesiology 1998;88:629-633.
69. Morisaki H, Masuda J, Kaneko S, et al. Transient neurological syndrome in one thousand forty-five patients after 3% lidocaine spinal anesthesia. Anesth Analg 1998;86:1023-1026.
70. Zaric D, Christiansen C, Pace NL, Punjasawadwong Y. Transient neurologic symptoms after spinal anesthesia with lidocaine versus other local anesthetics: a systematic review of randomized, controlled trials. Anesth Analg 2005;100:1811-1816.
71. Brown WU, Bell GC, Lurie AO, et al. Newborn blood levels of lidocaine and mepivacaine in the first postnatal day following maternal epidural anesthesia. Anesthesiology 1975;42:698-707.
72. Meffin P, Long GJ, Thomas J. Clearance and metabolism of mepivacaine in the human neonate. Clin Pharmacol Exp Ther 1972;14:218-222.
73. Cockings E, Moore PL, Lewis RC. Transarterial brachial plexus blockade using high doses of 1.5% mepivacaine. Reg Anesth 1987;12:159-164.
74. Vester-Andersen T, Eriksen C, Christiansen C. Perivascular axillary block III. Blockade following 40 ml of 0.5%, 1% or 1.5% mepivacaine with adrenaline. Acta Anaesthesiol Scand 1984;28:95-98.
75. Pitkanen M, Kytta J, Rosenberg PH. Comparison of 2-chloroprocaine and prilocaine for intravenous anaesthesia of the arm: a clinical study. Anaesthesia 1993;48:1091-1093.
76. Tham EJ, Morris S, Wright EM, et al. An assessment of prilocaine as a topical anaesthetic agent for fiberoptic bronchoscopy in comparison with lidocaine. Acta Anaesthesiol Scand 1994;38:442-447.
77. Ramanathan S, Chalon J, Richards M, et al. Prolonged spinal nerve involvement after epidural anesthesia with etidocaine. Anesth Analg 1978;57:361-364.
78. Nydahl PA, Axelsson K, Philipson L, et al. Motor blockade and EMG recordings in epidural anaesthesia: a comparison between mepivacaine 2%, bupivacaine 0.5% and etidocaine 1.5%. Acta Anaesthesiol Scand 1989;33:597-604.
79. Artru AA, Strumwasser TA. Intratracheal aerosolized etidocaine to attenuate cardiovascular and cough responses to laryngoscopy and intubation. Ann Emerg Med 1985;64:1069-1073.
80. Lund PC, Cwik JC, Gannon RT, Vassallo HG. Etidocaine for caesarean section—effects on mother and baby. Br J Anaesth 1977;49:457-460.
81. Madej THJ, Ellis FR, Halsall PJ. Prolonged femoral nerve block with 0.5% bupivacaine. Anaesthesia 1987;42:607-608.
82. Reynolds F, Taylor G. Maternal and neonatal concentrations of bupivacaine. Anesthesia 1970;25:14-23.
83. Scott DQA, Beilby DSN, McClytmont C. Postoperative analgesia using epidural infusions of fentanyl with bupivacaine. Anesthesiology 1995;83:727-737.
84. Friedman GA, Rowlingson JC, DiFazio CA, Donegan MF. Evaluation of the analgesic effect and urinary excretion of systemic bupivacaine in man. Anesth Analg 1982;61:23-27.

85. Fariss BL, Foresman PA, Rodeheaver GT, et al. Anesthetic properties and toxicity of bupivacaine and lidocaine for infiltration anesthesia. J Emerg Med 1987;5:275-282.
86. Bromage PR, Gertel M. An evaluation of two new local anaesthetics for major conduction blockade. Can Anaesth Soc J 1970;17:557-564.
87. Covino BG. Local anesthetic agents for peripheral nerve blocks. Anaesthetist 1980;29:33-37.
88. Casati A, Fanelli G, Cappelleri G, et al. Low dose hyperbaric bupivacaine for unilateral spinal anaesthesia. Can J Anaesth 1998;45:850-854.
89. Baumgarten RK. Labeling of bupivacaine solutions. Reg Anesth 1992;17:240-242.
90. Davies JAH, Gill SS, Weber JCP. Intravenous regional anesthesia using bupivacaine. Anaesthesia 1981;36:331.
91. Sztark F, Malgat M, Dabadie P, Mazat JP. Comparison of the effects of bupivacaine and ropivacaine on heart cell mitochondrial bioenergetics. Anesthesiology 1998;88:1340-1349.
92. Pitkanen M, Feldman HS, Arthur GR, et al. Chronotropic and inotropic effects of ropivacaine, bupivacaine and lidocaine in spontaneously beating and electrically paced, isolated, perfused rabbit heart. Reg Anesth 1992;17:183-192.
93. Scott DB, Lee A, Fagan D, et al. Acute toxicity of ropivacaine compared with that of bupivacaine. Anesth Analg 1989;69:563-569.
94. Selander D. Accidental IV injection of ropivacaine: clinical experiences of 6 cases. Reg Anesth 1997;22:S70.
95. Korman B, Riley RH. Convulsions induced by ropivacaine during interscalene brachial plexus block. Anesth Analg 1997;85:1128-1129.
96. Dahl JB, Simonsen L, Mogensen T, et al. The effect of 0.5% ropivacaine on epidural blood flow. Acta Anaesthesiol Scand 1990;34:308-310.
97. Wildsmith JAW. Peripheral nerve block and ropivacaine. Am J Anesthesiol 1997;24:14-17.
98. Kehlet H. Ropivacaine for postoperative pain relief and incisional anesthesia/analgesia. Am J Anesthesiol 1997;24:26-30.
99. Concepcion M, Arthur GR, Steele SM, et al. A new local anesthetic, ropivacaine: its epidural effect in humans. Anesth Analg 1990;70:80-85.
100. Zaric D, Axelsson K, Nydahl P-A, et al. Sensory and motor blockade during epidural analgesia with 1%, 0.75%, and 0.5% ropivacaine—a double blind study. Anesth Analg 1991;72:509-515.
101. Ng HP, Cheong KF, Lim A, et al. Intraoperative single-shot "3-in-1" femoral nerve block with ropivacaine 0.25%, ropivacaine 0.5% or bupivacaine 0.25% provides comparable 48-hour analgesia after unilateral knee replacement. Can J Anaesth 2001;48:1102-1108.
102. Senard M, Joris JL, Ledoux D, et al. A comparison of 0.1% and 0.2% ropivacaine and bupivacaine combined with morphine for postoperative patient-controlled epidural analgesia after major abdominal surgery. Anesth Analg 2002;95:444-449.
103. Ekatodramis G, Boreat A, Huledal G, et al. Continuous interscalene analgesia with ropivacaine 2 mg/ml after major shoulder surgery. Anesthesiology 2003;98:143-150.
104. Macias A, Monedero P, Adame M, et al. A randomized, double-blinded comparison of thoracic epidural ropivacaine, ropivacaine/fentanyl, or bupivacaine/fentanyl for postthoracotomy analgesia. Anesth Analg 2002;95:1344-1350.
105. De Jong RH. Ropivacaine: white knight or dark horse? Reg Anesth 1995;20:474-481.
106. Nau C, Strichartz GR. Drug chirality in anesthesia. Anesthesiology 2002;97:497-502.
107. Morrison SG, Dominguez JJ, Frascarolo P, Reiz S. A comparison of the electrocardiographic cardiotoxic effects of racemic bupivacaine, levobupivacaine, and ropivacaine in anesthetized swine. Anesth Analg 2000;90:1308-1314.
108. Chang DH, Ladd LA, Wilson KA, et al. Tolerability of large-dose intravenous levobupivacaine in sheep. Anesth Analg 2000;91:671-679.
109. Huang HF, Pryor ME, Mather LE, Veering AT. Cardiovascular and central nervous system effects of intravenous levobupivacaine and bupivacaine in sheep. Anesth Analg 1998;86:797-804.
110. Foster RH, Markham A. Levobupivacaine: a review of its pharmacology and use as a local anesthetic. Drugs 2000;59:551-559.
111. Mazoit JX, Decaux A, Bouaziz H, Edouard A. Comparative ventricular electrophysiologic effect of racemic bupivacaine, levobupivacaine, and ropivacaine on the isolated rabbit heart. Anesthesiology 2000;93:784-792.
112. Groban L, Deal DD, Vernon JC, et al. Cardiac resuscitation after incremental overdosage with lidocaine, bupivacaine, and ropivacaine in anesthetized dogs. Anesth Analg 2001;92:37-43.
113. Chang DH, Ladd LA, Copeland S, et al. Direct cardiac effects of intracoronary bupivacaine, levobupivacaine and ropivacaine in the sheep. Br J Pharmacol 2001;132:649-658.
114. Groban L, Deal DD, Vernon JC, et al. Ventricular arrhythmias with or without programmed electrical stimulation after incremental overdosage with lidocaine, bupivacaine, levobupivacaine, and ropivacaine. Anesth Analg 2000;91:1103-1111.
115. Groban L, Deal DD, Vernon JC, et al. Does local anesthetic stereospecificity or structure predict myocardial depression in anesthetized canines? Reg Anesth Pain Med 2002;27:460-468.
116. Graf BM, Abraham I, Eberbach N, et al. Differences in cardiotoxicity of bupivacaine and ropivacaine are the result of physiochemical and stereoselective properties. Anesthesiology 2002;96:1427-1434.
117. Foster RH, Markham A. Levobupivacaine: a review of its pharmacology and use as a local anesthetic. Drugs 2000;59:551-579.
118. McClellan KJ, Spencer CM. Levobupivacaine. Drugs 1998;56:355-362.
119. Murdoch JCA, Dickson UK, Wilson PA, et al. The efficacy and safety of three concentrations of levobupivacaine administered as a continuous epidural infusion in patients undergoing orthopedic surgery. Anesth Analg 2002;94:438-444.

60

GENERAL ANESTHESIA AND SEDATION

Joseph F. Foss and Marco A. Maurtua

OVERVIEW 873
INTRODUCTION 873
PHYSIOLOGY 873
THERAPEUTICS AND CLINICAL PHARMACOLOGY 873
Goals of Therapy 873
Therapeutics by Class 874
Inhalational Anesthetics 874
Intravenous Anesthetics and Sedatives 878

OVERVIEW

This chapter focuses on drugs that act in the central nervous system (CNS) to produce sedation and anesthesia. This includes inhalational and gaseous anesthetics, barbiturates, benzodiazepines, and other intravenous anesthetics. Opioids, often administered as a part of a balanced anesthetic, are not considered in this chapter, except to note their synergistic actions. The chapter explores the mechanisms of action of these drugs and the rapidly increasing understanding of the systems of the brain involved.

The chapter reviews approaches to providing anesthesia or conscious sedation for procedures and contrasts the use of available agents in a variety of clinical settings. All of the drugs discussed produce sedation. The differences in their secondary effects are discussed as these effects often guide selection and use in a clinical setting.

INTRODUCTION

Providing sedation and anesthesia for patients who are undergoing procedures or surgery, and for patients who are on ventilatory support for critical illness, is a complex process that has undergone continued evolution over the last one and one-half centuries. The initial exuberance at being able to perform surgery on an anesthetized patient was quickly tempered by the side effects and mortality associated with the anesthetics themselves. The practice of anesthesia and sedation is now recognized as a continuum, with many drugs being utilized in either situation with appropriate titration of dosing. Many surgeries that were once done as inpatient procedures under deep anesthesia may now be completed in patients who are able to go home within hours after a sedative technique with monitored care. The mortality directly related to anesthetic drugs, in spite of their narrow therapeutic index, is exceeding low when these drugs are administered by properly trained personnel.

The understanding of the mechanisms of interfering with consciousness, perception, and memory has advanced, but remains imperfect. However, tailoring the pharmacology of the different drug classes to provide agents with desirable pharmacokinetic and pharmacodynamic profiles has brought specific agents to clinical practice that have proven to be difficult to improve upon over the last decade.

It is worth considering that little more than a century and a half ago there was no anesthesia available for surgery. Crawford Long was documented to have first used ether in his rural practice about 1842. The first public demonstration of the practical use of ether as an anesthetic is credited to William Morton in the ether dome at Massachusetts General Hospital in 1846. Chloroform came into practice in Scotland and England in 1847, popularized by its use during labor for the Queen. Nitrous oxide (N_2O) was demonstrated as an effective anesthetic in 1845, but was not widely put into use until the 1860s, when it became available as a compressed gas. Each of these agents had a long period of use (N_2O continuing to today) in spite of being hindered by a variety of significant limitations. Ether, while easily made, potent, and relatively devoid of organ toxicity and depression of respiration or the cardiovascular system, was extremely flammable. Chloroform was not flammable but caused significant hepatotoxicity and cardiovascular depression. N_2O is relatively impotent and, when administered in a fashion to achieve high inspired concentrations, was often associated with hypoxic mixtures.

Intravenous anesthesia was launched with the discovery of the fast-acting barbiturate thiopental by Lundy in 1935. The use of barbiturates as sole anesthetic agents was hampered by their cardiovascular effects.

PHYSIOLOGY

The mechanisms that account for anesthesia have been under active investigation since the phenomenon was first described. Observations of the relationship of anesthetics to lipid solubility and the ability of increased atmospheric pressure to reverse the effects of some anesthetics, in spite of a wide variation in their molecular structures, drove investigators to search for a unitary theory of anesthesia. Modern molecular- and receptor-based models of sedation and anesthesia suggest that multiple targets in several anatomic locations best explain how widely different molecules can produce anesthetic effects and also may account for observed differences in efficacy and side effects.

Anesthetics appear to work by different approaches, including increasing the activity of inhibitory neurotransmission, direct inhibition of receptors, and the alteration of resting membrane potentials. A given drug may trigger more than one action, and there may be differential effects at different anatomic sites. Thus inhalational agents, which seem to have effects at the broadest number of receptors and sites, are "total anesthetics" providing analgesia, unconsciousness, amnesia, and immobility, while barbiturates, acting at a smaller subset of targets, produce primarily unconsciousness.

THERAPEUTICS AND CLINICAL PHARMACOLOGY

Goals of Therapy

Sedation is provided for patients to decrease, but not absolutely eliminate, their awareness, anxiety, and recall. Sedative techniques are typically thought of as being associated with shorter recovery periods. Selection of drugs and an awareness of the residual psychomotor effects, which may not be grossly evident, is important in achieving this rapid recovery profile. Sedative techniques must be supplemented by the use of local anesthesia and analgesics to decrease or eliminate the painful stimuli associated with the procedure.

Anesthesia is literally the absence of sensation. The term *general anesthesia* is taken to refer to a reversible depression of CNS function with a resultant decrease in response to stimuli such as a surgical incision. The responses that are suppressed include awareness of the stimulation, memory or recall of the stimulation, somatic movement, and physiologic responses such as increases in sympathetic tone associated with increased heart rate and blood pressure. Thus, general anesthesia may be characterized by unconsciousness, amnesia, lack of motion, and autonomic stability. Each of these factors may be measured separately, and different drugs may produce varying degrees of suppression for each axis.

Drugs used to produce sedation, such as propofol, are continuously administered and titrated to effect. The differentiation between light sedation, deep sedation, and general anesthesia is clinically determined, and the patient's level will be determined by an interplay between drug concentrations at the site of action and the stimulus of the procedure. Thus, a patient who is moderately sedated at one infusion rate, breathing spontaneously and responding to verbal and tactile stimulation, during the initial incision and dissection of a face lift may slide into general anesthesia and require airway support later in the case as the stimulation decreases if the infusion rate is not decreased.

Therapeutics by Class

Inhalational Anesthetics

From the use of N_2O by Horace Wells and Gardner Colton as an anesthetic in 1844 to William Morton's use of diethyl ether as an anesthetic at Massachusetts General Hospital in 1846 to the use of chloroform by Holmes Coote in 1847, inhalational anesthetics (IAs) available today have changed remarkably. In the last few decades, improved development of these agents has helped achieve a faster onset/offset of action, decreased airway irritability, and decreased toxicity (arrhythmogenicity, seizures, renal failure, hepatotoxicity, etc.), and has eliminated flammability, resulting in a safer way of delivering general anesthesia.[1,2]

Pharmacokinetics. IAs are a group of agents with different physical structures that induce general anesthesia (Fig. 60-1). Several factors affect the absorption and elimination of IAs.

Inspiratory Concentration. The inspiratory concentration of IAs is affected by:

1. Degree of fresh gas flow (FGF). By increasing the FGF, a higher concentration of the IA can be achieved in the alveoli and a faster onset will occur.
2. Volume of the breathing system. The smaller the breathing system, the less dilution of the IA, thus resulting in a higher concentration reaching the alveoli.
3. Degree of absorption of the IA by the breathing circuit, which can be decreased by the use of high FGFs. Increasing the inspiratory concentration of the IA speeds up the onset of IA action by increasing its concentration in the alveoli. This in turn leads to an increase in the IA transfer rate known as the *concentration effect*. Another phenomenon responsible for the concentration effect is the *augmented inflow effect*. Another effect of highly concentrated IAs is the rise of the alveolar concentration of a second gas when administered simultaneously. This is called the *second gas effect*. The concentration effect and the second gas effect are more noticeable with the use of N_2O since a higher concentration of this gas is generally used.[1]

Uptake. Three factors affect uptake:

1. Blood solubility of the IA
2. Alveolar blood flow
3. IA partial pressure difference between alveolar gas and venous blood

The solubility of inhalation anesthetics in blood, air, and different tissues is described by their partition coefficient (Table 60-1). Partition coefficient is the ratio of the concentrations of the anesthetic in two phases at equilibrium. Equilibrium is reached when equal partial pressures are achieved in the two phases. For example, desflurane is less soluble in blood when compared to isoflurane. This decreased solubility allows desflurane to achieve equilibrium (same partial pressure) in the two phases much faster when compared to isoflurane. In the case of isoflurane, its highest solubility requires more isoflurane molecules to be dissolved in blood to achieve equilibrium. Therefore, the lower the blood/gas partition coefficient, the lower the solubility of the IA. This leads to a faster increase in the alveolar partial pressure of the IA and a faster achievement of a therapeutic level[1,3-6] (Fig. 60-2).

Alveolar blood flow physiologically should be equal to cardiac output minus physiologic shunting. If the cardiac output decreases to zero, so will the IA uptake. This occurs with soluble and less soluble agents. If cardiac output increases, and a soluble IA is used, there is a delay in its onset of action because of an increase in the IA uptake, thereby decreasing the alveolar partial pressure. Ventilation-perfusion mismatch increases the alveolar partial pressure and decreases the arterial partial pressure of the IAs.[1,4]

The partial pressure difference between alveolar gas and venous blood generates a gradient between alveolar gas and the venous blood returning to the alveoli. This gradient depends on IA tissue uptake. Tissue uptake depends on:

- Tissue/blood partition coefficient
- Tissue blood flow
- Partial pressure difference between arterial blood and the tissue (see Fig. 60-2).

Tissues can be classified into four groups: vessel rich (brain, heart, kidney, liver, etc.), muscle (muscle and skin), fat, and vessel poor (bone, ligaments, cartilage, etc.). Each of these groups shows a different degree of IA uptake, with vessel rich being the most important and vessel poor least due to its negligible uptake.[1,4]

Ventilation. Increased ventilation has a greater impact in the uptake of soluble agents, since it will maintain higher partial pressures in the alveoli. It also helps replace the IAs transferred to blood more efficiently, speeding their onset of action. With less soluble agents such as desflurane, sevoflurane, and N_2O, an increase in ventilation has a lower effect when compared to more soluble agents.[1,3]

Elimination. Elimination of IAs depends on:

1. Degree of FGF. Increasing the FGF avoids rebreathing of IAs and speeds up their pulmonary elimination.
2. Anesthetic circuit volume. The lower the anesthetic circuit volume, the faster the IA elimination.
3. Solubility of the IA. The lower the solubility, the faster the elimination.
4. Ventilation. Increased ventilation increases IA pulmonary elimination.
5. Length of IA exposure. The longer the IA exposure, the more saturated the tissues become with the IA, thereby prolonging its elimination time.

Pharmacodynamics

Mechanism of Action. General anesthesia is a temporary, induced coma that consists of hypnosis, analgesia, and muscle relaxation. The brain is the main target organ for the IAs. The mechanism of action of IAs has yet to be elucidated, but several theories exist. These theories are summarized below.

The unitary hypothesis states that all IAs share a common mechanism of action at the molecular level due to the observation that the anesthetic potency of these agents correlates directly with their lipid solubility. This may lead to the conclusion that anesthesia results from molecules dissolving at specific hydrophobic sites in the neuronal membrane.

The critical volume hypothesis consists of the expansion of the neuronal membranes (phospholipid bilayer) to a critical degree, producing anesthesia by disrupting the neuronal membrane function.

The fluidization theory of anesthesia and *the lateral phase separation theory* both focus on how changes in the membrane form and conductance produced by IAs may inhibit intersynaptic communications.

The modulation of γ-aminobutyric acid (GABA) release is involved in the mechanism of action of several anesthetics. GABA receptor agonists enhance anesthesia by hyperpolarization of the neuronal membrane (Fig. 60-3).

Finally, the action of IAs on ion channels, second messengers, and neurotransmitter receptors may add to their highly effective anesthetic properties.[1,3]

Inhalation Anesthetic	Molecular Structure
Nitrous Oxide	Inorganic gas N≡N=O
Xenon	Inert gas Xe
Halothane	Halogenated alkane 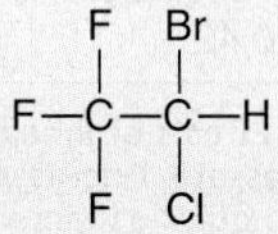 F Br F—C—C—H F Cl
Methoxyflurane	Halogenated methyl ethyl ether 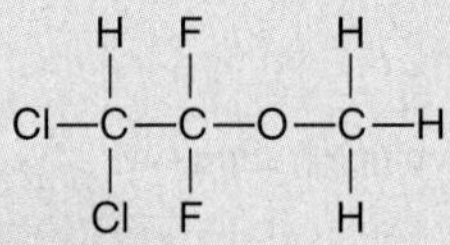 H F H Cl—C—C—O—C—H Cl F H
Enflurane	Halogenated methyl ethyl ether 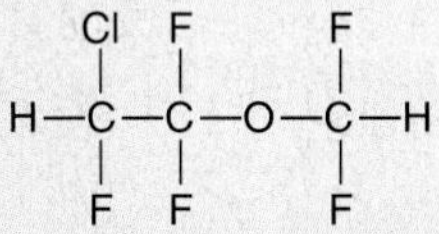 Cl F F H—C—C—O—C—H F F F
Isoflurane	Halogenated methyl ethyl ether 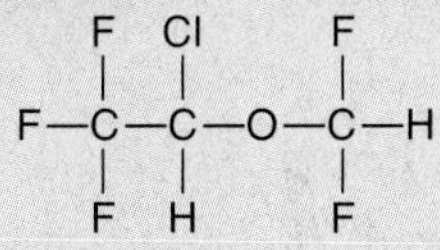 F Cl F F—C—C—O—C—H F H F
Sevoflurane	Fluorinated methyl isopropyl ether 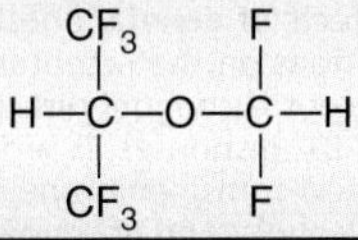 CF_3 F H—C—O—C—H CF_3 F
Desflurane	Fluorinated methyl ethyl ether 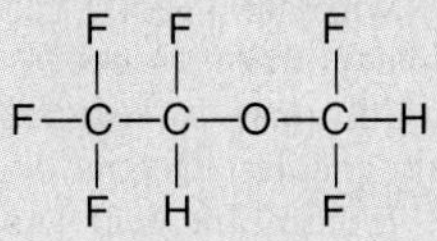 F F F F—C—C—O—C—H F H F

FIGURE 60-1 • Structures of liquid and gaseous inhalational anesthetics.

TABLE 60-1 PARTITION COEFFICIENTS OF VOLATILE ANESTHETICS AT 37° C AND MAC

Anesthetic	Blood/Gas	Brain/Blood	Muscle/Blood	Fat/Blood	Oil/Water	MAC (%)
Nitrous oxide	0.47	1.1	1.2	2.3	3	105.00
Xenon	0.12				20	71
Halothane	2.4	2.9	3.5	60	220	0.75
Methoxyflurane	12	2.0	1.3	49		0.16
Enflurane	1.9	1.5	1.7	36	120	1.7
Isoflurane	1.4	2.6	4.0	45	170	1.2
Sevoflurane	0.59	1.7	3.1	48	55	2.0
Desflurane	0.42	1.3	2.0	27	18.7	6.0

MAC, minimum alveolar concentration.

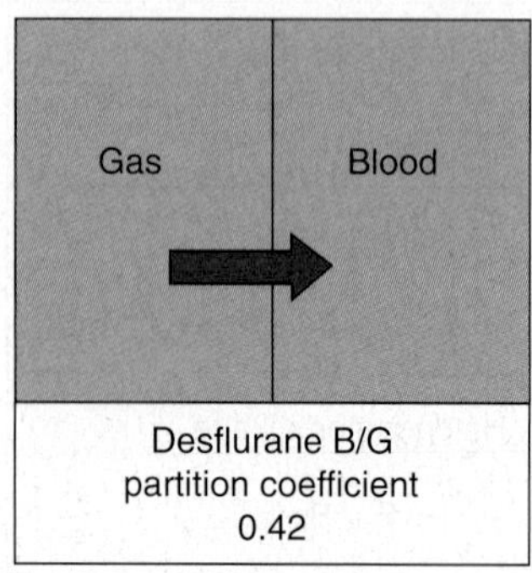

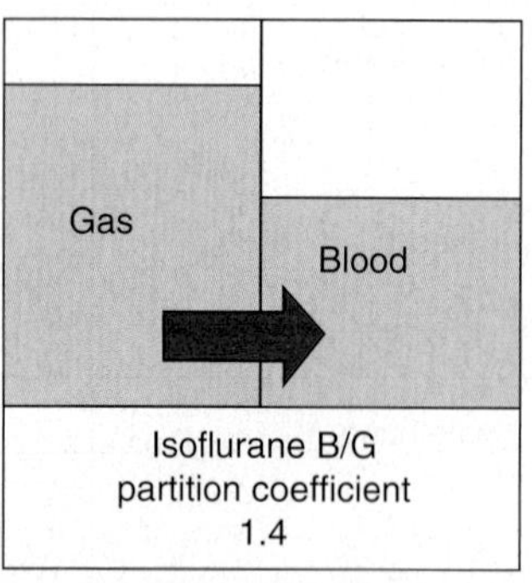

FIGURE 60-2 • Effects of inhalational anesthetic solubility on gas and blood partial pressure. Agents with a lower solubility (e.g., desflurane) will equilibrate more quickly than agents with a higher solubility (e.g., isoflurane), leading to a faster increase in alveolar partial pressure and earlier achievement of a therapeutic level.

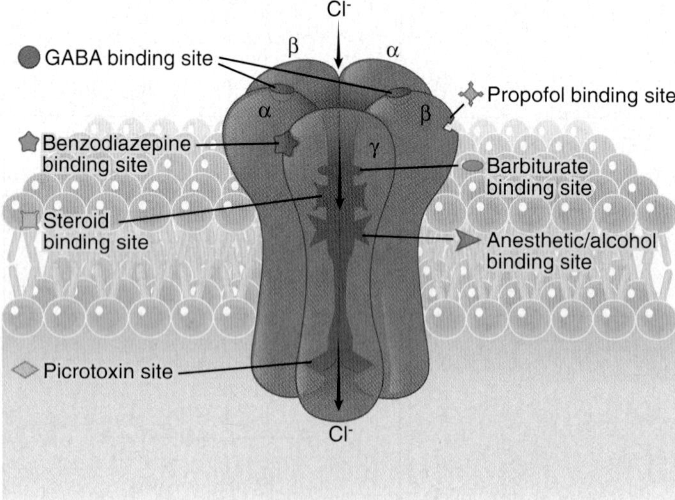

FIGURE 60-3 • Sites of activity at the $GABA_A$ receptor. The $GABA_A$ receptor is a transmembrane receptor with an anion channel permeable to Cl^-. The effects of general anesthetics and sedatives are mediated at different locations on the receptor, either by their ability to activate/gate the $GABA_A$ receptor channel directly or by modulating GABA binding to potentiate GABA responses. A separate site at the interface between the second and third transmembrane segments appears to interact with volatile anesthetics, alcohols, and etomidate.

Potency. Minimal alveolar concentration (MAC) is defined as the alveolar concentration of an IA that prevents movement in 50% of patients in response to surgical stimulation. The MAC concept is similar to the median effective dose concept for intravenous (IV) anesthetics. If we combine two IAs, their MACs will be additive. For example, the use of 0.5 MAC of N_2O and 0.5 MAC of isoflurane will achieve 1 MAC.[1,7]

The MAC concept helps to compare the potencies of different IAs (see Fig. 60-2) and is an indirect way to determine depth of anesthesia. IAs' MAC values will be different if the goal for depth of anesthesia changes, as occurs with MAC-Awake (the concentration of IA that suppresses appropriate response to commands in 50% of the patients) and MAC Bar (the concentration of IA that blocks autonomic response in 50% of the patients).[3,8]

Effects of IAs on Pulmonary Physiology. IAs produce a dose-dependent respiratory depression that consists of a decrease in tidal volume and an increase in the respiratory rate. However, the increase in respiratory rate does not occur to the same degree with all IAs. We will describe those changes by agent. In general, IAs produce bronchodilation and decrease hypoxic pulmonary vasoconstriction.[1-3,7]

N_2O triggers a pronounced increase in the respiratory rate due to CNS stimulation. When the minimal decrease in tidal volume and the increased respiratory rate are combined, minute ventilation and arterial partial pressure of carbon dioxide ($PaCO_2$) remain almost unchanged. The ventilatory response to hypoxia is mediated by chemoreceptors located in the carotid bodies. This physiologic response is called *hypoxic drive.* N_2O depresses hypoxic drive, which may lead to hypoxemia. N_2O does not irritate the airway during induction of anesthesia.[1-3,7]

Xenon does not affect respiratory mechanics and pulmonary function. Airway resistance is not increased.[6]

Isoflurane does not increase the respiratory rate. It produces a dose-dependent decrease in tidal volume, thereby producing a more acute decrease in minute ventilation and faster respiratory depression. Hypoxic drive and ventilatory response to hypercarbia are both depressed by isoflurane. Isoflurane's airway irritation prevents its use for inhalation induction. Relaxation of bronchial smooth muscle is a property shared with other IAs such as sevoflurane, desflurane, and halothane. This bronchodilator response can be helpful in patients with asthma, chronic obstructive pulmonary disease, airway hyperreactivity, and the like.[1-3,7]

Sevoflurane shares the effects on tidal volume and respiratory depression of isoflurane. The avoidance of airway irritation makes sevoflurane the IA of choice for inhalation induction, especially in pediatric patients. It also produces bronchodilation.[1-3,7]

Desflurane depresses the tidal volume and increases the respiratory rate, with an overall effect of dose-dependent respiratory depression that increases $PaCO_2$. It blunts hypoxic drive and the ventilatory response to hypercarbia. Its use may lead to airway irritation and laryngospasm, making it a poor choice for inhalation induction. At higher doses, a bronchodilator response is also seen.[8-10]

Halothane produces respiratory depression and blunting of hypoxic drive and ventilatory response to hypercarbia even at low concentrations. The nonpungency and bronchodilator properties of halothane make it useful during induction of anesthesia. However, due to its dysrhythmogenic effects, it has currently been displaced by sevoflurane.[1-3,7]

Methoxyflurane and *enflurane* produce changes in the respiratory system that are similar to those described for isoflurane. Currently, the use of these agents is reduced due to the renal toxicity exerted by their by-products, especially fluoride, and the CNS toxicity seen with the use of enflurane, consisting of seizures.[1-3,7]

Effects of IAs on Cardiac Physiology. All IAs show a dose-dependent decrease in arterial pressure. The mechanisms involved include vasodilation, which leads to a decrease in systemic vascular resistance, decreased cardiac output, and decreased sympathetic nervous system tone. IAs decrease myocardial oxygen consumption 10% to 15% due to myocardial depression. They also attenuate baroreflex responses, which are important because they help to compensate for hemodynamic changes produced by pathologic conditions such as hemorrhage and sepsis. Although coronary blood flow is preserved during general anesthesia, due to coronary artery vasodilation, the presence of coronary artery disease may produce coronary steal and ischemia.[1-3,7]

N_2O increases pulmonary artery pressures. Therefore, it should be avoided in patients with severe pulmonary hypertension. In vitro N_2O depresses myocardial contractility. However, the increase it elicits in endogenous catecholamine levels leads to a slight increase in blood pressure, cardiac output, and heart rate in the healthy patient that masks its myocardial depression. Careful titration in patients with severe coronary artery disease, low ejection fraction, or severe hypovolemia should be performed to avoid myocardial depression.[1-3,7]

Xenon does not produce cardiovascular depression because it does not affect the cardiomyocytes' calcium flow. These findings have been confirmed by transesophageal echocardiography.[5-7]

Isoflurane decreases systemic vascular resistance, while exerting minimal myocardial depression. A rapid increase in end-tidal isoflurane will produce a transient endogenous release of norepinephrine that will increase heart rate and blood pressure. Isoflurane's theoretical *coronary steal syndrome* is controversial since it was not confirmed by large outcome studies. Isoflurane decreases pulmonary vascular resistance to a lesser degree than it does systemic vascular resistance.[1-3,7]

Sevoflurane produces a decrease in myocardial contractility, systemic vascular resistance, and arterial blood pressure, although not as pronounced as with isoflurane or desflurane.[1-3,7]

Desflurane does not increase coronary artery blood flow. Cardiac output is slightly decreased. A rapid increase of end-tidal desflurane produces a transient increase of endogenous catecholamines resulting in an increase in arterial blood pressure and heart rate greater than that seen with isoflurane.[9-11]

Halothane produces a dose-dependent decrease in arterial blood pressure due to myocardial depression secondary to interference with intracellular calcium utilization. It does not decrease systemic vascular resistance. The overall negative effect of halothane on coronary artery circulation is due to a further decrease in blood pressure despite coronary artery vasodilation. However, myocardial perfusion is not compromised due to a simultaneous decrease in myocardial oxygen demand. Halothane blunts the physiologic baroreceptor reflexes. It not only sensitizes the myocardium to the dysrhythmogenic effects of catecholamines but also produces a conduction delay in the sinoatrial node and a prolongation of the QT interval.[1-3,7]

Effects of IAs on CNS Physiology. In general, IAs decrease cerebral metabolic rate of oxygen ($CMRO_2$) and cerebral electrical activity. The agent that decreases $CMRO_2$ the most is isoflurane. Once an isoelectric electroencephalographic tracing is achieved, further increase in the IA does not decrease the $CMRO_2$ any further.

In the awake state, cerebral blood flow (CBF) is directly related to $CMRO_2$. After the administration of IAs, cerebral vasodilation as well as an increase in cerebrospinal fluid (CSF) pressure occurs, leading to an increase in CBF and cerebral blood volume; $CMRO_2$ decreases. The increase in CBF and decrease in $CMRO_2$ by IAs is also known as *uncoupling*. This increase in CBF produces an increase in brain volume that may lead to suboptimal neurosurgical conditions and is one of the major reasons why, in modern neuroanesthesia, narcotic infusions are used to potentiate IAs to decrease their requirements and brain vasodilatory effects.

The cerebral vasodilation potency of IAs is described as follows[1-3,7]:

Halothane > enflurane > isoflurane = desflurane = sevoflurane

N_2O exposure for several months may cause patients to develop a condition called subacute combined degeneration of the spinal cord. Its symptoms consist of extremity numbness and paresthesias, loss of balance, and unsteady gate. N_2O increases CBF and increases $CMRO_2$. The latter is particular to N_2O since decreased $CMRO_2$ is a constant during the use of halogenated volatile anesthetics. The analgesic effects of N_2O are mediated by the stimulation of the α_{2B}-adrenergic receptors located in the CNS. At the level of the neuromuscular junction, N_2O does not produce muscle relaxation; instead it produces muscle rigidity, as seen during the delivery of higher doses of N_2O in hyperbaric chambers.

Xenon reduces the occurrence of intraoperative tissue hypoxia, maintaining regional blood flow in the brain, liver, kidney, and intestine. These properties make xenon the drug of choice for transplant surgery. Its analgesic effect is mediated by the inhibition of *N*-methyl-D-aspartate (NMDA) receptors located at the dorsal horns of the spinal cord.[4-6]

Isoflurane increases CBF and intracranial pressure (ICP). This can be prevented by hyperventilation. Isoflurane decreases $CMRO_2$ and, at 2 MAC, produces an isoelectric electroencephalogram. It produces skeletal muscle relaxation and potentiates the effects of nondepolarizing muscle relaxants.[1-3,7]

Sevoflurane increases CBF and ICP, both of which can be abolished by hyperventilation. $CMRO_2$ is decreased and may have a protective effect during focal brain ischemia. Skeletal muscle relaxation and potentiation of the nondepolarizing muscle relaxants also occurs during sevoflurane anesthesia.[1-3,7]

Desflurane shares the same properties with isoflurane and sevoflurane regarding CBF, ICP, $CMRO_2$, and skeletal muscle relaxation.[8-10]

Halothane is similar to isoflurane, sevoflurane, and desflurane with regard to having the same effects on CBF, ICP, $CMRO_2$, and skeletal muscle. It also blunts cerebral perfusion autoregulation.[1-3,7]

Effects of IAs on Renal Physiology. Renal blood flow is preserved during administration of IAs because renal perfusion autoregulation is well maintained. Therefore, a decrease in blood pressure will elicit a decrease in renal vascular resistance, maintaining renal blood flow. With IAs, glomerular filtration rate decreases during periods of hypotension. This may lead to a decrease in urine output that returns to normal as soon as normotension is reestablished.[1-3,9]

N_2O decreases renal blood flow because it increases renal vascular resistance, possibly leading to a decrease in urine output.[1-4]

Xenon has minimal effects on tissue perfusion, leading to a better preservation of renal perfusion and urine output.[5-7]

Isoflurane decreases renal blood flow, glomerular filtration rate, and urine output.[1-4]

Sevoflurane may lead to renal failure due to decreased renal blood flow and the potential formation of its by-products, compound A and fluoride. Compound A is a degradation product that is produced after the interaction of sevoflurane with soda lime or baralime. Since compound A formation occurs generally during the delivery of low FGF, the U.S. Food and Drug Administration recommends FGF greater than 2 L/min if sevoflurane is used.[1-4]

Desflurane does not produce renal toxicity.[11-13]

Halothane decreases renal blood flow to a greater degree than glomerular filtration rate. Therefore, the net effect is a decrease in urine output.[2,3,7,8]

Effects of IAs on Hepatic Physiology. Before discussing the effects that IAs have on hepatic physiology, it is important to recall that IAs are not the only ones that may have a deleterious effect on the liver; liver damage may also be caused by intraoperative surgical manipulation.[4]

N_2O decreases hepatic blood flow to a lesser degree than halogenated volatile anesthetics.[1-4]

Isoflurane decreases hepatic blood flow but, because hepatic artery perfusion is maintained, liver function is better preserved.[1-4]

Sevoflurane decreases portal vein blood flow but at the same time increases hepatic artery blood flow, keeping liver blood flow normal.[1-4]

Desflurane, in a small prospective study of patients with chronic hepatitis, showed no increase in liver enzymes or worsening of hepatitis in any patient. However, a few case reports exist that describe hepatitis as a complication of desflurane anesthesia in relation to the length of desflurane exposure.[8-10]

Halothane hepatitis has many etiologies, including localized liver hypoxia, disturbed calcium homeostasis, altered cellular metabolism, and immune-mediated injury. Consensus exists in that halothane hepatitis generally occurs after repetitive exposure to halothane. After the metabolism of halothane by cytochrome P-450, it forms trifluoroacetyl chloride, which binds to proteins contained in the endoplasmic reticulum, triggering an autoimmune response. Controversy still exists regarding what predisposes some patients to this autoimmune response.[1-4]

Biotransformation and Toxicity. *N_2O* is eliminated 99.9% through the lungs and has less than 0.01% metabolism by anaerobic bacteria in the gastrointestinal tract. N_2O inhibits enzymes that are vitamin B_{12} dependent, because it oxidizes the cobalt atom in the vitamin. Vitamin B_{12}-dependent enzymes include methionine synthetase, which is involved in the formation of myelin, and thymidylate synthetase, which is involved in DNA synthesis. Therefore, chronic exposure to N_2O will lead to bone marrow suppression, megaloblastic anemia, peripheral neuropathy, and pernicious anemia.[1-4]

Xenon is not metabolized, so it is completely eliminated through the lungs.[8-10]

Isoflurane metabolites include trifluoroacetic acid and fluoride. Their effects, although potentially deleterious to the liver and kidneys, are limited due to minimal isoflurane metabolism.[1-4]

Sevoflurane's by-products, fluoride and compound A, may lead to impaired renal function.[1-4]

Desflurane undergoes minimal liver metabolism. Despite this, case reports exist linking this agent to postoperative hepatitis.[8-10] No renal side effects have been described.

Halothane's main hepatic metabolites are trifluoroacetic acid and bromide. Autoimmune response to halothane's by-products and hepatic hypoxia due to decreased hepatic perfusion may lead to halothane hepatitis. The incidence of halothane hepatitis is 1 in 35,000 patients generally exposed on several occasions to halothane. Liver centrilobular necrosis is a common pathologic finding. Halothane interaction with catecholamines (endogenous or exogenous) and aminophylline may lead to ventricular dysrhythmias. β-Adrenergic blocking agents and calcium channel blockers potentiate halothane's myocardial depressant effect.[1-4]

Methoxyflurane is metabolized in the liver by cytochrome P-450, resulting in the formation of nephrotoxic by-products such as fluoride and oxalic acid. Its metabolites produce a vasopressin-resistant high-output renal failure. This condition leads to polyuria resistant to vasopressin and increased serum osmolality, sodium, creatinine, and blood urea nitrogen. Hepatotoxicity has also been reported after methoxyflurane exposure.[1-4]

Enflurane is metabolized to fluoride to a lesser degree than methoxyflurane. This decreases the likelihood of nephrotoxicity and hepatotoxicity. However, enflurane at high concentrations may induce seizures. Enflurane's induced epileptic activity can be treated by decreasing its dose and by inducing hypercarbia. Caution must be exercised in that this may have a deleterious effect in patients with increased ICP.[1-4]

Malignant Hyperthermia. Malignant hyperthermia (MH) is an inherited autosomal dominant metabolic disorder of the muscle. MH is triggered by succinylcholine and specific volatile anesthetics such as halothane, isoflurane, sevoflurane, desflurane, enflurane, and methoxyflurane. These agents produce a biochemical chain reaction that leads to a skeletal muscle hypermetabolic response. N_2O and xenon are not triggering agents for MH. Signs and symptoms include muscle rigidity, tachycardia, hyperthermia, combined metabolic and respiratory acidosis, and hyperkalemia.

The treatment of this lethal condition is carried out with the avoidance of triggering agents, IV administration of dantrolene, cold fluids, correction of the acidosis, oxygenation with a fractional concentration of oxygen of 1, and administration of mannitol to force diuresis and improve urine output since rhabdomyolysis results in myoglobinuria, and myoglobinuria will lead to renal failure. Another late complication can be disseminated intravascular coagulation and recurrence of MH.

Since MH is an inherited condition, it is imperative to perform a thorough preoperative anesthesiology exam and obtain the patient's family history and complications from previous anesthetics. It is important to remember that MH episodes have been reported even in patients who had no MH complications from previous anesthetics.[12]

Intravenous Anesthetics and Sedatives

Intravenous anesthetics are postulated to work primarily through three receptor systems. Sedative and hypnotic effects can be mediated through the GABA receptor system, an important inhibitory neurotransmitter system in the CNS. When the GABA type A ($GABA_A$) receptor is activated, it increases chloride conductance in the postsynaptic cell membrane, causing hyperpolarization and inhibition. Barbiturates, benzodiazepines, propofol, and etomidate, acting at different sites on the receptor, enhance the effect of GABA on the receptor (see Fig. 60-3).

The glutamate receptor, activated by glutamate or its analogue NMDA, increases the flux of cations (Na^+, K^+, and Ca^{2+}), leading to an excitatory response. The postsynaptic neuron becomes depolarized, and there is initiation of an action potential. Ketamine primarily acts as an antagonist at the NDMA receptor.

The α_2-adrenergic receptors in the CNS inhibit norepinephrine release. Dexmedetomidine, an α_2-agonist, produces sedation and analgesia.

Barbiturates. Barbiturates are a class of organic compounds that were developed in the late 19th century and first introduced for medical use in 1934. Barbiturates produce a wide spectrum of CNS depression, from mild sedation to coma, and have been used as sedatives, hypnotics, anesthetics, and anticonvulsants. The primary differences among many of these products are how fast they produce an effect and how long the effect lasts, so barbiturates have been classified as ultrashort, short, intermediate, and long-acting.

Thiopental (5-ethyl-5-[1-methylbutyl]-2-thiobarbituric acid; Pentothal), methohexital (1-methyl-5-allyl-5-[1-methyl-2-pentynyl]-barbituric acid; Brevital), and thiamylal (5-allyl-5-[1-methylbutyl]-2-thiobarbituric acid; Surital) are the three ultra-short-acting barbiturates in use for anesthesia. Other short-acting and intermediate-acting barbiturates include amobarbital (Amytal), pentobarbital (Nembutal), secobarbital (Seconal and Tuinal, an amobarbital/secobarbital combination product), butalbital (Fiorina), butabarbital (Butisol), talbutal (Lotusate), and aprobarbital (Alurate). Long-acting barbiturates include phenobarbital (Luminal) and mephobarbital (Mebaral).

Barbiturates for injection are formulated as sodium salts with 6% sodium carbonate and reconstituted in water or isotonic saline to produce 1% (methohexital), 2% (thiamylal), or 2.5% (thiopental) alkaline solutions with pHs of 10 to 11. The basic pH of the solutions can lead to precipitation of the barbiturate if it is coadministered with more acidic medications. In addition, these solutions can produce necrosis if they are inadvertently infiltrated into the subcutaneous tissues or intra-arterially. They should be injected into a freely running IV line, and a small test dose should be administered while observing the patient for evidence of pain on injection.

An induction dose of thiopental (3 to 5 mg/kg) produces unconsciousness in 10 to 30 seconds, with a peak effect in 1 minute and duration of anesthesia of 5 to 8 minutes (Table 60-2). Neonates and infants usually require a higher induction dose of 5 to 8 mg/kg, whereas elderly and pregnant patients require lower doses of 1 to 3 mg/kg.[13-15] Doses can be reduced by 10% to 50% after premedication with other hypnotics or opiates.[16-18] Thiamylal is approximately equipotent with thiopental, while methohexital is threefold more potent (induction dose of 1 to 2 mg/kg); both are otherwise similar to thiopental in onset and duration of action.

In addition to being used for induction of anesthesia, barbiturates have been used for the treatment of status epilepticus. However, methohexital may lower the seizure threshold and has been used as an anesthetic for electroconvulsive therapy.[19,20]

Thiopental decreases cerebral metabolism, cerebral oxygen consumption, CBF, and ICP.[21,22] This decrease in cerebral metabolism has been demonstrated to have potential effects in decreasing ischemic damage.[23,24] Thiopental is typically given as a single dose for induction of anesthesia. Thiopental has a beta-phase half-life of 12.1 hours, clearance of 3.4 ml/min per kilogram, is 85% protein bound, and has a volume of distribution at steady state of 2.3 L/kg. The minimal hypnotic level in plasma is 15.6 mcg/ml.

Methohexital is typically given as a single dose for induction of anesthesia. Methohexital has a beta-phase half-life of 3.6 hours, clearance of 10.9 ml/min per kilogram, is 85% protein bound, and has a volume of distribution at steady state of 2.2 L/kg. The minimal hypnotic level in plasma is 10 mcg/ml. Hepatic disease or other conditions that reduce serum protein concentration will decrease the volume of distribution and increase the initial free fraction and effect of a given dose. This can result in an increased effect.

Anesthetic duration after single doses is limited by redistribution of these hydrophobic drugs from the brain to other tissues. After multiple doses or infusions, the duration of action of the barbiturates depends on their clearances. Thiopental and thiamylal can produce unconsciousness for hours to days after long infusions or repeated boluses. Single induction doses of thiopental and to a lesser degree methohexital can produce measurable psychomotor impairment 8 hours later.[28]

Barbiturates are primarily eliminated by hepatic metabolism and renal excretion of inactive metabolites.

Barbiturates may produce excitement phenomena demonstrated as hypertonus or tremor. They produce dose-dependent decreases in blood pressure secondary to both vasodilation and decreased cardiac motility. There may be a reflex tachycardia. Barbiturates decrease respiratory response to hypercarbia and hypoxia and may produce apnea. They have minimal effect on bronchomotor tone. Barbiturates are contraindicated in patients with acute intermittent porphyria as they may produce fatal attacks of porphyria. Allergic reactions to barbitu-

TABLE 60-2 CHARACTERISTICS OF INTRAVENOUS ANESTHETICS AND SEDATIVES

Drug	Metabolism/Elimination	Dose	Therapeutic Considerations	Notes
Propofol (Diprivan and generic)	Hepatic hydroxylation to inactive metabolite; high clearance	Induction: 1.5-2.5 mg/kg Sedation: 40-100 mcg/kg/min Maintenance of anesthesia: 100-300 mcg/kg/min	May be used for long infusions or repeated bolus without prolonging recovery.	May cause burning at site of infusion.
Fospropofol (Aquavan)	Hepatic hydroxylation to inactive metabolite	Induction: 7.5-12.5 mg/kg	Perineal paresthesias.	Water-soluble prodrug of propofol; associated with lower peak concentrations.
Ketamine (Ketalar and generic)	Hepatic demethylation to active nor-ketamine; subsequent further metabolism and renal excretion	Induction: 0.5-1.5 mg/kg IV; 4-6 mg/kg IM Maintenance of anesthesia: 25-100 mcg/kg/min	Dissociative anesthesia; increases secretions; potent analgesia; maintains respiratory drive; increases HR and BP secondary to increased sympathetic tone.	Postoperative dysphoria may be decreased by coadministration with benzodiazepine or propofol.
Etomidate (Amidate)	Hepatic hydrolysis to inactive compounds	Induction: 0.2-0.4 mg/kg Maintenance of anesthesia: 5-10 mcg/kg/min	Stable hemodynamics; increased nausea and vomiting; inhibits adrenal synthesis of corticosteroids.	May cause pain on injection; frequent myoclonic movements.
Thiopental (Pentothal)	Hepatic oxidation, *N*-dealkylation, desulfuration, barbituric ring destruction	Induction: 3-5 mg/kg	Action after a single dose or short infusions terminated by redistribution. Longer infusions associated with prolonged time to awakening.	Can self-induce hepatic enzymes. Should not be used in patients with acute intermittent porphyria.
Thiamylal (Surital)	See Thiopental	Induction: 3-5 mg/kg	See Thiopental	See Thiopental
Methohexitol (Brevital)	See Thiopental; clearance 3 times thiopental	Induction: 1-2 mg/kg	See Thiopental	See Thiopental
Midazolam (Versed and generic)	Hepatic CYP 3A4 oxidation	Sedation: 0.3-0.7 mg/kg Induction: 0.3-0.35 mg/kg; Reduce initial dose by 50% if given with premedication, age >55, or ASA PS 3-4		
Dexmedetomidine (Precedex)	Hepatic glucuronidation and CYP-mediated hydroxylation	Loading dose: 1 mcg/kg over 20 min Maintenance of sedation: 0.2-0.7 mcg/kg/hr	Too rapid a loading dose causes hypertension.	Approved for ICU sedation up to 24 hr.

BP, blood pressure; CYP, cytochrome P-450; HR, heart rate; ICU, intensive care unit; IM, intramuscularly; IV, intravenously.

rates are rare, but they may release histamine via a direct drug action. Barbiturates are not triggering agents for MH.[26]

Benzodiazepines. Benzodiazepines have anxiolytic, sedative, amnestic, hypnotic, anticonvulsant, and muscle relaxant properties. The benzodiazepines act at specific binding sites on the $GABA_A$ receptor to increase sensitivity of the receptor to GABA. The commonly available parenteral drugs include midazolam (short acting), diazepam (intermediate acting), and lorazepam (long acting). Flumazenil is a benzodiazepine antagonist with a short duration of action. These drugs find broad use both as primary agents and as adjuncts to a balanced anesthetic technique.

Midazolam. Midazolam is a short-acting CNS depressant used for sedation/anxiolysis/amnesia for procedures. Sedation in adult and pediatric patients is achieved within 3 to 5 minutes after IV injection, and 15 minutes after intramuscular (IM) administration. When midazolam is given IV as an anesthetic induction agent, induction of anesthesia occurs in approximately 1.5 minutes when narcotic premedication has been administered and in 2 to 2.5 minutes without narcotic premedication.[26a]

Midazolam reliably produces amnesia in patients. In one adult study, when tested the following day, 73% of the patients who received midazolam IM had no recall of memory cards shown 30 minutes following drug administration; 40% had no recall of the memory cards shown 60 minutes following drug administration. In pediatric patients, up to 85% to 91% had no recall of pictures shown after receiving midazolam compared with 5% of the placebo controls and 35% with fentanyl alone. Seventy-one percent of the patients in endoscopy studies had no recall of introduction of the endoscope; 82% of the patients had no recall of withdrawal of the endoscope.

While classified as a short-acting agent, the effects may persist for some hours after administration. Midazolam, used as directed, does not delay awakening from general anesthesia in adults. Gross tests of recovery after awakening (orientation, ability to stand and walk, suitability for discharge from the recovery room, return to baseline Trieger competency) usually indicate recovery within 2 hours, but recovery may take up to 6 hours in some cases. When compared with patients who received thiopental, patients who received midazolam generally recovered at a slightly slower rate. Intravenous midazolam is associated with a moderate decrease in CSF pressure, but does not blunt the rise in ICP associated with intubation.

Midazolam's activity is primarily due to the parent drug. Elimination of the parent drug takes place via hepatic metabolism of midazolam to hydroxylated metabolites that are conjugated and excreted in the urine. Pharmacokinetic parameters for midazolam are in the following ranges: volume of distribution (Vd), 1.0 to 3.1 L/kg; elimination half-life, 1.8 to 6.4 hours (mean approximately 3 hours); total clearance, 0.25 to 0.54 L/hr per kilogram. Kinetics were linear up to 0.3 mg/kg, and clearance decreased by approximately 30% with doses of 0.45 to 0.6 mg/kg. The mean peak concentration (C_{max}) and time to peak concentration (T_{max}) following the IM dose was 90 ng/mL (20% coefficient of variation [CV]) and 0.5 hr (50% CV), respectively. Following IM administration, C_{max} for midazolam and its 1-hydroxy metabolite were approximately one half of those achieved after IV injection. The Vd determined in healthy adults ranged from 1.0 to 3.1 L/kg. Female gender, old age, and obesity are associated with increased values of midazolam Vd. In humans, midazolam has been shown to cross the placenta and enter into fetal circulation, and has been detected in human milk; CSF protein binding is approximately 97%.

The biotransformation of midazolam is mediated by cytochrome P-450 isoenzyme 3A4. 1-Hydroxymidazolam (also termed α-hydroxymidazolam) is 60% to 70% of the biotransformation products, while 4-hydroxy-midazolam constitutes 5% or less. Drugs that inhibit the activity of cytochrome P-450 isoenzyme 3A4 may inhibit midazolam clearance and elevate steady state midazolam concentrations. Clearance of midazolam is reduced in association with old age, congestive heart failure, liver disease (cirrhosis), or conditions that diminish cardiac output and hepatic blood flow. The principal urinary excretion product is 1-hydroxymidazolam in the form of a glucuronide conjugate; smaller amounts of the glucuronide conjugates of 4-hydroxymidazolam and dihydroxymidazolam are detected as well. Midazolam can accumulate in peripheral tissues with continuous infusion, and the effects are greater after long-term infusions than after short-term infusions.

In pediatric patients age 1 year and older, the pharmacokinetic properties following a single dose of midazolam are similar to those in adults. Weight-normalized clearance is similar to or higher (0.19 to 0.80 L/hr per kilogram) than in adults, and the terminal elimination half-life (0.78 to 3.3 hours) is similar to or shorter than in adults. In seriously ill neonates, however, the terminal elimination half-life of midazolam is substantially prolonged (6.5 to 12.0 hours) and the clearance reduced (0.07 to 0.12 L/hr per kilogram) compared to healthy adults or other groups of pediatric patients.

In a study comparing normal and obese patients, the mean half-life was greater in the obese group (5.9 vs. 2.3 hours). This was due to an increase of approximately 50% in the Vd corrected for total body weight. The clearance was not significantly different between groups. Plasma half-life is approximately twofold higher in the elderly. The mean Vd based on total body weight increased between 15% and 100% and mean clearance decreased approximately 25% in the elderly. In patients suffering from congestive heart failure, there appeared to be a twofold increase in the elimination half-life, a 25% decrease in the plasma clearance, and a 40% increase in the volume of distribution of midazolam. The mean half-life of midazolam increased 2.5-fold in patients with alchoholic cirrhosis. Clearance was reduced by 50% and the Vd increased by 20%.

Patients with renal impairment may have longer elimination half-lives for midazolam and its metabolites, which may result in slower recovery. Midazolam clearance was reduced (1.9 vs 2.8 ml/min per kilogram) and the half-life was prolonged (7.6 vs 13 hours) in patients with acute renal failure (ARF) who received a midazolam infusion. The renal clearance of the 1-hydroxymidazolam glucuronide was prolonged in the ARF group (4 vs. 136 ml/min) and the half-life was prolonged (12 vs. > 25 hours). Plasma levels accumulated in all ARF patients to about 10 times that of the parent drug. The relationship between accumulating metabolite levels and prolonged sedation is unclear. In a study of 15 chronic renal failure patients receiving a single IV dose, there was a twofold increase in the clearance and volume of distribution but the half-life remained unchanged.

Concentration-effect relationships (after an IV dose) have been demonstrated for a variety of pharmacodynamic measures (e.g., reaction time, eye movement, sedation). At plasma concentrations greater than 100 ng/mL, there is at least a 50% probability that patients will be sedated but responsive to verbal commands (sedation score = 3). At 200 ng/mL, there is at least a 50% probability that patients will be asleep but responsive to glabellar tap (sedation score = 4).

Caution is advised when midazolam is administered concomitantly with drugs that are known to inhibit the cytochrome P-450 3A4 isoenzyme system, such as cimetidine, erythromycin, diltiazem, verapamil, ketoconazole, and itraconazole. These drug interactions may result in prolonged sedation due to a decrease in plasma clearance of midazolam. Cimetidine 800 mg increased the mean midazolam steady state concentration from 57 to 71 ng/mL. Erythromycin administered as a 500-mg dose three times a day for 1 week reduced the clearance of midazolam following a single 0.5-mg/kg IV dose, and the half-life was approximately doubled. The half-life of midazolam increased from 5 to 7 hours when midazolam was taken in conjunction with verapamil or diltiazem.

Hypotension occurs more frequently in the sedation studies in patients premedicated with a narcotic. Reactions such as agitation, involuntary movements (including tonic-clonic movements and muscle tremor), hyperactivity, and combativeness have been reported in both adult and pediatric patients. These reactions may be due to inadequate or excessive dosing or improper administration of midazolam; however, consideration should be given to the possibility of cerebral hypoxia or true paradoxical reactions.

Diazepam and Lorazepam. Diazepam and lorazepam have a low solubility in water and are formulated in propylene glycol, which can irritate veins on administration. Diazepam is frequently administered orally 30 to 60 minutes prior to a procedure. A single sleep dose of diazepam, 0.3 to 0.6 mg/kg, will have a duration of 15 to 45 minutes while a lorazepam dose of 0.03 to 0.06 mg/kg will have a duration of 60 to 120 minutes. The amnestic effects of the lorazepam may last much longer.

As with midazolam, diazepam and lorazepam undergo hepatic metabolism (oxidation and glucuronidation). The primary metabolites of diazepam, desmethyldiazepam and 3-hydroxydiazepam, are active and may contribute to prolonged or residual drug effect. Liver disease and hepatic dysfunction are associated with decreased clearance of diazepam.

Reversal with Flumazenil. Flumazenil, a specific benzodiazepine receptor antagonist, is indicated for the complete or partial reversal of the sedative effects of benzodiazepines.[26b] There are anecdotal reports of reversal of adverse hemodynamic responses associated with midazolam following administration of flumazenil. Patients treated with flumazenil should be monitored for resedation, respiratory depression, and other residual benzodiazepine effects for an appropriate period after treatment. The reversal of benzodiazepine effects may be associated with the onset of seizures in certain high-risk patients, particularly in long-term benzodiazepine users.

α-Agonists. α_2-Adrenergic receptors in the brain are associated with sedation and analgesia.

Clonidine was demonstrated to act as an adjunct to anesthesia, providing sedation and decreased opioid requirements.[27,28] Dexmedetomidine was developed as an α_2-selective agent with a relatively short half-life. It is approved for use as a short-term sedative in critically ill adults. It produces a state of sedation that is characterized by the ability to easily arouse the patient, but is not a good amnestic agent. It can produce analgesia and significantly reduce the amount of opioid required for a procedure.[29] It does not produce significant respiratory depression at clinical doses.[30]

Dexmedetomidine is administered as a continuous infusion. The loading dose is 1 mcg/kg administered over 10 to 20 minutes, followed by an infusion at a rate of 0.2 to 0.7 mcg/kg per hour. The distribution and terminal half-lives are 6 minutes and 2 hours, respectively.[31] Dexmedetomidine is highly protein bound and is primarily hepatically metabolized; the glucuronide and methyl conjugates are renally excreted.[32] Use is associated with bradycardia and hypotension. Doses should be adjusted in patients at risk for severe hypotension. Administration of the initial loading dose too rapidly may activate α_{2B} receptors, causing a marked hypertension that may further aggravate the bradycardia through reflex systems. The drug has also been associated with nausea.

Atipamezole is a competitive α_2-antagonist that is in use in veterinary medicine for the reversal of sedation produced by drugs like dexmedetomidine. It has been shown to be able to reverse the effects of dexmedetomidine in human volunteers.[33,34]

Propofol. Propofol (2,6-diisopropylphenol; Diprivan and others) was developed in the 1970s and is now the most widely used IV anesthetic. It has many characteristics of an ideal agent, including rapid onset, predictable duration whether given as a bolus or by infusion, low organ toxicity, few residual effects on recovery, and compatibility with a wide range of drugs commonly used in the setting of anesthesia. Initially formulated in Cremophor EL due to its low solubility in water, the use of propofol was limited by reactions to this carrier. It was subsequently reformulated in a lipid emulsion of 10% soybean oil with egg phosphatide as an emulsifier.

When administered as an IV bolus of 1.5 to 2 mg/kg, onset of unconsciousness is within 30-60 seconds, with a duration of 6 to 8 minutes. The dose should be reduced in the elderly and when administered with other sedatives or opioids. Propofol may be used for the maintenance of anesthesia or for continuous sedation. An infusion of 100 to 300 mcg/kg per minute, adjusted to effect, will provide maintenance, and a dose of 20 to 100 mcg/kg per minute can provide good sedation and amnesia. The rapid clearance of propofol and lack of active metabolites contibute to a rapid recovery and lack of "hangover" after anesthesia.

Propofol may be given as a single dose for induction or by continuous infusion for sedation and maintenance of anesthesia. Propofol has a beta-phase half-life of 1.8 hours and a high clearance of 30 ml/min per kilogram, is 98% protein bound, and has a Vd at steady state of 2.3 L/kg. The minimal hypnotic level in plasma is 1.1 mcg/ml. Propofol is metabolized in the liver to less active metabolites that are renally excreted.[35] Anhepatic metabolism, with decreased levels across the pulmonary circulation, has been demonstrated.[36]

Propofol decreases $CMRO_2$, CBF, and intracranial and intraocular pressures.[37] There are no human outcome studies of the potential neuroprotectant effect of propofol, however. Propofol has not been shown to effectively treat seizures; some data even suggest it has proconvulsant activity.[19,20]

Grounds et al.[38] studied the hemodynamic changes following induction of anesthesia with equipotent doses of propofol and pentothal. Propofol caused a significant fall in arterial blood pressure and total peripheral resistance, with a slight fall in cardiac output and no changes in heart rate. These effects were somewhat greater than the changes with pentothal.[38]

Propofol is a respiratory depressant, and facilities for airway management and support of ventilation should be available when it is used for sedation or anesthesia. Propofol 2.5 mg/kg produces slightly more respiratory depression than thiopental 4 mg/kg.[39] It has no clinically significant effects on hepatic, renal, or endocrine organ systems.

Propofol has significant antiemetic action and reduces the risk for nausea and vomiting.[40,41] Propofol elicits pain on injection that can be severe. The pain can most effectively be reduced with preinjection of lidocaine 40 mg during venous occlusion, or by mixing lidocaine with the propofol.[42] Excitatory phenomena during induction with propofol are observed and occur at about the same frequency as with thiopental.[37]

Fospropofol. Fospropofol (GPI 15715, AQUAVAN injection) is a new water-soluble prodrug that is hydrolyzed to release propofol. Unlike propofol, which is formulated in an oil- or lipid-based emulsion, fospropofol is formulated in a clear aqueous solution and is rapidly converted by alkaline phosphatase into propofol after IV injection.

In a trial of healthy male volunteers (ages 19 to 35, 67 to 102 kg), all subjects experienced loss of consciousness after an infusion of 1160 mg, with propofol concentrations of 2.1 ± 0.6 mcg/ml. Compared with propofol lipid emulsion, the potency seemed to be higher with respect to plasma concentration but was apparently less with respect to dose. Pharmacokinetic simulations showed a longer time to peak propofol concentration after a bolus dose and a longer context-sensitive half-time.[43]

Fospropofol may be given as a single dose for induction or by continuous infusion for sedation and maintenance of anesthesia. Fospropofol has a beta-phase half-life of 0.75 hour and clearance of 70 ml/min per kilogram.[43]

Phencyclidines: Ketamine. Ketamine has unique properties, including intense analgesia while maintaining spontaneous respiration, and unique side effects such as dysphoria that limit its utility. These effects appear to be mediated in part through blockade of the NMDA receptor. An induction dose of 0.5 to 1.5 mg/kg IV produces rapid onset of a dissociative anesthesia characterized by analgesia, amnesia, and lack of responsiveness to commands. This state of catalepsy is mediated by inhibition of thalamocortical pathways and limbic stimulation. The patient may have his or her eyes open, may exhibit involuntary motions of the limbs, and generally will maintain an airway and spontaneous respiration. Ketamine may also be administered at doses of 4 to 6 mg/kg IM or 8 to 10 mg per rectum, with a slower onset and longer duration of action. The effect may be maintained by intermittent boluses or a continuous infusion of 25 to 100 mcg/kg per minute.[44]

Ketamine is typically given as a single dose for induction of anesthesia. Ketamine has a beta-phase half-life of 3 hours and a clearance of 19.1 ml/min per kilogram, is 27% protein bound, and has a Vd at steady state of 3.1 L/kg. The minimal hypnotic level in plasma is 1 mcg/ml.

The psychomimetic effects and dysphoria may be decreased by limiting the dose or by coadministration of benzodiazepines or propofol. Ketamine has been associated with increases in CBF and ICP, which can be blunted when administered with a barbiturate.

Etomidate. Etomidate was developed by Janssen Pharmaceutica in 1964 and came into clinical use in 1974. It is a substituted imidazole that is poorly soluble in water. It was formulated as a 2-mg/ml solution in 35% propylene glycol. Pain on administration and potential for hemolysis to the propylene glycol carrier have led to efforts to develop a lipid-based formulation in Europe.

Etomidate can be used for induction of anesthesia (0.2 to 0.4 mg/kg) and maintenance of short cases (10 mcg/kg per minute). Trials of the drug for intensive care unit sedation led to the discovery of adrenal suppression as a side effect. Etomidate augments GABA-gated chloride currents.

Etomidate is typically given as a single dose for induction of anesthesia and has a rapid onset. Redistribution (half-life 2 to 5 minutes) limits the duration of action of a single dose. The minimal hypnotic level in plasma is 0.3 mcg/ml. Etomidate has a beta-phase half-life of 2.9 hours and a clearance of 17.9 ml/min per kilogram, is 76% protein bound, and has a Vd at steady state of 2.5 L/kg. Hepatic metabolism is primarily to inactive compounds, with renal (78%) and biliary (22%) elimination.[45]

Etomidate is often selected over other induction agents when cardiovascular stability is important. Etomidate typically produces a small increase in heart rate and little or no decrease in blood pressure or cardiac output.[46]

Pain on injection and myoclonus are frequently observed.[47] Etomidate reduces CBF, metabolism, and intracranial and intraocular pressures.[48] Etomidate has been shown in some studies to be a proconvulsant.[20] Etomidate has been associated with nausea and vomiting.[49]

Etomidate inhibits adrenal biosynthetic enzymes required for the production of cortisol and some other steroids, possibly inhibiting the adrenocortical stress response.[50] Even single induction doses of etomidate may mildly and transiently reduce cortisol levels, but no differences in outcomes were observed.[51]

REFERENCES

1. Morgan GE, Mikhail MS. Clinical Anesthesiology, 2nd ed. Stamford, CT: Appleton & Lange, 1996.
2. Stoelting RK. Pharmacology and Physiology in Anesthetic Practice, 3rd ed. Philadelphia: Lippincott–Raven Publishers, 1999.
3. Miller RD, Fleisher LA, Johns RA, et al (eds). Miller's Anesthesia, 6th ed. Philadelphia: Elsevier Churchill Livingstone, 2005.
4. Goto T. Is there a future for xenon anesthesia? Can J Anaesth 2002;49:335-338.
5. Luttropp HH, Thomasson R, Dahm S, et al. Clinical experience with minimal flow xenon anesthesia. Acta Anaesthesiol Scand 1994;38:121-125.
6. Lynch C 3rd, Baum J, Tenbrinck R. Xenon anesthesia. Anesthesiology 2000;92:865-868.
7. Goodman Gilman A, et al. (eds). Goodman and Gilman's The Pharmacological Basis of Therapeutics, 8th ed. New York: Pergamon Press, 1990.
8. Eger EI 2nd. Age, minimum alveolar anesthetic concentration, and minimum alveolar anesthetic concentration–awake. Anesth Analg 2001;93:947-953.
9. Berghaus TM, Baron A, Geier A, et al. Hepatotoxicity following desflurane anesthesia. Hepatology 1999;29:613-614.
10. Suprane Volatile Liquid for Inhalation. Drugs.com, 2007. Available at *http://www.drugs.com/pro/suprane.html* (accessed May 15, 2007).
11. Martin JL, Plevak DJ, Flannery KD, et al. Hepatotoxicity after desflurane anesthesia. Anesthesiology 1995;83:1125-1129.
12. Malignant Hyperthermia Association of the United States (MHAUS) web site, 2007. Available at *http://www.mhaus.org/index.cfm/fuseaction/Content.Display/PagePK/Home.cfm* (accessed April 30, 2007).
13. Gin T, Mainland P, Chan MT, Short TG. Decreased thiopental requirements in early pregnancy. Anesthesiology 1997;86:73-78.
14. Homer TD, Stanski DR. The effect of increasing age on thiopental disposition and anesthetic requirement. Anesthesiology 1985;62:714-724.
15. Jonmarker C, Westrin P, Larsson S, Werner O. Thiopental requirements for induction of anesthesia in children. Anesthesiology 1987;67:104-107.
16. Nishina K, Mikawa K, Maekawa N, et al. Clonidine decreases the dose of thiamylal required to induce anesthesia in children. Anesth Analg 1994;79:766-768.
17. Short TG, Galletly DC, Plummer JL. Hypnotic and anaesthetic action of thiopentone and midazolam alone and in combination. Br J Anaesth 1991;66:13-19.
18. Wang LP, Hermann C, Westrin P. Thiopentone requirements in adults after varying pre-induction doses of fentanyl. Anaesthesia 1996;51:831-835.
19. Modica PA, Tempelhoff R, White PF. Pro- and anticonvulsant effects of anesthetics (Part I). Anesth Analg 1990;70:303-315.
20. Modica PA, Tempelhoff R, White PF. Pro- and anticonvulsant effects of anesthetics (Part II). Anesth Analg 1990;70:433-444.
21. Shapiro HM, Galindo A, Wyte SR, Harris AB. Rapid intraoperative reduction of intracranial pressure with thiopentone. Br J Anaesth 1973;45:1057-1062.
22. Stullken EH Jr, Milde JH, Michenfelder JD, Tinker JH. The nonlinear responses of cerebral metabolism to low concentrations of halothane, enflurane, isoflurane, and thiopental. Anesthesiology 1977;46:28-34.
23. Nussmeier NA, Arlund C, Slogoff S. Neuropsychiatric complications after cardiopulmonary bypass: cerebral protection by a barbiturate. Anesthesiology 1986;64:165-170.
24. Smith AL, Hoff JT, Nielsen SL, Larson CP. Barbiturate protection in acute focal cerebral ischemia. Stroke 1974;5:1-7.
25. Korttila K, Linnoila M, Ertama P, Hakkinen S. Recovery and simulated driving after intravenous anesthesia with thiopental, methohexital, propanidid, or alphadione. Anesthesiology 1975;43:291-299.
26. Rosenberger AD, Treudler R, Blume-Peytavi U, et al. [Allergies and pseudoallergic reactions to anesthetics: the clinical symptoms, risk factors and the diagnostic possibilities]. Hautarzt 1997;48:791-799.

26a. Reves JG, Fragen RJ, Vinik HR, Greenblatt DJ. Midazolam: pharmacology and uses. Anesthesiology 1985;62:24.

26b. Brogden RN, Goa KL. Flumazenil. A reappraisal of its pharmacological properties and therapeutic efficacy as a benzodiazepine antagonist. Drugs 1991;42:1061-1089.

27. Ghignone M, Quintin L, Duke PC, et al. Effects of clonidine on narcotic requirements and hemodynamic response during induction of fentanyl anesthesia and endotracheal intubation. Anesthesiology 1986;64:36-42.
28. Imai Y, Mammoto T, Murakami K, et al. The effects of preanesthetic oral clonidine on total requirement of propofol for general anesthesia. J Clin Anesth 1998;10:660-665.
29. Aho M, Lehtinen AM, Erkola O, et al. The effect of intravenously administered dexmedetomidine on perioperative hemodynamics and isoflurane requirements in patients undergoing abdominal hysterectomy. Anesthesiology 1991;74:997-1002.
30. Belleville JP, Ward DS, Bloor BC, Maze M. Effects of intravenous dexmedetomidine in humans. I. Sedation, ventilation, and metabolic rate. Anesthesiology 1992;77:1125-1133.
31. Khan ZP, Munday IT, Jones RM, et al. Effects of dexmedetomidine on isoflurane requirements in healthy volunteers. 1: Pharmacodynamic and pharmacokinetic interactions. Br J Anaesth 1999;83:372-380.
32. Bhana N, Goa KL, McClellan KJ. Dexmedetomidine. Drugs 2000;59:263-268; discussion 269-270.
33. Karhuvaara S, Kallio A, Salonen M, et al. Rapid reversal of alpha 2-adrenoceptor agonist effects by atipamezole in human volunteers. Br J Clin Pharmacol 1991;31:160-165.
34. Scheinin H, Aantaa R, Anttila M, et al. Reversal of the sedative and sympatholytic effects of dexmedetomidine with a specific alpha2-adrenoceptor antagonist atipamezole: a pharmacodynamic and kinetic study in healthy volunteers. Anesthesiology 1998;89:574-584.
35. Simons PJ, Cockshott ID, Douglas EJ, et al. Disposition in male volunteers of a subanaesthetic intravenous dose of an oil in water emulsion of ^{14}C-propofol. Xenobiotica 1988;18:429-440.
36. Veroli P, O'Kelly B, Bertrand F, et al. Extrahepatic metabolism of propofol in man during the anhepatic phase of orthotopic liver transplantation. Br J Anaesth 1992;68:183-186.
37. Langley MS, Heel RC. Propofol: a review of its pharmacodynamic and pharmacokinetic properties and use as an intravenous anaesthetic. Drugs 1988;35:334-372.
38. Grounds RM, Twigley AJ, Carli F, et al. The haemodynamic effects of intravenous induction: comparison of the effects of thiopentone and propofol. Anaesthesia 1985;40:735-740.
39. Blouin RT, Conard PF, Gross JB. Time course of ventilatory depression following induction doses of propofol and thiopental. Anesthesiology 1991;75:940-944.
40. Apfel CC, Korttila K, Abdalla M, et al. A factorial trial of six interventions for the prevention of postoperative nausea and vomiting. N Engl J Med 2004;350:2441-2451.
41. McCollum JS, Milligan KR, Dundee JW. The antiemetic action of propofol. Anaesthesia 1988;43:239-240.
42. Picard P, Tramer MR. Prevention of pain on injection with propofol: a quantitative systematic review. Anesth Analg 2000;90:963-969.
43. Fechner J, Ihmsen H, Hatterscheid D, et al. Pharmacokinetics and clinical pharmacodynamics of the new propofol prodrug GPI 15715 in volunteers. Anesthesiology 2003;99:303-313.
44. White PF, Way WL, Trevor AJ. Ketamine—its pharmacology and therapeutic uses. Anesthesiology 1982;56:119-136.
45. Heykants JJ, Meuldermans WE, Michiels LJ, et al. Distribution, metabolism and excretion of etomidate, a short-acting hypnotic drug, in the rat: comparative study of (R)-(+)-(−)-etomidate. Arch Int Pharmacodyn Ther 1975;216:113-129.
46. Criado A, Maseda J, Navarro E, et al. Induction of anaesthesia with etomidate: haemodynamic study of 36 patients. Br J Anaesth 1980;52:803-806.
47. Gooding JM, Corssen G. Etomidate: an ultrashort-acting nonbarbiturate agent for anesthesia induction. Anesth Analg 1976;55:286-289.
48. Modica PA, Tempelhoff R. Intracranial pressure during induction of anaesthesia and tracheal intubation with etomidate-induced EEG burst suppression. Can J Anaesth 1992;39:236-241.
49. Fragen RJ, Caldwell N. Comparison of a new formulation of etomidate with thiopental—side effects and awakening times. Anesthesiology 1979;50:242-244.
50. Ledingham IM, Watt I. Influence of sedation on mortality in critically ill multiple trauma patients. Lancet 1983;1:1270.
51. Wagner RL, White PF. Etomidate inhibits adrenocortical function in surgical patients. Anesthesiology 1984;61:647-651.

61

TREATMENT OF PAIN

Kishor Gandhi, James W. Heitz, and Eugene R. Viscusi

INTRODUCTION 883
THERAPEUTICS AND CLINICAL PHARMACOLOGY 883
Multimodal Therapy 883
Therapeutic Goals in Pain Management 883
Central Sensitization and Preemptive Analgesia 884
Barriers to Effective Analgesia 884
WHO Analgesic Ladder 884
Therapeutics by Class 885
Opioid Agonists 885
Mixed Opioid Agonist-Antagonists 888
Opioid Antagonists 888
Nonopioid Analgesics 889
Anticonvulsants 890
Antidepressants 891
Local Anesthetics 891
N-Methyl-D-Aspartate Receptor Antagonist 891
α_2-Adrenergic Receptor Agonist 891
CONCLUSION 892

"Divine is the work to subdue pain."

Hippocrates

INTRODUCTION

The amelioration of suffering is a therapeutic objective that crosses the traditional boundaries of medical specialties. To varying extents, most clinicians in medicine and allied medical professions will be confronted with the treatment of pain in one form or another. From the patient's perspective, the fear of pain when approaching surgery or illness may be as great as the fear of death, disfigurement, and disability. Many patients additionally fear the *treatment* of pain because of side effects or concerns regarding addiction to medication. From a societal perspective, pain costs the U.S. economy an estimated $61 billion each year in lost worker productivity.[1]

The word *pain* is derived from the Latin word *poena*, meaning penalty. Pain refers to any unpleasant sensation and can range from mild to agonizing. It is a subjective experience that defies objective measurement. The equivalent stimulus can produce very different perceptions of pain between individuals or even within the same individual at different times. In some conditions, normally nonpainful sensations such as light touch may be perceived as pain, a symptom referred to as allodynia.

Despite the complexity and subjectiveness of the pain experience, it is possible to divide pain into three broad categories: nociceptive pain, neuropathic pain, and psychogenic pain. Nociceptive pain is somatic or visceral pain caused by injury to body tissues. Neuropathic pain originates from abnormality of peripheral nerves or the central nervous system (CNS). Psychogenic pain is primarily or entirely related to a psychological disorder. Pain is also often referred to as acute (lasting less than 3 months) or chronic (lasting greater than 3 months), which can profoundly influence the choice of pharmacologic agents used for treatment.

Nociceptive pain is the most common type of pain seen in an acute care setting. Somatic nociceptive pain is classically described as stabbing or aching pain. It is usually well localized when it originates from skin or subcutaneous tissue and may be less well localized when it originates from bone, muscle, or other connective tissue. Bone fractures, bone metastases, surgical incisions, lacerations, and arthritic joint pain would all be examples of somatic pain. Visceral nociceptive pain originates from visceral organs or cavity linings. As such, it is much harder to localize and is often described as dull or crampy pain. Pain from distention of bowel or bladder and organ metastases are examples of visceral pain. Neuropathic pain is often described as a burning, tingling, or "electrical shock" sensation. Examples of neuropathic pain include peripheral neuropathies (diabetic, human immunodeficiency virus related, and alcoholic), postherpetic neuralgia, phantom limb pain, and reflex sympathetic dystrophy.

While these classifications are the foundation upon which an approach to the treatment of pain is constructed, they are not mutually exclusive. An individual's pain may simultaneously have acute and chronic components and nociceptive, neuropathic, or psychological components. For example, most cancer pain is somatic or visceral nociceptive pain, but patients may have cancer-related neuropathic pain, which can result from direct mechanical compression of nervous tissue or from injury to nervous tissue from cancer treatment (surgical or chemotherapy).

The therapeutic armamentarium of the clinician is similarly complex. A broad variety of dissimilar pharmacologic agents are employed in the treatment of pain, often in combination with physical modalities (heat, cold, acupuncture, transcutaneous electrical nerve stimulation, and physical therapy) or other nonpharmacologic therapies (biofeedback relaxation training, distraction techniques, and hypnosis). The purpose of this chapter is not to provide an exhaustive summary of every possible drug that has some analgesic action. Rather, the major classes of clinically useful pain drugs are discussed in some detail.

THERAPEUTICS AND CLINICAL PHARMACOLOGY

Multimodal Therapy

Although clinicians generally strive to simplify drug regimens and treat most disorders with as few pharmacologic agents as possible, multimodal approaches to pain management offer several potential advantages. With a multimodal approach to pain, different components of the pain syndrome may be treated individually. Moreover, it is sometimes possible to minimize the dose-related side effects of pharmacologic agents by treating with several agents from different classes. This is particularly true when the therapeutic aim is to limit the dose of opioid-class medications. Nonopioid medications and physical modalities may be used to achieve sufficient analgesia without the need for large doses of opioids.

Therapeutic Goals in Pain Management

Providing analgesia is one of the chief aims of pain management, and from a humanitarian viewpoint is sufficient reason to treat pain. The

Joint Commission (formerly known as the Joint Commission on the Accreditation of Healthcare Organizations) implemented standards to assess and manage pain in 2001. Partly in response to a perception that pain was largely undertreated, the Joint Commission defined pain relief as a basic patient right, and the U.S. Congress declared 2001-2010 the "Decade of Pain Control and Research."[2]

However, the therapeutic goals in pain management often transcend simply providing analgesia. The treatment of acute postsurgical pain often includes the attempt to reduce morbidity and mortality and length of hospitalization, thereby also reducing hospital expenditures. Preventing or minimizing the development of chronic pain may also be a component of a well-designed acute pain care plan. Similarly, the treatment goals in chronic pain often extend beyond analgesia and often focus upon functional improvement, including improving quality of life, ability to perform activities of daily living, and return to work. A survey of 7000 physicians (family practice, internal medicine, neurology, neurosurgery, orthopedic surgery, physical medicine and rehabilitation, and rheumatology) involved in the treatment of chronic nonmalignant pain revealed that the majority do not view improvement in pain control solely as justification for the prescribing of opioids unless there is a concurrent improvement in function.[3]

To do no harm to the patient is a therapeutic goal in every medical intervention. In pain management, this includes attempting to minimize side effects related to medications and to minimize the risk of addiction. Many practitioners also recognize an ethical responsibility to "do no harm" to society as well and seek to minimize the risk of drug diversion.

Central Sensitization and Preemptive Analgesia

It has long been known that tissue injury produces both continuing pain and an increased sensitivity to further noxious stimuli, a phenomenon once erroneously believed to be due solely to excitation of peripheral receptors (peripheral sensitization). In 1983 in the journal *Nature*, Woolf[4] implicated changes at the spinal cord level in what is now known as central sensitization. Central sensitization involves an increase in excitatory neurotransmitter function at a presynaptic and a postsynaptic level, as well as a reduction in inhibitory neurotransmitter function and the loss of inhibitory interneurons.[5] These changes at the spinal cord level facilitate the transmission of pain. Secondary hyperalgesia (tenderness outside the area of tissue injury) and allodynia (pain from normally nonpainful stimulation) are both believed to be related to central sensitization. Central sensitization is involved in the development of chronic pain from acute injury as well as in many of the chronic pain syndromes that develop without preceding acute injury, such as fibromyalgia.

Preemptive analgesia is the attempt to intervene in the process of central sensitization in order to reduce the severity of acute pain and the subsequent development of chronic pain. Chronic pain develops in approximately half of patients undergoing thoracotomy or breast surgery and may be even more frequent among patients undergoing a limb amputation.[6] Efforts to prevent centralization by utilizing preemptive analgesia have yielded mixed results.

Barriers to Effective Analgesia

A survey of 897 medical oncologists, hematologists, surgeons, and radiation therapists involved in the care of cancer patients reported that 86% of these physicians believed that the majority of their patients were undermedicated for pain.[7] The most common barrier to adequate analgesia was ascribed to poor pain assessment (76%), but there was also both a patient reluctance to take analgesics (62%) and a physician reluctance to prescribe opioids (61%).

The irrational fear of opioids, or opiophobia, is just one of the multiple barriers that exist to achieving analgesia. Physicians may be reluctant to prescribe adequate doses of opioids for fear of precipitating serious side effects, such as ventilatory depression or sedation, or of masking significant changes in the patient's condition. Patients may fear taking opioids for fear of addiction or other side effects. More recently, prosecution of several physicians in the United States for excessive OxyContin prescribing has made some physicians hesitant to prescribe opioids.

These difficulties are further compounded by cultural and religious or medical attitudes toward pain and suffering. Patients may perceive taking pain medicine as an admission of weakness or vulnerability; physicians may mistakenly prescribe analgesia on the basis of perceived severity of disease and not the severity of the pain the patient experiences.

WHO Analgesic Ladder

The World Health Organization (WHO) introduced a flexible framework of principles in the approach to the treatment of cancer pain in 1986. The WHO Analgesic Ladder is a simplified three-step strategy that emphasizes "around-the-clock" dosing of medications as opposed to "as-needed" dosing[8] (Fig. 61-1). Step 1 of the ladder treats mild pain with nonopioid agents such as acetylsalicylic acid or a nonsteroidal anti-inflammatory drug (NSAID). Step 2 treats moderate pain with a weak opioid. More recent modifications of the Analgesic Ladder allow substitution of small doses of a potent opioid in place of the weak opioid. Step 3 treats severe pain with a potent opioid. On each step of the ladder, adjuvant agents may be used to improve analgesia and treat anxiety.

Although developed specifically to address the undertreatment of pain in cancer patients, the principles of the WHO Analgesic Ladder apply equally well to pain caused by nonmalignant conditions.[9] However, modification of the principles may be necessary when extending this therapeutic framework to other patient populations. While avoiding agents contraindicated in renal insufficiency, the WHO Analgesic Ladder principles have been used to achieve substantial improvement in pain symptoms among 96% of one series of end-stage renal disease patients.[10]

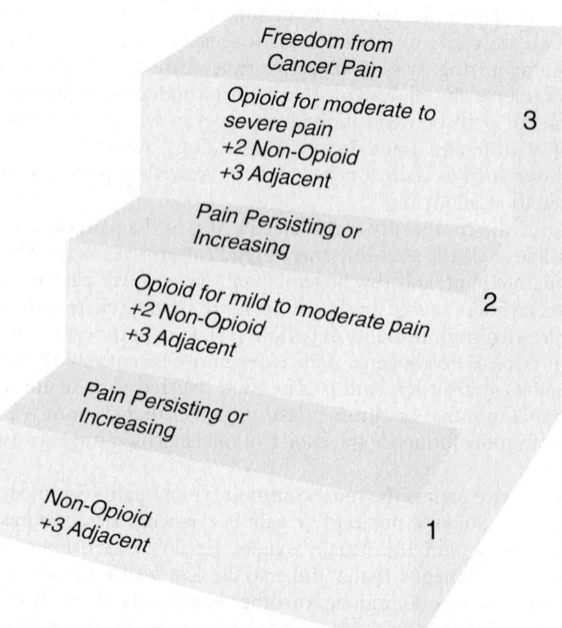

FIGURE 61-1 • World Health Organization stepwise approach to treatment of cancer pain. (From World Health Organization. Cancer Pain Relief and Palliative Care: Report of a WHO Expert Committee [Technical Report Series No. 804]. Geneva: World Health Organization, 1990.)

Therapeutics by Class

Opioid Agonists

Opioids form the second and third steps of the WHO Analgesic Ladder. Opioids mimic the actions of naturally occurring endogenous opioid ligands and bind to specific opioid receptors that were first identified in 1973. Since that time, a number of opioid receptors with various functions have been described.

Opioid receptors are divided into three classes: μ, δ, and κ. Previously identified σ- and γ-receptors are no longer considered to be opioid receptors. The binding of opioid agonists produces discrete effects depending upon the receptor involved. These receptors may be found in both ascending pain pathways and descending inhibitory pathways of the spinal cord and the brain and in the periphery. Spinal and supraspinal analgesia is produced by agonist binding to these receptors. Common opioid side effects are also produced by agonist binding to specific receptors, including depression of ventilation and physical dependence (μ_2, δ); constipation (μ_2); sedation (κ); miosis (μ_1, κ); and euphoria, bradycardia, and urinary retention (μ_1). Table 61-1 presents equianalgesic opioid dosing regimens for management of acute or chronic pain. These relative potencies can vary dramatically when converting from one opioid to another because of "incomplete cross-tolerance." Methadone potency varies dramatically in opioid-naive versus opioid-tolerant individuals. When converting from one opioid to another, as in opioid rotation, slow upward titration is generally practiced.

Morphine. Morphine derives its name from Morpheus, the Greek god of dreams. Although it was first isolated in the early 1800s, it was not until the development of the hypodermic needle in 1853 that morphine began to experience widespread clinical use. It is the prototype opioid to which other opioid agonists are compared. Although morphine has been used extensively in the treatment of pain, its use as an analgesic follows strong geographic prescribing patterns. A mere six nations account for 79% of the world's medical morphine consumption, with 120 nations consuming little or no morphine.[2] Morphine may be administered with efficacy in both acute and chronic pain and somatic and visceral nociceptive pain and some neuropathic pain. Depending upon the need, morphine may be administered orally in immediate-release or extended-release (ER) preparations, intramuscularly, intravenously (bolus or continuous infusion or patient-controlled analgesia), or via an epidural catheter (bolus or continuous infusion or patient-controlled epidural analgesia). Dosing requirements for morphine may differ between individuals by 1000-fold,[11] displaying significantly more dosing variability than most other classes of pharmacologic agents.

After intravenous or intramuscular administration, peak plasma concentrations correlate poorly with pharmacologic activity. The peak plasma–peak pharmacologic activity discordance, or hysteresis, is a reflection of morphine's low lipid solubility and slow movement across the blood-brain barrier. Peak pharmacologic effect after intravenous morphine administration occurs in 15 to 30 minutes, which coincides with peak cerebrospinal fluid (CSF) concentrations.[12] Intramuscular administration is associated with rapid absorption and peak pharmacologic effect in 45 minutes. The fraction of morphine entering the CNS is small. In addition to poor lipid solubility, morphine's movement across the blood-brain barrier is also limited by protein binding, ionization, and rapid conjugation with glucuronic acid. Alkalosis increases the nonionized fraction of morphine in the plasma, so CNS concentrations will increase with hypoventilation. Significant depression of ventilation can therefore progress to ventilatory arrest.

Oral administration of morphine results in slower and less predictable absorption than does intravenous or intramuscular administration. Peak plasma concentrations of a sustained-release morphine preparation in healthy volunteers can occur 142.5 minutes after oral ingestion.[13] Various preparations of sustained-release morphine tablets will achieve peak plasma concentrations with different rapidity depending upon their formulation.[14] Sustained-release preparations allow for daily or twice-daily dosing. In one study of cancer patients with chronic pain, peak plasma concentrations of morphine were achieved in 3.6 ± 2.3 hours after the oral administration of MSContin.[15] Morphine is a substrate for the efflux pump P-glycoprotein, and peak plasma concentrations after oral administration are increased in healthy volunteers after coadministration of quinidine, a P-glycoprotein pump inhibitor. Individual variations in the activity of the P-glycoprotein pump may have a role in explaining the individual variability seen in oral morphine absorption and bioavailability.[16] The role of P-glycoprotein affecting the CNS concentration of morphine in humans remains undetermined.

Morphine distributes to skeletal muscle, liver, kidneys, intestinal tract, lungs, spleen, and brain with a volume of distribution of 1 to 6 L/kg. Approximately 20% to 35% of morphine is reversibly bound to plasma proteins. Morphine metabolism occurs primarily by conjugation at hepatic and extrahepatic sites. Conjugation occurs primarily with D-glucuronic acid to form morphine 3-glucuronide (M3G) and smaller quantities of morphine 6-glucuronide (M6G), but also occurs with sulfuric acid to form morphine 3-etheral sulfate. M3G is the primary metabolite and lacks intrinsic analgesic activity. M6G has potent μ_1-receptor affinity with relatively low μ_2-receptor affinity and potentially exceeds morphine in its analgesic potential,[17] but has low permeability across the blood-brain barrier. M6G lacks analgesic efficacy when administered by intravenous bolus with short-term infusion because of its poor CNS penetration.[18] When administered orally, M6G undergoes gut hydrolysis and is absorbed as morphine with a bioavailability of 11% ± 3%.[19] Elimination of morphine is primarily by renal

TABLE 61-1 APPROXIMATE EQUIANALGESIC DOSES OF OPIOID AGONISTS

	Route and Dosage*			
Drug	**IM/SubQ/IV (mg)**	**PO/PR/SL (mg)**	**Duration (hr)**	**Half-life (hr)**
Morphine	10	20-30	3-6	1.5-3
Meperidine	75-100	300	2-4	2-3
Fentanyl	0.1	—	0.5-2	1.5-6
Codeine	75-100	300	4-6	3
Hydromorphone	2	4	3-4	2-3
Oxycodone	—	15-20	3-4	—
Oxymorphone	1	10	3-6	—
Hydrocodone	—	20-30	4-8	3.3-4.5
Methadone	Short term: 5-10 Chronic use: 1-4	Short term: 20 Chronic use: 2-4	4-6	15-30
Propoxyphene	—	130-200	4-6	6-12

*Routes: IM, intramuscular; IV, intravenous; PO, oral; PR, per rectum; SL, sublingual; SubQ, subcutaneous.

excretion of M3G and M6G, although approximately 10% is excreted unchanged in urine. There is a minor component of excretion of M3G and M6G in bile, and about 7% to 10% of morphine is eliminated via feces. Because of gut hydrolysis of glucuronides, a small fraction of M3G and M6G excreted in bile undergo enterohepatic recycling. The mean adult plasma clearance of morphine is 20 to 30 ml/min per kilogram. In addition to the common opioid side effects, morphine can trigger histamine release leading to flushing, pruritus, or bronchospasm.

Meperidine. Meperidine is a synthetic opioid derived from phenylpiperidine. It shares a structural similarity to atropine and was initially developed as an anticholinergic agent, but its analgesic properties were soon recognized to exceed its weak anticholinergic properties. It additionally contains the structural elements common to amine local anesthetics, including a tertiary amine, an ester group, and a lipophilic phenyl group. Meperidine produces effects similar to local anesthetics when administered into the intrathecal or intraperitoneal space.

Meperidine is approximately one tenth as potent as morphine. When introduced into clinical practice, meperidine received widespread use partly based upon the unfounded assumption that it produced less depression of ventilation than does morphine. However, in equianalgesic doses, its side effect profile is similar to morphine, including its ability to depress the ventilatory drive. Another myth was that meperidine caused less spasm of the sphincter of Oddi compared to other opioids, but this was disproven long ago. Claims that meperidine produces a longer duration of analgesia when administered by intramuscular injection as opposed to intravenously are also unfounded, with the pharmacokinetics of the two routes of administration being essentially the same.[20] Evidence-based medicine does not support the practice of administering intramuscular meperidine to patients with established intravenous access.

Meperidine is metabolized by two distinct pathways. The major metabolite is meperidinic acid, which is inactive. However, the secondary pathway produces normeperidine. Normeperidine has less analgesic potency than does meperidine, but greater potential to cause CNS excitation. Accumulation of normeperidine, which can occur in the setting of renal insufficiency, has been associated with anxiety, hyperreflexia, myoclonus, and seizures.[21]

Absorption after intramuscular injection has been demonstrated to have significant variability between patients and between injections in a single patient. The elimination half-life is approximately 3.6 hours. Bioavailability after oral ingestion is more predictable than that after parenteral administration and ranges from 41% to 61%. Because of significant first-pass hepatic metabolism, plasma normeperidine levels are greater with oral than with parenteral administration.

Meperidine is associated with less miosis than is morphine, which may hinder detection in cases of drug diversion. Drug interactions are numerous. The most significant is the ability of meperidine to precipitate serotonin crisis when used in combination with monoamine oxidase inhibitors.

Fentanyl. Fentanyl is a phenylpiperidine-derivative synthetic opioid. It has a potency approximately 100 times greater than morphine. After a single intravenous bolus administration, fentanyl has both a faster onset time and shorter duration of action than morphine. This triad of pharmacologic properties—high potency, quick onset, and short duration of action—makes intravenous fentanyl a particularly useful opioid in surgical anesthesia and as a component of procedural sedation.

Fentanyl has a shorter onset time than morphine primarily because of its greater lipid solubility. Fentanyl crosses the blood-brain barrier three to five times more rapidly than does morphine. Duration of action following a single intravenous dose is limited to 30 minutes. Although fentanyl undergoes extensive metabolism, its short duration of action is primarily a function of rapid redistribution to inactive tissues, including adipose tissue and muscle. First-pass metabolism occurs in the lungs and is extensive, accounting for 75% of an intravenous dose.[22] When delivered by continuous infusion or by repeated doses of sufficient quantity, the content-sensitive half-life of fentanyl increases substantially. Consequently, fentanyl administered by intravenous patient-controlled analgesia is an effective modality.

Transdermal administration of fentanyl (base) may be used with great efficacy in chronic pain, particularly in the treatment of cancer pain. Transdermal delivery takes advantage of the high lipid solubility and low molecular weight of fentanyl. Fentanyl transdermal patches allow for continuous delivery of fentanyl for 3 days. Since sustained high plasma levels are obtained, transdermal delivery is not suited for intermittent or acute pain or treatment of opioid-naive patients. Transdermal administration may be beneficial for patients with chronic pain when oral administration is difficult due to dysphagia, anorexia, nausea and vomiting, or an inability to comply with dosing regimens (poor memory, confusion, sedation). However, drug absorption via the skin varies between patients,[23] and transdermal delivery makes titration of the dose potentially cumbersome. Peak plasma concentrations are achieved approximately 17 hours after application, but can take as long as 2 days depending upon absorption. Absorption through the skin continues even after the patch is removed. Patch formulations may be either "reservoir" or "matrix" formulation. Matrix formulations allow the patch to be cut without "dose dumping."

Fentanyl is well absorbed after transmucosal administration. Use of the phrase "fentanyl lollipop" is discouraged since it is believed to place children at risk for accidental ingestion. Absorption is rapid after transmucosal administration, with peak plasma concentrations occurring in approximately 20 to 25 minutes.[24] Both the fentanyl lozenge and the recently introduced effervescent fentanyl buccal tablet provide rapid onset of analgesia and are useful "rescue" analgesics in opioid-tolerant patients.

Fentanyl Iontophoretic Transdermal System. In 2006, the U.S. Food and Drug Administration (FDA) gave approval to a transdermal delivery system for fentanyl hydrochloride that utilizes a low-intensity and imperceptible electric current to transport a preprogrammed predictable dose of fentanyl across the skin via a small needle-free device worn by the patient. Iontophoresis provides relatively rapid transdermal delivery of on-demand fentanyl. Absorption is only 41% during the first hour of therapy, but increases to nearly 100% by the 10th hour.[25] The device delivers fentanyl only when activated by the patient, with an hourly limit of six doses. Fentanyl (40 mcg) is delivered slowly over the 10-minute dosing interval, during which time the system is "locked out" to additional activation. The system automatically shuts off after 24 hours or 80 delivered doses, whichever comes first. The amount of fentanyl delivered is determined by the electric current delivered by device. There is no passive drug delivery. Plasma levels begin to fall almost immediately after the device is removed.

The fentanyl iontophoretic transdermal system has been compared to standard morphine in intravenous patient-controlled analgesia.[26] These studies demonstrate a comparable safety and efficacy profile. Investigations have focused upon the treatment of acute postoperative pain, and hence the device is currently approved for acute pain management in a medically supervised setting. A needle-free, preprogrammed system may provide ease of use and safety benefits compared to traditional invasive systems requiring programming and drug syringe placement. The iontophoretic transdermal system has not yet been studied in other clinical situations in which episodic pain occurs and intravenous access is difficult or impractical, such as breakthrough cancer pain or sickle cell crisis.

Fentanyl Analogues. Alfentanil has approximately one tenth the potency and one third the duration of action of fentanyl. Sufentanil is a thienyl analogue with approximately 10 times the potency of fentanyl and a duration of action intermediate to alfentanil and fentanyl. When delivered by continuous infusion, both may exhibit prolonged durations of action. Both are used primarily for perioperative or procedural analgesia. Intranasal sufentanil may be used in the treatment of moderate or severe pain.

Remifentanil is a newer fentanyl analogue. It is a selective μ-agonist with a unique ester linkage that is hydrolyzed by plasma and tissue esterases. It has a duration of action of approximately 6 minutes and, unlike fentanyl, sulfentanil, or alfentanil, this is unaffected by the duration of infusion. The ultrashort duration of action of remifentanil limits its usefulness in pain management, but makes it clinically useful during brief painful or unpleasant procedures. It has also been used effectively for analgesia during childbirth.

Codeine. Codeine, or methylmorphine, is an alkaloid found in opium, although most commercially available codeine is synthesized from morphine. Codeine is a prodrug that must be metabolized to its active metabolites, morphine and codeine 6-gluronide, to be effective. Up to 10% of patients do not have the enzymes necessary for this conversion; hence, codeine is not effective for everyone. It is less potent than morphine and may be useful for analgesia in moderate pain or for antidiarrhea or antitussive purposes. Metabolism to morphine occurs hepatically via the cytochrome P-450 (CYP) isoenzyme CDY6, and inhibitors of this enzyme, including the antidepressants fluoxetine and citalopram, may greatly diminish its analgesic potency.

Hydromorphone. Hydromorphone, a semisynthetic opioid, is a hydroxylated ketone derivative of morphine. Its potency is approximately five to eight times that of morphine.[27] It is indicated for the treatment of moderate to severe pain. Its side effect profile mimics that of morphine, but it produces more sedation and less euphoria.

The pharmacokinetics of hydromorphone is similar to morphine when administered intravenously, but its duration of action is slightly less. Like morphine, it has wide interindividual bioavailability and undergoes extensive first-pass metabolism when administered orally. Hydromorphone is administered orally every 4 hours, which limits its convenience in the treatment of chronic or terminal pain. One ER formulation of hydromorphone was briefly available in the United States, but had a significant drug interaction with alcohol that led to potentially lethal plasma concentrations of the drug. Hydromorphone ER was withdrawn from the U.S. market voluntarily by the manufacturer in 2005. Various forms of hydromorphone ER with other delivery systems remain available in other countries.

Intranasal administration of hydromorphone avoids the need for intravenous access and the significant first-pass hepatic metabolism. Bioavailability is more predictable than with oral administration. Onset of action is rapid with intranasal administration, although peak plasma concentrations are significantly less.[28]

Oxycodone. Oxycodone is a semisynthetic opioid derived from thebaine. It is available in oral formulation under numerous trade names, usually in combination with acetaminophen or aspirin. Bioavailability is 60% to 87% after oral administration. Orally administered oxycodone is approximately equianalgesic on a per-milligram basis with subcutaneously administered morphine. Anaglesic duration of action is 4 to 5 hours. Oxycodone may offer some analgesic benefit compared with other opioids in the treatment of pain in cancer patients.

Controlled-release (CR) oxycodone allows for a more convenient twice-daily dosing. Bioavailability of CR oxycodone after oral administration is 60% to 87%. Breaking, chewing, or crushing CR oxycodone may cause immediate release of the active drug. CR oxycodone was originally marketed as having a lower abuse potential due to its sustained-release formulation, which may mitigate the euphoria of the immediate-release form. However, the CR carrier can be defeated by intentional crushing of the tablet. Hence, CR oxycodone has significant abuse potential, and reports of drug diversion and illicit use are plentiful.[29]

Oxymorphone. Oxymorphone is a congener of morphine, although most commercially available oxymorphone is synthesized from thebaine. Oxymorphone is a metabolite of oxycodone and is twice as potent as the parent compound. It is available for injection or by oral administration. The bioavailability when taken orally is approximately 10%. It is hepatically metabolized with a half-life of 1.3 ± 0.7 hours. No drug interactions with other drugs metabolized by CYP isoenzymes have been identified. Oxymorphone (immediate release) requires dosing every 4 to 6 hours, but an ER formulation allows for twice-daily dosing. ER oxymorphone is intended for use in opioid-tolerant patients. Alcohol or alcohol-containing medications may cause disruption of the ER carrier leading to rapid release of oxymorphone, resulting in excessively high plasma levels.

Hydrocodone. Hydrocodone is a semisynthetic opioid derived from codeine and thebaine. It is available in tablets under a variety of trade names and is most commonly paired with either acetaminophen or aspirin. After oral administration, peak plasma concentrations occur in approximately 80 minutes. It is available in a volume-limiting concentrated form for parenteral administration. Analgesic potency and plasma half-life are similar to those of codeine.[30]

Tramadol. Tramadol is a nonscheduled synthetic centrally acting opioid. It displays a dual action of being a μ-receptor agonist and weak inhibiter of norepinephrine and serotonin neuronal reuptake, which augments the efficacy of inhibitory spinal pathways. Tramadol is a racemic mixture of two enantiomers, with one enantiomer blocking norepinephrine reuptake and the other blocking serotonin reuptake.[31] The effect of tramadol upon receptor reuptake contributes significantly to its analgesic properties. Its μ-receptor agonist properties occur primarily through its primary metabolite, *o*-desmethyltramadol.[32] However, individuals with diminished capacity to metabolize tramadol still experience analgesia,[33] and only approximately one third of analgesia from tramadol is reversible with the opioid receptor antagonist naxolone in healthy volunteers.[34]

Preparations of tramadol are available for oral, rectal, intravenous, intramuscular, and subcutaneous administration. After oral administration, peak plasma concentration is achieved within 2 hours. However, elimination is also rapid, with tramadol displaying a short elimination half-life of 5 to 6 hours.[32] The consequent four-times-a-day dosing of tramadol limits its convenience of administration in the therapy of chronic pain. A sustained-released preparation of tramadol (tramadol ER) is now available utilizing a semipermeable membrane (Smartcoat; Biovail Corporation) that allows for the slow osmotic diffusion of the active ingredient in a pH-independent manner. Bioavailability of tramadol ER 200 mg is equivalent to tramadol immediate release 50 mg taken every 6 hours.[35]

Methadone. Methadone is a synthetic opioid that is a racemic mixture of (*R*-) and (*S*-) enantiomers. The (*R*-) enantiomer has 10-fold greater affinity for the μ-receptor than does the (*S*-) enantiomer and believed to be primarily responsible for its analgesia. Methadone also blocks neuronal reuptake of norepinephrine and serotonin spinal descending inhibitory pathways, with the (*R*-) enantiomer demonstrating greater activity, but both enantiomers bind with equal affinity to presynaptic *N*-methyl-D-aspartate (NMDA) receptors.[36]

Methadone has long been utilized in therapy of opioid addiction, but its efficacy as an analgesic in chronic pain is gaining clinical popularity. Methadone has several properties that make it a desirable analgesic for chronic pain, including low cost, low potential for abuse, and a long elimination half-time allowing for convenient once-daily or twice-daily dosing. Its bioavailability after oral ingestion is approximately 85%, and its oral-to-parenteral potency is 1:2. Peak plasma concentrations occur 1 to 5 hours after oral administration and appear to be delayed with chronic administration, perhaps due to chronic effects on gastric emptying. Methadone is highly protein bound to α_1-acid glycoprotein. Concurrent administration of medications that also bind to α_1-acid glycoprotein (e.g., propranolol, phenothiazines) may increase the free plasma concentration of methadone. Disease states that increase the amount of α_1-acid glycoprotein, including some forms of cancer, may reduce the free plasma concentration of methadone.[37]

There is some evidence that methadone may be superior to other opioids in the treatment of neuropathic pain.[38] However, several factors limit its use in chronic pain. Some patients may object to a social stigma associated with methadone and its relationship to maintenance therapy for opioid addiction. Methadone displays important interindividual variability in pharmacokinetics, making conversion from other opioids to an equipotent dose of methadone challenging. Plasma half-life averages 24 hours, but ranges from 13 to 50 hours and greatly exceeds its duration of analgesia. Methadone can accumulate with repetitive dosing, causing sedation, somnolence, and, in extreme cases, death.[30] Methadone overdose was implicated in over 3100 fatalities in the United States in 2003, an increase of 275% since 1999.[39] Therefore, the use of methadone for therapy for chronic pain is often reserved for pain specialists and other physicians with extensive methadone prescribing experience.

Propoxyphene. Propoxyphene is a weak synthetic diphenyl heptane opioid with a structural similarity to methadone. It is most commonly prescribed in combination with acetaminophen. It is well absorbed in the small intestine after oral administration, with peak plasma concentrations occurring at roughly 2 hours depending upon the preparation of propoxyphene ingested. There is extensive first-pass metabolism by the liver. Propoxyphene is indicated for mild to moderate pain, with 120 mg of propoxyphene producing analgesia comparable to 650 mg of aspirin. Propoxyphene is extensively metabolized and undergoes both renal and biliary excretion. Nor-propoxyphene, the major metabolite, has been implicated in sedation, dizziness, and unsteady ambulation in geriatric populations as well as in more serious side effects, including pulmonary edema, QTc prolongation, and cardiac arrest.[40] The abuse potential of propoxyphene is believed to be comparable to that of codeine.

Mixed Opioid Agonist-Antagonists

Mixed opioid agonist-antagonists are compounds with agonist properties on at least one of the opioid receptor types while having antagonist properties on another. These drugs produce a partial agonism response at the μ-receptor and agonism at κ- and δ-receptors. This partial agonist property at the μ-receptor will result in some analgesia for the patient who has not received other opioids, but patients who have significant plasma levels of potent opioids will experience an antagonism of the analgesic effect by the partial agonist. These agents as a class provide limited analgesia while reducing undesirable opioid effects, particularly depression of the ventilatory drive, euphoria, and physical dependence. Some patients may experience dysphoria from the central κ-agonist effect. The attributes of mixed opioid agonist-antagonists have been represented by the colorful metaphor, "a bee without the stinger." As a class, these drugs typically display a ceiling effect for analgesia, but have a lower potential for addiction.

Pentazocine. Pentazocine is a mixed opioid agonist-antagonist that was originally developed with the hope that it would be free of abuse potential. Introduced into clinical practice in 1967, pentazocine was assigned as a Schedule IV controlled substance in 1979 due to reports of abuse. Pentazocine is a synthetic agonist-antagonist that is less potent than morphine. It provides analgesia with less ventilatory depression, nausea, vomiting, and constipation. An oral preparation of pentazocine combined with naxolone is marketed to limit the possibility of drug diversion and abuse. This drug is available in both oral and parenteral formulations.

Pentazocine is an antagonist at the μ-receptor, so there are limited side effects of the classic μ-receptor type. Agonist properties of pentazocine at κ- and δ-receptors produce altered perception of pain. Intravenous or oral pentazocine may be used in the treatment of moderate pain, with an oral dose of pentazocine 50 mg having an equivalent analgesic efficacy to codeine 60 mg orally. Common side effects include sedation, diaphoresis, dizziness, and severe dysphoria. Pentazocine may increase serum catecholamine levels, causing abrupt increases in heart rate and blood pressure. This drug may not be indicated in individuals who have a history of heart disease. Pentazocine is well absorbed after oral administration, but first-pass hepatic metabolism limits bioavailability to approximately 20%. The elimination half-life of pentazocine is 2 to 3 hours.

Butorphanol. Butorphanol is a mixed agonist-antagonist used to treat moderate to severe pain. Butorphanol shares a structural similarity to pentazocine, but possesses significantly greater agonist and antagonist qualities. Butorphanol is believed to have a low affinity for μ-opioid receptors and a moderate affinity for κ-receptors. Since it has a weak interaction at the μ-receptor, it produces less physical dependence and respiratory depression. The drug is well absorbed after intramuscular or intranasal administration, but poorly absorbed after oral administration. Bioavailability of butorphanol after intranasal administration is approximately 70% compared with 5% to 17% after oral administration.[41] Immediate effects are also seen with intravenous dosages (1 minute), and duration of action is 2 to 4 hours. Dysphoria is reported infrequently with butorphanol compared with other mixed agonist-antagonists. Common side effects include nausea, sedation, and diaphoresis. Butorphanol can increase systemic blood pressure. Butorphanol may be used to relieve the pruritus associated with other opioids.[42,43] Intranasal butorphanol is widely used in the treatment of migraine headaches. However, because of reports of abuse and dependence, butorphanol was classified as a Schedule IV controlled substance in 1997.

Nalbuphine. Nalbuphine is a mixed agonist-antagonist opioid with a structural similarity to both oxymorphone and naxolone. It has an analgesic equivalency and duration of action similar to morphine. Nalbuphine has potent μ-receptor antagonist activity that is 10 times that of pentazocine. Its agonistic activity on κ-receptors produces alteration in the perception of pain. Nalbuphine has a ceiling effect for depression of ventilation and may reverse the opioid-related depression of ventilation resulting from μ-agonists. It is also used to treat pain associated with biliary and renal colic, migraines, cancer, and surgical trauma.

After intravenous administration, onset of action is less than 3 minutes, but with intramuscular administration onset of action may be as long as 15 minutes. The duration of effective analgesia is 3 to 6 hours. Nalbuphine is less likely than pentazocine to cause dysphoria or other psychomimetic effects. Nalbuphine produces depression of ventilation up to a maximal dose of 30 mg, after which a ceiling effect is seen. Nalbuphine does not produce the increase in heart rate and blood pressure seen with pentazocine and butorphanol. Sedation is the most common side effect. Some of the other side effects of nalbuphine include decreased secretion in the gastrointestinal (GI) tract, constipation, urinary retention, and hypotension. Nalbuphine may also cause nausea and vomiting by stimulation of the chemoreceptor trigger zone.

Buprenorphine. Buprenorphine is an opium alkaloid derivative that has a high binding affinity for, but only partial agonist properties at, the μ-opioid receptor and antagonist properties at the κ-opioid receptor. It is indicated in the treatment of moderate to severe pain and treatment of opioid addiction. In animal models, it has 20 times the potency of morphine. There is a ceiling effect for depression of ventilation, but not for analgesia, in humans.[44] However, ventilatory depression can occur in opioid-naive or elderly individuals and, because of buprenorphine's high affinity for μ-receptors, it may be difficult to reverse this effect with opioid antagonists. Continuous infusion of the opioid antagonist naxolone may be more effective than a bolus administration when ventilatory depression develops.[45] Other common side effects, including drowsiness, nausea, and vomiting, occur with a frequency similar to morphine.

Buprenorphine is a potent analgesic when delivered by injection. Buprenorphine 0.3 mg intramuscularly has the analgesic potency of morphine 10 mg intramuscularly. After intramuscular injection, peak plasma levels occur in approximately 30 minutes and analgesia persists for 8 hours. Several preparations of buprenorphine have been developed for sublinguinal administration, with one preparation incorporating naxolone to limit its potential for drug diversion.[46] Intranasal and transdermal preparations are also currently being investigated.

Opioid Antagonists

Opioid antagonists bind to μ-receptors and displace agonists that may be bound to the receptor. Such antagonism results in the reversal of analgesia seen at the μ-, κ-, or δ-receptors as well as reversal of respiratory depression. These drugs have no agonist activity and produce abrupt reversal of opioid overdose, resulting in sudden pain and subsequent stimulation of the sympathetic nervous system.

Naloxone. Naloxone is a potent competitive antagonist of μ-, κ-, and δ-receptors. It quickly reverses the toxic effects of opioids during respiratory depression. Naloxone has a short duration of action and is quickly removed from the brain (within 30 to 45 minutes). Repeated doses or infusion (1 to 5 mcg/kg per minute) of the drug is required for treatment of long-acting opiates. Metabolism of naloxone takes place in the liver, and excretion is in the urine. Rapid reversal of opioids with naloxone results in reversal of analgesia. This will have the effect of increased stimulation of the sympathetic nervous system manifesting with rapid heart rate and increased blood pressure. Naxolone should be administered in small divided doses and titrated to the desired effect of reversing opioid-induced side effects, thus preserving analgesia.

Nalmefene. Nalmefene is an opiate receptor antagonist that has longer half-life than naloxone. It competitively antagonizes the effects of opioids at μ-, κ-, and δ-receptors. Due to its long duration of activity, nalmefene can be used in the reversal of methadone. It is available in parenteral formulations, and effects are seen within 5 to 15 minutes of administration. The half-life of nalmefene is 11 to 15 hours. It is metabolized in the liver and excreted in the kidneys. Side effects of this drug include rapid reversal of analgesia with stimulation of the sympathetic nervous system as seen with naloxone.

Nonopioid Analgesics

Nonsteroidal Anti-inflammatory Drugs. NSAIDs and cyclooxygenase-2 (COX-2) inhibitors are popular alternatives to opioids for control of acute and chronic pain. They form the first step of the WHO Analgesic Ladder and are used as adjuvant to opioids in steps 2 and 3 as part of multimodal analgesia for acute and chronic pain. Conventional NSAIDs are readily available over the counter with a multitude of brand names for the consumer. NSAIDs can come in a variety of forms and differ in their potency, duration of action, and metabolism in the body. Commonly used NSAIDs include aspirin, diclofenac, ibuprofen, naproxen, and ketorolac (Table 61-2).

Mechanism of Action. Any physical or chemical insults to the tissue will release inflammatory mediators from the cell membranes. The disruption of cell membranes from tissues will release phospholipids to the environment, causing them to be converted to arachidonic acid by phospholipase A_2 (Fig. 61-2). Arachidonic acid will follow a series of cascades of enzymatic reaction through two different pathways. In the cyclooxygenase (COX) pathway, arachidonic acid serves as a substrate for COX-1 and COX-2 to produce prostaglandins (PGs), prostacyclin, and thromboxane. Alternatively, the lipo-oxygenase pathway converts arachidonic acid to leukotrienes and HPETE. The release of prostaglandins, leukotrienes, and other inflammatory mediators at the injury site leads to inflammation and sensitization of pain receptors.[47] Such stimuli are carried by nociceptors to the brain, where they are interpreted as pain.

NSAIDs are nonspecific inhibitors of the COX pathway, and their use results in the inhibition of prostaglandin biosynthesis. Since PGE_2 is the primary agent responsible for reducing the pain threshold, inhibition of its synthesis will reduce nociception at the site of injury.[48] However, most of the side effects of NSAIDs are due to the nonspecific inhibition of both COX-1 and COX-2 enzymes. COX-1 is expressed predominantly in the gastric mucosa, renal parenchyma, and platelets. COX-2 is expressed at the site of injury and mediates inflammation and pain. Nonspecific inhibition of COX-1 leads to decreased production of prostaglandins in the stomach, resulting in loss of protection of the integrity of the gastric mucosa. Decreased prostaglandin production also leads to altered renal hemodynamics and renal insufficiency during decreased perfusion of the kidneys. NSAIDs, through inhibition of COX-1, cause inhibition of platelet aggregation and increase bleeding time.

Pharmacokinetics. Most NSAIDs are organic acids and are well absorbed in the GI tract without substantial decreases in their bioavailability. NSAIDs undergo phase I or phase II metabolism in the liver and are excreted through the kidneys. NSAIDs are largely bound to albumin in the blood and have low volume of distribution. NSAIDs are weakly acidic (pK_a: 3 to 5) and may cross the blood-brain barrier depending on lipid solubility.

Side Effects. The side effects of NSAIDs are associated with their inhibition of the COX pathway. The most common side effect seen with NSAIDs is the GI toxicity due to COX-1 inhibition and reduction in the gastric and duodenal mucus barrier. Chronic therapy with NSAIDs may lead to gastric and duodenal ulcers. Other side effects seen with NSAIDs include impaired platelet aggregation through the COX-1 enzyme. Aspirin will irreversibly inactivate platelets for the life of the platelet (7 to 10 days). The antiplatelet activity of nonselective NSAIDs may increase the bleeding time. For this reason, most NSAID therapy is customarily discontinued for a period of time prior to major surgical procedures. Renal toxicity may also be manifested in patients taking NSAIDs. Inhibition of prostaglandin synthesis leads to decreased renal blood flow, decreased glomerular filtration, and altered ion transport. Renal toxicity may manifest with renal medullary ischemia in susceptible individuals and lead to nephrotoxicity. NSAIDs may trigger asthma in susceptible individuals through inhibition of PGE_2 synthesis and increased production of leukotrienes (see Fig. 61-2), which lead to bronchoconstriction. Other side effects of NSAIDs include alterations in bone healing and, in rare instances, aseptic meningitis.

Acetylsalicylic Acid. Aspirin is a salicylate that has its mechanism of action through irreversible acetylation of the COX enzyme. Aspirin has

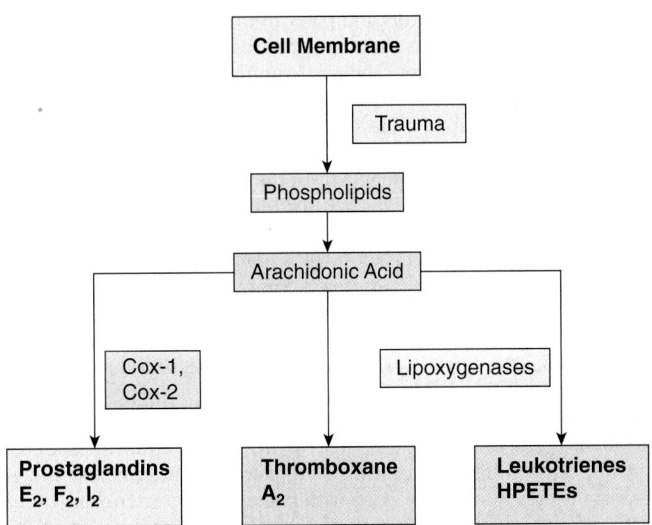

FIGURE 61-2 • Arachidonic acid cascade.

TABLE 61-2 CONVENTIONAL NSAIDS AND COX-2 INHIBITORS

Generic Name	Common Brand Name	Dosage (mg)	Route*	Half-life (hr)	Elimination
Acetylsalicylic acid	Aspirin	81-650	PO	0.25	Liver, kidney
Diclofenac	Cataflam Solaraze Voltaren	25-75	PO	1.9	Liver, kidney
Ibuprofen	Advil Motrin	200-400	PO	2-2.5	Liver, kidney
Indomethacin	Indocin	25-75	PO, IV, IM	4.5	Liver, kidney
Ketorolac	Toradol	10	PO, IV, IM	5	Liver, kidney
Acetaminophen	Tylenol	500-2000	PO	2-2.5	Liver
Celecoxib	Celebrex	100-200	PO	11-16	Liver, kidney

*Routes: IM, intramuscular; IV, intravenous; PO, oral.

important anti-inflammatory uses in the treatment of autoimmune disorders such as juvenile arthritis, rheumatoid arthritis, and osteoarthritis. Aspirin has an important antithrombotic function by irreversible inhibiting platelets for the life of the cell. Low-dose aspirin is helpful in preventing or reducing the risk of myocardial infarction in people with a history of coronary artery disease or cerebrovascular accidents.

Aspirin irreversibly inhibits the COX enzymes by acetylation of a serine moiety on the enzymes. It is more potent in inhibiting COX-1 than COX-2 enzyme. The antithrombotic actions of aspirin are due to its inhibition of the COX-1 enzyme and inhibition of production of thromboxane A_2 and prostacyclin (PGI_2). The antiplatelet effect of aspirin results in increased bleeding time. The anti-inflammatory actions of aspirin are due to the inhibition of cytokines and prostaglandins E and F. The inflammatory inhibition prevents prostaglandin-induced capillary wall permeability and influx of leukocytes. Aspirin's antipyretic actions are due to reduction in synthesis of PGE_2, which maintains the body temperature set point in the hypothalamus.

The side effects of aspirin are due to decreases in prostaglandin synthesis. Inhibition of the gastric prostaglandins, which have a protective role in the gastric mucosa, leads to increased permeability of gastric mucosa to acids. Over time, this results in aspirin-associated gastritis, ulceration, and bleeding. Other effects of aspirin include respiratory alkalosis and decreases in renal blood flow leading to impaired renal function in people with renal insufficiency.

Diclofenac. Diclofenac is a nonselective NSAID under the acetic acid class. Similar to other NSAIDs, it inhibits the COX-1 and COX-2 enzymes and has analgesic, antipyretic, and anti-inflammatory effects. Diclofenac is useful for the inhibition of COX-1 enzyme in the synovial lining of joints in patients with rheumatoid arthritis and osteoarthritis. With reduction in prostaglandin synthesis, diclofenac suppresses hyperalgesia at pain receptors and plays an important role in analgesia during inflammation. This drug also inhibits meiotic response in the eye during ocular surgery. Topical formulations of diclofenac are important for preventing the manifestation of ocular inflammation and vascular permeability. Diclofenac has GI, antiplatelet, and renal effects similar to those of other NSAIDs.

Ibuprofen. Ibuprofen is an NSAID of the proprionic acid class given in oral formulations. It is indicated for the treatment of rheumatoid arthritis, osteoarthritis, and dysmenorrheal pain. Other clinical uses of this drug include ankylosing spondylitis, gout, and psoriatic arthritis. Similar to other NSAIDs, ibuprofen has anti-inflammatory, analgesic, and antipyretic effects. It functions through nonspecific inhibition of COX-1 and COX-2 enzymes. Adverse effects of ibuprofen include decreased bleeding time, gastric ulcerations, and decreased renal perfusion in susceptible individuals.

Indomethacin. Indomethacin is an NSAID in the family of inoles or indene acetic acids. As with other NSAIDs, indomethacin produces a nonspecific inhibition of the COX enzymes. Indomethacin has important uses in neonates born with patent ductus arteriosus. Indomethacin reduces the production of prostaglandins that maintain the ductus in an open state and allows the patent ductus arteriosus to close. This NSAID has potent anti-inflammatory, analgesic, and antipyretic effects. Some of the non–FDA-approved uses of indomethacin include primary dysmenorrhea, pericarditis, juvenile arthritis, pseudogout, and Paget's disease. Side effects of indomethacin include the same reactions seen with NSAIDs, such as platelet inhibition, gastritis, renal dysfunction, and suppression of bone formation.

Ketorolac. Ketorolac belongs to the acetic acid class of NSAIDs and has potent analgesic, anti-inflammatory, and antipyretic effects. It suppresses the synthesis of prostaglandins E and F and reduces the sensitization of pain receptors after acute trauma. The use of ketorolac is limited to 5 consecutive days due to the increased incidence of GI side effects. This drug is also available in ophthalmic formulations for use after ocular surgery. Ocular application of topical ketorolac is efficacious in preventing inflammation of the eye and reducing subsequent rise in intraocular pressures. The side effects of ketorolac are similar to other NSAIDs.

Acetaminophen. Acetaminophen, a *para*-aminophenol derivative, is typically classified with conventional NSAIDs, but it does not have anti-inflammatory effects. Its site of action was presumed to be at the COX-3 enzyme within the CNS. However, this mechanism of action is controversial, and recent evidence suggests a central activity on serotonergic receptors.[49] Acetaminophen has analgesic and antipyretic properties comparable to some NSAIDs. Acetaminophen is currently available in oral and intravenous formulations worldwide; however, intravenous formulations are still in development in the United States. This drug is metabolized in the liver by conjugation and hydroxylation to inactive metabolites.

COX-2–Selective Inhibitors. COX-2–selective inhibitors were developed to minimize the side effects seen with traditional nonselective NSAIDs. COX-2 inhibitors block the activity of COX-2 more selectively than that of COX-1, which is located in the GI tract, kidneys, and platelets. COX-2 inhibitors have the benefits of analgesic, antipyretic, and anti-inflammatory effects, while the side effect profile compares with traditional NSAIDs. COX-2 inhibitors do not inhibit platelets and have a minimal role in antithrombotic effects in patients with atherosclerotic diseases. COX-2 inhibitors create a prothrombotic state by reducing prostacyclin production in the setting of sustained thromboxane production, causing platelet aggregation, vasoconstriction, and vascular proliferation. Furthermore, inhibition of PGI_2 causes fluid retention and worsening of heart failure. Findings of higher incidences of cardiovascular thrombotic events led to the withdrawal of rofecoxib. Celecoxib is currently the only COX-2 inhibitor available in the United States.

Celecoxib. Celecoxib (Celebrex) selectively inhibits the COX-2 enzyme by binding to its sulfonamide side chain. This active binding site is specific to the COX-2 enzymes. COX-2–mediated inhibition leads to analgesic, antipyretic, and anti-inflammatory effects. Celecoxib has proven efficacy in treating the symptoms of rheumatoid arthritis and osteoarthritis. Celecoxib is routinely used before and after surgery as part of multimodal therapy to reduce the need for postoperative opioids. Studies have found that patients had better outcomes after total knee arthroplasty and spinal fusion surgeries when celecoxib was used for pain relief. Patients have reduced opioid requirements, reduced postoperative nausea and vomiting, and quicker physical rehabilitation after surgery.[50,51]

Platelet activity is not altered with celecoxib since its inhibition is regulated by the COX-1 enzyme. COX-2 inhibitors do not completely avoid the GI side effects seen with NSAIDs.

Anticonvulsants

Antineuropathic agents are gaining popularity for the treatment of acute and chronic pain. Such drugs as gabapentin and pregabalin, normally used for antiseizure activity, are now used to treat such neuropathic pain syndromes as diabetic polyneuropathy, postherpetic neuralgia, and acute pain associated with surgical trauma. The hypothesized mechanism of action of these agents is binding to voltage-gated calcium channels in the CNS. Down-regulation of calcium channels by these agents prevents the release of excitatory neurotransmitters from dorsal root ganglia and the spinal cord. The stimulation of primary pain fibers and the subsequent hyperexcitability of dorsal horn neurons are eliminated with antineuropathic agents.[52]

Gabapentin. Gabapentin (Neurontin) is an oral anticonvulsant and an analogue of the neurotransmitter γ-aminobutyric acid. Besides being an effective antiseizure medication, it is approved for the treatment of postherpetic neuralgia. The drug prevents the central neuronal sensitization seen with chronic pain syndromes. Furthermore, gabapentin has important clinical uses in the prevention and treatment of acute postoperative pain. Studies have shown that preoperative administration of gabapentin leads to reduction in postoperative pain and morphine consumption.[53,54] It is a lipid-soluble drug with minimal protein binding in the blood and has a high degree of solubility in the CNS due to its lipophilicity. Its peak effects are seen within 3 hours, and gabapentin is not metabolized in the body. It is eliminated unchanged in the urine with an elimination half-life of 5 to 9 hours.

Pregabalin. Pregabalin (Lyrica) is a newer antineuropathic agent that has antiepileptic, analgesic, and anxiolytic properties similar to gabapentin. It is chemically similar to gabapentin and is approved by the FDA for the treatment of partial seizures, diabetic neuropathy, and postherpetic neuralgia. It is the first drug to be approved for the treatment of fibromyalgia. Pregabalin has greater potency than gabapentin and has limited protein binding in the plasma. It is also eliminated by the kidneys and has minimal hepatic clearance. Some patients may experience drowsiness and dizziness.

Antidepressants

Antidepressants can be classified according to their mechanism of action as monoamine oxidase inhibitors (MAOIs), tricyclic antidepressants (TCAs), and selective serotonin reuptake inhibitors (SSRIs). MAOIs increase the amount of norepinephrine through direct inhibition of the enzyme monoamine oxidase in the CNS and autonomic nervous system. This inhibition increases the amount of norepinephrine available for release from nerve endings. Common side effects of MAOIs include hypotension and sedation. Patients on MAOIs are restricted from eating tyramine-containing foods since interactions between the two compounds cause systemic hypertension. Overdose of MAOIs can result in tachycardia, hypertension, hyperthermia, seizures, and coma.

TCAs work by blocking the reuptake of serotonin and norepinephrine at the presynaptic terminal, thereby resulting in accumulation of amines in the CNS. Common TCAs include amitriptyline, imipramine, clomipramine, desipramine, and nortriptyline. TCAs have high incidences of anticholinergic (dry mouth, blurred vision, tachycardia, urinary retention), cardiovascular (orthostatic hypotension, cardiac dysrhythmias), and CNS (sedation, seizures) side effects.

SSRIs are among the most widely prescribed antidepressants in the United States due to their low side effect profile with respect to anticholinergic properties, postural hypotension, and lower seizure thresholds. SSRIs block the reuptake of serotonin and enhance its activity in the CNS. Typical SSRIs include fluoxetine, paroxetine, sertraline, fluvoxamine, citalopram, and escitalopram.

Antidepressants are thought to have central as well as peripheral analgesic effects.[55] Some central and peripheral effects of antidepressants include binding both directly and indirectly to the opioid system, inhibition of NMDA-induced spinal hyperalgesia, release of adenosine to produce analgesia, and inhibition of specific ion channels that cause pain. They reduce central sensitization and hyperexcitability of spinal and supraspinal pathways. Studies show TCAs to have better efficacy in treatment of neuropathic pain when compared to other classes of antidepressants.[56]

Duloxetine, a serotonin-norepinephrine receptor inhibitor, has been shown in clinical trials to reduce neuropathic pain associated with diabetic neuropathy.[57] This study showed duloxetine 60 mg and 120 mg/day for 12 weeks had better outcomes than placebo for treatment of pain associated with type 1 and type 2 diabetes described as "shooting, stabbing, hot-burning, and splitting." This antidepressant is proven to treat pain independent of existing depression in patients. Duloxetine 60 mg was also found in another study to be safe and effective in the treatment of fibromyalgia, a debilitating musculoskeletal pain disorder.[58]

Local Anesthetics

Mexiletine. Mexiletine is a local anesthetic agent that is structurally similar to lidocaine and traditionally used as a class IB antiarrhythmic agent in the treatment of ventricular arrhythmias. Studies have shown the benefit of mexiletine in the treatment of neuropathic pain syndromes such as diabetic neuropathy, alcoholic neuropathy, peripheral nerve injuries characterized by burning, aching, or lancinating pain, and sensory changes.[59-61] Mexiletine functions by blocking sodium channels in the depolarized state in the CNS and at peripheral nerve sites. Unlike other local anesthetics, mexiletine is available in oral formulation and has a high bioavailability after absorption in the GI tract. The majority of mexiletine is metabolized through the liver, and the normal half-life of the drug is 10 to 12 hours. Mexiletine in a dosage of 200 mg twice daily to three times daily has also been reported in case series to be effective in treatment of neuropathic cancer pain from lumbosacral plexus tumor infiltration.[62] Common side effects of this drug include GI (nausea and vomiting) and neurologic (dizziness, ataxia, and tremors) side effects. In addition, mexiletine at 600 mg/day after breast surgery reduces analgesic requirements 24 hours after surgery and reduces overall pain after day 3.[63]

Lidocaine Patch. The 5% lidocaine patch (Lidoderm) is an amide local anesthetic transdermal patch used for the treatment of acute and chronic pain. Lidoderm was approved in 1999 by the FDA as a transdermal agent for the treatment of pain associated with postherpetic neuralgia. As a local anesthetic, Lidoderm produces analgesia through diminishing direct nerve membrane permeability to sodium. It is most effective when applied directly over the area to be anesthetized. There is very little systemic absorption, since only 3% to 5% of the drug is absorbed transcutaneously, and limited interaction with other drugs. A Lidoderm patch is applied over an intact skin area for 12 hours (maximum of three patches in a 24-hour period). Lidocaine is metabolized in the liver and excreted through the kidneys. Recent randomized studies have shown efficacy of the lidocaine patch in the treatment of diabetic polyneuropathy, myofascial pain, and chronic low back pain.[64] Superior results were found when the lidocaine patch is combined with multimodal approaches for treatment of chronic pain.

N-Methyl-D-Aspartate Receptor Antagonist

Ketamine. Ketamine, a phencyclidine derivative, has been in clinical use since the 1970s. Ketamine in high doses (>2 mg/kg) produces profound hypnosis, amnesia, and anesthetic qualities for surgical procedures. Ketamine produces inhibitory activity on the thalamo-neocortical pathways and the receptors of the cortex and the limbic system. Low-dose ketamine is profoundly analgesic. In addition, it binds to NMDA receptors in the CNS. Ketamine is well known for its dissociative qualities and has a high potential for abuse. Drug diversion with ketamine may be a significant problem. High doses of ketamine produce sympathomimetic activity resulting in nystagmus, hypertension, increased myocardial oxygen consumption, cognitive dysfunction, hallucinations, and nightmares. The NMDA activity of ketamine has generated recent interest in an antihyperalgesic role of this drug in clinical practice.[65] When given in intravenous forms, ketamine works within seconds and the analgesic effects are seen for 20 to 45 minutes. The half-life of ketamine is 2 to 3 hours, and it is metabolized in the liver and excreted in the urine.

Low-dose ketamine (<1 mg/kg) has been used in the acute perioperative period as part of multimodal analgesia to reduce the need for opioids intraoperatively and postoperatively. Ketamine may also have a role in pain management of the opioid-tolerant patient in both acute and chronic pain settings.

α_2-Adrenergic Receptor Agonist

Clonidine. Clonidine is a specific α_2-agonist, traditionally used as an antihypertensive agent, with analgesic actions at low doses at the peripheral and central pain receptors. Analgesic effects of clonidine may be due to release of enkephalin-like substances and inhibition of norepinephrine from prejunctional α_2 receptors[65] and prevention of pain transmission to the brain. Clonidine (1 mcg/kg) has opioid-sparing effects when combined with morphine and local anesthetics during neuroaxial block in orthopedic procedures.[66] During epidural or peripheral nerve block, clonidine blocks the conduction of A delta and C pain fibers. With epidural administration of clonidine, the peak plasma and CSF levels are achieved within 30 minutes. The half-life of clonidine in the CSF is 1.3 hours.

Clonidine is also available in a transdermal preparation (Catapress TTS) consisting of four layers of a microporous polypropylene membrane that releases the drug over a 7-day period. Therapeutic plasma concentrations of transdermal clonidine are established within 2 to 3 days. Studies have shown reduced opioid requirements for treatment of chronic pain with transdermal clonidine.

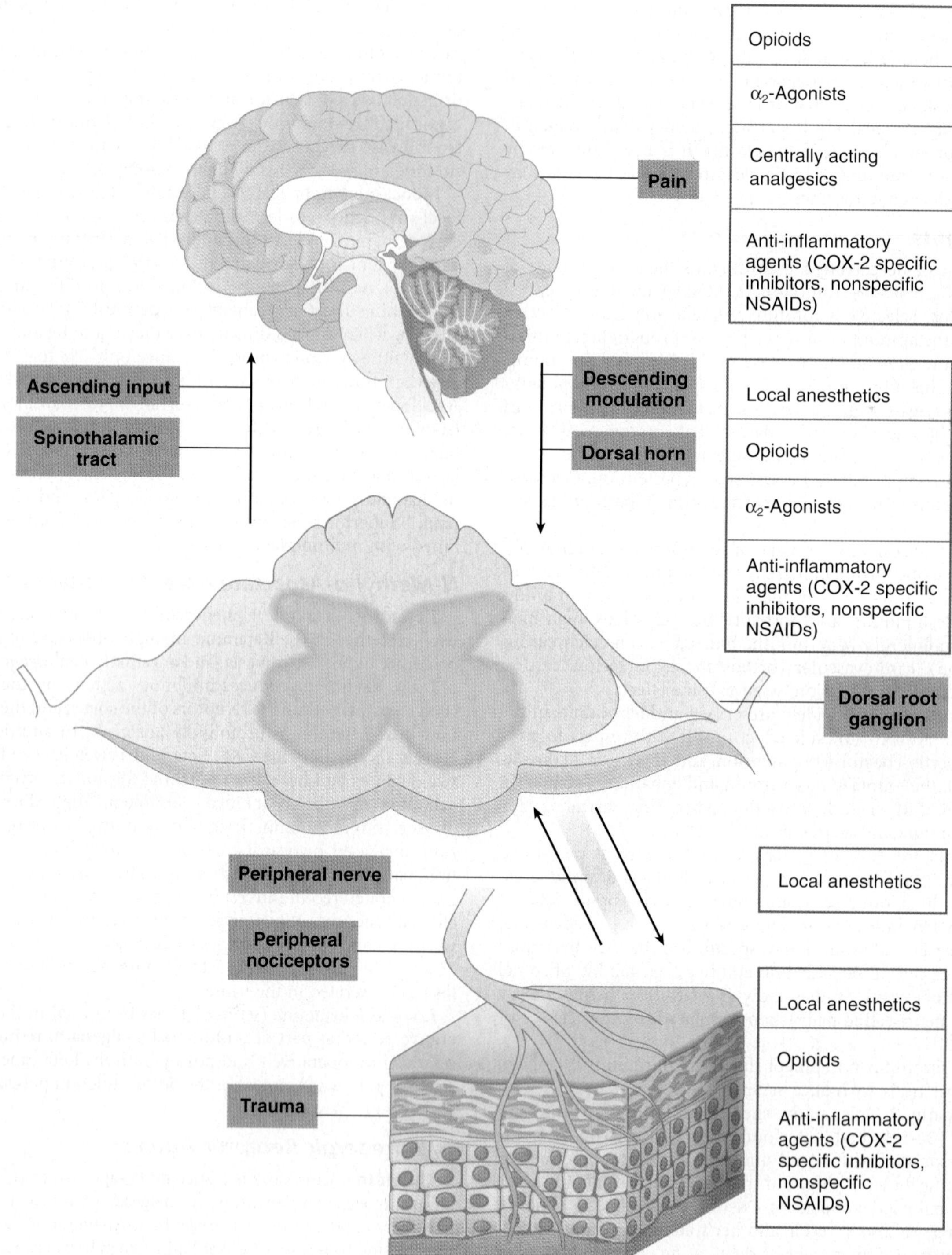

FIGURE 61-3 • Multimodal therapy for pain relief, with or without opioids, is now accepted as a more balanced approach to pain management in surgical patients. Such therapy aims to decrease the dose of any single agent, thus improving antinociception and reducing side effects. Multimodal therapy employs combinations of cyclooxygenase-2–specific inhibitors, local anesthetics, opioids, nonsteroidal anti-inflammatory drugs, and α_2-agonists. Opioid sparing is a key goal of multimodal therapy. Opioids—some of the most common drugs associated with hospital-administered medication-related complications—result in increased morbidity and length of stay. In addition, multimodal analgesia aims to avoid sedation and respiratory depression from excessive dosing. Constipation, pruritis, and postoperative nausea and vomiting should also be reduced with this therapeutic approach. This method of pain management also interrupts the pain transmission pathway at numerous points, from the peripheral to the central nervous system.

CONCLUSION

Numerous drugs are available for the treatment of pain. Effective pain management requires an understanding of the types of pain and the mechanisms of action of the various analgesic drugs. Multimodal analgesia requires an understanding of the molecular mechanisms of pain. A multimodal approach to pain management provides the best balance of side effects and efficacy (Fig. 61-3, Box 61-1).

BOX 61-1 MULTIMODAL ANALGESIA: RATIONAL POLYPHARMACY

- Reduced doses of each analgesic
- Improved antinociception due to synergistic/additive effects
- May reduce severity of side effects of each drug

REFERENCES

1. Stewart WF, Ricci JA, Chee E, et al. Lost productive time and cost due to common pain conditions in the US workforce JAMA 2003;290:2443-2454.
2. Brennan F, Carr DB, Cousins M. Pain management: a fundamental human right. Anesth Analg 2007;105:205-221.
3. Turk DC, Brody MC, Okifuji A. Physicians' attitudes and practices regarding long-term prescribing of opioids for non-cancer pain. Pain 1994;59:201-208.
4. Woolf CJ. Evidence for a component of post-injury pain hypersensitivity. Nature 1983;306:686-688.
5. Woolf CJ. Central sensitization: uncovering the relation between pain and plasticity. Anesthesiology 2007;106:864-867.
6. Perkins FM, Kehlet H. Chronic pain as an outcome of surgery—a review of predictive factors. Anesthesiology 2000;93:130-137.
7. Von Roenn JH, Cleeland CS, Gonin R, et al. Physician attitudes and practice in cancer pain management: a survey from the Eastern Cooperative Oncology Group. Ann Intern Med 1993;119:121-126.
8. World Health Organization. Cancer Pain Relief and Palliative Care: Report of a WHO Expert Committee (Technical Report Series No. 804). Geneva: World Health Organization, 1990.
9. O'Brien T, Welsh J, Dunn FG. ABC of palliative care: non-malignant conditions. BMJ 1998;316:286-289.
10. Barakzoy AS, Moss AH. Efficacy of the World Health Organization analgesic ladder to treat pain in end-stage renal disease. J Am Soc Nephrol 2006;17:3198-3203.
11. Expert Working Group of the European Association for Palliative Care. Morphine in cancer pain: modes of administration. BMJ 1996;312:823-826.
12. Murphy MR, Hug CC. Pharmacokinetics of intravenous morphine in patients anesthetized with enflurance–nitrous oxide. Anesthesiology 1981;54:187-192.
13. Vater M, Smith G, Aherne GW, Aitkenhead AR. Pharmacokinetics and analgesic effect of slow-release oral morphine sulphate in volunteers. Br J Anaesth 1984;56:821-827.
14. Bochner F, Somogyi AA, Christrup LL, et al. Comparative pharmacokinetics of two modified-release oral morphine formulations (Reliadol and Kapanol) and an immediate-release morphine tablet (Morfin 'DAK') in healthy volunteers. Clin Drug Invest 1999;17:59-66.
15. Thirlwell MP, Sloan PA, Maroun JA, et al. Pharmacokinetics and clinical efficacy of oral morphine solution and controlled-release morphine tablets in cancer patients. Cancer 1989;63:2275-2283.
16. Kharasch ED, Hoffer C, Whittington D, Sheffels P. Role of P-glycoprotein in the intestinal absorption and clinical effects of morphine. Clin Pharmacol Ther 2003;74:543-554.
17. Frances B, Gout R, Montsarrat B, et al. Further evidence that morphine-6-beta-glucuronide is a more potent opioid agonist than morphine. J Pharmacol Exp Ther 1992;262:25-31.
18. Motamed C, Mazoit X, Ghanouchi K, et al. Preemptive intravenous morphine-6-glucuronide is ineffective for postoperative pain relief. Anesthesiology 2000:92:355-360.
19. Penson RT, Joel SP, Roberts M, et al. The bioavailability and pharmacokinetics of subcutaneous, nebulized and oral morphine-6-glucuronide. Br J Clin Pharmacol 2001;53:347-354.
20. Stambaugh J, Wainer I, Sanstead J, Hemphill D. The clinical pharmacology of meperidine: comparison of routes of administration. Clin Pharmacol Ther 1981;30:619-628.
21. Latta KS, Ginsberg B, Barkin RL. Meperidine: a critical review. Am J Ther 2002;9: 53-68.
22. Roerig DL, Kotrly KJ, Vucins EJ, et al. First pass uptake of fentanyl, meperidine, and morphine in the human lung. Anesthesiology 1987;67:466-472.
23. Larsen RH, Nielsen F, Sorensen JA, et al. Dermal penetration of fentanyl: inter- and intraindividual variations. Pharmacol Toxicol 2003;93:244-248.
24. Streisand JB, Varvel JR, Stanski DR, et al. Absorption and bioavailability of oral transmucosal fentanyl citrate. Anesthesiology 1991;75:223-229.
25. Viscusi ER, Witkowski TA. Iontophoresis: the process behind noninvasive drug delivery. Reg Anesth Pain Med 2005;30:292-294.
26. Viscusi ER, Reynolds L, Chung F, et al. Patient-controlled transdermal fentanyl hydrochloride vs. intravenous morphine pump for postoperative pain. JAMA 2004;291:1333-1341.
27. Sarhill N, Walsh D, Nelson KA. Hydromorphone: pharmacology and clinical applications in cancer patients. Support Care Cancer 2001;9:84-96.
28. Davis GA, Rudy AC, Archer SM, et al. Bioavailability and pharmacokinetics of intranasal hydromorphone in patients experiencing vasomotor rhinitis. Clin Drug Invest 2004;24:633-639.
29. Lessons learned from OxyContin, after guilty plea by Purdue Pharma for fraud in marketing drug. Topics Pain Manage 2007;22:9-10.
30. Inturrisi CE. Clinical pharmacology of opioids for pain. Clin J Pain 2002;18:S3-S13.
31. Keeting GM. Tramadol sustained-release capsules. Drugs 2006;66:223-230.
32. Grond S, Sablotzki A. Clinical pharmacology of tramadol. Clin Pharmacokinet 2004;43:879-923.
33. Enggaard TP, Poulsen L, Arendt-Neilsen L, et al. The analgesic effect of tramadol after intravenous injection in healthy volunteers in relation to CYP2D6. Anesth Analg 2006;102:146-150.
34. Collart L, Luthy C, Drayer P. Multimodal analgesic effects of tramadol. Clin Pharmacol Ther 1993;53:223-226.
35. Hair PI, Curran MP, Keam SJ. Tramadol extended-release tablets in moderate to moderately severe chronic pain in adults. CNS Drugs 2007;21:259-263.
36. Auret K, Roger Goucke C, Ilett KF, et al. Pharmacokinetics and pharmacodynamics of methadone enantiomers in hospice patients with cancer pain. Ther Drug Monit 2006;28:359-366.
37. Brown R, Kraus C, Fleming M, Reddy S. Methadone: applied pharmacology and use as adjunctive treatment in chronic pain. Postgrad Med J 2004;80:654-659.
38. Morley J, Makin M. The use of methadone in cancer pain poorly responsive to other opiates. Pain Rev 1998;5:51-58.
39. Wysowski DK. Surveillance of prescription drug-related mortality using death certificate data. Drug Saf 2007;30:533-540.
40. Barkin RL, Barkin SJ, Barkin DS. Propoxyphene (dextropropoxyphene): a critical review of a weak opioid analgesic that should remain in antiquity. Am J Ther 2006;13:534-542.
41. Davis GA, Rudy AC, Archer SM, Wermeling P. Bioavailability of intranasal butorphanol administered from a single-dose sprayer. Am J Health Syst Pharm 2005;62:48-53.
42. Dunteman E, Karanikolas M, Filos KS. Transnasal butorphanol for the treatment of opioid-induced pruritus unresponsive to antihistamines. J Pain Symptom Manage 1996;12:255-260.
43. Gunter JB, McAuliffe J, Gregg T, et al. Continuous epidural butorphanol relieves pruritus associated with epidural morphine infusions in children. Paediatr Anaesth 2000;10:167-172.
44. Dahan A, Yassen A, Romberg R, et al. Buprenorphine induces ceiling in respiratory depression but not in analgesia. Br J Anaesth 2006;96:627-632.
45. Van Dorp E, Yassen A, Sarton E, et al. Naloxone reversal of buprenorphine-induced respiratory depression. Anesthesiology 2006;105:51-57.
46. Cowan J. Buprenorphine: basic pharmacology revisted. J Addiction Med 2007;1: 68-72.
47. Raja S, Meyer RA, Campbell JN. Peripheral mechanisms of somatic pain. Anesthesiology 1988;68:571-590.
48. Dahl JB, Kehlet H. Non-steroidal anti-inflammatory drugs: rationale for use in severe postoperative pain. Br J Anaesth 1991;66:703-712.
49. Pickering G, Loriot MA, Libert F, et al. Analgesic effect of acetaminophen in humans: first evidence of a central serotonergic mechanism. Clin Pharmacol Ther 2006;79:371-378.
50. Buvenendran A, Kroin JS, Tuman KJ, et al. Effects of perioperative administration of a selective cyclooxygenase 2 inhibitor on pain management and recovery of function after knee replacement: a randomized controlled trial. JAMA 2003;290:2411-2418.
51. Reuben SS, Connelly NR. Postoperative analgesic effects of celecoxib or rofecoxib after spinal fusion surgery. Anesth Analg 2000;91:1221-1225.
52. Tiippana EM, Hamunen K, Kontinen VK, Kalson E. Do surgical patients benefit from perioperative gabapentin/pregabalin? A systematic review of efficacy and safety. Anesth Analg 2007;104:1545-1556.
53. Turan A, Karamanliouglu B, Memis D, et al. Analgesic effects of gabapentin after spinal surgery. Anesthesiology 2004;100:935-938.
54. Turan A, Karamanliouglu B, Memis D, et al. The analgesic effects of gabapentin after total abdominal hysterectomy. Anesth Analg 2004;98:1370-1373.
55. Sawyonk J, Esser MJ, Reid AR. Antidepressants as analgesics: an overview of central and peripheral mechanisms of action. J Psychiatry Neurosci 2001;26:2001.
56. Collins SL, Moore RA, McQuay HJ, Wiffen P. Antidepressants and anticonvulsants for diabetic neuropathy and postherpetic neuralgia: a quantitative systemic review. J Pain Symptom Manage 2000;20:449-458.
57. Goldstein DJ, Lu Y, Detke MJ, et al. Duloxetine vs. placebo in patients with painful diabetic neuropathy. Pain 2005;116:109-118.
58. Arnold LM, Rosen A, Pritchett YL, et al. A randomized, double-blind, placebo-controlled trial of duloxetine in the treatment of women with fibromyalgia with or without major depressive disorder. Pain 2005;119:5-15.
59. Stracke H, Meyer UE, Schumacher HE, Federlin K. Mexiletine in the treatment of diabetic neuropathy. Diabetes Care 1992;15:1550-1555.
60. Nishiyama K, Sakuta M. Mexiletine for painful alcoholic neuropathy. Intern Med 1995;34:577-579.
61. Chabal C, Jacobson L, Mariano A, et al. The use of oral mexeletine for the treatment of pain after peripheral nerve injury. Anesthesiology 1992;76:513-517.
62. Sloan P, Basta M, Storey P, Von Gunten C. Mexiletine as an adjuvant analgesic for the management of neuropathic cancer pain. Anesth Analg 1999;89:760-761.
63. Fassoulaki A, Patris K, Sarantopoulos C, Hogan Q. The analgesic effect of gabapentin and mexiletine after breast surgery for cancer. Anesth Analg 2002;95:985-991.
64. White WT, Patel N, Drass M, Nalamachu S. Lidocaine patch 5% with systemic analgesics such as gabapentin: a rational polypharmacy approach for the treatment of chronic pain. Pain Med 2003;4:321-330.
65. Reuben SS, Buvanendran A. Current Concepts Review: Preventing the development of chronic pain after orthopaedic surgery with preventive multimodal analgesic techniques. J Bone Joint Surg 2007;89:1343-1358.
66. Reuben SS, Steinberg RB, Klatt JL, Klatt ML. Intravenous regional anesthesia using lidocaine and clonidine. Anesthesiology 1999;91:654-658.

62

ANEMIAS AND CYTOPENIAS

Nandi J. Reddy and Lionel D. Lewis

OVERVIEW 895
ANEMIAS 895
Introduction 895
Iron-Deficiency Anemia 895
Pathophysiology 896
Therapeutics and Clinical Pharmacology 897
Copper- and Zinc-Related Anemia 898
Vitamin-Deficiency Anemias 898
Vitamin B_{12} 898
Folic Acid 900
Other Vitamins 900
Drug-Related Anemia 901
Aplastic Anemia 901
Therapeutic Approach to Drug-Related Anemia 902
NEUTROPENIA AND LYMPHOPENIA 902
THROMBOCYTOPENIA 902
Introduction 902
Pathophysiology 902
Therapeutics and Clinical Pharmacology 902
Hematopoietic Growth Factors and Their Receptors 902
Erythroid Growth Factors 903
Myeloid Growth Factors 905
Thrombopoietic Growth Factors 905

OVERVIEW

Common hematologic disorders include anemia, neutropenia, and thrombocytopenia. These hematologic disorders can be due to deficient production, excessive loss or destruction, or redistribution of blood cells. The production of the different lineages of hematopoietic cells is complex and is influenced by the availability of certain vitamins, minerals, and a number of hematopoietic growth factors (Fig. 62-1). A deficiency in any of these moieties could potentially lead to various inherited or acquired disorders of hematopoiesis.

Drugs may adversely affect the bone marrow and peripheral blood cells. Although the risk from most drugs is very small, many cases are reported because of the millions of doses of drugs taken each year by patients. In order of frequency, neutropenia, thrombocytopenia, hemolytic anemia, aplastic anemia, and macrocytic anemia are the most common drug-induced adverse hematologic effects.[1,2] Drug-induced hematologic effects should always be considered as a possible cause in any acquired hematologic disorder.

ANEMIAS

Introduction

Anemia is a reduction in the circulating red blood cell (RBC) mass, and thus hemoglobin concentration, to below age-specific and gender-specific population-defined lower limits. Anemia can be due to a hypoproliferative bone marrow (low reticulocyte count), chronic inflammatory conditions leading to a normochromic normocytic anemia, or excessive red cell destruction with a hyperproliferative bone marrow as in hemolytic anemia (high reticulocyte count). Most patients with anemia are asymptomatic or only minimally symptomatic with vague constitutional symptoms. Anemia should be considered a physical state, not a disease,[3] as it may be caused by primary hematologic disorders or secondary to a variety of systemic diseases (Box 62-1 and Fig. 62-2).

Targets of therapy include

1. Replacement of nutritional deficiency (hematinics—iron, vitamin B_{12} [cyanocobalamin], folate)
2. Optimization of the management of other comorbid conditions
3. Discontinuation of the causative offending agent (i.e., medications, exposure to toxins)

Iron-Deficiency Anemia

An average 70-kg adult has a total body iron content of about 4000 mg. Most of the iron is circulating as hemoglobin within the erythrocytes (2500 mg). Approximately 1000 mg is in body stores as ferritin and hemosiderin, and about 300 mg is incorporated into myoglobin and respiratory enzymes. Humans absorb only 1 mg of iron daily from a diet containing 10 to 20 mg, in order to maintain equilibrium with body losses of iron in body secretions and exfoliated skin and gut epithelium. In females, iron losses through normal menstruation add an additional average daily incremental loss of 0.4 mg, giving a total daily loss of 1.3 mg. During pregnancy and lactation, additional demands of up to 4 mg/day are placed on maternal iron stores. Intercellular iron transport, as a part of the iron reutilization process, is quantitatively more important than intestinal absorption. The greatest mass of iron is found in erythrocytes, which contain about 80% of the total body iron. The reticuloendothelial system recycles a substantial amount of iron. Breakdown of erythrocytes releases iron back into plasma in the form of transferrin (Fig. 62-3).[4]

Most iron absorption takes place in the duodenum and jejunum. In order to be absorbed, iron must be in its reduced ferrous form. The acid pH of the stomach, along with reducing substances and vitamin C, enhance iron absorption by maintaining iron in its reduced, more soluble form, and by forming a chelate with ferric iron, which remains soluble as the pH rises in the small intestine. Iron absorption is largely carried out by the enterocytes, and a mucosal control mechanism has been proposed in which solubilized ionic iron in the intestinal lumen adsorbs to receptors in the brush border of the mucosal cells. Regulation of iron uptake into the body occurs at the apical and basolateral membranes of the intestinal epithelium (Fig. 62-4).

The apical membrane of the differentiated enterocyte is specialized for transport of heme and ferrous iron into the cell. The most extensively characterized uptake pathway is via divalent metal transporter 1, which is an energy-dependent process. The transferrin receptor–hereditary hemochromatosis protein complex, the basolateral iron transporter, and the ceruloplasmin homologue hephaestin are the proteins related to iron transport on the basolateral membrane of the enterocyte.[5-12] Transferrin transports iron from across the intestinal mucosal surface to plasma and ultimately to red cell precursors in the bone marrow.

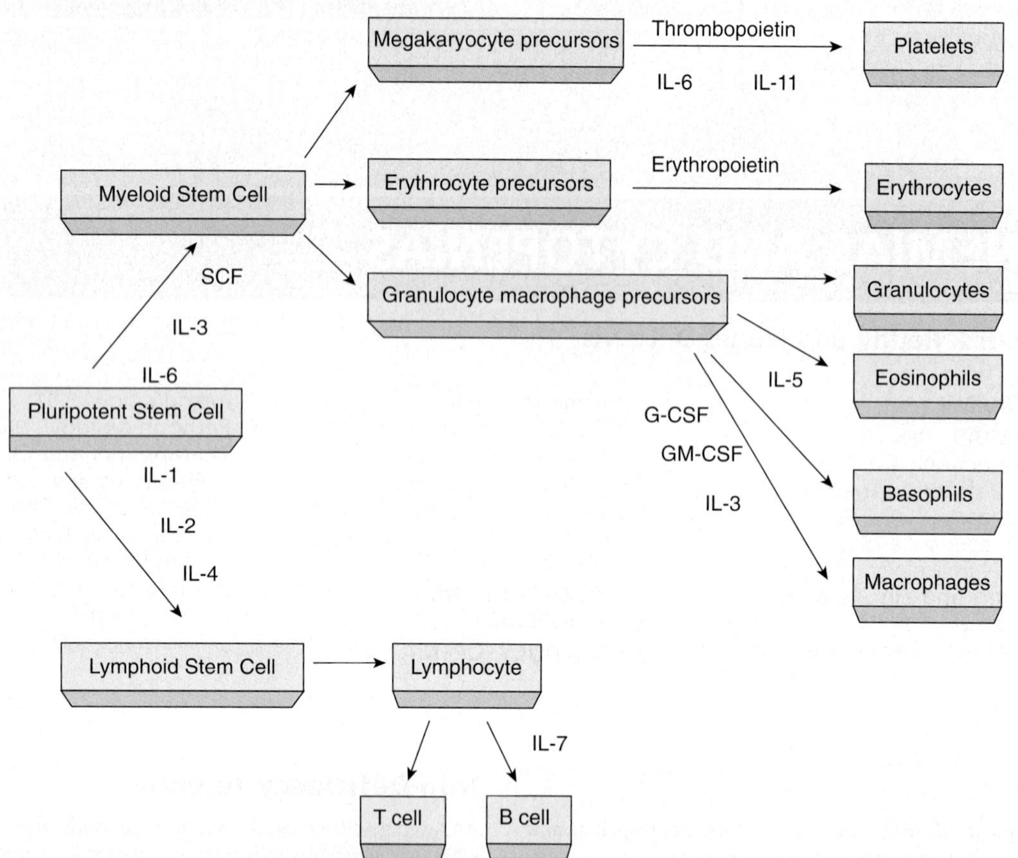

FIGURE 62-1 • Outline of hematopoiesis.

BOX 62-1 COMMON CAUSES OF ANEMIA

Nutritional Deficiency
- Iron
- Folate
- Cyanocobalamin (vitamin B_{12})

Anemia of Chronic Disease
- Chronic renal failure
- Chronic inflammatory conditions (e.g., systemic lupus erythematosus, rheumatoid arthritis, tuberculosis)
- Chronic liver disease
- Endocrine deficiency states (e.g., hypothyroidism)

Iatrogenic/Drug-Induced Anemia
- Most commonly cytotoxic chemotherapy agents

Hemolytic Anemia
- Hereditary glucose 6-phosphate deficiency
- Acquired—includes drug-induced (e.g., quinine, β-lactams)

Aplastic Anemia and Bone Marrow Suppression/Failure Syndromes
- Chloramphenicol
- Cytotoxic agents

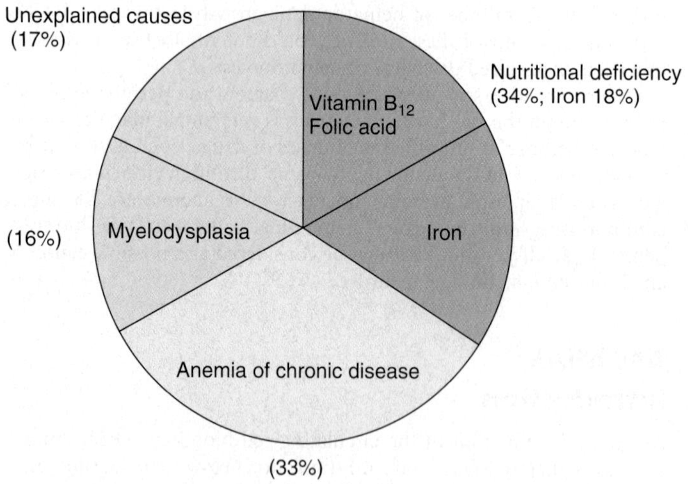

Unexplained causes (17%)
Nutritional deficiency (34%; Iron 18%)
Vitamin B_{12} Folic acid
Iron
(16%) Myelodysplasia
Anemia of chronic disease
(33%)

FIGURE 62-2 • Causes of anemia in the elderly (>65 years of age). (Data from Guralnick et al.,[13] Artz et al.,[14] and the Third National Health and Nutrition Examination Survey [NHANES III].[15])

Pathophysiology

Iron deficiency is the most common cause of anemia (Table 62-1).[13-15] According to National Institutes of Health statistics, 12% of women between the ages of 12 and 49 years in the United States have iron deficiency anemia,[15] and 8% of individuals over age 65 years have anemia from a number of other causes, as shown in Figure 62-2. Anemia results from inadequate dietary iron intake and/or increased demands on iron stores such as during pregnancy and lactation, and in premature infants. Chronic blood loss from the gastrointestinal tract, uterine bleeding, or other blood loss can also lead to iron deficiency anemia. Inadequate iron absorption (e.g., due to achlorohydria or following a partial gastrectomy) is another cause of iron deficiency anemia. A thorough diagnostic search in patients with iron deficiency anemia (microcytosis being a common indicator) for the underlying cause is of paramount importance, especially in men and postmenopausal women. The transferrin saturation, plasma ferritin, and total iron-binding capacity are useful in differentiating other causes of microcytic anemia.

Therapeutics and Clinical Pharmacology

Goals of Therapy. The goals of therapy for iron deficiency anemia include normalization of hemoglobin and restoration of iron stores. This may take up to 3 to 6 months of treatment with iron supplements.

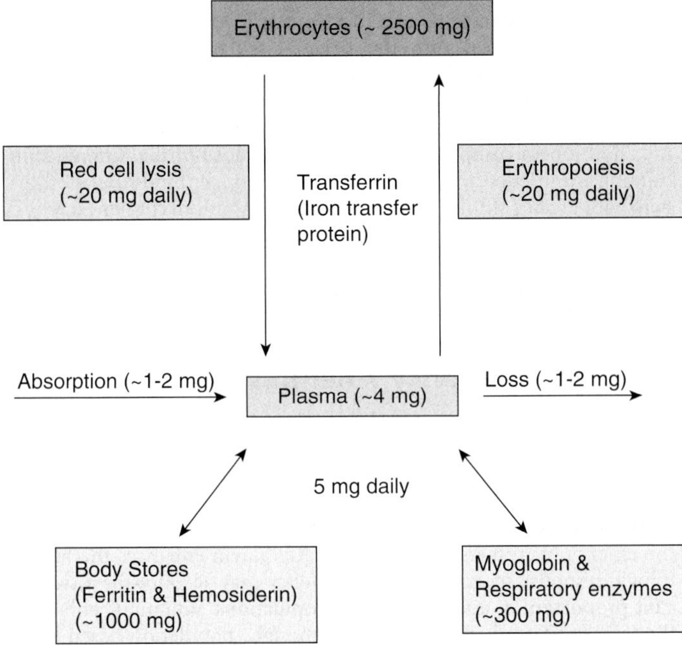

FIGURE 62-3 • Iron metabolism. (Modified from Conrad ME, Umbreit JN. Pathways of iron absorption. Blood Cells Mol Dis 2002;29:337.)

Therapeutics. During 4th century BC, Hippocrates first used iron as a therapeutic agent as "styptics," a practice that exists even today in the form of Monsel's solution (ferric subsulfate).[16] Iron plays a vital role in body homeostasis and is a pivotal component of several heme-containing proteins and enzymes (e.g., hemoglobin, myoglobin, cytochrome, catalases, and peroxidases).

Iron absorption takes place in the jejunum and upper ileum. Inorganic ferrous iron is better absorbed than ferric iron. Absorption of iron from orally administered salts is approximately 10%. Gastric acid, vitamin C, and ethanol facilitate iron absorption.

TABLE 62-1 PREVALENCE OF IRON DEFICIENCY ANEMIA—UNITED STATES

	1988-1994 (NHANES III)		*1999-2000*	
Sex/Age Group (yr)	**No.**	**%**	**No.**	**%**
Both Sexes				
1-2	1339	9	319	7
3-5	2334	3	363	5
6-11	2813	2	882	4
Males				
12-15	691	1	547	5
16-69	6635	1	2084	2
>70	1437	4	381	3
Females (nonpregnant only)				
12-49	5982	11	1950	12
50-69	2034	5	611	9
>70	1630	7	394	6

(Data from Guralnick et al.,[13] Artz et al.,[14] and the Third National Health and Nutrition Examination Survey [NHANES III].[15])

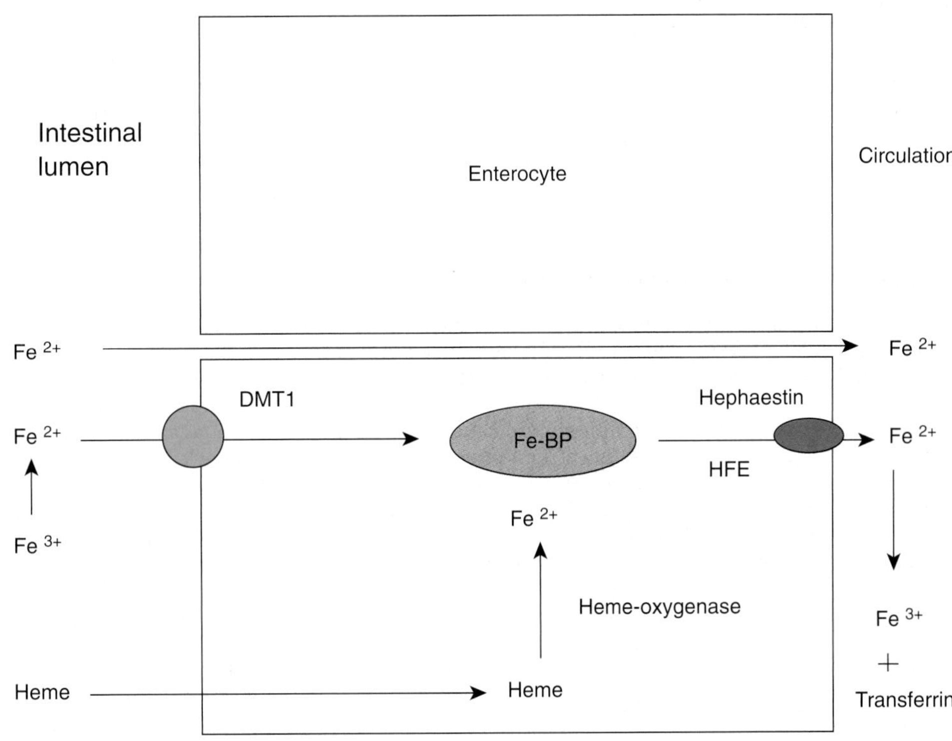

FIGURE 62-4 • Mechanisms of iron transport in the intestine. *1*, Inorganic iron is converted into its ferrous form (Fe^{2+}) at the intestinal epithelium brush border before it is transported into the cell. *2*, Divalent metal transporter 1 (DMT1) transports Fe^{2+} across the apical cell membrane. Within the cell, one or more iron-binding proteins (Fe-BP) take up iron and transfer it to the basolateral membrane. *3*, Transferrin receptor–hereditary hemochromatosis protein (HFE) complex and hephaestin transport Fe^{2+} across the basolateral membrane with subsequent binding to transferrin in the circulation. *4*, A small amount of inorganic iron may pass through via the paracellular route. (Adapted from Roy CN, Enns CA. Iron homeostasis: new tales from the crypt. Blood 2000;96:4020-4027.)

TABLE 62-2 IRON CONTENT IN SOME COMMERCIALLY AVAILABLE ORAL IRON PREPARATIONS

Iron Formulation	Dose	Iron Content
Ferrous sulfate	200 mg	60 mg
Ferrous fumarate	325 mg	106 mg
Ferrous gluconate	225 mg	27 mg
Polysaccharide-iron complex	2.5-5 ml	50-100 mg

Modified from Ritter JM, Lewis LD, Mant TGK. Anemia and hematological disorders (chapter 48). In Ritter JM, Lewis LD, Mant TGK (eds): Textbook of Clinical Pharmacology, 4th ed. New York: Oxford University Press, 1999, Ch 48.

Oral Iron. The most commonly prescribed treatment for iron deficiency anemia is oral iron salt preparations. The ferrous form of iron is the treatment of choice, because iron absorption from ferrous salts is three times greater than from ferric salts. Table 62-2 shows some of the common commercially available formulations of oral iron salts and their iron content.

Monitoring the hemoglobin (or the hematocrit) will guide the effectiveness of iron therapy. The average dose for the treatment of a patient with iron deficiency anemia is about 2 to 3 mg/kg per day of iron, administered in two to four divided doses; the iron is best absorbed in a fasting state. At this dose an increase in hemoglobin of 0.7 to 2 g/dl per day is expected.

Gastrointestinal side effects are common (12% to 25% of patients) and include nausea, heartburn, and constipation.[18-20] Iron poisoning by accidental ingestion in children can be fatal, leading to gastrointestinal hemorrhage, hepatic injury, and shock. Deferoxamine, an iron-chelating agent, is indicated in this situation.

Parenteral Iron. Parenteral iron is effective and used as an alternative[21,22] only when oral preparations are not tolerated, or in patients with malabsorption of iron, or to achieve rapid restoration of iron stores in pregnant women near term. Although iron stores are repleted faster with parenteral iron, the rate of increase in hemoglobin is about the same as with oral iron therapy. The rate-limiting factor is erythropoiesis in the bone marrow. Sodium ferric gluconate complex (Ferrlecit) is the commonly used parenteral formulation. It is given by deep intramuscular injection. It has a lower incidence of severe anaphylactoid reactions than iron dextran, which is the other commercially available parenteral formulation in the United States.

Copper- and Zinc-Related Anemia

Copper and zinc are available from a wide variety of food sources, and dietary deficiency of either is rare in a typical American diet. These are two essential trace elements whose role in iron metabolism has been investigated.[23]

Copper deficiency is associated with abnormalities in iron metabolism and iron deficiency anemia, due at least in part to the importance of the copper-containing ferroxidases ceruloplasmin and hephaestin.[24-27] Ceruloplasmin is a plasma glycoprotein containing six to seven copper atoms. Ceruloplasmin acts as an oxidase for a variety of substrates, one of which is ferrous iron. Ceruloplasmin probably acts by catalyzing the oxidation of ferrous iron to the ferric form, which is a prerequisite for iron binding by transferrin. The anemia of copper deficiency, however, is not explained solely by defective ceruloplasmin function. A second copper-containing ferroxidase, hephaestin, expressed in the duodenal enterocytes, has an important role in iron absorption (see Fig. 62-4).[28,29]

Copper deficiency secondary to excessive zinc intake has also been well described in patients taking large doses of supplemental zinc (e.g., for the treatment of sickle cell anemia, aphthous ulcers, and prostate cancer), as well as in zinc coin ingestion.[30-33] Zinc supplements gained popularity as a remedy for the common cold (zinc lozenges), to promote healing of skin ulcers, and to treat macular degeneration.[34] Patients ingesting excessive zinc present with signs and symptoms of anemia (microcytic or sideroblastic) and may have concurrent neutropenia.

Zinc and copper have a competitive absorption relationship within enterocytes mediated by metallothionein, a zinc- and copper-binding protein that binds copper with greater affinity than zinc. Zinc and copper are either bound to metallothionein and stored inside enterocytes, or exist in an unbound state. Bound complexes are shed intraluminally and excreted as enterocytes turn over. Unbound zinc and copper are absorbed into the portal circulation. Metallothionein expression is regulated by dietary zinc content alone. When large amounts of dietary zinc are ingested, metallothionein expression increases, more zinc is bound to metallothionein, and more zinc-metallothionein complexes are excreted. Because of the difference in binding affinities between zinc and copper (copper binds metallothionein with greater affinity), a potential for pronounced copper excretion exists. Therefore, a substantial increase in zinc ingestion potentially would cause a dramatic decrease in copper absorption.[35,36]

The treatment of copper deficiency is careful oral copper replacement, or, if this is due to excess zinc intake, reduction in zinc intake.

Vitamin-Deficiency Anemias

While iron deficiency is regarded as the major cause of nutritional anemia, deficiencies in vitamin B_{12} and folic acid can also lead to anemia. Both vitamin B_{12} and folate can treat and prevent megaloblastic anemia. More rarely, deficiency in other vitamins can be associated with anemia. Vitamin A can improve hematologic indices and enhance the efficacy of iron supplementation. Riboflavin enhances the hematologic response to iron, and its deficiency may account for a significant proportion of anemia in many populations. Vitamin C enhances the absorption of dietary iron, although population-based data showing its efficacy in reducing the prevalence of anemia or iron deficiency are lacking. Vitamin E supplementation given to preterm infants has not reduced the severity of the anemia of prematurity. Vitamin B_6 (pyridoxine) effectively treats sideroblastic anemia.[37]

Vitamin B_{12}

Deficiency of vitamin B_{12} leads to a macrocytic megaloblastic anemia. Vitamin B_{12} must be obtained from external sources in humans (and other mammals) because vitamin B_{12} is not synthesized in mammalian cells. The terms *vitamin B_{12}* and *cyanocobalamin* are used interchangeably for all cobamides active in humans. Vitamin B_{12} consists of a nucleotide linked to four pyrole rings with a cobalt atom attached. Linked to the cobalt atom may be a cyanide (cyanocobalamin; Fig. 62-5), hydroxyl (hydroxocobalamin), methyl (methylcobalamin), or 5′-deoxyadenosyl group.[37] The liver has the largest storage of vitamin B_{12} in the human body. The daily requirement of vitamin B_{12} is 0.6 to 1.2 mg, which is derived from animal products and bacterial flora in the intestine. Vegetable products contain no vitamin B_{12} but, interestingly, strict vegetarians rarely develop B_{12} deficiency. Vitamin B_{12} functions as an important cofactor for enzymes involved in DNA synthesis. Methylcobalamin is a cofactor in the methionine synthetase reaction, which is essential for the normal metabolism of folate. Methyl groups contributed by methyltetrahydrofolate are used to form methylcobalamin, which then acts as a methyl group donor for the conversion of homocysteine to methionine.

Pathophysiology. Vitamin B_{12} forms a complex with intrinsic factor (IF), which is secreted by the parietal cells of the stomach and is readily absorbed in the distal ileum. The most common cause of vitamin B_{12} deficiency is pernicious anemia. Formation of antibody to the gastric parietal cells or to IF leads to pernicious anemia. Other causes include gastric atrophy, gastric surgery, and loss of pancreatic protease secretion, bacterial overgrowth, and disease at the site of absorption in the distal ileum (e.g., inflammatory bowel disease).

Vitamin B_{12} deficiency is recognized clinically by its impact on hematopoiesis and the nervous system (causing dementia, neuropathy, and, if severe, a spastic lower limb weakness). As a result of vitamin B_{12} deficiency, DNA replication becomes highly abnormal, leading to ineffective erythropoiesis. Vitamin B_{12} is an essential cofactor in at least two key transmethylation reactions, one of which closely interrelates with folic acid in DNA biosynthesis and hematopoiesis. The conversion of homocysteine to the amino acid methionine requires a B_{12}-dependent enzyme as well as a methyl group donated by the folate compound 5-methyltetrahydrofolate. With deficiency of vitamin B_{12}, the enzyme function is impaired, methionine synthesis is compromised, and both 5-methyltetrahydrofolate and homocysteine accumulate. Through either the trapping of folate in the form of 5-methyltetrahydrofolate or the failure of methionine synthesis, the concentrations of 5,10-methylenetetrahydrofolate are reduced, ultimately leading to impaired synthesis of thymidine. An inadequate supply of thymidine, in turn, impairs cellular DNA biosynthesis (Fig. 62-6). In this situation, the peripheral blood smear and bone marrow show macrocytosis and hypersegmented neutrophils.[37]

Neuropathy commonly complicates vitamin B_{12} deficiency in humans. The neuropathy is characterized by demyelination of the posterolateral columns of the spinal cord (subacute combined degeneration). The lesion was thought to arise primarily from impairment of the adenosylcobalamin-dependent methylmalonyl-coenzyme A mutase reaction, leading to the formation of abnormal odd-chain and branched-chain fatty acids and their incorporation into myelin with resultant demyelination.[38]

The pathogenesis of subacute combined degeneration is thought to be related to interference with the methylation reactions in nerve cells. The methylation reactions are processed by *S*-adenosylmethionine, which is controlled by its product, *S*-adenosylhomocysteine. The relationship of these two compounds is termed the *methylation ratio.* It has been demonstrated that, if the ratio falls, the methylation reactions are inhibited, leading to a state of central nervous system (CNS) hypomethylation. The ratio can fall due to either a rise in *S*-adenosylhomocysteine or a fall in *S*-adenosylmethionine. It is suggested that, for clinical signs to develop in humans who are susceptible to the lesion, both events are usually required. Inhibition of the vitamin B_{12}-dependent enzyme methionine synthase leads to a rapid fall in the ratio in the CNS, since unlike other organs such as the liver, it does not have an alternative method of remethylating homocysteine to maintain the endogenous synthesis of *S*-adenosylmethionine. The supply of methyl groups necessary for the remethylation reactions is controlled by a series of enzymes, which include methionine synthase. Neurologic syndromes associated with deficiency of these enzymes have close associations with subacute combined degeneration.[39]

Measuring vitamin B_{12} concentrations can usually make the diagnosis, though a minority of B_{12}-deficient patients may have normal concentrations. Measurement of urine or serum methylmalonic acid is a more sensitive test for vitamin B_{12} deficiency. A Schilling test (with and without added IF) is performed to diagnose pernicious anemia.

Therapeutics and Clinical Pharmacology

Goals of Therapy. Goals of therapy for vitamin B_{12}-deficiency anemia include replacement of vitamin B_{12} stores, correction of anemia, and reversal of neurologic deficits, although the latter may not always be successful.

Therapeutics. Vitamin B_{12} is used to treat pernicious anemia and vitamin B_{12} deficiency, as well as to determine vitamin B_{12} absorption in the Schilling test. Vitamin B_{12} replacement therapy is available as parenteral cyanocobalamin and hydroxocobalamin. Cyanocobalamin is administered orally and parenterally, while hydroxocobalamin is administered only parenterally. Hydroxocobalamin given in doses of

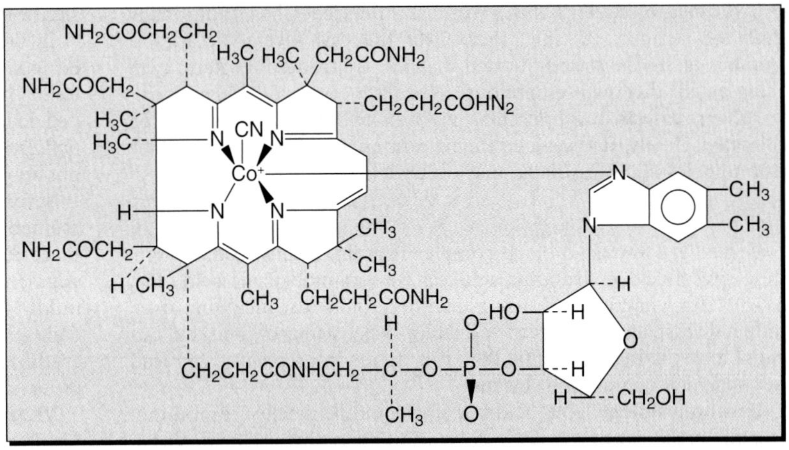

FIGURE 62-5 • Structure of cyanocobalamin.

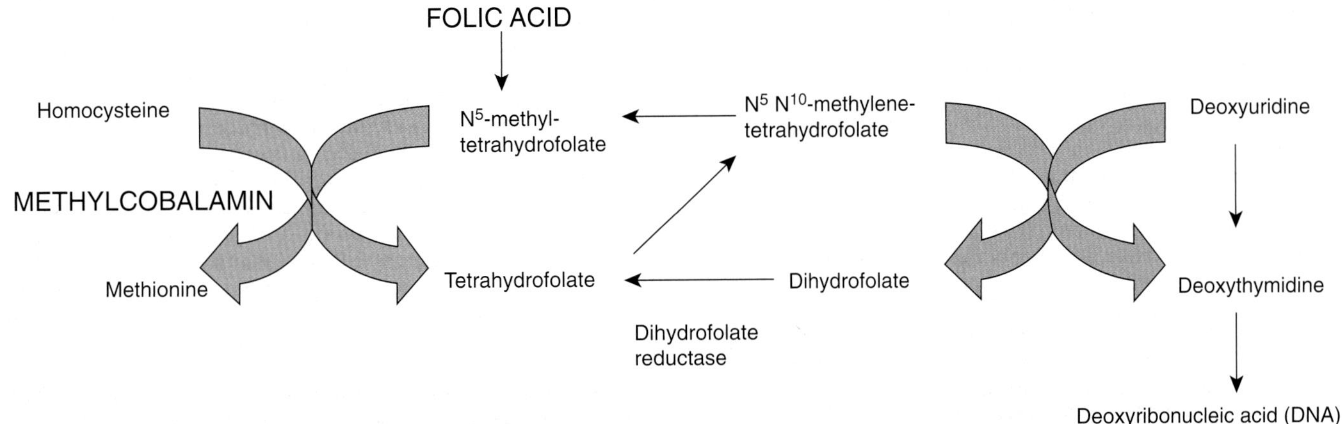

FIGURE 62-6 • Vitamin B_{12} and folic acid interaction in DNA synthesis. Cobalamin is a cofactor for homocysteine-methionine methyltransferase, which transfers a methyl group from methyltetrahydrofolate to homocysteine to make methionine. The folate compound 5,10-methylenetetrahydrofolate is the carbon donor for the conversion of deoxyuridine to deoxythymidine.

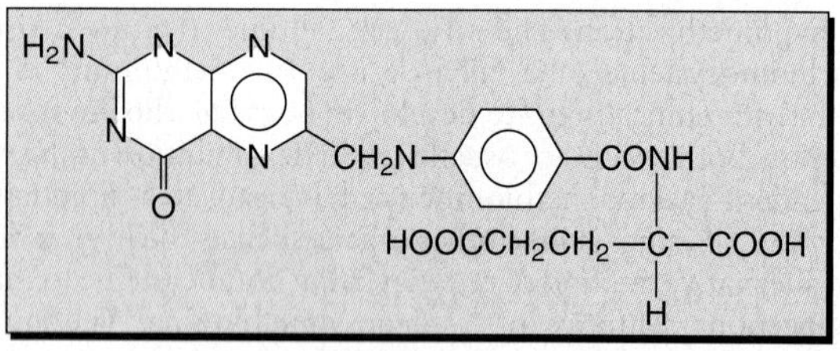

FIGURE 62-7 • Structure of folic acid.

100 μg intramuscularly (IM) has been reported to have a more sustained effect than cyanocobalamin, with a single dose maintaining plasma vitamin B_{12} concentrations for up to 3 months. For pernicious anemia, treatment with cyanocobalamin is 100 μg IM once daily for 1 week is recommended initially, followed by 100 μg IM or subcutaneously (subQ) on alternate days for seven doses, then every 3 to 4 days for another 2 to 3 weeks, then 100 μg IM monthly for life.

Pharmacokinetics. Oral absorption of vitamin B_{12} from the gastrointestinal tract depends on the presence of adequate IF, which is secreted from gastric parietal cells. Initially, oral doses of B_{12} and IF will increase cobalamin levels in patients with pernicious anemia. However, 50% of patients develop intestinal antibodies to IF. Once absorbed, vitamin B_{12} is highly bound to transcobalamin II, a specific β-globulin carrier protein, and is distributed and stored primarily in the liver as coenzyme B_{12}. The bone marrow also stores a significant amount of the absorbed vitamin B_{12}. Enterohepatic recirculation conserves systemic stores. The B_{12} plasma half-life is about 6 days (400 days in the liver). Elimination is primarily through the bile; however, excess cyanocobalamin is excreted unchanged in the urine.

Treatment of patients with vitamin B_{12} deficiency has traditionally been via periodic IM injections. Over the past several decades, a number of studies have indicated that the oral route for vitamin B_{12} replacement therapy is efficacious.[40-47]

Adverse Effects. Intramuscular injection of cyanocobalamin is well tolerated. Rarely, transient erythema and anaphylaxis thought to be immunoglobulin E mediated may occur.[48]

Folic Acid

Folic acid is a water-soluble, B-complex vitamin. It consists of a pteridine ring linked to glutamic acid via *para*-aminobenzoic acid (Fig. 62-7). This vitamin is found in a variety of foods, including liver, kidneys, yeast, and leafy green vegetables. A deficiency of folic acid can cause a megaloblastic anemia that, if it occurs in pregnancy, can lead to congenital neural tube defects.

Pathophysiology. Folic acid is a biochemically inactive compound. It is the precursor of tetrahydrofolic acid and methyltetrahydrofolate. Tetrahydrofolic acid, methyltetrahydrofolate, and other folic acid congeners are essential for the maintenance of normal erythropoiesis and are also required cofactors for the synthesis of purines and thymidylate. Folic acid congeners are transported across cell membranes by receptor-mediated endocytosis to their intracellular locations, where they function and are stored. Folate is also a cofactor for enzymes involved in the catabolism of formate and the methylation of transfer RNA. The impairment of thymidylate synthesis leads to impaired DNA synthesis, which in turn leads to megaloblastosis and a macrocytic anemia. Another important role of folic acid is the formation of methionine from homocysteine using vitamin B_{12} as a cofactor (see Fig. 62-6).

Folate deficiency may be due to poor nutrition (e.g., in alcoholics), malabsorption seen in diseases of the small intestine (celiac disease, prolonged biliary drainage), increased demand (pregnancy), or may be drug related (phenytoin). Patients with malabsorption may be deficient in both folic acid and vitamin B_{12}, and administration of folic acid alone may precipitate an acute vitamin B_{12} deficiency.

Therapeutics and Clinical Pharmacology

Goals of Therapy. Reversal of megaloblastic anemia and prevention of congenital neural tube defects are the major goals of folic acid replacement therapy. Patients with malabsorption may be deficient in both folic acid and vitamin B_{12}, and administration of folic acid alone may precipitate acute vitamin B_{12} deficiency. Indiscriminate use of folate alone may therefore mask the symptoms of vitamin B_{12} deficiency and lead to irreversible neurologic deficits.

Therapeutics. Folic acid is available for use both orally and parenterally. The usual daily requirement for folic acid is about 200 μg. In pregnancy, 400 to 500 μg as supplemental folic acid is recommended to prevent neural tube defects. For megaloblastic anemia, 1 mg once daily gives a satisfactory hematologic response. In conditions such as tropical sprue causing folic acid deficiency, larger doses (3 to 15 mg) are needed. Parenteral folic acid is indicated only when oral administration is not possible or if malabsorption is suspected.

Other Vitamins

Vitamin A. Vitamin A deficiency can be associated with anemia. Early animal studies of vitamin A deficiency suggested it caused loss of hematopoietic tissue in bone marrow, hypochromia, depressed hemoglobin concentration, and splenic accumulation of hemosiderin.[49,50] Vitamin A deficiency may induce anemia by impairing the differentiation and proliferation of pluripotent hematopoietic cells,[51,52] disturbing renal and hepatic erythropoietin synthesis,[53] reducing mobilization of body iron stores, and disturbing iron and heme metabolism[51,54] by sequestration of iron during the acute-phase response to infection.[55,56]

Riboflavin. Riboflavin (7,8-dimethyl-10-ribityl-isoalloxazine) is a water-soluble vitamin present in a wide variety of foods, and is mainly obtained from milk and dairy products in Western diets. Its most biologically active forms, flavin adenine dinucleotide and flavin mononucleotide, are involved in a range of redox reactions that are pivotal to the function of aerobic cells. Poor riboflavin status in Western countries seems to be of most concern for the elderly and adolescents, despite the diversity of riboflavin-rich foods available. Biochemical signs of depletion arise within only a few days of dietary deprivation.

Evidence suggests that poor riboflavin status modulates iron handling and contributes to the etiology of anemia when iron intakes are low.[57-59] The efficiency of iron utilization is impaired in riboflavin deficiency, but iron absorption is unaffected.[60,61] Thus, riboflavin deficiency appears to impair iron mobilization, globin synthesis, and possibly iron absorption (Fig. 62-8).

Several clinical trials have assessed the effects of riboflavin supplementation on anemia. Results have been mixed, but several have shown that riboflavin can significantly improve hematologic status and augment the response to iron supplementation. A European study of mildly anemic pregnant women showed that those who had received daily riboflavin (9 mg) along with iron (60 mg) maintained their erythrocyte counts, hemoglobin, and hematocrit while an iron-alone group showed significant reductions in all three indices.[61]

Vitamin C. Vitamin C deficiency has been associated with various forms of anemia, but it is still unclear whether vitamin C (ascorbic acid) is directly involved in hematopoiesis or if anemia arises indirectly through the interactions of vitamin C with folate and iron metabolism.[62] As an antioxidant (reducing agent), vitamin C can facilitate iron absorption from the gastrointestinal tract and enable its mobilization from storage (see Fig. 62-8). Iron and ascorbic acid form an iron chelate complex that is more soluble in the alkaline environment of the small intestine and, as a result, better absorbed.[63-66] The simultaneous consumption of 25 to 75 mg of vitamin C has been shown to enhance fourfold or more the absorption of the less bioavailable, but more common, nonheme iron.[67-69] Ascorbic acid also activates the enzyme folic acid reductase, to produce tetrahydrofolic acid, the active form of folic acid, which prevents megaloblastic anemia. Vitamin C deficiency is evident when serum ascorbate falls below 11.4 mmol/L. Patient groups at risk of vitamin C deficiency include pregnant and lactating women, infants fed exclusively cow's milk, elderly men, and smokers.[70,71]

Pyridoxine. Vitamin B_6 (pyridoxine) deficiency can impair heme synthesis and lead to a normocytic, microcytic, or sideroblastic anemia (see Fig. 62-8). Treatment of sideroblastic anemia with vitamin B_6 resulted in the restoration of activity of erythroblastic δ-aminolevulinic acid synthetase, the rate-limiting enzyme in heme

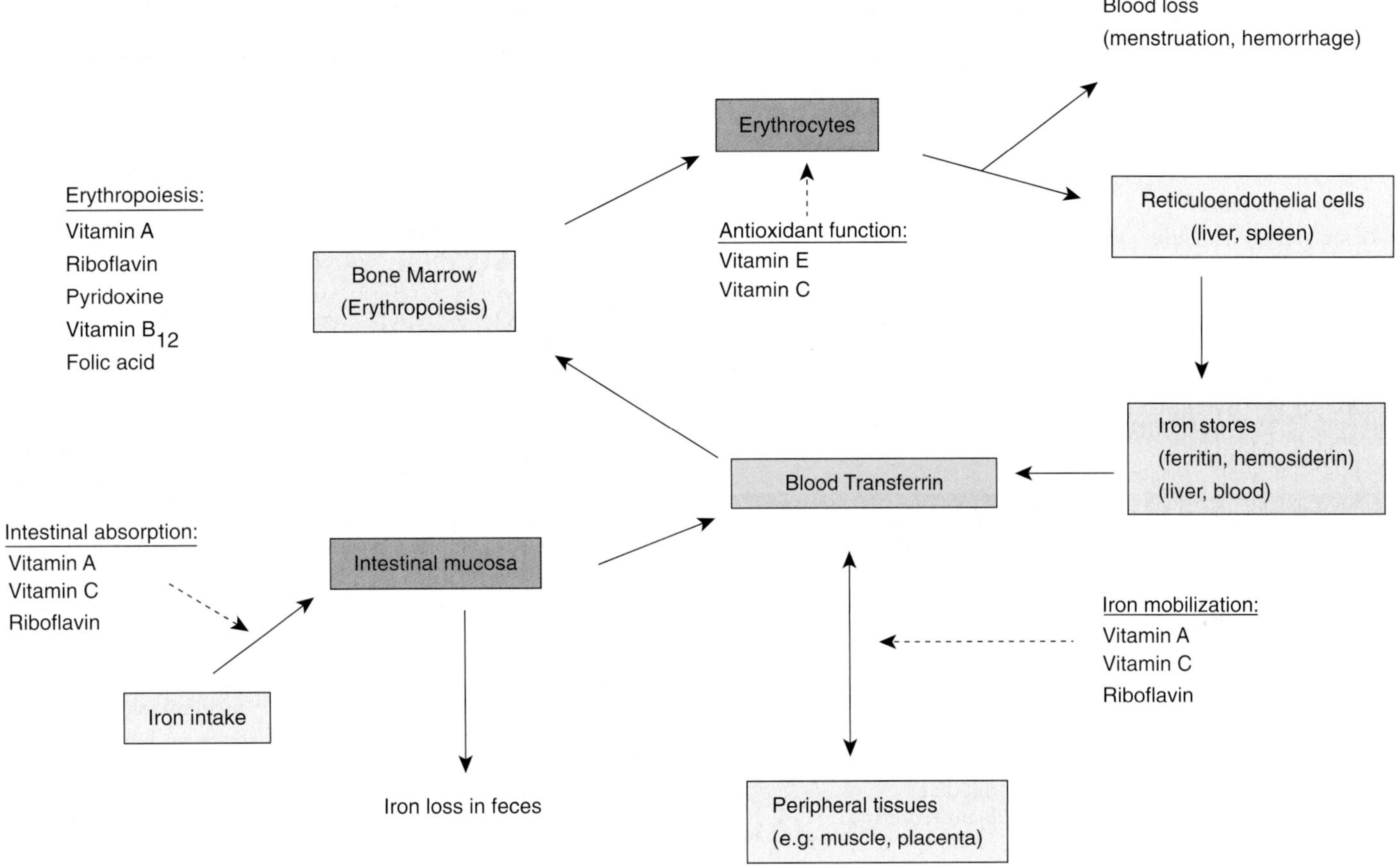

FIGURE 62-8 • Roles of vitamins in iron metabolism and erythropoiesis.

synthesis. In addition, pyridoxine increased red cell pyridoxine kinase and aspartate aminotransferase activity.[72-76]

Vitamin B_6 may also inhibit sickling of erythrocytes in sickle cell anemia, possibly increasing erythrocyte counts, hemoglobin concentrations, and hematocrit among sickle cell anemia patients.[77] In addition, the sideroblastic anemia associated with isoniazid and pyrazinamide responds to treatment with oral pyridoxine 50 mg daily. This is one reason why patients on treatment with antituberculosis drug regimens containing isoniazid and pyrazinamide are routinely prescribed supplemental pyridoxine. In the treatment of idiopathic acquired sideroblastic anemia, a trial of high-dose oral pyridoxine (300 mg/day) has been shown to benefit the occasional patient.[78]

Drug-Related Anemia

Several drugs in clinical practice are implicated in causing anemia. Drug-induced anemia can be due to several different mechanisms (Table 62-3). Drug-induced anemia is often associated with an immune-related increase in RBC destruction. The mechanism of immune-related destruction of RBCs varies and can involve direct antidrug antibodies, antibodies that are directed against the drug complexed with other protein(s), or antibodies against a component of the blood cell independent of the drug.[79] For example, in β-lactam–induced hemolytic anemia (including that induced by penicillin and cephalosporin), the β-lactam binds to plasma and RBC membrane proteins to form a complex in which the β-lactam molecule acts as a hapten in the immune response. Antibodies that are directed against the β-lactam can induce hemolytic anemia by binding to the penicillin that is bound to the RBC membrane. Other drugs, such as methyldopa, quinidine, and procainamide, induce antibodies that bind RBC membrane antigens and cause autoimmune hemolytic anemia independent of immune complex formation with drug or drug metabolite.[80]

TABLE 62-3 DRUG-RELATED ANEMIA

Type of Anemia	Causative Drug(s)
Drug-induced immune hemolytic anemia	Penicillins, cephalosporins, procainamide, quinidine, quinine, sulfonamides, α-methyldopa
Oxidant-induced hemolytic anemia (G6PDH deficient)	Fava beans, dapsone, primaquine, sulfonamides, methylene blue, nitrofurantoin
Bone marrow hypoplasia, myelodysplasia	Cancer chemotherapeutic drugs
Aplastic anemia	Chloramphenicol, trimethoprim-sulfamethaxazole, zidovudine, phenytoin, erythropoietin antibodies
Megaloblastic anemia	Methotrexate, azathioprine, pyrimethamine
Acute reversible bone marrow suppression	Ethanol

G6PDH, glucose-6-phosphate dehydrogenase.

Aplastic Anemia

Aplastic anemia is marrow failure due to an inadequate number of hematopoietic cells in the marrow, often due to injury of the pluripotent stem cell, leading to pancytopenia. Aplastic anemia was first recognized in the 1930s in industrial workers exposed to benzene. Later, chloramphenicol was one of the first drugs associated with this condition in the 1950s. Several other drugs (Box 62-2), chemicals, and viruses have been implicated as a cause for this rare but fatal condition.

TABLE 62-4 POSSIBLE MECHANISMS OF DRUG-RELATED NEUTROPENIA

Mechanism	Causative Drug(s)
Hapten-induced antibodies[81,82]	Aminopyrine, penicillin, gold compounds
Apoptosis[83,84]	Clozapine
Immune complexes[85]	Quinidine
Complement-mediated mechanism[86]	Propylthiouracil
Dose-dependent inhibition maturation of granulocyte precursors[87-89]	β-Lactam antibiotics, carbamazepine, valproic acid
Direct toxicity for myeloid precursors[90,91]	Ticlopidine, doxorubicin, cyclophosphamide, chlorpromazine

BOX 62-2 DRUGS COMMONLY ASSOCIATED WITH ACQUIRED APLASTIC ANEMIA

- **Cytotoxic agents**
  Alkylating agents: busulfan, melphalan, cyclophosphamide
  Antimitotics: vincristine, vinblastine, colchicine, daunorubicin, doxorubicin
- **Antimicrobials:** Chloramphenicol, chloroquine, sulfonamides, zidovudine
- **Antiseizure agents:** carbamazepine, ethosuximide, hydantoins
- **Antihyperglycemic agents:** tolbutamide, chlorpropamide
- **Thyroid agents:** methimazole, propylthiouracil
- **Miscellaneous agents:** gold, D-penicillamine, lindane

TABLE 62-5 POSSIBLE MECHANISMS OF DRUG-RELATED LYMPHOPENIA

Mechanism of Lymphopenia	Causative Drug(s)
Reduced production of lymphocytes	Cyclophosphamide, azathioprine, methotrexate
Altered distribution in body compartments of lymphocytes	Corticosteroids, interleukin-2
Direct dose-related effects	Fludarabine
Idiosyncratic drug reactions	Quinine, cimetidine, opioids, carbamazepine, bisphosphonates

From Gergely P. Drug-induced lymphopenia: focus on CD4+ and CD8+ cells. Drug Saf 1999;21:91-100.

BOX 62-3 DRUGS KNOWN TO BE ASSOCIATED WITH NEUTROPENIA

Cardiovascular drugs: procainamide, propranolol, quinidine, methyldopa, captopril, acetazolamide, hydrochlorothiazide, chlorthalidone
Anti-infective agents: chloramphenicol, penicillins, sulfonamides, vancomycin, isoniazid, nitrofurantoin, ganciclovir, dapsone, quinine, pyrimethamine, amphotericin B, zidovudine
Anticonvulsants: phenytoin, ethosuximide, carbamazepine
Endocrinologic agents: chlorpropamide, methimazole, propylthiouracil, aminoglutethimide
Anti-inflammatory agents: phenylbutazone, gold salts, penicillamine, nonsteroidal anti-inflammatory drugs
Psychotropic drugs: chlorpromazine, prochlorperazine, clozapine
Immunosuppressive agents: alkylating agents, antimetabolites

Therapeutic Approach to Drug-Related Anemia

Treatment primarily includes discontinuation of the putative offending drug and supportive care with transfusions if needed. In aplastic anemia, antithymocyte globulin, cyclosporine, corticosteroids, and androgens have been used with some success in improving survival, although they are not curative. Hematopoietic cell transplantation has been shown to be the most effective treatment in younger individuals with aplastic anemia.

NEUTROPENIA AND LYMPHOPENIA

Neutropenia is defined as an absolute neutrophil count of less than 1500/mm^3. Agranulocytosis is defined as an absolute neutrophil count of less than 500/mm^3. Neutropenia can be due to direct bone marrow injury or to maturation defects. The most common cause of leukopenia is drug-related bone marrow suppression.

Drug-induced neutropenia can be immune mediated or can occur as a result of direct toxicity to the myeloid precursors (Box 62-3 and Table 62-4).[81-91] Drug-related lymphopenia can be due to one of several mechanisms (Table 62-5).[92]

THROMBOCYTOPENIA

Introduction

Thrombocytes (or platelets) arise from the differentiation of megakaryocytes. The normal blood platelet count ranges from 150,000 to 450,000/mm^3. Thrombocytopenia stimulates an increase in the number of megakaryocytes, releasing additional platelets into the circulation. This process is regulated by thrombopoietin. A low platelet count is one of the most common causes of hemorrhage.

Pathophysiology

The pathophysiology of thrombocytopenia is similar in principle to that of anemia, but the latter is better understood. Deficient platelet production, accelerated platelet destruction, and abnormal distribution are the three principal mechanisms that lead to thrombocytopenia.

Many drugs can cause thrombocytopenia (Table 62-6). Cancer chemotherapeutic agents may depress megakaryocyte production. Ingestion of large quantities of ethanol has a marrow-suppressing effect leading to transient thrombocytopenia, particularly in binge drinkers. Thiazide diuretics, used to treat hypertension or congestive heart failure, impair megakaryocyte production and can produce mild thrombocytopenia (50,000 to 100,000/mm^3), which may persist for several months after the offending drug is discontinued. Several immune mechanisms are postulated to be involved in drug-induced thrombocytopenia (Table 62-7).

Therapeutics and Clinical Pharmacology

Growth factors are required for the survival and proliferation of hematopoietic cells at all stages of development (Fig. 62-1; see also Fig. 62-9). Of the factors that affect pluripotent hematopoietic cells, steel factor (also known as Fms-like tyrosine kinase 3 [FLT3] ligand or stem cell factor), granulocyte colony-stimulating factor (G-CSF), granulocyte-macrophage colony-stimulating factor (GM-CSF), interleukin (IL)-2, IL-3, and IL-7 are the best characterized. Each of these proteins supports the survival and proliferation of a number of distinct target hematopoietic lineage cells by binding to and activating specific cell membrane–bound receptors.

Hematopoietic Growth Factors and Their Receptors

The cytokine receptor superfamily consists of the cell surface receptors for erythropoietin, thrombopoietin, several colony-stimulating factors, and the interleukins.[93] Each of these receptors includes one or two extracellular cytokine-binding domains containing approximately 200 amino acids, a transmembrane domain of 20 to 25 residues, and an

Practice: Hematologic Therapeutics

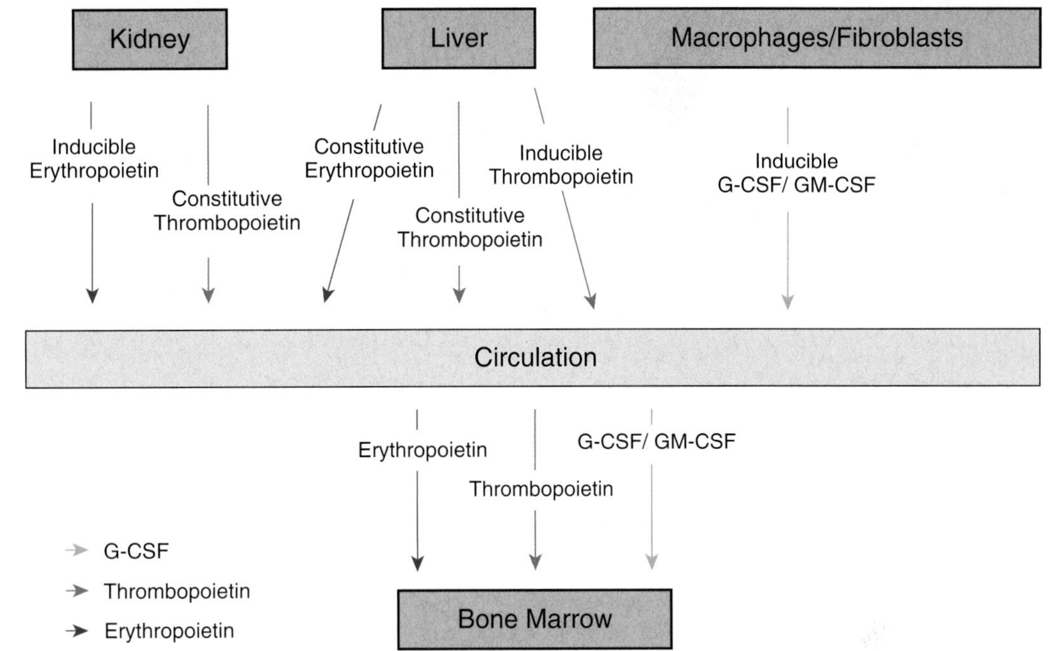

FIGURE 62-9 • **Production of hematopoietic growth factors.**

TABLE 62-6 DRUGS ASSOCIATED WITH THROMBOCYTOPENIA

	Mechanism	Causative Drug(s)
Quantitative platelet disorders	Bone marrow hypoplasia/suppression	Valproic acid (dose-dependent mechanism) Anagrelide
	Nonimmunologic mechanism	Amphotericin B, zidovudine; ethanol Chemotherapeutic drugs such as alkylating agents, antimetabolites (esp. 6-mercaptopurine), and anthracyclines
	Immunologic mechanism	Heparin and see Table 62-7 below
Qualitative platelet disorders	Diminished platelet function	Aspirin and nonsteroidal anti-inflammatory drugs

TABLE 62-7 POSSIBLE IMMUNE MECHANISMS INVOLVED IN DRUG-INDUCED THROMBOCYTOPENIA

Drugs	Immune Mechanism
Penicillin and penicillin derivatives	Hapten-induced antibody
Quinidine, quinine, NSAIDs	"Quinine-type" thrombocytopenia
Tirofiban, eptifibatide	Ligand mimetic GPIIb/IIIa inhibitor
Abciximab	Drug-specific antibody
Gold salts, procainamide	Drug-induced autoantibody
Heparin	Immune complex

GP, glycoprotein; NSAIDs, nonsteroidal anti-inflammatory drugs.

intracellular domain that recruit kinases of the Janus kinase (JAK) family (Fig. 62-10). The functional unit of the erythropoietin, G-CSF, and thrombopoietin receptors is a homodimer[94]; the engagement of a single molecule of hematopoietic growth factor by the homodimeric receptor then induces a major conformational shift in the ligand-receptor protein complex, bringing the two tethered cytoplasmic JAKs into close juxtaposition, thereby triggering activation of the receptor-located tyrosine kinases by mutual cross-phosphorylation.[95] Once the JAKs are activated by the lineage-specific hematopoietic growth factors, a number of secondary signaling molecules are phosphorylated, and these initiate numerous events that promote cell survival, proliferation, and differentiation. The cytokine-signaling pathways we know most about entail activation of the signal transducer and activator of transcription (STAT) factors, phosphoinositol-3-kinase, and mitogen-activated protein kinase, each of which activates an overlapping subgroup of tertiary signaling molecules (see Fig. 62-10).

Of these, transcription factors, cell cycle activators and inhibitors (p27Kip), antiapoptosis molecules (Bcl-xL an inhibitor of apoptosis), and other growth factors (transforming growth factor and vascular endothelial growth factor) are ultimately responsible for the effects induced by the binding of a hematopoietic growth factor to its receptor. In addition, the activation of hematopoietic growth factor receptors initiates self-regulatory mechanisms that terminate the growth signal, namely internalization of receptors, activation of phosphatases, and production of suppressors of cytokine signaling.[94-96]

In principle, there are four general indications for the administration of a hematopoietic growth factor: (i) correction of the cytopenia owing to the deficiency of the growth factor, (ii) stimulation of the recovery of hematopoietic stem and progenitor cells in iatrogenic and naturally occurring deficiency states, (iii) augmentation of hematopoiesis to compensate for pathologically rapid blood cell destruction, and (iv) activation of mature hematopoietic cells.

Erythroid Growth Factors

Erythropoietin. Erythropoietin is a glycosylated protein containing 166 amino acids, with a molecular weight of approximately 36,000 Da. It is encoded by human chromosome 7. Interstitial cells of the renal cortex account for 90% of the erythropoietin produced in the human body (the remaining 10% is produced by hepatocytes). The production of erythropoietin is stimulated by anemia via tissue hypoxia. The rate of RBC production is normally determined by the serum erythropoietin concentration. In the bone marrow, erythropoietin stimulates

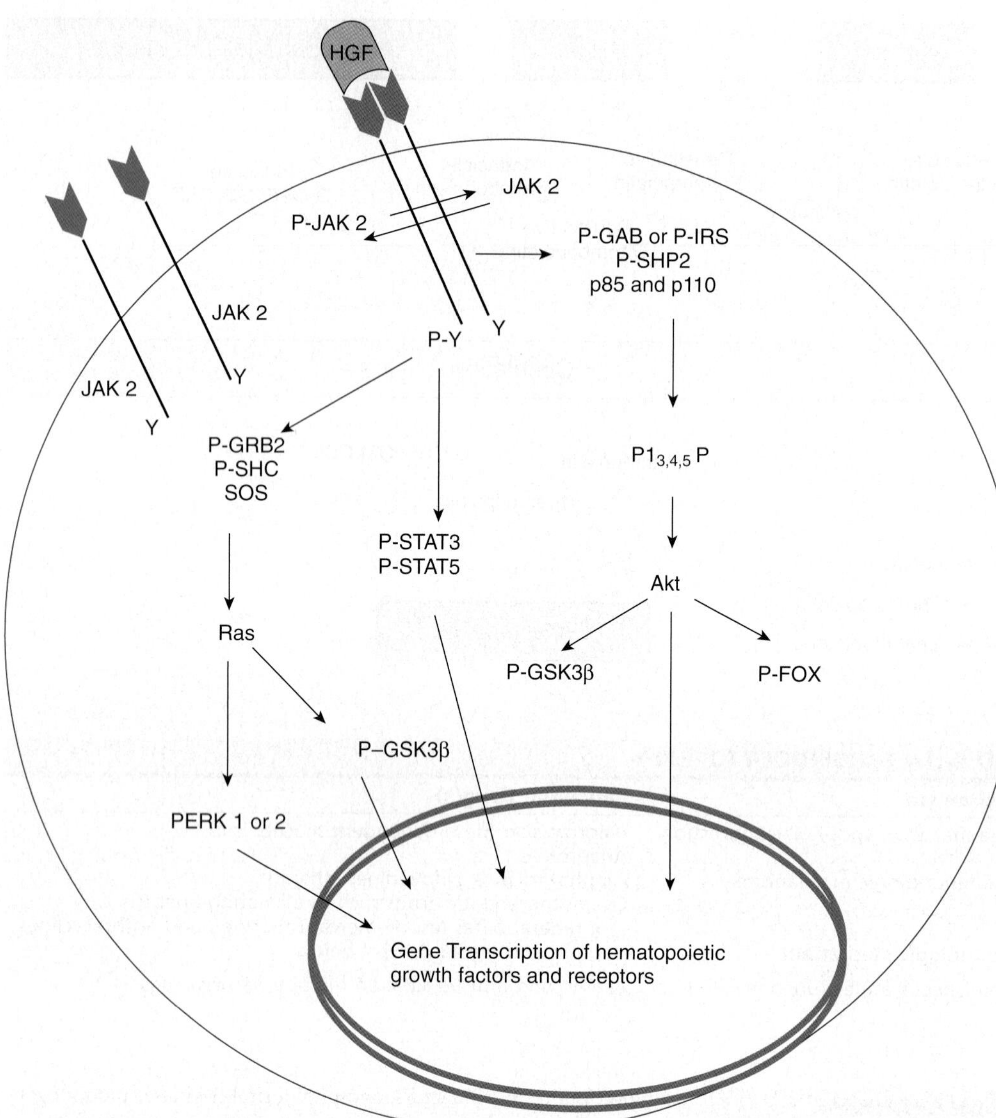

FIGURE 62-10 • Hematopoietic growth factor signaling. Hematopoietic growth factor–receptor dimers are composed of two subunits, which bind two molecules of Janus kinase 2 (JAK2) and are in an open conformation (left) when endogenous growth factor is not present. Ligand binding substantially changes the conformation of the receptor, bringing the cytoplasmic domains into close juxtaposition and allowing the tethered kinases to cross-phosphorylate (activate) each other. One of the first substrates for activation is the JAK2 receptor tyrosine (Y) residues; when these are phosphorylated (P), they serve as docking sites for adaptors (SHC [Src homology containing], GRB2 [growth factor receptor–bound protein 2], GAB [Grb binding], and IRS [insulin receptor substrate]) phosphatases (SHP2 [Shc homology domain containing phosphatase]), G-protein activators (SOS [son of sevenless]), and lipid kinases (p85 and p110 and phosphoinositol 3-kinase). Other signaling molecules include signal transducer and activator of transcription 3 and 5 (STAT3 and STAT5, respectively), phosphoinositol 3,4,5-phosphate [$PI_{3,4,5}P$]), the small guanine nucleotide–binding protein Ras, and the kinases AKT, p38 mitogen-activated protein kinase (MAPK), extracellular response–stimulated kinase (ERK) 1 and 2, phosphatase forkhead (P-FOX), and phosphatase glycogen synthase kinase 3β (P-GSK3β). Such signal transduction affects nuclear transcription of antiapoptosis molecules ($BCLX_L$), cell-cycle regulators (cyclins), and additional growth factors and their receptors. *Arrows* indicate signaling pathways. (Adapted from Kaushanky K. Lineage specific hematopoietic growth factors. N Engl J Med 2006;354:2034-2045.)

proliferation and maturation of erythroid precursors and promotes red cell production.

Mechanism of Action. Erythropoietin production is inversely related to oxygen availability (the level can increase up to 20,000 mU/ml in response to anemia or arterial hypoxemia),[97,98] so that an effective feedback loop is established that controls erythropoiesis. The juxtatubular interstitial cells of the renal cortex sense tissue oxygen through a newly identified, oxygen-dependent prolyl hydroxylase that regulates the stability of the primary transcription factor for erythropoietin, hypoxia-inducible factor 1 (HIF-1). Once hydroxylated, HIF-1 binds the von Hippel-Lindau (VHL) protein, thereby targeting it for ubiquitin-mediated destruction.[99,100] Under conditions of low tissue oxygen tension, the hydroxylase is inactive; consequently, HIF-1 is not hydroxylated and cannot bind VHL, thereby maintaining its stability and capacity to drive the production of erythropoietin. Although HIF-1α was the first transcription factor identified through its ability to bind to an enhancer sequence in the promoter region of the erythropoietin gene, more recent evidence suggests that HIF-2α is responsible for the regulation of erythropoietin.[101-103] This mechanism also accounts for the erythrocytosis associated with high-altitude heart or lung disease leading to hypoxemia and hemoglobin variants with a low affinity for oxygen.

Formulations. Epoetin, the recombinant human erythropoietin (rhEpo), is produced from Chinese hamster ovary cells transfected with the human erythropoietin gene.[104,105] It is available in three forms, epoetin alfa (Epogen, Procrit), epoetin beta (approved only in Europe), and epoetin delta (still in Phase III trials). Therapeutically, the actions are similar for all forms. Epoetin alfa first became available for clinical trials in 1985 and was approved by the U.S. Food and Drug Administration (FDA) in 1989.

Darbepoietin alfa (Aranesp) is a novel erythropoiesis-stimulating protein (NESP) with a longer plasma half-life. Darbepoietin possesses two additional *N*-glycans compared to endogenous erythropoietin or rhEpo. The composition of the *N*-glycans is important in determining the biologic activity and the rate of the degradation of erythropoietin and its analogues.[99,106]

Indications. The indications for administration of epoetin alfa include

1. Anemia in chronic renal failure patients (80 to 120 IU/kg epoetin alfa three times a week, conveniently given for patients getting hemodialysis three times a week). Epoetin alfa is not removed by hemodialysis.
2. Anemia of drug-induced bone marrow suppression, as in cancer chemotherapy (typical dosing is 40,000 U subcutaneously weekly for epoetin alfa). Zidovudine-treated human immunodeficiency virus (HIV) patients (50 to 100 IU/kg of epoetin alfa, given subcutaneously three times a week).
3. Anemia of chronic disease.

4. To reduce the need for blood transfusions in surgery patients (150 to 300 IU/kg of epoetin alfa once daily for 10 days preceding surgery), on the day of surgery, and for 4 days after surgery.

Pharmacokinetics. When administered subcutaneously, the epoetin alfa plasma half-life in patients with chronic renal failure is 4 to 13 hours with a volume of distribution of 50 ml/kg. It can also be given intravenously. Subcutaneous injection yields a systemic bioavailability of approximately 40%. Darbepoietin alfa has a half-life of 42 hours after subQ injection. The bioavailability of darbepoietin alfa in chronic renal failure patients after subQ administration is approximately 30% to 50%.

Adverse Effects. Adverse effects of epoetin alfa include hypertension and headaches,[107] thrombosis, heart failure, and transient flulike symptoms during initiation of therapy. The presence of neutralizing antibodies (i.e., antierythropoietin antibodies to native erythropoietin) has been associated with the development of pure red cell aplasia in patients receiving recombinant erythropoietin products. This effect has been observed predominantly with subQ use of epoetin alfa produced outside the United States after albumin was removed from the formulation.[108]

Iron deficiency anemia may be unmasked. Supplemental iron therapy is routinely used in patients who receive erythropoietin.

The Correction of Hemoglobin and Outcomes in Renal Insufficiency (CHOIR) study[109] showed that patients treated with erythropoietin and dosed to a target hemoglobin concentration of 13.5 g/dl were at a significantly increased risk for serious and life-threatening cardiovascular complications, as compared to use of the erythropoietin to target a hemoglobin concentration of 11.3 g/dl. The incidence of thrombovascular events was highest at 18.4%, followed by congestive heart failure at 11.2%.

Myeloid Growth Factors

The myeloid growth factors stimulate the production of myeloid cell lines. T cells, endothelial cells, fibroblasts, monocytes, and macrophages produce these growth factors. The proliferation and differentiation of neutrophils is regulated by G-CSF. G-CSF binds to its receptor, a member of the cytokine receptor superfamily with the downstream intracellular signaling processes described previously[110] (see Fig. 62-10).

Granulocyte Colony-Stimulating Factor. Endogenous G-CSF is involved in the regulation and production of neutrophils in response to host defense needs. Filgrastim [Neupogen] is an unglycosylated recombinant human G-CSF glycoprotein (molecular weight 18,800 Da) produced by *Escherichia coli* bacteria transfected with the human G-CSF gene.

Pharmacokinetics. Filgrastim is rapidly eliminated, with a short serum half-life (~3.5 hours).[111] The major routes of clearance are by binding to cell surface receptors and being internalized and, to a lesser extent, by renal elimination. G-CSF is administered daily, usually by subQ injection, but it may be given intravenously if necessary. The dose of filgrastim is between 5 and 10 μg/kg per day for a course of 14 to 21 days, which can be shortened once the neutrophil count exceeds 5000/mm^3. Lenograstim is a glycosylated recombinant human G-CSF.

The development of pegfilgrastim [Neulasta], a pegylated form of filgrastim, has advanced G-CSF therapy. Pegfilgrastim has a longer duration of action compared with filgrastim.[112-114] It is given as a fixed-dose, subQ injection (6 mg) only once per chemotherapy cycle.[114] Once-per-cycle dosing simplifies the management of chemotherapy-induced neutropenia for patients, their caregivers, and health care professionals, and may result in improved patient compliance. Pegfilgrastim should not be administered either 14 days before or 24 hours after administration of cytotoxic chemotherapy. Currently it is only FDA indicated for chemotherapy-induced neutropenia.

Indications and Uses. FDA-approved indications for G-CSF include

1. Chemotherapy-induced neutropenia
2. Febrile neutropenia
3. Peripheral blood stem cell mobilization and subsequent harvesting for transplant
4. Congenital and cyclical neutropenia
5. For patients with nonmyeloid malignancies following autologous or allogeneic bone marrow transplantation (BMT)

Non–FDA-approved uses of G-CSF include HIV-related zidovudine-induced neutropenia, ganciclovir-induced neutropenia, and aplastic anemia.

Adverse Effects. Adverse effects include mild to moderate bone pain and myalgias, splenomegaly, hyperuricemia, headache, skin rash, hypotension, and leukocytosis. Patients with history of hypersensitivity to proteins produced by *E. coli* should not receive this drug.

Granulocyte-Macrophage Colony-Stimulating Factor. Sargramostim (Leukine) is a recombinant human GM-CSF. GM-CSF is considered a multilineage growth factor that supports the survival and differentiation of progenitors in the granulocyte-macrophage lineage as well as megakaryocytic and erythroid progenitor cells. As opposed to G-CSF, the activity of GM-CSF is species specific (e.g., mouse GM-CSF has no activity in humans). Sargramostim is a glycoprotein of 127 amino acids that is variably glycosylated and is produced by a yeast (*Saccharomyces cerevisiae*) expression system. The amino acid sequence of sargramostim differs from native human GM-CSF by a substitution at the leucine position 23, and the carbohydrate moiety may be different from the native GM-CSF protein. Molgramostim, a nonglycosylated recombinant human GM-CSF (rhGM-CSF) protein that has a longer half-life than the glycosylated protein, is produced using *E. coli* and is available in Europe. Although glycosylation is not necessary for rhGM-CSF activity, the degree of glycosylation is important because it affects pharmacokinetics, activity, antigenicity, and toxicity. The nonglycosylated protein is associated with increased adverse reactions (e.g., capillary leak syndrome, fever, chills). GM-CSF primarily increases production and survival of neutrophils at lower doses; an increase in eosinophil and monocyte counts is seen at higher doses. GM-CSF is a potent regulator of eosinophil production and function, and promotes the survival of eosinophils by suppressing apoptosis.[115-117]

Pharmacokinetics. Sargramostim is administered subQ or by slow intravenous infusion. Cebon et al.[118] studied the pharmacokinetics of GM-CSF (0.3 to 30 μg/kg) after subQ bolus or intravenous bolus injection or 2-hour intravenous infusion. Highest peak serum concentrations (C_{max}) followed the intravenous bolus, and the time GM-CSF maintained a plasma concentration greater than 1 ng/ml was longer after a subQ than after an intravenous administration. The half-life of the terminal phase following an intravenous bolus ranged from 0.24 to 1.2 hours and, following intravenous infusion, from 0.6 to 9.1 hours. The apparent clearance was greatest following subcutaneous injection at doses below 3 μg/kg, suggesting a saturable mechanism or variable bioavailability.[119,120]

The recommended dose of sargramostim ranges from 0.3 to 10 μg/kg per day for a duration 7 to 10 days. With the initial dose of GM-CSF, there is a transient leukopenia due to margination and sequestration in lungs.

Indications. FDA-approved indications include chemotherapy-induced neutropenia, febrile neutropenia, and patients with nonmyeloid malignancies following autologous or allogeneic BMT. Other conditions in which it has been used but is not FDA approved include myelodysplastic syndrome, aplastic anemia, and HIV-related zidovudine- and ganciclovir-induced neutropenia.

Adverse Effects. Sargramostim can produce a first-dose reaction; dyspnea, flushing, hypoxia, hypotension, nausea, and vomiting have been reported. These reactions are probably due to sequestration of neutrophils in the pulmonary circulation and to capillary leak syndrome. Additional adverse effects include bone pain; fluid retention; fever, chills, myalgias and arthralgia; pleural and pericardial effusion; eosinophilia; and transaminitis.

Thrombopoietic Growth Factors

Interleukin-11. IL-11 stimulates the growth and proliferation of megakaryocytic progenitor cells, and induces megakaryocytic maturation. Oprelvekin is a recombinant version of human IL-11 derived from genetically altered *E. coli.* Unlike endogenous IL-11, oprelvekin lacks the amino-terminal proline residue. The biologic activity of oprelvekin and of endogenous IL-11 is essentially the same.

Mechanism of Action. At the molecular level, IL-11 binds to the IL-11 receptor (IL-11Rα) on megakaryocytes and megakaryocyte progenitor cells. Binding of IL-11 to IL-11Rα causes intracellular downstream signaling as described previously for the cytokine receptor superfamily (see Fig. 62-10). This stimulates the proliferation of hematopoietic stem cells and megakaryocyte progenitor cells, and induces megakaryocyte maturation resulting in increased platelet production. Platelets produced in response to oprelvekin are morphologically and functionally normal and possess a normal life span of 9 to 11 days.

Pharmacokinetics. Recombinant IL-11 showed linear pharamacokinetics in healthy males after both intravenous infusion and subQ administration. Subcutaneous administration yields 65% bioavailability and demonstrates absorption rate–dependent pharmacokinetics. In a study in which a single 50-μg/kg subcutaneous dose was administered to 18 healthy men, the C_{max} of 17.4 ± 5.4 ng/ml was reached at 3.2 ± 2.4 hours (time to peak serum concentration) following dosing. The terminal half-life was 6.9 ± 1.7 hours, and both the liver and kidneys play an important role in clearance.[121] Studies in patients with differing degrees of renal impairment revealed that the area under the curve for oprelvekin increased, although half-life remained unchanged as renal dysfunction increased.[122-126] Overall exposure to oprelvekin increased as renal function decreased, indicating that a 50% dose reduction of oprelvekin is warranted for patients with severe renal impairment.[122]

Indications. IL-11 is FDA approved for severe chemotherapy-induced thrombocytopenia (<20,000/mm^3). It is administered to patients at a dose of 50 μg/kg per day subcutaneously. Dosing should be initiated after the completion of chemotherapy and continued until the platelet count returns to more than 50,000/mm^3.

Adverse Effects.[122-124] Adverse effects of IL-11 include hypersensitivity reactions, including anaphylaxis; fluid retention, with an incidence rate as high as 66%; fever; dyspnea; dizziness; skin rash; and palpitations and tachycardia.

Thrombopoietin. A recombinant formulation of human thrombopoietin has been studied for preventing and/or treating chemotherapy-induced thrombocytopenia in cancer patients. The product used in clinical trials is a full-length glycosylated molecule produced in a genetically modified mammalian cell line. Thrombopoietin was shown to be effective in accelerating platelet recovery to baseline values after conventional doses of cancer chemotherapy and after BMT for breast cancer.[127] These successes provide the basis for optimism that thrombopoietin will prove effective in ameliorating thrombocytopenia.

Indications. Thrombopoietin is under investigation for the management of chemotherapy-induced thrombocytopenia. It may also be useful for thrombocytopenia due to other causes. It is currently undergoing clinical investigation following stem cell transplantation and to increase autologous platelet donations from healthy volunteers.

Pharmacokinetics. Thrombopoietin has a serum half-life of 20 to 30 hours and remains in the circulation for 5 to 6 days.[127,128]

REFERENCES

1. Lubran MM. Hematologic side effects of drugs. Ann Clin Lab Sci 1989;19:114-121.
2. Andersohn F, Bronder E, Klimpel A, Garbe E. Proportion of drug-related serious rare blood dyscrasias: estimates from the Berlin Case-Control Surveillance Study. Am J Hematol 2004;77:316-318.
3. Schnall SF, Berliner N, Duffy TP, Benz EF Jr. Approach to the adult and child with anemia. In Hoffman R, et al. (eds): Hematology: Basic Principles and Practice, 3rd ed. New York: Churchill Livingstone, 2000, pp 367-382.
4. Conrad ME, Umbreit JN. Pathways of iron absorption. Blood Cells Mol Dis 2002;29:336-355.
5. Roy CN, Enns CA. Iron homeostasis: new tales from the crypt. Blood 2000;96:4020-4027.
6. Andrews NC. The iron transporter DMT1. Int J Biochem Cell Biol 1999;31:991-994.
7. Andrews NC, Levy JE. Iron is hot: an update on the pathophysiology of hemochromatosis. Blood 1998;92:1845-1851.
8. Gunshin H, Mackenzie B, Berger UV, et al. Cloning and characterization of a mammalian proton-coupled metal-ion transporter. Nature 1997;388:482-488.
9. Waheed A, Parkkila S, Saarnio J, et al. Association of HFE protein with transferrin receptor in crypt enterocytes of human duodenum. Proc Natl Acad Sci U S A 1999;96:1579-1584.
10. Feder JN, Penny DM, Irrinki A, et al. The hemochromatosis gene product complexes with the transferrin receptor and lowers its affinity for ligand binding. Proc Natl Acad Sci U S A 1998;95:1472-1477.
11. Abboud S, Haile DJ. A novel mammalian iron-regulated protein involved in intracellular iron metabolism. J Biol Chem 2000;275:19906-19912.
12. Vulpe CD, Kuo YM, Murphy TL, et al. Hephaestin, a ceruloplasmin homologue implicated in intestinal iron transport, is defective in the sla mouse. Nat Genet 1999;21:195-199.
13. Guralnik JM, Eisenstaedt RS, Ferrucci L, et al. Prevalence of anemia in persons 65 years and older in the United States: evidence for a high rate of unexplained anemia. Blood 2004;104:2263-2268.
14. Artz AS, Fergusson D, Drinka PJ, et al. Mechanisms of unexplained anemia in the nursing home. J Am Geriatr Soc 2004;52:423-427.
15. Centers for Disease Control and Prevention, National Center for Health Statistics. Third National Health and Nutrition Examination Survey (NHANES III): Iron deficiency—United States, 1999-2000. Available at http://www.cdc.gov/nchs/fastats/anemia.htm
16. Beutler E. History of iron in medicine. Blood Cells Mol Dis 2002;29:297-308.
17. Ritter JM, Lewis LD, Mant TGK. Anemia and hematological disorders. In Ritter JM, Lewis LD, Mant TGK (eds): Textbook of Clinical Pharmacology, 4th ed. New York: Oxford University Press, 1999, Ch 48.
18. Makrides M, Crowther CA, Gibson RA, et al. Efficacy and tolerability of low-dose iron supplements during pregnancy: a randomized controlled trial. Am J Clin Nutr 2003;78:145-153.
19. Hyder SM, Persson LA, Chowdhury AM, Ekstrom EC. Do side effects reduce compliance to iron supplementation? A study of daily- and weekly-dose regimens in pregnancy. J Health Popul Nutr 2002;20:175-179.
20. Milman N, Byg KE, Bergholt T, Eriksen L. Side effects of oral iron prophylaxis in pregnancy—myth or reality? Acta Haematol 2006;115:53-57.
21. Laman CA, Silverstein SB, Rodgers GM. Parenteral iron therapy: a single institution's experience over a 5-year period. J Natl Compr Canc Netw 2005;3:791-795.
22. Silverstein SB, Rodgers GM. Parenteral iron therapy options. Am J Hematol 2004;76:74-78.
23. Prasad AS. Zinc: the biology and therapeutics of an ion [Editorial]. Ann Intern Med 1996;125:142-144.
24. Harless W, Crowell E, Abraham J. Anemia and neutropenia associated with copper deficiency of unclear etiology. Am J Hematol 2006;81:546-549.
25. Nagano T, Toyoda T, Tanabe H, et al. Clinical features of hematological disorders caused by copper deficiency during long-term enteral nutrition. Intern Med 2005;44:554-559.
26. Todd LM, Godber IM, Gunn IR. Iatrogenic copper deficiency causing anemia and neutropenia. Ann Clin Biochem 2004;41(Pt 5):414-416.
27. Xu X, Pin S, Gathinji M, et al. Aceruloplasminemia: an inherited neurodegenerative disease with impairment of iron homeostasis. Ann N Y Acad Sci 2004;1012:299-305.
28. Anderson GJ, Frazer DM, McKie AT, Vulpe CD. The ceruloplasmin homolog hephaestin and the control of intestinal iron absorption. Blood Cells Mol Dis 2002;29:367-367.
29. Cherukuri S, Potla R, Sarkar J, et al. Unexpected role of ceruloplasmin in intestinal iron absorption. Cell Metab 2005;2:309-319.
30. Forman WB. Zinc abuse—an unsuspected cause of sideroblastic anemia. West J Med 1990;152:190-192.
31. Simon SR, Branda RF, Tindle BF, Burns SL. Copper deficiency and sideroblastic anemia associated with zinc ingestion. Am J Hematol 1988;28:181-183.
32. Broun ER, Greist A, Tricot G, Hoffman R. Excessive zinc ingestion: a reversible cause of sideroblastic anemia and bone marrow depression [Letter]. JAMA 1990;264:1441-1443.
33. Hoffman HN II, Phyliky RL, Fleming CR. Zinc-induced copper deficiency. Gastroenterology 1988;94:508-512.
34. Hambidge M. Biomarkers of trace mineral intake and status. J Nutr 2003;133(Suppl 3):948S-955S.
35. Pawson R, Mehta A. Review article: the diagnosis and treatment of haematinic deficiency in gastrointestinal disease. Aliment Pharmacol Ther 1998;12:687-698.
36. McClain CJ. Trace metal abnormalities in adults during hyperalimentation. JPEN J Parenter Enteral Nutr 1981;5:424-429.
37. Fishman SM, Christian P, West KP. The role of vitamins in the prevention and control of anemia. Public Health Nutr 2000;3:125-150.
38. Metz J. Cobalamin deficiency and the pathogenesis of nervous system disease. Annu Rev Nutr 1992;12:59-79.
39. Weir DG, Scott JM. Brain function in the elderly: role of vitamin B_{12} and folate. Br Med Bull 1999;55:669-682.
40. Elia M. Oral or parenteral therapy for B_{12} deficiency. JAMA 1998;352:1721-1722.
41. Freeman AG, Nyholm ES, Snowden JA, et al. Oral or parenteral therapy for B_{12} deficiency. JAMA 1999;353:410-411.
42. Kuzminski AM, Del Giacco EJ, Allen RH, et al. Effective treatment of cobalamin deficiency with oral cobalamin. Blood 1998;92:1191-1198.
43. Berlin H, Berlin R, Brante G. Oral treatment of pernicious anemia with high doses of vitamin B_{12} without intrinsic factor. Acta Med Scand 1968;184:247-258.
44. McIntyre PA, Hahn R, Masters JM, Krevans JR. Treatment of pernicious anemia with orally administered cyancolobalamin (vitamin B_{12}). Arch Intern Med 1960;106:170-182.
45. Waife SO, Jansen CJ, Crabtree RE, Grinnan Fouts PJ. Oral vitamin B_{12} without intrinsic factor in the treatment of pernicious anemia. Ann Intern Med 1963;58:810-817.

46. Lederle FA. Oral cobalamin for pernicious anemia: medicine's best kept secret? JAMA 1991;265:94-95.
47. Wang X, Wei L, Kotra LP. Cyanocobalamin (vitamin B_{12}) conjugates with enhanced solubility. Bioorg Med Chem 2007;15:1780-1787.
48. Denis R, Amin S, Cummins D. Sensitivity reaction to parenteral vitamin B_{12}: recurrence of symptoms after Marmite ingestion. Clin Lab Haematol 1996;18(2):129-31.
49. Koessler KK, Maurer S, Loughlin R. The relation of anemia, primary and secondary, to vitamin A deficiency. J Am Med Assoc 1926;87:476-482.
50. Sure B, Kik MC, Walker DJ. The effect of avitaminosis on hematopoietic function. I. Vitamin A deficiency. J Biol Chem 1929;83;375-385.
51. Sommer A, West KP. Vitamin A Deficiency: Health, Survival and Vision. New York: Oxford University Press, 1996.
52. Amatruda TT, Koeffler HP. Retinoids and cells of the hematopoietic system. In Sherman MI (ed): Retinoids and Cell Differentiation. Boca Raton, FL: CRC Press, 1986, pp 80-103.
53. Jelkmann W, Pagel H, Hellwig T, Fandrey J. Effects of antioxidant vitamins on renal and hepatic erythropoietin production. Kidney Int 1997;51:497-501.
54. Mejia LA, Hodges RE, Rucker RB. Role of vitamin A in the absorption, retention, and distribution of iron in the rat. J Nutr 1979;109:129-137.
55. Semba RD. Vitamin A, immunity, and infection. Clin Infect Dis 1994;19:489-499.
56. Bloem MW. Interdependence of vitamin A and iron: an important association for programmes of anemia control. Proc Nutr Soc 1995;54:501-508.
57. Powers HJ. Riboflavin (vitamin B-2) and health. Am J Clin Nutr 2003;77:1352-1360.
58. Powers HJ, Bates CJ, Prentice AM, et al. The relative effectiveness of iron and iron with riboflavin in correcting a microcytic anemia in men and children in rural Gambia. Hum Nutr Clin Nutr 1983;37C:413-425.
59. Powers HJ, Bates CJ, Duerden JM. Effects of riboflavin deficiency in rats on some aspects of iron metabolism. Int J Vitam Nutr Res 1983;53:371-376.
60. Fairweather-Tait SJ, Powers HJ, Minski MJ, et al. Riboflavin deficiency and iron absorption in adult Gambian men. Ann Nutr Metab 1992;36:34-40.
61. Decker K, Dotis B, Glatzle D, Hinselmann M. Riboflavin status and anemia in pregnant women. Nutr Metab 1977;21(Suppl):17-19.
62. Oski FA. Anemia due to other nutritional deficiencies. In Williams WJ, Beutler E (eds): Hematology. New York: McGraw-Hill, 1995, pp 511-515.
63. Bothwell TH, Bradlow BA, Jacobs P. Iron metabolism in scurvy with special to erythropoiesis. Br J Haematol 1964;10:50-58.
64. Lynch SR, Cook JD. Interaction of vitamin C and iron. Ann N Y Acad Sci 1980;355:32-44.
65. Hallberg L, Brune M, Rossander-Hulthen L. Is there a physiological role of vitamin C in iron absorption? Ann N Y Acad Sci 1987;498:324-332.
66. Clark NG, Sheard NF, Kelleher JF. Treatment of iron-deficiency anemia complicated by scurvy and folic acid deficiency. Nutr Rev 1992;50:134-137.
67. Cook JD, Monsen ER. Vitamin C, the common cold, and iron absorption. Am J Clin Nutr 1977;30:235-241.
68. Stokes PL, Melikian V, Leeming RL, et al. Folate metabolism in scurvy. Am J Clin Nutr 1975;28:126-129.
69. Hodges RE, Hood J, Canham JE, et al. Clinical manifestations of ascorbic acid deficiency in man. Am J Clin Nutr 1971;24:432-443.
70. Sauberlich HE. Ascorbic acid. In Brown ML (ed): Present Knowledge in Nutrition, 6th ed. Washington, DC: International Life Sciences Institute/Nutrition Foundation, 1990, pp 132-141.
71. Garry PJ, Vanderjagt DJ, Hunt WC. Ascorbic acid intakes and plasma levels in healthy elderly. Ann N Y Acad Sci 1987;498:90-99.
72. Ofori-Nkansah N, Weissenfels I, Pribilla W. Vitamin B_6 deficiency anemia [in German]. Schweiz Med Wochenschr 1975;105:1319-1324.
73. Meier PJ, Giger U, Brandli O, Fehr J. Acquired, vitamin B_6-responsive, primary sideroblastic anemia, an enzyme deficiency in heme synthesis [in German]. Schweiz Med Wochenschr 1981;111:1533-1535.
74. Solomon LR, Hillman RS. Regulation of vitamin B_6 metabolism in human red cells. Am J Clin Nutr 1979;32:1824-1831.
75. Solomon LR, Hillman RS. Vitamin B_6 metabolism in idiopathic sideroblastic anemia and related disorders. Br J Haematol 1979;42:239-253.
76. Solomon LR, Hillman RS. Vitamin B_6 metabolism in human red cells. I. Variations in normal subjects. Enzyme 1978;23:262-273.
77. Natta CL, Reynolds RD. Apparent vitamin B_6 deficiency in sickle cell anemia. Am J Clin Nutr 1984;40:235-239.
78. Chillar RK, Johnson CS, Beutler E. Erythrocyte pyridoxine kinase levels in patients with sideroblastic anemia. N Engl J Med 1976;295:881-883.
79. Vandendries ER, Drews RE. Drug-associated disease: hematologic dysfunction. Crit Care Clin 2006;22:347-355.
80. Aster RH. Drug-induced immune cytopenias. Toxicology 2005;209:149-153.
81. Salama A, Schutz B, Kiefel V, et al. Immune mediated agranulocytosis related to drugs and their metabolites: mode of sensitization and heterogeneity of antibodies. Br J Haematol 1989;72:127-132.
82. Murphy MF, Chapman JF, Metcalf P, Waters AH. Antibiotic induced neutropenia. Lancet 1985;2:1306-1307.
83. Williams DP, Pirmohamed M, Naisbitt DJ, et al. Induction of metabolism-dependent and -independent neutrophil apoptosis by clozapine. Mol Pharmacol 2000;58:207-216.
84. Eisner EV, Carr RM, MacKinney AA. Quinidine induced agranulocytosis. JAMA 1977;238:884-886.
85. Akamizu T, Ozaki S, Hiratani H, et al. Drug-induced neutropenia associated with anti-neutrophil cytoplasmic antibodies (ANCA): possible involvement of complement in granulocyte cytoxicity. Clin Exp Immunol 2002;127:92-98.
86. Neftel KA, Hauser SP, Muller MR. Inhibition of granulopoiesis in vivo and in vitro by beta-lactam antibiotics. J Infect Dis 1985;152:90-98.
87. Irvine AE, French A, Daly A, et al. Drug induced neutropenia due to direct effects on CFU-C: ten years of culture experience. Eur J Haematol 1994;52:21-27.
88. Watts RG, Emanuel PD, Zuckerman KS, Howard TH. Valproic acid induced cytopenias: evidence of a dose related suppression of hematopoiesis. J Pediatr 1990;117:495-499.
89. Symeonidis A, Kouraklis-Symeonidis A, Seimeni U, et al. Ticlopidine-induced aplastic anemia: two new case reports, review, and meta-analysis of 55 additional cases. Am J Haematol 2002;71:24-32.
90. Pannacciulli IM, Lerza RA, Bogliolo GV, et al. Effect of diethyldithiocarbamate on toxicity of doxorubicin, cyclophosphamide, and *cis*-diamminedichloroplatinum (II) on mice hematopoietic progenitor cells. Br J Cancer 1989;59:371-374.
91. Pisciotta AV, Kaldahl J. Studies on agranulocytosis. IV. Effects of chlorpromazine on nucleic acid synthesis of bone marrow cells in vitro. Blood 1962;20:364-376.
92. Gergely P. Drug-induced lymphopenia: focus on CD4+ and CD8+ cells. Drug Saf 1999;21:91-100.
93. Cosman D. The hematopoietin receptor superfamily. Cytokine 1993;5:95-106.
94. Livnah O, Stura EA, Middleton SA, et al. Crystallographic evidence for preformed dimers of erythropoietin receptor before ligand activation. Science 1999;283:987-990.
95. Kaushanky K. Lineage specific hematopoietic growth factors. N Engl J Med 2006;354:2034-2045.
96. Dijkers PF, Medema RH, Pals C, et al. Forkhead transcription factor FKHR-L1 modulates cytokine-dependent transcriptional regulation of p27 (KIP1). Mol Cell Biol 2000;20:9138-9148.
97. Starr R, Willson TA, Viney EM, et al. A family of cytokine-inducible inhibitors of signalling. Nature 1997;387:917-921.
98. Krantz SB. Erythropoietin. Blood 1991;77:419-434.
99. Reichardt Dipl-Ing B. Cost comparison of epoetin alpha, epoetin beta and darbepoetin alpha for cancer patients with anaemia in the clinical practice setting. J Clin Pharm Ther 2006;31:5, 503-512.
100. Ratcliffe PJ. Understanding hypoxia signaling in cells—a new therapeutic opportunity? Clin Med 2006;6:573-578.
101. Eckardt KU, Kurtz A. Regulation of erythropoietin production. Eur J Clin Invest 2005;35(Suppl 3):13-19.
102. Stockmann C, Fandrey J. Hypoxia-induced erythropoietin production: a paradigm for oxygen-regulated gene expression. Clin Exp Pharmacol Physiol 2006;33:968-979.
103. Maxwell PH, Pugh CW, Ratcliffe PJ. The pVHL-hIF-1 system: a key mediator of oxygen homeostasis. Adv Exp Med Biol 2001;502:365-376.
104. Davis JM, Arakawa T, Strickland TW, Yphantis DA. Characterization of recombinant human erythropoietin produced in Chinese hamster ovary cells. Biochemistry 1987;26:2633-2638.
105. Lin FK, Suggs S, Lin CH, et al. Cloning and expression of the human erythropoietin gene. Proc Natl Acad Sci U S A 1985;82:7580-7584.
106. Jelkmann W. The enigma of the metabolic fate of circulating erythropoietin (Epo) in view of the pharmacokinetics of the recombinant drugs rhEpo and NESP. Eur J Haematol 2002;69:265-274.
107. Drueke TB, Locatelli F, Clyne N, et al, for the CREATE Investigators. Normalization of hemoglobin level in patients with chronic kidney disease and anemia. N Engl J Med 2006;355:2071-2084.
108. Deicher R, Horl WH. Differentiating factors between erythropoiesis-stimulating agents: a guide to selection for anemia of chronic kidney disease. Drugs 2004;64:499-509.
109. Singh AK, Szczech L, Tang KL, et al. Correction of anemia with epoetin alfa in chronic kidney disease. CHOIR study. N Engl J Med 2006;355:2085-2098.
110. Shimoda K, Feng J, Murakami H, et al. JAK1 plays an essential role for receptor phosphorylation and STAT activation in response to granulocyte colony-stimulating factor. Blood 1997;90:597-604.
111. Vincent ME, Foote M, Morstyn G. Pharmacology of filgrastim (r-metHuG-CSF). In Morstyn G, Dexter T (eds): Filgrastim (Royal-Methug-CSF) in Clinical Practice. New York: Marcel Dekker, 1994, pp 33-50.
112. Molineux G, Kinstler O, Briddell B, et al. A new form of filgrastim with sustained duration in vivo and enhanced ability to mobilize PBPC in both mice and humans. Exp Hematol 1999;27:1724-1734.
113. Waladkhani AR. Pegfilgrastim: a recent advance in the prophylaxis of chemotherapy-induced neutropenia. Eur J Cancer Care 2004;13:371-379.
114. Green MD, Koelbl H, Baselga J, et al. A randomized, double-blind, multicenter, Phase 3 study of fixed-dose, single-administration pegfilgrastim vs daily filgrastim in patients receiving myelosuppressive chemotherapy. Ann Oncol 2003;14:29-35.
115. Iversen PO, Robinson D, Ying S. The GM-CSF analogue E21R induces apoptosis of normal and activated eosinophils. Am J Respir Crit Care Med 1997;156:1628-1632.
116. Begley CG, Lopez AF, Nicola NA, et al. Purified colony-stimulating factors enhance the survival of human neutrophils and eosinophils in vitro: a rapid and sensitive microassay for colony-stimulating factors. Blood 1986;68:162-166.
117. Owen WF Jr, Rothenberg ME, Silberstein DS, et al. Regulation of human eosinophil viability, density, and function by granulocyte-macrophage colony-stimulating factor in the presence of 3T3 fibroblasts. J Exp Med 1987;166:129-141.
118. Cebon JS, Bury RW, Lieschke GJ, Morstyn G. The effects of dose and route of administration on the pharmacokinetics of granulocyte-macrophage colony-stimulating factor. Eur J Cancer 1990;26:1064-1069.
119. Hovgaard D, Mortensen BT, Schifter S, Nissen NI. Clinical pharmacokinetic studies of a human haemopoietic growth factor, GM-CSF. Eur J Clin Invest 1992;22:45-49.

120. Stute N, Furman WL, Schell M, Evans WE. Pharmacokinetics of recombinant human granulocyte-macrophage colony stimulating factor in children after intravenous and subcutaneous administration. J Pharm Sci 1995;84:824-828.
121. Aoyarna K, Uchida T, Takanuki F, et al. Pharmacokinetics of recombinant human IL-11 in healthy male subjects. Br J Clin Pharmacol 1997;43:571-578.
122. Neumega™ package insert. Philadelphia: Wyeth Pharmaceuticals Inc., revised September 2006.
123. Tepler I, Elias L, Smith W II, et al. A randomized placebo-controlled trial of recombinant human interleukin-11 in cancer patients with severe thrombocytopenia due to chemotherapy. Blood 1996;87:3607.
124. Gordon MS, McCaskill-Stevens WJ, Battiato LA, et al. A Phase I trial of recombinant human interleukin-11 (Neumega rhIL-11 growth factor) in women with breast cancer receiving chemotherapy. Blood 1996;87:3615.
125. Ault KA, Mitchell J, Knowles C, et al. Recombinant human interleukin eleven (Neumega™ rhIL-11 growth factor) increases plasma volume and decreases urine sodium excretion in normal human subjects. Blood 1994;84(Suppl 1):276a.
126. Isaacs C, Robert N, Loewy J, Kaye JA, for the Participating Investigators. Neumega® (rhIL-11) prevents platelet transfusions in up to 4 cycles of dose-intense chemotherapy in women with breast cancer. Blood 1996;88(Suppl 1):448a.
127. Kaushansky K. Thrombopoietin. N Engl J Med 1998;339:746-754.
128. Vadhan-Raj S, Kavanagh JJ, Freedman RS, et al. Safety and efficacy of transfusions of autologous cryopreserved platelets derived from recombinant human thrombopoietin to support chemotherapy-associated severe thrombocytopenia: a randomised cross-over study. Lancet 2002;359:2145-2152.

63

DISORDERS OF HEMOSTASIS AND THROMBOSIS

Erev E. Tubb and Steven E. McKenzie

OVERVIEW 909
PATHOPHYSIOLOGY 909
THERAPEUTICS AND CLINICAL PHARMACOLOGY 909
Disorders of Hemostasis 909
Goals of Therapy 909
Therapeutics by Class 909
Thrombotic Disorders 913
Goals of Therapy 913
Therapeutics by Class 913

OVERVIEW

Disorders of hemostasis and thrombosis are in many ways mirror images of each other. The physiologic components of hemostasis stop bleeding by forming a clot at the site of vascular injury. Deficiencies in these factors result in bleeding, and therapy requires replacement of the factor or substitution for its missing function. Conversely, imbalances in these components and their endogenous regulators can result in thrombosis, formation of a clot within a physically intact blood vessel. Therapy requires the blockade of the factors' actions.

The therapeutic agents in use also follow the mirror image principle. This chapter on the pharmacology and therapeutics of disorders of hemostasis and thrombosis revolves around a core set of physiologic components, approaching each from opposite directions—how to enhance a given function for hemostasis, and how to block that same function for treating thrombosis. It should come as no surprise that the primary complications of these therapeutic agents follow from their opposing pharmacodynamics. Agents promoting hemostasis often result in thrombosis; agents treating thrombosis often result in bleeding. A goal for emerging targets and drugs is to find those that treat bleeding without increased clotting, and vice versa.

PATHOPHYSIOLOGY

Hemostasis is the physiologic process in which blood loss from damaged blood vessels is halted. Disorders of hemostasis result from inherited or acquired deficiencies of one or more hemostatic components. These deficiencies may be quantitative or qualitative. Hemostatic disorders manifest as hemorrhage. The components of normal hemostasis are (i) the coagulation factor protein system; (ii) platelets; (iii) the vessel wall, especially its endothelial cell inner lining but also including surrounding smooth muscle and connective tissue; and (iv) the fibrinolytic protein system.[1] A schema for the hemostatic system is shown in Figure 63-1.

Thrombosis is the pathologic process in which blood clots when and where it should not. Thrombotic disorders can result from deficiency of natural anticoagulant factors and/or overabundance of prothrombotic factors. The components of thrombosis are the same as those of hemostasis (coagulation factor proteins, platelets, the vessel wall, and fibrinolytic proteins) but with the additional interaction of inflammatory cells (neutrophils and monocytes) and mediators (cytokines, chemokines). Thrombosis is the final common pathway of gene-environment interactions, and thus is multifactorial. Multiple behavioral factors impact on the likelihood and severity of thrombosis.

THERAPEUTICS AND CLINICAL PHARMACOLOGY

Disorders of Hemostasis

Goals of Therapy

Effective pharmacologic therapy for hemostatic disorders aims to replace or bypass the deficient components in order to achieve cessation of blood loss when and where it is needed. Therapy seeks to prevent bleeding from occurring, or to stop bleeding once it has occurred. Safe pharmacologic therapy for hemostatic disorders aims to avoid thrombotic side effects and the transmission of infectious agents.

Therapeutics by Class

The pharmacologic agents for disorders of hemostasis can be divided into (i) coagulation factor replacement or bypassing agents, (ii) prohemostatic drugs, and (iii) antifibrinolytics. We will avoid the discussion of transfusion therapy, wherein a blood component product is prescribed from a blood bank instead of taking a pharmacologic approach. Rather, we focus on drugs/agents regulated by the U.S. Food and Drug Administration (FDA).

Coagulation Factors. The coagulation factor proteins in plasma—fibrinogen and factors II, V, VII, VIII, IX, X, and XI—work as shown in Figure 63-1 to form a fibrin clot. Factor XIII (FVIII) works to stabilize fibrin clots. Currently pharmaceutical products exist for deficiencies of factors VIII, IX, and VII and von Willebrand factor (vWF).

Factor VIII. The most common inherited deficiency of coagulation factors is deficiency of FVIII in the disorder hemophilia A. As the FVIII gene is on the X chromosome, virtually all affected patients are male, with the rare exception of females with two defective FVIII genes or with markedly skewed X inactivation (lyonization). In 2007, the standard of care is to prevent or treat hemorrhage in hemophilia A patients with a recombinant FVIII protein preparation. Under certain circumstances, FVIII purified from human donor plasma may be used. Some patients have clinically significant antibody inhibitors of human FVIII action. As described at the end of this section, either porcine FVIII or protein factors that "bypass" the inhibited FVIII to complete hemostasis can be used for these patients with inhibitors.

Indications for use of FVIII are (i) treatment of spontaneous or traumatic bleeding in patients with severe and moderate disease, (ii) prevention of hemorrhage in the perioperative/procedure setting, and (iii) primary prophylaxis for prevention of spontaneous or minor trauma-related hemorrhage. Common bleeding sites are joints (especially the large joints), muscles, the retroperitoneum, and intracranial and mucosal sites (notably oropharyngeal, nasopharyngeal, genitourinary, and gastrointestinal).

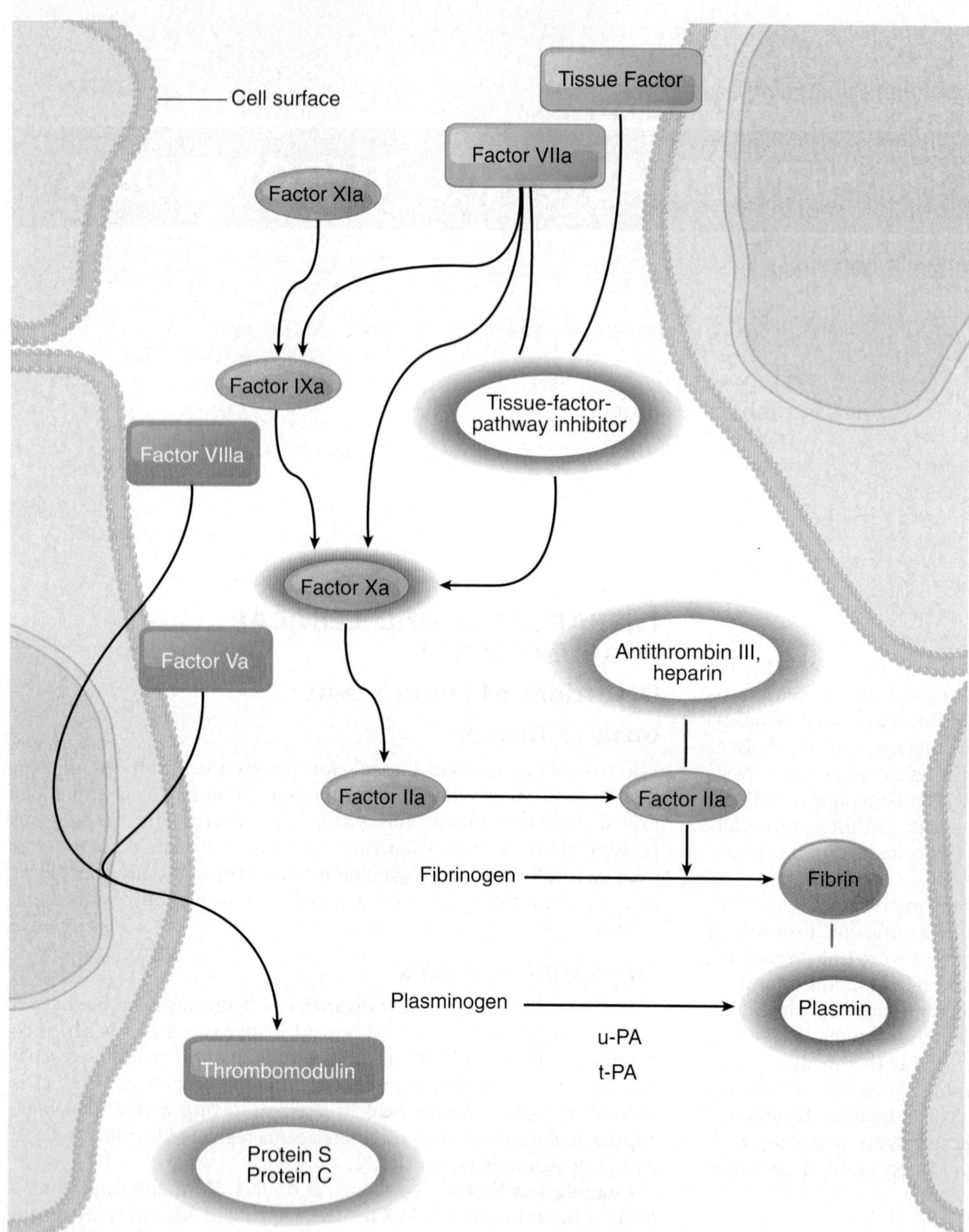

FIGURE 63-1 • The components of the hemostatic system are shown as they are employed to stop blood loss from a damaged blood vessel.

As its mechanism of action, recombinant or plasma-derived FVIII provides the deficient factor that enables propagation of the protein complexes into a fully formed clot.

Recombinant FVIII is a large (280-kDa) protein, produced from human FVIII complementary DNA in mammalian cell cultures. There are two major forms, one that is full length and one that has the B domain of the protein removed. The B domain is dispensable for hemostatic function, but its absence results in some manufacturing differences of potential advantage. Recombinant FVIII protein is purified from the culture supernatant either by antibody-based affinity purification or by biochemical methods. Human donor purified protein is resuspended in one of several solutions for administration (see later). Plasma-derived FVIII is now exclusively provided following both antibody-based purification and one or more additional viral inactivation steps, such as solvent-detergent treatment.

FVIII is prepared as a concentrate that is lyophilized. There are three "generations" of recombinant FVIII preparations with respect to formulation. In the first generation, the protein was grown, purified, and resuspended and/or stabilized as a concentrate in medium containing human or animal plasma-derived proteins, such as human serum albumin. Hypothetically, the presence of a human or animal plasma-derived protein (albumin, vWF, or a monoclonal antibody) could be associated with transmission of viruses, prions, or other agents. In the second generation, the concentrate is stabilized in a sugar nonprotein medium, but other steps may involve the presence of human or animal protein. Third-generation products are stabilized in a sugar nonprotein medium and are grown and formulated in the absence of human or animal proteins. However, within third-generation products, there can be a difference as to whether monoclonal anti-FVIII antibody is used in purification.

The dose of FVIII administered is based on the hemostatic correction desired in any single patient. This correction considers the pharmacokinetics of the drug, the severity of the hemostatic challenge, the severity of the patient's deficiency, the duration of correction needed, and the size of the patient. The lyophilized protein concentrate is provided with the label of units of activity. One unit of FVIII activity is defined as that present in 1 ml of a mixed pool of normal plasma. The "normal" activity level is thus 1 unit/ml. Therefore, each manufactured lot is tested for the specific activity of the preparation in units per milligram, and the number of units per vial is specified. Upon reconstitution in sterile diluent, FVIII is provided by intravenous infusion. The volume of distribution of FVIII is primarily within the vascular space, so that the dose is calculated based on a fixed fraction (0.5) of the patient's weight in kilograms. A dose of 1 unit/kg raises the plasma FVIII activity by 0.02 units/ml (2%). A dose of 40 units/kg is considered "full" correction, and is calculated to bring the FVIII activity level to 0.8 units/ml. The elimination half-time is 8 to 12 hours.

It is important to recognize that plasma FVIII activity of 0.3 units/ml, or 30% of the mean normal value, is associated with negligible spontaneous hemorrhage and low risk of surgical or traumatic hemorrhage. Therefore, when treating a significant hemorrhage or with major surgery, clinicians seek extended duration of hemostatic protection. The desired trough value of FVIII activity is ≥0.3 units/ml, except with high-risk areas such as the brain and spinal cord, where trough values in excess of 0.5 units/ml are the standard of care. In order to maintain plasma FVIII activity within the therapeutic range, a dose of 20 units/kg should be given 8 hours after the initial dose, and subsequent doses given every 8 to 12 hours. Laboratory monitoring of an individual patient's actual FVIII levels in comparison with the predicted values can be an important clinical management tool.

Successful prophylactic treatment is based on the observation that individuals with moderate hemophilia A, with activity levels between 1% and 5% of normal (0.01 to 0.05 units/ml), have minimal spontaneous hemorrhage. Therefore, FVIII is administered every other day, or three times per week, at individual doses of 20 to 40 units/kg. By the time the following dose is due, the desired nadir FVIII activity is greater than 0.01 units/ml. Prospective studies have validated the utility of this approach in minimizing recurrent joint bleeding episodes and the subsequent arthropathy.

FVIII protein is bound by vWF in the circulation. Cleavage by thrombin results in formation of the active disulfide linked coagulation factor, which dissociates from vWF and works as the requisite cofactor with activated factor IX (FIXa) on anionic phospholipid surfaces in the intrinsic Xase complex. Recall that the intrinsic Xase complex consists of activated factor VIII (FVIIIa) and FIXa, and it activates factor X (FX) to FXa. FVIII protein is catabolized in the intravascular space and in the reticuloendothelial system.

Use of FVIII as therapy for hemorrhage or during invasive procedures requires monitoring for efficacy and side effects. For hemorrhages at external surfaces, inspection for the cessation of bleeding is the major monitoring step. Serial physical examinations, radiologic studies, and laboratory tests for hemoglobin levels are all part of monitoring for control of internal hemorrhage. Interindividual differences in metabolism, or new development of inhibitors, may necessitate monitoring of the corrected activated partial thromboplastin time (aPTT) and/or of FVIII activity levels, particularly when the clinical course is unsatisfactory or the risks of uncontrolled hemorrhage, such as in the brain, are catastrophic. Side effects include allergic-type reactions, development of inhibitors, and thrombosis. FVIII products that are plasma derived, or prepared in the presence of human or animal proteins, may result in transmission of viruses or prions.

There are alternatives for treatment of patients with FVIII inhibitors. There are two broad types of patients with FVIII inhibitors: hemophilia A patients who have developed antibodies against the FVIII they have received as treatment, and patients born with normal FVIII but who acquire autoantibodies that inhibit FVIII, so-called acquired FVIII inhibitor patients. The principle of treatment for these patients is to overcome or bypass the blocked FVIII activity. Hemophilia A patients with inhibitors require treatment at comprehensive hemophilia treatment centers because of the intricacy and individualized nature of the management decisions. Therefore, rather than provide management recommendations, we review the available agents for clinicians who need products other than human FVIII itself. (Some hemophilia A patients with low-titer inhibitors and who do not manifest anamnestic responses to exposure to FVIII have been successfully treated with "overwhelming" amounts of FVIII.)

Historically, plasma-derived coagulation protein complex concentrates have been used to bypass the lack of FVIII activity. So-called prothrombin complex concentrates (PCCs) possess multiple coagulation factors, notably factors II, VII, IX, and X. Some are activated during the manufacturing process, and contain higher levels of activated factor VII (FVIIa). The dose is based on the measured factor IX (FIX) activity in each lot. Usual starting doses are 75 units/kg of FIX activity, and the timing of subsequent doses depends on the clinical severity of the hemorrhage and the risk of thrombosis.

Porcine FVIII has also been used to obtain hemostasis in patients with antibody inhibitors to human FVIII. It is the current standard of care to demonstrate lack of cross-reactivity of a patient's sample to porcine FVIII in the laboratory before it is given therapeutically. The dose is based on the desired units of activity in the patient, comparable to use of human FVIII. As this is currently a porcine plasma product, immunologic reactions and transmission of infectious agents are potential side effects.

Recombinant FVIIa is approved for treatment of patients with FVIII inhibitors (see later). It is most often administered by intermittent intravenous bolus infusion. The dose regimens have been empirically derived. The dose is calculated on a microgram per kilogram basis, with manufactured lots meeting specific activity measures. Monitoring is clinical, as there is no laboratory parameter of efficacy to follow.

Factor IX. The indications for use of FIX pharmacotherapy are treatment or prevention of hemorrhage in patients with inherited FIX deficiency, also known as hemophilia B. FIX deficiency is X-linked, so virtually all affected patients are male. The standard of care in 2007 is to use recombinant FIX. Plasma-derived FIX preparations are also available, some with solely FIX as a result of biochemical or affinity purification, and some as PCCs.

FIX therapy has as its mechanism of action the replacement of deficient FIX zymogen levels in order to provide FIXa activity. FIXa is the active enzyme in the VIIIa/IXa complex, which activates FX to FXa. The ultimate result is the successful generation of a stable fibrin clot.

FIX is a 56-kDa glycoprotein, and a vitamin K–dependent factor, in that it is synthesized in the liver with specifically modified glutamic acid residues, added by a vitamin K–dependent process called γ-carboxylation. The anionic glutamic acid residues facilitate association with Ca^{2+} cations and phosphatidylserine (PS) surfaces. This process to date has required use of mammalian cells for production of the recombinant protein.

The formulations of FIX depend on the source, recombinant or plasma derived. In general, FIX is provided as a lyophilized protein with a defined specific activity. Upon reconstitution in sterile diluent, it is provided by intravenous infusion. The dosage of FIX depends on the size of the patient, the volume of distribution, and the desired activity. In general, a bolus dose of 1 unit/kg raises the plasma level 0.01 unit/ml, due to a greater volume of distribution than FVIII. However, FIX has a longer elimination half-time of 18 hours, allowing intermittent dosage every 24 hours. As with FVIII, an alternative dosing strategy that has been used is the continuous intravenous infusion. This is most often used in high-risk perioperative situations for which prolonged hemostatic coverage is needed.

FIX protein is catabolized in the intravascular space and in the reticuloendothelial system. As with FVIII, monitoring for efficacy may be clinical in a minor hemorrhage in a patient with no inhibitors. If laboratory monitoring is used, it is based primarily on normalization of the aPTT. In prolonged use for serious hemorrhages, determination of the recipient's plasma FIX activity is performed. Side effects of therapeutic FIX replacement are similar to those of FVIII. Development of antibody inhibitors, transmission of viruses, thrombosis, and anaphylactic reactions have been observed. Though antibody inhibitors are slightly less common than in FVIII deficiency, the presence of immunoglobulin E anti-FIX antibodies in some patients may result in anaphylactic reactions. Treatment of FIX inhibitor patients in a center equipped to manage this complication is essential. Prion transmission and emerging viral pathogens not susceptible to the processing and purification steps remain hypothetical risks in plasma-derived products. Low-titer FIX inhibitors can sometimes be overwhelmed by higher FIX doses. Higher titer inhibitors require PCCs or recombinant FVIIa therapy (see later).

von Willebrand Factor. vWF deficiency is the most common hemostatic disorder. vWF is a large multimeric protein found in endothelial cells and platelets. It is secreted into both plasma and the subendothelial extracellular matrix. It has two major biologic functions: it carries plasma FVIII, and it binds the platelet glycoprotein (GP) Ib/IX receptor complex to enable platelet adhesion to a damaged blood vessel wall.

The biochemistry and physiology of vWF are complex. The monomeric polypeptide is processed within the cell to covalently linked multimeric forms, some of which can be several million Daltons in molecular weight. The stoichiometry of FVIII binding is 1 vWF monomer to 1 FVIII molecule. The interaction of vWF with the platelet GP Ib/IX complex depends on a conformational change in vWF induced by high shear stress under flow. This receptor-binding conformation is mimicked in vitro by the concurrent presence of the compound ristocetin. Large vWF multimers are more effective in stopping hemorrhage than smaller multimers.

There are several major forms of von Willebrand's disease (vWD) that differ in their severity and genetics. The most common form, type I, is a mild to moderate autosomal dominant hemorrhagic disorder characterized by low plasma levels of vWF. However, in most type I vWD patients, there is functional vWF protein in the storage granules (Weibel-Palade bodies) of the endothelial cells. As is discussed later, the vasopressin analogue desamino-D-arginine vasopressin (DDAVP) stimulates endothelial cells to secrete vWF. Therefore, replacement therapy with a source of vWF protein often can be avoided in such patients.

Some type I vWD patients, and virtually all type II and type III vWD patients, do not respond to or tolerate DDAVP therapy. For these patients, the current practice is to provide replacement vWF protein. Currently, only purified, plasma-derived vWF is available. The plasma-derived products contain both vWF and FVIII. Recently, these lyophilized protein concentrates have had the units of vWF ristocetin cofactor (vWF:RCo) activity determined in each lot, such that dosing for vWD patients could be more rational than the prior dosing based on the FVIII activity. Only those products containing measured vWF activity and the most hemostatically effective high-molecular-weight multimers should be used. Also, these products have been subjected to viral inactivation steps to reduce the likelihood of transmission.

One unit of vWF:RCo activity is defined as that equal to the amount found in 1 ml of pooled normal human plasma. For each 1 unit of vWF:RCo activity per kilogram infused, the expected rise in vWF:RCo activity is 0.02 units/ml (2% of the normal value). However, there is wide variability among individuals, such that testing of an individual's yield and recovery of vWF is recommended prior to elective use. The use of a loading bolus dose, followed by intermittent dosing at 8- to 12-hour intervals, is recommended. The dose depends on the specific type of vWD, its severity, and the nature of the hemorrhage or procedure.[2] In general, keeping the trough value above 0.5 units/ml improves efficacy.

Side effects of vWF replacement therapy are those common to all plasma-derived products, as detailed previously. vWF protein is catabolized intravascularly and in the reticuloendothelial system. One important protease in vWF processing and catabolism is ADAMTS13, which is responsible for cleaving high-molecular-weight vWF multimers. Inherited deficiency of ADAMTS13, or acquired inhibitors of ADAMTS13, are found in some cases of thrombotic thrombocytopenic purpura. This link between control of vWF multimer size and thrombosis underscores the critical role of the vWF protein in hemostasis.

Factor VIIa. Factor VII (FVII) circulates as a natural zymogen protein, with a small percentage in an activated form, FVIIa. The mechanism for the formation of the low level of circulating FVIIa is still under investigation. FVII/FVIIa binds to its cofactor tissue factor (TF) to form the extrinsic Xase complex. FVII bound to TF is converted to FVIIa by one of several mechanisms. The extrinsic Xase complex converts FX to FXa, the key factor in generating thrombin. Tissue factor pathway inhibitor is a major control point, because it binds avidly to the ternary complex of TF/FVIIa/FX to stop further conversion of FX to FXa.

Pharmacologic therapy with recombinant FVIIa was developed to treat hemophilia patients with inhibitors, specifically FVIII and FIX deficiency. It is administered intravenously and has a short half-life, approximately 2.5 hours. It can be used in these conditions for prevention of bleeding prior to surgical procedures, or for treatment of bleeding. The most common approach in hemophilia patients is to give a bolus dose of 90 mcg/kg and repeat this every 2 hours until hemostasis is achieved. If the result is inadequate, the dose and interval may need to be adjusted. It has also received FDA approval for treatment of FVII deficiency. In FVII deficiency, less is needed (15 to 30 mcg/kg) less often (every 4 to 6 hours) than in patients with hemophilia and inhibitors.

There are other indications for FVIIa therapy that have not received FDA approval. These include liver cirrhosis, acquired FXIII deficiency, and reversal of severe excessive anticoagulation. These indications have Category B evidence in adults. Studies of other uses, such as in intracerebral hemorrhage, have failed to find a survival advantage, and have raised the major issue of thrombotic events as a side effect.[3]

Prohemostatic Drugs

DDAVP. DDAVP is a synthetic analogue of the natural pituitary hormone vasopressin (also known as antidiuretic hormone). DDAVP works by causing the release of vWF and its associated FVIII from endothelial cells. Because the vWF is in the high-molecular-weight multimeric form, it is very hemostatic. The use of DDAVP in vWD was presented earlier. There are additional indications for its prohemostatic effects beyond vWD. These include mild hemophilia A and some inherited and acquired platelet function disorders. Each patient for whom future DDAVP treatment is contemplated should undergo a test dose and monitoring of the safety and efficacy. Efficacy needs to be assessed by shortening of the bleeding time test and/or increases in the plasma vWF concentrations.

DDAVP can be administered as a slow intravenous infusion of 30 mcg/kg. The major side effects are flushing, hypotension, and transient hyponatremia. Restriction of fluid intake during the anuretic phase that follows receipt of DDAVP, a period lasting several hours, can minimize serious hyponatremia and its consequences, such as seizures. DDAVP is also available in an intranasal form, although care must be used in distinguishing this formulation from that used to manage enuresis. Metered-dose sprays of the prohemostatic formulation, marketed as Stimate, provide a dose of 150 mcg/spray. For individuals weighing less than 50 kg, a 150-mcg dose is indicated; for larger individuals, a 300-mcg dose is used.

Antifibrinolytics. The major antifibrinolytics are aminocaproic acid and tranexamic acid. They each work by interfering with the generation, and to some extent the activity, of plasmin, which cleaves fibrin in clots. Antifibrinolytics can only be used as an adjunct to treatments that ensure the formation first of a platelet/fibrin clot. Therefore, they are used to accompany factor replacement or DDAVP treatments. They are not used concurrently with PCCs, however, because of the potential risk of thrombotic complications. Extended use is beneficial, because several days are needed after primary hemostasis for wound healing and tissue remodeling. In particular, in the oropharynx, where salivary proteases are present that can adversely affect clot integrity, 5 to 10 days of antifibrinolytic treatment is associated with better outcome.

Aminocaproic acid is provided as a tablet or a liquid for oral administration, and as a solution for intravenous administration. The half-life is 2 hours, and it is excreted renally. The oral or intravenous dose for dental surgical procedures in hemophilia is 75 mg/kg, up to 6 g. This is repeated every 6 hours for 5 to 10 days. Dose adjustment for renal impairment should be considered. Common side effects are nausea and dizziness. Aminocaproic acid is also used for surgical or nonsurgical hematuria at comparable doses, although if intravenous aminocaproic acid is used for hematuria, it may be provided as a continuous infusion of 1 g/hr until bleeding stops or up to 8 hours. The additional concern in hematuria use is thrombosis in the renal/urinary tract. In renal impairment or oliguria, the dose must be reduced. Aminocaproic acid is contraindicated in disseminated intravascular coagulation (DIC). Monitoring consists of physical examinations for bleeding or thrombosis, supplemented by hematologic studies (complete blood count, coagulation panel, DIC panel) and radiologic studies as needed.

Tranexamic acid is provided as a tablet or a liquid for oral administration, and as a solution for intravenous administration. On a molar basis, tranexamic acid is more potent than aminocaproic acid. The half-life is 2 hours, and it is excreted renally. The intravenous dose for dental surgical procedures in hemophilia is 10 mg/kg, while the oral dose is 25 mg/kg. The dose is repeated every 6 hours for 5 to 10 days. Common side effects are nausea and dizziness and hypotension (if infused too rapidly). Prolonged use can result in ophthalmologic impairment. In renal impairment the dose must be reduced. Tranexamic acid is contraindicated in DIC. Monitoring should be the same as for aminocaproic acid supplemented by ophthalmologic studies as needed.

Thrombotic Disorders

Goals of Therapy

Effective pharmacologic therapy for thrombotic disorders can be divided into prevention of thrombosis or treatment of existing thrombosis. Prevention can be primary, stopping a first thrombotic event in those at high risk, or secondary, stopping recurrence in those who have already had one or more thrombotic events. In the treatment of existing thrombosis, there are several goals. For thrombi in large to medium arteries, rapid restoration of blood flow is critical to minimizing ischemic damage to the tissue supplied by that arterial bed. In addition, avoidance of clot embolization is important. For thrombi in deep veins, avoidance of embolization to the pulmonary vasculature is of primary importance, with prevention of clot extension and restoration of blood flow of ongoing importance. Prevention of post-phlebitic complications, such as pain and skin compromise, is another major goal of treatment. Safe pharmacologic therapy for thrombotic disorders aims to minimize thrombosis and thromboemboli while avoiding hemorrhage and harmful immune reactions.

Therapeutics by Class

Thrombotic diseases are the leading cause of morbidity and mortality in Western countries, and therfore antithrombotics are among the most often-used drugs. It is helpful to segregate these drugs into classes according to their mechanism of action, as follows: (i) anticoagulants, (ii) antiplatelet agents, and (iii) fibrinolytics. Anticoagulants act primarily on the generation of thrombin to decrease fibrin formation. They are used in the treatment of atrial fibrillation, unstable angina, myocardial infarction, deep venous thrombosis (DVT), and pulmonary embolism. Antiplatelet agents act to decrease platelet function and are used in the treatment of arterial thromboses, notably ischemic stroke and coronary artery disease. Fibrinolytics accelerate clot breakdown by increasing the conversion of plasminogen to plasmin and are used in the treatment of acute myocardial infarction, stroke and pulmonary embolism, and massive DVT.

Anticoagulants. The most common adverse event encountered in the use of anticoagulant drugs is bleeding. It is therefore important to recognize the narrow therapeutic window of these agents and to use the minimal effective dose for the treatment of thromboses and the prophylaxis of high-risk patients.

Vitamin K Antagonists. The development of this class of agents was founded on the discovery by Karl Paul Link and Harold Campbell in the 1930s and 1940s at the University of Wisconsin that a substance, dicumarol, in moldy hay was responsible for a hemorrhagic cattle disease. Subsequently warfarin was developed by the Wisconsin Alumni Research Fund as a potent rodenticide. Numerous coumarin derivatives have been developed and are available around the world; however, warfarin is almost exclusively used in North America. In the 1950s, Coumadin (the brand name of warfarin) was first introduced as an oral antithrombotic for humans. These compounds, collectively referred to as vitamin K antagonists, remain the only oral anticoagulants currently approved for clinical use in the United States.

The 4-hydroxycoumarin residue, with a nonpolar carbon substituent at the 3 position, is the minimal structural requirement for anticoagulant activity. Many derivatives of 4-hydroxycoumarin have been synthesized, and all commercial preparations of these oral anticoagulants are racemic mixtures. The (*R*-) and (*S*-) enantiomers differ in anticoagulant potency, metabolism, elimination, and interactions with other drugs.

Coumarins are competitive inhibitors of vitamin K. They indirectly inhibit the γ-carboxylation reaction necessary for the hepatic synthesis of coagulant factors II, VII, IX, and X and the natural anticoagulant factors protein C and protein S. γ-Glutamyl carboxylase carboxylates 9 through 13 of the amino-terminal glutamate residues to form a calcium-binding γ-carboxyglutamate. Warfarin antagonizes vitamin K reductase, the enzyme responsible for converting the oxidized vitamin K epoxide, generated during the γ-carboxylation reaction, back to the reduced form of vitamin K (Fig. 63-2).

Warfarin causes a 30% to 50% decrease in vitamin K–dependent factor concentrations in the serum as well as leading to undercarboxylation of vitamin K–dependent factor, leading to a decreased biologic activity. Fully carboxylated factors retain their full activity; therefore, the clinical effectiveness of warfarin depends on the clearance of circulating vitamin K–dependent factors and the time to achieve a new steady state level. The maximum anticoagulation effect is not achieved for several days despite prolonged in vitro coagulation studies because of the long half-life of factor II (60 to 72 hours) relative to FVII (4 to 6 hours) (Table 63-1).

Dietary vitamin K intake and absorption affect the efficacy of warfarin. Therefore, high vitamin K–containing vegetables, diarrhea, broad-spectrum antibiotics, liver disease, vitamin K ingestion, and many pharmaceuticals can alter the bioavailability/metabolism and pharmacodynamics of warfarin. Additionally, aspirin, nonsteroidal anti-inflammatory drugs (NSAIDs), and heparins can potentiate bleeding by inhibiting complementary hemostatic pathways.

Warfarin is essentially completely bioavailable after oral, rectal, or intravenous administration. Different preparations of warfarin may affect the rate of dissolution and thereby affect the rate of absorption. After oral administration, warfarin is detectable in the plasma after 1 hour, achieving peak concentrations in 2 to 8 hours.

Warfarin is 99% bound to plasma albumin and other plasma proteins. Therefore, the drug distributes to a volume approximately equal to that of albumin (0.14 L/kg). The free form of warfarin is the biologically active compound. Fetal concentrations approximate maternal concentrations, but unlike other coumarin derivatives, warfarin is not found in breast milk.

Warfarin is a racemic mixture of (*R*-) (weak) and (*S*-) (potent) anticoagulant enantiomers in equal proportion that is stereoselectively metabolized by the cytochrome P-450 (CYP) enzymes. CYP2C9 is the principle enzyme that metabolizes *S*-warfarin, modulating warfarin's in vivo activity. *R*-warfarin is metabolized by the CYP1A2 and CYP3A4 enzymes. Genetic polymorphisms of CYP2C9 may be responsible for a significant part of the interpatient variability of response to warfarin and may predispose certain patients to more significant drug interactions. Up to 92% of the inactive metabolites of warfarin are excreted in urine; biliary excretion accounts for the rest. The half-life of warfarin ranges from 25 to 60 hours, with a mean of about 40 hours; the duration of action of a single dose of warfarin is 2 to 5 days. The effects

TABLE 63-1 APPROXIMATE HALF-LIFE OF SELECTED FACTORS

Factor	Half-Life
Factor II	60-72 hr
Factor VII	4-6 hr
Factor IX	24 hr
Factor X	48-72 hr
Protein C	8 hr
Protein S	30 hr

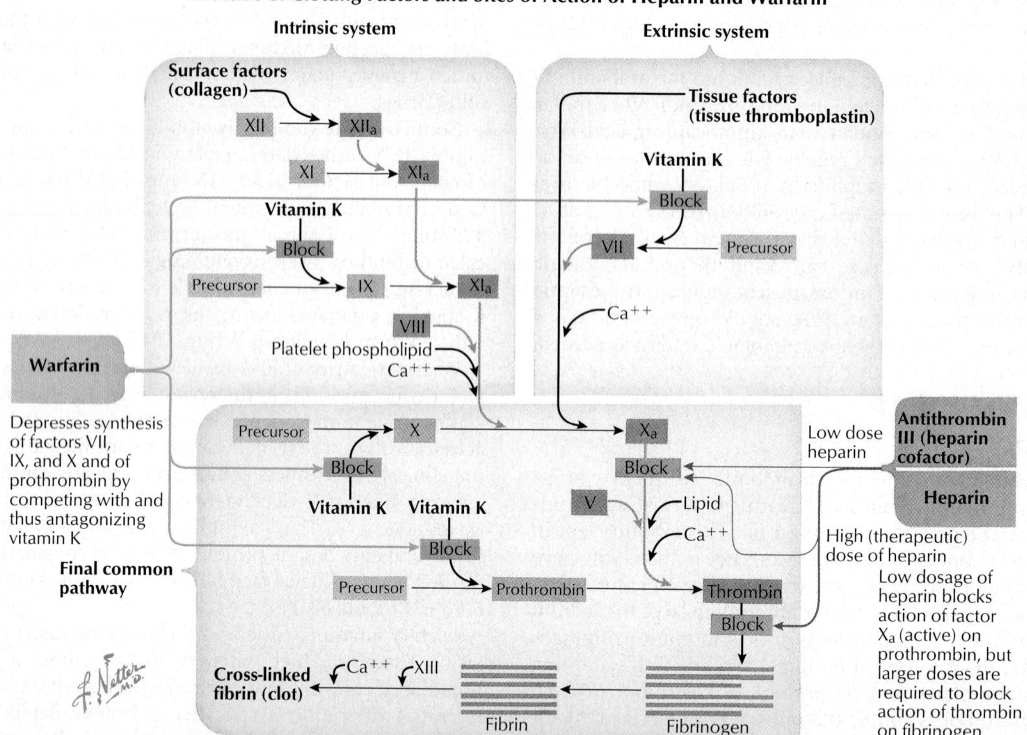

FIGURE 63-2 • Cascade of clotting factors and sites of action of heparin and warfarin. (Courtesy of Netterimages.com.)

of warfarin become more pronounced as effects of daily maintenance doses overlap.

Warfarin is indicated for the prophylaxis and/or treatment of venous thrombosis and its extension, pulmonary embolism; for the prophylaxis and/or treatment of thromboembolic complications associated with atrial fibrillation and/or cardiac valve replacement; and to reduce the risk of death, recurrent myocardial infarction, and thromboembolic events such as stroke or systemic embolization after myocardial infarction.[4]

An anticoagulation effect generally occurs within 24 hours after drug administration. Initiation of warfarin therapy should be concomitant with rapidly acting anticoagulation agents such as heparin, heparin derivatives, or direct thrombin inhibitors. The usual effective dose is 5 to 10 mg orally per day except in the frail, elderly, or profoundly malnourished patient, who may require a smaller dose. Loading doses are not recommended.[5]

Measurement of the international normalized ratio (INR) derived from the patient's prothrombin time (PT) is used to account for the variability in thromboplastin reagents between laboratories. The INR is an exponential mathematical transformation of the PT ratio into a corrected ratio value. The INR is based on the ratio of the patient's PT to the laboratory mean normal PT, along with the international sensitivity index (ISI) calculated by the manufacturer and provided in the thromboplastin package insert. The formula for calculation of the INR is as follows[6]:

$$\text{INR} = (\text{RT ratio})^{\text{ISI}}$$

During warfarin therapy initiation, the INR should be checked every 2 to 3 days for the first 1 to 2 weeks until a stable dose is achieved. Recent FDA-approved product insert labeling notifies precribers of the availability of CYP2C9/VKORC1 genetic testing to help guide initial warfarin dosing, though this practice is by no means routine currently. The goal of warfarin therapy is to reduce prothrombin activity to approximately 25% of baseline. The therapeutic INR will range between 2 and 3 for the treatment of thrombotic disease (DVT, pulmonary embolism, atrial fibrillation, and thromboprophylaxis) and between 2.5 and 3.5 for certain mechanical heart valves. INR monitoring can be done in the physician's office, in a clinical laboratory, and in the home. Home INR monitoring with physician supervision for dosing has been validated as a safe, efficient, and cost-effective alternative.[7]

Bleeding is the most serious and common side effect of oral anticoagulants. The risk of bleeding increases with increased INR, length of therapy, and certain patient characteristics such as old age, renal failure, recent surgery or trauma, prior history of intracerebral or gastrointestinal bleeding, hypertension, and concomitant use of interacting drug(s) that potentiate warfarin's anticoagulant effect. The risk of bleeding during a 6-month course of anticoagulation for venous thrombosis is approximately 3% to 5%.

The list of drugs that affect the oral anticoagulants is ever growing and expansive. Frequently cited drugs that enhance the risk of hemorrhage by inhibition of CYP2C9 in patients taking warfarin include amiodarone, azole antifungals, cimetidine, clopidogrel, cotrimoxazole, disulfiram, fluoxetine, isoniazid, lovastatin/metronidazole, sulfinpyrazone, tolcapone, and zafirlukast. Additionally, valproic acid and loop diuretics can displace warfarin from its plasma protein binding site, thereby increasing the free plasma warfarin concentration. Cholestyramine can reduce absorption of warfarin in the gastrointestinal tract, hypoproteinemia (e.g., as a result of nephrotic syndrome) can increase the volume of distribution of warfarin, and barbiturates, carbamazepine, or rifampin can shorten warfarin's half-life by increasing its metabolic clearance secondary to induction of hepatic enzymes, especially CYP2C9, all leading to decreased efficacy.

Warfarin skin necrosis is a rare complication associated with warfarin therapy with an incidence of 0.01% to 0.1%. Although the etiology of warfarin skin necrosis is still obscure, initiation of warfarin without heparin/direct thrombin inhibitor therapy appears to be the cause, especially in patients with low protein C/S levels. Clinical complaints usually involve tingling or burning in sites with large amounts of subcutaneous tissue (breast, buttock, and thigh) followed by full-thickness painful hemorrhagic skin infarction. Microscopic evaluation reveals thrombosis of dermal and subdermal venules as the underlying cause.

Warfarin crosses the placenta readily and is contraindicated in pregnancy. Warfarin can cause fetal hemorrhages as well as severe bone malformation. Fetal exposure to warfarin during organogenesis can lead to severe cranial cartilage/bone and limb malformations.

If complications of bleeding, trauma, overdosage, or the need for surgery is encountered, warfarin anticoagulation can be reversed. For the patient with supratherapeutic INR but no evidence of bleeding, withholding warfarin doses, frequent monitoring of INR, and reducing subsequent doses is usually effective. Additionally, a low dose (0.5 to 1 mg) of oral or subcutaneous vitamin K can be given. Patients with serious bleeding may require larger doses of vitamin K, which can be given orally, subcutaneously, or intravenously, and/or factor replacement by infusion of fresh frozen plasma. It is usually better to postpone elective surgery until several months of anticoagulation have been administered following an acute thrombosis, as the risk of recurrent thrombosis is greatest early and decreases with time.

Heparin and Heparin Derivatives. Heparin is the most widely used rapidly acting parenteral anticoagulant. Heparin is an indirect inhibitor of thrombin. It acts on antithrombin III to enhance its activity against FXa and activated factor IIa (FIIa) (activated clotting factors of the intrinsic and common pathway). Initially described as an aqueous extract of liver with an anticoagulant effect in vitro, heparin is commonly obtained by extraction from porcine intestinal mucosa or bovine lung (see Fig. 63-2).

Heparin is a mucopolysaccharide organic acid found in the secretory granules of mast cells, basophils, and the vascular endothelium. Heparin is composed of chains of alternating residues of D-glucosamine and iduronic acid that undergo a series of incomplete modifications, yielding a variety of oligosaccharide structures. After the heparin proteoglycan has been transported to the mast cell granule, an endo-β-D-glucuronidase degrades the glycosaminoglycan chains to fragments of 6 to 30 kDa (mean, about 15 kDa or 50 saccharide units) over a period of hours.

Although different commercial preparations of heparin are heterogeneous in composition, their biologic activities are standardized (approximately 120 USP units/mg). The USP unit defines the quantity of heparin that prevents 1 ml of citrated sheep plasma from clotting for 1 hour after the addition of 0.2 ml of 1% $CaCl_2$.

Low-molecular-weight heparins (LMWHs) are obtained from unfractionated heparin by gel filtration chromatography, chemical hydrolysis, or partial alkaline depolymerization with nitrous acid and other chemical or enzymatic reagents. LMWHs have different pharmacokinetic and pharmacodynamic properties than unfractionated heparin and from each other. The biologic activity of LMWH is generally measured by an antithrombin-mediated in vitro assay: the FXa inhibition assay.

The action of heparin is dependent on the activity of antithrombin III, FIIa, and FXa. Heparin acts as a cofactor to antithrombin III, a glycosylated, single-chain polypeptide composed of 432 amino acid residues, synthesized in the liver and circulating in plasma at a concentration of approximately 2.6 μmol/L. Heparin enhances antithrombin III activity by 1000-fold by inducing a conformational change in the active site such that the complex can more readily and rapidly bind to and inhibit proteases IIa and Xa. The inhibition of thrombin requires the formation of a ternary complex (heparin-antithrombin-thrombin) and requires a heparin molecule that consists of at least 19 or more saccharide units. The smaller heparin molecules and LMWHs are effective in inactivating FXa as the formation of a ternary complex is not necessary.

Factor II, FIXa, and FXa are rapidly inhibited by antithrombin when the concentration of heparin in plasma is 0.1 to 1 unit/ml. This prolongs both the aPTT and the thrombin time (the time required for plasma to clot when exogenous thrombin is added); the PT may be affected to a lesser degree. FXa bound to platelets in the prothrombinase complex and thrombin bound to fibrin are both protected from inhibition by antithrombin in the presence of heparin.

Heparin is not absorbed after oral ingestion, and is administered either intravenously or subcutaneously. The anticoagulation effect is immediate following intravenous injection, but with subcutaneous injection there is a delay of 1 to 2 hours in the onset of action and a bioavailability of 50% or less at low doses, which increases at higher doses.

In contrast, LMWHs (enoxaparin, dalteparin, tinzaparin) are uniformly absorbed after subcutaneous administration. After subcutaneous injection of enoxaparin, the maximum anti-FXa and antithrombin activities occur within 3 to 5 hours, and its volume of distribution is approximately 4.3 L. The mean absolute bioavailability of enoxaparin, after 1.5 mg/kg given subcutaneously, is approximately 100% in healthy patients. The mean peak levels of plasma anti-FXa activity following single subcutaneous doses of 5000 and 10,000 IU of dalteparin were 0.41 ± 0.07 and 0.82 ± 0.10 IU/ml, respectively, and were attained in about 4 hours in most healthy volunteers. Peak anti-FXa activity increased more or less linearly with dose over the same dose range. The absolute bioavailability in healthy volunteers was 87% ± 6%, and dalteparin's volume of distribution was 40 to 60 ml/kg. Tinzaparin's plasma levels of anti-FXa activity increased within the first 2 to 3 hours after subcutaneous administration and reached a maximum within 4 to 5 hours. The absolute bioavailability of tinzaparin was 86.7%, and its volume of distribution ranged from 3.1 to 5 L.

Heparin does not cross the placenta and does not appear to increase the incidence of fetal malformation, mortality, or premature delivery. Heparin is the drug of choice for anticoagulation during pregnancy. If possible, the drug should be discontinued 24 hours before delivery to minimize the risk of postpartum bleeding. The safety and efficacy of LMWH use during pregnancy is currently under investigation but has not been firmly established.

Heparin clearance is dose dependent. Heparin is cleared primarily by the reticuloendothelial system. Heparin is metabolized by a rapid, zero-order mechanism, followed by slower first-order renal clearance; a small amount of undegraded heparin also appears in the urine. The half-life of heparin may be shortened in patients with massive thromboembolic disease and prolonged in patients with hepatic cirrhosis. LMWHs have longer biologic half-lives than does unfractionated heparin and are cleared renally. The elimination half-life of enoxaparin was 4.5 hours after a single subcutaneous dose to about 7 hours after repeated dosing. Significant anti-FXa activity persisted in plasma for about 12 hours following a daily 40-mg subcutaneous dose, with a clearance of approximately 15 ml/min. The terminal half-life of dalteparin following subcutaneous administration was observed to be 3 to 5 hours. The elimination half-life of tinzaparin following subcutaneous administration was approximately 3 to 4 hours.

To achieve full and rapid anticoagulant effect, heparin is usually administered intravenously. A widely used dosing regimen is to administer an 80-unit/kg bolus, followed by an 18-unit/kg per hour continuous infusion. Because there is wide interindividual variability in response to heparin, laboratory monitoring of the aPTT is required. The usual therapeutic range is equivalent to a plasma heparin level of 0.3 to 0.7 units/ml as determined with an anti-FXa assay, or of 0.2 to 0.4 units/ml as determined by protamine titration (this is approximately between 1.5 and 2.5 times the mean of the normal aPTT range). LMWH's therapeutic range is between 0.4 and 1.1 units/ml for twice-daily dosing and between 1 and 2 units/ml for daily dosing.[8]

The risk of recurrence of thromboembolism is greater in patients who do not achieve a therapeutic level of anticoagulation within the first 24 hours. Initially, the aPTT should be measured and the infusion rate adjusted every 6 hours. Once a stable dose is established, daily monitoring is sufficient.

In patients with a baseline prolongation of their aPTT, as in patients with a lupus anticoagulant, the anti-FXa activity can be followed. During cardiopulmonary bypass, the activated clotting time is used to monitor heparin dosing as very high doses of heparin are used and the aPTT is indefinitely prolonged. No monitoring is required when standard heparin is used for thromboprophylaxis (usual dose is 5000 units every 8 to 12 hours administered subcutaneously), although a mild prolongation of the aPTT may be noted.

Patients who respond suboptimally to heparin anticoagulation may be labeled as heparin resistant. This is usually not due to low antithrombin concentrations, but rather to an increase in procoagulant proteins during the acute-phase response. In these cases, an anti-FXa assay can be performed and a plasma heparin concentration derived, allowing for a more reliable estimation of anticoagulation. Extremely low antithrombin concentrations can cause heparin resistance.

FDA-approved LMWH preparations, including enoxaparin, dalteparin, and tinzaparin, differ in composition. Two preparations that have similar anti-FXa activity may not produce equivalent antithrombotic effects. LMWHs are administered in a fixed or weight-adjusted dosage regimen once or twice daily by subcutaneous injection, as their pharmacokinetic properties are more predictable. In vitro monitoring is not done routinely since LMWHs have a minimal effect on in vitro clotting assays. Patients with end-stage renal failure may require monitoring with an anti-FXa assay because this condition may prolong the half-life of LMWH. Specific dosage recommendations for the LMWHs may be obtained from their package inserts.

Fondaparinux is a synthetic pentasaccharide that mediates inhibition of FXa by antithrombin. Due to its short polymer length, it does not cause thrombin inhibition. Its structure was derived from the structure of the antithrombin binding region of heparin. When fondaparinux binds to antithrombin, it induces a permanent conformational change in the antithrombin molecule that increases its affinity for FXa 300-fold. Fondaparinux is administered by subcutaneous injection, and peak plasma concentrations are achieved in 2 to 3 hours. It is excreted in the urine with a half-life of 17 to 21 hours and is contraindicated in patients with renal failure. Fondaparinux can be given once a day at a fixed dose without coagulation monitoring; it has minimal interaction with plasma proteins other than antithrombin. Fondaparinux is approved for the therapy of pulmonary embolism and DVT and for the thromboprophylaxis of patients undergoing hip or knee surgery.

Bleeding is the primary complication of heparin therapy. Major bleeding occurs in 1% to 5% of patients receiving heparin for the treatment of venous thromboembolism. The risk of bleeding increases with the total daily dose of heparin and is higher with supratherapeutic aPTT, although patients can bleed within a therapeutic aPTT range. Often an underlying cause of bleeding can be identified, such as recent surgery, trauma, or peptic ulcer disease.

Unfractionated heparin has a short half-life (60 to 90 minutes), and after discontinuation of the intravenous infusion, the anticoagulant effect disappears. If life-threatening bleeding is encountered while a patient is on heparin, rapid discontinuation of the infusion followed by protamine sulfate infusion can neutralize the heparin effect. The dose of protamine to be infused depends on the dose of heparin used for anticoagulation: 1 mg of protamine can neutralize 100 units of heparin. In overdosage of LMWHs, protamine may also be used, although one must refer to the manufacturer's literature for specific dosages. There is no antidote for fondaparinux.

Beyond bleeding, another major complication of heparin therapy is heparin-induced thrombocytopenia (HIT). Heparin can cause two types of HIT, type I and type II. Type I HIT occurs in about a quarter of patients treated with heparin and is usually mild and reversible within 4 to 7 days despite continued heparin treatment. It is caused by a direct interaction between platelets and heparin leading to a low level of platelet aggregation. Type II HIT is a more serious clinical diagnosis made when a patient develops a platelet count below 150,000/μl, or a 50% drop from baseline, or develops new thromboses during heparin therapy. The pathophysiology of this disorder is the development of an immunoglobulin G antibody against the heparin–platelet factor 4 (PF4) complex. The antibody-antigen complex binds to the platelet FcγRIIa receptor and leads to platelet activation and aggregation and thrombin formation.[9]

The incidence of HIT antibody development in the medical patient is approximately 8%. About 1% to 3% of patients receiving heparin will go on to develop thrombocytopenia, thrombosis, or both. The incidence of antibody development in the surgical patient is much higher: 20% in patients undergoing orthopedic surgery and 40% to 70% in patients undergoing cardiopulmonary bypass. The incidence of developing HIT with an LMWH is much lower.

Both venous and arterial thromboses occur. Though venous thromboembolism occurs more commonly, the arterial thromboses are often devastating (myocardial infarction, ischemic stroke, limb loss). Confirmation of the clinical diagnosis can be supported by use of an enzyme-linked immunosorbent assay for the anti-heparin/PF4 antibody, and confirmation can be made with a serotonin release assay (heparin-dependent platelet activation assay).

It was thought that the smaller pentasaccharide, fondaparinux, was unlikely to induce anti-PF4/heparin antibodies, and it has even been used to succesfully anticoagulate patients with HIT. However, in two large trials investigating the use of fondaparinux in the postoperative orthopedic patient, HIT antibodies were induced as frequently as in an LMWH group. Despite antibody formation, no patient has been reported to date to have developed HIT while receiving fondaparinux.[10]

The treatment of HIT involves immediate discontinuation of the heparin product and anticoagulation with a direct thrombin inhibitor such as lepirudin or agratroban. Single-agent warfarin is contraindicated in the treatment of HIT as it may exacerbate the prothrombotic state.

Other side effects of heparin include hyperkalemia caused by suppressing aldosterone secretion, and hypersensitivity reactions, including fever, chills, urticaria and anaphylaxis. Bone loss (osteoporosis) and elevated liver enzymes may occur with prolonged (>3 months') treatment.

Direct Thrombin Inhibitors. Lepirudin is a yeast-derived recombinant derivative of hirudin, a direct thrombin inhibitor present in the salivary glands of the medicinal leech (*Hirudo medicinalis*). Lepirudin is identical to natural hirudin except for substitution of leucine for isoleucine at the NH_2-terminal end of the molecule and the absence of a sulfate group on the tyrosine at position 63. Lepirudin was the first anticoagulant approved in the United States for the treatment of patients with HIT. It is a 65–amino acid polypeptide that forms a tight stoichiometric complex with both the catalytic site and the extended substrate recognition site of a single molecule of thrombin. Its action is independent of antithrombin, and therefore it can reach and inactivate fibrin bound thrombin in thrombi. It is administered intravenously, and the dose is adjusted to maintain the aPTT at 1.5 to 2.5 times the median of the laboratory's normal range for aPTT. Lepirudin is cleared by the kidneys and has a half-life of approximately 1.3 hours in healthy volunteers. Lepirudin should be used cautiously in patients with renal failure, since it can accumulate and cause bleeding in these patients. Up to 74% of patients may develop antihirudin antibodies when treated with lepirudin for more than 5 days. These antibodies may cause a decrease in anticoagulant activity by neutralization or an increase in anticoagulant activity by reducing renal clearance; therefore, daily monitoring of the aPTT is recommended. There is no antidote for lepirudin.

Bivalirudin is a synthetic, 20–amino acid peptide containing the sequence Phe_1-Pro_2-Arg_3-Pro_4 that is a specific and reversible direct thrombin inhibitor. It is a parenteral bivalent analogue of hirudin. Bivalirudin reversibly inhibits the catalytic site of thrombin, neutralizing the actions of thrombin, including thrombin entrapped within established clots. Thrombin slowly cleaves the Arg_3-Pro_4 peptide bond and regains activity. Bivalirudin is administered intravenously and is used as an anticoagulant in patients undergoing percutaneous coronary intervention. Bivalirudin is eliminated from plasma by a combination of renal excretion and proteolytic cleavage. The half-life of bivalirudin in patients with normal renal function is 25 minutes; dosage reductions are recommended for patients with moderate or severe renal impairment. Side effects include back pain, nausea, headaches, and hypotension.[11]

Argatroban is a synthetic intravenous direct thrombin inhibitor. It is an N2-substituted derivative of arginine. Argatroban is the second agent to be indicated for HIT. It binds reversibly to the catalytic site of thrombin, neutralizing the actions of thrombin, including thrombin entrapped within established clots. It is administered intravenously and has an immediate onset of action. Its elimination half-life is 40 to 50 minutes. Argatroban is metabolized by hepatic CYP450 and is excreted in the bile; therefore dosage reduction is required for patients with hepatic insufficiency. The dosage is adjusted to maintain an aPTT of 1.5 to 3 times the baseline value. Argatroban also prolongs the PT, thereby affecting the INR of patients on warfarin. A nomogram is useful in titrating the therapeutic dose of warfarin when the patient is also receiving argatroban.

Antiplatelet Agents. Platelets respond to endothelial injury by adhering via GP VI to exposed vascular collagen and via the GP Ib/IX/V complex to circulating vWF. Platelet adherence is followed by platelet activation/degranulation, and the synthesis and release of adenosine diphosphate (ADP), serotonin, and thromboxane A_2 (TXA_2). These mediators increase the expression of GP IIb/IIIa receptors on the surface of the platelet, causing platelet aggregation via the binding of fibrinogen. Aspirin, ticlopidine, clopidogrel, and dipyridamole act by inhibiting specific processes involved in platelet activation, whereas abciximab, tirofiban, and eptifibatide bind directly to the GP IIb/IIIa receptors.

Aspirin. Aspirin is an NSAID drug with multiple effects: analgesic, anti-inflammatory, antipyretic, and antiplatelet aggregation. It is used in a variety of clinical situations, including in the treatment and prevention of thromboembolic disease.

Eicosanoids are products of the oxygenation of polyunsaturated long-chain fatty acids. They are highly potent and ubiquitous and have a wide biologic activity. TXA_2 is synthesized by platelets and is a powerful vasoconstrictor and platelet aggregator derived from arachidonic acid (the most abundant eicosanoid) through the cyclooxygenase (COX) pathway. Prostaglandins are synthesized by vascular endothelial cells, and although also derived from arachidonic acid through the COX pathway, conversely inhibit platelet aggregation. Two unique COX isoenzymes (COX-1 and COX-2) convert arachidonic acid to thromboxanes and prostaglandins, and they are both inhibited to different extents by aspirin (200-fold greater inhibition of COX-1 than COX-2). Aspirin irreversibly acetylates serine 530 in the active site of the COX enzymes, thus inhibiting thromboxane synthesis at low doses and thromboxane and prostaglandin synthesis at higher doses. Since platelets lack a nucleus, platelet aggregation as mediated by TXA_2 is inhibited for the life of the platelet. The effect of aspirin on platelets is demonstrated by a prolonged bleeding time in patients taking aspirin.

Aspirin and other salicylates are readily absorbed after oral administration, but absorption after rectal administration is less predictable. Aspirin and salicylates can be absorbed through the skin. Nonionized aspirin is absorbed in the stomach and the small intestine and rapidly hydrolyzed in the liver by nonspecific esterases to salicylate (the half-life of aspirin is 20 minutes). Aspirin is 80% to 90% bound to albumin, and its volume of distribution is approximately 170 ml/kg in adults. As plasma protein-binding sites for aspirin become saturated, the volume of distribution increases. Salicylate is 90% to 95% protein bound but is distributed to all parts of the body, including the synovial cavity, central nervous system, saliva, breast milk, and placenta. Both aspirin and salicylate are active compounds; however, only aspirin has an antiplatelet effect.

The hepatic metabolites of salicylate are salicyluric acid, salicylphenolic glucuronide, salicylic acyl glucuronide, gentisic acid, and gentisuric acid. The formation of the major metabolites, salicyluric acid and salicylphenolic glucuronide, is easily saturated and follows Michaelis-Menten (zero-order) kinetics; the other metabolic routes are first-order processes.

Renal excretion of salicylate involves glomerular filtration, active renal tubular secretion, and passive tubular reabsorption. The amount of salicylate excreted increases with increasing dose and is pH dependent, 30% of a dose being excreted in alkaline urine compared with 2% of a dose in acidic urine. Salicylate can be removed by hemodialysis.

After a 325-mg aspirin dose, elimination is a first-order process and the plasma-salicylate elimination half-life is approximately 2 to 3 hours; at high aspirin doses, the half-life increases to 15 to 30 hours.

Aspirin's antiplatelet activity has led to its use for the treatment or prevention of a variety of disorders. It is used as part of the initial treatment of unstable angina and is given in the early treatment of myocardial infarction; it is also of benefit in the initial treatment of acute ischemic stroke.

In a meta-analysis conducted by the Antithrombotic Trialists' Collaboration, daily doses of 75 to 325 mg appeared to be equally effective for their antiplatelet effect; doses greater than 500 mg did not appear to be superior and caused more gastrointestinal adverse effects.[12] The meta-analysis concluded that, for the long-term prevention of serious vascular events in high-risk patients, a daily dose of aspirin in the range of 75 to 150 mg should be effective. In the initial treatment of acute myocardial infarction, acute ischemic stroke, or unstable angina, however, a loading dose of 150 to 300 mg may be given. Aspirin should be chewed or dispersed in water; chewing a tablet of aspirin ensures that some buccal absorption occurs.

The major adverse effect of aspirin is bleeding, especially in the gastrointestinal tract, where it inhibits synthesis of prostaglandin E_1, which protects gastric mucosal cells from the acidic and/or *Helicobacter pylori*–colonized environment. A systematic review of randomized, controlled studies found that, although low-dose aspirin (up to 325 mg daily) increased the risk of major bleeding (including gastrointestinal bleeding) by twofold when compared to placebo, the actual risk of bleeding was modest; for every 833 patients taking low-dose aspirin for cardiovascular prophylaxis, only one additional major bleeding episode will occur annually.[13] Underlying gastrointestinal risk factors such as age greater than 60 years might increase the risk of bleeding. It is estimated that up to 60% of aspirin users are in this higher risk group.

There appears to be no convincing evidence that the risk of major gastrointestinal bleeding associated with a 75-mg dose is reduced by using enteric-coated or modified-release formulations rather than soluble aspirin, although individual studies have reported a reduction in acute mucosal injury with enteric coating. All known NSAIDs have the potential for causing acute damage to the gastric mucosa. Comparative studies of acute gastric mucosal damage caused by NSAIDs consistently associate aspirin with the most severe lesions. Gastric mucosal injury can occur even with cutaneous application.

Other rare side effects of aspirin on the blood include thrombocytopenia, aplastic anemia, agranulocytosis, hemolytic anemia in patients with glucose-6-phosphate dehydrogenase deficiency, and hypoprothrombinemia.

Hypersensitivity to aspirin can be manifested clinically by asthma. The prevalence of aspirin-induced asthma in adults varies from 10% to 21% in the asthmatic population and 2.5% in nonasthmatics. There is a considerable cross-reactivity between aspirin and other NSAIDs, and it is advised to avoid the NSAID class of drugs altogether if aspirin-induced asthma develops.

ADP Receptor Blockade: Clopidogrel and Ticlopidine. Clopidogrel is a thienopyridine antiplatelet drug used in thromboembolic disorders. It is an analogue of ticlopidine and acts by inhibiting ADP-mediated platelet aggregation. Like aspirin, clopidogrel and ticlopidine irreversibly inhibit platelet aggregation and thereby prolong the bleeding time. Clopidogrel is given prophylactically as an alternative to aspirin in patients with atherosclerosis who are at risk of thromboembolic disorders such as myocardial infarction, peripheral arterial disease, and stroke. Clopidogrel is also used with aspirin in acute coronary syndromes, including acute myocardial infarction and unstable angina.

Clopidogrel is approximately 50% absorbed, whereas ticlopidine is almost completely absorbed, after oral administration. Clopidogrel is a prodrug that is metabolized by hepatic CYP3A4 and CYP2B6, and to a lesser extent by CYP1A2, CYP1A1, and CYP2C19, to its inactive carboxylic acid derivative. The active compound is a thiol derivative but has not been characterized in plasma. Clopidogrel is extensively protein bound. Parent drug and metabolite are excreted in the urine and feces in approximately equal ratios. Ticlopidine is also metabolized in the liver and mostly excreted in feces, with only 25% excretion in the urine.

For the prophylaxis of thromboembolic events, the usual dose of clopidogrel is 75 mg once daily. In the management of acute ST-elevation myocardial infarction, clopidogrel is used with aspirin as an adjunct in medically treated patients. It is given in a dose of 75 mg once daily; patients under 75 years of age may be given a loading dose of 300 mg. Treatment should be continued for at least 4 weeks. In the management of unstable angina and non–Q-wave myocardial infarction, clopidogrel is used with aspirin as an adjunct to either medical or interventional treatment. A single loading dose of 300 mg is given, followed by 75 mg once daily.

The dose of ticlopidine is 250 mg twice daily as a prophylactic alternative to aspirin in patients at high risk for thrombotic/thromboembolic stroke, in the management of intermittent claudication, and in ischemic heart disease. Ticlopidine is also approved to prevent subacute thrombosis of an intracoronary stent and is administered at 250 mg twice daily for 4 weeks following the placement of an intracoronary stent. Shorter courses (2 weeks) may be as effective in reducing rethrombosis rates with fewer side effects.

The risks of developing neutropenia, thrombotic thrombocytopenic purpura (TTP), and/or aplastic anemia are highest in the first 3 months of therapy. Ticlopidine can cause a reversible severe neutropenia in 2% to 4% of treated patients; the incidence of TTP is 1 in 2000 to 4000 treated patients, and the incidence of aplastic anemia may be as high as 1 in 4000 to 8000 treated patients. A complete blood count every 2 weeks starting the second week of treatment through the third month of treatment is required to monitor for these potentially life-threatening side effects.

Clopidogrel has fewer reported adverse effects and is the preferred agent over ticlopidine. Routine blood work is not required during clopidogrel therapy but should be ordered as soon as possible in the case of a suspected blood dyscrasia. Other adverse effects, reported rarely, include serum sickness, interstitial pneumonitis, erythema multiforme, Stevens-Johnson syndrome, lichen planus, and myalgia. Clopidogrel should be stopped 7 to 10 days prior to surgical procedures.

Dipyridamole. Dipyridamole is an adenosine reuptake inhibitor and a phosphodiesterase inhibitor with antiplatelet and vasodilatory effects. It is used in combination with aspirin for the management of thromboembolic stroke, with warfarin for the thromboprophylaxis of patients with prosthetic cardiac valves, and alone in cardiac perfusion imaging.

Dipyridamole is incompletely absorbed after oral administration and is more than 90% plasma protein bound. Its peak plasma level is attained 75 minutes after ingestion, and its serum half-life is 10 to 12 hours. Dipyridamole is primarily metabolized in the liver and excreted in the bile. A small proportion may be excreted in the urine, and it is found in breast milk

Dipyridamole may enhance the actions of anticoagulants, and dose reductions may be needed during concomitant administration. Nausea, vomiting, diarrhea, headache, dizziness, flushing, hypotension, and angina may occur after use of dipyridamole. It should be used with caution in patients with unstable angina, hypotension, aortic stenosis, recent myocardial infarction, and heart failure or coagulation disorders.

Glycoprotein IIb/IIIa Receptor Antagonists. The GP IIb/IIIa receptor binds fibrinogen, vitronectin, fibronectin, and vWF, acting as the final common pathway in platelet aggregation. The GP IIb/IIIa complex is a member of the integrin family of proteins, a cell surface transmembrane glycoprotein that links the cell surface to the cytoskeleton of the cell. There are approximately 50,000 copies of the GP IIb/IIIa receptor on the surface of normal platelets. Patients deficient in this receptor have a rare bleeding disorder called Glanzmann thrombasthenia (autosomal recessive) manifested clinically with mucosal bleeding, petechiae, ecchymoses, and menorrhagia. Rarely, patients with non-Hodgkin's lymphoma can develop autoantibodies against the GP IIb/IIIa receptor, resulting in a bleeding diathesis.

Abciximab is the Fab fragment of a chimeric human-murine monoclonal antibody, 7E3. Its target is the GP IIb/IIIa receptor on the surface of platelets, preventing fibrinogen, vWF, and other adhesive molecules from binding and thus cross-linking platelets. It was the first platelet integrin GP IIb/IIIa inhibitor and the only monoclonal antibody against GP IIb/IIIa receptor approved by the FDA. After intravenous doses of abciximab, free plasma concentrations fall rapidly due to binding to platelet receptors. Platelet function recovers over about 48 hours, although abciximab may remain in the circulation for 15 days or more in a platelet-bound state.

Abciximab is used as an adjunct to heparin and aspirin therapy for the prevention of acute myocardial ischemic complications in patients undergoing percutaneous transluminal coronary procedures, including angioplasty, atherectomy, and stenting. It is also used in patients with unstable angina who are candidates for such procedures.[14]

Abciximab is given intravenously as a bolus injection over 1 minute in a dose of 250 mcg/kg followed immediately by an infusion of 0.125 mcg/kg per minute (to a maximum dose of 10 mcg/min). For stabilization in patients with unstable angina, the bolus dose followed by the infusion should be started up to 24 hours before the possible intervention and continued for 12 hours after; for other patients the bolus should be given 10 to 60 minutes before the intervention followed by the infusion for 12 hours.

The most common adverse effect of abciximab is bleeding. Abciximab should not be given to patients who are actively bleeding or at high risk of hemorrhage from comorbid conditions. These include patients with thrombocytopenia, uncontrolled hypertension, recent history of hemorrhagic stroke, intracerebral neoplasm, cerebral aneurysm or arteriovenous malformations; patients having suffered from recent trauma or who have undergone recent surgery; and patients with severe hepatic failure or renal failure requiring hemodialysis. Other adverse effects include thrombocytopenia, development of antibodies 2 to 4 weeks after treatment, hypersensitivity reaction after prior monoclonal antibody treatment or upon readministration, hypotension, and bradycardia.

Tirofiban, a nonpeptide (peptidomimetic) tyrosine derivative, and eptifibatide, a cyclic heptapeptide derivative of the snake venom protein barbourin, are competitive antagonists at the GP IIb/IIIa receptor.

Tirofiban and eptifibatide are both administered intravenously as infusions and have short half-lives. Tirofiban is not tightly bound to plasma proteins, and the unbound fraction is approximately 35%. Its plasma elimination half-life is 2 hours, and it is renally excreted largely unchanged with minimal excretion in bile and feces. Tirofiban can be removed by hemodialysis. Its antiplatelet effect lasts about 4 to 8 hours after discontinuation of the infusion. Eptifibatide is approximately 25% plasma protein bound. Eptifibatide's antiplatelet effect persists 4 hours after discontinuation of an infusion. Its plasma elimination half-life is about 2.5 hours, and it is 50% cleared renally.

Tirofiban is given initially intravenously at a rate of 400 ng/kg per minute for 30 minutes, and then continued at 100 ng/kg per minute. The recommended duration of treatment is at least 48 hours. Tirofiban infusion may be continued during coronary angiography, and should be maintained for 12 to 24 hours after angioplasty or atherectomy. The entire duration of treatment should not exceed 108 hours. The dose of tirofiban should be reduced by half the standard infusion rate in patients with renal impairment (creatinine clearance <30 ml/min).

Eptifibatide for the management of unstable angina is given in an initial dose of 180 mcg/kg by intravenous injection, followed by 2 mcg/kg per minute by intravenous infusion, for up to 72 hours. If percutaneous coronary intervention is performed during eptifibatide therapy, the infusion should be continued for 18 to 24 hours after the procedure, to a maximum total duration of 96 hours of therapy. In patients undergoing angioplasty, but not presenting with unstable angina, eptifibatide is given in an initial dose of 180 mcg/kg by intravenous injection immediately before the procedure, followed by 2 mcg/kg per minute by intravenous infusion, with a second 180-mcg/kg intravenous injection given 10 minutes after the first. The infusion should be continued until hospital discharge or for up to 18 to 24 hours; a minimum of 12 hours is recommended.[15]

In patients with moderate renal failure (creatinine clearance <50 ml/min), the same initial bolus infusion dose is given but the maintenance infusion dose should be reduced to 1 mcg/kg per minute. Eptifibatide is contraindicated in dialysis-dependent renal failure.

Bleeding is the most common adverse effect of tirofiban and eptifibatide. Other side effects of tirofiban include nausea, headache, fever, rashes and other hypersensitivity reactions, and thrombocytopenia. Thrombocytopenia following eptifibatide therapy is rare but has been reported.

Fibrinolytics

Tissue-Type Plasminogen Activator. Alteplase is a recombinant tissue-type plasminogen activator (t-PA) with relatively little effect on circulating, unbound plasminogen and thus may be designated a fibrin-specific thrombolytic. Its initial plasma half-life is 4 to 5 minutes and its terminal elimination half-life is approximately 40 minutes; it is metabolized by the liver. It is used in the treatment of arterial and venous thromboembolism, catheter and cannula thrombosis, intracardiac thrombosis, microvessel thrombosis, ocular fibrinolysis, and peripheral arterial thromboembolism.

In the treatment of acute myocardial infarction, alteplase is given intravenously as soon as possible after the onset of symptoms at a total dose of 100 mg; the total dose should not exceed 1.5 mg/kg in patients weighing less than 65 kg. The total dose may be given either over 1.5 hours (accelerated) or over 3 hours. The accelerated schedule has been recommended where administration is within 6 hours of myocardial infarction, while the 3-hour schedule has been recommended where administration is more than 6 hours after myocardial infarction.

In the treatment of acute, massive pulmonary embolism, a total dose of 100 mg is given; the total dose should not exceed 1.5 mg/kg in patients weighing less than 65 kg. The first 10 mg is given as an intravenous bolus and the remainder by intravenous infusion over 2 hours.

In acute ischemic stroke, alteplase is given within 3 hours of the onset of symptoms in a dose of 0.9 mg/kg up to a maximum total dose of 90 mg. The dose is administered intravenously over 60 minutes, with 10% being given as a bolus during the first minute.

To restore function in central venous lines, alteplase is instilled into the catheter at a concentration of 1 mg/ml. The usual dose is 2 mg, repeated after 2 hours if necessary. A total dose of 4 mg should not be exceeded. Alteplase has been used, in a dose of 100 mg given intravenously over 2 hours, for thrombosis of prosthetic heart valves.

Tenecteplase is a modified recombinant human t-PA with a substitution of threonine 103 with asparagine, and a substitution of asparagine 117 with glutamine, both within the kringle 1 domain, and a tetra-alanine substitution at amino acids 296 through 299 in the protease domain. In patients with acute myocardial infarction, tenecteplase administered as a single bolus exhibits a biphasic disposition from the plasma. Tenecteplase is cleared from the plasma with an initial distribution half-life of 20 to 24 minutes. The terminal elimination half-life of tenecteplase is 90 to 130 minutes. The initial volume of distribution is weight related and approximates plasma volume. Liver metabolism is the major clearance mechanism for tenecteplase.

Tenecteplase is indicated for use in the reduction of mortality associated with acute myocardial infarction. The dosage of tenecteplase is based on patient weight and should not exceed a single dose of 50 mg.

Reteplase is another recombinant human t-PA that is less expensive to produce than alteplase. It lacks the major fibrin-binding domain due to the deletion of several amino acid sequences, and thus is less fibrin specific than alteplase. Reteplase is reported to have an initial plasma half-life of about 14 minutes and a terminal elimination half-life of 1.6 hours in patients with myocardial infarction; it is cleared primarily by the liver and kidneys. Reteplase is given intravenously as soon as possible after the onset of symptoms. The dose is 10 units given by slow intravenous injection (but not over more than 2 minutes), and this dose of 10 units is repeated once, 30 minutes after the initiation of the first injection.

Urokinase. Urokinase is a human enzyme derived from human neonatal kidney cells grown in culture. There are two forms of urokinase that differ in molecular weight. The low-molecular-weight form is used clinically and converts plasminogen to plasmin. Urokinase is cleared rapidly from the plasma by the liver, with a half-life of biologic activity of 12 minutes and a volume of distribution of 11.5 L. Urokinase is currently approved for the lysis of acute massive pulmonary emboli with or without unstable hemodynamics. In addition to the risk of life-threatening bleeding, rare cases of fatal anaphylaxis have been reported. Other allergic reactions, including bronchospasm, urticaria, and orolingual edema, have also been reported and respond to discontinuation of the infusion and/or the administration of intravenous corticosteroids, antihistamines, or α-adrenergic agonists.

REFERENCES

1. Mann KG. Thrombin formation. Chest 2003;124(3 Suppl):4S-10S.
2. Michiels JJ, Gadisseur A, van der Planken M, et al. Guidelines for the evaluation of intravenous desmopressin and von Willebrand factor/factor VIII concentrate in the treatment and prophylaxis of bleedings in von Willebrand disease types 1, 2, and 3. Semin Thromb Hemost 2006;32:636-645.
3. Mannucci PM, Levi M. Prevention and treatment of major blood loss. N Engl J Med 2007;356:2301-2311.
4. Ansell J, Hirsh J, Poller L, et al. The pharmacology and management of the vitamin K antagonists: the Seventh ACCP Conference on Antithrombotic and Thrombolytic Therapy. Chest 2004;126(3 Suppl):204S-233S.
5. Harrison L, Johnston M, Massicotte MP, et al. Comparison of 5-mg and 10-mg loading doses in initiation of warfarin therapy. Ann Intern Med 1997;126:133-136.
6. Loeliger EA, van den Besselaar AM, Lewis SM. Reliability and clinical impact of the normalization of the prothrombin times in oral anticoagulant control. Thromb Haemost 1985;53:148-154.
7. Gardiner C, Williams K, Mackie IJ, et al. Patient self-testing is a reliable and acceptable alternative to laboratory INR monitoring. Br J Haematol 2005;128:242-247.
8. Hirsh J, Dalen J, Anderson DR, et al. Oral anticoagulants: mechanism of action, clinical effectiveness, and optimal therapeutic range. Chest 2001;119(1 Suppl):8S-21S.
9. Arepally GM, Ortel TL. Clinical Practice. Heparin-induced thrombocytopenia. N Engl J Med 2006;355:809-817.
10. Warkentin TE, Cook RJ, Marder VJ, et al. Anti-platelet factor 4/heparin antibodies in orthopedic surgery patients receiving antithrombotic prophylaxis with fondaparinux or enoxaparin. Blood 2005;106:3791-3796.
11. Hirsh J, O'Donnell M, Weitz JI. New anticoagulants. Blood 2005;105:453-463.
12. Antithrombotic Trialists' Collaboration. Collaborative meta-analysis of randomised trials of antiplatelet therapy for prevention of death, myocardial infarction, and stroke in high risk patients. BMJ 2002;324:71-86.
13. Garcia Rodriguez LA, Hernandez-Diaz S, de Abajo FJ. Association between aspirin and upper gastrointestinal complications: systematic review of epidemiologic studies. Br J Clin Pharmacol 2001;52:563-571.
14. Montalescot G, Barragan P, Wittenberg O, et al. Platelet glycoprotein IIb/IIIa inhibition with coronary stenting for acute myocardial infarction. N Engl J Med 2001;344:1895-1903.
15. Novel dosing regimen of eptifibatide in planned coronary stent implantation (ESPRIT): a randomised, placebo-controlled trial. Lancet 2000;356:2037-2044.

64

LUNG CANCER

Sarah A. Holstein and Raymond J. Hohl

NON–SMALL CELL LUNG CANCER 921
Introduction 921
Therapeutics and Clinical Pharmacology 921
Chemotherapy Agents 921
Biologic Agents 923
Chemoradiation 923
SMALL CELL LUNG CANCER 925
Introduction 925
Therapeutics and Clinical Pharmacology 925
Single-Agent Therapies 925
Combination Therapies 926
New Agents 926

NON–SMALL CELL LUNG CANCER

Introduction

Lung cancer is the leading cause of cancer death. The majority of lung cancers fall into the broad category of non–small cell lung cancer (NSCLC), which includes adenocarcinoma, squamous cell carcinoma, and large cell carcinoma. Management of NSCLC may involve multiple modalities, including surgery, chemotherapy, and radiation therapy, depending on the extent of the disease. The biologic behavior of this disease is characterized by advancement of local disease through frank tumor growth and involvement of draining lymphatic nodes as well as by hematogenous dissemination to other visceral sites, bone, and brain. As a consequence, the staging for NSCLC is rather complex (Box 64-1). Briefly, stage I disease represents limited local disease without nodal involvement. Stage II disease is limited local disease with ipsilateral hilar and/or peribronchial lymph node invasion or limited local invasion without nodal involvement. Stage IIIA disease includes limited invasion of local structures and/or ipsilateral mediastinal nodal involvement. Stage IIIB disease is unresectable invasion of local structures and/or contralateral mediastinal nodal involvement. Finally, stage IV disease includes distant metastasis. Five-year survival ranges from 61% for stage IA disease down to a dismal 1% for stage IV disease.[1] For inoperable stage IIIB or metastatic stage IV disease, treatment includes palliative chemotherapy. An overview of the agents used in this setting is shown in Box 64-2, and a discussion is provided in the following section.

Therapeutics and Clinical Pharmacology

Chemotherapy Agents

A number of drugs have activity as single agents in NSCLC, including the platinum-containing agents (cisplatin and carboplatin), the taxanes (paclitaxel and docetaxel), gemcitabine, pemetrexed, vinorelbine, and the camptothecins (topotecan and irinotecan). However, with the exception of patients with poor performance status or the elderly, most first-line therapy consists of combination regimens. A meta-analysis that evaluated 65 trials comparing doublet therapy with single-agent therapy found that two-drug regimens yielded an increase in both response rate and 1-year survival.[2] Not unexpectedly, combination therapy is associated with higher toxicity.

Platinum-Containing Agents. The platinum-containing agents (cisplatin and carboplatin) are alkylating agents (Fig. 64-1). Cisplatin is associated with significant toxicities, including myelosuppression, nephrotoxicity, electrolyte abnormalities, and neuropathy, and is a highly emetogenic agent. While carboplatin is usually better tolerated, it may also cause neuropathy and thrombocytopenia. Single-agent cisplatin has been reported to have response rates in the 20% to 40% range,[3-5] while single-agent carboplatin has yielded response rates of 9% to 20%.[6]

Platinum-containing doublets are frequently chosen in the front-line setting. The combinations of carboplatin and paclitaxel or cisplatin and paclitaxel are widely used and have been shown to improve survival.[7-10] Other doublets include cisplatin and docetaxel,[11] carboplatin and docetaxel,[11] cisplatin and etoposide,[9,12] carboplatin and etoposide,[12] cisplatin and vinorelbine,[13,14] cisplatin and vindesine,[13] carboplatin and vinorelbine, cisplatin and gemcitabine,[15] carboplatin and gemcitabine,[15,16] cisplatin and irinotecan,[17,18] and carboplatin and pemetrexed.[19] Non–platinum containing regimens include gemcitabine and docetaxel,[20,21] paclitaxel and vinorelbine,[22] gemcitabine and paclitaxel,[23] and gemcitabine and vinorelbine.[24]

There appears to be some evidence to suggest that cisplatin is more active than carboplatin; however, the additional toxicity often outweighs the potential clinical benefit. In a meta-analysis that examined nine trials, use of carboplatin (as opposed to cisplatin) was associated with statistically significant lower response rates but no difference in survival.[25] Another meta-analysis suggested that cisplatin-containing regimens provide slightly higher 1-year survival than non–platinum-containing regimens.[26] Multiple trials have evaluated the use of three-drug combinations. While response rates are improved with the addition of a third drug, the hematologic toxicity is increased, and a meta-analysis of these trials has shown that overall survival does not improve.[2] Despite many clinical trials, no single regimen has been shown to be significantly more active than the rest for advanced NSCLC.

Taxanes. The taxanes, paclitaxel and docetaxel, are antimicrotubule agents (Fig. 64-2). These drugs prevent depolymerization of microtubules, thus interfering with progression through mitosis. Paclitaxel may induce an immune hypersensitivity reaction and requires premedications with acetaminophen, corticosteroids, and antihistamines. Other common toxicities include myelosuppression, peripheral neuropathy, and arthralgias/myalgias. Paclitaxel has been approved for first-line use in combination with cisplatin in patients who are not surgical candidates. Docetaxel is associated with edema, skin and nail changes, cytopenias, and neuropathy. Docetaxel is approved by the U.S. Food and Drug Administration (FDA) as single-agent therapy for those patients who have failed first-line therapy containing platinums. In Phase III trials in which patients were randomized to docetaxel (as second-line therapy) versus best supportive care, docetaxel led to improved survival.[27]

BOX 64-1 NON–SMALL LUNG CANCER STAGING

Stage I

Stage IA

- The tumor is in the lung only and is 3 cm or smaller.

Stage IB

- One or more of the following is true:
  - The tumor is larger than 3 cm.
  - Cancer has spread to the main bronchus of the lung, and is at least 2 cm from the carina (where the trachea joins the bronchi).
  - Cancer has spread to the innermost layer of the membrane that covers the lungs.
  - The tumor partly blocks the bronchus or bronchioles and part of the lung has collapsed or developed pneumonitis (inflammation of the lung).

Stage II

Stage IIA

- The tumor is 3 cm or smaller and cancer has spread to nearby lymph nodes on the same side of the chest as the tumor.

Stage IIB

- Cancer has spread to nearby lymph nodes on the same side of the chest as the tumor and one or more of the following is true:
  - The tumor is larger than 3 cm.
  - Cancer has spread to the main bronchus of the lung and is 2 cm or more from the carina (where the trachea joins the bronchi).
  - Cancer has spread to the innermost layer of the membrane that covers the lungs.
  - The tumor partly blocks the bronchus or bronchioles and part of the lung has collapsed or developed pneumonitis (inflammation of the lung).

  or
- Cancer has not spread to lymph nodes and one or more of the following is true:
  - The tumor may be any size and cancer has spread to the chest wall, the diaphragm, the pleura between the lungs, or membranes surrounding the heart.
  - Cancer has spread to the main bronchus of the lung and is no more than 2 cm from the carina (where the trachea meets the bronchi), but has not spread to the trachea.
  - Cancer blocks the bronchus or bronchioles and the whole lung has collapsed or developed pneumonitis (inflammation of the lung).

Stage III

Stage IIIA

- Cancer has spread to the lymph nodes on the same side of the chest as the tumor. Also:
  - The tumor may be any size.
  - Cancer may have spread to the main bronchus, the chest wall, the diaphragm, the pleura around the lungs, or the membrane around the heart, but has not spread to the trachea.
  - Part or all of the lung may have collapsed or developed pneumonitis (inflammation of the lung).

Stage IIIB

- The tumor may be any size and has spread:
  - To lymph nodes above the collarbone or in the opposite side of the chest from the tumor; and/or
  - To any of the following: heart, major blood vessels that lead to or from the heart, chest wall, diaphragm, trachea, esophagus, sternum (chest bone) or backbone, more than one place in the same lobe of the lung, or the fluid of the pleural cavity surrounding the lung.

Stage IV

- Cancer may have spread to lymph nodes and has spread to another lobe of the lungs or to other parts of the body, such as the brain, liver, adrenal glands, kidneys, or bone.

BOX 64-2 COMMON AGENTS USEFUL FOR LUNG CANCER

Traditional

- Platinums (cisplatin and carboplatin)
- Taxanes (paclitaxel and docetaxel)
- Gemcitabine
- Pemetrexed
- Vinorelbine
- Camptothecins (topotecan and irinotecan)
- Alkylating agents (cyclophosphamide, ifosfamide, and others)*
- Topoisomerase II inhibitors (etoposide and teniposide)
- Antimetabolites (gemcitabine)
- Anthracyclines (doxorubicin [Adriamycin] and others)*

Targeted

- Epidermal growth factor inhibitors (gefitinib, erlotinib, and cetuximab)
- Antiangiogensis inhibitors (bevacizumab)

*Primarily used for small cell lung cancers.

Vinca Alkaloids. Vinorelbine is a semisynthetic vinca alkaloid that interferes with formation of microtubules (Fig. 64-3). Toxicities include neutropenia, neurotoxicity, respiratory toxicity, and gastrointestinal toxicity. Vinorelbine is FDA approved for the first-line therapy of unresectable disease. As a single agent, vinorelbine has been associated with response rates of 14% to 33%.[28,29] Vinorelbine is frequently used in combination with cisplatin.

Antifolate Agents. Pemetrexed is an antifolate agent that inhibits enzymes required for de novo synthesis of thymidine and purine nucleotides (thymidylate synthase, dihydrofolate reductase, and glycinamide ribonucleotide formyltransferase). In the first-line setting, pemetrexed has been associated with response rates of 14% to 23%.[30,31] Toxicities include neutropenia, skin rash, and anorexia. Hematologic toxicity may be mitigated by supplementation with folate and vitamin B_{12}. Pemetrexed has been FDA approved for the treatment of NSCLC as second-line therapy. The use of pemetrexed in combination with other agents is being investigated.

Adjuvant Chemotherapy. Patients with early-stage disease, even after complete resection, have high risk of relapse. Thus there has been interest in the use of adjuvant chemotherapy. Earlier trials performed in the 1970s and 1980s did not provide conclusive evidence for the role of adjuvant chemotherapy. However, a meta-analysis from 1995 suggested that there was a 13% reduction in risk of death in those trials comparing surgery and chemotherapy with surgery alone.[32] More recent trials have focused on cisplatin-containing regimens. The majority of trials have used cisplatin and vinorelbine. In the ANITA trial, patients with stage IB, II, or IIIA NSCLC were randomized to adjuvant chemotherapy (cisplatin and vinorelbine) or observation. The chemotherapy arm was associated with increased overall survival, with an absolute overall survival benefit of 8.6% at 5 years.[33] In Japan, clinical trials have been performed to investigate the role of oral ftorafur, a 5-fluorouracil derivative, with uracil. A Phase III trial randomized patients with resected stage IA and IB disease to ftorafur and uracil versus observation.[34] Five year survival was slightly improved in the chemotherapy arm, although subgroup analysis showed improved survival only for patients with IB disease.

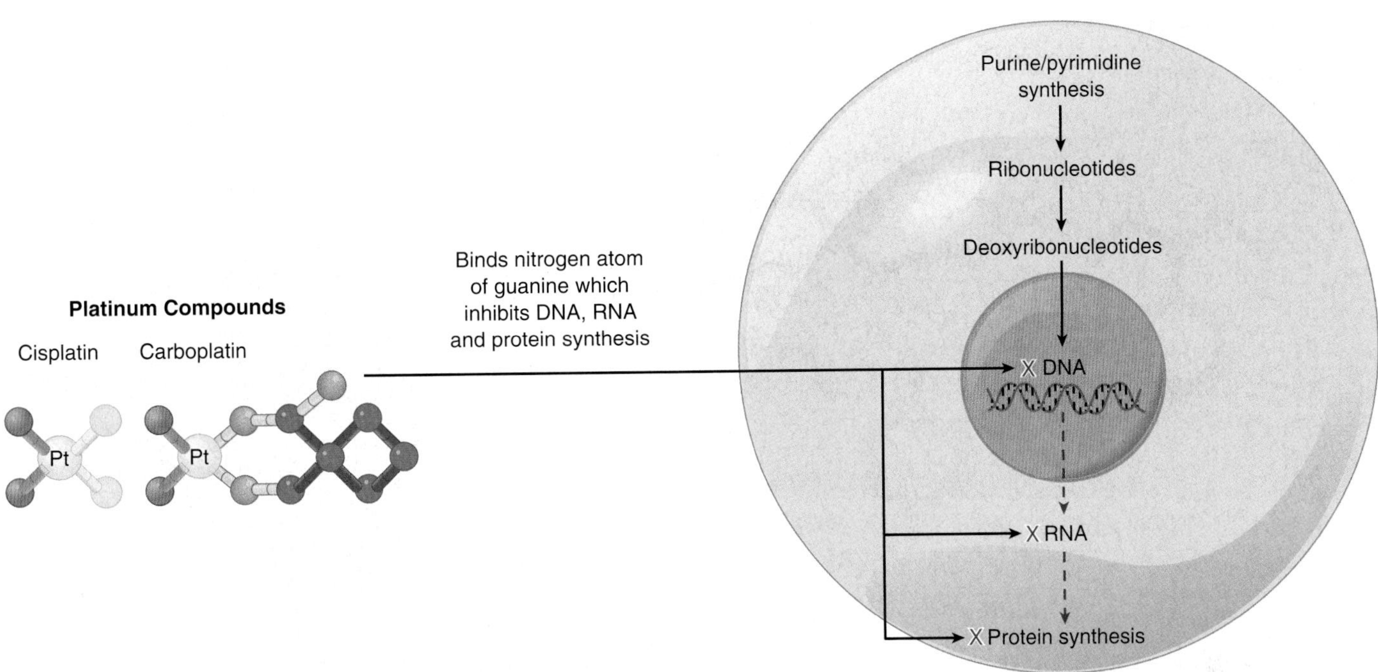

FIGURE 64-1 • Platinum-containing compounds: cisplatin and carboplatin. Platinum-containing compounds act as alkylating agents and form covalent bonds with the nitrogen atom of guanine to disrupt DNA, RNA, and protein synthesis.

Biologic Agents

Epidermal Growth Factor Receptor Inhibitors. The cell surface epidermal growth factor receptor (EGFR) activates multiple intracellular signaling cascades that regulate cell proliferation, motility, angiogenesis, and apoptosis. Overexpression of the EGFR protein or mutated EGFR has been reported in association with NSCLC. Two oral EGFR tyrosine kinase inhibitors—gefitinib and erlotinib—were initially approved for second-line therapy in NSCLC following Phase II trials. However, a follow-up Phase III trial that compared gefitinib to placebo in the second- or third-line setting did not show an improvement in survival.[35] The use of gefitinib has now been restricted to those patients already on therapy who are responding to treatment.

A randomized Phase III clinical trial compared erlotinib to placebo in patients with previously treated stage IIIB or IV disease.[36] A response rate of 8.9% was observed and there was a statistically significant improvement in survival. In the front-line setting, a Phase II trial with erlotinib has shown a response rate of 23%.[37] While Phase II studies suggested that EGFR overexpression or the presence of EGFR-activating mutations was associated with increased responsiveness,[38-41] analysis of samples from the Phase III trial led to the conclusion that survival after treatment with erlotinib was not influenced by those molecular abnormalities.[42] Toxicities associated with the EGFR inhibitors include an acneiform rash and diarrhea. Interestingly, the presence of the rash has been shown to correlate with response to treatment.[43,44]

Several trials have evaluated the combination of EGFR inhibitors with standard chemotherapy agents. In a Phase III trial, patients with advanced NSCLC were randomized to receive gemcitabine and cisplatin with or without erlotinib as first-line therapy.[45] No differences in overall survival, time to progression, response rate, or quality of life were observed. In another Phase III trial, patients with previously untreated advanced disease were randomized to receive carboplatin and paclitaxel with erlotinib or placebo followed by maintenance therapy with erlotinib.[46] There was no difference in overall survival or time to progression.

The precise role of the small-molecule EGFR inhibitors has yet to be determined. As indicated, there appears to be little value in combining erlotinib with traditional chemotherapy agents. The use of erlotinib as second-line therapy following failure of traditional cytotoxic agents may be a reasonable approach.

Monoclonal antibodies directed against EGFRs are currently being evaluated in NSCLC. In a Phase II trial involving previously treated patients, administration of cetuximab resulted in a 4.5% response rate and 30% stable disease.[47] The response rate for EGFR-positive tumors was 5%. Randomized Phase II trials have evaluated gemcitabine and cisplatin with or without cetuximab as front-line therapy,[48] and cisplatin and vinorelbine with or without cetuximab in patients with EGFR-expressing tumors.[49] As with the small-molecule tyrosine kinase inhibitors, cetuximab causes an acneiform rash.

Antiangiogenesis Inhibitors. Bevacizumab is a recombinant humanized monoclonal antibody that binds vascular endothelial growth factor (VEGF) and prevents interaction with the VEGF receptor. Bevacizumab has been approved in combination with paclitaxel and carboplatin for the treatment of advanced or metastatic recurrent nonsquamous NSCLC. A Phase III trial randomized patients to paclitaxel and carboplatin with or without bevacizumab.[50] Improved response rate, median overall survival, and progression-free survival were observed in the bevacizumab arm. Patients with brain lesions or hemoptysis were excluded from the trial. The addition of bevacizumab to other chemotherapy regimens is currently being investigated. Toxicities associated with bevacizumab include bleeding, proteinuria, thrombotic events, hypertension, impaired wound healing, diarrhea, asthenia, and headache. A clinical trial evaluating the role of bevacizumab in the adjuvant setting is underway.

There is interest in the potential role of the multitargeted kinase inhibitors sorafenib and sunitinib in NSCLC. In addition, there are ongoing clinical trials involving vandetanib, a dual inhibitor of the VEGF and EGFR receptors. As stated earlier, the biologic behavior for some NSCLCs is to disseminate in a hematogenous manner. It would seem that, if this feature could be predicted from a phenotype, the antiangiogenesis agents might have greater therapeutic and preventive activities than for disease whose spread appears to be through primarily lymphatic processes.

Chemoradiation

Combined-modality chemoradiation is used as definitive treatment for inoperable stage III disease and as preoperative induction therapy prior to surgery. Clinical trials have shown that sequential chemotherapy followed by radiation therapy led to improved survival com-

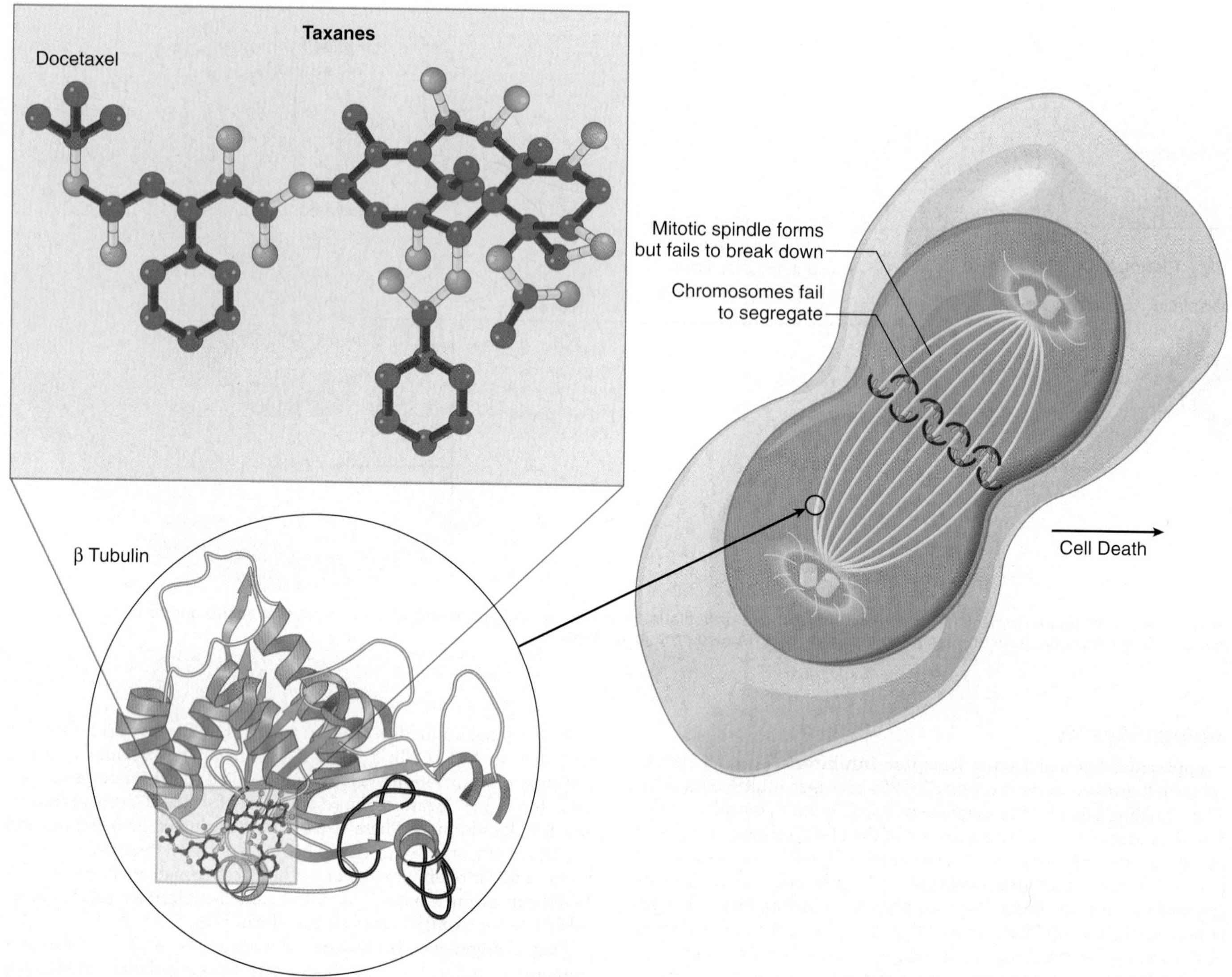

FIGURE 64-2 • Taxanes: docetaxel and paclitaxel. Paclitaxel is extracted from a rare Pacific yew tree while docetaxel is a semisynthetic analogue extracted from the European yew tree. The taxanes bind to tubulin but do not promote microtubule disassembly. Rather, they promote the assembly of microtubules from tubulin dimers and stabilize them by preventing depolymerization. The microtubules formed in the presence of taxanes are dysfunctional because they are too stable; cell death ultimately occurs.

pared to radiation alone. In a Phase III trial, patients with surgically unresectable (stages II, IIIA, and IIIB) NSCLC were randomized to chemotherapy (cisplatin and vinblastine) followed by radiation versus radiation alone.[51] Overall survival was improved in the chemotherapy plus radiation arm. In a similar trial, patients with stage III disease were randomized to chemotherapy (cisplatin and vinblastine) followed by radiation versus radiation alone. Response rates were significantly improved in the chemoradiation arm (56% vs. 43%), and median survival was improved as well (13.7 vs. 9.6 months).[52]

Concurrent chemoradiation therapy has been compared with sequential therapy. A Phase III trial randomized patients with unresectable stage III disease to concurrent therapy (cisplatin, vindesine, and mitomycin) with radiation therapy versus chemotherapy (the same agents) followed by radiation therapy.[53] The response rate in the concurrent arm was higher (84% vs. 66%), as was median survival (16.5 months vs. 13.3 months). There was increased myelosuppression in the concurrent arm. In another trial, patients with unresectable stage III NSCLC received either concurrent chemoradiation therapy consisting of cisplatin and etoposide followed by cisplatin and vinorelbine or sequential therapy comprising induction chemotherapy (cisplatin and vinorelbine) followed by radiation.[54] Survival rates appeared to be improved in the concurrent arm; however, this was not statistically significant.

Concurrent chemoradiation therapy can be associated with severe pulmonary toxicity, esophagitis, and hematologic toxicity. Amifostine is an agent that is converted to a free thiol metabolite that can serve as a free radical scavenger. This drug has been investigated as a means to prevent radiation-induced toxicity. In a randomized study including inoperable stage II/III NSCLC, patients were randomized to receive concurrent chemoradiation (with etoposide and cisplatin) with or without amifostine.[55] In this study, amifostine was associated with a reduction in severe esophagitis and pneumonitis. Hypotension was more frequent on the amifostine arm. Amifostine was shown to reduce esophagitis, acute pulmonary toxicity, and pneumonitis in a randomized trial utilizing concurrent chemoradiation (paclitaxel and carboplatin).[56] However, other trials have not shown clear benefit for amifostine.[57-59] While amifostine has been approved for use in patients receiving radiation therapy for head and neck cancer, it has not been approved for use in NSCLC.

Other chemotherapy agents that induce radiosensitization include the ribonucleotide reductase inhibitor hydroxyurea for head and neck cancers, the taxanes for head and neck cancers, 5-fluorouracil for rectal

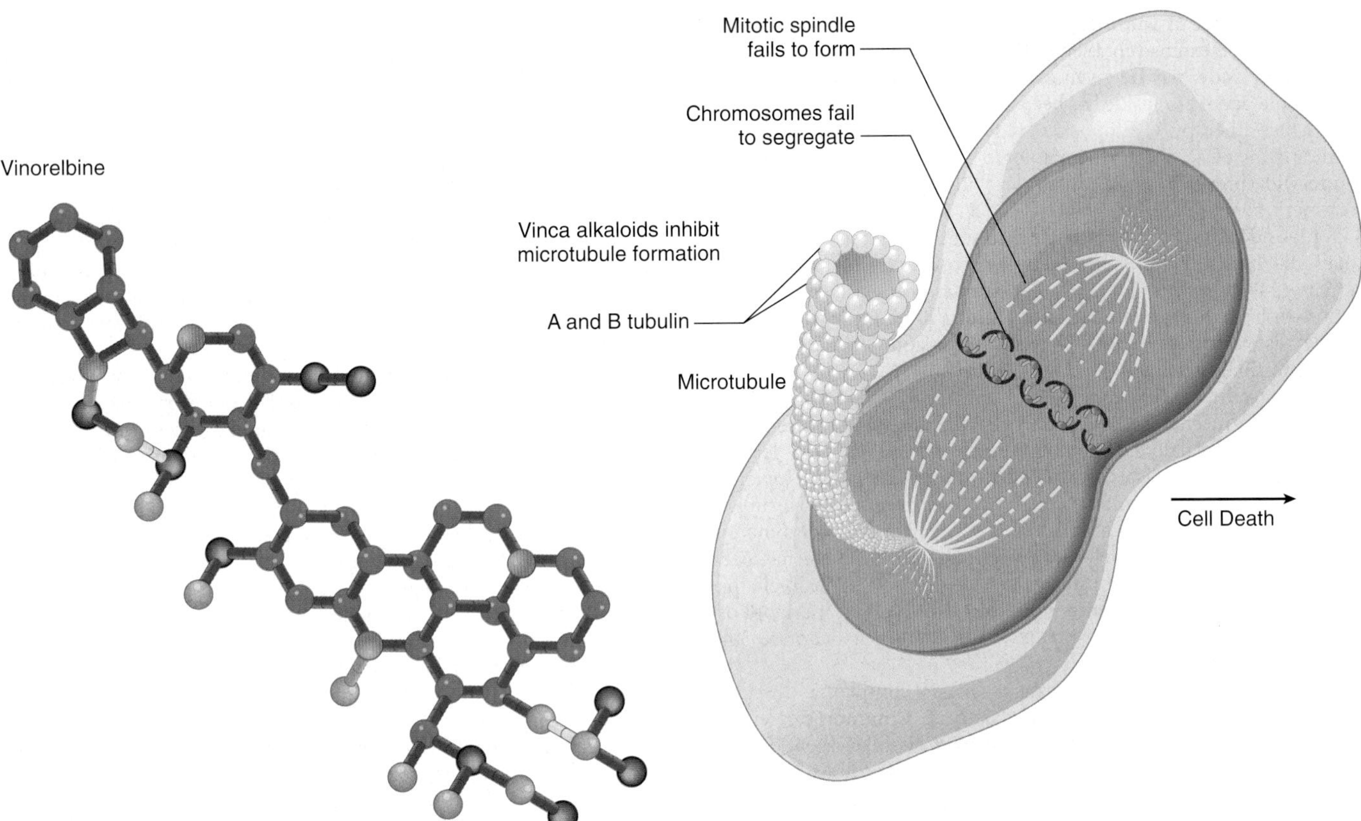

FIGURE 64-3 • Vinorelbine. A semisynthetic vinca alkaloid derived from the periwinkle, *Vinca rosea,* vinorelbine is a cell cycle–specific agent (inhibits mitosis). It binds to tubulin and prevents formation of microtubules (essential part of the mitotic spindle); chromosomes do not segregate correctly, and cell death ensues.

cancers, temozolamide for primary CNS tumors, and gemcitabine for pancreatic cancers. These have not yet been fully evaluated in NSCLC.

SMALL CELL LUNG CANCER

Introduction

Small cell lung cancer accounts for approximately 13% of all lung cancers and occurs primarily in smokers. Small cell lung cancer is characterized by early metastases and rapid growth. While initially very responsive to both chemotherapy and radiation therapy, the majority of patients will have recurrent disease or become refractory to treatment. The 5-year survival of patients with small cell lung cancer is only 5%. The staging of small cell lung cancer is divided into limited stage and extensive stage (Box 64-3). Limited stage refers to disease that can be confined to one radiation port. At the time of presentation, approximately 60% to 70% of patients will have advanced disease. Unlike NSCLC, surgery does not play a role in treatment. The treatment for limited-stage disease has been chemoradiation, while extensive stage disease is managed with chemotherapy.

Therapeutics and Clinical Pharmacology

A variety of chemotherapy agents have been used in the treatment of extensive stage small cell lung cancer, including platinum-containing agents (cisplatin, carboplatin), anthracyclines (doxorubicin, epirubicin), camptothecins (irinotecan, topotecan), podophyllotoxins (etoposide, teniposide), alkylating agents (ifosfamide, cyclophosphamide), and taxanes. In general, combination therapies are chosen in the first-line setting as clinical trials have shown survival benefit over single-agent therapies.[60]

BOX 64-3 SMALL CELL LUNG CANCER STAGING

Limited disease: cancer can only be seen in one lung, in nearby lymph nodes, or in fluid around the lung (pleural effusion).
Extensive disease: cancer has spread outside the lung to the chest or to other parts of the body.

Single-Agent Therapies

Alkylating Agents. One of the first drugs shown to have benefit in small cell lung cancer was the alkylating agent cyclophosphamide.[61] Combination regimens that have incorporated cyclophosphamide include the previously widely used cyclophosphamide, doxorubicin, and vincristine (CAV) regimen[62,63]; CAV and etoposide[64]; lomustine, cyclophosphamide, doxorubicin, and etoposide[65]; and cyclophosphamide, procarbazine, vincristine, and methotrexate.[66]

Ifosfamide, an alkylating agent that cross-links strands of DNA and RNA, yields response rates of approximately 50% as single-agent therapy.[67] Combinations incorporating ifosfamide have included etoposide, ifosfamide, and cisplatin[68] and ifosfamide, etoposide, and carboplatin.[69] Ifosfamide confers significant hematologic toxicity and may also cause neurotoxicity, nephrotoxicity, and cystitis.

Platinum-Containing Agents. Cisplatin and carboplatin are platinum-containing agents that are thought to act as alkylating agents (see Fig. 64-1). Both have been used extensively in the treatment of small cell lung cancer, primarily in combination with other agents. Cisplatin is highly emetogenic and causes myelosuppression, nephrotoxicity, ototoxicity, neuropathy, and electrolyte abnormalities. Carboplatin is generally better tolerated and is associated with thrombocytopenia and neuropathy.

Topoisomerase II Inhibitors. The topoisomerase II inhibitor etoposide has been extensively used in the management of small cell lung cancer. Etoposide may be given orally or by intravenous administration. Single-agent etoposide has been shown to be inferior to combination chemotherapy.[70] Etoposide has been associated with the development of secondary hematologic malignancies. Etoposide has found widespread use in combination with other agents as first-line treatment of small cell lung cancer.

Teniposide, also a topoisomerase II inhibitor, has been evaluated in small cell lung cancer. Single-agent teniposide has shown minimal activity (24% response rate).[71] Teniposide has been studied in combination with methotrexate, vincristine, and cyclophosphamide.[72] Teniposide is associated with myelosuppression, mucositis, and gastrointestinal toxicities.

Anthracyclines. Doxorubicin and epirubicin are anthracyclines. Their precise mechanisms of action remain unclear; however, these agents can intercalate DNA, alter mitochondrial function, lead to formation of free radicals, and inhibit topoisomerase II. Toxicities include myelosuppression and congestive heart failure. Doxorubicin is part of the CAV regimen and has also been used in combination with paclitaxel[73] and vinorelbine.[74] Single-agent epirubicin has been associated with a response rate of 40% to 50%.[75-77] Epirubicin has been used in combination with etoposide and cisplatin[78]; cyclophosphamide, etoposide, and cisplatin[79]; and cyclophosphamide and vincristine.[80]

Camptothecins. Topotecan forms a ternary complex with topoisomerase I and DNA, leading to DNA damage. Common side effects include cytopenias and gastrointestinal toxicity. As single-agent therapy in chemotherapy-naive patients with extensive-stage disease, topotecan has been reported to induce response rates of 39%.[81] In patients with previously treated disease, response rates of 6.4% (refractory patients) and 37.8% (sensitive patients) with single-agent topotecan have been observed.[82] The use of oral topotecan has also been investigated, and efficacy equivalent to the intravenous form has been reported.[83,84] In patients who had previously been treated with irinotecan and platinum, second-line single-agent topotecan showed minimal activity.[85] Topotecan has been extensively studied in combination with other agents, including topotecan and docetaxel[86]; topotecan and paclitaxel[87-89]; topotecan and etoposide[90,91]; paclitaxel, carboplatin, and etoposide[92]; topotecan and carboplatin[93]; topotecan and cisplatin[94,95]; and topotecan and cyclophosphamide.[96]

Irinotecan is a camptothecin derivative that also inhibits topoisomerase I. Common toxicities include myelosuppression, diarrhea, and pulmonary toxicity. As single-agent therapy in patients with refractory or relapsed disease, response rates as high as 47% have been observed.[97] Multiple combinations have been studied in the setting of first-line or relapsed/refractory disease, including irinotecan and cisplatin[98-103]; cisplatin, etoposide, and irinotecan[104,105]; irinotecan, cisplatin, and mitomycin[106]; gemcitabine and irinotecan[107-111]; irinotecan and carboplatin[112-115]; irinotecan and etoposide[116]; and irinotecan and ifosfamide.[117] The optimal irinotecan-containing regimen has yet to be determined.

Other Single Agents. Gemcitabine, an antimetabolite, has shown limited activity as a single agent in recurrent disease (0% to 12% response rates).[118,119] Despite this, there have been multiple trials using gemcitabine in combination with other agents. In a trial involving patients with relapsed disease, single-agent paclitaxel yielded a response rate of 29%.[120] Single-agent docetaxel has been reported to have a 25% response rate in patients with previously treated disease.[121] Other agents that have been evaluated include vinorelbine,[122] and methotrexate.[123]

Combination Therapies

The combination of cisplatin and etoposide (EP) was first reported in 1979.[124] In a small trial involving 38 patients, EP was given in an alternating fashion with CAV. In a Phase III trial that compared EP versus CAV versus CAV/EP, no significant differences in response rates or median survival were observed.[125] In a similar trial, patients were randomized to CAV versus EP versus CAV/EP.[126] Improved response rates were seen for the EP and CAV/EP arms, with slightly superior survival in the alternating arm. A trial comparing EP with CEV (cyclophosphamide, epirubicin, and vincristine) found no difference in survival between the two arms in patients with extensive-stage disease, although there was an improvement in survival for the EP arm in patients with limited-stage disease.[127]

While cisplatin and etoposide has emerged as the most frequently used combination, carboplatin is often substituted in an attempt to minimize toxicity. Only one randomized trial has compared EP to carboplatin and etoposide.[128] No differences in response rates or survival were seen, although the EP arm was associated with increased toxicity.

Several studies have compared the combination of cisplatin and irinotecan with EP. In one trial, the cisplatin plus irinotecan arm was associated with a statistically significant improvement in median survival.[129] However, in a second Phase III trial, no differences in response rates, median time to progression, or overall survival were observed.[130] The combination of topotecan and cisplatin also has been compared to EP. In this trial, there was no difference in response rates or overall survival.[131] Finally, in a trial comparing EP with epirubicin and cisplatin, no differences in response rate, time to progression, or survival were noted; however, the epirubicin plus cisplatin regimen had slightly less toxicity.[132]

Thus there is currently no definitive evidence that one combination is more effective than another in the first-line setting. However, a meta-analysis incorporating 19 randomized trials concluded that patients who received a cisplatin-containing regimen had significant reduction of risk of death as well as a higher likelihood of responding to therapy.[133] A clear standard of care does not exist for second-line therapy. As noted earlier, many agents have shown moderate activity. The choice is also dependent on the agent's specific toxicities and the patient's performance status.

New Agents

One study has reported the use of bortezomib, a proteasome inhibitor, in previously treated patients[134] (Fig. 64-4). Limited activity was seen, with only one partial response reported. There is some evidence that the tyrosine kinase KIT is expressed in small cell lung cancer. Imatinib, developed as an inhibitor of Bcr-Abl in chronic myelogenous leukemia, also inhibits KIT (Fig. 64-5). The combination of imatinib with irinotecan and carboplatin in patients with untreated extensive-stage disease has been studied.[135] While the regimen was generally well tolerated, the results were similar to historical control with chemotherapy alone.

Amrubicin, a topoisomerase II inhibitor, has shown promise in initial studies. A recent multicenter Phase II study involving previously treated patients reported an overall response rate of 50%.[136] In the front-line setting, a response rate of 76% was achieved.[137] Pemetrexed is currently being investigated in the treatment of small cell lung cancer.

Thalidomide, which is thought to have antiangiogenesic and immunomodulatory effects (Fig. 64-6), has been evaluated in a variety of settings. In a small Phase II trial, thalidomide was added to the combination of carboplatin and irinotecan in previously untreated patients.[138] The study was stopped early secondary to patients' inability to tolerate the thalidomide. In another Phase II trial, patients were started on thalidomide as maintenance therapy after receiving first-line chemotherapy.[139] Maintenance thalidomide was shown to be well tolerated. A Phase III trial has been performed that randomized patients to etoposide, cisplatin, cyclophosphamide, and 4′-epidoxorubicin with or without thalidomide.[140] An improvement in survival was not observed.

Traditional cytotoxic agents, while initially effective, fail in the long term as the vast majority of patients die of their disease. Further understanding of the molecular pathophysiology of small cell lung cancer is required for the development of targeted therapies. This is a very fertile field for drug development and thus for clinical pharmacology.

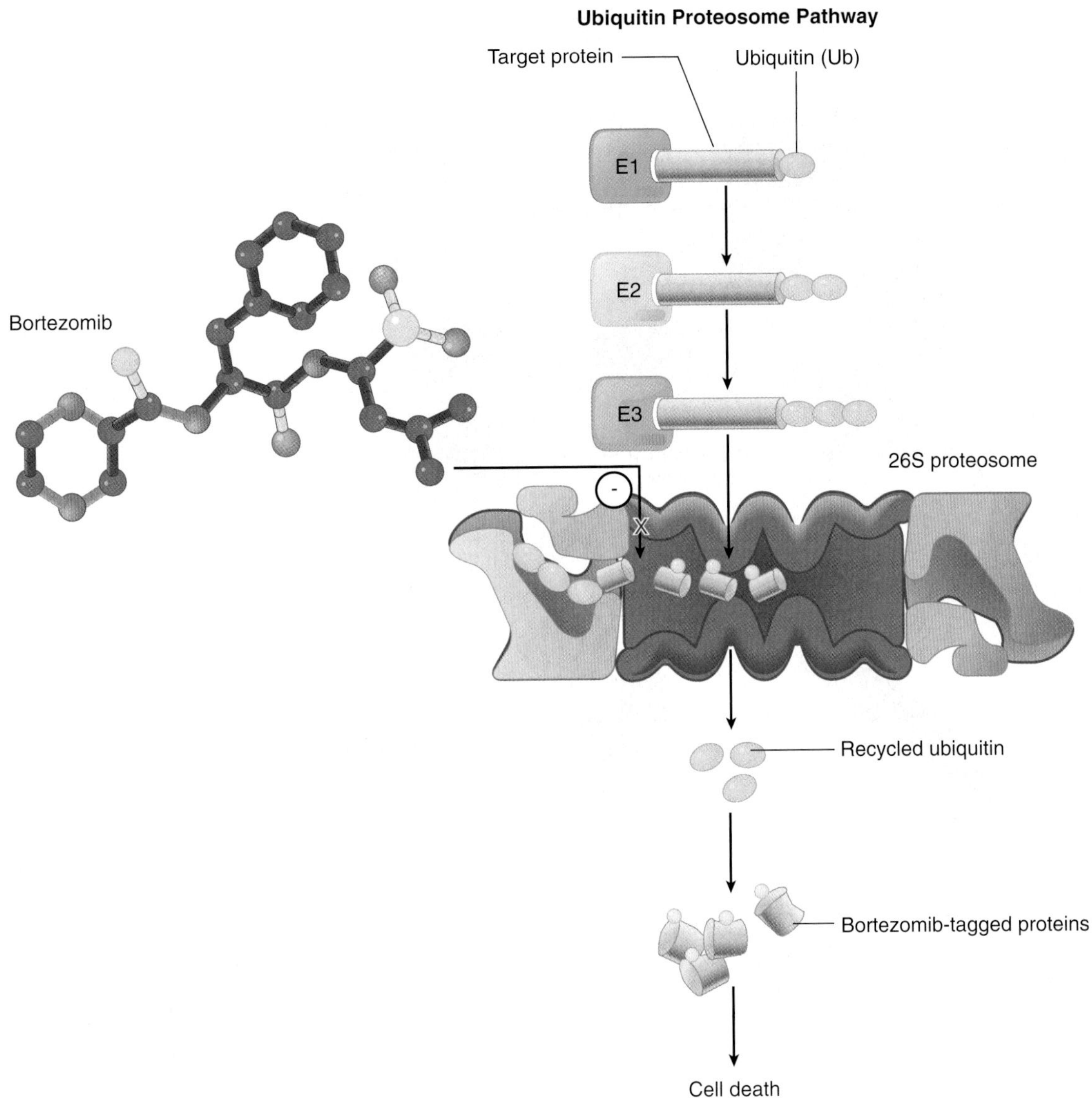

Ubiquitin Proteosome Pathway

Target protein

Ubiquitin (Ub)

Bortezomib

E1

E2

E3

26S proteosome

-

Recycled ubiquitin

Bortezomib-tagged proteins

Cell death

FIGURE 64-4 • Bortezomib. Bortezomib is a reversible inhibitor of the 26S proteosome, a large protein complex that degrades ubiquinated proteins. The ubiquitine-proteosome pathway is known to play a major role in intracellular degradation of numerous regulatory proteins involved in cell integrity, such as cell cycle control, cellular apoptosis, transcription factor activation, and tumor growth. Inhibition of the 26S proteosome disrupts cell proliferation and apoptosis, which leads to cell death.

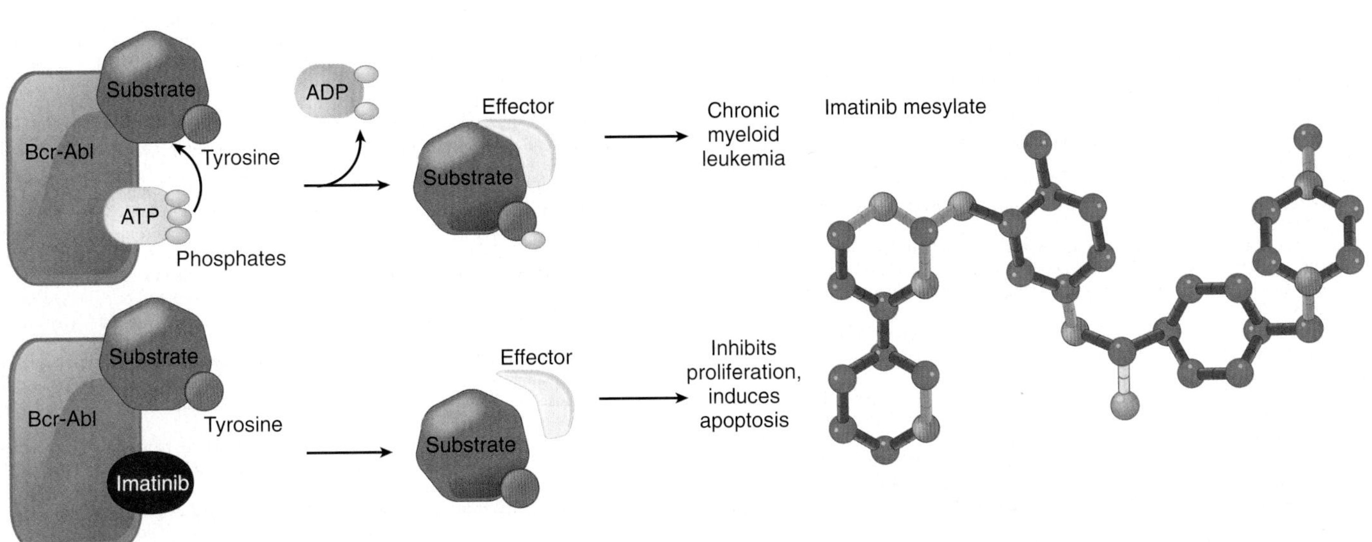

FIGURE 64-5 • Imatinib mesylate. Imatinib inhibits BCR-Abl tyrosine kinase.

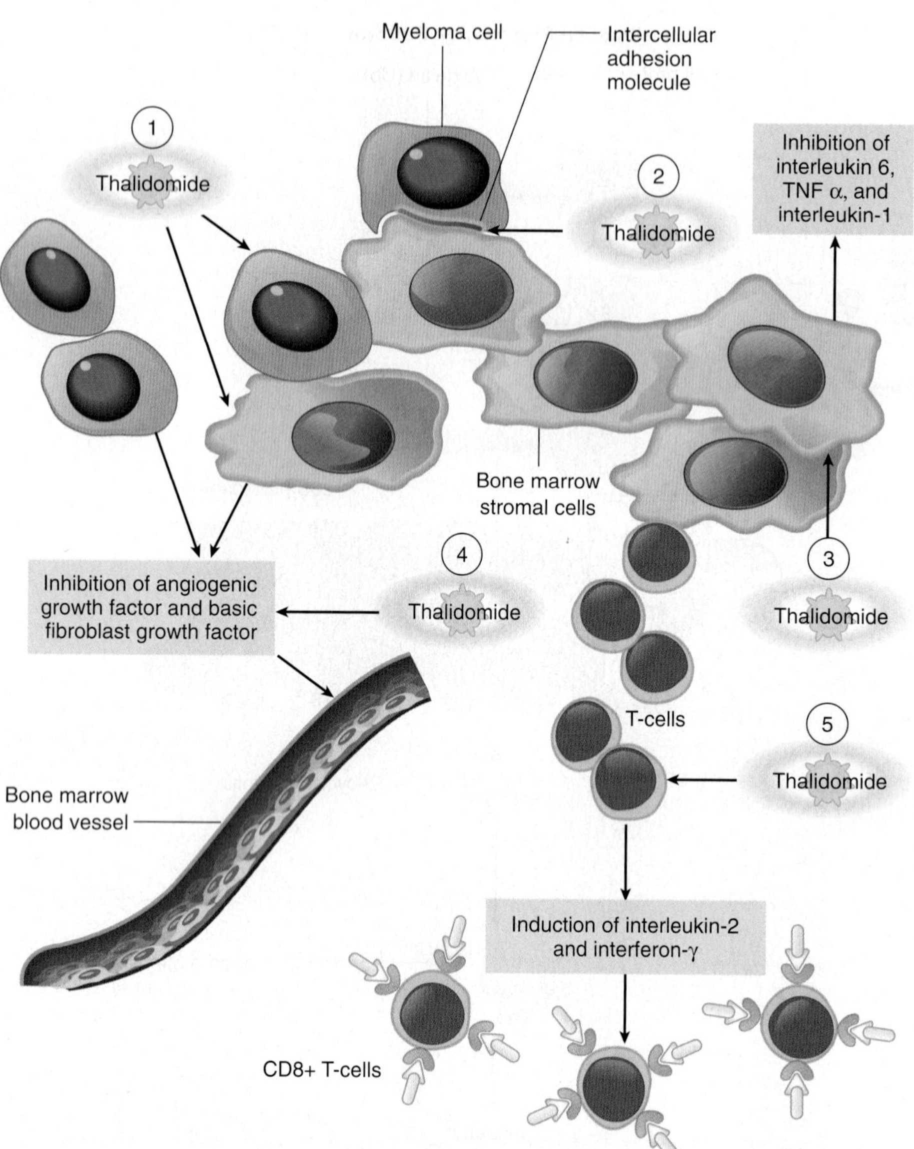

FIGURE 64-6 • Potential mechanisms of action of thalidomide and its in vivo metabolites. Thalidomide may (1) inhibit the growth and survival of tumor cells, bone marrow stromal cells, or both; (2) alter the profile of adhesion molecules and interactions between tumor cells and bone marrow stromal cells; (3) modulate the cytokine milieu and thereby affect the growth and survival of tumor cells, bone marrow stromal cells, or both; (4) inhibit angiogenesis; or (5) increase the number of $CD8^+$ T cells by means of its immunomodulatory effects.

REFERENCES

1. Mountain CF. Revisions in the International System for Staging Lung Cancer. Chest 1997;111:1710-1717.
2. Delbaldo C, Michiels S, Syz N, et al. Benefits of adding a drug to a single-agent or a 2-agent chemotherapy regimen in advanced non-small-cell lung cancer: a meta-analysis. JAMA 2004;292:470-484.
3. Gandara DR, Wold H, Perez EA, et al. Cisplatin dose intensity in non-small cell lung cancer: Phase II results of a day 1 and day 8 high-dose regimen. J Natl Cancer Inst 1989;81:790-794.
4. Saito Y, Mori K, Yokoi K, et al. [Pilot Phase II study of 5-day continuous infusion of cisplatin in treatment of non-small cell lung cancer]. Gan To Kagaku Ryoho 1989;16:2081-2086.
5. Sculier JP, Klastersky J, Giner V, et al. Phase II randomized trial comparing high-dose cisplatin with moderate-dose cisplatin and carboplatin in patients with advanced non-small-cell lung cancer. European Lung Cancer Working Party. J Clin Oncol 1994;12:353-359.
6. Bonomi P. Carboplatin in non-small cell lung cancer: review of the Eastern Cooperative Oncology Group trial and comparison with other carboplatin trials. Semin Oncol 1991;18:2-7.
7. Langer CJ, Leighton JC, Comis RL, et al. Paclitaxel and carboplatin in combination in the treatment of advanced non-small-cell lung cancer: a Phase II toxicity, response, and survival analysis. J Clin Oncol 1995;13:1860-1870.
8. Hainsworth JD, Gray JR, Morrissey LH, et al. Long-term follow-up of patients treated with paclitaxel/carboplatin-based chemotherapy for advanced non-small-cell lung cancer: sequential Phase II trials of the Minnie Pearl Cancer Research Network. J Clin Oncol 2002;20:2937-2942.
9. Bonomi P, Kim K, Fairclough D, et al. Comparison of survival and quality of life in advanced non-small-cell lung cancer patients treated with two dose levels of paclitaxel combined with cisplatin versus etoposide with cisplatin: results of an Eastern Cooperative Oncology Group trial. J Clin Oncol 2000;18:623-631.
10. Kelly K, Crowley J, Bunn PA Jr, et al. Randomized Phase III trial of paclitaxel plus carboplatin versus vinorelbine plus cisplatin in the treatment of patients with advanced non–small-cell lung cancer: a Southwest Oncology Group trial. J Clin Oncol 2001;19:3210-3218.
11. Fossella F, Pereira JR, von Pawel J, et al. Randomized, multinational, Phase III study of docetaxel plus platinum combinations versus vinorelbine plus cisplatin for advanced non-small-cell lung cancer: the TAX 326 study group. J Clin Oncol 2003;21:3016-3024.
12. Klastersky J, Sculier JP, Lacroix H, et al. A randomized study comparing cisplatin or carboplatin with etoposide in patients with advanced non-small-cell lung cancer: European Organization for Research and Treatment of Cancer Protocol 07861. J Clin Oncol 1990;8:1556-1562.
13. Le Chevalier T, Brisgand D, Douillard JY, et al. Randomized study of vinorelbine and cisplatin versus vindesine and cisplatin versus vinorelbine alone in advanced non-small-cell lung cancer: results of a European multicenter trial including 612 patients. J Clin Oncol 1994;12:360-367.
14. Wozniak AJ, Crowley JJ, Balcerzak SP, et al. Randomized trial comparing cisplatin with cisplatin plus vinorelbine in the treatment of advanced non-small-cell lung cancer: a Southwest Oncology Group study. J Clin Oncol 1998;16:2459-2465.
15. Zatloukal P, Petruzelka L, Zemanova M, et al. Gemcitabine plus cisplatin vs. gemcitabine plus carboplatin in stage IIIb and IV non-small cell lung cancer: a Phase III randomized trial. Lung Cancer 2003;41:321-331.
16. Sederholm C, Hillerdal G, Lamberg K, et al. Phase III trial of gemcitabine plus carboplatin versus single-agent gemcitabine in the treatment of locally advanced or metastatic non-small-cell lung cancer: the Swedish Lung Cancer Study Group. J Clin Oncol 2005;23:8380-8388.

17. Cardenal F, Domine M, Massuti B, et al. Three-week schedule of irinotecan and cisplatin in advanced non-small cell lung cancer: a multicentre Phase II study. Lung Cancer 2003;39:201-207.
18. Kakolyris S, Kouroussis C, Souglakos J, et al. Cisplatin and irinotecan (CPT-11) as second-line treatment in patients with advanced non-small cell lung cancer. Lung Cancer 2001;34(Suppl 4):S71-S76.
19. Scagliotti GV, Kortsik C, Dark GG, et al. Pemetrexed combined with oxaliplatin or carboplatin as first-line treatment in advanced non-small cell lung cancer: a multicenter, randomized, Phase II trial. Clin Cancer Res 2005;11:690-696.
20. Neubauer MA, Garfield DH, Kuerfler PR, et al. Results of a Phase II multicenter trial of weekly docetaxel and gemcitabine as first-line therapy for patients with advanced non-small cell lung cancer. Lung Cancer 2005;47:121-127.
21. Binder D, Schweisfurth H, Grah C, et al. Docetaxel/gemcitabine or cisplatin/gemcitabine followed by docetaxel in the first-line treatment of patients with metastatic non-small cell lung cancer (NSCLC): results of a multicentre randomized Phase II trial. Cancer Chemother Pharmacol 2007;60:143-150.
22. Ginopoulos P, Kontomanolis E, Kardamakis D, et al. A Phase II study of non-platinum based chemotherapy with paclitaxel and vinorelbine in non-small cell lung cancer. Lung Cancer 2002;38:199-203.
23. Douillard JY, Lerouge D, Monnier A, et al. Combined paclitaxel and gemcitabine as first-line treatment in metastatic non-small cell lung cancer: a multicentre Phase II study. Br J Cancer 2001;84:1179-1184.
24. Tan EH, Szczesna A, Krzakowski M, et al. Randomized study of vinorelbine–gemcitabine versus vinorelbine–carboplatin in patients with advanced non-small cell lung cancer. Lung Cancer 2005;49:233-240.
25. Ardizzoni A, Boni L, Tiseo M, et al. Cisplatin- versus carboplatin-based chemotherapy in first-line treatment of advanced non-small-cell lung cancer: an individual patient data meta-analysis. J Natl Cancer Inst 2007;99:847-857.
26. Rajeswaran A, Trojan A, Burnand B, Giannelli M. Efficacy and side effects of cisplatin- and carboplatin-based doublet chemotherapeutic regimens versus non-platinum-based doublet chemotherapeutic regimens as first line treatment of metastatic non-small cell lung carcinoma: a systematic review of randomized controlled trials. Lung Cancer 2008;59:1-11.
27. Shepherd FA, Fossella FV, Lynch T, et al. Docetaxel (Taxotere) shows survival and quality-of-life benefits in the second-line treatment of non-small cell lung cancer: a review of two Phase III trials. Semin Oncol 2001;28:4-9.
28. Gridelli C, Perrone F, Gallo C, et al. Vinorelbine is well tolerated and active in the treatment of elderly patients with advanced non-small cell lung cancer: a two-stage Phase II study. Eur J Cancer 1997;33:392-397.
29. Goss GD, Logan DM, Newman TE, Evans WK. Use of vinorelbine in non-small-cell lung cancer. Provincial Lung Disease Site Group. Cancer Prev Control 1997;1:28-38.
30. Postmus PE, Bunn PA Jr. Pemetrexed as a single agent in the therapy of advanced lung cancer. Semin Oncol 2002;29:17-22.
31. Rusthoven JJ, Eisenhauer E, Butts C, et al. Multitargeted antifolate LY231514 as first-line chemotherapy for patients with advanced non-small-cell lung cancer: a Phase II study. National Cancer Institute of Canada Clinical Trials Group. J Clin Oncol 1999;17:1194.
32. Chemotherapy in non-small cell lung cancer: a meta-analysis using updated data on individual patients from 52 randomised clinical trials. Non-small Cell Lung Cancer Collaborative Group. BMJ 1995;311:899-909.
33. Douillard JY, Rosell R, De Lena M, et al. Adjuvant vinorelbine plus cisplatin versus observation in patients with completely resected stage IB-IIIA non-small-cell lung cancer (Adjuvant Navelbine International Trialist Association [ANITA]): a randomised controlled trial. Lancet Oncol 2006;7:719-727.
34. Kato H, Ichinose Y, Ohta M, et al. A randomized trial of adjuvant chemotherapy with uracil-tegafur for adenocarcinoma of the lung. N Engl J Med 2004;350:1713-1721.
35. Thatcher N, Chang A, Parikh P, et al. Gefitinib plus best supportive care in previously treated patients with refractory advanced non-small-cell lung cancer: results from a randomised, placebo-controlled, multicentre study (Iressa Survival Evaluation in Lung Cancer). Lancet 2005;366:1527-1537.
36. Shepherd FA, Rodrigues Pereira J, Ciuleanu T, et al. Erlotinib in previously treated non-small-cell lung cancer. N Engl J Med 2005;353:123-132.
37. Giaccone G, Gallegos Ruiz M, Le Chevalier T, et al. Erlotinib for frontline treatment of advanced non-small cell lung cancer: a Phase II study. Clin Cancer Res 2006;12:6049-6055.
38. Pao W, Miller V, Zakowski M, et al. EGF receptor gene mutations are common in lung cancers from "never smokers" and are associated with sensitivity of tumors to gefitinib and erlotinib. Proc Natl Acad Sci U S A 2004;101:13306-13311.
39. Lynch TJ, Bell DW, Sordella R, et al. Activating mutations in the epidermal growth factor receptor underlying responsiveness of non-small-cell lung cancer to gefitinib. N Engl J Med 2004;350:2129-2139.
40. Paez JG, Janne PA, Lee JC, et al. EGFR mutations in lung cancer: correlation with clinical response to gefitinib therapy. Science 2004;304:1497-1500.
41. Cappuzzo F, Hirsch FR, Rossi E, et al. Epidermal growth factor receptor gene and protein and gefitinib sensitivity in non-small-cell lung cancer. J Natl Cancer Inst 2005;97:643-655.
42. Tsao MS, Sakurada A, Cutz JC, et al. Erlotinib in lung cancer—molecular and clinical predictors of outcome. N Engl J Med 2005;353:133-144.
43. Perez-Soler R. Rash as a surrogate marker for efficacy of epidermal growth factor receptor inhibitors in lung cancer. Clin Lung Cancer 2006;8(Suppl 1):S7-S14.
44. Wacker B, Nagrani T, Weinberg J, et al. Correlation between development of rash and efficacy in patients treated with the epidermal growth factor receptor tyrosine kinase inhibitor erlotinib in two large Phase III studies. Clin Cancer Res 2007;13:3913-3921.
45. Gatzemeier U, Pluzanska A, Szczesna A, et al. Phase III study of erlotinib in combination with cisplatin and gemcitabine in advanced non-small-cell lung cancer: the Tarceva Lung Cancer Investigation Trial. J Clin Oncol 2007;25:1545-1552.
46. Herbst RS, Prager D, Hermann R, et al. TRIBUTE: a Phase III trial of erlotinib hydrochloride (OSI-774) combined with carboplatin and paclitaxel chemotherapy in advanced non-small-cell lung cancer. J Clin Oncol 2005;23:5892-5899.
47. Hanna N, Lilenbaum R, Ansari R, et al. Phase II trial of cetuximab in patients with previously treated non-small-cell lung cancer. J Clin Oncol 2006;24:5253-5258.
48. Butts CA, Bodkin D, Middleman EL, et al. Randomized Phase II study of gemcitabine plus cisplatin, with or without cetuximab, as first-line therapy for patients with advanced or metastatic non small-cell lung cancer. J Clin Oncol 2007;25:5777-5784.
49. Rosell R, Robinet G, Szczesna A, et al. Randomized Phase II study of cetuximab plus cisplatin/vinorelbine compared with cisplatin/vinorelbine alone as first-line therapy in EGFR-expressing advanced non-small-cell lung cancer. Ann Oncol 2008;19:362-369.
50. Sandler A, Gray R, Perry MC, et al. Paclitaxel-carboplatin alone or with bevacizumab for non-small-cell lung cancer. N Engl J Med 2006;355:2542-2550.
51. Sause W, Kolesar P, Taylor SI, et al. Final results of Phase III trial in regionally advanced unresectable non-small cell lung cancer: Radiation Therapy Oncology Group, Eastern Cooperative Oncology Group, and Southwest Oncology Group. Chest 2000;117:358-364.
52. Dillman RO, Herndon J, Seagren SL, et al. Improved survival in stage III non-small-cell lung cancer: seven-year follow-up of cancer and leukemia group B (CALGB) 8433 trial. J Natl Cancer Inst 1996;88:1210-1215.
53. Furuse K, Fukuoka M, Kawahara M, et al. Phase III study of concurrent versus sequential thoracic radiotherapy in combination with mitomycin, vindesine, and cisplatin in unresectable stage III non-small-cell lung cancer. J Clin Oncol 1999;17:2692-2699.
54. Fournel P, Robinet G, Thomas P, et al. Randomized Phase III trial of sequential chemoradiotherapy compared with concurrent chemoradiotherapy in locally advanced non-small-cell lung cancer: Groupe Lyon-Saint-Etienne d'Oncologie Thoracique–Groupe Francais de Pneumo-Cancerologie NPC 95-01 Study. J Clin Oncol 2005;23:5910-5917.
55. Komaki R, Lee JS, Kaplan B, et al. Randomized Phase III study of chemoradiation with or without amifostine for patients with favorable performance status inoperable stage II-III non-small cell lung cancer: preliminary results. Semin Radiat Oncol 2002;12:46-49.
56. Antonadou D, Throuvalas N, Petridis A, et al. Effect of amifostine on toxicities associated with radiochemotherapy in patients with locally advanced non-small-cell lung cancer. Int J Radiat Oncol Biol Phys 2003;57:402-408.
57. Leong SS, Tan EH, Fong KW, et al. Randomized double-blind trial of combined modality treatment with or without amifostine in unresectable stage III non-small-cell lung cancer. J Clin Oncol 2003;21:1767-1774.
58. Senzer N. A Phase III randomized evaluation of amifostine in stage IIIA/IIIB non-small cell lung cancer patients receiving concurrent carboplatin, paclitaxel, and radiation therapy followed by gemcitabine and cisplatin intensification: preliminary findings. Semin Oncol 2002;29:38-41.
59. Movsas B, Scott C, Langer C, et al. Randomized trial of amifostine in locally advanced non-small-cell lung cancer patients receiving chemotherapy and hyperfractionated radiation: Radiation Therapy Oncology Group trial 98-01. J Clin Oncol 2005;23:2145-2154.
60. Lowenbraun S, Bartolucci A, Smalley RV, et al. The superiority of combination chemotherapy over single agent chemotherapy in small cell lung carcinoma. Cancer 1979;44:406-413.
61. Green RA, Humphrey E, Close H, Patno ME. Alkylating agents in bronchogenic carcinoma. Am J Med 1969;46:516-525.
62. Johnson DH, Einhorn LH, Birch R, et al. A randomized comparison of high-dose versus conventional-dose cyclophosphamide, doxorubicin, and vincristine for extensive-stage small-cell lung cancer: a Phase III trial of the Southeastern Cancer Study Group. J Clin Oncol 1987;5:1731-1738.
63. Shepherd FA, Evans WK, MacCormick R, et al. Cyclophosphamide, doxorubicin, and vincristine in etoposide- and cisplatin-resistant small cell lung cancer. Cancer Treat Rep 1987;71:941-944.
64. Messeih AA, Schweitzer JM, Lipton A, et al. Addition of etoposide to cyclophosphamide, doxorubicin, and vincristine for remission induction and survival in patients with small cell lung cancer. Cancer Treat Rep 1987;71:61-66.
65. Urban T, Baleyte T, Chastang CL, et al. Standard combination versus alternating chemotherapy in small cell lung cancer: a randomised clinical trial including 394 patients. "Petites Cellules" Group. Lung Cancer 1999;25:105-113.
66. Veronesi A, Magri MD, Tirelli U, et al. Chemotherapy of advanced non-small-cell lung cancer with cyclophosphamide, adriamycin, methotrexate, and procarbazine versus cisplatin and etoposide: a randomized study. Am J Clin Oncol 1988;11:566-571.
67. Ettinger DS. Overview of ifosfamide in small cell lung cancer. Semin Oncol 1992;19:59-67.
68. Loehrer PJ Sr, Rynard S, Ansari R, et al. Etoposide, ifosfamide, and cisplatin in extensive small cell lung cancer. Cancer 1992;69:669-673.
69. Wolff AC, Ettinger DS, Neuberg D, et al. Phase II study of ifosfamide, carboplatin, and oral etoposide chemotherapy for extensive-disease small-cell lung cancer: an Eastern Cooperative Oncology Group pilot study. J Clin Oncol 1995;13:1615-1622.
70. Souhami RL, Spiro SG, Rudd RM, et al. Five-day oral etoposide treatment for advanced small-cell lung cancer: randomized comparison with intravenous chemotherapy. J Natl Cancer Inst 1997;89:577-580.
71. Grozea PN, Crowley JJ, Canfield VA, et al. Teniposide (VM-26) as a single drug treatment for patients with extensive small cell lung carcinoma: a Phase II study of the Southwest Oncology Group. Cancer 1997;80:1029-1033.

72. Giaccone G, Schmidt G, Calciati A. Pilot study of teniposide in combination chemotherapy for small cell lung cancer. Eur J Cancer 1991;27:141-143.
73. Sonpavde G, Ansari R, Walker P, et al. Phase II study of doxorubicin and paclitaxel as second-line chemotherapy of small-cell lung cancer: a Hoosier Oncology Group Trial. Am J Clin Oncol 2000;23:68-70.
74. Johnson E, Lake D, Herndon JE 2nd, et al. Phase II trial of vinorelbine plus doxorubicin in relapsed small-cell lung cancer: CALGB 9332. Am J Clin Oncol 2004;27:19-23.
75. Macchiarini P, Danesi R, Mariotti R, et al. Phase II study of high-dose epirubicin in untreated patients with small-cell lung cancer. Am J Clin Oncol 1990;13:302-307.
76. Blackstein M, Eisenhauer EA, Wierzbicki R, Yoshida S. Epirubicin in extensive small-cell lung cancer: a Phase II study in previously untreated patients. A National Cancer Institute of Canada Clinical Trials Group Study. J Clin Oncol 1990;8: 385-389.
77. Quoix EA, Giaccone G, Jassem J, et al. Epirubicin in previously untreated patients with small cell lung cancer: a Phase II study by the EORTC Lung Cancer Cooperative Group. Eur J Cancer 1992;28A:1667-1670.
78. Jassem J, Karnicka-Mlodkowska H, Jassem E, et al. Combination chemotherapy with cyclophosphamide, epirubicin and etoposide in small cell lung cancer. Lung Cancer 1994;11:283-291.
79. Bamberga M, Michetti G, Bamberga P, et al. Cyclophosphamide, epirubicin, etoposide, cis platinum (CEVP) in combination with radiotherapy: evaluation of a protocol adopted for 6 years in 148 cases of small cell lung cancer. Tumori 1992;78: 333-337.
80. Kretzschmar A, Drings P. Epirubicin weekly in combination chemotherapy with cyclophosphamide and vincristine in untreated small cell lung cancer: a Phase II trial. Onkologie 1990;13:141-142.
81. Schiller JH, Kim K, Hutson P, et al. Phase II study of topotecan in patients with extensive-stage small-cell carcinoma of the lung: an Eastern Cooperative Oncology Group Trial. J Clin Oncol 1996;14:2345-2352.
82. Ardizzoni A, Hansen H, Dombernowsky P, et al. Topotecan, a new active drug in the second-line treatment of small-cell lung cancer: a Phase II study in patients with refractory and sensitive disease. The European Organization for Research and Treatment of Cancer Early Clinical Studies Group and New Drug Development Office, and the Lung Cancer Cooperative Group. J Clin Oncol 1997;15:2090-2096.
83. Eckardt JR. Feasibility of oral topotecan in previously untreated patients with small-cell lung cancer ineligible for standard therapy. Oncology 2001;61(Suppl 1):42-46.
84. von Pawel J, Gatzemeier U, Pujol JL, et al. Phase II comparator study of oral versus intravenous topotecan in patients with chemosensitive small-cell lung cancer. J Clin Oncol 2001;19:1743-1749.
85. Park SH, Cho EK, Kim Y, et al. Salvage treatment with topotecan in patients with irinotecan-refractory small cell lung cancer. Cancer Chemother Pharmacol 2008. [Epub ahead of print]
86. Morgensztern D, Perry MC, Govindan R. A Phase II study of topotecan and docetaxel in patients with sensitive relapse small cell lung cancer. Acta Oncol 2007:1-2.
87. Dy GK, Jett JR, Geoffroy FJ, et al. Topotecan and paclitaxel in previously treated patients with relapsed small cell lung cancer: Phase II trial of the North Central Cancer Treatment Group. J Thorac Oncol 2006;1:211-217.
88. Molina JR, Jett JR, Foster N, et al. Phase II NCCTG trial of oral topotecan and paclitaxel with G-CSF (filgrastim) support in patients with previously untreated extensive-stage small cell lung cancer. Am J Clin Oncol 2006;29:246-251.
89. Ramalingam S, Belani CP, Day R, et al. Phase II study of topotecan and paclitaxel for patients with previously untreated extensive stage small-cell lung cancer. Ann Oncol 2004;15:247-251.
90. Ciuleanu TE, Curca R, Iancu D, et al. First-line chemotherapy with topotecan and etoposide in advanced small cell lung cancer: a Phase II study. J BUON 2002;7:43-46.
91. Reck M, Groth G, Buchholz E, et al. Topotecan and etoposide as first-line therapy for extensive disease small cell lung cancer: a Phase II trial of a platinum-free regimen. Lung Cancer 2005;48:409-413.
92. Hesketh PJ, McCoy J, Dunphy FR 2nd, et al. Phase II trial of paclitaxel, carboplatin, and topotecan with G-CSF support in previously untreated patients with extensive stage small cell lung cancer: Southwest Oncology Group 9914. J Thorac Oncol 2006;1:991-995.
93. Seifart U, Fink T, Schade-Brittinger C, et al. Randomised Phase II study comparing topotecan/carboplatin administration for 5 versus 3 days in the treatment of extensive-stage small-cell lung cancer. Ann Oncol 2007;18:104-109.
94. Seifart U, Jensen K, Ukena J, et al. Randomized Phase II study comparing topotecan/ cisplatin administration for 5 days versus 3 days in the treatment of extensive stage small cell lung cancer (SCLC). Lung Cancer 2005;48:415-422.
95. Christodoulou C, Kalofonos HP, Briasoulis E, et al. Combination of topotecan and cisplatin in relapsed patients with small cell lung cancer: a Phase II study of the Hellenic Cooperative Oncology Group (HeCOG). Cancer Chemother Pharmacol 2006;57:207-212.
96. Hobdy EM, Kraut E, Masters G, et al. A Phase II study of topotecan and cyclophosphamide with G-CSF in patients with advanced small cell lung cancer. Cancer Biol Ther 2004;3:89-93.
97. Masuda N, Fukuoka M, Kusunoki Y, et al. CPT-11: a new derivative of camptothecin for the treatment of refractory or relapsed small-cell lung cancer. J Clin Oncol 1992;10:1225-1229.
98. Lee JE, Park HS, Jung SS, et al. Phase II study of a 3-week schedule of irinotecan combined with cisplatin in previously untreated extensive-stage small-cell lung cancer. Oncology 2008;73:76-80.
99. Kim HG, Lee GW, Kang JH, et al. Combination chemotherapy with irinotecan and cisplatin in elderly patients (≥65 years) with extensive-disease small-cell lung cancer. Lung Cancer 2008. [Epub ahead of print]
100. Bae SH, Ryoo HM, Do YR, et al. A Phase II study of biweekly irinotecan and cisplatin for patients with extensive stage disease small cell lung cancer. Lung Cancer 2008;59:76-80.
101. Hong YS, Lee HR, Park S, et al. Three-week schedule of irinotecan plus cisplatin in patients with previously untreated extensive-stage small-cell lung cancer. Br J Cancer 2006;95:1648-1652.
102. Masuda N, Matsui K, Negoro S, et al. Combination of irinotecan and etoposide for treatment of refractory or relapsed small-cell lung cancer. J Clin Oncol 1998;16:3329-3334.
103. Kudoh S, Fujiwara Y, Takada Y, et al. Phase II study of irinotecan combined with cisplatin in patients with previously untreated small-cell lung cancer. West Japan Lung Cancer Group. J Clin Oncol 1998;16:1068-1074.
104. Pectasides D, Samantas E, Fountzilas G, et al. Combination chemotherapy with cisplatin, etoposide and irinotecan in patients with extensive small-cell lung cancer: a Phase II study of the Hellenic Co-operative Oncology Group. Lung Cancer 2007;58:355-361.
105. Goto K, Sekine I, Nishiwaki Y, et al. Multi-institutional Phase II trial of irinotecan, cisplatin, and etoposide for sensitive relapsed small-cell lung cancer. Br J Cancer 2004;91:659-665.
106. Fennell DA, Steele JP, Shamash J, et al. Phase II trial of irinotecan, cisplatin and mitomycin for relapsed small cell lung cancer. Int J Cancer 2007;121:2575-2577.
107. Akerley W, McCoy J, Hesketh PJ, et al. Gemcitabine and irinotecan for patients with untreated extensive stage small cell lung cancer: SWOG 0119. J Thorac Oncol 2007;2:526-530.
108. Ohyanagi F, Horiike A, Okano Y, et al. Phase II trial of gemcitabine and irinotecan in previously treated patients with small-cell lung cancer. Cancer Chemother Pharmacol 2008;61:503-508.
109. Rocha-Lima CM, Herndon JE 2nd, Lee ME, et al. Phase II trial of irinotecan/ gemcitabine as second-line therapy for relapsed and refractory small-cell lung cancer: Cancer and Leukemia Group B Study 39902. Ann Oncol 2007;18:331-337.
110. Schuette W, Nagel S, Juergens S, et al. Phase II trial of gemcitabine/irinotecan in refractory or relapsed small-cell lung cancer. Clin Lung Cancer 2005;7:133-137.
111. Agelaki S, Syrigos K, Christophylakis C, et al. A multicenter Phase II study of the combination of irinotecan and gemcitabine in previously treated patients with small-cell lung cancer. Oncology 2004;66:192-196.
112. Laack E, Thom I, Krull A, et al. A Phase II study of irinotecan (CPT-11) and carboplatin in patients with limited disease small cell lung cancer (SCLC). Lung Cancer 2007;57:181-186.
113. Kinoshita A, Fukuda M, Soda H, et al. Phase II study of irinotecan combined with carboplatin in previously untreated small-cell lung cancer. Br J Cancer 2006;94:1267-1271.
114. Hirose T, Horichi N, Ohmori T, et al. Phase II study of irinotecan and carboplatin in patients with the refractory or relapsed small cell lung cancer. Lung Cancer 2003;40:333-338.
115. Naka N, Kawahara M, Okishio K, et al. Phase II study of weekly irinotecan and carboplatin for refractory or relapsed small-cell lung cancer. Lung Cancer 2002;37:319-323.
116. Kudoh S, Nakamura S, Nakano T, et al. Irinotecan and etoposide for previously untreated extensive-disease small cell lung cancer: a Phase II trial of West Japan Thoracic Oncology Group. Lung Cancer 2005;49:263-269.
117. Ichiki M, Gohara R, Rikimaru T, et al. Combination chemotherapy with irinotecan and ifosfamide as second-line treatment of refractory or sensitive relapsed small cell lung cancer: a Phase II study. Chemotherapy 2003;49:200-205.
118. Masters GA, Declerck L, Blanke C, et al. Phase II trial of gemcitabine in refractory or relapsed small-cell lung cancer: Eastern Cooperative Oncology Group Trial 1597. J Clin Oncol 2003;21:1550-1555.
119. Hoang T, Kim K, Jaslowski A, et al. Phase II study of second-line gemcitabine in sensitive or refractory small cell lung cancer. Lung Cancer 2003;42:97-102.
120. Smit EF, Fokkema E, Biesma B, et al. A Phase II study of paclitaxel in heavily pretreated patients with small-cell lung cancer. Br J Cancer 1998;77:347-351.
121. Smyth JF, Smith IE, Sessa C, et al. Activity of docetaxel (Taxotere) in small cell lung cancer. The Early Clinical Trials Group of the EORTC. Eur J Cancer 1994;30A:1058-1060.
122. Jassem J, Karnicka-Mlodkowska H, van Pottelsberghe C, et al. Phase II study of vinorelbine (Navelbine) in previously treated small cell lung cancer patients. EORTC Lung Cancer Cooperative Group. Eur J Cancer 1993;29A:1720-1722.
123. Hande KR, Oldham RK, Fer MF, et al. Randomized study of high-dose versus low-dose methotrexate in the treatment of extensive small cell lung cancer. Am J Med 1982;73:413-419.
124. Sierocki JS, Hilaris BS, Hopfan S, et al. cis-Dichlorodiammineplatinum(II) and VP-16-213: an active induction regimen for small cell carcinoma of the lung. Cancer Treat Rep 1979;63:1593-1597.
125. Roth BJ, Johnson DH, Einhorn LH, et al. Randomized study of cyclophosphamide, doxorubicin, and vincristine versus etoposide and cisplatin versus alternation of these two regimens in extensive small-cell lung cancer: a Phase III trial of the Southeastern Cancer Study Group. J Clin Oncol 1992;10:282-291.
126. Fukuoka M, Furuse K, Saijo N, et al. Randomized trial of cyclophosphamide, doxorubicin, and vincristine versus cisplatin and etoposide versus alternation of these regimens in small-cell lung cancer. J Natl Cancer Inst 1991;83:855-861.
127. Sundstrom S, Bremnes RM, Kaasa S, et al. Cisplatin and etoposide regimen is superior to cyclophosphamide, epirubicin, and vincristine regimen in small-cell lung cancer: results from a randomized Phase III trial with 5 years' follow-up. J Clin Oncol 2002;20:4665-4672.
128. Skarlos DV, Samantas E, Kosmidis P, et al. Randomized comparison of etoposide-cisplatin vs. etoposide-carboplatin and irradiation in small-cell lung cancer. A Hellenic Co-operative Oncology Group study. Ann Oncol 1994;5:601-607.

129. Noda K, Nishiwaki Y, Kawahara M, et al. Irinotecan plus cisplatin compared with etoposide plus cisplatin for extensive small-cell lung cancer. N Engl J Med 2002;346:85-91.
130. Hanna N, Bunn PA Jr, Langer C, et al. Randomized Phase III trial comparing irinotecan/cisplatin with etoposide/cisplatin in patients with previously untreated extensive-stage disease small-cell lung cancer. J Clin Oncol 2006;24:2038-2043.
131. Eckardt JR, von Pawel J, Papai Z, et al. Open-label, multicenter, randomized, Phase III study comparing oral topotecan/cisplatin versus etoposide/cisplatin as treatment for chemotherapy-naive patients with extensive-disease small-cell lung cancer. J Clin Oncol 2006;24:2044-2051.
132. Artal-Cortes A, Gomez-Codina J, Gonzalez-Larriba JL, et al. Prospective randomized Phase III trial of etoposide/cisplatin versus high-dose epirubicin/cisplatin in small-cell lung cancer. Clin Lung Cancer 2004;6:175-183.
133. Pujol JL, Carestia L, Daures JP. Is there a case for cisplatin in the treatment of small-cell lung cancer? A meta-analysis of randomized trials of a cisplatin-containing regimen versus a regimen without this alkylating agent. Br J Cancer 2000;83:8-15.
134. Lara PN Jr, Chansky K, Davies AM, et al. Bortezomib (PS-341) in relapsed or refractory extensive stage small cell lung cancer: a Southwest Oncology Group Phase II trial (S0327). J Thorac Oncol 2006;1:996-1001.
135. Spigel DR, Hainsworth JD, Simons L, et al. Irinotecan, carboplatin, and imatinib in untreated extensive-stage small-cell lung cancer: a Phase II trial of the Minnie Pearl Cancer Research Network. J Thorac Oncol 2007;2:854-861.
136. Onoda S, Masuda N, Seto T, et al. Phase II trial of amrubicin for treatment of refractory or relapsed small-cell lung cancer: Thoracic Oncology Research Group Study 0301. J Clin Oncol 2006;24:5448-5453.
137. Yana T, Negoro S, Takada M, et al. Phase II study of amrubicin in previously untreated patients with extensive-disease small cell lung cancer: West Japan Thoracic Oncology Group (WJTOG) study. Invest New Drugs 2007;25:253-258.
138. Riedel RF, Crawford J, Dunphy F, et al. Phase II study of carboplatin, irinotecan, and thalidomide combination in patients with extensive stage small-cell lung cancer. Lung Cancer 2006;54:431-432.
139. Dowlati A, Subbiah S, Cooney M, et al. Phase II trial of thalidomide as maintenance therapy for extensive stage small cell lung cancer after response to chemotherapy. Lung Cancer 2007;56:377-381.
140. Pujol JL, Breton JL, Gervais R, et al. Phase III double-blind, placebo-controlled study of thalidomide in extensive-disease small-cell lung cancer after response to chemotherapy: an intergroup study FNCLCC cleo04 IFCT 00-01. J Clin Oncol 2007;25:3945-3951.

65

BREAST CANCER

Vivek Roy and Edith A. Perez

INTRODUCTION 933
THERAPEUTICS AND CLINICAL PHARMACOLOGY 933
Rationale and Goals of Therapy 933
Primary Prevention 933
Adjuvant Therapy 933
Treatment of Metastatic Disease 934
Therapeutics by Class 934
Endocrine Therapy 934
Chemotherapy 935
Targeted Therapy 937
Therapeutic Approach 939
Adjuvant Therapy 939
Therapy for Metastatic Disease 941

INTRODUCTION

Breast cancer (BC) is one of the most common malignancies in women in the United States. In 2007, over 180,510 new cases were expected to be diagnosed.[1] Approximately 5% to 10% of BC patients have metastatic disease at presentation. Another 30% of patients who present with early-stage BC will later develop metastatic disease. The outlook for metastatic breast cancer (MBC) remains poor, with median survival of 18 to 24 months (at least utilizing older hormonal and chemotherapeutic agents), and only 6 to 12 months for patients with predominantly visceral disease.[1] In recent years there has been a decrease in mortality rates from BC, likely due to early detection as well as improvements in the treatment of early-stage BC.

The treatment of BC continues to evolve as the pathophysiology of cancer, including BC, is better understood. Elucidation of cellular pathways and molecules involved in cancer cell proliferation and apoptosis have presented opportunities for targeted interventions. Therapies directed at pathways that are uniquely or predominantly involved in malignant transformation may result in clinical benefit with minimal toxicities. Additionally, several new conventional chemotherapeutic agents that have increased efficacy and/or better tolerability have also been developed.

In this chapter we present an overview of the pharmacotherapy of BC. We discuss the various classes of agents used for the treatment of BC, the goals and philosophy of treatment of early- and late-stage BC, practical therapeutic approaches, and future directions. It is important to appreciate that BC is a heterogeneous disease with diverse tumor-specific characteristics and clinical presentations. A thorough understanding of these factors along with patients' specific characteristics and preferences determines the most appropriate therapeutic approach for any given patient.

THERAPEUTICS AND CLINICAL PHARMACOLOGY

Rationale and Goals of Therapy

Pharmacotherapy of BC can be considered in three broad categories:

1. Primary prevention
2. Adjuvant therapy
3. Treatment of metastatic disease

Primary Prevention

Several risk factors for BC have been identified in epidemiologic studies. However, even when the factors are potentially modifiable, a significant, sustained, and long-term behavioral or lifestyle change is required, limiting the practical utility of those interventions. Estrogen exposure is a well-known risk factor for causation of BC,[2] and reducing the exposure, such as by oophorectomy, has long been known to result in the reduction of risk of BC.[3,4] Prophylactic oophorectomy or mastectomy, although effective, is a highly invasive intervention suitable only for very high-risk circumstances.

The pharmacologic approach to preventing BC has utilized agents that block the synthesis or action of estrogen. Tamoxifen is a selective estrogen receptor modulator (SERM) that binds to the estrogen receptors and either mimics or antagonizes the action of estrogen in a tissue-dependent manner. In breast tissue, tamoxifen blocks estrogen-dependent proliferation. Tamoxifen was first used in the adjuvant setting in BC patients, in whom it was noted to prevent not only systemic recurrence but also the occurrence of new primary cancer in the contralateral breast. This laid the foundation for testing tamoxifen as a chemopreventive agent for primary prevention. A large randomized, controlled trial by the National Surgical Adjuvant Breast and Bowel Project (NSABP), in which women at high risk for BC received 5 years of tamoxifen or placebo, showed a 49% reduction in the incidence of invasive and noninvasive BC in the tamoxifen arm.[5] Long-term follow-up studies have shown that the risk reduction persists for at least 10 years.[6,7] Concerns about the side effects, such as endometrial proliferation leading to endometrial malignancy, have limited the widespread acceptance of tamoxifen for primary prevention of BC.[8]

Raloxifene (a SERM alternative to tamoxifen) was approved by the U.S. Food and Drug Administration (FDA) for prevention and treatment of osteoporosis. Both animal and human data also suggested its activity as a BC preventive agent. Unlike tamoxifen, raloxifene does not have estrogenic effects, making it an attractive agent to investigate for primary BC prevention. The Study of Tamoxifen and Raloxifene (STAR) trial was designed to compare the two drugs for BC prevention. It enrolled 19,747 postmenopausal women who were at increased risk for developing BC. Participants were randomly assigned to receive either 60 mg of raloxifene or 20 mg of tamoxifen daily for 5 years. Both drugs reduced the risk of developing invasive BC by about 50%. In addition, women assigned to take raloxifene had fewer uterine cancers (relative risk 0.62) and blood clots (relative risk 0.70) than the women who were assigned to take tamoxifen.[9] Thus, there was a minimal overall improvement with raloxifene compared to tamoxifen, but this was not a breakthrough study.

Aromatase inhibitors (AIs) have shown superiority over tamoxifen in the adjuvant treatment of BC in many studies.[10] In these studies, a reduced risk of contralateral breast cancer in AI-treated patients was also noted, raising the possibility of AIs being effective as primary preventive agents. These studies are currently ongoing.

Adjuvant Therapy

Adjuvant therapy is defined as treatment given to patients who remain at high risk of recurrence after all evidence of cancer has been surgically removed. It has long been observed that, even after adequate loco-regional treatment (surgical removal of breast tumor and axillary lymph node with or without radiation therapy), systemic recurrences can occur, suggesting that unrecognized micrometastases must be present in the body that later lead to systemic recurrence. The underlying rationale for adjuvant therapy is that cancer cells acquire additional genetic abnormalities and resistance to therapy with advancing disease burden, and chemotherapy may be able to eradicate micrometastatic disease but not established clinically evident metastases.

Adjuvant therapy for BC has evolved over the years as our understanding of BC biology has improved and newer agents have become available that are effective against BC. Estrogen is a potent promoter of BC growth. The ovaries are the predominant source of estrogen in premenopausal women, with only a small amount produced by aromatization in extragonadal tissues. In contrast, peripheral aromatase-mediated conversion of androgens is the main source of estrogen in postmenopausal women. This important physiologic difference supports the rationale for ovarian suppression therapy for premenopausal women with hormone-responsive BC. Oophorectomy was the first adjuvant therapeutic maneuver used based on its proven activity against demonstrable disease.[11] AIs can be used for postmenopausal women only, whereas tamoxifen is active in both pre- and postmenopausal women.

Agents for adjuvant therapy have traditionally been chosen based on their efficacy in metastatic settings, where responses can be readily observed. Bonadonna and colleagues were the first to demonstrate efficacy of combination chemotherapy for BC adjuvant therapy.[12] Since then, multiple studies have established the role of adjuvant therapy in BC, and newer, more effective agents have been introduced over time. Studies are ongoing to define the optimal agents, drug combinations, and schedules as well as to test novel approaches. Systemic adjuvant therapy (chemotherapy or endocrine therapy), while effective, is not without potentially serious side effects. Therefore, treatment decisions need to take into account individual patients' recurrence risks. Predictive and prognostic factors such as tumor size, grade, histologic type, hormone receptor expression, *HER2* status, and lymph node involvement are some of the factors that must be considered in addition to patient age, impairment of functional status that may alter the risk : benefit ratio, and patient's preference. Genetic profiling using gene expression analysis can be helpful in further refining risk stratification and predicting benefit from systemic hormonal or chemotherapy, but a lot of additional work is needed to identify the best profile to utilize in practice.[13,14]

Treatment of Metastatic Disease

The ideal goal of treatment of MBC is cure. However, that goal is currently unattainable for the vast majority of patients, and MBC remains essentially an incurable disease. In the absence of cure as a realistic possibility, the primary goal of MBC therapy is disease control, symptom palliation, improvement in quality of life, and, where possible, improvement in survival. Tumor regression often (but not always) correlates with symptom control and better quality of life.[15] There is also evidence of correlation between quality of life with time-to-progression and overall survival in patients with MBC.[16,17] On the other hand, chemotherapy itself can lead to a variety of toxicities. Potential beneficial effects of chemotherapy must be carefully balanced against the toxicities to maximize the possibility of net improvement in quality of life.

The biologic characteristics of BC in addition to the extent of disease, organs involved, and the patient's general health status influence the choice of agents. Hormonal therapy is generally the first consideration in patients with hormone receptor–positive MBC, especially if the disease is limited to the bones with no (or minimal) visceral organ involvement. Tamoxifen had been the drug of choice in this setting for many years.[18] AIs are now preferred agents in postmenopausal patients, with several trials showing improved outcomes and their generally better toxicity profile.[19-21] Chemotherapy remains the mainstay of treatment for the majority of patients with MBC at presentation or after progression on hormonal interventions.

Therapeutics by Class

Agents effective against BC can be categorized into distinct classes. In this section we describe the principal classes of agents in clinical use or under development. Their mechanisms of action, common side effects, and an overview of data supporting their use in BC are provided.

Endocrine Therapy

BC is an estrogen-driven cancer in the majority of women, and estrogen withdrawal is associated with retardation of tumor growth.

Oophorectomy/Gonadotropin-Releasing Hormone Analogues. Oophorectomy was recognized as a treatment option for MBC more than 100 years ago.[11] Gonadotropin-releasing hormone (GnRH) analogues can provide reversible ovarian function suppression. These agents act by binding to and down-regulating GnRH receptors on the pituitary, leading to suppression of luteinizing hormone and release of follicle-stimulating hormone and, finally, decrease in estradiol production by the ovaries. GnRH analogues result in tumor regression in hormone receptor–positive BC and are approved by the FDA for treatment of MBC in premenopausal women.[22,23] Postmenopausal levels of estrogen and progesterone are attained in 2 to 4 weeks after the start of therapy. Leuprolide and goserelin are the most commonly used agents in this class. Both are administered by intramuscular injection every month, although longer acting depot preparations are also available. They are generally well tolerated, but hot flashes and nausea occur in some women and their use is associated with bone mineral loss.

Selective Estrogen Receptor Modulators. SERMs are agents that bind to the estrogen receptors and either mimic or antagonize the action of estrogen in a tissue-dependent manner. Tamoxifen, the prototype SERM, is the most commonly used and most studied agent in this class. It is a nonsteroidal antiestrogen that acts by competitive binding to the estrogen receptor. Clinical trials with tamoxifen have been conducted in advanced disease and adjuvant settings as well as for chemoprevention. In MBC, response is seen in up to 50% to 60% of patients with estrogen receptor–positive disease.[24,25] It has an established role in adjuvant therapy, with many studies showing improvement in disease-free and overall survival.[26,27] Tamoxifen is generally well tolerated. The most frequent side effects are hot flashes, vaginal discharge or bleeding, and menstrual irregularities. There is a higher incidence of thromboembolic events, and a two to three times higher risk of endometrial cancer in tamoxifen-treated women.[26]

Raloxifene is another SERM that has no proliferative effects on the uterine endometrium, and consequently its use is not associated with risk of endometrial carcinoma. Its role as a potential primary preventive agent is being evaluated in the STAR trial. Preliminary results suggest that raloxifene has efficacy equivalent to tamoxifen in postmenopausal women and a better side effect profile.[9]

Aromatase Inhibitors. The enzyme aromatase converts androstenedione into estrone, and testosterone to estrogen, and is the primary source of estrogen in postmenopausal women. AIs block this enzyme and consequently decrease estrogen levels. The first AI to be clinically used was aminoglutethimide in the 1970s. Its lack of specificity for aromatase caused adrenal suppression and other toxicities, preventing its widespread use despite clinical efficacy. The second-generation agent formestane had more aromatase enzyme specificity and fewer side effects but required twice-weekly intramuscular administration.[28] Three newer "third-generation," highly specific AI agents are currently in clinical use. Anastrazole and letrozole are nonsteroidal compounds that cause reversible aromatase enzyme inhibition, and exemestane is a steroidal compound that causes nonreversible inhibition.

All AI agents have excellent oral bioavailability and offer significant advantages over previously available hormonal treatments for BC. They are generally well tolerated, with hot flashes, arthralgias, and loss of bone mineral density as the main side effects. Additionally, adverse effects on lipid profiles have been reported. There are pharmacokinetic differences between the three available AIs and also differences in their

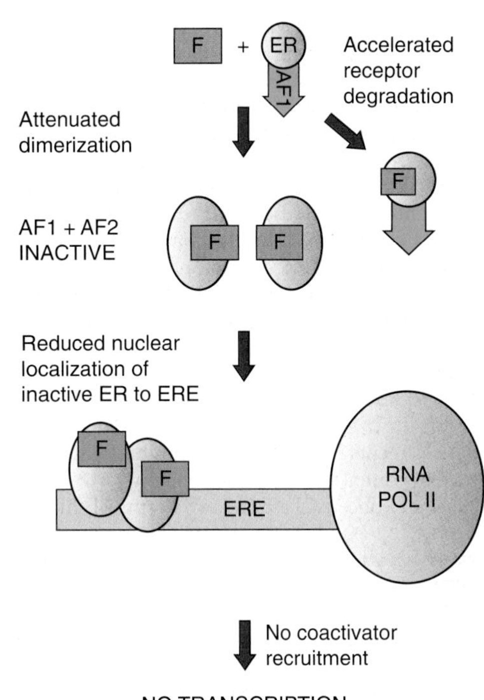

FIGURE 65-1 • **Fulvestrant.**

effects on bone health and lipid profiles, but any long-term effects of these differences are unclear.[29]

Estrogen Receptor Down-regulators. Fulvestrant is the prototype example of this class of drugs (Fig. 65-1). It is an estrogen receptor antagonist with no agonistic effects in any tissue. It binds to and causes down-regulation of estrogen receptors. The FDA has approved fulvestrant for women with MBC whose disease has progressed after antiestrogen treatment. It is approved for administration as a 250-mg intramuscular injection once a month. The role of a loading dose (500 mg) to rapidly achieve a therapeutic level is under investigation. Fulvestrant was at least as efficacious as anastrazole in two Phase III clinical trials in postmenopausal women with MBC that had progressed on prior endocrine therapy.[30,31] As a third-line agent after tamoxifen and AIs, fulvestrant was associated with stable disease or response in 35% of patients with MBC.[32] In a randomized, double-blind, double-dummy, multicenter Phase III trial comparing the efficacy and tolerability of fulvestrant versus exemestane in postmenopausal women with hormone receptor–positive advanced BC that had progressed or recurred after prior nonsteroidal AI therapy, fulvestrant was equally effective and well tolerated as exemestane. A loading-dose regimen was used for fulvestrant: a 500-mg intramuscular injection on day 0, 250 mg on days 14 and 28, and 250 mg every 28 days thereafter. A steady state level of fulvestrant was reached in 1 month.[33]

Chemotherapy

Breast cancer is one of the most chemosensitive solid tumors. A variety of chemotherapeutic agents that target different cell cycle processes vital for cell survival have been used. These include antimetabolites (methotrexate, 5-fluorouracil [5-FU], gemcitabine, pemetrexed), DNA alkylating agents (cyclophosphamide, platinum compounds), topoisomerase II inhibitors (anthracyclines, etoposide), a topoisimerase I inhibitor (irinotecan), and microtubule function inhibitors (taxanes, vinorelbine). Introduction of many agents over the past few years has been associated with meaningful improvement in outcomes. Salient features of commonly used chemotherapeutic agents are described in this section. Specific treatment approaches are reviewed later in the chapter.

Established Chemotherapy Agents

Cyclophosphamide. Alkylating agents were one of the first classes of drugs used for MBC or adjuvant treatment of BC. They cause cross-linking of DNA strands, which prevents further DNA replication and cell division. These agents can affect cells in all phases of the cell cycle (cell cycle nonspecific). Cyclophosphamide, the most commonly used drug in this class, is an inactive prodrug that is transformed via hepatic intracellular enzymes to the active alkylating metabolites 4-hydroxycyclophophosphamide, aldophosphamide, acrolein, and phosphoramide mustard. It has been the cornerstone of adjuvant therapy of BC as part of the CMF (cyclophosphamide, methotrexate, 5-FU) regimen or in combination with an anthracycline.[34] Objective responses are seen in 25% to 60% of MBC patients with single-agent cyclophosphamide or a combination.[34] In addition to side effects such as nausea, vomiting, alopecia, and myelosuppression that are seen with most chemotherapeutic agents, urinary bladder irritation causing hematuria, and risk of myelodysplasia and acute leukemia are important side effects with cyclophosphamide.

Platinum Compounds. Cisplatin and carboplatin are alkylating agents with significant activity against several malignancies, including BC. They have been used to treat BC either singly or in combination with other agents. Nausea, vomiting, alopecia, and myelosuppression are seen with both these agents; delayed nausea is a particularly bothersome side effect associated with cisplatinum use. Nephrotoxicity, ototoxicity, and neuropathy are other notable toxicities of cisplatinum and to a lesser extent of carboplatin. As a single agent, carboplatin results in responses in 20% to 35% of previously untreated patients with MBC.[35-37] There is also evidence of preclinical and potentially clinical synergism with other cytotoxic agents. Because of synergism, different mechanisms of action, and nonoverlapping toxicities, platinum compounds are often used in combination with taxanes, gemcitabine, or trastuzumab.[38-41]

Anthracyclines. Anthracyclines have long been an important component of BC therapy both in adjuvant and metastatic settings. Responses are seen in 35% to 50% of anthracycline-naive MBC patients. Doxorubicin and epirubicin are the two anthracyclines commonly used for BC therapy. In addition to nausea, vomiting, alopecia, and myelosuppression, myocardial damage resulting in heart failure is a major adverse effect. Cardiac toxicity is related to cumulative dose, a major factor limiting anthracycline use in MBC. Coadministration of anthracycline and trastuzumab results in potentiation of cardiotoxicity and is contraindicated. Liposomal formulation of doxorubicin reduces the cardiotoxicity while maintaining antitumor efficacy and allows a higher total dose to be administered.[42] Anthracyclines are a major component of many multidrug BC regimens such as AC (doxorubicin [Adriamycin], cyclophosphamide), FAC (5-FU, doxorubicin, cyclophosphamide), TAC (docetaxel [Taxotere], doxorubicin, cyclophosphamide), AT (doxorubicin, paclitaxel), and FEC (5-FU, epirubicin, cyclophosphamide). In general, multidrug combinations are more active than single agents but also have higher toxicity.

Taxanes. Paclitaxel and docetaxel are the two agents of this class in common use. They act by stabilization of cellular microtubule elements leading to mitotic arrest. They have both been used as single agents or in combination with other chemotherapeutic drugs. As single agents, the responses range from 20% to 60% in Phase II studies for MBC.[43] Side effects associated with docetaxel and paclitaxel include neutropenia, infection, asthenia, fatigue, myalgias, mucositis, nail changes, and neuropathy. There are also important differences in their toxicity profiles. Hypersensitivity reactions and neuropathy are most commonly described with paclitaxel, whereas asthenia, fatigue, fluid retention, and nail changes are predominantly associated with docetaxel. In a randomized trial comparing docetaxel and paclitaxel, docetaxel was found to be superior with better overall survival and time to progression but with significantly more toxicity, although global quality-of-life scores were similar.[44]

Both paclitaxel and docetaxel were initially developed and are commonly administered in an every-3-weeks schedule. Other dosing schedules have also been studied. A dose-dense, every-2-weeks schedule is also commonly utilized in adjuvant therapy for lymph node–positive breast cancer based on demonstrated benefit over an every-3-weeks schedule.[45] Weekly administration of paclitaxel as well as docetaxel appears to be better tolerated than an every-3-weeks schedule, with less hematologic toxicity.[46,47] In a recent study, weekly paclitaxel after doxorubicin and cyclophosphamide was found to be superior to every-3-weeks paclitaxel, or weekly or every-3-weeks docetaxel as adjuvant therapy for breast cancer.[47a]

Taxanes and anthracyclines are probably the most active agents against BC. The combination of doxorubicin and paclitaxel showed a higher response rate (RR) but was more toxic as first-line therapy of MBC compared with doxorubicin and cyclophosphamide. Moreover, overall survival was not significantly different.[48] The three-drug combination TAC (docetaxel, doxorubicin, cyclophosphamide) was shown to be active with manageable toxicity.[49] A Phase III trial comparing TAC with FAC (5-FU, doxorubicin, cyclophosphamide), reported in an abstract, showed a higher RR (54% vs. 43%) but not overall survival (21 vs. 21 months) with TAC. Neutropenia was six times more common in the TAC regimen. In contrast to docetaxel, paclitaxel in combination with other drugs has shown less consistent results. Higher RRs and toxicity were seen with doxorubicin compared to paclitaxel as a single agent.[50] Doxorubicin in combination with paclitaxel was associated with RRs and survival similar to doxorubicin and cyclophosphamide in a multicenter Phase III clinical trial.[51] A randomized three-arm trial in 739 patients compared doxorubicin (60 mg/m^2), paclitaxel (175 mg/m^2 per 24 hours), and the combination of doxorubicin and paclitaxel (AT; 50 mg/m^2 and 150 mg/m^2 per 24 hours, respectively) as first-line therapy for MBC. Patients who were originally assigned to the single agent crossed over to the second drug on progression. Doxorubicin and paclitaxel were equally effective, but the combination of AT resulted in superior overall RRs and time to treatment failure. However, the combination therapy with AT did not improve either survival or quality of life compared to sequential single-agent therapy.[52]

Capecitabine. 5-Fluorouracil is an antimetabolite that has long been used in the treatment of breast cancer. It is administered by the intravenous route, mostly as a bolus, in BC treatment. There is strong evidence from studies in colorectal carcinoma and other cancers that prolonged infusion is more effective than bolus administration. However, infusional 5-FU is rarely used in BC. Capecitabine is an oral fluoropyrimidine prodrug that is converted in the tumor cells to 5-FU by the enzyme thymidine phosphorylase. Because of sustained exposure, the overall effect on the cancer cell mimics that of infusional 5-FU. Capecitabine is approved by the FDA for use in MBC progressing after taxane therapy. In a Phase II trial of heavily pretreated patients with MBC, including those who had received both anthracycline and taxane therapy, a 20% to 25% RR was observed with capecitabine, and an additional 43% of patients maintained stable disease status. Eighty-two percent of these patients had previously been treated with 5-FU.[53]

The main side effects of capecitabine are nausea, diarrhea, oral mucositis, hand-foot syndrome, and myelosuppression. The oral route of administration is attractive to patients as this allows less time to be spent in the physician's office or clinic. Capecitabine is also approved in combination with docetaxel for treatment of MBC patients who have progressed after anthracycline treatment. A capecitabine and docetaxel combination was shown to result in a superior RR (42% vs. 30%) and survival (14.5 vs. 11.5 months) compared with docetaxel alone.[54,55] Combination therapy had more frequent but manageable side effects. Whether capecitabine and docetaxel used in sequence rather than in combination will result in similar outcomes is an important unanswered question.

Gemcitabine. Gemcitabine (difluorodeoxycytidine) is a novel pyrimidine nucleotide antimetabolite that is phosphorylated intracellularly to the active triphosphate, which inhibits DNA replication and RNA synthesis. Incorporation of gemcitabine triphosphate in the DNA makes it resistant to exonuclease excision leading to apoptosis. Gemcitabine has activity in a wide variety of malignancies, including cancer of the pancreas, lung, breast, bladder, and ovaries and lymphomas.

Typically, gemcitabine is administered as a weekly intravenous injection and is usually very well tolerated. Neutropenia and thrombocytopenia are the main dose-limiting toxicities, with a low incidence of nausea or alopecia. RRs in previously treated or newly diagnosed patients with MBC were similar (26%) in Phase II studies.[56,57] Based on minimal toxicity and potential synergism, combinations of gemcitabine and other chemotherapeutic agents with different mechanisms of action have been evaluated. In a Phase III trial that included 529 patients with previously untreated metastatic or locally recurrent inoperable BC, a gemcitabine and paclitaxel combination showed an RR (45.5 vs. 25.5%, $P < .00005$) and median overall survival (18.5 vs. 15.8 months) superior to paclitaxel alone.[58] More grade 3 and 4 neutropenia was seen in the combination arm (48% vs. 11%), but febrile neutropenia was infrequent in both arms (5% vs. 1%). A gemcitabine and docetaxel combination for MBC has been studied in Phase II trials, with RRs ranging from 36% to 79%.[59,60] A Phase III trial of 355 patients receiving first- or second-line treatment for MBC compared a gemcitabine and docetaxel combination with capecitabine and docetaxel and found similar frequency and duration of responses but lower toxicity with the gemcitabine-docetaxel combination (hand-foot syndrome: 0 vs. 26%; diarrhea, 8% vs. 29%; mucositis, 6% vs. 26%).[61]

Vinorelbine. Vinorelbine is a second-generation semisynthetic vinca alkaloid that, in contrast to earlier generation vinca alkaloids, has substitution in the catharanthine moiety of the molecule. It exerts cytotoxic effects by binding to tubulin and disrupting the mitotic spindle apparatus during metaphase. Antitumor activity of vinorelbine has been demonstrated in several preclinical studies against many cancer cell lines and xenograft tumor models, including BC. In Phase II and III studies in advanced BC, RRs of 40% to 59% were demonstrated.[62-64] Encouraging RRs have also been reported with a combination of vinorelbine and doxorubicin, docetaxel, or trastuzumab.[65-67] Nausea, vomiting, myelosuppression, alopecia, asthenia, and neuromyopathy are the main adverse effects. Vinorelbine is administered intravenously, although an orally bioavailable formulation has also been evaluated in a Phase II study in women with MBC over the age of 65.[68] Oral vinorelbine was well tolerated but has a low level of objective efficacy (complete response + partial response rate of 12%).

Etoposide. Etoposide is a semisynthetic podophyllotoxin derivative that exerts its anticancer effect through topoisomerase II inhibition. It was introduced in clinical trials in the 1970s. Initial studies with etoposide, which used intravenous administration on day 1 or days 1 through 3 (or 5) every 3 to 4 weeks, showed disappointing results in the treatment of BC.[69] Later in its evaluation, schedule dependency was observed, suggesting that more prolonged exposure via an oral route may be more effective.[70] Etoposide has approximately 50% bioavailability orally. In a Phase II study in previously treated MBC patients, an objective RR was observed in 15 of 43 patients (35%) with a schedule of 50 mg/m^2 daily for 21 days every 4 weeks.[71] Oral etoposide is generally well tolerated, with myelosuppression, alopecia, and mucositis as the main adverse effects.

Irinotecan. Irinotecan, a semisynthetic derivative of camptothecin, is a topoisomerase I inhibitor. Irinotecan is converted in the cell to SN-38, its active metabolite, which has 250 to 1000 times more potent topoisomerase I inhibitory activity. Irinotecan is active against a broad spectrum of malignancies, including breast, colorectal, lung, and ovarian. In a Phase II study of previously treated MBC patients, a 23% RR was noted at a dose of 100 mg/m^2 weekly for 4 weeks, given every 6 weeks.[72] Neutropenia and diarrhea were the main adverse effects. The active metabolite SN-38 is glucuronidated to an inactive product by UDP-glucuronosyltransferase (UGT1A1). Since irinotecan toxicity is inversely related to SN-38 glucuronidation rate, individuals with low UGT1A1 expression or function may experience severe toxicity.[73] Encouraging single-agent activity has led to its evaluation in combination with other agents such as docetaxel that act through different intracellular mechanisms and have nonoverlapping side effect profiles. Phase I studies showed that this combination is feasible with an acceptable toxicity profile.[74,75] Phase II studies are in progress.

Pemetrexed. Pemetrexed is a novel folate antimetabolite that inhibits a number of folate-dependent enzymes, including thymidylate synthase, dihydrofolate reductase, and glycinamide ribonucleotide formyltransferase involved in purine and pyrimidine synthesis.[76] The major toxicities of pemetrexed are myelosuppression, mucositis, skin rash, transient elevations of liver transaminases, and rise in homocystine level. Vitamin B_{12} and folate supplementation has been shown to ameliorate pemetrexed toxicity and is recommended from the start of treatment. Pemetrexed was approved for the treatment of malignant mesothelioma, but single-agent pemetrexed has activity against a variety of tumors, including lung, colorectal, head and neck, and breast. Response rate of 10% to 28% were observed in previously treated MBC patients, including those previously treated with anthracyclines and taxanes.[77,78] A combination of pemetrexed with gemcitabine had an overall RR of 24% (14 of 59 patients) in a Phase II trial of anthracycline- and taxane-treated MBC patients.[79]

Newer Chemotherapy Agents

Nanoparticle Albumin-Bound Paclitaxel (NAB-Paclitaxel; Abraxane). The poor solubility of paclitaxel requires the use of the lipid-based solvent polyoxyl castor oil (Cremophor EL; BASF, Ludwigshafen, Germany) as a vehicle, which can cause histamine-mediated hypersensitivity reactions. This necessitates the use of prophylactic premedications and slow infusion of the drug to minimize the risk of hypersensitivity reactions. Despite this, severe or fatal reactions can still occur.[80] Abraxane (Abraxis Oncology, Schaumburg, IL) is a polyoxyl castor oil–free formulation in which paclitaxel is delivered as a suspension of albumin nanoparticles (average size 130 nm), eliminating the need for premedication or special infusion sets, and allowing infusion to be safely given over 30 minutes. Additionally, drug transport into tumors may be enhanced by albumin receptor–mediated transport across endothelial cells.[81] A Phase II study testing the albumin-bound formulation of paclitaxel demonstrated the safety of a high dose of 300 mg/m^2 infused over 30 minutes without premedication. RRs (complete and partial responses) of 64% and 21% were seen in first-line and subsequent-line treatment of MBC, respectively.[82] In a Phase III trial comparison of NAB-paclitaxel (260 mg/m^2) given without premedication over 30 minutes every 3 weeks with paclitaxel (175 mg/m^2) every 3 weeks, no hypersensitivity reactions and a significantly higher RR, time to progression, and lower incidence of grade 4 neutropenia were seen with NAB-paclitaxel.[83] Preliminary data suggest superior activity of weekly NAB-paclitaxel compared to an every-3-weeks schedule. Every-3-weeks NAB-paclitaxel (300 mg/m^2) had RRs similar to docetaxel (100 mg/m^2 every 3 weeks) but less neutropenia.[84] Studies are ongoing to evaluate NAB-paclitaxel in combination with other agents and encouraging results have been presented.[84a]

Ixabepilone. Ixabepilone, a novel semisynthetic analogue of epothelone B, is a tubulin-polymerizing agent in development for the treatment of breast and other cancers. It binds to the same binding site on tubulin as paclitaxel, and leads to microtubule stabilization, causing cell cycle arrest and apoptosis.[85] It has demonstrated activity against BC, including in patients with taxane-refractory disease. An objective response was seen in 22% of previously taxane-treated MBC patients in a Phase II trial.[86] Ixabepilone demonstrated clear activity and a manageable safety profile in patients with MBC resistant to anthracycline, taxane, and capecitabine, including in patients who had not previously responded to multiple prior therapies.[86a] The activity of ixabepilone in taxane-refractory disease makes it an attractive alternative to paclitaxel in combination with other agents such as trastuzumab or carboplatin. A Phase II trial of trastuzumab with weekly carboplatin and ixabepilone in patients with HER2-overexpressing MBC is ongoing through the North Central Cancer Treatment Group. A multicenter, multinational Phase III trial sponsored by Bristol-Myers Squibb comparing ixabepilone plus capecitabine versus capecitabine alone is also in progress. Accrual of approximately 1200 patients is planned, with overall survival as the primary end point.

Vinflunine. Vinflunine is a new tubulin-targeted third-generation vinca alkaloid. It was developed by a semisynthetic process using superacidic chemistry to introduce two fluorine atoms into the vinorelbine molecule.[87] Vinflunine is freely water soluble, obviating the need for polyoxyl castor oil or other solvents, as well as the need for steroid premedication. Based on its activity on cell lines as well as human tumor xenograft models, human studies were conducted that showed activity in second- and third-line treatment of MBC (RR 30%; stable disease RR 36%; $N = 60$).[88] Further studies to define the role of vinflunine in BC are ongoing.

Targeted Therapy

Chemotherapy agents achieve their cytotoxic effects by disrupting critical cellular functions that are common to both malignant and normal cells. Consequently, they have a narrow therapeutic window. Improved understanding of the cellular biology of cancer has identified cellular pathways and molecules that are uniquely or predominantly altered in cancer cells. These alterations are responsible for causing, sustaining, or potentiating the cancer phenotype. Targeting these pathways for therapy (targeted therapy) offers the prospect of anticancer efficacy with minimal effect on the normal tissues (toxicities). Targeted therapies may also be able to synergize with conventional chemotherapy agents or other targeted agents. With improved techniques to identify deranged pathways or cellular proteins specific to a given tumor, it is hoped that targeted therapies can in the future be chosen to suit the unique phenotype of that tumor (individualized therapy). The following are some of the targeted therapy agents in use or in development for BC.

Epidermal Growth Factor Receptor Inhibitors. The epidermal growth factor receptor (EGFR) family of transmembrane tyrosine kinase (TK) receptors is important for the growth and survival of epithelial cells. Receptor activation leads to dimerization followed by sequential phosphorylation of downstream messenger molecules, culminating in transcription of the genes responsible for cell proliferation. In several human cancers, including BC, overexpression of EGFR has been shown to be associated with poor prognosis. Four members

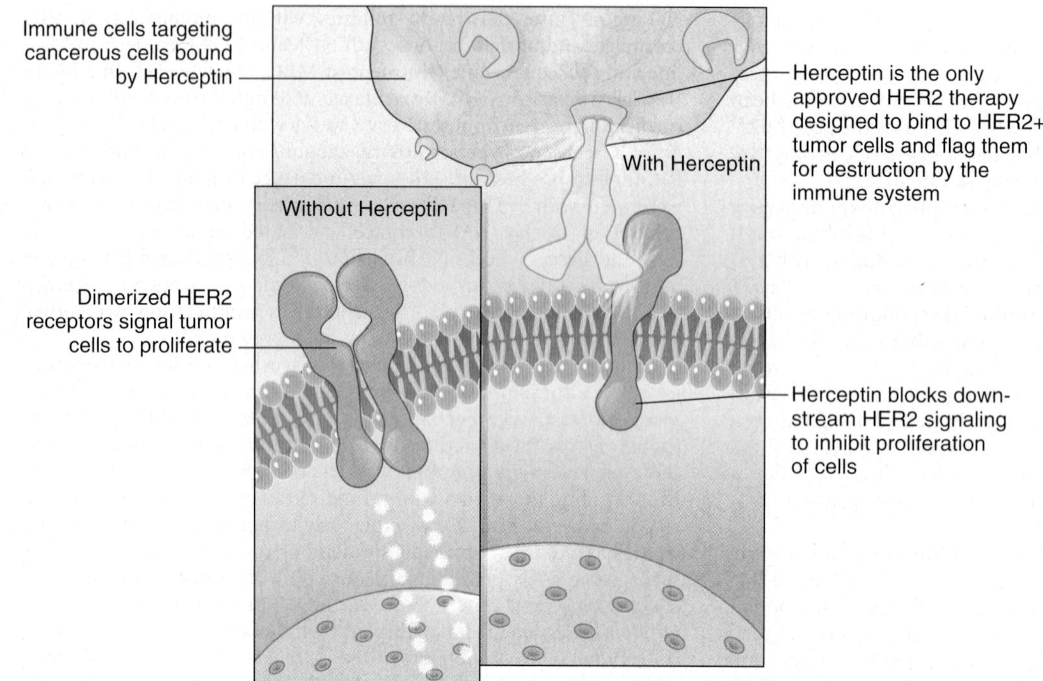

FIGURE 65-2 • Trastuzumab.

of the EGFR family are described: HER1, HER2 (neu/ErbB2), HER3, and HER4.[89] Expression of HER2 (the best-recognized EGFR in breast cancer) is amplified in 20% to 25% of invasive BCs (termed HER2 positive) and confers an adverse prognosis.

Trastuzumab. Trastuzumab, a humanized monoclonal antibody directed against the extracellular domain of HER2 (Fig. 65-2), is biologically active and has been shown to improve the survival of patients with HER2-positive MBC as evaluated by protein expression or gene amplification.[90,91] Accurate assessment of *HER2* status in all patients is critical in order to provide them with the opportunity to benefit from this life-prolonging therapy. It is important that this be performed in an appropriately experienced laboratory.[92] Preclinical data also suggests that trastuzumab may induce a receptor-enhanced chemosensitivity effect in the presence of activated HER2 signaling even without HER2 overexpression.[93] Trastuzumab is approved for weekly administration in the United States, but pharmacokinetics data and clinical experience suggest that an every-3-weeks schedule, which may be preferred by the patients, is safe and effective.[94] Multiple Phase II trials have shown that trastuzumab can be effectively combined with other chemotherapeutic agents, such as vinorelbine, gemcitabine, carboplatinum, or paclitaxel.[95-97] Despite the success of trastuzumab, less than 50% of patients who overexpress HER2 respond, and almost all eventually progress. Newer small-molecule or antibody inhibitors of HER2 are in development.

Lapatinib. Lapatinib is an orally active small-molecule inhibitor of HER1- and HER2-associated TK. It has shown efficacy, alone and with conventional chemotherapy, in patients with HER2-positive BC who had progressed during trastuzumab treatment.[98] A Phase II trial of lapatinib as first-line treatment of HER2-positive metastatic or locally advanced BC showed a 35% RR.[99] This agent is being actively investigated in several Phase III trials. In a randomized, controlled trial of capecitabine with or without lapatinib in HER2-positive locally advanced BC or MBC that had progressed after prior anthracycline, taxane, and trastuzumab therapy, significant prolongation in time to progression (8.4 vs. 4.4 months) and better overall RR (22% vs. 14%, $P = .09$) were observed with the combination arm. The study was closed on the recommendation of an independent Data Monitoring Committee based on the superior efficacy and acceptable toxicity of the combination regimen.[100] Trastuzumab does not cross the blood-brain barrier, and about a third of patients with HER2-positive MBC treated with trastuzumab develop central nervous system (CNS) metastasis. There is preliminary evidence that lapatinib can penetrate the CNS and may have activity in patients with HER2-positive CNS metastasis.[101] Lapatinib is generally well tolerated, with only rare decline in cardiac function that was nonprogressive or reversible.[102]

Angiogenesis Inhibitors. Angiogenesis is a critical factor in tumor progression. Vascular endothelial growth factor (VEGF) is an important angiogenic growth factor that has been implicated in the pathogenesis of a number of diseases, including BC. Higher levels of tumor VEGF expression correlate with a worse prognosis in BC. The angiogenic growth factor family, comprising five isoforms of VEGF (VEGF-A, -B, -C, -D, and -E) and placental growth factor, acts through three TK receptors: VEGF receptor (VEGFR)-1, VEGFR-2, and VEGFR-3. In addition to angiogenic activity, VEGF also has a powerful permeability-increasing effect on vasculature, which might contribute to tumor progression by enhancing nutrient exchange and easier intravasation of tumor cells during metastasis.

Bevacizumab, a recombinant humanized antibody, inhibits angiogenesis by binding to VEGF and preventing its binding to the receptor (Fig. 65-3). The ability of antiangiogenic agents to enhance the anticancer efficacy of conventional chemotherapeutic agents has been shown in randomized clinical trials in metastatic colorectal cancer and advanced non–small cell lung cancer, where the use of bevacizumab was associated with increased survival. A large randomized clinical trial in BC also showed a better RR (19.8%) with a combination of bevacizumab plus capecitabine compared with capecitabine alone (9.1%; $P = .001$), but without an associated survival benefit.[103] An interim planned analysis of a Phase III randomized, controlled, multicenter trial (E2100) of 722 women with previously untreated MBC showed marked improvement in progression-free survival in the bevacizumab plus paclitaxel arm compared with paclitaxel alone (11 vs. 6 months, respectively).[104] Multiple ongoing trials are evaluating the role of bevacizumab in MBC and high-risk early-stage BC. Hypertension, proteinuria, thromboembolic events, and hemorrhage are the main side effects of bevacizumab. Additionally, congestive heart failure in patients who had been exposed to anthracyclines, gastrointestinal perforations, and wound healing complications were observed as possible bevacizumab-associated adverse effects in recent Phase III trials.

Other small molecules that inhibit angiogenesis by disrupting VEGF signaling pathways are under investigation. In contrast to bevacizumab, they are orally active and some have the potential additional benefit of targeting multiple cellular pathways. Sunitinib (SU11248) is a multitargeted oral TK inhibitor with activity against VEGF, platelet-derived growth factor (PDGF), c-Kit, and Flt-3. A Phase II study ($N = 51$) of 50 mg a day for 28 days in a 42-day cycle in heavily pretreated patients with MBC found encouraging activity (partial response in 14% and stable disease in 2% of patients). About half the patients required dose reduction because of toxicity.[105] Further definitive studies are needed to clarify the role of these agents in BC therapy.

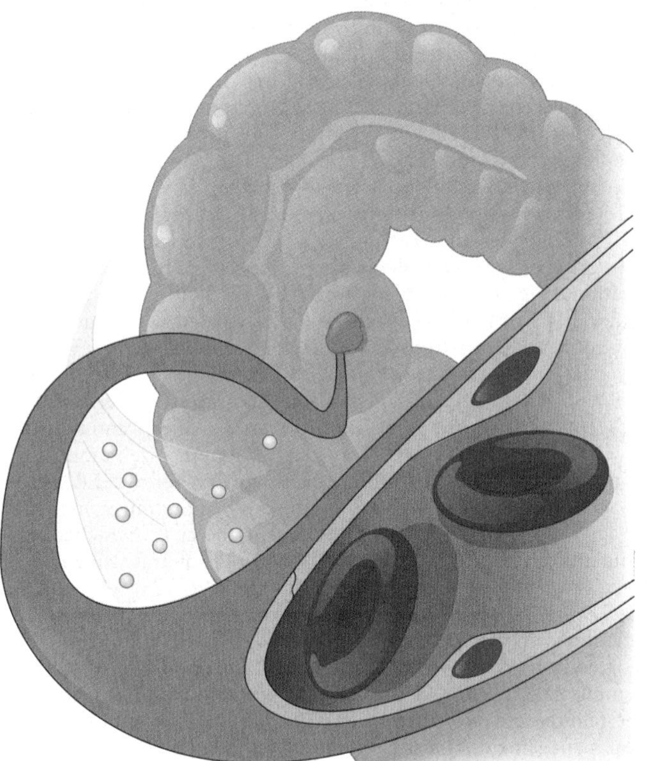

The angiogenesis-inhibiting monoclonal antibody bevacizumab blocks formation of blood vessels essential for tumor growth.

FIGURE 65-3 • Bevacizumab.

Ras/Raf/MEK/ERK Pathway Inhibitors. Activation of the Ras signaling pathway is considered an important mechanism of human oncogenesis. Ras regulates several pathways, including the Raf/mitogen-activated protein kinase (MAPK) and extracellular signal–regulated kinase (ERK) kinase (MEK)/ERK cascade, which synergistically induces cellular transformation. Ras-mediated activation of Raf leads to sequential phosphorylation and activation of MEK and ERK, which translocates from the cytoplasm to the nucleus and modulates the expression of growth-regulating genes. Therefore, inhibition of the Ras/Raf/MEK/ERK signaling pathway in tumors may be of clinical benefit.

Raf is a family of serine-threonine kinases that act as downstream effectors of the Ras pathway. Sorafenib (previously BAY43-9006) is a Raf kinase inhibitor with demonstrated activity in a broad spectrum of preclinical tumor models (Fig. 65-4). It also inhibits several receptor TKs that are involved in tumor progression, including VEGFR-2 and -3, PDGF receptor-β, Flt-3, c-Kit, and p38a (a member of the MAPK family). Sorafenib treatment resulted in reduction in tumor neovascularization in human tumor xenograft models. Only minimal single-agent activity was seen in previously anthracycline- and/or taxane-treated MBC patients.[106] However, given its broad spectrum of oral antitumor activity and inhibition of the Raf/MEK/ERK pathway and receptor TKs involved in tumor progression and angiogenesis, further evaluation of sorafenib in combination with other agents is ongoing.

Therapeutic Approach

Adjuvant Therapy

Adjuvant therapy in BC has been proven to improve disease-free and overall survival in multiple large, randomized, controlled clinical trials. It is thought to improve survival by eradicating micrometastatic disease that may later lead to systemic recurrence. Over the years, many hormonal agents and chemotherapy combinations and schedules have been studied with the aim of identifying the most efficacious treatment with the lowest possibility of toxicity. Several expert panels have published their recommendations to guide clinicians and place this vast body of data in context (Box 65-1). An important principle to appreciate when considering adjuvant therapy is that not all patients derive equal benefit from adjuvant therapy but all are equally exposed to the risks of therapy. It is important, therefore, to consider an individual

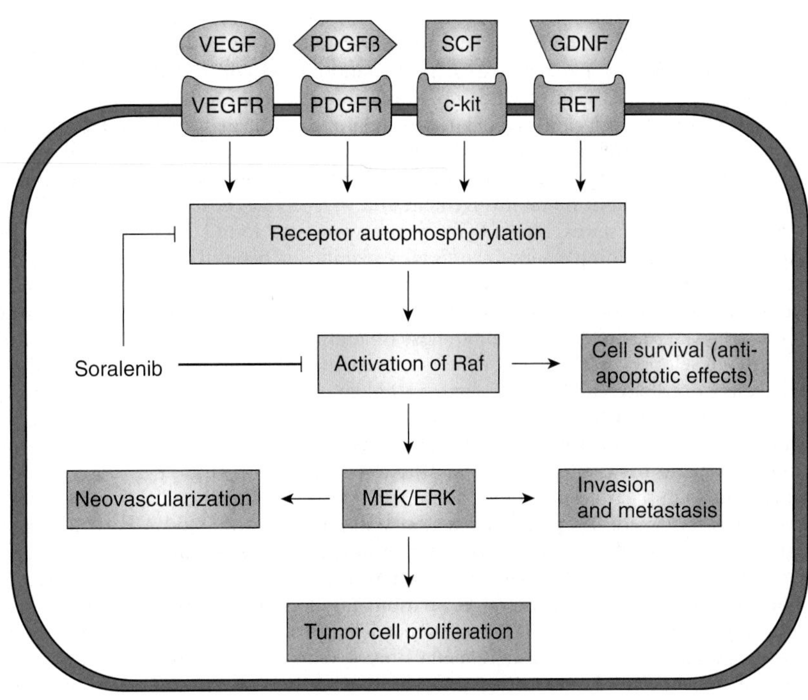

FIGURE 65-4 • Sorafenib.

BOX 65-1 ADJUVANT THERAPY OF BREAST CANCER: SUMMARY STATEMENTS

- Adjuvant therapy of BC leads to decreased relapse risk and improved survival.
- Adjuvant therapy should be considered in all patients with BC that is more than 1 cm or patients with lymph node metastasis, irrespective of tumor size. Some patients with smaller tumors may also be appropriate candidates for systemic adjuvant therapy.
- In postmenopausal women with hormone receptor–positive disease, antiestrogen therapy is the mainstay of adjuvant therapy.
- Aromatase inhibitors are preferred over tamoxifen for postmenopausal women because of better efficacy and favorable side effect profile.
- For premenopausal women or women with hormone receptor–negative disease, chemotherapy for 3 to 6 months should be considered.
- Anthracycline-containing regimens are more efficacious than non–anthracycline-containing regimens.
- Taxanes provide incremental benefit over anthracyclines but, because of increase in toxicity, their use should be limited to higher risk patients.
- Trastuzumab in conjunction with chemotherapy is recommended for women with HER2-overexpressing lymph node–positive disease or high-risk lymph node–negative disease.

patient's prognostic profile to estimate the recurrence risk and the expected reduction of the risk in absolute terms with adjuvant therapy. Factors such as tumor size, grade, lymph node metastasis, and hormone receptor and HER2 expression have been utilized to provide this valuable prognostic information. The relative and absolute improvement in risk can be estimated based on published results of adjuvant therapy clinical trials. In the last few years, evidence has emerged that tumor gene-expression profile can provide additional robust prognostic information[13,14] that can further refine the risk : benefit estimation. Validated instruments such as "adjuvantonline" that incorporate patient-specific prognostic information and data from published clinical trials to provide an individualized estimate of benefit with therapy are available online.

The Early Breast Cancer Trialists Collaborative Group (EBCTCG) undertakes a systematic review of all randomized, controlled clinical trials in early BC. In a review based on 47 randomized controlled trials involving 17,723 women with approximately 10 years of follow-up, they reported clear evidence of proportional reduction in recurrence risk with several months of combination chemotherapy.[107] The benefit of chemotherapy was seen in both pre- and postmenopausal women with or without nodal involvement and irrespective of tumor hormonal receptor status. The EBCTCG overview also found that anthracycline-containing regimens offered a significant benefit over non–anthracycline-containing regimens (such as cyclophosphamide, methotrexate, and 5-FU).[107] In 2000, the National Institutes of Health published a consensus statement on the use of adjuvant treatment for early BC developed by a panel of experts representing the disciplines of medical oncology, surgery, radiology, pathology, and public health as well as patient representatives.[108] In that report, the benefit of adjuvant endocrine therapy for hormone receptor–positive cancer, and of adjuvant chemotherapy for 4 to 6 months for women with tumors more than 1 cm regardless of nodal, menopausal, or tumor hormonal status, was affirmed. They concluded that anthracyclines offered a significant but small advantage over non–anthracycline-containing regimens, but the role of taxanes was not established.

Since these publications, new information has become available regarding adjuvant therapy. Taxanes, both paclitaxel and docetaxel, have been shown to provide incremental improvement in outcome either in sequence with or together with an anthracycline-containing regimen, but at the cost of additional toxicity.[109-112] Paclitaxel is approved by the FDA for adjuvant therapy of BC, and the combination of doxorubicin and cyclophosphamide followed by paclitaxel is one of the "standard" regimens for adjuvant therapy.

In the Gompertzian kinetic model of tumor growth, Norton[113] proposed that the rate of tumor growth is not constant but decreases as the tumor increases in size, eventually reaching a plateau. After cytoreductive chemotherapy, the residual tumor may reenter a period of rapid exponential growth, contributing to rapid relapse. Decreasing the period available for regrowth by more frequent administration of chemotherapy in a dose-dense schedule can be hypothesized to result in an improved response rate. The concept of dose-dense chemotherapy was tested in a clinical trial by the Cancer and Leukemia Group B (Intergroup trial C9741).[45] In this study, 2005 patients were randomized to receive doxorubicin and cyclophosphamide for four cycles followed by paclitaxel for four cycles or sequential single-agent use of these agents in a dose-dense every-2-weeks schedule with growth factor (granulocyte colony-stimulating factor) support, compared with the same drugs administered every 3 weeks (utilizing a 2 : 2 randomization design to evaluate the every-2-weeks vs. the every-3-weeks schedules). The dose-dense schedule was associated with significant improvement in disease-free survival (DFS) (risk ratio = 0.74, $P = .010$) and overall survival (risk ratio = 0.69, $P = .013$). The dose-dense arm was not associated with additional toxicity and was well tolerated.[45]

The *HER2*/neu gene is amplified in 20% to 25% of BCs and is associated with poor outcomes.[114,115] Trastuzumab, a humanized monoclonal antibody directed against the extracellular domain of HER2, has single-agent activity against HER2-positive BC and confers survival advantage in MBC in combination with chemotherapy.[90] Evidence has accumulated over the last few years of the role of trastuzumab in combination with chemotherapy for adjuvant therapy of HER2-positive BC. Three randomized studies found that trastuzumab in conjunction with adjuvant chemotherapy significantly reduced rates of recurrence and death.[91,116-118] Trastuzumab use is associated with risk of asymptomatic decline in cardiac ejection fraction, but congestive cardiac failure was very infrequent and almost always responsive to medical management. The risk of congestive heart failure is increased with concurrent use of anthracyclines, depending on the cumulative dose of the anthracycline used.[119] Several questions regarding the optimal chemotherapy accompaniment, schedule, and duration of therapy remain to be answered.

Aromatase Inhibitors. Until relatively recently, tamoxifen (Fig. 65-5) was the only choice for hormonal therapy for BC. Five years of adjuvant tamoxifen causes a 50% reduction in the risk of relapse and 28% reduction in the risk of death in estrogen receptor–positive BC patients irrespective of menopausal or lymph node status.[107] Tamoxifen use beyond 5 years is not recommended based on the NSABP B-14 trial, in which patients who had completed 5 years of tamoxifen were randomized to a further 5 years of tamoxifen or placebo. DFS after 7 years' follow-up was 78% in the tamoxifen arm and 82% in the placebo arm ($P = .07$).[26]

In the last few years, data have become available from randomized controlled clinical trials showing superior clinical outcomes for postmenopausal women who receive AIs compared to tamoxifen. The Anastrazole, Tamoxifen, and Combination (ATAC) trial enrolled 9366 women with estrogen receptor– and/or progesterone receptor–positive or unknown BC and randomized them to anastrazole, tamoxifen, or the combination for 5 years. The vast majority of patients did not receive chemotherapy. After 68 months of follow-up, when almost all patients had completed the planned 5 years of treatment, anastrazole was found to be superior to tamoxifen with prolonged DFS (hazard ratio [HR] 0.87, $P = .01$), longer time to recurrence (HR 0.79, $P = .0005$), significantly reduced incidence of distant metastases (HR 0.86, $P = .04$), and 42% reduction in contralateral BCs (35 vs. 59, $P = .01$).[10] The side effects profile also favored anastrazole, with fewer cases of endometrial carcinoma and thromboses but higher incidence of myalgias and arthralgias.[10]

Switching to an AI after 2 to 3 years of tamoxifen was studied in a 2362-patient randomized controlled clinical trial in which

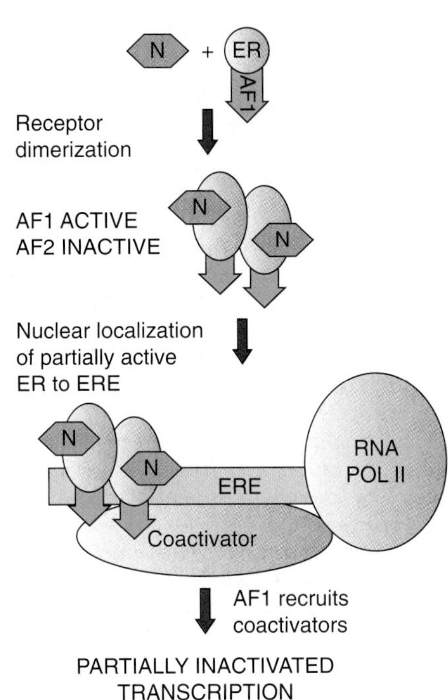

FIGURE 65-5 • Tamoxifen.

postmenopausal women who had received tamoxifen for 2 to 3 years were randomized to further tamoxifen or examustane to complete 5 years of therapy. There was a 32% reduction in relative risk of recurrence or death with the use of examustane.[120]

Duration of Adjuvant Hormonal Therapy. Since the risk of BC recurrence continues indefinitely after treatment, there is an interest in studying whether long-term adjuvant therapy will be beneficial. In the MA.17 trial, the National Cancer Institute of Canada investigated adding letrozole or placebo for 5 years in 5187 women who had completed 5 years of tamoxifen. After a median follow-up of 30 months, women in the letrozole arm had statistically significantly better DFS (HR = 0.58, $P < .001$) and distant DFS (HR = 0.60, $P = .002$) but not overall survival (HR = 0.82, $P = .3$). However, lymph node–positive patients also had overall survival benefit (HR = 0.61, $P = .04$). Letrozole treatment was associated with more hormonally related side effects, but the incidences of bone fractures and cardiovascular events were the same.[121] An extension trial is ongoing in which patients who have completed 5 years of letrozole are randomized to 5 more years of letrozole or placebo. From these data, it is clear that 5 years of tamoxifen is not optimal for postmenopausal women; 5 years of an AI or 5 years of tamoxifen followed by an AI has superior activity. However, the optimal agent, duration of AI treatment, or sequence of hormonal agents remain to be determined.

Therapy for Metastatic Disease

BC is one of the most chemosensitive solid tumors. However, despite chemosensitivity, MBC is not curable. Several chemotherapeutic agents that target different cell cycle components have activity against BC and can provide meaningful palliation and possibly improved survival. However, conclusive evidence proving improved survival of MBC patients with chemotherapy is lacking. Since MBC remains essentially incurable, the goal of therapy is palliation, and a guiding principle is to chose therapy that can provide the maximum chance of benefit for the longest period of time at the least cost in terms of toxicity. MBC should be thought of and approached as a chronic disease and various hormonal and chemotherapeutic agents utilized in a carefully thought-out sequence to maximize the likelihood of accomplishing the goal of palliation. The following sections provide general guidelines to the pharmacologic therapy for MBC (Box 65-2).

How to Choose Therapy for a Particular Patient. There is no single standard of care for treatment of MBC, and the choice of regimen should be individualized taking into account factors such as disease characteristics (extent of disease, organs involved, interval between initial diagnosis and relapse), patient characteristics (performance status, organ function impairment, comorbidities, side effect tolerance, previous treatments), and patient and physician preference. Because of its favorable side effect profile, endocrine therapy is the preferred initial treatment for patients with hormone receptor–positive disease, especially for relatively asymptomatic patients or those with disease confined to bone and soft tissues structures. Tamoxifen was the standard first-line therapy for many years. In the last few years, direct comparative studies of AIs and tamoxifen have shown AIs to be at least equivalent to and possibly more effective than tamoxifen for first-line treatment of postmenopausal women with MBC.[19-21] For previously untreated MBC, objective RRs of 32% to 44% and time to progression of 8 to 10 months can be expected.[19-21] Second- or third-line hormonal therapies are appropriate maneuvers at progression as they may provide additional responses or disease stability in some patients.

Patients who progress on hormonal therapy, have extensive visceral organ involvement, or have other extenuating circumstances are better served with chemotherapy. There are many chemotherapeutic agents with proven efficacy against BC, taxanes and anthracyclines being the most active. Coexisting medical conditions and the patient's ability to tolerate side effects are important factors that influence the choice of chemotherapeutic agent. For example, patients with diabetes mellitus

BOX 65-2 THERAPY OF METASTATIC BREAST CANCER: SUMMARY STATEMENTS*

- MBC remains essentially incurable, although long-term survival is possible in a minority of patients. The goal of MBC treatment is palliation.
- For patients with hormone receptor–positive disease, endocrine therapy is the preferred treatment unless there is extensive visceral disease or other extenuating circumstances.
- Second- or third-line antihormonal therapies may be appropriate after progression on first- or second-line treatments, respectively.
- When chemotherapy is necessary (hormone receptor–negative disease, progression on antihormonal therapy, extensive visceral metastatic disease), anthracyclines and taxanes are two of the most effective agents.
- Combination chemotherapy can result in higher response rates and improved survival but is associated with more toxicity. However, sequential single agents may be equally effective.
- Several second-line (and subsequent-line) therapies can be utilized as needed in succession after failure of previous chemotherapy regimens, after careful assessment of risks and benefits with a fully informed patient.
- Trastuzumab is recommended with first-line chemotherapy for patients with HER2-positive MBC. The role of trastuzumab with second- or subsequent-line chemotherapy remains to be defined.

*We would emphasize that the choice of therapy for any particular patient is a complex individual decision taking into account various factors discussed in the text.

are more suseptible to the neurotoxic side effects of agents such as cisplatin, the taxanes, and vinorelbine. Coexisting or previous cardiovascular disease increases the potential for cardiac toxicity with an anthracycline. Doxorubicin and paclitaxel, which depend on hepatic metabolism for clearance, must be used cautiously in patients with liver dysfunction and hyperbilirubinemia.

Taxanes are often chosen for the initial therapy of MBC because they are highly active, including in patients who have previously been treated with anthracyclines, and are relatively well tolerated. More recently, biologic therapy such as monoclonal antibodies against HER2 (trastuzumab) or VEGF (bevacizumab) have been incorporated along with chemotherapy agents with encouraging results. A randomized trial in previously untreated MBC showed marked improvement in progression-free survival in the bevacizumab plus paclitaxel arm compared with paclitaxel alone (11 vs. 6 months, respectively).[104] Firm recommendations about the use of bevacizumab must await completion of definitive clinical trials.

Trastuzumab should be strongly considered in patients with MBC whose tumors overexpress the HER2 protein or amplify the *HER2* gene. The benefit of adding trastuzumab to paclitaxel chemotherapy in patients with HER2-positive MBC was demonstrated in a randomized clinical trial.[90] Nonrandomized data are also available supporting the activity of a variety of agents such as docetaxel, vinorelbine, and platinum compounds in combination with trastuzumab.[95-97] Combination trastuzumab and doxorubicin chemotherapy is associated with a high frequency of significant cardiac dysfunction and is not recommended.[122]

An important clinical issue is whether to use a single chemotherapeutic agent at a time versus combination therapy. Many combination regimens have been studied and, in general, found to result in superior response rates and longer time to progression than single agents, but at the cost of greater toxicity. Two recent randomized trials showed improved survival with a combination of two agents than with one of the agent alone.[54,58] In a Phase III trial of 511 anthracycline-pretreated patients with MBC, a combination of docetaxel and capecitabine was associated with significantly superior RRs, time to progression, and overall survival than docetaxel alone.[54] Toxicities were more frequent but manageable. Whether similar results may be obtained with sequential use of the agents in a combination regimen is an important question.[55] Randomized comparisons of combination therapy with the same agents used in sequence do not show any difference in overall survival.[52,123-125] Nonetheless, a combination approach may be considered in patients in excellent performance status who have a large volume of visceral disease, in whom a regimen associated with a rapid and high response rate is particularly desirable.

Duration of Treatment. Therapy is generally continued in responding patients until there is evidence of disease progression. It is generally suggested that response to therapy be evaluated after 8 to 12 weeks of treatment. Failure to achieve any response by that time predicts a very low likelihood of response with further treatment. While chemotherapy is palliative in most patients, some patients achieve durable complete or partial remission. The duration of treatment in responding patients or those with stable disease is controversial. The general practice, also favored by National Comprehensive Cancer Network guidelines, is to continue therapy until progression. Comparative studies of a continuous chemotherapy approach (chemotherapy until progression) versus interrupted therapy (stopping therapy after an induction period and resuming it at the time of progression) showed improved time to progression with the continuous approach but with more toxicity and no difference in overall survival.[126] A recent study also did not find any benefit of maintenance with paclitaxel as first-line therapy for MBC.[127] Nonetheless, the continuous therapy approach was associated with better quality of life in one randomized trial.[128] The option of continuous or interrupted therapy should be carefully discussed and decided in partnership with a well-informed patient.

REFERENCES

1. Jemal A, Siegel R, Ward E, et al. Cancer statistics, 2007. CA Cancer J Clin 2007;57:43-66.
2. Clemons M, Goss P. Estrogen and the risk of breast cancer. N Engl J Med 2001;344:276-285.
3. Rebbeck TR, Lynch HT, Neuhausen SL, et al. Prophylactic oophorectomy in carriers of *BRCA1* or *BRCA2* mutations. N Engl J Med 2002;346:1616-1622.
4. Kauff ND, Satagopan JM, Robson ME, et al. Risk-reducing salpingo-oophorectomy in women with a *BRCA1* or *BRCA2* mutation. N Engl J Med 2002;346:1609-1615.
5. Fisher B, Costantino JP, Wickerham DL, et al. Tamoxifen for prevention of breast cancer: report of the National Surgical Adjuvant Breast and Bowel Project P-1 Study. J Natl Cancer Inst 1998;90:1371-1388.
6. Cuzick J, Forbes JF, Sestak I, et al. Long-term results of tamoxifen prophylaxis for breast cancer—96-month follow-up of the randomized IBIS-I trial. J Natl Cancer Inst 2007;99:272-282.
7. Powles TJ, Ashley S, Tidy A, et al. Twenty-year follow-up of the Royal Marsden randomized, double-blinded tamoxifen breast cancer prevention trial. J Natl Cancer Inst 2007;99:283-290.
8. Chlebowski RT, Collyar DE, Somerfield MR, Pfister DG. American Society of Clinical Oncology technology assessment on breast cancer risk reduction strategies: tamoxifen and raloxifene. J Clin Oncol 1999;17:1939-1955.
9. Vogel VG, Costantino JP, Wickerham DL, et al. Effects of tamoxifen vs raloxifene on the risk of developing invasive breast cancer and other disease outcomes: the NSABP Study of Tamoxifen and Raloxifene (STAR) P-2 trial. JAMA 2006;295:2727-2741.
10. Howell A, Cuzick J, Baum M, et al. Results of the ATAC (Arimidex, Tamoxifen, Alone or in Combination) trial after completion of 5 years' adjuvant treatment for breast cancer. Lancet 2005;365:60-62.
11. Beatson G. On the treatment of inoperable carcinoma of the mamma: suggestions for a new method of treatment, with illustrative cases. Lancet 1896;2:104-107.
12. Bonadonna G, Brusamolino E, Valagussa P, et al. Combination chemotherapy as an adjuvant treatment in operable breast cancer. N Engl J Med 1976;294:405-410.
13. Paik S, Shak S, Tang G, et al. A multigene assay to predict recurrence of tamoxifen-treated, node-negative breast cancer. N Engl J Med 2004;351:2817-2826.
14. Paik S, Tang G, Shak S, et al. Gene expression and benefit of chemotherapy in women with node-negative, estrogen receptor-positive breast cancer. J Clin Oncol 2006;24:3726-3734.
15. Geels P, Eisenhauer E, Bezjak A, et al. Palliative effect of chemotherapy: objective tumor response is associated with symptom improvement in patients with metastatic breast cancer. J Clin Oncol 2000;18:2395-2405.
16. Coates AS, Hurny C, Peterson HF, et al. Quality-of-life scores predict outcome in metastatic but not early breast cancer. International Breast Cancer Study Group. J Clin Oncol 2000;18:3768-3774.
17. Luoma ML, Hakamies-Blomqvist L, Sjostrom J, et al. Prognostic value of quality of life scores for time to progression (TTP) and overall survival time (OS) in advanced breast cancer. Eur J Cancer 2003;39:1370-1376.
18. Hortobagyi GN. Treatment of breast cancer. N Engl J Med 1998;339:974-984.
19. Nabholtz JM, Buzdar A, Pollak M, et al. Anastrozole is superior to tamoxifen as first-line therapy for advanced breast cancer in postmenopausal women: results of a North

American multicenter randomized trial. Arimidex Study Group. J Clin Oncol 2000;18:3758-3767.
20. Nabholtz JM, Bonneterre J, Buzdar A, et al. Anastrozole (Arimidex) versus tamoxifen as first-line therapy for advanced breast cancer in postmenopausal women: survival analysis and updated safety results. Eur J Cancer 2003;39:1684-1689.
21. Mouridsen H, Gershanovich M, Sun Y, et al. Phase III study of letrozole versus tamoxifen as first-line therapy of advanced breast cancer in postmenopausal women: analysis of survival and update of efficacy from the International Letrozole Breast Cancer Group. J Clin Oncol 2003;21:2101-2109.
22. Santen RJ, English H, Rohner T, et al. Androgen depletion/repletion in combination with chemotherapy: strategy for secondary treatment of metastatic prostatic cancer. Prog Clin Biol Res 1985;185A:359-371.
23. Harvey HA, Lipton A, Max DT, et al. Medical castration produced by the GnRH analogue leuprolide to treat metastatic breast cancer. J Clin Oncol 1985;3:1068-1072.
24. Jaiyesimi IA, Buzdar AU, Decker DA, Hortobagyi GN. Use of tamoxifen for breast cancer: twenty-eight years later. J Clin Oncol 1995;13:513-529.
25. Ward HW. Anti-oestrogen therapy for breast cancer: a trial of tamoxifen at two dose levels. Br Med J 1973;1:13-14.
26. Fisher B, Dignam J, Bryant J, et al. Five versus more than five years of tamoxifen therapy for breast cancer patients with negative lymph nodes and estrogen receptor-positive tumors. J Natl Cancer Inst 1996;88:1529-1542.
27. Organization NAT. Controlled trial of tamoxifen as a single adjuvant agent in the management of early breast cancer. 'Nolvadex' Adjuvant Trial Organisation. Br J Cancer 1988;57:608-611.
28. Venturino A, Comandini D, Granetto C, et al. Formestane is feasible and effective in elderly breast cancer patients with comorbidity and disability. Breast Cancer Res Treat 2004;62:217-222.
29. Ingle JN, Suman VJ. Aromatase inhibitors for therapy of advanced breast cancer. J Steroid Biochem Mol Biol 2005;95:113-119.
30. Osborne CK, Pippen J, Jones SE, et al. Double-blind, randomized trial comparing the efficacy and tolerability of fulvestrant versus anastrozole in postmenopausal women with advanced breast cancer progressing on prior endocrine therapy: results of a North American trial. J Clin Oncol 2002;20:3386-3395.
31. Howell A, Robertson JF, Quaresma Albano J, et al. Fulvestrant, formerly ICI 182,780, is as effective as anastrozole in postmenopausal women with advanced breast cancer progressing after prior endocrine treatment. J Clin Oncol 2002;20:3396-3403.
32. Ingle JN, Suman VJ, Rowland KM, et al. Fulvestrant in women with advanced breast cancer after progression on prior aromatase inhibitor therapy: North Central Cancer Treatment Group Trial N0032. J Clin Oncol 2006;24:1052-1056.
33. Chia S, Gradishar W, Mauriac L, et al. Double-blind, randomized placebo controlled trial of fulvestrant compared with exemestane after prior nonsteroidal aromatase inhibitor therapy in postmenopausal women with hormone receptor-positive, advanced breast cancer: results from EFECT. J Clin Oncol 2008;26:1664-1670.
34. Mouridsen HT, Palshof T, Brahm M, Rahbek I. Evaluation of single-drug versus multiple-drug chemotherapy in the treatment of advanced breast cancer. Cancer Treat Rep 1977;61:47-50.
35. Kolaric K, Vukas D. Carboplatin activity in untreated metastatic breast cancer patients—results of a Phase II study. Cancer Chemother Pharmacol 1991;27:409-412.
36. Martin M, Diaz-Rubio E, Casado A, et al. Carboplatin: an active drug in metastatic breast cancer. J Clin Oncol 1992;10:433-437.
37. O'Brien ME, Talbot DC, Smith IE. Carboplatin in the treatment of advanced breast cancer: a Phase II study using a pharmacokinetically guided dose schedule. J Clin Oncol 1993;11:2112-2117.
38. Decatris MP, Sundar S, O'Byrne KJ. Platinum-based chemotherapy in metastatic breast cancer: current status. Cancer Treat Rev 2004;30:53-81.
39. Perez EA, Suman VJ, Rowland KM, et al. Two concurrent Phase II trials of paclitaxel/carboplatin/trastuzumab (weekly or every-3-week schedule) as first-line therapy in women with HER2-overexpressing metastatic breast cancer: NCCTG study 983252. Clin Breast Cancer 2005;6:425-432.
40. Burch PA, Mailliard JA, Hillman DW, et al. Phase II study of gemcitabine plus cisplatin in patients with metastatic breast cancer: a North Central Cancer Treatment Group Trial. Am J Clin Oncol 2005;28:195-200.
41. Perez EA. Carboplatin in combination therapy for metastatic breast cancer. Oncologist 2004;9:518-527.
42. O'Brien ME, Wigler N, Inbar M, et al. Reduced cardiotoxicity and comparable efficacy in a Phase III trial of pegylated liposomal doxorubicin HCl (CAELYX/Doxil) versus conventional doxorubicin for first-line treatment of metastatic breast cancer. Ann Oncol 2004;15:440-449.
43. Sparano JA. Taxanes for breast cancer: an evidence-based review of randomized Phase II and Phase III trials. Clin Breast Cancer 2000;1:32-40; discussion 1-2.
44. Jones SE, Erban J, Overmoyer B, et al. Randomized Phase III study of docetaxel compared with paclitaxel in metastatic breast cancer. J Clin Oncol 2005;23:5542-5551.
45. Citron M, Berry D, Cirrincione C, et al. Randomized trial of dose-dense versus conventionally scheduled and sequential versus concurrent combination chemotherapy as postoperative adjuvant treatment of node-positive primary breast cancer: first report of intergroup trial C9741/Cancer And Leukemia Group B trial 9741. J Clin Oncol 2003;21:1-9.
46. Burstein HJ, Manola J, Younger J, et al. Docetaxel administered on a weekly basis for metastatic breast cancer. J Clin Oncol 2000;18:1212-1219.
47. Eniu A, Palmieri FM, Perez EA. Weekly administration of docetaxel and paclitaxel in metastatic or advanced breast cancer. Oncologist 2005;10:665-685.
47a. Sparano JA, Wang M, Martino S, et al. Weekly paclitaxel in the adjuvant treatment of breast cancer. N Engl J Med 2008;358:1663-1671.
48. Nabholtz JM, Falkson C, Campos D, et al. Docetaxel and doxorubicin compared with doxorubicin and cyclophosphamide as first-line chemotherapy for metastatic breast cancer: results of a randomized, multicenter, Phase III trial. J Clin Oncol 2003;21:968-975.
49. Nabholtz JM, Mackey JR, Smylie M, et al. Phase II study of docetaxel, doxorubicin, and cyclophosphamide as first-line chemotherapy for metastatic breast cancer. J Clin Oncol 2001;19:314-321.
50. Paridaens R, Biganzoli L, Bruning P, et al. Paclitaxel versus doxorubicin as first-line single-agent chemotherapy for metastatic breast cancer: a European Organization for Research and Treatment of Cancer randomized study with cross-over. J Clin Oncol 2000;18:724-733.
51. Biganzoli L, Cufer T, Bruning P, et al. Doxorubicin and paclitaxel versus doxorubicin and cyclophosphamide as first-line chemotherapy in metastatic breast cancer: The European Organization for Research and Treatment of Cancer 10961 Multicenter Phase III Trial. J Clin Oncol 2002;20:3114-3121.
52. Sledge GW, Neuberg D, Bernardo P, et al. Phase III trial of doxorubicin, paclitaxel, and the combination of doxorubicin and paclitaxel as front-line chemotherapy for metastatic breast cancer: an intergroup trial (E1193). J Clin Oncol 2003;21:588-92.
53. Blum JL, Dieras V, Lo Russo PM, et al. Multicenter, Phase II study of capecitabine in taxane-pretreated metastatic breast carcinoma patients. Cancer 2001;92:1759-1768.
54. O'Shaughnessy J, Miles D, Vukelja S, et al. Superior survival with capecitabine plus docetaxel combination therapy in anthracycline-pretreated patients with advanced breast cancer: Phase III trial results. J Clin Oncol 2002;20:2812-2823.
55. Miles D, Vukelja S, Moiseyenko V, et al. Survival benefit with capecitabine/docetaxel versus docetaxel alone: analysis of therapy in a randomized Phase III trial. Clin Breast Cancer 2004;5:273-278.
56. Spielmann M, Llombart-Cussac A, Kalla S, et al. Single-agent gemcitabine is active in previously treated metastatic breast cancer. Oncology 2001;60:303-307.
57. Blackstein M, Vogel CL, Ambinder R, et al. Gemcitabine as first-line therapy in patients with metastatic breast cancer: a Phase II trial. Oncology 2002;62:2-8.
58. Albain K, Nag S, Calderillo-Ruiz G, et al. Global Phase III study of gemcitabine plus paclitaxel (GT) vs. paclitaxel (T) as frontline therapy for metastatic breast cancer (MBC): first report of overall survival [Abstract 510]. J Clin Oncol 2004;22(14 Suppl).
59. Fountzilas G, Nicolaides C, Bafaloukos D, et al. Docetaxel and gemcitabine in anthracycline-resistant advanced breast cancer: a Hellenic Cooperative Oncology Group Phase II study. Cancer Invest 2000;18:503-509.
60. Laufman LR, Spiridonidis CH, Pritchard J, et al. Monthly docetaxel and weekly gemcitabine in metastatic breast cancer: a Phase II trial. Ann Oncol 2001;12:1259-1264.
61. Chan S, Romieu G, Huober J, et al. Gemcitabine plus docetaxel (GD) versus capecitabine plus docetaxel (CD) for anthracycline-pretreated metastatic breast cancer (MBC) patients (pts): results of a European Phase III study [Abstract 581]. J Clin Oncol 2005;23(16 Suppl).
62. Garcia-Conde J, Lluch A, Martin M, et al. Phase II trial of weekly IV vinorelbine in first-line advanced breast cancer chemotherapy. Ann Oncol 1994;5:854-857.
63. Weber BL, Vogel C, Jones S, et al. Intravenous vinorelbine as first-line and second-line therapy in advanced breast cancer. J Clin Oncol 1995;13:2722-2730.
64. Terenziani M, Demicheli R, Brambilla C, et al. Vinorelbine: an active, non cross-resistant drug in advanced breast cancer. Results from a Phase II study. Breast Cancer Res Treat 1996;39:285-291.
65. Spielmann M, Dorval T, Turpin F, et al. Phase II trial of vinorelbine/doxorubicin as first-line therapy of advanced breast cancer. J Clin Oncol 1994;12:1764-1770.
66. Romero Acuna L, Langhi M, Perez J, et al. Vinorelbine and paclitaxel as first-line chemotherapy in metastatic breast cancer. J Clin Oncol 1999;17:74-81.
67. Burstein HJ, Kuter I, Campos SM, et al. Clinical activity of trastuzumab and vinorelbine in women with HER2-overexpressing metastatic breast cancer. J Clin Oncol 2001;19:2722-2730.
68. Baweja M, Suman VJ, Fitch TR, et al. Phase II trial of oral vinorelbine for the treatment of metastatic breast cancer in patients > or = 65 years of age: an NCCTG study. Ann Oncol 2006;17:623-629.
69. Sledge GW Jr. Etoposide in the management of metastatic breast cancer. Cancer 1991;67(1 Suppl):266-270.
70. Slevin ML, Clark PI, Joel SP, et al. A randomized trial to evaluate the effect of schedule on the activity of etoposide in small-cell lung cancer. J Clin Oncol 1989;7:1333-1340.
71. Martin M, Lluch A, Casado A, et al. Clinical activity of chronic oral etoposide in previously treated metastatic breast cancer. J Clin Oncol 1994;12:986-991.
72. Perez EA, Hillman DW, Mailliard JA, et al. Randomized Phase II study of two irinotecan schedules for patients with metastatic breast cancer refractory to an anthracycline, a taxane, or both. J Clin Oncol 2004;22:2849-2855.
73. Ando Y, Saka H, Ando M, et al. Polymorphisms of UDP-glucuronosyltransferase gene and irinotecan toxicity: a pharmacogenetic analysis. Cancer Res 2000;60:6921-6926.
74. Adjei AA, Klein CE, Kastrissios H, et al. Phase I and pharmacokinetic study of irinotecan and docetaxel in patients with advanced solid tumors: preliminary evidence of clinical activity. J Clin Oncol 2000;18:1116-1123.
75. Couteau C, Risse ML, Ducreux M, et al. Phase I and pharmacokinetic study of docetaxel and irinotecan in patients with advanced solid tumors. J Clin Oncol 2000;18:3545-3552.
76. Shih C, Chen VJ, Gossett LS, et al. LY231514, a pyrrolo[2,3-D]pyrimidine-based antifolate that inhibits multiple folate-requiring enzymes. Cancer Res 1997;57:1116-1123.
77. Spielmann M, Martin M, Namer M, et al. Activity of pemetrexed (ALIMTA, multi-targeted antifolate, LY231514) in metastatic breast cancer patients previously treated with an anthracycline and a taxane: an interim analysis. Clin Breast Cancer 2001; 2:47-51.

78. Martin M, Spielmann M, Namer M, et al. Phase II study of pemetrexed in breast cancer patients pretreated with anthracyclines. Ann Oncol 2003;14:1246-1252.
79. Ma CX, Steen P, Rowland KM, et al. A Phase II trial of a combination of pemetrexed and gemcitabine in patients with metastatic breast cancer: an NCCTG study. Ann Oncol 2006;17:226-231.
80. Sparreboom A, van Zuylen L, Brouwer E, et al. Cremophor EL-mediated alteration of paclitaxel distribution in human blood: clinical pharmacokinetic implications. Cancer Res 1999;59:1454-1457.
81. John TA, Vogel SM, Tiruppathi C, et al. Quantitative analysis of albumin uptake and transport in the rat microvessel endothelial monolayer. Am J Physiol Lung Cell Mol Physiol 2003;284:L187-L196.
82. Ibrahim NK, Samuels B, Page R, et al. Multicenter Phase II trial of ABI-007, an albumin-bound paclitaxel, in women with metastatic breast cancer. J Clin Oncol 2005;23:6019-6026.
83. Gradishar WJ, Tjulandin S, Davidson N, et al. Phase III trial of nanoparticle albumin-bound paclitaxel compared with polyethylated castor oil-based paclitaxel in women with breast cancer. J Clin Oncol 2005;23:7794-7803.
84. Gradishar W, Krasnojon D, Cheporov S, et al. A randomized Phase 2 trial of qw or q3w ABI-007 (ABX) vs. q3W solvent-based docetaxel (TXT) as first-line therapy in metastatic breast cancer (MBC) [Abstract 46]. Breast Cancer Res Treat 2006; 100(Suppl 1).

84a. Roy V, LaPlant B, Gross G, et al. NCCTG phase II trial N0531 of weekly nab-paclitaxel (nab-p) in combination with gemcitabine (gem) in patients with metastatic breast cancer (MBC). J Clin Oncol 2007 ASCO Annual Meeting Proceedings Part I 2007;25(18S (June 20 Supplement)):Abstr 1048.

85. Lee FYF, Borzilleri R, Fairchild CR, et al. BMS-247550: A novel epothilone analog with a mode of action similar to paclitaxel but possessing superior antitumor efficacy. Clin Cancer Res 2001;7:1429-1437.
86. Low JA, Wedam SB, Lee JJ, et al. Phase II clinical trial of ixabepilone (BMS-247550), an epothilone B analog, in metastatic and locally advanced breast cancer. J Clin Oncol 2005;23:2726-2734.

86a. Perez EA, Lerzo G, Pivot X, et al. Efficacy and safety of ixabepilone (BMS-247550) in a phase II study of patients with advanced breast cancer resistant to an anthracycline, a taxane, and capecitabine. J Clin Oncol 2007;25:3407-3414.

87. Bennouna J, Campone M, Delord J, Pinel M. Vinflunine: a novel antitubulin agent in solid malignancies. Expert Opin Investig Drugs 2005;14:1259-1267.
88. Fumoleau P, Campone M, Vorobiof D, et al. Phase II study of i.v. vinflunine as second line in patients with metastatic breast cancer after anthracycline-taxane failure [Abstract 542]. J Clin Oncol 2004;22(14 Suppl).
89. Yarden Y, Sliwkowski MX. Untangling the ErbB signalling network. Nat Rev Mol Cell Biol 2001;2:127-137.
90. Slamon DJ, Leyland-Jones B, Shak S, et al. Use of chemotherapy plus a monoclonal antibody against HER2 for metastatic breast cancer that overexpresses HER2. N Engl J Med 2001;344:783-792.
91. Romond EH, Perez EA, Bryant J, et al. Trastuzumab plus adjuvant chemotherapy for operable HER2-positive breast cancer. N Engl J Med 2005;353:1673-1684.
92. Perez EA, Suman VJ, Davidson NE, et al. HER2 testing by local, central, and reference laboratories in specimens from the North Central Cancer Treatment Group N9831 Intergroup Adjuvant Trial. J Clin Oncol 2006;24:3032-3038.
93. Menendez JA, Mehmi I, Lupu R. Trastuzumab in combination with heregulin-activated Her-2 (erbB-2) triggers a receptor-enhanced chemosensitivity effect in the absence of Her-2 overexpression. J Clin Oncol 2006;24:3735-3746.
94. Baselga J, Carbonell X, Castaneda-Soto N-J, et al. Updated efficacy and safety analyses of 3-weekly Herceptin monotherapy in women with HER2-positive metastatic breast cancer: results from twelve months of follow-up to a Phase II study [Abstract 3042]. Breast Cancer Res Treat 2004;88(Suppl 1).
95. Pegram MD, Konecny GE, O'Callaghan C, et al. Rational combinations of trastuzumab with chemotherapeutic drugs used in the treatment of breast cancer. J Natl Cancer Inst 2004;96:739-749.
96. Burstein HJ, Harris LN, Marcom PK, et al. Trastuzumab and vinorelbine as first-line therapy for HER2-overexpressing metastatic breast cancer: multicenter Phase II trial with clinical outcomes, analysis of serum tumor markers as predictive factors, and cardiac surveillance algorithm. J Clin Oncol 2003;21:2889-2895.
97. O'Shaughnessy JA, Vukelja S, Marsland T, et al. Phase II study of trastuzumab plus gemcitabine in chemotherapy-pretreated patients with metastatic breast cancer. Clin Breast Cancer 2004;5:142-147.
98. Burris HA 3rd. Dual kinase inhibition in the treatment of breast cancer: initial experience with the EGFR/ErbB-2 inhibitor lapatinib. Oncologist 2004;9(Suppl 3):10-15.
99. Gomez H, Chavez M, Doval D, et al. A Phase II, randomized trial using the small molecule tyrosine kinase inhibitor lapatinib as a first-line treatment in patients with FISH positive advanced or metastatic breast cancer [Abstract 3046]. J Clin Oncol 2005;23(16 Suppl).
100. Geyer CE, Forster J, Lindquist D, et al. Lapatinib plus capecitabine for HER2-positive advanced breast cancer. N Engl J Med 2006;355:2733-2743.
101. Lin N, Carey L, Liu M, et al. Phase II trial of lapatinib for brain metastases in patients with HER2+ breast cancer [Abstract 503]. J Clin Oncol 2006;24(18 Suppl).
102. Perez EA, Koehler M, Byrne J, et al. Cardiac safety of lapatinib: pooled analysis of 3689 patients enrolled in clinical trials. Mayo Clin Proc 2008;83:679-686.
103. Miller KD, Chap LI, Holmes FA, et al. Randomized Phase III trial of capecitabine compared with bevacizumab plus capecitabine in patients with previously treated metastatic breast cancer. J Clin Oncol 2005;23:792-799.
104. Miller K, Wang M, Gralow J, et al. Paclitaxel plus bevacizumab versus paclitaxel alone for metastatic breast cancer. N Engl J Med 2007;357:2666-2676.
105. Miller KD, Burstein HJ, Elias A, et al. Phase II study of SU11248, a multitargeted receptor tyrosine kinase inhibitor (TKI), in patients (pts) with previously treated metastatic breast cancer (MBC) [Abstract 563]. J Oncol 2005;23(16 Suppl).
106. Moreno-Aspitia A, Hillman D, Wiesenfeld M, et al. BAY 43-9006 as single oral agent in patients with metastatic breast cancer previously exposed to anthracycline and/or taxane [Abstract 577]. J Clin Oncol 2006;24(18 Suppl).
107. Polychemotherapy for early breast cancer: an overview of the randomised trials. Early Breast Cancer Trialists' Collaborative Group. Lancet 1998;352:930-942.
108. Eifel P, Axelson JA, Costa J, et al. National Institutes of Health Consensus Development Conference Statement: adjuvant therapy for breast cancer, November 1-3, 2000. J Natl Cancer Inst 2001;93:979-989.
109. Henderson IC, Berry DA, Demetri GD, et al. Improved outcomes from adding sequential paclitaxel but not from escalating doxorubicin dose in an adjuvant chemotherapy regimen for patients with node-positive primary breast cancer. J Clin Oncol 2003;21:976-983.
110. Mamounas EP, Bryant J, Lembersky B, et al. Paclitaxel after doxorubicin plus cyclophosphamide as adjuvant chemotherapy for node-positive breast cancer: results from NSABP B-28. J Clin Oncol 2005;23:3686-3696.
111. Martin M, Pienkowski T, Mackey J, et al. Adjuvant docetaxel for node-positive breast cancer. N Engl J Med 2005;352:2302-2313.
112. Roy V, Perez EA. Adjuvant docetaxel plus doxorubicin and cyclophosphamide increases survival compared with fluorouracil plus doxorubicin and cyclophosphamide in women with operable node-positive breast cancer. Cancer Treat Rev 2006;32:55-58.
113. Norton L. A Gompertzian model of human breast cancer growth [Comment]. Cancer Res 1988;48:7067-7071.
114. Press MF, Pike MC, Chazin VR, et al. Her-2/neu expression in node-negative breast cancer: direct tissue quantitation by computerized image analysis and association of overexpression with increased risk of recurrent disease. Cancer Res 1993;53:4960-4970.
115. Slamon DJ, Clark GM, Wong SG, et al. Human breast cancer: correlation of relapse and survival with amplification of the HER-2/neu oncogene. Science 1987;235:177-182.
116. Piccart-Gebhart MJ, Procter M, Leyland-Jones B, et al. Trastuzumab after adjuvant chemotherapy in HER2-positive breast cancer. N Engl J Med 2005;353:1659-1672.
117. Hortobagyi GN. Trastuzumab in the treatment of breast cancer. N Engl J Med 2005;353:1734-1736.
118. Joensuu H, Kellokumpu-Lehtinen P-L, Bono P, et al. Adjuvant docetaxel or vinorelbine with or without trastuzumab for breast cancer. N Engl J Med 2006;354:809-820.
119. Perez EA, Rodeheffer R. Clinical cardiac tolerability of trastuzumab. J Clin Oncol 2004;22:322-329.
120. Coombes RC, Hall E, Gibson LJ, et al. A randomized trial of exemestane after two to three years of tamoxifen therapy in postmenopausal women with primary breast cancer. N Engl J Med 2004;350:1081-1092.
121. Goss PE, Ingle JN, Martino S, et al. Randomized trial of letrozole following tamoxifen as extended adjuvant therapy in receptor-positive breast cancer: updated findings from NCIC CTG MA.17. J Natl Cancer Inst 2005;97:1262-1271.
122. Seidman A, Hudis C, Pierri MK, et al. Cardiac dysfunction in the trastuzumab clinical trials experience. J Clin Oncol 2002;20:1215-1221.
123. Alba E, Martin M, Ramos M, et al. Multicenter randomized trial comparing sequential with concomitant administration of doxorubicin and docetaxel as first-line treatment of metastatic breast cancer: a Spanish Breast Cancer Research Group (GEICAM-9903) Phase III study. J Clin Oncol 2004;22:2587-2593.
124. Baldini E, Prochilo T, Salvadori B, et al. Multicenter randomized Phase III trial of epirubicin plus paclitaxel vs epirubicin followed by paclitaxel in metastatic breast cancer patients: focus on cardiac safety. Br J Cancer 2004;91:45-49.
125. Cresta S, Grasselli G, Mansutti M, et al. A randomized Phase II study of combination, alternating and sequential regimens of doxorubicin and docetaxel as first-line chemotherapy for women with metastatic breast cancer. Ann Oncol 2004;15:433-439.
126. Muss H, Case L, Richards F, et al. Interrupted versus continuous chemotherapy in patients with metastatic breast cancer. The Piedmont Oncology Association. N Engl J Med 1991;325:1342-1348.
127. Gennari A, Amadori D, De Lena M, et al. Lack of benefit of maintenance paclitaxel in first-line chemotherapy in metastatic breast cancer. J Clin Oncol 2006;24:3912-3918.
128. Coates A, Gebski V, Bishop J, et al. Improving the quality of life during chemotherapy for advanced breast cancer: a comparison of intermittent and continuous treatment strategies. N Engl J Med 1987;317:1490-1495.

66

HEMATOLOGIC MALIGNANCIES

Jasmine Nabi and Raymond J. Hohl

INTRODUCTION 945
THERAPEUTICS AND CLINICAL PHARMACOLOGY 945
Therapeutics by Class 945
Antimetabolites 945
Antitumor Antibiotics 945
Alkylating Agents 946
Other Chemotherapy Agents 946
Biologic Therapies 948
Therapeutic Approach 948

INTRODUCTION

Malignancy of the hematopoietic and lymphoid systems covers a broad range of diseases with variable presentations. These blood disorders can be divided into five general categories: leukemias, malignant lymphomas, myelodysplastic syndromes, myeloproliferative disorders, and plasma cell dyscrasias (Table 66-1). Leukemias are neoplasms of the hematopoietic stems cells (Fig. 66-1) characterized by diffuse replacement of the bone marrow by neoplastic cells. Malignant lymphomas are a group of diseases composed of neoplastic lymphocytes. Myelodysplastic syndromes are a heterogeneous group of clonal hematologic disorders characterized by ineffective hematopoiesis. Myeloproliferative disorders are neoplastic clonal proliferations of myeloid stem cells. Plasma cell dyscrasias are neoplastic proliferations of well-differentiated immunoglobulin-producing cells.[1-3] Numerous therapeutic agents are employed in the treatment of these diseases.

THERAPEUTICS AND CLINICAL PHARMACOLOGY

Therapeutics by Class

Antimetabolites

Cladribine (2-CdA or Chlorodeoxyadenosine). Cladribine is used in lymphoid malignancies, particularly hairy cell leukemia. This drug is a purine analogue of deoxyadenosine. The triphosphate form of cladribine does not readily exit the cell, which inhibits DNA synthesis and induces DNA strand breaks. Cladribine is mainly associated with myelosuppression.[4-6]

Cytarabine. Cytarabine has been used to treat leukemia and lymphoid malignancies. Cytarabine is a pyrimidine analogue of deoxycytidine. The triphosphate form of the drug inhibits DNA synthesis. Cytarabine can be administered by intravenous and intrathecal routes. The drug is associated with nausea, vomiting, diarrhea, and myelosuppression. Cerebellar toxicity is seen with high-dose cytarabine. Conjunctivitis and keratitis have also been noted with high-dose cytarabine. Prophylactic steroid eyedrops can reduce the ocular toxicities from the drug.[4,7-9]

Fludarabine. Fludarabine is primarily used to treat chronic lymphocytic leukemia. The drug is a purine nucleotide analogue. The triphosphate form of fludarabine inhibits DNA synthesis. Fludarabine is mainly associated with myelosuppression.[4,10]

Hydroxyurea (Hydrea). Hydroxyurea is used to treat leukemias and myeloproliferative disorders. The exact mechanism of action for hydroxyurea is not clear. The drug inhibits DNA synthesis. Toxicities associated with hydroxyurea include nausea, vomiting, diarrhea, mucosal ulcers, skin changes, and myelosuppression.[4,8,11]

Hypomethylating Agents (5-Azacytidine and Decitabine). 5-Azacytidine and decitabine have been used to treat myelodysplastic syndromes. These agents are analogues of the nucleoside cytosine. Once incorporated into DNA, they inhibit DNA methylation. The hypomethylated DNA may allow cellular differentiation to occur. Toxicities associated with 5-azacytidine include thrombocytopenia, leukopenia, arthralgias, and diarrhea. Decitabine is associated with neutropenia, thrombocytopenia, anemia, leukopenia, fever, and hyperbilirubinemia.[12,13]

6-Mercaptopurine. 6-Mercaptopurine is primarily used to treat acute lymphoblastic leukemia. This drug is a purine analogue of hypoxanthine and gets incorporated into DNA and RNA. Also, it inhibits de novo purine synthesis. Side effects from 6-mercaptopurine include nausea, vomiting, diarrhea, and myelosuppression. Hepatic dysfunction can be seen with this agent. Finally, it should be noted that allopurinol interferes with oral 6-mercaptopurine metabolism. Therefore, the dose of the drug should be reduced when given to patients also taking allopurinol.[4,7]

Methotrexate. Methotrexate is used in leukemia and malignant lymphoma therapy. The drug is structurally related to folic acid and has a strong affinity for dihydrofolate reductase. By inhibiting dihydrofolate reductase, methotrexate leads to decreased cellular thymidine levels. A decreased concentration of thymidine ultimately leads to depressed DNA synthesis. Methotrexate can be administered by oral, intravenous, and intrathecal routes.

The drug is associated with hair loss, rash, nausea, vomiting, diarrhea, stomatitis, and myelosuppression. Methotrexate can lead to hepatic and renal dysfunction. Intrathecal administration can cause neurologic toxicities. With high-dose methotrexate therapy, a leucovorin rescue is given to minimize toxicities and reduce bone marrow suppression. (Leucovorin bypasses dihydrofolate reductase and replenishes the folate pool.) To reduce renal toxicity with high-dose methotrexate, the urine should be alkalized to a pH greater than 7.0 and aggressive hydration should be administered. Finally, methotrexate should be avoided in patients with malignant effusions. Pleural, peritoneal, and pericardial fluids can sequester methotrexate, prolonging its half-life and increasing its toxic effects.[4,7,8,14,15]

Pentostatin. Pentostatin is used to treat lymphoid malignancies. Pentostatin inhibits adenosine deaminase, an enzyme involved in purine metabolism that is found in all lymphoid cells. Deoxyadenosine metabolites accumulate and lead to cytotoxic effects. Toxicities associated with pentostatin include nausea, vomiting, dry skin, fatigue, myelosuppression, and immunosuppression.[4,6]

6-Thioguanine. 6-Thioguanine has been used to treat leukemia. This drug is a purine analogue of guanine and gets incorporated into DNA and RNA. Also, it inhibits de novo purine synthesis. The major toxicity from 6-thioguanine is myelosuppression.[4,7]

Antitumor Antibiotics

Anthracyclines (Daunorubicin, Doxorubicin, and Idarubicin). Anthracyclines are used in a variety of hematologic malignancies, particularly leukemias and malignant lymphomas. Anthracyclines intercalate between base pairs of DNA, blocking DNA synthesis. Also, these

TABLE 66-1 MALIGNANT BLOOD DISORDERS

Blood Disorder Category	Disease Examples
Leukemias	Acute lymphoblastic leukemia Acute myeloid leukemia
Malignant lymphomas	Hodgkin's lymphoma Non-Hodgkin's lymphoma Chronic lymphocytic leukemia Diffuse large B-cell lymphoma Follicular lymphoma Hairy cell leukemia Mantle cell lymphoma Lymphoplasmacytic lymphoma (Waldenström's macroglobulinemia)
Myelodysplastic syndromes	Refractory anemia Refractory anemia with excess blasts Refractory anemia with excess blasts in transformation Refractory anemia with ringed sideroblasts
Myeloproliferative disorders	Chronic myeloid leukemia Essential thrombocythemia Idiopathic myelofibrosis Polycythemia vera
Plasma cell dyscrasias	Multiple myeloma Primary amyloidosis Waldenström's macroglobulinemia (lymphoplasmacytic lymphoma)

drugs lead to free radical formation and DNA fragmentation. Anthracyclines are associated with hair loss, nausea, vomiting, and bone marrow suppression. These drugs can cause cardiac toxicity. (The incidence of congestive heart failure depends on the cumulative dose of the drug.) Finally, anthracyclines are vesicants, and extravasation can cause tissue necrosis.[4,7,16,17]

Bleomycin. Bleomycin has been used in combination therapy for malignant lymphomas. Bleomycin leads to free radical formation and DNA fragmentation. This agent has been associated with fevers, chills, and anaphylactoid reactions. Also, hypertrophic skin changes and hyperpigmentation have been noted. Pulmonary fibrosis is the most concerning side effect of bleomycin.[4,7,18]

Alkylating Agents

Busulfan. Busulfan has been used for chronic myeloid leukemia. By forming DNA cross-links, busulfan inhibits DNA replication. Side effects include prolonged myelosuppression and pulmonary reactions (bronchopulmonary dysplasia with pulmonary fibrosis).[4,8,11]

Chlorambucil. Chlorambucil is used to treat chronic lymphocytic leukemia and lymphoplasmacytic lymphoma (Waldenström's macroglobulinemia). As an alkylating agent, chlorambucil forms covalent bonds with DNA. Myelosuppression is the most common toxicity associated with the drug.[4]

Cyclophosphamide (Cytoxan). Cyclophosphamide is used to treat leukemia and lymphoid malignancies. Its cytotoxicity results from forming DNA cross-links. The drug is associated with hair loss, nausea, vomiting, diarrhea, and bone marrow suppression. Additionally, cyclophosphamide can cause hemorrhagic cystitis and bladder fibrosis. Hydration with intravenous fluids, bladder irrigation with an indwelling catheter, and intravenous mesna have been used to reduce the risk of hemorrhagic cystitis. (Mesna inactivates the toxic metabolites in the urine, decreasing the risk of hemorrhagic cystitis.)[4,7,8,19]

Mechlorethamine. Mechlorethamine is used in combination therapy to treat Hodgkin's lymphoma. This drug forms DNA cross-links and facilitates DNA fragmentation. Mechlorethamine is associated with nausea, vomiting, and myelosuppression.[4,7]

Melphalan. Melphalan is used to treat multiple myeloma. Its cytotoxicity results from forming DNA cross-links. As an alkylating agent, this drug is associated with myelosuppression.[7,8]

Methylating Agents (Dacarbazine and Procarbazine). The methylating agents dacarbazine and procarbazine are used in combination therapy to treat Hodgkin's lymphoma. These drugs exert their cytotoxic effect by inhibiting DNA and RNA synthesis. Methylating agents are associated with nausea, vomiting, and myelosuppression. Procarbazine has been associated with paresthesias, peripheral neuropathy, and altered mental status. Procarbazine is a monoamine oxidase inhibitor and can cause a disulfiram-like reaction with alcohol ingestion.[4,7,8] (For more information on dacarbazine, please see Chapter 69, Melanoma.)

Nitrosoureas (Carmustine and Lomustine). Nitrosoureas have been used in combination therapy for malignant lymphomas and multiple myeloma. Nitrosoureas are alkylating agents that form DNA cross-links to inhibit DNA replication. These drugs are associated with nausea, vomiting, myelosuppression, renal toxicity, and pulmonary fibrosis.[4,7]

Other Chemotherapy Agents

All-Trans Retinoic Acid. All-*trans* retinoic acid (ATRA) is used in acute promyelocytic leukemia (APL). APL is associated with the translocation that fuses the promyelocytic leukemia (PML) gene on chromosome 15 to the retinoic acid receptor (RAR) gene on chromosome 17. By binding to the fusion product (PML/RARα), ATRA induces differentiation of the leukemic cells into mature granulocytes.[20,21] ATRA is associated with headaches, dry skin, xerostomia, cheilitis, arthralgias, bone pain, and leukocytosis.[22,23] The major toxicity of ATRA is retinoic acid syndrome (RAS). Signs and symptoms of RAS include fever, weight gain, respiratory distress, interstitial pulmonary infiltrates, pleural effusion, pericardial effusion, hypotension, and acute renal failure. RAS is treated with dexamethasone.[21,24]

Arsenic Trioxide. Arsenic trioxide has been used in APL and myelodysplastic syndromes. This agent acts by promoting differentiation and apoptosis. Also, it suppresses proliferation and angiogenesis. Common toxicities associated with arsenic trioxide include nausea, vomiting, fatigue, edema, hyperglycemia, dyspnea, cough, rash, headaches, and dizziness. Additionally, QT prolongation can occur with this drug.[25] When used to treat APL, arsenic trioxide can lead to APL differentiation syndrome and leukocytosis. Signs and symptoms of APL differentiation syndrome include fluid retention, fever, pulmonary infiltrates, and pleural effusions.[22,25]

BCR-Abl Tyrosine Kinase Inhibitors (Imatinib and Dasatinib). The balanced translocation between chromosomes 9 and 22 produces the Philadelphia chromosome. The fusion gene encodes a chimeric protein, BCR-Abl, which functions as a constitutively activated tyrosine kinase. The BCR-Abl tyrosine kinase inhibitors are effective in Philadelphia chromosome–positive leukemias (chronic myelogenous leukemia and acute lymphoblastic leukemia). Dasatinib is a dual Src and Abl kinase inhibitor and has activity in imatinib-resistant disease. Toxicities associated with these drugs include nausea, vomiting, diarrhea, fluid retention, and myelosuppression.[26,27]

Corticosteroids (Dexamethasone and Prednisone). Corticosteroids are often used in combination with other agents in a variety of hematologic malignancies. They are particularly useful in the management of certain malignant lymphomas and multiple myeloma. As a single agent, dexamethasone has activity in multiple myeloma.[28]

Etoposide. Etoposide is used in combination with other agents in the treatment of leukemia and malignant lymphoma. As a topoisomerase II inhibitor, etoposide results in single- and double-strand DNA breaks. Ultimately, this leads to apoptosis. Toxicities associated with etoposide include alopecia, nausea, vomiting, and myelosuppression.[4,7,8]

L-Asparaginase. L-Asparaginase is used in the treatment of acute lymphoblastic leukemia. This agent hydrolyzes L-asparagine to aspartic acid and ammonia. Sensitive tumor cells require exogenous sources of L-asparagine. When L-asparaginase hydrolyzes L-asparagine in the bloodstream, sensitive tumor cells are deprived of L-asparagine, without which they are unable to synthesize proteins. Toxicities associated with L-asparaginase include allergic reactions, hyperglycemia, pancreatitis, decrease in clotting factors, and increase in liver transaminases.[4,7,8]

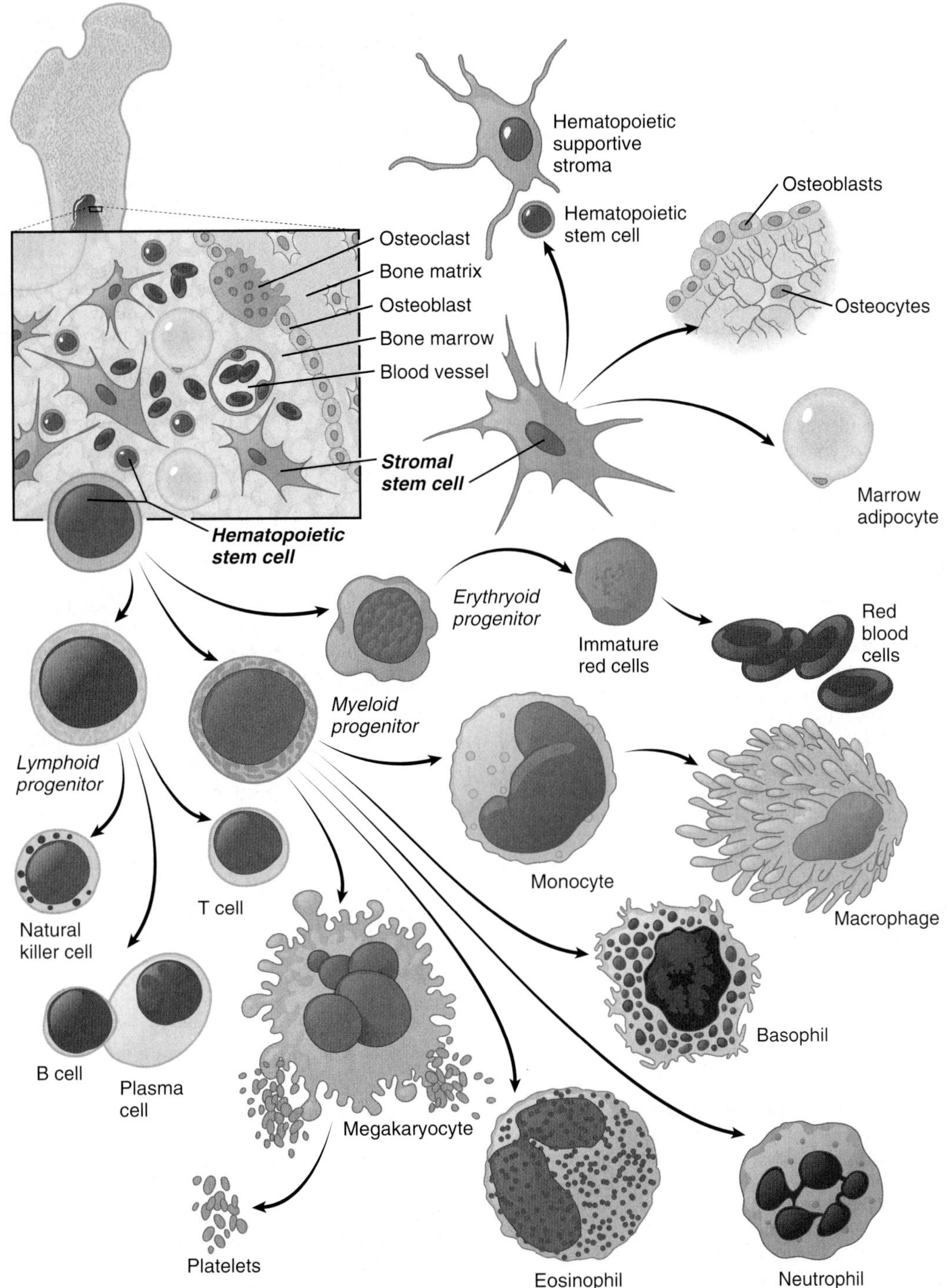

FIGURE 66-1 • Hematopoietic and stromal stem cell differentiation.

Thalidomide and Lenalidomide. Thalidomide and lenalidomide, an analogue of thalidomide, have been used in the treatment of myelodysplastic syndromes and multiple myeloma. The exact mechanism of action of these agents is not clear. Thalidomide and its analogues induce apoptosis or growth arrest of myeloma cells.[29,30] Also, these drugs are thought to have antiangiogenic effects, immunomodulatory properties, and anti-inflammatory activity.[31]

Thalidomide is most commonly associated with constipation, neuropathy, somnolence, fatigue, dry skin, and dry mouth.[32,33] In the treatment of multiple myeloma, thalidomide is often combined with dexamethasone. This combination is associated with a higher risk of deep vein thrombosis. Therefore, prophylactic anticoagulation is recommended for patients receiving thalidomide and dexamethasone. Lenalidomide is thought to be better tolerated than thalidomide. It is associated with neutropenia and thrombocytopenia. Again, there is an increased risk of thrombosis when lenalidomide is combined with corticosteroids.[28] (For more information on thalidomide, please see Chapter 69, Melanoma.)

Vinca Alkaloids (Vincristine and Vinblastine). A number of hematologic malignancies are treated with vinca alkaloids, including acute lymphoblastic leukemia, malignant lymphomas, and multiple myeloma.[4] Vinca alkaloids bind to tubulin and prevent microtubule formation. As a result, the mitotic spindle apparatus is disrupted. This prevents chromosome separation and cell proliferation. Major toxicities linked with vinca alkaloids include peripheral neuropathy and myelosuppression.[4,7,34]

Biologic Therapies

Antithymocyte Globulin. Antithymocyte globulin (ATG) has been used to treat aplastic anemia and myelodysplastic syndromes. By immunizing horses or other animals with human thoracic duct lymphocytes, ATG is produced. ATG suppresses T-cell function and may stimulate hematopoiesis by augmenting hematopoietic growth factor release by T cells and stromal cells. Toxicities associated with ATG include allergic reactions and serum sickness (fever, malaise, nausea, vomiting, and rash).[35-37]

Alemtuzumab (Campath-1H). Alemtuzumab is an anti-CD52 humanized monoclonal antibody that is used to treat chronic lymphocytic leukemia. CD52 is expressed on essentially all lymphocytes, natural killer cells, monocytes, macrophages, and eosinophils. Alemtuzumab is thought to induce cell death by various mechanisms, including antibody-dependent cellular cytotoxicity, complement-dependent cytotoxicity, and induction of apoptosis.[38-40]

Increased numbers of infections with *Pneumocystis jiroveci* and herpesviruses have been attributed to alemtuzumab. Therefore, antimicrobial prophylaxis with trimethoprim-sulfamethoxazole and famciclovir, acyclovir, or valacyclovir is recommended. Infusion-related toxicities with alemtuzumab include rigors, fevers, nausea, vomiting, and rash. Systemic reactions are less frequent with the subcutaneous mode of administration.[38]

Gemtuzumab Ozogamicin (Mylotarg). Gemtuzumab ozogamicin is a humanized anti-CD33 monoclonal antibody that is linked to the cytotoxic antibiotic calicheamicin. (Calicheamicin induces its cytotoxic effects by intercalation into DNA.) Gemtuzumab ozogamicin is used to treat acute myeloid leukemia. Approximately 80% to 90% of acute myeloid leukemia patients have myeloid blasts that express the CD33 antigen. Toxicities commonly associated with this agent include myelosuppression, hyperbilirubinemia, and elevated hepatic transaminases.[41-43]

Interferon Alfa. Interferon alfa is a cytokine that has been used in the treatment of certain hematologic malignancies, including hairy cell leukemia and chronic myeloid leukemia.[44,45] The exact mechanism by which interferons work is unclear. It is thought that interferon alfa has direct antiproliferative effects on tumor cells. Interferon alfa has indirect immune-mediated effects by stimulating T cells and natural killer cells.[46,47] Also, interferons enhance major histocompatibility complex expression, which may make malignant cells more antigenic.[48] Furthermore, interferon alfa may have antiangiogenic effects.[46]

With regard to toxicity, an influenza-like syndrome with fevers, rigors, headache, and myalgia is common with interferon alfa. Other notable side effects include fatigue, depression, anorexia, neutropenia, and liver function abnormalities. Most toxicity is rapidly reversible with dose reduction or cessation of the drug.[9,47,49] (For more details on interferon, please see Chapter 69, Melanoma.)

Radioimmunotherapy. Radioimmunoconjugates are monoclonal antibodies with an attached radioisotope. Currently, the two radioimmunoconjugates commercially available are [^{90}Y]ibritumomab tiuxetan (Zevalin; IDEC Pharmaceuticals, San Diego, CA) and [^{131}I]tositumomab (Bexxar; Corixa Corporation, Seattle, WA). Both these agents are directed against the CD20 antigen and have been used in B-cell malignancies. Radioimmunoconjugates provide radiation therapy to cells that bind the antibody. Also, they may affect neighboring cells that have insufficient antigen expression.[38]

Major complications of radioimmunotherapy are infusion reactions and myelosuppression. Myelotoxicity is delayed about 7 to 9 weeks after therapy. Also, [^{131}I]tositumomab therapy is associated with hypothyroidism in about 10% of patients.[50] To minimize the risk of severe myelotoxicity, radioimmunotherapy should be avoided in patients with greater than 25% of the bone marrow involved with disease. This therapy should also be avoided in patients with a hypocellular bone marrow (<15% cellular), platelet counts less than 100,000/mm^3, and neutrophil counts less than 1500/mm^3.[38]

TABLE 66-2 SELECTED COMBINATION CHEMOTHERAPY REGIMENS USED TO TREAT SPECIFIC HEMATOLOGIC MALIGNANCIES

Disease	Chemotherapy Regimen
Hodgkin's lymphoma	ABVD[53] • Doxorubicin 25 mg/m^2 IV days 1, 15 • Bleomycin 10 units/m^2 IV days 1, 15 • Vinblastine 6 mg/m^2 IV days 1, 15 • Dacarbazine 375 mg/m^2 IV days 1, 15 Stanford V[54] • Mechlorethamine 6 mg/m^2 IV day 1 • Doxorubicin 25 mg/m^2 IV days 1, 15 • Vinblastine 6 mg/m^2 IV days 1, 15 • Vincristine 1.4 mg/m^2 IV days 8, 22 (maximum 2 mg) • Bleomycin 5 units/m^2 IV days 8, 22 • Etoposide 60 mg/m^2 IV days 15, 16 • Prednisone 40 mg/m^2 PO every other day
Non-Hodgkin's lymphoma	CHOP[55] • Cyclophosphamide 750 mg/m^2 IV day 1 • Doxorubicin 50 mg/m^2 IV day 1 • Vincristine 1.4 mg/m^2 IV day 1 (maximum 2 mg) • Prednisone 100 mg PO days 1-5 EPOCH[56] • Etoposide 50 mg/m^2/day continuous IV infusion over 96 hr • Vincristine 0.4 mg/m^2/day continuous IV infusion over 96 hr • Doxorubicin 10 mg/m^2/day continuous IV infusion over 96 hr • Prednisone 60 mg/m^2 PO days 1-5 • Cyclophosphamide 750 mg/m^2 IV day 5
Acute myeloid leukemia	7+3 (Induction)[57] • Cytarabine 100 mg/m^2 continuous IV infusion days 1-7 • Daunorubicin 45 mg/m^2 IV days 1, 2, 3
Multiple myeloma	VAD[58] • Vincristine 0.4 mg/day continuous IV infusion days 1-4 • Doxorubicin 9 mg/m^2/day continuous IV infusion days 1-4 • Dexamethasone 40 mg PO days 1-4, 9-12, and 17-20

IV, intravenously; PO, orally.

Rituximab (Rituxan). Rituximab is a chimeric human-mouse monoclonal antibody that is directed against the CD20 antigen. CD20 is expressed on B lymphocytes. As such, rituximab is used in a variety of malignant lymphomas or B-cell malignancies. Rituximab induces cell death by antibody-dependent cellular cytotoxicity and complement-dependent cytotoxicity. Also, by binding to CD20, rituximab leads to high intracellular calcium levels and apoptosis. Infusion-related toxicities with rituximab include fevers, chills, nausea, vomiting, rash, orthostatic hypotension, and bronchospasm.[51,52]

Therapeutic Approach

This chapter is meant to give a basic foundation of the treatments utilized in hematopoietic and lymphoid malignancies. A number of drugs, both in combination and as single agents, are used to treat these diseases. In that context, algorithms for treating selected hematologic malignancies are presented as therapeutic prototypes in Table 66-2.

REFERENCES

1. Schneider AS, Szanto PA. Neoplastic and proliferative disorders of the hematopoietic and lymphoid systems. *In* Board Review Series: Pathology. Baltimore: Williams & Wilkins, 1993, pp 165-175.
2. Kumar V, Cotran RS, Robbins SL. The Hematopoietic and Lymphoid Systems: Basic Pathology. Philadelphia: WB Saunders, 1997, pp 362-383.

3. Cataland SR, Shannon K, Caligiuri MA. Myelodysplasia. *In* Williams ME, Kahn MJ (eds): American Society of Hematology Self-Assessment Program. Malden, CT: Blackwell Publishing, 2005, pp 200-209.
4. Perry MC (ed). The Chemotherapy Source Book, 3rd ed. Philadelphia: Lippincott Williams & Wilkins, 2001.
5. Saven A, Piro LD. 2-Chlorodeoxyadenosine: a newer purine analog active in the treatment of indolent lymphoid malignancies. Ann Intern Med 1994;120:784-791.
6. Tallman MS, Hakimian D, Variakojis D, et al. A single cycle of 2-chlorodeoxyadenosine results in complete remission in the majority of patients with hairy cell leukemia. Blood 1992;80:2203-2209.
7. Mycek MJ, Harvey RA, Champe PC (eds). Lippincott's Illustrated Reviews: Pharmacology, 2nd ed. Philadelphia: Lippincott–Raven, 1997.
8. USP DI, Vol I: Drug Information for the Health Care Professsional, 26th ed. Greenwood Village, CO: Thomson MICROMEDEX, 2006.
9. Baker WJ, Royer GL Jr, Weiss RB. Cytarabine and neurologic toxicity. J Clin Oncol 1991;9:679-693.
10. Tallman MS, Hakimian D. Purine nucleoside analogs: emerging roles in indolent lymphoproliferative disorders. Blood 1995;86:2463-2474.
11. Faderl S, Talpaz M, Estrov Z, Kantarjian HM. Chronic myelogenous leukemia: biology and therapy. Ann Intern Med 1999;131:207-219.
12. Gryn J, Zeigler ZR, Shadduck RK, et al. Treatment of myelodysplastic syndromes with 5-azacytidine. Leuk Res 2002;26:893-897.
13. Kantarjian H, Issa JP, Rosenfeld CS, et al. Decitabine improves patient outcomes in myelodysplastic syndromes: results of a Phase III randomized study. Cancer 2006;106:1794-1803.
14. Li J, Gwilt P. The effect of malignant effusions on methotrexate disposition. Cancer Chemother Pharmacol 2002;50:373-382.
15. Widemann BC, Balis FM, Kempf-Bielack B, et al. High-dose methotrexate-induced nephrotoxicity in patients with osteosarcoma. Cancer 2004;100:2222-2232.
16. Goolsby TV, Lombardo FA. Extravasation of chemotherapeutic agents: prevention and treatment. Semin Oncol 2006;33:139-143.
17. Shan K, Lincoff AM, Young JB. Anthracycline-induced cardiotoxicity. Ann Intern Med 1996;125:47-58.
18. Sleijfer S. Bleomycin-induced pneumonitis. Chest 2001;120:617-624.
19. Wong TM, Yeo W, Chan LW, Mok TS. Hemorrhagic pyelitis, ureteritis, and cystitis secondary to cyclophosphamide: case report and review of the literature. Gynecol Oncol 2000;76:223-225.
20. Appelbaum FR. Acute myeloid leukemia in adults. *In* Abeloff MD, et al (eds): Clinical Oncology. New York: Churchill Livingstone, 2004, p 2829.
21. Tallman MS, Nabhan C, Feusner JH, Rowe JM. Acute promyelocytic leukemia: evolving therapeutic strategies. Blood 2002;99:759-767.
22. Camacho LH, Soignet SL, Chanel S, et al. Leukocytosis and the retinoic acid syndrome in patients with acute promyelocytic leukemia treated with arsenic trioxide. J Clin Oncol 2000;18:2620-2625.
23. Warrell RP Jr, de The H, Wang ZY, Degos L. Acute promyelocytic leukemia. N Engl J Med 1993,329:177-189.
24. Sanz MA, Tallman MS, Lo-Coco F. Tricks of the trade for the appropriate management of newly diagnosed acute promyelocytic leukemia. Blood 2005;105:3019-3025.
25. List A, Beran M, DiPersio J, et al. Opportunities for Trisenox (arsenic trioxide) in the treatment of myelodysplastic syndromes. Leukemia 2003;17:1499-1507.
26. Quintas-Cardama A, Kantarjian H, Jones D, et al. Dasatinib (BMS-354825) is active in Philadelphia chromosome-positive chronic myelogenous leukemia after imatinib and nilotinib (AMN107) therapy failure. Blood 2007;109:497-499.
27. Talpaz M, Shah NP, Kantarjian H, et al. Dasatinib in imatinib-resistant Philadelphia chromosome-positive leukemias. N Engl J Med 2006;354:2531-2541.
28. Kumar S, Rajkumar SV. Thalidomide and lenalidomide in the treatment of multiple myeloma. Eur J Cancer 2006;42:1612-1622.
29. Hideshima T, Chauhan D, Shima Y, et al. Thalidomide and its analogs overcome drug resistance of human multiple myeloma cells to conventional therapy. Blood 2000;96:2943-2950.
30. Mitsiades N, Mitsiades CS, Poulaki V, et al. Apoptotic signaling induced by immunomodulatory thalidomide analogs in human multiple myeloma cells: therapeutic implications. Blood 2002;99:4525-4530.
31. Eleutherakis-Papaiakovou V, Bamias A, Dimopoulos MA. Thalidomide in cancer medicine. Ann Oncol 2004;15:1151-1160.
32. Pawlak WZ, Legha SS. Phase II study of thalidomide in patients with metastatic melanoma. Melanoma Res 2004;14:57-62.
33. Reiriz AB, Richter MF, Fernandes S, et al. Phase II study of thalidomide in patients with metastatic malignant melanoma. Melanoma Res 2004;14:527-531.
34. Brown CK, Kirkwood JM. Medical management of melanoma. Surg Clin North Am 2003;83:283-322, viii.
35. McEvoy GK (ed). AHFS Drug Information Essentials. Bethesda, MD: American Society of Health-System Pharmacists, 2006.
36. Steensma DP, Dispenzieri A, Moore SB, et al. Antithymocyte globulin has limited efficacy and substantial toxicity in unselected anemic patients with myelodysplastic syndrome. Blood 2003;101:2156-2158.
37. Yazji S, Giles FJ, Tsimberidou AM, et al. Antithymocyte globulin (ATG)-based therapy in patients with myelodysplastic syndromes. Leukemia 2003;17:2101-2106.
38. Cheson BD. Monoclonal antibody therapy for B-cell malignancies. Semin Oncol 2006;33(2 Suppl 5):S2-S14.
39. Faderl S, Coutre S, Byrd JC, et al. The evolving role of alemtuzumab in management of patients with CLL. Leukemia 2005;19:2147-2152.
40. Ginaldi L, De Martinis M, Matutes E, et al. Levels of expression of CD52 in normal and leukemic B and T cells: correlation with in vivo therapeutic responses to Campath-1H. Leuk Res 1998;22:185-191.
41. Burnett AK, Mohite U. Treatment of older patients with acute myeloid leukemia—new agents. Semin Hematol 2006;43:96-106.
42. Sievers EL, Larson RA, Stadtmauer EA, et al. Efficacy and safety of gemtuzumab ozogamicin in patients with CD33-positive acute myeloid leukemia in first relapse. J Clin Oncol 2001;19:3244-3254.
43. van der Heiden PL, Jedema I, Willemze R, Barge RM. Efficacy and toxicity of gemtuzumab ozogamicin in patients with acute myeloid leukemia. Eur J Haematol 2006;76:409-413.
44. Saven A, Piro LD. Treatment of hairy cell leukemia. Blood 1992;79:1111-1120.
45. Silver RT, Woolf SH, Hehlmann R, et al. An evidence-based analysis of the effect of busulfan, hydroxyurea, interferon, and allogeneic bone marrow transplantation in treating the chronic phase of chronic myeloid leukemia: developed for the American Society of Hematology. Blood 1999;94:1517-1536.
46. Jonasch E, Haluska FG. Interferon in oncological practice: review of interferon biology, clinical applications, and toxicities. Oncologist 2001;6:34-55.
47. Kefford RF. Adjuvant therapy of cutaneous melanoma: the interferon debate. Ann Oncol 2003;14:358-365.
48. Gray RJ, Pockaj BA, Kirkwood JM. An update on adjuvant interferon for melanoma. Cancer Control 2002;9:16-21.
49. Kirkwood JM, Bender C, Agarwala S, et al. Mechanisms and management of toxicities associated with high-dose interferon alfa-2b therapy. J Clin Oncol 2002;20:3703-3718.
50. Kaminski MS, Tuck M, Estes J, et al. ^{131}I-tositumomab therapy as initial treatment for follicular lymphoma. N Engl J Med 2005;352:441-449.
51. Boye J, Elter T, Engert A. An overview of the current clinical use of the anti-CD20 monoclonal antibody rituximab. Ann Oncol 2003;14:520-535.
52. Hainsworth JD. Monoclonal antibody therapy in lymphoid malignancies. Oncologist 2000;5:376-384.
53. Canellos GP, Anderson JR, Propert KJ, et al. Chemotherapy of advanced Hodgkin's disease with MOPP, ABVD, or MOPP alternating with ABVD. N Engl J Med 1992;327:1478-1484.
54. Horning SJ, Hoppe RT, Breslin S, et al. Stanford V and radiotherapy for locally extensive and advanced Hodgkin's disease: mature results of a prospective clinical trial. J Clin Oncol 2002;20:630-637.
55. Coiffier B, Lepage E, Briere J, et al. CHOP chemotherapy plus rituximab compared with CHOP alone in elderly patients with diffuse large-B-cell lymphoma. N Engl J Med 2002;346:235-242.
56. Wilson WH, Grossbard ML, Pittaluga S, et al. Dose-adjusted EPOCH chemotherapy for untreated large B-cell lymphomas: a pharmacodynamic approach with high efficacy. Blood 2002;99:2685-2693.
57. Wiernik PH, Banks PL, Case DC Jr, et al. Cytarabine plus idarubicin or daunorubicin as induction and consolidation therapy for previously untreated adult patients with acute myeloid leukemia. Blood 1992;79:313-319.
58. Alexanian R, Barlogie B, Tucker S. VAD-based regimens as primary treatment for multiple myeloma. Am J Hematol 1990;33:86-89.

67

PROSTATE CANCER

Sarah A. Holstein and Raymond J. Hohl

INTRODUCTION 951
THERAPEUTICS AND CLINICAL PHARMACOLOGY 951
Hormone-Dependent Prostate Cancer 951
Androgen Deprivation 951
Androgen Antagonists 953
Intermittent Androgen Deprivation 953
Complete Androgen Blockade 953
Hormone-Refractory Prostate Cancer 953
Mitoxantrone 954
Taxotere 954
Estramustine Phosphate 954
Other Single-Agent Chemotherapeutics 954
Combinations 954
Metastatic Bone Disease 954
Bisphosphonates 955
Radioisotopes 955
Emerging Targets and Therapeutics 955
Vitamin D 955
Histone Deacetylase Inhibitors 955
Sipuleucel-T 955
Growth Factor Receptor Antagonists 955
Epothilones 956
Atrasentan 956

INTRODUCTION

Prostate cancer is one of the most common malignancies in men, second only to nonmelanoma skin cancer. It was estimated that over 230,000 men in the United States would be diagnosed with prostate cancer in 2006 and that over 27,000 men would die of the disease.[1] In the United States, the lifetime risk of being diagnosed with prostate cancer is 1 in 6 and the risk of dying from prostate cancer is 1 in 30. The incidence of prostate cancer has been on the rise since the early 1990s, in part due to widespread screening with the blood prostate-specific antigen (PSA) level. This has led to earlier detection of the disease, and many men are asymptomatic at the time of diagnosis. When prostate cancer is symptomatic, it often mimics those symptoms caused by benign prostatic hyperplasia: urinary frequency or urgency, nocturia, or hesitancy. New-onset erectile dysfunction can also be a presenting symptom. Less commonly, men can present with symptoms secondary to metastatic disease such as bony pain, pathologic fractures, or spinal cord compression. Management of local disease includes watchful waiting, radical prostatectomy, external beam radiation therapy, and brachytherapy (Fig. 67-1). Once prostate cancer has progressed beyond local disease, it becomes an incurable disease, although there are many systemic therapeutic options.

The prostate gland is an accessory sexual organ that requires androgens for normal growth and development. Leydig cells in the testes produce approximately 90% to 95% of the total circulating testosterone. The adrenal glands are responsible for the remainder of the testosterone production. Testosterone is converted to the more potent 5α-dihydrotestosterone (DHT) via the enzyme 5α-reductase in the prostate. DHT then binds to androgen receptors that serve as transcription factors and induce the expression of genes with androgen response elements. The production of testosterone is regulated by luteinizing hormone (LH), which is produced in the pituitary, which in turn is regulated by the hypothalamic production of gonadotropin-releasing hormone (GnRH) (Fig. 67-2). DHT stimulates the growth of both malignant and benign prostate cells.

THERAPEUTICS AND CLINICAL PHARMACOLOGY

Hormone-Dependent Prostate Cancer

Androgen Deprivation

In 1941, Huggins and Hodges reported the use of androgen deprivation, via either surgical castration or medical castration with estrogens, in the treatment of prostate cancer.[2,3] They later won the Nobel Prize in Medicine for this work. Androgen deprivation has continued to be a mainstay of treatment for advanced prostate cancer. Androgen deprivation may be achieved through a number of methods, including surgical removal of the testes, inhibition of release of gonadotropins, or treatment with estrogens. Bilateral orchiectomy remains the fastest way to produce androgen deprivation and can result in an almost immediate improvement in bony pain. However, the majority of men are now choosing medical hormonal manipulation.

GnRH Agonists. The hypothalamus secretes the decapeptide GnRH in a pulsatile manner. While intermittent exposure of GnRH leads to release of LH, continuous exposure to GnRH leads to desensitization of the pituitary with subsequent suppression of GnRH secretion. Four GnRH agonists are currently in use in the United States: leuprolide acetate, goserelin acetate, triptorelin pamoate, and histrelin acetate (see Fig. 67-2). All are synthetic analogues of GnRH and are 15 to 210 times more potent than GnRH.[4] These analogues have increased affinity for the receptor as well as decreased susceptibility to enzymatic proteolysis.[4] They differ in their route of injection and dosing interval. Goserelin acetate can be given subcutaneously every 28 or 84 days. Leuprolide acetate may be given as a depot suspension via intramuscular injection or as a subcutaneous injection every 28, 84, or 112 days. In addition, both leuprolide acetate and histrelin acetate may be implanted every 365 days. Triptorelin pamoate is injected intramuscularly every 28 or 84 days.

The time to achieve a castration level of testosterone does not significantly differ among these agents and is generally within 3 to 4 weeks. After approximately 1 week of continuous exposure to a GnRH agonist, there is down-regulation of the GnRH receptor. This results in a decrease in LH secretion with subsequent decrease in testosterone levels. However, with the initial exposure to the GnRH agonist, there is a transient surge in testosterone levels that may exacerbate the symptoms of the prostate cancer.[5] Therefore, patients are often started on antiandrogen therapy 1 week prior to the initiation of treatment with the GnRH agonist and are continued on the antiandrogen therapy for 2 weeks.[6]

GnRH agonists are associated with significant side effects, including sexual dysfunction, loss of bone mineral density, hot flashes, anemia, fatigue, and decrease in lean body mass with an increase in fat mass.[7] The anemia is typically a mild normochromic, normocytic anemia and generally does not require treatment with erythropoietin.[8] Studies have shown benefit of several agents in treating hot flashes, including transdermal estrogen,[9] selective serotonin receptor inhibitors,[10,11] and megestrol acetate.[12]

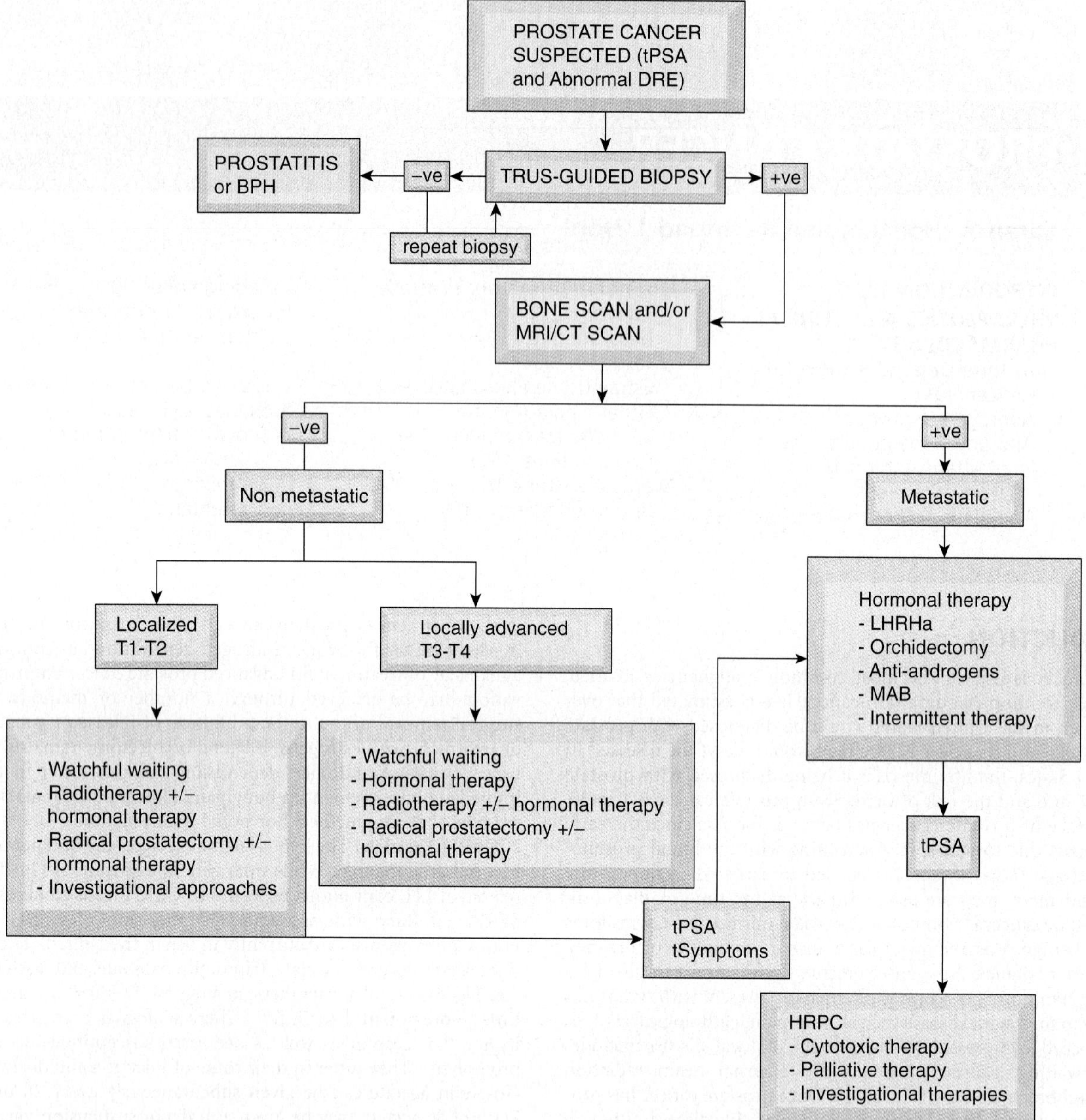

FIGURE 67-1 • Treatment algorithm for prostate cancer.

GnRH Antagonist. Abarelix is a synthetic decapeptide that competitively inhibits GnRH by binding to the GnRH receptor in the pituitary (see Fig. 67-2). Clinical trials have shown that, compared with leuprolide, abarelix does not cause a testosterone surge and causes testosterone suppression more rapidly.[13,14] Significant reductions in testosterone levels were seen by 1 day, and castration level was achieved after a median of 7 days. The drug is administered as an intramuscular injection, and its half-life is 13 days. Immediate-onset allergic reactions have been described.

Ketoconazole. Ketoconazole is an antifungal agent that, in high doses, has been shown to inhibit adrenal and testicular steroid synthesis[15] via inhibition of 17,20-desmolase (see Fig. 67-2).[16] Its benefit in prostate cancer is thought to be secondary to the further reduction in androgen levels. Direct cytotoxic effects of ketoconazole on prostate cancer cells have also been suggested in in vitro studies.[17] Adverse effects include skin rash, nausea, fatigue, and gynecomastia. High doses (200 to 400 mg three times a day) of ketoconazole can lead to adrenal insufficiency; therefore, patients are commonly given hydrocortisone or prednisone. As ketoconazole is a substrate and inhibitor of the cytochrome P-450 (CYP) isoenzyme CYP3A4 as well as an inhibitor of CYP1A2, CYP2A6, CYP2B6, CYP2C8, CYP2C9, and CYP2C19, there is the potential for a wide array of drug interactions. In addition, as the absorption of ketoconazole depends on gastric acidity,[18] patients should avoid concomitant use of antacids, histamine blockers, or proton pump inhibitors.

Aminoglutethimide. Aminogluthethimide inhibits CYP11A1, the enzyme that converts cholesterol to δ^5-pregnenolone and therefore inhibits the synthesis of adrenal steroids. This drug has the potential to cause many drug interactions as it is a strong inducer of CYP1A2, CYP2C19, and CYP3A4. Adverse effects include headache, lethargy, nausea, skin rash, myalgias, and abnormal liver function tests. Aminogluthethimide is usually given in conjunction with hydrocortisone.

Estrogens. High-dose estrogens can suppress testosterone levels by feedback inhibition of the hypothalamic-pituitary axis (see Fig. 67-2). Diethylstilbestrol (DES), a nonsteroidal estrogen, has been the estrogen most commonly used in the past. While long-term follow-up has suggested that DES may confer a survival advantage,[19] its significant cardiovascular toxicity (including myocardial infarction, pulmonary embolism, and stroke) has limited its use. Other estrogens that have been studied include ethinyl estradiol, conjugated estrogens (Prema-

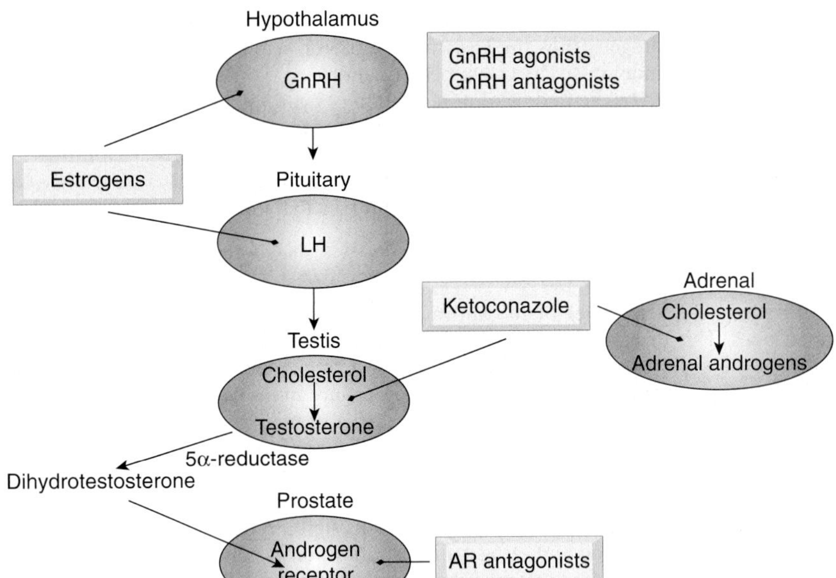

FIGURE 67-2 • The hypothalamic-pituitary-testicular axis. The normal pathway for androgen production is shown as are the sites of action for agents used in the treatment of hormone-sensitive prostate cancer.

rin), medroxyprogesterone, and chlorotrianisene. There is some initial evidence suggesting that transdermal estrogen could be effective in prostate cancer and may be associated with fewer side effects.[20] Side effects of high-dose estrogen therapy include gynecomastia, nipple tenderness, and sexual dysfunction. Prophylactic breast irradiation may decrease the risk of gynecomastia and nipple tenderness.[21]

Androgen Antagonists

Androgen antagonists bind to the androgen receptor and competitively inhibit testosterone and DHT (see Fig. 67-2). Three nonsteroidal agents are used in the United States: flutamide, bicalutamide, and nilutamide. Cyproterone is a steroid agent that has been used in Europe. These agents are not typically used as monotherapy, but instead are used in conjunction with a GnRH agonist. As noted earlier, antiandrogen therapy is commonly started prior to the initiation of GnRH agonist therapy in order to prevent the initial androgen surge. In addition, androgen antagonists are sometimes used in combination with GnRH agonists to achieve "combined androgen blockade" (see later).

Bicalutamide (Casodex) is a pure nonsteroidal antiandrogen that is administered once a day orally. It is a racemate; however, only the (*R*)-enantiomer is active. It is metabolized via glucuronidation. Daily dosing does result in increased circulating levels of testosterone and gonadotropins.[22] Breast tenderness, gynecomastia, and hot flashes are common side effects. Single-agent bicalutamide has been associated with inferior survival when compared with castration; however, quality of life was improved.[23]

Flutamide has a shorter half-life than bicalutamide and is generally given three times per day. It undergoes extensive metabolism and its active metabolite is 2-hydroxyflutamide.[24] Flutamide is a substrate of CYP1A2 and CYP3A4; therefore, drug-drug interactions must be considered. Monitoring of transaminases should be performed periodically as flutamide can cause hepatotoxicity. Common side effects include diarrhea, gynecomastia, nipple tenderness, nausea, and vomiting. A randomized clinical trial comparing orchiectomy and flutamide showed similar survival and time to progression.[25] A trial comparing single-agent flutamide with DES suggested inferiority of flutamide.[26]

Nilutamide is given once a day and is a substrate of CYP2C19. Side effects include nausea, impaired dark adaptation, hot flashes, gynecomastia, and disulfuram-like reaction. As its side effect profile appears less favorable, nilutamide is rarely used.[27] Cyproterone acetate is a steroidal antiandrogen that can either be given orally or as a depot intramuscular injection. It has been associated with increased risk of thromboembolism as well as liver toxicity.

Intermittent Androgen Deprivation

Intermittent androgen deprivation has been proposed as a strategy for delaying the development of hormone-refractory disease. Initial animal studies demonstrated that intermittent androgen suppression, achieved through cycles of treatment (>6 months) interrupted by no treatment (2 to 11 months), could induce multiple regressions in the tumor.[28] Initial clinical trials employing GnRH agonists with or without androgen antagonists have shown that patients can respond to re-treatment.[29] Typically the time between treatment cycles diminishes until hormone-refractory disease emerges. Studies have shown improved quality of life with intermittent androgen deprivation[30] but have not yet shown survival benefit.

Complete Androgen Blockade

Complete androgen blockade (CAB) involves the combination of GnRH agonist or orchiectomy with antiandrogen therapy. Clinical trials have yielded conflicting results. Several large trials have shown a benefit for CAB compared with androgen deprivation therapy alone,[31-33] while other trials have failed to show a benefit.[34,35] Several meta-analyses have been performed and have suggested small benefits in survival with CAB.[36,37]

Hormone-Refractory Prostate Cancer

While androgen deprivation therapy can ameliorate symptoms, it is not curative. Nearly all patients progress to develop androgen-independent cancer within 2 years. The median survival of men with hormone-refractory prostate cancer is approximately 12 months.[38]

Preclinical studies have suggested that, over time, androgen suppression therapy can create a population of clonogenic tumor cells that have evolved from an androgen-dependent to an androgen-independent state.[39] Other studies have shown that, regardless of continuous versus intermittent androgen suppression, conversion to androgen independence occurs in the stem cells.[40] A number of mechanisms for the development of androgen-independent disease have been proposed. Overexpression of the androgen receptor has been reported in 20% to 25% of recurrent primary tumors and metastatic tumors.[41,42] Mutations in the androgen receptor have also been reported, many of which result in gain-of-function. However, correlation of mutation with response to androgen deprivation or with survival has not been demonstrated.[43] While androgen suppression therapy can lead to castration levels of testosterone in the blood (<50 ng/ml), studies have shown that intratumoral androgen levels may be sufficient for continued androgen receptor signaling.[44] This may be due to adrenal production of androgen (thus the basis for the use of ketoconazole or aminoglutethimide) or to direct synthesis of androgens within the tumor, as evidenced by the finding of upregulation of hydroxymethylglutaryl coenzyme A reductase in hormone-refractory cancer.[45] Finally, a variety of growth factors, including human epidermal growth factor receptor 2 (HER2), insulin-like growth factor 1, and epidermal growth factor, can activate the androgen receptor in the absence of androgens.[46]

Mitoxantrone

Mitoxantrone is a member of the anthracycline class of antitumor antibiotics. This drug intercalates DNA and stimulates formation of DNA breaks via interaction with topoisomerase II. Compared to doxorubicin, mitoxantrone has a limited ability to produce quinone-type free radicals[47] and is less cardiotoxic. Major toxicities of mitoxantrone include myelosuppression and mucositis. Clinical trials involving mitoxantrone plus steroids have shown significant improvements in pain relief without an effect on PSA response rate or overall survival.[48,49] Mitoxantrone, in combination with corticosteroids, has been approved by the U.S. Food and Drug Administration for pain related to advanced hormone-refractory prostate cancer.

Taxotere

Taxanes, including paclitaxel and docetaxel, inhibit cell cycle progression. Unlike vinca alkaloids, which inhibit microtubule polymerization, taxanes inhibit microtubule depolymerization.[50] Docetaxel (Taxotere) is a more potent inhibitor of microtubule depolymerization than is paclitaxel.[50] The dose-limiting toxicity of Taxotere is neutropenia; other side effects include neuropathy, hypersensitivity reactions, skin changes, mucositis, peripheral edema, vomiting, and diarrhea. A landmark clinical trial comparing Taxotere plus prednisone with mitoxantrone plus prednisone revealed improved survival, PSA response, pain response, and quality of life in the Taxotere plus prednisone arm.[51] Taxotere plus prednisone is now the standard of care for hormone-refractory prostate cancer.

A Phase II trial has shown evidence for activity of single-agent paclitaxel in hormone-refractory prostate cancer.[52] Paclitaxel-based regimens have not been evaluated in Phase III trials. Paclitaxel-associated toxicities include neutropenia, neuropathy, arthralgias, and myalgias.

Estramustine Phosphate

Estramustine phosphate (EMP) is a prodrug of the nitrogen mustard derivative of estradiol-17β phosphate. Its effects in prostate cancer cells are thought to be secondary to both hormonal effects of the estrogen component as well as cytotoxic effects secondary to inhibition of microtubules and binding to the nuclear matrix. EMP as a single agent does not have significant activity in prostate cancer. However, in vitro studies have shown synergistic activity in combination with other antimicrotubule agents, including vinblastine, paclitaxel, and docetaxel.[53] A randomized clinical trial involving docetaxel plus EMP versus mitoxantrone plus prednisone showed statistically significant improvements in median survival (17.5 vs. 15.6 months) as well as median progression-free survival and PSA response rate.[54] The docetaxel plus EMP arm was associated with increased neurologic, gastrointestinal, and cardiac toxicities. In addition, EMP has been associated with increased risk of thromboembolic events.[55] Given the similar survival advantage seen with docetaxel plus prednisone over mitoxantrone plus prednisone[51] and the significant risk of thromboembolism with EMP, the combination of docetaxel plus EMP is generally not recommended over docetaxel plus prednisone.

Other Single-Agent Chemotherapeutics

A wide array of chemotherapy agents have been studied in the setting of androgen-independent prostate cancer. With the exception of the agents discussed previously, the measurable response rates have generally been less than 20%, although some studies have reported greater than 50% decline in PSA. A brief discussion of these agents is found in this section.

Cisplatin/Carboplatin. Cisplatin and carboplatin form DNA adducts and interfere with DNA replication and transcription. Cisplatin has significant toxicities, including nephrotoxicity, ototoxicity (tinnitus and high-frequency hearing loss), nausea and vomiting, peripheral neuropathy, electrolyte disturbances, mild myelosuppression, and anaphylactic reactions. Carboplatin is associated with less nausea, ototoxicity, nephrotoxicity, and neurotoxicity. However, the dose-limiting toxicity of carboplatin is myelosuppression, in particular, thrombocytopenia.

Cyclophosphamide. The cytotoxic effects of cyclophosphamide are due to alkylation of DNA. The drug undergoes metabolic activation via the CYP system. The active metabolites include phosphoramide mustard and acrolein, while 4-ketocyclophosphamide and carboxyphosphamide are the inactive metabolites. Toxicities include nausea and vomiting, cystitis (which may be counteracted by administration of mesna), and myelosuppression.

Doxorubicin. Doxorubicin is an anthracycline antibiotic. Its mechanism of action involves intercalation of DNA. In addition, doxorubicin, via CYP reductase, can form semiquinone radicals that can react with oxygen to produce superoxide radicals. Myelosuppression, mucositis, and cumulative dose-related congestive heart failure are the predominant toxicities.

Etoposide. Etoposide is a semisynthetic derivative of podophyllotoxin. Etoposide forms a ternary complex with DNA and topoisomerase II, resulting in accumulation of DNA breaks. Leukopenia is the dose-limiting toxicity. Other toxicities include nausea, vomiting, diarrhea, alopecia, allergic reactions, and hepatic toxicity. Of note is the development of acute myeloid leukemia, which can occur 1 to 3 years after treatment with etoposide in the absence of a preceding myelodysplastic syndrome.

5-Fluorouracil. 5-Fluorouracil is a halogenated pyrimidine whose cytotoxic activity is dependent on enzymatic conversion to a nucleotide. Formation of 5-fluoro-2′-deoxyuridine-5′-phosphate (F-dUMP) results in the inhibition of thymidine kinase. In addition, 5-fluorouracil may become incorporated into both DNA and RNA. Toxicities include mucositis, myelosuppression, and acute chest pain.

Vinblastine. Vinblastine is a vinca alkaloid that binds tubulin, blocking mitosis. Unlike vincristine, vinblastine is not associated with significant neurotoxicity. Toxic effects include leukopenia, nausea, vomiting, diarrhea, and syndrome of inappropriate secretion of antidiuretic hormone.

Vinorelbine. Vinorelbine is a semisynthetic member of the vinca alkaloid family. The mechanism of action is presumed to be similar to that of the vinca alkaloids, namely as an antimitotic agent via the disruption of microtubules. Vinorelbine causes mild neurotoxicity as well as myelosuppression. It can be given orally; however, the bioavailability is only 30%.[56]

Combinations

A variety of the agents listed previously have been tried in combination in hormone-refractory metastatic prostate cancer in small clinical trials. These combinations include estramustine and vinblastine[57]; estramustine and etoposide[58,59]; estramustine and paclitaxel[60]; estramustine, etoposide, and paclitaxel[61]; estramustine, etoposide, paclitaxel, and carboplatin[62]; estramustine and vinorelbine[63]; and doxorubicin and cyclophosphamide.[64] Combinations involving docetaxel have included docetaxel and vinorelbine,[65] docetaxel and calcitriol,[66] and docetaxel and capecitabine.[67,68]

Metastatic Bone Disease

Postmortem studies have shown that 70% of patients with prostate cancer will have metastatic bone disease. Bone metastases can cause significant morbidity, including pain, fractures, and spinal cord compression. These significantly affect quality of life, and patients often require narcotics, radiotherapy, or surgery for bony complications.

While metastatic prostate cancer lesions have classically been characterized as osteoblastic in nature, it is recognized that there is also dysregulation of osteolysis.

Bisphosphonates

The bisphosphonates are a group of small molecules that have found use clinically in a variety of settings, including osteoporosis and metastatic bone disease. Bisphosphonates avidly bind calcium and thus accumulate at the site of bone resorption. Osteoclasts endocytose bisphosphonates. Bisphosphonates prevent differentiation of macrophages into osteoclasts, block the activity of mature osteoclasts, and increase osteoclast apoptosis. While the net effect of bisphosphonates is the same, the underlying mechanism of action appears to depend on whether the bisphosphonate is a nitrogen-containing compound. Bisphosphonates such as etidronate and clodronate are converted to ATP analogues and are thought to induce apoptosis via inhibition of ATP-dependent processes.[69] Conversely, nitrogen-containing bisphosphonates such as zoledronic acid, pamidronate, ibandronate, and alendronate inhibit farnesyl pyrophosphate (FPP) synthase, an enzyme in the isoprenoid biosynthetic pathway.[70] Inhibition of this enzyme results in the depletion of both FPP and geranylgeranyl pyrophosphate, which in turn, leads to inhibition of farnesylation and geranylgeranylation. This inhibition has the potential to affect a wide array of targets, including those proteins in the Ras superfamily of small GTPases. Also, interesting preclinical data suggest that bisphosphonates may have anticancer activity. Bisphosphonates have been shown to induce apoptosis in human prostate cancer cell lines as well as inhibit adhesion.[71] Other preclinical studies have showed intriguing additive or synergistic effects when bisphosphonates are combined with agents such as Taxotere or doxorubicin.[72,73]

Only zoledronic acid (Zometa) has been approved in the setting of metastatic prostate cancer. Zometa is the most potent of the bisphosphonates. In the Zometa 039 trial, 643 men with androgen-independent prostate cancer and asymptomatic or minimally symptomatic bone metastases were randomized to Zometa versus placebo.[74] The primary end point was the number of skeletal-related events (SREs). There was a significant reduction in SREs in the Zometa arm (33% vs. 44% in the placebo arm) as well as a significant increase in the time to first SRE.[74] Significant effects on mortality have not been demonstrated. Clinical trials involving other intravenous bisphosphonates (pamidronate, clodronate) have not shown efficacy.[75]

The Zometa 039 trial did highlight the renal toxicity of Zometa. This renal toxicity was lessened by dose reduction and an increase in the time of infusion of the drug.[74] The current guidelines do not recommend use of Zometa if a patient has a serum creatinine greater than 3 or a creatinine clearance less than 30. Other toxicities include acute systemic inflammatory reactions involving fever, edema, myalgia, nausea, and ocular inflammation. More recently, bisphosphonate-induced osteonecrosis of the jaw (ONJ) has been reported. Over 700 cases have been described thus far in patients treated with bisphosphonate.[76] To date, only Zometa and pamidronate have been associated with ONJ. Risk factors appear to be duration of bisphosphonate therapy and previous dental procedures.[77] The median duration of therapy prior to development of ONJ may be shorter with Zometa than with pamidronate.[78]

Radioisotopes

Several radioisotopes have been used to provide palliation of pain from bony metastases. These radionuclides preferentially target the bone and provide local irradiation. In general, the radioisotopes provide pain relief within 2 to 3 weeks after injection, and responses can last for several months. The primary toxicity is marrow suppression. Contraindications include renal insufficiency and bone marrow suppression.

Strontium-89 chloride is a calcium analogue that concentrates in bone. Clinical trials have shown that 80% of patients experience some degree of pain relief, with 10% having complete relief.[79] The nadir of white blood cells and platelets generally occurs 4 to 8 weeks following the injection, and counts typically recover by 12 weeks.[79] Duration of response has been reported to be 3 to 6 months.[79] Samarium-153 is a beta particle and γ-photon emitter with a half-life of 46 hours. It has been chelated with ethylene diamine tetramethylene phosphonate, which allows for a stable complex that preferentially binds bone.[80] A clinical trial showed pain relief in approximately 70% of patients with a median duration of relief of 2.6 months.[81] Rhenium-186 is also a beta particle– and γ-photon–emitting radionuclide with a half-life of 3.7 days. It has been complexed with etidronate (hydroxyethylidene diphosphonate), and a placebo-controlled trial showed improved pain relief.[82]

Emerging Targets and Therapeutics

Vitamin D

Prostate cancer cells express vitamin D receptors, and exposure of cells to 1,25-dihydroxyvitamin D has been shown to induce differentiation and inhibit proliferation and invasiveness.[83] Interestingly, 1,25-dihydroxyvitamin D induces upregulation of the androgen receptor.[84] As administration of 1,25-dihydroxyvitamin D results in hypercalcemia and hypercalcuria, a number of analogues are being investigated.

Histone Deacetylase Inhibitors

Acetylation of histones allows for transcription while histone deacetylase results in stabilization between DNA and histones, repressing transcription. By increasing DNA acetylation, inhibitors of histone deacetylase are thought to induce the transcription of genes that were previously silent, such as tumor suppressors. Phenylbutyrate is an analogue of sodium butyrate. Treatment of prostate cancer cells with phenylbutyrate has been shown to have pleiotropic effects, including induction of apoptosis, G_1/G_1 cell cycle arrest, and increased expression of peroxisome proliferator activated receptor nuclear receptors.[85,86] Preclinical data have suggested a synergistic interaction with paclitaxel.[87] Suberoylanilide hydroxamic acid (SAHA) was initially found to induce differentiation of malignant cells[88] and was then noted to inhibit histone deacetylation.[89] In vitro studies have demonstrated a decrease in expression of androgen receptor in prostate cancer cells treated with SAHA.[90] Initial clinical trials have indicated that SAHA (either oral or intravenous) is relatively well tolerated, with toxicities including fatigue, cytopenias, and anorexia.[91,92]

Sipuleucel-T

Sipuleucel-T (the Provenge vaccine) is composed of autologous dendritic cells that have had ex vivo exposure to PA 2024. PA 2024 is a recombinant protein containing both human prostatic acid phosphatase and granulocyte-macrophage colony-stimulating factor. Initial clinical trials have had some promising results, with a Phase III trial in asymptomatic men with hormone-refractory prostate cancer showing a statistically significant improvement in median overall survival compared with the placebo arm.[93]

Growth Factor Receptor Antagonists

The erbB family of tyrosine kinase inhibitors consists of four members: ErbB1 (epidermal growth factor receptor [EGFR]), ErbB2 (HER2/neu), ErbB3, and ErbB4. EGFR is expressed in prostate cancer cells, and the level of expression appears to be higher in hormone-refractory prostate cancer.[94] Activation of EGFR via ligand binding has been shown to result in the proliferation of prostate cancer cells. Overexpression of HER2/neu has been found in association with hormone-refractory disease.[95] Cross talk between the HER2/neu pathway and the androgen receptor has been identified and may play a role in the development of androgen independence.[96] In addition, stimulation of cells with androgen results in the upregulation of EGFR.[97] Small-molecule inhibitors of EGFR, including gefitinib and erlotinib, are being studied in advanced prostate cancer. Investigation is underway on the use of monoclonal antibodies to EGFR (cetuximab) or HER2/neu (trastuzumab). Pertuzumab, a monoclonal antibody that binds HER2 and prevents receptor dimerization, has shown in vitro activity[98]; however, initial clinical studies have not demonstrated significant single-agent activity.[99,100]

Epothilones

Epothilones are a new class of macrolides that have been extracted from myxobacteria. Like the taxanes, epothilones bind to microtubules, resulting in microtubule bundling, formation of multipolar spindles, and mitotic arrest.[101] Preclinical studies have suggested activity of epothilones in taxane-resistant cells.[102] Four epothilone analogues are currently being investigated in clinical trials. In a Phase II trial of ixabepilone (aza-epothilone B), 16 of 41 patients had a greater than 50% decrease in PSA.[103] Toxicities included neutropenia and neuropathy.[103] The major toxicity of patupilone (epothilone B) appears to be diarrhea.[104]

Atrasentan

Atrasentan is an orally active inhibitor of the endothelin-A (ET_A) receptor. Endothelins are 21–amino acid peptides that play roles in regulating proliferation, hormone production, vasomotor tone, and nociception. There are two endothelin receptors, ET_A and endothelin-B (ET_B). In prostate cancer, there is loss of ET_B receptors and overexpression of endothelin-1, which results in inhibition of apoptosis via ET_A receptors.[105,106] In addition, increased expression of ET_A receptors has been found in high-grade prostate cancer and in prostate cancer that is metastatic to bone.[107] Initial clinical trials have suggested that atrasentan is well tolerated, with reported adverse events including rhinitis, headache, and peripheral edema.[108]

REFERENCES

1. Jemal A, Siegel R, Ward E, et al. Cancer statistics, 2007. CA Cancer J Clin 2007;57:43-66.
2. Huggins C, Hodges CV. Studies on prostatic cancer I: the effect of castration, of estrogen and of androgen injection on serum phosphatases in metastatic carcinoma of the prostate. Cancer Res 1941;19:293-297.
3. Huggins C, Hodges CV. Studies on prostatic cancer II: the effects of castration on advanced carcinoma of the prostate gland. AMA Arch Surg 1941, pp 209-223.
4. Conn PM, Crowley WF Jr. Gonadotropin-releasing hormone and its analogues. N Engl J Med 1991;324:93-103.
5. Waxman J, Man A, Hendry WF, et al. Importance of early tumour exacerbation in patients treated with long acting analogues of gonadotrophin releasing hormone for advanced prostatic cancer. Br Med J (Clin Res Ed) 1985;291:1387-1388.
6. Labrie F, Dupont A, Belanger A, et al. Simultaneous administration of pure antiandrogens, a combination necessary for the use of luteinizing hormone-releasing hormone agonists in the treatment of prostate cancer. Proc Natl Acad Sci U S A 1984;81:3861-3863.
7. Basaria S, Lieb J 2nd, Tang AM, et al. Long-term effects of androgen deprivation therapy in prostate cancer patients. Clin Endocrinol (Oxf) 2002;56:779-786.
8. Strum SB, McDermed JE, Scholz MC, et al. Anaemia associated with androgen deprivation in patients with prostate cancer receiving combined hormone blockade. Br J Urol 1997;79:933-941.
9. Gerber GS, Zagaja GP, Ray PS, Rukstalis DB. Transdermal estrogen in the treatment of hot flushes in men with prostate cancer. Urology 2000;55:97-101.
10. Quella SK, Loprinzi CL, Sloan J, et al. Pilot evaluation of venlafaxine for the treatment of hot flashes in men undergoing androgen ablation therapy for prostate cancer. J Urol 1999;162:98-102.
11. Loprinzi CL, Barton DL, Carpenter LA, et al. Pilot evaluation of paroxetine for treating hot flashes in men. Mayo Clin Proc 2004;79:1247-1251.
12. Loprinzi CL, Michalak JC, Quella SK, et al. Megestrol acetate for the prevention of hot flashes. N Engl J Med 1994;331:347-352.
13. Trachtenberg J, Gittleman M, Steidle C, et al. A Phase 3, multicenter, open label, randomized study of abarelix versus leuprolide plus daily antiandrogen in men with prostate cancer. J Urol 2002;167:1670-1674.
14. Tomera K, Gleason D, Gittelman M, et al. The gonadotropin-releasing hormone antagonist abarelix depot versus luteinizing hormone releasing hormone agonists leuprolide or goserelin: initial results of endocrinological and biochemical efficacies in patients with prostate cancer. J Urol 2001;165:1585-1589.
15. Pont A, Williams PL, Loose DS, et al. Ketoconazole blocks adrenal steroid synthesis. Ann Intern Med 1982;97:370-372.
16. Trachtenberg J, Zadra J. Steroid synthesis inhibition by ketoconazole: sites of action. Clin Invest Med 1988;11:1-5.
17. Eichenberger T, Trachtenberg J, Toor P, Keating A. Ketoconazole: a possible direct cytotoxic effect on prostate carcinoma cells. J Urol 1989;141:190-191.
18. Van Der Meer JW, Keuning JJ, Scheijgrond HW, et al. The influence of gastric acidity on the bio-availability of ketoconazole. J Antimicrob Chemother 1980;6:552-554.
19. Byar DP, Corle DK. Hormone therapy for prostate cancer: results of the Veterans Administration Cooperative Urological Research Group studies. NCI Monogr 1988;(7):165-170.
20. Ockrim JL, Lalani EN, Laniado ME, et al. Transdermal estradiol therapy for advanced prostate cancer—forward to the past? J Urol 2003;169:1735-1737.
21. Widmark A, Fossa SD, Lundmo P, et al. Does prophylactic breast irradiation prevent antiandrogen-induced gynecomastia? Evaluation of 253 patients in the randomized Scandinavian trial SPCG-7/SFUO-3. Urology 2003;61:145-151.
22. Cockshott ID. Bicalutamide: clinical pharmacokinetics and metabolism. Clin Pharmacokinet 2004;43:855-878.
23. Tyrrell CJ, Kaisary AV, Iversen P, et al. A randomised comparison of "Casodex" (bicalutamide) 150 mg monotherapy versus castration in the treatment of metastatic and locally advanced prostate cancer. Eur Urol 1998;33:447-456.
24. Schulz M, Schmoldt A, Donn F, Becker H. The pharmacokinetics of flutamide and its major metabolites after a single oral dose and during chronic treatment. Eur J Clin Pharmacol 1988;34:633-636.
25. Boccon-Gibod L, Fournier G, Bottet P, et al. Flutamide versus orchidectomy in the treatment of metastatic prostate carcinoma. Eur Urol 1997;32:391-395; discussion 395-396.
26. Chang A, Yeap B, Davis T, et al. Double-blind, randomized study of primary hormonal treatment of stage D2 prostate carcinoma: flutamide versus diethylstilbestrol. J Clin Oncol 1996;14:2250-2257.
27. Dole EJ, Holdsworth MT. Nilutamide: an antiandrogen for the treatment of prostate cancer. Ann Pharmacother 1997;31:65-75.
28. Akakura K, Bruchovsky N, Goldenberg SL, et al. Effects of intermittent androgen suppression on androgen-dependent tumors: apoptosis and serum prostate-specific antigen. Cancer 1993;71:2782-2790.
29. Bhandari MS, Crook J, Hussain M. Should intermittent androgen deprivation be used in routine clinical practice? J Clin Oncol 2005;23:8212-8218.
30. Mottet N, Prayer-Galetti T, Hammerer P, et al. Optimizing outcomes and quality of life in the hormonal treatment of prostate cancer. BJU Int 2006;98:20-27.
31. Dijkman GA, Janknegt RA, De Reijke TM, Debruyne FM. Long-term efficacy and safety of nilutamide plus castration in advanced prostate cancer, and the significance of early prostate specific antigen normalization. International Anandron Study Group. J Urol 1997;158:160-163.
32. Crawford ED, Eisenberger MA, McLeod DG, et al. A controlled trial of leuprolide with and without flutamide in prostatic carcinoma. N Engl J Med 1989;321:419-424.
33. Denis LJ, Keuppens F, Smith PH, et al. Maximal androgen blockade: final analysis of EORTC Phase III trial 30853. EORTC Genito-Urinary Tract Cancer Cooperative Group and the EORTC Data Center. Eur Urol 1998;33:144-151.
34. Eisenberger MA, Blumenstein BA, Crawford ED, et al. Bilateral orchiectomy with or without flutamide for metastatic prostate cancer. N Engl J Med 1998;339:1036-1042.
35. Iversen P, Rasmussen F, Klarskov P, Christensen IJ. Long-term results of Danish Prostatic Cancer Group trial 86: goserelin acetate plus flutamide versus orchiectomy in advanced prostate cancer. Cancer 1993;72:3851-3854.
36. Maximum androgen blockade in advanced prostate cancer: an overview of the randomised trials. Prostate Cancer Trialists' Collaborative Group. Lancet 2000;355:1491-1498.
37. Samson DJ, Seidenfeld J, Schmitt B, et al. Systematic review and meta-analysis of monotherapy compared with combined androgen blockade for patients with advanced prostate carcinoma. Cancer 2002;95:361-376.
38. Smaletz O, Scher HI, Small EJ, et al. Nomogram for overall survival of patients with progressive metastatic prostate cancer after castration. J Clin Oncol 2002;20:3972-3982.
39. Bruchovsky N, Rennie PS, Coldman AJ, et al. Effects of androgen withdrawal on the stem cell composition of the Shionogi carcinoma. Cancer Res 1990;50:2275-2282.
40. Akakura K, Bruchovsky N, Rennie PS, et al. Effects of intermittent androgen suppression on the stem cell composition and the expression of the TRPM-2 (clusterin) gene in the Shionogi carcinoma. J Steroid Biochem Mol Biol 1996;59:501-511.
41. Koivisto P, Visakorpi T, Kallioniemi OP. Androgen receptor gene amplification: a novel molecular mechanism for endocrine therapy resistance in human prostate cancer. Scand J Clin Lab Invest Suppl 1996;226:57-63.
42. Linja MJ, Savinainen KJ, Saramaki OR, et al. Amplification and overexpression of androgen receptor gene in hormone-refractory prostate cancer. Cancer Res 2001;61:3550-3555.
43. Taplin ME, Rajeshkumar B, Halabi S, et al. Androgen receptor mutations in androgen-independent prostate cancer: Cancer and Leukemia Group B Study 9663. J Clin Oncol 2003;21:2673-2678.
44. Titus MA, Schell MJ, Lih FB, et al. Testosterone and dihydrotestosterone tissue levels in recurrent prostate cancer. Clin Cancer Res 2005;11:4653-4657.
45. Holzbeierlein J, Lal P, LaTulippe E, et al. Gene expression analysis of human prostate carcinoma during hormonal therapy identifies androgen-responsive genes and mechanisms of therapy resistance. Am J Pathol 2004;164:217-227.
46. Culig Z, Hobisch A, Cronauer MV, et al. Androgen receptor activation in prostatic tumor cell lines by insulin-like growth factor-I, keratinocyte growth factor, and epidermal growth factor. Cancer Res 1994;54:5474-5478.
47. Doroshow JH, Davies KJ. Comparative cardiac oxygen radical metabolism by anthracycline antibiotics, mitoxantrone, bisantrene, 4′-(9-acridinylamino)-methanesulfon-*m*-anisidide, and neocarzinostatin. Biochem Pharmacol 1983;32:2935-2939.
48. Tannock IF, Osoba D, Stockler MR, et al. Chemotherapy with mitoxantrone plus prednisone or prednisone alone for symptomatic hormone-resistant prostate cancer: a Canadian randomized trial with palliative end points. J Clin Oncol 1996;14:1756-1764.
49. Kantoff PW, Halabi S, Conaway M, et al. Hydrocortisone with or without mitoxantrone in men with hormone-refractory prostate cancer: results of the Cancer and Leukemia Group B 9182 Study. J Clin Oncol 1999;17:2506-2513.
50. Gueritte-Voegelein F, Guenard D, Lavelle F, et al. Relationships between the structure of taxol analogues and their antimitotic activity. J Med Chem 1991;34:992-998.

51. Tannock IF, de Wit R, Berry WR, et al. Docetaxel plus prednisone or mitoxantrone plus prednisone for advanced prostate cancer. N Engl J Med 2004;351:1502-1512.
52. Trivedi C, Redman B, Flaherty LE, et al. Weekly 1-hour infusion of paclitaxel: clinical feasibility and efficacy in patients with hormone-refractory prostate carcinoma. Cancer 2000;89:431-436.
53. Kreis W, Budman DR, Calabro A. Unique synergism or antagonism of combinations of chemotherapeutic and hormonal agents in human prostate cancer cell lines. Br J Urol 1997;79:196-202.
54. Petrylak DP, Tangen CM, Hussain MH, et al. Docetaxel and estramustine compared with mitoxantrone and prednisone for advanced refractory prostate cancer. N Engl J Med 2004;351:1513-1520.
55. Lubiniecki GM, Berlin JA, Weinstein RB, Vaughn DJ. Thromboembolic events with estramustine phosphate-based chemotherapy in patients with hormone-refractory prostate carcinoma: results of a meta-analysis. Cancer 2004;101:2755-2759.
56. Leveque D, Jehl F. Clinical pharmacokinetics of vinorelbine. Clin Pharmacokinet 1996;31:184-197.
57. Hudes GR, Greenberg R, Krigel RL, et al. Phase II study of estramustine and vinblastine, two microtubule inhibitors, in hormone-refractory prostate cancer. J Clin Oncol 1992;10:1754-1761.
58. Pienta KJ, Redman B, Hussain M, et al. Phase II evaluation of oral estramustine and oral etoposide in hormone-refractory adenocarcinoma of the prostate. J Clin Oncol 1994;12:2005-2012.
59. Pienta KJ, Redman BG, Bandekar R, et al. A Phase II trial of oral estramustine and oral etoposide in hormone refractory prostate cancer. Urology 1997;50:401-406; discussion 406-407.
60. Hudes GR, Nathan FE, Khater C, et al. Paclitaxel plus estramustine in metastatic hormone-refractory prostate cancer. Semin Oncol 1995;22:41-45.
61. Smith DC, Esper P, Strawderman M, et al. Phase II trial of oral estramustine, oral etoposide, and intravenous paclitaxel in hormone-refractory prostate cancer. J Clin Oncol 1999;17:1664-1671.
62. Smith DC, Chay CH, Dunn RL, et al. Phase II trial of paclitaxel, estramustine, etoposide, and carboplatin in the treatment of patients with hormone-refractory prostate carcinoma. Cancer 2003;98:269-276.
63. Carles Galceran J, Bastus Piulats R, Martin-Broto J, et al. A Phase II study of vinorelbine and estramustine in patients with hormone-resistant prostate cancer. Clin Transl Oncol 2005;7:66-73.
64. Small EJ, Srinivas S, Egan B, et al. Doxorubicin and dose-escalated cyclophosphamide with granulocyte colony-stimulating factor for the treatment of hormone-resistant prostate cancer. J Clin Oncol 1996;14:1617-1625.
65. Koletsky AJ, Guerra ML, Kronish L. Phase II study of vinorelbine and low-dose docetaxel in chemotherapy-naive patients with hormone-refractory prostate cancer. Cancer J 2003;9:286-292.
66. Beer TM, Ryan CW, Venner PM, et al, for the ASCENT Investigators. Double-blinded randomized study of high-dose calcitriol plus docetaxel compared with placebo plus docetaxel in androgen-independent prostate cancer: a report from the ASCENT Investigators. J Clin Oncol 2007;25:669-674.
67. Ferrero JM, Chamorey E, Oudard S, et al. Phase II trial evaluating a docetaxel-capecitabine combination as treatment for hormone-refractory prostate cancer. Cancer 2006;107:738-745.
68. Kolodziej M, Neubauer MA, Rousey SR, et al. Phase II trial of docetaxel/capecitabine in hormone-refractory prostate cancer. Clin Genitourin Cancer 2006;5:155-161.
69. Frith JC, Monkkonen J, Blackburn GM, et al. Clodronate and liposome-encapsulated clodronate are metabolized to a toxic ATP analog, adenosine 5′-(beta, gamma-dichloromethylene) triphosphate, by mammalian cells in vitro. J Bone Miner Res 1997;12:1358-1367.
70. Bergstrom JD, Bostedor RG, Masarachia PJ, et al. Alendronate is a specific, nanomolar inhibitor of farnesyl diphosphate synthase. Arch Biochem Biophys 2000;373:231-241.
71. Coxon JP, Oades GM, Kirby RS, Colston KW. Zoledronic acid induces apoptosis and inhibits adhesion to mineralized matrix in prostate cancer cells via inhibition of protein prenylation. BJU Int 2004;94:164-170.
72. Ullen A, Lennartsson L, Harmenberg U, et al. Additive/synergistic antitumoral effects on prostate cancer cells in vitro following treatment with a combination of docetaxel and zoledronic acid. Acta Oncol 2005;44:644-650.
73. Neville-Webbe HL, Rostami-Hodjegan A, Evans CA, et al. Sequence- and schedule-dependent enhancement of zoledronic acid induced apoptosis by doxorubicin in breast and prostate cancer cells. Int J Cancer 2005;113:364-371.
74. Saad F, Gleason DM, Murray R, et al. A randomized, placebo-controlled trial of zoledronic acid in patients with hormone-refractory metastatic prostate carcinoma. J Natl Cancer Inst 2002;94:1458-1468.
75. Small EJ, Smith MR, Seaman JJ, et al. Combined analysis of two multicenter, randomized, placebo-controlled studies of pamidronate disodium for the palliation of bone pain in men with metastatic prostate cancer. J Clin Oncol 2003;21:4277-4284.
76. Dunstan CR, Felsenberg D, Seibel MJ. Therapy insight: the risks and benefits of bisphosphonates for the treatment of tumor-induced bone disease. Nat Clin Pract Oncol 2007;4:42-55.
77. Bamias A, Kastritis E, Bamia C, et al. Osteonecrosis of the jaw in cancer after treatment with bisphosphonates: incidence and risk factors. J Clin Oncol 2005;23: 8580-8587.
78. Durie BG, Katz M, Crowley J. Osteonecrosis of the jaw and bisphosphonates. N Engl J Med 2005;353:99-102.
79. Robinson RG, Preston DF, Schiefelbein M, Baxter KG. Strontium 89 therapy for the palliation of pain due to osseous metastases. JAMA 1995;274:420-424.
80. Ketring AR. ^{153}Sm-EDTMP and ^{186}Re-HEDP as bone therapeutic radiopharmaceuticals. Int J Rad Appl Instrum B 1987;14:223-232.
81. Collins C, Eary JF, Donaldson G, et al. Samarium-153-EDTMP in bone metastases of hormone refractory prostate carcinoma: a Phase I/II trial. J Nucl Med 1993;34:1839-1844.
82. Han SH, de Klerk JM, Tan S, et al. The PLACORHEN study: a double-blind, placebo-controlled, randomized radionuclide study with ^{186}Re-etidronate in hormone-resistant prostate cancer patients with painful bone metastases. Placebo Controlled Rhenium Study. J Nucl Med 2002;43:1150-1156.
83. Skowronski RJ, Peehl DM, Feldman D. Vitamin D and prostate cancer: 1,25 dihydroxyvitamin D3 receptors and actions in human prostate cancer cell lines. Endocrinology 1993;132:1952-1960.
84. Zhao XY, Ly LH, Peehl DM, Feldman D. Induction of androgen receptor by 1alpha,25-dihydroxyvitamin D3 and 9-cis retinoic acid in LNCaP human prostate cancer cells. Endocrinology 1999;140:1205-1212.
85. Melchior SW, Brown LG, Figg WD, et al. Effects of phenylbutyrate on proliferation and apoptosis in human prostate cancer cells in vitro and in vivo. Int J Oncol 1999;14:501-508.
86. Pineau T, Hudgins WR, Liu L, et al. Activation of a human peroxisome proliferator-activated receptor by the antitumor agent phenylacetate and its analogs. Biochem Pharmacol 1996;52:659-667.
87. Verheul HM, Qian DZ, Carducci MA, Pili R. Sequence-dependent antitumor effects of differentiation agents in combination with cell cycle-dependent cytotoxic drugs. Cancer Chemother Pharmacol 2007;60:329-339.
88. Richon VM, Webb Y, Merger R, et al. Second generation hybrid polar compounds are potent inducers of transformed cell differentiation. Proc Natl Acad Sci U S A 1996;93:5705-5708.
89. Richon VM, Emiliani S, Verdin E, et al. A class of hybrid polar inducers of transformed cell differentiation inhibits histone deacetylases. Proc Natl Acad Sci U S A 1998;95:3003-3007.
90. Marrocco DL, Tilley WD, Bianco-Miotto T, et al. Suberoylanilide hydroxamic acid (vorinostat) represses androgen receptor expression and acts synergistically with an androgen receptor antagonist to inhibit prostate cancer cell proliferation. Mol Cancer Ther 2007;6:51-60.
91. Kelly WK, Richon VM, O'Connor O, et al. Phase I clinical trial of histone deacetylase inhibitor: suberoylanilide hydroxamic acid administered intravenously. Clin Cancer Res 2003;9:3578-3588.
92. Kelly WK, O'Connor OA, Krug LM, et al. Phase I study of an oral histone deacetylase inhibitor, suberoylanilide hydroxamic acid, in patients with advanced cancer. J Clin Oncol 2005;23:3923-3931.
93. So-Rosillo R, Small EJ. Sipuleucel-T (APC8015) for prostate cancer. Expert Rev Anticancer Ther 2006;6:1163-1167.
94. Di Lorenzo G, Tortora G, D'Armiento FP, et al. Expression of epidermal growth factor receptor correlates with disease relapse and progression to androgen-independence in human prostate cancer. Clin Cancer Res 2002;8:3438-3444.
95. Shi Y, Brands FH, Chatterjee S, et al. Her-2/neu expression in prostate cancer: high level of expression associated with exposure to hormone therapy and androgen independent disease. J Urol 2001;166:1514-1519.
96. Craft N, Shostak Y, Carey M, Sawyers CL. A mechanism for hormone-independent prostate cancer through modulation of androgen receptor signaling by the HER-2/neu tyrosine kinase. Nat Med 1999;5:280-285.
97. Schuurmans AL, Bolt J, Mulder E. Androgens stimulate both growth rate and epidermal growth factor receptor activity of the human prostate tumor cell LNCaP. Prostate 1988;12:55-63.
98. Agus DB, Akita RW, Fox WD, et al. Targeting ligand-activated ErbB2 signaling inhibits breast and prostate tumor growth. Cancer Cell 2002;2:127-137.
99. de Bono JS, Bellmunt J, Attard G, et al. Open-label Phase II study evaluating the efficacy and safety of two doses of pertuzumab in castrate chemotherapy-naive patients with hormone-refractory prostate cancer. J Clin Oncol 2007;25:257-262.
100. Agus DB, Sweeney CJ, Morris MJ, et al. Efficacy and safety of single-agent pertuzumab (rhuMAb 2C4), a human epidermal growth factor receptor dimerization inhibitor, in castration-resistant prostate cancer after progression from taxane-based therapy. J Clin Oncol 2007;25:675-681.
101. Bollag DM, McQueney PA, Zhu J, et al. Epothilones, a new class of microtubule-stabilizing agents with a taxol-like mechanism of action. Cancer Res 1995;55:2325-2333.
102. Kowalski RJ, Giannakakou P, Hamel E. Activities of the microtubule-stabilizing agents epothilones A and B with purified tubulin and in cells resistant to paclitaxel (Taxol®). J Biol Chem 1997;272:2534-2541.
103. Hussain M, Tangen CM, Lara PN Jr, et al. Ixabepilone (epothilone B analogue BMS-247550) is active in chemotherapy-naive patients with hormone-refractory prostate cancer: a Southwest Oncology Group trial S0111. J Clin Oncol 2005;23:8724-8729.
104. Rubin EH, Rothermel J, Tesfaye F, et al. Phase I dose-finding study of weekly single-agent patupilone in patients with advanced solid tumors. J Clin Oncol 2005;23:9120-9129.
105. Nelson JB, Hedican SP, George DJ, et al. Identification of endothelin-1 in the pathophysiology of metastatic adenocarcinoma of the prostate. Nat Med 1995;1:944-949.
106. Nelson JB, Chan-Tack K, Hedican SP, et al. Endothelin-1 production and decreased endothelin β receptor expression in advanced prostate cancer. Cancer Res 1996;56:663-668.
107. Gohji K, Kitazawa S, Tamada H, et al. Expression of endothelin receptor α associated with prostate cancer progression. J Urol 2001;165:1033-1036.
108. Michaelson MD, Kaufman DS, Kantoff P, et al. Randomized Phase II study of atrasentan alone or in combination with zoledronic acid in men with metastatic prostate cancer. Cancer 2006;107:530-535.

68

COLON CANCER

Muhammad Wasif Saif and Robert B. Diasio

INTRODUCTION 959
Stages of Colon Cancer 959
THERAPEUTICS AND CLINICAL PHARMACOLOGY 959
Goals of Therapy 961
Stage III Colon Cancer 961
Stage II Colon Cancer 961
Metastatic Colon Cancer 962
Therapeutics by Class 962
Cytotoxic Agents 962
Novel Targeted Agents 965
Emerging Targets and Therapeutics 966

INTRODUCTION

Colorectal cancer (CRC) is the third most common cancer, with an estimated 150,000 new cases each year. More than 55,000 CRC-related deaths were estimated in 2006, making it the second leading cause of cancer-related death in the United States.[1] Among these patients, 19% present at stage IV, 37.2% present at stage III, 27.9% at stage II, and 11% at stage I.[2] In loco-regionally advanced CRC, surgery is the primary treatment modality and has a curative intent. However, as many as 40% to 50% of the patients will relapse and require additional treatment of their disease. Clinical failure following resection of CRC is predominantly secondary to the clinical progression of previously undetected distant metastatic disease.[3] Except for the patients who are candidates for resection of liver metastasis, the approach in treating metastatic colorectal cancer (mCRC) patients is palliative systemic chemotherapy. Since the late 1950s, 5-fluorouracil (5-FU) had been the only active anticancer agent in CRC, providing a modest clinical benefit with a median overall survival (OS) of 6 to 8 months.[4]

In the past 10 years, development of the topoisomerase I inhibitor irinotecan, the third-generation platinum analogue oxaliplatin, and the oral fluoropyrimidine capecitabine have changed the landscape of mCRC treatment. Optimizing the combination of these agents has improved the outlook of patients with mCRC, resulting in median OS consistently reaching approximately 20 months. More recently, the development of targeted agents such as bevacizumab, cetuximab, and panitumumab have advanced the treatment of mCRC even further. These monoclonal antibodies gave rise to more therapeutic options for oncologists and improved outcomes for mCRC patients as evidenced by an impressive median OS of 25.1 months reported in a study that added bevacizumab to irinotecan + 5-FU + leucovorin (IFL) combination therapy.[5] The future outlook on treatment of mCRC is ever promising as more targeted agents (vatalanib, etc.) are being introduced and more sophisticated combination regimens are being developed to optimize anticancer therapy.

Stages of Colon Cancer

The stage of CRC at the time of diagnosis plays a significant role in determining the course of treatment. Treatment decisions should be made with reference to the tumor-node-metastasis (TNM) classification rather than to the older Dukes' or the Modified Astler-Coller classification schema.[6] The American Joint Committee on Cancer and a National Cancer Institute–sponsored panel recommended that at least 12 lymph nodes be examined in patients with colon and rectal cancer to confirm the absence of nodal involvement by tumor.[7] This recommendation takes into consideration that the number of lymph nodes examined is a reflection of the aggressiveness of lymphovascular mesenteric dissection at the time of surgical resection and the pathologic identification of nodes in the specimen. Retrospective studies have demonstrated that the number of lymph nodes examined in colon and rectal surgery may be associated with patient outcome.

Independent of the stage of diagnosis, surgery is the standard of care for CRC. For patients with stage II or higher CRC, chemotherapy is considered in addition to surgery. Radiotherapy is not part of the standard of care for colon cancer, but is often administered in combination with 5-FU chemotherapy for patients with stage II or higher rectal cancer. In addition to surgery and chemotherapy, molecular targeted therapies are often used to treat tumors that have metastasized (stage IV).[3]

THERAPEUTICS AND CLINICAL PHARMACOLOGY

Studies from the National Surgical Adjuvant Breast and Bowel Project (NSABP) and other cooperative groups have clearly demonstrated that adjuvant chemotherapy has resulted in improvement in disease-free survival (DFS) and survival.[8-17] These adjuvant regimens included 5-FU + levamisole (LEV) and 5-FU + leucovorin (LV) (5-FU/LV). The Intergroup 0035 study using 5-FU and LEV for 1 year, the Intergroup study using 6 months of 5-FU/LV, and the IMPACT study using 5-FU/LV for 6 months demonstrated similar improvements in DFS and survival rates.[10-12] These encouraging results led to direct comparison of these regimens. Intergroup study (INT-0089) randomly assigned 3759 patients (20% with high-risk Dukes' stage B2 disease) to receive standard 5-FU + LEV for 12 months, 5-FU + high-dose LV, 5-FU + low-dose LV, or 5-FU + low-dose LV + LEV.[13] The latter three regimens were administered for approximately 6 months. The results affirmed that 6 months of therapy with 5-FU/LV should represent standard adjuvant treatment for patients with resected high-risk colon cancer (Table 68-1). The results of NSABP C-04, in which 2152 patients (41% Dukes' B) were randomized, were similar.[17a] The 5-year DFS was 74% for 5-FU/LV, 70% for 5-FU + LEV, and 73% for 5-FU + LV + LEV; therefore, LEV did not appear to add to the survival advantage associated with 5-FU/LV. Duration of therapy was approximately 1 year for all groups. No significant differences in toxicity were noticed. Based on data from these trials, adjuvant chemotherapy using 6 months of 5-FU/LV became a current standard of care in the United States.

The superior efficacy of oxaliplatin and 5-FU regimens in the treatment of advanced CRC provided the rationale for trials assessing oxaliplatin-based combination regimens in the adjuvant setting. A large trial conducted in Europe used an oxaliplatin + 5-FU/LV regimen as adjuvant therapy for stages II and III CRC. The MOSAIC trial randomized 2246 patients with stage II and stage III CRC to receive either 6 months of LV5FU2 (bolus plus infusional 5-FU/LV) or FOLFOX4 (folinic acid + 5-FU + oxaliplatin).[18] FOLFOX4 was found to be superior to LV5FU2 in terms of 3-year DFS, a parameter that is highly predictive of 5-year OS. A combined analysis for stage II and stage III patients demonstrated a 23% risk reduction for 3-year recurrence

TABLE 68-1 COMMON REGIMENS FOR ADJUVANT THERAPY OF COLON CANCER

Regimen	Dose
Mayo regimen	Leucovorin 20 mg/m^2 + 5-FU bolus 425 mg/m^2 qd × 5 (6 cycles)
Roswell Park regimen	5-FU 500 mg/m^2 + LV 500 mg/m^2 weekly × 6 every 8 wk for 3-4 cycles
GERCOR/LV5FU2	LV 200 mg/m^2 IV + FU 400 mg/m^2 IV bolus, followed by FU 600 mg/m^2 IV over 22 hr on days 1 and 2, every 2 wk
FOLFOX4	Oxaliplatin on day 1 at 85 mg/m^2 as a 2-hr infusion, concurrently with FA 200 mg/m^2/day, followed by bolus 5-FU 400 mg/m^2 and a 22-hr infusion of 5-FU 600 mg/m^2 for 2 consecutive days.
mFOLFOX6	A 2-hr infusion of L-LV 200 mg/m^2 or D,L-LV 400 mg/m^2 followed by an FU bolus of 400 mg/m^2 and a 46-hour infusion of 2400-3000 mg/m^2 every 46 hr every 2 wk, with oxaliplatin 85 mg/m^2 as a 2-hr infusion on day 1
FLOX	Oxaliplatin at 85 mg/m^2 every 2 wk on weeks 1, 3, and 5 of the 8-wk cycle with 5-FU/LV (500 mg/m^2 of both given weekly for 6 wk followed by 2 wk rest for 3 cycles)
PVI 5-FU	PVI 5-FU (300 mg/m^2/day for 12 wk)
Capecitabine	1250 mg/m^2 twice daily PO on days 1-14 every 21 days

FA, folinic acid; 5-FU, 5-fluorouracil; IV, intravenously; LV, leucovorin; PO, orally; PVI, protracted venous infusion.

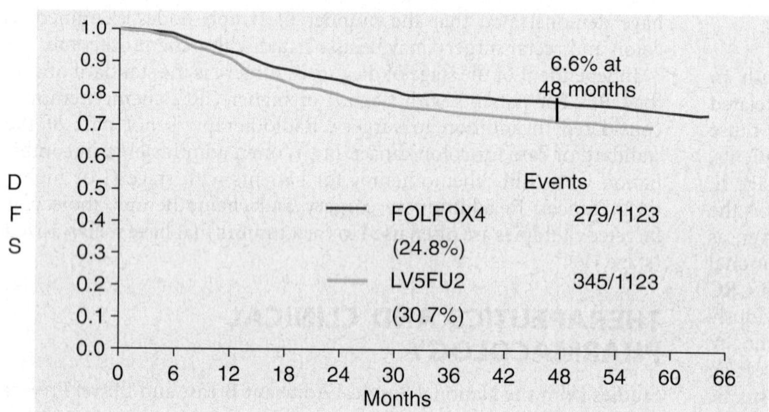

FIGURE 68-1 • Disease-free survival (DFS) of stage II and III CRC patients in the MOSAIC study.

(hazard ratio [HR] 0.77, 95% confidence interval [95% CI] 0.65 to 0.91, $P = .002$). DFS after 3 years was 78.2% in the FOLFOX4 arm and 72.9% in the LV5FU2 arm (Fig. 68-1). An updated DFS analysis at 4 years was reported at the 2005 meeting of the American Society for Clinical Oncology (ASCO 2005), and FOLFOX4 continues to demonstrate about a 24% reduction in relapse ($P = .0008$). However, a stage-based subgroup analysis showed that the difference in DFS was only significant for stage III patients (3-year DFS, 72.2% vs. 65.3%; HR 0.76, 95% CI 0.62 to 0.92) and not for stage II (87.0% vs. 84.3%; HR 0.80, 95% CI 0.56 to 1.15). As with previously reported studies with stage II patients, this result can be attributed to the study being statistically underpowered.

The main side effect of FOLFOX4 was anticipatory sensory neuropathy with grade 3 toxicity affecting 12.4% of patients overall and 18% of patients who received the entire planned 1020 mg/m^2 dose of oxaliplatin (Table 68-2). However, the neurotoxicity proved reversible in the vast majority of patients so that, 12 and 18 months after discontinuation of therapy, only 1.1% and 0.5% of patients, respectively, had residual grade 3 neurotoxicity. Based on the results of the MOSIAC trial, FOLFOX4 has emerged as the new standard of care in the adjuvant treatment of stage III and high-risk stage II patients.[18]

Another study conducted by the NSABP (NSABP C-07) and reported at ASCO 2005 supports the importance of oxaliplatin in the adjuvant setting.[19] In this study, 2407 patients were randomized to either the Roswell Park schedule of 5FU/LV (500 mg/m^2 of both given weekly for 6 weeks followed by 2 weeks rest for three cycles) versus the same 5FU/LV regimen and oxaliplatin (FLOX). The oxaliplatin was administered at 85 mg/m^2 every 2 weeks but only on weeks 1, 3, and 5 of the 8-week cycle (cumulative dose 765 mg/m^2). Seventy-three percent of patients received the planned oxaliplatin treatment. The primary end point, 3-year DFS, favored the FLOX arm (76.5% vs. 71.6%; HR 0.79, $P = .004$) (Fig. 68-2). Importantly, the regimen was tolerable as grade 3 and 4 toxicities were similar in the two arms (grade 3/4: 50%/10% with FLOX vs. 41%/9% with 5FU/LV). Only 8% of patients experienced grade 3 neurotoxicity and, after 12 months, this decreased to 0.5% of patients. Enteritis leading to diarrhea and dehydration was higher in the experimental arm (4.5% vs. 2.7%). Additional efficacy and toxicity data are awaited to fully define whether FLOX is as effective as but more tolerable than FOLFOX.

TABLE 68-2 ADVERSE EVENTS OBSERVED IN MOSAIC STUDY

	Percentage	
NCI Grade ≥3	**FOLFOX4 (*n* = 1108)**	**LV5FU2 (*n* = 1111)**
Neuropathy	12.4 (G3)	0
Thrombocytopenia	1.6	0.4
Neutropenia	41.0 (G4: 12.2)	4.7
Febrile neutropenia	0.7	0.1
Diarrhea	10.8	6.7
Stomatitis	2.7	2.2
Vomiting	5.9	1.4
Allergy	3.0	0.2
Alopecia (G2)	5.0	5.0
All-cause mortality	0.5	0.5

From De Graumont A, Banzi M, Navarro M, et al. Oxaliplatin/5-FU in adjuvant colon cancer: results of the international randomized MOSAIC trial [Abstract 1015]. Proc Am Soc Clin Oncol 2003;22.

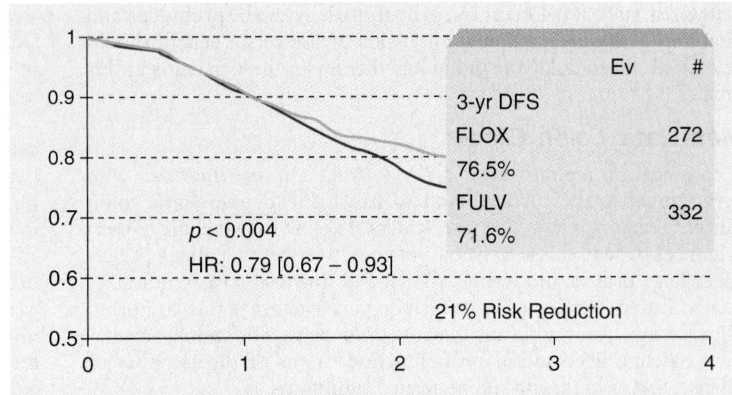

FIGURE 68-2 • **Disease-free survival (DFS) of CRC patients in the NSABP C-07 study (FLOX regimen).**

The results from these Phase III adjuvant trials demonstrate the superiority of oxaliplatin-containing arms over conventional 5FU/LV controls. This is in contrast to the less favorable results observed with irinotecan in this group of patients.

Recent Phase III studies have shown that targeted agents improved survival in patients with advanced CRC. Bevacizumab, a monoclonal antibody targeting vascular endothelial growth factor (VEGF), is the first antiangiogenic drug to show improved efficacy when used in combination with irinotecan and oxaliplatin for first- and second-line treatment of CRC. Cetuximab, another monoclonal antibody targeting epidermal growth factor receptor (EGFR), has shown efficacy in third-line therapy and promising results in first-line Phase II studies. There is great interest in whether the biologic agents bevacizumab and cetuximab can improve survival in the adjuvant therapy setting, and current studies (NSABP C-08, AVANT, ECOG 5202, US NO147) are evaluating the role of these agents.[3]

BOX 68-1 ASCO RECOMMENDATIONS FOR STAGE II DISEASE

- **There is no reason to routinely recommend adjuvant therapy.**
- **If there is any benefit in overall survival, it is on the order of 2% to 4%.**
- **To detect a 2% benefit, a randomized, controlled trial would have to enroll >9000 patients.**
- **High-risk subsets exist:**
  - Inadequate lymph node sampling
  - T_4 lesions
  - Perforation/obstruction
  - Poorly differentiated histology
- **After TNM staging:**
  - Number of lymph nodes
  - Grade
  - Signet-ring cell feature
  - Lymphovascular invasion

Goals of Therapy

Stage III Colon Cancer

Oxaliplatin-based chemotherapy (FOLFOX) is now the standard of care as adjuvant chemotherapy for stage III colon cancer and for patients with high-risk stage II disease.[18] Based on the clinical studies conducted to date, irinotecan cannot be recommended for use in the adjuvant setting.[20-22] The oral fluoropyrimidine capecitabine has demonstrated equivalent efficacy to bolus 5-FU/LV as adjuvant treatment, and is a standard of care when fluoropyrimidine therapy is being considered.[23] Presently, Phase III randomized studies are ongoing to determine the role of capecitabine in combination with oxaliplatin[24] and the biologic agents bevacizumab and cetuximab in the adjuvant setting.[3] The advent of monoclonal antibodies in metastatic CRC has set off a wave of adjuvant therapy trials focusing on the use of these new targeted agents in the adjuvant setting. However, aside from assessing the additional benefit of these monoclonal antibodies over cytotoxic agents, it will be important to address the long-term effects of these agents on cancer survivors, the optimal duration of these agents, and the costs associated with these treatments.

Six months of adjuvant treatment is the current standard duration, and treatment should start within 8 weeks following surgery.

Stage II Colon Cancer

The role of adjuvant chemotherapy for patients with stage II colon adenocarcinoma remains controversial.[25,26] The high surgical cure rate for patients with "low-risk" stage II CRC ranges from 75% to 80%, and the available clinical trials and meta-analyses provide conflicting recommendations for or against adjuvant chemotherapy for this group of patients (Box 68-1). For fit "high-risk" stage II patients with characteristics such as intestinal perforation, clinical obstruction, T_4 tumors, poorly differentiated tumors, and inadequately pathologically examined (<13) lymph node and extramural venous or lymphatic invasion, in whom the 5-year survival rate is 60% to 70%, there is little controversy, as these patients are routinely treated with adjuvant chemotherapy.[27] In addition to pathologic factors, some molecular factors considered potentially "high risk," including high histologic grade, microsatellite instability, and loss of 18q, have yet to be validated in prospective trials. Currently, more emphasis is placed on those patients with fewer than 12 regional lymph nodes identified in the surgical specimen—these patients have a statistically unclear risk of lymph node involvement.[28] These patients might be upgraded to stage III disease if more lymph nodes were sampled, and therefore should receive adjuvant therapy.

The decision to use adjuvant chemotherapy to treat low-risk stage II colon cancer patients (no obstruction or perforation) should be an informed decision weighing the magnitude of a net 2% to 5% survival benefit, a 0.5% to 1.0% risk of mortality with chemotherapy in addition to 6 months of chemotherapy-related toxicities, other coexisting patient morbidities, and the anticipated life expectancy of each patient. As adjuvant chemotherapy is therapy addressing local or metastatic microscopic disease, and the effectiveness of systemic and biologically targeted therapy for advanced macroscopic colon cancer continues to improve rapidly, it remains to be determined by clinical trials whether therapies including newer agents such as cetuximab and bevacizumab administered in the adjuvant setting may affect survival for stage II cancer patients.

Approximately 30% of stage II patients currently receive adjuvant chemotherapy in the United States. "High-risk" patients may be considered for 5-FU/LV or FOLFOX. For average-risk patients, a discussion of the small benefit of chemotherapy should be conducted, and the patient should be involved in the decision-making process. Oxaliplatin-based combination chemotherapy may be overtreatment in low-risk stage II colon cancer, as neurotoxicity can be prolonged and disabling. Therefore, an honest discussion of risk versus benefit should be carried out to tailor the individual therapy in these patients at this time.

Metastatic Colon Cancer

A combination regimen of 5-FU/LV + oxaliplatin or irinotecan with bevacizumab is the current standard treatment for metastatic colon cancer.[29] Factors involved in a treatment decision may include clinical evidence, patient characteristics, previous treatments, patient preferences (e.g., oral vs. intravenous [IV]), and financial costs/reimbursements. Patient's characteristics include performance status/comorbid illnesses, age, prior adjuvant therapy, prior pelvic/abdominal irradiation, baseline liver and/or renal function, status of disease, sites of disease, tumor bulk, and tumor-related symptoms.

Therapeutics by Class

Cytotoxic Agents

5-Fluorouracil. 5-FU is a fluoropyrimidine analogue that inhibits thymidylate synthase and ultimately inhibits DNA synthesis and function.[30] 5-FU had been the only anticancer drug proven to benefit patients with mCRC for 50 years. 5-FU has also been the backbone on which most regimens for treatment of mCRC are built.[31] 5-FU, when used alone, has limited activity in advanced disease, rendering a response rate (RR) ranging from 10% to 15%. A meta-analysis of data incorporating 3300 patients from 19 clinical trials demonstrated that combining LV (a biomodulating agent) with 5-FU was associated with improved RR up to 21% from 11% ($P < .0001$) and improved survival from 10.5 months to 11.7 months ($P < .004$).[32,33] The 5-FU/LV regimen was recognized as standard first-line treatment of mCRC until more advanced combination therapies containing irinotecan and oxaliplatin were developed. However, optimizing ways in which 5-FU/LV is delivered remains quite debatable.

Among several different regimens, the most common bolus schedules are the Mayo regimen, with 5-FU at a dose of 425 mg/m^2 and LV at 20 mg/m^2 every 4 weeks, and a weekly schedule developed by Roswell Park Cancer Institute, with 5-FU at 600 mg/m^2 and LV at 500 mg/m^2 weekly for 6 of 8 weeks. Two randomized trials have demonstrated similar RR, duration of response, progression-free intervals, and median OS between the monthly and weekly schedules of LV-modulated 5-FU.[34,35]

The clinical efficacy of 5-FU/LV has been improved upon by the use of infusional schedules. A meta-analysis that incorporated 1219 patients from six different randomized trials compared infusional 5-FU with bolus 5-FU revealed that infusional schedules of 5-FU resulted in higher RR than bolus schedules (22% vs. 14%; $P < .0002$). Infusional schedules were also associated with less hematologic toxicity compared to that of bolus regimens (4% vs. 31%, respectively; $P < .0001$) and less gastrointestinal toxicity.[36] Common infusional schedules include the protracted venous infusion (PVI) schedule with 5-FU at 300 mg/m^2 for 28 days; the AIO German regimen of 5-FU at 2000 to 2600 mg/m^2 over 24 hours with LV at 500 mg/m^2 administered once weekly for 6 weeks with 1 week of rest; LV5FU2 (the de Gramont regimen), which is a combination of bolus and infusional 5-FU/LV administered on days 1 and 2 on a biweekly schedule; and a simplified LV5FU2 schedule with LV 400 mg/m^2 and 5-FU 400 mg/m^2 on day 1, followed by a single 46-hour continuous infusion of 5-FU for a total 5-FU infusion dose of 2400 mg/m^2.[36-38] Based on recent National Comprehensive Cancer Network (NCCN) guidelines, the PVI 5-FU ± LV schedule is a reasonable first-line treatment option for patients who cannot tolerate intensive chemotherapy.[39]

Capecitabine. Capecitabine is an oral fluoropyrimidine carbamate prodrug of 5-FU designed to be reliably absorbed intact through the gastrointestinal tract. It then becomes activated by three successive enzymatic steps. The enzyme thymidylate phosphorylase is involved in the final step, and it is also thought to be expressed at a higher level in tumor tissue when compared to corresponding normal tissue. This tumor localization of thymidylate phosphorylase may be the basis for its selective activation of capecitabine in tumors and associated favorable tolerability.[40,41]

In two randomized Phase III trials comparing capecitabine with Mayo regimen bolus 5-FU/LV, capecitabine showed similar efficacy. An integrated analysis of the two trials revealed that the overall RR was higher with capecitabine than with bolus 5-FU/LV (25.7% vs. 16.7%; $P < .0002$) while time to progression (TTP) and survival were similar. Capecitabine also was associated with fewer side effects (Table 68-3).

TABLE 68-3 SUMMARY OF TOXICITIES OF APPROVED AGENTS FOR THE MANAGEMENT OF CRC

Agent	Toxicities
5-fluorouracil (5-FU)	The most commonly reported toxicities include myelosuppression, mucositis, diarrhea, and palmar-plantar erythrodysesthesia. Less common but clinically relevant toxicities include coronary vasospasms, which may result in cardiac ischemia, blepharitis, and photosensitivity. The presence of a deficiency of dihydropyrimidine dehydrogenase, a critical enzyme in the catabolic pathway of 5-FU, may lead to severe, life-threatening toxicities and should be clinically recognized by the early development of 5-FU toxicities.
Capecitabine	Similar to those for 5-FU; common toxicities include nausea, diarrhea, mucositis, and palmar-plantar erythrodysesthesia, which may be dose limiting. Myelosuppression is less frequently seen than with intravenous 5-FU. Capecitabine can increase the anticoagulant effect of warfarin.
Oxaliplatin	The most commonly reported toxicities include a dose-limiting peripheral sensory neuropathy with distal paresthesias, oropharyngeal dysesthesia, and nausea and vomiting. The cumulative sensory neuropathy appears to be reversible in the majority of patients, with a 10-14% grade 3-4 neuropathy with doses ≥850 mg/m^2. An acute hypersensitivity reaction manifesting as a rash, fever, and ocular and respiratory symptoms has been reported in up to 19% of patients.
Irinotecan	The most common dose-limiting toxicities include neutropenia and diarrhea. An acute cholinergic syndrome manifesting as diarrhea, diaphoresis, and abdominal cramping, often during the infusion, can be treated with atropine. Increased toxicities develop in the setting of hepatic dysfunction.
Bevacizumab	The most common toxicity is hypertension, which usually can be modulated and controlled with antihypertensive agents. Less common but clinically significant toxicities include arterial thromboembolic events, bleeding and bowel perforations, and proteinuria. The risk of serious arterial thromboembolic events appears to be highest in patients with underlying heart disease.
Cetuximab	The most common adverse effect is an acneiform rash seen in varying intensity in virtually all patients. Less common effects include weakness, malaise, fever, headache, nausea, and hypersensitivity reactions.
Panitumumab	Similar to cetuximab, the most common adverse effect is an acneiform rash seen in varying intensity in virtually all patients. Less common effects include paronychia, hypomagnesemia, stomatitis, and hypersensitivity reactions.

Gastrointestinal and hematologic toxicities were significantly lower in incidence in the capecitabine arm compared to that in the bolus 5-FU/LV arm. Hand-foot syndrome was the only side effect that was observed with higher incidence in the capecitabine arm. There have been no randomized clinical trials comparing the efficacy and toxicity of capecitabine with any infusional 5-FU schedules. When compared to historical controls of continuous infusion of 5-FU, capecitabine monotherapy appeared to have similar RR, TTP, and median survival.[41]

Capecitabine, at a dosage of 1250 mg/m^2 twice daily for 14 days of every 21-day cycle, was approved in the United States for first-line treatment of mCRC when fluoropyrimidine monotherapy is indicated. However, clinical experience and retrospective analysis indicate that 900 to 1000 mg/m^2 twice daily may be better tolerated with similar efficacy.[41]

Irinotecan. Irinotecan is a topoisomerase I poison.[42] Irinotecan monotherapy in 5-FU–refractory mCRC patients showed an improved 1-year OS (36% vs. 14%) and improved quality of life when compared with best supportive care. Severe diarrhea is the well-known dose-limiting toxicity of irinotecan.[43] Irinotecan was initially approved for second-line treatment by the U.S. Food and Drug Administration (FDA); however, three randomized Phase III trials provided evidence that a first-line combination regimen including irinotecan and 5-FU/LV rendered improved clinical efficacy, including OS, compared to 5-FU/LV alone.[43-45]

In Europe, Douillard et al. compared the clinical efficacy of infusional 5-FU plus irinotecan versus infusional 5-FU/LV alone. In this trial, the irinotecan group was superior in RR (35% vs. 22%; $P = .005$), time to treatment failure (6.7 vs. 4.4 months; $P = .001$), and OS (17.4 vs. 14.2 months; $P = .031$).[44] Kohne et al. compared weekly infusional 5-FU/LV with and without irinotecan and reported that addition of irinotecan improved RRs (54% vs. 31.5%; $P < .0001$) and TTP (8.5 vs. 6.4 months; $P = .0001$). However, the median survival benefit (10.1 vs. 16.9 months; $P = .2279$ log-rank) did not reach the level of statistical significance.[45]

In the United States, Saltz et al. compared an IFL (bolus 5-FU/LV) weekly schedule versus 5-FU/LV alone, and reported the superiority of the IFL regimen over 5-FU/LV alone in terms of RR (39% vs. 21%; $P < .001$), median progression-free survival (PFS) (7.0 vs. 4.3 months; $P = .004$), and OS (14.8 vs. 12.6 months; $P = .04$).[46] The weekly IFL regimen resulted in increased incidence of diarrhea, dehydration, and myelosuppression when compared to the infusional schedules of 5-FU/LV (the FOLFIRI or Douillard regimen). Based on this observation, the IFL regimen, which used to be preferred among U.S. oncologists due to their familiarity with it, are now used rarely or used with modification consisting of 2 weeks on and 1 week off. Conversely, the FOLFIRI strategies have been embraced by more U.S. oncologists recently. In fact, based on a recent randomized trial by Fuchs et al., even the modified IFL regimen (m-IFL) should be considered obsolete, and the FOLFIRI regimen should be the regimen of choice when 5-FU is combined with irinotecan in treatment of previously untreated mCRC. In this trial, FOLFIRI showed its superiority over m-IFL with respect to TTP (8.2 vs. 6.0 months; $P = .01$) and median OS (23.1 vs. 17.6 months; $P = .10$). FOLFIRI was also better tolerated than m-IFL.[47]

Capecitabine plus Irinotecan (CapeIri). Investigators are actively evaluating the combination of capecitabine + irinotecan (CapeIri) to take advantage of the convenience and tolerability of the oral capecitabine. Numerous Phase II studies have shown the efficacy of CapeIri with a manageable side effect profile.[48-50] In one Phase II study including 47 patients with metastatic or unresectable CRC, Ahn et al. investigated the combination of capecitabine (1000 mg/m^2 orally twice daily on days 2 to 15 of a 3-week cycle) + irinotecan (100 mg/m^2 IV on days 1 and 8). This trial reported an overall RR of 51.4% (19 partial responses; 95% CI 35.3 to 67.5%), median TTP of 7.1 months (95% CI 4.6 to 9.6 months), and median OS of 24.8 months (95% CI 10.5 to 39.1 months). This regimen was relatively well tolerated, with grade 3/4 diarrhea (24%) and grade 3/4 neutropenia (11%). There were no treatment-related deaths.[48] However, in a recent multicenter, randomized trial comparing FOLFIRI, m-IFL, and CapeIri in a first-line setting of mCRC, CapeIri was inferior in efficacy with a higher rate of toxicities compared to the other two regimens.[47]

Oxaliplatin. Oxaliplatin is a third-generation platinum compound with significant anticancer activity in CRC in combination with 5-FU. Its dose-limiting toxicity is acute and chronic sensory neuropathy. The chronic form is a dose-dependent sensory neuropathy that develops in up to 12% to 15% of patients when the cumulative dose is greater than 850 mg/m^2.[3,51]

The benefit of adding oxaliplatin to 5-FU/LV was reported in a randomized Phase III trial by de Gramont et al. The FOLFOX4 regimen (oxaliplatin at a dose of 85 mg/m^2 as a 2-hour infusion on day 1, every 2 weeks, plus LV5FU2) was compared with LV5FU2 alone in 420 patients with previously treated mCRC[52] (Fig. 68-3). FOLFOX4 resulted in a longer median PFS (9 vs. 6.2 months; $P = .0003$) and a higher RR (50.7% vs. 22.3%; $P = .0001$). The difference in median OS did not reach statistical significance (16.2 vs. 14.7 months; $P = .12$). However, this trial was not sufficiently powered to detect such a difference, and any potential survival difference may have been obscured as both treatment arms were able to receive salvage therapies. Grade 3/4 neutropenia and grade 3/4 diarrhea were more common with FOLFOX4 but were at clearly manageable levels.[52]

Capecitabine plus Oxaliplatin (CAPOX). Capecitabine's convenience of being an oral agent with better tolerability than 5-FU/LV led to a series of studies that compared combination of oxaliplatin with either capecitabine or 5-FU/LV. A Phase II trial investigated the combination of capecitabine (1000 mg/m^2 twice daily from day 1 to 14) and oxaliplatin (130 mg/m^2 IV on day 1) every 3 weeks. The regimen resulted in an overall RR of 55% and a median OS of 19.5 months, comparable to those observed with FOLFOX4. This trial showed that the CAPOX combination is efficacious and well tolerated, with common side effects being diarrhea, myelosuppression, and neurotoxicity. This result captured the potential of capecitabine becoming an alternative to 5-FU/LV in the first-line setting.[53,54]

Additional Trials Comparing Therapeutic Regimens

FOLFOX4 versus IFL. Intergroup trial N9741 was a randomized Phase III trial that compared FOLFOX, IFL, or oxaliplatin/irinotecan (IROX).[55] This pivotal trial showed that FOLFOX4 was superior to IFL in RR (45% vs. 31%; $P = .002$), TTP (8.7 vs. 6.9 months: $P = .0001$), and median OS (19.5 vs. 14.8 months: $P = .0001$). In addition, when compared to IFL or IROX, FOLFOX4 was associated with a significantly lower incidence of febrile neutropenia and fewer gastrointestinal side effects. Based on this trial, FOLFOX4 was approved in the United States as first-line treatment for patients with mCRC.[55]

FOLFIRI versus FOLFOX. Tournigand et al. conducted a randomized, multicenter, open-label prospective Phase III trial in order to answer the question of whether oxaliplatin is a more active agent than

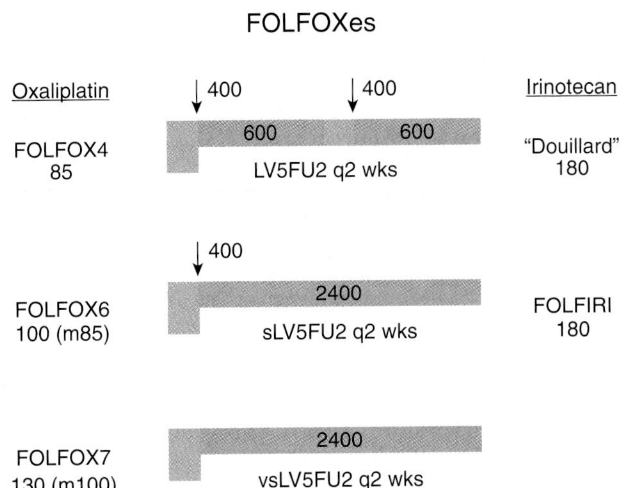

FIGURE 68-3 • Various modifications of FOLFOX regimens in clinical practice.

TABLE 68-4 PHASE III TRIAL OF FIRST-LINE FOLFIRI VERSUS FOLFOX6 (GERCOR C97-3)

	Arm A		*Arm B*		
	FOLFIRI (*n* = 109)	**FOLFOX6 (*n* = 81)**	**FOLFOX6 (*n* = 111)**	**FOLFIRI (*n* = 69)**	***P* Value**
ORR (%)	56	15	54	4	0.68
Median PFS (mo)	8.5	4.2	8	2.5	—
Median TTP (mo)	14.2		10.9		0.64
Median OS (mo)	21.5		20.6		0.99

ORR, overall response rate; OS, overall survival; PFS, progression-free survival; TTP, time to progression.
From Tournigand C, Andre T, Achille E, et al. FOLFIRI followed by FOLFOX6 or the reverse sequence in advanced colorectal cancer: a randomized GERCOR study. J Clin Oncol 2004;22:229.

irinotecan when an identical 5-FU–based schedule is used.[56] Patients had equal access to the alternative regimen at progression. This trial used a simplified LV5FU2 regimen with a single 46-hour infusion. In one arm, patients received FOLFIRI (biweekly irinotecan 180 mg/m^2, LV 200 mg/m^2, 5-FU 400 mg/m^2 on day 1 followed by a 46-hour continuous infusion of 5-FU at 2.4 to 3.0 g/m^2) followed at progression by FOLFOX6 (biweekly oxaliplatin 100 mg/m^2 and the same dose and schedule of 5-FU/LV), while patients in the second arm received the reverse sequence of FOLFOX6 as first-line therapy followed by FOLFIRI at the time of progression. The efficacy was similar in terms of RR (54% vs. 56% for FOLFOX6 and FOLFIRI, respectively), PFS (8 vs. 8.5 months) and median OS (20.6 vs. 21.5 months). Both treatment arms were relatively well tolerated. Patients treated with first-line FOLFIRI experienced a higher incidence of grade 3/4 nausea and mucositis. The first-line FOLFOX6 group experienced a higher incidence of grade 3/4 myelosuppression. Use of oxaliplatin was associated with grade 3/4 neurotoxicity (34%).

The Tournigand study was important as it demonstrated equivalent clinical efficacy between irinotecan and oxaliplatin in the first-line setting when used with the same de Gramont infusional 5-FU/LV regimen. It also demonstrated that there is not a superior sequence of the two regimens (Table 68-4).[56] This conclusion was further augmented by another randomized Phase III trial that reported no difference in overall RR, TTP, and OS for mCRC patients treated with the FOLFIRI or FOLFOX4 as first-line regimens.[57]

CAPIRI versus CAPOX and FUFOX versus CAPOX. Based on randomized trial data, CAPOX and a regimen consisting of weekly infusional 5-FU/LV + oxaliplatin (FUFOX) appeared to have similar antitumor activities, but CAPOX was associated with more significant gastrointestinal toxicities and myelosuppression.[58] A randomized Phase II trial by Grothey et al. compared the combination of capecitabine + irinotecan (CAPIRI) with CAPOX in the first-line setting. Patients from both arms were allowed to cross over at progression. There was no difference in OS, and the safety profiles of both regimens were equally manageable.[59] These trials further solidified the potential of capecitabine as an alternative to 5-FU/LV in the first-line setting. Intergroup study NO16966 is the first Phase III trial to evaluate the efficacy of bevacizumab in combination with FOLFOX4 and XELOX regimens in the first-line treatment of mCRC, as described later in the chapter.[60]

Sequential versus Combination Therapy. Grothey et al. have shown that exposure to all three main anticancer agents during the treatment course of mCRC is a critical predictor of OS.[61] A few studies were conducted to assess whether sequential administration of these agents is superior to up-front combination therapy or vice versa. The Fluorouracil, Oxaliplatin, CPT-11 Usage Study (FOCUS) trial was a five-arm randomized Phase III trial conducted to compare sequential therapy with up-front use of combination regimens.[62] The up-front use of combination regimens such as FOLFOX or FOLFIRI yielded higher RR, PFS, and median OS. Initiation of combination therapy up front would be reasonable in patients with good to excellent performance status, those with aggressive disease, and potential candidates for salvage surgical resection. Conversely, sequential therapy initiated with 5-FU/LV or capecitabine followed by FOLFOX or FOLFIRI as second-line options may be a reasonable approach in relatively asymptomatic patients with less aggressive and unresectable diseases.[62]

FOLFOXIRI. An approach of initiating combination therapy that contains all three cytotoxic agents (5-FU/LV, oxaliplatin, and irinotecan; FOLFOXIRI) together has been investigated. A Phase III trial by Falcone et al. compared FOLFOXIRI with FOLFIRI in a first-line setting followed by an oxaliplatin-containing regimen as a second-line therapy.[63] FOLFOXIRI was superior to FOLFIRI, yielding higher overall RR (66% vs. 41%; $P = .0002$), median PFS (9.8 vs. 6.9 months; $P = .0006$), and median OS (22.6 vs. 16.7 months; $P = .032$). More patients in FOLFOXIRI went on to have resection of liver-only metastasis (36% vs. 12%; $P = .017$). FOLFOXIRI was associated with higher incidence of grade 3/4 neuropathy and neutropenia.[63] Souglakos et al. conducted a similar trial but with lower FOLFOXIRI doses than Falcone et al.'s trial. This study reported no significant difference in RR, OS, or ability to resect liver-only metastasis.[64] FOLFOXIRI may become a reasonable first-line option for a selected group of patients, particularly for potential candidates for definitive liver metastasis resections or for patients in whom biologic agents are contraindicated.

Optimal Duration of Chemotherapy. Maughan et al. conducted a randomized study to show that, by treating patients intermittently, toxicities were reduced without difference in OS versus continuous chemotherapy. This was evidence that discontinuing chemotherapy after a treatment period and reinitiating the same regimen at disease progression may be an appropriate option in chemotherapy-sensitive disease.[65]

The OPTIMOX trial compared FOLFOX7 to FOLFOX4. Patients in the FOLFOX4 arm received the regimen continuously until disease progression, and patients in the FOLFOX7 arm received intermittent exposure to oxaliplatin, allowing a lower cumulative dose of neurotoxic oxaliplatin.[66] The FOLFOX7 arm rendered a similar clinical efficacy with improved safety profile when compared to the FOLFOX4 arm. While this trial's outcome may have been obscured by the fact that there was a series of protocol violations in relation to reintroduction of oxaliplatin, it was an important study suggesting that intermittent use of oxaliplatin-based chemotherapy may be a reasonable alternative with improved tolerability to continuous combination chemotherapy.[66]

The OPTIMOX2 trial was a large Phase II study that compared LV5FU maintenance therapy until progression to observation until progression after six cycles of FOLFOX7. The maintenance arm was reintroduced to modified FOLFOX7 at the time of progression, and the observation arm was reintroduced to modified FOLFOX7 before the tumor progression reached the baseline measures. The maintenance LV5FU arm showed longer PFS (8.7 vs. 6.9 months; $P = .09$). However, there was no difference in the duration of disease control (12.9 vs. 11.7 months; $P = .41$). In addition, the chemotherapy-free interval (CFI) was nearly 6 months.[67] Another trial was conducted to evaluate whether the same efficacy of continuous chemotherapy can be achieved with intermittent chemotherapy. Labianca et al. compared FOLFIRI scheduled every 2 weeks continuously versus an alternating schedule of FOLFIRI for 2 months and CFI for 2 months. This trial reported no significant difference in PFS or median OS between the two treatment arms, supporting the suggestion that intermittent chemotherapy may be a potential alternative to continuous chemotherapy.[68] CFI without significant compromise of PFS and OS can potentially have a significant impact on quality of life of mCRC patients.

Novel Targeted Agents

Bevacizumab. Bevacizumab is a recombinant humanized monoclonal antibody targeted against VEGF, which is a proangiogenic growth factor that is overexpressed in CRC as well as in a wide range of solid human cancers.[3] Bevacizumab monotherapy does not appear to have significant activity in mCRC. Conversely, it has considerable activity when used in combination with commonly used chemotherapies, including 5-FU, irinotecan, oxaliplatin, and possibly in combination with cetuximab.[5,69,70]

Hurwitz et al. reported Phase III trial data showing that addition of bevacizumab to IFL led to statistically significant improvement of OS (20.3 vs. 15.6 months; $P = .001$), RR (44.8% vs. 34.8%; $P = .004$), and PFS (10.6 vs. 6.2 months) in patients with mCRC (Fig. 68-4). Patients who progressed after IFL plus bevacizumab then went on to receive second-line therapy with an oxaliplatin-based regimen and achieved an OS of 25.1 months, which was the longest median OS rendered by any first- and second-line combination therapy at the time.[5] One can reasonably presume that an even better outcome might have resulted by using an infusional 5-FU/LV schedule (FOLFIRI), which now is a standard of care, rather than a bolus 5-FU/LV schedule (IFL).

The final analysis of the Three Regimen of Eloxatin Evaluation (TREE)-1 and -2 trials reported that addition of bevacizumab to bolus, infusional, or capecitabine regimens rendered improved RR in all groups. This important trial showed that FOLFOX plus bevacizumab treatment was a superior first-line regimen to FOLFOX alone, improving overall RR (44% vs. 53%), median TTP (8.7 vs. 9.9 months), and median OS (19.2 vs. 26 months). Bevacizumab is now recommended to be used with all five first-line therapy regimens outlined by the NCCN.[69]

The Eastern Cooperative Oncology Group 3200 study, including 820 patients who were previously treated with first-line 5-FU, irinotecan either separately or as a combination regimen without bevacizumab, reported that adding bevacizumab to a second-line FOLFOX4 regimen improved median OS when compared to FOLFOX4 alone (12.5 vs. 10.7 months; $P = .002$).[70]

NO16966 is the first Phase III trial to evaluate the efficacy of bevacizumab in combination with FOLFOX4 and XELOX regimens in the first-line treatment of MCRC. In this Intergroup study, 1401 patients were randomized to receive FOLFOX4 (oxaliplatin and 5-FU/LV as described previously[52]) or XELOX (oxaliplatin 130 mg/m^2 IV + capecitabine 1000 mg/m^2 twice daily orally on days 1 to 14, every 3 weeks) plus bevacizumab (5 mg/kg to FOLFOX, 7.5 mg/kg to XELOX) or placebo in a 2 × 2 factorial design.[60] The main end point of the recently presented results was PFS. Two primary objectives were:

1. XELOX is noninferior to FOLFOX (noninferiority concluded if upper limit of 97.5% CI = 1.23)
2. Bevacizumab + chemotherapy is superior to placebo + chemotherapy (superiority concluded if $P = .025$)

The results presented at the ASCO Gastrointestinal Cancers Symposium in January 2007 showed that the median PFS for XELOX-bevacizumab + FOLFOX4-bevacizumab was 9.3 months versus 8.0 months for XELOX-placebo + FOLFOX4-placebo (HR 0.83, 97.5% CI, 0.72 to 0.95, $P = .0023$). Although the protocol specified study drug treatment until progression of disease (PD), only 56% of patients were treated in this manner, and 50% of patients discontinued for reasons unrelated to PD. Median PFS on the specified study treatment was 10.4 months for chemotherapy + bevacizumab versus 8.1 months for chemotherapy + placebo (HR 0.63, $P < .0001$). Heterogeneity was detected in subgroups. No unexpected toxicity has been reported. Additional efficacy data, including independently reviewed data and subgroup analyses, will be presented at the annual meeting of ASCO 2007.[70a] In summary, this large, international Phase III trial provided evidence from a first-line CRC Phase III trial to show that the addition of bevacizumab to oxaliplatin-based chemotherapy regimens significantly improves PFS. This study further supports the use of bevacizumab in combination with standard first-line chemotherapy.[60]

	XELOX-Placebo + FOLFOX-Placebo	XELOX-Bev + FOLFOX-Bev	
PFS general approach	8.0	9.4	HR 0.83 (97.5% CI 0.72-0.95), p = 0.0023
PFS on treatment approach	7.9	10.4	HR 0.63 (97.5% CI 0.52-0.75), p < 0.0001
PFS based on IRC dataset	8.6	11.1	HR 0.70 (97.5% CI 0.58-0.83), p < 0.0001

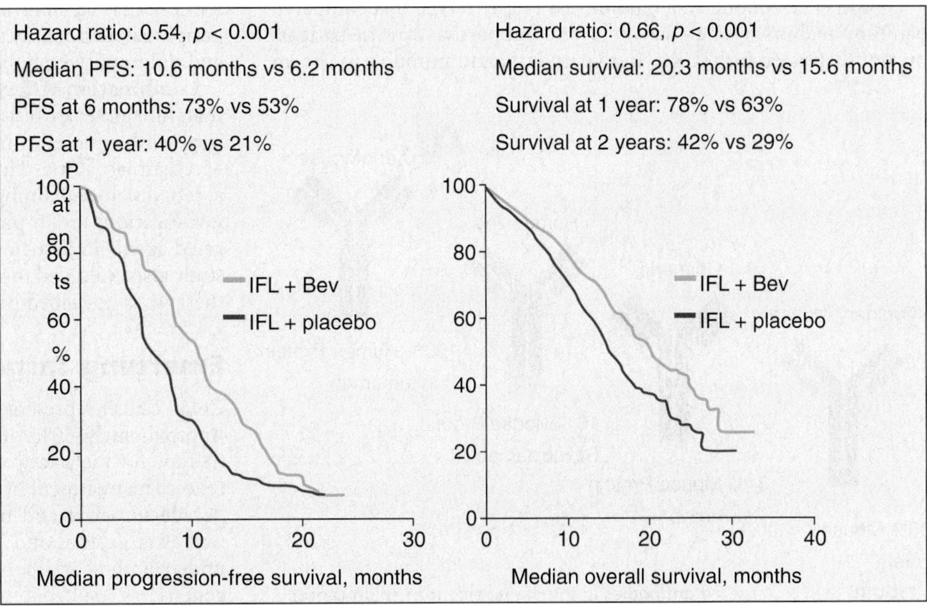

FIGURE 68-4 • Efficacy data of Phase III trial in first-line therapy for mCRC with IFL + bevacizumab.

Bevacizumab as a third-line therapy appears to have very limited activity in patients who failed previous treatment with oxaliplatin- or irinotecan-based regimens. Optimal duration of bevacizumab, particularly in patients who progressed on first-line combination therapy with bevacizumab, is unclear at this time. The Southwest Oncology Group is conducting a Phase II trial in an attempt to answer this question.[71]

Bevacizumab is generally well tolerated and has very few overlapping toxicities with chemotherapeutic agents. Hurwitz et al. reported grade 3 hypertension (11%), which was managed with oral medications, and increased risk of gastrointestinal perforation (1.5%). However, there was no significant difference in treatment-related hospitalization, in treatment delay due to toxicity, or in the 60-day rate of death from all causes.[5] Skillings et al., by reviewing 1745 patients who received bevacizumab, noted an approximately twofold increased risk of arterial thromboembolic events. Bevacizumab was also associated with bleeding (2% to 9.3%), proteinuria (1% to 2%), and poor wound healing (1% to 2%).[72] These side effects should be considered when clinicians evaluate patients for the use of bevacizumab. The recommended dose of bevacizumab in treating first-line mCRC is 5 mg/kg IV administered over 90 minutes, while 10 mg/kg IV is the dose for second-line treatment. A dose of 7.5 mg/kg IV every 3 weeks can be used when bevacizumab is used with capecitabine-containing regimens.[72,73]

Cetuximab. Cetuximab is a recombinant human/mouse chimeric EGFR monoclonal antibody. EGFR is overexpressed in CRC as well as in a broad range of solid tumors. Preliminary data on cetuximab in combination with FOLFIRI, FOLFOX, and XELOX first-line therapy is encouraging, and this area is under further investigation.[3,74-78]

Currently, cetuximab is a recommended second-line agent in mCRC patients who cannot tolerate, progressed on, or failed irinotecan-based chemotherapy. In the Bowel Oncology with cetuximab Antibody 007 (BOND-1) trial, a combination of cetuximab with irinotecan was found to be superior to cetuximab alone in patients who progressed on an irinotecan-based first-line regimen. Cetuximab is also recommended as a third-line therapy for patients who failed irinotecan- or oxaliplatin-based chemotherapies. Cetuximab was associated with acneiform rash (up to 88% of all patients), severe infusion reaction (3%), interstitial lung disease, and hypomagnesemia. Cetuximab is administered with a loading dose of 400 mg/m^2 IV over 90 minutes, followed by a maintenance dose of 200 mg/m^2 IV given weekly.[79]

Panitumumab. Panitumumab is a fully human monoclonal antibody (Fig. 68-5) targeting EGFR. Panitumumab monotherapy was recently approved by the FDA based on clinical trials that showed activity in mCRC patients with prior chemotherapy.[80,81]

Gibson et al. conducted a randomized Phase III trial that compared panitumumab as a single agent to best supportive care in patients previously treated for mCRC. In this study, panitumumub was shown to be efficacious (46% reduction in the risk of tumor progression and a partial RR of 8%) with a manageable side effect profile.[82]

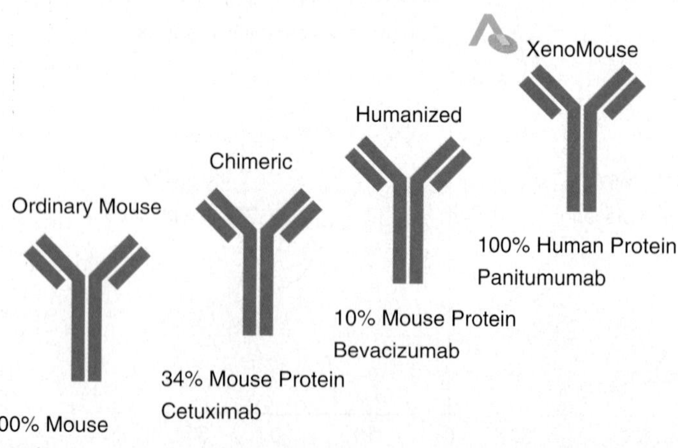

FIGURE 68-5 • **Targeted antibodies in the management of colon cancer.**

The use of panitumumab in combination with other cytotoxic agents in the first-line setting appears to be an option that is worthy of further investigation. In a Phase II trial, the combination of IFL and panitumumab as first-line therapy showed a disease control rate (overall response + stabilized disease) of 74% with a median PFS of 5.6 months and an OS of 17 months. In this trial, panitumumab was also combined with FOLFIRI and resulted in similar efficacy, with a disease control rate of 79% (33% partial response and 46% stabilized disease), and median PFS of 10.9 months. The survival data are still maturing. In terms of side effects, fewer patients experienced grade 3/4 diarrhea (25% vs. 47%). Skin-related toxicities were reported at up to 17% in the FOLFIRI group and 16% in the IFL group.[83]

The Panitumumab Advanced Colorectal Cancer Evaluation (PACCE) study is a Phase IIIb randomized, open-label clinical trial evaluating oxaliplatin- and irinotecan-based chemotherapy and bevacizumab with and without panitumumab in the first-line treatment of patients with mCRC.[84] The trial is powered to show a 30% reduction in PFS, the primary end point. The PACCE trial enrolled 1054 patients (824 patients were randomized to receive oxaliplatin-based chemotherapy, and 230 patients were randomized to receive irinotecan-based chemotherapy) at 240 trial sites in the United States between Q1 2005 and Q3 2006. Amgen announced on March 27, 2007, that it had discontinued panitumumab treatment in the PACCE trial evaluating the addition of panitumumab to standard chemotherapy and bevacizumab for the treatment of first-line mCRC. The decision to discontinue panitumumab treatment in the trial was based on a preliminary review of data from a preplanned interim efficacy analysis scheduled after the first 231 events (death or disease progression). This analysis revealed a statistically significant difference in PFS in favor of the control arm. An unplanned analysis of OS also demonstrated a statistically significant difference favoring the control arm. Additional analyses are ongoing, and the sponsor plans to present the results at the annual meeting of ASCO in June 2007.[84a]

Vatalanib. Vatalanib is an oral small-molecule VEGF receptor inhibitor that blocks the activity of the VEGF receptor tyrosine kinase. Preliminary results from the CONFIRM-1 study by Hecht et al. suggested an improved outcome of FOLFOX by adding vatalanib in treating chemotherapy-naive patients with mCRC.[85] The initial primary end point of the study, which was PFS time only, showed a modest statistically insignificant benefit of adding vatalanib to FOLFOX4. However, a subsequent analysis showed that there is a statistically significant improvement in PFS time with vatalanib in patients with elevated pretreatment lactate dehydrogenase. Final survival data on this trial are maturing. Common side effects of vatalanib were hypertension (21%), neutropenia (31%), diarrhea (15%), nausea (9%), peripheral neuropathy (9%), venous thrombosis (7%), dizziness (7%), and pulmonary embolism (6%).

Combination of Targeted Agents. The BOND-2 trial demonstrated that, in irinotecan-resistant mCRC, combining bevacizumab + cetuximab with irinotecan improved outcomes compared to bevacizumab + cetuximab alone. This trial suggested that adding bevacizumab to a cetuximab-containing regimen may improve the outcome. Active investigations are in progress to define a role for combination of targeted agents in first-line as well as second-line settings.[86] The PACCE study also evaluated the combination of two targeted agents in chemotherapy, as described previously.

Emerging Targets and Therapeutics

Colon cancer represents a major health problem in the Western world. Approximately 60% of patients with colon cancer require systemic therapy for metastatic disease, either at diagnosis or at disease recurrence. The treatment of colon cancer has definitely advanced in the last decade as newer and more active cytotoxic chemotherapy agents as well as targeted monoclonal antibodies have become available. Better understanding of different fundamental molecular changes in carcinogenesis has resulted in the emergence of such therapeutic targets in the treatment of colon cancer. Finally, intense efforts are attempting to identify the critical molecular biomarkers that can be used to predict for either clinical response to chemotherapy and/or targeted therapies and/or the drug-specific side effects.

REFERENCES

1. Jemal A, Siegel R, Ward E, et al. Cancer statistics, 2007. CA Cancer J Clin 2007;57: 43-66.
2. Wu X, Chen VW, Martin J, et al. Comparative Analysis of Incidence Rates Subcommittee, Data Evaluation and Publication Committee, North American Association of Central Cancer Registries. Subsite-specific colorectal cancer incidence rates and stage distributions among Asians and Pacific Islanders in the United States, 1995 to 1999. Cancer Epidemiol Biomarkers Prev 2004;13:1215-1222.
3. Saif MW. Targeted agents for adjuvant therapy of colon cancer. Clin Colorectal Cancer 2006;6:46-51.
4. Meta-Analysis Group in Cancer. Modulation of fluorouracil by leucovorin in patients with advanced colorectal cancer: an updated meta-analysis. J Clin Oncol 2004;22:3766-3775.
5. Hurwitz H, Fehrenbacher L, Novotny W, et al. Bevacizumab plus irinotecan, fluorouracil, and leucovorin for metastatic colorectal cancer. N Engl J Med 2004;350:2335-2342.
6. American Joint Committee on Cancer. Colon and rectum. *In* American Joint Committee on Cancer: AJCC Cancer Staging Manual, 6th ed. New York: Springer-Verlag, 2002, pp 113-124.
7. Compton CC, Greene FL. The staging of colorectal cancer: 2004 and beyond. CA Cancer J Clin 2004;54:295-308.
8. Smith RE, Colangelo L, Wieand HS, et al. Randomized trial of adjuvant therapy in colon carcinoma: 1-year results of NSABP protocol C-01. J Natl Cancer Inst 2004;96:1128-1132.
9. Moertel CG, Fleming TR, Macdonald JS, et al. Levamisole and fluorouracil for adjuvant therapy of resected colon carcinoma. N Engl J Med 1990;322:352-358.
10. Moertel CG, Fleming TR, Macdonald JS, et al. Intergroup study of fluorouracil plus levamisole as adjuvant therapy for stage II/Dukes B2 colon cancer. J Clin Oncol 1995;13:2936-2943.
11. O'Connell MJ. A Phase III trial of 5-fluorouracil and leucovorin in the treatment of advanced colorectal cancer. A Mayo Clinic/North Central Cancer Treatment Group study. Cancer 1989;63(6 Suppl):1026-1030.
12. International Multicentre Pooled Analysis of Colon Cancer Trials (IMPACT) Investigators. Efficacy of adjuvant fluorouracil and folinic acid in colon cancer. Lancet 1995;345:939-944.
13. Haller DG, Catalano PJ, Macdonald JS, et al. Phase III study of fluorouracil, leucovorin, and levamisole in high-risk stage II and III colon cancer: final report of Intergroup 0089. J Clin Oncol 2005;23:8671-8678.
14. Andre T, Cloin P, Louvet C, et al. Semimonthly versus monthly regimen of fluorouracil and leucovorin administered for 24 or 36 weeks as adjuvant therapy in stage II and III colon cancer: results of a randomized trial. J Clin Oncol 2003;21:2896-2903.
15. Andre T, Quinaux E, Louvet C, et al. Updated results at 6 year of the GERCOR C96.1 Phase III study comparing LV5FU2 to monthly 5FU-leucovorin (mFUfol) as adjuvant treatment for Dukes B2 and C colon cancer patients [Abstract 3522]. J Clin Oncol 2005;23(16 Suppl).
16. Chau I, Norman AR, Cunningham D, et al. A randomized comparison between 6 months of bolus fluorouracil/leucovorin and 12 weeks of protracted venous infusion fluorouracil as adjuvant treatment in colorectal cancer. Ann Oncol 2005;16:549-557.
17. Poplin EA, Benedetti JK, Estes NC, et al. Phase III Southwest Oncology Group 9415/ Intergroup 0153 randomized trial of fluorouracil, leucovorin, and levamisole versus fluorouracil continuous infusion and levamisole for adjuvant treatment of stage III and high-risk stage II colon cancer. J Clin Oncol 2005;23:1819-1825.

17a. Schumacher K. Comparison of 5-FU + folinic acid, 5-FU + levamisole and 5-FU + folinic acid + levamisole in Duke's B and C colon cancer. NSABP Trial C-04. Strahlenther Onkol 2000;176(5):239-240.

18. Andre T, Boni C, Mounedji-Boudiaf L, et al. Oxaliplatin, 5-fluorouracil and leucovorin as adjuvant treatment of colon cancer: results of the international randomized MOSAIC trial. N Engl J Med 2004;350:2343-2351.
19. Wolmark M, Wieand HS, Kuebler JP, et al. A Phase III trial comparing FULV to FULV + oxaliplatin in stage II or III carcinoma of the colon: results of NSABP Protocol C-07 [Abstract 3500]. J Clin Oncol 2005;23(16 Suppl).
20. Van Cutsem E, Labianca R, Hossfeld D, et al. Randomized Phase III trial comparing infused irinotecan/5-fluorouracil (5-FU) folinic acid (IF) versus 5-FU/FA (F) in stage III colon cancer patients (pts) (PETACC 3). [Abstract LBA8]. J Clin Oncol 2005;23(16 Suppl).
21. Ychou M, Raoul JL, Douillard JY, et al. A Phase III randomized trial of LV5FU2 + CPT-11 vs. LV5FU2 alone in adjuvant high risk colon cancer (FNCLCC Accord02/ FFCD9802) [Abstract 3502]. J Clin Oncol 2005;23(16 Suppl).
22. Rothernberg ML, Meropol NJ, Poplin EA, et al. Mortality associated with irinotecan plus bolus fluorouracil/leucovorin: summary finding of an independent panel. J Clin Oncol 2001;19:3801-3807.
23. Twelves C, Wong A, Nowacki MP, et al. Capecitabine as adjuvant treatment for stage III colon cancer. N Engl J Med 2005;352:2696-2704.
24. Schmoll HJ, Cartwright T, Tabernero J, et al. Phase III trial of capecitabine plus oxaliplatin as adjuvant therapy for stage III colon cancer: a planned safety analysis in 1,864 patients. J Clin Oncol 2007;25:102-109.
25. Gill S, Loprinzi CL, Sargent DJ, et al. Pooled analysis of fluorouracil-based adjuvant therapy for stage II and III colon cancer: who benefits and by how much? J Clin Oncol 2004;22:1797-1806.
26. Figueredo A, Charette ML, Maroun J, et al. Adjuvant therapy for stage II colon cancer: a systematic review from the Cancer Care Ontario Program in Evidence-Based Care's Gastrointestinal Cancer Disease Site Group. J Clin Oncol 2004;22:3395-3407.
27. Benson AB 3rd, Schrag D, Somerfield MR, et al. American Society of Clinical Oncology recommendations on adjuvant chemotherapy for stage II colon cancer. J Clin Oncol 2004;22:3408-3419.
28. Le Voyer T, Sigurdson E, Hanlon A, et al. Colon cancer survival is associated with increasing number of lymph nodes analyzed: a secondary survey of intergroup trial INT-0089. J Clin Oncol 2003;21:2912-2919.
29. Saif MW, Kang SP, Chu E. Treatment of metastatic colorectal cancer: from cytotoxic agents to molecular agents and multitargeted strategies. Oncology (Williston Park). 2006;20(14 Suppl 10):11-19.
30. Chu E, Devita VT Jr. Physician's Cancer Chemotherapy Drug Manual 2006. Sudbury, MA: Jones & Bartlett.
31. Meyerhardt JA, Mayer RJ. Systemic therapy for colorectal cancer. N Engl J Med 2005;352:476-487.
32. Poon MA, O'Connell MJ, Moertel CG, et al. Biochemical modulation of fluorouracil: evidence of significant improvement of survival and quality of life in patents with advanced colorectal carcinoma. J Clin Oncol 1989;7:1407-1418.
33. The Meta-Analysis Group in Cancer. Toxicity of fluorouracil in patients with advanced colorectal cancer: effect of administration schedule and prognostic factors. J Clin Oncol 1998;11:3537-3541.
34. Buroker TR, O'Connell MJ, Wieand HS, et al. Randomized comparison of two schedules of flurouracil and leucovorin in the treatment of advanced colorectal cancer. J Clin Oncol 1994;12:14.
35. Wang WS, Lin JK, Chiou TJ, et al. Randomized trial comparing weekly bolus 5-fluorouracil plus leucovorin versus monthly 5-day 5-fluororuacil plus leucovorin in metastatic colorectal cancer. Hepatogastroenterology 2000;47:1599.
36. The Meta-Analysis Group in Cancer. Efficacy of intravenous continuous infusion of fluorouracil compared with bolus administration in advanced colorectal cancer. J Clin Oncol 1998;16:301-308.
37. Weh HJ, Wilke HJ, Dierlamm J, et al. Weekly therapy with folinic acid (FA) and high-dose 5-fluorouracil (5-FU) 24-hour infusion in pretreated patients with metastatic colorectal carcinoma: a multicenter study by the Association of Medical Oncology of the German Cancer Society (AIO). Ann Oncol 1994;5:233-237.
38. de Gramont A, Bosset JF, Milan C, et al. Randomized trial comparing monthly low dose leucovorin and fluorouracil bolus with bimonthly high-dose leucovorin and fluorouracil bolus plus continuous infusion for advanced colorectal cancer: a French intergroup study. J Clin Oncol 1997;15:808.
39. National Comprehensive Cancer Network. Clinical Practice Guidelines in Oncology: Colon Cancer, Version 2. 2006. Available at: *http://nccn.org/professionals/physician_gls/PDF/colon.pdf*
40. Schuller J, Cassidy J, Dumont E, et al. Preferential activation of capecitabine in tumor following oral administration to colorectal cancer patients. Cancer Chemother Pharmacol 2000;45:291.
41. Saif MW. Capecitabine versus continuous-infusion 5-fluorouracil for colorectal cancer: a retrospective efficacy and safety comparison. Clin Colorectal Cancer 2005;5:89-100.
42. Vanhoefer U, Harstrick A, Achterrath W, et al. Irinotecan in the treatment of colorectal cancer: clinical overview. J Clin Oncol 2001;19:1501-1518.
43. Cunningham D, Pyrhonen S, James RD, et al. Randomised trial of irinotecan plus supportive care versus supportive care alone after fluorouracil failure for patients with metastatic colorectal cancer. Lancet 1998;352:1413.
44. Douillard JY, Cunningham D, Roth AD, et al. Irinotecan combined with fluorouracil compared with fluorouracil alone as first-line treatment for metastatic colorectal cancer: a multicenter randomised trial. Lancet 2000;355:1041.
45. Kohne CH, van Cutsem E, Wils J, et al. Phase III study of weekly high-dose infusional fluorouracil plus folinic acid with or without irinotecan in patients with metastatic colorectal cancer: European Organization for Research and Treatment of Cancer Gastrointestinal Group Study 40986. J Clin Oncol 2005;23:4856.
46. Saltz LB, Cox JV, Blanke C, et al. Irinotecan plus fluorouracil and leucovorin for metastatic colorectal cancer. Irinotecan Study Group. N Engl J Med 2000; 343:905.
47. Fuchs C, Marshall J, Mitchell E, et al. A randomized trial of first-line irinotecan/ fluoropyrimidine combinations with or without celecoxib in metastatic colorectal cancer (BICC-C) [Abstract 3506]. J Clin Oncol 2006;24(18 Suppl).
48. Ahn KH, Jung YS, Park YH, et al. Phase II trial of irinotecan and capecitabine in patients with advanced colorectal cancer [Abstract 3714]. J Clin Oncol 2005;23(16 Suppl):299s.
49. Patt YZ, Leibmann J, Diamondidis D, et al. Capicitabine (X) plus irinotecan (XELIRI) as first-line treatment for metastatic colorectal cancer (MCRC): final safety findings from a Phase II trial [Abstract 3602]. J Clin Oncol 2004;22(14 Suppl):271a.
50. Bajetta E, Di Bartolomeo M, Mariani L, et al. Randomized multicenter Phase II trial of two different schedules of irinotecan combined with capecitabine as first-line treatment in metastatic colorectal carcinoma. Cancer 2004;100:279.
51. Grothey A, Goldberg RM. A Review of oxaliplatin and its clinical use in colorectal cancer. Expert Opin Pharmacother 2004;5:2159-2170.
52. de Gramont A, Figer A, Seymour M, et al. Leucovorin and fluorouracil with or without oxaliplatin as first-line treatment in advanced colorectal cancer. J Clin Oncol 2000;18:2938.
53. Cassidy J, Tabernero J, Twelves C, et al. XELOX (capecitabine plus oxaliplatin): active first-line therapy for patients with metastatic colorectal cancer. J Clin Oncol 2004;22:2084.
54. Scheithauer W, Kornek GV, Raderer M, et al. Randomized multicenter Phase II trial of two different schedules of capecitabine plus oxaliplatin as first-line treatment in advanced colorectal cancer. J Clin Oncol 2003;21:1307.

55. Goldberg RM, Sargent DJ, Morton RF, et al. A randomized controlled trial of fluorouracil plus leucovorin, irinotecan, and oxaliplatin combinations in patients with previously untreated metastatic colorectal cancer. J Clin Oncol 2004;22:23.
56. Tournigand C, Andre T, Achille E, et al. FOLFIRI followed by FOLFOX6 or the reverse sequence in advanced colorectal cancer: a randomized GERCOR study. J Clin Oncol 2004;22:229.
57. Colucci G, Gebbia V, Paoletti G, et al. Phase III randomized trial of FOLFIRI versus FOLFOX4 in the treatment of advanced colorectal cancer: a multicenter study of the Gruppo Oncologico Dell'Italia Meridionale. J Clin Oncol 2005;23:4811-4814.
58. Arkenau H, Schmoll H, Kubicka S, et al. Infusional 5-fluorouracil/folinic acid plus oxaliplatin (FUFOX) versus capecitabine plus oxaliplatin (CAPOX) as first line treatment of metastatic colorectal cancer (MCRC): results of the safety and efficacy analysis [Abstract 3507]. J Clin Oncol 2005;23(16 Suppl):247s.
59. Grothey A, Jordan K, Kellner O, et al. Capecitabine/irinotecan (CapIri) and capecitabine/oxaliplatin (CapOx) are active second-line protocols in patients with advanced colorectal cancer after failure of first-line combination therapy: results of a randomized Phase II study [Abstract 3534]. J Clin Oncol 2004;22(14 Suppl).
60. Saltz LB, Clarke S, Diaz-Rubio E, et al. Bevacizumab (Bev) in combination with XELOX or FOLFOX4: efficacy results from XELOX-1/NO16966, a randomized Phase III trial in the first-line treatment of metastatic colorectal cancer (MCRC) [Abstract 238]. *In* Proceedings of the 2007 Gastrointestinal Cancers Symposium. Alexandria, VA: American Society of Clinical Oncology.
61. Grothey A, Sargent D, Goldberg RM, et al. Survival of patients with advanced colorectal cancer improves with the availability of fluorouracil-leucovorin, irinotecan, and oxaliplatin in the course of treatment. J Clin Oncol 2004;22:1209-1214.
62. Maughan T, on Behalf of the NCRI Colorectal Group. Fluorouracil, oxaliplatin, CPT-11 (irinotecan), use and sequencing, in advanced colorectal cancer: the UK MRC FOCUS Trial [Abstract 165]. J Clin Oncol 2005;23(16 Suppl).
63. Falcone A, Masi G, Murr R, et al. Biweekly irinotecan, oxaliplatin, and infusional 5FU/LV (FOLFOXIRI) versus FOLFIRI as first-line treatment of metastatic colorectal cancer (MCRC): results of a randomized, Phase III trial by the GONO [Abstract 227]. *In* Proceedings of the 2007 Gastrointestinal Cancers Symposium. Alexandria, VA: American Society of Clinical Oncology.
64. Souglakos J, Androulakis N, Syrigos K, et al. FOLFOXIRI (folinic acid, 5-fluorouracil, oxaliplatin and irinotecan) vs. FOLFIRI (folinic acid, 5-fluorouracil and irinotecan) as first-line treatment in metastatic colorectal cancer (MCC): a multicentre randomised Phase III trial from the Hellenic Oncology Research Group (HORG). Br J Cancer 2006;94:798-805.
65. Maughan TS, Kerr J, Ledermann M, et al. Comparison of intermittent and continuous palliative chemotherapy for advanced colorectal cancer: a multicenter randomized trial. Lancet 2003;361:457-464.
66. de Gramont A, Cervantes A, Andre T, et al. OPTIMOX study: FOLFOX/LV5FU2 compared to FOLFOX 4 in patients with advanced colorectal cancer [Abstract 3525]. J Clin Oncol 2004;22(14 Suppl):251.
67. Maindrault-Goebel F, Lledo G, Chibaudel B, et al. OPTIMOX2, a large randomized Phase II study of maintenance therapy or chemotherapy-free intervals (CFI) after FOLFOX in patients with metastatic colorectal cancer (MRC). A GERCOR study [Abstract 3504]. J Clin Oncol 2006;24(18 Suppl).
68. Labianca R, Floriani I, Cortesi E, et al. Alternating versus continuous "FOLFIRI" in advanced colorectal cancer (ACC): a randomized "GISCAD" trial [Abstract 3505]. J Clin Oncol 2006;24(18 Suppl).
69. Hochester HS, Welles L, Hart L, et al. Safety and efficacy of bevacizumab when added to oxaliplatin/fluoropyrimidine regimens as first line treatment of metastatic colorectal cancer: TREE 1 & 2 study [Abstract 3515]. J Clin Oncol 2005;23(16 Suppl).
70. Giantonio BJ, Catalano G, Meropol NJ, et al. High-dose bevacizumab improves survival when combined with FOLFOX4 in previously treated advanced colorectal cancer: results from the Eastern Cooperative Oncology Group (ECOG) study E3200 [Abstract 2]. J Clin Oncol 2005;23(16 Suppl).

70a. Saltz L, Clarke S, Diaz-Rubio E, et al. Bevacizumab (Bev) in combination with XELOX or FOLFOX4: Updated efficacy results from XELOX-1/NO16966, a randomized phase III trial in first-line metastatic colorectal cancer. J Clin Oncol 2007;25:4028 [Abstract].

71. Chen HX, Mooney M, Boron M, et al. Bevacizumab (BV) plus 5-FU/leucovorin (FU/LV) for advanced colorectal cancer (CRC) that progressed after standard chemotherapies: an NCI Treatment Referral Center trial (TRC-0301) [Abstract 3515]. J Clin Oncol 2004;22:249a.
72. Skillings JR, Johnson DH, Miller K, et al. Arterial thromboembolic events (ATEs) in a pooled analysis of 5 randomized, controlled trials (RCTs) of bevacizumab (BV) with chemotherapy [Abstract 3019]. J Clin Oncol 2005;23(16 Suppl).
73. Saif MW. Incidence and management of bevacizumab-related toxicities in colorectal cancer. Expert Opin Drug Saf 2006;5:553-566.
74. Rougier P, Raoul JL, van Laethem J-L, et al. Cetuximab + FOLFIRI as first line treatment for metastatic colorectal CA [Abstract 3513]. J Clin Oncol 2004;22(14 Suppl).
75. Borner M, Mingrone W, Koeberle D, et al. The impact of cetuximab on the capecitabine plus oxaliplatin (XELOX) combination in first-line treatment of metastatic colorectal cancer: a randomized Phase II trial of the Swiss Group for Clinical Cancer Research (SAKK) [Abstract 3551]. J Clin Oncol 2006;24(18 Suppl).
76. Venook A, Niedzwiecki D, Hollis D, et al. Phase III study of irinotecan/5FU/LV (FOLFIRI) or oxaliplatin/5FU/LV (FOLFOX) ± cetuximab for patients (pts) with untreated metastatic adenocarcinoma of the colon or rectum (MCRC): CALGB 80203 preliminary results [Abstract 3509]. J Clin Oncol 2006;24(18 Suppl).
77. Dakhil S, Cosgriff T, Headley D, et al. Cetuximab + FOLFOX6 as first line therapy for metastatic colorectal cancer (an International Oncology Network study, I-03-002) [Abstract 3557]. J Clin Oncol 2006;24(18 Suppl).
78. Heinemann V, Fischer Von Weikersthal L, Moosmann N, et al. Cetuximab + capecitabine + irinotecan (CCI) versus cetuximab + capecitabine + oxaliplatin (CCO) as first line therapy for patients with metastatic colorectal cancer (CRC): Preliminary results of a randomized Phase II trial of the AIO CRC Study Group [Abstract 3550]. J Clin Oncol 2006;24(18 Suppl).
79. Cunningham D, Humblet Y, Siena S, et al. Cetuximab monotherapy and cetuximab plus irinotecan in irinotecan-refractory metastatic colorectal cancer. N Engl J Med 2004;351:337-345.
80. Saif MW, Cohenuram M. Role of panitumumab in the management of metastatic colorectal cancer. Clin Colorectal Cancer 2006;6:118-124.
81. Malik JR, Hecht A, Patnaik A, et al. Safety and efficacy of panitumumab monotherapy in patients with metastatic colorectal cancer [Abstract 3520]. J Clin Oncol 2005;23(16 Suppl).
82. Gibson TB, Ranganathan A, Grothey A, et al. Randomized Phase III trial results of panitumumab, a fully human anti-epidermal growth factor receptor monoclonal antibody, in metastatic colorectal cancer. Clin Colorectal Cancer 2006;6:29-31.
83. Berlin J, Malik I, Picus J. Panitumumab therapy with irinotecan, 5-fluorouracil, and leukovorin (IFL) in metastatic colorectal patients [Abstract 265PD]. Ann Oncol 2004;15(Suppl 3):70.
84. National Cancer Institute. PACCE: a randomized, open-label, controlled, clinical trial of chemotherapy and bevacizumab with and without panitumumab in the first-line treatment of subjects with metastatic colorectal cancer. Available at: *http://www.clinicaltrials.gov.ct/show/NCT00115765*

84a. Hecht JR, Mitchell E, Chidiac T, et al. An updated analysis of safety and efficacy of oxaliplatin (Ox)/bevacizumab (bev) +/− panitumumab (pmab) for first-line treatment (tx) of metastatic colorectal cancer (mCRC) from a randomized controlled trial (PACCC). 2008 ACOG Abstract 273.

85. Hecht JR, Trarbach T, Jaeger E, et al. A randomized, double-blind, placebo-controlled, phase III study in patients with metastatic adenocarcinoma of the colon or rectum receiving first-line chemotherapy with oxaliplatin/5-FU/LV, and PTK 787/ZK222584 or placebo (CONFIRM-1) [Abstract LBA3]. J Clin Oncol 2005;23(16 Suppl).
86. Saltz LB, Lenz H, Hochster H, et al. Randomized phase II trial of cetuximab/bevacizumab/irinotecan (CBI) versus cetuximab/bevacizumab (CB) in irinotecan-refractory colorectal cancer [Abstract 3508]. J Clin Oncol 2005;23(16 Suppl).

69

MELANOMA

Jasmine Nabi and Raymond J. Hohl

INTRODUCTION 969
THERAPEUTICS AND CLINICAL PHARMACOLOGY 969
Chemotherapy 969
Dacarbazine 969
Temozolomide 969
Platinum-Containing Compounds 969
Nitrosoureas 969
Vinca Alkaloids 969
Taxanes 969
Tamoxifen 970
Thalidomide 970
Combination Chemotherapy 970
Immunotherapy 970
Interferon 970
Interleukin-2 970
Granulocyte-Macrophage Colony-Stimulating Factor 970
Therapeutic Approach 971

INTRODUCTION

Malignant melanoma is a relatively common neoplasm. Approximately 90,000 new cases of melanoma are diagnosed annually in the United States.[1] Generally, the disease is thought to arise from the skin (Fig. 69-1). However, other sites of origin include mucosal surfaces, esophagus, meninges, and eye.[2]

Melanoma arises from a malignant transformation of the melanocyte, a cell of neural crest origin that produces melanin pigment. Exposure to sunlight increases the risk of melanoma. It is thought that the initial event in the disease process is DNA injury by ultraviolet radiation. People who are fair-skinned, with a tendency to sunburn, are most susceptible to melanoma.[3,4]

When diagnosed early, melanoma can be cured with a wide surgical excision. However, patients with advanced disease involving regional lymph nodes or distant metastasis generally have a poor prognosis. The median survival is only 6 months in patients with distant metastatic disease. Chemotherapy and biologic therapies have been used to treat locally advanced and disseminated melanoma.[5,6]

THERAPEUTICS AND CLINICAL PHARMACOLOGY

Chemotherapy

Dacarbazine

Dacarbazine or dimethyltriazenoimidazole carboxamide (DTIC) is the only cytotoxic drug approved by the U.S. Food and Drug Administration (FDA) for the treatment of metastatic melanoma, and has a response rate of about 20%.[5,7] The exact mechanism of action of dacarbazine is not known. Its major action is through alkylation. Dacarbazine is activated by liver microsomal enzymes to form 5-(3-monomethyl-1-triazenyl)-1H-imidazole-4-carboxamide (MTIC).[8] It inhibits DNA and RNA synthesis by forming carbonium ions.[9]

As dacarbazine does not cross the blood-brain barrier, cerebral metastases do not respond to this drug.[10] The major side effects associated with dacarbazine are nausea and vomiting. Modest bone marrow suppression is also noted with this agent. Additionally, photosensitivity reactions are seen in patients receiving moderate to high doses of DTIC. Finally, dacarbazine causes pain with infusion and is a known vesicant.[5,8]

Temozolomide

Temozolomide is an analogue of dacarbazine. At physiologic pH, temozolomide spontaneously transforms to MTIC.[5] Temozolomide has shown efficacy equal to DTIC in the treatment of metastatic melanoma.[11] Unlike dacarbazine, temozolomide is orally administered, which may be more convenient. Also, temozolomide crosses the blood-brain barrier, and it has been used to treat brain metastases from melanoma.[12] Toxicities associated with temozolomide include nausea, vomiting, and myelosuppression.[11]

Platinum-Containing Compounds

The platinum-containing compounds cisplatin and carboplatin have shown modest activity in patients with metastatic melanoma.[13,14] These agents inhibit DNA synthesis by cross-linking DNA molecules.[8,10] In the treatment of melanoma, cisplatin has been evaluated more extensively than carboplatin. As described later, cisplatin has been used in combination chemotherapy regimens for metastatic melanoma.

Cisplatin is associated with nephrotoxicity, neurotoxicity, ototoxicity, nausea, vomiting, and myelosuppression. Generally, carboplatin is thought to be better tolerated than cisplatin. Myelosuppression, specifically thrombocytopenia, can be more pronounced with carboplatin.[5,8] (For more information on platinum-containing compounds, see Chapter 64, Lung Cancer.)

Nitrosoureas

Nitrosoureas that have been used in melanoma treatment include carmustine (BCNU), lomustine (CCNU), semustine (methyl CCNU), and fotemustine (FTMU).[10,15] Carmustine (BCNU) is one of the agents used in the Dartmouth regimen as described later. Nitrosoureas are alkylating agents that form DNA cross-links to inhibit DNA replication.[16] All these agents are able to penetrate into the central nervous system.[10] However, fotemustine is very lipophilic and is most effective at crossing the blood-brain barrier.[5,10,17] Therefore, fotemustine has activity in metastatic melanoma to the brain.[18-20] Fotemustine is associated with neutropenia, thrombocytopenia, nausea, and vomiting.[5,21]

Vinca Alkaloids

Single-agent vinca alkaloids (vindesine and vinblastine) have shown response rates of about 10% to 15% in metastatic melanoma.[5,10] These agents have been utilized in combination chemotherapy regimens for melanoma. Vinca alkaloids bind to tubulin and prevent microtubule formation. As a result, the mitotic spindle apparatus is disrupted. This prevents chromosome separation and cell proliferation. Major toxicities linked with vinca alkaloids include peripheral neuropathy and myelosuppression.[5,8,10,16]

Taxanes

As single agents, the taxanes (paclitaxel and docetaxel) have demonstrated response rates of approximately 15% in metastatic

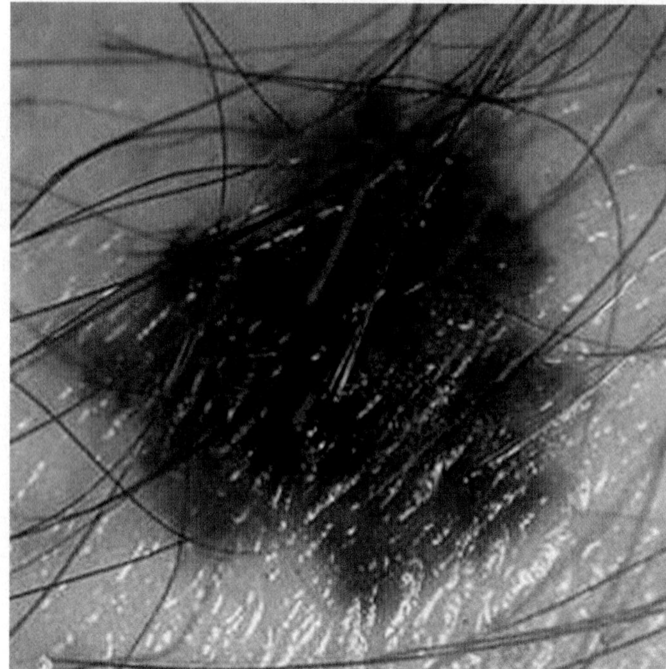

FIGURE 69-1 • Cutaneous melanoma.

melanoma.[22,23] These drugs have been used in combination with other agents in melanoma therapy. Taxanes bind to tubulin and stabilize microtubule formation. Dysfunctional microtubules ultimately inhibit cell proliferation.[16] (For further details regarding taxanes, see Chapter 64, Lung Cancer.)

Tamoxifen

It has been hypothesized that melanoma is estrogen dependent, given that melanoma cells expressed estrogen receptors. Therefore, tamoxifen (an antiestrogen agent) has been used in melanoma treatment.[5,24] However, several trials have been conducted and there is little support for the use of tamoxifen in this disease.[25-27] The National Cancer Institute of Canada conducted a double-blind, placebo-controlled trial comparing the Dartmouth regimen (see later) with and without tamoxifen. There was no statistically significant difference in overall response rates or survival.[27] (For more information on tamoxifen, see Chapter 65, Breast Cancer.)

Thalidomide

Thalidomide was initially introduced in Europe for the treatment of morning sickness. As limb defects were found in infants born to mothers who consumed thalidomide during pregnancy, the medication was withdrawn from the market in the 1960s.[28] Now it is thought that the limb deformities were likely secondary to inhibition of blood vessel growth in the developing fetal limb buds.[29] In addition to its antiangiogenic effects, thalidomide has immunomodulatory and anti-inflammatory properties.[28]

As a single agent, thalidomide has not shown efficacy in treating advanced melanoma.[30,31] However, a number of trials suggest that thalidomide may be active in melanoma when combined with temozolomide.[32-35] Thalidomide is most commonly associated with constipation, neuropathy, somnolence, fatigue, dry skin, and dry mouth.[30,31]

Combination Chemotherapy

Combination chemotherapy regimens have been used to treat metastatic melanoma. Two of the most commonly used polychemotherapy regimens include CVD (cisplatin, a vinca alkaloid, and DTIC) and CDBT (cisplatin, DTIC, BCNU, and tamoxifen).[5] It is important to recognize that neither the CVD regimen nor the CDBT regimen (Dartmouth regimen) has been shown to be superior to dacarbazine (DTIC) alone.[5,36]

Immunotherapy

The host immune system is able to generate a response to tumor cells. Cytokines are important regulatory proteins in the function of the immune system. Cytokines that have been used in the treatment of melanoma include interferon, interleukin-2 (IL-2), and granulocyte-macrophage colony-stimulating factor (GM-CSF).[6]

Interferon

Interferons were first described in 1957 by Isaacs and Lindenmann,[37] and were named as such due to their ability to "interfere" with viral replication in the infected cells.[10] In the 1960s, interferons were shown to have antitumor activity in laboratory models.[38] Initially, the interferons were classified according to their biochemical properties (interferon-α, interferon-β, and interferon-γ). Later, it was discovered that interferon-α was produced primarily by leukocytes, interferon-β by fibroblasts, and interferon-γ by immune cells.[10,39,40]

Interferon-α has been used most extensively in the clinical trial work for melanoma. Recombinant IFN alfa is produced by two pharmaceutical companies. Interferon alfa2a (Roferon A; Roche Laboratories, Nutley, NJ) and interferon alfa2b (Intron-A; Schering-Plough, Kenilworth, NJ) are both produced by recombinant DNA technology. Interferon alfa2a and interferon alfa2b have molecular sequences that differ from one another by a single amino acid at position 23.[39,41]

The exact mechanism by which interferons work is unclear. It is thought that interferon alfa has direct antiproliferative effects on tumor cells. Interferon has indirect immune-mediated effects by stimulating T cells and natural killer cells.[39,41] Also, interferons enhance major histocompatibility complex expression, which may make malignant cells more antigenic.[38] Furthermore, interferon may have antiangiogenic effects.[41]

The clinical trials using interferon in melanoma treatment have evaluated low-dose interferon and high-dose interferon. Although low-dose interferon may be better tolerated, it has not shown an improvement in overall survival following surgical resection of the primary disease.[10,42,43] In contrast, high-dose interferon alfa has shown prolongation of overall survival in high-risk patients with melanoma.[10,44] As a result, the FDA approved interferon alfa for the adjuvant treatment of patients with high-risk disease.[10]

With regard to toxicity, an influenza-like syndrome with fevers, rigors, headache, and myalgia is common with interferon. Other notable side effects include fatigue, depression, anorexia, neutropenia, and liver function abnormalities. Most toxicity is rapidly reversible with dose reduction or cessation of the drug.[39,45,46] Also, interferon alfa inhibits the activity of specific cytochrome P-450 isoenzymes, and this correlates with certain toxicities.[45]

Interleukin-2

IL-2 is an immunostimulatory cytokine that has been produced using recombinant technology. This agent does not have direct cytotoxic or cytostatic effects on melanoma cells.[7] Instead, IL-2 induces cytotoxic T lymphocytes, natural killer cells, and lymphokine-activated killer cells.[47,48] Additionally, IL-2 stimulates the secretion of other cytokines that may have antitumor activity.[47]

Common toxicities associated with IL-2 include nausea, vomiting, diarrhea, and malaise.[49] However, the dose-limiting toxicity with IL-2 is capillary leak syndrome. Capillary leak syndrome can lead to pulmonary edema, kidney failure, cardiac dysfunction, and hypotension.[5] Additionally, increased capillary permeability can lead to fluid extravasation into soft tissues and weight gain.[49] The significant toxicities linked with high-dose IL-2 have limited its use in treating melanoma.[24]

Granulocyte-Macrophage Colony-Stimulating Factor

GM-CSF is a cytokine with multiple actions. This factor is thought to stimulate the proliferation and maturation of antigen-presenting cells, known as dendritic cells.[50] Also, GM-CSF may stimulate monocytes to become cytotoxic.[51] Side effects associated with GM-CSF include myalagias, fatigue, and rash.[51]

Therapeutic Approach

Early-stage cutaneous melanoma can be cured with surgical resection. Although a number of agents have been used in the treatment of advanced or metastatic melanoma, the disease has a median survival between 2 and 8 months.[52] Both chemotherapy and biologic therapies, in combination and as single agents, have been used in melanoma treatment. Unfortunately, none of these approaches has made a major impact on overall survival.[52] Continued research is needed to find more effective therapeutic options.

REFERENCES

1. Wagner RF, Casciato DA. Skin cancers. *In* Casciato DA (ed): Manual of Clinical Oncology. Philadelphia: Lippincott Williams & Wilkins, 2004, pp 355-367.
2. Murphy GF. The skin. *In* Kumar V, Cotran RS, Robbins SL (eds): Basic Pathology. Philadelphia: WB Saunders, 1997, pp 711-712.
3. Lange JR, et al. Melanoma. *In* Abeloff MD, et al (eds): Clinical Oncology. Elsevier Philadelphia: Churchill Livingstone, 2004, pp 1561-1583.
4. Urist MM, Miller DM, Maddox WA. Malignant melanoma. *In* Murphy GP, Lawrence JW, Lenhard RE (eds): American Cancer Society Textbook of Clinical Oncology. Atlanta: American Cancer Society, 1995, pp 304-309.
5. Bajetta E, Del Vecchio M, Bernard-Marty C, et al. Metastatic melanoma: chemotherapy. Semin Oncol 2002;29:427-445.
6. Kim CJ, Dessureault S, Gabrilovich D, et al. Immunotherapy for melanoma. Cancer Control 2002;9:22-30.
7. Flaherty LE, Gadgeel SM. Biochemotherapy of melanoma. Semin Oncol 2002;29:446-455.
8. Perry MC (ed). The Chemotherapy Source Book, 3rd ed. Philadelphia: Lippincott Williams & Wilkins, 2001.
9. USP DI, Vol 1: Drug Information for the Health Care Professsional. Philadelphia: Thompson Scientific, 2006.
10. Brown CK, Kirkwood JM. Medical management of melanoma. Surg Clin North Am 2003;83:283-322, viii.
11. Middleton MR, Grob JJ, Aaronson N, et al. Randomized Phase III study of temozolomide versus dacarbazine in the treatment of patients with advanced metastatic malignant melanoma. J Clin Oncol 2000;18:158-166.
12. Agarwala SS, Kirkwood JM, Gore M, et al. Temozolomide for the treatment of brain metastases associated with metastatic melanoma: a Phase II study. J Clin Oncol 2004;22:2101-2107.
13. Al-Sarraf M, Fletcher W, Oishi N, et al. Cisplatin hydration with and without mannitol diuresis in refractory disseminated malignant melanoma: a Southwest Oncology Group study. Cancer Treat Rep 1982;66:31-35.
14. Chang A, Hunt M, Parkinson DR, et al. Phase II trial of carboplatin in patients with metastatic malignant melanoma: a report from the Eastern Cooperative Oncology Group. Am J Clin Oncol 1993;16:152-155.
15. Ahmann DL. Nitrosoureas in the management of disseminated malignant melanoma. Cancer Treat Rep 1976;60:747-751.
16. Mycek MJ, Harvey RA, Champe PC (eds). Lippincott's Illustrated Reviews: Pharmacology, 2nd ed. Philadelphia: Lippincott–Raven, 1997.
17. Li Y, McClay EF. Systemic chemotherapy for the treatment of metastatic melanoma. Semin Oncol 2002;29:413-426.
18. Douglas JG, Margolin K. The treatment of brain metastases from malignant melanoma. Semin Oncol 2002;29:518-524.
19. Falkson CI, Falkson G, Falkson HC. Phase II trial of fotemustine in patients with metastatic malignant melanoma. Invest New Drugs 1994;12:251-254.
20. Jacquillat C, Khayat D, Banzet P, et al. Final report of the French multicenter Phase II study of the nitrosourea fotemustine in 153 evaluable patients with disseminated malignant melanoma including patients with cerebral metastases. Cancer 1990;66:1873-1878.
21. Avril MF, Aamdal S, Grob JJ, et al. Fotemustine compared with dacarbazine in patients with disseminated malignant melanoma: a Phase III study. J Clin Oncol 2004;22:1118-1125.
22. Bedikian AY, Weiss GR, Legha SS, et al. Phase II trial of docetaxel in patients with advanced cutaneous malignant melanoma previously untreated with chemotherapy. J Clin Oncol 1995;13:2895-2899.
23. Einzig AI, Hochster H, Wiernik PH, et al. A Phase II study of taxol in patients with malignant melanoma. Invest New Drugs 1991;9:59-64.
24. O'Day SJ, Kim CJ, Reintgen DS. Metastatic melanoma: chemotherapy to biochemotherapy. Cancer Control 2002;9:31-38.
25. Creagan ET, Suman VJ, Dalton RJ, et al. Phase III clinical trial of the combination of cisplatin, dacarbazine, and carmustine with or without tamoxifen in patients with advanced malignant melanoma. J Clin Oncol 1999;17:1884-1890.
26. Falkson CI, Ibrahim J, Kirkwood JM, et al. Phase III trial of dacarbazine versus dacarbazine with interferon alpha-2b versus dacarbazine with tamoxifen versus dacarbazine with interferon alpha-2b and tamoxifen in patients with metastatic malignant melanoma: an Eastern Cooperative Oncology Group study. J Clin Oncol 1998;16:1743-1751.
27. Rusthoven JJ, Quirt IC, Iscoe NA, et al. Randomized, double-blind, placebo-controlled trial comparing the response rates of carmustine, dacarbazine, and cisplatin with and without tamoxifen in patients with metastatic melanoma. National Cancer Institute of Canada Clinical Trials Group. J Clin Oncol 1996;14:2083-2090.
28. Eleutherakis-Papaiakovou V, Bamias A, Dimopoulos MA. Thalidomide in cancer medicine. Ann Oncol 2004;15:1151-1160.
29. D'Amato RJ, Loughnan MS, Flynn E, Folkman J. Thalidomide is an inhibitor of angiogenesis. Proc Natl Acad Sci U S A 1994;91:4082-4085.
30. Pawlak WZ, Legha SS. Phase II study of thalidomide in patients with metastatic melanoma. Melanoma Res 2004;14:57-62.
31. Reiriz AB, Richter MF, Fernandes S, et al. Phase II study of thalidomide in patients with metastatic malignant melanoma. Melanoma Res 2004;14:527-531.
32. Hwu WJ, Krown SE, Menell JH, et al. Phase II study of temozolomide plus thalidomide for the treatment of metastatic melanoma. J Clin Oncol 2003;21:3351-3356.
33. Hwu WJ, Lis E, Menell JH, et al. Temozolomide plus thalidomide in patients with brain metastases from melanoma: a Phase II study. Cancer 2005;103:2590-2597.
34. Krown SE, Niedzwiecki D, Hwu WJ, et al. Phase II study of temozolomide and thalidomide in patients with metastatic melanoma in the brain: high rate of thromboembolic events (CALGB 500102). Cancer 2006;107:1883-1890.
35. Laber DA, Okeke RI, Arce-Lara C, et al. A Phase II study of extended dose temozolomide and thalidomide in previously treated patients with metastatic melanoma. J Cancer Res Clin Oncol 2006;132:611-616.
36. Chapman PB, Einhorn LH, Meyers ML, et al. Phase III multicenter randomized trial of the Dartmouth regimen versus dacarbazine in patients with metastatic melanoma. J Clin Oncol 1999;17:2745-2751.
37. Isaacs A, Lindenmann J. Virus interference: I. The interferon. Proc R Soc Lond 1957;147:258-267.
38. Gray RJ, Pockaj BA, Kirkwood JM. An update on adjuvant interferon for melanoma. Cancer Control 2002;9:16-21.
39. Kefford RF. Adjuvant therapy of cutaneous melanoma: the interferon debate. Ann Oncol 2003;14:358-365.
40. Pfeffer LM, Dinarello CA, Herberman RB, et al. Biological properties of recombinant alpha-interferons: 40th anniversary of the discovery of interferons. Cancer Res 1998;58:2489-2499.
41. Jonasch E, Haluska FG. Interferon in oncological practice: review of interferon biology, clinical applications, and toxicities. Oncologist 2001;6:34-55.
42. Cameron DA, Cornbleet MC, Mackie J, et al. for the Scottish Melanoma Group. Adjuvant interferon alpha 2b in high risk melanoma—the Scottish study. Br J Cancer 2001;84:1146-1149.
43. Grob JJ, Dreno B, de la Salmonière P, et al. Randomised trial of interferon alpha-2a as adjuvant therapy in resected primary melanoma thicker than 1.5 mm without clinically detectable node metastases. French Cooperative Group on Melanoma. Lancet 1998;351:1905-1910.
44. Kirkwood JM, Strawderman MH, Ernstoff MS, et al. Interferon alfa-2b adjuvant therapy of high-risk resected cutaneous melanoma: the Eastern Cooperative Oncology Group Trial EST 1684. J Clin Oncol 1996;14:7-17.
45. Kirkwood JM, Bender C, Agarwala S, et al. Mechanisms and management of toxicities associated with high-dose interferon alfa-2b therapy. J Clin Oncol 2002;20:3703-3718.
46. Weiss K. Safety profile of interferon-alpha therapy. Semin Oncol 1998;25(1 Suppl 1): 9-13.
47. Keilholz U, Gore ME. Biochemotherapy for advanced melanoma. Semin Oncol 2002;29:456-461.
48. Philip PA, Flaherty L. Treatment of malignant melanoma with interleukin-2. Semin Oncol 1997;24(1 Suppl 4): S32-S38.
49. Rosenberg SA, Lotze MT, Yang JC, et al. Experience with the use of high-dose interleukin-2 in the treatment of 652 cancer patients. Ann Surg 1989;210:474-484; discussion 484-485.
50. McClay EF. Adjuvant therapy for patients with high-risk malignant melanoma. Semin Oncol 2002;29:389-399.
51. Spitler LE, Grossbard ML, Ernstoff MS, et al. Adjuvant therapy of stage III and IV malignant melanoma using granulocyte-macrophage colony-stimulating factor. J Clin Oncol 2000;18:1614-1621.
52. Khayat D, Bernard-Marty C, Meric JB, Rixe O. Biochemotherapy for advanced melanoma: maybe it is real. J Clin Oncol 2002;20:2411-2414.

70

ACNE

Joseph Genebriera and Mark Davis

INTRODUCTION 973
PATHOPHYSIOLOGY 973
THERAPEUTICS AND CLINICAL PHARMACOLOGY 974
Therapeutics by Class 974
Topical Treatments 974
Oral Treatments 977
Therapeutic Approaches 978
Emerging Targets and Therapeutics 979
Laser Treatment 979
Topical Treatments 980
Nutrition 980

INTRODUCTION

Acne (From the Greek *akne,* or eruption of the face) is a disorder of the skin caused by inflammation of the skin glands and hair follicles. It is the most common skin disease worldwide, being especially common in teenagers and young adults (Figs. 70-1 and 70-2). It can, however, also affect infants and adults at any age. This chapter reviews the pathophysiology, topical and oral treatments, therapeutic approaches, and emerging therapeutics for acne.

The pathogenesis of acne vulgaris is multifactorial. The major pathogenic factors involved are obstruction of sebaceous follicles resulting from abnormal keratinization of the infundibular epithelium, stimulation of sebaceous gland secretion by androgens, and microbial colonization of pilosebaceous units. Acne vulgaris, a disease of pilosebaceous follicles, is an extremely common clinical problem. In westernized societies, acne vulgaris is a nearly universal skin disease, affecting 79% to 95% of the adolescent population. Though it is more prevalent among men than women at age 18, beyond the age of 23 clinical acne is more prevalent among women as the prevalence in men gradually declines. At 40 to 49 years, 3% of men and 5% of women still have definite, mild, clinical acne, and at 50 to 59 years, 6% of men and 8% of women have physiologic acne.[1,2] Epidemiologic evidence suggests that acne incidence rates are considerably lower in nonwesternized societies; the reason for this is not understood.[3,4]

There is a wide range of treatment options depending on skin type and acne severity. The preferred treatment for comedogenic acne is a topical retinoid. Acne with papulopustules is treated with a dual therapy of topical retinoids and benzoyl peroxide plus a topical antibiotic, which has shown the highest efficacy. In more severe or refractory cases an oral antibiotic can be added, and in cystic acne an oral isotretinoin is the treatment of choice in most patients. Antiandrogens and oral contraceptives can also be treatment options in certain patients. In the United States, the process of ensuring that pregnancy is avoided has been mandated by the federal government via the iPLEDGE program. The program strives to ensure that no female patient starts isotretinoin therapy if pregnant, and no female patient on isotretinoin therapy becomes pregnant.

Nutrition is also an important aspect in acne treatment as certain vitamins, minerals, and supplements can be taken in combination with the standard treatment to help clear up acne faster. Brewer's yeast, zinc, essential fatty acids, and vitamins A and B have been shown to reduce the severity of acne. Avoidance of chocolate, fats, sweets, and carbonated beverages was commonly recommended as part of the treatment for acne. However, these dietary restrictions are no longer part of standard medical treatment, as little evidence has been found to link the consumption of these foods to the incidence of acne.[5,6]

Certain drugs have also been noted to cause or exacerbate acne, including lithium, hydantoin, topical and systemic glucocorticoids, oral contraceptives, and androgens. Occlusion and pressure can exacerbate acne. Acne mechanica is a form of acne caused by heat, pressure, occlusion of the skin, and repetitive frictional rubbing against the skin. It is very common in people playing certain sports, such as hockey and soccer, or in people wearing tight uniforms.

Photodynamic therapy with blue (415 nm) and red light (633 nm) has shown to be effective as a coadjuvant in mild to moderate acne treatment. Other treatment options, such as dapsone 5% gel, are under investigation.

PATHOPHYSIOLOGY

The pathogenesis of acne vulgaris is multifactorial. The major pathogenic factors involved are hyperkeratinization, obstruction of sebaceous follicles resulting from abnormal keratinization of the infundibular epithelium, stimulation of sebaceous gland secretion by androgens, and microbial colonization of pilosebaceous units by *Propionibacterium acnes*, which promotes perifollicular inflammation.

There are several hypotheses that could explain why individuals with acne have an increased follicular epidermal hyperproliferation and hyperkeratinization. Androgens have been implicated in the pathogenesis of acne. Androgen levels in patients with acne are higher than those in controls, and people with the androgen insensitivity syndrome do not develop acne. The skin contains enzymes that convert precursor hormones to the more potent androgens such as testosterone and dihydrotestosterone. Androgen synthesis can therefore be regulated locally. The effects of androgens on the skin are the result of circulating androgens and enzyme activity in local tissues and androgen receptors.[7]

Sebum is produced by sebaceous glands (Fig. 70-3). Sebaceous glands on the mid-back, forehead, and chin are larger and more numerous than elsewhere. Sebum is produced when the sebaceous gland disintegrates. The cells take about a week from formation to discharge. Triglycerides produced by sebaceous glands are broken down by bacterial enzymes (lipases) in the sebaceous duct to form free fatty acids. Sebum production is under the control of androgens.[8,9] The most active androgens are testosterone, dihydrotestosterone, and 5-androstene-3,17-diol. Androgens stimulate the sebaceous glands to produce larger amounts of sebum. The increased activity of sebaceous glands elicited by androgen causes proliferation of *P. acnes*, an anaerobe present within the retained sebum in the pilosebaceous ducts. The organism possesses a ribosome-rich cytoplasm and a relatively thick cell wall, and produces several biologically active mediators that may contribute to inflammation, for instance, by promoting leukocyte

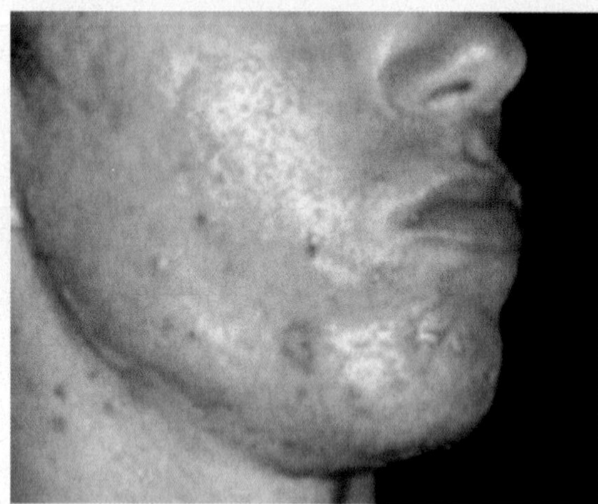

FIGURE 70-1 • Acne of an older teenager.

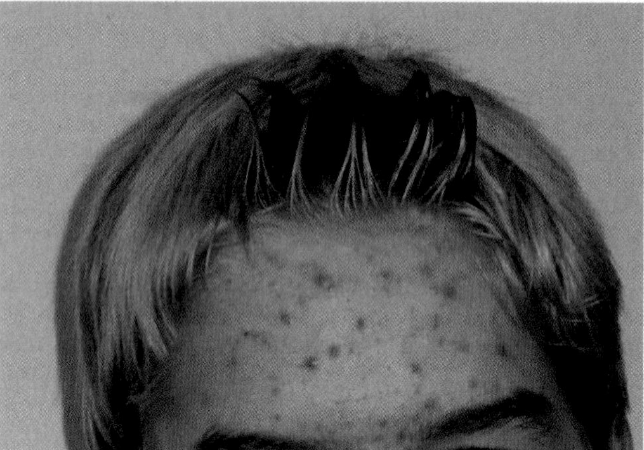

FIGURE 70-2 • Acne of a 14-year-old boy during puberty.

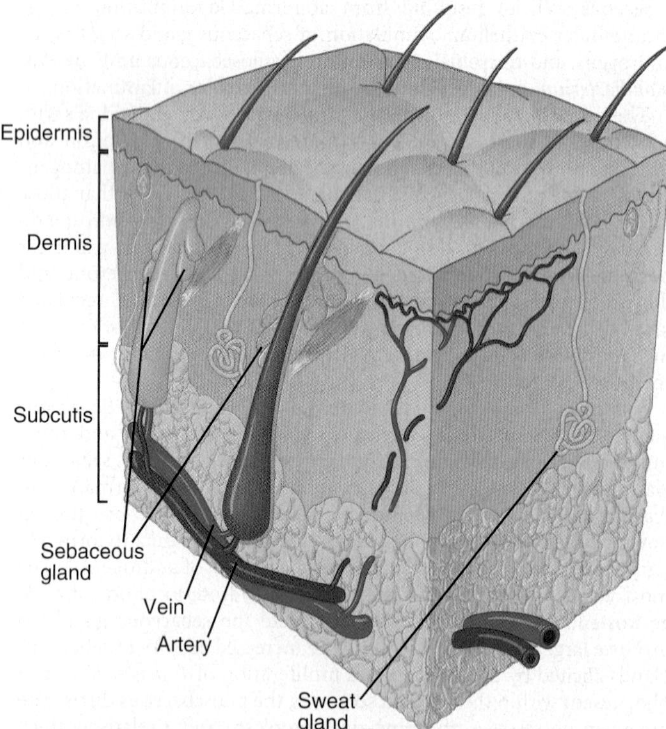

FIGURE 70-3 • Skin layers (epidermis, dermis, and subcutis), showing a hair follicle, sweat gland, and sebaceous gland.

migration and follicular rupture.[10] *Propionibacterium acnes* contains lipases that convert lipids into fatty acids, which promotes perifollicular inflammation. *Propionibacterium acnes* activates the toll-like receptor 2 on monocytes and neutrophils. Activation of the toll-like receptor 2 then leads to the production of multiple proinflammatory cytokines, including interleukins 12 and 8, and tumor necrosis factor.

Sebum and fatty acids cause an inflammatory response in the pilosebaceous unit that results in hyperkeratinization of the lining of the follicle with resultant plugging. The enlarged follicular lumen contains keratin and lipid debris forming the whitehead. When the follicle has a portal of entry at the skin, the semisolid mass protrudes, forming a plug (the blackhead). These lesions are called comedones, and they are usually 1 to 3 mm in diameter.

Papules and pustules are red lesions 2 to 5 mm in diameter. The follicular epithelium becomes damaged with accumulation of neutrophils and then lymphocytes. When the epithelium ruptures, the comedone contents elicit an intense inflammatory reaction in the dermis. Pustules are more superficial than papules. Nodules are larger, deeper, and more solid than papules. Cysts are suppurative nodules. Occasionally, cysts become infected and form abscesses. Long-term cystic acne can cause scarring that manifests as deep pits ("icepick scars") or areas of hypertrophic scar. Acne conglobata is a severe form of acne, found particularly in males, with comedones, papules, pustules, nodules, cysts, and draining sinuses. Scarring and keloid formation are frequent sequelae.

THERAPEUTICS AND CLINICAL PHARMACOLOGY

Therapeutics by Class

Topical Treatments (Table 70-1)

Topical Retinoids. Topical retinoids are comedolytic and anti-inflammatory. The retinoids are a class of chemical compounds that are related chemically to vitamin A (Fig. 70-4). There are three generations of retinoids:

First-generation retinoids, including retinol, tretinoin (Retin-A), isotretinoin, and alitretinoin

Second-generation retinoids, including etritinate and its metabolite acitretin

Third-generation retinoids, including tazarotene (Tazorac) and bexarotene

First- and second-generation retinoids are able to bind with several retinoid receptors due to the flexibility imparted by their alternating single and double bonds. Third-generation retinoids are less flexible than first- and second-generation retinoids and therefore interact with fewer retinoid receptors.

Retinoids act by normalizing the follicle cell life cycle, and appear to influence cell creation and death of cells in the follicle lining. This helps prevent the hyperkeratinization of these cells that can create a blockage.

It is preferable not to use them in topical form for pregnant women, although a pregnancy test is only compulsory for tazarotene.

Tretinoin (Retin-A). Tretinoin is the acid form of vitamin A and also known as all-*trans* retinoic acid (Fig. 70-5). It was the first retinoid developed for the topical treatment of acne. It has also been used for other dermatologic conditions such as keratosis pilaris, and to decrease wrinkle formation.

Although the exact mode of action of tretinoin is unknown, current evidence suggests that topical tretinoin decreases cohesiveness of follicular epithelial cells with decreased blackhead formation. Additionally, tretinoin stimulates mitotic activity and increased turnover of follicular epithelial cells, causing extrusion of the blackheads (comedones).

When used, dryness of the affected skin may occur. More sensitive patients may also experience redness, scaling, itching, and burning. It is best to gradually increase the frequency and amount of tretinoin application to allow the patient's skin to adjust. This product increases the risk of extreme sunburn. Application of sunscreens while using

TABLE 70-1 TOPICAL TREATMENT

Agent	Brand Name	Common Formulations	Dosage	Side Effects
RETINOIDS				
Tretinoin	Retin-A, Retin-A micro, Avita, Renova	0.025%, 0.05%, 0.1% gel and cream	Apply small amount once daily before bedtime.	Skin irritation, photosensitivity, initially may worsen acne
Isotretinoin	Isotrex, Isotrexin	0.05% gel	Apply small amount once daily before bedtime.	Skin irritation, photosensitivity, initially may worsen acne
Adapalene	Differin	0.1% gel and solution	Apply small amount once daily before bedtime.	Skin irritation, photosensitivity, initially may worsen acne
Tazarotene	Tazorac	0.05%, 0.1% gel and cream	Apply small amount once daily before bedtime.	Skin irritation, photosensitivity, initially may worsen acne
ANTIBIOTICS				
Clindamycin	Cleocin T, Clinda-Derm, Evoclin	1% foam, gel, solution, suspension	Apply once or twice daily.	Skin dryness, pseudomembranous colitis (extremely rare)
Erythromycin	Akne-Mycin, Emgel, Erycette, EryDerm, Erygel, Erymax, Ery-Sol, Erythra-Derm, Staticin, Theramycin Z, T-Stat	1.5%, 2% gel, ointment, solution	Apply once or twice daily.	Skin dryness
Azelaic acid	Azelex	20% cream	Apply once or twice daily.	May cause skin dryness, hypopigmentation
Benzoyl peroxide	Benzac AC, Benzac W, Desquam-X, Desquam-E, Clerasil, Benoxyl, Benzagel, BenzaShave, Brevoxyl, Clean & Clear, Clearplex, Del-Aqua-Gel, Fostex, Loroxide, Noxzema, Oxy Balance, PanOxyl, Triaz	2.5%, 5%, 10% lotion, gel, cream, facial mask, and cleansing bar	Apply once or twice daily.	Drying of skin, contact dermatitis (1%-2% of users) Can bleach clothing and bedding
Benzoyl peroxide/ erythromycin	Benzamycin	5% Benzoyl peroxide/3% erythromycin gel	Apply once or twice daily.	May cause skin irritation, needs refrigeration
Benzoyl peroxide/ clindamycin	Benzaclin, Duac	5% Benzoyl peroxide/1% clindamycin gel	Apply once or twice daily.	May cause skin irritation, needs refrigeration
Salicylic acid	Clearasil, Noxzema, Oxy Clean, Propa PH, Stri-Dex	2% gel, cream, lotion, ointment, pads, shampoo, and soap	Apply once or twice daily.	May cause irritation and dryness
Sodium sulfacetamide	Sulface-Rt, Novacet	10% sulfacetamide/5% sulfur lotion	Apply once or twice daily.	

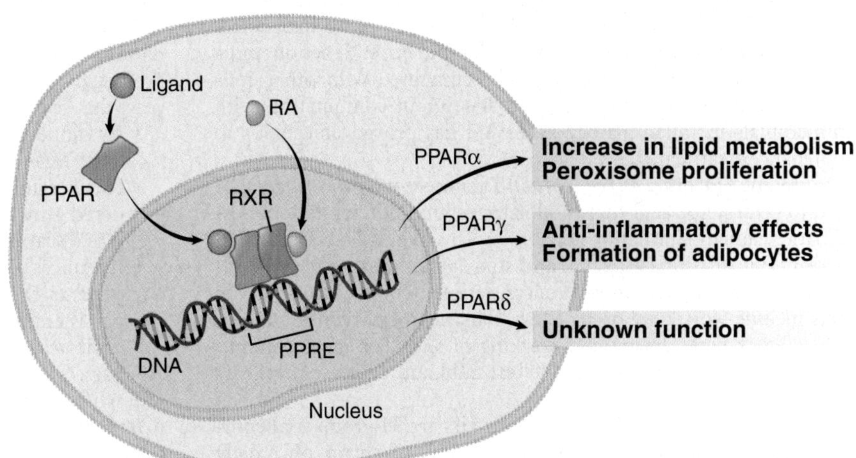

FIGURE 70-4 • Retinoids are derivatives of vitamin A and bind to nuclear retinoic acid receptors (RARs) and retinoid X receptors (RXRs) to directly modulate gene expression. Three isoforms of RARs and three isoforms of RXRs have so far been identified. The peroxisome proliferator activated receptors (PPARs) are also ligand-activated transcription factors, and heterodimerize with RXR isoforms to regulate gene expression. The exact mechanism of action is unknown; however, retinoids work by altering DNA transcription.

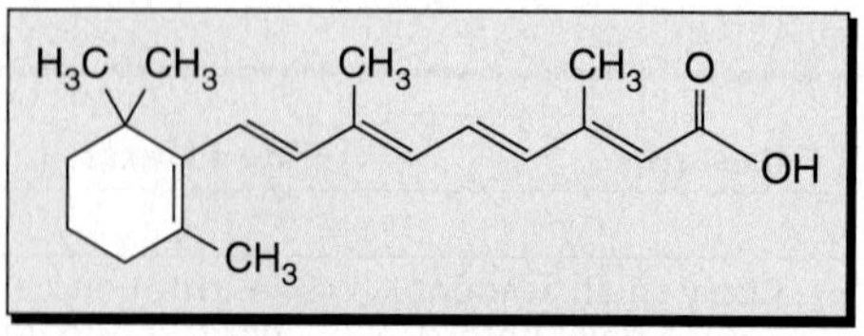

FIGURE 70-5 • Tretinoin.

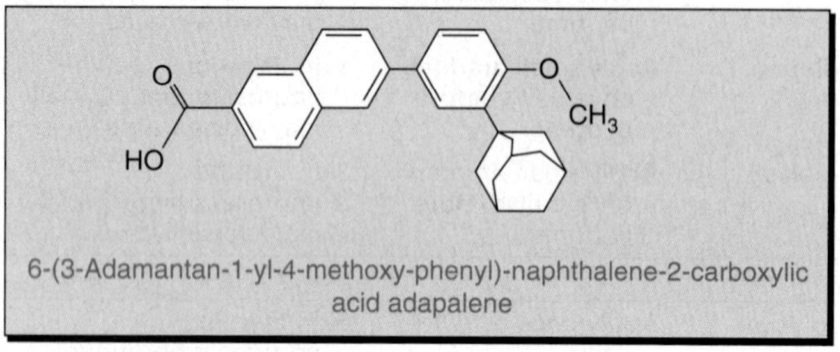

6-(3-Adamantan-1-yl-4-methoxy-phenyl)-naphthalene-2-carboxylic acid adapalene

FIGURE 70-6 • Adapalene.

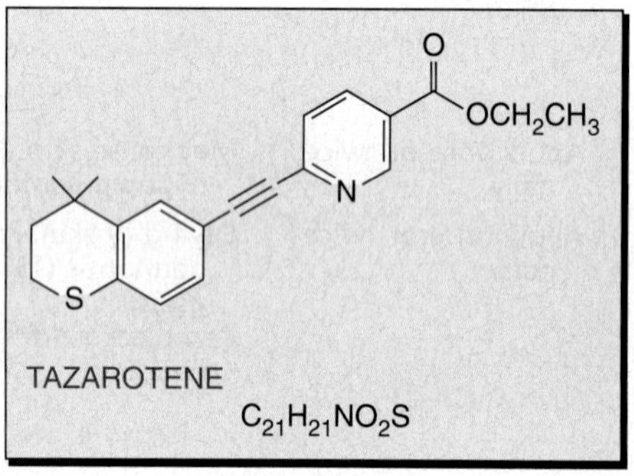

TAZAROTENE $C_{21}H_{21}NO_2S$

FIGURE 70-7 • Tazarotene.

tretinoin is strongly recommended. If sunscreen is not applied, there is minimal evidence of an increase in incidence of skin cancer.

Adapalene (Differin). Adapalene in small concentrations is a moderator of cellular differentiation, keratinization, and inflammatory processes. The exact mode of action of adapalene is unknown. Adapalene, a derivative of naphthoic acid, has comedolytic, antiproliferative, and anti-inflammatory properties (Fig. 70-6). Although adapalene is currently only available in a 0.1% formulation, Phase III clinical trials have shown that a 0.3% formulation is significantly more effective.[11]

In clinical trials, 0.1% adapalene gel has proved to be effective for the treatment of acne and was as effective as 0.025% tretinoin gel, 0.1% tretinoin microsphere gel, 0.05% tretinoin cream, and 0.1% tazarotene gel once every 2 days; however, the drug was less effective than once-daily 0.1% tazarotene gel. Adapalene has a rapid onset of action and a particularly favorable tolerability profile compared with other retinoids.[12] It can be used alone in mild acne or in combination with antimicrobials in inflammatory acne, and has proved efficacious as maintenance treatment.

Tazarotene (Tazorac, Avage, Zorac). Tazarotene is a prodrug metabolized to tazarotenic acid that modulates cellular differentiation, desquamation, and inflammation (Fig. 70-7). This medication is approved for treatment of psoriasis, acne, and sun-damaged skin (photodamage). It is commonly sold in two concentrations: 0.05% and 0.1%. Side effects include worsening of acne, dry skin, itchiness, redness, and in some cases extreme drying and cracking of skin. For most patients, these side effects are uncomfortable but mild and decrease markedly after the first 2 to 4 weeks of use.

A multicenter, double-blind, randomized, parallel-group trial compared tazarotene 0.1% cream with adapalene 0.1% cream, once daily for 12 weeks, in 173 patients with facial acne vulgaris. Tazarotene was associated with a significantly greater incidence of patients achieving 50% or greater global improvement (77% vs. 55%), and a significantly greater reduction in comedo count (median of 68% vs. 36%), compared with adapalene. The most common adverse events were dryness, peeling/flaking, itching, redness/erythema, burning, and facial irritation, with comparable incidences of each between groups. Mean peeling and burning levels were milder with adapalene, though they were trace or less in both groups throughout the study.[13]

Topical Antibiotics

Clindamycin and Erythromycin. Antibiotics have two main effects in acne: reduction of the number of bacteria on the skin surface and follicles, and anti-inflammatory action. The most commonly used topical antibiotics are clindamycin and erythromycin. Common side effects are as follows:

- Dryness of the treated area can be expected and is usually mild.
- Skin irritation is rarely severe. Occasionally, irritation results in discontinuation of the product. Lotions are less likely than solutions or gels to cause irritation.
- Contact dermatitis (red, dry, itchy skin) can be due to irritancy or allergy.
- Bacterial resistance most frequently arises with intermittent use of topical antibiotics. To reduce this, topical antibiotics should be applied liberally twice daily and ideally combined with benzoyl peroxide and/or a topical retinoid.

Clindamycin is a semisynthetic antibiotic derived from lincomycin; it has a bacteriostatic effect. Clindamycin interferes with bacterial protein synthesis in a way similar to erythromycin. It works by reducing *P. acnes* and decreasing inflammation. In topical form, clindamycin has proven safe and is well tolerated. Skin dryness and irritation are possible side effects.

Erythromycin is a macrolide antibiotic that has an antimicrobial spectrum similar to or slightly wider than that of penicillin. It prevents bacteria from growing by interfering with their protein synthesis. Erythromycin binds to the 23s ribosomal RNA molecule in the 50S portion of the bacterial ribosome, blocking the exit of the growing peptide chain and thus inhibiting the translocation of peptide.

Combined agents such as erythromycin/zinc, erythromycin/tretinoin, erythromycin/isotretinoin, erythromycin/benzoyl peroxide, and clindamycin/benzoyl peroxide are increasingly being used and have been proven to be effective. They generally demonstrate good overall tolerability and are useful in reducing the development of antibacterial resistance in *P. acnes.*

One hundred two patients with mild to moderate facial acne vulgaris completed a 12-week, investigator-masked, randomized, parallel-group comparison of a gel formation of erythromycin (2%) with clindamycin phosphate 1% solution. Both medications significantly reduced the numbers of papules and open and closed comedones. No significant differences in lesion count reductions were detected between the treatment groups after 8 and 12 weeks of treatment. By the end of 12 weeks, 48% of the patients in the erythromycin group and 47% in the clindamycin group had good or excellent responses to treatment.[14]

Azelaic Acid. Azelaic acid is a saturated dicarboxylic acid found naturally in wheat, rye, and barley. It is a natural substance that is produced by *Malassezia furfur* (also known as *Pityrosporum ovale*), a yeast that lives on normal skin. Azelaic acid has several properties:

- It is antibacterial; it reduces the growth of bacteria such as *P. acnes* and *Staphylococcus epidermidis* in the follicle.
- It is keratolytic and comedolytic; it returns to normal the disordered growth of the skin cells lining the follicle.
- It is a scavenger of free radicals and reduces inflammation.
- It reduces pigmentation; it is particularly useful for darker skinned patients, those who have melasma, or those whose acne spots leave persistent hyperpigmented brown macules.

Azelaic acid is well tolerated by most people and can be safely used for years. Side effects may include skin dryness and lightening of the skin where applied. It is normally used in a concentration of 20%.

Benzoyl Peroxide. Benzoyl peroxide is a chemical in the organic peroxide family. It consists of two benzoyl groups (benzaldehyde with the hydrogen of CHO removed) joined by a peroxide group (Fig. 70-8).

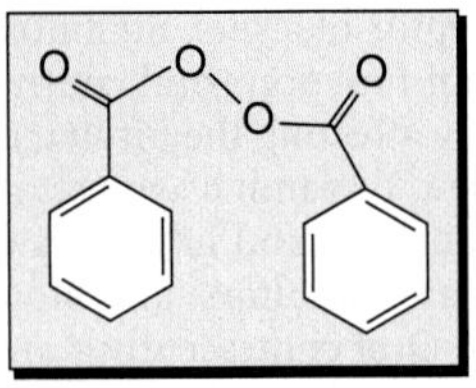

FIGURE 70-8 • Benzoyl peroxide.

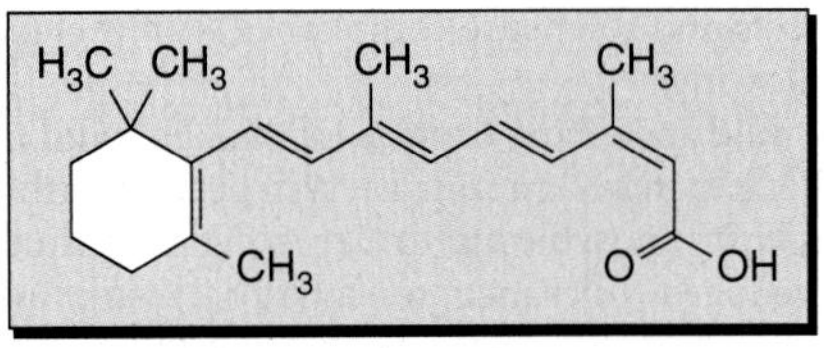

FIGURE 70-9 • Isotretinoin.

Benzoyl peroxide, like most peroxides, is a powerful bleaching agent. In the United States, the U.S. Food and Drug Administration (FDA) monograph for benzoyl peroxide is 2.5% to 10% for both prescription and over-the-counter use.

Benzoyl peroxide is effective in the treatment of most forms of acne. It is typically placed over the affected areas in gel or cream form, in concentrations beginning at 2.5% and increasing through the usually effective 5% to up to 10%. Research suggests that 5% and 10% concentrations are not significantly more effective than 2.5%, and 2.5% is usually better tolerated.[15,16] It commonly causes initial dryness and sometimes irritation, although skin tolerance usually occurs after a week or so. A small percentage of people are much more sensitive to it and liable to suffer burning, itching, peeling, and possibly swelling. Benzoyl peroxide works as a peeling agent, increasing skin turnover and clearing pores and thus reducing the bacterial count there, as well as directly as an antibacterial.

Combination products containing benzoyl peroxide and various topical antibiotics have been shown to both prevent the development of antibiotic resistance in acne patients and confer significant clinical improvement to patients who have already developed antibiotic resistance. Topical benzoyl peroxide and benzoyl peroxide 5%/erythromycin 3% combinations are similar in efficacy to oral oxytetracycline and minocycline and are not affected by propionibacterial antibiotic resistance.[17]

Benzoyl peroxide 5%/clindamycin 1% gel has demonstrated clinical efficacy in the treatment of acne vulgaris through both antibacterial and anti-inflammatory means. Several well-designed clinical trials have demonstrated that twice-daily application of benzoyl peroxide 5%/clindamycin 1% gel for 10 to 16 weeks was more effective in reducing the number of inflammatory lesions than benzoyl peroxide 5%, clindamycin 1%, or vehicle in patients with mild to moderately severe acne. Compared with benzoyl peroxide, benzoyl peroxide/clindamycin demonstrated significantly greater reductions in inflammatory lesions and significantly greater overall improvement as assessed by physicians and patients. Benzoyl peroxide/clindamycin demonstrated a nonsignificant trend for greater efficacy compared to benzoyl peroxide/erythromycin.[18]

Salicylic Acid. Salicylic acid is also known as 2-hydroxybenzoic acid (one of several β-hydroxy acids). It treats acne by causing skin cells to slough off more readily, preventing pores from clogging up as it is a keratolytic agent. Salicylic acid 1% to 2% preparations are usually well tolerated. Mild stinging may occur, especially on broken skin and when higher concentrations are used. Salicylic acid has been shown to exhibit the greatest keratolytic efficacy superficially as compared with retinoic acid or benzoyl peroxide, hence its clinical effectiveness in superficial conditions such as comedonal acne. Benzoyl peroxide is more effective at deeper levels, complementing its antimicrobial effects and enabling it to treat deeper, more inflammatory lesions.[19]

Sodium Sulfacetamide. Sodium sulfacetamide is a sulfonamide antibiotic. It inhibits *P. acnes* and opens clogged pores; it is effective in treating inflammatory acne. Many products containing sodium sulfacetamide include sulfur. Some patients do not like the smell of the sulfur or its grittiness. Usually, the newer products that contain sulfur do not have these problems.

Oral Treatments

Oral Antibiotics. For patients with moderate to severe and persistent acne, oral antibiotics have been a mainstay of therapy for years. Like topical antimicrobials, oral antibiotics work to reduce the *P. acnes* population (a contributing factor in acne), which, in turn, decreases inflammation. Treatment with oral antibiotics usually begins with a higher dosage, which is reduced as acne resolves. Generally, antibiotics are prescribed for 6 months or less.

Erythromycin. Erythromycin is a macrolide antibiotic, which has an antimicrobial spectrum similar to or slightly wider than that of penicillin, and is often used for people who have an allergy to penicillins. Erythromycin prevents bacteria from growing by interfering with their protein synthesis. Gastrointestinal disturbances such as diarrhea, nausea, abdominal pain, and vomiting are fairly common, so it tends not to be prescribed as a first-line drug. More serious side effects, such as reversible deafness, are rare. Bacteria frequently become resistant to erythromycin. Recommended dosage is 250 to 500 mg twice daily.

Tetracycline. Tetracycline is a broad-spectrum antibiotic produced by the *Streptomyces* bacterium, indicated for use against many bacterial infections. It works by inhibiting action of the prokaryotic 30S ribosome. It can stain developing teeth (even when taken by the mother during pregnancy), is not recommended to be taken with milk, and can induce photosensitivity. It can cause drug-induced lupus, hepatitis, and tinnitus. It is inexpensive and safe, but must be taken on an empty stomach, and sunscreen must be worn. Recommended dosage is 250 to 500 mg twice daily.

Doxycycline. Doxycycline is a member of the tetracycline antibiotics group and is commonly used to treat a variety of infections. Cautions and side effects are similar to those for other members of the tetracycline group. It is especially likely to induce photosensitivity; sunscreen and protective clothing must be worn while taking the drug. Doxycycline impairs the effectiveness of many types of contraceptive pills, and physicians recommend the use of barrier contraception for people taking the drug to prevent unwanted pregnancy. Recommended dosage is 50 to 100 mg twice daily.

Minocycline. Minocycline is a member of the broad-spectrum tetracycline antibiotics, and has a broader antibacterial coverage than the other members. As a result of its long half-life, it generally has a serum level two to four times that of most other tetracyclines. It is primarily used to treat acne and rosacea, as the once-daily 100-mg dosage is far easier for patients than the four times a day required with tetracycline or oxytetracycline. In addition to those side effects common to the tetracycline antibiotics group, minocycline may be used in patients with renal impairment, but may aggravate systemic lupus erythematosus. Also, more so than other tetracyclines, minocycline can cause the rare condition of secondary intracranial hypertension, which has initial symptoms of headache, visual disturbances, and confusion. It is considered by many to be the most effective antibiotic for acne but the most expensive. Recommended dosage is 50 to 100 mg twice daily.

Isotretinoin. Isotretinoin is a medication used for the treatment of severe cystic acne vulgaris. Isotretinoin (13-*cis*-retinoic acid) is an oral retinoid (meaning it is derived from vitamin A) that decreases the size and secretion of the sebaceous glands, normalizes follicular keratinization, inhibits *P. acnes* growth, and exerts an anti-inflammatory effect (Fig. 70-9). The exact mechanism of action is unknown; however, it is known that, like other retinoids, isotretinoin works by altering DNA transcription. Isotretinoin, when administered orally, is best absorbed when taken after a high-fat meal, as it has a high level of lipophilicity.

The potential side effects of isotretinoin are extensive, and physicians prescribing this medication should be advised about its potentially dangerous consequences. Patients should be evaluated frequently for adverse effects and to ensure compliance with therapy. Side effects include the following:

- *Common*: mild acne flare; dryness of skin, lips, and mucous membranes; cheilitis; itch; skin fragility, skin peeling, rash, and flushing; photosensitivity; nosebleeds; dry eyes, eye irritation, conjunctivitis, and reduced tolerance to contact lenses; hyperlipidemia; raised liver enzymes; headaches; hair thinning; myalgia and/or arthralgia
- *Infrequent*: severe acne flare, raised blood glucose level, increased erythrocyte sedimentation rate, fatigue and/or mood changes
- *Rare*: impaired night vision, cataracts, optic neuritis, menstrual disturbances, inflammatory bowel disease, pancreatitis, hepatitis, corneal opacities, papilloedema, idiopathic intracranial hypertension, skeletal hyperostosis, extraosseous calcification, moderate memory loss

The following adverse effects have been reported to persist, even after discontinuing therapy: alopecia, arthralgias, decreased night vision, degenerative disk disease, keloids, bone disease, and depression (in some cases). High dosages of isotretinoin have been reported to cause rosacea. While vitamin E supplements have been advocated by some to reduce the toxicity of high-dose retinoids without reducing drug efficacy, they do not appear to be effective. Patients receiving isotretinoin therapy are not permitted to donate blood during and for at least 1 month after discontinuation of isotretinoin therapy. Several studies have suggested a possible link between isotretinoin and clinical depression. However, no conclusive evidence has been produced.

Isotretinoin can cause birth defects in the developing fetus, including defects of the central nervous system, skull, eyes, and cardiovascular system. It is important that women of childbearing age are not pregnant and do not get pregnant while taking this medication. Women must sign consent forms and take a pregnancy test prior to initiation of isotretinoin. They must use two separate effective forms of birth control at the same time for 1 month before treatment begins, during the entire course of treatment, and for 1 full month after stopping the drug. In the United States, the process of ensuring that pregnancy is avoided has been mandated by the federal government via the iPLEDGE program. iPLEDGE is a computer-based risk management program designed to further the public health goal to eliminate fetal exposure to isotretinoin through a special restricted distribution program approved by the FDA. The program strives to ensure that

- No female patient starts isotretinoin therapy if pregnant
- No female patient on isotretinoin therapy becomes pregnant

Since March 1, 2006, the dispensing of isotretinoin in the United States has been controlled by an FDA-mandated web site for iPLEDGE. Dermatologists are required to register their patients on the iPLEDGE web site before prescribing isotretinoin. The dispensing pharmacist then interviews the patient about her sexual practices and checks the web site before filling the prescription. The stated goal is to prevent female patients "of childbearing potential" from receiving the drug if they are pregnant, and to prevent them from becoming pregnant if they are taking the drug.

The concurrent use of isotretinoin with tetracycline antibiotics or vitamin A supplementation is not recommended. Concurrent use of isotretinoin with tetracycline significantly increases the risk of idiopathic intracranial hypertension. Concurrent intake of vitamin A supplementation increases the risk of vitamin A toxicity.

Isotretinoin is available in 5-, 10-, and 20-mg pills. Brand names include Accutane, Amnesteem, Claravis, and Sotret. The dose of isotretinoin a patient receives is dependent on his or her weight and the severity of the condition. Generally it is prescribed at between 0.5 and 2 mg/kg per day (most often at 1 to 1.25 mg/kg per day) for 4 to 6 months. A second course may be used 2 months following the cessation of the initial course if severe acne recurs. Efficacy appears to be related to the cumulative dose of isotretinoin taken, with a total cumulative dose of 120 to 150 mg/kg used as a guideline.

Antiandrogens. Antiandrogen treatment targets the androgen-metabolizing follicular keratinocytes and the sebaceous glands leading to sebostasis, with a reduction of the sebum secretion rate of 12.5% to 65%. Antiandrogens can be classified based on their mechanism of action as androgen receptor blockers, inhibitors of circulating androgens by affecting ovarian function (oral contraceptives), inhibitors of circulating androgens by affecting the pituitary (gonadotropin-releasing hormone agonists and dopamine agonists in hyperprolactinemia), inhibitors of adrenal function, and inhibitors of peripheral androgen metabolism (5α-reductase inhibitors, inhibitors of other enzymes).[20]

Oral Contraceptives. Oral contraceptives are used to prevent pregnancy. The most commonly reported adverse effects are weight gain; nausea; variations in menstrual flow; breast changes such as tenderness, discomfort, or swelling; depression or mood disturbances; decreased sexual desire or response; and acne. However, oral contraceptives have also been shown to effectively treat acne in women. Open-label and comparative studies beginning in the 1980s were the first to demonstrate objective and subjective reductions in the incidence of acne, as well as the severity of existing acne and seborrhea. Placebo-controlled trials have corroborated these findings with a trend toward effective acne treatment with declining doses of ethinyl estradiol. The combinations of cyproterone acetate (2 mg)/ethinyl estradiol (35 mcg), drospirenone (3 mg)/ethinyl estradiol (30 mcg), and desogestrel (25 mcg)/ethinyl estradiol (40 mcg) for 1 week, followed by desogestrel (125 mcg)/ethinyl estradiol (30 mcg) for 2 weeks, showed the strongest antiacne activity.

Oral contraceptives for the treatment of acne can be used in women who have worsening acne during premenstrual or menstrual periods or when other options have failed and there are no contraindications for their use. Rare but serious potential side effects include cardiovascular diseases, such as stroke, and an increased risk for breast cancer, liver tumors, and gallbladder disease. Hormonal contraceptive use should be avoided in women at risk for blood clots, by heavy smokers, and in women with breast or other cancers.

Therapeutic Approaches

The first step in the management of the acne should be the patient's acne classification. There are different ways to classify acne patients, based on the severity (mild, moderate, severe), localization of the lesions (face, chest, back), type of lesions (comedones, papulopustules, cystic lesions), gender of the patient (male, female), and type of skin (oily, dry, sensitive). Most of the time the classification is based on physician judgment rather than an exact method. However, the classification shown in Box 70-1 can be useful to determine mild, moderate, and severe cases.

If the patient has mild acne, usually single-agent therapy is recommended. Topical retinoids are the treatment of choice. Follicular hyperkeratinization is a key element in the pathogenesis of acne and a main target of retinoid activity (Box 70-2). Products with retinoid activity normalize follicular keratinization, inhibit formation of microcomedones, decrease formation of inflammatory lesions, and speed resolution of comedones. Adverse effects include erythema, burning, stinging, and peeling. Several retinoids can be used as monotherapy agents: adapalene, tretinoin, and tazarotene. The choice among the different retinoids can be based on the severity of acne and the skin type of the patient. Tazarotene can be more irritating to the skin than the other retinoids; however, it is slightly more effective. Most of the time for a patient with comedonal acne the treatment can be initiated with adapalene, and if after 6 to 8 weeks there is no improvement, tretinoin or tazarotene can be initiated in escalating concentrations as tolerated (Table 70-2). Tazarotene is sometimes used in rotation if it is

BOX 70-1 CLASSIFICATION OF ACNE SEVERITY

Mild: <20 comedones, <15 inflammatory lesions, or <30 total lesions

Moderate: 20-100 comedones, 15-50 inflammatory lesions, or 30-125 total lesions

Severe: >5 cysts, >100 comedones, >50 inflammatory lesions, or >125 total lesions

TABLE 70-2 SUMMARY OF TREATMENT

Type of Acne (Main Type of Lesions)	Type of Treatment	Treatment of Choice	Alternative Treatments	Comments
1. Comedones	Single-agent therapy	Topical retinoids (can be chosen depending on skin type and severity of acne) Adapalene ↓ Tretinoin ↓ Tazarotene	Azelaic acid Salicylic acid	If treatment fails after at least 6 wk, increase dosage or go to number 2.
2. Papulopustules	Dual therapy	Topical retinoids + benzoyl peroxide/clindamycin or benzoyl peroxide/erythromycin	Topical retinoids or azelaic acid + benzoyl peroxide, topical clindamycin or erythromycin	If treatment fails after at least 6 wk, add oral antibiotics.
3. Cystic lesions: mild (face and few lesions back)	Dual therapy + oral antibiotics			If treatment fails after at least 12 wk, consider if patient is candidate for oral isotretinoin.
4. Cystic lesions: moderate-severe	Oral isotretinoin			

BOX 70-2 PROPERTIES OF TREATMENTS

Normalize Follicular Keratinization
Isotretinoin
Tazarotene
Tretinoin
Adapalene
Salicylic acid
Azelaic acid
Benzoyl peroxide
Vitamins A and B

Anti-Inflammatory
Antibiotics
Zinc, essential fatty acids, nicotinamide, brewer's yeast

Antibacterial
Antibiotics
Benzoyl peroxide
Azelaic acid
Sodium sulfacetamide
Isotretinoin (indirect effect)

Inhibit Sebaceous Gland Function
Antiandrogens
Estrogens (oral contraceptives)
Isotretinoin
Zinc, vitamins B_6 and A, brewer's yeast

too irritating and the patient cannot tolerate it in consecutive treatments. Azelaic acid and salicylic acid can also been used if the topical retinoids cannot be tolerated. They are not as effective as topical retinoids, but sometimes can be better tolerated by certain patients and can be very effective in very mild comedonal acne. Physical extraction of comedones using a comedone extractor is an option for patients unresponsive to topical treatment. Comedone extraction may be performed by a physician, nurse, or physician assistant.

In patients with a combination of comedones and papulopustules or with only papulopustules, combination therapy is necessary. The most effective combination is topical retinoids at bedtime and either benzoyl peroxide alone or a combination of benzoyl peroxide and a topical antibiotic in the morning. The combination of benzoyl peroxide and a topical antibiotic such as clindamycin or erythromycin has been shown to decrease bacterial resistance to the antibiotic. These combinations also have no significant adverse effects other than drying and irritation (and rare allergic reactions to benzoyl peroxide). This therapy achieves anti-inflammatory activity with the topical antibiotics, normalizes follicular keratinization with the topical retinoids and benzoyl peroxide, and is antibacterial with the topical antibiotics and benzoyl peroxide. Other treatment options include substitution of azelaic acid for the topical retinoid and combining it with benzoyl peroxide and a topical antibiotic. This option is useful in cases in which the initial combination is too irritating or cannot be tolerated. If this treatment combination fails or there is no improvement in 6 to 8 weeks, oral antibiotics can be added to the treatment.

Tetracycline, doxycycline, or minocycline can be chosen as an oral antibiotic. Doxycycline is very photosensitizing: sunscreen must be worn and the sun avoided during summer months. Minocycline is the treatment of choice of many dermatologists. It produces fewer gastrointestinal adverse effects, is easier to take, and is less likely to cause photosensitization, but it is the most costly option.

If the treatment with dual therapy and oral antibiotics fails, or the patient has cystic acne or moderate to severe acne, especially on the back, treatment with oral isotretinoin is recommended. Dosage of isotretinoin is usually 1 mg/kg once daily for 16 to 20 weeks, but the dosage may be increased to 2 mg/kg once daily in occasional cases. If adverse effects make this dosage intolerable, it may be reduced to 0.5 mg/kg once daily. After therapy, acne may continue to improve. Most patients do not require a second course of treatment. However, when needed, isotretinoin should be resumed only after the drug has been stopped for 4 months. Re-treatment is required more often if the initial dosage is low (0.5 mg/kg). The new iPLEDGE program makes the prescription for and follow-up of patients taking isotretinoin stricter, especially for women.

For women with premenstrual acne flare-ups, oral contraceptives can be an alternative treatment option.

Emerging Targets and Therapeutics

Laser Treatment

Over the past decade, lasers and light-based systems have become a common modality to treat a wide variety of skin-related conditions, including acne vulgaris. In spite of the various oral and topical treatments available for the treatment of acne, many patients fail to respond adequately or may develop side effects.[21]

Photodynamic therapy is based on the tissue-selective accumulation of a photosensitizer that is generally a porphyrin derivative. Following illumination with light of an appropriate wavelength, and in the presence of oxygen, the photosensitizer generates active molecular species, such as free radicals and singlet oxygen, that are toxic to cells and tissues.

Near-infrared (NIR) diode laser low-intensity (soft) phototherapy with the topical application of indocyanine green (ICG) has been suggested for treatment of acne vulgaris. Observations 1 month after the completion of the treatment showed that only multiple treatments with a combination of ICG and NIR irradiation reduced inflammation and improved the state of the skin for a month without any side effects. A month after treatment, the improvement was about 80% for the group receiving multiple treatments.[22]

Several research studies have shown the efficacy of combination therapy with blue (415 nm) and red (633 nm) light. Subjects were treated over eight sessions, two per week 3 days apart, alternating between blue light (20 minutes/session, 48 J/cm^2) and red light (20 minutes/session, 96 J/cm^2) from a light-emitting diode–based therapy system. At the 4-week follow-up, the mean lesion count reduction was significant at 46%. At the 12-week follow-up, the mean lesion count reduction was also significant at 81%.[23]

Topical Treatments

Dapsone 5% Gel. A gel formulation of dapsone has been developed that allows clinically effective doses of dapsone to be administered topically with minimal systemic absorption. Patients 12 years of age and older with acne vulgaris participated in two identically designed 12-week, randomized, double-blind studies of twice-daily monotherapy with dapsone gel 5%, versus a vehicle gel. Dapsone gel–treated patients achieved superior results in terms of the investigator's global acne assessment and the mean percentage reduction in inflammatory, noninflammatory, and total lesion counts at week 12. Reductions in inflammatory lesion counts were apparent as early as 2 weeks and reached statistical significance by 4 weeks. No clinically significant changes in laboratory parameters, including hemoglobin, even among glucose-6-phosphate dehydrogenase–deficient patients, were observed. Adverse events were comparable between the treatment groups and rarely led to discontinuation.[24]

Nutrition

***Saccharomyces cerevisiae* (Brewer's Yeast).** *Saccharomyces cerevisiae* is a species of budding yeast. It is perhaps the most important yeast owing to its use since ancient times in baking and brewing. In a randomized, controlled, double-blind study involving 139 patients with various forms of acne, the effectiveness and tolerance of *S. cerevisiae* Hansen CBS 5926 (Perenterol) were studied in comparison with a placebo over a maximum period of 5 months. The results of therapy were assessed by a physician as very good/good in 74.3% of the patients receiving the preparation, as compared with 21.7% in the placebo group. In more than 80% of the former patients, the condition was considered to be healed or considerably improved, while the corresponding figure for the placebo group was only 26%.[25]

Zinc. Zinc is the most abundant trace element in the body, and is a necessary component of many enzymes involved in DNA, RNA, protein, and collagen synthesis and cell proliferation. Zinc has anti-inflammatory activity by inhibiting polynuclear leukocyte chemotaxis.

Zinc has shown to decrease seborrhea by inhibiting the activity of 5α-reductase; at high concentrations, zinc could completely inhibit the enzyme activity. Vitamin B_6 potentiated the inhibitory effect of zinc.[26] 5α-Reductase converts testosterone to the more potent dihydrotestosterone, an androgen that increases the production of sebum. Free fatty acids in sebum arise from lipolytic action of bacterial lipases. Zinc also has an inhibitory effect on the lipase of the three *Propionibacterium* species found in human pilosebaceous follicles.[27]

Essential Fatty Acids. The concentrations of essential fatty acids and their metabolites in plasma phospholipids were measured by gas chromatography in normal individuals and in patients with acne vulgaris. In acne patients, concentrations of arachidonic acid (20 : 4 ν-6) and docosapentaenoic acid (22 : 5 ν-6) were significantly below those in controls.[28]

The proportion of linoleic acid is markedly decreased in acne comedones. Linoleic acid significantly suppresses reactive oxygen species (ROS) generated by neutrophils. The ability of neutrophils to produce ROS was significantly increased in patients with acne inflammation. These results seem to reveal the involvement of ROS generated by neutrophils in the disruption of the integrity of the follicular epithelium, which is responsible for the inflammatory processes of acne.[29]

Vitamin A. *Vitamin A* is a generic term for a large number of related compounds. Retinol (an alcohol) and retinal (an aldehyde) are often referred to as "preformed vitamin A." Retinal can be converted by the body to retinoic acid, the form of vitamin A known to affect gene transcription. Retinol, retinal, retinoic acid, and related compounds are known as retinoids. β-Carotene and other carotenoids that can be converted by the body into retinol are referred to as "provitamin A carotenoids." Hundreds of different carotenoids are synthesized by plants, but only about 10% of them are provitamin A carotenoids. Vitamin A is needed by all epithelial tissue. It helps protect the skin and tissues inside and outside of the body.

B Vitamins. B vitamins are related to the activity of sebaceous glands and the keratinization process. Nicotinamide (vitamin B_3, niacin) is essential for the synthesis of sexual hormones. It has anti-inflammatory properties inhibiting the chemotaxis of neutrophils; it inhibits lymphocytic transformation and mast cell degranulation.[30] Biotin enhances the niacin effect, regulates sebum production by the sebaceous glands, and improves the skin quality (acne), hair, and nails.

According to a study published in 1997 by Dr. Lit-Hung Leung, high doses of panthotenic acid (vitamin B_5) resolved acne and decreased pore size. Dr. Leung also proposes a mechanism, stating that coenzyme A (CoA) regulates both hormones and fatty acids, and without sufficient quantities of pantothenic acid, CoA will preferentially produce androgens. This causes fatty acids to build up and be excreted through sebaceous glands, causing acne.[31]

Vitamin B_6 has antiseborrheic properties, enhancing zinc's activity inhibiting 5α-reductase. In women, a potential cause for vitamin B_6 deficiency is use of oral contraceptives and other medications containing estro-progestational hormones (such as those prescribed as part of hormone replacement therapy). Other contraceptive medications that may cause vitamin B_6 deficiency include the patch (Ortho Evra), vaginal ring (Nuvaring), hormonal IUD (Mirena), and shot (Depo Provera). Specifically, habitual use of estro-progestational hormones inhibits absorption of vitamin B_6 (due to a disturbance of tryptophan metabolism), necessitating a larger daily dosage of B_6 into the bloodstream. Signs of a vitamin B_6 deficiency include depression, anxiety, loss of libido, insomnia, water retention, and inability to process glucose (weight loss/gain). Vitamin B_6 has been useful treating premenstrual acne.

REFERENCES

1. Goulden V, Stables GI, Cunliffe WJ. Prevalence of facial acne in adults. J Am Acad Dermatol 1999;41:577-580.
2. Cunliffe WJ, Gould DJ. Prevalence of facial acne vulgaris in late adolescence and in adults. Br Med J 1979;1:1109-1110.
3. Cordain L, Lindeberg S, Hurtado M, et al. Acne vulgaris: a disease of Western civilization. Arch Dermatol 2002;138:1584-1590.
4. Schäfer T, Nienhaus A, Vieluf D, et al. Epidemiology of acne in the general population: the risk of smoking. Br J Dermatol 2001;145:100-104.
5. Bershad SV. The modern age of acne therapy: a review of current treatment options. Mt Sinai J Med 2001;68:279.
6. Webster GF. Acne vulgaris. BMJ 2002;325:475.
7. Dekkers OM, Thio BH, Romijn JA, Smit JW. Acne vulgaris: endocrine aspects. Ned Tijdschr Geneeskd 2006;150:1281-1285.
8. Essah PA, Wickham EP 3rd, Nunley JR, Nestler JE. Dermatology of androgen-related disorders. Clin Dermatol 2006;24:289-298.
9. Aizawa H, Nakada Y, Niimura M. Androgen status in adolescent women with acne vulgaris. J Dermatol 1995;22:530-532.
10. Toyoda M, Morohashi M. Pathogenesis of acne. Med Electron Microsc 2001;34:29-40.
11. Thiboutot D, Pariser D, Egan N, et al. Adapalene gel 0.3% for the treatment of acne vulgaris: a multicenter, randomized, double-blind, controlled, Phase III trial. J Am Acad Dermatol 2006;54:242-250.
12. Waugh J, Noble S, Scott LJ. Spotlight on adapalene in acne vulgaris. Am J Clin Dermatol 2004;5:369-371.

13. Shalita A, Miller B, Menter A, et al. Tazarotene cream versus adapalene cream in the treatment of facial acne vulgaris: a multicenter, double-blind, randomized, parallel-group study. J Drugs Dermatol 2005;4:153-158.
14. Leyden JJ, Shalita AR, Saatjian GD, Sefton J. Erythromycin 2% gel in comparison with clindamycin phosphate 1% solution in acne vulgaris. J Am Acad Dermatol 1987;16:822-827.
15. Mills OH Jr, Kligman AM, Pochi P, Comite H. Comparing 2.5%, 5%, and 10% benzoyl peroxide on inflammatory acne vulgaris. Int J Dermatol 1986;25:664-667.
16. Yong CC. Benzoyl peroxide gel therapy in acne in Singapore. Int J Dermatol 1979;18:485-488.
17. Ozolins M, Eady EA, Avery AJ, et al. Comparison of five antimicrobial regimens for treatment of mild to moderate inflammatory facial acne vulgaris in the community: randomised controlled trial. Lancet 2004;364:2188-2195.
18. Leyden JJ, Hickman JG, Jarratt MT, et al. The efficacy and safety of a combination benzoyl peroxide/clindamycin topical gel compared with benzoyl peroxide alone and a benzoyl peroxide/erythromycin combination product. J Cutan Med Surg 2001;5:37-42.
19. Waller JM, Dreher F, Behnam S, et al. "Keratolytic" properties of benzoyl peroxide and retinoic acid resemble salicylic acid in man. Skin Pharmacol Physiol 2006;19:283-289.
20. Zouboulis CC. Treatment of acne with antiandrogens—an evidence-based review. J Dtsch Dermatol Ges 2003;1:535-546.
21. Divaris DXG, Kennedy JC, Pottier RH. Phototoxic damage to sebaceous glands and hair follicles of mice after systemic administration of 5-aminolevulinic acid correlates with localized protoporphyrin IX fluorescence. Am J Pathol 1990;136:891-897.
22. Genina EA, Bashkatov AN, Simonenko GV, et al. Low-intensity indocyanine-green laser phototherapy of acne vulgaris: pilot study. J Biomed Opt 2004;9:828-834.
23. Goldberg DJ, Russell BA. Combination blue (415 nm) and red (633 nm) LED phototherapy in the treatment of mild to severe acne vulgaris. J Cosmet Laser Ther 2006;8:71-75.
24. Draelos ZD, Carter E, Maloney JM, et al, for the United States/Canada Dapsone Gel Study Group. Two randomized studies demonstrate the efficacy and safety of dapsone gel, 5% for the treatment of acne vulgaris. J Am Acad Dermatol 2007; 56:439.
25. Weber G, Adamczyk A, Freytag S. Treatment of acne with a yeast preparation. Fortschr Med 1989;107:563-566.
26. Stamatiadis D, Bulteau-Portois MC, Mowszowicz I. Inhibition of 5 alpha-reductase activity in human skin by zinc and azelaic acid. Br J Dermatol 1988;119:627-632.
27. Rebello T, Atherton DJ, Holden C. The effect of oral zinc administration on sebum free fatty acids in acne vulgaris. Acta Derm Venereol 1986;66:305-310.
28. Grattan C, Burton JL, Manku M, et al. Essential-fatty-acid metabolites in plasma phospholipids in patients with ichthyosis vulgaris, acne vulgaris and psoriasis. Clin Exp Dermatol 1990;15:174-176.
29. Akamatsu H, Horio T. The possible role of reactive oxygen species generated by neutrophils in mediating acne inflammation. Dermatology 1998;196:82-85.
30. Ungerstedt JS, Blomback M, Soderstrom T. Nicotinamide is a potent inhibitor of proinflammatory cytokines. Clin Exp Immunol 2003;131:48-52.
31. Leung LH. Pantothenic acid deficiency as the pathogenesis of acne vulgaris. Med Hypotheses 1995;44:490-492.

71

PSORIASIS

Mark R. Pittelkow and Joseph Genebriera

INTRODUCTION 983
EPIDEMIOLOGY 983
PATHOPHYSIOLOGY 984
Disease Assessments 985
Clinical Types of Psoriasis 985
Plaque Psoriasis 985
Guttate Psoriasis 985
Flexural (Inverse) Psoriasis 986
Erythroderma 986
Localized and Generalized Pustular Psoriasis 986
Palmoplantar Pustulosis 986
Psoriatic Nail Disease 986
Psoriatic Arthritis 986
THERAPEUTICS AND CLINICAL PHARMACOLOGY 986
Therapeutics by Class 986
Topical Treatments 986
Phototherapy 990
Oral Treatments 991
Biologics 995
Laser 998
Therapeutic Approaches 999
Mild Psoriasis 999
Moderate to Severe Psoriasis 1000
Pregnancy and Psoriasis 1002
Psoriatic Arthritis 1002
Emerging Targets and Therapeutics 1004
ShK(L5) and PAP-1 1004
Apremilast (CC-10004) 1004
ABT-874 1004
MEDI-545 1004
Essential Fatty Acids (ω-3) 1004

INTRODUCTION

Psoriasis is an inflammatory skin disorder with hyperproliferation and abnormal differentiation of the stratified epidermis that also affects the enthesium and joints in some patients. It commonly causes discrete, red, scaly plaques to appear on the skin, and thus is classified as a papulosquamous disorder (Fig. 71-1). The indurated and elevated plaques caused by psoriasis are due to enlargement and coalescence of papules with epidermal thickening and inflammation. Scale rapidly accumulates on the surface of these affected sites and typically appears silvery white with mica-like desquamation. Plaques most often occur on extensor regions of the skin, especially the elbows and knees, but can affect any areas including the scalp, skinfolds, and genital skin.

The disorder is a chronic, recurring condition that affects approximately 2% to 3% of various genetically susceptible populations around the world and varies in severity from minor, localized lesions to complete body coverage, designated erythroderma. Fingernails and toenails are frequently affected (psoriatic nail dystrophy). Psoriasis can also cause inflammation of the joints and adjacent enthesial attachments and has the potential for articular destruction. This associated condition, psoriatic arthritis, affects up to 30% to 40% of the psoriatic population.

Psoriasis became known as Willan's lepra in the late 18th century when English dermatologists Drs. Robert Willan and Thomas Bateman differentiated it from other common skin diseases. They assigned names to the condition based on the appearance of lesions. Willan identified two categories: leprosa graecorum and psora leprosa. It was not until 1841 that the condition was finally given the New Latin name "psoriasis" by the Viennese dermatologist Ferdinand von Hebra, from the Greek *psorian*, "to have the itch."

In 1876 Balmanno Squire accidentally, but fortuitously, identified a treatment for psoriasis using Goa powder, a tree extract that contained anthralin (dithranol), which is still used to the present time in skin-directed, topical therapies.

In 1925, Dr. William Goeckerman, a dermatologist at Mayo Clinic, developed a highly effective, skin-directed treatment regimen that combined crude coal tar ointment with gradually increasing exposure to ultraviolet B (UVB) radiation from hot quartz, mercury vapor lamps. This therapeutic regimen still bears his name and remains one of the most effective topical treatments administered in courses for psoriasis.

In the 1950s, Dr. John Ingram developed the "Ingram regimen," combining UVB radiation and topically applied anthralin to the plagues. By the late 1950s, following the discovery of cortisone a decade earlier, topical corticosteroid formulations started to be developed and applied to affected lesions of psoriasis, sometimes with occlusive dressings to enhance penetration and effectiveness.

Following the synthesis and development of aminopterin in the late 1940s and, subsequently, the folate acid antagonist methotrexate, these agents were administered in psoriasis patients to reverse epidermal hyperproliferation. Methotrexate was the first parenterally administered drug approved for use in psoriasis and remains a widely used systemic medication for treatment of the skin and joint manifestations of the disease. Over the past decade, however, the mechanism of action of methotrexate has come to be known to principally target and diminish the inflammatory, T-lymphocytic infiltrate within skin and, in turn, the hyperproliferation, abnormal scaling, and disrupted differentiation of the epidermis.

In the 1980s, the oral agent cyclosporine, which attenuates T cell–specific immune responses, was observed to be effective in the treatment of psoriasis during chronic immune suppression of solid organ transplant recipients or rheumatoid arthritis patients who also had psoriasis. With this discovery and the findings that the epidermal and dermal lymphocytes were predominantly T cells, psoriasis was beginning to be recognized as a cell-mediated autoimmune disorder.

In the past decade, extensive research and biotechnology efforts have been leveraged to develop biologic agents that act primarily on the immune system, target specific molecules that appear to be key in propagating the immunopathogenesis of psoriasis, and reestablish epidermal regulation of the abnormal hyperproliferation and differentiation of skin that typify various forms of psoriasis.

EPIDEMIOLOGY

The prevalence of psoriasis varies considerable among world populations and geography, especially latitude. It is essentially a disease of Caucasians (2% to 3%), being much less common in Asians (0.1%) and native Africans. In the United States, approximately 2% of the population is affected.[1] High rates of psoriasis have been reported in people of the Faroe Islands, where one study found 2.8% of the population to be affected. Prevalence of psoriasis is low in certain ethnic groups such as the Japanese, and may be virtually absent in aboriginal

Australians[2] and Indians from South America.[3] Psoriasis affects the genders almost equally. Studies of monozygotic twins suggest a 70% chance of the twin developing psoriasis if the index twin has psoriasis. The concordance is much less, approximately 20%, for dizygotic twins. These findings were early evidence for both a genetic predisposition and environmental factors in the development of psoriasis.

The course and progress of psoriasis is unpredictable. Psoriasis presents at any age and has been reported rarely at birth and, more commonly, in the advanced age population. The mean age of initial onset of psoriasis ranges from 15 to 20 years of age, with a second peak occurring at 55 to 60 years. Henseler and Christophers examined a series of 2147 patients and reported two clinical presentations of psoriasis, type I and II, distinguished by a bimodal age at onset. Type I begins at or before age 40 years; type II begins after the age of 40 years. Type I disease accounts for more than 75% of cases.[4] Patients with early-onset, or type I, psoriasis tend to have more relatives affected and more severe disease than patients who have later-onset, type II psoriasis. In addition, strong associations have been reported with human leukocyte antigen (HLA)-Cw6 in patients with early onset, compared with later onset, of psoriasis. Recent genetic studies of psoriasis have identified several risk loci for the disease, but the strongest risk allele remains on chromosome 6, within the Cw6 locus.

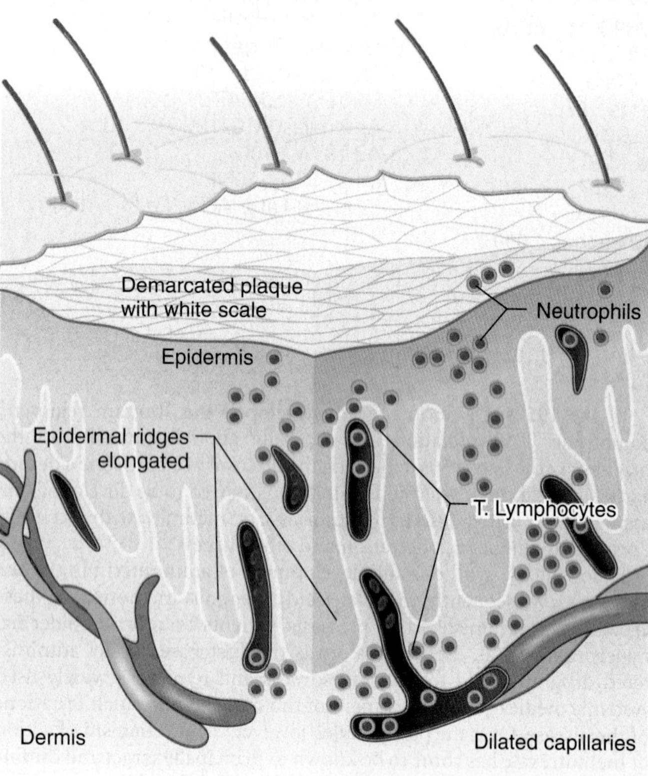

FIGURE 71-1 • Psoriasis pathophysiology.

PATHOPHYSIOLOGY

Psoriasis is characterized by hyperproliferation and abnormal differentiation of epidermal keratinocytes, lymphocyte infiltration consisting principally of T lymphocytes, and specific endothelial vascular changes within the dermal microvasculature, including limited neoangiogenesis, capillary dilation, and high endothelial venule formation, all this contributing to the visible redness (erythema) of psoriatic skin lesions. T lymphocytes, especially $CD4^+$ cells in the dermis and T helper type 17 (Th17) and $CD8^+$ cells within the epidermis, in conjunction with the characteristic cytokines and chemokines released by these cells and the epidermis and other resident cells appear to be the primary mediators of lesion development and persistence, although endothelial cells, neutrophils, and natural killer (NK) T cells also likely play modulating or exacerbating roles along with other inflammatory cell–specific cytokines and adhesion molecules/selectins/integrins, such as intracellular adhesion molecule-1 and integrin $\alpha_1\beta_1$.[5,6]

Histologically, there is marked thickening (acanthosis) of the epidermis, due to increased proliferation of keratinocytes in the interfollicular epidermis. Epidermal rete pegs elongate and form long, thin downward projections into the dermis. Normal differentiation of stratified keratinocytes is extensively altered in psoriasis. Psoriatic plaques have surface scale, which is caused by aberrant terminal differentiation of keratinocytes (Fig. 71-2). Scaling and the consequent disruption of the protective epidermal barrier are caused by failure of psoriatic corneocytes (terminally differentiated keratinocytes) to form normally, develop tight junctions, synthesize and secrete the normal extracellular complement of lipids, and adhere efficiently to one another. In psoriatic lesions, the granular layer of the epidermis is reduced or absent, creating a stratum corneum with incompletely differentiated keratinocytes that retain a remnant of the cell nucleus (parakeratosis). Often, there are neutrophils in the stratum corneum and mononuclear cell infiltrates in the epidermis as well as specific

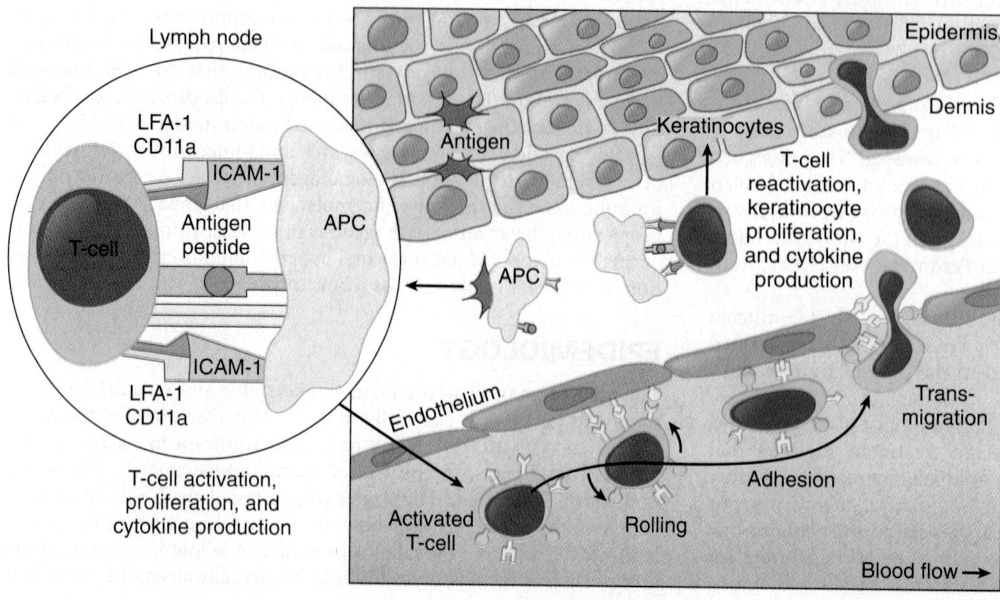

FIGURE 71-2 • Dendritic-antigen presentation, T-cell activation and localization in skin.

pathogenic leukocytes (T cells and dendritic cells [DCs]) within the dermis. Endothelial cells appear activated in psoriatic lesions, and specific subtypes of peripheral blood leukocytes enter into the lesional skin by transmigration through these activated vessels. It is increasingly being recognized that even normal skin contains a significant population and number of T lymphocytes[7] as well as resident populations of DCs,[8] suggesting that skin might be a potential site for the direct triggering of recall immune responses.

The role of T lymphocytes in the pathogenesis of psoriasis can be summarized by three primary events: (i) the initial innate immune response(s), followed by specific sensitization and activation of T lymphocytes within skin; (ii) the transit, amplification, and migration of pathogenic T cells into skin sites where psoriasis will develop; and (iii) the pathogenic roles played by specific cytokines-chemokines released from T lymphocytes and cooperating cell types, including epidermal keratinocytes that provide the environment to sustain and propagate psoriasis. The initial signal is provided by binding of the T-cell receptor to peptide(s) presented by the major histocompatibility complex (MHC) on plasmacytoid DCs. This sensitization step characterizes the specificity of the immune response in psoriasis. The antigen-presenting cell (APC) is the plasmacytoid DC that is co-stimulated by specific peptides within the epidermis that serve as innate immune signals, specifically LL-37 among others, in the case of naive responses, although B cells and macrophages may also serve as APCs. The peptides presented to $CD8^+$ T cells by MHC class I molecules are typically eight to nine amino acids in length; the peptides presented to $CD4^+$ cells by MHC class II molecules are longer, as the ends of the binding cleft of the MHC class II molecule are more accessible. The second signal comes from co-stimulation, in which surface receptors on the APC are induced by a relatively small number of stimuli, usually products of pathogens but sometimes breakdown products of cells, such as necrotic bodies or heat-shock proteins. The only co-stimulatory receptor expressed constitutively by naive T cells is CD28, with co-stimulation for these cells by CD80 and CD86 on APCs. The activated T lymphocytes, via cell-cell interactions with vascular endothelial cells, migrate to inflamed skin.[9,10]

Once at the inflamed skin site, activated T lymphocytes encounter the potential initiating antigen, and release T helper type 1 (Th1) cytokines, which play a central role in the phenotypic expression of psoriasis. Both $CD4^+$ and $CD8^+$ T lymphocytes produce Th1 cytokines. Principal Th1 cytokines involved in the pathogenesis of psoriasis are interferon (IFN)–γ, interleukin (IL)–2, and tumor necrosis factor (TNF)–α. Interleukin-2 stimulates T-lymphocyte replication, and IL-2 treatment is associated with psoriatic flares.[11] Interferon-γ may inhibit apoptosis of keratinocytes by stimulating expression of the antiapoptotic protein Bcl-x in these cells.[12] Keratinocyte antiapoptotic signals may contribute to the overall hyperproliferative response and increase in epidermal cell mass of psoriatic lesions.

TNF-α appears to promote psoriasis development by several mechanisms, including enhancing proliferation of keratinocytes and augmenting the production of proinflammatory cytokines from T lymphocytes and macrophages, as well as chemokines from macrophages and adhesion molecules on vascular endothelial cells.[13,14] Th1 cytokines also induce the release of cytokines from other cells, producing a cascade of chemical messengers that, together, create the distinctive features of psoriatic lesions.

Psoriasis is inherited as a complex trait; thus the genetic basis of psoriasis has been challenging to dissect, with evidence of multiple genetic loci. To date, between 15 and 20 chromosome regions have been proposed to harbor psoriasis risk alleles, but only a small number of genes have been identified.[15,16] One locus consistently identified in studies of psoriasis is the class I region of the major histocompatibility locus antigen cluster (MHC). The exact identity of the psoriasis susceptibility 1 (PSORS1) locus remains controversial. Whether PSORS1 is a classical MHC allele or a regulatory variant within this region remains to be established. Other predisposing genes likely affect disease severity and onset, including those regulating the immune system and keratinocyte differentiation, barrier function, and innate immune responses. Common variants in the SLC9A3R1/NAT9 region and loss of a potential RUNX binding site have been identified as loci affecting regulation of the immune synapse.[17] Association of psoriasis with variant alleles of the lymphoid phosphatase PTPN22 have been reported. PTPN22 also regulates the immune synapse, and a R620W polymorphism is associated with at least four other autoimmune diseases. Associations with alleles encoding other components of the immune system, such as IL-12, IL-23 receptor, IL-19/20, IL-20/24, and IRF2 have also been described. Genetic variants within the epidermal differentiation complex (EDC) might also affect keratinocyte proliferation or differentiation and development of psoriasis.[18]

The challenge to validate psoriasis susceptibility loci also likely relates, in part, to heterogeneity among different populations. More sophisticated analyses, including genome-wide association studies and the HapMap project phase 2, will hopefully provide more definitive characterization. Though the genetic underpinnings of psoriasis are certain, the exact locations of the genes involved remain to be fully defined.[19]

Disease Assessments

Psoriasis is usually graded as mild (affecting less than 2% of the body surface area [BSA]), moderate (affecting 2% to 10% of BSA) or severe (>10% of BSA). Several scales exist for measuring the severity of psoriasis. The degree of severity is generally based on the following factors: the proportion of BSA affected; disease activity (redness, thickness, and scaling of plaques); response to previous therapies; and the impact of the disease on the individual.

The Psoriasis Area and Severity Index (PASI) score remains the most accepted and widely used index in clinical trials. PASI combines the assessment of the severity of lesions and the area affected into a single score ranging from 0 (no disease) to 72 (maximal disease) based on clinical features such as erythema, scaling, and surface area affected. The major drawback is that the objective signs of erythema—scale and induration—are scored equally and assume linearity, but exceptions often occur in clinical practice. Percent improvement is routinely determined in clinical trials to assess efficacy of investigational agents. For example, PASI 75 designates 75% improvement in PASI score from baseline.

The Physician Global Assessment (PGA) scale is the physician's overall assessment of the severity of psoriasis. This is a 7-point scale with 0 being clear, 1 almost clear, 2 mild, 3 mild to moderate, 4 moderate, 5 moderate to severe, and 6 severe psoriasis.

To more accurately capture both the PASI and the PGA, the lattice system-PGA (LS-PGA) has been recently developed. This is an 8-point scale (1 to 8) with 1 being clear and 8 very severe. It incorporates BSA (measured by palm surface) of seven "percent " groupings as well as a matrix system to capture average plaque qualities (erythema, scale, and elevation).

The Psoriasis Disability Index (PDI) is another quantitative measure aimed to standardize and accurately capture the overall quality of life in adult patients with psoriasis. Several other assessment instruments also are used in psoriasis, including the Dermatology Quality of Life Index (DLQI) and the SF-36.

Clinical Types of Psoriasis

Plaque Psoriasis

Chronic plaque psoriasis or vulgaris-type disease is the most common form of psoriasis. It is typically symmetric and bilateral. Plaques are well demarcated (Fig. 71-3) and typically exhibit Auspitz sign (punctate bleeding after the removal of the scale) as well as manifesting Köbner's phenomenon (lesions induced by trauma). The most common distribution is the extensor surfaces (elbows and knees). The lower back, scalp, and nails are also frequently affected. Nail changes include onycholysis, pitting, oil spots, and nail dystrophy.

Guttate Psoriasis

The word "guttate" is derived from the Latin word *gutta,* meaning "drop." This variant primarily occurs on the trunk and the proximal

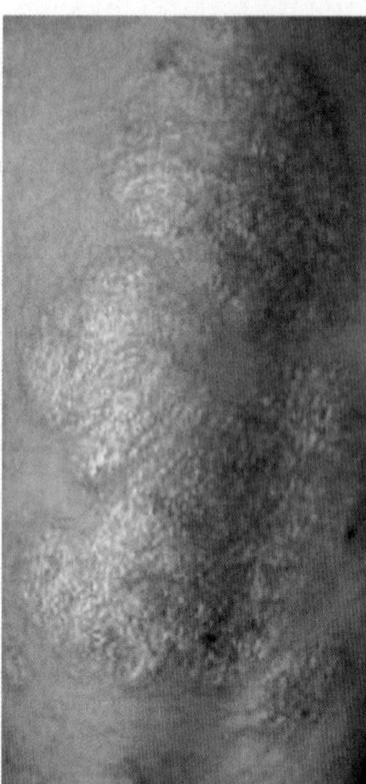

FIGURE 71-3 • Psoriasis plaque.

extremities, but it may have a generalized distribution. Guttate psoriasis is characterized by small, droplike, 1- to 10-mm diameter, salmon pink papules, usually with a fine scale. This form is more common in individuals after a history of upper respiratory infection secondary to group A β-hemolytic streptococci and precedes the eruption by 2 to 3 weeks. In children, an acute episode of guttate psoriasis is usually self-limiting; in adults, guttate flares may complicate chronic plaque disease. Compared with control populations, a significant excess of HLA-Bw17 and increased prevalence of HLA-Cw6 have been found in patients with guttate psoriasis.

Flexural (Inverse) Psoriasis

Psoriasis affecting the flexures, particularly the inframammary, perineal, and axillary folds, is distinct morphologically from traditional plaques elsewhere on the trunk and limbs. Flexural lesions are devoid of scale and appear as red, shiny, well-demarcated plaques occasionally confused with candida, intertrigo, and dermatophyte infections.

Erythroderma

Erythroderma usually occurs in the setting of known worsening or unstable psoriasis but may uncommonly be the first presentation of psoriasis; it is characterized by total or near-total involvement of the skin by active psoriasis. It can be precipitated by infections, low calcium, withdrawal of oral corticosteroids, discontinuation of extensive topical corticosteroids, and certain medications, including lithium, antimalarials and IL-2. Complications may include dehydration, heart failure, infection, anemia (due to loss of iron, vitamin B_{12}, and folate), hypothermia, protein loss, and malnutrion.

Localized and Generalized Pustular Psoriasis

This is an uncommon form of psoriasis, with the generalized form also known as von Zumbusch's psoriasis. It is characterized by the development of erythema and pustules in flexural areas as well as their appearance within established plaques of psoriasis. The pustules rupture easily and may become secondarily infected. This condition can be fatal if the patient becomes dehydrated, or complications of infections ensue. Precipitants include withdrawal of systemic or potent topical corticosteroids and infections.

Palmoplantar Pustulosis

Palmoplantar pustulosis affects the palms and soles and is associated with psoriasis in some individuals. It is characterized by groups of sterile pustules occurring in crops on one or both hands and/or feet. Pustulosis is associated with thickened, scaling, red skin that easily develops painful fissures. A considerably higher prevalence of smoking, in patients with palmoplantar pustulosis has been reported.[20] Approximately 25% of cases are associated with classical psoriasis vulgaris, but palmoplantar pustulosis may also represent a distinct entity.[21] This conclusion is derived from genetic studies showing no association with HLA-Cw6 or other markers on chromosome 6p- that are linked to chronic plaque and guttate psoriasis. The demographics of palmoplantar pustulosis are also different than classical plaque psoriasis, more commonly affecting women (9 : 1) and an older age group (onset 40 to 60 years), and having a strong association with smoking, either current or past, in up to 95% of subjects.

Psoriatic Nail Disease

Psoriatic nail dystrophy mainly occurs in patients suffering from psoriatic skin involvement. Fewer than 5% of patients solely manifest psoriasis of the nails. It is commonly seen in patients with psoriatic arthritis, especially when the arthritis affects the fingers and toes. Signs of nail psoriasis vary according to the part of the nail affected and the nature of the deformity. Oil drop sign, pitting, Beau's lines (transverse lines in nails due to intermittent inflammation causing growth arrest lines), leukonychia (areas of white nail plate due to foci of parakeratosis within the body of the nail plate), subungueal hyperkeratosis, onycholysis, and nail plate crumbling are characteristic abnormalities of psoriatic nail disease.

Psoriatic Arthritis

Psoriatic arthritis is a type of inflammatory arthritis that affects up to 30% to 40% of people with psoriasis. It may have very mild symptoms, and more severe forms occur more commonly in patients harboring HLA-B27. Treatment of psoriatic arthritis is similar to that of rheumatoid arthritis. More than 80% of patients with psoriatic arthritis will have psoriatic nail lesions characterized by pitting of the nails or onycholysis. Psoriatic arthritis is categorized as a seronegative spondyloarthropathy.

Psoriatic arthritis can develop at any age; however, on average, it tends to appear about a decade after the first signs of psoriasis. For the majority of individuals, onset is between the ages of 30 and 50 years, but it can rarely affect children. Men and women appear to be equally affected. In about one in seven cases, the arthritis symptoms occur before any skin involvement. It can also cause tendonitis, bursitis, and dactylitis.

Psoriatic arthritis has been subdivided into five distinct groups. The symmetric type (50% of cases) affects joints bilaterally and may be mistaken for rheumatoid arthritis. The asymmetric type (35% of cases) usually involves fewer than three joints (pauciarticular). Arthritis mutilans (<5% of cases) is a severe, deforming, and destructive arthritis of small and large joints. The spondylitis type causes stiffness of the spine and/or neck but can also affect the hands and feet. The distal interphalangeal predominant type (5% of cases) is less frequent.

In the very early stages of the disease, radiographs usually do not reveal signs of arthritis and often are not helpful in establishing the diagnosis. At later stages, radiographs may show changes that are characteristic of psoriatic arthritis not found with other types of arthritis, such as the "pencil-in-cup" phenomenon wherein the end of one bone is whittled and abuts an adjacent joint that forms the cup.

THERAPEUTICS AND CLINICAL PHARMACOLOGY

Therapeutics by Class

Topical Treatments

Topical Corticosteroids. Corticosteroids are a class of steroid hormones that are produced by the adrenal cortex. They are involved in a wide range of physiologic systems such as stress response, immune response and regulation of inflammation, carbohydrate metabolism, protein catabolism, blood electrolyte levels, and behavior. Glucocorticoids such as cortisol control carbohydrate, fat, and protein metabolism and are anti-inflammatory by preventing phospholipid release, decreasing eosinophil action, and a number of other mechanisms. Mineralocorticoids such as aldosterone control electrolyte and water levels, mainly by promoting sodium retention in the kidney.

The corticosteroids are synthesized from cholesterol within the adrenal cortex. Most steroidogenic reactions are catalyzed by enzymes of the cytochrome P-450 family. They are located within the mitochondria and require adrenodoxin as a cofactor (except 21-hydroxylase and 17α-hydroxylase). Aldosterone and corticosterone share the first part of their biosynthetic pathway. The last part is mediated either by aldosterone synthase or by 11β-hydroxylase. These enzymes are nearly identical (they share 11β-hydroxylation and 18-hydroxylation functions), but aldosterone synthase is also able to perform an 18-oxidation. Moreover, aldosterone synthase is found within the zona glomerulosa at the outer edge of the adrenal cortex; 11β-hydroxylase is found in the zonae fasciculata and reticularis.

Topical corticosteroids are absorbed at different rates and extent from different parts of the body. For example, a steroid having efficacy on the face may be ineffective on the palm. Extent of absorption from body areas includes

- Forearm: 1%
- Axilla: 4%
- Face: 7%
- Eyelids and genitals: 30%
- Palm: 0.1%
- Sole: 0.05%

Despite their demonstrated effectiveness as treatment for psoriasis, topical corticosteroids are associated with various side effects that may limit their use. The risk of these side effects depends on the strength of the steroid, the duration of application, the site treated, and the nature of the skin problem.

Local reactions usually occur when corticosteroids are used either with excessive frequency or duration or on particularly steroid-sensitive areas such as the face and intertriginous areas; they include atrophy, striae, telangiectases, acneiform eruption, rosacea, and contact dermatitis.[22] A potent steroid applied elsewhere on the body may cause side effects on the face. Systemic side effects, although uncommon, may occur when locally applied corticosteroids become absorbed through the skin and enter the general circulatory system. For example, if more than 50 g of clobetasol propionate (equivalent to 500 g of hydrocortisone) is used per week, sufficient steroid may be absorbed through the skin to result in adrenal gland suppression and/or eventually Cushing's syndrome. The greatest risk of systemic side effects occurs when ultra-high-potency or high-potency agents (Table 71-1) are used over a wide surface area for a prolonged period. Infants and small children are at elevated risk with any corticosteroid potency because of their increased skin surface–to–body mass ratio. Systemic effects of most concern are suppression of the hypothalamic-pituitary-adrenal axis, growth retardation in children, cataract formation, and glaucoma development. Proper use of superpotent topical corticosteroids is imperative. They should be used cautiously in patients with a history of diabetes mellitus, hypertension, liver failure, glaucoma, or positive tuberculin test results.[23]

In addition to localized and systemic side effects, tachyphylaxis has been reported to occur after long-term treatment with topical corticosteroids,[24] and this appears to be a major limiting factor in their use for psoriasis.

Calcipotriene. Calcipotriene (Dovonex), or calcipotriol, is a sythetic derivative of calcitriol or vitamin D. The exact mechanism by which calcipotriene improves psoriasis is not well understood. Calcipotriene has been shown to have comparable affinity with calcitriol for the vitamin D receptor (VDR), while being less than 1% as active as calcitriol in regulating calcium metabolism. VDR belongs to the steroid/thyroid receptor superfamily, and is expressed by cells of many different tissues including the thyroid, bone, kidney, and T cells of the immune system. T cells are known to play a role in psoriasis, and it is thought that the binding of calcipotriol to the VDR modulates the T cells' gene transcription of cell differentiation– and cell proliferation–related genes.

Available as a cream, ointment, or scalp solution, calcipotriene is applied twice daily to plaque psoriasis on the body or scalp, but not the face. Improvement is usually detectable within 2 weeks. It is also available in combination with the synthetic glucocorticoid betamethasone under the trade name Dovobet.

Calcipotriol has been shown in clinical trials to have an excellent safety profile. Reports of hypercalcemia are rare. However, less than 120 g should be used weekly. Other vitamin D analogues such as tacalcitol are also being used for psoriasis.

Tazarotene. Tazarotene (Tazorac, Avage, Zorac) is a prescription topical retinoid formulated as a cream or gel. This medication is approved for treatment of psoriasis, acne, and sun-damaged skin (photodamage). It is commonly prepared in two concentrations: 0.05% and 0.1%. The retinoids are a class of chemical compounds that are related chemically to vitamin A. Retinoids are used in medicine primarily to regulate epithelial cell growth and gene expression. Tazarotene belongs to the third generation of retinoids.

Tazarotene is a synthetic acetylenic retinoid that is hydrolyzed to its active form, tazarotenic acid. Unlike other retinoids, tazarotenic acid has selective affinity for the retinoic acid receptors. The exact molecular mechanism of action of topical tazarotene in the treatment of psoriasis has not been determined. Tazarotene appears to modulate the three main pathologic features of psoriasis: abnormal differentiation of keratinocytes, increased keratinocyte proliferation, and inflammation.[25]

Monotherapy of once-daily topical tazarotene 0.05% or 0.1% cream or gel effectively controlled signs and symptoms of plaque psoriasis in adult patients in randomized, single- or double-blind studies of 12 weeks' duration.[26] In these trials, topical tazarotene was significantly more effective than vehicle in terms of global treatment success rates, reduction in plaque elevation, and reduction in scaling scores. The efficacy of tazarotene was maintained over a 12-week posttreatment period. The addition of some, but not all, mid- to high-potency topical corticosteroids to tazarotene 0.1% gel monotherapy significantly improved global success rates and reduction in plaque elevation, scaling, and erythema.[26]

The penetration across human skin and, consequently, systemic absorption are limited. Low plasma concentrations of tazarotene were detected in 1% to 3% of patients in 12-week, Phase III clinical trials of tazarotene 0.05% or 0.1% gel or cream monotherapy in patients with plaque psoriasis.

Common side effects include dry skin, pruritus, redness, and, in some cases, extreme drying and cracking of skin. For most patients, these side effects are uncomfortable but mild and decrease markedly after the first 2 to 4 weeks of use. In clinical trials, 9% to 20% of tazarotene gel recipients discontinued treatment because of adverse effects. The addition of a corticosteroid to tazarotene monotherapy generally reduces the incidence of adverse effects. Tazarotene has also been shown to ameliorate the skin atrophy induced by a corticosteroid as it has been shown to increase epidermal thickness.

Tars. Tar is a viscous black liquid derived from the destructive distillation of organic matter. Most tar is produced from coal as a by-product of coke production, but it can also be produced from petroleum, peat, or wood. In English and French convention, "tar" is a substance primarily derived from coal. It was formerly one of the products of gasworks. Tar made from coal or petroleum is considered toxic and carcinogenic because of its high benzene and aromatic hydrocarbon content. However, coal tar in low concentrations is used as a topical medicament. Coal and petroleum tar has a pungent odor.

According to the International Agency for Research on Cancer, preparations that include more than 5% crude coal tar are Group 1 carcinogens. Despite this, the National Psoriasis Foundation claims coal tar is a valuable, safe, and inexpensive treatment option for millions of people with psoriasis and other scalp conditions. The U.S. Food and Drug Administration (FDA) agrees, and states that coal tar

TABLE 71-1 TOPICAL CORTICOSTEROIDS

Brand Name	Generic Name
CLASS 1—SUPERPOTENT (UP TO 600 TIMES AS POTENT AS HYDROCORTISONE)	
Clobex Lotion/Spray/Shampoo, 0.05%	Clobetasol propionate
Cormax Cream/Solution, 0.05%	Clobetasol propionate
Diprolene Gel/Ointment, 0.05%	Betamethasone dipropionate
Olux Foam, 0.05%	Clobetasol propionate
Psorcon Ointment, 0.05%	Diflorasone diacetate
Temovate Cream/Ointment/Solution, 0.05%	Clobetasol propionate
Ultravate Cream/Ointment, 0.05%	Halobetasol propionate
Vanos Cream, 0.1%	Fluocinonide
CLASS 2—POTENT (50-100 TIMES AS POTENT AS HYDROCORTISONE)	
Cyclocort Ointment, 0.1%	Amcinonide
Diprolene Cream AF, 0.05%	Betamethasone dipropionate
Diprosone Ointment, 0.05%	Betamethasone dipropionate
Elocon Ointment, 0.1%	Mometasone furoate
Florone Ointment, 0.05%	Diflorasone diacetate
Halog Ointment/Cream, 0.1%	Halcinonide
Lidex Cream/Gel/Ointment, 0.05%	Fluocinonide
Maxiflor Ointment, 0.05%	Diflorasone diacetate
Maxivate Ointment, 0.05%	Betamethasone dipropionate
Psorcon Cream, 0.05%	Diflorasone diacetate
Taclonex Ointment, 0.064%	Betamethasone dipropionate and calcipotriene
Topicort Cream/Ointment, 0.25%	Desoximetasone
Topicort Gel, 0.05%	Desoximetasone
CLASS 3—UPPER MID-STRENGTH (2-25 TIMES AS POTENT AS HYDROCORTISONE)	
Aristocort A Ointment, 0.1%	Triamcinolone acetonide
Cutivate Ointment, 0.05%	Fluticasone propionate
Cyclocort Cream/Lotion, 0.1%	Amcinonide
Diprosone Cream, 0.05%	Betamethasone dipropionate
Florone Cream, 0.05%	Diflorasone diacetate
Lidex-E Cream, 0.05%	Fluocinonide
Luxiq Foam, 0.12%	Betamethasone valerate
Maxiflor Cream, 0.05%	Diflorasone diacetate
Maxivate Cream/Lotion, 0.05%	Betamethasone dipropionate
Topicort Cream, 0.05%	Desoximetasone
CLASS 4—MID-STRENGTH	
Aristocort Cream, 0.1%	Triamcinolone acetonide
Cordran Ointment, 0.05%	Flurandrenolide
Elocon Cream, 0.1%	Mometasone furoate
Kenalog Cream/Ointment/Spray, 0.1%	Triamcinolone acetonide
Synalar Ointment, 0.025%	Fluocinolone acetonide
Uticort Gel, 0.025%	Betamethasone benzoate
Westcort Ointment, 0.2%	Hydrocortisone valerate
CLASS 5—LOWER MID-STRENGTH	
Cordran Cream/Lotion/Tape, 0.05%	Flurandrenolide
Cutivate Cream, 0.05%	Fluticasone propionate
DermAtop Cream, 0.1%	Prednicarbate
DesOwen Ointment, 0.05%	Desonide
Diprosone Lotion, 0.05%	Betamethasone dipropionate
Kenalog Lotion, 0.1%	Triamcinolone acetonide
Locoid Cream, 0.1%	Hydrocortisone
Pandel Cream, 0.1%	Hydrocortisone
Synalar Cream, 0.025%	Fluocinolone acetonide
Uticort Cream/Lotion, 0.025%	Betamethasone benzoate
Valisone Cream/Ointment, 0.1%	Betamethasone valerate
Westcort Cream, 0.2%	Hydrocortisone valerate
CLASS 6—MILD	
Aclovate Cream/Ointment, 0.05%	Aclometasone dipropionate
Derma-Smoothe/FS Oil, 0.01%	Fluocinolone acetonide
DesOwen Cream, 0.05%	Desonide
Synalar Cream/Solution, 0.01%	Fluocinolone acetonide
Tridesilon Cream, 0.05%	Desonide
CLASS 7—LEAST POTENT	
Topicals with hydrocortisone, dexamethasone, methylprednisolone, and prednisolone	

Modified from National Psoriasis Foundation, 2006.

Practice: Dermatologic Therapeutics

concentrations between 0.5% and 5% are safe and effective for psoriasis and that no scientific evidence suggests that the coal tar in the concentrations used in nonprescription treatments is overtly carcinogenic.

Exactly how coal tar exerts its activity in these conditions is not completely understood. It appears to have antimicrobial, antipruritic, and keratoplastic (normalizes epidermal growth and reduce scaling) effects.

Most patients tolerate coal tar preparations well. Coal tar may initially cause mild burning or skin irritation. When used on the scalp, it may temporarily discolor bleached, tinted, light blond, or grey hair. Coal tar also stains skin and clothing. Skin staining fades after the treatment has been stopped. Coal tar may cause photosensitivity (ultraviolet A [UVA] range), hence the need to stay out of direct sunlight when using these preparations.

Goeckerman Regimen. The Goeckerman regimen was described by Dr. Goeckerman in 1925 at the Mayo Clinic. Once- or twice-daily skin applications of crude coal tar for at least 4 hr/day are performed, followed by vegetable oil removal before the patient is exposed to total body UVB radiation. This is followed by a cleansing bath or shower to remove the residual tar and scales. The regimen can be supplemented with steroid medications and keratolytics, particularly in the early stages of treatment. In a modification of the Goeckerman regimen, anthralin is used instead of coal tar (this is called the Ingram regimen).

Compared with the original Goeckerman method, the modern, modified Goeckerman therapy in use in the 21st century shows significantly enhanced efficacy through improvements in technology (e.g., narrowband UVB [NB-UVB]) and the possibility of adding other relatively safe therapeutic options for more resistant cases to enhance efficacy without compromising the basic safety profile. Studies have demonstrated attainment of PASI 75 within 3 to 4 weeks of intensive treatment.[27] The Goeckerman regimen is one of the most effective treatments for psoriasis. It is regarded as messy, inconvenient, and time consuming compared to most newer therapies, and, thus, has limited utility in modern psoriasis treatment, even in day care programs that formerly offered this treatment option to many patients.

Anthralin. Anthralin or dithranol (Dithrocream, Micanol, Psorlin) is a hydroxyanthrone (anthracene derivative) medicine applied to the skin of people with psoriasis. It is available as creams, ointment, or pastes in 0.1 to 2% strengths. This substance has been used to treat psoriasis for more than 100 years.

Several mechanisms of action have been identified. Dithranol accumulates in mitochondria, where it interferes with the supply of energy to the cell, probably by the oxidation of dithranol releasing free radicals. This impedes DNA replication and so slows the excessive cell division that occurs in psoriatic plaques. Dithranol has also been shown to cause apoptosis and cell death of lymphocytes with significantly greater sensitivity than keratinocytes, effectively eliminating these pathogenic immune-inflammatory cells from lesional skin. In addition, dithranol may act by reducing the elevated levels of cyclic GMP that occurs in psoriasis.

More dithranol penetrates into impaired skin in 30 minutes than into intact skin over 16 hours. For this reason, weaker 0.1% to 0.5% preparations are applied overnight, but stronger 1% to 2% products are applied for between 30 minutes and 1 hour (short-contact anthralin therapy) depending upon the formulation. Short-contact therapy is designed for patients with localized areas of psoriasis. Anthralin is left on the involved skin for a short period of time, ranging from 10 minutes to an hour. Patients may be instructed to gradually increase the amount of contact time as their skin becomes accustomed to the medication.

Dithranol has a slower onset of action in controlling psoriasis, typically several weeks, compared to glucocorticoid steroids, but has far less potential for rebound reactions on withdrawal or tachyphylaxis. It cannot be used on the face or genitalia. It temporarily stains the skin a yellowish brown and permanently stains clothing fabrics. It may cause a local burning sensation and irritation; this can be minimized by careful attention to the details of treatment application and gradually increasing the strengths of dithranol formulations applied. Much of the irritation and staining from anthralin use can be prevented with the application of triethanolamine, a nonsteroidal chemical used for many years as a stabilizer in soaps and cosmetics.

Psoriatec is an anthralin formulation designed to reduce the risk of staining and irritation. It is a 1% anthralin cream in which the active ingredient is surrounded by a protective layer of lipids. These layers melt at body temperature, releasing the anthralin only on the skin where it is applied, not on clothes, bedding, or bathroom fixtures.

The Ingram regimen combines anthralin paste and UVB exposure. Anthralin is applied to lesions as a thick paste. Once the anthralin is removed, the patient is then exposed to UVB and may also take coal tar baths. Generally, a patient using the Ingram regimen in the hospital or a day treatment program will require 3 weeks of therapy, with clearing in an average of 20 days.

Salicylic Acid. Salicylic acid is the chemical compound with the formula $C_6H_4(OH)CO_2H$, where the OH group is adjacent to the carboxyl group. It is also known as 2-hydroxybenzoic acid. Salicylic acid belongs to a group of medicines known as keratolytics. Salicylic acid works by softening keratin, a protein that forms the major part of the outer skin structure. This helps to loosen dry, scaly skin, making it easier to remove. When salicylic acid is used in combination with other medicines, it desquamates the upper layer of skin, allowing the additional medicines to penetrate more effectively. Salicylic acid is available over the counter in concentrations up to 3%; concentrations greater than 3% are only available by prescription.

Salicylic acid preparations are usually well tolerated. Mild stinging may occur, especially on broken skin and when higher concentrations are used. Salicylic acid can irritate or burn healthy skin, so it is important to keep the medicine confined to the affected area(s).

Tacrolimus. Tacrolimus (Prograf, Protopic) and Pimecrolimus (Elidel) is an immunosuppressive drug whose main use is after allogenic organ transplant to reduce the activity of the patient's immune system and so the risk of organ rejection. It is a 23-membered macrolide lactone discovered in 1984 from the fermentation broth of a Japanese soil sample that contained the bacteria *Streptomyces tsukubaensis*.

It is also used in a topical preparation in the treatment of severe atopic dermatitis, vitiligo and other skin conditions. Topically, it suppresses inflammation similar to steroids, and is equally as effective as a mid-potency steroid. An important advantage of tacrolimus is that, unlike steroids, it does not cause skin atrophy or other steroid related side-effects. It has been approved for the treatment of atopic dermatitis, however it can be used topically to treat mild psoriasis in pediatric patients and/or treat areas where a topical steroid is not recommended. Long-term efficacy and safety of topical tacrolimus solely or in combination in the treatment of psoriasis must be evaluated. It can be used 0.3% ointment daily or 0.1% ointment twice per day. Similarly, pimecrolimus (Elidel) can be used as the 1% formulation twice per day.

Tacrolimus is chemically known as a macrolide. It reduces peptidylprolyl isomerase activity by binding to the immunophilin FKBP-12 (FK506 binding protein) creating a new complex. This FKBP12-FK506 complex interacts with and inhibits calcineurin, thus inhibiting both T-lymphocyte signal transduction and IL-2 transcription.[28] Although this activity is similar to cyclosporine, studies have shown that the incidence of acute rejection is reduced by tacrolimus versus cyclosporine.

Pimecrolimus is an ascomycin macrolactam derivative. It has been shown in vitro that pimecrolimus binds to macrophilin-12 and inhibits calcineurin. Thus, pimecrolimus inhibits T-cell activation by inhibiting the synthesis and release of cytokines from T-cells. Pimecrolimus also prevents the release of inflammatory cytokines and mediators from mast cells. Topical pimecrolimus is also used in mild psoriasis in areas where other topical treatments are contraindicated, even though it has been approved for atopic dermatitis.

Tacrolimus and pimecrolimus have been suspected of carrying a cancer risk, though the matter is still a subject of controversy. The FDA issued a health warning in March 2005 for the topical formulations of these drugs, based on animal models and a small number of patients. Until further human studies yield more conclusive results, the FDA recommends that users be advised of the potential risks.

The European FK506 Multi-Center Psoriasis Study Group randomized 50 patients with recalcitrant plaque-type psoriasis to receive either oral tacrolimus or placebo in a double-blind, prospective study.[29] The initial dose of tacrolimus was 0.05 mg/kg per day and increased gradually to 1.5 mg/kg per day at week 6 to improve efficacy. At 9 weeks, tacrolimus-treated patients experienced greater reductions in PASI compared to placebo. The group determined that oral tacrolimus was an effective treatment for recalcitrant plaque-type psoriasis, and that most side-effects were mild to moderate in severity.

Phototherapy

Light therapy or phototherapy consists of exposure to specific wavelengths of light using lasers, light-emitting diodes, fluorescent lamps, dichroic lamps, or very bright, full-spectrum light (radiation) for a prescribed amount of time.

Ultraviolet (UV) radiation (light) is electromagnetic radiation with a wavelength shorter than that of visible light, but longer than soft x-rays. UVA, long-wave, or black light has a wavelength of 400 to 320 nm. UVB or medium-wave radiation has a wavelength of 320 to 280 nm, and ultraviolet C (UVC), short-wave, or germicidal radiation has a wavelength of less than 280 nm. The sun emits UV radiation in the UVA, UVB, and UVC band ranges, but because of absorption in the atmosphere's ozone layer, 99% of the ultraviolet radiation that reaches the Earth's surface is UVA. The primary advantageous biologic effect of UVB exposure for humans is that it induces the production of vitamin D in the skin.

UVA, UVB, and UVC each have several target chromogens in skin. UV has the potential to damage proteins, including collagen fibers, and thereby accelerate aging of the skin. In general, UVA is the least harmful, but can contribute to the aging of skin, DNA damage, and possibly skin cancer. UVB radiation can cause skin cancer. The radiation alters DNA molecules in skin cells, causing covalent bonds to form between adjacent thymine bases, producing thymidine dimers. Thymidine dimers do not base pair normally, which can cause distortion of the DNA helix, stalled replication, gaps, and mis-incorporation. These lead to mutations, which can result in cancer development.

Phototherapy, especially UVB light therapy and photochemotherapy, remains an essential treatment option for patients with moderate to severe psoriasis. Natural sunlight for the treatment of psoriasis has been used for centuries. A mainstay of therapy for psoriasis during the midportion of the 20th century was the use of UVB produced by an artificial light source. The current mainstay for office-based UV light therapy is fluorescent lamp sources, which produce a wide range of UV radiation emissions. UVB sources contain higher energy, lower frequency UV radiation and carry a greater potential for erythemogenic responses and sunburning reactions. UVB treatment can be administered to adults and children, and is effective in treating psoriasis for at least two thirds of patients who meet these criteria: thinner plaques, moderate to severe disease (involving >2% of the skin), and/or responsive to natural sunlight.

The most efficient approach is first to determine the minimal erythema dose (MED), which is a biologic response (pink-red appearance) of the skin to that particular UVB radiation source or unit. The MED is determined and phototherapy is initiated at 70% to 75% MED, increasing steadily (as much as 50% MED) at each visit. A patient generally will receive treatments three to five times per week. It takes an average of 30 treatments to reach maximum improvement of psoriasis lesions.

NB-UVB refers to a specific wavelength of UV radiation, 311 to 312 nm. Compared with broadband UVB (BB-UVB), exposure times are shorter but of higher intensity. The course of treatment is typically shorter, and efficacy of NB-UVB is typically greater. Longer periods of remission also have been shown for NB-UVB. The long-term safety of NB- versus BB-UVB phototherapy is uncertain. "Selective" BB-UVB lamps, which have little emission less than 290 nm, are also available but have not been adequately compared to NB-UVB lamps. Dosing of NB-UVB has been compared by a half-body treatment study with either 70% or 35% MED. A total of 55% of patients in the 70% MED group and 27% in the 35% MED group achieved PASI 75 or greater at 3 weeks.[30]

A randomized comparison of NB-UVB and selective BB-UVB in 100 patients with psoriasis has been performed. Side effects, including the development of erythema during phototherapy, were similar for the two lamp types. Risk estimates based on the human photocarcinogenesis action spectrum predict that NB-UVB lamps will be 50% more carcinogenic for equal erythemal doses than selective BB-UVB lamps. As these two lamp types appear to be of similar efficacy, phototherapy using a selective BB-UVB source may be a safer option than use of NB-UVB.[31]

Combination Photochemotherapy

UVA (Psoralen + UVA). PUVA photochemotherapy has been in routine clinical use since the 1970s. Psoralen is applied topically or taken orally to sensitize the skin, followed by UVA exposure. Long-term use has been associated with higher rates of skin cancer. Psoralens are photosensitizing agents found in plants. 8-Methoxypsoralen is used in the United States, and, in Europe, 5-methoxypsoralen is also used as it has fewer gastrointestinal (GI) side effects. Therapeutic benefits of psoralens have been known since ancient Egypt but have only been available in chemically synthesized forms since the 1970s. Psoralens are taken systemically or can be applied directly to the skin. The psoralens are photosensitizing and allow a much lower dose of UVA to achieve a biologic response. When they are combined with exposure to UVA in PUVA, they are highly effective at clearing psoriasis. The full mechanism(s) of action of the psoralen molecule and UVA in the treatment of psoriasis have not been entirely clear but likely involve targeting the pathogenic T cells within psoriatic lesions.

The psoralen molecule intercalates between DNA base pairs but also has effects on the cell membrane. There is no biochemical interaction between the psoralen molecule and DNA itself without activation or absorption of photons of UV radiation as a photodynamic effect. A photochemical reaction results with the psoralen molecule and a pyrimidine base, and DNA cross-links occur. Formation of the cyclobutane ring requires an additional photochemical reaction. In addition to its therapeutic effects, DNA alterations likely account for the increased development of squamous cell and basal cell carcinomas with repetitive therapy over years.

A second mechanism of action of PUVA therapy on inflammatory skin disorders is oxygen-dependent photochemical reactions. This type of reaction causes membrane and cell damage and may be central to the observable effects of UV light on the skin. APCs and T lymphocytes are more susceptible to these oxygen-dependent reactions than keratinocytes, and the underlying mechanism of action of PUVA photochemotherapy appears to be inhibition of immunocyte activation and immune recruitment of additional T cells into the skin.[32]

The duration of remission following clearing with PUVA is more durable than with UVB therapy. However, with new treatment alternatives and the increased risk of squamous cell carcinoma (SCC), especially in fair-skinned individuals with greater than 250 treatments over time, PUVA has diminished popularity. PUVA is considered for moderate to severe cases of psoriasis in adults. Stable plaque psoriasis, guttate psoriasis, and psoriasis of the palms and soles are especially responsive to PUVA treatments.

PUVA is not normally recommended for children or teenagers. However, it can be used by young people to avoid unwanted side effects of other treatments or if other treatments have not been successful.

Choosing the proper dose for PUVA is similar to the procedure followed with UVB. A starting dose is typically selected based on the patient's skin type. Often, however, a small area of the patient's skin is exposed to UVA after ingestion of psoralen. The dose of UVA that produces uniform redness 48 to 72 hours later, called the minimum phototoxic dose, becomes the starting dose for treatment. One of the most common side effects of psoralen is nausea.

The primary long-term risk of PUVA treatment is a higher risk of skin cancer, particularly SCC as well as basal cell carcinoma. Some

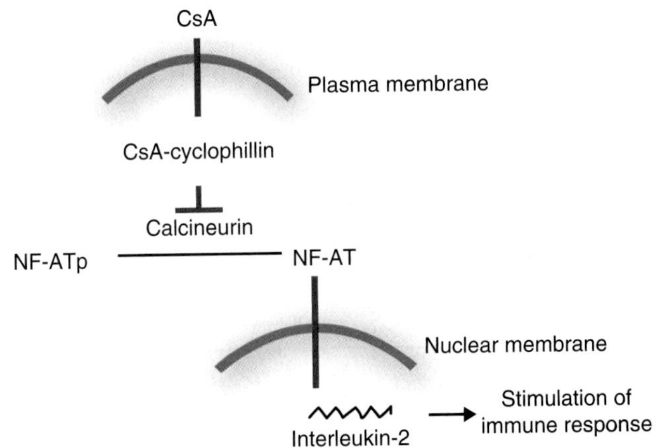

FIGURE 71-4 • Mechanism of action of cyclosporine.

studies have shown that oral retinoid use during PUVA treatment decreases the risk of developing SCCs.[33] There is a potential for PUVA to induce cataracts if the eyes are not protected. Psoralen remains in the eye lens for a period of time following ingestion of the drug. To date, no increase in cataracts has been noted in patients using proper eye protection.

Other Combinations. Combination photochemotherapy for treatment of psoriasis has gained popularity over the past several decades as more therapeutic agents become clinically available. Topical steroids are still the most common treatment for mild plaque-type psoriasis and can be used safely in combination with phototherapy. When superpotent topical corticosteroids are used, a regimen of using the initial treatment for induction followed by tapering and discontinuation of topical steroids should be used. Calcipotriene can also be used with phototherapy. However, it should be applied after phototherapy as UV will inactivate the compound. Topical retinoids also should be used a few hours after phototherapy.

Another effective combination therapy with UV radiation is use of systemic retinoids.[34] The treatment rationale for combining retinoids with UV light is to reduce the total energy delivered to the skin and enhance the therapeutic regimen by decreasing the total number of treatments needed. Retinoids also have antitumorigenic activities and suppress carcinogenic progression.

The approach of this treatment is to initiate therapy with the retinoid for at least 7 to 14 days to establish the retinoid effect on the skin and its modification on the psoriatic plaques. The effect of the retinoids is to decrease the thickness of the plaques and the scaling, allowing the UV therapy to be more effective. Retinoids also increase susceptibility to erythema from UVB and enhance the phototoxic effects from PUVA. Nowadays acitretin is the most widely used retinoid in combination with phototherapy.

Other systemic treatments can be used in combination with phototherapy. Methotrexate and cyclosporine have both been used. Cyclosporine and phototherapy should be used cautiously because, in combination with PUVA, cyclosporine further increases the risk of SCC development.[35]

Calcipotriol-PUVA has shown to be more effective than PUVA alone. A randomized, multicenter, vehicle-controlled, double-blind, 12-week comparative study examined 120 patients with psoriasis covering 20% to 50% of BSA. The study consisted of a washout phase followed by a 10-week treatment phase. PUVA therapy three times weekly was added within 1 week after randomization. At baseline, the mean PASI scores were 17.5 and 19.2 in the calcipotriol and vehicle (placebo) groups, respectively. At the end of treatment, the mean PASI scores were 2.65 and 7.03, respectively. A reduction in PASI score greater than 90% was observed in 69% of the patients in the calcipotriol-treated group and in 36.4% of the patients in the vehicle group.[36]

Oral Treatments

Methotrexate. Methotrexate (Folex, Mexate, Amethopterin, Rheumatrex, Trexall) was the first systemic therapy for patients with moderate to severe psoriasis and remains one of the most prescribed systemic agents. Methotrexate replaced the more powerful and toxic antifolate aminopterin, and the two should not be confused with each other.

Methotrexate competitively and reversibly inhibits dihydrofolate reductase (DHFR), an enzyme that is part of the folate synthesis metabolic pathway. The affinity of methotrexate for DHFR is about 1000-fold that of folate for DHFR. DHFR catalyses the conversion of dihydrofolate to the active tetrahydrofolate. Folic acid is required for the de novo synthesis of the nucleoside thymidine, required for DNA synthesis. Methotrexate, therefore, inhibits the synthesis of DNA, RNA, thymidylates, and proteins (Fig. 71-4).

Methotrexate acts specifically during DNA and RNA synthesis and, thus, is cytotoxic during the S phase of the cell cycle. It therefore has a greater toxic effect on rapidly dividing cells (such as malignant and myeloid cells as well as GI and oral mucosa) and, thus, inhibits the growth and proliferation of these noncancerous cells as well as causing the side effects noted later.

Lower doses of methotrexate have been shown to be very effective for the management of rheumatoid arthritis and psoriasis. In these cases, inhibition of DHFR is not thought to be the main mechanism. Rather, there is inhibition of enzymes involved in purine metabolism like amidophosphoribosyltransferase, leading to accumulation of adenosine, or the inhibition of T-cell activation and suppression of intracellular adhesion molecule expression by T cells.[37]

Mean oral bioavailability is 33% (range 13% to 76%), and there is no clear benefit to subdividing an oral dose. Mean intramuscular bioavailability is 76%. Methotrexate is metabolized by intestinal bacteria to the inactive metabolite 4-amino-4-deoxy-*N*-methylpteroic acid, which accounts for less than 5% loss of the oral dose. Factors that decrease absorption include food, oral nonabsorbable antibiotics (e.g., vancomycin, neomycin, and bacitracin), and more rapid transit through the GI tract (e.g., with diarrhea), while slower transit time in the GI tract (e.g., with constipation) will increase absorption.

Possible side effects include anemia, neutropenia, increased risk of bruising, nausea and vomiting, dermatitis and diarrhea with blood in the stools, headache and alopecia. A small percentage of patients develop hepatitis, and there is an increased risk of pulmonary fibrosis. If sores appear in the mouth, the dose may be too high. The higher doses of methotrexate often used in cancer chemotherapy can cause toxic effects to the rapidly dividing cells of bone marrow and GI mucosa. The resulting myelosuppression and mucositis are often prevented (termed methotrexate "rescue") by using folinic acid supplements (not to be confused with folic acid).

Methotrexate is a highly teratogenic drug and is categorized in Pregnancy Category X by the FDA. Women must not take the drug during pregnancy, if there is a risk of becoming pregnant, or if they are breastfeeding. Men who are trying to get their partner pregnant must also not take the drug. To safely engage in any of these activities (after discontinuing the drug), women must wait until the end of a full ovulation cycle and men must wait 3 months.

The main risk of long-term methotrexate treatment is the potential for liver damage. A small percentage of patients (0.5%) will develop reversible liver scarring. This is a risk after a cumulative dose of 1.5 g. How long it takes to reach 1.5 g depends on the patient's dose, treatment schedule and rest periods from the drug. When a patient reaches a cumulative dose of 1 to 1.5 g, liver biopsy to test for liver damage is often recommended. If significant liver damage is observed, methotrexate is usually discontinued.

Anti-inflammatory medications should be avoided while the patient is receiving methotrexate. These drugs elevate the effects of methotrexate to potentially harmful levels. Vaccines should be avoided due to the immunosuppressive action of methotrexate, and ethanol consumption should be strictly avoided to reduce the risk of liver complications.

Methotrexate is indicated for use in adults with severe psoriasis. Methotrexate is often prescribed for severe plaque psoriasis, ery-

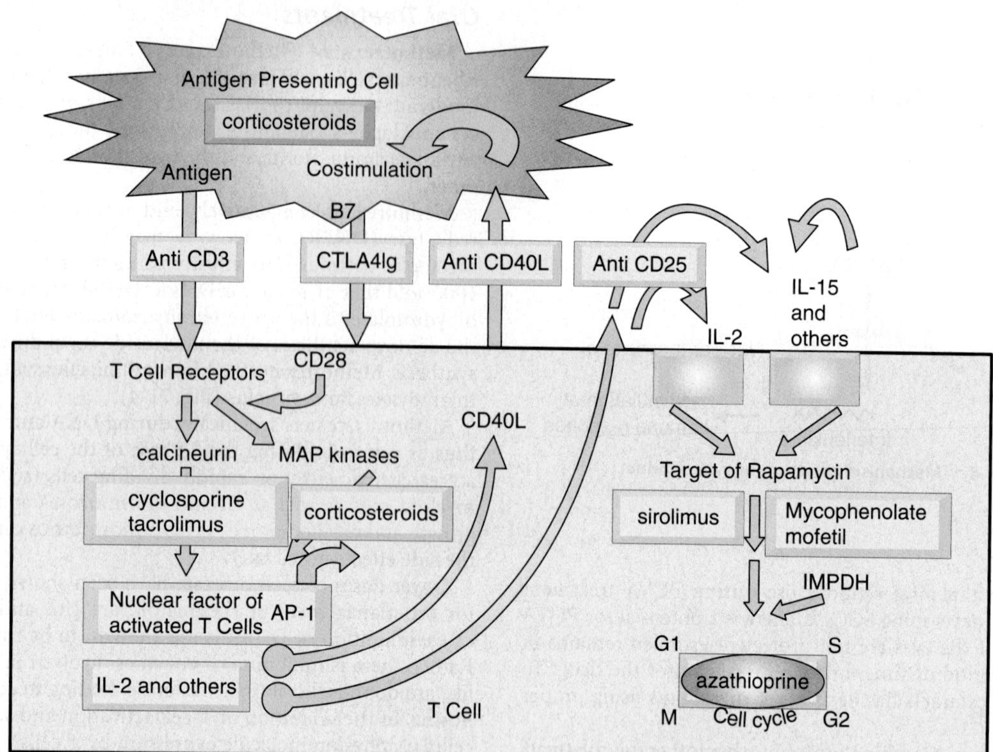

FIGURE 71-5 • Mechanism of action of different biologics and systemic treatments.

throdermic psoriasis, and acute pustular psoriasis. The drug can also be used to treat psoriatic arthritis. Methotrexate is sometimes used on a rotational basis with other treatments such as PUVA, acitretin, or cyclosporine in order to decrease treatment duration side effects or improve results. It is usually taken once per week, either orally or by injection. In psoriasis, the weekly dose is often divided into three doses given at 12-hour intervals each week. There is evidence that this dosing schedule increases efficacy.

In psoriasis, the recommended starting dose schedule is weekly single oral, intramuscular, or intravenous administration of 10 to 25 mg/wk until an adequate response is achieved. The divided oral dose schedule is 2.5 to 5 mg at 12-hour intervals for three doses. Dosages in each schedule may be gradually adjusted to achieve optimal clinical response, and the minimum effective dose should be sought for long-term control of skin disease; however, 30 mg/wk should not ordinarily be exceeded.

Folic acid supplementation 1 mg/day is recommended because it mitigates the GI effects of methotrexate (nausea, diarrhea, elevated liver enzymes) without altering its efficacy. It also prevents megaloblastic anemia due to folic acid deficiency.

A randomized, controlled trial comparing methotrexate and cyclosporine was conducted with an average dose of cyclosporine 4.5 mg/kg per day and methotrexate 22.5 mg/wk for 16 weeks, with a 36-week follow up. By week 16, PASI 75 was achieved by 60% of the methotrexate group and 71% of cyclosporine group.[38]

Cyclosporine. Cyclosporine (Sandimmune, Cicloral, Gengraf, Neoral) is an immunosuppressant drug widely used in postallogeneic organ and bone marrow transplantation to reduce the activity of the patient's immune system and the risk of organ rejection. Cyclosporin A, the main form of the drug, is a cyclic peptide of 11 amino acids produced by the fungus *Tolypocladium inflatum* Gams, initially isolated from a Norwegian soil sample.

Cyclosporine is thought to bind to the cytosolic protein cyclophilin of immunocompetent lymphocytes, especially T lymphocytes (Fig. 71-5). This complex of cyclosporine and cyclophilin inhibits calcineurin, which activates transcription of IL-2. It also inhibits lymphokine production and interleukin release and, therefore, leads to a reduced function of effector T cells. It does not affect cytostatic activity. It has also an effect on mitochondria. Cyclosporin A also prevents mitochondrial PT pore opening, thus inhibiting release of cytochrome *c*, a potent apoptotic stimulation factor. However, this is not the primary mode of action in clinical use. An alternate form of the drug, cyclosporin G, has been found to be much less nephrotoxic than the standard cyclosporin A. Cyclosporin G differs from cyclosporin A in the amino acid 2 position, where an L-nor-valine replaces the α-aminobutyric acid.

Cyclosporine side effects include gum hyperplasia, convulsions, peptic ulcers, pancreatitis, fever, vomiting, diarrhea, confusion, breathing difficulties, numbness and tingling, pruritus, high blood pressure, potassium retention and possibly hyperkalemia, nephrotoxicity, hepatotoxicity, and obviously an increased vulnerability to opportunistic fungal and viral infections. Cyclosporine interacts with a wide variety of other drugs and other substances, including grapefruit juice, although there have been studies using grapefruit juice to increase the blood level of cyclosporine.

Extended use of cyclosporine by transplantation patients is well established. However, long-term use as a treatment for psoriasis is more limited. Therefore, use of the drug is not currently recommended by the FDA for longer than 1 year. A risk of long-term cyclosporine treatment is kidney damage/toxicity. In some cases, the damage to the kidneys can be irreversible. People taking cyclosporine have an increased risk of developing skin malignancies, particularly if they have a history of nonmelanoma skin cancers.

Oral Retinoids. Retinoids have a structure similar to vitamin A and regulate normal growth and differentiation of skin cells. Acitretin acts by inhibiting the excessive cell growth and aberrant keratinization seen in psoriasis. It reduces acanthosis of the epidermis as well as plaque formation and scaling. Acitretin is the only oral retinoid approved by the FDA specifically for treating psoriasis. Isotretinoin is sometimes used as an alternative. Isotretinoin is cleared from the body much faster than acitretin, often making it a safer choice for young women of childbearing potential. However, both have the potential for severe birth defects if a woman becomes pregnant and drug remains in the system.

Side effects of oral retinoids are extensive, and physicians prescribing this medication should recognize its potentially serious consequences.

Patients should be evaluated frequently for adverse effects and to ensure compliance with therapy. Side effects include

Common: dryness of skin, lips, and mucous membranes; cheilitis, itch, skin fragility, skin peeling, rash, flushing, photosensitivity; nosebleeds; dry eyes, eye irritation, conjunctivitis, reduced tolerance to contact lenses; hyperlipidemia, raised liver enzymes; headaches; hair thinning; myalgia and/or arthralgia

Infrequent: raised blood glucose level, increased erythrocyte sedimentation rate, fatigue and/or mood changes

Rare: impaired night vision, cataracts, optic neuritis, menstrual disturbances, inflammatory bowel disease, pancreatitis, hepatitis, corneal opacities, papilloedema, idiopathic intracranial hypertension, skeletal hyperostosis, extraosseous calcification, moderate memory loss

The following adverse effects have been reported to persist, even after discontinuing therapy: alopecia (hair loss), arthralgias, decreased night vision, degenerative disk disease, keloids, bone disease, and depression (in some cases). Patients receiving oral retinoid therapy are not permitted to donate blood during and for at least 1 month after discontinuation of therapy. Several studies have suggested a possible link between oral retinoids and clinical depression. However, no conclusive evidence has been produced.

Oral retinoids can cause birth defects in the developing fetus, including defects of the central nervous system, skull, eyes, and cardiovascular system. It is important that women of childbearing age are not pregnant and do not become pregnant while taking this medication. Women must sign consent forms and take a pregnancy test prior to initiation of retinoids. Women must use two separate effective forms of birth control at the same time for 1 month before treatment begins, during the entire course of treatment, and for 1 full month after stopping the drug. In the United States, the process of ensuring that pregnancy is avoided has been mandated by the U.S. government via the iPLEDGE program. iPLEDGE is a computer-based risk management program designed to further the public health goal to eliminate fetal exposure to isotretinoin through a special restricted distribution program approved by the FDA. The program strives to ensure that

- No female patient starts isotretinoin therapy if pregnant
- No female patient on isotretinoin therapy becomes pregnant

Since March 2006, the dispensing of isotretinoin in the United States has been controlled by an FDA-mandated website called iPLEDGE. Dermatologists are required to register their patients before prescribing, and pharmacists are required to check the web site before dispensing the drug.

The concurrent use of oral retinoids with tetracycline antibiotics or vitamin A supplementation is not recommended. Concurrent use of oral retinoids with tetracycline significantly increases the risk of idiopathic intracranial hypertension. Concurrent intake of vitamin A supplementation increases the risk of vitamin A toxicity.

Acitretin. Acitretin (Soriatane) is a second-generation retinoid. It is a metabolite of etretinate, which was marketed prior to the introduction of acitretin. Etretinate was discontinued because it had a narrow therapeutic index as well as a long elimination half-life of 120 days, making dosing difficult. In contrast, acitretin's half-life is approximately 2 days. The mechanism of action of acitretin likely involves targeting specific retinoid receptors in the skin to normalize the abnormal growth cycle of psoriatic skin cells. It is taken orally and typically used for psoriasis. It is usually taken at a dose of 0.25 to 1 mg/kg of body weight per day.

Acitretin is particularly effective for pustular psoriasis, erythrodermic psoriasis, and psoriasis affecting hands and feet. It is not effective for psoriatic arthritis. Acitretin is a convenient once-a-day oral medication that is available in 10- and 25-mg capsules approved for both the initial and maintenance treatment of severe psoriasis (BSA > 10%) in adults. It can be considered one of the treatments of choice for pustular and erythrodermic psoriasis. However, the efficacy of acitretin as a monotherapy for plaque psoriasis is less, although it is often used in combination therapy with other systemic psoriasis therapies, especially UVB or PUVA phototherapy, to increase efficacy. Such combination treatments may potentially minimize toxicity by using lower doses of each of the two agents.

Women must avoid becoming pregnant for at least 3 years after discontinuing acitretin. In comparison, etretinate was not recommended at all for women who planned to become pregnant. Clinical evidence has shown that etretinate can be formed with concurrent ingestion of acitretin and ethanol. Because the longer elimination half-life of etretinate would increase the duration of teratogenic potential for female patients, ethanol must not be ingested by female patients either during treatment with acitretin or for 2 months after cessation of therapy. This allows for elimination of acitretin, thus removing the substrate for transesterification to etretinate.

Acitretin may also be prescribed in rotation with other systemic medications, such as cyclosporine or methotrexate. Soriatane is most effective for treating psoriasis when it is used with phototherapy rather than by itself. Combination therapy can speed clearing and help reduce the amount of phototherapy needed to clear symptoms, thereby reducing risks and side effects.

Isotretinoin. Isotretinoin (13-*cis*-retinoic acid) is used primarily to treat cystic nodular acne. Isotretinoin (Accutane, Amnesteem, Claravis, Sotret) comes in dosages of 5, 10, 20 and 40 mg. Isotretinoin dosing is dependent on weight and the severity of the condition. Generally it is prescribed at a dose of 0.5 to 2 mg/kg per day (most often 1 to 1.25 mg/kg per day) and tapered to a dose that maintains control of disease with minimum side effects.

Hydroxyurea (Hydrea). Hydroxyurea is an oral anticancer medication that, in the 1960s, was found to be effective for psoriasis. It is an antineoplastic drug used primarily in hematologic malignancies. It is also used as an antiretroviral agent. Its mechanism of action is believed to be based on its inhibition of the enzyme ribonucleotide reductase by scavenging tyrosyl free radicals as they are involved in the reduction of nucleotide diphosphates.

Hydroxyurea is a second-line modality for the treatment of psoriasis. It is usually reserved for cases in which other second-line agents have failed or are contraindicated. The dose used has generally been 0.5 to 1.5 g daily, give orally either as a single dose or divided into two doses (morning and evening). Hydroxyurea avoids the hepatotoxicity associated with methotrexate and the nephrotoxicity associated with cyclosporine, and can often be useful when other drugs are contraindicated, although it should be avoided, if possible, when renal function is markedly impaired.

Reported side effects are drowsiness, nausea and vomiting, diarrhea, constipation, mucositis, anorexia, stomatitis, bone marrow toxicity (which may take 7 to 21 days to recover after the drug has been discontinued), alopecia, skin changes, and abnormal liver enzymes, creatinine, and blood urea nitrogen. The main concern regarding toxicity of hydroxyurea has been over myelosuppression, which may manifest as megaloblastic anemia, thrombocytopenia, or leukopenia. These side effects may develop after several months of treatment. They have generally been reversible after discontinuation of the drug. Due to its effect on the bone marrow, regular monitoring of the complete blood count is vital, as well as close monitoring for possible infections. In addition, renal function, uric acid and electrolytes, and liver enzymes are commonly checked. Hydroxyurea is a cytotoxic drug with potential for teratogenic effects and is best avoided in women of childbearing age.

There is reported experience with severe psoriasis using a combination of hydroxyurea (500 mg daily) with methotrexate (12.5 to 15 mg weekly).[39] An adequate response was obtained in the vast majority of patients, and hydroxyurea appeared to reduce the quantity of methotrexate required. Successful treatment of recalcitrant psoriasis with a combination of infliximab and hydroxyurea has been reported. The combination was used to treat psoriasis that proved resistant to conventional therapy, including vitamin D analogues, topical steroids, dithranol, crude coal tar, NB-UVB, bath PUVA, and acitretin. Hydroxyurea 1 g daily combined with infliximab infusions repeated at 3-month intervals led to satisfactory control of psoriasis and psoriatic arthritis.[40]

Mycophenolate Mofetil. Introduced in the 1970s as a treatment for psoriasis, mycophenolic acid has since been reformulated as mycophe-

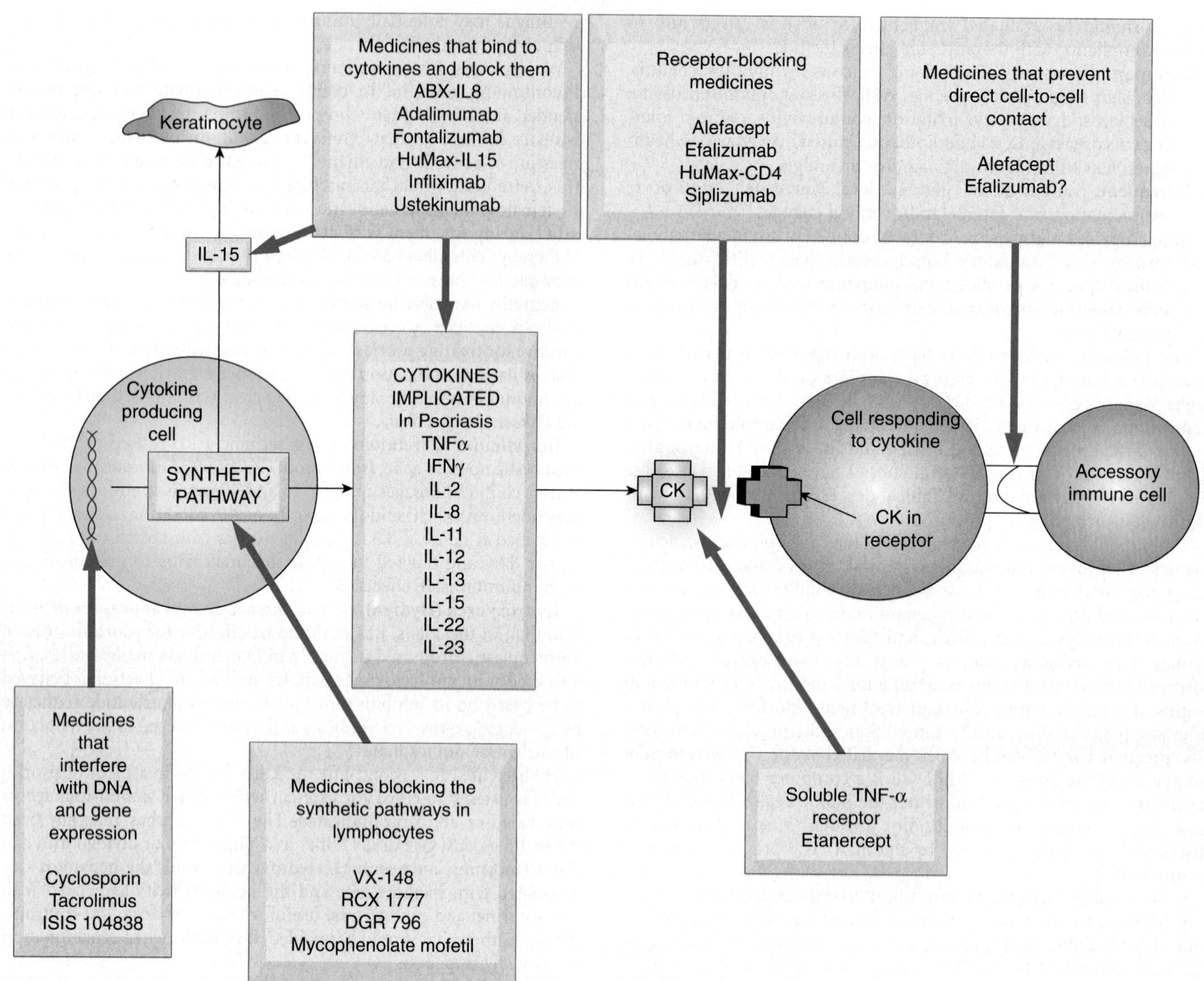

FIGURE 71-6 • Mechanism of action for different biologics and systemic treatments for psoriasis.

nolate mofetil. More recently, the salt mycophenolate sodium has also been introduced. Mycophenolate is derived from the fungus *Penicillium stoloniferum.* Mycophenolate mofetil is metabolized in the liver to the active moiety mycophenolic acid. It inhibits inosine monophosphate dehydrogenase, the enzyme that controls the rate of synthesis of guanine monophosphate in the de novo pathway of purine synthesis used in the proliferation of B and T lymphocytes.

Mycophenolate mofetil (CellCept, Myfortic) is an immunosuppressant drug used to prevent rejection in organ transplantation, as well as in the treatment of several inflammatory or autoimmune skin diseases. It can be used in combination with cyclosporine, and some doctors use it when tapering patients off of cyclosporine. Its relative lack of hepatonephrotoxicity and seemingly low risk of carcinogenicity offer important therapeutic advantages. Doses range from 1 to 1.5 g twice daily for the treatment of psoriasis and most other skin diseases (typically up to a maximum dose of 3 g daily). As psoriasis begins to improve, the dose can be decreased to 1 g daily in divided doses.

Common adverse drug reactions (≥1% of patients) associated with mycophenolate therapy include diarrhea, nausea, vomiting, infections, leukopenia, and/or anemia. Mycophenolate sodium is also commonly associated with fatigue, headache, and/or cough. Intravenous administration of mycophenolate mofetil is also commonly associated with thrombophlebitis and thrombosis. Infrequent adverse effects (0.1% to 1% of patients) include esophagitis, gastritis, GI tract hemorrhage, and/or invasive cytomegalovirus infection.

A sequential study comparing the efficacy and toxicity of mycophenolate mofetil and cyclosporine in the treatment of moderate to severe chronic plaque psoriasis showed cyclosporine being more effective, fast, and predictable in its effect than mycophenolate mofetil to control moderate to severe chronic plaque psoriasis[41] (Fig. 71-6). Both drugs were well tolerated in short courses of treatment. Patients were treated with oral mycophenolate mofetil (30 mg/kg per day) over a period of 16 weeks. Following a variable washout period and after a new outbreak of the disease, oral cyclosporine was introduced at a dose of 4 mg/kg per day.

Sulfasalazine. Sulfasalazine is a sulfa drug, a derivative of mesalazine (5-aminosalicylic acid [5-ASA]), used primarily as an anti-inflammatory agent in the treatment of inflammatory bowel disease as well as for rheumatoid arthritis. Sulfasalazine, and its metabolite 5-ASA, are poorly absorbed. Its main mode of action is therefore believed to be within the intestine. It is significantly less effective than methotrexate. However, sulfasalazine tends to have less serious systemic side effects.

Sulfasalazine (Azulfidine) is a second-line treatment for psoriatic arthritis. Sulfasalazine can be used in the treatment of moderate to severe psoriasis in patients whose disease severity does not justify use of methotrexate, etretinate, or PUVA, but whose disease is too widespread for safe and practical use of topical corticosteroids.[42] Response to therapy with sulfasalazine is low compared to methotrexate or cyclosporine; typically only 30% to 40% of patients respond.

The most common side effect is nausea, but often this can be controlled by a reduction in dose. Sometimes other medications may be needed. Occasionally mouth ulcers, a sore mouth, or loose bowel movements may occur. Certain patients may develop a headache or slight dizziness, but adjusting the dosage may bring things under control.

Drug eruptions can develop that may be pruritic, but usually resolve quite quickly once the drug is stopped. Sulfasalazine can in rare cases cause a drop in the numbers of white blood cells, which are needed to fight infection. If the blood count is monitored closely, it is unusual for this to be serious. Sulfasalazine can cause thrombocytopenia, but it is rare for this to actually cause problems. Easy bruising, nosebleeds, or bleeding gums are infrequent side effects.

The other potential problem is that sulfasalazine can cause a type of hepatitis. This is most commonly minor and does not cause symptoms. Most often, liver function tests may become slightly elevated, but these soon return to normal if the treatment is stopped. Sulfasalazine may cause a decrease in the sperm count, which may result in temporary infertility. This reverses when the drug is stopped. Temporary infertility may also occur in women.

Mercaptopurine and Azathioprine. Mercaptopurine (6-mercaptopurine; Purinethol) is an immunosuppressive drug used to treat leukemia. It is also used for pediatric non-Hodgkin's lymphoma, polycythemia vera, psoriatic arthritis, and inflammatory bowel disease. Azathioprine (Azasan, Imuran) is a prodrug that is converted in the body to the active metabolites 6-mercaptopurine and 6-thioinosinic acid. Azathioprine acts to inhibit purine synthesis necessary for proliferation of cells, especially leukocytes and lymphocytes.

Some of the adverse effects of taking mercaptopurine include diarrhea, nausea, vomiting, loss of appetite, abdominal pain, weakness, skin rash, darkening of the skin, and hair loss. Serious adverse effects include mouth sores, fever, sore throat, easy bruising or bleeding, petechiae (pinpoint red spots on the skin), yellowing of eyes or skin, dark urine, and painful or difficult urination. Unlikely but serious side effects include black or tarry stools, bloody stools, and bloody urine.

Mercaptopurine causes myelosuppression, suppressing the production of white blood cells. Weekly blood counts are recommended for patients on mercaptopurine. Caution should be taken when it is used in conjunction with purine analogues such as allopurinol. Patients who exhibit myelosuppression or bone marrow toxicity should be tested for thiopurine methyltransferase (TPMT) enzyme deficiency. Patients with TPMT deficiency are much more likely to develop dangerous myelosuppression. In such patients, it may be possible to continue using mercaptopurine, but at a lower dose. Screening of the TPMT blood level, therefore, is often performed prior to starting mercaptopurine or azathioprine.

This drug is traditionally not recommended during pregnancy, but this issue has been debated, and current evidence indicates that pregnant women on mercaptopurine show no increase in fetal abnormalities. However, women receiving mercaptopurine during the first trimester of pregnancy have an increased incidence of abortion.

Azathioprine can be used as a second-line agent to treat severe psoriasis and/or psoriatic arthritis if other treatment options have failed. It is usually given at a dosage of 2 to 4 mg/kg per day, with an upper limit of 300 mg/day.

Azathioprine is listed as a human carcinogen in the *11th Report on Carcinogens* of the U.S. Department of Health and Human Services. The risks involved seem to be related both to the duration and dosage used. People who have previously been treated with an alkylating agent may have an excessive risk of cancers if treated with azathioprine. It is used mostly in patients requiring transplantation. Those patients with increased risk of malignancies, especially nonmelanoma skin cancers, may have further increased risk with azathioprine.

Fumaric Acid Esters. Fumaric acid esters (FAEs) are marketed in some European countries and constitute a mixture of dimethylfumarate, calcium, magnesium, and zinc salts of monoethyl hydrogen fumarate. They were first introduced in the late 1950s by the German chemist Schweckendiek. Dimethylfumarate, the main ingredient of the marketed mixture, is the active compound. Currently, FAE (Fumaderm) is only available for use in Europe and is undergoing clinical trials in the United States.

Although the mode of action of FAEs in the treatment of psoriasis is not fully understood, they seem to shift a Th1-type cytokine response to a T helper type 2 (Th2)-type pattern whereby IL-10 inhibits Th1 cytokines IL-2, IL-12, and IFN-γ, and act by inhibiting translocation of nuclear factor-κB (NF-κB) and inhibiting proliferation of keratinocytes. It has been demonstrated that the nuclear translocation of the activated transcription factor NF-κB is inhibited in human endothelial cells and fibroblasts activated with TNF-α. The NF-κB pathway plays a major role in regulating inflammatory cytokine production as well as in cell differentiation and apoptosis. The influence of FAEs on the expression of nuclear transcription factors in T cells has not yet been investigated.[43]

Patients tolerating the therapy can expect a 75% reduction in PASI in 4 months. FAEs are being used in combination with second-line drugs such as cyclosporine, methotrexate, and hydroxyurea for additional benefit or to facilitate dose reduction of the second-line agent. However, all studies of the mixture of esters have a high dropout rate due to GI complaints of diarrhea and stomach pain and complaints of flushing, which is worse at the onset of therapy and can occur in up to 60% of patients. Headaches may be associated with sudden flushing. The frequency of flushing is greatest at the onset of therapy and decreases with prolonged treatment time.

Laboratory monitoring is required monthly particularly for lymphopenia, transient eosinophilia, and lymphocytopenia. Liver enzymes are frequently raised and reverse on stopping therapy, and there is an increase in triglycerides, cholesterol, potassium, and serum creatinine; however, there is no evidence of significant nephrotoxicity as seen with cyclosporine.

It is important to emphasise the difference between fumaric acid and FAEs. Fumaric acid formulations are available as health supplements and often marketed as a natural alternative medicine to treat psoriasis. They are, in fact, poorly absorbed and basically excreted via the urine without having any therapeutic effect.

Biologics

Biologics include a wide range of medicinal products such as vaccines, blood and blood components, allergenics, somatic cells, gene therapy, tissues, and recombinant therapeutic proteins (Fig. 71-7). Biologics can be composed of sugars, proteins, or nucleic acids or complex combinations of these substances, or may be living components such

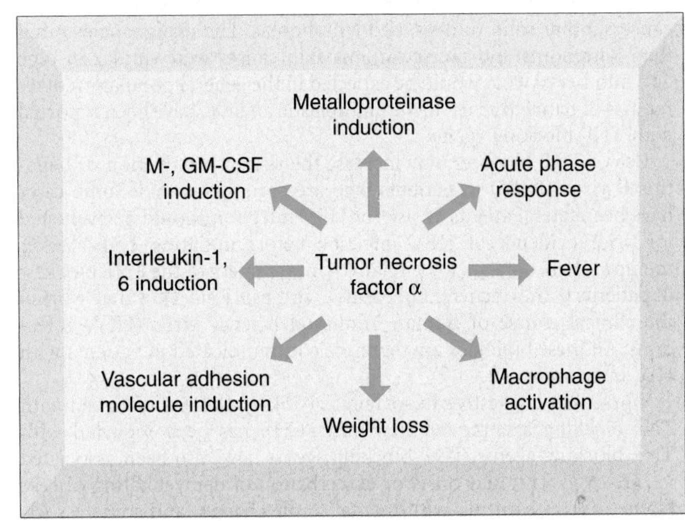

FIGURE 71-7 • TNF-α actions.

as cells and tissues. Biologics are isolated from a variety of natural sources—human, animal, and microorganism—and may be produced by biotechnological methods and other advanced technologies.

The current biologics manufactured by recombinant DNA technology, and approved or available for use in the treatment of psoriasis, are adalimumab, alefacept, efalizumab, etanercept, and infliximab. Infliximab and adalimumab are in the subclass of "anti-TNF antibodies," and are capable of neutralizing all forms (extracellular, transmembrane, and receptor-bound) of TNF-α. Etanercept, a third TNF antagonist, is in a different subclass (receptor-construct fusion protein), and, because of its modified form, cannot neutralize receptor-bound TNF-α. Additionally, the anti-TNF antibodies infliximab and adalimumab have the capability of lysing cells involved in the inflammatory process, whereas etanercept apparently lacks this capability. Although the clinical significance of these differences have not been firmly established, they may account for the differential actions of these drugs in both efficacy and side effects.

Various common side effects such as pharyngitis, cough, dizziness, nausea, pruritus, myalgias, chills, and reactions at injection sites were observed quite frequently. Urticaria and angioedema were also observed. If an anaphylactic reaction should occur, symptomatic treatment should be initiated at once. Since these biologics share many side effects and cautions in their use, common or general observations regarding these agents are reviewed and summarized together here.

In clinical studies, 0.9% of patients experienced significant infections compared to 0.2% in the placebo group. Among the infections were more serious events such as sepsis, pneumonia, abscesses, wound infections, and toxic shock syndrome. Many of these infections occurred in patients predisposed to infections because of concomitant immunosuppressive therapy in addition to their underlying disease. Caution should be taken in patients with a history of recurrent infection or with underlying conditions that may predispose patients to infections, or patients who have resided in regions where tuberculosis and histoplasmosis are endemic. Serious infections were seen in studies with concurrent use of anakinra and another TNF-blocking agent; therefore, the combination of biologics and anakinra is not recommended.

Patients currently undergoing immunosuppressive therapy should not receive biologics in order to avoid the risks of excessive immunosuppression. The efficacy of concomitant application of live vaccines has not been fully examined yet. However, the effect of tetanus toxoid was well preserved in selected clinical trials where tested.

$CD4^+$ cell counts should be obtained before initiation of therapy and during the course of therapy in intervals of 2 weeks for alefacept. Most common in clinical trials was a significant and dose-related reduction of $CD4^+$ and $CD8^+$ counts, again for alefacept versus the other biologics. Consequences of lymphopenia may be infections and/or treatment-related malignancies. Most malignancies observed in patients receiving these biologics were nonmelanoma and melanoma skin cancers, other solid tumors, and lymphomas. The malignancies other than lymphoma and nonmelanoma skin cancer were similar in type and number to what would be expected in the general population. Rare reports of pancytopenia, including aplastic anemia, have been reported with TNF-blocking agents.

Use of TNF blockers may increase the risk of reactivation of hepatitis B virus (HBV) in patients who are chronic carriers. Some cases have been fatal. Patients at risk for HBV infection should be evaluated for prior evidence of HBV infection before initiating TNF-blocker therapy. There appears to be relatively more safety of the TNF blockers in patients with concurrent hepatitis C and psoriasis. They may worsen the clinical course of human immunodeficiency virus (HIV) infections. All these biologics are therefore contraindicated in patients with HIV infections.

Worsening congestive heart failure (CHF) has been observed with TNF-blocking agents, and new-onset CHF has been reported with TNF-blocking agents. TNF-blocking agents have also been associated in rare cases with new onset or exacerbation of demyelinating disease (some cases presenting with mental status changes and some associated with permanent disability), transverse myelitis, optic neuritis, multiple sclerosis, and new onset or exacerbation of seizure disorders.

A variable percentage of patients receiving infliximab developed low- to higher titer antibodies with potential importance for the clinical efficiency of the drug. Neutralizing antibodies may affect the activity and doses required for achieving and maintaining clinical responses. Many fewer reports of antibodies have been reported for etanercept and the other biologics. Long-term immune effects have begun to be investigated in more detail, especially for infliximab, Rarely, development of a lupus-like syndrome and other autoimmune disorders have been reported for anti-TNF agents. Treatment should be discontinued if symptoms of lupus-like syndrome develop.

It may be desirable to monitor liver function studies in patients at high risk to develop liver toxicity. Postmarketing reports revealed asymptomatic increases in transaminases, fatty liver degeneration, decompensation of preexisting liver cirrhosis, and acute treatment-related liver failure. It is not known if some or all of these manifestations are attributable to alefacept therapy, but it is recommended to discontinue therapy as soon as any sign of liver toxicity develops.

Etanercept. Etanercept (Enbrel) is a recombinant human soluble TNF-α receptor fusion protein. It is a large molecule, with a molecular weight of 150 kDa, that binds to TNF-α and decreases its activity in disorders involving excess inflammation in humans and other animals, including autoimmune diseases such as ankylosing spondylitis, juvenile rheumatoid arthritis, psoriasis, psoriatic arthritis, rheumatoid arthritis, and, potentially, a variety of other disorders mediated by excess TNF-α. This therapeutic potential is based on the fact that TNF-α is one of the "master regulators" of the inflammatory response in many organ systems.

Etanercept is a dimeric molecule, and this dimeric structure is necessary for its proper therapeutic activity. It is made from the combination of two naturally occurring soluble human 75-kDa TNF receptors linked to an Fc portion of immunoglobulin G (IgG)1. The effect is an artificially engineered dimeric fusion protein. Etanercept mimics the inhibitory effects of naturally occurring soluble TNF receptors, the difference being that etanercept, because it is a fusion protein rather than a simple TNF receptor, has a greatly extended half-life in the bloodstream, and therefore a more profound and long-lasting biologic effect than a naturally occurring soluble TNF receptor.

Enbrel is marketed as a lyophylized powder in 25-mg vials that must be reconstituted with a diluent and then injected subcutaneously, typically by the patient at home. (It cannot be administered orally, because the digestive system would destroy the drug.) Because patients with arthritis found the reconstitution procedure difficult, Enbrel was made available as prefilled 50-mg/ml syringes in late 2004, and a single-use 50-mg autoinjector "pen" was brought to market in mid-2006. the FDA-approved dose is 25 mg twice weekly or 50 mg once weekly.

Enbrel is an approved treatment for rheumatoid arthritis, polyarticular-course juvenile rheumatoid arthritis, ankylosing spondylitis, psoriatic arthritis, and chronic moderate to severe plaque psoriasis. It has shown to be effective in about 50% of psoriatic arthritis patients who used it. Clinical responses were apparent at the time of the first visit (4 weeks) and were maintained through 6 months of therapy. Enbrel is indicated for the treatment of adult patients (18 years or older) with chronic moderate to severe plaque psoriasis who are candidates for systemic therapy or phototherapy. One of the major side effects was injection site reaction.

A multicenter 24-week study with 583 patients with stable plaque psoriasis involving at least 10% of BSA has been reported. During the first 12 weeks of the study, patients were randomly assigned to receive by subcutaneous injection etanercept twice weekly (BIW) at a dose of 50 mg or 25 mg, or placebo BIW in a double-blind fashion. During the second 12 weeks, all patients received etanercept 25 mg BIW. At week 12, a PASI 75 was achieved by 49% of patients in the etanercept 50 mg BIW group, 34% in the 25 mg BIW group, and 3% in the placebo group. At week 24 (after 12 weeks of open-label 25 mg etanercept BIW), a PASI 75 was achieved by 54% of patients whose dose was reduced from 50 mg BIW to 25 mg BIW, by 45% of patients in the continuous 25 mg BIW group, and by 28% in the group that received

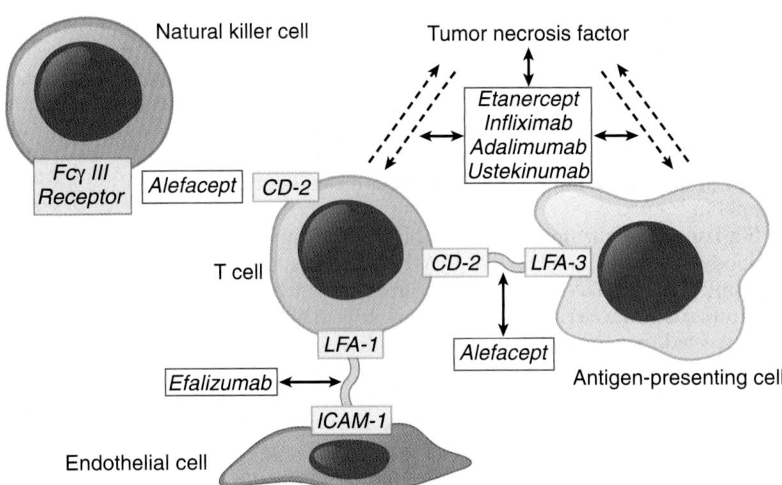

FIGURE 71-8 • Mechanisms of action for different biologics.

placebo followed by etanercept 25 mg BIW. Etanercept was well tolerated throughout the study.[44]

Infliximab. Infliximab is known as a chimeric monoclonal antibody. Infliximab neutralizes the biologic activity of TNF-α by binding with high affinity to the soluble and transmembrane forms of TNF-α and inhibits or prevents the effective binding of TNF-α with its receptors. Infliximab has high specificity for TNF-α, and does not neutralize TNF-β (also called lymphotoxin a), a related but less inflammatory cytokine that utilizes the same receptors as TNF-α. Biologic activities that are attributed to TNF-α (Fig. 71-8) include induction of proinflammatory cytokines such as IL-1 and IL-6, enhancement of leukocyte movement or migration from the blood vessels into the tissues by increasing the permeability of endothelial layer of blood vessels, and increasing the release of adhesion molecules.

Infliximab prevents disease in transgenic mice (a special type of mice that are biologically engineered to produce a human form of TNF-α and that are used to test the results of these drugs that might be expected in humans). These experimental mice develop arthritis as a result of their production of human TNF-α, and, when administered after disease onset, infliximab allows eroded joints to heal.

Infliximab (Remicade) has been approved by the FDA for the treatment of psoriasis, pediatric and adult Crohn's disease, ankylosing spondylitis, psoriatic arthritis, rheumatoid arthritis, and ulcerative colitis. Remicade is administered by intravenous infusion at infusion centers established within a clinic or hospital. (It cannot be administered orally, because the digestive system would destroy the drug.) It is administered typically every 6 to 8 weeks, with an initial start-up period requiring smaller time frames between infusions. In psoriasis and psoriatic arthritis, the dose is typically initiated at 5 mg/kg.

A Phase III multicenter, double-blind trial was conducted in which 378 patients with moderate to severe plaque psoriasis were allocated in a 4:1 ratio to receive infusions of either infliximab 5 mg/kg or placebo at weeks 0, 2, and 6, then every 8 weeks to week 46. At week 24, placebo-treated patients crossed over to infliximab treatment. At week 10, 80% of patients treated with infliximab achieved PASI 75 and 57% achieved at least PASI 90, compared with 3% and 1% in the placebo group, respectively. At week 50, 61% achieved PASI 75 and 45% achieved PASI 90 in the infliximab group. Infliximab was generally well tolerated in most patients.[45]

Adalimumab. Adalimumab (Humira) is the third TNF antagonist (after infliximab and etanercept) to be approved in the United States. Adalimumab was constructed from a fully human monoclonal antibody, while infliximab is a mouse-human chimeric antibody and etanercept is a TNF receptor–IgG fusion protein. Like infliximab and etanercept, adalimumab binds to TNF-α, preventing it from activating TNF receptors. TNF-α inactivation has proven to be important in down-regulating the inflammatory reactions associated with autoimmune diseases. Adalimumab has been approved for the treatment of rheumatoid arthritis, psoriatic arthritis, ankylosing spondylitis, and Crohn's disease, and data have been submitted to the FDA for expanding the label to include the treatment of plaque psoriasis.

Humira is marketed in both preloaded 0.8-ml syringes and also in preloaded pen devices, both injected subcutaneously, typically by the patient at home. It cannot be administered orally, as the digestive system destroys the protein. The most frequent adverse effects versus placebo from rheumatoid arthritis placebo-controlled studies were injection site reactions (20% vs. 14%), upper respiratory infection (17% vs. 13%), injection site pain (12% vs. 12%), headache (12% vs. 8%), rash (12% vs. 6%), and sinusitis (11% vs. 9%). Discontinuations due to adverse events were 7% for Humira versus 4% for placebo.

A clinical trial of 147 patients with moderate to severe psoriasis received adalimumab 80 mg at week 0, followed by 40 mg every other week; or 80 mg at weeks 0 and 1, followed by 40 mg/wk; or placebo. The number of patients achieving PASI 75 at week 12 was 53%, 80%, and 4%, respectively. The responses were maintained for 60 weeks.[46]

Alefacept. Alefacept is a genetically engineered immunosuppressive drug that seems to inhibit the activation of $CD2^+$, $CD4^+$, and $CD8^+$ T cells, which stimulate hyperproliferation of keratinocytes resulting in the typical psoriatic symptoms. It is a fusion protein composed of the external domain of LFA-3 and a human IgG1 Fc region. It eliminates pathogenic T cells by binding to NK cells; it also blocks T-cell activation.

Alefacept (Amevive) is the first biologic approved by the FDA for the treatment of moderate to severe chronic plaque psoriasis in adults who are candidates for systemic therapy or phototherapy. The standard dosing regimen is the weekly application of either 7.5 mg intravenously or 15 mg intramuscularly for a course of 12 weeks. The drug was approved based upon studies involving 1869 patients with plaques covering at least 10% of BSA. Either 7.5 mg intravenously or 15 mg intramuscularly once a week was administered. The long-term results (reduction of at least 75% in pretreatment PASI scores) were 14% and 21%, respectively. Additional improvements ensuing after completion of the 12-week treatment phase or after completion of a second alefacept treatment were also seen. Often the remissions were maintained for 7 to 12 months after end of treatment.

Commonly observed side effects with Amevive include sore throat, dizziness, cough, nausea, itching, muscle aches, chills, injection site reactions, and accidental injury. Alefacept has been assigned to Pregnancy Category B in the United States and to Category C in Australia. It is not known if the drug is excreted into human milk. Either the drug or breast-feeding should be terminated, taking into account the importance of treatment to the mother.

An international, randomized, double-blind, placebo-controlled, parallel-group trial with 507 patients with chronic plaque psoriasis was conducted. Placebo, 10 mg of alefacept, or 15 mg of alefacept was administered once weekly for 12 weeks, followed by 12 weeks of observation. Throughout the study, a greater percentage of patients in the 15-mg group than in the placebo group achieved a significant reduction in PASI. Of patients in the 15-mg group who achieved at least 75% PASI reduction 2 weeks after the last dose, 71% maintained at least 50% improvement in PASI throughout the 12-week follow-up.[47]

Efalizumab. Efalizumab is a recombinant humanized monoclonal antibody that binds to CD11a of LFA-1 and acts as an immunosuppressant. It blocks T-cell activation and reactivation, also blocking T-cell trafficking into dermis and epidermis. It is the only biologic that is a targeted, reversible T-cell modulator. It does not bind TNF or induce T-cell apoptosis.

Efalizumab (Raptiva) is indicated for the treatment of adult patients (18 years or older) with chronic moderate to severe plaque psoriasis who are candidates for systemic therapy or phototherapy. The recommended dose of Raptiva is 1 mg/kg by subcutaneous injection once weekly, following an initial conditioning dose of 0.7 mg/kg. The maximum dose should not exceed a total of 200 mg.

In Raptiva clinical trials, there were no signals for demyelinating disorders or for new-onset or exacerbated CHF, no pancytopenia or aplastic anemia was observed, and there was a low incidence of granulomatous infections such as tuberculosis, histoplasmosis, or *Listeria*. Reports of immune-mediated hemolytic anemia, some serious, diagnosed 4 to 6 months after the start of Raptiva treatment have been received. Raptiva should be discontinued if hemolytic anemia occurs.

The most common adverse reactions associated with Raptiva were a symptom complex that included headache, chills, fever, nausea, and myalgia within 48 hours following the first two injections. These events were largely mild to moderate when a conditioning dose of 0.7 mg/kg was given, and by the third dose acute adverse affects were no different than placebo. Less than 1% of patients discontinued Raptiva treatment because of these adverse events.

Worsening of psoriasis can occur during or after treatment with Raptiva. During clinical studies, 19 of 2589 Raptiva-treated patients (0.7%) had serious worsening of psoriasis during treatment (n = 5, 0.2%) or after discontinuation of Raptiva (n = 14, 0.5%). Some patients required hospitalization (n = 17, 0.7%).

Infrequent new-onset or recurrent severe arthritis events, including psoriatic arthritis events, have been reported in clinical trials and postmarketing. Infrequent cases (0.3%) of immune-mediated thrombocytopenia were observed during clinical trials, and reports of severe thrombocytopenia have been received postmarketing; therefore, platelet monitoring is recommended.

A multinational, randomized, double-blind, placebo-controlled, parallel-group trial was designed to evaluate the safety and efficacy of subcutaneous efalizumab 1.0 mg/kg once weekly for 12 weeks compared with placebo. Patients with moderate to severe plaque psoriasis were randomized in a 2 : 1 ratio to receive efalizumab or placebo. A total of 793 patients were enrolled (529 received efalizumab and 264 placebo), including 526 high-need patients (342 received efalizumab and 184 placebo). At week 12, PASI 75 rates were 29.5% for efalizumab compared with 2.7% for placebo among high-need patients and 31.4% for efalizumab compared with 4.2% for placebo in the full study population.[48]

CNTO 1275. CNTO 1275 (Ustekinumab) is an antagonist to interleukins 12 and 23, two key cytokines known to be involved in type 1 immune responses. The Biologics License Application (BLA) for ustekinumab (CNTO 1275) has been accepted for review by the U.S. Food and Drug Administration (FDA) for the treatment of adult patients with chronic moderate to severe plaque psoriasis.

The study performed by Centocor was a 52-week, double-blind and placebo-controlled trial. The investigators enrolled 320 patients and randomized them to placebo or one of four doses of CNTO 1275 administered subcutaneously: one injection of 50 mg; one injection of 100 mg; four weekly injections of 50 mg; four weekly 100-mg injections. Each of the five groups had 64 subjects. CNTO 1275 subjects also received an additional dose at week 16 if they did not achieve an excellent or complete response (75% clearing) as measured by the standard Physician's Global Assessment (PGA). Subjects in the placebo group also received 100 mg of CNTO 1275 at week 20.

At week 12, more than 75% improvement in PASI score was achieved by 52%, 59%, 67%, and 81% of subjects treated with 50 mg, 100 mg, four weekly 50-mg injections, or four weekly 100-mg injections of CNTO 1275, respectively. This compared to 2% of placebo subjects, the researchers reported. There was also at least a 90% improvement in PASI score, or virtual clearing of disease, in 23%, 30%, 44%, and 52% of subjects in the respective CNTO 1275 groups, versus 2% of placebo. Only 87 patients were re-treated with CNTO 1275 at week 16. No uncommon adverse events were reported during treatment in any of the CNTO 1275 groups.

Laser

Excimer Laser. An excimer laser is a form of UV chemical laser that is commonly used in eye surgery and semiconductor manufacturing. The excimer laser delivers high-energy monochromatic UVB at 308 nm. An excimer laser typically uses a combination of an inert gas (argon, krypton, or xenon) and a reactive gas (fluorine or chlorine). Under the appropriate conditions of electrical stimulation, a pseudo-molecule called a dimer is created, which can only exist in an energized state and can give rise to laser light in the UV range. The UV light from an excimer laser is well absorbed by biologic matter and organic compounds. Rather than burning or cutting material, the excimer laser adds enough energy to disrupt the molecular bonds of the surface tissue, which effectively disintegrates into the air in a tightly controlled manner through ablation rather than burning. Thus excimer lasers have the useful property of being able to remove exceptionally fine layers of surface material or interact with and target cells within tissues with almost no heating or change to the remainder of the material, which is left intact.

Pulsed Dye Laser. A dye laser is a laser that uses an organic dye as the lasing medium, usually as a liquid solution. Compared to gases and most solid-state lasing media, a dye can usually be used for a much wider range of wavelengths. The wide bandwidth makes dyes particularly suitable for tunable lasers and pulsed lasers. Moreover, one dye can be replaced by another in order to generate different wavelengths with the same laser, although this usually requires replacing other optical components in the laser as well.

Taibjee et al. conducted a prospective trial comparing excimer and pulsed dye lasers in the treatment of psoriasis.[49] Twenty-two adult patients with a mean PASI of 7.1 were recruited. Fifteen patients completed the full treatment, of which 13 were followed up to 1 year. Two selected plaques were treated, one with an excimer laser twice weekly and the other with V Beam pulsed dye laser (PDL), following pretreatment with salicylic acid, every 4 weeks. Two additional plaques, treated with salicylic acid alone or untreated, served as controls. The mean improvement in PASI was 4.7 with excimer laser and 2.7 with PDL. PASI improvement was significantly greater in excimer laser than PDL or both control plaques. Thirteen patients responded best with excimer laser, two patients best with PDL, and in seven patients there was no difference between the two lasers. Nine patients (41%) cleared with excimer laser, after a mean 8.7 weeks (median 10 weeks) of treatment. Seven of these nine patients were followed up to 1 year; four remained clear, two relapsed at 1 month, and one relapsed at 6 months. Six patients (27%) cleared with PDL, after a mean 3.3 (median 4) treatments. All six patients were followed up to 1 year; four remained clear, one relapsed at 4 months, and one relapsed at 9 months. Despite common side effects including blistering and hyperpigmentation, patient satisfaction was high.[49]

PDL requires fewer treatments and has fewer side effects; in addition, it might be useful in excimer laser–resistant cases as some of these patients did not respond to the excimer laser but did respond to the PDL. The two systems target different parts of the psoriasis pathway, with the PDL targeting the abnormal microvasculature of psoriatic plaques versus the excimer laser, which targets the immune-inflammatory cells within the lesions.

Therapeutic Approaches

There can be substantial variation between individuals in the effectiveness of specific psoriasis treatments. Because of this, dermatologists often resort to an empirical or trial-and-error approach to finding the most appropriate treatment for their patients with psoriasis. The decision to employ a particular treatment is based on the type of psoriasis and its location, extent, and severity. The patient's age, gender, quality of life, comorbidities, and attitude toward risks associated with the treatment are also taken into consideration, as well as availability of the therapy at specific sites and accessibility of the patient to return for ongoing therapies.

Medications with the least potential for adverse reactions are preferentially employed. If the treatment goal is not achieved, then therapies with greater potential toxicity may be used. Medications with significant toxicity are reserved for severe, unresponsive psoriasis. This is called the psoriasis treatment ladder (Fig. 71-9). In the first step, medicated ointments or creams are applied to the skin (Table 71-2). If topical treatment fails to achieve the desired goal, then the next step would be to expose the skin to UV radiation. The third step involves the use of medications that are administered orally or by injection (Table 71-3).

An alternative algorithmic approach to psoriasis therapy has been developed by the National Psoriasis Foundation, in conjunction with a panel of dermatology experts. Rather than designing a more linear decision tree or "ladder" approach, therapeutic decisions and initiation of treatment are determined by the extent of psoriasis as well as disease severity based on specific patient criteria (Fig. 71-10). Topical therapeutics are initially employed, and therapeutics are advanced to the next levels of phototherapy or systemics, including biologics, based on these patient characteristics and relative toxicities of agents. This has been a widely adopted algorithmic approach and continues to undergo revisions and updating as newer agents become available and more clinical experience and safety data on newer agents are reported and assimilated.

Mild Psoriasis

Most patients with psoriasis have skin lesions limited to localized areas such as the elbows or knees, affecting less than 2% of BSA. For these patients, topical therapy may remain part of their therapeutic regimen

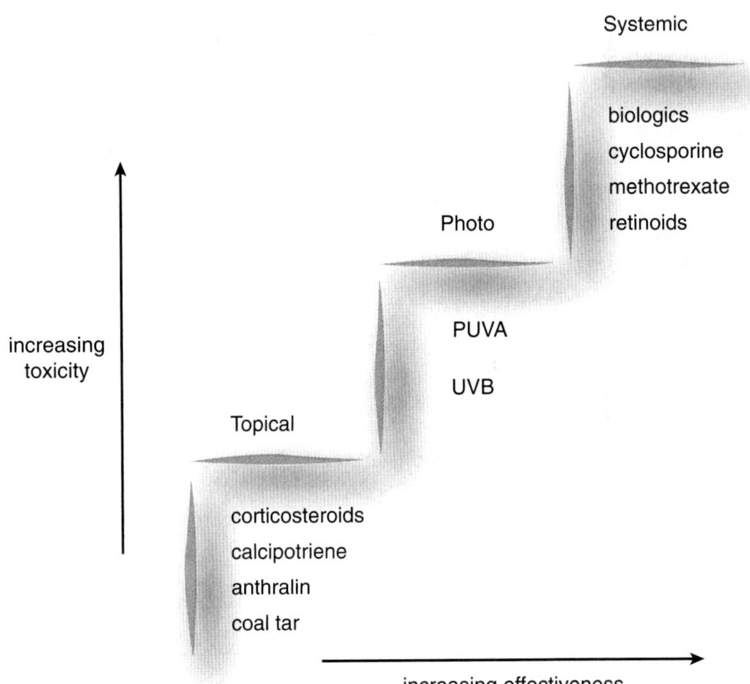

FIGURE 71-9 • Psoriasis treatment ladder.

TABLE 71-2 TOPICAL TREATMENTS SIDE EFFECTS

Drug	Most Common Side Effects	Other Side Effects
Topical corticosteroids	Atrophy, striae, telangiectases, acneiform eruption, rosacea, contact dermatitis, infections.	Very rare and only with prolonged use of superpotent corticosteroids, suppression of the HPA axis, growth retardation in children, cataract formation, and glaucoma development
Calcipotriene	Burning, itching, skin irritation.	Hyperpigmentation, hypercalcemia, folliculitis
Tazarotene	Dry skin, pruritus, redness and in some cases extreme drying and cracking of skin.	
Tars	Mild burning or skin irritation. When used on the scalp, it may temporarily discolor bleached, tinted, or light blond or gray hair. Stains skin and clothing.	Potential skin carcinogenicity
Anthralin	It temporarily stains the skin a yellowy-brown and permanently stains clothing fabrics. Burning sensation and irritation.	
Salicyclic acid	Mild stinging and burning.	Salicylism (systemic absortion)

HPA, hypothalamic-pituitary-adrenal.

TABLE 71-3 SYSTEMIC TREATMENTS AND PHOTOTHERAPY SIDE EFFECTS

Drug	Most Common Side Effects	Other Side Effects
Adalimumab	Increased risk of tuberculosis reactivation, injection site reaction.	Lymphoma, CHF, demyelinating process, lupus-like syndrome, opportunistic infections
Efalizumab	Rebound effect and flare-up during therapy.	Hemolytic anemia, decreased platelets, arthritis
Infliximab	Increased risk of tuberculosis reactivation, injection site reaction.	Lymphoma, CHF, demyelinating process, lupus-like syndrome, opportunistic infections
Etanercept	Injection site reaction.	CHF, demyelinating process, lupus-like syndrome, bone marrow suppresssion, opportunistic infections
Alefacept	Injection site reaction, $CD4^+$ count to <250 cells/µl.	Liver inflammation
NB-UVB, 311 nm	Phototoxicity.	
PUVA	Phototoxicity, photoaging.	Cutaneous carcinogenesis
RePUVA	Phototoxicity, photoaging.	Cutaneous carcinogenesis (less risk than with PUVA alone)
Goeckerman regimen	Skin irritation, folliculitis, phototoxicity.	
Acitretin	Teratogenicity, liver inflammation, hyperlipidemia, mucous membrane side effects.	Osteoporosis, pseudotumor cerebri
Methotrexate	Teratogenicity, bone marrow suppression, cirrhosis, alopecia, fatigue, GU symptoms.	Lymphoma
Cyclosporine	Nephrotoxicity, high blood pressure; increased uric acid, potassium, and magnesium.	Paresthesias
Hydroxyurea	Drowsiness, nausea and vomiting, diarrhea, constipation, mucositis, anorexia, stomatitis, alopecia, skin changes; abnormal liver enzymes, creatinine, and blood urea nitrogen.	Myelosuppression (megaloblastic anemia, thrombocytopenia, or leukopenia)
Mycophenolate mofetil	Diarrhea, nausea, vomiting, infections, leukopenia, anemia, fatigue, headache, cough. IV administration can cause thrombophlebitis and thrombosis.	Esophagitis, gastritis, gastrointestinal tract hemorrhage, invasive cytomegalovirus infection
Sulfasalazine	Nausea, diarrhea, mouth ulcers, headache or slight dizziness, skin rash, bruising.	Decreased platelets, liver inflammation, infertility
Mercaptopurine	Diarrhea, nausea, vomiting, loss of appetite, abdominal pain, weakness, skin rash, darkening of the skin, alopecia.	Myelosuppression
Fumaric acid esters	Increased liver enzymes, triglycerides, cholesterol, potassium, and serum creatinine.	Lymphopenia, transient eosinophilia
Leflunomide	Skin reactions up to life-threatening forms (Stevens-Johnson syndrome and toxic epidermal necrolysis), heart problems, alopecia.	Hepatitis, liver cirrhosis, myelosuppression, myeloid/lymphatic malignancies, solid cancers, interstitial lung disease, infections

CHF, congestive heart failure; GU, genitourinary; IV, intravenous; NB-UVB, narrow-band ultraviolet B; PUVA, psoralen plus ultraviolet A; RePUVA, retinoid plus psoralen plus ultraviolet A.

whether or not they require additional treatments for psoriatic arthritis. Patients receiving systemic therapies and/or phototherapy may also require the use of topical treatments.[50] Topical therapies may be used in combination, rotational, or sequential treatment strategies for patients with more severe disease.

Topical corticosteroids continue to be the cornerstone of mild to moderate psoriasis treatment, despite the introduction of newer nonsteroidal drugs. Topical corticosteroids are effective and provide superior results compared with vitamin D derivatives such as calcipotriene.[51] The age of the patient, disease severity, type, and extent of surface area involvement must be considered when deciding which topical corticosteroid to prescribe and in what vehicle. Low-potency corticosteroids are typically used on the face, groin, and axillary areas and areas with thin skin, and in infants.[52] In other areas and in adult patients, initial therapy usually involves mid-potency agents, with higher potency corticosteroids used on thick chronic plaques resistant to lower potency agents. Topical corticosteroids are best used to treat psoriasis affecting less than 20% of total BSA.[53]

There are other topical treatments that can be used depending on the severity of psoriasis, age of the patient, and area affected. Tazarotene is also very effective and can be combined or alternated with topical corticosteroids for higher efficacy. Angelo et al. compared the efficacy of once-daily tazarotene 0.1% cream and clobetasol propionate 0.05% in psoriatic plaques during 12 weeks of treatment.[54] Patients with bilaterally symmetric lesions were enrolled in this double-blind, randomized, controlled study. Clobetasol cream was better than tazarotene cream in reducing the erythema and scaling, and tazarotene was better in reducing the induration. Treatment success rate was 100% with clobetasol and 88% with tazarotene at the end of week 12, with clobetasol achieving 100% success at the end of week 6.

Moderate to Severe Psoriasis

Moderate (2% to 10% BSA) to severe (>10% BSA) psoriasis patients initially undergo topical treatment in the mildest cases and topical treatment plus phototherapy in cases with higher percentage of BSA affected (Table 71-4). If topical treatments plus phototherapy fail, acitretin can be added to the regimen. If the BSA is greater or the previous treatment fails, the Goeckerman regimen or PUVA plus acitretin is a common treatment of choice. In more severe cases or when previous treatments fail, methotrexate or cyclosporine alone can be started, depending on the comorbidities of the patient; if this treatment fails, a combination with acitretin or biologics can be used. Methotrexate and cyclosporine can also be used in combination with topicals and/or phototherapy.

Treatment Algorithm
Moderate (2%–10% BSA) to
Severe (>10% BSA)
Mild (<2% BSA)
Topical tx*
If topical tx fails, follow
therapy for mild to moderate
UVB phototherapy or UVB + adjunct
topical tx* ± acitretin (especially if
plaque is thick)
If patient lives too far away for phototherapy,
can go directly to systemic tx
Goeckerman*
PUVA ± acitretin*
Biologics, MTX or CsA* ± acitretin†
• Once stable, transition to maintenance tx
• If resistant, initiate combination tx
Maintenance tx* (sequential
or rotational) ± acitretin
Combination therapy* using
Systemic + topical tx or
Systemic + phototherapy or
Systemic + topical + phototherapy
*Topical therapy may be added to any regimen.
† No currently available biologic tx is approved or available for psoriasis at the time of writing. (Etanercept is approved for psoriatic arthritis.) These algorithms may be updated as more data become available.
† Preliminary data suggest that tumor necrosis factor (TNF) inhibitors may be safe and highly effective treatments for plaque psoriasis. Although these and other biologics are not yet approved for psoriasis, they may be considered for patients with severe, resistant disease.
BSA = body surface area, tx = therapy, MTX = methotrexate,
CsA = cyclosporine A.

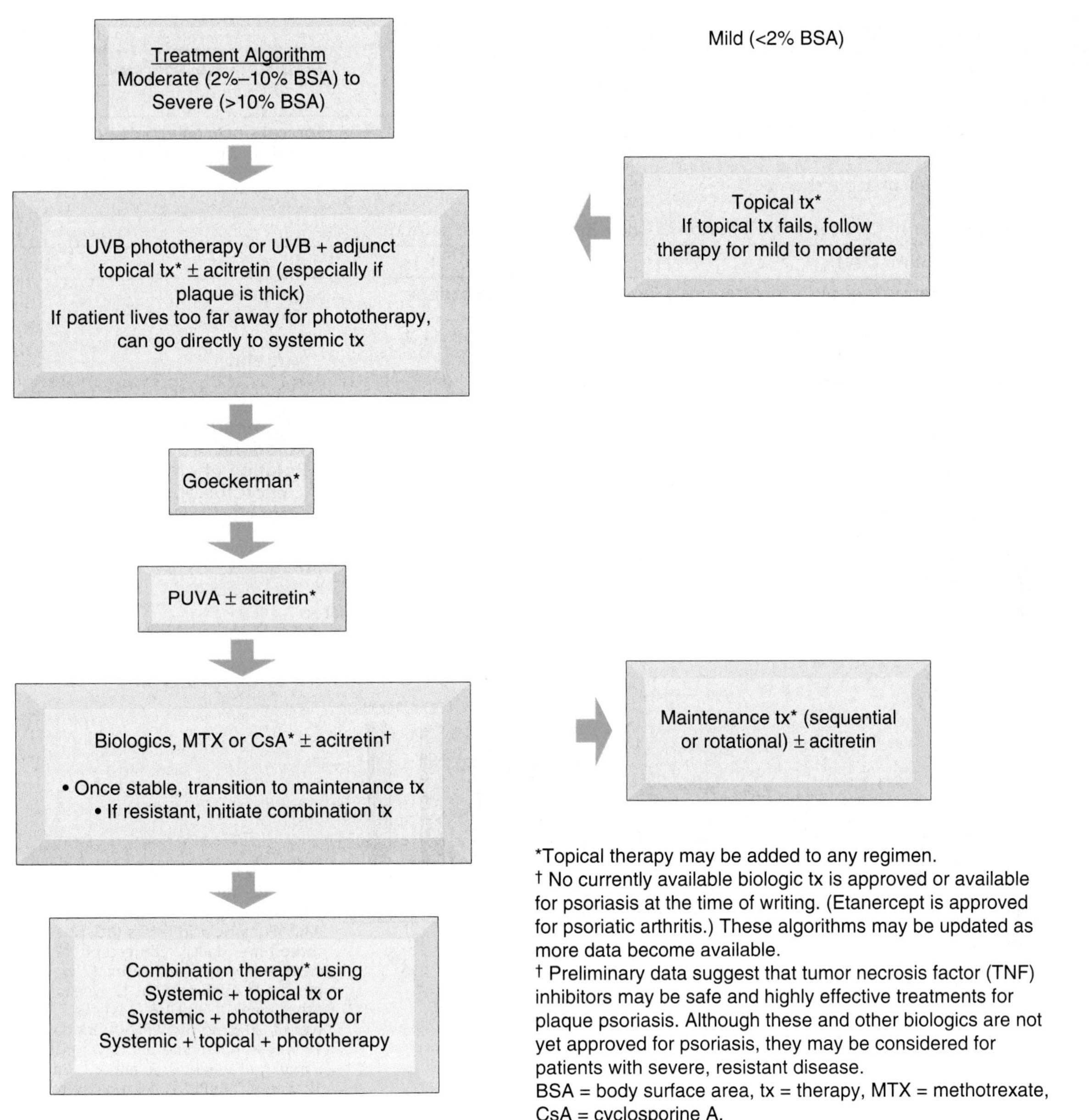

FIGURE 71-10 • Psoriatic treatment algorithm. (From National Psoriasis Foundation. Psoriasis: Treatment Options and Patient Management. City: National Psoriasis Foundation, 2002.)

Once the treatment has achieved a clearance or improvement of the BSA affected, the patient can initiate a maintenance therapy that can be either rotational or sequential. Rotational therapy minimizes the risk of cumulative toxicity by switching from one therapy to another before the initial agent or more toxic agent can create adverse effects. Sequential therapy is a sequence of specific therapies to maximize the rate of initial improvement, minimize long-term adverse effects, and improve clearance. This therapy entails three phases: a clearing phase using a rapidly acting therapy; a transitional phase once the patient improves, to taper the initial therapy; and a maintenance phase.

A recent review of treatments, with the percentage of PASI 75 reduction at approximately 12 weeks, showed the following outcomes: Goeckerman regimen and retinoids plus PUVA (RePUVA), 100%; calcipotriene plus PUVA, 87%; cyclosporine, 78.2% to 80.3%; infliximab, 80%; adalimumab 40 mg every other week, 53%, and 40 mg/week, 80%; PUVA, 63%; methotrexate, 60%; NB-UVB, 55%; acitretin 52%; etanercept 50 mg twice weekly, 49%, and 25 mg twice weekly, 34%; efalizumab, 31.4%; and alefacept, 21% (Fig. 71-11). Psoriatic treatments with safer profiles compared with other agents include bath PUVA, the Goeckerman regimen, and RePUVA. Based on the literature review of efficacy and safety of biologics and prebiologic treatment options for moderate to severe psoriasis, the risk:benefit ratio seems most favorable for the Goeckerman regimen and RePUVA, followed by either etanercept or adalimumab.[55]

There are other considerations besides the PASI 75. The treatment should be individualized depending on the severity, the areas affected, the age of the patient, and other comorbidities. Infliximab is noted to have the highest PASI 75 among biologics; however, its efficacy decreases over time, in part due to the formation of anti-infliximab antibodies. Efalizumab has shown to have a "rebound" effect in 13.8% of patients. Adalimumab, unlike etanercept, is not expected to need a decrease in dosage after 3 months of therapy, which will give adalimumab better long-term efficacy.

Cyclosporine is one of the most effective traditional systemic drugs. The traditional dosage of less than 5 mg/kg per day seems to have an acceptable side effect profile. Cyclosporine is not recommended for long-term use; however, it is highly effective in achieving fast clearing in psoriasis. Methotrexate was the first systemic therapy for patients

TABLE 71-4 TREATMENT OF PSORIASIS

Severity	Treatment	Maintenance Therapy
MILD PSORIASIS (<2% BSA)		
Localized	Topical Corticosteroids (high potency) + Tazarotene or Calcipotriene	Topical Corticosteroids (low/medium potency) and/or Tazarotene or Calcipotriene
Scalp	Tar or Ketoconazole shampoo ↓ High-potency Corticosteroid solution or foam ± Calcipotriene solution	
MODERATE TO SEVERE (BSA > 2%)		
	High-potency Topical Corticosteroids + Tazarotene or Calcipotriene ↓ UVB + Topicals ± Acitretin ↓ Goeckerman regimen ↓ PUVA + Acitretin ↓ MTX, CsA, Biologics ± Acitretin ↓ Combination therapy: • Systemic + Topicals • Systemic + Phototherapy • Systemic + Topicals + Phototherapy	Sequential: CsA or MTX ↓ Acitretin ↓ Topicals Phototherapy Rotational: Rotation of different systemic and/or phototherapy treatments to avoid toxicity

BSA, body surface area; CsA, cyclosporin A; MTX, methotrexate; PUVA, psoralen plus ultraviolet A; UVB, ultraviolet B.

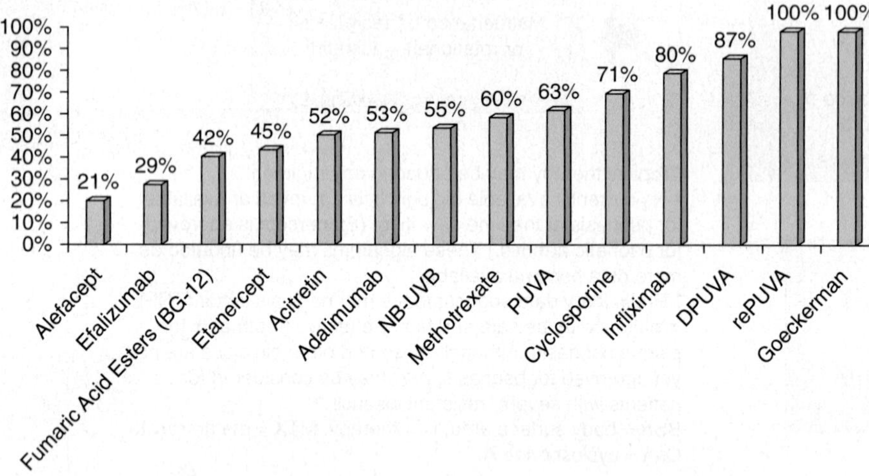

FIGURE 71-11 • PASI 75 of different treatments for moderate to severe psoriasis. Alefacept: 14 weeks, 15 mg/wk.[47] Efalizumab: 12 weeks, 1 mg/wk.[48] Fumaric acid esters (BG-12): 12 weeks, 720 mg three times daily.[65] Etanercept: 12 weeks, 25 mg twice per week.[45] Acitretin: 12 weeks, 0.54 mg/kg per day.[66] Adalimumab: 12 weeks, 40 mg every other week.[44] NB-UVB: 3 weeks.[28] Methotrexate: 16 weeks, 20.6 mg/wk.[36] PUVA: 34 days.[67] Cyclosporine: 16 weeks, 4.5 mg/kg per day.[36] Infliximab: 10 weeks, 5 mg/kg at weeks 0, 2, and 6.[46] Calcipotriol-PUVA: 12 weeks.[34] RePUVA: 20 mg/day retinoid + PUVA three times per week.[68] Goeckerman regimen: 12 weeks, 5 days per week.[27]

with moderate to severe psoriasis and is one of the most frequently prescribed treatments nowadays.

The treatment of moderate to severe psoriasis in healthy children younger than 18 years old would consist of an initial treatment of UVB; if the treatment with light is not enough, tar, calcipotriene, or tazarotene can be added in combination. If this treatment fails, the Goeckerman regimen can be chosen. PUVA can be considered only in selected cases, and a low-dose retinoid (consider isotretinoin in females) can be added to the treatment. If all these treatments fail or the case is severe, a systemic treatment can be initiated.

Pregnancy and Psoriasis

Topical corticosteroids and topical calcipotriene as well as topical anthralin and topical tacrolimus appear to be safe choices for control of localized psoriasis in pregnancy. UVB is the safest treatment for extensive psoriasis during pregnancy, particularly when topical application of other agents is not practical. Short-term use of cyclosporine during pregnancy is probably the safest option for management of severe psoriasis that has not responded to topical or UVB treatment.[56]

Psoriatic Arthritis

The treatments used in psoriatic arthritis are directed at reducing and controlling inflammation. Nonsteroidal anti-inflammatory drugs (NSAIDs) such as diclofenac and naproxen are usually the first-line medication. Other treatment options for this disease include joint injections with corticosteroids; however, this is only practical if just a few joints are affected. If acceptable control is not achieved using NSAIDs or joint injections, then second-line treatments with immunosuppressants such as methotrexate are added to the treatment regimen. An advantage of immunosuppressive treatment is that it also treats the psoriasis in addition to the arthropathy.

Some NSAIDs, when taken in high doses or over long periods of time, carry a risk of causing stomach problems, including ulcers and GI bleeding. The risk depends on the strength of the NSAID and how long it is taken. The NSAIDs known as cyclooxygenase-2 (COX-2) inhibitors have proven to be less problematic for the stomach than other NSAIDs. The COX-2 inhibitor Celebrex has been approved for treating the symptoms of rheumatoid arthritis and osteoarthritis.

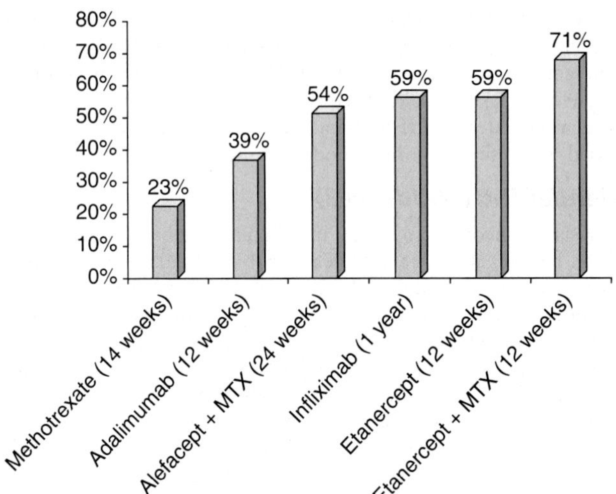

FIGURE 71-12 • American College of Rheumatology core criteria (ACR20) of different treatments of psoriatic arthritis.

Antimalarial treatment, commonly used with success in rheumatoid arthritis, has sometimes been used to treat psoriatic arthritis. Steroid medications taken orally are not generally recommended for long-term treatment of psoriatic arthritis, although in some circumstances they may be needed for relief of acute, severe joint inflammation and swelling. Cyclosporine is an immunosuppressive drug that is FDA approved for treating psoriasis, and it may produce improvement in psoriatic arthritis. Sulfasalazine is sometimes used for psoriatic arthritis. Approximately one-third of psoriatic arthritis patients respond rapidly to this treatment (usually within 4 to 8 weeks).

Biologics. The FDA approved the use of etanercept for patients with moderate to severe psoriatic arthritis in January 2002. Adalimumab was approved by the FDA in October 2005, and infliximab was approved in May 2005. The primary efficacy end point to evaluate the efficacy of treatment was the percentage of patients who met the American College of Rheumatology (ACR) core criteria (ACR20) (Fig. 71-12), 20% improvement in tender and swollen joint counts and 20% improvement in at least three of the following five ACR core set measures: pain, patient global assessment, physician global assessment, self-assessed physical disability, and acute-phase reactant.

Etanercept plus methotrexate combination therapy is generally superior to either monotherapy in reducing disease activity and structural joint damage, as well as improving health-related quality of life. Etanercept monotherapy is superior to placebo and at least as effective as methotrexate monotherapy in reducing disease activity and improving health-related quality of life in patients with early or refractory disease.[57]

In patients with psoriatic arthritis, etanercept 25 mg twice weekly significantly reduced disease activity and improved skin lesions in two double-blind, placebo-controlled, 12- to 24-week trials. In the 24-week study, ACR20 response rates (50% vs. 13%), psoriatic arthritis response rates (70% vs. 23%), and the median improvement in skin lesions (33% vs. 0%) were significantly greater in etanercept than in placebo recipients. Furthermore, etanercept has been shown to inhibit radiographic progression in those patients with early disease.[58]

Genovese et al. conducted a double-blind, randomized, multicenter study in which patients were treated for 12 weeks with subcutaneous injections of adalimumab 40 mg every other week or placebo.[59] Secondary efficacy measures included the modified Psoriatic Arthritis Response Criteria (PsARC) and assessments of disability, psoriatic lesions, and quality of life. A total of 100 patients received a study drug (51 adalimumab, 49 placebo). At week 12, an ACR20 response was achieved by 39% of adalimumab patients versus 16% of placebo patients and a PsARC response was achieved by 51% with adalimumab versus 24% with placebo. No serious infections occurred during adalimumab therapy.

Kavanaugh et al. conducted a double-blind, placebo-controlled, Phase III study of 200 patients with active psoriatic arthritis who were randomized to receive infusions of infliximab 5 mg/kg or placebo at weeks 0, 2, 6, and every 8 weeks thereafter through 1 year. Through 1 year of treatment, 58.9% and 61.4% of patients in the randomized infliximab and placebo/infliximab groups, respectively, achieved ACR20; corresponding figures for PASI 75 were 50.0% and 60.3%. At week 54, major clinical response was achieved by 12.1% of patients in the infliximab group.[60]

To evaluate the efficacy of alefacept in combination with methotrexate (MTX) a randomized, double-blind, placebo-controlled trial was performed by Mease et al.[61] Alefacept (15 mg) or placebo was administered intramuscularly once weekly for 12 weeks in combination with MTX, followed by 12 weeks of observation during which only MTX treatment was continued. A total of 185 patients were randomly assigned to receive alefacept plus MTX or placebo plus MTX. At week 24, 54% of patients in the alefacept plus MTX group achieved an ACR20 response, compared with 23% of patients in the placebo plus MTX group. Mean reductions in tender and swollen joint counts in patients receiving alefacept plus MTX were −8.0 and −6.3, respectively. A 50% reduction from the baseline PASI at week 14 was achieved by 53% of patients receiving alefacept plus MTX compared with 17% of those receiving placebo plus MTX. Most adverse events were mild to moderate in severity.

Disease-Modifying Antirheumatic Drugs. Disease-modifying antirheumatic drugs (DMARDs) may relieve more severe symptoms and attempt to slow or stop joint and tissue damage and progression of psoriatic arthritis. Leflunomide (Arava) is a pyrimidine synthesis inhibitor belonging to the DMARD class of drugs. It is an immunomodulatory drug inhibiting dihydroorotate dehydrogenase (an enzyme involved in de novo pyrimidine synthesis). Antiproliferative and anti-inflammatory activity has been shown. An oral loading dose of 100 mg is followed by a once-daily administration of 10 to 20 mg as determined. The onset of clinical improvement can be expected after 4 to 6 weeks of continued therapy.

Aspirin or other NSAIDs and/or low-dose corticosteroids may be continued during treatment with leflunomide. The combined use of leflunomide with antimalarials, intramuscular or oral gold, D penicillamine, azathioprine, or methotrexate has not been adequately studied and is therefore contraindicated. The concomitant use of methotrexate may lead to severe or even fatal liver or hematotoxicity.

Important contraindications are preexisting pregnancy, or women of childbearing potential not using reliable contraceptive methods. Finally, women should not become pregnant before 2 years after termination of therapy have elapsed or should undergo a rapid washout procedure. Men wishing to father a child should discontinue leflunomide after consultation with their prescribing physician and also undergo the washout procedure.

Due to its potent immunosuppression, leflunomide has the potential to promote myeloid/lymphatic malignancies or solid cancers. In rheumatoid arthritis patients, a several-fold increase of lymphoma is already present in those patients not treated with any DMARD.

The most serious side effect is symptomatic liver damage ranging from jaundice to hepatitis, which can be fulminant, severe liver necrosis, and liver cirrhosis. Fatalities have occurred. Abnormal liver function studies may or may not preceede the outbreak of clinical disease. The total incidence of severe liver damage is estimated to be as high as 0.5%, according to an internal report of the FDA.

Also very important is a relatively high incidence of myelosuppression with leukopenia, and/or hypoplastic anemia, and/or thrombocytopenia. Infections, sometimes as severe as development of active tuberculosis, pneumonia (including *Pneumocystis jiroveci* pneumonia), and severe viral or mycotic infections, possibly leading to sepsis, death, or permanent damage, have been seen. Anemia or bleeding episodes may also lead to serious complications.

Interstitial lung disease may occasionally be noticed and is recognized by progressive dyspnea and typical radiographic findings. This disease may or may not be reversible upon treatment, and may lead to permanent disability or death. Other adverse effects are skin reactions ranging up to life-threatening forms (Stevens-Johnson syndrome and toxic epidermal necrolysis), heart problems, and alopecia (17%).

If severe side effects are encountered, leflunomide can be readily removed from the body with oral cholestyramine or activated charcoal to slow or reverse the noted side effects.

Emerging Targets and Therapeutics

ShK(L5) and PAP-1

ShK(L5) is a synthetic version of a component of sea anemone venom. PAP-1 is derived from a shrub, the common rue. Both compounds act to block channels that allow potassium ions to flow into or out of cells. These ion channels appear to play an important role in regulating the activity of cells in the immune system and are especially abundant on a type of immune cell implicated in diseases such as multiple sclerosis and psoriasis.

In effector memory T cells, $K_v1.3$ potassium channel traffic moves to the immunologic synapse during antigen presentation, where it co-localizes with $K_v\beta2$, SAP97, ZIP, p56(lck), and CD4. Although $K_v1.3$ inhibitors [ShK(L5) amide (SL5) and PAP1] do not prevent immunologic synapse formation, they suppress Ca^{2+} signaling, cytokine production, and proliferation of autoantigen-specific T cells at pharmacologically relevant concentrations while sparing other classes of T cells.[62]

Apremilast (CC-10004)

CC-10004 is a novel, orally available small molecule with anti-inflammatory activities that inhibits the production of multiple pro-inflammatory mediators, including phosphodiesterase-4, TNF-α, IL-2, IFN-γ, leukotrienes, and nitric oxide synthase. CC-10004 (Apremilast) is the lead investigational drug in this class of anti-inflammatory compounds, and is being studied in Phase II clinical trials by Celgene Corporation for the treatment of psoriasis and other chronic inflammatory diseases.

ABT-874

Abbott Laboratories reported significant results in Phase II testing for its experimental biologic currently known as ABT-874. ABT-874 is a fully human monoclonal antibody designed to target and neutralize IL-12 and IL-23, two proteins associated with inflammation in psoriasis and other autoimmune disorders. It reduced psoriasis symptoms significantly in the majority of patients treated.

One hundred eighty patients with moderate to severe psoriasis were enrolled in a 12-week, double-blind, placebo-controlled study. Patients were randomized evenly to six treatment groups: a single, subcutaneous 200-mg injection of ABT-874 at week zero; 100 mg every other week for 12 weeks; 200 mg weekly for 4 weeks; 200 mg every other week for 12 weeks; 200 mg weekly for 12 weeks; or placebo. The primary end point was the proportion of patients achieving 75% improvement in the degree and severity of skin lesions after 12 weeks, as measured by the PASI. At 12 weeks, 90% of patients achieved 75% improvement in psoriasis signs and symptoms in four of the five dosing groups receiving ABT-874, versus 3% of patients receiving placebo. Also, more than half of patients achieved 90% improvement, in the same four of five ABT-874 dosing groups, versus 0% of those receiving placebo.

ABT-874 represents a novel approach to treating psoriasis, targeting a part of the inflammatory response that is not addressed by any therapy available today. The most common adverse events observed were injection site reactions, nasopharyngitis, upper respiratory infections, and headache.

MEDI-545

MedImmune has initiated a Phase I trial with its monoclonal antibody targeting IFN-α, known as MEDI-545, in patients with psoriasis. The psoriasis treatment trial marks a second clinical study underway with MEDI-545, which is also being evaluated in an ongoing Phase I trial in patients with systemic lupus erythematosus.

Elevated type-1 interferon messenger RNA levels have been found in preclinical models of psoriasis, and inhibition of type 1 interferon in these models has been shown to block the development of psoriasis mediated by plasmacytoid dendritic cells. Preclinical study results have also demonstrated that IFN-α–induced genes and proteins are overexpressed in the skin in animal models of psoriasis.

Essential Fatty Acids (ω-3)

Psoriasis is uncommonly seen in Africans, probably partly due to genetic factors. However, the dietary habits of Africans may provide another explanation. Maize, the staple diet in most parts of Africa, is high in linoleic acid but low in other polyunsaturated fatty acids and riboflavin. Linoleic acid is a precursor of prostaglandin E_2, and its high intake, especially in the absence of other polyunsaturated fatty acids and riboflavin, results in high tissue production of prostaglandin E_2.[63]

The ω-3 fatty acids are a family of polyunsaturated fatty acids that have in common a carbon-carbon double bond in the ω-3 position. Important ω-3 fatty acids in nutrition are α-linolenic acid, eicosapentaenoic acid (EPA), and docosahexaenoic acid (DHA). The human body cannot synthesize ω-3 fatty acids de novo, but can synthesize all the other necessary ω-3 fatty acids from the simpler ω-3 fatty acid α-linolenic acid. Therefore, α-linolenic acid is an essential nutrient that must be obtained from food, and the other ω-3 fatty acids that can be either synthesized from it within the body or obtained from food are sometimes also referred to as essential nutrients.

Mayser et al. conducted a double-blind, randomized, parallel group study performed in eight European centers.[64] Eighty-three patients hospitalized for chronic plaque-type psoriasis were randomly selected to receive daily infusions with either a ω-3 fatty acid–based lipid emulsion (Omegavenous; 200 ml/day with 4.2 g of both EPA and DHA; 43 patients) or a conventional ω-6 lipid emulsion (Lipovenous; EPA + DHA < 0.1 g/100 ml; 40 patients). The total PASI score decreased by 11.2 ± 9.8 in the ω-3 group and by 7.5 ± 8.8 in the ω-6 group. In addition, the ω-3 group was superior to the ω-6 group with respect to change in severity of psoriasis per body area, change in overall erythema, overall scaling, and overall infiltration, as well as change in overall assessment by the investigator and self-assessment by the patient. Thirty-seven percent of patients receiving the ω-3 emulsion and 23% of those receiving the ω-6 emulsion had a decrease in total PASI of at least 50% between admission and last value. No major side effects were observed.

REFERENCES

1. Lomholt G. Prevalence of skin disease in a population: a census study from the Faroe Islands. Dan Med Bull 1964;11:1-7.
2. Green AC. Australian Aborigines and psoriasis. Australas J Dermatol 1984;25:18-24.
3. Convit J. Investigation of the incidence of psoriasis amongst Latin-American Indians. *In* Proceedings of 13th Congress on Dermatology. Amsterdam: Excerpta Medica, 1962, p 196.
4. Henseler T, Christophers E. Psoriasis of early and late onset: characterization of two types of psoriasis vulgaris. J Am Acad Dermatol 1985;13:450-456.
5. Guenther LC, Ortonne J-P. Pathophysiology of psoriasis: science behind therapy. J Cutan Med Surg 2002;6(Suppl 3):2-7.
6. Cameron AL, Kirby B, Fei W, Griffiths CEM. Natural killer and natural killer-T cells in psoriasis. Arch Dermatol Res 2002;294:363-369.
7. Clark RA, Chong B, Mirchandani N, et al. The vast majority of CLA^+ T cells are resident in normal skin. J Immunol 2006;176:4431-4439.
8. Boyman O, Conrad C, Dudli C, et al. Activation of dendritic antigen-presenting cells expressing common heat shock protein receptor CD91 during induction of psoriasis. Br J Dermatol 2005;152:1211-1218.
9. Mehlis SL, Gordon KB. The immunology of psoriasis and biologic immunotherapy. J Am Acad Dermatol 2003;49:S44-S50.
10. Lebwohl M. Psoriasis. Lancet 2003;361:1197-1204.
11. Lee RE, Gaspari AA, Lotze MT, et al. Interleukin 2 and psoriasis. Arch Dermatol 1988;124:1811-1815.
12. Chaturvedi V, Qin J-Z, Denning MF, et al. Apoptosis in proliferating, senescent, and immortalized keratinocytes. J Biol Chem 1999;274:23358-23367.
13. Victor FC, Gottlieb AB. TNF-alpha and apoptosis: implications for the pathogenesis and treatment of psoriasis. J Drugs Dermatol 2002;1:264-275.
14. Goffe B, Cather JC. Etanercept: an overview. J Am Acad Dermatol 2003;49:S105-S111.
15. Bowcock AM, Krueger JG. Getting under the skin: the immunogenetics of psoriasis. Nature Rev Immunol 2005;5:699-711.
16. Liu Y, Krueger JG, Bowcock AM. Psoriasis: genetic associations and immune system changes. Genes Immun 2007;8:1-12.

17. Helms C, Cao L, Krueger JG, et al. A putative RUNX1 binding site variant between SLC9A3R1 and NAT9 is associated with susceptibility to psoriasis. Nature Genet 2003;35:349-356.
18. Lowes MA, Bowcock AM, Krueger JG. Pathogenesis and therapy of psoriasis. Nature 2007;445:866-873.
19. Langley RG, Krueger GG, Griffiths CE. Psoriasis: epidemiology, clinical features, and quality of life. Ann Rheum Dis 2005;64(Suppl 2):ii18-ii23; discussion ii24-ii5.
20. O'Doherty CJ, MacIntyre C. Palmoplantar pustulosis and smoking. Br Med J (Clin Res Ed) 1985;289:861-864.
21. Asumalahti K, Ameen M, Suomela S, et al. Genetic analysis of PSORS1 distinguishes guttate psoriasis and palmoplantar pustulosis. J Invest Dermatol 2003;120:627-632.
22. Callis KP, Krueger GG. Topical agents in the treatment of moderate-to-severe psoriasis. *In* Weinstein GD, Gottlieb AB (eds): Therapy of Moderate-to-Severe Psoriasis, 2nd ed. New York: Marcel Dekker, 2003, pp 29-51.
23. Trozak DJ. Topical corticosteroid therapy in psoriasis vulgaris. Cutis 1990;46:341-350.
24. Du Vivier A, Stoughton RB. Tachyphylaxis to the action of topically applied corticosteroids. Arch Dermatol 1975;111:581-583.
25. Foster RH, Brogden RN, Benfield P. Tazarotene. Drugs 1998;55:705-711.
26. Dando TM, Wellington K. Topical tazarotene: a review of its use in the treatment of plaque psoriasis. Am J Clin Dermatol 2005;6:255-272.
27. Lee E, Koo J. Modern modified "ultra" Goeckerman therapy: a PASI assessment of a very effective therapy for psoriasis resistant to both prebiologic and biologic therapies. J Dermatolog Treat 2005;16:102-107.
28. Liu J, Farmer J, Lane W, et al. Calcineurin is a common target of cyclophilin-cyclosporin A and FKBP-FK506 complexes. Cell 1991;66:807-815.
29. The European FK506 Multicentre Psoriasis Study Group. Systemic tacrolimus (FK506) for the treatment of psoriasis in a double-blind, placebo-controlled study Arch Dermatol 1996;132:419-423.
30. Hofer A, Fink-Puches R, Kerl H, Wolf P. Comparison of phototherapy with near vs. far erythemogenic doses of narrow-band ultraviolet B in patients with psoriasis. Br J Dermatol 1998;138:96-100.
31. Kirke SM, Lowder S, Lloyd JJ, et al. A randomized comparison of selective broadband UVB and narrowband UVB in the treatment of psoriasis. J Invest Dermatol 2007;127:1641-1646.
32. Coven TR, Walters IB, Cardinael I, Krueger JG. PUVA-induced lymphocyte apoptosis: mechanism of action in psoriasis. Photodermatol Photoimmunol Photomed 1999;15:22-27.
33. Nijsten TE, Stern RS. Oral retinoid use reduces cutaneous squamous cell carcinoma risk in patients with psoriasis treated with psoralen-UVA: a nested cohort study. J Am Acad Dermatol 2003;49:644-650.
34. Lebwohl M, Drake L, Menter A, et al. Consensus conference: acitretin in combination with UVB or PUVA in the treatment of psoriasis. J Am Acad Dermatol 2001;45:544-553.
35. Zanolli M. Phototherapy arsenal in the treatment of psoriasis. Dermatol Clin 2004;397-406.
36. Torras H, Aliaga A, López-Estebaranz JL, et al. A combination therapy of calcipotriol cream and PUVA reduces the UVA dose and improves the response of psoriasis vulgaris. J Dermatolog Treat 2004;15:98-103.
37. Johnston A, Gudjonsson JE, Sigmundsdottir H, et al. The anti-inflammatory action of methotrexate is not mediated by lymphocyte apoptosis, but by the suppression of activation and adhesion molecules. Clin Immunol 2005;14:154-163.
38. Heydendael VM, Spuls PI, Opmeer BC, et al. Methotrexate versus cyclosporine in moderate-to-severe chronic plaque psoriasis. N Engl J Med 2003;349:658-665.
39. Sauer GC. Combined methotrexate and hydroxyurea therapy for psoriasis. Arch Dermatol 1973;107:369-370.
40. Gach JE, Berth-Jones J. Successful treatment of recalcitrant psoriasis with a combination of infliximab and hydroxyurea. J Dermatolog Treat 2003;14:226-228.
41. Pedraz J, Daudén E, Delgado-Jiménez Y, et al. Sequential study on the treatment of moderate-to-severe chronic plaque psoriasis with mycophenolate mofetil and cyclosporin. J Eur Acad Dermatol Venereol 2006;20:702-706.
42. Gupta AK, Ellis CN, Siegel MT, et al. Sulfasalazine improves psoriasis: a double-blind analysis. Arch Dermatol 1990;126:487-493.
43. Gerdes S, Shakery K, Mrowietz U. Dimethylfumarate inhibits nuclear binding of nuclear factor kappaB but not of nuclear factor of activated T cells and CCAAT/enhancer binding protein beta in activated human T cells. Br J Dermatol 2007;156:838-842.
44. Papp KA, Tyring S, Lahfa M, et al, for the Etanercept Psoriasis Study Group. A global Phase III randomized controlled trial of etanercept in psoriasis: safety, efficacy, and effect of dose reduction. Br J Dermatol 2005;152:1304-1312.
45. Reich K, Nestle FO, Papp K, et al, for the EXPRESS study investigators. Infliximab induction and maintenance therapy for moderate-to-severe psoriasis: a Phase III, multicentre, double-blind trial. Lancet 2005;366:1367-1374.
46. Gordon KB, Langley RG, Leonardi C, et al. Clinical response to adalimumab treatment in patients with moderate to severe psoriasis: double-blind, randomized controlled trial and open-label extension study. J Am Acad Dermatol 2006;55:598-606.
47. Lebwohl M, Christophers E, Langley R, et al, for the Alefacept Clinical Study Group. An international, randomized, double-blind, placebo-controlled Phase 3 trial of intramuscular alefacept in patients with chronic plaque psoriasis. Arch Dermatol 2003;139:719-727.
48. Dubertret L, Sterry W, Bos JD, et al, for the CLEAR Multinational Study Group. Clinical experience acquired with the efalizumab (Raptiva) (CLEAR) trial in patients with moderate-to-severe plaque psoriasis: results from a Phase III international randomized, placebo-controlled trial. Br J Dermatol 2006;155:170-181.
49. Taibjee SM, Cheung ST, Laube S, Lanigan SW. Controlled study of excimer and pulsed dye lasers in the treatment of psoriasis. Br J Dermatol 2005;153:960-966.
50. Lebwohl M, Ting PT, Koo JYM. Psoriasis treatment: traditional therapy. Ann Rheum Dis 2005;64(Suppl II):83-86.
51. Mason J, Mason AR, Cork MJ. Topical preparations for the treatment of psoriasis: a systematic review. Br J Dermatol 2002;146:351-364.
52. Pardasani AG, Feldman SR, Clark AR. Treatment of psoriasis: an algorithm-based approach for primary care physicians. Am Fam Physician 2000;61:725-733, 736.
53. Del Rosso J, Friedlander SF. Corticosteroids: options in the era of steroid-sparing therapy. J Am Acad Dermatol 2005;53(1 Suppl 1):S50-S58.
54. Angelo JS, Kar BR, Thomas J. Comparison of clinical efficacy of topical tazarotene 0.1% cream with topical clobetasol propionate 0.05% cream in chronic plaque psoriasis: a double-blind, randomized, right-left comparison study. Indian J Dermatol Venereol Leprol 2007;73:65.
55. Leon A, Nguyen A, Letsinger J, Koo J. An attempt to formulate an evidence-based strategy in the management of moderate-to-severe psoriasis: a review of the efficacy and safety of biologics and prebiologic options. Expert Opin Pharmacother 2007;8:617-632.
56. Tauscher AE, Fleischer AB, Phelps KC, Feldman SR. Psoriasis and pregnancy. J Cutan Med Surg 2002;6:561-570.
57. Dhillon S, Lyseng-Williamson KA, Scott LJ. Etanercept: a review of its use in the management of rheumatoid arthritis. Drugs 2007;67:1211-1241.
58. Culy CR, Keating GM. Spotlight on etanercept in rheumatoid arthritis, psoriatic arthritis and juvenile rheumatoid arthritis. BioDrugs 2003;17:139-145.
59. Genovese MC, Mease PJ, Thomson GT, et al, for the M02-570 Study Group. Safety and efficacy of adalimumab in treatment of patients with psoriatic arthritis who had failed disease modifying antirheumatic drug therapy. J Rheumatol 2007;34:1040-1050.
60. Kavanaugh A, Krueger GG, Beutler A, et al, for the IMPACT 2 Study Group. Infliximab maintains a high degree of clinical response in patients with active psoriatic arthritis through 1 year of treatment: results from the IMPACT 2 trial. Ann Rheum Dis 2007;66:498-505.
61. Mease PJ, Gladman DD, Keystone EC, for the Alefacept in Psoriatic Arthritis Study Group. Alefacept in combination with methotrexate for the treatment of psoriatic arthritis: results of a randomized, double-blind, placebo-controlled study. Arthritis Rheum 2006;54:1638-1645.
62. Beeton C, Wulff H, Standifer NE, et al. $K_v1.3$ channels are a therapeutic target for T cell-mediated autoimmune diseases. Proc Natl Acad Sci U S A 2006;103:17414-17419.
63. Namazi MR. Why is psoriasis uncommon in Africans? The influence of dietary factors on the expression of psoriasis. Int J Dermatol 2004;43:391-392.
64. Mayser P, Mrowietz U, Arenberger P, et al. Omega-3 fatty acid-based lipid infusion in patients with chronic plaque psoriasis: results of a double-blind, randomized, placebo-controlled, multicenter trial. J Am Acad Dermatol 1998;38:539-547.
65. Langner A, Roszkiewicz J, Baran E, Placek W. Results of a Phase II study of a novel oral fumarate, BG-12 in the treatment of severe psoriasis [Abstract P075]. J Eur Acad Dermatol Venereol 2004;18:798.
66. Geiger JM. Efficacy of acitretin in severe psoriasis. Skin Therapy Lett 2003;8:1-3, 7.
67. Frappaz A, Thivolet J. Calcipotriol in combination with PUVA: a randomized double blind placebo study in severe psoriasis. Eur J Dermatol 1993;3:351-354.
68. Lauharanta J, Geiger JM. A double-blind comparison of acitretin and etretinate in combination with bath PUVA in the treatment of extensive psoriasis. Br J Dermatol 1989;121:107-112.
00a. Tiilikainen A, Lassus A, Karvonen J, et al. Psoriasis and HLA-Cw6. Br J Dermatol 1980;102:179-184.

Practice: Dermatologic Therapeutics

72

DERMATITIS

Mark Davis

INTRODUCTION 1007
Phases of Dermatitis 1007
Dermatitis Types 1007
Asteatotic Dermatitis 1007
Atopic Dermatitis (Eczema) 1007
Seborrheic Dermatitis 1007
Contact Dermatitis 1008
Nummular Dermatitis 1008
Dyshidrotic Eczema (Pompholyx or Dyshidrosis) 1008
Stasis Dermatitis 1009
Dermatitis of Unknown Cause 1009
Perioral Dermatitis 1009
Infectious Eczematoid Dermatitis 1009
PATHOPHYSIOLOGY 1009
Overview 1009
Asteatotic Dermatitis 1010
Atopic Dermatitis (Eczema) 1010
Seborrheic Dermatitis 1011
Contact Dermatitis 1011
Stasis Dermatitis 1011
Infectious Eczematoid Dermatitis 1011
Diagnosis 1011
THERAPEUTICS AND CLINICAL PHARMACOLOGY 1011
Goals of Therapy 1011
Moisturizers and Lubricants 1011
Management of Contributing Factors: Dry Skin, Infection, Contact Factors 1012
Topical Medications 1012
Wet Dressings 1012
Therapeutics by Class 1012
Topical Treatments 1012
Antihistamines 1013
Antibiotics 1013
Phototherapy 1013
Systemic Corticosteroids 1014
Other Immunosuppressive Medications 1014
Therapeutic Approach 1014
General Treatment Guidelines 1014
Treatment Guidelines for Specific Forms of Dermatitis 1014
Emerging Targets and Therapeutics 1014

INTRODUCTION

Dermatitis is derived from "derm," meaning skin and "itis," meaning inflammation, thus inflammation of the skin. The term is used synonymously with the term *eczema,* although others emphasize that it is important to specify that "eczematous dermatitis" better describes inflammation of the skin characterized by erythema, scale, and vesicles.

Phases of Dermatitis

Arbitrarily, dermatitis has been divided into three phases based on its duration: dermatitis that is less than 6 weeks old is termed *acute dermatitis,* that between 6 weeks and 3 months old is termed *subacute dermatitis,* and dermatitis lasting for more than 3 months is termed *chronic dermatitis.* Each of these phases has a characteristic morphologic appearance. In the acute phase, skin typically has vesicles and bullae (Fig. 72-1). In the subacute phase, vesicles and bullae are less prominent, and red (erythematous) patches are apparent (Fig. 72-2). In the chronic phase, the red patches appear lichenified (with exaggerated skin lines; Fig. 72-3). Because delineation of these phases is arbitrary, the morphologic appearance often does not correspond directly with the phase of the dermatitis. For example, in chronic dermatitis, one can occasionally observe vesicles and blisters.

Dermatitis Types

The skin forms an important barrier against the outside world that must be maintained to function properly. Any factor that removes water, lipids, or protein from the skin, specifically from the epidermis, disrupts the integrity of this barrier and compromises its function. Inflammation of the skin (dermatitis) has many causes, and for that reason, a descriptor is usually used in association with the term *dermatitis.* For example, "seborrheic dermatitis" denotes a particular type of inflammation of the skin, "contact dermatitis" describes another type of inflammation of the skin, and "nummular dermatitis" denotes a further type. The most common types are discussed in this section.

Asteatotic Dermatitis

Dermatitis due to dry skin is extremely common, especially in the winter months, when humidity is low. The areas commonly involved are the legs, flanks, and hands. As the skin dries, water and often epidermal lipids and proteins that help contain epidermal moisture are lost. To restore the barrier, these must be restored. The skin becomes irritated by the dryness and inflamed. Patients complain of itching and burning. Clinically, skin is rough and associated with fine white scale; then scaling pruritic pink patches are noted on the legs and posterior flank. In cases of severe dryness, one may notice a "crazy paving" type of appearance to the skin, termed *eczema craquele;* the skin may be crisscrossed with shallow red fissures.

Atopic Dermatitis (Eczema)

Atopic dermatitis is a chronic inflammatory skin disease that is often associated with other atopic disorders such as allergic rhinitis and asthma. It is often familial, and it is being increasingly recognized that genetic factors may be contributory. The incidence of atopic dermatitis appears to be increasing, particularly in urban areas and in developed countries. Present estimates are that between 25% and 30% of children in Western societies have atopic dermatitis. Most atopic dermatitis presents before age 5 years, but it can present later.[1]

In children, pruritic erythematous patches can be seen anywhere on the body (Fig. 72-4). Interestingly, diaper areas are often spared. In adults, flexor areas such as the neck, antecubital fossa, and popliteal fossa are more commonly involved, although wrists, forearms, and face can also be involved. In severe cases, any area of the body can be involved.

The diagnosis of atopic dermatitis is a clinical one. An association of pruritus, recurrent dermatitis, and a positive personal or family history of atopy (asthma, allergic rhinitis) are important factors in establishing the diagnosis. Criteria have been established to make the diagnosis.[2,3]

Seborrheic Dermatitis

Seborrheic dermatitis is an extremely common problem that affects areas of the body that are rich in sebaceous glands (scalp, face, upper trunk). *Seborrhea* is a term meaning excess oil secretion. In infants,

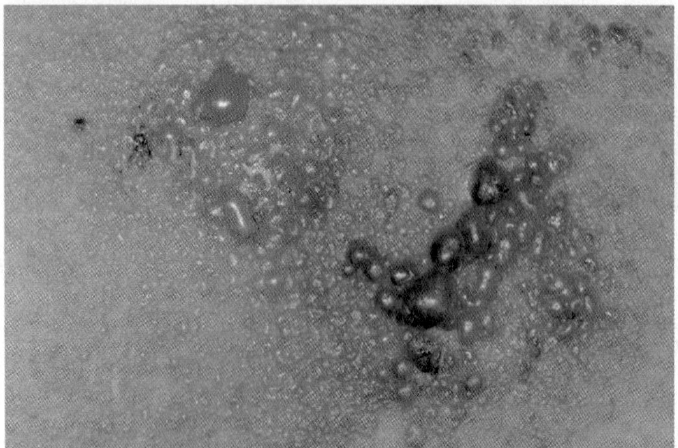

FIGURE 72-1 • **Acute dermatitis.** Note vesicles and bullae.

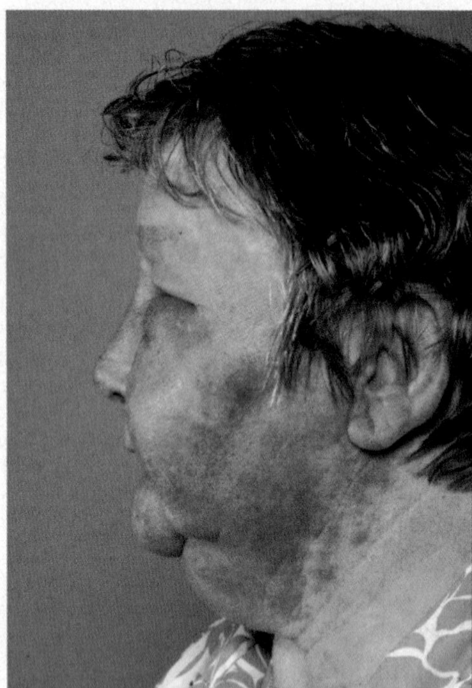

FIGURE 72-2 • **Subacute dermatitis.** Note red (erythematous) patches.

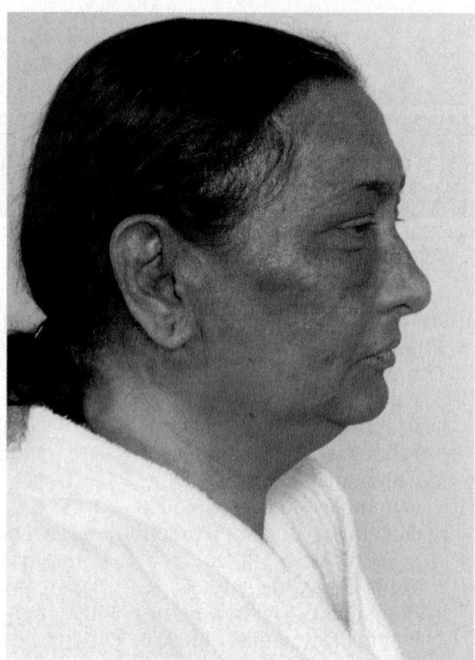

FIGURE 72-3 • **Chronic dermatitis.** The red patches appear lichenified.

seborrheic dermatitis of the scalp is called "cradle cap" (Fig. 72-5). The clinical manifestations of seborrheic dermatitis are erythematous (red) scaling patches involving the central forehead, eyebrows, glabella, nasolabial folds, and scalp; the upper trunk may also be involved. The lay term for involvement of the scalp is "dandruff," the name given to the scaling from the scalp. Seborrheic dermatitis can also occur under mustaches and beards.

Contact Dermatitis

Contact dermatitis is inflammation of the skin induced by contact with an external agent. The dermatitis can be irritant (the substance coming in contact with the skin irritates the skin by directly damaging it) or allergic (the substance coming in contact with the skin induces a type IV hypersensitivity reaction). Contact dermatitis is a relatively frequent cause of occupational disability.

Irritant Contact Dermatitis. When a substance comes in contact with the skin, it can cause mechanical, physical, or chemical irritation to the skin. Irritant contact dermatitis may be caused by common exposures such as water in patients doing "wet work," or be due to irritants at home or in the workplace such as bleach, acids, or alkalis. Since irritants are directly damaging the skin, dermatitis often occurs soon after exposure (Fig. 72-6). The skin becomes inflamed. When the irritant is removed, the dermatitis gradually fades. Soon after exposure, an acute dermatitis is clinically apparent with vesicles, bullae, oozing, and serous crust observed.

Allergic Contact Dermatitis. If any particular substance comes in contact with the skin, it may lead to an allergic contact dermatitis, a delayed-type hypersensitivity reaction. This is termed *allergic contact dermatitis.* Typically, the allergic contact dermatitis does not occur soon after exposure; it starts usually 2 days following exposure and continues for up to 1 or 2 weeks following the exposure and sometimes longer. For example, the most common sensitizer in North America is urushiol, which is found in poison oak, poison ivy, and poison sumac. When any of these plants comes in contact with the skin of a person who has been sensitized, no immediate reaction is noted. However, approximately 24 to 48 hours later, a rash starts at the site. The reaction often presents with an extremely itchy rash, which is characterized by vesicles and bullae and oozing, that corresponds directly to the area where the leaves of the plant came in contact with the skin. The rash progresses and persists for up to 3 to 4 weeks after exposure.

Many substances can induce an allergic contact dermatitis. The only way to determine what might be causing the reaction is to perform patch testing. Common sensitizers in the United States include metals (e.g., nickel), preservatives, and nearly everything we come in contact with in the environment (e.g., formaldehyde, fragrances). Patch testing is not generally performed to urushiol as it may sensitize a patient to this allergen. However, in general, patch testing can be performed for other allergens.

Nummular Dermatitis

Patients with nummular dermatitis present with coin-shaped, red, scaling patches scattered on the trunk and extremities (Fig. 72-7). The cause of these patches is generally unknown, and this form of dermatitis is often stubborn to treat.

Dyshidrotic Eczema (Pompholyx or Dyshidrosis)

Patients with dyshidrotic eczema present with a very pruritic, chronic recurrent dermatitis involving the palms and soles and lateral aspects of the fingers (Fig. 72-8). Patients complain that they experience ini-

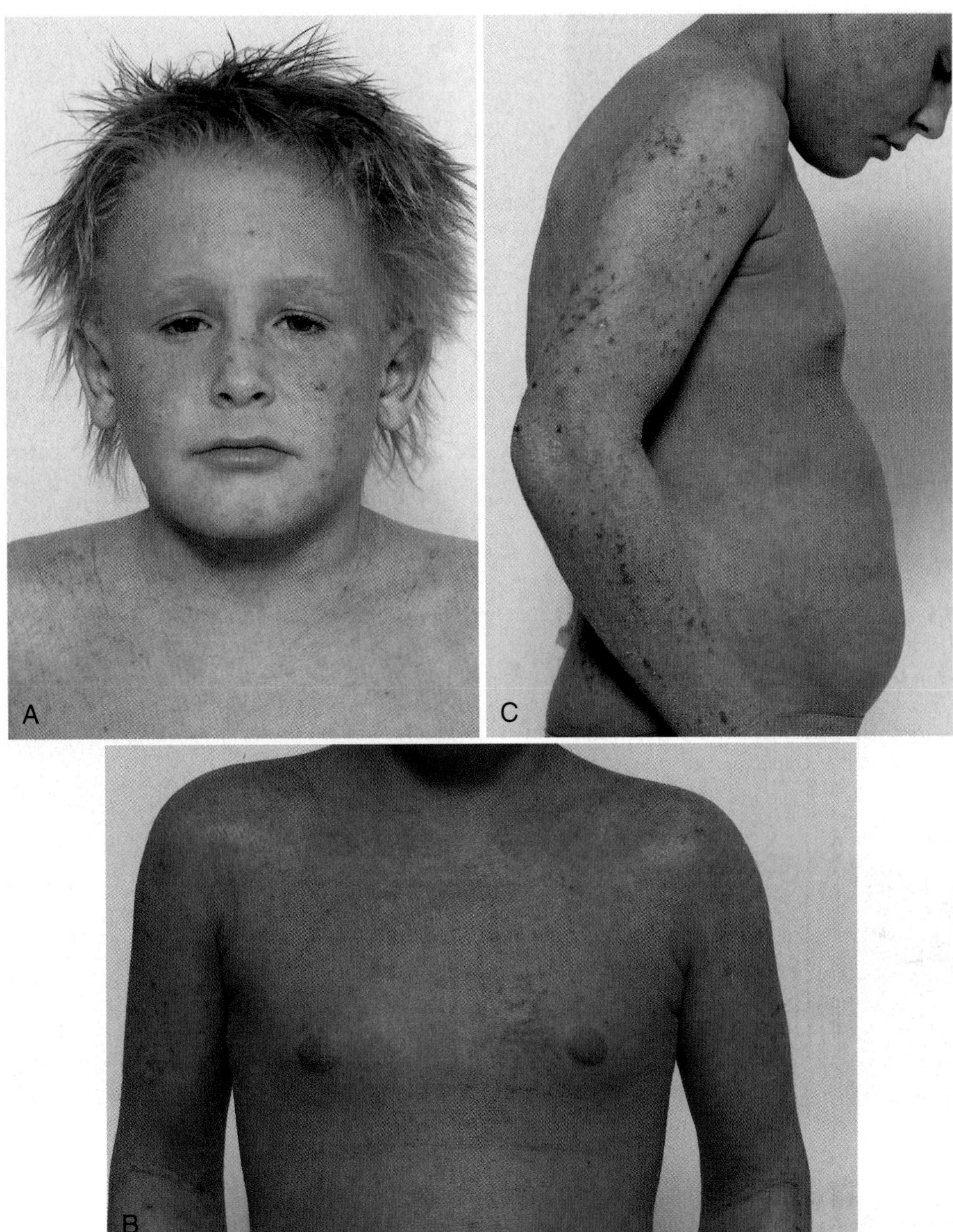

FIGURE 72-4 • Atopic dermatitis with pruritic erythematous patches. A, Atopic dermatitis with involvement of the face and shoulders. **B,** Atopic dermatitis with involvement of the upper extremity. **C,** Atopic dermatitis with involvement of the chest.

tially severe itching in these areas and then start to notice small vesicles, which then desquamate over a period of 1 to 2 weeks.

Stasis Dermatitis

Patients with stasis dermatitis present with a rash, which is itchy, on the legs (Fig. 72-9). On investigation, venous insufficiency will be found. Theoretically, red blood cells extravasate from the veins and venules, leading to inflammation of the skin of the lower legs.

Dermatitis of Unknown Cause

Occasionally, dermatitis does not fit into any of these recognized patterns. It is important to recognize that many forms of dermatitis, particularly severe dermatitis, fit into the "unknown cause" category.

Perioral Dermatitis

Perioral dermatitis is a form of dermatitis that has been increasingly recognized in the last couple of decades. Its prevalence seems to be rising. The condition appears to be related to exposure to cosmetics. It presents characteristically as pink confluent patches in a periorifacial distribution, particularly around the mouth with sparing of the immediate perioral area. Papules and pustules may be associated with this from of dermatitis.

Infectious Eczematoid Dermatitis

In infectious eczematoid dermatitis, inflammation of the skin is caused by infection, most often with staphylococcus or streptococcus. This form of dermatitis may complicate any of the other forms of dermatitis if they become "superinfected." For example, if dermatitis becomes superinfected with herpes simplex infection, this is termed *eczema herpeticum.* In all of these forms of dermatitis, it is important to treat the superinfection.

PATHOPHYSIOLOGY

Overview

In dermatitis, the classic signs of inflammation are present: rubor, calor, tumor, and dolor—redness, heat, swelling, and pain, most com-

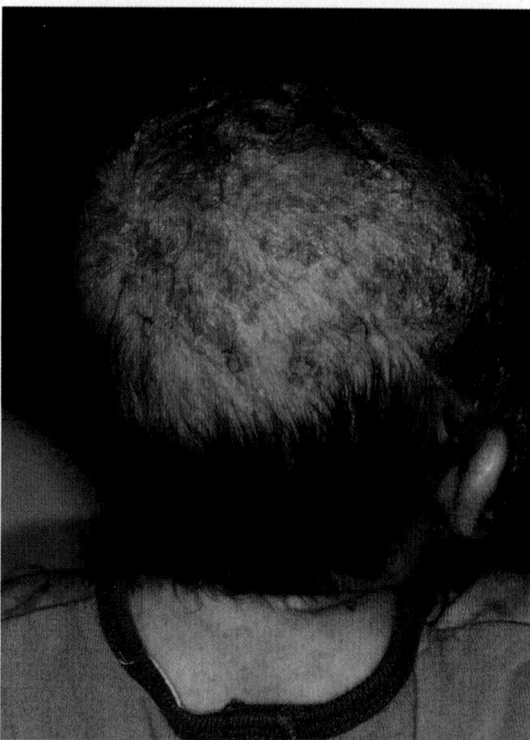

FIGURE 72-5 • Cradle cap.

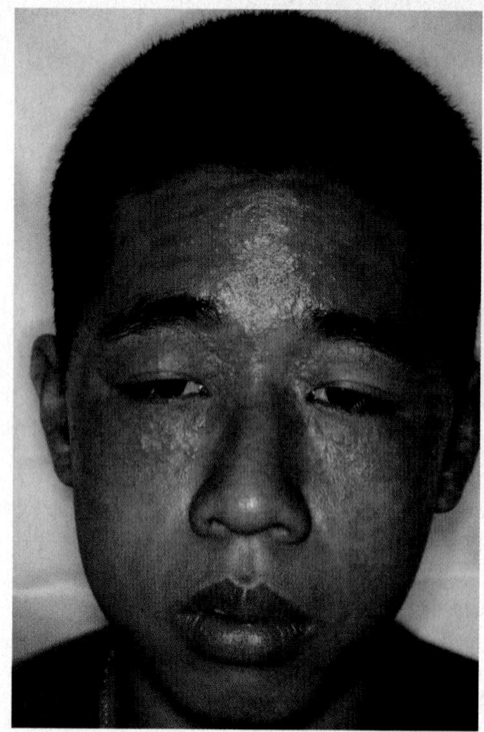

FIGURE 72-6 • Irritant contact dermatitis.

monly reported by the patient as itch. Different factors are therefore involved in different types of dermatitis. The mechanisms by which these factors lead to dermatitis are not fully understood. The mechanisms of dyshidrotic dermatitis and nummular dermatitis have not been elicited, but advances have been made in our understanding of the mechanisms of other types.

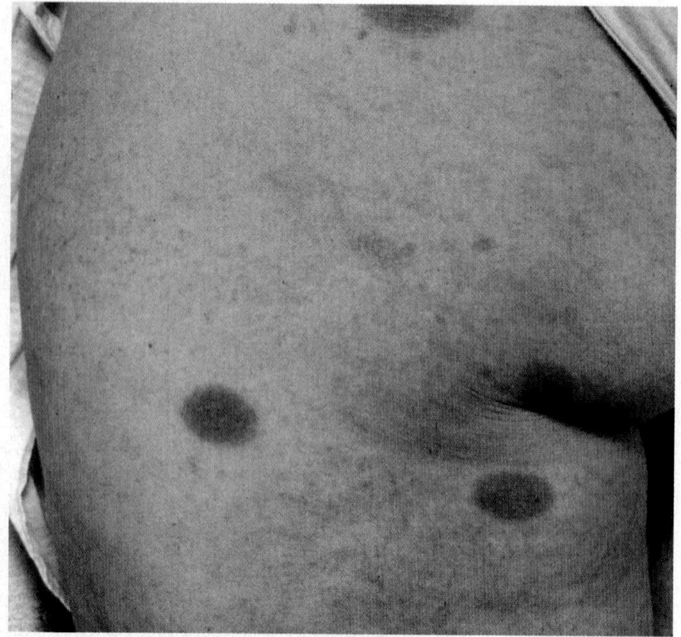

FIGURE 72-7 • Nummular dermatitis.

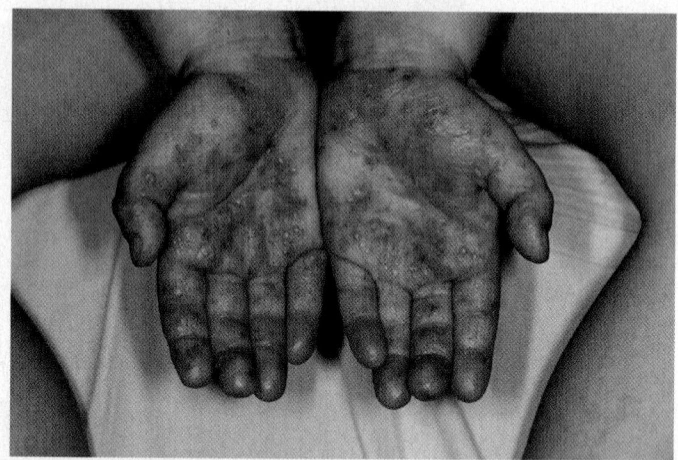

FIGURE 72-8 • Dyshidrotic eczema.

Asteatotic Dermatitis

Asteatotic dermatitis is the most common form of dermatitis. Dryness of the skin leads to inflammation of the skin through an unknown mechanism.

Atopic Dermatitis (Eczema)

Atopic dermatitis denotes a recurrent inflammatory skin condition that is often associated with other "atopic disorders" such as allergic rhinitis and asthma. It is thought that there is a genetic basis for this disorder, but the exact genes involved have not yet been identified. Immunologic disturbances characterize atopy with a predominance of T cells of the T helper type 2 (Th2) type, high interleukin 4 levels, high concentrations of serum immunoglobulin E (IgE). Also noted are reduced cell-mediated immunity, decreased numbers of immunoregulatory T cells, and defective antibody-dependent cellular cytotoxicity. Compromise of the skin barrier is thought to predispose greatly to atopic dermatitis.

It is thought that infections with antigens such as *Staphylococcus aureus* may precipitate and exacerbate atopic dermatitis. These antigens can react as "superantigens." Bacterial infections (such as *S. aureus*) or a viral infection (such as herpes simplex) can complicate atopic

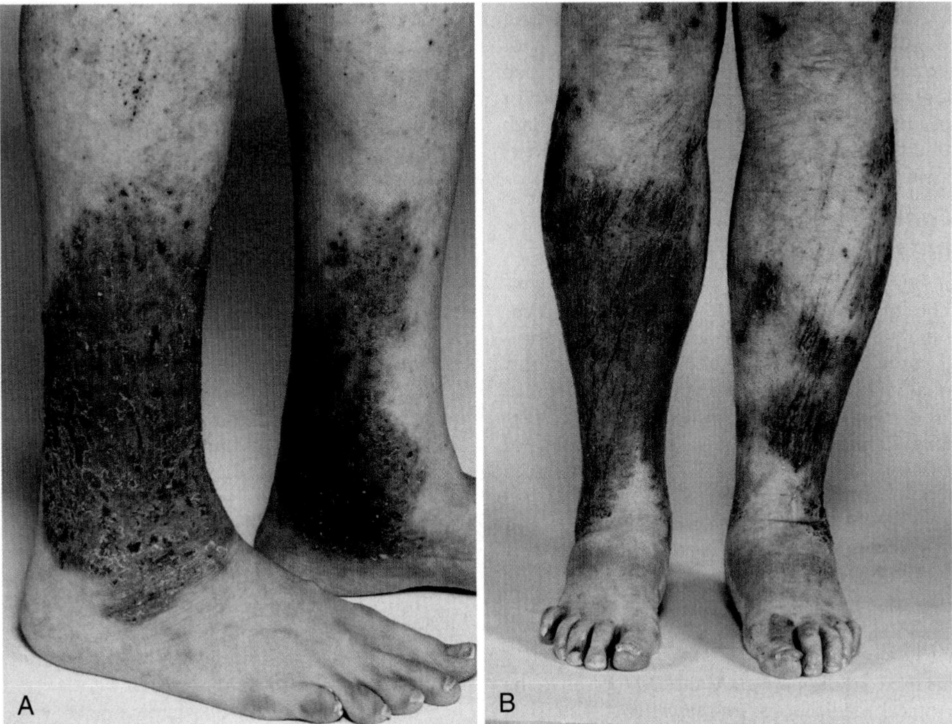

FIGURE 72-9 • **Stasis dermatitis. A,** Stasis dermatitis involves both legs. **B,** Stasis dermatitis involving both legs, worse on the right.

dermatitis. Local deficiencies of antimicrobial peptides have been demonstrated to contribute and reduce the ability to kill *S. aureus.*

Seborrheic Dermatitis

Malassezia furfur has been identified as colonizing the skin of patients with seborrheic dermatitis. It is not known whether this is a secondary or a primary factor. The cause of seborrheic dermatitis is not completely understood.

Contact Dermatitis

In allergic contact dermatitis, an antigen comes in contact with epidermal antigen-presenting cells such as Langerhans cells. It is processed and engulfed by the Langerhans cell, and then moves to regional lymph nodes, where it is presented to T lymphocytes. In the nodes, populations of sensitized T lymphocytes of both CD4 and CD8 subtypes are produced and released into the circulation. These lymphocytes move to the areas where the antigen is present. This is the process of sensitization, which takes approximately 10 to 14 days to occur. Upon reexposure, the antigen is now presented to sensitized lymphocytes, which release cytokines leading to inflammation. This latter process takes 24 to 48 hours.

Stasis Dermatitis

Although the cause of stasis dermatitis is not precisely known, it does seem that venous hypertension leads to some leaking of red cells from the blood vessels, leading to inflammation of the skin by unknown mechanisms. This results in dermatitis patches involving the lower extremities.

Infectious Eczematoid Dermatitis

Infection, usually bacterial, complicates or directly leads to inflammation of the skin. When the infection is herpes simplex virus, the dermatitis is called eczema herpeticum.

Diagnosis

In most circumstances the diagnosis can be made clinically. If there is doubt about the diagnosis, a biopsy will show typical changes. Patch testing may help elicit contact factors that contribute to dermatitis. In cases where allergic contact dermatitis is suspected, patch testing is performed, and the patient is educated on allergen avoidance. In the setting of irritant contact dermatitis, protecting the skin from the irritating substance is extremely important. For example, if soap and water are thought to be the irritant, decrease in exposure to soap and water would be useful.

THERAPEUTICS AND CLINICAL PHARMACOLOGY

Goals of Therapy

Dermatitis is characterized by the signs of inflammation: a rash that is red, hot, swollen, and above all painful and itchy. The goal of therapy is to suppress the inflammation and remove the reason for the inflammation. Clinically this translates to relieving the itch, suppressing the rash, and removing the cause if possible.

The inflammation of dermatitis can be suppressed by:

- Moisturizers and lubricants to restore and maintain the epidermal barrier
- Management of factors contributing to dermatitis: dry skin, infection, contact factors
- Topical medications
- Wet dressings
- Phototherapy
- Immunosuppressant medications

Moisturizers and Lubricants

Emollient creams and lotions restore water and lipids to the epidermis and are an integral part of restoring the normal epidermal barrier, which is disrupted in the setting of dermatitis or other dermatoses. They should be applied frequently to skin and are most effective applied to moist skin, when they "seal in" the moisture (e.g., following a bath or shower). Creams and lotions contain water and are the most effective moisturizers; creams are thicker and more lubricating than lotions.

This is a simple but essential part of therapy. Inflamed skin becomes dry and is more susceptible to further irritation and inflammation.

Resolved dry areas may easily relapse into subacute eczema if proper lubrication is neglected. Lubricants should be continued for days or weeks even after the dermatitis has cleared. Frequent application (up to four times a day) should be encouraged. Lotions or creams with or without the hydrating chemicals urea and lactic acid may be used. Bath oils are very useful if used in amounts sufficient to make the skin feel oily when the patient leaves the tub.[4]

Management of Contributing Factors: Dry Skin, Infection, Contact Factors

Many of the therapeutic approaches are successful in temporarily controlling the itching patches of dermatitis, but the dermatitis will recur if the underlying cause and contributing factors are not treated appropriately. Control of all factors contributing to the dermatitis is important. For example, adequate moisturizing of the skin is a key factor in controlling dermatitis as dry skin can contribute to any form of dermatitis. Thus moisturizers form an important part of prevention of dermatitis. If a contact factor is leading to irritation of the skin or to an allergic contact reaction, that contact factor should be identified and removed if possible. Infection can complicate any dermatitis, and this should be treated if it is thought that this is contributing to perpetuation of the dermatitis; this is especially true in the case of atopic dermatitis.

Topical Medications

Many of the medications used for dermatitis are applied topically. The most commonly used topical medications are topical corticosteroids and the new calcineurin inhibitors (see Therapeutics by Class). Topical medications, especially the topical corticosteroids, are available in cream, ointment, gel, or more recently foam preparations. Each of these has advantages and disadvantages:

- *Creams* are semisolid emulsions of oil and 20% to 50% water; they are considered cosmetically appealing.
- *Ointments* consist primarily of water suspended in oil; these are the most potent vehicles due to their occlusive effect, but they are considered to be greasy.
- *Gels* are an oil-and-water emulsion with alcohol in the base; they are generally used to treat hair-bearing areas and for treating acne.
- *Lotions* consist of powder and water; they are useful in conditions where large areas have to be treated.
- *Solutions* consist of water or water in combination with various medications or substances; they are useful in places such as the scalp.
- *Foams* are pressurized collections of gaseous bubbles in the matrix of liquid film. They spread easily and are easily used on the scalp or on inflamed skin. They are expensive preparations but generally considered the optimum preparation for the scalp.

Wet Dressings

In the setting of severe dermatitis, wet dressings are very effective in obtaining control of the dermatitis. They work in many ways:

- Cooling the skin, thereby decreasing inflammation—A wet dressing rapidly cools, and the cool dressing directly cools the inflamed skin. Cooled skin is associated with vasoconstriction; thus inflammation is suppressed.
- Moisturizing of the skin—The moisture of the wet dressing moisturizes the skin.
- Mechanical débridement—Wet dressings lead to maceration of crusts associated with dermatitis; when the wet dressing is removed, scale, crust (dried serum), and pus are removed with the dressing.
- Antimicrobial action—The diluent effect of water used in wet dressings lessens impetiginization; additionally, anti-infective solutions such as acetic acid and Sweitzer's solution can be used in wetting the dressing for antimicrobial effect in infected dermatitis.
- Occlusion—Wet dressings act as occlusive dressings, leading to increased absorption and penetration of any creams placed underneath (e.g., topical corticosteroids or moisturizers).

The technique of application of wet dressings (also called compresses) may be quite simple: a damp to wet cotton cloth is placed over the patches of dermatitis and left on for various periods of time. For example, in cases of widespread dermatitis, this may take the form of damp to wet pajamas. The damp to wet cloth may be left on for anywhere from 5 minutes to hours. It is important that the temperature of the room be high enough so the patient does not feel chilled.

Specifics of the use of wet dressings include the following:

What should be used to wet the dressings? Tap water, normal saline, or anti-infective solutions such as acetic acid. For antibacterial action, aluminum acetate, acetic acid, or silver nitrate may be added to the water to provide an additional antibacterial effect.

How long should wet dressings be left on? For minutes to hours—protocols vary.

How many times a day should they be applied? Protocols vary: they can be applied from once daily to continuously.

When should they be discontinued? When the acuity of the dermatitis has diminished.

Therapeutics by Class

Topical Treatments

Topical Corticosteroids. Topical corticosteroids are the most important and commonly used anti-inflammatory medications for controlling dermatitis. The armamentarium of topical corticosteroids available to the clinician is large.

Potency. Topical corticosteroids have various potencies as anti-inflammatory agents. They also induce cutaneous vasoconstriction to various extents. Interestingly, the degree of vasoconstriction correlates well with clinical anti-inflammatory efficacy. For that reason, a standard vasoconstriction bioassay is used to measure potency. Therefore, topical corticosteroids are subdivided into four groups:

- Superpotent (class 1)
- Potent (classes 2 to 3)
- Intermediate (classes 4 to 5)
- Mild (classes 6 to 7)

A class 1 agent (e.g., clobetasol propionate ointment) is approximately 1000 times more potent than hydrocortisone 1% (which is the only corticosteroid that is available over the counter in the United States).

Mechanisms of Action. Topical corticosteroids, like systemic corticosteroids, produce an anti-inflammatory response in the skin by many different mechanisms:

- Stabilizing the lysosomes in neutrophils, which prevents degranulation and the resulting inflammatory response.
- Inducing the anti-inflammatory protein lipocortin. This protein inhibits the enzyme phospholipase A_2, which inhibits synthesis of prostaglandins and lipoxygenase products.
- Binding to glucocorticoid receptors (GRs) located in the cytoplasm. After binding occurs, the activated GR moves from the cytoplasm to the nucleus, where upregulation of anti-inflammatory genes (e.g., lipocortin, neutral endopeptidase, inhibitors of plasminogen activator) occurs. This effect results from binding of the GRs to glucocorticoid response elements.
- Decreasing the stability of selected messenger RNA molecules, which alter gene transcription. Genes affected by this action include those involved in synthesis of collagenase, elastase, plasminogen activator, nitric oxide synthase, cyclooxygenase-2, cytokines, and chemokines.[5]
- Inhibiting the cytokines involved with allergic reactions; they thus reduce the inflammatory response elicited by these cytokines.[5]

Application. Topical corticosteroids are applied generally one to three times daily. They are most commonly prescribed in cream or ointment forms.

Selection. Generally a mid-potency type of corticosteroid (intermediate potency) is adequate to control dermatitis if applied regularly (two to three times daily) to affected areas of the trunk and extremities. In severe cases, this can be used in conjunction with wet dressings. For areas of thinner skin, such as the face and body folds (axillae, groin), a corticosteroid of mild potency can be used. When the dermatitis is under control, the medication should be weaned (to prevent rebound) and stopped. Superpotent corticosteroids are generally reserved for areas of severe dermatitis involving the trunk and extremities for short periods of time (up to 3 weeks).[6]

Side Effects. Generally, topical corticosteroids are safe, but they may occasionally be associated with atrophy, telangiectasia, and striae, especially with potent and superpotent forms. To avoid these side effects, it is generally recommended that topical corticosteroids be used for a relatively short time. It is also important to realize that allergic sensitization to topical corticosteroids can occur either to the vehicle preservative or the corticosteroid itself. This should be suspected in patients with dermatitis who do not respond to topical corticosteroids. Suppression of the hypothalamic-pituitary axis can occur with the prolonged use of potent or superpotent corticosteroids especially if used on widespread areas of the body, but this is rare.[7]

Calcineurin Inhibitors. In the past decade, calcineurin inhibitors (tacrolimus ointment [Protopic] and pimecrolimus cream [Elidel]) have been introduced and are finding their place in the armaterium of treatment options used for dermatoses, including dermatitis. They are macrolide immune suppressants that inhibit the production of inflammatory cytokines in T cells and mast cells, and thus act as effective immunosuppressants. A major advantage of these agents is that they do not cause the atrophy associated with the use of topical corticosteroids. They are approximately similar in clinical effectiveness as immunosuppressants to corticosteroids of mild to intermediate potency.[8]

The long-term safety of topical calcineurin inhibitors has not been established. Although a causal relationship has not been established, rare cases of malignancy (e.g., skin and lymphoma) have been reported in patients treated with topical calcineurin inhibitors, including tacrolimus ointment and pimecrolimus cream. In March 2005, the U.S. Food and Drug Administration issued an alert to health care professionals concerning a potential link between topical pimecrolimus and tacrolimus and cancer (mainly lymphoma and skin cancer) on the basis of studies in animals, case reports, and knowledge of how these drugs work. The alert emphasizes the importance of using these preparations only as labeled and when first-line treatment has failed or cannot be tolerated.

Continuous long-term use of topical calcineurin inhibitors, including tacrolimus ointment and pimecrolimus cream, in any age group should be avoided, and application limited to areas of involvement with atopic dermatitis. Tacrolimus ointment and pimecrolimus cream are not indicated for use in children less than 2 years of age. Only 0.03% tacrolimus ointment is indicated for use in children 2 to 15 years of age

Tacrolimus. Tacrolimus is a macrolide immunosuppressant 10 to 100 times more potent than cyclosporine. Its lower molecular weight and higher potency suggest that it might be a better topical agent than cyclosporine. Although chemically unrelated to cyclosporine, tacrolimus suppresses the immune response through a similar mechanism of action by preventing nuclear translocation of the transcription factor nuclear factor-AT and inhibiting the expression of early T-cell activation genes. The exact mechanism of action of tacrolimus in atopic dermatitis is not known. Tacrolimus inhibits T-lymphocyte activation by first binding to the intracellular protein FK506 binding protein 12 (FKBP-12), by forming a complex with FKBP-12, calcium, calmodulin, and calcineurin, inhibiting the phosphatase activity of calcineurin. This is believed to prevent the formation of lymphokines such as interleukin (IL)–2 and interferon-γ. Tacrolimus also inhibits the transcription of genes that encode IL-3, IL-4, IL-5, granulocyte-macrophage colony-stimulating factor, and tumor necrosis factor-α; inhibits the release of preformed mediators from skin mast cells and basophils; and down-regulates FcεRI expression on Langerhans cells.

Tacrolimus is effective in the treatment of children (ages 2 years and older) and adults with atopic dermatitis. The most common adverse effect of tacrolimus is a sensation of pruritus and a burning sensation involving the skin to which it is applied. Systemic problems are rare as there is little absorption of this large molecule.[8]

Pimecrolimus. The mechanism of action of pimecrolimus in atopic dermatitis is not known. It has been demonstrated that pimecrolimus binds with high affinity to macrophilin-12 (FKBP-12) and inhibits the calcium-dependent phosphatase calcineurin. As a consequence, it inhibits T-cell activation by blocking the transcription of early cytokines. Pimecrolimus at nanomolar concentrations inhibits IL-2 and interferon-γ (T helper type 1) and IL-4 and IL-10 (Th2 type) cytokine synthesis in human T cells. Also, pimecrolimus prevents the release of inflammatory cytokines and mediators from mast cells in vitro after stimulation by antigen/IgE.

Pimecrolimus permeates through skin at a lower rate than tacrolimus, indicating a lower potential for percutaneous absorption. The cream is applied twice a day and may be used on the face. There are no restrictions on duration of use. Adverse effects include a burning sensation in the skin; rarely, a headache and fever have been described.[9]

Tar. Prior to the availability of topical corticosteroids in the 1950s, tars were used for dermatitis. Preparations included tar ointments, baths, and soaps. Tar preparations are occasionally still used in the setting of recalcitrant dermatitis or between short courses of topical steroids.

Antihistamines

Antihistamines are useful in the context of dermatitis primarily to control the sensation of itch. Sedating antihistamines such as diphenhydramine (Benadryl) and hydroxyzine (Atarax) are beneficial because of their sedative properties that permit patients to sleep; in general, these are used at night but can be used during the daytime in cases of severe itching. Nonsedating anthistamines are often used during the daytime to suppress the itch sensation.

Doxepin hydrochloride, a dibenzoxepin derivative with antipruritic and antidepressant effects, belongs to a class of psychotherapeutic agents called dibenzoxepin tricyclic compounds. It has no known mechanism of action, although its antidepressant effect is believed to be partly due to its influences on the adrenergic activity at the synapses, where it prevents norepinephrine deactivation through reuptake into the nerve terminals. It is also known to have anticholinergic, antiserotonin, and antihistamine effects. It is considered a very effective antipruritic.

Antibiotics

Antibiotics are useful in the control of infected dermatitis. Signs of infected dermatitis include pustules, purulent material, and crusting of the dermatitis. Systemic antibiotics are favored in the treatment of infected dermatitis; topical antibiotics are much less effective. Superinfection of dermatitis is most often caused by *Staphylococcus.* The choice of antibiotic should be guided by the results of culture and susceptibility studies of a skin culture. Empirically, systemic antibiotic therapy including that with cephalexin, erythromycin, or one of the tetracyclines is used pending the results of culture/susceptibility studies. Although combinations of topical corticosteroids and antibiotics are used for atopic dermatitis, no good evidence suggests that they offer additional benefits as compared with topical corticosteroids alone.[6]

Phototherapy

Phototherapy is a useful therapeutic modality in dermatitis that is recalcitrant to topical treatments of the skin, including the use of topical corticosteroids, moisturizers, calcineurin, and calcineurin inhibitors. Modalities of ultraviolet (UV) light treatment include broadband ultraviolet B (UVB), narrowband UVB (NB-UVB), and psoralen plus ultraviolet A (PUVA). All of these have been found to be useful in the setting of atopic dermatitis in particular, but can also be used for any type of widespread dermatitis. How UVB phototherapy works is not fully understood, although the overall effect is local immunosuppression in the skin. It has been demonstrated that, with UV light, a decrease in the number of Langerhans cells in the skin occurs. Ultraviolet light has been found to induce T-cell apoptosis.

Conventional UV phototherapy involves treatment of both diseased and normal skin, which are exposed to UV light usually in the setting of a cabinet. In cases of widespread dermatitis, generally low doses of

UV light are used and then gradually advanced. With repetitive exposures, normal human skin gradually photoadapts or acquires tolerance to UV light; the rate at which this develops in normal skin has been established empirically through clinical practice. The concept of UV tolerance guides any course of phototherapy, and detailed insights into its biologic basis and kinetics are still under active systematic study.

Over the past one or two decades, NB-UVB treatments have become very popular, and their use is now surpassing that of PUVA. This is in part because NB-UVB is convenient. It is said to be as effective as PUVA for dermatitis involving the skin; however, robust studies have not been performed comparing these modalities.[10]

Systemic Corticosteroids

Oral corticosteroids such as prednisone are useful for controlling intense acute dermatitis. For example, in the context of poison ivy dermatitis, prednisone is prescribed for 3 weeks to suppress the allergic contact dermatitis, which is known to persist for up to 3 weeks but generally not beyond that.

Most forms of dermatitis persist for longer periods of time, however, and for that reason treatment of dermatitis with systemic corticosteroids is generally not favored. In addition, there is a lack of data supporting this practice. If this modality of treatment is used for most forms of dermatitis, high doses of corticosteroids over prolonged periods will be necessary, predisposing the patients to all the side effects of systemic corticosteroids.

In cases of severe intractable dermatitis, systemic corticosteroids can be used for short periods of time, generally combined with other steroid-sparing immunosuppressive drugs.

Other Immunosuppressive Medications

In rare circumstances, it is not possible to control severe dermatitis with topical corticosteroids, wet dressings, and phototherapy. Azathioprine, cyclosporine, and mycophenolate mofetil can be used as immunosuppressive drugs in this circumstance.[11]

Therapeutic Approach

General Treatment Guidelines

General guidelines for treatment of dermatitis follow a progression:

- Adequate lubrication of the skin is the cornerstone of management of any dermatitis.
- In general, the first line of treatment for dermatitis is the application of topical corticosteroids. Generally a mid-potency type of corticosteroid is adequate to control dermatitis if applied regularly (two to three times daily). In severe cases, this can be used in conjunction with wet dressings. Adequate moisturizing of the skin using lubricants is extremely important also.
- If widespread dermatitis proves to be recalcitrant to this regimen, then the addition of UV light treatments can be considered, and either PUVA, NB-UVB, or broadband UVB can be added.
- If the dermatitis does not respond to these measures, consideration can be given to initiation of an immunosuppressive medication.

Treatment Guidelines for Specific Forms of Dermatitis

Specific types of dermatitis can be treated with specific treatment intervention.[12]

- For atopic dermatitis, the previously mentioned regimens can be used with aggressive moisturizing of the skin, the use of topical corticosteroids, and the use of UV light treatments. Systemic immunosuppressives can also be used.
- For seborrheic dermatitis, an antifungal shampoo can be added to the use of topical corticosteroids. This has also been used alone in some cases.
- The management of contact dermatitis entails removal of the agent causing the contact allergy or irritation.
- The management of nummular dermatitis can be difficult. This is often a recalcitrant type of dermatitis. Sometimes a higher potency topical corticosteroid is necessary to control nummular dermatitis.
- For dyshidrotic eczema, class I topical corticosteroids may be necessary. This form of dermatitis can also be very recalcitrant to treatment.
- For stasis dermatitis, in addition to the use of topical corticosteroids, compression is necessary, and sometimes treatment of the varicose veins.
- For dermatitis of unknown cause, topical corticosteroids, moisturizing, and phototherapy can be used.
- For the most common type of dermatitis, asteatotic dermatitis, the above measures can be initiated, with particular emphasis on adequate moisturizing of the skin.

Emerging Targets and Therapeutics

Much of the research in new treatments for dermatitis has focused on atopic dermatitis. Many new treatments are currently under investigation, including IL-11, thymopentin, thalidomide, probiotics, and phosphodiesterase inhibitors. It has recently been realized that, in atopic dermatitis, there is decreased capacity to produce antimicrobial peptides (AMPs), and this is associated with an increased susceptibility to skin infection. Current research continues to discover novel AMPs, and how they function and are regulated. It is possible that, in the future, drugs that would upregulate AMPs in the skin may be available.

REFERENCES

1. Trepka MJ, Heinrich J, Wichmann HE. The epidemiology of atopic diseases in Germany: an East-West comparison. Rev Environ Health 1996;11:119.
2. Hanifin JM, Rajka G. Diagnostic features of atopic dermatitis. Acta Dermatol Venereol 1980;92:44.
3. Leung DY, Bieber T. Atopic dermatitis. Lancet 2003;361:151-160.
4. Lucky AW, Leach AD, Laskarzewski P, Wenck H. Use of an emollient as a steroid-sparing agent in the treatment of mild to moderate atopic dermatitis in children. Pediatr Dermatol 1997;14:321-324.
5. Schwiebert LM, Beck LA, Stellato C, et al. Glucocorticosteroid inhibition of cytokine production: relevance to antiallergic actions [Review]. J Allergy Clin Immunol 1996;97(1 Pt 2):143-152.
6. Hoare C, Li Wan Po A, Williams H. Systematic review of treatments for atopic eczema. Health Technol Assess 2000;4:1-191.
7. Drake LA, Dinehart SM, Farmer ER, et al. Guidelines of care for the use of topical glucocorticosteroids. American Academy of Dermatology. J Am Acad Dermatol 1996;35:615.
8. Ashcroft DM, Dimmock P, Garside R, et al. Efficacy and tolerability of topical pimecrolimus and tacrolimus in the treatment of atopic dermatitis: meta-analysis of randomised controlled trials. BMJ 2005;330:516.
9. Eichenfield LF, Lucky AW, Boguniewicz M, et al. Safety and efficacy of pimecrolimus (ASM 981) cream 1% in the treatment of mild and moderate atopic dermatitis in children and adolescents. J Am Acad Dermatol 2002;46:495.
10. Jekler J, Larko O. Combined UVA-UVB versus UVB phototherapy for atopic dermatitis: a paired-comparison study. J Am Acad Dermatol 1990;22:49.
11. Meggitt SJ, Gray JC, Reynolds NJ. Azathioprine dosed by thiopurine methyltransferase activity for moderate-to-severe atopic eczema: a double-blind, randomised controlled trial. Lancet 2006;367:839.
12. Hanifin JM, Cooper KD, Ho VC, et al. Guidelines of care for atopic dermatitis, developed in accordance with the American Academy of Dermatology (AAD)/American Academy of Dermatology Association "Administrative Regulations for Evidence-Based Clinical Practice Guidelines." J Am Acad Dermatol 2004;50:391-404.

SECTION 17 Rheumatologic Therapeutics

73 OSTEOARTHRITIS

William F. Harvey and David J. Hunter

OVERVIEW 1015
INTRODUCTION 1015
NORMAL PHYSIOLOGY 1015
Articular Cartilage 1015
Bone 1016
Synovium 1016
Meniscus 1016
Ligaments 1016
Muscle 1016
PATHOPHYSIOLOGY 1016
THERAPEUTICS AND CLINICAL PHARMACOLOGY 1017
Goals of Therapy 1017
Therapeutics by Class 1018
Analgesics 1018
Nonsteroidal Anti-inflammatory Medications 1019
Topical Agents 1020
Intra-articular Corticosteroids 1021
Hyaluronic Acid Derivatives 1021
Glucosamine and Chondroitin 1021
Therapeutic Approach 1021
Emerging Targets and Therapeutics 1022
Interleukin-1 1022
Matrix Metalloproteinases 1023
Cyclooxygenase-2 Isoenzymes 1023
Bradykinin and Nitric Oxide 1023
SUMMARY 1023

OVERVIEW

This chapter covers the clinical pharmacology of osteoarthritis. It begins by discussing the impact of osteoarthritis and then covers the normal physiology of the joint. Each structure within the joint is reviewed to provide a framework for discussing the pathophysiology of osteoarthritis, with reference to drug targets.

The goals of therapy are discussed, followed by a detailed review of the major therapeutic options, by class. The classes covered include analgesics, anti-inflammatory medications, topical agents, and intra-articular agents. Included in each section is history, pharmacokinetics and pharmacodynamics, and typical dosages of each agent as well as common toxicities. We conclude by discussing a rational therapeutic approach followed by an overview of emerging therapeutic targets.

INTRODUCTION

Osteoarthritis (OA) is the most prevalent form of arthritis and one of the leading causes of chronic disability among older individuals.[1] The societal burden imposed (in terms of both personal suffering and health resource utilization) by this highly prevalent condition is expected to increase even further with the increasing prevalence of obesity and the aging of the community.[1] By 2020, the number of people with OA will have doubled, due in large part to the exploding prevalence of obesity and the aging of the "baby boomer" generation.[2] The largest increases will occur among older adults, for whom OA also has the greatest functional impact.

Osteoarthritis is a multifactorial process in which mechanical factors play a central role and is characterized by changes in structure and function of the whole joint.[3] The etiopathogenesis of OA is widely believed to be the result of local mechanical factors acting within the context of systemic susceptibility. These systemic factors that increase the vulnerability of the joint to OA include age, gender, bone density, nutritional factors, and genetic predisposition.[4] In persons vulnerable to the development of OA, local mechanical factors such as malalignment, muscle weakness, or alterations in the structural integrity of the joint environment (such as meniscal damage or bone marrow lesions) facilitate the progression of OA.

The pharmacologic treatment of OA focuses on the components of this whole joint, with targets as small as individual cells and the cytokines they produce and as large as joint components such as cartilage and bone and their innervations and blood supply. The aims of management of patients with OA are patient education about both the disease and its management, pain control, improvement of function and reduction in disability, and alteration of the disease process and its consequences. With these goals and targets in mind, a detailed understanding of the structure, function, and pathology of joints is critical.

NORMAL PHYSIOLOGY

Osteoarthritis can be viewed as the clinical and pathologic outcome of a range of disorders that result in structural and functional failure of synovial joints.[5] Osteoarthritis occurs when the dynamic equilibrium between the breakdown and repair of joint tissues is overwhelmed.[6] Traditionally, OA has been considered a disease of articular cartilage. The current concept holds that OA involves the entire joint organ, including the subchondral bone, menisci, ligaments, periarticular muscle, capsule, and synovium. The pathology reflects the result of and response to joint failure, with loss and erosion of articular cartilage, subchondral bone alterations, meniscal degeneration, synovitis, and bone and cartilage growth (osteophytes).

Articular Cartilage

The cartilage present at the articular surface of synovial joints is made up of hyaline cartilage. The name "hyaline" is derived from the Greek word *hyalos*, meaning glass. This refers to the translucent matrix or ground substance. Hyaline cartilage is found lining bones in joints (articular cartilage). The main constituents of hyaline cartilage are type II collagen, water, chondrocytes, and a proteoglycan matrix.

Type II collagen makes up 40% of the dry weight of hyaline cartilage, and is arranged in cross-striated fibers, 15 to 45 nm in diameter, that do not assemble into large bundles. Cartilage is a specialized form of connective tissue containing chondrocytes that secrete, and are surrounded by, the intercellular matrix. Chondrocytes occur singly or in isogenous groups, composed of two to eight cells derived by mitosis from a single chondrocyte. The cells are in lacunae (cavities) within the matrix.

The strength and durability of cartilage are properties of the matrix, which is an interlaced network of collagenous and/or elastic fibers in a ground substance, a gel of complex proteoglycans. The water and proteoglycan provide the cartilage with elasticity, and the orientation of the collagen promotes resistance to wear. Cartilage matrix is a homogeneous material principally composed of proteoglycans (macromolecules with a proteinaceous backbone), to which are attached complex carbohydrates known as glycosaminoglycans (GAGs). The GAGs radiate from the protein core like the bristles of a bottle brush. The principal GAGs of cartilage are chondroitin sulfate and keratin sulfate.

Articular cartilage lacks a blood supply and gains its nutrients from the surrounding synovial fluid. It also lacks lymphatic drainage and has no innervations, and therefore is unlikely to be responsible for the symptoms experienced by persons affected by OA. Chondrocytes, in response to various cytokines such as interleukin (IL)-1 and tumor necrosis factor (TNF), degrade and rebuild cartilage to maintain a homeostatic thickness of 2 to 4 mm in joints such as the knee and hip.

Bone

Underlying the articular cartilage is the subchondral bone. Bone is made up of a combination of inorganic components such as calcium hydroxyapatite and organic components such as protein matrix and osteocytes, which control the metabolism of bone. Osteoblasts, under the influence of various hormones and cytokines, work to build bone, while osteoclasts erode it. Normally there is a homeostasis that maintains bone strength and health. The hormones and cytokines involved in this process include parathyroid hormone, IL-1, IL-3, IL-6, IL-11, fibroblast growth factor, platelet-derived growth factor, and transforming growth factor-β.

Synovium

The synovium is the inner lining of the joint space and is responsible for producing the synovial fluid, which provides nutrients as well as lubrication for the cartilage. Hyaluronic acid is an important constituent of joint fluid. Synovial tissue is highly vascular and also has some innervations. Synoviocytes also produce cytokines to help control the normal biochemical processes in the joint.

Meniscus

Several joints in the body, most notably the knee, contain an additional cartilaginous structure called the meniscus. Made up primarily of fibrocartilage, the meniscus serves to provide additional cushioning and alignment to the joint. The menisci have a limited amount of vascular supply and innervations.

Ligaments

The ligaments and joint capsule are composed of collagen and function to provide stability to the joint. The various joints have varying degrees of mobility related to their function. In order to maintain this mobility, a sacrifice must be made in stability, and the ligaments and periarticular muscle maintain this stability. The joint capsule also serves to contain the synovial fluid within the joint space. The capsule has a rich blood supply and is well innervated.

Muscle

The muscles provide additional strength and stability to the joint through coordinated contraction. For example, flexion of the knee requires the paired contraction of the hamstring muscles with relaxation of the quadriceps. Muscles also help to maintain alignment of the articular surfaces throughout the range of mobility. The more mobile a joint is, the more important a role muscle health plays. In the shoulder, the rotator cuff helps prevent dislocation and impingement caused by misalignment. Tears of the rotator cuff are a well-described risk factor for OA in that joint.

PATHOPHYSIOLOGY

Osteoarthritis can occur in any synovial joint in the body, but is most common in the hands, knees, hips, and spine. Research into the etiology and progression of knee OA has focused on the destruction of articular cartilage. However, it is clear that knee OA is an organ-level failure of the joint and involves pathologic changes in articular cartilage as well as in subchondral bone, menisci, ligaments, periarticular muscle, capsule, and synovium.[7] The pathology reflects the result of and response to joint failure, with loss and erosion of articular cartilage, subchondral bone alterations, meniscal degeneration, synovitis, and bone and cartilage growth (osteophytes) (Fig. 73-1).

One of the earliest recognized changes in a joint with OA is fibrillation of the articular cartilage. This presumably occurs when the mechanical forces on the cartilage exceed the tensile strength and cause microdamage. In addition to mechanical forces, various cytokines (IL-1, TNF-α) also play a role by stimulating the production of metalloproteinases, which assist in degrading cartilage and also inhibit the production of collagen and matrix. Injuries to the meniscus and/or ligaments are also known risk factors for the incidence and progression of disease.[8]

It has been suggested that the health and integrity of the joint cartilage is dependent upon the mechanical properties of the underlying subchondral bone. Thick, dense bone is thought to be incapable of dissipating the forces on the joint during ambulation, leading to cartilage breakdown. It may also inhibit nutrition from the marrow space to the joint cartilage. However, the exact role of bony changes in the initiation and progression of knee OA is unclear—in particular, whether the observed changes occur prior to, simultaneously with, or secondary to the deterioration of articular cartilage.[7] Indeed, there do appear to be some changes that occur within the bone prior to cartilage destruction, including the thickening of the subchondral cortical plate.[9]

Changes in subchondral bone are well described in established OA, in both human and animal models.[10] These changes include remodeling of the subchondral trabeculae,[11] stiffening of the subchondral bone,[12,13] thickening of the subchondral plate,[14] a steep stiffness gradient,[13] and a decrease of the ability to absorb energy. Changes in subchondral bone may be caused by mechanical,[7,15] genetic,[16] hormonal,[17] or other metabolic factors.[18,19]

Subjacent to the thickened cortical plate, studies have reported hypomineralization of trabecular bone.[14,20,21] This osteoporosis is possibly linked to abnormal bone cell behavior in osteoarthritic joints, reported as imbalances in bone resorption, formation, or both.[22] In addition to bone being lost locally within the diseased joint, altered bone tissue content has been reported in OA patients at sites distant from weight-bearing joints.[23]

Osteoarthritis is characterized by hypertrophic bone changes with osteophyte formation and subchondral plate thickening. The bone sclerosis may be due to dysregulation of bone remodeling. These variations in osteoarthritic subchondral bone structure may significantly affect the biomechanical competence of bone.

The bone also undergoes changes in response to cytokines. These cytokines cause the formation of osteophytes, bony protrusions that theoretically serve to strengthen the mechanics of the joint, but that also affect the structures surrounding the joint and can cause pain.

Eventually, the articular cartilage erodes completely and the bones come in direct contact with each other. This leads to additional deformities and decreased function of the joint. The end stage of this deterioration is complete loss of the joint space, with little to no joint function. It is important to note that, while cytokines certainly play an important role in pathophysiology, true inflammation with recruitment of inflammatory cells and systemic inflammatory symptoms occurs only as a minor component of the disease process.

Contributing to the milieu of pathology are the muscles, the synovium, and the presence of effusions. As noted previously, the muscles help maintain joint stability and, when diseased, may play a role in the initiation of cartilage damage. The inflamed synovium produces cytokines and fluid that contribute to the symptoms experienced by persons affected by OA. While effusions are a response to injury that makes some biomechanical sense (decreasing the friction within joints), this can be maladaptive because of the cytokine-producing cells contained within the effusion.

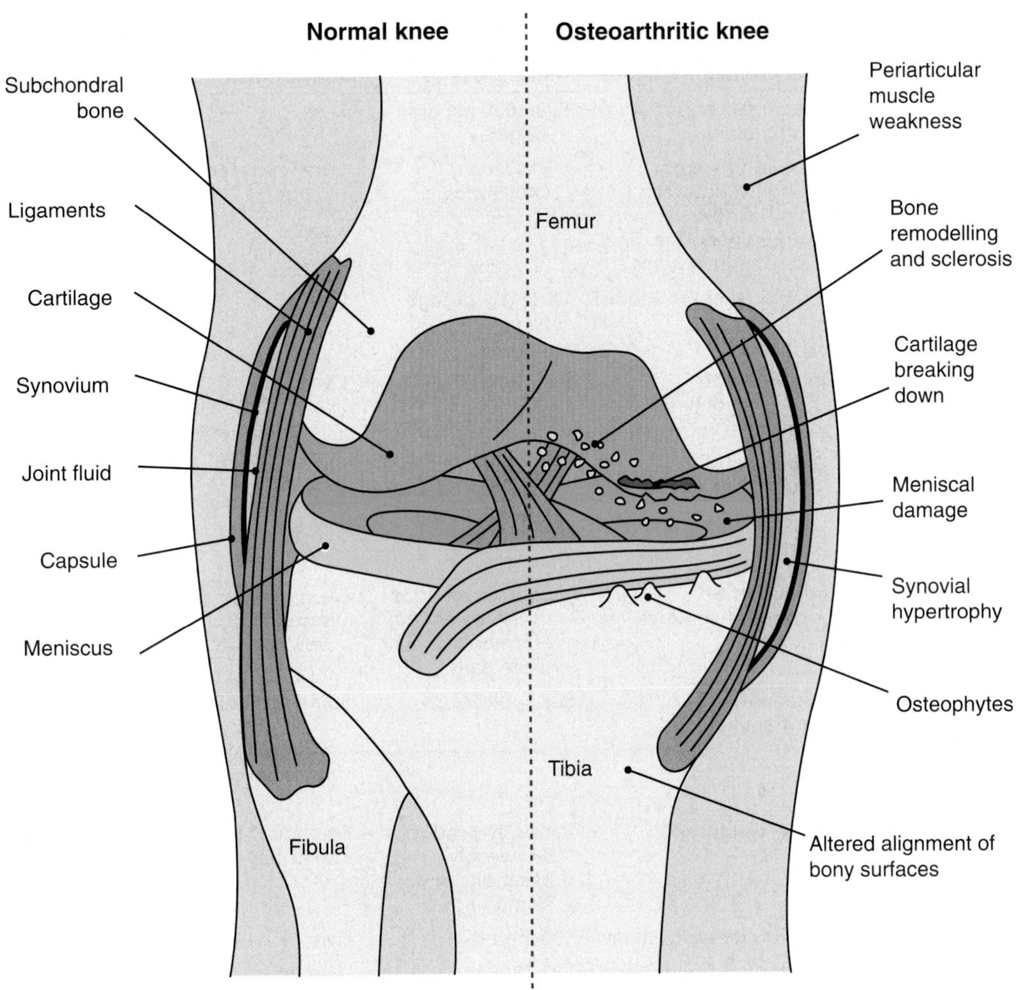

FIGURE 73-1 • Schematic demonstrating the characteristic pathologic changes that occur in joints affected by osteoarthritis.

BOX 73-1 GOALS OF PHARMACOTHERAPY

- Patient education
- Pain control
- Improvement of function
- Reduction of disability
- Alteration of disease progression
- Individualizing the treatment plan

THERAPEUTICS AND CLINICAL PHARMACOLOGY

Goals of Therapy (Box 73-1)

The goals of therapy in OA are patient education about the disease and its management, pain control, improvement in function and reduction in disability, and altering the disease process and its consequences. The management of OA should be individualized for the person presenting, and likely will consist of a combination of treatment options. It should be modified according to the response obtained. Comprehensive management always includes a combination of treatment options that are directed toward the common goal of improving the patient's pain and tolerance for functional activity.

The majority of interventions currently tested and prescribed for knee OA involve either drugs or surgery.[24] Options for the conservative care of patients with knee OA are often overlooked.[25] However, given the known toxicity and adverse event profiles of therapies such as nonsteroidal anti-inflammatory drugs (NSAIDs), cyclooxygenase (COX)-2 inhibitors, and total joint replacement surgery, we recommend that primary care for knee OA place far greater emphasis on nonpharmacologic treatments. Only when more conservative efforts fail to improve function should pharmaceuticals be offered. Surgery should be a last resort.

Prevention is based on management of known risk factors, the most important of which are obesity and injury.[26] Modification of these factors is largely nonpharmacologic and will not be discussed in further detail here. Likewise, the management of end-stage OA with the goal of restoring normal function is largely a surgical issue and will not be discussed in detail. As we learn more about the pathogenesis of OA, these two areas may see the advent of novel therapies for prevention and cure of OA.

Mechanical factors play a predominant role in the progression of OA. Attention to these factors (especially obesity, malalignment, and muscle weakness) in managing the patient with OA is critical if we are to impact the increasing burden of OA among older adults.[27] Nonpharmacologic modalities of therapy, including weight control, physical therapy, exercise, braces, shoes, and devices, are helpful in reducing the impact of mechanical factors.

Symptom management in OA can also be achieved through the use of analgesic medications of various classes. These include several routes of administration such as oral, topical, and intra-articular. Symptom management, while not altering the disease course, will improve an individual's functional status, with the goal of allowing continued participation in work, activities of daily living, and recreation. Delaying disease progression is a challenging part of the management of OA. With the goal of delaying the need for surgical intervention, several therapeutics show potential in this area. This area also represents a focus of intense investigation for new pharmacologic interventions.

TABLE 73-1 OVERVIEW OF PHARMACOLOGIC THERAPY FOR OSTEOARTHRITIS

Drug Name	Mechanism of Action	Usual Dosage	Metabolism	Side Effects	Comments
Acetaminophen	Exact mechanism unknown	500-1000 mg qid, <4 g/day	Liver	Hepatotoxicity if >4 g/day or with alcohol	Analgesic of choice.
Tramadol	μ-Opioid receptor agonist, interacts with GABA, norepinephrine, and serotonin systems	50-100 mg qid, <400 mg/day	Liver, excreted in urine	Nausea, CNS depression; may potentiate seizures in combination with other drugs	May be expensive.
Narcotics	Opioid receptor agonist	Varies by dosage form	Liver	CNS and respiratory depression	Requires license to prescribe, high addiction potential.
NSAIDs	Inhibition of cyclooxygenase enzymes	See Table 73-2	Liver	Gastrointestinal, renal, cardiovascular	
Capsaicin	Depletion of substance P	Very thin layer topically tid–qid, 0.025% or 0.075%	Not absorbed	Local skin irritation and burning	Wear gloves to apply, wash hands with soap and water, avoid contact with sensitive areas of the body.
Lidocaine	Inhibition of nociceptive nerve fibers	Moderate amount of 5% cream or ointment for 2 hr twice daily	Liver, but minimal systemic absorption	Local irritation, numbness	Transdermal patch is expensive.
Intra-articular steroids	Local anti-inflammatories	See Table 73-3	Some systemic absorption, multiple sites of metabolism	Local skin atrophy and depigmentation, risk for muscle and tendon rupture	Generally less beneficial when no joint is effusion present. Limit to ≤4 injections per site per year.
Hyaluronic acid	Surface lubricant	Varies by product, 3-5 weekly injections of 16-30 mg each	Remains intra-articular	Pain at injection site	Very expensive, benefit is controversial.
Glucosamine	Nutritional supplement	500 mg tid–qid	Liver	Mild GI discomfort	Benefit is controversial.
Chondroitin	Nutritional supplement	300-1500 mg/day	Liver	Mild GI discomfort	Benefit is controversial.

CNS, central nervous system; GABA, γ-aminobutyric acid; GI, gastrointestinal; qid, four times daily; tid, three times daily.

Therapeutics by Class (Table 73-1)

Analgesics

Acetaminophen (paracetamol) is the analgesic of choice for mild to moderate pain in OA.[28] It is a purely analgesic drug with no anti-inflammatory properties. Paracetamol was first discovered in the late 1800s, but its utility was not recognized until the 1950s, when it was recognized as the active metabolite of the more toxic compound acetanilide.[29] Its mechanism of action is not completely understood, but it is believed the drug interacts with the COX system without affecting the inflammatory cascade. The onset of action is typically less than 1 hour and duration of action is typically 4 to 6 hours, but this may vary with extended-release formulations.[30] Acetaminophen is metabolized by the liver, and care must be taken in patients with liver disease or people who regularly consume moderate amounts of alcohol. The dosage must be adjusted in renal failure to prevent the accumulation of toxic metabolites. The dose should be limited to 4 g/day in divided doses in healthy adult individuals. In acetaminophen overdose, toxic metabolites cause severe hepatotoxicity, and this toxicity is the leading cause of emergency liver transplantations in the United States. In standard doses, the drug is usually very well tolerated, causing few gastrointestinal (GI) or hematologic side effects.[31]

Tramadol is a non-narcotic opioid analgesic that is useful in the treatment of moderate to severe pain in OA. It was introduced in 1977 by the German company Grünenthal. Its mechanism of action is different from and synergistic with that of acetaminophen. Combination of this drug with acetaminophen allows a lower dosage of tramadol with the same analgesic benefit. Tramadol interacts with the serotonergic, γ-aminobutyric acidergic, and noradrenergic systems centrally to produce its effect. Its half-life is 5 to 7 hours, and it has active metabolites. Tramadol is metabolized in the liver and excreted in the urine; therefore, dosage must be adjusted in both hepatic and renal impairment.[32] It must be used with some caution in the elderly due to central nervous system (CNS) depression. In combination with other CNS depressants, this effect is amplified. Tramadol does not raise the seizure threshold but should be used with caution in patients with a seizure disorder or in combination with other medications that raise the seizure threshold. There is also an increased risk of serotonin syndrome when used in combination with monoamine oxidase inhibitor and selective serotonin reuptake inhibitor medications. The most common side effects are nausea, flushing, and drowsiness. Typical dosage is 50 to 100 mg every 4 to 6 hours. Total 24-hour dosing should not exceed 400 mg/day.

Numerous preparations of narcotic-containing medications are available on the market, each with different potency. Rather than describe several of their number here, we address the general strategy for prescribing narcotic medications. They should be restricted to the treatment of severe pain that is refractory to non-narcotic medications. They all cause CNS depression and respiratory depression, and have addiction potential. In general, short-acting narcotics are useful for short-term management of severe pain. Long-acting narcotics are more useful in the treatment of long-term chronic pain refractory to other treatments. Despite the caveats mentioned here, these medications are extremely effective at controlling pain. The authors recommend that institutions or physicians prescribing these medications institute a strict written policy or "narcotics contract" with patients governing narcotic distribution, both to minimize potential for abuse and to assist with government oversight. Prescribing these medications in the United States requires a license from the federal government and some state governments.

Nonsteroidal Anti-inflammatory Drugs

NSAIDs are a large group of drugs with both analgesic and anti-inflammatory properties. The first to be discovered was salicylic acid, which was isolated from the bark of the willow tree. The use of willow bark as a remedy dates as far back as Ancient Greece and the early Middle East. In the late 1800s, acetylsalicylic acid (aspirin) was the first successfully marketed NSAID.

All NSAIDs inhibit the COX isoenzymes that convert arachadonic acid into prostaglandins, major mediators of inflammation. There are two isoenzymes, referred to as COX-1 and COX-2, and NSAIDs inhibit each to varying degrees. The COX-1 isoenzyme is found in almost all cells. Of particular importance, gastric mucosal cells use the COX-1 enzyme to produce the protective prostaglandins that limit damage from acids in the stomach. COX-2 is only expressed in cells activated by inflammatory cytokines, and inhibition of this isoenzyme is thought to be most relevant to systemic anti-inflammatory effects (Fig. 73-2).

There are six major classes of NSAID medications (Table 73-2).[33] There is a great deal of individual variation in response within each group. A general therapeutic strategy when prescribing these medications is to start with a medication that is easily dosed and low in cost. If one NSAID fails to improve pain, a switch can be made to an NSAID of a different class. It is not uncommon for an individual to respond to a particular NSAID after having failed several others. There are no clear clinical data regarding relative potency of the various medications. Table 73-2 shows the major classes of NSAIDs with examples of each, including generic and brand names and usual dosage. Various trials comparing the use of NSAIDs versus acetaminophen for treatment of knee OA have been mixed, with several more recent studies showing a greater benefit with NSAID use. The potential benefits must be weighed, however, against the more significant side effect profile of this class of medications. NSAIDs alone cause over 16,500 deaths and over 103,000 hospitalizations per year in the United States.[34] In addition, these drugs rarely relieve symptoms completely. In clinical trials, all NSAIDs performed similarly, with participants reporting approximately 30% reduction in pain and 15% improvement in function.[35]

There is no evidence that NSAIDs alter the natural history of OA. In fact, commensurate with reductions in pain, NSAIDs also offer improvements in a person's walking speed, with increased potential for structural deterioration.[36] Of particular concern is the fact that anti-inflammatory or analgesic therapy may actually be associated with an increase in joint forces and possibly a reduction in the adaptive strategies that protect the joint from excessive loading. Whether this is the mechanism that explains the potential for increased structural damage associated with NSAID use remains unclear.[37]

The most common toxicity is that to the GI tract.[38,39] Due to the mechanism of COX-1 inhibition noted earlier, gastritis and ulceration are common. The highest risk of gastric toxicity is for patients with prior history of ulcer or GI bleeding, age over 60, more than twice the normal dosage of NSAID, concurrent use of corticosteroids, and concurrent use of anticoagulants. Evidence from clinical trials indicates that primary prevention of adverse GI events can be accomplished with misoprostil, a prostaglandin analogue. In a large clinical trial, the absolute risk reduction for misoprostil in preventing GI complications was 0.57%, thus requiring the treatment of 175 patients to prevent 1 GI event.[40] Proton pump inhibitors are also useful in preventing NSAID-induced ulceration. A study of esomeprazole showed an absolute risk reduction of 11.8% with a 20-mg dose, requiring the treatment of eight patients to prevent one GI event.[41] Histamine$_2$ blockers such as famotidine have not been shown to prevent gastric ulceration in persons on concomitant NSAIDs.[42] Use of COX-2–selective NSAIDs showed a relative risk reduction of 0.49 in large trials as distinct from use of standard NSAIDs.[43] For secondary prevention of gastric ulceration in patients who must remain on NSAID therapy, proton pump inhibitors have the strongest evidence for healing and prevention of further ulceration.[44]

Nephrotoxicity is also a significant problem with use of NSAIDs.[45] There are two major mechanisms of this toxicity. The first is mediated by the hemodynamic effects of prostaglandin inhibition in the kidney. Prostaglandins play a small role in normal individuals. However, in patients with renal insufficiency or other causes of elevated angiotensin, the kidney becomes much more dependent on the counterbalancing effect of prostaglandins, and their inhibition can lead to decreased glomerular filtration and reversible renal ischemia. NSAIDs must therefore be used with extreme caution in patients with preexisting renal insufficiency. Rarely, NSAIDs can also cause interstitial nephritis and nephritic syndrome by unknown mechanisms.[46] The result is an infiltration of T lymphocytes in the kidney as well as pyuria,

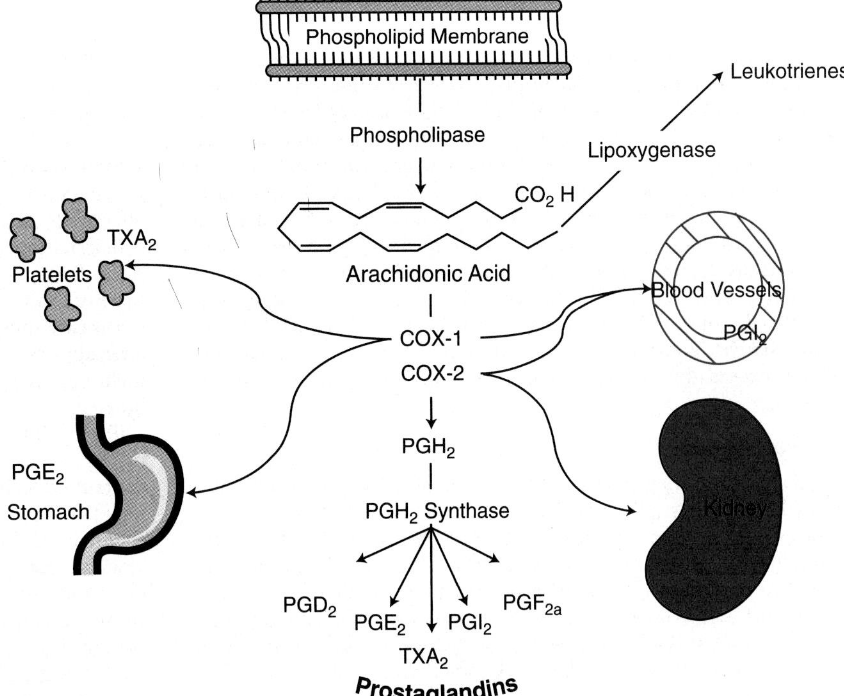

FIGURE 73-2 • Cyclooxygenase-derived eicosanoids and other arachidonic acid metabolites and their respective actions on relevant end organs.

TABLE 73-2 OVERVIEW OF NONSTEROIDAL ANTI-INFLAMMATORY DRUGS

NSAID	Trade Name	Dosage	Relative Cost* Generic	Relative Cost* Brand	COX-1/COX-2 Ratio†
CARBOXYLIC ACIDS					
Aspirin	Multiple	650-1500 mg qid	$	—	166
Trisalicylate	Trilisate	500 mg–1.5 g tid	$$$	—	
Diflunisal	Dolobid	500 mg bid–tid	$$$	$$$$	
Salsalate	Amigesic	500-1500 mg bid	$	—	
PROPRIONIC ACIDS					
Naproxen	Naprosyn, Alleve	500-750 mg bid	$	$$$$$	–1.2
Ibuprofen	Advil, Motrin	400-800 mg tid-qid	$	$$	15
Oxaprozin	Daypro	600-1200 mg daily	$$	$$$$$	
ACEDIC ACIDS					
Idomethacin	Indocin	25-50 mg bid–tid	$	$$$	60
Sulindac	Clinoril	150-200 mg bid	$$$	$$$$	100
Etodolac	Lodine	200-400 mg tid–qid	$$$	$$$$	
Diclofenac	Voltarin	50-75 mg bid	$$$	$$$$$	–1.4
ENOLIC ACIDS					
Piroxicam	Feldene	10-20 mg daily	$	$$$	350
Meloxicam	Mobic	7.5-15 mg daily	$$	$$$$$	–3
NAPTHYLKANONES					
Nabumetone	Relafen	500-1000 mg bid	$$	$$$$$	
SELECTIVE COX-2S					
Celecoxib	Celebrex	100-200 mg daily	—	$$$$$	

*Based on Drugstore.com listings, August 2006.
†Data from Tannenbaum et al. (1996).
COX, cyclooxygenase; NSAID, nonsteroidal anti-inflammatory drug.

eosinophilia, eosinuria, rash, and fever. Typically all the manifestations are not present. The effects are usually self-limited with cessation of the drug.

Cardiovascular complications are now a more recognized complication of NSAID use, particularly with the newer COX-2–selective medications. Because prostaglandins are vasodilatory, their inhibition can cause hypertension. In addition, the antiplatelet effects of aspirin are reduced by coadministration of NSAIDs, which compete with aspirin in the binding of COX in platelets. Early studies showing the possible cardiovascular benefits of NSAIDs have been called into question after a recent study involving long-term use of naproxen and celecoxib showed an increase in cardiovascular event rates.[47] Two of the three COX-2–specific drugs (rofecoxib, valdecoxib) previously approved for use in the United States were pulled from the market in 2004 and 2005, respectively, because of concerns regarding cardiovascular toxicity. Current American Heart Association guidelines regarding COX-2–selective NSAID use recommends use of these agents in patients with or at risk for cardiovascular disease only when there are no alternatives, and for as short a duration as possible.[48] Many investigators extend this warning to all NSAIDs until further evidence is gathered.

Topical Agents

The use of topical agents in the treatment of OA has been a poorly studied area. The studies that have been done indicate that, for most agents, there may be significant but short-term benefit. All of these agents have as their main side effect local skin irritation. There are several compounds on the market that warrant specific discussion.

Topical NSAIDs have been studied and are available, although primarily outside the United States. Topical diclofenac has been shown to have good short-term pain relief, with less GI and renal toxicity.[49] It is available in Canada and Europe.

Topical salicylate-containing compounds work as rubefacients that presumably reduce pain while increasing local blood flow. Studies involving these agents also show short-term benefit.[50] Some examples are methyl salicylate, diethylamine salicylate, and hydroxyethyl salicylate. These medications provide an alternative to systemically absorbed compounds. Many of these compounds have a strong menthol odor that may be objectionable to some.

Capsaicin is a topical product made from the oils from various hot pepper plants. Its proposed mechanism of action is to produce local pain and irritation that depletes substance P, a powerful pain stimulus, from local neurons. When applied, it causes a burning sensation on the skin that, with time, helps to relieve pain from the nearby musculoskeletal branches of neurons. It has been shown to be effective for hand and knee OA.[51] This compound produces significant skin irritation and must be applied in very small amounts initially, and once daily. As tolerance to the burning occurs, the amount can be increased and the frequency increased to three to four times daily. Great care must be taken to use gloves or wash the hands thoroughly after application. Getting the compound on any mucous membrane, including the eyes, nose, mouth, and genitals, can cause severe burning.

Topical lidocaine is another method of pain relief that can be tried in OA. There are numerous creams and patches on the market that contain lidocaine or other local anesthetics. Lidocaine works by altering the depolarization of sensory nerve fibers by blocking fast sodium channels in the neuron membrane. Effectiveness has been demonstrated in patients with OA of the spine.[52] Commercial patch preparations may be expensive; alternatives can be made by applying the cheaper creams and ointments under an occlusive dressing. The preparation should be applied once daily and left for 2 hours, then removed for 12 hours. This prevents tolerance to the medication as well as significant systemic absorption. Care must also be taken with applying

TABLE 73-3 OVERVIEW OF INTRA-ARTICULAR STEROIDS

Agent	Relative Anti-inflammatory Potency	Solubility	Dose
Hydrocortisone acetate	1	High	10-25 mg
Methylprednisolone acetate	5	Medium	20-80 mg
Triamcinolone acetonide	5	Medium	10-40 mg
Triamcinolone hexacetonide	5	Medium	10-20 mg
Betamethasone sodium phosphate and acetate	20	Low	0.25-2 ml

these compounds with the fingers, as digital numbness with subsequent loss of dexterity can occur.

Intra-articular Corticosteroids

There is a long history of injection of steroids into joints for the purpose of pain relief and anti-inflammatory effect. Many studies show the efficacy of various preparations.[53] As noted previously, OA is not primarily an inflammatory disease, although there does seem to be a response in OA patients to anti-inflammatory medications, including intra-articular preparations. Triamcinolone acetonide (Kenalog) and methylprednisolone acetate (Depo-Medrol) are the two most common preparations. Injectable corticosteroids can be thought of in terms of solubility and duration of action (Table 73-3). High-solubility preparations have a short duration of action, and low-solubility compounds have a long duration. Triamcinolone hexacetonide (Aristospan) was designed to be less soluble and therefore longer acting.

Care must be taken with injectable corticosteroids to ensure intra-articular placement as significant soft tissue inflammation can result if the injection is misplaced. The dosage varies based on the preparation and joint size. Many practitioners also mix the steroid with local anesthetic such as lidocaine or bupivocaine, both as a diluent and to provide some immediate pain relief as the steroid typically takes 24 to 48 hours for effect.[54] There is a theoretical risk of decreasing the bioavailability of steroid when mixed with anesthetic because of flocculation of the steroid with the parabens preservatives in the anesthetic. A recent survey indicated that most rheumatologists mix the steroid with anesthetic, and no clinical trial has shown a decrease in efficacy with this method.

There are several risks associated with injection of corticosteroid. There is often a postinjection flare of pain induced by the crystalline composition of the preparations. This typically lasts less than 48 hours, but patients should be counseled regarding this. Steroids can also cause atrophy of tissues, including skin and tendon structures. Recommended frequency of injection varies, but it is generally accepted that intra-articular injections can be given four times a year per joint. There is some systemic absorption of the steroid, and there have been reports of adrenal insufficiency, osteoporosis, and diabetes complications from frequent high-dose steroid injections. There is a small risk of iatrogenic infection that is less than 1%.

Typically we reserve the use of intra-articular steroid injections to subjects with exacerbations of pain with effusions. The pain relief varies dramatically from weeks to several months. It is also our experience that repeated injections gradually lose efficacy, presumably due to disease progression. There is no evidence that injection of corticosteroids alters the natural history of the disease. Where not otherwise contraindicated, intra-articular corticosteroids are of short-term benefit (1 week) for pain and function.[55]

Hyaluronic Acid Derivatives

There has been a great deal of focus in recent years on synovial fluid supplementation as a method for restoring viscoelasticity and flow of synovial fluid. Hyaluronic acids are large carbohydrate polymers made of disaccharides linked by glycosidic bonds. The polymers range in size from 100 to 10,000 kDa. Studies of the use of hyaluronic acid in humans indicate a half-life of about 4 weeks.[56] Unlike previously mentioned strategies, this may theoretically alter the natural history of the disease. In vitro studies of hyaluronic acid in bovine cartilage media showed a trophic dose-related response, suggesting that exogenous hyaluronic acid may promote cartilage growth.[57] There are now several products on the market, including Hylan G-F 20 and sodium hyaluronate. They are administered as a series of weekly injections for three to five doses. Two meta-analyses have been able to demonstrate a statistically significant improvement in pain and function.[58,59] The clinical significance was small (largely a placebo effect), however, and response rates, time to response, and duration of response have been varied. These compounds are expensive and all have, to date, shown no benefit in rate of disease progression in clinical trials. These compounds are currently approved only for knee and hip OA.

Glucosamine and Chondroitin

Glucosamine and chondroitin are compounds that have been advocated recently in the treatment of OA. Strictly speaking, they are nutritional supplements and are not controlled by the U.S. Food and Drug Administration (FDA). These two compounds are important constituents of cartilage. By increasing the amount of substrate available for the production of cartilage, it is theorized that they may help slow the progression of disease and even help repair damaged cartilage. A 2005 meta-analysis did indicate a modest benefit for slowing joint space narrowing with the use of glucosamine sulfate.[60] Likewise, chondroitin has been shown in several studies to improve pain and function in patients with OA.[61] Although numerous studies purportedly show this benefit, there are methodologic problems with all of these studies. In a meta-analysis of trials with adequate blinding, no benefit was found for glucosamine or chondroitin.[60] Although expensive and not covered by insurance, the side effect profile is not significantly different from placebo. Certainly future investigations will continue to examine their efficacy. Because of concerns with cost and quality assurance (these compounds are not FDA regulated), we do not currently recommend glucosamine or chondroitin to our patients.

Therapeutic Approach

There are a number of well-written guidelines available describing the management of OA that are based on evidence from trials and expert consensus.[62-64] The recommended hierarchy of management should consist of nonpharmacologic modalities first, then drugs, and then surgery. Too frequently the first step is forgotten or not emphasized sufficiently, to patients' detriment. Typically, the first agent of choice is a simple analgesic such as acetaminophen or tramadol. Although the evidence is weak, use of glucosamine and chondroitin may provide additional pain relief. If these are ineffective, one can proceed to topical agents such as capsaicin or nonsteroidal medications. If an effusion is present, the patient may benefit from joint aspiration and injection with an intra-articular corticosteroid. Many experts recommend proceeding to injection of a hyaluronic acid derivative as a final step before referral to surgery. As previously noted, the evidence for the benefit of these medications is weak, but ongoing studies will help to clarify their usefulness. Some patients are not surgical candidates, and will eventually require use of narcotic analgesics for chronic pain management (Fig. 73-3).

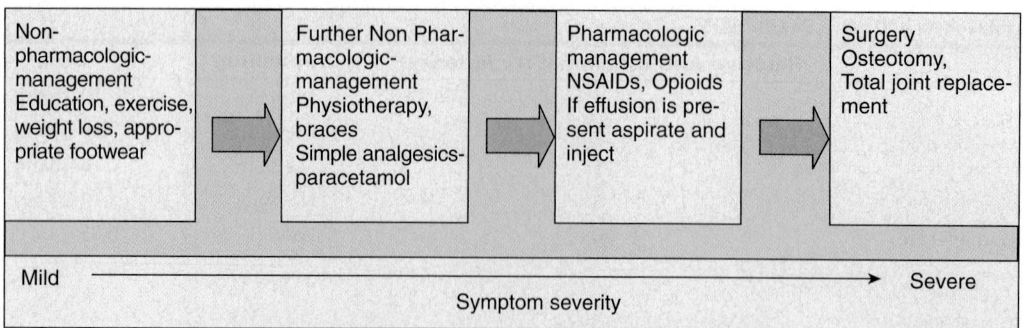

FIGURE 73-3 • A stepwise algorithm for the management of the patient with osteoarthritis. This is an example of a treatment algorithm that is modified according to the patient's response and the clinician's preference. It highlights the encompassing need to consider nonpharmacologic management as first line for all patients.

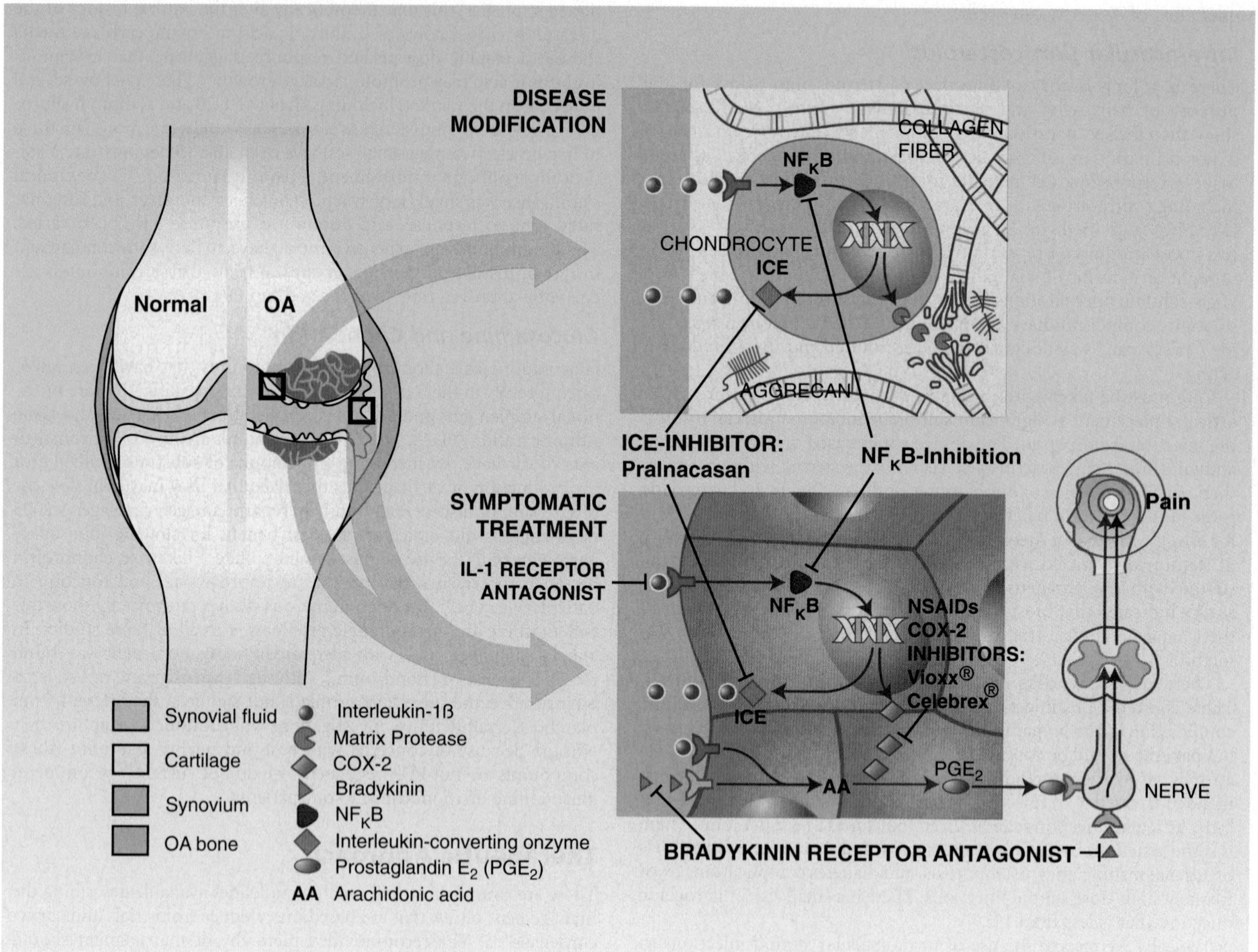

FIGURE 73-4 • Molecular targets of emerging therapeutics.

Emerging Targets and Therapeutics

A vast number of agents are currently under development for treatment of OA. They can generally be grouped together by their molecular target (Fig. 73-4). By affecting different targets, drugs can be developed either to primarily enhance symptomatic control or to actually modify the structure and thereby the overall disease process (disease-modifying drugs).

Interleukin-1

As noted in the physiology discussion, IL-1 has been noted to play a role in the pathophysiology of OA.[65] Interleukin-1 interacts with its receptor to cause the stimulation of transcription factors such as nuclear factor-κB (NF-κB), which promotes the production of the matrix metalloproteinases (MMPs) that degrade cartilage. In addition to MMPs, there is up-regulation of interleukin-1β (IL-1β)–converting enzyme (ICE), which converts IL-1β into its active form, thereby further stimulating the degradation process through positive feedback. Attempts have been made in the past to use IL-1 receptor antagonists (anakinra) to block the first step in that process. The clinical trials of anakinra showed no benefit, but other formulations and IL-1 receptor antagonist agents are being developed.[66] Inhibition of ICE is another potential target, and agents such as pralnacasan (Aventis) are undergoing investigation.[67] NF-κB is another potential target in the biochemical pathway. Blocking this enzyme could decrease the production of both ICE and MMPs, but the systemic effects of doing so are currently unknown. All of these drugs are being developed to improve symptoms but, based on their targets, are hoped to be disease-modifying drugs.

Matrix Metalloproteinases

MMPs represent the final common pathway in cartilage degradation, and therefore represent a promising target for therapy. There are currently at least seven MMP inhibitors under investigation, including the antibiotic doxycycline,[68] which has showed some promise in treating rheumatoid arthritis, presumably by the same mechanism. These drugs are being developed as disease-modifying drugs.

Cyclooxygenase-2 Isoenzymes

Despite the problems with toxicity mentioned earlier, a large number of COX-2–specific drugs are being developed to symptomatically treat OA. These drugs will need to be examined carefully in clinical trials to determine the extent of their cardiotoxicity.

Bradykinin and Nitric Oxide

Bradykinin is a molecule that has a variety of physiologic roles, including vasodilation, increased vascular permeability, and pain.[69] There are ongoing investigations of drugs that block various bradykinin receptors and thereby improve symptoms. Nitric oxide (NO) is also a potent vasodilator and is involved in the mechanism of pain. New NO analgesics are also under development.

SUMMARY

- OA is a chronic, progressive disease affecting many structures within the joint.
- Pharmacologic therapy is part of a comprehensive, individualized treatment plan.
- Simple analgesics are the first-line drugs, followed by topical agents and NSAIDs.
- Injection of corticosteroids or hyaluronic acid derivatives can be adjunctive.
- Surgical referral is reserved for the end stages of disease.
- Future therapeutic targets will seek to modify disease progression on a molecular level.

REFERENCES

1. Centers for Disease Control. Arthritis prevalence and activity limitations—United States, 1990. MMWR Morb Mortal Wkly Rep 1994;43:433-438.
2. Badley E, DesMeules M. Arthritis in Canada: an ongoing challenge. Ottawa: Health Canada, 2003.
3. Martin JA, Buckwalter JA. Roles of articular cartilage aging and chondrocyte senescence in the pathogenesis of osteoarthritis. Iowa Orthop J 2001;21:1-7.
4. Felson DT. An update on the pathogenesis and epidemiology of osteoarthritis. Radiol Clin North Am 2004;42:1-9, v.
5. Nuki G. Osteoarthritis: a problem of joint failure. Z Rheumatol 1999;58:142-147.
6. Eyre DR. Collagens and cartilage matrix homeostasis. Clin Orthop Relat Res 2004;(427 Suppl):S118-S122.
7. Burr DB. The importance of subchondral bone in the progression of osteoarthritis. J Rheumatol Suppl 2004;70:77-80.
8. Dieppe PA, Lohmander LS. Pathogenesis and management of pain in osteoarthritis. Lancet 2005;365:965-973.
9. Buckland-Wright JC, MacFarlane DG, Jasani MK, Lynch JA. Quantitative microfocal radiographic assessment of osteoarthritis of the knee from weight bearing tunnel and semiflexed standing views. J Rheumatol 1994;21:1734-1741.
10. Burr DB, Radin EL. Microfractures and microcracks in subchondral bone: are they relevant to osteoarthrosis? Rheum Dis Clin North Am 2003;29:675-685.
11. Messent EA, Ward RJ, Tonkin CJ, Buckland-Wright C. Tibial cancellous bone changes in patients with knee osteoarthritis: a short-term longitudinal study using Fractal Signature Analysis. Osteoarthritis Cartilage 2005;13:463-470.
12. Hayami T, Pickarski M, Wesolowski GA, et al. The role of subchondral bone remodeling in osteoarthritis: reduction of cartilage degeneration and prevention of osteophyte formation by alendronate in the rat anterior cruciate ligament transection model. Arthritis Rheum 2004;50:1193-1206.
13. Radin EL, Rose RM. Role of subchondral bone in the initiation and progression of cartilage damage. Clin Orthop Relat Res 1986;(213):34-40.
14. Grynpas MD, Alpert B, Katz I, et al. Subchondral bone in osteoarthritis. Calcif Tissue Int 1991;49:20-26.
15. Burr DB. Increased biological activity of subchondral mineralized tissues underlies the progressive deterioration of articular cartilage in osteoarthritis. J Rheumatol 2005;32:1156-1158.
16. Spector TD, Cicuttini F, Baker J, et al. Genetic influences on osteoarthritis in women: a twin study. BMJ 1996;312:940-943.
17. Sowers MF, Hochberg M, Crabbe JP, et al. Association of bone mineral density and sex hormone levels with osteoarthritis of the hand and knee in premenopausal women. Am J Epidemiol 1996;143:38-47.
18. McAlindon TE, Felson DT, Zhang Y, et al. Relation of dietary intake and serum levels of vitamin D to progression of osteoarthritis of the knee among participants in the Framingham Study. Ann Intern Med 1996;125:353-359.
19. Uchino M, Izumi T, Tominaga T, et al. Growth factor expression in the osteophytes of the human femoral head in osteoarthritis. Clin Orthop Relat Res 2000;(377):119-125.
20. Karvonen RL, Miller PR, Nelson DA, et al. Periarticular osteoporosis in osteoarthritis of the knee. J Rheumatol 1998;25:2187-2194.
21. Li B, Aspden RM. Material properties of bone from the femoral neck and calcar femorale of patients with osteoporosis or osteoarthritis. Osteoporos Int 1997;7:450-456.
22. Hunter DJ, Spector TD. The role of bone metabolism in osteoarthritis. Curr Rheumatol Rep 2003;5:15-19.
23. Dequeker J, Mohan S, Finkelman RD, et al. Generalized osteoarthritis associated with increased insulin-like growth factor types I and II and transforming growth factor beta in cortical bone from the iliac crest: possible mechanism of increased bone density and protection against osteoporosis. Arthritis Rheum 1993;36:1702-1708.
24. Tallon D, Chard J, Dieppe P. Relation between agendas of the research community and the research consumer. Lancet 2000;355:2037-2040.
25. Glazier RH, Dalby DM, Badley EM, et al. Management of common musculoskeletal problems: a survey of Ontario primary care physicians. CMAJ 1998;158:1037-1040.
26. Felson DT, Zhang Y. An update on the epidemiology of knee and hip osteoarthritis with a view to prevention. Arthritis Rheum 1998;41:1343-1355.
27. Hunter DJ, Felson DT. Osteoarthritis. BMJ 2006;332:639-642.
28. Hochberg MC, Altman RD, Brandt KD, et al. Guidelines for the medical management of osteoarthritis. Part II. Osteoarthritis of the knee. American College of Rheumatology. Arthritis Rheum 1995;38:1541-1546.
29. Brodie BB, Axelrod J. The fate of acetanilide in man. J Pharmacol Exp Ther 1948;94:29-38.
30. Clissold SP. Paracetamol and phenacetin. Drugs 1986;32(Suppl 4):46-59.
31. Graham GG, Scott KF, Day RO. Tolerability of paracetamol. Drug Saf 2005;28:227-240.
32. Dayer P, Collart L, Desmeules J. The pharmacology of tramadol. Drugs 1994;47(Suppl 1):3-7.
33. Tannenbaum H, Davis P, Russell AS, et al. An evidence-based approach to prescribing NSAIDs in musculoskeletal disease: a Canadian consensus. Canadian NSAID Consensus Participants. CMAJ 1996;155:77-88.
34. Wolfe MM, Lichtenstein DR, Singh G. Gastrointestinal toxicity of nonsteroidal antiinflammatory drugs. N Engl J Med 1999;340:1888-1899.
35. Todd PA, Clissold SP. Naproxen: a reappraisal of its pharmacology, and therapeutic use in rheumatic diseases and pain states. Drugs 1990;40:91-137.
36. Blin O, Pailhous J, Lafforgue P, Serratrice G. Quantitative analysis of walking in patients with knee osteoarthritis: a method of assessing the effectiveness of non-steroidal anti-inflammatory treatment. Ann Rheum Dis 1990;49:990-993.
37. Huskisson EC, Berry H, Gishen P, et al. Effects of antiinflammatory drugs on the progression of osteoarthritis of the knee. LINK Study Group. Longitudinal Investigation of Nonsteroidal Antiinflammatory Drugs in Knee Osteoarthritis. J Rheumatol 1995;22:1941-1946.
38. Flower RJ. Studies on the mechanism of action of anti-inflammatory drugs: a paper in honour of John Vane. Thromb Res 2003;110:259-263.
39. Flower RJ. The development of COX2 inhibitors. Nat Rev Drug Discov 2003;2:179-191.
40. Silverstein FE, Graham DY, Senior JR, et al. Misoprostol reduces serious gastrointestinal complications in patients with rheumatoid arthritis receiving nonsteroidal anti-inflammatory drugs: a randomized, double-blind, placebo-controlled trial. Ann Intern Med 1995;123:241-249.
41. Scheiman JM, Yeomans ND, Talley NJ, et al. Prevention of ulcers by esomeprazole in at-risk patients using non-selective NSAIDs and COX-2 inhibitors. Am J Gastroenterol 2006;101:701-710.
42. Taha AS, Hudson N, Hawkey CJ, et al. Famotidine for the prevention of gastric and duodenal ulcers caused by nonsteroidal antiinflammatory drugs. N Engl J Med 1996;334:1435-1439.
43. Silverstein FE, Faich G, Goldstein JL, et al. Gastrointestinal toxicity with celecoxib vs nonsteroidal anti-inflammatory drugs for osteoarthritis and rheumatoid arthritis. The CLASS study: a randomized controlled trial. Celecoxib Long-term Arthritis Safety Study. JAMA 2000;284:1247-1255.
44. Lai KC, Chu KM, Hui WM, et al. Esomeprazole with aspirin versus clopidogrel for prevention of recurrent gastrointestinal ulcer complications. Clin Gastroenterol Hepatol 2006;4:860-865.
45. Huerta C, Castellsague J, Varas-Lorenzo C, García-Rodríguez LA. Nonsteroidal anti-inflammatory drugs and risk of ARF in the general population. Am J Kidney Dis 2005;45:531-539.
46. Abraham PA, Keane WF. Glomerular and interstitial disease induced by nonsteroidal anti-inflammatory drugs. Am J Nephrol 1984;4:1-6.
47. Hippisley-Cox J, Coupland C. Risk of myocardial infarction in patients taking cyclo-oxygenase-2 inhibitors or conventional non-steroidal anti-inflammatory drugs: population based nested case-control analysis. BMJ 2005;330:1366-1369.

48. Bennett JS, Daugherty A, Herrington D, et al. The use of nonsteroidal anti-inflammatory drugs (NSAIDs): a science advisory from the American Heart Association. Circulation 2005;111:1713-1716.
49. Lin J, Zhang W, Jones A, Doherty M. Efficacy of topical non-steroidal anti-inflammatory drugs in the treatment of osteoarthritis: meta-analysis of randomised controlled trials. BMJ 2004;329:324.
50. Mason L, Moore RA, Edwards JE, et al. Systematic review of efficacy of topical rubefacients containing salicylates for the treatment of acute and chronic pain. BMJ 2004;328:995.
51. Mason L, Moore RA, Derry S, et al. Systematic review of topical capsaicin for the treatment of chronic pain. BMJ 2004;328:991.
52. Burch F, Codding C, Patel N, Sheldon E. Lidocaine patch 5% improves pain, stiffness, and physical function in osteoarthritis pain patients: a prospective, multicenter, open-label effectiveness trial. Osteoarthritis Cartilage 2004;12:253-255.
53. Arroll B, Goodyear-Smith F. Corticosteroid injections for osteoarthritis of the knee: meta-analysis. BMJ 2004;328:869.
54. Centeno LM, Moore ME. Preferred intraarticular corticosteroids and associated practice: a survey of members of the American College of Rheumatology. Arthritis Care Res 1994;7:151-155.
55. Bellamy N, Campbell J, Robinson V, et al. Intraarticular corticosteroid for treatment of osteoarthritis of the knee. Cochrane Database Syst Rev 2006;(2):CD005328.
56. Lindqvist U, Tolmachev V, Kairemo K, et al. Elimination of stabilised hyaluronan from the knee joint in healthy men. Clin Pharmacokinet 2002;41:603-613.
57. Akmal M, Singh A, Anand A, et al. The effects of hyaluronic acid on articular chondrocytes. J Bone Joint Surg Br 2005;87:1143-1149.
58. Arrich J, Piribauer F, Mad P, et al. Intra-articular hyaluronic acid for the treatment of osteoarthritis of the knee: systematic review and meta-analysis. CMAJ 2005;172:1039-1043.
59. Lo GH, LaValley M, McAlindon T, Felson DT. Intra-articular hyaluronic acid in treatment of knee osteoarthritis: a meta-analysis. JAMA 2003;290:3115-3121.
60. Towheed TE, Maxwell L, Anastassiades TP, et al. Glucosamine therapy for treating osteoarthritis. Cochrane Database Syst Rev 2005;(2):CD002946.
61. Richy F, Bruyere O, Ethgen O, et al. Structural and symptomatic efficacy of glucosamine and chondroitin in knee osteoarthritis: a comprehensive meta-analysis. Arch Intern Med 2003;163:1514-1522.
62. Recommendations for the medical management of osteoarthritis of the hip and knee: 2000 update. American College of Rheumatology Subcommittee on Osteoarthritis Guidelines. Arthritis Rheum 2000;43:1905-1915.
63. Jordan KM, Arden NK, Doherty M, et al. EULAR Recommendations 2003: an evidence based approach to the management of knee osteoarthritis. Report of a Task Force of the Standing Committee for International Clinical Studies Including Therapeutic Trials (ESCISIT). Ann Rheum Dis 2003;62:1145-1155.
64. Zhang W, Doherty M, Arden N, et al. EULAR evidence based recommendations for the management of hip osteoarthritis: report of a task force of the EULAR Standing Committee for International Clinical Studies Including Therapeutics (ESCISIT). Ann Rheum Dis 2005;64:669-681.
65. Jacques C, Gosset M, Berenbaum F, Gabay C. The role of IL-1 and IL-1Ra in joint inflammation and cartilage degradation. Vitam Horm 2006;74:371-403.
66. Domagala F, Martin G, Bogdanowicz P, et al. Inhibition of interleukin-1beta-induced activation of MEK/ERK pathway and DNA binding of NF-kappaB and AP-1: potential mechanism for Diacerein effects in osteoarthritis. Biorheology 2006;43:577-587.
67. Rudolphi K, Gerwin N, Verzijl N, et al. Pralnacasan, an inhibitor of interleukin-1beta converting enzyme, reduces joint damage in two murine models of osteoarthritis. Osteoarthritis Cartilage 2003;11:738-746.
68. Brandt KD, Mazzuca SA, Katz BP, et al. Effects of doxycycline on progression of osteoarthritis: results of a randomized, placebo-controlled, double-blind trial. Arthritis Rheum 2005;52:2015-2025.
69. Bond AP, Lemon M, Dieppe PA, Bhoola KD. Generation of kinins in synovial fluid from patients with arthropathy. Immunopharmacology 1997;36:209-216.

74

RHEUMATOID ARTHRITIS

Richard M. Keating

INTRODUCTION 1025
Epidemiology 1025
Diagnosis 1025
Differential Diagnosis 1026
Treatment History and Goals 1027
PATHOPHYSIOLOGY 1027
THERAPEUTICS AND CLINICAL PHARMACOLOGY 1030
Goals of Therapy 1030
Therapeutics by Class 1030
Anti-inflammatory Agents 1031
Disease-Modifying Antirheumatic Drugs 1031
Biologic Response Modifiers 1033
Therapeutic Approach 1035
Recommended Approach 1035
Emerging Targets and Therapeutics 1035
CONCLUSION 1036

INTRODUCTION

Rheumatoid arthritis (RA) is a common, incurable, and serious disease. Although much attention is devoted to the management of its articular features, it should be appreciated that RA is a systemic disorder with wide-ranging organ manifestations. The word *rheum* roughly translates from the Greek for "flowing" and was applied to this condition with the premise that the disease was secondary to the "bad humors" disseminated throughout the body.

Epidemiology

RA is clearly the most common of the inflammatory arthritidies, affecting almost 1% of the adult population worldwide. Interestingly, this is a statistic that holds true across many "developed" population groups.[1,2] It is seen across all ethnic groups and cultures. Its onset is often in the peak of adulthood, bringing with it the threat of disability and, more recently recognized, early death. Incidence in the United States is estimated at 25 per 100,000 population for men and almost doubles that (54 per 100,000) for women.[3] It is estimated that RA results, directly or indirectly, in 250,000 hospitalizations and up to 9 million physician office visits per year.[4]

Of even more consequence than the need for hospitalization or office visits is the cost of RA on an individual's lifestyle and work effort. Ten years after the onset of RA, more than half of all patients will demonstrate significant disability, and as the disease advances to the 15-year mark, only 40% are still working.[5] As recently as 20 years ago, more than half of 100 RA patients treated in a London referral center were either dead or severely disabled at the 20-year mark despite receiving the accepted "standard of care" treatment regimen for RA available at that time.[6]

Not only is disability an ever-looming threat, but early mortality is a real feature. Life expectancy is reduced by an average of 3 to 18 years with established RA.[7-9] More recent work has demonstrated that a significant reason for the higher mortality seen in RA population groups is directly attributable to excess cardiovascular disease. As a group, RA patients suffer more myocardial infarction, cerebrovascular accidents, and even heart failure than those without RA.[10-12] The direct and indirect costs of this disease, to the individual patient and to a larger society, are simply staggering.

Diagnosis

The diagnosis of RA is a clinical one. No laboratory test, physical examination finding, or imaging modality result alone can provide the diagnosis. A clinician must take the time and effort to obtain a careful history, perform a detailed examination, and review all ancillary studies to arrive at the diagnosis of RA. Although the disease may begin in one or a limited number of joints, it will eventually become symmetric and polyarticular. The systemic features of the disease, with its attendant malaise, fatigue, and lethargy, are often as significant for the patient in terms of symptoms as is the articular pain and swelling. The pattern of joint involvement usually evolves more than 6 to 8 weeks with eventual symmetry and persistence of symptoms, although this can be quite variable. As well, the disease can take on periods of inexplicable increased activity, only to "quiet" again without explanation. The location of the involved joints is critical to making the correct diagnosis. Wrist, proximal interphalangeal (PIP) joint, and metacarpophalangeal (MCP) joint involvement is very typical of rheumatoid arthritis. The distribution of joint involvement is quite different from that seen in osteoarthritis, with its predilection for hips, knees, and the lumbosacral spine. The involved joints in RA are swollen and mildy tender to palpation. Functional impairment is a common patient complaint. Morning stiffness is a classic feature.[13] Far too often, clinicians depend on the presence or absence of rheumatoid factor (RF) in the blood to make or negate the diagnosis of RA. This is a mistake. It is quite often the case that RF positivity will not manifest until the patient has been symptomatic for 1 or even 2 years.

The American College of Rheumatology has developed classification criteria for the diagnosis of RA (Table 74-1). An important nuance to appreciate is that these classification criteria are just that—criteria for classifying patients who have similar clinical characteristics and thus meet a predefined definition of a disease entity. The classification criteria for RA were developed to ensure that patients enrolled in studies of RA met an agreed-upon set of criteria. These criteria were not designed to apply to individual patients to make a diagnosis of RA, although they are frequently used in just such a manner in clinical practice. Care must be exercised by clinicians. The fact that a patient does not yet meet the requisite number of classification criteria should not dissuade the clinician from applying the diagnosis of RA. Simply put, a patient can have RA although "criteria" are not met. Although not developed to make an individual diagnosis, these criteria do offer the clinician a framework for approaching the individual patient with inflammatory arthritis. One caveat: Waiting for bone erosion on plain film to make the diagnosis of RA ensures nothing more than a lost opportunity in attempting disease control and is strongly discouraged.

An inflammatory arthritis lasting more than 6 weeks, symmetry in joint involvement, involvement of the wrists, MCPs, and PIPs, and supporting laboratory or plain film evaluation should raise the very distinct possibility of RA. Synovitis is a clinical descriptor; it implies a joint effusion that, if aspirated, would demonstrate more than 2000 white blood cells/mm^3, an inflammatory fluid. More recently, rheumatologists have been diagnosing synovitis earlier with the use of

TABLE 74-1 1987 CRITERIA FOR THE CLASSIFICATION OF ACUTE ARTHRITIS OF RHEUMATOID ARTHRITIS*

Criterion	Definition
1. Morning stiffness	Morning stiffness in and around the joints, lasting at least 1 hr before maximal improvement.
2. Arthritis of three or more joint areas	At least three joint areas simultaneously have had soft tissue swelling or fluid (not bony overgrowth alone) observed by a physician. The 14 possible areas are right or left PIP, MCP, wrist, elbow, knee, ankle, and MTP joints.
3. Arthritis of hand joints	At least one joint area swollen (as defined in criterion 2) in a wrist, MCP, or PIP joint.
4. Symmetric arthritis	Simultaneous involvement of the same joint areas (as defined in criterion 2) on both sides of the body (bilateral involvement of PIPs, MCPs, or MTPs is acceptable without absolute symmetry).
5. Rheumatoid nodules	Subcutaneous nodules over bony prominences, or extensor surfaces, or in juxta-articular regions, observed by a physician.
6. Serum rheumatoid factor	Demonstration of abnormal amounts of serum rheumatoid factor by any method for which the result has been positive in <5% of normal control subjects.
7. Radiographic changes	Radiographic changes typical of rheumatoid arthritis on posteroanterior hand and wrist radiographs, which must include erosions or unequivocal bony decalcification localized in or most marked adjacent to the involved joints (osteoarthritis changes alone do not qualify).

*For classification purposes, a patient shall be said to have rheumatoid arthritis if he or she has satisfied at least four of these seven criteria. Criteria 1 through 4 must have been present for at least 6 weeks. Patients with two clinical diagnoses are not excluded. Designation as classic, definite, or probable rheumatoid arthritis is *not* to be made.

MCP, metacarpophalangeal; MTP, metatarsophalangeal; PIP, proximal interphalangeal.

Adapted from Arnett FC, Edworthy SM, Bloch DA, et al. The American Rheumatism Association 1987 revised criteria for the classification of rheumatoid arthritis. Arthritis Rheum 1988;31:315-324. © 2006 American College of Rheumatology.

magnetic resonance imaging (MRI), a modality that is capable of demonstrating synovitis early and one that may well prove to be more sensitive than physical examination.

The joint presentation of RA can be quite varied; the disease clearly is capable of taking on many faces in its presentation. Some patients will present with a symmetric polyarthritis, and some will have a prolonged period of a monoarthritis or oligoarthritis before developing a typical polyarthritis. Some will have an insidious onset of swelling and tenderness in their joints; others will have a fulminant onset with severe disability. Morning stiffness is an important and characteristic finding in the history. Osteoarthritis may cause some brief "gelling" in an affected joint, but this type of stiffness usually resolves promptly after taking the joint through a few range-of-motion exercises. The morning stiffness of RA is quite different in that it lasts so much longer, usually measured in hours.

Rheumatoid factor (RF), typically an immunoglobulin M antibody that reacts with human immunoglobulin G (IgG), is a frequently employed laboratory test used by clinicians when evaluating a patient with joint complaints. The test is "positive" in a majority of patients with RA, but several caveats apply. First, as previously noted, it often does not turn "positive" for many months if not years after the onset of symptoms. The absence of RF early in the disease course should not dissuade one from considering the diagnosis of RA when the other features of RA are present. Second, RF presence can be seen in a number of disease entities, including interstitial lung disease, chronic hepatitis C, subacute bacterial endocarditis, and other chronic inflammatory conditions. The presence of RF argues for a more aggressive course of RA with an increased risk for extra-articular manifestations.

A recent addition to the serologic diagnosis of RA has been the introduction of anti–cyclic citrullinated peptide (CCP) antibody testing. Citrulline is a posttranslationally modified arginine residue. Early-generation anti-CCP antibody testing was more specific for RA than was RF but at a loss in terms of sensitivity. Newer generation assays for anti-CCP antibody have equal sensitivity to RF, better specificity than RF, and improved positive and negative predictive values.[14] Anti-CCP antibody status is proving useful in identifying patients with early RA among the larger population of inflammatory polyarthritis patients. Most rheumatologists now order an anti-CCP antibody test routinely when ordering an RF test.

Anemia, thrombocytosis, and other nonspecific markers of inflammation are characteristic of RA, as they are in myriad other autoimmune diseases. Extra-articular manifestations can include low-grade fever, weight loss, and fatigue. Other features extending beyond the articular region in patients with RA may include subcutaneous nodules, small-vessel vasculitis, pyoderma gangrenosum, pericardial effuions, pleural effusions, interstitial lung disease, Sjögren's syndrome, scleritis, mononeuritis multiplex, and Felty's syndrome (the triad of RA, splenomegaly, and neutropenia). Table 74-2 lists the more common extra-articular manifestations of RA.

TABLE 74-2 EXTRA-ARTICULAR FEATURES OF RHEUMATOID ARTHRITIS

Organ System	Features
Hematologic	Anemia of chronic disease (most commonly seen) Iron deficiency anemia from occult GI bleed with NSAIDs Felty's syndrome
Ophthalmologic	Episcleritis and/or scleritis
Pulmonary	Lung (rheumatoid) nodules Interstitial lung disease Pleuritis
Vascular	Vasculitis
Cutaneous	Rheumatoid nodules
Cardiac	Pericarditis
Neurologic	Peripheral neuropathy
Lymphatic	Increased risk of lymphoma

GI, gastrointestinal; NSAID, nonsteroidal anti-inflammatory drug.

Differential Diagnosis

Although the differential diagnosis of inflammatory arthritis is beyond the scope of this chapter, a mention of other etiologies for inflammatory polyarthritis that might mimic RA is called for. Table 74-3 lists possible alternative diagnoses to be considered in patients with a polyarthritis.

As noted in the classification criteria, the arthritis of RA should last for more than 6 weeks to differentiate it from the numerous viral causes for polyarthritis that resolve within 6 weeks in the vast majority of cases. The common forms of viral polyarthritis include infection with parvovirus, rubella, hepatitis B and C, and Epstein-Barr virus.

TABLE 74-3 DIFFERENTIAL DIAGNOSIS OF RHEUMATOID ARTHRITIS (RA)

Diagnosis	Comments
Diffuse connective tissue disease	Involvement of organ systems other than MSK and positive serologies seen.
Fibromyalgia syndrome (FMS)	No synovitis or inflammatory findings on physical examination in FMS.
Generalized osteoarthritis	Location of involved joints different from distribution seen in RA.
Crystalline arthropathy	More often mono- or oligoarticular; history of brief but intensely painful episodes that recur.
Polymyalgia rheumatica	Proximal muscle pain predominant feature and usually seen in population >65 yr.
Sarcoidosis	Organ involvement other than MSK is common.
Seronegative spondyloarthropathies (psoriatic arthritis, IBD-associated arthritis, reactive arthritis, ankylosing spondylitis)	Inflammatory low back pain seen; more asymmetric joint involvement than RA.
Still's disease	Fever, pharyngitis, RF negativity, organomegaly, rash.
Viral arthritis	Can mimic RA but usually resolves before 6 weeks; consider parvovirus B19 and hepatitis B serologies.

IBD, inflammatory bowel disease; MSK, medullary sponge kidney; RF, rheumatoid factor.

Systemic lupus erythematosus (SLE) may include a polyarthritis as a feature of its multiorgan involvement, but the arthritis of SLE is usually self-limited and nonerosive. The spondyloarthropathies include reactive arthritis (formerly known as Reiter's syndrome), psoriatic arthritis, arthritis attendant to inflammatory bowel disease, and ankylosing spondylitis. Each of these conditions can have a peripheral (extra-axial) inflammatory arthritis. Paraneoplastic arthritis and crystalline arthritis are also sometimes "mimickers" of RA.

Treatment History and Goals

As recently as the mid-1980s, RA was treated via the "pyramid approach."[15] The bottom of the pyramid included time-tested anti-inflammatory agents such as aspirin and nonsteroidal anti-inflammatory drugs (NSAIDs), which were prescribed in conjunction with rest and physical therapy. Second-line therapy, using agents that were "higher up" in the pyramid, was initiated only after the patient had proven radiographic damage or had developed serious extra-articular features of RA such as vasculitis. The presumption at the time of the pyramid approach was that RA was a benign disease and its sufferers should not be exposed to potentially dangerous medications unless they "really" needed them. The pyramid was a faulty treatment construct that advised clinicians to provide treatment that was very much symptom-oriented. The guiding premise underlying this approach was the concept that RA was more a "nuisance" to its sufferer than a significant disease.

The "old" approach to rheumatoid arthritis as a "nuisance disease" was certainly misplaced with its presumption that the treatment of the disease was worse than its natural course. Although we still can offer no cure for RA, the approach of clinicians has very much evolved. This change in approach was due, in no small part, to a better understanding of the long-term morbidity and mortality resulting from RA. Treatment constructs have thus moved far away from the old pyramid approach. Although there is no one treatment paradigm that fits all patients with RA, certain overriding themes in approaching the treatment of RA have taken hold in the past 10 to 15 years. These include

1. RA is not a benign condition—it cripples and kills.
2. Pharmacologic intervention is necessary early to prevent structural damage.
3. Multidrug therapy is not only well tolerated, it is also necessary.
4. Combination drug therapy has become the standard of care in treating RA.

Rheumatologists are now approaching the disease of RA in a fashion analogous to that of the oncologist. Pannus, the growth of synovium that invades surrounding bone and damages articular and periarticular structure, is viewed as if it is a localized cancer. As the reader will learn, polypharmacy, not unlike that used in combination chemotherapy for the oncologic diseases, is the standard of care for RA treatment.

The goal of therapy for RA is to put the disease into remission—defined by the absence of active inflammatory joint pain, morning stiffness, fatigue, synovitis on joint examination, progression of radiographic damage on sequential radiographs, and elevation of the erythrocyte sedimentation rate (ESR) or C-reactive protein (CRP). The purpose of this chapter, then, is to place this newer understanding of the need for early/combined treatment for RA into its clinical context and to describe in more detail the exciting development and rapid deployment of the newer RA pharmacotherapies.

PATHOPHYSIOLOGY

Before proceeding to a discussion of the varied medications employed to treat RA, a review of the pathophysiology of RA is necessary. This will also allow the reader to better integrate the mechanism of action of the RA medications with the pathophysiology of the disease itself. A better understanding of key features in the mechanism of disease perpetuation has led to exciting developments in the last decade in drug treatment for this disease.

A full understanding of the pathogenesis of RA has not yet been developed, but many of the details have been unraveled. As is true of many rheumatologic diseases, a dynamic interplay of genetics and environment occurs, resulting eventually in the patient having the disease we recognize as RA. In RA, as in most inflammatory conditions, the mediators that perpetuate inflammation and those that temper inflammation are in a state of imbalance, with inflammation going unchecked with resultant bone, cartilage, and periarticular destruction. Much of the recent success in pharmacotherapy for RA has resulted from a clearer understanding of the roles of various inflammatory mediators and therapies that target these processes.

The pathogenesis of RA is pictorially explained in Figure 74-1. Note that the synovial membrane in patients with RA demonstrates hyperplasia, hypervascularity, and an inflammatory cell infiltrate. $CD4^+$ T cells play a key role in pathogenesis through their ability to recognize antigens presented via class II human leukocyte antigen (HLA) molecules. A more detailed description of downstream cytokine signaling is seen in Figure 74-2. In particular, RA is strongly linked to the major histocompatibility complex class II antigens HLA-DRB1*0404 and DRB1*0401.[16]

The current understanding is that RA is caused by an antigen that is arthritogenic. This antigen can be either exogenous, such as a viral product, or endogenous, such as citrullinated protein (the basis for the anti-CCP antibody test). T-cell activation requires that an antigen be presented to it, in conjunction with a major histocompatibility

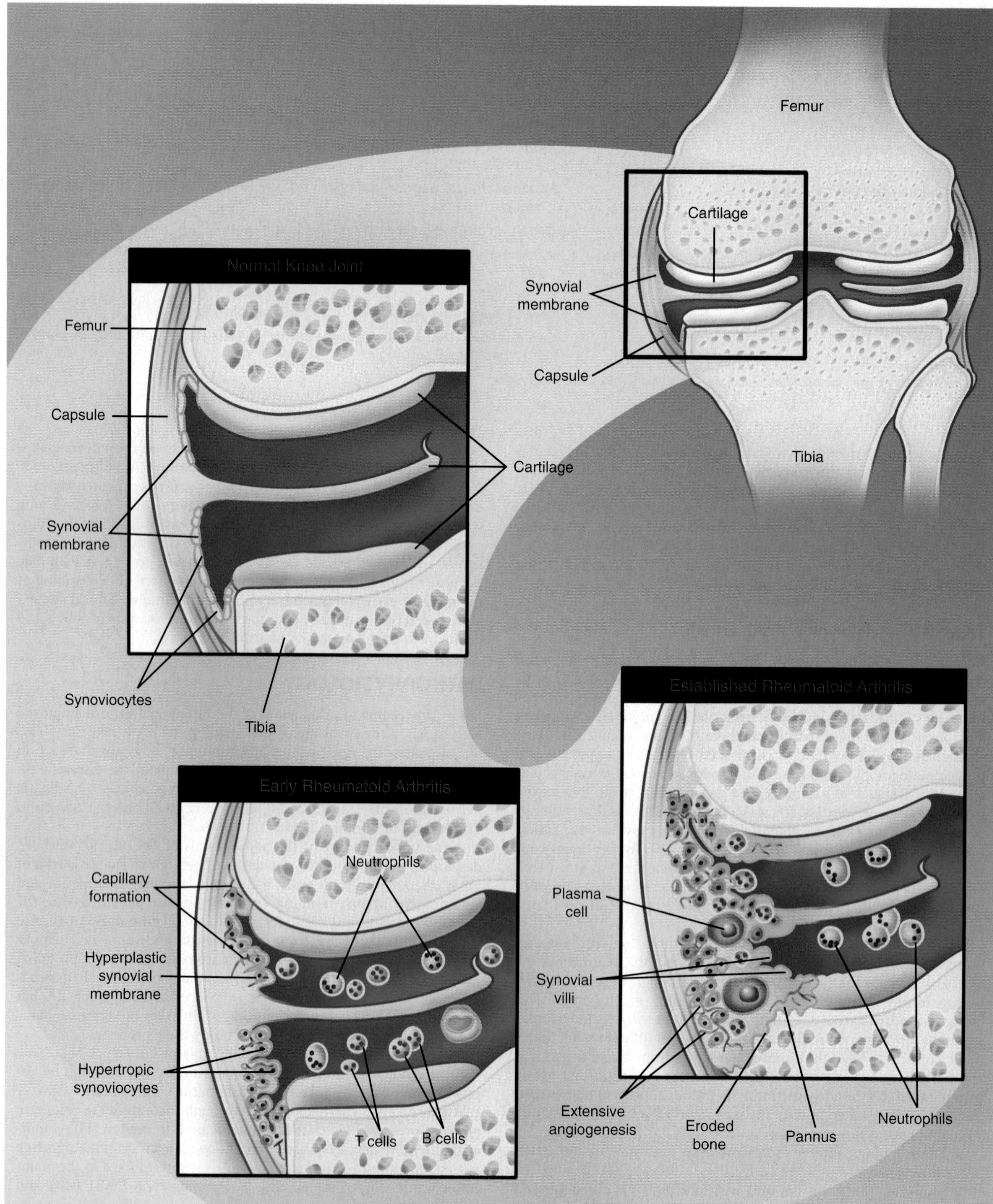

FIGURE 74-1 • Pathogenesis of rheumatoid arthritis. In the normal knee joint, the synovium consists of a synovial membrane (usually one or two cells thick) and underlying loose connective tissue. Synovial-lining cells are designated type A (macrophage-like synoviocytes) or type B (fibroblast-like synoviocytes). In early rheumatoid arthritis, the synovial membrane becomes thickened because of hyperplasia and hypertrophy of the synovial-lining cells. An extensive network of new blood vessels is formed in the synovium. T cells (predominantly $CD4^+$) and B cells (some of which become plasma cells) infiltrate the synovial membrane. These cells are also found in the synovial fluid, along with large numbers of neutrophils. In the early stages of rheumatoid arthritis, the synovial membrane begins to invade the cartilage. In established rheumatoid arthritis, the synovial membrane becomes transformed into inflammatory tissue, the pannus. This tissue invades and destroys adjacent cartilage and bone. The pannus consists of both type A and type B synoviocytes and plasma cells.

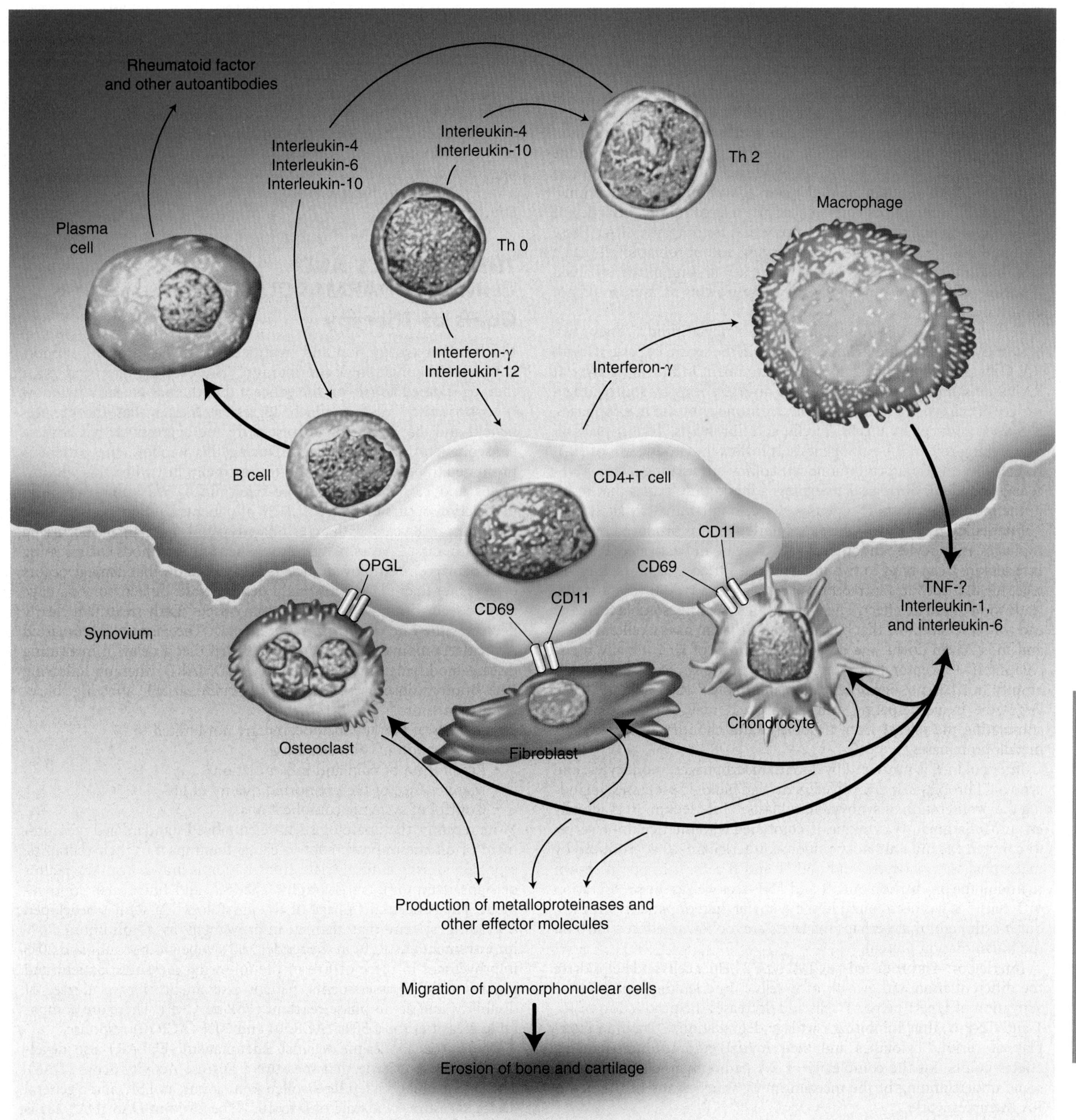

FIGURE 74-2 • Cytokine signaling pathways involved in inflammatory arthritis. The major cell types and cytokine pathways believed to be involved in joint destruction mediated by TNF-α and interleukin-1 are shown. OPGL, osteoprotegerin ligand; Th0, precursor of type 1 and type 2 helper T cells; Th2, type 2 helper T cells. (Reproduced from Choy EHS, Panayi GS. Cytokine pathways and joint inflammation in rheumatoid arthritis. N Engl J Med 2001;344:907-916.)

complex molecule. It also requires costimulation or a "second stimulus" such as occurs when CD28 on the T-cell surface interacts with CD80 or CD86 on the antigen-presenting cell. The CD80/86 interaction with CD28 on the T cell initiates production of interleukin (IL)-2 via IL-2 receptor up-regulation and T-cell proliferation.[17] At the same time, T-cell activation stimulates the expression of cytotoxic T-lymphocyte–associated antigen 4 (CTLA4, a co-inhibitory molecule) that dampens down the T-cell response by interfering with the interaction between CD28 and CD80 or CD86. CTLA4 thus interrupts the T-cell activation and cytokine production pathway.[18]

Once CD4$^+$ T cells are activated by antigenic presentation, they incite other inflammatory cells in the synovium. These antigenically stimulated T cells are thought to be the driving force responsible for the synovitis seen in RA. This synovitis is characterized by infiltration of

T cells, B cells, and macrophages and is also characterized by an abnormal local cytokine profile.[19] Monocytes, macrophages, and synovial fibroblasts then produce IL-1, IL-6, and tumor necrosis factor-α (TNF-α) as well as matrix metalloproteinases and other effector molecules. Interleukin-1, IL-6, and TNF-α are key cytokine mediators in the pathogenesis of RA, and thus serve as specific foci of therapy.

Activated $CD4^+$ T cells also stimulate B cells with resultant production of RF and other immunoglobulins. The precise role of RF in the perpetuation of synovitis is not entirely clear, but it may form immune complexes with resultant complement activation. Finally, activated $CD4^+$ T cells stimulate osteoclasts that play a large role in periarticular bone erosions and in the osteoporosis that accompanies RA. These activated cells (macrophages, lymphocytes, and fibroblasts) all play a role in stimulating angiogenesis, another key finding in the inflamed synovium of RA. Without angiogenesis, the growing pannus would not be sustainable.

IL-1 and TNF-α are found in the RA synovial fluid.[20] These two cytokines are also found in large quantity in the serum of patients with RA. Cells producing TNF-α are quite prominent in the lining layer of RA tissue samples.[21] TNF-α can have diverse effects by stimulating a variety of cell types. Produced mainly by monocytes and macrophages, it is also produced by B cells, T cells, and fibroblasts. TNF-α plays an overarching role in RA pathogenesis: It fosters the production of IL-1, IL-6, IL-8, and granulocyte-monocyte colony-stimulating factor. TNF-α also stimulates fibroblasts to express adhesion molecules that result in the increased transport of leukocytes into inflammatory sites.

Interleukin-1 biology is complex. Interleukin-1 is produced by macrophages, monocytes, endothelial cells, B cells, and activated T cells.[22] Interleukin-1 can bind to two different cell surface receptors: a type I receptor that activates intracellular signaling or a type II receptor that leads to no biologic effect. There are also circulating, soluble forms of each of these receptors that bind IL-1 before it can have a cellular effect and thus "tamp down" the downstream effects of IL-1. Finally, a circulating IL-1 receptor antagonist binds to the type I receptor with high affinity but has no signal activation internally.[23] Interleukin-1 has a large role in perpetuating joint damage. It may cause damage by stimulating the release from fibroblasts and chondrocytes of matrix metalloproteinases.

Interleukin-6 is produced by T cells, macrophages, monocytes, and synovial fibroblasts. It is involved in myriad biologic processes, including the proliferation of synovial fibroblasts.[24] Interleukin-10 is actually an anti-inflammatory cytokine. It, combined with interleukin-4, serves to dampen the inflammatory response. Interleukin-10 is produced by macrophages, monocytes, and both T and B cells. It has been shown to inhibit the production of IL-1 and TNF-α as well as the proliferation of T cells.[25] It has been found in the synovial fluid of patients with RA, but it is thought that perhaps the levels are too low to effect a curb on the inflammation present.[26]

Interleukin-4 is produced by $CD4^+$ type 2 helper cells and helps drive the differentiation and growth of B cells.[25] Interleukin-4 inhibits the activation of type 1 helper T cells and decreases the production of IL-1 and TNF-α, thus inhibiting cartilage degradation.[27] The fine interplay of various cytokines and their myriad and counterbalancing effects points out the complexity of RA pathophysiology, and offers some understanding of the mechanism by which many of the newer RA therapies work.

To summarize, $CD4^+$ T cells initiate the RA inflammatory cascade via stimulation/activation of mononuclear cells, synovial fibroblasts, chondrocytes, and osteoclasts. A proliferating pannus erodes through bone cartilage and bone. At the interface of pannus and cartilage is a cellular advance populated by activated macrophages and synovial fibroblasts that produce matrix metalloproteinases and catharsis. Major effector cytokines include TNF-α, IL-1, and IL-6. Interleukin-1 and TNF-α act on endothelial cells to express adhesion molecules. This results in recruitment of neutrophils into the joint space. Neutrophils subsequently release elastase and proteases, which degrade proteoglycan in the superficial cartilage layer.[28] The depletion of proteoglycan is followed by the deposition of immune complexes in the superficial layer of collagen, and chondrocytes are exposed.[29] The chondrocytes and synovial fibroblasts then release matrix metalloproteinases that degrade the connective tissue matrix. Joint damage ensues, both from the effects of released metalloproteinases and the activation of osteoclasts.

The past decade has seen a truly revolutionary approach to the treatment of RA. An understanding of the cytokine cascade and its role in RA has enabled basic scientists and clinical researchers to collaborate in the development and application of anticytokine therapy as a therapeutic modality in RA. Cytokine-based therapies for RA now include a variety of agents that variously inhibit normal cytokine pathways or effects.

THERAPEUTICS AND CLINICAL PHARMACOLOGY

Goals of Therapy

Much earlier recognition and treatment of RA has growing support within the rheumatologic community.[30] This evolving approach to RA therapy is based largely on the concept that there is an early "window of opportunity" during which aggressive therapy has the greatest benefit and that hesitancy to treat early and aggressively has adverse consequences for the patient.[31] During this window, the patient is presumed to be more responsive to treatment. Just when this window opens and closes remains to be determined. We know that joint destruction occurs early in RA; 70% of patients have erosions seen on plain film by 8 years, with an estimated half of that damage occurring within the first 2 years.[32] When more sensitive methods for assessing joint damage are employed, such as MRI, we know that damage occurs even earlier than plain films might demonstrate. In fact, bone damage may be seen within weeks of symptom onset.[33] Early treatment clearly decreases the rate of disease progression.[34] The Finnish Rheumatoid Arthritis Combination Therapy trial noted that a delay in instituting disease-modifying antirheumatic drug (DMARD) therapy following RA symptom onset was the most important variable affecting subsequent remission.[35]

The goals of therapy include, but are not limited to

- Preservation of joint structures
- Eradication of pain and inflammation
- Maintenance of the premorbid quality of life
- Control of systemic complications

More recently, rheumatologists have employed standardized measurement of disease improvement to gauge the impact of their therapies, especially during clinical trials. Information is drawn from the realms of signs, symptoms, radiographic changes, and functional improvement. The American College of Rheumatology (ACR) has developed a grading system that defines improvement as a minimum 20% improvement (ACR20) in the tender and swollen joint count and 20% improvement in three of five of the following measures: patient and physician global assessments, patient assessment of pain, degree of disability, and acute-phase reactant (ESR or CRP). There are comparable measures for a 50% (ACR50) and 70% (ACR70) response.[36]

The European League Against Rheumatism (EULAR) also developed response criteria that measure a Disease Activity Score (DAS). The DAS evaluates a tender/swollen joint count, an ESR, and a general health measure on a scale of 0 to 10.[37] The 28-joint DAS (DAS 28) is commonly used to measure RA severity. Scores higher than 5.1 are considered severe, scores between 3.2 and 5.1 are moderate, those between 2.6 and 3.2 are low, and those lower than 2.6 indicate "remission." A good EULAR response to treatment is a DAS improvement of greater than 1.2.[38]

Therapeutics by Class

Although the emphasis of this chapter is on pharmacologic therapy, it should be appreciated that nonpharmacologic therapy is a major determinant of outcome in RA. In particular, patient education that emphasizes the nature of RA, its various manifestations beyond joint pain or swelling, coping mechanisms, and counseling is needed.

Physical and occupational therapy are too often overlooked as adjunctive treatment. Training the patient on joint protection, the use of adaptive devices, safe exercises, and the importance of strengthening exercises will greatly benefit the individual patient's outcome.

Attention must also be directed toward osteoporosis prevention in the RA patient. The disease itself leads to bone mineral density loss. Elemental calcium at 1000 to 1500 mg/day and vitamin D at 400 to 800 IU/day should be offered. Importantly, antiresorptive therapy with a bisphosphonate should be considered in those patients who receive chronic corticosteroids.[39]

Pharmacologic therapy for RA may be imprecisely divided into three large categories:

1. Anti-inflammatory agents (NSAIDs and corticosteroids).
2. DMARDs (immunosuppressants and immunomodulators). DMARDs are also known imprecisely as second-line drugs or slow-acting antirheumatic drugs (SAARDs). These agents reduce or retard the expected joint damage of untreated RA.
3. Biologics or biologic response modifiers (TNF-α inhibitors, IL-1 inhibitors, CD20 inhibition, CTLA4-mediated costimulation blockade). Biologic response modifiers are agents developed and deployed to have specific actions on specific targets in the immune cascade. They share the fact that they modify the immune response in RA.

Anti-inflammatory Agents

The most frequently employed initial therapy for a patient complaining of musculoskeletal pain is an NSAID. NSAIDs can be subdivided into salicylates, nonselective cyclooxygenase (COX) inhibitors, and COX-2 inhibitors. These agents are not described here in depth as they are covered in greater detail elsewhere. Furthermore, their use in RA really should be limited to symptom control alone and as adjuncts to DMARDs. They have no impact on the disease process, nor do they serve any disease-modifying purpose. The era of using NSAIDs as a primary therapy for RA is over. NSAIDs do serve a useful function in RA via their ability to inhibit proinflammatory prostaglandins; this does serve to diminish pain and swelling in affected joints. However, joint damage can march right through NSAID usage.

Corticosteroids are highly effective in symptom control in RA. Usually prescribed at "low dose" of less than 10 mg/day, prednisone can potentially impact on bone erosions and actually serve a disease-modifying function.[40] Corticosteroids are often employed as a so-called bridge therapy to offer immediate symptom control while other agents are begun but have not yet shown their effect. Long-term corticosteroid use has a number of deleterious side effects well known to any clinician who prescribes them: osteoporosis, cataract formation, hyperglycemia, cushingoid phenotype, avascular necrosis, acne, and others. Intra-articular corticosteroids are a useful, temporizing measure that the rheumatologist will employ to address a particularly problematic joint that needs more immediate synovitis control. Injection of a steroid preparation into an inflamed joint will often offer immediate relief while systemic therapy from other medications takes effect.

Disease-Modifying Antirheumatic Drugs

The large number of agents that are grouped into the category of DMARDs are prescribed for RA patients to mitigate joint damage in addition to offering necessary symptom control. Included in this category are methotrexate, leflunomide, sulfasalazine, and hydroxychloroquine. Several older agents are almost never used now. The risk: benefit ratio of these previously used agents, such as injectable gold salts, penicillamine, cyclosporine, and cyclophosphamide, argues against including these older agents for RA in the current therapeutic armamentarium.

Tetracyclines, in particular doxycycline and minocycline, have shown a small but modest effect in patients with RA. These drugs decrease collagenase activity and diminish bone resorption, and may offer anti-inflammatory benefit. Meta-analysis has shown that tetracyclines, particularly minocycline, are associated with an improvement in disease control in RA.[41] Control of erosions was not demonstrated. In general, the tetracyclines are best viewed as adjunctive agents in early disease.

Methotrexate. Methotrexate (MTX) is quite effective in RA and has been approved by the U.S. Food and Drug Administration (FDA) for treatment of the same. Methotrexate inhibits leukotriene synthesis and dihydrofolate reductase and decreases TNF-α concentrations. The net result is a decrease in the proliferation of T and B cells, a decrease in rapidly dividing synoviocytes, and a promotion of apoptosis of activated peripheral T cells.[42] The exact mechanism of action of MTX in RA is unknown, but appears to be more that of an anti-inflammatory agent and less that of an antimetabolite.

The ususal dosing regimen is 7.5 to 20 mg given weekly, either orally, intramuscularly, or subcutaneously. It may be dosed at one time or in divided doses on 1 day of each week. For the rare patient who has poor tolerability of oral MTX, it can be taken in three equal doses received every 12 hours over 36 hours. Dose escalation usually is in 2.5- or 5.0-mg increments per week. The maximum oral dose of MTX is thought to be 20 mg/wk. If the dose is increased beyond this range, it usually is given subcutaneously or intramuscularly but usually at no greater a dose than 30 mg/wk. Efficacy is often not seen for 6 to 8 weeks after starting MTX.

Oral absorption averages 70% but is quite variable. It is readily absorbed from the gastrointestinal tract when dosed at less than about 25 mg/m^2. Approximately 50% of MTX is bound to plasma proteins and may be displaced from albumin by sulfonamides, tetracycline, chloramphenicol, phenytoin, and NSAIDs. At least for NSAIDs, this displacement has little clinical significance.[43] Most of the drug is excreted unchanged in the urine within 48 hours. A much smaller quantity is excreted in the stool. Methotrexate clearance is reduced in the elderly or in those with diminished renal function. Impaired renal function can result in myelosuppression from delayed drug excretion. Its clearance is increased by hemodialysis.

Methotrexate is contraindicated in pregnancy. It does not appear to have an impact on female fertility but may cause reversible male sterility.[44] Men should probably discontinue MTX 3 months before attempting impregnation, and women should discontinue it for at least one menstrual cycle prior to pregnancy.

Adverse effects from MTX can include stomatitis, hair thinning, gastrointestinal upset, hepatotoxicity (including fibrosis and cirrhosis), accelerated rheumatoid nodulosis, bone marrow suppression, rare B-cell non-Hodgkin's lymphoma, and an elevation of the mean corpuscular volume, indicative of folate deficiency. Folic acid supplementation, usually prescribed at 1 mg/day orally, may diminish the stomatitis, macrocytic changes, and other side effects. Severe bone marrow suppression is usually only seen in those with underlying renal disease or hypoalbuminemia, and the elderly. Patients should be cautioned to avoid alcohol while taking MTX to diminish the risk of hepatotoxicity. Most surgeons prefer to see MTX discontinued 1 to 2 weeks prior to any surgical procedure to mitigate wound infections. It may also cause pulmonary toxicity as a pneumonitis with cough, shortness of breath, and fever, with possible progression to fibrosis.[45]

Patients considered for MTX use should be screened for underlying renal or hepatic disease (Table 74-4); MTX should be avoided in those with alcoholic liver disease or chronic viral hepatitis. Most rheumatologists screen for chronic hepatitis B and C before administering MTX. Caution is advised for those with concomitant obesity or diabetes but it certainly is not contraindicated in this group. Monitoring for toxicity is recommended, with a complete blood count (CBC) and liver enzymes examined every 6 to 8 weeks. In its earlier years of use for RA, liver biopsies were recommended after a cumulative dose, but this is no longer considered necessary.

Leflunomide. Leflunomide (Arava), an isoxazole derivative, competitively inhibits dihydroorotate dehydrogenase, the rate-limiting intracellular enzyme required for the de novo synthesis of pyrimidines.[46] Activated lymphocytes depend on de novo synthesis of pyrimidines to function. By blocking pyrimidine production, the proliferative lymphocyte response is interrupted. Leflunomide is an alternative to MTX as an initial DMARD. It is FDA approved for the treatment of adults with RA and to retard structural damage. It has clinical efficacy similar to that of MTX and is useful as a replacement agent for those unable to tolerate MTX. It can be combined with MTX for MTX

TABLE 74-4 RECOMMENDED MONITORING OF DMARD MEDICATIONS

Drug	Toxicity	Monitoring	
		Baseline	Routine
Hydroxychloroquine	Macular damage	Ophthalmologic examination if age >40 G6PD	Ophthalmologic examination to include funduscopy and visual fields every 6-12 mo
Sulfasalazine	Myelosuppression Hepatotoxicity Rash	CBC Liver enzymes G6PD	CBC, liver enzymes q mo for 3 mo CBC, liver enzymes q 3 mo
Methotrexate	Myelosuppression Hepatotoxicity Pulmonary fibrosis Oral ulcers GI tract upset	CBC Liver enzymes and albumin Renal function Viral hepatitis serologies CXR	CBC, albumin, and liver enzymes every 4-8 wk
Leflunomide	Hepatotoxicity GI tract upset	CBC Liver enzymes and albumin Renal function Viral hepatitis serologies	CBC, albumin, and liver enzymes every 4-8 wk

CBC, complete blood count; CXR, chest radiograph; DMARD, disease-modifying antirheumatic drug; G6PD, glucose-6-phosphate dehydrogenase; GI, gastrointestinal.

nonresponders, but hepatotoxicity is increased and close monitoring is important.

Leflunomide is a prodrug that undergoes conversion to its active metabolite, A77 1726, found in the circulation. A77 1726 is highly protein bound with a half-life of 15 to 18 days.[47,48] When leflunomide was first marketed, a loading dose of 100 mg/day for 3 days was recommended. More recently, clinicians have started this agent at its usual daily dosing of 10 mg/day with the understanding that its steady state concentration may not be achieved for several months. Its usual dosing range is 10 to 20 mg/day. The active metabolite undergoes extensive enterohepatic recirculation, with persisting drug detectable for 1 to 2 years after discontinuation. It is not recommended in patients with advanced renal disease.

Leflunomide inhibits cytochrome P-450 isoenzyme 2C9, theoretically increasing the anticoagulant activity of warfarin. Rifampin can raise leflunomide's active metabolite and requires dosage adjustment.

Adverse effects from leflunomide are primarily hepatic. Approximately 5% of patients in the initial clinical trials demonstrated elevated transaminase levels, but usually less than twice the upper limit of normal, and these elevations were reversible with drug discontinuation.[49] Postmarketing evaluation demonstrated similar rates of transaminase elevation. Although cases of hepatocellular necrosis were reported, these cases were all confounded by concomitant use of hepatotoxins or underlying liver disease.[50]

Although the most common side effect is diarrhea, hypertension, reversible alopecia, rash, thrombocytopenia, pancytopenia, interstitial pneumonitis, and peripheral neuropathy have all been reported with this agent.[51] Leflunomide is teratogenic, and women of childbearing potential should have a negative pregnancy test prior to its use and ensure adequate contraception. Two years between discontinuation of the drug and attempts at pregnancy is recommended. An alternative strategy to help ensure drug clearance prior to attempting pregnancy is the use of oral cholestyramine, 8 g taken three times a day for 11 days, followed by an assay of plasma drug level to ensure the drug is below 0.02 mg/L on two separate occasions, 2 weeks apart. It is recommended that the same protocol be followed by men who wish to father a child.[52]

The current monitoring recommendation for leflunomide is to obtain a CBC along with transaminase measurements at baseline, monthly until stable, and then at 2- to 3-month intervals (see Table 74-4).

Sulfasalazine. Probably more popular in Europe than in the United States for the treatment of RA, sulfasalazine (Azulfidine) has both anti-inflammatory and antimicrobial effects and is approved for the treatment of RA.

Sulfasalazine is quickly absorbed by the small bowel and promptly recycled via the enterohepatic circulation into bile. It reaches the large intestine, where it is reduced to sulfapyridine and 5-aminosalicylic acid (5-ASA) by the enteric bacterial enzyme azoreductase. It is thought that sulfapyridine is the active moiety in the treatment of RA.[53] The 5-ASA is mostly excreted in stool and the sulfapyridine is absorbed. Sulfapyridine is then metabolized in the liver via hydroxylation and acetylation. The half-life of these components is prolonged in slow acetylators, which affects toxicity but not efficacy. No major drug-drug interactions have been found, although the combination of sulfasalazine and etanercept led to a greater decrement in the neutrophil count.[54]

The particular mechanism of action of sulfapyridine has not been fully elucidated.[55] Nuclear factor-κ, which induces transcription of mediators of the immune response, can be inhibited by corticosteroids and sulfasalazine.[56] TNF-α has been inhibited in macrophages and macrophage-like cell lines after exposure to sulfasalazine, likely through apoptosis and activation of caspase.[57]

The usual dosing regimen is 500 mg/day for the first week, with subsequent dosing increases every week until a standard dose of 2.0 g/day is reached, usually in divided doses. Adverse effects include skin reactions, hepatitis, pneumonitis, aplastic anemia, and agranulocytosis—all idiosyncratic in etiology. Typical dose-related adverse effects include headache, gastrointestinal upset, leukopenia, and megaloblastic anemia. A CBC, liver testing, and viral hepatitis serologies should be obtained as baseline studies. Subsequent monitoring is recommended monthly for 3 months and then every 3 months (see Table 74-4). Men prescribed sulfasalazine may experience oligospermia and temporary infertility. It is believed to be safe for use during pregnancy (FDA Pregnancy Category B).

Although MTX is the preferred initial or baseline therapy for the treatment of RA, sulfasalazine does have an important role in management either in combination with MTX or in the time-tested triple combination of MTX-sulfasalazine-hydroxychloroquine.

Hydroxychloroquine. Hydroxychloroquine (Plaquenil) has been used to treat RA and other rheumatologic diseases such as SLE, discoid lupus, a variety of photosensitive diseases, and sarcoidosis for decades. It has a very favorable safety profile. Hydroxychloroquine interferes with antigen processing, concentrates in lysosomes, and has anti-inflammatory properties. Its actual mechanism of action in RA is poorly understood. There is no compelling evidence that it stops structural damage to joints. It is dosed at 200 to 400 mg/day orally.

Hydroxychloroquine is easily absorbed orally, with peak levels seen in 1 to 3 hours. It is approximately 45% bound to serum albumin, distributes well into tissues, and has a half-life of about 40 days. It does not need to be dose adjusted for renal disease. Its efficacy is usually seen after 3 or 4 months of administration.

Hydroxychloroquine shares the toxicity of other 4-aminoquinoline antimalarials. Its major toxicity is that of irreversible damage to vision via retinal toxicity. This is a relatively rare event, especially if dosing does not exceed 6.5 mg/kg. As well, there can be visual disturbances from corneal deposition. Regular ophthalmologic evaluation is required[58] (see Table 74-4). Retinopathy is likely secondary to accumulation of the drug in melanin-rich tissues and can be avoided if dosing guidelines are followed.[59] Adverse effects may include gastrointestinal disturbance, rash, and rarely neuromuscular toxicity. It is safe to continue during pregnancy. Hydroxychloroquine as effective monotherapy for RA is distinctly uncommon.

Biologic Response Modifiers

Biologic therapy has entered the therapeutic armamentarium in the past decade. The biologic agents have very focused methods of action in the cytokine cascade. The current FDA-approved biologic response modifiers include those that impact on TNF-α, CD20, CTLA4, and IL-2.

Tumor Necrosis Factor-α Inhibitors. Activated macrophages, monocytes, and T cells all release TNF-α as part of the inflammatory cascade intrinsic to RA. TNF-α in turn promotes the release of downstream proinflammatory cytokines, including IL-1, IL-6, and IL-8, and stimulates protease production. Patients with RA have high levels of TNF-α in their synovial fluid. TNF-α bind to two cell surface receptors: TNF-α type 1 receptor (p55) and TNF-α type 2 receptor (p75), which are found on many cell types. Blocking TNF-α improves the signs and symptoms of RA. Three TNF-α–blocking agents are now in use, and all have been approved for use in RA (Table 74-5): etanercept (Enbrel), a dimer of two recombinant soluble p75 TNF-α receptors covalently bound to the Fc portion of human IgG1; infliximab (Remicade), a chimeric (mouse-human) IgG1 anti–TNF-α antibody; and adalimumab (Humira), a recombinant humanized monoclonal anti–TNF-α antibody. Each is described here in detail.

The TNF-α inhibitors have been evaluated in many series of clinical trials, either as cotherapy with MTX or in comparison to MTX. The consensus is that a TNF-α inhibitor given in combination with MTX is more effective than monotherapy with MTX or a TNF-α inhibitor alone. In contrast to DMARDs, their onset of action is measured in days to weeks.

Etanercept. Etanercept (Enbrel) binds to TNF-α, preventing it from linking to its usual receptor. It might be thought of as a "sponge" for TNF-α in the extracellular milieu. It also, unlike the other two agents in this category, targets tumor necrosis factor-β (lymphotoxin). It is approved for the reduction of signs and symptoms of RA as well as for the inhibition of structural damage in patients with moderate or severe RA.

After subcutaneous administration, etanercept is slowly absorbed and peak concentrations are realized in about 2 days. The half-life of the agents is 4 days. The initial dosing regimen is 25 mg subcutaneously twice weekly, but more recently it has been approved for once-weekly administration at 50 mg subcutaneously and is self-administered.

Etanercept may be given as monotherapy or along with MTX if MTX does not provide enough response when given alone. Injection site reactions, usually urticarial, are common but usually self-limited and do not result in discontinuation of the agent. They also tend to diminish with time as the injections are continued.

Infliximab. Infliximab (Remicade) was first approved for Crohn's disease. It is also approved for reduction in the signs and symptoms of moderate or severe RA in combination with MTX in patients who have had an inadequate response to monotherapy with MTX. Infliximab is also approved for the inhibition of structural damage from RA. It is a chimeric IgG1 antibody, with the antigen-binding region of mouse origin and the constant region from a human antibody. It can bind to both cell surface and soluble TNF-α with very high affinity and thus impairs the binding of TNF-α to its receptor. Infliximab also leads to cell death of those cells that express TNF-α through both antibody-dependent and complement-dependent cytotoxicity.

The frequent development of anti-infliximab antibodies led to the recommendation that it be administered with MTX to abrogate the development of antichimeric antibodies. A standard regimen of infliximab has evolved, and it is given as an intravenous infusion administered at 3 mg/kg of body weight at 0, 2, and 6 weeks for the first three doses and then readministered every 8 weeks. If response is incomplete, the maintenance dose may be increased up to 10 mg/kg of body weight or the frequency of administration may be shortened to every 4 to 6 weeks. Infliximab has a half-life of 8 to 12 days.

Infusion reactions with infliximab may include urticaria, chills, pruritus, headache, rash, pharyngitis, cough, and even noncardiac chest pain. Infliximab administration has also been associated with the development of anti–double-stranded DNA antibodies, but this does not usually result in clinical features of SLE.[60] Coadministration of infliximab with MTX is effective at diminishing this autoantibody response as well as in controlling infusion reactions. Human anti–chimeric molecule antibody response to infliximab is found often in treated patients. These antibodies are found more often in those patients who receive infliximab without concomitant MTX, and their presence may result in the need to increase either the infliximab dose or its frequency.[61]

Adalimumab. Adalimumab (Humira) is a fully humanized monoclonal antibody that binds directly to TNF-α with a result that both type 1 and type 2 TNF-α receptors are blocked. Adalimumab has a half-life of about 2 weeks following its usual subcutaneous administration.

Adalimumab may be administered alone or in combination with MTX. The coadministration with MTX does offer better disease control. This was demonstrated in the PREMIER study, which showed that a combination of MTX and adalimumab was more effective in

TABLE 74-5 COMPARISON OF TNF-α BLOCKING AGENTS

	Etanercept	Adalimumab	Infliximab
Class	Soluble TNF-α receptor	Monoclonal antibody to TNF-α	Monoclonal antibody to TNF-α
Form	Recombinant fusion protein	Human monoclonal antibody	Chimeric (mouse-human) monoclonal antibody
Able to neutralize soluble and cell-bound TNF-α	Yes	Yes	Yes
Able to neutralize TNF-β	Yes	No	No
Able to lyse TNF-producing cells in vivo	No	Yes	Yes
Origin	Human	Mouse-human	Human
Half-life (days)	4.8	12-14	9.5
Antibodies directed against agent	<5%	<1%-12%	13%
Requires concomitant methotrexate	No	No	Yes

Adapted from Haraoui B. Is there a rationale for switching from one anti-tumor necrosis factor agent to another? J Rheumatol 2004;31:1021-1022.

preventing radiologic progression of erosions and symptoms than either agent given singly.[62] The standard dose is 40 mg subcutaneously given every 2 weeks. Some rheumatologists prescribe this dose weekly in poor responders.

Efficacy and Adverse Effects of TNF-α Inhibitors. There have been no studies directly comparing the various TNF-α inhibitors to each other in the treatment of RA. Clinical consensus after many years of use would indicate that they are similarly effective. Although both etanercept and adalimumab may be prescribed as monotherapy, concomitant administration of MTX, as with infliximab, offers the best outcome. Injection site reactions with etanercept and adalimumab occur commonly but usually are self-limited.

Disseminated infections are the most feared adverse effect from the use of TNF-α inhibitors. The most common infectious complication is that of mycobacterial disease, often a reactivation of latent tuberculosis. When it occurs, it usually does so within the first several months of treatment.[63] As well, *Listeria, Pneumocystis*, and fungal infections have been seen.[64,65] Patients with advanced RA are the very group that most need aggressive therapy, which often includes biologic agents. Unfortunately, this is also the group that more often experiences an infectious complication, even in the absence of a biologic agent! For this reason, teasing out the relationship of these newer agents to the true risk of an infectious complication is difficult.

Current practice mandates screening for latent tuberculosis prior to prescribing a TNF-α inhibitor. Minimal evaluation should include skin testing with purified protein derivative (PPD) and a chest film. Induration of more than 0.5 mm or more on the skin test is considered "positive." If the screening reveals latent tuberculosis, treatment should be promptly initiated prior to administration of a TNF-α inhibitor. Recommendations for rescreening while receiving a TNF-α inhibitor are not well formulated.

Malignancy risk with the use of TNF-α inhibitors is controversial. Patients with aggressive RA are at an already increased risk for lymphoma and define a population most likely to receive a TNF-α inhibitor. As is true with the infectious complication risk, trying to define the contribution of the TNF-α inhibitor to the increased lymphoma risk is very difficult.[66] To date, national registries and databases show no overall increased risk for solid tumors or cancers other than lymphoma.[67]

There are concerns regarding a link between TNF-α inhibitors and demyelinating disease. Although the data are not conclusive, most rheumatologists will not prescribe a TNF-α inhibitor to anyone with a known demyelinating disease, and remain very attentive to the possible evolution of the same for those patients who are indeed receiving such treatment.

Infliximab increases mortality in heart failure patients such that TNF-α inhibitors are usually avoided in RA patients with concomitant heart failure. It is not thought that TNF-α inhibitors will induce new heart failure in RA patients.[68]

Although no adverse outcomes have been documented in those patients who conceived and delivered while on a TNF-α inhibitor, it is recommended that these agents be avoided during pregnancy and lactation.[69]

Cost is a limiting factor to the ready employment of all TNF-α inhibitors. Monthly expenses for each of these drugs exceed $1200. This puts the availability of these agents beyond the means of some patients.

Abatacept. Abatacept (Orencia) is approved for moderate to severe RA in patients who have not responded to one or more DMARDs or to a TNF-α inhibitor. Abatacept is a fusion protein of CTLA4 linked to IgG1. Functionally similar to CTLA4, abatacept selectively inhibits T cells. CD80 and CD86 ligands on the surface of antigen-presenting cells must bind to the T-cell receptor CD28 for subsequent T-cell activation to occur. Abatacept has a high affinity for CD80 or CD86 and prevents them from binding to CD28, thus inhibiting T-cell activation.[70] Abatacept is considered a costimulation modulator of the immune response and allows other signaling pathways to remain intact.

The dosage of abatacept is based on weight. It is given intravenously over 30 minutes on day 1 and repeated at 2 and 4 weeks. It is then readministered every 4 weeks. It is supplied in 250-mg vials and dosed at 500 mg if the patient's weight is less than 60 kg, 750 mg for a weight of 60 to 100 kg, and 1 g if weight is more than 100 kg. The mean serum half-life is 13 days. The effect of diminished renal or hepatic function on drug clearance is not known. Clearance increases with increasing body weight.

As with the TNF-α inhibitors, patients on abatacept are at increased risk for disseminated infections. A pretreatment PPD and chest radiograph to evaluate for latent tuberculosis are important. The incidence of infections was much higher when abatacept was combined with a TNF-α inhibitor, and for this reason coadministration is contraindicated. Patients may take standard DMARDs with abatacept, but it should not be taken with a TNF-α inhibitor or anakinra. No known drug interactions have been reported. It should be avoided in patients with chronic obstructive pulmonary disease. Common adverse events include headache, nasopharyngitis, and nausea.

Abatacept has been studied in patients who had an inadequate response to MTX in the AIM (Abatacept in Inadequate responders to Methotrexate) trial. Patients who were not responding to MTX were randomized to placebo or abatacept and continued on MTX. At 1 year, those patients receiving both abatacept and MTX demonstrated significant slowing of structural joint damage and improvement in signs and symptoms of RA.[71] Additionally, abatacept has been evaluated in those patients with RA who did not respond to a TNF-α inhibitor. The ATTAIN trial (Abatacept Trial in Treatment of Anti-TNF Inadequate Responders) studied patients who had already failed a DMARD in addition to a TNF-α inhibitor. The TNF-α inhibitor was "washed out" and the patients were randomized to either placebo or abatacept. The group receiving abatacept had a clearly superior response without significant adverse effects.[72]

Rituximab. Rituximab (Rituxan) is approved for use with MTX to treat moderate to severe RA in patients who have not responded adequately to one or more TNF-α agents. Rituximab is a chimeric, anti-CD20 monoclonal antibody that was originally developed to treat B-cell non-Hodgkin's lymphoma and has been used for that purpose successfully since 1997. $CD20^+$ B cells play a critical role in perpetuating synovitis and inflammation in RA. B cells can function as antigen-presenting cells, produce cytokines, regulate T cells, and produce antibodies. Rituximab binds to the CD20 cell surface receptor with resultant interference in the activation and development of circulating B cells. The end result is depletion of circulating B cells. These cells may remain reduced for up to 1 year in the circulation. Regardless, retreatment is often required at an interval of 6 to 9 months.

The standard protocol for administration in RA is that of two 1000-mg intravenous doses given 2 weeks apart. The original studies of its use in RA found that coadministration with MTX offered the best outcome, and it is approved for use in this manner.[73] The initial infusion should be started at 50 mg/hr. If no reaction is noted, the infusion rate can be gradually increased to 400 mg/hr. The infusion typically lasts 4 to 5 hours.

Acute infusion reactions include rigors, fever, nausea, angioedema, headache, cough, dyspnea, and blood pressure fluctuations; these reactions occur frequently but are usually not severe. Most occur with the first infusion and then diminish with subsequent infusions. Premedication with acetaminophen, antihistamines, or corticosteroids controls most such reactions. For example, intravenous methylprednisolone, 100 mg, can be given 30 minutes before each infusion to reduce the incidence and severity of reactions. Should a hypersensitivity or infusion reaction develop, the infusion should be slowed or interrupted. It should be restarted, if the patient improves, at half the infusion rate that precipitated the reaction.

Although serious infections are a consideration in the setting of B-cell depletion, only 2% of patients treated with rituximab versus 1% of patients treated with placebo in a study of 520 RA patients developed an infection. No opportunistic infections were noted. All the patients in this study received background MTX and failed a TNF-α agent.[74] Caution and close observation, however, are still required. Reactivation of hepatitis B has been seen in those patients receiving rituximab for malignancies. Women should be cautioned against pregnancy while on rituximab and for 12 months following its discontinuation.

Anakinra. Interleukin-1 has proinflammatory effects that include the induction of IL-6 and COX-2. It is produced by a variety of cells, including monocytes and macrophages. Interleukin-1 is naturally dampened by the presence of IL-1 receptor antagonist (IL-1RA), an inhibitor that competes for binding to cell surface IL-1β receptors but does not activate the cell. The effects of inhibiting IL-1 include a decrease in mononuclear cell infiltration into the synovium, decreased prostaglandin production by synovial cells and chondrocytes, and decreased matrix metalloproteinase production by activated synovial cells and articular chondrocytes.[75]

The only currently available IL-1 inhibitor is the recombinant IL-1RA, anakinra (Kineret). As with the naturally occurring form of IL-1RA, it binds to the IL-1 receptor and blocks IL-1 from locating its receptor without activating the receptor itself. It has been approved by the FDA for the treatment of RA, either alone or in combination with DMARDs such as MTX for the reduction of signs and symptoms of moderate or severe RA. It differs from the naturally occurring form of IL-1RA only by the addition of one N-terminal methionine.[76]

Anakinra has its onset of efficacy within 1 month usually. Patient comorbidities, including diabetes, cardiovascular disease, and pulmonary disease, do not seem to adversely impact the efficacy of this agent or lead to an increase in opportunistic infections.[77] The usual dose is 100 mg/day administered as a subcutaneous injection. It has a short half-life and requires daily administration subcutaneously. Adjustments in dose or frequency may be indicated in the setting of chronic kidney disease.[78]

As with the TNF-α inhibitors, injection site reactions do occur but are usually self-limited and resolve over several weeks. The risk of infection in patients receiving anakinra is controversial, with some reporting an increase in bacterial infections and others finding no increased risk.[79,80] Anakinra should not be combined with a TNF-α inhibitor because of the increased infectious risk attendant to this potent combination.

Most rheumatologists now view anakinra as a "second tier" biologic agent, to be considered for use after failure of anti–TNF-α agents. The dramatic response seen frequently in patients who receive a TNF-α inhibitor is not as often seen with anakinra.

Therapeutic Approach

The ACR Subcommittee on Rheumatoid Arthritis recommends that patients with suspected RA be referred within 3 months of presentation for confirmation of the diagnosis and to initiate directed therapy.[4] As noted earlier, the older pyramid approach to RA therapy (treating symptoms at presentation with NSAIDs and adding additional medications only when damage to the joint structures was documented) has been supplanted by the "reverse pyramid" approach that advocates early and aggressive therapy.[81] The current therapeutic approach is based upon several important and overlapping concepts that include[82]

- An understanding that RA causes damage early and that treatment early, during a "window of opportunity," is paramount.
- Prompt DMARD employment has greater benefit than late employment.
- Combination DMARDs offer greater benefit than single-agent use.

A time-tested regimen has been triple therapy with MTX, hydroxychloroquine, and sulfasalazine. Occasionally, corticosteroids are added. The Finnish Rheumatoid Arthritis Combination Therapy Trial showed that triple therapy combined with low-dose prednisone (5 to 10 mg/day) was superior to single-agent therapy in those patients with early RA.[83] Triple therapy was also proven effective in a U.S. study that showed this three-drug regimen was more effective than monotherapy or dual therapy in patients with RA.[84]

Recommended Approach

In most patients with RA, rheumatologists will begin treatment with a "baseline" of MTX at 7.5 to 10.0 mg/wk and increase the dose by 2.5 to 5.0 mg/wk each month until there is adequate "disease control" or a maximum oral dose of 20 mg/wk has been achieved. Low-dose prednisone (7.5 mg/day or less) is often used as a bridge to control signs and symptoms while awaiting MTX efficacy, with an aim to taper and discontinue the steroid. MTX can occasionally suffice as monotherapy for RA, but this is not common. Most patients will require combination therapy. An incomplete response to MTX is often followed by escalation to combination therapy with other DMARDs (hydroxychloroquine, sulfasalazine, or leflunomide) or the addition to MTX of a biologic agent. The "right" initial approach to RA is based on patient comorbidities and patient/physician characteristics. The use of RA agents continues to evolve with study and the introduction of ever more agents. The current role for biologic agents in those patients who have had a suboptimal response to MTX or other DMARDs is under continued study and refinement.

BeSt (*Behandel Strategieen*, or "treatment strategy") is a Dutch acronym for an important study that enrolled over 500 patients with early RA. Four groups were assigned to different treatment arms. The first group was treated with one drug at a time, sequentially, starting with MTX and switching to another DMARD if there was no improvement. The second group was a "step-up therapy" group that received MTX and then had other DMARDs added as necessary. The third group started immediately on a combination of MTX and sulfasalazine as well as a tapering dose of high-dose prednisone. The fourth and final group received initial combination MTX and infliximab at the outset. Although the patients in groups three and four showed greater functional recovery early on, the clinical outcome at 2 years was similar in all four treatment groups. Importantly, patients in groups three and four showed significantly less radiographic damage. Finally, the patients in groups three and four were best able to taper their treatment to monotherapy (36% in group three and 54% in group four) after 2 years because of excellent disease control.[85]

Several points can be drawn. The "right" drug(s) to prescribe for a patient with RA are very much patient specific. Patient preference, how aggressive the disease is in a particular patient, cost, convenience of monitoring, toxicity concerns, and so forth all weigh on the patient's and physician's decision-making. We do know that early treatment is very important and that damage that occurs before appropriate therapy is initiated does not repair. Various combinations of traditional DMARDs and combinations of traditional DMARDs and biologic agents have been used to treat both active early RA and established, moderate to severe disease. We know that MTX is effective and should be the baseline therapy in this disease. We know that triple DMARD therapy is more effective than single-agent therapy. We know that low-dose prednisone may a very useful adjunct therapy, and there is some evidence that it prevents erosions in early RA.[41,86] Finally, a combination of methotrexate with a TNF-α inhibitor is often very effective in reducing disease activity as well as in reducing the progressive radiographic damage seen in RA.

Figure 74-3 depicts a rational treatment approach to drug therapy in RA developed by the ACR.

Emerging Targets and Therapeutics

Although the development of the biologic agents has greatly augmented the efficacy of MTX in treating patients with RA, there is still a subpopulation of patients who do not have adequate control of their disease with the currently available medications. New agents on the horizon may offer some hope for these patients, or perhaps even demonstrate an agent superior to those already in use. Brief mention is given here to just a few of these emerging therapies:

- HuMax-CD20 is a fully humanized B-cell tropic agent that has efficacy, in preliminary studies, comparable to rituximab.[87]
- Tocilizumab is an anti–IL-6 monoclonal antibody that acts on the IL-6 receptor. Interleukin-6 is involved in synovial proliferation in RA. Tocilizumab has shown early promise in patients with active RA despite treatment with MTX.[88]
- Belimumab, also known as LymphoStat-B, inhibits B-cell stimulation. It is frequently referred to as BlyS in view of its effects on B-cell stimulation.[89,90]

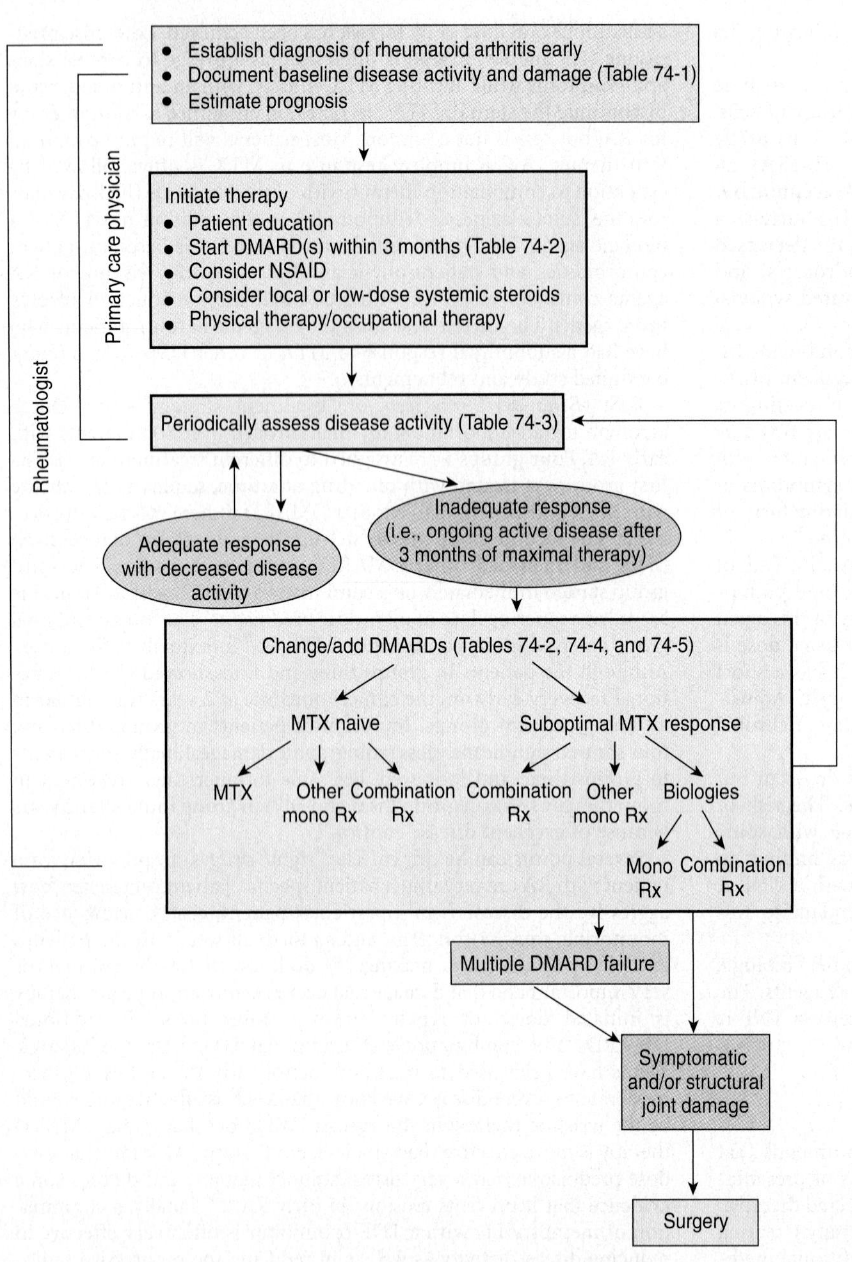

DMARD, disease-modifying antirheumatic drug; NSAID, nonsteroidal anti-inflammatory drug; mono Rx, monotherapy; combination Rx, combination therapy.

FIGURE 74-3 • Approach to rheumatoid arthritis therapy.

CONCLUSION

Several themes permeate the current literature on RA treatment and are worth summarizing:

- RA requires early and aggressive therapy to avert erosions of the subchondral bone and hence disability.
- MTX is an anchor drug around which other therapies are added.
- Corticosteroids do serve well as adjunct therapy, especially in early RA.
- Combination therapy offers greater disease control than monotherapy.
- Clinical research studies infrequently reflect "real-world" patient care, where patients have comorbidities that influence drug use, variable drug cost coverage by insurance, and other issues that preclude entry into studies.
- RA cannot be cured, but it can be exceptionally well controlled with newer therapies.

REFERENCES

1. Gabriel SE. The epidemiology of rheumatoid arthritis. Rheum Dis Clin North Am 2001;27:269-281.
2. Abdel-Nasser A, Rasker J, Valkenburg H. Epidemiological and clinical aspects relating to the variability of rheumatoid arthritis. Semin Arthritis Rheum 1997;27:123-140.
3. Firestein GS. Etiology and pathogenesis of rheumatoid arthritis. In Ruddy S, Harris ED, Sledge CB, Kelley WN (eds): Kelley's Textbook of Rheumatology, 7th ed. Philadelphia: Elsevier Saunders, 2005, pp 996-1042.
4. American College of Rheumatology Subcommittee on Rheumatoid Arthritis Guidelines. Guidelines for the management of rheumatoid arthritis: 2002 update. Arthritis Rheum 2002;46:328-346.
5. Callahan L. The burden of rheumatoid arthritis: facts and figures. J Rheumatol 1998;25(Suppl):8-12.
6. Scott DL, Symmons DP, Coulton BL, Popert AJ. Long-term outcome of treating rheumatoid arthritis: results after 20 years. Lancet 1987;1:1108-1111.
7. Pincus T, Callhan LF. Taking mortality in rheumatoid arthritis seriously—predictive markers, socioeconomic status and comorbidity. J Rheumatol 1986;13:841-845.
8. Gabriel SE, Crowson SC, Kremers HM, et al. Survival in rheumatoid arthritis: a population based analysis of trends over 40 years. Arthritis Rheum 2003;48:54-58.

9. Doran MF, Pond GR, Crowson CS, et al. Trends in incidence and mortality in rheumatoid arthritis in Rochester, Minnesota over a forty-year period. Arthritis Rheum 2002;46:625-631.
10. del Rincón ID, Williams K, Stern MP, et al. High incidence of cardiovascular events in a rheumatoid arthritis cohort not explained by traditional cardiac risk factors. Arthrits Rheum 2001;44:2737-2745.
11. Wolfe F, Freundlich B, Straus WL. Increase in cardiovascular and cerebrovascular disease prevalence in rheumatoid arthritis. J Rheumatol 2003;30:36-40.
12. Nicola PJ, Maradit-Kremers H, Roger VL, et al. The risk of congestive heart failure in rheumatoid arthritis: a population-based study over 46 years. Arthritis Rheum 2005;52:412-420.
13. Harris ED. Clinical features of rheumatoid arthritis. In Ruddy S, Harris ED, Sledge CB, Kelley WN (eds): Kelley's Textbook of Rheumatology, 7th ed. Philadelphia: Elsevier Saunders, 2005, pp 1043-1078.
14. Avouac J, Gossec L, Dougados M. Diagnostic and predictive value of anti-cyclic citrullinated protein antibodies in rheumatoid arthritis: a systematic literature review. Ann Rheum Dis 2006;65:845-851.
15. Weinblatt ME. Rheumatoid arthritis: treat now, not later! Ann Intern Med 1996;124:773-774.
16. Launchbury JS. The HLA association with rheumatoid arthritis. Clin Exp Rheumatol 1992;10:301-304.
17. Arcuto O, Michel F. CD28-mediated co-stimulation: a quantitative support for TCR signaling. Nat Rev Immunol 2003;3:939-951.
18. Solomon B, Bluestone JA. Complexes of CD28/B7:CTLA4 costimulatory pathways in autoimmunity and transplantation. Annu Rev Immunol 2001;19:225-252.
19. Choy EH, Panayi GS. Cytokine pathways and joint inflammation in rheumatoid arthritis. N Engl J Med 2001;344:907-916.
20. Houssiau FA. Cytokines in rheumatoid arthritis. Clin Rheumatol 1995;14(Suppl 2):10-13.
21. Ulfgren A-K, Lindblad S, Klareskog L, et al. Detection of cytokine producing cells in the synovial membrane from patients with rheumatoid arthritis. Ann Rheum Dis 1995;54:654-661.
22. Koch AE, Kunkel SL, Strieter RM. Cytokines in rheumatoid arthritis. J Invest Med 1995;43:28-38.
23. Svenson M, Nedergaard S, Heegaard PMH, et al. Differential binding of human interleukin-1 (IL-1) receptor antagonist to natural and recombinant soluble and cellular IL-1 type receptors. Eur J Immunol 1995;25:2842-2850.
24. Van Snick J. Interleukin-6: an overview. Annu Rev Immunol 1990;8:253-278.
25. Isomaki P, Punnonen J. Pro- and anti-inflammatory cytokines in rheumatoid arthritis. Annu Rev Med 1997;29:499-507.
26. Katsikis PD, Chu C-Q, Brennan FM, et al. Immunoregulatory role of interleukin 10 in rheumatoid arthritis. J Exp Med 1994;179;1517-1527.
27. van Roon JA, van Roy JL, Duits A, et al. Proinflammatory cytokine production and cartilage damage due to rheumatoid synovial T helper-1 activation is inhibited by interleukin-4. Ann Rheum Dis 1995;54:836-840.
28. Moore AR, Iwamura H, Larbre JP, et al. Cartilage degradation by polymorphonuclear leucocytes: in vitro assessment of the pathogenic mechanisms. Ann Rheum Dis 1995;54:836-840.
29. Jasin HE, Taurog JD. Mechanism of disruption of the articular cartilage surface in inflammation: neutrophil elastase increases availability of collagen type II epitopes for binding with antibody on the surface of articular cartilage. J Clin Invest 1991;87:1531-1536.
30. Kim JM, Weisman MH. When does rheumatoid arthritis begin and why do we need to know? Arthritis Rheum 2000;43:473-484.
31. Quinn MA, Emery P. Window of opportunity in rheumatoid arthritis: possibility of altering the disease process with early intervention. Clin Exp Rheumatol 2003;21(5 Suppl 31):S154-S157.
32. Ryan L, Brooks P. Disease-modifying antirheumatic drugs. Curr Opin Rheumatol 1999;11:161-165.
33. McGonagale D, Conaghan PG, O'Connor P, et al. The relationship between synovitis and bone changes in early untreated rheumatoid arthritis: a controlled magnetic resonance imaging study. Arthritis Rheum 1999;42:1706-1711.
34. Emery P, Breedveld FC, Dougados M, et al. Early referral recommendation for newly diagnosed rheumatoid arthritis: evidence based development of a clinical guide. Ann Rheum Dis 2002;61:290-297.
35. Mottonen T, Hannonen P, Korpela M, et al. Delay to institution of therapy and induction of remission using single-drug or combination-disease-modifying antirheumatic drug therapy in early rheumatoid arthritis. Arthritis Rheum 2002;46:894-898.
36. Felson DT, Anderson JJ, Boers M, et al. for the American College of Rheumatology. Preliminary definition of improvement in rheumatoid arthritis. Arthritis Rheum 1995;38:727-735.
37. van Gestel M, Prevoo ML, van't Hof MA, et al. Development and validation of the European League Against Rheumatism response criteria for rheumatoid arthritis: comparison with the preliminary American College of Rheumatology and the World Health Organization/International League Against Rheumatism criteria. Arthritis Rheum 1996;39:34-40.
38. Prevoo ML, van't Hof MA, Kuper HH, et al. Modified disease activity scores that include twenty-eight joint counts: development and validation in a prospective longitudinal study of patients with rheumatoid arthritis. Arthritis Rheum 1995;38:44-48.
39. Recommendations for the prevention and treatment of glucocorticoid-induced osteoporosis. American College of Rheumatology Task Force on Osteoporosis Guidelines. Arthritis Rheum 1996;39:1791.
40. Kirwan JR, for the Arthritis and Rheumatism Council Low Dose Glucocorticoid Study Group. The effect of glucocorticoids on joint destruction in rheumatoid arthritis. N Engl J Med 1995;333:142-146.
41. Stone M, Fortin PR, Pacheco-Tena C, Inman RD. Should tetracycline treatment be used more extensively for rheumatoid arthritis? Metaanalysis demonstrates clinical benefit with reduction in disease activity. J Rheumatol 2003;30:2112-2122.
42. Genestier L, Paillot R, Fournel S, et al. Immunosuppressive properties of methotrexate: apoptosis and clonal deletion of activated peripheral T cells. J Clin Invest 1998;102:322-328.
43. Iqbal MP, Baig JA, Ali AA, et al. The effects of non-steroidal anti-inflammatory drugs on the disposition of methotrexate in patients with rheumatoid arthritis. Biopharm Drug Dispos 1998;19;163-167.
44. Bresnihan B. Treatment of early rheumatoid arthritis in the younger patient. J Rheumatol 2001;28(Suppl 62):4-9.
45. Kremer JM, Alarcon GS, Weinblatt ME, et al. Clinical, laboratory, radiographic, and histopathologic features of methotrexate-associated lung injury in patients with rheumatoid arthritis: a multicenter study with literature review. Arthritis Rheum 1997;39:1711-1719.
46. Kremer JM. Methotrexate and leflunomide: biochemical basis for combination therapy in the treatment of rheumatoid arthritis. Semin Arthritis Rheum 1999;29:14-26.
47. Breedveld FC, Dayer JM. Leflunomide mode of action in the treatment of rheumatoid arthritis. Ann Rheum Dis 2000;59:841-849.
48. Rozman B. Clinical pharmacokinetics of leflunomide. Clin Pharmacokinet 2002;41:421-430.
49. Schuna AA, Megeff C. New drugs for the treatment of rheumatoid arthritis. Am J Health Syst Pharm 2000;57:225-234.
50. American College of Rheumatology. Hotline. FDA meeting March 2003: update on the safety of new drugs for rheumatoid arthritis. Part III: safety and efficacy update on leflunomide (Arava®). Available at http://www.rheumatology.org/publications/hotline/0503leffda.asp?aud=mem
51. Olsen NJ, Stein M. New drugs for rheumatoid arthritis. N Engl J Med 2004;350:2167-2179.
52. Brent RL. Teratogen Update: Reproductive risks of leflunomide (Arava): a pyrimidine synthesis inhibitor. Counseling women taking leflunomide before or during pregnancy and men taking leflunomide who are contemplating fathering a child. Teratology 2001;63:106-112.
53. Bird HA. Sulphasalazine, sulphapyridine or 5-aminosalicylic acid—which is the active moiety in rheumatoid arthritis? Br J Rheumatol 1995;34(Suppl 2):16-19.
54. Box A, Pullar T. Sulphasalazine in the treatment of rheumatoid arthritis. Br J Rheumatol 1997;36:382-386.
55. Smedegard G, Bjork J. Sulphasalazine: mechanism of action in rheumatoid arthritis. Br J Rheumatol 1995;34(Suppl 2):7-15.
56. Wahl C, Liptay S, Adler G, Schmid RM. Sulfasalazine: a potent and specific inhibitor of nuclear factor kappa B. J Clin Invest 1998;101:1163-1174.
57. Rodenburg RJ, Ganga A, van Lent PL, et al. The anti-inflammatory drug sulfasalazine inhibits tumor necrosis factor alpha expression in macrophages by inducing apoptosis. Arthritis Rheum 2000;43:1941-1950.
58. American College of Rheumatology Committee on Rheumatologic Care. Position Statement: Screening for hydroxychloroquine retinopathy. Available at *http://www.rheumatology.org/publications/position/hydroxy.asp?aud=mem*
59. Rennie IG. Clinically important ocular reactions to systemic drug therapy. Drug Saf 1993;45:430-475.
60. De Rycke L, Baeten D, Kruithof E, et al. Infliximab, but not etanercept, induces IgM anti-double-stranded DNA autoantibodies as main antinuclear reactivity: biologic and clinical implications in autoimmune arthritis. Arthritis Rheum 2005;52:2192-2201.
61. Haraoui B, Cameron L, Ouellet M, White B. Anti-infliximab antibodies in patients with rheumatoid arthritis who require higher doses of infliximab to achieve or maintain a clinical response. J Rheumatol 2006;33:31-36.
62. Breedveld FC, Weisman MH, Kavanaugh AF, et al. The PREMIER study: a multicenter, randomized, double-blind clinical trial of combination therapy with adalimumab plus methotrexate versus methotrexate alone or adalimumab alone in patients with early, aggressive rheumatoid arthritis who had not had previous methotrexate treatment. Arthritis Rheum 2006;54:26-37.
63. Keane J, Gershon S, Wise RP, et al. Tuberculosis associated with infliximab, a tumor necrosis factor alpha-neutralizing agent. N Engl J Med 2001;345:1098-1104.
64. Hamilton CD. Infectious complications of treatment with biologic agents. Curr Opin Rheumatol 2004;16:393-398.
65. Khanna D, McMahon M, Furst DE. Safety of tumour necrosis factor-alpha antagonists. Drug Saf 2004;27:307-324.
66. Baecklund E, Iliadou A, Askling J, et al. Association of chronic inflammation, not its treatment, with increased lymphoma risk in rheumatoid arthritis. Arthritis Rheum 1996;54:692-701.
67. Wolfe F, Michaud K. Lymphoma in rheumatoid arthritis: the effect of methotrexate and anti-tumor necrosis factor therapy in 18,572 patients. Arthritis Rheum 2004;50:1740-1751.
68. Wolfe F, Michaud K. Heart failure in rheumatoid arthritis: rates, predictors, and the effect of anti-tumor necrosis factor therapy. Am J Med 2004;116:305-311.
69. Chakravarty EF, Sanchez-Yamamoto D, Bush TM. The use of disease modifying antirheumatic drugs in women with rheumatoid arthritis of childbearing age: a survey of practice patterns and pregnancy outcomes. J Rheumatol 2003;30:241-246.
70. Teng GG, Turkiewicz AM, Moreland LW. Abatacept: a costimulatory inhibitor for treatment of rheumatoid arthritis. Expert Opin Biol Ther 2005;5:1245-1254.
71. Kremer JM, Genant HK, Moreland LW, et al. Effects of abatacept in patients with methotrexate-resistant active rheumatoid arthritis. Ann Intern Med 2006;144:865-876.

72. Genovese MC, Becker JC, Schiff M, et al. Abatacept for rheumatoid arthritis refractory to tumor necrosis factor alpha inhibition. N Engl J Med 2005;353:1114-1123.
73. Edwards JC, Szczepanski L, Szechinski J, et al. Efficacy of B-cell-targeted therapy with rituximab in patients with rheumatoid arthritis. N Engl J Med 2004;350:2572-2581.
74. Cohen S, Emery P, Greenwald M, et al. Prolonged efficacy of rituximab in rheumatoid arthritis patients with inadequate response to one or more TNF inhibitors: 1-year follow-up of a subset of patients receiving a single course in a controlled trial (REFLEX study). Ann Rheum Dis 2006;65(Suppl 2):183.
75. Cunnane G, Madigan A, Murphy E, et al. The effects of treatment with interleukin-1 receptor antagonist on the inflamed synovial membrane in rheumatoid arthritis. Rheumatology (Oxford) 2001;40:62-69.
76. Breshihna B, Cunnane G. Interleukin-1 receptor antagonist. Rheum Dis Clin North Am 1998;24:615-628.
77. Schiff MH, DiVittorio G, Tesar J, et al. The safety of anakinra in high-risk patients with active rheumatoid arthritis: six-month observations of patients with comorbid conditions. Arthritis Rheum 2004;50:1752-1760.
78. Yang BB, Baughman S, Sullivan JT. Pharmacokinetics of anakinra in subjects with different levels of renal function. Clin Pharmacol Ther 2003;74:85-94.
79. Fleischmann RM, Schechtman J, Bennett R, et al. Anakinra, a recombinant human interleukin-1 receptor antagonist (r-metHuIL-1ra), in patients with rheumatoid arthritis: a large, international, multicenter placebo-controlled trial. Arthritis Rheum 2003;48:927-934.
80. Cohen S, Hurd E, Cush J, et al. Treatment of rheumatoid arthritis with anakinra, a recombinant human interleukin-1 receptor antagonist. Arthritis Rheum 1999;41:2196-2204.
81. Boers M. Rheumatoid arthritis: treatment of early disease. Rheum Dis Clin North Am 2001;27:407-415.
82. Pincus T, O'Dell JR, Kremer JM. Combination therapy with multiple disease-modifying antirheumatic drugs in rheumatoid arthritis: a preventive strategy. Ann Intern Med 1999;131:768-774.
83. Mottonen T, Hannonen P, Leirisalo-Repo M, et al., for the FIN-RACo Trial Group. Comparison of combination therapy with single-drug therapy in early rheumatoid arthritis: a randomized trial. Lancet 1999;353:1568-1573.
84. O'Dell JR, Leff R, Paulsen G, et al. Treatment of rheumatoid arthritis with methotrexate and hydroxychloroquine, methotrexate and sulfasalazine, or a combination of the three medications: results of a two year, randomized, double-blind, placebo-controlled trial. Arthritis Rheum 2002;46:1164-1170.
85. Goekoop-Ruiterman UP, de Vries-Bouwstra JK, Allaart CF, et al. Clinical and radiographic outcomes of four different treatment strategies in patients with early rheumatoid arthritis (the BeSt study): a randomized, controlled trial. Arthritis Rheum 2005;52:3381-3390.
86. Smolen JS, Aletaha D, Keystone E. Superior efficacy of combination therapy for rheumatoid arthritis: fact or fiction? Arthritis Rheum 2005;52:2975-2983.
87. Ostergaard M, Wiell C, Dawes PT, et al. First clinical results of HuMax CD20 fully humanized monoclonal IgG1 antibody treatment in rheumatoid arthritis. Ann Rheum Dis 2006;65:58.
88. Miyasaka N, Yamamoto K, Kawai S, et al. Efficacy and safety of tocilizumab in monotherapy, an anti-IL-6 receptor monoclonal antibody, in patients with active rheumatoid arthritis: results from a 24 week double blind Phase III study. Ann Rheum Dis 2006;65:175.
89. McKay J, Chwalinska-Sadowska H, Boling E, et al. Belimumab, a fully human monoclonal antibody to B-lymphocyte stimulator (BLyS), combined with standard care of therapy reduces the signs and symptoms of rheumatoid arthritis in a heterogeneous subject population. 2005 ACR/ARHP Annual Scientific Meeting; Nov. 12-17, 2005; San Diego, CA. Abstract 1920.
90. Stohl W, Chatham W, Weisman M, et al. Belimumab, a novel fully human monoclonal antibody to B-lymphocyte stimulator (BLyS), selectively modulates B-cell subpopulations and immunoglobulins in a heterogeneous rheumatoid arthritis subject population. 2005 ACR/ARHP Annual Scientific Meeting; Nov. 12-17, 2005; San Diego, CA. Abstract 1160.

75

GOUT

Michael P. Keith, William R. Gilliland, and Kathleen Uhl

INTRODUCTION 1039
PATHOPHYSIOLOGY 1039
THERAPEUTICS AND CLINICAL PHARMACOLOGY OF ACUTE GOUT 1039
Therapeutics by Class 1039
Colchicine 1039
Nonsteroidal Anti-inflammatory Drugs 1041
Corticosteroids and Related Compounds 1041
THERAPEUTICS AND CLINICAL PHARMACOLOGY OF CHRONIC GOUT 1041
Therapeutics by Class 1041
Xanthine Oxidase Inhibitors 1041
Uricosuric Agents 1042
Probenecid 1042
Sulfinpyrazone 1042
Therapeutic Approach 1043
Practical Initiation of Urate-Lowering Therapy 1043
Lifestyle Considerations 1043
Adjunctive Therapies 1043
Emerging Therapies 1044
Febuxostat 1044
Benzbromarone 1044
Uricase 1044
SUMMARY 1044

INTRODUCTION

Gout is the prototypical crystalline arthritis and is among the most common causes of inflammatory arthritis, especially in men. Gout is associated with obesity and the metabolic syndrome.[1] The incidence and prevalence of gout appears to be rising,[2] possibly related to the increase in the metabolic syndrome. Gout is likely to be encountered in all specialty areas, particularly primary care.

PATHOPHYSIOLOGY

Gout is a metabolic disease associated with hyperuricemia, a biochemical abnormality defined by elevated serum urate concentrations. Under normal circumstances, serum uric acid levels reflect a balance between filtration at the glomerulus and reabsorption and secretion at the proximal tubule. Consequently, hyperuricemia results from either increased production of uric acid, decreased excretion of uric acid, or a combination of both. Over the course of a day, approximately 10 g of urate are filtered, greater than 9 g are absorbed, and a much smaller amount is secreted. This critical reabsorptive role is performed by the urate anion exchanger URAT1, while other transporters such as UAT, OAT1, and OAT3 play smaller roles.[3]

Uric acid is the normal end product of the degradation of purine-containing compounds such as nucleic acids. Supersaturation of uric acid in extracellular fluids or deposition of monosodium urate crystals in tissues lead to the clinical manifestations of gout such as arthritis, tophi, uric acid nephrolithiasis, and interstitial nephropathy. The clinical manifestations in humans result from the lack of the enzyme uric acid oxidase, or uricase. In most other mammals, uricase oxidizes uric acid to the highly soluble allantoin. The lack of this enzyme subjects humans to the potential risk of tissue deposition of uric acid crystals. While a complete discussion of purine metabolism is beyond the scope of this chapter, Figure 75-1 provides an overview of purine production. It also provides a biochemical rationale for the use of several of the medications discussed later in the chapter.

Classically, the course of gout passes through various stages: asymptomatic hyperuricemia, intermittent attacks of acute gout, and chronic tophaceous gout. Asymptomatic hyperuricemia is a very common biochemical abnormality that occurs in approximately 5% of the population.[4] Increasing levels of uric acid correspond to a higher risk of developing gouty arthritis, with a risk of 3% for uric acid levels between 7.0 and 8.0 mg/dl and 22% for uric acid levels of 9.0 mg/dl or more.[5] Despite these percentages, the vast majority of patients with hyperuricemia do not develop gout.

Acute intermittent gouty arthritis is generally the first clinical manifestation of gout. Classically described as an acute monoarthritis with severe pain escalating over a 6- to 12-hour period, swelling, and erythema, it is easily recognized by physicians and patients. Since systemic features such as fevers and chills sometimes accompany an attack, it is important to make a definitive diagnosis of gout by aspiration and demonstration of characteristic monosodium urate crystals in synovial fluid.

The transition from acute intermittent gout to chronic tophaceous gout develops over 10 or more years. This transition is characterized by shortening of the intercritical periods between gout attacks, diminished pain intensity, and persistent joint abnormalities. Though dietary and lifestyle modifications have a positive impact on gout,[6] the majority of patients will require pharmacologic management to arrest the progression of disease.

THERAPEUTICS AND CLINICAL PHARMACOLOGY OF ACUTE GOUT

Acute gouty arthritis most commonly presents as monoarthritis of the lower extremities, and involvement of the first metatarsophalangeal joint (podagra) is classic. Appropriate therapy is associated with decreased duration of the attack and reduced pain and disability. Currently available treatment options for acute gout include colchicine, nonsteroidal anti-inflammatory drugs (NSAIDs), and corticosteroids. Urate-lowering agents such as allopurinol or probenecid should neither be started nor discontinued during acute gout because this may prolong the attack. A summary of treatment options for acute gout is presented in Table 75-1.

Therapeutics by Class

Colchicine

Colchicine is an alkaloid derived from two plants of the lily family, *Colchicum autumnale* and *Gloriosa superba*, that was first recommended for the treatment of gout in the sixth century A.D.[7] It remains widely in use today for the treatment of acute gout. In fact, some authors advocate its use in patients when gout is suspected but not confirmed; if the patient does not respond after up to 10 hourly doses of colchicine, then the diagnosis of gout should be reconsidered.[8]

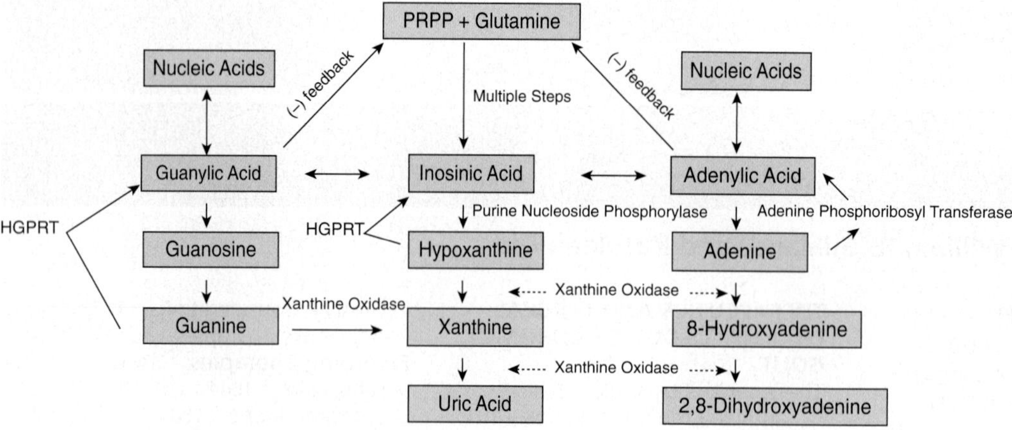

FIGURE 75-1 • Overview of purine metabolism in humans.

TABLE 75-1 TREATMENT OF ACUTE GOUTY ARTHRITIS

Medication	Dosage	Comments
NSAIDs (indomethacin)	200 mg/day in divided doses on the first day followed by 150 mg/day in divided doses, until the attack subsides, then taper.	Other NSAIDs in anti-inflammatory doses are probably equally efficacious.
Colchicine	0.6 mg qh until pain and inflammation are alleviated, gastrointestinal side effects develop, or a maximum of 10 tablets/24 hr is reached.	Gastrointestinal complaints common. Must adjust dose for creatinine clearance. IV form potentially more toxic and rarely indicated.
Oral corticosteroids	Starting doses of 30-50 mg of prednisone or equivalent daily with subsequent taper over 10 days.	Especially useful when NSAIDs and colchicine are contraindicated or in polyarticular flares.
IA corticosteroids (sample doses given for triamcinolone)	40 mg IA with lidocaine for large joints, 10-20 mg for small joints or bursae.	Treatment of choice for monoarthritic flare or for patients in whom NSAIDs, colchicine, and systemic corticosteroids are contraindicated.
Parenteral corticosteroids	IV corticosteroids such as methylprednisolone 100 mg daily with taper, or IM corticosteroids such as triamcinolone 40 mg, repeated in 12 hr if needed.	May be especially useful in hospitalized patients who cannot take oral medications.
Adrenocorticotropic hormone (ACTH)	40-80 USP units IM q8-12h (usually 2-3 injections required).	More costly than alternative therapies.

IA, intra-articular; IM, intramuscular; IV, intravenous; NSAID, nonsteroidal anti-inflammatory drug.

Colchicine is available orally as 0.5- or 0.6-mg tablets or intravenously (IV) as a 0.5-mg/ml solution, although the oral form is most widely used. The typical dose used in normal patients for acute gout is 0.6 mg orally every hour until relief of joint symptoms, occurrence of gastrointestinal side effects, or the patient has taken 10 doses.[8] Initial pharmacokinetic studies used IV colchicine,[9] whereas subsequent reports employed the oral formulation.[10] When given IV, colchicine is rapidly cleared from plasma in the first 10 to 20 minutes and declines in logarithmic fashion thereafter.[9] Oral administration of colchicine leads to a maximum concentration in approximately 1 hour, with an estimated bioavailability of 50%.[10] Following oral administration, 50% of colchicine in the plasma is protein bound.[7]

Up to 30% of an IV dose of colchicine is excreted in the urine, and there is evidence of enterohepatic circulation with 10% of the drug metabolized in the liver.[7] The half-life for an IV dose is 19 minutes, whereas for an oral dose the half-time ranges from 9 to 16 hours.[7] Although it was reported that there is no significant difference in elimination half-times between patients and normal controls and that patients with liver impairment have increased clearance of colchicine,[9] subsequent studies demonstrate that colchicine clearance is impaired in patients with renal and hepatic dysfunction.[7]

Colchicine exerts its effect in gout by inhibiting leukocyte activation and migration. Colchicine is thought to be most effective when given in the first 24 to 48 hours of an attack. In the only controlled study of colchicine in acute gout, it was twice as effective as placebo at 48 hours.[11] However, all patients given colchicine developed diarrhea at a median time of 24 hours, and diarrhea preceded pain relief in the majority of colchicine-treated patients.[11]

Gastrointestinal symptoms are the most common manifestations of colchicine toxicity when it is used in appropriate doses for gout. Typical gastrointestinal toxicity of colchicine includes abdominal pain, nausea, vomiting, and diarrhea.[7] More serious manifestations of colchicine toxicity include bone marrow suppression, disseminated intravascular coagulation, and hepatic, renal, cardiopulmonary, and nervous system failure.[7] These manifestations are most likely to occur with massive doses of colchicine, as in attempted suicide. These patients have traditionally had a poor prognosis, but treatment with colchicine-specific Fab fragments has been reported to be effective.[12]

Severe colchicine toxicity occasionally occurs through routine use of colchicine, especially in the setting of hepatic or renal impairment.[13] In addition, colchicine neuromyopathy with reversible symmetric proximal muscle weakness and elevated serum creatine kinase occurs in patients with renal insufficiency.[13,14] Therefore colchicine must be used with caution in patients with renal and hepatic insufficiency.

Guidelines for the appropriate use of colchicine in patients with gout and renal impairment have been proposed. Colchicine should be avoided in hemodialysis patients and the dose reduced in those with impaired creatinine clearance.[13] Doses of 0.6 mg twice daily are not recommended in patients with serum creatine levels of 1.6 mg/dl or more.[13] This dose has resulted in toxicity and death in a patient with a creatinine level only as high as 2.3 mg/dl.[15]

Intravenous colchicine is less commonly used in the acute management of gout due to the potential for severe toxicity. The maximum recommended cumulative dose for IV colchicine is 4 mg; exceeding this dose has been associated with increased mortality.[16] Furthermore, use of IV colchicine in patients on chronic oral colchicine is associated with bone marrow failure and death.[16] Currently IV colchicine is rarely indicated due to the availability of more efficacious and less toxic alternatives.

Nonsteroidal Anti-inflammatory Drugs

NSAIDs are frequently used to treat acute gout. They share common side effects and generally should not be used in patients with renal impairment and a history of or risk factors for gastrointestinal bleeding. The pharmacologic properties of individual NSAIDs are described in detail in Chapter 11.

Indomethacin is often considered the NSAID of choice for treating acute gout. The typical oral dose of indomethacin for acute gout is 150 to 200 mg daily in divided doses. Indeed, many studies of NSAIDs in acute gout compare the effectiveness of the study drug to indomethacin.[17] Intramuscular ketorolac[18] and oral ketoprofen[19] performed equally well as indomethacin in the treatment of acute gout. Etodolac and naproxen appear to have similar efficacy based on direct comparison.[17] However, any NSAID used at a full anti-inflammatory dose is likely to be efficacious in gout.

Cyclooxygenase-2 (COX-2) has been implicated in the inflammatory response induced by monosodium urate,[20] providing a basis for the use of COX-2 inhibitors in gout. These agents could be used as an alternative to traditional NSAIDs because of reduced gastrointestinal toxicity. The COX-2 inhibitors are discussed in detail in Chapter 11. Rofecoxib, now withdrawn by the manufacturer in the United States, was more effective than diclofenac and meloxicam in acute gout.[21] Etoricoxib has been shown to be safe in acute gout and is as effective as indomethacin.[22]

Corticosteroids and Related Compounds

Corticosteroids are effective in acute gout and are an excellent treatment choice when the patient has renal impairment or gastrointestinal bleeding that would contraindicate the use of colchicine or NSAIDs. They are also useful in hospitalized patients who cannot receive medication by mouth. The pharmacologic properties of corticosteroids are reviewed in detail in Chapter 11. Routes of corticosteroid administration include oral, intramuscular (IM), IV, and intra-articular.

In acute monoarthritis due to gout, intra-articular corticosteroids are the treatment of choice, and small doses have been claimed to be effective.[23] Oral corticosteroids should be considered when patients decline arthrocentesis or have an inadequate response or contraindication to colchicine or NSAIDs. Systemic corticosteroids are preferred in oligo- and polyarticular presentations. Prednisone is effective when started at 30 to 50 mg or its equivalent and tapered over 10 days.[24]

Intravenous or IM steroids are useful in patients who cannot take medications by mouth. Triamcinolone acetonide 60 mg IM is as safe and effective as indomethacin 50 mg three times daily in acute gouty arthritis.[25] IM corticosteroids for acute gout are likely to improve treatment outcomes when patient compliance is problematic.

Adrenocorticotropic hormone (ACTH) has been used in the treatment of acute gout[26] and is thought to exert its beneficial effect through the stimulated release of adrenal corticosteroids.[24] However, ACTH is also effective in patients with adrenal insufficiency, possibly via its effects on a melanocortin receptor described in a rat model of gouty arthritis.[27]

ACTH may be given IM, IV or subcutaneously and is effective for gout with comorbid congestive heart failure, chronic renal insufficiency, and gastrointestinal bleeding.[28] Moreover, intramuscular ACTH was more rapidly effective than indomethacin with fewer side effects in a study of 100 male gout patients with no major organ system dysfunction.[29] Although ACTH 40 units IM was as efficacious as triamcinolone acetonide 60 mg IM in acute gout, ACTH resulted in more rebound attacks and treatment failures requiring repeat injections.[30]

THERAPEUTICS AND CLINICAL PHARMACOLOGY OF CHRONIC GOUT

The long-term management of gout consists of antihyperuricemic or urate-lowering therapy. In general, indications for urate-lowering therapy include two or more gout attacks per year, tophaceous gout, erosive arthritis on radiographs, and kidney disease due to elevated uric acid including urate nephropathy, uric acid nephropathy, and/or uric acid nephrolithiasis. A serum uric acid level of less than 6.0 mg/dl is recommended as the initial target for antihyperuricemic therapy because a serum uric acid below this level has demonstrated a reduced frequency or elimination of gout attacks.[31,32]

Two classes of urate-lowering drugs, xanthine oxidase inhibitors and uricosurics, are available for use in chronic gout. Xanthine oxidase inhibitors block metabolic steps in the synthetic pathway of uric acid. Currently available xanthine oxidase inhibitors include allopurinol and its metabolite oxypurinol. Uricosurics, including probenecid and sulfinpyrazone, increase renal uric acid clearance. A summary of current treatment options for chronic gout is presented in Table 75-2.

Therapeutics by Class

Xanthine Oxidase Inhibitors

Allopurinol is a purine analogue inhibitor of xanthine oxidase that blocks the conversion of xanthine to uric acid. Allopurinol is probably the agent most commonly used for urate-lowering therapy

TABLE 75-2 TREATMENT OF CHRONIC GOUT

Medication	Class	Dosage	Comments
Allopurinol	Xanthine oxidase inhibitor	100-300 mg/day, but may require up to 800 mg/day.	Adjust dosage in patients with renal insufficiency.
Probenecid	Uricosuric	Starting dose of 250 mg bid, increased slowly to doses not to exceed 1 g bid.	Ineffective for patients with a glomerular filtration rate of <50-60 ml/min and contraindicated in patients with renal stones.
Sulfinpyrasone	Uricosuric	Starting dose of 50 mg PO bid; can be increased to 200 mg PO bid.	Promotes urate nephrolithiasis and causes gastrointestinal side effects in approximately 5% of patients.

PO, orally.

by practicing rheumatologists, despite the fact that approximately 90% of gout patients are uric acid underexcreters. This is because it is effective in both uric acid underexcreters and normal excretors,[33] and a 24-hour measurement of urine uric acid is not required prior to its use.

Allopurinol was first used as a hypouricemic drug in the 1960s. Both allopurinol and its major metabolite, oxypurinol, inhibit xanthine oxidase and prevent the conversion of hypoxanthine to xanthine and the conversion of xanthine to uric acid. Another mechanism of action appears to be feedback inhibition of amidophosphoribosyltransferase, and therefore de novo purine synthesis, by the allopurinol and oxypurinol ribonucleotides generated by the purine salvage pathway.[34]

Allopurinol is readily absorbed following an oral dose. Average bioavailability is reported to be approximately 70%, and peak concentrations are achieved in 1 hour.[34] Oxypurinol is detectable 15 minutes following administration of allopurinol, and peak oxypurinol concentrations are achieved within 4 hours.[34] Allopurinol is negligibly protein bound, and its high volume of distribution (1.6 L/kg) indicates extensive uptake in the tissues.[34]

Elimination of allopurinol does not appear dose dependent and, for a 300-mg dose, occurs rapidly with a half-life of 1.1 to 1.6 hours.[34] In contrast, the oxypurinol generated by an allopurinol dose of 300 mg has a half-life of 13 to 21 hours.[34] Because oxypurinol is predominantly eliminated unchanged in the urine and its half-life may be extended up to 7 days in the presence of renal dysfunction,[34] renal impairment is a major determinant of the risk for drug toxicity.

Side effects may occur in up to 20% of allopurinol-treated patients.[8] The most common include gastrointestinal intolerance and skin rash. More severe reactions include fever, myelosuppression, toxic epidermal necrolysis, hepatitis, and vasculitis.[35] The most severe reaction is the allopurinol hypersensitivity syndrome, which includes fever, rash, eosinophilia, progressive kidney failure, and even death.[35,36] While this may occur in any patient treated with allopurinol, it is most common in patients with chronic kidney disease or receiving diuretics.[8] The dose of allopurinol should be reduced based on the patient's creatinine clearance,[8,36] and patients should be advised to stop the medication and contact their physician should fever or rash develop.

Several drug-drug interactions with respect to allopurinol deserve mention. Allopurinol raises the plasma levels of theophylline and warfarin, potentiating the risk for toxicity. Allopurinol impairs the metabolism of 6-mercaptopurine (6-MP) and its prodrug azathioprine (AZA) by blocking the xanthine oxidase–mediated conversion of 6-MP to 6-thiouric acid. In cases in which both allopurinol and 6-MP/AZA are required, the dose of 6-MP/AZA should be reduced by at least 50%[8] and up to 75%[34] in order to avoid life-threatening myelosuppression.

Typical doses of allopurinol range from 100 mg daily to 300 mg daily in patients with normal renal function, but higher doses are sometimes required to achieve the target serum uric acid concentration. Oxypurinol sodium demonstrated similar efficacy in reducing serum uric acid compared to allopurinol when used in amounts equimolar to 300 mg of allopurinol.[37] The initial dose should be reduced in patients with impaired renal function due to the increased rate of adverse events at higher starting doses in these patients.[8] Periodic laboratory monitoring for patients on allopurinol should include a complete blood count, hepatic enzymes, and serum uric acid. One approach is to start allopurinol at 100 mg daily and increase by 100 mg daily every 2 to 4 weeks as needed based on the serum uric acid level until the target uric acid level is reached.[38]

Patients who develop a cutaneous reaction to allopurinol may be considered for allopurinol desensitization when the drug is required for management of their gout. Desensitization has been shown to be effective and can be conducted by oral[39] or parenteral administration. Oxypurinol is available on a compassionate use basis and is another option in patients allergic to allopurinol who do not exhibit cross-reactivity to oxypurinol,[40] although 40% of patients allergic to allopurinol are intolerant of oxypurinol.[8]

Uricosuric Agents

Though sometimes overlooked, uricosuric drugs are ideal antihyperuricemic agents for young gout patients with normal renal function who are underexcreters of uric acid and have no history of nephrolithiasis. Available uricosuric drugs include probenecid, sulfinpyrazone, and benzbromarone, although probenecid is most commonly used. Each of these agents inhibits the action of URAT1 in the kidneys, thus blocking proximal tubular reabsorption of uric acid.[41]

These agents may be relatively more cumbersome than allopurinol in clinical use because of associated laboratory testing. Measurement of a 24-hour urine uric acid concentration should be performed in patients for whom uricosuric therapy is considered. Patients on a regular purine diet who excrete less than 800 mg of uric acid in the urine per day are considered underexcreters and are candidates for a uricosuric agent.

Physicians should counsel their patients that uricosurics can cause nephrolithiasis and that they should therefore maintain an adequate urine output. It has been reported that doses of aspirin greater than 81 mg/day will diminish the efficacy of uricosurics[8]; however a trial of 325 mg aspirin used with probenecid did not demonstrate significant degradation of the uricosuric effect.[42] Addition of a xanthine oxidase inhibitor is necessary if the patient cannot achieve a serum urate level of less than 6 mg/dl on uricosurics alone.[8]

Probenecid

Probenecid first entered clinical use in 1950 as a means to slow the renal elimination of penicillin.[43] Probenecid has a potent uricosuric effect, and doses of 1 to 2 g daily cause four- to sixfold increases in uric acid clearance.[43] It has since been used for the treatment of chronic gout and remains the most widely used uricosuric agent in the United States. The recommended starting dose is 250 mg twice daily, and a typical maintenance dose is 1 g twice daily.[44]

Probenecid is well absorbed when given orally and provides drug levels equivalent to the IV form, no longer available in the United States.[43] Peak concentrations are reached in 1 to 5 hours, and the peak action occurs about 2 hours after an oral dose with effects lasting up to 8 hours.[43] Probenecid is extensively protein bound, ranging from 83% to 95% depending on the dose.[43]

In human studies, probenecid is primarily metabolized via oxidation of its alkyl side chains, with a smaller fraction undergoing glucuronidate conjugation.[43] The half-life of probenecid is dose dependent and ranges from 2 to 6 hours for doses of 0.5 to 1 g and from 4 to 12 hours for doses of 2 g.[43] Renal clearance appears to be the major route of elimination of probenecid and its metabolites in humans and, although enterohepatic circulation has been described in rats, it is unknown if probenecid is excreted in bile in humans.[43] Side effects include nephrolithiasis, precipitation of acute gout, and the risk of bleeding when used in patients on heparin.[44]

Sulfinpyrazone

Sulfinpyrazone is a pyrazolidine-derived uricosuric agent. In addition to its potent uricosuric effects, reported by Burns et al. in 1957, sulfinpyrazone inhibits prostaglandin synthesis and reduces platelet activity.[45] Though related to the NSAID phenylbutazone, sulfinpyrazone has no anti-inflammatory properties.[46] The typical starting dose is 50 mg twice daily, and maintenance doses of up to 200 mg twice daily are used to obtain a target serum uric acid level of 6.0 mg/dl or less.[44]

Sulfinpyrazone is readily absorbed following an oral dose, and peak plasma concentration is achieved in 1 to 2 hours.[47,48] The half-life is 1 to 3 hours, and the drug is highly protein bound.[47] Sulfinpyrazone caused a dose-dependent increase in renal uric acid clearance and decrease in plasma uric acid concentration in healthy volunteers.[48] The majority of drug is excreted in the urine as a parahydroxyl metabolite, possessing uricosuric activity of its own.[47]

Common side effects include uric acid nephrolithiasis and decreased platelet aggregation.[47] Rare but serious side effects include bone marrow suppression[47] and induction of peptic ulcer.[44] The side effect of decreased platelet aggregation led to its past use in myocardial infarction as an antiplatelet agent. However, acute renal failure was not infrequently reported following the use of sulfinpyrazone subsequent to an acute myocardial infarction.[46,49]

Sulfinpyrazone has been used successfully in lieu of allopurinol in heart transplant patients with cyclosporine-associated gout.[50] However, this treatment was associated with reduced plasma cyclosporine levels, increasing the possibility of transplant rejection. The use of sulfinpyrazone in other transplant settings has not been reported.

Therapeutic Approach

Practical Initiation of Urate-Lowering Therapy

Gout should be in remission prior to starting urate-lowering therapy. However, the optimal duration of remission before embarking on a course of antihyperuricemic therapy has not been determined. Prophylaxis of gout is an important concern when initiating antihyperuricemic therapy. The initiation of xanthine oxidase inhibitors or uricosurics often causes gout to flare. Indeed, recent experience demonstrates that 64% of patients treated with allopurinol experienced a flare during the first year of therapy.[51]

Agents that are available for gout prophylaxis in this setting include colchicine or an NSAID. Colchicine decreases the number of gout flares when used for prophylaxis when initiating allopurinol therapy.[52] When given for prophylaxis, colchicine should be given at a dose of no more than 0.6 mg twice daily, and lower doses are required in patients with chronic renal insufficiency. Similarly, low doses of an NSAID are commonly used for prophylaxis of gout after starting urate-lowering therapy. Currently, no randomized trial has been conducted to demonstrate the efficiency of NSAIDs for this purpose, nor have NSAIDs been compared to colchicine for the prophylaxis of gout when initiating urate-lowering therapy.[53] Low-dose prednisone (10 mg or less daily) may also be considered in patients for whom colchicine or NSAIDs are contraindicated due to comorbidities.

Management of a gout flare in a patient on concomitant antihyperuricemic therapy is the same as for acute gout except that urate-lowering agents *should not* be stopped. The duration of prophylactic therapy varies widely among practicing rheumatologists, with recommendations ranging from 3 to 12 months. Colchicine is effective for prophylaxis for up to 6 months.[52] A common practice is to continue prophylactic therapy until the serum uric acid level has been below goal for 3 to 6 months and the patient has had no acute attacks during this period.[8]

Lifestyle Considerations

Lifestyle and medication changes should be considered in the optimal management of gout (Box 75-1). The role of low-purine diets has been less emphasized in the chronic management of gout because of the increased use of potent uric acid–lowering agents. Although it is difficult to manage gout by diet alone, patients should be advised to limit their consumption of foods that contribute to hyperuricemia, especially alcohol (beer and liquor), meat, and seafood.[6] Vegetables, even those containing purines, wine, and low-fat dairy products do not appear to contribute to gout and are possibly protective.[6]

Through a variety of mechanisms, excessive alcohol intake is associated with increased frequency of gout attacks. Beer and liquor, but not wine, raise serum uric acid levels[54] and thus increase the risk of gout. Ketoacids produced during alcohol consumption activate URAT1, thus increasing proximal tubular reabsorption of urate and compounding the hyperuricemic effect of alcohol.[6]

Physicians should be aware that several medications cause hyperuricemia due to their effects on URAT1 and resultant decreased renal excretion of urate. These include cyclosporine, nicotinic acid, furosemide, thiazide diuretics, ethambutol, pyrazinamide, and aspirin.[41] When possible, alternative medications should be considered.

Adjunctive Therapies

In addition to the standard agents discussed in the chronic management of gout, certain drugs used in the treatment of hypertension or hypertriglyceridemia have been found to have salutary effects on serum uric acid. These agents are beneficial in gout patients with other manifestations of the metabolic syndrome. The use of these agents in lieu of the standard agents indicated for urate lowering used in the chronic management of gout is not recommended.

Fenofibrate. Fenofibrate is a fibric acid derivative that is used in the treatment of hypertriglyceridemia. Fenofibrate has been shown to exert a modest uricosuric effect, enough to lower the serum uric acid concentration. Treatment of hypertriglyceridemic men with fenofibrate resulted in lowering of serum uric acid with a concomitant increase in renal uric acid clearance of 30%.[55] In addition, fenofibrate blunted the increased hepatic production of urate seen in response to an infusion of fructose.[55] Treatment of 64 dyslipidemic patients with micronized fenofibrate led to a statistically significant drop in serum uric acid levels of 27.9% accompanied by an increase in the fractional excretion of urate.[56] Fenofibrate 300 mg daily led to a reduction in mean uric acid concentration in Japanese hyperlipidemic patients from 7.0 ± 1.58 mg/dl to 5.2 ± 1.57 mg/dl ($P < 0.01$) after 12 weeks.[57] These studies suggest benefit of the use of fenofibrate in gout patients with hypertriglyceridemia.

Fenofibrate is also effective for urate lowering in patients with both gout and hyperuricemia. The addition of fenofibrate to allopurinol in chronic gout patients produced a mean reduction of serum uric acid concentration of 19% following 3 weeks of treatment, an effect that was reversed when fenofibrate was withdrawn.[58] In addition to uric acid, fenofibrate increased the fractional excretion of xanthine and oxypurinol.[59] Although it was claimed that fenofibrate may decrease the effectiveness of allopurinol therapy by increasing clearance of its active metabolite, oxypurinol,[59] this has not been confirmed.

Fenofibrate has important drug interactions that are described in detail in Chapter 23. Briefly, important drug interactions of fenofibrate include those with oral hypoglycemic agents, hydroxymethylglutaryl coenzyme A reductase inhibitors, and cyclosporine.[60] Clinically important bleeding has resulted from concurrent use of fenofibrate and warfarin.[61]

Losartan. Losartan is first in the class of angiotensin receptor antagonists now commonly used for the treatment of hypertension, especially in patients who require but are intolerant of

BOX 75-1 TEN PRINCIPLES FOR THE MANAGEMENT OF GOUT

1. The definitive diagnosis of gout is made by visualizing intracellular monosodium urate crystals in synovial fluid.
2. Asymptomatic hyperuricemia usually does not require treatment.
3. Although colchicine, NSAIDs, and corticosteroids are equally efficacious in the management of acute gout, patient considerations will dictate the choice of therapy.
4. Consider uric acid–lowering therapy in patients with two or more attacks per year.
5. The initial target serum uric acid level when using uric acid–lowering therapy is less than 6.0 mg/dl.
6. Urate-lowering agents should neither be stopped nor started during an acute gout flare.
7. Oral colchicine or low-dose NSAIDs should be used for prophylaxis for a period of 3 to 12 months when initiating urate-lowering therapy.
8. Allopurinol, rather than uricosurics, should be used in patients with renal stones, tophaceous gout, or a glomerular filtration rate of less than 50 ml/min, or those who are urate overproducers.
9. Febuxostat, a novel nonpurine xanthine oxidase inhibitor, may be a useful alternative medication in patients with renal insufficiency once it is approved by the FDA.
10. Lifestyle modification and avoidance of medications that raise uric acid levels play an adjunctive management role, but do not replace urate-lowering therapy in most cases.

FDA, U.S. Food and Drug Administration; NSAID, nonsteroidal anti-inflammatory drug.

angiotensin-converting enzyme inhibitors. Losartan is unique in the class of angiotensin receptor blockers in that it is uricosuric. A comparison of losartan 50 mg daily to eprosartan 600 mg daily for 4 weeks in hypertensive patients demonstrated that uric acid excretion was increased in the losartan group but not in the eprosartan group.[62] Neither drug, however, significantly decreased the serum uric acid concentration. Losartan but not irbesartan had a uricosuric effect that caused decreased serum uric acid levels in hypertensive patients with gout.[63] These results demonstrate the potential for losartan as an attractive agent to treat comorbid hypertension in patients with gout.

The combination of fenofibrate and losartan provides additional uric acid lowering in gout patients with both hypertriglyceridemia and hypertension.[64,65] Amlodipine, a dihydropyridine class calcium channel blocker discussed in detail in Chapter 22, also exerts a modest uricosuric effect in hypertensive renal transplant recipients receiving cyclosporine.[66] However, this effect has not been evaluated in typical gout patients alone or in combination therapy with fenofibrate or losartan.

Vitamin C. Although not indicated for treatment of comorbid conditions of the metabolic syndrome, vitamin C has been suggested for the treatment of gout. The ingestion of 4 g ascorbic acid daily led to doubling of the fractional excretion of uric acid in 9 of 14 patients.[67] Vitamin C demonstrated a mild urate-lowering effect in nonsmokers at a daily dose of 500 mg for 2 months.[68] The effect of higher doses for prolonged periods in patients with gout has not been studied, although the tight control of plasma concentrations despite increasing oral doses of vitamin C[69] suggests that higher doses are not likely to be more effective in reducing uric acid.

Emerging Therapies

Fortunately, several new medications show promise for the treatment of chronic gout. Several of these agents were developed for the treatment of chronic gout. It is important to note that, since the development of allopurinol in the 1960s,[8] no new medications have been developed for this indication. Therefore, considerable excitement has been generated about these new agents in the armamentarium to treat gout. These include a nonpurine inhibitor of xanthine oxidase (febuxostat), a potent uricosuric (benzbromarone), and uricase.

Febuxostat

Febuxostat is a novel nonpurine inhibitor of xanthine oxidase awaiting U.S. Food and Drug Administration approval for the management of gout. Febuxostat inhibits both oxidized and reduced forms of xanthine oxidase and, unlike allopurinol and oxypurinol, does not impair other enzymes involved in purine and pyrimidine metabolism.[70] Febuxostat is rapidly absorbed and, at doses of 10 to 120 mg, has a half-life of 4 to 12 hours.[71] Conjugation and oxidation are the major pathways of drug elimination, and neither renal clearance[8] nor the cytochrome P-450 system are important in the elimination of the drug.

Safety and efficacy have been demonstrated for febuxostat in patients with varying degrees of renal dysfunction. After a single dose of 20 mg, there were no significant differences in the area under the curve of febuxostat in patients with mild or moderate renal impairment compared to normal controls.[72] A dose of 80 mg was well tolerated and effective in mild, moderate, and severe renal dysfunction, and produced comparable decreases in serum uric acid concentration across all levels of renal function.[73] Likewise, dose reductions were not required in mild and moderate hepatic impairment compared to controls, although febuxostat-induced reduction of uric acid was lower in groups with hepatic dysfunction.[74]

Currently, few comparisons of febuxostat to allopurinol are available. Febuxostat was more effective than fixed-dose allopurinol in reducing serum urate levels and has a favorable safety profile.[51] Febuxostat also performed equally well as allopurinol in reducing gout flares and the area of tophi.[51]

Although its exact role in the management of gout has not been determined, febuxostat is a welcome addition to the therapeutic armamentarium available for chronic gout. It will be useful in patients who are intolerant of allopurinol or in patients who, due to chronic renal insufficiency, are not candidates for uricosurics. The use of febuxostat in place of allopurinol will avoid possible drug interactions in patients who require therapy with azathioprine or 6-mercaptopurine. Likewise, it may prove to be useful as add-on therapy in those patients who cannot achieve a target serum uric acid level of less than 6.0 mg/dl because of dose limitations to allopurinol due to chronic kidney disease. The recommended dose of febuxostat is likely to be 80 mg or 120 mg once daily.[51]

Benzbromarone

Benzbromarone is a benzofuran-derived uricosuric drug that is more likely to be encountered in Europe than in the United States. Its urate-lowering properties were first described in the late 1960s. Single-dose studies have confirmed its profound uricosuric effect.[75]

Peak serum concentrations are reached by 6 hours following a single oral dose of 100 mg benzbromarone. This is followed by an extended period of benzbromarone activity persisting up to 48 hours,[76] confirming the suitability of once-daily dosing. Benzbromarone is primarily eliminated through the intestinal tract, and 50% of a single 100-mg dose is excreted unchanged in the feces after 2 to 3 days.[76] In contrast, only 8% of the drug is excreted in the urine.[76]

Benzbromarone has been shown to be effective hypouricemic therapy when administered alone or in combination with allopurinol. Benzbromarone causes a rapid fall in plasma urate concentrations when given daily at 40 or 80 mg, and this effect persisted during a study period of up to 1 year.[77] Benzbromarone does not inhibit xanthine oxidase or affect the activity of purine phosphoribosyltransferase,[77] indicating that its mechanism of action is via a uricosuric effect. Despite the lower plasma concentration of oxypurinol observed during concomitant administration of allopurinol with benzbromarone, the combination was more effective than allopurinol alone at reducing the plasma uric acid concentration.[78]

Benzbromarone appears safe and well tolerated. In patients treated with benzbromarone observed for up to 18 months, no skin rash or renal colic developed.[79] Moreover, there were no signficiant abnormalities in serum creatinine, liver enzymes, or blood counts observed.[79] Unlike probenecid and sulfinpyrazone, benzbromarone maintains effectiveness in patients with creatinine clearance as low as 25 ml/min.[8]

Uricase

Uricase was purified from the fungus *Aspergillus flavus*. Since all mammals except great apes and humans have this enzyme, they are able to convert uric acid to the more soluble allantoin. However, humans lack the enzyme and are therefore more vulnerable to develop gout. A recombinant uricase (rasburicase) genetically synthesized from *A. flavus* has been used successfully to rapidly lower uric acid levels in tumor lysis syndrome.[80] Adverse events include antibody formation, anaphylaxis, hemolysis in patients who are glucose-6-phosphate dehydrogenase deficient, neutropenia, and sepsis.[81] Case reports suggest that doses of 0.15 mg/kg IV monthly for 3 months may be effective in treating tophaceous gout in transplant patients.[82]

Because of the immunogenicity and to extend the biologic half-life of rasburicase, a porcine uricase with polyethylene glycol (PEG) groups added (PEG-uricase) was developed. It has been given IV or subcutaneously.[83,84] PEG-uricase has shown significant promise and is currently in Phase III trials for refractory or tophaceous gout.

SUMMARY

Gout is a common inflammatory arthritis that is gratifying for physicians to manage because of the dramatic response to prompt, appropriate therapy. Though common, gout remains one of the most frequently suboptimally managed diseases in both emergency rooms[85] and primary care settings.[86] The management approach needs to be comprehensive and individualized, taking into account factors unique to the patient such as comorbidities and disease manifestations and potential side effects of the medications.

A summary of basic principles for managing gout is outlined in Box 75-1. NSAIDs, colchicine, and corticosteroids are useful in the treatment of acute gout. The majority of chronic gout patients should receive urate-lowering therapy, including xanthine oxidase inhibitors or uricosuric agents. Therapies used for comorbid medical conditions may have an adjunctive role in patients with gout but do not replace standard hypouricemic medications.

REFERENCES

1. Fam AG. Gout, diet, and the insulin resistance syndrome. J Rheumatol 2002;29:1350-1355.
2. Choi H. Epidemiology of crystal arthropathy. Rheum Dis Clin North Am 2006;32:255-273.
3. Enomoto A, Kimura H, Chairoungdua A, et al. Molecular identification of a renal urate anion exchanger that regulates blood urate levels. Nature 2002;417:447-452.
4. Hall AP, Barz PE, Dawber TR, McNamara PM. Epidemiology of gout and hyperuricemia: a long-term population study. Am J Med 1967;42:27-37.
5. Champion EW, Glynn RJ, DeLabry LO. Asymptomatic hyperuricemia: risks and consequences in the Normative Aging Study. Am J Med 1987;82:421-426.
6. Lee SJ, Terkeltaub RA, Kavanaugh A. Recent developments in diet and gout. Curr Opin Rheumatol 2006;18:193-198.
7. Ben-Chitrit E, Levy M. Colchicine: 1998 update. Semin Arthritis Rheum 1998;28:48-59.
8. Wortmann RL. Recent advances in the management of gout and hyperuricemia. Curr Opin Rheumatol 2005;17:319-324.
9. Wallace SL, Omokoku B, Ertel NH. Colchicine plasma levels: implications as to pharmacology and mechanism of action. Am J Med 1970;48:443-448.
10. Ferron GM, Rochdi M, Jusko WJ, Scherrmann JM. Oral absorption characterics and pharmacokinetics of colchicine in healthy volunteers after single and multiple doses. J Clin Pharmacol 1996;36:874-883.
11. Ahern MJ, Reid C, Gordon TP, et al. Does colchicine work? The results of the first controlled study in acute gout. Aust N Z J Med 1987;17:301-304.
12. Baud FJ, Sabouraud A, Vicaut E, et al. Brief report: treatment of severe colchicine overdose with colchicine specific Fab fragments. N Engl J Med 1995;332:642-645.
13. Wallace SL, Singer JZ, Duncan GJ, et al. Renal function predicts colchicine toxicity: guidelines for the prophylactic use of colchicine in gout. J Rheum 1991;18:264-269.
14. Wilbur K, Makowsky M. Colchicine myotoxicity: case reports and literature review. Pharmacotherapy 2004;24:1784-1792.
15. Neuss MN, McCallum RM, Brenckman WD, Silberman HR. Long-term colchicine administration leading to colchicine toxicity and death. Arthritis Rheum 1986;29:448-449.
16. Bonnel RA, Villalba ML, Karwoski CB, Beitz J. Deaths associated with inappropriate intravenous colchicine administration. J Emerg Med 2002;22:385-387.
17. Sutaria S, Katbamna R, Underwood M. Effectiveness of interventions for the treatment of acute and prevention of recurrent gout—a systematic review. Rheumatology 2006;45:1422-1431.
18. Shresta M, Morgan DL, Moreden JM, et al. Randomized double-blind comparison of the analgesic efficacy of intramuscular ketorolac and oral indomethacin in the treatment of acute gouty arthritis. Ann Emerg Med 1995;26:682-686.
19. Altman RD, Honig S, Levin JM, Lightfoot RW. Ketoprofen versus indomethacin in patients with acute gouty arthritis: a multicenter, double blind comparative study. J Rheumatol 1988;15:1422-1426.
20. Pouliot M, James MJ, McColl SR, et al. Monosodium urate microcrystals induce cyclooxygenase-2 in human monocytes. Blood 1998;91:1769-1776.
21. Cheng TT, Lai HM, Chiu CK, Chem YC. A single-blind, randomized, controlled trial to assess the efficacy and tolerability of rofecoxib, diclofenac sodium, and meloxicam in patients with acute gouty arthritis. Clin Ther 2004;26:399-406.
22. Rubin BR, Burton R, Navarra S, et al. Efficacy and safety profile of treatment with etoricoxib 120 mg once daily compared with indomethacin 50 mg three times daily in acute gout: a randomized controlled trial. Arthritis Rheum 2004;50:598-606.
23. Fernandez C, Noguera R, Gonzalez JA, Pascual E. Treatment of acute attacks of gout with a small dose of intraarticular triamcinolone acetonide. J Rheumatol 1999;26:2285-2286.
24. Groff GD, Franck WA, Raddatz DA. Systemic steroid therapy for acute gout: a clinical trial and review of the literature. Semin Arthritis Rheum 1990;19:329-336.
25. Alloway JA, Moriarty MJ, Hoogland YT, Nashel DJ. Comparison of triamcinolone acetonide with indomethacin in the treatment of acute gouty arthritis. J Rheumatol 1993;20:111-113.
26. Taylor CT, Brooks NC, Kelley KW. Corticotropin for acute management of gout. Ann Pharmacother 2001;35:365-368.
27. Getting SJ, Christian HC, Flower RJ, Perretti M. Activation of melanocortin type 3 receptor as a molecular mechanism for adrenocorticotropic hormone efficacy in gouty arthritis. Arthritis Rheum 2002;46:2765-2775.
28. Ritter J, Kerr LD, Valeriano-Marcet J, Spiera H. ACTH revisited: effective treatment for acute crystal induced synovitis in patients with multiple medical problems. J Rheumatol 1994;21:696-699.
29. Axelrod D, Preston S. Comparison of parenteral adrenocorticotropic hormone with oral indomethacin in the treatment of acute gout. Arthritis Rheum 1988;31:803-805.
30. Siegel LB, Alloway JA, Nashel DJ. Comparison of adrenocorticotropic hormone and triamcinolone acetonide in the treatment of acute gouty arthritis. J Rheumatol 1994;21:1325-1327.
31. Li-Yu J, Clayburne G, Sieck M, et al. Treatment of chronic gout: can we determine when urate stores are depleted enough to prevent attacks of gout? J Rheumatol 2001;28:577-580.
32. Shoji A, Yamanaka H, Kamatani N. A retrospective study of the relationship between serum urate level and recurrent attacks of gouty arthritis: evidence for reduction of recurrent gouty arthritis with antihyperuricemic therapy. Arthritis Rheum 2004;51:321-325.
33. Perez-Ruiz F, Alonso-Ruiz A, Calabozo M, et al. Efficacy of allopurinol and benzbromarone for the control of hyperuricaemia: a pathogenic approach to the treatment of primary chronic gout. Ann Rheum Dis 1998;57:545-549.
34. Murrell GA, Rapeport WG. Clinical pharmacokinetics of allopurinol. Clin Pharmacokinet 1986;11:343-353.
35. Singer JZ, Wallace SL. The allopurinol hypersensitivity syndrome: unnecessary morbidity and mortality. Arthritis Rheum 1986;29:82-87.
36. Hande KR, Noone RM, Stone WJ. Severe allopurinol toxicity: description and guidelines for prevention in patients with renal insufficiency. Am J Med 1984;76:47-56.
37. Walter-Sack I, de Vries JX, Ernst B, et al. Uric acid lowering effect of oxypurinol sodium in hyperuricemic patients—therapeutic equivalence to allopurinol. J Rheumatol 1996;23:498-501.
38. Zhang W, Doherty M, Bardin T, et al. EULAR evidence based recommendations for gout. Part II: management. Report of a task force of the EULAR Standing Committee for International Clinical Studies Including Therapeutics (ESCISIT). Ann Rheum Dis 2006;65:1312-1324.
39. Fam AG, Dunne SM, Iazzetta J, et al. Efficacy and safety of desensitization to allopurinol following cutaneous reactions. Arthritis Rheum 2001;44:231-238.
40. Earll JM, Saavedra M. Oxipurinol therapy in allopurinol allergic patients. Am Fam Physician 1983;28(5):147-148.
41. Choi HK, Mount DB, Reginato AM. Pathogensis of gout. Ann Intern Med 2005;143:499-516.
42. Harris M, Bryant LR, Danaher P, Alloway J. Effect of low dose daily aspirin on serum urate levels and urinary excretion in patients receiving probenecid for gouty arthritis. J Rheumatol 2000;27:2873-2876.
43. Cunningham RF, Israili ZH, Dayton PG. Clinical pharmacokinetics of probenecid. Clin Pharmacokinet 1981;6:135-151.
44. Terkeltaub RA. Clinical Practice: Gout. N Engl J Med 2003;349:1647-1655.
45. Marguiles EH, White AM, Sherry S. Sulfinpyrazone: a review of its pharmacological properties and therapeutic use. Drugs 1980;20:179-197.
46. Boelaert J, Schurgers M, Daneels R, et al. Sulfinpyrazone: risk for renal insufficiency [Letter]. Arch Intern Med 1984;144:648-649.
47. Kelley WN. Effects of drugs on uric acid in man. Annu Rev Pharmacol 1975;15:327-350.
48. Pfister B, Imhof P, Wirz H. Effect of sulphinpyrazone (Anturan) on uric acid excretion and plasma uric acid concentration in healthy volunteers. Eur J Clin Pharmacol 1978;13:263-265.
49. Docci D, Mambelli M, Manzoni G, et al. Acute renal failure secondary to sulfinpyrazone treatment after myocardial infarction [Letter]. Nephron 1984;37:213-214.
50. Caforio AL, Gambino A, Tona F, et al. Sulfinpyrazone reduces cyclosporine levels: a new drug interaction in heart transplant recipients. J Heart Lung Transplant 2000;19:1205-1208.
51. Becker MA, Schumacher HR Jr, Wortmann RL, et al. Febuxostat compared with allopurinol in patients with hyperuricemia and gout. N Engl J Med 2005;353:2450-2461.
52. Borstad GC, Bryant LR, Abel MP, et al. Colchicine for prophylaxis of acute flares when initiating allopurinol for chronic gouty arthritis. J Rheumatol 2004;31:2429-2432.
53. Schlesinger N. Management of acute and chronic gouty arthritis: present state of the art. Drugs 2004;64:2399-2416.
54. Choi HK, Curhan G. Beer, liquor, and wine consumption and serum uric acid level: the Third National Health and Nutrition Examination Survey. Arthritis Care Res 2004;51:1023-1029.
55. Bastow MD, Durrington PN, Ishola M. Hypertriglyceridemia and hyperuricemia: effects of two fibric acid derivatives (bezafibrate and fenofibrate) in a double-blind, placebo-controlled trial. Metabolism 1988;37:217-220.
56. Liamis G, Bairataki ET, Elisaf MS. Effect of fenofibrate on serum uric acid levels [Letter]. Am J Kidney Dis 1999;34:594.
57. Noguchi Y, Tatsuno I, Suyama K, et al. Effect of fenofibrate on uric acid metabolism in Japanese hyperlipidemic patients. J Atheroscler Thromb 2004;11:335-340.
58. Feher MD, Hepburn AL, Hogarth MB, et al. Fenofibrate enhances urate reduction in men treated with allopurinol for hyperuricaemia and gout. Rheumatology 2003;42:321-325.
59. Yamamoto T, Moriwaki Y, Takahashi S, et al. Effect of fenofibrate on plasma concentration and urinary excretion of purine bases and oxypurinol. J Rheumatol 2001;28:2294-2297.
60. Miller DB, Spence JD. Clinical pharmacokinetics of fibric acid derivatives (fibrates). Clin Pharmacokinet 1998;34:155-162.
61. Aldridge MA, Ito MK. Fenofibrate and warfarin interaction. Pharmacotherapy 2001;21:886-889.
62. Puig JG, Mateos F, Buno A, et al. Effect of eprosartan and losartan on uric acid metabolism in patients with essential hypertension. J Hypertens 1999;17:1033-1039.
63. Wurzner G, Gerster JC, Chiolero A, et al. Comparative effects of losartan and irbesartan on serum uric acid in hypertensive patients with hyperuricaemia and gout. J Hypertens 2001;19:1855-1860.
64. Elisaf M, Tsimichodimos V, Bairaktair E, Siamopoulos KC. Effect of micronized fenofibrate and losartan combination on uric acid metabolism in hypertensive patients with hyperuricemia. J Cardiovasc Pharmacol 1999;34:60-63.
65. Takahashi S, Moriwaki Y, Yamamoto T, et al. Effect of combination treatment using anti-hyperuricaemic agents with fenofibrate and/or losartan on uric acid metabolism. Ann Rheum Dis 2003;62:572-575.

66. Chanard J, Toupance O, Lavaud S, et al. Amlodipine reduces cyclosporin-induced hyperuricaemia in hypertensive renal transplant recipients. Nephrol Dial Transplant 2003;18:2147-2153.
67. Stein HB, Hasan A, Fox IH. Ascorbic acid-induced uricosuria: a consequence of megavitamin therapy. Ann Intern Med 1976;84:385-388.
68. Huang HY, Appel LJ, Choi MJ, et al. The effects of vitamin C supplementation on serum concentrations of uric acid: results of a randomized controlled trial. Arthritis Rheum 2005;52:1843-1847.
69. Padayatty SJ, Sun H, Wang Y, et al. Vitamin C pharmacokinetics: implications for oral and intravenous use. Ann Intern Med 2004;140:533-537.
70. Takano YT, Hase-Aoki K, Horiuchi H, et al. Selectivity of febuxostat, a novel nonpurine inhibitor of xanthine oxidase/xanthine dehydrogenase. Life Sci 2005;76:1835-1847.
71. Becker MA, Kisicki J, Khosravan R, et al. Febuxostat (TMX-67), a novel, non-purine, selective inhibitor of xanthine oxidase, is safe and decreases serum urate in healthy volunteers. Nucleosides Nucleotides Nucleic Acids 2004;23:1111-1116.
72. Hoshide S, Takahashi Y, Ishikawa T, et al. PK/PD and safety of a single dose of TMX-67 (febuxostat) in subjects with mild and moderate renal impairment. Nucleosides Nucleotides Nucleic Acids 2004;23:1117-1118.
73. Mayer MD, Khosravan R, Vernillet L, et al. Pharmacokinetics and pharmacodynamics of febuxostat, a new non-purine selective inhibitor of xanthine oxidase in subjects with renal impairment. Am J Ther 2005;12:22-34.
74. Khosravan R, Grabowski BA, Mayer MD, et al. The effect of mild moderate hepatic impairment on pharmacokinetics, pharmacodynamics, and safety of febuxostat, a novel nonpurine selective inhibitor of xanthine oxidase. J Clin Pharmacol 2006;46:88-102.
75. Jain AK, Ryan JR, McMahon FG, Noveck RJ. Effect of single oral doses of benzbromarone on serum and urinary uric acid. Arthritis Rheum 1974;17:149-157.
76. Broekhuysen J, Pacco M, Sion R, et al. Metabolism of benzbromarone in man. Eur J Clin Pharmacol 1972;4:125-130.
77. Sorensen LB, Levinson DJ. Clinical evaluation of benzbromarone. Arthritis Rheum 1976;19;183-190.
78. Muller FO, Schall R, Groenewoud G, et al. The effect of benzbromarone on allopurinol/oxypurinol kinetics in patients with gout. Eur J Clin Pharmacol 1993;44:69-72.
79. Yu TF. Pharmacokinetic and clinical studies of a new uricosuric agent—benzbromarone. J Rheumatol 1976;3;305-312.
80. Navolanic PM, Pui CH, Larson RA, et al. Elitek-rasburicase: an effective means to prevent and treat hyperuricemia associated with tumor lysis syndrome. Leukemia 2003;17:499-514.
81. Bomalaski JS, Clark MA. Serum uric acid-lowering therapies: where are we heading in management of hyperuricemia and the potential role of uricase? Curr Rheumatol Rep 2004;6:240-247.
82. Vogt B. Urate oxidase (rasburicase) for treatment of severe tophaceous gout. Nephrol Dial Transplant 2005;20:431-433.
83. FDA Office of Orphan Products Development. Pegylated recombinant mammalian uricase (PRG-uricase) as treatment for refractory gout. Available at *http://www.clinicaltrials.gov/ct/show/NCT00111657* (accessed February 14, 2007).
84. Ganson NJ, Kelly SJ, Scarlett E, et al. Control of hyperuricemia in subjects with refractory gout, and induction of antibody against poly(ethylene) glycol (PEG), in a Phase I trial of subcutaneous PEGylated urate oxidase. Arthritis Res Ther 2005;8:R12.
85. Chin MH, Wang LC, Jin L, et al. Appropriateness of medication selection for older persons in an urban academic emergency department. Acad Emerg Med 1999;6:1189-1193.
86. Sarawate CA, Brewer KK, Yang W, et al. Gout medication treatment patterns and adherence to standards of care from a managed care perspective. Mayo Clin Proc 2006;81:925-934.

76

SYSTEMIC LUPUS ERYTHEMATOSUS

William R. Gilliland, Michael P. Keith, and Kathleen Uhl

OVERVIEW 1047
INTRODUCTION 1047
PATHOPHYSIOLOGY 1047
THERAPEUTICS AND CLINICAL PHARMACOLOGY 1047
Goals of Therapy 1047
Therapeutics by Class 1048
Renal 1048
Cutaneous 1053
Musculoskeletal 1056
Hematologic 1056
Cardiac 1057
Pulmonary 1057
Gastrointestinal 1057
Neuropsychiatric 1057
Antiphospholipid Antibody Syndrome 1058
Reproductive Issues 1059
Emerging Targets and Therapeutics 1060
CONCLUSION 1061

OVERVIEW

Systemic lupus erythematosus (SLE) is a prototypic inflammatory autoimmune disorder characterized by multisystem involvement and fluctuating disease activity. For the million or more patients who have SLE in the United States,[1] symptoms may range from rather mild manifestations such as rash or arthritis to life-threatening manifestations such as glomerulonephritis or thrombosis. Essentially no organ system is spared from potential damage as a result of this disorder. Unfortunately, even though symptoms typically wax and wane over the course of the disease, many patients with SLE will experience a slow decline in their health because of the ongoing systemic inflammation.

Therefore, treatment is based on the specific manifestations that are seen in each patient. Effective treatment must be individualized, taking into account patient demographics, organ system involvement, and severity of the manifestations. Similarly, prognosis is also dependent on the severity and the specific organ systems involved.

INTRODUCTION

The overall prevalence of SLE has been reported to range from 14.6 to 50.8 cases per 100,000 persons.[2,3] While it can affect individuals of all age groups, the typical patient is a female between the ages of 15 and 45. Black women are three times more likely than white women to get lupus.[4] A detailed discussion of the pathogenesis of SLE is beyond the scope of this book. However, susceptibility is multifactorial. A number of susceptibility genes, genetic factors, and environmental exposures may predispose the individual to SLE. The loss of immune tolerance, increased antigenic load, excess T-cell help, and defective B-cell suppression lead to cytokine imbalance, B-cell hyperactivity, and the production of autoantibodies. Ultimately, immune complex formation and complement activation cause immunologically mediated tissue injury[5] (Fig. 76-1).

Because of the variable manifestations and course of this disease, the American College of Rheumatology (ACR) created classification criteria that allowed the comparison of patients across research centers and clinical studies. The ACR Criteria for the Classification of SLE were originally created in 1982 and revised in 1997 (Table 76-1).[6] Any person having 4 of the 11 criteria, serially or simultaneously, during the interval of observation is considered to have SLE for the purposes of clinical studies. While many clinicians use the classification criteria to diagnose patients with SLE, it is important to note that these criteria were not designed for this purpose.[7]

PATHOPHYSIOLOGY

While the vast majority of tissue injury in SLE is secondary to inflammation related to aberrant immunologic mechanisms, some of the morbidity may also be due to nonimmunologic processes such as atherosclerotic, infectious, or degenerative processes. The complexity of the disease and uniqueness of each patient make it difficult for clinical researchers to obtain sufficient information on the precise elements leading to the tissue destruction. In addition, it is difficult to sort out the effects of individual cellular defects when so many interrelated abnormalities are seen in SLE patients. Defects in the function or amount of monocytes, neutrophils, natural killer cells, T cells, B cells, complements, Fc γ receptors, and cytokines have all been described.[8]

SLE is one of the most common systemic inflammatory diseases; capable of unleashing a wide variety of cell-killing forces against the host. Unlike some organ-specific autoimmune diseases such as diabetes mellitus or myasthenia gravis, in which the pancreas and thymus, respectively, are targeted by the inflammatory process, SLE is not organ specific, affecting virtually any organ in the body with varying frequencies throughout the course of the disease[9] (Fig. 76-2). Antigen-specific and antigen-nonspecific immunologic mechanisms cause damage and lead to a broad range of pathologic manifestations and potential targets of therapy.

THERAPEUTICS AND CLINICAL PHARMACOLOGY

Goals of Therapy

Since the majority of the manifestations of SLE are inflammatory in nature, most of the medications aim to control either the systemic inflammatory or organ-specific symptoms. As mentioned previously, the treatment of SLE must be individualized and it is not a disease that is easily approached with treatment algorithms. That said, Figure 76-3 provides a simple algorithm in order to give the reader an idea of which medications are used in organ-threatening and non–organ-threatening disease.

The most common classes of medications used to treat SLE include nonsteroidal anti-inflammatory drugs (NSAIDs), antimalarials, corticosteroids, and immunosuppressive agents, primarily azathioprine, cyclophosphamide, and mycophenolate mofetil. Since much of the therapy for SLE is based on the specific disease manifestation, the bulk of the chapter is arranged by organ involvement. Table 76-2 provides an overview of medications used in the treatment of SLE based on the specific manifestation. Interestingly, none of these medications except for aspirin, systemic corticosteroids, and hydroxychloroquine is approved by the U.S. Food and Drug Administration (FDA) for treatment of SLE. Currently, the medications commonly used have numerous effects on the immune system, making it difficult to determine the precise mechanism of action in SLE. However, targeted biologic

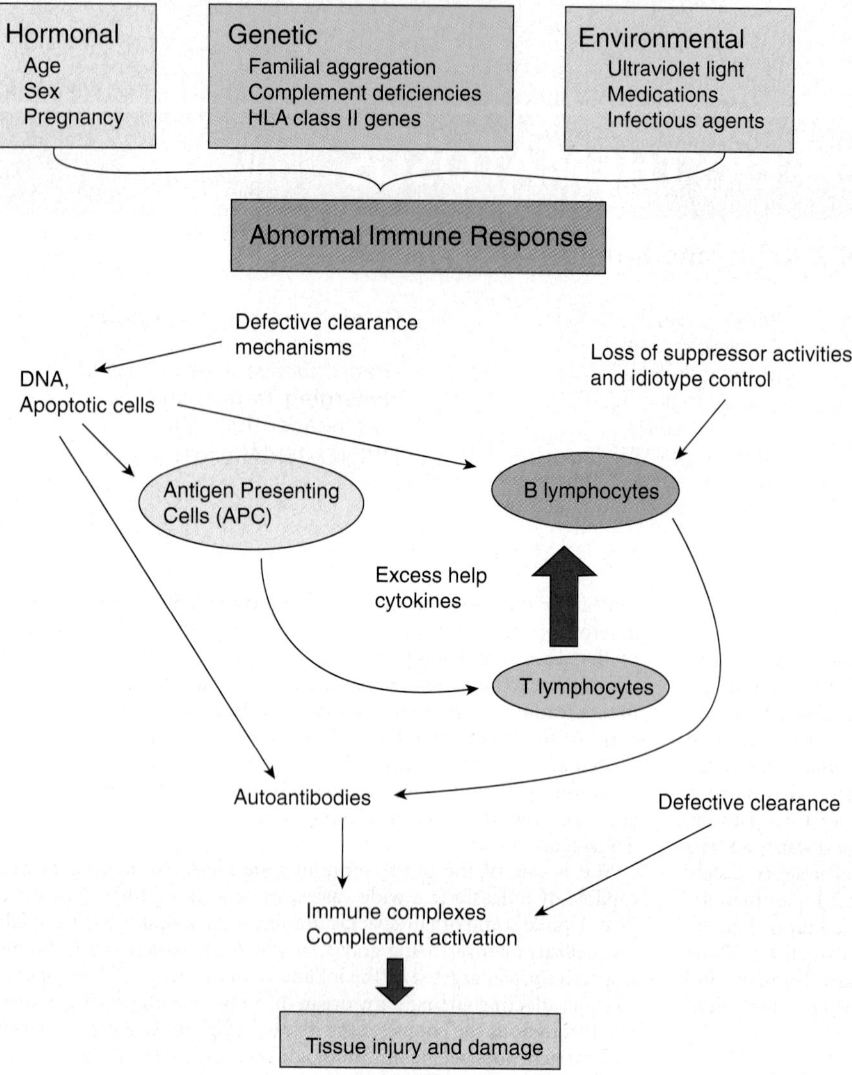

FIGURE 76-1 • Overview of the pathogenesis of systemic lupus erythematosus.

therapies are being used with more frequency to treat SLE, and more of these medications are in development. Some of these agents are discussed at the end of this chapter.

Therapeutics by Class

Renal

Kidney involvement is the most feared complication of SLE, and is associated with significant morbidity and mortality. More than half of patients in many large centers will present with asymptomatic urine abnormalities, including hematuria or proteinuria. Therefore, a urinalysis should be done at each patient visit.

While a complete discussion of the pathology of lupus nephritis is beyond the scope of this chapter, proper treatment is based primarily on the clinical presentation and biopsy findings. The histologic classification most commonly used is the World Health Organization (WHO) system[10] (Table 76-3). Additional histologic information obtained from the biopsy can be used to calculate activity and chronicity indices that may also help to determine prognosis and response to therapy.[11] Although the clinical presentation and urinalysis do not always correlate with the renal biopsy, several generalizations can be made. Mesangial nephritis is usually associated with a small amount of proteinuria (<1 g/day) and mild hematuria, but typically no cellular casts. Proliferative disease is associated with nephritic urinary sediment, a variable degree of proteinuria, hypertension, low complement levels, and high double-stranded DNA (dsDNA) antibody titers. In contrast, membranous nephritis presents with proteinuria (often in the nephrotic range, >3.5 g/day), normal complement levels, and negative or low dsDNA titers.

Fortunately, the vast majority of randomized controlled studies of SLE patients have addressed the treatment of lupus nephritis. However, many of these studies are limited by short-term follow-up, small numbers of patients, and diverse racial and economic backgrounds. Additionally, studies have almost exclusively addressed the treatment of proliferative nephritis. Therefore, the vast majority of the information in this section addresses treatment of WHO Classes III and IV disease.

Treatment of lupus nephritis depends not only on the severity of the disease, but also on access to care and patient choice after a candid discussion of potential side effects of the various medications and severity of the nephritis. It is also important to recognize that the therapy should include an induction phase aimed at improving disease activity and a maintenance phase aimed at maximizing the therapeutic effect, reducing relapses, and minimizing adverse effects. Treatment options include corticosteroids and various immunosuppressive agents, in many ways akin to regimens to treat certain cancers. The key to improved renal survival is early, aggressive treatment when dealing with proliferative lesions.

While controlled studies of the use of corticosteroids in lupus nephritis have never been performed, corticosteroids are included in all induction regimens because of their rapidity of action. They are typically administered as intravenous (IV) boluses of methylpredniso-

TABLE 76-1 CLASSIFICATION OF SYSTEMIC LUPUS ERYTHEMATOSUS—REVISED CRITERIA

Criterion	Definition
1. Malar rash	Fixed erythema, flat or raised over the malar eminences, tending to spare the nasolabial folds
2. Discoid rash	Erythematous raised patches with adherent keratotic scaling and follicular plugging; atrophic scarring occurring in older lesions
3. Photosensitivity	Skin rash as a result of unusual reaction to sunlight, by patient history or physician observation
4. Oral ulcers	Oral or nasopharyngeal ulceration, usually painless, observed by physician
5. Arthritis	Nonerosive arthritis involving 2 or more peripheral joints, characterized by tenderness, swelling, or effusion
6. Serositis	(a) Pleuritis—convincing history of pleuritic pain or rub heard by physician or evidence of pleural effusion *or* (b) Pericarditis—documented by ECG or rub or evidence of pericardial effusion
7. Renal disorder	(a) Persistent proteinuria greater than 0.5 g/day or greater than 3+ if quantification not performed *or* (b) Cellular casts—may be red cell, hemoglobin, granular, tubular, or mixed
8. Neurologic disorder	(a) Seizures—in the absence of offending drugs or known metabolic derangements (e.g., uremia, ketoacidosis, or electrolyte imbalance) *or* (b) Psychosis—in the absence of offending drugs or known metabolic derangements (e.g., uremia, ketoacidosis, or electrolyte imbalance)
9. Hematologic disorder	(a) Hemolytic anemia—with reticulocytosis *or* (b) Leukopenia—less than 4000/mm^3 total on 2 or more occasions *or* (c) Lymphopenia—less than 1500/mm^3 on 2 or more occasions *or* (d) Thrombocytopenia—less than 100,000/mm^3 in the absence of offending drugs
10. Immunologic disorder	(a) Anti-DNA—antibody to native DNA in abnormal titer *or* (b) Anti-Sm—presence of antibody to Sm nuclear antigen *or* (c) Positive finding of antiphospholipid antibodies based on (1) an abnormal serum concentrated of IgG or IgM anticardiolipin antibodies, (2) a positive test result for lupus anticoagulant using a standard measure, and (3) a false-positive serologic test for syphilis known to be positive for at least 6 months and confirmed by *Treponema pallidum* immobilization or fluorescent treponemal antibody absorption test
11. Antinuclear antibody	An abnormal titer of antinuclear antibody by immunofluorescence or an equivalent assay at any point in time and in the absence of drugs known to be associated with "drug-induced lupus" syndrome

Note: For the purpose of identifying patients in clinical studies, a person must have SLE if any 4 or more of the 11 criteria are present, serially or simultaneously, during any interval of observation.
IgG, immunoglobulin G; IgM, immunoglobulin M; ECG, electrocardiogram.
From Hochberg MC. Updating the American College of Rheumatology revised criteria for the classification of systemic lupus erythematosus. Arthritis Rheum 1997;40:1725.

lone (i.e., 1000 mg IV daily for 3 days, or 1 g/m^2), followed by 1 mg/kg of prednisone orally daily.[12]

Cyclophosphamide. Cyclophosphamide (Cytoxan) is the most common immunosuppressive agent used to treat Class IV nephritis, and has been championed by researchers at the National Institutes of Health (NIH). Intermittent IV cyclophosphamide is the preferred route of administration because it is as efficacious as daily oral cyclophosphamide and has fewer side effects.[13] In a follow-up study, an extended course of intermittent cyclophosphamide (monthly pulses for 6 months followed by quarterly pulses for an additional 2 years) reduced the rate of renal exacerbation compared to a shorter course (monthly pulses for 6 months).[14] According to NIH protocol,[15] the dosage for the intermittent cyclophosphamide is 0.75 to 1.0 g/m^2. The dose of subsequent pulses is adjusted to maintain the total white blood cell count above 1500 cells/mm^3. A later NIH study found that extended courses of pulse methylprednisolone administered for at least 1 year (up to 3 years) were not as effective in terms of inducing a renal remission as pulse cyclophosphamide for longer periods (3 to 5 years).[16] Results from a randomized multicenter study suggest that low-dose cyclophosphamide (six biweekly pulses at a fixed dose of 500 mg), when used as an induction agent, induces remission at the same rate as a high-dose pulse regimen used in NIH protocols.[17]

Cyclophosphamide is an alkylating agent, antineoplastic agent, and nitrogen mustard. It is a mechlorethamine derivative that is inactive as administered. It is FDA approved for the treatment of 16 cancers, and is most commonly used for treatment of breast cancer and numerous types of lymphomas and leukemias. It is not FDA approved for lupus nephritis. The cytotoxic action is manifested by cross-linking strands of DNA and RNA, as well as inhibiting protein synthesis. These direct effects also contribute to its role as a potent immunosuppressive agent. Other immunosuppressive mechanisms may include alteration of macrophage function, alteration in gene transcription, and direct functional and quantitative effects on leukocytes.[18]

Cyclophosphamide is available in oral and intravenous forms. The typical dose for the treatment of lupus nephritis is 0.75 to 1.0 g/m^2 administered IV no more frequently than monthly. The doses and treatment schedules differ for treating malignancies (e.g., 40 to 50 mg/kg IV over a 2- to 5-day period for chronic lymphoid leukemia). Cyclophosphamide is well absorbed following oral administration, with a bioavailability of 85% to 100% with peak concentrations occurring in 1 to 3 hours. It is a prodrug that is extensively metabolized to several active and inactive metabolites. The majority of an administered dose is activated by various hepatic cytochrome P-450 (CYP) isoenzymes, including CYP2A6, 2B6 (highest activity), 3A4, 3A5, 2C9, 2C18, and 2C19. Less than 20% of the administered dose is eliminated unchanged in the urine, with complete elimination of parent drug and metabolites 24 hours following a dose. The elimination half-life of cyclophosphamide ranges between 5 and 9 hours over a large concentration range.

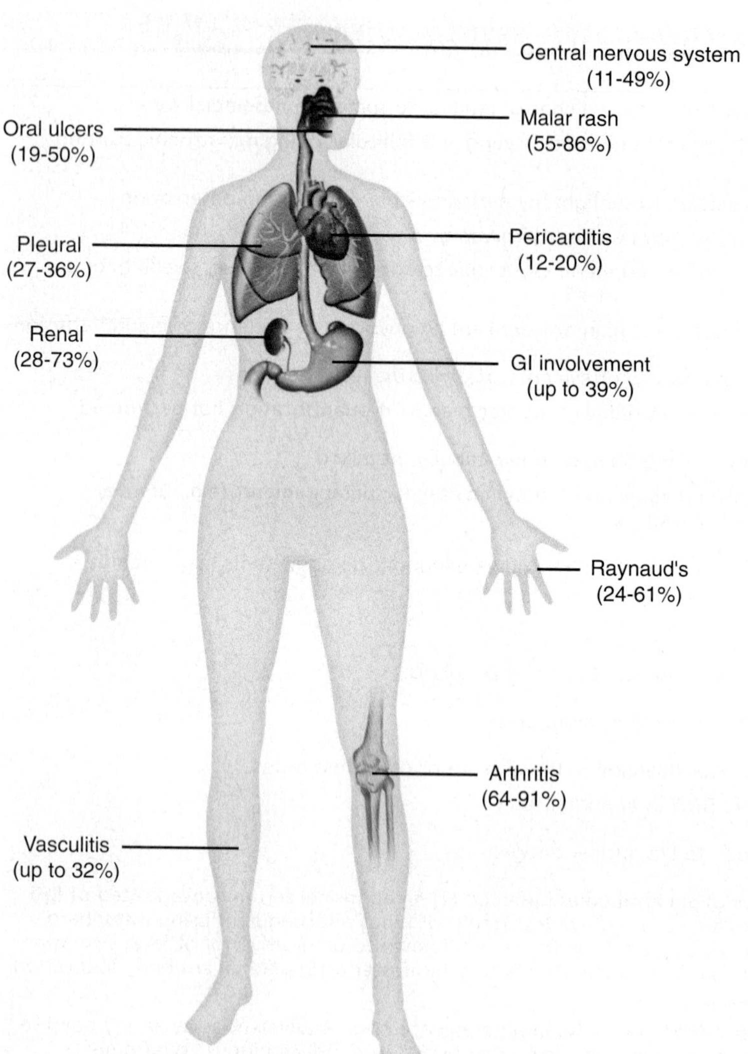

FIGURE 76-2 • Organ involvement in systemic lupus erythematosus.

It exhibits a low degree of plasma protein binding. Cyclophosphamide distributes to body water with a volume of distribution of 30 to 50 L.[19]

Cyclophosphamide is a potent inducer of CYP2C8, 2C9, and 3A4 and induces its own metabolism after several days of dosing that may have implications for its toxic and therapeutic effects. Autoinduction is due to activation of the orphan nuclear receptor pregnane X receptor.[20] Drugs that have demonstrated inhibition of cyclophosphamide metabolism in humans include allopurinol, busulfan, chloramphenicol, chlorpromazine, ciprofloxacin, fluconazole, and thiotepa. Drugs that have been demonstrated to induce cyclophosphamide metabolism in humans include dexamethasone, ondansetron, phenobarbital, phenytoin, prednisone/prednisolone, and rifampin. Active uptake and efflux of parent drug, active metabolites, inactive metabolites, and conjugated metabolites are mediated through several drug transporters such as breast cancer resistant protein and multidrug resistance proteins (MRP1, MRP2, MRP4).[20] Because several CYP isoenzymes are involved in the metabolism of cyclophosphamide and several transporters mediate movement of the drug and metabolites, the clinical relevance of most drug-drug interactions with cyclophosphamide is not clear and is likely to be less important with monthly dosing.[19]

Clearance of cyclophosphamide is decreased in patients with hepatic and renal dysfunction. There is no evidence that hepatic impairment requires dose adjustment; however, the dose may need adjustment for patients with renal impairment.[19] In patients with end-stage renal disease, cyclophosphamide is incompletely cleared by dialysis; therefore, the dose should be lowered in dialysis patients.[21]

Cyclophosphamide is contraindicated in those patients with severely depressed bone marrow function or who have a known hypersensitivity to cyclophosphamide products. Daily oral dosing causes more bone marrow suppression than monthly IV therapy.[22] Common adverse effects include alopecia, nausea, vomiting, leukopenia, and amenorrhea. Serious adverse effects include cardiomyopathy, Stevens-Johnson syndrome, toxic epidermal necrolysis, hemorrhagic cystitis, azoospermia, oligospermia, myelosuppression, interstitial pneumonia, and numerous infectious complications. Other significant concerns include carcinogenesis, impairment of fertility, mutagenesis, and interference with wound healing. Recommended monitoring for monthly IV dosing includes a complete blood count (CBC) with urinalysis before each dose followed by a CBC 10 to 14 days after each dose. Since the risk of bone marrow suppression is higher with daily oral cyclophosphamide, a CBC should be drawn every 1 to 2 weeks until the dose is stable, and then repeated monthly. With oral dosing, a urinalysis should be performed monthly while on the medication and a urinalysis with cytology should be performed every 12 months for life even after cessation of the medication.[23]

Azathioprine. While it has not been as extensively studied in the treatment of proliferative nephritis as has cyclophosphamide, azathioprine may be an alternative immunosuppressive agent in certain situations. In particular, it may be an option in patients who are opposed to the use of cyclophosphamide or have milder degrees of nephritis. At the doses of 2 to 3 mg/kg per day, it is remarkably safe when compared to cyclophosphamide. However with rare exception, azathioprine is used strictly as a maintenance therapy in lupus nephritis. In

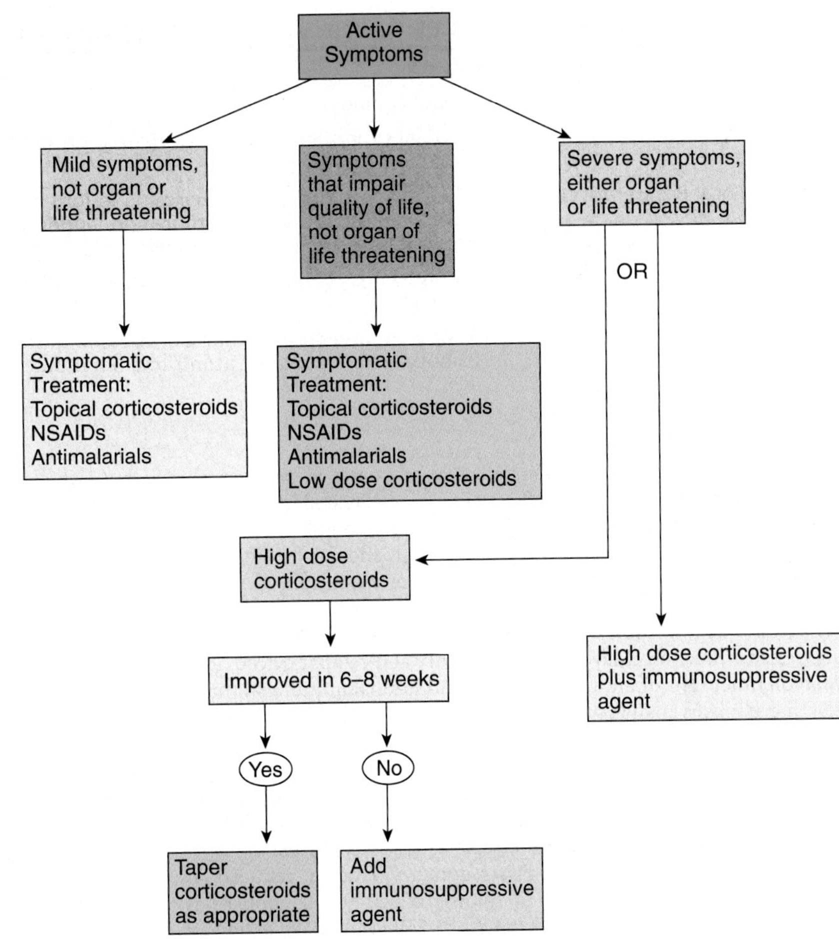

FIGURE 76-3 • Treatment algorithm for systemic lupus erythematosus.

TABLE 76-2 DRUGS USED IN THE MANAGEMENT OF SYSTEMIC LUPUS ERYTHEMATOSUS

	Constitutional	Cutaneous	Musculoskeletal	Major Organ (Kidney, Nervous System, Hematologic)	aPL Antibody
NSAIDs	X		X		
Corticosteroids					
Topical		X			
Low dose	X	X	X		
High dose				X	X
Antimalarials	X	X	X		
Dapsone		X			
Thalidomide		X			
Analgesics	X		X		
Retinoids		X			
Immunosuppressives					
Azathioprine	X	X	X	X	
Cyclophosphamide				X	X
Cyclosporin A				X	
Methotrexate			X	X	
MMF				X	
TNF-α agents			X		
Rituximab	X		X	X	
DHEA			X		
Danazol				X	
IVIG				X	
Anticoagulants					X

aPL, antiphospholipid antibody; DHEA, dehydroepiandrosterone; IVIG, intravenous immune globulin; MMF, mycophenolate mofetil; NSAIDs, nonsteroidal anti-inflammatory drugs; TNF, tumor necrosis factor.

TABLE 76-3 HISTOLOGIC FEATURES OF THE VARIOUS TYPES OF LUPUS NEPHRITIS

WHO Type	Histology
Class I	Normal histology
Class II (Mesangial)	Mesangial expansion with cell or matrix: preservation of mostly intact capillary loops. Mesangial immune deposits.
Class III (Focal Proliferative)	Proliferative, necrotizing or sclerosing lesions of less than 50% of glomeruli. Compromised capillary loop lumens by leukocyte infiltration, endocapillary proliferation, and endothelial swelling and proliferation. Subendothelial immune deposits.
Class IV (Diffuse Proliferative)	Same as in Class III but affecting more than 50% of glomeruli. Loss of the capillary space is the hallmark.
Class V (Membranous)	Widespread basement membrane thickening. Numerous immune deposits early on at epimembranous (subepithelial) and later at intramembranous locations.

fact, several recent studies looking at renal outcomes in proliferative nephritis demonstrated similar efficacy in patients treated in the maintenance phase with azathioprine, mycophenolate mofetil, or quarterly cyclophosphamide after cyclophosphamide induction.[24,25]

Azathioprine is an antimetabolite, or more specifically a purine metabolism antagonist. While the exact mechanism of the immunosuppressive action is not known, azathioprine has a greater immunosuppressive effect on delayed hypersensitivity and cellular cytotoxicity than on other tests of antibody response. Additional immunosuppressive mechanisms may include inhibition of synthesis of DNA, RNA, and proteins. It also has a steroid-sparing effect that may allow a reduction in corticosteroid dose in patients with chronic inflammatory diseases. It is FDA approved for prophylaxis against renal transplant rejections and rheumatoid arthritis. It is not FDA approved for the treatment of inflammatory bowel disease or lupus nephritis.

Azathioprine is a prodrug that is nonenzymatically reduced to 6-mercaptopurine (6-MP) and a thiomidazole; its metabolism is complex and incompletely understood. 6-MP undergoes extensive metabolism by numerous enzymes including thiopurine methyltransferase (TPMT), hypoxanthine-guanine phosphoribosyltransferase, aldehyde oxidase, and xanthine oxidase. TPMT varies in activity with known genetic polymorphism and is the main enzyme responsible for metabolism of 6-MP. Patients with TPMT deficiency are susceptible to severe myelosuppression when treated with azathioprine, and patients with the heterozygous phenotype have been reported to suffer severe hepatotoxicity and reduction of total leukocyte count.[26]

After an oral dose, azathioprine is well absorbed, with intestinal absorption ranging from 50% to 72%, and once absorbed, 88% is converted to 6-MP and the thiomidazole. Following a 2-mg/kg per day dose of azathioprine, peak concentrations of 6-MP are 75 ng/ml with a plasma half-life of less than 2 hours. Twelve percent is excreted in the urine as *S*-methyl 4-nitro-5-thiomidazole.[26] Pharmacokinetic studies in SLE are lacking. In the treatment of systemic lupus, the dose ranges between 1 and 3 mg/kg depending on the clinical manifestation. In addition to its role as a maintenance therapy in lupus nephritis, it can be used for a number of nonrenal manifestations such as cutaneous and musculoskeletal. As previously mentioned, it also has a steroid-sparing effect and may be especially useful in patients with multiple manifestations of SLE who are unable to taper their dose of corticosteroids.

Common side effects include nausea, vomiting, and gastritis medicamentosa. Serious side effects include pancreatitis, leukopenia, megaloblastic anemia, thrombocytopenia, hepatotoxicity, increased risk of infections, and rare cases of cancer. TPMT is strongly inhibited by benzoic acid derivatives. Coadministration of azathioprine or 6-MP with allopurinol, mesalamine, sulfasalazine, or olsalazine results in increased frequency of clinically important leukopenia.[26] Increased concentrations of azathioprine have been reported with coadministration of allopurinol, sulfasalazine, and salicylic acid.[27] A recommendation for monitoring of toxicity includes a CBC every 1 to 2 weeks with changes in dose and every 1 to 3 months thereafter. Liver-associated enzymes should be checked yearly. TPMT activity can be measured, but whether this is necessary prior to starting azathioprine is controversial.[23]

Mycophenolate Mofetil. Mycophenolate mofetil (MMF; Cellcept), an immunosuppressive agent initially developed for the prevention of liver and kidney transplant rejection, has also been used successfully off label to treat lupus nephritis. In a study of 75 patients with diffuse proliferative nephritis who failed traditional therapy (corticosteroids and cyclophosphamide), MMF at a dose of 0.5 to 2.0 g/day combined with corticosteroids was effective in controlling lupus activity on a number of parameters, including renal function, hemoglobin, proteinuria, disease activity scores, and biopsies.[28] Other studies that included patients with diffuse proliferative glomerulonephritis, along with other patients who had other SLE manifestations who failed traditional therapy, also suggest improvement in renal parameters.[29,30] As these studies suggest, it is reasonable to consider MMF as a maintenance medication in those patients who are refractory to pulse cyclophosphamide, although it has not been approved by the FDA for this use. Its role as an induction agent is unknown. A controlled study comparing MMF to pulse cyclophosphamide is near completion. The role of MMF in treating nonrenal manifestations is unclear at this time. A recent case report also suggested that it may be useful in treating patients with membranous nephropathy.[31]

Mycophenolic acid (MPA), the active metabolite of MMF, inhibits the de novo synthesis of guanosine nucleotides without being incorporated into DNA. It is a reversible inhibitor of the enzyme inosine monophosphate dehydrogenase. Because T and B lymphocytes are critically dependent for their proliferation on de novo synthesis of proteins, MPA has potent cytostatic effects on lymphocytes. When used in combination with cyclosporine and corticosteroids, it is FDA approved for preventing cardiac, liver, and renal transplant rejection. When used to prevent transplant rejection, the typical dose is 750 to 1000 mg orally twice daily. In treatment of SLE, the initial dose is usually 1 g daily, and it may be increased to 3 g daily.

Following oral administration, MMF is rapidly metabolized to MPA. Bioavailability is greater than 90%, with maximum concentrations of MPA achieved in less than 1 hour. MPA is glucoronidated to an inactive metabolite that undergoes enterohepatic circulation. Over 90% of the drug is eliminated in the urine as the MPA glucoronide. The elimination half-life in healthy volunteers was reported to be 17.9 hours. MPA binds to serum albumin, independent of MPA concentration. Free, or non–protein-bound, MPA is the active form, the extent of which can be affected by hypoalbuminemia, uremia, and hyperbilirubinemia. Significant drug-drug interactions occur with coadministration of other immunosuppressive agents, particularly cyclosporine and tacrolimus, which is clinically more relevant to transplant recipients than to SLE patients. Only acyclovir and cholestyramine have been demonstrated to alter MPA pharmacokinetics in humans. Drugs that alter gastrointestinal flora may potentially disrupt enteropathic recirculation of MPA glucoronide.[32]

Patients with impaired renal or hepatic function achieve maximal concentrations of MPA as rapidly as normal volunteers; however, data are lacking on the pharmacokinetics in patients with SLE. An increased

TABLE 76-4 RECOMMENDED TREATMENT STRATEGIES FOR LUPUS NEPHRITIS

Histology/Severity	Induction*	Maintenance*
PROLIFERATIVE		
Mild: Class III without severe histologic features (e.g., crescents, fibrinoid necrosis; low chronicity index; normal renal function; non–nephrotic range proteinuria)	High-dose CS (oral or by bolus); if no remission in 8 wk, treat as moderate/severe	Low-dose CS
Moderate/severe: Mild disease failing to achieve remission; marked delay (i.e., >2 yr) in remission; abnormal creatinine and/or proteinuria >1 g/day after 6-12 mo of treatment Type III or IV with severe histologic features or abnormal renal function Type III or IV with moderate to high chronicity index (i.e., >3) Mixed membranous and proliferative lupus nephritis Rapidly progressive glomerulonephritis (i.e., doubling of serum creatinine in 3 mo)	Monthly pulse CY (alone or with MP) (MMF)	Quarterly pulse CY (AZ, MMF)
MEMBRANOUS		
Mild: Non–nephrotic range proteinuria, normal renal function	High-dose CS	Low-dose CS
Moderate/severe: Nephrotic range proteinuria and/or impaired renal function at presentation	Bimonthly pulse CY (MMF; boluses of MP alternating with oral chlorambucil or CY for 3-6 mo; CsA)	Low-dose CS (quarterly pulse CY; AZ; MMF; CsA)

*Alternative agents are shown in parentheses.
AZ, azathioprine; CS, corticosteroids; CsA, cyclosporin A; CY, cyclophosphamide; MMF, mycophenolate mofetil; MP, methylprednisolone.

free fraction of MPA has been seen in patients with impaired renal or hepatic function.[27] Therapeutic drug monitoring, adjusting dose based on MPA plasma concentrations or area under the curve, has been advocated for patients receiving MMF for prevention of organ transplant rejection.[32] However, no such expertise has been developed for lupus nephritis.

Common adverse events include constipation, diarrhea, nausea, vomiting, and headache. Serious complications include hypertension, peripheral edema, gastrointestinal hemorrhage, leukopenia, myelosuppression, infections, lymphoma, confusion, tremor, and cough. Recommendations for laboratory monitoring to prevent toxicity include a CBC and liver-associated enzymes weekly with dosage changes and then every 1 to 3 months.[23]

Treatment of Other Classes of Renal Pathology. Less is known about the treatment of the other renal pathology classes (WHO Classes II, III, and V). Fortunately, mesangial disease (WHO type II) rarely requires therapy. Over the last decade, Class III disease has been treated more aggressively since many cases progress to Class IV disease. Since membranous disease (Class V) is less likely to progress to end-stage renal disease, it is less studied and does not typically require aggressive therapy unless severe. Table 76-4 shows one approach to the treatment of lupus nephritis,[33] taking into account histologic and clinical information that helps to determine if aggressive therapy is warranted.

Cutaneous

Involvement of the skin and mucous membranes results in some of the most common manifestations of SLE, occurring in upward of 80% of patients.[2] Before considering the various treatment options, it is important to recognize that many rashes have been described in association with SLE. The most common SLE-specific lesions are listed in Box 76-1. SLE is also associated with many nonspecific skin lesions as well, including vasculitis, alopecia, urticaria, bullous lesions, and Raynaud's phenomenon. The goal of therapy is to prevent telangiectasias, pigmentary changes, alopecia, and scarring.

The malar rash, or "butterfly rash," is perhaps the most recognizable acute rash associated with SLE. Generally, it along with other acute and subacute rashes does not lead to scarring and usually does not require aggressive therapy. Preventive measures such as avoiding sun exposure, wearing light-blocking clothing, and the use of sunscreens of at least SPF15 will prevent rashes in most patients.[34]

BOX 76-1 SLE-SPECIFIC SKIN LESIONS

Acute
Localized (malar rash)
Generalized

Subacute
Annular
Papulosquamous

Chronic
Discoid (localized or generalized)
Hypertrophic (verrucous)
Lupus panniculitis
Lupus tumidus
Chilblain lupus

Topical corticosteroids also provide benefit in these rashes. Although these topical agents are discussed in great detail in Chapter 8, some important guidelines are included in this section. As a general guideline, the least potent preparation should be used. Twice-daily application of 1% hydrocortisone is generally safe, effective, and well tolerated. Moderately potent preparations such as 0.1% triamcinolone may be required for resistant lesions or early discoid lesions. Fluorinated preparations such as 0.05% fluocinonide may be used for thicker lesions and established discoid lesions. Fluorinated compounds should be used cautiously in facial lesions in order to avoid telangiectasias, atrophy, and depigmentation. Patients with persistent rashes should be treated briefly with systemic corticosteroids or more chronically with an antimalarial such as hydroxychloroquine or quinacrine. Discoid and other chronic cutaneous lesions generally require treatment with an antimalarial, intralesional corticosteroids, or immunosuppressive agents.

Antimalarials. Antimalarials were first used as antipyretics in the 17th century.[35] In 1894, quinine became the first antimalarial to be used to treat cutaneous lupus.[36] Quinacrine, an antimalarial still in use, was used to successfully treat discoid lupus in 1941.[37] Several years later, chloroquine and hydroxychloroquine were found to be equally effective and less toxic. Hydroxychloroquine, chloroquine, and quinacrine

TABLE 76-5 COMPARISON OF CLINICALLY IMPORTANT ANTIMALARIAL AGENTS

	Hydroxychloroquine	Chloroquine	Quinacrine
Trade name	Plaquenil	Aralen	Atabrine
Structure	Cl, N (quinoline ring); HN—CH(CH$_2$)$_3$N(C$_2$H$_4$OH)(C$_2$H$_5$); CH$_3$	Cl, N (quinoline ring); HN—CH(CH$_2$)$_3$N(C$_2$H$_5$)$_2$; CH$_3$	Cl, N, OCH$_3$ (acridine ring); HN—CH(CH$_2$)$_3$N(C$_2$H$_5$)$_2$; CH$_3$
Dosage	200-400 mg/day (≤6.5 mg/kg of IBW)	250 mg/day (≤3.5 mg/kg of IBW)	100-200 mg/day
Hepatic metabolism	CYP450s (variety, exact isoforms unknown)	CYP3A4 (substrate & inhibitor) CYP2D6 (inhibitor)	CYP3A4/3A5 (substrate)
Renal elimination	10-45%	10-58%	Insignificant
Drug-drug interactions	Aurothioglucose Digoxin Hypoglycemic agents Cyclosporin A D-Penicillamine	Aurothioglucose Acetaminophen D-Penicillamine Cimetidine Methotrexate	Aurothioglucose

CYP, cytochrome P-450; IBW, ideal body weight.

BOX 76-2 POSSIBLE MECHANISMS OF ACTION OF ANTIMALARIAL DRUGS

Immunologic actions
- Block antigen processing by raising intracytoplasmic pH
- Inhibit natural killer cell activity, mitogenic stimulation
- Impede formation of and help to dissolve immune complexes

Anti-inflammatory effects
- Inhibit phospholipase A_2 and C
- Protaglandin antagonism
- Stabilize lysosomal membranes
- Decrease fibronectin release by macrophages
- Block superoxide release

Ultraviolet light absorption

Hormonal actions
- Hypoglycemic, impair insulin release

Antiproliferative properties
- Intercalate with DNA
- DNA, RNA polymerase inhibition
- Decrease tumor size and chemotherapy resistance

Inhibit platelet aggregation and adhesion

Antimicrobial effects, decrease antibody resistance

Anticholinesterase and sympatholytic actions

Quinidine-like cardiac effects, reduction of infarct size

Lower cholesterol and low-density lipoprotein levels by 15% to 20%

are chiral compounds and are administered as racemic mixtures. No studies have directly examined the effects of the individual enantiomers on the pharmacokinetics in SLE, the effects on SLE, or mediators of arthritis.[38] Despite decades of use, the pharmacokinetics of these drugs have been poorly studied. In general, the drugs are readily absorbed from the gastrointestinal tract, have low hepatic extraction ratios (<0.3) and low clearance, extensively distribute into tissues with resultant large volumes of distribution, and have long terminal elimination half-lives (up to 1 month or longer) with little drug recovered unchanged in urine.[38]

Hydroxychloroquine sulfate (Plaquenil) is the prototypic 4-aminoquinolone used for the treatment of SLE. It is FDA approved for the treatment of SLE, as well as rheumatoid arthritis and malaria. It is by far the most commonly used antimalarial for the treatment of SLE (Table 76-5). Several mechanisms of action have been proposed[39] (Box 76-2). The contribution of each mechanism may vary depending on which clinical manifestation is being treated.

A 200-mg tablet contains 155 mg of the hydroxychloroquine base with equal amounts of *R*- (−) and *S*- (+) enantiomers. The dose for SLE is typically 200 to 400 mg daily. Its active metabolites are desethylchloroquine, desethylhydroxychloroquine, and bidesethylchloroquine. Metabolism is probably mediated by hepatic CYP enzymes, although the mechanism in humans is not entirely clear.[40] Hydroxychloroquine is well absorbed orally, with bioavailability of 75% to 100% and peak concentrations in 3 to 4 hours. The drug distributes slowly into a very large volume of distribution reflecting extensive tissue binding, with the highest levels achieved in the adrenal and pituitary glands. It binds moderately (50% to 60%) to plasma proteins. The drug and metabolites are primarily excreted via the kidneys. Elimination occurs in two phases: a rapid one with a half-life of 3 days and a slower one with an overall half-life of 40 days, reflecting the extensive tissue distribution.[38]

In vitro data suggest that chloroquine is an inhibitor of CYP2D6, a CYP3A substrate and/or inhibitor; however, no inhibitory effect was shown with CYP1A2, CYP2C19, CYP2E1, and CYP3A4 in vivo. Quinacrine is metabolized by hepatic CYP3A4 and CYP3A5 and is a P-glycoprotein substrate.[41] No drug-drug interactions have been identified when administered with other antimalarials for the treatment of malaria.[40] Increased serum digoxin levels may result with concomitant use of hydroxychloroquine. Hydroxychloroquine has been reported to reduce the requirement for hypoglycemic agents, and patients taking these medications should have blood glucose monitored more closely with initiation of hydroxychloroquine. One report suggested increased renal toxicity with coadministration of cyclosporin A.[42] Potentially important kinetic drug-drug interactions have been reported with coadministration of chloroquine with acetaminophen, D-penicillamine, methotrexate (reduced methotrexate levels) and cimetidine, although no interactions were reported with aspirin, ranitidine, and imipramine.[43]

Generally, hydroxychloroquine is considered to be useful in treating mild manifestations of SLE such as rashes, serositis, fatigue, and arthritis. Improvement in cutaneous disease and other non–major organ manifestations may not be seen for several months. However, there are no randomized, placebo-controlled studies using antimalarials to treat cutaneous disease. Much of the popularity of hydroxychloroquine is based on older review articles[44] and observational studies.[45] However, it remains the most popular therapeutic agent for management of cutaneous SLE according to an international survey, with 85% of physician respondents choosing it as their drug of choice.[46] In regard to arthritis, one placebo-controlled study showed improvement of subjective joint pain in those patients treated with hydroxychloroquine.[47] Older studies suggest that hydroxychloroquine has a steroid-sparing effect[48] and that its discontinuation was associated with disease exacerbations.[49] In the Canadian Hydroxychloroquine Study Group, 47 patients whose SLE was controlled on hydroxychloroquine were randomized into two groups in which one group continued on the hydroxychloroquine and the other was switched to a placebo. The hydroxychloroquine group had fewer disease flares and lower risk of major organ disease.[50] Therefore, most rheumatologists believe that in patients with a prior history or who are at risk of major organ disease should be treated with hydroxychloroquine.

Hydroxychloroquine and other antimalarials are well tolerated in the majority of patients. Common side effects are drug-induced pigmentation, nausea, vomiting, diarrhea, myopathy, and headache. Serious side effects include torsades de pointes, agranulocytosis, ototoxicity, and retinal toxicity. Retinopathy is the most feared complication of antimalarials and is more common with chloroquine than hydroxychloroquine, and is usually asymptomatic. If symptomatic, the most common presenting symptoms are difficulty reading, photophobia, blurring, and visual field defects. Fortunately, these symptoms are rare especially when hydroxychloroquine is dosed according to ideal body weight, but the actual frequency is controversial. While older reports suggested the incidence was 1% to 2%, more recent studies suggest it is much less. In a prospective cohort study of 526 patients treated with hydroxychloroquine for either rheumatoid arthritis or SLE, no retinal toxicity was noted on ophthalmic examinations conducted every 6 to 12 months in any patients in the first 6 years of therapy. Only two cases of retinopathy were seen in patients treated with hydroxychloroquine for a period of longer than 6 years.[51] Traditionally, the frequency for ophthalmologic screening was for one to be performed within 6 months of starting an antimalarial and then every 12 months thereafter. However given the low incidence of this complication, many rheumatologists and ophthalmologists are recommending examinations every 2 years.

The use of hydroxychloroquine in pregnancy remains controversial because data are limited. However, two recent studies suggest that it may be used in pregnancy with few, if any, adverse effects in doses used to treat SLE. Because of the long half-life, stopping the drug as soon as pregnancy is recognized will not eliminate fetal exposure for months. A small randomized, controlled study to assess safety of hydroxychloroquine during pregnancy suggested that those mothers treated with hydroxychloroquine required less prednisone and had fewer flares, while outcomes for the newborns were identical.[52] A larger study of 133 pregnancies in women treated with hydroxychloroquine found no difference in the percentage of successful pregnancies (88%) versus a control group (84%).[53] Additional potential benefits of the antimalarials include an antiplatelet effect that may decrease the risk of thrombosis, and a lipid-lowering effect.

Systemic Immunosuppressive Agents. Systemic corticosteroid or immunosuppressive agents may be required to treat some of the chronic cutaneous rashes. In one double-blind, randomized, placebo-controlled study of 41 patients, methotrexate (15 to 20 mg/wk) was effective in controlling cutaneous and articular activity and permitted a reduction in the prednisone dose.[54] In addition, thalidomide, dapsone, azathioprine, retinoids, cyclophosphamide, chlorambucil, intravenous immune globulin (IVIG), and clofazimine have all been used with variable success. With the exception of antimalarials and methotrexate, there is a paucity of data derived from adequately powered, randomized, controlled trials for any of these medications used for cutaneous SLE.[55] Since many of these agents are discussed in other chapters, only dapsone and thalidomide are discussed in this section. While both of these agents show promise in the treatment of cutaneous SLE, they are seldom used by physicians because of fear of adverse events and unfamiliarity with their use.

Thalidomide. Thalidomide was synthesized in 1953 and was marketed as a sedative (not in the United States) in the 1950s. While its original marketing strategy emphasized its safety in animals, its teratogenic (limb deformities) and neuropathic side effects were recognized in humans soon after its release. Any interest in its use was lost until reports surfaced about its benefits in treating erythema nodosum leprosum, a reactive lepromatous state.[56] Ultimately, the WHO conducted a controlled trial of its use in this condition and established it as the drug of choice.[57] Subsequently, it has been used in a number of diseases, including Behçet's syndrome, graft-versus-host disease, sarcoidosis, pyoderma gangrenosum, rheumatoid arthritis, and SLE. It is FDA approved for the treatment of erythema nodosum leprosum and newly diagnosed multiple myeloma.

Thalidomide (Thalomid) is a racemate composed of two equal amounts of *S*- and *R*- enantiomers. It is an immunomodulatory agent with a spectrum of activity that is not fully characterized, but may in part be due to suppression of tumor necrosis factor-α (TNF-α) production, down-modulation of selected cell adhesion molecules involved in leukocyte migration, and potent co-stimulation of human T cells in vivo. The standard dose of thalidomide in SLE is 100 to 300 mg/day, administered once daily with water, preferably at bedtime due to its sedative properties or at least 1 hour after the evening meal.

Thalidomide is slowly and extensively absorbed following oral administration. Peak concentrations are achieved 3 to 4 hours after administration. It is minimally metabolized by the hepatic CYP system but undergoes nonenzymatic hydrolysis into numerous metabolites. Less than 1% of the total dose is found in the urine over 24 hours following a dose. Most of an oral dose is eliminated in the excreta; however, it is not known how much is eliminated through urine and feces. The extent of hydrolysis is estimated to be 80% 24 hours following dosing. The elimination half-life is 6 hours, which represents absorption and not elimination because thalidomide has rate-limited absorption from the gastrointestinal tract due to low solubility. Thalidomide interconverts between *R*- and *S*- enantiomers in plasma, with protein binding of 55% and 65%, respectively, and the enantiomers have different pharmacokinetic and pharmacodynamic properties. The pharmacokinetics of thalidomide are not expected to be altered with renal or hepatic impairment since it is principally hydrolyzed and excreted passively. No pharmacokinetic data are available in SLE patients. Drug-drug interactions have not been extensively studied with thalidomide; no pharmacokinetic interactions were observed in two studies with oral contraceptives. There is no information on the potential interaction with warfarin.[58]

In a Brazilian case series of 23 patients who were unresponsive to conventional therapy (chloroquine, photoprotectors, and corticosteroids in doses of <0.5 mg/kg per day), patients were treated with 300 mg/day of thalidomide. Ninety percent of the patients had complete remission of their disease, and the average dose of prednisone was tapered from 40.5 mg/day to 17.4 mg/day.[59] Eighteen of the patients who had relapsed when the thalidomide was discontinued were later treated with 25 to 100 mg of thalidomide daily for 6 months; a complete remission in 72% and a partial remission in 28% of patients were observed.[60] A more recent case series of 65 patients treated with thalidomide reported a partial or complete response in 98.9%.[61] Less common SLE skin lesions, such as lupus profundus and hypertrophic lesions, have also been reported to improve.

Common side effects include edema, rash, hypocalcemia, constipation, nausea, leukopenia, confusional state, somnolence, and tremor. Serious side effects of thalidomide include teratogenicity (FDA Pregnancy Category X), Stevens-Johnson syndrome, toxic epidermal necrolysis, neutropenia, thrombosis, peripheral neuropathy, and pulmonary embolus. The peripheral neuropathy is characterized by symmetric painful paresthesias of the hands and feet. The incidence of peripheral neuropathy seems to vary with the disease being treated; in the case of SLE, it has been reported in 21% to 27% of patients.[62] Medications known to cause peripheral neuropathy should be avoided when using thalidomide. The drowsiness associated with thalidomide may potentiate the sedative properties of barbituates, alcohol, chloropromazine, and reserpine. Drug interactions include darbepoetin alfa (theoretical), dexamethasone (probable), and docetaxel (established).

A Mandatory Safety Program for the clinical use of thalidomide was established in 1999 when thalidomide was approved in the

United States. This program is known by the acronym STEPS (System for Thalidomide Education and Prescribing Safety).[63] The goals of the program are to control access to the drug; educate pharmacists, physicians, and patients; and monitor compliance. Clinicians who prescribe thalidomide are also required to be registered in the STEPS program.

Dapsone. Dapsone is a sulfone derivative. It is FDA approved for the treatment of acne vulgaris, dermatitis herpetiformis, and leprosy. It is used off label for treatment and prophylaxis for *Pneumocystis jiroveci* (formerly *carinii*) pneumonia and prophylaxis for toxoplasmosis. In SLE, it has not been studied in a controlled fashion. Case reports suggest that it may be useful in the treatment of vasculitis[64] and discoid lupus.[65] In SLE, the dose frequently used is 50 to 100 mg daily.

Dapsone is slowly and almost completely absorbed following oral administration, with bioavailability of 70% to 80%. Peak concentrations are achieved 4 hours after administration, and 70% to 85% of the drug is slowly eliminated in the urine as dapsone and metabolites. The drug is extensively metabolized via hydroxylation and conjugation to glucoronides and sulfates. Acetylation shows a genetic bimodal distribution with slow and rapid acetylators. CYP3A4 has been determined to be an important mediator of *N*-hydroxylation.[40] Enteropathic circulation occurs with the metabolites as well as dapsone, resulting in their persistence in the plasma for several weeks after therapy is discontinued. The elimination half-life is approximately 30 hours. Dapsone is about 70% to 90% protein bound, and its monoacetylated metabolite is almost completely protein bound. Dose adjustment is recommended for patients with renal impairment.[66] No pharmacokinetic data are available in SLE patients.

Serious side effects include dermatologic (erythema multiforme, erythema nodosum, and toxic epidermal necrolysis), gastrointestinal (abdominal pain and pancreatitis), hematologic (acquired Heinz body anemia, aplastic anemia, agranulocytosis, and hemolysis), and hepatic (cholestasis and hepatitis) effects as well as peripheral neuropathy and psychosis. Important drug-drug interaction can occur with rifampin (increases the plasma clearance of dapsone) and probenecid (reduces excretion of dapsone), and probable interactions with multiple antiretroviral agents are possible. Recommendations for laboratory monitoring to prevent toxicity include a CBC and reticulocyte count every month for 3 months, then every 3 months with renal and liver panels.[67]

Musculoskeletal

Both arthralgias and arthritis are common symptoms of SLE. Arthralgias can generally be managed with NSAIDs or analgesics such as acetaminophen (see Chapters 61 and 73). For patients with arthritis, the addition of hydroxychloroquine should also be considered. Hormonal therapies such as dehydroepiandrosterone at a dose of 200 mg/day have also shown promising preliminary results in treating arthritis,[68] but their role in the management of SLE is not yet known. Low-dose corticosteroids (10 to 20 mg of prednisone orally per day) are also helpful in managing acute synovitis.

For refractory arthritis, medications such as those used to treat rheumatoid arthritis (methotrexate and azathioprine) should be considered (see Chapter 74). Because of concern of antibody production with anti–TNF-α blocking agents, these medications have not been widely used in the treatment of SLE. However, an open-label study using infliximab in six SLE patients concluded that its use led to clinical improvement and did not lead to any increased SLE activity despite an increase in autoantibody formation.[69]

Hematologic

Autoimmune cytopenias may be seen in all three cell lines and, when present, usually do not require treatment. Anemia is a common laboratory abnormality in SLE patients, with a prevalence of 78% when defined as a hemoglobin of 12 g/dl.[70] The anemia can generally be divided into two groups: non–immune mediated (anemia of chronic disease, iron deficiency anemia, sideroblastic anemia, drug-induced anemia, and anemia secondary to other disorders) and immune mediated (hemolytic anemia, drug-induced hemolytic anemia, aplastic anemia, pure red cell aplasia, and pernicious anemia). While only the treatment of hemolytic anemia is discussed, it is important to consider the multitude of potential etiologies when evaluating an SLE patient with anemia.

Hemolytic anemia typically responds to high-dose corticosteroids (1 mg/kg per day of prednisone). Once hemolysis is controlled, the dose can be rapidly tapered. If it does not respond, other therapeutic considerations include pulse IV corticosteroids, azathioprine (1 to 2 mg/kg per day), or cyclophosphamide in doses similar to those used to treat renal disease. In a series of 26 patients, danazol was also found to be effective in the management of hemolytic anemia.[71] MMF has also been shown to be effective in a case of refractory hemolytic anemia.[72]

Except in the presence of recurrent infections, leukopenia does not require treatment. In the evaluation of leukopenia, it is incumbent on clinicians to examine the patient's medication list to make sure that one of the medications, in particular the immunosuppressives, is not causing or contributing to the cytopenia. Although lymphopenia is the most common leukopenia in SLE patients, any type of white blood cells may be decreased. Severe neutropenia may respond to systemic corticosteroid therapy[73] or recombinant human granulocyte colony-stimulating factor.[74]

Thrombocytopenia, defined as a platelet count of less than 150,000 cells/ml, has a prevalence between 7% and 52%.[75] While the degree of thrombocytopenia is highly variable, profound thrombocytopenia (<20,000 cells/ml) is unusual. According to one prospective study of outcomes in SLE patients with less than 100,000 cells/ml, two distinct clinical groups were noted: those who developed profound thrombocytopenia with multisystem flares and those who had chronic thrombocytopenia with intermittent mild flares of their disease. Severe bleeding was not seen in either group.[76]

However, two syndromes associated with thrombocytopenia deserve special consideration, idiopathic thrombocytopenic purpura (ITP) and thrombotic thrombocytopenic purpura (TTP). Typically, young females are the most prone to develop ITP, and a significant percentage (5% to 15%) of those who present with ITP ultimately are diagnosed as having SLE.[77] Many patients with ITP are asymptomatic, but symptoms such as purpura, increased bruising, and heavy menstrual flow can be associated with platelet counts of less than 50,000 cells/ml. Counts lower than 20,000 cells/ml may be associated with oozing from gums, spontaneous epistaxis, and petechiae. Corticosteroids, such as 1 mg/kg per day of prednisone for several weeks with a rapid taper when the counts recover to greater than 80,000 cells/ml, are the mainstay of management. In case reports and series, corticosteroid-resistant cases have been treated with danazol (see later), an androgenic steroid with few virilizing effects.[78,79] Unfortunately, thrombocytopenia may recur after the danazol is stopped. Other medications used successfully in case reports include vincristine, azathioprine, cyclophosphamide, dapsone, cyclosporine, MMF, and rituximab. IVIG may also be effective, but its effects may not be long lasting, so it may be considered in life-threatening bleeding or impending fetal loss prior to surgery.

TTP is a life-threatening disorder of the microcirculation characterized by the pentad of fever, microangiopathic hemolytic anemia, neurologic dysfunction, thrombocytopenic purpura, and renal dysfunction. It is increasingly common that TTP is being diagnosed in the absence of all five of these findings. Fortunately, it is a rare disorder. While the strength of the association of TTP and SLE has been debated, it is clear that more cases of this association are being reported. The treatment of TTP in SLE patients is the same as for other patients with TTP, namely systemic corticosteroids, IVIG, and/or plasma exchange.

Danazol. Danazol (Danocrine) is a synthetic steroid derived from ethisterone that suppresses the pituitary-ovarian axis via at least three mechanisms: decreased hypothalamic-pituitary response to lowered estrogen production, alteration of sex steroid metabolism, and interaction with sex hormone receptors. It is FDA approved for the treatment of endometriosis, fibrocystic breast disease, and hereditary angioedema. In SLE, it has been used off label to treat hemolytic anemia, pure red cell aplasia, ITP, and Evans' syndrome (immune hemolytic anemia and thrombocytopenia).

The typical dose in SLE is 200 mg orally, three to four times a day. Publications of danazol pharmacokinetics are quite old and use a variety of analytic techniques that are no longer employed in current pharmacokinetic studies. Danazol is well absorbed following oral administration and is metabolized via a hepatic mechanism, the specifics of which are not known, to approximately 60 different metabolites. The circulating half-life in women is approximately 15 hours, with tissue half-life of metabolites in the range of days.[80] No pharmacokinetic data are available in SLE patients. In a recent study that examined the long-term effectiveness of danazol, corticosteroids, cytotoxics, and dapsone in the treatment of hematologic manifestations of SLE, danazol had one of the highest rates of continuation, presumably because of less frequent adverse effects and better efficacy.[81]

The most common side effects include edema, acne, flushing, hirsutism, seborrhea, sweating, weight gain, nervousness, abnormal menstruation, vaginal dryness, and change in voice. Serious side effects include thrombophlebitis, thromboembolic disorder, hepatotoxicity, stroke, and pseudotumor cerebri. Because danazol is metabolized predominantly via a hepatic mechanism, it should be used cautiously if at all in patients with hepatic dysfunction. Additionally, patients with congestive heart failure and renal dysfunction may experience clinical deterioration due to fluid retention. However, discontinuation of danazol due to adverse side effects is uncommon.[80]

Cardiac

Many patients with SLE develop cardiac complications during the course of their disease. The most common are pericardial disease, valvular heart disease, myocarditis, and coronary artery disease. Treatment of cardiac manifestations has never been studied using controlled methodology.

Pericardial disease is reported to occur in up to 60% of SLE patients.[82] In the vast majority of patients, the course is generally benign, although large effusions, tamponade, and constrictive pericarditis can rarely be seen. Symptomatic pericarditis typically responds to treatment with an NSAID or prednisone (0.5 to 1 mg/kg in divided doses). IVIG has been used to treat life-threatening pericarditis.[83] Depending on the method of detection, valvulopathy can be seen in up to 77% of patients.[82] No therapy is required unless the lesion is hemodynamically significant, although subacute bacterial endocarditis prophylaxis should be considered in those patients undergoing procedures associated with bacteremia. Fortunately, myocarditis is an uncommon manifestation, occurring in 8% to 25% of patients.[84] Typically, it is treated with prednisone (1 mg/kg per day in divided doses). Premature coronary artery disease is increasingly recognized in SLE patients, and its prevalence may not be explained by traditional cardiac risk factors.[85] Nevertheless, it is prudent to advise patients to exercise, stop smoking, and aggressively treat hyperlipidemia if present.

Pulmonary

Pulmonary manifestations of SLE include costochondritis, pleural disease, pneumonitis, pulmonary hemorrhage, pulmonary hypertension, and "shrinking lung" syndrome. Costochondritis typically responds to local therapies such as heat, topical analgesics, and rarely corticosteroid injections, NSAIDs, and analgesics such as acetaminophen.

The prevalence of symptomatic serositis in a cohort of 310 Chinese SLE patients was 12%. Pleural involvement was the most common pulmonary manifestation, seen in 44% of the patients, while peritoneal (30%) and pericardial (26%) involvement were less frequent. In this observational study, 35% were treated with NSAIDs alone and 76% were treated with moderate to high doses of oral prednisolone. All episodes of serositis resolved completely within 2 months of therapy.[86]

Fortunately acute lupus pneumonitis is an uncommon manifestation of SLE; it presents with dyspnea, fever, pleurisy, cough, tachycardia, and pulmonary infiltrates on radiographs. This clinical presentation, especially in patients being treated with immunosuppressive agents, may be confused with serious infections. It is associated with 50% mortality within weeks if corticosteroid therapy is not started promptly. The mainstay of therapy is high-dose prednisone administered at a dose of 1 mg/kg per day. The administration of high-dose pulse IV methylprednisolone (500 to 1000 mg/day for 3 days), similar to treatment for SLE nephritis, may also be considered.

Interstitial lung disease is seen in 3% of SLE patients and clinically presents much more gradually than acute pneumonitis. Symptoms and signs include dyspnea on exertion, nonproductive cough, and tachypnea. High-resolution computed tomography scans, pulmonary function testing measurement of carbon monoxide diffusion in the lungs, and bronchoalveolar lavage are helpful in determining whether the symptoms are secondary to inflammation, scarring, or alveolitis. If the process is thought to be inflammatory in nature, oral prednisone (1 mg/kg per day) is the first-line therapy, with consideration of other immunosuppressive therapy if no significant improvement is seen. A recent case series of 34 patients with pulmonary disease who underwent hematopoietic stem cell transplantation showed significant improvement in their pulmonary function testing and symptoms.[87]

Pulmonary alveolar hemorrhage is a rare complication of SLE and anecdotally should be treated with a combination of corticosteroids, cyclophosphamide, and mechanical ventilation if necessary. Pulmonary hypertension may also occur in SLE, although it more commonly occurs in scleroderma. Treatment options include calcium channel blockers, anticoagulation, bosentan, or infusions of prostacyclin analogues.

Gastrointestinal

While gastrointestinal complaints are common (25% to 40%) in patients with SLE,[88] most are nonspecific and may represent medication side effects such as dyspepsia secondary to NSAIDs. However, three gastrointestinal syndromes are potentially serious if not recognized and treated promptly: pancreatitis, mesenteric vasculitis, and protein-losing enteropathy. No controlled clinical trials exist in the treatment of any of these syndromes.

Pancreatitis occurs in 2% to 8% of patients with SLE.[89] The majority of cases are due to medication side effects, as with azathioprine and corticosteroids, or lifestyle choices (e.g., alcoholism), but 8% are thought to be due to vasculitis of the pancreatic blood supply.[90] It is important to rule out common causes of pancreatitis such as gallstones and alcoholism before concluding the pancreatitis is secondary to SLE. One useful clinical observation is that, if a patient has pancreatitis secondary to SLE activity, the patient usually has other active manifestations of SLE. Regardless of the cause, standard medical therapy (bowel rest, volume resuscitation, and analgesics) should be initiated. If conservative therapy does not work, and especially if there is evidence of active disease elsewhere, corticosteroids may be considered (1 mg/kg per day).

Mesenteric vasculitis is the feared gastrointestinal complication of SLE; it is associated with a mortality rate of 50%. Typically, abdominal pain starts insidiously prior to the development of an acute abdomen. Pathologically, it is thought to be due to arteriolar vasculitis and/or clots secondary to antiphospholipid antibodies. Owing to the rarity of this condition, treatment is anecdotal, with one expert recommending a combination of pulse methylprednisolone (1000 to 1500 mg IV daily for 1 to 3 days) and a single IV dose of cyclophosphamide (1000 mg), with reassessment after 7 to 10 days to determine whether another cyclophosphamide bolus is indicated.[90]

Another uncommon manifestation of SLE is a protein-losing enteropathy. It typically occurs in young women and presents with hypoalbuminemia, edema, and diarrhea. Treatment consists of corticosteroids and, anecdotally, immunosuppressive agents.[91,92]

Neuropsychiatric

SLE can affect the nervous system in many ways. It is useful to divide the manifestations into diffuse and focal manifestations. Diffuse manifestations are mostly mediated through autoantibodies directed toward neural cells that affect neural function in a generalized manner through mechanisms such as immune complexes, vasculitis, and vasculopathies. Focal manifestations are likely related to intravascular occlusion secondary to antiphospholipid antibodies or vasculitis. It is

BOX 76-3 CENTRAL NERVOUS SYSTEM INVOLVEMENT IN SLE

Diffuse Manifestations
Headache
Cognitive defects
Seizures
Organic brain syndrome
Behavioral disorders
Psychoses
Mood disorders
Myelopathy
Peripheral neuropathies
Aseptic meningitis

Focal Manifestations
Stroke
Chorea
Myelopathy
Behavioral disorders (secondary to stroke)

Indirect Factors
Medication side effects
Electrolyte imbalances
Infection
Complications of renal disease
Complications of hypertension

also important to recognize the numerous neuropsychiatric manifestations in SLE patients that are not due to active disease, such as medication side effects (e.g., steroid-induced psychosis or ibuprofen-induced aseptic meningitis), uremia leading to mental status changes, and meningitis leading to delirium (Box 76-3).

Approximately 10% of SLE patients have central nervous system vasculitis that may progress from lethargy and headaches to stupor and coma in a matter of days if not appropriately recognized and treated. To complicate matters, infections with common and opportunistic organisms must always be considered in febrile SLE patients who have neurologic syndromes.

Neuropsychiatric manifestations such as organic brain syndrome, psychoses, myelopathy, peripheral neuropathies, and some headaches may respond to immunosuppressive agents, most commonly high-dose oral corticosteroids (1 mg/kg per day of prednisone or its equivalent) or pulses of IV methylprednisolone (1000 mg/day for 3 days) similar to how it is used in renal disease. In a case series of seven pediatric patients with severe neuropsychiatric lupus, the combination of IV methylprednisolone and IV cyclophosphamide led to clinical improvement in all of the patients.[93] More recently, in a study of 60 patients with primary neuropsychiatric manifestations comparing low-dose IV cyclophosphamide (200 to 400 mg/mo) plus oral prednisone with hydroxychloroquine ± prednisone, statistically significant clinical and electrophysiologic improvement was noted in the group treated with cyclophosphamide and prednisone.[94] A controlled multicenter clinical trial for severe neurologic involvement was completed that used an induction treatment with 3 g of IV methylprednisolone in both groups. This was followed by either methylprednisolone 1 g daily for 3 days, monthly for 4 months, then bimonthly for 6 months, and subsequently every 3 months or cyclophosphamide 0.75 g/m^2 body surface monthly for 1 year, then every 3 months for a year. Overall, a response rate of 75% was observed, with the primary end point (a 20% improvement in basal conditions on clinical, laboratory, or specific neurologic variables) favoring the cyclophosphamide group.[95] In refractory cases, plasmapheresis may be useful.[96]

Ischemic central nervous system events secondary to antiphospholipid antibodies should be treated with lifelong anticoagulation; this is discussed in the next section. The role for chronic anticoagulation in those patients believed to have progressive cognitive defects is unknown.

BOX 76-4 PRELIMINARY CLASSIFICATION CRITERIA FOR ANTIPHOSPHOLIPID ANTIBODY SYNDROME*

Vascular Thrombosis
a) One or more clinical episodes of arterial, venous, or small-vessel thrombosis in any tissue or organ *and*
b) Thrombosis confirmed by imaging or Doppler studies or histopathology, with the exception of superficial thrombosis *and*
c) For histopathologic confirmation, thrombosis present without significant evidence of inflammation in the vessel wall.

Pregnancy Morbidity
a) One or more unexplained deaths of a morphologically normal fetus at or beyond the 10th week of gestation, with normal fetal morphology documented by ultrasound or by direct examination of the fetus *or*
b) One or more premature births of a morphologically normal neonate at or before the 34th week of gestation because of severe preeclampsia or severe placental insufficiency *or*
c) Three or more unexplained consecutive spontaneous abortions before the 10th week of gestation, with maternal anatomic or hormonal abnormalities and paternal and maternal chromosomal causes excluded.

Laboratory Criteria
a) Anticardiolipin antibody of IgG and/or IgM isotype in blood, present in medium or high titer on two or more occasions at least 6 weeks apart, measured by standard enzyme-linked immunosorbent assay for β_2 glycoprotein-1–dependent anticardiolipin antibodies *or*
b) Lupus anticoagulant present in plasma on two or more occasions at least 6 weeks apart, detected according to the guidelines of the International Society on Thrombosis and Hemostasis.

*Definite APS is considered to be present if at least one of the clinical and one of the laboratory criteria are met.
IgG, immunoglobulin G; IgM, immunoglobulin M.
From Wilson WA, Gharavi AE, Koike T, et al. International consensus statement on preliminary classifications criteria for definite antiphospholipid syndrome. Arthritis Rheum 1999;42:1309-1311.

Antiphospholipid Antibody Syndrome

The antiphospholipid antibody syndrome (APS) is commonly seen in association with SLE and other diffuse connective tissue diseases. It is diagnosed by the demonstration of persistent antiphospholipid antibodies (anticardiolipin antibodies and/or lupus anticoagulants) when associated with evidence of venous or arterial thrombotic events. The criteria used to diagnose APS are listed in Box 76-4.[97] Some of the more common manifestations are listed in Table 76-6.

Consensus opinion for the treatment of APS is hindered by the lack of controlled studies and the diverse manifestations of this disorder. Certainly, anticoagulation remains the treatment of choice for patients who have had thombotic events in association with antiphospholipid antibodies. Choices include unfractionated heparin, low-molecular-weight heparin, and warfarin. The recommended duration of therapy is generally lifelong. This is based on a study that demonstrated a marked increase in risk of venous thrombosis recurrence in those patients not anticoagulated long term (50% recurrence rate of venous thrombosis at 2 years vs. 0% in those treated with long-term warfarin).[98]

No consensus has been established for the optimal international normalized ratio (INR) in these patients. Older studies suggested that intensive warfarin therapy to maintain an INR of 3 or greater was the most effective therapy.[99] However, in a recent randomized, controlled study, a moderate intensity of anticoagulation (INR range 2.0 to 3.0) was just as effective in preventing recurrent thrombosis as a high intensity (INR 3.0 to 4.0) therapy and was associated with fewer bleeding complications.[100] The role of low-molecular-weight heparin is not clear, but a case series suggests that it may also be safe and effective therapy.[101] The role of antiplatelet therapy, cyclophosphamide, corticosteroids, and IVIG is unknown.

Since warfarin crosses the placenta and is a known teratogen, it is contraindicated in pregnancy. The approach to the management of APS in pregnancy is fairly well accepted and delineated.[102] The combination of aspirin and heparin, adjusted to a higher dose than the 5000 IU twice daily used in nonpregnant thrombotic prophylaxis, is a common treatment. Low-molecular-weight heparin may be as effective and equally safe as unfractionated heparin in this group of patients.[103]

TABLE 76-6 CLINICAL PRESENTATIONS OF ANTIPHOSPHOLIPID ANTIBODY SYNDROME

Organ System	Clinical Manifestations
Dermatologic	Livedo reticularis, leg ulceration, distal cutaneous ischemia, superficial thrombophlebitis
Vascular	Deep venous thrombosis, intra-abdominal venous thrombosis
Neurologic	Transient ischemic attacks, cerebral infarction, transverse myelitis, migraine, amaurosis fugax, chorea
Cardiac	Angina, myocardial infarction, valvular vegetations, intracardiac thrombus
Renal	Glomerular thrombi, accelerated hypertension, renal artery thrombosis
Pulmonary	Pulmonary emboli, pulmonary hypertension
Hematologic	Thrombocytopenia, hemolytic anemia
Reproductive	Recurrent fetal loss

Reproductive Issues

SLE is a disease of women in the childbearing years. Pregnancy is fraught with potential problems for the mother (e.g., hypertension, disease flare, diabetes mellitus, thrombosis, and preeclampsia) and fetus (e.g., fetal loss, preterm birth, neonatal lupus, and intrauterine growth retardation). Disease flares can occur at any time during the pregnancy or the postpartum period, so frequently monitoring women during pregnancy is prudent and requires special attention from both the rheumatologist and the obstetrician.

While the FDA Pregnancy Category drug labeling is useful, it is important to note that very little is known about the use of many of these agents during pregnancy in humans. As with the use of any drugs during pregnancy, "safety" is a relative term as the background rate for adverse pregnancy outcomes is much higher in SLE patients compared with the general population. While it makes sense to use as few drugs as possible during pregnancy, it is also important to recognize that medications may help to prevent a systemic flare in the mother. The FDA drug labeling categories for pregnancy of most of the medications discussed in this chapter are shown in Table 76-7.

TABLE 76-7 FDA PREGNANCY LABELING CATEGORIES FOR DRUGS USED IN THE TREATMENT OF SYSTEMIC LUPUS ERYTHEMATOSUS

Drug	FDA Pregnancy Category	Fetal Effects	Compatible with Lactation	Recommendations
Azathioprine	D	IUGR; neonatal leukopenia, lymphopenia, hypogammaglobulinemia; infections (CMV and gram-negative)	No	Use with caution if needed to suppress disease activity; consider decreasing dose at 32 wk
COX-2 inhibitors	C	Risk of fetal hemorrhage; premature closure of ductus arteriosus	Insufficient data	Discontinue 6-8 wk prior to delivery, preferably by week 32
Cyclophosphamide	D	Embryopathy with growth deficiency; developmental delay; craniosynostosis, craniofacial defects; distal limb defects	No	Avoid during pregnancy, especially during first trimester
Cyclosporin A	C	Abnormal T, B, and NK cell development and maturation	No	Use with caution to suppress disease activity
Glucocorticoids	B	Oral clefts with first trimester exposure	Yes, breast-feed 4 hr after last dose	Evaluate need for stress dosing, avoid during first trimester
Hydroxychloroquine	C	Probably none	Yes	May continue through pregnancy
Methotrexate	X	Cranial abnormalities; limb defects; CNS abnormalities	No	Discontinue 4 mo prior to conception; supplement with folic acid during those 4 mo and through pregnancy
Mycophenolate mofetil	C	Teratogenic; craniofacial, distal limb, and other fetal malformations	No	Avoid if possible during pregnancy
NSAIDs	B	Risk of fetal hemorrhage; premature closure of ductus arteriosus	Yes, but increased potential of jaundice and kernicterus	Discontinue 6-8 wk prior to delivery, preferably by week 32
Rituximab	C	Insufficient data; case reports of granulocytopenia and lymphopenia	Insufficient data, no	Avoid if possible during pregnancy

CMV, cytomegalovirus; CNS, central nervous system; COX, cyclooxygenase; FDA, U.S. Food and Drug Administration; IUGR, intrauterine growth retardation; NK, natural killer; NSAIDs, nonsteroidal anti-inflammatory drugs.

Corticosteroids, NSAIDs, antimalarials, and immunosuppressive agents are the most common drugs used during pregnancy. Depending on the symptoms treated and the severity of the flares, oral corticosteroids up to 1 mg/kg per day may be used during pregnancy with few adverse fetal effects. While many corticosteroid preparations have been shown to cross the placenta, fetal levels are approximately less than 10% of maternal levels. While intrauterine growth retardation and low birth weight have been reported with maternal corticosteroid therapy, a prospective study of 102 pregnancies in SLE patients suggested that these complications may instead be due to active SLE rather than to the corticosteroid use.[104]

NSAIDs interfere with prostaglandin formation through inhibition of cyclooxygenase, thereby potentially inhibiting uterine contractility and prolonging labor. In addition, salicylates and other NSAIDs can also complicate pregnancy by causing maternal, fetal, and neonatal bleeding due to their effects on platelets. The use of salicylates and NSAIDs in pregnancy has been studied extensively in diseases other than SLE and is discussed in Chapter 18. From these data, it is prudent to avoid NSAIDs and anti-inflammatory doses of salicylates during the last 6 to 8 weeks of pregnancy to avoid prolonged labor, excessive bleeding, and premature closure of the ductus arteriosus. On the other hand, low-dose salicylates have been suggested for SLE patients with recurrent fetal loss secondary to antiphospholipid antibodies.[105]

Antimalarial use during pregnancy has been controversial as several studies suggested that stopping these agents may be associated with exacerbations in SLE, often with major organ involvement.[106] A recent randomized, double-blind, placebo-controlled study of 20 patients on hydroxychloroquine for either SLE or discoid lupus noted beneficial effects of hydroxychloroquine during pregnancy as measured by activity indices and a decrease in prednisone use with no detriment to the infant or mother.[52] In a review of over 250 live births of mothers maintained on hydroxychloroquine throughout pregnancy, there was no increase in birth defects, retinal toxicity, or ototoxicity. Data concerning lactation were rare. These authors concluded that hydroxychloroquine should be continued throughout pregnancy and did not advise stopping it when breast-feeding.[107]

The continuation of cytotoxic or immunosuppressive therapies during pregnancy demands that the physician and patient carefully examine the need for disease control and potential risk to the woman and child. Most medical centers use azathioprine when needed in SLE pregnancies complicated by major organ involvement and unresponsive to corticosteroids. Cyclophosphamide, methotrexate, and MMF should not be used during pregnancy. The information on outcomes of pregnant women is limited, and there are no controlled studies of any these medications during pregnancy. Therefore, groups such as the Organization of Teratology Information Specialists (OTIS) have been formed to stimulate and encourage research, education, patient counseling, and the dissemination of knowledge in the field of teratology and to collect data regarding pregnancy outcomes while on these and other medications (*http://www.otispregnancy.org*).

The management of APS during pregnancy largely depends on the number of prior miscarriages. If a woman has no history of miscarriages, no therapy or therapy with 81 mg daily of aspirin may be considered. If a woman has had one prior first trimester miscarriage, 81 mg of daily aspirin is appropriate. Multiple prior early miscarriages or one late miscarriage should be treated with prophylactic heparin (either unfractionated or fractionated) with aspirin (81 mg daily). Patients already on warfarin for manifestations of APS should be switched to therapeutic doses of heparin as soon as pregnancy is detected.

Many drugs are excreted in trace or variable amounts in breast milk. Although concentrations of various corticosteroids in the milk of lactating women may vary, in one study looking at long-term therapy of women taking up to 80 mg/day of prednisolone, the milk concentrations were 5% to 25% of those found in maternal serum. These researchers concluded that, from a quantitative standpoint, maternal doses of prednisolone of 20 mg twice daily were safe.[108] While the use of antimalarials is generally thought to be safe, small amounts are found in human milk. While the concentration of cytotoxic agents discussed in this chapter varies in breast milk, little is known about the clinical consequences for the nursing infant. Therefore, breast-feeding is best avoided if the mother is on these medications.

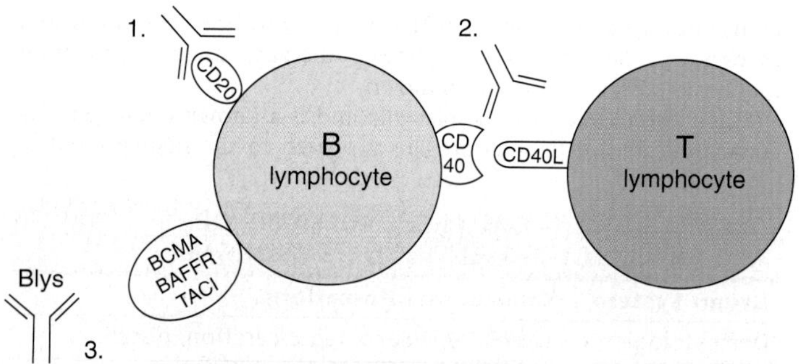

FIGURE 76-4 • Rationale and strategy for targeting B and T lymphocytes in the treatment of systemic lupus erythematosus. *1*, B-cell surface antigens. Monoclonal antibodies against CD20 (rituximab) cause death of B lymphocytes. *2*, Inhibition of co-stimulation. Monoclonal antibodies against CD40 ligand block co-stimulatory signals, thus inhibiting B-lymphocyte activation. *3*, Inhibition of B-lymphocyte survival. Monoclonal antibodies against the cytokine BlyS disrupt the survival signals through the BAFF receptor family.

While in the general population estrogen-containing oral contraceptives are the preferred and most popular method of birth control, barrier methods and progesterone-only contraceptive methods have been the preferred methods in women with SLE. This is primarily because of fears about inducing an SLE flare or thrombotic event. However, the results of a recent randomized double-blind, placebo-controlled study (Safety of Estrogen in Lupus: National Assessment [SELENA] study) suggest that combination oral contraceptives do not increase the risk of flare among women with SLE or thrombosis.[109] However, it seems prudent that those women who have antiphospholipid antibodies should avoid estrogen-containing birth control pills.

Emerging Targets and Therapeutics

The success of the biologic response modifiers such as the use of TNF-α blockers to treat rheumatoid arthritis has paved the way for the introduction of similar strategies for the treatment of SLE. The advantage of these biologic agents is that they target specific pathways that contribute to the inflammatory response. The presence of autoantibodies, hence autoimmunity, is a hallmark of SLE and many other chronic inflammatory diseases. These autoantibodies may be present years before the clinical onset of disease. In addition to the production of antibodies, B lymphocytes also take up and present autoantigens via specific cell surface immunoglobulins to T lymphocytes and thereby regulate inflammatory responses.

Numerous biologic agents are now in development for the treatment of SLE and other inflammatory diseases. Potential targets include cytokine-directed therapies, interference with T- and B-cell interactions, B-cell depletion, induction of tolerance, interference with immune complex formation, and chemokine modulation. To illustrate the rationale and mechanisms of action, three medications utilizing different mechanisms are discussed[110] (Fig. 76-4).

Rituximab (Rituxan) is a chimeric mouse/human monoclonal antibody directed against the B lymphocyte surface antigen CD20. Since CD20 is expressed early in the development of B lymphocytes, it is an ideal target for the treatment of B-cell lymphomas, and indeed that was the reason for its development. However, it has also been used successfully to treat rheumatoid arthritis, and more Phase I/II studies have been completed to determine the safety, efficacy, and dose response in the treatment of SLE. As part of a Phase I/II dose-ranging trial of rituximab in the treatment of SLE, rituximab dramatically improved abnormalities in B-cell homeostasis and tolerance that are characteristic of SLE.[111] In an open study of 24 SLE patients who had failed conventional immunosuppression, considerable improvement was noted in both laboratory markers and disease scores.[112] However, in a

French retrospective study of 11 female children with SLE treated with rituximab combined with a variety of other immunosuppressive agents, clinical remission was achieved in 8 of 11 children. Eight of the children had class IV or V lupus nephritis, two had severe autoimmune cytopenias, and one had antiprothrombin antibody. However, 45% had severe adverse events, including septicemia and severe hematologic toxicity.[113]

CD40 binding to CD154 (CD40 ligand) is an important co-stimulatory signal to B cells inducing activation, proliferation, and class switching. There have been three well-designed studies using anti-CD154 in SLE. The first study of 85 patients with mild to moderate severe SLE demonstrated improvement in serologies but had to be discontinued because of unexpected vascular complications.[114] The second study of 85 patients with nephritis failed to show any benefit.[115] While this particular molecular target is hampered by significant toxicity, other co-stimulatory factors as targets are being investigated.

B-lymphocyte activating factor (BAFF, BlyS) is a survival factor for B cells, belonging to the tumor necrosis factor family of cytokines. Its receptors (BCMA, BAFFR, and TACI) are largely restricted to B cells. Serum BAFF levels have been found to be elevated in SLE, and neutralization of BAFF has been suggested as a therapeutic approach.[116] LymphoStat-B, a fully human IgG1λ monoclonal antibody that neutralizes BlyS, reduced B cells in blood and tissue with minimal toxicity when administered to cynomolgus monkeys.[110,117]

CONCLUSION

The prognosis of SLE is unpredictable due to the wide variability of clinical expression, ranging from relatively benign manifestations to major organ-threatening manifestations. Effective treatment must be individualized, taking into account patient demographics, organ system involvement, and severity of the manifestations. Fortunately, the survival rate in SLE patients has improved dramatically over the past 60 years at least in part due to prompt recognition and treatment of SLE. However, patients with SLE are still at risk for significant morbidity and mortality because of active disease or complications related to its treatment. Serious infections and other complications of current immunosuppressive therapies make it essential that new classes of pharmaceutical agents be developed. Innovative, targeted therapy aimed at molecules that modify the inflammatory response seems to be a practical approach.

REFERENCES

1. National Women's Health Information Center. Lupus—frequently asked questions. Available at *http://www.4woman.gov/faq/lupus.pdf* (accessed October 10, 2006).
2. Siegel M, Lee SL. The epidemiology of systemic lupus erythematosus. Semin Arthritis Rheum 1973;3:1-54.
3. Fessel WJ. Systemic lupus erythematosus in the community: incidences, prevalence, outcome, and first symptoms; the high prevalence in black women. Arch Intern Med 1974;134:1027-1035.
4. Manzi SM, Stark VE, Ramsey-Goldman R. Systemic lupus erythematosus: epidemiology and classification of systemic lupus erythematosus. In Hochberg MC, Silman AJ, Smolen JS, et al (eds): Rheumatology, 3rd ed. St. Louis: CV Mosby, 2003, pp 1291-1296.
5. Mok CC, Lau CS. Pathogenesis of systemic lupus erythematosus. J Clin Pathol 2003;56:481-490.
6. Hochberg MC. Updating the American College of Rheumatology revised criteria for the classification of systemic lupus erythematosus. Arthritis Rheum 1997;40:1725.
7. Tan EM, Cohen AS, Fries JF, et al. The 1982 revised criteria for the classification of systemic lupus erythematosus (SLE). Arthritis Rheum 1982;25:1271-1277.
8. Karim MY. Immunodeficiency in the lupus clinic. Lupus 2006;15:127-131.
9. Gladman DD, Urowitz MB. Systemic lupus erythematosus: clinical features. In Hochberg MC, Silman AJ, Smolen JS, et al (eds): Rheumatology, 3rd ed. St. Louis: CV Mosby, 2003, pp 1359-1379.
10. Golbus J, McCune WJ. Lupus nephritis: classification, prognosis, immunopathogenesis and treatment. Rheum Dis Clin North Am 1994;20:213-242.
11. Nossent HC, Nenzen-Logmans SC, Vroom TM, et al. Contribution of renal biopsy data in predicting outcome in lupus nephritis. Arthritis Rheum 1990;33:970-977.
12. Boumpas DT, Sidiropoulos P, Bertsias G. Optimum therapeutic approaches for lupus nephritis: what therapy and for whom. Nat Clin Pract Rheumatol 2005;1:22-30.
13. Austin HA 3rd, Klippel JH, Balow JE, et al. Therapy of lupus nephritis: controlled trial of prednisone and cytotoxic drugs. N Engl J Med 1986;314:614-619.
14. Boumpas DT, Austin HA 3rd, Vaughn EM, et al. Controlled trial of pulse methylprednisolone versus two regimens of pulse cyclophosphamide in severe lupus nephritis. Lancet 1992;340:741-745.
15. Balow JE, Boumpas DT, Austin HA. Systemic lupus erythematosus and the kidney. In Lahita RG (ed): Systemic Lupus Erythematosus, 4th ed. Amsterdam: Elsevier, 2004, pp 877-907.
16. Gourley MF, Austin HA 3rd, Scott D, et al. Methylprednisolone and cyclophosphamide, alone or in combination, in patients with lupus nephritis: a randomized, controlled study. Ann Intern Med 1996;125:549-557.
17. Houssiau FA, Vasconcelos C, D'Cruz D, et al. Immunosuppressive therapy in lupus nephritis: the Euro-Lupus Nephritis Trial, a randomized trial of low-dose versus high-dose intravenous cyclophosphamide. Arthritis Rheum 2002;46:2121-2131.
18. Fox DA, McCune WJ. Immunosuppressive drug therapy of systemic lupus erythematosus. Rheum Dis Clin North Am 1994;20:265-299.
19. De Jonge ME, Huitema AD, Rodenhuis S, et al. Clinical pharmacokinetics of cyclophosphamide. Clin Pharmacokinet 2005;44:1135-1164.
20. Zhang J, Tian Q, Yung CS, et al. Metabolism and transport of oxazaphosphorines and the clinical implications. Drug Metab Rev 2005;37:611-703.
21. McCune WJ, Riskalla M. Immunosuppressive drug therapy. In Wallace DJ, Hahn BH (eds): Dubois' Lupus Erythematosus, 6th ed. Baltimore: Williams & Wilkins, 2002, pp 1195-1218.
22. Haubitz M, Schellong S, Gobel U, et al. Intravenous pulse administration of cyclophosphamide versus daily oral treatment in patients with antineutrophil cytoplasmic antibody-associated vasculitis and renal involvement: a prospective, randomized study. Arthritis Rheum 1998;41:1835-1844.
23. Cannella A, O'Dell J. Cytotoxic, immunoregulatory, and biologic agents. In West SG (ed): Rheumatology Secrets, 2nd ed. Philadelphia: Hanley & Belfus, 2002, pp 588-598.
24. Yee CS, Gordon C, Dostal C, et al. EULAR randomized controlled trial of pulse cyclophosphamide and methylprednisolone versus continuous cyclophosphamide and prednisolone followed by azathioprine and prednisolone in lupus nephritis. Ann Rheum Dis 2004;63:525-529.
25. Contreras G, Tozman E, Nahar N, et al. Maintenance therapies for proliferative lupus nephritis: mycophenolate mofetil, azathioprine and intravenous cyclophosphamide. Lupus 2005;14(Suppl 1):s33-s38.
26. Coulthard S, Hogarth L. The thioprines: an update. Invest New Drugs 2005;23:523-532.
27. Warrington JS, Shaw LM. Pharmacogenetic differences and drug-drug interactions in immunosuppressive therapy. Expert Opin Drug Metab Toxicol 2005;1:487-503.
28. Li L, Wang H, Lin S, et al. Mycophenolate mofetil treatment for diffuse proliferative lupus nephritis: a multicenter clinical trial in China. Zhonghua Nei Ke Za Zhi 2002;41:476-479.
29. Gaubitz M, Schorat A, Schotte H, et al. Mycophenolate mofetil for the treatment of systemic lupus erythematosus: an open pilot trial. Lupus 1999;8:731-736.
30. Pisoni CN, Sanchez FJ, Karim Y, et al. Mycophenolate mofetil in systemic lupus erythematosus: efficacy and tolerability in 86 patients. J Rheumatol 2005;32:967-970.
31. Spetie DN, Tang Y, Rovin BH, et al. Mycophenolate therapy of SLE membranous nephropathy. Kidney Int 2004;66:2411-2415.
32. van Gelder T, Shaw LM. The rationale for and limitations of therapeutic drug monitoring for mycophenolate mofetil in transplantation. Transplantation 2005;80(2 Suppl):s244-s253.
33. Boumpas DT, Illei GG, Balow JE. Systemic lupus erythematosus: treatment—renal involvement. In Hochberg MC, Silman AJ, Smolen JS, et al (eds): Rheumatology, 3rd ed. St. Louis: CV Mosby, 2003, pp 1405-1417.
34. Schur PH, Kammer GM. Treatment of systemic lupus erythematosus. In Tsokos GC (ed): Modern Therapeutics in Rheumatic Diseases. Totowa, NJ: Humana Press, 2002, pp 259-296.
35. Leden I. Antimalarial drugs: 350 years. Scand J Rheumatol 1981;10:307-312.
36. Payne JF. A postgraduate lecture on lupus erythematosus. Clin J 1894;4:223-229.
37. Prokopchuk AI. Treatment of lupus with quinacrine. Vestn Dermatol Venerol 1940;2-3:23-26.
38. Brocks DR, Mehvar R. Stereoselectivity in the pharmacodynamics and pharmacokinetics of the chiral antimalarial drugs. Clin Pharmacokinet 2003;42:1359-1382.
39. Wallace DJ. Antimalarial therapies. In Wallace DJ, Hahn BH (eds): Dubois' Lupus Erythematosus, 6th ed. Baltimore: Williams & Wilkins, 2002, pp 1149-1172.
40. Giao PT, de Vries PJ. Pharmacokinetics interactions of antimalarial agents. Clin Pharmacokinet 2001;40:343-373.
41. Huang Y, Okochi H, May BCH, et al. Quinicrine is mainly metabolized to mono-desethyl quinacrine by CYP3A4/5 and its brain accumulation is limited by P-glycoprotein. Drug Metab Disp 2006;34:1136-1144.
42. Canadian Rheumatology Association. Canadian consensus conference on hydroxychloroquine. J Rheumatol 2000;27:2919-2921.
43. Furst DE. Pharmacokinetics of hydroxychloroquine and chloroquine during treatment of rheumatic diseases. Lupus 1996;5(Suppl 1):s11-s15.
44. Dubois EL, Martel S. Antimalarials in the management of discoid and systemic lupus erythematosus. Semin Arthritis Rheum 1978;8:33-51.
45. Callen JP. Chronic cutaneous lupus erythematosus: clinical, laboratory, therapeutic and prognostic examination of 62 patients. Arch Dermatol 1982;118:412-416.
46. Vitali C, Doria A, Tincani A, et al. International survey on the management of patients with SLE: I. General data on the participating centers and the results of a questionnaire regarding mucocutaneous involvement. Clin Exp Rheumatol 1996;14(Suppl 16):S17-S22.
47. Williams HJ, Egger MJ, Singer JZ, et al. Comparison of hydroxychloroquine and placebo in the treatment of the arthropathy of mild systemic lupus erythematosus. J Rheumatol 1994;21:1457-1462.
48. Ziff M, Esserman P, McEwen C. Observations on the course and treatment of SLE. Arthritis Rheum 1956;7:332-350.
49. Rothfield N. Efficacy of antimalarials in systemic lupus erythematosus. Am J Med 1988;85(Suppl 4A):53-56.

50. Canadian Hydroxychloroquine Study Group. A randomized study of the effect of withdrawing hydroxychloroquine sulfate in systemic lupus erythematosus. N Engl J Med 1991;324:150-154.
51. Mavrikakis M, Papazoglou S, Sfikakis PP, et al. Retinal toxicity in long term hydroxychloroquine treatment. Ann Rheum Dis 1996;55:187-189.
52. Levy RA, Vilela VS, Cataldo MJ, et al. Hydroxychloroquine (HCQ) in lupus pregnancy: double-blind and placebo-controlled study. Lupus 2001;10:401-404.
53. Costedoat-Chalumeau N, Amoura Z, et al. Safety of hydroxychloroquine in pregnant patients with connective tissue diseases: a study of one hundred thirty-three cases compared with a control group. Arthritis Rheum 2004;48:3207-3211.
54. Carneiro JR, Sato EI. Double blind, randomized, placebo controlled clinical trial of methotrexate in systemic lupus erythematosus. J Rheumatol 1999;26:1275-1279.
55. Heath M, Raugi GJ. Evidence-based evaluation of immunomodulatory therapy for the cutaneous manifestation of lupus. Adv Dermatol 2004;20:257-291.
56. Sheskin J. Thalidomide in the treatment of lepra reactions. Clin Pharmacol Ther 1965;6:303-306.
57. Iyer CG, Languillon J, Ramanujam K, et al. WHO co-ordinated short-term double-blind trial with thalidomide in the treatment of acute lepra reactions in male lepromatous patients. Bull World Health Organ 1971;45:719-732.
58. Teo SK, Colburn WA, Tracewall WG, et al. Clinical pharmacokinetics of thalidomide. Clin Pharmacokinet 2004;43:311-327.
59. Atra E, Sato EJ. Treatment of the cutaneous lesions of systemic lupus erythematosus with thalidomide. Clin Exp Rheumatol 1993;11:487-493.
60. Sato EI, Assis LS, Lourenzi VP, et al. Long-term thalidomide use in refractory cutaneous lesions of systemic lupus erythematosus. Rev Assoc Med Bras 1998;44:289-293.
61. Coehlo A, Souto MI, Cardoso CR, et al. Long-term thalidomide use in refractory cutaneous lesions of lupus erythematosus: a series of 65 Brazilian patients. Lupus 2005;14:434-439.
62. Calabrese L, Fleischer AB. Thalidomide: current and potential clinical applications. Am J Med 2000;108:487-495.
63. Zeldis JB, Williams BA, Thomas SD, et al. S.T.E.P.S.®: a comprehensive program for controlling and monitoring access to thalidomide. Clin Ther 1999;21:319-330.
64. Nishijima C, Hatta N, Inaoki M, et al. Urticarial vasculitis in systemic lupus erythematosus: fair response to prednisolone/dapsone and persistent hypocomplementemia. Eur J Dermatol 1999;9:54-56.
65. Neri R, Mosca M, Bernacchi E, et al. A case of SLE with acute, subacute and chronic cutaneous lesions successfully treated with dapsone. Lupus 1999;8:240-243.
66. Auidema J, Hilbers-Modderman ES, Merkus FW. Clinical pharmacokinetics of dapsone. Clin Pharmacokinet 1986;11:299-315.
67. Bird K, O'Dell J. Systemic antirheumatic drugs. In West SG (ed): Rheumatology Secrets, 2nd ed. Philadelphia: Hanley & Belfus, 2002, pp 579-587.
68. van Vollenhoven RF, Morabito LM, Engleman EG, et al. Treatment of systemic lupus erythematosus with dehydroepiandrosterone: 50 patients treated up to 12 months. J Rheumatol 1998;25:285-289.
69. Aringer M, Graninger WB, Steiner G, et al. Safety and efficacy of tumor necrosis factor alpha blockade in systemic lupus erythematosus: an open-label study. Arthritis Rheum 2004;50:3161-3169.
70. Michael SR, Vural IL, Bassen FA, et al. The hematologic aspects of disseminated (systemic) lupus erythematosus. Blood 1951;6:1059-1072.
71. Gomard-Mennesson E, Ruivard M, Koenin M, et al. Treatment of isolated severe immune hemolytic anaemia associated with systemic lupus erythematosus: 26 cases. Lupus 2006;15:223-231.
72. Mak A, Mok CC. Mycophenolate mofetil for refractory haemolytic anemia in systemic lupus erythematosus. Lupus 2005;14:856-858.
73. Kondo H, Date Y, Sakai Y, et al. Effective simultaneous rhG-CSF and methylprednisolone "pulse" therapy in agranulocytosis associated with systemic lupus erythematosus. Am J Hematol 1994;46:157-158.
74. Eular HH, Schwab UM, Schroeder JO. Filgrastim for lupus neutropenia. Lancet 1994;344:1513-1514.
75. Quismorio FP. Hematologic and lymphoid abnormalities in systemic lupus erythematosus. In Wallace DJ, Hahn BH (eds): Dubois' Lupus Erythematosus, 6th ed. Baltimore: Williams & Wilkins, 2002, pp 793-820.
76. Miller MH, Urowitz MB, Gladman DD. The significance of thrombocytopenia in systemic lupus erythematosus. Arthritis Rheum 1983;26:1181-1186.
77. Rabinowitz Y, Dameshek W. Systemic lupus erythematosus after "idiopathic" thrombocytopenic purpura: clinical study and evaluation of 381 cases over a period of 28 years. Ann Intern Med 1960;51:1-28.
78. Tiede MP, Ahn ER, Jy W, et al. Life-threatening hypercoagulable state following splenectomy in ITP: successful management with aggressive antithrombotic therapy and danazol. Clin Appl Thromb Hemost 2005;11:347-352.
79. Arnal C, Piette JC, Leone J, et al. Treatment of severe immune thrombocytopenia associated with systemic lupus erythematosus. J Rheumatol 2002;29:75-83.
80. Barbieri RL, Ryan KJ. Danazol: endocrine pharmacology and therapeutic applications. Am J Obstet Gynecol 1981;141:453-463.
81. Avina-Zubeat JA, Galindo-Rodriguez G, Robledo I, et al. Long-term effectiveness of danazol, corticosteroids and cytotoxic drugs in the treatment of hematologic manifestations of systemic lupus erythematosus. Lupus 2003;12:52-57.
82. Bijl M, Brouwer J, Kallenberg GG. Cardiac abnormalities in SLE: pancarditis. Lupus 2000;9:236-240.
83. Meissner M, Sherer Y, Levy Y, et al. Intravenous immunoglobulin therapy in a patient with lupus serositis and nephritis. Rheumatol Int 2000;19:199-201.
84. Mandell BF. Cardiovascular involvement in systemic lupus erythematosus. Semin Arthritis Rheum 1987;17:126-141.
85. Karadag O, Calguneri M, Atalar E, et al. Novel cardiovascular risk factors and cardiac event predictor in female inactive systemic lupus erythematosus patients. Clin Rheumatol 2007;26:695-699.
86. Man BL, Mok CC. Serositis related to systemic lupus erythematosus: prevalence and outcome. Lupus 2005;14:822-826.
87. Traynor AE, Corbridge TC, Eagan AE, et al. Prevalence and reversibility of pulmonary dysfunction in refractory systemic lupus: improvement correlates with disease remission following hematopoietic stem cell transplantation. Chest 2005;127:1680-1689.
88. Hoffman BI, Katz WA. The gastrointestinal manifestations of systemic lupus erythematosus: a review of the literature. Semin Arthritis Rheum 1980;9:237-247.
89. Saab S, Corr MP, Weisman MH. Corticosteroids and systemic lupus erythematosus pancreatitis: a case series. J Rheumatol 1998;25:801-806.
90. Petri M. Gastrointestinal manifestations. In Schur PH (ed): The Clinical Management of Systemic Lupus Erythematosus, 2nd ed. Philadelphia: JB Lippincott, 1996, pp 127-140.
91. Werner de Castro GR, Appenzeller S, Bertolo MB, et al. Protein-losing enteropathy associated with systemic lupus erythematosus: response to cyclophosphamide. Rheumatol Int 2005;25:135-138.
92. Mok CC, Ying KY, Mak A, et al. Outcome of protein-losing gastroenteropathy in systemic lupus erythematosus treated with prednisolone and azathioprine. Rheumatology (Oxford) 2006;45:425-429.
93. Baca V, Lavalle C, Garcia R, et al. Favorable response to intravenous methylprednisolone and cyclophosphamide in children with severe neuropsychiatric lupus. J Rheumatol 1999;26:432-439.
94. Stovanovich L, Stovanovich R, Kostich V, et al. Neuropsychiatric lupus favourable response to low dose i.v. cyclophosphamide and prednisolone (pilot study). Lupus 2003;12:3-7.
95. Barile-Fabris L, Ariza-Andraca R, Olguin-Ortega L, et al. Controlled clinical trial of IV cyclophosphamide versus IV methylprednisolone in severe neurological manifestations in systemic lupus erythematosus. Ann Rheum Dis 2005;64:620-625.
96. Neuwalt CM, Lacks S, Kaye BR, et al. Role of intravenous cyclophosphamide in the treatment of severe neuropsychiatric systemic lupus erythematosus. Am J Med 1995;98:32-41.
97. Wilson WA, Gharavi AE, Koike T, et al. International consensus statement on preliminary classifications criteria for definite antiphospholipid syndrome. Arthritis Rheum 1999;42:1309-1311.
98. Derksen RH, de Groot PG, Kater L, et al. Patients with antiphospholipid antibodies and venous thrombosis should receive long term anticoagulant treatment. Ann Rheum Dis 1993;52:689-692.
99. Khamashta MA, Cuadrado MJ, Mujic F, et al. The management of thrombosis in the antiphospholipid-antibody syndrome. N Engl J Med 1995;332:993-997.
100. Finazzi G, Marchioli R, Brancaccio V, et al. A randomized clinical trial of high-intensity warfarin vs. conventional antithrombotic therapy for the prevention of recurrent thrombosis in patients with the antiphospholipid syndrome (WAPS). J Thromb Haemost 2005;3:848-853.
101. Bick RL, Rice J. Long-term outpatient dalteparin (Fragmin) therapy for arterial and venous thrombosis: efficacy and safety—a preliminary study. Clin Appl Thromb Hemost 1999;5(Suppl 1):s67-s71.
102. Welsch S, Branch DW. Antiphospholipid syndrome in pregnancy: obstetric concerns and treatment. Rheum Dis Clin North Am 1997;23:71-84.
103. Sanson BJ, Lensing AW, Prins MH, et al. Safety of low-molecular-weight heparin in pregnancy: a systemic review. Thromb Haemost 1999;81:668-672.
104. Mintz G, Niz J, Gutierrez G, et al. Prospective study of pregnancy in systemic lupus erythematosus: results of a multidisciplinary approach. J Rheumatol 1986;13:732-739.
105. Merrill JT. Treatment of antiphospholipid syndrome. In Tsokos GC (ed): Modern Therapeutics in Rheumatic Diseases. Totowa, NJ: Humana Press, 2002, pp 297-314.
106. Parke A, West B. Hydroxychloroquine in pregnant patients with systemic lupus erythematosus. J Rheumatol 1996;23:1715-1718.
107. Costedoat-Chalumeau N, Amoua Z, Huong DL, et al. Safety of hydroxychloroquine in pregnant patients with connective tissue disease: a review of the literature. Autoimmun Rev 2005;4:111-115.
108. Ost L, Wettrell G, Bjorkhem I, et al. Prednisolone excretion in human milk. J Pediatr 1985;106:1008-1011.
109. Petri M, Kim MY, Kalunian KC, et al. Combined oral contraceptives in women with systemic lupus erythematosus. N Engl J Med 2005;353:2550-2558.
110. Looney RJ, Anolik J, Sanz I. B cells as therapeutic targets for rheumatic diseases. Curr Opin Rheumatol 2004;16:180-185.
111. Anolik JH, Barnard J, Cappione A, et al. Rituximab improves peripheral B cell abnormalities in human systemic lupus erythematosus. Arthritis Rheum 2004;50:3580-3590.
112. Leandro MJ, Cambridge G, Edwards JC, et al. B-cell depletion in the treatment of patients with systemic lupus erythematosus: a longitudinal analysis of 24 patients. Rheumatology (Oxford) 2005;44:1542-1545.
113. Willems M, Haddad E, Niaadet P, et al. Rituximab therapy for childhood-onset systemic lupus erythematosus. J Pediatr 2006;148:623-627.
114. Boumpas DT, Furie R, Manzi S, et al. A short course of BG9588 (anti-CD40 ligand antibody) improves serologic activity and decreases hematuria in patients with proliferative lupus glomerulonephritis. Arthritis Rheum 2003;48:719-727.
115. Kalunian KC, Davis JC Jr, Merrill JT, et al. Treatment of systemic lupus erythematosus by inhibition of T cell costimulation with anti-CD154: a randomized, double-blind, placebo-controlled study. Arthritis Rheum 2002;46:3251-3258.
116. Toubi E, Kessel A, Rosner I, et al. The reduction of serum B-lymphocyte activating factor levels following quinicrine add-on therapy in systemic lupus erythematosus. Scand J Immunol 2006;63:299-303.
117. Baker KP, Edwards BM, Main SH, et al. Generation and characterization of LymphoStat-B, a human monoclonal antibody that antagonizes the bioactivities of B lymphocyte stimulator. Arthritis Rheum 2003;48:3253-3265.

77

INFLUENZA AND VIRAL RESPIRATORY INFECTIONS

Joseph P. Lynch, III

INFLUENZA 1063
Virology 1063
Epidemiology 1063
Clinical Features 1064
Diagnosis 1065
Treatment 1065
  Adamantanes (M2 Inhibitors) 1065
  Neuraminidase Inhibitors 1066
Prevention 1067
AVIAN INFLUENZA 1068
Virology 1068
Epidemiology 1069
Clinical Features 1069
Diagnosis 1069
Treatment 1069
Prevention 1069
RESPIRATORY SYNCYTIAL VIRUS 1070
Virology 1070
Epidemiology 1071
Clinical Features 1071
Diagnosis 1071
Treatment 1071
Prevention 1071
PARAINFLUENZA VIRUS 1071
Virology 1072
Epidemiology 1072
Clinical Features 1072
Diagnosis 1072
Treatment 1072
Prevention 1072
HUMAN METAPNEUMOVIRUS 1072
Virology 1072
Epidemiology 1072
Clinical Features 1073
Diagnosis 1073
Treatment 1073
Prevention 1073
RHINOVIRUS AND CORONAVIRUS INFECTIONS 1073
Virology 1073
Epidemiology 1073
Clinical Features 1073
Diagnosis 1073
Treatment and Prevention 1073
SEVERE ACUTE RESPIRATORY SYNDROME-RELATED CORONAVIRUS 1073
Virology 1073
Epidemiology 1074
Clinical Features 1074
Diagnosis 1074
Treatment 1074
Prevention 1074
HANTAVIRUS 1074
Virology 1074
Epidemiology 1074
Clinical Features 1075
Diagnosis 1075
Treatment 1075
ADENOVIRUS 1075
Virology 1075
Epidemiology 1075
Clinical Features 1076
Diagnosis 1076
Treatment 1076
Prevention 1076

Community-acquired respiratory viruses (CARVs) are a diverse group of viruses belonging to several families, including the Orthomyxoviridae (influenza A and B), Paramyxoviridae (respiratory syncytial virus, parainfluenza virus, human metapneumovirus), Coronaviridae (coronavirus), Picornaviridae (rhinovirus), and Adenoviridae (adenovirus). CARVs are generally transmitted directly from person to person, through fomites in respiratory secretions or via direct contact with infected secretions.[1] Most infections arise in the community, but nosocomial transmission can occur.[1] Infection control measures are critical to contain the spread of these viruses.[1] In the sections that follow, each of these viruses is discussed in depth.

INFLUENZA

Influenza A and B viruses infect on average 10% to 15% of the population annually (all age groups are affected).[2,3] Influenza causes seasonal outbreaks globally, and (rarely) pandemics.[4] Seasonal influenza epidemics from 1976 through 2001 were responsible for more than 200,000 annual hospitalizations and more than 30,000 influenza-associated deaths (IADs) (all causes) in the United States[5] (Fig. 77-1). The toll is considerably higher during pandemics.[4]

Virology

Influenza virus belongs to the virus family Orthomyxoviridae, which includes *Influenzavirus* A, B, and C.[6] Influenza A and B cause most human infections.[6] Most seasonal epidemics and all recognized pandemics in humans are due to influenza A. Influenza A viruses are characterized by their antigenicity, according to hemagglutinin (H) and neuraminidase (N) proteins; there are 16 H and 9 N subtypes.[6] All antigen subtypes circulate among avian species.[6] Globally, the most common circulating influenza A viruses from 1994 to 2005 included H3N2 (90.6%), H1N1 (8%), and H1N2 (1.1%).[7] There is significant variability among seasons, with H3N2-dominant years being worse than H1N1 years.[2,8]

Influenza viruses have evolved mechanisms that promote antigenic variability. Point mutations in the H gene give rise to new influenza strains of the same H type (termed *antigenic drift;* Fig. 77-2).[3] In this context, existing antibodies may fail to cover the new variant. Antigenic drift mandates modification of influenza vaccines annually.[3] A second mechanism, known as *antigenic shift,* is more dramatic and allows one influenza strain (such as H3N2) to acquire a completely new H or N gene (such as H1 or N1), resulting in a new virus (such as H3N1 or H1N2) (Fig. 77-3).

Pandemic influenza results when the antigenic mutations are dramatically different from previously circulating strains; this could occur by *antigenic shift* or by cross-species transmission of novel H- or N-type viruses.[3] The recent emergence of the highly pathogenic avian viruses (H5N1)[4] is discussed later.

Epidemiology

Influenza is one of the most common and important respiratory illnesses, affecting all ages. In temperate climates, influenza exhibits a

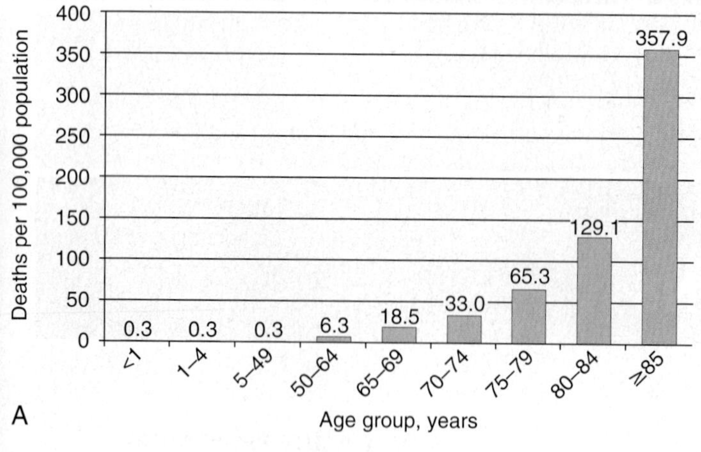

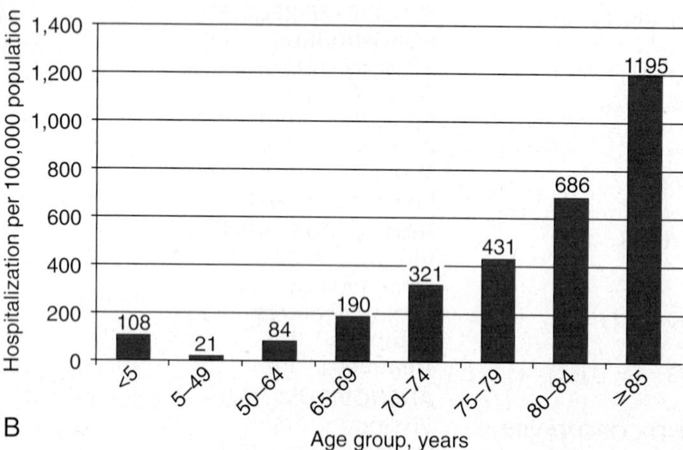

FIGURE 77-1 • A, Influenza-associated mortality rates, by age group, during 1976-2000. **B,** Influenza-associated hospitalization rates, by age group, during 1979-2001. (Data from Thompson et al.[5])

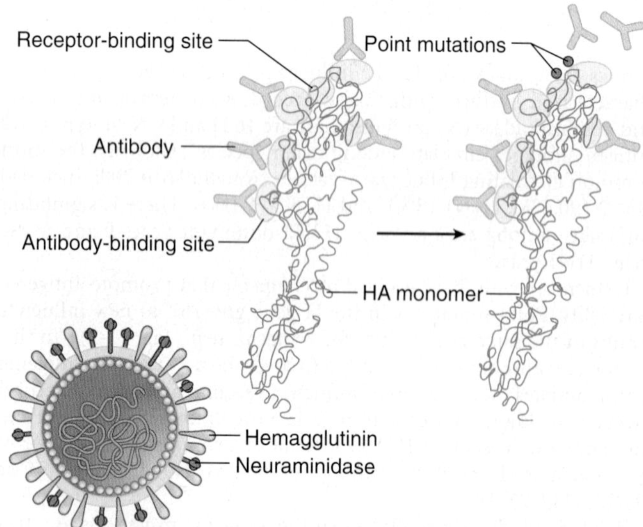

FIGURE 77-2 • Antigenic drift. Structure of a hemagglutinin monomer and location of the five known antibody-binding sites in the HA1 subunit. (Adapted from Treanor J: Influenza virus—outmaneuvering antigenic drift and shift. N Engl J Med 2004;350:218.)

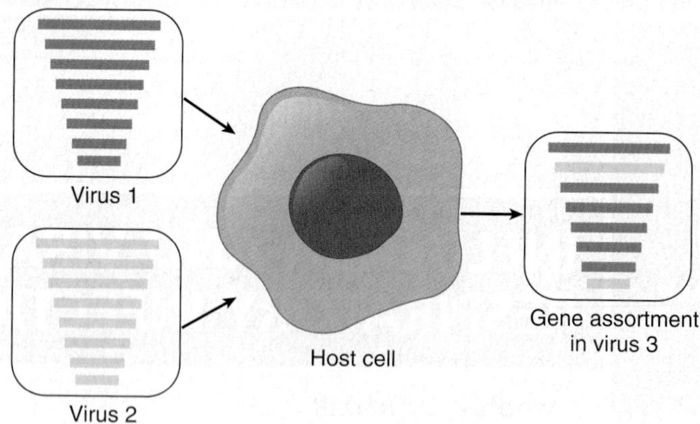

FIGURE 77-3 • Antigenic shift.

seasonal pattern, with peak activity during the winter months (December through March).[2] Local outbreaks abate after 6 to 8 weeks.[2] Influenza A predominates in most seasons, but epidemics of influenza B occur.[9]

The virus is present in high titer in respiratory secretions and is transmitted as a small-particle aerosol generated by coughing and sneezing.[2] Person-to-person spread by direct contact with respiratory secretions may also occur. Children are important as vectors for transmission to adult populations.[10] Spread throughout the general population often includes nosocomial outbreaks in nursing homes and other closed communities.[1]

The severity of influenza epidemics varies among seasons, depending upon the virulence and antigenicity of the predominant circulating strain and immune status of the population at risk. The 1984-1985 influenza season was severe, with an estimated 51,000 IADs in the United States compared to fewer than 8000 IADs during the 1978-1979 season.[8] Approximately 90% of deaths occur among the elderly, in contrast to approximately 150 annual deaths in the United States in children under age 5 years.[8] Influenza and serious complications of influenza are more common in the elderly (age >65 years), children under age 2 years, adults or children with concurrent illness (e.g., pulmonary, cardiac, metabolic), residents of chronic care facilities, and pregnant women.[2,11]

Pandemics occur infrequently but can be devastating.[12] The most recent global pandemics included 1918-1919 (Spanish flu, H1N1; responsible for up to 50 to 100 million deaths worldwide); 1957-1958 (Asian flu, H2N2; >1 million deaths); and 1968-1970 (Hong Kong flu, H3N2; >700,000 deaths).[4] Given the considerable growth of the population worldwide and exponential growth in foreign travel over the past 50 years, another pandemic could be catastrophic (Fig. 77-4).

Clinical Features

Following an incubation period of 2 to 5 days, symptom onset is generally abrupt, distinguishing influenza from other viral respiratory infections. Fever is present in more than 90% of cases; other symptoms include a dry, nonproductive cough, nasal congestion or rhinorrhea, headache, sore throat, and constitutional complaints (e.g., myalgias, malaise, fatigue, prostration).[10,13] Influenza is an important cause of respiratory illness in children.[10] Most influenza infections in children are self-limited, but influenza may be severe in young children (age <2 years) or those with chronic medical conditions.[2] Influenza is associated with increased hospitalizations,[14] outpatient visits,[15] and health care costs[15] in children.

In previously healthy individuals (children or adults), symptoms resolve spontaneously within 5 to 8 days. The course may be protracted, and complications more frequent, in high-risk or immunocompromised patients.[2,16,17] Primary influenza pneumonia, characterized by diffuse interstitial infiltrates and severe hypoxemia, is unusual except during pandemics or in individuals with specific risk factors.[2] Secondary bacterial pneumonia may complicate influenza, usually 7 to

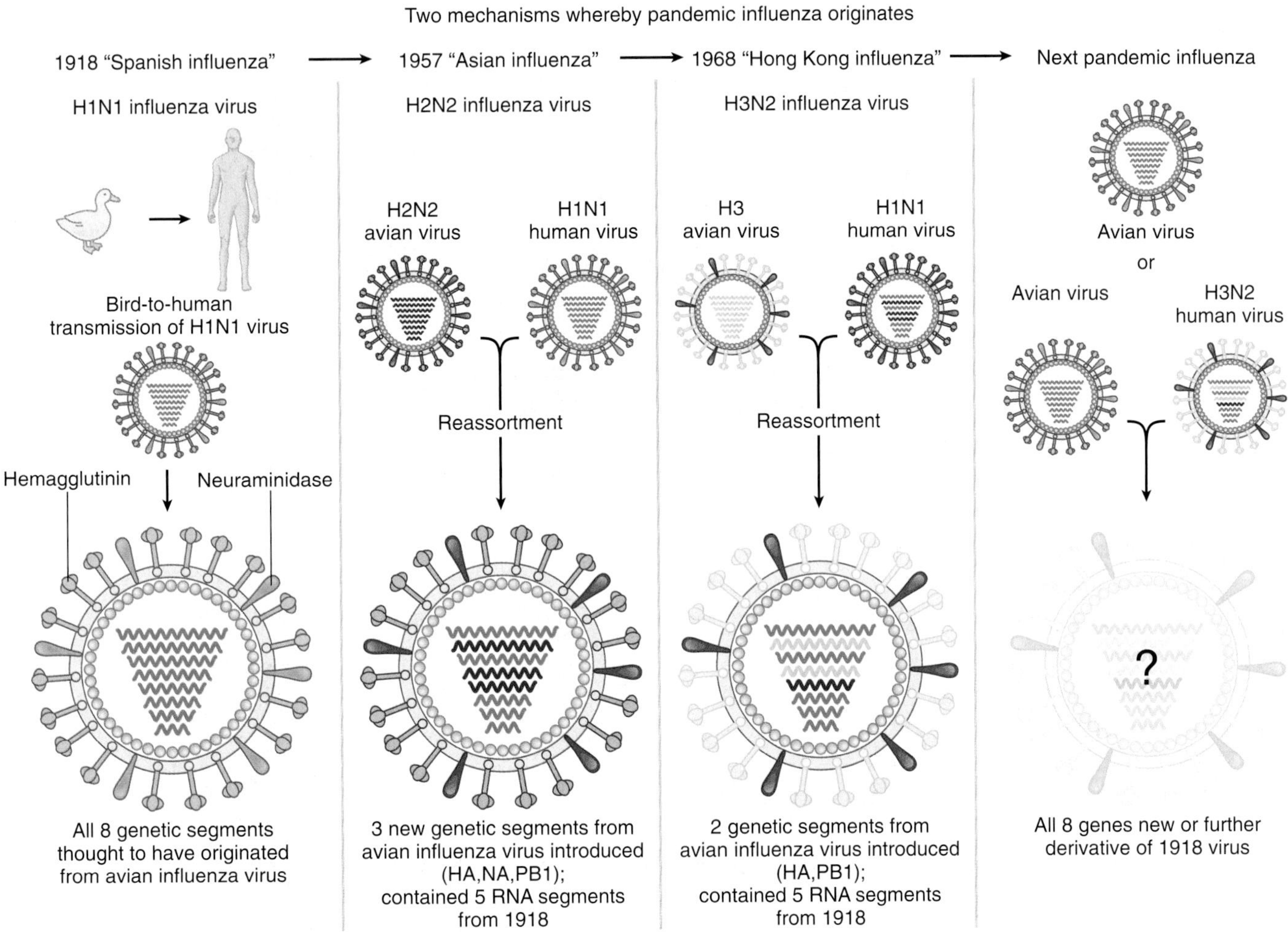

FIGURE 77-4 • The two mechanisms whereby pandemic influenza originates. In 1918, an H1N1 virus closely related to avian viruses adapted to replicate efficiently in humans. In 1957 and in 1968, reassortment events led to new viruses that resulted in pandemic influenza. The 1957 influenza virus (Asian influenza, an H2N2 virus) acquired three genetic segments from an avian species (a hemagglutinin, a neuraminidase, and a polymerase gene, PB1), and the 1968 influenza virus (Hong Kong influenza, an H3N2 virus) acquired two genetic segments from an avian species (hemagglutinin and PB1). Future pandemic strains could arise through either mechanism. (Adapted from Belshe RB. The origins of pandemic influenza—lessons from the 1918 virus. N Engl J Med 2005;353:2209-2211.)

21 days following resolution of the initial illness.[2] Acute respiratory distress syndrome may occur with some influenza strains, likely mediated by a virus-induced cytokine storm.[18]

Serious nonrespiratory complications of influenza are rare, but include encephalopathy, pericarditis, rhabdomyolysis, and renal failure.[2,19] Central nervous system complications are more common in children than adults.[19] Reye's syndrome, a severe neurologic complication of influenza in children, has largely disappeared since the link between aspirin use and Reye's syndrome was discovered.[20]

Diagnosis

Clinical features of influenza are nonspecific.[21] Laboratory confirmation of influenza is necessary if infection control measures and treatment are to be optimized. Culture of respiratory secretions is the gold standard, but can take 3 to 5 days and is expensive and often not available in an outpatient setting. Virus titers are high early in the illness, but fall rapidly in adults. In one study, only 48% of hospitalized elderly persons with confirmed influenza had a positive culture.[21] Commercialized kits allow rapid detection of influenza antigens in less than 1 hour with a sensitivity of 40% to 80%.[6,21] Reverse transcriptase–polymerase chain reaction (RT-PCR) is more sensitive than viral cultures or antigen detection tests, but is less readily available.[10] Rapid diagnostic tests may be invaluable during epidemics in emergency departments and outpatient and inpatient settings.

Treatment

Currently, four drugs are licensed in the United States for the treatment or prophylaxis of influenza.[22] These include the adamantanes (i.e., amantadine and rimantadine) and the neuraminidase inhibitors (NAIs) (e.g., oseltamivir and zanamivir).[23] Currently, NAIs are the therapeutic agents of choice for *treatment or prevention* of influenza infections. Treatment should be considered for patients with influenza-like illness (ILI) in communities where influenza has been documented, especially those with underlying high-risk conditions.[22] Further, patients hospitalized with acute respiratory illness during an epidemic period may be candidates for treatment. Prophylaxis with NAIs is appropriate during influenza seasons for household contacts or asymptomatic high-risk patients such as nursing home residents or staff during an outbreak, or for unvaccinated persons at high risk (e.g., with chronic lung disease, immunosuppressed, etc.).[23,24]

Adamantanes (M2 Inhibitors)

The adamantanes block the influenza A virus M2 ion channel protein, thereby preventing replication within infected cells; these agents have no activity against influenza B[2,22] (Fig. 77-5).

In early studies, both amantadine (Symmetrel; licensed in 1966) and rimantadine (Flumadine; licensed in 1993) were shown to be effective to treat[22,25] or prevent[22] uncomplicated infections due to sensitive influenza A. Amantadine or rimantadine are equally effective, provided that

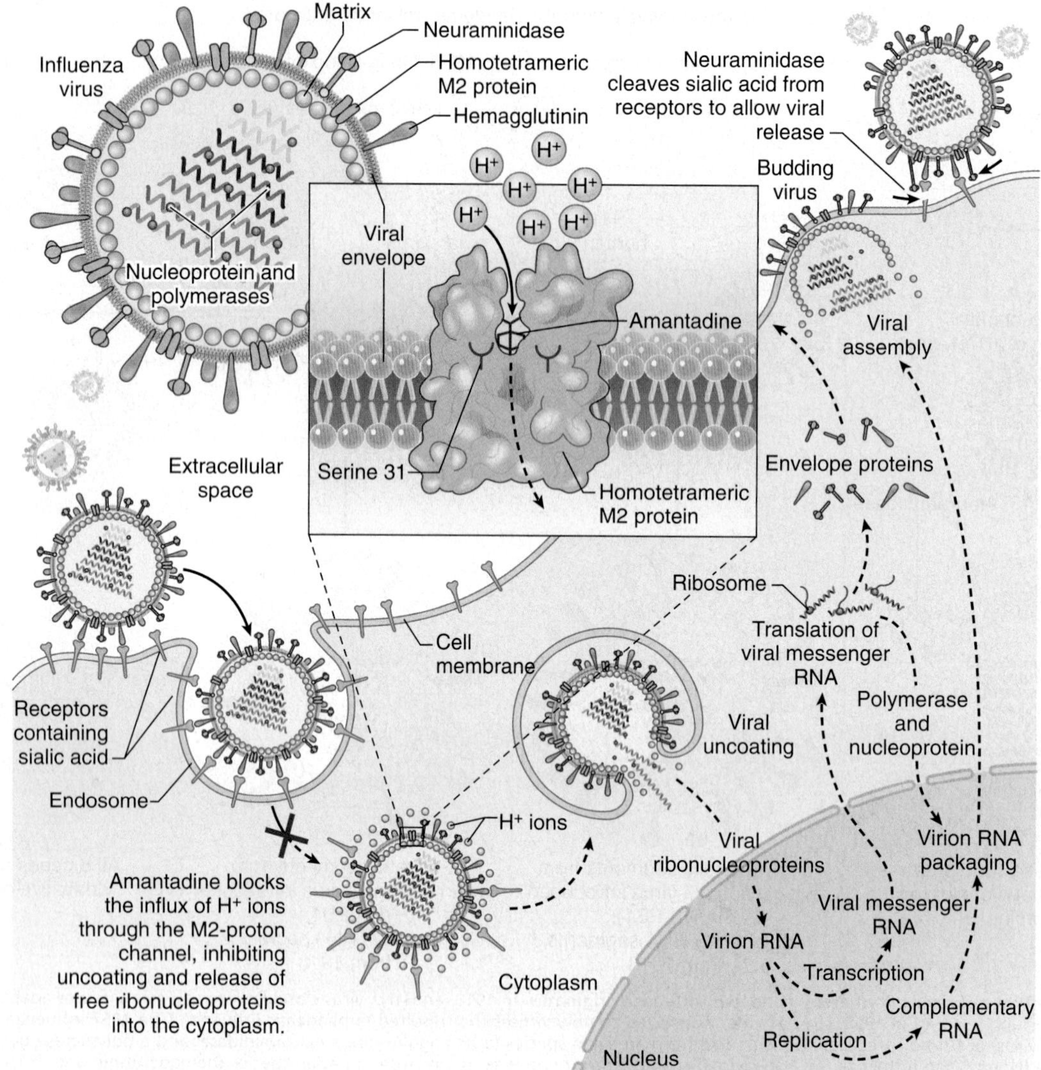

FIGURE 77-5 • Mechanism of action of and development of resistance to M2 inhibitors. In the absence of amantadine, the proton channel mediates an influx of H^+ ions into the infecting virion early in the viral replication cycle, which facilitates the dissociation of the ribonucleoproteins from the virion interior and allows them to be released into the cytoplasm and transported into the cell nucleus. In highly pathogenic avian viruses (H5 and H7), the matrix protein 2 (M2) proton channel protects the hemagglutinin from acid-induced inactivation in the trans-Golgi network during transport to the cell surface. In the presence of amantadine, the channel is blocked and replication is inhibited. The serine at position 31 lies partially in the protein-protein interface and partially in the channel (*inset*). Replacement of serine by a larger asparagine leads to the loss of amantadine binding and the restoration of channel function. Depending on the particular amino acid, other mutations at position 26, 27, 30, or 34 may inhibit amantadine binding or allow binding without the loss of ion channel function. (Adapted from Hayden FG. Antiviral resistance in influenza viruses—implications for management and pandemic response. N Engl J Med 2006;354:785-788.)

the drug is administered within 48 hours of onset of symptoms.[22,25] Importantly, resistance to adamantanes may emerge rapidly.[7,26,27] Resistance to adamantanes is due to single amino acid substitutions within the viral M2 protein[7] that confer cross-resistance to both agents.[22,26] Although resistance to adamantanes among *untreated* individuals has remained low (<1%) through the 1990s,[7] resistance rates to influenza A viruses (H3N2, H1N1, or H1N2) have skyrocketed within the past few years.[7,26] The increase in resistance was weighted heavily by isolates from Asia.[7,28] By 2004-2005, rates of adamantane resistance in selected Asian locales included 96% (China), 72% (Hong Kong), 42% (Singapore), and 36% (South Korea).[27]

Resistance to adamantanes has also escalated dramatically in North America.[7] By the 2005-2006 influenza season in the United States, greater than 90% of isolates of influenza A (H3N2) from the United States or Canada submitted to the Centers for Disease Control and Prevention (CDC) were resistant to adamantanes.[27] In view of these extraordinarily high rates of resistance, adamantanes should not be used for the treatment or prophylaxis of influenza A in the United States.[29] Currently, adamantanes have little role to treat or prevent influenza.

Neuraminidase Inhibitors

NAIs are analogues of *N*-acetylneuraminic acid (the cell surface receptor for influenza viruses) and inhibit the enzyme neuraminidase, reducing viral replication[22,23] (Fig. 77-6). Inhibition of neuraminidase reduces viral replication.[22] NAIs are active against both influenza A and B, but activity against influenza B is less.[9,23] Currently available NAIs include oseltamivir and zanamivir.

Oseltamivir. Oral oseltamivir (Tamiflu) is approved to *treat* infections due to influenza A or B and for *prophylaxis* of influenza among persons greater than 1 year old. Oseltamivir is not approved for infants less than 1 year of age since studies are lacking in this age group.[23] For treating acute influenza, the dose in adults or children greater than 12 years old is 75 mg twice daily for 5 days; the dose is lower in children 1 to 12 years old (adjusted for weight).[22,30] For prophylaxis, the dose is 75 mg daily for 10 days.[22,30]

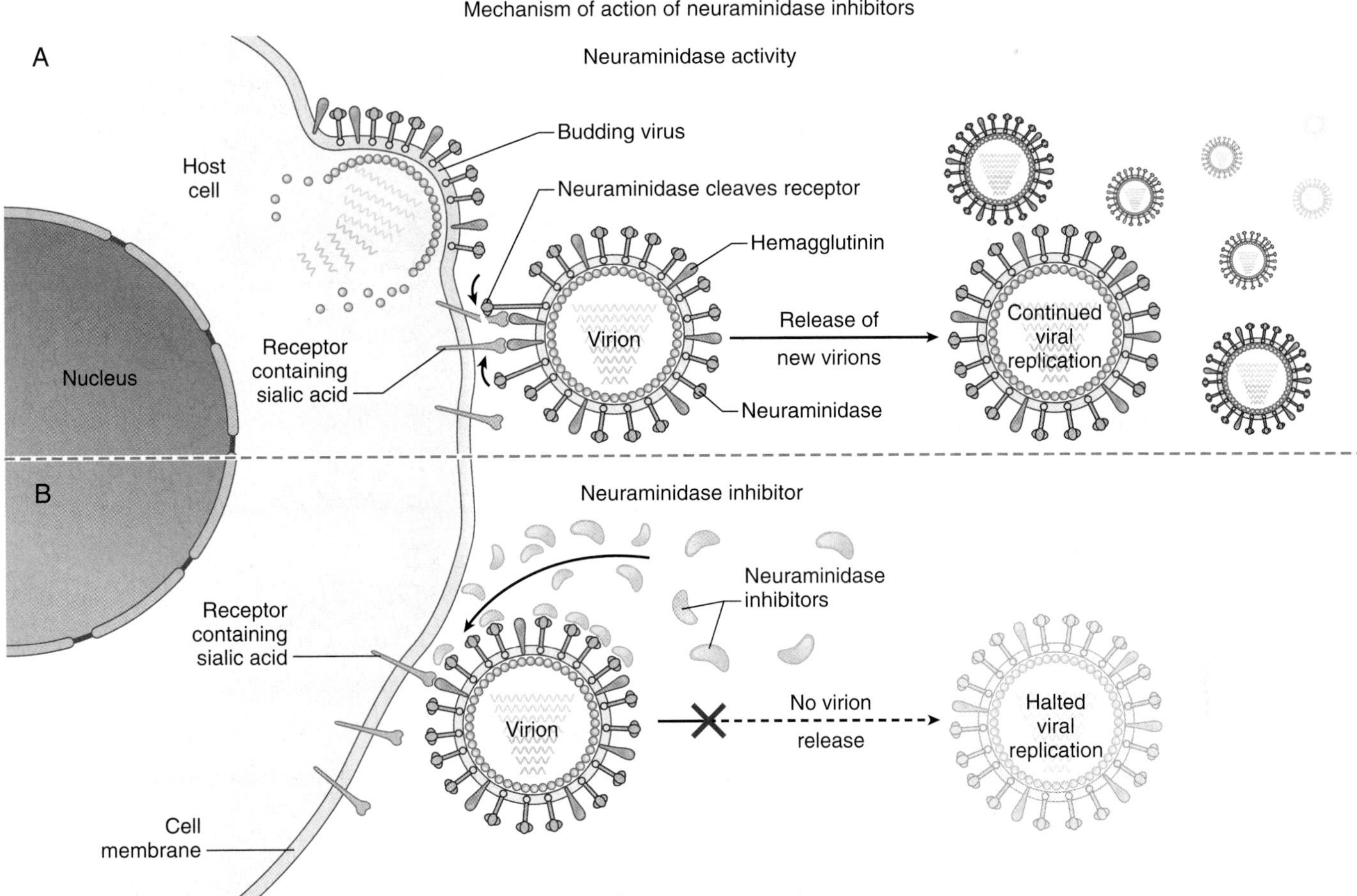

FIGURE 77-6 • Mechanism of action of neuroaminidase inhibitors. A, Action of neuraminidase in the continued replication of virions in influenza infection. The replication is blocked by neuraminidase inhibitors **(B)**, which prevent virions from being released from the surface of infected cells. (From Moscona A. Neuraminidase inhibitors for influenza. N Engl J Med 2005;353:1363-1373.)

Early treatment with oral oseltamivir in patients with acute influenza (A or B) shortens the course and reduces complications in previously healthy children or adults and high-risk patients.[9,25,31] NAIs are efficacious only if administered within 48 hours of onset of symptoms.[23,25] Duration of symptoms is shortened by 1 to 2 days in patients receiving NAIs (compared to placebo).[23] Large studies in North America found that patients with ILI treated with oseltamivir during the influenza seasons from 1999 to 2004 had lower rates of pneumonia, hospitalizations, or deaths (within 30 days) compared to untreated patients.[31,32]

In controlled, randomized trials, administration of oseltamivir as prophylaxis reduced the risk of influenza in unvaccinated healthy adults, household contacts, nursing home residents, and the elderly.[30,33] Oseltamivir prophylaxis was efficacious in a cohort of 45 hematopoietic stem cell transplant recipients at high risk.[24] The use of oseltamivir during influenza outbreaks in nursing homes was associated with reductions in hospitalizations, deaths, and antibiotic use compared to patients receiving either amantadine or no therapy.[34]

Zanamivir. Zanamivir (Relenza) is approved to *treat* infections due to influenza A or B and for *prophylaxis* of influenza in children greater than 5 years of age.[22,23] Zanamivir is administered by a dry powder inhaler (Diskhaler) delivered directly to the respiratory tract.[23] For treating acute influenza, the dose is 10 mg twice daily for 5 days (children or adults).[22] For prophylaxis (e.g., contacts of index cases), the dose is 10 mg once daily for 10 days.[22] Zanamivir achieves high concentrations in the respiratory tract (1000 times the 50% inhibitory concentration for neuraminidase).[23] The inhibitory effect starts within 10 seconds.[23] These properties reduce the chance for emergence of resistant viruses. The major drawback to zanamivir is the inability of young children or adults with neurologic or muscular deficits to use the Diskhaler.

Zanamivir (10 mg twice daily for 5 days) is effective therapy for influenza A or B in adults and children (age >5 years) and has minimal toxicity.[22] The duration of symptoms was shorted by 1 to 2.5 days, and complications were reduced, provided zanamivir was initiated within 30 hours of the onset of symptoms.[22] Inhaled zanamivir (10 mg once daily for 10 days) was effective (55% to 80%) as chemoprophylaxis of influenza in healthy adults and healthy household contacts (children >5 years old or adults).[2,35]

Adverse Effects with NAIs. Adverse effects with NAIs are uncommon.[22,23,29] Resistance to NAIs is rare[36-38] but can arise by single amino acid substitutions at N or H residues.[39] Mutations at N residues are more clinically relevant.[39] Mutations in N that prevent oseltamivir from binding to the N active do *not* affect zanamivir.[37] Resistance to oseltamivir was noted in 4% to 8% of children and less than 1% of adults after treatment with oseltamivir.[2,40] Higher rates of oseltamivir-resistant mutants were detected in Japan (18%) in children treated with oseltamivir (possibly reflecting subtherapeutic doses).[41] The recent epidemic of avian influenza A (H5N1) infection in Asia[42] raises the possibility that NAI-resistant mutants could emerge as a result of increasing exposure to oseltamivir.[43] Importantly, most oseltamivir-resistant isolates remain susceptible to zanamivir.[37]

Prevention

Vaccines are the cornerstone for control of influenza.[22,44,45] Influenza vaccines are developed annually, with input from the World Health Organization (WHO) and national authorities.[46] Viruses must be

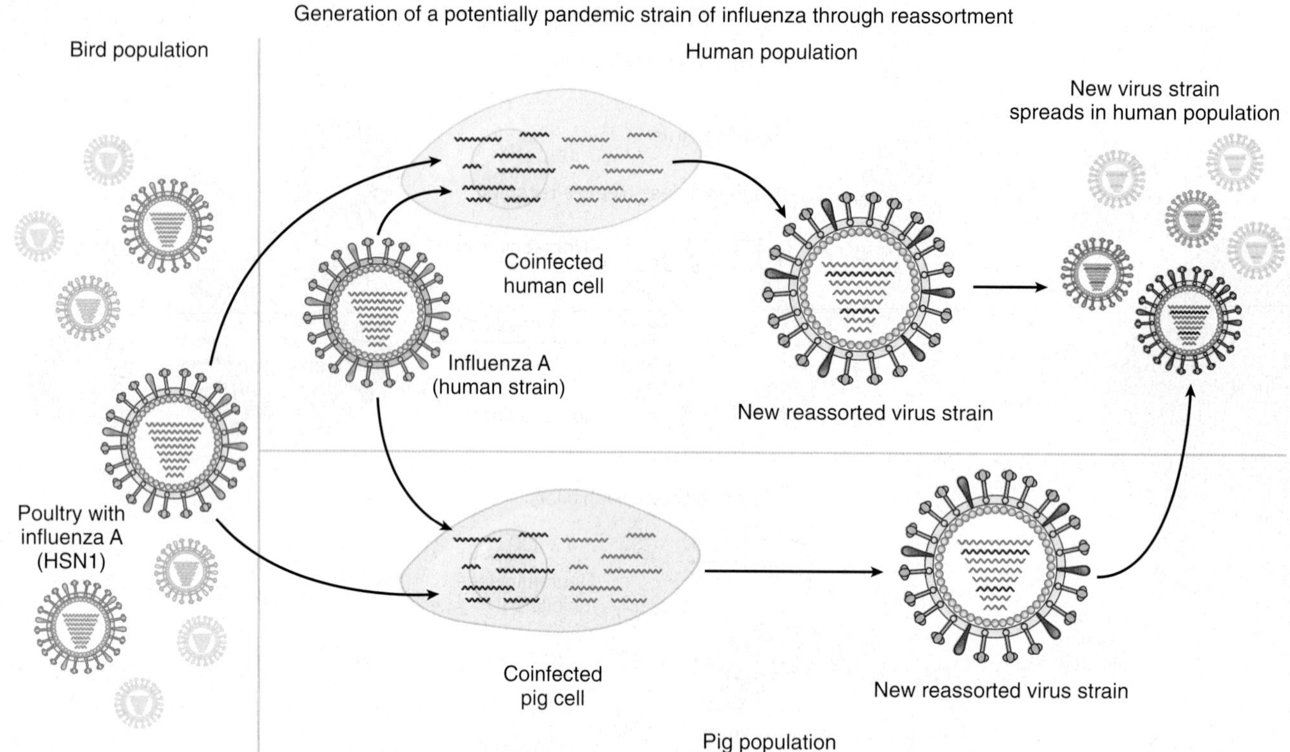

FIGURE 77-7 • Generation of a potentially pandemic strain of influenza through reassortment. (From Hien T, de Jong M, Farrar J. Avian influenza—a challenge to global health care structures. N Engl J Med 2004;351:2363-2365.)

reformulated annually, since genetic mutations arise continuously in influenza viruses in a process termed *antigenic drift.*[46] Given the potential for pandemic influenza (e.g., with the antigen shift or the avian H5N1 strain) (Fig. 77-7),[12] the WHO has developed an action plan to increase vaccine supply.[46] However, current technologies for developing vaccines (i.e., egg-based manufacturing process) are slow, and existing supplies of vaccines would be inadequate in the face of a global pandemic.[12]

Currently available influenza vaccines include the trivalent inactivated vaccines (TIVs) and live, attenuated influenza vaccine (LAIV).[47] Both vaccines contain the predicted antigenic variants of influenza A (H3N2, H1N1) and influenza B viruses.[3] The inactivated vaccine is administered intramuscularly; LAIV is given as an intranasal spray (FluMist; MedImmune).[3] TIV evokes a higher systemic response (i.e., serum immunoglobulin G antibody response) whereas LAIV elicits a better immunoglobulin A mucosal response at the site where viruses enter the body.[3] In the United States, TIV is approved for individuals greater than 6 months of age; LAIV is approved for healthy persons 5 to 49 years of age.[48] No vaccines are approved for infants under the age of 6 months.

Provided the strains encompassed by the vaccine match the circulating epidemic strain, inactivated vaccines provided 70% to 100% protection among healthy adults and 30% to 60% protection among the elderly or young children.[22,47] Serum antibody responses to influenza vaccination may be blunted in the elderly, immunocompromised individuals, and preschool children.[22] In adults, LAIV may be less effective than TIV, which may reflect reduced activity against influenza B viruses.[47]

Influenza vaccination is beneficial in adults greater than 65 years old living in the community[45,49] or nursing homes.[13] Benefits of vaccination include lower mortality (all causes), hospitalizations, and pneumonias.[2,45,49] Further, influenza vaccination reduced mortality, hospitalizations, and outpatient visits for patients less than 65 years of age with concurrent medical conditions.[50] Additionally, vaccination of health care workers is highly effective in protecting high-risk patients.[44,51,52]

Influenza vaccination (either TIV or LAIV) in healthy children reduces the incidence of laboratory-confirmed cases of influenza and acute otitis media (AOM).[53-55] Vaccination of children in day care centers or schools reduced the incidence of ILI among family contacts or in the community at large.[2,55] Indirect benefits of vaccinating children include fewer parental days lost from work and less impaired work productivity.[3]

Recommendations for annual influenza vaccination are published annually by the CDC. In 2007, the CDC recommended annual influenza vaccination for the following populations: children or adults at high risk for complications of influenza, close contacts of high-risk persons, all children ages 6 to 59 months, and all adults greater than 50 years old (regardless of health status)[29] (Box 77-1). Indications for vaccination continue to evolve. Many experts favor expanding influenza vaccination, potentially toward universal vaccination.[44]

Adverse effects from influenza vaccination are minimal.[22] With the inactivated vaccine, mild soreness of the arm at the site of vaccination may persist for 1 to 2 days.[22] Serious adverse effects are rare. The vaccine is contraindicated in patients who are allergic to eggs, but even in this context serious hypersensitivity reactions to the vaccine are rare. LAIV is well tolerated[3,47,56] but should *not* be administered to immunocompromised individuals.

AVIAN INFLUENZA

Avian influenza is a highly virulent H5N1 subtype of influenza.[4] The ongoing global epidemic of epizootic avian influenza infection has been responsible for the death or destruction of greater than 140 million birds.[4] Infections due to avian influenza viruses are rare in humans, but the antigenic novelty of H5N1 suggests the potential for pandemic spread.[4]

Virology

Infections in humans due to H7 and H9 avian influenza viruses are typically mild. By contrast, the H5N1 avian virus causes serious respi-

BOX 77-1 ANNUAL VACCINATION AGAINST INFLUENZA

Annual vaccination against influenza is recommended for

- All persons, including school-aged children, who want to reduce the risk of becoming ill with influenza or of transmitting influenza to others;
- All children aged 6-59 months (i.e., 6 months-4 years);
- All persons aged 50 years and older;
- Children and adolescents (aged 6 months-18 years) receiving long-term aspirin therapy who therefore might be at risk for experiencing Reye's syndrome after influenza virus infection;
- Women who will be pregnant during the influenza season;
- Adults and children who have chronic pulmonary (including asthma), cardiovascular (except hypertension), renal, hepatic, hematological or metabolic disorders (including diabetes mellitus);
- Adults and children who have immunosuppression (including immunosuppression caused by medications or by human immunodeficiency virus);
- Adults and children who have any condition (e.g., cognitive dysfunction, spinal cord injuries, seizure disorders, or other neuromuscular disorders) that can compromise respiratory function or the handling of respiratory secretions or that can increase the risk for aspiration;
- Residents of nursing homes and other chronic-care facilities;
- Health-care personnel;
- Healthy household contacts (including children) and caregivers of children aged <5 years and adults aged 50 years and older, with particular emphasis on vaccinating contacts of children aged <6 months; and
- Healthy household contacts (including children) and caregivers of persons with medical conditions that put them at higher risk for severe complications from influenza.

From Prevention and control of influenza—recommendations of the Advisory Committee on Immunization Practices (ACIP). MMWR Recomm Rep 2007;56(RR06):1-54.

ratory infections, with case fatality rates of greater than 50%.[4] Sequence analysis suggests that the current H5N1 virus originated by reassortment between multiple co-circulating avian influenza strains prevalent in Hong Kong in 1997.[57] Certain unique structural features in the H5N1 virus are present among highly pathogenic viruses infecting chickens but are not common among the avian viruses circulating among wild birds.[4] This suggests that transmission to humans originated from poultry rather than wild birds. The avian viruses exhibit preferential binding to sialic acid α2-3 linkages, which are sparse in the human upper respiratory tract.[58] This may explain the absence of human-to-human transmission.

Epidemiology

Outbreaks of severe influenza in humans with highly virulent H5N1 strains derived from infected poultry were reported in China and Southeast Asia in 2003.[59] The first known transmission of H5N1 viruses from birds to humans took place in 1997, shortly following an outbreak of sick geese on a farm in Guangdong Province of China.[60] A fatal infection in May 1997 in Hong Kong was followed by 17 cases (5 died) in November-December 1997.[4] The outbreak ceased after Hong Kong culled 1.5 million poultry in 3 days and banned the import of poultry from mainland China.[57] No further human cases were recognized until February 2003, when at least two confirmed cases were identified in Hong Kong.[61] Subsequent cases in China, Vietnam, Thailand, Cambodia, and other Southeast Asian countries were followed by human cases in Europe, Russia, the Middle East, and Africa[4,59] (Fig. 77-8). The virus has spread along the flyways of migratory birds to more than 30 countries worldwide.[4] By August 2006, 238 cases had been cited in humans, with 139 deaths (58%).[4,59] Large-scale culling operations and intensified surveillance led to eradication of H5N1 infection in poultry in some countries. However, in many countries, H5N1 infection is endemic in wild birds and poultry.[4] In countries where human contact with poultry is common, the likelihood of further adaptation of the virus to humans and transmission between humans is high.

Clinical Features

H7 and H9 avian influenza viruses are highly lethal in poultry, but typically cause mild symptoms in humans (e.g., conjunctivitis with subtype H7[62,63] or mild ILI with H9N2).[59,64] In sharp contrast, human cases of H5N1 have been characterized by severe pneumonia with high fatality rates (58%).[59] Ninety percent of cases occurred in individuals less than 40 years old.[59] Most cases had close contact with poultry in the week preceding the illness.[42] Human-to-human transmission has been rare.[65]

The most common symptoms among documented cases of H5N1 include fever (98%), cough (88%), dyspnea (62%), rhinorrhea (55%), sore throat (52%), diarrhea (39%), myalgias (29%), headache (28%), and abdominal pain (23%).[42] Diarrhea may precede the onset of respiratory symptoms. Pulmonary infiltrates on chest radiographs were noted in 88% of cases[42]; this likely overestimates the true incidence since asymptomatic or mild cases may have been missed. Elevated liver enzymes, lymphopenia, and thrombocytopenia were noted in 50% to 67% of cases.[4,42] Pathology revealed diffuse alveolar damage, reactive hemophagocytosis in the bone marrow, and lymphoid depletion in the spleen and lymph nodes.[4]

Diagnosis

Cultures of pharyngeal or nasal swabs or respiratory secretions may confirm the diagnosis,[42] but should be performed only in laboratories meeting biosafety level III or higher requirements.[4] Rapid antigen tests are insensitive.[4] RT-PCR methods are more sensitive and specific, and do not require handling of live virus.[4]

Treatment

Because of the high risk of nosocomial spread, patients with suspected H5N1 should be isolated and placed in negative pressure rooms (if available).[4] Strict infection control measures among health care workers and all contacts are mandatory. Antiviral treatment should be initiated as early as possible, and should be continued if active viral replication continues.[42] Controlled trials evaluating adamantanes to treat H5N1 infections in humans are lacking. However, resistance to adamantanes is considerable in some regions. Point mutations in the M2 region (conferring resistant to adamantanes) were detected in greater than 95% of H5N1 isolates from Vietnam and Thailand but fewer than 10% of isolates from Indonesia and China.[66] Because of the potential for rapid emergence of resistance, adamantanes should not be used irrespective of in vitro susceptibility.[4]

NAIs display in vitro activity against H5N1, but controlled trials assessing these agents in humans are lacking. Currently, the WHO recommends oseltamivir as the first-line drug to treat suspected H5N1 infections.[4] Because humans lack immunity against H5N1, a higher dose (150 mg twice daily) and longer duration (7 to 10 days) should be considered.[4] Resistance to oseltamivir has been detected in some treated patients.[4] Some oseltamivir-resistant isolates displaying the H274Y mutation remain susceptible to zanamivir.[37]

Prevention

Chemoprophylaxis with oseltamivir or zanamivir should be considered for patients at high risk for transmission (e.g., household or close contact, exposure to infected poultry or environmental source, health care workers or laboratory personnel without appropriate protec-

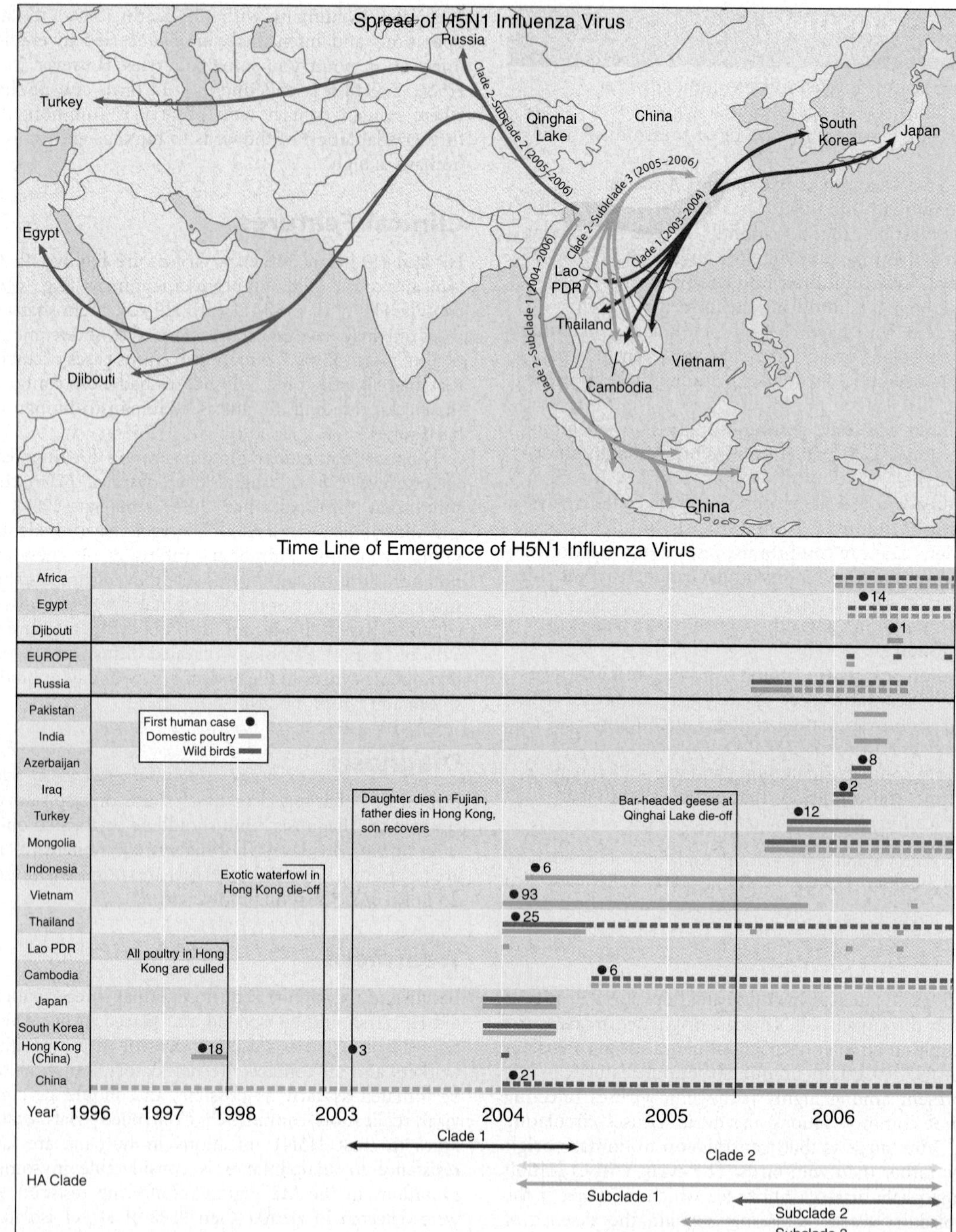

FIGURE 77-8 • The spread of H5N1 influenza virus and time line showing its emergence. The *shaded area* across southern China is the hypothetical epicenter for the emergence of H5N1 clades and subclades. The H5N1 viruses are being perpetuated in the domestic birds of the region, despite the use of universal vaccination of all domestic poultry. The *red dot* in the time line denotes the occurrence of the first human case, followed by the number of confirmed human cases in that country. The *green and blue solid bars* represent documented H5N1 infection in domestic poultry and wild birds, and *dashed bars* indicate that H5N1 in the avian population is suspected. These limited surveillance data are adapted from the World Health Organization and the U.N. Food and Agriculture Organization (*http://www.fao.org*). HA, hemagglutinin. (Adapted from Webster RG, Govorkova EA. H5N1 influenza—continuing evolution and spread. N Engl J Med 2006;355:2174-2177.)

tion).[4] Vaccines against H5N1 are not currently available, but research and development in this area are ongoing.[67]

RESPIRATORY SYNCYTIAL VIRUS

Respiratory syncytial virus (RSV) is a common respiratory virus affecting persons of all ages.[68,69] The spectrum of RSV disease ranges from a mild "cold" to severe respiratory failure.[68,69] RSV is the leading cause of lower respiratory tract infection in young children but is also an important pathogen in adults,[70] particularly in the elderly[71] or patients with comorbidities.[68,70,72]

Virology

RSV is an enveloped RNA virus within the family Paramyxoviridae and the genus *Pneumovirus*.[68] Human RSV isolates are classified into two major groups (A and B) based primarily upon antigenic differences in the G protein.[68] Both A and B strains circulate concurrently, with A

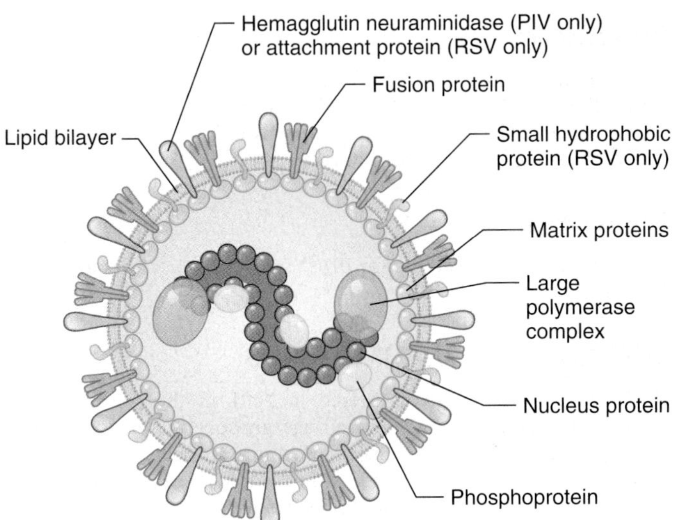

FIGURE 77-9 • Structure of respiratory syncytial virus (RSV) and parainfluenza virus (PIV).

strains usually predominating.[69] Several distinct genotypes exist; annual changes in the dominant strains may evade immune defenses, leading to frequent reinfections[69] (Fig. 77-9).

Epidemiology

RSV is the chief cause of hospitalization for respiratory tract infections (RTIs) in children,[69] and is second to influenza as a cause of serious viral RTIs in adults.[68,71,73,74] Primary RSV infection is nearly universal by age 2; due to incomplete immunity, reinfections are common throughout life.[68,69] In adults, RSV infections are more common in those with comorbidities (e.g., pulmonary or cardiac disorders), impaired immunity, or advanced age.[68,71] However, RSV may infect previously healthy adults.[75] Epidemiologic studies implicated RSV in 3% to 5% of cases of community-acquired pneumonia in adults and in 6% to 22% of acute exacerbations of chronic obstructive pulmonary disease (COPD).[68,73] Outbreaks of RSV infections have been described in closed populations (e.g., nursing homes, senior day care centers, health care workers,[68] and military recruits in training[75]).

Clinical Features

The spectrum of RSV (in both children and adults) ranges from a trivial cold to severe (sometimes fatal) respiratory failure.[68] In infants, RSV typically presents as bronchiolitis, with low-grade fever, rhinorrhea, cough, wheezing, and poor feeding.[68,69] Physical examination reveals crackles and expiratory wheezing. In severe cases, intercostal retraction, hypoxemia, and respiratory failure may ensue. The disease usually resolves spontaneously, but cough or bronchial hyperreactivity may persist for days or even weeks. In young adults, RSV typically gives rise to mild upper respiratory tract (URT) symptoms (e.g., nasal congestion, rhinorrhea, sore throat) that resolve over 4 to 10 days.[68] However, cough, wheezing, dyspnea, and a protracted course may occur.[68,69] Symptoms of RSV and influenza overlap, but nasal symptoms, cough, wheezing, and sputum are more common with RSV, whereas myalgias are more common with influenza.[76] Even in previously healthy adults, RSV may cause missed work days and incurs economic costs.[68,69] Severe RSV pneumonia is uncommon, but can occur in elderly patients or those with comorbidities[71,76] or (rarely) in previously normal adults.[68,70]

Chest radiographs in RSV pneumonia are variable, and range from faint interstitial opacities (mimicking heart failure) to lobar consolidation.[68,76] Concomitant infection with bacterial pathogens has been noted in 15% to 30% of patients with RSV pneumonia.[68,76] RSV may be a cause of exacerbations of asthma[68,71] or COPD[77,78] in adults (particularly during the winter months) and was linked to a more rapid decline in lung function in a cohort of COPD patients.[79]

Diagnosis

Laboratory diagnosis of RSV can be established via four methods: viral culture, antigen detection by immunofluorescence assay (IFA) or enzyme immune assay (EIA), RNA detection by RT-PCR, and serologies.[68] Sensitivity of cultures or antigen detection ranges from 9% to 45%; sensitivity of RT-PCR is higher (60% to 90%).[68] RT-PCR is sensitive (>70%) and specific (99%),[68] and is the preferred method to detect RSV. RT-PCR may be obtained from nasal swabs, nasal washes, sputum, or bronchoalveolar lavage fluid (BALF).[68] In adults, sputum or BALF are more sensitive than nasal specimens.[68] Unfortunately, RT-PCR is complex, expensive, and not available in many hospitals. Serologies are useful in epidemiologic surveys, but are of limited practical value in individual patients.[68] Given the limitations of diagnostic methods, and limited therapeutic options (discussed later), an aggressive diagnostic evaluation for RSV is rarely performed in clinical practice. However, nasal or BALF cultures and antigen detection assays should be considered for patients with severe disease or immunocompromised status.[68] RT-PCR is reserved for research or commercial laboratories in selected high-risk patients.

Treatment

Treatment is supportive. Bronchodilators may be useful in patients with wheezing or a history of asthma or COPD.[71] Aerosolized ribavirin is approved for RSV infections in infants, but not all studies cited benefit.[68] Ribavirin is difficult to administer, requiring continuous inhalation by face mask or tent for 18 hr/day.[68] Alternatively, high-dose ribavirin (i.e., 2 g aerosolized for 2 hr three times daily) may be considered.[80] One multicenter trial randomized 14 hematopoietic stem cell transplant (HSCT) recipients with RSV URT infections to aerosolized ribavirin (2 gm t.i.d.) or standard care.[80] Progression to pneumonia was noted in one of nine patients receiving ribavirin compared to two of five patients receiving supportive care ($P = 0.51$). At 10 days, viral loads were lower in ribavirin recipients ($P = 0.07$). These data are insufficient to judge efficacy. Currently the role of ribavirin (either aerosolized or intravenous) in adults remains controversial. In a nonrandomized trial, RSV-IVIG (a human polyclonal immunoglobulin with high neutralizing antibody titers), combined with inhaled ribavirin, decreased viral shedding and was associated with lower mortality in HSCT recipients with RSV pneumonia.[81]

Palivizumab (Synagis) (a humanized monoclonal antibody directed against the fusion protein of RSV) is approved for prophylaxis against RSV (once monthly for 5 months during winter season) in high-risk infants.[68] However, in a randomized trial of 43 immunocompetent children with RSV infection, palivizumab ($n = 22$) was no better than placebo ($n = 21$).[82] Further, a retrospective study of 40 allogeneic HSCT recipients (mostly adolescents) with symptomatic RSV infection found that palivizumab (administered to 19 patients) had no effect on survival or clinical end points.[83]

Prevention

No RSV vaccine is currently available, but several candidate vaccines are under development.[67,68] Data regarding passive immunization with intravenous immune globulin (IVIG) or palivizumab in adults are lacking. Since RSV is transmitted by fomites and large droplets, infection control (particularly handwashing) is important to limit the spread of nosocomial RSV.[68] Masks are not required because RSV is not transmitted via aerosol.[68]

PARAINFLUENZA VIRUS

Parainfluenza viruses (PIVs) cause a spectrum of respiratory illnesses similar to those caused by RSV, but are usually milder.[69] Infection is limited to the URT in 40% to 60% of cases, and croup (laryngotracheobronchitis) is a cardinal symptom, noted in 10% to 44%; lower respiratory tract infections (LRTI) are infrequent (<10%) in immunocompetent patients.[69,84] PIV typically infects children less than 3 years of age, but reinfections may occur in adults, particularly the elderly or those with pulmonary disease[77,78] or immunosuppression.[16,69]

Virology

PIV types 1, 2, 3, and 4 are enveloped RNA virus within the family Paramyxoviridae[69] (see Fig. 77-9).

Epidemiology

Most children are infected with PIV within the first 2 years of life. While URT symptoms predominate, parainfluenza is second only to RSV (and possibly human metapneumovirus [hMPV]) as a cause of viral bronchiolitis and pneumonia in children.[67,69] Most children are infected with PIV type 3 by age 2 years and by types 1 and 2 by age 5 years.[69] PIV type 4 is rare.[16,69] Pneumonia or bronchitis from type 3 PIV occurs primarily in infants less than 6 months old.[69]

PIV infections exhibit distinct seasonal patterns.[69] Type 1 PIV causes the largest outbreaks, with sharp rises in autumn of odd-numbered years.[69] PIV type 2 infections are less predictable but usually follow type 1 outbreaks. Type 3 PIV infections occur annually, usually in the spring and summer. A seasonal pattern has not been noted for PIV type 4.

PIV replicates in the nasopharyngeal epithelium and spreads to the lower respiratory tract 1 to 3 days later.[69] Transmission occurs by close or direct contact with large droplets or fomites.[69] The duration of viral shedding in healthy people is approximately 1 week, but PIV shedding for greater than 4 weeks has been noted in immunocompromised patients.[16,85]

Infections with PIV are less common than RSV in children and adults, and are typically milder. PIV can infect COPD patients during peak seasons[77,78] and can infect the elderly or healthy adults. In a cohort of senior day care attendees, PIV was implicated in 2.7% of acute respiratory infections; RSV accounted for 21%.[86] In a study of respiratory infections in 256 military recruits, PIV was isolated by culture in 3%; adenovirus (AdV) was detected in 48% and influenza in 11%.[75] PIV infections were cited in 2% to 7% of adult and pediatric HSCT recipients.[16,85,87,88] Data on solid organ transplant (SOT) recipients are limited.

Clinical Features

PIVs cause a spectrum of respiratory illnesses similar to those caused by RSV, but are milder.[69] Most are upper respiratory tract infections (URTIs); 30% to 50% are complicated by AOM.[69] Croup is the cardinal symptom of PIV infections (noted in 10% to 44%), and is the main cause of hospitalization from PIV infections in children 2 to 6 years of age.[69] The lower respiratory tract is involved in only 15% of cases; 2.8 of 1000 children with such infections require hospitalization.[69] Similar to RSV, PIV may precipitate exacerbations of asthma in children and adults.[69] Reinfections may occur in adults, particularly the elderly.[69] PIV may cause bronchitis or pneumonia in organ transplant recipients[87] and human immunodeficiency virus–infected or immunocompromised[16] patients. However, even among HSCT recipients, PIV infections are often confined to the URT. In a series of 198 HSCT patients with PIV-3 infection, 87% presented with URTI symptoms only; 6% had simultaneous URTI and LRTI symptoms.[88] The disease progressed from URTI to LRTI in 25 patients (13%). Progression was more likely among patients receiving corticosteroids.[88] PIV is a risk factor for airflow decline in HSCT recipients and a cause of long-term pulmonary complications.[89]

Diagnosis

As with other viruses, laboratory diagnosis of PIV can be established by viral culture, antigen detection (by IFA or EIA), RT-PCR, or serologies.[69] Given the low prevalence of PIV in adults, and the lack of effective therapy, diagnostic assays are rarely performed in clinical practice.

Treatment

No licensed or proven therapy for PIV is available. Ribavirin has in vitro activity against PIV, and aerosolized or intravenous ribavirin has been used to treat or prevent PIV infections in immunocompromised hosts,[87,88,90] but efficacy remains uncertain.[16,69]

Prevention

Currently there is no vaccine for PIV,[16] but several vaccines are being developed.[67]

HUMAN METAPNEUMOVIRUS

hMPV, a paramyxovirus discovered in 2001 in the Netherlands,[91] causes upper and lower RTIs in all age groups, but predominantly affects young children[92,93] and immunocompromised or frail, elderly patients.[94] The spectrum of hMPV is similar to RSV, ranging from mild URTIs to severe bronchiolitis and pneumonia.[91,92,95,96]

Virology

hMPV is a member of the Paramyxoviridae family, Pneumovirinae subfamily, and *Metapneumovirus* genus[94] (Fig. 77-10). Two major genotypes (A and B) and four subgroups (A1, A2, B1, and B2) are recognized.[93,97] One research group suggested that genotype A may be more virulent than genotype B,[97] but others found no difference between genotypes.[93] The predominant genotype (A or B) may vary between seasons.[93,94]

Epidemiology

hMPV has a global distribution.[93,94,98] It was first identified in 2001,[91] but has been circulating (based on serologic studies) for 50 years in the Netherlands[98] and at least 15 to 20 years in North America.[99] hMPV accounts for 5% to 12% of acute RTIs in children (next to RSV and influenza).[93,97,98,100] Serologic studies suggest that virtually all children are infected by the age of 5 to 10 years.[91,94] More than three quarters of hMPV infections are in children less than 2 years old,[101] but all ages may be affected.[95,98] Infections due to hMPV (both children and adults) are more common in immunosuppressed individuals.[102-104] In adults, hMPV accounts for 2% to 7% of acute RTIs[101,105] or ILIs and may be implicated in 5% to 10% of acute exacerbations of asthma,[92] COPD,[106] or congestive heart failure.[106]

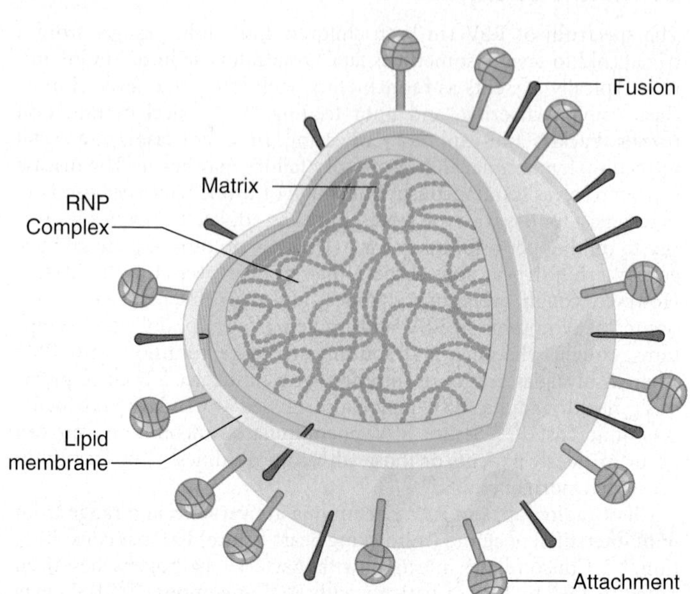

FIGURE 77-10 • Human metapneumovirus.

Transmission of hMPV is similar to RSV (i.e., via respiratory droplets and hand-to-mouth or hand-to-eye contact with contaminated surfaces).[94] Outbreaks of hMPV respiratory infections have been described in long-term care facilities[95,107] and health care workers (i.e., case contacts).[107] Like other respiratory viruses, hMPV predominates in winter and spring in temperate climates.[97,98,101] However, outbreaks may occur in the late spring[93] or summer.[107]

Clinical Features

Clinical symptoms of hMPV infections in infants and young children are indistinguishable from RSV.[92,97,98,100,101,108] In previously healthy children, the most common features of hMPV were bronchiolitis (59%), croup (18%), exacerbation of asthma (14%), and pneumonia (8%).[101] Vomiting was less common in hMPV infections (10%) compared to RSV (31%) or influenza (28%).[101] Hospitalization is rarely required in previously healthy children,[101] but severe pneumonia can occur in children with comorbidities or immunosuppression.[97,98] Co-infection with RSV and hMPV occurs in 4% to 6% of cases.[101,109] Like other respiratory viruses, hMPV may evoke exacerbations of asthma in children.[94] In young children, AOM occurs in one third to one half of cases.[92,94,101] Conjunctivitis was noted in 4% of children with hMPV versus 22% of children with influenza infections.[101] In adults, hMPV may cause exacerbations of asthma[92] or COPD.[110]

Infections due to hMPV are usually self-limited (in children and adults),[94,101] but fatal pneumonia may occur.[94,95] Among fatal cases, diffuse alveolar hyaline membrane damage and peribronchiolitis have been observed.[94,95] Because of the presence of multiple viral genotypes and waning immunity,[95] reinfections may occur throughout life.[94] Reinfections are typically milder than primary infections.[94]

Diagnosis

hMPV exhibits fastidious growth requirements in culture and may require 14 to 21 days to grow.[93,94] A rapid antigen test is not available. RT-PCR is the preferred means to diagnose hMPV.[93,95,98] No sensitive anti-hMPV antibody tests are currently available.[93]

Treatment

No antiviral or antibody preparation is approved for the treatment of hMPV. Intravenous ribavirin has shown promise in vitro and in animal models.[111,112] Inhaled ribavirin was ineffective in one HSCT recipient[104]; however, in a lung transplant recipient, intravenous ribavirin was associated with a favorable response.[103] Intravenous polyclonal antibodies inhibit hMPV, and have a plausible (albeit untested) role in treating serious cases.[112]

Prevention

Live, attenuated vaccines have shown efficacy in animals, but vaccines are not yet available in humans.[67]

RHINOVIRUS AND CORONAVIRUS INFECTIONS

Rhinovirus and coronavirus infections account for more than 50% of common colds.[113,114] Symptoms include rhinitis, pharyngitis, sneezing, hoarseness, sinusitis, and cough; bronchopneumonia is rare.[113,115] These viral infections usually are self-limited,[113] but complications may arise in immunosuppressed individuals[16,116] or patients with cardiac or pulmonary disease.[113,117]

Virology

Both are single-stranded RNA viruses (Fig. 77-11). Rhinoviruses are members of the Picornaviridae family; more than 100 serotypes exist.[113] Variations in surface proteins account for antigenic diversity.[113] Coronaviruses are divided into three genera and can infect humans, animals, and birds.[113]

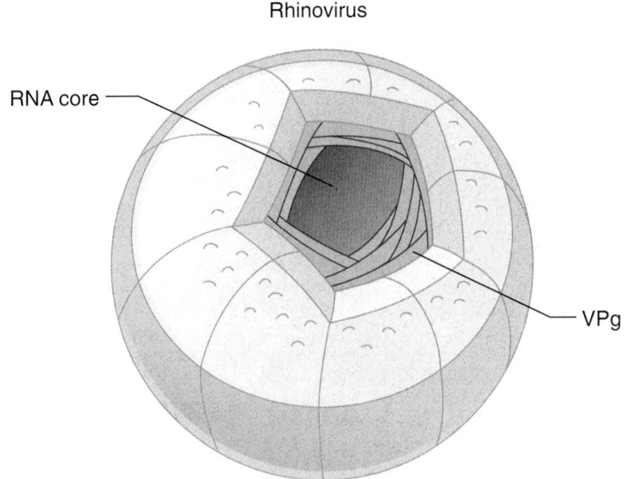

FIGURE 77-11 • Rhinovirus and coronavirus.

Epidemiology

Both rhinoviruses and coronaviruses cause respiratory infections (predominantly URTIs) in all age groups.[113,115] In temperate climates, rhinoviral illnesses peak in the early fall and spring[115]; coronaviruses peak in the late fall, winter, and early spring.[113] Schools, day care centers, family members, and businesses are sources of transmission.[113]

Clinical Features

Rhinoviruses account for approximately 50% of common colds; coronaviruses, 15%.[113,114] Rhinoviruses or coronaviruses may also cause exacerbations of asthma[115] or COPD.[117] In children, these viruses may serve as cofactors for AOM.[118,119] These viral infections usually are self-limited,[113,115] but complications (including fatal pneumonias) may arise in immunosuppressed individuals.[16,116]

Diagnosis

Conventional virus culture methods are sensitive for rhinoviruses, but insensitive for coronaviruses.[113,120] RT-PCR is more sensitive than cultures for rhinovirus and coronavirus.[120] Serologies are not helpful in clinical practice and are not available in most centers.[113] Given the mild and self-limited course observed with these viruses, cultures or RT-PCT are rarely performed, except in epidemiologic or research studies.

Treatment and Prevention

No proven therapy for rhinoviruses or coronaviruses is available. Vaccines are not available.[113]

SEVERE ACUTE RESPIRATORY SYNDROME–RELATED CORONAVIRUS

Severe acute respiratory syndrome (SARS) emerged in the Guangdong Province of southern China in 2002[121] and was followed by a pandemic. In less than one year, more than 8000 cases were identified in 26 countries, with a case fatality rate of 9.6%.[122] The epidemic was over by July 2003, and human-to-human transmission of the SARS virus globally has not been reported since.[122]

Virology

The etiologic agent of SARS is a novel human coronavirus (SARS-CoV) that is *not* closely related to other human or animal coronavi-

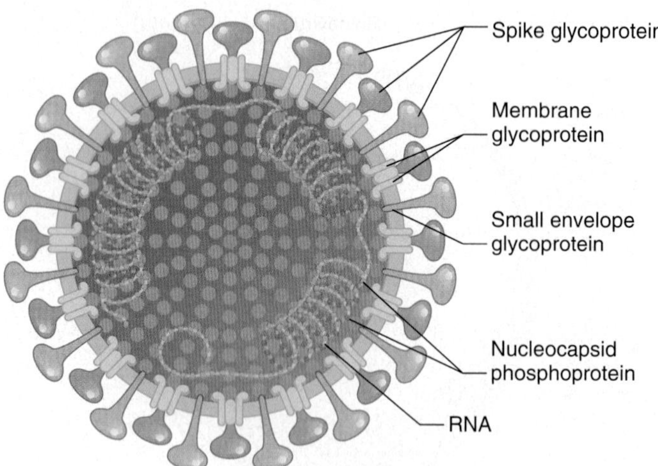

FIGURE 77-12 • SARS-related coronavirus. (Adapted from Drazen JM. SARS—looking back over the first 100 days. N Engl J Med 2003;349:319-320.)

ruses[122] (Fig. 77-12). SARS-CoV exhibits 99.8% homology between SARS-like coronaviruses found in animal markets.[122,123]

Epidemiology

SARS is a zoonotic disease that can be transmitted by droplet or contact routes.[122,124,125] The virus was transmitted from exotic animals to food handlers or workers in the food markets in Guangdong Province and other Asian countries.[122]

The incubation period of SARS ranges from 2 to 14 days (mean 5 days).[122,126] Maximal infectivity occurs in the second week of illness, at the time of rapid clinical deterioration, which correlates with the peak viral load.[126] It is important to emphasize that a single case of SARS could trigger a global pandemic. Vigilant surveillance and *strict* infection control measures among suspected cases and contacts are critical to minimize spread.[122]

Clinical Features

Presenting symptoms include chills, myalgias, malaise, and headache.[127,128] Fever is present in greater than 95% of cases.[122,127,128] Rhinorrhea and sore throat are uncommon in SARS.[128] Diarrhea occurs in up to 70% of patients.[126,127] Lymphopenia, thrombocytopenia, and elevations in creatine kinase (CK) and lactate dehydrogenase (LDH) are early findings.[127,128] During the first few days of the illness, respiratory symptoms are absent and chest radiographs may be normal. By 7 to 10 days, respiratory symptoms develop or worsen.[126] Pulmonary infiltrates, ground-glass opacities, and multifocal consolidation are usually evident on chest computed tomography scans.[126] Most patients recover spontaneously by the second or third week of illness.[122] However, 20% to 30% develop progressive respiratory failure requiring mechanical ventilation (similar to acute respiratory distress syndrome [ARDS]).[122,129] The median time from disease onset to mechanical ventilation among patients who developed respiratory failure was 9 days (range 7 to 13 days).[122] Mortality in this subset is approximately 50%.[122] SARS is uncommon in children, and has a milder course.[122] Atypical presentations of SARS (e.g., fever and diarrhea without respiratory manifestations[130,131] or lack of symptoms) may result in delayed diagnosis.

Diagnosis

Given the potential for pandemic spread of SARS, rapid diagnostic confirmation is essential for suspected cases. SARS should be considered in patients with pneumonia and ARDS of unknown etiology and one of the following risk factors: travel to mainland China or Asia (within 10 days) or employment in occupations at high risk (e.g., exposure to wildlife or other animals that may be reservoirs; health care workers or laboratory workers with close contact to SARS-CoV).[122] Even a single case mandates immediate efforts to identify the source and potential contacts.[122] When a case of SARS is suspected, public health authorities should be contacted *immediately* and can guide appropriate diagnostic workup and infection control measures.

Samples of nasopharyngeal aspirates, respiratory secretions, and stool should be sent for cultures and RT-PCR.[122] However, virus isolation using cell culture is relatively insensitive, requires several days, and must be performed in a laboratory with biosafety level III capability.[132] Detection of viral RNA by RT-PCR provides rapid results, with sensitivity rates greater than 80% at days 9 to 12 of the illness, but less than 50% at earlier or later time points.[122] Serologic detection of an antibody response to SARS-CoV is the gold standard.[122] Acute and convalescent (3 to 4 weeks) sera should be obtained.[122] Seroconversion occurs in 50% of patients by day 10 and greater than 90% by day 28.[122] Serologies are useful for epidemiologic investigations, but are less valuable in individual patients because of the time lag between infection and seroconversion. Personal protective equipment, handwashing, and infection control measures are essential when collecting, transporting, and handling specimens.[122]

Treatment

Because of the potential for rapid epidemic spread, patients with SARS should be admitted to the hospital, and rigorous infection control measures are essential.[122] Droplet and Contact Precautions are mandatory.[122] Hypoxemic patients require careful monitoring, and in severe cases, mechanical ventilation.[122] Procedures that involve airway manipulation (e.g., intubation, bronchoscopy, suctioning, nebulized therapy) should be performed only when essential, and under tightly controlled conditions.[122]

No treatment has been shown to influence mortality or clinical outcomes in SARS.[122] Intravenous ribavirin was ineffective and had significant toxicity.[133] Corticosteroids were used in uncontrolled studies, but were of unproven benefit.[122] Other strategies employed include interferon alfa, lopinavir/ritonavir, and Chinese herbal medications[122]; none is of proven efficacy.

Prevention

Vaccines are not yet available in humans.[67]

HANTAVIRUS

Hantavirus is an RNA virus that causes the hantavirus pulmonary syndrome (HPS) or hantavirus cardiopulmonary syndrome (HCPS) in the Americas[134-136] and hemorrhagic fever renal syndrome (HFRS) in Asia and Europe.[136]

Virology

Hantavirus is a genus of RNA viruses in the Bunyaviridae family and is the only group in this family that is not a naturally arthropod-borne virus[136] (Fig. 77-13). More than 25 viruses have been identified within the genus *Hantavirus.*[36] Hantaviruses are hosted in nature by rodents (the source of transmission to humans).[135,136]

Epidemiology

Three distinct groups of hantaviruses have been recognized, and result in distinct clinical presentations. The Hantaan virus (HTN), first isolated in Korea in 1978, is a cause of HFRS in Asia and Europe.[136] The second group of viruses, primarily found in the Americas, is associated with a severe pulmonary capillary leak syndrome and high mortality.[137] The first cases of HPS, due to the Sin Nombre (SN) virus, were described in the Four Corners region of New Mexico in 1993.[137] In North America, the SN virus is by far the most common, but other types have been described (e.g., Bayou virus, Black Creek Canal virus, New York virus, Monongahela virus).[135,136] The first cases of HPS in

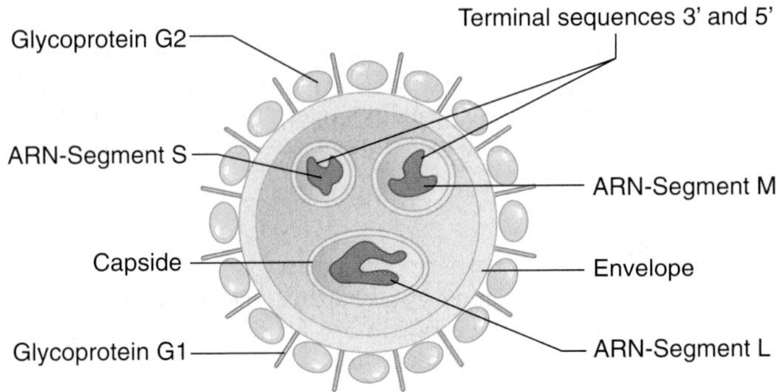

FIGURE 77-13 • Hantavirus.

South America were described in 1997.[138] By 2002, HPS had been confirmed in at least six countries in South America (Argentina, Bolivia, Brazil, Chile, Uruguay, and Paraguay).[135] The first case of human hantavirus infection in Central America was described in Panama in February 2000.[135] Several types of hantavirus were described in those outbreaks. The Andes virus was the predominant species in Chile and Argentina, whereas other subtypes were identified in other countries (e.g., Laguna Negra virus in Paraguay; Choclo virus in Panama; Juquitiba virus in Brazil).[135,136] A third group of hantaviruses, associated with the subfamily Arvicolinae, has been detected in North America and Europe, and may result in less severe forms of HFRS.[139]

In this chapter, we restrict our discussion to respiratory infections due to hantaviruses in North America (principally the SN virus). Hantaviral infections in North America remain exceedingly rare, with a seroprevalence of less than 0.1%.[136] Since the initial report of HCPS in New Mexico in 1993, fewer than 500 cases have been reported in North America.[136] Inhalation of aerosolized virus particles present in urine, feces, or saliva of rodents is the most important route of human infection.[136] Following excretion by rodents, hantaviruses may remain infectious for several days.[136] Outbreaks of hantavirus infections in humans are related to variations in rodent density (e.g., due to climate and food supply) and rodents invading peridomestic environments.[135,136,139] Person-to-person transmission has not been described in North America, Europe, or Asia,[136] but was described in several cases in Argentina and Chile.[138,140] Incubation period ranges from 7 to 39 days.[136,141]

Clinical Features

In the most severe cases, hantavirus elicits a pulmonary capillary leak syndrome, producing ARDS and cardiogenic shock.[136] Typically, HCPS is characterized by three phases: prodromal, cardiopulmonary, and recovery.[136] In the prodromal phase (1 to 5 days), nonspecific symptoms of fever, headache, malaise, and myalgia are present.[136] Gastrointestinal symptoms (e.g., nausea, vomiting, diarrhea, abdominal pain) may be present.[136] Importantly, rhinorrhea or nasal congestion (often the presenting features of other respiratory viral syndromes) are absent in this early phase.[136] During the next (cardiopulmonary) phase, dyspnea, cough, and pulmonary infiltrates develop.[136] Thrombocytopenia occurs in 80% to 95% of patients with HCPS, and is usually present even in the early (prodromal phase).[136] Other laboratory aberrations may include hypoalbuminemia and elevations in transaminases, creatinine, CK, and LDH.[136] With the onset of the cardiopulmonary phase, dyspnea, hypoxemia, hypotension, or cardiovascular collapse may develop.[136] During this phase, hematocrit and leukocyte counts rise.[136] Rapid progression to fulminant pulmonary and/or cardiac failure may occur over the next 8 to 24 hours, with mortality rates exceeding 30% to 50%.[136] Pulmonary hemorrhage is rare with SN virus, but may complicate severe HCPS due to Andes virus.[136] Pulmonary edema may reflect capillary leak as well as severe myocardial depression.[136] As myocardial function worsens, pulmonary capillary wedge pressure rises and cardiac index is low and resistant to fluid resuscitation.[136] In addition, arrhythmias and cardiogenic shock may develop. Interestingly, at least one third of patients with SN infection do well, with modest or no pulmonary edema.[136]

No clinical or laboratory features during the prodromal or early cardiopulmonary phases predict the ultimate severity of the disease.[136] Further, serologic epidemiologic studies cited serum antibodies to hantavirus in up to 13% of local community residents with no clinical evidence for illness,[135] suggesting that mild or asymptomatic hantavirus infections occur in humans.

Diagnosis

A careful history is critical. Hantavirus exposure should be considered in individuals who reside in or visit rural locations, even if an overt history of rodent exposure is lacking. Laboratory criteria suggestive of HCPS include thrombocytopenia ($<150 \times 10^3/\mu L$), hemoconcentration (hematocrit >50% in men or >48% in women), lack of toxic granulations in neutrophils, left shift of myeloid series, and greater than 10% immunoblasts.[136] A definitive diagnosis is made by serologies; serum antibodies are usually present on the first day of symptoms.[136] Viral antigen detection in fixed tissue by immunohistochemistry is sensitive and specific.[136] Viral RNA can be detected from serum or tissues by RT-PCR.[136]

Treatment

No specific antiviral therapy for HCPS exists.[136] Treatment is supportive and directed toward treating shock and acute respiratory, cardiac, or renal failure.[136] Because HCPS is associated with severe myocardial depression, aggressive fluid resuscitation is *discouraged.*[136] Early use of vasopressors should be initiated. Extracorporeal membrane oxygenation may be efficacious in extreme, fulminant cases of HPS.[136] Hyperimmune serum from convalescent patients is promising.[136] High levels of neutralizing antibodies correlated with improved survival and persist for years in survivors.[136]

ADENOVIRUS

Adenoviruses typically cause mild, self-limited infections involving the URT, gastrointestinal tract, or conjunctivae.[142] Adenovirus infections are more common in children, owing to lack of humoral immunity.[16,142] The disease is more severe and dissemination is more likely in immunocompromised hosts.[16,142-144] Pneumonia develops in fewer than 1% of immunocompetent patients with AdV infections,[145,146] but in up to 10% of immunocompromised patients.[16,142] Fatality rates for severe AdV pneumonia range from 10% to 70%.[16,142]

Virology

Human AdV is a family of double-stranded nonenveloped DNA viruses[147] (Fig. 77-14). Fifty-one serotypes and six species (A through F) are recognized; one third of serotypes are associated with human disease.[147] Manifestations of AdV are related to specific species and strains.[142,144] In immunocompetent children, species B and C predominate (>95%), typically AdV strains 1 to 7.[144,148] Most infections among military recruits are due to AdV strains 4 and 7.[145,146] Gastroenteritis is associated with enteric AdV strains 40 and 41, and hemorrhagic gastritis with AdV 11, 33, 34, and 35.[16] Among HSCT recipients, most infections are due to AdV species B and C,[142,149] but significant diversity[144] and even multiple serotypes in individual patients[144,150] have been noted.

Epidemiology

Adenovirus is a common pathogen among children and adults, and accounts for at least 5% to 10% of pediatric and 1% to 7% of adults RTIs.[142] Infections occur throughout the year, with no seasonal variation.[142] Transmission of AdV can occur via inhalation of aerosolized droplets, direct conjunctival inoculation, fecal-oral spread, or exposure

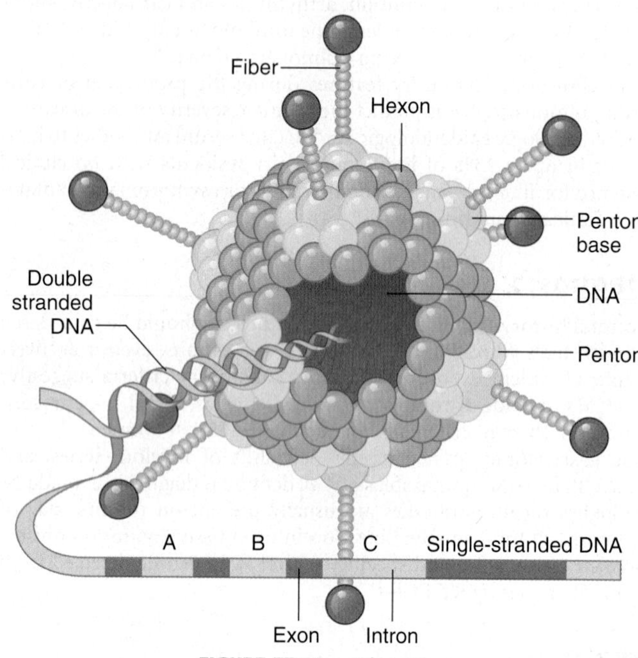

FIGURE 77-14 • Adenovirus.

to infected tissue or blood.[142] The incubation period ranges from 2 to 14 days, and depends upon viral serotype and mechanism of transmission.[142] Infection can be by reactivation or new acquisition from exogenous sources.[142,144] Rates of AdV infection are higher among children (due to lack of immunity) and immunosuppressed patients.[16,142,151] The incidence of AdV infections is 5% to 22% among SOT recipients[142,152,153] and 3% to 47% among HSCT recipients.[16,142-144,148,150,153-155] Risk factors for AdV infections among HSCT recipients include pediatric age group, allogeneic HSCT, severe T-cell depletion, and graft-versus-host disease.[142,143,153-155] Severe lymphopenia is associated with disseminated and often fatal disease.[142] Among SOT recipients, risk factors include pediatric age group, receipt of antilymphocyte antibodies, and donor-positive/recipient-negative AdV status.[142]

Epidemic AdV infections may spread rapidly in closed environments such as military recruit barracks,[145,156] civilian job training facilities, long-term care facilities,[151] and psychiatric care facilities,[157] as well as among hospitalized or institutionalized civilians.[158] Adenovirus accounts for greater than 50% of febrile respiratory illnesses among healthy military recruits.[145,146,156] Surveillance of U.S. recruits in training from 1999 to 2004 cited greater than 73,000 AdV infections, with peak illness rates in weeks 3 to 5 of training.[156] Serotype 4 accounted for greater than 95% of infections.[156] Importantly, the annual rate of AdV infections rose more than threefold after vaccine usage ceased.[156] High baseline immunity against AdV (titer of >1:32) confers substantial protection.[146]

Clinical Features

Adenoviral infections typically cause self-limited respiratory, gastrointestinal, or conjunctival disease.[142] Less common manifestations of AdV infections include hepatitis, hemorrhagic cystitis, nephritis, encephalitis, pancreatitis, and disseminated disease.[159,160] Respiratory symptoms range from mild coldlike symptoms to severe (sometimes lethal) pneumonia and ARDS.[142,157] Pneumonia due to AdV is rare in immunocompetent adults, but life-threatening cases have been described.[146] Gastrointestinal symptoms range from mild diarrhea to hemorrhagic colitis.[142] Hepatitis is often associated with subgroup C viruses (types 1, 2, and 5), and hemorrhagic cystitis with AdV types 11, 34, and 35.[142] The presence of AdV in urine is usually associated with hemorrhagic cystitis.[142] Severe AdV infections are rare among immunocompetent hosts, but dissemination occurs in 10% to 30% of HSCT recipients.[16,142-144,150,154,155] Adenovirus infections in SOT recipients may lead to graft loss or death.[161] Among HSCT recipients with *symptomatic* AdV disease, fatality rates range from 19% to 65%.[16,142,143,153,154] Case fatality rates for untreated AdV pneumonia may exceed 50%.[16,142]

Diagnosis

Viral cultures are difficult and may take up to 21 days to isolate AdV.[16,142] The commercially available AdV EIA test for stool specimens detects only serotypes 40 and 41.[16] Adenovirus nuclear inclusions may be observed in tissue.[142] RT-PCT of AdV DNA in plasma or infected sites is the preferred technique[142] and is highly sensitive for disseminated disease.[160,162] Persistently high titers correlate with clinical disease.[160] Serial RT-PCR assays of blood and stool weekly may detect AdV disease prior to the onset of symptoms, and facilitate early "preemptive" therapy.[144,152,154,163] However, the role of routine surveillance is controversial.[142]

Treatment

No antiviral drug has been approved to treat adenovirus. Prospective randomized controlled trials are lacking. Cidofovir, a cytosine nucleotide analogue that inhibits DNA polymerase, has the greatest in vitro activity; most, but not all, species are resistant to ribavirin.[164,165] Ganciclovir displays in vitro activity against AdV, but has no role to treat AdV infections.[142] While not all AdV infections require treatment, cidofovir (available only intravenously) is the preferred therapeutic agent.[142] Numerous studies of HSCT and SOT recipients have documented favorable responses to cidofovir.[143,144,154,163,166,167] Major dosing regimens include intravenous cidofovir 5 mg/kg once weekly or 1 mg/kg thrice weekly for 4 to 6 weeks.[163] Cidofovir is generally well tolerated,[154,163] but may cause nephrotoxicity.[142] Hydration and probenacid may minimize nephrotoxicity.[142,154,167,168] Newer lipid formulations of cidofovir exhibit increased activity against AdV and are less toxic, but not yet available.[169]

Reduction of immunosuppression[154] or immune reconstitution of HSCT recipients[143] may have adjunctive roles. IVIG has been used (together with cidofovir), but data are insufficient to assess efficacy.[143] Not all patients with AdV infections require treatment.[142] Interestingly, in a cohort of SOT recipients, all 19 with AdV infection recovered spontaneously.[152] Similarly, in one study of pediatric HSCT recipients, AdV viremia was detected in 42% and cleared without therapy in 64%.[170]

Prevention

Oral vaccines against AdV types 4 and 7 were developed for the U.S. military, and routine vaccination began at U.S. recruit training camps in 1971.[156] These vaccines were safe and highly efficacious,[145] but production ceased in 1996, and available stores were depleted by 1999.[156] Restoration of an effective AdV vaccine is anticipated in 2008.[156]

REFERENCES

1. Hall CB. The spread of influenza and other respiratory viruses: complexities and conjectures. Clin Infect Dis 2007;45:353-359.
2. Lynch JP 3rd, Walsh EE. Influenza: evolving strategies in treatment and prevention. Semin Respir Crit Care Med 2007;28:144-158.
3. Nichol KL, Treanor JJ. Vaccines for seasonal and pandemic influenza. J Infect Dis 2006;194(Suppl 2):S111-S118.
4. Rajagopal S, Treanor J. Pandemic (avian) influenza. Semin Respir Crit Care Med 2007;28:159-170.
5. Thompson WW, Comanor L, Shay DK. Epidemiology of seasonal influenza: use of surveillance data and statistical models to estimate the burden of disease. J Infect Dis 2006;194(Suppl 2):S82-S91.
6. Petric M, Comanor L, Petti CA. Role of the laboratory in diagnosis of influenza during seasonal epidemics and potential pandemics. J Infect Dis 2006;194(Suppl 2): S98-S110.
7. Bright RA, Medina MJ, Xu X, et al. Incidence of adamantane resistance among influenza A (H3N2) viruses isolated worldwide from 1994 to 2005: a cause for concern. Lancet 2005;366:1175-1181.

8. Thompson WW, Shay DK, Weintraub E, et al. Mortality associated with influenza and respiratory syncytial virus in the United States. JAMA 2003;289:179-186.
9. Sugaya N, Mitamura K, Yamazaki M, et al. Lower clinical effectiveness of oseltamivir against influenza B contrasted with influenza A infection in children. Clin Infect Dis 2007;44:197-202.
10. Poehling KA, Edwards KM, Weinberg GA, et al. The underrecognized burden of influenza in young children. N Engl J Med 2006;355:31-40.
11. Nichols WG, Guthrie KA, Corey L, Boeckh M. Influenza infections after hematopoietic stem cell transplantation: risk factors, mortality, and the effect of antiviral therapy. Clin Infect Dis 2004;39:1300-1306.
12. Osterholm MT. Preparing for the next pandemic. N Engl J Med 2005;352:1839-1842.
13. Whitley RJ, Monto AS. Prevention and treatment of influenza in high-risk groups: children, pregnant women, immunocompromised hosts, and nursing home residents. J Infect Dis 2006;194(Suppl 2):S133-S138.
14. Grijalva CG, Craig AS, Dupont WD, et al. Estimating influenza hospitalizations among children. Emerg Infect Dis 2006;12:103-109.
15. O'Brien MA, Uyeki TM, Shay DK, et al. Incidence of outpatient visits and hospitalizations related to influenza in infants and young children. Pediatrics 2004;113(3 Pt 1):585-593.
16. Kim Y-J, Boeckh M, Englund J. Community respiratory virus infections in immunocompromised patients: hematopoietic stem cell and solid organ transplant recipients, and individuals with human immunodeficiency virus infection. Semin Respir Crit Care Med 2007;28:222-242.
17. Ison MG, Gubareva LV, Atmar RL, et al. Recovery of drug-resistant influenza virus from immunocompromised patients: a case series. J Infect Dis 2006;193:760-764.
18. Kobasa D, Takada A, Shinya K, et al. Enhanced virulence of influenza A viruses with the haemagglutinin of the 1918 pandemic virus. Nature 2004;431:703-707.
19. Peltola V, Ziegler T, Ruuskanen O. Influenza A and B virus infections in children. Clin Infect Dis 2003;36:299-305.
20. Starko KM, Ray CG, Dominguez LB, et al. Reye's syndrome and salicylate use. Pediatrics 1980;66:859-864.
21. Walsh EE, Cox C, Falsey AR. Clinical features of influenza A virus infection in older hospitalized persons. J Am Geriatr Soc 2002;50:1498-1503.
22. Couch RB. Prevention and treatment of influenza. N Engl J Med 2000;343:1778-1787.
23. Moscona A. Neuraminidase inhibitors for influenza. N Engl J Med 2005;353:1363-1373.
24. Vu D, Peck AJ, Nichols WG, et al. Safety and tolerability of oseltamivir prophylaxis in hematopoietic stem cell transplant recipients: a retrospective case-control study. Clin Infect Dis 2007;45:187-193.
25. Kawai N, Ikematsu H, Iwaki N, et al. Factors influencing the effectiveness of oseltamivir and amantadine for the treatment of influenza: a multicenter study from Japan of the 2002-2003 influenza season. Clin Infect Dis 2005;40:1309-1316.
26. Weinstock DM, Zuccotti G. Adamantane resistance in influenza A. JAMA 2006;295:934-936.
27. Bright RA, Shay DK, Shu B, et al. Adamantane resistance among influenza A viruses isolated early during the 2005-2006 influenza season in the United States. JAMA 2006;295:891-894.
28. Ilyushina NA, Govorkova EA, Webster RG. Detection of amantadine-resistant variants among avian influenza viruses isolated in North America and Asia. Virology 2005;341:102-106.
29. Smith NM, Bresee JS, Shay DK, et al. Prevention and control of influenza: recommendations of the Advisory Committee on Immunization Practices (ACIP). MMWR Recomm Rep 2006;55(RR-10):1-42.
30. Hayden FG, Belshe R, Villanueva C, et al. Management of influenza in households: a prospective, randomized comparison of oseltamivir treatment with or without postexposure prophylaxis. J Infect Dis 2004;189:440-449.
31. Hayden FG, Pavia AT. Antiviral management of seasonal and pandemic influenza. J Infect Dis 2006;194(Suppl 2):S119-S126.
32. Nordstrom BL, Sung I, Suter P, Szneke P. Risk of pneumonia and other complications of influenza-like illness in patients treated with oseltamivir. Curr Med Res Opin 2005;21:761-768.
33. Monto AS, Rotthoff J, Teich E, et al. Detection and control of influenza outbreaks in well-vaccinated nursing home populations. Clin Infect Dis 2004;39:459-464.
34. Bowles SK, Lee W, Simor AE, et al. Use of oseltamivir during influenza outbreaks in Ontario nursing homes, 1999-2000. J Am Geriatr Soc 2002;50:608-616.
35. Cooper NJ, Sutton AJ, Abrams KR, et al. Effectiveness of neuraminidase inhibitors in treatment and prevention of influenza A and B: systematic review and meta-analyses of randomised controlled trials. BMJ 2003;326:1235.
36. Moscona A. Oseltamivir-resistant influenza? Lancet 2004;364:733-734.
37. Moscona A. Oseltamivir resistance—disabling our influenza defenses. N Engl J Med 2005;353:2633-2636.
38. Brett AS, Zuger A. The run on Tamiflu—should physicians prescribe on demand? N Engl J Med 2005;353:2636-2637.
39. Yen HL, Herlocher LM, Hoffmann E, et al. Neuraminidase inhibitor-resistant influenza viruses may differ substantially in fitness and transmissibility. Antimicrob Agents Chemother 2005;49:4075-4084.
40. McKimm-Breschkin J, Trivedi T, Hampson A, et al. Neuraminidase sequence analysis and susceptibilities of influenza virus clinical isolates to zanamivir and oseltamivir. Antimicrob Agents Chemother 2003;47:2264-2272.
41. Kiso M, Mitamura K, Sakai-Tagawa Y, et al. Resistant influenza A viruses in children treated with oseltamivir: descriptive study. Lancet 2004;364:759-765.
42. Beigel JH, Farrar J, Han AM, et al. Avian influenza A (H5N1) infection in humans. N Engl J Med 2005;353:1374-1385.
43. de Jong MD, Tran TT, Truong HK, et al. Oseltamivir resistance during treatment of influenza A (H5N1) infection. N Engl J Med 2005;353:2667-2672.
44. Schwartz B, Hinman A, Abramson J, et al. Universal influenza vaccination in the United States: are we ready? Report of a meeting. J Infect Dis 2006;194(Suppl 2): S147-S154.
45. Nichol KL, Nordin JD, Nelson DB, et al. Effectiveness of influenza vaccine in the community-dwelling elderly. N Engl J Med 2007;357:1373-1381.
46. Fukuda K, Kieny MP. Different approaches to influenza vaccination. N Engl J Med 2006;355:2586-2587.
47. Ohmit SE, Victor JC, Rotthoff JR, et al. Prevention of antigenically drifted influenza by inactivated and live attenuated vaccines. N Engl J Med 2006;355:2513-2522.
48. Harper SA, Fukuda K, Uyeki TM, et al. Prevention and control of influenza: recommendations of the Advisory Committee on Immunization Practices (ACIP). MMWR Recomm Rep 2005;54(RR-8):1-40.
49. Jefferson T, Rivetti D, Rivetti A, et al. Efficacy and effectiveness of influenza vaccines in elderly people: a systematic review. Lancet 2005;366:1165-1174.
50. Hak E, Buskens E, van Essen GA, et al. Clinical effectiveness of influenza vaccination in persons younger than 65 years with high-risk medical conditions: the PRISMA study. Arch Intern Med 2005;165:274-280.
51. Pearson ML, Bridges CB, Harper SA. Influenza vaccination of health-care personnel: recommendations of the Healthcare Infection Control Practices Advisory Committee (HICPAC) and the Advisory Committee on Immunization Practices (ACIP). MMWR Recomm Rep 2006;55(RR-2):1-16.
52. Burls A, Jordan R, Barton P, et al. Vaccinating healthcare workers against influenza to protect the vulnerable—is it a good use of healthcare resources? A systematic review of the evidence and an economic evaluation. Vaccine 2006;24:4212-4221.
53. Jefferson T, Smith S, Demicheli V, et al. Assessment of the efficacy and effectiveness of influenza vaccines in healthy children: systematic review. Lancet 2005;365:773-780.
54. Negri E, Colombo C, Giordano L, et al. Influenza vaccine in healthy children: a meta-analysis. Vaccine 2005;23:2851-2861.
55. Piedra PA, Gaglani MJ, Kozinetz CA, et al. Herd immunity in adults against influenza-related illnesses with use of the trivalent-live attenuated influenza vaccine (CAIV-T) in children. Vaccine 2005;23:1540-1548.
56. King JC Jr, Stoddard JJ, Gaglani MJ, et al. Effectiveness of school-based influenza vaccination. N Engl J Med 2006;355:2523-2532.
57. Chan PK. Outbreak of avian influenza A (H5N1) virus infection in Hong Kong in 1997. Clin Infect Dis 2002;34(Suppl 2):S58-S64.
58. Matrosovich MN, Matrosovich TY, Gray T, et al. Human and avian influenza viruses target different cell types in cultures of human airway epithelium. Proc Natl Acad Sci U S A 2004;101:4620-4624.
59. Epidemiology of WHO-confirmed human cases of avian influenza A (H5N1) infection. Wkly Epidemiol Rec 2006;81:249-257.
60. Shortridge KF, Zhou NN, Guan Y, et al. Characterization of avian H5N1 influenza viruses from poultry in Hong Kong. Virology 1998;252:331-342.
61. Peiris JS, Yu WC, Leung CW, et al. Re-emergence of fatal human influenza A subtype H5N1 disease. Lancet 2004;363:617-619.
62. Koopmans M, Wilbrink B, Conyn M, et al. Transmission of H7N7 avian influenza A virus to human beings during a large outbreak in commercial poultry farms in the Netherlands. Lancet 2004;363:587-593.
63. Tweed SA, Skowronski DM, David ST, et al. Human illness from avian influenza H7N3, British Columbia. Emerg Infect Dis 2004;10:2196-2199.
64. Butt KM, Smith GJ, Chen H, et al. Human infection with an avian H9N2 influenza A virus in Hong Kong in 2003. J Clin Microbiol 2005;43:5760-5767.
65. Ungchusak K, Auewarakul P, Dowell SF, et al. Probable person-to-person transmission of avian influenza A (H5N1). N Engl J Med 2005;352:333-340.
66. Cheung CL, Rayner JM, Smith GJ, et al. Distribution of amantadine-resistant H5N1 avian influenza variants in Asia. J Infect Dis 2006;193:1626-1629.
67. Schmidt A. Progress in respiratory virus vaccine development. Semin Respir Crit Care Med 2007;28:243-252.
68. Falsey AR. Respiratory syncytial virus infection in adults. Semin Respir Crit Care Med 2007;28:171-181.
69. Hall CB. Respiratory syncytial virus and parainfluenza virus. N Engl J Med 2001;344:1917-1928.
70. Hall CB, Long CE, Schnabel KC. Respiratory syncytial virus infections in previously healthy working adults. Clin Infect Dis 2001;33:792-796.
71. Falsey AR, Hennessey PA, Formica MA, et al. Respiratory syncytial virus infection in elderly and high-risk adults. N Engl J Med 2005;352:1749-1759.
72. Beckham JD, Cadena A, Lin J, et al. Respiratory viral infections in patients with chronic, obstructive pulmonary disease. J Infect 2005;50:322-330.
73. Falsey AR, Formica MA, Hennessey PA, et al. Detection of respiratory syncytial virus in adults with chronic obstructive pulmonary disease. Am J Respir Crit Care Med 2006;173:639-643.
74. Mullooly JP, Bridges CB, Thompson WW, et al. Influenza- and RSV-associated hospitalizations among adults. Vaccine 2007;25:846-855.
75. O'Shea MK, Ryan MA, Hawksworth AW, et al. Symptomatic respiratory syncytial virus infection in previously healthy young adults living in a crowded military environment. Clin Infect Dis 2005;41:311-317.
76. Walsh EE, Peterson DR, Falsey AR. Is clinical recognition of respiratory syncytial virus infection in hospitalized elderly and high-risk adults possible? J Infect Dis 2007;195:1046-1051.
77. Johnston NW. The similarities and differences of epidemic cycles of chronic obstructive pulmonary disease and asthma exacerbations. Proc Am Thorac Soc 2007;4:591-596.
78. Martinez FJ. Pathogen-directed therapy in acute exacerbations of chronic obstructive pulmonary disease. Proc Am Thorac Soc 2007;4:647-658.

79. Wilkinson TM, Donaldson GC, Johnston SL, et al. Respiratory syncytial virus, airway inflammation, and FEV1 decline in patients with chronic obstructive pulmonary disease. Am J Respir Crit Care Med 2006;173:871-876.
80. Boeckh M, Englund J, Li Y, et al. Randomized controlled multicenter trial of aerosolized ribavirin for respiratory syncytial virus upper respiratory tract infection in hematopoietic cell transplant recipients. Clin Infect Dis 2007;44:245-249.
81. DeVincenzo JP, Hirsch RL, Fuentes RJ, Top FH Jr. Respiratory syncytial virus immune globulin treatment of lower respiratory tract infection in pediatric patients undergoing bone marrow transplantation—a compassionate use experience. Bone Marrow Transplant 2000;25:161-165.
82. Saez-Llorens X, Moreno MT, Ramilo O, et al. Safety and pharmacokinetics of palivizumab therapy in children hospitalized with respiratory syncytial virus infection. Pediatr Infect Dis J 2004;23:707-712.
83. de Fontbrune FS, Robin M, Porcher R, et al. Palivizumab treatment of respiratory syncytial virus infection after allogeneic hematopoietic stem cell transplantation. Clin Infect Dis 2007;45:1019-1024.
84. Reed G, Jewett PH, Thompson J, et al. Epidemiology and clinical impact of parainfluenza virus infections in otherwise healthy infants and young children <5 years old. J Infect Dis 1997;175:807-813.
85. Nichols WG, Erdman DD, Han A, et al. Prolonged outbreak of human parainfluenza virus 3 infection in a stem cell transplant outpatient department: insights from molecular epidemiologic analysis. Biol Blood Marrow Transplant 2004;10:58-64.
86. Falsey AR, McCann RM, Hall WJ, et al. Acute respiratory tract infection in daycare centers for older persons. J Am Geriatr Soc 1995;43:30-36.
87. Dignan F, Alvares C, Riley U, et al. Parainfluenza type 3 infection post stem cell transplant: high prevalence but low mortality. J Hosp Infect 2006;63:452-458.
88. Nichols WG, Corey L, Gooley T, et al. Parainfluenza virus infections after hematopoietic stem cell transplantation: risk factors, response to antiviral therapy, and effect on transplant outcome. Blood 2001;98:573-578.
89. Erard V, Chien JW, Kim HW, et al. Airflow decline after myeloablative allogeneic hematopoietic cell transplantation: the role of community respiratory viruses. J Infect Dis 2006;193:1619-1625.
90. Wright JJ, O'Driscoll G. Treatment of parainfluenza virus 3 pneumonia in a cardiac transplant recipient with intravenous ribavirin and methylprednisolone. J Heart Lung Transplant 2005;24:343-346.
91. van den Hoogen BG, de Jong JC, Groen J, et al. A newly discovered human pneumovirus isolated from young children with respiratory tract disease. Nat Med 2001;7:719-724.
92. Williams JV, Crowe JE Jr, Enriquez R, et al. Human metapneumovirus infection plays an etiologic role in acute asthma exacerbations requiring hospitalization in adults. J Infect Dis 2005;192:1149-1153.
93. Agapov E, Sumino KC, Gaudreault-Keener M, et al. Genetic variability of human metapneumovirus infection: evidence of a shift in viral genotype without a change in illness. J Infect Dis 2006;193:396-403.
94. Deffrasnes C, Hamelin ME, Boivin G. Human metapneumovirus. Semin Respir Crit Care Med 2007;28:213-221.
95. Boivin G, De Serres G, Hamelin ME, et al. An outbreak of severe respiratory tract infection due to human metapneumovirus in a long-term care facility. Clin Infect Dis 2007;44:1152-1158.
96. Sumino KC, Agapov E, Pierce RA, et al. Detection of severe human metapneumovirus infection by real-time polymerase chain reaction and histopathological assessment. J Infect Dis 2005;192:1052-1060.
97. Vicente D, Montes M, Cilla G, et al. Differences in clinical severity between genotype A and genotype B human metapneumovirus infection in children. Clin Infect Dis 2006;42:e111-e113.
98. van den Hoogen BG, van Doornum GJ, Fockens JC, et al. Prevalence and clinical symptoms of human metapneumovirus infection in hospitalized patients. J Infect Dis 2003;188:1571-1577.
99. Boivin G, Abed Y, Pelletier G, et al. Virological features and clinical manifestations associated with human metapneumovirus: a new paramyxovirus responsible for acute respiratory-tract infections in all age groups. J Infect Dis 2002;186:1330-1334.
100. Williams JV, Wang CK, Yang CF, et al. The role of human metapneumovirus in upper respiratory tract infections in children: a 20-year experience. J Infect Dis 2006;193:387-395.
101. Williams JV, Harris PA, Tollefson SJ, et al. Human metapneumovirus and lower respiratory tract disease in otherwise healthy infants and children. N Engl J Med 2004;350:443-450.
102. Larcher C, Geltner C, Fischer H, et al. Human metapneumovirus infection in lung transplant recipients: clinical presentation and epidemiology. J Heart Lung Transplant 2005;24:1891-1901.
103. Raza K, Ismailjee SB, Crespo M, et al. Successful outcome of human metapneumovirus (hMPV) pneumonia in a lung transplant recipient treated with intravenous ribavirin. J Heart Lung Transplant 2007;26:862-864.
104. Englund JA, Boeckh M, Kuypers J, et al. Brief communication: fatal human metapneumovirus infection in stem-cell transplant recipients. Ann Intern Med 2006;144:344-349.
105. Falsey AR, Erdman D, Anderson LJ, Walsh EE. Human metapneumovirus infections in young and elderly adults. J Infect Dis 2003;187:785-790.
106. Hamelin ME, Cote S, Laforge J, et al. Human metapneumovirus infection in adults with community-acquired pneumonia and exacerbation of chronic obstructive pulmonary disease. Clin Infect Dis 2005;41:498-502.
107. Louie JK, Schnurr DP, Pan CY, et al. A summer outbreak of human metapneumovirus infection in a long-term-care facility. J Infect Dis 2007;196:705-708.
108. Boivin G, De Serres G, Cote S, et al. Human metapneumovirus infections in hospitalized children. Emerg Infect Dis 2003;9:634-640.
109. Semple MG, Cowell A, Dove W, et al. Dual infection of infants by human metapneumovirus and human respiratory syncytial virus is strongly associated with severe bronchiolitis. J Infect Dis 2005;191:382-386.
110. Martinello RA, Esper F, Weibel C, et al. Human metapneumovirus and exacerbations of chronic obstructive pulmonary disease. J Infect 2006;53:248-254.
111. Hamelin ME, Prince GA, Boivin G. Effect of ribavirin and glucocorticoid treatment in a mouse model of human metapneumovirus infection. Antimicrob Agents Chemother 2006;50:774-777.
112. Wyde PR, Chetty SN, Jewell AM, et al. Comparison of the inhibition of human metapneumovirus and respiratory syncytial virus by ribavirin and immune serum globulin in vitro. Antiviral Res 2003;60:51-59.
113. Greenberg SB. Rhinovirus and coronavirus infections. Semin Respir Crit Care Med 2007;28:182-192.
114. Wat D. The common cold: a review of the literature. Eur J Intern Med 2004;15:79-88.
115. Hayden FG. Rhinovirus and the lower respiratory tract. Rev Med Virol 2004;14:17-31.
116. Ison MG, Hayden FG, Kaiser L, et al. Rhinovirus infections in hematopoietic stem cell transplant recipients with pneumonia. Clin Infect Dis 2003;36:1139-1143.
117. Wedzicha JA. Role of viruses in exacerbations of chronic obstructive pulmonary disease. Proc Am Thorac Soc 2004;1:115-120.
118. Bulut Y, Guven M, Otlu B, et al. Acute otitis media and respiratory viruses. Eur J Pediatr 2007;166:223-228.
119. Chantzi FM, Papadopoulos NG, Bairamis T, et al. Human rhinoviruses in otitis media with effusion. Pediatr Allergy Immunol 2006;17:514-518.
120. Loens K, Goossens H, de Laat C, et al. Detection of rhinoviruses by tissue culture and two independent amplification techniques, nucleic acid sequence-based amplification and reverse transcription-PCR, in children with acute respiratory infections during a winter season. J Clin Microbiol 2006;44:166-171.
121. Zhong NS, Zheng BJ, Li YM, et al. Epidemiology and cause of severe acute respiratory syndrome (SARS) in Guangdong, People's Republic of China, in February, 2003. Lancet 2003;362:1353-1358.
122. Muller MP, McGeer A. Severe acute respiratory syndrome (SARS) coronavirus. Semin Respir Crit Care Med 2007;28:201-212.
123. Song HD, Tu CC, Zhang GW, et al. Cross-host evolution of severe acute respiratory syndrome coronavirus in palm civet and human. Proc Natl Acad Sci U S A 2005; 102:2430-2435.
124. Kan B, Wang M, Jing H, et al. Molecular evolution analysis and geographic investigation of severe acute respiratory syndrome coronavirus-like virus in palm civets at an animal market and on farms. J Virol 2005;79:11892-11900.
125. Li W, Shi Z, Yu M, et al. Bats are natural reservoirs of SARS-like coronaviruses. Science 2005;310:676-679.
126. Peiris JS, Yuen KY, Osterhaus AD, Stohr K. The severe acute respiratory syndrome. N Engl J Med 2003;349:2431-2441.
127. Peiris JS, Chu CM, Cheng VC, et al. Clinical progression and viral load in a community outbreak of coronavirus-associated SARS pneumonia: a prospective study. Lancet 2003;361:1767-1772.
128. Muller MP, Richardson SE, McGeer A, et al. Early diagnosis of SARS: lessons from the Toronto SARS outbreak. Eur J Clin Microbiol Infect Dis 2006;25:230-237.
129. Yu IT, Wong TW, Chiu YL, et al. Temporal-spatial analysis of severe acute respiratory syndrome among hospital inpatients. Clin Infect Dis 2005;40:1237-1243.
130. Ho KY, Singh KS, Habib AG, et al. Mild illness associated with severe acute respiratory syndrome coronavirus infection: lessons from a prospective seroepidemiologic study of health-care workers in a teaching hospital in Singapore. J Infect Dis 2004;189:642-647.
131. Christian MD, Poutanen SM, Loutfy MR, et al. Severe acute respiratory syndrome. Clin Infect Dis 2004;38:1420-1427.
132. Chan KH, Poon LL, Cheng VC, et al. Detection of SARS coronavirus in patients with suspected SARS. Emerg Infect Dis 2004;10:294-299.
133. Chiou HE, Liu CL, Buttrey MJ, et al. Adverse effects of ribavirin and outcome in severe acute respiratory syndrome: experience in two medical centers. Chest 2005;128:263-272.
134. Mertz GJ, Hjelle B, Crowley M, et al. Diagnosis and treatment of New World hantavirus infections. Curr Opin Infect Dis 2006;19:437-442.
135. Bayard V, Kitsutani PT, Barria EO, et al. Outbreak of hantavirus pulmonary syndrome, Los Santos, Panama, 1999-2000. Emerg Infect Dis 2004;10:1635-1642.
136. Chang B, Crowley M, Campen M, Koster F. Hantavirus cardiopulmonary syndrome. Semin Respir Crit Care Med 2007;28:193-200.
137. Nichol ST, Spiropoulou CF, Morzunov S, et al. Genetic identification of a hantavirus associated with an outbreak of acute respiratory illness. Science 1993;262:914-917.
138. Toro J, Vega JD, Khan AS, et al. An outbreak of hantavirus pulmonary syndrome, Chile, 1997. Emerg Infect Dis 1998;4:687-694.
139. Rosa ES, Mills JN, Padula PJ, et al. Newly recognized hantaviruses associated with hantavirus pulmonary syndrome in northern Brazil: partial genetic characterization of viruses and serologic implication of likely reservoirs. Vector Borne Zoonotic Dis 2005;5:11-19.
140. Martinez VP, Bellomo C, San Juan J, et al. Person-to-person transmission of Andes virus. Emerg Infect Dis 2005;11:1848-1853.
141. Vial PA, Valdivieso F, Mertz G, et al. Incubation period of hantavirus cardiopulmonary syndrome. Emerg Infect Dis 2006;12:1271-1273.
142. Ison MG. Adenovirus infections in transplant recipients. Clin Infect Dis 2006;43:331-339.
143. Neofytos D, Ojha A, Mookerjee B, et al. Treatment of adenovirus disease in stem cell transplant recipients with cidofovir. Biol Blood Marrow Transplant 2007;13: 74-81.

144. Zheng X, Lu X, Erdman DD, et al. Identification of adenoviruses from high risk pediatric stem cell transplant recipients and controls. J Clin Microbiol 2008;46:317-320.
145. Sanchez JL, Binn LN, Innis BL, et al. Epidemic of adenovirus-induced respiratory illness among US military recruits: epidemiologic and immunologic risk factors in healthy, young adults. J Med Virol 2001;65:710-718.
146. Kolavic-Gray SA, Binn LN, Sanchez JL, et al. Large epidemic of adenovirus type 4 infection among military trainees: epidemiological, clinical, and laboratory studies. Clin Infect Dis 2002;35:808-818.
147. Lu X, Erdman DD. Molecular typing of human adenoviruses by PCR and sequencing of a partial region of the hexon gene. Arch Virol 2006;151:1587-1602.
148. Ebner K, Rauch M, Preuner S, Lion T. Typing of human adenoviruses in specimens from immunosuppressed patients by PCR-fragment length analysis and real-time quantitative PCR. J Clin Microbiol 2006;44:2808-2815.
149. Suparno C, Milligan DW, Moss PA, Mautner V. Adenovirus infections in stem cell transplant recipients: recent developments in understanding of pathogenesis, diagnosis and management. Leuk Lymphoma 2004;45:873-885.
150. Kroes AC, de Klerk EP, Lankester AC, et al. Sequential emergence of multiple adenovirus serotypes after pediatric stem cell transplantation. J Clin Virol 2007;38:341-347.
151. James L, Vernon MO, Jones RC, et al. Outbreak of human adenovirus type 3 infection in a pediatric long-term care facility—Illinois, 2005. Clin Infect Dis 2007;45:416-420.
152. Humar A, Kumar D, Mazzulli T, et al. A surveillance study of adenovirus infection in adult solid organ transplant recipients. Am J Transplant 2005;5:2555-2559.
153. de Mezerville MH, Tellier R, Richardson S, et al. Adenoviral infections in pediatric transplant recipients: a hospital-based study. Pediatr Infect Dis J 2006;25:815-818.
154. Sivaprakasam P, Carr TF, Coussons M, et al. Improved outcome from invasive adenovirus infection in pediatric patients after hemopoietic stem cell transplantation using intensive clinical surveillance and early intervention. J Pediatr Hematol Oncol 2007;29:81-85.
155. Robin M, Marque-Juillet S, Scieux C, et al. Disseminated adenovirus infections after allogeneic hematopoietic stem cell transplantation: incidence, risk factors and outcome. Haematologica 2007;92:1254-1257.
156. Russell KL, Hawksworth AW, Ryan MA, et al. Vaccine-preventable adenoviral respiratory illness in US military recruits, 1999-2004. Vaccine 2006;24:2835-2842.
157. Klinger JR, Sanchez MP, Curtin LA, et al. Multiple cases of life-threatening adenovirus pneumonia in a mental health care center. Am J Respir Crit Care Med 1998;157:645-649.
158. Singh-Naz N, Brown M, Ganeshananthan M. Nosocomial adenovirus infection: molecular epidemiology of an outbreak. Pediatr Infect Dis J 1993;12:922-925.
159. Bateman CM, Kesson AM, Shaw PJ. Pancreatitis and adenoviral infection in children after blood and marrow transplantation. Bone Marrow Transplant 2006;38:807-811.
160. Erard V, Huang ML, Ferrenberg J, et al. Quantitative real-time polymerase chain reaction for detection of adenovirus after T cell-replete hematopoietic cell transplantation: viral load as a marker for invasive disease. Clin Infect Dis 2007;45:958-965.
161. Bridges ND, Spray TL, Collins MH, et al. Adenovirus infection in the lung results in graft failure after lung transplantation. J Thorac Cardiovasc Surg 1998;116:617-623.
162. Lankester AC, Heemskerk B, Claas EC, et al. Effect of ribavirin on the plasma viral DNA load in patients with disseminating adenovirus infection. Clin Infect Dis 2004;38:1521-1525.
163. Yusuf U, Hale GA, Carr J, et al. Cidofovir for the treatment of adenoviral infection in pediatric hematopoietic stem cell transplant patients. Transplantation 2006;81:1398-1404.
164. Naesens L, Lenaerts L, Andrei G, et al. Antiadenovirus activities of several classes of nucleoside and nucleotide analogues. Antimicrob Agents Chemother 2005;49:1010-1016.
165. Morfin F, Dupuis-Girod S, Mundweiler S, et al. In vitro susceptibility of adenovirus to antiviral drugs is species-dependent. Antivir Ther 2005;10:225-229.
166. Wallot MA, Dohna-Schwake C, Auth M, et al. Disseminated adenovirus infection with respiratory failure in pediatric liver transplant recipients: impact of intravenous cidofovir and inhaled nitric oxide. Pediatr Transplant 2006;10:121-127.
167. Doan ML, Mallory GB, Kaplan SL, et al. Treatment of adenovirus pneumonia with cidofovir in pediatric lung transplant recipients. J Heart Lung Transplant 2007;26:883-889.
168. Keswani M, Moudgil A. Adenovirus-associated hemorrhagic cystitis in a pediatric renal transplant recipient. Pediatr Transplant 2007;11:568-571.
169. Hartline CB, Gustin KM, Wan WB, et al. Ether lipid-ester prodrugs of acyclic nucleoside phosphonates: activity against adenovirus replication in vitro. J Infect Dis 2005;191:396-399.
170. Walls T, Hawrami K, Ushiro-Lumb I, et al. Adenovirus infection after pediatric bone marrow transplantation: is treatment always necessary? Clin Infect Dis 2005;40:1244-1249.

78

COMMUNITY-ACQUIRED PNEUMONIA

Andrew R. Haas and Paul E. Marik

INTRODUCTION 1081
PATHOPHYSIOLOGY 1081
Risk Stratification and Treatment Setting 1082
CLINICAL PHARMACOLOGY AND THERAPEUTICS 1083
Specific Pharmacologic Considerations for CAP 1083
Antimicrobial Resistance 1083
Pulmonary Bioavailability of Antibiotics 1084
Time to First Dose of Antibiotics 1084
Intravenous Versus Oral Therapy and Duration of Therapy 1084
Treatment Recommendations for CAP 1084
Outpatients without Prior Cardiopulmonary Disease or Modifying Factors 1084
Outpatients with Cardiopulmonary Disease and/or Modifying Factors 1085
Inpatients without Cardiopulmonary Disease or Modifying Factors 1085
Inpatients with Cardiopulmonary Disease and/or Modifying Factors 1085
Inpatients Requiring ICU Admission and without *Pseudomonas aeruginosa* Risk Factors 1085
Special Considerations 1086
Community-Acquired MRSA Pneumonia 1086
Health Care–Associated Pneumonia 1086
Supportive and Emerging Therapies for CAP 1086
CONCLUSIONS 1086

INTRODUCTION

Community-acquired pneumonia (CAP) is an infection of the lung parenchyma acquired outside of hospitals or extended-care facilities. Even with the advent of and continuing advances in antimicrobial therapy, CAP remains a major health problem in the United States. It is the seventh leading cause of death in the United States, and the number one cause of death from infectious disease. Nearly 1 million hospitalizations with an estimated cost of $12 billion for therapy alone can be attributed to CAP.[1-3] These estimates do not factor in the associated costs of lost productivity, rehabilitation, and potential disability. Therefore, the health care and economic impact of CAP is readily evident.

Over the last 60 years, our armamentarium to battle pneumonia has expanded dramatically. This expansion in therapeutic options for CAP is driven by changes in the pathogenic organisms and the ever-evolving antimicrobial resistance acquired by these pathogens. This chapter provides an overview of CAP and recommendations for the use of the various antimicrobial agents available for its treatment.

PATHOPHYSIOLOGY

CAP development and prognosis is defined by the route of infection, host, and microbial factors. Identification of the offending organism in CAP is important to guide therapy and predict complications and outcomes. Unfortunately, even with extensive diagnostic evaluation, the etiologic agent is not identified in as many as 50% of patients.[4-16] For all patients presenting with CAP, *Streptococcus pneumoniae* is the most common pathogen isolated (Fig. 78-1) and accounts for 5% to 11% of CAP patients treated on an ambulatory basis, 5% to 43% of patients requiring hospitalization, and 11% to 38% of patients requiring intensive care unit (ICU) admission.[4,6,17,18] Other "typical" pathogens that account for CAP include the gram-negative coccobacillus *Haemophilus influenzae* and the gram-negative diplococcus *Moraxella catarrhalis*. The classically described "atypical" pathogens that cause CAP include *Chlamydia pneumoniae, Mycoplasma pneumoniae,* and *Legionella* species. The "atypical" moniker is an inaccurate description of the clinical features of the pneumonia associated with these organisms and is retained more as a classification than a specific descriptor of the disease process or clinical presentation. *Mycoplasma pneumoniae* has been shown to be the most common of the atypical pathogens and accounts for 17% to 37% of outpatient CAP and 2% to 33% of CAP requiring hospitalization.[4,6,18] *Chlamydia pneumoniae* is more common than *Legionella* species; however, *Legionella* species can lead to rapidly progressive and fatal pneumonia.

Although 90% or more of CAP can be explained by the previously mentioned organisms, other organisms can be encountered. In certain patient populations, aerobic gram-negative infections (*Pseudomonas aeruginosa*), enteric gram-negative infections, and anaerobic infections must be considered (see Box 78-1 later). Furthermore, it has recently been demonstrated that age greater than 65 alone is a specific epidemiologic risk factor for drug-resistant *S. pneumoniae* (DRSP), but not other organisms.[19,20] Of particular interest and concern in the last several years have been several reports of methicillin-resistant *Staphylococcus aureus* (MRSA) CAP. Traditionally, MRSA infection and/or pneumonia had been isolated to health care settings or high-risk groups such as intravenous drug abusers; however, since 2003, there have been several reports of severe, fulminant necrotizing MRSA pneumonia in young, healthy individuals without typical risk factors.[21,22] In addition, the clinician must also take into consideration any unusual exposure or occupational hazards that would predispose a patient to unusual pathogens such as *Chlamydia psittaci* (birds), *Coxiella burnetii* (ungulates), *Leptospira* species (rats), and *Francisella tularensis* (rabbits).

The mortality rate from CAP varies dramatically depending on the patient's severity of illness at presentation and underlying comorbid conditions. In the outpatient setting, the mortality rate is less than 1% to 5%; however, once patients require hospitalization, the mortality rate approaches 12%.[4-9] In more seriously ill patients with bacteremia who require ICU admission, the mortality rate can approach more than 40%.[10,11] The presence of underlying comorbid conditions such as chronic obstructive pulmonary disease (COPD), asthma, diabetes mellitus, renal insufficiency, congestive heart failure (CHF), coronary artery disease, malignancy, alcoholism, age greater than 70 years,

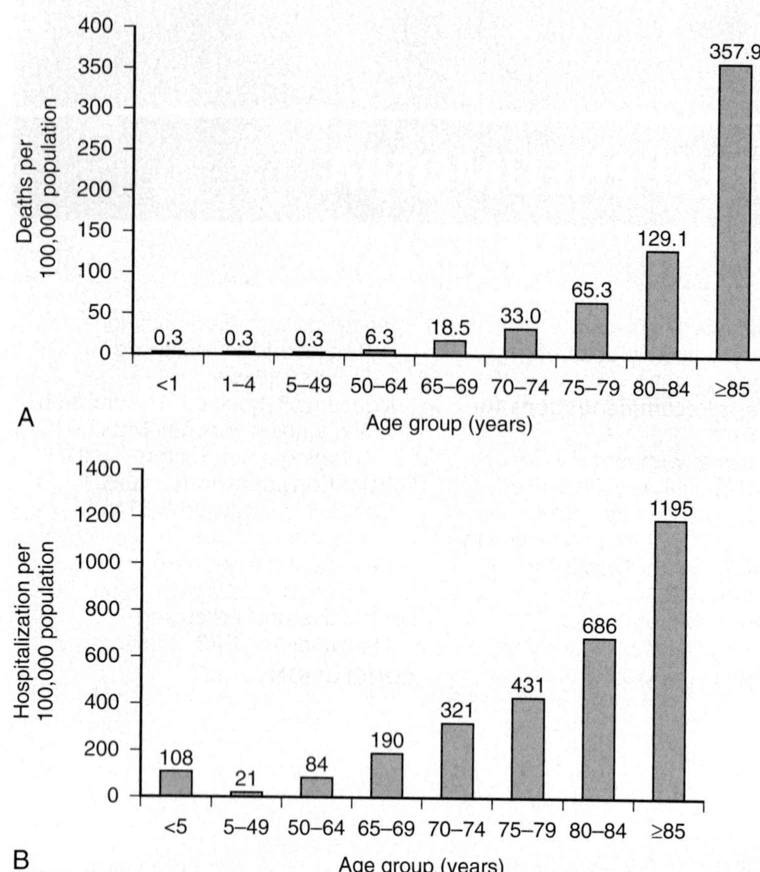

FIGURE 78-1 • Portable chest radiograph (**A**) and computed tomography scan (**B**) of patient with bacteremic multilobar pneumococcal pneumonia.

chronic neurologic disease, and/or chronic liver disease not only can contribute significantly to CAP mortality, but also may alter the etiologic organisms underlying the infection (Box 78-1).[12-14]

Risk Stratification and Treatment Setting

When CAP is strongly suspected on the basis of history, physical examination, and chest radiography, the next critical management decision is whether the patient will require hospital admission. The American Thoracic Society and Infectious Disease Society of America have defined four groups in their 2001 management of CAP consensus statement[3,23]:

1. Outpatients with no prior cardiopulmonary disease or modifying factors
2. Outpatients with cardiopulmonary disease (CHF or COPD) and/or other modifying factors (risk factors for specific organisms; see Box 78-1)
3. Inpatients, not admitted to the ICU, with or without cardiopulmonary disease or modifying factors
4. ICU-admitted patients with or without risk factors for *P. aeruginosa*

These stratification groups were defined by the expert panels in order to try to ensure adequate antimicrobial coverage of the most common organisms encountered in each group based on their risk factors and severity of illness. As discussed later in the section on Treatment Recommendations for CAP, there are specific organisms of concern for each group.

The difficulty with this stratification system is the lack of an objective quantification of severity of illness to predict if a patient needs inpatient versus outpatient care or general medical admission versus ICU admission. Therefore, more recently, many groups have attempted to apply multivariate analyses to patients' objective data to predict the need for admission and to ascertain their level of care. Two of the most

BOX 78-1 SPECIFIC PATHOGENS ASSOCIATED WITH UNDERLYING COMORBID CONDITIONS

Streptococcus pneumoniae
- Dementia
- Congestive heart failure
- Chronic obstructive pulmonary disease
- Cerebrovascular disease
- Institutional overcrowding
- Seizures

Penicillin-resistant and drug-resistant *S. pneumoniae*
- Age > 65 years
- Alcoholism
- Immunomodulating illness or therapy (including corticosteroid therapy)
- Previous β-lactam therapy within 3 months
- Multiple medical comorbidities
- Exposure to child in day care center

Enteric gram-negatives
- Residence in a long-term care facility
- Underlying cardiopulmonary disease
- Recent antibiotic therapy
- Multiple medical comorbidities

Pseudomonas aeruginosa
- Broad-spectrum antibiotic treatment for >7 days in past month
- Structural lung disease (bronchiectasis)
- Corticosteroid therapy
- Malnutrition
- Undiagnosed human immunodeficiency virus infection
- Neutropenia

Legionnaires' disease (*Legionella* species)
- Acquired immunodeficiency syndrome
- Hematologic malignancy
- End-stage renal disease

TABLE 78-1 BRITISH THORACIC SOCIETY RESEARCH COMMITTEE PREDICTION RULE FOR COMMUNITY-ACQUIRED PNEUMONIA

Clinical Factor	Points
Confusion	1
Blood urea nitrogen > 19 mg/dl	1
Respiratory rate ≥ 30 breaths/min	1
Systolic blood pressure < 90 mm Hg *or* Diastolic blood pressure ≤ 60 mm Hg	1
Age ≥ 65 yr	1
Total points	
CURB-65 SCORE	
0	Low risk; consider outpatient treatment
1	
2	Short inpatient stay or closely supervised outpatient treatment
3	High risk; inpatient hospitalization and consider admission to intensive care unit
4 or 5	

TABLE 78-2 PNEUMONIA SEVERITY INDEX FOR COMMUNITY-ACQUIRED PNEUMONIA AS DEVELOPED BY PORT

Risk Factor	Points*
DEMOGRAPHIC	
Men	Age (yr):
Women	Age (yr) − 10:
Nursing home resident	+10
COMORBIDITIES	
Neoplasm	+30
Liver disease	+20
Congestive heart failure	+10
Stroke	+10
Renal failure	+10
PHYSICAL EXAMINATION FINDINGS	
Altered mental status	+20
Respiratory rate > 30 breaths/min	+20
Systolic blood pressure < 90 mm Hg	+20
Temperature < 95° F or ≥ 104° F	+15
Pulse rate ≥ 125 beats/min	+10
LABORATORY AND RADIOGRAPHIC FINDINGS	
Arterial pH < 7.35	+30
Blood urea nitrogen > 30 mg/dl	+20
Sodium < 130 mmol/L	+20
Glucose ≥ 250 mg/dl	+10
Hematocrit < 30%	+10
Partial pressure of arterial oxygen < 60 mm Hg	+10
Pleural effusion	+10
Total points	

Total Points	Risk Class	Recommendation
<51	I	Outpatient therapy should be considered, especially Class I and II
51-70	II	
71-90	III	
91-130	IV	Inpatient hospitalization
>130	V	

*Total score is determined by beginning with the patient age and adding graded points based on objective data and findings. A risk class is then defined by the total of points to assist in determining severity of illness.

widely accepted prediction rules are the British Thoracic Society (BTS) Research Committee rule (Table 78-1) and the Pneumonia Patient Outcomes Research Team (PORT) rule (Table 78-2). Interestingly, these two prediction rules are meant to serve complementary roles as they attempt to identify different patients. The BTS rule aims to identify high-risk patients who require not only admission, but ICU admission; therefore, it is meant to prevent underestimation of severity of illness.[24,25] In contrast, the PORT rule separates patients into high and low risk of death and is meant to identify patients at low risk of death so as not to overestimate their severity of illness.[8] Many investigators have studied the role of these prediction rules in various settings and support the ability of these prediction rules to assist in the triage of patients with CAP,[26-29] while other studies reinforce that, while these prediction rules may have a role, clinicians still need to use their clinical judgment when stratifying patient care.[30]

CLINICAL PHARMACOLOGY AND THERAPEUTICS

Specific Pharmacologic Considerations for CAP

Antimicrobial agents are the cornerstone of treatment in patients with CAP. While a randomized, placebo-controlled study in patients with CAP has never been performed (nor is one likely to be performed), the overwhelming preponderance of evidence suggests that the timely administration of an antibiotic(s) to which the offending pathogens(s) are sensitive reduces the complications and improves the survival of patients with CAP. Following its discovery and introduction into clinical medicine, penicillin G was the drug of choice for CAP for almost half a century. However, with the recognition that pathogens other than *S. pneumoniae* may cause CAP and with the emergence of DRSP, penicillin G is no longer recommended in the management strategy of patients with CAP. Macrolides, quinolones, and second- and/or third-generation cephalosporins are now considered the antimicrobial agents of first choice in patients with CAP. As discussed later, the treatment recommendations depend upon the patient's comorbidities, risk stratification, and treatment setting.

Antimicrobial Resistance

Resistance to antibiotics has been an increasingly recognized problem in the therapy for CAP. Many factors contribute to resistance, including overutilization of antibiotics, patient comorbidities, and a higher percentage of the population residing in long-term care facilities. Since *S. pneumoniae* is the most common etiologic agent of CAP, resistance to this pathogen is a major concern and increasing problem. According to the Tracking Resistance in the US Today study in 2004 (TRUST-8), 19% to 25% of *S. pneumoniae* has in vitro resistance to penicillin and/or macrolides, 1.4% to ceftriaxone, and 1.1% to levofloxacin. The current definition of "intermediate-level" in vitro resistance to penicillin is a minimum inhibitory concentration (MIC) value of 0.12 mcg/ml, while "high-level" in vitro resistance is defined by MIC values of 2.0 mcg/ml.[31] Interestingly, when high-level penicillin resistance was present, in vitro resistance to cefotaxime (42%), meropenem (52%), erythromycin (61%), and trimethoprim-sulfamethoxazole (92%) was also present.[32] A Centers for Disease Control and Prevention study has demonstrated that the breakpoint for clinically relevant resistance to penicillin is a MIC value of 4.0 mcg/ml.[33]

Significant controversy exists about the clinical relevance of these in vitro resistance patterns as few clinical failures (in the absence of meningitis) are documented, especially with macrolides and fluoroquinolones, which are commonly used to treat CAP in the outpatient setting. The unanswered question is whether continued use of these antibiotic classes for outpatient management of CAP will further push selection pressure and increase the virulence of these in vitro resistant organisms such that clinical treatment failures become more prevalent. Although the resistance patterns of *S. pneumoniae* appear to have changed the greatest, increased antimicrobial resistance is a universal phenomenon of all organisms associated with CAP. Moreover, it should be noted that resistance patterns vary considerably among geographic areas, and clinicians should be familiar with their local resistance patterns in order to adjust their therapeutic decisions accordingly.

Pulmonary Bioavailability of Antibiotics

The pulmonary vasculature and parenchyma filter the entire blood volume; however, not all antibiotics have the same degree of penetration into the lung parenchyma so as to achieve appropriate dose levels for adequate killing and prevention of resistance. With the development of the fluoroquinolones, effective high levels of lung penetration have been achieved without the development of resistance to treat even those patients with severe pneumonia using a single agent once a day (except those with risk factors for *P. aeruginosa*). In fact, levels of fluoroquinolones are greater in the epithelial lining fluid and alveolar macrophages than in serum.[34,35] These agents (levofloxacin, moxifloxacin, gatifloxacin) have excellent antipneumococcal activity as well as activity against gram-positive, gram-negative, and atypical pathogens; thus, they are ideal single agents for many patients, except those with severe CAP requiring ICU admission.

Macrolides are another highly effective class of antibiotics with excellent lung and alveolar macrophage penetration and good coverage for gram-positive and atypical organisms. As discussed previously, there has been increasing in vitro *S. pneumoniae* resistance to macrolides, which has many concerned about the clinical effectiveness of these agents in the years ahead.

Although vancomycin is not recommended for initial empirical therapy of CAP due to adequate antibiotic coverage of DRSP and methicillin-sensitive *S. aureus* with currently recommended agents, in the appropriate patient population (long-term care facility or young healthy individuals with aggressive pneumonia), failure of initial treatment should raise the suspicion of MRSA pneumonia. In these patients, vancomycin therapy has been considered the drug of choice, but recently the question of what constitutes adequate serum levels to provide appropriate lung penetration of vancomycin to treat MRSA has been raised.[36] In this setting, linezolid may have better penetration into lung tissue and be more active against MRSA.[37,38]

Time to First Dose of Antibiotics

Two retrospective analyses of large Medicare databases identified that the time between presentation to the hospital and the time to the first antibiotic dose (TFAD) is a predictor of patient outcome when patients require hospital admission. These studies demonstrated a 15% reduction in 30-day mortality when the TFAD was either 8 hours or a more stringent 4 hours.[39,40] Based on the findings in these two retrospective studies, the National Pneumonia Project of the Centers for Medicare & Medicaid Services has decided that patients (age > 65) who require hospitalization should receive antibiotics within 4 hours of hospital presentation as a quality-of-care benchmark for CAP. Many third-party payers have extrapolated these data to all patients presenting to the hospital with CAP and have begun to use it for hospital-level public reporting and "pay-for-performance" programs. Consequently, much controversy has arisen surrounding the benchmark of 4 hours to TFAD. Two recent prospective cohort studies of patients admitted to the hospital with CAP demonstrated that the delay to TFDA was strongly associated with altered mental status, absence of fever and/or hypoxia, lack of infiltrates on chest radiograph, and increasing age.[41,42] Since diagnostic uncertainty can be a barrier to TFAD, an excessive number of patients will be treated with antibiotics in order to comply with the TFAD 4-hour benchmark, thus leading to the potential for increased antibiotic resistance, costs, and adverse events. Investigators in this field believe that the benchmark should be applied to the population from which the data were derived—persons age 65 or older with radiographic evidence of CAP and no antibiotic pretreatment.[43]

With our understanding that early aggressive antibiotic therapy is one of the cornerstones in management of septic shock,[44] it seems intuitive that early recognition and antibiotic administration for CAP could improve outcomes; however, within what time frame and in what populations remain to be determined. This clearly will be an area of intense investigation and debate in the forthcoming years.

Intravenous Versus Oral Therapy and Duration of Therapy

The traditional therapeutic period for CAP had been 14 days of intravenous antibiotics until a study in 1996 demonstrated that 48 hours of intravenous antibiotic therapy followed by 12 days of oral therapy had similar outcomes to 14 days of intravenous therapy.[45] This study and several subsequent studies have confirmed that the conversion from intravenous to oral antibiotics decreases hospital length of stay, costs, and incidence of phlebitis and intravenous line infection without impacting on mortality or outcomes.[46,47] The improved pharmacokinetic profile of newer generation antibiotics due to their high degree of bioavailability, rapid gastrointestinal absorption, and equivalent blood and tissue levels regardless of oral or intravenous administration (particularly the antipneumococcal fluoroquinolones) has enhanced the ability to treat patients with moderate to moderately severe CAP with oral therapy. In fact, several studies have demonstrated that short-course high-dose therapy with antibiotics has equivalency to traditional antibiotic regimens with better patient compliance, less cost and fewer adverse events, and a possible reduction in selection pressure for resistance.[48-51]

Interestingly, in a recent randomized trial in the Netherlands, patients with mild to moderately severe CAP were randomized to 3 days versus 8 days of high-dose ampicillin therapy. There was no difference in clinical success rate or radiographic success at day 10 or day 28 between the two groups.[52] Consequently, patients with mild to moderately severe CAP requiring hospitalization can likely be treated for much shorter durations than the traditional 7- to 10-day time period without an impact on patient outcomes. These shorter durations of therapy would surely represent cost savings, reduce the number of adverse events, and decrease the selection pressure for antibiotic resistance. The conversion from the traditional 2-week treatment period to much shorter time frames will give some clinicians trepidation of treatment failure, but the data have not demonstrated differences in outcome. Therefore, as more data become available, clinicians should strongly reconsider shorter treatment courses for CAP.

Treatment Recommendations for CAP

Outpatients without Prior Cardiopulmonary Disease or Modifying Factors

In this patient population without underlying cardiopulmonary disease, and no risk factors for DRSP, aspiration, or enteric gram-negative organisms (see Box 78-1), the most likely pathogens are *S. pneumoniae*, atypical pathogens, respiratory viruses, and possibly *H. influenzae* (especially in smokers). For these patients, initial therapy with an advanced-generation macrolide (azithromycin or clarithromycin) is optimal, with doxycycline as a second choice if patients are intolerant of or allergic to macrolides (Table 78-3). Advanced-generation macrolides are preferred over erythromycin due to fewer gastrointestinal side effects and less frequent dosing, which may improve patient compliance. Although an antipneumococcal fluoroquinolone would be equally effective, use of one of these agents in this

TABLE 78-3 OUTPATIENTS WITHOUT CARDIOPULMONARY DISEASE OR MODIFYING RISK FACTORS

Organisms	Recommended Therapy
Streptococcus pneumoniae *Mycoplasma pneumoniae* *Chlamydia pneumoniae* *Haemophilus influenzae* *Legionella* spp. Respiratory viruses *Mycobacterium tuberculosis* Endemic fungi	Advanced-generation macrolide: azithromycin or clarithromycin *or* Doxycycline

TABLE 78-4 OUTPATIENT WITH CARDIOPULMONARY DISEASE AND/OR MODIFYING FACTORS

Organisms	Recommended Therapy
Streptococcus pneumoniae (including DRSP) *Mycoplasma pneumoniae* *Chlamydia pneumoniae* Mixed infection (bacteria plus atypical pathogen or virus) *Haemophilus influenzae* Enteric gram-negatives Respiratory viruses *Moraxella catarrhalis, Legionella* spp., aspiration, *Mycobacterium tuberculosis*, endemic fungi	β-Lactam (oral cefpodoxime, cefuroxime, high-dose ampicillin, amoxicillin-clavulanate; or parenteral ceftriaxone followed by oral cefpodoxime) *plus* Macrolide or doxycycline *or* Antipneumococcal fluoroquinolone alone

low-risk patient population is likely unnecessary and may promote selection pressure for resistance.

Outpatients with Cardiopulmonary Disease and/or Modifying Factors

Although these patients are at risk for the usual CAP pathogens, they are at increased risk for CAP due to DRSP, enteric gram-negatives, and aspiration; consequently, the empirical coverage of CAP in these patients must be adjusted accordingly to take these organisms into consideration (Table 78-4). An oral β-lactam agent may be used in combination with an advanced-generation macrolide (or doxycycline if the patient is intolerant of macrolides) in these patients. The oral β-lactam agent is chosen to be effective against DRSP (MIC = 2 mg/L), but should be administered at high doses to overcome drug resistance. Options for β-lactam agents include cefuroxime or cefpodoxime, high-dose ampicillin (1 g every 8 hours), or amoxicillin-clavulanate (2 g twice daily). Alternatively, a more appealing choice for these patients with risk factors for DRSP is the new-generation antipneumococcal fluoroquinolones. Due to the very low incidence of resistance of these agents to DRSP and their once-daily administration, patient compliance and cost may be reduced compared to the combination of a β-lactam agent and a macrolide. Moreover, if the patient has risks for aspiration or resides in a long-term care facility, coverage for anaerobes should be considered with amoxicillin-clavulanate or amoxicillin with a macrolide. If anaerobes are documented or a lung abscess is present, clindamycin or metronidazole should be incorporated into the regimen.

Inpatients without Cardiopulmonary Disease or Modifying Factors

This category of patients likely represents a small population as most patients without cardiopulmonary disease or modifying factors likely can be treated effectively on an outpatient basis. The most common organisms in this group are similar to those of the outpatient without cardiopulmonary disease: *S. pneumoniae*, atypicals, *H. influenzae*, and respiratory viruses (Table 78-5). If the severity of illness entails hospitalization (not to an ICU), these patients are effectively treated with intravenous azithromycin alone at 500 mg daily for 2 to 5 days followed by oral therapy at 500 mg daily for a total of 7 to 10 days.[53,54] If the patient is intolerant of macrolides due to adverse events, then therapy should be initiated with doxycycline and a β-lactam or an antipneumococcal fluoroquinolone.

TABLE 78-5 INPATIENTS NOT REQUIRING INTENSIVE CARE UNIT ADMISSION

Organisms	Recommended Therapy
A. No cardiopulmonary disease or modifying factors	
Streptococcus pneumoniae *Haemophilus influenzae* *Mycoplasma pneumoniae* *Chlamydia pneumoniae* Mixed infection (bacteria plus atypical pathogen) Respiratory viruses *Legionella* spp. Miscellaneous (*Mycobacterium tuberculosis*, endemic fungi)	Intravenous (IV) azithromycin alone If macrolide allergic: doxycycline ***and*** a β-lactam *or* Antipneumococcal fluoroquinolone alone
B. Cardiopulmonary disease and/or modifying factors	
S. pneumoniae (including DRSP) *H. influenzae* *M. pneumoniae* *C. pneumoniae* Mixed infection (bacteria plus atypical pathogen) Enteric gram-negatives Aspiration (anaerobes) Respiratory viruses *Legionella* spp. Miscellaneous (*M. tuberculosis*, endemic fungi)	IV β-Lactam (cefotaxime, ceftriaxone, ampicillin-sulbactam, high-dose ampicillin) *plus* IV or oral macrolide or doxycycline *or* IV antipneumococcal fluoroquinolone alone

Inpatients with Cardiopulmonary Disease and/or Modifying Factors

Therapy for these patients should include coverage for DRSP and enteric gram-negatives as this population is at risk for these pathogens. Similar to outpatients with similar risk factors, therapy with a β-lactam agent and macrolide can be initiated (see Table 78-5). The β-lactam agent should be administered at the high dose level discussed earlier to ensure adequate coverage of DRSP. A macrolide is added to cover atypical pathogens and can be administered orally or intravenously depending on the severity of illness. Doxycycline is the alternative if the patient is intolerant of macrolide therapy. Similar to outpatients with DRSP risk factors, an alternative to the β-lactam–macrolide regimen is to use an antipneumococcal fluoroquinolone alone. Once again, the fluoroquinolones simplify the regimen to once daily and may improve compliance and decrease costs. If the patient has risk factors for aspiration or lives in a long-term care facility, coverage for anaerobes should be considered with the addition of ampicillin-sulbactam, high-dose ampicillin, or other active β-lactams. The documentation of anaerobes or the presence of a lung abscess should prompt the addition of clindamycin or metronidazole to the regimen.

Inpatients Requiring ICU Admission and without *Pseudomonas aeruginosa* Risk Factors

Patients with severe CAP with admission to the ICU should have therapy directed against *S. pneumoniae*, *H. influenzae*, and *Legionella* and other atypicals, but stratification based on risk factors for *P. aeruginosa* infection must be considered (Table 78-6). If no *P. aeruginosa*

TABLE 78-6 INTENSIVE CARE UNIT–ADMITTED PATIENTS

Organisms	Recommended Therapy
A. No *Pseudomonas aeruginosa* risk factors	
Streptococcus pneumoniae (including DRSP) *Legionella* spp. *Haemophilus influenzae* Enteric gram-negative bacilli *Staphylococcus aureus* *Mycoplasma pneumoniae* Respiratory viruses Miscellaneous (*Chlamydia pneumoniae, Mycobacterium tuberculosis*, endemic fungi)	Intravenous (IV) β-lactam (cefotaxime, ceftriaxone) ***plus either*** IV macrolide (azithromycin) *or* IV fluoroquinolone
B. *Pseudomonas aeruginosa* risk factors	
All of the above organisms plus *P. aeruginosa*	Selected IV antipseudomonal: β-lactam (cefepime, imipenem, meropenem, piperacillin-tazobactam) ***plus*** IV antipseudomonal quinolone (ciprofloxacin) *or* Selected IV antipseudomonal: β-lactam ***plus*** IV aminoglycoside ***plus*** either IV macrolide or IV nonpseudomonal fluoroquinolone

risk factors are present, initial therapy with a β-lactam active against DRSP in combination with either azithromycin or a fluoroquinolone should be instituted. The β-lactam agent that is chosen should have activity against DRSP (cefotaxime, ceftriaxone, ampicillin-sulbactam), but those β-lactam agents that also have antipseudomonal activity (cefepime, piperacillin-tazobactam, imipenem, meropenem) are not recommended for primary treatment when *P. aeruginosa* is not suspected.

If *P. aeruginosa* risk factors are present, therapy should always include two agents with antipseudomonal activity and also cover DRSP and *Legionella* species. Therapeutic options include select β-lactams (cefepime, piperacillin-tazobactam, imipenem, meropenem) plus an antipseudomonal quinolone (ciprofloxacin), or select β-lactams with an aminoglycoside plus either azithromycin or a nonpseudomonal fluoroquinolone. If the patient has *P. aeruginosa* risk factors and is β-lactam allergic, aztreonam can replace the β-lactam agent and should be combined with an antipneumococcal fluoroquinolone and an aminoglycoside.

Special Considerations

Community-Acquired MRSA Pneumonia

As mentioned previously, an increasing incidence of community-acquired MRSA infection has been reported throughout the country. Although this clearly represents a small number of patients with CAP, it tends to affect young, healthy individuals with devastating effects. Therefore, in the appropriate patient population—a resident of a long-term care facility; a young, healthy person with rapidly progressive necrotizing pneumonia; or a person with a post–influenza syndrome pneumonia—serious consideration should be given to the addition of vancomycin or linezolid to cover MRSA, especially if there is minimal to no clinical response to initial treatment. With recent reports clearly documenting the increasing incidence of MRSA cutaneous infections,[55] it is likely that MRSA CAP will become more prevalent, and clinicians must be aware of the possibility of this organism as a community-acquired pathogen.

Health Care–Associated Pneumonia

Patients who develop pneumonia in the setting of an acute or chronic health care facility must be distinguished from those who develop pneumonia in the community; the former patients are referred to as having health care–associated pneumonia, which includes hospital-acquired pneumonia and ventilator-associated pneumonia. This distinction is important as these patients are at high risk of having infection with MRSA and multidrug-resistant (MDR) bacterial pathogens. The MDR pathogens include *P. aeruginosa*, extended-spectrum β-lactamase–producing *Klebsiella pneumoniae, Acinetobacter baumanii, Enterobacter* species, and *Enterococcus* species.[56] Health care–associated pneumonia contributes significantly to morbidity, length of hospitalization, increased health care costs, and increased mortality. Early broad-spectrum antimicrobial coverage with multiple antibiotics is recommended in these patients, with de-escalation once the implicated pathogen has been identified. In general, this requires the combination of an antipseudomonal cephalosporin (cefepime, ceftazidime), carbapenem (imipenem, meropenem), or penicillin (piperacillin-tazobactam) plus either an antipseudomonal fluoroquinolone or an aminoglycoside.

Supportive and Emerging Therapies for CAP

Supplemental oxygen is usually required for those patients with CAP admitted to a hospital. The oxygen saturation of these patients should be closely followed. Patients with CAP who progress to develop severe sepsis and septic shock will require resuscitation with intravenous fluids and vasopressor agents. Drotrecogin alfa activated (activated protein C) should be considered in patients with CAP who develop organ failure or septic shock. The Recombinant Human Activated Protein C Worldwide Evaluation in Severe Sepsis (PROWESS) study demonstrated a reduction in 28-day all-cause mortality in patients with CAP and severe sepsis who were treated with this agent.[57]

The role of corticosteroids in patients with severe CAP is controversial. Confalonieri and colleagues, in a small randomized, placebo-controlled study, demonstrated that hydrocortisone given as a bolus of 200 mg followed by an infusion of 10 mg/hr for 7 days reduced the complication rate and mortality in patients with severe CAP.[58] Additional studies are required to determine the role of corticosteroids and other immunomodulating agents in the management of patients with severe CAP.

CONCLUSIONS

Community-acquired pneumonia is the leading cause of infectious mortality in the United States. Recognition of the clinical syndrome consistent with pneumonia, assessing patients' risk factors for specific organisms, determining their medical comorbidities, and evaluating their severity of illness will allow the clinician to ascertain pertinent pathogens and choose appropriate empirical coverage for CAP. Clinicians should have an understanding of their local resistance patterns as this may alter the empirical coverage chosen. When and if specific pathogens are isolated, empirical coverage should be de-escalated as guided by microbiologic data to maximize kill and minimize the development of resistance. Due to the evolution of existing infectious pathogens and newly discovered pathogens (e.g., that causing severe acute respiratory syndrome), the recommendations included herein will invariably change with time to address these factors.

As our armamentarium for the treatment of CAP has rapidly evolved over the last 60 years since the discovery of penicillin, so has the ability of the bacterial pathogens evolved to develop resistance mechanisms to thwart the effectiveness of these new antibiotics. Therefore, judicious use of antibiotics to cover appropriate organisms for each individual patient will minimize the risk of developing resistance. In this manner, it is hoped the medical profession can offer curative therapy to all patients with CAP and continue to decrease morbidity and mortality from "the old man's friend."

REFERENCES

1. Mandell LA, Bartlett JG, Dowell SF, et al. Update of practice guidelines for the management of community-acquired pneumonia in immunocompetent adults. Clin Infect Dis 2003;37:1405-1433.
2. Colice GL, Morley MA, Asche C, et al. Treatment costs of community-acquired pneumonia in an employed population. Chest 2004;125:2140-2145.
3. Niederman MS, Mandell LA, Anzueto A, et al. Guidelines for the management of adults with community-acquired pneumonia: diagnosis, assessment of severity, antimicrobial therapy, and prevention. Am J Respir Crit Care Med 2001;163:1730-1754.
4. Marrie TJ, Durant H, Yates L. Community-acquired pneumonia requiring hospitalization: 5-year prospective study. Rev Infect Dis 1989;11:586-599.
5. Woodhead MA, Macfarlane JT, McCracken JS, et al. Prospective study of the aetiology and outcome of pneumonia in the community. Lancet 1987;1:671-674.
6. Torres A, Serra-Batlles J, Ferrer A, et al. Severe community-acquired pneumonia: epidemiology and prognostic factors. Am Rev Respir Dis 1991;144:312-318.
7. Pachon J, Prados MD, Capote F, et al. Severe community-acquired pneumonia: etiology, prognosis, and treatment. Am Rev Respir Dis 1990;142:369-373.
8. Fine MJ, Smith MA, Carson CA, et al. Prognosis and outcomes of patients with community-acquired pneumonia: a meta-analysis [see comment]. JAMA 1996;275:134-141.
9. Marston BJ, Plouffe JF, File TM Jr, et al. Incidence of community-acquired pneumonia requiring hospitalization: results of a population-based active surveillance study in Ohio. The Community-Based Pneumonia Incidence Study Group. Arch Intern Med 1997;157:1709-1718.
10. Ortqvist A, Sterner G, Nilsson JA. Severe community-acquired pneumonia: factors influencing need of intensive care treatment and prognosis. Scand J Infect Dis 1985;17:377-386.
11. Leroy O, Santre C, Beuscart C, et al. A five-year study of severe community-acquired pneumonia with emphasis on prognosis in patients admitted to an intensive care unit. Intensive Care Med 1995;21:24-31.
12. Koivula I, Sten M, Makela PH. Risk factors for pneumonia in the elderly. Am J Med 1994;96:313-320.
13. Ruiz M, Ewig S, Marcos MA, et al. Etiology of community-acquired pneumonia: impact of age, comorbidity, and severity. Am J Respir Crit Care Med 1999;160:397-405.
14. Marrie TJ. Community-acquired pneumonia. Clin Infect Dis 1994;18:501-513.
15. Bates JH, Campbell GD, Barron AL, et al. Microbial etiology of acute pneumonia in hospitalized patients [see comment]. Chest 1992;101:1005-1012.
16. Fang GD, Fine M, Orloff J, et al. New and emerging etiologies for community-acquired pneumonia with implications for therapy: a prospective multicenter study of 359 cases. Medicine (Baltimore) 1990;69:307-316.
17. File TM Jr, Tan JS, Plouffe JF. The role of atypical pathogens: *Mycoplasma pneumoniae, Chlamydia pneumoniae*, and *Legionella pneumophila* in respiratory infection. Infect Dis Clin North Am 1998;12:569-592.
18. Burman LA, Trollfors B, Andersson B, et al. Diagnosis of pneumonia by cultures, bacterial and viral antigen detection tests, and serology with special reference to antibodies against pneumococcal antigens. J Infect Dis 1991;163:1087-1093.
19. Ewig S, Ruiz M, Torres A, et al. Pneumonia acquired in the community through drug-resistant *Streptococcus pneumoniae*. Am J Respir Crit Care Med 1999;159:1835-1842.
20. Clavo-Sanchez AJ, Giron-Gonzalez JA, Lopez-Prieto D, et al. Multivariate analysis of risk factors for infection due to penicillin-resistant and multidrug-resistant *Streptococcus pneumoniae*: a multicenter study. Clin Infect Dis 1997;24:1052-1059.
21. Kollef MH, Micek ST. Methicillin-resistant *Staphylococcus aureus*: a new community-acquired pathogen? Curr Opin Infect Dis 2006;19:161-168.
22. Francis JS, Doherty MC, Lopatin U, et al. Severe community-onset pneumonia in healthy adults caused by methicillin-resistant *Staphylococcus aureus* carrying the Panton-Valentine leukocidin genes [see comment]. Clin Infect Dis 2005;40:100-107.
23. Mandell LA, Bartlett JG, Dowell SF, et al. Update of practice guidelines for the management of community-acquired pneumonia in immunocompetent adults [see comment]. Clin Infect Dis 2003;37:1405-1433.
24. Farr BM, Sloman AJ, Fisch MJ. Predicting death in patients hospitalized for community-acquired pneumonia [see comment]. Ann Intern Med 1991;115:428-436.
25. Neill AM, Martin IR, Weir R, et al. Community acquired pneumonia: aetiology and usefulness of severity criteria on admission. Thorax 1996;51:1010-1016.
26. Aujesky D, Auble TE, Yealy DM, et al. Prospective comparison of three validated prediction rules for prognosis in community-acquired pneumonia. Am J Med 2005;118:384-392.
27. Marrie TJ, Lau CY, Wheeler SL, et al. A controlled trial of a critical pathway for treatment of community-acquired pneumonia. CAPITAL Study Investigators. Community-Acquired Pneumonia Intervention Trial Assessing Levofloxacin. JAMA 2000;283:749-755.
28. Atlas SJ, Benzer TI, Borowsky LH, et al. Safely increasing the proportion of patients with community-acquired pneumonia treated as outpatients: an interventional trial. Arch Intern Med 1998;158:1350-1356.
29. Lim WS, van der Eerden MM, Laing R, et al. Defining community acquired pneumonia severity on presentation to hospital: an international derivation and validation study [see comment]. Thorax 2003;58:377-382.
30. Smyrnios NA, Schaefer OP, Collins RM, et al. Applicability of prediction rules in patients with community-acquired pneumonia requiring intensive care: a pilot study. J Intensive Care Med 2005;20:226-232.
31. Heffelfinger JD, Dowell SF, Jorgensen JH, et al. Management of community-acquired pneumonia in the era of pneumococcal resistance: a report from the Drug-Resistant Streptococcus pneumoniae Therapeutic Working Group. Arch Intern Med 2000; 160:1399-1408.
32. Whitney CG, Farley MM, Hadler J, et al. Increasing prevalence of multidrug-resistant *Streptococcus pneumoniae* in the United States. N Engl J Med 2000;343:1917-1924.
33. Feikin DR, Schuchat A, Kolczak M, et al. Mortality from invasive pneumococcal pneumonia in the era of antibiotic resistance, 1995-1997. Am J Public Health 2000;90:223-229.
34. Capitano B, Mattoes HM, Shore E, et al. Steady-state intrapulmonary concentrations of moxifloxacin, levofloxacin, and azithromycin in older adults. Chest 2004;125:965-973.
35. Niederman MS. The quinolones. In Andriole V (ed): Treatment of Respiratory Infections with Quinolones. San Diego, CA: McGraw-Hill, 1998, pp 229-250.
36. Lamer C, de Beco V, Soler P, et al. Analysis of vancomycin entry into pulmonary lining fluid by bronchoalveolar lavage in critically ill patients. Antimicrob Agents Chemother 1993;37:281-286.
37. Honeybourne D, Tobin C, Jevons G, et al. Intrapulmonary penetration of linezolid. J Antimicrob Chemother 2003;51:1431-1434.
38. Conte JE Jr, Golden JA, Kipps J, et al. Intrapulmonary pharmacokinetics of linezolid. Antimicrob Agents Chemother 2002;46:1475-1480.
39. Houck PM, Bratzler DW, Niederman M, et al. Pneumonia treatment process and quality. Arch Intern Med 2002;162:843-844.
40. Meehan TP, Fine MJ, Krumholz HM, et al. Quality of care, process, and outcomes in elderly patients with pneumonia. JAMA 1997;278:2080-2084.
41. Metersky ML, Sweeney TA, Getzow MB, et al. Antibiotic timing and diagnostic uncertainty in Medicare patients with pneumonia: is it reasonable to expect all patients to receive antibiotics within 4 hours? Chest 2006;130:16-21.
42. Waterer GW, Kessler LA, Wunderink RG. Delayed administration of antibiotics and atypical presentation in community-acquired pneumonia. Chest 2006;130:11-15.
43. Houck PM. Antibiotics and pneumonia: is timing everything or just a cause of more problems? Chest 2006;130:1-3.
44. Dellinger RP, Carlet JM, Masur H, et al. Surviving Sepsis Campaign guidelines for management of severe sepsis and septic shock. Crit Care Med 2004;32:858-873.
45. Siegel RE, Halpern NA, Almenoff PL, et al. A prospective randomized study of inpatient iv. antibiotics for community-acquired pneumonia: the optimal duration of therapy. Chest 1996;110:965-971.
46. Ramirez JA, Srinath L, Ahkee S, et al. Early switch from intravenous to oral cephalosporins in the treatment of hospitalized patients with community-acquired pneumonia. Arch Intern Med 1995;155:1273-1276.
47. Cunha BA. Oral or intravenous-to-oral antibiotic switch therapy for treating patients with community-acquired pneumonia. Am J Med 2001;111:412-413.
48. File TM Jr. Shorter course therapy of serious respiratory infections: new data for new approaches to management. Curr Opin Infect Dis 2004;17:105-107.
49. File TM Jr. A new dosing paradigm: high-dose, short-course fluoroquinolone therapy for community-acquired pneumonia. Clin Cornerstone 2003;Suppl 3:S21-S28.
50. Ruhe JJ, Hasbun R. *Streptococcus pneumoniae* bacteremia: duration of previous antibiotic use and association with penicillin resistance. Clin Infect Dis 2003;36:1132-1138.
51. Dunbar LM, Wunderink RG, Habib MP, et al. High-dose, short-course levofloxacin for community-acquired pneumonia: a new treatment paradigm. Clin Infect Dis 2003;37:752-760.
52. el Moussaoui R, de Borgie CA, van den Broek P, et al. Effectiveness of discontinuing antibiotic treatment after three days versus eight days in mild to moderate-severe community acquired pneumonia: randomised, double blind study. BMJ 2006;332: 1355.
53. Vergis EN, Indorf A, File TM Jr, et al. Azithromycin vs cefuroxime plus erythromycin for empirical treatment of community-acquired pneumonia in hospitalized patients: a prospective, randomized, multicenter trial. Arch Intern Med 2000;160:1294-1300.
54. Plouffe J, Schwartz DB, Kolokathis A, et al. Clinical efficacy of intravenous followed by oral azithromycin monotherapy in hospitalized patients with community-acquired pneumonia. The Azithromycin Intravenous Clinical Trials Group. Antimicrob Agents Chemother 2000;44:1796-1802.
55. Moran GJ, Krishnadasan A, Gorwitz RJ, et al. Methicillin-resistant *S. aureus* infections among patients in the emergency department. N Engl J Med 2006;355:666-674.
56. American Thoracic Society and Infectious Diseases Society of America. Guidelines for the management of adults with hospital-acquired, ventilator-associated, and healthcare-associated pneumonia. Am J Resp Crit Care Med 2005;171:388-416.
57. Bernard GR, Vincent JL, Laterre PF, et al. Efficacy and safety of recombinant human activated protein C for severe sepsis. N Engl J Med 2001;344:699-709.
58. Confalonieri M, Urbino R, Potena A, et al. Hydrocortisone infusion for severe community-acquired pneumonia: a preliminary randomized study. Am J Respir Crit Care Med 2005;171:242-248.

79

TUBERCULOSIS

Ying Zhang

OVERVIEW 1089
PATHOPHYSIOLOGY RELATED TO CHEMOTHERAPY 1089
THERAPEUTICS AND CLINICAL PHARMACOLOGY 1090
Goals of Therapy 1090
Therapeutics by Class 1090
Inhibitors of Cell Wall Synthesis 1092
Inhibitors of Nucleic Acid Synthesis 1095
Inhibitors of Protein Synthesis 1096
Inhibitors of Membrane Energy Metabolism 1097
Others 1098
Therapeutic Approach 1098
Treatment of TB Caused by Drug-Susceptible Organisms 1098
Alternative Regimens Used in Drug Intolerance or Drug Resistance 1099
Re-treatment Regimen 1100
Recommended Doses 1100
Treatment of Latent TB Infection: Preventive Therapy 1100
Treatment of Extrapulmonary TB 1100
Treatment of TB Patients with HIV Infection 1100
Treatment of MDR-TB 1104
Emerging Targets and Therapeutics 1104
New Fluoroquinolones 1104
Oxazolidinones (Linezolid) 1105
Nitroimidazopyran (PA-824) 1105
Diarylquinoline 1105

OVERVIEW

Mycobacterium tuberculosis is a particularly successful pathogen that latently infects about one third of the world's population (2 billion people). Despite the availability of chemotherapy and bacille Calmette-Guérin vaccine, the bacillus caused 9 million new tuberculosis (TB) cases and nearly 2 million deaths in 2004.[1] The increasing emergence of drug-resistant TB—especially multidrug-resistant TB (MDR-TB) (resistant to at least isoniazid and rifampin) and most recently, extensively or extreme drug-resistant TB (i.e., MDR-TB plus resistance to three other second-line drugs)—is particularly alarming.[2] Already 50 million people have been infected with MDR-TB.[2] There is much concern that the TB situation may become even worse with the spread of the human immunodeficiency virus (HIV) pandemic worldwide, which weakens the host immune system and allows latent TB to reactivate or makes the person more susceptible to re-infection with drug-susceptible and even drug-resistant strains.[3] The current control of TB is compromised by drug-resistant TB and HIV infection, a lethal combination that presents a serious challenge for effective TB control.

The current recommended standard TB chemotherapy, part of the DOTS (*d*irectly *o*bserved *t*herapy, *s*hort-course) strategy, is a 6-month therapeutic regimen consisting of an initial phase of treatment with four drugs, isoniazid (INH), rifampin (RIF), pyrazinamide (PZA), and ethambutol (EMB) for 2 months, followed by a continuation phase of treatment with INH and RIF for another 4 months.[4] DOTS is currently the best TB treatment strategy, with a cure rate of 78% to 95%, and is recommended by the World Health Organization (WHO) for treating every TB patient.[4] However, the lengthy therapy is often associated with significant side effects and makes patient compliance difficult, which frequently selects drug-resistant TB bacteria. Moreover, DOTS may not work in areas where there is a high incidence of MDR-TB, with a cure rate as low as 50%. In such situations, the WHO recommends the use of DOTS-Plus, which is DOTS plus second-line TB drugs for the treatment of MDR-TB and TB.[4] However, treatment of MDR-TB with DOTS-Plus can take up to 24 months and is not only costly but also has significant toxicity. Despite the fact that TB chemotherapy renders a patient noninfectious a few weeks after the initiation of the therapy, the complete 6-month regimen is necessary to kill a population of slowly metabolizing, persistent bacilli and to allow the host to develop sufficient immunity to prevent relapse.

There is renewed interest in developing new TB drugs that not only are active against drug-resistant TB but, more importantly, also shorten the TB therapy.[5-8] New progress is being made in this area, and there is hope that more effective TB therapy may be in sight in the near future. This chapter addresses the goals and principles of TB therapy, based on the pathophysiology of the disease. Individual TB drugs and their discovery, mechanisms of action, and resistance, along with guidelines for treatment, are reviewed. Finally, new promising TB drug candidates are briefly discussed.

PATHOPHYSIOLOGY RELATED TO CHEMOTHERAPY

During the course of infection by *M. tuberculosis*, host cells and tissues respond by producing typical pathologic lesions. The bacilli initially replicate inside host macrophages that then burst to release the bacilli, which spread to other cells or replicate in more host cells to form granulomas. Development of immunity and host inflammation halts the bacterial replication but also causes granuloma formation and central caseous necrosis and subsequent liquefaction and cavity formation.[9] The varying types of lesions where the tubercle bacilli reside produce different microenvironments (sufficient oxygen in a cavity, low oxygen inside host macrophages, and acid pH during active inflammation) and dictate different metabolic statuses of tubercle bacilli in vivo; these microenvironments are the basis for the generation of different bacterial populations. These different bacterial populations have varying susceptibility to different TB drugs. According to Mitchison,[10] tubercle bacilli in lesions consist of at least four different subpopulations:

1. Those that are actively growing, such as those in cavities exposed to sufficient oxygen, which are killed primarily by INH (in cases of INH resistance, the bacilli are killed by RIF or streptomycin [SM] or inhibited by EMB)
2. Those that have spurts of metabolism, which are killed by RIF
3. Those that have low metabolic activity in acid pH environment, which are killed by PZA
4. Those that are "dormant," which are not killed by current TB drugs

A modified version of the Mitchison hypothesis is shown in Figure 79-1, where the speed of growth in the original Mitchison hypothesis is replaced with metabolic status.

Different bactericidal drugs (INH, RIF, PZA) are used in combination to kill different populations of bacilli in different types of lesions (see Fig. 79-1), and to reduce the number of viable bacilli in the lesions

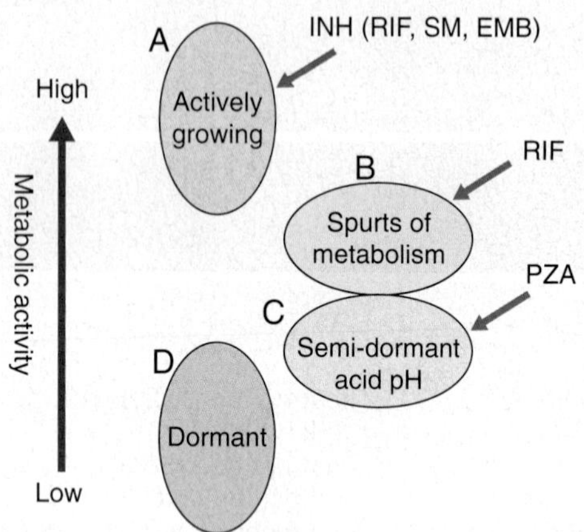

FIGURE 79-1 • Special bacterial populations theory and TB therapy.

to quickly achieve sputum negativity and prevent drug resistance. The rapidly growing extracellular bacilli that reside mainly in cavities are the largest bacterial population, which is most likely to contain organisms with random mutations that confer resistance to any single drug. The frequency of mutations that confer resistance is about 10^{-6} for INH and 10^{-8} for RIF[11]; thus, the frequency of concurrent mutations to resistance to both INH and RIF would be 10^{-14}, which is a highly unlikely event. Therefore, drug combinations can prevent drug resistance. RIF and PZA have the greatest sterilizing activity, followed by INH and SM.[10] The sterilizing activity of RIF persists throughout the therapy, but the sterilizing activity of PZA is confined to the first 2 months of the initial phase of treatment since giving PZA longer than 2 months does not provide any added benefit,[12] presumably because local tissue pH becomes neutral due to resolution of inflammation after 2 month of therapy. Importantly, in RIF-containing regimens, PZA provides additional sterilizing activity by killing a special population of bacilli not killed by other TB drugs.[10] The inclusion of the bacteriostatic drug EMB is mainly to replace the injection drug SM (which is often classified as a front-line agent but used essentially like a second-line drug as it is an injection drug) for convenient oral administration of TB therapy and to prevent drug resistance in case the bacilli are resistant to INH.

Besides prevention of drug resistance, drug combination also improves the efficacy of the treatment as shown by shortening of the therapy. Several factors underlie lengthy therapy. First, the nature of the disease pathology can influence the efficacy and duration of chemotherapy. For example, open cavities containing large numbers of bacilli present a particular problem for eradication of the bacilli by chemotherapy.[13] Second, the phenotypic resistance in nonreplicating persisters presents a major problem for the current TB therapy. It is well known that antibiotics are active against growing bacteria but are ineffective against nongrowing bacteria.[14] The rapidly growing bacterial population is eliminated early in therapy such that about 80% of patients are cleared of viable bacilli from the sputum at the end of the 2-month initial phase of treatment.[15] The remaining bacterial subpopulations that are growing more slowly account for treatment failures and relapses, especially when the duration of therapy is inadequate.

There are at least three types of nongrowing bacteria that are phenotypically resistant to antibiotics: the stationary-phase bacteria, residual survivors or persisters not killed during antibiotic exposure but that can grow in regular media, and dormant bacteria that do not grow in regular media.[16] RIF and PZA are important sterilizing drugs that significantly reduce the number of persistent bacilli in the lesions and play an important role in shortening the therapy from 12 to 18 months to 6 months.[10,12] However, there are still other persister populations that are not killed by RIF or PZA.[8] Little is known about the biology of these persisters[16] despite significant interest in this area and interest in developing drugs targeting persisters.[8,17] The intracellular location of the bacilli could render some drugs such as SM inactive against intracellular bacilli. However, most drugs do penetrate the necrotic tissues[13] but cannot effectively kill nonreplicating bacilli in the lesions.

The third factor in lengthy therapy for TB is that the host immune system may not effectively eliminate tubercle bacilli in the lesions. In many bacterial infections, small numbers of residual bacteria after antibiotic therapy can be effectively eliminated or controlled by the immune system. However, in TB, it appears that the host immune system is not very effective in controlling the residual bacteria not killed by TB chemotherapy. Thus the current chemotherapy while achieving clinical cure, cannot achieve a bacteriologic cure—that is, the therapy cannot completely eradicate all bacilli in the lesion.[13,14] However, if the number of persisters or dormant bacilli is sufficiently small, and the immune response is adequate, the small number of persisters may die off and a stable cure can be achieved without relapse.

THERAPEUTICS AND CLINICAL PHARMACOLOGY

Goals of Therapy

The goals of TB therapy are to kill tubercle bacilli rapidly, prevent the emergence of drug resistance, and eliminate persistent bacilli from the host tissues to prevent relapse.[15] From the perspective of disease control in patients, the goals of therapy are to cure individual patients by sterilizing lesions quickly and completely without relapse using first-line TB drugs, and to minimize the transmission of *M. tuberculosis* to other people.[4]

During the therapy, three factors—drugs, bacteria, and host factors—come into play. The action of TB drugs can be divided into three phases according to these factors. In Phase 1, which lasts 2 to 3 days, over 90% of actively growing bacilli in cavities with sufficient oxygen are killed by INH. In Phase 2, which lasts 2 months, the surviving bacilli (which grow quite slowly) not killed by INH exposure are now killed by RIF and PZA, which kill a population of persister bacilli at acid pH. In Phase 3, lasting 4 months (the continuation phase with INH and RIF), the intracellular persister bacilli are killed very slowly primarily by RIF and only marginally by INH.[12] The mechanism underlying the use of INH and RIF in the continuation phase of treatment is not well understood, despite clinical experience supporting this practice. INH is known to be active only against growing tubercle bacilli,[8] but after the initial phase of treatment with INH, RIF, PZA, and EMB for 2 months, the residual bacilli are supposed to be nongrowing and metabolically quiescent and thus not susceptible to INH or RIF. However, it is quite likely that the main role of INH and RIF in the continuation phase is to prevent the reversion of persister bacilli (the urge of life) and kill occasionally growing bacilli derived from reverted persisters.

The symptoms associated with TB (fever, night sweats, cough, etc.) disappear in a few weeks after the start of TB therapy. Directly observed therapy (DOT) and appropriate patient compliance to therapy are essential for the success of TB chemotherapy.

To prevent early-stage TB infection (also called latent TB infection [LTBI]) from developing into active disease in contacts and recent tuberculin converters, INH is used singly for 6 or 9 months. LTBI can also be treated with rifampin for 4 months.[15] However, treatment with rifampin and PZA for 2 months, a regimen initially found to be as effective as 6-month INH treatment in HIV-positive individuals,[18] is not recommended by the Centers for Disease Control and Prevention (CDC) due to severe hepatoxicity.[19]

The current TB therapeutic regimens are discussed later in the chapter.

Therapeutics by Class

The current TB drugs can be divided into first-line drugs and second-line drugs. The first-line drugs (Fig. 79-2) include INH, RIF (and its derivative rifapentine), PZA, and EMB, and the second-line drugs (Fig. 79-3) include SM (sometimes considered a first-line drug), kana-

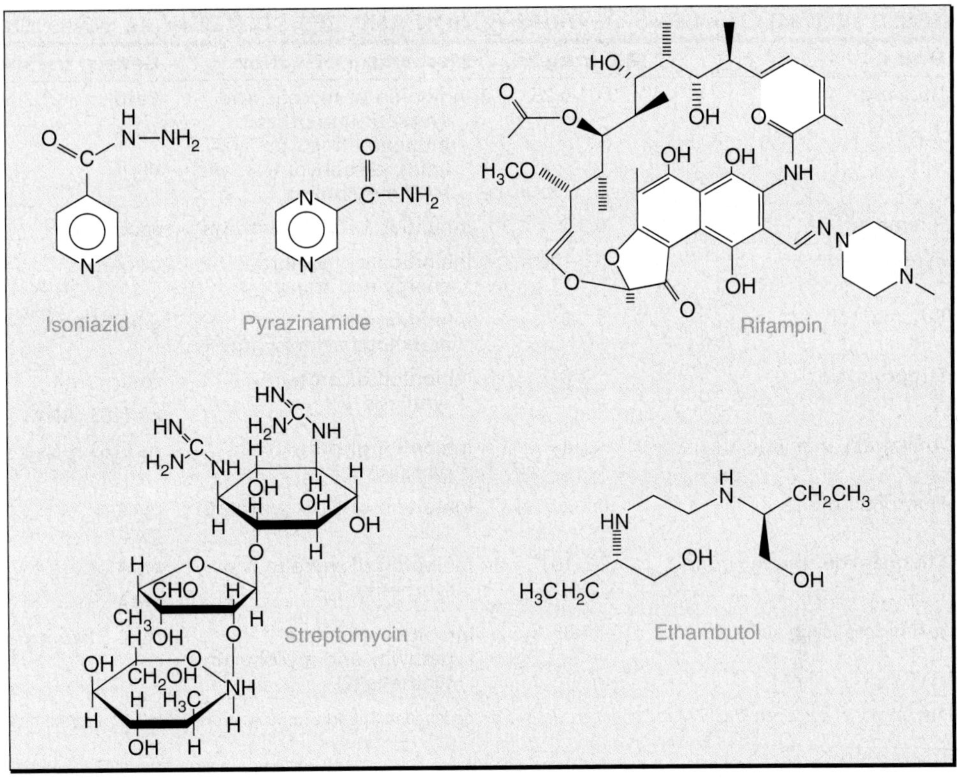

Isoniazid

Pyrazinamide

Rifampin

Streptomycin

Ethambutol

FIGURE 79-2 • Structures of front-line antituberculosis drugs.

Cycloserine

p-Aminosalicylic acid

Ethionamide (R=C2H5)/
Prothionamide (R=C3H7)

Capreomycin

Kanamycin

Ciprofloxacin

Thiacetazone

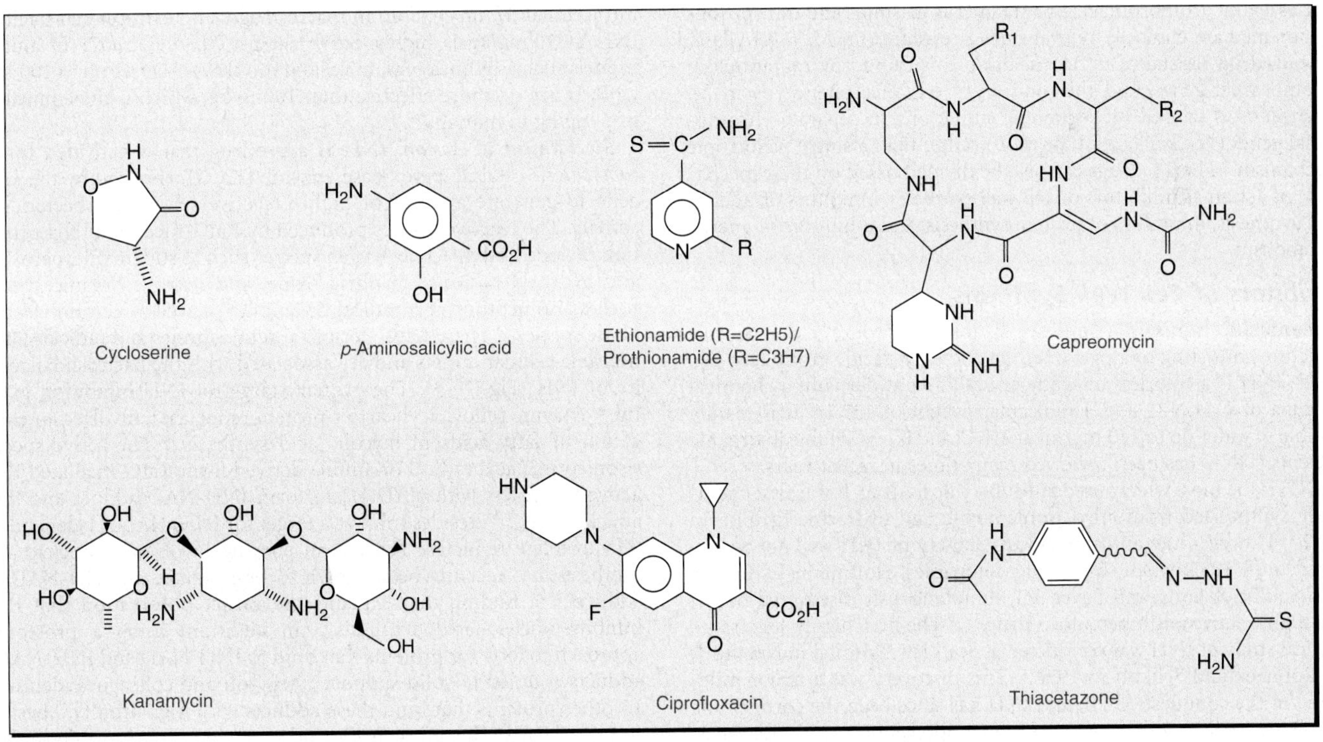

FIGURE 79-3 • Structures of commonly used second-line antituberculosis drugs.

mycin, amikacin, capreomycin, cycloserine (CS), *p*-aminosalicylic acid (PAS), ethionamide (ETH)/prothionamide (PTH), thiacetazone, and the fluoroquinolones.[15] First-line drugs are used in combination to prevent drug resistance and also improve therapeutic efficacy for the treatment of all newly diagnosed TB patients, whereas second-line drugs are used in combination with first-line drugs for the treatment of MDR-TB.

According to their specificity, TB drugs can also be grouped into TB-specific or mycobacteria-specific drugs such as INH, PZA, EMB, PAS, ETH, and thiacetazone, and broad-spectrum antibiotics such as RIF, SM, kanamycin, amikacin, capreomycin, CS, and the fluoroquinolones. The mechanisms of action and resistance to TB-specific drugs are specific to *M. tuberculosis* (Table 79-1), whereas mechanisms of action and resistance of the broad-spectrum drugs in *M. tuberculosis*

TABLE 79-1 MECHANISMS OF DRUG ACTION AND RESISTANCE IN *M. TUBERCULOSIS*

Drugs	MIC (mcg/ml)	Mechanism of Action	Gene(s) Involved in Resistance	Role in Resistance
Isoniazid	0.01-0.25	Inhibition of mycolic acid synthesis and other multiple effects on DNA, lipids, carbohydrates, and NAD metabolism	*katG* *inhA* *ahpC*	Prodrug conversion Drug target Marker of resistance
Rifampin	0.5-2	Inhibition of RNA synthesis	*rpoB*	Drug target
Pyrazinamide	16-100*	Inhibition of membrane energy and transport	*pncA*	Prodrug conversion
Ethambutol	1-5	Inhibition of arabinogalactan synthesis	*embCAB*	Drug target
Streptomycin	2-8	Inhibition of protein synthesis	*rpsL* *rrs* (16S rRNA)	Drug target Drug target
Amikacin/kanamycin	2-4	Inhibition of protein synthesis	*rrs* (16S rRNA)	Drug target
Fluoroquinolones	0.5-2.5	Inhibition of DNA synthesis	*gyrA* *gyrB*	Drug target
Ethionamide, thiacetazone	2.5-101	Inhibition of mycolic acid synthesis	*etaA or ethA* *inhA*	Prodrug conversion Drug target
p-Aminosalicylic acid	1-8	Inhibition of folate pathway and mycobactin synthesis (?)	*thyA* (thymidylate synthase)?	Drug target?

*The activity of pyrazinamide (PZA) for *M. tuberculosis* is pH dependent. The MIC of PZA at pH 6.0 is 100 mcg/ml, but is in the range of 16 to 50 mcg/ml at pH 5.5.

are the same as in other bacterial species. Unlike many other bacterial species, extrachromosomal elements such as plasmids and transposons do not mediate clinically relevant drug resistance in *M. tuberculosis*. Instead, drug resistance in *M. tuberculosis* is caused by mutations in chromosomal genes, and the multidrug-resistance phenotype in *M. tuberculosis* is caused by sequential mutations in separate chromosomal genes (i.e., *katG, inhA*, or *rpoB*) rather than a single pleiotropic mechanism.[8] The TB drugs can also be divided based on their mechanism of action as inhibitors of cell wall synthesis, inhibitors of nucleic acid synthesis, inhibitors of protein synthesis, and inhibitors of energy metabolism.

Inhibitors of Cell Wall Synthesis

Isoniazid. Isoniazid (isonicotinic acid hydrazide) has a simple structure consisting of a pyridine ring and a hydrazide group (see Fig. 79-2). INH is a colorless or white crystalline powder with a chemical formula of $C_6H_7N_3O$ and a molecular weight of 137.14. It is readily soluble in water up to 140 mg/ml at 25° C, and is less soluble in organic solvents.[20] INH has been reviewed many times in recent years.[11,20-22]

INH is the most widely used antituberculosis drug. It was first chemically synthesized from ethyl isonicotinate and hydrazine hydrate in 1912.[23] However, the antituberculosis activity of INH was not recognized until 1952, when three drug companies, Hoffmann-La Roche, E.R. Squibb & Sons, and Bayer AG, simultaneously discovered that it is a highly active antituberculosis drug.[24-26] The first, highly successful, clinical study of INH was conducted at Sea View Hospital in New York by Robitzek and Selikoff in 1952.[27] This discovery was a major milestone in the conquest of TB, and INH has since been the cornerstone of all effective regimens for the chemoprevention and treatment of TB.

Mycobacterium tuberculosis is highly susceptible to INH, with minimum inhibitory concentrations (MICs) in the range of 0.01 to 0.25 mcg/ml. Other mycobacteria, such as *M. smegmatis, M. phlei*, and *M. avium*, are less susceptible, with MICs in the range of 10 to 100 mcg/ml INH.[11] However, *M. kansasii, M. gastri*, and *M. xenopi* (MICs = 1 to 5 mcg/ml)[20] are more susceptible to INH than are other nontuberculous mycobacteria. Other non-*Mycobacterium* bacterial species are highly resistant to INH (MIC > 600 mcg/ml).[28] INH is only active against growing tubercle bacilli and not active against nonreplicating bacilli or under anaerobic conditions.[29] INH is active against both intracellular *M. tuberculosis* in macrophages and extracellular bacilli.[30] INH at 10 mg/kg is highly active against *M. tuberculosis* in animal models such as guinea pigs, mice, and monkeys.[30] Doses up to 100 mg/kg INH are no more effective than 10 mg/kg, which is the equivalent of 5 mg/kg in humans.[30]

Mechanism of Action. INH is a prodrug that is activated by *M. tuberculosis* catalase-peroxidase enzyme (KatG), encoded by the *katG* gene to generate a range of highly reactive species for bactericidal activity. The reactive species produced by KatG-mediated INH activation include both reactive oxygen species such as superoxide, peroxide, and hydroxyl radicals,[31,32] nitric oxide, and reactive organic species such as isonicotinic acyl radical or anion,[22] as well as certain electrophilic species.[33] These KatG-derived reactive species and radicals affect multiple cellular targets and are associated with the bactericidal activity of INH (Fig. 79-4). The primary target of INH inhibition is the InhA enzyme (enoyl acyl carrier protein reductase), involved in elongation of fatty acids in mycolic acid synthesis.[34] The active species (isonicotinic acyl radical or anion) derived from KatG-mediated INH activation reacts with NAD(H) to form INH-NAD adduct and then attacks InhA.[35,36] Besides InhA as a target for INH, NADPH-dependent dihydrofolate reductase (DfrA), an enzyme involved in nucleic acid synthesis, has recently been shown to be inhibited by INH-NAD(P) adducts,[37] a finding that explains the earlier observation that INH inhibits nucleic acid synthesis.[38] In addition, using a proteomic approach to look for proteins that bind to INH-NAD and INH-NADP adducts coupled to solid supports, Argyrou and colleagues identified 16 other proteins that bind these adducts with high affinity,[39] besides InhA and DfrA. These proteins include pyridine nucleotide–dependent dehydrogenases/reductases, *S*-adenosylmethionine–dependent methyl transfer reactions, and proteins involved in pyrimidine and valine catabolism, the arginine degradative pathway, proton and potassium transport, stress response, lipid metabolism, and riboflavin biosynthesis.[39] Further biochemical and genetic studies that demonstrate inhibition by INH and increased resistance upon overexpression of these putative targets would be necessary to assess their role in INH's mode of action.

Mechanism of Resistance. Resistance to INH occurs more frequently than to most TB drugs, at a frequency of 1 in 10^6 bacilli in vitro.[11] The

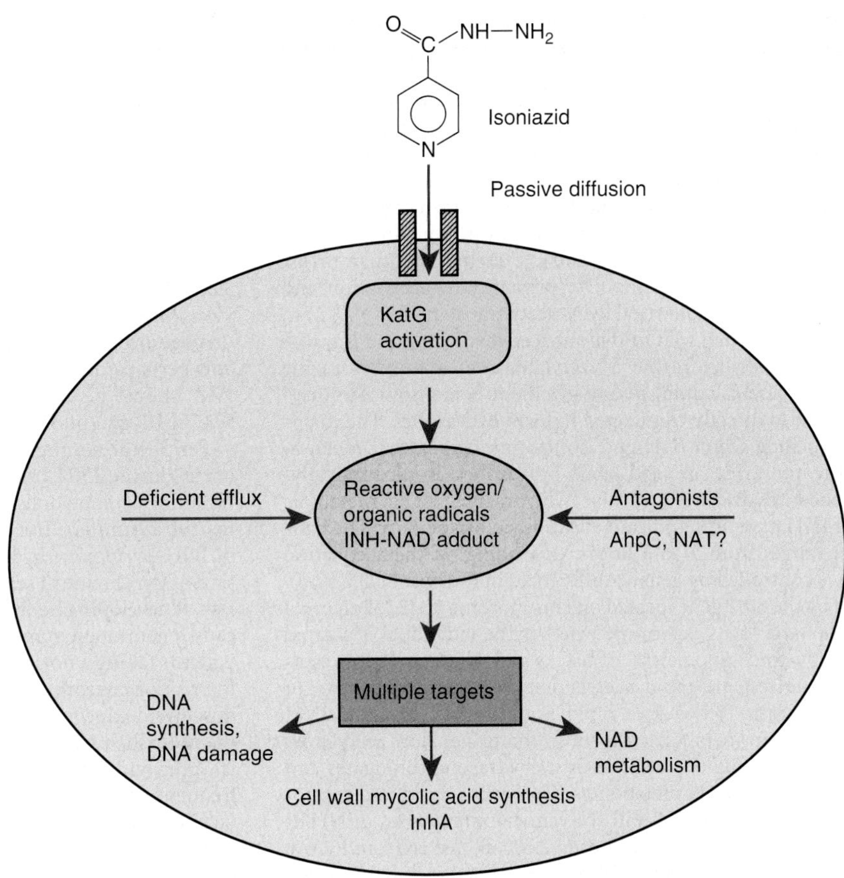

FIGURE 79-4 • Mechanism of INH action. INH gets into tubercle bacilli by passive diffusion where it is activated by KatG to a range of reactive radicals (peroxide, superoxide, peroxynitrite, hydroxyl radical) and INH-NAD adduct. These radicals then attract multiple targets, e.g., mycolic acid synthesis, DNA synthesis, DNA damage, lipid peroxidation, and NAD metabolism in the cell. Deficient efflux of INH radicals, defective antioxidative defense or insufficient inactivation of INH may underlie the unique susceptibility of *M. tuberculosis* to INH.

degree of INH resistance varies from 0.2 to more than 100 mcg/ml. INH resistance is most prevalent among TB drug resistances. INH-resistant clinical isolates of *M. tuberculosis* often lose catalase and peroxidase enzyme[40] encoded by *katG*, especially in high-level resistant strains (MIC > 5 mcg/ml).[11] Low-level resistant strains (MIC < 1 mcg/ml) often still possess catalase activity.[11] Mutation in *katG* is the major mechanism of INH resistance.[41] About 50% to 80% of INH-resistant *M. tuberculosis* strains contain a mutation in the *katG* gene.[42] Although various mutations in *katG* have been identified in INH-resistant strains, the *katG* S315T mutation is the most common mutation, accounting for 50% to 92% of INH-resistant clinical isolates.[42] Resistance to INH can also occur by mutations in the promoter region of the *mabA/inhA* operon, causing overexpression of InhA, or by mutations at the InhA active site, lowering the InhA affinity to NADH.[34,35] Mutations in the *inhA* promoter region are more frequent than mutations in the *inhA* structural gene in INH-resistant strains.[42,43] Mutations in *inhA* or the promoter region of the *mabA/inhA* operon occur in 15% to 34% of resistant strains and are usually associated with low levels of INH resistance (MICs = 0.2 to 1 mcg/ml).[42] INH-resistant *M. tuberculosis* harboring *inhA* mutations could have additional mutations in *katG* conferring a higher level of INH resistance.[44] Mutations in *inhA* not only cause INH resistance but also confer resistance to the structurally related second-line drug ETH.[34] Mutations in *ndh*, encoding NADH dehydrogenase, initially identified in *M. smegmatis* as involved in INH resistance,[45] have subsequently been found in some INH-resistant clinical isolates.[46] Decreased activity of Ndh supposedly increases the NADH/NAD ratio, which could possibly compete for the binding of activated INH (isonicotinic acyl radical) to the target InhA, or may promote displacement of the isonicotinic acyl NADH from InhA.[45] However, it appears that, although *ndh* mutations could be found in initial clinical isolates in mixed cultures, subsequent in vitro culture seems to select against mutants with *ndh* mutations such that strains with *ndh* mutations cannot compete with the sensitive bacilli and therefore are lost upon subculture.[47] In KatG-negative INH-resistant strains, mutations in the promoter region of *ahpC*, encoding an alkylhydroperoxide reductase, have been observed as a compensation for the lack of catalase-peroxidase activity in such strains.[48-50] Overexpression of AphC did not appear to confer significant INH resistance.[51]

Some low-level INH-resistant strains do not have mutations in *katG* or *inhA* and may be due to new mechanism(s) of resistance. It must be emphasized that the report by Stoeckle et al. that 35 (90%) of 39 INH-sensitive clinical isolates had the 282 bp *katG* fragment by polymerase chain reaction (PCR) or 4 INH-sensitive strains lacked the *katG* PCR product[52] is misleading, because no strains have been found that lack the *katG* sequence and yet are sensitive to INH. This is clearly due to technical problems with PCR, and therefore an artifact, and should not be taken as valid. This point is clarified here because this incorrect claim[52] has confused the literature and contributed to erroneous understanding on this topic.[53]

INH-resistant strains with defective catalase activity due to *katG* mutations can be attenuated for virulence, but mutations in *inhA* do not cause attenuation of virulence.[54] However, low-level INH-resistant strains with catalase activity may not lose virulence. The highly successful MDR-TB strain W, which harbors the common *katG* S315T mutation and still retains significant catalase activity, is clearly capable of causing active transmission of the disease, mainly in HIV-positive individuals, as seen in the MDR-TB outbreak in New York City.[55]

Pharmacokinetics and Metabolism. INH is readily absorbed after oral or parenteral administration and distributes into all body fluids and intracellular compartments.[56] After oral administration of the usual dose of 5 mg/kg INH or 300 mg/day, a peak serum concentration of 5 mcg/ml is achieved in 1 to 2 hours.[56] INH is minimally bound to serum proteins, crosses the placenta, and is excreted in human breast milk.[56] INH is metabolized in the liver primarily by acetylation and dehydrazination. INH is converted by *N*-acetyltransferase 2 (NAT2) to acetyl-INH, which is then split into monoacetylhydrazine and isonicotinic acid. Monoacetylhydrazine is acetylated into diacetylhydrazine and isonicotinic acid is conjugated to glycine to form isonicotinoylglycine. INH is also directly conjugated to form hydrazones. The major metabolites include acetyl-INH and isonicotinic acid. Other metabolites found in the urine are acid-labile hydrazones, isonicotinoylglycine, monoacetylhydrazine, and diacetylhydrazine.[56] The metabolic products of INH have no significant antituberculosis activity. The half-life of INH ranges from 1 to 3 hours, depending on the acetylation rate, which is controlled by genetic differences in the host NAT2 activity encoded by the *nat2* gene located on chromosome 8p22.[57] Polymorphisms at the *nat2* locus determine whether the individual is a rapid or a slow acetylator.[57] About 50% of blacks and whites are "slow acetylators" and the rest are rapid acetylators, whereas the majority of Eskimos and Asians (85%) are "rapid acetylators."[57] Most of INH (70%) is excreted in metabolized form in the urine. Slow acetylators excrete 37% of the drug as free INH or its hydrazone conjugates and 63% as acetyl-INH and its metabolites (isonicotinic acid and monoacetylhydrazine). In contrast, rapid acetylators excrete 94% of INH as acetyl-INH and its metabolites and only 2.8% as free INH and 3.6% as hydrazone conjugates.[56] Liver disease can reduce acetylation rates. The rate of acetylation does not significantly alter the efficacy of the drug with current INH dosage.

Clinical Use. INH is usually given by the oral route but can be given intramuscularly or intravenously when oral administration is not feasible. The recommended daily dose of INH is 10 to 20 mg/kg for children and 5 mg/kg for adults, with a maximum dosage of 300 mg.[56] For most children, the daily 10 mg/kg is sufficient, but a 20-mg/kg daily dose should be used for tuberculous meningitis.[56] INH can be safely used in pregnant women. INH has a high early bactericidal activity and kills actively growing bacterial populations, which causes a rapid fall in the number of bacilli in the patient's sputum during the first 2 weeks of treatment.[10] Its activity slows down for the nongrowing bacterial populations. Although INH is a powerful TB drug, it is not used singly for the treatment of TB except for chemoprophylaxis. INH is used in combination with RIF, PZA, and EMB in the DOTS strategy for the treatment of TB to improve efficacy and avoid emergence of drug resistance. INH is used singly for 6 to 9 months in the chemoprophylaxis of early-stage TB infection (LTBI) to prevent the development of active disease in contacts and recent tuberculin converters (see "Treatment of Latent TB Infection: Preventive Therapy" in the Therapeutic Approach section later in the chapter).

INH is also used in combination with other antimycobacterial drugs for the treatment of infections caused by *M. kansasii* and *M. xenopi*[56] because of the INH sensitivity of these two organisms. For both *M. kansasii* and *M. xenopi* infections, treatment with INH, RIF, and EMB for 12 to 24 months may be needed.[56] However, *M. avium* infection cannot be treated with INH due to its high level of resistance.

Adverse Effects. INH is well tolerated in most instances. The most frequent side effects are hepatoxicity and nervous system toxicity. The most serious adverse effect is damage to the liver and potentially fatal hepatitis. INH-associated hepatotoxicity results from the toxic effect of an intermediate product produced by *N*-hydroxylation of monoacetyl hydrazine by the liver cytochrome P-450 oxidase system.[58] The frequency of liver damage increases with age and is in general less than 2%.[56] In the United States, during 1-year INH treatment, INH-associated hepatitis occurred in no persons under age 20, 2.4 persons ages 20 to 34, and 19.2 persons ages 50 to 64 years of age, per 1000 subjects.[59] Those who are slow INH acetylators due to mutant *nat2* have a higher risk of hepatoxicity.[60] Other factors that predispose to INH-associated liver damage include excessive alcohol consumption, drug abuse, and a history of previous liver disease. Asymptomatic elevations of serum transaminase levels may occur in some cases during the first few months of INH therapy. In most instances, abnormal enzyme levels return to normal with no need to discontinue medication.[56] Routine monitoring of serum transaminase is not necessary except in high-risk individuals, such as those who are over 35 years of age, those who take alcohol daily or take hepatoxic medications, or those who have a previous history of liver disease.[56] In occasional instances, progressive liver damage occurs, with accompanying symptoms. In these cases, INH, and perhaps other potentially liver-damaging drugs such as RIF and PZA, should be stopped. Drugs that cause no liver toxicities, such as SM, EMB, and ofloxacin, can be used instead.[56]

Peripheral neuropathy and central nervous system symptoms can occur during INH treatment due to its interference with pyridoxine (vitamin B_6) metabolism. Vitamin B_6 is a cofactor for the synthesis of neurotransmitters. INH can cause vitamin B_6 deficiency by formation of INH-pyridoxine hydrazones, which lowers the effective concentration of pyridoxine in serum and tissues. Slow acetylators are at a higher risk of developing neurotoxicity. INH, at a daily dose of 5 mg/kg, rarely causes neurologic symptoms, and pyridoxine is not given routinely to patients taking a normal dosage of INH. Higher doses of INH increase the risk of neurotoxicity. Symptoms can be prevented by adding low-dose pyridoxine at 10 to 25 mg/day when prescribing INH therapy for malnourished patients, diabetic and uremic patients, chronic alcoholics, pregnant patients, and persons with seizure disorders.[56] Other less frequent neurologic adverse effects include toxic encephalopathy, convulsions, optic neuritis and atrophy, memory impairment, restlessness and insomnia, and psychiatric disturbances (psychosis).[56] INH overdose should be treated promptly with pyridoxine in a dose that is similar to the estimated overdose of INH.[56]

Gastrointestinal (GI) reactions such as nausea, vomiting, and epigastric distress are uncommon.[56] Hypersensitivity to INH is occasionally encountered, manifesting as fever, pruritus, skin eruptions, lymphadenopathy, and vasculitis.[56] Hematologic reactions include agranulocytosis; hemolytic, sideroblastic, or aplastic anemia; thrombocytopenia; and eosinophilia. Metabolic and endocrine reactions such as pellagra, hyperglycemia, metabolic acidosis, and gynecomastia could occur.[56] Rheumatic syndrome and systemic lupus erythematosus–like syndrome occur infrequently. Local irritation has been observed at the site of intramuscular injection. INH is contraindicated in patients who have had previous severe INH-associated hepatitis, acute liver diseases, and INH hypersensitivity reactions.[56]

Drug Interactions. INH inhibits the metabolism of the anticonvulsant drug phenytoin, which can cause phenytoin toxicity, especially in slow inactivators. INH may interfere with the metabolism of the anticonvulsant drug carbamazepine, causing carbamazepine toxicity. INH inhibits histaminase and can cause histamine toxicity when patients eat foods (such as cheese and fish) that are rich in histamine.[56] In addition, due to its structural similarity to iproniazid, a known inhibitor of monoamine oxidase used in treatment of certain mental illnesses, INH may inhibit monoamine oxidase and cause hypertensive crisis in patients who consume substances (e.g., cheese and red wine) rich in monoamines.[56] INH may increase the anticoagulant activity of warfarin.[56] The half-life of INH can be increased by drugs such as PAS, procainamide, and chlorpromazine and reduced by ethanol and other drugs that increase microsomal enzyme activity in the liver.[56] No known interactions exist between INH and antiretroviral drugs for the treatment of HIV infection.

Ethambutol. Ethambutol [(*S,S′*)-2,2′(ethylenediimino)di-1-butanol] (see Fig. 79-2) was discovered in 1961 at Lederle based on the observation that polyamines and diamines had activity against *M. tuberculosis*, and subsequent synthesis of diamine analogues led to the identification of EMB.[61] EMB is active primarily against mycobacteria, with *Nocardia* being slightly less sensitive and other bacteria completely resistant.[62] The MIC of EMB for *M. tuberculosis* is in the range of 0.5 to 2 mcg/ml. EMB is a bacteriostatic agent that is active against growing bacilli and has no effect on nonreplicating bacilli. EMB interferes with the biosynthesis of arabinogalactan, a major polysaccharide of the mycobacterial cell wall.[63] It inhibits the polymerization of cell wall arabinan of arabinogalactan and of lipoarabinomannan, and induces accumulation of D-arabinofuranosyl-*p*-decaprenol, an intermediate in arabinan biosynthesis.[64,65] Arabinosyl transferase, encoded by *embB*, an enzyme involved in synthesis of arabinogalactan, has been proposed as the target of EMB in *M. tuberculosis*[66] and *M. avium*.[67] In *M. tuberculosis, embB* is organized into an operon with *embC* and *embA* in the order *embCAB*. *embC, embB*, and *embA* share over 65% amino acid identity with each other and are predicted to encode transmembrane proteins.[66] Strains resistant to EMB have MICs greater than 7.5 mcg/ml.[62,68] Mutation to EMB resistance occurs at a frequency of 10^{-5}.[62] Mutations in the *embCAB* operon, in particular in *embB* and occasionally *embC*, are responsible for resistance to EMB.[66] *embB* codon 306 mutation is most frequent in clinical isolates of *M. tuberculosis* resistant to EMB.[69] EMB is active against intracellular *M. tuberculosis* and also in the mouse model.[62]

EMB is a bacteriostatic first-line drug that is used in combination with other TB drugs (INH, RIF, PZA) to prevent emergence of drug resistance. EMB is well distributed in body fluids after oral ingestion. A dose of 15 to 25 mg/kg by the oral route is recommended for treating TB in humans. A peak serum concentration of 3 to 5 mcg/ml is reached after 1 to 2 hours when EMB is given at 20 mg/kg orally.[70] The main metabolites of EMB include dialdehyde, dicarboxylic acid, and a glucuronide of EMB.[71] About 60% to 80% of ingested EMB is eliminated in urine as an unaltered form in 24 hours, 15% in the form of the aldehyde and carboxylic acid metabolites, and 20% is eliminated in feces as unchanged drug. The side effects of EMB include optic neuritis manifested by decreased visual acuity, hyperuricemia, nephrotoxicity, and hypersensitivity.[56] Because of the difficulty in measuring visual acuity in children, EMB is usually not used in children. EMB is contraindicated in cases of hypersensitivity and any prior optic neuritis.[15,72]

Cycloserine and Terizidone. CS (see Fig. 79-3) was first identified from *Streptomyces* by Kurosawa in 1952.[73] Terizidone is a combination of two molecules of CS. CS is readily soluble in water but not in organic solvents. CS is active against a broad range of bacterial species (including *Escherichia coli* and *Staphylococcus aureus*) and is more active against mycobacteria than other bacteria. The MIC of CS for *M. tuberculosis* ranges widely from 1.5 to 30 mcg/ml depending on the culture medium. The MIC is quite high, up to 20 to 30 mcg/ml, in Lowenstein-Jensen medium and 7H11 agar. The cutoff for resistance in 7H11 agar is 60 mcg/ml.[68] CS inhibits the synthesis of cell wall peptidoglycan by blocking the action of D-alanine racemase (Alr) and D-alanine:D-alanine ligase (Ddl).[74,75] Alr is involved in conversion of L-alanine to D-alanine, which then serves as a substrate for Ddl. The D-alanine racemase encoded by *alrA* from *M. smegmatis* was cloned, and its overexpression in *M. smegmatis* and *M. bovis* bacille Calmette-Guérin caused resistance to CS.[76] In *M. smegmatis*, inactivation of *alrA*[77] or *ddl*[78] resulted in increased sensitivity to CS. Overexpression of Alr conferred higher resistance to CS than Ddl overexpression in *M. smegmatis*, suggesting Alr might be the primary target of CS.[79] However, the mechanism of CS resistance in *M. tuberculosis* is unknown.

CS and terizidone are second-line agents that are used in combination with other second-line agents for the treatment of MDR-TB. CS is mainly a bacteriostatic drug and can be used to prevent resistance to other second-line drugs. The maximum dose of CS is 15 to 20 mg/kg per day. The usual dose is 500 to 750 mg CS, or 600 mg terizidone.[80] CS 250 mg is given in the morning, and 500 mg is given 12 hours later. Terizidone 300 mg is given twice a day at 12-hour intervals. After oral ingestion, CS is well distributed in the body and penetrates into the cerebrospinal fluid. A peak serum concentration of 10 mcg/ml is achieved in 3 to 4 hours when 250 mg CS is given orally.[70] About 60% to 70% of CS is excreted from urine and 35% is metabolized in the body. The side effects of CS include primarily neurotoxicity (dizziness, headache, slurred speech, convulsions, tremor, depression, insomnia),[72] and rarely drug fever, rashes, or cardiac arrythmias. The neurotoxicity may be prevented by pyridoxine or nicotinamide. Patients with a history of epilepsy, mental illness, and alcoholism should not take CS.[72]

Thioamides: Ethionamide and Prothionamide. Research on the nicotinamides led to discovery of not only INH and PZA, but also ethionamide (2-ethylisonicotinamide)[81] (see Fig. 79-3). ETH is a derivative of isonicotinic acid, which was synthesized in France in 1956.[81] ETH is slightly soluble in water and more soluble in organic solvents. ETH is a bactericidal agent that is active only against *M. tuberculosis, M. avium-intracellulare*, and *M. leprae*.[56] The MIC of ETH for *M. tuberculosis* is 0.5 to 2 mcg/ml in liquid medium, 2.5 to 10 mcg/ml in 7H11 agar, and 5 to 20 mcg/ml in Lowenstein-Jensen medium.[70] ETH, which is structurally related to INH (see Fig. 79-2), is also a prodrug that is activated by EtaA (a monooxygenase also called EthA)[82,83] and inhibits the same target as INH, the InhA of the mycolic acid synthesis pathway.[34] Prothionamide (2-ethyl-4-pyridinecarbothioamide) shares almost identical structure and activity with ETH (the *R*- group in ETH is C_2H_5 and the *R*- group in PTH is C_3H_7; see Fig. 79-3) and works in the same way as ETH. EtaA or EthA is a FAD-containing enzyme that oxidizes ETH to the corresponding *S*-oxide, which is further oxidized to 2-ethyl-4-amidopyridine, presumably via the unstable oxidized sulfinic acid intermediate.[84] EtaA also activates thiacetazone, thiocarlide, thiobenzamide, and perhaps other thioamide drugs,[84] which explains the cross-resistance between ETH and thiacetazone, thiocarlide, and other thioamides. Mutations in the drug-activating enzyme EtaA/EthA[82,83] and in the target InhA[34] cause resistance to ETH.

ETH is a second-line TB drug used to treat drug-resistant TB and also leprosy. ETH is given orally at a dose of 15 to 20 mg/kg per day, with a peak serum concentration of 1 to 2 mcg/ml 2 hours after oral ingestion.[56] The recommended dose for the treatment of human TB is 15 to 20 mg/kg per day (1.0 g/day maximum), usually 500 to 750 mg/day in a single daily dose or two doses.[15,72] ETH is widely distributed in the body and is metabolized to sulfoxides, which are active against *M. tuberculosis*. The sulfoxides are then converted to inactive metabolites. The side effects of ETH include GI tract symptoms (nausea, anorexia, vomiting, excessive salivation), metallic taste, hepatotoxicity, peripheral neuropathy, and rashes.[56] Other rare side effects include gynecomastia, menstrual disturbance, impotence, acne, and headache. PTH is better tolerated than ETH, and both drugs have similar side effects.[15,72]

Thiacetazone. Thiacetazone (Conteban, with empirical formula of $C_{10}H_{12}N_4OS$, molecular weight 236.29) (see Fig. 79-3) is one of the many thiosemicarbazones developed by Domagk in 1946. Initially it was considered to be too toxic for clinical use,[85] but subsequent clinical study in East Africa showed that thiacetazone had its value in clinical treatment of TB. Because of its low cost, thiacetazone is still used in developing countries as a first-line drug but rarely used in technologically advanced countries.[86] Thiacetazone is a bacteriostatic drug that is active against *M. tuberculosis* with a MIC of 1 mcg/ml.[56] There is cross-resistance between thiacetazone and ETH and other thioamides and thioureas (e.g., Isoxyl).[87] Recently, it was shown that thiacetazone and ETH are both activated by the mycobacterial enzyme EtaA/EthA, a flavin-containing monooxygenase that is responsible for the oxidative activation of both drugs in *M. tuberculosis*. EtaA oxidizes thiacetazone to sulfinic acid and carbodiimide as metabolites, which may be related to the toxic action of the drug.[88]

After oral administration of 150 mg, the peak serum concentration is 1 to 2 mcg/ml.[56] The serum half-life is about 12 hours. Thiacetazone (150 mg) is used with INH (300 mg) for 12 months, supplemented with SM for the treatment of TB in the initial phase of therapy in developing countries. Thiacetazone is also used along with INH for the continuation phase of treatment for 6 months in place of INH and for 4 months in place of RIF to lower cost in developing countries.[86]

Inhibitors of Nucleic Acid Synthesis

Rifampin. Rifampin (see Fig. 79-2) is a semisynthetic derivative of rifamycin, which was first isolated from *Streptomyces mediterranei* in the late 1950s.[89] RIF was developed in the Dow-Lepetit Research Laboratories in Italy, and was first used to treat TB in 1968.[90] RIF is a broad-spectrum antibiotic active against a wide range of bacteria, including *M. tuberculosis, M. leprae, M. kansasii, M. avium-intracellulare, M. marinum*, and *Neisseria meningitidis*. RIF is bactericidal for *M. tuberculosis* with MICs ranging from 0.005 to 1 mcg/ml in agar or liquid medium. However, in Lowenstein-Jensen medium the MIC of RIF is very high due to inactivation of RIF by egg yolk phospholipids.[91] Strains with MICs less than 0.4 mcg/ml in liquid or agar medium or less than 40 mcg/ml in Lowenstein-Jensen medium are considered RIF sensitive. RIF is poorly soluble in water but can be dissolved in organic solvents such as dimethyl sulfoxide or ethanol. RIF is as active as INH for intracellular and extracellular tubercle bacilli. RIF is active against growing and also stationary-phase bacilli with low metabolic activity. The activity against the latter bacterial population is related to its high sterilizing activity in vivo and its ability to shorten the treatment from 12 to 18 months to 9 months.[10] However, there is still a subpopulation of persisters in old stationary-phase cultures that are tolerant to RIF.[92]

RIF interferes with RNA synthesis by binding to the beta subunit of the RNA polymerase. The RNA polymerase is an oligomer consisting of a core enzyme formed by four chains ($\alpha_2\beta\beta'$) in association with a sigma subunit to specifically initiate transcription from promoters. The RIF binding site is located upstream of the catalytic center[93] and physically blocks the elongation of the RNA chain.[94] In *M. tuberculosis*, resistance to RIF occurs at a frequency of 10^{-7} to 10^{-8} bacilli. As in other bacteria, mutations in a defined 81-bp region of the *rpoB* are found in about 96% of RIF-resistant *M. tuberculosis* isolates.[95] Resistance to RIF in *M. leprae* follows the same mechanism.[96] Although *rpoB* mutations have been described in RIF-resistant *M. avium*, any isolates from the *M. avium-intracellulare* complex present a significant level of natural resistance to RIF, probably due to a decreased permeability[97] or increased efflux. Mutation in *rpoB* generally results in high-level resistance (MIC > 32 mcg/ml) and cross-resistance to all rifamycins.

RIF is used to treat TB in combination with INH, PZA, and EMB, and to treat leprosy and other mycobacterial infections such as those caused by *M. avium-intracellulare, M. kansasii*, and *M. marinum*. RIF is readily absorbed from the GI tract. After oral intake of 600 mg RIF, peak serum concentration of 8 to 10 mcg/ml is reached after 2 to 4 hours.[70] About 50% of the serum concentration reaches the cerebrospinal fluid. The elimination half-life is about 3 hours. RIF is metabolized in the liver to 25-*O*-deacetylated RIF, which is excreted into bile and not reabsorbed. However, a small portion of free RIF is eliminated in the bile and reabsorbed by the GI tract. RIF is generally a well-tolerated drug, but some side effects such as hepatotoxicity, hypersensitivity, GI tract symptoms, and the like can occur.[56] RIF induces cytochrome P-450 enzyme activity and may reduce the therapeutic efficacy of some drugs such as oral anticoagulants, contraceptives, glucocorticoids, oral antidiabetic drugs, immune suppressors (cyclosporine), and methadone. RIF also interacts with co-trimoxazole, reducing the area under the curve for trimethoprim by 63% and that for sulfamethoxazole by 23%.[86] RIF can reduce the serum concentration of anti-HIV protease inhibitors through induction of the P-450 isoenzyme CYP3A4, involved in metabolizing the protease inhibitors.[86]

Rifapentine is a semisynthetic derivative of rifamycin SV with MICs of 0.02 to 0.2 mcg/ml for *M. tuberculosis*. Rifapentine, with a longer half-life and more active than RIF, was approved by the U.S. Food and Drug Administration (FDA) in 1998 for treatment of TB. Rifapentine (10 mg/kg) is approved by the FDA for the twice-weekly treatment of TB in intensive-phase therapy and once-weekly treatment in the continuation phase in place of RIF. Rifapentine can reduce the frequency of drug dosage required, but it is not active against RIF-resistant *M. tuberculosis* due to cross-resistance.[98] Rifabutin is not approved by the FDA for the treatment of TB in the United States[15] but is approved for the treatment of *M. avium* complex disease in acquired immunodeficiency syndrome (AIDS) patients.[15]

Fluoroquinolones. Fluoroquinolone drugs are broad-spectrum antibacterial agents and show bactericidal activity against a wide range of bacterial species, including mycobacteria. The first quinolone drug, nalidixic acid, was obtained as an impurity during the manufacture of quinine in the early 1960s.[99] Since then, many derivatives have been synthesized and evaluated for antibacterial activity. Fluoroquinolones inhibit DNA synthesis by targeting the DNA gyrase A and B subunits. Fluoroquinolones bind to DNA gyrase, thereby inhibiting DNA supercoiling.[80] Two C8-methoxyfluoroquinolone drugs, moxifloxacin (MXF) and gatifloxacin, are highly active against gram-positive bacteria and mycobacteria.[80] Ciprofloxacin, ofloxacin, levofloxacin, sparfloxacin, and MXF (see Fig. 79-3) are the best studied of these agents, and are highly active against *M. tuberculosis*.[80] Their activity against *M. tuberculosis* in vitro and in animal studies is in the following order: MXF = gatifloxacin > levofloxacin > ofloxacin = ciprofloxacin.[80] While the fluoroquinolones are primarily active against growing tubercle bacilli, ofloxacin and levofloxacin had some activity against a 100-day-old culture, while MXF and gatifloxacin had the highest activities.[100] In particular, MXF was found to kill nongrowing RIF-tolerant tubercle bacilli and was suggested to be able to shorten TB therapy.[100]

Strains of *M. tuberculosis* can develop resistance to fluoroquinolones by mutations primarily in *gyrA* and sometimes also in *gyrB*.[101,102] The frequency of mutants resistant to quinolones in mycobacteria is in the range of 10^{-7} to 10^{-8}.[80] Mutations in *gyrB* are associated with low-level resistance but mutations in *gyrA* are associated with high-level resistance. Mutations in *gyrA* at positions 90, 91, and 94 are associated with fluoroquinolone resistance and can cause cross-resistance to different fluoroquinolones.[103] Although topoisomerase IV (*parC*) mutations cause quinolone resistance in other bacteria,[80] no such homologues are present in the genome of *M. tuberculosis*.[104] Some low-level resistant mutants do not involve DNA gyrase, and the mechanism of such resistance is not clear.[80] Recently, a new mechanism of quinolone resistance mediated by MfpA was identified.[105] MfpA is a member of the pentapeptide repeat family of proteins from *M. tuberculosis*, whose expression causes resistance to fluoroquinolones. MfpA binds to DNA gyrase and inhibits its activity in the form of a DNA mimicry, which explains its inhibitory effect on DNA gyrase and quinolone resistance.[105]

Fluoroquinolones are currently used to treat MDR-TB as second-line drugs, but MDR-TB strains are becoming resistant to fluoroquinolones.[106] Levofloxacin is used at 500 to 1000 mg daily, and after oral intake of 500 mg levofloxacin, its peak serum concentration reached about 5 mcg/ml in 1.3 hours.[107] Levofloxacin is the preferred fluoroquinolone for the treatment of TB due to its good safety profile in long-term use.[15] However, data on long-term safety and tolerability of MXF and gatifloxacin in humans, especially at doses above 400 mg/day, are limited.[15] A recent clinical study showed that MXF did not affect 2-month sputum culture conversion when added to INH, RIF, and PZA in comparison to EMB, but appeared to show increased activity at early time points.[108] In another clinical study, it was found that the combination of MXF and INH is not antagonistic, but the combination did not enhance the bactericidal activity above that of INH alone.[109] Additional ongoing clinical studies will reveal in the near future whether MXF and gatifloxacin can be used to shorten TB therapy, and also their value in treating MDR-TB. A preliminary study from India appeared to show some promise of ofloxacin in combination with first-line drugs in a shorter course of TB treatment in 3 months,[110] but more study is needed to confirm this. Adverse reactions to fluoroquinolones are uncommon but consist of GI disturbance (anorexia, nausea, vomiting) or central nervous system symptoms (such as dizziness, headache, mood changes and rarely convulsions). Due to drug-drug interaction, antacids, iron, and zinc should not be used together with quinolone drugs.[72] Fluoroquinolones should not be used in pregnant women or children because they may impair growth and produce injury to growing cartilage.[72]

Inhibitors of Protein Synthesis

Aminoglycosides: Streptomycin and Kanamycin/Viomycin/Capreomycin. Streptomycin (see Fig. 79-3) was the first effective TB drug discovered in 1944.[111] Aminoglycosides are bactericidal broad-spectrum antibiotics that are active against a variety of bacterial species, including *M. tuberculosis*. SM inhibits protein synthesis by binding to the 16S ribosomal RNA (rRNA) of the 30S subunit of the bacterial ribosome, causing misreading of the messenger RNA message during translation,[112,113] and can also cause damage to the cell membrane.[114] SM is a bactericidal drug that kills actively growing tubercle bacilli at neutral or alkaline pH with MICs of 2 to 4 mcg/ml,[68] but is inactive against nongrowing or intracellular bacilli.[10] Resistance to SM is caused by mutations in the S12 protein encoded by the *rpsL* gene and in 16S rRNA encoded by the *rrs* gene.[115] Mutations in *rpsL* and *rrs* are the major mechanism of SM resistance,[115-117] accounting for about 50% and 20% of SM-resistant strains, respectively.[115-117] The most common mutation in *rpsL* is a substitution in codon 43 from lysine to arginine,[115-117] causing high-level resistance to SM. Mutation in codon 88 is also common.[115-117] Mutations of the *rrs* gene occur in the loops of 16S rRNA and are clustered in two regions around nucleotides 530 and 915.[115-117] An SM-dependent SM-resistant *M. tuberculosis* strain appears to be caused by a "C" insertion in the 530 loop of 16S rRNA.[118]

Like streptomycin, kanamycin (see Fig. 79-3) and its derivative amikacin are inhibitors of protein synthesis through modification of ribosomal structures at 16S rRNA.[119,120] Kanamycin was originally isolated from a *Streptomyces* species later called *Streptomyces kanamyceticus*.[121] Mutations at 16S rRNA (*rrs*) position 1400 are associated with high-level resistance to kanamycin and amikacin.[119,120] Capreomycin is a polypeptide antibiotic isolated from *Streptomycin capreolus* in 1960.[122] A new gene called *tlyA* encoding rRNA methyltransferase was shown to be involved in resistance to capreomycin.[123] The rRNA methyltransferase modifies nucleotide C1409 in helix 44 of 16S rRNA and nucleotide C1920 in helix 69 of 23S rRNA.[124] Variable cross-resistance may be observed between kanamycin, amikacin, capreomycin, and viomycin.[11] Mutants resistant to capreomycin and viomycin could have *tlyA*, C1402T, or G1484T *rrs* mutations, while mutants resistant to capreomycin but not viomycin could have A1401G *rrs* mutation.[125] Mutants with A1401G mutation could cause resistance to kanamycin and capreomycin but not viomycin.[125] Mutants resistant to capreomycin, kanamycin, and viomycin could have either a C1402T or a G1484T mutation in the *rrs* gene.[125] Multiple mutations may occur in the *rrs* gene in one strain, conferring cross-resistance among these agents.[125] SM-resistant strains are usually still susceptible to kanamycin and amikacin.

SM has been found to have efficacy equivalent to EMB in the initial phase of therapy. Because SM is an injection drug and not convenient to administer, it is relegated to a second-line drug.[15] The usefulness of SM is limited due to relatively high resistance to SM in high-incidence countries.[15] SM, kanamycin, amikacin, and capreomycin are used as second-line agents for the treatment of drug-resistant TB. All these aminoglycosides are administered by single daily intramuscular (or occasionally intravenous) injection at 15 mg/kg, but should be reduced to 10 mg/kg in people over 60 years old. The peak serum concentration of the aminoglycosides ranges from 15 to 25 mcg/ml with a half-life of about 2 hours.[70] The aminoglycosides are poorly distributed to host cells. The biotransformation of aminoglycosides is very limited, and most of the drug is excreted in an unchanged bioactive form in the urine in 24 hours.[70] A minor proportion (0.5% to 2%) is excreted through the biliary route with no enterohepatic cycle.[70] The side effects of the aminoglycosides include ototoxicity, nephrotoxicity, and hypersensitivity reactions. The aminoglycosides are contraindicated in pregnant women.[15,56]

Inhibitors of Membrane Energy Metabolism

Pyrazinamide. Pyrazinamide, a nicotinamide analogue (see Fig. 79-2), was first synthesized in 1936 but its antituberculosis activity was not recognized until 1952. Its discovery was based on a serendipitous observation that nicotinamide had certain activity against mycobacteria in animal models.[126] Subsequent synthesis of nicotinamide analogues and direct testing in the mouse model led to the identification of PZA as the most active agent.[127,128] PZA has a formula of $C_5H_5N_3O$ with a molecular weight of 123.1 and dissolves in water at no more than 15 mg/ml at room temperature. PZA dissolves relatively poorly in organic solvents.

PZA is an unconventional and paradoxical drug that has high in vivo sterilizing activity involved in shortening TB therapy,[129] but has no activity against TB bacteria at normal culture conditions near neutral pH.[130] PZA is only active against *M. tuberculosis* at acid pH (e.g., 5.5),[131] an environment that is produced during active inflammation. PZA is active only against *M. tuberculosis* complex organisms (*M. tuberculosis, M. africanum*, and *M. microti*) but not against *M. bovis* due to a characteristic mutation (C to G change at nucleotide position 169, causing amino acid substitution of His57Asp) in its *pncA* gene.[132] The PZA MIC for *M. tuberculosis* is in the range of 6.25 to 50 mcg/ml at pH 5.5,[129] whereas nontuberculous bacteria such as *E. coli* and *M. smegmatis* are resistant to at least 2000 mcg/ml PZA at pH 5.5[129] due to a highly active pyrazinoic acid (POA) efflux mechanism in the nonsusceptible bacteria.[133] The activity of PZA is closely related to the acidity of the medium, that is, the lower the pH and the lower the MIC, the higher the PZA activity.[134] PZA has little activity against young and actively growing bacilli and primarily shows bacteriostatic activity for such bacilli, but has more activity against nonreplicating bacilli in old cultures and can show bactericidal activity.[134] PZA activity is adversely affected by bovine serum albumin and high inoculum size.[134] PZA is more active under low-oxygen or anaerobic conditions than aerobic conditions.[135] PZA activity is enhanced by agents that compromise the membrane energy status, such as the weak acids benzoic acid and sorbic acid[136] and energy inhibitors such as *N,N'*-dicyclohexyl carbodiimide, azide, and rotenone.[137]

PZA is a prodrug that requires conversion to its active form, POA (Fig. 79-5), by the PZase/nicotinamidase enzyme encoded by the *pncA* gene of *M. tuberculosis*.[132] Mutation in *pncA* is a major mechanism of PZA resistance in *M. tuberculosis*,[132] although some low-level resistant strains do not have *pncA* mutations.[138] The POA produced intracellularly gets to the cell surface through passive diffusion and a defective efflux.[133] The extracellular acid pH facilitates the formation of uncharged protonated POA, which then permeates through the membrane and causes accumulation of POA and disrupts membrane potential in *M. tuberculosis*.[137] The protonated POA brings protons into the cell and could eventually cause cytoplasmic acidification and de-energize the membrane by collapsing the proton motive force, which affects membrane transport[137] (see Fig. 79-5). The target of PZA is the membrane energy metabolism, though the specific cellular target is yet to be identified. More details on PZA can be found in a recent review by Zhang and Mitchison.[129]

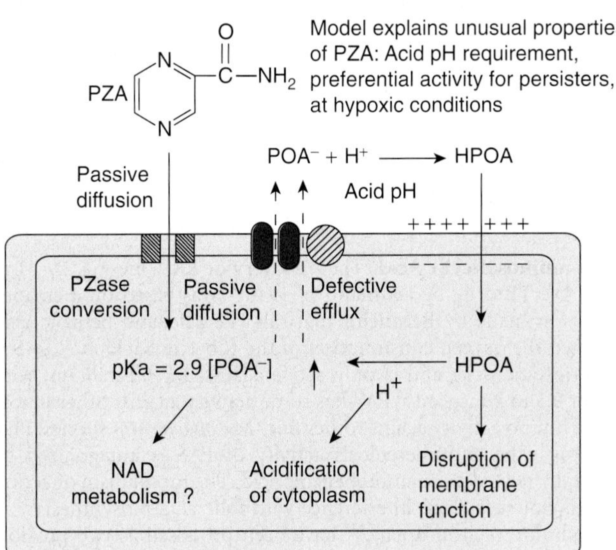

PZA enters tubercle bacilli by passive diffusion where it is converted to the active form pyrazinoic acid (POA) by the bacterial enzyme pyrazinamidase (PZase). POA then gets to the cell surface by passive diffusion and a defective efflux and at acid pH forms protonated HPOA which permeates back into the cell through passive diffusion, which can disrupt membrane energy, cause acidification and potentially NAD metabolism of the bacilli.

FIGURE 79-5 • Mechanism of action of PZA.

PZA is an important front-line drug used in the initial phase of treatment along with INH and RIF. These three drugs form the cornerstone of modern short-course TB chemotherapy. PZA plays a unique role in shortening the therapy from 9 to 12 months to 6 months because it kills a population of persister tubercle bacilli in the acidic pH environment in the lesions and inside macrophages that are not killed by other TB drugs.[10] Studies of early bactericidal activity (EBA), in which drug activity is measured by serial colony-forming unit (CFU) counts of bacilli in sputum, have shown that PZA has little or no activity during the first 2 days of treatment, but over the next 12 days there is a steady fall in sputum CFU counts comparable to the effect of other antituberculosis drugs.[139] During the 2 months of treatment, the sterilizing activity of PZA is only evident as a reduction in CFU counts between days 15 and 56.[140]

Before the 1970s, PZA was mainly used as a second-line TB drug for the treatment of drug-resistant TB or in treatment of relapsed TB because of the liver toxicity caused by higher PZA dosage (3.0 g) and longer treatment used in earlier clinical studies. However, largely encouraged by the impressive mouse studies by McDermott and colleagues that demonstrated high sterilizing activity of PZA in combination with INH,[141] the British Medical Research Council conducted clinical trials in East Africa with lower PZA doses (1.5 to 2.0 g daily), which are not hepatotoxic. PZA is almost as effective as RIF as a sterilizing drug as judged by more frequent sputum conversion at 2 months and by the relapse rates. The effects of RIF and PZA were synergistic. It was shown that treatment could be shortened from 12 months or more to 9 months if either RIF or PZA was added to the regimen, but to 6 months if both were included.[12] PZA is now used as a first-line TB drug. PZA only acts as a sterilizing drug during the first 2 months of therapy, and giving PZA longer than 2 months does not provide any additional benefit.[12] This is presumably because inflammation leading to an acid environment in the lesions had decreased after 2 months.

PZA is well absorbed from the GI tract after oral intake and reaches a serum concentration of 33 mcg/ml after 2 hours with a 1.5-g dose.[56] The recommended dose is 2 g/day or 15 to 30 mg/kg.[15,72] The half-life of PZA is 6 to 8 hours. PZA is widely distributed throughout the body tissues and easily penetrates into cells. PZA is mainly metabolized in the liver.[72] The major pathway of PZA metabolism is hydrolysis to POA. POA is then oxidized by xanthine oxidase to 5-hydroxypyrazinoic acid, which is excreted in the urine. The side effects of PZA include hepatotoxicity, arthralgia, and gout associated with elevated serum uric acid levels. POA competes with uric acid during elimination through the kidney and causes increased blood levels of uric acid, and can cause hyperuricemia. Gastrointestinal tract symptoms and hypersensitivity may also occur.[15] PZA is contraindicated in cases of hypersensitivity and severe liver disease.[56]

Others

Para-aminosalicylic Acid. The discovery of PAS (see Fig. 79-3) as an effective TB drug by Lehmann in 1946[142] was based on a curious observation made by Bernheim that salicylic acid and benzoic acid stimulated the oxygen consumption of the tubercle bacillus.[143] PAS is a bacteriostatic drug and is only active against *M. tuberculosis*, with MICs of 0.5 to 2 mcg/ml.[56] PAS has some activity against other mycobacteria but no activity against other non-*Mycobacterium* species. Like sulfa drugs, the antituberculosis activity of PAS is antagonized by structurally related *para*-aminobenzoic acid. The mechanism of action of PAS is not very clear. Interference with folic acid biosynthesis[144,145] and inhibition of iron uptake[146] have been proposed as two possible mechanisms of action for PAS.[11] Mutation to PAS resistance occurs at a frequency of 10^{-5} to 10^{-9}.[145] The mechanism of PAS resistance is not well understood. Recently, *thyA* encoding thymidylate synthase was found to be involved in PAS resistance in a small number of clinical isolates of *M. tuberculosis*.[144] However, the frequency of *thyA* mutations in a relatively large number of PAS-resistant strains is not yet available.

PAS is a second-line TB drug used to treat MDR-TB in combination with other TB drugs. The daily dosage is 150 mg/kg or 10 to 12 g daily in two divided doses. The recommended schedule is 5 to 6 g (10 to 12 tablets) every 12 hours.[72] PAS is well absorbed from the GI tract. After absorption, PAS is well distributed in body fluids. At an oral dose of 4 g, peak serum concentration of 7 to 8 mcg/ml is achieved after 1 to 2 hours.[56] The half-life is about 0.75 hour.[56] PAS is metabolized by acetylation to *N*-acetylaminosalicylic acid in the liver and is mainly excreted in urine. The side effects of PAS include GI tract disturbance, hypersensitivity reactions, and hypokalemia.[56] Gastrointestinal symptoms may improve if PAS is taken after meal or milk.[72] Prolonged use in large doses may also result in hypothyroidism and goiter.[72] PAS is not used in renal failure as it may cause acidosis.

Therapeutic Approach

Treatment of TB Caused by Drug-Susceptible Organisms

Appropriate treatment of TB rapidly renders the patient noninfectious, prevents drug resistance, minimizes the risk of disability or death from TB, and nearly eliminates the possibility of relapse. Patients are rendered noninfectious during the first 2 weeks of TB therapy,[139] and the positive sputum smear in most patients converts to negative after 2 months of initial-phase treatment.[72] It is emphasized in the recent American Thoracic Society (ATS)/CDC guidelines for the treatment of TB that the responsibility for successful treatment of TB is placed primarily on the health care provider or program initiating therapy rather than on the patient and that TB chemotherapy is both a personal and a public health measure that is different from the treatment of other noninfectious diseases.[15] The following TB drugs are approved by the FDA to treat TB in the United States: first-line drugs INH, RIF, rifapentine, PZA, and EMB, and second-line drugs CS, ETH, PAS, SM, and capreomycin.[15]

The CDC/ATS, the WHO, and the International Union Against Tuberculosis and Lung Diseases (IUATLD) have set clear guidelines for the treatment of TB.[15,147,148] The WHO recently established the International Standards for Tuberculosis Care to better manage and treat TB and drug-resistant TB.[147,149] A single combined approach is synthesized here from the CDC/ATS, WHO, and IUATLD guidelines, which share a great deal of similarity with some differences. TB chemotherapy, when used appropriately, can have cure rates as high as 95%. In all treatment regimens, attempts should be made to include more effective first-line TB drugs whenever possible and to ensure patient adherence to therapy.

All patients (both HIV negative and positive) who have not been treated previously should take the internationally accepted first-line treatment regimen, consisting of an initial phase of treatment of 2 months with INH, RIF, PZA, and EMB, followed by the continuation phase of treatment of 4 months with INH and RIF (Table 79-2).[15,72] The WHO recommends inclusion of the fourth drug EMB in the initial phase of treatment for most patients who are HIV negative with drug-susceptible bacilli due to a relatively high incidence of INH resistance.[72] EMB may be omitted in the initial phase of treatment in smear-negative cases, or in HIV-negative patients who do not have extensive pulmonary TB or severe forms of extrapulmonary TB,[72] or if drug susceptibility test results are known and the organisms are fully susceptible.[15] INH and EMB given for 6 months is an alternative regimen in place of INH and RIF for 4 months for the continuation phase when adherence cannot be assessed, but this regimen is associated with a higher rate of failure and relapse, especially in patients with HIV infection.[149] The rationale for the INH and EMB for 6 months instead of INH and RIF for 4 months is to save cost in low- to middle-income countries and to reduce resistance to RIF in case of nonadherence.[149] EMB is usually not recommended for children, whose visual acuity cannot be monitored, except when there is an increased likelihood of the disease being caused by INH-resistant organisms.[15] Patients who have cavitation on an initial chest radiograph and who have a positive culture at the end of 2 months of therapy are at substantially higher risk of relapse, and it is recommended that the continuation phase be prolonged to 7 months, making a total treatment of 9 months.[15] INH and EMB daily for 6 months for the continuation phase of

TABLE 79-2 DRUG REGIMENS FOR CULTURE-POSITIVE PULMONARY TUBERCULOSIS CAUSED BY DRUG-SUSCEPTIBLE ORGANISMS

Initial Phase			*Continuation Phase*			Range of Total Doses (Minimal Duration)	Rating* (Evidence)†	
Regimen	Drugs	Interval and Doses‡,§ (Minimal Duration)	Regimen	Drugs	Interval and Doses‡,§,¶ (Minimal Duration)		HIV⁻	HIV⁺
1	INH RIF PZA EMB	7 days/wk for 56 doses (8 wk) *or* 5 days/wk for 40 doses (8 wk)¶	1a	INH/RIF	7 days/wk for 126 doses (18 wk) *or* 5 days/wk for 90 doses (18 wk)¶	182-130 (26 wk)	A (I)	A (II)
			1b	INH/RIF	Twice weekly for 36 doses (18 wk)	92-76 (26 wk)	A (I)	A (II)#
			1c	INH/RPT	Once weekly for 18 doses (18 wk)	74-58 (26 wk)	B (I)	E (I)
2	INH RIF PZA EMB	7 days/wk for 14 doses (2 wk), then twice weekly for 12 doses (6 wk) *or* 5 days/wk for 10 doses (2 wk),¶ then twice weekly for 12 doses (6 wk)	2a	INH/RIF	Twice weekly for 36 doses (18 wk)	62-58 (26 wk)	A (II)	B (II)#
			2b**	INH/RPT	Once weekly for 18 doses (18 wk)	44-40 (26 wk)	B (I)	E (I)
3	INH RIF PZA EMB	Three times weekly for 24 doses (8 wk)	3a	INH/RIF	Three times weekly for 54 doses (18 wk)	78 (26 wk)	B (I)	B (II)
4	INH RIF EMB	7 days/wk for 56 doses (8 wk) *or* 5 days/wk for 40 doses (8 wk)¶	4a	INH/RIF	7 days/wk for 217 doses (31 wk) or 5 days/wk for 155 doses (31 wk)¶	273-195 (39 wk)	C (I)	C (II)
			4b	INH/RIF	Twice weekly for 62 doses (31 wk)	118-102 (39 wk)	C (I)	C (II)

*Definitions of strength of recommendation ratings: A, preferred; B, acceptable alternative; C, offer when A and B cannot be given; E, should never be given.
†Definitions of quality of evidence ratings: I, randomized clinical trial; II, data from clinical trials that were not randomized or were conducted in other populations; III, expert opinion.
‡When DOT is used, drugs may be given 5 days/wk and the necessary number of doses adjusted accordingly. Although there are no studies that compare five with seven daily doses, extensive experience indicates this would be an effective practice.
§The WHO recommends three-times-weekly treatment as an alterative to both daily treatment for the initial phase and continuation phase. The WHO does not recommend once- or twice-weekly treatment for the continuation phase.[149]
¶Patients with cavitation on initial chest radiograph and positive cultures at completion of 2 months of therapy should receive a 7-month (31-week; either 217 doses [daily] or 62 doses [twice weekly]) continuation phase.
¶Five-days-a-week administration is always given by DOT. The rating for 5-days-a-week regimens is AIII.
#Not recommended for HIV-infected patients with CD4⁺ cell counts less than 100 cells/ml.
**Options 1c and 2b should be used only in HIV-negative patients who have negative sputum smears at the time of completion of 2 months of therapy and who do not have cavitation on initial chest radiograph (see text). For patients started on this regimen and found to have a positive culture from the 2-month specimen, treatment should be extended an extra 3 months.
DOT, directly observed therapy; EMB, ethambutol; HIV, human immunodeficiency virus; INH, isoniazid; PZA, pyrazinamide; RIF, rifampin; RPT, rifapentine; WHO, World Health Organization.
Adapted from American Thoracic Society, CDC, and Infectious Diseases Society of America. Treatment of tuberculosis. MMWR Recomm Rep 2003;52(RR11):1-77.

treatment is associated with a higher rate of treatment failure and relapse; this regimen should generally not be used in patients with HIV infection.

The IUATLD recommends a 2-month initial phase of INH, RIF, PZA, and EMB given by DOT, followed by a 6-month continuation phase of daily INH and thiacetazone (thiacetazone is not effective when used intermittently), for a total duration of 8 months.[86] The replacement of RIF by thiacetazone is less efficacious but reduces the cost of therapy for low-income countries and preserves RIF for re-treatment regimens. The WHO and the CDC do not recommend the use of thiacetazone due to its toxicity, especially in AIDS patients,[15,72] but it is still used in some low-income countries where there is low incidence of HIV infection.[86] For patients with HIV infection, the IUATLD recommends EMB in place of thiacetazone.[86]

Intermittent treatment has the advantage of improving patient compliance and reducing costs and drug toxicity without compromising efficacy. Patients who are managed by DOT administered 5 days/wk have a rate of successful therapy equivalent to those being given drugs 7 days/wk.[15] However, the WHO recommends INH, RIF, PZA, and EMB treatment three times per week as an alterative to the daily treatment regimen for the initial phase, and INH and RIF three times per week for the continuation phase.[72] However, the WHO does not recommend intermittent treatment in the initial phase if INH and EMB (in place of RIF) are used in the continuation phase.[72] In contrast, the ATS/CDC recommend only daily or 5 days/wk treatment for the initial phase.[15] Another difference is that the WHO does not recommend once- or twice-weekly treatment for the continuation phase,[149] which is recommended by the ATS/CDC[15] (see Table 79-2). Rifapentine (10 mg/kg), a rifamycin derivative with a longer half-life, is approved by the FDA for twice-weekly treatment of TB in the intensive phase and once-weekly treatment in the continuation phase in place of RIF. Thiacetazone is the only drug that is ineffective when given intermittently.[72]

Alternative Regimens Used in Drug Intolerance or Drug Resistance

If INH cannot be used due to drug intolerance, or the bacilli are resistant to INH, a 6-month regimen of RIF, PZA, and EMB is almost as efficacious as the INH-containing regimen (rating BI; see Table 79-2).[15] Alternatively, RIF and EMB for 12 months may be used, preferably with PZA included during the initial 2-month treatment (rating BII).[15] If RIF is not used, INH, EMB, and fluoroquinolones should be given for a minimum of 12 to 18 months supplemented with PZA during the initial 2 months (rating BIII).[15] Levofloxacin, MXF, or gatifloxacin may be useful in alternative regimens, but their role and optimal length of therapy have not been defined.[15] If PZA cannot be included in the initial phase of treatment (as in severe liver disease, gout, and, pregnancy), or if the isolate is resistant to PZA, the initial phase should consist of INH, RIF, and EMB given daily for 2 months (regimen 4; see Table 79-2) followed by INH and RIF for 7 months, with a total duration of 9 months when PZA cannot be used.[15] If patients have cavitation on the initial chest radiograph and the 2-month culture is positive, the minimum duration of treatment should be 9 months.[15] If EMB cannot be used, 2 months of INH, RIF, PZA, and SM followed by 4 months of INH and RIF is recommended.[86]

Re-treatment Regimen

For patients who have relapsed, interrupted treatment, or failed treatment, the WHO and the IUATLD recommend a standardized regimen consisting of an initial phase of five drugs (INH, RIF, PZA, EMB, and SM) given daily for 2 months, and then 1 month of daily INH, RIF, PZA, and EMB, and a continuation phase of 5 months of daily INH, RIF, and EMB.[72,86] An alternative regimen is to give the above drugs three times weekly instead of daily for the same duration of treatment as above.[72]

Recommended Doses

The dosages for the first-line and commonly used second-line TB drugs used for the treatment of TB are listed in Tables 79-3 and 79-4, respectively. The WHO recommends 10 mg/kg as the dose for three-times-weekly INH,[72] whereas the ATS/CDC/Infectious Diseases Society of America (IDSA) recommend 15 mg/kg.[15] While there is no difference in the daily doses recommended for adults (5 mg/kg per day to a maximum of 300 mg/day), the ATS/CDC/IDSA recommend a higher dose for children (10 to 15 mg/kg per day), based primarily on the expert opinion of pediatricians.[15] According to the WHO guideline, the recommended dose of EMB is higher in children (20 mg/kg) than in adults (15 mg/kg), because the pharmacokinetics are different (peak serum concentration of EMB is lower in children than in adults receiving the same milligram per kilogram dose).[72]

Fixed-dose combinations of two (INH and RIF; Rifamate), three (INH, RIF, and PZA; Rifater), and four (INH, RIF, PZA, and EMB) drugs are highly recommended by the WHO, IUATLD, and CDC for improved compliance, especially when medication ingestion is not observed.[149] Patients with smear- and culture-negative TB can be treated with INH and RIF for 4 months.[150]

Adverse effects, especially GI upset, are relatively common in the first few weeks of therapy. However, first-line TB drugs, particularly RIF, must not be discontinued because of minor side effects. If patients have epigastric distress or nausea with the first-line drugs, dosing with meals or changing the hour of dosing is recommended. Administration with food is preferable to splitting a dose or changing to second-line drugs.[15]

Treatment of Latent TB Infection: Preventive Therapy

LTBI refers to initial early TB infection that has not yet developed into disease but has the potential to do so. It has been demonstrated that preventive treatment with INH can significantly reduce the risk of active disease in individuals with LTBI.[15,151] INH used singly for 6 or 9 months is recommended for preventive therapy for LTBI[151] (Table 79-5). LTBI is diagnosed by tuberculin skin test positivity. However, INH prophylaxis is not commonly used in developing countries. For people who are at highest risk of developing active TB—those who are HIV positive, receiving immunosuppressant therapy, or in close contact with TB patients, or who have abnormal chest radiographs consistent with prior TB—a skin test result of greater than 5 mm of induration is considered positive. For other people with an increased probability of recent infection or with other clinical conditions that increase the risk for progression to active TB, greater than 10 mm of induration is considered positive. These include recent immigrants from high-prevalence countries; injection drug users; health care workers with exposure to TB; TB lab personnel; persons with clinical conditions such as silicosis, diabetes, and chronic renal failure; children; and adolescents exposed to adults in high-risk categories. For people at low risk for TB, greater than 15 mm of induration is considered positive. INH chemoprophylaxis should be offered to persons with LTBI at increased risk for TB (active disease should be ruled out) unless there is a strong contraindication.[151]

Chemoprophylaxis with INH 5 mg/kg of body weight for adults and 10 mg/kg of body weight for children (maximum 300 mg/day) is given daily for 6 to 9 months[151] for high-risk populations. The recently updated CDC guideline recommends that INH be given daily for 9 months regardless of HIV status.[151] The 9-month INH regimen is the preferred regimen, with a recommendation level of A. The 6-month INH daily regimen is an acceptable alternative with a recommendation level of B (alternative, acceptable to offer) for HIV-negative individuals but a level of C (offer when preferred or alternative regimens cannot be given) for HIV-positive individuals.[151] The current ATS/CDC recommendation for preventive therapy in HIV-positive individuals includes the use of INH 300 mg/day for 12 months with a positive tuberculin test and no evidence of TB.[15] This INH preventive therapy should be supplemented with pyridoxine (25 to 50 mg/day) to help prevent INH-associated peripheral neuropathy.[15]

Persons infected with INH-resistant organisms are unlikely to benefit from INH prophylaxis, and use of other TB drugs such as RIF and PZA should be considered. For persons who are likely infected with MDR-TB and at a high risk of developing TB, treatment with PZA and EMB or PZA and a fluoroquinolone for 6 to 12 months is recommended.[151]

Patients treated for LTBI should receive clinical evaluation at least monthly. Clinical monitoring during treatment is indicated for all patients, which includes education of patients about signs and symptoms of side effects of INH, including unexplained anoxia, nausea, vomiting, dark urine, rash, and persistent fatigue.[151] Laboratory testing (e.g., serum aspartate aminotransferase, alanine aminotransferase, and bilirubin) is not usually recommended at the start of the prophylaxis except in HIV-infected people, pregnant women, persons with history of liver disease, or persons who regularly use alcohol.[151] The risk of liver damage by INH, especially in patients over 35 years of age, resulted in conflicting views in the United States on the benefits of INH prophylaxis in low-risk tuberculin reactors.[59] Because of this potential problem, many physicians use decision analysis on the benefits and drawbacks of "to treat or not to treat" with INH.

LTBI can also be treated with RIF for 4 months[151] (see Table 79-5). However, treatment with RIF and PZA for 2 months, a regimen initially found to be as effective as 6 months of INH treatment in HIV-positive individuals,[18] is not recommended by the CDC for the treatment of LTBI in HIV-negative individuals due to severe hepatoxicity. The latter regimen can be used in HIV-positive individuals only as a second choice, with a BI rating[15] (see Table 79-5).

Treatment of Extrapulmonary TB

Extrapulmonary TB can be treated with the same principles as those for pulmonary TB, with some slight modifications in some cases (Table 79-6). The 6-month therapeutic regimen is recommended for the treatment of all forms of extrapulmonary TB except tuberculous meningitis, which requires a 9- to 12-month regimen.[15] Prolonged treatment may be needed if the extrapulmonary TB is slow to respond. The addition of corticosteroids is recommended in cases of tuberculous pericarditis and meningitis.[15]

Treatment of TB Patients with HIV Infection

Recommendations for the treatment of TB patients with HIV infection are essentially the same as those for the treatment of HIV-negative patients, with a few exceptions[15] (see Table 79-2). Thiacetazone is contraindicated in AIDS patients.[72,86] INH and rifapentine once weekly are contraindicated in HIV-positive TB patients due to high relapse rates and frequent emergence of rifamycin resistance.[15] In advanced AIDS patients (CD4 count < 100 cells/mm^3) with TB, daily or three-times-weekly treatment is recommended. DOT is important for HIV-related TB. Rifamycins may adversely interact with certain antiretroviral agents. However, RIF can be used for the treatment of TB with certain combinations of antiretroviral agents. Rifabutin, which has fewer unwanted drug interactions, may also be used in place of RIF. Coadministration of TB therapy and antiretroviral therapy is complex, and

TABLE 79-3 DOSE, SERUM CONCENTRATION AND TOXICITY OF THE FIRST-LINE TB DRUGS

Drug	*Dose in mg/kg (Maximum Dose)*			Peak Serum Concentration (μg/ml) (Dose)	Toxicity	Comments
	Daily	**Twice Weekly**	**Three Times Weekly**			
Isoniazid	*Adults:* 5 (300 mg) *Children:* 10-20 (300 mg)	*Adults:* 15 (900 mg) *Children:* 20-40 (900 mg)	*Adults:* 15 (900 mg) *Children:* 20-40 (900 mg)	3-5 (300 mg)	Hepatoxicity, peripheral neuropathy, central nervous system (mild), lupus-like syndrome, hypersensitivity	Hepatoxicity increases with age and alcohol consumption; pyridoxine can prevent peripheral neuropathy.
Rifampin	*Adults:* 10 (600 mg) *Children:* 10-20 (600 mg)	*Adults:* 10 (600 mg) *Children:* 10-20 (600 mg)	*Adults:* 10 (600 mg) *Children:* 10-20 (600 mg)	8-29 (600 mg)	Gastrointestinal upset, hepatoxicity, flulike symptoms, cutaneous reactions, severe immunologic reactions causing thrombocytopenia and bleeding	Drug interaction with methadone, birth control pills, and some other drugs; colors body fluids orange.
Pyrazinamide	*Adults:* 15-30 (2 g) *Children:* 15-30 (2 g)	*Adults:* 50-70 (3 g) *Children:* 50 (2 g)	*Adults:* 50 (2–3 g)* *Children:* 50*	20-60 (30 mg/kg)	Hepatoxicity, rash, gastrointestinal upset, joint aches, hyperuricemia, gout (rare)	Treat hyperuricemia only if patient has symptoms.
Ethambutol	*Adults:* 15-25 (2.5 g) *Children:* 15-25 (2.5 g)	*Adults:* 50 (2.5 g) *Children:* 50 (2.5 g)	*Adults:* 25-30 (2.5 g) *Children:* 25-30 (2.5 g)	3-5 (15-25 mg/kg)	Optic neuritis, cutaneous reactions, peripheral neuritis	Not recommended for children too young to monitor changes in vision unless TB is drug resistant.
Streptomycin	*Adults:* 15 (1 g) *Children:* 20-30 (1 g)	*Adults:* 25-30 (1 g) *Children:* 25-30 (1 g)	*Adults:* 25-30 (1.5 g) *Children:* 25-30 (1.5 g)	35-45 (15 mg/kg)	Ototoxicity, nephrotoxicity, hypersensitivity	Avoid or reduce dose in adults over 60 years old. Not recommended in pregnancy.

*WHO recommends 30-40 mg/kg PZA.[149]

Adapted from American Thoracic Society, CDC, and Infectious Diseases Society of America. Treatment of tuberculosis. MMWR Recomm Rep 2003;52(RR11):1-77.

TABLE 79-4 DOSE, SERUM CONCENTRATION AND TOXICITY OF SECOND-LINE TB DRUGS

Drug	Daily Dose		Peak Serum Concentration (mcg/ml) (Dose)	Toxicity	Comments	Contraindications
	Adults	Children				
Cycloserine	10-15 mg/kg (1 g in two doses/day)	10-15 mg/kg (1 g in two doses/day)	20-35 (250 mg bid)	Psychosis, headaches, convulsions, rash, depression	Start with low dose and increase as tolerated. Assess mental status. Pyridoxine may decrease CNS effects.	Should be avoided in patients with a history of epilepsy, mental illness, or alcoholism.
Ethionamide	15-20 mg/kg (1 g/day)	15-20 mg/kg (1 g/day)	1-5 (250 mg bid)	GI upset, metallic taste, hepatoxicity, bloating, hypersensitivity	Start with low dose and increase as tolerated. May cause hypothyroid condition. Measure hepatic enzymes.	Not recommended in pregnancy.
Amikacin*/ Kanamycin*	15 mg/kg (0.75-1 g/day)†	15-30 mg/kg (1 g) intravenous or intramuscular injection as single dose	35-45 (15 mg/kg)	Ototoxicity, nephrotoxicity	Assess hearing function. Measure renal function.	Amikacin and kanamycin are contraindicated in pregnant women because of risk of fetal nephrotoxicity and congenital hearing loss.
Capreomycin	15 mg/kg (1 g/day)†	15-30 mg/kg (1 g)	35-45 (15 mg/kg)	Ototoxicity, nephrotoxicity	Assess hearing function. Measure renal function.	Should be avoided in pregnancy.
p-Aminosalicylic acid	8-12 g/day, in two to three doses	200-300 mg/kg/day in two to four doses	40-70 (3 g qid)	GI upset, hypersensitivity, hepatoxicity, sodium overload	Start with low dose and increase as tolerated. Measure hepatic enzymes. Monitor cardiac patients for sodium load.	The only available formulation in the United States is granules in 4-g packets (Paser Granules). A solution for intravenous use is available in Europe.
Levofloxacin*	500-1000 mg/day	Not known	9 (1000 mg)	GI disturbance, neurotoxicity, psychosis, allergic reaction, phototoxicity		Fluoroquinolones should be avoided in pregnancy because of teratogenic effects.
Moxifloxacin*	400 mg/day	Not known	3-4 (400 mg)	Allergic reaction, central nervous system side effects, tendinopathy, GI disturbance, phototoxicity		Fluoroquinolones should be avoided in pregnancy because of teratogenic effects.
Gatifloxacin*	400 mg/day	Not known	5-6 (400 mg)	Allergic reaction, central nervous system side effects, GI disturbance, phototoxicity		Fluoroquinolones should be avoided in pregnancy because of teratogenic effects.

*Not approved by the U.S. Food and Drug Administration in the United States to treat TB.
†10 mg/kg (0.75 g/day) for persons aged 59 years or older IM or IV.
bid, twice daily; CNS, central nervous system; GI, gastrointestinal; IM, intramuscularly; IV, intravenously; qid, four times per day.
Adapted from American Thoracic Society, CDC, and Infectious Diseases Society of America. Treatment of tuberculosis. MMWR Recomm Rep 2003;52(RR11):1-77.

TABLE 79-5 ATS/CDC/IDSA REVISED REGIMENS FOR TREATMENT OF LATENT TUBERCULOSIS INFECTION (LTBI) IN ADULTS

Drug	Interval and Duration	Comments*	Rating[†] (Evidence)[‡] HIV⁻	Rating[†] (Evidence)[‡] HIV⁺
Isoniazid	Daily for 9 mo[§]	In HIV-infected persons, INH may be administered concurrently with nucleoside reverse transcriptase inhibitors (NRTIs), protease inhibitors, or non-nucleoside reverse transcriptase inhibitors (NNRTIs).	A (II)	A (II)
	Twice weekly for 9 mo[§,¶]	Directly observed therapy (DOT) must be used with twice-weekly dosing.	B (II)	B (II)
Isoniazid	Daily for 6 mo[¶]	Not indicated for HIV-infected persons, those with fibrotic lesions on chest radiographs, or children.	B (I)	C (I)
	Twice weekly for 6 mo[¶]	DOT must be used with twice-weekly dosing.	B (II)	C (I)
Rifampin[¶]	Daily for 4 mo	Used for persons who are contacts of patients with INH-resistant, RIF-susceptible TB. In HIV-infected persons, most protease inhibitors or delavirdine should not be administered concurrently with rifampin. Rifabutin, with appropriate dose adjustments, can be used with protease inhibitors (saquinavir should be augmented with ritonavir) and NNRTIs (except delavirdine). Clinicians should consult web-based updates for the latest specific recommendations.	B (II)	B (III)
Rifampin plus pyrazinamide (R+Z)	Daily for 2 mo	R+Z generally should not be offered for treatment of LTBI for HIV-infected or HIV-negative persons.	D (II)	D (II)
	Twice weekly for 2-3 mo		D (III)	D (III)

*Interactions with HIV-related drugs are updated frequently and are available at *http://www.aidsinfo.nih.gov/guidelines.*
†Strength of the recommendation:
A. Both strong evidence of efficacy and substantial clinical benefit support recommendation for use. Should always be offered.
B. Moderate evidence for efficacy or strong evidence for efficacy but only limited clinical benefit supports recommendation for use. Should generally be offered.
C. Evidence for efficacy is insufficient to support a recommendation for or against use, or evidence for efficacy might not outweigh adverse consequences (e.g., drug toxicity, drug interactions) or cost of the treatment or alternative approaches. Optional.
D. Moderate evidence for lack of efficacy or for adverse outcome supports a recommendation against use. Should generally not be offered.
E. Good evidence for lack of efficacy or for adverse outcome support a recommendation against use. Should never be offered.
‡Quality of evidence supporting the recommendation:
I. Evidence from at least one properly randomized controlled trial.
II. Evidence from at least one well-designed clinical trial without randomization from cohort or case-controlled analytic studies (preferably from more than one center), from multiple time-series studies, or from dramatic results from uncontrolled experiments.
III. Evidence from opinions of respected authorities based on clinical experience, descriptive studies, or reports of expert committees.
§Recommended regimen for persons age less than 18 years.
¶Recommended regimens for pregnant women.
¶The substitution of rifapentine for rifampin is not recommended because rifapentine's safety and effectiveness have not been established for patients with LTBI.
ATS, American Thoracic Society; CDC, Centers for Disease Control and Prevention; HIV, human immunodeficiency virus; IDSA, Infectious Diseases Society of America; INH, isoniazid; RIF, rifampin.
Adapted from Centers for Disease Control and Prevention. Update: Adverse event data and revised American Thoracic Society/CDC recommendations against the use of rifampin and pyrazinamide for treatment of latent tuberculosis infection—United States, 2003. MMWR Morb Mortal Wkly Rep 2003;52:735-739.

TABLE 79-6 EVIDENCE-BASED GUIDELINES FOR THE TREATMENT OF EXTRAPULMONARY TUBERCULOSIS AND ADJUNCTIVE USE OF CORTICOSTEROIDS

Site	Duration of Therapy (Mo)*	Rating (Duration)[†]	Corticosteroids	Rating (Corticosteroids)[†]
Lymph node	6	AI	Not recommended	DIII
Bone and joint	6-9	AI	Not recommended	DIII
Pleural disease	6	AII	Not recommended	DI
Pericarditis	6	AII	Strongly recommended	AI
Central nervous system, including meningitis	9-12	BII	Strongly recommended	AI
Disseminated disease	6	AII	Not recommended	DIII
Genitourinary	6	AII	Not recommended	DIII
Peritoneal	6	AII	Not recommended	DIII

*Duration of therapy for extrapulmonary tuberculosis caused by drug-resistant organisms is not known.
†For rating system, see Table 79-2.
From American Thoracic Society, CDC, and Infectious Diseases Society of America. Treatment of tuberculosis. MMWR Recomm Rep 2003;52(RR11):1-77.

consultation with experts in this area is recommended. The WHO recommends inclusion of co-trimoxazole as prophylaxis for other infections for HIV/TB patients.[149]

Due to drug interactions, RIF is not recommended for patients who (i) will start treatment with an antiretroviral regimen that includes a protease inhibitor or a non-nucleoside reverse transcriptase inhibitor or (ii) have established HIV infection and are on antiretroviral therapy when TB is newly diagnosed and needs to be treated. Two options are currently recommended for such patients: (i) a 6-month rifabutin-based regimen and (ii) a 9-month SM-based regimen when rifamycin is contraindicated (such as intolerance to rifamycins or patient/physician decision not to combine antiretroviral and TB therapy together). For patients who have delayed response (lack of bacterial conversion from positive to negative, or lack of resolution or progression of signs and symptoms of TB), the 6-month DOTS should be prolonged to 9 months, whereas the 9-month SM-containing regimen should be prolonged to 12 months. For TB that is resistant to INH only, a 6- to 9-month therapeutic regimen with RIF, PZA, and EMB should be given.[15]

Treatment of MDR-TB

MDR-TB is defined as strains resistant to at least INH and RIF. In addition to patient noncompliance, which is frequently the cause of MDR-TB, clinical errors that commonly lead to the emergence of drug resistance include failure to provide effective treatment support and assurance of adherence, failure to recognize and address patient nonadherence, inadequate drug regimens, adding a single new drug to a failing regimen, and failure to recognize existing drug resistance.[149]

The standard TB therapy is ineffective in controlling MDR-TB in areas of high MDR-TB incidence.[152] DOTS-Plus, which is DOTS plus second-line TB drugs, is required for the treatment of MDR-TB.[72] The dosage and side effects of commonly used second-line drugs are listed in Table 79-4. DOTS-Plus is not intended as a universal TB treatment but should be implemented in selected areas with moderate to high levels of MDR-TB in order to combat an emerging epidemic (*http://www.who.int/tb/dots/dotsplus/management/en/index.html*). DOTS-Plus is still under development, and treatment of MDR-TB is complex and controversial. Recently, the WHO outlined new standards, mainly in the form of treatment principles, for the treatment of drug-resistant TB and MDR-TB (Table 79-7). Patients with drug-resistant (especially MDR) TB should be treated with specialized regimens containing second-line drugs. Treatment of MDR-TB is more expensive and more toxic and takes longer (at least 18 months).[72] At least four drugs to which the organisms are susceptible should be used. As in HIV-related TB, patient adherence to therapy is critical. Consultation with a provider experienced in treatment of patients with MDR-TB should be obtained.[149]

Since randomized controlled treatment trials for MDR-TB are difficult to design, no data are available to serve as a reliable basis for objective recommendation. Current recommendations (see Table 79-7) are based on observational studies, general microbiologic and therapeutic principles, extrapolation from available evidence from pilot MDR-TB treatment projects, and expert opinion.[149] Three strategic options for treatment of MDR-TB are currently recommended by the WHO[149]: standardized regimens, empirical regimens, and individualized treatment regimens. The choice among these should be based on availability of second-line drugs and drug susceptibility testing for first- and second-line drugs, local drug resistance patterns, and the history of use of second-line drugs. The basic principles involved in the design of any regimen include the use of at least four drugs with either certain or highly likely effectiveness, drug administration at least 6 days a week, drug dosage determined by patient weight, the use of an injectable agent (kanamycin, amikacin, capreomycin) and a fluoroquinolone for at least 6 months in the initial phase of treatment followed by a continuation phase of 12 to 18 months (with total treatment duration of 18 to 24 months), and DOT throughout the treatment.[72,149] Drug susceptibility testing is critical for choosing drugs for treatment of MDR-TB. Patients with localized MDR-TB disease who have failed chemotherapy and who have adequate pulmonary reserves may be considered for resectional surgery.[153]

Extremely drug-resistant TB (XDR-TB) is defined as resistance to at least INH and RIF from the first-line antituberculosis drugs (which is the definition of MDR-TB) in addition to resistance to any fluoroquinolone, and to at least one of three injectable second-line antituberculosis drugs used in TB treatment (capreomycin, kanamicin, and amikacin).[2,4] XDR-TB was identified in all regions of the world, though it is still thought to be relatively uncommon.[2] The previously described guidelines for the treatment of MDR-TB would be applicable for the treatment of XDR-TB, and specific treatment regimens will have to be designed according to the specific situation of the patient and drug susceptibility data about the drug-resistant TB strain that caused the disease.

Emerging Targets and Therapeutics

The increasing emergence of drug-resistant TB has highlighted the need for new and more effective TB drugs. Recent years have seen renewed interest and efforts in this area.[5-8] Various drug candidates and active compounds have been identified. For a more detailed review on this topic, please refer to the recent reviews.[5-8] Here only the most promising drug candidates that are in clinical trials are briefly discussed. The structures of these TB drug candidates are shown in Figure 79-6.

New Fluoroquinolones

The new C-8-methoxyfluoroquinolines MXF (see Fig. 79-6) and gatifloxacin, with a longer half-life, are more active against *M. tuberculosis* (MICs of 0.125 and 0.06 mcg/ml, respectively) than ofloxacin and

TABLE 79-7 SUGGESTED REGIMENS FOR TREATMENT OF MDR-TB

	Initial Phase		Continuation Phase	
Susceptibility Testing to Drugs	**Drugs**	**Duration**	**Drugs**	**Duration**
Not available*	KM† + ETH + FQ‡ + PZA + EMB	At least 6 mo	ETH + FQ + PZA + EMB	12-18 mo
Resistance to INH + RIF	SM§ + ETH + FQ‡ + PZA + EMB	At least 6 mo	ETH + FQ + PZA + EMB	12-18 mo
Resistance to all essential drugs	1 injectable + 1 FQ‡ + 2 of the 3 oral drugs: PAS, CS, ETH	At least 6 mo	Same drugs except the injectable	18 mo
Susceptibility testing to reserve drugs available	Tailored regimen according to drug susceptibility pattern	At least 6 mo		

*Use of a standardized regimen could be feasible in resource-limited countries with a high burden of TB and a strong and efficient NTP.
†Amikacin or capreomycin could also be used. However, since there is cross-resistance between KM and amikacin, if either drug was used previously or if resistance to them is suspected, capreomycin is the preferred choice.
‡Fluoroquinolone (ciprofloxacin or ofloxacin).
§If resistance to SM is confirmed, replace this drug with KM, amikacin, or capreomycin.
CS, cycloserine; EMB, ethambutol; ETH, ethionamide; FQ, fluoroquinolone; INH, isoniazid; KM, kanamycin; NTP, National Tuberculosis Control Program; PAS, *para*-aminosalicylic acid; PZA, pyrazinamide; RIF, rifampin; SM, streptomycin.
From World Health Organization. Treatment of Tuberculosis: Guidelines for National Programmes. Geneva: World Health Organization, 2003.

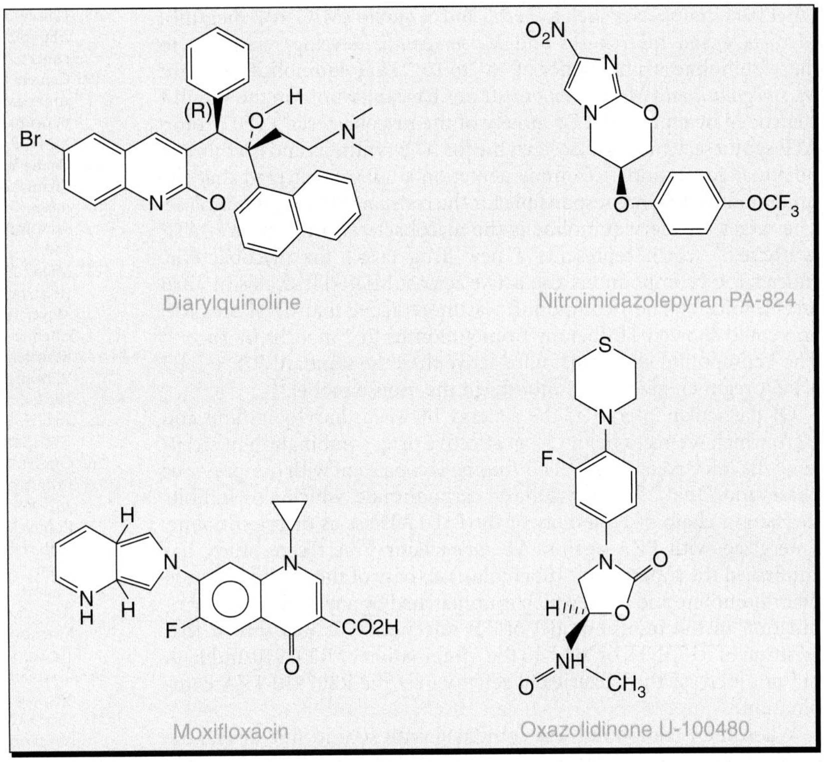

FIGURE 79-6 • **Structures of some promising TB drug candidates.**

ciprofloxacin (MICs of 2 and 4 mcg/ml, respectively).[154,155] MXF appeared to kill a subpopulation of tubercle bacilli not killed by RIF (i.e., RIF-tolerant persisters) in vitro.[100] MXF was active against *M. tuberculosis* comparable to INH in a mouse model.[156] A recent study showed that MXF in combination with RIF and PZA killed the bacilli more effectively than the INH + RIF + PZA combination in mice.[157] The higher activity of MXF + RIF + PZA than INH + RIF + PZA raises the hope that MXF may replace INH in combination with RIF and PZA to shorten TB therapy in humans. However, there is also concern about the potential toxicity of the MXF + RIF + PZA combination in the absence of INH, as seen in the treatment of LTBI with RIF-PZA.[18] MXF has early bactericidal activity against tubercle bacilli comparable to INH in a preliminary human study,[158] and was well tolerated, and combination therapy with MXF seems to be as effective as current standard drug combinations.[159] However, in a recent study, addition of MXF to IHN, RIF, and PZA did not affect 2-month sputum culture status but did show increased activity at earlier time points.[108] In another study to evaluate the EBA of the new quinolones in TB patients, while day 0 to 2 EBA of levofloxacin, MXF, and gatifloxacin is not as high as INH, day 2 to 7 EBA for the quinolones was higher than INH.[160] More studies are needed to further evaluate these new quinolones for possible improved treatment of TB and MDR-TB.

Oxazolidinones (Linezolid)

Oxazolidinones (see Fig. 79-6) are a new class of antibiotics approved by the FDA for the treatment of drug-resistant gram-positive bacterial infections.[161] Oxazolidinones inhibit an early step of protein synthesis by binding to ribosomal 50S subunits, most likely within domain V of the 23S rRNA peptidyltransferase, and forming a secondary interaction with the 30S subunit.[161] Oxazolidinones had significant activity against *M. tuberculosis*, with MICs of 0.125 to 0.5 mcg/ml, and against *M. avium* complex, with MICs of 0.5 to 4 mcg/ml.[162] One derivative, PNU100480, was active against tubercle bacilli comparable to that of INH and RIF in mice.[163] Linezolid has been used to treat MDR-TB in a few isolated cases in combination with other TB drugs.[164] Limited experience suggests linezolid in combination with other TB drugs was effective but appeared to have significant side effects such as peripheral neuropathy, optic neuropathy, and anemia.[165] Oxazolidinones may have potential for the treatment of MDR-TB and other mycobacterial infections.

Nitroimidazopyran (PA-824)

Nitroimidazopyran PA-824 (see Fig. 79-6) is a new nitroimidazole derivative[166] based on an earlier observation that 5-nitroimidazole had good in vitro and in vivo activity against *M. tuberculosis.*[167,168] PA-824 is highly active against *M. tuberculosis*, with MICs of 0.015 to 0.25 mcg/ml.[166] PA-824 is also active against nonreplicating tubercle bacilli. PA-824 is a prodrug that is activated by F420-dependent glucose-6-phosphate dehydrogenase and a nitroreductase activity in the bacilli.[166] The resulting active metabolites interfere with cell wall lipid biosynthesis by inhibiting an enzyme responsible for the oxidation of hydroxymycolic acid to ketomycolate.[166] PA-824 was also active against MDR-TB strains, suggesting that it inhibits a new target in tubercle bacilli. PA-824 was as active as INH in animal models of TB infection.[166] A preliminary toxicity study indicated that mice tolerated a single dose of PA-824 at 1000 mg/kg or 500 mg/kg daily for 28 days.[166] In the mouse model, PA-824's minimal effective dose was 12.5 mg/kg per day and minimal bactericidal dose was 100 mg/kg per day.[169] PA-824 had bactericidal activity in the initial and continuation phases of treatment in mice.[169] Although PA-824 in combination with RIF and PZA led to higher sterilizing activity compared with the standard INH + RIF + PZA combination during the first 2 months of treatment in mice, PA-824 did not do any better than the standard INH + RIF + PZA combination to shorten the 6-month therapeutic regimen.[170] No other PA-824–containing regimen tested was superior to the standard regimen of INH + RIF + PZA.[170] A Phase I clinical trial is being conducted by the TB Alliance.

Diarylquinoline

Diarylquinoline (see Fig. 79-6) is a promising TB drug that can shorten TB therapy.[171] Diarylquinoline was identified in an in vitro drug screen for activity against the fast-growing mycobacterium *M. smegmatis.*[171] Modification of the diarylquinolines led to the identification of diarylquinoline R207910 (J compound) as the most active agent, with MICs for *M. smegmatis* and *M. tuberculosis* being 0.003 mcg/ml and 0.03 mcg/ml, respectively. The J compound is much less active against other bacterial species such as *E. coli* and *S. aureus* (MIC > 32 mcg/ml). *Mycobacterium tuberculosis* and *M. smegmatis* develop resistance to diarylquinoline at a frequency of 10^{-7} to 10^{-8}. Diarylquinoline-resistant *M. smegmatis* and *M. tuberculosis* strains have mutations in the subunit c encoded by *atpE* in the F0 moiety of the mycobacterial F1F0 proton ATP synthase, which is a key enzyme for ATP synthesis and membrane potential generation.[171] Complementation studies confirmed that the mutations in *atpE* are responsible for the resistance to diarylquinoline. The target for diarylquinoline is the mycobacterial F1F0 proton ATP synthase,[171] which represents a new drug target for mycobacteria. Indeed, the J compound is also active against MDR-TB strains in vitro and in mice.[172] The J compound was more active than INH and RIF and could shorten TB therapy from 4 months to 2 months in mice.[171] The J compound alone was more active than the standard RIF + INH + PZA regimen given for 2 months in the mouse model.[172]

Of particular interest is the synergy between diarylquinoline and PZA, which seems to be the most effective drug combination in sterilizing the infected organs.[171] This finding is consistent with our previous observation that *N,N′*-dicyclohexyl carbodiimide, which also inhibits the same c chain of F0 moiety of the F1F0 ATPase as diarylquinoline, synergized with PZA against *M. tuberculosis*.[137] A recent study has confirmed the superior antituberculosis activity of the combination of diarylquinoline and PZA, which is unmatched by any other drug combination in the mouse model of TB infection.[173] It was shown that addition of RIF, INH, or MXF to the combination of R207910 and PZA did not increase the bactericidal activity over the R207910-PZA combination.[173]

When the J compound was combined with second-line drugs, the combinations were more active than the currently recommended regimen for MDR-TB (amikacin + ETH + MXF + PZA), with culture negativity for both the lungs and spleen after 2 months of treatment.[172] The J compound had excellent early and late bactericidal activity in the mouse model, good pharmacokinetic and pharmacodynamic properties with a long half-life, and absence of significant toxicity in mice and in preliminary human safety testing, raising the hope that diarylquinoline may be used for shortening the therapy of TB in humans. The J compound is currently under clinical testing.

REFERENCES

1. World Health Organization. 2006 Tuberculosis Facts. Geneva: World Health Organization, 2006.
2. World Health Organization. XDR-TB, Extensively Drug-Resistant Tuberculosis. Geneva: World Health Organization, 2006.
3. Small PM, Shafer RW, Hopewell PC, et al. Exogenous reinfection with multidrug-resistant *Mycobacterium tuberculosis* in patients with advanced HIV infection. N Engl J Med 1993;328:1137-1144.
4. World Health Organization. The World Health Organization Global Tuberculosis Program. Geneva: World Health Organization, 2006.
5. Duncan K, Barry CE 3rd. Prospects for new antitubercular drugs. Curr Opin Microbiol 2004;7:460-465.
6. Tuberculosis: scientific blueprint for tuberculosis drug development. Tuberculosis (Edinb) 2001;81(Suppl 1):1-52.
7. O'Brien R, Nunn P. The need for new drugs against tuberculosis: obstacles, opportunities, and next steps. Am J Respir Crit Care Med 2001;163:1055-1058.
8. Zhang Y. The magic bullets and tuberculosis drug targets. Annu Rev Pharmacol Toxicol 2005;45:529-564.
9. Dannenberg A. Pathogenesis of Human Pulmonary Tuberculosis: Insights from the Rabbit. Washington, DC: ASM Press, 2006.
10. Mitchison DA. The action of antituberculosis drugs in short course chemotherapy. Tubercle 1985;66:219-225.
11. Winder F. Mode of action of the antimycobacterial agents and associated aspects of the molecular biology of mycobacteria. *In* Ratledge C, Stanford J (eds): The Biology of Mycobacteria. New York: Academic Press, 1982, pp 354-438.
12. Fox W, Ellard GA, Mitchison DA. Studies on the treatment of tuberculosis undertaken by the British Medical Research Council tuberculosis units, 1946-1986, with relevant subsequent publications. Int J Tuberc Lung Dis 1999;3:S231-S279.
13. Canetti G. The Tubercle Bacillus in the Pulmonary Lesion of Man. New York: Springer Publishing Company, 1955.
14. McDermott W. Microbial persistence. Yale J Biol Med 1958;30:257-291.
15. American Thoracic Society, CDC, and Infectious Diseases Society of America. Treatment of tuberculosis. MMWR Recomm Rep 2003;52(RR11):1-77.
16. Zhang Y. Persistent and dormant tubercle bacilli and latent tuberculosis. Front Biosci 2004;9:1136-1156.
17. Mitchison D. The search for new sterilizing anti-tuberculosis drugs. Front Biosci 2004;9:1059-1072.
18. Halsey NA, Coberly JS, Desormeaux J, et al. Randomised trial of isoniazid versus rifampicin and pyrazinamide for prevention of tuberculosis in HIV-1 infection. Lancet 1998;351:786-792.
19. Centers for Disease Control and Prevention. Update: Adverse event data and revised American Thoracic Society/CDC recommendations against the use of rifampin and pyrazinamide for treatment of latent tuberculosis infection—United States, 2003. MMWR Morb Mortal Wkly Rep 2003;52:735-739.
20. Zhang Y. Isoniazid. New York: Lippincott Williams & Wilkins, 2004, pp 739-758.
21. Zhang Y, Vilcheze C, Jacobs WR. Mechanisms of drug resistance in *Mycobacterium tuberculosis*. *In* Cole ST, Eisenach KD, McMurray DN, Jacobs WR Jr (eds): Tuberculosis and the Tubercle Bacillus, 2nd ed. Washington, DC: ASM Press, 2005, pp 115-140.
22. Miesel L, Rozwarski DA, Sacchettini JC, et al: Mechanisms for isoniazid action and resistance. Novartis Found Symp 1998;217:209-220; discussion 220-221.
23. Meyer H, Malley J. Uber hydrazinderivate de pyridincarbonsauren. Montashefte fur Chemie 1912;33:393-414.
24. Bernstein J, Lott W, Steinberg B, et al. Chemotherapy of experimental tuberculosis. V. Isonicotinic acid hydrazide (Nydrazid) and related compounds. Am Rev Tuberc 1952;65:357-364.
25. Fox H. The chemical approach to the control of tuberculosis. Science 1952;116: 129-134.
26. Offe H, Siefken W, Domagk G. The tuberculostatic activity of hydrazine derivatives from pyridine carboxylic acids and carbonyl compounds. Z Naturforsch 1952;7b: 462-468.
27. Robitzek E, Selikoff I. Hydrazine derivatives of isonicotinic acid (Rimifon, Marsilid) in the treatment of active progressive caseous-pneumonic tuberculosis: a preliminary report. Am Rev Tuberc 1952;65:402-428.
28. Pansy F, Stander H, Donovick R. In vitro studies on isonicotinic acid hydrazide. Am Rev Tuberc 1952;65:761-764.
29. Mitchison D, Selkon J. The bactericidal activities of antituberculosis drugs. Am Rev Tuberc 1956;74(Suppl):109-116.
30. Bartmann K. Isoniazid. *In* Bartmann K (ed): Handbook of Experimental Pharmacology, Vol 84: Antituberculosis Drugs. Berlin: Springer-Verlag, 1988, pp 113-134.
31. Shoeb HA, Bowman BU Jr, Ottolenghi AC, et al. Peroxidase-mediated oxidation of isoniazid. Antimicrob Agents Chemother 1985;27:399-403.
32. Shoeb HA, Bowman BU Jr, Ottolenghi AC, et al. Evidence for the generation of active oxygen by isoniazid treatment of extracts of *Mycobacterium tuberculosis* H37Ra. Antimicrob Agents Chemother 1985;27:404-407.
33. Johnsson K, King DS, Schultz PG. Studies on the mechanism of action of isoniazid and ethionamide in the chemotherapy of tuberculosis. J Am Chem Soc 1995;117:5009-5010.
34. Banerjee A, Dubnau E, Quemard A, et al. *inhA*, a gene encoding a target for isoniazid and ethionamide in *Mycobacterium tuberculosis*. Science 1994;263:227-230.
35. Rozwarski DA, Grant GA, Barton DH, et al. Modification of the NADH of the isoniazid target (InhA) from *Mycobacterium tuberculosis*. Science 1998;279:98-102.
36. Rawat R, Whitty A, Tonge PJ. The isoniazid-NAD adduct is a slow, tight-binding inhibitor of InhA, the *Mycobacterium tuberculosis* enoyl reductase: adduct affinity and drug resistance. Proc Natl Acad Sci U S A 2003;100:13881-13886.
37. Argyrou A, Vetting MW, Aladegbami B, et al. *Mycobacterium tuberculosis* dihydrofolate reductase is a target for isoniazid. Nat Struct Mol Biol 2006;13:408-413.
38. Gangadharam P, Harold F, Schaefer W. Selective inhibition of nucleic acid synthesis in *Mycobacterium tuberculosis* by isoniazid. Nature 1963;198:712-714.
39. Argyrou A, Jin L, Siconilfi-Baez L, et al. Proteome-wide profiling of isoniazid targets in *Mycobacterium tuberculosis*. Biochemistry 2006;45:13947-13953.
40. Middlebrook G. Isoniazid resistance and catalase activity of tubercle bacilli. Am Rev Tuberc 1954;69:471-472.
41. Zhang Y, Heym B, Allen B, et al. The catalase-peroxidase gene and isoniazid resistance of *Mycobacterium tuberculosis*. Nature 1992;358:591-593.
42. Zhang Y, Telenti A. Genetics of Drug Resistance in *Mycobacterium tuberculosis*. Washington, DC: ASM Press, 2000, pp 235-254.
43. Musser JM, Kapur V, Williams DL, et al. Characterization of the catalase-peroxidase gene (*katG*) and *inhA* locus in isoniazid-resistant and -susceptible strains of *Mycobacterium tuberculosis* by automated DNA sequencing: restricted array of mutations associated with drug resistance. J Infect Dis 1996;173:196-202.
44. Heym B, Alzari PM, Honore N, et al. Missense mutations in the catalase-peroxidase gene, *katG*, are associated with isoniazid resistance in *Mycobacterium tuberculosis*. Mol Microbiol 1995;15:235-245.
45. Miesel L, Weisbrod TR, Marcinkeviciene JA, et al. NADH dehydrogenase defects confer isoniazid resistance and conditional lethality in *Mycobacterium smegmatis*. J Bacteriol 1998;180:2459-2467.
46. Lee A, Teo A, Wong S. Novel mutations in *ndh* in isoniazid-resistant *Mycobacterium tuberculosis* isolates. Antimicrob Agents Chemother 2001;45:2157-2159.
47. Guo H, Seet Q, Denkin S, et al. Molecular characterization of isoniazid-resistant clinical isolates of *Mycobacterium tuberculosis* from the USA. J Med Microbiol 2006;55:1527-1531.
48. Deretic V, Philipp W, Dhandayuthapani S, et al. *Mycobacterium tuberculosis* is a natural mutant with an inactivated oxidative stress regulatory gene: implications for sensitivity to isoniazid. Mol Microbiol 1995;17:889-900.
49. Sherman DR, Sabo PJ, Hickey MJ, et al. Disparate responses to oxidative stress in saprophytic and pathogenic mycobacteria. Proc Natl Acad Sci U S A 1995;92:6625-6629.
50. Wilson TM, Collins DM. *ahpC*, a gene involved in isoniazid resistance of the *Mycobacterium tuberculosis* complex. Mol Microbiol 1996;19:1025-1034.
51. Heym B, Stavropoulos E, Honore N, et al. Effects of overexpression of the alkyl hydroperoxide reductase AhpC on the virulence and isoniazid resistance of *Mycobacterium tuberculosis*. Infect Immun 1997;65:1395-1401.

52. Stoeckle MY, Guan L, Riegler N, et al. Catalase-peroxidase gene sequences in isoniazid-sensitive and -resistant strains of *Mycobacterium tuberculosis* from New York City. J Infect Dis 1993;168:1063-1065.
53. Scholar E, Pratt W. The Antimicrobial Drugs. Oxford, UK: Oxford University Press, 2000, p 287.
54. Wilson TM, de Lisle GW, Collins DM. Effect of *inhA* and *katG* on isoniazid resistance and virulence of *Mycobacterium bovis*. Mol Microbiol 1995;15:1009-1015.
55. Bifani PJ, Plikaytis BB, Kapur V, et al. Origin and interstate spread of a New York City multidrug-resistant *Mycobacterium tuberculosis* clone family. JAMA 1996;275:452-457.
56. Kucers A, Crowe S, Grayson M, et al. The Use of Antibiotics. Oxford: Butterworth Heinemann, 1997.
57. van Soolingen D, de Haas PE, van Doorn HR, et al. Mutations at amino acid position 315 of the *katG* gene are associated with high-level resistance to isoniazid, other drug resistance, and successful transmission of *Mycobacterium tuberculosis* in the Netherlands. J Infect Dis 2000;182:1788-1790.
58. Holdiness M. Clinical pharmacokinetics of the antituberculosis drugs. Clin Pharmacokinet 1984;9:511-544.
59. Comstock G, Edwards P. The competing risks of tuberculosis and hepatitis for adult tuberculin reactors. Am Rev Respir Dis 1975;111:573-577.
60. Ohno M, Yamaguchi I, Yamamoto I. Slow *N*-acetyltransferase 2 genotype affects the incidence of isoniazid and rifampicin-induced hepatotoxicity. Int J Tuberc Lung Dis 2000;4:256-261.
61. Thomas J, Baughn C, Wilkinson R, et al. A new synthetic compound with antituberculous activity in mice: ethambutol (dextro-2,2′-(ethylenediimino)-di-butanol). Am Rev Respir Dis 1961;83:891-893.
62. Otten H. Ethambutol. *In* Bartmann K (ed): Handbook of Experimental Pharmacology, Vol 84: Antituberculosis Drugs. Berlin: Springer-Verlag, 1988, pp 197-203.
63. Takayama K, Kilburn J. Inhibition of synthesis of arabinogalactan by ethambutol in *Mycobacterium smegmatis*. Antimicrob Agents Chemother 1989;33:1493-1499.
64. Mikusov K, Slayden R, Besra G, et al. Biogenesis of the mycobacterial cell wall and the site of action of ethambutol. Antimicrob Agents Chemother 1995;39:2484-2489.
65. Wolucka B, McNeil M, de Hoffmann E, et al. Recognition of the lipid intermediate for arabinogalactan/arabinomannan biosynthesis and its relation to the mode of action of ethambutol on mycobacteria. J Biol Chem 1994;269:23328-23335.
66. Telenti A, Philipp W, Sreevatsan S, et al. The *emb* operon, a unique gene cluster of *Mycobacterium tuberculosis* involved in resistance to ethambutol. Nat Med 1997;3:567-570.
67. Belanger A, Besra G, Ford M, et al. The *embAB* genes of *Mycobacterium avium* encode an arabinosyl transferase involved in cell wall arabinan biosynthesis that is the target for the antimycobacterial drug ethambutol. Proc Natl Acad Sci U S A 1996;93:11919-11924.
68. Heifets L, Desmond E. Clinical mycobacteriology laboratory. In Cole S, Eisenach K, McMurray D, Jacobs W Jr (eds): Tuberculosis and the Tubercle Bacillus. Washington, DC: ASM Press, 2005, pp 49-70.
69. Sreevatsan S, Stockbauer K, Pan X, et al. Ethambutol resistance in *Mycobacterium tuberculosis:* critical role of *embB* mutations. Antimicrob Agents Chemother 1997;41:1677-1681.
70. Bryskier A, Grosset J. Antituberculosis agents. *In* Bryskier A (ed): Antimicrobial Agents. Washington, DC: ASM Press, 2005, pp 1088-1123.
71. Peets EA, Sweeney WM, Place VA, et al. The absorption, excretion, and metabolic fate of ethambutol in man. Am Rev Respir Dis 1965;91:51-58.
72. World Health Organization. Treatment of Tuberculosis: Guidelines for National Programmes. Geneva: World Health Organization, 2003.
73. Kurosawa H. Studies on the antibiotic substances from *Actinomyces*. XXIII. The isolation of an antibiotic produced by a strain of *Streptomyces* "K 30." J Antibiot Ser B 1952;5:682-688.
74. David HL, Takayama K, Goldman D. Susceptibility of mycobacterial D-alanyl-D-alanine synthetase to D-cycloserine. Am Rev Respir Dis 1969;100:579-581.
75. Strych U, Penland R, Jimenez M, et al. Characterization of the alanine racemases from two mycobacteria. FEMS Microbiol Lett 2001;196:93-98.
76. Caceres N, Harris N, Wellehan J, et al. Overexpression of the D-alanine racemase gene confers resistance to D-cycloserine in *Mycobacterium smegmatis*. J Bacteriol 1997;179:5046-5055.
77. Chacon O, Feng Z, Harris N, et al. *Mycobacterium smegmatis* D-alanine racemase mutants are not dependent on D-alanine for growth. Antimicrob Agents Chemother 2002;46:47-54.
78. Belanger A, Porter J, Hatfull G. Genetic analysis of peptidoglycan biosynthesis in mycobacteria: characterization of a *ddlA* mutant of *Mycobacterium smegmatis*. J Bacteriol 2000;182:6854-6856.
79. Feng Z, Barletta R. Roles of *Mycobacterium smegmatis* D-alanine : D-alanine ligase and D-alanine racemase in the mechanisms of action of and resistance to the peptidoglycan inhibitor D-cycloserine. Antimicrob Agents Chemother 2003;47:283-291.
80. Drlica K, Malik M. Fluoroquinolones: action and resistance. Curr Top Med Chem 2003;3:249-282.
81. Liebermann D, Moyeux M, Rist N, et al. Sur la preparation de nouveaux thioamides pyridineques acitifs dans la tubercolose experimentale. C R Acad Sci 1956;242:2409-2412.
82. DeBarber A, Mdluli K, Bosman M, et al. Ethionamide activation and sensitivity in multidrug-resistant *Mycobacterium tuberculosis*. Proc Natl Acad Sci U S A 2000;97:9677-9682.
83. Baulard A, Betts J, Engohang-Ndong J, et al. Activation of the pro-drug ethionamide is regulated in mycobacteria. J Biol Chem 2000;275:28326-28331.
84. Vannelli T, Dykman A, Ortiz de Montellano P. The antituberculosis drug ethionamide is activated by a flavoprotein monooxygenase. J Biol Chem 2002;277:12824-12829.
85. Hinshaw H, McDermott W. Thiosemicarbazone therapy of tuberculosis in humans. Am Rev Tuberc 1950;61:145-157.
86. Luna JC. A Tuberculosis Guide for Specialist Physicians. Paris: International Union Against Tuberculosis and Lung Disease, 2004.
87. Trnka L. Thiosemicarbazones. *In* Bartmann K (ed): Handbook of Experimental Pharmacology, Vol 84: Antituberculosis Drugs. Berlin: Springer-Verlag, 1988, pp 92-103.
88. Qian L, Ortiz de Montellano P. Oxidative activation of thiacetazone by the *Mycobacterium tuberculosis* flavin monooxygenase EtaA and human FMO1 and FMO3. Chem Res Toxicol 2006;19:443-449.
89. Sensi P, Margalith P, Timbal M. Rifomycin, a new antibiotic: preliminary report. Farmaco Sci 1959;14:146-147.
90. Sensi P. History of the development of rifampin. Rev Infect Dis 1983;5(Suppl 3): S402-S406.
91. Stottmeier KD, Kubica GP, Woodley CL. Antimycobacterial activity of rifampin under in vitro and simulated in vivo conditions. Appl Microbiol 1969;17:861-865.
92. Hu Y, Mangan JA, Dhillon J, et al. Detection of mRNA transcripts and active transcription in persistent *Mycobacterium tuberculosis* induced by exposure to rifampin or pyrazinamide. J Bacteriol 2000;182:6358-6365.
93. Mustaev A, Zaychikov E, Severinov K, et al. Topology of the RNA polymerase active center probed by chimeric rifampicin-nucleotide compounds. Proc Natl Acad Sci U S A 1994;91:12036-12040.
94. McClure WR, Cech CL. On the mechanism of rifampicin inhibition of RNA synthesis. J Biol Chem 1978;253:8949-8956.
95. Telenti A, Imboden P, Marchesi F, et al. Detection of rifampicin-resistance mutations in *Mycobacterium tuberculosis*. Lancet 1993;341:647-650.
96. Honore N, Cole ST. Molecular basis of rifampin resistance in *Mycobacterium leprae*. Antimicrob Agents Chemother 1993;37:414-418.
97. Guerrero C, Stockman L, Marchesi F, et al. Evaluation of the *rpoB* gene in rifampicin-susceptible and -resistant *Mycobacterium avium* and *Mycobacterium intracellulare*. J Antimicrob Chemother 1994;33:661-663.
98. Williams DL, Spring L, Collins L, et al. Contribution of *rpoB* mutations to development of rifamycin cross-resistance in *Mycobacterium tuberculosis*. Antimicrob Agents Chemother 1998;42:1853-1857.
99. Deitz WH, Bailey JH, Froelich EJ. In vitro antibacterial properties of nalidixic acid, a new drug active against gram-negative organisms. Antimicrobial Agents Chemother (Bethesda) 1963;161:583-587.
100. Hu Y, Coates AR, Mitchison DA. Sterilizing activities of fluoroquinolones against rifampin-tolerant populations of *Mycobacterium tuberculosis*. Antimicrob Agents Chemother 2003;47:653-657.
101. Takiff H, Salazar L, Guerrero C, et al. Cloning and nucleotide sequence of *Mycobacterium tuberculosis gyrA* and *gyrB* genes and detection of quinolone resistance mutations. Antimicrob Agents Chemother 1994;38:773-780.
102. Kocagoz T, Hackbarth C, Unsal I, et al. Gyrase mutations in laboratory selected, fluoroquinolone-resistant mutants of *Mycobacterium tuberculosis* H37Ra. Antimicrob Agents Chemother 1996;40:1768-1774.
103. Cambau E, Sougakoff W, Basson M, et al. Selection of a *gyrA* mutant of *Mycobacterium tuberculosis* resistant to fluoroquinolones during treatment with ofloxacin. J Infect Dis 1994;170:479-483.
104. Cole S, Brosch R, Parkhill J, et al. Deciphering the biology of *Mycobacterium tuberculosis* from the complete genome sequence. Nature (Lond) 1998;393:537-544.
105. Hegde SS, Vetting MW, Roderick SL, et al. A fluoroquinolone resistance protein from *Mycobacterium tuberculosis* that mimics DNA. Science 2005;308:1480-1483.
106. Grimaldo E, Tupasi T, Rivera A, et al. Increased resistance to ciprofloxacin and ofloxacin in multidrug-resistant *Mycobacterium tuberculosis* isolates from patients seen at a tertiary hospital in the Philippines. Int J Tuberc Lung Dis 2001;5:546-550.
107. Bryskier A. Fluoroquinolones. *In* Bryskier A (ed): Antimicrobial Agents. Washington, DC: ASM Press, 2005, pp 668-788.
108. Burman WJ, Goldberg S, Johnson JL, et al. Moxifloxacin versus ethambutol in the first 2 months of treatment for pulmonary tuberculosis. Am J Respir Crit Care Med 2006;174:331-338.
109. Gillespie SH, Gosling RD, Uiso L, et al. Early bactericidal activity of a moxifloxacin and isoniazid combination in smear-positive pulmonary tuberculosis. J Antimicrob Chemother 2005;56:1169-1171.
110. Tuberculosis Research Center, Chennai. Shortening short course chemotherapy: a randomised clinical trial for treatment of smear positive pulmonary tuberculosis with regimens using oflaxacin in the intensive phase. Indian J Tuberc 2002;49:27-38.
111. Schatz A, Bugie E, Waksman S. Streptomycin, a substance exhibiting antibiotic activity against gram-positive and gram-negative bacteria. Proc Soc Exp Biol Med 1944;55:66-69.
112. Davies J, Gorini L, Davis B. Misreading of RNA codewords induced by aminoglycoside antibiotics. Mol Pharmacol 1965;1:93-106.
113. Garvin RT, Biswas DK, Gorini L. The effects of streptomycin or dihydrostreptomycin binding to 16S RNA or to 30S ribosomal subunits. Proc Natl Acad Sci U S A 1974;71:3814-3818.
114. Anand N, Davis B. Effect of streptomycin on *Escherichia coli*. Nature 1960;185:22-23.
115. Finken M, Kirschner P, Meier A, et al. Molecular basis of streptomycin resistance in *Mycobacterium tuberculosis:* alterations of the ribosomal protein S12 gene and point mutations within a functional 16S ribosomal RNA pseudoknot. Mol Microbiol 1993; 9:1239-1246.
116. Honore N, Cole ST. Streptomycin resistance in mycobacteria. Antimicrob Agents Chemother 1994;38:238-242.
117. Nair J, Rouse DA, Bai GH, et al. The *rpsL* gene and streptomycin resistance in single and multiple drug-resistant strains of *Mycobacterium tuberculosis*. Mol Microbiol 1993;10:521-527.

118. Honore N, Marchal G, Cole ST. Novel mutation in 16S rRNA associated with streptomycin dependence in *Mycobacterium tuberculosis*. Antimicrob Agents Chemother 1995;39:769-770.
119. Alangaden G, Kreiswirth B, Aouad A, et al. Mechanism of resistance to amikacin and kanamycin in *Mycobacterium tuberculosis*. Antimicrob Agents Chemother 1998;42:1295-1297.
120. Suzuki Y, Katsukawa C, Tamaru A, et al. Detection of kanamycin-resistant *Mycobacterium tuberculosis* by identifying mutations in the 16S rRNA gene. J Clin Microbiol 1998;36:1220-1225.
121. Umezawa H, Ueda M, Maeda K, et al. Production and isolation of a new antibiotic, kanamycin. J Antibiot Jpn Ser A 1957;10:181-188.
122. Herr E, Haney M, Pittenger G, et al. Isolation and characterization of a new peptide antibiotic. Proc Indiana Acad Sci 1960;69:134.
123. Maus CE, Plikaytis BB, Shinnick TM. Mutation of *tlyA* confers capreomycin resistance in *Mycobacterium tuberculosis*. Antimicrob Agents Chemother 2005;49:571-577.
124. Johansen S, Maus C, Plikaytis B, et al. Capreomycin binds across the ribosomal subunit interface using *tlyA*-encoded 2′-*O*-methylations in 16S and 23S rRNAs. Mol Cell 2006;23:173-182.
125. Maus CE, Plikaytis BB, Shinnick TM. Molecular analysis of cross-resistance to capreomycin, kanamycin, amikacin, and viomycin in *Mycobacterium tuberculosis*. Antimicrob Agents Chemother 2005;49:3192-3197.
126. Chorine V. Action de l'amide nicotinique sur les bacilles du genre *Mycobacterium*. C R Acad Sci (Paris) 1945;220:150-151.
127. Malone L, Schurr A, Lindh H, et al. The effect of pyrazinamide (Aldinamide) on experimental tuberculosis in mice. Am Rev Tuberc 1952;65:511-518.
128. Solotorovsky M, Gregory FJ, Ironson EJ, et al. Pyrazinoic acid amide—an agent active against experimental murine tuberculosis. Soc Exp Biol Med Proc 1952;79:563-565.
129. Zhang Y, Mitchison D. The curious characteristics of pyrazinamide: a review. Int J Tuberc Lung Dis 2003;7:6-21.
130. Tarshis M, Weed W. Lack of significant in vitro sensitivity of *Mycobacterium tuberculosis* to pyrazinamide on three different solid media. Am Rev Tuberc 1953;67:391-395.
131. McDermott W, Tompsett R. Activation of pyrazinamide and nicotinamide in acidic environment in vitro. Am Rev Tuberc 1954;70:748-754.
132. Scorpio A, Zhang Y. Mutations in *pncA*, a gene encoding pyrazinamidase/nicotinamidase, cause resistance to the antituberculous drug pyrazinamide in tubercle bacillus. Nat Med 1996;2:662-667.
133. Zhang Y, Scorpio A, Nikaido H, et al. Role of acid pH and deficient efflux of pyrazinoic acid in unique susceptibility of *Mycobacterium tuberculosis* to pyrazinamide. J Bacteriol 1999;181:2044-2049.
134. Zhang Y, Permar S, Sun Z. Conditions that may affect the results of susceptibility testing of *Mycobacterium tuberculosis* to pyrazinamide. J Med Microbiol 2002;51:42-49.
135. Wade MM, Zhang Y. Anaerobic incubation conditions enhance pyrazinamide activity against *Mycobacterium tuberculosis*. J Med Microbiol 2004;53:769-773.
136. Wade MM, Zhang Y. Effects of weak acids, UV and proton motive force inhibitors on pyrazinamide activity against *Mycobacterium tuberculosis* in vitro. J Antimicrob Chemother 2006;58:936-941.
137. Zhang Y, Wade MM, Scorpio A, et al. Mode of action of pyrazinamide: disruption of *Mycobacterium tuberculosis* membrane transport and energetics by pyrazinoic acid. J Antimicrob Chemother 2003;52:790-795.
138. Scorpio A, Lindholm-Levy P, Heifets L, et al. Characterization of *pncA* mutations in pyrazinamide-resistant *Mycobacterium tuberculosis*. Antimicrob Agents Chemother 1997;41:540-543.
139. Jindani A, Aber V, Edwards E, et al. The early bactericidal activity of drugs in patients with pulmonary tuberculosis. Am Rev Respir Dis 1980;121:939-949.
140. Brindle R, Odhiambo J, Mitchison D. Serial counts of *Mycobacterium tuberculosis* in sputum as surrogate markers of the sterilising activity of rifampicin and pyrazinamide in treating pulmonary tuberculosis. BMC Pulm Med 2001;1:2.
141. McCune R, Tompsett R, McDermott W. The fate of *Mycobacterium tuberculosis* in mouse tissues as determined by the microbial enumeration technique. II. The conversion of tuberculous infection to the latent state by administration of pyrazinamide and a companion drug. J Exp Med 1956;104:763-802.
142. Lehmann J. Determination of pathogenicity of tubercle bacilli by their intermediate metabolism. Lancet 1946;250:14-15.
143. Bernheim F. The effect of salicylate on the oxygen uptake of the tubercle bacillus. Science 1940;92:204.
144. Rengarajan J, Sassetti CM, Naroditskaya V, et al. The folate pathway is a target for resistance to the drug *para*-aminosalicylic acid (PAS) in mycobacteria. Mol Microbiol 2004;53:275-282.
145. Trnka L, Mison P. *p*-Aminosalicylic acid (PAS). In Bartmann K (ed): Handbook of Experimental Pharmacology, Vol 84: Antituberculosis Drugs. Berlin: Springer-Verlag, 1988, pp 51-68.
146. Ratledge C. Iron, mycobacteria and tuberculosis. Tuberculosis (Edinb) 2004;84:110-130.
147. Tuberculosis Coalition for Technical Assistance. International Standards for Tuberculosis Care (ISTC). Geneva: World Health Organization, 2006.
148. World Care Council. The Patients' Charter for Tuberculosis Care. Viols en Laval, France: World Care Council, 2006.
149. Hopewell PC, Pai M, Maher D, et al. International standards for tuberculosis care. Lancet Infect Dis 2006;6:710-725.
150. Dutt AK, Moers D, Stead WW. Smear- and culture-negative pulmonary tuberculosis: four-month short-course chemotherapy. Am Rev Respir Dis 1989;139:867-870.
151. American Thoracic Society, CDC. Targeted tuberculin testing and treatment of latent tuberculosis infection. Am J Respir Crit Care Med 2000;161:S221-S247.
152. De Cock K, Chaisson R. Will DOTS do it? A reappraisal of tuberculosis control in countries with high rates of HIV infection. Int J Tuberc Lung Dis 1999;3:457-465.
153. Iseman MD, Madsen L, Goble M, et al. Surgical intervention in the treatment of pulmonary disease caused by drug-resistant *Mycobacterium tuberculosis*. Am Rev Respir Dis 1990;141:623-625.
154. Ji B, Lounis N, Maslo C, et al. In vitro and in vivo activities of moxifloxacin and clinafloxacin against *Mycobacterium tuberculosis*. Antimicrob Agents Chemother 1998;42:2066-2069.
155. Alvirez-Freites E, Carter J, Cynamon M. In vitro and in vivo activities of gatifloxacin against *Mycobacterium tuberculosis*. Antimicrob Agents Chemother 2002;46:1022-1025.
156. Miyazaki E, Miyazaki M, Chen J, et al. Moxifloxacin (BAY12-8039), a new 8-methoxyquinolone, is active in a mouse model of tuberculosis. Antimicrob Agents Chemother 1999;43:85-89.
157. Nuermberger E, Yoshimatsu T, Tyagi S, et al. Moxifloxacin-containing regimen greatly reduces time to culture conversion in murine tuberculosis. Am J Respir Crit Care Med 2004;169:421-426.
158. Pletz M, De Roux A, Roth A, et al. Early bactericidal activity of moxifloxacin in treatment of pulmonary tuberculosis: a prospective, randomized study. Antimicrob Agents Chemother 2004;48:780-782.
159. Valerio G, Bracciale P, Manisco V, et al. Long-term tolerance and effectiveness of moxifloxacin therapy for tuberculosis: preliminary results. J Chemother 2003;15:66-70.
160. Johnson JL, Hadad DJ, Boom WH, et al. Early and extended early bactericidal activity of levofloxacin, gatifloxacin and moxifloxacin in pulmonary tuberculosis. Int J Tuberc Lung Dis 2006;10:605-612.
161. Barrett J. Linezolid (Pharmacia Corp). Curr Opin Investig Drugs 2000;1:181-187.
162. Barbachyn MR, Hutchinson DK, Brickner SJ, et al. Identification of a novel oxazolidinone (U-100480) with potent antimycobacterial activity. J Med Chem 1996;39:680-685.
163. Cynamon MH, Klemens SP, Sharpe CA, et al. Activities of several novel oxazolidinones against *Mycobacterium tuberculosis* in a murine model. Antimicrob Agents Chemother 1999;43:1189-1191.
164. Fortun J, Martin-Davila P, Navas E, et al. Linezolid for the treatment of multidrug-resistant tuberculosis. J Antimicrob Chemother 2005;56:180-185.
165. von der Lippe B, Sandven P, Brubakk O. Efficacy and safety of linezolid in multidrug resistant tuberculosis (MDR-TB)—a report of ten cases. J Infect 2006;52:92-96.
166. Stover CK, Warrener P, VanDevanter DR, et al. A small-molecule nitroimidazopyran drug candidate for the treatment of tuberculosis. Nature 2000;405:962-966.
167. Nagarajan K, Shankar R, Rajappa S, et al. Nitroimidazoles XXI. 2,3-Dihydro-6-nitroimidazo [2,1-b] oxazoles with antitubercular activity. Eur J Med Chem 1989; 24:631-633.
168. Ashtekar DR, Costa-Perira R, Nagrajan K, et al. In vitro and in vivo activities of the nitroimidazole CGI 17341 against *Mycobacterium tuberculosis*. Antimicrob Agents Chemother 1993;37:183-186.
169. Tyagi S, Nuermberger E, Yoshimatsu T, et al. Bactericidal activity of the nitroimidazopyran PA-824 in a murine model of tuberculosis. Antimicrob Agents Chemother 2005;49:2289-2293.
170. Nuermberger E, Rosenthal I, Tyagi S, et al. Combination chemotherapy with the nitroimidazopyran PA-824 and first-line drugs in a murine model of tuberculosis. Antimicrob Agents Chemother 2006;50:2621-2625.
171. Andries K, Verhasselt P, Guillemont J, et al. A diarylquinoline drug active on the ATP synthase of *Mycobacterium tuberculosis*. Science 2005;307:223-227.
172. Lounis N, Veziris N, Chauffour A, et al. Combinations of R207910 with drugs used to treat multidrug-resistant tuberculosis have the potential to shorten treatment duration. Antimicrob Agents Chemother 2006;50:3543-3547.
173. Ibrahim M, Andries K, Lounis N, et al. Synergistic activity of R207910 combined with pyrazinamide in murine tuberculosis. Antimicrob Agents Chemother 2006;51:1011-1015.

80

BACTERIAL MENINGITIS

Diederik van de Beek, Martijn Weisfelt, and Jan de Gans

INTRODUCTION 1109
PATHOGENESIS AND PATHOPHYSIOLOGY 1109
THERAPEUTICS AND CLINICAL PHARMACOLOGY 1109
Goals of Therapy 1109
Epidemiologic Aspects 1109
Clinical Aspects 1110
Differential Diagnosis 1110
Therapeutics by Class 1110
Antimicrobial Agents 1110
Anti-inflammatory Agents 1112
Other Adjunctive Therapies 1114
Hyperventilation 1115
Osmotic Agents 1115
Lund Concept 1115
Activated Protein C 1115
Heparin 1115
Therapeutic Approach 1115
Computed Tomography before Lumbar Puncture 1116
Timing of Empirical Therapy 1116
Duration of Antimicrobial Therapy 1116
Duration of Dexamethasone Therapy 1116
Emerging Targets and Therapeutics 1116

INTRODUCTION

The association of headache and tinnitus with lethal inflammation of the brain was described by Hippocrates. It was not before the 19th century that lumbar puncture (LP) was introduced as diagnostic procedure. Soon thereafter, the use of cerebrospinal fluid (CSF) drainage was advised in patients with bacterial meningitis; however, it did not have clinical efficacy. Most important in the treatment of bacterial meningitis was the introduction of penicillin in 1940, which reduced the mortality rates of bacterial meningitis to an overall fatality rate of approximately 20%.[1-3] Ever since, advances in medical care such as the introduction of cranial computed tomography (CT) and improvements in intensive care support, as well as the global emergence of multidrug-resistant bacteria, have influenced our approach of patients with bacterial meningitis. Recent changes in pharmacotherapy of bacterial meningitis include the implementation of adjunctive dexamethasone therapy and the anticipation of infection with antibiotic-resistant organisms.[4] This chapter provides a brief overview of pathogenesis and pathophysiology, epidemiology, and clinical features of bacterial meningitis, but focuses on pharmacology and therapeutics in patients with community-acquired bacterial meningitis. Patients with meningitis after neurosurgical operation are beyond the scope of this chapter.

PATHOGENESIS AND PATHOPHYSIOLOGY

The central nervous system (CNS) is protected against microbial entry from the bloodstream by the blood-brain/CSF barrier and by an external barrier that is formed by the leptomeninges and skull[4] (Fig. 80-1). As a consequence, the pathogen enters the CNS via the bloodstream or by direct invasion through the external barrier (e.g., dural leakage, ear or sinus infection).[5] Nasopharyngeal colonization generally leads to asymptomatic carriage.[6] However, in response to the local generation of inflammatory factors, as seen in the presence of viral infections, the composition of surface components on target epithelial and endothelial cells is changed.[6] Binding of bacteria to up-regulated receptors (e.g., platelet-activating-factor receptors) promotes migration through the respiratory epithelium and vascular endothelium, resulting in invasive disease.[6] Once the bacterium invades the bloodstream, the host can react with massive activation of inflammatory cascades.[5] The main cascade pathways that are involved are the complement system, the inflammatory response, and the coagulation and fibrinolysis pathways.[4] These pathways do not act independently but are able to interact with each other.[7] Genetic polymorphisms among components of these pathways (e.g., complement deficiencies and defects in sensing or opsonophagocytic pathways) are involved in the susceptibility to infection, as well as in severity of disease and outcome.[8] Cytokines coordinate a wide variety of inflammatory reactions and play an important role in the initiation, maintenance, and termination of inflammatory reactions.[9] Prominent proinflammatory cytokines include tumor necrosis factor-α, interleukin-1 and interleukin-6.[10] Essential parts of the inflammatory response include activation of coagulation and fibrin deposition, shifting the hemostatic balance toward thrombosis.[7]

The blood-brain barrier is formed by cerebral microvascular endothelial cells that restrict blood-borne pathogen invasion.[5] Cytokines stimulate cell surface expression of receptors, which allows binding to activated endothelial cells and invasion of bacteria into the subarachnoid space.[10] Physiologically, concentrations of leukocytes, antibodies, and complement components in the subarachnoid space are low.[10] This condition facilitates multiplication of bacteria, which undergo autolysis under conditions such as growth to stationary phase or exposure to antibiotics. Lysis of bacteria leads to the release of immunostimulatory and/or toxic bacterial products. Bacterial cell wall products (e.g., lipopolysaccharide and lipoteichoic acid), bacterial toxins (e.g., pneumolysin), and bacterial DNA induce a severe inflammatory response via binding to Toll-like receptors, which are key elements in the innate immune system.[11]

THERAPEUTICS AND CLINICAL PHARMACOLOGY

Goals of Therapy

Epidemiologic Aspects

The estimated incidence of bacterial meningitis is four to six cases per 100,000 adults per year in developed countries, and the most common pathogens are *Streptococcus pneumoniae* and *Neisseria meningitidis*, which are responsible for 80% of cases.[1,12] Neonatal meningitis is caused by specific causative organisms and is beyond the scope of this review.[12] Vaccination strategies have substantially changed the epidemiology of bacterial meningitis during the past 2 decades.[13,14] The routine vaccination of children against *Haemophilus influenzae* type B has virtually eradicated bacterial meningitis due to this bacterium in the developed world (Fig. 80-2).[14] As a consequence, *S. pneumoniae* has become the most common pathogen beyond the neonatal period, and bacterial meningitis has become a disease predominantly of adults rather than of infants and children.[15] The introduction of conjugate

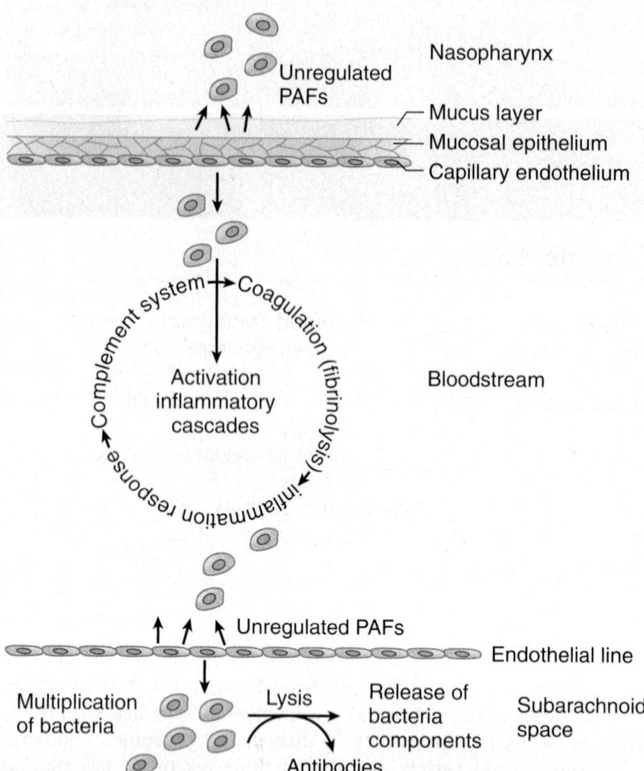

FIGURE 80-1 • Pathogenic steps of bacterial meningitis. In response to inflammatory factors, the viscosity of the mucus is decreased and receptors on epithelial cells are exposed. Up-regulation of receptors facilitates binding of bacteria, which induces migration of bacteria through the respiratory epithelium and vascular endothelium. Once bacteria are in the bloodstream, the host can react with massive activation of inflammatory cascades. Activated endothelial cells up-regulate receptors, enabling bacteria to invade the subarachnoid space, where the poor local host defense facilitates multiplication of bacteria. Antibiotics induce lysis of bacteria, resulting in release of immunostimulatory and toxic bacterial compounds within the subarchnoid space.

vaccines against seven serotypes of *S. pneumoniae* that are among the most prevalent in children ages 6 months to 2 years and include most antibiotic-resistant types has reduced the rate of antibiotic-resistant invasive pneumococcal infections in young children as well as in older persons.[13] The integration of the meningococcal protein-polysaccharide conjugate vaccines into vaccination programs in several countries of the developed world is expected to further reduce the disease burden of bacterial meningitis in high- and medium-income countries.[16]

Another important epidemiologic trend that influenced pharmacotherapy in bacterial meningitis is the increase of drug-resistant strains of *S. pneumoniae,* which now pose an emerging problem worldwide.[17] Depending on geographic region, the prevalence of antibiotic-resistant strains in the United States is as high as 50% to 70%. In response to this epidemiologic trend, recommendations for the treatment of bacterial meningitis have necessarily evolved.[1,18,19]

Clinical Aspects

Early diagnosis and rapid initiation of appropriate therapy are vital in the treatment of patients with bacterial meningitis.[1,15,19,20] Bacterial meningitis is often considered in a differential diagnosis but may be difficult to recognize.[15] The clinical presentation of a patient with bacterial meningitis may vary depending on age, underlying conditions, and severity of illness. Infants may become irritable or lethargic, stop feeding, and are found to have a bulging fontanelle, separation of the cranial sutures, meningism, and opisthotonos, and they may develop convulsions. These findings are uncommon in neonates, who sometimes present with respiratory distress, diarrhea, or jaundice.

Clinical findings of meningitis in young children are often minimal, and in childhood bacterial meningitis and in elderly patients classical symptoms such as headache, fever, nuchal rigidity, and altered mental status may be less common than in younger and middle-aged adults.[12,15,21,22] In a prospective study on adults with bacterial meningitis, the classic triad of signs and symptoms consisting of fever, nuchal rigidity, and altered mental status was present in only 44% of the patients.[3] Certain clinical features may predict the bacterial cause of meningitis. Predisposing conditions such as ear or sinus infections, pneumonia, immunocompromised status, and dural fistulas are estimated to be present in 68% to 92% of adults with pneumococcal meningitis.[5,23] Rashes occur more frequently in patients with meningococcal meningitis, with reported sensitivities of 63% to 80% and with specificities of 83% to 92%.

Fatality rates in adults with pneumococcal meningitis (15% to 33%) and meningococcal meningitis (7% to 10%) are significant, and overall, neurologic sequelae are estimated to occur in 15% to 40% of surviving patients.[1-3,12,24] Meningitis due to *S. pneumoniae* is especially associated with considerable disability; hearing loss occurs in 22% of surviving patients as compared to 8% of those after meningococcal meningitis. Even in patients with apparent good recovery, cognitive impairment occurs frequently. In a prospective study, cognitive impairment was detected in 27% of adults who had a good recovery from pneumococcal meningitis.[25] Results of a more recent study that pooled data from three previous studies on cognitive outcome after bacterial meningitis showed that about one third of adult survivors of bacterial meningitis experience subtle long-term cognitive impairment, which consists mainly of slight mental slowness (median time between meningitis and cognitive testing was 49.5 months).[26] In this study, the prevalence of cognitive impairment in patients after pneumococcal and meningococcal meningitis was similar.

Posttraumatic bacterial meningitis is often indistinguishable clinically from spontaneous meningitis. However, in obtunded or unconscious patients who have suffered a recent head injury, few clinical signs may be present. A fever and deterioration in the level of consciousness or loss of vital functions may be the only signs of meningitis. Finding a CSF leak adds support to the possibility of meningitis in such patients, but this is undetectable in many cases.

Patients with infections of CSF shunts may present with clinical features typical of spontaneous meningitis, especially if virulent organisms are involved. The more usual presentation is insidious, with features of shunt blockage such as headache, vomiting, fever, and a decreasing level of consciousness. Fever is a helpful sign, but is not a constant feature and may be present in as few as 20% of cases.

Differential Diagnosis

The differential diagnosis of the triad of fever, headache, and stiff neck is bacterial or viral meningitis, fungal meningitis, tuberculous meningitis, drug-induced aseptic meningitis, carcinomatous or lymphomatous meningitis, aseptic meningitis associated with inflammatory diseases (systemic lupus erythematosus, sarcoidosis, Behçet's syndrome, Sjögren syndrome), and, when temperature is only moderately elevated and onset of headache is acute, subarachnoid hemorrhage. When an impaired level of consciousness, focal neurologic deficits, or new-onset seizure activity are added to the classic triad, the differential diagnosis includes viral encephalitis, venous sinus thrombosis, tick-borne bacterial infections (depending on geographic area: *Borrelia* and *Ehrlichia* infections in North America and Europe, Rocky Mountain spotted fever in North America), brain abscess, and subdural empyema.

Therapeutics by Class

Antimicrobial Agents

Cerebrospinal Fluid Penetration. Penetration of the blood-brain barrier into the subarachnoid space is the first pharmacologic factor that determines whether an antimicrobial agent is able to clear bacteria from the CSF. Blood-brain barrier penetration is affected by

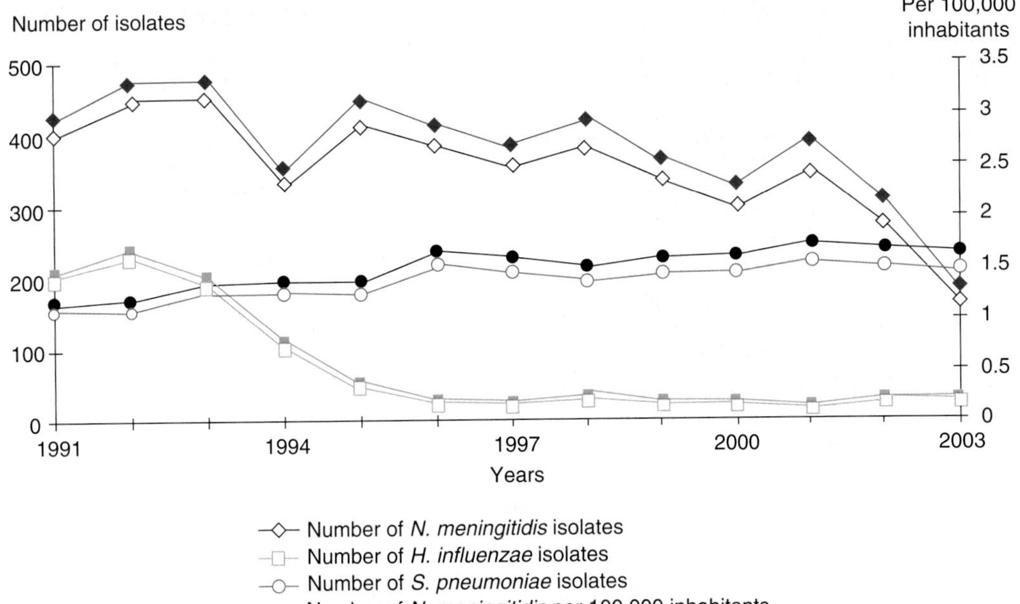

FIGURE 80-2 • Change in epidemiology after the introduction of routine use of the conjugate vaccine against *Haemophilus influenzae*. Number of cerebrospinal fluid isolates from meningitis patients as received by the Netherlands Reference Laboratory for Bacterial Meningitis from 1991 through 2003. In the Netherlands, routine vaccination with the conjugate *Haemophilus influenzae* type b vaccine started in 1993.

lipophilicity, molecular weight and structure, and protein-bound fraction.[27] Lipophilic agents with a low molecular weight and simple structure penetrate relatively well and reach peak CSF concentrations quickly even if the meninges are not inflamed. Fluoroquinolones and rifampin have these characteristics, in contrast to hydrophilic agents (β-lactams) or large molecules (vancomycin).[27] Highly protein-bound antimicrobial agents may also have diminished CSF penetration, because only the unbound fraction of the drug is available to cross the blood-brain barrier.[27] It is important to realize that bacterial meningitis is a dynamic process and CSF penetration of antimicrobials is highly depended on the breakdown of the blood-brain barrier. Anti-inflammatory drugs, such as dexamethasone, might influence the breakdown of the blood-brain barrier and thereby interfere with CSF penetration of antimicrobial agents (see later).[28]

Antimicrobial Activity in Cerebrospinal Fluid. The activity of an individual antimicrobial drug in infected purulent CSF depends on a number of factors, such as activity in an environment of decreased pH, protein-bound fraction, bacterial growth rate and density, and metabolism in the CSF.[27] Mechanisms of antibiotic action are targeting of the bacterial cell wall (block synthesis, digest enzymatically, break down surface), targeting of the bacterial cell membrane (loss of permeability barrier), or targeting biosynthetic processes (block protein synthesis or prevent DNA replication). Whereas bacteriostatic activity involves inhibition of growth of microorganisms (chloramphenicol), bactericidal antimicrobials cause bacterial cell death (penicillin, cephalosporins, vancomycin). Antibiotic-induced lysis of bacteria leads to the release of immunostimulatory cell wall components and toxic bacterial products that induce a severe inflammatory response through binding to Toll-like receptors.

Empirical Antimicrobial Therapy. Empirical treatment should be based on the most common bacterial species that cause the disease according to the patient's age group or clinical setting, and on local antibiotic susceptibility patterns of the predominant pathogens (Table 80-1).[29] Neonatal meningitis is largely caused by group B streptococci, *Escherichia coli*, and *Listeria monocytogenes*. Initial treatment, therefore, should consist of penicillin or ampicillin plus a third-generation cephalosporin, preferably cefotaxime or ceftriaxone, or penicillin or ampicillin and an aminoglycoside.

Spontaneous meningitis in children and adults is likely due to *S. pneumoniae* and *N. meningitidis*. Empirical coverage with a third-generation cephalosporin (cefotaxime or ceftriaxone) at appropriate doses for meningitis is recommended, based on a broad spectrum of activity and excellent penetration into the CSF during inflammatory conditions.[1,18] Due to the worldwide emergence of multidrug-resistant strains of *S. pneumoniae*, most experts recommend the addition of vancomycin to the initial empirical antimicrobial regimen in adult patients. Vancomycin has been evaluated in case series of patients with bacterial meningitis caused by penicillin- and cephalosporin-resistant pneumococci. Additionally, in patients over 50 years of age, treatment with ampicillin should be added to the above antibiotic regimen for additional coverage of *L. monocytogenes*, which is more prevalent among this age group.[30] Although no clinical data on the efficacy of rifampin in patients with pneumococcal meningitis are currently available, some experts recommend the use of this agent in combination with a third-generation cephalosporin, with or without vancomycin, in patients with pneumococcal meningitis caused by bacterial strains that, on the basis of local epidemiology, are likely to be highly resistant to penicillin or a cephalosporin.[18,28]

Nosocomial posttraumatic meningitis is mainly caused by multidrug-resistant hospital-acquired organisms such as *Klebsiella pneumoniae*, *E. coli*, *Pseudomonas aeruginosa*, and *Staphylococcus aureus*. Depending on the pattern of susceptibility in a given hospital unit, ceftazidime (2 g intravenously every 8 hours), cefotaxime, ceftriaxone, or meropenem should be chosen. If *P. aeruginosa* infection seems likely, ceftazidime or meropenem is the preferred antibiotic.

Device- and ventriculoperitoneal shunt–associated meningitis is caused by a wide range of organisms, including methicillin-resistant staphylococci (mostly coagulase-negative staphylococci) and multi-drug-resistant aerobic bacilli. Cases with cerebral shunts and an insidious onset are probably caused by organisms of low pathogenicity, and empirical therapy is a less urgent requirement. For post-operative meningitis, the first-line empirical therapy should be cefotaxime or ceftriaxone or meropenem. If the patient has received broad-spectrum antibiotics recently or if *P. aeruginosa* is suspected, ceftazidime or meropenem should be given. Meropenem should be used if an extended-spectrum β-lactamase organism is suspected,

TABLE 80-1 RECOMMENDATIONS FOR EMPIRICAL ANTIMICROBIAL THERAPY IN SUSPECTED COMMUNITY-ACQUIRED BACTERIAL MENINGITIS

Predisposing Factor	Common Bacterial Pathogens	Initial Intravenous Antibiotic Therapy
Age		
<1 mo	*Streptococcus agalactiae, Escherichia coli, Listeria monocytogenes*	Ampicillin plus cefotaxime or an aminoglycoside
1-3 mo	*Streptococcus pneumoniae, Neisseria meningitidis, S. agalactiae, Haemophilus influenzae, E. coli, L. monocytogenes*	Ampicillin plus vancomycin plus ceftriaxone or cefotaxime*
3-23 mo	*S. pneumoniae, N. meningitidis, S. agalactiae, H. influenzae, E. coli*	Vancomycin plus ceftriaxone or cefotaxime*
2-50 yr	*N. meningitidis, S. pneumoniae*	Vancomycin plus ceftriaxone or cefotaxime*
>50 yr	*N. meningitidis, S. pneumoniae, L. monocytogenes*, aerobic gram-negative bacilli	Vancomycin plus ceftriaxone or cefotaxime plus ampicillin†
With risk factor present‡	*S. pneumoniae, L. monocytogenes, H. influenzae*	Vancomycin plus ceftriaxone or cefotaxime plus ampicillin†
Posttraumatic	*S. pneumoniae, H. influenzae*	Vancomycin plus ceftriaxone or cefotaxime plus ampicillin
Postneurosurgery	Coagulase-negative staphylococci, *Staphylococcus aureus*, aerobic gram-negative bacilli (including *Pseudomonas aeruginosa*)	Vancomycin plus ceftazidime
CSF shunt	Coagulase-negative staphylococci, *S. aureus*, aerobic gram-negative bacilli (including *P. aeruginosa*), *Propionibacterium acnes*	Vancomycin plus ceftazidime

*In areas with very low penicillin resistance rates, monotherapy penicillin may be considered.
†In areas with very low penicillin resistance and cephalosporin resistance rates, combination therapy of amoxicillin and third-generation cephalosporin may be considered.
‡Alcoholism, altered immune status.
CSF, cerebrospinal fluid.
Adapted from van de Beek D, de Gans J, Tunkel AR, Wijdicks EF. Community-acquired bacterial meningitis in adults. N Engl J Med 2006;354:44-53.

and flucloxacillin or vancomycin if *S. aureus* is likely. The infected shunt or drain will almost certainly have to be removed urgently.

Antimicrobial Therapy Directed to Specific Organisms. Empirical antimicrobial treatment can be modified once culture results and in vitro susceptibility testing of the isolated microorganisms become available.[29] Recommendations directed to common specific organisms in adults are described here, and general recommendations based on the isolated microorganism are listed in Table 80-2.

Streptococcus pneumoniae. Due to the global increase in multidrug-resistant strains of *S. pneumoniae*, monotherapy with penicillin should only be considered in areas with very low penicillin resistance rates (<1%), although many experts recommend combination therapy for all patients pending results of in vitro susceptibility testing.[1] Combination therapy with vancomycin plus a third-generation cephalosporin (either ceftriaxone or cefotaxime) has become the standard approach to empirical antimicrobial therapy in suspected pneumococcal meningitis.[18] Once the organism and its in vitro antimicrobial susceptibilities are known, therapy may be appropriately modified.

Neisseria meningitidis. Penicillin G and ampicillin have long been accepted as the standard for empirical therapy of meningococcal meningitis, but the increasing emergence and spread of penicillin resistance may require modification of this antibiotic regimen. A Spanish study on the evolution of penicillin resistance in a children's hospital described a rise in penicillin resistance in strains of *N. meningitidis* from 9.1% in 1986 to 71.4% in 1997.[31] Although the majority of patients with penicillin-intermediate-resistant *N. meningitidis* described in the literature have responded well to penicillin therapy, another Spanish study described an association between reduced susceptibility to penicillin and an increased risk of death or neurologic sequelae in children with meningococcal meningitis.[32] Based on these data, some authorities recommend the use of a third-generation cephalosporin as empirical therapy for meningococcal meningitis until the results of susceptibility testing are known.

Anti-inflammatory Agents

Dexamethasone. Animal models of bacterial meningitis showed that bacterial lysis, induced by antibiotic therapy, leads to inflammation in the subarachnoid space.[33,34] The severity of this inflammatory response is associated with outcome and can be attenuated by treatment with steroids (Fig. 80-3). On the basis of experimental meningitis studies, several clinical trials have been undertaken to determine the effects of adjunctive steroids in children and adults with bacterial meningitis.[24,28,35] Of several corticosteroids, the use of dexamethasone in bacterial meningitis has been investigated most extensively.[28] Dexamethasone is a glucocorticosteroid with anti-inflammatory as well as immunosuppressive properties and has excellent penetration in the CSF. In a meta-analysis of randomized trials since 1988, adjunctive dexamethasone was shown to reduce meningitis-associated hearing loss in children with meningitis due to *H. influenzae* type B.[36]

As most available studies on adjunctive dexamethasone therapy in adults with bacterial meningitis were limited by methodologic flaws, its value in adults remained a long-standing subject of debate.[37] In 2002, results of the European Dexamethasone Study were published.[38] This randomized, placebo-controlled trial of 301 adults with bacterial meningitis showed that adjunctive treatment with dexamethasone, given before or with the first dose of antimicrobial therapy, was associated with a reduction in the risk for unfavorable outcome (relative risk [RR] 0.6; 95% confidence interval [CI], 0.3 to 0.9) and with a reduction in mortality (RR 0.48; 95% CI, 0.2 to 0.96). This beneficial effect was most apparent in patients with pneumococcal meningitis, in whom mortality was decreased from 34% to 14%. The benefits of adjunctive dexamethasone therapy were not undermined by an increase of severe neurologic disability in patients who survived or by any corticosteroid-induced complication. In a post hoc analysis, which included only patients with pneumococcal meningitis who died within 14 days after admission, the mortality benefit of dexamethasone therapy was entirely due to reduced mortality from systemic causes such as septic shock, pneumonia, or acute respiratory distress syndrome (2% vs. 16% without dexamethasone); there was no significant reduction in

TABLE 80-2 SPECIFIC ANTIMICROBIAL THERAPY IN COMMUNITY-ACQUIRED BACTERIAL MENINGITIS*

Microorganism, Susceptibility	Standard Therapy†	Alternative Therapies
Streptococcus pneumoniae		
Penicillin MIC		
<0.1 mg/L	Penicillin G or ampicillin	Cefotaxime or ceftriaxone, chloramphenicol
0.1-1.0 mg/L	Cefotaxime or ceftriaxone	Cefepime, meropenem
≥2.0 mg/L	Vancomycin plus cefotaxime or ceftriaxone‡	Fluoroquinolone§
Cefotaxime or ceftriaxone MIC		
≥1.0 mg/L	Vancomycin plus cefotaxime or ceftriaxone¶	Fluoroquinolone§
Neisseria meningitidis		
Penicillin MIC		
<0.1 mg/L	Penicillin G or ampicillin	Cefotaxime or ceftriaxone, chloramphenicol
0.1-1.0 mg/L	Cefotaxime or ceftriaxone	Chloramphenicol, fluoroquinolone, meropenem
Listeria monocytogenes	Penicillin G or ampicillin‖	Trimethoprim-sulfamethoxazole, meropenem
Group B streptococcus	Penicillin G or ampicillin‖	Cefotaxime or ceftriaxone
Escherichia coli and other Enterobacteriaceae	Cefotaxime or ceftriaxone‖	Aztreonam,‖ fluoroquinolone, meropenem,‖ trimethoprim-sulfamethoxazole, ampicillin‖
Pseudomonas aeruginosa	Ceftazidime‖ or cefepime‖	Aztreonam,‖ ciprofloxacin,‖ meropenem‖
Haemophilus influenzae		
β-Lactamase negative	Ampicillin	Cefotaxime or ceftriaxone, cefepime, chloramphenicol, fluoroquinolone
β-Lactamase positive	Cefotaxime or ceftriaxone	Cefepime, chloramphenicol, fluoroquinolone
Chemoprophylaxis#		
Neisseria meningitidis	Rifampicin (rifampin), ceftriaxone, ciprofloxacin, azithromycin	

*Based on CSF culture results and in vitro susceptibility testing; this material was previously published as part of an online supplementary appendix to van de Beek et al.[1]

†General recommendations for intravenous empirical antibiotic treatment have included penicillin (2 million units every 4 hours); amoxicillin or ampicillin (2 g every 4 hours); vancomycin (15 mg/kg every 6 hours); a third-generation cephalosporin: ceftriaxone (2 g every 12 hours) or cefotaxime (2 g every 4 to 6 hours) or cefepime (2 g every 8 hours) or ceftazidime (2 g every 8 hours) or meropenem (2 g every 8 hours); chloramphenicol (1 to 1.5 g every 6 hours); a fluoroquinolone: gatifloxacin (400 mg every 24 hours) or moxifloxacin (400 mg every 24 hours, although no data are available on optimal dose needed in patients with bacterial meningitis) or ciprofloxacin (400 mg every 8 to 12 hours); trimethoprim-sulfamethoxazole (5 mg/kg every 6 to 12 hours); aztreonam (2 g every 6 to 8 hours); rifampicin (rifampin) (600 mg every 12 to 24 hours); and an aminoglycoside: gentamicin (1.7 mg/kg every 8 hours).

‡Consider addition of rifampicin (rifampin) if dexamethasone is given.

§Gatifloxacin or moxifloxacin; no clinical data on use in patients with bacterial meningitis.

¶Consider addition of rifampicin (rifampin) if the MIC of ceftriaxone is ≥2 mg/L.

‖Consider addition of an aminoglycoside.

#Prophylaxis is indicated for close contacts, who are defined as those with intimate contact, which covers those eating and sleeping in the same dwelling as well as those having close social and kissing contacts; or health care workers who perform mouth-to-mouth resuscitation, endotracheal intubation, or endotracheal tube management. Patients with meningococcal meningitis who are treated with monotherapy of penicillin or amoxicillin (ampicillin) should also receive chemoprophylaxis, since carriage is not reliably eradicated by these drugs. The preferred dose for chemoprophylaxis is rifampicin (rifampin), 600 mg orally twice daily for 2 days; ceftriaxone, 250 mg intramuscularly; ciprofloxacin, 500 mg orally; or azithromycin, 500 mg orally.

CSF, cerebrospinal fluid; MIC, minimum inhibitory concentration.

Adapted from van de Beek D, de Gans J, Tunkel AR, Wijdicks EF. Community-acquired bacterial meningitis in adults. N Engl J Med 2006;354:44-53.

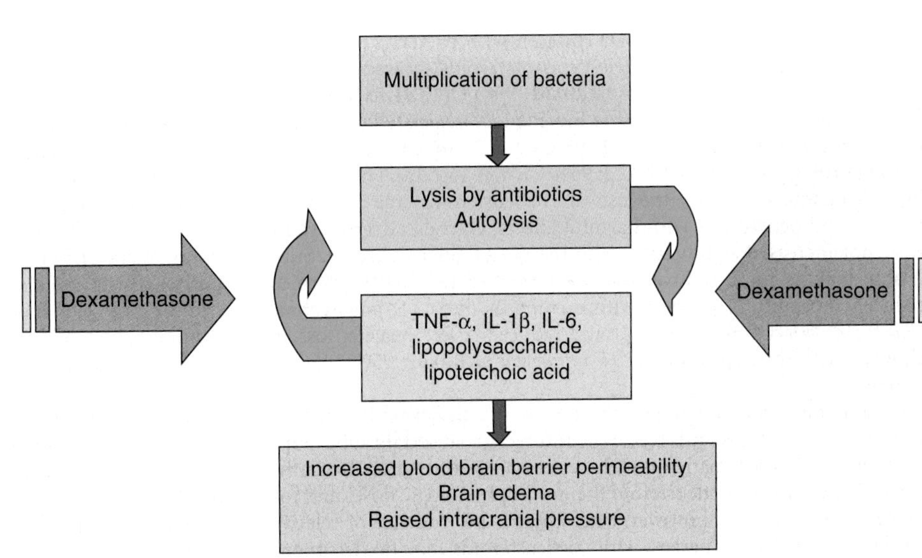

FIGURE 80-3 • Mechanisms of action of dexamethasone in bacterial meningitis: inflammatory reaction in the subarachnoid space and pathophysiologic alterations.

Dexamethasone 10 mg (4 times daily, 4 days) before or with first dose of antibiotic in:
1. Adults with bacterial meningitis
2. Adults with suspected bacterial meningitis

No dexamethasone:
1. Pre-treatment with parenteral antibiotics
2. Hypersensitivity to steroids
3. Recent head injury
4. CSF shunt
5. Hospital-acquired bacterial meningitis

No dexamethasone, but low dose corticosteroids (hydrocortisone 50 mg) if:
1. Adults with septic shock with bacterial meningitis
2. Adults with septic shock and suspected bacterial meningitis

FIGURE 80-4 • Recommendations for adjunctive corticosteroid treatment in adults.

mortality due to neurologic causes (7% vs. 10%).[39] Results of a subsequent quantitative review on this topic, which included five clinical trials, confirmed that treatment with corticosteroids was associated with a significant reduction in mortality (RR 0.6; 95% CI, 0.4 to 0.8) and in neurologic sequelae (RR 0.6; 95% CI, 0.4 to 1.0).[35] The reduction in case fatality in patients with pneumococcal meningitis was 21% (RR 0.5; 95% CI, 0.3 to 0.8). In meningococcal meningitis, mortality (RR 0.9; 95% CI, 0.3 to 2.1) and neurologic sequelae (RR 0.5; 95% CI, 0.1 to 1.7) were both reduced, but not significantly. Adverse events were equally divided between the treatment and placebo groups (RR 1.0; 95% CI, 0.1 to 1.7). Since publications of these results, adjunctive dexamethasone has become routine therapy in most adults with suspected bacterial meningitis (Fig. 80-4).[1,18,40]

In 2007, an updated Cochrane analysis was published on the efficacy and safety of adjunctive corticosteroids, including 20 randomized, controlled trials involving 2750 people.[24] In this analysis, adjuvant corticosteroids were associated with lower case fatality (RR 0.83; 95% CI, 0.71 to 0.99), lower rates of severe hearing loss (RR 0.65; 95% CI, 0.47 to 0.91), and fewer long-term neurologic sequelae (RR 0.67; 95% CI, 0.45 to 1.00). The use of corticosteroids was not associated with an increase of adverse events. Again, the effect of corticosteroids was evident in adults with bacterial meningitis. Subanalyses for high-income and low-income countries of the effect of corticosteroids on mortality showed RRs of 0.83 (95% CI, 0.52 to 1.05) and 0.87 (95% CI, 0.72 to 1.05), respectively. For children with bacterial meningitis admitted in high-income countries, corticosteroids showed a protective effect on severe hearing loss (RR 0.61; 95% CI, 0.41 to 0.90) and favorable point estimates for severe hearing loss associated with non–*H. influenzae* meningitis (RR 0.51; 95% CI, 0.23 to 1.13) and short-term neurologic sequelae (RR 0.72; 95% CI, 0.39 to 1.33). For children in low-income countries, the use of corticosteroids was associated neither with benefit nor with harmful effects. Overall, adverse events were not increased significantly with the use of corticosteroids. Subgroup analysis for causative organisms showed that corticosteroids reduced mortality in patients with meningitis due to *S. pneumoniae* (RR 0.59; 95% CI, 0.45 to 0.77) and reduced severe hearing loss in children with meningitis due to *H. influenzae* (RR 0.37; 95% CI, 0.20 to 0.68).

Despite these encouraging results, the use of adjunctive dexamethasone in bacterial meningitis remains controversial in certain subgroups of patients.[24,28] First, patients with septic shock and adrenal insufficiency benefit from corticosteroid therapy in physiologic doses and for longer than 4 days[41,42]; however, when there is no evidence of relative adrenal insufficiency, therapy with corticosteroids may be detrimental.[43] Results of a subsequent quantitative review on this topic that included nine studies comparing mortality rates of corticosteroid treatment in sepsis or septic shock showed a trend toward increased mortality associated with their administration (RR 1.13; 95% CI, 0.99 to 1.29).[44] There was a trend toward increased mortality in four trials with a lower methodologic quality score (RR 1.20; 95% CI, 0.94 to 1.52) as well as the five trials receiving higher methodologic scores (RR 1.10; 95% CI, 0.94 to 1.29). As controlled studies of the effects of corticosteroid therapy in a substantial number of patients with both meningitis and septic shock are not available at present, treatment with corticosteroids cannot be unequivocally recommended for such patients, although the use of low doses seems reasonable at present.[1,24] Animal studies of bacterial meningitis suggest that the initiation of steroid therapy before or with the first dose of antibiotics is more effective than starting corticosteroids after the first dose of antimicrobial therapy, although the time point beyond which dexamethasone loses its effectiveness has not been clearly defined.[24,28]

Second, by reducing the permeability of the blood-brain barrier, steroids can impede penetration of antibiotics into the CSF, as was shown for vancomycin in animal studies,[45] which can lead to treatment failures, especially in patients with meningitis due to drug-resistant pneumococci in whom antibiotic regimens often include vancomycin. However, in an observational study that included 14 adult patients admitted to the intensive care unit because of suspected pneumococcal meningitis, appropriate concentrations of vancomycin in the CSF were obtained even when concomitant steroids were used.[46] The dose of vancomycin used in this study was 60 mg/kg per day. These results suggest that dexamethasone can be used without fear of impeding vancomycin penetration into the CSF of patients with pneumococcal meningitis, provided that vancomycin dosage is adequate.

Third, corticosteroids may potentiate ischemic and apoptotic injury to neurons. In animal studies of bacterial meningitis, corticosteroids aggravated hippocampal neuronal apoptosis and learning deficiencies in dosages similar to those used in clinical practice.[47] Therefore, concerns existed about the effects of steroid therapy on long-term cognitive outcome. To examine the potential harmful effect of treatment with adjunctive dexamethasone on long-term neuropsychological outcome in adults with bacterial meningitis, a follow-up study of the European Dexamethasone Study was conducted.[48] In 87 of 99 eligible patients, 46 (53%) of whom were treated with dexamethasone and 41 (47%) of whom received placebo, no significant differences in outcome were found between patients in the dexamethasone and placebo groups (median time between meningitis and testing was 99 months). Therefore, treatment with adjunctive dexamethasone does not worsen long-term cognitive outcome in adults after bacterial meningitis.

Other Adjunctive Therapies

The management of adults with bacterial meningitis can be complex, and common complications are meningoencephalitis, systemic compromise, stroke, and increased intracranial pressure (ICP). Various adjunctive therapies have been described to improve outcome in such patients, including anti-inflammatory agents, anticoagulant therapies, and strategies to reduce ICP.[4] Few randomized clinical studies are available for other adjunctive therapies in adults with bacterial meningitis.

The inflammatory response in the CNS results in blood-brain barrier permeability, cerebral edema, and increased ICP. There are two major types of brain edema. Vasogenic edema is due to blood-brain barrier disruption resulting in extracellular water accumulation, while cytotoxic or cellular edema is due to sustained intracellular water collection.[49] A third type, osmotic brain edema, is caused by osmotic imbalances between blood and tissue.

The Dutch Cohort Study[3] evaluated the effects of complications on mortality in patients with pneumococcal meningitis and compared these findings among different age groups. In older patients (≥60 years), death was usually a result of systemic complications, whereas death in younger patients (<60 years) was predominantly due to neurologic complications such as brain herniation.[22] This observation may be explained by age-related cerebral atrophy, which allows elderly patients to tolerate brain swelling.[50] These findings suggest that supportive treatments that aim to reduce ICP could be most beneficial in younger adults with pneumococcal meningitis. Methods available to reduce ICP range from simple (e.g., elevation of the head of the bed to 30 degrees) to aggressive strategies (e.g., the "Lund concept"; see later), although there is no evidence that ICP monitoring and treatment of increased ICP is beneficial in patients with bacterial meningitis.

Hyperventilation

The rationale of hyperventilation in patients with bacterial meningitis is the relation between cerebral arteriolar dilation, increased cerebral blood flow, and a subsequent rise in ICP. Hyperventilation-induced hypocapnia causes vasoconstriction and a reduction in cerebral blood flow, resulting in lowering of ICP. This approach has been used in patients with traumatic brain injury as well; however, the enthusiasm for hyperventilation was greatly tempered after a study on prophylactic hyperventilation in patients with severe brain injury showed a worse outcome.[51] In bacterial meningitis, patients are often hypocapnic at the time of admission, suggesting that there is spontaneous hyperventilation.[52] A Danish study in adults with bacterial meningitis found a decline of cerebral blood flow with hyperventilation without change in regional cerebral blood flow pattern.[53] Therefore, experts recommend that the arterial partial pressure of CO_2 be maintained slightly below "normal" (i.e., 30 to 35 mm Hg) during the first 24 hours in patients with bacterial meningitis. However, there are no published controlled trials on the effect of hyperventilation in bacterial meningitis, so recommendations in this area are based only on expert opinion.

Osmotic Agents

In patients with traumatic brain injury, studies have shown that mannitol decreases blood viscosity and reduces the diameter of pial arterioles in a manner similar to the vasoconstriction produced by hyperventilation.[54] Although osmotic tissue dehydration may still play some role, mannitol works primarily through its immediate rheologic effect, by diluting the blood and increasing the deformability of erythrocytes, thereby decreasing blood viscosity and increasing cerebral blood flow. This sudden increase in cerebral blood flow causes autoregulatory vasoconstriction of cerebral arterioles, decreasing the intracerebral blood volume, thereby lowering ICP.[55]

In bacterial meningitis, because blood-brain barrier permeability has been increased, the effect of mannitol is uncertain. There is little information from clinical and experimental studies concerning the use of mannitol in bacterial meningitis. A single dose of mannitol reduced ICP for approximately 3 hours in a meningitis model.[56] Continuous intravenous infusion of mannitol attenuated the increases of regional cerebral blood flow, brain water content, and ICP in a pneumococcal meningitis model. Other hyperosmolar agents are glycerol and hypertonic saline.[57] One study assessed the value of adjunctive intravenous dexamethasone and oral glycerol for the treatment of bacterial meningitis in 122 infants and children.[58] Overall 4 (7%) of the glycerol-treated patients, compared with 11 (19%) of those not given glycerol, developed audiologic or neurologic sequelae ($P = .052$); however, the study was not blinded. No experimental studies have been performed on the use of glycerol in bacterial meningitis, and clinical data in adults are lacking. Nevertheless, data on glycerol are quite promising and results of clinical studies are awaited. The effects of hypertonic (7%) saline in bacterial meningitis have been tested in one experimental study, in which decreased ICP and lower CSF white cell counts were reported.[59]

Lund Concept

Continuous ICP and cerebral perfusion pressure measurements in patients with severe bacterial meningitis have been attempted. In one study from Sweden, ICP was successfully lowered in most meningitis patients by a broad range of measures and using unconventional volume-targeted ("Lund concept") ICP management: sedation, steroids, normal fluid and electrolyte homeostasis, blood transfusion, albumin infusion, decrease of mean arterial pressure, treatment with a prostacyclin analogue, and eventually thiopental, ventriculostomy, and dihydroergotamine.[60] In nonsurvivors, mean ICP was significantly higher and cerebral perfusion pressure was markedly decreased despite treatment; however, this was not a comparative study and the results should be interpreted with caution.

Activated Protein C

Activated protein C (APC) is an endogenous protein that promotes fibrinolysis and inhibits thrombosis and inflammation. A large multicenter, placebo-controlled trial reported a beneficial effect of APC in patients with severe sepsis and organ failure. [61] Another large clinical trial showed that APC cannot be recommended in patients with sepsis who are at low risk for death, such as those with single-organ failure.[62] Although life-threatening bleeds and intracranial hemorrhage appeared to be uncommon in APC-treated patients in controlled and open-label trials (0.4% to 0.5%), concern exists about intracranial hemorrhage in patients with meningitis. A retrospective analysis of multiple trials showed a high rate of intracranial hemorrhage in adults with meningitis.[63] Of the 4096 adults included, 128 patients with meningitis were identified. Of these patients, 111 (87%) had a CSF culture result available with *N. meningitidis* identified in 46% and *S. pneumoniae* identified in 33% of patients. Twenty-one patients received placebo and one patient was lost to follow-up. Intracranial hemorrhage occurred in 6 of 106 patients (6%). This is substantially higher than reported rates of intracranial hemorrhage in patients with bacterial meningitis (<1%). Therefore, APC should not be administered to patients with bacterial meningitis.

Heparin

Anecdotic observations have suggested an improved clinical outcome of heparin-treated patients with bacterial meningitis.[4] In addition to its well-characterized effect on blood coagulation, heparin has been found to modulate the inflammatory process. In an experimental model of pneumococcal meningitis, heparin interfered with leukocyte-endothelium interaction, resulting in lower CSF white cell counts.[64] However, heparin should not be used as routine treatment in meningitis because of the risk of intracranial hemorrhage.

Therapeutic Approach

Controversies remain for emergency medicine and primary care providers who need to accurately diagnose patients with bacterial meningitis and administer antibiotics and adjunctive therapies rapidly for this life-threatening disease. Once an initial patient evaluation has been completed with history and physical findings, LP is the diagnostic procedure of choice if the diagnosis of bacterial meningitis cannot be ruled out. Characteristic findings in the CSF are typically used to make the diagnosis of meningitis (Table 80-3).[15] As classically described, the white blood cell count in bacterial meningitis is typically greater than 1000 cells/µl, while in viral meningitis it is less than 300 cells/µl—although considerable overlap exists in these categories.[65-70] The neutrophil count is typically elevated in bacterial meningitis compared with viral meningitis. The measurement of protein and glucose is an important aspect of CSF analysis to complement the cell counts because abnormal protein and glucose levels are typically found in

TABLE 80-3 CLASSICALLY DESCRIBED CSF FINDINGS IN BACTERIAL AND VIRAL MENINGITIS

CSF Findings	Bacterial Meningitis	Viral Meningitis
WBC count (cells/mm^3)	1000-10,000 Range <100 to >10,000	<300 Range <100-1000
Neutrophils	>80%	<20%
Protein	Elevated	Normal
Glucose	Reduced	Normal

WBC, white blood cell.

- Signs of brain shift
  - Papilledema
  - Focal neurologic signs, not including cranial nerve palsy
- Glasgow Coma Scale score below 10
- Severe immunocompromised state
- New onset seizures

FIGURE 80-5 • Indications for imaging before lumbar puncture.

bacterial disease but are relatively normal in many cases of viral meningitis.

One should keep in mind that there are several problems with using a chart such as Table 80-3 for clinical decisions on individual patients, particularly when determining whether patients require admission or can be discharged home. Much of the data in the literature concerning guidelines for predicting bacterial disease are derived from pediatric patients,[71-75] with several multiple retrospective models using logistic equations and other mathematical modeling; however, none has yet proved robust enough for widespread clinical practice. Practice guidelines for the management of bacterial meningitis have been published by the Infectious Diseases Society of America[18] suggesting that these prediction rules should not be used for clinical decisions in individual patients. There are no well-designed studies available to assist clinicians with this particular disposition decision, and individual clinicians will have to decide what level of risk is tolerable when diagnosing someone with viral meningitis and considering them as a possible candidate for discharge home with outpatient follow-up.

Computed Tomography before Lumbar Puncture

With the urgent nature of testing to make the diagnosis of meningitis, one of the issues physicians are faced with in an emergency department setting is whether neuroimaging, either CT or magnetic resonance imaging, is required before LP. One set of recommendations for emergency department brain CT scanning prior to LP are based on a prospective study in 2001 that included 301 adult patients with suspected meningitis.[76] Findings associated with an abnormal CT scan included age greater than 60 years, altered mental status, gaze or facial palsy, abnormal language or inability to answer two questions or follow two commands, immunocompromised status, history of CNS disease, seizure in the past week, visual field abnormalities, and arm or leg drift. In this cohort of patients, if none of these features was present, there was a negative predictive value of 97% for an intracranial abnormality, confirming that clinical features can be used to identify patients who are unlikely to have abnormal findings on brain CT. It is reasonable to proceed with LP without a CT scan if the patient does not meet any of the following criteria: new-onset seizures, an immunocompromised state, signs that are suspicious for space-occupying lesions (papilledema or focal neurologic signs not including cranial nerve palsy), or moderate to severe impairment of consciousness (Fig. 80-5).

Timing of Empirical Therapy

While there has not yet been a definitive study demonstrating a clear beneficial time frame for antibiotics, there have been findings concerning for worsening patient outcome with increased delays between presentation and antibiotic administration, and a suggestion that early antibiotic treatment in the emergency department may contribute to increased survival when compared to patients who did not receive antibiotics until after admission to the hospital. There are no prospective clinical data on the relationship of the timing of administration of antimicrobial agents to clinical outcome in patients with bacterial meningitis; however, there have been results that suggest a link between delay in the administration of antimicrobial therapy and adverse outcome.[19,20,77] In a retrospective case record study of adults with acute bacterial meningitis, delay in antibiotic treatment (because of cranial imaging or hospital transfer) was a significant risk factor for mortality.[77] In another retrospective cohort study of adults with community-acquired bacterial meningitis, patients were stratified into three stages of prognostic severity.[20] Delay in treatment was associated with adverse outcome when the patient's condition deteriorated to the highest stage of prognostic severity before the first dose of antibiotics was administered. A prospective study involving 156 patients with pneumococcal meningitis who were admitted to the intensive care unit indicated that a delay of more than 3 hours after presentation to the hospital before the initiation of antimicrobial therapy was associated with an increased 3-month mortality.[19]

In patients with suspected bacterial meningitis in whom immediate LP is postponed due to the presence of coagulation disorders (e.g., disseminated intravascular coagulation) or severe septic shock or in whom cranial imaging is indicated before LP, antimicrobial therapy should be initiated without delay (Fig. 80-6). In patients who have not undergone prior imaging and in whom disease progression is apparent, as well as in all patients with cloudy CSF (suggestive of bacterial meningitis), therapy should be started directly after LP. In patients without apparent progression of disease and no cloudy CSF on LP, antimicrobial therapy should be initiated once CSF analysis confirms the diagnosis.

Duration of Antimicrobial Therapy

General recommendations for empirical antibiotic treatment have included ceftriaxone administered intravenously every 12 hours or intravenous cefotaxime every 4 to 6 hours, and/or ampicillin at 4-hour intervals, or penicillin G every 4 hours.[1,12,18,27] There are no randomized comparative clinical studies of the various dosing regimens. In general, 7 days of antimicrobial therapy are given for meningitis caused by *N. meningitidis* and *H. influenzae*, 10 to 14 days for *S. pneumoniae*, and at least 21 days for *L. monocytogenes*.[1,12,18] As these guidelines are not standardized, it must be emphasized that the duration of therapy may need to be individualized on the basis of the patient's response.[1,29]

Duration of Dexamethasone Therapy

The consistency and degree of benefit identified for steroids merits the use of steroids in adults with acute bacterial meningitis and in children with acute bacterial meningitis in high-income countries with good access to services (see previous discussion).[1,24,28,35,38,40,78] We recommend a 4-day regimen of dexamethasone (0.6 mg/kg daily in children, 10 mg four times daily in adults) given before or with the first dose of antibiotics. The beneficial effect of corticosteroids was most apparent in meningitis due to *H. influenzae* and *S. pneumoniae*.[1,24,28,35,38,40,78] There were no adverse effects in the meningococcal subgroup.[24,28,35,38] In clinical practice, the causative organisms in many cases will not be known when treatment is started. On basis of the overall benefit and absence of excess of adverse events, if corticosteroids are indicated, a 4-day regimen of dexamethasone therapy should be given, regardless of bacterial etiology.

Emerging Targets and Therapeutics

Experimental research has increased our knowledge about the pathophysiology of bacterial meningitis and the mechanisms involved in neuronal injury.[5,10,11] Recent animal studies in experimental lipopolysaccharide-induced meningitis demonstrated that europium is a useful marker for quantifying blood-brain barrier permeability.[79] Understanding and quantifying the mechanisms by which the blood-brain barrier is altered is paramount to identifying new treatment strategies. In addition, animal studies are used to evaluate the effect of potential adjunctive therapies and the possible role of neuroprotective substances.[80-86] A number of adjunctive strategies for treatment have been considered, but, thus far, all of the therapies described here have been tested only in experimental bacterial meningitis models.

Administration of antibodies to the proinflammatory cytokines tumor necrosis factor-α and interleukin-1β decreased pleocytosis and reduced blood-brain barrier permeability in experimental bacterial meningitis. Pharmacologic interference with activation of nuclear

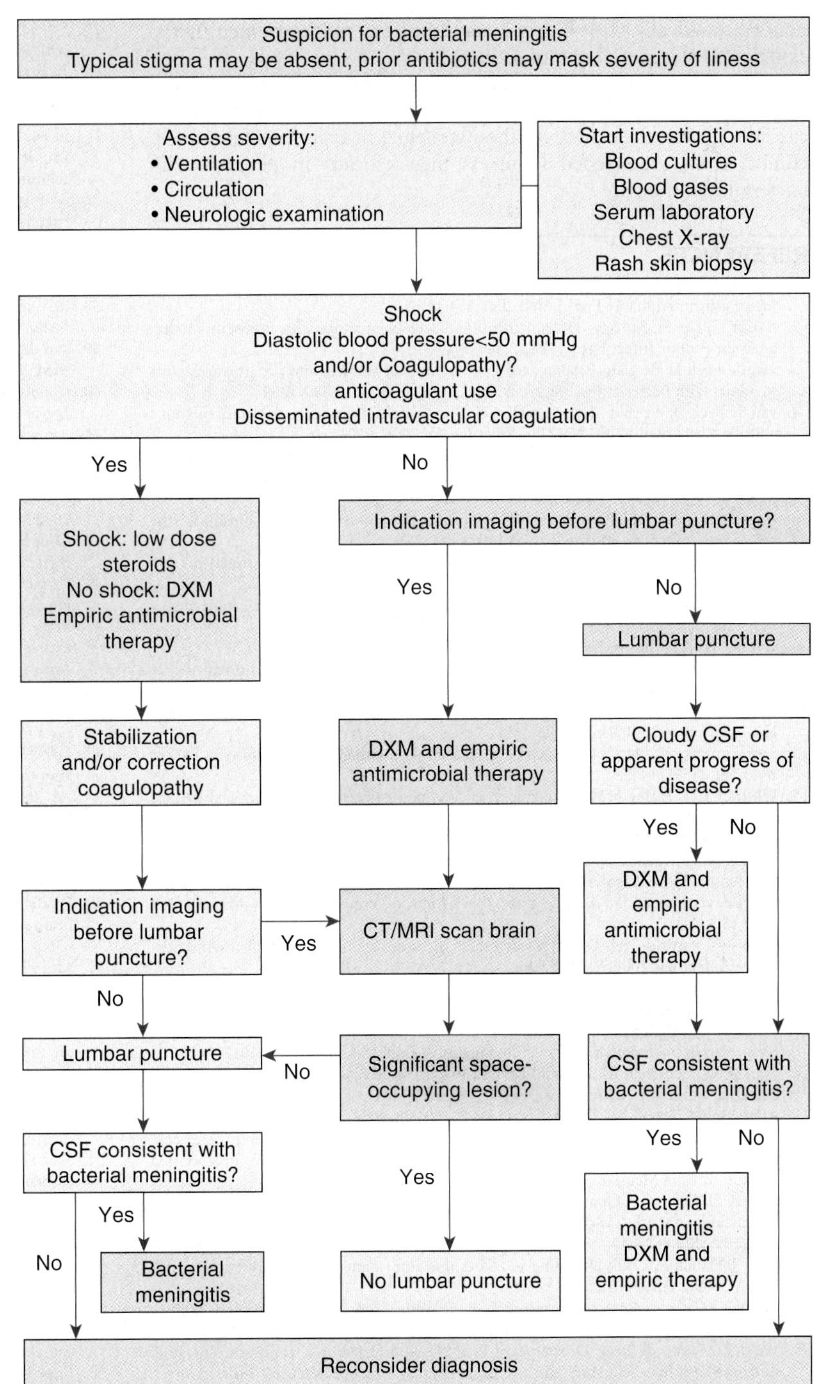

FIGURE 80-6 • An algorithm for the management of the patient with suspected bacterial meningitis. CSF, cerebrospinal fluid. (This material was previously published as part of an online supplementary appendix to van de Beek D et al.[4] Copyright 2006 Massachusetts Medical Society. All rights reserved.)

factor-κB, a transcription factor involved in the activation of many genes during bacterial meningitis, has reduced meningitis-induced CNS inflammation. Matrix metalloproteinases are a family of zinc-dependent matrix-degrading enzymes that can disrupt the blood-brain barrier and thereby facilitate leukocyte extravasation and brain edema. Inhibition of matrix metalloproteinases reduced blood-brain barrier permeability and the extent of cortical damage in experimental meningitis.[87]

Reactive oxygen species and reactive nitrogen intermediates are involved in several aspects of the host response to bacterial infections.[86] Antioxidants attenuate early events associated with neurologic injury in bacterial meningitis and are a promising strategy in the treatment of bacterial meningitis; among these therapies, the antioxidant *N*-acetylcysteine seems to be closest to a clinical application.[86,88] *N*-acetylcysteine reduced meningeal inflammation, oxidative brain damage, cortical neuronal injury, brain edema, ICP, cochlear injury, and hearing loss in animal models of pneumococcal meningitis.[86,88,89] Simultaneous production of oxygen-centered and nitrogen-centered free radicals favors the production of a toxic reaction product, an oxidant called peroxynitrite.[86] Peroxynitrite induces cytotoxicity and thereby initiates lipid peroxidation and induction of DNA single-strand breakage.[86] Damaged DNA activates poly(ADP-ribose) polymerase (PARP) and thereby induces an energy-consuming cycle that can result in cellular energy depletion and necrotic cell death.[90] Treatment with peroxynitrite scavengers and PARP inhibitors are other potential effective strategies in bacterial meningitis.

Caspases are a family of proteases that are involved in inflammation, upstream signaling, and most forms of apoptosis.[91] Apoptosis can pharmacologically be blocked, leading to reduced meningitis-associated intracranial complications.[92]

Potentially, the efficacy of therapeutic interventions may be enhanced by simultaneous intervention at several levels of the inflammatory cascade. Despite the benefits of these strategies in experimental models, clinical trials are needed to assess their efficacy in patients with bacterial meningitis.

REFERENCES

1. van de Beek D, de Gans J, Tunkel AR, Wijdicks EF. Community-acquired bacterial meningitis in adults. N Engl J Med 2006;354:44-53.
2. Baraff LJ, Lee SI, Schriger DL. Outcomes of bacterial meningitis in children: a meta-analysis. Pediatr Infect Dis J 1993;12:389-394.
3. van de Beek D, de Gans J, Spanjaard L, et al. Clinical features and prognostic factors in adults with bacterial meningitis. N Engl J Med 2004;351:1849-1859.
4. van de Beek D, Weisfelt M, de Gans J, et al. Drug Insight: Adjunctive therapies in adults with bacterial meningitis. Nat Clin Pract Neurol 2006;2:504-516.
5. Weisfelt M, de Gans J, van der Poll T, van de Beek D. Pneumococcal meningitis in adults: new approaches to management and prevention. Lancet Neurol 2006;5:332-342.
6. Bogaert D, De Groot R, Hermans PWM. *Streptococcus pneumoniae* colonisation: the key to pneumococcal disease. Lancet Infect Dis 2004;4:144-154.
7. Levi M, Van Der Poll T, Buller HR. Bidirectional relation between inflammation and coagulation. Circulation 2004;109:2698-2704.
8. Emonts M, Hazelzet JA, De Groot R, Hermans PWM. Host genetic determinants of *Neisseria meningitidis* infections. Lancet Infect Dis 2003;3:565-577.
9. van der Poll T. Immunotherapy of sepsis. Lancet Infect Dis 2001;1:165-174.
10. Koedel U, Scheld WM, Pfister HW. Pathogenesis and pathophysiology of pneumococcal meningitis. Lancet Infect Dis 2002;2:721-736.
11. Kim KS. Pathogenesis of bacterial meningitis: from bacteraemia to neuronal injury. Nat Rev Neurosc 2003;4:376-385.
12. Saez-Llorens X, McCracken GH Jr. Bacterial meningitis in children. Lancet 2003;361:2139-2148.
13. Whitney CG, Farley MM, Hadler J, et al. Decline in invasive pneumococcal disease after the introduction of protein-polysaccharide conjugate vaccine. N Engl J Med 2003;348:1737-1746.
14. Peltola H. Worldwide *Haemophilus influenzae* type b disease at the beginning of the 21st century: global analysis of the disease burden 25 years after the use of the polysaccharide vaccine and a decade after the advent of conjugates. Clin Microb Rev 2000;13:302-317.
15. Fitch MT, van de Beek D. Emergency diagnosis and treatment of adult meningitis. Lancet Infect Dis 2007;7:191-200.
16. Snape MD, Pollard AJ. Meningococcal polysaccharide-protein conjugate vaccines. Lancet Infect Dis 2005;5:21-30.
17. Whitney CG, Farley MM, Hadler J, et al. Increasing prevalence of multidrug-resistant *Streptococcus pneumoniae* in the United States. N Engl J Med 2000;343:1917-1924.
18. Tunkel AR, Hartman BJ, Kaplan SL, et al. Practice guidelines for the management of bacterial meningitis. Clin Infect Dis 2004;39:1267-1284.
19. Auburtin M, Wolff M, Charpentier J, et al. Detrimental role of delayed antibiotic administration and penicillin-nonsusceptible strains in adult intensive care unit patients with pneumococcal meningitis: the PNEUMOREA prospective multicenter study. Crit Care Med 2006;34:2758-2765.
20. Aronin SI, Peduzzi P, Quagliarello VJ. Community-acquired bacterial meningitis: risk stratification for adverse clinical outcome and effect of antibiotic timing. Ann Intern Med 1998;129:862-869.
21. Attia J, Hatala R, Cook DJ, Wong JG. Does this adult patient have acute meningitis? JAMA 1999;282:175-181.
22. Weisfelt M, van de Beek D, Spanjaard L, et al. Community-acquired bacterial meningitis in older people. J Am Geriatr Soc 2006;54:1500-1507.
23. Weisfelt M, van de Beek D, Spanjaard L, et al. Clinical features, complications, and outcome in adults with pneumococcal meningitis: a prospective case series. Lancet Neurol 2006;5:123-129.
24. van de Beek D, de Gans J, McIntyre P, Prasad K. Corticosteroids for acute bacterial meningitis. Cochrane Database Syst Rev 2007;(1):CD004405.
25. van de Beek D, Schmand B, de Gans J, et al. Cognitive impairment in adults with good recovery after bacterial meningitis. J Infect Dis 2002;186:1047-1052.
26. Hoogman M, van de Beek D, Weisfelt M, et al. Cognitive outcome in adults after bacterial meningitis. J Neurol Neurosurg Psychiatry 2007;78:1092-1096.
27. Sinner SW, Tunkel AR. Antimicrobial agents in the treatment of bacterial meningitis. Infect Dis Clin North Am 2004;18:581-602.
28. van de Beek D, de Gans J. Dexamethasone in adults with community-acquired bacterial meningitis. Drugs 2006;66:415-427.
29. van de Beek D, de Gans J, Spanjaard L, et al. Antibiotic guidelines and antibiotic use in adult bacterial meningitis in The Netherlands. J Antimicrob Chemother 2002;49:661-666.
30. Brouwer MC, van de Beek D, Heckenberg SG, et al. Community-acquired *Listeria monocytogenes* meningitis in adults. Clin Infect Dis 2006;43:1233-1238.
31. Latorre C, Gene A, Juncosa T, et al. *Neisseria meningitidis*: evolution of penicillin resistance and phenotype in a children's hospital in Barcelona, Spain. Acta Paediatr 2000;89:661-665.
32. Luaces Cubells C, Garcia Garcia JJ, Roca Martinez J, Latorre Otin CL. Clinical data in children with meningococcal meningitis in a Spanish hospital. Acta Paediatr 1997;86:26-29.
33. Scheld WM, Dacey RG, Winn HR. Cerebrospinal fluid outflow resistance in rabbits with experimental meningitis: alterations with penicillin and methylprednisolone. J Clin Invest 1980;66:243-253.
34. Tauber MG, Khayam-Bashi H, Sande MA. Effects of ampicillin and corticosteroids on brain water content, cerebrospinal fluid pressure, and cerebrospinal fluid lactate levels in experimental pneumococcal meningitis. J Infect Dis 1985;151:528-534.
35. van de Beek D, de Gans J, McIntyre P, Prasad K. Steroids in adults with acute bacterial meningitis: a systematic review. Lancet Infect Dis 2004;4:139-143.
36. McIntyre PB, Berkey CS, King SM, et al. Dexamethasone as adjunctive therapy in bacterial meningitis: a meta-analysis of randomized clinical trials since 1988. JAMA 1997;278:925-931.
37. van de Beek D. Brain teasing effect of dexamethasone. Lancet Neurol 2007;6:203-204.
38. de Gans J, van de Beek D. Dexamethasone in adults with bacterial meningitis. N Engl J Med 2002;347:1549-1556.
39. van de Beek D, de Gans J. Dexamethasone and pneumococcal meningitis. Ann Intern Med 2004;141:327.
40. Chaudhuri A. Adjunctive dexamethasone treatment in acute bacterial meningitis. Lancet Neurol 2004;3:54-62.
41. Annane D, Bellissant E, Bollaert PE, et al. Corticosteroids for severe sepsis and septic shock: a systematic review and meta-analysis. BMJ 2004;329:480-484.
42. Annane D, Sebille V, Charpentier C, et al. Effect of treatment with low doses of hydrocortisone and fludrocortisone on mortality in patients with septic shock. JAMA 2002;288:862-871.
43. Cooper MS, Stewart PM. Corticosteroid insufficiency in acutely ill patients. N Engl J Med 2003;348:727-734.
44. Cronin L, Cook DJ, Carlet J, et al. Corticosteroid treatment for sepsis: a critical appraisal and meta-analysis of the literature. Crit Care Med 1995;23:1430-1439.
45. Paris MM, Hickey SM, Uscher MI, et al. Effect of dexamethasone on therapy of experimental penicillin- and cephalosporin-resistant pneumococcal meningitis. Antimicrob Agents Chemother 1994;38:1320-1324.
46. Ricard JD, Wolff M, Lacherade JC, et al. Levels of vancomycin in cerebrospinal fluid of adult patients receiving adjunctive corticosteroids to treat pneumococcal meningitis: a prospective multicenter observational study. Clin Infect Dis 2007;44:250-255.
47. Leib SL, Heimgartner C, Bifrare YD, et al. Dexamethasone aggravates hippocampal apoptosis and learning deficiency in pneumococcal meningitis in infant rats. Pediatr Res 2003;54:353-357.
48. Weisfelt M, Hoogman M, van de Beek D, et al. Dexamethasone and long-term outcome in adults with bacterial meningitis. Ann Neurol 2006;60:456-468.
49. Unterberg AW, Stover J, Kress B, Kiening KL. Edema and brain trauma. Neuroscience 2004;129:1021-1029.
50. Wijdicks EFM, Diringer MN. Middle cerebral artery territory infarction and early brain swelling: progression and effect of age on outcome. Mayo Clin Proc 1998;73:829-836.
51. Muizelaar JP, Marmarou A, Ward JD, et al. Adverse effects of prolonged hyperventilation in patients with severe head injury: a randomized clinical trial. J Neurosurg 1991;75:731-739.
52. Møller K, Skinhøj P, Knudsen GM, Larsen FS. Effect of short-term hyperventilation on cerebral blood flow autoregulation in patients with acute bacterial meningitis. Stroke 2000;31:1116-1122.
53. Møller K, Strauss GI, Thomsen G, et al. Cerebral blood flow, oxidative metabolism and cerebrovascular carbon dioxide reactivity in patients with acute bacterial meningitis. Acta Anaesthesiol Scand 2002;46:567-578.
54. Muizelaar JP, Wel EP, Kontos HA, Becker DP. Mannitol causes compensatory cerebral vasoconstriction and vasodilation in response to blood viscosity changes. J Neurosurg 1983;59:822-828.
55. Schrot RJ, Muizelaar JP. Mannitol in acute traumatic brain injury. Lancet 2002;359:1633-1634.
56. Syrogiannopoulos GA, Olsen KD, McCracken GH Jr. Mannitol treatment in experimental *Haemophilus influenzae* type b meningitis. Pediatr Res 1987;22:118-122.
57. Lorenzl S, Koedel U, Pfister H-W. Mannitol, but not allopurinol, modulates changes in cerebral blood flow, intracranial pressure, and brain water content during pneumococcal meningitis in the rat. Crit Care Med 1996;24:1874-1880.
58. Kilpi T, Peltola H, Jauhiainen T, Kallio MJ. Oral glycerol and intravenous dexamethasone in preventing neurologic and audiologic sequelae of childhood bacterial meningitis. The Finnish Study Group. Pediatr Infect Dis J 1995;14:270-278.
59. Choi CW, Hwang JH, Chang YS, et al. Effects of hypertonic (7%) saline on brain injury in experimental *Escherichia coli* meningitis. J Korean Med Sci 2005;20:870-876.
60. Lindvall P, Ahlm C, Ericsson M, et al. Reducing intracranial pressure may increase survival among patients with bacterial meningitis. Clin Infect Dis 2004;38:384-390.
61. Bernard GR, Vincent J-L, Laterre P-F, et al. Efficacy and safety of recombinant human activated protein C for severe sepsis. N Engl J Med 2001;344;699-709.
62. Abraham E, Laterre P-F, Garg R, et al. Drotrecogin alfa (activated) for adults with severe sepsis and a low risk of death. N Engl J Med 2005;353:1332-1341.
63. Vincent JL, Nadel S, Kutsogiannis DJ, et al. Drotrecogin alfa (activated) in patients with severe sepsis presenting with purpura fulminans, meningitis, or meningococcal disease: a retrospective analysis of patients enrolled in recent clinical studies. Crit Care 2005;9:331-343.
64. Weber JR, Angstwurm K, Rosenkranz T, et al. Heparin inhibits leukocyte rolling in pial vessels and attenuates inflammatory changes in a rat model of experimental bacterial meningitis. J Cereb Blood Flow Metab 1997;17:1221-1229.
65. Straus SE, Thorpe KE, Holroyd-Leduc J. How do I perform a lumbar puncture and analyze the results to diagnose bacterial meningitis? JAMA 2006;296:2012-2022.
66. Nigrovic LE, Kuppermann N, Macias CG, et al. Clinical prediction rule for identifying children with cerebrospinal fluid pleocytosis at very low risk of bacterial meningitis. JAMA 2007;297:52-60.

67. Sigurdardottir B, Bjornsson OM, Jonsdottir KE, et al. Acute bacterial meningitis in adults: a 20-year overview. Arch Intern Med 1997;157:425-430.
68. Pizon AF, Bonner MR, Wang HE, Kaplan RM. Ten years of clinical experience with adult meningitis at an urban academic medical center. J Emerg Med 2006;30:367-370.
69. Hussein AS, Shafran SD. Acute bacterial meningitis in adults: a 12-year review. Medicine 2000;79:360-368.
70. Spanos A, Harrell FE Jr, Durack DT. Differential diagnosis of acute meningitis: an analysis of the predictive value of initial observations. JAMA 1989;262:2700-2707.
71. Negrini B, Kelleher KJ, Wald ER. Cerebrospinal fluid findings in aseptic versus bacterial meningitis. Pediatrics 2000;105:316-319.
72. Oostenbrink R, Moons CGM, Derksen-Lubsen AG, et al. A diagnostic decision rule for management of children with meningeal signs. Eur J Epidemol 2004;19:109-116.
73. Hoen B, Viel JF, Paquot C, et al. Multivariate approach to differential diagnosis of acute meningitis. Eur J Clin Microb Infect Dis 1995:267-274.
74. Jaeger F, Leroy J, Duchêne F, et al. Validation of a diagnosis model for differentiating bacterial from viral meningitis in infants and children under 3.5 years of age. Eur J Clin Microb Infect Dis 2000;19:418-421.
75. Brivet FG, Ducuing S, Jacobs F, et al. Accuracy of clinical presentation for differentiating bacterial from viral meningitis in adults: a multivariate approach. Intensive Care Med 2005;31:1654-1660.
76. Hasbun R, Abrahams J, Jekel J, Quagliarello VJ. Computed tomography of the head before lumbar puncture in adults with suspected meningitis. N Engl J Med 2001;345:1727-1733.
77. Proulx N, Frechette D, Toye B, et al. Delays in the administration of antibiotics are associated with mortality from adult acute bacterial meningitis. QJM 2005;98:291-298.
78. van de Beek D, de Gans J. Adjunctive corticosteroids in adults with bacterial meningitis. Curr Infect Dis Rep 2005;7:285-291.
79. Ivey NS, Martin EN Jr, Scheld WM, Nathan BR. A new method for measuring blood-brain barrier permeability demonstrated with europium-bound albumin during experimental lipopolysaccharide (LPS) induced meningitis in the rat. J Neurosci Methods 2005;142:91-95.
80. Grandgirard D, Schürch C, Cottagnoud P, Leib SL. Prevention of brain injury by the nonbacteriolytic antibiotic daptomycin in experimental pneumococcal meningitis. Antimicrob Agents Chemother 2007;51:2173-2178.
81. Meli DN, Coimbra RS, Erhart DG, et al. Doxycycline reduces mortality and injury to the brain and cochlea in experimental pneumococcal meningitis. Infect Immun 2006;74:3890-3896.
82. Bifrare YD, Kummer J, Joss P, et al. Brain-derived neurotrophic factor protects against multiple forms of brain injury in bacterial meningitis. J Infect Dis 2005;191:40-45.
83. Grandgirard D, Leib SL. Strategies to prevent neuronal damage in paediatric bacterial meningitis. Curr Opin Pediatr 2006;18:112-118.
84. Angstwurm K, Hanisch UK, Gassemi T, et al. Tyrosine kinase inhibition reduces inflammation in the acute stage of experimental pneumococcal meningitis. Infect Immun 2004;72:3294-3298.
85. Kastenbauer S, Koedel U, Weih F, et al. Protective role of NF-κB1 (p50) in experimental pneumococcal meningitis. Eur J Pharmacol 2004;498:315-318.
86. Klein M, Koedel U, Pfister HW. Oxidative stress in pneumococcal meningitis: a future target for adjunctive therapy? Prog Neurobiol 2006;80:269-280.
87. Leib SL, Clements JM, Lindberg RLP, et al. Inhibition of matrix metalloproteinases and tumour necrosis factor converting enzyme as adjuvant therapy in pneumococcal meningitis. Brain 2001;125:1734-1742.
88. Kastenbauer S. Pneumococcal meningitis: a 21st century perspective. Lancet Neurol 2006;5:104-105.
89. Klein M, Koedel U, Pfister HW, Kastenbauer S. Meningitis-associated hearing loss: protection by adjunctive antioxidant therapy. Ann Neurol 2003;54:451-458.
90. Koedel U, Winkler F, Angele B, et al. Meningitis-associated central nervous system complications are mediated by the activation of poly(ADP-ribose) polymerase. J Cereb Blood Flow Metab 2002;22:39-49.
91. Koedel U, Winkler F, Angele B, et al. Role of caspase-1 in experimental pneumococcal meningitis: evidence from pharmacologic caspase inhibition and caspase-1-deficient mice. Ann Neurol 2002;51:319-329.
92. Braun JS, Novak R, Herzog K-H, et al. Neuroprotection by a caspase inhibitor in acute bacterial meningitis. Nat Med 1999;5:298-302.

81

ENDOCARDITIS

Lisa G. Winston, Daniel Deck, and Ann F. Bolger

OVERVIEW 1121
INTRODUCTION 1121
PATHOGENESIS AND PATHOPHYSIOLOGY 1122
CLINICAL MANIFESTATIONS AND COMPLICATIONS 1123
THERAPEUTICS AND CLINICAL PHARMACOLOGY 1123
Bactericidal Versus Bacteriostatic Antimicrobials 1123
Cell Wall–Active Antibiotics 1124
β-Lactam Antibiotics 1124
Vancomycin 1127
Cell Membrane–Active Antibiotic 1128
Daptomycin 1128
Protein Synthesis Inhibitors 1128
Aminoglycosides 1128
Oxazolidinones 1129
Streptogramins 1129
Tetracyclines 1129
Ribonucleic Acid Synthesis Inhibitor 1129
Rifamycins (Rifampin) 1129
Deoxyribonucleic Acid Synthesis Inhibitors 1130
Fluoroquinolones 1130
Antifungals 1130
Amphotericin B Preparations 1130
Triazoles (Fluconazole) 1130
Nonantibiotic Interventions 1130
Therapeutic Approach 1131
Viridans Group Streptococci, *Streptococcus bovis, Abiotrophia defectiva, Granulicatella* Species, and *Gemella* Species 1131
Streptococcus pneumoniae, S. pyogenes, and Groups B, C, and G Streptococci 1132
Enterococci 1132
Staphylococci 1134
HACEK Organisms 1135
Enterobacteriaceae and *Pseudomonas aeruginosa* 1136
Fungi 1136
Culture-Negative Endocarditis 1136
Prophylaxis 1137
Areas of Uncertainty and Future Directions 1138

OVERVIEW

Infective endocarditis (IE) is defined as an infection of the endothelial surface of the heart, most commonly involving one or more of the cardiac valves. While this infection is not as common as some of the others covered in this text, it is associated with high morbidity and mortality. Given the serious consequences of developing this disease, antimicrobial prophylaxis for IE has been the standard in specific circumstances for a number of years. In addition, our knowledge of many therapeutic agents has been shaped by animal models of this infection and by studies in humans.

The goal of this chapter is to examine IE from a pharmacologic standpoint. The chapter briefly reviews the epidemiology of IE and discusses pathophysiology and pathogenesis. The pharmacology of antibiotics commonly used for IE is considered, with an emphasis on principles specific to IE. Nonantibiotic interventions are included, where appropriate. Guidelines for prophylaxis are reviewed. Finally, emerging drugs for resistant gram-positive infections and their potential applicability to IE treatment, as well as other areas needing further study, are discussed.

INTRODUCTION

The epidemiology of IE has evolved over recent years. Health care–associated infections seem to account for a much larger proportion of cases than previously reported, with *Staphylococcus aureus* as the predominant organism in patients with catheter- and other device-associated IE.[1] However, at least one population-based assessment emphasizes the continuing contribution of typical, community-acquired viridans group streptococcal infection to the overall burden of IE.[2] IE remains a relatively uncommon disease with an annual incidence between 1.5 and 6.2 cases per 100,000 person-years.[3,4] In-hospital mortality, however, remains high, with an overall risk for unselected patients of about 15%.[4] However, certain organisms such as *S. aureus,* gram-negative rods, and fungi are associated with higher mortality in most studies.

Certain groups have a much higher risk for IE than the general population. The most significant risk factors include device- and health care–associated risks (e.g., in hemodialysis patients), structural cardiac abnormalities, and injection drug use. For example, with injection drug use, the risk for IE is estimated to be greater than 150 cases per 100,000 person-years,[5] at least 100 times the risk for the average population. Presence of a prosthetic valve is also an important risk factor; in one retrospective study spanning more than 20 years, 3.7% of prosthetic valves developed infection.[6] Mitral valve prolapse, while associated with a smaller relative increase in risk, is important due to the frequency with which it occurs, and rheumatic heart disease remains an important risk factor in countries where the disease is prevalent.[7]

There are several important concepts that strongly influence therapeutic decision making. One of the key issues is accurately ruling in and ruling out the diagnosis of IE. Currently, the modified Duke criteria constitute the most commonly used method for making the diagnosis of IE. Both the original Duke criteria and the modified Duke criteria have been validated as clinically useful diagnostic approaches and have largely replaced other diagnostic criteria.[8] The Duke criteria place patients initially suspected of having IE into three categories after diagnostic evaluation: definite IE, possible IE, and rejected diagnosis of IE. Definite IE can be established by pathologic criteria with the demonstration of microorganisms associated with a cardiac valve or valvular vegetation either by culture or by histopathology or by other pathologic examination consistent with active IE. Definite IE can also be established by clinical criteria, which are divided into major and minor criteria. Major criteria are either microbiologic or provide evidence of endocardial involvement. Microbiologic findings meeting the major criteria are finding typical organisms in two separate blood cultures, finding consistent organisms in persistently positive blood cultures, or a single positive blood culture for *Coxiella burnetii* or antiphase I immunoglobulin G antibody titer greater than 1:800. Evidence of endocardial involvement can be demonstrated by an echocardiogram with an oscillating valvular mass, endocardial abscess, or new dehiscence of a prosthetic valve. Presence of new valvular regurgitation is also a major criterion that provides evidence of endocardial involvement. Minor criteria include having a predisposing condition or risk factor, fever, evidence of vascular or embolic phenomena consistent with IE, immunologic phenomena, and culture of organisms from blood or serologic evidence of infection with an IE-causing organism without meeting the microbiologic major criteria. Definite IE by clinical criteria is said to be present when 2 major criteria, 1 major and 3 minor criteria, or all 5 minor criteria are met. Possible IE is said to be present when 1 major criterion and 1 minor criterion or 3 minor criteria are met. The diagnosis of IE is otherwise rejected.

Blood cultures are a critical component of the diagnosis of IE, and blood culture results also direct the therapeutic strategy. However, negative blood cultures are not uncommon in patients who meet diagnostic criteria for IE. One study estimated that about 20% of patients with IE had negative blood cultures and that about half of these patients received antibiotics before blood cultures were drawn.[9] The most common organisms that cause disease in the particular population to which the patient belongs should be covered with the therapeutic regimen selected. While special studies, especially serologic tests, are helpful in some patients, the tests are not available in all settings and do not provide immediate information. Also, testing for all possible pathogens is frequently impractical. Therefore, stratification according to epidemiologic risk is important when considering such organisms as *C. burnettii, Brucella* species, fungi, and *Tropheryma whippleii. Bartonella* species may be among the most common pathogens causing IE that are not easily cultured. *Chlamydophila* and *Legionella* organisms should also be considered.

The location of the infection within the heart is also fundamentally important to the therapeutic strategy. Right-sided IE usually involving the tricuspid valve is frequently seen in injection drug users (IDUs) but is uncommon in patients without this risk factor. Tricuspid valve endocarditis has a more favorable prognosis than IE involving the mitral or aortic valves. Right-sided IE may be associated with septic pulmonary emboli, does not usually require surgery, and can often be treated with a shorter course of antibiotic therapy. *Staphylococcus aureus* is by far the most common pathogen. Left-sided IE involving the mitral valve, aortic valve, or both can occur in IDUs and non-IDUs. It may be associated with systemic emboli and has high morbidity and mortality. Although *S. aureus* is a common organism in left-sided disease, particularly in patients with health care–associated infections and in IDUs, other organisms, especially viridans group streptococci, play a major role.

Echocardiography provides essential diagnostic and prognostic information when the diagnosis of IE is suspected. Specific echocardiographic findings, as discussed previously, are a major diagnostic feature according to the Duke criteria. While transesophageal echocardiography is more sensitive for left-sided valvular pathology than transthoracic echocardiography, it is also more invasive and more expensive. Transthoracic echocardiography alone may be appropriate for certain patients in whom there is low suspicion of disease or in whom initial transthoracic echocardiography shows findings consistent with IE but the patient is at low risk for complications and surgical intervention is unlikely to be required.[10] The indications for surgery are discussed later in this chapter.

The chief therapeutic goal in the pharmacologic treatment of IE is to eradicate infection and sterilize the heart valve. Antibiotics with bactericidal activity are preferred for this serious infection given clinical experience and the concern that the heart valves are a "privileged site," where the host response may be unable to eliminate residual disease. Ideally, therapy will prevent the onset of heart failure by stemming progressive valvular dysfunction. Although the efficacy is unproven, antibiotics are also used in an effort to prevent IE in persons at high risk, including those with a previous history of IE.

PATHOGENESIS AND PATHOPHYSIOLOGY

IE results when organisms with the propensity to cause this disease enter the bloodstream and then seed the endocardium. However, transient bacteremia with certain organisms that cause IE, especially oral flora, is probably common, yet leads to IE in only a small minority of cases.[11] Undamaged endothelium is quite resistant to seeding by most bacteria and fungi. Therefore, persons with preexisting endothelial abnormalities have a higher risk of developing IE when the endocardium is exposed to microorganisms. Presence of a prosthetic heart valve confers a particularly high risk. A previous episode of IE, complex cyanotic congenital heart disease, unrepaired ventricular septal defect or patent ductus arteriosus, and surgical systemic pulmonary shunts also confer substantial risk. A number of other conditions, including mitral valve prolapse with regurgitation, are thought to confer moderate risk. Mitral valve prolapse without regurgitation is considered low risk. Some estimates suggest that up to 75% of patients with IE have underlying cardiac disorders,[11] but these estimates are probably more applicable to non–health care–associated disease. Implanted cardiac devices such as pacemakers and defibrillators are also considered low risk, but infection originating in any part of the device can lead to intracardiac infection and the development of IE.

Microorganisms can access the bloodstream through mucous membranes or the skin, and increased opportunity for access leads to higher risk of IE. Viridans group streptococci were traditionally the most common organisms implicated in IE and are a component of normal oral flora. Even minor disruptions of oral mucosa can lead to bacteremia. Edentulous patients are at lower risk for IE due to dental organisms.[12] Enterococci may enter the bloodstream via the gastrointestinal or genitourinary tract. *Staphylococcus aureus* may now be the most common organism causing IE and usually enters the bloodstream through breaks in the skin. Increased use of intravascular catheters and other health care–associated devices has been associated with a larger proportion of IE cases due to *S. aureus,* as these devices provide a portal of entry.[1]

Hemodynamic factors contribute to the likelihood and location of endothelial damage. The aortic and mitral valves are subjected to higher pressures than the right-sided cardiac valves. This results in higher blood flow velocities and greater turbulence when left-sided valves are insufficient. These factors are postulated to contribute to the higher incidence of left-sided IE. The common locations for vegetations correspond to the turbulent zones and endothelial activation created by valve leakage; mitral and tricuspid vegetations most commonly occur on the atrial side of the valve, while aortic and pulmonic (rare) vegetations are more frequent on the ventricular side.[13,14] The high-velocity jet through a ventricular septal defect may also cause endothelial damage and predispose to the formation of vegetations at the site of jet contact with cardiac walls or valvular structures.[15]

Microthrombi are thought to play an important role in the development of IE. These deposits are initially sterile but can serve as attachment sites for circulating microorganisms.[16] Thrombus formation is initiated by the binding of platelets to damaged endothelium. Endothelial attachment results in platelet activation, which precipitates a conformational change in the glycoprotein (GP) IIb/IIIa receptor permitting binding of soluble fibrinogen. Thromboxane A_2 is released from activated platelets and activates other platelets. Fibrinogen can bind to two GPIIb/IIIa receptors, which results in cross-linking of platelets and aggregation at the site of endothelial abnormalities.[17]

Platelet interactions with microorganisms are complex, and platelets act as inflammatory cells in host defense. Platelets can internalize microorganisms, probably facilitating clearance of pathogens in most cases, but may also permit intracellular persistence and avoidance of the immune system and antimicrobial agents. Platelets contain microbicidal proteins active against a range of pathogens that are released in conjunction with platelet activation.[18,19] *Staphylococcus aureus,* coagulase-negative staphylococci, and viridans streptococci with in vitro resistance to platelet microbicidal proteins are associated with endovascular sources of infection.[20,21] *Staphylococcus aureus* that are resistant in vitro to the effects of platelet microbicidal proteins proliferated more vigorously in vegetations in a rabbit model of IE.[22] Microorganisms can also adhere to platelets, activate platelets, and facilitate platelet aggregation. This may allow for initial organism adherence to sterile microthrombi at sites of endothelial injury and for the propagation of valvular vegetations.

The observation that viridans streptococci and *S. aureus* are the most common organisms implicated in IE has led to investigations of the particular pathogenic mechanisms involved. Both viridans streptococci and *S. aureus* carry surface molecules referred to as microbial surface components recognizing adhesive matrix molecules (MSCRAMMs). MSCRAMMs bind to host extracellular matrix proteins, and several MSCARMMs have been implicated in experimental models of IE.[23] Glucan polysaccharides were among the earliest surface molecules implicated in IE caused by certain species of viridans streptococci.[24] Adherence to fibronectin is also associated with pathogenicity in an animal model.[25] Other adhesins probably also play a role, although some have not yet been evaluated in vivo.

While viridans streptococci usually cause a subacute syndrome and rarely infect valves without preexisting abnormalities, *S. aureus* typically causes acute disease and can infect apparently normal endothelium. *Staphylococcus aureus* carries a number of virulence factors, the coordinated expression of which is mediated by several global regulators, including the accessory gene regulator locus (*agr*). The interactions between the various factors are complex, and in vitro and in vivo experiments have sometimes produced contradictory results as to the role of individual determinants in IE pathogenesis.[23] Clumping factor A, which binds fibrinogen and fibrin, is probably important in the development of *S. aureus* IE, as is the ability to bind fibronectin.

Coagulase-negative staphylococci, especially *Staphylococcus epidermidis,* can cause native valve IE but are particularly implicated in prosthetic valve endocarditis (PVE). Infection with *S. epidermidis* is most common in the first year following valve replacement, and so-called early PVE typically results from contamination during surgery. The virulence factors for coagulase-negative staphylococci have not been investigated to the same extent as those of *S. aureus,* but the ability of *S. epidermidis* to infect foreign materials has long been appreciated. Many strains of *S. epidermidis* produce a "slime" layer that coats foreign material; capsular PS/A (polysaccharide/adhesion), which is also involved in the initial attachment of *S. epidermidis* to plastic surfaces, forms one component of this layer. *Staphylococcus epidermidis* colonies live within the slime layer, which presumably helps to protect the bacteria from host defenses.[26]

Another feature of IE is the apparent lack of effective killing of microorganisms in vegetations by polymorphonuclear leukocytes (PMNLs). Microorganisms appear to be physically sequestered from the PMNLs by the vegetation matrix.[27] In at least one study of experimental IE, leukocytes were found very early in vegetation formation, but few were present in vegetations at least 24 hours old.[28] Those PMNLs that were present in mature vegetations had limited contact with colonies of streptococcal bacteria. However, in the earliest lesions, streptococci were mostly contained within phagocytic cells. Virulence in experimental IE has been linked to the ability to survive in PMNLs.[29] Additionally, reversible defects in PMNL intracellular killing may be present in untreated patients with IE.[30] Monocytes may also play a role in the maturation of the vegetation, thereby allowing microorganisms to persist and evade host defenses. Streptococci and staphylococci can induce monocytes to produce tissue factor.[31,32] Tissue factor, a key component in the coagulation cascade, is needed for vegetation growth and also serves to activate platelets.[23]

In addition to the limited impact of PMNLs in IE, some of the organisms within infected vegetations may be metabolically inactive, leading to decreased killing by antibiotics. This was classically demonstrated to be the case in experimental streptococcal IE in rabbits, where bacterial deposits deep within the vegetation were largely composed of dead and inactive bacteria. Inactivity was determined by the failure of organisms to take up tritium-labeled L-alanine, a component of the cell wall.[27,33] These metabolically inactive bacteria may form a reservoir that, if not killed by adequate antibiotic therapy, can lead to relapses of infection. Taken together, the lack of an effective PMNL response and the presence of bacterial colonies that are not metabolically active support the therapeutic approach of using bactericidal antibiotics for a prolonged period of time in an attempt to completely eradicate infection.[27] This concept is discussed in more detail later.

CLINICAL MANIFESTATIONS AND COMPLICATIONS

IE can present with acute or subacute symptoms. *Staphylococcus aureus* is the prototypical organism in acute IE, while viridans streptococcal infection usually presents subacutely, as do infections with a number of other organisms. Fever is the most common manifestation, and, even with initiation of appropriate therapy, may persist for up to 2 weeks. Fever lasting more than 2 weeks after the start of appropriate therapy is associated with a complicated course.[34] Other nonspecific systemic symptoms such as malaise and weight loss may be present. Heart murmur is typically discernable, although it is preexisting in many cases. With left-sided IE, evidence of peripheral embolic phenomena may be present, including splinter hemorrhages under the fingernails or toenails, conjunctival petechiae, and Janeway lesions (flat, erythematous, painless lesions on the palms or soles). With right-sided IE, peripheral embolic phenomona are absent, but septic pulmonary emboli are common. Due to the persistent antigenic challenge to the immune system, circulating immune complexes can develop in IE. Rheumatoid factor is frequently positive in patients after several weeks of symptoms. Glomerulonephritis can develop with deposition of immune complexes and complement along the glomerular basement membrane. Osler's nodes are painful, nodular lesions usually found on the digits whose etiology is not entirely clear. They are traditionally described as secondary to immune complex deposition, but reports of positive cultures from the lesions raise the possibility that they result from septic emboli. Roth's spots are white-centered retinal hemorrhages that are suggestive of the presence of IE but can also be found in a number of other conditions.

Complications of IE can be divided into cardiac and systemic categories. Valvular insufficiency is common and can be associated with congestive heart failure. Tricuspid valve regurgitation is usually tolerated fairly well and rarely requires surgical repair. However, refractory heart failure can develop with left-sided disease, especially related to aortic insufficiency, and is one of the clearest indications for valve replacement in IE. Valvular and perivalvular abscesses can also develop and usually require surgery. Myocarditis and pericarditis are uncommon complications.

Systemic complications usually relate to emboli from the vegetation. Involvement of the cerebral vasculature is one of the most feared complications, and morbidity and mortality can result from embolic cerebrovascular accidents and from rupture of infected mycotic aneurysms. Emboli can also involve the spleen, liver, and kidney, leading to infarcts or frank abscesses. Osteomyelitis and septic arthritis may also be present in patients with IE, especially in disease due to *S. aureus* in IDUs.[35]

THERAPEUTICS AND CLINICAL PHARMACOLOGY

Bactericidal Versus Bacteriostatic Antimicrobials

Strictly speaking, bactericidal antibiotics are those which kill bacteria, while bacteriostatic antibiotics inhibit bacterial growth. These characteristics are determined by in vitro testing, and data regarding correlation with clinical efficacy are sparse. A given antibiotic may be bactericidal for one organism and bacteriostatic for another. In vitro testing is used to compare the minimum bactericidal concentration (MBC) of an antibiotic with the minimum inhibitory concentration (MIC). The MBC is determined by performing serial dilutions of an antibiotic to determine the lowest concentration that results in a ≥99.9% reduction of the original organism inoculum upon subculture to an antibiotic-free medium. The MIC is the lowest concentration of antibiotic that prevents visible growth of the organism. Antibiotics are typically considered to be bacteriostatic if the ratio of the MBC to the MIC is greater than 4. However, technical aspects of testing can have a significant impact on the results. While the use of bactericidal antibiotics has long been the "gold standard" in IE therapy, there are instances in which cidal drugs may not be available or tolerated. Cases of successful therapy with bacteriostatic antibiotics have been reported, and alternative approaches may need to be considered in certain circumstances.

Cell Wall–Active Antibiotics

β-Lactam Antibiotics

Since the discovery of penicillin over 70 years ago, the β-lactam antibiotics have been used extensively in the treatment of bacterial infections, including IE. The clinically available β-lactam antibiotics comprise four closely related yet structurally unique classes: penicillins, cephalosporins, carbapenems, and monobactams. These compounds are classified as β-lactam antibiotics because of their unique four-membered lactam ring, which is essential for their antimicrobial activity.

β-Lactam antibiotics inhibit bacterial growth by interfering with a specific step in bacterial cell wall synthesis (Fig. 81-1). Bacterial penicillin-binding proteins (PBPs) catalyze the transpeptidase reaction that cross-links glycopeptides in the cell wall. β-Lactam antibiotics are structural analogues of the natural cell wall substrate and are covalently bound by PBPs. After a β-lactam antibiotic has attached to the PBP, the transpeptidase reaction is inhibited, peptidoglycan synthesis is blocked, and the bacterium dies. β-Lactam antibiotics are bactericidal only if bacteria are actively growing and synthesizing cell wall.

While β-lactam antibiotics share the same mechanism of action, their antimicrobial spectrum may vary greatly across classes and also within the same class. The activity of a β-lactam antibiotic is in part determined by various chemical side chains that are attached to the basic ring structure. These side chains affect the affinity for the target PBPs, the ability to penetrate the outer membrane of gram-negative bacteria, and the stability against β-lactamase enzymes that may be produced by the bacteria. Additionally, cephalosporins are inherently more stable against hydrolysis by most of the common β-lactamases than are the penicillins. Therefore, penicillins are frequently combined with β-lactamase inhibitors to protect them from hydrolysis, thereby increasing the spectrum of activity of the penicillin antibiotic. β-Lactamase inhibitors are also β-lactam compounds but have only weak antibacterial activity themselves.

Penicillins and cephalosporins have activity against many of the bacteria that frequently cause IE. They are also remarkably nontoxic in the absence of a history of allergy. As a result, prolonged courses of high-dose, intravenously administered penicillins and cephalosporins have historically been the cornerstone of therapy for bacterial IE. While recent changes in the epidemiology of IE have limited the empirical use of penicillins and cephalosporins, once a pathogen is identified and known to be susceptible, they are usually the preferred treatment option.

β-Lactam antibiotics are well tolerated, with most serious adverse effects due to hypersensitivity reactions. In the general population, 5% to 8% of persons report allergies to penicillin, but only 5% to 10% of those with a history of allergy will have a reaction when given a penicillin antibiotic.[36] Given the potential for anaphylaxis, penicillin and all other members of the penicillin family should be administered with caution or a substitute drug should be given if there is a history of an immediate-type hypersensitivity reaction. In penicillin-allergic patients, cross reactivity to cephalosporins is low; less than 10% of patients with a penicillin allergy will have a reaction to cephalosporins.[37,38] However, there have been reports of anaphylaxis following administration of a cephalosporin to patients allergic to penicillin. Therefore, patients reporting a severe penicillin allergy should only be administered a cephalosporin in a monitored setting where appropriate precautions are taken for managing a hypersensitivity reaction. In

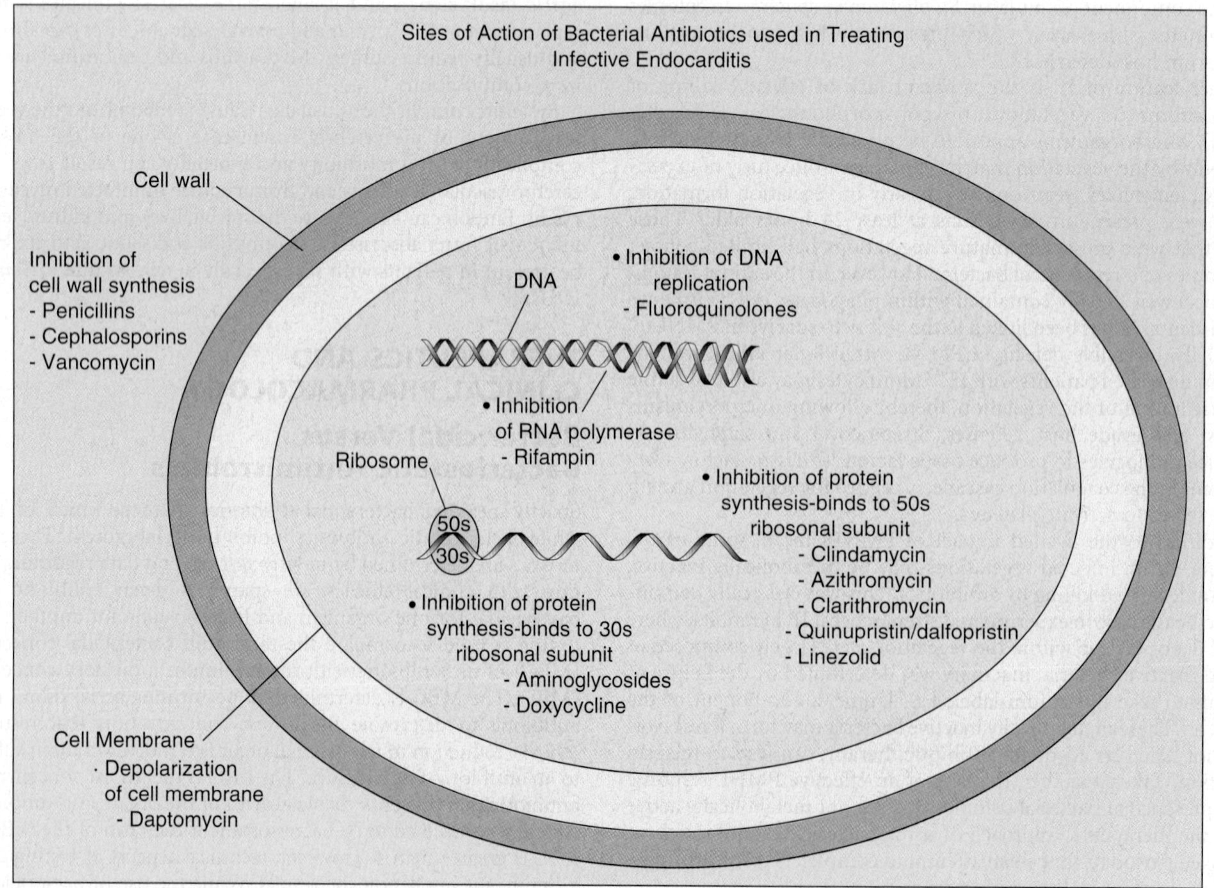

FIGURE 81-1 • **Sites of action of antibacterical antibiotics used in treating infective endocarditis.**

patients reporting only a mild reaction to penicillin, such as a typical maculopapular drug rash, cephalosporins may be administered. Vancomycin is generally the preferred alternative for IE caused by gram-positive pathogens when there is a documented serious allergy to penicillin. In situations such as enterococcal IE, when a penicillin is clearly the preferred treatment option, treatment with a penicillin may be started with graduated doses of antibiotic according to a desensitization protocol.

Penicillins. All penicillins have the basic structure shown in Figure 81-2. A thiazolidine ring (A) is attached to a β-lactam ring (B) that carries a secondary amino group. Substituents (R) can be attached to the amino group to produce compounds with varied spectra of activity. Integrity of the 6-aminopenicillanic acid is essential for antibacterial activity. If the β-lactam ring is cleaved by bacterial β-lactamases, the resulting product lacks antibacterial activity. The penicillins most commonly used for IE treatment can be classified into three groups: the natural penicillins (e.g., penicillin G), the antistaphylococcal penicillins (e.g., nafcillin), and the extended-spectrum penicillins (e.g., ampicillin).

Penicillin G. Penicillin G has been in clinical use since the 1940s and continues to have an important role in the treatment of bacterial IE. While penicillin G is a narrow-spectrum antibiotic, it is reliably active against many gram-positive pathogens that cause IE, most notably streptococci and enterococci. Penicillin G resistance may occur in streptococci and enterococci through alterations in the PBPs that decrease the binding affinity of penicillin. Isolates with altered PBPs often have modest elevations in their penicillin G MICs and are not fully resistant to penicillin. IE caused by these isolates may still be treated successfully with penicillin G, although higher doses are needed, and penicillin is frequently combined with an aminoglycoside to achieve synergistic killing (see later). While penicillin G was historically active against staphylococci, most current clinical isolates produce a β-lactamase that confers resistance to penicillin. However, IE due to susceptible staphylococci can still be treated with penicillin G.

In the treatment of IE penicillin G is administered intravenously at total daily doses that range from 12 to 30 million units per day. The total daily dose must be divided and administered at frequent intervals, usually every 4 to 6 hours, because of the short half-life (~30 minutes). Alternatively, the total daily dose of penicillin may be administered as a continuous infusion over 24 hours. Penicillin G is rapidly excreted by the kidneys into the urine in patients with normal renal function. In patients with renal failure, the half-life may be as long as 10 hours; therefore, the dose of penicillin must be adjusted based on renal function. In general, patients with a creatinine clearance of 10 to 50 ml/min should receive 50% of the normal recommended dose and patients with a creatinine clearance of less than 10 ml/min should receive 25% of the normal recommended dose. Dose reduction with renal failure is imperative as high doses of penicillin G may cause seizures.

Ampicillin, Amoxicillin, and Ampicillin-Sulbactam. The aminopenicillins, ampicillin and amoxicillin, retain the gram-positive spectrum of penicillin G with increased gram-negative activity due to their ability to penetrate the outer membrane of gram-negative bacteria. Like penicillin G, they are inactivated by β-lactamases. This is problematic as many gram-negative pathogens that were once uniformly

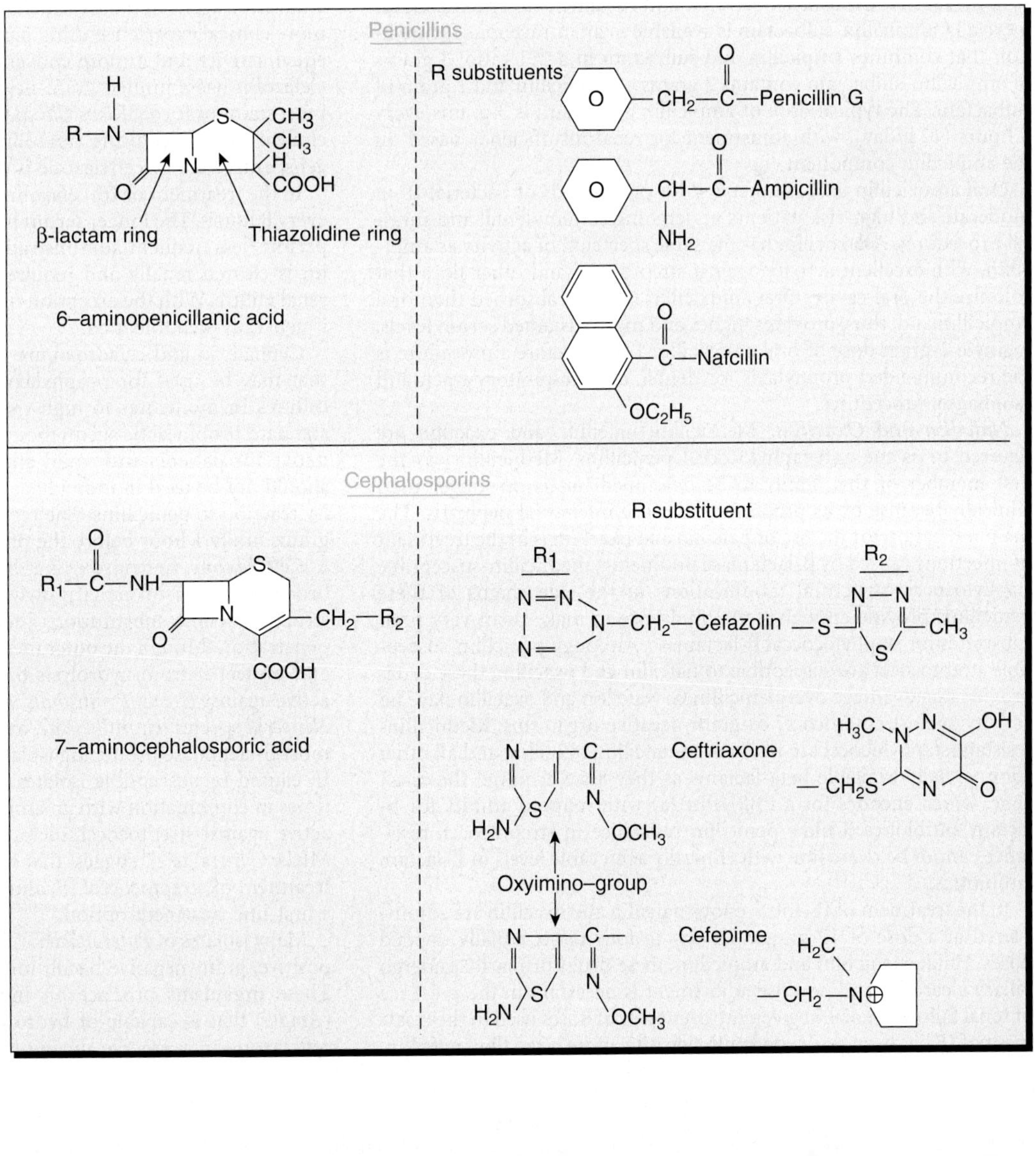

FIGURE 81-2 • Structures of selected penicillins and cephalosporins.

susceptible have acquired β-lactamases that confer resistance to the aminopenicillins. Ampicillin and amoxicillin are active against non-β-lactamase–producing strains of *Escherichia coli, Proteus mirabilis,* and *Salmonella* species. The aminopenicillins are not active against many of the gram-negative pathogens encountered in health care settings, including *Klebsiella, Enterobacter, Citrobacte*r, *Serratia,* and *Pseudomonas* species.

Ampicillin, but not amoxicillin, is available as an intravenous formulation in the United States. High-dose intravenous ampicillin is useful in treating IE caused by penicillin-susceptible organisms, including anaerobes, enterococci, *Listeria monocytogenes,* and susceptible strains of gram-negative cocci and bacilli. Ampicillin is often favored over penicillin in the treatment of enterococcal IE as the MIC of ampicillin is usually slightly lower than that of penicillin G. Ampicillin may also be used as an alternative to penicillin G when penicillin is not available because of supply problems. Like penicillin, ampicillin has a short half-life that requires multiple daily doses to achieve adequate therapeutic levels. Up to 12 grams of ampicillin per day given in divided doses every 4 hours is a standard regimen. Ampicillin is also renally cleared, and doses must be adjusted for patients with renal failure. Ampicillin is generally well tolerated but may cause a skin rash that is not allergic in nature. Ampicillin has also been associated with pseudomembranous colitis.

The combination of ampicillin with a β-lactamase inhibitor, sulbactam, restores the activity of ampicillin against certain β-lactamase–producing pathogens, including methicillin-susceptible *S. aureus, Haemophilus influenzae, E. coli, Salmonella* species, *Klebsiella* species, the HACEK organisms, and many anaerobes. Sulbactam is not an effective inhibitor of chromosomally encoded β-lactamases produced by *Enterobacter, Citrobacter, Serratia,* and *Pseudomonas* species. Commercially, ampicillin-sulbactam is available in an intravenous formulation that combines ampicillin and sulbactam in a 2:1 ratio; 3 grams of ampicillin-sulbactam contains 2 grams of ampicillin and 1 gram of sulbactam. The typical dose of ampicillin-sulbactam is 3 grams every 6 hours (12 g/day), with adjustment for renal insufficiency based on the ampicillin component.

Oral amoxicillin is recommended for prophylaxis of bacterial IE in moderate and high-risk patients undergoing certain dental and surgical procedures. Amoxicillin has the same spectrum of activity as ampicillin, with excellent activity against streptococci and other flora that colonize the oral cavity. Oral amoxicillin is better absorbed than oral ampicillin and, thus, provides higher and more sustained serum levels. A single 2-gram dose of oral amoxicillin 1 hour before a procedure is the recommended prophylaxis for dental, oral, respiratory tract, and esophageal procedures.

Nafcillin and Oxacillin. Methicillin, nafcillin, and oxacillin are referred to as the antistaphylococcal penicillins. Methicillin was the first member of this family to be developed but is no longer used clinically because of its propensity to cause interstitial nephritis. The main indication for the use of nafcillin and oxacillin is in the treatment of infections caused by β-lactamase producing, methicillin-susceptible staphylococci. Structural modifications in the side chains of these penicillins provide enough steric hindrance to make them very poor substrates for staphylococcal β-lactamase. Although penicillin-susceptible streptococci are susceptible to nafcillin and oxacillin, these drugs provide no advantage over penicillin G. Nafcillin and oxacillin have no activity against enterococci or gram-negative organisms. Methicillin-resistant staphylococci are resistant to nafcillin, oxacillin, and all other commercially available beta-lactams as they have acquired the *mecA* gene, which encodes for a PBP (PBP2a) with reduced affinity for β-lactam antibiotics. Unlike penicillin resistance in streptococci, resistance cannot be overcome with clinically achievable levels of β-lactam antibiotics.

In the treatment of IE, intravenous nafcillin and oxacillin are administered at a dose of 12 grams per day in four to six equally divided doses. Unlike penicillin and ampicillin, these drugs primarily undergo biliary clearance and no dose adjustment is necessary in the presence of renal failure. Oxacillin given intravenously at doses used in the treatment of IE has been associated with hepatitis more often than nafcillin. Intravenous nafcillin frequently causes reversible bone marrow suppression that manifests primarily as neutropenia.

Cephalosporins. Cephalosporins have the basic 7-aminocephalosporic acid structure shown in Figure 81-2. The antimicrobial activity of natural cephalosporins is low, but substitution of various R1 and R2 groups yields drugs with potent activity and low toxicity. Cephalosporins are more stable than penicillins against many bacterial β-lactamases and have a broad spectrum of activity. Cephalosporins are not active against enterococci or *L. monocytogenes.* Cephalosporins are classified into four generations based on their spectra of activity. First-generation cephalosporins are generally used for their gram-positive activity, while later generation cephalosporins have excellent activity against aerobic gram-negative pathogens.

Cefazolin, Cephalexin, and Cefadroxil. Cefazolin, a first-generation cephalosporin, has activity against methicillin-susceptible staphylococci, as the β-lactamase produced by these pathogens is primarily a penicillinase. Notably, cefazolin is not as stable against inactivation by the staphylococcal β-lactamase as the antistaphylococcal penicillins.[39] Clinically, this is an issue as there have been reports of cefazolin failure in high-inoculum staphylococcal infections such as IE.[40] For this reason, the antistaphylococcal penicillins are generally preferred over cefazolin in the treatment of staphylococcal IE, with cefazolin reserved for patients who are penicillin allergic but are able to tolerate cephalosporins. While several of the later generation cephalosporins also have activity against staphylococci, the first-generation cephalosporins are generally preferred in the treatment of serious staphylococcal infections such as IE on the basis of in vitro activity, clinical experience, and narrower spectrum of activity.

Cefazolin is active against streptococci. However, it is not considered a first-line agent in the treatment of streptococcal IE, as there is much more clinical experience using penicillin G, while ceftriaxone provides equal activity and a more convenient dosing regimen than cefazolin. Cefazolin has a limited gram-negative spectrum but is active against most stains of *E. coli, Klebsiella* species, and *P. mirabilis.* There is limited clinical experience using cefazolin to treat IE caused by these pathogens; ampicillin or ceftriaxone is generally preferred.

In the treatment of IE, cefazolin is administered at a dose of 2 grams every 8 hours. The longer serum half-life of cefazolin (1.4 to 2.2 hours) permits less frequent administration compared to penicillins. Cefazolin is cleared renally and requires dose adjustment in patients with renal failure. With the exception of hypersensitivity reactions, cefazolin is generally well tolerated.

Cephalexin and cefadroxil are oral first-generation cephalosporins that may be used for prophylaxis prior to dental and surgical procedures in moderate- to high-risk patients. While amoxicillin is the standard prophylactic agent, these oral cephalosporins may be an alternative for patients with mild allergic reactions to amoxicillin. They should not be used in individuals with immediate-type hypersensitivity reaction to penicillins. The recommended dose for prophylaxis is 2 grams orally 1 hour before the procedure.

Ceftriaxone. Ceftriaxone is a third-generation cephalosporin with a broad spectrum of activity owing to substitutions to its basic ring structure. These substitutions increase its affinity for PBPs, increase penetration through the outer membrane of gram-negative organisms, and protect it from hydrolysis by many β-lactamases. Ceftriaxone is active against *E. coli, P. mirabilis, Klebsiella* species, *Salmonella* species, *Neisseria* species, *H. influenzae,* and the HACEK organisms, including most β-lactamase producing isolates. Ceftriaxone may be used to treat IE caused by susceptible isolates of gram-negative pathogens, sometimes in combination with an aminoglycoside. Ceftriaxone is also very active against streptococci, including isolates with elevated penicillin MICs. Clinical trials suggest that ceftriaxone is an effective agent in the treatment of streptococcal IE, and current guidelines recommend it as a first-line treatment option.[10,41,42]

Many isolates of *Enterobacter, Citrobacter, Serratia,* and other indole-positive, gram-negative bacilli initially test susceptible to ceftriaxone. These organisms produce an inducible, chromosomal β-lactamase (*AmpC*) that is capable of hydrolyzing cephalosporins. Resistance to ceftriaxone may emerge during treatment of these infections due to selection of mutants that constitutively produce β-lactamase.[43] Given the dire consequence of treatment failure, ceftriaxone should be avoided in cases of IE caused by these pathogens. Additional pathogens that are not reliably covered by ceftriaxone include *Pseudomonas aeruginosa* and *Bacteroides fragilis.*

In addition to its broad spectrum of activity, ceftriaxone has pharmacokinetic properties that make it an attractive agent for the treatment of IE. Ceftriaxone has a half-life of 7 to 8 hours that allows for treatment with a single daily intravenous injection. In the treatment of IE, ceftriaxone is usually administered at a dose of 2 grams once daily. The once-daily dose may be advantageous for home IV therapy in select patients with IE. Ceftriaxone has a dual mechanism of excretion, with 40% of the drug eliminated by the biliary system. As a result of its mixed elimination, ceftriaxone does not require dose adjustment in renal failure. High doses of ceftriaxone may cause pseudocholelithiasis, which is generally asymptomatic and occurs more frequently in children than adults. Therapy with broad-spectrum cephalosporins such as ceftriaxone may predispose patients to superinfection with resistant pathogens such as methicillin-resistant staphylococci, enterococci, and resistant gram-negative pathogens.[44]

Cefepime. Cefepime, a so-called fourth-generation cephalosporin, shares many of the characteristics of the third-generation cephalosporins. It has a spectrum of activity similar to ceftriaxone with added activity against *P. aeruginosa.* The substitutions to the basic cephem ring structure at position 7 make cefepime a poor inducer of chromosomal β-lactamase and more stable against hydrolysis compared to the third-generation compounds. As a result, cefepime may be used in the treatment of infections caused by pathogens with an inducible, chromosomal β-lactamase. In the context of IE, cefepime may be useful as an empirical agent when gram-negative pathogens are suspected and as directed therapy for IE caused by health care–associated gram-negative organisms.

Cefepime is cleared renally and has a half-life of 2 hours. In the treatment of IE, the recommended dose of cefepime is 2 grams every 8 hours. Like ceftriaxone, cefepime therapy may predispose patients to superinfection with resistant organisms.

Vancomycin

Vancomycin is a glycopeptide antibiotic produced by *Streptomyces orientalis.* Vancomycin was first isolated in 1952, with clinical use starting in 1956. It initially showed promise in treating infections caused by β-lactamase–producing staphylococci. The first semisynthetic penicillin, methicillin, was marketed in 1958 and thus replaced vancomycin as the drug of choice for infections caused by β-lactamase–producing staphylococci, as methicillin was considered to be less toxic and equally or more efficacious. Vancomycin use was relegated to patients with serious β-lactam allergies or infections caused by organisms resistant to the newer β-lactam agents. Clinical use of vancomycin began to increase in the 1980s with the emergence of methicillin-resistant *S. aureus* (MRSA) as an important health care–associated pathogen. The widespread use of vancomycin has continued over the past decade as MRSA has been increasingly associated with community-acquired infections. After a half-century of use, vancomycin remains a controversial agent, with debate over its place in therapy, its optimal dosing, the value of therapeutic monitoring, and its potential to cause toxicity.

Vancomycin inhibits cell wall synthesis by tightly binding the D-Ala–D-Ala terminus of the precursor peptidoglycan pentapeptide. Once bound, vancomycin blocks the transglycosylase reaction, preventing further elongation and cross-linking of peptidoglycan. As a result, the cell wall is weakened and the cell becomes susceptible to lysis. Vancomycin is primarily active against gram-positive pathogens as it does not readily pass through the outer membrane of gram-negative bacteria. It is active against *S. aureus* and coagulase-negative staphylococci, including methicillin-resistant strains. Vancomycin is also active against most clinical isolates of streptococci and enterococci, although vancomycin-resistant enterococci (VRE) are a notable exception.

VRE were first reported in Europe in 1986 and in the United States in 1987.[45] Vancomycin resistance occurs primarily through acquisition of the *vanA* gene present on a mobile genetic element. VanA confers inducible, high-level resistance to vancomycin and a similar glycopeptide antibiotic, teicoplanin. VanA catalyzes the formation of D-Ala–D-lactate, which is substituted for D-Ala–D-Ala as the terminal building block in the peptidoglycan precursor. Vancomycin affinity for the D-Ala–D-lactate terminus is 1000-fold less than for D-Ala–D-Ala, accounting for the observed resistance.[46] Sixteen years after the isolation of VRE, the first case of vancomycin-resistant *S. aureus* (VRSA) was reported in a patient in Michigan.[47] At least two subsequent cases of VRSA have been documented in the literature.[48,49] In each reported case, it appears that the resistant *S. aureus* isolate acquired the *vanA* gene from VRE, conferring high-level vancomycin resistance (MIC > 16 mcg/ml).[50,51] The relative rarity of this mechanism of resistance in staphylococci may be explained by inefficient replication of enterococcal plasmids in staphylococci.[52] A second type of vancomycin resistance in staphylococci has been described that results in "intermediate" levels of resistance (MIC 4 to 8 mcg/ml). The first vancomycin-intermediate *S. aureus* (VISA) was isolated in Japan in 1997.[53] The underlying mechanism of this resistance is poorly understood but appears to be related to a thickening of the cell wall with overexpression of D-ala–D-ala binding sites.[54] Many of these binding sites are nonproductive; vancomycin binding does not hamper the continued synthesis of the necessary cell wall components. Clinical VISA isolates are rare, and more commonly encountered are strains of MRSA that are "heteroresistant" to vancomycin (hVISA). The vancomycin MIC of hVISA is within the susceptible range (<2 mcg/ml), but these strains contain subpopulations that exhibit reduced susceptibility. The clinical consequence of hVISA is still a matter of debate. However, there are data to suggest that bloodstream infections caused by hVISA strains have been associated with a poor clinical response to vancomycin therapy.[55,56]

Vancomycin is bactericidal against many gram-positive pathogens, although vancomycin kills staphylococci relatively slowly and only if they are actively dividing. The rate of vancomycin killing for staphylococci is less than that of the antistaphylococcal penicillins both in vitro and in vivo.[57] This observation is consistent with clinical data that suggest vancomycin is inferior to β-lactam antibiotics in the treatment of staphylococcal IE.[58,59] In these studies, patients treated with vancomycin had a prolonged time to clearance of bacteremia and rates of treatment failure that were higher than those observed with the antistaphylococcal penicillins. As a single agent, vancomycin is often not bactericidal versus enterococci.[60] However, it produces synergistic killing when combined with gentamicin or streptomycin in susceptible enterococci.[61] In the treatment of enterococcal IE, vancomycin plus gentamicin or streptomycin is an alternative to a penicillin-based regimen, but there is less clinical experience using vancomycin. Clinical data and experience suggest that β-lactam antibiotics are favored over vancomycin for the treatment of IE caused by susceptible pathogens. Vancomycin should only be used in the treatment of IE caused by β-lactam–resistant organisms (MRSA, ampicillin-resistant enterococci) or in patients with a serious β-lactam allergy. In the latter case, desensitization to the β-lactam antibiotic may be considered in patients who have a poor response to vancomycin.

The dose of parenteral vancomycin should be based on the total body weight of the patient, taking into account renal function. In patients with normal renal function, the total daily dose of vancomycin is 30 mg/kg typically divided in two to three evenly spaced doses. Vancomycin is renally eliminated with a half-life in adults that ranges from 5 to 11 hours; in anephric patients, the half-life may be as long as 7 days. Several nomograms for modification of the initial vancomycin dose according to creatinine clearance have been published.[62,63] Monitoring of vancomycin serum levels may be helpful in preventing toxicity and assuring adequate therapeutic drug concentrations. However, there are no definitive studies relating vancomycin levels to treatment outcome or toxicity. Monitoring peak serum concentrations does not provide valuable data as vancomycin does not exhibit concentration-dependent killing. Monitoring of a steady state trough concentration is recommended when using vancomycin to treat serious infections such as IE. The vancomycin dose should be adjusted to achieve a target trough value of at least 10 to 15 mcg/ml. Once a target trough is obtained, continued monitoring of levels is not required except when there are changes in renal function.

Initial studies in the 1950s showed vancomycin to be ototoxic and nephrotoxic, although this is now thought to be related to impurities in the vancomycin product that earned it the nickname "Mississippi mud." In later studies with a more purified form of vancomycin, auditory toxicity was not seen, drug fever and rash were uncommon, and nephrotoxicity was seen infrequently and often occured with coadministration of aminoglycosides.[64,65] Vancomycin rarely causes interstitial nephritis. Reversible neutropenia may occur in up to 5% of patients receiving vancomycin, especially those receiving an extended course of therapy.[66] Vancomycin may cause thrombocytopenia more rarely. Rapid infusion of vancomycin has been associated with "red man" syndrome: a histamine-like response characterized by erythema, pruritis, hypotension, and angioedema. It can be prevented largely by prolonging the infusion time to 1 to 2 hours.[67] Pretreatment with antihistamines may also be helpful in preventing this reaction.[68]

Cell Membrane–Active Antibiotic

Daptomycin

Daptomycin, a fermentation product of *Streptomyces roseosporus,* is a cyclic lipopeptide with a highly lipophilic side chain linked to a cyclic 13-member peptide. Daptomycin is rapidly bactericidal against gram-positive organisms, including strains resistant to β-lactams and vancomycin. It is active against streptococci, enterococci (including VRE), and staphylococci (including MRSA). It is not active against gram-negative pathogens as it does not penetrate their outer membrane. The precise mechanism of action is not fully understood. Daptomycin is known to bind to the bacterial cell membrane via a calcium-dependent insertion of its lipid tail. Current understanding implies that it then forms an ion conduction structure, resulting in efflux of potassium ions with subsequent loss of the ion concentration gradient. Cell death occurs from widespread dysfunction in cellular processes, but cell lysis does not occur.

Daptomycin, at a dose of 6 mg/kg administered intravenously once daily, has been studied in the treatment of bacteremia and IE caused by *S. aureus.* In this study, daptomycin alone was found to be noninferior to standard therapy consisting of either nafcillin or vancomycin plus gentamicin for the first 4 days of treatment.[69] Based on the results of this trial, daptomycin was granted an indication by the U.S. Food and Drug Administration for bacteremia and right-sided IE caused by *S. aureus,* including MRSA. Approval for left-sided IE was not granted as there were small numbers of patients with this infection and failures were common regardless of therapy. Of concern, there were several cases of daptomycin treatment failure associated with the development of resistance during therapy. The mechanism of daptomycin resistance has not been fully elucidated. There have also been reports of daptomycin resistance in MRSA isolates with intermediate susceptibility to vancomycin (VISA).[70] The thickened cell wall that characterizes these isolates may interfere with the antimicrobial activity of daptomycin.[71] Daptomycin has not been rigorously evaluated for the treatment of IE caused by other pathogens.

Daptomycin was originally studied in the early 1990s. Skeletal muscle toxicity was observed in the early clinical trials, and further human studies were halted.[72] These adverse effects were seen with twice-daily dosing. Subsequent animal studies suggested the muscle toxicity correlated with high trough values seen with the twice-daily dosing regimen.[73] Several years later, the drug was re-licensed and clinical studies were started using a once-daily dosing regimen that sought to minimize potential for toxicity. In trials using the once-daily dosing regimen, the skeletal muscle toxicity has been seen but at much lower incidence (~3%).[74] Patients receiving daptomycin should have serum creatine phosphokinase (CPK) levels monitored weekly, and the patient should be monitored for signs and symptoms of myopathy. Daptomycin therapy should be discontinued in patients who develop myopathy with an elevated CPK (>5 times the upper limit of normal or >1000 units/L) or an isolated increase in CPK (>10 times the upper limit of normal). Daptomycin is renally eliminated with a half-life of 8 to 9 hours. In patients with a creatinine clearance less than 30 ml/min, the dosing interval should be extended to 48 hours.

Protein Synthesis Inhibitors

Aminoglycosides

Gentamicin and Streptomycin. Aminoglycosides are a group of structurally related polycationic antibiotics derived from different species of *Streptomyces* and *Micromonosporum.* These drugs inhibit protein synthesis by irreversibly binding to the 30S subunit of the bacterial ribosome. They demonstrate concentration-dependent bactericidal activity as well as a postantibiotic effect, demonstrated by residual bactericidal activity after the concentration has fallen below the MIC. Aminoglycosides passively diffuse through porins in the outer membrane of gram-negative bacteria. They are then actively transported across the cell membrane into the cytoplasm, where they bind to their ribosomal target. As a result of this process, aminoglycosides are primarily active against aerobic gram-negative organisms. They do not readily cross the cell wall of gram-positive organisms; hence, they are not active when administered as a single agent. However, aminoglycosides show synergistic killing against gram-positive pathogens when administered with a cell wall–active agent such as penicillin or vancomycin. Inhibition of cell wall synthesis permits the entry of aminoglycosides into the cytoplasm.

In the treatment of IE, the combination of a β-lactam and an aminoglycoside is frequently used to achieve synergisitic killing.[75] In enterococcal IE, the combination of penicillin and gentamicin is necessary to achieve bactericidal activity. Streptomycin may be used as an alternative if the enterococcus demonstrates high-level gentamicin resistance. In the treatment of viridans streptococcal IE, the addition of gentamicin to penicillin may shorten the duration of treatment for highly sensitive isolates or may be required for treatment of isolates with reduced susceptibility to penicillin. While gentamicin demonstrates in vitro synergy with nafcillin against *S. aureus,* its addition is considered optional in most cases of staphylococcal IE, with benefit limited to faster clearance of blood cultures. The exception is in uncomplicated right-sided IE caused by methicillin-susceptible *S. aureus* (MSSA), where the addition of gentamicin to nafcillin allows for a 2-week course of therapy. The recommended treatment of IE caused by gram-negative pathogens is generally a combination of an active β-lactam and an aminoglycoside. Gentamicin is recommended in the treatment of IE caused by *Bartonella* species.

Factors that must be considered for proper dosing of aminoglycosides in the treatment of IE include whether they are being used for gram-positive synergy and whether multiple-daily or once-daily dosing regimens should be used. When used for gram-positive synergy, the total daily dose of gentamicin in a person with normal renal function is 3 mg/kg per day. Traditionally, this dose has been administered in three equally divided doses (1 mg/kg every 8 hours) to achieve a peak serum level of 3 mcg/ml and trough level ≤1 mcg/ml. This method of dosing is recommended in the treatment of IE caused by staphylococci and enterococci. In vitro and clinical studies support the use of a once-daily dosing regimen (3 mg/kg as a single daily infusion) in the treatment of IE caused by viridans streptococci and *Streptococcus bovis.*[42,76] Target peak and trough concentrations have not been standardized for this regimen. In the treatment of IE caused by gram-negative pathogens, higher doses of gentamicin (5 to 8 mg/kg per day) are recommended. Multiple-daily dosing regimens (1.7 mg/kg every 8 hours) are administered to achieve peak levels of 6 to 8 mcg/ml and trough levels less than 2 mcg/ml. Once-daily, high-dose (8 mg/kg per day) regimens of gentamicin or tobramycin have been used in the treatment of *P. aeruginosa* IE with maintenance of peak and trough levels of 15 to 20 mcg/ml and ≤2 mcg/ml, respectively.[77]

Aminoglycosides are cleared by the kidney, and excretion is directly proportional to creatinine clearance. The normal half-life is 2 to 3 hours, increasing to 24 to 48 hours in patients with renal failure. Close monitoring of serum levels with appropriate dose adjustments must be made to prevent the accumulation of drug and subsequent toxicity. All aminoglycosides are nephrotoxic and ototoxic. Nephrotoxicity is generally reversible upon discontinuation of the aminoglycoside, while ototoxicity is irreversible. Risk factors for toxicity include advanced age, therapy for more than 5 days, use of higher doses, and preexisting renal insufficiency. Concurrent use of other nephrotoxic drugs increases the risk of nephrotoxicity. In very high doses, aminoglycosides may produce neuromuscular blockage resulting in respiratory paralysis.

Oxazolidinones

Linezolid. Linezolid is a synthetic oxazolidinone antibiotic that binds to the bacterial ribosome, preventing protein synthesis. Linezolid has a unique binding site located on the 23S ribosomal RNA of the 50S subunit; thus no cross-resistance is seen with other classes of antibiotics that act at the bacterial ribosome. Linezolid has bacteriostatic activity against gram-positive pathogens. Gram-negative bacteria are not susceptible due to an efflux mechanism. Resistance in gram-positive pathogens has been encountered but remains rare. Linezolid is active against MRSA, including isolates with reduced susceptibility to vancomcyin. It is one of the few antibiotics with reliable activity versus enterococci, both *Enterococcus faecalis* and *Enterococcus faecium*, including VRE.

Linezolid has been used primarily in the treatment of complicated skin and skin-structure infections and health care–associated pneumonia. Generally, bactericidal antibiotics have been used in the treatment IE, and linezolid is bacteriostatic. Linezolid has not been rigorously studied for the treatment of IE, but it has been used to treat cases caused by organisms resistant to conventional antibiotics and in patients allergic to first-line therapies. Linezolid is available in a highly bioavailable oral formulation, prompting its use in treating IE in situations in which intravenous therapy is not possible. There are case reports of both success and failure using linezolid alone or in combination with other active antibiotics for the treatment of IE.[78] Given the lack of proven efficacy in IE, linezolid should be considered an alternate therapy when conventional antibiotics cannot be used due to resistance or allergy.

Linezolid is available in both intravenous and oral formulations. The standard dose for both formulations is 600 mg administered twice daily. Linezolid is cleared hepatically, and no dose adjustment is necessary in renal failure. While short courses of linezolid were well tolerated in clinical studies, longer courses (>2 weeks) used in clinical practice are associated with several important adverse effects. Linezolid may cause reversible bone marrow suppression that usually manifests as thrombocytopenia.[79] More rarely, there have been case reports of peripheral neuropathy and optic neuritis.[80,81] Linezolid is also a weak monoamine oxidase inhibitor, and serotonin syndrome can occur when linezolid is coadminstered with drugs such as selective serotonin reuptake inhibitors.[82]

Streptogramins

Quinupristin-Dalfopristin. This antibiotic is a 70:30 mixture of quinupristin and dalfopristin, semisynthetic derivatives of streptogramin B and A, respectively. The streptogramin antibiotics are protein synthesis inhibitors that share the same ribosomal binding site as the macrolide and lincosamide antibiotics. Each component alone is bacteriostatic. When the two are combined, they may display bactericidal activity against susceptible pathogens. Quinupristin-dalfopristin is active against most gram-positive pathogens, including those that are resistant to multiple classes of antibiotics. A notable exception is *E. faecalis*, as it possesses an efflux pump that confers resistance. In contrast, most isolates of vancomycin-resistant *E. faecium* are susceptible to this agent.

Quinupristin-dalfopristin is approved for the treatment of serious infections due to vancomycin-resistant *E. faecium* associated with bacteremia. It has been used in the treatment of IE caused by this pathogen with case reports of both success and failure.[83,84] The recommended dose is 7.5 mg/kg administered parenterally via a central venous catheter every 8 hours. Patients with hepatic failure may not tolerate the standard dose due to increased serum levels seen in this patient population, and dose reduction may be necessary. Quinupristin-dalfopristin is often not well tolerated as many patients develop myalgias and/or arthralgias that may be severe. In one report, more than 50% of patients reported experiencing these symptoms.[85] Also of note, this agent inhibits the cytochrome P-450 3A4 enzyme, interfering with the clearance of drugs that are metabolized via this system.

Tetracyclines

Doxycycline. Doxycycline, a member of the tetracycline family of antibiotics, is a semisynthetic derivative of oxytetracycline. Doxycycline is a broad-spectrum, bacteriostatic antibiotic that reversibly binds to the 30S subunit of the bacterial ribosome. The spectrum of activity includes many gram-positive and gram-negative organisms. Doxycycline is particularly active against intracellular pathogens. The role of doxycycline in the therapy of IE is limited to "culture-negative" cases caused by fastidious organisms such as *Bartonella* species, *Brucella* species, and *C. burnetti* (Q fever). Doxycycline is frequently combined with another active agent such as an aminoglycoside or rifampin in these difficult-to-treat infections.[86]

The recommended dose of doxycycline is 100 mg administered intravenously or orally every 12 hours. When administered orally, absorption is impaired by di- and trivalent cations, including dairy products and antacids that contain these compounds; hence, it should not be coadministered with these products. Doxycycline is eliminated by nonrenal mechanisms and does not require dose adjustment in renal failure. Doxycycline is generally well tolerated. The most common side effects are gastrointestinal, such as nausea, vomiting, and diarrhea. Less common side effects include vestibular reactions and photosensitivity. Doxycycline is readily deposited in growing bones and teeth and should be avoided during pregnancy and childhood.

Ribonucleic Acid Synthesis Inhibitor

Rifamycins (Rifampin)

Rifampin is a semisynthetic derivative of rifamycin, an antibiotic produced by *Streptomyces mediterranei.* Rifampin binds tightly to the beta subunit of bacterial DNA-dependent RNA polymerase, thereby inhibiting RNA synthesis. It is active in vitro against gram-positive and gram-negative cocci, mycobacteria, and chlamydia. Rifampin is less active against gram-negative bacilli as it does not readily penetrate the outer membrane of these organisms. When used as a single agent, rifampin readily selects for highly resistant isolates. These isolates have a single point mutation in their RNA polymerase that confers high-level rifampin resistance.[87] To prevent the emergence of resistance, rifampin is combined with a second active antibiotic when used clinically.[88]

Rifampin has a unique role in the treatment of prosthetic device infections. Rifampin is able to penetrate into the biofilm that forms on prosthetic material and is active against slowly replicating intracellular organisms found therein.[89] As a result, rifampin is including in regimens for the treatment of prosthetic valve IE caused by staphylococci. While rifampin is generally bactericidal against staphylococci, the in vivo effect when combined with other antistaphylococcal agents is highly variable.[90-92] Routine addition of rifampin to the regimens used in the treatment of native valve IE caused by staphylococci is not recommended as studies have not demonstrated a clear benefit.[58] The predominantly oral regimen of rifampin plus ciprofloxacin has been used to successfully treat right-sided IE caused by *S. aureus* in IDUs.[93]

Rifampin is available in intravenous and oral formulations, and the oral formulation is well absorbed. Rifampin is metabolized by the liver, and dose adjustment for renal insufficiency is unnecessary. Patients should be informed that rifampin may turn bodily fluids such as sweat, urine, and tears an orange color. Adverse effects include rash, thrombocytopenia, and nephritis. In addition, rifampin may cause cholestatic jaundice and more rarely hepatitis. Rifampin is also a potent inducer of cytochrome P-450 enzymes, and close attention must be paid to potential drug interaction.

Deoxyribonucleic Acid Synthesis Inhibitors

Fluoroquinolones

Ciprofloxacin, Levofloxacin, and Moxifloxacin. The fluoroquinolones are synthetic analogues of nalidixic acid that act by disrupting bacterial DNA synthesis through inhibition of topoisomerase II (DNA gyrase) and topoisomerase IV. They exhibit bactericidal activity against many gram-positive and gram-negative bacteria. As use of these agents has increased, resistance has become a major problem. While these compounds are active against many of the typical pathogens that cause IE, clinical data supporting their use are sparse. They may be considered as alternative agents for IE caused by gram-negative pathogens when a β-lactam antibiotic cannot be administered. Ciprofloxacin in combination with rifampin is an oral regimen that has been used with some success in the treatment of right-sided IE cause by *S. aureus.*[93] The combination of these two drugs results in synergistic killing and also prevents the emergence of resistance to either agent.[94]

The fluoroquinolones may be administered intravenously and are also well absorbed when given orally. They have relatively long half-lives that permit once- or twice-daily dosing. The fluoroquinolones have varied routes of elimination. Levofloxacin is predominantly renally eliminated, ciprofloxacin is eliminated by both renal and hepatic routes, while moxifloxacin is mainly hepatically eliminated. These agents are generally very well tolerated. Adverse effects include gastrointestinal upset, headache, dizziness, photosensitivity, and skin rash. As fluoroquinolones may damage growing cartilage, they are not recommended for use during pregnancy or in childhood. There have also been reports of tendinitis in adults receiving fluoroquinolones. Absorption of oral fluoroquinlones may be impaired when coadministered with products containing di- and trivalent cations.

Antifungals

Amphotericin B Preparations

Amphotericin B is an amphoteric polyene antifungal produced by *Streptomyces nodosus.* It is a highly lipophilic molecule that is prepared as a colloidal suspension with sodium dexoxycholate for intravenous injection. Amphotericin B binds to ergosterol, a component of the fungal cell membrane. Upon binding, amphotericin alters the permeability of the cell by forming pores in the fungal cell membrane. The pores allow leakage of intracellular ions and macromolecules, leading to cell death. Amphotericin B has a broad spectrum of activity against clinically relevant fungi, including most *Candida* and *Aspergillus* species. It may be fungicidal or fungistatic depending on the drug concentration and sensitivity of the organism.

Until the early 1990s, amphotericin B was the only antifungal available for the treatment of serious, systemic fungal infections. As a result, clinical experience in treating fungal IE has been almost exclusively with amphotericin B.[95] It is still considered the preferred treatment option despite its propensity to cause nephrotoxicity. Administration of amphotericin B causes a decline in glomerular filtration rate and renal blood flow in addition to impaired proximal and distal tubular reabsorption of electrolytes. Patients with fungal IE commonly require high doses and prolonged treatment courses, placing them at high risk for amphotericin B–related nephrotoxicity. Newer lipid-associated formulations of amphotericin B are considered equally efficacious and have lower rates of renal toxicity. For these reasons, the lipid-associated formulations may be preferable for the treating fungal IE. Nephrotoxicity may be minimized by reversing sodium depletion with normal saline boluses administered before and after each infusion.[96] Close monitoring for hypokalemia and hypomagnesemia is also warranted, with repletion when necessary. Amphotericin B infusion-related reactions such as chills, fevers, and phlebitis at the injection site are also common. Premedication with meperidine and/or hydrocortisone has been shown to be helpful in alleviating these symptoms.[97,98] Acetaminophen and diphenhydramine are also frequently prescribed as part of the pretreatment regimen, but clinical evidence does not support this practice.

Triazoles (Fluconazole)

The triazole antifungals are synthetic compounds that inhibit the fungal cytochrome P-450 enzyme 14α-demethylase. This enzyme is responsible for the biosynthesis of ergosterol, an essential component of the fungal cell membrane. The triazoles are considered to be fungistatic agents. Fluconazole, the triazole with which there is most clinical experience, has activity against most *Candida* species, including *Candida albicans.* However, some non-*albicans* species such as *Candida krusei* and *Candida glabrata* may be resistant. Fluconazole has been used for long-term treatment of IE caused by *Candida* as it can be administered orally and is very well tolerated.[95] Adverse effects include upper gastrointestinal adverse effects, headache, skin rash, and mild elevations in hepatic enzymes. Rare cases of hepatic toxicity have been reported; therefore, hepatic enzymes should be checked at the start of fluconazole therapy and intermittently thereafter.

Nonantibiotic Interventions

While prolonged antibiotic therapy is curative in many patients with IE, surgery plays a key role in a substantial subset. Valve replacement surgery, in conjunction with appropriate antimicrobials, is associated with lower mortality in observational studies of patients with complicated left-sided IE.[7,99] However, no randomized trials have been performed to identify indications for surgery. Congestive heart failure unresponsive to medical therapy is an indication for valve replacement, and moderate to severe congestive heart failure is a strong predictor of mortality.[100] Other cardiac complications of IE, including valvular dehiscence, rupture, or fistula or perivalvular abscess, probably benefit from surgery as well.

Another potential role for surgery is to prevent embolic complications. However, the relationship between features of the vegetation as seen on echocardiogram and the risk for clinical events is not clear. Vegetations greater than 10 mm and mitral valve vegetations, particularly those on the anterior leaflet, are associated with higher risk for emboli.[101] Vegetations greater than 15 mm in length and highly mobile vegetations may be particularly prone to embolize.[102] Since embolization is most likely to occur before beginning antibiotics and the risk decreases over the first 2 weeks of treatment, surgery with the aim of preventing embolization should be performed early. Unfortunately, embolic complications already may be present before or during evaluation for IE. In patients with stroke secondary to septic emboli and indications for valve surgery, the timing of surgery has been controversial. Due to risks of bleeding with cardiopulmonary bypass and concerns for exacerbating acute neurologic injury, delaying surgery several weeks, when possible, has been recommended.[103] Other studies suggest that early surgery can be performed safely in patients with uncomplicated strokes when otherwise indicated,[104] and may even be preferred.[105]

Microbiologic considerations may also lead to valve replacement. Uncontrolled infection and persistently positive blood cultures despite appropriate antibiotic therapy should prompt consideration for surgery. The infecting organism can influence the need for intervention. Fungi and aerobic gram-negative bacilli, such as *Pseudomonas,* are difficult to eradicate with antibiotics alone. Patients with *Brucella* and *C. burnetti* IE often require valve replacement and prolonged courses of antibiotics.

Use of aspirin could be of theoretical benefit in the treatment of IE because it has both antiplatelet and antimicrobial properties.[106] However, a randomized, placebo-controlled trial of daily aspirin in conjunction with antibiotic treatment failed to show any therapeutic benefit and resulted in a trend toward increased incidence of bleeding.[107] Therefore, aspirin is not recommended for treatment of IE. Anticoagulation is relatively contraindicated in patients with left-sided IE due to concerns about central nervous system (CNS) hemorrhage. In patients with mechanical prosthetic valves who are maintained on anticoagulation, the management is more difficult. For *S. aureus* prosthetic valve IE in which a CNS embolic event has occurred, anticoagulation should be discontinued for at least the first 2 weeks of antibiotic therapy.[10,108]

Therapeutic Approach

Viridans Group Streptococci, Streptococcus bovis, Abiotrophia defectiva, Granulicatella *Species, and* Gemella *Species*

Overview. The viridans group streptococci include a variety of α-hemolytic streptococcal species that are part of the normal human respiratory and gastrointestinal flora. They are a common cause of subacute IE in patients with congenital valvular abnormalities who are not IDUs. *Streptococcus bovis* is a non-enterococcal penicillin-susceptible group D streptococcus that is also part of the normal human gastrointestinal flora. *Streptococcus bovis* may also cause subacute IE that is clinically indistinguishable from infection caused by viridans streptococci. *Abiotrophia defectiva* and *Granulicatella* species (formerly known as nutritionally variant streptococci) have nutritional deficiencies that hinder their growth in routine laboratory culture media. *Gemella* species share some physiologic characteristics with the nutritionally variant streptococci and are treated with the same antibiotic regimen. These pathogens cause IE that has been more difficult to cure in comparison to disease caused by highly penicillin-susceptible viridans streptococci and *S. bovis.*[109]

Antimicrobial therapy for IE caused by viridans streptococci and *S. bovis* is dictated by the penicillin MIC of the clinical isolate. Many isolates are exquisitely sensitive to penicillin and can be treated successfully with penicillin or ceftriaxone alone. The addition of gentamicin to penicillin or ceftriaxone results in synergistic killing of viridans streptococci and *S. bovis* in vitro.[110] The optional addition of gentamicin may allow for an abbreviated course of therapy in certain patients with IE caused by highly susceptible isolates. Of concern, isolates with elevated penicillin MICs are being encountered with increasing frequency. Higher doses of penicillin with addition of synergistic doses of gentamicin may be required for successful treatment of IE caused by isolates with elevated penicillin MICs.

When gentamicin is included in the treatment regimen, monitoring of serum levels may be warranted in patients with renal insufficiency. The target peak and trough concentrations with the recommended once-daily gentamicin dose are not defined. Current treatment guidelines reference a gentamicin dosing nomogram to assist in adjusting the dose; however, this nomogram is not valid for the recommended 3-mg/kg once-daily dose.[111] A reasonable approach would be to check a trough level just before the next dose is scheduled. If the trough is undetectable, then no dose adjustment is necessary. If there is a detectable level, the dosing interval should be extended to every 36 or 48 hours. Alternatively, the conventional regimen of multiple daily doses may be used to target a peak of 3 mcg/ml and a trough ≤1 mcg/ml.

Viridans Group Streptococci and *S. bovis* with Penicillin MIC ≥ 0.12 mcg/ml. Treatment recommendations for highly penicillin-susceptible viridans streptococci and *S. bovis* are presented in Table 81-1.[10] Clinical studies have shown high cure rates (≥98%) in patients who receive 4 weeks of intravenous penicillin G or ceftriaxone for IE caused by highly penicillin-susceptible isolates.[41,112] These cure rates are comparable to those achieved with combined penicillin-aminoglycoside regimens, suggesting that the addition of a synergistic aminoglycoside is not warranted when 4 weeks of treatment is administered. The 4-week penicillin and ceftriaxone regimens are equally efficacious, yet each has different potential benefits and drawbacks. Penicillin has a narrower spectrum of activity but is typically administered in multiple daily doses. Outpatient therapy with penicillin may be possible if administered as a continuous infusion via a programmed pump. Ceftriaxone offers the convenience of a once-daily infusion; however, it has a broad spectrum of activity that may predispose patients to superinfection with resistant pathogens.

Several clinical studies have examined the efficacy of shorter treatment durations using 2 weeks of combination therapy with penicillin G or ceftriaxone and an aminoglycoside.[42,113,114] These studies have shown similar cure rates for 2-week combination regimens when compared to 4 weeks of penicillin G or ceftriaxone monotherapy. In two of these studies, once-daily ceftriaxone was combined with a once-daily dose of aminoglycoside (netilmicin or gentamicin). The once-daily ceftriaxone-aminoglycoside regimens demonstrated efficacy equivalent to a regimen consisting of multiple daily doses of penicillin G and an aminoglycoside. The 2-week regimen of penicillin G or

TABLE 81-1 TREATMENT FOR INFECTIVE ENDOCARDITIS DUE TO VIRIDANS GROUP STREPTOCOCCI, *STREPTOCOCCUS BOVIS, ABIOTROPHIA DEFECTIVA, GRANULICATELLA* SPECIES, AND *GEMELLA* SPECIES

Organism	Regimen*
Viridans group streptococci and *Streptococcus bovis* with penicillin MIC ≤ 0.12 mcg/ml	**1.** Penicillin G 2-3 million units every 4 hr × 2 wk *or* Ceftriaxone 2 g every 24 hr × 2 wk *plus* Gentamicin 3 mg/kg every 24 hr × 2 wk (regimen #1 not for prosthetic valve IE) **2.** Penicillin G 2-3 million units every 4 hr × 4 wk (for prosthetic valve IE: 4 million units every 4 hr × 6 wk) *or* Ceftriaxone 2 g every 24 hr × 4 wk (for prosthetic valve IE: ×6 wk) **3.** Vancomycin 15 mg/kg every 12 hr × 4 wk (regimen #3 only if β-lactams not tolerated; for prosthetic valve IE: ×6 wk)
Viridans group streptococci and *Streptococcus bovis* with penicillin MIC > 0.12 mcg/ml and ≤0.5 mcg/ml	**1.** Penicillin G 4 million units every 4 hr × 4 wk (for prosthetic valve IE: ×6 wk) *or* Ceftriaxone 2 g every 24 hr × 4 wk (for prosthetic valve IE: ×6 wk) *plus* Gentamicin 3 mg/kg every 24 hr × 2 wk (for prosthetic valve IE: ×6 wk) **2.** Vancomycin 15 mg/kg every 12 hr × 4 wk (regimen #2 only if β-lactams not tolerated; for prosthetic valve IE: ×6 wk)
Viridans group streptococci with penicillin MIC > 0.5 mcg/ml and *Abiotrophia defectiva, Granulicatella* species, *Gemella* species	See regimen for enterococci susceptible to penicillin, gentamicin, and vancomycin (Table 81-2)

*Specific points:
- Adult dosing only.
- Doses are for normal renal function.
- All regimens are intravenous (IV) unless specifically noted.
- Ceftriaxone, gentamicin, and streptomycin can be dosed intramuscularly, if necessary.
- For situations in which there are alternate, first-line regimens without gentamicin, gentamicin should be avoided in patients at elevated risk for toxicity.
- Penicillin can be dosed routinely every 4 hours or as a continuous infusion; every-6-hour dosing may be acceptable in certain circumstances.

MIC, minimum inhibitory concentration.

ceftriaxone plus gentamicin may be considered for uncomplicated cases of IE in patients who are at low risk for adverse effects caused by gentamicin. This regimen is relatively simple and may allow for earlier hospital discharge.

Vancomycin is the recommended treatment for patients with a serious β-lactam allergy. Vancomycin should not be used in the absence of a convincing allergy history. There are no clinical data that support using shorter courses of vancomycin in combination with an aminoglycoside in this situation. A 4-week regimen of vancomycin monotherapy should be administered.

Treatment of prosthetic valve IE is similar to that of native valve IE, but the treatment duration should be extended to 6 weeks. Some clinicians would add gentamicin for the first 2 weeks of therapy. There are no clinical data to support this practice, and patients may be placed at unnecessary risk for gentamicin-related toxicities. For this reason, the routine addition of 2 weeks of gentamicin is not recommended.

***Viridans Group Streptococci* and *S. bovis* with Penicillin MIC Greater Than 0.12 to ≥0.5 mcg/ml.** Treatment recommendations for viridans streptococci and *S. bovis* with a penicillin MIC greater than 0.12 to ≤0.5 mcg/ml are presented in Table 81-1.[10] Published data for treatment of IE caused by viridans streptococci with a penicillin MIC greater than 0.12 mcg/ml are limited. Current treatment guidelines recommend combination therapy with penicillin or ceftriaxone and gentamicin. Gentamicin should be administered for the first 2 weeks of the 4-week treatment regimen.

***Abiotrophia defectiva* and *Granulicatella* Species, *Gemella* Species, and Viridans Group Streptococci with Penicillin MIC Greater Than 0.5 mcg/ml.** Determination of antimicrobial susceptibilities for the nutritionally variant streptococci is technically difficult and may be inaccurate. Elevated pencillin MICs are common in these organisms. In a recent report, 50% of clinical isolates had intermediate susceptibility to penicillin (i.e., MICs of 0.25 to 2 mcg/ml). In addition, 33% of isolates were fully resistant to the third-generation cephalosporin cefotaxime.[115] Given microbiologic data and clinical experience that suggest IE caused by these organisms is more difficult to treat, current guidelines recommend a regimen used for treatment of enterococcal IE.[10] Penicillin or ampicillin should be given in combination with gentamicin for the entire 4 to 6 weeks of treatment. Patients with a serious β-lactam allergy should receive vancomycin plus gentamicin for a full 6 weeks. Prosthetic valve IE should be treated with 6 weeks of therapy.

Streptococcus pneumoniae, Streptococcus pyogenes, *and Groups B, C, and G Streptococci*

IE caused by these organisms is relatively uncommon, and therefore treatment recommendations are based on case series and expert opinion. Of concern, IE caused by these pathogens is associated with a much higher mortality rate (24% to 47%) in comparison to IE caused by viridans streptococci.[116-118] There are data that suggest that valve replacement surgery in addition to medical therapy may improve treatment outcomes when compared to medical therapy alone.[119,120] Accordingly, prompt evaluation for valve replacement surgery is recommended.

For strains of *S. pneumoniae* that are fully susceptible to penicillin (MIC ≤ 0.06 mcg/ml), 4 weeks of therapy with a highly active β-lactam antibiotic is recommended. Penicillin G (12 to 24 million units/day), ampicillin (12 g/day), or ceftriaxone (2 g/day) may be used in this situation. Strains of *S. pneumoniae* with reduced susceptibility to penicillin are being encountered with increasing frequency.[121] The majority of strains are intermediately susceptible (MIC 0.1 to 1.0), while a smaller number are resistant (MIC ≥ 2 mcg/ml). A retrospective case series of patients with pneumococcal IE compared treatment outcomes for strains that were fully sensitive to those with reduced susceptibility.[116] In this study, reduced susceptibility to penicillin did not impact treatment outcomes, suggesting that treatment with high-dose penicillin (24 to 30 million units/day) or ceftriaxone (2 g/day) is appropriate in patients who do not have concurrent meningitis.

Streptococcus pyogenes is universally susceptible to penicillin, and IE caused by this pathogen should be treated with intravenous penicillin G for 4 weeks. Ampicillin and ceftriaxone are acceptable alternatives to penicillin G. Vancomycin therapy should be reserved for patients with a serious allergic response to β-lactam antibiotics. Groups B, C, and G streptococci are generally penicillin susceptible, but there are reports of infection caused by isolates with reduced susceptibility to penicillin.[117,118] IE caused by groups B, C, and G streptococci should also be treated with penicillin, ampicillin, or ceftriaxone for 4 to 6 weeks; some experts would add gentamicin at synergistic doses for the first 2 weeks of therapy.

Enterococci

Overview. Enterococci are gram-positive pathogens that are part of the normal flora of the human gastrointestinal tract. While there are numerous species of enterococci, *E. faecalis* and *E. faecium* are responsible for the majority of enterococcal infections in humans. Enterococci are the third most common cause of native valve IE in patients who are not IDUs. Treatment of enterococcal IE is problematic as these pathogens are relatively resistant to penicillin, ampicillin, and vancomycin. In general, monotherapy with these antibiotics does not result in bactericidal activity at clinically achievable concentrations.[60] Historical studies have demonstrated poor outcomes (40% to 50% cure rate) when penicillin G or ampicillin is used as monotherapy for enterococcal IE. As a result, cell wall–active antibiotics are administered in combination with synergistic doses of aminoglycosides to achieve bactericidal activity and improve clinical outcomes (>80% cure rate).[122]

While enterococci are resistant to standard concentrations of aminoglycosides, the combination of synergistic doses of gentamicin or streptomycin with an active cell wall agent may result in bactericidal killing of these pathogens.[61,123] Enterococci must be screened for high-level aminoglycoside resistance as synergistic killing does not occur if this mechanism of resistance is present. High-level aminoglycoside resistance is defined as a MIC ≥ 500 mcg/ml for gentamicin or ≥1000 mcg/ml for streptomycin and is mediated by the presence of aminoglycoside-modifying enzymes. Isolates that are highly gentamicin resistant are also resistant to other aminoglycosides, except some strains may remain susceptible to streptomycin. Other aminoglycosides (e.g., tobramycin) should not be substituted for gentamicin or streptomycin as they may not provide synergistic activity even in the absence of high-level resistance. Animal studies of enterococcal IE that have compared once-daily aminoglycoside dosing regimens to every-8-hour dosing regimens have not conclusively demonstrated the effectiveness of the once-daily regimen.[124,125] Therefore, gentamicin and streptomycin should be administered in multiple daily doses when treating enterococcal IE.

Enterococci Susceptible to Penicillin, Vancomycin, and Gentamicin. Treatment recommendations for enterococcal IE caused by isolates susceptible to penicillin, vancomycin, and gentamicin are presented in Table 81-2.[10] The recommended regimen for native valve enterococcal IE is penicillin G or ampicillin combined with gentamicin for a full 4 to 6 weeks of therapy. Ampicillin is generally preferred over penicillin G as it is more active in vitro against enterococci. Both penicillin G and ampicillin may be administered as a continuous 24-hour infusion, but in vivo studies in animals have not demonstrated a clear benefit to this practice.[126,127] The duration of treatment is based on the length of symptoms prior to initiation of therapy. Patients with less than 3 months of symptoms may be treated with 4 weeks of therapy, while patients with at least 3 months of symptoms should be treated with 6 weeks of therapy.[128] Patients with prosthetic valve IE should be treated with a full 6 weeks of therapy.

There are no demonstrated differences in treatment outcomes between regimens containing gentamicin or streptomycin.[128] A major advantage of using gentamicin is the ability to routinely monitor serum concentrations. For this reason, when an isolate is susceptible to both drugs, gentamicin should be used. In patients with normal renal function, gentamicin is dosed at 1 mg/kg every 8 hours to target a peak level of approximately 3 mcg/ml and a trough ≤1 mcg/ml. For patients with preexisting renal insufficiency or those who develop treatment-related nephrotoxicity, target levels may be obtained by

TABLE 81-2 TREATMENT FOR INFECTIVE ENDOCARDITIS DUE TO ENTEROCOCCI

Organism	Regimen*
Enterococci susceptible to penicillin, gentamicin, and vancomycin	**1.** Ampicillin 2 g every 4 hr × 4-6 wk (for symptoms >3 mo or prosthetic valve IE: ×6 wk) *or* Penicillin G 3-5 million units every 4 hr × 4-6 wk (for symptoms >3 mo or prosthetic valve IE: ×6 wk) *plus* Gentamicin 1 mg/kg every 8 hr × 4-6 wk (for symptoms >3 mo or prosthetic valve IE: ×6 wk) **2.** Vancomycin 15 mg/kg every 12 hr × 6 wk *plus* Gentamicin 1 mg/kg every 8 hr × 6 wk (regimen #2 only if penicillins not tolerated)
Enterococci susceptible to penicillin, vancomycin, and streptomycin; resistant to gentamicin	**1.** Ampicillin 2 g every 4 hr × 4-6 wk (for symptoms >3 mo or prosthetic valve IE: ×6 wk) *or* Penicillin G 4 million units every 4 hr × 4-6 wk (for symptoms >3 mo or prosthetic valve IE: ×6 wk) *plus* Streptomycin 15 mg/kg every 12 hr × 4-6 wk (for symptoms >3 mo or prosthetic valve IE: ×6 wk) **2.** Vancomycin 15 mg/kg every 12 hr × 6 wk *plus* Streptomycin 15 mg/kg every 12 hr × 6 wk (regimen #2 only if penicillins not tolerated)

*Specific points:
- Adult dosing only.
- Doses are for normal renal function.
- All regimens are intravenous (IV) unless specifically noted.
- Ceftriaxone, gentamicin, and streptomycin can be dosed intramuscularly, if necessary.
- For situations in which there are alternate, first-line regimens without gentamicin, gentamicin should be avoided in patients at elevated risk for toxicity.
- Penicillin can be dosed routinely every 4 hours or as a continuous infusion; every-6-hour dosing may be acceptable in certain circumstances.

extending the dosing interval to every 12 or 24 hours. If patients develop acute renal failure, consideration can be given to discontinuing the gentamicin. This approach is supported by a prospective study in which many patients had the aminoglycoside discontinued 2 to 3 weeks into therapy.[129] In these patients, early discontinuation of the aminoglycoside did not adversely affect treatment outcomes. Further studies supporting an abbreviated course of gentamicin are needed before this practice can be routinely recommended in patients who do not experience significant treatment-related toxicities.

Vancomycin should be used only when there is a convincing history of a serious allergic reaction to penicillin. The combination of penicillin or ampicillin plus gentamicin is more active than vancomycin plus gentamicin in vitro and in animal models of IE.[75,130] There is also less clinical experience using the vancomycin-gentamicin combination. Additionally, vancomycin may increase the potential nephrotoxicity and ototoxicity associated with gentamicin therapy. For these reasons, penicillin desensitization may be considered for patients with a serious allergy. When the vancomycin-gentamicin regimen is used, the treatment duration for native valve IE is 6 weeks, while the duration for prosthetic valve endocarditis should be a minimum of 6 weeks and potentially longer based on clinical response.

Enterococci Susceptible to Penicillin, Vancomycin, and Streptomycin; Resistant to Gentamicin. Treatment recommendations for enterococcal IE caused by isolates susceptible to penicillin, vancomycin, and streptomycin are presented in Table 81-2.[10] The approach to treatment is essentially the same as that described previously with streptomycin substituted in place of gentamicin. In patients with normal renal function, streptomycin is dosed at 7.5 mg/kg every 12 hours to target a peak concentration of 20 to 35 mcg/ml and a trough concentration of less than 10 mcg/ml. Streptomycin serum concentration monitoring is not routinely available at most medical centers, but samples may be sent to an outside laboratory that has this capacity. Streptomycin has been associated with more ototoxicity than other aminoglycosides, so special consideration should be given to obtaining a baseline audiometric exam. Patients should be monitored closely for signs and symptoms of ototoxicity throughout an extended course of therapy with any aminoglycoside.

Enterococci Susceptible to Vancomycin and Aminoglycosides; Resistant to Penicillin. *Enterococcus faecium* isolates may be highly resistant to penicillin and ampicillin and retain susceptibility to vancomycin. This resistance is mediated by changes in the target PBP that dramatically reduce the binding affinity of penicillin and ampicillin. In vitro synergy studies do not support the use of penicillin-aminoglycoside combinations when high-level penicillin resistance is present.[131] *Enterococcus faecalis* isolates are generally more susceptible to penicillin; however, resistant strains have been encountered. Rarely, strains of *E. faecalis* may produce an inducible β-lactamase that is difficult to detect by routine susceptibility testing.[132,133] Detection of this β-lactamase requires screening for resistance with an inoculum that is 100-fold greater than what is typically used to detect β-lactamase production. This enterococcal β-lactamase is inhibited by the available β-lactamase inhibitors. Accordingly, ampicillin-sulbactam plus an aminoglycoside may be used to treat IE caused by isolates that produce β-lactamase.

Enterococci Susceptible to Penicillin and Vancomycin; Resistant to Gentamicin and Streptomycin. There are few well-documented cases of IE due to enterococci highly resistant to both gentamicin and streptomycin. Nevertheless, strains with high-level resistance to both streptomycin and gentamicin are now sufficiently common that the number of cases of IE due to these organisms will continue to increase. Treatment recommendations for these strains are based on limited case reports as well as in vitro and animal model data. Monotherapy with ampicillin or vancomycin may be attempted as there is no benefit to combination therapy with gentamicin or streptomycin. In this situation, some experts recommend administration of ampicillin as a continuous 24-hour infusion to provide sustained high levels of antibiotic. Novel synergistic combinations of antibiotics may be useful in patients who do not have an adequate clinical response to ampicillin monotherapy. In patients who fail to respond to therapy, valve replacement surgery may afford the best chance of cure.

Synergistic bactericidal activity has been demonstrated in vitro and in vivo for *E. faecalis* using a double β-lactam regimen containing ampicillin and ceftriaxone or cefotaxime.[134,135] While enterococci are intrinsically resistant to cephalosporins, synergy occurs when administered with ampicillin as a result of the saturation of different PBP targets. The ampicillin-cephalosporin regimen has been successfully used to treat IE caused by aminoglycoside-resistant strains in experimental models and in a small number of patients.[136] The combination of ampicillin and ciprofloxacin has demonstrated synergistic in vitro activity against isolates of *E. faecalis* and *E. faecium* with ciprofloxacin MICs ≤ 8 mcg/ml.[137] There is a single case report of two patients with aminoglycoside-resistant IE that were successfully treated with the combination of ampicillin and a fluoroquinolone.[138] If either of these novel regimens is used, consideration may be given to performing in vitro time-kill studies to test for the presence of synergistic killing.

Enterococci Resistant to Penicillin, Vancomycin, and Aminoglycosides. Few therapeutic options are available for the treatment of IE caused by VRE. Treatment recommendations are based on in vitro data, animal models of IE, and case reports. While antibiotic therapy is limited, a recent review of the literature showed a relatively high success rate in curing IE caused by VRE with a minority of patients requiring valve replacement surgery.[139] Linezolid and daptomycin are generally active against vancomycin-resistant strains of *E. faecalis* and *E. faecium*, while quinupristin-dalfopristin is active against *E. faecium* but not *E. faecalis*. There have been reports of both success and failure when linezolid or quinupristin-dalfopristin has been used to treat IE caused by VRE.[78,83,84] Quinupristin-dalfopristin has significant toxicities that may limit its use. Linezolid also has increased potential for toxicity when given for extended courses. Daptomycin has excellent in vitro activity against enterococci, including those resistant to vancomycin.[140] In vitro and animal models support the use of daptomycin in the treatment of enterococcal IE, but clinical data are lacking.[141,142]

Staphylococci

Overview. Staphylococci are a frequent cause of both native and prosthetic valve IE. *Staphylococcus aureus* has traditionally been associated with right-sided, native valve disease in IDUs.[143,144] Cure rates for right-sided IE caused by *S. aureus* are high and may be achieved with a short treatment course (2 weeks) for uncomplicated disease caused by methicillin-susceptible isolates. However, recent studies show that *S. aureus* has become the most common cause of IE in the developed world, largely as a result of contact with the health care system.[1] In health care–associated IE, *S. aureus* frequently causes left-sided disease of both native and prosthetic valves. Left-sided disease is associated with a significant risk of embolic complications, metastatic infection, perivalvular abscess, and death. In left-sided disease, treatment courses are prolonged (4 to 6 weeks) and valve replacement surgery may be necessary to prevent embolic complications and achieve cure.

Coagulase-negative staphylococci (CoNS) are one of the most frequent causes of prosthetic valve IE, but they may cause native valve disease as well.[145,146] IE caused by CoNS may have a more subacute presentation than IE caused by *S. aureus*. An exception is IE caused by *Staphylococcus lugdunensis*, a more virulent species of CoNS. This organism causes IE that has a presentation much like that with *S. aureus*, with high rates of metastatic infection and perivalvular disease.[147] Unlike other CoNS, *S. lugdunensis* is very susceptible to most antibiotics and can be treated based on in vitro sensitivities with a standard regimen recommended for other staphylococci. Many microbiology labs do not routinely speciate CoNS. If there is a high clinical suspicion that *S. lugdunensis* is the causative pathogen, the microbiology lab should be notified so they may perform the appropriate tests to identify this species.

The antistaphylococcal penicillins, nafcillin and oxacillin, are considered the preferred treatment choices for IE caused by methicillin-susceptible staphylococci. Cefazolin is more susceptible to hydrolysis by the staphylococcal β-lactamase and is less effective in the treatment of experimental endocarditis caused by MSSA.[39,148] The clinical significance of these observations is unknown, as cefazolin has been used to successfully treat IE caused by MSSA. For these reasons, cefazolin should be considered a second-line agent for patients with a penicillin allergy that is not anaphylactic in nature. Vancomycin may be used in patients with an anaphylactic reaction to β-lactams, but data from animal models of IE and clinical studies in humans suggest that vancomycin is inferior to β-lactams in the treatment of *S. aureus* IE.[57,58] Therefore, desensitization and treatment with a β-lactam may be considered. Occasionally staphylococcal isolates do not produce a β-lactamase and are sensitive to pencillin. IE caused by susceptible isolates may be treated with penicillin G.

Increasing rates of methicillin resistance have complicated the treatment of IE caused by staphylococci. MRSA was once almost exclusively a hospital-acquired infection. Over the last decade, community-acquired MRSA has been encountered with increasing frequency. In fact, methicillin-resistant strains are more prevalent than methicillin-sensitive strains in some communities.[149-151] As the burden of disease caused by MRSA increases, a greater portion of the cases of IE will also be caused by MRSA. Vancomycin is still considered the gold standard treatment for IE caused by MRSA, although in vitro data, animal studies, and clinical experience show that it is less effective than β-lactam antibiotics against MSSA. Daptomycin is approved for the treatment of right-sided IE caused by MSSA and MRSA and represents an alternative to vancomycin.[69] Clinical experience in treating IE with other antibiotics active against MRSA is limited, and none of these drugs can be recommended on the basis of available data.

Right-Sided, Native Valve IE. Treatment recommendations for right-sided, native valve IE caused by staphylococci are presented in Table 81-3.[10] When gentamicin is combined with an antistaphylococcal penicillin, synergistic killing is observed in vitro.[152] Several studies have

TABLE 81-3 TREATMENT FOR INFECTIVE ENDOCARDITIS DUE TO STAPHYLOCOCCI

Organism and Infection Characteristics	Regimen*
Methicillin-sensitive staphylococci, right-sided IE	Nafcillin or oxacillin 2 g every 4 hr × 2 wk *plus* Gentamicin 1 mg/kg every 8 hr × 2 wk
Methicillin-resistant staphylocci, right-sided IE	Vancomycin 15 mg/kg every 12 hr × 4-6 weeks
Methicillin-sensitive staphylococci, left-sided IE	Nafcillin or oxacillin 2 g every 4 hr × 6 wk *optionally add* Gentamicin 1 mg/kg every 8 hr × first 3-5 days
Methicillin-resistant staphylocci, left-sided IE	Vancomycin 15 mg/kg every 12 hr × 6 wk
Methicillin-sensitive staphylococci, prosthetic valve IE	Nafcillin or oxacillin 2 g every 4 hr × ≥ 6 wk *plus* Rifampin 300 mg PO/IV every 8 hr × ≥ 6 wk *plus* Gentamicin 1 mg/kg every 8 hr × 2 wk
Methicillin-resistant staphylocci, prosthetic valve IE	Vancomycin 15 mg/kg every 12 hr × 6 wk *plus* Rifampin 300 mg PO/IV every 8 hr × 6 wk *plus* Gentamicin 1 mg/kg every 8 hr × 2 wk

*Specific points:
- Adult dosing only.
- Doses are for normal renal function.
- All regimens are intravenous (IV) unless specifically noted.
- Ceftriaxone, gentamicin, and streptomycin can be dosed intramuscularly, if necessary.
- For situations in which there are alternate, first-line regimens without gentamicin, gentamicin should be avoided in patients at elevated risk for toxicity.

demonstrated the effectiveness of short-course (2 weeks), combined β-lactam–aminoglycoside therapy for uncomplicated right-sided IE caused by MSSA.[153,154] Here uncomplicated disease is defined as the absence of renal failure, extrapulmonary metastatic infection, involvement of aortic or mitral valves, or meningitis. The short-course combination regimen achieves cure rates similar to those of 4 weeks of β-lactam monotherapy. In a more recent study, 2 weeks of β-lactam monotherapy resulted in cure rates equivalent to those achieved with 2 weeks of bβ-lactam–aminoglycoside combination therapy.[155] As a result, patients with uncomplicated right-sided disease caused by MSSA may be treated with an antistaphylococcal β-lactam with or without gentamicin for 2 weeks. Current evidence supports a multiple-daily dosing schedule for gentamicin. In patients with normal renal function, 3 mg/kg per day of gentamicin is divided in three doses to achieve target peak concentrations of approximately 3 mcg/ml and target trough concentrations of less than 1 mcg/ml. Many authorities would attempt to use combination therapy given a greater amount of data and clinical experience with this regimen. If patients fail to tolerate gentamicin, β-lactam monotherapy may be considered. Complicated right-sided IE caused by MSSA should be treated with 4 to 6 weeks of β-lactam monotherapy. The available evidence does not support the addition of an aminoglycoside for complicated right-sided IE.[156]

Vancomycin monotherapy is the recommended treatment for right-sided IE caused by MRSA or MSSA when patients have serious β-lactam allergy. Vancomycin plus gentamicin regimens are less effective than β-lactam–aminoglycoside combinations for right-sided IE caused MSSA.[157] The available data do not support using vancomycin plus gentamicin for an abbreviated course of therapy. Moreover, the addition of an aminoglycoside to vancomycin offers no proven therapeutic benefit. Therefore, vancomycin monotherapy should be administered for 4 to 6 weeks. Daptomycin may also be considered in this clinical situation. One study demonstrated that daptomycin is not inferior to vancomycin in the treatment of right-sided IE caused by MSSA or MRSA.[69] Daptomycin may be considered in patients who fail to respond to or are intolerant of vancomycin. Daptomycin offers the advantage of once-daily dosing but is significantly more expensive than vancomycin.

Oral therapy may be an option for certain patients who are unable to receive parenteral therapy. Two studies have demonstrated the effectiveness of a predominantly oral 4-week regimen of ciprofloxacin plus rifampin in the treatment of uncomplicated right-sided *S. aureus* IE in IDUs.[93,158] In these two studies, the ciprofloxacin plus rifampin regimen achieved cure rates of over 90%. Of note, fluoroquinolone resistance in staphylococci is increasingly common, so susceptibility to ciprofloxacin must be confirmed if this regimen is used.

Left-Sided, Native Valve IE. Treatment recommendations for left-sided, native valve IE caused by staphylococci are presented in Table 81-3.[10] The recommended treatment for left-sided IE caused by MSSA is an antistaphylococcal β-lactam, preferably nafcillin or oxacillin, administered for 6 weeks. If patients have uncomplicated disease and an excellent response to therapy, a total of 4 weeks of therapy may be sufficient. In a prospective study of left-sided IE caused by *S. aureus*, the addition of gentamicin to nafcillin for the first 2 weeks of therapy did not reduce mortality.[156] The nafcillin-gentamicin therapy reduced the duration of *S. aureus* bacteremia by approximately 1 day in comparison to nafcillin monotherapy, but combination therapy resulted in increased frequency of nephrotoxicity. The administration of gentamicin for the first 3 to 5 days of therapy is considered optional. Gentamicin therapy should not be continued beyond 5 days given the lack of proven benefit and potential for toxicity. If gentamicin is administered, it should be administered in a multiple-daily dosing regimen as discussed in the previous section.

Left-sided IE caused by MRSA should be treated with vancomycin monotherapy for a total of 6 weeks. Many strains of MRSA are resistant to aminoglycosides, and the combination of vancomcyin-gentamicin may be associated with an increased risk of ototoxicity and nephrotoxicity. Given these potential drawbacks and no clear evidence of improved efficacy, the routine administration of gentamicin in the treatment of left-sided IE caused by MRSA is not recommended. Although most staphylococci are sensisitive to rifampin, the efficacy of vancomycin-rifampin combinations is variable. In a prospective trial of patients with MRSA IE who did not adequately respond to vancomycin, the addition of rifampin did not decrease the duration of bacteremia or mortality.[58] Therefore, the routine addition of rifampin to vancomycin is not recommended for native valve disease caused by MRSA. For patients who do not tolerate vancomycin, there is no alternative with proven efficacy. Daptomycin is a promising agent, but, at this time, experience using it to treat left-sided IE caused by *S. aureus* is limited. MRSA isolates that exhibit intermediate resistance to vancomycin (VISA) are being encountered with greater frequency, and there have been several cases of MRSA isolates that are fully resistant to vancomycin.[47-49,159] The optimal treatment for MRSA strains with decreased susceptibility to vancomycin is unknown at this time.

Prosthetic Valve IE. Treatment recommendations for prosthetic valve IE caused by staphylococci are presented in Table 81-3.[10] CoNS that cause prosthetic valve infection are frequently methicillin resistant.[145] Evidence from experimental models and limited human data suggest that optimal treatment of prosthetic valve IE caused by methicillin-resistant CoNS is vancomycin plus rifampin and gentamicin.[160,161] Vancomycin and rifampin should be administered for a full 6 weeks of therapy, while gentamicin should be administered for the first 2 weeks of therapy. If the isolate is methicillin sensitive, an antistaphylococcal β-lactam should be administered in place of vancomycin. If the isolate is resistant to gentamicin, another aminoglycoside to which the isolate is susceptible should be administered in place of gentamicin. If the isolate is resistant to all aminoglycosides but sensitive to fluoroquinolones, then a fluoroquinolone may be administered. Based on the limited available data, these regimens are also recommended for the treatment of prosthetic valve IE caused by *S. aureus*.

HACEK Organisms

Treatment recommendations for IE caused by the HACEK organisms are presented in Table 81-4.[10] IE caused by the fastidious gram-negative bacilli of the HACEK group (*Haemophilus parainfluenzae, Haemophilus aphrophilus, Actinobacillus actinomycetemcomitans, Cardiobacterium hominis, Eikenella corrodens,* and *Kingella kingae*) accounts for approximately 5% to 10% of native valve IE in patients who are not IDUs.[162] These organisms grow slowly but are usually detected in blood cultures held for the standard time period. Routine antimicrobial sus-

TABLE 81-4 TREATMENT FOR INFECTIVE ENDOCARDITIS DUE TO HACEK ORGANISMS

Organism	Regimen*
Haemophilus parainfluenzae, H. aphrophilus, Actinobacillus actinomycetemcomitans, Cardiobacterium hominis, Eikenella corrodens, and *Kingella kingae*	1. Ceftriaxone 2 g every 24 hr × 4 wk (for prosthetic valve IE: ×6 wk) 2. Ampicillin-sulbactam 2 g every 4 hr × 4 wk (for prosthetic valve IE: ×6 wk) 3. Ciprofloxacin 500 mg PO every 12 hr or 400 mg IV every 12 hr × 4 wk (regimen #3 only if β-lactam not tolerated; for prosthetic valve IE: ×6 wk)

*Specific points:
- Adult dosing only.
- Doses are for normal renal function.
- All regimens are intravenous (IV) unless specifically noted.
- Ceftriaxone, gentamicin, and streptomycin can be dosed intramuscularly, if necessary.

ceptibility testing for these organisms is difficult to perform given their fastidious nature. In recent years, β-lactamase production has been detected in a significant portion of isolates. Therefore, all HACEK organisms should be assumed to be resistant to ampicillin; however, they remain susceptible to third- and fourth-generation cephalosporins and ampicillin-sulbactam. Ceftriaxone should be considered the drug of choice given its excellent activity and ease of administration. Other third- or fourth-generation cephalosporins or ampicillin-sulbactam may be used if patients do not tolerate ceftriaxone. While the flouroquinolones have in vitro activity against the HACEK organisms, there are limited data on their use in the treatment of IE caused by HACEK organisms. Therefore, they should only be used when patients cannot tolerate β-lactam antibiotics.

Enterobacteriaceae and Pseudomonas aeruginosa

Aerobic gram-negative bacilli are a relatively rare cause of IE, accounting for less than 5% of all cases.[162] Risk factors for IE caused by gram-negative bacteria include presence of a prosthetic valve, injection drug use, and cirrhosis. The presentation of the disease is often severe, with heart failure a common finding. As left-sided disease carries a high mortality, antibiotic therapy combined with early valve replacement may afford the best chance of cure. Right-sided disease may sometimes be cured by antibiotics alone. In general, treatment regimens should consist of a β-lactam in combination with an aminoglycoside and should be based on the results of susceptibility testing. Aminoglycosides should be administered at full doses used for the treatment of gram-negative infections. For the aminoglycoside, both once-daily and multiple-daily dosing regimens are acceptable, but the once-daily regimen may be associated with less nephrotoxicity. (See earlier section on aminoglycosides for the dosing recommendations.)

Fungi

Fungal IE is rare and occurs primarily in patients with known risk factors such as the presence of a prosthetic valve or central venous catheter. *Candida* and *Aspergillus* species account for the majority of cases, with *Candida*-related disease being much more common. The mortality of fungal IE is high, and cure is unlikely with medical therapy alone.[95] Therefore, a combined medical-surgical approach to treatment is generally indicated. Initial control of the infection may be achieved with antifungal therapy, usually an amphotericin B product, and valve replacement surgery. Parenteral therapy is generally administered for greater than 6 weeks, putting patients at high risk for amphotericin B–related nephrotoxicity. For this reason, initiating therapy with a lipid-based amphotericin formulation is reasonable. Relapse rates are high in fungal IE, so lifelong suppressive therapy with an oral azole is recommended by some experts, even after surgery. Fluconazole is the preferred oral azole for most *Candida*, but some isolates, especially non-*albicans* species, are resistant. *Aspergillus* species are resistant to fluconazole. Newer azoles such as voriconazole may be active against fluconazole-resistant fungi, but clinical experience in fungal IE is limited.

Culture-Negative Endocarditis

Positive blood cultures are a hallmark of IE and part of the diagnostic criteria. Blood culture results allow the clinician to target antimicrobial therapy against the appropriate pathogen, taking into account antimicrobial susceptibility results. However, in up to 20% of cases of IE, blood cultures may not yield a pathogen.[163] The first clinical situation in which blood cultures may be negative is when antibiotics are administered prior to obtaining cultures. This situation should be confirmed by obtaining an accurate history of prior antibiotic exposure. Clinicians should be aware that prior receipt of antibiotics may cause blood cultures to remain negative for days to weeks. The second scenario in which blood cultures are negative is when the infection is caused by fastidious organisms. Some of these organisms are harder to culture using routine microbiologic techniques, and others do not grow at all on standard media. Patients will often have risk factors that raise the clinical suspicion for IE caused by specific pathogens in this group. Classifying patients into one of these two groups may help to determine which pathogens need to be covered by the empirical antibiotic regimen. Other clinical factors such as the acuity of infection and whether a prosthetic valve is involved also influence the pathogens that should be covered.

Treatment recommendations for culture-negative IE are presented in Table 81-5.[10] The first group of patients, those who received antibi-

TABLE 81-5 TREATMENT FOR CULTURE-NEGATIVE INFECTIVE ENDOCARDITIS

Infection Characteristics	Regimen*
Native valve: enterococcal IE considered; *Bartonella* not suspected *or* Prosthetic valve (late, >1 yr)	**1.** Ampicillin-sulbactam 3 g IV every 6 hr × 4-6 wk (for prosthetic valve IE: ×6 wk) *plus* Gentamicin 1 mg/kg every 8 hr × 4-6 wk (for prosthetic valve IE: ×6 wk) **2.** Vancomycin 15 mg/kg every 12 hr × 4-6 wk (for prosthetic valve IE: ×6 wk) *plus* Gentamicin 1 mg/kg every 8 hr × 4-6 wk (for prosthetic valve IE: ×6 wk) *plus* Ciprofloxacin 500 mg PO every 12 hr or 400 mg IV every 12 hr × 4-6 wk (regimen #2 only if penicillins not tolerated; for prosthetic valve IE: ×6 wk)
Prosthetic valve (early, ≤1 yr)	Vancomycin 15 mg/kg every 12 hr × 6 wk *plus* Gentamicin 1 mg/kg every 8 hr × 2 wk *plus* Cefepime 2 g every 8 hr × 6 wk *plus* Rifampin 300 mg PO/IV every 8 hr × 6 wk
Bartonella suspected but not confirmed	Ceftriaxone 2 g every 24 hr × 6 wk *plus* Gentamicin 1 mg/kg every 8 hr × 2 wk *optionally add* Doxycycline 100 mg PO/IV every 12 hr × 6 wk

*Specific points:
- Adult dosing only.
- Doses are for normal renal function.
- All regimens are intravenous (IV) unless specifically noted.
- Ceftriaxone, gentamicin, and streptomycin can be dosed intramuscularly, if necessary.
- For situations in which there are alternate, first-line regimens without gentamicin, gentamicin should be avoided in patients at elevated risk for toxicity.

otics prior to blood cultures, are at risk for infection with many of the typical pathogens that cause IE. Patients who have an acute presentation involving a native valve should receive a regimen that includes coverage for *S. aureus*. Considering the increasing prevalence of MRSA, treatment with vancomycin is warranted in this situation. For patients with a subacute presentation, *S. aureus*, viridans group streptococci, enterococci, and HACEK organisms should be covered. These same organisms should be covered in the setting of prosthetic valve disease if symptom onset is greater than 1 year after valve replacement. One treatment option is ampicillin-sulbactam combined with gentamicin. This regimen provides good empirical coverage for these organisms with the notable exception of MRSA. An alternative regimen for patients unable to tolerate penicillins is vancomycin plus gentamicin plus ciprofloxacin. Vancomycin plus ceftriaxone is another regimen with which there is some clinical experience. Patients with culture-negative prosthetic valve IE that occurs within 1 year of valve replacement should receive coverage against methicillin-resistant staphylococci and aerobic gram-negative bacilli. A regimen of vancomycin plus gentamicin plus rifampin plus cefepime may be considered.

The second group of patients with culture-negative IE are those with infection caused by fastidious organisms. *Bartonella* species are the most commonly identified fastidious pathogens that cause culture-negative IE. Patients with suspected *Bartonella* IE should receive ceftriaxone plus gentamicin with the optional addition of doxycycline. If *Bartonella* infection is confirmed by culture or serology, patients should receive doxycycline plus gentamicin.[86] In each instance, gentamicin should be administered for 2 weeks. If patients cannot tolerate gentamicin, rifampin may be substituted in its place. Other fastidious organisms that have been implicated in culture-negative IE include *C. burnetii*, *Brucella* species, *Chlamydia* species, *Legionella* species, *Tropheryma whippleii*, and non-*Candida* fungi. Appropriate treatment of IE caused by each of these pathogens is based on limited data, and the optimal regimens are not well defined.

Prophylaxis

Antibiotic prophylaxis to prevent IE is routine in many parts of the world yet remains controversial. IE is a very serious disease, and certain groups at elevated risk have been identified clearly. Organisms that typically cause IE and may cause bacteremia following procedures that disrupt mucosal barriers are usually susceptible to narrow-spectrum antibiotics, particularly penicillins. Administration of antibiotics may reduce the frequency of bacteremia following dental procedures.[11] Therefore, it would be an attractive strategy to give inexpensive, well-tolerated antibiotics to prevent a life-threatening disease. However, no trials have been performed that demonstrate that antimicrobial prophylaxis is effective in preventing IE. In addition, IE is uncommon and, when it occurs, usually does not follow an invasive procedure.[12,164] The magnitude of risk from prophylaxis has not been well defined in terms of allergy, drug resistance, and complications, including *Clostridium difficile* colitis. Given these uncertainties regarding prophylaxis, it is difficult to weigh the costs versus benefits.

In the United States, many clinicians follow the prophylaxis guidelines developed by the American Heart Association in conjunction with several other organizations.[165] These guidelines were substantially revised in 2007 and now recommend prophylaxis only for those persons with the highest risk of adverse outcome from IE who undergo particular procedures. The cardiac indications for prophylaxis adapted from the guidelines are outlined in Box 81-1. Prophylaxis is no longer recommended for many cardiac conditions, including mitral valve prolapse, which increase the lifetime risk of IE but are associated with less morbidity if IE occurs. The dental procedures for which prophylaxis is recommended are reviewed in Box 81-2. Antibiotic prophylaxis is also recommended for patients at highest risk for adverse outcomes who undergo an invasive procedure of the respiratory tract that involves an incision, such as tonsillectomy or adenoidectomy.

The prophylactic antibiotic regimens suggested for dental and respiratory procedures are listed in Table 81-6. However, one recent study found that clindamycin, which is recommended as alternative antibiotic in patients with penicillin allergy, was not effective in preventing bacteremia after dental extractions.[166] In addition, for patients with a cardiac condition listed in Box 81-1 who undergo drainage of a respiratory tract infection, an antibiotic regimen is recommended that is active against viridans group streptococci and against *S. aureus*, if this organism is known or suspected to be present. For patients with a cardiac condition listed in Box 81-1 who are treated surgically for a skin or soft tissue infection, an antimicrobial regimen active against *S. aureus* and β-hemolytic streptococci should be considered.

Finally, antibiotic prophylaxis is no longer recommended for gastrointestinal and genitourinary tract procedures in most cases. For patients

BOX 81-1 CARDIAC CONDITIONS ASSOCIATED WITH HIGHEST RISK OF ADVERSE OUTCOME FROM INFECTIVE ENDOCARDITIS

- Prosthetic valve
- Previous IE
- Congenital heart disease (CHD) only as follows:
  - Unrepaired cyanotic CHD, including palliative shunts and conduits
  - CHD completely repaired using prosthetic material or device during the first 6 months after the procedure
  - Repaired CHD with residual defects at the site or adjacent to the site of prosthetic material
- Cardiac transplantation with development of valvulopathy

BOX 81-2 DENTAL SITUATIONS AND INFECTIVE ENDOCARDITIS PROPHYLAXIS

Prophylaxis Recommended

- All procedures that involve manipulation of gingiva or periapical region of teeth or perforation of oral mucosa

Prophylaxis Not Recommended

- Anesthetic injections through uninfected tissue
- Radiographs
- Placement of removable prosthodontic or orthodontic appliances
- Adjustment of orthodontic devices
- Placement of orthodontic brackets
- Shedding of deciduous teeth
- Bleeding from trauma to lips or oral mucosa

TABLE 81-6 PROPHYLACTIC ANTIBIOTIC REGIMENS FOR DENTAL AND RESPIRATORY TRACT PROCEDURES

Situation	Regimen*
Routine	Amoxicillin 2 g PO
Unable to take oral medications	Ampicillin 2 g IM or IV *or* Cefazolin† or ceftriaxone† 1 g IM or IV
Penicillin allergy	Cephalexin† 2 g PO *or* Clindamycin 600 mg PO *or* Azithromycin or clarithromycin 500 mg PO
Penicillin allergy and unable to take oral medications	Cefazolin† or ceftriaxone† 1 g IM or IV *or* Clindamycin 600 mg IM or IV

*All regimens are for a single dose 30 to 60 minutes prior to the procedure.
†Cephalosporins should be avoided in patients with immediate-type hypersensitivity reactions to penicillins.

with a cardiac condition listed in Box 81-1 who have an active gastrointestinal or genitourinary infection or urinary colonization with enterococci, an antimicrobial regimen active against enterococci may be considered prior to a gastrointestinal or genitourinary procedure. It should be noted that the guidelines are not a substitute for clinical judgment, nor are they intended to set a standard of care given the limited evidence available.

Areas of Uncertainty and Future Directions

Despite changes in the epidemiology of IE and possible increases in overall cases due to health care–associated infections, IE remains fairly uncommon and challenging to study. Patients with IE are often quite ill with comorbid conditions, and this poses problems for recruitment into clinical trials. Prolonged duration of therapy, though largely empirical in many situations, is required. Moreover, different organisms necessitate different pharmacotherapeutic approaches, and some organisms are rare and/or difficult to diagnose. Therefore, the lack of high-quality clinical trials in IE is perhaps not surprising but leaves many areas of uncertainty. Guidelines rely largely on data gathered from experimental IE, retrospective observational studies of patients, and small clinical trials. Expert opinion is an important component underlying the recommendations. Through international collaboration, investigators are attempting to study IE in larger numbers of patients using standardized methodologies with an eye toward future randomized clinical trials.[167,168]

As stated previously, antibiotic prophylaxis for IE in patients with cardiac risk factors undergoing certain procedures remains an area of considerable controversy. This, too, is difficult to study, as IE following procedures is devastating but rare. A very large clinical trial would be required to definitively answer this question. However, collection of observational, population-based data encompassing large numbers of people may advance understanding of the risks and benefits.

Surgery is recognized as a critical treatment modality, but the indications have not been fully clarified. Randomized trials are not available, making comparisons challenging because patients who undergo valve replacement are quite different from those who do not. However, the use of specific analytic techniques has advanced our knowledge in this area and has provided strong support for the notion that patients with complicated left-sided IE benefit from valve replacement surgery, particularly when moderate or severe congestive heart failure is present.[99]

Finally, resistant gram-positive infections, particularly those due to *S. aureus*, are increasingly prevalent and notoriously difficult to treat. While vancomycin has been the standard of care for serious infections due to MRSA, clinical failures are common. Daptomycin has been evaluated for right-sided IE and bacteremia and provides an alternative to vancomycin but not a clear advantage.[69] New agents active against MRSA, including the lipoglycopeptides dalbavancin and telavancin and the cephalosporin ceftobiprole, may have a future role in the treatment of IE.

REFERENCES

1. Fowler VG Jr, Miro JM, Hoen B, et al. *Staphylococcus aureus* endocarditis: a consequence of medical progress. JAMA 2005;293:3012-3021.
2. Tleyjeh IM, Steckelberg JM, Murad HS, et al. Temporal trends in infective endocarditis: a population-based study in Olmsted County, Minnesota. JAMA 2005;293:3022-3028.
3. Quagliarello V. Infective endocarditis: global, regional, and future perspectives. JAMA 2005;293:3061-3062.
4. Hoen B, Alla F, Selton-Suty C, et al. Changing profile of infective endocarditis: results of a 1-year survey in France. JAMA 2002;288:75-81.
5. Frontera JA, Gradon JD. Right-side endocarditis in injection drug users: review of proposed mechanisms of pathogenesis. Clin Infect Dis 2000;30:374-379.
6. Agnihotri AK, McGiffin DC, Galbraith AJ, et al. The prevalence of infective endocarditis after aortic valve replacement. J Thorac Cardiovasc Surg 1995;110:1708-1720; discussion 1720-1724.
7. Mylonakis E, Calderwood SB. Infective endocarditis in adults. N Engl J Med 2001;345:1318-1330.
8. Li JS, Sexton DJ, Mick N, et al. Proposed modifications to the Duke criteria for the diagnosis of infective endocarditis. Clin Infect Dis 2000;30:633-638.
9. Werner M, Andersson R, Olaison L, et al. A clinical study of culture-negative endocarditis. Medicine (Baltimore) 2003;82:263-273.
10. Baddour LM, Wilson WR, Bayer AS, et al. Infective endocarditis: diagnosis, antimicrobial therapy, and management of complications. A statement for healthcare professionals from the Committee on Rheumatic Fever, Endocarditis, and Kawasaki Disease, Council on Cardiovascular Disease in the Young, and the Councils on Clinical Cardiology, Stroke, and Cardiovascular Surgery and Anesthesia, American Heart Association—executive summary. Endorsed by the Infectious Diseases Society of America. Circulation 2005;111:3167-3184.
11. Durack DT. Prevention of infective endocarditis. N Engl J Med 1995;332:38-44.
12. Strom BL, Abrutyn E, Berlin JA, et al. Risk factors for infective endocarditis: oral hygiene and nondental exposures. Circulation 2000;102:2842-2848.
13. Rodbard S. Blood velocity and endocarditis. Circulation 1963;27:18-28.
14. Lepeschkin E. On the relation between the site of valvular involvement in endocarditis and the blood pressure resting on the valve. Am J Med Sci 1952;224:318-319.
15. Bashore TM, Cabell C, Fowler V Jr. Update on infective endocarditis. Curr Probl Cardiol 2006;31:274-352.
16. Thiene G, Basso C. Pathology and pathogenesis of infective endocarditis in native heart valves. Cardiovasc Pathol 2006;15:256-263.
17. Fitzgerald JR, Foster TJ, Cox D. The interaction of bacterial pathogens with platelets. Nat Rev Microbiol 2006;4:445-457.
18. Tang YQ, Yeaman MR, Selsted ME. Antimicrobial peptides from human platelets. Infect Immun 2002;70:6524-6533.
19. Yeaman MR. The role of platelets in antimicrobial host defense. Clin Infect Dis 1997;25:951-968.
20. Wu T, Yeaman MR, Bayer AS. In vitro resistance to platelet microbicidal protein correlates with endocarditis source among bacteremic staphylococcal and streptococcal isolates. Antimicrob Agents Chemother 1994;38:729-732.
21. Bayer AS, Cheng D, Yeaman MR, et al. In vitro resistance to thrombin-induced platelet microbicidal protein among clinical bacteremic isolates of *Staphylococcus aureus* correlates with an endovascular infectious source. Antimicrob Agents Chemother 1998;42:3169-3172.
22. Dhawan VK, Yeaman MR, Cheung AL, et al. Phenotypic resistance to thrombin-induced platelet microbicidal protein in vitro is correlated with enhanced virulence in experimental endocarditis due to *Staphylococcus aureus.* Infect Immun 1997;65:3293-3299.
23. Moreillon P, Que YA, Bayer AS. Pathogenesis of streptococcal and staphylococcal endocarditis. Infect Dis Clin North Am 2002;16:297-318.
24. Scheld WM, Valone JA, Sande MA. Bacterial adherence in the pathogenesis of endocarditis: interaction of bacterial dextran, platelets, and fibrin. J Clin Invest 1978;61:1394-1404.
25. Lowrance JH, Baddour LM, Simpson WA. The role of fibronectin binding in the rat model of experimental endocarditis caused by *Streptococcus sanguis.* J Clin Invest 1990;86:7-13.
26. Huebner J, Goldmann DA. Coagulase-negative staphylococci: role as pathogens. Annu Rev Med 1999;50:223-236.
27. Freedman LR, Valone J Jr. Experimental infective endocarditis. Prog Cardiovasc Dis 1979;22:169-180.
28. Durack DT. Experimental bacterial endocarditis. IV. Structure and evolution of very early lesions. J Pathol 1975;115:81-89.
29. Young Lee S, Cisar JO, Bryant JL, et al. Resistance of *Streptococcus gordonii* to polymorphonuclear leukocyte killing is a potential virulence determinant of infective endocarditis. Infect Immun 2006;74:3148-3155.
30. Repine JE, Clawson CC, Burchell HB, et al. Reversible neutrophil defect in patients with bacterial endocarditis. J Lab Clin Med 1976;88:780-787.
31. Bancsi MJ, Veltrop MH, Bertina RM, et al. Influence of monocytes and antibiotic treatment on tissue factor activity of endocardial vegetations in rabbits infected with *Streptococcus sanguis.* Infect Immun 1996;64:448-451.
32. Bancsi MJ, Veltrop MH, Bertina RM, et al. Role of monocytes and bacteria in *Staphylococcus epidermidis* endocarditis. Infect Immun 1998;66:448-450.
33. Durack DT, Beeson PB. Experimental bacterial endocarditis. II. Survival of a bacteria in endocardial vegetations. Br J Exp Pathol 1972;53:50-53.
34. Blumberg EA, Robbins N, Adimora A, et al. Persistent fever in association with infective endocarditis. Clin Infect Dis 1992;15:983-990.
35. Lamas C, Boia M, Eykyn SJ. Osteoarticular infections complicating infective endocarditis: a study of 30 cases between 1969 and 2002 in a tertiary referral centre. Scand J Infect Dis 2006;38:433-440.
36. Salkind AR, Cuddy PG, Foxworth JW. The Rational Clinical Examination. Is this patient allergic to penicillin? An evidence-based analysis of the likelihood of penicillin allergy. JAMA 2001;285:2498-2505.
37. Kelkar PS, Li JT. Cephalosporin allergy. N Engl J Med 2001;345:804-809.
38. Romano A, Gueant-Rodriguez RM, Viola M, et al. Cross-reactivity and tolerability of cephalosporins in patients with immediate hypersensitivity to penicillins. Ann Intern Med 2004;141:16-22.
39. Zygmunt DJ, Stratton CW, Kernodle DS. Characterization of four beta-lactamases produced by *Staphylococcus aureus.* Antimicrob Agents Chemother 1992;36:440-445.
40. Nannini EC, Singh KV, Murray BE. Relapse of type A beta-lactamase-producing *Staphylococcus aureus* native valve endocarditis during cefazolin therapy: revisiting the issue. Clin Infect Dis 2003;37:1194-1198.
41. Francioli P, Etienne J, Hoigne R, et al. Treatment of streptococcal endocarditis with a single daily dose of ceftriaxone sodium for 4 weeks: efficacy and outpatient treatment feasibility. JAMA 1992;267:264-267.
42. Francioli P, Ruch W, Stamboulian D. Treatment of streptococcal endocarditis with a single daily dose of ceftriaxone and netilmicin for 14 days: a prospective multicenter study. Clin Infect Dis 1995;21:1406-1410.

43. Chow JW, Fine MJ, Shlaes DM, et al. *Enterobacter* bacteremia: clinical features and emergence of antibiotic resistance during therapy. Ann Intern Med 1991;115:585-590.
44. Paterson DL. "Collateral damage" from cephalosporin or quinolone antibiotic therapy. Clin Infect Dis 2004;38(Suppl 4):S341-S345.
45. Murray BE. Vancomycin-resistant enterococcal infections. N Engl J Med 2000;342:710-721.
46. Walsh CT. Vancomycin resistance: decoding the molecular logic. Science 1993;261:308-309.
47. *Staphylococcus aureus* resistant to vancomycin—United States, 2002. MMWR Morb Mortal Wkly Rep 2002;51:565-567.
48. Vancomycin-resistant *Staphylococcus aureus*—Pennsylvania, 2002. MMWR Morb Mortal Wkly Rep 2002;51:902.
49. Vancomycin-resistant *Staphylococcus aureus*—New York, 2004. MMWR Morb Mortal Wkly Rep 2004;53:322-323.
50. Chang S, Sievert DM, Hageman JC, et al. Infection with vancomycin-resistant *Staphylococcus aureus* containing the *vanA* resistance gene. N Engl J Med 2003;348:1342-1347.
51. Whitener CJ, Park SY, Browne FA, et al. Vancomycin-resistant *Staphylococcus aureus* in the absence of vancomycin exposure. Clin Infect Dis 2004;38:1049-1055.
52. Courvalin P. Vancomycin resistance in gram-positive cocci. Clin Infect Dis 2006;42(Suppl 1):S25-S34.
53. Hiramatsu K, Hanaki H, Ino T, et al. Methicillin-resistant *Staphylococcus aureus* clinical strain with reduced vancomycin susceptibility. J Antimicrob Chemother 1997;40:135-136.
54. Hiramatsu K. Vancomycin-resistant *Staphylococcus aureus:* a new model of antibiotic resistance. Lancet Infect Dis 2001;1:147-155.
55. Liu C, Chambers HF. *Staphylococcus aureus* with heterogeneous resistance to vancomycin: epidemiology, clinical significance, and critical assessment of diagnostic methods. Antimicrob Agents Chemother 2003;47:3040-3045.
56. Wong SS, Ho PL, Woo PC, et al. Bacteremia caused by staphylococci with inducible vancomycin heteroresistance. Clin Infect Dis 1999;29:760-767.
57. Small PM, Chambers HF. Vancomycin for *Staphylococcus aureus* endocarditis in intravenous drug users. Antimicrob Agents Chemother 1990;34:1227-1231.
58. Levine DP, Fromm BS, Reddy BR. Slow response to vancomycin or vancomycin plus rifampin in methicillin-resistant *Staphylococcus aureus* endocarditis. Ann Intern Med 1991;115:674-680.
59. Chang FY, MacDonald BB, Peacock JE Jr, et al. A prospective multicenter study of *Staphylococcus aureus* bacteremia: incidence of endocarditis, risk factors for mortality, and clinical impact of methicillin resistance. Medicine (Baltimore) 2003;82:322-332.
60. Kaye D. Enterococci: biologic and epidemiologic characteristics and in vitro susceptibility. Arch Intern Med 1982;142:2006-2009.
61. Watanakunakorn C, Bakie C. Synergism of vancomycin-gentamicin and vancomycin-streptomycin against enterococci. Antimicrob Agents Chemother 1973;4:120-124.
62. Matzke GR, McGory RW, Halstenson CE, et al. Pharmacokinetics of vancomycin in patients with various degrees of renal function. Antimicrob Agents Chemother 1984;25:433-437.
63. Moellering RC Jr, Krogstad DJ, Greenblatt DJ. Vancomycin therapy in patients with impaired renal function: a nomogram for dosage. Ann Intern Med 1981;94:343-346.
64. Farber BF, Moellering RC Jr. Retrospective study of the toxicity of preparations of vancomycin from 1974 to 1981. Antimicrob Agents Chemother 1983;23:138-141.
65. Rybak MJ, Albrecht LM, Boike SC, et al. Nephrotoxicity of vancomycin, alone and with an aminoglycoside. J Antimicrob Chemother 1990;25:679-687.
66. Pai MP, Mercier RC, Koster SA. Epidemiology of vancomycin-induced neutropenia in patients receiving home intravenous infusion therapy. Ann Pharmacother 2006;40:224-228.
67. Healy DP, Sahai JV, Fuller SH, et al. Vancomycin-induced histamine release and "red man syndrome": comparison of 1- and 2-hour infusions. Antimicrob Agents Chemother 1990;34:550-554.
68. Sahai J, Healy DP, Garris R, et al. Influence of antihistamine pretreatment on vancomycin-induced red-man syndrome. J Infect Dis 1989;160:876-881.
69. Fowler VG Jr, Boucher HW, Corey GR, et al. Daptomycin versus standard therapy for bacteremia and endocarditis caused by *Staphylococcus aureus.* N Engl J Med 2006;355:653-665.
70. Patel JB, Jevitt LA, Hageman J, et al. An association between reduced susceptibility to daptomycin and reduced susceptibility to vancomycin in *Staphylococcus aureus.* Clin Infect Dis 2006;42:1652-1653.
71. Cui L, Tominaga E, Neoh HM, et al. Correlation between reduced daptomycin susceptibility and vancomycin resistance in vancomycin-intermediate *Staphylococcus aureus.* Antimicrob Agents Chemother 2006;50:1079-1082.
72. Tally FP, DeBruin MF. Development of daptomycin for gram-positive infections. J Antimicrob Chemother 2000;46:523-526.
73. Oleson FB Jr, Berman CL, Kirkpatrick JB, et al. Once-daily dosing in dogs optimizes daptomycin safety. Antimicrob Agents Chemother 2000;44:2948-2953.
74. Carpenter CF, Chambers HF. Daptomycin: another novel agent for treating infections due to drug-resistant gram-positive pathogens. Clin Infect Dis 2004;38:994-1000.
75. Le T, Bayer AS. Combination antibiotic therapy for infective endocarditis. Clin Infect Dis 2003;36:615-621.
76. Francioli PB, Glauser MP. Synergistic activity of ceftriaxone combined with netilmicin administered once daily for treatment of experimental streptococcal endocarditis. Antimicrob Agents Chemother 1993;37:207-212.
77. Reyes MP, Brown WJ, Lerner AM. Treatment of patients with *Pseudomonas* endocarditis with high dose aminoglycoside and carbenicillin therapy. Medicine (Baltimore) 1978;57:57-67.
78. Falagas ME, Manta KG, Ntziora F, et al. Linezolid for the treatment of patients with endocarditis: a systematic review of the published evidence. J Antimicrob Chemother 2006;58:273-280.
79. Gerson SL, Kaplan SL, Bruss JB, et al. Hematologic effects of linezolid: summary of clinical experience. Antimicrob Agents Chemother 2002;46:2723-2726.
80. Lee E, Burger S, Shah J, et al. Linezolid-associated toxic optic neuropathy: a report of 2 cases. Clin Infect Dis 2003;37:1389-1391.
81. Bishop E, Melvani S, Howden BP, et al. Good clinical outcomes but high rates of adverse reactions during linezolid therapy for serious infections: a proposed protocol for monitoring therapy in complex patients. Antimicrob Agents Chemother 2006;50:1599-1602.
82. Lawrence KR, Adra M, Gillman PK. Serotonin toxicity associated with the use of linezolid: a review of postmarketing data. Clin Infect Dis 2006;42:1578-1583.
83. Moellering RC, Linden PK, Reinhardt J, et al. The efficacy and safety of quinupristin/dalfopristin for the treatment of infections caused by vancomycin-resistant *Enterococcus faecium.* Synercid Emergency-Use Study Group. J Antimicrob Chemother 1999;44:251-261.
84. Linden PK, Moellering RC Jr, Wood CA, et al. Treatment of vancomycin-resistant *Enterococcus faecium* infections with quinupristin/dalfopristin. Clin Infect Dis 2001;33:1816-1823.
85. Olsen KM, Rebuck JA, Rupp ME. Arthralgias and myalgias related to quinupristin-dalfopristin administration. Clin Infect Dis 2001;32:e83-e86.
86. Rolain JM, Brouqui P, Koehler JE, et al. Recommendations for treatment of human infections caused by *Bartonella* species. Antimicrob Agents Chemother 2004;48:1921-1933.
87. Wehrli W. Rifampin: mechanisms of action and resistance. Rev Infect Dis 1983;5(Suppl 3):S407-S411.
88. Mandell GL, Moorman DR. Treatment of experimental staphylococcal infections: effect of rifampin alone and in combination on development of rifampin resistance. Antimicrob Agents Chemother 1980;17:658-662.
89. Chuard C, Herrmann M, Vaudaux P, et al. Successful therapy of experimental chronic foreign-body infection due to methicillin-resistant *Staphylococcus aureus* by antimicrobial combinations. Antimicrob Agents Chemother 1991;35:2611-2616.
90. Ein ME, Smith NJ, Aruffo JF, et al. Susceptibility and synergy studies of methicillin-resistant *Staphylococcus epidermidis.* Antimicrob Agents Chemother 1979;16:655-659.
91. Watanakunakorn C, Guerriero JC. Interaction between vancomycin and rifampin against *Staphylococcus aureus.* Antimicrob Agents Chemother 1981;19:1089-1091.
92. Hackbarth CJ, Chambers HF, Sande MA. Serum bactericidal activity of rifampin in combination with other antimicrobial agents against *Staphylococcus aureus.* Antimicrob Agents Chemother 1986;29:611-613.
93. Heldman AW, Hartert TV, Ray SC, et al. Oral antibiotic treatment of right-sided staphylococcal endocarditis in injection drug users: prospective randomized comparison with parenteral therapy. Am J Med 1996;101:68-76.
94. Kang SL, Rybak MJ, McGrath BJ, et al. Pharmacodynamics of levofloxacin, ofloxacin, and ciprofloxacin, alone and in combination with rifampin, against methicillin-susceptible and -resistant *Staphylococcus aureus* in an in vitro infection model. Antimicrob Agents Chemother 1994;38:2702-2709.
95. Ellis ME, Al-Abdely H, Sandridge A, et al. Fungal endocarditis: evidence in the world literature, 1965-1995. Clin Infect Dis 2001;32:50-62.
96. Branch RA. Prevention of amphotericin B-induced renal impairment: a review on the use of sodium supplementation. Arch Intern Med 1988;148:2389-2394.
97. Burks LC, Aisner J, Fortner CL, et al. Meperidine for the treatment of shaking chills and fever. Arch Intern Med 1980;140:483-484.
98. Tynes BS, Utz JP, Bennett JE, et al. Reducing amphotericin B reactions: a double-blind study. Am Rev Respir Dis 1963;87:264-268.
99. Vikram HR, Buenconsejo J, Hasbun R, et al. Impact of valve surgery on 6-month mortality in adults with complicated, left-sided native valve endocarditis: a propensity analysis. JAMA 2003;290:3207-3214.
100. Hasbun R, Vikram HR, Barakat LA, et al. Complicated left-sided native valve endocarditis in adults: risk classification for mortality. JAMA 2003;289:1933-1940.
101. Rohmann S, Erbel R, Gorge G, et al. Clinical relevance of vegetation localization by transoesophageal echocardiography in infective endocarditis. Eur Heart J 1992;13:446-452.
102. Di Salvo G, Habib G, Pergola V, et al. Echocardiography predicts embolic events in infective endocarditis. J Am Coll Cardiol 2001;37:1069-1076.
103. Gillinov AM, Shah RV, Curtis WE, et al. Valve replacement in patients with endocarditis and acute neurologic deficit. Ann Thorac Surg 1996;61:1125-1129; discussion 1130.
104. Ruttmann E, Willeit J, Ulmer H, et al. Neurological outcome of septic cardioembolic stroke after infective endocarditis. Stroke 2006;37:2094-2099.
105. Piper C, Wiemer M, Schulte HD, et al. Stroke is not a contraindication for urgent valve replacement in acute infective endocarditis. J Heart Valve Dis 2001;10:703-711.
106. Kupferwasser LI, Yeaman MR, Nast CC, et al. Salicylic acid attenuates virulence in endovascular infections by targeting global regulatory pathways in *Staphylococcus aureus.* J Clin Invest 2003;112:222-233.
107. Chan KL, Dumesnil JG, Cujec B, et al. A randomized trial of aspirin on the risk of embolic events in patients with infective endocarditis. J Am Coll Cardiol 2003;42:775-780.
108. Tornos P, Almirante B, Mirabet S, et al. Infective endocarditis due to *Staphylococcus aureus:* deleterious effect of anticoagulant therapy. Arch Intern Med 1999;159:473-475.
109. Wilson WR, Zak O, Sande MA. Penicillin therapy for treatment of experimental endocarditis caused by viridans streptococci in animals. J Infect Dis 1985;151:1028-1033.

110. Watanakunakorn C, Glotzbecker C. Synergism with aminoglycosides of penicillin, ampicillin and vancomycin against non-enterococcal group-D streptococci and viridans streptococci. J Med Microbiol 1977;10:133-138.
111. Nicolau DP, Freeman CD, Belliveau PP, et al. Experience with a once-daily aminoglycoside program administered to 2,184 adult patients. Antimicrob Agents Chemother 1995;39:650-655.
112. Karchmer AW, Moellering RC Jr, Maki DG, et al. Single-antibiotic therapy for streptococcal endocarditis. JAMA 1979;241:1801-1806.
113. Wilson WR, Thompson RL, Wilkowske CJ, et al. Short-term therapy for streptococcal infective endocarditis: combined intramuscular administration of penicillin and streptomycin. JAMA 1981;245:360-363.
114. Sexton DJ, Tenenbaum MJ, Wilson WR, et al. Ceftriaxone once daily for four weeks compared with ceftriaxone plus gentamicin once daily for two weeks for treatment of endocarditis due to penicillin-susceptible streptococci. Endocarditis Treatment Consortium Group. Clin Infect Dis 1998;27:1470-1474.
115. Liao CH, Teng LJ, Hsueh PR, et al. Nutritionally variant streptococcal infections at a University Hospital in Taiwan: disease emergence and high prevalence of beta-lactam and macrolide resistance. Clin Infect Dis 2004;38:452-455.
116. Martinez E, Miro JM, Almirante B, et al. Effect of penicillin resistance of *Streptococcus pneumoniae* on the presentation, prognosis, and treatment of pneumococcal endocarditis in adults. Clin Infect Dis 2002;35:130-139.
117. Lefort A, Lortholary O, Casassus P, et al. Comparison between adult endocarditis due to beta-hemolytic streptococci (serogroups A, B, C, and G) and *Streptococcus milleri:* a multicenter study in France. Arch Intern Med 2002;162:2450-2456.
118. Smyth EG, Pallett AP, Davidson RN. Group G streptococcal endocarditis: two case reports, a review of the literature and recommendations for treatment. J Infect 1988;16:169-176.
119. Lefort A, Mainardi JL, Selton-Suty C, et al. *Streptococcus pneumoniae* endocarditis in adults: a multicenter study in France in the era of penicillin resistance (1991-1998). The Pneumococcal Endocarditis Study Group. Medicine (Baltimore) 2000;79:327-337.
120. Sambola A, Miro JM, Tornos MP, et al. *Streptococcus agalactiae* infective endocarditis: analysis of 30 cases and review of the literature, 1962-1998. Clin Infect Dis 2002;34:1576-1584.
121. Yu VL, Chiou CC, Feldman C, et al. An international prospective study of pneumococcal bacteremia: correlation with in vitro resistance, antibiotics administered, and clinical outcome. Clin Infect Dis 2003;37:230-237.
122. Megran DW. Enterococcal endocarditis. Clin Infect Dis 1992;15:63-71.
123. Moellering RC Jr, Wennersten C, Weinberg AN. Synergy of penicillin and gentamicin against enterococci. J Infect Dis 1971;124(Suppl):S207-S209.
124. Fantin B, Carbon C. Importance of the aminoglycoside dosing regimen in the penicillin-netilmicin combination for treatment of *Enterococcus faecalis*-induced experimental endocarditis. Antimicrob Agents Chemother 1990;34:2387-2391.
125. Marangos MN, Nicolau DP, Quintiliani R, et al. Influence of gentamicin dosing interval on the efficacy of penicillin-containing regimens in experimental *Enterococcus faecalis* endocarditis. J Antimicrob Chemother 1997;39:519-522.
126. Thauvin C, Eliopoulos GM, Willey S, et al. Continuous-infusion ampicillin therapy of enterococcal endocarditis in rats. Antimicrob Agents Chemother 1987;31:139-143.
127. Eliopoulos GM, Thauvin-Eliopoulos C, Moellering RC Jr. Contribution of animal models in the search for effective therapy for endocarditis due to enterococci with high-level resistance to gentamicin. Clin Infect Dis 1992;15:58-62.
128. Wilson WR, Wilkowske CJ, Wright AJ, et al. Treatment of streptomycin-susceptible and streptomycin-resistant enterococcal endocarditis. Ann Intern Med 1984;100:816-823.
129. Olaison L, Schadewitz K. Enterococcal endocarditis in Sweden, 1995-1999: can shorter therapy with aminoglycosides be used? Clin Infect Dis 2002;34:159-166.
130. Sande MA, Scheld WM. Combination antibiotic therapy of bacterial endocarditis. Ann Intern Med 1980;92:390-395.
131. Torres C, Tenorio C, Lantero M, et al. High-level penicillin resistance and penicillin-gentamicin synergy in *Enterococcus faecium.* Antimicrob Agents Chemother 1993;37:2427-2431.
132. Rice LB, Eliopoulos GM, Wennersten C, et al. Chromosomally mediated beta-lactamase production and gentamicin resistance in *Enterococcus faecalis.* Antimicrob Agents Chemother 1991;35:272-276.
133. Wells VD, Wong ES, Murray BE, et al. Infections due to beta-lactamase-producing, high-level gentamicin-resistant *Enterococcus faecalis.* Ann Intern Med 1992;116:285-292.
134. Mainardi JL, Gutmann L, Acar JF, et al. Synergistic effect of amoxicillin and cefotaxime against *Enterococcus faecalis.* Antimicrob Agents Chemother 1995;39:1984-1987.
135. Gavalda J, Torres C, Tenorio C, et al. Efficacy of ampicillin plus ceftriaxone in treatment of experimental endocarditis due to *Enterococcus faecalis* strains highly resistant to aminoglycosides. Antimicrob Agents Chemother 1999;43:639-646.
136. Tascini C, Doria R, Leonildi A, et al. Efficacy of the combination ampicillin plus ceftriaxone in the treatment of a case of enterococcal endocarditis due to *Enterococcus faecalis* highly resistant to gentamicin: efficacy of the "ex vivo" synergism method. J Chemother 2004;16:400-403.
137. Tripodi MF, Utili R, Rambaldi A, et al. Unorthodox antibiotic combinations including ciprofloxacin against high-level gentamicin resistant enterococci. J Antimicrob Chemother 1996;37:727-736.
138. Tripodi MF, Locatelli A, Adinolfi LE, et al. Successful treatment with ampicillin and fluoroquinolones of human endocarditis due to high-level gentamicin-resistant enterococci. Eur J Clin Microbiol Infect Dis 1998;17:734-736.
139. Stevens MP, Edmond MB. Endocarditis due to vancomycin-resistant enterococci: case report and review of the literature. Clin Infect Dis 2005;41:1134-1142.
140. Jorgensen JH, Crawford SA, Kelly CC, et al. In vitro activity of daptomycin against vancomycin-resistant enterococci of various *van* types and comparison of susceptibility testing methods. Antimicrob Agents Chemother 2003;47:3760-3763.
141. Cha R, Rybak MJ. Daptomycin against multiple drug-resistant staphylococcus and enterococcus isolates in an in vitro pharmacodynamic model with simulated endocardial vegetations. Diagn Microbiol Infect Dis 2003;47:539-546.
142. Vouillamoz J, Moreillon P, Giddey M, et al. Efficacy of daptomycin in the treatment of experimental endocarditis due to susceptible and multidrug-resistant enterococci. J Antimicrob Chemother 2006;58:1208-1214.
143. El-Khatib MR, Wilson FM, Lerner AM. Characteristics of bacterial endocarditis in heroin addicts in Detroit. Am J Med Sci 1976;271:197-201.
144. Sklaver AR, Hoffman TA, Greenman RL. Staphylococcal endocarditis in addicts. South Med J 1978;71:638-643.
145. Whitener C, Caputo GM, Weitekamp MR, et al. Endocarditis due to coagulase-negative staphylococci: microbiologic, epidemiologic, and clinical considerations. Infect Dis Clin North Am 1993;7:81-96.
146. Arber N, Militianu A, Ben-Yehuda A, et al. Native valve *Staphylococcus epidermidis* endocarditis: report of seven cases and review of the literature. Am J Med 1991;90:758-762.
147. Anguera I, Del Rio A, Miro JM, et al. *Staphylococcus lugdunensis* infective endocarditis: description of 10 cases and analysis of native valve, prosthetic valve, and pacemaker lead endocarditis clinical profiles. Heart 2005;91:e10.
148. Steckelberg JM, Rouse MS, Tallan BM, et al. Relative efficacies of broad-spectrum cephalosporins for treatment of methicillin-susceptible *Staphylococcus aureus* experimental infective endocarditis. Antimicrob Agents Chemother 1993;37:554-558.
149. Fridkin SK, Hageman JC, Morrison M, et al. Methicillin-resistant *Staphylococcus aureus* disease in three communities. N Engl J Med 2005;352:1436-1444.
150. King MD, Humphrey BJ, Wang YF, et al. Emergence of community-acquired methicillin-resistant *Staphylococcus aureus* USA 300 clone as the predominant cause of skin and soft-tissue infections. Ann Intern Med 2006;144:309-317.
151. Moran GJ, Krishnadasan A, Gorwitz RJ, et al. Methicillin-resistant *S. aureus* infections among patients in the emergency department. N Engl J Med 2006;355:666-674.
152. Watanakunakorn C, Tisone JC. Synergism between vancomycin and gentamicin or tobramycin for methicillin-susceptible and methicillin-resistant *Staphylococcus aureus* strains. Antimicrob Agents Chemother 1982;22:903-905.
153. Chambers HF, Miller RT, Newman MD. Right-sided *Staphylococcus aureus* endocarditis in intravenous drug abusers: two-week combination therapy. Ann Intern Med 1988;109:619-624.
154. Torres-Tortosa M, de Cueto M, Vergara A, et al. Prospective evaluation of a two-week course of intravenous antibiotics in intravenous drug addicts with infective endocarditis. Grupo de Estudio de Enfermedades Infecciosas de la Provincia de Cadiz. Eur J Clin Microbiol Infect Dis 1994;13:559-564.
155. Ribera E, Gomez-Jimenez J, Cortes E, et al. Effectiveness of cloxacillin with and without gentamicin in short-term therapy for right-sided *Staphylococcus aureus* endocarditis: a randomized, controlled trial. Ann Intern Med 1996;125:969-974.
156. Korzeniowski O, Sande MA. Combination antimicrobial therapy for *Staphylococcus aureus* endocarditis in patients addicted to parenteral drugs and in nonaddicts: a prospective study. Ann Intern Med 1982;97:496-503.
157. Fortun J, Navas E, Martinez-Beltran J, et al. Short-course therapy for right-side endocarditis due to *Staphylococcus aureus* in drug abusers: cloxacillin versus glycopeptides in combination with gentamicin. Clin Infect Dis 2001;33:120-125.
158. Dworkin RJ, Lee BL, Sande MA, et al. Treatment of right-sided *Staphylococcus aureus* endocarditis in intravenous drug users with ciprofloxacin and rifampicin. Lancet 1989;2:1071-1073.
159. Fridkin SK, Hageman J, McDougal LK, et al. Epidemiological and microbiological characterization of infections caused by *Staphylococcus aureus* with reduced susceptibility to vancomycin, United States, 1997-2001. Clin Infect Dis 2003;36:429-439.
160. Karchmer AW, Archer GL, Dismukes WE. *Staphylococcus epidermidis* causing prosthetic valve endocarditis: microbiologic and clinical observations as guides to therapy. Ann Intern Med 1983;98:447-455.
161. Karchmer AW, Archer GL, Dismukes WE. Rifampin treatment of prosthetic valve endocarditis due to *Staphylococcus epidermidis.* Rev Infect Dis 1983;5(Suppl 3):S543-S548.
162. Geraci JE, Wilson WR. Symposium on infective endocarditis. III. Endocarditis due to gram-negative bacteria: report of 56 cases. Mayo Clin Proc 1982;57:145-148.
163. Werner AS, Cobbs CG, Kaye D, et al. Studies on the bacteremia of bacterial endocarditis. JAMA 1967;202:199-203.
164. Strom BL, Abrutyn E, Berlin JA, et al. Dental and cardiac risk factors for infective endocarditis: a population-based, case-control study. Ann Intern Med 1998;129:761-769.
165. Wilson W, Taubert KA, Gewitz M, et al. Prevention of infective endocarditis: guidelines from the American Heart Association. Rheumatic Fever, Endocarditis, and Kawasaki. Disease Committee, Council on Cardiovascular Disease in the Young, and the Council on Clinical Cardiology, Council on Cardiovascular Surgery and Anesthesia, and the Quality of Care and Outcomes Research Interdisciplinary Working Group. Circulation 2007;116:1736-1754.
166. Diz Dios P, Tomas Carmona I, Limeres Posse J, et al. Comparative efficacies of amoxicillin, clindamycin, and moxifloxacin in prevention of bacteremia following dental extractions. Antimicrob Agents Chemother 2006;50:2996-3002.
167. Cabell CH, Abrutyn E. Progress toward a global understanding of infective endocarditis: lessons from the International Collaboration on Endocarditis. Cardiol Clin 2003;21:147-158.
168. Cabell CH, Abrutyn E. Progress toward a global understanding of infective endocarditis: early lessons from the International Collaboration on Endocarditis investigation. Infect Dis Clin North Am 2002;16:255-272, vii.

82

MALARIA

Myaing Nyunt and Christopher V. Plowe

OVERVIEW 1141
INTRODUCTION 1141
PATHOPHYSIOLOGY 1141
Biology of Malaria 1141
Development in Humans 1142
Development in the Mosquito Vector 1143
Malaria Disease and Mechanisms of Disease 1143
Epidemiology 1145
Transmission Intensity and Acquired Immunity 1145
Malaria and Human Immunodeficiency Virus 1145
THERAPEUTICS AND CLINICAL PHARMACOLOGY 1145
Goals of Therapy 1145
Clinical Spectrum of Malaria Disease and Principles of Malaria Therapy 1145
Uncomplicated Malaria 1145
Severe Malaria 1146
Malaria in Pregnancy 1146
Intermittent Preventive Treatment 1147
Malaria Chemoprophylaxis for Travelers 1147
Therapeutics by Class 1147
Quinolines and Related Compounds 1147
Antifolates 1155
Artemisinin Derivatives 1158
Drugs That Interfere with Mitochondrial Function 1160
Antibiotics with Antimalarial Activity 1161
Malaria Vaccines 1162
Therapeutic Approaches 1162
Combination Therapy in Malaria 1163
Uncomplicated Malaria 1163
Severe Malaria 1164
Chemoprophylaxis for Travelers 1164
Malaria in Pregnancy 1164
Emerging Targets and Therapeutics 1165

OVERVIEW

Malaria is one of the world's most important infectious diseases, causing an estimated 350 to 500 new clinical cases and approximately 1 million deaths each year.[1-3] Safe, effective and inexpensive antimalarial drugs developed during the Second World War contributed to a sense of optimism that malaria could be defeated. A global malaria eradication campaign led by the World Health Organization (WHO) in the mid-20th century failed, in large part due to the emergence and spread of drug resistance to chloroquine. Today malaria remains a major health problem throughout the tropics and subtropics, where 3.2 billion people live at risk of acquiring malaria[4] (Fig. 82-1).

Four species of *Plasmodium* cause malaria in humans: *P. falciparum*, *P. vivax*, *P. ovale*, and *P. malariae*. Most of the severe disease and death caused by malaria is attributable to *P. falciparum*, which is most prevalent in sub-Saharan Africa, although *P. vivax* also causes substantial morbidity in Asia and parts of Central and South America. Approximately 60% of clinical malaria cases and 80% of deaths occur in Africa.[5] Most of the disease burden in Africa is borne by young children and pregnant women. Severe disease is also common in nonimmune adults such as travelers and those living in areas of unstable malaria transmission. Malaria's lifelong effects on cognitive development, education, productivity, and life expectancy impose a large economic cost on the developing world.[6] For practitioners in the developed world, malaria represents a serious risk to the health and life of their traveling patients and a febrile illness in returned travelers that is frequently diagnosed and treated inadequately, resulting in severe disability and death.

INTRODUCTION

Malaria is both a parasitic infection and a set of clinical syndromes involving several organ systems, most notably the circulatory and central nervous systems. In thinking about preventing and treating malaria, it is important to distinguish between infection and disease.[7] Infection with malaria parasites may or may not be associated with clinical symptoms, depending on the stage of infection and the immune status of the host. The obligate intracellular parasites go through complex, multistage development and modification in two hosts, the mosquito and the human. The four human malaria species and their different life stages have different morphologies and behaviors and are differentially susceptible to drugs. This biologic complexity has to be taken into account in targeting drug treatment to specific preventive and therapeutic objectives such as preventing malaria infection, treating severe falciparum malaria, or providing radical cure of vivax malaria. Increasing the complexity of malaria therapeutics, drug therapies that combine multiple antimalarial agents are now recommended and widely used to overcome or prevent drug resistance. The recent shift to combination therapies has resulted in greater risks of drug toxicity and higher costs.

Because of the limitations of vector control methods and the lack of an effective malaria vaccine, prompt and effective drug treatment remains a mainstay of malaria control. Nevertheless, our understanding of antimalarial drug behaviors in the body in relation to clinical and parasitologic responses is limited. The list of safe, effective, and affordable antimalarial drugs is still very short, and the list of drugs that can be used safely in infants and pregnant women is shorter still. Antimalarial drugs are commonly introduced into widespread use with inadequate information about pharmacokinetics and pharmacodynamics and with insufficient evidence of drug safety in target populations.

PATHOPHYSIOLOGY

Biology of Malaria

Malaria parasites belong to the genus *Plasmodium*. Malaria infection in humans is caused by four species of obligate intracellular protozoa: *P. falciparum*, *P. vivax*, *P. malariae*, and *P. ovale*. Hundreds of other *Plasmodium* species infect other mammals, reptiles, and birds, generally in a species-restricted fashion. To complete its life cycle, the parasite requires two hosts, the female anopheline mosquito vector and the vertebrate host. The infection is usually transmitted by the bite of infected mosquitoes, and rarely by transfusion of infected blood, sharing needles, and transplacental transfer to the fetus.

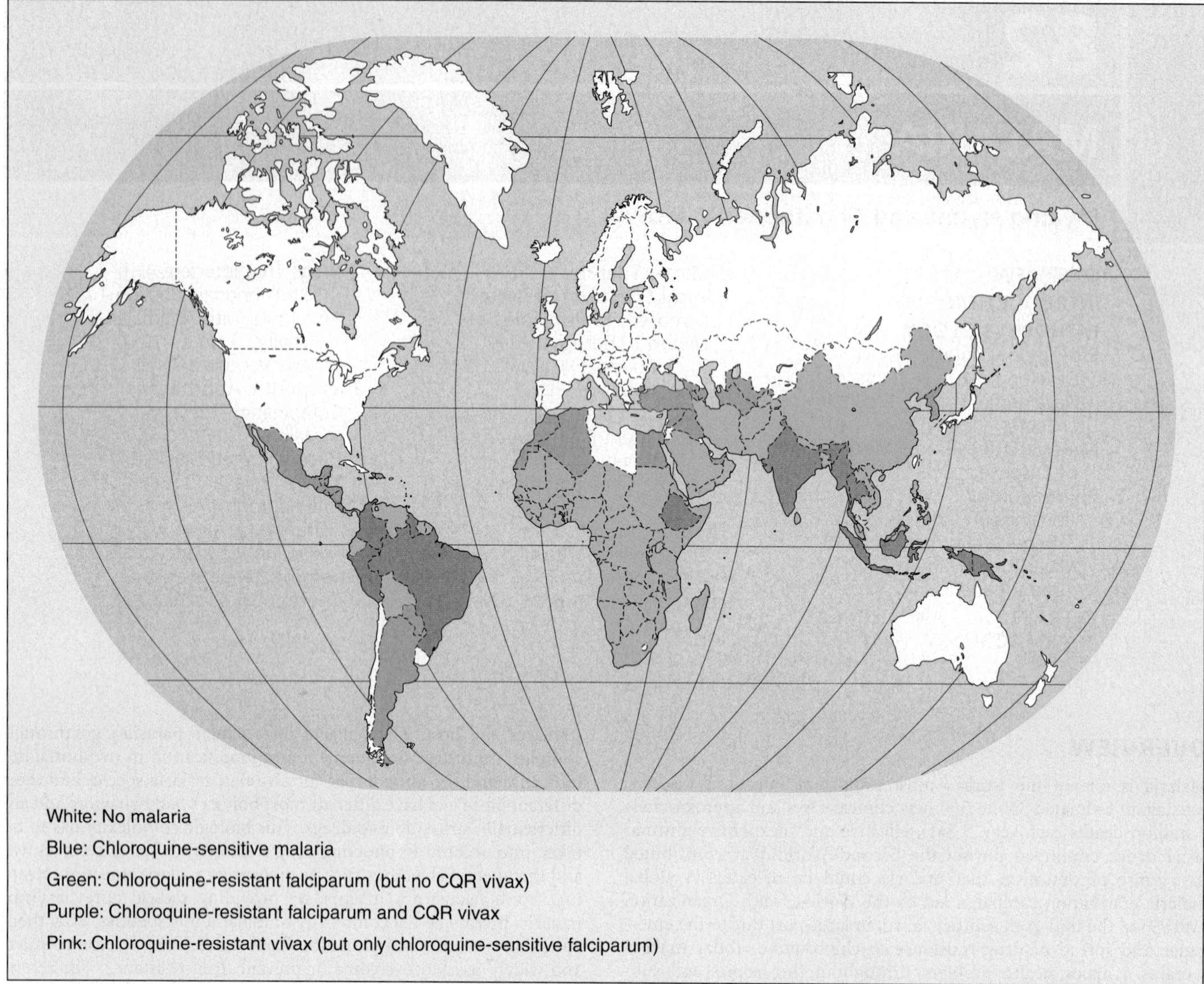

FIGURE 82-1 • Global distribution of malaria and chloroquine-resistant *Plasmodium falciparum* and *Plasmodium vivax* malaria.

TABLE 82-1 CHARACTERISTICS OF HUMAN *PLASMODIUM* INFECTION

Characteristics	*P. falciparum*	*P. vivax*	*P. ovale*	*P. malariae*
Minimum duration of hepatic development (days)	6.5	8	9	15
Merozoites released per hepatocyte	30,000	10,000	15,000	Variable
Duration of erythrocytic development (hr)	48	48	48	72
Presence of latent form in liver (relapse)	No	Yes	Yes	No
Red cell preference	Young cells (invade all)	Up to 14 days old	Reticulocytes	Old cells

Development in Humans

The malaria life cycle in humans begins when sporozoites are injected from the female mosquito's salivary gland as she takes a blood meal. Each mosquito bite may inoculate five to seven sporozoites, which are motile, wormlike single-celled organisms approximately 7 μm in length, or about as long as an erythrocyte is wide. Sporozoites rapidly enter the circulation and invade hepatocytes, where the parasites develop and multiply. Over the next 5 to 15 days, depending on the *Plasmodium* species (Table 82-1), the infected hepatocyte develops into a tissue schizont containing as many as 10,000 to 30,000 merozoites that have developed from a single sporozoite. The infected hepatocytes rupture, each releasing a shower of merozoites into the circulation, where these small (1- to 2-μm diameter), briefly extracellular parasites initiate the blood stage of the infection, which is responsible for disease manifestations. The liver stage of malaria is clinically asymptomatic. In *P. vivax* and *P. ovale* infection, some tissue parasites can develop into latent forms called hypnozoites, which persist in the liver for as long as 3 to 5 years. These "sleeping parasites," which do not produce any clinical manifestations, can be reactivated and cause relapses long after the disease-causing blood-stage parasites have been eliminated by drug cure.

Merozoites released from hepatocytes enter the bloodstream, where they invade erythrocytes. In erythrocytes, the parasites undergo another set of morphologic changes, and asexual multiplication. Most develop from compact ring forms to larger but still unicellular trophozoites, and then multiply to become multicellular blood schizonts. Once mature, the schizonts rupture, releasing 6 to 32 merozoites that in turn invade more erythrocytes in a process known as schizogony. This process continues in a periodic cycle until it is interrupted by host immunity, drug treatment, or the death of the host. Clinical symptoms may develop during this blood stage of infection. The cycle of invasion, multiplication, and reinvasion takes place over 48 hours for *P. falciparum*, *P. vivax*, and *P. ovale*, and 72 hours for *P. malariae*. When the infecting parasites cycle in a synchronized fashion, the classic malaria symptoms of fever and chills followed by a period of relative relief can follow the same periodicity, although a more chaotic fever pattern is typical of *P. falciparum*, which tends not to be synchronized, especially in endemic populations.

In their different stages of development, malaria parasites are antigenically, biologically, and morphologically distinct, and their susceptibility to chemical therapeutics is also highly variable. Examples of antimalarial drugs and vaccines that target these different developmental and functional stages in the parasites are shown in Figure 82-2. Most antimalarial drugs can effectively kill the erythrocytic stage (e.g., quinolines, artemisinin derivatives, and antifolates). Some drugs are effective for only the hepatic stage (e.g., primaquine) and some are active against both (e.g., atovaquone). The only drug that can eradicate hypnozoites is primaquine. No antimalarial drug is known to effectively kill sporozoites or halt their development. For this reason, malaria infection cannot be entirely prevented by chemoprophylaxis, which is instead intended to prevent infection from progressing to malaria disease. Prophylaxis of malaria disease by eliminating liver-stage parasites is called "causal prophylaxis," whereas "suppressive prophylaxis" refers to using drugs to eliminate erythrocytic-stage parasites.

Development in the Mosquito Vector

During erythrocytic development in humans, some parasites develop into sexual forms, male and female gametocytes. Gametogenesis is increased when the parasite is stressed by drug treatment or clinical deterioration of the host. These sexual forms are taken up by the mosquito vector, emerge from the erythrocyte in the mosquito midgut, and fertilize to form diploid zygotes. The zygotes differentiate into ookinetes that burrow across the wall of the midgut and develop into oocysts, where haploid asexual reproduction occurs until each oocyst contains up to 1000 sporozoites. The sporozoites emerge from the midgut, carried by the mosquito hemolymph, and invade the salivary glands, from which they will be injected into the human host to complete the parasite life cycle. This extrinsic incubation period takes about 1 to 2 weeks depending on ambient temperature and humidity.

Malaria Disease and Mechanisms of Disease

Malaria is a set of complex clinical syndromes involving several of the body's vital systems. Depending on the infecting species and on the immunologic status of the human host, the severity of clinical manifestations varies widely, ranging from a complete lack of clinical symptoms to a mild febrile illness, to severe disease and death. (Note: Because uncomplicated clinical malaria is similar for all four human malaria species and most manifestations of severe malaria are associated only with *P. falciparum*, the reader should assume discussion of malaria disease refers to falciparum malaria unless otherwise specified.) Our understanding of the pathophysiology of malaria disease has evolved greatly in the last decade, although application of this knowledge to the development of new antimalarial therapeutics has been limited.

Some of the clinical features of severe malaria are specific to malaria, but many features are shared with other sepsis syndromes. Clinical studies of severe malaria[8-11] conducted in the 1990s expanded understanding of the pathophysiology of malaria beyond the well-known syndromes of fever, severe malarial anemia, and cerebral malaria. Severe metabolic derangements including acidosis and systemic inflammation induced by the interaction between host cells parasite are now known to play critical roles. As in many other infectious diseases, the most important common final pathway of severe malaria pathology is a disruption of tissue perfusion.

The clinical syndrome of falciparum malaria originates with changes in the infected erythrocytes. After they invade, malaria parasites effectively hijack the host cell and its machinery, and express their own proteins on the surface of the erythrocyte. Strain-specific, antigenically variant large protein receptors (e.g. *P. falciparum* erythrocyte membrane proteins [PfEMPs]) are expressed on the surface of infected red blood cells in clumps known as "knobs" that are visible by electron microscopy on the surface of the infected cells. These sticky knobs are responsible for adherence of parasitized erythrocytes to the vascular endothelium (cytoadherence), to other infected red cells (agglutination), and to uninfected red cells (rosetting). Several vascular receptors have been recognized as important in cytoaherence: intercellular adhesion molecule 1 in the brain, and chondroitin sulfate A and halyuronic acid in the placenta. Cytoadherence and agglutination result in sequestration of infected red cells in the microcirculatory compartments of organs, most importantly in the brain and placenta, leading to disease, and most abundantly in the spleen, causing splenomegaly. Sequestered infected red cells not only interfere with microcirculatory blood flow and thus with critical metabolic functions and tissue perfusion (including maternal support to the fetus in the case of placental malaria), but also hide outside the reach of host defense mechanisms. Infected red cells lose their deformability and compromise blood flow in small capillaries and venules. The ability of falciparum malaria to sequester plays a critical role in disease severity—the other human malarias (*P. vivax*, *P. ovale*, and *P. malariae*) do not sequester, and therefore are not associated with the severe manifestations seen with falciparum malaria. The life spans of infected red blood cells and agglutinated uninfected red cells are shortened by rapid splenic removal, a factor that contributes to anemia. The destruction of infected red blood cells during schizont rupture and malaria-induced suppression of the hematopoietic system (reduced production of erythropoietin, reduced hemopoietic response from bone marrow and spleen) as well as immune-mediated hemolysis are also increasingly appreciated as important factors in malarial anemia.

The clinical impact of malaria-specific events taking place in the red blood cells is augmented by activated nonspecific body defense mechanisms, as seen in clinical syndromes caused by other infectious organisms. Severe malaria is associated with overactivation of host immune factors and inflammatory cytokines such as interleukin-1β, interleukin-6, and tumor necrosis factor-α.[12-15] The involvement of oxygen free radicals and reactive nitrogen species in malaria disease is a matter of some controversy, and limited experience with therapeutics targeting these mediators has been unsuccessful. (High-dose steroids have no benefit in Asian adults with severe malaria,[16] but have not been assessed in African children, whose clinical presentation is somewhat different.) It is fair to conclude that disturbances in these immune mediators are associated with the features seen in vital organs of patients with severe malaria, including endothelial damage, massive vasodilation, and increased vascular permeability. Pathologic hemodynamic consequences include hypovolemia, late hypotension, and subsequent cardiac failure. These hemodynamic derangements are more common in adults in low-transmission areas than in African children, who tend to have primary respiratory failure not related to cardiovascular compromise.

Malaria-specific and nonspecific abnormalities are manifested clinically as a wide range of clinical syndromes. Anemia is one of the most common and prominent presenting features in children with malaria in endemic countries. Microcirculatory disturbances are seen in the brain (cerebral hypoxia, inflammation, and edema), liver (dysgluconeogenesis and hypoglycemia, hepatocyte injury, cholestasis and jaundice), kidneys (acute tubular and cortical necrosis and renal failure), and lungs (noncardiogenic pulmonary edema and acute respiratory distress syndrome). Multiple factors (reduced tissue perfusion and organ failure, hypermetabolic state, anemia, increased glycolysis and hypovolemia) contribute to a metabolic acidosis that often presents

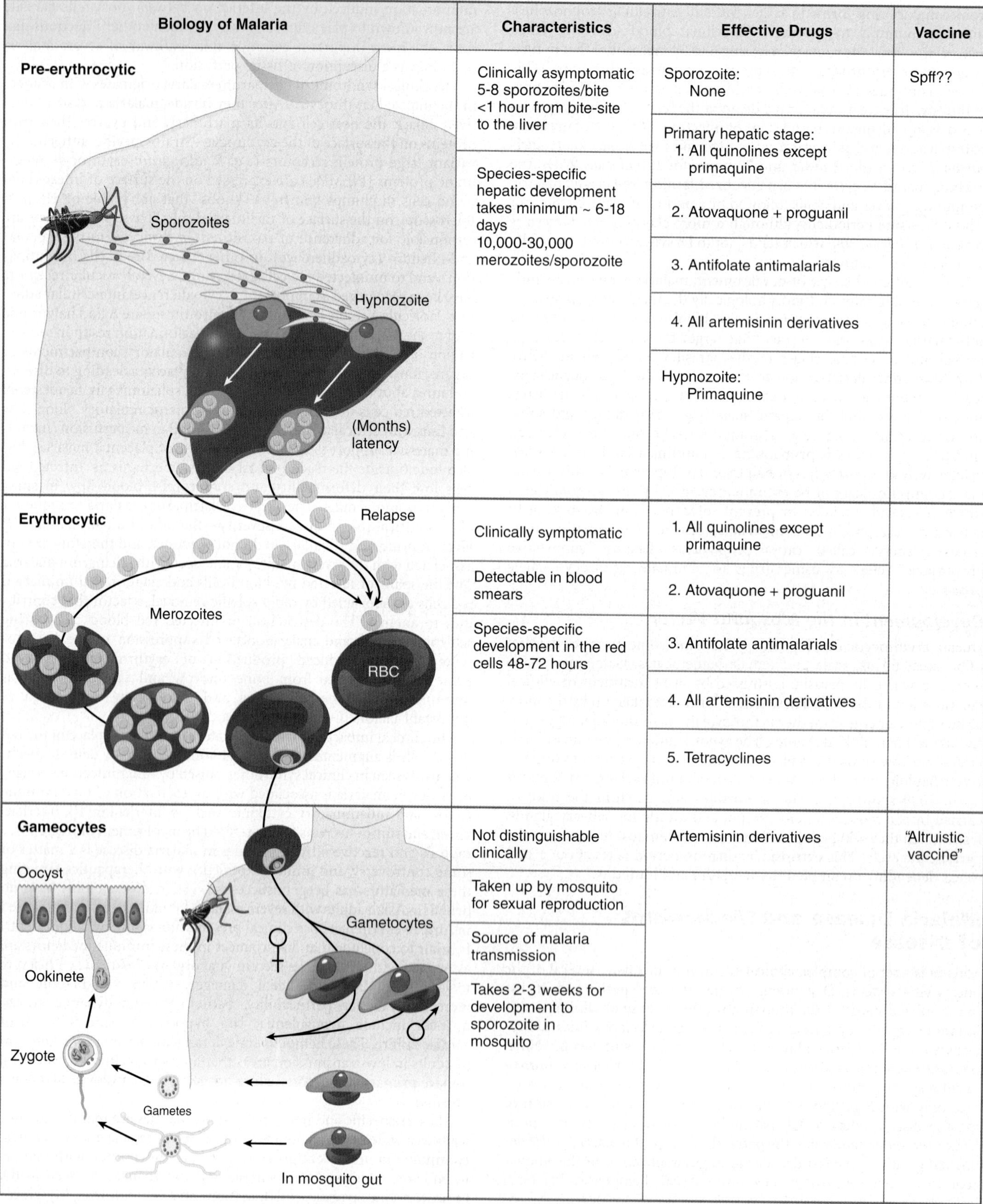

Biology of Malaria	Characteristics	Effective Drugs	Vaccine
Pre-erythrocytic	Clinically asymptomatic 5-8 sporozoites/bite <1 hour from bite-site to the liver	Sporozoite: None	Spff??
	Species-specific hepatic development takes minimum ~ 6-18 days 10,000-30,000 merozoites/sporozoite	Primary hepatic stage: 1. All quinolines except primaquine	
		2. Atovaquone + proguanil	
		3. Antifolate antimalarials	
		4. All artemisinin derivatives	
		Hypnozoite: Primaquine	
Erythrocytic	Clinically symptomatic	1. All quinolines except primaquine	
	Detectable in blood smears	2. Atovaquone + proguanil	
	Species-specific development in the red cells 48-72 hours	3. Antifolate antimalarials	
		4. All artemisinin derivatives	
		5. Tetracyclines	
Gameocytes	Not distinguishable clinically	Artemisinin derivatives	"Altruistic vaccine"
	Taken up by mosquito for sexual reproduction		
	Source of malaria transmission		
	Takes 2-3 weeks for development to sporozoite in mosquito		

FIGURE 82-2 • Malaria biology, stage-specific characteristics, and antimalarial therapeutics.

with respiratory distress and disturbances in the central nervous system and carries high morbidity and mortality.[17]

Epidemiology

Transmission Intensity and Acquired Immunity

Malaria is endemic in most of the tropics and subtropics (140 countries and territories), and 3.2 billion people live at risk of acquiring malaria infection.[4] Of the four *Plasmodium* species that cause disease in humans, *P. falciparum* is responsible for the most disease and death and is the most common cause of malaria in Africa, Haiti, Papua New Guinea, and Indonesia. *Plasmodium vivax* is the most prevalent species in Southeast Asia and Central America. Both *P. vivax* and *P. falciparum* are commonly found in South America, East Asia, and Oceania, and can occur together in the same individual, complicating diagnosis and treatment. *Plasmodium ovale* is seen mostly in Africa. *Plasmodium malariae* can be found in all endemic regions but is less common than other species.

The epidemiology of malaria is determined primarily by the intensity of malaria transmission, which in turn drives the prevalence of malaria infection and the incidence of different forms of malaria disease. Malaria transmission is measured by the entomologic inoculation rate (EIR), an estimate of the number of infected mosquito bites per person per unit of time. Annual entomologic inoculation rates range from less than 1 in parts of Latin America and Southeast Asia to more than 300 in some parts of Africa. In high-transmission areas (typical of much of sub-Saharan Africa), neonates and infants in the first 3 to 6 months of life are protected by immunity acquired from the mother. Older infants and young children are not immune to malaria, and carry a high burden of severe malaria morbidity and mortality. If these children survive the first few years of the high-risk period in which they are repeatedly exposed to malaria, they gradually acquire natural immunity and become protected against malaria disease while remaining susceptible to malaria infection. This acquired immunity is hard won and short lived, and wanes in the absence of continued exposure. In areas where malaria transmission is unstable or sporadic, protective immunity is never established and symptomatic and severe malaria are seen in all age groups. The same is true for nonimmune travelers, who may succumb rapidly to a severe, often fatal disease without prompt, appropriate treatment.

Both humoral and cellular immune factors contribute to protection against clinical malaria. In general, cellular immune responses are thought to be more important in controlling the pre-erythrocytic stages of malaria infection, and antibodies are thought to block erythrocyte invasion to suppress blood-stage infection. However, protective immunity against malaria is poorly understood and no specific immune response has been established as an essential correlate of clinical protection, complicating malaria vaccine development. In addition to acquired immunity, several host genetic factors offer some degree of protection against malaria. Sickle cell trait and some other hemoglobinopathies are more prevalent in populations living at risk of malaria because they afford protection against clinical malaria. Various other human genetic polymorphisms associated with the host immune response and with host-parasite binding have also been correlated with susceptibility to clinical malaria in genetic association studies.

Malaria and Human Immunodeficiency Virus

The distributions of human immunodeficiency virus (HIV) and malaria overlap, especially in sub-Saharan Africa. Not surprisingly, some clinical and pharmacologic interactions between these two infections have been described.[18-20] The most important and best established of these are seen in pregnancy. Mothers infected with HIV have higher rates of malaria infection and disease, and deliver babies with lower birth weights. These differences are more pronounced in multigravid women, who appear to have an impaired ability to develop the antibody-mediated immunity that is usually acquired by the second or third pregnancy in women living in high-transmission areas. Other adults living with HIV in high-transmission settings have some increased risk of malaria infection and more frequent episodes of fever in the presence of malaria infection. These effects are modest in comparison with the increased risks to other opportunistic infections, and some of the apparent increase in clinical malaria is likely attributable to more frequent fevers from nonmalaria causes occurring in the presence of incidental malaria infection and leading to misdiagnosis of malaria illness. Where malaria transmission is low or has unstable transmission, HIV infection is associated with an increased risk of severe malaria disease.

Daily chemoprophylaxis with sulfamethoxazole-trimethoprim, which is recommended to prevent HIV-related opportunistic infections (mainly enteric bacteria in sub-Saharan Africa), is also highly effective at preventing malaria.[21,22] Chloroquine appears to have some antiretroviral activity in vitro, although the clinical significance of this observation, if any, is unknown. Numerous potential and known interactions between antimalarial and antiretroviral drugs have been described.[19] The most important of these interactions is reduced metabolism of lumefantrine and halofantrine by the cytochrome P-450 (CYP) isoform 3A4 in the presence of protease inhibitors and nonnucleoside reverse transcriptase inhibitors, resulting in prolonged QT intervals and possible increased risk of sudden cardiac death from ventricular arrhythmias. Antiretroviral drugs of various classes that induce or inhibit CYP activities may either increase or decrease blood levels of quinine and other antimalarial drugs, leading to increased toxicity or diminished efficacy, respectively, but these potential interactions are not well studied and their clinical impact is unknown.

THERAPEUTICS AND CLINICAL PHARMACOLOGY

Goals of Therapy

The clinical management of malaria differs in different settings depending on the clinical severity, age of the patient, presence or absence of acquired immunity, drug resistance patterns and availability of drugs. Antimalarial drugs are used for four main purposes: (i) treatment of uncomplicated malaria, (ii) treatment of severe malaria, (iii) prevention of malaria disease and its complications in vulnerable populations such as infants and pregnant women, and (iv) prevention of malaria in nonimmune travelers.

Clinical Spectrum of Malaria Disease and Principles of Malaria Therapy

Uncomplicated Malaria

Uncomplicated malaria refers to clinically symptomatic malaria without signs of severe malaria disease. The clinical presentation of uncomplicated malaria tends to be nonspecific, resembling the symptoms of a viral syndrome, and is similar for all four species of *Plasmodium* that cause malaria in humans. Common symptoms include headache, body aches, chills, fever, rigors, nausea, and abdominal discomfort. In malaria-endemic countries, the local languages often have only one word to connote both "malaria" and "fever," and fevers are routinely treated with antimalarial drugs, usually without any other diagnostic evaluation. A classic pattern of cyclical fevers punctuated by periods of relative relief (known as malaria paroxysms), corresponding to the waves of merozoites released into the bloodstream during schizogony, is characteristic of malaria, but continuous and chaotic fever patterns are also seen.[23] Common physical findings include mild anemia and splenomegaly. Thrombocytopenia is common but rarely associated with bleeding even when profound. Leukocytosis is not caused by malaria, and its presence suggests alternative sources of fever or concurrent bacterial infection.

The objective of treatment in uncomplicated malaria is to eradicate the blood stages of infection as quickly as possible, to prevent the progression of disease and complications, and secondarily to decrease transmission. If treated promptly with effective drugs, uncomplicated

TABLE 82-2 CLINICAL FEATURES OF SEVERE MALARIA AND PROGNOSTIC INDICATORS

Clinical or Laboratory Findings	Diagnostic Criteria for Severe Malaria
Neurologic abnormality (other causes of encephalopathy must be excluded)	Cerebral malaria (coma with *P. falciparum* parasitemia) Generalized convulsion (≥2 in 24 hr) Impaired consciousness* Cerebral malaria/coma following generalized seizure*
Hematologic and bleeding abnormality	Severe anemia* (hemoglobin <5 g/dl) in the presence of parasites >100,000/μl Leukocytosis (WBC count >12,000/μl) Coagulopathy* (platelets <50,000/μl, prolonged PT/PTT, increased fibrinogen) and disseminated intravascular coagulation*
Metabolic dysfunction	
Hypoglycemia*	Plasma glucose <40 mg/dl
Acidosis* (often presented as respiratory distress)	Arterial pH < 7.3, plasma bicarbonate <15 mmol/L
Hyperlactesemia*	Lactate >15 mmol/L
Jaundice/hyperbilirubinemia	Serum bilirubin >3 mg/dl
Hepatic enzyme abnormality	Elevation of AST and ALT
Muscle enzyme abnormality	Elevated CPK
Respiratory abnormality*	Noncardiogenic pulmonary edema Acute respiratory distress syndrome
Renal dysfunction*	Decreased urine output Acute renal failure (serum creatinine >3 mg/dl)
Cardiovascular dysfunction*	Hypotension Circulatory collapse
Malaria blood smear	Hyperparasitemia* (>100,000/μl: increased mortality; >500,000/μl: ~50% mortality; hemozoin in >20% of trophozoites and schizonts or >5% of neutrophils)†

*Clinical and laboratory parameters associated with poor prognosis.
†Represent the threshold in nonimmune individuals; these threshold may be higher in immune or semi-immune individuals.
ALT, alanine aminotransferase; AST, aspartate aminotransferase; CPK, creatine phosphokinase; PT, prothrombin time; PTT, partial thromboplastin time; WBC, white blood cell.

malaria can be effectively prevented from progressing to severe or fatal malaria. Cure is rapid, with clearance of parasites and fever in 1 to 3 days. Uncomplicated malaria should be diagnosed and treated without delay, especially in vulnerable groups such as young children, pregnant women, and nonimmune individuals whose clinical condition can deteriorate quickly.

Severe Malaria

While serious complications and death are relatively uncommon in non-falciparum malaria, *P. falciparum*, the most common species in Africa, carries a high risk of morbidity and mortality. The defining features of severe malaria and those that are associated with a poor prognosis are shown in Table 82-2. The progression of falciparum malaria from uncomplicated to severe disease can be extremely rapid, and death may occur within hours of presentation, especially in young children, nonimmune individuals, and pregnant women. The case fatality rate for untreated severe malaria is estimated at 50% and is about 10% to 15% with appropriate treatment. Severe malaria is a medical emergency, and the major objective of treatment is to prevent death. Aggressive supportive care and monitoring in an intensive care setting are required. Among several factors that determine survival, achieving therapeutic concentrations of effective antimalarial drug(s) as quickly as possible using parenteral administration of fast-acting schizonticides is most important.

Malaria in Pregnancy

Pregnant women are at a higher risk of acquiring malaria infection, and of developing symptomatic and severe disease such as severe anemia. Malaria during pregnancy also carries a risk of adverse birth outcomes such as spontaneous abortion, stillbirth, and premature birth or intrauterine growth restriction, both contributing to low birth weight, which is the single most important indicator of infant mortality. Physiologic alteration or suppression of immune functions essential to maintain stability and growth of the fetus may be partially responsible for this heightened vulnerability during pregnancy. The pathophysiology of malaria in pregnancy involves a massive sequestration of parasitized red blood cells in the placenta. Interaction between the parasite ligand *P. falciparum* erythrocyte membrane protein 1 (PfEMP1)[24,25] on the surface of infected erythrocytes and specific endothelial receptors in placental tissue, particularly chondroitin sulfate A and hyaluronic acid,[26] appears to be an important mechanism of placental sequestration. Adverse effects of malaria in pregnancy seem to stem from this sequestration interfering with placenta nutrient transfer between the mother and fetus.[27] Chronic inflammatory responses, proinflammatory cytokines, and other immune mediators likely also play important roles. Malaria-induced adverse outcomes in pregnancy are most pronounced in the first and second pregnancy, with acquired immunity protecting multigravid women.[28]

The clinical presentation of malaria in pregnancy depends on the degree of malaria transmission. In areas of low transmission, acute symptomatic cases are common and the development of severe disease is rapid. Once severe malaria develops, the case fatality rate of falciparum malaria in pregnancy approaches 50%, even with treatment.[29] In areas of moderate to high transmission, acute clinical episodes and severe malaria are relatively uncommon; instead the infection tends to be chronic, leading to maternal anemia and complications to the fetus. In this setting, minimizing the adverse impact of malaria on pregnancy outcome (such as reduction of the number of newborns with low birth weight) is an important objective.

Management of malaria in pregnancy includes the treatment of acute malaria episodes and intermittent preventive treatment (IPT). The management of malaria in pregnancy is challenging for several reasons: limited choices of safe and effective antimalarial drugs, difficult diagnosis because of low placental parasitemia (despite heavy parasite sequestration in the placenta), and the high rate of recrudescence. The objective of treatment in uncomplicated malaria is to eradicate the infection as rapidly as possible, while protecting the fetus. The objective of treatment of severe malaria in pregnancy is to save the mother's life; it is imperative to use effective treatment even if the drugs are not known to be safe for the fetus.

Intermittent Preventive Treatment

IPT of pregnant women refers to the administration of treatment doses of antimalarial drugs, usually sulfadoxine-pyrimethamine, at intervals during pregnancy, irrespective of the presence or absence of peripheral parasitemia. Several clinical trials have demonstrated that IPT improves maternal health (e.g., correction of maternal anemia) and birth outcome (reductions in premature births and low birth weight).[29a] In 2000, the WHO recommended that all pregnant women in areas with moderate to high malaria transmission be treated with sulfadoxine-pyrimethamine (1.5 g sulfadoxine and 75 mg pyrimethamine) at least twice after the end of the first trimester. This dosing regimen for IPT is based on the pharmacokinetics information obtained in nonpregnant groups, mostly adult males. The pharmacokinetics of these compounds are likely to be different in pregnancy due to dramatic physiologic shifts in renal function and fluid volume and distribution. IPT in pregnancy retains significant therapeutic benefit even in the face of substantially reduced sulfadoxine-pyrimethamine efficacy for treating acute malaria in children.[29b]

Following the idea of IPT in pregnancy, IPT in infancy has been shown to reduce clinical malaria episodes and malarial anemia in high-transmission settings. IPT is also being evaluated in children who remain vulnerable to severe malaria in areas of seasonal malaria transmission.

Malaria Chemoprophylaxis for Travelers

Nonimmune travelers are at high risk of rapid deterioration and death from malaria. Most years, over 1000 cases of malaria in returned travelers in the United States are reported to the Centers for Disease Control and Prevention (CDC). In addition to measures to reduce exposure to malaria such as covering exposed skin with clothing, sleeping under a bed net (preferably impregnated with insecticide), avoiding the outdoors during prime mosquito biting times (dusk and dawn), and using insect repellents containing DEET (diethylmetatoluamide), preventing malaria in travelers relies on effective chemoprophylaxis. The choice of prophylactic drug depends on whether travel is to areas with chloroquine-resistant malaria, convenience, tolerability, cost, and convenience. Detailed recommendations for malaria chemotherapy for travelers are provided in the Therapeutic Approaches section of this chapter.

Therapeutics by Class

Quinolines and Related Compounds

Quinolines and related compounds are the largest group of antimalarials used effectively and the longest surviving antimalarials in the modern history of malaria treatment and prophylaxis. After almost 400 years of therapeutic use, quinine, the oldest quinoline antimalarial, is still used for the treatment of chloroquine-resistant falciparum malaria. Chloroquine, its 4-amino derivative, is probably still the most widely used antimalarial drug in the world, despite widespread chloroquine-resistant *P. falciparum*, as well as *P. vivax* in some regions, and recommendations against the use of chloroquine in the treatment of falciparum malaria in many endemic areas. The major determinant of drug use in malaria-endemic areas is often the cost. Chloroquine is very inexpensive, often costing well under $0.50 for a treatment regimen, and well tolerated, and its antipyretic effect also favors its use even when its antiparasitic activity is curtailed by resistance. Chemical structures of some important quinolines are shown in Figure 82-3.

Mechanism of Action. Quinolines interfere with the processing of toxic heme in the parasites' digestive food vacuoles. After infection of the red blood cell, hemoglobin degradation takes place in the parasites' acidic food vacuoles. Heme is toxic to the parasite, and is sequestered as an insoluble nontoxic molecule hemozoin, also known as malaria pigment. Chloroquine is concentrated in the parasite food vacuole and binds to heme, interfering with heme polymerization. It is believed that drug-heme complexes cause oxidative damage to the food vacuole membrane and to the proteases essential for hemoglobin digestion, leading to the death of the parasite. This mechanism of killing may be common to other quinolines (quinine, mefloquine, amodiaquine, piperaquine), as well as aminoalcohol analogues (halofantrine, lumefantrine) and Mannich base analogues (pyronaridine).[30] Other possible specific mechanisms of quinoline activity include blocking heme polymerization and/or crystallization,[31] inhibition of synthesis of proteinases essential in hemoglobin digestion,[32] and blockade of tumor necrosis factor release from macrophage.[33]

Mechanism of Resistance. Resistance in *P. falciparum* to quinolines, particularly to chloroquine, is increasingly common in most endemic areas (see Fig. 82-1). The common pathway that parasites use to develop drug resistance against many quinolines involves interference with drug transporters such as *P. falciparum* chloroquine resistance transporter (PfCRT) or P-glycoprotein transporter.

Chloroquine Resistance. The first clinical cases of chloroquine-resistant *P. falciparum* were reported in South America and Southeast Asia in the late 1950s, and these reports were later confirmed by in vitro testing.[34,35] Chloroquine resistance spread slowly but inexorably from these initial foci throughout most of the malaria-endemic world, rendering chloroquine ineffective against falciparum malaria in all but a few limited geographic regions. Chloroquine resistance is one of two best understood mechanisms of antimalarial drug resistance (the other being antifolate resistance). Chloroquine is concentrated less in the digestive vacuoles of resistant *P. falciparum* than in those of chloroquine-sensitive parasites.[36] This reduction in chloroquine concentration is conferred by mutations in a highly conserved transporter, PfCRT, encoded by the *pfcrt* gene located on chromosome 7 and expressed on the membrane of digestive vacuole.[37] The key mutation is a change from lysine to threonine in the 76th amino acid (K76T).[37] This mutant PfCRT is strongly associated with clinical treatment failure[38] and has been used as a molecular marker for surveillance of chloroquine resistance.[39] A variable set of additional mutations that do not themselves confer resistance without K76T always accompanies the PfCRT K76T mutation, and these additional mutations are thought to compensate for a fitness cost associated with K76T.[40] Once chloroquine resistance has been conferred by PfCRT mutation, mutations in P-glycoprotein transporter, encoded by the gene *pfmdr1* on chromosome 5, can modulate the level of resistance, although the relevance of this effect on clinical treatment outcome remains unclear.[41,42] The mechanism of chloroquine resistance in *P. vivax* is not yet known.

Resistance to Other Quinolines. Mefloquine resistance is prevalent in Southeast Asia and is associated with amplification of *pfmdr1* (increased copy number of the gene), which encodes energy-dependent P-glycoprotein transporter.[43] Quinine (and quinidine) resistance remains rare in most areas, although it was first documented in Brazil in the early 20th century and has become widespread in Southeast Asia. Decreased susceptibility to quinine may be associated with resistance to other structurally related quinolines such as mefloquine and halofantrine.[44,45] Genetic changes associated with quinine resistance are likely to be more complex and/or come at a significant cost to fitness, based on the continuous range of quinine susceptibility measured in resistant isolates and on the failure of pronounced resistance to spread beyond Southeast Asia as resistance to other drugs has done. Some resistance mechanisms share some common genetic events, others do not. For instance, chloroquine-resistant *P. falciparum* usually remains sensitive to amodiaquine,[40] which is structurally closely related to chloroquine.

Chloroquine

History. Chloroquine was first synthesized in the 1930s in Germany but was prematurely abandoned owing to concerns about toxicity observed in an avian model. It was reexamined by Americans during World War II as a part of an extensive search for antimalarial compounds. Thousands of compounds were synthesized, and chloroquine became the lead compound among 4-aminoquinolines, superior to the others, quinacrine and quinine. With its low cost, good tolerability, and excellent efficacy against sensitive parasites, chloroquine became the first-line drug for treating malaria worldwide and was the linchpin of the global campaign to eradicate malaria in the 1960s. The rise and spread of resistance has led to its withdrawal from most of the malaria-endemic world, at least as a matter of policy, although it continues to be used and sold through private sources even where it has been

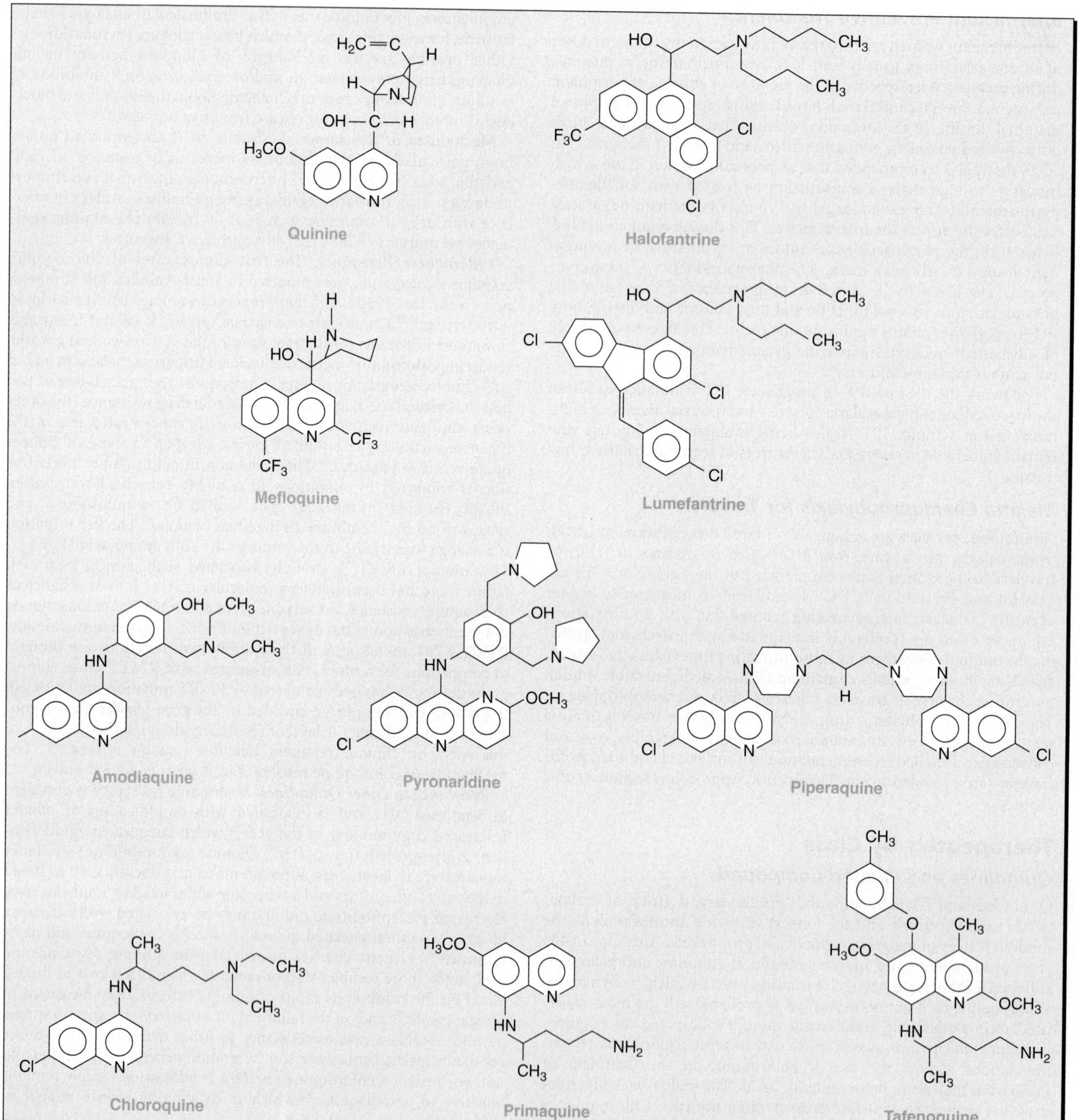

Quinine

Halofantrine

Mefloquine

Lumefantrine

Amodiaquine

Pyronaridine

Piperaquine

Chloroquine

Primaquine

Tafenoquine

FIGURE 82-3 • Chemical structures of quinolines and related compounds.

replaced with more effective but also more expensive drugs. One country that effectively withdrew chloroquine, Malawi in Central Africa, experienced a complete return of chloroquine-susceptible malaria several years later, suggesting a high fitness cost of resistance leading to its loss in the absence of drug pressure, and raising the possibility of rotating antimalarial drugs.[46,47]

Chemistry. The chemical structure of chloroquine is shown in Figure 82-3. Chloroquine is structurally derived directly from quinine. Stereoisomers of chloroquine—D (+), L (−), and DL—have been identified and are all active against sensitive falciparum parasites, but the D-isomer is less toxic and more active against resistant parasites.[48]

Antimalarial Activity. Chloroquine is effective against sensitive strains of blood-stage parasites (*P. falciparum*, *vivax*, *ovale*, and *malariae*) but has no activity against the primary hepatic or the latent stage of any *Plasmodium* species. Prolonged therapy with primaquine is required to prevent relapse of latent forms of malaria infection following cure of the blood stages with chloroquine (see Primaquine section below).

Pharmacokinetics. The pharmacokinetics of chloroquine have been extensively reviewed by Krishna and White.[49] Chloroquine is formulated as sulfate, phosphate, and hydrochloride salts. It is usually prescribed based on the weight of the base content and is available in

TABLE 82-3 TREATMENT REGIMEN FOR UNCOMPLICATED MALARIA

Drug	Dosing Regimen	Comment
Chloroquine phosphate*	Oral; 1000 mg salt (600 mg base) at diagnosis followed by 500 mg (300 mg base) at 6, 24, and 48 hr *Pediatric dosing:* 10 mg base/kg followed by 5 mg base/kg at 6, 24, and 48 hr	Only for the treatment of chloroquine-sensitive *P. falcipaum, P. vivax, P. ovale*, and *P. malariae*.
Quinine sulfate*	Oral; 650 mg salt (542 mg base) every 8 hr for 7 days for monotherapy or for 3 days when used with adjunct therapy *Pediatric dosing:* 8.3 mg base/kg every 8 hr or 3-7 days	Common unpleasant side effects, poor tolerability and compliance; shorter course used in combination with adjunct therapy.
Artesunate (not registered in the United States)	Consult WHO treatment guidelines for dosing regimens as part of artemisinin-based combination therapies	Can be effective if given for 7 days if used as monotherapy, but strongly recommended to be used in combination with longer-acting partner drugs in 3-5 day regimens; recrudescence common with monotherapy; highly variable blood concentrations.
Artemether-lumefantrine (not registered in the United States)	Four tablets at diagnosis followed by same dose at 8, 24, 36, 48, and 60 hr for adults; consult WHO treatment guidelines for weight-based pediatric dosing	Each tablet contains 20 mg artemether and 120 mg lumefantrine; should be taken with fatty food to enhance absorption.
Mefloquine hydrochloride*	Oral; 750 mg salt followed by 500 mg 6-12 hr later (total 1250 mg) *Pediatric dosing:* 15 mg salt/kg as initial dose, followed by 10 mg salt/kg 6-12 hr after initial dose	May be used in combination with artesunate; early vomiting is common; must repeat the dose if vomiting occurs within 1 hr of dosing; split dose regimen may be suitable; should not be given if recurrent use of other quinolines (quinine or halofantrine) is suspected.
Sulfadoxine-pyrimethamine	Oral; 3 tablets single dose for adults; consult WHO treatment guildelines for pediatric dosing as part of artemisinin-based combination therapy	Increasing resistance limits usefulness; combination with artesunate or amodiaquine recommended where no other effective drugs available.
Atovaquone-proguanil*	Four tablets once a day for 3 days *Pediatric dosing:* by weight—1 adult tablet for 11-20 kg, 2 for 21-30 kg, and 3 for 31-40 kg, daily for 3 days	Each tablet contains 250 mg atovaquone and 100 mg proguanil. Should be taken with fatty food to enhance absorption and to reduce gastrointestinal side effects.
Primaquine phosphate*	Oral; 30 mg base daily for 14 days *Pediatric dosing:* 0.6 mg base/kg daily for 14 days	Used for radical therapy to eradicate *P. vivax* or *ovale* hypnozoites; start 3-4 days after primary treatment; contraindicated in severe G6PD deficiency.
Adjunct Therapy		
Tetracycline*	250 mg 4 times daily for 7 days (6.25 mg/kg for children >8 yr)	Used only in combination with quinine/artemisinin derivative. Not for children <8 and pregnant women.
Doxycycline*	100 mg twice daily for 7 days (2.2 mg/kg for children >8 yr)	Used only in combination with quinine/artemisinin derivative. Not for children <8 and pregnant women.
Clindamycin*	20 mg base/kg/day in 3-4 divided doses for 7 days	Used only in combination with quinine/artemisinin derivative. Safe in children and pregnancy.

*Recommended by the U.S. Centers for Disease Control and Prevention.
WHO, World Health Organization.

oral, rectal, and injectable forms. A liquid formulation is also available for children, but its extremely bitter taste limits its use. Information on another chloroquine formulation used to treat rheumatologic diseases, hydroxychloroquine, can be found in Chapter 74 (Rheumatoid Arthritis).

Chloroquine is well absorbed from the gastrointestinal tract when administered orally (more than 80% bioavailability). It peaks in 3 to 5 hours. It is rapidly absorbed via intramuscular or subcutaneous injection. These routes provide a rate of absorption faster than distribution and can result in a transiently high, potentially toxic peak blood concentration.[50]

Chloroquine is distributed slowly but extensively in the body. Although its predominant distribution is in the liver, chloroquine has no activity against hepatic stages of malaria parasites. Other major tissue distribution includes the spleen, kidney, lungs, and melanin-containing tissue such as skin and retina. Its distribution in the central nervous system is small. This extensive distribution influences the drug concentrations in the small central compartment.[49] Chloroquine is approximately 50% to 60% protein bound. Chloroquine disposition is similar in healthy and malaria-infected individuals, and disease severity dose not alter its disposition. More than 50% of chloroquine is eliminated unchanged by the kidneys and 25% of urinary chloroquine represents metabolites. Urinary elimination can be increased by urine acidification. The rest of absorbed chloroquine is biotransformed by the liver to desethyl- and bisdesethylchloroquine, whose concentrations reach 40% and 10% of measured chloroquine, respectively. Tissue elimination of chloroquine is slower than central elimination, resulting in a very long terminal half-life ranging from 30 to 60 days. Elimination half-life is even longer for the metabolites. Traces of chloroquine can be found in the urine years after dosing.

Relationship between Pharmacokinetics and Clinical Response. A few attempts have been made to identify the minimal inhibitory concentrations (MIC at a 99% effective concentration [EC_{99}] in vitro) of chloroquine for the in vivo clinical response.[51] More than a fivefold difference in the median range of the estimated MIC value for *P. falciparum* was observed for low-level in vivo resistance (initial clearance of parasites followed by recrudescence in 7 to 28 days) versus moderate in vivo resistance (parasitemia fails to clear by day 7 of therapy) (44 mcg/ml and 237 mcg/ml, respectively).

Therapeutic Considerations. The therapeutic indication for chloroquine is now restricted to limited areas that remain free of chloroquine resistance. Chloroquine is safe at therapeutic doses. It is inexpensive and its antipyretic nature favors clinical use. It is one of the most rapidly acting drugs against asexual parasites, mainly mature ring forms and trophozoites. If parasites are sensitive, fever usually clears within 1 to 2 days and parasites disappear from the blood within 2 to 3 days. Therefore, failure to respond or rising parasitemia on the second or third day after treatment suggests resistance and the need for rescue therapy with quinine or another rapidly acting schizonticide.

Adverse Effects, Precautions, and Contraindications. Although extraordinarily safe within the therapeutic range, chloroquine overdose carries the highest mortality of all antimalarial drug overdoses, with a fatality rate of more than 30%.[52] Acute toxicity is seen mainly in overdose or rapid parenteral administration. Primary toxicity is in seen in the cardiovascular (vasodilation, hypotension, arrhythmias, QRS and QTc prolongation, torsade de pointes ventricular arrhythmias, and cardiac arrest) and central nervous (confusion, convulsion, and coma) systems. Prompt treatment with epinephrine, diazepam, and supportive treatment is required.

The most common adverse effect at indicated oral doses to treat an acute malaria episode is pruritis, which is more frequent in dark-skinned individuals. Other adverse effects include gastrointestinal upset, headache, and visual disturbances. In long-term therapy, chloroquine is associated with retinal injury due to the drug's deposition in melanin-rich tissues. Therefore, an annual ophthalmologic examination is indicated for persons on long-term chemoprophylaxis with chloroquine. Other side effects include bleaching of hair, headache, skin eruption, cardiac rhythm abnormalities, and rarely blood dyscrasias. A high cumulative dose of chloroquine in prolonged use (>250 mg/day) is also associated with toxic myopathy, cardiopathy, peripheral neuropathy, and rarely neuropsychiatric disturbances. The use of chloroquine in individuals with any of these conditions is recommended only if the benefits outweigh the risks.

Chloroquine is contraindicated in those individuals with known hypersensitivity to aminoquinolines, epilepsy, or myasthenia gravis or with psoriasis or other exfoliative skin disorders. Careful monitoring and precautions are indicated for persons with preexisting retinal or auditory damage, and history of seizure disorder.

Drug Interactions. Chloroquine absorption may be reduced by concomitant administration of antacids and ampicillin. Cimetidine inhibits chloroquine metabolism by CYP3A4, leading to increased plasma levels of chloroquine. Chloroquine inhibits CYP2D6 and can increase the plasma level of cyclosporine and digoxin. Concomitant administration of chloroquine with mefloquine increases the risk of seizure, and coadministration with halofantrine or amodiaquine may increase the risk of cardiac arrhythmias.

Chloroquine in Pregnancy and Breast-feeding. Chloroquine was, and still is in some areas, commonly used to treat malaria in pregnancy. For the prevention of malaria disease and complications in pregnancy, chloroquine has been increasingly replaced by sulfadoxine-pyrimethamine and other more effective drugs. Chloroquine crosses the placenta and is deposited in fetal eye tissue[53]; however, no significant increase in fetal abnormalities associated with the drug has been reported and it is considered safe in pregnancy. Chloroquine is secreted into the breast milk (milk:plasma ratio 0.27 to 0.46) and this small quantity is reported to be harmless in the infant.[54] Knowledge of pharmacokinetics of chloroquine in pregnancy is limited. In comparison with historical data obtained mainly from adult males and children, an increase in chloroquine clearance was reported in a small group of women.[55]

Future of Chloroquine. A recent report of the return of chloroquine efficacy in Malawi several years after its withdrawal raised the possibility of a second life for this drug.[47] However, in other settings where chloroquine is still used to treat vivax malaria and where low malaria transmission affords few opportunities for direct competition between sensitive and resistant parasites in the same host, this phenomenon has not been observed to the same degree.[56] While it is possible that chloroquine could eventually be re-introduced for limited indications such as intermittent preventive treatment, the likelihood of a rapid re-emergence of resistance calls for a cautious approach. Studies assessing chloroquine in combination with other drugs intended to block the return of resistance are underway.

Quinine and Quinidine

History. Quinine has been in therapeutic use to treat "fever" for at least four centuries. It is a bitter powder obtained from the bark of the cinchona tree, as reported in descriptions of the cure of a febrile illness in the Countess of Chinchon in Lima, Peru, in the 17th century. It was probably brought to and distributed in Europe by the Jesuit Fathers. By 1640 it was widely used to treat febrile illnesses there, where it was also known as Peruvian's or Jesuit's bark. Quinine was initially employed as a powder, extract, or infusion, and the active compound was isolated from cinchona in 1820. A complete synthesis of quinine was achieved in 1945. Its synthesis, however, is complex and natural products are still used to produce quinine.

Chemistry. Chemical structures of quinine and quinidine are shown in Figure 82-3. Cinchona contains a mixture of four major cinchona alkaloids: quinine, quinidine, cinchonine, and cindhonidine, the first two of which are presently used as antimalarials. Both quinine and quinidine contain a quinoline group linked by a quinuclidine ring. A methoxy side chain is attached to the quinoline ring and a vinyl to the quinuclidine ring. The only difference between quinine and quinidine is the steric configuration of two of the three asymmetric centers at C-8 and C-9, carbon atoms at the quinuclidine junction and bearing the secondary alcohol group. The direction of aliphatic N-H and O-H bond linking to these carbons and their directional relation to each other are believed to influence the potency of antimalarial activity.[57] Quinidine is more potent as an antimalarial and more toxic than quinine.

Antimalarial Activity. Quinine and quinidine are active primarily against asexual erythrocytic forms, more so for mature schizonts and trophozoites than the young ring forms. They are not active against primary hepatic stages or latent hypnozoites of vivax malaria or gametocytes.

Pharmacokinetics. The pharmacokinetics of quinine are extensively described by Krishna and White.[49] Quinine and quinidine are formulated as dihydrochloride salt for the parenteral form, and as sulfate, bisulfate, dihydrochloride, ethylcarbonate, hydrochloride, and hydrobromide salts for oral administration. In the United States, only quinidine is available in parenteral form. Both oral and parenteral salts are absorbed similarly well, with more than 76% bioavailability, and peak in 3 to 8 hours when given orally.

Quinine is not concentrated in red blood cells, unlike other quinolines such as chloroquine. Concentration is actually higher in the plasma.[58] Quinine is primarily bound to α1-acid glycoprotein (an acute-phase reactant), approximately 80% in healthy individuals and more than 90% in patients with malaria. When given intravenously, quinine is distributed from the central compartment quickly, resulting in a large apparent volume of distribution. The major route of elimination is hepatic biotransformation, mainly by CYP3A4 to hydroxylated metabolites, with approximately 20% eliminated unchanged in the urine. Quinidine is also metabolized by one of the major drug-metabolizing enzymes, CYP2D6. The predominant metabolite is 3-hydroxyquinine, which retains antimalarial activity. These metabolites can accumulate in the body and may be associated with toxicity in patients with renal failure. The mean half-life is approximately 10 to 12 hours, which may be increased in the elderly and malnourished and in hepatic failure. Dose adjustment is recommended in only those patients with severe hepatic or renal failure.

Disease severity influences the pharmacokinetic behaviors of quinine (see Therapeutic Considerations). With increasing severity and volume contraction during acute infection, the plasma half-life of quinine is prolonged to up to 18 hours due primarily to a reduction in its clearance. Despite elevated total plasma concentration, often up to 50%, quinine toxicity is unusual in patients with malaria since the majority of drug is bound due to an increase in the acute-phase reactant α1-acid glycoprotein, a major plasma protein for basic drugs. Therefore, dose reduction is not recommended in initial treatment. Dose modification may be necessary during convalescence when the unbound fraction may be increasing. Acute cardiac, ocular, and auditory toxicities, are common with a high plasma concentration of quinine in patients with overdose.

Rectal administration of quinine results in a lower bioavailability, but clinical outcomes are similar compared with the intramuscular route.[59] There may be renal tubular secretion of these drugs reflected by a significant difference in renal clearance between bound and unbound fractions.[60] The main pharmacokinetic difference between quinine and quinidine is plasma protein binding.[61] Quinidine has a lower protein binding (about 80%). Quinidine also has a smaller volume of distribution, and higher total and renal clearance than quinine.[61]

Relationship Between Pharmacokinetics and Clinical Response. The concentration of quinine required to maintain adequate antiparasitic activity and clinical response has been suggested.[62-64] In these studies, a targeted therapeutic unbound concentration of quinine was derived from in vitro dose-response studies. Despite achieving the target, the clinical and parasitologic responses were less than optimal in those patients who did not receive a loading dose. In general, a direct relationship may not exist between the in vitro MICs (at 50% effective concentration [EC_{50}] or 90% effective concentration [EC_{90}]) and in vivo clinical response for quinine. Direct extrapolation of in vivo drug concentrations from the in vitro data cannot be justified since many factors are not comparable in the two situations, including background immunity in the host, protein binding and pH of in vitro culture medium, and the polyclonal nature of many natural infections versus a single strain typically used in in vitro experiments. It is estimated that any dosing regimen (with or without a loading dose) achieving less than 5 mg/L of total quinine concentrations in the first 12 hours of treatment may result in inadequate antimalarial effect.[49] A pharmacodynamic model based on findings in patients with uncomplicated falciparum malaria suggests that the average plasma concentration of free quinine required is at least 3.4 mg/L and that this concentration must be maintained over at least four asexual cycles (more than 6 days).[65] Maintaining a target concentration of 8 to 15 mg/L for quinine and 3.5 to 8 mg/L for quinidine in the first 2 days is generally recommended.

The total concentration of quinine associated with the development of cinchonism (predictable quinine toxicity comprised of hearing and visual impairment, headache, nausea, vomiting, and dysphoria) is approximately 5 mg/L. Therefore, at least a mild form of cinchonism is expected with successful therapy of an acute malaria episode with quinine. These data are derived from a study of a large number of prisoners using induced malaria treated with quinine,[66] and later in healthy volunteers.[67] It has been recommended that plasma quinine concentrations should be monitored and optimized to reduce the risk of quinine toxicity, although this is not often done in practice. Quinidine has a narrower therapeutic window for inducing cardiovascular toxicity. Although QTc prolongation is concentration dependent, there is no specific guideline for a targeted therapeutic concentration. Quinidine is more potent than quinine at prolonging the electrocardiographic QTc interval, both in healthy volunteers[67] and in malaria patients,[68] and at increasing the risk of hypotension.[69]

Therapeutic Considerations. Due to common toxicities and a short half-life, quinine and quinidine are not used for prophylaxis. Quinine is still widely used orally to treat uncomplicated malaria in endemic areas, despite very poor compliance due to unpleasant and predictable toxicity. Quinine (with an adjunct treatment) remains the first choice of therapy for severe malaria where no other effective antimalarial drugs (e.g., intravenous artesunate) are available. Both intravenous and intramuscular quinine are commercially available in many countries. Intravenous quinidine is used to treat severe malaria in countries where intravenous quinine is not available, including the United States and Canada.

A loading dose of quinine is highly recommended in treating severe malaria to achieve an adequate therapeutic concentration rapidly, even when it cannot be ascertained whether quinine treatment might have been started before presentation.[49] The dose may be modified in the convalescence phase. Quinine should never be given in intravenous bolus. The other clinical uses of quinidine and quinine include for cardiac indications and nocturnal leg cramps, respectively. Marketing of over-the-counter quinine product for the latter indication was discontinued since data on clinical efficacy and safety of quinine for this treatment are insufficient, according to a ruling issued by the U.S. Food and Drug Administration (FDA) in 1995.

Adverse Effects, Precautions, and Contraindications. Quinine is poorly tolerated. It is associated with a triad of dose-related toxicity: cinchonism, hypoglycemia, and hypotension. Cinchonism is very common: the mild form includes headache; vasodilation; sweating; nausea; vertigo or dizziness; disturbance in visual, auditory, and color perception; and dysphoria. The more severe form of cinchonism includes abdominal pain, vomiting, diarrhea, deafness, blindness, and disturbances in cardiac rhythm. Visual and auditory disturbances are caused by a direct neurotoxicity of the VIIIth cranial nerve and possibly secondary vascular changes. Cinchonism is reversible and resolves if the drug is discontinued. Hypoglycemia is due to stimulation of pancreatic release of insulin, seen with both quinine and quinidine. It is particularly dangerous in patients with severe malaria in sepsis and pregnancy. Hypotension is less common but serious and often life threatening, usually associated with rapid intravenous infusion.

Despite its propensity to prolong the QTc interval, cardiovascular complications with quinine are uncommon in patients with uncomplicated or severe malaria treated with therapeutic doses, and cardiac monitoring is not recommended. Acute overdose does carry a high risk of serious, often fatal, cardiac dysrhythmia such as atrioventricular block, junctional rhythm, sinus arrest, ventricular tachycardia, and fibrillation. The fatal oral dose of quinine in adult is about 2 to 8 g. Cardiac risks, particularly for QTc prolongation and ventricular arrhythmias, are higher with quinidine than with quinine, and continuous cardiac monitoring is advised for intravenous quinidine therapy.

Quinine hypersensitivity may present with skin rash, pruritis, flushing, fever, ringing in the ear, asthma-like symptoms, dyspnea, and visual changes. A rare and serious type of hypersensitivity is known as "blackwater fever," consisting of a triad of massive hemolysis, hemoglobinemia, and hemoglobinuria. This can result in rapid development of anuria, renal failure, and death. Mild hemolysis may occur in those with more severe forms of glucose-6-phosphate dehydrogenase (G6PD) deficiency. Infused intravenously, quinine is an irritant, and intramuscular injection can cause tissue abscesses. Quinine is contraindicated in patients with preexisting prolonged QTc interval, optic neuritis, and previous history of hypersensitivity. Package inserts assert contraindication in patients with G6PD deficiency, but this caution is virtually never followed in practice.

Drug Interactions. Drugs that may induce quinine and quinidine metabolism and clearance include phenobarbitone, phenytoin, and rifampin, a CYP3A4 inducer.[70] Drugs that may inhibit their metabolism and clearance include cimetidine, amiodarone, and erythromycin, all CYP3A4 inhibitors.[70,71] Quinine, more so than quinidine, may elevate the plasma levels of digoxin and other cardiac glycosides by interfering with absorption.[72] Metabolism of warfarin and other vitamin K–dependent anticoagulants may be delayed and their plasma levels may be raised by quinine.[73] Smoking can increase quinine clearance as much as 77%, through a suspected mechanism of induction of CYP4501A.[74] The renal clearance of quinine is increased by urine acidification. Drugs with potential for cardiac toxicity, such as halofantrine, mefloquine, and prochlorperazine, can amplify quinine's cardiotoxicity.[75]

Quinine in Pregnancy and Breast-feeding. Quinine is the drug of choice to treat severe malaria in pregnancy. Quinine at therapeutic doses is relatively safe in pregnancy.[76] The most concerning risk of quinine in pregnancy is the risk of severe hyperinsulinemia and hypoglycemia, via increased insulin release and glucose clearance by quinine.[77] Glucose, along with quinine infusion, is recommended. Quinine crosses the placenta and a small quantity is secreted in the breast milk. Quinine is, however, considered harmless in pregnancy and breast-feeding,[78] except for a theoretical risk of hypersensitivity in the newborn. Quinine does not alter uterine activity and does not induce abortion (contrary to common belief), but high doses of quinine used in an attempt to terminate pregnancy can cause fetal abnormalities and are associated with high maternal mortality and morbidity.[79]

Pharmacokinetic data on quinine in pregnancy are limited, but historical comparison with nonpregnant adult patients suggests that the volume of distribution of quinine may be lower in the third trimester, while clearance may be similar.[78] No dose adjustment is recommended. Both quinine and quinidine unbound fractions are higher in pregnant women with malaria than nonpregnant women, likely due to a physiologic fall in albumin and α1-acid glycoprotein concentrations in pregnancy.[80]

Mefloquine

History. The origin of mefloquine can be traced to World War II when a chemical designated SN10275 was selected as the most promising lead compound in a U.S. government–supported program to develop new antimalarial drugs. SN10275 was not further developed due to phototoxicity. In the 1960s, the Malaria Research Program established by the Walter Reed Army Institute of Research re-examined SN10275 to combat emerging chloroquine-resistant falciparum malaria, and synthesized a closely related compound, which did not cause phototoxicity, termed WR30090. Due to its poor bioavailability and erratic absorption, the next compound, WR142490, later named mefloquine, was chosen for clinical development. Mefloquine was first tested and deployed in Thailand in the early 1970s and enjoyed initial efficacy for the prophylaxis and treatment of chloroquine-resistant malaria until early 1980s. Unfortunately, mefloquine resistance then emerged rapidly. In an unsuccessful attempt to delay mefloquine resistance, mefloquine was formulated in a combination with sulfadoxine and pyrimethamine. Mefloquine resistance is now firmly established in Thailand and surrounding areas and increasing in other parts of the world, although use of mefloquine combined with artesunate appears to have arrested and even reversed resistance in Thailand.[81] To prolong the usefulness of this valuable drug, it has been strictly recommended that mefloquine alone be used only in malaria prophylaxis in travelers and in the treatment of multidrug-resistant malaria in combination with artemisinin derivatives.

Chemistry. Mefloquine, a fluorinated 4-quinlinemethanol, is structurally related to quinine (see Fig. 82-3). It contains an equal racemic mixture of four optical isomers with similar antimalarial potency but with different pharmacokinetic profiles.[82]

Antimalarial Activity. Mefloquine is a highly effective blood schizonticide against *P. falciparum* and *P. vivax*. It is more active against the more mature trophozoites and schizonts, and less against younger ring forms. It has no activity against primary-stage or latent hepatic stage parasites or gametocytes.

Pharmacokinetics. Mefloquine is formulated as hydrochloride salt in a tablet form, and there is no parenteral or liquid formulation available. The pharmacokinetics of mefloquine have been widely studied in both healthy individuals and patients with malaria, and are extensively reviewed by Karbwang and White.[83] It is highly insoluble in water and its oral absorption is moderate. Bioavailability is unknown since there is no intravenous formulation. Food enhances the rate and extent of absorption significantly.[84] Mefloquine enters extensive enterogastric and enterohepatic circulation, resulting in a biphasic rise in the plasma concentrations. It peaks in about 17 hours (ranging from 6 to 24 hours). The drug is widely distributed, highly protein bound (~98%), and slowly eliminated. Its terminal elimination half-life is about 20 days, ranging from 14 to 28 days. Mefloquine is metabolized to a major inactive metabolite, a 4-carboxylic acid derivative. The peak concentrations of this metabolite exceed that of the parent compound, and it is eliminated at a rate similar to mefloquine. Both the parent compound and the metabolites are excreted mainly in bile and feces, and less than 10% is excreted unchanged in the urine. Large interindividual variations and ethnic differences in mefloquine pharmacokinetics have been reported.[85] There are conflicting reports on the effects of malaria infection on the pharmacokinetics of mefloquine, but these are likely to be clinically insignificant except in severe malaria, in which oral absorption is significantly compromised.[83]

Relationship between Pharmacokinetics and Clinical Response. A therapeutic concentration for mefloquine has not been established for malaria treatment or prophylaxis. Considerable differences in effective drug concentrations are likely to exist for parasites with different drug resistance profiles. Cardiac and neuropsychiatric toxicity seem to be dose related; however, the association between these toxicities and blood or tissue concentrations of mefloquine remains uncertain due to the paucity of pharmacokinetic data, conflicting findings from some studies, and a large interindividual variability in drug concentrations.

Therapeutic Considerations. Mefloquine is used for malaria prophylaxis in travelers, and is used in combination with artemisinin derivatives for the treatment of multidrug-resistant *P. falciparum* and *P. vivax* infection in Asia. Mefloquine as a single agent given as 25 mg/kg in two to three doses is an acceptable alternative for treating uncomplicated falciparum or vivax malaria in settings such as the United States where more effective artemisinin-based treatments are not available.

Early vomiting induced by mefloquine is seen commonly, particularly in young children.[86] This significantly reduces the drug concentrations and total exposure.[87] Early vomiting seems to be dose dependent, and split-dose regimens consisting of three daily doses of 8 mg/kg (500 mg in the typical adult) or 15 mg/kg (1000 mg typical adult dose) followed by 10 mg/kg (750 mg adult dose) in 24 hours have been evaluated.[88,89] When compared with the conventional single-dose regimen, the split-dose regimen results in better bioavailability, comparable area under the time-concentration curve (AUC) (total drug exposure), and an equivalent therapeutic response but less early vomiting. A lower treatment dose of a total of 1250 mg for adults given in one or two doses was found to be less effective, leading to the higher treatment dose of 1750 mg that is presently recommended for adults.

Adverse Effects, Precautions, and Contraindications. Although mefloquine is generally well tolerated, particularly at prophylactic doses, mild adverse reactions such as nausea, dizziness, sleep disturbance, restlessness, and dysphoria, usually not resulting in the need to stop therapy, are common, occurring in about 10% to 15% of persons. More severe reactions such as psychosis are rare. These mainly neuropsychiatric side effects of mefloquine have been widely publicized in the media and on the Internet, leading some travelers to stop taking mefloquine based on advice from fellow travelers, putting themselves at high risk of malaria. The reported frequency and severity of reactions vary greatly due partly to differences in study designs (retrospective questionnaires vs. controlled trials) and the nature of population studied, and in several studies mefloquine has had an incidence of side effects similar to that of chloroquine. The estimated risk of severe neuropsychiatric side effects (confusion, altered sensorium, seizure, acute psychosis, and severe vertigo) from malaria prophylaxis is about 1 in 1000, comparable to that of chloroquine. Mild to moderate gastrointestinal disturbances (abdominal pain, diarrhea), headache, and dizziness may occur at a prophylactic dose. Mefloquine-related adverse effects are usually reversible, often occur after the second or third dose, and frequently resolve completely even with continued use of drug. Long-term prophylaxis is generally well tolerated, and many long-term expatriates take weekly mefloquine for years and tolerate it well.

Mefloquine-induced toxicities are reviewed in detail by Taylor and White.[76] Among patients with malaria who are treated with mefloquine, the most important adverse effect seems to be early vomiting. Other important adverse effects include dose-dependent nausea, late vomiting, and dizziness. The frequency of central nervous system side effects is increased at the higher doses used for treatment, especially in young children, and in those who are re-treated due to vomiting or those recovering from severe malaria. Ethnic differences in vulnerability to the central nervous system effects have been reported, with these effects being more common in Caucasians and Africans and less common in Asians. Other cutaneous, cardiovascular, hepatic, and hematologic side effects are rare.

Mefloquine is contraindicated in individuals with known allergy or serious toxicity related to mefloquine or related compounds. Mefloquine is not recommended for those recovering from cerebral malaria because of the possibility of confounding neurologic assessments. Alternative drugs are preferred for individuals with a history of epilepsy controlled by anticonvulsant medications; a current or past history of major psychiatric disorder such as major depression, bipolar disorder, or anxiety disorder; or with a history of severe hepatic disease. The use of mefloquine is also cautioned in those who require great dexterity, such as pilots.

Drug Interactions. Limited data are available on drug-drug interaction with mefloquine. Mefloquine seems to lower the plasma levels of the anticonvulsants phenytoin, valproic acid, and phenobarbital, and therapeutic concentration monitoring of anticonvulsants is advised if coadministered with mefloquine. The risk of cardiac dysrrhythmias may be increased if mefloquine is used concomitantly with drugs that can disrupt cardiac conduction or repolarization. These include antimalarial drugs (quinine, quinidine, chloroquine, and halofantrine) and antiarrhythmic drugs, calcium channel and β-blocking agents, antihistamines, and tricyclic antidepressant drugs. Treatment with mefloquine after halofantrine or treatment with halofantrine within 2 months after mefloquine therapy is contraindicated because of a possible risk of sudden cardiac death. Vaccination with live, attenuated bacterial vaccines (e.g., typhoid vaccine) is recommended to be completed 3 days before initiation of mefloquine therapy because of its possible antibacterial effects on the vaccines.

Mefloquine in Pregnancy and Breast-feeding. High-dose mefloquine is teratogenic in animals. Mefloquine is recommended by the CDC for the prophylaxis and treatment of malaria in pregnancy after the first trimester. There have been no adequate well-controlled studies of mefloquine in pregnancy, and some data suggested an increased rate of stillbirths during the first trimester.[90,91] It is recommended that pregnancy be avoided at least for 3 months after mefloquine treatment.

As for many other antimalarial drugs, data on pharmacokinetic properties of mefloquine in pregnancy are inadequate. A few studies suggest that, in late pregnancy, mefloquine absorption is unchanged but there may an increase in systemic clearance resulting in a shorter elimination half-life.[92] The clinical implications of these changes, if any, are unknown. Mefloquine is secreted in breast milk in a small quantity and is unlikely to have any clinically relevant impact on the infant.[93]

Primaquine

History. Primaquine is the only registered antimalarial drug capable of preventing relapses after infection with *P. vivax* and *P. ovale*. Although it was first approved by the FDA in 1952, its history goes back more than a century when the weak antimalarial activity of methylene blue was discovered by Ehrlich in 1891. Methylene blue was the origin of the 8-aminoquinolines. Primaquine is the product of the search for new antimalarials in World War II, and one of a large series of quinolines synthesized with methoxy and 8-amino substitution. G6PD deficiency, the first X-linked genetic disorder associated with an enzyme, was discovered following the observation of significant hemolysis after primaquine therapy in African American soldiers.

As old as the drug is, understanding of its mechanism of action is still very limited. Its antimalarial activity is probably related to the conversion of primaquine to reactive oxygen species and metabolites toxic to the intracellular parasites.[94] Another potential mechanism involves in the disturbances to the function of ubiquinone, an essential electron carrier in the respiratory chain of mitochondria.[95] The chemical structure of primaquine is shown in Figure 82-3.

Antimalarial Activity. Primaquine is active against primary-stage and latent hepatic stage parasites and gametocytes of *P. vivax* and *P. ovale*. Its activity against erythrocytic-stage parasites is inconsistent. Primaquine can kill only hepatic-stage parasites and gametocytes of *P. falciparum*, but not erythrocytic forms. Thus, primaquine plays a vital role in preventing relapses of vivax and ovale malaria and primary infections with falciparum malaria, but it cannot be used reliably for the treatment of acute malaria episodes.

Pharmacokinetics. Primaquine is formulated as primaquine phosphate tablets, and its dosage is expressed in terms of the base. Detailed pharmacokinetic properties of primaquine can be found in a series of articles published in the 1980s with data collected from healthy and malaria-infected subjects.[96-99] Briefly, primaquine is absorbed almost completely from the oral route with bioavailability of approximately 96%. Primaquine is commonly taken with food to minimize gastrointestinal side effects; however, the effects of food on its pharmacokinetics have not been evaluated. It is extensively distributed in many tissues, reaching an apparent volume of distribution much larger than the total body water. It binds preferentially to α1-acid glycoprotein, an acute-phase reactant elevated during microbial infections. Primaquine does not accumulate in infected red blood cells. It reaches its maximal concentrations within about 3 hours and declines with an elimination half-life of about 6 to 7 hours. Primaquine is metabolized rapidly to several oxidative metabolites, and the major metabolite is carboxyprimaquine. Only a very small portion of primaquine (less than 10%) is excreted unchanged in the urine.

Relationship between Pharmacokinetics and Clinical Response. The dose-related effects of primaquine in malaria therapy (radical cure of *P. vivax* or effective prophylaxis of *P. falciparum*)[100,101] or toxicity (e.g., hemolysis and gastrointestinal side effects)[102-104] are well described. However, the plasma concentrations of primaquine that are associated with these clinical responses have not been established. The lack of a clear relationship between plasma primaquine pharmacokinetics and the degree of hemolysis has been reported.[105]

Therapeutic Considerations. Primaquine is primarily used for the treatment of relapsed malaria infection caused by *P. vivax* and *P. ovale*. Patients are treated with a schizonticidal drug initially (commonly chloroquine), followed by primaquine for a "radical cure." Different geographic strains of *P. vivax* vary considerably in their susceptibility to primaquine. *Plasmodium vivax* strains acquired in Papua New Guinea, areas of Oceania, and some other parts of the world require a higher dose to prevent relapse effectively. There has been debate over what the effective dosing regimen should be for radical cure or prophylaxis with primaquine. Efficacy of primaquine chemoprophylaxis has been shown in both *P. vivax* and *P. falciparum* prophylaxis for persons with normal G6PD status.[106-108] Its prophylactic efficacy ranges between 80% and 90% for both species, and primaquine can be used as an alternative chemoprophylaxis agent, though it is not yet approved for this indication by the FDA. A recent recommendation from a CDC expert meeting on malaria chemoprophylaxis is to increase the dose of primaquine from 15 to 30 mg daily for 14 days for both radical cure and prophylaxis.[109] G6PD testing is required before the initiation of treatment or prophylaxis.

Adverse Effects, Precautions, and Contraindications. The most commonly encountered side effect of primaquine at recommended doses in G6PD-normal individuals is mild to moderate gastrointestinal distress (10% to 12%), which can be prevented by taking the drug with food. Gastrointestinal side effects are dose dependent. At doses higher than 30 mg/day, the side effects of abdominal cramps, nausea, and vomiting occur in the majority of patients. The most serious side effect of primaquine in G6PD-deficient individuals is intravascular hemolysis.

Primaquine-induced hemolysis is a well-recognized adverse reaction in individuals with G6PD enzyme deficiency. It is an X-linked hereditary disorder caused by an amino acid substitution in the G6PD enzyme. It is associated with an increased vulnerability to hemolysis induced by pro-oxidant drugs such as primaquine. Drug-induced hemolysis is also seen in other enzyme deficiencies and hemoglobinopathies. G6PD deficiency affects more than 200 million worldwide and is seen fairly commonly in African populations (11%). There are many variants of this enzyme deficiency with varying degrees of severity. The most prevalent variant (A–) is associated with mild hemolysis, and this is the variant most common in African populations. Hemolysis in this variant is reversible, resolving within a few days of drug withdrawal. It can also be self-limited with continued use of the drug, after reaching equilibrium between red cell destruction and bone marrow recovery (reticulocyte release and maturation) within 1 to 2 weeks. Normal hemoglobin levels are usually recovered after 4 weeks of continued primaquine therapy.[110]

In general, daily primaquine therapy or weekly regimens with higher doses of primaquine in individuals with mild G6PD deficiency are well tolerated. Other variants of G6PD deficiency, collectively known as Mediterranean (B–) forms, are seen in Caucasian and Asian populations, cause more severe hemolysis, and carry the risk of high morbidity and mortality. The risk of hemolysis is not consistently dose dependent or self-limiting in these populations.

Asymptomatic methemoglobinemia is another adverse effect observed with primaquine. This results from an oxidation of hemoglobin by the drug to methemoglobin. This is also dose dependent and self-limited at therapeutic doses. Clinical symptoms and cyanosis are rare. Thresholds for clinically significant methemoglobinemia may be lower in patients with low cardiopulmonary reserve such as in pulmonary disease or heart failure. Coadministration of other pro-oxidant drugs such as dapsone or chloroquine can worsen the problem and should be avoided.

Primaquine is contraindicated in individuals deficient in G6PD or NADH methemoglobin reductase enzyme, or who are allergic to other 8-aminoquinolines, and in pregnant women. Although primaquine is contraindicated in all persons with G6PD deficiency, according to the FDA label, the weight of the evidence suggests that the benefits may outweigh the risk in those with mild variants of G6PD deficiency. Repeated monitoring of blood count and hemoglobin, and confirmation of hemoglobin recovery, must be done to ensure safety. In the FDA package insert, primaquine use is also warned against in persons with immune suppression or with the potential for immune suppression. The label also includes a warning for those who are using other drugs with myeloid suppressive effects. This warning is based on earlier in vitro and animal findings that primaquine has myeloid suppression effects. These findings, however, were not supported in human trials with long-term use of primaquine, where no such toxicity was observed.[106,111]

The experience with primaquine overdose is limited. Doses above 60 to 240 mg/day are associated with more severe gastrointestinal side effects, cyanotic methemoglobinemia, and hemolysis.[112] Urgent treatment with oxygen, gastric lavage, or activated charcoal may be needed, and intravenous administration of methylthioninium chloride and blood transfusion may be necessary in some cases.

Drug Interactions. There may be a higher risk of hemolysis and symptomatic methemoglobinemia if primaquine is administered with other drugs with hemolytic potentials, such as dapsone, sulfonamides, or chloroquine.

Primaquine in Pregnancy and Breast-feeding. Primaquine is contraindicated in pregnancy due to the risk of hemolysis in the fetus with unknown G6PD status. Those who require primaquine radical therapy must wait until after delivery. No information is available regarding primaquine secretion into breast milk.

Amodiaquine. Amodiaquine is a congener of chloroquine, developed by the U.S. Army Malaria Research Program in the 1960s. It was withdrawn from the market in 1986 due to a high risk (1 in 2000) of developing drug-induced agranulocytosis or/and hepatotoxicity observed in travelers who were taking amodiaquine for malaria prophylaxis. It is no longer recommended for malaria prophylaxis. The mechanism of amodiaquine toxicity is incompletely understood. These severe reactions were seen at an alarming rate in nonimmune travelers taking prophylaxis, but not in persons treated with amodiaquine for acute clinical malaria in endemic areas. These reactions are not concentration or dose related and seem to have a strong immunologic basis,[113] and may be associated with the formation of a reactive metabolite, quinine imine, in the liver or white blood cells.[114,115]

In the last decade, amodiaquine has made a comeback in Africa since it is active against most chloroquine-resistant falciparum malaria, is easy to administer, is generally well tolerated, and is inexpensive. In combination with an artemisinin derivative, it is one of the WHO-recommended drugs for the treatment of uncomplicated falciparum malaria. Although cross-resistance with chloroquine can occur, amodiaquine's efficacy against chloroquine-resistant falciparum malaria remains relatively good.

Amodiaquine is absorbed orally. It enters hepatic first-pass metabolism and is extensively metabolized primarily to an active metabolite, desethylamodiaquine, and a few other metabolites. The main metabolite has a mean half-life of approximately 12 hours.[116,117] Its metabolism may be predominantly mediated by the polymorphic CYP2C8,[118] and the involvement of other hepatic and nonhepatic CYP isoenzymes in its metabolism is likely. Information about the metabolic interaction of amodiaquine and other antimalarial drugs is limited. A few clinical trials have assessed the role of amodiaquine in combination therapy of malaria in Africa, and found superior efficacy of amodiaquine as a component of combination therapies over amodiaquine alone or sulfadoxine-pyrimethamine alone,[119-122] and equal or better efficacy than artemether-lumefantrine.[123,124] These recent studies found no strong evidence of serious hepatic toxicity relating to amodiaquine; however, a significant decline of neutrophil counts over time was observed in a few patients in some studies. Amodiaquine remains a valuable antimalarial drug, and is being promoted in combination with artesunate for widespread use in Africa. However, the possibility of serious, potentially life-threatening, toxicity associated with this drug, particularly when dosed repeatedly as will occur if it becomes used widely in Africa, cannot be ignored. Careful surveillance for hepatic and hematologic toxicity is imperative as amodiaquine-artesunate and other amodiaquine combinations are deployed in Africa.

Halofantrine. Two important pharmacologic factors that have limited the clinical use of halofantrine are its highly erratic and unreliable absorption and its potential for inducing cardiac rhythm abnormalities. Halofantrine is a phenanthrene methanol and is active against multidrug-resistant *P. falciparum*, particularly the late trophozoite stages, and against *P. vivax*. Following oral administration, its absorption is slow and incomplete and is improved by coadministration with fatty food. Reported pharmacokinetic parameters of halofantrine are highly variable, with its elimination half-life ranging from 14 hours to days. It is metabolized to desbutyl-halofantrine, which also has antimalarial activity. Hepatic CYP3A4 and CYP3A5 play a major role in its metabolism. Halofantrine-associated cardiac toxicity is serious and has been associated with sudden death. Toxicity is unpredictable due to unpredictable absorption and may be more likely in patients who have recently taken mefloquine. Concentration-dependent QTc prolongation occurs at the standard or higher dose and correlates well with plasma halofantrine concentration. It is primarily associated with the parent compound, not with its metabolite, which accumulates with repeated dosing. Due to these drawbacks and the extensive cross-resistance with mefloquine, clinical use of halofantrine is restricted to patients who have no adequate alternative treatment.

Lumefantrine. Lumefantrine (also known as benflumetol) is used in malaria treatment only in a fixed-dose combination with artemether, containing 20 mg of β-artemether and 120 mg of lumefantrine. This combination was developed jointly by the Academy of Military Medical Sciences (Beijing, China) and Novartis Pharma (Basel, Switzerland), and is now registered and used in many countries outside the United States. Lumefantrine is structurally similar to halofantrine and arylaminoalcohols such as mefloquine; however lumefantrine, unlike halofantrine, seems to have no effects on cardiac conduction. It contains a racemic mixture of *dextro-* and *levo-* enantiomers. They are equally active against *P. falciparum* and *P. vivax*. Lumefantrine resistance can be induced readily in rodents,[125] and late treatment failures with artemether-lumefantrine have been associated with decreased in vitro susceptibility to lumefantrine and increased copy number and/or expression of the *pfmdr1* gene that encodes the transporter protein P-glycoprotein homologue-1.

Lumefantrine is very lipophilic. Its oral absorption is erratic and slow—the peak may take up to 10 hours—and is improved significantly by concomitant fatty food intake. Lumefantrine is highly protein bound, mainly to high-density lipoproteins (~99%), is metabolized in the liver and mainly excreted in the bile and feces. CYP3A4 is likely involved in lumefantrine metabolism, and the major metabolite is desbutyl benflumetol, which is also active against malaria parasites. Similar to halofantrine, reported pharmacokinetic parameters for lumefantrine are highly variable and its elimination half-life ranges from 33 hours to 6 days, likely reflected by variability in food intake. Its pharmacokinetics are similar when administered alone or in combination with artemether. Although synergistic activity of lumefantrine and artemether in vitro has been observed when the drugs are combined at different ratios,[126] detailed pharmacologic interactions among metabolites of the two components have not been fully elucidated.

Multiple dosing of artemether-lumefantrine is required for the treatment of falciparum malaria, and different dosing regimens for the combination have been evaluated in several clinical trials. The bioavailability of lumefantrine increases with repeated dosing,[127] likely reflecting improved oral intake and gut absorption as the patient recovers from an acute attack of malaria. The clinical efficacy of the lumefantrine-artemether combination generally relies on the total drug exposure (AUC) of lumefantrine and initial degree of parasitemia,[127] and duration of dosing (5- vs. 2- or 3-day regimens).[128] Artemether is believed to be responsible for the initial reduction in parasitemia, and the day 7 plasma concentration of lumefantrine has been used as predictor of clinical failure; above 500 ng/ml is associated with 94% cure and below 280 ng/ml with almost 50% recrudescence. This combination has also been investigated for the treatment of vivax malaria and does not prevent *P. vivax* relapse, suggesting the lack of activity against hypnozoites.[129]

The lumefantrine-artemether combination is generally well tolerated and shows good safety profiles in clinical trials conducted in Asia. Unlike the related compounds halofantrine and mefloquine, lumefantrine lacks evidence of producing cardiotoxicity in humans.[130] The potential for adverse drug reactions to lumefantrine related to its high lipophilicity, high protein binding, and metabolic profiles needs further study. One small study suggested an increased clearance of lumefantrine in mid- and late pregnancy,[131] but information on this drug is in pregnancy and breast-feeding is lacking.

Piperaquine. Piperaquine is a bisquinoline synthesized in the 1960s, used extensively to treat *P. falciparum* and *P. vivax* in the 1960s to 1980s in China. Its use declined in the late 1980s due to the development of drug resistance and the increasing popularity of artemisinin derivatives. Piperaquine was rediscovered in the last decade during the search for appropriate partner drugs for artemisinin-based combination therapy. Piperaquine was chosen on the basis of good tolerability, low cost, its requirement of a short-course treatment regimen, and its relatively sustained activity against multidrug-resistant parasites. Piperaquine has been tested in combination with dihydroartemisinin (DHA), trimethoprim, and primaquine; with DHA and primaquine; and with DHA alone. Piperaquine-containing products have not been registered with the FDA or equivalent regulatory entities, but serious effort are being made to improve the standard of production and manufacturing of these compounds in preparation for such licensure.[132]

The mechanism of piperaquine action is not fully understood, and there is some evidence that it lacks cross-resistance with other quinolines such as chloroquine and amodiaquine.[133] It may inhibit the transporters that efflux chloroquine from digestive food vacuoles of the parasite.[134] Piperaquine is active against blood-stage *P. falciparum* and *P. vivax* in vitro. The clinical efficacy of piperaquine in artemisinin-based combination therapy is high for the treatment of both falciparum and vivax malaria.[135,136] Although piperaquine has been in clinical use for more than 30 years, data on its pharmacokinetics are very limited. Recent studies suggest that it is absorbed well orally, and has a large volume of distribution and long terminal half-life of greater than 10 days.[137,138] Fatty foods may facilitate its oral absorption.[138]

Safety data on piperaquine are also limited. Piperaquine is associated with hepatotoxicity in chronic dosing in animals, but its potential for adverse effects on the cardiovascular system (commonly seen with other aminoquinolines) is less than chloroquine.[139] Early studies conducted in China reported no hematologic, biochemical, cardiac, or hepatic abnormalities; however, the extent to which these toxicities were specifically assessed has been questioned.[139] Recent efficacy trials of piperaquine as a component of artemisinin-based combination therapy also reported only minor, self-limited side effects.[135,136] No information is available on the safety, efficacy, and pharmacokinetics of piperaquine in pregnancy and breast-feeding. Considering its structural similarities with other aminoquinolines and troubling animal safety data, this potentially valuable drug deserves a careful and thorough evaluation of safety, particularly for potential cardiac and hepatic toxicity, as well as proper pharmacokinetic-pharmacodynamic assessments and the development of rational dosing regimens for target populations.

Pyronaridine. Pyronaridine (also known as malaridine) is chemically related to chloroquine. It is a Mannich base, a synthetic 1-aza-9-aminoacridine and a derivative of benzonaphthyridine. Pyronaridine was first synthesized in China in the 1970s and has been used clinically for more than 20 years. It is available in oral, intramuscular, and intravenous forms. The oral formulation has been shown to have 100% clinical efficacy in a small clinical trial in Cameroon.[140] Pyronaridine is registered only in China, and preclinical toxicology data are not available outside of China. Information on its clinical safety, pharmacokinetics, and efficacy are still very limited, and the dosing regimen was designed empirically.

Antifolates

History. Major categories of antifolate drugs with antimalarial activity include the sulfonamides and sulfones, diaminopyrimidines, and metabolites of biguanides (Fig. 82-4). The antimalarial activity of sulfonamides was discovered soon after their introduction into clinical use as antifolate agents. Intensive investigation to develop effective antimalarial drugs during World War II in North America and Europe led to the development of the sulfone dapsone and the biguanide proguanil, and later pyrimethamine (the diaminopyrimidine) based on its structural similarity to cycloguanil (active metabolite of proguanil with antifolate activity). Proguanil and pyrimethamine were widely used for malaria chemoprophylaxis in the 1940s, and the development of parasite resistance to the drugs followed very quickly, within months to a few years in areas where they were deployed. Today these antifolate drugs are used mainly in combination with drugs from other classes for the treatment of uncomplicated falciparum malaria. Combining antifolate compounds was once thought to be an ideal rational antimalarial combination because of their synergistic killing activity, complementary mechanism of action, and matched pharmacokinetic properties. The most popular formulation is a fixed-dose combination of the long-acting sulfonamide sulfadoxine and pyrimethamine. Although this combination replaced chloroquine in many areas after resistance developed to chloroquine, the clinical use of this combination is declining due to increasing resistance and the recent availability of more efficacious combination therapies.

Another antifolate combination used to treat uncomplicated malaria is chlorproguanil-dapsone, two short-acting drugs combined in hopes of reducing selection pressure for antifolate resistance seen with the longer acting combination sulfadoxine-pyrimethamine, which continues to select pyrimethamine-resistant parasites for about 8 weeks after a treatment dose.[141]

Trimethoprim is another inhibitor of folate metabolism with antimalarial properties, and is widely used as a fixed-dose combination with sulfamethoxazole for the prevention of HIV-related opportunistic infections and for the treatment of other bacterial infections (see Chapter 84, HIV Infection and AIDS). Recently the daily use of this combination in children for the prevention of HIV-related opportu-

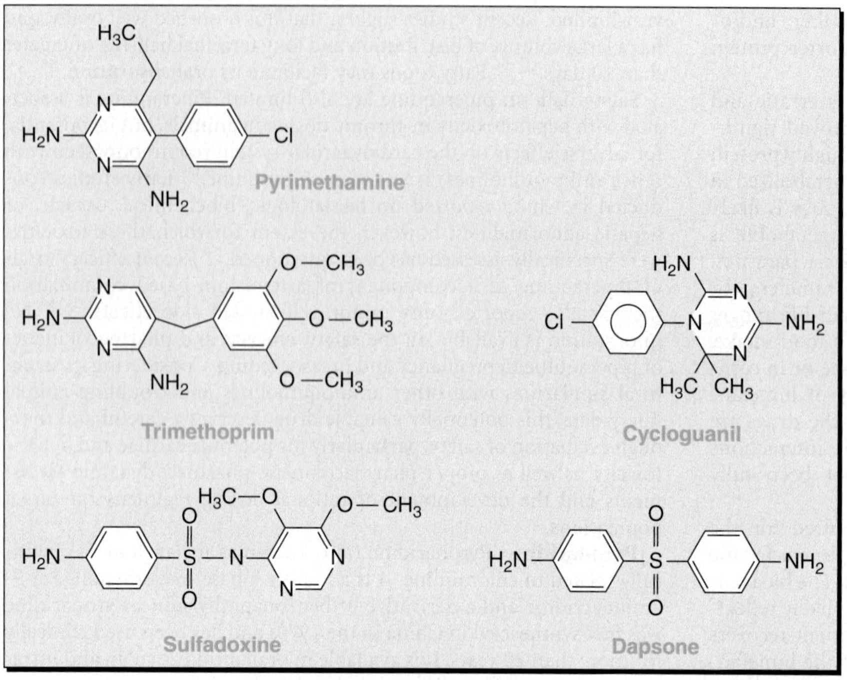

FIGURE 82-4 • Chemical structures of antifolate antimalarials.

nistic infection was shown to be associated with a reduction in the incidence of falciparum malaria.[142,143] Despite a seemingly bleak future of the antifolate compounds in clinical practice, they are still widely used in many endemic countries, alone or in combination with more effective drugs (e.g., an artemisinin derivative), due to the lack of available alternatives.

Antimalarial Activity. Antifolate antimalarials are slow-acting schizonticides effective at killing sensitive strains of *P. falciparum* and *P. vivax*. They are active against erythrocytic forms, and against primary hepatic forms to varying degrees. Cycloguanil, for an example, is more active than pyrimethamine against hepatic-stage parasites, and sulfa drugs are more active against *P. falciparum* than against *P. vivax*. None of these compounds is effective in eradicating the latent hepatic parasites (hypnozoites) or gametocytes. Other antiparasitic activities (e.g., *Toxoplasma gondii*) of these compounds are described in Chapter 83 (Helminthic and Protozoan Infections).

Mechanism of Action and Resistance. The enzymes dihydrofolate reductase (DHFR) and dihydropteroate synthase (DHPS) are sequentially involved in the synthesis of folate for the production of nucleic acids. Malaria parasites were first thought to require de novo synthesis of folate[144] and later discovered to be capable of salvaging folate or folate metabolites, at least in some strains.[145] DHFR, along with thymidylate synthase (TS), is encoded by a single copy gene on chromosome 4, and DHPS along with 7,8-dihydro-6-hydroxymethylpterin pyrophosphokinase (PPPK) is encoded by a gene on chromosome 8. Both DHFR-TS and DHPS-PPPK function as bifunctional enzymes in the parasite folate pathway.

All antifolate antimalarial compounds act to interfere with the metabolic pathway of folate synthesis. Sulfa and sulfone compounds are analogues of *para*-aminobenzoic acid, and reversibly and competitively inhibit DHPS, interfering with the utilization of *para*-aminobenzoic acid for the synthesis of dihydropteroic acid, which is catalyzed by DHPS. Pyrimethamine and cycloguanil block reduction of dihydrofolate to tetrahydrofolate, which is catalyzed by DHFR. The biguanide proguanil (or chloroguanide) is cyclized in the liver to produce a triazine metabolite, cycloguanil. Although proguanil itself possesses antimalarial activity by a mechanism other than folate antagonism,[146] cycloguanil is the active product that is capable of interfering with folate pathway.

Several different mutations in DHFR and DHPS are responsible for pyrimethamine and sulfadoxine resistance, respectively. These mutations are acquired in a stepwise fashion, in that primary mutation is required for subsequent mutations. The key mutation is a substitution of asparagine for serine at codon 108 in DHFR. Other clinically important mutations in DHFR occur at codons 50, 51, 59, and 164. Although cross-resistance may occur between structurally related pyrimethamine and cycloguanil, different patterns and degrees of resistance to cycloguanil are observed in association with these DHFR mutations. The key mutations in DHPS associated with sulfa resistance occur at codons 436, 613, 437, 540, and 581.[147,148] These mutations accumulate sequentially and progressively in the presence of drug pressure, correlating with an increasing prevalence of clinical treatment failure in many geographic areas.[149-151] Parasites with "triple mutant" DHFR (Asn108, Ile51, Arg59) are associated with increased risk of sulfadoxine-pyrimethamine treatment failure. The DHFR/DHPS "quintuple mutant," consisting of the DHFR triple mutant and two DHPS mutations (Gly437, Glu540) that are commonly found in Africa, is associated with an almost 20-fold increased risk of sulfadoxine-pyremethamine treatment failure but has a minimal effect on the outcome of treatment with chlorproguanil-dapsone.[150] The outcome of malaria drug treatment depends not only on mutations in DHFR and DHPS but also on the host background immunity and host plasma level of folate and *para*-aminobenzoic acid. Molecular evolutionary studies have shown that, while DHFR and DHPS mutations conferring low-level resistance arise frequently under drug pressure, the highly mutated forms causing high-level resistance share common ancestry, suggesting global genetic sweeps of the most resistant parasites.[151,152]

Sulfadoxine and Pyrimethamine. The sulfonamide most commonly used as an antimalarial agent is the long-acting sulfadoxine, used in a fixed-dose combination with pyrimethamine. Sulfalene and sulfamethoxazole have also been used in some formulations. These sulfonamides are absorbed rapidly and completely after oral administration, reaching the maximal concentration in 2 to 6 hours. Sulfadoxine undergoes metabolic clearance to some extent, mainly acetylation and glucuronidation. It is largely bound to plasma protein albumin (~80% to 90%). Sulfadoxine and its metabolites are predominantly eliminated via the kidneys, with a terminal elimination half-life of approximately 200 hours. Pyrimethamine is slowly but completely absorbed orally, with a time to peak concentration ranging from 2 to 12 hours. It is highly protein bound (~90%) and has a large tissue accumulation (liver, kidneys, lungs, and spleen). It is metabolized in the liver to several metabolites. The parent compound and metabolites are predominantly excreted in the urine. The elimination half-life of pyrimethamine is quite long, approximately 100 hours.

When used in acute malaria treatment, sulfadoxine-pyrimethamine is well tolerated and serious adverse reactions are rare. Commonly reported adverse effects include mild and reversible gastrointestinal symptoms and pruritis (up to 12% in Africans). A megaloblastic anemia (resembling folate deficiency) may be seen with high-dose and/or long-term therapy with pyrimethamine alone. Sulfadoxine accounts for most serious toxicity, namely severe cutaneous reactions. These include Stevens-Johnson syndrome, erythema multiforme, erythroderma, and toxic epidermal necrolysis and associated fatality, which were documented in persons taking weekly malaria prophylaxis with sulfadoxine-pyrimethamine or weekly prophylaxis of nonmalaria infections with sulfadoxine alone (estimated risk of severe cutaneous reactions in travelers is 1 in 5000 to 1 in 8000; risk of fatal reaction is 1 in 11,000 to 1 in 35,000). Other rare but serious adverse effects reported in travelers taking the sulfadoxine-pyrimethamine combination for weekly malaria prophylaxis include hepatic toxicity (acute or chronic hepatitis, focal hepatic necrosis), hypersensitivity reactions (systemic vasculitis, glomerulonephritis, pulmonary reactions), and hematologic abnormalities (thrombocytopenia, methemoglobinemia, hemolysis, white blood cell dyscrasias, and disseminated intravascular coagulation). Due to these risks, sulfadoxine-pyrimethamine is no longer recommended for weekly malaria prophylaxis. Sulfonamides may cause kernicterus in newborns, particularly if premature (encephalopathy caused by a large deposition of unbound bilirubin in the basal ganglia and subthalamic nuclei in the brain displaced from plasma protein albumin by sulfonamides).

Sulfones (Dapsone). Dapsone has been used in combination with pyrimethamine for malaria prophylaxis and in combination with chlorproguanil for the treatment of uncomplicated malaria. Oral absorption of dapsone is rapid and improved by concomitant food intake, and it reaches its maximal concentration in 2 to 8 hours.[153] It is metabolized to mono-acetyldapsone (major metabolite with antimalarial activity) and dapsone hydroxylamine. The *N*-hydroxylation process of dapsone may be mediated by CYP3A, CYP2C9, and CYP2E1.[154] The dapsone metabolite hydroxylamine is suspected to be associated with common hematologic toxicities of dapsone, including methemoglobinemia, agranulocytosis, and hemolytic anemia.[155] The plasma half-life of dapsone is approximately 24 hours, and excretion is mainly via the fecal route.[153]

Biguanides and Their Metabolites. Proguanil and chlorproguanil (the chloro derivative of proguanil) are commonly used biguanides in the treatment of malaria. Although both have intrinsic antimalarial activity, the antifolate activity of these compounds against malarial parasites relies on their cyclic triazine active metabolites cycloguanil and cyclochlorproguanil, respectively. Proguanil's separate non-antifolate activity when used in combination with atovaquone is discussed in the section on atovaquone and proguanil.

Proguanil is absorbed well orally and peaks within 2 to 5 hours. The transformation of proguanil to cycloguanil is fast, with the concentration of active metabolite cycloguanil peaking within 1 hour of the proguanil peak. This metabolism is mediated by CYP3A4 and CYP2C19. Polymorphism in CYP2C19 (involving mephentoin oxidation)[156] associated with variable proguanil metabolism is seen in up to 20% of Asian and some African descendents and in about 3% of Caucasians, and this may result in an inadequate cycloguanil exposure and failure of prophylaxis in poor metabolizers.[157,158] Forty percent to 60% of absorbed proguanil and cycloguanil is excreted in the urine. The half-life of proguanil ranges from 12 to 20 hours, and the half-life of cycloguanil is approximately 12 hours.

Chlorproguanil is a chloro derivative of proguanil, and both chlorproguanil and its active antifolate metabolite cyclochlorproguanil have more intrinsic antimalarial activity than proguanil and cycloguanil. Chlorproguanil is well absorbed orally and peaks in about 4 hours. Although the mean half-life of chlorproguanil is long (17 to >30 hours), cyclochlorproguanil has a shorter half-life, an attractive feature to reduce the time when subtherapeutic concentration may select for drug resistance. The combination of dapsone-chlorproguanil was registered in the United Kingdom but is not used despite extensive clinical testing for safety and efficacy because of persistent concerns about hemolytic anemia in G6PD-deficient persons.

These biguanides at prophylactic doses (200 to 300 mg daily) may cause occasional diarrhea and nausea and more severe gastrointestinal discomfort with a higher dose. Proguanil is very well tolerated and remarkably safe, and no serious toxicity has been documented even with gross overdose.

Relationship between Pharmacokinetics and Clinical Response. The in vivo efficacy of an antimicrobial drug is determined by the correlation between pharmacokinetic and pharmacodynamic parameters. These are most commonly measured as the ratio between peak drug level and MIC, the ratio between the 24-hour AUC and MIC, and the percentage of time of the dosing interval that the drug level exceeds the MIC (time above MIC). Those values are well studied and established for many antibacterial agents, and knowledge of the killing mechanism (time vs. concentration dependent) is helpful in determining the dose and the dosing interval for a given antimicrobial.[159] Knowledge of pharmacokinetic-pharmacodynamic relationships and the mechanism of killing in antimalarial drugs, however, is very limited. Several studies have explored these relationships for antifolate antimalarial drugs, particularly for the most popular combination, sulfadoxine and pyrimethamine. The antiparasitic activity of this combination likely depends on the time during which drug concentrations are maintained above the MIC. Clinically effective minimal concentrations or clinical therapeutic ranges are not established for either of these compounds. The in vitro concentration of sulfadoxine that is effective against resistant *P. falciparum* was found to be 60 mcg/ml.[160] Several pharmacokinetic-pharmacodynamic studies of sulfadoxine-pyrimethamine in parasitemic patients were conducted in different endemic areas where susceptibility of *P. falciparum* varied. The concentration of sulfadoxine associated with 100% in vitro inhibition was less than 2 mcg/ml (as low as 0.39 mcg/ml) in earlier studies.[161,162] More recent studies showed that maintaining concentrations of sulfadoxine of 62 to 115 mcg/ml was associated with treatment success and that concentrations below this range were associated with recrudescence within 28 days.[163-167]

The synergistic antiparasitic activity of the combination of sulfadoxine and pyrimethamine, however, is dictated primarily by parasites' sensitivity to pyrimethamine. This is due to the pharmacokinetic nature of the two constituents, such as the elimination half-life and availability of the free drug fraction.[168] This predominance of pyrimethamine in sulfadoxine-pyrimethamine synergy has been observed both in vitro and in vivo.[160,167,169] Watkins and colleagues have estimated the duration of synergy of sulfadoxine-pyrimethamine in the presence of different levels of drug-resistant molecular markers in the parasite population.[168] It has been postulated that the MIC (or the 50% inhibitory concentration) will be increased significantly by the presence of one or more drug-resistance-conferring mutations in the parasite. The presence of the single point mutation in DHFR (DHFR Asn108) decreases parasites' sensitivity to pyrimethamine 10-fold. DHFR triple mutants, which are increasingly common in many endemic African countries, reduce pyrimethamine susceptibility approximately 1000-fold. The duration of in vivo inhibitory concentration above the synergistic effective concentration was also found to be significantly shorter for the pyrimethamine-resistant strain than the sensitive one (7 days vs. more than 52 days).[168] Despite these elegant pharmacokinetic studies, clinical studies show that resistance to sulfadoxine mediated by DHPS mutations clearly and substantially increases the risk of clinical treatment failure.[150] The failure of pharmacokinetic models to predict treatment outcomes may be because the concentrations of both drugs remain above the MIC long enough to eradicate most initial infections and because background host immunity plays an important role in clearing infections, particularly in hyperendemic areas where frequent infection maintains protective immunity.

The concept of IPT with sulfadoxine-pyrimethamine is different from acute treatment of malaria. The efficacy of sulfadoxine-pyrimethamine in IPT relies mainly on the prolonged effective antiparasitic activity of sulfadoxine-pyrimethamine during the interval between doses, which is usually about 30 days. The duration of this period of "posttreatment prophylaxis" is loosely defined as the time taken for sulfadoxine-pyrimethamine concentrations to fall from the peak levels to the MIC values. It is recommended conservatively that the dosing interval should not be a week longer than the time taken for the peak plasma concentration to fall to the MIC.[170] It was hypothesized that, for each doubling of the MIC, the duration of posttreatment prophylaxis is shortened by one half-life of the drug; in the face of high prevalence of triple mutant resistance markers, the shortening of posttreatment prophylaxis may be approximately three half-lives or at least 10 days for pyrimethamine.

Drug Interactions. High plasma protein binding of sulfonamides is suspected to be the potential source of interaction with other drugs, although clinical significance is likely to be minimal.[171] There has been no clinically important pharmacokinetic drug interaction reported in the combined use of sulfonamides with other antifolates[171] or other drugs such as mefloquine.[172] Limited clinical data suggest no kinetic interaction between dapsone and pyrimethamine or chlorproguanil.[173,174] Information on drug interaction between these antifolate compounds and artemisinin derivatives is very limited.

Antifolates in Pregnancy and Breast-feeding. Sulfadoxine-pyrimethamine still plays an important role in the reduction of malaria-related complications in pregnancy and its outcomes in endemic areas where efficacy is retained. This combination is administered as monthly dosing of 1.5 g of sulfadoxine and 75 mg of pyrimethamine, at least twice during the second and third trimesters. Both compounds cross the placenta, and a large pool of clinical data[76] suggests a lack of serious maternal or fetal adverse effects such as drug toxicity and congenital malformation. Sulfonamides are not known to be teratogenic. There are no available pharmacokinetic data on sulfadoxine, pyrimethamine, or dapsone in pregnant women. Sulfonamides and pyrimethamine are both secreted into breast milk.[175] Although anecdotal clinical evidence is favorable, solid clinical data are needed to assess the effects of these compounds on the newborn. Ingestion of sulfadoxine by the newborn via breast milk was a theoretical concern for the development of kernicterus; however, the clinical data are reassuring.

Proguanil, alone or in combination with other antifolates or atovaquone, is considered safe in pregnancy. Limited clinical data suggest reduction in the concentrations and total drug exposure of the active metabolite cycloguanil in the third trimester of pregnancy,[176,177] and its clinical significance needs further exploration.

Artemisinin Derivatives

Many artemisinin derivatives are described in the literature. This chapter discusses only compounds that are in common clinical use, namely artemisinin, artesunate, dihydroartemisinin (DHA), and artemether.

History. Artemisinin derives from the plant *qinghao (Artemesia annua)*, also known as sweet wormwood or annual wormwood. The medical use of this plant has been described in traditional Chinese medicine for more than 200 years. The infusion of *qinghao* in tea was prescribed by Ge Hong in 340 A.D. to treat fever, and later it was specifically recommended for the symptoms of malaria. The active component of the plant, *qinghaosu* or artemisinin, was extracted and crystallized by a group of Chinese scientists in 1972. A complete description of the synthesis and preclinical and clinical data on artemisinin and its several derivatives was published in a large series in 1982.[178-183] These compounds were in wide clinical use in China in the 1980s, and by the 1990s in most of Southeast Asia, where *P. falciparum* resistant to quinolines and antifolate drugs is widespread. Their introduction to the rest of the malaria-endemic world has been slowly increasing in the last decade, following increasing resistance to most other antimalarial drugs. Although their availability in most African countries has been limited by cost and limited supplies, a recent surge of international donor support for malaria control is rapidly increasing the rate at which countries in Africa adopt artemisinin-based combination therapies (ACTs) as their first-line drugs. The commonly used artemisinin derivatives are artesunate, artemether, artemisinin, and

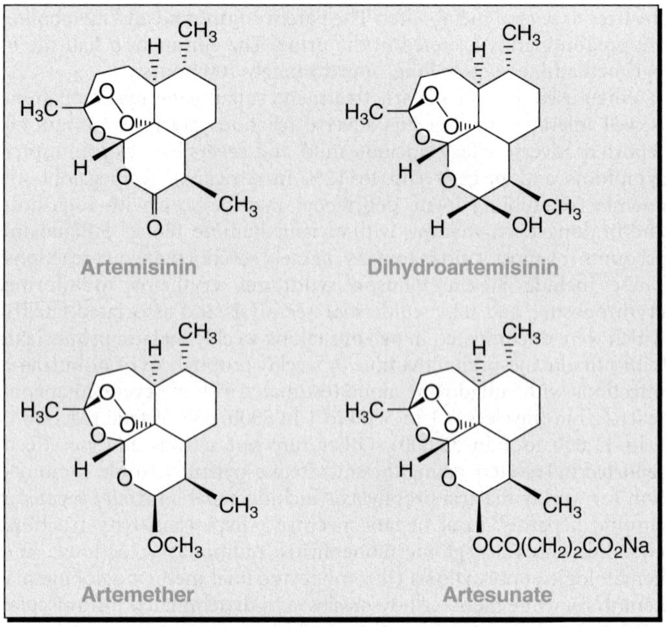

FIGURE 82-5 • Chemical structures of artemisinin derivatives.

DHA, and these drugs are now increasingly manufactured and marketed by Western pharmaceutical companies. Arteether and artelinic acid are no longer under development or clinical investigation, although they are still in limited use in some areas. Despite their extensive use and worldwide popularity, these agents have not yet been approved by the regulatory agencies in the United States.

Chemistry. Artemisinin is a semisynthetic sesquiterpene (formed from three isoprene units—trioxane) lactone endoperoxide derived from the plant *qinghao* (Fig. 82-5).

Less than 1% (ranging from 0.01% to 0.8%) of the dry weight of the plant (leaves, stems, flowers, and seeds) represents active artemisinin. Artemisinin is a crystalline compound with poor dissolution in water or oil. It is chemically modified to produce more soluble derivatives for clinical use. The descriptive biosynthetic pathway of artemisinin is described by Liu and colleagues.[184] Chemical structures of the derivatives are shown in Figure 82-5. They contain a peroxide bridge that is believed to be essential for antiparasitic activity. Lactone is readily reduced to DHA, which has the highest antiparasitic activity and from which most derivatives under investigation (artesunate, artemether) are derived.

Antimalarial Activity. Artemisinin derivatives are potent and rapidly acting antimalarial compounds, and active against all asexual stages of chloroquine-sensitive and -resistant *P. falciparum* and *P. vivax*. They are also active against sexual forms (gametocytes) of *P. falciparum*,[185] with important implications for reducing malaria transmission.[186] The major disadvantage of artemisinin derivatives as monotherapy is a high rate of late parasite recrudescence. Resistance does not account for these late recrudescences, which are just as susceptible to artemisinins in vitro and in vivo as the initial infection. The mechanism of recrudescence suggests that some parasites escape the short action of artemisinins through a mechanism other than stable resistance. These compounds have no activity against primary or latent hepatic forms. They also have a broad spectrum of antiparasitic activity, including *Leishmania major*, *Toxoplasma gondii*, and *Schistosoma* species.

Mechanism of Action and Resistance. The mechanisms of antimalarial action of artemisinin derivatives have been investigated extensively. It is generally accepted that the mode of action comprises multiple steps: covalent binding of artemisinin to globin protein in the parasite food vacuole, heme-catalyzed irreversible cleavage of the endoperoxide bridge, and production of carbon-centered free radicals. These carbon-centered free radicals that alkylate and damage the parasite macromolecules are essential to parasite killing.[187] An alternative mechanism has also been proposed: a potent inhibition of sarcoplasmic endoplasmic reticulum calcium ATPase located outside the parasite food vacuole.[188] It has been shown in vitro in an isolated oocyte system that a single amino acid on this protein determines susceptibility to the drug.[189] The specificity of these compounds to particular parasitic molecules and selectivity to parasite versus host are still subject to debate. An increase in the copy number of *pfmdr1*,[190] the likely principal determinant of mefloquine resistance, and a reduction in plasma lumefantrine concentration are associated with treatment failure of the artemether-lumefantrine combination.[191] Clinically significant drug resistance, however, has not been clearly documented for artemisinin derivatives. The frequent late recrudescences do not represent drug resistance, in that the recrudescent parasites are easily cleared by repeat treatment and do not have decreased in vitro susceptibility to artemisinins.[192]

Pharmacokinetics. Elucidating the pharmacokinetic properties of artemisinins has been limited by difficulties in developing reliable and accurate drug assays, although recent advances have improved the understanding of pharmacokinetics, pharmacodynamics, and toxicologic properties of these compounds. Several formulations are available in clinical practice: oral (artesunate, artemisinin, DHA), intramuscular (artesunate and artemether), intravenous (artesunate), and rectal (artesunate and artemisinin). All of the artemisinin derivatives have poor oral absorption and bioavailability, with the exception of artesunate, which has approximately 60% bioavailability.[193,194] All artemisinin derivatives (except artemisinin itself) are rapidly hydrolyzed in biologic systems to the principal active metabolite DHA. Parent compounds and metabolites (e.g., DHA) contribute varying degrees of antimalarial activity: artemisinin itself exerts significant antimalarial activity and artesunate relies on its conversion to DHA, while artemether probably contributes to an equal share with DHA. All artemisinins are likely subjected to the first-pass effect when given orally.

In vitro and animal studies suggest a wide tissue distribution (including brain, liver, kidney, heart, lung, muscle, and fat)[195] and selective binding to parasitized red blood cells.[196] All artemisinins, to varying degrees, cross the blood-brain barrier and some the blood-placental barrier.[197] These compounds bind to both albumin and α1-acid glycoprotein (artemether to several lipoproteins), and the extent of protein binding varies (~40% to 90%).[198] All artemisinin derivatives reach their peak concentrations very rapidly (less than 1 to 2 hours), are biotransformed mostly in the liver, and are quickly eliminated in feces and, to a lesser extent, as urine glucuronide. Their elimination half-life ranges from 2 to 5 hours. They have a complex metabolic profile, and many of them (artemisinin, artesunate, and artemether) exhibit a phenomenon of autoinduction, suggested by a decline in the AUC after repeated oral dosing.[199-201] The pharmacokinetics and metabolic degradation of artemisinin and its derivatives are complex and yet incompletely understood. Readers are referred to excellent available reviews.[171,198,202] Despite their similarities, the pharmacokinetic and pharmacodynamic properties of these compounds are surprisingly different, likely due to differences in formulation and in the intrinsic lipophilicity of the compounds. These differences contribute to the toxicity characteristics of the individual compounds, particularly neurotoxicity.

Artemisinin. Artemisinin is formulated in oral, rectal, and intramuscular preparations. All formulations have a poor bioavailability of about 30%, and food does not seem to change its absorption.[203] Its rapid metabolism likely takes place in the liver,[197] with an elimination half-life of about 2 to 3 hours. Its metabolism is mediated primarily by CYP2B6 and to a lesser extent by CYP3A4.[204] Increased activity of CYP2C19 by artemisinin has also been reported.[205] Knowledge of the metabolic interaction of artemisinin and its derivatives has been expanding quickly in the last decade, and it is likely that multiple metabolic enzymes are involved.

Artesunate. Artesunate (artesunic acid) is available in oral, intravenous, intramuscular, and rectal forms. It is a water-soluble derivative of artemisinin. Artesunate is rapidly absorbed, and extensively and almost completely hydrolyzed to DHA before reaching the systemic circulation. The bioavailability of oral artesunate is highly variable, particularly in patients with acute malaria, ranging from 15% to 60%.[206,207] The rate of conversion from artesunate to DHA depends on the rate of dissolution in the gastrointestinal tract and the pH of intraluminal fluid, and therefore is likely affected by the route of administration. The absorption of DHA, after an oral dosing of artesunate, takes about an hour. The elimination half-life of artesunate is less than 3 hours and that of its active metabolite DHA less than 1 hour (~45 minutes) with either oral or intravenous dosing of artesunate. Although the rectal formulation of artesunate has a high clinical value for its convenience, its highly variable absorption and bioavailability in patients with malaria, particularly severe malaria, should be carefully considered.

Artemether. Artemether is a lipid-soluble derivative of artemisinin. It is available in oral and intramuscular preparations. It is also coformulated with lumefantrine as a fixed-dose combination. Artemether-lumefantrine is one of the ACTs recommended by the WHO and the one being adopted by most countries switching from less effective drugs to ACTs.

The pharmacokinetics of artemether, alone or in combination, have been evaluated in several clinical trials.[208-214] Absorption of artemether is rapid when administered orally, reaching its maximal concentrations within 2 hours and entering extensive first-pass metabolism. Its principal active metabolite is DHA. Artemether is highly protein bound (>90%) to α1-acid glycoprotein, albumin, and lipoproteins.[215] The elimination half-life is approximately 2 to 4 hours. Absorption of artemether from the intramuscular route in patients with malaria is very poor and highly variable, may take many hours to reach maximal concentrations, and has been shown to be associated with impaired parasite clearance.[211,213,216] Artemether is probably metabolized by several hepatic and intestinal CYP enzymes, including CYP3A4, 2C11, and 2B6.[198] It is likely to be a substrate of intestinal CYP3A4, suggested by a rise in artemether bioavailability when administered with grapefruit juice (a potent inhibitor of CYP3A4).[217] However, grapefruit juice does not prevent a fall in the AUC of artemether in repeated dosing, suggesting the lack of its effect in the hepatic processes.[218] CYP2D6 and CYP2C9, common drug-metabolizing enzymes with ethnic polymorphism, are probably not involved in artemether metabolism.[219] These findings have raised concerns about the possibility of drug interactions, although there has been no report of significant interaction between artemether with lumefantrine or other quinolines antimalarials.[220] The impact of artemether on the pharmacokinetics of other drugs needs to be further explored.

Dihydroartemisinin. DHA is a principal active metabolite of artemisinin and artesunate and is also formulated in a direct oral preparation. DHA information is obtained mostly from studies of patients or volunteers dosed with artesunate or artemether (see earlier), and rarely from dosing directly with DHA.[221] The bioavailability of DHA is higher than artemisinin. With repeated dosing with artesunate or artemether, regardless of route, the time to reach maximal DHA concentration is approximately 1 to 2 hours. It is mainly eliminated by a glucuronidation with a half-life of less than 1 hour. It is excreted mainly in bile, and in urine in a small percentage. Glucuronidation is mediated primarily by UDP-glucuronosyltransferases (UGTs), probably UGT1A9 and UGT2B7.[222] The clinical development of DHA has been retarded by concerns about neurotoxicity and advanced development of more suitable artemisinin derivatives.

Relationship between Pharmacokinetics and Clinical Response. Artemisinins are probably the most widely studied antimalarial compounds in the areas of pharmacokinetics, pharmacodynamics, and their interactions in humans. Artemisinins are potent and rapidly acting antimalarials effective in killing all asexual stages of *P. falciparum* and *P. vivax*. Their 50% inhibitory concentration values in vitro remain in the low nanomolar range consistently.[223] Artemisinin compounds quickly attenuate parasite growth, particularly the young ring forms, seen as a rapid and early decline in parasitemia following artemisinin treatment.[224] The pattern of reduction in parasitemia is similar to that of chloroquine in chloroquine-sensitive infections; however, parasite reduction is significantly faster and steeper than that induced by other antimalarials such as quinine or mefloquine.[225] A unique pharmacologic property of artemisinins is a continued and sustained decline in parasitemia with decreasing drug levels in the blood. There is no concentration-response relationship observed with these compounds. The action of artemisinins is also independent of dose at doses higher than 2 mg/kg, probably because of limited metabolic capacity of the liver. In a study with intravenous artesunate,[193] a rapid 20% reduction in parasitemia was observed while the drug concentration was about 400 nM, close to the assay sensitivity limit. This was followed by a slower 60% decline in parasitemia at a drug concentration of 2 nM and finally a 95% reduction when no drug was detectable in the blood at 24 hours. This pharmacodynamic profile is described as a postantibiotic-like effect of artemisinins. The recommendation is to dose these compounds daily, instead of twice a day, based on the fact that there is no difference in clinical efficacy between the two dosing schedules.[226]

As with all other antimalarial drugs, it is not known which pharmacokinetic parameter of artemisinin compounds (peak concentration, AUC, or time above MIC) determines their therapeutic efficacy. Attention must be paid to the importance of large interindividual variability in the pharmacokinetics of any of artemisinin compounds and their metabolites in choosing dosing regimens. The widely accepted general concept that the concentrations of antimalarial drugs above therapeutic level need to be maintained during the whole period of dosing interval is clearly challenged by artemisinins.

Therapeutic Considerations. Artemisinin treatment of less than 7 days, or less than 3 days when combined with long-acting partner drugs, is associated with high rates of late recrudescence. Although artemisinin derivatives as monotherapy have been marketed and remain available in some settings, the WHO has strongly recommended that they be used only in combination with a longer acting antimalarial drugs, to deter the emergence of resistance to artemisinins and prevent late treatment failures. Current combination regimens were developed based variously on clinical findings, empirical results, or limited pharmacokinetic data. Rational dosing regimens for these compounds in a variety of formulations for different malaria syndromes require further study, with careful consideration of risk:benefit ratios and of the wide range of pharmacokinetic variability seen with artemisinins. The rationale for combination therapy is discussed in more detail later in this chapter.

Adverse Effects, Precautions, and Contraindications. Although artemisinin derivatives enjoy a reputation of good tolerability, they are associated with dose-related reversible hematologic changes (reduction in reticulocytes and neutrophils and acute hemolysis) and transient increase in hepatic transaminases. There have been a few cases of acute allergic urticaria and anaphylaxis (estimated risk is 1 in 3000).[227] Although cardiovascular side effects are uncommon with these compounds, some clinically silent electrocardiographic changes (transient bradycardia, PR or QTc prolongation, and extrasystole) have been reported.

A safety concern with artemisinins has been neurotoxicity. There has been a large debate over the safety and toxicity of artemisinin compounds in the last decade, without a clear consensus to reassure practicing clinicians. Concerns with artemisinins' neurotoxicity originate primarily from in vitro and animal data, which were thoroughly reviewed by Toovey in 2006.[228] Briefly, in vitro studies showed mitochondrial dysfunction, energy depletion, and inhibition of outgrowth in brainstem neurons.[229-231] Principal targets in animals include the central nervous system, liver, bone marrow, and fetus. Thirteen of 16 animal studies showed a dose-dependent but delayed neuropathology in brainstem nuclei.[232] These findings were more pronounced with repeated administration of lipophilic derivatives such as artemether, and much less evident with water-soluble artesunate.

Issues of safety in humans are more complex. Many clinical trials have assessed the efficacy of artemisinins in children and adults since the early 1990s, and measured safety as a secondary outcome. Many small trials comparing intramuscular artemether and intravenous quinine fail to show a clinically meaningful difference in neurologic adverse effects, measured as coma recovery time. Neurologic complications have been reported following treatment with artemether, including tremor, ataxic gait, nystagmus, decreased coordination, anxiety, and slurred speech. Retrospective studies that specifically assessed neurologic sequelae in patients repeatedly treated with artemisinins reported conflicting results: two of them showed no difference between cases and controls,[233,234] while one study showed drug-related high-frequency hearing loss in cases more than controls.[235] The strength of the evidence from these data is weak due to small sample sizes, possible bias, and the presence of multiple confounders, including direct effects of malaria. A compilation of data from various studies with prospective neurologic assessment[236] attempted to compare artesunate and artemether alone and in combination with mefloquine, and showed no evidence of drug-related neurologic adverse effects in patients treated with artesunate or artemether alone, but a higher risk of neurologic manifestations in those treated with the combination, implicating mefloquine. In two large prospective, well-designed and adequately powered studies of cerebral malaria, longer neurologic recovery was reported in the artemisinin group compared with those receiving intravenous quinine. Intramuscular artemether was used in one study,[237] and in the other intravenous artesunate was used.[238] These findings, however, are confounded by the fact that severe malaria itself can produce many neurologic consequences, and the relevance of use of coma recovery time as a measure of drug toxicity was questioned. Moreover, no systemic neurologic changes attributable to the drugs were described. Giving these uncertainties in available data, artemisinin compounds must be used with caution in individuals with preexisting neurologic illness or those who are taking concomitant medications with potentials for neurotoxicity.

There are no safety data on artemisinins in infants. Artemisinins are contraindicated in those with known previous allergic reaction and pregnant women in the first trimester, unless the benefit outweighs the risk.

Drug Interactions. Limited data exist for interaction between artemisinins and their common partners such as quinolines and related compounds. Some data suggest a synergistic effect of neurotoxicity with the known neurotoxin mefloquine,[236] and of cardiotoxicity with quinine,[239] although the clinical significance of this is questionable. Due to the structural similarities, the combination of artemisinins and quinoline antimalarials must be used with caution. Multiple drug-metabolizing enzymes—including CYP3A4, which metabolizes the majority of commonly used drugs—are involved in artemisinin disposition, and the clinical impact of interaction between these compounds and other drugs such as antiretroviral drugs has not been adequately assessed.

Artemisinin Derivatives and Pregnancy. These compounds are potent embryotoxins in animal. In humans, very limited data are available for safety in pregnancy. Available data do not provide evidence of fetal or maternal toxicity of artemisinins used in the second or third trimester of pregnancy.[240-243] In mothers who were treated with artemisinins during the first trimester, the rate of stillbirth, spontaneous abortion, and congenital malformation is similar to the background rate in the community.[244] The risks of death and complications from falciparum malaria are high in pregnancy and the choice of drugs is very limited, particularly in the areas where multidrug resistance is extremely common, such as in specific areas of Southeast Asia. The risk:benefit balance must be carefully considered in deciding whether to use these compounds in pregnancy, but where no suitable alternatives are available, artemisinins should be and are used to treat malaria in pregnancy. The clearance of DHA following oral artesunate seems to be higher in pregnancy when compared with that in nonpregnant adults historically,[245] although the clinical implication of this needs to be further assessed. There are no data available on the breast milk secretion of artemisinin derivatives, or on effects on the nursing infant.

Drugs That Interfere with Mitochondrial Function

Atovaquone and Proguanil

History. The history of atovaquone can be traced to Hooker's discovery of the presence of naphthoquinones in plant extracts, leading

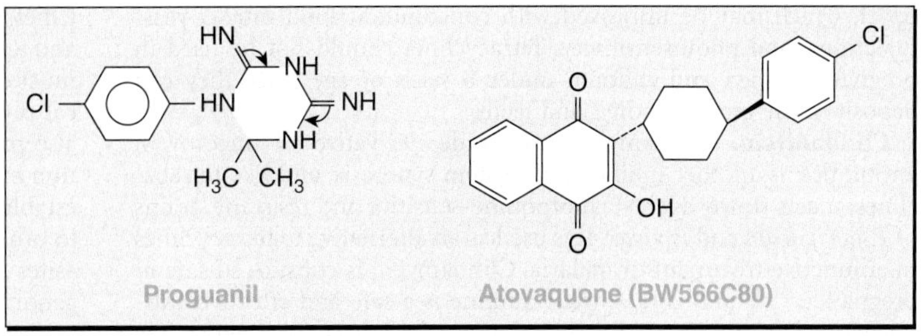

FIGURE 82-6 • Chemical structures of atovaquone and proguanil.

to the synthesis of lapachol in 1936. Naphthoquinones were one of the antimalarial compounds investigated during World War II, but their development was curtailed by the advent of highly effective chloroquine. Interest was renewed in the 1960s as chloroquine resistance emerged and spread. Several synthetic derivatives of hydroxynapththoquinone were developed and tested (Fig. 82-6), and many faced problems with metabolic instability and oral availability. Atovaquone was subsequently selected as the most metabolically stable and the one with a broad antiprotozoal spectrum. It was first approved by the FDA as a second-line agent to treat the opportunistic infection *Pneumocystis jiroveci*. Atovaquone is also highly potent against *Plasmodium* species. The rapid development of atovaquone resistance and high relapse in clinical outcome when used alone led to its use in combination with proguanil.[246] A fixed-dose combination of atovaquone with proguanil was approved by the FDA in 2000 for the prophylaxis and treatment of malaria. The potential role of atovaquone in the treatment of *Toxoplasma gondii* is currently under clinical evaluation.

Antimalarial Activity. Atovaquone is highly active against sensitive strains of erythrocytic- and hepatic-stage *P. falciparum*,[247] and atovaquone-proguanil is used for both prophylaxis and treatment of uncomplicated falciparum malaria. The relapse rate of atovaquone-proguanil treatment of *P. vivax* is high due to the lack of atovaquone activity against hypnozoites; therefore, radical therapy with primaquine is required.[248]

Mechanism of Action and Resistance. Atovaquone selectively binds to the cytochrome bc_1 complex located on the inner membrane of mitochondria and inhibits electron transport and collapses the parasite mitochondrial membrane potential,[249] at a concentration significantly lower than what is required to inhibit mammalian mitochondria. Synergistic activity is seen with proguanil, which enhances the antimalarial action of atovaquone specifically through mitochondria membrane collapsing ability, though proguanil alone does not possesses this ability.[146] Proguanil acts in this synergism as a biguanide, rather than its metabolite cycloguanil, although the DHFR inhibitory activity of cycloguanil presumably contributes to the antimalarial activity of atovaquone-proguanil.

Atovaquone resistance develops readily in vitro and in vivo[250] when it is used as a single agent. A mutation in the mitochondria-associated cytochrome *b* gene has been shown to be responsible for the resistance. Combination with proguanil may not overcome atovaquone resistance once it has emerged, and atovaquone action in the mitochondria itself may promote drug resistance by generating mutagenic reactive oxygen species.[251] Several cases of prophylaxis failure with atovaquone-resistant parasites have been reported,[252-254] but the efficacy of atovaquone-proguanil for preventing and treating malaria has been consistently high in clinical trials.

Pharmacokinetics. The pharmacokinetic features of proguanil are discussed in a previous section in this chapter. The oral absorption of atovaquone is slow and erratic and improved by coadministration with fatty foods. It is highly protein bound (~99%) and may undergo enterohepatic circulation, represented by the appearance of double peaks in its pharmacokinetic profile (the first one at 1 to 8 hours and the second at 1 to 4 days). The majority of atovaquone is excreted unchanged in the bile, with a very small quantity present in the urine. It has a long half-life, ranging from 1.5 to 3 days, and shows no significant accumulation in long-term administration. Atovaquone clearance may be variable in different ethnic groups,[255] and its clearance has been shown to be higher in young children.[256] There is no reported clear relationship between the pharmacokinetics of atovaquone or proguanil and clinical response.

Therapeutic Considerations. Atovaquone-proguanil is one of four recommended malaria prophylaxis drugs for travelers to malaria-endemic areas. It is highly effective in the prevention of falciparum malaria, with clinical efficacy ranging from 90% to 100%,[257] and is preferred for short-term travel because it need only be continued for a week after the last malaria exposure due to its causal prophylactic efficacy. Atovaquone-proguanil is also effective in the treatment of uncomplicated falciparum and vivax malaria (with radical therapy with primaquine for vivax).[258,259] Limited availability and high cost limit the use of this combination in malaria-endemic countries, but atovaquone-proguanil is preferred by some practitioners over quinine for treating uncomplicated malaria in returned travelers because of its much more favorable side effect profile.

Adverse Effects, Precautions, and Contraindications. Atovaquone-proguanil is well tolerated, and the few side effects (gastrointestinal discomfort and headache) were reported at a frequency similar to that reported with placebo. Vomiting may be associated with therapeutic failure, since atovaquone is poorly absorbed. Readministration within 1 hour of vomiting is recommended to ensure clinical efficacy. Mild and transient abnormalities in serum transaminases and amylase have been reported in association with atovaquone treatment. To date, no serious toxicity has been reported. Atovaquone-proguanil is contraindicated in persons with known allergy and in severe renal failure, and no adequate data exist on liver impairment.

Drug Interactions. Although the high protein binding of atovaquone was a source of concern about possible drug interactions, there have been no clinical data to support this concern. A modest decrease in the AUC of atovaquone was reported when administered with tetracycline, rifampicin, rifabutin, or metoclopramide[257]; however, clinical significance is unlikely. Limited data showed no significant interaction between atovaquone or proguanil and artesunate.[260]

Atovaquone/Proguanil in Pregnancy and Breast-feeding. Atovaquone is not teratogenic or embryotoxic in animal studies. The use of atovaquone-proguanil in pregnancy is considered safe, although clinical data for the safety and pharmacokinetics of these compounds are very limited in the pregnant population. It is not known whether atovaquone is secreted in breast milk; proguanil is secreted in the milk in a small quantity. Atovaquone-proguanil is not recommended for pregnant women or nursing mothers; however, careful consideration of the risk:benefit ratio must be made on an individual basis.

Antibiotics with Antimalarial Activity

Tetracycline and Doxycycline. Tetracyclines are slow-acting schizonticides effective against multidrug-resistant strains of *P. falciparum* as well as *P. vivax*. Tetracyclines act classically by inhibiting ribosomal protein synthesis. They are used as adjunctive therapy to the faster acting antimalarials quinine or quinidine in the treatment of falciparum malaria, although the use of tetracyclines as single agents is not effective in the treatment of acute malaria due to their slow action. They are also used for short-term malaria prophylaxis for travel to areas with chloroquine and mefloquine resistance. Doxycycline, a modified form of tetracycline with a longer half-life (~16 hours), is one of four prophylactic antimalarial agents recommended by the FDA. Commonly encountered adverse effects include gastrointestinal upset, which may be improved with concomitant food intake; yeast infections, and photosensitivity. Tetracyclines should not be used in pregnant women and children under 8 years of age since they can deposit in the growing bones and teeth.

Clindamycin. Clindamycin, an amide derivative of lincomycin antibiotics, is another inhibitor of protein synthesis, and like tetracyclines, it acts slowly against chloroquine-sensitive and resistant strains of *P. falciparum* and *P. vivax*. It is used as an alternative to tetracyclines in adjunctive treatment of malaria. Clindamycin is considered safe in pregnancy,[261,262] and clindamycin-quinine is a safe and effective antimalarial treatment for this population. Its pharmacokinetics are unchanged during pregnancy, and it crosses the placenta and is secreted in the breast milk.[263] It is available in both oral and parenteral salt forms. Clindamycin has a short half-life (~3 hours). The common adverse effects include diarrhea (up to 20%) and skin rash, particularly common in HIV-infected patients. It is also associated with rare but serious pseudomembranous colitis caused by toxin released from *Clostridium difficile*.

Macrolides: Azithromycin. Azithromycin is a semisynthetic second-generation azalide broad-spectrum antibacterial agent derived from erythromycin. Its antibacterial activity is based on interference with bacterial protein synthesis, and limited data suggest that it may target 50S ribosomal subunits in the apicoplasts of *P. falciparum*.[264] Its antimalarial activity in vitro[265] and in animals[266] against chloroquine-sensitive and chloroquine-resistant *Plasmodium* was first discovered in the early 1990s. Subsequent clinical trials showed both prophylactic[267,268] and treatment[269-272] efficacy against uncomplicated *P. falciparum* and *P. vivax*, although azithromycin has generally been less efficacious than other drugs in comparative clinical trials. Its efficacy is improved when combined with fast-acting antimalarial agents such as quinine, chloroquine, or artemisinin.

Azithromycin displays better oral availability and pharmacokinetic profiles than older macrolides such as erythromycin. Azithromycin is absorbed rapidly after oral administration, and has a concentration-dependent plasma protein binding (decreasing binding with increasing concentration).[273] It is widely distributed in many tissues (liver, lungs, spleen, and kidneys but not in the cerebrospinal fluid), and its liver concentration is more than 200 to 300 times higher than that in the plasma.[274] It is also deposited in blood cells, with uptake in leukocytes thousands-fold higher than in red blood cells and plasma.[275] Azithromycin is predominantly eliminated unchanged in the bile, with its urinary elimination approximately 10%. It has a long plasma half-life ranging from 40 to 60 hours, likely owing to the tissue binding. Data suggest that azithromycin may have very limited involvement in hepatic CYP metabolism, unlike other macrolides.[276,277]

Azithromycin is used worldwide in pregnancy for the treatment of various infections, including sexually transmitted disease, and enjoys a good reputation for safety in this population. Pharmacokinetic data are very limited in pregnancy. Azithromycin crosses the placenta to a limited degree (about 10% to 40% of the maternal dose), and accumulates in the placenta at up to 10-fold higher concentration than in the serum, and is eliminated slowly, with an estimated half-life in the placenta of approximately 70 hours in contrast to its serum half-life of 12 hours.[278,279] Because of its record of safety in pregnant women and fetuses, the nature of its pharmacokinetic disposition, and its ability to deposit itself in the placenta without crossing through it, azithromycin may come to play a role in the prevention and treatment of malaria in pregnancy, including IPT. The somewhat inferior efficacy compared to other drugs makes it unlikely that azithromycin will be used for prophylaxis in travelers, which requires complete eradication of parasites, or as monotherapy for acute malaria. Azithromycin is, however, being tested in combination with chloroquine for the treatment of chloroquine-resistant falciparum malaria. Its possible action against hepatic-stage parasites should also be investigated, as this would affect the dosing regimen of malaria prophylaxis.

Malaria Vaccines

Despite major advances in understanding the molecular and cellular biology of malaria, an effective malaria vaccine has remained elusive. Chief among the obstacles to developing malaria vaccines is the partial and temporary nature of natural immunity, which means that vaccines must do better than nature, or at least achieve more quickly the clinical protection that takes years to develop naturally. Parasite biology also presents challenges. The extreme efficiency of parasite amplification means that a vaccine that allows even a few parasites to escape and establish infection may only delay but not prevent disease. Compared to other organisms against which effective vaccines exist, malaria parasites are monstrously large and complex. For example, the polio genome consists of 0.8 Mb of DNA and *Haemophilus influenzae* 1.8 Mb, but the *P. falciparum* genome contains 30 Mb of DNA spread across 14 chromosomes containing 5000 genes that control a highly complex set of morphologically distinct stages. Furthermore, *P. falciparum* maintains extreme genetic polymorphism through both mutation and sexual recombination, and has the ability to switch expression of the cytoadherence antigens it expresses on the surface of infected erythrocytes, thus evading memory immune responses. Clear correlates of immune protection have yet to be identified, making it difficult to assess likely efficacy of vaccine candidates short of expensive field trials. Finally, the key role host immune responses play in pathogenesis raises a concern that a potent vaccine could actually worsen disease.

Despite these obstacles, malaria vaccine development efforts have been intense since advances in recombinant DNA technologies in the 1970s and 1980s made it possible to identify, characterize, and express parasite surface proteins in heterologous systems. Renewed attention to malaria as a global problem has produced a new surge of support for vaccine development activity in recent years, resulting in more than 45 malaria vaccine candidates being in various, mostly early, stages of development. Most malaria vaccines are based on recombinant versions of antigenic targets from specific stages of the parasite life cycle, although DNA vaccines and viral vector expression approaches have been used with limited success to date.[280] The most advanced malaria vaccine is based on the circumsporozoite protein, which coats the surface of the infectious sporozoites. In recent trials, the RTS,S vaccine reduced malaria disease by 30% and severe malaria by 58% for at least 18 months.[281,282] This vaccine uses the hepatitis B surface antigen as a carrier matrix for the T- and B-cell epitopes of circumsporozoite protein from the 3D7 clone of *P. falciparum*. The vaccine antigen is expressed in *E. coli* and formulated with a proprietary adjuvant system, AS02A. RTS,S is the first and thus far only malaria vaccine to prevent malaria and reduce severe disease in field trials. This pre-erythrocytic vaccine appears to reduce malaria disease by delaying parasite amplification, but it does not block infection, and efforts to improve the efficacy of RTS,S by adding additional antigens and improving the adjuvant are underway,[283] even as this modestly effective vaccine moves toward licensure in its present form.

Blood-stage vaccines are intended not to prevent infection but to prevent disease by blocking parasite amplification in the blood. Several blood-state vaccines are in various stages of development, and vaccines based on *P. falciparum* merozoite surface protein-1[284,285] and apical membrane antigen-1[286] are presently being evaluated in clinical trials in Africa. Transmission-blocking vaccines would inhibit development of the sexual stages of the parasite in the mosquito, but would not directly benefit vaccinated individuals. The only highly effective malaria vaccines have been live, radiation-attenuated whole sporozoite vaccines, delivered by infected mosquitoes in experimental challenge studies.[287] This seemingly impractical approach has recently been resurrected by Luke and Hoffman,[288] whose controversial plan is to develop a live vaccine by mass-producing sporozoites in mosquitoes raised in sterile conditions and harvesting the attenuated sporozoites by manual dissection for freezing, thawing, and injection. All predictions of when an effective malaria vaccine will be ready have been proven overly optimistic.

Therapeutic Approaches

Therapeutic approaches and objectives in malaria management are different in different settings. The objective of malaria treatment in a nonimmune traveler with falciparum malaria is to eradicate the infection completely and to prevent further disease progression and complications. In contrast, the treatment of malaria in endemic areas may have multiple objectives beyond eradicating the initial infection, such as preventing or delaying the development of drug resistance, providing a period of posttreatment prophylaxis, and blocking transmission. Based on these considerations, the WHO recommendations for malaria treatment emphasize combination therapy, particularly artemisinin-based combination therapy (ACT).

The recommended treatment algorithm and guidelines provided by the CDC for preventing and treating malaria in the United States[289] differ substantially from the WHO recommendations for endemic regions. The CDC recommendation for uncomplicated malaria includes three treatment options: (i) oral quinine with an adjunct therapy with tetracycline, doxycycline, or clindamycin; (ii) atovaquone-proguanil; or (iii) mefloquine. The disadvantages of these options are several. The predictable, highly noxious adverse effects and the need for 7 days of therapy compromise compliance with quinine regimens. Quinine resistance is also common in limited parts of Southeast Asia. Mefloquine has well-known neuropsychiatric adverse reactions and mefloquine resistance is also common in some parts of Southeast Asia. Although most guidelines relegate atovaquone-proguanil to alternative status for treating malaria in nonimmune travelers, its efficacy and tolerability make it a reasonable first choice for this indication. However, its high cost and the potential for rapid selection of atovaquone resistance has limited its use in endemic areas.

Parenteral quinidine is the only initial treatment for severe malaria recommended by the CDC, because intravenous quinine is not commercially available in the United States and the CDC no longer provides it. Likewise, intravenous artesunate, now preferred because of better efficacy than quinine, is not yet licensed in the United States, although this process is underway and intravenous artesunate can be obtained under an Investigational New Drug protocol from the CDC. Quinidine is cardiotoxic, and the rest of its toxicity profile is similar to quinine (hypotension, hypoglycemia). Once the patient with severe malaria is able to take oral medication, intravenous quinine should be switched to oral quinine to complete the 7-day course along with adjunctive therapy. The CDC recommendation for treating severe malaria is likely to be changed when intravenous artesunate is licensed in the United States.

WHO recommendations for the treatment of uncomplicated malaria emphasize drug combinations that include at least two drugs with different mechanisms of action. The objective is to enhance the therapeutic efficacy of any given drug and, more importantly, to delay or prevent the development of drug resistance. The recommended combinations are artemether-lumefantrine, or artesunate with mefloquine, amodiaquine, or sulfadoxine-pyrimethamine. Other partner drugs under investigation for ACT include piperaquine, chlorproguanil-dapsone (concern: adverse effects and background antifolate resistance), halofantrine (concern: adverse effects), and atovaquone-proguanil (concern: cost). Artemisinins are rapidly acting blood schizonticides and they induce a remarkable reduction in parasitemia, the most important feature of treatment success. They are also active against gametocytes, interrupting transmission. The most concerning issue of artemisinin compounds is a common recrudescence when used alone, and monotherapy is strongly discouraged in malaria treatment. Other concerns and practical issues with artemisinins as components of ACTs include inadequate knowledge of toxicity (particularly neurotoxicity with repeated dosing and safety in pregnancy), limited understanding of the impact of their complex metabolism on partner drugs and other drugs commonly used in endemic areas (e.g., antiretroviral drugs), highly variable pharmacokinetic profiles, poor standardization and regulation of manufacturing (counterfeit drugs are very common in parts of Asia and Africa), and availability and sustainability of their supply for global markets.

Combination Therapy in Malaria

Combination therapy will likely dominate the treatment of malaria in the future, and artemisinin derivatives have been and likely will to continue to be the major component of antimalarial combinations, despite their pitfalls. All artemisinin derivatives have a very short half-life, and the initial choices of partner drugs in ACT have been opportunity-based rather than based on rational considerations of pharmacokinetics and pharmacodynamics. The use of long-acting antimalarial drugs (e.g., piperaquine) as partner drugs has been recently shown to be superior to shorter acting partner drugs (amodiaquine and lumefantrine) in reducing the risk of new infection in high-transmission settings (posttreatment prophylaxis).[290,291] The advantage of a long-acting partner drug is clearly its ability to protect the other component of the combination and to prevent subsequent infection in endemic areas, while the main disadvantage is the likelihood of remaining in the blood at a subtherapeutic concentration, a factor believed to contribute to the development of drug resistance. A similar but opposite argument can be made for a short-acting partner—it will not offer posttreatment prophylaxis but may result in less selection for resistance.

This illustrates the impact of pharmacokinetic comparability of combining drugs on the long-term usefulness of a drug combination, and in the past pharmacokinetic matching was required by the FDA in the development of anti-infective drug combinations. The choice of partner drug should depend on two factors: (i) the objective of drug treatment (e.g., acute treatment or IPT) and/or (ii) the risk of recurrent malaria in a given population. A long-acting partner in ACT may be more valuable if the treatment objective is not only to treat acute infection but also to provide a long-term suppressive drug concentration to prevent new infections in settings where the probability of a new infection is high. A short-acting partner may be more appropriate to treat acute infection in areas where the probability of a new infection is very low. Matching pharmacokinetic profiles of partner drugs to protect each other from the development of drug resistance may be the most important feature for a combination therapy in IPT (both for pregnant women and infants).

Uncomplicated Malaria

Recommended dosing regimens for uncomplicated malaria are displayed in Table 82-3. Chloroquine is still the drug of choice for *P. vivax*, *P. ovale*, *P. malariae*, and chloroquine-sensitive *P. falciparum*. The oral route of chloroquine is preferred, although intramuscular and intravenous formulations are available outside the United States. Chloroquine-resistant *P. vivax* occurs in parts of Asia and Oceania, and is treated with artemisinin-based combinations, quinine followed by doxycycline or clindamycin, mefloquine, or atovaquone-proguanil. Because treatment with blood schizonticides does not eradicate the liver hypnozoites of *P. vivax* and *P. ovale*, initial treatment of these malaria species must be followed with primaquine for 14 days to prevent relapse. More than one course of primaquine may be required to achieve a complete, or radical, cure.

Chloroquine-resistant *P. falciparum* is now widespread virtually throughout the malaria-endemic world with the exception of Latin America north of the Panama Canal and the Caribbean. Although chloroquine-susceptible *P. falciparum* is still relatively common in many areas where chloroquine resistance is present, all cases of falciparum malaria should be considered to be chloroquine resistant unless acquired in an area that is known to be free of resistance. To counter the rising resistance to multiple antimalarial drugs, combination therapy with two or more individual drugs with different modes of action is increasingly recommended. The rationale for combination therapy is to sustain or improve the effectiveness of individual drug components and to delay the emergence of drug resistance. The disadvantages are the higher risk of adverse effects, reduced adherence to multiple-day dosing regimens, and cost.

The earliest form of antimalarial combination therapy to be used widely was a fixed-dose combination of two antifolate drugs, sulfadoxine and pyrimethamine, although the current definition of combination therapy does not include drugs that target against the same pathway. Sulfadoxine-pyrimethamine was the initial replacement for chloroquine in many areas, but its usefulness has been compromised in most regions by the relatively rapid rise of resistance. Atovaquone-proguanil is safe and efficacious, but high cost limits its use.

ACT is now recommended as the first line against *P. falciparum* malaria in most of the world. Rapid-acting artemisinin derivatives are paired with longer acting partner drugs, including lumefantrine, mefloquine, amodiaquine, sulfadoxine-pyrimethamine, and piperaquine. Artemisinins alone are very effective at initial parasite and fever clearance, but treatment for less than 7 days is associated with a high rate of recrudescence, and artemisinin monotherapy has been condemned by the WHO, mainly because of concerns about the possible emergence of resistance.

Where ACTs are unavailable (such as in the United States, where they are not yet licensed), alternative drugs must be used to treat uncomplicated falciparum malaria. Choices include atovaquone-proguanil and mefloquine as well as quinine, which should be followed by adjunct therapy with tetracycline, doxycycline, or clindamycin. Quinine is often recommended as the first choice for treating chloroquine-resistant malaria in the United States, but its poor tolerability and 7-day regimen represent significant drawbacks.

Severe Malaria

Parenteral chloroquine is no longer recommended by the WHO due to widespread chloroquine resistance, although there are a few areas where the drug is still effective. Intravenous quinine/quinidine is still used widely and highly effective. Recent studies have demonstrated lower mortality rates for severe malaria with intravenous artesunate than with standard intravenous quinine treatment,[238] and artesunate should be considered the first-line treatment where it is available. In addition to intravenous quinine or quinidine, intramuscular artemether is another alternative. Rectal artesunate is being investigated as an interim treatment in situations in which parenteral treatment is not immediately available. Other highly lipid-soluble artemisinin derivatives (artemotil, DHA) are not widely used and are advised against because of neurotoxicity concerns unless there is no alternative available. Detailed dosing regimens for the treatment of severe malaria are shown in Table 82-4.

When the patient can tolerate oral treatment, adjunct therapy with doxycycline, tetracycline, or clindamycin should be given for 7 days, while continuing the initial therapy (quinine or artesunate or artemether) in oral form. Mefloquine should be avoided in patients with an initial presentation including impaired consciousness or neurologic dysfunction because of the potential for neuropsychiatric side effects that could confuse the diagnosis.

Other aspects of managing severe malaria include respiratory support and careful fluid management to avoid heart failure, and blood transfusion for severe anemia. Based on clinical experience, exchange transfusion has been recommended for very high parasitemias (>5% to 10%) in the presence of other severe manifestations, but this intervention has not been assessed in clinical trials. Other adjunctive treatments that have been assessed but thus far show no benefit and are not recommended include biologics (such as tumor necrosis factor antagonists or hyperimmune serum), iron chelators (desferrioxamine), antioxidants, *N*-acetylcysteine, low- or high-dose corticosteroids, heparin, pentoxifylline, low-molecular-weight dextran, urea, prostacyclin, adrenaline, and cyclosporine.

Chemoprophylaxis for Travelers

Travelers to malaria-endemic areas should consult a travel clinic or travel medicine specialist well in advance of travel. A website (*http://www.cdc.gov/travel/*) maintained by the CDC provides frequently updated information on malaria risk and drug resistance in all countries. Drugs recommended by the CDC (Table 82-5) for malaria prophylaxis include chloroquine, atovaquone-proguanil, doxycycline, and mefloquine. Primaquine is used in limited settings. Due to a risk of hemolysis in persons with G6PD deficiency, primaquine must be used only after testing for G6PD deficiency. Dosing regimens are based on the mechanism of drug action. Some travel medicine practitioners prefer to have travelers start prophylaxis before traveling to establish adequate drug concentrations in the blood. Experience with the drug of choice before departure is also useful to assess individual tolerability and to give time to modify the drug regimen as necessary. Duration of postexposure prophylaxis is dictated by the site of drug action (hepatic vs. erythrocytic stage). A shorter duration is required if a drug that acts against hepatic schizonts is used than when using a drug that acts against the erythrocytic stage only (i.e., 1 week for atovaquone-proguanil and 4 weeks for mefloquine, doxycycline, or chloroquine).

Malaria in Pregnancy

Severe malaria in pregnancy is a medical and obstetric emergency. Effective antimalarial treatment must be instituted rapidly. Sepsis, aspiration, pulmonary edema, renal failure, and severe hypoglycemia are particularly common in pregnancy. In addition to standard supportive therapy, pregnant women with severe malaria require close monitoring of blood glucose, aggressive ventilatory support, and continuous fetal monitoring. Intravenous artesunate, intramuscular artemether, and intravenous quinine are the treatments of choice for severe malaria. Dosing regimens for pregnant women are generally the same as for nonpregnant adults. Pharmacokinetic-based dose adjustment

TABLE 82-4 TREATMENT REGIMEN FOR SEVERE MALARIA

Drug (Parenteral)	Dosing Regimen	Comment
Quinine dihydrochloride* (not available in the United States)	IV infusion; 20 mg salt/kg over 4 hr (loading), followed by 10 mg/kg over 2-8 hr every 8h (maintenance) *Pediatric dosing:* 10 mg salt/kg over 2-8 hr q8h	Loading dose is required; target plasma quinine level is 8-15 mg/L; dose adjustment only in convalescence or if acute renal failure >2 days; cardiac monitoring not recommended, except for those with underlying cardiac rhythm abnormality; frequent blood glucose monitoring required; must be followed by an adjunct therapy† with tetracycline, doxycycline, or clindamycin
Quinidine gluconate*	Constant IV infusion; 10 mg salt/kg over 1-2 hr (loading), followed by 0.02 mg/kg/min *Pediatric dose:* same as adult	Blood pressure, ECG (widening of QRS complex and lengthening of QTc interval), and blood glucose monitoring required; target blood concentration 3.5-8 mg/L; must be followed by an adjunct therapy†
Artesunate (not available in the United States)	2.4 mg/kg IV or IM injection, followed by same dose at 12 hr & 24 hr, and then daily	Must be followed by adjunct therapy† in severe malaria; lower rate of hypoglycemia than quinine; common recrudescence in monotherapy; highly variable blood concentration
Artemether (not available in the United States)	3.2 mg/kg IM injection first day, followed by 1.6 mg/kg daily for 5-7 days in total	Alternative to quinine where artesunate is unavailable; highly variable blood concentration; must be followed by an adjunct therapy† to prevent recrudescence

*Centers for Disease Control and Prevention recommended treatment regimen for severe malaria. Parenteral dosing must be converted to oral dosing as soon as the patient can tolerate it and the reduction in parasitemia is satisfactory, and adjunct therapy with tetracycline, doxycycline, or clindamycin must be completed. Intravenous artesunate can be obtained from CDC under an Investigational New Drug protocol.
†Adjunct therapy is described in Table 82-3.
ECG, electrocardiogram; IM, intramuscular; IV, intravenous.

TABLE 82-5 MALARIA CHEMOPROPHYLAXIS*

Drug	Prophylaxis	Comment
Chloroquine phosphate	Oral; 300 mg base/500 mg salt weekly (from 1-2 wk before entering to 4 wk after leaving an endemic country)	Used only in limited region of chloroquine-sensitive *P. falcipaum*, and for the prophylaxis of *P. vivax*, *P. ovale*, and *P. malariae*.
Atovaquone-proguanil	Oral; one tablet daily (from 1-2 days before entering to 1 wk after leaving an endemic country) *Pediatric dosing:* by weight—1 tablet for 11-20 kg, 2 for 21-30 kg, and 3 for 31-40 kg daily	Well tolerated; high cost.
Doxycycline	Oral; 100 mg daily (from 1 day before entering to 4 wk after leaving endemic country)	Not for children <8 yr and pregnant women; GI side effects and photosensitivity limit its usefulness.
Mefloquine	Oral; 250 mg salt weekly (from 1-2 wk before entering to 4 wk after leaving an endemic country)	Chemoprophylaxis of choice for pregnant women going to endemic area with chloroquine-resistant *P. falciparum* (see more in Malaria in Pregnancy section in text); widely publicized neuropsychiatric side effects, high cost.
Primaquine phosphate	Oral; 30 mg daily (from a few days before entering to 1 wk after leaving an endemic country)	Should be used only as an alternative to one of above regimens; should be used with caution; G6PD testing is required before therapy; expert opinion should be sought.

*These dosing regimens are frequently updated by the Centers for Disease Control and Prevention (CDC). The reader is advised to review the updated recommendation from the CDC at *www.cdc.gov/travel/*.
GI, gastrointestinal; G6PD, glucose-6-phosphate dehydrogenase.

may be needed to ensure therapeutic drug levels, but the data on pharmacokinetics of malaria drugs in pregnancy are very limited. Safety information on most antimalarial drugs in the first trimester is also very limited. If possible, artemisinin-containing combination therapies should be avoided in the first trimester due to the possibility of teratogenicity and neurotoxicity (see the Artemisinin Derivatives section). A 7-day course of quinine plus clindamycin is the treatment of choice in the first trimester. Other drugs that are considered safe, though limited in efficacy due to drug resistance, include chloroquine, proguanil, and sulfadoxine-pyrimethamine. Recently the WHO has recommended using artemisinin derivatives to treat malaria in the second and third trimesters. The choice of partner drug is scant, and clindamycin may be the only safe option. In late pregnancy, quinine is not recommended unless there is no effective alternative, because of its potential to induce life-threatening hypoglycemia. Mefloquine has been associated with an increased risk of stillbirth[91] and should be avoided in pregnancy if possible. When safer alternatives are not available, effective drugs must be used to treat malaria in pregnancy even if not known to be safe.

Emerging Targets and Therapeutics

Historically, the discovery of antimalarial agents has been serendipitous or empirical. Major classes of these agents, notably the quinolines and artemisinins, which were used as herbal remedies for centuries, were in large-scale use long before their mechanisms of action, which are still incompletely understood today, were explored. The main classes of established antimalarial drugs are also the focus of most new development efforts, namely, the quinolines, the antifolates, and artemisinin derivatives. Several new and old compounds related to quinolines (amodiaquine and other chloroquine analogues, piperaquine, isoquine, pyronaridine, lumefantrine, and tafenoquine, a long-acting primaquine analogue) are under clinical assessment, mostly as components of ACT. Chlorproguanil-dapsone represents an antifolate combination with good potential for clinical use, and has been tested alone and in combination with artesunate. Newer DHFR inhibitors active against parasites resistant to pyrimethamine and the active biguanide metabolites have been under development for many years but have been slow to move into clinical trials. Several synthetic artemisinin derivatives are in various stages of development, including some in Phase II clinical efficacy trials.

The pace at which promising compounds move through the steps of clinical development and become commercial products has been agonizingly slow since the winding down of the massive effort by the U.S. Army in the mid-20th century to address the need to prevent and treat malaria in overseas World War II troops. The malaria drug discovery program at the Walter Reed Army Institute of Research, which had a Manhattan Project–like urgency and support when it began, has suffered from neglect for decades, although the U.S. Army malaria drug program remains a vital kernel of drug discovery expertise with a significant archive of potentially promising compounds. As with malaria vaccine development, a surge of private donor interest and support in the last few years has revitalized malaria drug discovery and development, with the creation of a new public-private partnership, the Medicines for Malaria Venture, to sponsor development of drugs for a market that has historically attracted little interest from private pharmaceutical companies.

The first malaria genome was sequenced in 2002,[292] and genomic and proteomic (and metabolomic) analyses are beginning to yield new drug and vaccine targets with potentially improved safety and efficacy. Excellent reviews published recently provide detailed descriptions of new agents in antimalarial drug development.[293-297] Novel biochemical and metabolic pathways (such as fatty acid biosynthesis, isoprenoid synthesis, phospholipid metabolism and membrane transport, glycolysis and electron transport chain, and DNA synthesis) are being explored, and new compounds are in various stages of preclinical and clinical development. Several new compounds are also being investigated that target pathways that have been previously exploited, including folate metabolism, hemoglobin degradation, and protein metabolism. Classes of drugs used to treat other infections, such as protease inhibitors, have been evaluated for their antimalarial effects, yielding promising leads. Many drug combinations, most of which include artemisinin derivatives, are being evaluated in clinical trials to assess their efficacy and potential for delaying or preventing drug resistance. These efforts will be greatly enhanced by prospective consideration of pharmacokinetic and pharmacodynamic properties of drugs and careful assessments of these properties in clinical trials in settings with different levels of malaria transmission and host immunity.

As new drugs and drug combinations are assessed for use in Africa, where repeated treatment is common, longitudinal clinical trials will be an important tool for assessing safety and efficacy with repeated dosing.[298] In these trials, the same drug is used for all episodes of malaria experienced by participants over the course of a year, and the primary end point is the cumulative incidence of all clinical malaria episodes, reflecting not only efficacy against the initial infection but prevention of subsequent episodes. Importantly, safety with repeated dosing, which is virtually never assessed for these ubiquitous drugs that are used to treat all fevers in many populations, can be measured in longitudinal trials. As promising new antimalarial drugs and drug combinations are developed, more emphasis is needed on assessing not only safety but pharmacokinetics, especially in understudied populations such as pregnant women, and with repeated dosing.

REFERENCES

1. Korenromp EL for the Roll Back Malaria Monitoring and Evaluation Reference Group & MERG Task Force on Malaria Morbidity. Malaria Incidence Estimates at Country Level for the Year 2004—Proposed Estimates and Draft Report. Geneva: Roll Back Malaria/World Health Organization, 2004.
2. Rowe AK, Rowe SY, Snow RW, et al. The burden of malaria mortality among African children in the year 2000. Int J Epidemiol 2006;35:691-704.
3. Morris SS, Black RE, Tomaskovic L. Predicting the distribution of under-five deaths by cause in countries without adequate vital registration systems. Int J Epidemiol 2003;32:1041-1051.
4. World Health Organization. The World Malaria Report. Geneva: World Health Organization, 2005.
5. World Health Organization. The World Health Report 2003: Shaping the Future. Geneva: World Health Organization, 2003.
6. Gallup JL, Sachs JD. The economic burden of malaria. Am J Trop Med Hyg 2001;64:85-96.
7. Marsh K. Malaria—a neglected disease? Parasitology 1992;104(Suppl):S53-S69.
8. Allen SJ, O'Donnell A, Alexander ND, et al. Severe malaria in children in Papua New Guinea. Q J Med 1996;89:779-788.
9. Krishna S, Waller DW, ter Kuile F, et al. Lactic acidosis and hypoglycaemia in children with severe malaria: pathophysiological and prognostic significance. Trans R Soc Trop Med Hyg 1994;88:67-73.
10. Marsh K, Forster D, Waruiru C, et al. Indicators of life-threatening malaria in African children. N Engl J Med 1995;332:1399-1404.
11. Taylor TE, Borgstein A, Molyneux ME. Acid-base status in paediatric *Plasmodium falciparum* malaria. Q J Med 1993;86:99-109.
12. Grau GE, Taylor TE, Molyneux ME, et al. Tumor necrosis factor and disease severity in children with falciparum malaria. N Engl J Med 1989;320:1586-1591.
13. Kern P, Hemmer CJ, Van Damme J, et al. Elevated tumor necrosis factor alpha and interleukin-6 serum levels as markers for complicated *Plasmodium falciparum* malaria. Am J Med 1989;87:139-143.
14. Kwiatkowski D, Hill AV, Sambou I, et al. TNF concentration in fatal cerebral, non-fatal cerebral, and uncomplicated *Plasmodium falciparum* malaria. Lancet 1990;336:1201-1204.
15. Thuma PE, Weiss G, Herold M, et al. Serum neopterin, interleukin-4, and interleukin-6 concentrations in cerebral malaria patients and the effect of iron chelation therapy. Am J Trop Med Hyg 1996;54:164-168.
16. Hoffman SL, Rustama D, Punjabi NH, et al. High-dose dexamethasone in quinine-treated patients with cerebral malaria: a double-blind, placebo-controlled trial. J Infect Dis 1988;158:325-331.
17. Day NP, Phu NH, Mai NT, et al. The pathophysiologic and prognostic significance of acidosis in severe adult malaria. Crit Care Med 2000;28:1833-1840.
18. Hewitt K, Steketee R, Mwapasa V, et al. Interactions between HIV and malaria in non-pregnant adults: evidence and implications. Aids 2006;20:1993-2004.
19. Khoo S, Back D, Winstanley P. The potential for interactions between antimalarial and antiretroviral drugs. AIDS 2005;19:995-1005.
20. Laufer MK, Plowe CV. The interaction between HIV and malaria in Africa. Curr Infect Dis Rep 2007;9:47-54.
21. Anglaret X, Chene G, Attia A, et al. Early chemoprophylaxis with trimethoprim-sulphamethoxazole for HIV-1-infected adults in Abidjan, Cote d'Ivoire: a randomised trial. Cotrimo-CI Study Group. Lancet 1999;353:1463-1468.
22. Thera MA, Sehdev PS, Coulibaly D, et al. Impact of trimethoprim-sulfamethoxazole prophylaxis on falciparum malaria infection and disease. J Infect Dis 2005;192:1823-1829.
23. Church LW, Le TP, Bryan JP, et al. Clinical manifestations of *Plasmodium falciparum* malaria experimentally induced by mosquito challenge. J Infect Dis 1997;175:915-920.
24. Beeson JG, Brown GV. Pathogenesis of *Plasmodium falciparum* malaria: the roles of parasite adhesion and antigenic variation. Cell Mol Life Sci 2002;59:258-271.
25. Scherf A, Pouvelle B, Buffet PA, et al. Molecular mechanisms of *Plasmodium falciparum* placental adhesion. Cell Microbiol 2001;3:125-131.
26. Fried M, Duffy PE. Adherence of *Plasmodium falciparum* to chondroitin sulfate A in the human placenta. Science 1996;272:1502-1504.
27. Yamada M, Steketee R, Abramowsky C, et al. *Plasmodium falciparum* associated placental pathology: a light and electron microscopic and immunohistologic study. Am J Trop Med Hyg 1989;41:161-168.
28. Okoko BJ, Enwere G, Ota MO. The epidemiology and consequences of maternal malaria: a review of immunological basis. Acta Trop 2003;87:193-205.
29. WHO Expert Committee on Malaria. World Health Organ Tech Rep Ser 2000;892: i-v, 1-74.

29a. Shulman CE, Dorman EK, Cutts F, et al. Intermittent sulphadoxine-pyrimethamine to prevent severe anaemia secondary to malaria in pregnancy: a randomised placebo-controlled trial. Lancet 1999;353:632-636.

29b. ter Kvile FO, van Eijk AM, Filler SJ. Effect of sulfadoxine-pyrimethamine resistance on the efficacy of intermittent preventive therapy for malaria control during pregnancy: a systematic review. JAMA 2007;297:2603-2616.

30. Ayad F, Tilley L, Deady LW. Synthesis, antimalarial activity and inhibition of haem detoxification of novel bisquinolines. Bioorg Med Chem Lett 2001;11:2075-2077.
31. Chou AC, Chevli R, Fitch CD. Ferriprotoporphyrin IX fulfills the criteria for identification as the chloroquine receptor of malaria parasites. Biochemistry 1980;19:1543-1549.
32. Ginsburg H, Krugliak M. Effects of quinoline-containing antimalarials on the erythrocyte membrane and their significance to drug action on *Plasmodium falciparum*. Biochem Pharmacol 1988;37:2013-2018.
33. Kwiatkowski D, Bate C. Inhibition of tumour necrosis factor (TNF) production by antimalarial drugs used in cerebral malaria. Trans R Soc Trop Med Hyg 1995;89:215-216.
34. Rieckmann KH, Campbell GH, Sax LJ, et al. Drug sensitivity of *Plasmodium falciparum*. An in-vitro microtechnique. Lancet 1978;1:22-23.
35. Rieckmann KH, McNamara JV, Frischer H, et al. Effects of chloroquine, quinine, and cycloguanil upon the maturation of asexual erythrocytic forms of two strains of *Plasmodium falciparum* in vitro. Am J Trop Med Hyg 1968;17:661-671.
36. Fitch CD, Chan RL, Chevli R. Chloroquine resistance in malaria: accessibility of drug receptors to mefloquine. Antimicrob Agents Chemother 1979;15:258-262.
37. Fidock DA, Nomura T, Talley AK, et al. Mutations in the *P. falciparum* digestive vacuole transmembrane protein PfCRT and evidence for their role in chloroquine resistance. Mol Cell 2000;6:861-871.
38. Djimde A, Doumbo OK, Cortese JF, et al. A molecular marker for chloroquine-resistant falciparum malaria. N Engl J Med 2001;344:257-263.
39. Djimde AA, Dolo A, Ouattara A, et al. Molecular diagnosis of resistance to antimalarial drugs during epidemics and in war zones. J Infect Dis 2004;190:853-855.
40. Sidhu AB, Verdier-Pinard D, Fidock DA. Chloroquine resistance in *Plasmodium falciparum* malaria parasites conferred by *pfcrt* mutations. Science 2002;298:210-213.
41. Babiker HA, Pringle SJ, Abdel-Muhsin A, et al. High-level chloroquine resistance in Sudanese isolates of *Plasmodium falciparum* is associated with mutations in the chloroquine resistance transporter gene *pfcrt* and the multidrug resistance gene *pfmdr1*. J Infect Dis 2001;183:1535-1538.
42. Ngo T, Duraisingh M, Reed M, et al. Analysis of *pfcrt*, *pfmdr1*, *dhfr*, and *dhps* mutations and drug sensitivities in *Plasmodium falciparum* isolates from patients in Vietnam before and after treatment with artemisinin. Am J Trop Med Hyg 2003;68:350-356.
43. Price RN, Uhlemann AC, Brockman A, et al. Mefloquine resistance in *Plasmodium falciparum* and increased *pfmdr1* gene copy number. Lancet 2004;364:438-447.
44. Cowman AF, Galatis D, Thompson JK. Selection for mefloquine resistance in *Plasmodium falciparum* is linked to amplification of the *pfmdr1* gene and cross-resistance to halofantrine and quinine. Proc Natl Acad Sci U S A 1994;91:1143-1147.
45. Reed MB, Saliba KJ, Caruana SR, et al. *Pgh1* modulates sensitivity and resistance to multiple antimalarials in *Plasmodium falciparum*. Nature 2000;403:906-909.
46. Kublin JG, Cortese JF, Njunju EM, et al. Reemergence of chloroquine-sensitive *Plasmodium falciparum* malaria after cessation of chloroquine use in Malawi. J Infect Dis 2003;187:1870-1875.
47. Laufer MK, Thesing PC, Eddington ND, et al. Return of chloroquine antimalarial efficacy in Malawi. N Engl J Med 2006;355:1959-1966.
48. Ducharme J, Farinotti R. Clinical pharmacokinetics and metabolism of chloroquine: focus on recent advancements. Clin Pharmacokinet 1996;31:257-274.
49. Krishna S, White NJ: Pharmacokinetics of quinine, chloroquine and amodiaquine: clinical implications. Clin Pharmacokinet 1996;30:263-299.
50. White NJ, Miller KD, Churchill FC, et al. Chloroquine treatment of severe malaria in children: pharmacokinetics, toxicity, and new dosage recommendations. N Engl J Med 1988;319:1493-1500.
51. Hellgren U, Kihamia CM, Mahikwano LF, et al. Response of *Plasmodium falciparum* to chloroquine treatment: relation to whole blood concentrations of chloroquine and desethylchloroquine. Bull World Health Organ 1989;67:197-202.
52. Neuvonen PJ, Kivisto KT, Laine K, et al. Prevention of chloroquine absorption by activated charcoal. Hum Exp Toxicol 1992;11:117-120.
53. Ullberg S, Lindquist NG, Sjostrand SE. Accumulation of chorio-retinotoxic drugs in the foetal eye. Nature 1970;227:1257-1258.
54. Akintonwa A, Gbajumo SA, Mabadeje AF. Placental and milk transfer of chloroquine in humans. Ther Drug Monit 1988;10:147-149.
55. Massele AY, Kilewo C, Aden Abdi Y, et al. Chloroquine blood concentrations and malaria prophylaxis in Tanzanian women during the second and third trimesters of pregnancy. Eur J Clin Pharmacol 1997;52:299-305.
56. Wang X, Mu J, Li G, et al. Decreased prevalence of the *Plasmodium falciparum* chloroquine resistance transporter 76T marker associated with cessation of chloroquine use against *P. falciparum* malaria in Hainan, People's Republic of China. Am J Trop Med Hyg 2005;72:410-414.
57. Karle JM, Karle IL, Gerena L, et al. Stereochemical evaluation of the relative activities of the cinchona alkaloids against *Plasmodium falciparum*. Antimicrob Agents Chemother 1992;36:1538-1544.
58. White NJ, Looareesuwan S, Silamut K. Red cell quinine concentrations in falciparum malaria. Am J Trop Med Hyg 1983;32:456-460.
59. Barennes H, Kahiatani F, Pussard E, et al. Intrarectal Quinimax (an association of *Cinchona* alkaloids) for the treatment of *Plasmodium falciparum* malaria in children in Niger: efficacy and pharmacokinetics. Trans R Soc Trop Med Hyg 1995;89:418-421.

60. Notterman DA, Drayer DE, Metakis L, et al. Stereoselective renal tubular secretion of quinidine and quinine. Clin Pharmacol Ther 1986;40:511-517.
61. Karbwang J, Davis TM, Looareesuwan S, et al. A comparison of the pharmacokinetic and pharmacodynamic properties of quinine and quinidine in healthy Thai males. Br J Clin Pharmacol 1993;35:265-271.
62. Pasvol G, Newton CR, Winstanley PA, et al. Quinine treatment of severe falciparum malaria in African children: a randomized comparison of three regimens. Am J Trop Med Hyg 1991;45:702-713.
63. Winstanley P, Newton C, Watkins W, et al. Towards optimal regimens of parenteral quinine for young African children with cerebral malaria: the importance of unbound quinine concentration. Trans R Soc Trop Med Hyg 1993;87:201-206.
64. Winstanley PA, Mberu EK, Watkins WM, et al. Towards optimal regimens of parenteral quinine for young African children with cerebral malaria: unbound quinine concentrations following a simple loading dose regimen. Trans R Soc Trop Med Hyg 1994;88:577-580.
65. Pukrittayakamee S, Wanwimolruk S, Stepniewska K, et al. Quinine pharmacokinetic-pharmacodynamic relationships in uncomplicated falciparum malaria. Antimicrob Agents Chemother 2003;47:3458-3463.
66. Powell R, McNamara J. Quinine: side effects and plasma levels. Proc Helm Soc Wash 1972;39:331-338.
67. Alvan G, Karlsson KK, Hellgren U, et al. Hearing impairment related to plasma quinine concentration in healthy volunteers. Br J Clin Pharmacol 1991;31:409-412.
68. White NJ, Looareesuwan S, Warrell DA. Quinine and quinidine: a comparison of EKG effects during the treatment of malaria. J Cardiovasc Pharmacol 1983;5:173-175.
69. Phillips RE, Warrell DA, White NJ, et al. Intravenous quinidine for the treatment of severe falciparum malaria: clinical and pharmacokinetic studies. N Engl J Med 1985;312:1273-1278.
70. Wanwimolruk S, Wong SM, Zhang H, et al. Metabolism of quinine in man: identification of a major metabolite, and effects of smoking and rifampicin pretreatment. J Pharm Pharmacol 1995;47:957-963.
71. Spinler SA, Cheng JW, Kindwall KE, et al. Possible inhibition of hepatic metabolism of quinidine by erythromycin. Clin Pharmacol Ther 1995;57:89-94.
72. Aronson JK, Carver JG. Interaction of digoxin with quinine. Lancet 1981;1:1418.
73. Dozal A, Keyzer H, Kim HK, et al. Charge transfer complexes of K vitamins with several classes of antimicrobials. Int J Antimicrob Agents 2000;14:261-265.
74. Wanwimolruk S, Wong SM, Coville PF, et al. Cigarette smoking enhances the elimination of quinine. Br J Clin Pharmacol 1993;36:610-614.
75. Halliday RC, Jones BC, Smith DA, et al. An investigation of the interaction between halofantrine, CYP2D6 and CYP3A4: studies with human liver microsomes and heterologous enzyme expression systems. Br J Clin Pharmacol 1995;40:369-378.
76. Taylor WR, White NJ. Antimalarial drug toxicity: a review. Drug Saf 2004;27:25-61.
77. Phillips RE, Looareesuwan S, White NJ, et al. Hypoglycaemia and antimalarial drugs: quinidine and release of insulin. Br Med J (Clin Res Ed) 1986;292:1319-1321.
78. Phillips RE, Looareesuwan S, White NJ, et al. Quinine pharmacokinetics and toxicity in pregnant and lactating women with falciparum malaria. Br J Clin Pharmacol 1986;21:677-683.
79. Dannenberg AL, Dorfman SF, Johnson J. Use of quinine for self-induced abortion. South Med J 1983;76:846-849.
80. Mihaly GW, Ching MS, Klejn MB, et al. Differences in the binding of quinine and quinidine to plasma proteins. Br J Clin Pharmacol 1987;24:769-774.
81. Brockman A, Price RN, van Vugt M, et al. *Plasmodium falciparum* antimalarial drug susceptibility on the north-western border of Thailand during five years of extensive use of artesunate-mefloquine. Trans R Soc Trop Med Hyg 2000;94:537-544.
82. Hellgren U, Berggren-Palme I, Bergqvist Y, et al. Enantioselective pharmacokinetics of mefloquine during long-term intake of the prophylactic dose. Br J Clin Pharmacol 1997;44:119-124.
83. Karbwang J, White NJ. Clinical pharmacokinetics of mefloquine. Clin Pharmacokinet 1990;19:264-279.
84. Crevoisier C, Handschin J, Barre J, et al. Food increases the bioavailability of mefloquine. Eur J Clin Pharmacol 1997;53:135-139.
85. Looareesuwan S, White NJ, Warrell DA, et al. Studies of mefloquine bioavailability and kinetics using a stable isotope technique: a comparison of Thai patients with falciparum malaria and healthy Caucasian volunteers. Br J Clin Pharmacol 1987;24:37-42.
86. Luxemburger C, Price RN, Nosten F, et al. Mefloquine in infants and young children. Ann Trop Paediatr 1996;16:281-286.
87. Karbwang J, Bangchang KN, Bunnag D, et al. Pharmacokinetics and pharmacodynamics of mefloquine in Thai patients with acute falciparum malaria. Bull World Health Organ 1991;69:207-212.
88. Ashley EA, Stepniewska K, Lindegardh N, et al. Population pharmacokinetic assessment of a new regimen of mefloquine used in combination treatment of uncomplicated falciparum malaria. Antimicrob Agents Chemother 2006;50:2281-2285.
89. Simpson JA, Aarons L, Price R, et al. The influence of body weight on the pharmacokinetics of mefloquine. Br J Clin Pharmacol 2002;53:337-338.
90. Nosten F, ter Kuile F, Maelankiri L, et al. Mefloquine prophylaxis prevents malaria during pregnancy: a double-blind, placebo-controlled study. J Infect Dis 1994;169:595-603.
91. Nosten F, Vincenti M, Simpson J, et al. The effects of mefloquine treatment in pregnancy. Clin Infect Dis 1999;28:808-815.
92. Nosten F, Karbwang J, White NJ, et al. Mefloquine antimalarial prophylaxis in pregnancy: dose finding and pharmacokinetic study. Br J Clin Pharmacol 1990;30:79-85.
93. Edstein MD, Veenendaal JR, Hyslop R. Excretion of mefloquine in human breast milk. Chemotherapy 1988;34:165-169.
94. Bates MD, Meshnick SR, Sigler CI, et al. In vitro effects of primaquine and primaquine metabolites on exoerythrocytic stages of *Plasmodium berghei*. Am J Trop Med Hyg 1990;42:532-537.
95. Krungkrai J, Burat D, Kudan S, et al. Mitochondrial oxygen consumption in asexual and sexual blood stages of the human malarial parasite, *Plasmodium falciparum*. Southeast Asian J Trop Med Public Health 1999;30:636-642.
96. Mihaly GW, Ward SA, Edwards G, et al. Pharmacokinetics of primaquine in man: identification of the carboxylic acid derivative as a major plasma metabolite. Br J Clin Pharmacol 1984;17:441-446.
97. Mihaly GW, Ward SA, Edwards G, et al. Pharmacokinetics of primaquine in man. I. Studies of the absolute bioavailability and effects of dose size. Br J Clin Pharmacol 1985;19:745-750.
98. Ward SA, Mihaly GW, Edwards G, et al. Pharmacokinetics of primaquine in man. II. Comparison of acute vs chronic dosage in Thai subjects. Br J Clin Pharmacol 1985;19:751-755.
99. Bhatia SC, Saraph YS, Revankar SN, et al. Pharmacokinetics of primaquine in patients with *P. vivax* malaria. Eur J Clin Pharmacol 1986;31:205-210.
100. Arnold J, Alving AS, Hockwald RS, et al. The antimalarial action of primaquine against the blood and tissue stages of falciparum malaria (Panama, P-F-6 strain). J Lab Clin Med 1955;46:391-397.
101. Arnold J, Alving AS, Hockwald RS, et al. The effect of continuous and intermittent primaquine therapy on the relapse rate of Chesson strain vivax malaria. J Lab Clin Med 1954;44:429-438.
102. Clayman CB, Arnold J, Hockwald RS, et al. Toxicity of primaquine in Caucasians. J Am Med Assoc 1952;149:1563-1568.
103. Clyde DF, McCarthy VC. Radical cure of Chesson strain vivax malaria in man by 7, not 14, days of treatment with primaquine. Am J Trop Med Hyg 1977;26:562-563.
104. Edgcomb JH, Arnold J, Yount EH Jr, et al. Primaquine, SN 13272, a new curative agent in vivax malaria: a preliminary report. J Natl Malar Soc 1950;9:285-292.
105. Bangchang KN, Songsaeng W, Thanavibul A, et al. Pharmacokinetics of primaquine in G6PD deficient and G6PD normal patients with vivax malaria. Trans R Soc Trop Med Hyg 1994;88:220-222.
106. Fryauff DJ, Baird JK, Basri H, et al. Randomised placebo-controlled trial of primaquine for prophylaxis of falciparum and vivax malaria. Lancet 1995;346:1190-1193.
107. Soto J, Toledo J, Rodriquez M, et al. Primaquine prophylaxis against malaria in non-immune Colombian soldiers: efficacy and toxicity. A randomized, double-blind, placebo-controlled trial. Ann Intern Med 1998;129:241-244.
108. Weiss WR, Oloo AJ, Johnson A, et al. Daily primaquine is effective for prophylaxis against falciparum malaria in Kenya: comparison with mefloquine, doxycycline, and chloroquine plus proguanil. J Infect Dis 1995;171:1569-1575.
109. Hill DR, Baird JK, Parise ME, et al. Primaquine: report from CDC expert meeting on malaria chemoprophylaxis I. Am J Trop Med Hyg 2006;75:402-415.
110. Clyde DF. Clinical problems associated with the use of primaquine as a tissue schizontocidal and gametocytocidal drug. Bull World Health Organ 1981;59:391-395.
111. Baird JK, Lacy MD, Basri H, et al. Randomized, parallel placebo-controlled trial of primaquine for malaria prophylaxis in Papua, Indonesia. Clin Infect Dis 2001;33:1990-1997.
112. Jaeger A, Sauder P, Kopferschmitt J, et al. Clinical features and management of poisoning due to antimalarial drugs. Med Toxicol Adverse Drug Exp 1987;2:242-273.
113. Christie G, Breckenridge AM, Park BK. Drug-protein conjugates—XVIII. Detection of antibodies towards the antimalarial amodiaquine and its quinone imine metabolite in man and the rat. Biochem Pharmacol 1989;38:1451-1458.
114. Harrison AC, Kitteringham NR, Clarke JB, et al. The mechanism of bioactivation and antigen formation of amodiaquine in the rat. Biochem Pharmacol 1992;43:1421-1430.
115. O'Neill PM, Harrison AC, Storr RC, et al. The effect of fluorine substitution on the metabolism and antimalarial activity of amodiaquine. J Med Chem 1994;37:1362-1370.
116. Hombhanje FW, Hwaihwanje I, Tsukahara T, et al. The disposition of oral amodiaquine in Papua New Guinean children with falciparum malaria. Br J Clin Pharmacol 2005;59:298-301.
117. Winstanley PA, Simooya O, Kofi-Ekue JM, et al. The disposition of amodiaquine in Zambians and Nigerians with malaria. Br J Clin Pharmacol 1990;29:695-701.
118. Li XQ, Bjorkman A, Andersson TB, et al. Amodiaquine clearance and its metabolism to *N*-desethylamodiaquine is mediated by CYP2C8: a new high affinity and turnover enzyme-specific probe substrate. J Pharmacol Exp Ther 2002;300:399-407.
119. Tagbor H, Bruce J, Browne E, et al. Efficacy, safety, and tolerability of amodiaquine plus sulphadoxine-pyrimethamine used alone or in combination for malaria treatment in pregnancy: a randomised trial. Lancet 2006;368:1349-1356.
120. Dorsey G, Njama D, Kamya MR, et al. Sulfadoxine/pyrimethamine alone or with amodiaquine or artesunate for treatment of uncomplicated malaria: a longitudinal randomised trial. Lancet 2002;360:2031-2038.
121. Staedke SG, Kamya MR, Dorsey G, et al. Amodiaquine, sulfadoxine/pyrimethamine, and combination therapy for treatment of uncomplicated falciparum malaria in Kampala, Uganda: a randomised trial. Lancet 2001;358:368-374.
122. Adjuik M, Agnamey P, Babiker A, et al. Amodiaquine-artesunate versus amodiaquine for uncomplicated *Plasmodium falciparum* malaria in African children: a randomised, multicentre trial. Lancet 2002;359:1365-1372.
123. Guthmann JP, Cohuet S, Rigutto C, et al. High efficacy of two artemisinin-based combinations (artesunate + amodiaquine and artemether + lumefantrine) in Caala, Central Angola. Am J Trop Med Hyg 2006;75:143-145.
124. Meremikwu M, Alaribe A, Ejemot R, et al. Artemether-lumefantrine versus artesunate plus amodiaquine for treating uncomplicated childhood malaria in Nigeria: randomized controlled trial. Malar J 2006;5:43.

125. Wernsdorfer WH, Landgraf B, Kilimali VA, et al. Activity of benflumetol and its enantiomers in fresh isolates of *Plasmodium falciparum* from East Africa. Acta Trop 1998;70:9-15.
126. Hassan Alin M, Bjorkman A, Wernsdorfer WH. Synergism of benflumetol and artemether in *Plasmodium falciparum*. Am J Trop Med Hyg 1999;61:439-445.
127. Ezzet F, Mull R, Karbwang J. Population pharmacokinetics and therapeutic response of CGP 56697 (artemether + benflumetol) in malaria patients. Br J Clin Pharmacol 1998;46:553-561.
128. Vugt MV, Wilairatana P, Gemperli B, et al. Efficacy of six doses of artemether-lumefantrine (benflumetol) in multidrug-resistant *Plasmodium falciparum* malaria. Am J Trop Med Hyg 1999;60:936-942.
129. Li X, Li C, Che L, et al. [Observation on efficacy of artemether compound against vivax malaria]. Zhongguo Ji Sheng Chong Xue Yu Ji Sheng Chong Bing Za Zhi 1999;17:175-177.
130. Bakshi R, Hermeling-Fritz I, Gathmann I, et al. An integrated assessment of the clinical safety of artemether-lumefantrine: a new oral fixed-dose combination antimalarial drug. Trans R Soc Trop Med Hyg 2000;94:419-424.
131. McGready R, Stepniewska K, Lindegardh N, et al. The pharmacokinetics of artemether and lumefantrine in pregnant women with uncomplicated falciparum malaria. Eur J Clin Pharmacol 2006;62:1021-1031.
132. Olliaro P, Smith PG. The European and developing countries clinical trials partnership. J HIV Ther 2004;9:53-56.
133. Guan WB, Huang WJ, Zhou YC, et al. [Effect of piperaquine and hydroxypiperaquine on a chloroquine-resistant strain of *Plasmodium falciparum*]. Ji Sheng Chong Xue Yu Ji Sheng Chong Bing Za Zhi 1983;1:88-90.
134. Vennerstrom JL, Ellis WY, Ager AL Jr, et al. Bisquinolines. 1. *N,N*-bis(7-chloroquinolin-4-yl)alkanediamines with potential against chloroquine-resistant malaria. J Med Chem 1992;35:2129-2134.
135. Denis MB, Davis TM, Hewitt S, et al. Efficacy and safety of dihydroartemisinin-piperaquine (Artekin) in Cambodian children and adults with uncomplicated falciparum malaria. Clin Infect Dis 2002;35:1469-1476.
136. Tran TH, Dolecek C, Pham PM, et al. Dihydroartemisinin-piperaquine against multidrug-resistant *Plasmodium falciparum* malaria in Vietnam: randomised clinical trial. Lancet 2004;363:18-22.
137. Hung TY, Davis TM, Ilett KF, et al. Population pharmacokinetics of piperaquine in adults and children with uncomplicated falciparum or vivax malaria. Br J Clin Pharmacol 2004;57:253-262.
138. Sim IK, Davis TM, Ilett KF. Effects of a high-fat meal on the relative oral bioavailability of piperaquine. Antimicrob Agents Chemother 2005;49:2407-2411.
139. Davis TM, Hung TY, Sim IK, et al. Piperaquine: a resurgent antimalarial drug. Drugs 2005;65:75-87.
140. Ringwald P, Bickii J, Basco L. Randomised trial of pyronaridine versus chloroquine for acute uncomplicated falciparum malaria in Africa. Lancet 1996;347:24-28.
141. Watkins WM, Mosobo M. Treatment of *Plasmodium falciparum* malaria with pyrimethamine-sulfadoxine: selective pressure for resistance is a function of long elimination half-life. Trans R Soc Trop Med Hyg 1993;87:75-78.
142. van Oosterhout JJ, Laufer MK, Graham SM, et al. A community-based study of the incidence of trimethoprim-sulfamethoxazole-preventable infections in Malawian adults living with HIV. J Acquir Immune Defic Syndr 2005;39:626-631.
143. Mermin J, Ekwaru JP, Liechty CA, et al. Effect of co-trimoxazole prophylaxis, antiretroviral therapy, and insecticide-treated bednets on the frequency of malaria in HIV-1-infected adults in Uganda: a prospective cohort study. Lancet 2006;367:1256-1261.
144. Ferone R. Folate metabolism in malaria. Bull World Health Organ 1977;55:291-298.
145. Krungkrai J, Webster HK, Yuthavong Y. De novo and salvage biosynthesis of pteroylpentaglutamates in the human malaria parasite, *Plasmodium falciparum*. Mol Biochem Parasitol 1989;32:25-37.
146. Srivastava IK, Vaidya AB. A mechanism for the synergistic antimalarial action of atovaquone and proguanil. Antimicrob Agents Chemother 1999;43:1334-1339.
147. Brooks DR, Wang P, Read M, et al. Sequence variation of the hydroxymethyldihydropterin pyrophosphokinase: dihydropteroate synthase gene in lines of the human malaria parasite, *Plasmodium falciparum*, with differing resistance to sulfadoxine. Eur J Biochem 1994;224:397-405.
148. Wang P, Read M, Sims PF, et al. Sulfadoxine resistance in the human malaria parasite *Plasmodium falciparum* is determined by mutations in dihydropteroate synthetase and an additional factor associated with folate utilization. Mol Microbiol 1997;23:979-986.
149. Cortese JF, Caraballo A, Contreras CE, et al. Origin and dissemination of *Plasmodium falciparum* drug-resistance mutations in South America. J Infect Dis 2002;186:999-1006.
150. Kublin JG, Dzinjalamala FK, Kamwendo DD, et al. Molecular markers for failure of sulfadoxine-pyrimethamine and chlorproguanil-dapsone treatment of *Plasmodium falciparum* malaria. J Infect Dis 2002;185:380-388.
151. Roper C, Pearce R, Bredenkamp B, et al. Antifolate antimalarial resistance in southeast Africa: a population-based analysis. Lancet 2003;361:1174-1181.
152. Roper C, Pearce R, Nair S, et al. Intercontinental spread of pyrimethamine-resistant malaria. Science 2004;305:1124.
153. Edstein MD, Rieckmann KH, Veenendaal JR. Multiple-dose pharmacokinetics and in vitro antimalarial activity of dapsone plus pyrimethamine (Maloprim) in man. Br J Clin Pharmacol 1990;30:259-265.
154. Gill HJ, Tingle MD, Park BK. *N*-Hydroxylation of dapsone by multiple enzymes of cytochrome P450: implications for inhibition of haemotoxicity. Br J Clin Pharmacol 1995;40:531-538.
155. Mahmud R, Tingle MD, Maggs JL, et al. Structural basis for the haemotoxicity of dapsone: the importance of the sulphonyl group. Toxicology 1997;117:1-11.
156. Ward SA, Helsby NA, Skjelbo E, et al. The activation of the biguanide antimalarial proguanil co-segregates with the mephenytoin oxidation polymorphism—a panel study. Br J Clin Pharmacol 1991;31:689-692.
157. Kaneko A, Bergqvist Y, Taleo G, et al. Proguanil disposition and toxicity in malaria patients from Vanuatu with high frequencies of CYP2C19 mutations. Pharmacogenetics 1999;9:317-326.
158. Watkins WM, Mberu EK, Nevill CG, et al. Variability in the metabolism of proguanil to the active metabolite cycloguanil in healthy Kenyan adults. Trans R Soc Trop Med Hyg 1990;84:492-495.
159. Drusano GL, Craig WA. Relevance of pharmacokinetics and pharmacodynamics in the selection of antibiotics for respiratory tract infections. J Chemother 1997;9(Suppl 3):38-44.
160. Spencer HC, Watkins WM, Sixsmith DG, et al. A new in vitro test for pyrimethamine/sulfadoxine susceptibility of *Plasmodium falciparum* and its correlation with in vivo resistance in Kenya. Bull World Health Organ 1984;62:615-621.
161. Hellgren U, Kihamia CM, Bergqvist Y, et al. Standard and reduced doses of sulfadoxine-pyrimethamine for treatment of *Plasmodium falciparum* in Tanzania, with determination of drug concentrations and susceptibility in vitro. Trans R Soc Trop Med Hyg 1990;84:469-472.
162. Nguyen-Dinh P, Payne D, Teklehaimanot A, et al. Development of an in vitro microtest for determining the susceptibility of *Plasmodium falciparum* to sulfadoxine-pyrimethamine: laboratory investigations and field studies in Port-au-Prince, Haiti. Bull World Health Organ 1985;63:585-592.
163. Aubouy A, Bakary M, Keundjian A, et al. Combination of drug level measurement and parasite genotyping data for improved assessment of amodiaquine and sulfadoxine-pyrimethamine efficacies in treating *Plasmodium falciparum* malaria in Gabonese children. Antimicrob Agents Chemother 2003;47:231-237.
164. Bustos DG, Lazaro JE, Gay F, et al. Pharmacokinetics of sequential and simultaneous treatment with the combination chloroquine and sulfadoxine-pyrimethamine in acute uncomplicated *Plasmodium falciparum* malaria in the Philippines. Trop Med Int Health 2002;7:584-591.
165. Dua VK, Dev V, Phookan S, et al. Multi-drug resistant *Plasmodium falciparum* malaria in Assam, India: timing of recurrence and anti-malarial drug concentrations in whole blood. Am J Trop Med Hyg 2003;69:555-557.
166. Dzinjalamala FK, Macheso A, Kublin JG, et al. Blood folate concentrations and in vivo sulfadoxine-pyrimethamine failure in Malawian children with uncomplicated *Plasmodium falciparum* malaria. Am J Trop Med Hyg 2005;72:267-272.
167. Schapira A, Bygbjerg IC, Jepsen S, et al. The susceptibility of *Plasmodium falciparum* to sulfadoxine and pyrimethamine: correlation of in vivo and in vitro results. Am J Trop Med Hyg 1986;35:239-245.
168. Watkins WM, Mberu EK, Winstanley PA, et al. The efficacy of antifolate antimalarial combinations in Africa: a predictive model based on pharmacodynamic and pharmacokinetic analyses. Parasitol Today 1997;13:459-464.
169. Lamont G, Darlow B. Comparison of in vitro pyrimethamine assays and in vivo response to sulphadoxine-pyrimethamine in *Plasmodium falciparum* from Papua New Guinea. Trans R Soc Trop Med Hyg 1982;76:797-799.
170. White NJ. Intermittent presumptive treatment for malaria. PLoS Med 2005;2:e3.
171. Giao PT, de Vries PJ. Pharmacokinetic interactions of antimalarial agents. Clin Pharmacokinet 2001;40:343-373.
172. Weidekamm E, Schwartz DE, Dubach UC, et al. Single-dose investigation of possible interactions between the components of the antimalarial combination Fansimef. Chemotherapy 1987;33:259-265.
173. Edstein MD, Veenendaal JR, Rieckmann KH. Multiple-dose kinetics in healthy volunteers and in vitro antimalarial activity of proguanil plus dapsone. Chemotherapy 1990;36:169-176.
174. Winstanley P, Watkins W, Muhia D, et al. Chlorproguanil/dapsone for uncomplicated *Plasmodium falciparum* malaria in young children: pharmacokinetics and therapeutic range. Trans R Soc Trop Med Hyg 1997;91:322-327.
175. Edstein MD, Veenendaal JR, Newman K, et al. Excretion of chloroquine, dapsone and pyrimethamine in human milk. Br J Clin Pharmacol 1986;22:733-735.
176. McGready R, Stepniewska K, Edstein MD, et al. The pharmacokinetics of atovaquone and proguanil in pregnant women with acute falciparum malaria. Eur J Clin Pharmacol 2003;59:545-552.
177. Na-Bangchang K, Manyando C, Ruengweerayut R, et al. The pharmacokinetics and pharmacodynamics of atovaquone and proguanil for the treatment of uncomplicated falciparum malaria in third-trimester pregnant women. Eur J Clin Pharmacol 2005;61:573-582.
178. The chemistry and synthesis of qinghaosu derivatives. China Cooperative Research Group on Qinghaosu and Its Derivatives as Antimalarials. J Tradit Chin Med 1982;2:9-16.
179. Clinical studies on the treatment of malaria with qinghaosu and its derivatives. China Cooperative Research Group on Qinghaosu and Its Derivatives as Antimalarials. J Tradit Chin Med 1982;2:45-50.
180. Studies on the toxicity of qinghaosu and its derivatives. China Cooperative Research Group on Qinghaosu and Its Derivatives as Antimalarials. J Tradit Chin Med 1982;2:31-38.
181. Chemical studies on qinghaosu (artemisinine). China Cooperative Research Group on Qinghaosu and Its Derivatives as Antimalarials. J Tradit Chin Med 1982;2:3-8.
182. Metabolism and pharmacokinetics of qinghaosu and its derivatives. China Cooperative Research Group on Qinghaosu and Its Derivatives as Antimalarials. J Tradit Chin Med 1982;2:25-30.
183. Antimalarial efficacy and mode of action of qinghaosu and its derivatives in experimental models. China Cooperative Research Group on Qinghaosu and Its Derivatives as Antimalarials. J Tradit Chin Med 1982;2:17-24.
184. Liu C, Zhao Y, Wang Y. Artemisinin: current state and perspectives for biotechnological production of an antimalarial drug. Appl Microbiol Biotechnol 2006;72:11-20.

185. Kumar N, Zheng H. Stage-specific gametocytocidal effect in vitro of the antimalaria drug qinghaosu on *Plasmodium falciparum*. Parasitol Res 1990;76:214-218.
186. Price R, Nosten F, Simpson JA, et al. Risk factors for gametocyte carriage in uncomplicated falciparum malaria. Am J Trop Med Hyg 1999;60:1019-1023.
187. Posner GH, Oh CH, Wang D, et al. Mechanism-based design, synthesis, and in vitro antimalarial testing of new 4-methylated trioxanes structurally related to artemisinin: the importance of a carbon-centered radical for antimalarial activity. J Med Chem 1994;37:1256-1258.
188. Eckstein-Ludwig U, Webb RJ, Van Goethem ID, et al. Artemisinins target the SERCA of *Plasmodium falciparum*. Nature 2003;424:957-961.
189. Uhlemann AC, Cameron A, Eckstein-Ludwig U, et al. A single amino acid residue can determine the sensitivity of SERCAs to artemisinins. Nat Struct Mol Biol 2005;12:628-629.
190. Sisowath C, Stromberg J, Martensson A, et al. In vivo selection of *Plasmodium falciparum pfmdr1* 86N coding alleles by artemether-lumefantrine (Coartem). J Infect Dis 2005;191:1014-1017.
191. Price RN, Uhlemann AC, van Vugt M, et al. Molecular and pharmacological determinants of the therapeutic response to artemether-lumefantrine in multidrug-resistant *Plasmodium falciparum* malaria. Clin Infect Dis 2006;42:1570-1577.
192. Ittarat W, Pickard AL, Rattanasinganchan P, et al. Recrudescence in artesunate-treated patients with falciparum malaria is dependent on parasite burden not on parasite factors. Am J Trop Med Hyg 2003;68:147-152.
193. Batty KT, Thu LT, Davis TM, et al. A pharmacokinetic and pharmacodynamic study of intravenous vs oral artesunate in uncomplicated falciparum malaria. Br J Clin Pharmacol 1998;45:123-129.
194. Newton P, Suputtamongkol Y, Teja-Isavadharm P, et al. Antimalarial bioavailability and disposition of artesunate in acute falciparum malaria. Antimicrob Agents Chemother 2000;44:972-977.
195. Li QG, Peggins JO, Lin AJ, et al. Pharmacology and toxicology of artelinic acid: preclinical investigations on pharmacokinetics, metabolism, protein and red blood cell binding, and acute and anorectic toxicities. Trans R Soc Trop Med Hyg 1998;92:332-340.
196. Li Q, Xie LH, Si Y, et al. Toxicokinetics and hydrolysis of artelinate and artesunate in malaria-infected rats. Int J Toxicol 2005;24:241-250.
197. Niu XY, Ho LY, Ren ZH, et al. Metabolic fate of Qinghaosu in rats: a new TLC densitometric method for its determination in biological material. Eur J Drug Metab Pharmacokinet 1985;10:55-59.
198. Navaratnam V, Mansor SM, Sit NW, et al. Pharmacokinetics of artemisinin-type compounds. Clin Pharmacokinet 2000;39:255-270.
199. Ashton M, Hai TN, Sy ND, et al. Artemisinin pharmacokinetics is time-dependent during repeated oral administration in healthy male adults. Drug Metab Dispos 1998;26:25-27.
200. Khanh NX, de Vries PJ, Ha LD, et al. Declining concentrations of dihydroartemisinin in plasma during 5-day oral treatment with artesunate for falciparum malaria. Antimicrob Agents Chemother 1999;43:690-692.
201. van Agtmael MA, Cheng-Qi S, Qing JX, et al. Multiple dose pharmacokinetics of artemether in Chinese patients with uncomplicated falciparum malaria. Int J Antimicrob Agents 1999;12:151-158.
202. Woodrow CJ, Haynes RK, Krishna S. Artemisinins. Postgrad Med J 2005;81:71-78.
203. Dien TK, de Vries PJ, Khanh NX, et al. Effect of food intake on pharmacokinetics of oral artemisinin in healthy Vietnamese subjects. Antimicrob Agents Chemother 1997;41:1069-1072.
204. Svensson US, Ashton M. Identification of the human cytochrome P450 enzymes involved in the in vitro metabolism of artemisinin. Br J Clin Pharmacol 1999;48:528-535.
205. Svensson US, Ashton M, Trinh NH, et al. Artemisinin induces omeprazole metabolism in human beings. Clin Pharmacol Ther 1998;64:160-167.
206. Batty KT, Ashton M, Ilett KF, et al. The pharmacokinetics of artemisinin (ART) and artesunate (ARTS) in healthy volunteers. Am J Trop Med Hyg 1998;58:125-126.
207. Benakis A, Paris M, Loutan L, et al. Pharmacokinetics of artemisinin and artesunate after oral administration in healthy volunteers. Am J Trop Med Hyg 1997;56:17-23.
208. Hien TT, Davis TM, Chuong LV, et al. Comparative pharmacokinetics of intramuscular artesunate and artemether in patients with severe falciparum malaria. Antimicrob Agents Chemother 2004;48:4234-4239.
209. Karbwang J, Na-Bangchang K, Congpuong K, et al. Pharmacokinetics and bioavailability of oral and intramuscular artemether. Eur J Clin Pharmacol 1997;52:307-310.
210. Karbwang J, Na-Bangchang K, Congpuong K, et al. Pharmacokinetics of oral artemether in Thai patients with uncomplicated falciparum malaria. Fundam Clin Pharmacol 1998;12:242-244.
211. Karbwang J, Na-Bangchang K, Thanavibul A, et al. Plasma concentrations of artemether and its major plasma metabolite, dihydroartemisinin, following a 5-day regimen of oral artemether, in patients with uncomplicated falciparum malaria. Ann Trop Med Parasitol 1998;92:31-36.
212. Karbwang J, Na-Bangchang K, Tin T, et al. Pharmacokinetics of intramuscular artemether in patients with severe falciparum malaria with or without acute renal failure. Br J Clin Pharmacol 1998;45:597-600.
213. Silamut K, Newton PN, Teja-Isavadharm P, et al. Artemether bioavailability after oral or intramuscular administration in uncomplicated falciparum malaria. Antimicrob Agents Chemother 2003;47:3795-3798.
214. Teja-Isavadharm P, Nosten F, Kyle DE, et al. Comparative bioavailability of oral, rectal, and intramuscular artemether in healthy subjects: use of simultaneous measurement by high performance liquid chromatography and bioassay. Br J Clin Pharmacol 1996;42:599-604.
215. Colussi D, Parisot C, Legay F, et al. Binding of artemether and lumefantrine to plasma proteins and erythrocytes. Eur J Pharm Sci 1999;9:9-16.
216. Murphy SA, Mberu E, Muhia D, et al. The disposition of intramuscular artemether in children with cerebral malaria: a preliminary study. Trans R Soc Trop Med Hyg 1997;91:331-334.
217. van Agtmael MA, Gupta V, van der Wosten TH, et al. Grapefruit juice increases the bioavailability of artemether. Eur J Clin Pharmacol 1999;55:405-410.
218. van Agtmael MA, Gupta V, van der Graaf CA, et al. The effect of grapefruit juice on the time-dependent decline of artemether plasma levels in healthy subjects. Clin Pharmacol Ther 1999;66:408-414.
219. van Agtmael MA, Van Der Graaf CA, Dien TK, et al. The contribution of the enzymes CYP2D6 and CYP2C19 in the demethylation of artemether in healthy subjects. Eur J Drug Metab Pharmacokinet 1998;23:429-436.
220. Na-Bangchang K, Karbwang J, Ubalee R, et al. Absence of significant pharmacokinetic and pharmacodynamic interactions between artemether and quinoline antimalarials. Eur J Drug Metab Pharmacokinet 2000;25:171-178.
221. Le NH, Na-Bangchang K, Le TD, et al. Phamacokinetics of a single oral dose of dihydroartemisinin in Vietnamese healthy volunteers. Southeast Asian J Trop Med Public Health 1999;30:11-16.
222. Ilett KF, Ethell BT, Maggs JL, et al. Glucuronidation of dihydroartemisinin in vivo and by human liver microsomes and expressed UDP-glucuronosyltransferases. Drug Metab Dispos 2002;30:1005-1012.
223. ter Kuile F, White NJ, Holloway P, et al. *Plasmodium falciparum:* in vitro studies of the pharmacodynamic properties of drugs used for the treatment of severe malaria. Exp Parasitol 1993;76:85-95.
224. White NJ, Waller D, Crawley J, et al. Comparison of artemether and chloroquine for severe malaria in Gambian children. Lancet 1992;339:317-321.
225. White NJ. Clinical pharmacokinetics and pharmacodynamics of artemisinin and derivatives. Trans R Soc Trop Med Hyg 1994;88(Suppl 1):S41-S43.
226. Nosten F, Luxemburger C, ter Kuile FO, et al. Treatment of multidrug-resistant *Plasmodium falciparum* malaria with 3-day artesunate-mefloquine combination. J Infect Dis 1994;170:971-977.
227. Leonardi E, Gilvary G, White NJ, et al. Severe allergic reactions to oral artesunate: a report of two cases. Trans R Soc Trop Med Hyg 2001;95:182-183.
228. Toovey S. Safety of artemisinin antimalarials. Clin Infect Dis 2006;42:1214-1215.
229. Fishwick J, Edwards G, Ward SA, et al. Morphological and immunocytochemical effects of dihydroartemisinin on differentiating NB2a neuroblastoma cells. Neurotoxicology 1998;19:393-403.
230. Schmuck G, Roehrdanz E, Haynes RK, et al. Neurotoxic mode of action of artemisinin. Antimicrob Agents Chemother 2002;46:821-827.
231. Smith SL, Fishwick J, McLean WG, et al. Enhanced in vitro neurotoxicity of artemisinin derivatives in the presence of haemin. Biochem Pharmacol 1997;53:5-10.
232. Toovey S. Are currently deployed artemisinins neurotoxic? Toxicol Lett 2006;166:95-104.
233. Hutagalung R, Htoo H, Nwee P, et al. A case-control auditory evaluation of patients treated with artemether-lumefantrine. Am J Trop Med Hyg 2006;74:211-214.
234. Kissinger E, Hien TT, Hung NT, et al. Clinical and neurophysiological study of the effects of multiple doses of artemisinin on brain-stem function in Vietnamese patients. Am J Trop Med Hyg 2000;63:48-55.
235. Toovey S, Jamieson A. Audiometric changes associated with the treatment of uncomplicated falciparum malaria with co-artemether. Trans R Soc Trop Med Hyg 2004;98:261-267; discussion 268-269.
236. Price R, van Vugt M, Phaipun L, et al. Adverse effects in patients with acute falciparum malaria treated with artemisinin derivatives. Am J Trop Med Hyg 1999;60:547-555.
237. Tran TH, Day NP, Nguyen HP, et al. A controlled trial of artemether or quinine in Vietnamese adults with severe falciparum malaria. N Engl J Med 1996;335:76-83.
238. Dondorp A, Nosten F, Stepniewska K, et al. Artesunate versus quinine for treatment of severe falciparum malaria: a randomised trial. Lancet 2005;366:717-725.
239. Lefevre G, Carpenter P, Souppart C, et al. Interaction trial between artemether-lumefantrine (Riamet) and quinine in healthy subjects. J Clin Pharmacol 2002;42:1147-1158.
240. Deen JL, von Seidlein L, Pinder M, et al. The safety of the combination artesunate and pyrimethamine-sulfadoxine given during pregnancy. Trans R Soc Trop Med Hyg 2001;95:424-428.
241. McGready R, Brockman A, Cho T, et al. Randomized comparison of mefloquine-artesunate versus quinine in the treatment of multidrug-resistant falciparum malaria in pregnancy. Trans R Soc Trop Med Hyg 2000;94:689-693.
242. McGready R, Cho T, Cho JJ, et al. Artemisinin derivatives in the treatment of falciparum malaria in pregnancy. Trans R Soc Trop Med Hyg 1998;92:430-433.
243. McGready R, Cho T, Samuel, et al. Randomized comparison of quinine-clindamycin versus artesunate in the treatment of falciparum malaria in pregnancy. Trans R Soc Trop Med Hyg 2001;95:651-656.
244. McGready R, Cho T, Keo NK, et al. Artemisinin antimalarials in pregnancy: a prospective treatment study of 539 episodes of multidrug-resistant *Plasmodium falciparum*. Clin Infect Dis 2001;33:2009-2016.
245. McGready R, Stepniewska K, Ward SA, et al. Pharmacokinetics of dihydroartemisinin following oral artesunate treatment of pregnant women with acute uncomplicated falciparum malaria. Eur J Clin Pharmacol 2006;62:367-371.
246. Looareesuwan S, Viravan C, Webster HK, et al. Clinical studies of atovaquone, alone or in combination with other antimalarial drugs, for treatment of acute uncomplicated malaria in Thailand. Am J Trop Med Hyg 1996;54:62-66.
247. Shapiro TA, Ranasinha CD, Kumar N, et al. Prophylactic activity of atovaquone against *Plasmodium falciparum* in humans. Am J Trop Med Hyg 1999;60:831-836.
248. Berman JD, Nielsen R, Chulay JD, et al. Causal prophylactic efficacy of atovaquone-proguanil (Malarone) in a human challenge model. Trans R Soc Trop Med Hyg 2001;95:429-432.

249. Fry M, Pudney M. Site of action of the antimalarial hydroxynaphthoquinone, 2-[trans-4-(4′-chlorophenyl) cyclohexyl]-3-hydroxy-1,4-naphthoquinone (566C80). Biochem Pharmacol 1992;43:1545-1553.
250. Vaidya AB, Mather MW. Atovaquone resistance in malaria parasites. Drug Resist Updat 2000;3:283-287.
251. Srivastava IK, Morrisey JM, Darrouzet E, et al. Resistance mutations reveal the atovaquone-binding domain of cytochrome b in malaria parasites. Mol Microbiol 1999;33:704-711.
252. Fivelman QL, Butcher GA, Adagu IS, et al. Malarone treatment failure and in vitro confirmation of resistance of *Plasmodium falciparum* isolate from Lagos, Nigeria. Malar J 2002;1:1.
253. Legrand E, Demar M, Volney B, et al. First case of emergence of atovaquone resistance in *Plasmodium falciparum* during second-line atovaquone-proguanil treatment in South America. Antimicrob Agents Chemother 2007;51:2280-2281.
254. Wichmann O, Muehlen M, Gruss H, et al. Malarone treatment failure not associated with previously described mutations in the cytochrome b gene. Malar J 2004;3:14.
255. Hussein Z, Eaves J, Hutchinson DB, et al. Population pharmacokinetics of atovaquone in patients with acute malaria caused by *Plasmodium falciparum*. Clin Pharmacol Ther 1997;61:518-530.
256. Sabchareon A, Attanath P, Phanuaksook P, et al. Efficacy and pharmacokinetics of atovaquone and proguanil in children with multidrug-resistant *Plasmodium falciparum* malaria. Trans R Soc Trop Med Hyg 1998;92:201-206.
257. McKeage K, Scott L. Atovaquone/proguanil: a review of its use for the prophylaxis of *Plasmodium falciparum* malaria. Drugs 2003;63:597-623.
258. Looareesuwan S, Wilairatana P, Chalermarut K, et al. Efficacy and safety of atovaquone/proguanil compared with mefloquine for treatment of acute *Plasmodium falciparum* malaria in Thailand. Am J Trop Med Hyg 1999;60:526-532.
259. Looareesuwan S, Wilairatana P, Glanarongran R, et al. Atovaquone and proguanil hydrochloride followed by primaquine for treatment of *Plasmodium vivax* malaria in Thailand. Trans R Soc Trop Med Hyg 1999;93:637-640.
260. van Vugt M, Edstein MD, Proux S, et al. Absence of an interaction between artesunate and atovaquone–proguanil. Eur J Clin Pharmacol 1999;55:469-474.
261. Chow AW, Jewesson PJ. Pharmacokinetics and safety of antimicrobial agents during pregnancy. Rev Infect Dis 1985;7:287-313.
262. Czeizel AE, Rockenbauer M, Sorensen HT, et al. A teratological study of lincosamides. Scand J Infect Dis 2000;32:579-580.
263. Lell B, Kremsner PG. Clindamycin as an antimalarial drug: review of clinical trials. Antimicrob Agents Chemother 2002;46:2315-2320.
264. Sidhu AB, Sun Q, Nkrumah LJ, et al. In vitro efficacy, resistance selection, and structural modeling studies implicate the malarial parasite apicoplast as the target of azithromycin. J Biol Chem 2007;282:2494-2504.
265. Gingras BA, Jensen JB. Activity of azithromycin (CP-62,993) and erythromycin against chloroquine-sensitive and chloroquine-resistant strains of *Plasmodium falciparum* in vitro. Am J Trop Med Hyg 1992;47:378-382.
266. Gingras BA, Jensen JB. Antimalarial activity of azithromycin and erythromycin against *Plasmodium berghei*. Am J Trop Med Hyg 1993;49:101-105.
267. Andersen SL, Oloo AJ, Gordon DM, et al. Successful double-blinded, randomized, placebo-controlled field trial of azithromycin and doxycycline as prophylaxis for malaria in western Kenya. Clin Infect Dis 1998;26:146-150.
268. Taylor WR, Richie TL, Fryauff DJ, et al. Malaria prophylaxis using azithromycin: a double-blind, placebo-controlled trial in Irian Jaya, Indonesia. Clin Infect Dis 1999;28:74-81.
269. Dunne MW, Singh N, Shukla M, et al. A multicenter study of azithromycin, alone and in combination with chloroquine, for the treatment of acute uncomplicated *Plasmodium falciparum* malaria in India. J Infect Dis 2005;191:1582-1588.
270. Dunne MW, Singh N, Shukla M, et al. A double-blind, randomized study of azithromycin compared to chloroquine for the treatment of *Plasmodium vivax* malaria in India. Am J Trop Med Hyg 2005;73:1108-1111.
271. Noedl H, Krudsood S, Chalermratana K, et al. Azithromycin combination therapy with artesunate or quinine for the treatment of uncomplicated *Plasmodium falciparum* malaria in adults: a randomized, Phase 2 clinical trial in Thailand. Clin Infect Dis 2006;43:1264-1271.
272. Miller RS, Wongsrichanalai C, Buathong N, et al. Effective treatment of uncomplicated *Plasmodium falciparum* malaria with azithromycin-quinine combinations: a randomized, dose-ranging study. Am J Trop Med Hyg 2006;74:401-406.
273. Lalak NJ, Morris DL. Azithromycin clinical pharmacokinetics. Clin Pharmacokinet 1993;25:370-374.
274. Cárceles CM, Fernández-Varón E, Marin NP, Escudero E. Tissue disposition of azithromycin after intravenous and intramuscular administration to rabbits. Vet J 2007;174:154-159.
275. Wildfeuer A, Laufen H, Zimmermann T. Uptake of azithromycin by various cells and its intracellular activity under in vivo conditions. Antimicrob Agents Chemother 1996;40:75-79.
276. Honig PK, Woosley RL, Zamani K, et al. Changes in the pharmacokinetics and electrocardiographic pharmacodynamics of terfenadine with concomitant administration of erythromycin. Clin Pharmacol Ther 1992;52:231-238.
277. Peters DH, Friedel HA, McTavish D. Azithromycin: a review of its antimicrobial activity, pharmacokinetic properties and clinical efficacy. Drugs 1992;44:750-799.
278. Heikkinen T, Laine K, Neuvonen PJ, et al. The transplacental transfer of the macrolide antibiotics erythromycin, roxithromycin and azithromycin. BJOG 2000;107:770-775.
279. Ramsey PS, Vaules MB, Vasdev GM, et al. Maternal and transplacental pharmacokinetics of azithromycin. Am J Obstet Gynecol 2003;188:714-718.
280. Ballou WR, Arevalo-Herrera M, Carucci D, et al. Update on the clinical development of candidate malaria vaccines. Am J Trop Med Hyg 2004;71:239-247.
281. Alonso PL, Sacarlal J, Aponte JJ, et al. Duration of protection with RTS,S/AS02A malaria vaccine in prevention of *Plasmodium falciparum* disease in Mozambican children: single-blind extended follow-up of a randomised controlled trial. Lancet 2005;366:2012-2018.
282. Alonso PL, Sacarlal J, Aponte JJ, et al. Efficacy of the RTS,S/AS02A vaccine against *Plasmodium falciparum* infection and disease in young African children: randomised controlled trial. Lancet 2004;364:1411-1420.
283. Heppner DG Jr, Kester KE, Ockenhouse CF, et al. Towards an RTS,S-based, multistage, multi-antigen vaccine against falciparum malaria: progress at the Walter Reed Army Institute of Research. Vaccine 2005;23:2243-2250.
284. Thera MA, Doumbo OK, Coulibaly D, et al. Safety and allele-specific immunogenicity of a malaria vaccine in Malian adults: results of a Phase I randomized trial. PLoS Clin Trials 2006;1:e34.
285. Withers MR, McKinney D, Ogutu BR, et al. Safety and reactogenicity of an MSP-1 malaria vaccine candidate: a randomized Phase Ib dose-escalation trial in Kenyan children. PLoS Clin Trials 2006;1:e32.
286. Polhemus ME, Magill AJ, Cummings JF, et al. Phase I dose escalation safety and immunogenicity trial of *Plasmodium falciparum* apical membrane protein (AMA-1) FMP2.1, adjuvanted with AS02A, in malaria-naive adults at the Walter Reed Army Institute of Research. Vaccine 2007;25:4203-4212.
287. Clyde DF. Immunization of man against falciparum and vivax malaria by use of attenuated sporozoites. Am J Trop Med Hyg 1975;24:397-401.
288. Luke TC, Hoffman SL. Rationale and plans for developing a non-replicating, metabolically active, radiation-attenuated *Plasmodium falciparum* sporozoite vaccine. J Exp Biol 2003;206:3803-3808.
289. Griffith KS, Lewis LS, Mali S, et al. Treatment of malaria in the United States: a systematic review. JAMA 2007;297:2264-2277.
290. Hasugian AR, Purba HL, Kenangalem E, et al. Dihydroartemisinin-piperaquine versus artesunate-amodiaquine: superior efficacy and posttreatment prophylaxis against multidrug-resistant *Plasmodium falciparum* and *Plasmodium vivax* malaria. Clin Infect Dis 2007;44:1067-1074.
291. Ratcliff A, Siswantoro H, Kenangalem E, et al. Two fixed-dose artemisinin combinations for drug-resistant falciparum and vivax malaria in Papua, Indonesia: an open-label randomised comparison. Lancet 2007;369:757-765.
292. Gardner MJ, Hall N, Fung E, et al. Genome sequence of the human malaria parasite *Plasmodium falciparum*. Nature 2002;419:498-511.
293. Rathore D, McCutchan TF, Sullivan M, et al. Antimalarial drugs: current status and new developments. Expert Opin Investig Drugs 2005;14:871-883.
294. Ridley RG, Hudson AT. Chemotherapy of malaria. Curr Opin Infect Dis 1998;11:691-705.
295. Rosenthal PJ. Antimalarial drug discovery: old and new approaches. J Exp Biol 2003;206:3735-3744.
296. Wiesner J, Ortmann R, Jomaa H, et al. New antimalarial drugs. Angew Chem Int Ed Engl 2003;42:5274-5293.
297. Mital A. Recent advances in antimalarial compounds and their patents. Curr Med Chem 2007;14:759-773.
298. Plowe CV. Antimalarial drug resistance in Africa: strategies for monitoring and deterrence. Curr Top Microbiol Immunol 2005;295:55-79.

83

PROTOZOAN AND HELMINTHIC INFECTIONS

Eric R. Houpt and Omer Chaudhry

INTRODUCTION 1171
THERAPEUTICS AND CLINICAL PHARMACOLOGY 1171
Drugs for Helminths 1171
Albendazole 1171
Mebendazole 1172
Thiabendazole 1174
Pyrantel Pamoate 1174
Diethylcarbamazine 1174
Ivermectin 1175
Praziquantel 1177
Additional Drugs 1178
Drugs for Protozoa 1178
Metronidazole 1178
Tinidazole 1178
Nitazoxanide 1178
Paromomycin 1179
Iodoquinol 1180
Diloxanide Furoate 1181
Furazolidone 1181
Atovaquone 1181
Pyrimethamine 1181
Trimethoprim-Sulfamethoxazole 1184
Additional Drugs 1185

INTRODUCTION

Parasitic infections, particularly common in the developing world, affect between 1 and 3 billion humans worldwide and many more domestic animals. In industrial nations, parasitic infection typically arises in those who have traveled to epidemic areas, have been exposed to an area of poor hygiene (some day care and nursing home settings), or have impaired immunity. While the term *parasite* may be applied to all of infectious disease, the term is typically restricted to helminths (worms, such as the tapeworms) and protozoa (single-cell organisms such as amebas). Chemotherapeutic agents targeting helminths and protozoa are the focus of this chapter.

The usual portals of entry for parasites are the mouth or skin. Parasites that enter through the skin are introduced through the bites of an infected vector (e.g., mosquito for malaria) or bore directly through the skin (often due to walking barefoot or bathing in contaminated water). Parasites that enter through the mouth (typically through undercooked meet from infected livestock) are swallowed and can either remain in the intestine or burrow through the intestinal wall to invade other organs.

THERAPEUTICS AND CLINICAL PHARMACOLOGY

Drugs for Helminths

Helminths that infect humans produce eggs or larvae that develop in the external environment, which may involve development in another animal (an intermediate host). The site of entry is typically oral, and helminths may either reside in the gastrointestinal tract or tunnel from there into tissues. The toxic effects of these parasites may either be due to the worm itself or a secondary inflammatory action.

Drugs targeting helminths have quite diverse structures and modes of action. Some target helminth microtubule synthesis while others target the reproductive cycle. Albendazole is a broad-spectrum intestinal nematode antimicrobial with activity against *Ascaris* (hookworm), *Enterobius* (pinworm), and *Strongyloides* (threadworm). It also is the first-line agent for the cestode *Echinococcus* (hydatid disease). Mebendazole may be superior for *Trichuris.* The medical treatment of neurocysticercosis and echinococcus is controversial, although albendazole is used for adjunctive medical therapy in many patients. Diethylcarbamazine is used in the microfilarial disease caused by *Wuchereria bancrofti, Brugia malayi,* and *Brugia timori.* Ivermectin is the drug of choice for *Strongyloides* and onchocerciasis. Praziquantel treats schistosomiasis and is useful for several other trematodes and cestodes. Triclabendazole is the drug of choice for treatment of fascioliasis.

Albendazole (Fig. 83-1)

Pharmacology. Albendazole is a benzimidazole derivative and a broad-spectrum anthelmintic agent. Benzimidazoles bind to β-tubulin to prevent the formation of microtubules and also prevent the uptake of glucose, leading to depletion of glycogen stores and consequently paralysis and death of the helminth.[1] Oral absorption of albendazole is increased after a fatty meal,[2] is superior to that of mebendazole, and is metabolized in the liver to albendazole sulfoxide.[3]

Therapeutic Approaches

***First-Line Therapy for* Ascaris, *Hookworm, or* Enterobius.** For *Ascaris* (Fig. 83-2), albendazole is administered as a single dose of 400 mg[1] and has a 96% cure rate.[4] This convenience has allowed its use in global community-based deworming campaigns. Single-dose albendazole is also superior to mebendazole or pyrantel in the treatment of human hookworm infection, with cure rates of 92% to 99%.[5] Albendazole or mebendazole are the treatments of choice for infection with *Enterobius vermicularis,* with cure rates up to 100%.[6,7] It is recommended to repeat the treatment after 1 week due to potential autoinfection from eggs that are deposited in the perianal region.

***Second-Line Therapy for* Trichuris *or* Strongyloides.** Single-dose 500-mg mebendazole was superior to single-dose 400-mg albendazole in the treatment of *Trichuris trichiura* infection in a study of South African children.[8] The addition of ivermectin to albendazole is associated with higher *Trichuris* cure and egg reduction rates.[9] Others advocate multiple doses of albendazole for trichuriasis.

Albendazole is an alternative to ivermectin for treatment of strongyloidiasis, although with a 3-day course of albendazole, the cure rate was only 38% versus 83% for ivermectin ($P < .01$).[10] Two courses of albendazole 400 mg/day for 3 days given 2 weeks apart has been 66% to 88% curative for *Strongyloides*[11] (Fig. 83-3).

Trichinella *and* Toxocara canis. Albendazole has been used in the treatment of the systemic nematode *Trichinella spiralis* (Fig. 83-4) at a dose of 800 mg/day in two cycles of 10 to 15 days.[12] Albendazole is also used for visceral larva migrans (*Toxocara canis*) and cutaneous larval migrans (dog and cat hookworms).

***Role in* Echinococcus.** Echinococcal infection (Fig. 83-5) of the liver is generally treated either with surgical resection or with prolonged medical therapy. Albendazole has been used at doses of 400 mg twice a day for up to 6 months.[13] In a study comparing albendazole 400 mg twice daily in three 6-week cycles to placebo, 82% of hydatid patients had cure or improvement in their cysts versus 14% of placebo-treated patients.[14] Albendazole has also been used as an adjunct to surgical resection or to percutaneous drainage procedures. Percutaneous drainage combined with albendazole treatment for 8 weeks was found to decrease hospital stay, decrease procedure-related complications, and have a similar outcome in terms of curing cysts compared to surgical resection alone.[15]

Role in Neurocysticercosis. Neurocysticercosis is caused by the larval form of *Taenia solium* (Fig. 83-6) after ingestion of *T. solium* eggs, and is clinically marked by seizures, headaches, and/or focal neurologic deficits.[16] Therapy for symptomatic disease may involve antiepileptic drugs, and potentially mannitol and corticosteroids. Neurosurgery is needed in cases of hydrocephalus for ventriculoperitoneal shunting, for racemose cysts in the basal cistern, and for intraventricular cysts.[16] Treatment recommendations for neurocysticercosis remain controversial. As of 2000, there was insufficient evidence to assess whether anthelmintic therapy in neurocysticercosis was associated with beneficial effects, either in persistence of cysts after 6 months follow-up, in the occurrence of seizures after 1 to 2 years of follow-up, or in the presence of hydrocephalus.[16,17] However, more recent studies have reported that albendazole plus dexamethasone decreased seizures when administered for between 10 and 30 days.[18,19] High-dose albendazole (30 mg/kg/day) plus dexamethasone has been advocated in the presence of ventricular cysts or subarachnoid involvement.[20]

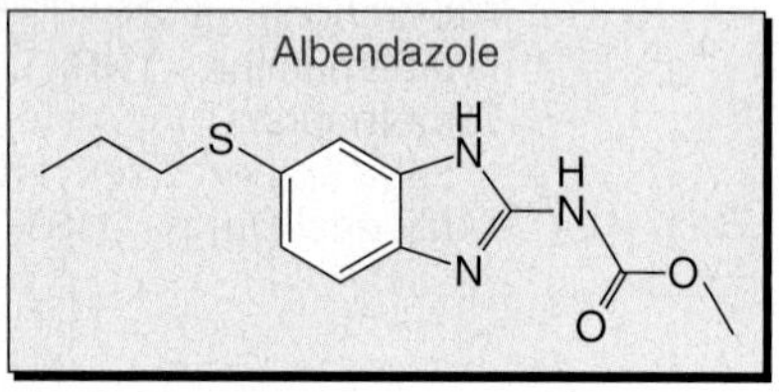

Side Effects. The side effects of albendazole include rash, alopecia, dizziness, abdominal discomfort, and diarrhea. High-dose, prolonged albendazole can result in reversible elevations in hepatic transaminases and bone marrow suppression, and therefore requires monitoring of complete blood counts and liver function tests.[2] Its use is contraindicated in pregnancy.

Albendazole

FIGURE 83-1 • Albendazole.

Mebendazole (Fig. 83-7)

Mebendazole is also a benzimidazole derivative with activity similar to albendazole but poorer oral absorption (<10% of the drug is absorbed systemically). As mentioned earlier, single-dose 500-mg mebendazole was superior to single-dose 400-mg albendazole in the treatment of *T. trichiura* infection in a study of South African children.[8] Mebendazole can be used for the intestinal nematodes *Ascaris, Trichuris,* and *Enterobius* and the hookworms *Ancylostoma* and *Necator.* A single dose is

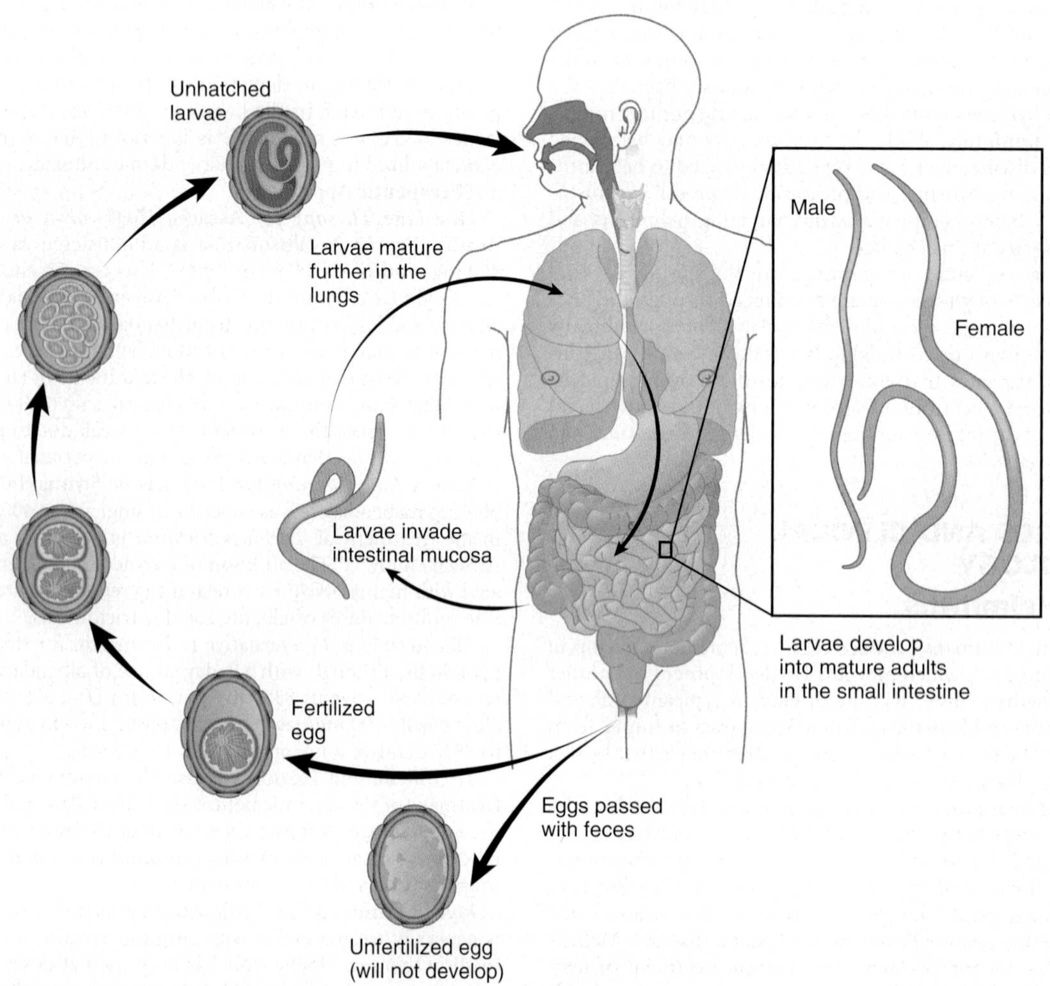

FIGURE 83-2 • Adult *Ascaris* worms live in the lumen of the small intestine. A female may produce approximately 200,000 eggs per day, which are passed with the feces. Unfertilized eggs may be ingested but are not infective. Fertile eggs embryonate and become infective after 18 days to several weeks, depending on the environmental conditions (optimum: moist, warm, shaded soil). After infective eggs are swallowed, the larvae hatch, invade the intestinal mucosa, and are carried via the portal and then the systemic circulation to the lungs. The larvae mature further in the lungs (10 to 14 days), penetrate the alveolar walls, ascend the bronchial tree to the throat, and are swallowed. Upon reaching the small intestine, they develop into adult worms. Between 2 and 3 months are required from ingestion of the infective eggs to oviposition by the adult female. Adult worms can live 1 to 2 years. (From Division of Parasitic Diseases, Centers for Disease Control and Prevention. Laboratory identification of parasites of public health concern: image library. 2008. Available at: *http://www.dpd.cdc.gov/dpdx*)

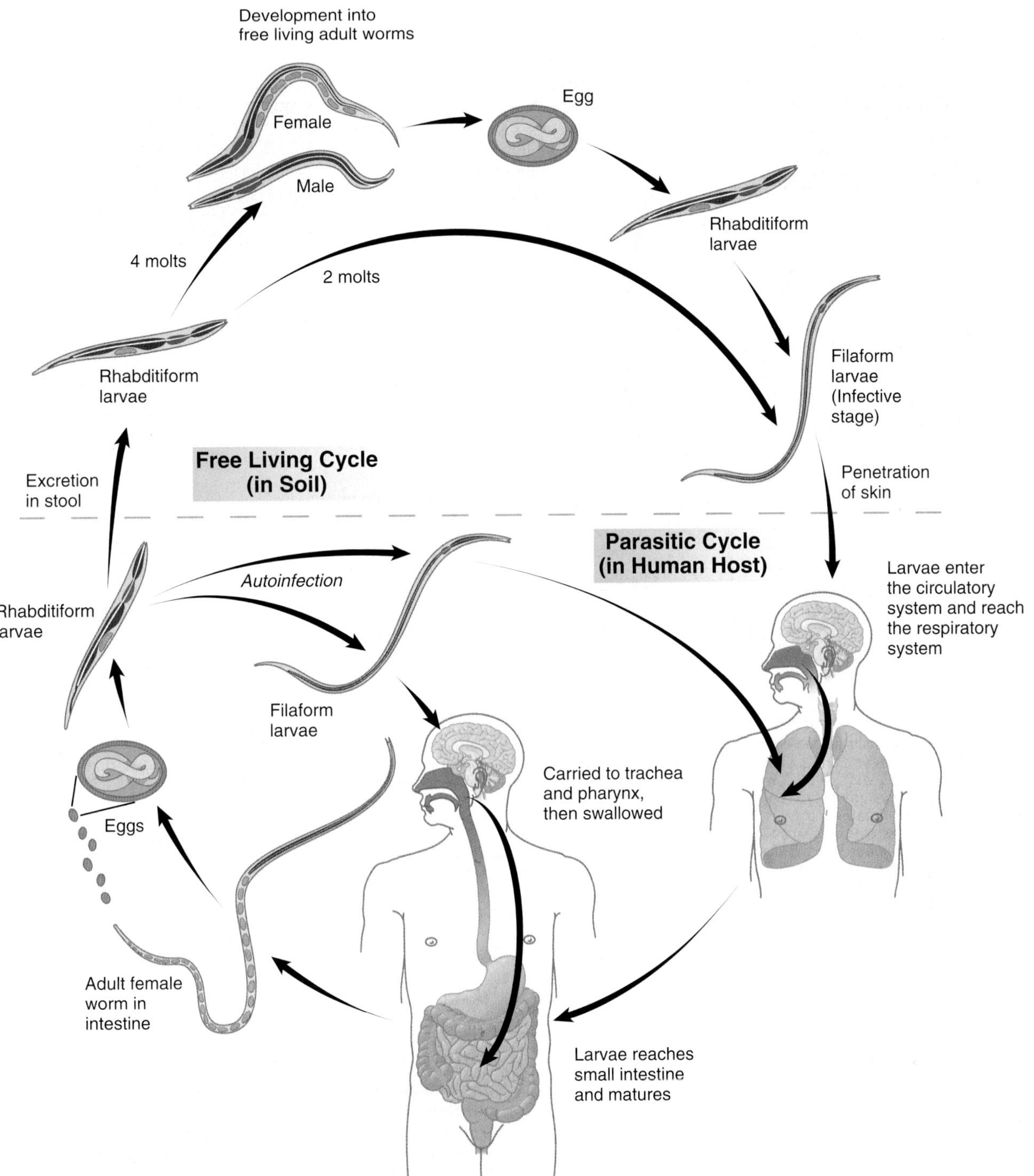

FIGURE 83-3 • The *Strongyloides* life cycle is more complex than that of most nematodes with its alternation between free-living and parasitic cycles, and its potential for autoinfection and multiplication within the host. Two types of cycles exist:

Free-living cycle: The rhabditiform larvae passed in the stool (see "Parasitic cycle" below) can either molt twice and become infective filariform larvae (direct development) or molt four times and become free-living adult males and females that mate and produce eggs from which rhabditiform larvae hatch. The latter in turn can either develop into a new generation of free-living adults or into infective filariform larvae. The filariform larvae penetrate the human host skin to initiate the parasitic cycle.

Parasitic cycle: Filariform larvae in contaminated soil penetrate the human skin and are transported to the lungs, where they penetrate the alveolar spaces; they are carried through the bronchial tree to the pharynx, are swallowed, and then reach the small intestine. In the small intestine, they molt twice and become adult female worms. The females live threaded in the epithelium of the small intestine and by parthenogenesis produce eggs, which yield rhabditiform larvae. The rhabditiform larvae can either be passed in the stool (see "Free-living cycle" above), or can cause autoinfection. In autoinfection, the rhabditiform larvae become infective filariform larvae, which can penetrate either the intestinal mucosa (internal autoinfection) or the skin of the perianal area (external autoinfection). In either case, the filariform larvae may follow the previously described route, being carried successively to the lungs, the bronchial tree, the pharynx, and the small intestine, where they mature into adults; or they may disseminate widely in the body. To date, occurrence of autoinfection in humans with helminthic infections is recognized only in *Strongyloides stercoralis* and *Capillaria philippinensis* infections. In the case of *Strongyloides,* autoinfection may explain the possibility of persistent infections for many years in persons who have not been in an endemic area and of hyperinfections in immunodepressed individuals. (From Division of Parasitic Diseases, Centers for Disease Control and Prevention. Laboratory identification of parasites of public health concern: image library. 2008. Available at: http://www.dpd.cdc.gov/dpdx)

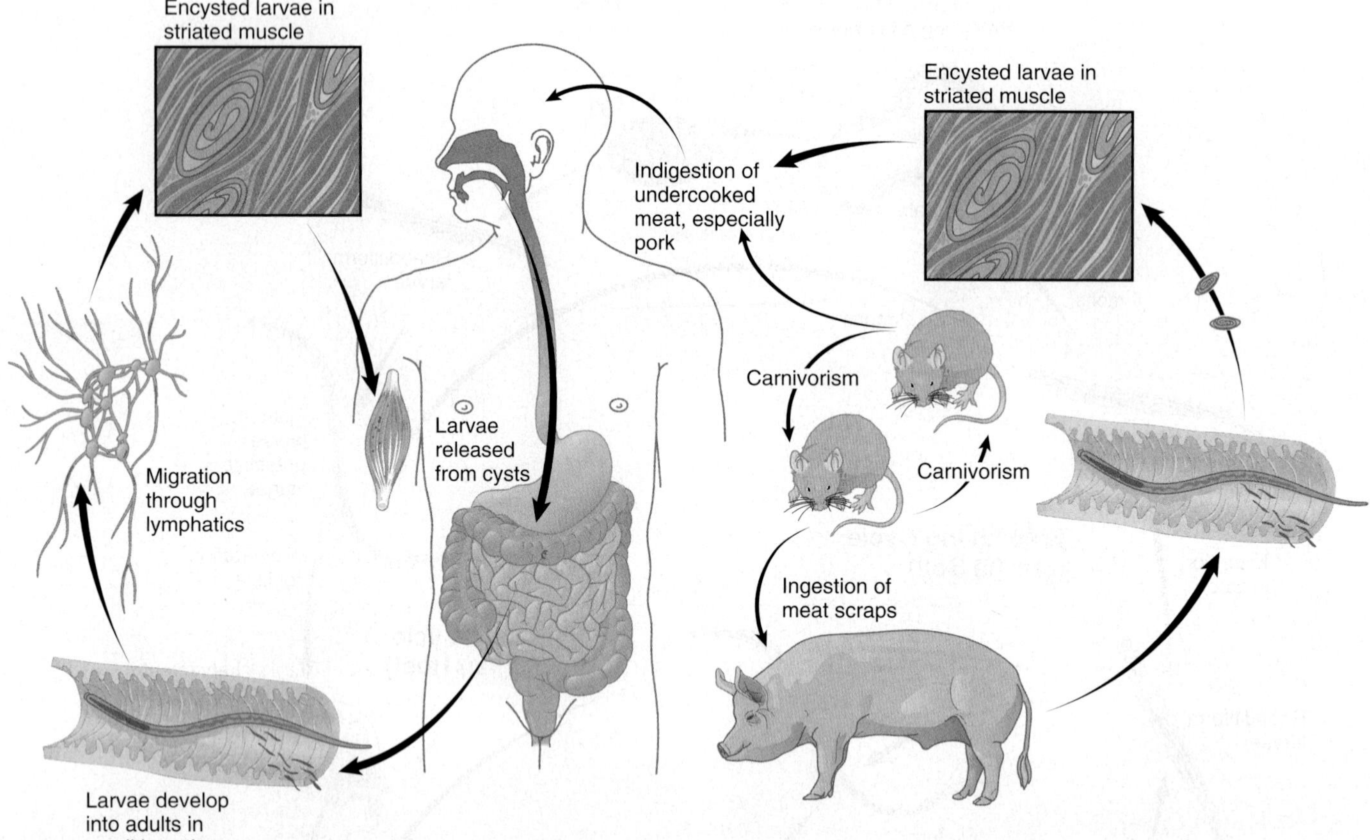

FIGURE 83-4 • Trichinellosis is acquired by ingesting meat containing cysts (encysted larvae) of *Trichinella*. After exposure to gastric acid and pepsin, the larvae are released from the cysts and invade the small bowel mucosa, where they develop into adult worms (females 2.2 mm in length, males 1.2 mm; life span in the small bowel: 4 weeks). After 1 week, the females release larvae that migrate to the striated muscles, where they encyst. *Trichinella pseudospiralis*, however, does not encyst. Encystment is completed in 4 to 5 weeks, and the encysted larvae may remain viable for several years. Ingestion of the encysted larvae perpetuates the cycle. Rats and rodents are primarily responsible for maintaining the endemicity of this infection. Carnivorous/omnivorous animals, such as pigs or bears, feed on infected rodents or meat from other animals. Different animal hosts are implicated in the life cycle of the different species of *Trichinella*. Humans are accidentally infected when eating improperly processed meat of these carnivorous animals (or eating food contaminated with such meat). (From Division of Parasitic Diseases, Centers for Disease Control and Prevention. Laboratory identification of parasites of public health concern: image library. 2008. Available at: *http://www.dpd.cdc.gov/dpdx*)

administered for *Ascaris* and *Trichuris*, a single dose is followed by repeat dosing in 1 week for *Enterobius*,[21] and 3 days of mebendazole treatment is used for the hookworms.[3] Mebendazole is not generally used for *Strongyloides* infection due to the use of ivermectin, and its role against hydatid disease has been replaced by albendazole.[22] Its side effect profile is similar to that of albendazole, and it is also contraindicated during pregnancy.

Thiabendazole

Thiabendazole is an older benzimidazole compound with even more limited use due to significant adverse effects and the availability of other agents. Its role for many decades as the treatment for *Strongyloides* has been replaced by ivermectin. It is still used at times as a topical suspension for the treatment of cutaneous larva migrans, with cure rates of 80% to 98% after 10 days of treatment.[23,24] Due to the requirement for multiple daily applications and the possible presence of several skin lesions, oral therapy with ivermectin or albendazole may be preferred. Approximately 50% of people who take thiabendazole develop side effects, including diarrhea, headache, tinnitus, hypotension, bradycardia, liver function abnormalities, allergic manifestations, and crystalluria.[13]

Pyrantel Pamoate (Fig. 83-8)

Pyrantel is a cyclic amidine derivative that has anticholinesterase activity leading to neuromuscular blockade and paralysis of the worm. It has been used successfully as an alternative treatment for ascariasis, hookworm, and *Enterobius* infections. Treatment for ascariasis and hookworm is given at 11 mg/kg for 3 days. Pyrantel is not effective against *Trichuris*.[3] It may cause some gastrointestinal symptoms and lead to liver function test abnormalities.[25] It is contraindicated during pregnancy.

Diethylcarbamazine (Fig. 83-9)

Pharmacology. Diethylcarbamazine (DEC) is derived from the anthelmintic compound piperazine. The mechanism of action of the drug is unclear, but paralysis of the worm has been proposed.[13] Diethylcarbamazine also alters the surface membrane of the worm and may disrupt the formation of helminth microtubules. In the United States, it is only available through the Centers for Disease Control and Prevention (CDC).

Therapeutic Approach. DEC is the drug of choice for lymphatic filariasis caused by *Wuchereria bancrofti* (Fig. 83-10), *Brugia malayi*, and *Brugia timori*. A single annual dose of DEC reduces microfilaremia by 90%,[13] and it is frequently used as part of mass drug administration campaigns at a dose of 6 mg/kg. Single-dose DEC led to an 85% reduction in microfilaria counts and a 23% cure rate at 12 months,[26] while a 7-day treatment regimen led to a 99.6% reduction in counts and a 75% cure rate. Many mass drug treatment campaigns have consisted of annual treatments for 4 to 6 years. DEC has also been used for treatment and prophylaxis for *Loa loa* infection.[27] A dose of 8 to 10 mg/kg per day for 21 days cures 50% of patients, although multiple courses may be necessary.

Side Effects. DEC can cause headaches, malaise, and vomiting.[13] In cases of onchocerciasis, it can precipitate an inflammatory reaction

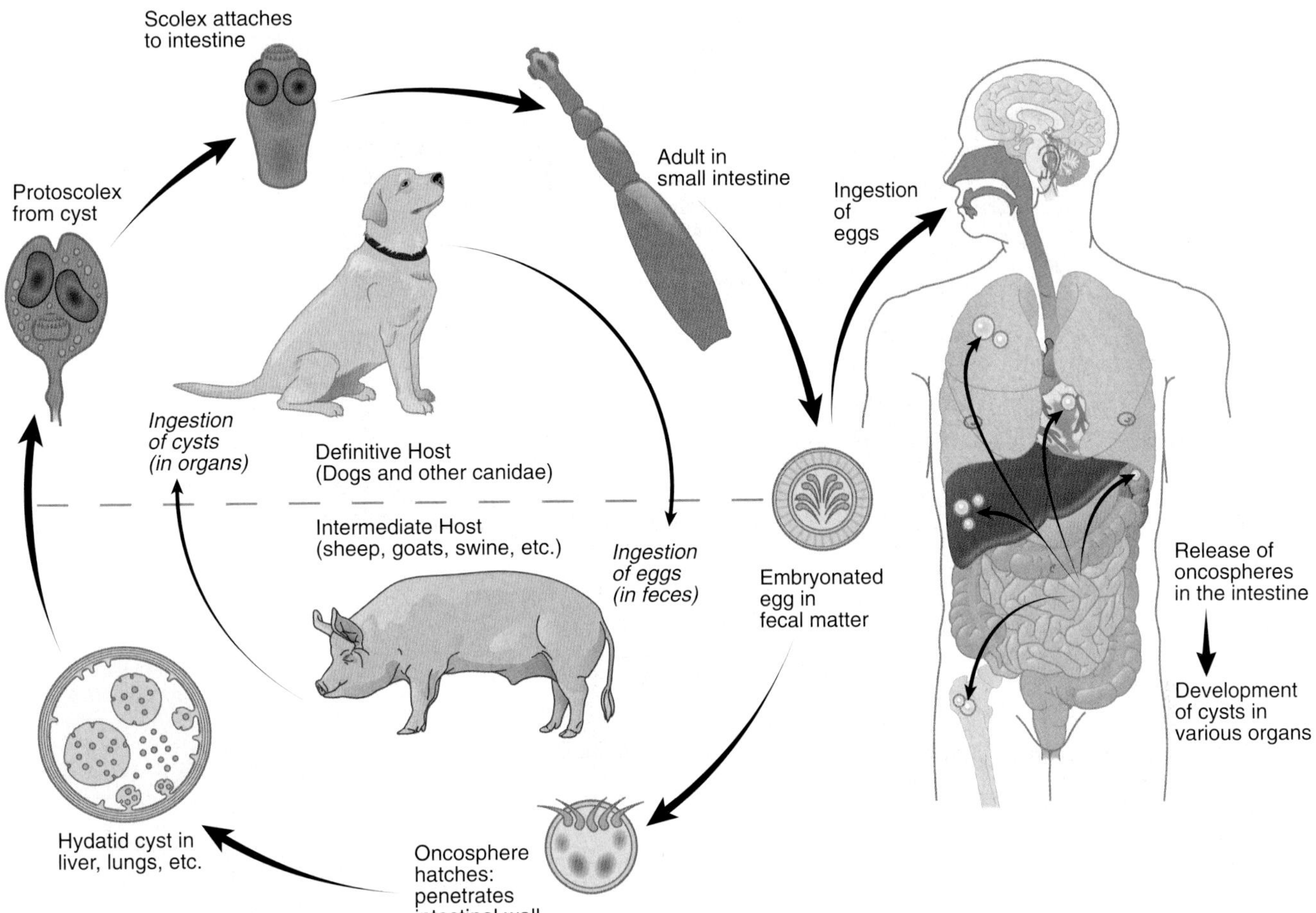

FIGURE 83-5 • The adult *Echinococcus granulosus* (3 to 6 mm long) resides in the small bowel of the definitive hosts, dogs or other canids. Gravid proglottids release eggs that are passed in the feces. After ingestion by a suitable intermediate host (under natural conditions: sheep, goats, swine, cattle, horses, camels), the egg hatches in the small bowel and releases an oncosphere that penetrates the intestinal wall and migrates through the circulatory system into various organs, especially the liver and lungs. In these organs, the oncosphere develops into a cyst that enlarges gradually, producing protoscolices and daughter cysts that fill the cyst interior. The definitive host becomes infected by ingesting the cyst-containing organs of the infected intermediate host. After ingestion, the protoscolices evaginate, attach to the intestinal mucosa, and develop into adult stages in 32 to 80 days. The same life cycle occurs with *E. multilocularis* (1.2 to 3.7 mm), with the following differences: the definitive hosts are foxes and to a lesser extent dogs, cats, coyotes, and wolves; the intermediate host are small rodents; and larval growth (in the liver) remains indefinitely in the proliferative stage, resulting in invasion of the surrounding tissues. With *E. vogeli* (up to 5.6 mm long), the definitive hosts are bush dogs and dogs; the intermediate hosts are rodents; and the larval stage (in the liver, lungs and other organs) develops both externally and internally, resulting in multiple vesicles. *E. oligarthrus* (up to 2.9 mm long) has a life cycle that involves wild felids as definitive hosts and rodents as intermediate hosts. Humans become infected by ingesting eggs, with resulting release of oncospheres in the intestine and the development of cysts in various organs. (From Division of Parasitic Diseases, Centers for Disease Control and Prevention. Laboratory identification of parasites of public health concern: image library. 2008. Available at: http://www.dpd.cdc.gov/dpdx)

within the eye leading to permanent damage, as well as systemic effects such as hypotension, fever, splenomegaly, and proteinuria. Patients with *L. loa* infection may develop encephalopathy when treated with DEC.[13]

Ivermectin (Fig. 83-11)

Pharmacology. Ivermectin acts by binding to and increasing the permeability of chloride channels in nematode nerve and muscle cells, causing hyperpolarization and paralysis and death of the worm.[11] The drug may also cause the release of the inhibitory neurotransmitter γ-aminobutyric acid. It is a broad-spectrum anthelmintic (see below) but has not been effective for dracunculiasis.[28]

Therapeutic Approach

***Intestinal Nematodes:* Strongyloides, Ascaris, Trichuris.** Ivermectin is the drug of choice for strongyloidiasis. When given as a single dose of 200 mcg/kg for intestinal strongyloides, it has cured 83% of cases.[10,29] Treatment failures have occurred in cases of disseminated disease, and multiple doses (e.g., daily doses for a week) are recommended. Co-infection with human T-lymphotropic virus 1 is also associated with treatment resistance and merits a prolonged course. Ivermectin has also cured 78% of ascariasis and 35% of trichuriasis cases, similar to cure rates in studies with albendazole.[9]

Onchocerciasis. Ivermectin is also the drug of choice for onchocerciasis. The standard protocol for mass eradication programs consists of 150 mcg/kg given once per year. In some cases doxycycline 100 mg daily for 6 weeks is given to kill the symbiotic organism *Wolbachia*, which is usually present. This can then be followed by a dose of ivermectin to suppress the development of microfilariae by the adult worms. Because the adult worm is not killed by ivermectin, annual treatments are often given to suppress the level of microfilariae. Increased dose frequency (every 3 to 6 months) has produced improved outcomes,[30] while increased dose quantity has not. The potential for ocular inflammatory effects with treatment of onchocerciasis with ivermectin exists but is much less compared to the effects of DEC.

Scabies. Ivermectin has been used successfully in the treatment of ectoparasitic infections with *Sarcoptes scabies*, particularly Norwegian scabies.[31]

Side Effects. Ivermectin has been associated with fever, headache, arthralgias, pruritis, and cutaneous edema.[13] Treatment of *L. loa* infection can also lead to encephalopathy.

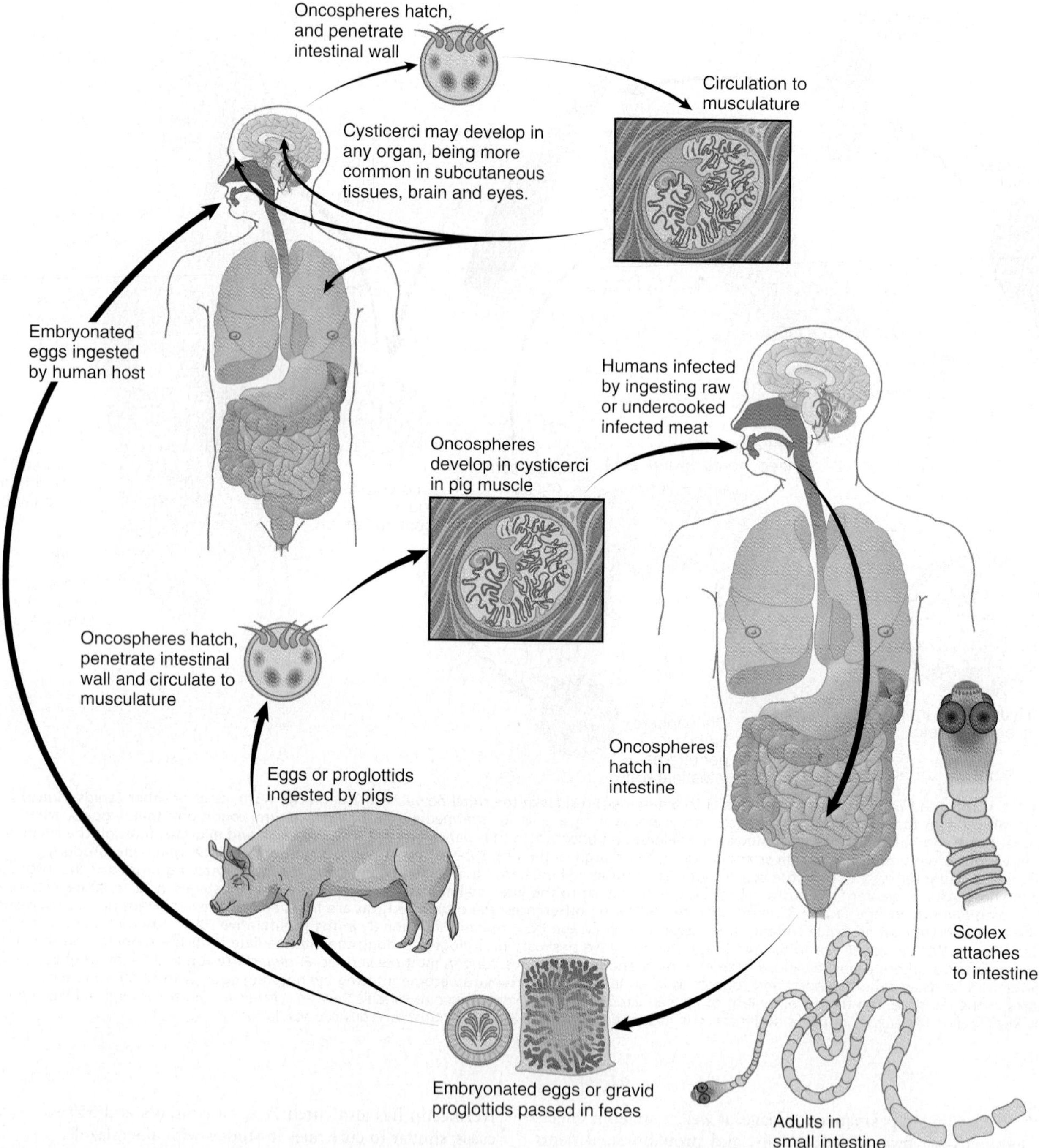

FIGURE 83-6 • Cysticercosis is an infection of both humans and pigs with the larval stages of the parasitic cestode *Taenia solium.* This infection is caused by ingestion of eggs shed in the feces of a human tapeworm carrier. Pigs and humans become infected by ingesting eggs or gravid proglottids. Humans are infected either by ingestion of food contaminated with feces, or by autoinfection. In the latter case, a human infected with adult *T. solium* can ingest eggs produced by that tapeworm, either through fecal contamination or, possibly, from proglottids carried into the stomach by reverse peristalsis. Once eggs are ingested, oncospheres hatch in the intestine, invade the intestinal wall, and migrate to striated muscles as well as the brain, liver, and other tissues, where they develop into cysticerci. In humans, cysts can cause serious sequelae if they localize in the brain, resulting in neurocysticercosis. The parasite life cycle is completed, resulting in human tapeworm infection, when humans ingest undercooked pork containing cysticerci. Cysts evaginate and attach to the small intestine by their scolex. Adult tapeworms develop (up to 2 to 7 m in length and producing <1000 proglottids, each with approximately 50,000 eggs) and reside in the small intestine for years. (From Division of Parasitic Diseases, Centers for Disease Control and Prevention. Laboratory identification of parasites of public health concern: image library. 2008. Available at: http://www.dpd.cdc.gov/dpdx)

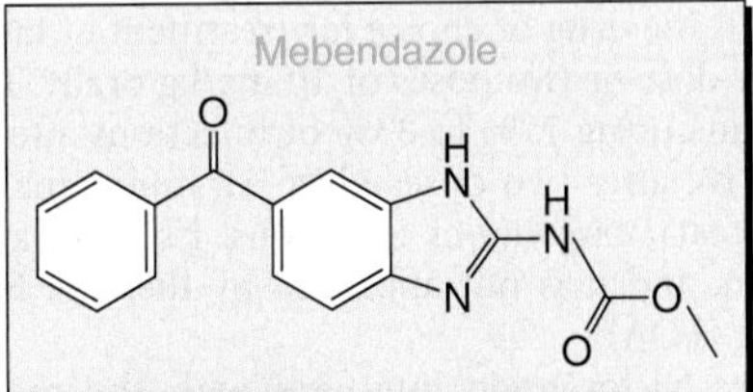

FIGURE 83-7 • Mebendazole.

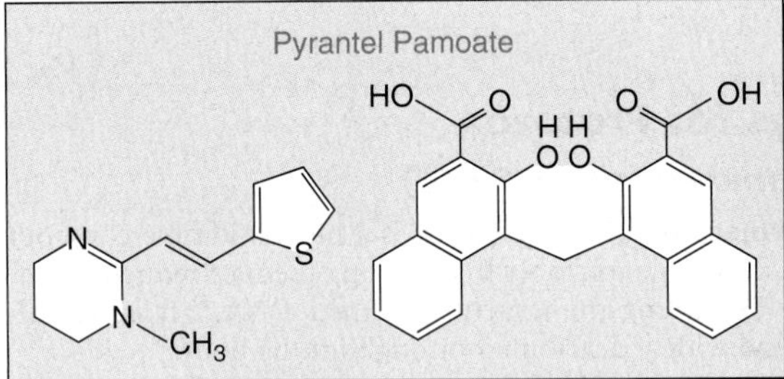

FIGURE 83-8 • Pyrantel pamoate.

Praziquantel (Fig. 83-12)

Pharmacology. Praziquantel disrupts calcium homeostasis and leads to stimulation of worm muscular activity, tegumental damage, and metabolic changes.[32] The oral absorption is almost complete and rapidly achieved in 1 to 2 hours.

Therapeutic Approach

Schistosomiasis. Praziquantel is the drug of choice for schistosomiasis, with broad activity against essentially all *Schistosoma* species (Fig. 83-13). It is given in a dose of 40 to 60 mg/kg as a single or a divided daily dose and results in high parasitologic cure and egg reduction rates.[32] It is also approved for pregnant women at risk for morbidity from schistosomiasis.[33]

Other Trematodes. Praziquantel is an effective drug for several other trematode infections, including *Opisthorchis, Clonorchis, Paragonimus,*

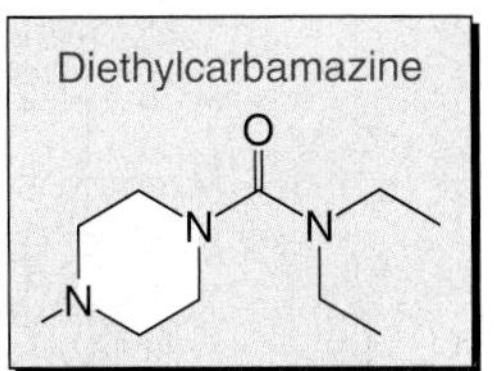

FIGURE 83-9 • Diethylcarbamazine.

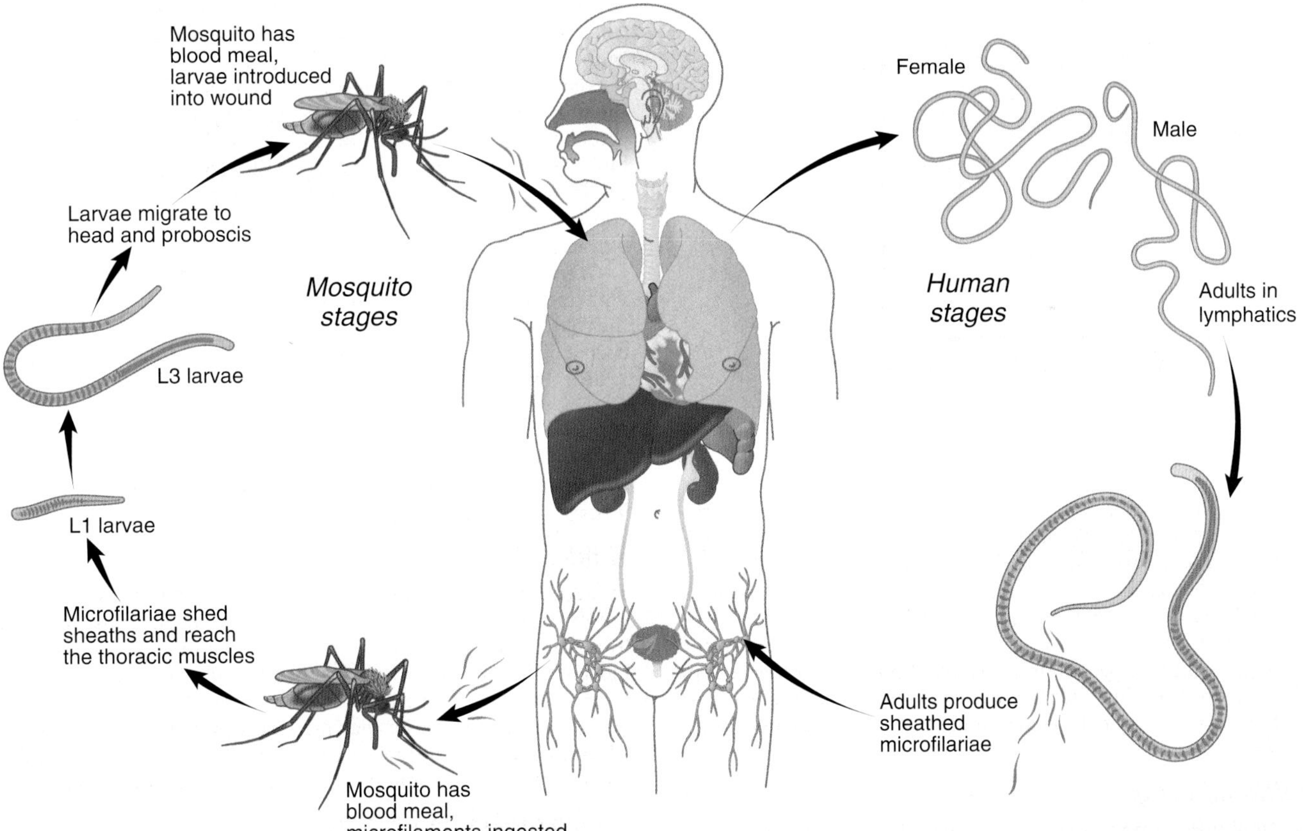

FIGURE 83-10 • Different species of the following genera of mosquitoes are vectors of *Wuchereria bancrofti* filariasis, depending on geographical distribution: *Culex* (*C. annulirostris, C. bitaeniorhynchus, C. quinquefasciatus,* and *C. pipiens*); *Anopheles* (*A. arabinensis, A. bancroftii, A. farauti, A. funestus, A. gambiae, A. koliensis, A. melas, A. merus, A. punctulatus,* and *A. wellcomei*); *Aedes* (*A. aegypti, A. aquasalis, A. bellator, A. cooki, A. darlingi, A. kochi, A. polynesiensis, A. pseudoscutellaris, A. rotumae, A. scapularis,* and *A. vigilax*); *Mansonia* (*M. pseudotitillans* and *M. uniformis*); and *Coquillettidia* (*C. juxtamansonia*). During a blood meal, an infected mosquito introduces third-stage filarial larvae onto the skin of the human host, where they penetrate into the bite wound. They develop into adults that commonly reside in the lymphatics. The female worms measure 80 to 100 mm in length and 0.24 to 0.30 mm in diameter, while the males measure about 40 mm by 0.1 mm. Adults produce microfilariae measuring 244 to 296 μm by 7.5 to 10 μm that are sheathed and have nocturnal periodicity, except the South Pacific microfilariae, which have the absence of marked periodicity. The microfilariae migrate into lymph and blood channels, moving actively through lymph and blood. A mosquito ingests the microfilariae during a blood meal. After ingestion, the microfilariae lose their sheaths and some of them work their way through the wall of the proventriculus and cardiac portion of the mosquito's midgut and reach the thoracic muscles. There the microfilariae develop into first-stage larvae and subsequently into third-stage infective larvae. The third-stage infective larvae migrate through the hemocele to the mosquito's proboscis and can infect another human when the mosquito takes a blood meal. (From Division of Parasitic Diseases, Centers for Disease Control and Prevention. Laboratory identification of parasites of public health concern: image library. 2008. Available at: *http://www.dpd.cdc.gov/dpdx*)

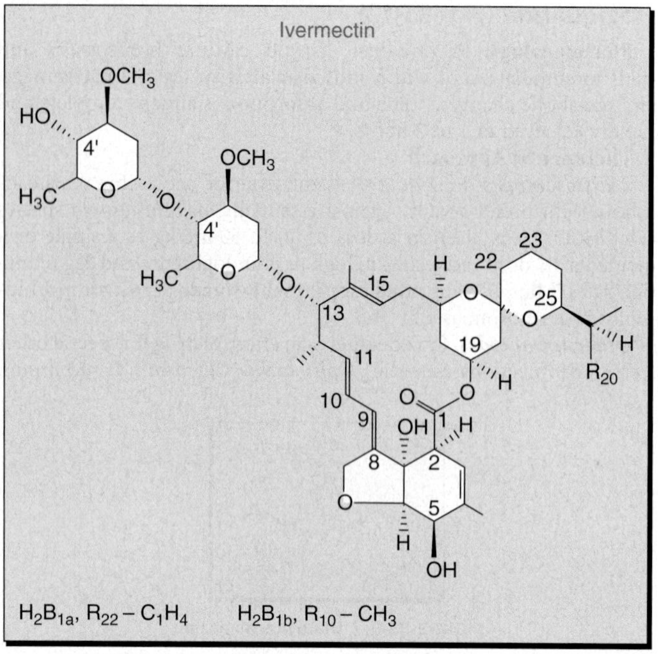

FIGURE 83-11 • Ivermectin.

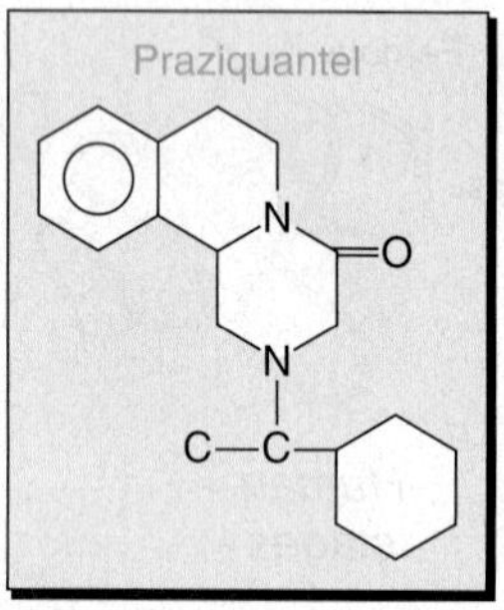

FIGURE 83-12 • Praziquantel.

and *Fasciolopsis buski*[13,33-35]; however, it is not effective for *Fasciola hepatica.*

Cestodes. Praziquantel is effective against the cestodes *Taenia saginata, Hymenolepis, Diphyllobothrium,* and *T. solium*[13] (Fig. 83-14). It has also been used for neurocysticercosis; however, most studies have shown that albendazole is either more successful than or equivalent to praziquantel at decreasing the number of cysts.[36,37]

Side Effects. There are no major adverse effects of praziquantel, and it is frequently used as part of mass treatment programs. Minor effects include abdominal pain, headache, fever, and rash.[33] The frequency and severity of adverse events is related to the intensity of the underlying infection.

Additional Drugs

Oxamniquine. Oxamniquine works by inhibition of nucleic acid synthesis of the target helminth.[33] It is used in a dosage of 20 to 60 mg/kg in divided doses. Its main use is as an alternative agent for the treatment of *Schistosoma mansoni.*[32]

Bithionol. Bithionol is an older drug used for the treatment of *Fasciola hepatica* and *Paragonimus.*[38] It has been generally replaced by triclabendazole for the treatment of *Fasciola* and by praziquantel for the treatment of *Paragonimus.* It has significant adverse effects, including photosensitivity, vomiting, diarrhea, abdominal pain, and urticaria.[39]

Triclabendazole. Triclabendazole is a benzimidazole that may function by binding to β-tubulin and disrupting the helminthic microtubule system. It is the drug of choice for treatment of fascioliasis and is used as a single dose or two doses of 10 mg/kg orally. Triclabendazole was successful in curing 79% to 83% of infections after one dose and was 92% effective after two doses given 12 hours apart.[39] It has also been used to treat *Paragonimus* infections. Its main adverse effect is abdominal pain, and it is not approved by the U.S. Food and Drug Administration (FDA).

Niclosamide. Niclosamide interferes with the metabolic system of the worm. It is effective against most of the intestinal tapeworm infections. It should be avoided in infections with *T. solium* because it can theoretically lead to an increased risk of autoinfection. It is generally well tolerated, with occasional gastrointestinal symptoms and rash.[13]

Drugs for Protozoa

Metronidazole (Fig. 83-15)

Pharmacology. Metronidazole is a nitroimidazole compound that acts on anaerobic microbes by depleting them of reducing equivalents and by disrupting the structure of their DNA.[40] It is well absorbed orally and widely distributed throughout the body.

Therapeutic Approach

Entamoeba histolytica. Metronidazole is used in the treatment of colitis or liver abscess due to *Entamoeba histolytica* (Fig. 83-16) at a dose of 750 mg orally three times daily for 7 to 10 days. Metronidazole is active only against the trophozoite stage of the parasite; therefore, following therapy with a cysticidal agent such as paromomycin is recommended.[41]

Giardia lamblia. Metronidazole is commonly used for the treatment of giardiasis in the United States (Fig. 83-17), although it is not actually FDA approved for this indication. It can be given as 250-mg tablets two to three times a day for 5 to 10 days.[40] This longer treatment results in a successful treatment in 60% to 100% of cases. Shorter courses from 1 to 3 days have also been given but usually are less efficacious.

Other. Vaginitis due to *Trichomonas vaginalis* is effectively treated with metronidazole.[42] The pathogenicity of *Blastocystis hominis* and the role of medical treatment remain controversial; however, metronidazole or iodoquinol has been used.[43]

Side Effects. Adverse effects of metronidazole include headache, nausea, metallic taste, and potentially pancreatitis and neutropenia.[40] Alcohol use must also be avoided due to the potential for a disulfiram-like reaction. It is contraindicated in the first trimester of pregnancy and should be used with caution in the second and third trimesters as it is an FDA Pregnancy Category B agent.

Tinidazole

Tinidazole is another nitroimidazole compound and has been used for the treatment of trichomoniasis, giardiasis, amebic colitis, and amebic liver abscess. It was recently FDA approved for these indications,[44] and indeed tinidazole may emerge as the drug of choice since it appears to have equivalent or superior cure rates for amebiasis (2 g per day for 5 days) and giardia (2 g per day for 1 dose) versus metronidazole. The adverse effects of tinidazole are generally less than metronidazole and include vertigo, gastrointestinal symptoms, and bitter taste.[40]

Nitazoxanide (Fig. 83-18)

Pharmacology. Nitazoxanide is a broad-spectrum antiprotozoal agent. It has an unclear mechanism of action but is thought to inhibit electron transport reactions within the microbe.[13]

Therapeutic Approach

Cryptosporidium. Nitazoxanide is FDA approved for the treatment of *Cryptosporidium* (Fig. 83-19) and *Giardia.* In a study of children in Zambia, 3 days of treatment with nitazoxanide for cryptosporidiosis was found to improve diarrhea and oocyst shedding in the stool in human immunodeficiency virus (HIV)–negative patients,[45] but no benefit was seen in HIV-positive children. A different study that enrolled adults and children without acquired immunodeficiency syn-

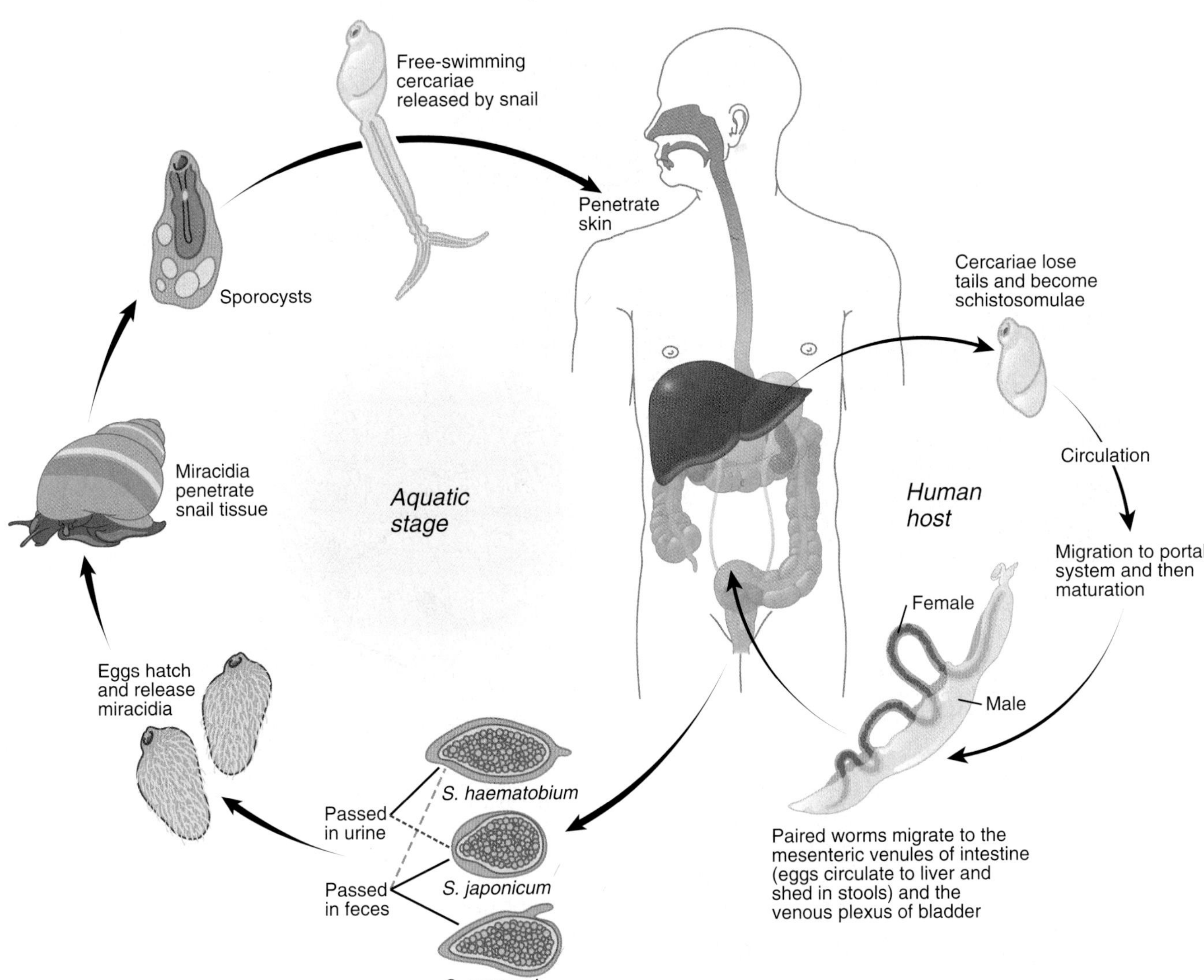

FIGURE 83-13 • *Schistosoma* eggs are eliminated with feces or urine. Under optimal conditions, the eggs hatch and release miracidia, which swim and penetrate specific snail intermediate hosts. The stages in the snail include two generations of sporocysts and the production of cercariae. Upon release from the snail, the infective cercariae swim, penetrate the skin of the human host, and shed their forked tail, becoming schistosomulae. The schistosomulae migrate through several tissues and stages to their residence in the veins. Adult worms in humans reside in the mesenteric venules in various locations, which at times seem to be specific for each species. For instance, *S. japonicum* is more frequently found in the superior mesenteric veins draining the small intestine, and *S. mansoni* occurs more often in the superior mesenteric veins draining the large intestine. However, both species can occupy either location, and they are capable of moving between sites, so it is not possible to state unequivocally that one species only occurs in one location. *S. haematobium* most often occurs in the venous plexus of bladder, but it can also be found in the rectal venules. The females (size 7 to 20 mm; males slightly smaller) deposit eggs in the small venules of the portal and perivesical systems. The eggs are moved progressively toward the lumen of the intestine (*S. mansoni* and *S. japonicum*) and of the bladder and ureters (*S. haematobium*), and are eliminated with feces or urine, respectively. Pathology of *S. mansoni* and *S. japonicum* schistosomiasis includes Katayama fever, hepatic perisinusoidal egg granulomas, Symmers' (pipestem) periportal fibrosis, portal hypertension, and occasional embolic egg granulomas in the brain or spinal cord. Pathology of *S. haematobium* schistosomiasis includes hematuria, scarring, calcification, squamous cell carcinoma, and occasional embolic egg granulomas in the brain or spinal cord.

Human contact with water is necessary for infection by schistosomes. Various animals, such as dogs, cats, rodents, pigs, horses, and goats, serve as reservoirs for *S. japonicum,* and dogs for *S. mekongi.* (From Division of Parasitic Diseases, Centers for Disease Control and Prevention. Laboratory identification of parasites of public health concern: image library. 2008. Available at: *http://www.dpd.cdc.gov/dpdx*)

drome (AIDS) found that a 3-day course of nitazoxanide compared to placebo was found to have a clinical response of 91% versus 36%, respectively, and a parasitologic response of 71% versus 0%, respectively.[46] An earlier study of HIV-infected patients from Mexico found that nitazoxanide for 2 weeks decreased diarrhea and cryptosporidial oocyst shedding only in patients with a CD4 count over 50 cells/mm^3.[47] Nitazoxanide therefore needs further study to clarify its role in patients with HIV.

Other. Though not approved for these indications, nitazoxanide has been reported to have activity against *Trichuris, E. histolytica, Toxocara, Ascaris, Enterobius, T. saginata,* and *Hymenolepis,* and variable activity with *Fasciola.*[48]

Side Effects. The adverse effects of nitazoxanide are mild and have been found to be similar to placebo.[46] They include abdominal pain, dyspepsia, nausea, and headache.

Paromomycin

Pharmacology. Paromomycin is a nonabsorbable aminoglycoside agent that acts like other aminoglycosides by binding to the 30S ribosomal RNA and inhibiting protein synthesis.

Therapeutic Approach. Paromomycin is used in the treatment of asymptomatic *E. histolytica* cyst passers and after metronidazole treatment of invasive amebiasis.[41] It has also been used in the treatment of *G. lamblia* at a dosage of 500 mg three times daily for 10 days, for which

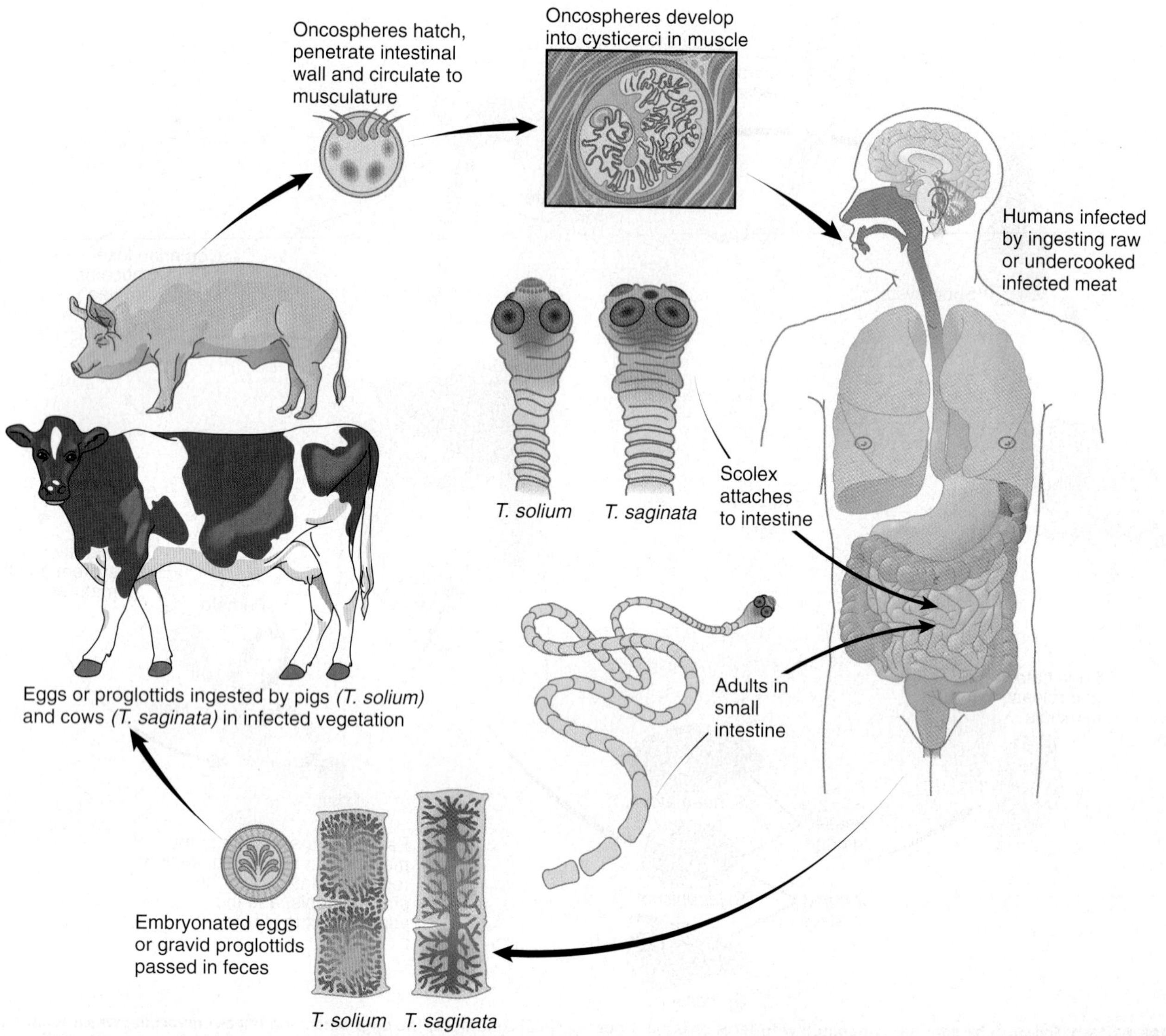

Oncospheres hatch, penetrate intestinal wall and circulate to musculature

Oncospheres develop into cysticerci in muscle

Humans infected by ingesting raw or undercooked infected meat

T. solium *T. saginata*

Scolex attaches to intestine

Adults in small intestine

Eggs or proglottids ingested by pigs *(T. solium)* and cows *(T. saginata)* in infected vegetation

Embryonated eggs or gravid proglottids passed in feces

T. solium *T. saginata*

FIGURE 83-14 • Taeniasis is the infection of humans with the adult tapeworm of *Taenia saginata* or *Taenia solium*. Humans are the only definitive hosts for *T. saginata* and *T. solium*. Eggs or gravid proglottids are passed with feces; the eggs can survive for days to months in the environment. Cattle (*T. saginata*) and pigs (*T. solium*) become infected by ingesting vegetation contaminated with eggs or gravid proglottids. In the animal's intestine, the oncospheres hatch, invade the intestinal wall, and migrate to the striated muscles, where they develop into cysticerci. A cysticercus can survive for several years in the animal. Humans become infected by ingesting raw or undercooked infected meat. In the human intestine, the cysticercus develops over 2 months into an adult tapeworm, which can survive for years. The adult tapeworms attach to the small intestine by their scolex and reside in the small intestine. Length of adult worms is usually 5 m or less for *T. saginata* (however, it may reach up to 25 m) and 2 to 7 m for *T. solium*. The adults produce proglottids that mature, become gravid, detach from the tapeworm, and migrate to the anus or are passed in the stool (approximately 6 worms/day). *T. saginata* adults usually have 1000 to 2000 proglottids, while *T. solium* adults have an average of 1000 proglottids. The eggs contained in the gravid proglottids are released after the proglottids are passed with the feces. *T. saginata* may produce up to 100,000 and *T. solium* may produce 50,000 eggs per proglottid, respectively. (From Division of Parasitic Diseases, Centers for Disease Control and Prevention. Laboratory identification of parasites of public health concern: image library. 2008. Available at: *http://www.dpd.cdc.gov/dpdx*)

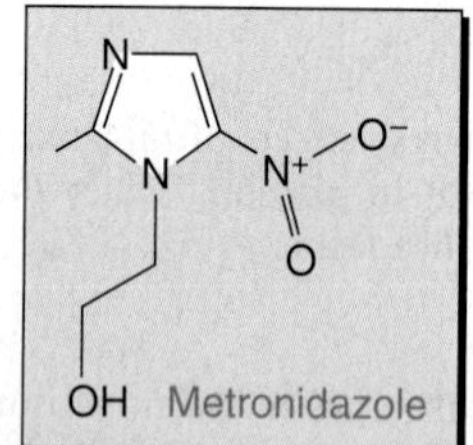

FIGURE 83-15 • **Metronidazole.**

it has had an efficacy of 55% to 90%.[40] A topical form has been used to treat cutaneous leishmaniasis and a parenteral form has been suggested for treatment of visceral leishmaniasis.[49,50] The topical form has also been applied in the treatment of resistant trichomoniasis.[13] Paromomycin has been suggested as a treatment option for *Cryptosporidium*, but some trials have found no benefit compared to placebo.[51]

Side Effects. Paromomycin may cause gastrointestinal side effects. Systemic administration can lead to ototoxicity and nephrotoxicity. Although poorly absorbed, oral paromomycin is still considered to be contraindicated in renal failure.[40]

Iodoquinol

Iodoquinol can be used as an intraluminal agent to eradicate the cyst form of *E. histolytica*. It has also been used in the treatment of *Dient-*

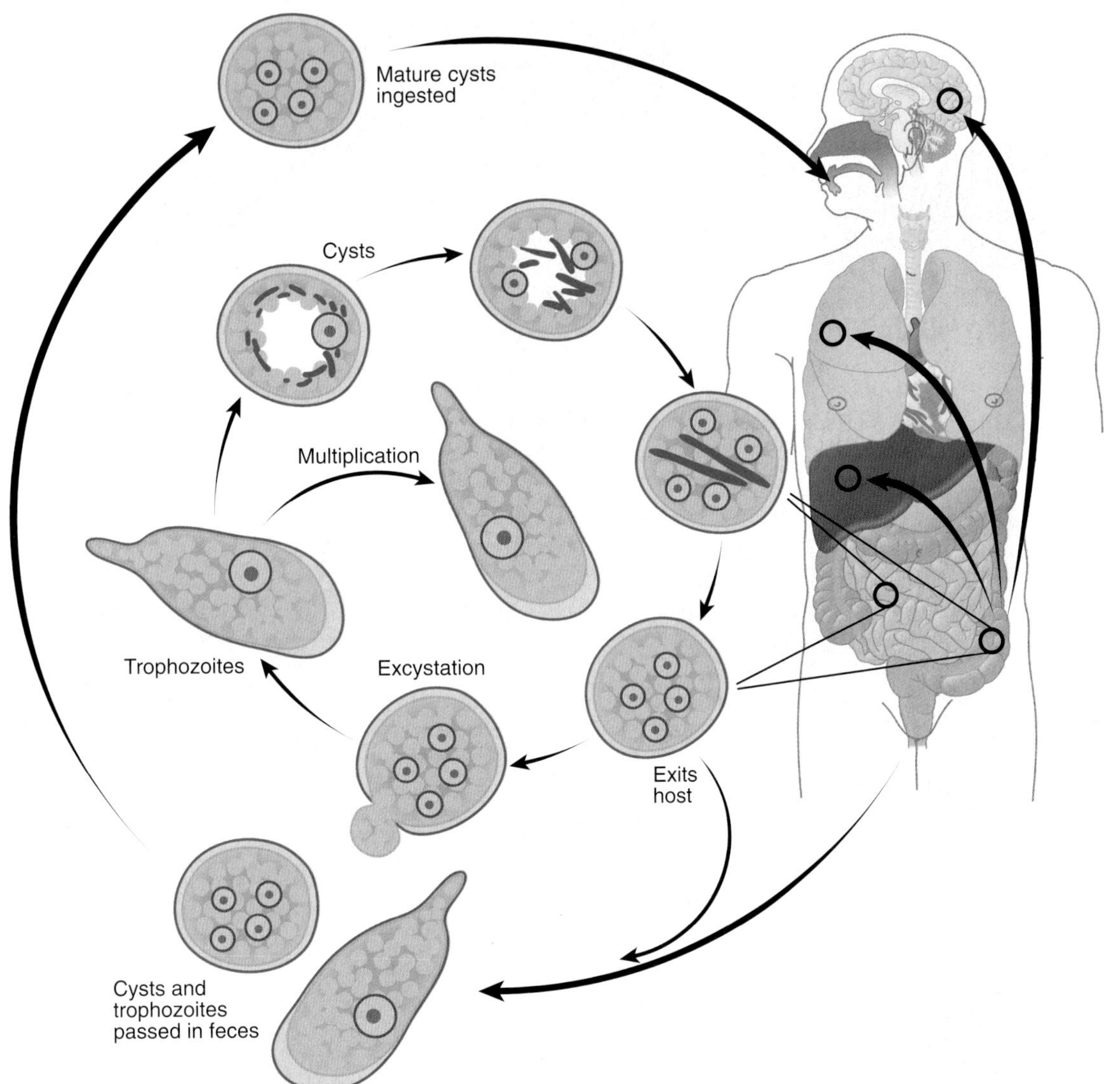

FIGURE 83-16 • *Entamoeba* cysts and trophozoites are passed in feces. Cysts are typically found in formed stool, whereas trophozoites are typically found in diarrheal stool. Infection by *Entamoeba histolytica* occurs by ingestion of mature cysts via fecally contaminated food, water, or hands. Excystation occurs in the small intestine, and trophozoites are released that migrate to the large intestine. The trophozoites multiply by binary fission and produce cysts, and both stages are passed in the feces. Because of the protection conferred by their walls, the cysts can survive days to weeks in the external environment and are responsible for transmission. Trophozoites passed in the stool are rapidly destroyed once outside the body, and if ingested would not survive exposure to the gastric environment. In many cases, the trophozoites remain confined to the intestinal lumen (noninvasive infection) of individuals who are asymptomatic carriers, passing cysts in their stool. In some patients the trophozoites invade the intestinal mucosa (intestinal disease), or, through the bloodstream, extraintestinal sites such as the liver, brain, and lungs (extraintestinal disease), with resultant pathologic manifestations. It has been established that the invasive and noninvasive forms represent two separate species, respectively *E. histolytica* and *E. dispar*. These two species are morphologically indistinguishable unless *E. histolytica* is observed with ingested red blood cells (erythrophagocystosis). Transmission can also occur through exposure to fecal matter during sexual contact (in which case not only cysts but also trophozoites could prove infective). (From Division of Parasitic Diseases, Centers for Disease Control and Prevention. Laboratory identification of parasites of public health concern: image library. 2008. Available at: *http://www.dpd.cdc.gov/dpdx*)

amoeba fragilis, *B. hominis*, and *Balantidium coli*.[13,52] Its mechanism of action is unknown. Rare side effects can include seizures, encephalopathy, and abdominal pain.

Diloxanide Furoate

Diloxanide furoate can be used to treat the cyst form of *E. histolytica*. The mechanism of action of the drug is unknown, and it is generally well tolerated.

Furazolidone

Furazolidone is used as an alternative treatment for giardiasis, with an efficacy of 80% to 96%.[40] It has several potential side effects, including gastrointestinal symptoms, monoamine oxidase inhibitory effects, and disulfiram-like reactions.

Atovaquone

Atovaquone in combination with pyrimethamine has been used to treat toxoplasmosis, and it is an alternate agent for babesiosis.

Pyrimethamine

Pyrimethamine is a dihydrofolate reductase inhibitor used in combination with sulfadiazine and leucovorin for the treatment of acute toxoplasmosis. Duration of treatment is typically for 4 to 6 weeks after the resolution of signs and symptoms.[53] It is also used in combination with dapsone for prophylaxis against toxoplasmosis in HIV-infected patients with CD4 counts less than 100 cells/mm^3. It has also been used as an alternative to trimethoprim-sulfamethoxazole in the treatment of *Isospora*. Leucovorin is given to mitigate the bone marrow suppression of pyrimethamine.

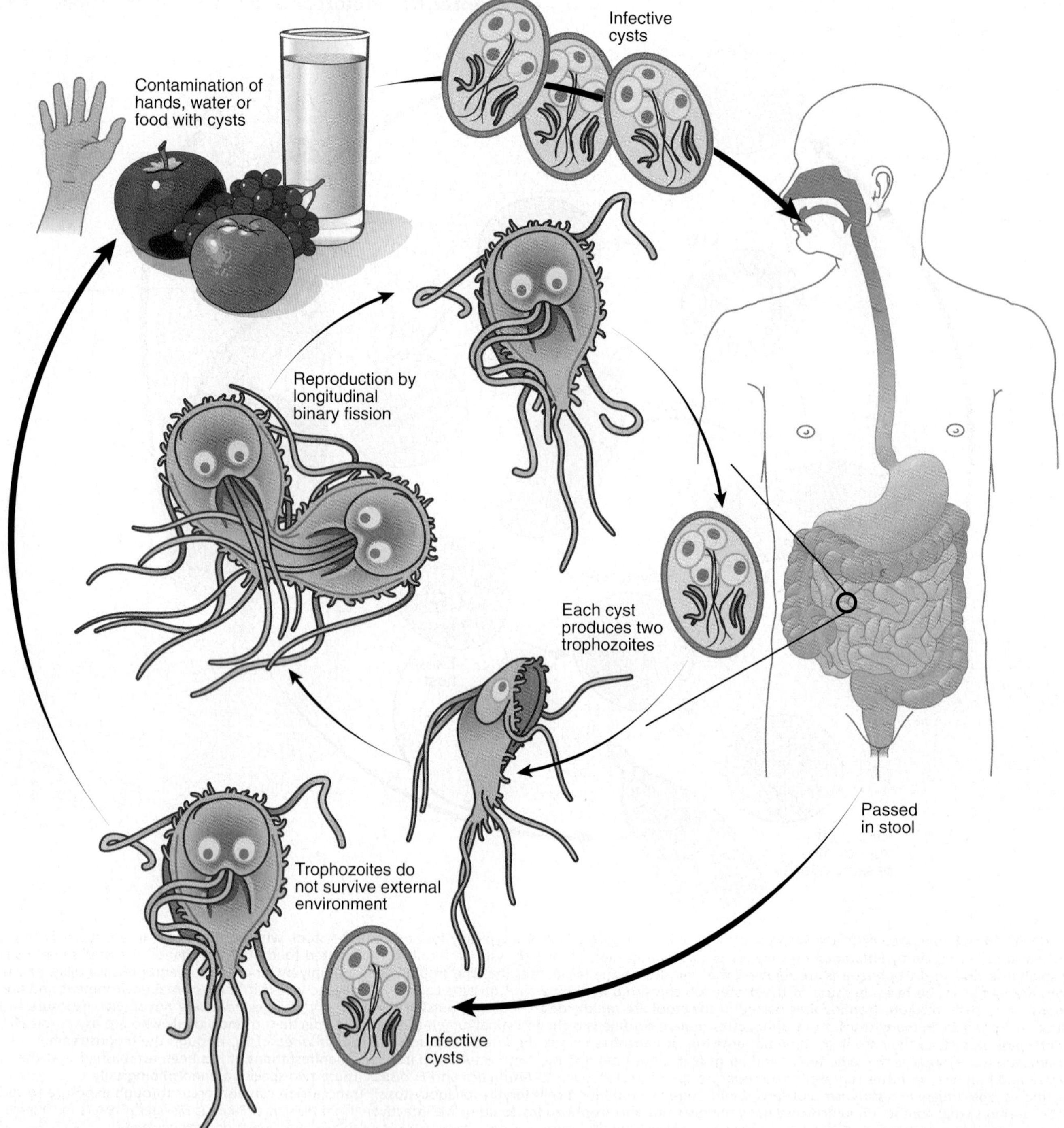

FIGURE 83-17 • *Giardia* cysts are resistant forms and are responsible for transmission of giardiasis. Both cysts and trophozoites can be found in the feces (diagnostic stages). The cysts are hardy and can survive several months in cold water. Infection occurs by the ingestion of cysts in contaminated water or food, or by the fecal-oral route (hands or fomites). In the small intestine, excystation releases trophozoites (each cyst produces two trophozoites). Trophozoites multiply by longitudinal binary fission, remaining in the lumen of the proximal small bowel, where they can be free or attached to the mucosa by a ventral sucking disk. Encystation occurs as the parasites transit toward the colon. The cyst is the stage found most commonly in nondiarrheal feces. Because the cysts are infectious when passed in the stool or shortly afterward, person-to-person transmission is possible. While animals are infected with *Giardia,* their importance as a reservoir is unclear. (From Division of Parasitic Diseases, Centers for Disease Control and Prevention. Laboratory identification of parasites of public health concern: image library. 2008. Available at: *http://www.dpd.cdc.gov/dpdx*)

Nitazoxanide

FIGURE 83-18 • Nitazoxanide.

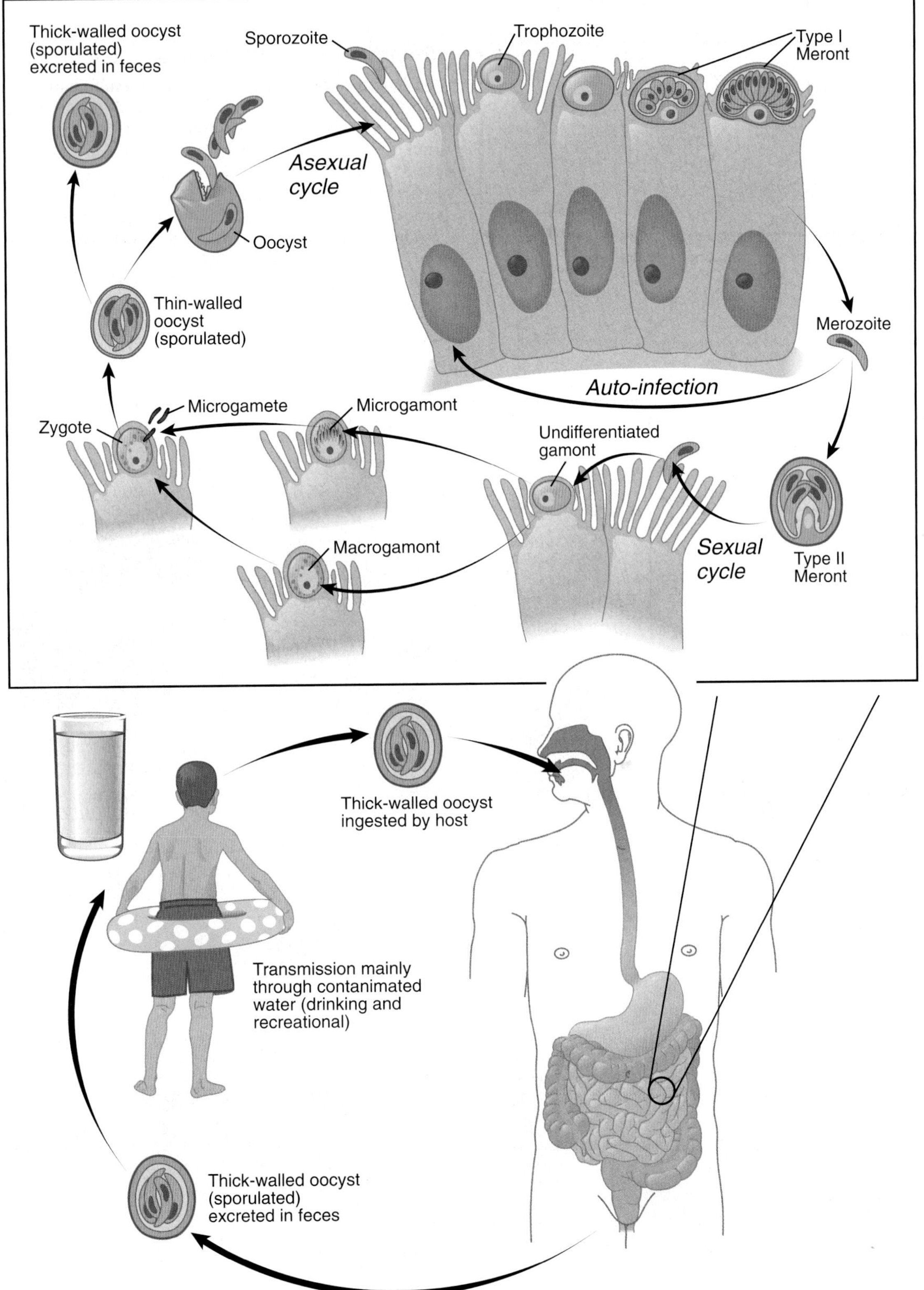

FIGURE 83-19 • Life cycle of *Cryptosporidium parvum* and *C. hominis.* Sporulated oocysts, containing four sporozoites, are excreted by the infected host through feces and possibly other routes such as respiratory secretions. Transmission of *C. parvum* and *C. hominis* occurs mainly through contact with contaminated water (e.g., drinking or recreational water). Occasionally food sources, such as chicken salad, may serve as vehicles for transmission. Many outbreaks in the United States have occurred in waterparks, community swimming pools, and day care centers. Zoonotic and anthroponotic transmission of *C. parvum* and anthroponotic transmission of *C. hominis* occur through exposure to infected animals or exposure to water contaminated by feces of infected animals. Following ingestion (and possibly inhalation) by a suitable host, excystation occurs. The sporozoites are released and parasitize epithelial cells of the gastrointestinal tract or other tissues such as the respiratory tract. In these cells, the parasites undergo asexual multiplication (schizogony or merogony) and then sexual multiplication (gametogony), producing microgamonts (male) and macrogamonts (female). Upon fertilization of the macrogamonts by the microgamonts, oocysts develop that sporulate in the infected host. Two different types of oocysts are produced, the thick-walled oocyst, which is commonly excreted from the host, and the thin-walled oocyst, which is primarily involved in autoinfection. Oocysts are infective upon excretion, thus permitting direct and immediate fecal-oral transmission. (Note that oocysts of *Cyclospora cayetanensis,* another important coccidian parasite, are unsporulated at the time of excretion and do not become infective until sporulation is completed.) (From Division of Parasitic Diseases, Centers for Disease Control and Prevention. Laboratory identification of parasites of public health concern: image library. 2008. Available at: *http://www.dpd.cdc.gov/dpdx.* Cryptosporidium stages were reproduced from Juranek DD. Cryptosporidiosis. In Strickland GT [ed]: Hunter's Tropical Medicine and Emerging Infectious Diseases, 8th ed. Philadelphia: WB Saunders, 2000. Originally adapted from the life cycle that appears in Current WL, Garcia LS. Cryptosporidiosis. Clin Microbiol Rev 1991;4:325-358.)

a) Trimethoprim b) Sulfamethoxazole

FIGURE 83-20 • Trimethoprim and sulfamethoxale.

Trimethoprim-Sulfamethoxazole (Fig. 83-20)

Pharmacology. Sulfamethoxazole is a sulfonamide that prevents the incorporation of *para*-aminobutyric acid into tetrahydropteroic acid. Trimethoprim inhibits dihydrofolate reductase, preventing the conversion of dihydrofolate to tetrahydrofolate and leading to inhibition of DNA synthesis. These two agents are combined in a 1 : 5 formulation of trimethoprim-sulfamethoxazole because trimethoprim has a five times higher volume of distribution than sulfamethoxazole.[13]

Therapeutic Approach. Trimethoprim-sulfamethoxazole is the drug of choice for *Isospora belli* (Fig. 83-21) and *Cyclospora cayatenensis* infection and has been used for prophylaxis or as an alternate treatment of *Toxoplasma gondii* in AIDS patients.[53]

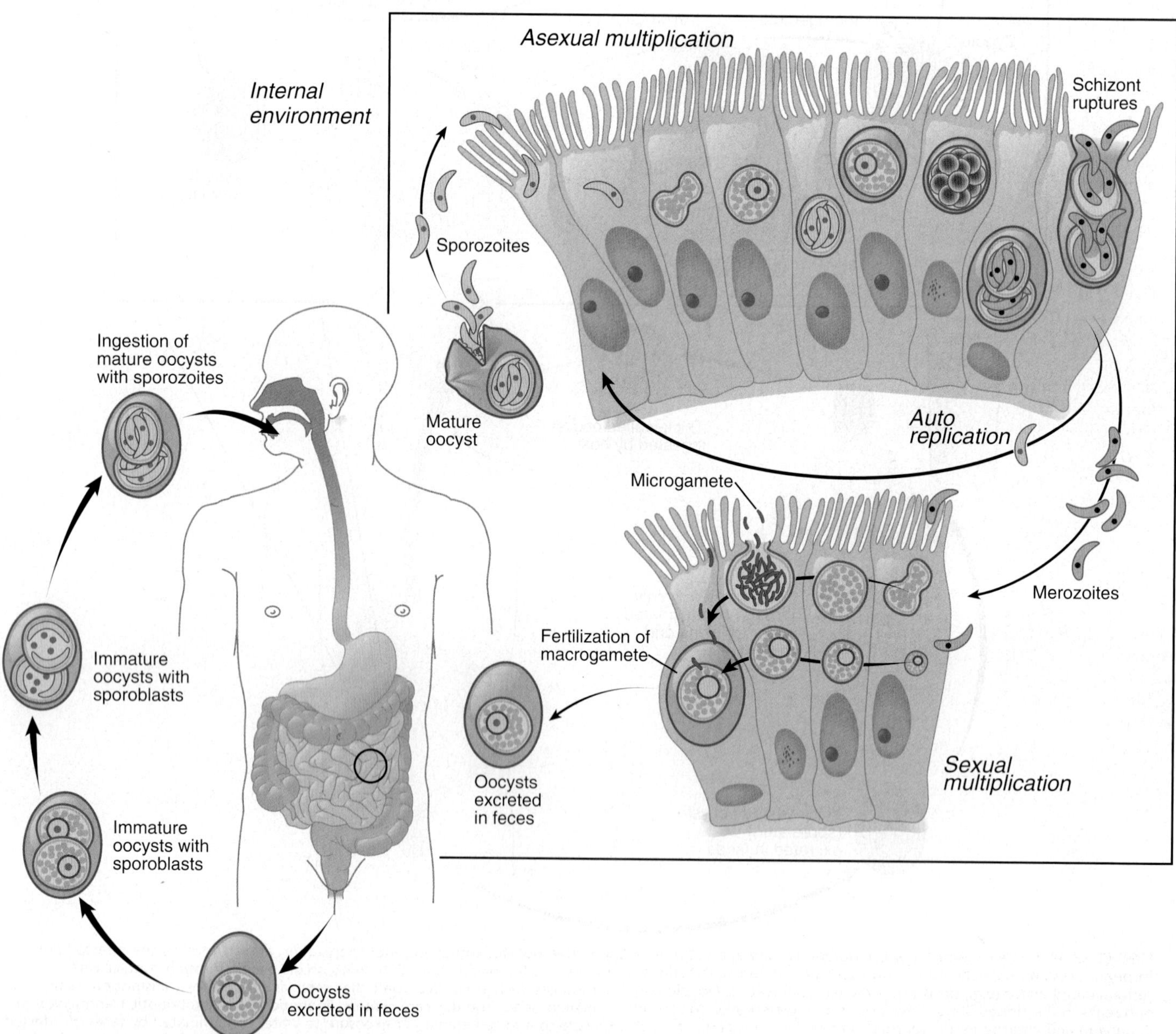

FIGURE 83-21 • At time of excretion, the immature *Isospora* oocyst contains usually one sporoblast (more rarely two). In further maturation after excretion, the sporoblast divides in two (the oocyst now contains two sporoblasts); the sporoblasts secrete a cyst wall, thus becoming sporocysts; and the sporocysts divide twice to produce four sporozoites each. Infection occurs by ingestion of sporocyst-containing oocysts: the sporocysts excyst in the small intestine and release their sporozoites, which invade the epithelial cells and initiate schizogony. Upon rupture of the schizonts, the merozoites are released, invade new epithelial cells, and continue the cycle of asexual multiplication. Trophozoites develop into schizonts that contain multiple merozoites. After a minimum of 1 week, the sexual stage begins with the development of male and female gametocytes. Fertilization results in the development of oocysts that are excreted in the stool. *Isospora belli* infects both humans and animals. (From Division of Parasitic Diseases, Centers for Disease Control and Prevention. Laboratory identification of parasites of public health concern: image library. 2008. Available at: *http://www.dpd.cdc.gov/dpdx*)

Side Effects. Trimethoprim-sulfamethoxazole can lead to the development of allergic reactions and gastrointestinal symptoms.

Additional Drugs

Dapsone. Dapsone can been combined with pyrimethamine for the prophylaxis of toxoplasmosis. Dapsone should not be used in patients who are glucose-6-phosphate dehydrogenase deficient. Its side effects include hemolytic anemia and bone marrow suppression.[13]

Clindamycin. Clindamycin is combined with pyrimethamine for prophylaxis and treatment of toxoplasmosis and is as effective as treatment with pyrimethamine and sulfadiazine.[54] It has also been used in the treatment of several other infections, including *Pneumocystis* and babesiosis.[13]

Spiramycin. This macrolide antibiotic has activity against toxoplasmosis. It is not an antifolate drug and can be used in pregnancy. It may lead to cardiac problems in neonates.[53]

Azithromycin. Azithromycin combined with atovaquone for 7 days was found to be as effective as clindamycin plus quinine for 7 days for the treatment of babesiosis,[55] but was associated with significantly fewer side effects.

Pentamidine. Pentamidine has been used in the treatment of antimony-resistant leishmaniasis and the hemolymphatic stages of *Trypanosoma brucei*.[56,57] Some of its significant side effects are renal failure, hypoglycemia, and tachycardia.

Suramin. Suramin is the drug of choice for early stages of African trypanosomiasis. It binds to and inhibits various trypanosomal enzymes, but its exact mechanism of action is unclear. Suramin must be given intravenously. There are several possible side effects, including rashes, renal failure, and anaphylaxis.[58] In the United States, it is available from the CDC.

Melarsoprol. Melarsoprol is an arsenical compound that is used to treat the late stage of both *T. brucei gambiense* and *T. brucei rhodesiense* infections. It has a significant complication of reactive encephalopathy in about 5% to 15% of patients that is lethal in 50% of cases.[59] Other reactions include polyneuropathy, exfoliative dermatitis, and fevers.[58]

Eflornithine. Eflornithine is used in the treatment of the hemolymphatic stage of *T. brucei gambiense*. It inhibits the *T. brucei gambiense* ornithine decarboxylase. It only is effective in those patients with an intact immune system.[57] It can cause bone marrow suppression, seizures, and diarrhea.

Nifurtimox. Nifurtimox is reported to be active against both stages of *T. brucei gambiense* infections. The adverse reactions to this medication include seizures, psychotic reactions, neuropathy, and weight loss.[57]

Benzinidazole. Benzinidazole can be used for therapy of acute Chagas' disease but is not available in the United States.

Stibogluconate. Stibogluconate is used to treat leishmaniasis. It is a pentavalent antimony that may cause cardiac toxicity, hepatic toxicity, and muscle aches.[60] It is only available from the CDC.

Amphotericin B. Amphotericin can be used in the treatment of leishmaniasis. It can cause chills, hypokalemia, and thrombophlebitis.

Miltefosine. Miltefosine is used in the treatment of leishmaniasis. Its side effects include gastrointestinal symptoms and elevation of hepatic transaminases.[60]

REFERENCES

1. Albanese G, Venturi C. Albendazole: a new drug for human parasitoses. Dermatol Clin 2003;21:283-290.
2. Venkatesan P. Albendazole. J Antimicrob Chemother 1998;41:145-147.
3. Bethony J, Brooker S, Albonico M, et al. Soil-transmitted helminth infections: ascariasis, trichuriasis, and hookworm. Lancet 2006;367:1521-1532.
4. Pene P, Mojon M, Garin JP, et al. Albendazole: a new broad spectrum anthelmintic. Double-blind multicenter clinical trial. Am J Trop Med Hyg 1982;31:263-266.
5. Sacko M, De Clercq D, Behnke JM, et al. Comparison of the efficacy of mebendazole, albendazole and pyrantel in treatment of human hookworm infections in the southern region of Mali, West Africa. Trans R Soc Trop Med Hyg 1999;93:195-203.
6. Cook GC. *Enterobius vermicularis* infection. Gut 1994;35:1159-1162.
7. Georgiev VS. Parasitic infections: treatment and developmental therapeutics. 1. Necatoriasis. Curr Pharm Des 1999;5:545-554.
8. Jackson TF, Epstein SR, Gouws E, Cheetham RF. A comparison of mebendazole and albendazole in treating children with *Trichuris trichiura* infection in Durban, South Africa. S Afr Med J 1998;88:880-883.
9. Belizario VY, Amarillo ME, de Leon WU, et al. A comparison of the efficacy of single doses of albendazole, ivermectin, and diethylcarbamazine alone or in combinations against *Ascaris* and *Trichuris* spp. Bull World Health Organ 2003;81:35-42.
10. Datry A, Hilmarsdottir I, Mayorga-Sagastume R, et al. Treatment of *Strongyloides stercoralis* infection with ivermectin compared with albendazole: results of an open study of 60 cases. Trans R Soc Trop Med Hyg 1994;88:344-345.
11. Satoh M, Kokaze A. Treatment strategies in controlling strongyloidiasis. Expert Opin Pharmacother 2004;5:2293-2301.
12. Dupouy-Camet J, Kociecka W, Bruschi F, et al. Opinion on the diagnosis and treatment of human trichinellosis. Expert Opin Pharmacother 2002;3:1117-1130.
13. Pearson R. Agents active against parasites and pneumocystis. *In* Mandell G, Bennett J, Dolin R (eds): Priniciples and Practice of Infectious Diseases, 6th ed. Philadelphia: Churchill Livingstone, 2005, pp 568-603.
14. Keshmiri M, Baharvahdat H, Fattahi SH, et al. Albendazole versus placebo in treatment of echinococcosis. Trans R Soc Trop Med Hyg 2001;95:190-194.
15. Khuroo MS, Dar MY, Yattoo GN, et al. Percutaneous drainage versus albendazole therapy in hepatic hydatidosis: a prospective, randomized study. Gastroenterology 1993;104:1452-1459.
16. Carpio A. Neurocysticercosis: an update. Lancet Infect Dis 2002;2:751-762.
17. Salinas R, Prasad K. Drugs for treating neurocysticercosis (tapeworm infection of the brain). Cochrane Database Syst Rev 2000;(2):CD000215.
18. Garcia HH, Pretell EJ, Gilman RH, et al. A trial of antiparasitic treatment to reduce the rate of seizures due to cerebral cysticercosis. N Engl J Med 2004;350:249-258.
19. Kalra V, Dua T, Kumar V. Efficacy of albendazole and short-course dexamethasone treatment in children with 1 or 2 ring-enhancing lesions of neurocysticercosis: a randomized controlled trial. J Pediatr 2003;143:111-114.
20. Gongora-Rivera F, Soto-Hernandez JL, Gonzalez Esquivel D, et al. Albendazole trial at 15 or 30 mg/kg/day for subarachnoid and intraventricular cysticercosis. Neurology 2006;66:436-438.
21. St. Georgiev V. Chemotherapy of enterobiasis (oxyuriasis). Expert Opin Pharmacother 2001;2:267-275.
22. Smego RA Jr, Bhatti S, Khaliq AA, Beg MA. Percutaneous aspiration-injection-reaspiration drainage plus albendazole or mebendazole for hepatic cystic echinococcosis: a meta-analysis. Clin Infect Dis 2003;37:1073-1083.
23. Blackwell V, Vega-Lopez F. Cutaneous larva migrans: clinical features and management of 44 cases presenting in the returning traveller. Br J Dermatol 2001;145:434-437.
24. Caumes E. Treatment of cutaneous larva migrans. Clin Infect Dis 2000;30:811-814.
25. St. Georgiev V. Pharmacotherapy of ascariasis. Expert Opin Pharmacother 2001;2:223-239.
26. El Setouhy M, Ramzy RM, Ahmed ES, et al. A randomized clinical trial comparing single- and multi-dose combination therapy with diethylcarbamazine and albendazole for treatment of bancroftian filariasis. Am J Trop Med Hyg 2004;70:191-196.
27. Nutman TB, Miller KD, Mulligan M, et al. Diethylcarbamazine prophylaxis for human loiasis: results of a double-blind study. N Engl J Med 1988;319:752-756.
28. Cairncross S, Muller R, Zagaria N. Dracunculiasis (Guinea worm disease) and the eradication initiative. Clin Microbiol Rev 2002;15:223-246.
29. Marti H, Haji HJ, Savioli L, et al. A comparative trial of a single-dose ivermectin versus three days of albendazole for treatment of *Strongyloides stercoralis* and other soil-transmitted helminth infections in children. Am J Trop Med Hyg 1996;55:477-481.
30. Gardon J, Boussinesq M, Kamgno J, et al. Effects of standard and high doses of ivermectin on adult worms of *Onchocerca volvulus:* a randomised controlled trial. Lancet 2002;360:203-210.
31. Dourmishev AL, Dourmishev LA, Schwartz RA. Ivermectin: pharmacology and application in dermatology. Int J Dermatol 2005;44:981-988.
32. Utzinger J, Keiser J, Shuhua X, et al. Combination chemotherapy of schistosomiasis in laboratory studies and clinical trials. Antimicrob Agents Chemother 2003;47:1487-1495.
33. Utzinger J, Keiser J. Schistosomiasis and soil-transmitted helminthiasis: common drugs for treatment and control. Expert Opin Pharmacother 2004;5:263-285.
34. Rim HJ. Clonorchiasis: an update. J Helminthol 2005;79:269-281.
35. Harinasuta T, Bunnag D, Radomyos P. Efficacy of praziquantel on fasciolopsiasis. Arzneimittelforschung 1984;34(9B):1214-1215.
36. Takayanagui OM, Jardim E. Therapy for neurocysticercosis: comparison between albendazole and praziquantel. Arch Neurol 1992;49:290-294.
37. Del Brutto OH, Campos X, Sanchez J, Mosquera A. Single-day praziquantel versus 1-week albendazole for neurocysticercosis. Neurology 1999;52:1079-1081.
38. Bacq Y, Besnier JM, Duong TH, et al. Successful treatment of acute fascioliasis with bithionol. Hepatology 1991;14:1066-1069.
39. Keiser J, Utzinger J. Chemotherapy for major food-borne trematodes: a review. Expert Opin Pharmacother 2004;5:1711-1726.
40. Gardner TB, Hill DR. Treatment of giardiasis. Clin Microbiol Rev 2001;14:114-128.
41. Haque R, Huston CD, Hughes M, et al. Amebiasis. N Engl J Med 2003;348:1565-1573.
42. Spence MR, Harwell TS, Davies MC, Smith JL. The minimum single oral metronidazole dose for treating trichomoniasis: a randomized, blinded study. Obstet Gynecol 1997;89(5 Pt 1):699-703.
43. Stenzel DJ, Boreham PF. *Blastocystis hominis* revisited. Clin Microbiol Rev 1996;9:563-584.
44. Fung HB, Doan TL. Tinidazole: a nitroimidazole antiprotozoal agent. Clin Ther 2005;27:1859-1884.
45. Amadi B, Mwiya M, Musuku J, et al. Effect of nitazoxanide on morbidity and mortality in Zambian children with cryptosporidiosis: a randomised controlled trial. Lancet 2002;360:1375-1380.

46. Rossignol JF, Ayoub A, Ayers MS. Treatment of diarrhea caused by *Giardia intestinalis* and *Entamoeba histolytica* or *E. dispar:* a randomized, double-blind, placebo-controlled study of nitazoxanide. J Infect Dis 2001;184:381-384.
47. Rossignol JF, Hidalgo H, Feregrino M, et al. A double-'blind' placebo-controlled study of nitazoxanide in the treatment of cryptosporidial diarrhoea in AIDS patients in Mexico. Trans R Soc Trop Med Hyg 1998;92:663-666.
48. Davila-Gutierrez CE, Vasquez C, Trujillo-Hernandez B, Huerta M. Nitazoxanide compared with quinfamide and mebendazole in the treatment of helminthic infections and intestinal protozoa in children. Am J Trop Med Hyg 2002;66:251-254.
49. Asilian A, Jalayer T, Nilforooshzadeh M, et al. Treatment of cutaneous leishmaniasis with aminosidine (paromomycin) ointment: double-blind, randomized trial in the Islamic Republic of Iran. Bull World Health Organ 2003;81:353-359.
50. Thakur CP, Kanyok TP, Pandey AK, et al. Treatment of visceral leishmaniasis with injectable paromomycin (aminosidine): an open-label randomized Phase-II clinical study. Trans R Soc Trop Med Hyg 2000;94:432-433.
51. Hewitt RG, Yiannoutsos CT, Higgs ES, et al. Paromomycin: no more effective than placebo for treatment of cryptosporidiosis in patients with advanced human immunodeficiency virus infection. AIDS Clinical Trial Group. Clin Infect Dis 2000;31:1084-1092.
52. Johnson EH, Windsor JJ, Clark CG. Emerging from obscurity: biological, clinical, and diagnostic aspects of *Dientamoeba fragilis.* Clin Microbiol Rev 2004;17:553-570.
53. Montoya JG, Liesenfeld O. Toxoplasmosis. Lancet 2004;363:1965-1976.
54. Dedicoat M, Livesley N. Management of toxoplasmic encephalitis in HIV-infected adults (with an emphasis on resource-poor settings). Cochrane Database Syst Rev 2006 19;(3):CD005420.
55. Krause PJ, Lepore T, Sikand VK, et al. Atovaquone and azithromycin for the treatment of babesiosis. N Engl J Med 2000;343:1454-1458.
56. Murray HW, Berman JD, Davies CR, Saravia NG. Advances in leishmaniasis. Lancet 2005;366:1561-1577.
57. Nok AJ. Effective measures for controlling trypanosomiasis. Expert Opin Pharmacother 2005;6:2645-2653.
58. Docampo R, Moreno SN. Current chemotherapy of human African trypanosomiasis. Parasitol Res 2003;90(Suppl 1):S10-S13.
59. Jannin J, Cattand P. Treatment and control of human African trypanosomiasis. Curr Opin Infect Dis 2004;17:565-571.
60. Sundar S, Rai M. Treatment of visceral leishmaniasis. Expert Opin Pharmacother 2005;6:2821-2829.

84

HIV INFECTIONS AND AIDS

Paul A. Pham and Charles W. Flexner

INTRODUCTION 1187
THERAPEUTICS AND CLINICAL PHARMACOLOGY 1187
Therapeutics by Class 1187
Nucleoside/Nucleotide Reverse Transcriptase Inhibitors 1187
Non-nucleoside Reverse Transcriptase Inhibitors 1188
Protease Inhibitors 1191
Entry Inhibitors 1193
Therapeutic Approach 1196
Emerging Targets and Therapeutics 1197
CCR5 Antagonists 1197
Integrase Inhibitors 1198
Maturation Inhibitors 1198
Anti-CD4 Monoclonal Antibody 1198

INTRODUCTION

Globally, there were 40.3 million people living with human immunodeficiency virus (HIV) and 3.1 million acquired immunodeficiency syndrome (AIDS) deaths in 2005.[1] The introduction of protease inhibitors and highly active antiretroviral therapy (HAART) in the mid-1990s revolutionized the treatment of HIV infection, transforming it from an almost universally fatal disease into a chronic, manageable illness. However, despite its profound effects on HIV-related morbidity and mortality, the use of HAART is associated with a number of problems that limit our ability to maintain durable virologic responses in a proportion of HIV-infected patients.

The pharmacotherapy of HIV infection is a dynamic and rapidly moving field, presenting a daunting task for clinicians who wish to keep their knowledge base up-to-date. Barriers to durable virologic suppression include adherence, resistance, and toxicity associated with antiretrovirals. In 2008, there were 25 antiretroviral drugs available in the United States: 7 nucleoside and 1 nucleotide reverse transcriptase inhibitors (NRTIs), 4 non-nucleoside reverse transcriptase inhibitors (NNRTIs), 10 protease inhibitors (PIs), 1 integrase inhibitor, and 2 entry inhibitors. Although there can be many potential antiretroviral combinations, understanding the pharmacology, side effect profile, and genotypic resistance pattern of these antiretrovirals can help clinicians develop a rational regimen that is convenient and well tolerated, has durable virologic suppression, and is tailored to the needs of the individual patient. Overviews of these antiretrovirals are summarized categorically.

THERAPEUTICS AND CLINICAL PHARMACOLOGY

Therapeutics by Class

Nucleoside/Nucleotide Reverse Transcriptase Inhibitors

Mechanism of Action. The RNA-dependent DNA polymerase of HIV, known as the reverse transcriptase, converts viral RNA into proviral DNA, which is then incorporated into the chromosome of the host cell. Inhibitors of this enzyme are either nucleoside/nucleotide analogues or non-nucleoside inhibitors. These drugs block infection of susceptible cells by HIV, but have no impact on cells that already harbor the virus. The NRTIs (abacavir, didanosine, emtricitabine, lamivudine, stavudine, tenofovir, zalcitabine, and zidovudine) must undergo intracellular phosphorylation to generate synthetic substrates for this enzyme. Triphosphorylated nucleoside analogues block replication of the virus in two ways: (i) by competitively inhibiting incorporation of native nucleotides into the nascent viral RNA-DNA duplex, and (ii) by terminating elongation of proviral DNA due to the absence of the 3′-hydroxyl group otherwise needed for chain elongation.

Tenofovir disoproxil fumarate (DF), a nucleotide analogue that belongs to the NRTI class, will be used in this discussion as a prototype for the NRTI class. It is an orally bioavailable prodrug of tenofovir, an acyclic nucleoside phosphonate diester analogue of adenosine 5′-monophosphate (Fig. 84-1). Tenofovir DF requires initial diester hydrolysis in the intestine for conversion to tenofovir, and subsequent phosphorylations by cellular enzymes to form tenofovir diphosphate. Tenofovir diphosphate inhibits the activity of HIV reverse transcriptase by competing with the natural substrate, deoxyadenosine 5′-triphosphate, and causing DNA chain termination. In vitro, tenofovir's 50% inhibitory concentration (IC_{50}) was in the range of 0.04 to 8.5 μM. The median reduction in HIV RNA was 1.6 $\log_{10}$ copies/ml in naive patients given monotherapy with tenofovir DF for 21 days.[2] Tenofovir DF appears to be more or as potent as other NRTIs, which decrease plasma concentrations of HIV RNA by 3- to 100-fold.[3]

Pharmacokinetics. The absolute bioavailability of tenofovir DF is 25% under fasting conditions. Bioavailability is approximately 40% higher when administered with a high-fat (1000 kcal, 50% fat) meal. In comparison, zidovudine absorption is decreased by 24% with a fatty meal and didanosine absorption is decreased by 55% with food.[4] Tenofovir DF is rapidly hydrolyzed to tenofovir via plasma esterases following oral absorption. Tenofovir is well distributed, with a volume of distribution of 1.2 L/kg and a low protein binding of less than 7%. Similar to other NRTIs (with the exception of zidovudine and abacavir), tenofovir undergoes minimal systemic metabolism; it is cleared by glomerular filtration and active tubular secretion, therefore the dose should be decreased in patients with renal insufficiency. Tenofovir DF has the longest plasma and intracellular half-life (approximately 17 and 60 to over 175 hours, respectively) of any NRTI.[5] The intracellular half-lives of other NRTIs range from 3 to 40 hours, which allows for once-a-day or twice-a-day dosing.

Drug-Drug Interactions. Similar to other NRTIs, tenofovir is not a substrate, inducer, or inhibitor of the cytochrome P-450 (CYP) enzyme system; therefore, there are only limited numbers of drug interactions of clinical relevance. Didanosine concentrations are increased when coadministered with tenofovir DF. This interaction may increase the risk of pancreatitis and has been associated with a paradoxical CD4 cell decline in treated patients.[6-9] The proposed mechanism of this interaction is an interference with didanosine breakdown by direct inhibition of purine nucleoside phosphorylase by tenofovir DF.[10] It is recommended to reduce the dose of didanosine (250 mg of the enteric-coated formulation in patients weighing ≥60 kg, or 200 mg in patients weighing <60 kg) with tenofovir DF coadministration.[11] However, the combination of tenofovir DF with dose-reduced didanosine plus efavirenz is not recommended due to high

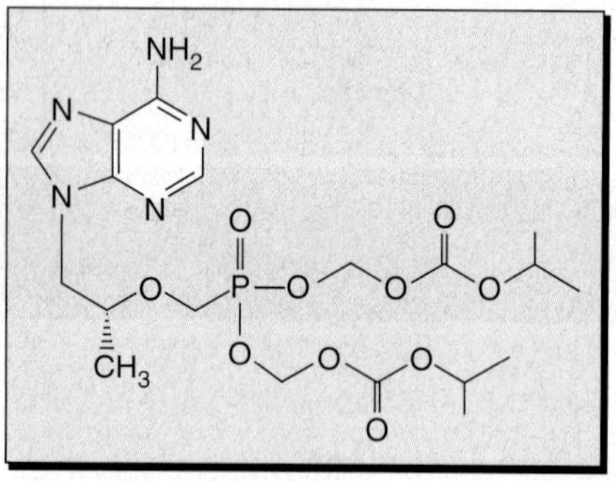

FIGURE 84-1 • Chemical structure of tenofovir disoproxil fumarate.

rates of early virologic failure.[12,13] Atazanavir's plasma concentrations are lower when administered with tenofovir DF. Although most pharmacokinetic parameters did not reach statistical significance, the area under the concentration-time curve (AUC) of atazanavir was significantly reduced by 25%.[14] This interaction is not likely to be clinically significant when atazanavir is also coadministered with ritonavir, since the inhibitory effect of ritonavir on atazanavir metabolism results in a threefold increase in the atazanavir AUC, which more than compensates for the effect of tenofovir DF on atazanavir concentrations.

Resistance. NRTI resistance generally follows several mutational patterns. Resistance to thymidine analogue mutations (zidovudine and stavudine) is associated with mutations at reverse transcriptase codons 41, 44, 67, 70, 118, 210, 215, and 219.[15] Two clusters of resistance mutations occur commonly. The pattern of 41L (leucine), 210W (tryptophan), and 215Y (tyrosine) is associated with high-level resistance to zidovudine as well as cross-resistance to other drugs in this class, including tenofovir and abacavir. The pattern 67N (asparagine), 70R (arginine), 215F (phenylalanine), and 219Q (glutamine) is less common and is also associated with lower levels of resistance and cross-resistance. Mutations accumulated gradually when zidovudine was used as the sole antiretroviral agent, and clinical resistance developed in only 31% of patients after 1 year of zidovudine monotherapy.[16] Cross-resistance to multiple nucleoside analogues has been reported following prolonged therapy and has been associated with a mutation cluster involving codons 62, 75, 77, 116, and 151. In addition, a mutation at codon 69 (typically T69S) followed by a two-amino acid insertion produces cross-resistance to all current nucleoside/nucleotide analogues.[15] On the other hand, tenofovir's signature mutation, K65R, results in variably reduced susceptibility to tenofovir as well as to didanosine, abacavir, and lamivudine. Susceptibility to zidovudine is preserved or increased, and susceptibility to stavudine is decreased, with K65R. Patients failing initial regimens containing tenofovir DF may develop this mutation; however, this was not consistently seen in all trials, with 0 to 2.7% of patients developing the K65R with virologic failure.[17,18]

Safety and Tolerability. The selective toxicity of NRTIs is a consequence of their ability to inhibit the HIV reverse transcriptase without inhibiting human cellular DNA polymerases. The intracellular triphosphates for these drugs generally have low affinity for human DNA polymerases-α and -β. However, some are capable of inhibiting human DNA polymerase-γ, the mitochondrial enzyme, resulting in several important toxicities common to this class of drugs.[19] This in turn impairs the ability of the respiratory chain to recycle NAD^+ from its reduced form, NADH. Reduction of NAD^+ ultimately shifts the equilibrium toward lactate and away from its precursor, pyruvate. Common examples of mitochondrial toxicity include peripheral neuropathy and lipoatrophy. Lactic acidosis, which may be accompanied by hepatosteatosis, can be fatal.

In vitro studies suggest that tenofovir DF, abacavir, emtricitabine, and lamivudine are less toxic to mitochondria than the other NRTIs (e.g., stavudine, didanosine, and zidovudine).[20,21] Results of in vitro and animal studies are consistent with findings in clinical studies, in which peripheral neuropathy, lipodystrophy (predominantly lipoatrophy), and lactic acidosis were reported in 83 (28%) of 301 stavudine-treated patients and only 17 (6%) of 299 tenofovir DF–treated patients ($P < .001$).[17]

Proximal renal tubular dysfunction, interstitial nephritis, nephrogenic diabetes insipidus, and acute tubular necrosis have been reported rarely in patients taking tenofovir DF.[22] However, clinical trials have not shown a significantly higher rate of renal insufficiency compared to patients on control arms.[17,18]

Clinical Efficacy of NRTI-Based Regimens. Clinical efficacy of emtricitabine or lamivudine when combined with tenofovir plus a PI or an NNRTI is well established and is one of the recommended initial combinations in the U.S. Department of Health and Human Services (DHHS) guidelines[24] (see Table 84-6). These recommendations are based on a randomized, multicenter, double-blind trial comparing tenofovir DF and stavudine, both administered in combination with lamivudine and efavirenz, in 602 antiretroviral therapy (ART)–naive patients.[17] Patients had a mean HIV RNA of 81,300 copies/ml, and 45% of participants had a baseline HIV RNA greater than 100,000 copies/ml. At 144 weeks, 71% of patients in the tenofovir DF arm and 64% in the stavudine arm achieved an HIV RNA less than 400 copies/ml by intent-to-treat, missing, or switch-equals-failure analysis, with no significant difference in response by baseline HIV RNA or CD4 cell count. HIV RNA suppression to below 50 copies/ml was achieved in 68% of tenofovir DF recipients and 63% of stavudine recipients. Through week 144, mean CD4 cell increases were 263 and 283 cells/mm^3 in the tenofovir DF and stavudine arms, respectively.

In another 144-week multicenter, open-label trial comparing tenofovir DF plus emtricitabine vs. coformulated zidovudine/lamivudine, both administered in combination with efavirenz, in 509 treatment-naive patients,[18] mean baseline HIV RNA was 5.0 $\log_{10}$ copies/ml. At 48 weeks, 84% of the 487 evaluable subjects in the tenofovir DF + emtricitabine arm had an HIV RNA below 400 copies/ml compared to 73% in the zidovudine/lamivudine arm ($P = .002$) by the U.S. Food and Drug Administration (FDA)–mandated time to loss of viral response analysis. Suppression to less than 50 copies/ml was achieved in 80% and 70% of subjects, respectively ($P = .02$).[18] The higher intent-to-treat success rate in the tenofovir DF + emtricitabine arm was due to a higher rate of discontinuation as a result of adverse events in the zidovudine/lamivudine arm (9% vs. 4%; $P = .016$), with 6% discontinuing due to anemia.

Certain NRTI combinations should be avoided due to in vivo antagonism (e.g., zidovudine plus stavudine), high rate of virologic failure (e.g., tenofovir plus abacavir or didanosine), or increased risk of toxicity (e.g., didanosine plus stavudine).[24] The most important combinations to be avoided are summarized in Box 84-1. Table 84-1 summarizes the pharmacokinetics parameters, advantages, and disadvantages of the available NRTIs.

Non-nucleoside Reverse Transcriptase Inhibitors

Mechanism of Action. NNRTIs do not affect the active site of the viral reverse transcriptase, but bind to a nonessential hydrophobic pocket in the p66 subunit of the enzyme. This binding pocket is distant from the active site. These drugs induce a conformational change in the reverse transcriptase that greatly reduces its efficiency, and act

BOX 84-1 REGIMENS THAT SHOULD NOT BE USED

- AZT combined with d4T in any regimen
- ddI combined with d4T in any regimen
- 3TC combined with FTC
- TDF + ddI + 3TC once daily
- TDF + ddI + EFV *or* NVP

AZT, zidovudine; ddI, didanosine; d4T, stavudine; EFV, efavirenz; FTC, emtricitabine; NVP, nevirapine; TDF, tenofovir disoproxil fumarate; 3TC, lamivudine.
Adapted from references 24 and 60.

TABLE 84-1 PROPERTIES OF NUCLEOSIDE/NUCLEOTIDE REVERSE TRANSCRIPTASE INHIBITORS (NRTIs)

NRTI	Dose	Pharmacokinetics	Comments
Abacavir (ABC; Ziagen)	*ABC:* 300 mg bid *Coformulated product:* Epzicom (ABC 600 mg + 3TC 300 mg), 1 tab qd Trizivir (AZT 300 mg + 3TC 110 mg + ABC 300 mg), 1 tab bid	*Absorption:* Well absorbed with 83% oral bioavailability. *Metabolism and Excretion:* 81% metabolized by alcohol dehydrogenase and glucuronyl transferase with renal excretion of metabolites; 16% recovered in stool and 1% unchanged in urine. *Protein Binding:* Low (50%) C_{max}: 3 mcg/ml; AUC: 6 mcg/ml/hr. Intracellular levels of carbovir triphosphate: 100 FM/million cells. $T^1/_2$: serum, 1.5 hr; intercellular (carbovir triphosphate), 12-20 hr.	**Pros:** One of the most potent NRTIs, with VL reduction of 1.5-2.0 logs in monotherapy; coformulated with 3TC (Epzicom) and with AZT/3TC (Trizivir); good data on ABC/3TC as well-tolerated and effective. **Cons:** Hypersensitivity reaction; must screen for HLA-B*5701 requires detailed pretreatment counseling/education; can be fatal with rechallenge.
Didanosine (ddI; Videx)	*Weight > 60 kg:* 400 mg qd (tabs and enteric-coated caps) or 500 mg qd (powder) *Weight < 60 kg:* 250 mg qd (tabs) or 334 mg qd (powder) Dose can also be taken in two divided doses. Must be taken on an empty stomach.	*Absorption:* 30-40% absorption on an empty stomach. *Metabolism and Excretion:* 50% excreted unchanged in the urine via glomerular filtration and tubular secretion. *Protein Binding:* Low (<5%) C_{max}: 1.6 mcg/ml after a single dose of 375 mg. $T^1/_2$: serum, 1.6 hr; intracellular, 25-40 hr.	**Pros:** good clinical track record; qd administration. **Cons:** GI intolerance with powder; need to be taken on an empty stomach; pancreatitis and mitochondrial toxicity; relative lack of controlled data in HAART era for ddI + 3TC or ddI + FTC compared to other dual-NRTI backbones.
Emtricitabine (FTC; Emtriva)	*FTC (cap):* 200 mg qd *FTC (liquid):* 240 mg qd *Coformulated products:* Truvada (TDF 300 mg + FTC 200 mg), 1 tab qd Atripla (TDF 300 mg + FTC 200 mg + EFV 600 mg), 1 tab qd	*Absorption:* Well absorbed with an absolute bioavailability of 93%. *Metabolism and Excretion:* Only 13% of administered dose is metabolized to sulfadoxide and glucuronide metabolites. Metabolites and unchanged drug are excreted primarily via glomerular filtration and tubular secretion. *Protein Binding:* Low (<4%) Mean C_{max}: 1.8 mcg/ml; C_{min}: 0.09 g/ml; AUC: 10 mcg/ml/hr after 200-mg qd at steady state. $T^1/_2$: 10 hr.	**Pros:** Activity against HBV; well tolerated; qd dosing; coformulation with TDF; similar to 3TC with respect to activity, tolerability, and resistance profile. **Cons:** Hyperpigmentation in some patients; high-level resistance for single point mutation (184V); risk of fulminant hepatitis if FTC is withdrawn in HBV co-infected patients.
Lamivudine (3TC; Epivir)	*3TC:* 150 mg bid *Coformulated products:* Epzicom (ABC 600 mg + 3TC 300 mg), 1 tab qd Combivir (AZT 300 mg + 3TC 150 mg), 1 tab bid Trizivir (AZT 300 mg + 3TC 150 mg + ABC 300 mg), 1 tab bid	*Absorption:* 86% absorption. *Metabolism and Excretion:* Renal excretion accounts for 71%. *Protein Binding:* Low (36%); high volume of distribution (1.3 L/kg) C_{max}: 3 mcg/ml. Intracellular levels of carbovir triphosphate: 100 FM/million cells. $T^1/_2$: serum, 5-7 hr; intracellular, 12 hr.	**Pros:** very well tolerated; active against HBV; qd dosing; 3TC or FTC are essential components of all recommended initial regimens; coformulated with AZT (Combivir), ABC (Epzicom), and AZT + ABC (Trizivir). **Cons:** high-level resistance with single point mutation (184V); risk of fulminant hepatitis if 3TC is withdrawn in co-infected patients; high rate of HBV resistance with prolonged therapy of HBV.
Stavudine (d4T; Zerit)	*Weight > 60 kg:* 40 mg bid *Weight < 60 kg:* 30 mg bid Lower dose of d4T (30 mg bid) is as effective*	*Absorption:* 86% absorption with or without food. *Metabolism and Excretion:* 50% excreted unchanged in the urine via glomerular filtration and tubular secretion. C_{max}: 1.4 mcg/ml after a single dose of 70 mg. C_{max} for the Triomune (NVP/3TC/d4T) formulation is 40% higher than Zerit (d4T). $T^1/_2$: serum, 1.0 hr; intracellular, 3.5 hr.	**Pros:** well-studied NRTI, well tolerated in the short term. **Cons:** NRTI most commonly associated with mitochondrial toxicity that can result in fatal lactic acidosis, peripheral neuropathy, and lipoatrophy.
Zidovudine (AZT; Retrovir)	*AZT:* 300 mg bid *Coformulated products:* Combivir (AZT 300 mg + 3TC 150 mg), 1 tab bid Trizivir (AZT 300 mg + 3TC 150 mg + ABC 300 mg), 1 tab bid	*Absorption:* 60% absorption; high-fat meals may decrease absorption (clinical significance unknown). *Metabolism and Excretion:* Metabolized by liver to glucuronide (G-ZVD) that is renally excreted. *Protein Binding:* Low (34-38%) Mean steady state C_{max}: 1.5 mcg/ml. AZT triphosphate intracellular levels: 0.19 mcg/ml. $T^1/_2$: plasma, 1.1 hr; intracellular, 3 hr.	**Pros:** Extensive long-term data and clinical experience; documented efficacy in preventing perinatal and occupational transmission; effective in treating thrombocytopenia. High-level resistance requires multiple mutations. **Cons:** bid dosing; GI intolerance (especially nausea), headaches, fatigue, asthenia, anemia, neutropenia; mitochondrial toxicity, including lipoatrophy, lactic acidosis, hepatic steatosis; AZT/3TC less effective than TDF/FTC at 48 wk, primarily because of greater dropout due to anemia and other side effects.

TABLE 84-1 PROPERTIES OF NUCLEOSIDE/NUCLEOTIDE REVERSE TRANSCRIPTASE INHIBITORS (NRTIs)—cont'd

NRTI	Dose	Pharmacokinetics	Comments
Zalcitabine (ddC; Hivid)	*ddC:* 0.75 mg tid	*Absorption:* 70-88% absorption. *Metabolism and Excretion:* 70% excreted unchanged in the urine via glomerular filtration and tubular secretion. *Protein Binding:* Low (<4%) C_{max}: 25.2 ng/ml; AUC: 72 ng/ml/hr (ddC 1.5 mg). Intracellular levels: no data. $T^1/_2$: plasma, 1.2 hr; intracellular, 3 hr.	**Pros:** None. Pulled from the US market. **Cons:** tid administration; low potency; high incidence of ADRs, including mitochondrial toxicity; not well studied; rarely used for these reasons.
Tenofovir (TDF; Viread)	*TDF:* 300 mg qd *Coformulated products:* Truvada (TDF 300 mg + FTC 200 mg), 1 tab qd Atripla (TDF 300 mg + FTC 200 mg + EFV 600 mg), 1 tab qd	*Absorption:* 30% absorption fasting and 40% absorption with fatty meal. *Metabolism and Excretion:* Undergoes renal elimination. *Protein Binding:* Low (<7.2%) Mean C_{max}: 296 ± 90 ng/ml; AUC: 2287 ± 685 ng/ml/hr.	**Pros:** qd administration; well tolerated with few short-term side effects and no clear mitochondrial or other long-term toxicity; activity against some NRTI-resistant strains; longer intracellular half-life than most NRTIs; active against HBV. Coformulations available, including the only single-pill, once-daily regimen (TDF/FTC/EFV). **Cons:** potential for nephrotoxicity.

*Milinkovic A, López S, Miro O, et al. A randomized open study comparing the impact of reducing stavudine dose vs. switching to tenofovir on mitochondrial function, metabolic parameters, and subcutaneous fat in HIV-infected patients receiving antiretroviral therapy containing stavudine. CROI 2005 abstract 857. *In* Program and Abstracts of the 12th Conference on Retroviruses and Opportunistic Infections, Boston, MA, February 22-25, 2005.

ADRs, adverse drug reactions; AUC, area under the concentration-time curve; bid, twice daily; C_{max}, peak concentration; C_{min}, trough concentration; GI, gastrointestinal; HAART, highly active antiretroviral therapy; HBV, hepatitis B virus; qd, daily.

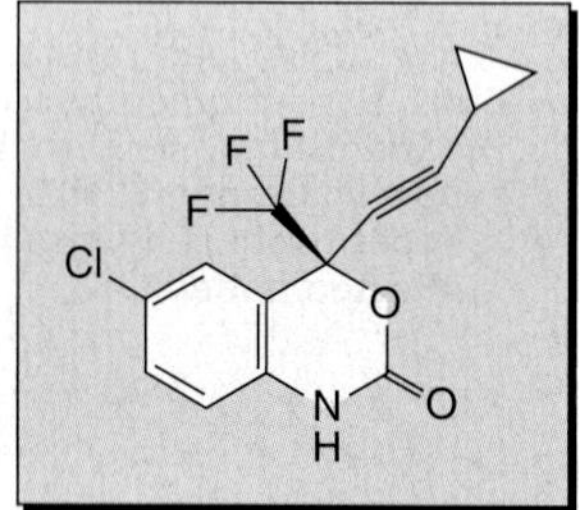

FIGURE 84-2 • Chemical structure of efavirenz.

as noncompetitive inhibitors of the enzyme.[25] There are currently four approved NNRTIs (delavirdine, efavirenz, nevirapine, and etravirine) in the United States; however, due to the frequent dosing requirement of delavirdine (thrice daily), it is not routinely recommended.[24]

Efavirenz, a 1,4-dihydro-2H-3,1-benzoxazin-2-one NNRTI (Fig. 84-2) with an in vitro IC_{50} that ranges from 3 to 9 nM,[26] will be used here as the prototype for the NNRTI class. Like all NNRTIs, efavirenz has no activity against HIV-2 and should not be used to treat HIV-2 infection.[27] Unlike NRTIs, NNRTIs do not require intracellular phosphorylation to become active. These compounds have no activity against human DNA polymerases, and are not associated with mitochondrial toxicity. The two most commonly used agents in this class, efavirenz and nevirapine, could transiently decrease plasma HIV RNA concentrations by 100-fold or greater when used as sole agents in early studies.[28]

Pharmacokinetics. Efavirenz has excellent oral bioavailability and is well absorbed from the gastrointestinal tract, reaching peak plasma concentrations within 5 hours after administration. The bioavailability is increased by a high-fat meal (22% mean increase in AUC). Efavirenz is greater than 99% bound to plasma proteins, and has a low cerebrospinal fluid (CSF):plasma ratio of 0.01, presumably as a consequence of high protein binding.[29] Since the major toxicities of efavirenz involve the central nervous system (CNS), the clinical significance of this low CNS penetration is unclear. The 516T/T genotype of the human CYP isoenzyme 2B6 gene, more frequently found in African Americans, was associated with higher plasma efavirenz concentrations, slower clearance, and increased early CNS toxicity.[30] It is recommended that the drug be taken on an empty stomach at bedtime to reduce these side effects.

Similar to other approved NNRTIs, efavirenz is eliminated from the body by hepatic metabolism. Nevirapine and delavirdine are primarily substrates for the CYP 3A4 isoform, while efavirenz is primarily a substrate for CYP 2B6[29] and to a lesser extent 3A4. The parent drug is not renally excreted to a significant extent.[29] Efavirenz is slowly cleared, with an elimination half-life of 40 to 55 hours at steady state; this allows once-daily dosing.

Drug-Drug Interactions. Similar to nevirapine, efavirenz is a moderate inducer of hepatic drug-metabolizing enzymes, especially CYP3A4. As a consequence, efavirenz may decrease the concentrations of coadministered anticonvulsants such as phenobarbital, phenytoin, and carbamazepine. Efavirenz also reduces the steady state AUC of methadone by an average of 33% to 66%.[23] Rifampin concentrations are not changed by concurrent efavirenz, but rifampin reduces efavirenz concentrations. In contrast, efavirenz reduced the AUC of rifabutin by 38% on average. With the exception of nelfinavir and ritonavir, efavirenz induces the metabolism of all other HIV PIs: amprenavir, indinavir, atazanavir, saquinavir, lopinavir, darunavir, tipranavir, and fosamprenavir concentrations are reduced. However, if PIs are pharmacokinetically boosted with low doses of ritonavir, the coadministration of efavirenz is possible with dose adjustment. Carbamazepine decreased the AUC of efavirenz by 34%; similarly, other anticonvulsants that induce CYP2B6 and/or CYP3A4 (e.g., phenobarbital and phenytoin) would be expected to increase the clearance of efavirenz and should be avoided.[23]

Resistance. The development of resistance to nucleoside analogues and PIs develops gradually over months. However, efavirenz and nevirapine can induce resistance and virologic relapse within days or weeks if given as monotherapy.[31] Exposure to only a single dose of nevirapine to prevent mother-to-child transmission of HIV is associated with resistance mutations in up to one third of patients.[32] These agents are potent and highly effective, but must be combined with at least two other active agents to avoid resistance. The most common resistance mutation seen clinically is at codon 103 of reverse transcriptase (K103N), and this decreases susceptibility by greater than 100-fold.[33] Additional resistance mutations have been seen at reverse transcriptase codons 100, 106, 108, 181, 188, 190, and 225. With the exception of 181C, where efavirenz sensitivity is retained, cross-resistance extends to nevirapine and delavirdine.[33] Any patient who fails treatment with one NNRTI because of a specific resistance mutation should be considered to have failed the entire class, with the exception of etravirine (TMC-125), a newly approved NNRTI.

Safety and Tolerability. Similar to other drugs in this class, rash occurs frequently with efavirenz and is reported in up to 27% of patients.[34] The median time to the onset of the rash is 11 days and the rash lasts about 2 weeks. However, in contrast to nevirapine, rash due to efavirenz is not as severe, requiring discontinuation in only 1.7% of cases, compared to a 7% discontinuation rate with nevirapine. Life-threatening skin eruptions such as Stevens-Johnson syndrome have been reported with nevirapine, and rarely with efavirenz; however, this remains a theoretical concern with all NNRTIs.

The most common reported adverse effects of efavirenz involve the CNS. CNS or psychiatric side effects are reported in up to 53% of patients, but fewer than 5% discontinue the drug because of this. CNS symptoms may occur with the first dose, and are most commonly reported within the first 2 weeks of treatment. Severe symptoms may sometimes persist for several weeks. It is not unusual for patients to report dizziness, impaired concentration, dysphoria, vivid or disturbing dreams, and insomnia. Rarely, frank psychosis (including depression, hallucinations, and/or mania) has been associated with initiating efavirenz. Most CNS side effects diminish or resolve within the first 4 weeks of therapy.

False-positive screening tests for marijuana metabolites can also occur.[33] Other side effects reported with efavirenz include hepatitis and elevated serum cholesterol. However, unlike nevirapine's severe acute hepatitis, which is reported in up to 11% of treatment-naive women with CD4 counts greater than 250 cells/mm^3 and 6.4% of men with CD4 counts greater than 400 cells/mm^3, the hepatitis associated with efavirenz is generally mild and does not require drug discontinuation. Efavirenz is the only antiretroviral drug that is teratogenic in nonhuman primates. When administered to pregnant cynomolgus monkeys, 25% of fetuses developed significant malformations. In cases in which women were exposed to efavirenz during the first trimester of pregnancy, significant fetal malformations, mainly of the brain and spinal cord, have been reported.[35] *Women of childbearing potential should therefore use two methods of birth control and avoid pregnancy while taking efavirenz.*

Clinical Efficacy of NNRTI-Based Regimens. The use of efavirenz or nevirapine, in combination with other antiretroviral drugs, is associated with favorable long-term suppression of viremia and elevation of CD4 lymphocyte counts.[27] In a large, prospective, randomized trial comparing nevirapine 400 mg daily, nevirapine 200 mg twice daily, efavirenz 600 mg daily, or nevirapine 400 mg + efavirenz 800 mg daily, in combination with stavudine and lamivudine, for 48 weeks in 1216 treatment-naive patients, the efavirenz and nevirapine regimens were comparable, with plasma HIV RNA (viral load [VL]) less than 50 copies/ml in 65% versus 60% of treated patients, respectively, at 48 weeks ($P = .193$). This difference did not meet study criteria for noninferiority.[36] Hepatotoxicity was more common in the nevirapine arm (9.6% vs. 3.5%).

In clinical studies in ART-naive patients in which efavirenz was compared to a PI, both combined with two NRTIs, efavirenz-based regimens outperformed indinavir, nelfinavir, and lopinavir/ritonavir (LPV/r)–based regimens. Compared to unboosted indinavir, 70% of patients treated with efavirenz, zidovudine, and lamivudine achieved undetectable plasma HIV-1 RNA as compared to 48% of those receiving indinavir plus zidovudine and lamivudine.[37] However, much of this difference appeared to be the consequence of improved patient adherence and fewer adverse drug reactions with the efavirenz regimen. In a recently completed study, 753 ART-naive patients were randomized to receive one of three regimens: LPV/r plus NRTIs, efavirenz plus NRTIs, or LPV/r plus efavirenz. At 96 weeks, 89% of patients in the efavirenz + two NRTIs arm had a VL less than 50 copies/ml compared to 77% in the LPV/r + two NRTIs arm ($P = .003$). The LPV/r + efavirenz arm had similar virologic efficacy compared to efavirenz + two NRTIs. There was no difference between the three arms in time to first treatment-limiting toxicity.[38] Despite superior virologic response with the efavirenz + two NRTIs regimen, the LPV/r-containing regimen resulted in an unexplained higher increase in CD4 cell counts (241 vs. 285 cells/mm^3; $P = .01$). In patients with virologic failure, development of resistance was more common in the NNRTI + two NRTIs arm than in either LPV/r-containing arm. Efavirenz has also been used effectively in patients who have failed previous ART, in combination with other active drugs.[39] As a result of these studies, an efavirenz-based regimen is one of the DHHS preferred regimens for treatment-naive patients (see Table 84-6 later). Efavirenz is also available as part of a three-drug coformulation: one pill (efavirenz + tenofovir DF + emtricitabine) taken once daily.[24]

Table 84-2 summarizes the pharmacokinetics, advantages, and disadvantages of the available NNRTIs.

Protease Inhibitors

Mechanism of Action. HIV PIs (amprenavir, fosamprenavir, atazanavir, indinavir, lopinavir, ritonavir, nelfinavir, saquinavir, tipranavir, and darunavir) are transition-state peptidomimetics that block the proteolytic cleavage of HIV Gag and Pol polyproteins, including essential structural (p17, p24, p9, and p7) and enzymatic (reverse transcriptase, protease, and integrase) components of the virus. The HIV aspartyl protease is a homodimer that consists of two 99–amino acid monomers; each contributes an aspartic acid residue essential for catalysis.[40] The most common cleavage site for this enzyme is the N-terminal side of a proline residue, especially between phenylalanine and proline, although other sites are recognized. Human aspartyl proteases such as renin, pepsin, gastricsin, and cathepsin D contain only one polypeptide chain and are not inhibited by HIV PIs to a significant degree. These drugs prevent the maturation of HIV virus particles into their infectious form.[41]

Infected patients treated with HIV PIs as sole agents experience a 100- to 1000-fold mean decrease in plasma viral RNA concentrations within 12 weeks; this is similar in magnitude to VL changes produced by NNRTIs such as efavirenz.[41] Atazanavir, an azapeptide with a C_2-symmetric chemical structure (Fig. 84-3), will be used here as the prototype for the PI class. In various in vitro assays, the IC_{50} for HIV-1 ranges from 2 to 15 nM. The in vitro IC_{50} is increased three- to fourfold in the presence of 40% human serum.[42]

Pharmacokinetics. Atazanavir is rapidly absorbed after oral administration, and reaches peak plasma concentrations about 2 hours after dosing. A light, low-fat meal increases the AUC of atazanavir by 70%, while a high-fat meal increases the AUC by 35%.[42] It is recommended that this drug be administered with food, which also decreases interindividual variability in pharmacokinetics.

Like most HIV PIs, atazanavir undergoes oxidative metabolism in the liver primarily by CYP3A4, accounting for most of its elimination. With the standard 400-mg daily dose (without ritonavir pharmacokinetic enhancement), the mean elimination half-life of atazanavir is approximately 7 hours; this allows for once-daily dosing. Atazanavir is 86% bound to plasma proteins, both to albumin and α_1-acid glycoprotein. CSF concentrations are less than 3% of plasma concentrations. However, the drug has excellent penetration into seminal fluid, with a semen : plasma concentration ratio of 11% to 440%.[42] Atazanavir pharmacokinetic parameters are characterized by high interindividual

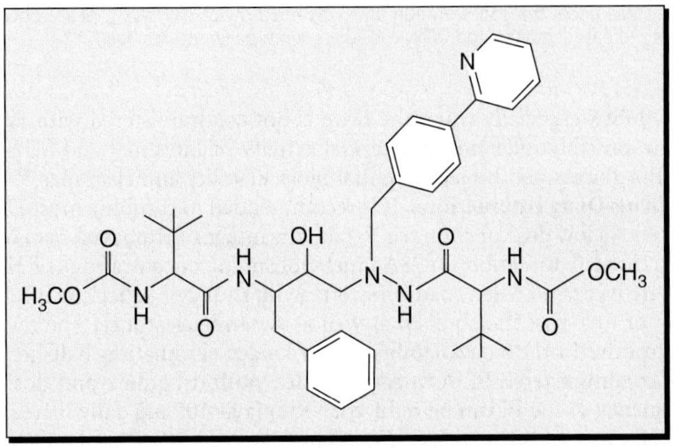

FIGURE 84-3 • Chemical structure of atazanavir.

TABLE 84-2 PROPERTIES OF NON-NUCLEOSIDE REVERSE TRANSCRIPTASE INHIBITORS (NNRTIs)

NNRTI	Dose	Pharmacokinetics	Comments
Delavirdine (DLV; Rescriptor)	*DLV:* 400 mg tid	*Absorption:* Bioavailability 85%. Absorption highly dependent on gastric acidity. *Metabolism and Excretion:* Metabolized by CYP3A4 to several hydroxylated metabolites, which undergo subsequent glucuronidation. Both unchanged drug and metabolites are excreted in the feces. *Protein Binding:* 98-99% Steady state mean AUC: 83 mcg/ml/hr; C_{max}: 16 mcg/ml; C_{min}: 7 mcg/ml (400 mg tid). $T^1/_2$: 5.8 hr.	**Pros:** May still have activity with G190A, G190S, P225H, and F227L mutations, but few clinical data; increases drug levels of some PIs. **Cons:** Low potency; fewer clinical data than for other NNRTIs; tid dosing.
Efavirenz (EFV; Sustiva)	*EFV:* 600 mg at bedtime. May be taken with or without meals but administer on an empty stomach during the first 2 wk to minimize the risk of CNS side effects. *Coformulated product:* Atripla (TDF 300 mg + FTC 200 mg + EFV 600 mg), 1 tab qd	*Absorption:* 40-45% absorption with or without food; high-fat meals increase absorption by 39% (caps) to 79% (tabs) *Metabolism and Excretion:* Metabolized by CYP3A4 and CYP2D6 to several hydroxylated metabolites, which undergo subsequent glucuronidation. Both unchanged drug and metabolites are excreted in the feces. *Protein Binding:* 99.5-99.75% Steady state (600 mg) mean C_{max}: 13 μmol/ml; C_{min}: 5.6 μmol/ml; AUC: 184 μmol/ml/hr. $T^1/_2$: 36-100 hr. The 516T/T genotype (more frequently found in African Americans) is associated with higher plasma EFV concentrations, slower clearance, and increased CNS toxicity.[30]	**Pros:** Unbeaten NNRTI with multiple studies demonstrating potency and durability, including in patients with high VL and/or low CD4 count; convenient (1 pill qd), including coformulated with TDF and FTC (Atripla); generally well tolerated; minimal long-term toxicity; less hepatotoxicity and less severe rash than with NVP. **Cons:** Early CNS side effects common and require significant patient education/ counseling; more hyperlipidemia than with NVP (though less than with most PIs); low genetic barrier (single point mutation) to resistance; long-half life may increase risk of resistance in patients who abruptly discontinue therapy.
Nevirapine (NVP; Viramune)	*NVP:* 200 mg qd × 14 days, then 200 mg bid	*Absorption:* 93% absorption with or without food. *Metabolism and Excretion:* Metabolized by CYP3A4 to several hydroxylated metabolites, which undergo subsequent glucuronidation. Both unchanged drug and metabolites are excreted in the feces. *Protein Binding:* 50-60% Median AUC: 55.95 mcg/ml/hr; C_{max}: 5.86 mcg/ ml; C_{min}: 3.72 mcg/ml at steady state. $T^1/_2$: 25-30 hr.	**Pros:** Efficacy comparable to EFV at 1 yr in 2NN trial; more favorable lipid profiles than EFV; safety and efficacy of single dose to prevent perinatal transmission is established. **Cons:** Fewer clinical data than for EFV; potential for severe hepatotoxicity and sometimes lethal rash reaction; low barrier (single point mutation) to high-level resistance to NNRTIs.
Etravirine (ETR; Intelence)	*ETR:* 200 mg twice daily with food.	*Absorption:* (with DRV/r co-administration): AUC_{12h} (GM +/– SD): 4531 +/– 4543 ng•h/m; C_{min} (GM +/– SD): 296 +/– 377 ng/mL *Metabolism and Excretion:* Etravirine undergoes oxidative metabolism by CYP3A4, CYP2C9, and CYP2C19 in vitro. Etravirine's methylhydroxylated metabolites have 90% less activity against wild-type virus compared to etravirine. Primarily excreted in the feces with only 1.2% recovered in the urine. *Protein binding:* 99.9% $T_{1/2}$ 41 (+/– 20) hours	**Pros:** Active against most EFV- and NVP-resistant HIV strains, generally well tolerated, higher genetic barrier to resistance compared to EFV and NVP. **Cons:** Bid dosing, rash, not as extensively studied compared to EFV, and many complex drug-drug interactions. In vitro, ETR is a mild inducer of CYP3A4, 2B6, and glucuronidation. In addition, it also inhibits 2C9 and 2C19.

AUC, area under the concentration-time curve; bid, twice daily; C_{max}, peak concentration; C_{min}, trough concentration; CNS, central nervous system; CYP, cytochrome P-450; PIs protease inhibitors; qd, daily; tid, three times daily; VL, viral load.

variability, especially when the drug is not coadministered with ritonavir, possibly reflecting differential activity of intestinal and hepatic CYP isoforms and thus differential bioavailability and clearance.[43]

Drug-Drug Interactions. It is recommended to combine most HIV PIs with a low dose of ritonavir to take advantage of ritonavir's remarkable capacity to inhibit CYP3A4 metabolism.[41] Concentrations of HIV PIs are increased when coadministered with ritonavir, reflecting inhibition of first-pass metabolism as well as systemic clearance. The result is improved oral bioavailability and a longer elimination half-life of the coadministered PI. As a consequence, both drug dose and dosing frequency of the PI can be reduced.[44] Ritonavir 100 mg daily increases the atazanavir 300 mg daily steady state AUC by 2.5-fold, and increases the trough concentration 6.5-fold.[42] Low-dose ritonavir also counters the adverse pharmacokinetic effects of efavirenz on the atazanavir AUC; the AUC of atazanavir 300 mg with ritonavir 100 mg plus efavirenz 600 mg is 30% higher than the AUC of atazanvir 400 mg alone when given with efavirenz. Efavirenz 600 mg daily reduced the AUC of atazanavir by 74% when coadministered without ritonavir boosting. Other PIs such as lopinavir, saquinavir, fosamprenavir, tipranavir, and darunavir are coadministered with low-dose ritonavir to take advantage of this beneficial pharmacokinetic drug interaction.

Like most other HIV PIs, atazanavir inhibits CYP3A4 at clinically achieved concentrations.[45] Atazanavir is a moderate inhibitor of CYP3A4 and may alter plasma concentrations of other drugs. Concentrations of midazolam, triazolam, ergot derivatives, amiodarone, and quinidine as well as other CYP3A4 substrates with a narrow therapeutic index may be significantly increased by atazanavir. Coadministration of these drugs should therefore be avoided. Since atazanavir is metabolized by CYP3A4, concomitant administration of agents that induce this enzyme (e.g., rifampin) is contraindicated due to a reduction of up to 80% in atazanavir concentrations.[46]

Unique to atazanavir, nelfinavir, and possibly tipranavir, an increase in gastric pH significantly affects its absorption. The atazanavir trough concentration was decreased by 78% and 28% with coadministration of omeprazole and famotidine, respectively.[47] The pharmacokinetic interaction with proton pump inhibitors cannot be overcome with higher atazanavir doses, dose separation, or "boosting" with ritonavir. If patients require acid suppression, histamine$_2$ blockers can be given 2 hours after or 10 hours before unboosted atazanavir administration; alternatively, "boosting" with ritonavir can minimize the decrease in atazanavir serum level observed with histamine$_2$ blockers. Patients and care providers must be vigilant about the possibility of clinically significant pharmacokinetic drug interactions in patients receiving PIs.

Drug transporters such as P-glycoprotein (Pgp) may affect the pharmacokinetics and distribution of HIV PIs, most of which are substrates for Pgp. Pgp in capillary endothelial cells of the blood-brain barrier limits the penetration of some HIV PIs into the CSF.[48] This low CSF : plasma drug concentration ratio may also reflect extensive binding of these drugs to plasma proteins. Many HIV PIs penetrate less well into semen than do NRTIs and NNRTIs. Although there have been case reports of ongoing viral replication in these sanctuary sites despite an undetectable plasma VL, the majority of patients will have concordant virologic responses in plasma, CSF, and semen.[49] The clinical significance of Pgp and protein binding effects on these drugs remains to be defined under most circumstances.

Adverse Drug Reactions. Nausea, vomiting, and diarrhea are the most common PI adverse effects, although these symptoms are less severe with atazanavir. Similar to indinavir, atazanavir frequently causes unconjugated hyperbilirubinemia. This is mainly a cosmetic side effect and is not associated with hepatotoxicity. In initial clinical trials, 41% of subjects receiving 400 mg of atazanavir daily developed a significant increase in total bilirubin,[42] although only 5% developed clinical jaundice. Overall, 6% of patients discontinued atazanavir because of side effects during 48 weeks of treatment. Patients treated with unboosted atazanavir in randomized clinical trials had lower fasting triglycerides and cholesterol than patients treated with nelfinavir or efavirenz,[42] indicating a reduced likelihood of causing these side effects. When atazanavir is combined with ritonavir, lipids are somewhat higher, although few patients required lipid-lowering therapy.[50] In contrast to indinavir, atazanavir is not known to cause glucose intolerance or changes in insulin sensitivity.

Resistance. HIV PIs promote drug resistance at a rate that is intermediate between that of NRTIs and NNRTIs. The median time to rebound in HIV plasma RNA concentrations of one log or greater was 3 to 4 months in initial monotherapy trials with these drugs.[41] High-level resistance to PIs requires accumulation of a minumum of four to five codon substitutions, which generally takes several months. Primary resistance mutations in the enzymatic active site are the first to emerge; these confer only a three- to fivefold drop in sensitivity to the drug.

HIV replication in the presence of atazanavir selects for drug-resistant virus. The primary atazanavir resistance mutation occurs at HIV protease codon 50, and confers approximately a ninefold decrease in susceptibility. This is an isoleucine-to-leucine substitution (I50L) that is distinct from the isoleucine-to-valine substitution selected by amprenavir. This mutation was present in 100% of viruses isolated from patients failing therapy in one clinical trial.[42] Fortunately, isolates with only this mutation are still susceptible to inhibition by other HIV PIs. However, this mutation is followed by secondary mutations often distant from the active site that compensate for the reduction in proteolytic efficiency and increase the likelihood of cross-resistance.[51] Until recently, the likelihood of virologic suppression in highly treatment-experienced patients was low.

Patients with resistance to atazanavir may be successfully treated with newer agents such as tipranvir and darunavir. Ritonavir-boosted darunavir and tipranavir are two PIs that have recently been FDA approved for the treatment of PI-experienced patients. A 24-week pooled analysis of two ongoing randomized trials involving highly treatment-experienced patients with 8 recognized PI resistance mutations showed that an undetectable (<50 copies/ml) VL was achieved in 45% and 12% of darunavir/ritonavir-treated and control patients, respectively.[52]

Clinical Efficacy of PI-Based Regimens. Numerous clinical studies have shown that HIV PIs produce favorable long-term suppression of viremia, increase CD4 lymphocyte counts, reduce disease progression, and improve long-term survival when combined with other active antiretroviral drugs.[41] PI-based regimens are commonly used for both treatment-naive and treatment-experienced patients. With the exception of nelfinavir, all approved PI-based regimens are comparable in terms of efficacy in treatment-naive patients when combined with ritonavir. However, efficacy will differ between different PIs in treatment-experienced patients with genotypic resistance. In addition, short-term and long-term toxicities, including gastrointestinal intolerance, the risk of insulin resistance, hyperlipidemia, and lipodystrophy will vary significantly (Table 84-3).

In randomized clinical trials in treatment-naive patients, unboosted atazanavir produced virologic and CD4 benefits similar to those of a nelfinavir combination regimen.[42] A separate study showed that unboosted atazanavir produced benefits similar to those of efavirenz plus nucleoside analogues.[53] The combination of atazanavir and low-dose ritonavir also had a VL effect similar to the LPV/r coformulation in treatment-experienced patients. A total of 358 patients who had failed at least two HAART regimens containing at least one PI, one NNRTI, and one NRTI were randomized to atazanavir/ritonavir 300/100 mg daily, atazanavir/saquinavir 400/1200 mg daily, or LPV/r 400 mg/100 mg twice daily combined with tenofovir plus one NRTI. At 48 weeks, 58% versus 56% achieved a VL less than 400 copies/ml in the LPV/r and atazanavir/ritonavir arms, respectively. There was a nonsignificant trend favoring LPV/r, with 46% versus 38% achieving the VL end point of less than 50 copies/ml. The atazanavir/saquinavir arm did not perform as well as the other two groups.[54] However, in treatment-experienced patients, atazanavir 400 mg daily without ritonavir was inferior to the LPV/r coformulation given twice daily; at 24 weeks, the LPV/r arm showed a better virologic response (50% vs. 34% with VL <50 copies/ml).[55] This study suggests that atazanavir should be combined with ritonavir in treatment-experienced patients—and in treatment-naive patients with high baseline VLs—in order to take advantage of the enhanced pharmacokinetic profile.

Table 84-3 summarizes the pharmacokinetics, advantages, and disadvantages of the available PIs.

Entry Inhibitors

Mechanisms of Action. Of all antiretrovirals, enfuvirtide is the only approved entry inhibitor and has a unique mechanism of action. This peptide blocks the interaction between the N36 and C34 sequences of the gp41 glycoprotein by binding to a hydrophobic groove in the N36 coil[56] (Fig. 84-4). This prevents the formation of a six-helix bundle necessary for membrane fusion and subsequent viral entry into the host cell. Because of its unique mechanism of action and target, enfuvirtide retains activity against viruses that have become resistant to antiretroviral agents of the NRTI, NNRTI, and PI classes.

CH_3CO-Tyr-Thr-Ser-Leu-Ile-His-Ser-Leu-Ile-Glu-Glu-Ser-Gln-Asn-Gln-Gln-Glu-Lys-
Asn-Glu-Gln-Glu-Leu-Leu-Glu-Leu-Asp-Lys-Trp-Ala-Ser-Leu-Trp-Asn-Trp-Phe-H_2N

FIGURE 84-4 • Chemical structure of enfuvirtide.

TABLE 84-3 PROPERTIES OF PROTEASE INHIBITORS (PIs)

PI	Dose	Pharmacokinetic	Comments
Atazanavir (ATV; Reyataz)	*ATV:* 400 mg qd *or* *ATV/r:* 300 mg/ 100 mg qd	*Absorption:* Well absorbed with food. *Metabolism and Excretion:* CYP3A4 substrate and inhibitor. Metabolized to two inactive metabolites and excreted primarily via biliary excretion. 13% of ATV and/or its metabolites is excreted in the urine. *Protein Binding:* 86%. Mean C_{max}: 3.152 mcg/ml; C_{min}: 0.273 mcg/ml; AUC: 22.3 mcg/ml/hr (ATV 400 mg qd at steady state). C_{min}: 0.15-0.85 mcg/ml associated with good response. $T^1/_2$: 6.5 hr.	**Pros:** Good potency, especially when boosted with RTV (ATV/r); lowest pill burden for a PI regimen; qd regimen; no effects on lipids; good GI tolerability; less likely to cause insulin resistance and fat accumulation (limited data). **Cons:** jaundice or scleral icterus may be problematic for some patients; drug interactions with PPIs, H_2 blockers, and antacids (not recommended with PPIs); food requirement. RTV boosting may improve potency, but with slight increase in lipids and jaundice vs. unboosted ATV.
Amprenavir (APV; Agenarase)	*APV (liquid):* 1400 mg bid	*Absorption:* Estimated 89% absorption with or without food. Formulated with vitamin E for improved absorption. Absorption decreased by 21% with high-fat meal. *Metabolism and Excretion:* Metabolized by CYP3A4 to several hydroxylated metabolites, which undergo subsequent glucuronidation. Both unchanged drug and metabolites excreted in the feces. *Protein Binding:* 90%. APV 1200 mg bid at steady state: mean C_{max}: 7.66 mcg/ml; C_{min}: 0.32 mcg/ml; AUC: 17.7 mcg/ml/hr. $T^1/_2$: 7-10 hr.	**Pros:** May retain activity against some viral strains resistant to other PIs. **Cons:** rash; propylene glycol content, higher cross-resistance rate with DRV/r. Avoid in ESRD and ESLD.
Fosamprenavir (FPV; Lexiva)	*FPV:* 1400 mg bid *or* *FPV/r:* 700/100 mg bid *or* *FPV/r:* 1400 mg/ 100-200 mg qd (PI-naive patients only)	*Absorption:* Well absorbed independent of food. *Metabolism and Excretion:* Metabolized by CYP3A4. The metabolite is excreted primarily in feces (75%), with 14% excreted in urine *Protein Binding:* 90%. C_{max}: 4.85 mcg/ml, C_{min}: 0.35 mcg/ml after 1400-mg dose. $T^1/_2$: 7.7 hr.	**Pros:** improved formulation with decreased pill burden and GI side effects compared to old APV capsules; good lipid profile, especially if used unboosted; option for qd administration (with RTV in PI-naive patients); can be taken with or without food **Cons:** Fewer long-term data than LPV/r; higher pill burden than ATV or ATV/r; may not be as effective as LPV/r in PI-experienced patients.
Indinavir (IDV; Crixivan)	*IDV:* 800 mg tid with light meal *or* *IDV/r:* 800/100 mg bid	*Absorption:* 65% absorption in fasting state (food decreases absorption by 77%). *Metabolism and Excretion:* Metabolized by CYP3A4 to several hydroxylated metabolites, which undergo subsequent glucuronidation. Both unchanged drug and metabolites are excreted in the feces. *Protein Binding:* 60% (variable). Mean steady state AUC: 18.8 mcg/ml/hr; C_{max}: 7.7 mcg/ml; C_{min}: 0.154 mcg/ml. Serum levels significantly decreased in pregnancy. $T^1/_2$: 1.5-2 hr.	**Pros:** Long-term clinical data supporting durability and potency **Cons:** Variable PK and inconvenient dosing without RTV boosting; nephrolithiasis (unique to IDV); GI side effects; retinoid effects (unique to IDV); insulin resistance (more common than with other PIs).
Lopinavir/ ritonavir (LPV/r; Kaletra)	*LPV/r:* 400/100 mg bid *or* *LPV/r:* 800/200 mg qd (PI-naive patients only)	*Absorption:* Tabs: food increases bioavailability by 27%. *Metabolism and Excretion:* Primarily biliary excretion with less than 3% excreted unchanged in the urine. *Protein Binding:* 98-99%. LPV/r 400 mg bid at steady state: mean C_{max}: 9.8 (±3.7) mcg/ml; C_{min}: 7.1 (±2.9) mcg/ml; AUC: 92.6 (±36.7) mcg/ml/hr $T^1/_2$: 5-6 hr.	**Pros:** Long-term efficacy as initial therapy with potency retained at VL >100,000; good PK profile; active against PI-resistant strains. Decreased pill burden with new tablet formulation. **Cons:** GI intolerance and elevated triglyceride and cholesterol in some patients; inferior to EFV-based regimen in treatment-naive patients.
Nelfinavir (NFV; Viracept)	*NFV:* 750 mg tid *or* *NFV:* 1250 mg bid Administer with a minimum of 500 kcal with 20% fat meal.	*Absorption:* Variable absorption (20-80%); high-fat food (20% and 50% fat content) increases absorption by 3- to 4-fold, respectively. *Metabolism and Excretion:* Converted to its major active metabolite (M8) by CYP2C19; M8 is metabolized by CYP3A4. Both unchanged drug and metabolites are excreted in the feces. *Protein Binding:* 99%. Mean steady state C_{max}: 3-4 mcg/ml; C_{min}: 1-3 mcg/ ml; AUC: 53 mcg/ml/hr. $T^1/_2$: 3.5-5 hr.	**Pros:** Extensive experience in pregnancy but no longer recommended due to carcinogen contaminated lot; reduced pill burden with 625-mg formulation. **Cons:** Unboostable PI; less potent than NNRTIs and boosted PIs; high variability in absorption with dependence on fatty foods; more diarrhea compared to the other PIs.

TABLE 84-3 PROPERTIES OF PROTEASE INHIBITORS (PIs)—cont'd

PI	Dose	Pharmacokinetic	Comments
Ritonavir (RTV; Norvir)	*RTV:* 100-200 mg qd–bid to enhance PK of the coadministered PI.*	*Absorption:* 60-80% absorption; levels increased 15% with food. *Metabolism and Excretion:* Metabolized by CYP3A4 and 2D6 to several hydroxylated metabolites, which undergo subsequent glucuronidation. Both unchanged drug and metabolites are excreted in the feces. *Protein Binding:* 98-99%. Mean steady state AUC: 61 mcg/ml/hr; C_{max}: 11.2 mcg/ml; C_{min}: 3 mcg/ml. $T^1/_2$: 3-5 hr.	**Pros:** The most reliable "booster" of all PIs: typically used to enhance PK of all PIs except NFV. **Cons:** Costly; dose-dependent GI side effects, hepatitis, cholesterol and triglyceride elevation; many significant drug interactions.
Saquinavir (SQV; Invirase)	*SQV/r:* 1000/ 100 mg bid	*Absorption:* Only 4% absorption with food. Absorption not influenced by food when combined with RTV. *Metabolism and Excretion:* Extensive first-pass metabolism; over 90% of SQV is metabolized by hepatic and intestinal CYP3A4 isoenzyme. *Protein Binding:* 98%. Mean steady state (with SQV/RTV) AUC: 29,214 ng/ ml/hr; C_{max}: 1420 ng/ml, C_{min}: 371 ng/ml. $T^1/_2$: 1-2 hr. *Distribution:* 700 L.	**Pros:** Moderate effect on lipid profile, improved pill burden with the 500-mg tablet, a reasonable alternative choice in PI-naive patients. **Cons:** Inferior to LPV/r in PI-experienced patients; higher pill burden than with ATV/r or FPV/r; must be boosted with RTV.
Tipranavir (TPV; Aptivus)	*TPV/r:* 500/200 mg bid with food	*Absorption:* Bioavailability improved by 31% with high-fat meal *Metabolism and Excretion:* Substrate and potent inducer of CYP3A4. Excreted primarily in feces (82.3%), with only 4.4% recoved in the urine. *Protein Binding:* >99.9%. C_{max}: approx. 120 mcg/ml; C_{min}: approx. 35 mcg/ml (Dose TPV/r 500/200 mg bid at steady state). $T^1/_2$: 6 hr.	**Pros:** Active against many PI-resistant strains. **Cons:** Requires boosting with RTV 200 mg bid. More transaminase and lipid elevation than with comparator PIs. Cannot be combined with other PIs because of potent CYP3A4/Pgp induction. Case reports of intracranial hemorrhage and severe hepatitis.
Darunavir (DRV; Prezista)	*DRV/r:* 600/ 100 mg bid with food	*Absorption:* With RTV coadministration, DRV is well absorbed with an absolute bioavailability of 82%. Food (a light snack or a full meal) increases DRV AUC by 30%. *Metabolism and Excretion:* DRV undergoes extensive oxidative metabolism via CYP3A4 to weakly active oxidative metabolites that are primarily excreted in the feces. At steady state, the geometric mean DRV, AUC: 62.35 mcg/ml/hr; C_{min}: 3.54 mcg/ml. $T^1/_2$: 15 hr.	**Pros:** The most active against PI-resistant strains; comparable tolerance to comparator PI. **Cons:** Requires boosting with RTV 100 mg bid. Severe hepatitis reported in 0.5% of patients.

*Gallant JE, DeJesus E, Arribas JR, et al. Tenofovir DF, emtricitabine and efavirenz vs. zidovudine, lamivudine and efavirenz for HIV. N Engl J Med 2006;354:251-260.
AUC, area under the concentration-time curve; bid, twice daily; C_{max}, peak concentration; C_{min}, trough concentration; GI, gastrointestinal; H_2, histamine$_2$; Pgp, P-glycoprotein; PK, pharmacokinetics; PPIs, proton pump inhibitors; qd, daily; tid, three times daily; /r, low dose RTV used for PK enhancement; VL, viral load.

Enfuvirtide is a 36–amino acid synthetic peptide with a sequence derived from a part of the transmembrane gp41 protein of HIV-1 involved in the fusion of the virus membrane with that of the host cell. Enfuvirtide is not active against HIV-2, but has a broad range of potencies against HIV-1 isolates. The in vitro IC_{50} for this drug is 0.1 nM to 1.7 μM, depending on the HIV-1 strain used and the laboratory testing method.[57]

Pharmacokinetics. Enfuvirtide is the only approved antiretroviral drug that must be given parenterally.[57] Following subcutaneous administration, peak plasma concentrations occur approximately 4 hours after dosing. There is a deamidated metabolite of enfuvirtide at the C-terminal phenylalanine whose AUC is 2% to 15% that of the parent drug,[57] but no other metabolites are detected. The major route of elimination for enfuvirtide has not been determined. Enfuvirtide must be given twice daily, because its mean elimination half-life is less than 4 hours.

Drug-Drug Interactions. Enfuvirtide is not metabolized to a significant extent, and is not known to alter the concentrations of any coadministered drugs. Enfuvirtide concentrations were not changed in the presence of ritonavir, rifampin, or ritonavir plus saquinavir.[58]

Adverse Drug Reactions. Injection site reactions are the most common adverse effect associated with enfuvirtide use; 98% of patients experience one or more injection site complaints, including pain, erythema, and induration. Up to 80% of patients may develop nodules or cysts at injection sites.[57] However, only 4% to 5% of patients discontinue treatment due to these local skin reactions. Use of enfuvirtide was associated with a higher incidence of lymphadenopathy and pneumonias in one study.[57] Whether these are directly and mechanistically related to drug exposure remains to be determined.

Resistance. Resistance to enfuvirtide is associated with specific amino acid mutations in the enfuvirtide binding domain of the transmembrane protein gp41. Ninety-four percent of patients developing virologic failure while taking enfuvirtide had resistance mutations in the gp41 region.[57] This usually consisted of a valine-to-alanine substitution at codon 38, or an asparagine-to–aspartic acid substitution at codon 43 of gp41. Single amino acid substitutions can produce up to 450-fold resistance to enfuvirtide in vitro. High-level resistance in patients is usually associated with two or more amino acid changes.[57]

Clinical Efficacy. Enfuvirtide is only approved by the FDA for use in treatment-experienced adults who have failed prior antiretroviral regimens. Phase III clinical trials have been conducted in heavily treatment-experienced patients with documented resistance to multiple antiretroviral drugs. In such patients, enfuvirtide given 90 mg subcutaneously twice daily in combination with an optimized background

TABLE 84-4 PROPERTIES OF THE HIV ENTRY INHIBITOR ENFUVIRTIDE

Fusion Inhibitor	Dose	Pharmacokinetics	Comments
Enfuvirtide (ENF, T-20; Fuzeon)	*ENF:* 90 mg q12h	*Absorption:* Well absorbed from subQ site with bioavailability of 84.3% (±15.5%). *Metabolism and Excretion:* Undergoes catabolism. Exact pathway of ENF metabolism is unknown. In vitro, undergoes a non-NADPH–dependent hydrolysis. *Protein Binding:* 92%. Following 90 mg subQ, mean C_{max}: 5.0 ± 1.7 mcg/ml; C_{min}: 3.3 ± 1.6 mcg/ml; AUC: 48.7 ± 19.1 mcg/ml/hr. C_{min}: 2.2 mcg/ml was associated with virologic suppression.* $T^1/_2$: 3.8 ± 0.6 hr. *Distribution:* 5.5 ± 1.1 L.	**Pros:** Active against PI-, NNRTI-, and NRTI-resistant virus; good response if background regimen includes ≥2 active ARTs; well studied in ART-experienced patients. **Cons:** SubQ administration; injection site reactions; time-consuming reconstitution process; expensive; requires extensive patient education and training. Only short-term benefit if not combined with an active background regimen.

*Bonora S, Gonzalez de Requena D, Castagna A, et al. Pharmacokinetic and pharmacodynamic determinants of virologic response to enfuvirtide regimens. CROI 2005 abstract 643. *In* Program and Abstracts of the 12th Conference on Retroviruses and Opportunistic Infections, Boston, MA, February 22-25, 2005.
ART, antiretroviral therapy; AUC, area under the concentration-time curve; C_{max}, peak concentration; C_{min}, trough concentration; subQ, subcutaneously.

TABLE 84-5 DHHS AND IAS GUIDELINES FOR INITIATING THERAPY IN TREAMENT-NAIVE HIV-INFECTED PATIENTS, 2008: WHOM TO TREAT

Clinical Category	CD4 Cell Count	DHHS Recommendations	IAS Recommendations
Symptomatic	Any value	Treat at any VL value.	Treat at any VL value.
Asymptomatic, AIDS	<200 cells/mm³	Treat at any VL value.	Treat at any VL value.
Asymptomatic	>200 cells/mm³, but ≤350 cells/mm³	Treat at any VL value, the optimal time to initiate therapy in asymptomatic patients with CD4 count >350 is not well defined, patient comorbidities and scenario should be taken into consideration.	Consider ART, especially if CD4 is close to 200/mm³, the VL is 100,000 or there is a rapid decline in CD4 (>100/g).
Asymptomatic	350-500 cells/mm³	Consider or observe: VL >100,000 copies/ml Defer therapy with VL <100,000 copies/ml	Consider if VL >100,000 copies/ml or CD4 decline is >100 cells/mm³/yr.
Asymptomatic	>500 cells/mm³	Consider or observe: VL >100,000 copies/ml Defer therapy with VL <100,000 copies/ml	ART generally not recommended.

DHHS, U.S. Department of Health and Human Services; IAS, International AIDS Society–USA Panel; VL, viral load.
Adapted from Panel on Clinical Practices for Treatment of HIV Infection, Department of Health and Human Services[24] and Hammer SM et al.[60]

TABLE 84-6 DHHS AND IAS GUIDELINES FOR INITIATING THERAPY IN TREAMENT-NAIVE HIV-INFECTED PATIENTS, 2008: PREFERRED INITIAL ANTIRETROVIRAL THERAPY

	Boosted PI-Based Regimen	NNRTI-Based Regimen
DHHS	LPV/r + TDF + FTC *or* ABC* + 3TC FPV/r + TDF + FTC *or* ABC* + 3TC ATV/r + TDF + FTC *or* ABC* + 3TC	EFV + TDF + FTC EFV + ABC* + 3TC
IAS-USA	ATV/r *or* FPV/r *or* LPV/r *or* SQV/r *plus* AZT/3TC *or* TDF/FTC *or* ABC*/3TC	EFV or NVP *plus* AZT/3TC *or* TDF/FTC *or* ABC*/3TC

*Patient should be screened for HLA-B*5701.
DHHS, U.S. Department of Health and Human Services; IAS, International AIDS Society–USA Panel.
Adapted from Panel on Clinical Practices for Treatment of HIV Infection, Department of Health and Human Services[24] and Hammer SM et al.[60]

antiretroviral regimen (OBR) produced a VL of less than 50 copies/ml after 24 weeks of treament in about twice the number of patients as those treated with the OBR alone (19.6% to 12.2% vs. 7.3% to 5.3%).[59] Of note, treatment responses were much more likely in patients who received at least two other active drugs, based on treatment history and HIV genotype.

Enfuvirtide is generally reserved for patients who have failed most other available antiretroviral regimens, because of its cost, inconvenience, and injection site toxicity. Clinicians must keep in mind that, like other antiretrovirals, the efficacy of enfuvirtide depends on combining it with other active antiretroviral drugs.

Table 84-4 summarizes the pharmacokinetic properties, advantages, and disadvantages associated with the use of enfuvirtide.

Therapeutic Approach

The DHHS and the International AIDS Society–USA periodically issue guidelines of whom to treat and what drugs to start treatment with; these are summarized in Tables 84-5 and 84-6, respectively.[24,60] It is important to note that recommendations are based on a consensus assessment of the results of published clinical trials, with consideration given to regimens with the best published clinical evidence for antiviral efficacy, safety, and tolerability. In addition to clinical data, guidelines from the World Health Organization (WHO) intended for resource-poor countries are restricted by drug availability and costs, which may outweigh the importance of long-term toxicities in some circumstances.[61] Clinicians need to be aware that guidelines are intended to inform therapy for an average uncomplicated patient, but may need to be modified based on intercurrent disease, medications (Table 84-7), and other circumstances.

Although recommendations vary slightly, the combination of two NRTIs plus a ritonavir-boosted PI or an NNRTI is recommended for all symptomatic patients and/or those with a CD4 count less than 200 cells/mm³. These recommendations emphasize combination therapy in order to prevent the emergence of resistant virus; regimen convenience, tolerability, and adherence in order to chronically suppress HIV replication; and finally the expected need for lifelong treatment.

TABLE 84-7 CLINICALLY SIGNIFICANT DRUG INTERACTIONS IN HIV-INFECTED PATIENTS

Affected Drug	Interacting Drug	Effect	Comments
Midazolam, triazolam	All PIs, DLV, and potentially EFV	May significantly increase midazolam and triazolam serum levels.	Coadministration is contraindicated. *Alternative:* lorazepam or temazepam
Fentanyl	All PIs and DLV	May significantly increase fentanyl serum levels.	Avoid coadministration. *Alternative:* morphine
PIs and NNRTIs	Phenytoin, carbamazepine, phenobarbital	LPV AUC decreased by 33% and phenytoin AUC decreased by 31%.	Levels of all PIs and NNRTIs may be decreased. *Alternatives:* valproic acid, levetiracetam, topiramate
All PIs (except NFV)	EFV, NVP	Significant decrease in PI serum level when not coadministered with RTV.	Coadminister protease inhibitor with RTV.
Antiarrhythmics (amiodarone, disopyramide, dofetilide, flecainide, lidocaine, mexiletine, propafenone, quinidine)	All PIs and DLV	May significantly increase antiarrhythmic serum levels.	Avoid coadministration.
Clarithromycin, erythromycin	All PIs and DLV	Clarithromycin AUC increased by 94% with ATV coadministration.	QTc prolongation observed. Use 50% of clarithromycin dose. *Alternative:* azithromycin
Calcium channel blockers	All PIs and DLV	Diltiazem AUC increased by 125% with ATV coadministration.	Increase in PR interval observed. Start with 50% diltiazem dose and titrate slowly.
ATV, DLV, itraconazole, ketoconazole	Proton pump inhibitors and antacids	ATV AUC decreased by 75%. DLV, itraconazole, and ketoconazole AUC may be significantly decreased.	Coadministration should be avoided. ATV may be given 2 hr before or 10 hr after H_2 blockers.
Rifampin	All PIs	PI AUC decreased by 70-92%.	Coadministration contraindicated. *Alternative:* dose-adjusted rifabutin
Rifabutin	RTV-boosted PIs	Rifabutin AUC increased 3- to 4-fold.	Decrease rifabutin to 150 mg every other day.
Methadone	NVP, EFV	Methadone AUC decreased by 46-57%.	Monitor for withdrawal symptoms and titrate methadone dose to effect.
Simvastatin, lovastatin	All PIs and DLV	Simvastatin AUC increased 32-fold with RTV-boosted PI.	Coadministration contraindicated. *Alternatives:* pravastatin and possibly atorvastatin and rosuvastatin.
Erectile dysfunction agents (sildenafil, tadalafil, vardenafil)	All PIs and DLV	Significant increase in AUC of erectile dysfunction agents.	Do not exceed the following doses: sildenafil, 25 mg q48h; tadalafil, 10 mg q72h; vardenafil, 2.5 mg q72h.
Ergot alkaloid	All PIs, DLV, and EFV	May result in acute ergot toxicity.	Coadministration contraindicated. *Alternative:* sumatriptan

AUC, area under the concentration-time curve; ATV, atazanavir; DLV, delavirdine; EFV, efavirenz; H_2, histamine$_2$; LPV, lopinavir; NFV, nelfinavir; NNRTIs, non-nucleoside reverse transcriptase inhibitors; NVP, nevirapine; PIs, protease inhibitors; RTV, ritonavir.

Emerging Targets and Therapeutics

Identification of drugs that block other steps in the HIV life cycle is a major goal of new drug development. Drugs for new targets will not likely be cross-resistant with those in existing classes. Several promising new drug classes are in the pipeline: CCR5 and CXCR4 antagonists, integrase inhibitors, maturation inhibitors, and an anti-CD4 monoclonal antibody.

CCR5 Antagonists

The first selective oral CCR5 antagonist, maraviroc, was recommended for FDA approval in the second quarter of 2007. Approval was based on two double-blind, randomized, placebo-controlled Phase III trials (MOTIVATE 1 and 2) that evaluated maraviroc 300 mg daily or twice daily with optimized background therapy (OBT) in over 1000 treatment-experienced patients infected with CCR5-tropic HIV-1. Heavily treatment-experienced HIV-1–infected patients who were failing their current ART, had at least 6 months of prior treatment with at least one agent (two agents for PIs) from three of the four antiretroviral drug classes, and/or documented resistance to three of the four antiretroviral drug classes and plasma HIV-1 RNA ≥5000 copies/ml were considered for study participation. OBT was administered as open-label therapy and could consist of three to six agents, not including ritonavir used for pharmacokinetic enhancement, based on individual susceptibility results, prior treatment, or safety/tolerability considerations. Patients were stratified by enfuvirtide use and HIV-1 RNA less than 100,000 or ≥100,000 copies/ml. The primary efficacy end point was change in $\log_{10}$ HIV-1 RNA from baseline. Patients enrolled had a median VL of 4.86 $\log_{10}$ copies/ml and median CD4 cell count of 167 cells/mm^3. Forty-one percent of patients enrolled had baseline VLs of ≥100,000 copies/ml and 58% had baseline CD4 cell count less than 200 cells/mm^3. Approximately two thirds of patients were infected with virus, with an overall susceptibility score of less than 3. The Week 24 intention-to-treat analysis in both studies demonstrated significantly greater reduction of HIV-1 RNA from baseline in both maraviroc daily or twice-daily groups compared to placebo. Mean changes in VL were −1.87, −1.96, and −0.99 $\log_{10}$ copies/ml in the daily, twice daily, and placebo-treated groups, respectively. VL suppression to less than 50 copies/ml was achieved in 44.0%, 45.3%, and 23.0% of the respective groups.[62]

Although controversial, concern has been raised with regard to the possibility of selection of CXCR4-tropic or dual-tropic virus with the use of maraviroc, which has been associated with detrimental treatment outcomes. Change in viral tropism from greater than 80% CCR5-tropic to less than 50% CCR5-tropic has been observed in treatment-naive patients, with low CD4 counts predicting greater prevalence of dual-mixed or CXCR4-tropic virus.[63] Combined data from the week 24 analysis of MOTIVATE 1 and 2 revealed that, of 1042 patient enrolled with CCR5 tropism at baseline, among those who experienced treatment failure ($n = 204$) at week 24, change in tropism from baseline CCR5 to dual/mixed or CXCR4 was observed in 4%, 46%, and 42% of patients in the placebo, maraviroc daily, and maraviroc twice-daily groups, respectively.

Maraviroc does not inhibit or induce CYP3A4. Maraviroc does not affect the pharmacokinetics of oral contraceptives, zidovudine, lamivudine, or midazolam. As maraviroc is a substrate for CYP3A4 and Pgp, the dose of maraviroc should be halved when coadministered with CYP3A4 and/or Pgp inhibitors. Coadministration of HIV PIs (with the exception of tipranavir/ritonavir) resulted in a two- to eightfold elevation of maraviroc's AUC. Efavirenz and rifampin, CYP3A4 inducers, decreased the AUC of maraviroc by 45% and 63%, respectively. Maraviroc's dose should be doubled (600 mg twice daily) when it is coadministered with CYP3A4 and/or Pgp inducers in the absence of other potent CYP3A4 inhibitors.

Integrase Inhibitors

Integrase is an HIV enzyme that catalyzes a strand transfer reaction essential for the integration of proviral DNA into the host chromosome. Raltegravir (MK-0518) is one of the first integrase inhibitors that has been FDA approved. In a double-blind, randomized trial in 198 ART-naive patients, raltegravir was compared to efavirenz in combination with tenofovir and lamivudine. Undetectable VL was achieved in 85% to 100% of patients across all arms, with comparable efficacy between the efavirenz and raltegravir arms. However, a surprising finding was a more rapid reduction in HIV RNA to less than 50 copies/ml in the raltegravir group compared to the efavirenz groups at weeks 4 and 8. After 24 weeks of treatment, the mean increase in CD4 count from baseline ranged from 139 to 175 cells/mm^3 in the raltegravir group compared to 112 cells/mm^3 in the efavirenz group.[64]

In highly treatment-experienced patients, a randomized, double-blind, placebo-controlled trial of raltegravir at 200 mg, 400 mg, or 600 mg twice daily demonstrated unprecedented virologic suppression.[65] All patients were genotypically or phenotypically resistant to one or more drugs in each of three classes (NNRTI, NRTI, PI). Baseline characteristics of the 124 patients randomized to raltegravir plus OBR were VL = 4.7 $\log_{10}$ copies/ml, CD4 count = 226 to 244 cells/mm^3, and 9 to 11 years of prior ARTs. Optimized background regimens contained a median of four antiretrovirals, with 45 patients (36%) receiving enfuvirtide. An undetectable (<50 copies/ml) VL was achieved in 56% to 72% and 20% of raltegravir and control patients, respectively.

Raltegravir is mainly metabolized by glucuronidation (like zidovudine), and thus is less susceptible to drug interactions. Its metabolism is partially blocked by atazanavir, a selective inhibitor of the UGT-glucuronosyltransferase enzyme UGT1A1; this resulted in a 41% increase in the AUC of raltegravir.

Maturation Inhibitors

PA-457 is the first in a new class of molecules called maturation inhibitors. These agents have the same effect on the virus as PIs, by blocking the processing of the Gag precursor polyprotein that must be cleaved in order for the virus to become infectious. But unlike PIs, PA-457 achieves this by binding directly to the Gag polyprotein; it does not bind to the protease. By applying a pharmacokinetic/pharmacodynamic model to data from the first PA-457 proof-of-concept studies, investigators found that higher concentrations of PA-457 continued to produce greater reductions in VL without reaching a plateau in activity, even at the highest doses studied.[66] Unfortunately, some PA-457 recipients even at the highest doses showed little change in VL, and an explanation for that observation is lacking. Although resistance to PA-457 occurs in vitro through specific amino acid changes at the capsid (CA)/SP1 binding site, no resistance has been detected in patients, even those who failed to respond to the drug in monotherapy studies.[67] Since the PA-457 binding site is highly conserved, it has been suggested that resistance may occur with a substantial cost in terms of viral fitness.

Anti-CD4 Monoclonal Antibody

TNX-355 is a humanized monoclonal antibody that binds to a part of the CD4 receptor that is essential for HIV entry. This antibody does not block the HIV outer envelope protein gp120 from binding to CD4; rather, it interferes with a conformational change in CD4 that is essential for access of gp120 to the chemokine receptors CCR5 or CXCR4. The antibody is equally active against CCR5- and CXCR4-tropic virus isolates.

Highly treatment-experienced patients who receive an injection of TNX-355 every 2 weeks have a sustained average drop in VL of about 1.0 $\log_{10}$ copies/ml after 24 weeks. There has been hope that resistance would not develop with this agent, since it targets the host rather than a virus-encoded protein. However, some treated patients show little virologic benefit, suggesting the possibility of resistance. Investigators examined the TNX-355 sensitivity of baseline HIV isolates from 82 patients participating in an ongoing Phase II treatment trial.[68] They reported that TNX-355–resistant strains have modifications in their envelope proteins that result in altered envelope conformation. The gp120 trimers that normally form during the process of HIV entry are more open in these strains, allowing access to co-receptors even in the presence of the antibody.

REFERENCES

1. AIDS Epidemic Update December 2005. UNAIDS Publication CP125. Available at: *http://www.unaids.org* (accessed January 5, 2006).
2. Louie M, Hogan C, Hurley A, et al. Determining the antiviral activity of tenofovir disoproxil fumarate in treatment-naïve chronically HIV-1-infected individuals. AIDS 2003;17:1151-1156.
3. Hervey PS, Perry CM. Abacavir: a review of its clinical potential in patients with HIV infection. Drugs 2000;60:447-479.
4. Kearney BP, Flaherty JF, Sayre JR, et al. Effect of formulation and food on the pharmacokinetics of tenofovir DF [Abstract 3]. Presented at the 2nd International Workshop on Clinical Pharmacology of HIV Therapy, Noordwijk, The Netherlands, April 2-4, 2001.
5. Hawkins T, Veikley W, St Claire RL, et al. Intracellular pharmacokinetics of tenofovir diphosphate, carbovir triphosphate, and lamivudine triphosphate in patients receiving triple-nucleoside regimens. J Acquir Immune Defic Syndr 2005;39:406-411.
6. Blanchard JN, Wohlfeiler M, Canas A, et al. Pancreatitis with didanosine and tenofovir disoproxil fumarate. Clin Infect Dis 2003;37:e57-e62.
7. Karrer U, Ledergerber B, Furrer H, et al. Dose-dependent influence of didanosine on immune recovery in HIV-infected patients treated with tenofovir. AIDS 2005;19:1987-1994.
8. Negredo E, Bonjoch A, Paredes R, et al. Compromised immunologic recovery in treatment-experienced patients with HIV infection receiving both tenofovir disoproxil fumarate and didanosine in the TORO studies. Clin Infect Dis 2005;41:901-905.
9. Barrios A, Rendón A, Negredo E, et al. Paradoxical CD4+ T-cell decline in HIV-infected patients with complete virus suppression taking tenofovir and didanosine. AIDS 2005;19:569-575.
10. Ray AS, Olson L, Fridland A. Role of purine nucleoside phosphorylase in interactions between 2′,3′-dideoxyinosine and allopurinol, ganciclovir, or tenofovir. Antimicrob Agents Chemother 2004;48:1089-1095.
11. Kearney BP, Sayre JR, Flaherty JF, et al. Drug-drug and drug-food interactions between tenofovir disoproxil fumarate and didanosine. J Clin Pharmacol 2005;45:1360-1367.
12. Maitland D, Moyle G, Hand J, et al. Early virologic failure in HIV-1 infected subjects on didanosine/tenofovir/efavirenz: 12-week results from a randomized trial. AIDS 2005;19:1183-1188.
13. Torti C, Quiros-Roldon E, Regazzi M, et al. Early virological failure after tenofovir + didanosine + efavirenz combination in HIV-positive patients upon starting antiretroviral therapy. Antivir Ther 2005;10:505-513.
14. Taburet AM, Piketty C, Chazallon C, et al. Interactions between atazanavir-ritonavir and tenofovir in heavily pretreated human immunodeficiency virus-infected patients. Antimicrob Agents Chemother 2004;48:2091-2096.
15. Gallant JE, Gerondelis PZ, Wainberg MA, et al. Nucleoside and nucleotide analogue reverse transcriptase inhibitors: a clinical review of antiretroviral resistance. Antivir Ther 2003;8:489-506.
16. Fischl MA, Richman DD, Grieco MH, et al. The efficacy of azidothymidine (AZT) in the treatment of patients with AIDS and AIDS-related complex: a double-blind, placebo-controlled trial. N Engl J Med 1987;317:185-191.

17. Gallant JE, Staszewski S, Pozniak AL, et al. Efficacy and safety of tenofovir DF vs. stavudine when used in combination with lamivudine and efavirenz in antiretroviral naïve patients: a 3-year randomized trial. JAMA 2004;292:191-201.
18. Gallant JE, DeJesus E, Arribas JR, et al. Tenofovir DF, emtricitabine and efavirenz vs. zidovudine, lamivudine and efavirenz for HIV. N Engl J Med 2006;354:251-260.
19. Lee H, Hanes J, Johnson KA. Toxicity of nucleoside analogues used to treat AIDS and the selectivity of the mitochondrial DNA polymerase. Biochemistry 2003;42:14711-14719.
20. Birkus G, Hitchcock MJM, Cihlar T. Assessment of mitochondrial toxicity in human cells treated with tenofovir: comparison with other nucleoside analog transcriptase inhibitors. Antimicrob Agents Chemother 2002;46:716-723.
21. Feng JY, Murakami E, Zorca SM, et al. Relationship between antiviral activity and host toxicity: comparison of the incorporation efficiencies of 2′,3′-dideoxy-5-fluoro-3′-thiacytidine-triphosphate analogs by human immunodeficiency virus type 1 reverse transcriptase and human mitochondrial DNA polymerase. Antimicrob Agents Chemother 2004;48:1300-1306.
22. Rifkin BS, Perazella MA. Tenofovir-associated nephrotoxicity: Fanconi syndrome and renal failure. Am J Med 2004;117:282-284.
23. Adkins JC, Noble S. Efavirenz. Drugs 1998;56:1055-1064.
24. Panel on Clinical Practices for Treatment of HIV Infection, Department of Health and Human Services. Guidelines for the use of antiretroviral agents in HIV-1-infected adults and adolescents, January 29, 2008. HIV/AIDS Treatment Information Service web site. Available at: *http://www.hivatis.org*
25. Spence RA, Kati WM, Anderson KS, Johnson KA. Mechanism of inhibition of HIV-1 reverse transcriptase by nonnucleoside inhibitors. Science 1995;267:988-993.
26. Young SD, Britcher SF, Tran LO, et al. L-743,726 (DMP-266): a novel, highly potent nonnucleoside inhibitor of the human immunodeficiency virus type 1 reverse transcriptase. Antimicrob Agents Chemother 1995;39:2602-2605.
27. Harris M, Montaner JS. Clinical uses of non-nucleoside reverse transcriptase inhibitors. Rev Med Virol 2000;10:217-229.
28. Havlir D, McLaughlin MM, Richman DD. A pilot study to evaluate the development of resistance to nevirapine in asymptomatic human immunodeficiency virus-infected patients with CD4 cell counts of >500/mm^3: AIDS Clinical Trials Group Protocol 208. J Infect Dis 1995;172:1379-1383.
29. Smith PF, DiCenzo R, Morse GD. Clinical pharmacokinetics of non-nucleoside reverse transcriptase inhibitors. Clin Pharmacokinet 2001;40:893-905.
30. Haas DW, Ribaudo HJ, Kim RB, et al. Pharmacogenetics of efavirenz and central nervous system side effects: an Adult AIDS Clinical Trials Group study. AIDS 2004;18:2391-2400.
31. Wei X, Ghosh SK, Taylor ME, et al. Viral dynamics in human immunodeficiency virus type 1 infection. Nature 1995;373:117-122.
32. Eshleman SH, Guay LA, Mwatha A, et al. Comparison of nevirapine (NVP) resistance in Ugandan women 7 days vs. 6-8 weeks after single-dose NVP prophylaxis: HIVNET 012. AIDS Res Hum Retroviruses 2004;20:595-599.
33. Kuritzkes DR. Preventing and managing antiretroviral drug resistance. AIDS Patient Care STDs 2004;18:259-273.
34. Adkins JC, Noble S. Efavirenz. Drugs 1998;56:1055-1064.
35. Jeantils V, Khuong MA, Delassus JL, et al. Efavirenz (Sustiva) in pregnancy: a study about 12 HIV patients. Gynecol Obstet Fertil 2006;34:593-596.
36. van Leth F, Phanuphak P, Ruxrungtham K, et al. Comparison of first-line antiretroviral therapy with regimens including nevirapine, efavirenz, or both drugs, plus stavudine and lamivudine: a randomised open-label trial, the 2NN Study. Lancet 2004;363:1253-1263.
37. Staszewski S, Morales-Ramirez J, Tashima KT, et al. Efavirenz plus zidovudine and lamivudine, efavirenz plus indinavir, and indinavir plus zidovudine and lamivudine in the treatment of HIV-1 infection in adults. Study 006 Team. N Engl J Med 1999;341:1865-1873.
38. Riddler SA, et al. A prospective, randomized, Phase III trial of NRTI-, PI-, and NNRTI-sparing regimens for initial treatment of HIV-1 infection—ACTG 5142 [Abstract ThLB0204]. *In* Program and Abstracts of the 16th International AIDS Conference, Toronto, 2006.
39. Falloon J, Piscitelli S, Vogel S, et al. Combination therapy with amprenavir, abacavir, and efavirenz in human immunodeficiency virus (HIV)-infected patients failing a protease-inhibitor regimen: pharmacokinetic drug interactions and antiviral activity. Clin Infect Dis 2000;30:313-318.
40. Pearl LH, Taylor WR. A structural model for the retroviral proteases. Nature 1987;329:351-354.
41. Flexner C. HIV-protease inhibitors. N Engl J Med 1998;338:1281-1292.
42. Goldsmith DR, Perry CM. Atazanavir. Drugs 2003;63:1679-1693.
43. Back D, Gatti G, Fletcher C, et al. Therapeutic drug monitoring in HIV infection: current status and future directions. AIDS 2002;16(Suppl 1):S5-S35.
44. Flexner C. Dual protease inhibitor therapy in HIV-infected patients: pharmacologic rationale and clinical benefits. Annu Rev Pharmacol Toxicol 2000;40:649-674.
45. Piscitelli SC, Gallicano KD. Interactions among drugs for HIV and opportunistic infections. N Engl J Med 2001;344:984-996.
46. Burger D, Agarwala S, Child M, et al. Effect of rifampin on steady-state pharmacokinetics of ATV and RTV in healthy subjects [Abstract 657]. *In* Program and Abstracts of the 12th Conference on Retroviruses and Opportunistic Infections, Boston, MA, February 22-25, 2005.
47. Agarwala S, Gray K, Wang Y, et al. Pharmacokinetic effect of omeprazole and atazanavir co-administered with ritonavir in healthy subjects [Abstract 658]. *In* Program and Abstracts of the 12th Conference on Retroviruses and Opportunistic Infections, Boston, MA, February 22-25, 2005.
48. Kim RB, Fromm MF, Wandel C, et al. The drug transporter P-glycoprotein limits oral absorption and brain entry of HIV-1 protease inhibitors. J Clin Invest 1998;101:289-294.
49. Taylor S, Back DJ, Workman J, et al. Poor penetration of the male genital tract by HIV-1 protease inhibitors. AIDS 1999;13:859-860.
50. Malan N, Krantz E, David N, et al. Efficacy and Safety of Atazanavir-based Therapy in Antiretroviral Naive HIV-1 Infected Subjects, Both with and without Ritonavir: 48-week Results from AI424-089 [Abstract 107LB]. Presented at the 13th Conference on Retroviruses and Opportunistic Infections, Denver, CO, February 5-8, 2006.
51. Kuritzkes DR. Preventing and managing antiretroviral drug resistance. AIDS Patient Care STDs 2004;18:259-273.
52. Katlama C, Berger D, Bellos N, et al. Efficacy of TMC114/r in 3-class experienced patients with limited treatment options: 24-week planned interim analysis of 2 96-week multinational dose-finding trials [Oral Abstract 164LB]. *In* Program and Abstracts of the 12th Conference on Retroviruses and Opportunistic Infections, Boston, MA, February 22-25, 2005.
53. Squires K, Lazzarin A, Gatell JM, et al. Comparison of once-daily atazanavir with efavirenz, each in combination with fixed-dose zidovudine and lamivudine, as initial therapy for patients infected with HIV. J Acquir Immune Defic Syndr 2004;36:1011-1019.
54. Johnson M, Grinsztejn B, Rodriguez C, et al. Atazanavir plus ritonavir or saquinavir, and lopinavir/ritonavir in patients experiencing multiple virological failures. AIDS 2005;19:685-694.
55. Cohen C, Nieto-Cisneros L, Zala C, et al. Comparison of atazanavir with lopinavir/ritonavir in patients with prior protease inhibitor failure: a randomized multinational trial. Curr Med Res Opin 2005;21:1683-1692.
56. Sodroski JG. HIV-1 entry inhibitors in the side pocket. Cell 1999;99:243-246.
57. Dando TM, Perry CM. Enfuvirtide. Drugs 2003;63:2755-2766.
58. Braun MC, Wang JM, Lahey E, et al. Activation of the formyl peptide receptor by the HIV-derived peptide T-20 suppresses interleukin-12 p70 production by human monocytes. Blood 2001;97:3531-3536.
59. Lalezari JP, Henry K, O'Hearn M, et al. Enfuvirtide, an HIV-1 fusion inhibitor, for drug-resistant HIV infection in North and South America (TORO1). N Engl J Med 2003;348:2175-2185.
60. Hammer SM, Saag MS, Schechter M, et al. Treatment of adult HIV infection: 2006 recommendations of the International AIDS Society–USA Panel. JAMA 2006;296:827-843.
61. Gilks CF, Crowley S, Ekpini R, et al. The WHO public-health approach to antiretroviral treatment against HIV in resource-limited settings. Lancet 2006;368:505-510.
62. U.S. Food and Drug Administration. Pfizer Inc, maraviroc tablets NDA 22-128, Antiviral Drugs Advisory Committee (AVDAC) briefing document, April 24, 2007. Available at: *http://www.fda.gov/ohrms/dockets/ac/07/briefing/2007-4283b1-01-Pfizer.pdf*
63. Brumme ZL, Goodrich J, Mayer HB, et al. Molecular and clinical epidemiology of CXCR4-using HIV-1 in a large population of antiretroviral-naive individuals. J Infect Dis 2005;192:466-474.
64. Markowitz M, Nguyen B-Y, Gotuzzo F, et al. Potent antiretroviral effect of MK-0518, a novel HIV-1 integrase inhibitor, as part of combination ART in treatment-naïve HIV-1 infected patients [Abstract THLB0214]. *In* Program and Abstracts of the 16th International AIDS Conference, Toronto, 2006.
65. Grinsztejn B, Nguyen B-Y, Katlama C, et al. Potent antiretroviral effect of MK-0518, a novel HIV-1 integrase inhibitor, in patients with triple-class resistant virus [Abstract]. Presented at the 13th Conference on Retroviruses and Opportunistic Infections, Denver, CO, February 5-8, 2006.
66. Smith P, Forrest A, Beatty G, et al. Pharmacokinetics/pharmacodynamics of PA-457 in a 10-day multiple dose monotherapy trial in HIV-infected patients [Abstract 52]. *In* Program and Abstracts of the 13th Conference on Retroviruses and Opportunistic Infections, Denver, CO, February 5-8, 2006.
67. Adamson C, Salzwedel K, Castillo A, et al. Viral resistance to PA-457, a novel inhibitor of HIV-1 maturation [Abstract 156]. *In* Program and Abstracts of the 13th Conference on Retroviruses and Opportunistic Infections, Denver, CO, February 5-8, 2006.
68. Duensing T, Fung M, Lewis S, Weinheimer S. In vitro characterization of HIV isolated from patients treated with the entry inhibitor TNX-355 [Abstract 158LB]. *In* Program and Abstracts of the 13th Conference on Retroviruses and Opportunistic Infections, Denver, CO, February 5-8, 2006.

85

SEXUALLY TRANSMITTED DISEASES

Kristine E. Johnson and Anne M. Rompalo

INTRODUCTION 1201
THERAPEUTICS AND CLINICAL PHARMACOLOGY 1201
Genital Ulcer Disease 1201
Chancroid 1201
Lymphogranuloma Venereum 1201
Granuloma Inguinale (Donovanosis) 1202
Herpes Simplex Virus 1202
Syphilis 1204
Gestational Syphilis 1204
Urethritis 1206
Treatment 1207
Cervicitis 1207
Vaginitis 1207
Trichomoniasis 1208
Bacterial Vaginosis 1208
Vulvovaginal Candidiasis 1208
Special Considerations 1209
Pelvic Inflammatory Disease 1209
Human Papillomavirus Infection 1210

INTRODUCTION

Sexually transmitted infections (STIs) can be caused by a variety of bacterial, viral, parasitic, and ectoparasitic pathogens. It is easiest to approach this broad topic by grouping pathogens according to the symptoms or syndromes they cause. Recommended therapy is targeted toward symptom relief, biologic cure when possible, and prevention of transmission to others. Therapeutic choices listed in this chapter are based on current evidence-based recommendations by the Centers for Disease Control and Prevention (CDC) for the treatment of sexually transmitted diseases.

THERAPEUTICS AND CLINICAL PHARMACOLOGY

Genital Ulcer Disease

Chancroid

Noted most commonly among men, chancroid is characterized by genital ulceration due to infection with the gram-negative organism *Haemophilus ducreyi.* It is an uncommon disease in the Western world, but cases are found among individuals who have contact with commercial sex workers or have recently traveled to indigenous areas. Transmission is presumed to be mechanical, secondary to microabrasions during sexual intercourse. Ulcers are classically associated with buboes and tender lymphadenitis. The ulcers are typically painful, with irregular borders. Ulcer distribution is primarily on the foreskin and frenulum in men. In women, ulcers may be seen on the vulva and cervix and in the perianal region. In the natural history of infection without treatment, lesions may resolve after weeks to months. In men, chronic infection can result in phimosis, a scarring and constriction of the foreskin over the glans, which may predispose the individual to future genital and urinary tract infections.[1] Although rare, penile cancer has been associated with phimosis.[2] Of note, 10% of individuals infected within chancroid in the United States are co-infected with *Treponema pallidum* or herpes simplex virus (HSV). Frequency of co-infection is even greater if chancroid infection develops outside the United States.

Haemophilus ducreyi culture has been the mainstay of diagnosis. Serologic tests are unreliable, in part due to cross-reactivity with *H. ducreyi* antigens. Direct immunofluorescence targeted at the outer membrane protein, indirect immunofluorescence for the lipo-oligosaccharide, and nucleic acid–based testing have been developed but are not in clinical use.[3]

Multiple options for therapy exist, including macrolides, quinolones, and third-generation cephalosporins. Table 85-1 presents agent and dosing information.

Lymphogranuloma Venereum

Lymphogranuloma venereum (LGV) induces painless genital ulcers and is caused by the L1, L2, and L3 serovars of *Chlamydia trachomatis.* These serovars preferentially infect monocytes and macrophages after crossing the epithelium of the genital tract. In the local lymph nodes, LGV may lead to disseminated infection and is often associated with unilateral, painful lymphadenitis. Inflammation associated with LGV lesions can be substantial, whether in the genital or colorectal regions. Fevers and lymphadenopathy outside the genitalia indicate a systemic component of the disease. Although rare in westernized countries, LGV is indigenous to various regions in Africa, Asia, South America, and the Caribbean. Recent outbreaks of LGV have been associated with men who have sex with men (MSM), engage in receptive anal intercourse, and are human immunodeficiency virus (HIV) seropositive.[4,5] LGV infection moves through three stages, advancing from primary infection at epithelial contact, where a painless papule forms that may ulcerate. This stage may go unnoticed by the patient. Infection then migrates to the regional lymph nodes, where painful, usually unilateral, inguinal and/or femoral lymphadenopathy occurs. The final stage involves the genitals and/or rectum. Untreated, LGV induces dramatic connective tissue changes, including rectal fistulas and/or strictures and lymphatic scarring leading to elephantiasis.

Proctitis from LGV has been a common manifestation of recent outbreaks among MSM and is seen in receptive anal intercourse in men and women, and may present with acute hemorrhagic discharge, rectal pain, and/or systemic symptoms. LGV-associated proctitis may be mistaken for inflammatory bowel disease, delaying diagnosis[5] and leading to an increased risk for chronic genitourinary or bowel complications. LGV should be included in the differential diagnosis among patients presenting with proctitis who are found to have sexual risk factors (MSM, unprotected sexual intercourse, HIV infection). Untreated infection may lead to lymphatic fibrosis, associated lymphatic obstruction and elephantiasis, and colorectal fistulas; the latter are more common in women.[6]

Diagnosis of LGV in general is based upon clinical history and examination, as serology may detect other, non-LGV serovars of *C. trachomatis.* Currently, there are no U.S. Food and Drug Administration (FDA)–approved laboratory-based diagnostic methods.[7] Available useful diagnostic techniques include serology for *C. trachomatis* using whole inclusion immunoassay. Recent development of a multiplex polymerase chain reaction (PCR) method allows detection of LGV and distinction between *C. trachomatis* and LGV.[8] This technique appears promising as a screening tool as well. A rectal swab or biopsy identifying *C. trachomatis* on nucleic acid amplification is considered diagnostic of LGV proctocolitis in particular. Overall, as the development of

TABLE 85-1 TREATMENT REGIMENS FOR CHANCROID, LYMPHOGRANULOMA VENEREUM, AND DONOVANOSIS

Disease	Medication	Dose	Duration
Chancroid	Azithromycin	1.0 g PO	Once
	Ceftriaxone	250 mg IM	Once
	Ciprofloxacin	500 mg PO bid	3 days
	Erythromycin base	500 mg PO tid	7 days
Lymphogranuloma venereum	Doxycycline	100 mg PO bid	21 days
	Erythromycin base	500 mg PO 4 × daily	21 days
Granuloma inguinale (donovanosis)	Doxycycline	100 mg PO bid	At least 21 days and until all lesions are healed
	Azithromycin	1.0 g PO weekly	Once weekly × 3 wk until all lesions are healed
	Ciprofloxacin	750 mg PO bid	At least 21 days and until all lesions are healed
	Erythromycin base	500 mg PO 4 × daily	At least 21 days and until all lesions are healed
	Trimethoprim-sulfamethoxazole	1 DS (160/800) PO bid	At least 21 days and until all lesions are healed

bid, twice daily; DS, double strength; IM, intramuscularly; PO, orally; tid, three times daily.

new testing and screening strategies for LGV continues, the clinical diagnosis of LGV mandates a full evaluation for other STIs, as co-infection with other STIs is common among patients with LGV.

Therapeutic choices for all chlamydial infections include tetracyclines and macrolides, which inhibit bacterial protein synthesis by binding to subunits of the bacterial ribosome (see Table 85-1).

Granuloma Inguinale (Donovanosis)

Although recognized as a rare disease in the United States, granuloma inguinale (also called donovanosis) is caused by the intracellular pleomorphic gram-negative rod Klebsiella formally called *Calymmatobacterium granulomatis.* Donovanosis causes friable, painless genital ulceration, often described as "beefy red," that may be progressive. Variants of presentation in donovanosis include hypertrophic or verrucous ulcers and necrotic, or dry and sclerotic lesions. Lesions may occur in extragenital areas as well. Locations of historical endemicity include India, Papua New Guinea, Brazil, the Caribbean, central Australia, and southern Africa. Chronic ulcers may become progressively larger and have a foul odor. Lesions may be mistaken for chancroid, primary syphilitic chancres, or, in HIV infection, large HSV lesions. The index of suspicion must be high for a diagnosis of donovanosis, given the lack of clinical experience with this disease in Western countries and its resemblance to other ulcerative STIs.

Klebsiella granulomatis may be grown in culture, but diagnosis typically follows visualization of Donovan's bodies within the cytoplasm of infected lymphoctyes on a scraping or tissue sample of a lesion. In time-limited clinical encounters where it is uncertain if the patient will return for follow-up, swabbing the top of the wound with smear onto slide and staining is a reasonable strategy. When the provider is convinced the patient will return, a biopsy is optimal as it allows for greater sampling and histologic evaluation. Serologic methods of diagnosis are not validated or well developed.[9]

Therapeutic choices vary as listed in Table 85-1, but the duration of therapy is generally 3 weeks regardless of antibiotic choice and may be longer depending on speed of lesion resolution.

Herpes Simplex Virus

HSV types 1 and 2 induce a chronic, recurrent anogenital viral infection characterized by painful, vesicular genital ulcers. The disease is incurable, but can be treated in the setting of acute flares. First flares with minor lesions may escalate to increasingly painful lesions prior to resolution; therefore, initial episodes warrant therapy. In many individuals, infection may be controlled via suppression of viral replication and shedding by directed antiviral therapy (Table 85-2).

Viral shedding may occur in the absence of symptoms, and for this reason, infected persons may not be aware of the risk to their sexual partners. Historically, HSV-1 was typically associated with oral ulcers, while HSV-2 was associated with genital ulcers. Given the increased frequency of oral-genital sex, it is necessary to consider HSV-1 in any new presentations of genital vesicular or denuded lesions. In fact, HSV-1 surpasses HSV-2 in number of new cases of HSV within selected populations. Among 499 university students with newly diagnosed HSV between 1993 and 2001, 78% of cases were due to HSV-1.[10] First episodes of genital herpes due to HSV-2 may be mild, with escalation to more severe symptoms with subsequent episodes. In contrast, first episodes of genital herpes with HSV-1 tend to be more severe, and recurrent episodes are often less frequent than those seen with HSV-2.[11] The severity of first-episode HSV-2 has been associated with more frequent recurrences.[11] Viral shedding (and the associated risk for infection of sexual partners) occurs during asymptomatic periods, and such shedding is more common in genital HSV-2 infection during the first year following infection.

Vulnerable immunologic status tends to complicate HSV infection. Immunocompromised patients may have more severe episodes of ulceration with longer duration. Further, vertical transmission resulting in neonatal HSV infection may be devastating to the infant. Severe manifestations include acute encephalitis, death, or chronic disability. Pregnant women without known prior HSV infection should be cautioned to avoid receptive oral-genital sex if the partner is known to have oral HSV infection. Pregnant women should also abstain from intercourse with partners with genital HSV infection during the third trimester, as the risk of vertical transmission is greatest in primary infection during this period.

Patients with newly diagnosed HSV infection should be counseled regarding HIV testing. Further, all individuals with new diagnoses should be educated about the chronic and recurrent nature of the disease, the availability of multiple treatment options for suppression and episodic flares, to abstain from sexual activity when lesions are present, and to inform any current or future sexual partners about their disease. Emphasis should be placed on the phenomenon of asymptomatic shedding and concurrent risk for disease transmission, even when lesions are not present.

Diagnosis of HSV-1 and HSV-2 may be elusive, if the classical history and presentation of painful vesicular or ulcerative lesions is absent. In their presence, providers may elect to diagnose active HSV infection based upon clinical features alone without adjunctive testing. The clinical course differs between HSV-1 and HSV-2, as HSV-2 tends to induce recurrence and asymptomatic viral shedding more often than HSV-1. Cell culture of virus is the "gold standard" diagnostic technique, but is unreliable due to poor sensitivity. Viral PCR may provide rapid results with improved test characteristics (better sensitivity and specificity),[12,13] but PCR-based testing is FDA-approved for cerebrospinal fluid (CSF) analysis only. The CDC now recommends PCR testing from swabs of active lesions. Ulcer sampling with microscopic examination for evidence of cytologic change (the Tzanck preparation) also has poor sensitivity and specificity.

Type-specific serologic testing greatly improves upon the limitations of the previously mentioned methods. Qualitative identification of glycoprotein immunoglobulin G (IgG) for HSV-1 and HSV-2 are enzyme-linked immunosorbent assay (ELISA) or immunoblot based. FDA-approved ELISA-based tests in the United States include HerpeSelect-1 and HerpeSelect-2 (Focus Tech., Herndon, VA), and HSV-2

(Trinity Biotech USA, Berkley Heights, NJ). Other tests available are the HerpeSelect HSV 1 and 2 Immunoblot IgG (Trinity Biotech), and Biokit HSV-2 and SureVue HSV-2 (Biokit USA, Lexington, MA).

Treatment of HSV Infection. Clinical management is based primarily upon the use of three agents active against HSV-1 and HSV-2: acyclovir, valacyclovir, and famciclovir. Acyclovir is an acyclic purine nucleoside analogue that inhibits HSV-1 and HSV-2 replication by selective binding of acyclovir triphosphate to the viral DNA polymerase. The drug is highly concentrated in infected as compared to uninfected cells, for only infected cells have the viral thymidine kinase that converts acyclovir monophosphate to acyclovir triphosphate. The latter active metabolite binds to the viral DNA polymerase and, via exposure of the 3′-end of the DNA strand, prevents continued DNA replication. Valacyclovir is equivalent to acyclovir, as it is metabolized to acyclovir by valine hydrolase once inside the cell. Valacyclovir is a convenient agent for patient use, as it allows a longer dosing interval than acyclovir.

Famciclovir is an analogue of penciclovir. In a fashion similar to acyclovir, penciclovir binds the viral-encoded thymidine kinase and is then metabolized to penciclovir triphosphate. This active metabolite inhibits the viral DNA polymerase. Penciclovir triphosphate has a longer intracellular half-life than acyclovir. Like valacyclovir, this characteristic allows greater dosing intervals and improved ease of patient self-administration.

Suppressive Therapy. Suppressive therapy should be considered in patients with six or more flares per year. Suppression may be appropriate for a subset of individuals with a lower frequency of flares who have uninfected partner(s) and/or a history of prior severe episodes and/or either of the following: immunosuppression or high-risk sexual activity (e.g., MSM, multiple partners). Providers should review the need to continue suppressive therapy with patients at least once annually, with consideration given to the general trend toward decreased frequency of flares as duration of infection increases. Prior data suggested that valacyclovir and famciclovir are equivalent to acyclovir in efficacy with a single exception noted to date: Valacyclovir dosed at 500 mg by mouth once daily appears to be a less efficacious suppressive regimen than acyclovir or famciclovir in patients with 10 or greater recurrences per year; therefore, a 1-g dose of valacyclovir is recommended in these cases. One recent study evaluating the performance of famciclovir against valacyclovir for suppression indicated that valacyclovir may induce decreased asymptomatic viral shedding compared to famciclovir.[14] Therapeutic options for suppressive therapy[15-20] are listed in Table 85-2.

Special Considerations

- If flare is severe, consider acyclovir therapy dosed at 5 to 10 kg/mg intravenously (IV) every 8 hours.
- In recurrent infection, consider HSV culture isolation with susceptibility testing, if treatment of prior flares has failed.
- If resistance to acyclovir and valacyclovir is present, susceptibility to famciclovir is questionable. Foscarnet IV or topical cidofovir may be effective when famciclovir is no longer a therapeutic option.
- Pregnant women should be interviewed for history of prior HSV infection or clinical episodes suggestive of undiagnosed HSV infection.
- If lesions are present at the time of labor, delivery by cesarean section is recommended.
- Pregnant women with known prior HSV may be given IV acyclovir during severe episodes. Likewise, pregnant women with first episodes may be treated with oral acyclovir.
- HSV discordance between couples and/or a partner with known oral herpes appear to increase the risk of new HSV infection in pregnant women.[21]
- Antiviral administration after the 36th week of pregnancy can reduce outbreaks prior to delivery, reducing the need for additional therapy and cesarean section.[22,23]

Herpes Encephalitis and Neonatal HSV Therapy. Herpes encephalitis and neonatal herpes may be devastating, leading to death or severe disability in the patient, even when antiviral therapy is used. Neonatal herpes should be treated with IV acyclovir 20 mg/kg every 8 hours; duration is 10 to 14 days for mucocutaneous disease and 21 days for disseminated or encephalitic HSV. Herpes encephalitis in children and adults should be treated with IV acyclovir, as this therapy has been associated with improved morbidity and mortality.[24]

TABLE 85-2 TREATMENT OF HSV IN NONPREGNANT ADULTS[14-18] (CDC 2006 STD TREATMENT GUIDELINES)*

	Drug	Dosage
First clinical episode of genital herpes	Acyclovir *or* Famciclovir *or* Valacyclovir	400 mg orally 3 times a day for 7-10 days *or* 200 mg orally 5 times a day for 7-10 days 250 mg orally 3 times a day for 7-10 days 1 g orally 2 times a day for 7-10 days
Daily suppressive therapy	Acyclovir *or* Famciclovir *or* Valacyclovir	400 mg orally 2 times a day† 250 mg orally 2 times a day‡ 500 mg orally once a day *or* 1 g orally once a day§
Episodic recurrent infection	Acyclovir *or* Famciclovir *or* Valacyclovir	800 mg orally 2 times a day for 5 days *or* 400 mg orally 3 times a day for 5 days *or* 800 mg orally 3 times a day for 2 days 125 mg orally 2 times a day for 5 days *or* 1000 mg orally 2 times a day for 1 day 500 mg orally 2 times a day for 3 days *or* 1 g orally once a day for 5 days

*See CDC 2006 guidelines for the management of herpes in pregnancy and in the neonate.
†Dose range 400-800 mg recommended for patients with HIV infection and HSV.
‡Increase dose to 500 mg by mouth twice daily in patients with HIV infection and HSV.
§Increase frequency of administration to twice daily in HIV infection.
CDC, Centers for Disease Control and Prevention; HIV, human immunodeficiency virus; HSV, herpes simplex virus.

Syphilis

Syphilis is caused by the spirochete *Treponema pallidum* subsp. *pallidum.* Untreated, syphilis causes chronic infection that may induce cardiovascular, orthopedic, and neurologic complications. Primary syphilis is characterized by one or more painless chancres, often initially indurated and occurring at the site of contact inoculation. The chancre matures to ulceration and is associated with local lympadenopathy. In heterosexual men, primary chancres usually occur on the penis, while MSM may have chancres in other locations, such as the rectum and mouth. In women, the primary chancre is most often found on the labia or cervix, but oral lesions may occur. Primary chancres are often painless, remaining undetected by the host and resulting in a diagnosis during later stages of disease, when morbidity may be higher. However, syphilis has been reported to cause painful chancres; therefore, a painful lesion should be evaluated as a possible manifestation of primary disease. Other atypical presentations of primary syphilis have been described in the perianal area, and in HIV-infected individuals may include painful and/or multiple chancres. In such cases, the lesion may have an irregular border.

During primary infection, treponemes disperse throughout the body and lodge in various tissues. If untreated, the natural history of infection is progression to secondary and tertiary syphilis. Secondary syphilis may manifest itself by any one or a combination of the following: generalized rash, pharyngitis, myalgias, weight loss, and/or nontender generalized lymphadenopathy. Rash is the most common manifestation of secondary syphilis. The rash may be macular, maculopapular, papular, pustular, or any combination thereof. In most patients, the rash involves the palms and soles. During the secondary stage of infection, HIV-positive patients in particular may present with simultaneous primary and secondary syphilis.

Syphilis diagnosed in the absence of clinical manifestations is latent disease. Early latent disease is defined as positive serology without clinical symptoms that may be linked to an exposure during the last 12 months, including a diagnosed partner, clinical history suggestive of primary and/or secondary disease, or stabilization of titer without a fourfold drop after initial therapy. Late latent disease is defined by positive serology without evidence of clinical disease, where exposure, infection, or lack of treatment response cannot be identified as events during the last 12 months.

Tertiary syphilis reveals the end-organ destruction induced by treponemal persistence in various tissues. Hallmarks of tertiary disease include (among others) iritis, retinitis, optic neuritis, auditory dysfunction, neurosyphilis, gummatous skin or bone lesions, and aortitis. The latter may result in ascending aortic aneurysm. Patients with tertiary syphilis require thorough evaluation for evidence of end-organ disease.

Considerations

- In all cases of syphilis, HIV testing is strongly recommended.
- Some providers equate auditory complaints in the setting of syphilis with neurosyphilis, independent of CSF findings.
- If abnormal CSF parameters are noted, patients should undergo repeat evaluation of CSF via lumbar puncture at 6 months of follow-up. Follow-up should be pursued until any noted pleocytosis has resolved. Re-treatment may be warranted if CSF parameters do not normalize after 2 years.
- Doxycycline may be used in patients with penicillin allergy. This should be done in consultation with an infectious disease specialist.

Diagnosis. The gold standard techniques for diagnosis of early syphilis are darkfield microscopic examination and direct fluorescent antibody tests (DFA) of lesion material. In the absence of direct testing, diagnosis may be pursued via serologic methods.

Testing for syphilis is based upon serologic reactivity in the Venereal Disease Research Laboratory (VDRL) and rapid plasma reagin (RPR) tests, which are considered nontreponemal tests. Two techniques for detection of the humoral immune response to treponemal antigens are the fluorescent treponemal antibody, absorbed (FTA-Abs) and the *T. pallidum* particle agglutination tests. A single positive nontreponemal serologic test must be confirmed via additional testing, as nontreponemal tests may be falsely positive due to cross-reactivity with antigens present in other disease states.

Disease activity may be linked to nontreponemal titers levels, and since *T. pallidum* cannot be cultured in vitro, cure is determined by falling titers from the time of therapy. A fourfold reduction in titer is the minimum acceptable titer change to indicate a clinically acceptable response to therapy when nontreponemal tests are used. With primary and secondary disease, appropriate titer decline is expected within 6 to 12 months after treatment. Titer decline with treatment of latent infection may take longer, and there is a subset of patients who will have persistent, low titers on VDRL or RPR testing, even after full and appropriate therapy. Finally, in contrast to nontreponemal tests, treponemal serologies are not associated with degree or stage of illness and generally remain positive over the lifetime of the patient.

Treatment. Penicillin G, given parenterally, is the preferred treatment for syphilis (Table 85-3). However, there has never been a well-controlled, carefully planned, prospective study to determine the optimal dose or duration of therapy. Since *T. pallidum* cannot be cultured in vitro, true susceptibility patterns to antibiotics are not known. Because syphilis responds well to penicillin and perceived clinical cure rates have changed little over decades, there are limited data to support the use of other antibiotic classes in the treatment of this disease. Among alternate agents, azithromycin has received the greatest study. A recent randomized, controlled trial of azithromycin versus benzathine penicillin G to treat early syphilis among 328 individuals in Tanzania suggests that azithromycin is not inferior to penicillin.[25] Emergence of azithromycin-resistant treponemal strains discovered by molecular testing raises concern that this drug may not remain effective, particularly in North America.[26,27] Limited clinical studies, along with biologic and pharmacologic evidence, suggest that ceftriaxone is effective for treating early syphilis and neurosyphilis. However, use of this drug is not endorsed unless other options have been excluded. As penicillin is the only demonstrated effective treatment for neurosyphilis and congenital or gestational syphilis, in cases of penicillin allergy, desensitization under close monitoring is strongly recommended.

Of note, it has been shown that a level equivalent to more that 0.03 mcg/ml of penicillin is needed to ensure killing of *T. pallidum,* and that maintenance of an effective blood level for at least 7 days is necessary to cure early syphilis. Further, increasing the dose to more than 0.6 mg/kg over a period of 9 hours does not clear treponemes from chancres at an increased rate.[28] Therefore, treatment recommendations using injectable benzathine penicillin, which provides circulation of penicillin at low levels for a minimum of 14 days and does not depend upon patient compliance, is the cornerstone of therapy, with shorter courses recommended for early, more active, infections. Longer courses are used in latent or late, and presumably less active, disease. Because benzathine penicillin G does not reliably produce detectable levels of penicillin in the CSF, aqueous penicillin G given IV is the drug of choice.

Special Considerations

- To ensure prompt detection of treatment failure, HIV patients with primary or secondary syphilis should be assessed clinically with serologic testing at 3, 6, 9, 12, and 24 months after treatment (see Table 85-3).
- In HIV-infected individuals, CSF evaluation is suggested if nontreponemal titers fail to decrease fourfold at 6 to 12 months after initial treatment. In this case, even if CSF studies are normal, the majority of care providers treat with benzathine penicillin, 2.4 million units intramuscularly (IM) weekly for 3 weeks.
- Patients may experience acute onset of fever, headache, and muscle pain within the initial 24 hours after treatment is started. This phenomenon, described as the "Jarisch-Herxheimer reaction," is more frequent among patients with early syphilis.

Gestational Syphilis

Evaluation, treatment, and follow-up of infants with suspected or confirmed syphilis is clinically challenging. Congenital syphilis is due to

TABLE 85-3 TREATMENT OF SYPHILIS*

Disease	Recommended Treatment	Alternatives
Primary (1°), secondary (2°) or early latent (<1 yr)		
Adults	Benzathine penicillin G 2.4 million units IM in a single dose	(For penicillin allergic *nonpregnant adult* patients) Doxycycline 100 mg orally 2 times a day for 14 days *or* Ceftriaxone 1 g daily IV or IM for 8-10 days *or* Azithromycin 2 g orally once†
Children	Benzathine penicillin G 50,000 units/kg IM, up to the adult dose of 2.4 million units, in a single dose	
Late latent (>1 yr) or latent of unknown duration		
Adults	Benzathine penicillin G 2.4 million units IM for 3 doses, 1 wk apart (total 7.2 million units)	Doxycycline 100 mg orally 2 times a day for 28 days for adults only
Children	Benzathine penicillin G 50,000 units/kg IM up to the adult dose of 2.4 million units, administered as 3 doses at 1-wk intervals (total 150,000 units up to the adult total dose of 7.2 million units)	
Neurosyphilis	Aqueous crystalline penicillin G 18-24 million units per day, administered as 3-4 million units IV every 4 hr or continuous infusion, for 10-14 days	Procaine penicillin 2.4 million units IM once daily plus probenecid 500 mg orally 4 times a day, both for 10-14 days
HIV infection	*For 1°, 2°, and early latent syphilis:* Treat as above. Some specialists recommend 3 doses. *For late latent syphilis or latent syphilis of unknown duration:* Perform CSF examination before treatment	The use of any alternative therapy in HIV-infected persons has not been well studied; therefore, the use of doxycycline, ceftriaxone, and azithromycin must be undertaken with caution.
Pregnancy	Penicillin is the only recommended treatment for syphilis during pregnancy. Women who are allergic should be desensitized and then treated with penicillin. Dosages are the same as in nonpregnant patients for each stage of syphilis.‡	

*See 2006 CDC guidelines for follow-up recommendations and management of congenital syphilis.
†Treatment failure with azithromycin has been reported.
‡Data insufficient to recommend azithromycin or ceftriaxone.
CDC, Centers for Disease Control and Prevention; CSF, cerebrospinal fluid; HIV, human immunodeficiency virus; IM, intramuscularly; IV, intravenously.

transplacental migration of treponemes. Management requires close consideration of maternal disease stage, serologies, and prior treatment, in addition to clinical assessment of the infant. All pregnant women should be evaluated for syphilis and HIV infection. During clinical assessment of the infant, credence is given to maternal serology, as a negative serologic test in the infant does not exclude infection in the infant (Table 85-4).[29] This is particularly true if the mother has a low titer or was recently infected during pregnancy. Due to transplacental IgG, neonatal diagnosis requires a thorough clinical evaluation in infants of mothers with *both* positive nontreponemal (VDRL, RPR) and treponemal (FTA-Abs) serologies. Evaluation for congenital syphilis includes assessment for hydrops, jaundice, hepatosplenomegaly, rhinitis, rash, or limb neurologic dysfunction. Placental or umbilical cord testing using FTA-Abs is suggestive of congenital infection if positive. Other recommended tests include darkfield microscopy and/or DFA of rhinorrhea or cutaneous abnormalities.

Evaluation and Treatment of Infants with Demonstrated or Suspected Disease. Evaluation of infants with demonstrated or suspected syphilis includes the following:

- Lumbar puncture for CSF VDRL, cell count, and protein assessment. (Keep in mind that baseline normal parameters for CSF cell count and protein are higher among infants as compared to adults.)
- Complete blood count (CBC) with differential.
- As necessary, limb and/or chest radiograph, liver function tests, cranial ultrasound, ophthalmologic evaluation, and auditory brainstem function.

Treatment of these infants is aqueous crystalline penicillin G 100,000 to 150,000 units/kg per day, given as 50,000 units/kg per dose IV every 12 hours for the first 7 days of life, then the same dose every 8 hours to complete a duration of 10 days. Alternatively, infants can be treated with procaine penicillin G 50,000 units/kg per dose IM once daily for 10 days. *If even one day is missed* during the therapeutic course, full therapy should be re-initiated, starting at day 1. If other β-lactam agents were used in initial management prior to the diagnosis of congenital syphilis, a complete 10-day course of penicillin is recommended.

Evaluation and Treatment of Clinically Normal Infants. Evaluation of clinically normal infants with nontreponemal titer equal to or less than four times the maternal titer is the same as for infants with confirmed or probable disease, but should include limb radiographs. If a full 10-day course of penicillin is administered empirically, the above-described evaluation is unnecessary. However, documentation of abnormal CSF parameters, CBC (including platelet count), and a long bone radiograph would inform vigilant follow-up. Treatment is the same as for infants with confirmed or probable disease, or benzathine penicillin G 50,000 units/kg per dose IM once (Box 85-1).

In clinically normal infants with nontreponemal titer equal to or less than four times the maternal titer *and*

1. Mother received appropriate treatment during pregnancy more than 4 weeks prior to delivery, or
2. Mother demonstrates no evidence of repeat infection or relapse, no additional evaluation of the infant is necessary. The recommended therapy is benzathine penicillin G 50,000 units/kg per dose IM once. However, if close follow-up is planned and the mother's nontreponemal antibody titers decreased by at least four times after appropriate treatment for early syphilis or titers were stable or low for late syphilis (i.e., VDRL <1 : 2, RPR < 1 : 4), some providers elect to perform sequential serologic testing. *In this setting, no treatment of the infant is pursued, provided there*

TABLE 85-4 GUIDE FOR INTERPRETATION OF SEROLOGIC TEST RESULTS FOR SYPHILIS IN MOTHERS AND THEIR NEWBORN INFANTS WHO ARE CLINICALLY NORMAL

Nontreponemal Test Result (e.g., VDRL, RPR)		*Treponemal Test Results (e.g., FTA-Abs, TP-PA)*		
Mother	**Infant**	**Mother**	**Infant**	**Interpretation**
–	–	–	–	No syphilis or incubating syphilis in the mother or infant
+	+	–	–	No syphilis in mother (false-positive result in mother with passive transfer to infant)
+	+ or –	+	+	Maternal syphilis with possible infant infection; mother treated; mother with latent syphilis and possible infant infection
+	+	+	+	Recent or previous syphilis in mother; possible infant infection
–	–	+	+	Mother successfully treated before or early in pregnancy

FTA-Abs, fluorescent treponemal antibody, absorbed; RPR, rapid plasma reagin; TP-PA, Treponema pallidum particle agglutination; VDRL, Venereal Disease Research Laboratory.

From Pickering LK, Baker CJ, Long SS, et al (eds): 2006 Red Book: Report of the Committee on Infectious Diseases, 27th ed. Elk Grove Village, IL: American Academy of Pediatrics, 2006.

BOX 85-1 ADDITIONAL CONSIDERATIONS IN THE TREATMENT OF CONGENITAL SYPHILIS

- If benzathine penicillin G is used, then full infant evaluation must be verified as normal during follow-up. Any abnormality on follow-up evaluation mandates a full 10-day course of penicillin in addition to the benzathine penicillin already administered to the infant.
- Consideration should be given to a full 10-day course of penicillin if the mother is diagnosed with untreated early syphilis at time of delivery.
- Mothers with penicillin allergy should be desensitized and treated with benzathine penicillin.

is no change in the serologic testing of the infant during careful follow-up.

Diagnosis and Treatment of Postneonatal Infants and Children. Maternal serology and clinical history should be reviewed for infants age greater than 4 weeks with positive serologic tests. Such infants and children should undergo complete clinical evaluation (see "Evaluation and Treatment of Infants with Demonstrated or Suspected Disease" earlier) and HIV testing. Additional follow-up considerations are listed in Box 85-2. In children beyond infancy, sexual assault or abuse should be considered.

When evaluation of infants or children results in diagnosis of or high suspicion for syphilis, the following treatment is recommended: aqueous crystalline penicillin G 200,000 to 300,000 units/kg per day IV, given as 50,000 units/kg every 4 to 6 hours for 10 days. Children with any evidence of neurologic involvement may be given additional therapy of one dose of benzathine penicillin G at 50,000 units/kg IM after the 10-day course of aqueous penicillin.

Urethritis

Urethritis is a syndrome of urethral inflammation clinically characterized by penile discharge urethral pruritis, and/or dysuria. Diagnosis follows two categories: urethritis due to (i) gonococcal infection and (ii) other infectious and noninfectious sources. Laboratory diagnosis includes ≥5 polymorphonuclear lymphocytes per high-power field and/or greater than 10 white blood cells (WBCs) per high-power field from first-void urine. Urinary leukocyte esterase is also an indicator of urethritis. Infection with *Neisseria gonorrheae* (gonococcus; GC) is responsible for an estimated 35% of all cases.[30] Gonococcal urethritis is diagnosed via the presence of intracellular gram-negative diplococci on urethral swab smear.

BOX 85-2 ADDITIONAL FOLLOW-UP RECOMMENDATIONS: CONGENITAL SYPHILIS

- Any seroreactive infants should be closely followed, regardless of whether treatment was administered.
- Nontreponemal test(s) should be followed every 2 to 3 months until the test is negative or titer is at a minimum of fourfold decline.
- If congenital syphilis was not present (rather, transplacental maternal antibody led to positive serology in the infant), infant serology should be negative by age 6 months but may persist until 15 months.
- Infants with positive treponemal tests indicating stable or increasing titers after age 18 months should undergo complete evaluation. These patients should be treated with IV penicillin G for 10 days.
- A positive treponemal test after age 18 months indicates congenital syphilis.
  - If the nontreponemal test is negative, no treatment is required.
  - If the nontreponemal test is positive, the infant should be completely evaluated and treated for congenital syphilis.

Uncomplicated gonococcal infections of the urethra, cervix, or rectum can no longer be treated with quinolones. The evolution of antimicrobial resistance in *N. gonorrhoeae* has been persistant, and resistance to new therapeutic agents has generally developed within a few years after the introduction of a new agent. Strains with chromosomal resistance to penicillin, tetracycline, erythromycin, and cefoxitin have been identified worldwide. Fluoroquinolone resistance, which is due to mutations in the DNA gyrase gene, *gyrA*, and/or the topoisomerase IV gene, *parC*, rapidly spreading and this class of antibiotics can no longer be used for the treatment of gonorrhea. Table 85-5 presents the current CDC recommendations for gonococcal infection therapeutic choices.

Nongonococcal urethritis (NGU) is considerably more common, and *Chlamydia trachomatis* (CT) is a frequent cause, inducing up to 20% of all NGU cases in one study[31] and 30% to 50% in other reports. Some fastidious organisms have been recently implicated in NGU, which also has been linked to *Ureaplasma urealyticum* and *Mycoplasma genitalium*. However, the low frequency of detection of these organisms has slowed the description of their role in pathogenesis. Other recognized etiologies of NGU include atypical sources, such as *Trichomonas vaginalis*,[32] *Mycoplasma hominis*, HSV,[33] and adenovirus. NGU attributed to any of these microbes remains a diagnosis of exclusion when GC and CT are not detected. Implication of one or more of the

TABLE 85-5 RECOMMENDED TREATMENT FOR GONOCOCCAL INFECTIONS

Location	Recommended Treatment	Alternatives
Adults		
Cervix, urethra, rectum	Ceftriaxone 125 mg IM in a single dose *or* Cefixime 400 mg orally in a single dose	Spectinomycin[‡] 2 g IM in a single dose *or* Single-dose cephalosporins regimens See 2006 CDC guidelines for discussion of alternative regimens.
Pharynx	Ceftriaxone 125 mg IM in a single dose	
Men who have sex with men or heterosexuals with a history of recent travel		
Cervix, urethra, rectum	Ceftriaxone 125 mg IM in a single dose *or* Cefixime 400 mg orally in a single dose	
Pharynx	Ceftriaxone 125 mg IM in a single dose	
Conjunctiva	Ceftriaxone 1 g IM once plus lavage the infected eye with saline solution once	
Children (<45 kg): vagina, cervix, urethra, pharynx, rectum	Ceftriaxone 125 mg IM once	Spectinomycin[‡] 40 mg/kg IM once (maximum 2 g)
Pregnancy	Ceftriaxone 125 mg IM once *or* Cefixime 400 mg orally in a single dose	Spectinomycin[‡] 2 g IM once

*Quinolones are contraindicated in pregnant women. No joint damage attributable to quinolone therapy has been observed in children treated with prolonged ciprofloxacin regimens. Thus children who weigh more than 45 kg can be treated with any regimen recommended for adults.

†Quinolones should not be used for infections in men who have sex with men or in those with a history of recent foreign travel or partner's travel, infections acquired in California or Hawaii, or infections acquired in other areas with increased quinolone-resistant *Neisseria gonorrhoeae*.

‡Unreliable to treat pharyngeal infections. Patients who have suspected or known pharyngeal infection should have a pharyngeal culture 3 to 5 days after treatment to verify eradication of infection.

CDC, Centers for Disease Control and Prevention; IM, intramuscularly.

atypical etiologies may occur in the setting of poor response to empirical therapy for GC and CT, or where partner tracing reveals a link between the affected patient and a partner with known, recently diagnosed *Trichomonas* or HSV.

Nucleic acid amplification testing (NAAT) for GC/CT from a urethral swab is a sensitive and specific technique. Microscopic evaluation of a urethral smear diluted in normal saline may reveal occult trichomoniasis. As this method is very insensitive, diagnosis by culture remains the standard. When present, appropriate antibiotic therapy for one or more of these infections, with partner tracing and treatment, is necessary. If patient follow-up is uncertain or unreliable, syndromic management with treatment for GC/CT and trichomoniasis is a reasonable strategy.

Treatment

All patients should abstain from sexual activity for 7 days after initiation of therapy to avoid possible reinfection. Sex partners should be informed by the patient and encouraged to seek evaluation even if asymptomatic. Therapy is chosen from the options among tetracyclines, macrolides, or quinolones (Table 85-6). In general, therapy for NGU follows the recommendations by the CDC for uncomplicated *C. trachomatis* infections.

If urethritis continues, patients may be treated again with the same regimen if medication adherence during therapy was in question. Likewise, the initial treatment may be repeated if the patient was exposed to a sex partner thought to be infected. In the absence of lack of adherence or reinfection, the presence of *T. vaginalis* should be excluded using culture after intraurethral swab collection or first-void urine sample. If the patient successfully completed the initial treatment regimen and has continued symptoms, two regimens are suggested: metronidazole 2 g by mouth once *or* tinidazole 2 g by mouth once and azithromycin 1 g by mouth once.

Cervicitis

Cervicitis is characterized by mucopus (purulent or mucopurulent cervical discharge visualized in the os) and/or readily provoked endocervical bleeding. Other associated signs include leukorrhea (>10 WBCs per high-power field in vaginal fluid) and irregular bleeding (or "spotting"), including postcoital bleeding. In addition, evidence of upper reproductive tract infection, such as cervical motion tenderness and adnexal pain, may be present. Women with these signs should be evaluated for pelvic inflammatory disease (PID) (see later section). While GC and CT may induce cervicitis, in many cases, a source is not determined upon clinical laboratory testing. When present, gram-negative diplococci on an endocervical fluid stain are diagnostic, but Gram stain is an insensitive test for GC. NAAT for GC and CT is the most sensitive and specific technique in the detection of these organisms. However, if these tests are uninformative, the differential diagnosis should include other infectious etiologies associated with cervicitis. These include *T. vaginalis,* HSV-2, *M. genitalium,* and bacterial vaginosis (BV).

If women are diagnosed with any of the above-mentioned causes, they should be treated and educated to return if symptoms persist. Assessment and treatment of sexual partner(s) should be pursued. Cervicitis attributed to noninfectious etiologies has been associated with an imbalance among the normal vaginal flora. Possible sources of such imbalance include douching and other irritant agents. Therapeutic options for treatment of gonococcal cervicitis and chlamydial cervicitis are presented in Tables 85-5 and 85-6, respectively. Additional information regarding gonococcal and chlamydial pharyngitis, proctitis, conjunctivitis, and treatment during pregnancy is also provided.[34]

Women with persistent cervicitis should be re-evaluated for GC/CT and partner treatment assessed. If GC/CT is absent and partner(s) have been appropriately treated, few recommendations exist to guide the clinical approach. In some cases, extended courses of antibiotics have been used, but there are no clear data to endorse such an approach. Referral to a gynecologist for ablative therapy may be warranted if continued symptoms are clearly attributed to cervicitis.

Vaginitis

Vulvar pruritis, discharge, irritation, and/or odor are syndromically defined as vaginitis. Like cervicitis, vaginitis may be due to a sexually

TABLE 85-6 RECOMMENDED TREATMENT FOR UNCOMPLICATED *CHLAMYDIA TRACHOMATIS* INFECTIONS, NONGONOCOCCAL URETHRITIS, AND CERVICITIS

	Recommended Treatment	Alternatives
Adult	Azithromycin 1 g orally single dose *or* Doxycycline 100 mg orally 2 times a day for 7 days	Erythromycin base 500 mg orally 4 times a day for 7 days *or* Erythromycin ethylsuccinate 800 mg orally 4 times a day for 7 days *or* Ofloxacin* 300 mg orally 2 times a day for 7 days *or* Levofloxacin* 500 mg orally once a day for 7 days
Pregnancy	Azithromycin 1 g orally single dose *or* Amoxicillin 500 mg orally 3 times a day for 7 days	Erythromycin base 500 mg orally 4 times a day for 7 days *or* Erythromycin 250 mg orally 4 times a day for 14 days *or* Erythromycin ethylsuccinate 800 mg orally 4 times a day for 7 days *or* Erythromycin ethylsuccinate 400 mg 4 times a day for 14 days

*Quinolones are contraindicated in pregnant women. No joint damage attributable to quinolone therapy has been observed in children treated with prolonged ciprofloxacin regimens. Thus children who weigh more than 45 kg can be treated with any regimen recommended for adults.

transmitted disease; however, it is also found in women without STIs or risk factors for STIs. Organisms commonly associated with vaginitis include anaerobes, *Mycoplasma* species, *Gardnerella vaginalis, T. vaginalis,* and *Candida* species. BV, a state of disruption of the normal vaginal flora, is a common cause of vaginitis as well. Recent data suggest that this may be a sexually transmitted disorder, but further investigation is required to determine causality.

Frequently, laboratory testing reveals the cause of vaginitis, including a basic vaginal fluid pH of greater than 4.5, which may be secondary to BV or trichomoniasis. Although this method is unreliable, dilution of vaginal fluid in normal saline and microscopic examination may allow visualization of active *T. vaginalis* or "clue cells" (bacteria adherent to the walls of epithelial cells), suggestive of BV. An amine, or "fishy," odor after application of a 10% potassium hydroxide (KOH) solution (a "whiff test") is also suggestive of BV infection. Yeast hyphae may also be visualized on a KOH slide, indicative of candidal vaginitis. Again, consideration should be given to microscopy as an insensitive method of detection. Culture or PCR may yield additional diagnostic information. Additionally, vaginal inflammation may be a result of local chemical or mechanical irritation; therefore, a thorough patient history may provide diagnostic clues.

Trichomoniasis

Infection with *T. vaginalis* may vary from complete lack of symptoms to vulvar inflammation and malodorous and prolific discharge, classically yellow-green. Microscopy of vaginal secretions is of poor sensitivity and specificity. Culture remains the gold standard. New technologies in enzymatic and PCR-based testing are promising for rapid diagnostics. FDA-approved tests for *T. vaginalis* in women only include the immunochromatographic capillary-flow dipstick (OSOM Trichomonas Rapid Test; Genzyme Diagnostics, Cambridge MA), and a nucleic acid probe for *T. vaginalis, G. vaginalis,* and *Candida albicans* (Affirm VP III; Becton Dickinson, Sparks, MD). The results from these tests are rapidly available.

The mainstay of trichomonas therapy has been metronidazole (Box 85-3). The drug is activated with reduction of the nitro group by ferredoxin-like proteins possessed only by anaerobic organisms. The other 5-nitroimidazole used to treat trichomonas infections is tinidazole, which has a longer half-life than metronidazole.

BOX 85-3 TREATMENT OPTIONS FOR TRICHOMONIASIS

- Metronidazole 2 g orally once *or* tinidazole 2 g orally once *or* (alternative)
- Metronidazole 500 mg orally twice daily for 7 days

Bacterial Vaginosis

The most frequent cause of vaginal malodor and discharge, BV is caused by disruption of the normal vaginal flora *Lactobacillus* species by *G. vaginalis, M. hominis,* and anaerobic bacteria (*Prevotella* species, *Atopobioum* species, *Mobiluncus* species). Diagnosis of BV requires three of the four diagnostic criteria listed in Box 85-4. Gram stain may be used to evaluate vaginal flora for quantity of gram-negative and gram-variable rods and cocci (also called Amsel's criteria). Rapid tests include the Affirm VP III (Becton Dickinson, Sparks, MD) DNA probe, the QuickVue Advance (Quidel, San Diego, CA) for pH measurement, and the Pip Activity Test Card (Quidel) for proline aminopeptidase.

BV may have implications for pregnancy and women undergoing invasive gynecologic procedures. Untreated BV in pregnant women is associated with preterm labor and delivery. This is of particular importance in women who are already considered at high risk for preterm delivery. Second, data suggest that treatment of BV reduces the risk of endometritis, PID, and vaginal cuff cellulitis after procedures such as biopsy, intrauterine device insertion, or cesarean section, among others.

Therapeutic strategies are aimed toward decreasing the anaerobic burden associated with BV in hopes of restoring the bacterial balance (Table 85-7). Women should be advised that the clindamycin cream is petroleum-based and therefore may disrupt condom and diaphragm structural integrity, with risk for device failure. The various regimens using metronidazole are equivalent in treatment success. Women should be advised to return for evaluation if symptoms continue after the treatment period. Persistent BV may require long-term (i.e., 6 months) treatment with metronidazole gel 0.75% twice weekly.[35]

Vulvovaginal Candidiasis

Features characteristic of vulvovaginal candidiasis (VVC) include vaginal discharge, pruritus, vaginal discomfort, dyspareunia, and dysuria. Cases are typically due to *C. albicans,* but other yeasts may play a role as well. Diagnosis is based upon visualization of yeast hyphae on a KOH slide of vaginal fluid. In the absence of hyphae, clinical history may indicate underlying infection. *Uncomplicated VVC* is found in women with normal immunity, occurs infrequently in the host, and is generally due to *C. albicans.* After diagnosis and treatment (Table 85-8), patients should return for repeat evaluation if symptoms continue or return within 2 months after original symptoms. *Complicated VVC,* or recurrent vulvovaginal candidiasis (RVVC), may occur in normal hosts but is described in immunosuppressed populations according to any of the following criteria: recurrent VVC, severe VVC, and non-*albicans* candidal species. Additional criteria include candidiasis in women with decreased immunity, in particular patients with

TABLE 85-7 TREATMENT OPTIONS FOR BACTERIAL VAGINOSIS

Agent	Dose	Duration
Metronidazole	500 mg orally	Twice daily × 7 days
Metronidazole 0.75%	5 g intravaginally	Once daily × 5 days
Clindamycin cream 2%	5 g intravaginally*	7 days
Clindamycin	300 mg orally	Twice daily × 7 days
Clindamycin	100-g ovules intravaginally*	Once daily × 3 days
Metronidazole + Clindamycin cream 2%	750-mg extended-release tablets + 5 g intravaginally*	Once daily × 7 days (metronidazole) *and* Once (clindamycin cream)

*Clindamycin cream is oil-based and may weaken latex condoms and diaphragms for 5 days after use.

BOX 85-4 DIAGNOSTIC CRITERIA FOR BACTERIAL VAGINOSIS

Patient must have at least three of the following criteria:

- White discharge coating vaginal walls
- Clue cells on microscopic examination of vaginal fluid
- Vaginal fluid pH > 4.5
- Fishy odor pre- or post-KOH (10%) (whiff test)

poor diabetic control, chronic immobility, chronic immunosuppression (autoimmune disorders, posttransplant patients, and/or HIV), or during pregnancy.

RVVC is present when the patient presents with four or more cases of VVC annually. Often, each individual case has responded to standard therapy, yet the source of RVVC is not identified in many cases. In RVVC, vaginal culture for possible etiologic organisms is encouraged. Non-*albicans* species, such as *C. glabrata,* may be the cause. However, this is not common, as non-*albicans* candida are observed in only 10% to 20% of patients with RVVC.

Special Considerations

Treatment of RVVC. After treatment for each recurrent infection, providers may elect to start extended therapy with oral fluconazole dosed at 100, 150, or 200 mg once every third day for 7 to 14 days for reduction of organism load. This treatment is followed by oral fluconazole once weekly. Alternatives to this therapy are clotrimazole 200 mg topically twice weekly or clotrimazole 500-mg vaginal suppositories once weekly.

Severe VVC. Characterized by significant vulvar erythema, edema, and fissures, severe VVC may respond poorly to traditional regimens. The physician should consider 7 to 14 days of treatment with topical azoles, or oral fluconazole 150 mg dosed once with repeat oral dosing once 3 days after the first dose.

Treatment of Non-*albicans* VVC. Clear treatment guidelines do not exist. If evidence of infection continues, an option is boric acid 600 mg in gelatin capsules given vaginally once daily for 7 to 14 days. Should symptoms remain after extensive and extended therapy, evaluation by a specialist may be warranted.

Pregnancy and HIV Infection. Pregnancy and HIV infection may complicate VVC or RVVC management. For example, in pregnancy, only topical agents should be used given the risk of azole-associated teratogenicity. Treatment of VVC is associated with poorer outcomes in HIV-infected women as compared to their HIV-negative peers. Rates of vaginal candidal colonization are greater in HIV-positive women, and colonization increases as immune status declines. More frequent use of azole agents among these patients is also associated with non-*albicans* vaginal colonization.

Pelvic Inflammatory Disease

PID may affect any portion of the upper female reproductive tract. A state of acute or chronic inflammation, PID includes endometritis, salpingitis, tubo-ovarian abscess, and pelvic peritonitis. GC and CT induce PID, yet a variety of commensal organisms within the vagina may lead to PID as well. These include, among others, anaerobes, *G. vaginalis, Haemophilus influenzae,* gram-negative rods, and *Streptococcus agalactiae.* Other etiologies include cytomegalovirus, *M. hominis, U. urealyticum,* and *M. genitalium.* In all circumstances, women given a diagnosis of PID should be evaluated for GC, CT, and HIV infection.

TABLE 85-8 REGIMENS FOR TREATMENT OF UNCOMPLICATED VULVOVAGINAL CANDIDIASIS*

Agent	Dose (Administered Daily)	Duration
Butoconazole 2% cream	5 g 5 g sustained release	3 days Once
Clotrimazole vaginal tablet	100 mg 100 mg × 2 (200 mg)	7-14 days 3 days
Miconazole		
2% cream	5 g	7 days
Vaginal suppository	100 mg 200 mg 1299 mg	7 days 3 days Once
Nystatin vaginal tablet	100,000 units	14 days
Tioconazole 6.5% ointment	5 g	Once
Terconazole		
0.4% cream	5 g	7 days
0.8% cream	5 g	3 days
Vaginal suppository	80 mg	3 days
Fluconazole oral tablet	150 mg	Once

*All agents are intravaginal unless otherwise noted.

Clinical presentation of PID may vary broadly, from minimal symptoms to acute febrile illness. Signs suggestive of PID include intermenstrual bleeding, abnormal vaginal discharge, and dyspareunia. Empirical antibiotic therapy for PID is suggested when any of three minimum findings are noted on physical examination: cervical motion tenderness, uterine tenderness, or adnexal tenderness. Evidence of lower tract involvement should increase clinical suspicion for PID. Box 85-5 presents the additional findings that increase the specificity of the minimum criteria and the likelihood of PID.

As presentations of PID vary widely, some patients with moderate to severe PID may require hospitalization, while other patients may reach satisfactory outcomes with oral therapy alone. There also exist multiple therapeutic options for inpatient management with transition to continued oral regimens (Box 85-6). It is recommended that any woman with a tubo-ovarian abscess be admitted and observed for a minimum of 24 hours after diagnosis, as should patients with acute illness, pregnancy, inability to follow or tolerate an outpatient regimen, or lack of response to oral treatment. Although a clear link has not been demonstrated between anaerobic infection and PID, consideration of anaerobic coverage should be given in each case. The addition of either metronidazole or clindamycin to treatment offers broad coverage against genital tract anaerobes.

Human Papillomavirus Infection

Human papillomavirus (HPV) is a sexually transmitted, circular DNA virus. The majority of sexually active individuals will have the HPV at some point during their adult lives. At least 100 known types of HPV infection have been identified to date, and viral types are identified by the genetic sequence of the capsid protein L1. HPV types are classified according to their link to cervical cancer. HPV types associated with oncogenesis (16, 18, 31, 33, 35, 39, 45, 51, 52, 56, 58, 59, 68, 73, 82) are identified as "high-risk" types, while the "low-risk" types, such as 6 and 11, are associated with genital warts.[36] "Indeterminate-risk" types have no clarified association with neoplastic or verrucous presentations. The mechanism of HPV infection is thought to occur via viral entry to the suprabasal layer of epithelial keratinocytes via microtears in tissue.

The hypothesized mechanism leading to cervical cancer is neoplastic transformation mediated through the viral oncogenes E6 and E7, which bind and inactivate the tumor suppressor proteins p53 and Rb, respectively. It remains unclear why certain individuals will go on to develop chronic HPV infection, while others clear the infection. On

BOX 85-5 DIAGNOSTIC CRITERIA FOR PELVIC INFLAMMATORY DISEASE (PID)

Minimum Criteria
Cervical motion tenderness
Uterine tenderness
Adnexal tenderness

Additional Criteria
Oral temperature <101° F (or >38.3° C)
Abnormal cervicovaginal mucopurulent discharge*
Many WBCs on saline microscopic examination of vaginal fluid*,†
High ESR or CRP
Cervical test positive for GC or CT

Highly Specific Criteria
Endometritis by endometrial biopsy
Thickened, fluid-filled fallopian tubes ± free pelvic fluid *or* tubo-ovarian lesion *or* tubal hyperemia on pelvic ultrasound
Laparoscopic evidence of PID

*Found in the majority of women with PID.
†Microscopic examination also permits evaluation for BV and trichomoniasis.
BV, bacteria vaginosis; CRP, C-reactive protein; CT, *Chlamydia trachomatis;* ESR, erythrocyte sedimentation rate; GC, *Neisseria gonorrhoeae;* WBCs, white blood cells.

BOX 85-6 OUTPATIENT TREATMENT OPTIONS FOR PID, BY CLINICAL IMPRESSION OF DISEASE STATUS*,†

Regimen
Ceftriaxone 250 mg IM once
or
Cefoxitin 2 g IM once plus probenicid 1 g orally once
or
Other third-generation cephalosporin
plus
Doxycycline 100 mg orally 2 times a day for 14 days

*This regimen is to be used with or without metronidazole 500 mg orally twice a day for 14 days.
†Pregnancy and PID: Patients should be hospitalized and treated with the appropriate recommended parenteral intravenous treatments (see CDC guidelines).
CDC, Centers for Disease Control and Prevention; IM, intramuscularly; PID, pelvic inflammatory disease.

BOX 85-7 TREATMENT OPTIONS FOR GENITAL WARTS

External
Provider-Administered
Cryotherapy with liquid nitrogen or cryoprobe. Repeat applications every 1 to 2 weeks if necessary.
or
Trichloroacetic acid (TCA) or bichloroacetic acid (BCA), 80% to 90%. Apply small amount only to warts. Allow to dry. If excess amount applied, powder with talc, baking soda, or liquid soap. Repeat weekly if necessary.
or
Podophyllin resin 10% to 25%* in a compound tincture of benzoin. Allow to air dry. Limit application to less than 10 cm^2 and to less than 0.5 ml. Wash off 1 to 4 hours after application. Repeat weekly if necessary.
or
Surgical removal.

Patient-Applied
Podofilox 0.5% solution or gel.*Apply two times a day for 3 days, followed by 4 days of no therapy. This cycle can be repeated as necessary for up to four times. Total wart area should not exceed 10 cm^2 and total volume applied daily should not exceed 0.5 ml.
or
Imiquimod 5% cream.*Apply once daily at bedtime three times a week for up to 16 weeks. Wash treatment area with soap and water 6 to 10 hours after application.

Urethral Meatus
Cryotherapy with liquid nitrogen.
or
Podophyllin 10% to 25%* in a compound tincture of benzoin. Treatment area must be dry before contact with normal mucosa. Repeat weekly if necessary.

Vaginal
Cryotherapy with liquid nitrogen. Cryoprobe is not recommended (risk of perforation and fistula formation).
or
TCA or BCA, 80% to 90%. Apply small amount only to warts. If excess amount applied, powder with talc, baking soda, or liquid soap. Repeat weekly if necessary.

Anal
Cryotherapy with liquid nitrogen.
or
TCA or BCA, 80% to 90%. Apply small amount only to warts. If excess amount applied, powder with talc, baking soda, or liquid soap. Repeat weekly if necessary.

Many persons with anal warts may also have them in the rectal mucosa. Inspect rectal mucosa by digital examination or anoscopy. Warts on the rectal mucosa should be managed in consultation with a specialist.

Oral
Cryotherapy with liquid nitrogen.
or
Surgical removal.

*Safety during pregnancy not established.

average, clearance occurs in women over a 18-month period. Data on the natural history of infection and time to clearance among men are limited. Identified risks for HPV infection include young age at sexual debut and multiple and/or new sexual partners.[37]

The clinical course of HPV varies. Persistence of high-risk HPV infection, most commonly types 16 and 18, is associated with cervical neoplasia that may progress to cervical cancer in women. Among men, persistent infection with high-risk HPV may lead to penile neoplasia and cancer. Infection with low-risk types leading to genital warts (condylomas) in men and women may motivate individuals to seek medical care. In the normal host, condylomas are typically a cosmetic, rather than functional disorder. As the treatment of cervical dysplasia and cancer is outside the realm of this chapter, we focus here on the treatment of genital warts. In most cases, repeat treatments for a course of therapy, typically over 3 months, are warranted to lead to resolution of lesions. Patients should be educated that treatment may lead to hypopigmented or scarred areas, chronic pelvic pain disorders, and, among those with rectal warts, painful bowel movements and/or rectal fistulas.

Patient-applied therapies include podophilox 0.5% solution or gel applied twice daily for 3 days, then followed by 4 days of no application. Podophilox prevents mitosis in replicating cells, inducing cell death. This treatment alternation may be followed up to four cycles. Imiquimod 5% cream once daily, 3 times weekly for up to 16 weeks, is another option for patient-applied therapy. Imiquimod acts by inducing a local immunologic response against the lesion.

Provider-administered therapies include cryotherapy, podophyllin resin 10% to 25%, trichloroacetic acid 80% to 90%, bichloroacetic acid 80% to 90%, surgical excision, intralesional interferon, or laser surgery. These agents work against warts via antimitotic, immunologic, or architectural mechanisms to destroy undesirable lesions. Women with cervical warts must be evaluated for evidence of high-grade dysplasia prior to wart therapy. The CDC 2006 STD Treatment Guidelines recommend different approaches to therapy, depending upon lesion location.[34] Box 85-7 presents these recommendations.

REFERENCES

1. Lewis DA. Chancroid: clinical manifestations, diagnosis, and management. Sex Transm Infect 2003;79:68-71.
2. Reddy CR, Devendranath V, Pratap S. Carcinoma of penis—role of phimosis. Urology 1984;24:85-88.
3. Lewis DA. Diagnostic tests for chancroid. Sex Transm Infect 2000;76:137-141.
4. Gotz HM, Ossewaarde JM, Nieuwenhuis RF, et al. [A cluster of lymphogranuloma venereum among homosexual men in Rotterdam with implications for other countries in Western Europe]. Ned Tijdschr Geneeskd 2004;148:441-442.
5. Tinmouth J, Rachlis A, Wesson T, Hsieh E. Lymphogranuloma venereum in North America: case reports and an update for gastroenterologists. Clin Gastroenterol Hepatol 2006;4:469-473.
6. Mabey D, Peeling RW. Lymphogranuloma venereum. Sex Transm Infect 2002;78:90-92.
7. Blank S, Schillinger JA, Harbatkin D. Lymphogranuloma venereum in the industrialised world. Lancet 2005;365:1607-1608.
8. Chen CY, Chi KH, Alexander S, et al. The molecular diagnosis of lymphogranuloma venereum: evaluation of a real-time multiplex polymerase chain reaction test using rectal and urethral specimens. Sex Transm Dis 2007;34:451-455.
9. O'Farrell N. Donovanosis. Sex Transm Infect 2002;78:452-457.
10. Roberts CM, Pfister JR, Spear SJ. Increasing proportion of herpes simplex virus type 1 as a cause of genital herpes infection in college students. Sex Transm Dis 2003;30:797-800.
11. Engelberg R, Carrell D, Krantz E, et al. Natural history of genital herpes simplex virus type 1 infection. Sex Transm Dis 2003;30:174-177.
12. Wald A, Huang ML, Carrell D, et al. Polymerase chain reaction for detection of herpes simplex virus (HSV) DNA on mucosal surfaces: comparison with HSV isolation in cell culture. J Infect Dis 2003;188:1345-1351.
13. Scoular A, Gillespie G, Carman WF. Polymerase chain reaction for diagnosis of genital herpes in a genitourinary medicine clinic. Sex Transm Infect 2002;78:21-25.
14. Wald A, Selke S, Warren T, et al. Comparative efficacy of famciclovir and valacyclovir for suppression of recurrent genital herpes and viral shedding. Sex Transm Dis 2006;33:529-533.
15. Conant MA, Schacker TW, Murphy RL, et al. Valaciclovir versus aciclovir for herpes simplex virus infection in HIV-infected individuals: two randomized trials. Int J STD AIDS 2002;13:12-21.
16. Patel R, Bodsworth NJ, Woolley P, et al. Valaciclovir for the suppression of recurrent genital HSV infection: a placebo controlled study of once daily therapy. International Valaciclovir HSV Study Group. Genitourin Med 1997;73:105-109.
17. az-Mitoma F, Sibbald RG, Shafran SD, et al. Oral famciclovir for the suppression of recurrent genital herpes: a randomized controlled trial. Collaborative Famciclovir Genital Herpes Research Group. JAMA 1998;280:887-892.
18. Mertz GJ, Loveless MO, Levin MJ, et al. Oral famciclovir for suppression of recurrent genital herpes simplex virus infection in women: a multicenter, double-blind, placebo-controlled trial. Collaborative Famciclovir Genital Herpes Research Group. Arch Intern Med 1997;157:343-349.
19. Reitano M, Tyring S, Lang W, et al. Valaciclovir for the suppression of recurrent genital herpes simplex virus infection: a large-scale dose range-finding study. International Valaciclovir HSV Study Group. J Infect Dis 1998;178:603-610.
20. DeJesus E, Wald A, Warren T, et al. Valacyclovir for the suppression of recurrent genital herpes in human immunodeficiency virus-infected subjects. J Infect Dis 2003;188:1009-1016.
21. Gardella C, Brown Z, Wald A, et al. Risk factors for herpes simplex virus transmission to pregnant women: a couples study. Am J Obstet Gynecol 2005;193:1891-1899.
22. Sheffield JS, Hollier LM, Hill JB, et al. Acyclovir prophylaxis to prevent herpes simplex virus recurrence at delivery: a systematic review. Obstet Gynecol 2003;102:1396-1403.
23. Watts DH, Brown ZA, Money D, et al. A double-blind, randomized, placebo-controlled trial of acyclovir in late pregnancy for the reduction of herpes simplex virus shedding and cesarean delivery. Am J Obstet Gynecol 2003;188:836-843.
24. Whitley RJ, Alford CA, Hirsch MS, et al. Vidarabine versus acyclovir therapy in herpes simplex encephalitis. N Engl J Med 1986;314:144-149.
25. Riedner G, Rusizoka M, Todd J, et al. Single-dose azithromycin versus penicillin G benzathine for the treatment of early syphilis. N Engl J Med 2005;353:1236-1244.
26. Centers for Disease Control and Prevention. Azithromycin treatment failures in syphilis infections—San Francisco, California 2002-2003. MMWR 2004;53:197-198.
27. Lukehart SA, Godornes C, Molini BJ, et al. Macrolide resistance in *Treponema pallidum* in the United States and Ireland. N Engl J Med 2004;351:154-158.
28. Mandel GL, Bennet JE, Dolin R (eds). Principles and Practice of Infectious Diseases, 6th ed. Philadelphia: Elsevier Saunders, 2005, p 2780.
29. Pickering LK, Baker CJ, Long SS, et al (eds): 2006 Red Book: Report of the Committee on Infectious Diseases, 27th ed. Elk Grove Village, IL: American Academy of Pediatrics, 2006.
30. Lau CS, Sant GR. Urethritis, prostatitis, epididymitis, and orchitis. *In* Gorbach SL, Bartlett JG, Blacklow NR (eds): Infectious Diseases, 3rd ed. Philadelphia: Lippincott Williams & Wilkins, 2004, pp 872-877.
31. Bradshaw CS, Tabrizi SN, Read TR, et al. Etiologies of nongonococcal urethritis: bacteria, viruses, and the association with orogenital exposure. J Infect Dis 2006;193:336-345.
32. Schwebke JR, Hook EW III. High rates of *Trichomonas vaginalis* among men attending a sexually transmitted diseases clinic: implications for screening and urethritis management. J Infect Dis 2003;188:465-468.
33. Madeb R, Nativ O, Benilevi D, et al. Need for diagnostic screening of herpes simplex virus in patients with nongonococcal urethritis. Clin Infect Dis 2000;30:982-983.
34. Centers for Disease Control and Prevention. Sexually transmitted diseases treatment guidelines, 2006. MMWR Morb Mortal Wkly Rep 2006;55(11):1-66.
35. Sobel JD, Ferris D, Schwebke J, et al. Suppressive antibacterial therapy with 0.75% metronidazole vaginal gel to prevent recurrent bacterial vaginosis. Am J Obstet Gynecol 2006;194:1283-1289.
36. Muñoz N, Bosch FX, de Sanjosé S, et al. Epidemiologic classification of human papillomavirus types associated with cervical cancer. N Engl J Med 2003;348:518-527.
37. Dunne EF, Markowitz LE. Genital human papillomavirus infection. Clin Infect Dis 2006;43:624-629.

86

MEDICAL TOXICOLOGY AND ANTIDOTES

Thomas P. Moyer

INTRODUCTION 1213
ANTIDOTES 1213
Acetaminophen 1213
Alcohols and Glycols 1213
Methanol 1214
Ethylene Glycol 1214
Treatment 1214
Cyanide 1215
Digitalis Alkaloids 1216
Amanita phalloides 1216
Transition Metals 1216
Aluminum 1217
Arsenic 1218
Iron 1218
Lead 1218
Manganese 1218
Mercury 1218
Opioids 1219
Vitamin K Inhibitors 1219

INTRODUCTION

Antidotes are drugs designed to counteract toxins. They act by altering the chemical nature of the toxin, or by interfering with toxin binding to biologic sites; in either case, the antidote interferes with the toxin to reduce morbidity or mortality.

This chapter reviews antidotes in common use in medical practice in the United States and Europe. The chapter is organized alphabetically by toxin or toxin group. Readers will also be interested in the excellent chapter on antidotes in *Ellenhorn's Medical Toxicology*.[1] Antivenins are not covered in this chapter. Readers are referred to the excellent book by Meier and White (*Handbook of Clinical Toxicology of Animal Venoms and Poisons*)[2] and to *Ellenhorn's Medical Toxicology*.[1] Cholinesterase inhibitors (see Chapter 9, Autonomic Pharmacology) and malignant hyperthermia (see Chapter 60, General Anesthesia and Sedation) are also discussed elsewhere.

ANTIDOTES

Acetaminophen

Acetaminophen toxicity is a major cause of hepatic failure in the United States, representing 40% of all cases of hepatic failure presenting to tertiary care hospitals. In 2003, poison control centers reported 127,000 potentially intoxicating acetaminophen exposures, with 65,000 patients receiving some form of treatment in a medical facility; 16,500 receiving the recommended antidote, *N*-acetylcysteine (NAC); and 214 deaths directly associated with acetaminophen overdose.[3] Of these patients, 39,000 were children under the age of 6. It is estimated that 30,000 to 40,000 adolescents and adults intentionally overdose on acetaminophen each year. Acetaminophen toxicity caused 15,000 adolescents and adults to be hospitalized an average of 2.7 days in 1995 because of acetaminophen overdose. This group of patients required 50 liver transplantations as a form of therapy. It is estimated that intentional acetaminophen overdose cost the U.S. health care system $90 million in 1995.[4]

Toxicity due to acetaminophen ingestion is associated with the formation of a metabolite, *N*-acetyl-*p*-benzoquinone imine (NAPQI). In the condition of normal dosage, the majority of acetaminophen is metabolized via phase II conjugation to form either glucuronide or sulfate (Fig. 86-1). A small fraction of acetaminophen is metabolized by the hepatic cytochrome P-450 (CYP) isoenzymes (CYP2E1, CYP1A2, and CYP3A4) in a phase I reaction to produce NAPQI, which is rapidly detoxified by conjugation with glutathione to nontoxic metabolites. However, acetaminophen overdose diverts more acetaminophen into the CYP metabolic pathway, producing NAPQI at concentrations that exceed the availability of glutathione. In the absence of glutathione, NAPQI acts as an electrophile, binding covalently to cysteine sulfhydryl groups on protein. These protein conjugates are inactive, leading to cell death.

Chronic consumption of ethanol induces CYP isoenzymes, resulting in increased diversion of acetaminophen down the CYP metabolic pathway and thus predisposing a patient to acetaminophen toxicity at usual doses. Malnutrition depletes glutathione stores and can also predispose an individual to acetaminophen toxicity with normal dosing.

The Rumack-Matthew nomogram is used to guide treatment after acetaminophen overdose.[5] The nomogram (Fig. 86-2) relates the serum acetaminophen concentration to time after ingestion to predict potential for hepatotoxicity. For example, an acetaminophen concentration greater than 200 mcg/ml in a specimen collected 4 hours after ingestion indicates high probability of hepatotoxicity. A serum acetaminophen concentration of 125 mcg/ml in a specimen collected 12 hours after ingestion also indicates high probability of hepatotoxicity. In the absence of acetaminophen levels, or if time of ingestion is unknown, hepatotoxicity is likely with doses greater than 150 mg/kg in children or 15 g in otherwise healthy adults.

N-Acetylcysteine is the antidote of choice for treating severe acetaminophen intoxication. *N*-acetylcysteine serves as a precursor of glutathione, increasing cellular glutathione concentrations (see Fig. 86-1). There are two accepted approaches to NAC treatment. In the United States, a loading dose of NAC of 140 mg/kg, followed by a maintenance dose of 70 mg/kg every 4 hours for 72 hours, is an accepted practice. In Europe, the standard of practice is a loading dose of 150 mg/kg intravenous NAC in 200 ml of 5% glucose over 15 minutes, followed by 50 mg/kg intravenous NAC in 500 ml of 5% glucose over 4 hours, followed by 100 mg/kg intravenous NAC in 100 ml of 5% glucose for 16 hours. Intravenous administration is the therapy of choice in the United States for patients with intractable vomiting.[4,6,7]

Alcohols and Glycols

Poisonings with methanol and ethylene glycol occur with sufficient frequency to justify specific antidotes and treatment protocols. In the United States, from a population base of 271 million in 2000, 2418 reports of methanol toxicity resulted in 193 patients suffering from moderate or major toxicity. There were 12 deaths, all occurring in adults. The province of Ontario, Canada, with a population of 11 million, reported 43 methanol-related deaths during the 7-year period of 1986 to 1991.[8] Twenty-two of these deaths were suicides, and 14

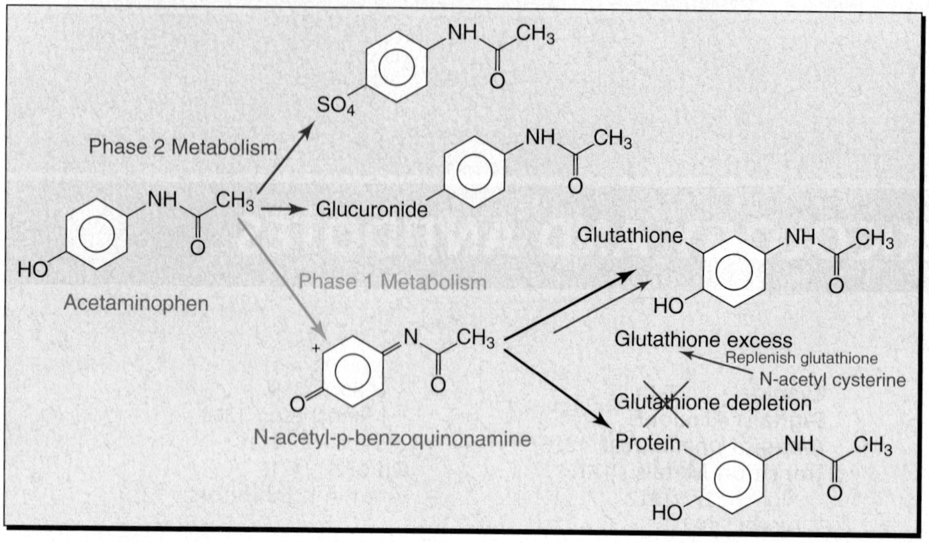

FIGURE 86-1 • Formation of *N*-acetyl-*p*-benzoquinone imine, the toxic metabolite of acetaminophen.

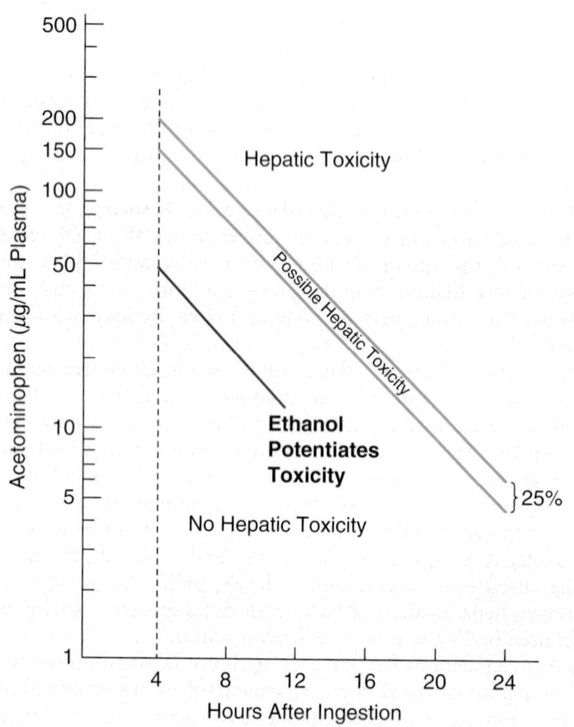

FIGURE 86-2 • Rumack-Matthew nomogram.

were the result of using methanol as a substitute for ethanol. All subjects were over the age of 18, and 91% were men.

Throughout the United States, 5816 cases of ethylene glycol poisoning were reported in 2002. Of these cases, 82% were unintentional, 12% involved children under the age of 6, 75% occurred in the home, and 10% occurred in the workplace. In 2003, 2241 cases of ethylene glycol exposure were reported, with 23% deaths. In fact, ethylene glycol was the most common chemical agent responsible for deaths reported by United States poison control centers in that year.[9]

Methanol

In the United States alone, over a billion gallons of methanol are produced annually. Methanol is used as a solvent in the manufacture of other chemicals, as an octane booster, and as a major component of cleaning solutions, printing and duplicating solutions, adhesives, enamels, stains, dyes, varnishes, thinners, and paint removers commonly found in the home. Methanol is the most common agent in

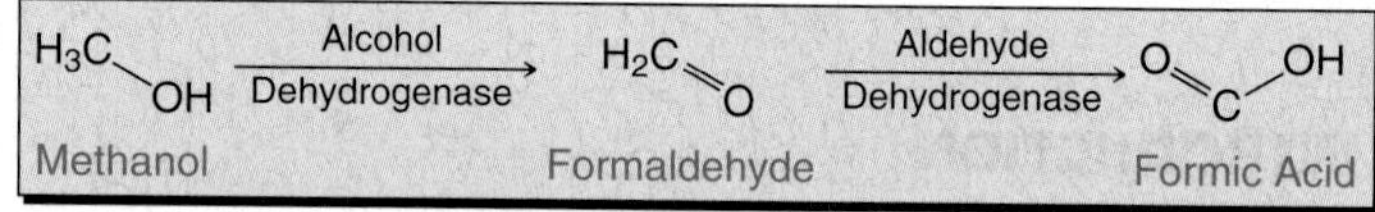

FIGURE 86-3 • Methanol metabolism.

windshield and gas line antifreeze and is the fuel most frequently used for heating chafing dishes. Methanol is absorbed rapidly following oral intake, with a mean absorption half-life of 5 minutes. Following ingestion, peak absorption occurs within 30 to 60 minutes. Methanol is readily absorbed through the skin and pulmonary epithelium. Methanol distributes throughout body water with a distribution volume of 0.6 to 0.77 L/kg.

Methanol itself has little toxicity; its metabolites are responsible for the toxicity associated with methanol exposure. Methanol undergoes metabolism by alcohol dehydrogenase to form formaldehyde (Fig. 86-3). Subsequent oxidation of formaldehyde to formic acid occurs very rapidly, with a half-life of 1 to 2 minutes, and is catalyzed by aldehyde dehydrogenase. Formic acid is metabolized slowly in the presence of tetrahydrofolate to form 10-formaltetrahydrofolate that then decomposes to carbon dioxide and water. The apparent half-life of formate metabolism can be as long as 20 hours. At concentrations associated with clinical toxicity, methanol elimination is characterized by apparent zero-order kinetics with a typical elimination rate of 150 to 200 mg/L per hour.[8]

Ethylene Glycol

Ethylene glycol is rapidly and completely absorbed from the gastrointestinal tract to achieve peak serum concentrations in 20 to 30 minutes after ingestion. Twenty percent of absorbed ethylene glycol is eliminated unchanged in the urine, while 80% is metabolized in the liver by alcohol dehydrogenase to form glycoaldehyde, which is subsequently metabolized by aldehyde dehydrogenase to glycolic acid, glyoxylic acid, and oxalic acid (Fig. 86-4). Following ethylene glycol ingestion, glycolic acid accumulates in serum and is primarily responsible for anion gap metabolic acidosis, and oxalic acid binds calcium to form calcium oxalate crystals that precipitate in urine and cause renal injury.[9,10]

Treatment

Two antidotes for methanol exposure are commonly used: ethanol and fomepizole. Both antidotes work to block the metabolism of methanol by alcohol dehydrogenase. Ethanol has approximately 10 times greater affinity for this enzyme than methanol and, by competitive inhibition, diverts methanol metabolism into alternative pathways that do not create formic acid (Fig. 86-5). Ethanol is rapidly absorbed from the

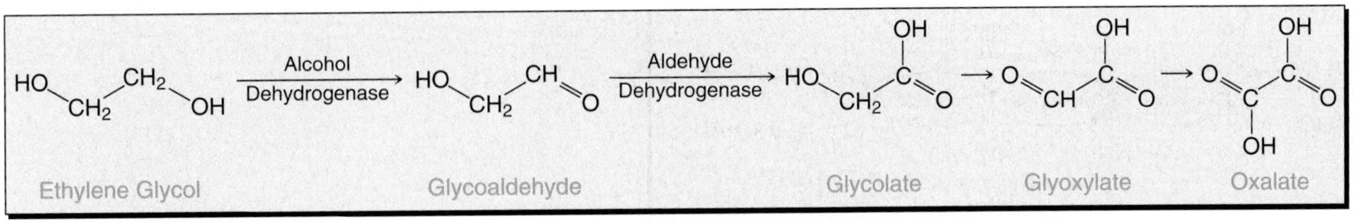

FIGURE 86-4 • Ethylene glycol metabolism.

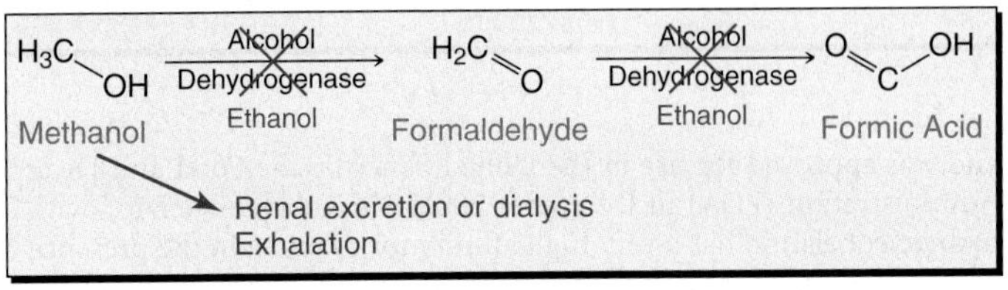

FIGURE 86-5 • Ethanol inhibits methanol metabolism, reducing toxicity.

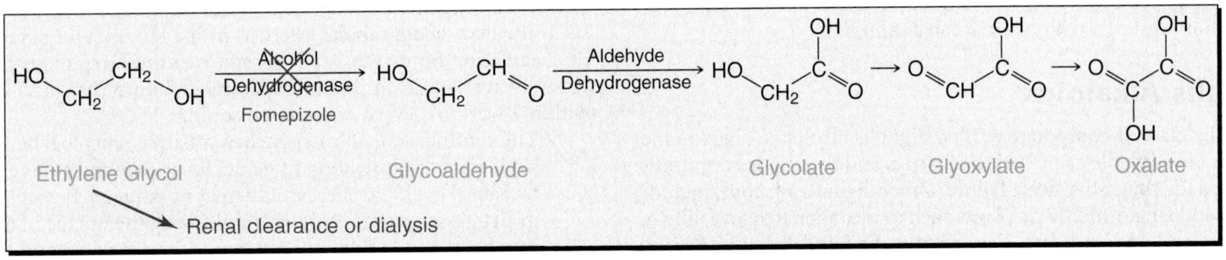

FIGURE 86-6 • Fomepizole inhibits ethylene glycol metabolism, reducing toxicity.

gastrointestinal tract and distributes into the total body water with an apparent volume of distribution of 0.6 to 0.7 L/kg. More than 90% of absorbed ethanol is metabolized in the liver, with the remainder excreted via kidneys and lungs. For treatment of methanol toxicity, ethanol is administered at a loading dose of 600 to 800 mg/kg to achieve serum concentrations in the range of 0.1 to 0.15 g/dl.[8]

Fomepizole distributes rapidly into total body water with a distribution volume of 0.6 to 1.0 L/kg and has an affinity for alcohol dehydrogenase 500 to 1000 times higher than that of ethanol. Fomepizole is a potent inhibitor of alcohol dehydrogenase, and plasma fomepizole concentrations greater than 0.8 mg/L completely inhibit metabolism of methanol to formaldehyde and formic acid (Fig. 86-6). Accordingly, it has become the standard of care in treating patients who have ingested either methanol or ethylene glycol.

Fomepizole is administered with a loading dose of 15 mg/kg, followed by 10-mg/kg doses at 10, 24, and 36 hours. Duration of fomepizole dose is determined by the methanol concentration. However, greater than 95% of fomepizole is eliminated via hepatic metabolism, and repeated dosing with fomepizole induces CYP2B1, resulting in increased metabolism of fomepizole. Therefore, to compensate for this enhanced metabolism, fomepizole doses must be increased if administered longer than 48 hours.[11]

Hemodialysis is effective and should be considered as an integral part of treatment of toxic methanol and ethylene glycol poisonings to expedite elimination. Hemodialysis effectively extracts both ethanol and fomepizole. If treatment includes fomepizole plus hemodialysis, the fomepizole dosing interval could be reduced from 12 hours to 4 hours. In Europe, the recommended fomepizole IV infusion rate during hemodialysis is 1 to 1.5 mg/kg per hr.

Cyanide

Cyanide is used in metal extraction, electroplating, pesticides, metal hardening, photography, and printing, and as a dye. Cyanide is an acute toxin producing complete blockade of oxidative phosphory-lation in just a few moments. While cyanide exposure is rare, cyanide recently has been deployed by terrorists in Tokyo, London, Rome, and Paris.[12]

The mechanism of action of cyanide, outlined in Figure 86-7, involves uncoupling of oxidative phosphorylation. Cyanide avidly binds to ferric iron (Fe^{3+}) associated with a wide array of proteins. Perhaps the most critical enzyme affected is cytochrome a_3, a key enzyme in the oxidative phosphorylation pathway. In the presence of cyanide, cytochrome a_3 becomes nonfunctional, resulting in loss of ATP synthesis, and all cells reliant upon the oxidative process for energy cease to function.

Two distinctly different cyanide antidotes are available. The Cyanide Antidote Kit, also known as the Lilly or Pasadena, or Taylor Cyanide Antidote Package, contains ammonium nitrite, sodium nitrite, and sodium thiosulfate. Nitrite oxidizes ferrous iron (+2) to ferric iron (+3), converting hemoglobin to methemoglobin. Methemoglobin has a very high affinity for cyanide and acts as a carrier protein to facilitate its elimination. Sodium thiosulfate coupled with the ubiquitous enzyme, rhodanase, converts cyanide to nontoxic thiocyanate, which is eliminated via renal excretion. Because the production of methemoglobin reduces the oxygen-carrying capacity of the blood, careful monitoring of oxygenation is required and high-dose oxygen should be administered as soon as possible to compensate for the effects of cyanide toxicity and methemoglobin formation.[13]

Immediately upon diagnosis of cyanide poisoning, ammonium nitrite is administered by allowing the subject to inhale ammonium nitrite fumes for 15 seconds followed by breathing regular air for 15 seconds until such time that a sodium nitrite intravenous infusion can be started. For adults, a 3% solution of sodium nitrite should be infused at a rate of 2.5 ml/min. For children, sodium nitrite should be infused at a rate of 6 to 8 ml/m^2 or 0.2 ml/kg body weight. As soon as the sodium nitrite infusion is completed, adults should receive 50 ml of an intravenous solution containing 25% sodium thiosulfate. For children, 7 g/m^2 of this solution should be administered. Blood pressure should be monitored carefully during nitrite administration because nitrites are potent vasodilators that can produce severe hypotension, compounding shock commonly associated with cyanide poisoning.

Hydroxycobalamin (vitamin B_{12}) is also an effective cyanide antidote. Hydroxycobalamin has been available in Europe for many years,

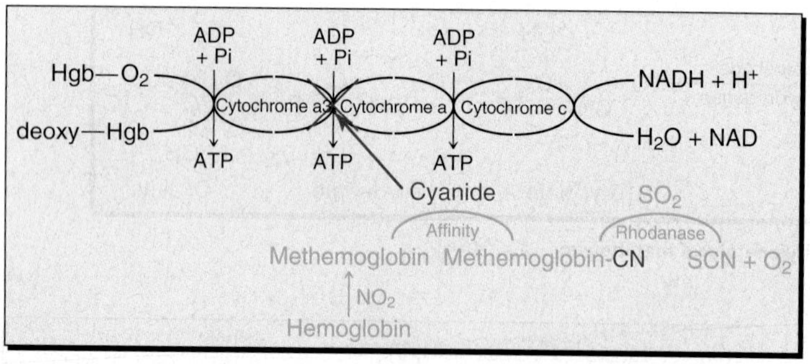

FIGURE 86-7 • Mechanism of cyanide blockade of oxidative phosphorylation, and methemoglobin scavenging to facilitate cyanide clearance as thiocyanate.

and was approved for use in the United States by the Food and Drug Administration (FDA) in December 2006. The cobalt associated with hydroxycobalamin has a very high affinity for cyanide; in the presence of cyanide, nontoxic cyanocobalamin is formed. Cyanocobalamin is administered to adults as an intravenous infusion of 5 g over 20 to 30 minutes. The pediatric dose is 17 mg/kg. Sodium thiosulfate is routinely coadministered with hydroxycobalamin.[12,14]

Digitalis Alkaloids

Within the class of compounds called digitalis alkaloids, digoxin and digitoxin are available as prescription drugs and digoxin is commonly prescribed for congestive heart failure. Other digitalis alkaloids include ouabain and lanatoside. Toxic plants such as oleander, foxglove, lilly of the valley, and Indian hemp also contain digitalis alkaloids. Several species of toad venom contain chemically related cardioactive sterols of the bufadienolides class, notably bufalin, cinobufotalin, and cinobufagin. All of these compounds interact with Na/K transporters and have a narrow therapeutic index. Cardiotoxicity with any of these compounds results from impaired cardiac conduction and enhanced automaticity, typically manifesting as supraventricular tachycardia, ventricular ectopy, and potentially fatal ventricular tachycardia.

An antidote for digoxin or digitoxin toxicity is a digoxin-specific antibody fragment, the Fab fragment, that is produced by papaine digestion of antibodies raised in sheep against digoxin–human albumin conjugate.[15] There are several commercial versions of antidigoxin Fab: Digibind (GlaxoSmithKline), Digitalis Antidote (Boehringer-Mannheim), and DigiFab (Protherics). These digoxin Fab fragments bind digoxin on a mole-to-mole basis. An adult dose of antidigoxin Fab fragment is 380 mg administered intravenously over 15 to 30 minutes in 250 ml of isotonic plasma protein solution. An 80-mg Fab fragment dose binds approximately 1 mg of digoxin or digitoxin. If the ingested dose is not known, the dose can be estimated from the plasma digoxin concentration using the following formula:

$$\text{Digoxin body burden} = \text{plasma digoxin (mcg/L)} \times 5\ \text{(L/kg)} \times \text{body weight (kg)} \div 1000$$

Pediatric administration also is guided by this relationship.

Antidigoxin Fab fragments have a volume of distribution of 0.4 L/kg and a plasma half-life of 12 to 20 hours, and the Fab-digoxin conjugate is eliminated via both renal and hepatic processes. In renal failure, the half-life of Fab fragments is prolonged by 10-fold.[16,17] It is important to recognize that, once doses of antidigoxin Fab fragment are administered, the standard immunoassays used by clinical laboratories to generate plasma digoxin levels are no longer accurate because the antidigoxin Fab fragment interferes with these immunoassays. A detailed discussion of this phenomenon has been presented by Jortani et al.[18]

Amanita phalloides

Wild mushrooms in the *Amanita* family are responsible for a number of fatal mushroom poisonings. Ingestion of 50 g (three mushrooms) of *Amanita phalloides*, also known as Death Cap, accounts for the majority of deaths due to mushroom poisoning. The principle toxic agent is α-amanitin, a cytotoxic cyclic peptide that acts by inhibiting transcription of DNA to RNA and is exacerbated by tumor necrosis factor-α, which, at the gene transcription level, inhibits mitogen-activating protein kinase type INK. Most affected are the liver, kidney, and blood coagulation mechanism, resulting in central lobular necrosis in the liver, acute tubular necrosis in the kidney, and derangement of coagulation homeostasis.[19,20] Several treatment regimens have successfully averted death due to hepatorenal failure that usually occurs within 1 week of severe *Amanita* poisoning:

1. The combination of intensive hemodialysis, charcoal hemoperfusion, and administration of penicillin and silibinin was employed by Sabeel et al.[19] to successfully treat 41 patients. Penicillin inhibits drug transporter proteins, minimizing the uptake of amatoxin into hepatocytes. Silibinin interrupts the enterohepatic recirculation of amatoxin, facilitating amatoxin clearance.
2. *N*-Acetylcysteine has been used to successfully treat 11 cases of *Amanita* poisoning following the treatment protocol for acetaminophen (see previous section). *N*-acetylcysteine is an oxygen free radical scavenger that rapidly distributes into many cells, thereby increasing intracellular oxygen and facilitating platelet aggregation.[20]
3. When patients cannot be treated quickly enough, orthotopic liver transplantation is an option.[21]

Transition Metals

In one group of 329,000 general medical outpatients that included a broad spectrum of all disease types, 1986 patients (0.6% of the total population) were identified as having some physical finding or exposure concern warranting further examination for heavy metal exposure. Of these, 152 cases (0.05% of the original population) were identified by laboratory testing as cases of high suspicion that heavy metals were involved in causing toxic symptoms. Of these, 32 cases (0.01% of the population, or 1 in 9700) ultimately were proven to have heavy metal toxicity. Eighteen of these cases were arsenic related, two were cadmium related, seven were lead related, and five were mercury related.[22]

Treatment of metal-based toxicity relies on administration of metal chelators that form electrostatic bonds with transition metal ions. Frequently, chelators form two or more bonds with the transition metal to form a ring structure. The most common chelating agents used are listed in Table 86-1.[23,24]

Dimercaprol (British Anti-Lewisite, 2,3-dimercapto-1-propanol) forms a five-member heterocyclic chelate ring with heavy metals. It is administered by deep intramuscular injection of 2 to 5 mg/kg per dose one to four times per day for up to 10 days. Peak serum concentrations of dimercaprol occur within 60 minutes. The most common adverse effects of dimercaprol observed in humans are nausea, vomiting, hypertension, and tachycardia and less frequently nephrotoxicity, seizures, hyperpyrexia, sweating, lacrimation, urticaria, and paresthesias. Although no human lethality data have been reported, dimercaprol has a median lethal dose (LD_{50}) of 0.85 mmol/kg in rats. Dimercaprol is contraindicated in treating poisonings by alkylmercury, cadmium, iron, or selenium.[25] The mechanism of dimercaprol binding is shown in Figure 86-8.

TABLE 86-1 COMMON CHELATING AGENTS

Transition Metal Ion	Chelating Agent
Aluminum	Deferoxamine (desferrioxamine; polyketo-tetraazaheptaeicosane)
Arsenic	Dimercaprol (British Anti-Lewisite [BAL]; 2,3-dimercapto-1-propanol) 2,3-dimercapto-1-propanesulfonic acid (DMPS) D-Penicillamine
Copper	D-Penicillamine, succimer, dimercaprol
Iron	Deferoxamine
Lead	Succimer, DMPS, ethylenediaminetetra-acetic acid (EDTA), D-penicillamine
Manganese	EDTA
Mercury	Succimer, D-penicillamine, dimercaprol
Thallium	Prussian Blue

Adapted from Blanuša M, Varnai VM, Piasek M, Kostial K. Chelators as antidotes of metal toxicity: therapeutic and experimental aspects. Curr Med Chem 2005;12:2771-2794; and Aposhian HV, Maiorino RM, Gonzalez-Ramirez D, et al. Mobilization of heavy metals by newer, therapeutically useful chelating agents. Toxicology 1995;97:23-38.

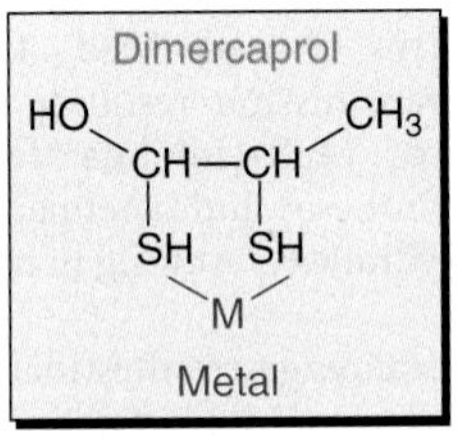

FIGURE 86-8 • Mechanism of action of dithiol chelators.

Succimer (*meso*-2,3-dimerptosuccinic acid) is a water soluble, orally active, and less toxic analogue of dimercaprol. A 10-mg/kg dose every 8 hours for 5 days is the recommended treatment for lead poisoning in children. Follow-up treatment of 10 mg/kg every 12 hours for an additional 14 days is recommended. In adults, 30 mg/kg per day for 5 days is the usual dose. Peak plasma levels of succimer occur within 2 hours of administration. Succimer has an LD_{50} of 18 mmol/kg in rats, considerably higher than doses administered during therapy. Side effects include mild and transient gastrointestinal cramps, nausea, vomiting, and diarrhea. Because succimer is eliminated by hepatic metabolism and renal clearance, patients with renal or liver impairment require careful dosing. Caution also is required when treating patients with neutropenia or with glucose-6-phosphate dehydrogenase deficiency. Use of succimer during pregnancy has not been associated with identifiable birth defects.

Another dimercaprol derivative, 2,3-dimercapto-1-propanesulfonic acid (DMPS), is available in Europe but not in the United States. A typical adult dose is 200 to 400 mg administered orally every 4 to 6 hours. No pediatric dosing guidelines have been established. Peak plasma concentration is achieved within 4 hours of administration, and the elimination half-life is 10 hours.

D-Penicillamine forms a divalent chelate with transition elements. The adult oral dose of D-penicillamine is 2 g/day. Peak plasma concentrations are reached within 4 hours, and D-penicillamine does not undergo significant metabolism. A variant of D-penicillamine, *N*-acetyl-D-penicillamine, is also available as a chelating agent. The dose and pharmacokinetic profile of *N*-acetyl-D-penicillamine are similar to those of D-penicillamine. Toxicity of D-penicillamine and *N*-acetyl-D-penicillamine is typified by hematologic disorders such as thrombocytopenia and occasionally aplastic anemia. Both compounds are considered teratogenic.

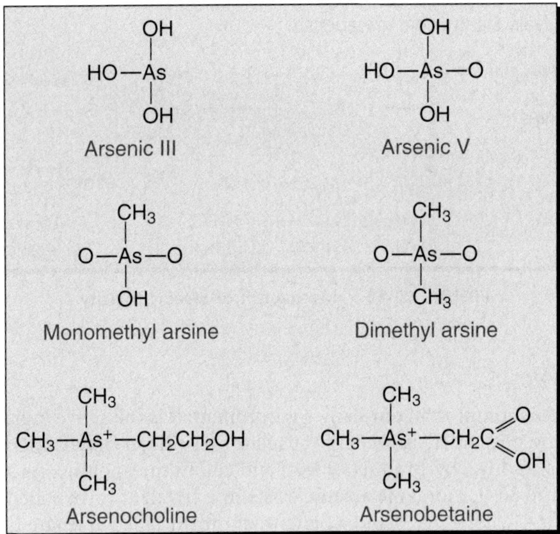

FIGURE 86-9 • Arsenic species.

Ethylenediaminetetra-acetic acid (EDTA), in either the dicalcium or tricalcium form, is administered parenterally for 5 days in doses of 50 to 75 mg/kg per day to adults or 1000 to 1500 mg/m^2 per day to children. Repeated 5-day courses may be required. EDTA reaches peak plasma levels in less than 3 hours and is completely excreted within 24 hours. Because EDTA has a high affinity for calcium and can rapidly chelate serum calcium, administration of the dicalcium version can induce hypocalcemic tetany. The principle toxic side effect of EDTA is nephrotoxicity, which is usually reversible following cessation of therapy. Renal tubular injury is dose related, and it is recommended that the daily dose be maintained less than 75 mg/kg per day. Zinc depletion could be anticipated during EDTA therapy, so zinc supplementation should be considered. Because EDTA is such an avid complexor of calcium and zinc, it is teratogenic.

Deferoxamine is administered parenterally at a daily dose not to exceed 50 mg/kg. Peak serum concentrations are achieved in less than 2 hours, and the drug is completely eliminated within 6 hours. Adverse effects of deferoxamine include hypotension, respiratory distress syndrome, thrombocytopenia, tachycardia, tinnitus, and retinal damage with vision loss. Allergic reactions are common. Deferoxamine is not known to be teratogenic.

Prussian Blue is the preferred antidote for thallium and cesium intoxication. Prussian Blue is normally administered orally to adults at 3 g three times per day; the pediatric dose is 1 g orally three times per day. Treatment should be continued for a minimum of 30 days. Prussian Blue has relatively low toxicity, but the possibility of potassium depletion should be monitored.

Chelation challenge testing has been reported as a tool to diagnose metal intoxication.[26] There is considerable skepticism about the value of chelation challenge testing. Results must be interpreted very carefully, and only in the context of baseline testing performed before the chelator is administered.[27]

Aluminum

While aluminum is commonly found in consumer products and has many industrial applications, it is not consider toxic. However, before deionizers were routinely used to prepare kidney dialysis fluid, and when aluminum-containing compounds still were used to reduce hyperphosphatemia, aluminum accumulation in brain and bone tissue was a frequent cause of dialysis encephalopathy and osteomalacia. A relationship between aluminum and Alzheimer's disease has been proposed but is unproven. Normal serum aluminum concentrations are below 10 mcg/L, and serum aluminum concentrations over 100 mcg/L can be associated with toxicity. Serum aluminum concentrations do not accurately reflect total body burden because aluminum is highly protein bound. Deferoxamine is the preferred chelating agent.[25]

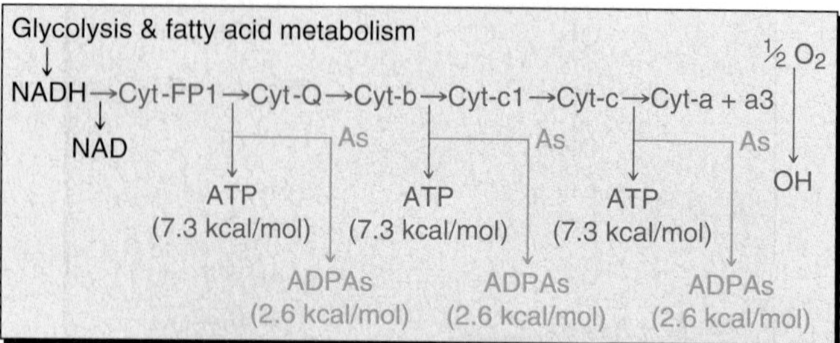

FIGURE 86-10 • Mechanism of arsenic toxicity.

Arsenic

Arsenic is common in our daily environment. It is the active ingredient in many pesticides, is a charge insulator in silicon-based microelectronics, and is a by-product of lead and cadmium smelting. As shown in Figure 86-9, inorganic arsenic exists in a trivalent form called arsenite (As_2O_3, AsIII, As^{3+}) and a pentavalent form called arsenate (As_2O_5, AsV, As^{5+}); both forms are toxic. Arsine (AsH_3) is a toxic, colorless, nonirritating gas that evolves from arsenic-containing metal alloys exposed to acidic conditions during smelting of various ores. Arsenic in food, particularly seafood, occurs predominantly as nontoxic organic compounds (arsenobetaine and arsenocholine). The organic arsenicals contain trivalent or pentavalent arsenic linked to a carbon atom by a covalent bond.

Toxic effects of arsenic are expressed in biologic systems through two different mechanisms of action: (i) arsenic uncouples oxidative phosphorylation in the glycolytic pathway, interfering with the synthesis of ATP (Fig. 86-10); and (ii) arsenic binds avidly to dihydrolipoic acid, an important cofactor in the coenzyme A–catalyzed synthesis of acetyl coenzyme A in the tricarboxylic acid cycle. Both of these mechanisms interrupt energy formation in oxidative cells, resulting in cell damage and death. Endothelial cells in the gastrointestinal tract and the kidney glomerulus are affected, as are cardiac and nerve cells. The most common symptoms of chronic arsenic exposure are hyperpigmentation, keratosis, hepatomegaly, neuropathy, weakness, and chronic respiratory disease.[28]

Chelation therapy is indicated in the treatment of symptomatic arsenic poisoning after confirmed acute ingestion with urinary arsenic levels greater than 50 mcg/L, and in asymptomatic patients with urinary arsenic levels greater than 200 mcg/L. In the United States, intramuscular injection of dimercaprol is the standard chelation therapy for arsenic poisoning. It is estimated that 30 mg of arsenic are eliminated for every 50 mg of dimercaprol administered. Succimer has been reported ineffective in treating arsenic intoxication.[29-31] However, DMPS (Unithiol) is another water-soluble analogue of dimercaprol that forms a complex with methylated arsenic species (see Fig. 86-10). DMPS can be administered orally, intravenously, or intramuscularly. DMPS is available in Europe for arsenic chelation, but is not approved by the FDA in the United States. However, reports of successful arsenic treatment with DMPS in the United States on a compassionate use basis suggest that DMPS is an effective arsenic chelator.[28-30]

Iron

It is estimated that there are 5000 cases of significant iron poisoning per year,[32-34] most frequently occurring as unintentional exposures in children. Pediatric exposure very likely occurs because many iron-containing vitamin and nutritional supplements look like candy. Excessive exposure to iron causes erosion of the gastrointestinal mucosa, resulting in stomach and intestinal ulcerations, hemorrhage, and disrupted coagulation. Excessive iron circulating in blood also damages vascular epithelium, leading to plasma loss, decreased blood volume, and impaired tissue perfusion. Circulating unbound iron accumulates in hepatic Kupffer cells that facilitate transport of iron into hepatic mitochondria, where resulting free radical formation and lipid peroxidation result in altered membrane permeability and loss of aerobic respiration. Iron also acts as an electron sink, shunting electrons away from the electron transport system and thereby reducing ATP production.

Deferoxamine, also known as desferrioxamine, was developed as an antidote for iron intoxication. Deferoxamine is a polyketotetraazaheptaeicosane that is an avid chelator of ferrous iron. Deferoxamine is available in two forms, a formulation intended for subcutaneous infusion and a formulation intended for oral administration. The subcutaneous formulation is administered at a dose of 40 mg/kg per day. The oral formulation is administered at 70 mg/kg per day in three divided doses. Several reports[35-37] suggest that the subcutaneous administration is potentially more effective than oral administration; however, compliance with oral administration is better. Simultaneous administration of both formulations also has been proven effective. Recently, deferoxamine has shown value in treating transfusion iron overload in patients with β-thalassemia major[35,37] and juvenile hemochromatosis.[36]

Lead

Inorganic forms of lead are absorbed through the gastrointestinal tract or lungs while organic forms of lead are absorbed through the skin. Children absorb lead more efficiently than adults. Calcium or iron deficiency can increase the amount of lead absorbed. Lead circulates in the blood bound to erythrocytes. Glomerular filtration is the primary route of lead excretion, subjecting proximal renal tubular epithelial cells to high lead concentrations, resulting in shedding of these cells. Lipid-rich tissues such as nerves are particularly sensitive to the organic forms of lead. Lead affects voltage-gated ion channels and synaptic transmission, resulting in damage to the endothelial microvasculature. Lead inhibits ferrochelatase, resulting in diminished heme synthesis and anemia. Lead also inhibits δ-aminolevulinic acid dehydratase, resulting in increased aminolevulinic acid excretion.

Acute lead exposure requires gastrointestinal lavage, including endoscopic removal if lead is visualized on abdominal radiographs. The American Academy of Pediatrics recommends that chelation not be prescribed for children with blood lead concentrations less than 45 mcg/dl.[38] Children with blood lead concentrations between 45 and 65 mcg/dl may benefit from the use of succimer.[39] Workers with a blood lead concentration over 50 mcg/dl must be removed from exposure, and active treatment is indicated when blood lead concentration exceeds 65 mcg/dl. In severe lead poisoning, dimercaprol should be administered, followed by $CaNa_2EDTA$, to prevent the latter from increasing the distribution of lead into the brain. A rebound in blood lead concentrations is common after chelation therapy is terminated because lead re-equilibrates from tissues into erythrocytes. Therefore, 10 to 14 days should be allowed after chelation therapy before obtaining another blood lead concentration to guide additional chelation.[25]

Manganese

Manganese is widely distributed in the environment and is an essential trace element. Miners and welders are at the highest risk of manganese toxicity. Manganese exposure in miners and during processing of manganese ore and ferromanganese is known to cause an extrapyramidal syndrome characterized by progressive parkinsonism, dystonia, and neuropsychiatric symptoms. Potassium permanganate is used in water purification, manganese dioxide in the manufacture of dry batteries and fireworks, manganese chloride in animal feed, and manganese sulfate as a fertilizer. Manganese toxicity from foods does not occur, but manganese toxicity may be seen in patients with chronic liver disease and may be caused by excessive manganese concentration in parenteral nutrition. Accordingly, it has been suggested that manganese supplementation in children on long-term parenteral nutrition not exceed 0.018 μmol/kg per day. Attempts to chelate manganese with $CaNa_2EDTA$ have not been successful. *N*-acetylcysteine has been used in potassium permanganate poisoning.[25]

Mercury

We live in an environment that contains mercury. It is present in the water we drink, the air we breath, and the food we eat. In nature, mercury vapor evaporates from granite rock, is emitted by volcanoes, municipal incinerators, coal-burning power stations, and in the effluent from paper manufacturing. Mercury has also been used as a medication. In the last century, mercury was used to treat syphilis and dysentery. Mercury is still used today in the topical antiseptic known as merthiolate (thimerisol). Much of what we know about the neurotoxicity of organic mercury is from the Minamata Bay incident in Japan in the 1950s that resulted from consumption of fish with a high methyl mercury content. In recent times, there has been considerable public interest in mercury toxicity due to concerns regarding possible toxicity from mercury vapor released from dental amalgam and from consumption of fish with a high mercury content.

The clinical presentation of mercury toxicity depends on the chemical state of the element to which the patient was exposed. Elemental mercury vaporizes easily at room temperature; mercury vapor may be inhaled or absorbed through the skin and mucous membranes. Exposure to mercury vapor may cause gastrointestinal, pulmonary, or, if chronic, neurologic symptoms. The target organs of inorganic mercury are the gastrointestinal tract and kidneys. Organic forms of mercury are more toxic to nerves.

No chelating agent has been conclusively documented to consistently affect clinical outcome. Succimer has a low toxicity and is the treatment of choice in methyl mercury poisoning.[40] D-Penicillamine, dimercaprol, and DMPS have been used to treat mercury poisoning with varied success. The prominent gastrointestinal effects of inorganic mercury poisoning may prompt use of parenteral dimercaprol. Dialysis may be required to remove the dimercaprol-mercury complex when inorganic mercury poisoning is associated with renal failure. Treatment begun after development of serious neurotoxicity due to organic mercury is of little benefit.[25]

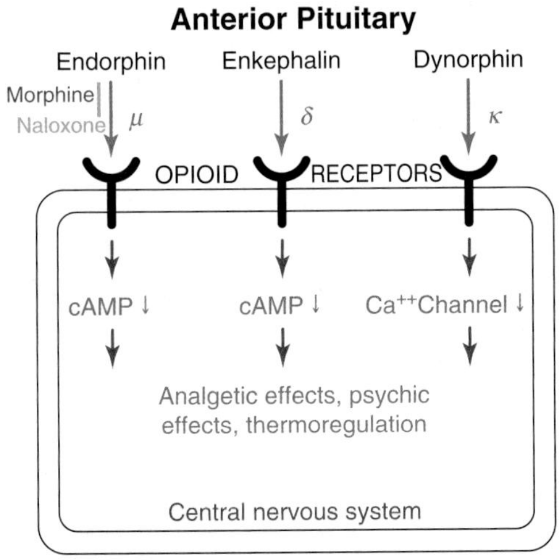

Anterior Pituitary

Endorphin Enkephalin Dynorphin

Morphine Naloxone μ δ κ

OPIOID RECEPTORS

cAMP ↓ cAMP ↓ Ca++Channel ↓

Analgetic effects, psychic effects, thermoregulation

Central nervous system

FIGURE 86-11 • Opioid receptors and actions.

Opioids

Opioids, most notably represented by the opiates morphine and heroin, bind to natural opioid receptors to inhibit response to painful stimuli, modulate gastrointestinal contraction, and have a profound effect on emotion (Fig. 86-11). Naturally circulating endogenous opioid peptides, known as endorphins, participate in a complex biologic system modulating sensation throughout the nervous system. Opioid receptors belong to the G protein–coupled receptor family that function by inhibiting adenylate cyclase activity, receptor-operated potassium currents, and suppression of voltage-gated calcium currents to control analgesia, mood, reward behavior, and respiratory, cardiovascular, gastrointestinal, and neuroendocrine function.

Opiate intoxication is the fourth most common emergency department drug-related event reported in U.S. databases,[41] with more than 164,000 cases reported in 2005. The most obvious sign of opiate toxicity is miosis (constriction of pupils to a pinpoint), caused by excitation of the parasympathetic nervous system. Opiates depress respiration rate and tidal volume, and intoxication results in hypoxia. The classical presentation of a patient with an opiate overdose is known as the opiate triad: coma, miosis, and suppressed respiration. Opiates also produce peripheral vasodilation, reduce peripheral resistance, and inhibit baroreceptor reflexes, resulting in orthostatic hypotension.

The toxic effects of opiates are readily reversed by administering opioid antagonists. Naloxone is a pure opioid antagonist that will block morphine binding to the μ-opioid receptor, reversing miosis, respiratory depression, and orthostatic hypotension associated with opioid overdose. Small doses (0.4 to 0.8 mg) of naloxone administered intramuscularly will reverse the effects of opioid receptor agonists within 1 to 2 minutes.[42]

Vitamin K Inhibitors

Anticoagulation therapy with warfarin is the most common mode of treatment and prophylaxis for venous and arterial thromboembolic conditions. As many as 2 million people in the United States may start warfarin therapy annually.[43,44] Because of its narrow therapeutic index, warfarin is a leading cause of iatrogenic bleeding and a cause of disabling and fatal hemorrhagic events. The incidence of warfarin-related intracerebral hemorrhage ranges from 1% to 4% in the entire population of patients administered warfarin. During 2002, 18% of all patients diagnosed with intracerebral hemorrhage were being anticoagulated. On this basis, it is projected that there are 8000 to 10,000 cases of warfarin-associated intracerebral hemorrhages per year in the United States.[45,46]

The efficacy and safety of warfarin are assessed by monitoring the international normalized ratio (INR), the ratio of the patient's prothrombin time to that of a sample of normal pooled plasma, after adjusting for the sensitivity of the laboratory's thromboplastin. A number of studies have shown a significant increase in bleeding when the INR is above the upper limit of normal and a significantly increased risk of thromboembolic events when the INR falls below the therapeu-

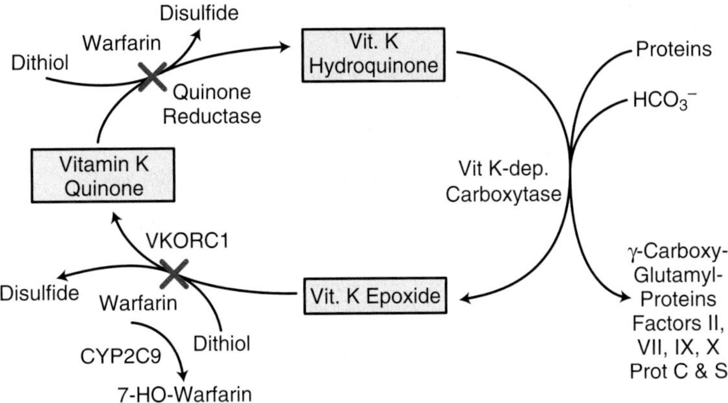

FIGURE 86-12 • Warfarin inhibition of the vitamin K cycle.

tic range. An INR of 1 is normal, an INR of 2 to 3 describes optimal anticoagulation therapy, an INR greater than 5 identifies a patient as predisposed to excessive bleeding, and an INR greater than 10 indicates a potential for severe bleeding.

Warfarin acts by inhibiting the vitamin K cycle (Fig. 86-12), reducing activity of coagulation factor–dependent clotting functions. Warfarin and other vitamin K antagonists, such as procoumarone, acecoumarone, and super-warfarins such as brodifacoum and difenacoum, inhibit regeneration of vitamin K, a cofactor in the γ-carboxylation of coagulation factors II, VII, IX, and X. Specifically, these compounds inhibit the enzymes vitamin K epoxide reductase C1 and quinone reductase. The end result of this inhibition is diminished vitamin K hydroquinone, a key cofactor in the formation of coagulation factors.

Replenishment of vitamin K by administration of either intravenous or oral formulations of vitamin K (phytonadione, phytomenadion) is the preferred antidote for treating excessive anticoagulation with warfarin and should be considered whenever the INR is greater than 6. Although the half-life of vitamin K in plasma is 1.5 to 3 hours, the full effect of vitamin K is only achieved 12 to 24 hours after administration. Therefore, patients presenting with major hemorrhage due to excessive warfarin anticoagulation require more rapid treatment to restore normal clotting function, and vitamin K administration should be accompanied by infusion of fresh frozen plasma.[46] Oral vitamin K administration provides more variable responses than intravenous administration,[47,48] and is ineffective in patients with biliary obstruction.[49] However, anaphylactoid reactions to intravenous vitamin K therapy occur in 3 of 10,000 doses administered.

A single intravenous dose of 0.5 mg vitamin K is usually administered, with a repeat dose at 24 hours if the INR has not normalized. In cases of severe bleeding, an intravenous dose of 2.5 mg may be considered.[49] Oral vitamin K (Konakion) is typically administered at a dose of 2 mg, although up to 5 mg may be indicated in treating severe bleeding. Two thirds of patients respond to a single 2-mg oral dose of vitamin K. One third of patients require a second dose of vitamin K to correct over-anticoagulation.[46]

REFERENCES

1. Ellenhorn MJ, Schonwald S, Ordog G, Wasserberger J. Ellenhorn's Medical Toxicology: Diagnosis and Treatment of Human Poisoning, 2nd ed. Baltimore: Williams & Wilkins, 1997.
2. Meier J, White J. Handbook of Clinical Toxicology of Animal Venoms and Poisons. New York: CRC Press, 1995.
3. Rowden AK, Norvell J, Eldridge DL, Kirk MA. Updates on acetaminophen toxicity. Med Clin North Am 2005;89:1145-1159.
4. Dart RC, Erdman AR, Olson KR, et al. Acetaminophen poisoning: an evidence-based consensus guideline for out-of-hospital management. Clin Toxicol 2006;44:1-18.
5. Rumack BH, Matthew H. Acetaminophen poisoning and toxicity. Pediatrics 1975;55: 871-876.
6. Tsai C-L, Chang W-T, Weng T-I, et al. A patient-tailored N-acetylcysteine protocol for acute acetaminophen intoxication. Clin Ther 2005;27:336-341.
7. Kerr F, Dawson A, Whyte IM, et al. The Australasian Clinical Toxicology Investigators Collaboration randomized trial of different loading infusion rates of N-acetylcysteine. Ann Emerg Med 2005;45:402-408.
8. Barceloux DG, Bond GR, Krenzelok EP, et al. American Academy of Clinical Toxicology practice guidelines on the treatment of methanol poisoning. Clin Toxicol 2002;40:415-446.
9. Caravati EM, Erdman AR, Christianson G, et al. Ethylene glycol exposure: an evidence-based consensus guideline for out-of-hospital management. Clin Toxicol 2005;43:327-345.
10. Battistella M. Fomepizole as an antidote for ethylene glycol poisoning. Ann Pharmacother 2002;36:1085-1089.
11. Mégarbane B, Borron SW, Baud FJ. Current recommendations for treatment of severe toxic alcohol poisonings. Intensive Care Med 2005;31:189-195.
12. Morrocco AP. Cyanides. Crit Care Clin 2005;21:691-705.
13. Koschel MJ. Management of the cyanide-poisoned patient. J Emerg Nurs 2006;32: S19-S26.
14. Mannaioni G, Vannacci A, Marzocca C, et al. Acute cyanide intoxication treated with a combination of hydroxycobalamin, sodium nitrite, and sodium thiosulfate. Clin Toxicol 2002;40:181-183.
15. Pullen MA, Brooks DP, Edwards RM. Characterization of the neutralizing activity of digoxin-specific Fab toward ouabain-like steroids. J Pharmacol Exp Ther 2004;310:319-325.
16. Flanagan RJ, Jones AL. Fab antibody fragments—some applications in clinical toxicology. Drug Saf 2004;27:1115-1133.
17. Chillet P, Korach JM, Petitpas D, et al. Digoxin poisoning and anuric acute renal failure: efficiency of the treatment associating digoxin-specific antibodies (Fab) and plasma exchanges. Int J Artif Organs 2002;25:538-541.
18. Jortani SA, Pinar A, Johnson NA, et al. Validity of unbound digoxin measurements by immunoassays in presence of antidote (Digibind®). Clin Chim Acta 1999;283:159-169.
19. Sabeel AI, Kurkus J, Lindholm T. Intensive hemodialysis and hemoperfusion treatment of *Amanita* mushroom poisoning. Mycopathologia 1995;131:107-114.
20. Montanini S, Sinardi D, Praticò C, et al. Use of acetylcysteine as the life-saving antidote in *Amanita phalloides* (death cap) poisoning. Drug Res 1999;49:1044-1047.
21. Broussard CN, Aggarwal A, Lacey SR, et al. Mushroom poisoning—from diarrhea to liver transplantation. Am J Gastroenterol 2001;96:3195-3198.
22. Moyer TP. Toxic metals. *In* Burtis CA, Ashwood ER, Bruns DA (eds): Tietz Textbook of Clinical Chemistry, 4th ed. Philadelphia: Elsevier Saunders, 2005, pp 1371-1390.
23. Blanuša M, Varnai VM, Piasek M, Kostial K. Chelators as antidotes of metal toxicity: therapeutic and experimental aspects. Curr Med Chem 2005;12:2771-2794.
24. Aposhian HV, Maiorino RM, Gonzalez-Ramirez D, et al. Mobilization of heavy metals by newer, therapeutically useful chelating agents. Toxicology 1995;97:23-38.
25. Kumar N, Moyer TP. Neurotoxic metals. *In* Noseworthy JH (ed): Neurological Therapeutics: Principles and Practice, Vol 2, 2nd ed. Abingdon, UK: Informa Healthcare, 2006, pp 1716-1735.
26. Frumkin H, Manning CC, Williams PL, et al. Diagnostic chelation challenge with DMSA: a biomarker of long-term mercury exposure? Environ Health Perspect 2001;109:167-171.
27. Risher JF, Amler SN. Mercury exposure: evaluation and intervention—the inappropriate use of chelating agents in the diagnosis and treatment of putative mercury poisoning. Neurotoxicology 2005;26:691-699.
28. Guha Mazumder DN. Chronic arsenic toxicity: clinical features, epidemiology, and treatment: experience in West Bengal. J Environ Sci Health A Tox Hazard Subst Environ Eng 2003;38:141-163.
29. Lai MW, Boyer EW, Kleinman ME, et al. Acute arsenic poisoning in two siblings. Pediatrics 2005;116:249-257.
30. Wax PM, Thornton CA. Recovery from severe arsenic-induced peripheral neuropathy with 2,3-dimercapto-1-propanesulphonic acid. Clin Toxicol 2000;38:777-780.
31. Hantson P, Haufroid V, Buchet J-P, Mahieu P. Acute arsenic poisoning treated by intravenous dimercaptosuccinic acid (DMSA) and combined extrarenal epuration techniques. J Toxicol Clin Toxicol 2003;41:1-6.
32. Gossel TA, Bricker JD. Principles of Clinical Toxicology, 3rd ed. New York: Raven Press, 1994, p 187.
33. Tran T, Wax JR, Philput C, et al. Intentional iron overdose in pregnancy—management and outcome. J Emerg Med 2000;18:225-228.
34. Wood JC, Otto-Duessel M, Gonzalez I, et al. Deferasirox and deferiprone remove cardiac iron in the iron-overloaded gerbil. Transl Res 2006;148:272-280.
35. Darr S, Pathare AV. Combined therapy with desferrioxamine and deferiprone in beta thalassemia major patients with transfusional iron overload. Ann Hematol 2006;85:315-319.
36. Fabio G, Minonzio F, Delbini P, et al. Reversal of cardiac complications by deferiprone and deferoxamine combination therapy in a patient affected by a severe type of juvenile hemochromatosis (JH). Blood 2007;109:362-364.
37. Galanello R, Kattamis A, Piga A, et al. A prospective randomized controlled trial on the safety and efficacy of alternating deferoxamine and deferiprone in the treatment of iron overload in patients with thalassemia. Haematologica 2006;91:1241-1243.
38. American Academy of Pediatrics Policy Statement: Lead exposure in children: prevention, detection, and management. Pediatrics 2005;116:1036-1046.
39. Farrar HC, McLeane LR, Wallace M, et al. A comparison of two dosing regimens of succimer in children with chronic lead poisoning. J Clin Pharmacol 1999;39:180-183.
40. Garza-Ocañas L, Torres-Alanís O, Piñeyro-López A. Urinary mercury in twelve cases of cutaneous mercurous chloride (calomel) exposure: effect of sodium 2,3-dimercaptopropane-1-sulfonate (DMPS) therapy. Clin Toxicol 1997;35:653-655.
41. Office of Applied Studies, Substance Abuse & Mental Health Services Administration. Drug Abuse Warning Network, 2005: National Estimates of Drug-Related Emergency Department Visits. March 13, 2007. Available at *http://www.oas.samhsa.gov/DAWN/2k5ed.cfm*.
42. Gutstein HH, Akil H. Opioid analgesics. *In* Hardman JG, Limbird LE (eds): Goodman & Gilman's The Pharmacologic Basis of Therapeutics, 10th ed. New York: McGraw-Hill, 2001, pp 569-619.
43. McWilliam A, Lutter R, Nardinelli C. Health care saving from personalizing medicine using genetic testing: the case of warfarin. AEI-Brookings Joint Center for Regulatory Studies, Working Paper 06-23. Washington, DC: AEI-Brookings Joint Center for Regulatory Studies, 2006.
44. Flaherty M, Kissela B, Woo D, et al. The increasing incidence of anticoagulant-associated intracerebral hemorrhage. Neurology 2007;68:116-121.
45. Aguilar M, Hart RG, Kase C, et al. Treatment of warfarin-associated intracerebral hemorrhage: literature review and expert opinion. Mayo Clin Proc 2007;82:82-92.
46. Sconce EA, Kamali F. Appraisal of current vitamin K dosing algorithms for the reversal of over-anticoagulation with warfarin: the need for a more tailored dosing regimen. Eur J Haematol 2006;77:457-462.
47. Dentali F, Ageno W, Crowther M. Treatment of coumarin-associated coagulopathy: a systematic review and proposed treatment algorithms. J Thromb Haemost 2006;4:1853-1863.
48. DeZee K, Shimeall W, Douglas K, et al. Treatment of excessive anticoagulation with phytonadione (vitamin K). Arch Intern Med 2006;166:391-397.
49. Schulman S, Bijsterveld NR. Anticoagulants and their reversal. Transfus Med Rev 2007;21:37-48.

87

OVER-THE-COUNTER MEDICATIONS

Barbara A. Levey

OVERVIEW 1221
INTRODUCTION 1221
THE OTC MONOGRAPH SYSTEM 1221
THERAPEUTICS AND CLINICAL PHARMACOLOGY 1221
OTC Medications 1221
OTC Therapeutic Considerations 1223
Excipients 1223
Acetaminophen and Aspirin 1223
Phenylpropanolamine—Removed from the OTC Market 1223
OTC Statins—Unapproved 1223
Pediatrics and Obstetrics/Gynecology 1223
Plan B OTC 1224
CONCLUSION 1224

OVERVIEW

The defining characteristic of over-the-counter (OTC) medications is availability without a prescription. The U.S. Food and Drug Administration (FDA) Center for Drug Evaluation and Research (CDER) Office of Nonprescription Products[1] employs a system analogous to the drug development process for prescription medications. The CDER provides oversight for a broad range of OTC products. The Office of Nonprescription Products also maintains a wealth of information for health professionals and the public on the center's rich and informative website.

The history[2-6] of significant FDA regulatory pharmaceutical legislation enactment has frequently been accompanied by therapeutic disasters. Regulation of medications in the United States emerged with importation restrictions in the 19th century and was inaugurated officially in 1906 with the first Federal Food and Drugs Act, after a tetanus outbreak was traced to contaminated vaccines and antitoxins. Legislation that followed included the Harrison Narcotics Act of 1914 and the Federal Food, Drug and Cosmetic Act of 1938, the latter in the wake of more than 100 deaths due to Elixir of Sulfanilamide prepared with diethylene glycol as solvent. In 1951, the Durham-Humphrey Amendment to the Food, Drug and Cosmetic Act distinguished three criteria for prescription drugs, thereby defining OTC drugs by exclusion. A noted incident occurred in 1962, when Dr. Frances Kelsey, an FDA officer, barred prenatal marketing of the teratogenic hypnotic drug thalidomide, thus avoiding in the United States a duplication of the neonatal anomalies reported in Europe and Africa. The Kefauver-Harris Drug Amendments of 1963 mandated broad regulation of pharmaceutical products, including proof of safety and efficacy in drug development. In 1968, the Drug Efficacy Study Implementation directed retrospective review of drugs, including 420 OTC medications introduced from 1938 to 1962. Regulatory requirements continue to evolve steadily. In 2004, the FDA issued a Final Rule requiring bar codes on specified OTC and prescription drugs.[7] Updates on OTC products are published regularly in the *Federal Register*.[8,9]

INTRODUCTION

Available pharmacokinetic and pharmacogenetic advances applied to OTC medications offer new opportunities for interindividual therapeutics and decline of adverse drug reactions. The goals of this chapter are to increase appreciation for the background and process of the OTC oversight system; to increase the reader's knowledge base of OTC drugs; to provide cogent examples of significant OTC topics of concern; and to suggest tools to enable evaluation of present and future OTC medications as they become available in therapeutics.

THE OTC MONOGRAPH SYSTEM

OTC drug review was initiated by the FDA in 1972. OTC drug development has progressed to a stepwise process of CDER evaluations by the Office of Nonprescription Products. OTC medications are recognized to be safe, effective, and not misbranded if they have met the conditions of the OTC Drug Monograph review process. This organizational structure impacts positively the safety, efficacy, and labeling of OTC products.

The three-step Monograph system[10,11] is in place to determine that OTC products meet conditions "generally recognized as safe and effective" (GRASE). This system applies both to new OTC preparations and to applications by drug sponsors to transfer prescription products to OTC status.[12] A special CDER Advisory Review Panel is constituted to conduct the review. The steps to OTC approval are the Advanced Notice of Proposed Rulemaking (ANPR), the Tentative Final Monograph (TFM), and the Final Monograph (Table 87-1). The OTC Drug Advisory Review Panel classifications are ranked categorically.

The Final Monograph for OTC medications is analogous to the New Drug Application for prescription drugs. The ANPR in the OTC medication development process invites public comments and requires uniform, clear labeling according to criteria defined. Final Rules are published in the *Federal Register*[8] with corresponding Final Monographs. OTC labeling provides a model of clarity and detail for the consumer.

For information on dietary supplements, which are sold over-the-counter but regulated under the Dietary Supplement Health and Education Act of 1994, see Chapter 90, Complementary and Alternative Medicine, Nutraceuticals, and Dietary Supplements.

THERAPEUTICS AND CLINICAL PHARMACOLOGY

OTC Medications

The scope of OTC medication regulations is large and growing. Recent analyses[13-17] catalogue more than 2700 OTC medication ingredients, 138 dosage forms, 93 routes of administration, 82 different units, 58 types of packing, and 81 Milestone[18] categories of *Federal Register* publication dates for major OTC rulemakings.

The following alphabetical list of examples is derived from the Food and Drug Administration's compilations of Over-the-Counter Ingredients.[15-17] Indications for ANPR and PR categories are designated. S represents Safety and E, Efficacy, justifications for classification as ANPR or PR II or III. Where the ANPR or PR is marked *n/a*, the OTC Drug Advisory Review Panel did not evaluate the product. Prescrip-

TABLE 87-1 FDA OVER-THE-COUNTER (OTC) MEDICATION DEVELOPMENT PROCESS: STEPS TO MARKET

Action	Comment
OTC Drug Advisory Review Panel appointed for each product.	Panel members are selected for **expertise** appropriate to OTC product reviewed. **Panel applies uniform Criteria:** Category I: GRASE (generally recognized as safe and effective) and not misbranded Category II: not GRASE or misbranded Category III: insufficient evidence to classify
Step 1: ANPR (Advanced Notice of Proposed Rulemaking)	Category I: ↔ *Federal Register*
Step 2: TFM (Tentative Final Monograph)	Category I: ↔ *Federal Register*
Step 3: FM (Final Monograph)	Category I: ↔ *Federal Register*

Adapted from Hilfiker D; Division of Over the Counter Drug Products. OTC 101. U.S. Food and Drug Administration, Center for Drug Evaluation and Research, 2005. Available at *http://www.fda.gov/cder/about/smallbiz/Presentations/4.ppt*; and U.S. Food and Drug Administration, Center for Drug Evaluation and Research. Food and Drug Administration Guide: OTC Drug Review Ingredient Report. Available at *www.fda.gov/cder/Offices/OTC/Ingredient_List_Guide.pdf.*

tion-to-OTC approvals[19] are also available, provided by the CHPA (Consumer Healthcare Providers Association).

A

Aluminum Carbonate Gel (basic)—antacid (ANPR I, PR I)
Aminobenzoic Acid (PABA)—sunscreen (ANPR I, PR I)
Aminophylline—(cough/cold)—bronchodilator (ANPR I, PR IIS)

B

Bacitracin—first aid antibiotic—(ANPR n/a, PR I)
Bacitracin—skin wound antibiotic—(ANPR IIIE, PR defer)
Brompheniramine Maleate—antihistamine (H1 antagonist)—(ANPR I, PR I)

C

Chlorpheniramine Maleate—antihistamine (H1 antagonist)—(ANPR I, PR I)
Codeine—antitussive—(ANPR I, PR I)
Codeine—internal analgesic—(ANPR IISE, PR IISE)

D

Denatonium Benzoate—topical thumbsucking deterrent (ANPR IIIE, PR IIIE)
Dextromethorphan—antitussive (ANPR I, PR I)
Docusate Calcium—stool softeners, laxative—(ANPR I, PR I)

E

Ephedrine—bronchodilator—(ANPR I, PR I)
Ephedrine—topical nasal decongestant—(ANPR I, PR I)
Epinephrine—oral nasal decongestant—(ANPR IIIE, PR IIIE)

F

Ferric Ammonium Citrate—weight control, anorectic—(ANPR IISE, PR IISE)
Ferric Chloride—skin protectant *et al*—(ANPR IISE, PR IISE)
Frangula—stimulant laxative (ANPR IIISE, PR IIISE)

G

Gamboge—stimulant laxative—(ANPR IISE, PR IISE)
Glutamic Acid Hydrochloride—digestive aid—(ANPR IIE, PR IIE)
Guaifenesin—expectorant—(ANPR IIIE, PR IIIE)

H

Haloprogin—antifungal—(ANPR I, PR I)
Hydrochloric Acid Diluted—stomach acidifier—(ANPR IIE, PR IIE)
Hydrocodone bitartrate—antitussive—(ANPR IIS, PR IIS)

I

Ibuprofen—internal analgesic/antipyretic—(ANPR n/a, PR I)
Ichthammol—boil treatment/corn/callus remover—(ANPR IISE, PR IISE)
Ipecac—emetic, poison treatment—(ANPR I, PR I)

J

Jalap—stimulant laxative—(ANPR IIS, PR IIS)
Jojoba Oil—hair grower—(ANPR n/a, PR IIE)
Juniper Extract—weight control, anorectic—(ANPR IISE, PR IISE)

K

Karaya Gum—bulk laxative—(ANPR I, PR I)
Karaya Gum—weight control, anorectic—(ANPR IIIE, PR IISE)
Kelp—weight control, anorectic—(ANPR IIIE, PR IISE)

L

Lactobacillus Acidophilus—antdiarrheal, fever blister/oral—(ANPR IIIE, PR IIIE)
Lidocaine—intrarectal anesthetic—(ANPR IIIE, PR IIIE)
Lidocaine—topical analgesic—(ANPR I, PR I)

M

Meclizine Hydrochloride—laxative, antiemetic—(ANPR I, PR I)
Metaproterenol Sulfate—cough, cold (bronchodilator)—(ANPR n/a, PR III)
Miconazole Nitrate—antifungal—(ANPR I, PR I)

N

Naphazoline Hydrochloride—topical/inhalant, ophthalmic vasoconstrictor—(ANPR I, PR I)
Neomycin Sulfate—cream/ointment, first aid antibiotic—(ANPR n/a, PR I)
Noscapine—cough/cold, antitussive—(ANPR IIIE, PR IIIE)

O

Octinoxate—sunscreen—(ANPR I, PR I)
Opium Tincture or Powdered—antidiarrheal—(ANPR I, PR IIISE)
Oxymetalozine Hydrochloride—nasal decongestant (topical/inhalant)—(ANPR I, PR I)

P

Pancreatin—exocrine pancreatic insufficiency—(ANPR I, PR I)
Pancreatin—digestive aid, intestinal distress—(ANPR IIIE, PR IIIE)
Pseudoephedrine Sulfate—nasal decongestant (oral)—(ANPR I, PR I)

Q

Quinine—internal analgesic/antipyretic—(ANPR IISE, PR IISE)
Quinine Ascorbate—smoking deterrent—(ANPR IIE, PR IIE)
Quinine Sulfate—nocturnal leg muscle cramps—(ANPR IIISE, PR IIISE)

R

Resorcinol Monoacetate—acne—(ANPR IIE, PR IIE)
Rhubarb, Chinese—stimulant laxative—(ANPR IIISE, PR IIISE)
Rice Polishings—weight control, anorectic—(ANPR IISE, PR IISE)

S

Saccharin—weight control, anorectic—(ANPR IISE, PR IISE)
Selenium Sulfide Micronized—dandruff, seborrheic dermatitis—(ANPR I, PR I)
Stannous Fluoride anticavity dental dentifrice, gel, rinse—(ANPR I, PR I)

T

Terpin Hydrate—cough/cold, (expectorant)—(ANPR IIIE, PR IIIE)
Thimerosal (external mercury)—antiseptic—(ANPR IISE, PR IISE)
Tryptophan—weight control, anorectic—(ANPR IISE, PR IISE)

U

Urea—hair grower—(ANPR n/a, PR IIE)
Urea—ingrown toenail—(ANPR IISE, PR IISE)
Uva Ursi, Extract—weight control, anorectic—(ANPR IIIE, PR IIIE)

V

Valine—weight control, anorectic—(ANPR IISE, PR IISE)
Vegetable Oil—hair grower—(ANPR IISE, PR n/a)
Vitamin E—acne—(ANPR IIE, PR IIE)

W

Wax, White—ophthalmic emollient—(ANPR I, PR I)
Wheat Germ—weight control, anorectic—(ANPR IIISE, PR IIISE)
Witch Hazel—external, skin protectant, astringent—(ANPR I, PR I)

X

Xanthan Gum—weight control, anorectic—(ANPR IIIE, PR IISE)
Xylometalozine Hydrochloride—cough/cold, nasal decongestant—(ANPR I, PR I)

Y

Yeast—weight control, anorectic—(ANPR IISE, PR IISE)
Yeast Cell Derivative, Live—wound healing agent—(ANPR IIISE, PR IIISE)
Yohimbine—internal aphrodisiac—(ANPR IISE, PR IISE)

Z

Zinx Oxide—topical anorectal astringent/protectant—(ANPR I, PR I)
Zinc Sulfide—antibiotic II—acne—(ANPR IIIE, PR IIE)
Zirconium Oxide—insect bite/sting—(ANPR IISE, PR IISE)

OTC Therapeutic Considerations

OTC regulations mandate standards recognized to be safe and effective, yet the safety of OTC products depends ultimately on several human factors. Accurate self-diagnosis, appropriate self-medication, recognition of adverse effects, and awareness of new information are important consumer responsibilities. The pharmacist and the physician, as the health care providers, are in positions to prevent adverse effects. The pharmacist, on site to provide expert information on OTC medications, should advise in the context of concurrent prescription drugs and orient consumers to the new FDA labeling system. The practicing physician should document OTC medications and prescription drugs in the medication history. Among the factors to evaluate to prevent adverse reactions are content of active ingredients and excipients, metabolic pathways of products, and genetic phenotypes of consumers.

Excipients

Excipients as well as active drugs are of potential significance in therapeutics. A relevant FDA publication demonstrates that the excipient sorbitol decreases the bioavailability (mean peak concentration [C_{max}] and area under the concentration-time curve) of ranitidine significantly, and decreases the C_{max} of metoprolol to a lesser degree.[20] Some excipients added for bulk cause hypersensitivity. The common excipient mannitol caused anaphylaxis, proven by demonstration of expression of mannitol-specific human immunoglobulin E.[21] In a second report, two of seven patients tested for skin reactions to the steroids triamcinolone and methylprednisolone succinate had confirmed skin reactions to the excipient carboxymethylcellulose rather than the active component.[22]

Acetaminophen and Aspirin

The widely used analgesics/antipyretics acetaminophen and acetylsalicylic acid (aspirin) offer vivid examples of potential toxicities of commonly used OTC active medications. Acetaminophen is favored in pediatrics for its safety profile and because of the association of aspirin with Reye's syndrome in children. Acetaminophen is readily available in a variety of compounds and dosages, and in tablet, chewable, and liquid forms. Safe at recommended dosages, acetaminophen overdose can lead to severe liver toxicity.[23] Acetaminophen undergoes hepatic metabolism by cytochrome P-450 isoenzymes 1A2 and 2E1, and acetaminophen toxicity is mediated by the active acetaminophen metabolite *N*-acetyl-*p*-benzoquinone imine, which causes glutathione depletion. (See Chapter 86, Medical Toxicology and Antidotes, for information on glutathione regeneration in the treatment of acetaminophen toxicity.)

Aspirin is an analgesic/antipyretic agent that has anti-inflammatory and cyclooxygenase inhibitory properties. Daily low-dose aspirin is used extensively for primary prevention of cardiovascular disease and stroke. Reports based on large studies indicate association of aspirin with increased risk of major bleeding in women, and of major bleeding and hemorrhagic stroke in men.[24-26]

Phenylpropanolamine—Removed from the OTC Market

Phenylpropanolamine, a common component of OTC decongestants and appetite suppressants, has been reclassified in status from OTC Approved Monograph to Nonmonograph. While individual reports of fatalities secondary to phenylpropanolamine date to 1983, a study conducted in 2000 concluded that there is increased risk for hemorrhagic stroke in women.[27] Phenylpropanolamine, an OTC ingredient with allegedly weak catecholamine properties, has been removed from the OTC market.

OTC Statins—Unapproved

The statins, or 3-hydroxy-3-methylglutaryl coenzyme A reductase inhibitors, are recognized and extensively used for their cardioprotective value and relatively benign side effect profiles.[28-30] Defined toxicities have made statins the topic of two unsuccessful proposals to the FDA for transfer from prescription to OTC status, in 2000 and in 2005. Among the issues discussed in evaluating the risk:benefit ratio was the proposal that muscle (rhabdomyolysis) and hepatic (hepatocellular) toxicities associated with administration of statins may be precipitated by drug interactions at the site of their hepatic metabolism by the cytochrome P450 3A4 isozyme. In 2004, the United Kingdom approved simvastatin behind-the-counter, for distribution under the oversight of pharmacists. Reports emerged suggesting increased morbidity and mortality risk upon abrupt discontinuation of statins during hospitalization for acute coronary episodes.[31,32]

Pediatrics and Obstetrics/Gynecology

Knowledge of drug safety in the areas of pediatrics and obstetrics/gynecology has lagged historically due to the traditional elimination of children and women of childbearing age from clinical research studies. (See Chapter 2, Drug Development, for further information.)

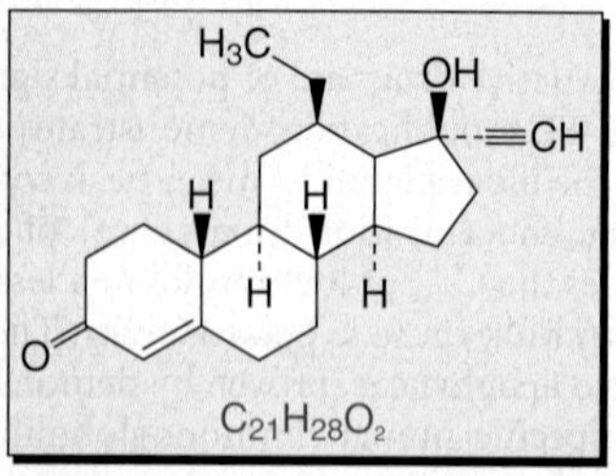

FIGURE 87-1 • Plan B OTC: 0.75-mg tablet levonorgestrel. (From RxList. Plan B. Available at *http://www.rxlist.com/cgi/generic/levonorgestrel.htm*).

Although currently being corrected, the available body of information being collected for these populations favors prescription medications. OTC medications tend to be perceived generally as safe. One noteworthy exception is aspirin, a recognized risk factor in late-term pregnancy for neonatal intracranial hemorrhage. The use of OTC medications during pregnancy is being recorded in two current projects: the Boston University Slone Epidemiology Center Birth Defects Study and the National Birth Defect Prevention Study.[33]

Plan B OTC

Levonorgestrel, or Plan B,[34] is the first emergency OTC contraceptive packet. The Plan B packet contains two 0.75-mg tablets of levonorgestrel to be taken 12 hours apart, the first within 72 hours after intercourse (Fig. 87-1). Plan B approval is restricted to behind-the-counter distribution by pharmacists. Sales of Plan B are limited to women with photo identification proof that they are at least 18 years of age.

CONCLUSION

The magnitude of information regulated as OTC ingredients presents a challenge to the consumer and the health care provider. This chapter proposes a framework on the subject of OTC medications with references as a source of future information. The FDA Center for Drug Evaluation and Research provides the evolving OTC oversight process. Specific OTC ingredients and medications transferred from prescription to OTC status are presented and referenced. Current OTC topics of concern are discussed. Because individual therapeutics pertain to OTC drugs, suggestions are offered for responsible self-medication behavior by the consumer and for evaluation by health care providers, on-site pharmacists, and practicing physicians.

OTC medications deserve to be among those recommended in the Institute of Medicine Report proposal for a comprehensive policy of postmarketing surveillance.[35]

REFERENCES

1. U.S. Food and Drug Administration, Center for Drug Evaluation and Research. Office of Nonprescription Products. Available at *http://www.fda.gov/cder/Offices/OTC/default.htm*.
2. Swann JP. Food and Drug Administration. Available at http://www.fda.gov/oc/history/historyoffda/fulltext.html
3. U.S. Food and Drug Administration. Milestones in U.S. Food and Drug Law History. FDA Backgrounder, May 3, 1999; updated August 2005. Available at *http://www.fda.gov/opacom/backgrounders/miles.html*.
4. FDAReview.org. History of Federal Regulation: 1902–Present. Available at *http://www.fdareview.org/history.shtml*.
5. U.S. Food and Drug Administration, Center for Drug Evaluation and Research. Time Line: Chronology of Drug Regulation in the United States. Available at *http://www.fda.gov/cder/about/history/time1.htm#1968*.
6. Kaplan AH: Fifty years of drug amendments revisited: in easy-to-swallow capsule form. Food Drug Law J 1995;50(Spec):179-196.
7. U.S. Food and Drug Administration. FDA Issues Bar Code Regulation. February 25, 2004. Available at *http://www.fda.gov/oc/initiatives/barcode-sadr/fs-barcode.html*.
8. Federal Register. Department of Health and Human Services Food and Drug Administration 21 CFR Parts 201, 330, 331, 341, 346, 355, 358, 369, and 701. Over-The-Counter Human Drugs: Labeling Requirements. March 17, 1999. Available at *http://www.fda.gov/cder/otc/label/label-fr-reg.htm*.
9. U.S. Food and Drug Administration, Center for Drug Evaluation and Research. Index of Significant OTC Drug Federal Register Publications 2000 through 2006, Volumes 65 through 71. Updated August 2006. Available at *http://www.fda.gov/cder/Offices/OTC/significant%20publications_2000-2009.pdf*.
10. Hilfiker D; Division of Over the Counter Drug Products. OTC 101. U.S. Food and Drug Administration, Center for Drug Evaluation and Research, 2005. Available at *http://www.fda.gov/cder/about/smallbiz/Presentations/4.ppt*.
11. U.S. Food and Drug Administration, Center for Drug Evaluation and Research. OTC Drug Monograph Review Process. Available at *http://www.fda.gov/cder/handbook/otc.htm*.
12. Brass EP. Changing the status of drugs from prescription to over-the-counter availability. N Engl J Med 2001;345:810-816.
13. U.S. Food and Drug Administration, Center for Drug Evaluation and Research. Drug Registration and Listing Instructions. Available at *http://www.fda.gov/cder/drls/default.htm*.
14. U.S. Food and Drug Administration, Center for Drug Evaluation and Research. Food and Drug Administration Guide: OTC Drug Review Ingredient Report. Available at *http://www.fda.gov/cder/Offices/OTC/Ingredient_List_Guide.pdf*.
15. U.S. Food and Drug Administration, Center for Drug Evaluation and Research. OTC Ingredient List A-C. Updated August 2006. Available at *http://www.fda.gov/cder/Offices/OTC/Ingredient_List_A-C.pdf*.
16. U.S. Food and Drug Administration, Center for Drug Evaluation and Research. OTC Ingredient List D-O. Updated August 2006. Available at *http://www.fda.gov/cder/Offices/OTC/Ingredient_List_D-O.pdf*.
17. U.S. Food and Drug Administration, Center for Drug Evaluation and Research. OTC Ingredient List P-Z. Updated August 2006. Available at *http://www.fda.gov/cder/Offices/OTC/Ingredient_List_P-Z.pdf*.
18. U.S. Food and Drug Administration, Center for Drug Evaluation and Research. Milestone Status of OTC Drug Review Documents as of August 3, 2006. Available at *http://www.fda.gov/cder/offices/otc/milestone.pdf*.
19. Consumer Healthcare Products Association. Rx-to-OTC Switch. September, 2005. Available at: *http://www.chpa-info.org/ChpaPortal/Issues/RxOTCSwitch*.
20. Chen ML, Straughn AB, Sadrieh N, et al. A modern view of excipient effects on bioequivalence: case study of sorbitol. Pharm Res 2007;24:73-80.
21. Hegde VL, Venkatesh YP. Anaphylaxis to excipient mannitol: evidence for an immunoglobulin E-mediated mechanism. Clin Exp Allergy 2004;34:1602.
22. Venturini M, Lobera T, del Pozo MD, et al. Immediate hypersensitivity to corticosteroids. J Investig Allergol Clin Immunol 2006;16:51-56.
23. James LP, Mayeux PR, Hinson JA. Acetaminophen-induced hepatotoxicity. Drug Metab Dispos 2003;31:1499-1506.
24. Ridker PM, Cook NR, Lee IM, et al. A randomized trial of low-dose aspirin in the primary prevention of cardiovascular disease in women. N Engl J Med 2005;352:1293-1304.
25. Berger JS, Roncaglioni MC, Avanzini F, et al. Aspirin for the primary prevention of cardiovascular events in women and men: a sex specific meta-analysis of randomized controlled trials. JAMA 2006;295:306-313.
26. Aspirin for primary prevention of cardiovascular disease (revisited). Med Lett Drugs Ther 2006;48(1238):53.
27. Kernan WN, Viscoli CM, Brass LM, et al. Phenylpropanolamine and the risk of hemorrhagic stroke in women. N Engl J Med 2000;343:1826-1832.
28. Gotto AM Jr. Over-the-counter statins and cardiovascular prevention: prospective challenges and opportunities. Clin Pharmacol Ther 2005;78:213-217.
29. Davidoff F. Primary prevention with over-the-counter statins: a cautionary tale. Clin Pharmacol Ther 2005;78:218-220.
30. Choudry NK, Avorn J. Over-the-counter statins. Ann Intern Med 2005;142:910-913.
31. Cubeddy LX, Seamon MJ. Statin withdrawal: clinical implications and molecular mechanisms. Pharmacotherapy 2006;26:1288-1296.
32. Heeschen C, Hamm CW, Laufs U, et al for the Platelet Receptor Inhibition in Ischemic Syndrome Management (PRISM) Investigators. Withdrawal of statins increases event rates in patients with acute coronary syndromes. Circulation 2002;105:1446-1452.
33. Werler MM, Mitchell AA, Hernandez-Diaz S, Honein MA. Use of over-the-counter medications during pregnancy. Am J Obstet Gynecol 2005;193:771-777.
34. Plan B OTC. Med Lett Drugs Ther 2006;48(1243):75.
35. Psaty BM, Burke SP. Protecting the health of the public—Institute of Medicine recommendations on drug safety. N Engl J Med 2006;355:1753-1755.

88

PRESCRIPTION AND ORDER WRITING

Carol L. Beck

OVERVIEW 1225
A RATIONAL APPROACH TO DRUG SELECTION 1225
Evidence-Based Information 1225
Patient-Specific Information 1225
Allergies 1225
Acute and Chronic Medical Conditions/Pharmacokinetic Alterations 1225
Genetic Differences in Drug-Metabolizing Enzymes 1225
Drug Interactions 1226
Patient-Specific Undesirable Side Effects 1226
Other Precautions 1226
Cost/Availability of the Drug 1226
Patient Adherence to Medication Regimen 1226
Summary 1226
CONVERTING THE DRUG SELECTION INTO A PRESCRIPTION 1226
History of Prescriptions 1227
Prescription and Nonprescription Medications 1227
Controlled Substances 1227
DEA Registration Numbers and NPI Numbers 1228
What Is the Purpose of a Prescription? 1228
The Use of Abbreviations 1228
Elements of a Prescription 1229
Patient Information 1229
Date Issued 1229
Drug Information 1229
Refill Authorization (If Any) 1230
Genetic Substitution 1230
Prescriber Information 1230
Other Elements 1230
Differences Between Prescriptions and Medication Orders 1231
THE ELECTRONIC FUTURE 1231
Electronic Prescriptions 1231
Electronic Medical Records (EMR) and Computerized Physician Order Entry (CPOE) 1231
SUMMARY 1231

OVERVIEW

Previous sections of this text have provided the intellectual framework of pharmacology. This chapter demonstrates how these principles are applied in the setting of acute and chronic medical conditions. The first part of this chapter outlines a rational approach to selecting the best drug for each individual patient, based on available evidence. The second part of the chapter discusses practical issues related to prescription and order writing in the outpatient and inpatient settings.

A RATIONAL APPROACH TO DRUG SELECTION

Rational drug selection, like the process of arriving at a diagnosis, is an iterative process. The process starts with the diagnosis and consideration of all possible therapeutic options. The list of choices is eventually reduced to the single best drug for a particular patient at that point in time. The risk:benefit analysis is a key factor in each part of the process and the benefit of receiving the selected drug needs to be greater than the risks associated with receiving it.

Evidence-Based Information

- Based on available evidence, what medications (if any) are appropriate for treating the patient's medical condition?
- What is the current standard-of-care treatment for a particular condition?
- If a drug is not approved by the U.S. Food and Drug Administration (FDA) for a specific condition, would this affect whether or not the patient could afford the drug? (Medicare and some third party payers will not cover "unlabeled uses" of medications.)

Patient-Specific Information

- Does the patient have any condition(s) that would make one drug (or one drug in a class) preferable to another drug?

Allergies

If a patient reports a drug allergy, it is important to inquire about the nature of the reaction: was it difficulty breathing (possibly anaphylaxis) or mild gastrointestinal upset (probably not anaphylaxis and not an immune-mediated response)?

Acute and Chronic Medical Conditions/ Pharmacokinetic Alterations

Some drugs may be contraindicated in specific disease states. Also, a variety of acute and chronic disease states can result in alterations in the absorption, distribution, metabolism, or elimination of a drug. For example, a drug that is renally eliminated would be a disadvantage in a patient with decreased renal function, but an advantage in a patient with decreased hepatic function.

For more information, see Chapter 13, Pharmacokinetics.

Genetic Differences in Drug-Metabolizing Enzymes

Genetic differences (polymorphisms) in key metabolic enzymes for a drug may put patients at risk for either decreased efficacy or increased risk of toxicities. Genetic testing will ultimately be most useful in drugs that have a low therapeutic index, a clear association between drug concentration and therapeutic effect, or severe concentration-related adverse effects, and in which the polymorphism results in dramatic changes in the levels of all active compounds in the pathway.[1] Although not yet routinely done, there is clinical evidence to support a recommendation to genotype (or phenotype) thiopurine methyltransferase activity in patients prior to their being started on azathioprine and 6-mercaptopurine to detect the 0.3% to 0.6% of patients who would develop life-threatening myelosuppression with standard doses.[1] Genotyping of butylcholinesterase in evaluating patients and families with prolonged responses to the neuromuscular blocking drugs succinylcholine (suxamethonium) or mivacurium is also accepted.[1] Prospective genotyping of cytochrome P-450 (CYP) isoenzymes CYP2C9 (for warfarin and phenytoin metabolism) and CYP2C19 for the metabolism of the proton pump inhibitors omeprazole or lansoprazole metabolism may also be useful.[1]

For more information, see Chapter 15, Pharmacogenetics and Pharmacogenomics.

Drug Interactions

To effectively assess the likelihood of drug interactions, a complete and current list of all of a patient's medications is essential, including over-the-counter medications, complementary and alternative medicines, neutraceuticals, and vitamins. If a patient is taking other medications, are any of them metabolized primarily by the CYP system? Is the potential new drug also metabolized by the same enzyme(s)? For a patient on multiple medications, the drug in the class with the fewest drug interactions (or least effect on the CYP enzymes) would be preferable. If all of the potential drugs could result in drug interactions, new drugs must be added carefully and with monitoring and observation when possible. If drug interactions are probable, the prescriber should consult a drug interaction database or reference to assess the possibility of a clinically significant interaction. Even if the interaction is not believed to be clinically significant, patient response after adding a new drug should be watched. Prescribers must remember that clinically significant drug interactions can result in additive and synergistic effects of the drug or drugs (increased responses), or they can have antagonistic effects on the drug or drugs (decreased responses).

For more information, see Chapter 20, Adverse Drug Reactions and Interactions; Chapter 87, Over-the Counter Medications; and Chapter 90, Complementary and Alternative Medicine, Nutraceuticals, and Dietary Supplements.

Patient-Specific Undesirable Side Effects

What are the side effects associated with the drugs being considered? For example, causing drowsiness would be an unacceptable side effect for a patient who operates heavy equipment, but acceptable in a patient who can take the medication at bedtime. Minor gastrointestinal upset caused by a drug might be acceptable in a patient without existing gastrointestinal problems, but unacceptable in a patient with inflammatory bowel disease.

For more information, see Chapter 16, Heterogeneity of Drug Responses and Individualization of Therapy.

Other Precautions

Are there any precautions about the use of this particular drug? Will it require monitoring with serum levels or therapeutic end points, scheduling of follow-up laboratory testing to watch for adverse events (which tests and how often?), or registering with a pharmaceutical company for tracking? Is this a high-alert drug in terms of having a greater risk of causing serious patient harm when used in error? "High-alert" medications can be classes or categories of drugs, such as anesthetic agents, oral hypoglycemics, or intrathecal medications, or specific medications, such as insulin, magnesium sulfate injection, or nitroprusside.[2]

Cost/Availability of the Drug

- For hospitalized patients, is the drug on the hospital formulary? Also, some drugs are available on a restricted use basis; use is restricted to patients on a specific service or the drug must be recommended by that service in a consult. (For more information, see Chapter 89, Pharmacy and Therapeutics Committees and the Hospital Formulary.)
- For patients on third-party or Medicare plans, is the drug on the formulary?
- For medications that are not on the formularies, can a case be made to the appropriate committee or service for an exception?
- If the patient does not have insurance, can he or she afford the medication? Are there local or other resources to cover the drug costs?

Patient Adherence to Medication Regimen

The thought processes applied up to this point in rational drug selection are ultimately meaningless unless the patient actually receives the selected medication, either by the filling of a prescription as an outpatient or by a drug being ordered for an inpatient. To quote former U.S. Surgeon General C. Everett Koop, "Drugs don't work in patients who don't take them."[3] Many factors can produce a net result of a patient not taking a medication as prescribed. These can range from medication costs or drugs not covered by insurance to errors in the prescription or order to errors in the distribution process to annoying effects of the drug. Cognitive abilities of the patient also play an important role. The study of patient adherence to medication regimens is an entire field of research. Some of the factors predicting poor patient adherence (also called compliance) are summarized in Box 88-1.[3] As much as possible, these factors should be considered an important part of the drug selection process. Simplifying dosing regimens, either by reducing the number of daily doses or with the use of pills containing two (or more) medications, is the approach that seems to be the most effective in increasing adherence to medication regimens.[4] An additional concern related to nonadherence to medication regimens is when nonadherence could create public health risks such as the development of resistance to antiviral drugs or resistant strains of tuberculosis.

BOX 88-1 MAJOR PREDICTORS OF POOR ADHERENCE TO MEDICATION REGIMENS

- Psychological problems (particularly depression)
- Cognitive impairment
- Treatment of asymptomatic disease
- Inadequate follow-up or discharge planning
- Side effects of medication
- Patient's lack of belief in benefit of treatment
- Presence of barriers to care or medications
- Poor provider-patient relationship
- Patient's lack of insight into the illness
- Missed appointments
- Complexity of treatment
- Cost of medication, copayment, or both

Adapted from Osterberg L, Blaschke T. Adherence to medication. N Engl J Med 2005;353:487-497.

Summary

The selection of the appropriate medication for a particular patient requires the consideration of multiple issues, with an underlying theme of the drug providing more benefits than risks to the patient.

CONVERTING THE DRUG SELECTION INTO A PRESCRIPTION

As important as is the intellectual process of rational drug selection, the processes of prescription and order writing to convert the choice of drug into medication received by the patient is of almost equal importance. Although many parts of the drug distribution process have become automated, the actual completion (or "writing") of the prescription or medication order is the one aspect of the process that is still mostly under the control of the prescriber. The task of prescription and medication order writing sounds relatively straightforward; however, the sheer number of prescriptions written and filled makes the overall impact of the task large. In 2006, 3.3 billion prescriptions were filled by retail pharmacies in the United States.[5] This number does not include medication orders written for inpatients, or prescriptions filled for mail-order, long-term or managed care, or government facilities. The potential for patient injury if even a small percentage of this number of prescriptions contained errors is frightening. The remainder of this chapter provides a brief history of prescriptions and the components required for a prescription or medication order, with a special focus on patient safety.

History of Prescriptions

Throughout history, communities have identified members with special expertise or training in the healing arts. These individuals have been called many things, including shaman, healer, medicine man or woman, midwife, barber-surgeon, nurse, and doctor. Patients were treated with herbs and other preparations that were in most cases prepared or provided either by the healer or, in some settings, by an apothecary. The art of mixing compounds specific to the needs of a patient goes back to at least 2200 to 3000 BC in China. This art spread to Baghdad in the late 8th century and later to Europe. In 1241, Frederick II, King of Sicily, issued the Edict of Salerno. Among other things, this edict officially separated the roles of physician and apothecary. This separation of roles became the basis of the two modern-day health care professions of medicine and pharmacy. Since then, apothecaries or pharmacies have been responsible for maintaining supplies of ever-growing numbers of drugs. More recently, pharmacists have also become involved in filling needs in patient education and medication regimen management.

Prescription and Nonprescription Medications

In the United States, the concept of a prescription for medication was formalized by the Durham-Humphrey Amendment of 1951 (also known as the Prescription Drug Amendment). This act divided medications into two categories: drugs that could be safely used without medical supervision (nonprescription or "over the counter"), and drugs that were not safe for unsupervised use but that could be used safely with appropriate monitoring (prescription or "legend"). (For more about this, see Chapter 87, Over-the-Counter Medications.) Prescriptions existed prior to this legislation, but the consequences of this act eventually led to standardization of the elements of a prescription.

The Durham-Humphrey Amendment was a necessary adjustment to the Food, Drug, and Cosmetic Act of 1938, which required that drugs be tested to demonstrate their safety. The original act effectively made many drugs illegal, as safety could not be demonstrated in all cases. However, many useful drugs that could not be shown to be "safe" could be used safely with medical supervision. Drugs with a small therapeutic index (or a small difference between the therapeutic and toxic doses) require medical supervision to avoid dose-related toxicities. Drugs used to treat infections require medical supervision not because of the inherent toxicity of the drugs, but because medical advice is needed for the diagnosis and selection of a drug to treat a specific infection. Still other drugs exhibit cumulative dose-related toxicities and require tracking of the total dose received and often monitoring of specific laboratory tests.

Controlled Substances

The Controlled Substances Act (CSA) was one part of the Comprehensive Drug Abuse Control Act of 1970. The provisions of the CSA were to be administered and enforced by the Bureau of Narcotics and Dangerous Drugs in the Department of Justice. In 1973, the Drug Enforcement Administration (DEA) was created as a "superagency" to coordinate all federal efforts related to drug abuse. The Controlled Substances Act also created a "schedule" for certain prescription drugs that would be most closely tracked for abuse and diversion. Table 88-1 lists representative compounds in each of the classes and compares the classes based on whether or not the drugs have accepted medical uses and their relative abilities to lead to either psychological or physical dependence in users. Schedule I drugs are not available for clinical use. Schedule II drugs have high potential to cause physical and psychological dependence if abused and are the most tightly regulated of Schedules II through IV. Medications on the list of scheduled drugs

TABLE 88-1 REPRESENTATIVE LIST OF SCHEDULED DRUGS BASED ON THE CONTROLLED SUBSTANCES ACT

Schedule	Representative Drugs or Compounds
I • Abuse potential: High • No accepted medical use • Lack of accepted safety as a drug	γ-Hydroxybutyric acid (GHB), heroin, "synthetic heroin," lysergic acid diethylamide (LSD), marijuana, mescaline, methaqualone, methylenedioxymethamphetamine (MDMA; "ecstasy"), peyote, psilocybin, tetrahydrocannabinols
II • Abuse potential: High • Current accepted medical use • Abuse may lead to psychological or physical dependence	Alfentanil, amobarbital, amphetamine, cocaine, codeine, fentanyl, glutethimide, hydromorphone, levorphanol, meperidine, methadone, methamphetamine, methylphenidate, morphine, nabilone, opium (various forms), oxycodone, oxymorphine, pentobarbital, phencyclidine, phenmetrazine, secobarbital, sufentanil
III • Abuse potential: Less than I or II • Current accepted medical use • Moderate or low potential for physical dependence • High potential for psychological dependence	Amobarbital, anabolic steroids (dihydrotestosterone, fluoxymesterone, methandrostenolone, methyltestosterone, stanolone, stanozolol, others), buprenorphine, butabarbital, butalbital, chlorphentermine, codeine or dihydrocodeine combination products (90 mg per dosing unit), dronabinol, hydrocodone combination products (15 mg per dosing unit), ketamine, pentobarbital or secobarbital combination products, phendimetrazine, thiopental
IV • Abuse potential: Less than III • Current accepted medical use • Limited potential for dependence	Alprazolam, barbital, butorphanol, chloral hydrate, chlordiazepoxide, clonazepam, clorazepate, dexfenfluramine, dextropropoxyphene dosage forms, diazepam, diethylpropion, estazolam, fenfluramine, flunitrazepam, flurazepam, halazepam, lorazepam, mazindol, mefenorex, meprobamate, methohexital, midazolam, modafinil, oxazepam, pentazocine, phenobarbital, phenteramine, prazepam, temazepam, triazolam, zaleplon, zolpidem
V • Abuse potential: Less than IV • Current accepted medical use. • Limited dependence possible With a few exceptions, these are combination products for cough suppression or for treating diarrhea. Schedule V status limits the amount of the compound, and it must be given in combination with other drugs in the specified ratios.	Codeine preparations (200 mg per 100 ml or 100 g); dihydrocodeine preparations (10 mg per 100 ml or 100 g), difenoxin preparations (0.5 mg per 25 mcg atropine sulfate), diphenoxylate preparations (2.5 mg per 25 mcg atropine sulfate), ethylmorphine preparations (100 mg per 100 ml or 100 g), opium preparations (100 mg per 100 ml or g)

For more information on the Controlled Substances Act and a listing of additional drugs and compounds, see http://www.usdoj.gov/dea/pubs/scheduling.html

require additional information on the prescription and are subject to other restrictions. Not all scheduled drugs are narcotics. In 1990, Congress added anabolic steroids to the list of Schedule III drugs. The list primarily includes the marketed drug, but the precursor compounds, parent compounds, metabolites, isomers, salts, and other derivatives may also be classified as controlled substances.

DEA Registration Numbers and NPI Numbers

As part of the process of tracking scheduled drugs, the DEA created identification numbers for prescribers, pharmacies, hospitals, manufacturers, and others involved in the production, transfer, prescribing, or dispensing of scheduled drugs or compounds. Specifically, prescriptions for the controlled drugs are required to have the DEA registration number of the prescriber included on the prescription. Although the numbers were originally designed to be used specifically for forms related to controlled substances, the prescriber numbers became the preferred identification numbers for many other purposes, such as serving as the provider numbers for third-party payments.

Congress recently passed legislation that should return the prescriber DEA number to its original function. Part of the confidentiality measures included in the Health Insurance Portability and Accountability Act of 1996 (HIPAA) was the mandate that a system for a National Provider Identifier (NPI) number be established. This is a new 10-digit "intelligence-free" permanent number that will be assigned by the National Provider System. These numbers will be provided to any entity that will need to bill for Medicare services, including individual providers, clearinghouses and health plans, and large and small health provider organizations. Examples of individual providers are physicians, dentists, nurses, chiropractors, and therapists. Provider organizations may include hospitals, medical or dental group practices, nursing homes, pharmacies, and laboratories. The NPI will be used as the only identifier for providers filing HIPAA electronic transactions such as electronic claims and claim status inquiries.[6] Once fully implemented, this identifier number will be required when billing for Medicare services, and it is likely that third-party providers will follow this example. DEA registration and state license numbers have often been used as the identifiers; these numbers will still be used for their respective original purposes, but will not be acceptable as identifiers for Medicare billing. (For more information about the NPI, see *http://www.cms.hhs.gov/*.)

What Is the Purpose of a Prescription?

The standard means of giving permission for a medication to be provided (or dispensed) to a patient remains the *prescription* (for outpatients) or the *medication order* (for inpatients). Prescriptions and medication orders contain the information necessary to provide a patient with a supply of medication. Certain information is required by law and other sets of information are helpful in avoiding errors. Historically, prescriptions were handwritten and given to the patient, who then took the prescriptions to a pharmacy to be filled. Starting with the telephone, then the fax machine, and continuing to electronic submission of prescriptions and electronic medical records, the handing of an actual paper prescription to the patient happens less and less. Several nationwide pharmacy chains now share prescription information between stores in the chain. The format of the paper document, however, is replicated in the other technologies, so this is the format discussed here.

The Use of Abbreviations

Abbreviations have been used in prescriptions and medication orders since the early days when details of a prescription were written using abbreviations of Latin words and phrases. These abbreviations are still seen; however, their use is increasingly discouraged in the interest of promoting patient safety and preventing medication errors. The Institute of Medicine report "To Err is Human," released in 1999, contained startling statistics about the number of medication errors in the United States. The study projected that medication errors lead to 98,000 deaths per year and that most of these errors are preventable.[7] The publicity surrounding that report led to a number of patient and medication safety initiatives. Decreasing the numbers of errors, injuries, and deaths has become a priority reinforced by policies implemented by the Joint Commission on Accreditation of Healthcare Organizations (JCAHO; or referred to as the Joint Commission) and insurers.

The Joint Commission now has an annual set of National Patient Safety Goals. Because abbreviations are responsible for a significant segment of medication errors, as part of the 2004 National Patient Safety Goals, each hospital was required to standardize abbreviations and acronyms that could be used throughout the hospital and to also designate a set of abbreviations that were not to be used and then monitor the level of adherence to this.[8] In each subsequent year, there have been additional patient safety goals, at least some of which relate to the safe use of medications and reducing if not eliminating medication errors. The "do not use" abbreviation list contains some suggested abbreviations and allows a hospital to add other abbreviations that have caused problems (Tables 88-2 and 88-3). The Institute for Safe Medication Practices (ISMP) also maintains a list of abbreviations, symbols, and dose designations that have been involved in serious medication errors. (More information about the ISMP is presented in Box 88-2.) All of the abbreviations have caused problems, often due to sloppy or difficult-to-read handwriting or decimal points that were not visible on carbon on fax copies of medication orders. The Official "Do Not Use" List bans the use of

- The abbreviation U for unit or IU for International Unit
- All variations of QD and QOD
- A trailing zero (X.0 mg)
- Lack of a leading zero (.25 mg)
- Abbreviations for morphine sulfate and magnesium sulfate

TABLE 88-2 JOINT COMMISSION OFFICIAL "DO NOT USE LIST"*

Do Not Use	Potential Problem	Use Instead
U (unit)	Mistaken for "0" (zero), the number "4" (four), or "cc"	Write "unit"
IU (international units)	Mistaken for IV (intravenous) or the number 10 (ten)	Write "International Unit"
Q.D., QD, q.d., qd (daily) Q.O.D., QOD, q.o.d., qod (every other day)	Mistaken for each other Period after Q mistaken for "I" and "O" mistaken for "I"	Write "daily" Write "every other day"
Trailing zero (X.0 mg)† Lack of leading zero (.X mg)	Decimal point is missed	Write X mg Write 0.X mg
MS MSO_4 and $MgSO_4$	Can mean morphine sulfate or magnesium sulfate Confused for one another	Write "morphine sulfate" Write "magnesium sulfate"

*Applies to all orders and all medication-related documentation that is handwritten (including free-text computer entry) or on preprinted forms.
†**Exception:** A "trailing zero" may be used only where required to demonstrate the level of precision of the value being reported, such as for laboratory results, imaging studies that report size of lesions, or catheter/tube sizes. It may not be used in medication orders or other medication-related documentation.
From Joint Commission on Accreditation of Healthcare Organizations. (2005). The official "do not use" list. Available at *http://www.jointcommission.org/PatientSafety/DoNotUseList*

TABLE 88-3 ADDITIONAL ABBREVIATIONS, ACRONYMS AND SYMBOLS (FOR POSSIBLE FUTURE INCLUSION IN THE OFFICIAL "DO NOT USE" LIST

Do Not Use	Potential Problem	Use Instead
> (greater than) < (less than)	Misinterpreted as the number "7" (seven) or the letter "L" Confused for one another	Write "greater than" Write "less than"
Abbreviations for drug names	Misinterpreted due to similar abbreviations for multiple drugs	Write drug names in full
Apothecary units	Unfamiliar to many practitioners Confused with the metric unit	Use metric units
@	Mistaken for the number "2" (two)	Write "at"
cc	Mistaken for U (units) when poorly written	Write "ml" or "milliliters"
µg	Mistaken for mg (milligrams), resulting in one thousand-fold overdose	Write "mcg" or "micrograms"

From Joint Commission on Accreditation of Healthcare Organizations. (2005). The official "do not use" list. Available at *http://www.jointcommission.org/PatientSafety/DoNotUseList*

BOX 88-2 ABOUT THE INSTITUTE FOR SAFE MEDICATION PRACTICES

The Institute for Safe Medication Practices (ISMP) is a nonprofit organization promoting safe medication use and facilitating the reporting of medication errors and adverse drug events to create awareness and prevent future medication error occurrences. Information about medication errors and adverse drug events are analyzed and summaries are shared with the health care community (and regulatory agencies, if appropriate) via the web site, newsletters, and educational programs.

The web site (*http://www.ismp.org/*) maintains lists of error-prone abbreviations, symbols, and dose designations, as well as easily confused drug names (look alike/sound alike). The site also has a secured web page form for reporting medication errors to the USP-ISMP Medication Errors Reporting program, operated by the ISMP and the United States Pharmacopeia (USP), and links to the reporting form for MedWatch, the FDA Safety Information and Adverse Event Reporting program.

The complete National Patient Safety Goals and the Official "Do Not Use" list can be found at *http://www.jointcommission.org/PatientSafety/NationalPatientSafetyGoals/*. Rather than learn lists of abbreviations that are not allowed to be used or to have to change prescription writing habits in the future, new clinicians can simply choose not to use abbreviations. It may be more efficient to write out all instructions and drug names.

Drug names should never be abbreviated. If the prescriber is uncertain of the spelling of a particular drug name, it can be looked up in readily available pocket drug references, handheld personal computers, or personal digital assistant (PDA) databases. When this is not possible, both the generic and trade names can be written out to avoid confusion in case of misspelling. For example, using just the trade names Celebrex (the cyclooxygenase-2–specific inhibitor celecoxib), Celexa (the selective serotonin reuptake inhibitor citalopram), or Cerebryx (the seizure medication fosphenytoin) can and has led to medication errors with the confusion resulting from a misspelled or sloppily written name. In these three examples, errors could have been avoided by using the generic names of the drugs, using both the trade and the generic names, or including the indication for the use of the drug. Listing the indication for a medication, either in a prescription or a medication order, is recommended for all medications, but this is especially important when there is a potential for confusion.

On another level, the FDA, ISMP, and pharmaceutical companies are now working together to avoid look-alike/sound-alike names for drugs, sometimes analyzing potential names prior to marketing or even changing the names of marketed medications, if warranted. As an example, in July 2007, Reliant Pharmaceuticals changed the name of its ω-3 acid ethyl esters from Omacor to Lovaza in response to a request from the FDA and reports of prescribing and dispensing errors between Omacor and the antifibrinolytic drug Amicar (aminocaproic acid).

Elements of a Prescription

The purpose of both prescriptions and medication orders is to accurately convey the intent for a particular medication to be provided to a specific patient. The elements of a prescription are described in this section. Figure 88-1 shows how these elements would be organized on a prescription blank.

Patient Information

The patient's full name is best. In the case of common names, writing out the full name and address is the best way to make sure that the correct patient receives the medication and that the correct third party is billed (if applicable). The age of the patient or the date of birth can further identify a patient.

Date Issued

This should include the month, day, and year. Prescriptions should not be postdated for later use.

Drug Information

Drug Name. The generic name should be used whenever possible, and abbreviations should be avoided. If unsure of the spelling, the prescriber should write out both the generic and trade names.

Strength. This refers to the amount of drug per dosing unit, usually in units of mass (milligrams or grams) or volume (milliliters or liters), or mass per volume (e.g., 15 mg/ml or 10%).

Dosage Form. This refers to the form of the dosage (e.g., capsule, tablet, suspension, cream, suppository).

Route. This refers to how the drug is to be administered. Examples are: by mouth (oral); under the tongue (sub-lingual); intravenous; and intramuscular. Drugs are produced in multiple dosage forms and are even used for multiple routes. (For example, an intravenous preparation of a drug might be given orally if an oral liquid form is not available.) Thus, inclusion of the route of administration on the prescription is increasing in importance.

Directions for Use. The directions often follow an "Rx" symbol. It may also be printed on prescription forms as "Sig.," a shortening of the Latin *Signatur* or "give thou." The prescriber should write out directions for the patient or caregiver on how to take the medication. This information is typically brief because it appears on the label for the prescription (Box 88-3).

Duration. This information is usually provided for short courses of therapy and should reinforce the importance of taking the full course of medication. Examples include "Take one tablet every six hours for ten days," and "Take one tablet every six hours until gone."

Quantity. This specifies the number of doses that should be dispensed. This may be determined by the intended duration of therapy

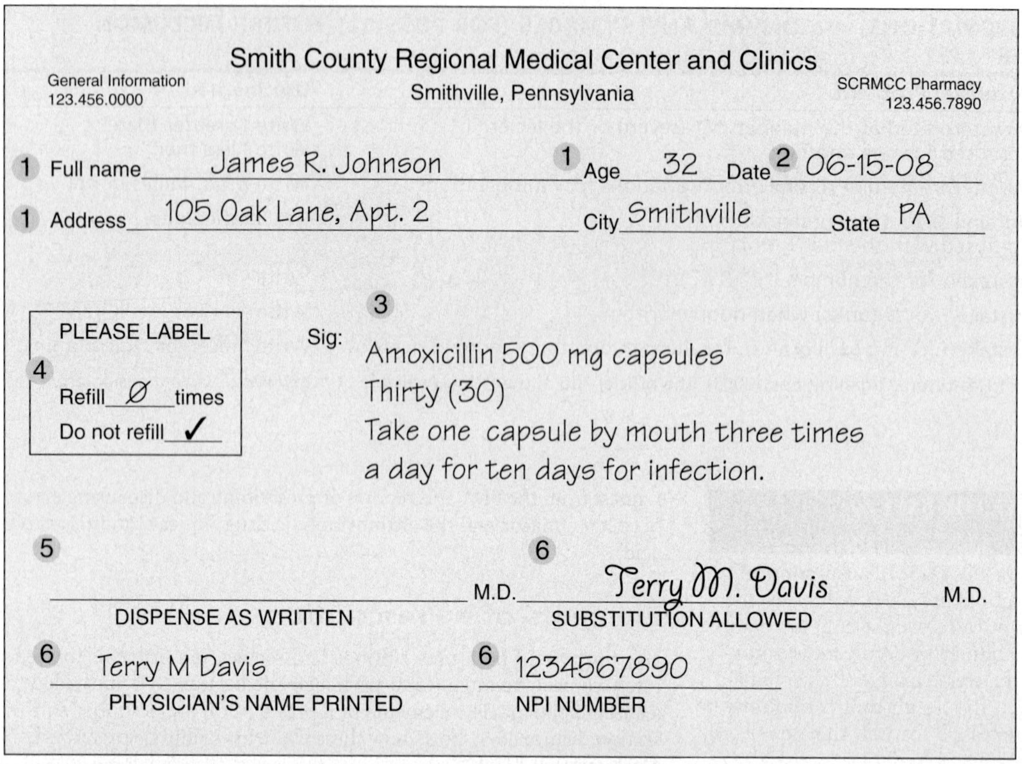

Smith County Regional Medical Center and Clinics

General Information
123.456.0000

Smithville, Pennsylvania

SCRMCC Pharmacy
123.456.7890

① Full name James R. Johnson ① Age 32 Date ② 06-15-08

① Address 105 Oak Lane, Apt. 2 City Smithville State PA

③

PLEASE LABEL
④
Refill Ø times
Do not refill ✓

Sig:
Amoxicillin 500 mg capsules
Thirty (30)
Take one capsule by mouth three times
a day for ten days for infection.

⑤ ⑥

M.D. Terry M. Davis M.D.

DISPENSE AS WRITTEN SUBSTITUTION ALLOWED

⑥ Terry M Davis ⑥ 1234567890

PHYSICIAN'S NAME PRINTED NPI NUMBER

FIGURE 88-1 • Sample prescription blank showing components of a prescription. ① Patient Information; ② Date Issued; ③ Drug Information; ④ Refill Authorization (If Any); ⑤ Generic Substitution and ⑥ Prescriber Information.

BOX 88-3 EXAMPLE OF DIRECTIONS FOR USE IN A PRESCRIPTION

Example: Take (or give, if to a child) one tablet by mouth every six hours for pain.

Summarized, this would be:

- Take/Give/Insert: Take
- (quantity): one
- (dosage form): tablet
- (route): by mouth
- (frequency): every 6 hours
- (Other information: duration, indication): for pain

or by the number of doses per day required for a 1-month or 3-month supply (for maintenance medications). While it is possible to write "10-day supply" or "1-month supply" and let the pharmacist calculate the number of doses, doing the calculation and writing a number provides a double check and helps avoid errors.

Refill Authorization (If Any)

This depends on the nature of the prescription. Antibiotics to treat an infection are typically prescribed for set durations with limited refills, if any. Schedule II prescriptions cannot be refilled. Prescriptions are usually valid for 1 year. If refills are allowed, the maximum is typically five refills within a 6-month period, even if the number indicated on the prescription is greater than this. Many states no longer allow prescriptions with unlimited refills.

Genetic Substitution

Many states require that the generic form of a drug be dispensed unless (i) no generics are available (i.e., the drug is still under patent); (ii) no approved generics are available (generic formulations must demonstrate bioequivalence to the original proprietary formulation); or (iii) the prescription is marked "do not substitute." The mechanism for marking a prescription "do not substitute" may vary between states. In some cases, the prescriber may still be contacted for a justification if an insurer or third party will not cover the proprietary form of the drug.

Prescriber Information

With the exception of the signature, prescriber information can be printed or stamped on the prescription blank.

General Information. Prescriber information always includes the prescriber name, address, phone number, and NPI number.

DEA Registration Number (for Controlled Substances). While having the DEA registration number printed on the prescription blank is discouraged, in practice, many insurers use DEA registration numbers (or state license numbers) to identify prescribers in their systems. Once the NPI system is fully implemented, DEA numbers should once again only be used on prescriptions for controlled substances.

NPI Number. This ten digit number will be required on any forms requesting Medicare reimbursement. It is anticipated that many insurers will convert to use the NPI number.

Signature. The signature MUST be legible. If a prescriber chooses to use a stylized, but illegible personal signature, the name should be printed neatly beneath the signature. In an earlier era, the local pharmacists might recognize the signatures of all local prescribers (regardless of legibility of the signature), but multiple factors now make this impractical and not in the best interests of patient care. Again, if the prescriber's signature tends to be illegible, the name should be printed legibly beneath the signature.

Other Elements

What is the indication or purpose of the medication? There may not be adequate space on a prescription pad or a prescription label to be grammatically correct, but it does help patients and/or their caregivers when the purpose of the medication is included on the prescription. The statement may be something such as "for blood pressure" or "for infection" or "heart pill." In the inpatient setting, the indication for a medication must be somewhere in the chart; including the indication when the order for the drug is first written simplifies the search process.

Legal Elements. Prescriptions for controlled or scheduled drugs must include the DEA registration number. Schedule II prescriptions are typically written on separate, tamper-proof paper (these regulations vary by state and institution). Schedule II prescriptions cannot be refilled and cannot be phoned in to the pharmacy. (In emergency situations, a 72-hour supply can be dispensed, with the paper copy to be submitted as soon as possible.)

Clarity and Completeness. Finally, to make sure that patients receive the intended medication, the prescriber should be as clear as possible when writing prescriptions. This effort will help cut down on medication errors and will save everyone involved significant amounts of time. The pharmacist has a legal obligation to contact the prescriber for missing information before filling a prescription. The extra few seconds spent making sure that a prescription—or an inpatient medication order—is written exactly right could save large amounts of time for prescribers, patients, and pharmacists.

Differences Between Prescriptions and Medication Orders

In the inpatient setting, medication orders are typically used instead of prescriptions. Order sheets with the patient's name, room number, and identification number (sometimes also the date of birth) are filed with the patient's chart. These are used instead of rewriting the name, address, and age information at the top of multiple prescription blanks. The same dangers of abbreviating drug names and information are present in the hospital setting and may be even more prevalent because of the larger volume and multiple types of orders being processed at the same time. The prescriber should write out both drug names and instructions, thus avoiding all abbreviations, and write as legibly as possible. The importance of legible handwriting in the prescription- and order-writing process cannot be overemphasized. At worst, poor handwriting can result in deadly or life-threatening medical errors. At best, it may results in delays in filling a prescription or medication order while information is verified.

THE ELECTRONIC FUTURE

Electronic Prescriptions

The Institute of Medicine report issued in July 2006, "Preventing Medication Errors," recommended that by 2010 all prescribers and pharmacies be using electronic prescriptions, or e-prescriptions.[9] In addition to avoiding problems created by illegible handwriting, other advantages include computer prompts to complete all fields and the ability to link the e-prescriptions with the patient's medical history to screen for drug allergies; drug-drug, drug-food, and other interactions; and inappropriate doses. As of August 2007, all 50 of the United States are part of a national network that will allow electronic prescriptions to be delivered to pharmacies. The transition of prescribers to e-prescriptions will be more gradual.

Electronic Medical Records (EMR) and Computerized Physician Order Entry (CPOE)

The process of converting medical records from paper to electronic format has been slow but steady. The delays are a function of the many details to resolve, systems to integrate with each other, and the financial costs of the conversion to the electronic format.

An early phase of the transition to electronic medical records (also called electronic health records or EHR) has been the introduction of computerized order entry systems. Many hospitals use computerized physician order entry systems for medication and care instructions. With these systems, orders are entered directly into the computer, either by physicians or by pharmacists or nurses transcribing handwritten orders. Latin abbreviations are still part of many order and prescription entry screens, but more and more include both the abbreviations and the written-out versions. Direct entry by prescribers avoids many of the issues related to illegible handwriting, but it also creates other issues. Other systems transcribe handwritten orders into the computerized system for generation of medication administration records and other records.

Advantages of CPOE systems include fewer errors related to illegible handwriting or transcription, the ability to check for duplicate or incorrect doses, and access to drug allergy, drug-drug interaction, or drug-disease interaction databases, plus clinical support features ranging from basic to advanced. Default values can be set, and the system can prompt for incomplete sections of the order or include reminders for related monitoring or automatic stop dates.

SUMMARY

The process of prescription and medication order writing is the culmination of the intellectual work of arriving at a diagnosis and selecting the appropriate medication for the patient. However, it is no less important than the other steps, and care should be taken to do a thorough job to avoid medication errors. Technological advances and shifts toward electronic medical records will soon change the way prescriptions and orders are recorded from pen and paper to keyboards, touchpads, and monitors, but the basic required elements will remain the same.

REFERENCES

1. Gardiner SJ, Begg EJ. Pharmacogenetics, drug-metabolizing enzymes, and clinical practice. Pharmacol Rev 2006;58:521-590.
2. Institute for Safe Medication Practices. List of High-Alert Medications. Available at *http://www.ismp.org/Tools/highalertmedications.pdf* (accessed January 3, 2008).
3. Osterberg L, Blaschke T. Adherence to medication. N Engl J Med 2005;353:487-497.
4. Schroeder K, Fahey T, Ebrahim S. How can we improve adherence to blood pressure-lowering medication in ambulatory care? Systematic review of randomized controlled trials. Arch Intern Med 2004;164:722-732.
5. Gebhart F. 2006 Rx market flashback. Drug Topics 2007;April 6.
6. Federal Register 2004;69(15):3434-3469.
7. Kohn LT, Corrigan JM, Donaldson MS (eds), for the Committee on Quality of Health Care in America, Institute of Medicine. To Err is Human: Building a Safer Health System. Washington, DC: National Academy Press, 2000.
8. Special Report: 2004 JCAHO National Patient Safety Goals: practical strategies and helpful solutions for meeting these goals. Available at *http://www.jcrinc.com/26813/newsletters/5308/*
9. Aspden P, Wolcott JA, Bootman JL, Cronenwett LR (eds). Preventing Medication Errors: Quality Chasm Series. Washington, DC: Institute of Medicine, 2006.

89

PHARMACY AND THERAPEUTICS COMMITTEES AND THE HOSPITAL FORMULARY

Joseph S. Bertino, Jr.

INTRODUCTION 1233
THE P&T COMMITTEE 1233
Functions of the P&T Committee 1233
Membership 1233
Chair 1233
Secretary 1233
Pharmacists and Pharmacologists 1233
Physicians 1234
Nurses 1234
Administrator 1234
House Staff 1234
Risk Manager 1234
Subcommittees 1234
Meetings 1234
Role of the Subspecialist on the P&T Committee 1235
Conflicts of Interest for P&T Committee Members 1235
Communication and Implementation of P&T Committee Decisions 1235
Other Functions of the P&T Committee 1235
THE FORMULARY 1235
SUMMARY 1236

INTRODUCTION

Almost every patient who is admitted to a hospital receives drug therapy. Drug therapy accounts for a substantial percentage of cost to an institution. While drugs are life saving, they also have the potential to cause morbidity and mortality. The Pharmacy and Therapeutics (P&T) Committee stands as the decision-making body concerning drug use for most institutions.

The concept of a P&T Committee has been around for decades; however, the committee has become substantially more important over the past 20 years. This committee is paramount to the drug decision process in hospitals. Formularies stem from P&T Committees and help provide useful, cost-effective, and safe therapeutic choices to clinicians. This chapter explores in detail the P&T Committee and the use of formularies in an institutional setting.

THE P&T COMMITTEE

Functions of the P&T Committee

The P&T Committee has a number of functions in an institution. These include objective appraisal and evaluation of drugs for the formulary, and reviews and updates of the appropriateness of the formulary system in light of new drugs and new indications, uses, or warnings affecting existing drugs. The most important aspect is the use of evidence-based principles to assess safety, efficacy, ease of dosing, impact on pharmacy and nursing time, potential for medication errors, and, lastly, economic impact of decisions. More functions of the P&T Committee are discussed later.

Membership

The P&T Committee is a compilation of members from a variety of general practice and subspecialty areas in the hospital (Fig. 89-1). P&T Committees are generally included as part of the medical staff bylaws and, thus, a committee that is essential and mandated. The members of the committee are very diverse, including physicians, pharmacists, nurses, and administrators. Importantly, it is essential that the P&T Committee be manageable in size. Too many members make decision making slow and difficult. While there is no "correct" number of members, 9 to 15 voting members (always an odd number) seems appropriate. A survey in the 1990s suggested that, for a teaching hospital, the average number of members was 19.3, with approximately 65% being physicians.[1] A somewhat typical composition of the committee would be as follows.

Chair

The chair is a physician, generally with high standing among members of the medical staff and administration. Often a subspecialist is selected, but this is not a prerequisite. Generally, the physician does not have formal clinical pharmacology training, however. The P&T Committee chair's job is to provide leadership, resolve disputes, and set an example for the use of rational drug therapy in the institution. In addition, the chair recommends to the Chief Executive Officer, Director, or medical staff which individuals should be appointed to the P&T Committee. The P&T Committee may be the most important hospital committee because its decisions affect patient care, length of stay, and cost of care for almost every patient. The decisions of the committee also affect anyone prescribing, monitoring, or administering drugs to patients. For these reasons, the actions of the committee may be very controversial among some individuals. The P&T Committee chair functions as the public representative to members of the institution to deal with these political issues.

Secretary

Generally this individual has been the Director of Pharmacy. The reasoning for this is that the Director of Pharmacy oversees (but does not control) the pharmaceutical budget for the institution. The secretary's job is to schedule meetings, assist in setting the agenda, contact individuals to present data to the committee, write the minutes for the meetings, and coordinate follow-up. Unfortunately, since the Director of Pharmacy often reports to an administrator with business training and not a clinician, the overseeing administrator sometimes feels the need to be more involved than appropriate in the decision-making process for drug use. This is clearly inappropriate and must be avoided.

Pharmacists and Pharmacologists

Clinical pharmacists and clinical pharmacologists, often MDs and PharmDs, serve as the "workhorses" for the P&T Committee. These individuals gather data, coordinate medical utilization reviews, and

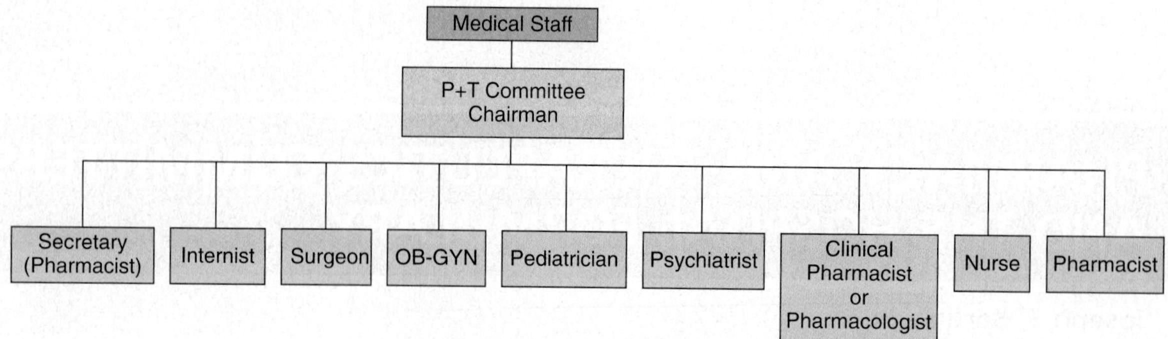

FIGURE 89-1 • Structure of the P&T committee.

present evidence-based information on efficacy, toxicity, comparative therapeutic use, and pharmacoeconomic data. Unfortunately, recent information suggests that pharmacoeconomic data available are sparse, often not timely, and not often used.[2] However, there are some data to dispute this assessment.[3]

Other representatives from the Pharmacy Department may be included as members.

Physicians

Individuals from each department, including medicine, surgery, pediatrics, psychiatry, obstetrics-gynecology, and others are essential. In addition, subspecialists from areas with high-cost or high-risk drug use, such as oncology, infectious diseases, critical care, and cardiology, should be included in committee decisions at least on an ad hoc basis.

Nurses

Representatives of nursing are important members of the P&T Committee. While often the Chief Nursing Executive is suggested as a representative to the committee, it is essential for a nurse who practices at the bedside or who directly supervises nurses practicing at the bedside to be included. Oftentimes the nurse member will offer insight into the impact of formulary decisions on nursing time and nursing care.

Administrator

An administrator, to whom *none* of the P&T Committee members directly reports (in an effort to avoid potential conflicts of interest), is a useful addition to the committee. This individual should serve as a nonvoting member or an ad hoc, nonvoting member. Many problems can arise when an individual such as the Director of Pharmacy, serving as the P&T Committee secretary, reports to the administrator on the P&T Committee. This sometimes presents a significant conflict of interest.

House Staff

House staff (such as chief residents) may be included, but should function in a nonvoting capacity. House staff are often the individuals targeted by pharmaceutical company representatives with "freebies." Thus, house staff should generally serve as nonvoting representatives on the P&T Committee to avoid potential conflicts of interest.

Risk Manager

In recent years, with the concern over medication errors, a risk manager has often been appointed as a member of the P&T Committee. While these individuals can offer useful input, caution must be exercised in having the "risk" override the potential for benefit for formulary additions. Often risk managers have limited (or outdated) clinical experience that causes undue work burden for the committee and delays implementation of important drug-related decisions for patient care. While patient safety is very important, this aspect has sometimes overshadowed the other important functions of the P&T Committee. The risk manager should provide useful and practical insight into the "risks" involved with medication selection and use. However, the scenario in which every possibility for medication error is considered, while being of interest, may sidetrack decision making for an institution. Risk, as with any other decision on the use of drugs, must be balanced. No drug will ever be 100% safe to use.

Subcommittees

In addition to the main P&T Committee, given the complexity of many drug therapies, P&T Committees often develop subcommittees (e.g., oncology and infectious diseases) to review formulary addition requests and make recommendations to the full committee. Oftentimes, subspecialists assist in these assessments but do not serve as members of the P&T Committee.

Meetings

Meeting frequency should be based on the institution size and need. This is generally written into the medical staff bylaws. For small institutions (<100 beds), quarterly meetings may be appropriate. For larger institutions that have more complex patients and many subspecialties, meetings one or two times a month are appropriate. This entails a substantial amount of work by the secretary, clinical pharmacist, and clinical pharmacologist members in particular. In large hospitals, almost a full-time equivalent (FTE) position (or more than one) can be dedicated to this. Administration in particular needs to recognize this and provide adequate financial support to the P&T Committee as a separate line item. Traditionally, the function of the P&T Committee is done by volunteers with no budget for the committee. Just as Institutional Review Boards have found that, in order to do their job, there is a need for dedicated FTEs and a budget, P&T Committees must have the personnel and financial support to function at the high level expected.

The format of meetings needs to be standardized, with time limits put on presentations and discussion as directed by the chair. Meeting duration of over 90 minutes shows decreasing return in terms of productivity.

In the past, discussion of new drugs proposed were preceded by a lengthy (5 to 20 pages) written review by the clinical pharmacist/pharmacologist. In the opinion of this writer, with 25 years of P&T Committee experience, these reviews are rarely read by the committee members and are extremely time consuming to prepare (unless one uses a therapeutic review subscription service). Better use of this time would be a short (5- to 10-minute) slide presentation using evidence-based information, with discussion of important points in order to facilitate decision making. The discussion points should include therapeutic efficacy, drug toxicity, assessment of risks of therapy, drug administration issues, and any agent-specific issues (e.g., for an antibiotic, whether its use should be restricted to reduce the potential for resistance). In addition, cost implications must be considered. Unfortunately, very few pharmacoeconomic data that are not generated "in house" are available in the literature to assist in this decision-making process.[3] Additionally, it is inappropriate for representatives from a pharmaceutical company to attend P&T Committee or subcommittee meetings.

Role of the Subspecialist on the P&T Committee

While subspecialists may not be regular members of the P&T Committee, their input is important in decision making for drugs that will be used in patients whom they either treat or consult on. Unfortunately, in some therapeutic areas, agents are often added to the hospital formulary based on anecdotal experience, drug company promotion, and availability of samples with few hard data.[4] Use of drugs for unlabeled indications should be evaluated using an evidence-based approach. Thus, it is essential for the subspecialist to provide objective input into the decision-making process. This is an extremely difficult area to deal with, and many institutions have struggled with this.

Conflicts of Interest for P&T Committee Members

In reality, it is difficult for any P&T Committee member to be objective all of the time. Important considerations for revealing conflicts of interest in an attempt to bring as much objectivity to the P&T Committee as possible include the following:

- Yearly financial disclosure following U.S. Food and Drug Administration (FDA) guidelines for investigators.[5] These should be filed with the P&T Committee chair. The chair should file his or her disclosure statement with the President of the medical staff.
- Full disclosure at the beginning of each meeting for any member who may have a conflict of interest for any agenda item. The member in conflict should refrain from any discussion and should not vote on the item. In theory, the member should be excused from the discussion and this documented in the meeting minutes. Conflicts include receipt of any financial support, trips, junkets, academic materials (e.g., textbooks), and the like from a drug company that markets the drug under consideration.

Communication and Implementation of P&T Committee Decisions

The absolute importance of prompt, accurate communication of P&T Committee decisions on drug therapy cannot be ignored. Following a P&T Committee meeting and finalization of the minutes (which should be complete and outline the entire decision-making process), decisions made should be immediately conveyed to physicians, house staff, nurses, pharmacists, and others involved with patient care. This can be in the form of e-mail, short written communications, flyers, and personal interactions with groups. These communications need to be concise and informative and cover important points or they will be ignored. Lengthy communications will result in a large amount of work being wasted and create new problems for individuals such as pharmacists who have to implement decisions of the P&T Committee. This is the area where full support of the chair, department chairs, and the medical staff is an absolute. The P&T Committee chair has the responsibility to facilitate this support. In addition, access to the P&T Committee minutes for anyone in the institution to review is important.

Pharmacists often bear the brunt of P&T Committee decision making with prescribers and nurses. These negative interactions take away from the team environment essential to patient care and must be dealt with immediately by the P&T Committee chair or the department chair. Once decisions are made, it is imperative for all members of the house staff, medical staff, pharmacists, and nurses to support these decisions and work as a team to carry them out and optimize patient care.

Other Functions of the P&T Committee

Besides reviewing drugs and selecting them for addition to the hospital formulary, the P&T Committee also has other important functions. These include

1. Formulating and maintaining ongoing review of drug safety policies. This includes involvement in Physician Order Entry software, pharmacy software systems, use of approved abbreviations, order writing, and establishment of policies for improving drug safety.
2. Assisting in standardization of instrumentation for drug delivery (e.g., intravenous infusion pumps).
3. Maintaining ongoing review of medication usage, adverse effects, and so forth. These medical use evaluations or drug utilization reviews should be performed on drugs that are expensive, those with narrow therapeutic-to-toxic ratios, or those used for unlabeled indications. These reviews provide information on whether the drugs are being used properly, appropriately, safely, and in a cost-effective fashion. Often data for these reviews are collected by students, pharmacy residents, or pharmacists and presented in a concise fashion to the P&T Committee.
4. Providing support for the Pharmacy Department. In many institutions, the Pharmacy Department is administratively placed under a nonclinician administrator with business training but no clinical training. In some instances, this individual puts cost considerations first and disregards the more important functions of the Pharmacy Department, including clinical services and efficient medication delivery. Oftentimes, the P&T Committee is the only clinical oversight and the initial support for the Pharmacy Department. In addition, the P&T Committee can use its influence to change policy and institute new programs in the Pharmacy Department. For example, in some institutions, a pharmacist serves as an "antibiotic stewart," reviewing antibiotic use and changing things according to protocols.[6] In some instances, these programs were the result of P&T Committee recommendations.
5. Reviewing the Formulary, with publication either on line or in a hard copy format.
6. Formulating policy on the use of drugs in an institution.
7. Formulating treatment guidelines for drug use and disease treatment in an institution.
8. Reviewing all medication incidents of a certain level of severity to look for trends and make recommendations for improvement.
9. Establishing and planning educational programs for members of the medical staff, house staff, pharmacists, nurses, and others.
10. Establishing policy for the conduct of business by representatives of pharmaceutical companies in an institution. This is a particularly sensitive issue because of the pervasiveness of "entitlement" of individuals in the medical field or gifts from pharmaceutical company representatives. Some institutions have stopped completely the provision of education, meals, giveaways, and the like from pharmaceutical company representatives.
11. Establishing policy for the acquisition and use of sample medications in an institution. It is important to note that sample medications must be handled in the same way as other medications and need to be obtained, stored, labeled, tracked, and dispensed properly (following pertinent state pharmacy laws).

Overall, the P&T Committee is very important to the functioning of the institution. Since nearly 100% of patients admitted to the hospital receive some drug therapy, a group that objectively evaluates efficacy, toxicity, safety, and cost considerations is essential.

THE FORMULARY

The Formulary is often a misunderstood concept. To some, the Formulary represents a "list" of drugs available in the institution. However, the Formulary is a concept that translates to a document that regulates drug use in the institution and guides clinicians in the proper use of drugs. An institution can have either an open or closed Formulary. An open Formulary (very unusual nowadays) allows any drug to be available in the institution for use. Since many drugs duplicate the pharmacologic effects and indications of other agents, the need for an open Formulary is essentially outdated.

A closed formulary is one that restricts drugs in each category to the most efficacious, safe, cost-effective agent(s). For example, if six β-blockers are available commercially, the P&T Committee will often pick one or two that are effective, can be used via multiple routes of administration, can be used with relative safety, and are cost effective. In addition, in a closed formulary system, some drugs will be restricted for use to certain groups because of potential for adverse effects or cost. An example would be the drug drotecogin, which might be restricted to use by intensivists or infectious disease physicians. This agent would be restricted because of its potential for toxicity, specificity of use, and cost. Additionally, some drugs may be available for use by all in the institution, but require approval by specific groups before they can be used. An example is the need for approval for certain broad-spectrum antibiotics by an infectious diseases physician or pharmacist before the drug can be ordered for a patient.[6] The rationale behind this type of restriction has to do with antibiotic "stewardship"—promoting rational use of the drug, controlling antibiotic-resistant organisms, and controlling costs.[6]

Other facets of a closed formulary may be the broad restriction of large numbers of drugs based on the potential for toxicity. In these cases, only certain clinicians can use these agents, and in many circumstances, these clinicians must write the specific orders for these agents before they can be administered to a patient. An example in many institutions is that of oncologic drugs. Because of tragedies with inappropriate dosing and administration of these drugs to patients in the past, many institutions allow only board-certified oncologists or oncologic surgeons to order these drugs and only certified oncology nurses to administer these agents. In many instances, no other clinician is allowed to write the orders for these agents, unless they are being used for nononcologic indications (i.e., methotrexate for rheumatoid arthritis).

Thus, in the closed Formulary, drugs can be classified as either "formulary" or "nonformulary." Formulary drugs are subject to the restrictions noted earlier. Nonformulary drugs encompass the rest. As one might expect, when the P&T Committee has objectively evaluated a Formulary choice and admitted the drug to the Formulary, there may be individuals who are upset at the P&T Committee choice. This can set into motion a series of events where the clinician writes a prescription for a nonformulary drug, and the order is sent to the pharmacist, who is then pressured to fill the nonformulary order. This defeats the formulary process and must be quickly addressed.

Reasons given for ordering nonformulary drugs include:

1. The patient has been on the nonformulary drug prior to admission and the clinician wants to continue it despite having appropriate formulary alternatives.
2. The patient believes that a generic equivalent of the drug he or she is taking is less effective than the brand name (an inappropriate argument given the process that is in place by the FDA for approval of generic medications).
3. The clinician, using anectodotal data, believes that the nonformulary drug is "better" than the formulary agent (not evidence based).[7,8]

These scenarios should be avoided through education of clinicians and patients and support by clinicians of the P&T Committee decision-making process. This support must start with the medical staff and chiefs of service. In addition, making the obtaining of nonformulary medications difficult (not stocking them in the institution, requiring that a written form be filled out along with the order, allowing up to 48 hours to obtain a nonformulary medication) is a way of forcing the use of formulary medications. In no instance should the patient be allowed to use his or her own medications, as the pharmacist and prescriber cannot assume that the medication has been stored properly or is not expired. While this may seem draconian to the reader, these techniques, in the face of a valid P&T Committee Formulary process, are appropriate. Another method is to allow "therapeutic substitution" of one formulary agent for a nonformulary agent. This has been commonly done with proton pump inhibitors, fluoroquinolones, oral cephalosporins, and histamine$_2$ blockers, to name a few of the categories.

Other ways to enforce the formulary process without relying on the above-mentioned tactics is the incorporation of clinical pharmacists into day-to-day patient care. Pharmacists rounding with teams, seeing patients, and working with nurses has been shown to be cost effective and result in more appropriate drug use.[9-11] Unfortunately, with the shortage of pharmacists, these individuals may be relegated to dispensing rather than clinical activities. With the availability of highly sophisticated automatic dispensing systems and the broad and appropriate use of pharmacy technicians, there is little reason for the pharmacist to be involved with dispensing activities in the pharmacy. This is an area that needs to be acutely addressed; while many institutions have been far ahead on this issue, others remain in the past in this regard. The use of pharmacists for dispensing functions is antiquated, is not cost-effective, and should be discouraged. Time is better spent in being at the bedside, guiding clinicians in appropriate drug use, writing orders (to reduce the writing of inappropriate orders), and monitoring patients' drug therapy for efficacy, adverse events, and safety. There is a significant body of literature showing the utility of clinical pharmacists in medication use.[9-11]

As noted, the Formulary is not a document but a process. Besides the list of available medications in the institution, the Formulary should contain the following:

1. Information on how drugs can be requested for P&T Committee review
2. Compilation of drug treatment guidelines
3. Drug information useful for day-to-day patient care
4. Conversion tables for medications
5. Generic-to–brand name conversions
6. Specific state laws for prescribing medications

In the recent past, institutions have moved from a paper Formulary document to on-line documents that can be accessed at the bedside and updated continuously. When coupled with a good Physician Order Entry system, safe and effective prescribing can be implemented. These steps should result in greater patient safety, economic benefits, and a greater degree of implementation of P&T Committee recommendations with the resultant benefits.

SUMMARY

The P&T Committee is essential in formulating drug policy in an institution. The Formulary is a process developed by the P&T Committee that directs individuals in how to use drugs.

REFERENCES

1. Tordoff JM, Murphy JE, Norris PT, Reith DM. Use of centrally developed pharmacoeconomic assessments for local formulary decisions. Am J Health Syst Pharm 2006; 63:1613-1618.
2. Odedina FT, Sullivan J, Nash R, Clemmons CD. Use of pharmacoeconomic data in making hospital formulary decisions. Am J Health Syst Pharm 2002;59:1441-1444.
3. Mannebach MA, Ascione FJ, Gaither CA, et al. Activities, functions, and structure of pharmacy and therapeutics committees in large teaching hospitals. Am J Health Syst Pharm 1999;56:622-628.
4. Schumock GT, Walton SM, Park HY, et al. Factors that influence prescribing decisions. Ann Pharmacother 2004;38:557-562.
5. Code of Federal Regulations. Title 21, Vol 1, Part 54—Financial Disclosure by Clinical Investigators. Revised as of April 1, 2000.
6. Dellit TH, Owens RC, McGowan JE, et al. Infectious Diseases Society of America and the Society for Healthcare Epidemiology of America guidelines for developing an institutional program to enhance antimicrobial stewardship. Clin Infect Dis 2007;44:159-177.
7. Rucker TD, Schiff G. Drug formularies: myths-in-formation. Med Care 1990;28:928-942.
8. Institute for Safe Medication Practices. The truth about hospital formularies. ISMP Med Saf Alert 2005;10:2-3.
9. Bond CA, Raehl CL. Clinical pharmacy services, pharmacy staffing, and adverse drug reactions in United States hospitals. Pharmacotherapy 2006;26:735-747.
10. Bond CA, Raehl CL, Franke T. Clinical pharmacy services, hospital pharmacy staffing, and medication errors in United States hospitals. Pharmacotherapy 2002;22:134-147.
11. Bond CA, Raehl CL, Franke T. Clinical pharmacy services, pharmacy staffing, and the total cost of care in United States hospitals. Pharmacotherapy 2000;20:609-621.

90

COMPLEMENTARY AND ALTERNATIVE MEDICINE, NUTRACEUTICALS, AND DIETARY SUPPLEMENTS

Christine A. Haller

INTRODUCTION 1237
REGULATION 1237
EPIDEMIOLOGY OF USE 1238
THERAPEUTICS AND CLINICAL PHARMACOLOGY 1238
Dietary Supplements with Demonstrated Therapeutic Benefit 1238
Black Cohosh 1238
Garlic 1238
Ginkgo biloba 1238
Milk Thistle 1240
St John's Wort 1240
Herb-Drug Interactions 1240
Pharmacokinetic Interactions 1240
Pharmacodynamic Interactions 1241
Toxicities of Dietary Supplements 1241
Ephedra 1242
Kava 1242
Yohimbine 1242
Dieter's Teas 1243
FUTURE OF DIETARY SUPPLEMENTS 1243

INTRODUCTION

Few therapeutic classes can match the enormity and diversity of the category of products known in the United States as nutraceuticals or dietary supplements. Also unrivaled in medicine is the dearth of premarketing and postmarketing scientific data that exists for the majority of these products that are consumed daily by millions of Americans. Nutraceuticals and dietary supplements are a subset of complementary and alternative medicine (CAM), which also includes a diversity of other therapeutic modalities such as mind-body interventions (e.g., hypnosis, yoga) and manipulative therapies (e.g., acupuncture, massage). The term *nutraceutical* is synonymous with "functional food" and refers to dietary products that are used for health benefits other than nutrition. In the United States, these products are classified as dietary supplements and regulated as foods instead of drugs. Throughout the rest of the world, however, botanicals and other natural products are heavily utilized as medications. The World Health Organization estimates that 75% to 80% of the developing world relies on CAM therapies to meet primary health needs.[1-3] Throughout history, as many as 70,000 plants have been used for medicinal purposes, and 25% of today's widely used pharmaceuticals were originally derived from plants.[1] For instance, clinical use of foxglove in ancient times led to the modern-day use of the cardioactive drug digoxin, morphine and codeine were originally derived from the poppy plant *Papaver somniferum*, the antimalarial drug quinine was obtained from the bark of *Cinchona* species, and salicylate was originally isolated from the bark of the willow tree.

The use of herbal medicines and other dietary supplements in the United States increased dramatically in the 1990s, peaking at the end of the decade amid growing reports of toxicity of some products (ephedra, kava) and ineffectiveness of many popular products (echinacea, saw palmetto), and consumer use has since slowly declined. Nonetheless, many people regularly take dietary supplements for preventive health (e.g., fish oils and garlic to lower cholesterol); to treat medical conditions (e.g., glucosamine for osteoarthritis, black cohosh for hot flashes); and to boost athletic performance (e.g., creatine, guarana) and enhance sexual function (e.g., yohimbe, horny goat weed). Although few premarket controlled clinical trials have been conducted on these agents, several popular dietary supplements have recently been scientifically evaluated, and reports on clinical benefits, pharmacokinetics, metabolism, and drug interactions are increasing. However, lack of standardization of active constituents, delays in implementation of good manufacturing practices, and inadequate postmarketing surveillance practices continue to be major deficiencies that hinder scientific and regulatory efforts to improve the safety and efficacy of dietary supplements.

In this chapter, the therapeutic indications, clinical pharmacology, and reported toxicities of the most commonly used dietary supplements are covered. Herb-drug interactions and regulatory issues, including labeling requirements and adverse event monitoring, are also discussed. For brevity and focus, homeopathic products, vitamin and mineral supplements, and traditional or cultural therapies such as traditional Chinese medicine and ayurveda will not be covered.

REGULATION

The regulatory framework of dietary supplements in the United States changed with the passage of the 1994 Dietary Supplement Health and Education Act (DSHEA). Dietary supplements include vitamins, minerals, herbs, amino acids, glandular extracts, and any other naturally occuring product that is taken orally for the purpose of promoting health and nutrition. Ingredients that meet these criteria that were in use prior to October 15, 1994, are allowed as dietary supplements. Manufacturers of new dietary supplements that were not available prior to 1994 are required to submit a New Dietary Ingredient application (NDI) to the U.S. Food and Drug Administration (FDA) and receive approval before marketing. Notification of the FDA must occur at least 75 days in advance of marketing the product. During this period, the FDA reviews the proposed dietary ingredient and its intended use and determines if it is reasonably safe for marketing. However, clinical data on the effectiveness and safety of the ingredient are not required as part of the NDI submission.

The primary determinant of the regulatory classification of a natural product is its intended use, which is largely determined by its labeling information.[4] "Structure/function" claims are permissible, but label statements that convey or imply that a dietary supplement prevents, cures, or mitigates disease are not allowed.[5] For instance, a label on a glucosamine supplement can state that it improves joint function and mobility, but the label cannot state that the product relieves symptoms of osteoarthritis. Some natural substances are allowed to be marketed as both drugs and dietary supplements with the distinction made only in the product labeling, such as senna, which is both an over-the-counter laxative drug and an herbal slimming product ingredient. The formulation of the ingredient also determines the regulatory category. For instance, caffeine is marketed as an over-the-counter drug (e.g., No-Doz capsules), a food product (e.g., Red Bull drinks), and a dietary supplement ingredient (guarana, yerba mate herbal extracts).

Postmarketing surveillance and FDA reporting of adverse events associated with dietary supplements is not required of manufacturers under DSHEA; however, federal legislation mandating adverse event reporting is currently being considered. Sporadic cases and clusters of serious adverse events have been published in the past decade, raising concern about the safety of some dietary supplements and the adequacy of regulatory oversight and monitoring. In 2005, the U.S. Institute of Medicine published a report that provides a framework for establishing the safety of dietary supplements.[5a] This approach includes three stepwise components of response to spontaneous reports of adverse events, consisting of (i) signal detection, (ii) systematic review of available data, and (iii) integrative evaluation to identify level of risk. Further efforts are needed to establish and implement a systematic approach for rapid notification of regulatory authorities in instances of serious dietary supplement toxicity.

EPIDEMIOLOGY OF USE

Use of nutraceuticals and dietary supplements increased rapidly in the United States in the mid- to late 1990s, with various surveys determining regular use of one or more nonvitamin supplements by approximately 20% of adults.[6,7] Sales of dietary supplements reached a peak in 1999 of approximately $4 billion, with steady decreases reported in each subsequent year. The drop in use of nutraceuticals and supplements is possibly attributed to increased negative reports, including adverse effects of products such as ephedra and kava, and lack of evidence of benefit for some popular supplements such as echinacea and St. John's wort (SJW).[8,9] In a recent report of herbal dietary supplement sales in food, drug, and mass market stores, sales for the calendar year 2004 decreased 7.4% overall, with large plummets in sales of kava (−68.7%), guarana (−77.3%), and siberian ginseng (−64.4%).[9a] According to the *Nutrition Business Journal*, 49% of supplements are purchased via direct-to-consumer sales, such as mail order, Internet, and network marketers; 32% of sales occur in specialty supplement or natural food stores; and 19% are sold in mass market or chain retail stores such as Wal-Mart.

The 20 top-selling dietary supplements in the United States based on 2004 major retail outlet sales figures, along with major indications for use, strength of supportive evidence of benefit, and common adverse effects, are shown in Table 90-1.

THERAPEUTICS AND CLINICAL PHARMACOLOGY

Dietary Supplements with Demonstrated Therapeutic Benefit

In this section, the pharmacology of some of the top-selling dietary supplements that have some demonstrated therapeutic benefit is discussed, including black cohosh, ginkgo biloba, SJW, garlic, and milk thistle.

Black Cohosh

With results of the Women's Health Initiative showing that hormone replacement therapy is associated with increased risk of cardiovascular adverse events, health care providers and women have sought alternative treatments for menopause-related symptoms, including several CAM therapies. Black cohosh (*Cimicifuga racemosa*) is sometimes recommended as an effective herbal supplement for relief of vasomotor symptoms of menopause, including hot flashes. These endorsements, including those of the American College of Obstetrics and Gynecology, are based on several short-term clinical trials showing some clinical benefit.[10,11] However, there are no human pharmacokinetic studies on black cohosh, and the active constituents responsible for its beneficial effects have not been identified. Recent systematic reviews of animal and in vitro studies suggest that black cohosh has central activity rather than an estrogenic effect, and thus may be useful in relieving symptoms in women with hormone receptor–positive breast cancer. Further investigations are needed to define the mechanism of action and identify the active components responsible for the observed effects.

Although adverse events are mild and consist primarily of gastrointestinal upset and rash, there are rare reports of hepatitis associated with black cohosh use. To date, there are five published cases of severe liver injury in women using black cohosh alone, including three cases requiring liver transplant and one death.[12-16] However, a causal association is questioned in several of these cases.[17,18] Descriptions of the cases suggest that it is a subacute drug-induced liver injury with autoimmune features including inflammatory cell infiltrates. Caution is advised in use of black cohosh in pregnancy because it could induce labor.[19]

Garlic

Garlic (*Allium sativum*) has a multitude of culinary and medicinal uses, but its major modern-day purpose as a CAM therapy is for lowering serum triglycerides and low-density lipoprotein (LDL) cholesterol, treating hypertension, and reducing the risk of coronary artery disease. The majority of clinical evidence indicates that garlic modestly lowers total cholesterol, LDL, and triglyceride levels, but does not affect high-density lipoprotein cholesterol levels.[20-24] There is some evidence that long-term garlic supplementation lowers blood pressure by 2% to 7%,[20,25] and slows development of arteriosclerosis,[26] as well as inhibiting platelet aggregation.[27] However, long-term benefits of garlic supplementation have not been demonstrated, and the overall impact of garlic on reducing cardiovascular disease risk is not known.[28] Garlic may also reduce the risk of colorectal cancer.[23,29]

Lack of reproducibility of study results dampens the field of garlic research. Discrepancies in the literature on cardiovascular and other health benefits of garlic may be due to differences in garlic preparations in addition to other factors. Studies have been conducted on aged garlic, raw garlic, fresh garlic juice, pressed garlic oil, and dried powdered extract, with several hundred-fold differences in concentration.

The pharmacologic actions of garlic are attributed to its major sulfur-containing constituent allicin, which is formed when fresh garlic bulbs are cut or crushed, compromising cell walls and allowing the enzyme alliinase to contact and convert the substrate alliin into the active chemical, which is responsible for the pungent garlic odor. Allicin readily degrades within hours, and is destroyed by boiling and cooking. Thus, only raw garlic and dried garlic extracts have biologic antiatherogenic, antilipidemic, antiplatelet, and antihypertensive activity.

Few human clinical studies have been performed on the pharmacology of allicin. The metabolism and mechanism of action in the body are not well understood. Allicin is well absorbed after oral consumption, as indicated by garlicky odor on the skin and breath of persons who consume it, but neither allicin nor its major transformation products, ajoene, vinydithiin, and diallyl disulfide, can be detected in blood, urine, or stool. In animals, wide variability in metabolites and kinetic parameters of allicin are observed among various species.[30-32] Rapid absorption (within 10 to 60 minutes) and abundance of metabolites in several tissues, including kidneys, liver, and stomach, suggests excellent bioavailability and distribution of allicin.

Ginkgo biloba

Concentrated extracts of the leaves of *Gingko biloba* are used for treatment of mild to moderate Alzheimer's disease and other forms of dementia, and to alleviate symptoms associated with peripheral and cerebrovascular disorders, such as intermittent claudication and vertigo and tinnitus, respectively. The herbal extract has been shown in trials lasting 3 months to 1 year to modestly improve caregiver assessment scores and short-term memory in patients with mild to moderate dementia,[33,34] but has no therapeutic benefit in improving cognitive performance in persons without dementia. Ginkgo extracts have also improved dizziness, vertigo, and pain-free walking distance in studies

TABLE 90-1 SUMMARY OF POSSIBLE BENEFITS AND ADVERSE EFFECTS OF SOME TOP-SELLING DIETARY SUPPLEMENTS IN THE UNITED STATES

Common Name	Scientific Name	Major Indications for Use	Strength of Evidence of Benefit*	Adverse Effects
Garlic	*Allium sativum*	Hyperlipidemia, hypertension	+	Gastroenteritis; contact dermatitis; antiplatelet actions
Echinacea	*E. purpurea* *E. angustifolia*	Prevent and shorten cold and flu duration	–	Allergic reaction
Saw palmetto	*Serenoa repens*	Male urinary dysfunction	–	Headache; diarrhea; antiandrogenic
Ginkgo	*Ginkgo biloba*	Dementia, peripheral vascular disease; tinnitus	++	Antiplatelet effect; bleeding
Soy	*Glycine max*	Menopausal symptoms; high cholesterol	+	Phytoestrogens may increase breast cancer risk
Cranberry	*Vaccinium macrocarpon*	Urinary tract infections	+	None reported
Ginseng	*Panax ginseng*	Weakness, fatigue, boost immune system	+	CNS/cardiac stimulation; hypoglycemia; bleeding
Black cohosh	*Cimicifuga racemosa*	Menopausal symptoms	+	Gastroenteritis; hepatitis
St. John's wort	*Hypericum perforatum*	Mild to moderate depression	++	Gastroenteritis; dizziness; sedation; photodermatitis
Milk thistle	*Silybum marianum*	Viral, alcoholic, and toxin-induced hepatitis	+	Gastroenteritis; possible allergic reaction
Evening primrose	*Oenothera biennis*	Rheumatoid arthritis; diabetes; PMS; hot flashes, mastalgia	+	Nausea, loose stools; headache; possible bleeding
Valerian	*Valerian officinale*	Insomnia; anxiety	++	Sedation; potentiation of alcohol effects
Green tea	*Camellia sinensis*	Lower cholesterol; weight loss; improve cognition; decrease cancer risk	++	Inhibits platelet function; GI upset; irritability, tremor, palpitations; diarrhea
Bilberry	*Vaccinium myrtillus*	Improve visual acuity; diabetic and hypertensive retinopathy	+	None reported
Grape seed	*Vitis vinifera*	Venous insufficiency; hemorrhoids; atherosclerosis	+	Inhibits platelet function
Horny goat weed	*Epimedium sagittatum*	Erectile dysfunction	0	Dry mouth, dizziness; vomiting
Yohimbine	*Pausinystalia yohimbe*	Erectile dysfunction	0	Hypertension; anxiety, tremor; headache; insomnia; palpitations
Horse chestnut	*Aesculus hippocastaneum*	Hemorrhoids, varicose veins, phlebitis	+	GI irritation; nephropathy
Siberian ginseng	*Eleutherococcus senticosus*	Weakness, fatigue; boost immune system	+	None reported
Ginger	*Zingiber officinale*	Motion sickness; postanesthesia, chemotherapy, and pregnancy-related nausea	++	Heartburn, diarrhea; bleeding; mouth/throat irritation; allergic dermatitis

*Strength of evidence based on:
(–), controlled clinical trials failed to demonstrate significant effect for major indications.
(0), no published clinical trial data.
(+), some evidence from clinical trials of a modest benefit or efficacy for limited indications, but with some conflicting data.
(++), controlled clinical trials demonstrate consistent, moderate benefit for major indications.
CNS, central nervous system; GI, gastrointestinal; PMS, premenstrual syndrome.

of patients with circulatory diseases,[35,36] but the majority of evidence indicates that ginkgo is ineffective in patients with tinnitus.[37-39]

Dried ginkgo leaf extracts contain 22% to 27% flavonol glycosides (quercetin, kaempferol, and isorhamnetin), and 5% to 7% terpene lactones (ginkgolide A, ginkolide B, and bilobalide), all of which have pharmacologic activity. The mechanism of effect of ginkgo for the various disease states is not well understood, but the properties of the active constitutents appear to work synergistically to prevent oxidative stress and inflammatory damage to various tissues,[34] improve vascular flow by inhibiting platelet aggregation and vascular smooth muscle contraction,[37] and possibly influence various neurotransmitter systems.[33] Dried extracts containing standardized quantities of flavone glycosides and terpenoids used in pharmacokinetic studies include EGb 761 and LI 1370, which are found in many commercial ginkgo supplements. Human pharmacokinetic studies of ginkgolides A and B and bilobalide after oral administration showed that twice-daily 40-mg ginkgo leaf extract dosing results in stable plasma concentrations with an elimination half-life of approximately 12 hours versus 4 hours with a single 80-mg dose regimen.[40] Food consumption does not affect pharmacokinetic parameters.[41] The ginkgo flavonoids quercetin, isorhamnetin, and kaempferol are rapidly absorbed after oral dosing with capsule, liquid, and tablet formulations.[42] Peak plasma concentrations are reached within 2 to 3 hours with half-lives of 2 to 4 hours.

Ginkgo biloba is associated with several published case reports of clinical bleeding events. A recent systematic review of the literature identified 15 published case reports of bleeding associated with ginkgo, including 8 episodes of intracranial bleeding, 4 cases of ocular bleeding, 2 cases of extensive bleeding postoperatively, and 1 case of superficial bruising and bleeding.[43] In 13 of the 15 case reports, patients had risk factors other than ginkgo (including advanced age, use of a medication known to increase bleeding risk, mechanical fall, advanced cirrhosis, and surgery) that might have caused the bleeding event. Six of the cases clearly described that ginkgo was stopped and bleeding did not recur. Three cases reported bleeding times that all were elevated when patients were taking ginkgo. Taken in summary, these case reports suggest, but do not prove, that ginkgo increases the risk of bleeding. However, recent human studies have failed to document signficant anticoagulant effects of ginkgo. In two separate placebo-controlled trials involving healthy men, the standard extract EGb 761 was found to have no effect on coagulation, fibrinolysis, or platelet aggregation.[44,45]

Milk Thistle

Extracts of the milk thistle plant (*Silybum marianum*) have been used for centuries to treat liver and gallbladder disorders, including cholestasis, jaundice, cirrhosis, chronic hepatitis, and toxin-induced liver injury.[46,47] Extracts are also taken orally to treat prostate cancer,[48] and to stimulate lactation and menstruation. The extract of the above-ground plant parts contains 70% to 80% of the active flavonoid silymarin, which is composed chiefly of silybins A and B. The seed is most often used for medicinal purposes. The hypothesized mechanism of action of silymarin demonstrated by in vitro and animal studies includes alteration of hepatocyte cell membrane permeability and increased ribosomal protein synthesis promoting hepatocyte regeneration.[46] Although the efficacy of milk thistle in treatment of liver disease in humans has not been definitively established, it appears to reduce mortality in patients with hepatic cirrhosis,[49] improve liver function tests in patients with subacute hepatitis,[47] and may be effective as adjuvant therapy when administered within 48 hours of *Amanita phalloides* mushroom ingestion[50] and other hepatotoxins such as acetaminophen. There is preliminary evidence that milk thistle constituents may also protect against the nephrotoxic effects of drugs such as acetaminophen, cisplatin, and vincristine.

Pharmacokinetic studies of the active silymarin component, silibinin, have been conducted in humans. Bioavailability of silibinin is low and depends on the content of accompanying constituents in the extract and the oral formulation.[51] Mean peak concentration (C_{max}) is reached in approximately 2 hours, and the total elimination half-life averages 6 hours.[52] Silibinin undergoes enterohepatic recirculation with 100-fold higher concentrations found in bile than peak levels reached in serum.[53] Biliary excretion continues for 24 hours after a single dose.

In addition to milk thistle dietary supplements that are easily available for oral use, parenteral formulations are available by prescription in Europe, with limited availability in the United States as well.

Adverse effects of milk thistle are few and generally include mild nausea, diarrhea, abdominal fullness, flatulence, and anorexia. Because milk thistle is a member of the *Asteraceae* (daisy) family, it may cause allergic reactions including rash, urticaria, pruritus, and anaphylaxis in sensitive individuals. There is some evidence that milk thistle affects drug concentrations of cytochrome P-450 (CYP) enzyme substrates (see "Toxicities of Dietary Supplements" section).

St. John's Wort

Extracts of the above-ground plant parts of *Hypericum perforatum*, known as St. John's wort (SJW) are used orally to treat depression. Several clinical studies have shown that SJW is superior to placebo, and as effective as low-dose tricyclic antidepressants and selective serotonin reuptake inhibitors in improving symptoms of mild to moderate depression.[54-57] However, one well-conducted study showed it is ineffective in treating major depression.[58] Other reported uses of SJW include treatment of obsessive-compulsive disorder, premenstrual syndrome, and polyneuropathies, and as an antiretroviral in people infected with human immunodeficiency virus. Few data exist on the clinical benefits of SJW for these indications; however, it appears to be poorly effective as an antiretroviral agent and for relieving neuropathic pain.[59,60]

Human pharmacokinetic studies have been conducted on SJW extracts standardized for two major active components, hypericin and hyperforin.[58] Most studies have utilized preparations of SJW standardized with a hypericin content of 0.2% to 0.3%; however, recent evidence suggests that hyperforin may be the primary constituent that modulates neurotransmitter reuptake.[61,62] Administration of 300 to 1800 mg of dried SJW extract containing 0.24% to 0.32% hypericin in single- and multiple-dose studies revealed elimination half-lives averaging 25 hours, time to peak concentration (T_{max}) values of 2.0 to 2.6 hours, and a time to steady state concentration of 4 days after thrice-daily dosing.[63-65] Kinetics parameters after intravenous administration are similar to those after oral dosing, and systemic bioavailability of hypericin is estimated to be about 14%.[65] Hyperforin kinetics were examined in healthy volunteers receiving 300 mg SJW extract containing 14.8 mg hyperforin in doses up to 3 times per day (900 mg total).[66] Hyperforin half-life was 9 hours, and no accumulation was observed after ingestion of 900 mg/day for 7 days. C_{max} was achieved 3.5 hours after oral intake; however, the absorption characteristics vary with SJW formulation. Ethanol extracts of SJW in soft gelatin capsules exhibit shorter average T_{max} of 2.5 hours and twofold higher peak hyperforin plasma concentrations compared to hard gelatin capsule formulations.[67]

SJW is generally well tolerated after oral use, with few associated adverse effects that include mild gastrointestinal distress, dizziness, and sedation.[68] Rarely, photodermatitis has been reported,[69-71] but only doses of SJW in excess of 1800 mg/day are thought to increase the risk of severe phototoxic skin reactions.[63] Although not absolutely contraindicated, caution is warranted in use of SJW during pregnancy because few human reproductive data exist on the herbal extract.[72] Animal studies indicate SJW use during pregnancy may lower birth weight but is not associated with long-term cognitive or behavioral deficits.[73] A study in lactating women showed SJW use was associated with increased drowsiness and colic in breast-fed infants.[74]

Herb-Drug Interactions

Dietary supplements are commonly used by patients with various chronic medical conditions, including breast cancer (12% use),[75] liver disease (21% use),[76] human immunodeficiency virus infection (22% use),[77] asthma (24% use),[78] and rheumatologic disorders (26% use).[79] Therefore, the likelihood of concomitant use of dietary supplements with prescription medications is high. Pharmacokinetic and pharmacodynamic interactions between dietary supplements and medications are of clinical concern and of increased scientific interest. Approximately 40 cases of supplement-drug interactions are reported in the medical literature, the majority involving SJW.[43,80-91] Such reports should be interpreted with caution, however, since definitive conclusions about adverse drug effects and interactions cannot be made from individual case events.[92]

Several recent investigations have characterized in vitro and in vivo effects of commonly used dietary supplements on CYP drug-metabolizing enzymes and the MDR1 drug transporter P-glycoprotein (Pgp) (Table 90-2). Unfortunately, many published studies show conflicting results. Factors that might be responsible for discrepancies in these study results include variability in dietary supplement content and concentrations of active phytochemicals, low bioavailability of supplement constituents, and individual differences in drug metabolism enzyme activity due to other factors such as genetic and environmental influences.

Pharmacokinetic Interactions

St. John's Wort. Oral use of SJW strongly induces CYP isoenzyme 3A, which is involved in the metabolism of approximately 50% of common medications. As shown in Table 90-3, numerous studies have reported decreased plasma concentrations of many drugs, including indinavir, simvastatin, and amitriptyline, due to co-ingestion of this herbal antidepressant.[81,85,86,88,89,93] Decreased efficacy is reported for

TABLE 90-2 SUMMARY OF DIETARY SUPPLEMENT EFFECTS ON DRUG-METABOLIZING ENZYMES AND DRUG TRANSPORTERS

	Pgp	CYP3A4	CYP2C9	CYP2C19	CYP2D6	CYP2E1	CYP1A2
St. John's wort	↑	↑	↑	↑		↑	↑
Goldenseal		↓			↓		
Kava		↔		↔	↔	↕	↕
Echinacea		↕	↔		↔		↓
Garlic oil						↓	
Milk thistle	↕	↔					
Black cohosh	↔	↔			↓	↔	↔

↑, Increased activity; ↓, decreased activity; ↕, mixed results; ↔, no effect on activity.

TABLE 90-3 SUMMARY OF EFFECT OF ST. JOHN'S WORT ON PLASMA LEVELS OF COMMON DRUGS

Medication	Enzyme/Transporter	Alteration in Plasma Levels
Alprazolam	3A4	41%
Amitryptiline	2C19, 3A4	22%
Cyclosporine	3A4, Pgp	30-60%
Digoxin	Pgp	25%
Fexofenadine	Pgp	20-40%
Imatinib mesylate	3A4	30%
Indinavir	3A4	57%
Irinotecan	Pgp	42%
Methadone	3A4	47%
Oral contraceptives	3A4	13-41%
Simvastatin	3A4	52%
Tacrolimus	3A4, Pgp	58%
Warfarin	2C9	Case reports

oral contraceptives because of induction of ethinyl estradiol–norethindrone metabolism,[94,95] and for post–organ transplantation immunosuppression due to increased clearance of tacrolimus and cyclosporine.[81,89] SJW also induces Pgp, an intestinal cell membrane transporter that decreases bioavailability and therapeutic efficacy for drug substrates such as irinotecan and digoxin.[88,93] SJW has further been reported to induce the metabolizing activity of CYP2E1, 2C9, 2C19, and 1A2.[88,96] The degree of enzyme induction correlates with the hyperforin content of the formulation.[97] The risk of drug interactions with use of SJW is considered to be clinically significant, prompting the FDA to issue a public health advisory in 2000 warning against its concomitant use with indinavir and other medications.

Other Dietary Supplements. Consumption of traditional kava preparations inhibited CYP1A2 but not 2C19, 2D6, 2E1, or 3A4, in one human study.[98] However, in another clinical investigation, kava root extract taken as a 1-g supplement twice daily for 28 days reduced CYP2E1 activity by 40%, but had no effect on CYP1A2 or 3A4.[99]

A study involving use of 900 mg goldenseal root extract thrice daily for 28 days showed that it significantly reduced CYP3A4/5 and CYP2D6 activity by approximately 40%.[99] Garlic oil was shown in one study to inhibit CYP2E1 activity.[100] Milk thistle flavonoids, including silibinin, were shown to inhibit Pgp in in vitro studies, but no change in digoxin pharmacokinetics was seen in a recent milk thistle human clinical trial.[101] Echinacea and black cohosh appear to have weak inhibitory effects on some CYP isoenzymes.[99,101,102] A number of other dietary supplements have been evaluated, including valerian, *Ginkgo biloba*, *Panax ginseng*, saw palmetto, and *Citrus aurantium*, and appear to have no significant effect on CYP isoenzyme activities.[99,101,103]

Pharmacodynamic Interactions

Pharmacodynamic interactions of dietary supplements with medications have not been well investigated, but there are a few reports of clinical adverse drug events related to concomitant supplement and medication use. Bleeding episodes are described with use of *Ginkgo biloba*, dong quai, and vitamin E in combination with warfarin, but not substantiated by clinical studies.[43,104,105] Combined use of SJW with pharmaceutical antidepressants is not advised because of the risk of central serotonergic excess characterized by autonomic instability, mental status changes, tremor, and clonus. Cases of serotonin syndrome have been described with use of SJW and selective serotonin reuptake inhibitors.[85,88]

Kava kava and valerian are herbal sedatives taken as sleep aids and anxiolytics. Lethargy and disorientation was reported in a 54-year-old woman taking kava kava and alprazolam together.[80] There are no other literature reports of cases of serious sedative interactions for kava or valerian; however, concomitant use with ethanol and prescription sedatives should be avoided. Sedative effects induced by alcohol were potentiated by kava in one rodent study,[106] but humans showed no impairment in motor performance skills in a clinical kava-ethanol interaction study.[107]

Toxicities of Dietary Supplements

A number of well-known toxins have been found in herbal preparations at various times throughout history, sometimes resulting in significant human injury. For example, root extracts of *Aconitum* species (e.g., chuan-wu, cao-wu), have sometimes been identified as adulterants in Chinese herbal medicines and can cause serious poisonings, including profound muscle weakness and cardiac dysrhythmias.[108] An outbreak of progressive renal fibrosis associated with a Belgian slimming herbal formulation, and sporadically found in other herbal preparations, was traced to misidentification and substitution of the herbal product *Stephania tetranda* by *Aristolchia fangchi*, which contains the cytotoxin aristolochic acid.[109] Pennyroyal (*Mentha pulegium*) produces dose-dependent liver injury through generation of a reactive metabolite, pulegone. Inadvertent ingestion of pennyroyal as an essential oil or tea is associated with cases of hepatoxicity, including fatal liver failure.[110-112] These cases illustrate that some herbal preparations are intrinsically toxic and cause predictable adverse effects in exposed persons. Fortunately, rapid identification of these herbal toxins is possible through laboratory testing, which limits human exposures to some known dangerous CAM therapies.

Of concern, however, is the incidence of sporadic dietary supplement–related adverse events that are not readily predictable, including idiosyncratic reactions and adverse effects in unknowingly susceptible people, such as those with underlying disease or genetic variants in drug transporters or metabolizing enzymes. Because of regulatory limitations imposed by DSHEA, such adverse events may occur for months or years before appropriate action is taken to minimize consumer risk.

BOX 90-1 DIETARY SUPPLEMENT-INDUCED TOXICITIES BY BODY SYSTEM

Central Nervous System

Stimulation
- Ephedra
- Guarana/yerba mate

Sedation
- Kava

Cardiovascular

Vasopressive
- Ephedra
- Guarana
- Yohimbine
- C. aurantium

Electrophysiologic
- Ephedra
- Hawthorn

Hypotension
- Hawthorn
- Ginseng

Dermatologic

Skin Rash
- Kava

Photodermatitis
- St. John's wort
- Goldenseal

Immune

Allergic Reaction
- Echinacea
- Bee pollen
- Milk thistle

Hematologic

Antiplatelet/Anticoagulant
- Feverfew
- Ginkgo biloba
- Garlic
- Ginseng
- Willow bark

Hepatic

Hepatitis
- Black cohosh
- Chaparral
- Comfrey
- Kava
- Pennyroyal
- Lipokinetix (usinic acid)

Metabolic

Hypokalemia
- Licorice
- Aloe
- Senna
- Cascara

Hyperglycemia
- Glucosamine
- Ephedra
- Licorice

Hypoglycemia
- Fenugreek
- Garlic
- Ginseng

Mutagenic/ Carcinogenic

Urothelial
- Aristolochic acid

Hepatocellular
- Pyrrolizidine alkaloids

Renal

Renal Failure
- Aristolochic acid

Many available dietary supplements possess intrinsic properties that could affect physiologic functions such as blood coagulation, glucose homeostasis, and immune response (Box 90-1), but relatively few available products have been associated with significant adverse events in humans. In this section, well-described toxicities of several dietary supplements are discussed.

Ephedra

Ephedra sinica is a plant that contains six sympathomimetic amines, known collectively as ephedra alkaloids, with ephedrine and pseudoephedrine as the two primary constituents. Ephedra was a popular weight loss dietary supplement ingredient available in products such as Metabolife 356, Xenadrine RFA, and Ripped Fuel, until the FDA banned ephedra-containing products in April 2004 because of peer-reviewed scientific reports on the effects of ephedra alkaloids, and reported cases of ephedra-related toxicity.[113,114] Adverse events included seizures, psychiatric disorders, cardiac dysrhythmias, myocardial infarctions, hemorrhagic and ischemic stroke, and sudden death.[115-119] The toxicity of ephedra-containing dietary supplements was enhanced by the sympathomimetic effects of caffeine co-ingredients, including guarana, yerba mate, and kola nut.[120,121] Ephedra can still be obtained from practitioners of alternative medicine as the traditional Chinese herbal medicine ma huang, for short-term treatment of wheezing and nasal congestion associated with asthma, allergies, and colds or flu.

Kava

Kava is an herbal anxiolytic with a long-standing history of traditional use in South Pacific cultures as a social/recreational beverage, similar to ethanol. Over 25 cases of hepatitis have been reported in association with use of kava in the United States, Europe, and Australia,[122-132] including 8 cases requiring liver transplant and several deaths[133,134]; however, kava hepatitis is unknown in South Pacific nations. The duration of kava use ranged from 8 weeks to 12 months, with reported doses of 60 to 240 mg/day. The clinical course of kava hepatotoxicity is characterized by an indolent onset of fatigue, nausea, jaundice, and weight loss with elevation of liver enzymes including alanine aminotransferase, aspartate aminotransferase, and γ-glutamyl transferase. Biopsy of the liver shows hepatocellular necrosis with or without inflammatory cell infiltrate and cholestasis. Discontinuation of kava and supportive care results in recovery of liver function in some cases, but in others, a fulminant course follows with progressive liver failure resulting in encephalopathy and death unless liver transplantation is performed.

Several countries, including Germany, France, Switzerland, Canada, and Australia, have restricted or banned the sale of kava-containing products based on reported adverse events.[133,134] In response to five case reports, the FDA in 2002 issued an advisory to health care providers and a warning to consumers about the potential risk of liver injury associated with use of kava-containing products.[21]

The pathogenesis of kava-induced hepatic injury remains unknown, but an idiosyncratic immune-mediated mechanism is postulated.[135,136] Kava supplements are typically derived from the ethanol or acetone extraction of kava pyrones known collectively as kavalactones. The hepatotoxin may be the kava alkaloid pipermethystin, found in the stem and aerial parts of the plant. Although traditional formulations of kava used in Polynesian cultures utilize the plant root, dietary supplement manufacturers may not differentiate plant parts in kava raw materials. Recent observations about kava hepatotoxicity show a disproportionate gender distribution, with threefold higher number of hepatitis cases in women than men, and the possibility that genetic polymorphisms in CYP drug-metabolizing enzymes may be involved, with two reported cases of liver failure in patients with CYP2D6 deficiency.[132]

Yohimbine

Dietary supplements that contain the botanical yohimbine are widely promoted for their sympathomimetic and aphrodisiac properties. Yohimbine is an indole alkaloid that occurs naturally in the bark of the West African tree *Pausinystalia yohimbe*. Yohimbe bark contains up to 5.9% total alkaloids, consisting chiefly of yohimbine.[137] Yohimbine has selective antagonist activity at α_2-adrenergic receptors, resulting in increased central and peripheral sympathetic activity. Yohimbine is available as an FDA-approved drug to treat xerostomia and orthostatic hypotension secondary to antidepressant therapy, and as a treatment for impotence, and is sometimes used to reverse adverse effects of clonidine.

Yohimbine is frequently combined with caffeine and other herbs, such as horny goat weed, in dietary supplements and marketed to increase energy, build lean body mass, and enhance sexual performance, despite a lack of scientific data demonstrating safety or efficacy of these combinations. A number of reports of yohimbine supplement-related toxicity suggest that these products have significant health risks. Several clinical studies indicate that yohimbine induces a dose-dependent increase in blood pressure and plasma norepinephrine with variable effects on heart rate.[138-144] There are several case reports in the medical literature of yohimbine-associated toxicity, including hypertension, anxiety, headache, tachycardia, tremor, weakness, and mania.[145]

Dieter's Teas

Among the myriad of weight loss dietary supplements are "dieter's teas" that frequently contain herbal constituents that have a stimulant cathartic action, including senna (*Cassia angustifolia*), Cascara (*Cascara sagrada*), aloe, and buckthorn. Senna is also available as an over-the-counter laxative. The use of dieter's teas in the setting of reduced food intake can produce profound fluid loss and electrolyte imbalance. Several cases of dehydration, hypokalemia, and sudden cardiac death have been reported, prompting the FDA to require label warnings on dieter's teas in 1995.

FUTURE OF DIETARY SUPPLEMENTS

The dietary supplement landscape has changed dramatically in the years since DSHEA was enacted. There has been a transformation from an early explosive growth in the number of dietary supplements products and consumers, to growing concern over potential health risks and drug interactions, and increased consumer skepticism about the truthfulness of product claims for safety and effectiveness. These changes have been fueled by greater public awareness of serious cases of supplement-related health injuries, and growing numbers of published scientific studies showing little or no effect of some popular supplements.

Full implementation of DSHEA is still ongoing amid calls by some for reform of the initially enacted legislation. Increased regulatory efforts include implementing good manufacturing practices, greater efforts to curb availability of supplements marketed without NDI approval, and mandatory reporting of adverse events. On the scientific side, efforts are underway to improve standardization of dietary supplements used in clinical trials to enable validation and reproducibility of results. Ultimately, botanicals and other natural products that are intended to treat or prevent disease will be developed as drugs, and a new Botanical Review Team established at the FDA's Center for Drug Evaluation and Research is dedicated to review botanical new drug applications. Ideally, dietary supplements will someday encompass true nutritional products such as vitamins, minerals, amino acids, and other essential substances that improve overall human health and well-being, and botanicals that are intended to treat human illness or cure disease will rightfully find a home in the drug world.

REFERENCES

1. Barrett B, Kiefer D, Rabago D. Assessing the risks and benefits of herbal medicine: an overview of scientific evidence. Altern Ther Health Med 1999;5(4):40-49.
2. Homsy J, King R, Balaba D, Kabatesi D. Traditional health practitioners are key to scaling up comprehensive care for HIV/AIDS in sub-Saharan Africa. AIDS 2004;18:1723-1725.
3. Gedif T, Hahn HJ. Epidemiology of herbal drugs use in Addis Ababa, Ethiopia. Pharmacoepidemiol Drug Saf 2002;11:587-591.
4. Ross S. Functional foods: the Food and Drug Administration perspective. Am J Clin Nutr 2000;71(6 Suppl):1735S-1738S; discussion 1739S-1742S.
5. Hathcock J. Dietary supplements: how they are used and regulated. J Nutr 2001;131(3 Suppl):1114S-1117S.

5a. Dietary Supplements: A Framework for Evaluating Safety. Washington, DC: The National Academies Press, 2005.

6. Ni H, Simile C, Hardy AM. Utilization of complementary and alternative medicine by United States adults: results from the 1999 National Health Interview Survey. Med Care 2002;40:353-358.
7. Eisenberg DM, Davis RB, Ettner SL, et al. Trends in alternative medicine use in the United States, 1990-1997: results of a follow-up national survey. JAMA 1998;280:1569-1575.
8. Bent S, Ko R. Commonly used herbal medicines in the United States: a review. Am J Med 2004;116:478-485.
9. Ernst E. Risks of herbal medicinal products. Pharmacoepidemiol Drug Saf 2004;13:767-771.

9a. Dietary supplements. Accessed March 8, 2008. Available at www.nutritionbusiness.com/data.htm.

10. Borrelli F, Izzo AA, Ernst E. Pharmacological effects of *Cimicifuga racemosa*. Life Sci 2003;73:1215-1229.
11. Huntley A, Ernst E. A systematic review of the safety of black cohosh. Menopause 2003;10:58-64.
12. Lynch CR, Folkers ME, Hutson WR. Fulminant hepatic failure associated with the use of black cohosh: a case report. Liver Transpl 2006;12:989-992.
13. Whiting PW, Clouston A, Kerlin P. Black cohosh and other herbal remedies associated with acute hepatitis. Med J Aust 2002;177:440-443.
14. Lontos S, Jones RM, Angus PW, Gow PJ. Acute liver failure associated with the use of herbal preparations containing black cohosh. Med J Aust 2003;179:390-391.
15. Levitsky J, Alli TA, Wisecarver J, Sorrell MF. Fulminant liver failure associated with the use of black cohosh. Dig Dis Sci 2005;50:538-539.
16. Cohen SM, O'Connor AM, Hart J, et al. Autoimmune hepatitis associated with the use of black cohosh: a case study. Menopause 2004;11:575-577.
17. Huntley A. The safety of black cohosh (*Actaea racemosa, Cimicifuga racemosa*). Expert Opin Drug Saf 2004;3:615-623.
18. Thomsen M, Schmidt M. Hepatotoxicity from *Cimicifuga racemosa?* Recent Australian case report not sufficiently substantiated. J Altern Complement Med 2003;9:337-340.
19. Dugoua JJ, Seely D, Perri D, et al. Safety and efficacy of black cohosh (*Cimicifuga racemosa*) during pregnancy and lactation. Can J Clin Pharmacol 2006;13:e257-e261.
20. Auer W, Eiber A, Hertkorn E, et al. Hypertension and hyperlipidaemia: garlic helps in mild cases. Br J Clin Pract Suppl 1990;69:3-6.
21. Jain AK, Vargas R, Gotzkowsky S, McMahon FG. Can garlic reduce levels of serum lipids? A controlled clinical study. Am J Med 1993;94:632-635.
22. Warshafsky S, Kamer RS, Sivak SL. Effect of garlic on total serum cholesterol: a meta-analysis. Ann Intern Med 1993;119(7 Pt 1):599-605.
23. Ariga T, Seki T. Antithrombotic and anticancer effects of garlic-derived sulfur compounds: a review. Biofactors 2006;26:93-103.
24. Rahman K, Lowe GM. Garlic and cardiovascular disease: a critical review. J Nutr 2006;136(3 Suppl):736S-740S.
25. Silagy CA, Neil HA. A meta-analysis of the effect of garlic on blood pressure. J Hypertens 1994;12:463-468.
26. Koscielny J, Klüssendorf D, Latza R, et al. The antiatherosclerotic effect of *Allium sativum*. Atherosclerosis 1999;144:237-249.
27. Lawson LD, Ransom DK, Hughes BG. Inhibition of whole blood platelet-aggregation by compounds in garlic clove extracts and commercial garlic products. Thromb Res 1992;65:141-156.
28. Ackermann RT, Mulrow CD, Ramirez G, et al. Garlic shows promise for improving some cardiovascular risk factors. Arch Intern Med 2001;161:813-824.
29. Matsuura N, Miyamae Y, Yamane K, et al. Aged garlic extract inhibits angiogenesis and proliferation of colorectal carcinoma cells. J Nutr 2006;136(3 Suppl):842S-846S.
30. Lachmann G, Lorenz D, Radeck W, Steiper M. [The pharmacokinetics of the S35 labeled garlic constituents alliin, allicin and vinyldithiine]. Arzneimittelforschung 1994;44:734-743.
31. Germain E, Auger J, Ginies C, et al. In vivo metabolism of diallyl disulphide in the rat: identification of two new metabolites. Xenobiotica 2002;32:1127-1138.
32. Nagae S, Ushijima M, Hatono S, et al. Pharmacokinetics of the garlic compound S-allylcysteine. Planta Med 1994;60:214-217.
33. Le Bars PL, Katz MM, Berman N, et al. A placebo-controlled, double-blind, randomized trial of an extract of *Ginkgo biloba* for dementia. North American EGb Study Group. JAMA 1997;278:1327-1332.
34. Oken BS, Storzbach DM, Kaye JA. The efficacy of *Ginkgo biloba* on cognitive function in Alzheimer disease. Arch Neurol 1998;55:1409-1415.
35. Pittler MH, Ernst E. *Ginkgo biloba* extract for the treatment of intermittent claudication: a meta-analysis of randomized trials. Am J Med 2000;108:276-281.
36. Cesarani A, Meloni F, Alpini D, et al. *Ginkgo biloba* (EGb 761) in the treatment of equilibrium disorders. Adv Ther 1998;15:291-304.
37. Diamond BJ, Shiflett SC, Feiwel N, et al. *Ginkgo biloba* extract: mechanisms and clinical indications. Arch Phys Med Rehabil 2000;81:668-678.
38. Drew S, Davies E. Effectiveness of *Ginkgo biloba* in treating tinnitus: double blind, placebo controlled trial. BMJ 2001;322:73.
39. Holgers KM, Axelsson A, Pringle I. *Ginkgo biloba* extract for the treatment of tinnitus. Audiology 1994;33:85-92.
40. Drago F, Floriddia ML, Cro M, Giuffrida S. Pharmacokinetics and bioavailability of a *Ginkgo biloba* extract. J Ocul Pharmacol Ther 2002;18:197-202.
41. Fourtillan JB, Brisson AM, Girault J, et al. [Pharmacokinetic properties of Bilobalide and Ginkgolides A and B in healthy subjects after intravenous and oral administration of *Ginkgo biloba* extract (EGb 761)]. Therapie 1995;50:137-144.
42. Kressmann S, Biber A, Wonnemann M, et al. Influence of pharmaceutical quality on the bioavailability of active components from *Ginkgo biloba* preparations. J Pharm Pharmacol 2002;54:1507-1514.
43. Bent S, Goldberg H, Padula A, Avins AL. Spontaneous bleeding associated with ginkgo biloba: a case report and systematic review of the literature. J Gen Intern Med 2005;20:657-661.
44. Bal Dit Sollier C, Caplain H, Drouet L. No alteration in platelet function or coagulation induced by EGb761 in a controlled study. Clin Lab Haematol 2003;25:251-253.
45. Kohler S, Funk P, Kieser M. Influence of a 7-day treatment with *Ginkgo biloba* special extract EGb 761 on bleeding time and coagulation: a randomized, placebo-controlled, double-blind study in healthy volunteers. Blood Coagul Fibrinolysis 2004;15:303-309.
46. Saller R, Meier R, Brignoli R. The use of silymarin in the treatment of liver diseases. Drugs 2001;61:2035-2063.
47. Salmi HA, Sarna S. Effect of silymarin on chemical, functional, and morphological alterations of the liver: a double-blind controlled study. Scand J Gastroenterol 1982;17:517-521.
48. Sharma Y, Agarwal C, Singh AK, Agarwal R. Inhibitory effect of silibinin on ligand binding to erbB1 and associated mitogenic signaling, growth, and DNA synthesis in advanced human prostate carcinoma cells. Mol Carcinog 2001;30:224-236.
49. Ferenci P, Dragosics B, Dittrich H, et al. Randomized controlled trial of silymarin treatment in patients with cirrhosis of the liver. J Hepatol 1989;9:105-113.

50. Hruby K, Csomos G, Fuhrmann M, Thaler H. Chemotherapy of *Amanita phalloides* poisoning with intravenous silibinin. Hum Toxicol 1983;2:183-195.
51. Schulz HU, Schürer M, Krumbiegel G, et al. [The solubility and bioequivalence of silymarin preparations]. Arzneimittelforschung 1995;45:61-64.
52. Lorenz D, Lücker PW, Mennicke WH, Wetzelsberger N. Pharmacokinetic studies with silymarin in human serum and bile. Methods Find Exp Clin Pharmacol 1984;6:655-661.
53. Flory PJ, Krug G, Lorenz D, Mennicke WH. [Studies on elimination of silymarin in cholecystectomized patients. I. Biliary and renal elimination after a single oral dose]. Planta Med 1980;38:227-237.
54. Brenner R, Azbel V, Madhusoodanan S, Pawlowska M. Comparison of an extract of hypericum (LI 160) and sertraline in the treatment of depression: a double-blind, randomized pilot study. Clin Ther 2000;22:411-419.
55. Philipp M, Kohnen R, Hiller KO. Hypericum extract versus imipramine or placebo in patients with moderate depression: randomised multicentre study of treatment for eight weeks. BMJ 1999;319:1534-1538.
56. Schrader E. Equivalence of St John's wort extract (Ze 117) and fluoxetine: a randomized, controlled study in mild-moderate depression. Int Clin Psychopharmacol 2000;15:61-68.
57. Woelk H. Comparison of St John's wort and imipramine for treating depression: randomised controlled trial. BMJ 2000;321:536-539.
58. Shelton RC, Keller MB, Gelenberg A, et al. Effectiveness of St John's wort in major depression: a randomized controlled trial. JAMA 2001;285:1978-1986.
59. Sindrup SH, Jensen TS. Pharmacologic treatment of pain in polyneuropathy. Neurology 2000;55:915-920.
60. Gulick RM, McAuliffe V, Holden-Wiltse J, et al. Phase I studies of hypericin, the active compound in St. John's wort, as an antiretroviral agent in HIV-infected adults. AIDS Clinical Trials Group Protocols 150 and 258. Ann Intern Med 1999;130:510-514.
61. Chatterjee SS, Bhattacharya SK, Wonnemann M, et al. Hyperforin as a possible antidepressant component of hypericum extracts. Life Sci 1998;63:499-510.
62. Laakmann G, Schüle C, Baghai T, Kieser M. St. John's wort in mild to moderate depression: the relevance of hyperforin for the clinical efficacy. Pharmacopsychiatry 1998;31(Suppl 1):54-59.
63. Brockmöller J, Reum T, Bauer S, et al. Hypericin and pseudohypericin: pharmacokinetics and effects on photosensitivity in humans. Pharmacopsychiatry 1997;30(Suppl 2):94-101.
64. Staffeldt B, Kerb R, Brockmöller J, et al. Pharmacokinetics of hypericin and pseudohypericin after oral intake of the hypericum perforatum extract LI 160 in healthy volunteers. J Geriatr Psychiatry Neurol 1994;7(Suppl 1):S47-S53.
65. Kerb R, Brockmöller J, Staffeldt B, et al. Single-dose and steady-state pharmacokinetics of hypericin and pseudohypericin. Antimicrob Agents Chemother 1996;40:2087-2093.
66. Biber A, Fischer H, Römer A, Chatterjee SS. Oral bioavailability of hyperforin from hypericum extracts in rats and human volunteers. Pharmacopsychiatry 1998;31(Suppl 1):36-43.
67. Agrosi M, Mischiatti S, Harrasser PC, Savio D. Oral bioavailability of active principles from herbal products in humans: a study on *Hypericum perforatum* extracts using the soft gelatin capsule technology. Phytomedicine 2000;7:455-462.
68. Ernst E, Rand JI, Barnes J, Stevinson C. Adverse effects profile of the herbal antidepressant St. John's wort (*Hypericum perforatum L.*). Eur J Clin Pharmacol 1998;54:589-594.
69. Bowers AG. Phytophotodermatitis. Am J Contact Dermat 1999;10:89-93.
70. Lane-Brown MM. Photosensitivity associated with herbal preparations of St John's wort (*Hypericum perforatum*). Med J Aust 2000;172:302.
71. Golsch S, Vocks E, Rakoski J, et al. [Reversible increase in photosensitivity to UV-B caused by St. John's wort extract]. Hautarzt 1997;48:249-252.
72. Freeman MP, Helgason C, Hill RA. Selected integrative medicine treatments for depression: considerations for women. J Am Med Womens Assoc 2004;59:216-224.
73. Dugoua JJ, Mills E, Perri D, Koren G. Safety and efficacy of St. John's wort (hypericum) during pregnancy and lactation. Can J Clin Pharmacol 2006;13:e268-e276.
74. Lee A, Minhas R, Matsuda N, et al. The safety of St. John's wort (*Hypericum perforatum*) during breastfeeding. J Clin Psychiatry 2003;64:966-968.
75. Burstein HJ, Gelber S, Guadagnoli E, Weeks JC. Use of alternative medicine by women with early-stage breast cancer. N Engl J Med 1999;340:1733-1739.
76. Strader DB, Bacon BR, Lindsay KL, et al. Use of complementary and alternative medicine in patients with liver disease. Am J Gastroenterol 2002;97:2391-2397.
77. Kassler WJ, Blanc P, Greenblatt R. The use of medicinal herbs by human immunodeficiency virus-infected patients. Arch Intern Med 1991;151:2281-2288.
78. Blanc PD, Trupin L, Earnest G, et al. Alternative therapies among adults with a reported diagnosis of asthma or rhinosinusitis: data from a population-based survey. Chest 2001;120:1461-1467.
79. Rafferty AP, McGee HB, Miller CE, Reyes M. Prevalence of complementary and alternative medicine use: state-specific estimates from the 2001 Behavioral Risk Factor Surveillance System. Am J Public Health 2002;92:1598-1600.
80. Almeida JC, Grimsley EW. Coma from the health food store: interaction between kava and alprazolam. Ann Intern Med 1996;125:940-941.
81. Barone GW, Gurley BJ, Ketel BL, et al. Drug interaction between St. John's wort and cyclosporine. Ann Pharmacother 2000;34:1013-1016.
82. Coon JT, Ernst E. *Panax ginseng:* a systematic review of adverse effects and drug interactions. Drug Saf 2002;25:323-344.
83. Cupp MJ. Herbal remedies: adverse effects and drug interactions. Am Fam Physician 1999;59:1239-1245.
84. Fessenden JM, Wittenborn W, Clarke L. *Gingko biloba:* a case report of herbal medicine and bleeding postoperatively from a laparoscopic cholecystectomy. Am Surg 2001;67:33-35.
85. Fugh-Berman A. Herb-drug interactions. Lancet 2000;355:134-138.
86. Hu Z, Yang X, Ho PC, et al. Herb-drug interactions: a literature review. Drugs 2005;65:1239-1282.
87. Izzo AA, Ernst E. Interactions between herbal medicines and prescribed drugs: a systematic review. Drugs 2001;61:2163-2175.
88. Izzo AA. Drug interactions with St. John's wort (*Hypericum perforatum*): a review of the clinical evidence. Int J Clin Pharmacol Ther 2004;42:139-148.
89. Moschella C, Jaber BL. Interaction between cyclosporine and *Hypericum perforatum* (St. John's wort) after organ transplantation. Am J Kidney Dis 2001;38:1105-1107.
90. Smolinske SC. Dietary supplement-drug interactions. J Am Med Womens Assoc 1999;54:191-192, 195.
91. Vaes LP, Chyka PA. Interactions of warfarin with garlic, ginger, ginkgo, or ginseng: nature of the evidence. Ann Pharmacother 2000;34:1478-1482.
92. Fugh-Berman A, Ernst E. Herb-drug interactions: review and assessment of report reliability. Br J Clin Pharmacol 2001;52:587-595.
93. Dürr D, Stieger B, Kullak-Ublick GA, et al. St John's Wort induces intestinal P-glycoprotein/MDR1 and intestinal and hepatic CYP3A4. Clin Pharmacol Ther 2000;68:598-604.
94. Hall SD, Wang Z, Huang SM, et al. The interaction between St John's wort and an oral contraceptive. Clin Pharmacol Ther 2003;74:525-535.
95. Murphy PA, Kern SE, Stanczyk FZ, Westhoff CL. Interaction of St. John's wort with oral contraceptives: effects on the pharmacokinetics of norethindrone and ethinyl estradiol, ovarian activity and breakthrough bleeding. Contraception 2005;71:402-408.
96. Wang Z, Gorski JC, Hamman MA, et al. The effects of St John's wort (*Hypericum perforatum*) on human cytochrome P450 activity. Clin Pharmacol Ther 2001;70:317-326.
97. Mueller SC, Majcher-Peszynska J, Uehleke B, et al. The extent of induction of CYP3A by St. John's wort varies among products and is linked to hyperforin dose. Eur J Clin Pharmacol 2006;62:29-36.
98. Russmann S, Lauterburg BH, Barguil Y, et al. Traditional aqueous kava extracts inhibit cytochrome P450 1A2 in humans: protective effect against environmental carcinogens? Clin Pharmacol Ther 2005;77:453-454.
99. Gurley BJ, Gardner SF, Hubbard MA, et al. In vivo effects of goldenseal, kava kava, black cohosh, and valerian on human cytochrome P450 1A2, 2D6, 2E1, and 3A4/5 phenotypes. Clin Pharmacol Ther 2005;77:415-426.
100. Brady JF, Ishizaki H, Fukuto JM, et al. Inhibition of cytochrome P-450 2E1 by diallyl sulfide and its metabolites. Chem Res Toxicol 1991;4:642-647.
101. Gurley BJ, Barone GW, Williams DK, et al. Effect of milk thistle (*Silybum marianum*) and black cohosh (*Cimicifuga racemosa*) supplementation on digoxin pharmacokinetics in humans. Drug Metab Dispos 2006;34:69-74.
102. Tsukamoto S, Aburatani M, Ohta T. Isolation of CYP3A4 inhibitors from the black cohosh (*Cimicifuga racemosa*). Evid Based Complement Alternat Med 2005;2:223-226.
103. Donovan JL, De Vane CL, Chavin KD, et al. Multiple night-time doses of valerian (*Valeriana officinalis*) had minimal effects on CYP3A4 activity and no effect on CYP2D6 activity in healthy volunteers. Drug Metab Dispos 2004;32:1333-1336.
104. Corrigan JJ Jr, Marcus FI. Coagulopathy associated with vitamin E ingestion. JAMA 1974;230:1300-1301.
105. Page RL 2nd, Lawrence JD. Potentiation of warfarin by dong quai. Pharmacotherapy 1999;19:870-876.
106. Jamieson DD, Duffield PH. Positive interaction of ethanol and kava resin in mice. Clin Exp Pharmacol Physiol 1990;17:509-514.
107. Stevinson C, Huntley A, Ernst E. A systematic review of the safety of kava extract in the treatment of anxiety. Drug Saf 2002;25:251-261.
108. Ko R. Adulterants in asian patent medicines. N Engl J Med 1998;339:847.
109. Yang CS, Lin CH, Chang SG, Hsu HC. Rapidly progressive fibrosing interstitial nephritis associated with Chinese herbal drugs. Am J Kidney Dis 2000;35:313-318.
110. Anderson IB, Mullen WH, Meeker JE, et al. Pennyroyal toxicity: measurement of toxic metabolite levels in two cases and review of the literature. Ann Intern Med 1996;124:726-734.
111. Sullivan JB Jr, Rumack BH, Thomas H Jr, et al. Pennyroyal oil poisoning and hepatotoxicity. JAMA 1979;242:2873-2874.
112. Bakerink JA, Gospe SM Jr, Dimand RJ, Eldridge MW. Multiple organ failure after ingestion of pennyroyal oil from herbal tea in two infants. Pediatrics 1996;98:944-947.
113. Final rule declaring dietary supplements containing ephedrine alkaloids adulterated because they present an unreasonable risk. Final rule. Fed Regist 2004;69:6787-6854.
114. Shekelle PG, Hardy ML, Morton SC, et al. Efficacy and safety of ephedra and ephedrine for weight loss and athletic performance: a meta-analysis. JAMA 2003;289:1537-1545.
115. Haller CA, Benowitz NL. Adverse cardiovascular and central nervous system events associated with dietary supplements containing ephedra alkaloids. N Engl J Med 2000;343:1833-1838.
116. Haller CA, Meier KH, Olson KR. Seizures reported in association with use of dietary supplements. Clin Toxicol (Phila) 2005;43:23-30.
117. Chen C, Biller J, Willing SJ, Lopez AM. Ischemic stroke after using over the counter products containing ephedra. J Neurol Sci 2004;217:55-60.
118. Maglione M, Miotto K, Iguchi M, et al. Psychiatric effects of ephedra use: an analysis of Food and Drug Administration reports of adverse events. Am J Psychiatry 2005;162:189-191.
119. Samenuk D, Link MS, Homoud MK, et al. Adverse cardiovascular events temporally associated with ma huang, an herbal source of ephedrine. Mayo Clin Proc 2002;77:12-16.

120. Haller CA, Jacob P, Benowitz NL. Enhanced stimulant and metabolic effects of ephedrine and caffeine. Clin Pharmacol Ther 2004;75:259-273.
121. Haller CA, Jacob P, Benowitz NL. Short-term metabolic and hemodynamic effects of ephedra and guarana combinations. Clin Pharmacol Ther 2005;77:560-571.
122. Kraft M, Spahn TW, Menzel J, et al. [Fulminant liver failure after administration of the herbal antidepressant Kava-Kava]. Dtsch Med Wochenschr 2001;126:970-972.
123. Escher M, Desmeules J, Giostra E, Mentha G. Hepatitis associated with Kava, a herbal remedy for anxiety. BMJ 2001;322:139.
124. Estes JD, Stolpman D, Olyaei A, et al. High prevalence of potentially hepatotoxic herbal supplement use in patients with fulminant hepatic failure. Arch Surg 2003;138:852-858.
125. Humberston CL, Akhtar J, Krenzelok EP. Acute hepatitis induced by kava kava. J Toxicol Clin Toxicol 2003;41:109-113.
126. Russmann S, Barguil Y, Cabalion P, et al. Hepatic injury due to traditional aqueous extracts of kava root in New Caledonia. Eur J Gastroenterol Hepatol 2003;15:1033-1036.
127. Stickel F, Baumüller HM, Seitz K, et al. Hepatitis induced by Kava (*Piper methysticum* rhizoma). J Hepatol 2003;39:62-67.
128. Strahl S, Ehret V, Dahm HH, Maier KP. [Necrotizing hepatitis after taking herbal remedies]. Dtsch Med Wochenschr 1998;123:1410-1414.
129. Bujanda L, Palacios A, Silvariño R, et al. [Kava-induced acute icteric hepatitis]. Gastroenterol Hepatol 2002;25:434-435.
130. Campo JV, McNabb J, Perel JM, et al. Kava-induced fulminant hepatic failure. J Am Acad Child Adolesc Psychiatry 2002;41:631-632.
131. Wooltorton E. Herbal kava: reports of liver toxicity. CMAJ 2002;166:777.
132. Russmann S, Lauterburg BH, Helbling A. Kava hepatotoxicity. Ann Intern Med 2001;135:68-69.
133. Hepatic toxicity possibly associated with kava-containing products—United States, Germany, and Switzerland, 1999-2002. MMWR Morb Mortal Wkly Rep 2002;51:1065-1067.
134. From the Centers for Disease Control and Prevention. Hepatic toxicity possibly associated with kava-containing products—United States, Germany, and Switzerland, 1999-2002. JAMA 2003;289:36-37.
135. Anke J, Ramzan I. Kava hepatotoxicity: are we any closer to the truth? Planta Med 2004;70:193-196.
136. Musch E, Chrissafidou A, Malek M. [Acute hepatitis due to kava-kava and St John's wort: an immune-mediated mechanism?]. Dtsch Med Wochenschr 2006;131:1214-1217.
137. Zanolari B, Ndjoko K, Ioset JR, et al. Qualitative and quantitative determination of yohimbine in authentic yohimbe bark and in commercial aphrodisiacs by HPLC-UV-API/MS methods. Phytochem Anal 2003;14:193-201.
138. Charney DS, Heninger GR, Sternberg DE. Assessment of alpha 2 adrenergic autoreceptor function in humans: effects of oral yohimbine. Life Sci 1982;30:2033-2041.
139. Charney DS, Woods SW, Goodman WK, Heninger GR. Neurobiological mechanisms of panic anxiety: biochemical and behavioral correlates of yohimbine-induced panic attacks. Am J Psychiatry 1987;144:1030-1036.
140. Krystal JH, McDougle CJ, Woods SW, et al. Dose-response relationship for oral idazoxan effects in healthy human subjects: comparison with oral yohimbine. Psychopharmacology (Berl) 1992;108:313-319.
141. Le Corre P, Parmer RJ, Kailasam MT, et al. Human sympathetic activation by $alpha_2$-adrenergic blockade with yohimbine: bimodal, epistatic influence of cytochrome P450-mediated drug metabolism. Clin Pharmacol Ther 2004;76:139-153.
142. Grasing K, Sturgill MG, Rosen RC, et al. Effects of yohimbine on autonomic measures are determined by individual values for area under the concentration-time curve. J Clin Pharmacol 1996;36:814-822.
143. Hedner T, Edgar B, Edvinsson L, et al. Yohimbine pharmacokinetics and interaction with the sympathetic nervous system in normal volunteers. Eur J Clin Pharmacol 1992;43:651-656.
144. Guthrie SK, Hariharan M, Grunhaus LJ. Yohimbine bioavailability in humans. Eur J Clin Pharmacol 1990;39:409-411.
145. Ruck B, Shih RD, Marcus SM. Hypertensive crisis from herbal treatment of impotence. Am J Emerg Med 1999;17:317-318.

91

VACCINES

Paul V. Targonski, Inna G. Ovsyannikova, Pritish K. Tosh, Robert M. Jacobson, and Gregory A. Poland

INTRODUCTION AND HISTORY 1247
MECHANISMS OF VACCINE RESPONSE 1248
VACCINE TECHNOLOGY 1249
Adjuvants 1249
Virosomes 1249
Cell-Based Vaccines 1249
Universal Vaccines 1250
VACCINES OF THE FUTURE 1250
DNA Vaccines 1250
Anticancer Vaccines 1250
CURRENTLY LICENSED VACCINES 1251
Anthrax 1251
Haemophilus influenzae Type b 1251
Hepatitis A 1252
Hepatitis B 1253
Human Papillomavirus 1253
Influenza 1254
Japanese Encephalitis Virus 1255
Measles, Mumps, and Rubella 1255
Meningococcus 1255
Pneumococcus 1256
Polio 1256
Rotavirus 1257
Smallpox 1257
Tetanus, Diphtheria, and Pertussis 1257
Typhoid Fever 1258
Varicella-Zoster Virus 1258
Yellow Fever 1259
SPECIAL POPULATIONS 1259
VACCINE REGULATION 1260
COMMON MISPERCEPTIONS ABOUT VACCINE SAFETY 1260
Disease Disappearance Before the Use of Vaccine 1261
Absence of Risk Related to Vaccine Use 1261
Vaccine "Hot Lots" 1261
Vaccine Failures 1261
Safety Profile 1262
Multiple Dosing 1262
Thimerosal 1262
OFFICE PRACTICE 1262

INTRODUCTION AND HISTORY

Vaccination can be defined as a deliberate attempt to induce protection against disease with the goal of inducing active immunity. The term *vaccination* was actually invented by Louis Pasteur in honor of the work done by Edward Jenner,[1] who first scientifically evaluated active immunization against smallpox using cowpox.

The earliest vaccinations in history took place long before Edward Jenner. Historical references indicate the Indian Buddhists of the seventh century drank snake venom to prevent reactions to the bites of venomous snakes. The history of vaccinations otherwise begins with smallpox. This dreaded disease was recognized as highly contagious and had a fatality rate exceeding 20%.[2] Although difficult to verify, the Chinese are credited with using dried pus as a form of vaccination against smallpox around 1000 BC.[3] This approach, called variolation, occurs when a healthy person is exposed to infected material from smallpox sufferers to provoke mild disease and stimulate immune protection. Cotton nasal plugs coated with powdered scabs were inserted into the noses of healthy individuals, and powdered scabs were also blown into the nose.[4] A similar description of variolation dating back to 1000 BC can be found in east Indian literature as well,[5] with records indicating the use of dried pus from smallpox pustules introduced into the skin.

In time, the use of variolation spread to other parts of the world, and in fact was adopted in Edward Jenner's homeland of England. Variolation was promulgated by Lady Mary Wortley Montagu, who had observed the practice in her travels to Istanbul.[6] She introduced the practice to England in 1721. While variolation was successful in preventing smallpox, 2% to 3% of patients died from smallpox as a result of the variolation itself.[7] Despite this, the success of variolation moved across the Atlantic into the Americas. George Washington is recognized as requiring variolation for recruits to the Continental Army.[8]

The use of cowpox as a vaccine against smallpox in England did not actually begin with Edward Jenner, but in fact originated with Benjamin Jesty, a cattle breeder from Dorcette County. He made himself immune through cowpox exposure and vaccinated his wife and two children with cowpox material.[9] The resulting immunity appeared to last 15 years or more by his accounts.

The occurrence of cowpox among cattle was actually relatively limited, and local wisdom regarding cowpox and its protective abilities against smallpox were not well known or widely appreciated. It was Edward Jenner who made the first scientific attempt to demonstrate that one could pass cowpox from person to person and that cowpox inoculation actually protected against smallpox. In 1796, he demonstrated that one could gain immunity through inoculation.[10] While he is widely credited for discovering the immunizing properties of cowpox, late in life Jenner acknowledged Jesty's work. It was at that time Jenner also recognized that cowpox inoculation did not convey lifelong immunity to smallpox. He demonstrated this lack of durability in 1810.

In 1836, Edward Ballard was credited with attenuating cowpox, resulting in a more predictable vaccine. In the 1850s, the Germans demonstrated the ability to sterilize calf lymph and decrease infections associated with cowpox administration.

It is said that Edward Jenner invented vaccination and Louis Pasteur invented vaccines. In the 1880s, Louis Pasteur first demonstrated the use of attenuation (rendering a disease-causing agent less virulent) instead of substitution (using a related agent for protection against disease caused by another) with vaccination against cholera in chickens using attenuated virus.[11] He similarly demonstrated this for anthrax and rabies. In addition to substitution and attenuation, work was done with inactivated germs as well. In 1886, Salmon and Smith demonstrated the use of killed hog cholera to prevent cholera infection.[12]

The end of the 19th century was marked by the rapid development of our understanding of immunity. Ilya Mechnikov published works regarding phagocytes, which won him the Nobel Prize in Physiology and Medicine in 1908. Paul Ehrlich demonstrated the receptor theory of immunity and characterized active versus passive immunity, and was a co-winner of the 1908 Nobel Prize along with Mechnikov. Meanwhile, Pfeiffer and Kolle in Germany as well as Wright in England developed a vaccine from killed typhoid bacteria.[13] Waldemar Haffkine developed a vaccine made from killed plague bacteria,[14] and Wilhelm Kolle developed a killed cholera vaccine.[15]

The development of routine vaccinations is often heralded as one of the most important public health accomplishments of the 20th century. The early 20th century was marked by work with toxin and antitoxin related to diphtheria as well as the chemical inactivation of toxins to form toxoids. These toxoids were demonstrated to generate immunity in 1923 against diphtheria and in 1928 against tetanus. The bacille Calmette-Guérin bacteria was developed in 1927 as a live vaccine from substitution similar to Jenner's work with cowpox,[16] and Madsen reported the use of a pertussis vaccine in 1933.[17]

The year 1949 marks the beginning of the golden age of vaccine development with the introduction of the ability to propagate virus in cell cultures. In 1955, Jonas Salk developed an inactivated polio vaccine that was effective against polio,[18] and within the next decade, Albert Sabin developed a live, attenuated polio vaccine.[19] These two vaccines were credited with the widespread control of polio and eventually led to our current status with the imminent eradication of polio. Many other live virus vaccines followed the development of the Sabin polio vaccine, including measles in the 1950s, mumps in 1967, rubella in 1970, varicella in 1980s, rotavirus in the 1990s, and human papillomavirus (HPV) in the 2000s.

The 1990s heralded new technologies that led to advances in vaccine design, and many vaccine design technologies matured, including reassortment (the combining of viruses), reverse genetics, and the development of cold adaptation. Examples of products of these technologies include novel live intranasal flu vaccines and live rotavirus vaccines. Other technologies have also been successfully deployed in the last decades, including protein conjugation of polysaccharide antigens and harnessing recombinant strains of yeast to make protein vaccines such as hepatitis B virus (HBV) and HPV vaccines.

The threat of bioterrorism, and specifically the use of anthrax in October of 2001 in the United States, demonstrated that elimination or control of disease may be an impossible goal in modern times, as any viral or bacterial disease might be engineered and used as a bioweapon. Proper therapies beyond prevention by vaccination might only evolve when dose-response models are studied and understood. To this end, it is critical that exposure metrics are used to determine median lethal dose (LD_{50}) exposures as well as those of subclinical significance.

Of note, centuries of vaccine development have also been marked by concerns with public reactions to vaccinations and concerns with safety. Jenner's vaccination with cowpox and the recognition of its relative safety compared to variolation led to variolation being outlawed in England by 1950. Doctor Louis Pasteur is well recognized as a leader in the field of vaccination, but in fact there was a vociferous outcry over his use of a vaccine against rabies in a 5-year-old human victim of a dog bite. The Mulkowal disaster in 1902, resulting in 19 deaths from a contaminated plague vaccine, marred the development of vaccines and indeed temporarily derailed it.[20] These historical notes with regard to public outcry resonate with regard to acceptance of and concern with vaccines even today.

The remarkable effect of vaccinations is recognized now at the beginning of the 21st century. Smallpox has been eradicated, and the incidence of pertussis has been dramatically reduced by 96.3% annually, from approximately 147,000 cases prior to the introduction of pertussis vaccine. Similar reductions in disease incidence, in some instances from 97.9% to nearly 100%, have been seen for tetanus, diphtheria, polio, measles, mumps, rubella, and congenital rubella syndrome. As a result, the annual mortality suffered from vaccine-preventable diseases has been dramatically reduced as well. The World Health Organization (WHO) estimated that vaccines prevented the deaths of 2 million children globally in 2003, yet at least 2.5 million deaths among children less than 5 years of age resulted from diseases for which vaccines are available but not used.[21] A WHO Global Immunization and Vision Strategy has been created to serve as a template for national vaccination strategies, with the ultimate goal of extending vaccination to all eligible persons.[22] The introduction of new vaccines and vaccine technologies is a key component of the WHO's vision.

This chapter reviews mechanisms of vaccine response as well as vaccine technology and vaccines of the future. The use of routine vaccines in preventive care and a brief description of the use of vaccines in special populations are also discussed. The development of vaccine regulations, pharmaceutical vigilance, and common misperceptions regarding the use of vaccines are addressed, along with a description of the tools and techniques of modern vaccine delivery in the practice setting.

MECHANISMS OF VACCINE RESPONSE

Pharmacologic studies of the immune response to biologics such as vaccines offer evidence-based recommendations for advances in vaccinology. Vaccination is the most effective tool known to date for disease prevention caused by infectious agents. Effective vaccination against human diseases depends on the vaccine's capacity to stimulate protective immune responses to pathogens and to produce neutralizing antibodies and/or cellular immunity. In humoral immunity, B lymphocytes secrete antibodies responsible for specific recognition and neutralization of pathogen-derived antigens. Many viruses and bacteria stimulate strong B cell responses, and virus-specific antibodies (e.g., immunoglobulin M) can be induced in the absence of T helper (Th) cells.[23,24] Cellular immunity is mediated by T lymphocytes that are instrumental in protection against infectious diseases and often determine recovery from infections. T lymphocytes express cell surface T-cell antigen receptors (TCRs) that specifically recognize human leukocyte antigen (HLA) molecules presenting naturally processed pathogen-derived peptides, 9 to 30 amino acids in length, on the surface of antigen-presenting cells (APCs) (Fig. 91-1).[25] The HLA genes are classified into the class I (A, B, and C) and class II (DR, DQ, and DP) genes, and genes within the class II cluster (TAP, DM, and others). The polymorphic residues of these HLA molecules contribute to determining the specificity of peptide binding and to determining the HLA-peptide structure recognized by TCRs. Both CD4 and CD8 T-cell surface molecules bind to nonpolymorphic regions of HLA molecules on APCs at the time of antigen recognition and are called co-receptors. $CD8^+$ cytotoxic T lymphocytes (CTLs) generally recognize class I HLA-presented peptides processed from endogenous proteins in the cytosol, while class II HLA molecules bind peptides on the surface of the APCs and present them for immune recognition to $CD4^+$ T lymphocytes.[26,27] The activation of TCRs on the surface of naive $CD4^+$ T cells requires the presence of additional cell surface co-stimulatory molecules, such as CD28, that interact with B7.1 and B7.2 expressed on the APCs.[28] The activation of $CD4^+$ T cells is further facilitated by autosecretion of interleukin (IL)–2 by $CD4^+$ T lymphocytes.[28] Two main T helper subsets have been recognized: type 1 helper (Th1) T cells producing cytokines favoring cell-mediated immunity (interferon-γ, IL-2, and tumor necrosis factor-α), and type 2 helper (Th2) T cells producing cytokines necessary for humoral immune responses (IL-4, IL-5, IL-6, IL-10, and IL-13).[29,30] As shown in Figure 91-1, depending on the nature of the cytokine milieu of the host cells, the $CD4^+$ T cell may differentiate into a Th1 or a Th2 type cell.[31]

B and T lymphocytes are known to be the main mediators of adaptive immunity; however, their function is under the control of dendritic cells that are also important in the initiation and modulation of the immune response. Dendritic cells are efficient stimulators of B and T lymphocytes and play a role in antigen processing and presentation.[32] Both $CD4^+$ and $CD8^+$ T cells are activated by infection or vaccination, and cytokine production by these two T-cell subsets is essential for the development and regulation of cellular and humoral immunity.[33-36] Alterations in cytokine levels during vaccination can have dramatic effects on vaccine efficacy.[37-39]

Progress has been achieved in understanding the mechanisms of both innate (natural) and adaptive (specific) immune responses to foreign antigens. In this regard, Toll-like receptors (TLRs) represent a critical bridge between innate and adaptive immunity.[40-44] For example, members of poxvirus, herpesvirus, retrovirus, and paramyxovirus families have the ability to activate T cells through TLRs to trigger

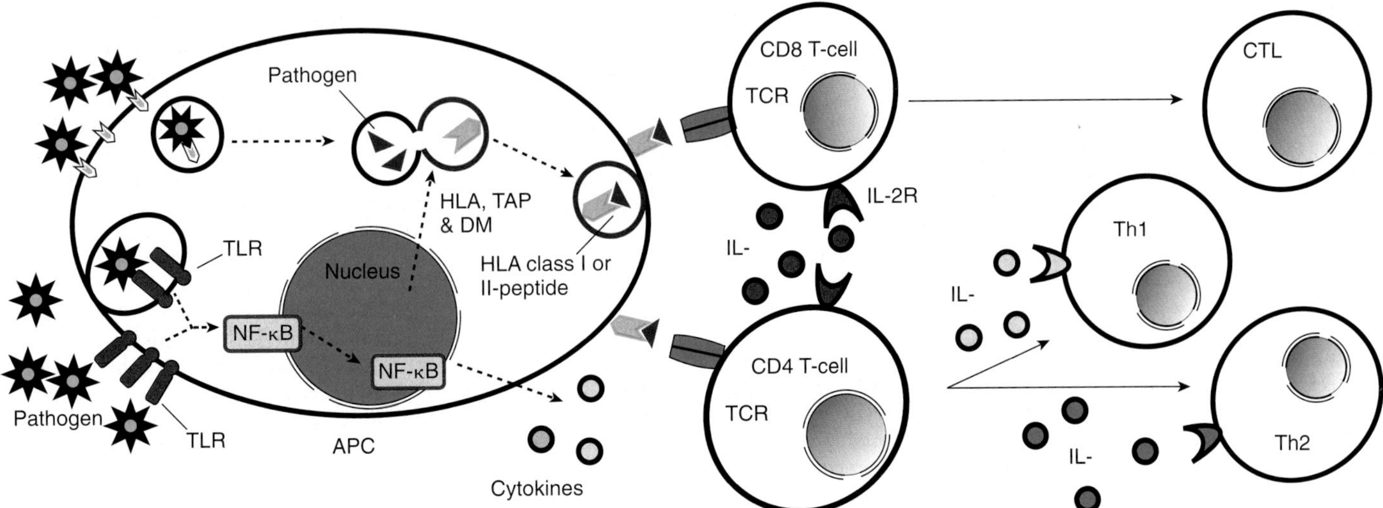

FIGURE 91-1 • Toll-like receptors (TLRs) recognize pathogenic products during infection or vaccination and initiate signaling pathways leading to the increased expression of immune genes. Pathogens are internalized by antigen-presenting cells (APCs) through receptor-mediated cytosolic and endocytic pathways. Transporter in antigen processing (TAP) molecules transport fragments of foreign proteins (peptides) into endoplasmic reticulum, and the HLA-DM molecules assist with loading of peptides on the human leukocyte antigen (HLA) class II molecules to form HLA-peptide complexes, which are then exported to the cell surface. The HLA class II peptide complexes are recognized by circulating $CD4^+$ T cells through a T-cell receptor (TCR) expressed on the cell surface, whereas $CD8^+$ T cells recognize antigen in association with the HLA class I peptide complexes and function as cytotoxic T cells (CTLs). The HLA peptide complex–TCR interaction activates the $CD4^+$ T cell to secrete interleukin (IL)–2, which promotes its growth and differentiation. The activated $CD4^+$ T cell may differentiate into a T helper type 1 (Th1)–like cell in the presence of IL-12 or a T helper type 2 (Th2)–like cell in the presence of IL-4. Both $CD4^+$ and $CD8^+$ T cells are activated by infection and produce cytokines that are essential for the development and regulation of cellular and humoral immune responses.

antiviral innate immune responses.[40,43,45,46] To date, 10 human TLRs have been identified.[46] In fact, each member of the TLR family recognizes a distinct pathogen-associated molecular pattern.[46] TLRs use several intracellular adaptor and signaling molecules, such as MyD88, TIRAP/MAL, TRIF, and TICAM-1, to induce signaling and cellular activation via up-regulation of HLA class II molecules, signaling molecules (such as nuclear factor-κB), and co-stimulatory molecules (CD80 and CD86) to induce expression of cytokines and their receptors.[44,46-51] This TLR-mediated signaling cascade leads to T-cell activation and differentiation.[42,44] It is now established that TLRs induce dendritic cell maturation required for activation and differentiation of Th cells, which can then provide help to B cells for the generation of specific antibody responses to microbial antigens.[52] By this mechanism, the generation of T-cell–dependent antigen-specific antibody responses requires activation of TLRs in B cells.[52]

Thus, the genes that appear to be particularly prominent in shaping human immune responses to vaccines include the HLA genes, cytokines and their receptor genes, TLR genes and their associated intracellular signaling molecules, and other immune response genes. Understanding the genetic factors that influence variations in vaccine immune response will provide further insight into the factors that influence both cellular and humoral immunity to infectious agents, and inform future vaccine development.

VACCINE TECHNOLOGY

Adjuvants

Adjuvants act to improve the immune response against specific antigens, and have been an important technology for vaccine development.[53,54] While not having any specific antigenic effect by itself, an adjuvant may stimulate the immune system, increasing the host response to vaccine antigens. The widely used licensed vaccine adjuvants, such as aluminum salts (hydroxide or phosphate), have been shown to be effective in promoting a Th2-type humoral immune response to some pathogens (*Bordetella pertussis*, HBV, and others).[55-57] However, aluminum salts are not particularly helpful in applications where inducing a Th1-type cellular immune response is required for protection against a disease.[54] Therefore, many compounds (QS21, MF59), chemicals (detergents), biochemicals, lipids (AS04, MALP-2), and proteins (hepatitis B surface antigen [HBsAg]/AS04, lipopolysaccharide, bacterial toxins, cytokines) with potential immunologic activity have been studied as potential adjuvants.[58-63]

Virosomes

A promising adjuvant and delivery system for prophylactic and therapeutic vaccines are virosomes. Virosomes are lipidic virus-like particles engineered to bear in their membrane specific viral proteins. For example, with influenza vaccines the influenza virus spike protein hemagglutinin is inserted, but the virosome lacks the genetic material of the native influenza virus.[64] Importantly, virosomes retain the antigenic profile as well as the cell binding and membrane fusion properties of their viral origin and are appropriate carriers for the delivery of encapsulated materials (recombinant proteins, synthetic peptides, lipophilic adjuvants) into the cytosol of target cells.[64-67] Influenza virosomes can also be administered by different routes (muscular, nasal, or dermal) and were found to be effective in inducing both humoral and cellular immune responses, including CTL activity.[65,66,68] Early clinical studies in humans have shown that virosomal influenza vaccines induce significant hemagglutination-inhibition antibody titers and also prime cell-mediated immune responses.[65,69-71]

Cell-Based Vaccines

Limitations of conventional egg-based production of vaccines and enhancements in reverse genetics have led to strategies for cell culture–based protein vaccine production.[72,73] Instead of fertilized chicken eggs, cell-based vaccine manufacture employs laboratory-adapted mammalian cell lines that are capable of hosting a replicating virus (influenza, polio).[74,75] For example, a virus is injected into mammalian kidney cells, the cells' external walls are disrupted, and the virus is then harvested, purified, and inactivated, allowing a vaccine that can be manufactured in a matter of days to weeks. The Madin-Darby Canine Kidney epithelial cell–based assay has also been used as a tool for determination of temperature-sensitive and cold-adapted phenotypes associated with live, attenuated influenza viruses.[76] Influenza hemagglutinin, neuraminidase, matrix, and nucleoproteins have been identified as potential targets for the development of cell-based protein vaccines.[74] These cell-based influenza vaccines may offer the potential to develop an effective avian influenza virus (H5N1 and H7N7 subtypes) pandemic vaccine.[77]

Universal Vaccines

Influenza is a recurrent global threat that affects millions of people in the world annually. Current vaccines must be administered every year to protect against infection as changes in circulating virus, viral drift, and potentially shift may alter vaccine and circulating strain match, effectively limiting effective vaccination. Therefore, it would be ideal to develop a universal vaccine candidate that could protect against A and B strains of influenza but, more significantly, one that would not require the yearly changes to vaccine formulation now necessary. The most promising universal vaccine approaches are based on developing protective antibodies specific for the relatively conserved ecto-domain of matrix protein 2 (M2), the inter-subunit region of hemagglutinin glycoprotein of influenza A and B viruses,[78] and highly conserved regions of the nucleoprotein. Various studies have been conducted to investigate the possibility of designing more cross-protective vaccines for use during interpandemic and pandemic years. Neirynck et al. designed a universal influenza A vaccine based on the conserved extracellular portion of the M2 protein, which is nearly invariant in all influenza A strains, fused to the HBV core (HBc) protein.[79] Intraperitoneal or intranasal administration of M2HBc vaccine to mice provided 90% to 100% protection against a lethal influenza virus challenge.[79] These data suggest that the M2 extracellular domain exposed on HBc may induce a cross-reactive response in the vaccinated host.

Increasing effort has been made to develop a universal vaccine for serogroup B meningococcus, which causes severe meningitis and sepsis. Conventional approaches have not been effective in preventing these infections.[80] A recent study in mice has demonstrated that a vaccine, developed using novel antigens identified by reverse vaccinology, covers 78% of a panel of 85 meningococcal strains using aluminum hydroxide as adjuvant.[80] Thus universal protein-based vaccines potentially can be developed against a variety of pathogens, such as pneumococcus, *Staphylococcus*, group A *Streptococcus*, and other microorganisms.

VACCINES OF THE FUTURE

DNA Vaccines

DNA vaccines or DNA-based immunization represents a novel means of expressing antigens in vivo for the generation of antibody and cell-mediated immune responses capable of protecting the host against infections.[81,82] To be useful, DNA immunization must elicit cellular and humoral immunity in a population with a heterogeneous genetic background. Free (naked) DNA vaccines consist of a bacterial DNA plasmid carrying a protein-coding gene of interest that transfects cells in vivo and expresses an antigen, resulting in an immune response. The plasmid is grown in *Escherichia coli*, purified, dissolved in saline, and then injected into the host. The DNA vaccine is taken up by host cells, transferred to the nucleus, translated into messenger RNA, and transcribed into protein antigen. This endogenously created antigen is then processed primarily through the HLA class I–restricted CTL system.

In addition to the practical advantages of construction, purification, and stability, DNA-mediated vaccination has several other potential advantages compared to conventional vaccination in terms of the following: (i) long-term expression of antigens in their native form, improving processing, presentation, and recognition in the host immune system; (ii) the ability to combine vaccines; and (iii) the possibility of reducing the number of doses because of prolonged antigen expression. In addition, vaccine "cocktails" containing DNA encoding multiple antigens, as well as immune response–enhancing lymphokine genes such as granulocyte-macrophage colony-stimulating factor (GM-CSF) or IL-12 and co-stimulatory molecules such as B7.1 and B7.2,[83] could theoretically be developed.

Several routes of administration have been tested, but direct intramuscular (IM) injection leading to transfection of muscle cells results in the highest levels of protein expression.[84,85] Administration of toxic agents intended to cause muscle necrosis and repair (such as repeated IM saline injections) prior to injection of DNA has been used to increase expression, resulting in an earlier antibody response. The magnitude of B- and T-cell responses generated after IM injection is equal to or greater than that observed after other routes of injection. Another approach is ballistic transfection of epidermal cells with plasmid DNA–coated gold microparticles. Skin cells can take up and express free foreign DNA and induce cellular and humoral immune responses against the encoded protein.[86] The method of DNA inoculation and the form of the DNA-expressed antigen (cell-associated vs. secreted) determine whether Th cells will be primarily of the Th1 or Th2 phenotype. For IM immunization with plasmid DNA, bone marrow–derived APCs were found to be responsible for the induction of $CD8^+$ CTL responses to the expressed antigen,[87] whereas "gene gun"–mediated epidermal immunization appears to favor Th2 responses by keratinocytes and antigen-bearing epidermal Langerhans cells.[85]

The efficacy of DNA immunization has been demonstrated in several different viral, bacterial, parasitic, and cancer models.[88,89] For example, plasmid constructs encoding carcinoembryonic antigen or artificial tumor antigens have been shown to elicit alloimmune and protective immune responses to tumors expressing the antigen gene.[90] DNA vaccines were shown to be effective in inducing immune responses and/or protection in selected animal models against human immunodeficiency virus (HIV), HBV, influenza virus, bovine herpesvirus, rabies virus, herpes simplex virus, *Leishmania*, malaria, and *Mycobacterium tuberculosis* antigens.[91] From these preclinical studies, DNA-based vaccination appears to induce diverse immune responses and formation of long-lasting specific antibody, Th cell responses of the Th1 phenotype, and CTLs. A study by Deck et al.[92] using the influenza A virus model demonstrated that influenza hemagglutinin DNA vaccine protected animals against lethal doses of the virus. A novel DNA vaccine against HBV was administered intraepidermally by particle-mediated epidermal delivery to human subjects who demonstrated absent or nonsustainable responses to conventional HBV vaccination. This DNA vaccine elicited antibody responses in 75% of subjects after a licensed subunit vaccine failed to induce a lasting response after three or more vaccinations.[93] Thus, the use of DNA vaccines may become an effective means of immunization against infectious diseases and may be a useful approach for vaccine development in the future. Multiple clinical trials of candidate DNA vaccines are in progress.

Anticancer Vaccines

Progress has been achieved in understanding the etiology of certain cancers and issues of tumor immunogenicity. Innovative vaccine strategies are currently being developed and studied for tumor vaccine design, which can be divided into two categories: (i) methods that use the tumor cells as antigens, and (ii) antigen-specific vaccine strategies that are designed to generate immune responses against specific gene products.

Whole-cell tumor experimental vaccines have been used to treat patients with renal cell carcinoma and melanoma.[94,95] Vaccines consisted of either irradiated autologous tumor cells, cell lysates, or irradiated virus-infected tumor cells co-injected with bacterial adjuvants that can be employed as a tool to augment antitumor responsiveness. The recent identification of defined tumor-specific T-cell epitopes renewed interest in the possibility of inducing anticancer immunity. While tumor cells are generally poorly immunogenic, T cells, including CTLs, have been recognized as a critical component of the immune response to tumors.[96,97] Therefore, inducing strong antigen-specific CTL responses is the goal of many current cancer vaccine strategies. Limitations exist in the capacity of CTL-mediated immunity to eliminate established tumors, such as the existence of the major histocompatibility complex (MHC) class I–negative tumor cells, the problem of access of CTLs to large malignant targets and cancer cell immune evasion strategies,[98] and poorly differentiated tumors in which an antigenic target is not readily identifiable.

For the development of cancer vaccines, the tumor-associated antigens (TAAs) recognized by CTLs must be identified.[99] CTLs recognize peptides derived from proteins synthesized within the tumor target cell. Peptide antigens have been defined for several human tumors. TAAs include differentiation antigens (carcinoembryonic antigen, prostate-specific antigen), oncogene-encoded antigens (p53, ras), structural or nonstructural proteins from oncogenic viruses (retrovirus, HPV), polymorphic epithelial mucins, and abnormal tumor-specific antigens that are mutated or posttranslationally modified.[97,100] The human MAGE genes encode proteins that can be recognized by autologous CTLs and, therefore, represent candidate targets for immunotherapy. Proteins of the MAGE family are not expressed in normal tissues with the exception of testis and placenta and are possibly developmental antigens reexpressed during the process of tumorigenesis. The human MAGE1 antigen is one of the best characterized tumor antigens. It contains at least two antigenic epitopes and is expressed in 50% of melanomas, representing a potential vaccine target.[101] Most of these altered proteins are intracellular, so that recognition by monoclonal antibodies is not likely to be of immunotherapeutic value. After a tumor antigen is identified, strong CTL-associated immunity is necessary for tumor eradication.

The strategy of peptide-based vaccines is theoretically attractive because it provides access for exogenously administered synthetic peptide antigens into the endogenous MHC class I presentation pathway.[102,103] Also, individual peptides will only have general therapeutic value if they can be efficiently presented by common HLA alleles such as HLA-A2 in populations of varying HLA allelic distributions. The advantage of the use of peptides as immunogens is that the T-cell–mediated immune response can be directed against preselected HLA-binding T-cell epitopes derived from TAAs, including functional oncogenes required by the tumor for growth.

In several experimental models, peptide antigen administered in vivo, with or without adjuvant, can stimulate antigen-specific CTL-mediated immunity. TAAs expressed by tumor cells could produce T-cell–based vaccines using a live vector, such as recombinant vaccinia virus or adenoviruses encoding multiple CTL epitopes.[104] Immunization with heat shock proteins (hsps) has been shown to prime effective CTL-mediated antitumor immunity.[105] Li[106] has reviewed the immunologic principles and the practical vaccination strategy of hsps (gp96/grp94 and hsp70) in antigen presentation by MHC class I molecules through professional APCs, and the application of this idea for vaccination against cancer. Targeting the phagocytic pathway can be an alternative approach because phagocytic cells may play an important role in the induction of CTL-mediated immunity and in the natural immune response to tumors.[107]

Genetic modification of tumor cells can produce vaccines with more defined biologic effects. This strategy includes the introduction of autologous MHC class I and class II genes into tumor cells and introduction of the co-stimulatory B7 gene to make tumor cells more like APCs (tumor-as-APC approach). Tumor cells can also potentially be transfected with cytokines (GM-CSF, IL-4, and IL-12), which enhance host APC function and make tumor vaccines more immunogenic by making the tumor cells more immunologically "presentable."[108-111] Analyses of immunoregulatory T cells and genetically modified tumor vaccines demonstrate that $CD4^+$ T cells are also necessary for generating efficient antitumor responses, as are $CD8^+$ cells.[96,99,100] Linkages between class I and class II HLA-restricted epitopes produce the most efficient interaction between $CD4^+$ and $CD8^+$ T cells, and it is likely that effective cancer vaccines will use antigens containing both MHC class I and class II epitopes.[112] Vaccines engineered on a molecular basis for the prevention and treatment of cancer now appear to be within our grasp.

CURRENTLY LICENSED VACCINES

Anthrax

Background. Anthrax is caused by a bacterium, *Bacillus anthracis*. Historically, anthrax has been a zoonotic disease largely affecting domestic mammals and causing cutaneous, gastrointestinal, and inhalational disease in humans exposed to spores of infected animals or animal products. More recent emphasis has been placed on anthrax as a biologic weapon. Weaponized anthrax would largely cause inhalational disease, for which the mortality is 86% to 89% among unimmunized persons; however, exposure intensity and duration for LD_{50} are not known.[113-115]

Vaccine Administration. Anthrax Vaccine Adsorbed (AVA; BioPort) is the only vaccine licensed in the United States against anthrax. The vaccine is created from a cell-free filtrate of a toxigenic, nonencapsulated strain of *B. anthracis*. The filtrate contains a mixture of cellular proteins adsorbed to an aluminum hydroxide adjuvant. The three anthrax toxoids (lethal factor, edema factor, and protective antigen) are contained in each 0.5-ml subcutaneous dose of the vaccine, though the protective antigen is the primary immunogen.[116]

Indications. Immunization is recommended for persons at high risk of exposure to aerosolized *B. anthracis* spores, including persons working with large quantities of *B. anthracis* cultures, veterinarians working in areas of high disease incidence, and persons working in the processing of animal wool or hide for whom precautions are not considered to prevent occupational exposure. Vaccination is also indicated for military personnel who may be at higher risk of exposure to agents of biologic warfare in high-threat areas. The currently recommended vaccination schedule involves subcutaneous injections at 0, 2, and 4 weeks followed by three booster injections at 6, 12, and 18 months and subsequent annual booster injections.[113]

Immunogenicity and Efficacy. A controlled human trial demonstrated 95% seroconversion after 3 injections.[117] It is unclear if seroconversion correlates with clinical protection, though animal studies suggest efficacy. A trial of alum-precipitated vaccine, a precursor to AVA vaccine, in mill workers showed 93% efficacy against cutaneous and inhalation anthrax.[113]

Adverse Effects and Contraindications. Vaccine receipt is commonly associated with local injection site reactions, including erythema, swelling, and pain, though they occur at the same frequency and intensity as with other vaccines. Systemic reactions including fevers, malaise, and myalgias are rare and also occur at the same frequency and intensity as observed with the receipt of other vaccines.[113] The safety data regarding this vaccine have been evaluated by the Institute of Medicine (IOM), which found "no evidence that life-threatening or permanently disabling immediate-onset adverse events occur at higher rates in individuals who have received AVA than in the general population."[118] Vaccination is contraindicated in persons who have a prior history of anthrax infection or persons who have had anaphylactic reaction to a previous dose of anthrax vaccine or vaccine component.[113]

Haemophilus influenzae Type b

Background. *Haemophilus influenzae* is a bacterium that causes infections predominantly in children, including meningitis, epiglottitis, and pneumonia. Of the six serotypes (a-f) of *H. influenzae*, type b (Hib) is associated with 95% of cases of invasive disease.[119] Prior to routine vaccination in the United States, Hib was the most common cause of invasive bacterial disease in children. Hib meningitis is fatal in 2% to 5% of cases, and long-term neurologic sequelae develop in 20% to 30% of cases. Since the incorporation of Hib vaccination in the routine childhood vaccination schedule, the incidence of invasive Hib infection has decreased by over 95%.[119-121]

Vaccine Administration. The vaccine is created by conjugating the polyribosylribitol phosphate (PRP) capsule of Hib to a T-cell–stimulating antigen, though the four licensed conjugate vaccines use different proteins for conjugation. HbOC (HibTiter; Lederle) uses PRP conjugated to mutant diphtheria protein CRM_{197}, PRP-OMP (PedvaxHib; Merck) uses PRP conjugated to the outer membrane protein complex of *Neisseria meningiditis*, PRP-D (ProHIBit; Connaught) uses PRP conjugated to diphtheria toxoid, and PRP-T (Act-HIB; Aventis Pasteur) uses PRP conjugated to tetanus toxoid. The vaccines are administered as 0.5-ml IM injections. Two combination Hib vaccines

Practice: Emerging Therapeutics

TABLE 91-1 CDC RECOMMENDED CHILDHOOD IMMUNIZATION SCHEDULE

United States Centers for Disease Control and Prevention

Recommended Childhood Immunization Schedule

Vaccine ▼ Age ▶	Birth	1 month	2 months	4 months	6 months	12 months	15 months	18 months	19–23 months	2–3 years	4–6 years
Hepatitis B	HepB	HepB				HepB					
Rotavirus			Rota	Rota	Rota						
Diphtheria, Tetanus, Pertussis			DTaP	DTaP	DTaP		DTaP				DTaP
Haemophilus influenzae type b			Hib	Hib	Hib	Hib					
Pneumococcal			PCV	PCV	PCV	PCV				PPV	
Inactivated Poliovirus			IPV	IPV		IPV					IPV
Influenza								Influenza (Yearly)			
Measles, Mumps, Rubella						MMR					MMR
Varicella						Varicella					Varicella
Hepatitis A								HepA (2 doses)		HepA Series	
Meningococcal										MCV4	

Range of recommended ages

Certain high-risk groups

are available: Hib conjugate vaccine with HBV vaccine (Comvax; Merck) and Hib conjugate vaccine with diphtheria, tetanus, and acellular pertussis vaccine (TriHIBit; Aventis Pasteur).[121]

Indications. Hib vaccination is part of the routine childhood immunization schedule, with administration of the four-dose regimen recommended at 2, 4, 6, and 12 to 15 months of age (Table 91-1). Persons over 5 years of age not previously vaccinated should receive vaccination if they are asplenic or are immunosuppressed, including those with HIV, sickle cell disease, and complement deficiencies.[122]

Immunogenicity and Efficacy. The serologic response to the different vaccines varies between vaccines and between populations studied, although 94% to 99% of vaccine recipients develop protective antibody levels. Clinical trials have demonstrated an efficacy of 87% to 100% in preventing invasive Hib infection.[119,122]

Adverse Effects and Contraindications. The vaccines are usually well tolerated, though some recipients have developed low-grade fever and transient injection site reactions. No serious adverse events have been associated with vaccine administration. The vaccines are contraindicated in those with prior anaphylactic responses to the vaccine or vaccine components.[122]

Hepatitis A

Background. Hepatitis A virus (HAV) causes acute hepatitis infections with significant morbidity worldwide. Though the infection rarely manifests as fulminant liver failure, mortality is seen in infections of persons with underlying conditions, including chronic liver disease.[123] Community outbreaks from food or water sources are more common in areas of low socioeconomic status and poor sanitation. Routine vaccination of at-risk individuals and children living in areas of high HAV incidence has decreased the disease burden in the United States by 76%.[124]

Vaccine Administration. HAV vaccine is prepared by formalin inactivation of whole virus. Havrix (GlaxoSmithKline) and Vaqta (Merck) are commercially available HAV vaccines and Twinrix (GlaxoSmithKline) is a combination of Havrix and Engerix-B, a recombinant HBV vaccine. Havrix is delivered as an IM injection of 720 EL. U. in 0.5 ml in children and 1440 EL. U. in 1.0 ml in adults, with a booster of the same dose 6 to 12 months later. Vaqta is delivered through an IM injection of 25 U in 0.5 ml in children and 50 U in 1.0 ml in adults, with a booster of the same dose after 6 to 18 months.[125]

Indications. Though initially recommended for children age 12 months or older living in areas of high incidence, HAV vaccination was incorporated into the routine childhood vaccine schedule in 2006[126] (see Table 91-1). HAV vaccination is recommended for adults traveling to areas of the world with high or intermediate HAV endemicity.[125] The initial dose of vaccine should be given at least 2 weeks prior to travel. Vaccination has also been recommended for people at higher risk of infection or at higher risk for morbidity and mortality with infection, including persons with occupational exposures, illegal drug users, men who have sex with men, and persons with chronic liver diseases or clotting-factor disorders[125] (Tables 91-2 and 91-3).

Immunogenicity and Efficacy. Protective antibody levels (>20 mIU/ml) were detected in 90% to 96% of adults and 96% of children following a single vaccine dose.[127,128] Protection in children and adults was found to be nearly 100% after administration of a booster 6 months following initial vaccination.[125] A study comparing Havrix and Vaqta in adults showed similar immunogenicity but fewer local side effects in those receiving Vaqta.[129]

Adverse Effects and Contraindications. HAV vaccines are well tolerated, and no serious adverse events have been reported.[130,131] The safety of HAV vaccines has not been established in pregnancy or in immunocompromised patients, but as it is an inactivated vaccine, the risk is thought to be low.[125] HAV vaccine should not be administered

TABLE 91-2 CDC RECOMMENDED ADOLESCENT IMMUNIZATION SCHEDULE, BY VACCINE AND AGE GROUP

United States Centers for Disease Control and Prevention
Recommended Adolescent Immunization Schedule

Vaccine ▼ / Age ▶	7–10 years	11–12 years	13–18 years
Diphtheria, Tetanus, Pertussis		Tdap	Tdap
Human Papillomavirus		HPV (3 doses)	HPV Series
Meningococcal	MCV4	MCV4	MCV4
Pneumococcal		PPV	
Influenza		Influenza (Yearly)	
Hepatitis A		HepA Series	
Hepatitis B		HepB Series	
Inactivated Poliovirus		IPV Series	
Measles, Mumps, Rubella		MMR Series	
Varicella		Varicella Series	

Range of recommended ages

Catch-up immunization

Certain high-risk groups

to those who have demonstrated a severe reaction to a prior dose of HAV vaccine or to a vaccine component.

Hepatitis B

Background. The preponderance of the morbidity and mortality associated with this viral infection is through chronic infection of the liver. An estimated 2 billion people worldwide have been infected by the virus, causing chronic infection in approximately 400 million people. Of these, 500,000 to 1 million people will die from complications of chronic infection, most commonly cirrhosis and hepatocellular carcinoma.[132,133] Infection is acquired through percutaneous or mucosal exposure to infected blood, semen, saliva, or other body fluids.[134]

Vaccine Administration. The HBV vaccine is created by expression of hepatitis B surface antigen (HBsAg) by yeast using recombinant DNA technology. Two licensed single-antigen vaccines are available in the United States, Recombivax HB (Merck) and Engerix-B (Glaxo SmithKline). Three combination vaccines are also available: Twinrix (GlaxoSmithKline) combines recombinant HBsAg vaccine with inactivated HAV vaccine; Comvax (Merck) contains recombinant HBsAg vaccine with conjugated Hib vaccine; and Pediarix (GlaxoSmithKline) contains recombinant HBsAg, inactivated poliovirus vaccine (IPV), and diphtheria and tetanus toxoids and acellular pertussis adsorbed (DTaP). In infants and young children (<10 years of age), 0.5 ml of 20-mcg/ml Engerix-B or 0.5 ml of 10-mcg/ml Recombivax should be used for each dose, in adolescents the dose is 1.0 ml of Engerix-B or 0.5 ml of Recombivax, and in adults the dose is 1.0 ml of Engerix-B or 1.0 ml of Recombivax.[134]

Indications. Immunization is now recommended for all infants as part of the routine childhood immunization schedule[126] (see Table 91-1). Vaccination is also recommended for persons at increased risk for infection or complications, including men who have sex with men, individuals with multiple sex partners, household contacts of hepatitis B patients, intravenous drug users, health care workers, patients on dialysis or receiving numerous blood products, and patients with chronic liver disease. Immunization is achieved by IM administration of three doses of the vaccine at 0, 1, and 6 months[134] (see Tables 91-2 and 91-3).

Immunogenicity and Efficacy. Successful seroconversion occurs in over 95% of healthy children and young adults receiving the three-dose vaccine regimen.[135] Immunologic response is poorer in smokers, obese patients, immunocompromised patients, cirrhotics, and patients with chronic kidney disease.[135-138] Lower rates of seroconversion are associated with vaccination later in life, with seroconversion rates of 86% in the fourth decade and 47% in the sixth decade.[135,139]

Adverse Effects and Contraindications. HBV vaccine is very safe. Anaphylactic reactions to HBV vaccine have been reported at an incidence of 1 per 1.1 million recipients.[140] Persons having such reactions or with known hypersensitivity to the yeast or vaccine components should not be given the vaccine.[134]

Human Papillomavirus

Background. Human papillomaviruses (HPV) are viruses that infect epithelial cells. Over 100 different HPV types exist, most of which cause benign warts but some of which cause squamous cell cancer. Cervical cancer is the second most common malignancy among women worldwide and is caused by HPV; 70% of these cases are caused by HPV types 16 and 18. In addition, HPV 6 and 11 are implicated in 80% of genital warts, which is the most common sexually transmitted disease.[141]

Vaccine Administration. Gardasil (Merck) is a quadrivalent vaccine licensed in 2006 for the prevention of cervical cancer and genital warts. The vaccine uses virus-like particles of HPV types 6, 11, 16, and 18. Virus-like particles are generated by using the L1 major capsid protein of each virus type, which self-assembles into a highly immunogenic structure that does not contain any viral DNA.[142] The virus-like particles are produced using recombinant *Saccharomyces cerevisiae*. Each 0.5-ml IM dose contains 20 mcg of HPV 6 L1 protein, 40 mcg of HPV 11 L1 protein, 40 mcg of HPV 16 L1 protein, and 20 mcg of HPV 18 L1 protein.

Indications. The three-dose regimen (0, 2, and 6 months) is recommended for routine vaccination of females ages 11 to 12. The vaccine

TABLE 91-3 CDC RECOMMENDED ADULT IMMUNIZATION SCHEDULE, BY VACCINE AND AGE GROUP

United States Centers for Disease Control and Prevention
Recommended Adult Immunization Schedule

Vaccine ▼ / Age ▶	19–49 years	50–64 years	≥65 years
Tetanus, Diphtheria, Pertussis (Td/Tdap)	1 dose Td booster every 10 yrs Substitute 1 dose of Tdap for Td	1 dose Td booster every 10 yrs Substitute 1 dose of Tdap for Td	1 dose Td booster every 10 yrs
Human Papillomavirus (HPV)	3 doses females (0, 2, 6 mos)		
Measles, Mumps, Rubella (MMR)	1 or 2 doses	1 dose	1 dose
Varicella	2 doses (0, 4–8 wks)	2 doses (0, 4–8 wks)	2 doses (0, 4–8 wks)
Influenza	1 dose annually	1 dose annually	1 dose annually
Pneumococcal (polysaccharide)	1–2 doses	1–2 doses	1 dose
Hepatitis A	2 doses (0, 6–12 mos or 0, 6–18 mos)	2 doses (0, 6–12 mos or 0, 6–18 mos)	2 doses (0, 6–12 mos or 0, 6–18 mos)
Hepatitis B	3 doses (0, 1–2, 4–6 mos)	3 doses (0, 1–2, 4–6 mos)	3 doses (0, 1–2, 4–6 mos)
Meningococcal	1 or more doses	1 or more doses	1 or more doses
Zoster		1 dose	1 dose

(Light bar) For all persons in this category who meet the age requirements and who lack evidence of immunity (e.g., lack documentation of vaccination or have no evidence of prior infection)

(Dark bar) Recommended if some other risk factor is present (e.g., on the basis of medical, occupational, lifestyle, or other indications)

can be given to females from age 9 years to 26 years (see Tables 91-2 and 91-3). The vaccine is recommended prior to the onset of sexual activity, but can benefit women who are sexually active.[143]

Immunogenicity and Efficacy. Thirty-six months after vaccination, protective antibodies are found for HPV 6 in 94% of recipients, for HPV 11 in 96%, for HPV 16 in 100%, and for HPV 18 in 76%.[144] The vaccine was found to be 95% effective in preventing cervical intraepithelial neoplasia and 95% effective in preventing genital warts 3 years after vaccination.[144] As the vaccine was recently licensed, long-term efficacy trial data are not available.

Adverse Effects and Contraindications. The vaccine has been well tolerated, with only mild local reactions.[144,145] There have been no serious adverse events encountered with the vaccine. The safety of the vaccine has not been assessed in pregnancy, and it is contraindicated in persons with anaphylactic response to prior vaccinations or to vaccine components.[146]

Influenza

Background. Influenza is a virus that is responsible for annual winter epidemics of viral pneumonia worldwide. The virus is spread through large droplet, fomites, and respiratory droplet transmission and causes 36,000 deaths annually in the United States, mostly in infants and the elderly. Influenza is categorized into types A, B, and C, with influenza A being subtyped based on the two surface antigens (hemagglutinin and neuraminidase, e.g., H1N2) expressed. Vaccines are effective but must be updated annually to reflect mutations in the surface antigens of the circulating viruses, called antigenic drift. Occasionally, changes in the circulating viruses are dramatic and result in the emergence of new subtypes (antigenic shift), causing pandemic infection and large-scale mortality worldwide. Two types of vaccines are currently licensed for prevention of annual epidemic influenza, an injectable inactivated vaccine and an intranasal live, attenuated vaccine.[147]

Vaccine Administration. Trivalent inactivated influenza vaccine (TIV) is composed of the inactivated subvirion hemagglutinin and neuraminidase of the two circulating influenza A viruses and the influenza B virus. Live, attenuated influenza vaccine (LAIV) is created from the incorporation of the circulating surface antigens to a cold-adapted influenza virus that replicates in the nares, but not at higher temperatures of the body. The virus is grown in eggs for the development of both vaccines. Each 0.5-ml IM dose of TIV contains 15 mcg of surface antigen of each subtype. TIV is commercially available as Fluzone (Aventis Pasteur), Fluvirin (Evans), and Fluarix (GlaxoSmithKline). LAIV (FluMist; MedImmune) is administered as a 0.5-ml intranasal spray, with administration divided between the two nares. LAIV must be stored at −15° C or colder, and can be thawed and refrigerated at 2° C to 8° C for up to 60 hours before use.[147]

Indications. Annual influenza vaccination is recommended for children ages 6 to 59 months; pregnant women; persons older than 50 years of age; persons with chronic cardiopulmonary disorders, persons with chronic disease of the blood or kidneys, diabetes, or immunosuppression (including HIV); persons at increased risk for aspiration or compromised ability to handle respiratory secretions; persons living in chronic care facilities; health care workers; and household contacts of persons at high risk of influenza-related complications (see Tables 91-1, 91-2 and 91-3). There are persons for whom TIV is preferred over LAIV (see Adverse Effects and Contraindications). Administration of two doses 1 month apart is recommended for the vaccination of previously unvaccinated children under 9 years of age.[147]

Immunogenicity and Efficacy. The immunogenicity of both vaccines is dependent on the age and medical condition of the recipient and how closely the vaccine matches the circulating influenza virus. TIV induced protective antibody levels in 89% of children ages 6 to 24 months.[148] The vaccine was 77% to 91% effective in preventing influenza infection in children ages 1 to 15 years, though the efficacy in children between 3 and 9 years was lower (56%).[149] TIV was 70% to 90% efficacious in preventing influenza infection in adults under age 65 when the vaccine was well matched, but only 52% effective when the vaccine was not well matched. The vaccine was 30% to 40% effective in preventing influenza infection in the elderly.[147] Two doses of LAIV were found to be 93% effective in preventing influenza infection in children when the vaccine was well matched and also 86% effective when the vaccine was not well matched.[150,151] One dose of LAIV was found to be 85% effective in preventing influenza infection in healthy adults.[152]

Adverse Effects and Contraindications. TIV is associated with injection site soreness, but is otherwise well tolerated. Although controversial, the 1976 swine influenza vaccine may have been associated with a higher risk of Guillain-Barré syndrome (GBS), but this has not been encountered since that time. LAIV is well tolerated, but is associated with self-limited low-grade fevers, nasal congestion, and sore throat. LAIV should not be administered to persons younger than 5 years or older than 50; immunocompromised persons; persons with chronic heart, lung, or kidney disease; persons with diabetes; children or adolescents taking aspirin; pregnant women; persons with a history of GBS; and persons with severe allergy to prior LAIV vaccinations, vaccine components, or eggs. TIV is contraindicated in persons with severe allergic reaction to prior vaccine administration or to vaccine components, including egg protein.[147]

Japanese Encephalitis Virus

Background. Japanese encephalitis (JE) is caused by a virus and is transmitted by *Culex* mosquitoes in Asia. Encephalitis is seen in only 0.1% to 5% of infections, but is fatal in 25% when present. The risk for infection in a traveler is increased with duration of stay, location of travel, season of travel, and activities.[153]

Vaccine Administration. The JE vaccine is made from formalin inactivation of the Nakayama-NIH strain of the JE virus grown in mouse brains. The vaccine is administered as a three-dose regimen of 1.0-ml IM injections on days 0, 7, and 30. A smaller dose of 0.5 ml should be used in children ages 1 to 3 years.[153]

Indications. The vaccine is recommended for persons traveling to or living in an area that is endemic for JE for over a month. Booster doses may be given 2 years after primary vaccination if the person remains at high risk.[153]

Immunogenicity and Efficacy. Protective antibodies are generated in nearly 100% of recipients of the three-dose regimen. The duration of protection conferred by the vaccine is not known. The vaccine was found to be 91% effective in preventing infection in children.[153,154]

Adverse Effects and Contraindications. Local reactions occur in 20% of recipients, and systemic side effects, including fever, headache, nausea, and vomiting, occur in 10% of vaccine recipients. Cases of hypersensitivity with urticaria and angioedema have been reported with the vaccine up to 2 weeks following vaccination. Vaccine recipients should be observed following vaccine administration and should remain in areas of ready access to medical care for 10 days following administration. Vaccination is contraindicated in persons with a history of severe allergic reaction to the vaccine or vaccine components, including mouse proteins and thimerosal.[153]

Measles, Mumps, and Rubella

Background. Measles, mumps, and rubella are viral diseases that were commonly acquired in childhood that have been nearly eliminated in developed countries due to successful vaccination programs. Measles infection is characterized by severe otitis media, bronchopneumonia, encephalitis, and death. Mortality in underdeveloped countries has been as high as 25%. Mumps infection is characterized by parotitis and fevers. The most serious complications are orchitis and meningitis, which can lead to sterility or deafness. Although rubella infections are usually subclinical or cause low-grade fever, rash, and arthralgias, congenital rubella syndrome can be severe. Congenital rubella syndrome has been associated with miscarriages, stillbirths, and numerous congenital anomalies, including auditory, ophthalmic, cardiac, and neurologic defects.[155]

Vaccine Administration. The vaccines for the three viruses are created from attenuated live viruses and are available separately, but are most commonly administered as a single combination vaccine (MMR). The attenuated measles vaccine is made from the Enders-Edmonston virus strain grown in chick embryo fibroblast cell culture; attenuated mumps vaccine is made from the Jeryl-Lynn strain grown in chick embryo cell culture, and attenuated rubella vaccine is prepared from virus strain RA 27/3 grown in human diploid cell culture. Monovalent measles vaccine (Attenuvax; Merck), mumps vaccine (Mumpsvax; Merck), and rubella vaccine (Meruvax; Merck) are available, as are bivalent measles-rubella vaccine (M-R-Vax; Merck) and rubella-mumps vaccine (Biovax II; Merck). However, the trivalent MMR II (Merck) has been most commonly used. In 2005, a tetravalent measles, mumps, rubella, and varicella vaccine was licensed (ProQuad; Merck), combining MMR II and Varivax (Merck), a single-antigen varicella vaccine.[156] These live vaccines must be refrigerated for storage and transport. They are supplied in lyophilized form and require reconstitution prior to administration. Although efficacy is high for all three vaccines with one injection, two doses given at least 4 weeks apart are recommended to ensure immunization of those who may not respond to a single dose. Administration involves subcutaneous injections of 0.5 ml of the combined vaccine or of each constituent vaccine.[156]

Indications. MMR vaccination is recommended as part of the childhood immunization schedule and is usually given at 12 to 15 months and repeated at 4 to 6 years (see Table 91-1). In addition, immunization is recommended for women who could become pregnant, college students, health care workers, and international travelers who were born after 1957 if they have not received previous vaccination and do not have laboratory evidence of immunity[155] (see Tables 91-2 and 91-3).

Immunogenicity and Efficacy. Protective antibodies were generated from a single measles vaccination in 95% of recipients, with greater than 99% having achieved seroconversion after a second dose.[155,157] Seropositivity following vaccination has been correlated with long-term clinical protection from disease.[155] Mumps vaccination resulted in seropositivity in 97% of recipients after one dose,[156] correlating with a similar long-term rate of clinical protection from disease.[155] A single dose of rubella vaccine generated a protective antibody response in over 95% of recipients,[158,159] and the protection is likely lifelong.[155,160]

Adverse Effects and Contraindications. The vaccines are usually well tolerated, and side effects are less often seen with revaccination. Fevers and local reactions have been associated with the vaccines, and transient arthralgias and arthritis have been associated with the rubella component. Transient rashes are seen in 5% of recipients of measles- or rubella-containing vaccines and occur 7 to 12 days following vaccination. Though rare, febrile seizures, thrombocytopenia, and anaphylaxis have also been associated with vaccination. The vaccines are contraindicated in pregnancy, persons who are severely immunocompromised, and persons with allergic reactions to a previous vaccine dose or component.[155]

Meningococcus

Background. *Neisseria meningitidis* causes meningitis in persons of all ages, but largely affects children and adolescents. Most cases are sporadic, though outbreaks in college dormitories have raised concern. The mortality of the disease is 10% to 14% even though *N. meningitidis* has largely remained sensitive to most antimicrobial agents. Serotypes A, B, C, Y, and W-135 are associated with invasive disease, with types B, C, and Y each causing approximately one third of cases in the United States. A polysaccharide vaccine has been available since the 1970s, and a conjugate vaccine was licensed for use in the

United States in 2005. Vaccine development thus far has not led to a vaccine that confers protection against serotype B in the United States.[161,162]

Vaccine Administration. The polysaccharide vaccine, Menomune (Aventis Pasteur), contains the bacterial capsular polysaccharide of *N. meningitidis* serotypes A, C, Y, and W-135. Each 0.5-ml IM or subcutaneous dose contains 50 mcg of each of the four capsular polysaccharides. The conjugate vaccine, Menactra (Aventis Pasteur), contains the same capsular polysaccharides but conjugates them with diphtheria toxoid. Each 0.5-ml IM or subcutaneous dose contains 4 mcg of each of the four vaccine conjugates.[161]

Indications. Conjugate meningococcal vaccine is recommended as part of the routine childhood vaccination schedule. A single dose should be administered to all children at 11 to 12 years of age (see Table 91-2). Vaccination is also recommended for college freshmen living in dormitories, persons with frequent occupational exposure to *N. meningitidis*, military recruits, persons traveling to or living in endemic areas, persons with complement deficiencies, and persons who are asplenic. Revaccination after 3 to 5 years may be indicated for persons who had received polysaccharide vaccination and remain at high risk of infection (see Table 91-3). Long-term data regarding protective antibodies after immunization with conjugate meningococcal vaccine is insufficient at this time to recommend routine revaccination.[161]

Immunogenicity and Efficacy. The polysaccharide vaccine was found to elicit a protective immune response to serotype A in 85% to 92% of recipients, to serotype C in 89%, to serotype Y in 80%, and to serotype W-135 in 95%.[161] The polysaccharide vaccine was poorly immunogenic in children less than 2 years of age, and protective immunity was found to wane significantly 3 years after vaccination. Clinical protection was conferred by the vaccine in over 85% of children and adults.[161] The conjugate vaccine elicited an initial immunologic response similar to that of the polysaccharide vaccine, with 90% to 93% having developed protective immunity to serotype A, 89% to 92% to serotype C, 74% to 82% to serotype Y, and 89% to 97% to serotype W-135. The presence of protective antibody levels 3 years after vaccination was more likely in those receiving conjugate vaccine than those receiving polysaccharide vaccine.[161,162]

Adverse Effects and Contraindications. Approximately half of polysaccharide or conjugate vaccine recipients will experience at least one systemic side effect, though less than 5% will experience a severe systemic side effect. Fever and local reactions are more common in those receiving conjugate vaccines, though they also occur in those receiving polysaccharide vaccine. Cases of adverse events, including GBS, have been reported following vaccine administration, but in reviewing the available safety data, serious adverse events were encountered with these vaccines at the same rate as was expected from healthy, unvaccinated persons. The safety of the vaccine has not been assessed in pregnancy, and the vaccine is contraindicated in persons with severe hypersensitivity reactions to prior administration of the vaccine or to vaccine components.[161]

Pneumococcus

Background. *Streptococcus pneumoniae* is a bacterial pathogen that is a leading cause of morbidity and mortality among children and older adults worldwide. It is the most common cause of pneumonia and meningitis in the United States and is a substantial cause of otitis media and sinusitis. Invasive pneumococcal disease, in the form of bacteremia and meningitis, is fatal in 20% of adults and 40% of elderly persons and is responsible for over 10,000 deaths annually in the United States.[162] Emerging antimicrobial resistance in pneumococcus is increasing worldwide and complicates management, and hence provides further impetus for prevention, rather than treatment. There are over 90 serotypes of pneumococcus, though serotypes 6, 14, 18, 19, and 23 account for 60% to 70% of infections.[163]

Vaccine Administration. One polysaccharide vaccine, Pneumovax 23 (Merck), is available for pneumococcal vaccination in adults and one conjugate vaccine, Prevnar 7 (Lederle), is available for vaccination in children. The polysaccharide vaccine contains 25 mcg of each of the capsular polysaccharide antigens of the 23 pneumococcal serotypes that cause 90% of invasive disease (1, 2, 3, 4, 5, 6B, 7F, 8, 9N, 9V, 10A, 11A, 12F, 14, 15B, 17F, 18C, 19A, 19F, 20, 22F, 23F, and 33F).[163-165] The vaccine is administered as a 0.5-ml subcutaneous or IM injection. Since children under 2 years of age do not have immunologic responses to polysaccharide vaccines, a conjugate pneumococcal vaccine was developed. This vaccine contains the capsular polysaccharide antigens of the seven serotypes that most commonly cause invasive disease in children (4, 6B, 9V, 14, 18C, 19F, and 23F). These antigens are conjugated to a mutated diphtheria toxin and complexed with an aluminum phosphate adjuvant. The vaccine is administered as a 0.5-ml IM injection.[166,167]

Indications. A single dose of polysaccharide pneumococcal vaccine is indicated in all persons over age 65; persons ages 2 to 64 years with a chronic medical illness, including the immunosuppressed; persons with functional or anatomic asplenia; and those who live in social environments at high risk for invasive pneumococcal disease (e.g., Alaskan natives). Revaccination is recommended as a single booster 5 years after the first dose in persons with asplenia and immunocompromised persons[163] (see Table 91-3). The conjugate pneumococcal vaccine is recommended as part of the schedule of routine immunizations for children under 24 months of age. The four-dose regimen is given at months 2, 4, 6, and 12 to 15 (see Table 91-1). In addition to vaccination of all children under 24 months, conjugate pneumococcal vaccine is recommended for children ages 24 to 59 months with chronic diseases, HIV or other immunocompromised states, and asplenia. Though polysaccharide pneumococcal vaccine is licensed for those over 2 years of age, conjugate pneumococcal vaccine should be administered preferentially to persons under 6 years of age.[167]

Immunogenicity and Efficacy. Polysaccharide vaccines induce a serologic response in 80% of healthy adult recipients, though it is unclear how well seropositivity correlates with protection from disease.[163,168] Immunocompromised persons and persons with chronic medical conditions have lower immune responses to the vaccine than healthy adults. Serologic evidence of immunity wanes after approximately 10 years, though the data are not conclusive.[163] The vaccine was found to be 56% to 81% effective in preventing invasive disease in adults, though there are not sufficient data to conclude that the vaccine reduces noninvasive pneumococcal pneumonia in older adults.[163,169] The conjugate vaccine induces a serologic response in 90% to 100% of recipients, though it is unclear how well this correlates with clinical protection.[170,171] A prelicensure study showed that the vaccine was 97% effective in preventing invasive pneumococcal disease, mostly from serotypes contained in the vaccine.[169] However, since universal vaccination of infants was started, the proportion of invasive pneumococcal disease caused by serotypes not contained in the vaccine has increased by 6% to 50%, though the overall rate of invasive pneumococcal disease has decreased by 50%. It is unclear at this time if there will be an eventual resurgence of invasive pneumococcal disease caused by serotypes not contained in the vaccine.[172]

Adverse Effects and Contraindications. Local reactions are seen in one third of polysaccharide and conjugate vaccine recipients, though fever and more severe local reactions have been seen. The vaccines have not been well studied in pregnancy and are contraindicated in persons with hypersensitivity to prior vaccine doses or to vaccine components.[163]

Polio

Background. Poliomyelitis is caused by poliovirus. Though most polio infections are asymptomatic, central nervous system infection can occur, resulting in paralysis in 0.1% to 1% of those infected. Aggressive immunization campaigns have been successful in eliminating polio infection from the Western Hemisphere.[173,174]

Vaccine Administration. Oral poliovirus vaccine (OPV), an attenuated live virus vaccine, and inactivated poliovirus vaccine (IPV) are the available vaccines for this disease. After the eradication of polio from the Western Hemisphere, OPV is no longer in production in the

United States but is available to control outbreaks. OPV is composed of the Sabin strains of the three poliovirus serotypes and propagated through monkey kidney cell culture. A 0.5-ml dose is administered orally. Ipol (Aventis Pasteur) is the IPV licensed and distributed in the United States. The vaccine is created by growing poliovirus serotypes 1 (Mahoney strain), 2 (MEF-1 strain), and 3 (Saukett strain) in monkey kidney cell culture and then inactivating them using formaldehyde. IPV is administered as a 0.5-ml subcutaneous injection.[175]

Indications. IPV is recommended as part of the routine childhood vaccination schedule and is given as a four-dose vaccine series at 2 months, 4 months, 6 to 18 months, and 4 to 6 years (see Table 91-1). IPV vaccination is also recommended for adults traveling to polio endemic countries, persons with occupational exposure to polioviruses, health care workers, and unvaccinated parents of children who will be receiving OPV. OPV is available for use in outbreak control and in special circumstances.[175]

Immunogenicity and Efficacy. After three doses of IPV, 99% to 100% of recipients developed protective antibodies.[176,177] Long-term studies of IPV protection are not available, but a Swedish study of a similar vaccine showed that 90% of recipients of four doses of vaccine retained protective serum antibody levels 25 years after vaccination.[174,176] OPV induced long-term immunity in over 95% of vaccine recipients. OPV is favored for use in controlling outbreaks due to superior induction of mucosal immunity compared to IPV.[178]

Adverse Effects and Contraindications. The most concerning side effect of OPV is vaccine-associated paralytic poliomyelitis (VAPP) which affects 1 in 2 million vaccine recipients. The highest risk of VAPP is among immunodeficient recipients, especially those with immune globulin deficiencies. Among immunocompetent persons, the risk of VAPP is 7 to 21 times lower with subsequent doses than with the initial dose.[175] IPV is largely well tolerated, and no serious adverse events have been encountered with its use, though local reactions do occur. IPV and OPV are contraindicated in persons with anaphylactic response to prior vaccinations or to vaccine components, including streptomycin, polymyxin B, and neomycin. OPV is also contraindicated in immunosuppressed persons.[175]

Rotavirus

Background. Rotavirus is the cause of 5% to 10% of gastroenteritis among children in the United States and is the most common cause of severe gastroenteritis in children worldwide. Though the infection is usually mild and self-limited, rotavirus infection can cause dehydration, shock, and death. Globally, it is responsible for the death of half a million children annually. Rotashield (Wyeth-Lederle), a rotavirus vaccine, was withdrawn from the market in 1999 due to its association with intussusception. A new vaccine, RotaTeq (Merck), was licensed in the United States in 2006, and intussusception does not appear to be associated with this vaccine.[179]

Vaccine Administration. RotaTeq is a live, attenuated oral vaccine composed of five reassortant rotaviruses. Four of the vaccine viruses express a bovine rotavirus attachment protein (P7[5] from the Wistar Calf 3 strain) and one of four outer capsid proteins (G1, G2, G3, and G4) from a human rotavirus strain. The fifth vaccine virus expresses an attachment protein (P1A[8]) from human rotavirus and outer capsid protein G6 from the bovine rotavirus. The reassortant viruses are propagated in monkey kidney epithelial cells. Each 2-ml oral vaccine dose contains at least 2.2×10^6 infectious units of the G1 component, 2.8×10^6 infectious units of the G2 component, 2.2×10^6 infectious units of the G3 component, 2.0×10^6 infectious units of the G4 component, and 2.3×10^6 infectious units of the G6 component.[179]

Indications. The three-dose vaccine regimen is recommended for administration at 2, 4, and 6 months of age. Due to insufficient safety and efficacy data, the vaccine series should not be started in infants older than 12 weeks and vaccine doses should not be administered to infants older than 32 weeks.[179]

Immunogenicity and Efficacy. Serologic correlates of protective immunity are unclear, but rotavirus vaccination resulted in seroconversion in 93% to 100% of vaccine recipients following a three-dose vaccine regimen.[179,180] The vaccine was found to be 74% effective in preventing rotavirus gastroenteritis and 98% effective in preventing severe rotavirus infections 3 years after vaccine administration.[180]

Adverse Effects and Contraindications. Prelicensure data suggest that the vaccine is well tolerated and is not associated with intussusception. Vaccine recipients did experience a small, but statistically significant, increase in the rate of vomiting, diarrhea, nasopharyngitis, otitis media, and bronchospasm. The vaccine is contraindicated in persons with severe allergic reactions to prior rotavirus vaccinations or to vaccine components. The vaccine should be used with caution in the immunocompromised as well as children with a history of intussusception until postlicensure data are available.[179]

Smallpox

Background. Smallpox virus is responsible for variola outbreaks causing an extensive rash, high fever, pneumonia, and death. Variola major can present in four types: ordinary, modified, flat, and hemorrhagic. The disease is fatal in 30% of cases and is fatal in most all cases of flat and hemorrhagic variola major. A worldwide vaccination effort was successful in eradicating the disease. Smallpox remains a concern due to its potential as a biologic weapon.[181]

Vaccine Administration. Dryvax (Wyeth) is the smallpox vaccine licensed in the United States. It is a live virus preparation of the New York City Board of Health (NYCBOH) strain of vaccinia virus (cowpox). The vaccine is administered by multiple skin punctures using a bifurcated needle that delivers approximately 2.5×10^5 pock-forming units of vaccine virus.[181]

Indications. Since global smallpox eradication, routine vaccination has not been recommended. Its use is largely limited to outbreak control measures and bioterrorism preparedness. Routine vaccination is recommended for certain military personnel and laboratory workers in contact with vaccinia or another orthopoxvirus. For these persons at risk of infection, routine revaccination is recommended at least every 10 years and can be given as frequently as every 3 years in persons working with more virulent nonvariola orthopoxviruses such as monkeypox.[181]

Immunogenicity and Efficacy. Over 95% of vaccine recipients developed a neutralizing antibody titer greater than 1:10, though it is unclear how well this correlates with protection.[181]

Adverse Effects and Contraindications. Smallpox vaccination is expected to result in a pustular skin eruption at the site of inoculation lasting up to 3 weeks. Fever and tenderness at local lymph nodes are common side effects. Vaccine virus can be cultured from the vaccination site from the time a skin lesion develops until the time the scab separates from the skin. Inadvertent inoculation of other body sites causes half of the vaccine complications, and great care must be taken to ensure that the vaccination site is covered. The vaccine virus can also be transmitted from recent recipients to susceptible persons, further stressing the importance of covering the vaccination site. Severe reactions after vaccination are not common but do occur and are more likely after primary vaccination. These include eczema vaccinatum (occurring in 40 per million primary recipients), generalized vaccinia (240 per million), progressive vaccinia (1.5 per million), myopericarditis (80 per million), and postvaccinial encephalitis (12 per million).[181-183] The vaccine is contraindicated in persons with eczema or other skin conditions, pregnant women, immunocompromised persons, persons with cardiac disease or three major risk factors for cardiac disease, and persons allergic to the vaccine or vaccine components.[181]

Tetanus, Diphtheria, and Pertussis

Background. Tetanus is a disease caused by a toxin produced by the bacterium *Clostridium tetani*, and is characterized by trismus (lockjaw) and generalized rigidity that can lead to death through respiratory failure and autonomic instability.[184] The bacterium is ubiquitous in the environment and most often produces infection after puncture trauma. Tetanus is fatal in nearly 20% of cases.[185] Diphtheria is a lower and upper respiratory tract infection most often caused by *Corynebacterium diphtheriae* and its toxin, with case mortality of 5% to 10%.[186] Pertussis is a highly communicable lower respiratory tract infection caused by the bacterium *Bordetella pertussis* and characterized by a prolonged, spasmodic cough and post-tussive emesis. Due to successful immunization programs, tetanus and diphtheria have largely been eliminated from the United States. Although pertussis vaccination has been widespread, waning immunity from vaccination has been associated with a resurgence of pertussis outbreaks, including among health care workers.[184]

Vaccine Administration. Several formulations of vaccine for these diseases have been licensed for use in children and adults. The vaccine components that induce immunity to tetanus and diphtheria are created by formaldehyde inactivation of tetanus toxin (T) and diphtheria toxin (D). The acellular pertussis (aP) component of the vaccines is made from formaldehyde-inactivated pertussis toxin (P), filamentous hemagglutinin, and pertactin. The components are adsorbed to aluminum hydroxide salt in the final vaccine preparation. DTaP is recommended for IM injection in children under 7 years of age and is available as three commercial products, Daptacel (Aventis Pasteur), Infanrix (GlaxoSmithKline), and Tripedia (Aventis Pasteur), each containing different concentrations of the component elements.[187] DTP vaccine, which used inactivated whole-cell *B. pertussis* as the pertussis component, is no longer available due to an improved side effect profile with the acellular pertussis preparations.[187] DT vaccine for diphtheria and tetanus is available for IM injection in children under 7 with contraindication to pertussis vaccination.

Booster vaccination in children over 7 and adults is provided using IM Td and Tdap vaccines. Td contains a reduced concentration of diphtheria toxoid compared to the DT vaccine used in children, as higher concentrations are associated with increased toxicity in adults without conferring a higher level of immunity.[186] Two Tdap vaccines, Boostrix (GlaxoSmithKline) and Adacel (Aventis Pasteur), were licensed in 2005 to provide adults with booster immunity against pertussis as well as tetanus and diphtheria. Boostrix is similar in composition to Infanrix and Adacel is similar in composition to Daptacel, but both Tdap preparations have reduced concentrations of diphtheria toxoid and detoxified pertussin toxin compared to their DTaP counterpart.[184]

Indications. DTaP is recommended as part of the childhood vaccination schedule and is given at 2, 4, 6, and 12 to 18 months and 4 to 6 years of age (see Table 91-1). Tdap is recommended as a single onetime booster to be given between ages 11 and 64. Td boosters should be given every 10 years, but can be given after 5 years after the previous vaccination in cases of puncture trauma or other injury that may result in a higher risk of tetanus infection (see Table 91-3). Tdap can be given within 2 years of the last Td booster.[184]

Immunogenicity and Efficacy. The vaccine efficacy of the tetanus and diphtheria components has been well established, but limited data are available regarding correlates of protective immunity against pertussis.[184] Protective immunity against tetanus and diphtheria was generated in 95% to 100% of recipients by the vaccines, and the immunity was maintained for the duration of the 10-year interval between booster immunizations.[184,186-188] Trials to assess the efficacy of the vaccines in the prevention of pertussis have demonstrated an efficacy of 85% for DTaP as well as Tdap.[184,187-189] The long-term efficacy of primary DTaP vaccination is unclear, but pertussis infections of individuals previously vaccinated with DTP suggest waning immunity over time as well as the need for booster vaccination with Tdap.[184]

Adverse Effects and Contraindications. The most common side effects of the vaccines are local reactions, including pain, erythema, and swelling at the injection site. Myalgias and headache are less common, but have been associated with vaccination more commonly than with placebo.[184,186] Vaccination with DTaP, Tdap, Td, and DT is contraindicated in persons with allergic reaction to a previous vaccine dose or to a vaccine component. Additionally, DTaP and Tdap are contraindicated in persons with encephalopathy within 7 days of prior vaccine administration or persons with a progressive neurologic disorder, including uncontrolled epilepsy.[184,186]

Typhoid Fever

Background. Typhoid fever is a systemic illness caused by *Salmonella typhi*. The bacterium is most often encountered in contaminated food and water and is common in most parts of the world with poor sanitation. In industrialized countries, the infection is most often seen in travelers returning from endemic regions.[190]

Vaccine Administration. Three vaccines are licensed for use in the United States. Vivotif (Berna) is an oral live, attenuated vaccine made from the Ty21a strain of *S. typhi*, Typhoid Vaccine (Wyeth) is an injectable vaccine made by heat- and phenol-inactivated bacterium, and Typhim Vi (Aventis Pasteur) is an injectable vaccine made from the capsular polysaccharide. Oral typhoid vaccine is administered as four capsules taken one every other day, and the vaccine must be kept refrigerated. Capsular polysaccharide typhoid vaccine is administered as a single 0.5-ml IM injection. Inactivated typhoid vaccine is administered as two 0.5-ml subcutaneous injections at least 4 weeks apart.[190]

Indications. The vaccines are indicated for persons traveling to typhoid-endemic areas and to persons with occupational exposure to *S. typhi*. The dose should be given at least a week prior to travel to the endemic region. Oral typhoid vaccine is indicated for persons over 6 years of age, and booster doses are recommended every 5 years for persons at risk. Polysaccharide vaccine is indicated for persons over 2 years of age, and booster doses are recommended every 2 years for persons remaining at risk. Inactivated typhoid vaccine is indicated for persons over 6 months of age, and booster doses are recommended every 3 years for those remaining at risk.[190]

Immunogenicity and Efficacy. Randomized prospective trials have not been conducted, but efficacy data have been derived from field trials of persons in endemic areas. The efficacy of oral typhoid vaccine has ranged from 53% to 66% in persons older than 10 years to 17% in persons ages 5 to 9 years. Inactivated typhoid vaccine was found to be 51% to 77% effective over 3 years, and capsular polysaccharide typhoid vaccine was 55% to 74% effective.[190]

Adverse Effects and Contraindications. Side effects are rare with oral typhoid vaccine, but can include fever, abdominal discomfort, nausea, vomiting, headache, and rash. Inactivated typhoid vaccine was associated with fever and severe local reactions in up to 25% of recipients. Capsular polysaccharide typhoid vaccine is better tolerated, with fever and local reactions occurring in less than 7% of recipients. Oral typhoid vaccine should not be used in immunocompromised patients or persons taking antimicrobials. All typhoid vaccines should be avoided in persons with a history of severe allergic reactions to previous typhoid vaccination or vaccine components.[190]

Varicella-Zoster Virus

Background. Varicella-zoster virus (VZV) is a herpesvirus that causes significant global morbidity through primary infection (varicella, i.e., chickenpox) and through reactivation disease (zoster, i.e., shingles). Primary infection is usually a self-limited disease consisting of fever, malaise, and a generalized pustular rash. Eighty percent of infections occur in healthy children and adolescents, but primary disease of older or immuncompromised persons can cause severe pneumonia, encephalitis, and hepatitis.[191,192] After recovery from primary infection, VZV remains dormant in sensory nerve ganglia, which can reactivate, often later in life or during immunosuppression, causing herpes zoster. This disease most often results in a self-limited pustular eruption limited to a single dermatome, but can lead to chronically painful herpetic neuralgia.[191,192]

Vaccine Administration. Varivax (Merck) is a live, attenuated vaccine used for the prevention of primary VZV infection. It is created by attenuating the Oka strain of VZV by passaging through different cell lines and growth in human diploid cell cultures. The vaccine is lyophilized and must be reconstituted prior to administration. As a live virus vaccine, it must be frozen for storage and transport. Each 0.5-ml subcutaneous dose of the vaccine contains at least 1350 plaque-forming units of virus, and the two doses of the vaccine regimen are given 4 weeks apart.[191,192] ProQuad (Merck), a combination varicella, measles, mumps, and rubella vaccine, was licensed in 2005. Zostivax (Merck) is a similar live, attenuated vaccine made from the Oka strain of VZV. It is intended for use in older patients to prevent zoster. Each 0.65-ml subcutaneous injection contains at least 19,400 plaque-forming units of vaccine virus. It was licensed in 2005 and is indicated for those persons older than 60 years for the prevention of herpes zoster. As a live, lyophilized vaccine it must be stored and reconstituted in a fashion similar to that of Varivax.[192]

Indications. Varicella vaccination is recommended as part of the routine vaccination schedule, and two doses are given to children between 12 and 18 months of age. In addition, it is recommended for the following persons if they have not had evidence of past varicella infection: health care workers, household contacts of immunocompromised persons, those over 13 years of age at high risk of exposure or transmission, children with altered immunity; it is also recommended in postexposure outbreak control.[191,192] Zostavax is recommended for use in those persons over age 60 years (see Table 91-3).[193]

Immunogenicity and Efficacy. Vaccination with Varivax induced an antibody response in 97% of recipients under 12 years of age after a single dose.[191] For those 13 years and older, 78% had a serologic response after a single dose, but 99% had serologic response after two doses.[191] The protection conferred by the vaccine appeared to decrease over time, with efficacy decreasing from 97% to 84% eight years after vaccination.[194,195] Studies of efficacy in adults and long-term efficacy in children are not available. Zostavax was found to be 51% efficacious in preventing herpes zoster in those persons older than 60 years, and 39% effective in preventing postherpetic neuralgia in those who did develop zoster.[196]

Adverse Effects and Contraindications. Varivax and Zostavax are well-tolerated vaccines. Only local reactions, including pain and erythema, are seen more often than with placebo.[197,198] The vaccines are contraindicated in persons with a history of anaphylaxis in response to the vaccine or vaccine components (including neomycin and gelatin), persons who are immunocompromised, persons with active untreated tuberculosis, and persons who are or could be pregnant.[191]

Yellow Fever

Background. Yellow fever is a virus found in Africa and South America and transmitted by *Aedes aegypti* mosquitoes. Infection can result in severe systemic illness characterized by fever, joint pain, headache, photophobia and vomiting that can progress to hemorrhagic fever accompanied by liver and renal failure.[199]

Vaccine Administration. Yellow fever vaccine, YF-Vax (Aventis Pasteur), is a live, attenuated vaccine made from the 17D yellow fever virus strain and grown in chick embryos. Each 0.5-ml dose is administered as an IM injection. The vaccine should be stored at 2° C to 8° C until reconstituted in saline for administration.[199]

Indications. The vaccine is recommended for persons over 9 months of age traveling to highly endemic regions of Africa or South America. Booster doses may be required every 10 years if a person remains at high risk.[199]

Immunogenicity and Efficacy. Yellow fever vaccine induced protective antibodies in over 95% of recipients, correlating with substantial clinical protection from infection.[199,200]

Adverse Effects and Contraindications. Mild side effects, including low-grade fevers, headaches, and myalgias, have been seen in less than a quarter of recipients. More severe reactions, including yellow fever vaccine-associated neurotropic disease and yellow fever vaccine-associated viscerotropic disease, are extremely rare but can be fatal. Administration of yellow fever vaccine should be avoided in pregnant women, nursing mothers, and immunocompromised persons.[199]

SPECIAL POPULATIONS

A discussion of each of the special populations to whom vaccines should be directed or contraindicated is beyond the scope of this chapter. However, health care providers administering vaccines should familiarize themselves with U.S. Food and Drug Administration (FDA, or equivalent oversight agencies in other countries) and manufacturer (package insert) information regarding the use of specific vaccines in order to safely use these biologic agents.

In general, special attention should be paid to characteristics of the vaccine and the recipient in order to determine if vaccine administration is appropriate.[201] Examples of specific vaccine characteristics that would influence a vaccine's use for a particular patient may include inactivated versus live virus formulation and inclusion of specific components that may be associated with allergic reactions, such as egg protein, porcine gelatin, or latex used in vials or syringes. Examples of patient characteristics that would influence use of a particular vaccine may include factors such as age, pregnancy, history of anaphylaxis, reaction to previous vaccine or component allergy, and various states of immunosuppression, including HIV infection or household contact with an immunodeficient person. The Centers for Disease Control and Prevention's (CDC's) "Guide to Contraindications to Vaccinations" provides specific details regarding vaccine and patient characteristics related to vaccine use.[202]

Extremes of age also may pose particular problems with vaccine use and efficacy. Vaccination is routinely administered to infants and children, and the overwhelming majority of routine vaccines are directed at this age group. Vaccinating infants in the first months of life serves them well for diseases for which they do not suffer exposure or morbidity until an older age. Maternal immunity provides protection for many of these diseases in the interim—protection against tetanus and measles are cases in point. In other situations, such as in HBV exposure, neonatal vaccination combined with maternal immunity is necessary.

The very young do pose a number of difficulties with respect to successful vaccination. Infant vaccination can be blocked or impaired by maternal immunity transmitted via immunoglobulins delivered placentally and perhaps, in the case of oral vaccines, via secretory immunoglobulin A delivered through lactation. The live virus vaccines directed against measles, mumps, rubella, and varicella are scheduled at 12 months of age, when maternal immunity no longer has significant blocking effects.

Very young infants may suffer from a lack of immune response to vaccines when that immaturity is coupled with low body weight. For example, small-for–gestational age, premature infants weighing less than 2000 g appear to respond poorly to vaccines against HBV when administered neonatally. Low-birth-weight infants, and especially small-for–gestational age premature infants, were also central to the theoretical concerns expressed regarding the use of thimerosal in vaccines. These children were thought to be at risk of mercury exposures that exceeded acceptable levels based on body weight for at least one federal standard.[203] However, no direct evidence substantiates these concerns.

For some diseases, vaccination after birth fails to protect. Infants less than 2 years of age lack a T-cell–dependent immune response to polysaccharide antigens and therefore develop transient immunity to polysaccharide vaccines such as the meningococcal, pneumococcal, and Hib vaccines. Conjugation of the polysaccharide antigens with immunoreactive proteins such as diphtheria CRM_{197} permits a durable immune response in infants less than 2 years of age. In other cases, disease exposure has already occurred in utero or at least at the time of the rupture of placental membranes, and thus vaccination after birth cannot prevent exposure. Work is underway to develop vaccines to be given to the mother-to-be to protect the fetus; group B streptococcus and *Listeria* provide obvious targets for such work.

Age-related challenges with immunity are not limited to the very young. Inadequate vaccine response and elevated risk for adverse vaccine-preventable disease outcomes following immunization in the elderly are thought, in part, to be due to the ineffectiveness of an aging immune system[204] rather than an underdeveloped immune system as seen in infants. Immunosenescence is defined as a decline in the body's ability to fight infection or mount novel immune responses. The changes associated with immunosenescence adversely affect the function of the immune system, appear to be progressive, and impact both the innate and adaptive immune compartments, as well as cell signaling and the cytokine milieu.[205] Increases in the proportion of CTLs to Th cells, along with expansion of dysfunctional memory cells, are observed.[206,207] Concomitant loss of CD28$^+$ co-stimulatory cell surface marker expression in cytotoxic T cells[208,209] and associated decreases in telomerase enzyme activity[210] appear to signal replicative senescence.[211] These ineffectual T cells essentially "clog" the immune system and restrict the T-cell repertoire.[212]

Trivalent inactivated influenza vaccine response in the elderly provides an example in which immunosenescence may have a role. Poorer influenza vaccine–related protection against influenza illness is frequently observed in elderly persons relative to that seen in children and younger adults.[147] In particular, T-cell immunosenescence and related low telomerase activity appear to be associated with poorer antibody response to influenza vaccine and increased risk of influenza and overall respiratory illness outcomes among the elderly.[213,214] Future studies may further elucidate the factors inciting and promoting this condition, as well as identify potential opportunities for augmenting a failing immune system or circumventing immunosenescence.

VACCINE REGULATION

Eradication of smallpox occurred worldwide in 1980, and eradication of polio worldwide is nearing. The number of measles cases in the United States is at an all-time low, and we now have control of many other important vaccine-preventable diseases. However, the success of vaccines has in some ways been its own worst enemy in terms of public opinion. The successful suppression and eradication of disease has created an atmosphere of indifference and in some cases misinformed opposition by the public regarding the value of continued vaccination. For many laypersons, there are concerns that vaccines produce many adverse events that outweigh the benefits of vaccination itself. In fact, it was the well-known reactivity of the diphtheria, tetanus, and whole-cell pertussis vaccine (DTP) that was used for more than 50 years that led to a major revolution in how the United States managed vaccination. The number of transient, local, and systemic effects that resulted from the whole-cell pertussis component of the vaccine was linked in the public's mind to a belief that the vaccine resulted in major neurologic disorders, permanent disability, and sudden infant death. While scientific evidence rejected those hypotheses in the 1980s, in 1986, lawsuits related to pertussis vaccine in the United States began to grow—255 lawsuits had been filed. Manufacturers withdrew from the marketplace, supplies diminished, and vaccine prices rose dramatically from 45 cents a dose to $10.10 a dose over a 10-year period.

As a result, Congress passed a law in 1986 entitled the National Childhood Vaccine Injury Act (PL 99-660), which provided a compensation program to replace existing litigation. The National Vaccine Injury Compensation Program pays for those serious injuries from rare events resulting from vaccination and removes the adjudication of vaccine injury from traditional civil torts. It rescued the industry as well as childhood vaccinations and resulted in renewed vaccine development and innovation. The year 1986 represented the highest number of DTP-related lawsuits, with a continued reduction ever since. While there have been more than 7800 claims to the Vaccine Injury Compensation Program since it began on October 1, 1988, 4260 claims were for doses given before that date. The program continues to protect against the liability threat but is only one of the features of that public law. Other features of the act were the development of the Vaccine Adverse Event Reporting System (VAERS) and Vaccine Information Statements.

VAERS was established by the National Childhood Vaccine Injury Act of 1986 as a cooperative program of the CDC and the FDA. It serves as the primary postmarketing safety surveillance program to collect information about vaccine-related adverse events. Participation is required for providers of vaccines and their manufacturers, although parents and others may report to this system. The system includes active surveillance for certain reactions and events among specific vaccines, but the passive event reporting system also permits reporting of additional events associated with other vaccines. Web-based forms, paper forms, and a toll-free phone number are provided to facilitate reporting.

Another aspect of PL 99-660 was the creation of a standard Vaccine Information Statement developed for each vaccine. The regulation requires that the parent or legal representative of a child scheduled to receive a vaccine must first receive the statement prior to administration of the vaccine dose. Vaccine Information Statements are written in an understandable form and are available through the CDC for all health care professionals and the public. These statements discuss why one should get vaccinated as well as risks from the vaccine, when an individual should receive the vaccine, and what can be done to reduce discomfort associated with vaccination. The Vaccine Information Statements also provide information regarding the Vaccine Injury Compensation Program and provide directions for obtaining additional information.

Grade school requirements for children to receive vaccination are legislated by states and vary by state. Requirements also exist in many states for day care, junior high school, and high school attendance, as well as for college matriculation. Most of these requirements permit nonparticipation secondary to religious or philosophical objections, and many provide a forced reminder system. School requirements that permit informed refusal actually facilitate completion of scheduled vaccination. When confronted, most families will vaccinate their children.

COMMON MISPERCEPTIONS ABOUT VACCINE SAFETY

Among the reasons for noncompliance with recommended vaccines are, as previously noted, concerns and misperceptions about the safety and efficacy of vaccines.[215] It is important for health care workers to thoroughly understand these concerns, and to be able to articulate clear answers to the legitimate questions patients and family members may have.[216]

It is also important to realize that legitimate concerns arise, even when not familiar to the clinician, that deserve to be heard and investigated. At some point, however (after appropriate studies have been completed), safety concerns must be dismissed and resources allocated to other areas of inquiry. As previously noted, pertussis vaccines were popularly believed by the lay public to be associated with severe adverse outcomes, such as sudden infant death syndrome.[217] Multiple studies, by multiple investigators, using multiple study designs failed to reveal such an association.[217-223] Nonetheless, pertussis-containing vaccine use plummeted, with the result of untold human tragedy due to pertussis infections, hospitalizations, and even deaths.[217] Similarly, in France, concerns arose that HBV vaccine was associated with the development of multiple sclerosis, particularly in adolescent females. The French health authorities halted HBV immunizations. The incidence of multiple sclerosis did not change, while HBV infections continued to occur.[224-229] As a result, the vaccine was reinstated by French government officials. More recent controversies have included unfounded concerns about "hot lots" of anthrax vaccine, as well as autistic spectrum disorder due to measles vaccine, MMR vaccine, or thimerosal—primarily fueled by speculation and poor science. No studies that have passed expert peer review, in any country, have provided data demonstrating that these concerns are warranted.

In particular, the debate about vaccines and autism has had tremendous negative effects. Parents now question whether their children should receive MMR or other thimerosal-containing vaccines,[230] with the result that outbreaks of these diseases now occur in areas previously free of these infections. This has occurred in developed countries such as England, where outbreaks of measles and rubella have occurred, resulting in death, hospitalizations, and long-term sequelae. In response to such concerns, the IOM published a full report from an independent group of experts in 2004, examining the published and available unpublished data.[231] Their conclusions were that the biologic plausibility supporting a claim between the association of MMR or thimerosal-containing vaccines and autism was only theoretical, and that the available epidemiologic evidence favored rejecting the hypothesis of such an association.[231] Multiple other studies, in multiple study settings, have reached the same conclusion.[232-239]

A contrary example is also worth noting. Since its development, OPV (Sabin vaccine) was the generally recommended polio vaccine in the United States. While appropriate at inception, as the incidence and risk of polio exposure fell in the United States, the rate of VAPP rose.[240,241] More as a result of the prompting of lay public groups urging a change in vaccine recommendation to IPV (Salk vaccine), rather than a proactive approach by vaccinologists, the CDC's Advisory Committee on Immunization Practices (ACIP) changed its recommendation for routine use of Sabin vaccine in the United States, instead recommending the use of IPV, which carries no risk for VAPP.[242] Thus, as scientists and physicians, we must not be arrogant in our knowledge or recommendations, and must be willing to hear and investigate legitimate concerns. At the same time, science, reasoning, and data must ultimately triumph over emotion and unsubstantiated concerns, or poor public health recommendations will be the result.

Disease Disappearance Before the Use of Vaccine

Various authors and critics have questioned the need for vaccines given that the incidence of many infectious diseases has decreased. For example, some have pointed to the decrease in HAV infections prior to the introduction of HAV vaccine and wondered whether the vaccine is really needed. The same questions arose regarding other diseases such as hepatitis B and polio. However, such observations and interpretations are incomplete. The incidence of hepatitis A did indeed decrease in the United States prior to the introduction of vaccine, related to improved sanitation, decreased crowding, and improved food handling and public health practices. Such practices can and do assist in reaching a certain decreased level of risk of subsequent exposure/infection, but will be insufficient to entirely protect against disease at the individual level. To further decrease infection, given the influx of new immigrants, increased adventure travel to poorer areas of the world, and food handling practice errors, prophylaxis with vaccination is necessary to further reduce the incidence of disease.

Absence of Risk Related to Vaccine Use

It is an absolute that risk cannot be reduced to zero. It simply is not possible to completely and absolutely eliminate risk for any vaccine, any drug, or any human activity. In part, this relates to the fact that allergies and hypersensitivities, some understood and calculable and others unknown, will always exist; in part, it is because interactions with other vaccines, drugs, medical conditions, and so forth are inherently unknowable in advance of vaccine receipt.[216] In addition, some side effects are unknowable in advance of receiving vaccine. For example, a side effect that occurs once in a million doses of administered vaccine will likely not be detectable until millions of doses are utilized, and even then is likely to escape detection, or be misattributed to something else.[243-245] These issues relate to the fact that there is no known method to develop an absolutely risk-free vaccine, and, in part, to the fact that economic and research feasibility prevents clinical trials of sufficient size to detect rare or idiosyncratic events. Excellent reviews on the issues surrounding vaccine safety are available.[215,216,245-249]

Vaccine "Hot Lots"

Concerns have been voiced regarding so-called hot lots of vaccine—by which proponents imply that certain lots of vaccine are inadequately inactivated, or contaminated, or associated with some other issue that causes an increase in local or systemic side effects. Most recently, this concern was raised by opponents of the anthrax vaccine. This is also a potentially complex issue. For one, it is impossible to produce absolutely identical lots of any biologic product; this is an inherent property of any biologic process that is dynamic and not static. Regardless, it may not be fully appreciated that, prior to FDA approval for release in the United States, each lot of vaccine must undergo sterility and purity testing. A recent review by an author expert in anthrax vaccine,[250] as well as an independent IOM committee, failed to find any evidence supporting such concerns.[118]

Nonetheless, concern over the safety of anthrax vaccine reached the point where Congress directed the IOM to independently examine the issue. The full report was published in 2002, and concluded that the vaccine is effective and safe without evidence of life-threatening or long-term adverse effects, and that anthrax vaccine recipients were not at increased risk of permanently disabling adverse events.[118] In addition, other groups also examined the data and reached similar conclusions.[250,251]

As an example of the relative effectiveness of the current vaccine surveillance and safety mechanisms, multiple lots of influenza vaccine manufactured at a plant in England by Chiron Corporation were found, prior to release during routine testing, to be contaminated with a bacteria. Production was shut down, and the lots discarded prior to any distribution, thus preventing any risk to humans.

Vaccine Failures

Primary and secondary vaccine failures are often held up as reasons to forgo immunization with recommended vaccines. The data, however, would argue for the opposite action, that is, one is statistically better off getting most vaccines than not getting them, if the goal is protection from disease. It is important to also realize that what the public may define as vaccine failure may not be legitimately called a scientific failure. Several examples are worthwhile. Perhaps the most common concern is "I get the influenza vaccine and yet I get the flu anyway." This common concern is complex and actually has several subissues within it. For example, the trivalent influenza vaccine is not designed to prevent influenza symptoms; rather, it is designed to prevent the morbidity and mortality that result from influenza infection. An excellent meta-analysis provides data illustrating this point.[252] Suppose we examine an influenza season in which the vaccine strains and the circulating wild virus strains are closely matched (the best possible scenario). Among healthy, young adults the vaccine will prevent symptoms of influenza 70% to 90% of the time.[253] Among frail elderly adults, prevention of symptoms may be as low as 30% to 50%.[252] However, among healthy adults and frail elderly, the efficacy of the vaccine in preventing death from all-cause mortality is approximately 50%, and prevention of lower respiratory tract involvement is in the 70% to 90% range. Thus, while symptoms of influenza may result, the vaccine does protect against complications of infection such as pneumonia, hospitalization, and death. To the uninformed, however, what is "visible" is the up to 70% of the elderly who will nevertheless experience influenza-related symptoms, rather than the protective effect against pneumonia and death. In addition, many members of the public and health professions habitually use the term "flu" to refer to any of a myriad of noninfluenza illnesses occurring from September to April, thereby falsely "blaming" the vaccine for failure to protect. Put starkly, the influenza vaccine only protects against influenza A and B (its components), and not, for example, rhinoviruses, respiratory syncytial virus, picornaviruses, and the like.

Another issue with popular experience among the public and health care workers is that of varicella vaccine failure. Indeed, after one dose of varicella vaccine, approximately 2% to 3% of vaccinated children will experience vaccine failure after exposure to the virus and develop chickenpox.[254,255] However, even after just one dose, the vaccine still provides protection against severe varicella and its complications, including hospitalizations for varicella-related complications.[194,256-260] Nonetheless, with increasing experience and knowledge of vaccine failure, the ACIP recently made new recommendations to administer two doses of varicella vaccine to children.

Thus, two major issues emerge: that of true vaccine failure, and that of misperceived vaccine failure. The "cure" would seem to be to first insist on high-quality clinical trials that provide pre- and postmarketing data on the incidence of vaccine failure, as well as clarity regarding the clinical outcomes of interests. Second, this requires that, as health care professionals, we need to be well informed and precise in our communications, and we must carefully educate the public. To do otherwise invites continued misperceptions and, worse, noncompliance with vaccine recommendations—to the peril of the individual's and, more broadly, the public's health.

Safety Profile

In order to be approved by the FDA for marketing and use in the United States, and similarly for use in Western Europe, vaccines must undergo preclinical and clinical investigations designed to demonstrate safety, immunogenicity, effectiveness, and efficacy. In turn, data generated by these clinical trials are closely examined and vetted by outside, independent experts. However, as mentioned earlier, the only side effects that can be elucidated are those for which adequate statistical power exists.[243,244] For this reason, a variety of postapproval mechanisms are in place to assist in determining side effects that may exist once the vaccine is used by millions under "field" (i.e., not strict clinical protocol conditions) conditions. Such mechanisms include individual reporting to the vaccine manufacturer, reporting to a national database such as VAERS, and studies commissioned by the manufacturer or other funding bodies—for example, studies funded by the Vaccine Safety Link projects in large health maintenance organizations or group practices in which data on hundreds of thousands to millions of recipients can be captured and analyzed. The VAERS system has been operational since 1990, and while it has the primary limitation of being a passive reporting system, nonetheless has contributed important data regarding intussusception after rotavirus vaccine, the link between influenza vaccine and GBS, safety after whole-cell pertussis vaccine, safety of OPV versus IPV, and safety assessment after the introduction of any new vaccine.[261-263]

The issue of influenza vaccine safety deserves specific comment. Influenza remains a disease that continues to kill more Americans than all other vaccine-preventable diseases combined. Despite 6 decades of clinical use and ample safety and efficacy studies, controversy about its safety continues and results in decreased vaccine uptake. In particular, concerns about the association of the 1976 swine flu vaccine with GBS[264] have generalized to concern about GBS with any influenza vaccine, despite studies that have been unable to demonstrate a causal relationship.[265,266]

Multiple Dosing

Occasional safety concerns are generated over receiving multiple doses of vaccines. This issue concerns both repeat doses of the same vaccine and, more often, the idea of receiving multiple different vaccines simultaneously or within a short time frame. Most often the concern is wrapped around concerns of "overstimulation" of the immune system. To date, there are no data suggestive of any long-term adverse consequences of the receipt of multiple vaccine antigens.[267]

Thimerosal

Thimerosal is an ethylmercury-containing preservative previously used in some multidose vaccine vials in order to prevent fungal or bacterial contamination. Although thimerosal had been used since the 1930s as a preservative, it came under renewed scrutiny in the 1990s when the FDA Modernization Act of 1997 required the FDA to review the risk of mercury in food and drugs. Thimerosal was used in concentrations of 0.01% to 0.003% in vaccines, and the FDA determined that these amounts might exceed Environmental Protection Agency (EPA) guidelines for mercury intake in infants less than 6 months of age based upon the recommended immunization schedule. Of note, EPA guidelines are based on data regarding methylmercury, for which more information is available. However, with existing high-dose exposure studies of ethylmercury and methylmercury at the time suggesting similar toxicity,[268] and the chemical similarity of the two compounds, low-dose toxicity was assumed to be similar between these agents as well.[269] Recent studies of thimerosal excretion in infants have since observed that ethylmercury is removed via the gastrointestinal route much more rapidly than is methylmercury,[270] and the most commonly cited review of the risks of thimerosal in childhood vaccines[203] found evidence only for elevated risk of local hypersensitivity reactions.

Nonetheless, in 1999 the American Academy of Pediatrics and the U.S. Public Health Service called for the reduction or elimination of thimerosal in childhood vaccines.[271] Mercury is neurotoxic, and concerns were raised regarding an increased risk of neurodevelopmental disorders in infants associated with exposure to thimerosal, including autism, attention-deficit/hyperactivity disorder (ADHD), and speech/language delays. The IOM responded to these concerns with a review of thimerosal-containing vaccines in 2001. This report concluded that "although the hypothesis that exposure to thimerosal-containing vaccines could be associated with neurodevelopmental disorders is not established and rests on indirect and incomplete information, primarily from analogies with methylmercury and levels of maximum mercury exposure from vaccines given in children, the hypothesis is biologically plausible" and "that the evidence is inadequate to accept or reject a causal relationship between thimerosal exposures from childhood vaccines and the neurodevelopmental disorders of autism, ADHD, and speech or language delay."[272] A subsequent IOM report updated these conclusions and determined that thimerosal-containing vaccines were not associated with autism, and that postulated biologic mechanisms for causality in this relationship are hypothetical only.[273] A subsequent systematic review has also observed no conclusive link between receipt of thimerosal-containing vaccines and the development of autistic spectrum disorder.[274]

Currently, thimerosal has been either completely removed or substantially reduced to trace amounts in vaccines directed at children 6 years of age or younger in the United States, with the exception of inactivated influenza vaccine. The FDA published and updates lists of thimerosal and other preservative-containing vaccines,[275] and thimerosal-free vaccines continue to be produced in greater quantities. Development of policies for immediate universal elimination of thimerosal as a vaccine preservative, however, would threaten to increase cost and potentially create logistical barriers for immunization delivery that, particularly for the global population, could result in a rise in vaccine-preventable diseases. We must rely upon preservative substitution and new technologies for the development of nontoxic, low-cost, mercury-free preservatives to replace this decades-old compound in newer vaccine formulations.

OFFICE PRACTICE

Even in the absence of new vaccine technologies and formulations, there are many existing opportunities to improve the practical benefits of vaccination for the U.S. and world populations. The most efficacious vaccine is ineffective if the right vaccine cannot be provided to the right individual at the right time. As such, recent opportunities for more rigorous and scientific evaluation of clinical practice systems, health care delivery, patient safety, and clinical outcomes afforded by practice-based, applied, and translational research serve to improve the effectiveness of all vaccines.

Critical to any discussion of improving prevention and control of vaccine-preventable illness is improved vaccination coverage, regardless of the type or number of vaccinations provided.[276] The U.S. Department of Health and Human Services Healthy People 2010 influenza vaccine coverage target, for example, is 90% for institutionalized persons and noninstitutionalized persons age 65+ years, and 60% for noninstitutionalized adults ages 18 to 64 years.[277] However, examination of national Medicare data revealed that, in a 3-month period in 1998, only 2.6% of fee-for-service Medicare patients age 65 years and older who were previously unvaccinated that year received influenza vaccination during hospitalization[278] in accordance with ACIP guidelines.[279] The CDC has provided estimates of population sizes and receipt rates for influenza vaccine target groups in 2006 (Table 91-4), and the overwhelming impression is of suboptimal vaccination rates

TABLE 91-4 ESTIMATES OF INFLUENZA VACCINATION TARGET POPULATION SIZES IN 2006 AND RECENT VACCINE UPTAKE LEVELS

	2006		
	Population (millions)*	**Percent Vaccinated†**	**Doses Used (millions)†**
Total Target	281.1	32.3	70.4
High Risk	91.2	47.2	43.0
≥65 yr‡	37.2	64.6	24.0
Chronic illness§	44.0	35.4	15.6
50–64 yr	17.1	45.5	7.8
18–49 yr	20.1	26.0	5.2
5–17 yr	5.5	36.3	2.0
24–59 mo	1.3	41.5	0.6
Pregnant women¶	4.0	12.9	0.5
All children ages 6–23 mo¶	6.0	48.4	2.9
Other Target Groups	126.9	21.6	27.4
Health care personnel <65 yr#	7.0	41.9	2.9
Healthy household contacts**	94.8	17.9	16.9
50–64 yr	15.0	33.2	4.9
18–49 yr	55.1	15.4	8.5
5–17 yr	21.2	10.8	2.3
24–59 mo	3.5	35.0	1.2
Healthy 24- to 59-month-olds who are not household contacts of high-risk persons or contacts of other persons ages 24–59 mo	7.1	24.5	1.8
Healthy 50- to 64-year-olds who are not household contacts of high-risk persons or contacts of other persons ages 24–59 mo	18.0	32.1	5.8
Total, Persons Age ≥6 mo	296.2	27.7	82.0
Total, all persons (U.S. population)	298.2		
Target persons (73.1% of U.S. population)	218.1	32.3	70.5
Nontarget persons (ages 5 to <50 yr)	78.1	14.8	11.5

*Based on U.S. interim population projections by age, sex, race, and Hispanic origin: 2000–2050 (Population Projections Branch, U.S. Census Bureau, released 5/11/04).
†Vaccination rates and doses used in adult groups based on 2004 National Health Interview Survey (NHIS) vaccine coverage estimates (CDC unpublished data). Vaccination rates in pediatric groups based on estimates from February 2005 BRFSS (Centers for Disease Control and Prevention. Estimated influenza vaccination coverage among adults and children—United States, September 1, 2004–January 31, 2005. MMWR Morb Mortal Wkly Rep 2005;54:304–307).
‡Includes approximately 1.6 million institutionalized persons.
§Estimated number of persons at high risk for influenza complications because of chronic illness based on age-specific population estimate and estimated proportion of persons (or parents for persons age <18 years) reporting selected medical conditions for the NHIS (33.0% for persons ages 50 to 64 years, 14.9% for persons ages 18 to 49 years, 10.2% for children 5 to 17 years of age, and 11.3% for children 24 to 59 months of age based on NHIS 2002). Not all high-risk conditions for influenza are included in the NHIS. For persons ages 18 to 64 years, reported medical conditions included in the NHIS that were used to estimate the number of high-risk persons included ever having been told by a physician they have diabetes, emphysema, coronary artery disease, angina, heart attack, or other heart conditions; being diagnosed with cancer in the past 12 months (exluding nonmelanoma skin cancer) or ever being told by a physician they had lymphoma, leukemia, or blood cancer; in the past 12 months being told by a physician they have chronic bronchitis or weak or failing kidneys; or reporting an asthma attack or episode in the past 12 months. Also, several neuromuscular conditions are included in the high-risk definition (stroke, senility, multiple sclerosis, Parkinson's disease, and seizures). For children age less than 18 years, high-risk conditions included ever having been diagnosed by a physician as having diabetes, cystic fibrosis, sickle cell anemia, congenital heart disease, other heart disease, current asthma, or neuromuscular conditions (seizures, cerebral palsy, and muscular dystrophy).
¶Estimate of women who would be pregnant at any time during the influenza season is based on 4 million births in the United States.
¶The 2004–2005 population estimate does not include approximately 2 million children who would turn age 6 months during October through March, but would include children who would turn 24 months during this period.
#Based on self-reported occupation from the 2004 NHIS.
**Estimates of healthy household contacts of either high-risk persons or healthy persons ages 24 to 59 months, based on multiplying the estimated number of persons not at increased risk, excluding health care personnel, by the estimated proportion of such persons living in a household with at least one person at increased risk (45.5% for persons ages 50 to 64 years, 50.1% for persons ages 18 to 49 years, 39.6% for persons ages 5 to 17 years, and 29.0% for persons ages 24 to 59 months). Proportions were estimated from the 2002 NHIS using Monte Carlo imputation of chronic illness and health care occupational status; persons ages less than 5 years or ≥65 years were considered at increased risk. Out-of-home caregivers of children age less than 5 years are not included, because estimates of population size and vaccination coverage are not available.
Adapted from Centers for Disease Control and Prevention. Estimates of influenza vaccination target population sizes in 2006 and recent vaccine uptake levels. July 17, 2006. Available at *http://www.cdc.gov/flu/professionals/vaccination/pdf/targetpopchart.pdf*

among the at-risk populations relative to the Healthy People 2010 goals.[280] Low compliance with recommended annual vaccination against influenza in the elderly, and inadequate programs to increase immunization rates in children and adults, are clear limitations of current vaccination strategies.[281]

One effective strategy for improving vaccination coverage rates is simply recommending vaccination to patients when appropriate. A health care provider's recommendation is among the strongest determinants for inducing adult patients to receive vaccinations.[282] Recommending and offering influenza vaccination consistently throughout the influenza season presents another opportunity—a three-state, 13-site study of vaccine receipt among individuals presenting for nonvaccination health care visits observed an increased rate of missed vaccination opportunities as the flu season progressed from October to January.[283] As noted earlier, the updated recommendations from the CDC specifically address this issue.[147]

System-based opportunities to improve vaccination coverage exist as well. Both immunization registries and recall and reminder systems can be effective in improving vaccination coverage for children and adults, yet remain underutilized.[284-286] Many studies have shown standing orders to be a valuable system approach to vaccine delivery,[287-289] and computer-based standing orders have demonstrated utility as well.[289] In the hospital setting, physicians with the highest volume of pneumonia care in their hospital practices may actually do significantly worse (35% to 40%) than their lower pneumonia volume colleagues with completing vaccine provision to their hospitalized patients,[290] further supporting the rationale for taking vaccine delivery out of physician's hands and utilizing standing orders. Additional information on standing order templates and other programs to improve vaccination rates, including patient education, drop-in clinics, recall and reminder systems, performance feedback, and other programs, may be found at the Vaccines & Immunization web site.[291]

There are also clear racial and socioeconomic disparities in the quality and delivery of health care and preventive services in the United States,[292,293] and vaccination metrics are not immune to these differences.[294,295] Among persons age 65 years or older in the 1999 Behavioral Risk Factor Surveillance Survey, non-Hispanic black and Hispanic respondents were 30% to 60% less likely than non-Hispanic white respondents to report vaccination against influenza or pneumococcal disease[295] after adjustment for age, sex, education level, length of time since last checkup, self-reported health, and diabetes status. Subsequent studies have observed the persistence of racial disparities in influenza vaccination among adults in managed care and fee-for-service settings,[296] and there is no evidence to suggest that these disparities do not extend to other vaccine recommendations. Clearly, additional efforts are necessary to better understand and reduce these differences.

Provider attention to optimizing the prevention and control of medical conditions predisposing to vaccine-preventable illness, such as diabetes, chronic obstructive pulmonary disease, cardiovascular disease, and chronic kidney disease, may shrink the "at-risk" population for vaccine-preventable illness. Wider and more aggressive use of smoking cessation programs may also provide benefits, as smoking and second-hand smoke exposure are recognized as risk factors for pneumococcal and influenza illness.[297-299] Analogous arguments can be made for improved education and risk counseling regarding other vaccine-preventable illnesses such as hepatitis B, HPV, Lyme disease, and tetanus for which exposure-specific risk might be reasonably mitigated.

REFERENCES

1. Plotkin SA. A hundred years of vaccination: the legacy of Louis Pasteur. Pediatr Infect Dis J 1996;15:391-394.
2. Radetsky M. Smallpox: a history of its rise and fall. Pediatr Infect Dis J 1999;18:85-93.
3. Ma B. [Variolation, pioneer of modern immunology]. Zhonghua Yi Shi Za Zhi 1995;25:139-144.
4. Klebs AC. The historic evolution of variolation. Bull Johns Hopkins Hosp 1913;(24):69-83.
5. Bourzac K. Smallpox: historical review of a potential bioterrorist tool. J Young Investigators 2002;(3).
6. Stewart AJ, Devlin PM. The history of the smallpox vaccine. J Infect 2006;52:329-334.
7. Parish HJ. A History of Immunization. Edinburgh: E&S Livingstone, 1965.
8. Stark RB. Immunization saves Washington's army. Surg Gynecol Obstet 1977;144:425-431.
9. Crookshank EM. History and Pathology of Vaccination, Vol 1: A Critical Inquiry. London: HK Lewis, 1889.
10. Moore J. The History and Practice of Vaccination. London: J Callow, 1817.
11. Wilson GS, Miles A. Topley and Wilson's Principles of Bacteriology, Virology, and Immunity. Baltimore: Williams & Wilkins, 1975, pp 2208-2224.
12. Salmon DE, Smith T. On a new method of producing immunity from contagious diseases. Proc Biol Soc Washington, 1884-1886 1886;(3):29-33.
13. Ravenel MP. The control of typhoid fever by vaccination. Proc Am Philos Soc 1913;(5):226-233.
14. Shafrir E. Waldemar Mordechai Wolf Haffkine—vaccine developer. Isr J Med Sci 1994;(30):249.
15. Stevenson LG. Exemplary disease: the typhoid pattern. J Hist Med Allied Sci 1982;37:159-181.
16. Petroff SA, Branch A. Bacillus Calmette-Guerin (BCG): animal experimentation and prophylactic immunization of children. An analysis and critical review. Am J Publ Health Nations Health 1928;(18):843-864.
17. Mille JJ Jr. The present status of immunization against pertussis. Calif West Med 1940;(53):25-28.
18. Francis T Jr, Korns RF, Voight RB, et al. An evaluation of the 1954 poliomyelitis vaccine trials. Am J Public Health 1955;45(5 Pt 2):1-63.
19. Sabin AB. Recent studies and field tests with a live attenuated poliovirus vaccine. *In* Live Poliovirus Vaccines. Washington, DC: Pan American Health Organization, 1959, p 33.
20. Chernin E. Ross defends Haffkine: the aftermath of the vaccine-associated Mulkowal disaster of 1902. J Hist Med Allied Sci 1991;46:201-218.
21. World Health Organization and United Nation's Children's Fund. Global Immunization Vision and Strategy, 2006-2015. Geneva: World Health Organization, 2005.
22. World Health Organization. Draft global immunization strategy (WHA 58.15, agenda item 13.8). Geneva: World Health Organization, 2005.
23. Zinkernagel RM. Immunology taught by viruses. Science 1996;271:173-178.
24. Zinkernagel RM. Immunity to viruses. *In* Paul WE (ed): Fundamental Immunology. New York: Raven Press, 1993, pp 1211-1250.
25. Pamer EG. Antigen presentation in the immune response to infectious diseases. Clin Infect Dis 1999;28:714-716.
26. Rammensee H-G, Friede T, Stevanovic S. MHC ligands and peptide motifs: first listing. Immunogenetics 1995;41:178-228.
27. Cox AL, Skipper J, Chen Y, et al. Identification of a peptide recognized by five melanoma-specific human cytotoxic T cell lines. Science 1994;264:716-719.
28. Harris NL, Ronchese F. The role of B7 costimulation in T-cell immunity. Immunol Cell Biol 1999;77:304-311.
29. Mosmann TR, Coffman RL. Heterogeneity of cytokine secretion patterns and functions of helper T cells. Adv Immunol 1989;46:111-147.
30. Mosmann TR, Coffman RL. TH1 and TH2 cells: different patterns of lymphokine secretion lead to different functional properties. Annu Rev Immunol 1989;7:145-173.
31. Romagnani S. Th1/Th2 cells. Inflamm Bowel Dis 1999;5:285-294.
32. Banchereau J, Steinman RM. Dendritic cells and the control of immunity. Nature 1998;392:245-252.
33. Howard MC, Miyajima A, Coffman R. T-cell-derived cytokines and their receptors. *In* Paul WE (ed): Fundamental Immunology. New York: Raven Press, 1993, pp 763-800.
34. Biron CA. Cytokines in the generation of immune responses to, and resolution of, virus infection. Curr Opin Immunol 1994;6:530-538.
35. Paul WE, Seder RA. Lymphocyte responses and cytokines. Cell 1994;76:241-251.
36. Mosmann TR. Cytokine secretion patterns and cross-regulation of T cell subsets. Immunol Res 1991;10:183-188.
37. Esser MT, Marchese RD, Kierstead LS, et al. Memory T cells and vaccines. Vaccine 2003;21:419-430.
38. Griffin DE, Ward BJ. Differential CD4 T cell activation in measles. J Infect Dis 1993;168:275-281.
39. van Den Broek M, Bachmann MF, Kohler G, et al. IL-4 and IL-10 antagonize IL-12-mediated protection against acute vaccinia virus infection with a limited role of IFN-γ and nitric oxide synthetase 2. J Immunol 2000;164:371-378.
40. Kawai T, Akira S. Pathogen recognition with Toll-like receptors. Curr Opin Immunol 2005;17:338-344.
41. Matsumoto M, Funami K, Oshiumi H, et al. Toll-like receptor 3: a link between Toll-like receptor, interferon and viruses. Microbiol Immunol 2004;48:147-154.
42. Medzhitov R. Toll-like receptors and innate immunity. Nat Rev Immunol 2001;1:135-145.
43. Pasare C, Medzhitov R. Toll-like receptors and acquired immunity. Semin Immunol 2004;16:23-26.
44. Takeda K, Kaisho T, Akira S. Toll-like receptors. Annu Rev Immunol 2003;21:335-376.
45. Bowie AG, Haga IR. The role of Toll-like receptors in the host response to viruses. Mol Immunol 2005;42:859-867.
46. Boehme KW, Compton T. Innate sensing of viruses by Toll-like receptors. J Virol 2004;78:7867-7873.
47. Rassa JC, Ross SR. Viruses and Toll-like receptors. Microbes Infect 2003;5:961-968.
48. Horng T, Barton GM, Medzhitov R. TIRAP: an adapter molecule in the Toll signaling pathway. Nat Immunol 2001;2:835-841.
49. Fitzgerald KA, Palsson-McDermott EM, Bowie AG, et al. Mal (MyD88-adapter-like) is required for Toll-like receptor-4 signal transduction. Nature 2001;413:78-83.
50. Yamamoto M, Sato S, Mori K, et al. Cutting edge: a novel Toll/IL-1 receptor domain-containing adapter that preferentially activates the IFN-beta promoter in the Toll-like receptor signaling. J Immunol 2002;169:6668-6672.
51. Oshiumi H, Matsumoto M, Funami K, et al. TICAM-1, an adaptor molecule that participates in Toll-like receptor 3-mediated interferon-beta induction. Nat Immunol 2003;4:161-167.
52. Pasare C, Medzhitov R. Control of B-cell responses by Toll-like receptors. Nature 2005;438:364-368.
53. Powell MF, Newman MJ, Burdman JR. Vaccine Design: The Subunit and Adjuvant Approach. New York: Plenum Press, 1995.
54. Moingeon P, Haensler J, Lindberg A. Towards the rational design of Th1 adjuvants. Vaccine 2001;19:4363-4372.
55. Ellis RW, Douglas RG Jr. New vaccine technologies. JAMA 1994;271:929-931.
56. Skea DL, Barber BH. Adhesion-mediated enhancement of the adjuvant activity of alum. Vaccine 1993;11:1018-1026.
57. Shirodkar S, Hutchinson RL, Perry DL, et al. Aluminum compounds used as adjuvants in vaccines. Pharm Res 1990;7:1282-1288.
58. Jacques P, Moens G, Desombere I, et al. The immunogenicity and reactogenicity profile of a candidate hepatitis B vaccine in an adult vaccine non-responder population. Vaccine 2002;20:3644-3649.
59. Smith KM, Garside P, McNeil RC, et al. Analysis of costimulatory molecule expression on antigen-specific T and B cells during the induction of adjuvant-induced Th1 and Th2 type responses. Vaccine 2006;24:3035-3043.
60. de Roux A, Marx A, Burkhardt O, et al. Impact of corticosteroids on the immune response to a MF59-adjuvanted influenza vaccine in elderly COPD-patients. Vaccine 2006;24:1537-1542.
61. Luhrmann A, Tschernig T, Pabst R, et al. Improved intranasal immunization with live-attenuated measles virus after co-inoculation of the lipopeptide MALP-2. Vaccine 2005;23:4721-4726.
62. Stephenson I, Bugarini R, Nicholson KG, et al. Cross-reactivity to highly pathogenic avian influenza H5N1 viruses after vaccination with nonadjuvanted and MF59-adjuvanted influenza A/Duck/Singapore/97 (H5N3) vaccine: a potential priming strategy. J Infect Dis 2005;191:1210-1215.

63. Lin R, Tarr PE, Jones TC. Present status of the use of cytokines as adjuvants with vaccines to protect against infectious diseases. Clin Infect Dis 1995;21:1439-1449.
64. de Jonge J, Holtrop M, Wilschut J, et al. Reconstituted influenza virus envelopes as an efficient carrier system for cellular delivery of small-interfering RNAs. Gene Ther 2006;13:400-411.
65. Huckriede A, Bungener L, Stegmann T, et al. The virosome concept for influenza vaccines. Vaccine 2005;23(Suppl 1):S26-S38.
66. Westerfeld N, Pluschke G, Zurbriggen R. Optimized malaria-antigens delivered by immunostimulating reconstituted influenza virosomes. Wien Klin Wochenschr 2006;118(Suppl 3):50-57.
67. Westerfeld N, Zurbriggen R. Peptides delivered by immunostimulating reconstituted influenza virosomes. J Peptide Sci 2005;11:707-712.
68. Cusi MG. Applications of influenza virosomes as a delivery system. Hum Vaccin 2006;2:1-7.
69. Glueck R. Review of intranasal influenza vaccine. Adv Drug Deliv Rev 2001;51:203-211.
70. de Bruijn IA, Nauta J, Cramer WC, et al. Clinical experience with inactivated, virosomal influenza vaccine. Vaccine 2005;23(Suppl 1):S39-S49.
71. Conne P, Gauthey L, Vernet P, et al. Immunogenicity of trivalent subunit versus virosome-formulated influenza vaccines in geriatric patients. Vaccine 1997;15:1675-1679.
72. Webby RJ, Perez DR, Coleman JS, et al. Responsiveness to a pandemic alert: use of reverse genetics for rapid development of influenza vaccines. Lancet 2004;363:1099-1103.
73. Ozaki H, Govorkova EA, Li C, et al. Generation of high-yielding influenza A viruses in African green monkey kidney (Vero) cells by reverse genetics. J Virol 2004;78:1851-1857.
74. Cox MM. Cell-based protein vaccines for influenza. Curr Opin Mol Ther 2005;7:24-29.
75. Palker T, Kiseleva I, Johnston K, et al. Protective efficacy of intranasal cold-adapted influenza A/New Caledonia/20/99 (H1N1) vaccines comprised of egg- or cell culture-derived reassortants. Virus Res 2004;105:183-194.
76. Kiseleva I, Su Q, Toner TJ, et al. Cell-based assay for the determination of temperature sensitive and cold adapted phenotypes of influenza viruses. J Virol Methods 2004;116:71-78.
77. Webby RJ, Webster RG. Are we ready for pandemic influenza? Science 2003;302:1519-1522.
78. Gerhard W, Mozdzanowska K, Zharikova D. Prospects for universal influenza virus vaccine. Emerg Infect Dis 2006;12:569-574.
79. Neirynck S, Deroo T, Saelens X, et al. A universal influenza A vaccine based on the extracellular domain of the M2 protein. Nat Med 1999;5:1157-1163.
80. Giuliani MM, Adu-Bobie J, Comanducci M, et al. A universal vaccine for serogroup B meningococcus. Proc Natl Acad Sci U S A 2006;103:10834-10839.
81. Donnelly JJ, Ulmer JB, Shiver JW, et al. DNA vaccines. Annu Rev Immunol 1997;15:617-648.
82. Hooper JW, Thompson E, Wilhelmsen C, et al. Smallpox DNA vaccine protects nonhuman primates against lethal monkeypox. J Virol 2004;78:4433-4443.
83. Iwasaki A, Torres CAT, Ohashi PS, et al. The dominant role of bone marrow-derived cells in CTL induction following plasmid DNA immunization at different sites. J Immunol 1997;159:11-14.
84. Wolff JA, Ludtke JJ, Acsadi G, et al. Long-term persistence of plasmid DNA and foreign gene expression in mouse muscle. Hum Mol Genet 1992;1:363-369.
85. Torres CA, Yang K, Mustafa F, et al. DNA immunization: effect of secretion of DNA-expressed hemagglutinins on antibody responses. Vaccine 1999;18:805-814.
86. Raz E, Carson DA, Parker SE, et al. Intradermal gene immunization: the possible role of DNA uptake in the induction of cellular immunity to viruses. Proc Natl Acad Sci U S A 1994;91:9519-9523.
87. Ulmer JB, Donnelly JJ, Parker SE, et al. Heterologous protection against influenza by injection of DNA encoding a viral protein. Science 1993;259:1745-1749.
88. Ulmer JB, Deck RR, DeWitt CM, et al. Protective immunity by intramuscular injection of low doses of influenza virus DNA vaccines. Vaccine 1994;12:1541-1544.
89. Morris S, Kelley C, Howard A, et al. The immunogenicity of single and combination DNA vaccines against tuberculosis. Vaccine 2000;18:2155-2163.
90. Horn NA, Meek JA, Budahazi G, et al. Cancer gene therapy using plasmid DNA: purification of DNA for human clinical trials. Hum Gene Ther 1995;6:565-573.
91. Donnelly JJ, Ulmer JB, Liu MA. Immunization with DNA. J Immunol Methods 1994;176:145-152.
92. Deck RR, DeWitt CM, Donnelly JJ, et al. Characterization of humoral immune responses induced by an influenza hemagglutinin DNA vaccine. Vaccine 1997;15:71-78.
93. Rottinghaus ST, Poland GA, Jacobson RM, et al. Hepatitis B DNA vaccine induces protective antibody responses in human non-responders to conventional vaccination. Vaccine 2003;21:4604-4608.
94. Berd D, Maguire HC Jr, Schuchter LM, et al. Autologous hapten-modified melanoma vaccine as postsurgical adjuvant treatment after resection of nodal metastases. J Clin Oncol 1997;15:2359-2370.
95. Petricciani J, Egan W, Vicari G, et al. Potency assays for therapeutic live whole cell cancer vaccines. Biologicals 2007;35:107-113.
96. Terabe M, Berzofsky JA. Immunoregulatory T cells in tumor immunity. Curr Opin Immunol 2004;16:157-162.
97. Maeurer MJ, Martin DM, Storkus WJ, et al. TCR usage in CTLs recognizing melanoma/melanocyte antigens. Immunol Today 1995;16:603-604.
98. Celluzzi CM, Falo LD Jr. Epidermal dendritic cells induce potent antigen-specific CTL-mediated immunity. J Invest Dermatol 1997;108:716-720.
99. Pardoll DM. Cancer vaccines. Nat Med 1998;4(Vaccine Suppl):525-531.
100. Pardoll DM. Tumour antigens: a new look for the 1990s. Nature 1994;369:357.
101. Visseren MJW, van der Burg SH, van der Voort EIH, et al. Identification of HLA-A*0201-restricted CTL epitopes encoded by the tumor-specific *MAGE-2* gene product. Int J Cancer 1997;73:125-130.
102. Melief CJM, Offringa R, Toes REM, et al. Peptide-based cancer vaccines. Curr Opin Immunol 1996;8:651-657.
103. Knutson KL, Schiffman K, Disis ML. Immunization with a HER-2/neu helper peptide vaccine generates HER-2/neu CD8 T-cell immunity in cancer patients. J Clin Invest 2001;107:477-484.
104. Bronte V, Carroll MW, Goletz TJ, et al. Antigen expression by dendritic cells correlates with the therapeutic effectiveness of a model recombinant poxvirus tumor vaccine. Proc Natl Acad Sci U S A 1997;94:3183-3188.
105. Udono H, Levey DL, Srivastava PK. Cellular requirements for tumor-specific immunity elicited by heat shock proteins: tumor rejection antigen gp96 primes CD8+ T cells in vivo. Proc Natl Acad Sci U S A 1994;91:3077-3081.
106. Li Z. Priming of T cells by heat shock protein-peptide complexes as the basis of tumor vaccines. Semin Immunol 1997;9:315-322.
107. Ohtani H, Naito Y, Saito K, et al. Expression of costimulatory molecules B7-1 and B7-2 by macrophages along invasive margin of colon cancer: a possible antitumor immunity? Lab Invest 1997;77:231-241.
108. Paquette RL, Hsu NC, Kiertscher SM, et al. Interferon-α and granulocyte-macrophage colony-stimulating factor differentiate peripheral blood monocytes into potent antigen-presenting cells. J Leukoc Biol 1998;64:358-367.
109. Dranoff G, Jaffee E, Lazenby A, et al. Vaccination with irradiated tumor cells engineered to secrete murine granulocyte-macrophage colony-stimulating factor stimulates potent, specific, and long-lasting anti-tumor immunity. Proc Natl Acad Sci U S A 1993;90:3539-3543.
110. Pippin BA, Rosenstein M, Jacob WF, et al. Local IL-4 delivery enhances immune reactivity to murine tumors: gene therapy in combination with IL-2. Cancer Gene Ther 1994;1:35-42.
111. Tahara H, Lotze MT, Robbins PD, et al. IL-12 gene therapy using direct injection of tumors with genetically engineered autologous fibroblasts. Hum Gene Ther 1995;6:1607-1624.
112. Blattman JN, Greenberg PD. Cancer immunotherapy: a treatment for the masses. Science 2004;305:200-205.
113. Centers for Disease Control and Prevention. Use of anthrax vaccine in the United States. MMWR Recomm Rep 2000;49(RR-15).
114. Meselson M, Guillemin J, Hugh-Jones M, et al. The Sverdlovsk anthrax outbreak of 1979. Science 1994;266:1202-1207.
115. Brachman PS, Plotkin SA, Bumford FH, et al. An epidemic of inhalation anthrax: the first in the twentieth century. II. Epidemiology. Am J Hyg 1960;72:6-23.
116. Kimman TG, Koopmans MPG, van der Avoort HGAM. Ending polio immunization: when and how are we sure that the needle is out of the haystack? Vaccine 1999;17:624-627.
117. Turnbull PCB, Broster MG, Carman JA, et al. Development of antibodies to protect antigen and lethal factor components of anthrax toxin in humans and guinea pigs and their relevance to protective immunity. Infect Immun 1986;52:356-363.
118. Institute of Medicine. The Anthrax Vaccine: Is It Safe? Does It Work? Washington, DC: National Academy Press, 2002.
119. Kelly DF, Moxon ER, Pollard AJ. *Haemophilus influenzae* type b conjugate vaccines. Immunology 2004;113:163-174.
120. Centers for Disease Control and Prevention. Progress toward eliminating *Haemophilus influenzae* type b disease among infants and children—United States, 1987-1997. MMWR Morb Mortal Wkly Rep 1998;47:993-998.
121. Centers for Disease Control and Prevention. Recommendations for use of *Haemophilus* b conjugate vaccines and a combined diphtheria, tetanus, pertussis, and *Haemophilus* b vaccine. Recommendations of the Advisory Committee on Immunization Practices (ACIP). MMWR Recomm Rep 1993;42(RR-13):1-15.
122. Centers for Disease Control and Prevention. *Haemophilus* b conjugate vaccines for prevention of *Haemophilus influenzae* type b disease among infants and children two months of age and older: recommendations of the Immunization Practices Advisory Committee (ACIP). MMWR Morb Mortal Wkly Rep 1991; 40:1-7.
123. Vento S, Garofano T, Renzini C, et al. Fulminant hepatitis associated with hepatitis A virus superinfection in patients with chronic hepatitis C. N Engl J Med 1998;338:286-290.
124. Wasley A, Samandari T, Bell BP. Incidence of hepatitis A in the United States in the era of vaccination. JAMA 2005;294:194-201.
125. Fiore AE, Wasley A, Bell BP. Prevention of hepatitis A through active or passive immunization: recommendations of the Advisory Committee on Immunization Practices (ACIP). MMWR Recomm Rep 2006;55:1-23.
126. Recommended childhood and adolescent immunization schedule—United States, 2006. Pediatrics 2006;117:239-240.
127. Andre FE, D'Hondt E, Delem A, et al. Clinical assessment of the safety and efficacy of an inactivated hepatitis A vaccine: rationale and summary of findings. Vaccine 1992;10(Suppl 1):S160-S168.
128. McMahon BJ, Williams J, Bulkow L, et al. Immunogenicity of an inactivated hepatitis A vaccine in Alaska Native children and Native and non-Native adults. J Infect Dis 1995;171:676-679.
129. Braconier JH, Wennerholm S, Norrby SR. Comparative immunogenicity and tolerance of Vaqta and Havrix. Vaccine 1999;17:2181-2184.
130. Innis BL, Snitbhan R, Kunasol P, et al. Protection against hepatitis A by an inactivated vaccine. JAMA 1994;271:1328-1334.
131. Black S, Shinefield H, Hansen J, et al. A post-licensure evaluation of the safety of inactivated hepatitis A vaccine (VAQTA, Merck) in children and adults. Vaccine 2004;22:766-772.

132. McMahon BJ. Epidemiology and natural history of hepatitis B. Semin Liver Dis 2005;25(Suppl 1):3-8.
133. Lavanchy D. Hepatitis B virus epidemiology, disease burden, treatment, and current and emerging prevention and control measures. J Viral Hepat 2004;11:97-107.
134. Mast EE, Margolis HS, Fiore AE, et al. A comprehensive immunization strategy to eliminate transmission of hepatitis B virus infection in the United States: recommendations of the Advisory Committee on Immunization Practices (ACIP), Part 1. Immunization of infants, children, and adolescents. MMWR Recomm Rep 2005;54(RR-16):1-31.
135. Poland GA. Hepatitis B immunization in health care workers: dealing with vaccine nonresponse. Am J Prev Med 1998;15:73-77.
136. Shaw FE Jr, Guess HA, Roets JM, et al. Effect of anatomic injection site, age and smoking on the immune response to hepatitis B vaccination. Vaccine 1989;7:425-430.
137. Assad S, Francis A. Over a decade of experience with a yeast recombinant hepatitis B vaccine. Vaccine 1999;18:57-67.
138. Propst T, Propst A, Lhotta K, et al. Reinforced intradermal hepatitis B vaccination in hemodialysis patients is superior in antibody response to intramuscular or subcutaneous vaccination. Am J Kidney Dis 1998;32:1041-1045.
139. Miller ER, Alter MJ, Tokars JI. Protective effect of hepatitis B vaccine in chronic hemodialysis patients. Am J Kidney Dis 1999;33:356-360.
140. Bohlke K, Davis RL, Marcy SM, et al. Risk of anaphylaxis after vaccination of children and adolescents. Pediatrics 2003;112:815-820.
141. Munoz N, Bosch FX, Castellsague X, et al. Against which human papillomavirus types shall we vaccinate and screen? The international perspective. Int J Cancer 2004;111:278-285.
142. Kirnbauer R, Booy F, Cheng N, et al. Papillomavirus L1 major capsid protein self-assembles into virus-like particles that are highly immunogenic. Proc Natl Acad Sci U S A 1992;89:12180-12184.
143. Centers for Disease Control and Prevention. Press Release: Advisory Committee recommends human papillomavirus virus vaccination. Atlanta: Centers for Disease Control and Prevention, June 29, 2006.
144. Villa LL, Costa RL, Petta CA, et al. Prophylactic quadrivalent human papillomavirus (types 6, 11, 16, and 18) L1 virus-like particle vaccine in young women: a randomised double-blind placebo-controlled multicentre Phase II efficacy trial. Lancet Oncol 2005;6(5):271-278.
145. Harper DM, Franco EL, Wheeler C, et al. Efficacy of a bivalent L1 virus-like particle vaccine in prevention of infection with human papillomavirus types 16 and 18 in young women: a randomised controlled trial. Lancet 2004;364(9447):1757-1765.
146. Advisory Committee on Immunization Practices. Provisional Recommendations for the Use of Quadrivalent HPV Vaccine. Atlanta: Advisory Committee on Immunization Practices, August 14, 2006.
147. Smith NM, Bresee JS, Shay DK, et al. Prevention and control of influenza: recommendations of the Advisory Committee on Immunization Practices (ACIP). MMWR Recomm Rep 2006;55(RR-10):1-42.
148. Hoberman A, Greenberg DP, Paradise JL, et al. Effectiveness of inactivated influenza vaccine in preventing acute otitis media in young children: a randomized controlled trial. JAMA 2003;290:1608-1616.
149. Clover RD, Crawford S, Glezen WP, et al. Comparison of heterotypic protection against influenza A/Taiwan/86 (H1N1) by attenuated and inactivated vaccines to A/Chile/83-like viruses. J Infect Dis 1991;163:300-304.
150. Belshe RB, Gruber WC, Mendelman PM, et al. Efficacy of vaccination with live attenuated, cold-adapted, trivalent, intranasal influenza virus vaccine against a variant (A/Sydney) not contained in the vaccine. J Pediatr 2000;136:168-175.
151. Belshe RB, Mendelman PM, Treanor J, et al. The efficacy of live attenuated, cold-adapted, trivalent, intranasal influenzavirus vaccine in children. N Engl J Med 1998;338:1405-1412.
152. Treanor JJ, Kotloff K, Betts RF, et al. Evaluation of trivalent, live, cold-adapted (CAIV-T) and inactivated (TIV) influenza vaccines in prevention of virus infection and illness following challenge of adults with wild-type influenza A (H1N1), A (H3N2), and B viruses. Vaccine 1999;18:899-906.
153. Centers for Disease Control and Prevention. Inactivated Japanese encephalitis virus vaccine: recommendations of the Advisory Committee on Immunization Practices (ACIP). MMWR Recomm Rep 1993;42(RR-1):1-15.
154. Hoke CH, Nisalak A, Sangawhipa N, et al. Protection against Japanese encephalitis by inactivated vaccines. N Engl J Med 1988;319:608-614.
155. Watson JC, Hadler SC, Dykewicz CA, et al. Measles, mumps, and rubella—vaccine use and strategies for elimination of measles, rubella, and congenital rubella syndrome and control of mumps: recommendations of the Advisory Committee on Immunization Practices (ACIP). MMWR Recomm Rep 1998;47(RR-8):1-57.
156. Centers for Disease Control and Prevention. Licensure of a combined live attenuated measles, mumps, rubella, and varicella vaccine. MMWR Morb Mortal Wkly Rep 2005;54:1212-1214.
157. Watson JC, Pearson JA, Markowitz LE, et al. An evaluation of measles revaccination among school-entry-aged children. Pediatrics 1996;97:613-618.
158. Weibel RE, Villarejos VM, Klein EB, et al. Clinical and laboratory studies of live attenuated RA 27/3 and HPV 77-DE rubella virus vaccines. Proc Soc Exp Biol Med 1980;165:44-49.
159. Balfour HH Jr, Groth KE, Edelman CK. RA27/3 rubella vaccine: a four-year follow-up. Am J Dis Child 1980;134:350-353.
160. Maes EF, Stehr-Green PA, Steward SS, et al. Rubella antibody persistence 20 years after immunization. *In* Program and abstracts of the 31st Interscience Congress on Antimicrobial Agents and Chemotherapy. Washington, DC: American Society for Microbiology, 1991.
161. Bilukha OO, Rosenstein N. Prevention and control of meningococcal disease: recommendations of the Advisory Committee on Immunization Practices (ACIP). MMWR Recomm Rep 2005;54(RR-7):1-21.
162. Gardner P. Clinical Practice: Prevention of meningococcal disease. N Engl J Med 2006;355:1466-1473.
163. Centers for Disease Control and Prevention. Prevention of pneumococcal disease: recommendations of the Advisory Committee on Immunization Practices (ACIP). MMWR Morb Mortal Wkly Rep 1997;46:1-24.
164. Robbins JB, Austrian R, Lee CJ, et al. Considerations for formulating the second-generation pneumococcal capsular polysaccharide vaccine with emphasis on the cross-reactive types within groups. J Infect Dis 1983;148:1136-1159.
165. Butler JC, Breiman RF, Campbell JF, et al. Pneumococcal polysaccharide vaccine efficacy: an evaluation of current recommendations. JAMA 1993;270:1826-1831.
166. Overturf GD; American Academy of Pediatrics, Committee on Infectious Diseases. Technical Report: Prevention of pneumococcal infections, including the use of pneumococcal conjugate and polysaccharide vaccines and antibiotic prophylaxis. Pediatrics 2000;106(2 Pt 1):367-376.
167. Centers for Disease Control and Prevention. Preventing pneumococcal disease among infants and young children: recommendations of the Advisory Committee on Immunization Practices (ACIP). MMWR Morb Mortal Wkly Rep 2000;49:1-38.
168. Musher DM, Luchi MJ, Watson DA, et al. Pneumococcal polysaccharide vaccine in young adults and older bronchitics: determination of IgG responses by ELISA and the effect of adsorption of serum with non-type-specific cell wall polysaccharide. J Infect Dis 1990;161:728-735.
169. Black S, Shinefield H, Fireman B, et al. Efficacy, safety and immunogenicity of heptavalent pneumococcal conjugate vaccine in children. Pediatr Infect Dis 2000;19:187-195.
170. Rennels MB, Edwards KM, Keyserling HL, et al. Safety and immunogenicity of heptavalent pneumococcal vaccine conjugated to CRM197 in United States infants. Pediatrics 1998;101(4 Pt 1):604-611.
171. Shinefield HR, Black S, Ray P, et al. Safety and immunogenicity of heptavalent pneumococcal CRM_{197} conjugate vaccine in infants and toddlers. Pediatr Infect Dis J 1999;18:757-763.
172. Centers for Disease Control and Prevention. Direct and indirect effects of routine vaccination of children with 7-valent pneumococcal conjugate vaccine on incidence of invasive pneumococcal disease—United States, 1998-2003. MMWR Morb Mortal Wkly Rep 2005;54:893-897.
173. Centers for Disease Control and Prevention. Poliomyelitis prevention in the United States: introduction of a sequential vaccination schedule of inactivated poliovirus vaccine followed by oral poliovirus vaccine. Recommendations of the Advisory Committee on Immunization Practices (ACIP). MMWR Recomm Rep 1997;46(RR-3):1-25.
174. Hull HF, Ward NA, Hull BP, et al. Paralytic poliomyelitis: seasoned strategies, disappearing disease. Lancet 1994;343:1331-1337.
175. Prevots DR, Burr RK, Sutter RW, et al. Poliomyelitis prevention in the United States: updated recommendations of the Advisory Committee on Immunization Practices (ACIP). MMWR Recomm Rep 2000;49(RR-5):1-22.
176. Faden H, Duffy L, Sun M, et al. Long-term immunity to poliovirus in children immunized with live attenuated and enhanced-potency inactivated trivalent poliovirus vaccines. J Infect Dis 1993;168:452-454.
177. Robertson SE, Traverso HP, Drucker JA, et al. Clinical efficacy of a new, enhanced-potency, inactivated poliovirus vaccine. Lancet 1988;1:897-899.
178. Onorato IM, Modlin JF, McBean AM, et al. Mucosal immunity induced by enhance-potency inactivated and oral polio vaccines. J Infect Dis 1991;163:1-6.
179. Parashar UD, Alexander JP, Glass RI. Prevention of rotavirus gastroenteritis among infants and children: recommendations of the Advisory Committee on Immunization Practices (ACIP). MMWR Recomm Rep 2006;55(RR-12):1-13.
180. Vesikari T, Matson DO, Dennehy P, et al. Safety and efficacy of a pentavalent human-bovine (WC3) reassortant rotavirus vaccine. N Engl J Med 2006;354:23-33.
181. Rotz LD, Dotson DA, Damon IK, et al. Vaccinia (smallpox) vaccine: recommendations of the Advisory Committee on Immunization Practices (ACIP), 2001. MMWR Recomm Rep 2001;50(RR-10):1-25.
182. Halsell JS, Riddle JR, Atwood JE, et al. Myopericarditis following smallpox vaccination among vaccinia-naive US military personnel. JAMA 2003;289:3283-3289.
183. Poland GA, Grabenstein JD, Neff JM. The US smallpox vaccination program: a review of a large modern era smallpox vaccination implementation program. Vaccine 2005;23:2078-2081.
184. Kretsinger K, Broder KR, Cortese MM, et al. Preventing tetanus, diphtheria, and pertussis among adults: use of tetanus toxoid, reduced diphtheria toxoid and acellular pertussis vaccine: recommendations of the Advisory Committee on Immunization Practices (ACIP), and recommendation of ACIP, supported by the Healthcare Infection Control Practices Advisory Committee (HICPAC), for use of Tdap among health-care personnel. MMWR Recomm Rep 2006;55(RR-17):1-37.
185. Pascual FB, McGinley EL, Zanardi LR, et al. Tetanus surveillance—United States, 1998-2000. Mor Mortal Wkly Rep CDC Surveill Summ 2003;52:1-8.
186. Centers for Disease Control and Prevention. Diphtheria, tetanus, and pertussis: recommendations for vaccine use and other preventive measures. Recommendations of the Immunization Practices Advisory Committee (ACIP). MMWR Recomm Rep 1991;40(RR-10):1-28.
187. Centers for Disease Control and Prevention. Use of diphtheria toxoid-tetanus toxoid-acellular pertussis vaccine as a five-dose series: supplemental recommendations of the Advisory Committee on Immunization Practices (ACIP). MMWR Recomm Rep 2000;49(RR-13):1-8.
188. Pichichero ME, Casey JR. Acellular pertussis vaccines for adolescents. Pediatr Infect Dis J 2005;24(6 Suppl):S117-S126.

189. Rothstein EP, Anderson EL, Decker MD, et al. An acellular pertussis vaccine in healthy adults: safety and immunogenicity. Pennridge Pediatric Associates. Vaccine 1999;17:2999-3006.
190. Centers for Disease Control and Prevention. Typhoid immunization: recommendations of the Immunization Practices Advisory Committee (ACIP). MMWR Recomm Rep 1990;39(RR-10):1-5.
191. Centers for Disease Control and Prevention. Prevention of varicella: recommendations of the Advisory Committee on Immunization Practices (ACIP). MMWR Morb Mortal Wkly Rep 1996;45:1-27.
192. Centers for Disease Control and Prevention. Prevention of varicella: updated recommendations of the Advisory Committee on Immunization Practices (ACIP). MMWR Morb Mortal Wkly Rep 1999;48:1-5.
193. Centers for Disease Control and Prevention. Press Release: Advisory Committee recommends "shingles" vaccination. Atlanta: Centers for Disease Control and Prevention, October 26, 2006.
194. Vazquez M, LaRussa PS, Gershon AA, et al. Effectiveness over time of varicella vaccine. JAMA 2004;291:851-855.
195. Vazquez M, Shapiro ED. Varicella vaccine and infection with varicella-zoster virus. N Engl J Med 2005;352:439-440.
196. Oxman MN, Levin MJ, Johnson GR, et al. A vaccine to prevent herpes zoster and postherpetic neuralgia in older adults. N Engl J Med 2005;352:2271-2284.
197. Kuter BJ, Weibel RE, Guess HA, et al. Oka/Merck varicella vaccine in healthy children: final report of a 2-year efficacy study and 7-year follow-up studies. Vaccine 1991;9:643-647.
198. Weibel RE, Neff BJ, Kuter BJ, et al. Live attenuated varicella virus vaccine: efficacy trial in healthy children. N Engl J Med 1984;310:1409-1415.
199. Centers for Disease Control and Prevention. Yellow fever vaccine: recommendations of the Immunization Practices Advisory Committee (ACIP). MMWR Morb Mortal Wkly Rep 1990;39:1-6.
200. Monath TP, Nichols R, Archambault WT, et al. Comparative safety and immunogenicity of two yellow fever 17D vaccines (ARILVAX and YF-VAX) in a Phase III multicenter, double-blind clinical trial. Am J Trop Med Hyg 2002;66:533-541.
201. Atkinson WL, Pickering LK, Schwartz B, et al. General recommendations on immunization: recommendations of the Advisory Committee on Immunization Practices (ACIP) and the American Academy of Family Physicians (AAFP). MMWR Recomm Rep 2002;51(RR-2):1-35.
202. Centers for Disease Control and Prevention. Guide to Contraindications to Vaccinations. 2006. Available at *http://www.cdc.gov/vaccines/recs/vac-admin/contraindications.htm*
203. Ball LK, Ball R, Pratt RD. An assessment of thimerosal use in childhood vaccines. Pediatrics 2001;107:1147-1154.
204. Webster RG. Immunity to influenza in the elderly. Vaccine 2000;18:1686-1689.
205. Burns EA. Effects of aging on immune function. J Nutr Health Aging 2004;8:9-18.
206. Kudlacek S, Jahandideh-Kazempour S, Graninger W, et al. Differential expression of various T cell surface markers in young and elderly subjects. Immunobiology 1995;192:198-204.
207. Effros RB, Pawelec G. Replicative senescence of T cells: does the Hayflick Limit lead to immune exhaustion? Immunol Today 1997;18:450-454.
208. Effros RB, Boucher N, Porter V, et al. Decline in CD28+ T cells in centenarians and in long-term T cell cultures: a possible cause for both in vivo and in vitro immunosenescence. Exp Gerontol 1994;29:601-609.
209. Posnett DN, Edinger JW, Manavalan JS, et al. Differentiation of human CD8 T cells: implications for in vivo persistence of CD8+. Int Immunol 1999;11:229-241.
210. Monteiro J, Batliwalla F, Ostrer H, et al. Shortened telomeres in clonally expanded CD28-CD8+ T cells imply a replicative history that is distinct from their CD28+CD8+ counterparts. J Immunol 1996;156:3587-3590.
211. Effros RB, Dagarag M, Spaulding C, et al. The role of CD8+ T-cell replicative senescence in human aging. Immunol Rev 2005;205:147-157.
212. Franceschi C, Valensin S, Fagnoni F, et al. Biomarkers of immunosenescence within an evolutionary perspective: the challenge of heterogeneity and the role of antigenic load. Exp Gerontol 1999;34:911-921.
213. Targonski PV, Peterson LG, Stansroud M, et al. Risk of respiratory infection in elderly persons with diminished white blood cell telomerase levels [Abstract]. Gerontologist 2006;46(SI 1).
214. McElhaney JE, Xie D, Hager WD, et al. T cell responses are better correlates of vaccine protection in the elderly. J Immunol 2006;176:6333-6339.
215. Jacobson RM. Vaccine safety. Immunol Allergy Clin North Am 2003;23:589-603.
216. Jacobson RM, Zabel KS, Poland GA. The challenge of vaccine safety. Semin Pediatr Infect Dis 2002;13:215-220.
217. Gangarosa EJ, Galazka AM, Wolfe CR, et al. Impact of anti-vaccine movements on pertussis control: the untold story. Lancet 1998;351:356-361.
218. Jonville-Bera AP, Autret-Leca E, Barbeillon F, et al. Sudden unexpected death in infants under 3 months of age and vaccination status—a case-control study. Br J Clin Pharmacol 2001;51:271-276.
219. Griffin MR, Ray WA, Livengood JR, et al. Risk of sudden infant death syndrome after immunization with the diphtheria-tetanus-pertussis vaccine. N Engl J Med 1988;319:618-623.
220. Flahault A, Messiah A, Jougla E, et al. Sudden infant death syndrome and diphtheria/tetanus toxoid/pertussis/poliomyelitis immunisation. Lancet 1988;1:582-583.
221. Mitchell EA, Stewart AW, Clements M. Immunisation and the sudden infant death syndrome. New Zealand Cot Death Study Group. Arch Dis Child 1995;73:498-501.
222. American Academy of Pediatrics, Committee on Infectious Diseases. The relationship between pertussis vaccine and central nervous system sequelae: continuing assessment. Pediatrics 1996;97:279-281.
223. Centers for Disease Control and Prevention. Update: vaccine side effects, adverse reactions, contraindications, and precautions. Recommendations of the Advisory Committee on Immunization Practices (ACIP). MMWR Recomm Rep 1996;45(RR-12):1-35.
224. Dittmann S. Special address: safety of hepatitis B vaccination. Vaccine 2000; 18(Suppl 1).
225. Stratton K, Almario DA, McCormick MC, for the Immunization Safety Review Committee, Board on Health Promotion and Disease Prevention. Immunization Safety Review: Hepatitis B Vaccine and Demyelinating Neurological Disorders. Washington, DC: The National Academies Press, 2002.
226. Duclos P. Safety of immunisation and adverse events following vaccination against hepatitis B. Expert Opin Drug Saf 2003;2:225-231.
227. Sadovnick AD, Scheifele DW. School-based hepatitis B vaccination programme and adolescent multiple sclerosis. Lancet 2000;355:550.
228. Halsey NA, Duclos P, Van Damme P, et al, for the Viral Hepatitis Prevention Board. Hepatitis B vaccine and central nervous system demyelinating diseases. Pediatr Infect Dis J 1999;18:23-24.
229. Ascherio A, Zhang SM, Hernán MA, et al. Hepatitis B vaccination and the risk of multiple sclerosis. N Engl J Med 2001;344:327-332.
230. Casiday R, Cresswell T, Wilson D, et al. A survey of UK parental attitudes to the MMR vaccine and trust in medical authority. Vaccine 2006;24:177-184.
231. Institute of Medicine. Immunization Safety Review: Vaccines and Autism. Washington, DC: National Academies Press, 2006.
232. Farrington CP, Miller E, Taylor B. MMR and autism: further evidence against a causal association. Vaccine 2001;19:3632-3635.
233. Madsen KM, Hviid A, Vestergaard M, et al. A population-based study of measles, mumps, and rubella vaccination and autism. N Engl J Med 2002;347:1477-1482.
234. Kastner JL, Gellin BG. Measles-mumps-rubella vaccine and autism: the rise (and fall?) of a hypothesis. Pediatr Ann 2001;30:408-415.
235. Dales L, Hammer SJ, Smith NJ. Time trends in autism and in MMR immunization coverage in California. JAMA 2001;285:1183-1185.
236. Taylor B, Miller E, Farrington CP, et al. Autism and measles, mumps, and rubella vaccine: no epidemiological evidence for a causal association. Lancet 1999;353:2026-2029.
237. Wilson K, Mills E, Ross C, et al. Association of autistic spectrum disorder and the measles, mumps, and rubella vaccine: a systematic review of current epidemiological evidence. Arch Pediatr Adolesc Med 2003;157:628-634.
238. Hviid A, Stellfeld M, Wohlfahrt J, et al. Association between thimerosal-containing vaccine and autism. JAMA 2003;290:1763-1766.
239. Madsen KM, Lauritsen MB, Pedersen CB, et al. Thimerosal and the occurrence of autism: negative ecological evidence from Danish population-based data. Pediatrics 2003;112(3 Pt 1):604-606.
240. Nkowane BM, Wassilak SGF, Orenstein WA, et al. Vaccine-associated paralytic poliomyelitis, United States: 1973 through 1984. JAMA 1987;257:1335-1340.
241. Querfurth H, Swanson PD. Vaccine-associated paralytic poliomyelitis: regional case series and review. Arch Neurol 1994;47:541-544.
242. Wattigney WA, Mootrey GT, Braun MM, et al. Surveillance for poliovirus vaccine adverse events, 1991 to 1998: impact of a sequential vaccination schedule of inactivated poliovirus vaccine followed by oral poliovirus vaccine. Pediatrics 2001;107:E83.
243. Jacobson RM, Adegbenro A, Pankratz VS, et al. Adverse events and vaccination—the lack of power and predictability of infrequent events in pre-licensure study. Vaccine 2001;19:2428-2433.
244. Jacobson RM, Poland GA. Sample sizes and negative studies in clinical vaccine research. Vaccine 2005;23:2318-2321.
245. Chen RT. Vaccine risks: real, perceived and unknown. Vaccine 1999;17:S41-S46.
246. Chen RT. Safety of vaccines. *In* Plotkin SA, Orenstein WA (eds): Vaccines, 3rd ed. Philadelphia: WB Saunders, 1999, pp 1144-1163.
247. Ward BJ. Vaccine adverse events in the new millennium: is there reason for concern? Bull World Health Organ 2000;78:205.
248. Chen RT, DeStefano F, Pless R, et al. Challenges and controversies in immunization safety. Infect Dis Clin North Am 2001;15:21-39.
249. Jacobson RM, Zabel KS, Poland GA. The overall safety profile of currently available vaccines directed against infectious diseases. Expert Opin Drug Saf 2003;2:215-223.
250. Grabenstein JD. Anthrax vaccine: a review. Immunol Allergy Clin North Am 2003;23:713-730.
251. Sever JL, Brenner AI, Gale AD, et al. Safety of anthrax vaccine: a review by the Anthrax Vaccine Expert Committee (AVEC) of adverse events reported to the Vaccine Adverse Event Reporting System (VAERS). Pharmacoepidemiol Drug Safety 2002;11:189-202.
252. Gross PA, Hermogenes AW, Sacks HS, et al. The efficacy of influenza vaccine in elderly persons: a meta-analysis and review of the literature. Ann Intern Med 1995;123:518-527.
253. Centers for Disease Control and Prevention. 2006-07 Influenza prevention & control recommendations: comparison of live, attenuated influenza vaccine (LAIV) with inactivated influenza vaccine. MMWR Recomm Rep 2006;55(RR10):1-42
254. Johnson CE, Stancin T, Fattlar D, et al. A long-term prospective study of varicella vaccine in healthy children. Pediatrics 1997;100:761-766.
255. Brisson M, Edmunds WJ, Gay NJ, et al. Analysis of varicella vaccine breakthrough rates: implications for the effectiveness of immunisation programmes. Vaccine 2000;18:2775-2778.
256. Davis MM, Patel MS, Gebremariam A. Decline in varicella-related hospitalizations and expenditures for children and adults after introduction of varicella vaccine in the United States. Pediatrics 2004;114:786-792.
257. Izurieta HS, Strebel PM, Blake PA. Postlicensure effectiveness of varicella vaccine during an outbreak in a child care center. JAMA 1997;278:1495-1499.

258. Clements DA, Armstrong CB, Ursano AM, et al. Over five-year follow-up of Oka/Merck varicella vaccine recipients in 465 infants and adolescents. Pediatr Infect Dis J 1995;14:874-879.
259. Bernstein HH, Rothstein EP, Watson BM, et al. Clinical survey of natural varicella compared with breakthrough varicella after immunization with live attenuated Oka/Merck varicella vaccine. Pediatrics 1993;92:833-837.
260. Galil K, Lee B, Strine T, et al. Outbreak of varicella at a day-care center despite vaccination. N Engl J Med 2002;347:1909-1915.
261. Zhou W, Pool V, Iskander JK, et al. Surveillance for safety after immunization: Vaccine Adverse Event Reporting System (VAERS)—United States, 1991-2001. MMWR Morb Mortal Wkly Rep 2003;52:1-24.
262. Chen RT, Rastogi SC, Mullen JR, et al. The Vaccine Adverse Event Reporting System (VAERS). Vaccine 1994;12:542-550.
263. Iskander JK, Miller ER, Pless RP, et al. Vaccine Safety Post-Marketing Surveillance: The Vaccine Adverse Event Reporting System. Atlanta: Centers for Disease Control and Prevention, National Immunization Program, Epidemiology and Surveillance Division, Vaccine Safety and Development Activity, 2004.
264. Safranek TJ, Lawrence DN, Kurland LT, et al. Reassessment of the association between Guillain-Barré syndrome and receipt of swine influenza vaccine in 1976-1977: results of a two-state study. Am J Epidemiol 1991;133:940-951.
265. Hughes RA, Charlton J, Latinovic R, et al. No association between immunization and Guillain-Barre syndrome in the United Kingdom, 1992 to 2000. Arch Intern Med 2006;166:1301-1304.
266. Lasky T, Terracciano GJ, Magder L, et al. The Guillain-Barré syndrome and the 1992-1993 and 1993-1994 influenza vaccines. N Engl J Med 1998;339:1797-1802.
267. Gregson AL, Edelman R. Does antigenic overload exist? The role of multiple immunizations in infants. Immunol Allergy Clin North Am 2003;23:649-664.
268. Zhang J. Clinical observations in ethyl mercury chloride poisoning. Am J Ind Med 1984;5:251-258.
269. Clarkson TW. The pharmacology of mercury compounds. Annu Rev Pharmacol 1972;12:375-406.
270. Pichichero ME, Cernichiari E, Lopreiato J, et al. Mercury concentrations and metabolism in infants receiving vaccines containing thiomersal: a descriptive study. Lancet 2002;360:1737-1741.
271. Thimerosal in vaccines: a joint statement of the American Academy of Pediatrics and the Public Health Service. MMWR Morb Mortal Wkly Rep 1999;48:563-565.
272. Stratton K, Gable A, McCormick M. Immunization Safety Review: Thimerosal-Containing Vaccines and Neurodevelopmental Disorders. Immunization Safety Review Committee, Board on Health Promotion and Disease Prevention. Washington, DC: National Academies Press, 2001.
273. Immunization Safety Review Committee. Immunization Safety Review: Vaccines and Autism. Washington, DC: National Academies Press, 2004.
274. Parker SK, Schwartz B, Todd J, et al. Thimerosal-containing vaccines and autistic spectrum disorder: a critical review of published original data. Pediatrics 2004;114:793-804.
275. U.S. Food and Drug Administration. Thimerosal in vaccines: Table 3. Thimerosal and expanded list of vaccines. 2007. Available at *http://www.fda.gov/cber/vaccine/thimerosal htm#t3*
276. Poland GA. If you could halve the mortality rate, would you do it? Clin Infect Dis 2002;35:378-380.
277. U.S. Department of Health and Human Services. Healthy People 2010 Immunization Goals. Rockville, MD: U.S. Department of Health and Human Services, 2000.
278. Bratzler DW, Houck PM, Jiang H, et al. Failure to vaccinate Medicare inpatients: a missed opportunity. Arch Intern Med 2002;162:2349-2356.
279. Bridges CB, Fukuda K, Cox NJ, et al. Prevention and control of influenza: recommendations of the Advisory Committee on Immunization Practices (ACIP). MMWR Recomm Rep 2001;50(RR-4):1-44.
280. Centers for Disease Control and Prevention. Estimates of influenza vaccination target population sizes in 2006 and recent vaccine uptake levels. July 17, 2006. Available at *http://www.cdc.gov/flu/professionals/vaccination/pdf/targetpopchart.pdf*
281. van Essen GA, Kuyvenhoven MM, de Melker RA. Why do healthy elderly people fail to comply with influenza vaccination? Age Ageing 1997;26:275-279.
282. Centers for Disease Control and Prevention. Adult immunization: knowledge, attitudes, and practices—DeKalb and Fulton Counties, Georgia, 1988. MMWR Morb Mortal Wkly Rep 1988;37:657-661.
283. Fishbein DB, Fontanesi J, Kopald D, et al. Why do not patients receive influenza vaccine in December and January? Vaccine 2006;24:798-802.
284. Tierney CD, Yusuf H, McMahon SR, et al. Adoption of reminder and recall messages for immunizations by pediatricians and public health clinics. Pediatrics 2003;112:1076-1082.
285. Centers for Disease Control and Prevention. Immunization information system progress—United States, 2003. MMWR Morb Mortal Wkly Rep 2005;54:722-724.
286. Gyorkos TW, Tannenbaum TN, Abrahamowicz M, et al. Evaluation of the effectiveness of immunization delivery methods. Can J Public Health 1994;85(Suppl 1):S14-S30.
287. Shefer A, McKibben L, Bardenheier B, et al. Characteristics of long-term care facilities associated with standing order programs to deliver influenza and pneumococcal vaccinations to residents in 13 states. J Am Med Dir Assoc 2005;6:97-104.
288. deHart MP, Salinas SK, Barnette LJ Jr, et al. Project Protect: pneumococcal vaccination in Washington State nursing homes. J Am Med Dir Assoc 2005;6:91-96.
289. Dexter PR, Perkins SM, Maharry KS, et al. Inpatient computer-based standing orders vs physician reminders to increase influenza and pneumococcal vaccination rates: a randomized trial. JAMA 2004;292:2366-2371.
290. Lindenauer PK, Behal R, Murray CK, et al. Volume, quality of care, and outcome in pneumonia. Ann Intern Med 2006;144:262-269.
291. Centers for Disease Control and Prevention. Vaccines & Immunization web site. 2006. Available at *http://www.cdc.gov/vaccines/recs/reminder-sys.htm*
292. Fiscella K, Franks P, Gold MR, et al. Inequality in quality: addressing socioeconomic, racial, and ethnic disparities in health care. JAMA 2000;283:2579-2584.
293. Gornick ME, Eggers PW, Reilly TW, et al. Effects of race and income on mortality and use of services among Medicare beneficiaries. N Engl J Med 1996;335:791-799.
294. O'Malley AS, Forrest CB. Immunization disparities in older Americans: determinants and future research needs. Am J Prev Med 2006;31:150-158.
295. Centers for Disease Control and Prevention. Health objectives for the nation: race-specific differences in influenza vaccination levels among Medicare beneficiaries—United States. MMWR Morb Mortal Wkly Rep 1995;44:24-27, 33.
296. Schneider EC, Cleary PD, Zaslavsky AM, et al. Racial disparity in influenza vaccination: does managed care narrow the gap between African Americans and whites? JAMA 2001;286:1455-1460.
297. Nuorti JP, Butler JC, Farley MM, et al. Cigarette smoking and invasive pneumococcal disease. N Engl J Med 2000;342:681-689.
298. Arcavi L, Benowitz NL. Cigarette smoking and infection. Arch Intern Med 2004;164:2206-2216.
299. Murin S, Bilello KS. Respiratory tract infections: another reason not to smoke. Cleve Clin J Med 2005;72:916-920.

92

TRANSPLANT MEDICINE

Mark Chaballa, Joanne Filicko-O'Hara, Dorothy Holt, Adam M. Frank, John L. Wagner, Dolores Grosso, and Neal Flomenberg

INTRODUCTION 1269
Tissue Sources Used for Transplantation 1269
Transplantation Antigens and Transplantation Immunology 1269
Graft Rejection and Graft-Versus-Host Disease 1270
Inducing Tolerance 1271
Cellular and Molecular Events in T-Cell Activation—Targets for Interventions to Prevent the Development of Alloresponses 1271
CLINICAL OVERVIEW 1272
Clinical Goals for Transplantation 1272
Solid Organ Transplantation 1273
Hematopoietic Stem Cell Transplantation 1274
Prevention of Rejection 1274
GVHD Prophylaxis 1275
GVHD Treatment 1275
Infection 1275
THERAPEUTICS AND CLINICAL PHARMACOLOGY 1275
Specific Agents and Modalities Used to Control Alloresponses 1275
Corticosteroids 1275
Cyclosporine 1276
Tacrolimus 1278
Sirolimus 1279
Mycophenolic Acid 1279
Antithymocyte Globulin (Equine) 1281
Antithymocyte Globulin (Rabbit) 1281
Muromonab-CD3 1282
Alemtuzumab 1282
Daclizumab 1283
Basiliximab 1283
Denileukin Diftitox 1283
Azathioprine 1284
Methotrexate 1284
Cyclophosphamide 1285
Purine Nucleoside Analogues 1285
Rituximab 1286
Immune Globulin 1286
Extracorporeal Photoimmune Therapy 1286
T-Cell Depletion 1287
Tumor Necrosis Factor-α Inhibitors 1287
Thalidomide 1287
Total Lymphoid Irradiation 1287
Leflunomide 1287
Belatacept 1288
Investigational Agents 1288
Future Directions 1288

INTRODUCTION

Transplantation of organs or tissues into a genetically distinct recipient triggers the activation of the host's immune system as well as activation of any donor lymphocytes deliberately or inadvertently introduced into the recipient as part of the transplant procedure. In the solid organ transplantation field, the primary immunologic issue of clinical significance is graft rejection mediated by host lymphocytes toward the transplanted organ (host-versus-graft response). In the case of hematopoietic stem cell transplantation (HSCT) using either marrow- or peripheral blood–derived hematopoietic progenitor cells, graft rejection can occur, but the more significant clinical problem is graft-versus-host disease (GVHD) mediated by donor-derived lymphocytes immunologically attacking the host. Graft rejection and GVHD represent a diversion of the immune system from its primary function of protecting the host against infection. Transplantation outcome is limited primarily by the incidence and severity of these problems and by the interventions required to try to prevent them, the subjects of this chapter.

Tissue Sources Used for Transplantation

The immunologic nature of graft rejection and GVHD is illustrated by experiments using alternate tissue sources. Transplants can be categorized based on the source of the transplanted tissue or organ. Autologous or "self" tissues can be utilized for a variety of purposes in which the tissues are harvested and utilized at remote sites (e.g., blood vessels and tendons) or utilized to repopulate the same target sites at a later time (autologous HSCT). Autologous tissues do not stimulate rejection episodes or cause classical GVHD. Failure of an autologous graft is usually related to damage to the organ or tissue during harvest or storage or to surgical or procedural complications, but not to rejection or GVHD. In animal models, tissues derived from inbred strains will be genetically identical with the exception of the products of genes encoded on the sex chromosomes. Such genetically identical tissues from a distinct donor are known as syngeneic or isogeneic tissues. In humans, syngeneic tissues can be obtained only for those rare individuals who have an identical twin. Syngeneic or isogeneic tissues behave like autologous tissues in that they do not lead to classical rejection episodes or GVHD. Transplants from genetically distinct donors are known as allogeneic transplants. These make up the overwhelming majority of solid organ transplants and about one third of hematopoietic stem cell (HSC) or marrow transplants. It is in the setting of an allograft that rejection and GVHD become problematic.

Transplantation Antigens and Transplantation Immunology

The mechanisms underlying graft rejection and GVHD are complex, including elements of innate as well as humoral and cellular adaptive immunity. Consequently, some aspects of alloresponses are highly specific, while others are nonspecific. Nonetheless, T lymphocytes represent the most problematic effector cell population mediating rejection and GVHD and, consequently, most efforts attempting to overcome these problems are focused on the T cell.

Antigenic determinants leading to graft rejection or GVHD can be classified as major or minor transplantation antigens. In mice, over 30 different loci triggering graft rejection have been demonstrated. These were designated as H or histocompatibility (tissue compatibility) loci and were sequentially numbered as they were identified.[1] Depending on the strength of the response evoked by disparity for a particular transplantation antigen, the kinetics of rejection can be more or less rapid. Mismatches for gene products of the H-2 complex led to the most rapid rejection events, and this gene complex thus became known as the major histocompatibility complex (MHC). The numerous other loci leading to rejection events in murine transplantation became known as minor transplantation antigens. These antigens produced much slower rejection events unless transplantation was performed across multiple minor antigen barriers. In humans, the MHC complex gene products are known as human leukocyte antigens (HLA).

The difference between major and minor transplantation antigens and their function as transplantation antigens is based on normal T-cell physiology. T lymphocytes respond to small antigenic peptide fragments presented by MHC molecules. MHC molecules have a groove on their surface, composed of a beta pleated sheet on the bottom and two alpha helices on the sides, in which the peptide fragments bind.[2,3] T cells interact, through their clonally unique receptors, with the peptide as well as portions of the adjacent MHC molecule, particularly the alpha helices.[4,5] Polymorphisms in MHC molecules lead to a different array of peptides binding to each distinct MHC molecule for presentation to T lymphocytes. Even if the same peptide is presented by different MHC molecules, differences in the MHC products may cause the peptide to be presented in conformationally distinct ways. These conformational differences or differences in the adjacent alpha helices of the MHC molecule may be recognized by T lymphocytes, leading to their activation.[6-8]

Two distinct forms of MHC molecules participate in presenting peptide antigens to T lymphocytes. Class I MHC molecules (HLA-A, -B, and -C or H-2 K, D, and L) consist of a larger alpha chain and a smaller invariant molecule, β_2-microglobulin, which is not encoded in the MHC region. These molecules typically present peptides of 8 to 10 amino acids derived from catabolism of endogenously produced proteins to CD8$^+$ T cells, though mechanisms for processing and presentation of internalized antigens also exist.[9,10] Class II MHC molecules (HLA-DR, -DQ, and -DP or H-2 IA and IE) consist of two peptide chains both of which are encoded within the MHC. These molecules typically present CD4$^+$ T cells with peptides of 8 to 15 amino acids derived primarily from exogenously produced proteins that are taken up and catabolized within the cell.[11,12] MHC class I molecules are fairly ubiquitously expressed on nucleated cells throughout the body, though levels of expression may vary. In contrast, MHC class II molecules have a narrower expression pattern, and are normally expressed on dendritic cells, monocytes, and B cells. However, after exposure to interferon-γ, MHC class II expression can be induced on many other somatic cells and MHC class I expression can be increased above basal levels. In the setting of allograft rejection, interferon-γ can thus boost MHC I and II expression on the allograft parenchyma and increase expression of MHC class II molecules on the organ's vascular endothelium, stimulating allorecognition and increasing target antigen expression.

During their maturation in the thymus, T cells undergo both positive and negative selection to produce a T-cell repertoire that is tolerant toward self peptide-MHC complexes so as to avoid autoimmunity yet be able to respond to foreign peptide-self MHC complexes.[13,14] Teleologically, one can think of the T-cell system as constantly sampling the peptides produced by normal cellular catabolism via their cell surface coexpression with MHC molecules. So long as the cell is healthy, the proteins are produced, and thus the peptide array will remain relatively constant and the T lymphocytes remain inactive. In contrast, in the setting of infection, peptides derived from the pathogen may compete with self peptides for MHC binding. These complexes of "non-self" peptides and self MHC molecules lead subsets of T cells to become activated in an effort to eliminate the infected population of cells.

Introduction of a genetically distinct tissue into the body triggers T-cell activation in a number of ways. Minor transplantation antigens are now understood to be natural polymorphisms in cellular or circulating proteins that lead to polymorphisms in one or at most a small number of distinct peptides that can be presented by MHC molecules, thus triggering an immune response.[15,16] In contrast, when MHC polymorphisms are introduced, the system becomes more complex with multiple potential mechanisms for immunologic activation. Expression of a different set of MHC molecules allows a different set of both donor and host peptides to be presented. Even self peptides to which the host is tolerant when presented by self MHC molecules may now be presented in conformationally distinct ways by donor MHC molecules, which may lead to activation of host T cells. Additionally, MHC and all other polymorphic allogeneic proteins from the transplanted cells have the potential to be catabolized and presented by self MHC molecules. Transplantation across an MHC difference thus can lead to activation of a larger number of T cells (up to 10% of the total T-cell repertoire) and a more rapid, vigorous immune response. For minor antigens to provoke a response of comparable magnitude, it would be necessary to transplant across multiple minor antigens rather than one.

Both donor and host antigen-presenting cells (APCs) can thus trigger an immune response to the transplanted organ. APCs of donor origin, such as interstitial dendritic cells, when transferred along with the graft, can directly activate host T cells in what is known as the direct pathway of allorecognition. In addition, host APCs in draining lymph nodes can take up and process shed protein antigens, leading to activation of host T cells through the indirect pathway of allorecognition.[17] While both pathways are important, the direct pathway can provide a stronger, more immediate stimulus, illustrating the importance of donor APCs in triggering alloresponses.

In the vast majority of transplant scenarios, better matching for the MHC is preferred when possible. The impact of MHC mismatching varies from organ to organ, with the biggest impact seen in HSCT, where the immune system itself is effectively being transplanted along with the hematopoietic progenitor cells. In contrast to solid organ transplantation, transplantation of completely MHC-mismatched HSC grafts is not feasible, and transplantation of even half-matched grafts (haploidentical transplantation) is conducted only in investigational settings.

Once activated, T cells may mediate their damage in a number of ways, including direct cytolytic damage or secretion of toxic cytokines such as tumor necrosis factor (TNF). The inflammatory milieu created by the cytokines released by T cells and other cells, such as dendritic cells or macrophages, can modulate the strength of the response. Interleukin (IL)–2 produced by T helper cells will be necessary for the activation and expansion of effector T cells. Interferon-γ induces MHC expression, increases APC activity, activates natural killer (NK) cells, and, together with lymphotoxin, activates macrophages. Interferon-γ can increase MHC I and II expression on the allograft parenchyma and increase expression of MHC class II molecules on the organ's vascular endothelium, stimulating allorecognition and increasing target antigen expression. Interferon-γ and lymphotoxin also increase adhesion molecules on vascular endothelium, which facilitates leukocyte entry into the transplanted organ.

In addition to T-cell–mediated damage to the target organ, other effector mechanisms can participate in alloresponses. T-cell–derived cytokines can recruit and activate antigen-independent cellular effector populations such as macrophages or NK cells and can provide help to antigen-specific B cells in generating a humoral response to the transplanted organ. Preexisting antibodies generated as a consequence of prior transplantation, transfusion, or fetal maternal blood exchanged during labor and delivery can bind to allogeneic tissues and lead to humoral-mediated immunologic injury. T cells, however, are important in the generation of these responses as well, and their central role in rejection and GVHD has strong experimental support. Rejection is not seen in mice lacking functional T cells due to either being congenitally athymic, neonatally thymectomized, or undergoing adult thymectomy and T-cell–depleted marrow transplantation. Introduction of T cells into such animals restores their ability to trigger rejection and GVHD, implying that T cells are necessary though not ruling out roles for antibody or other cellular populations in these pathophysiologic events.[18]

Graft Rejection and Graft-Versus-Host Disease

In virtually all transplantation scenarios, some donor lymphocytes will be introduced into the host along with the transplanted tissue or organ. In an immunologically intact recipient, the number of donor immune cells is usually tiny compared to the number of cells in the host's immune system. Therefore, although both donor antihost and host antidonor immune responses may be set in motion, the much smaller population of donor immune cells is eliminated by the host's immune system as described previously. If the recipient is immunologically vulnerable and/or the number of donor immune cells introduced is large, however, then the donor's immune system can become predominant. Instead of a host-versus-graft (rejection) response evolving, the reciprocal process, GVHD, can develop. Donor T cells now target recipient tissues, most commonly the skin, gastrointestinal tract, and liver.

Rejection events and graft-versus-host reactions are classified clinically and experimentally as to when they are seen and the end event causing tissue damage. Hyperacute rejection occurs from minutes to hours after the organ is surgically introduced. This event is caused by preformed antibodies that may have been stimulated by prior pregnancy, transfusion, or transplantation, or may represent naturally occurring antibodies such as anti-ABO isohemagglutinins. These antibodies lead to endothelial damage and vascular injury and, if present in sufficient quantity, can lead to rapid, catastrophic damage to the transplanted organ, even before the surgical procedure is completed. Efforts are made to prevent these events by transplanting ABO-compatible, crossmatch-negative organs, although some groups are actively working to circumvent this barrier. Natural antibodies also can serve as barriers to the use of xenogeneic organs from other species.

Acute graft rejection occurs days to weeks after transplantation and is the consequence of primary T-cell (or very rarely B-cell) activation and attack of the graft. When T and B cells have already been activated from prior transplantation, transfusion, or pregnancy, a secondary immune response is generated more quickly, leading to more rapid destruction of the graft, known as accelerated rejection.

The pathophysiologic events in chronic rejection are even more complex and less well understood. This process can take months or years to develop. While it can be seen de novo, its frequency rises once an acute rejection event has occurred, even after successful treatment. Blood vessel walls thicken and become blocked. Low-grade cell-mediated responses or deposition of antibody-antigen complexes damage the blood vessel lining and trigger inappropriate repair responses. The vessel lumen can be obliterated from proliferation of smooth muscle cells migrating from the vessel wall and increased production and deposition of matrix proteins. Parenchymal damage and interstitial fibrosis of the transplanted organ can also occur. Although great progress has been made in control of acute rejection, less progress has been made in the control of chronic rejection.[19]

GVHD also is seen in acute or chronic forms. Transplantation of haploidentical hematopoietic progenitor or marrow grafts without laboratory removal of the passenger T lymphocytes can lead to a rapid GVHD syndrome with fever, rash, and diarrhea occurring in less than 48 hours. In more conventional transplantation of HLA-matched grafts using conventional approaches to immune suppression, acute GVHD typically arises within a few weeks to a few months after transplantation. Chronic forms of GVHD can occur with vascular compromise and fibrous tissue deposition. Similar to chronic rejection of solid organs, the pathogenesis of chronic GVHD is more complex and less well defined.

Inducing Tolerance

The ideal goal of therapeutic efforts to prevent or treat graft rejection or GVHD would be the establishment of permanent but selective immunologic tolerance toward the transplanted organ (rejection) or host tissues (GVHD). Ideally, approaches that achieved specific tolerance, eliminating only alloreactive lymphocytes, would be most desirable to avoid rendering the host vulnerable to opportunistic infection. Tolerance to self antigens is mediated by several mechanisms, including induction of anergy, deletion of alloreactive cells, or active suppression of alloreactive populations.

Animal models provide insights into tolerance. Permanent chimerism, wherein an organism contains two or more different populations of genetically distinct cells, can lead to clonal deletion of alloreactive populations. This is seen in freemartins, genetically distinct animals sharing a single placental circulation. These animals contain hematopoietic and immunologic cells from both animals and are nonreactive to tissues of both animals while remaining immunologically competent to third-party alloantigens. Achievement of microchimerism of donor lymphohematopoietic elements after allografting is associated with high long-term graft survival, even if immune suppression is discontinued. However, achievement of microchimerism is inconsistent, and approaches to induce it remain investigational at this time.[20,21]

In mice, pups are born just before mature T cells begin emigration from the thymus. Exposure to allogeneic cells before thymic emigration leads to tolerance to the expressed alloantigens.[22,23] Immune responses by T helper cells can be steered into one of two pathways, T helper type 1 (Th1) or T helper type 2 (Th2). Th1 cells produce IL-2 and interferon-γ and are typically associated with graft rejection. In contrast, Th2 cells produce other cytokines that may suppress Th1 responses.[24,25] Animals rendered neonatally tolerant tend to have fewer Th1 and more Th2 cells recognizing the alloantigens in question.[26] In addition, such animals may have larger numbers of T suppressor or regulator populations, which may help to maintain tolerance. In humans, T cells begin to leave the thymus at 16 to 20 weeks of gestation, so a similar induction of tolerance is thus not possible. Nonetheless, understanding the mechanisms involved provides insights for potential therapeutic targets.

Blood transfusions administered prior to solid organ transplantation have led to increased survival of recipient allografts compared to patients who did not receive transfusion. The mechanisms remain controversial, though it has been demonstrated that rats receiving blood intravenously achieve donor-specific tolerance to subsequently transplanted kidneys, while administration of the blood subcutaneously leads to accelerated rejection. Donor-specific transfusion in humans leads to 20% of the recipients developing antidonor antibodies, confounding the transplant effort. The remaining 80% have a transplant success rate in excess of 95% at 1 year. Random transfusion may also provide some clinical benefit. Whether this occurs through mechanisms similar to neonatally induced tolerance, induction of microchimerism, or other mechanisms is under active investigation.[27]

Although cells with suppressive or regulatory functions used to be quite controversial in immunology, their existence is now firmly established. They are associated with a $CD4^+/CD25^+$ surface phenotype and with expression of the FOXP3 transcription factor. These cells are important in self tolerance and may be important in the induction of tolerance to foreign antigens as well.[28]

Cellular and Molecular Events in T-Cell Activation—Targets for Interventions to Prevent the Development of Alloresponses

T-cell receptor engagement with an appropriate peptide-MHC complex does not, by itself, lead to T-cell activation. The T-cell receptor is not directly coupled to signaling molecules inside the cell. The CD3 complex, consisting of at least five proteins, is noncovalently associated with the receptor and contributes to signal transduction when the receptor is cross-linked by antigen-MHC on APCs. CD4 and CD8 serve as co-receptors for class II and class I MHC molecules, respectively, and their cytoplasmic tails are associated with tyrosine kinases that participate in signaling events. In addition to the signals provided through the T-cell receptor, CD3, and CD4/8 (collectively referred to as signal 1), T cells require additional signals provided by a variety of additional co-stimulatory molecules that are not associated with the T-cell receptor–peptide-MHC complex (signal 2) in order to undergo primary activation by APCs. The best defined of the co-stimulatory molecules are the B7 proteins (including CD80 and CD86), which interact with CD28 on T cells. Expression of co-stimulatory molecules is upregulated when APCs are exposed to inflammatory cytokines.[29]

Activation begins in specialized subregions of the T-cell membrane known as lipid rafts, leading to reorganization of the cytoskeleton such that the rafts coalesce to form tight junctions with the APC, known as the immunologic synapse.[30] The membrane events of T-cell receptor engagement and cross-linking lead to phosphorylation of components of the T-cell receptor complex; recruitment and/or activation of membrane-associated kinases such as Lck, Fyn, and ZAP-70; inhibition of membrane phospatases such as CD45; and the consequent activation of various downstream kinases such as extracellular signal-regulated kinase (ERK), c-Jun N-terminal kinase (JNK), and protein kinase C (PKC) as well as phosphatases such as calcineurin. These events in turn lead to activation of transcription factors including nuclear factor of activated T cells (NF-AT), AP-1, and nuclear factor-κB (NF-κB). These transcription factors contribute to the production of IL-2 and other important cytokines, cytokine receptors such as the IL-2 receptor (IL-2R), and other immunologically important molecules. Co-stimulatory engagement leads to activation of phosphatidylinositol-3 (PI-3) kinase and activation of the Ras/ERK myelin-associated protein (MAP) kinase pathway as well as activation of Akt kinase. These pathways lead to inactivation of proapoptotic molecules and may independently activate JNK and lead to NF-κB binding to a unique site on the IL-2 promoter not activated via T-cell receptor signaling. There are also a variety of inhibitory second signals as well as the positive signals mediated by CD28. The best known of these is the inhibitory receptor for the B7 family of molecules known as cytotoxic T-lymphocyte–associated antigen 4 (CTLA4).[31]

Functional triggering of the T-cell receptor together with appropriate second signals leads to T-cell activation. One of the primary effects of activation of Th1 T cells is the production of IL-2, which serves as an autocrine growth factor for Th1 T cells as well as for a variety of other T-cell subsets. The IL-2R consists of a complex of three noncovalently associated proteins. The α chain of the complex (CD25) is unique to IL-2 binding, while the β and γ chains also participate in the receptors for other cytokines. The β and γ chains are expressed at low levels on resting T cells. α Chain expression and upregulation of β chain expression occur as a consequence of T-cell activation. Engagement of IL-2 with its receptor leads to activation of the Jak3 STAT5, MAP kinase, and PI-3 kinase signal transduction pathways. These effects lead to T-cell survival through induction of anti-apoptotic proteins such as Bcl-2 and progression through the cell cycle by induction of synthesis of cyclins and through p27 degradation, which relieves a block in cell cycle progression.[32] Although IL-2 drives proliferation of the effector cells of rejection, it is important to note that it is also essential for the survival and growth of $CD4^+/CD25^+$ regulatory T cells. Thus IL-2 is important in driving both the effector and regulatory arms of the immune response.[33]

Additionally, T cells may be steered into a type 1 or type 2 pathway (e.g., Th1 or Th2 cells) depending on the environmental milieu and signals present during activation. This will also influence whether the immune response is more likely to proceed in a rejection (type 1) or tolerance (type 2) direction when antigen is encountered.

All of these intercellular interactions and intracellular events, schematically represented in Figure 92-1, can theoretically be manipulated to promote graft survival. Box 92-1 attempts to categorize many of the current immunosuppressive agents as to where in lymphocyte biology they exert their effects.

However, improved patient survival would benefit most from approaches that are not only highly effective but also highly selective in blunting alloresponses while leaving the remainder of the immune system intact. Among our current armamentarium are agents that lyse all T cells or block proliferation of activated T cells indiscriminately. Patients with poorly controlled human immunodeficiency virus disease can illustrate all too well the problems that can arise as a consequence of being too effective at eliminating T cells. Rigorously immune-suppressed patients suffer from opportunistic infections that can be as or even more threatening to patient survival than GVHD or graft rejection. Thus, in the absence of establishment of true tolerance, the clinical goal of patient management is to find a degree of immune suppression that can control rejection or GVHD but that will not be too heavy handed, thus minimizing the number and severity of opportunistic infections.

BOX 92-1 TARGETS OF IMMUNOSUPPRESSIVE AGENTS

Inhibition of Antigen-Presenting Cell Function
- Corticosteroids

T-Cell Receptor/Signal 1 Disruption
- Muromonab-CD3
- CD4 or CD8 inhibitors
- AEB071

Co-stimulatory/Signal 2 Disruption
- Belatacept
- CD40 or CD156 inhibitors

Cytokine Transcription Inhibition
- Corticosteroids
- Calcineurin inhibitors
  - Cyclosporine
  - Tacrolimus
  - ISA247

Interleukin-2 Receptor (IL-2R) Targeting/Signaling
- Antibodies to IL-2R
  - Daclizumab
  - Basiliximab
- IL-2R–directed toxin
  - Denileukin diftitox
- IL-2/IL-2R signal disruption
  - Sirolimus
  - JAK3 inhibitors

Production of Tolerance-Inducing Signals
- Extracorporeal photoimmune therapy
- Total lymphoid irradiation

Agents Inhibiting Cellular Proliferation, DNA/RNA Synthesis
- Alkylating agents
  - Cyclophosphamide
- Purine metabolism
  - Azathioprine
  - Mycophenolic acid
  - Fludarabine, cladrabine, pentostatin
  - Methotrexate
- Pyrimidine metabolism
  - Methotrexate
  - Leflunomide

Broadly Acting Lympholytic Agents/ Lymphocyte Removal
- Antithymocyte globulins
- Muromonab-CD3
- Alemtuzumab
- Rituximab
- T-cell depletion

CLINICAL OVERVIEW

Clinical Goals for Transplantation

The clinical events leading to therapeutic transplantation differ between the solid organ and HSCT communities. The majority of solid organ transplants attempt to replace a functionally defective organ with a well-functioning substitute. Occasionally, solid organ transplantation may be performed as a means of surgically eliminating a malignancy such as a hepatocellular carcinoma. In contrast, the vast majority of

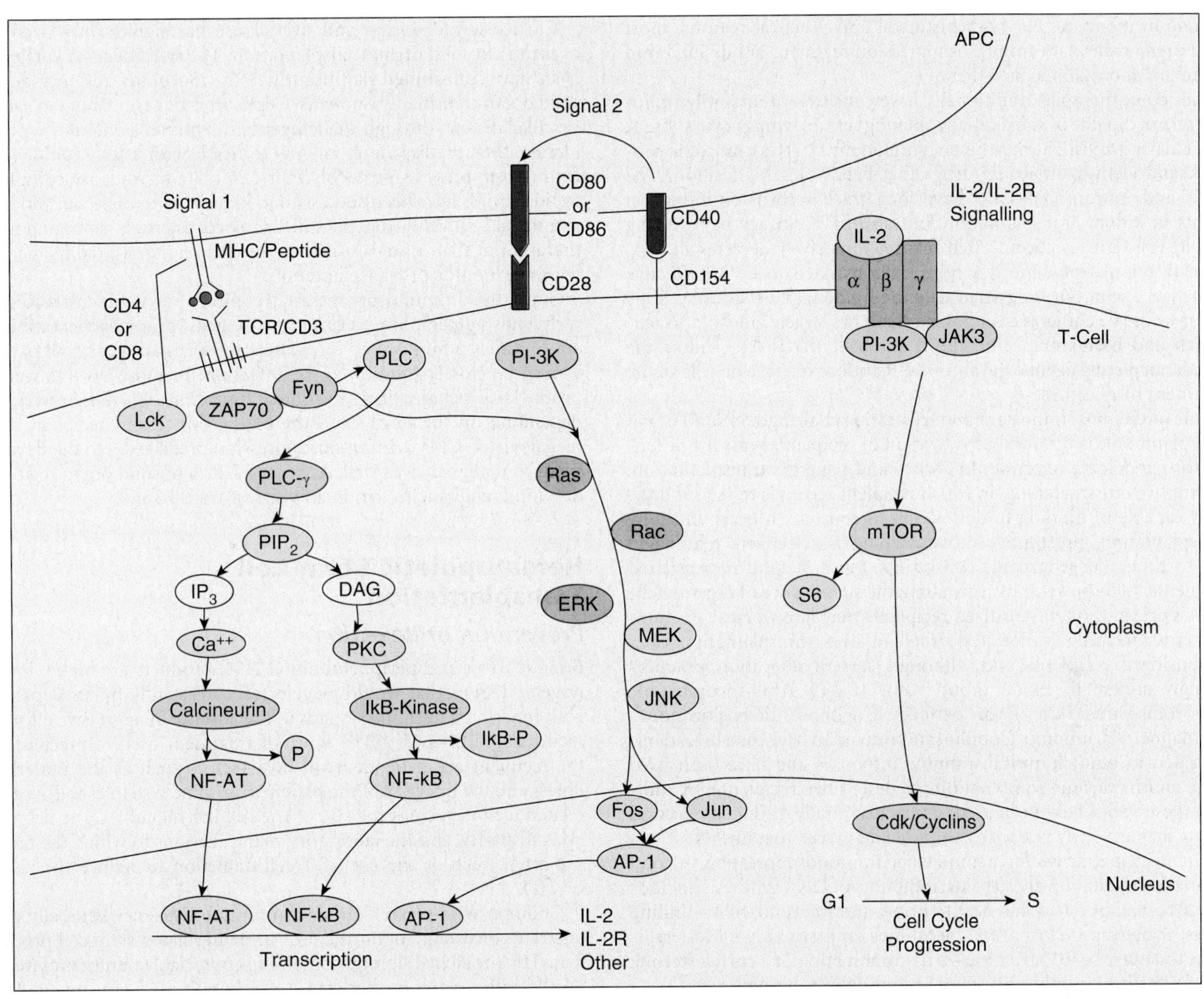

FIGURE 92-1 • The three cell surface signals to T cells and the intracellular downstream events which they trigger are illustrated. The antigen presenting cell (APC) is shown at the top of the figure with the T cell at the bottom. Signal 1 is transduced by the T cell receptor/CD3 complex along with the CD4 or CD8 co-receptor. Signal 2 is transduced by CD28 after engagement of CD80 or CD86. Engagement of CD40 by CD154 helps to upregulate CD80/86 expression and function. Signals induced by engagement of interleukin 2 (IL-2) with its receptor (IL-2R) are also illustrated. AP-1, activator protein-1; Ca^{++}, calcium; Cdk/Cyclins, cyclin dependent kinase/cyclins; DAG, diacyglycerol; ERK, extracellular signal-regulated kinase; Fos, FBJ osteosarcoma oncogene; Fyn, FYN oncogene related to SRC, FGR, YES; IκB-Kinase, IκB family of inhibitory proteins; IκB-P, IκB family of inhibitory proteins-phosphorylated; IL-2, interleukin-2; IL-2R, interleukin-2 receptor; IP_3, inositol triphosphate; JAK3, janus kinase 3; JNK, jun N-terminal kinase; Jun, JUN oncogene; Lck, Leukocyte-specific protein tyrosine kinase; MEK, http://www.wormbase.org/db/gene/gene_class?name=mek;class=Gene_class MAP kinase kinase or Erk kinase; MHC, major histocompatibilty complex; mTOR, mammalian target of rapamycin; NF-AT, nuclear factor of activated cells; NF-κB, nuclear factor kappa B; P, phosphate; PI-3K, phosphoinositide-3 kinase; PKC, protein kinase C; PLC, phospholipase C; PIP_2, phosphatidylinositol 4,5-bisphosphate; Ras, RAS family of proteins; Rac, Ras-related C3 botulinum toxin substrate; S6, ribosomal protein S6 kinase; TCR, T-cell receptor; ZAP 70, 70 kDa zeta-associated protein.

HSC transplants are performed as part of the treatment of malignancy, while less commonly they are used to treat nonmalignant disorders such as severe aplastic anemia or a variety of congenital disorders of lymphohematopoiesis or metabolism.

Solid Organ Transplantation

The principle purpose of solid organ transplantation is to restore organ function in the face of end-stage disease of the native organs. Even when alternative organ replacement therapy options are available, transplantation is usually the best and preferred approach. Kidney transplantation has the longest history and is established as the best treatment of end-stage renal disease. Pancreas transplantation is performed to treat insulin-dependent diabetes, most often in conjunction with a kidney transplant in type 1 diabetics with renal failure. Liver transplantation is the only viable long-term alternative for end-stage liver disease, with the majority of transplants performed for virus-induced injury. It is also routinely performed in patients with stage II hepatocellular cancer and is the only solid organ transplantation used frequently for the treatment of cancer. While ventricular assist devices are a potential option for many patients with cardiac failure, they have a shorter track record of use and have significant limitations in comparison to heart transplantation. In contrast, lung transplantation is the only viable long-term option for patients with end-stage pulmonary disease. For most patients with short gut syndrome, intestinal transplantation has significant advantages over parenteral nutrition. For all organs other than small bowel, there is a significant shortage of donor organs relative to need, and considerable efforts are made to ensure fair allocation.

Ideally, one would like the solid organ recipient to become selectively and permanently tolerant of the graft. Unfortunately, this is only rarely achieved,[34] and consequently, in the vast majority of cases, complete withdrawal of immunosuppression is accompanied by graft rejection. Acute rejection occurs most frequently early after transplantation, and thus, while immunosuppression cannot be stopped, in most cases it can be significantly decreased to lower levels as the time from transplantation increases. For both historical and practical reasons, most solid organ transplant immunosuppression regimens are divided into induction and maintenance therapies.

Induction therapies traditionally have consisted of an antilymphocyte serum capable of substantially ablating certain lymphocyte subsets, particularly T cells. The antithymocyte globulins (ATGs), muromonab-CD3, and alemtuzumab are drugs that behave in this fashion. The ATGs and muromonab-CD3 have long track records as induction agents in kidney transplantation, but also have efficacy in reversing steroid-resistant rejection.[35] Alemtuzumab massively depletes all lymphocyte populations and has been demonstrated to be an effective induction agent, but long-term data are limited, and the initial hope that it would be a tolerance-inducing agent has largely faded.[36,37] Daclizumab and basiliximab bind the α chain of the IL-2R. Unlike the broader depleting agents, the anti–IL-2R antibodies have no role in the treatment of rejection.

One of the most important and frustrating challenges in solid organ transplantation is humoral sensitization of recipients with the potential for hyperacute rejection. In kidney and pancreas transplantation, preemptive crossmatching, in which recipient serum is tested for antibody capable of binding to donor cells, is routine. In heart and lung transplantation, preemptive crossmatching is selectively performed due to time and geographic constraints, but is helpful in sensitized recipients.[38] For bowel transplantation, the significance of crossmatching is unclear, though sensitized recipients may fare worse.[39] Preemptive crossmatching is not performed in liver transplantation even in sensitized recipients and, although current allocation practices strongly adhere to blood group compatibility, ABO-incompatible liver transplants have been performed without desensitization.[40] Plasmapheresis, immune globulin, and rituximab have each been demonstrated to blunt humoral immune responses and have been used alone and in various combinations to desensitize recipients. In addition, these agents have been used to treat humorally mediated rejection events that are likely refractory to pure anti–T-cell therapy.[41,42]

The principal drugs for maintenance immunosuppression in solid organ transplantation are steroids; inhibitors of DNA synthesis, including mycophenolic acid and azathioprine; and immunophilin-binding drugs, including cyclosporine, tacrolimus, and sirolimus. Most regimens today are based on a three-drug combination of a corticosteroid, a DNA synthesis inhibitor, and an immunophilin-binding agent.

Mycophenolic acid has largely displaced azathioprine based on randomized trials conducted in kidney transplant recipients receiving cyclosporine-based immunosuppression. Mycophenolic acid has a relatively benign side effect profile when compared to the other components of maintenance immunosuppression, and most current research is directed toward finding effective substitutes for the other more toxic agents used in maintenance regimens.

Both tacrolimus and cyclosporine are still considered the backbone of most immunosuppressive regimens, and the two are considered highly interchangeable. In the early posttransplantation period, these drugs can contribute to delayed resumption of kidney graft function, further complicating this diagnostic dilemma. During the transplantation of other solid organs, their adverse renal effects may render the recipient's kidneys more vulnerable to other perioperative stresses, thus compromising native renal function. Long term, these drugs have been demonstrated to cause chronic renal injury that can lead to kidney failure in both kidney and nonkidney solid organ recipients.[43,44] For these reasons, regimens that avoid these agents are increasingly popular and the subject of considerable research.

Sirolimus, because of its different side effect profile, has been a particularly useful agent in regimens that attempt to avoid cyclosporine and tacrolimus or as an alternative to DNA synthesis inhibitors. Unfortunately, sirolimus can also be problematic in the early postoperative period largely because its antifibrotic effect inhibits normal wound healing.[45,46] Consequently, an alternative is to begin with cyclosporine or tacrolimus and transition to sirolimus at a later time point to exploit both its renal-sparing and its antitumor effects. For the same reasons, sirolimus is often used in liver transplant recipients with advanced hepatocellular cancer.

Corticosteroid dosing and overall use has significantly decreased over time in solid organ transplantation. The side effects of corticosteroids have contributed significantly to the morbidity and mortality of solid organ transplant recipients. Corticosteroids contribute to cardiovascular disease through diabetogenesis, hypertension, and hyperlipidemia, thus predisposing patients to death with a functioning graft. Immunosuppressive protocols that eliminate steroids or completely avoid steroids have been successful in kidney, pancreas, liver, and heart recipients.[47-50] Many centers still use corticosteroids as maintenance therapy, but their dose is usually reduced to 5 mg of prednisone daily within 6 months of transplantation.

Since the immunosuppression required inevitably increases the recipient's vulnerability to certain pathogens, prophylactic antibiotics are routinely administered early after transplantation, and all patients should be closely monitored for infection. In most cases, infectious prophylaxis includes drugs to combat fungi, *Pneumocystis jiroveci*, and, depending on the prior exposure of the donor and recipient, cytomegalovirus (CMV). Immunosuppression predisposes to the development of malignancy as well. As many as 20% of solid organ recipients develop malignancies within 10 years of transplant.[51]

Hematopoietic Stem Cell Transplantation

Prevention of Rejection

Bone marrow and peripheral blood HSC products are highly immunogenic tissues that would be rejected consistently by most patients with functional immune systems in the absence of aggressive efforts to secure engraftment.[52,53] The types of treatment used to precondition the recipient are dependent on host factors such as the underlying illness and the integrity of the patient's immune system as well as graft-related factors such as the size of the cellular inoculum, the degree of HLA disparity, and the laboratory manipulations to which the graft is subjected, such as the use of T-cell depletion to reduce the risk of GVHD.

Children with severe combined immunodeficiency generally demonstrate consistent engraftment of unmanipulated stem cell products from HLA-matched siblings containing appreciable numbers of mature T cells without any further steps to precondition the recipient. These patients can, however, reject HLA-mismatched products that have been depleted of mature T cells, presumably by an NK cell–mediated mechanism, and thus require some degree of conditioning to secure consistent engraftment in this setting.[54]

Patients with aplastic anemia have a damaged, but not malignant, bone marrow to be replaced in the transplantation process. These patients originally received a preparatory regimen consisting of high-dose cyclophosphamide (160 to 200 mg/kg divided in four daily doses), a potently immune-suppressive chemotherapeutic agent. This approach was sufficiently immunosuppressive to produce consistent engraftment in untransfused and thus unsensitized recipients. However, after exposure to even a few units of red blood cells or platelets, nearly one third of patients would demonstrate graft rejection. The use of ATG in addition to cyclophosphamide led to more consistent rates of engraftment in this disorder.[55]

Patients with hematopoietic malignancies typically received slightly smaller doses of cyclophosphamide (120 to 160 mg/kg divided in two to four daily doses) combined with other agents in an effort both to immune suppress the recipient and to eradicate the malignancy. The two original approaches developed, total body irradiation plus cyclophosphamide[56] and busulfan plus cyclophosphamide,[57] remain in clinical use today, though many additional and derivative approaches are used as well. These approaches are known as ablative transplantation regimens in that the regimens would lead to permanent marrow aplasia if the graft were not administered or were rejected. More recently, gentler approaches have been developed, including non-myeloablative transplantation regimens that would lead to autologous hematopoietic recovery in the absence of successful donor engraftment. Key steps in the successful development of nonmyeloablative transplantation have included the use of fludarabine or other purine nucleoside analogues, which are potently immune-suppressive chemotherapeutics, as part of the conditioning regimen, and the use of cyclosporine (or tacrolimus) plus mycophenolate mofetil posttransplantation.[58]

GVHD Prophylaxis

In contrast to solid organ recipients, most patients undergoing HSCT ultimately do achieve a state of tolerance and can eventually taper off their immunosuppressive regimens. The initial agent used for GVHD prophylaxis was low-dose methotrexate. Methotrexate was originally given at a dose of 15 mg/m^2 the day after transplantation, followed by doses of 10 mg/m^2 on days 3, 6, and 11 after transplantation and weekly thereafter until day 100. Cyclosporine was subsequently shown to have comparable efficacy, and may be used as a single agent or combined with a short course of methotrexate (consisting of the day 1, 3, 6, and 11 doses only). Tacrolimus has comparable efficacy to cyclosporine, though some studies suggest a slight advantage when tacrolimus is substituted for cyclosporine.[59,60]

More recently, mycophenolate mofetil and sirolimus have been combined with cyclosporine or tacrolimus in place of methotrexate.[61] These approaches avoid the increased mucositis and delayed count recovery associated with methotrexate. Use of calcineurin inhibitors can be associated with microangiopathic hemolytic anemia and thrombocytopenia with or without associated renal dysfunction. The incidence and severity of this problem may be increased using the combination of tacrolimus plus sirolimus.[62]

T-cell depletion may be used as GVHD prophylaxis, either as a sole modality or combined with pharmacoprophylaxis.[63,64] The incidence of immunologically mediated graft rejection increases when T-cell depletion is utilized.[65] Incorporation of ATG into the immunosuppressive regimen can help promote consistent engraftment but at the price of further delays in immune reconstitution and a higher frequency of infectious events, including Epstein-Barr virus (EBV)–associated posttransplantation lymphoproliferative disorder (PTLD).[66]

GVHD Treatment

Corticosteroids are the most commonly used agents as front-line therapy for GVHD. Minor skin-only disease is occasionally treated topically, but most clinically significant GVHD is treated with prednisone or methylprednisolone, most often starting at doses of 2 mg/kg per day in divided doses, tapering as the clinical course allows.[67] Other immunosuppressive agents may be continued or added if GVHD persists or progresses through corticosteroid treatment, or if GVHD recurs during steroid taper. Cyclosporine, tacrolimus, mycophenolate mofetil (CellCept), sirolimus, ATG, muromonab-CD3 (OKT3), photopheresis, and other agents have been combined with steroids or used in an effort to facilitate weaning steroids to avoid steroid-related side effects. None of these agents would be considered to represent a second-line standard of care. The approach to chronic GVHD is similar.

Infection

Like their solid organ counterparts, HSCT recipients are very infection prone. This predisposition correlates with the CD4 count posttransplantation. Prophylaxis against fungi, *P. jiroveci,* and herpesviruses is commonly employed in many centers.

THERAPEUTICS AND CLINICAL PHARMACOLOGY

Specific Agents and Modalities Used to Control Alloresponses

Corticosteroids

Corticosteroids (Solu-Medrol, Medrol, Deltasone; multiple generic equivalents) have played an important role in immunosuppressive therapy since the early days of transplantation. They are widely considered the first-line treatment for acute rejection and still play an important role for the prevention of rejection and GVHD, albeit a diminishing one. The combination of corticosteroids with the other maintenance immunosuppressive agents has been studied extensively in kidney, heart, liver, pancreas, lung, and HSC transplant patients. Due to numerous short- and long-term side effects, frequent attempts have been made to eliminate corticosteroids from immunosuppressive regimens. Although the earliest attempts at withdrawal were not very successful, subsequent attempts with a combination of the newer, more potent immunosuppressive agents have made corticosteroid withdrawal feasible while maintaining acceptable efficacy in the prevention of rejection.[68-70]

Mechanism of Action. Corticosteroids have a variety of anti-inflammatory and immunosuppressive effects. Although high doses of corticosteroids have been thought to produce a lympholytic effect, lymphocytopenia appears more related to redistribution than lysis, with a rapid but temporary reduction in circulating lymphocytes. This effect can, in some cases, resolve within a day.

The mechanism of action of corticosteroids is schematically represented in Figure 92-2. Due to their hydrophobic properties, corticosteroids diffuse easily into cells and bind specifically to cytoplasmic receptors.[71] Binding of corticosteroids to their receptors dissociates the

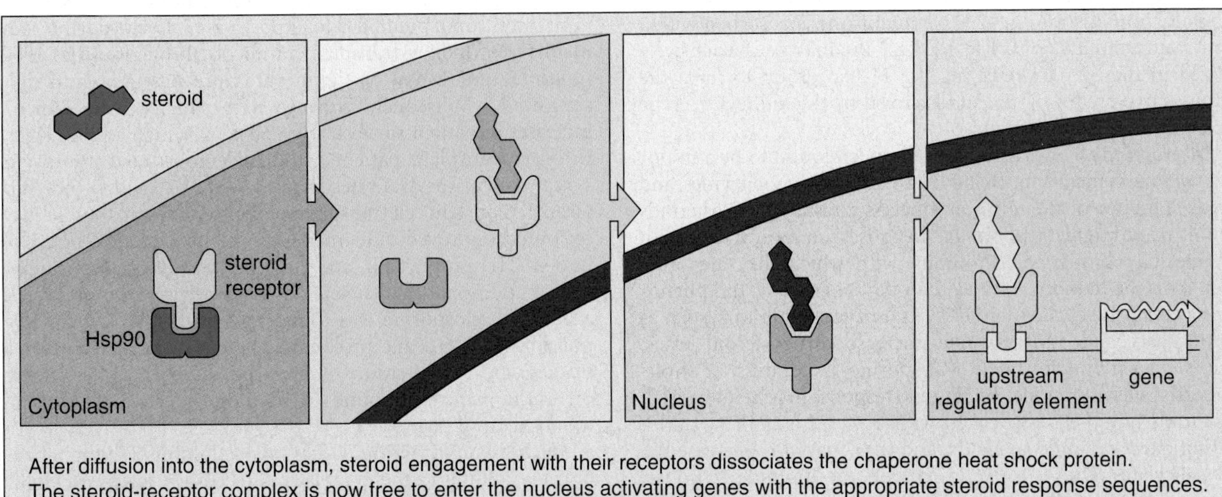

FIGURE 92-2 • Corticosteroid mechanism of action. After diffusion into the cytoplasm, engagement of steroids with their receptors dissociates the chaperone heat-shock protein. The steroid-receptor complex is now free to enter the nucleus-activating genes with the appropriate steroid response sequences. (From Janeway C. Immunobiology: The Immune System in Health and Disease, 5th ed. London: Garland Science with permission from the publisher, Taylor & Francis, 2001.)

receptor from heat-shock protein chaperones, allowing translocation of the drug-receptor complex to the nucleus. In the nucleus, the drug-receptor complex attaches to a variety of DNA sites with the consequent inhibition of transcription of certain cytokine genes.[71,72] As a result of decreased production of several proinflammatory cytokines, the inflammatory response is dampened. Specific cytokines inhibited by steroids include IL-1, IL-2, IL-6, interferon-γ, and TNF-α, leading to a blunted Th1 response. Macrophage functions, including chemotactic and phagocytic properties, are also inhibited. Additionally, high-dose corticosteroids for treatment of rejection can decrease the expression of HLA antigens and thereby decrease the immunogenicity of transplanted organs, antagonizing the effects of interferon-γ.[73,74] They also can inhibit the function of APCs. Corticosteroids are also commonly used to minimize the adverse effects occurring during infusion of polyclonal and monoclonal antibodies.

Dosing and Administration. The two main oral corticosteroids used are prednisolone (Europe) and prednisone (United States). Prednisone is metabolized in the liver to its active moiety, prednisolone. For induction therapy, treatment of acute rejection, or treatment of visceral GVHD, higher doses are usually given in the form of intravenous (IV) methylprednisolone. The dosing of corticosteroids varies widely depending on the transplant center and organ transplanted. If steroids are used for maintenance immunosuppression, initial doses at the time of transplantation usually range from 250 to 1000 mg of methylprednisolone followed by a rapid taper over the next few days to a maintenance dose of prednisone of 5 to 30 mg daily. Many patients are tapered off of their steroids by 3 to 6 months, though some patients may stay on low doses indefinitely. For treatment of acute rejection, doses of 5 to 10 mg/kg of methylprednisolone administered for 3 days are common, although some centers may opt for a fixed rather than weight-based dose for all patients. Small IV doses of methylprednisolone may be administered by bolus injection over a period of several minutes. Moderate IV doses (250 to 500 mg) should be infused over 15 to 30 minutes, while doses over 500 mg should be infused over 30 minutes or more. Oral doses should be administered after meals or with food as all corticosteroids may cause gastrointestinal disturbances. Corticosteroids are also available in alternative dosage forms such as oral solution, intramuscular injection, and dissolvable tablets.

Pharmacokinetics. The pharmacokinetics of corticosteroids in transplant patients demonstrate large interindividual variability. This may be due to differences in patient weight, renal and hepatic function, circadian rhythm, age, gender, and underlying disease state. For methylprednisolone, the time to peak concentration (T_{max}) is 31 minutes, with a volume of distribution (V_d) of 1.5 L/kg.[75,76] Methylprednisolone is extensively metabolized in the liver by reversible oxidation of the 11-hydroxyl group, and largely excreted by the kidneys.[77] The elimination half-life ($t_{1/2}$) is 2 to 3 hours with a clearance of 16 to 21 L/hr.[75,76] Following oral administration, 92% of prednisone is absorbed with a T_{max} of 1.3 hours and a V_d of 0.4 to 1 L/kg.[78] Prednisone is extensively metabolized in the liver by reducing the 11-oxo group to form the biologically active prednisolone, and excreted by the kidneys.[78,79] The $t_{1/2}$ of prednisone is 2.6 to 3 hours.[78]

Drug Interactions. Corticosteroids have been found to be a minor substrate for the cytochrome P-450 3A4 (CYP3A4) isoenzymes and also a weak inhibitor of the same enzyme. As a result, corticosteroids may exhibit drug interactions similar to those commonly seen with cyclosporine, tacrolimus, and sirolimus, with which they are often combined. Enzyme inducers such as rifampin, phenytoin, and phenobarbital may decrease corticosteroid levels. Enzyme inhibitors, such as azole antifungals, and diltiazem may increase corticosteroid levels. When given in combination with cyclosporine, tacrolimus, or sirolimus, the cortisosteroid elimination rate and response may be altered.[80,81] Corticosteroids have been associated with both an enhancing and a diminishing effect on anticoagulants, and they may also decrease the effect of salicylates. Due to their impact on the immune response, steroids can reduce the effectiveness of vaccines and toxoids.

Adverse Drug Reactions. Corticosteroids are associated with an enormous variety of short- and long-term side effects. Common adverse effects include cushingoid appearance, hypertension, fluid retention, dyslipidemia, weight gain, peptic ulcer formation, gastrointestinal bleeding, hyperglycemia progressing to diabetes, osteoporosis, avascular necrosis of bone, proximal muscle weakness, delayed wound healing, growth retardation, mental status changes, adrenal insufficiency, infection, cataracts, and glaucoma. Corticosteroids may also increase white blood cells (WBCs) by increasing polymorphonuclear leukocyte release from the marrow and decreasing margination. Although many of these adverse effects are dose and duration related, patients have wide variations in the frequency and severity of these effects in part due to large variations in the pharmacokinetics.

Monitoring. Therapeutic drug monitoring is not a routine part of corticosteroid treatment. The primary monitoring includes clinical and laboratory evaluation for adverse reactions. Routine monitoring should include blood pressure, blood glucose, electrolytes, lipids, and weight.

Cyclosporine

Cyclosporine (Sandimmune, Neoral, Gengraf; multiple generics) is a cyclic polypeptide agent consisting of 11 amino acids that is produced as a metabolite by the fungus species *Beauveria nivea* (also called *Tolypocladium inflatum*).[82] Cyclosporine was discovered in 1972 and was found to have potent immunosuppressive properties in 1976.[83] Although the molecular structure is completely different from that of tacrolimus, the immunosuppressive properties, use, and mechanism of action are similar. The original formulation of cyclosporine, Sandimmune, had very incomplete and unpredictable absorption along with large inter- and intrapatient variability. Neoral (cyclosporine modified) has a more consistent and reliable absorption profile, and was developed as a means to make dosing, administration, and monitoring more reliable.[84,85] Subsequently, multiple generic formulations (e.g., Gengraf) have been introduced throughout the world. Although the bioequivalence of the various formulations has been questioned, the generic cyclosporine modified formulations currently on the market are considered equivalent.[86,87]

Cyclosporine is indicated for rejection prophylaxis in kidney, liver, and heart transplant recipients, though its use in pancreas, lung, small bowel, and HSC transplant recipients is also common. Cyclosporine is also indicated for treatment of severe active rheumatoid arthritis and for severe, recalcitrant plaque psoriasis. Cyclosporine is also used for treatment of atopic dermatitis, Crohn's disease, and a number or other immune-mediated diseases. It is also commonly combined with ATG for the treatment of severe aplastic anemia.

Cyclosporine was first investigated for use in kidney and HSC transplant patients and was responsible for improving the success rate for all types of transplantation. It generally is credited with being the single factor most responsible for establishing kidney transplantation as a viable option for end-stage renal disease since it improved 3-year survival rates from about 50% to almost 80%.[87] Cyclosporine became the mainstay of kidney transplant protocols throughout the 1980s, with multiple studies showing significant improvement in graft and patient survival.[88,89] Subsequent trials in liver patients have shown similar increases in patient survival from 60% to as high as 80% at 1 year.[90,91] In heart transplant patients, studies demonstrated improvements in 1-year patient survival rates from 61% to 81%, with 5-year survival of 60%.[92,93] For stem cell transplant patients, numerous studies have demonstrated improved outcomes with the introduction of cyclosporine into GVHD prophylaxis, and combinations of cyclosporine with one to two additional agents generally have been even more effective. For example, cyclosporine was found to be superior to methotrexate in preventing GVHD and prolonging patient survival. However, in other studies, the combination of cyclosporine with either methotrexate or azathioprine was found to be more effective than cyclosporine monotherapy.[94-97]

Mechanism of Action. Cyclosporine inhibits T-lymphocyte activation by binding to the cytoplasmic receptor protein cyclophilin. The complex binds to calcineurin, which inhibits the calcium-stimulated phosphatase activity of calcineurin critical for dephosphorylation of NF-AT, a cytosolic component of a transcriptional activator that is important for a number of important lymphokines such as IL-2 and

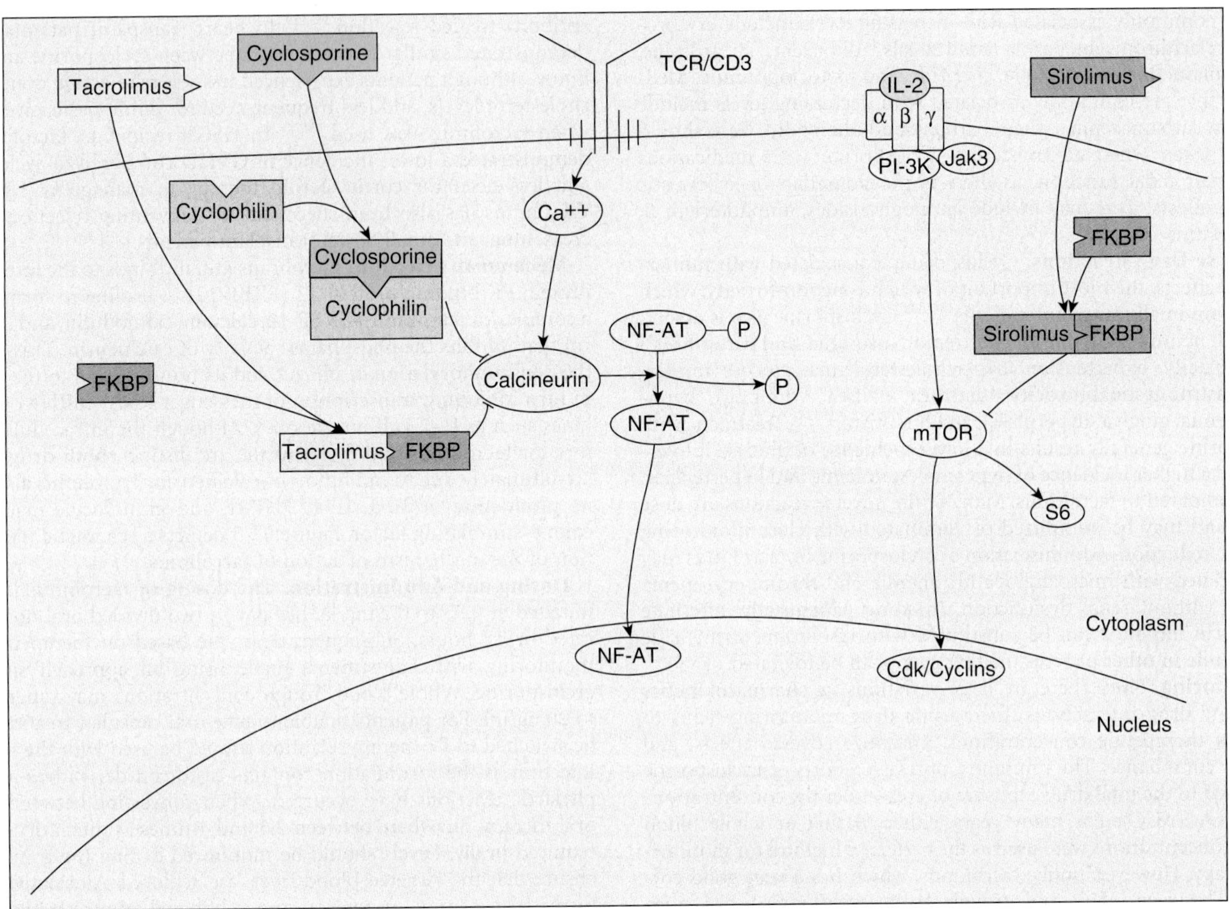

FIGURE 92-3 • The mechanisms of action of three immunophilin binding drugs, cyclosporine, tacrolimus, and sirolimus, are illustrated. Cyclosporine and tacrolimus bind to distinct immunophilins but both have similar inhibitory effects on calcineurin. Although sirolimus binds to the same immunophilin as tacrolimus, the intracellular effects of sirolimus are distinct and mediated primarily through the mammalian target of rapamycin (mTOR) rather than calcineurin. Ca^{++}, calcium; FKBP, FK binding protein-12; Cdk/Cyclins, cyclin dependent kinase/cyclins; IL-2, interleukin-2; Jak3, janus kinase 3; NF-AT, nuclear factor of activated T-cells; PI-3K, phosphoinositide-3 kinase; S6, ribosomal protein S6, TCR, T-cell receptor.

interferon-γ.[98,99] As a result of the failure to dephosphorylate NF-AT and its inability to migrate to the nucleus, there is inhibition of T-lymphocyte activation along with inhibition of the proinflammatory cytokines IL-2, IL-3, IL-4, granulocyte colony-stimulating factor, interferon-γ, and TNF-α. Cyclosporine may also increase expression of transforming growth factor-β, which is a potent inhibitor of IL-2 and T-cell proliferation.[100] It has been suggested that cyclosporine may inhibit Th1 cells to a greater degree than Th2 cells, thus promoting graft tolerance. Figure 92-3 depicts a schematic representation of the mechanism of action of cyclosporine.

Dosing and Administration. The dosing of cyclosporine is usually initiated at 5 to 10 mg/kg per day in two divided oral doses separated by 12 hours. Subsequent doses are adjusted based on therapeutic drug monitoring, efficacy, and toxicity. Therapeutic drug monitoring should be initiated within a few days of starting treatment, whenever dosage adjustments are made, when potentially interacting medications are started, or when otherwise clinically indicated. Whole blood trough concentrations, the most commonly employed monitoring method, may range from 50 to 450 ng/ml depending on organ type, concurrent immunosuppressants, and time from transplantation as well as patient response to therapy. In contrast to solid organ transplant programs, which typically monitor parent cyclosporine levels, many HSC transplant programs monitor combined levels of parent drug and common metabolites although this practice is becoming less frequent. No consensus levels have been established, though many centers will endeavor to maintain trough levels of 350 to 500 ng/ml. For patients unable to take oral capsules, treatment may be switched to IV therapy, which has a conversion rate of 1:3 (IV:oral). Alternative dosage forms such as oral suspension, inhalation, and rectal administration have also been effectively used in patients unable to tolerate the traditional routes of administration.

Pharmacokinetics. Multiple factors have been reported to affect cyclosporine pharmacokinetics, such as age, race, diet, disease, time posttransplantation, liver and gut function, transplant type, and concomitant drug therapy. Like many of the immunosuppressive medications, cyclosporine has large inter- and intrapatient variability, with additional variation between the original Sandimmune formulation and the newer Neoral formulation. The following summary of the pharmacokinetic data is combined for both Neoral and Sandimmune. After oral administration, the T_{max} is approximately 1.5 to 4 hours, with the bioavailability ranging from 10% to 89%.[101] An advantage of cyclosporine modified over the original formulation is that bile is not necessary for absorption, which may be important in liver transplant recipients who have T-tubes with bile diversion early after transplantation. Cyclosporine is highly protein bound and distributes widely throughout the body, with the liver being the primary site along with fat, blood, kidney, heart, lung, and pancreas.[102] The V_d is 3 to 5 L/kg and the $t_{1/2}$ varies from 5 to 27 hours.[103] The clearance of cyclosporine ranges from 4 to 13 ml/min per kilogram.[104]

Cyclosporine is metabolized by the CYP3A4 isoenzyme in the liver, kidney, and intestinal mucosa and is also a substrate for P-glycoprotein (Pgp) in the intestinal mucosa. At least 25 cyclosporine metabolites have been identified, although their biologic activity is considerably less than the parent compound.[105,106] The majority of cyclosporine is excreted in the feces with only a minor amount excreted in the urine.

Drug Interactions. Since cyclosporine is a substrate for both CYP3A4 and Pgp, it exhibits numerous drug interactions. Medications that are commonly associated with increasing levels include erythromycin, clarithromycin, azole antifungals, diltiazem, nicardipine, verapamil, methylprednisolone, cisapride, and metoclopramide. Medications that are commonly associated with decreasing levels include rifampin, carbamazepine, phenobarbital, and phenytoin. Care should also be taken when administering cyclosporine with medications that impair renal function, as there is the potential for synergistic negative effects. This may include aminoglycosides, amphotericin B, and cisplatin.

Adverse Drug Reactions. Cyclosporine is associated with numerous side effects, the most important of which is nephrotoxicity, which is common in all transplant patients.[107-109] Cyclosporine also is associated with neurotoxicity (headache, tremor, insomnia, and paresthesia), hepatotoxicity, hypertension, hypercholesterolemia, glucose intolerance, gastrointestinal toxicity (diarrhea, nausea, vomiting), hypomagnesemia, gingival hyperplasia, and hirsutism.[110,111] Treatment with cyclosporine generally results in a lower incidence of glucose intolerance and a higher incidence of hypercholesterolemia and hypertension when compared to tacrolimus. Many of the adverse reactions are dose related and may be minimized or eliminated with close monitoring and dose reduction. Administration of cyclosporine or tacrolimus may be associated with microangiopathic anemia and thrombocytopenia with or without renal dysfunction. In some patients, the alternate calcineurin inhibitor can be substituted with resolution of this side effect, while in other patients, neither agent can be tolerated.

Monitoring. Since there are large variations in pharmacokinetics and many drug interactions, therapeutic drug monitoring helps to maintain therapeutic concentrations, minimize adverse effects, and monitor compliance. The immunosuppressive effects of cyclosporine are related to the total drug exposure or area under the concentration-time curve (AUC). For many years, either plasma or whole blood trough concentrations were used as the preferred method for monitoring therapy. However, unlike tacrolimus, which has a very good correlation between AUC and trough level, cyclosporine has poor correlation between trough concentration and AUC and ultimately with clinical outcomes.[112] In recent years, numerous groups have reported more accurate methods for monitoring cyclosporine therapy, such as abbreviated AUCs or 2-hour postdose levels.[113,114] However, these alternative methods of monitoring patients may be difficult to practice due to the number or timing of the levels required. Therefore, many centers still rely heavily on whole blood trough level monitoring alone. Whichever method is used, levels should be initiated within a few days after starting or changing treatment, whenever side effects are suspected, or when otherwise clinically indicated. Whole blood trough concentrations may range from 50 to 450 ng/ml depending on organ type, concurrent immunosuppressants, and time from transplantation as well as patient response to therapy. Patients should also be monitored for renal dysfunction, hypercholesterolemia, hypertension, glucose intolerance, and signs and symptoms of infection.

Tacrolimus

Tacrolimus (Prograf), commonly referred to by its developmental code number FK506, is a macrolide antibiotic derived from the fermentation broth of *Streptomyces tsukubaensis*,[115,116] discovered in a soil sample from the foot of Mount Tsukuba in Tokyo. Although the molecular structure and intracellular binding protein of tacrolimus are completely different from those of cyclosporine, the immunosuppressive properties, use, and mechanism of action are strikingly similar. Tacrolimus has been demonstrated to be 10 to 100 times more potent than cyclosporine in vitro and in vivo. Tacrolimus is indicated for the prophylaxis of organ rejection in patients receiving kidney, liver, or heart transplants. However, use in pancreas, lung, small bowel, and HSC transplantation is also common. Tacrolimus is also available in a topical ointment for the treatment of moderate to severe atopic dermatitis.

Tacrolimus was first investigated for use in liver transplantation and was found to be equivalent to cyclosporine-based regimens.[117] Subsequent trials in kidney transplant patients have shown potential advantages over cyclosporine, with reduced incidences of acute rejection and antibody-treated rejection.[118,119] In heart transplant patients, studies demonstrated similar rejection rates between cyclosporine and tacrolimus, although patients experienced less severe rejection events, lower cholesterol levels, and less frequent need for antihypertensive therapy when tacrolimus was used.[120,121] In HSCT recipients, tacrolimus has demonstrated a lower incidence of GVHD compared to cyclosporine and less need for corticosteroid therapy to manage GVHD.[59,122,123] Tacrolimus has also been successful for preventing rejection in pancreas, lung, and small bowel transplant patients.[124-126]

Mechanism of Action. Tacrolimus initially binds to the intracellular protein FK binding protein-12 (FKBP-12),[127] leading to formation of a complex of tacrolimus–FKBP-12, calcium, calmodulin, and calcineurin that inhibits the phosphatase activity of calcineurin. This prevents the dephosphorylation of NF-AT and its translocation to the nucleus, in turn inhibiting transcription of messenger RNA (mRNA) for cytokines such as IL-2 and interferon-γ. Although the intracellular receptors for tacrolimus and cyclosporine are distinct, both drugs' effects are ultimately due to inhibition of calcineurin. Tacrolimus also inhibits production of IL-3, IL-4, TNF-α, and granulocyte-macrophage colony-stimulating factor. Figure 92-3 depicts a schematic representation of the mechanism of action of tacrolimus.

Dosing and Administration. The dosing of tacrolimus is usually initiated at 0.05 to 0.2 mg/kg per day in two divided oral doses separated by 12 hours. Subsequent doses are based on therapeutic drug monitoring with adjustments made using an approach similar to cyclosporine. Whole blood trough concentrations may range from 3 to 20 ng/ml. For patients unable to take oral capsules, treatment may be switched to IV therapy. Caution should be used with the initial IV injection as the formulation contains castor oil derivatives and anaphylactic reactions have occurred. When converting between IV and oral therapy, anywhere between 2.5 and 4 times as much drug will be required orally. Levels should be monitored during the transition to ensure that the targeted blood levels are achieved. Alternative dosage forms such as oral suspension and sublingual administration of the oral capsule powder have also been effectively used in patients unable to tolerate the traditional routes of administration.

Pharmacokinetics. Tacrolimus has large inter- and intrapatient variability. After oral administration, tacrolimus' T_{max} is approximately 1 to 4 hours, with the bioavailability ranging from 6% to 56%.[128,129] Tacrolimus is highly bound to red blood cells, with the plasma portion highly bound to albumin and α1-acid glycoprotein. The V_d is 0.85 to 1.91 L/kg and the $t_{1/2}$ varies from 3.5 to 40.5 hours.[130,131] Plasma clearance following IV administration ranges from 87 to 269 L/hr, while systemic clearance ranges from 0.6 to 5.4 L/hr per kilogram.[129-131]

Tacrolimus is metabolized by the CYP3A4 isoenzyme in the liver and intestinal mucosa and is also a substrate for Pgp in the intestinal mucosa.[131a] This pattern of metabolism leads to numerous drug-drug interactions. Demethylation and hydroxylation serve as the primary mechanisms of biotransformation. At least nine tacrolimus metabolites have been identified, although only two have been shown to possess immunosuppressive activity.[132] The majority of tacrolimus is excreted in the feces with only a minor amount excreted in the urine.

Drug Interactions. Since tacrolimus, like cyclosporine, is a substrate for both CYP3A4 and Pgp, it too has numerous potential drug interactions that may alter blood concentrations due to effects on drug metabolism or bioavailability. The medications that commonly alter tacrolimus levels are essentially the same as those altering cyclosporine levels. Like cyclosporine, care should be taken when administering tacrolimus with medications that impair renal function to avoid synergistic nephrotoxicity.

Adverse Drug Reactions. Tacrolimus has a toxicity profile very similar to that of cyclosporine. Tacrolimus use is associated with nephrotoxicity, neurotoxicity (headache, tremor, insomnia, and paresthesia), hypertension, hypercholesterolemia, glucose intolerance, gastrointestinal toxicity (diarrhea, nausea, vomiting), hyperkalemia, hypomagnesemia, and alopecia.[132-135] Treatment with tacrolimus generally results in a lower incidence of hypercholesterolemia and hypertension and a higher incidence of glucose intolerance when compared to cyclosporine. Many of the adverse reactions are dose related and may be minimized or eliminated with close monitoring and dosage reduction. Similar to cyclosporine, tacrolimus administration may be associated with microangiopathic anemia and thrombocytopenia with or without renal dysfunction.

Monitoring. Due to the large variations in pharmacokinetics and numerous potential drug interactions, therapeutic drug monitoring helps maintain appropriate blood levels, minimize adverse effects, and monitor compliance as with tacrolimus therapy. Although plasma concentrations of tacrolimus more closely reflect the pharmacologic activity of the drug, whole blood levels have become the clinical standard. Whole blood trough concentrations may range from 3 to 20 ng/ml.

Sirolimus

Sirolimus (Rapamune), formerly known as rapamycin, is a macrocyclic lactone produced by *Streptomyces hygroscopicus.* It was isolated from a soil sample from the island Rapa Nui, also known as Easter Island, and has potent immunosuppressive, antifungal, and antitumor properties.[136-139] Sirolimus is indicated for the prophylaxis of organ rejection in patients ages 13 years or older following renal transplantation. The combination of sirolimus with cyclosporine and/or corticosteroids has been studied extensively in renal transplantation. Fewer clinical trials of its use in heart, liver, and HSC transplant patients have been conducted.

Sirolimus and the immunosuppressive agent tacrolimus are structural analogues of one another and bind to the same cytoplasmic immunophilin binding protein, FKBP-12. However, despite these similarities, the mechanisms of action of these two drugs are quite distinct.[140,141] Despite initial concerns that binding to FKBP-12 would result in tacrolimus and sirolimus showing competition or antagonism for one another, this has not proved to be the case. The combination of sirolimus with tacrolimus in place of cyclosporine has become widely practiced in solid organ transplantation, although few studies of this combination of agents have been performed. In HSCT, a single-institution study has suggested that the combination of tacrolimus and sirolimus is highly effective in preventing acute GVHD, and a multicenter study is underway to try to confirm this finding.[142]

Mechanism of Action. Sirolimus inhibits T-lymphocyte activation and proliferation by a mechanism that is distinct from other immunosuppressants. The sirolimus–FKBP-12 complex binds to and inhibits the activation of the mammalian Target of Rapamycin (mTOR). Unlike the tacrolimus–FKBP-12 complex, the sirolimus–FKBP-12 complex has no effect on calcineurin activity (and thus cytokine transcription) but instead inhibits signal transduction pathways activated by cytokines such as IL-2, engaging with their receptors and thus inhibiting cytokine-mediated proliferation with consequent arrest in the G_1-S phase junction of the cell cycle.[140,143,144] Sirolimus thus acts synergistically with cyclosporine and tacrolimus at a later stage in the T-cell cycle activation pathway by blocking cytokine-mediated signal transduction pathways rather than cytokine production.[140,144] It also acts to inhibit IL-2–dependent and Il-2–independent proliferation of B lymphocytes and their production of immunoglobulins G, A, and M. Figure 92-3 depicts a schematic representation of the mechanism of action of sirolimus.

Sirolimus is also a potent inhibitor of smooth muscle cell migration and proliferation and may help reduce the rate of restenosis when employed in drug-eluting stents.[145-147] It has been shown that FKBP-12 is upregulated in smooth muscle cells involved in neointimal growth.[148] Sirolimus and the related compound temsirolimus also inhibit proliferation of nonlymphoid tumor cells and are being studied for treatment of cancers and for autoimmune diseases.

Dosing and Administration. When administered with cyclosporine and corticosteroids, sirolimus should be initiated with a single loading dose of either 6 or 15 mg, followed by a daily maintenance dose of 2 or 5 mg. The higher dose is generally used for high-risk patients. Therapeutic drug monitoring is used to adjust dosing and should be initiated 5 to 7 days after starting treatment. Whole blood trough concentrations may range from 5 to 24 ng/ml. Sirolimus is available as both an oral solution and tablets. To avoid potential drug interactions, it is recommended that sirolimus be administered 4 hours after administration of cyclosporine. Timing of administration when combined with tacrolimus has not been defined.

Pharmacokinetics. After oral administration, the sirolimus T_{max} is approximately 1 to 2 hours.[149-152] The bioavailability is approximately 14% with the oral solution and about 27% higher with the tablet. The V_d is 5.6 to 16.7 L/kg.[150,153] Sirolimus is extensively partitioned in red blood cells, resulting in higher whole blood concentrations compared to plasma concentrations. The binding of sirolimus is mainly associated with serum albumin (97%), α1-acid glycoprotein, and lipoproteins. The $t_{1/2}$ of sirolimus is 57 to 68 hours[149,150,152,153] with a clearance of 127 to 240 ml/hr per kilogram.[150,153]

Sirolimus is also a substrate for both CYP3A4 and Pgp. Sirolimus is extensively metabolized in the intestinal wall and the liver and undergoes counter-transport from the enterocytes in the small intestine into the gut lumen by the Pgp drug efflux pump. Sirolimus is potentially recycled between the enterocytes and the gut lumen, allowing multiple opportunies for metabolism by CYP3A4. Sirolimus is extensively metabolized by O-demethylation and/or hydroxylation. At least seven sirolimus metabolites have been identified, although they have been shown to possess less than 10% of the immunosuppressive activity of sirolimus.[150] The majority of sirolimus is excreted in the feces with only a minor amount excreted in the urine.

Drug Interactions. Similar to cyclosporine and tacrolimus, sirolimus is a substrate for both CYP3A4 and Pgp, with the potential for numerous drug interactions. Medications that may commonly alter sirolimus bioavailability, metabolism, and blood levels are similar to those that interact with both cyclosporine and tacrolimus.

Adverse Drug Reactions. Sirolimus is associated with numerous side effects, the most common and clinically important of which are thrombocytopenia and increases in triglycerides and cholesterol values. These dose-related lipid elevations are often controllable through diet and drug therapy; however, discontinuation is sometimes required.[154] Rare but troublesome reactions have included the development of lymphoceles, a decrease in wound healing, and pneumonitis. Other adverse reactions include peripheral edema, dizziness, nausea, vomiting, diarrhea, arthralgia, headache, leucopenia, anemia, acne, and aphthous ulcers.[151,152] It has been suggested that the frequency of microangiopathic hemolysis and thrombocytopenia is increased when sirolimus is combined with tacrolimus for prophylaxis of GVHD.[155]

Monitoring. Since there are large variations in pharmacokinetics and potential drug interactions, therapeutic drug monitoring helps to maintain concentrations as well as minimize adverse effects. Whole blood levels should be initiated 5 to 7 days after starting or changing treatment, whenever side effects are suspected, or when otherwise clinically indicated. Whole blood trough concentrations may range from 5 to 24 ng/ml. Patients should also be monitored for thrombocytopenia, leukopenia, hypertriglyceridemia, and hypercholesterolemia.[153]

Mycophenolic Acid

Mycophenolic acid (MPA; mycophenolate mofetil [CellCept], mycophenolate sodium [Myfortic]) was first isolated from a *Penicillium* culture in 1896, though its immunosuppressive properties were not recognized until 1969.[156,157] Mycophenolate mofetil (MMF), a prodrug of MPA, was the initial formulation of MPA approved for human use, although mycophenolate sodium (MPS) is now also available. The initial efficacy data in transplantation were obtained from a single-center study using MMF as maintenance therapy and a multicenter study using it to treat biopsy-proven acute rejection.[158,159] In a subsequent trial in renal transplant recipients, patients were randomized to receive either azathioprine (100 to 150 mg/day) or MMF (2 g/day or 3 g/day). Biopsy-proven rejection was demonstrated in 35.5% of the azathioprine group versus 19.7% and 15.9% of the 2-g/day and 3-g/day MMF groups.[160] A study of heart transplant patients receiving MMF or azathioprine also demonstrated improved mortality and decreased severity of rejection events in the MMF group.[161] More recent studies using the modified, more consistently bioavailable forms of cyclosporine failed to demonstrate differences between MMF and azathioprine

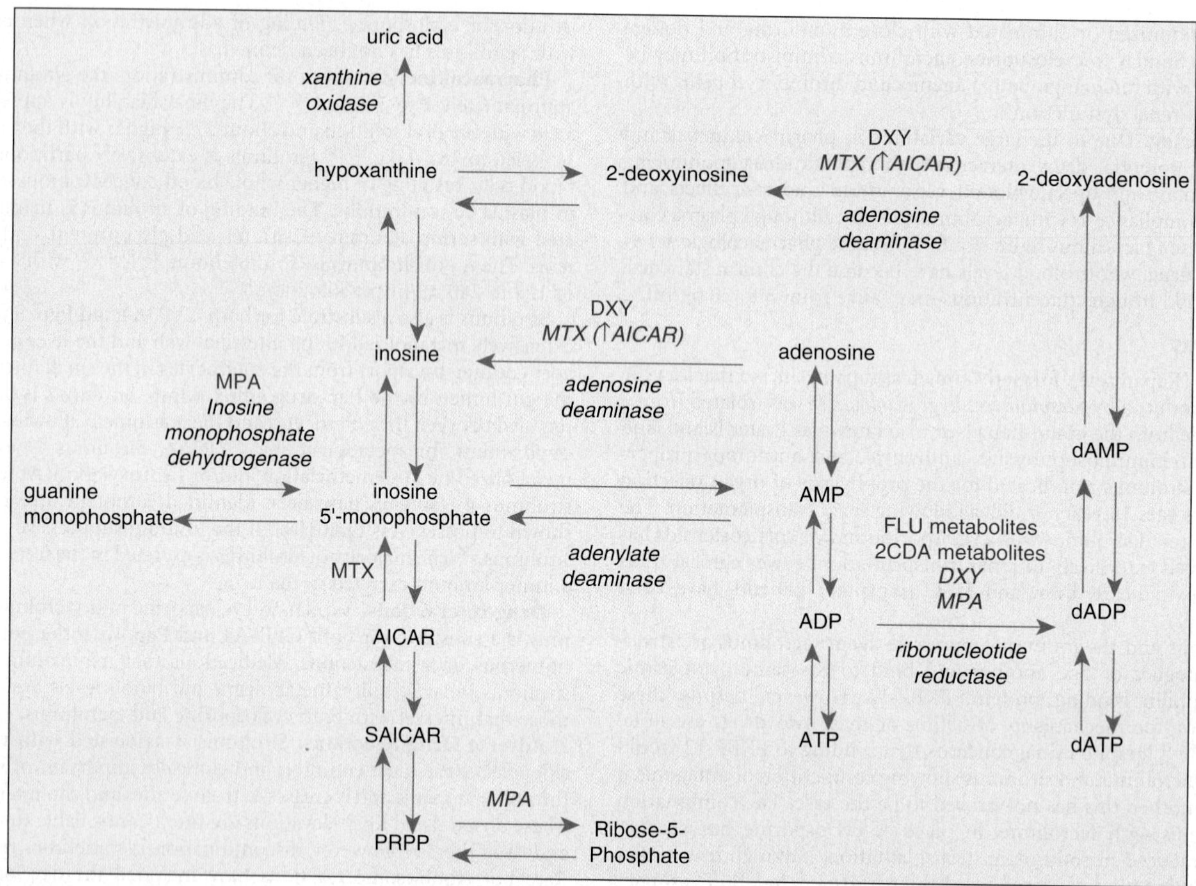

FIGURE 92-4 • Drugs affecting purine synthesis. Primary inhibitory effects of these agents or their direct metabolites are shown in red and secondary (downstream) inhibitory effects due to accumulation of other purine precursors or products are shown in blue. Methotrexate blocks the conversion of inosine 5′-monophosphate, leading to increased AICAR with the secondary effect of adenosine deaminase inhibition. 2-Chlorodeoxyadenosine is metabolized to 2-chlorodoxy ATP, which inhibits ribonucleotide reductase. Deoxycoformycin directly inhibits adenosine deaminase and, with the downstream result of increased dATP, has a secondary inhibition of ribonucleotide reductase. Fludarabine is metabolized to F-ara-ATP, which blocks DNA polymerase, inhibits DNA ligase and polymerase, and also inhibits ribonucleotide reductase. Mycophenolic acid inhibits inosine monophosphate dehydrogenase with an increase in adenosine versue guanine phosphates, in turn inhibiting PRPP synthetase and ribonucleotide reductase. The accumulation of adenosine leads to apoptosis of lymphocytes. (ADP, adenosine diphosphate; AICAR, aminoimidazole carboxamide ribonucleotide; AMP, adenosine monophosphate; ATP, adenosine triphosphate; dADP, deoxy adenosine diphosphate; dAMP, deoxy adenosine monophosphate; dATP, deoxy adenosine triphosphate; DXY, deoxyconformycin; FLU, fludarabine; MTX, methotrexate; PRPP, phosphoribosylpyrophosphate; SAICAR, succinylaminoimidazolecarboxamide riboside; 2CDA, 2-chlorodeoxyadenosine.)

with regard to rates of rejection in kidney transplantation or rates of bronchiolitis obliterans in lung transplantation.[162,163] MMF has also been used for GVHD prophylaxis after HSCT, particularly after non-myeloablative transplantation.[164] MMF is also used in the treatment of lupus nephritis.[165] Recently, increased concern has been raised about the teratogenicity of MPA suggesting that this drug should be avoided in female patients expecting to become pregnant in the near future if other treatment options are available.[165a]

Mechanism of Action. MPA inhibits T- and B-cell proliferation through potent, selective, noncompetitive, reversible inhibition of the enzyme inosine monophosphate dehydrogenase (IMPDH). This enzyme catalyzes the conversion of inosine monophosphate to guanosine monophosphate, leading to increased concentrations of guanosine phosphates that, in turn, activate the two rate-limiting enzymes of DNA synthesis, 5-phosphoribosyl-1-pyrophosphate (PRPP) synthetase and ribonucleotide reductase. Adenosine phosphates exert the opposite affect, inhibiting these two enzymes. When IMPDH is inhibited, adenosine phosphate concentrations increase relative to guanine phosphates, thus inhibiting PRPP synthetase and ribonucleotide reductase and slowing DNA synthesis. Figure 92-4 depicts a schematic representation of the mechanism of action of MPA as well as other drugs affecting purine metabolism.

The selectivity of MPA for lymphocytes is based on two factors. First, while most cells have both a de novo and a salvage pathway for purine synthesis, lymphocytes are dependent on the de novo pathway. Second, MPA has a nearly fivefold stronger affinity for the type II isoform of IMPDH, which is expressed in activated T and B lymphocytes, versus the type I isoform, which is constitutively expressed.[166,167] It has been postulated that this impairment in DNA synthesis traps lymphocytes in the early G_1 phase of the cell cycle and significantly increases the proportion of lymphocytes that undergo apoptosis.[166]

Dosing and Administration. MMF is rapidly absorbed from the gastrointestinal tract and is hydrolyzed to MPA in the bloodstream. MMF is also rapidly de-esterified in the gut. Peak concentrations of MPA occur about 1 hour after dosing. MPA can also be administered orally as the sodium salt (MPS) using enteric-coated tablets, which results in absorption lower in the intestine and a later peak blood concentration. Typically both drugs are administered in twice-daily dosing regimens, with 500 mg of MMF being equivalent to 360 mg of MPS.

In initial trials, 1 g of MMF administered twice daily had nearly the same efficacy as 1.5 g twice daily but with better tolerability. Tacrolimus results in a slightly increased AUC of MPA, allowing for slightly lower dosing. When MPA levels have been monitored, AUC levels of greater than 30 mg*hr/L appear associated with a lower incidence of rejection, but there does not appear to be any benefit of AUC levels greater than 60 mg*hr/L.

Pharmacokinetics. The $t_{1/2}$ of MPA is between 16.6 and 17.9 hours. MPA is highly protein bound, with 97.5% bound to albumin. MPA is typically metabolized to glucuronidated metabolites, and the major metabolite, mycophenolic acid glucuronide (MPAG), is inactive. A minor acyl glucuronide metabolite has pharmacologic activity comparable to MPA. Over 60% of MPAG is excreted in the urine, but a considerable amount enters the bile and becomes potentially reavailable as MPA through deconjugation by gut flora and enterohepatic circulation. This can produce a second MPA peak between 6 and 8 hours after dosing.

Drug Interactions. Cyclosporine appears to impair secretion of MPAG into bile and thus results in somewhat lower patient exposure to MPA than if tacrolimus is used.[168] Cholestyramine can bind MPAG in the intestinal lumen, reducing the enterohepatic circulation and significantly lowering total MPA exposure.

Adverse Drug Reactions. The principle side effects of MPA are a result of the drug's effect on rapidly dividing cell lineages. Gastrointestinal side effects (nausea, vomiting, diarrhea) predominate, followed closely by hematologic cytopenias (leukopenia, anemia, thrombocytopenia). Many of the adverse effects are dose related and may be minimized or eliminated with close monitoring and dosage reduction. MPA does not appear to increase the incidence of PTLD.[169]

Monitoring. MPA concentrations can be monitored in either MMF- or MPS-treated patients. In contrast to cyclosporine, tacrolimus, or sirolimus, routine monitoring of MPA levels is not routinely performed. Patients should be monitored for hematologic cytopenias as well as for signs and symptoms of infection.

Antithymocyte Globulin (Equine)

Equine ATG (Atgam), also referred to as lymphocyte immune globulin, is a γ-globulin preparation purified from the serum of horses hyperimmunized with human thymus lymphocytes. Atgam is indicated for the management of renal allograft rejection and for the treatment of moderate to severe aplastic anemia. Atgam has been used as an adjunct to other immunosuppressive therapy to delay the onset of the first rejection episode. Atgam as well as OKT3 and rabbit ATG (Thymoglobulin) have been used to delay introduction of calcineurin inhibitors to avoid early nephrotoxic effects following renal transplantation. The drug has also been used in conditioning regimens for patients receiving allogeneic HSCT as well as for treatment of acute GVHD.

Mechanism of Action. There has been much debate about the mechanism of action of Atgam and similar antithymocyte and antilymphocyte immune globulins. Similar to other polyclonal and monoclonal anti–T-cell antibodies, there appear to be a number of distinct mechanisms. Atgam contains antibodies to the cell surface antigens CD2, CD3, CD4, CD5, CD8, CD11a, CD14, CD18, CD19, CD20, and CD45.[170] Atgam appears to facilitate depletion of T cells by complement-mediated lysis, by antibody-dependent cell-mediated cytotoxicity, and by opsonization with subsequent T-cell clearance by the spleen, liver, and lungs.[171]

Dosing and Administration. Prior to the first Atgam infusion, the manufacturer recommends that patients be tested with an intradermal injection of 0.1 ml of a 1 : 1000 dilution. However, the predictive value of this test has not been proven, and many centers opt to simply initiate the first dose at a very low rate, escalating as tolerated. Atgam should be administered as a continuous IV infusion into a high-flow vein through an in-line filter with a pore size of 0.2 to 1.0 micron over no less than 4 hours. Lysis of leukocytes may release many inflammatory mediators, leading to fever and chills in some patients, despite coadministration of corticosteroids, acetaminophen, and diphenhydramine. With each subsequent dose, the severity of these reactions often declines, presumably as there are fewer leukocytes undergoing lysis with each successive treatment. The dosing of Atgam for the treatment of rejection is 10 to 15 mg/kg per day for 14 days. Dosing for treatment of aplastic anemia has included similar regimens of 10 to 20 mg/kg for 8 to 14 days, though shorter courses at a higher dose are now more often employed (40 mg/kg per day for 4 days). For rejection conditioning regimens, doses have ranged from 20 to 40 mg/kg for 2 to 5 days. Many alternative dosing regimens, such as shorter courses with or without higher daily doses, have also been used.

Appropriate resuscitation equipment should be available for anaphylactic reactions. It is important to distinguish between true severe allergic reactions, which are infrequent, versus the fever and chill reactions (occasionally with a lowering of the blood pressure), which are more commonly seen with the first dose due to white cell lysis. In the absence of desensitization or other measures, allergic reactions will persist with subsequent doses, while reactions due to white cell lysis typically become less pronounced.

Pharmacokinetics. The metabolism and elimination are complex, and the pharmacokinetics of Atgam have wide variations due to individual differences in patient clearance of immunoglobulins. The V_d is 0.12 L/kg and the $t_{1/2}$ is 5.7 hours.[172,173] However, one third of patients have a $t_{1/2}$ of less than 3.5 days.

Adverse Drug Reactions. Common adverse reactions include fever, skin reactions, chills, arthralgia, headache, myalgia, nausea, chest pain, phlebitis, leukopenia, and thrombocytopenia. These reactions occur more frequently with the first dose and often can be minimized with premedication as described previously. With mild leukopenia or thrombocytopenia, treatment may be continued, sometimes with reduced dosage. Less frequent reactions include rash, pruritis, anaphylaxis, edema, dyspnea, flank pain, hypotension, and stomatitis. ATG-treated patients are particularly prone to both infections and secondary lymphomas.[174,175] Serum sickness with rash, arthralgia, and proteinuria may be seen several weeks later as with administration of any foreign protein.

Monitoring. Since Atgam decreases the number of circulating T cells, enumeration of T cells can be used as a guide for determining the appropriate dose and duration of treatment. The absolute lymphocyte count can be determined from a complete blood count, or more precise measurements of CD2- and CD3-positive T cells can be determined by flow cytometric analysis.[176] It is also feasible to measure functional Atgam levels in serum using patient serum as the antibody source for immunofluorescent measurements by flow cytometry.[177]

Antithymocyte Globulin (Rabbit)

Rabbit ATG (Thymoglobulin) is a polyclonal immune globulin purified from the serum of rabbits immunized with human thymocytes. Like Atgam, Thymoglobulin contains cytotoxic antibodies directed against T cell and other antigens expressed on lymphocytes. Thymoglobulin is indicated for the treatment of acute rejection in renal transplant recipients when used in combination with other immune-suppressing agents. Thymoglobulin, similar to OKT3 and Atgam, has also been used to delay the onset of rejection in renal transplant patients and to delay introduction of a calcineurin inhibitor.[178,179] It has been used to prevent and treat rejection in other solid organ transplants, including liver,[180] lung,[181] pancreas,[182,183] intestine,[184] and heart.[185,186] Thymoglobulin, like Atgam, has also been used to treat aplastic anemia. It has been used in the HSCT setting to prevent and to treat GVHD.[177,187,188]

Mechanism of Action. Thymoglobulin contains antibodies against CD2, CD3, CD4, CD8, CD11a, CD18, CD25, CD44, CD45, HLA-DR, HLA class I heavy chains, and β_2-microglobulin. However, the mechanism of action of polyclonal lymphocyte immune globulins, such as Thymoglobulin or Atgam, is not completely understood. Several mechanisms of action have been proposed and are of varying importance based on the serum concentration. These include T-cell clearance from the circulation, apoptosis, modulation of T-cell activation and T-cell homing, antibody-dependent cytotoxicity, and suppression of dendritic cell function.[189,190]

Dosing and Administration. Thymoglobulin should be administered as a continuous IV infusion over at least 6 hours for the first infusion, and at least 4 hours subsequently. It must be given through an in-line 0.22-micron filter. Although the manufacturer recommends that it be infused through a high-flow vein, a number of groups have reported success with peripheral administration.[191,192] Just as with Atgam, infusion reactions may occur and premedication with corticosteroids, acetaminophen, and diphenhydramine is recommended. Appropriate resuscitation equipment should be available for anaphylactic reactions. As with Atgam, it is important to distinguish between true allergic reactions versus fever and chill reactions.

The dosing of Thymoglobulin for the treatment of acute renal allograft rejection is 1.5 mg/kg per day for 10 to 14 days,[193-196] whereas dosing to prevent rejection in solid organ transplant recipients is usually 1 to 1.5 mg/kg per day for 3 to 7 days.[197-199] In HSCT, Thymoglobulin has been used particularly in mismatched related and unrelated donor pairs, in whom doses have ranged from 4 to 10.5 mg/kg total dose, with the lowest treatment-related mortality associated with doses in the 6- to 8-mg/kg range.[187,192,200,201] Originally, the dosing equivalence between Atgam and Thymoglobulin was believed to be about 10:1, though more recently it has been suggested to be higher.

Pharmacokinetics. After an IV infusion of 1.25 to 1.5 mg/kg per day, Thymoglobulin levels were 21.5 mcg/ml at 4 to 8 hours postinfusion, with a $t_{1/2}$ of 2 to 3 days. In HSCT patients, in whom larger doses are given, $t_{1/2}$ is reported at 6 to 8 days, with a time to clearance to subtherapeutic levels (<1 mcg/ml) of 15 to 47 days (range 8 to 83).[177,192] There are two phases of clearance of Thymoglobulin, with an early alpha clearance during the first 4 weeks after administration, followed by a slower beta clearance during the subsequent 4 weeks.[177,192] Levels of Thymoglobulin can be checked using either enzyme-linked immunosorbent assay or flow-based assays, but neither is routinely available to the clinician.

Adverse Drug Reactions. Common adverse reactions to Thymoglobulin include fever, chills, leukopenia, pain, headache, abdominal pain, diarrhea, hypertension, nausea, thrombocytopenia, peripheral edema, dyspnea, asthenia, hyperkalemia, tachycardia, leucopenia, malaise, and dizziness. As with Atgam, these reactions occur more frequently with the first dose and often can be minimized with premedication and slow infusion as described previously. Serum sickness may also occur.[202,203]

Monitoring. The approach to monitoring Thymoglobulin is similar to that for Atgam and may include a total WBC, absolute lymphocyte count, platelet count, and T-cell enumeration by flow cytometry. It is also feasible to measure functional Thymoglobulin levels in serum using patient serum as the antibody source for immunofluorescent flow cytometric measurements.[177,204]

Muromonab-CD3

Muromonab-CD3 (Orthoclone OKT3), commonly referred to as OKT3, is a murine monoclonal anti–T-cell antibody directed against the CD3 complex. OKT3 is indicated for the treatment of acute allograft rejection in renal transplant patients and steroid-resistant acute allograft rejection in cardiac and hepatic transplant patients. OKT3 has been widely used as induction treatment at the time of transplantation in an attempt to block the initial immune response as well as reducing both the frequency and severity of rejection episodes. OKT3 has also been used to delay introduction of a calcineurin inhibitor, similar to Atgam and Thymoglobulin.

Mechanism of Action. CD3 is a complex of at least five proteins noncovalently associated with the T-cell receptor. Neither the CD3 complex nor the T-cell receptor will be expressed on the cell surface without the other. CD3 is involved in the transduction of signals from the T-cell receptor after cross-linking by antigen-MHC. Most CD3 antibodies, including OKT3, bind to the ε chain of the complex. OKT3 binds to circulating T lymphocytes and causes an immediate reduction due to opsonization with phagocytosis and removal by the reticuloendothelial system. Some T lymphocytes return to the circulation but, due to modulation of the antigen receptor–CD3 complex, these cells are rendered immunologically nonfunctional despite their persistence. Finally, due to close molecular proximity, binding of OKT3 to CD3 interferes with the ability of the adjacent T-cell receptor to bind ligand and thus prevents T-lymphocyte recognition of antigen and consequent activation.[205,206]

Dosing and Administration. The dosing of OKT3 for the treatment of rejection is 5 mg/day in a single IV injection over less than 1 minute for 10 to 14 days. Immunomonitoring of target cells and measurement of serum concentrations has allowed alterations in the traditional dosing methods. Several studies have demonstrated that reduced dosing is still efficacious for both the prevention and treatment of rejection episodes.[207,208] Due to a cytokine release syndrome commonly associated with the first few doses of OKT3 administration, patients should be monitored in a facility equipped for cardiopulmonary resuscitation. The patient's volume status should be assessed to make sure that weight gain is no more than 3% above the minimum weight for the week preceding treatment. Premedication is strongly recommended 1 to 4 hours prior to treatment and should include methylprednisolone for the first dose along with acetaminophen and diphenhydramine for all doses. Pentoxifylline and indomethacin have also been added to the premedication regimen.

Pharmacokinetics. Following IV administration of OKT3, a rapid decrease of CD3-positive cells occurs within minutes. After discontinuation of therapy, the function of T lymphocytes reappears rapidly and usually returns to normal within a week in solid organ transplant recipients, though this may be delayed far longer in patients receiving HSCT. The V_d is 6.5 L.[209,210] The metabolism and elimination of OKT3 is not well establsihed, as it may be removed by opsonization as previously described or by human antimurine antibody production induced by the recipient immune system in a small percentage of patients.[211-213] High serum anti-OKT3 antibody levels can neutralize the effect of OKT3 and limit the ability to receive a second course. The $t_{1/2}$ of OKT3 is approximately 18 hours and remains constant unless anti-OKT3 antibodies are produced, leading to more rapid elimination of OKT3.[214]

Adverse Drug Reactions. The majority of adverse reactions from OKT3 use are commonly associated with the cytokines released from activated lymphocytes or monocytes. These reactions occur more frequently with the first and second doses and often can be prevented or minimized with premedication as described previously. Typical symptoms include pyrexia, chills, dyspnea, nausea, vomiting, chest pain, diarrhea, tremor, wheezing, headache, tachycardia, rigor, and hypertension. Patients have also reported rash, pruritis, angioedema, serum sickness, arthritis, confusion, and nervousness. Rare cases of fatal cardiorespiratory manifestations have occurred. A number of groups have reported an increased risk of lymphoproliferative disorders with OKT3 use.[215-217]

Monitoring. Therapeutic drug monitoring has been extensively used to determine the appropriate dose, duration, and efficacy of OKT3 as well as to determine whether or not re-treatment is possible. Parameters monitored may include serum OKT3 levels, enumeration of CD3-positive T cells, and detection and quantitation of human antimurine antibodies.[207,209,211,212,218]

Alemtuzumab

Alemtuzumab (Campath-1H, Campath) is a humanized immunoglobulin G1 monoclonal antibody directed against the CD52 glycoprotein, which is found on T and B lymphocytes, NK cells, monocytes, and macrophages. Alemtuzumab is approved for the treatment of chronic B-cell lymphocytic leukemia (B-CLL). Due to its potent lymphocyte-depleting effects, it has also been used to treat rheumatoid arthritis, scleroderma, and multiple sclerosis.[219-221] In recent years, alemtuzumab has also become more commonly used in transplant patients for both the treatment and prevention of organ rejection as well as for prevention of GVHD.[222-225] Alemtuzumab has been used primarily as an induction agent similar to other T-cell antibody preparations. Numerous studies—mostly small, single-center, retrospective trials—have evaluated the use of alemtuzumab.[37,226-229] However, these studies have been conducted using a wide range of organ types, doses, concomitant immunosuppressive agents, and follow-up time points. Combined, the studies support alemtuzumab as a potentially valuable agent in transplantation. However, based on the current data, it is uncertain if alemtuzumab is superior in potency or efficacy to other agents.

Alemtuzumab causes cell death through complement-mediated cytolysis, antibody-mediated cytotoxicity, and induction of apoptosis. The dosing of alemtuzumab used in transplant patients has varied between centers and the organ being transplanted. Some of the common dosing schemes consist of 20 or 30 mg at the time of transplantation followed by an additional dose within 1 to 4 days. Others have used weight-based dosing of 0.3 mg/kg for two to four doses spaced out over the first week following the transplant.

Alemtuzumab should be administered as a continuous IV infusion over 2 hours, although, in the treatment of B-CLL, subcutaneous rather than IV therapy is currently preferred. Alemtuzumab use has been associated with many allergic- and anaphylactic-type reactions, and prophylactic premedication is recommended. Appropriate resuscitation equipment should also be kept nearby. The $t_{1/2}$ is approximately 12 days, though the depletional effects can persist for months or even years.[227,230] While head-to-head comparisons are lacking, many believe that alemtuzumab produces longer lasting immunosuppression than other lympholytic antibodies. Since the long-term cellular recovery and clinical outcomes remain unknown, few centers have gained extensive experience with alemtuzumab and few have initiated routine use of the drug.

In HSCT, alemtuzumab was originally used primarily for ex vivo T-cell depletion of stem cell products. More commonly now, alemtuzumab is added to the stem cell product at a dose of 20 mg per product to produce in vivo elimination of many of the T cells contained in the product.[231] The drug is also administered either pre- or posttransplant in a wide range of doses to accomplish the same effect.[224,232,233] Elimination of many remaining host T cells also occurs, which may simultaneously reduce the risks of graft rejection. Immune suppression may be long lasting.

In B-CLL, the most common side effects included infusion reactions (fever, rigors, hypotension, and nausea), lymphopenia, neutropenia, rash, diarrhea, anemia, thrombocytopenia, and infection. Many of these same effects can also be seen in transplant patients, although they tend to be less prominent and severe because of the reduced dosages used. Given the limited experience in transplantation, particularly regarding long-term follow-up, patients should be followed closely. Monitoring should include complete blood counts and $CD4^+$ cell counts.

Daclizumab

Daclizumab (Zenapax) was the first genetically engineered, humanized monoclonal antibody targeting the α chain of the IL-2R (also referred to as CD25 or Tac) expressed on activated but not resting T cells.[234] The DNA sequence of daclizumab is 90% human and 10% murine, thus improving upon complications associated with murine antibodies such as shorter half-life and increased immunogenicity.[235] Daclizumab is indicated for prophylaxis of acute rejection in renal transplant recipients in combination with cyclosporine and corticosteroids. Unlike antibodies targeted to both resting and activated T cells (OKT3, Atgam, Thymoglobulin), which are commonly used to delay introduction of a calcineurin inhibitor, daclizumab is not effective when used in this fashion.[236] Daclizumab has been commonly used in combination with tacrolimus, MMF, sirolimus, and azathioprine. Daclizumab has also been used for the prevention of rejection in liver, pancreas, heart, lung, and intestinal transplant patients as well as for treatment of acute GVHD.[236-242] Because IL-2 is a major stimulus for T-cell growth, blockade of the IL-2R has potential utility in treating T-cell–mediated (autoimmune) diseases such as uveitis and psoriasis.[243,244] Daclizumab has undergone some investigation in HSCT, but is not currently commonly utilized for the prevention or treatment of GVHD in these patients.

Mechanism of Action. Daclizumab is a genetically engineered monoclonal antibody in which the binding regions of a murine antibody have been grafted onto a human immunoglobulin G1 backbone. Daclizumab binds to the alpha subunit of the IL-2R expressed on the surface of activated T cells, thus preventing IL-2 binding and signal transduction and competitively antagonizing IL-2–mediated lymphocyte activation and IL-2–induced T-cell proliferation.[245] Daclizumab has slightly lower affinity than other murine monoclonal anti-Tac antibodies, but it is less immunogenic, has more immunosuppressive properties, and has a longer half-life.[234,235,245,246]

Dosing and Administration. The recommended dose of daclizumab in patients 11 months of age and older is 1 mg/kg by IV infusion over 15 minutes less than 24 hours prior to kidney transplantation. Treatment is repeated every 14 days for a total of five doses. Numerous studies evaluating alternative doses and schedules have shown promise both in terms of safety and efficacy.[247,248]

Pharmacokinetics. The estimated $t_{1/2}$ of daclizumab is about 20 days, which is comparable to the $t_{1/2}$ of human immunoglobulin G (IgG) (18 to 23 days). There is a significant decrease in the percentage of circulating $CD25^+$ cells starting 10 hours after transplantation and lasting up to 4 months following daclizumab administration.[246] In vitro and in vivo data suggest that serum levels of 1 to 10 mcg/ml are necessary for saturation of the Tac subunit of the IL-2R to block IL-2–mediated responses of T-cell lymphocytes.[247,249] The approved dosing regimen sustains serum concentrations that saturate IL-2Rs and inhibit T-cell proliferation for 90 days following transplantation.[250]

Adverse Effects and Monitoring. The incidence of adverse effects from daclizumab is comparable to placebo, perhaps reflecting that most of the molecule is human IgG1. However, since 10% of the molecule is of murine origin, there is a small potential risk of hypersensitivity reactions.[247,250]

Basiliximab

Basiliximab (Simulect) is a recombinant DNA monoclonal antibody similar to daclizumab that also targets the IL-2R α chain. Basiliximab is indicated for prophylaxis of acute rejection following renal transplantation when used in combination with cyclosporine and corticosteroids. Basiliximab has also been studied in prophylaxis of organ rejection in liver transplantation, GVHD, psoriasis, and atopic dermatitis.[251-255] Like daclizumab, basiliximab is also a chimeric (humanized/murine) monoclonal antibody, resulting in a prolonged half-life and reduced immunogenicity.[256-258]

Mechanism of Action. By binding to the α chain of the IL-2R, basiliximab, like daclizumab, inhibits IL-2–mediated lymphocyte activation and proliferation.[256,259] Since the receptors for IL-2 and IL-15 form a supramolecular complex, binding of basiliximab to the IL-2R α chain may also cause down-regulation of signaling by IL-15.[260,261]

Dosing and Administration. The recommended dose of basiliximab for renal transplant rejection prophylaxis in adults is 20 mg IV 2 hours prior to transplantation (day 0), followed by a second 20-mg dose given IV on day 4 following transplantation.[261,262] For pediatric patients, weight-based doses have been studied.[263] For patients less than 35 kg, a dose of 10 mg IV is given 2 hours prior to transplantation on day 0 and is repeated on day 4. For patients ≥35 kg, the adult dosing regimen can be administered. Basiliximab can be given as an IV bolus injection or can be further diluted in normal saline or 5% dextrose solution and infused over 20 to 30 minutes. Dose adjustments are not necessary based on age, gender, or renal function.[260,262]

Pharmacokinetics. Saturation of IL-2 α receptors has been shown to occur when basiliximab serum concentrations are greater than 0.2 mcg/ml.[262] If concentrations of basiliximab fall below this threshold, the number of circulating activated T lymphocytes expressing the IL-2R returns to normal in 1 to 2 weeks.[260] After administration of the approved dosing regimen in combination with cyclosporine and corticosteroids, the mean duration of IL-2R suppression is from 36 to 49 days. Basiliximab exhibits a slow clearance of 17.3 to 36.7 ml/hr and a long $t_{1/2}$ of 7.4 to 8.2 days.[264]

Adverse Effects and Monitoring. Since basiliximab is a humanized antibody, the incidence of adverse effects is very low, though patients should be monitored for cytokine release syndrome and anaphylaxis. Other adverse events reported in clinical trials are similar to placebo and include nonspecific cutaneous and gastrointestinal effects.[251,256-260,262]

Denileukin Diftitox

Denileukin diftitox (Ontak) is a genetically engineered protein consisting of portions of IL-2 and diphtheria toxin. IL-2 is the targeting moiety, which leads to internalization into cells expressing the IL-2R. After entry, the diphtheria toxin causes ADP-ribosylation of EF-2 which inhibits protein synthesis.[265] Ontak preferentially binds to cells expressing the high-affinity IL-2R, such as activated T cells. Although the use of Ontak in GVHD treatment is still being defined, two studies have shown that this agent is active in the treatment of steroid-resistant GVHD.[61,266,267] Side effects of the drug include infection and vascular leak syndrome.[266,267]

Azathioprine

Azathioprine (Imuran) was one of the original drugs used as an immunosuppressant in clinical transplantation, often in combination with corticosteroids prior to the availability of drugs such as MMF. Azathioprine is no longer one of the core transplantation medications, but still is widely used in autoimmune diseases such as rheumatoid arthritis, systemic lupus erythematosus, and multiple sclerosis.[268-270] Azathioprine is an antimetabolite purine analogue that is cleaved in vivo to produce 6-mercaptopurine (6-MP). In transplantation, azathioprine is used primarily as prophylaxis of organ rejection following renal transplantation.[268]

Mechanism of Action. Azathioprine is a prodrug that is metabolized in the liver to produce 6-MP, a purine analogue,[268] but it is less toxic than native 6-MP. Its precise mechanism of action is unknown. Azathioprine interferes with purine synthesis and is incorporated into DNA and RNA, thus interfering with DNA, RNA, and protein synthesis.[268] Due to its antiproliferative effects, T- and B-cell function are inhibited and the number of circulating leukocytes is reduced. Azathioprine is only effective if administered prior to antigenic stimulation. Therefore, it is effective in the prophylaxis but not treatment of acute rejection.[268,271]

Dosing and Administration. The initial dosing of azathioprine for prophylaxis of renal transplant rejection is 3 to 5 mg/kg IV or orally as a single dose given on the day of transplantation. Maintenance treatment for organ rejection prophylaxis is usually 1 to 3 mg/kg per day given orally. Azathioprine can be given in two divided doses with food to reduce gastrointestinal side effects.[272] Dose adjustments should be made based upon hematologic and hepatic adverse effects and based on creatinine clearance.

Pharmacokinetics. Azathioprine is well absorbed following oral administration.[268] The absolute oral bioavailability is estimated to be between 41% and 47%. Protein binding of azathioprine is approximately 30% and it is partially dialyzable. Azathioprine undergoes metabolism to 6-MP in the liver by sulfhydryl compounds such as glutathione. 6-MP undergoes further metabolism via oxidation and methylation in the liver and in erythrocytes. Metabolites of azathioprine are primarily excreted via the kidney, with very small amounts of the parent compound excreted intact. The $t_{1/2}$ of azathioprine is approximately 3 hours.[270]

Adverse Effects. The major dose-limiting toxicity of azathioprine is bone marrow suppression, so frequent hematologic monitoring is required.[273] The toxicity is dose dependent and is usually manifested as leukopenia, macrocytic anemia, and thrombocytopenia. Gastrointestinal effects such as nausea, vomiting, and diarrhea have been reported after large doses of azathioprine. Severe hepatotoxicity, characterized by increased serum levels of hepatic enzymes and bilirubin, is not dose dependent. Liver toxicity usually occurs within 6 months of starting azathioprine and is reversible if azathioprine is discontinued promptly.[274] Other adverse effects include rash and fever.

Drug Interactions. Because azathioprine is normally inactivated by xanthine oxidase, caution and substantial dose reduction are required when patients require concomitant xanthine oxidase inhibitors such as allopurinol. Allopurinol can potentiate azathioprine toxicity, manifested by severe anemia, leukopenia, nausea, and vomiting. Typically patients require only one fourth to one third of the normal dose of azathioprine when allopurinol is coadministered.

Monitoring. Complete blood counts, including platelets, should be monitored every 2 weeks for the first month of treatment and monthly thereafter. More frequent monitoring should be performed if the dose is changed or if leukopenia occurs. Azathioprine therapy should be discontinued if the WBC count falls below 3000 cells/mm^3. Hepatic function tests should be conducted every 2 weeks for the first month of treatment and monthly thereafter.[270]

Methotrexate

Methotrexate (4-amino-10-methyl pteroylglutamic acid), a folic acid analogue, was originally synthesized in 1948 and has undergone widespread use in the treatment of cancer.[275] Methotrexate was also found to have inhibitory effects on activated T cells, resulting in their apoptosis.[276] This led to use of the drug for treatment of immunologic disorders, including rheumatoid arthritis,[277] lupus,[278] and psoriasis.[279] In transplantation, methotrexate has been used primarily for the prophylaxis of GVHD in HSCT. Based upon its effectiveness in preventing GVHD in canine models,[280,281] methotrexate became the gold standard for GVHD prophylaxis in the 1970s and early 1980s, initially as a single agent and subsequently combined with cyclosporine.[282] By 1998, there were reports that the combination of methotrexate and tacrolimus was superior to that of methotrexate and cyclosporine.[283]

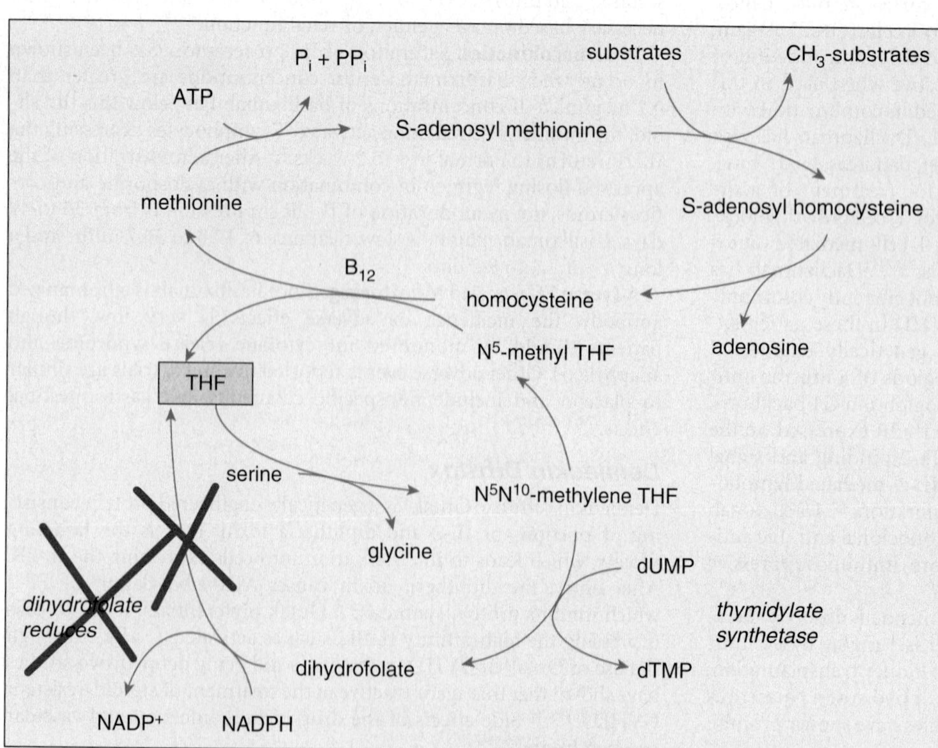

FIGURE 92-5 • The inhibitory effect of methotrexate on dihydrofolate reductase blocking conversion of dihydrofolate to tetrahydrofolate (THF) is illustrated. ATP, adenosine triphosphate; dUMP, deoxyuridylate monophosphate; dTMP, thymidylate monophosphate; NADPH, nicotinamide adenine dinucleotide phosphate; P_i, orthophosphate; PP_i, pyrophosphate.

Mechanism of Action. Methotrexate is an antimetabolite that works through inhibition of dihydrofolate reductase (DHFR), an enzyme required in the synthesis of thymidylate, purines, methionine, and serine.[284] In normal thymine synthesis, a methyl group is delivered to the enzyme thymidylate synthase by folate. The methyl group is then transferred to uracil to produce thymine. In this process, the folate molecule is oxidized, and must be restored to its reduced state by DHFR to continue thymine synthesis. When DHFR is inhibited by methotrexate, folate is not restored to its reduced state, and thymine synthesis is inhibited.[285] Figure 92-5 depicts a schematic representation of the effects of methotrexate on folate metabolism. Inflammatory effects and cell injury appear to be dose dependent. Patients receiving the drug posttransplantation develop more severe mucositis and delayed blood count recovery compared to other regimens for GVHD prophylaxis.

The immune-suppressive effects of methotrexate are thought to be due to the ability of the drug to inhibit 5-aminoimidazole-4-carboxamide ribonucleotide transformylase,[276] which catalyzes the last step of de novo biosynthesis of inosine biophosphate in purine nucleotide synthesis. Inhibition of this enzyme leads to the accumulation of aminoimidazole carboxamide riboside, an adenosine deaminase inhibitor. Inhibition of adenosine deaminase, in turn, produces increased concentrations of adenosine that inhibit lymphocyte proliferation,[276] consistent with the fact that congenital deficiency of adenosine deaminase leads to a severe combined immunodeficiency syndrome. Figure 92-4 depicts a schematic representation of the mechanism of action of methotrexate. In addition, methotrexate can directly suppress the secretion of proinflammatory cytokines such as interferon-γ and TNF.[286]

Dosing and Administration. Methotrexate was originally administered for GVHD prophylaxis on days 1, 3, 6, 11, and weekly thereafter until day 100 after allogeneic transplantation.[282] Typically, 15 mg/m^2 is given on day 1, and 10 mg/m^2 is given for the remaining doses. Single-agent methotrexate use is rare today. Most commonly, it is now combined with tacrolimus or cyclosporine, and, in these combinations, only the day 1, 3, 6, and 11 doses are given. The drug is administered by slow IV push. Dose attenuation is usually done for elevations of bilirubin and creatinine, or for grade III-IV mucositis.[286] Elimination of the day 11 dose of methotrexate has been associated with worse clinical outcomes.[287] An alternate strategy for methotrexate prophylaxis is termed *minidose methotrexate,* in which methotrexate is combined with a calcineurin inhibitor at a dose of 5 mg/m^2 on days 1, 3, 6, and 11 after transplantation. This regimen has been associated with decreased toxicity.[60]

Pharmacokinetics. Methotrexate is exclusively administered IV for GVHD prophylaxis. In the blood, 30% to 70% of methotrexate is bound to proteins, mostly albumin. Methotrexate can slowly diffuse into third-space fluids, causing prolongation of the $t_{1/2}$ and making its administration in patients with effusions or ascites problematic. After absorption, methotrexate is subject to hepatic and intracellular conversion to its polyglutamated form. Retention of methotrexate varies among tissues, accounting for its varying effects upon different organ systems. Methotrexate elimination occurs in three phases. The first two phases correlate with distribution and renal clearance. The terminal $t_{1/2}$ of methotrexate lasts about 10 to 12 hours, and is thought to reflect enterohepatic circulation.[288] Renal elimination is the primary route of IV methotrexate excretion, with 80% to 90% excreted unchanged in the urine. At higher doses, rapid excretion can result in high urinary concentrations of the drug and its metabolite, 7-hydroxymethotrexate, requiring alkalinization of the urine to prevent crystallization, though this does not occur at the doses used for GVHD prophylaxis.[286]

Drug Interactions. Methotrexate has a large spectrum of potential drug interactions. Discussion here is limited to medications that are likely to be used concomitantly with methotrexate in its short administration period from transplant to day 11. Oral sulfonylureas and hydantoin anticonvulsants such as phenytoin can displace methotrexate from plasma proteins, resulting in greater methotrexate-induced toxicity. Trimethoprim can be associated with additive antifolate effects and bone marrow suppression. Penicillin, vancomycin, probenecid, and ciprofloxicin may reduce renal elimination of methotrexate, causing increased toxicity. Finally, because rapidly dividing cells are more sensitive to the toxic effects of methotrexate, the coadministration of methotrexate and hematopoietic growth factors can result in cytopenias.[286]

Adverse Drug Reactions. In the posttransplantation setting, mucositis, suppression of blood cell counts, and hepatic and renal toxicity are the major adverse reactions associated with the use of methotrexate.[286] The administration of methotrexate can worsen hepatic or renal insufficiency, conditions that may occur posttransplantation due to sepsis with hypotension, veno-occlusive disease of the liver, or coadministration of potentially organ-toxic agents such as calcineurin inhibitors, amphotericin preparations, aminoglycosides, or various azole antifungals.

Monitoring. Alkalinization of the urine to prevent crystallization, monitoring of serum methotrexate levels, and leucovorin rescue, which are commonly used in cancer therapy, are not required with the small doses of methotrexate used for GVHD prophylaxis. However, close monitoring of the complete blood count, liver enzymes, and creatinine is recommended. Finally, mucositis initiated by the conditioning regimen may be severely exacerbated by methotrexate.

Cyclophosphamide

Cyclophosphamide (Cytoxan) is an alkylating agent approved for the treatment of multiple malignancies. In HSCT, it is a common component of conditioning regimens both for its antineoplastic effects and its potent immunosuppressive properties.[289-291] It is used with ATG to prevent graft rejection in patients with aplastic anemia and plays a similar role in other HSCT conditioning regimens.[292] Phosphoramide mustard, an activated form of cyclophosphamide, alkylates intracellular molecular structures, including nucleic acids.[293] The cytotoxic action is due to cross-linking of DNA and RNA and inhibition of protein synthesis. The DNA in proliferating cells is particularly sensitive to cyclophosphamide, including not only malignant cells but also proliferating alloreactive lymphocytes, thus promoting their preferential clonal elimination.

Dosing of cyclophosphamide varies from low doses of 25 to 50 mg taken orally for the treatment of autoimmune processes to doses of up to 200 mg/kg over 5 days in HSCT preparative regimens.[165,289,293-297] At low doses, the most worrisome adverse event is the development of secondary leukemia in up to 10% of patients. In higher doses, precautions must be taken to avoid pulmonary and cardiac toxicity. At the intermediate and higher doses, growth factor or stem cell transplant support is required because of myelotoxicity. The emetogenic potential is very high at these doses as well, and prophylaxis with antiemetics is required. Monitoring of blood counts during therapy is necessary to assess the need for transfusion support. Long-term monitoring should be performed for the development of myelodysplasia or acute leukemia. Hemorrhagic cystitis has been reported, and prophylaxis with mesna or hydration (>3 L/m^2 per day) is required at the highest doses. Voriconazole and related drugs may interfere with activation of cyclophosphamide in the liver.

Purine Nucleoside Analogues

Drugs that affect purine metabolism include fludarabine (Fludara), cladribine (Leustatin), and pentostatin (Elmiron). Like cyclophosphamide, they are utilized in HSCT both for their antineoplastic effects and potent immunosuppressive properties.[298-300] These drugs are structural analogues of adenosine. They are dephosphorylated, transported into cells, and rephosphorylated by deoxynucleoside salvage pathways and thereby interfere with normal purine metabolism, and thus with DNA synthesis and repair.[301-303] Decreased mRNA and protein synthesis also occur. Pentostatin is also a potent inhibitor of adenosine deaminase, producing elevated levels of adenosine with consequent strong antilymphoproliferative and lymphocytotoxic effects, as is also seen with congenital deficiency of this enzyme. Figure 92-4 depicts a schematic representation of the mechanism of action of the purine nucleoside analogues.

These drugs are primarily used in the treatment of low-grade lymphoproliferative disorders. While still capable of causing myelosuppression, the more profound lymphosuppressive effect of these agents has allowed the development of non-myeloablative and reduced-intensity preparative regimens that prevent graft rejection and facilitate HSC engraftment with less toxicity. Pentostatin has also been used in clinical trials to treat GVHD, though its role in this setting remains to be clarified.[304-306] Patients who receive these agents will remain lymphosuppressed for months and require prophylaxis and monitoring for opportunistic infections. Blood counts, including absolute lymphocyte counts, should be followed. Neurotoxicity has been reported, particularly at higher doses of fludarabine and pentostatin.

Rituximab

Rituximab (Rituxan) is a chimeric anti-CD20 monoclonal antibody containing human IgG1 heavy and light chain constant regions and murine variable regions.[307] CD20 is a hydrophobic transmembrane phosphoprotein present on pre-B and mature B lymphocytes and on greater than 90% of B-cell non-Hodgkin's lymphomas, but not on hematopoietic stem cells, pro-B cells, normal plasma cells, or other normal cells.[307,308] Rituximab is able to inhibit B cells by augmenting complement-mediated lysis and antibody-dependent cell-mediated cytotoxicity and cell death.[307,309] Rituximab is approved for the treatment of relapsed or refractory B-cell non-Hodgkin's lymphoma as well as refractory rheumatoid disease. It has also been used in the transplant community for various autoimmune disorders, desensitization protocols, and treatment of humoral rejection and PTLD.[310-315]

Although T-cell–mediated rejection has long been the primary target of immunosuppressive therapy in transplantation, there is a growing concern regarding humoral or B-cell–mediated rejection, which does not usually respond to the traditional treatments. Rituximab has been used alone or in combination with intravenous immume globulin (IVIG) or plasmapheresis for treatment of B-cell rejection.[310] Rituximab has also been successful in lowering pretransplantation HLA antibodies and transplanting patients despite a positive crossmatch.[316,317] ABO-incompatible patients are another high-risk group for whom rituximab may serve as a "chemical" splenectomy to help improve outcomes in this transplantation setting.[312,318]

Treatment of PTLD has often consisted of reduction in overall immunosuppression and chemotherapy. The outcomes and tolerability of these approaches have been poor, with significant morbidity. Recent reports have demonstrated success with the use of rituximab for treatment of PTLD in either the HSC or solid organ transplant setting.[313,315,319]

The dosing of rituximab varies widely depending on the disease, severity, and patient tolerance. Following the standard four-dose treatment for patients with lymphoma, B-cell depletion persists for 6 to 9 months in the majority of patients.[320] Rituximab use has been associated with infusion-related side effects such as fever and chills that may be related, in part, to B cell lysis, though true allergic/anaphylactic reactions may also occur. Other side effects have included pruritis, nausea, vomiting, asthenia, headache, and dizziness.

Immune Globulin

IVIG (multiple branded products) is a sterilized solution obtained from pooled human blood. Unselected IVIG preparations include IgG (including subclasses IgG1, IgG2, IgG3, and IgG4), and immunoglobulins A, M, and E, similar to normal human serum. There are also multiple selected IVIG preparations containing high titers of a specific antibody (e.g., CMV immune globulin [CMVIG] and hepatitis B immune globulin). There are currently more than 10 approved IVIG products available in the United States, each with distinct indications, although the products are used interchangeably. Some of the approved indications include primary immune deficiency, idiopathic thrombocytopenic purpura, chronic lymphocytic leukemia, Kawasaki disease, GVHD, bone marrow transplantation, and pediatric human immunodeficiency virus. However, IVIG is commonly used in unapproved settings, including systemic lupus erythematosus, chronic infection with immune disorder, myasthenia gravis, and many others.

Focusing on transplantation, donor-specific antibody (DSA) may be neutralized and eliminated by anti-idiotypic antibodies present in the IVIG preparation.[321-323] IVIG has been demonstrated to lower panel reactive antibodies in highly sensitized patients and permit transplantation in the setting of a positive crossmatch or ABO blood group mismatch.[42,324-326] IVIG is commonly used in combination with plasmapheresis or rituximab in these settings. IVIG also causes reversal of inflammation and organ dysfunction by decreasing circulating levels of DSA and inhibiting B-cell production of DSA.[327] Although IVIG is often used in combination with or in place of other immunosuppressive strategies, it is better regarded as an immunomodulator since it is not associated with lymphopenia, lymphocyte dysfunction, or the common infectious complications of immunosuppressive therapy. IVIG therapy has also been used in both solid organ and HSC transplantation to either prevent or treat viral infections, which may include CMV, hepatitis B, polyomavirus, adenovirus, and others.[328-330]

The dosing of IVIg varies widely depending on the disease, patient tolerance and specific product used (IVIG or CMVIG). Adverse reactions are commonly associated with infusion of IVIg and may include flushing, headache, nausea, myalgia and arthralgia. Other adverse effects may include anxiety, stomach cramps, dizziness and rash. Evidence suggests that IVIG products that contain sucrose may present a higher risk of acute renal failure especially in patients with underlying renal dysfunction. This is particularly important for the transplant community since these products are primarily used for kidney transplant recipients.

Extracorporeal Photoimmune Therapy

Extracorporeal phototherapy (ECP) is a type of photoactivated drug therapy utilized for the treatment of GVHD and to a much lesser extent for organ rejection. ECP has some features in common with psoralen plus ultraviolet A (UVA) light (PUVA) therapy of the skin, which has been used for the treatment of a number of dermatologic disorders, including skin GVHD. ECP, which can be thought of as a systemic version of PUVA, was first utilized to treat cutaneous T-cell lymphoma (CTCL).[331] The technique involves the infusion of autologous peripheral blood leukocytes that have been previously collected by apheresis and exposed to 8-methoxypsoralen or methoxsalen and long-wave UVA light.

Mechanism of Action. The precise events in tolerance induction are unknown, but the photoactivated drug can bind to single- and double-stranded DNA and some proteins, leading to apoptosis of the treated cells. After reinfusion, the treated cells are taken up by resident APCs. After the APCs engage the treated cells, they become tolerogenic rather than immunogenic.[332,333] Tolerogenic APCs are poor stimulators of effector immune responses and demonstrate increased production of anti-inflammatory cytokines and reciprocally decreased production of proinflammatory cytokines.[334,335] Tolerogenic APCs can also induce the generation of regulatory T cells. In addition to CTCL, ECP has been used for chronic GVHD especially of the skin and, to a much lesser extent, for acute GVHD.[336] ECP has been used for a variety of other autoimmune disorders, including Crohn's disease, pemphigus vulgaris, systemic sclerosis, systemic lupus erythematosus, rheumatoid arthritis, and chronic erosive lichen planus.[337-339] ECP has had limited use for the prevention and treatment of renal and cardiac allograft rejection.[340,341]

Dosing and Administration. Methoxsalen (UVADEX) is a naturally occurring photoactive substance found in the seed of the *Ammi majus* plant and belongs to a class of compounds known as psoralens. For each ECP treatment, peripheral blood leukocytes are first collected by apheresis using the ECP apparatus, after which methoxsalen is injected into the recirculation bag. Commonly, 0.34 mcg of methoxsalen will be added per milliliter of apheresis product to be treated, with treatment volumes commonly around 250 ml in adults. The buffy coat–plasma-methoxsalen mixture is then irradiated with UVA light in the ECP apparatus and subsequently reinfused into the patient. Various treatment schedules have been published, though no single standard has emerged. Most often, ECP is initiated two or three times a week (not on consecutive days) with decreasing frequency as treatment progresses. Treatment may be continued for up to 12 weeks or longer depending on the disease being treated and the patient's response.

Pharmacokinetics. One advantage of ECP is that there is minimal systemic exposure to methoxsalen. The total dose used is less than 1/200th of the oral dose used for PUVA treatments. For a typical treatment, an average 70-kg adult receives a systemic dose of methosaxlen of only 1.2 mcg/kg. Consequently, there is no detectable drug 30 minutes after cell reinfusion.

Adverse Effects and Monitoring. The small doses of methoxsalen required for ECP help to reduce potential toxicities. Higher doses of oral methosaxlen (such as for PUVA therapy) can, with exposure to sunlight or ultraviolet irradiation, cause serious sunburn or premature aging of the skin. This is far less problematic with the small doses required for ex vivo treatment. Nonetheless, patients should be monitored closely for the formation of basal cell carcinomas. Treatments can cause hypotension due to changes in the intravascular blood volume, anemia related to blood loss from the procedure, and infections related to the catheter required for repeated aphereses. Patients considered candidates for this therapy should have platelet counts greater than 20,000 and a WBC count greater than 1.5. The procedure is not effective with a bilirubin over 22, so plasma exchange is needed before ECP is carried out in patients with significant hyperbilirubinemia.

Care should be taken to avoid other photosensitizing agents either topically or systemically. Agents such as anthralin, coal tar and its derivatives, griseofulvin, phenothiazines, nalidixic acid, halogenated salicylanilides (found in bacteriostatic soaps), sulfonamides, tetracyclines, thiazides, and certain organic staining dyes such as methylene blue should be avoided. Patients should wear UVA-absorbing wrap-around sunglasses (in order to prevent the formation of cataracts) and cover exposed skin or use a sunblock (SPF 15 or higher) for the 24-hour period following treatment, whether exposed to direct or indirect sunlight in the open or through window glass.

T-Cell Depletion

Allogeneic marrow or peripheral stem cell products consist of complex cellular mixtures that include both hematopoietic stem/progenitor cells, best currently identified by expression of CD34 and T cells, best identified by expression of CD3. In rodent models, it has been straightforward to prevent GVHD by depleting the graft of mature T cells.[342,343] In humans, this is also possible but more difficult. Host T cells can survive the most aggressive chemoradiotherapy preparative regimens. In the setting of an unmanipulated graft, the large number of donor T cells overwhelms the few remaining host T cells and engraftment occurs. With a T-cell–depeleted product, the balance between donor and host T cells is more even and, consequently, immunologic rejection is seen more often, particularly as HLA disparity between donor and recipient increases.[65,344] The addition of ATG or similar reagents into the immunosuppressive regimen can prevent rejection and further reduce the likelihood of developing GVHD. However, this is associated with more profound and long-lasting T-cell deficiency, particularly in adults with high rates of EBV-associated PTLD and other infectious complications.[177,345-347]

T-cell depletion has been performed ex vivo using soybean agglutinin combined with sheep red blood cell resetting, elutriation, monoclonal antibodies, and a variety of other approaches.[64,348,349] These approaches vary as to whether they remove other cell populations besides T cells and whether they remove all T-cell subsets or have a preferential specificity for one or another subgroup. They also vary with regard to the log reduction achieved. As a consequence, some require additional immunosuppressives to prevent GVHD while others do not. Increasingly, T-cell depletion is being performed using positive selection of $CD34^+$ cells with immunomagnetic beads rather than using negative selection techniques targeted at the T cell.[350-353]

Tumor Necrosis Factor-α Inhibitors

TNF-α has been identified as a mediator of GVHD, particularly GVHD of the gastrointestinal tract. TNF contributes to the activation of macrophages, lymphocytes, eosinophils, and neutrophils; facilitates production of other inflam-matory cytokines; upregulates expression of HLA molecules; and facilitates lysis by T lymphocytes.[354] Infliximab (Remicade), an IgG1 murine/human chimeric monoclonal antibody, and etanercept (Enbrel), a recombinant human TNF-α receptor type II fusion protein, have shown activity in the treatment of GVHD.[355,356] Both agents, when combined with other GVHD therapy, have shown activity in skin, liver, and gut GVHD.[355,357] Infectious sequelae are the major side effect of these drugs.[357,358] Infliximab, like other monoclonal antibodies, has the potential to induce allergic reactions and should be monitored similar to other antibody-based therapies.

Thalidomide

Thalidomide (Thalomid) was first synthesized in 1954 and utilized as a sedative in the late 1950s. It was withdrawn from use because of severe teratogenic effects.[359] It was subsequently found to have immune-modulating effects, which led to its application in leprosy and GVHD.[360-362] Thalidomide was also found to have activity against multiple myeloma, which accounts for most of its use today. In transplantation, it is used primarily as part of multidrug treatment of difficult cases of chronic GVHD.[363,364]

Thalidomide's mechanism of action is not completely understood and is most likely multifactorial. The drug inhibits TNF-α production by monocytes and inhibits the activation of NF-κB, a transcription promoter of TNF-α and other cytokines.[365] The drug has been shown to induce Th2 cytokine production, which may inhibit GVHD and promote tolerance.[366] Thalidomide has been shown to interfere with the upregulation of the adhesion molecules E-selectin and vascular cell adhesion molecule, which may affect T-cell migration and trafficking.

Thalidomide has poor solubility and is only available in oral form. The drug undergoes rapid hydrolysis to multiple metabolites that are excreted in the urine. The mean $t_{1/2}$ is about 4.5 hours.[359] In the treatment of chronic GVHD, doses of thalidomide have ranged from 100 to 1200 mg/day, though more recent usage has favored lower doses.[363,367] In addition to its teratogenic effects, the major side effects of the drug include drowsiness, constipation, fatigue, skin rash, and peripheral neuropathy, the latter often limiting the dose of drug or duration of therapy that can be tolerated.[360] Deep venous thrombosis is a less common but important side effect of the drug and its analogues, though this is most often seen when thalidomide is administered together with corticosteroids.[368]

Total Lymphoid Irradiation

In total lymphoid irradiation (TLI), major lymphoid organs, including the lymph nodes, thymus, and spleen, are irradiated, though portions of the marrow are spared. In addition to producing partial lymphoablation, TLI increases the ratio of NK-T cells compared to conventional T cells because of the relative radioresistance of the NK-T cell population. NK-T cells perform regulatory functions, including suppressive activity in mixed lymphocyte reactions and GVHD assays.[369] In contrast to classical T cells, NK-T cells interact with the antigen-presenting molecule CD1d rather than classical MHC molecules, and secrete IL-4 and interferon-γ. They polarize immune responses to a Th2 pattern, which may promote tolerance and decrease inflammation.

TLI has been used for prophylaxis and treatment of graft rejection in solid organ transplant recipients.[370,371] In allogeneic HSCT, it has been used as part of conditioning regimens to prevent graft rejection,[372] for treatment of aplastic anemia,[373,374] and as part of non-myeloablative conditioning regimens.[375] In the latter setting, its use has been associated with reduced GVHD as well as consistent engraftment.[376]

Leflunomide

Leflunomide (Arava) belongs to a class of drugs known as malonitrilamides, which have immunosuppressive activity. Leflunomide is approved for the treatment of adults with active rheumatoid arthritis. Due to its immunomodulatory effects, leflunomide has been studied in autoimmune diseases as well as for the prevention and treatment of acute and chronic rejection following transplantation.[377-379] Leflunomide has also shown antiviral activity against CMV, herpes simplex virus, and, perhaps most important in transplantation, against polyomavirus.[377,380,381] Polyomavirus (BK virus), which is present in 80% of the population, may develop into an aggressive, destructive nephropathy in immunosuppressed patients.[382-384] Although there is no standard of care, treatment with leflunomide has become widely used.

Leflunomide acts by reversibly blocking dihydroorotate dehydrogenase, an enzyme required for de novo pyrimidine synthesis in lymphocytes and other cells, and by inhibition of selected tyrosine kinases.[385-387] The dosing of leflunomide varies widely depending on the indication as well as the immunosuppressive or antiviral agents with which it is combined. Following oral administration, leflunomide is rapidly metabolized to the active metabolite A77 1726, which is responsible for all its activity and toxicity. One limitation has been the long terminal half-life of 15 to 18 days, which makes titration very difficult.

In rheumatoid arthritis studies, the most common side effects included diarrhea, elevated liver enzymes, alopecia, hypertension, headache, nausea, rash, and bronchitis. Anemia was a common finding when used in transplant patients. With limited long-term experience in transplantation, patients should be followed closely.

Belatacept

Belatacept (CTLA4Ig, LEA29Y) is a selective inhibitor directed against the co-stimulatory ligands CD80 and CD86 found on APCs. Belatacept is a human fusion protein composed of the constant region (Fc) of human IgG1 combined with the extracellular portion of CTLA4. CTLA4 is a close molecular relative of CD28, but it binds to CD80 and CD86 with about a 20-fold higher affinity. Binding of belatacept to CD80 and CD86 renders them unavailable to engage CD28, thus blocking the second signal of T-cell activation. Belatacept was derived from abatacept (Orencia), which is approved for the treatment of rheumatoid arthritis.[388] Belatacept differs from abatacept by two amino acids, which enables higher affinity binding to CD80 and CD86 and greater inhibition of T-cell activation.[389]

Long-term studies are currently being conducted to better define belatacept's role.[390-393] Early results suggest that belatacept is similar in efficacy to cyclosporine while preserving kidney function.[394-396]

Due to its unique characteristics, belatacept has both advantages (long half-life, potent blockade of T-cell activation) and disadvantages (IV formulation only). Belatacept has been associated with very few adverse reactions. The one concern is the incidence of cancers, particularly PTLD. Although PTLD is associated with many immunosuppressive drugs, the incidence observed in Phase II studies of belatacept warrants close surveillance.[397,398]

Investigational Agents

A number of investigational agents have shown promise in initial trials and have moved into Phase II/III studies. ISA247 is a novel cyclosporine analogue that also works by inhibiting calcineurin. However, nephrotoxicity, hypercholesterolemia, and diabetes appear to be absent with ISA247. A Phase IIb study in kidney patients comparing use against tacrolimus is ongoing, and a Phase III study in psoriasis has been completed. JAK3 inhibitors represent new selective immunosuppressive drugs that are under investigation by a number of companies. JAK3 is activated by multiple cytokines, including IL-2, IL-4, IL-7, IL-9, IL-15, and IL-21, through engagement of the IL-2R common γ chain in both T and B cells. PKC, and more specifically the α and θ isoforms, play a key role in T-lymphocyte activation. AEB071 is a novel immunosuppressant that inhibits PKC and potently and selectively blocks a non–calcineurin-dependent pathway downstream from signal 1 and 2. Equally critical to the initial studies testing these drugs as single agents will be trials to evaluate their use in combination with the other commonly used agents for both prevention and treatment of rejection and GVHD.

Future Directions

Clinical transplantation has evolved greatly since the days when methotrexate, azathioprine, and corticosteroids were the only immunosuppressive drugs available. Newer agents have helped to improve outcome and reduce toxicity. Nonetheless, much remains to be done to enhance transplant survival while minimizing infection, malignancy, or other morbidity.

The ideal goal would be to develop approaches that ablate the allogeneic response to the transplanted organ selectively or at least preferentially. While the majority of HSC transplant recipients are eventually able to successfully discontinue immunosuppression, most solid organ transplant recipients cannot. Establishment of true tolerance through any mechanism would be highly desirable. Experimental efforts using TLI or new pharmacologic agents remain of interest.

The simplest way to envision establishing selective tolerance for transplantation would be to develop agents that have selective but permanent effects only on those T cells responding to antigen while the drug was present. Other T cells that did not encounter antigen at this time would be unaffected. Early after transplantation, alloreactive lymphocytes mediating rejection or GVHD would be expected to be disproportionately activated. Consequently, during this brief window of time, the alloimmune response to the transplanted organ would be disproportionately blunted by drugs that shift signals from stimulatory to inhibitory or block selected intracellular pathways, thus inducing inhibition rather than activation of T cells. Whether the mechanism is clonal deletion, clonal anergy, induction of regulatory T cells, or something else is not important so long as it exhibits the desired selectivity. One would be able to use such an agent only over a brief time frame early after transplantation when the bulk of alloreactive lymphocytes are encountering antigen. Once the agent was eliminated, other T cells encountering antigen at later time points would not undergo a similar fate. Thus the response to infectious pathogens would remain intact. Further understanding of the immunologic pathogenesis of graft rejection and GVHD and the mechanisms underlying immunologic activation and tolerance should allow the targeted development of immunosuppressive agents with the requisite properties to meet these clinical goals.

REFERENCES

1. Little C. The genetics of tumor transplantation. *In* Snell GD (ed): Biology of the Laboratory Mouse. Philadelphia: Blakiston, 1941, pp 279-309.
2. Bjorkman PJ, Saper MA, Samraoui B, et al. Structure of the human class I histocompatibility antigen, HLA-A2. Nature 1987;329:506-512.
3. Brown JH, Jardetzky TS, Gorga JC, et al. Three-dimensional structure of the human class II histocompatibility antigen HLA-DR1. Nature 1993;364:33-39.
4. Garboczi DN, Ghosh P, Utz U, et al. Structure of the complex between human T-cell receptor, viral peptide and HLA-A2. Nature 1996;384:134-141.
5. Rudolph MG, Stanfield RL, Wilson IA. How TCRs bind MHCs, peptides, and coreceptors. Annu Rev Immunol 2006;24:419-466.
6. Rudolph MG, Speir JA, Brunmark A, et al. The crystal structures of K_{bm1} and K_{bm8} reveal that subtle changes in the peptide environment impact thermostability and alloreactivity. Immunity 2001;14:231-242.
7. Reiser JB, Darnault C, Guimezanes A, et al. Crystal structure of a T cell receptor bound to an allogeneic MHC molecule. Nat Immunol 2000;1:291-297.
8. Obst R, Netuschil N, Klopfer K, et al. The role of peptides in T cell alloreactivity is determined by self-major histocompatibility complex molecules. J Exp Med 2000;191:805-812.
9. Androlewicz MJ. Peptide generation in the major histocompatibility complex class I antigen processing and presentation pathway. Curr Opin Hematol 2001;8:12-16.
10. Germain RN, Margulies DH. The biochemistry and cell biology of antigen processing and presentation. Annu Rev Immunol 1993;11:403-450.
11. Newcomb JR, Carboy-Newcomb C, Cresswell P. Trimeric interactions of the invariant chain and its association with major histocompatibility complex class II alpha beta dimers. J Biol Chem 1996;271:24249-24256.
12. Thery C, Amigorena S. The cell biology of antigen presentation in dendritic cells. Curr Opin Immunol 2001;13:45-51.
13. Sebzda E, Mariathasan S, Ohteki T, et al. Selection of the T cell repertoire. Annu Rev Immunol 1999;17:829-874.
14. Hogquist KA. Signal strength in thymic selection and lineage commitment. Curr Opin Immunol 2001;13:225-231.
15. Simpson E, Scott D, James E, et al. Minor H antigens: genes and peptides. Transpl Immunol 2002;10:115-123.
16. Simpson E, Roopenian D, Goulmy E. Much ado about minor histocompatibility antigens. Immunol Today 1998;19:108-112.
17. Braun MY, Grandjean I, Feunou P, et al. Acute rejection in the absence of cognate recognition of allograft by T cells. J Immunol 2001;166:4879-4883.
18. Hutchinson IV. Cellular mechanisms of allograft rejection. Curr Opin Immunol 1991;3:722-728.
19. Libby P, Pober JS. Chronic rejection. Immunity 2001;14:387-397.
20. Sykes M. Mixed chimerism and transplant tolerance. Immunity 2001;14:417-424.

21. Starzl TE, Demetris AJ, Murase N, et al. The lost chord: microchimerism and allograft survival. Immunol Today 1996;17:577-584; discussion 588.
22. Roser BJ. Cellular mechanisms in neonatal and adult tolerance. Immunol Rev 1989;107:179-202.
23. Streilein JW. Neonatal tolerance of H-2 alloantigens: procuring graft acceptance the "old-fashioned" way. Transplantation 1991;52:1-10.
24. Abbas AK, Murphy KM, Sher A. Functional diversity of helper T lymphocytes. Nature 1996;383:787-793.
25. Mosmann TR, Sad S. The expanding universe of T-cell subsets: Th1, Th2 and more. Immunol Today 1996;17:138-146.
26. Donckier V, Wissing M, Bruyns C, et al. Critical role of interleukin 4 in the induction of neonatal transplantation tolerance. Transplantation 1995;59:1571-1576.
27. Brennan DC, Mohanakumar T, Flye MW. Donor-specific transfusion and donor bone marrow infusion in renal transplantation tolerance: a review of efficacy and mechanisms. Am J Kidney Dis 1995;26:701-715.
28. Sakaguchi S. Naturally arising CD4+ regulatory T cells for immunologic self-tolerance and negative control of immune responses. Annu Rev Immunol 2004;22:531-562.
29. Baxter AG, Hodgkin PD. Activation rules: the two-signal theories of immune activation. Nat Rev Immunol 2002;2:439-446.
30. Davis DM, Dustin ML. What is the importance of the immunological synapse? Trends Immunol 2004;25:323-327.
31. Marsden VS, Strasser A. Control of apoptosis in the immune system: Bcl-2, BH3-only proteins and more. Annu Rev Immunol 2003;21:71-105.
32. Demoulin JB, Renauld JC. Signalling by cytokines interacting with the interleukin-2 receptor gamma chain. Cytokines Cell Mol Ther 1998;4:243-256.
33. Malek TR, Bayer AL. Tolerance, not immunity, crucially depends on IL-2. Nat Rev Immunol 2004;4:665-674.
34. Starzl TE. The mystique of organ transplantation. J Am Coll Surg 2005;201:160-170.
35. Webster A, Pankhurst T, Rinaldi F, et al. Polyclonal and monoclonal antibodies for treating acute rejection episodes in kidney transplant recipients. Cochrane Database Syst Rev 2006;(2):CD004756.
36. Halloran PF. Immunosuppressive drugs for kidney transplantation. N Engl J Med 2004;351:2715-2729. [published erratum appears in N Engl J Med 2005;352:1056.]
37. Kaufman DB, Leventhal JR, Gallon LG, Parker MA. Alemtuzumab induction and prednisone-free maintenance immunotherapy in simultaneous pancreas-kidney transplantation: comparison with rabbit antithymocyte globulin induction—long-term results. Am J Transplant 2006;6:331-339.
38. Lau CL, Palmer SM, Posther KE, et al. Influence of panel-reactive antibodies on post-transplant outcomes in lung transplant recipients. Ann Thorac Surg 2000;69:1520-1524.
39. Ruiz P, Garcia M, Pappas P, et al. Mucosal vascular alterations in isolated small-bowel allografts: relationship to humoral sensitization. Am J Transplant 2003;3:43-49.
40. Gordon RD, Iwatsuki S, Esquivel CO, et al. Liver transplantation across ABO blood groups. Surgery 1986;100:342-348.
41. Faguer S, Kamar N, Guilbeaud-Frugier C, et al. Rituximab therapy for acute humoral rejection after kidney transplantation. Transplantation 2007;83:1277-1280.
42. Montgomery RA, Zachary AA, Racusen LC, et al. Plasmapheresis and intravenous immune globulin provides effective rescue therapy for refractory humoral rejection and allows kidneys to be successfully transplanted into cross-match-positive recipients. Transplantation 2000;70:887-895.
43. Ojo AO, Held PJ, Port FK, et al. Chronic renal failure after transplantation of a non-renal organ. N Engl J Med 2003;349:931-940.
44. Sis B, Dadras F, Khoshjou F, et al. Reproducibility studies on arteriolar hyaline thickening scoring in calcineurin inhibitor-treated renal allograft recipients. Am J Transplant 2006;6:1444-1450.
45. Groetzner J, Kur F, Spelsberg F, et al. Airway anastomosis complications in de novo lung transplantation with sirolimus-based immunosuppression. J Heart Lung Transplant 2004;23:632-638.
46. Kuppahally S, Al-Khaldi A, Weisshaar D, et al. Wound healing complications with de novo sirolimus versus mycophenolate mofetil-based regimen in cardiac transplant recipients. Am J Transplant 2006;6(5 Pt 1):986-992.
47. Matas AJ, Kandaswamy R, Humar A, et al. Long-term immunosuppression, without maintenance prednisone, after kidney transplantation. Ann Surg 2004;240:510-516; discussion 516-517.
48. Kaufman DB, Leventhal JR, Axelrod D, et al. Alemtuzumab induction and prednisone-free maintenance immunotherapy in kidney transplantation: comparison with basiliximab induction—long-term results. Am J Transplant 2005;5:2539-2548.
49. O'Grady JG. Corticosteroid-free strategies in liver transplantation. Drugs 2006;66:1853-1862.
50. Al-khaldi A, Robbins RC. New directions in cardiac transplantation. Annu Rev Med 2006;57:455-471.
51. Buell JF, Gross TG, Woodle ES. Malignancy after transplantation. Transplantation 2005;80(2 Suppl):S254-S264.
52. Thomas E, Storb R, Clift RA, et al. Bone-marrow transplantation (first of two parts). N Engl J Med 1975;292:832-843.
53. Thomas ED, Storb R, Clift RA, et al. Bone-marrow transplantation (second of two parts). N Engl J Med 1975;292:895-902.
54. van Leeuwen JE, van Tol MJ, Joosten AM, et al. Relationship between patterns of engraftment in peripheral blood and immune reconstitution after allogeneic bone marrow transplantation for (severe) combined immunodeficiency. Blood 1994;84:3936-3947.
55. Kahl C, Leisenring W, Deeg HJ, et al. Cyclophosphamide and antithymocyte globulin as a conditioning regimen for allogeneic marrow transplantation in patients with aplastic anaemia: a long-term follow-up. Br J Haematol 2005;130:747-751.
56. Clift RA, Buckner CD, Appelbaum FR, et al. Allogeneic marrow transplantation in patients with chronic myeloid leukemia in the chronic phase: a randomized trial of two irradiation regimens. Blood 1991;77:1660-1665.
57. Santos GW, Tutschka PJ, Brookmeyer R, et al. Marrow transplantation for acute nonlymphocytic leukemia after treatment with busulfan and cyclophosphamide. N Engl J Med 1983;309:1347-1353.
58. Champlin R, Khouri I, Giralt S. Use of nonmyeloablative preparative regimens for allogeneic blood stem cell transplantation: induction of graft-vs.-malignancy as treatment for malignant diseases. J Clin Apheresis 1999;14:45-49.
59. Nash RA, Antin JH, Karanes C, et al. Phase 3 study comparing methotrexate and tacrolimus with methotrexate and cyclosporine for prophylaxis of acute graft-versus-host disease after marrow transplantation from unrelated donors. Blood 2000;96:2062-2068.
60. Przepiorka D, Ippoliti C, Khouri I, et al. Tacrolimus and minidose methotrexate for prevention of acute graft-versus-host disease after matched unrelated donor marrow transplantation. Blood 1996;88:4383-4389.
61. Ferrara JL. Novel strategies for the treatment and diagnosis of graft-versus-host-disease. Baillieres Best Pract Clin Haematol 2007;20:91-97.
62. Couriel DR, Saliba R, Escalon MP, et al. Sirolimus in combination with tacrolimus and corticosteroids for the treatment of resistant chronic graft-versus-host disease. Br J Haematol 2005;130:409-417.
63. Kawanishi Y, Passweg J, Drobyski WR, et al. Effect of T cell subset dose on outcome of T cell-depleted bone marrow transplantation. Bone Marrow Transplant 1997; 19:1069-1077.
64. O'Reilly RJ, Collins N, Dinsmore R, et al. Transplantation of HLA-mismatched marrow depleted of T-cells by lectin agglutination and E-rosette depletion. Tokai J Exp Clin Med 1985;10:99-107.
65. Kernan NA, Flomenberg N, Dupont B, O'Reilly RJ. Graft rejection in recipients of T-cell-depleted HLA-nonidentical marrow transplants for leukemia: identification of host-derived antidonor allocytotoxic T lymphocytes. Transplantation 1987;43:842-847.
66. van Esser JW, van der Holt B, Meijer E, et al. Epstein-Barr virus (EBV) reactivation is a frequent event after allogeneic stem cell transplantation (SCT) and quantitatively predicts EBV-lymphoproliferative disease following T-cell–depleted SCT. Blood 2001;98:972-978.
67. Chao NJ, Chen BJ. Prophylaxis and treatment of acute graft-versus-host disease. Semin Hematol 2006;43:32-41.
68. Ratcliffe PJ, Dudley CR, Higgins RM, et al. Randomised controlled trial of steroid withdrawal in renal transplant recipients receiving triple immunosuppression. Lancet 1996;348:643-648.
69. Hollander AA, Hene RJ, Hermans J, et al. Late prednisone withdrawal in cyclosporine-treated kidney transplant patients: a randomized study. J A Soc Nephrol 1997;8:294-301.
70. Opelz G, Dohler B, Laux G, for the Collaborative Transplant S. Long-term prospective study of steroid withdrawal in kidney and heart transplant recipients. Am J Transplant 2005;5(4 Pt 1):720-728.
71. Hollenberg SM, Giguere V, Segui P, Evans RM. Colocalization of DNA-binding and transcriptional activation functions in the human glucocorticoid receptor. Cell 1987;49:39-46.
72. Scheinman RI, Cogswell PC, Lofquist AK, Baldwin AS Jr. Role of transcriptional activation of I kappa B alpha in mediation of immunosuppression by glucocorticoids. Science 1995;270:283-286.
73. Cupps TR, Fauci AS. Corticosteroid-mediated immunoregulation in man. Immunol Rev 1982;65:133-155.
74. Dupont E, Wybran J, Toussaint C. Glucocorticosteroids and organ transplantation. Transplantation 1984;37:331-335.
75. Derendorf H, Mollmann H, Krieg M, et al. Pharmacodynamics of methylprednisolone phosphate after single intravenous administration to healthy volunteers. Pharm Res 1991;8:263-268.
76. Al-Habet SM, Rogers HJ. Methylprednisolone pharmacokinetics after intravenous and oral administration. Br J Clin Pharmacol 1989;27:285-290.
77. Gilman AG, Rall TW, Nies AS, et al (eds). Goodman and Gilman's The Pharmacological Basis of Therapeutics, 8th ed. New York: Pergamon Press, 1990.
78. Ferry JJ, Horvath AM, Bekersky I, et al. Relative and absolute bioavailability of prednisone and prednisolone after separate oral and intravenous doses. J Clin Pharmacol 1988;28:81-87.
79. Frey BM, Frey FJ. Clinical pharmacokinetics of prednisone and prednisolone. Clin Pharmacokinet 1990;19:126-146.
80. de Mattos AM, Olyaei AJ, Bennett WM. Pharmacology of immunosuppressive medications used in renal diseases and transplantation. Am J Kidney Dis 1996;28:631-667.
81. Jusko WJ, Ferron GM, Mis SM, et al. Pharmacokinetics of prednisolone during administration of sirolimus in patients with renal transplants. J Clin Pharmacol 1996;36:1100-1106.
82. Borel JF, Kis ZL. The discovery and development of cyclosporine (Sandimmune). Transplant Proc 1991;23:1867-1874.
83. Borel JF. Comparative study of in vitro and in vivo drug effects on cell-mediated cytotoxicity. Immunology 1976;31:631-641.
84. Farber L, Maibucher A, Geissler F, et al. Favourable clinical results of Sandimmun-Neoral in malabsorbing liver and heart transplant recipients. Transplant Proc 1994;26:2988-2993.
85. Belli LS, De Carlis L, Rondinara GF, et al. Sandimmun-Neoral in liver transplantation: a remarkable improvement in long-term immunosuppression. Transplant Proc 1994;26:2983-2984.
86. Pollard S, Nashan B, Johnston A, et al. A pharmacokinetic and clinical review of the potential clinical impact of using different formulations of cyclosporin A. Berlin, Germany, November 19, 2001. Clin Ther 2003;25:1654-1669.

87. Sabatini S, Ferguson RM, Helderman JH, et al. Drug substitution in transplantation: a National Kidney Foundation White Paper. Am J Kidney Dis 1999;33:389-397.
88. Ponticelli C, Tarantino A, Montagnino G, et al. A randomized trial comparing triple-drug and double-drug therapy in renal transplantation. Transplantation 1988;45:913-918.
89. Fries D, Hiesse C, Charpentier B, et al. Triple combination of low-dose cyclosporine, azathioprine, and steroids in first cadaver donor renal allografts. Transplant Proc 1987;19(1 Pt 3):1911-1914.
90. de Groen PC, Aksamit AJ, Rakela J, et al. Central nervous system toxicity after liver transplantation: the role of cyclosporine and cholesterol. N Engl J Med 1987;317:861-866.
91. Dunn SP, Falkenstein K, Lawrence JP, et al. Monotherapy with cyclosporine for chronic immunosuppression in pediatric liver transplant recipients. Transplantation 1994;57:544-547.
92. Radovancevic B, Birovljev S, Frazier OH, et al. Long-term follow-up of cyclosporine-treated cardiac transplant recipients. Transplant Proc 1990;22(3 Suppl 1):21-24.
93. Grattan MT, Moreno-Cabral CE, Starnes VA, et al. Eight-year results of cyclosporine-treated patients with cardiac transplants. J Thorac Cardiovasc Surg 1990;99:500-509.
94. Storb R, Deeg HJ, Whitehead J, et al. Methotrexate and cyclosporine compared with cyclosporine alone for prophylaxis of acute graft versus host disease after marrow transplantation for leukemia. N Engl J Med 1986;314:729-735.
95. Gluckman E, Devergie A, Poros A, Degoulet P. Results of immunosuppression in 170 cases of severe aplastic anaemia: report of the European Group of Bone Marrow Transplant (EGBMT). Br J Haematol 1982;51:541-550.
96. Storb R, Leisenring W, Deeg HJ, et al. Long-term follow-up of a randomized trial of graft-versus-host disease prevention by methotrexate/cyclosporine versus methotrexate alone in patients given marrow grafts for severe aplastic anemia. Blood 1994;83:2749-2750.
97. Chao NJ, Schmidt GM, Niland JC, et al. Cyclosporine, methotrexate, and prednisone compared with cyclosporine and prednisone for prophylaxis of acute graft-versus-host disease. N Engl J Med 1993;329:1225-1230.
98. Hess AD, Tutschka PJ, Santos GW. Effect of cyclosporin A on human lymphocyte responses in vitro. III. CsA inhibits the production of T lymphocyte growth factors in secondary mixed lymphocyte responses but does not inhibit the response of primed lymphocytes to TCGF. J Immunol 1982;128:355-359.
99. Larsson EL. Cyclosporin A and dexamethasone suppress T cell responses by selectively acting at distinct sites of the triggering process. J Immunol 1980;124:2828-2833.
100. Suthanthiran M, Strom TB. Renal transplantation. N Engl J Med 1994;331:365-376.
101. Kovarik JM, Mueller EA, Johnston A, et al. Bioequivalence of soft gelatin capsules and oral solution of a new cyclosporine formulation. Pharmacotherapy 1993;13:613-617.
102. McMillan MA. Clinical pharmacokinetics of cyclosporine. Pharmacol Ther 1989; 42:135-156.
103. Grevel J, Nuesch E, Abisch E, Kutz K. Pharmacokinetics of oral cyclosporin A (Sandimmun) in healthy subjects. Eur J Clin Pharmacol 1986;31:211-216.
104. Ptachcinski RJ, Venkataramanan R, Burckart GJ. Clinical pharmacokinetics of cyclosporin. Clin Pharmacokinet 1986;11:107-132.
105. Fahr A. Cyclosporin clinical pharmacokinetics. Clin Pharmacokinet 1993;24:472-495.
106. Christians U, Spiekermann K, Bader A, et al. Cyclosporine metabolite pattern in blood from patients with acute GVHD after BMT. Bone Marrow Transplant 1993;12:27-33.
107. Klintmalm GB, Iwatsuki S, Starzl TE. Nephrotoxicity of cyclosporin A in liver and kidney transplant patients. Lancet 1981;1:470-471.
108. Hamilton DV, Calne RY, Evans DB, et al. The effect of long-term cyclosporin A on renal function. Lancet 1981;1:1218-1219.
109. Shulman H, Striker G, Deeg HJ, et al. Nephrotoxicity of cyclosporin A after allogeneic marrow transplantation: glomerular thromboses and tubular injury. N Engl J Med 1981;305:1392-1395.
110. Klintmalm GB, Iwatsuki S, Starzl TE. Cyclosporin A hepatotoxicity in 66 renal allograft recipients. Transplantation 1981;32:488-489.
111. Scott JP, Higenbottam TW. Adverse reactions and interactions of cyclosporin. Med Toxicol Adverse Drug Exp 1988;3:107-127.
112. Nankivell BJ, Hibbins M, Chapman JR. Diagnostic utility of whole blood cyclosporine measurements in renal transplantation using triple therapy. Transplantation 1994; 58:989-996.
113. Levy G, Burra P, Cavallari A, et al. Improved clinical outcomes for liver transplant recipients using cyclosporine monitoring based on 2-hr post-dose levels (C2). Transplantation 2002;73:953-959.
114. Cantarovich M, Barkun JS, Tchervenkov JI, et al. Comparison of Neoral dose monitoring with cyclosporine through levels versus 2-hr postdose levels in stable liver transplant patients. Transplantation 1998;66:1621-1627.
115. Warty V, Diven W, Cadoff E, et al. FK506: a novel immunosuppressive agent. Characteristics of binding and uptake by human lymphocytes. Transplantation 1988;46:453-455.
116. Thomson AW, Woo J. Immunosuppressive properties of FK-506 and rapamycin. Lancet 1989;2:443-444.
117. Randomised trial comparing tacrolimus (FK506) and cyclosporin in prevention of liver allograft rejection. European FK506 Multicentre Liver Study Group. Lancet 1994;344:423-428.
118. Johnson C, Ahsan N, Gonwa T, et al. Randomized trial of tacrolimus (Prograf) in combination with azathioprine or mycophenolate mofetil versus cyclosporine (Neoral) with mycophenolate mofetil after cadaveric kidney transplantation. Transplantation 2000;69:834-841.
119. Pirsch JD, Miller J, Deierhoi MH, et al. A comparison of tacrolimus (FK506) and cyclosporine for immunosuppression after cadaveric renal transplantation. FK506 Kidney Transplant Study Group. Transplantation 1997;63:977-983.
120. Taylor DO, Barr ML, Radovancevic B, et al. A randomized, multicenter comparison of tacrolimus and cyclosporine immunosuppressive regimens in cardiac transplantation: decreased hyperlipidemia and hypertension with tacrolimus. J Heart Lung Transplant 1999;18:336-345.
121. Reichart B, Meiser B, Vigano M, et al. European Multicenter Tacrolimus (FK506) Heart Pilot Study: one-year results—European Tacrolimus Multicenter Heart Study Group. J Heart Lung Transplant 1998;17:775-781.
122. Ratanatharathorn V, Przepiorka D, Devine SM, et al. Phase III study comparing methotrexate and tacrolimus (Prograf, FK506) with methotrexate and cyclosporine for graft-versus-host disease prophylaxis after HLA-identical sibling bone marrow transplantation. Blood 1998;92:2303-2314.
123. Hiraoka A, Ohashi Y, Okamoto S, et al, for the Japanese FK506 BMT (Bone Marrow Transplantation) Study Group. Phase III study comparing tacrolimus (FK506) with cyclosporine for graft-versus-host disease prophylaxis after allogeneic bone marrow transplantation. Bone Marrow Transplant 2001;28:181-185.
124. Jordan ML, Shapiro R, Gritsch HA, et al. Long-term results of pancreas transplantation under tacrolimus immunosuppression. Transplantation 1999;67:266-272.
125. Gruessner RW, Sutherland DE, Najarian JS, et al. Solitary pancreas transplantation for nonuremic patients with labile insulin-dependent diabetes mellitus. Transplantation 1997;64:1572-1577.
126. Keenan RJ, Konishi H, Kawai A, et al. Clinical trial of tacrolimus versus cyclosporine in lung transplantation. Ann Thorac Surg 1995;60:580-584; discussion 584-585.
127. Liu J, Farmer JD Jr, Lane WS, et al. Calcineurin is a common target of cyclophilin-cyclosporin A and FKBP-FK506 complexes. Cell 1991;66:807-815.
128. Venkataramanan R, Jain A, Warty VW, et al. Pharmacokinetics of FK 506 following oral administration: a comparison of FK 506 and cyclosporine. Transplant Proc 1991;23(1 Pt 2):931-933.
129. Venkataramanan R, Jain A, Cadoff E, et al. Pharmacokinetics of FK 506: preclinical and clinical studies. Transplant Proc 1990;22:52-56.
130. Spencer CM, Goa KL, Gillis JC. Tacrolimus: an update of its pharmacology and clinical efficacy in the management of organ transplantation. Drugs 1997;54:925-975.
131. Venkataramanan R, Swaminathan A, Prasad T, et al. Clinical pharmacokinetics of tacrolimus. Clin Pharmacokinet 1995;29:404-430.
131a. Christians U, Jacobsen W, Benet LZ, Lampen A. Mechanisms of clinically relevant drug interactions associated with tacrolimus. Clin Pharmacokinet 2002;41:813-851.
132. Fung JJ, Todo S, Jain A, et al. Conversion from cyclosporine to FK 506 in liver allograft recipients with cyclosporine-related complications. Transplant Proc 1990;22:6-12.
133. Plosker GL, Foster RH. Tacrolimus: a further update of its pharmacology and therapeutic use in the management of organ transplantation. Drugs 2000;59:323-389.
134. Starzl TE, Jordan M, Shapiro R, et al. Kidney transplantation under FK 506. JAMA 1990;264:63-67.
135. McCauley J, Jain A, Todo S, Starzl TE. The effects of FK 506 on renal function after liver transplantation. Transplant Proc 1990;22:17-20.
136. Sehgal SN, Baker H, Vezina C. Rapamycin (AY-22,989), a new antifungal antibiotic. II. Fermentation, isolation and characterization. J Antibiot 1975;28:727-732.
137. Vezina C, Kudelski A, Sehgal SN. Rapamycin (AY-22,989), a new antifungal antibiotic. I. Taxonomy of the producing streptomycete and isolation of the active principle. J Antibiot 1975;28:721-726.
138. Douros J, Suffness M. New antitumor substances of natural origin. Cancer Treat Rev 1981;8:63-87.
139. Eng CP, Sehgal SN, Vezina C. Activity of rapamycin (AY-22,989) against transplanted tumors. J Antibiot 1984;37:1231-1237.
140. Sehgal SN. Rapamune (sirolimus, rapamycin): an overview and mechanism of action. Ther Drug Monit 1995;17:660-665.
141. Molnar-Kimber KL. Mechanism of action of rapamycin (sirolimus, Rapamune). Transplant Proc 1996;28:964-969.
142. Cutler C, Li S, Ho VT, et al. Extended follow-up of methotrexate-free immunosuppression using sirolimus and tacrolimus in related and unrelated donor peripheral blood stem cell transplantation. Blood 2007;109:3108-3114.
143. Brazelton TR, Morris RE. Molecular mechanisms of action of new xenobiotic immunosuppressive drugs: tacrolimus (FK506), sirolimus (rapamycin), mycophenolate mofetil and leflunomide. Curr Opin Immunol 1996;8:710-720.
144. Sehgal SN. Rapamune (RAPA, rapamycin, sirolimus): mechanism of action immunosuppressive effect results from blockade of signal transduction and inhibition of cell cycle progression. Clin Biochem 1998;31:335-340. [reprint in Clin Biochem 2006;39:484-489.]
145. Vasquez EM. Sirolimus: a new agent for prevention of renal allograft rejection. Am J Health Syst Pharm 2000;57:437-448.
146. Marx SO, Jayaraman T, Go LO, Marks AR. Rapamycin-FKBP inhibits cell cycle regulators of proliferation in vascular smooth muscle cells. Circ Res 1995;76:412-417.
147. Poon M, Marx SO, Gallo R, et al. Rapamycin inhibits vascular smooth muscle cell migration. J Clin Invest 1996;98:2277-2283.
148. Sousa JE, Serruys PW, Costa MA. New frontiers in cardiology: drug-eluting stents: Part I. Circulation 2003;107:2274-2279.
149. Ferron GM, Mishina EV, Zimmerman JJ, Jusko WJ. Population pharmacokinetics of sirolimus in kidney transplant patients. Clin Pharmacol Ther 1997;61:416-428.
150. Zimmerman JJ, Kahan BD. Pharmacokinetics of sirolimus in stable renal transplant patients after multiple oral dose administration. J Clin Pharmacol 1997;37:405-415.
151. Johnson EM, Zimmerman J, Duderstadt K, et al. A randomized, double-blind, placebo-controlled study of the safety, tolerance, and preliminary pharmacokinetics of ascending single doses of orally administered sirolimus (rapamycin) in stable renal transplant recipients. Transplant Proc 1996;28:987.

152. Brattstrom C, Tyden G, Sawe J, et al. A randomized, double-blind, placebo-controlled study to determine safety, tolerance, and preliminary pharmacokinetics of ascending single doses of orally administered sirolimus (rapamycin) in stable renal transplant recipients. Transplant Proc 1996;28:985-986.
153. Kelly PA, Gruber SA, Behbod F, Kahan BD. Sirolimus, a new, potent immunosuppressive agent. Pharmacotherapy 1997;17:1148-1156.
154. Brattstrom C, Wilczek HE, Tyden G, et al. Hypertriglyceridemia in renal transplant recipients treated with sirolimus. Transplant Proc 1998;30:3950-3951.
155. Cutler C, Henry NL, Magee C, et al. Sirolimus and thrombotic microangiopathy after allogeneic hematopoietic stem cell transplantation. Biol Blood Marrow Transplant 2005;11:551-557.
156. Sollinger HW. A few memories from the beginning . . . Transplantation 2005;80(2 Suppl):S178-S180.
157. Franklin TJ, Cook JM. The inhibition of nucleic acid synthesis by mycophenolic acid. Biochem J 1969;113:515-524.
158. Deierhoi MH, Kauffman RS, Hudson SL, et al. Experience with mycophenolate mofetil (RS61443) in renal transplantation at a single center. Ann Surg 1993;217:476-482; discussion 482-484.
159. Sollinger HW, Belzer FO, Deierhoi MH, et al. RS-61443 (mycophenolate mofetil): a multicenter study for refractory kidney transplant rejection. Ann Surg 1992;216:513-518; discussion 518-519.
160. A blinded, randomized clinical trial of mycophenolate mofetil for the prevention of acute rejection in cadaveric renal transplantation. The Tricontinental Mycophenolate Mofetil Renal Transplantation Study Group. Transplantation 1996;61:1029-1037.
161. Kobashigawa J, Miller L, Renlund D, et al. A randomized active-controlled trial of mycophenolate mofetil in heart transplant recipients. Mycophenolate Mofetil Investigators. Transplantation 1998;66:507-515.
162. Remuzzi G, Lesti M, Gotti E, et al. Mycophenolate mofetil versus azathioprine for prevention of acute rejection in renal transplantation (MYSS): a randomised trial. Lancet 2004;364:503-512.
163. McNeil K, Glanville AR, Wahlers T, et al. Comparison of mycophenolate mofetil and azathioprine for prevention of bronchiolitis obliterans syndrome in de novo lung transplant recipients. Transplantation 2006;81:998-1003.
164. Carella AM, Champlin R, Slavin S, et al. Mini-allografts: ongoing trials in humans. Bone Marrow Transplant 2000;25:345-350.
165. Ginzler EM, Dooley MA, Aranow C, et al. Mycophenolate mofetil or intravenous cyclophosphamide for lupus nephritis. N Engl J Med 2005;353:2219-2228.
165a. Sifontis NM, Coscia LA, Constantinescu S, et al. Pregnancy outcomes in solid organ transplant recipients with exposure to mycophenolate mofetil or sirolimus. Transplantation 2006;82:1698-1702.
166. Carr SF, Papp E, Wu JC, Natsumeda Y. Characterization of human type I and type II IMP dehydrogenases. J Biol Chem 1993;268:27286-27290.
167. Allison AC, Eugui EM. Mechanisms of action of mycophenolate mofetil in preventing acute and chronic allograft rejection. Transplantation 2005;80(2 Suppl):S181-S190.
168. van Gelder T, Klupp J, Barten MJ, et al. Comparison of the effects of tacrolimus and cyclosporine on the pharmacokinetics of mycophenolic acid. Ther Drug Monit 2001;23:119-128.
169. Funch DP, Ko HH, Travasso J, et al. Posttransplant lymphoproliferative disorder among renal transplant patients in relation to the use of mycophenolate mofetil. Transplantation 2005;80:1174-1180.
170. Henell KR, Norman DJ. In vivo pharmacodynamics of Atgam induction immunosuppression in renal transplantation. Transplant Proc 1995;27:1052-1053.
171. Burdick JF. Biology of immunosuppression medicated by antilymphocyte antibodies. *In* Burdick JF (ed): Kidney Transplant Rejection: Diagnosis and Treatment, 2nd ed. New York: Marcel Dekker.
172. Bunn D, Lea CK, Bevan DJ, et al. The pharmacokinetics of anti-thymocyte globulin (ATG) following intravenous infusion in man. Clin Nephrol 1996;45:29-32.
173. Grabenstein JD. Immunofacts: Vaccines & Immunologic Drugs. St. Louis: Facts and Comparisons, 1994.
174. Nash RA, Johnston L, Parker P, et al. A Phase I/II study of mycophenolate mofetil in combination with cyclosporine for prophylaxis of acute graft-versus-host disease after myeloablative conditioning and allogeneic hematopoietic cell transplantation. Biol Blood Marrow Transplant 2005;11:495-505.
175. Hibberd AD, Trevillian PR, Wlodarzcyk JH, et al. Cancer risk associated with ATG/OKT3 in renal transplantation. Transplant Proc 1999;31:1271-1272.
176. Buchler M, Thibault G, al Najjar A, et al. Monitoring of ATG therapy by flow cytometry and lymphocyte counts in renal transplantation. Transplant Proc 1996;28:2817-2818.
177. Kakhniashvili I, Filicko J, Kraft WK, Flomenberg N. Heterogeneous clearance of antithymocyte globulin after CD34+-selected allogeneic hematopoietic progenitor cell transplantation. Biol Blood Marrow Transplant 2005;11:609-618.
178. Goggins WC, Pascual MA, Powelson JA, et al. A prospective, randomized, clinical trial of intraoperative versus postoperative Thymoglobulin in adult cadaveric renal transplant recipients. Transplantation 2003;76:798-802.
179. Hardinger KL, Schnitzler MA, Koch MJ, et al. Thymoglobulin induction is safe and effective in live-donor renal transplantation: a single center experience. Transplantation 2006;81:1285-1289.
180. Tchervenkov J, Flemming C, Guttmann RD, des Gachons G. Use of Thymoglobulin induction therapy in the prevention of acute graft rejection episodes following liver transplantation. Transplant Proc 1997;29(7A):13S-15S.
181. Krasinskas AM, Kreisel D, Acker MA, et al. CD3 monitoring of antithymocyte globulin therapy in thoracic organ transplantation. Transplantation 2002;73:1339-1341.
182. Schulz T, Papapostolou G, Schenker P, Kapischke M. Single-shot antithymocyte globulin (ATG) induction for pancreas/kidney transplantation: ATG-Fresenius versus Thymoglobulin. Transplant Proc 2005;37:1301-1304.
183. Kuypers DR, Malaise J, Claes K, et al. Secondary effects of immunosuppressive drugs after simultaneous pancreas-kidney transplantation. Nephrol Dial Transplant 2005;20(Suppl 2):33-39.
184. Wu T, Bond G, Martin D, et al. Histopathologic characteristics of human intestine allograft acute rejection in patients pretreated with Thymoglobulin or alemtuzumab. Am J Gastroenterol 2006;101:1617-1624.
185. Schnetzler B, Leger P, Volp A, et al. A prospective randomized controlled study on the efficacy and tolerance of two antilymphocytic globulins in the prevention of rejection in first-heart transplant recipients. Transplant Int 2002;15:317-325.
186. De Santo LS, Della Corte A, Romano G, et al. Midterm results of a prospective randomized comparison of two different rabbit-antithymocyte globulin induction therapies after heart transplantation. Transplant Proc 2004;36:631-637.
187. Lacerda JF, Martins C, Lourenco F, et al. Unrelated stem cell transplantation after a reduced intensity conditioning regimen containing high-dose thymoglobulin leads to controllable graft-versus-host disease. Biol Blood Marrow Transplant 2007;13:494-497.
188. Kang HJ, Shin HY, Choi HS, Ahn HS. Fludarabine, cyclophosphamide plus thymoglobulin conditioning regimen for unrelated bone marrow transplantation in severe aplastic anemia. Bone Marrow Transplant 2004;34:939-943.
189. Preville X, Flacher M, LeMauff B, et al. Mechanisms involved in antithymocyte globulin immunosuppressive activity in a nonhuman primate model. Transplantation 2001;71:460-468.
190. Michallet MC, Saltel F, Preville X, et al. Cathepsin-B-dependent apoptosis triggered by antithymocyte globulins: a novel mechanism of T-cell depletion. Blood 2003; 102:3719-3726.
191. Remberger M, Svahn BM, Mattsson J, Ringden O. Dose study of Thymoglobulin during conditioning for unrelated donor allogeneic stem-cell transplantation. Transplantation 2004;78:122-127.
192. Waller EK, Langston AA, Lonial S, et al. Pharmacokinetics and pharmacodynamics of anti-thymocyte globulin in recipients of partially HLA-matched blood hematopoietic progenitor cell transplantation. Biol Blood Marrow Transplant 2003;9:460-471.
193. De Santo LS, Della Corte A, Romano G, et al. Midterm results of a prospective randomized comparison of two different rabbit-antithymocyte globulin induction therapies after heart transplantation. Transplant Proc 2004;36:631-637.
194. Daoud AJ, Schroeder TJ, Kano J, et al. The US compassionate experience with Thymoglobulin for the treatment of resistant acute rejection. Transplant Proc 1997;29(7A):18S-20S.
195. Colleen Hastings M, Wyatt RJ, Lau KK, et al. Five years' experience with Thymoglobulin induction in a pediatric renal transplant population. Pediatr Transplant 2006;10:805-810.
196. Schroeder TJ, Moore LW, Gaber LW, et al. The US multicenter double-blind, randomized, Phase III trial of Thymoglobulin versus ATGAM in the treatment of acute graft rejection episodes following renal transplantation: rationale for study design. Transplant Proc 1999;31(3B Suppl):1S-6S.
197. Hardinger KL, Schnitzler MA, Koch MJ, et al. Thymoglobulin induction is safe and effective in live-donor renal transplantation: a single center experience. Transplantation 2006;81:1285-1289.
198. Khositseth S, Matas A, Cook ME, et al. Thymoglobulin versus ATGAM induction therapy in pediatric kidney transplant recipients: a single-center report. Transplantation 2005;79:958-963.
199. Requiao-Moura LR, Durao MS, Tonato EJ, et al. Effect of Thymoglobulin in graft survival and function 1 year after kidney transplantation using deceased donors. Transplant Proc 2006;38:1895-1897.
200. Bacigalupo A, Lamparelli T, Bruzzi P, et al. Antithymocyte globulin for graft-versus-host disease prophylaxis in transplants from unrelated donors: 2 randomized studies from Gruppo Italiano Trapianti Midollo Osseo (GITMO). Blood 2001;98:2942-2947.
201. Duggan P, Booth K, Chaudhry A, et al. Unrelated donor BMT recipients given pretransplant low-dose antithymocyte globulin have outcomes equivalent to matched sibling BMT: a matched pair analysis. Bone Marrow Transplant 2002;30:681-686.
202. Lundquist AL, Chari RS, Wood JH, et al. Serum sickness following rabbit antithymocyte-globulin induction in a liver transplant recipient: case report and literature review. Liver Transplant 2007;13:647-650.
203. Busani S, Rinaldi L, Begliomini B, et al. Thymoglobulin-induced severe cardiovascular reaction and acute renal failure in a patient scheduled for orthotopic liver transplantation. Minerva Anestesiol 2006;72:243-248.
204. Preville X, Nicolas L, Flacher M, Revillard J. A quantitative flow cytometry assay for the preclinical testing and pharmacological monitoring of rabbit antilymphocyte globulins (rATG). J Immunol Methods 2000;245:45-54.
205. Caillat-Zucman S, Blumenfeld N, Legendre C, et al. The OKT3 immunosuppressive effect: in situ antigenic modulation of human graft-infiltrating T cells. Transplantation 1990;49:156-160.
206. Hooks MA, Wade CS, Millikan WJ Jr. Muromonab CD-3: a review of its pharmacology, pharmacokinetics, and clinical use in transplantation. Pharmacotherapy 1991;11:26-37.
207. Norman DJ, Barry JM, Bennett WM, et al. OKT3 for induction immunosuppression in renal transplantation: a comparative study of high versus low doses. Transplant Proc 1991;23(1 Pt 2):1052-1054.
208. Midtvedt K, Tafjord AB, Hartmann A, et al. Half dose of OKT3 is efficient in treatment of steroid-resistant renal allograft rejection. Transplantation 1996;62:38-42.
209. Goldstein G, Norman DJ, Henell KR, Smith IL. Pharmacokinetic study of orthoclone OKT3 serum levels during treatment of acute renal allograft rejection. Transplantation 1988;46:587-589.
210. Roitt IM. OKT3: immunology, production, purification, and pharmacokinetics. Clin Transplant 1993;7:367-373.

211. A randomized clinical trial of OKT3 monoclonal antibody for acute rejection of cadaveric renal transplants. Ortho Multicenter Transplant Study Group. N Engl J Med 1985;313:337-342.
212. Shield CF 3rd, Norman DJ, Marlett P, et al. Comparison of antimouse and antihorse antibody production during the treatment of allograft rejection with OKT3 or antithymocyte globulin. Nephron 1987;46(Suppl 1):48-51.
213. Jaffers GJ, Fuller TC, Cosimi AB, et al. Monoclonal antibody therapy: anti-idiotypic and non-anti-idiotypic antibodies to OKT3 arising despite intense immunosuppression. Transplantation 1986;41:572-578.
214. Goldstein G, Norman DJ, Henell KR, Smith IL. Pharmacokinetic study of orthoclone OKT3 serum levels during treatment of acute renal allograft rejection. Transplantation 1988;46:587-589.
215. Swinnen LJ, Costanzo-Nordin MR, Fisher SG, et al. Increased incidence of lymphoproliferative disorder after immunosuppression with the monoclonal antibody OKT3 in cardiac-transplant recipients. N Engl J Med 1990;323:1723-1728.
216. Morgan G, Superina RA. Lymphoproliferative disease after pediatric liver transplantation. J Pediatr Surg 1994;29:1192-1196.
217. Melosky B, Karim M, Chui A, et al. Lymphoproliferative disorders after renal transplantation in patients receiving triple or quadruple immunosuppression. J Am Soc Nephrol 1992;2(12 Suppl):S290-S294.
218. Alloway R, Kotb M, Hathaway DK, et al. Randomized double-blind study of standard versus low-dose OKT3 induction therapy in renal allograft recipients. Am J Kidney Dis 1993;22:36-43.
219. Matteson EL, Yocum DE, St. Clair EW, et al. Treatment of active refractory rheumatoid arthritis with humanized monoclonal antibody CAMPATH-1H administered by daily subcutaneous injection. Arthritis Rheum 1995;38:1187-1193.
220. Isaacs JD, Hazleman BL, Chakravarty K, et al. Monoclonal antibody therapy of diffuse cutaneous scleroderma with CAMPATH-1H. J Rheumatol 1996;23:1103-1106.
221. Moreau T, Thorpe J, Miller D, et al. Preliminary evidence from magnetic resonance imaging for reduction in disease activity after lymphocyte depletion in multiple sclerosis. Lancet 1994;344:298-301.
222. Heit W, Bunjes D, Wiesneth M, et al. Ex vivo T-cell depletion with the monoclonal antibody Campath-1 plus human complement effectively prevents acute graft-versus-host disease in allogeneic bone marrow transplantation. Br J Haematol 1986;64:479-486.
223. Friend PJ, Hale G, Waldmann H, et al. Campath-1M—prophylactic use after kidney transplantation: a randomized controlled clinical trial. Transplantation 1989;48:248-253.
224. Hale G, Cobbold S, Novitzky N, et al. CAMPATH-1 antibodies in stem-cell transplantation. Cytotherapy 2001;3:145-164.
225. Friend PJ, Waldmann H, Hale G, et al. Reversal of allograft rejection using the monoclonal antibody, Campath-1G. Transplant Proc 1991;23:2253-2254.
226. Ciancio G, Burke GW, Gaynor JJ, et al. The use of Campath-1H as induction therapy in renal transplantation: preliminary results. Transplantation 2004;78:426-433.
227. Knechtle SJ, Pirsch JD, Fechner JH Jr, et al. Campath-1H induction plus rapamycin monotherapy for renal transplantation: results of a pilot study. Am J Transplant 2003;3:722-730.
228. Knechtle SJ, Fernandez LA, Pirsch JD, et al. Campath-1H in renal transplantation: The University of Wisconsin experience. Surgery 2004;136:754-760.
229. Shapiro R, Basu A, Tan H, et al. Kidney transplantation under minimal immunosuppression after pretransplant lymphoid depletion with Thymoglobulin or Campath. J Am Coll Surg 2005;200:505-515.
230. Bloom DD, Hu H, Fechner JH, Knechtle SJ. T-lymphocyte alloresponses of Campath-1H-treated kidney transplant patients. Transplantation 2006;81:81-87.
231. Morris EC, Rebello P, Thomson KJ, et al. Pharmacokinetics of alemtuzumab used for in vivo and in vitro T-cell depletion in allogeneic transplantations: relevance for early adoptive immunotherapy and infectious complications. Blood 2003;102:404-406.
232. Morris E, Mackinnon S. Outcome following alemtuzumab (CAMPATH-1H)-containing reduced intensity allogeneic transplant regimen for relapsed and refractory non-Hodgkin's lymphoma (NHL). Transfus Apheresis Sci 2005;32:73-83.
233. Kottaridis PD, Milligan DW, Chopra R, et al. In vivo CAMPATH-1H prevents GvHD following nonmyeloablative stem-cell transplantation. Cytotherapy 2001;3:197-201.
234. Queen C, Schneider WP, Selick HE, et al. A humanized antibody that binds to the interleukin 2 receptor. Proc Natl Acad Sci U S A 1989;86:10029-10033.
235. Anasetti C, Hansen JA, Waldmann TA, et al. Treatment of acute graft-versus-host disease with humanized anti-Tac: an antibody that binds to the interleukin-2 receptor. Blood 1994;84:1320-1327.
236. Vincenti F, Grinyo J, Ramos E, et al. Can antibody prophylaxis allow sparing of other immunosuppressives? Transplant Proc 1999;31:1246-1248.
237. Heffron TG, Smallwood GA, Pillen T, et al. Liver transplant induction trial of daclizumab to spare calcineurin inhibition. Transplant Proc 2002;34:1514-1515.
238. Emre S, Gondolesi G, Polat K, et al. Use of daclizumab as initial immunosuppression in liver transplant recipients with impaired renal function. Liver Transplant 2001;7:220-225.
239. Stratta RJ, Alloway RR, Hodge E, Lo A, for the Pancreas Investigators Vital Outcomes Trial (PIVOT) Study Group. A multicenter, open-label, comparative trial of two daclizumab dosing strategies versus no antibody induction in simultaneous kidney-pancreas transplantation: 6-month interim analysis. Transplant Proc 2002;34:1903-1905.
240. Garrity ER Jr, Villanueva J, Bhorade SM, et al. Low rate of acute lung allograft rejection after the use of daclizumab, an interleukin 2 receptor antibody. Transplantation 2001;71:773-777.
241. Carreno MR, Kato T, Weppler D, et al. Induction therapy with daclizumab as part of the immunosuppressive regimen in human small bowel and multiorgan transplants. Transplant Proc 2001;33:1015-1017.
242. Przepiorka D, Kernan NA, Ippoliti C, et al. Daclizumab, a humanized anti-interleukin-2 receptor alpha chain antibody, for treatment of acute graft-versus-host disease. Blood 2000;95:83-89.
243. Nussenblatt RB, Fortin E, Schiffman R, et al. Treatment of noninfectious intermediate and posterior uveitis with the humanized anti-Tac mAb: a Phase I/II clinical trial. Proc Natl Acad Sci U S A 1999;96:7462-7466.
244. Krueger JG, Walters IB, Miyazawa M, et al. Successful in vivo blockade of CD25 (high-affinity interleukin 2 receptor) on T cells by administration of humanized anti-Tac antibody to patients with psoriasis. J Am Acad Dermatol 2000;43:448-458.
245. Wiseman LR, Faulds D. Daclizumab: a review of its use in the prevention of acute rejection in renal transplant recipients. Drugs 1999;58:1029-1042. [published erratum appears in Drugs 2000;59:476.]
246. Vincenti F, Kirkman R, Light S, et al. Interleukin-2-receptor blockade with daclizumab to prevent acute rejection in renal transplantation. Daclizumab Triple Therapy Study Group. N Engl J Med 1998;338:161-165.
247. Vincenti F, Pace D, Birnbaum J, Lantz M. Pharmacokinetic and pharmacodynamic studies of one or two doses of daclizumab in renal transplantation. Am J Transplant 2003;3:50-52.
248. Soltero L, Carbajal H, Sarkissian N, et al. A truncated-dose regimen of daclizumab for prevention of acute rejection in kidney transplant recipients: a single-center experience. Transplantation 2004;78:1560-1563.
249. Stock PG, Lantz M, Light S, Vincenti F. In vivo (Phase I) trial and in vitro efficacy of humanized anti-Tac for the prevention of rejection in renal transplant recipients. Transplant Proc 1996;28:915-916.
250. Vincenti F, Nashan B, Light S. Daclizumab: outcome of Phase III trials and mechanism of action. Double Therapy and the Triple Therapy Study Groups. Transplant Proc 1998;30:2155-2158.
251. Kagi MK, Heyer G. Efficacy of basiliximab, a chimeric anti-interleukin-2 receptor monoclonal antibody, in a patient with severe chronic atopic dermatitis. Br J Dermatol 2001;145:350-351.
252. Massenkeil G, Rackwitz S, Genvresse I, et al. Basiliximab is well tolerated and effective in the treatment of steroid-refractory acute graft-versus-host disease after allogeneic stem cell transplantation. Bone Marrow Transplant 2002;30:899-903.
253. Lee KH, Da Costa M, Lim SG, Tan KC. Delayed tacrolimus is safe with basiliximab induction therapy. Liver Transplant 2002;8:732.
254. Neuhaus P, Clavien PA, Kittur D, et al. Improved treatment response with basiliximab immunoprophylaxis after liver transplantation: results from a double-blind randomized placebo-controlled trial. Liver Transplant 2002;8:132-142.
255. Salim A, Emerson RM, Dalziel KL. Successful treatment of severe generalized pustular psoriasis with basiliximab (interleukin-2 receptor blocker). Br J Dermatol 2000;143:1121-1122.
256. Nashan B, Moore R, Amlot P, et al. Randomised trial of basiliximab versus placebo for control of acute cellular rejection in renal allograft recipients. CHIB 201 International Study Group. Lancet 1997;350:1193-1198.
257. Amlot PL, Rawlings E, Fernando ON, et al. Prolonged action of a chimeric interleukin-2 receptor (CD25) monoclonal antibody used in cadaveric renal transplantation. Transplantation 1995;60:748-756.
258. Kovarik JM, Rawlings E, Sweny P, et al. Prolonged immunosuppressive effect and minimal immunogenicity from chimeric (CD25) monoclonal antibody SDZ CHI 621 in renal transplantation. Transplant Proc 1996;28:913-914.
259. Lebranchu Y, Bridoux F, Buchler M, et al. Immunoprophylaxis with basiliximab compared with antithymocyte globulin in renal transplant patients receiving MMF-containing triple therapy. Am J Transplant 2002;2:48-56.
260. Chapman TM, Keating GM. Basiliximab: a review of its use as induction therapy in renal transplantation. Drugs 2003;63:2803-2835.
261. Baan CC, van Riemsdijk-Overbeeke IC, Boelaars-van Haperen MJ, et al. Inhibition of the IL-15 pathway in anti-CD25 mAb treated renal allograft recipients. Transpl Immunol 2002;10:81-87.
262. Kovarik J, Wolf P, Cisterne JM, et al. Disposition of basiliximab, an interleukin-2 receptor monoclonal antibody, in recipients of mismatched cadaver renal allografts. Transplantation 1997;64:1701-1705.
263. Grenda R, Watson A, Vondrak K, et al. A prospective, randomized, multicenter trial of tacrolimus-based therapy with or without basiliximab in pediatric renal transplantation. Am J Transplant 2006;6:1666-1672.
264. Kovarik JM, Kahan BD, Rajagopalan PR, et al. Population pharmacokinetics and exposure-response relationships for basiliximab in kidney transplantation. The U.S. Simulect Renal Transplant Study Group. Transplantation 1999;68:1288-1294.
265. Foss FM. DAB(389)IL-2 (ONTAK): a novel fusion toxin therapy for lymphoma. Clin Lymphoma 2000;1:110-116; discussion 117.
266. Ho VT, Zahrieh D, Hochberg E, et al. Safety and efficacy of denileukin diftitox in patients with steroid-refractory acute graft-versus-host disease after allogeneic hematopoietic stem cell transplantation. Blood 2004;104:1224-1226.
267. Shaughnessy PJ, Bachier C, Grimley M, et al. Denileukin diftitox for the treatment of steroid-resistant acute graft-versus-host disease. Biol Blood Marrow Transplant 2005;11:188-193.
268. Mueller XM. Drug immunosuppression therapy for adult heart transplantation. Part 1: Immune response to allograft and mechanism of action of immunosuppressants. Ann Thorac Surg 2004;77:354-362.
269. Contreras G, Pardo V, Leclercq B, et al. Sequential therapies for proliferative lupus nephritis. N Engl J Med 2004;350:971-980.
270. Gaffney K, Scott DG. Azathioprine and cyclophosphamide in the treatment of rheumatoid arthritis. Br J Rheumatol 1998;37:824-836.
271. Morris PJ, Chan L, French ME, Ting A. Low dose oral prednisolone in renal transplantation. Lancet 1982;1:525-527.
272. Singh G, Fries JF, Williams CA, et al. Toxicity profiles of disease modifying antirheumatic drugs in rheumatoid arthritis. J Rheumatol 1991;18:188-194.

273. Connell WR, Kamm MA, Ritchie JK, Lennard-Jones JE. Bone marrow toxicity caused by azathioprine in inflammatory bowel disease: 27 years of experience. Gut 1993;34:1081-1085.
274. Romagnuolo J, Sadowski DC, Lalor E, et al. Cholestatic hepatocellular injury with azathioprine: a case report and review of the mechanisms of hepatotoxicity. Can J Gastroenterol 1998;12:479-483.
275. Jukes TH. The history of methotrexate. Cutis 1978;21:396-398.
276. Cronstein BN, Naime D, Ostad E. The antiinflammatory mechanism of methotrexate: increased adenosine release at inflamed sites diminishes leukocyte accumulation in an in vivo model of inflammation. J Clin Invest 1993;92:2675-2682.
277. Mitchell KL, Pisetsky DS. Early rheumatoid arthritis. Curr Opin Rheumatol 2007;19:278-283.
278. Wenzel J, Tuting T. Identification of type I interferon-associated inflammation in the pathogenesis of cutaneous lupus erythematosus opens up options for novel therapeutic approaches. Exp Dermatol 2007;16:454-463.
279. Leon A, Nguyen A, Letsinger J, Koo J. An attempt to formulate an evidence-based strategy in the management of moderate-to-severe psoriasis: a review of the efficacy and safety of biologics and prebiologic options. Expert Opin Pharmacother 2007;8:617-632.
280. Storb R, Epstein RB, Graham TC, Thomas ED. Methotrexate regimens for control of graft-versus-host disease in dogs with allogeneic marrow grafts. Transplantation 1970;9:240-246.
281. Deeg HJ, Storb R, Weiden PL, et al. Cyclosporin A and methotrexate in canine marrow transplantation: engraftment, graft-versus-host disease, and induction of intolerance. Transplantation 1982;34:30-35.
282. Storb R, Deeg HJ, Thomas ED, et al. Marrow transplantation for chronic myelocytic leukemia: a controlled trial of cyclosporine versus methotrexate for prophylaxis of graft-versus-host disease. Blood 1985;66:698-702.
283. Nash RA, Antin JH, Karanes C, et al. Phase 3 study comparing methotrexate and tacrolimus with methotrexate and cyclosporine for prophylaxis of acute graft-versus-host disease after marrow transplantation from unrelated donors. Blood 2000;96:2062-2068.
284. Chabner BA, Allegra CJ, Curt GA, et al. Polyglutamation of methotrexate: is methotrexate a prodrug? J Clin Invest 1985;76:907-912.
285. Goodsell DS. The molecular perspective: methotrexate. Stem Cells 1999;17:314-315.
286. Methotrexate. *In* Brunton LL, Parker KL, Buxton IL, et al (eds): Goodman & Gilman's The Pharmacological Basis of Therapeutics, 11th ed. New York: McGraw-Hill, 2007. Available at *http://www.AccessMedicine.com*
287. Bensinger W, for the Stem Cell Trialists' Collaborative Group. Individual patient data meta-analysis of allogeneic peripheral blood stem cell transplant vs bone marrow transplant in the management of hematological malignancies: indirect assessment of the effect of day 11 methotrexate administration. Bone Marrow Transplant 2006;38:539-546.
288. Grim J, Chladek J, Martinkova J. Pharmacokinetics and pharmacodynamics of methotrexate in non-neoplastic diseases. Clin Pharmacokinet 2003;42:139-151.
289. Ferry C, Socie G. Busulfan-cyclophosphamide versus total body irradiation-cyclophosphamide as preparative regimen before allogeneic hematopoietic stem cell transplantation for acute myeloid leukemia: what have we learned? Exp Hematol 2003;31:1182-1186.
290. Gluckman E, Auerbach A, Ash RC, et al. Allogeneic bone marrow transplants for Fanconi anemia: a preliminary report from the International Bone Marrow Transplant Registry. Bone Marrow Transplant 1992;10(Suppl 1):53-57.
291. Laurence V, Pierga JY, Barthier S, et al. Long-term follow up of high-dose chemotherapy with autologous stem cell rescue in adults with Ewing tumor. Am J Clin Oncol 2005;28:301-309.
292. Geissler K. Pathophysiology and treatment of aplastic anemia. Wien Klin Wochenschr 2003;115:444-450.
293. de Jonge ME, Huitema AD, Rodenhuis S, Beijnen JH. Clinical pharmacokinetics of cyclophosphamide. Clin Pharmacokinet 2005;44:1135-1164.
294. Ahmed AR, Hombal SM. Cyclophosphamide (Cytoxan): a review on relevant pharmacology and clinical uses. J Am Acad Dermatol 1984;11:1115-1126.
295. Brodsky RA. High-dose cyclophosphamide for aplastic anemia and autoimmunity. Curr Opin Oncol 2002;14:143-146.
296. Dhaygude A, Griffith M, Cairns T, et al. Prolonged treatment with low-dose intravenous pulse cyclophosphamide may reduce rate of relapse in ANCA-associated vasculitis. Nephron 2004;97:154-159.
297. Weiner HL, Cohen JA. Treatment of multiple sclerosis with cyclophosphamide: critical review of clinical and immunologic effects. Mult Scler 2002;8:142-154.
298. Foss FM. The role of purine analogues in low-intensity regimens with allogeneic hematopoietic stem cell transplantation. Semin Hematol 2006;43(2 Suppl 2):S35-S43.
299. Miller KB, Roberts TF, Chan G, et al. A novel reduced intensity regimen for allogeneic hematopoietic stem cell transplantation associated with a reduced incidence of graft-versus-host disease. Bone Marrow Transplant 2004;33:881-889.
300. Pavletic SZ, Bociek RG, Foran JM, et al. Lymphodepleting effects and safety of pentostatin for nonmyeloablative allogeneic stem-cell transplantation. Transplantation 2003;76:877-881.
301. Tallman MS, Hakimian D. Purine nucleoside analogs: emerging roles in indolent lymphoproliferative disorders. Blood 1995;86:2463-2474. [published erratum appears in Blood 1996;87:2093.]
302. Steurer M, Pall G, Richards S, et al. Purine antagonists for chronic lymphocytic leukaemia. Cochrane Database Syst Rev 2006;(3):CD004270.
303. Pettitt AR. Mechanism of action of purine analogues in chronic lymphocytic leukaemia. Br J Haematol 2003;121:692-702.
304. Bolanos-Meade J, Vogelsang GB. Novel strategies for steroid-refractory acute graft-versus-host disease. Curr Opin Hematol 2005;12:40-44.
305. Goldberg JD, Jacobsohn DA, Margolis J, et al. Pentostatin for the treatment of chronic graft-versus-host disease in children. J Pediatr Hematol Oncol 2003;25:584-588.
306. Higman M, Vogelsang GB, Chen A. Pentostatin—pharmacology, immunology, and clinical effects in graft-versus-host disease. Expert Opin Pharmacother 2004;5:2605-2613.
307. Maloney DG, Grillo-Lopez AJ, White CA, et al. IDEC-C2B8 (Rituximab) anti-CD20 monoclonal antibody therapy in patients with relapsed low-grade non-Hodgkin's lymphoma. Blood 1997;90:2188-2195.
308. Maloney DG, Liles TM, Czerwinski DK, et al. Phase I clinical trial using escalating single-dose infusion of chimeric anti-CD20 monoclonal antibody (IDEC-C2B8) in patients with recurrent B-cell lymphoma. Blood 1994;84:2457-2466.
309. Reff ME, Carner K, Chambers KS, et al. Depletion of B cells in vivo by a chimeric mouse human monoclonal antibody to CD20. Blood 1994;83:435-445.
310. Garrett HE Jr, Duvall-Seaman D, Helsley B, Groshart K. Treatment of vascular rejection with rituximab in cardiac transplantation. J Heart Lung Transplant 2005;24:1337-1342.
311. Levine TD, Pestronk A. IgM antibody-related polyneuropathies: B-cell depletion chemotherapy using rituximab. Neurology 1999;52:1701-1704.
312. Tyden G, Kumlien G, Genberg H, et al. ABO incompatible kidney transplantations without splenectomy, using antigen-specific immunoadsorption and rituximab. Am J Transplant 2005;5:145-148.
313. Choquet S, Leblond V, Herbrecht R, et al. Efficacy and safety of rituximab in B-cell post-transplantation lymphoproliferative disorders: results of a prospective multicenter phase 2 study. Blood 2006;107:3053-3057.
314. Yoshizawa A, Sakamoto S, Ogawa K, et al. New protocol of immunosuppression for liver transplantation across ABO barrier: the use of rituximab, hepatic arterial infusion, and preservation of spleen. Transplant Proc 2005;37:1718-1719.
315. Cook RC, Connors JM, Gascoyne RD, et al. Treatment of post-transplant lymphoproliferative disease with rituximab monoclonal antibody after lung transplantation. Lancet 1999;354:1698-1699.
316. Vieira CA, Agarwal A, Book BK, et al. Rituximab for reduction of anti-HLA antibodies in patients awaiting renal transplantation: 1. Safety, pharmacodynamics, and pharmacokinetics. Transplantation 2004;77:542-548.
317. Gloor JM, DeGoey SR, Pineda AA, et al. Overcoming a positive crossmatch in living-donor kidney transplantation. Am J Transplant 2003;3:1017-1023.
318. Sonnenday CJ, Warren DS, Cooper M, et al. Plasmapheresis, CMV hyperimmune globulin, and anti-CD20 allow ABO-incompatible renal transplantation without splenectomy. Am J Transplant 2004;4:1315-1322.
319. Blaes AH, Peterson BA, Bartlett N, et al. Rituximab therapy is effective for posttransplant lymphoproliferative disorders after solid organ transplantation: results of a Phase II trial. Cancer 2005;104:1661-1667.
320. McLaughlin P, Grillo-Lopez AJ, Link BK, et al. Rituximab chimeric anti-CD20 monoclonal antibody therapy for relapsed indolent lymphoma: half of patients respond to a four-dose treatment program. J Clin Oncol 1998;16:2825-2833.
321. Kazatchkine MD, Kaveri SV. Immunomodulation of autoimmune and inflammatory diseases with intravenous immune globulin. N Engl J Med 2001;345:747-755.
322. Kurtzberg J, Friedman HS, Kinney TR, et al. Treatment of platelet alloimmunization with intravenous immunoglobulin: two case reports and review of the literature. Am J Med 1987;83(4A):30-33.
323. Kickler T, Braine HG, Piantadosi S, et al. A randomized, placebo-controlled trial of intravenous gammaglobulin in alloimmunized thrombocytopenic patients. Blood 1990;75:313-316.
324. Tyan DB, Li VA, Czer L, et al. Intravenous immunoglobulin suppression of HLA alloantibody in highly sensitized transplant candidates and transplantation with a histoincompatible organ. Transplantation 1994;57:553-562.
325. Warren DS, Zachary AA, Sonnenday CJ, et al. Successful renal transplantation across simultaneous ABO incompatible and positive crossmatch barriers. Am J Transplant 2004;4:561-568.
326. Jordan SC, Vo A, Bunnapradist S, et al. Intravenous immune globulin treatment inhibits crossmatch positivity and allows for successful transplantation of incompatible organs in living-donor and cadaver recipients. Transplantation 2003;76:631-636.
327. Jordan SC, Quartel AW, Czer LS, et al. Posttransplant therapy using high-dose human immunoglobulin (intravenous gammaglobulin) to control acute humoral rejection in renal and cardiac allograft recipients and potential mechanism of action. Transplantation 1998;66:800-805.
328. Sener A, House AA, Jevnikar AM, et al. Intravenous immunoglobulin as a treatment for BK virus associated nephropathy: one-year follow-up of renal allograft recipients. Transplantation 2006;81:117-120.
329. Snydman DR, Werner BG, Heinze-Lacey B, et al. Use of cytomegalovirus immune globulin to prevent cytomegalovirus disease in renal-transplant recipients. N Engl J Med 1987;317:1049-1054.
330. Nymann T, Shokouh-Amiri MH, Vera SR, et al. Prevention of hepatitis B recurrence with indefinite hepatitis B immune globulin (HBIG) prophylaxis after liver transplantation. Clin Transplant 1996;10(6 Pt 2):663-667.
331. Gasparro FP, Chan G, Edelson RL. Phototherapy and photopharmacology. Yale J Biol Med 1985;58:519-534.
332. Savill J, Dransfield I, Gregory C, Haslett C. A blast from the past: clearance of apoptotic cells regulates immune responses. Nat Rev Immunol 2002;2:965-975.
333. Aubin F, Mousson C. Ultraviolet light-induced regulatory (suppressor) T cells: an approach for promoting induction of operational allograft tolerance? Transplantation 2004;77(1 Suppl):S29-S31.
334. Morelli AE, Larregina AT, Shufesky WJ, et al. Internalization of circulating apoptotic cells by splenic marginal zone dendritic cells: dependence on complement receptors and effect on cytokine production. Blood 2003;101:611-620.

335. Fadok VA, Henson PM. Apoptosis: giving phosphatidylserine recognition an assist—with a twist. Curr Biol 2003;13:R655-R657.
336. Greinix HT, Volc-Platzer B, Kalhs P, et al. Extracorporeal photochemotherapy in the treatment of severe steroid-refractory acute graft-versus-host disease: a pilot study. Blood 2000;96:2426-2431.
337. Rook AH, Jegasothy BV, Heald P, et al. Extracorporeal photochemotherapy for drug-resistant pemphigus vulgaris. Ann Intern Med 1990;112:303-305.
338. Rook AH, Freundlich B, Jegasothy BV, et al. Treatment of systemic sclerosis with extracorporeal photochemotherapy: results of a multicenter trial. Arch Dermatol 1992;128:337-346.
339. Knobler RM, Graninger W, Graninger W, et al. Extracorporeal photochemotherapy for the treatment of systemic lupus erythematosus: a pilot study. Arthritis Rheum 1992;35:319-324.
340. Barr ML, Meiser BM, Eisen HJ, et al. Photopheresis for the prevention of rejection in cardiac transplantation. Photopheresis Transplantation Study Group. N Engl J Med 1998;339:1744-1751.
341. Sunder-Plassman G, Druml W, Steininger R, et al. Renal allograft rejection controlled by photopheresis. Lancet 1995;346:506.
342. Ferrara J, Mauch P, Murphy G, Burakoff SJ. Bone marrow transplantation: the genetic and cellular basis of resistance to engraftment and acute graft-versus-host disease. Surv Immunol Res 1985;4:253-263.
343. Shlomchik WD. Graft-versus-host disease. Nat Rev Immunol 2007;7:340-352.
344. O'Reilly RJ, Keever C, Kernan NA, et al. HLA nonidentical T cell depleted marrow transplants: a comparison of results in patients treated for leukemia and severe combined immunodeficiency disease. Transplant Proc 1987;19(6 Suppl 7):55-60.
345. Dey BR, Spitzer TR. Current status of haploidentical stem cell transplantation. Br J Haematol 2006;135:423-437.
346. Frere P, Pereira M, Fillet G, Beguin Y. Infections after CD34-selected or unmanipulated autologous hematopoietic stem cell transplantation. Eur J Haematol 2006;76:102-108.
347. Waller EK, Langston AA, Lonial S, et al. Pharmacokinetics and pharmacodynamics of anti-thymocyte globulin in recipients of partially HLA-matched blood hematopoietic progenitor cell transplantation. Biol Blood Marrow Transplant 2003;9:460-471.
348. Samijn JP, te Boekhorst PA, Mondria T, et al. Intense T cell depletion followed by autologous bone marrow transplantation for severe multiple sclerosis. J Neurol Neurosurg Psychiatry 2006;77:46-50.
349. Frame JN, Collins NH, Cartagena T, et al. T cell depletion of human bone marrow: comparison of Campath-1 plus complement, anti-T cell ricin A chain immunotoxin, and soybean agglutinin alone or in combination with sheep erythrocytes or immunomagnetic beads. Transplantation 1989;47:984-988.
350. Perseghin P, Gaipa G, Dassi M, et al. CD34+ stem cell recovery after positive selection of "overloaded" immunomagnetic columns. Stem Cells Dev 2005;14:740-743.
351. Vij R, Brown R, Shenoy S, et al. Allogeneic peripheral blood stem cell transplantation following CD34+ enrichment by density gradient separation. Bone Marrow Transplant 2000;25:1223-1228.
352. Bensinger WI, Buckner CD, Shannon-Dorcy K, et al. Transplantation of allogeneic CD34+ peripheral blood stem cells in patients with advanced hematologic malignancy. Blood 1996;88:4132-4138.
353. Ruggeri L, Capanni M, Mancusi A, et al. Natural killer cell alloreactivity in haploidentical hematopoietic stem cell transplantation. Int J Hematol 2005;81:13-17.
354. Couriel DR, Hicks K, Giralt S, Champlin RE. Role of tumor necrosis factor-alpha inhibition with inflixiMAB in cancer therapy and hematopoietic stem cell transplantation. Curr Opin Oncol 2000;12:582-587.
355. Uberti JP, Ayash L, Ratanatharathorn V, et al. Pilot trial on the use of etanercept and methylprednisolone as primary treatment for acute graft-versus-host disease. Biol Blood Marrow Transplant 2005;11:680-687.
356. Kobbe G, Schneider P, Rohr U, et al. Treatment of severe steroid refractory acute graft-versus-host disease with infliximab, a chimeric human/mouse antiTNFalpha antibody. Bone Marrow Transplant 2001;28:47-49.
357. Couriel D, Saliba R, Hicks K, et al. Tumor necrosis factor-alpha blockade for the treatment of acute GVHD. Blood 2004;104:649-654.
358. Marty FM, Lee SJ, Fahey MM, et al. Infliximab use in patients with severe graft-versus-host disease and other emerging risk factors of non-*Candida* invasive fungal infections in allogeneic hematopoietic stem cell transplant recipients: a cohort study. Blood 2003;102:2768-2776.
359. Eleutherakis-Papaiakovou V, Bamias A, Dimopoulos MA. Thalidomide in cancer medicine. Ann Oncol 2004;15:1151-1160.
360. Singhal S, Mehta J. Thalidomide in cancer: potential uses and limitations. Biodrugs 2001;15:163-172.
361. Vogelsang GB, Hess AD, Santos GW. Thalidomide for treatment of graft-versus-host disease. Bone Marrow Transplant 1988;3:393-398.
362. Vogelsang GB, Farmer ER, Hess AD, et al. Thalidomide for the treatment of chronic graft-versus-host disease. N Engl J Med 1992;326:1055-1058.
363. Kulkarni S, Powles R, Sirohi B, et al. Thalidomide after allogeneic haematopoietic stem cell transplantation: activity in chronic but not in acute graft-versus-host disease. Bone Marrow Transplant 2003;32:165-170.
364. Arora M, Wagner JE, Davies SM, et al. Randomized clinical trial of thalidomide, cyclosporine, and prednisone versus cyclosporine and prednisone as initial therapy for chronic graft-versus-host disease. Biol Blood Marrow Transplant 2001;7:265-273.
365. Corral LG, Kaplan G. Immunomodulation by thalidomide and thalidomide analogues. Ann Rheum Dis 1999;58(Suppl 1):107-113.
366. Fowler DH, Breglio J, Nagel G, et al. Allospecific CD8+ Tc1 and Tc2 populations in graft-versus-leukemia effect and graft-versus-host disease. J Immunol 1996;157:4811-4821.
367. Parker PM, Chao N, Nademanee A, et al. Thalidomide as salvage therapy for chronic graft-versus-host disease. Blood 1995;86:3604-3609.
368. Dimopoulos MA, Anagnostopoulos A, Weber D. Treatment of plasma cell dyscrasias with thalidomide and its derivatives [Comment]. J Clin Oncol 2003;21:4444-4454.
369. Zeng D, Lan F, Hoffmann P, Strober S. Suppression of graft-versus-host disease by naturally occurring regulatory T cells. Transplantation 2004;77(1 Suppl):S9-S11.
370. Trachiotis GD, Johnston TS, Vega JD, et al. Single-field total lymphoid irradiation in the treatment of refractory rejection after heart transplantation. J Heart Lung Transplant 1998;17:1045-1048.
371. Diamond DA, Michalski JM, Lynch JP, Trulock EP 3rd. Efficacy of total lymphoid irradiation for chronic allograft rejection following bilateral lung transplantation. Int J Radiat Oncol Biol Phys 1998;41:795-800.
372. Castro-Malaspina H, Childs B, Laver J, et al. Hyperfractionated total lymphoid irradiation and cyclophosphamide for preparation of previously transfused patients undergoing HLA-identical marrow transplantation for severe aplastic anemia. Int J Radiat Oncol Biol Phys 1994;29:847-854.
373. McGlave PB, Haake R, Miller W, et al. Therapy of severe aplastic anemia in young adults and children with allogeneic bone marrow transplantation. Blood 1987;70:1325-1330.
374. Gaziev D, Giardini C, Galimberti M, et al. Bone marrow transplantation for transfused patients with severe aplastic anemia using cyclophosphamide and total lymphoid irradiation as conditioning therapy: long-term follow-up from a single center. Bone Marrow Transplant 1999;24:253-257.
375. Maris MB, Sandmaier BM, Storer BE, et al. Allogeneic hematopoietic cell transplantation after fludarabine and 2 Gy total body irradiation for relapsed and refractory mantle cell lymphoma. Blood 2004;104:3535-3542.
376. Lowsky R, Takahashi T, Liu YP, et al. Protective conditioning for acute graft-versus-host disease. N Engl J Med 2005;353:1321-1331.
377. Williams JW, Javaid B, Kadambi PV, et al. Leflunomide for polyomavirus type BK nephropathy. N Engl J Med 2005;352:1157-1158.
378. Hardinger KL, Wang CD, Schnitzler MA, et al. Prospective, pilot, open-label, short-term study of conversion to leflunomide reverses chronic renal allograft dysfunction. Am J Transplant 2002;2:867-871.
379. Williams JW, Xiao F, Foster P, et al. Leflunomide in experimental transplantation: control of rejection and alloantibody production, reversal of acute rejection, and interaction with cyclosporine. Transplantation 1994;57:1223-1231.
380. Waldman WJ, Knight DA, Lurain NS, et al. Novel mechanism of inhibition of cytomegalovirus by the experimental immunosuppressive agent leflunomide. Transplantation 1999;68:814-825.
381. Knight DA, Hejmanowski AQ, Dierksheide JE, et al. Inhibition of herpes simplex virus type 1 by the experimental immunosuppressive agent leflunomide. Transplantation 2001;71:170-174.
382. Randhawa PS, Finkelstein S, Scantlebury V, et al. Human polyoma virus-associated interstitial nephritis in the allograft kidney. Transplantation 1999;67:103-109.
383. Hussain S, Bresnahan BA, Cohen EP, Hariharan S. Rapid kidney allograft failure in patients with polyoma virus nephritis with prior treatment with antilymphocyte agents. Clin Transplant 2002;16:43-47.
384. Stolt A, Sasnauskas K, Koskela P, et al. Seroepidemiology of the human polyomaviruses. J Gen Virol 2003;84(Pt 6):1499-1504.
385. Bartlett RR, Brendel S, Zielinski T, Schorlemmer HU. Leflunomide, an immunorestoring drug for the therapy of autoimmune disorders, especially rheumatoid arthritis. Transplant Proc 1996;28:3074-3078.
386. Fox RI. Mechanism of action of leflunomide in rheumatoid arthritis. J Rheumatol Suppl 1998;53:20-26.
387. Elder RT, Xu X, Williams JW, et al. The immunosuppressive metabolite of leflunomide, A77 1726, affects murine T cells through two biochemical mechanisms. J Immunol 1997;159:22-27.
388. Kremer JM, Westhovens R, Leon M, et al. Treatment of rheumatoid arthritis by selective inhibition of T-cell activation with fusion protein CTLA4Ig. N Engl J Med 2003;349:1907-1915.
389. Larsen CP, Pearson TC, Adams AB, et al. Rational development of LEA29Y (belatacept), a high-affinity variant of CTLA4-Ig with potent immunosuppressive properties. Am J Transplant 2005;5:443-453.
390. Clinical Study Protocol: A study of BMS-224818 (Belatacept) in patients who have undergone a kidney transplant and are currently on stable cyclosporine or tacrolimus regimen with or without corticosteroids. Available at *http://clinicaltrials.gov/ct2/show/NCT00402168* (accessed July 13, 2007).
391. Clinical Study Protocol: A Phase II study comparing the safety and efficacy of BMS-224818 to cyclosporine, in patients receiving a kidney transplant, when used in combination with CellCept, Simulect, and corticosteroids. Available at *http://clinicaltrials.gov/ct2/show/NCT00035555* (accessed July 13, 2007).
392. Clinical Study Protocol: Study of belatacept (BMS-224818) with a steroid-free regimen in subjects undergoing kidney transplantation. Available at *http://clinicaltrials.gov/ct2/show/NCT00455013* (accessed July 13, 2007).
393. Clinical Study Protocol: Belatacept evaluation of nephroprotection and efficacy as first-line immunosuppression (BENEFIT). Available at *http://clinicaltrials.gov/ct2/show/NCT00256750* (accessed July 13, 2007).
394. Vincenti F, Larsen C, Durrbach A, et al. Costimulation blockade with belatacept in renal transplantation. N Engl J Med 2005;353:770-781.
395. Ojo AO, Hanson JA, Wolfe RA, et al. Long-term survival in renal transplant recipients with graft function. Kidney Int 2000;57:307-313.
396. Nankivell BJ, Borrows RJ, Fung CL, et al. The natural history of chronic allograft nephropathy. N Engl J Med 2003;349:2326-2333.
397. Boubenider S, Hiesse C, Goupy C, et al. Incidence and consequences of post-transplantation lymphoproliferative disorders. J Nephrol 1997;10:136-145.
398. Opelz G, Dohler B. Lymphomas after solid organ transplantation: a collaborative transplant study report. Am J Transplant 2004;4:222-230.

93

GENE THERAPY

Stephen J. Russell and Kah Whye Peng

OVERVIEW 1295
INTRODUCTION 1295
GOALS OF GENE THERAPY 1296
Compensating for Gene Defects 1296
Tissue Engineering 1296
Cytoreductive/Antiproliferative Gene Therapy 1297
Immunostimulatory Gene Therapy 1297
GENE ADDITION 1297
Genes as Drugs 1297
Genes 1297
Delivery Vehicles (Vectors) 1298
Vector Choice 1300
Pharmacokinetics and Pharmacodynamics 1300
In Vivo Barriers to Gene Delivery 1300
Barriers to Gene Expression 1301
Noninvasive Expression Monitoring 1302
Safety Considerations 1302
Clinical Status and Prospects 1303
SCID Gene Therapy Trials 1304
Suicide Gene Therapy for Adoptively Transferred T Cells 1304
Hemophilia Gene Therapy 1304
Adp53 for Cancer Gene Therapy 1304
Proangiogenic Gene Therapy 1304
GENE SUPPRESSION 1305
Noncoding Nucleic Acids as Drugs 1305
Mechanism of Action 1305
Delivery Strategies 1305
Pharmacokinetics and Pharmacodynamics 1306
Barriers to Delivery 1306
Barriers to Gene Suppression 1306
Clinical Status and Prospects 1307
Cytomegalovirus Retinitis 1307
Antisense to Bcl-2 for Cancer Therapy 1307
GENE REPAIR 1308
Autologous, Corrected Cells as Drugs 1308
Mechanism of Homologous Recombination 1308
Homologous Recombination Vectors 1308
Pharmacokinetics and Pharmacodynamics 1308
Barriers to Delivery 1308
Clinical Status and Prospects 1308
Mesenchymal Stem Cell Therapy for Osteogenesis Imperfecta 1308
ONCOLYTIC VIROTHERAPY 1308
Replicating Viruses as Drugs 1308
Mechanism of Action 1309
Targeting Mechanism 1309
Pharmacokinetics and Pharmacodynamics 1311
Barriers to Delivery 1311
Barriers to Spread 1312
Noninvasive Monitoring 1312
Clinical Status and Prospects 1312

OVERVIEW

Gene therapy encompasses a broad range of emerging treatments that use nucleic acids to modulate gene function in somatic cells. This definition excludes genetic modification of the germline for therapeutic gain, which is currently banned in all countries. Great care is taken to avoid inadvertent germline gene transfer when gene therapy is administered. Therapeutic nucleic acids range in size from 20 to 20,000 bases and can be used to repair genetic defects (homologous recombination), to suppress the function of harmful genes (antisense approaches) or to deliver functional copies of a beneficial gene (gene addition). Also, replication-competent viruses that propagate selectively or exclusively in tumors can be used for cancer treatment (oncolytic virotherapy). Preclinical and clinical research in these areas has been progressing rapidly during the past 15 years such that gene therapy now offers a highly promising new therapeutic modality for the treatment of numerous human disorders. Since the first clinical test of gene therapy in 1989, more than 1200 gene therapy protocols have been approved, more than 4000 patients have received gene therapy, and marketing approvals are finally being granted for the most promising agents.

This chapter is divided into five sections, the first providing a brief overview of the aims and scope of gene therapy, followed by four sections, each dealing with a different category of gene therapy intervention (gene addition, gene suppression, gene repair, and oncolytic virotherapy). Each of the intervention-specific sections starts with a description of the therapeutic agents of relevance to the specific approach, followed by a section on their pharmacology (delivery, durability of action, and monitoring approaches) and finishing with a discussion of the current status of their clinical development and future prospects. Due to space limitations, we focus on a limited number of illustrative examples for each category of product.

INTRODUCTION

Previously, gene therapy has been defined as "any therapeutic procedure in which genes are intentionally introduced into human somatic cells."[1] However, the definition used in this chapter has been broadened to "any therapeutic procedure that uses nucleic acids to modulate gene function." This revised definition encompasses not just gene addition therapy, but also homologous recombination, wherein nucleic acids are used to repair disease-causing mutations in the chromosomes of somatic cells; antisense approaches, wherein short oligonucleotides are used to inhibit gene expression; and the use of oncolytic viruses to destroy tumor tissue.

In contrast to conventional small-molecule drug therapies, which usually have a transient effect on their molecular targets, gene therapy often results in a permanent change to the genetic constitution of the targeted somatic cells. Therapeutic nucleic acids may be delivered directly to target cells in the body (in vivo gene therapy) or, alternatively, the target cells may be explanted and exposed to nucleic acids outside the body before they are reimplanted in the patient (ex vivo gene therapy) (Fig. 93-1). Ex vivo gene therapy requires access to advanced laboratory facilities in which human cells or tissues can be processed in compliance with U.S. Food and Drug Administration (FDA) regulations.

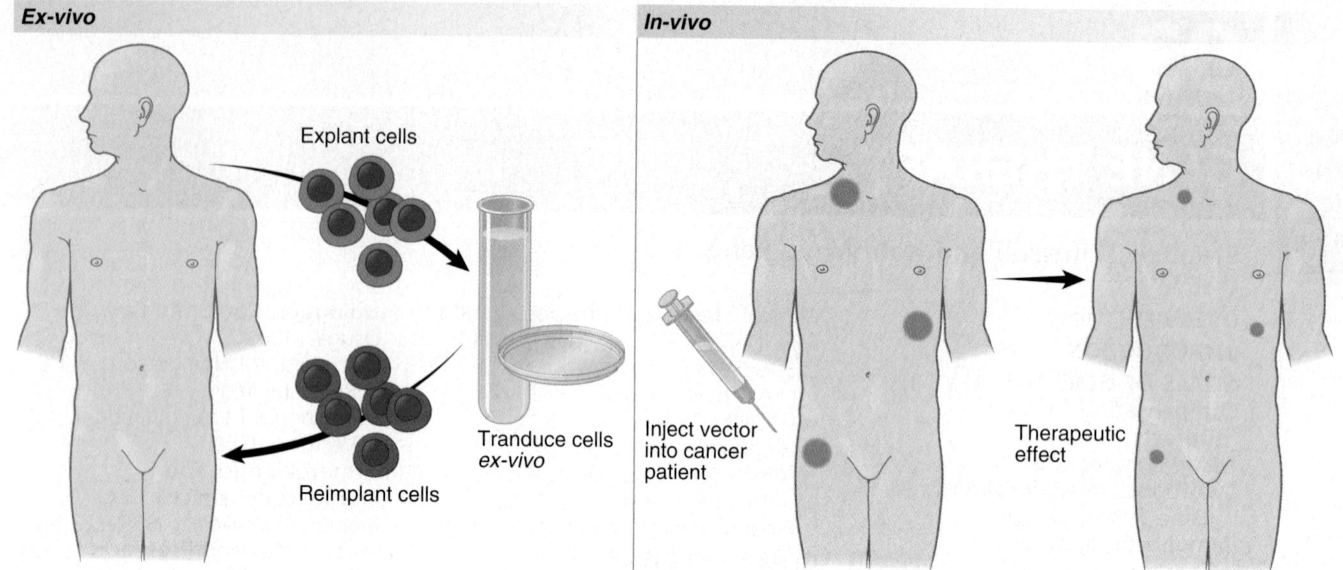

FIGURE 93-1 • Ex vivo and in vivo gene delivery strategies. (See text for details.)

GOALS OF GENE THERAPY

As outlined previously, gene therapy aims to change the genetic constitution of somatic cells, either by gene repair, gene suppression, or gene addition. Homologous recombination (HR) is the process by which gene defects can be repaired.[2] The abnormal gene segment containing a mutation, insertion, or deletion is excised and replaced; however, with current technology, the process is very inefficient such that only occasional cells are correctly repaired.[3] Gene suppression can be achieved through the use of short nucleic acid sequences that target specific messenger RNAs (mRNAs) in the cell. Ribozymes are more efficient than antisense oligonucleotides in this regard because they have catalytic activity and are able to cleave the target mRNA.[4] Similarly, RNA interference (RNAi) is highly efficient because it recruits cellular enzyme complexes to degrade the targeted mRNA.[5] In gene addition therapy, normal copies of a therapeutic gene are added into a cell without disrupting the expression of other genes. This can be achieved with reasonably high efficiency and provides the basis for most current gene therapy approaches.

In principle, all human diseases are potentially amenable to gene therapy approaches. Four broad categories of gene therapy are recognized as follows: compensating for gene defects, tissue engineering, cytotoxic or antiproliferative gene therapy, and immunostimulatory gene therapy. Each of these categories is further discussed in the next sections.

Compensating for Gene Defects

Gene therapy has obvious appeal for the treatment of inherited single gene disorders, particularly those for which current therapies are unsatisfactory or nonexistent.[6] There are more than 4000 known single gene disorders, and gene therapy for any one of these requires a detailed knowledge of the genetic basis and pathogenesis of the disease. Certain mutations lead only to protein deficiency (e.g., severe hemophilia) and are potentially amenable to treatment simply by adding normal copies of the damaged genes.[7] Other mutations lead to production of a harmful mutant protein (e.g., hemoglobin S in sickle cell anemia) and may not be corrected unless the harmful protein can be suppressed.[8]

In theory, HR could be extremely useful for the treatment of numerous single gene disorders. For example, in cystic fibrosis it might be used to repair the *CFTR* gene in airway epithelium, thereby correcting the chloride transport defect that is responsible for production of hyperviscous mucus in this condition.[9] In sickle cell anemia, HR might be used to repair the β-globin mutation that causes this disease, thereby terminating production of the cytotoxic protein, hemoglobin S, and simultaneously reinstating the production of normal hemoglobin A.[10] Alternatively, HR might be used in an autosomal dominant single gene disorder to inactivate a mutant gene that codes for a damaging protein. Osteogenesis imperfecta is a good example of this, wherein a mutation in the *COL1A1* gene leads to the synthesis of a mutant collagen polypeptide whose incorporation into collagen (with the nonmutant polypeptide) leads to formation of very brittle bones.[11] HR could therefore be used in osteogenesis imperfecta to disrupt the mutant *COL1A1* gene, leaving the normal *COL1A1* gene intact to synthesize normal collagen from which strong bones can be formed.[12]

However, as discussed in the introduction, gene repair is technically challenging and inefficient. An additional factor to be considered when compensating for single gene disorders is the reversibility of tissue pathology. For example, gene therapy for lysosomal storage disorders should be implemented before irreversible brain damage has occurred,[13] and gene therapy for cystic fibrosis should be implemented prior to the development of bronchiectasis.[14]

Tissue Engineering

Tissue engineering is a very broad term covering biomaterials science, cell and tissue culture methods, stem cell technology, and gene transfer technology. A central theme is the creation of genetically engineered cells or tissues with novel properties through the expression or suppression of intracellular proteins, membrane proteins, or secreted proteins having either short- or long-range activities. Examples include

- Erythropoietin (Epo) gene transfer (e.g., into muscle) or creation of Epo-secreting neo-organs to regulate red cell production in renal failure.[15]
- Expression of interleukin (IL)-1 antagonists in inflamed joints to suppress inflammation.[16]
- Expression of vascular endothelial growth factor (VEGF) or fibroblast growth factor (FGF) in ischemic tissues to promote angiogenesis.[17]
- Expression of nerve growth factor in neural stem cells implanted into the substantia nigra for treatment of Parkinson's disease.[18]
- Expression of chimeric T-cell receptors in cytotoxic T lymphocytes to target them against cancer antigens.[19]
- Expression of chemotherapy resistance genes in normal bone marrow progenitors to protect against chemotherapy-induced myelosuppression.[20]

- Manipulating the homing properties of autologous immune cells by suppressing the expression of homing receptors that direct them into nontarget tissues.[21]

Cytoreductive/Antiproliferative Gene Therapy

Cytoreductive gene therapy has particular relevance not only in cancer but also in cardiovascular disease, where it can be used to prevent restenosis and vessel reocclusion by combating vascular smooth muscle proliferation after angioplasty. Genes used for cytoreduction include drug sensitivity genes, also known as suicide genes, that render cells sensitive to an otherwise nontoxic prodrug. The most widely used suicide gene is thymidine kinase (TK) from the herpes simplex virus (HSV), which phosphorylates the prodrug ganciclovir to a toxic drug, ganciclovir triphosphate.[22] Under certain circumstances, death by apoptosis is preferred to necrotic cell death and can be achieved through proapoptotic gene transfer using, for example, p53[23] or a dominant negative mutant of cyclin-G.[24] Additional cytotoxic gene products being explored for cancer therapy include ribosomal toxins; fusogenic viral glycoproteins, which fuse tumor cells into large nonviable syncytia; or the thyroidal sodium iodide symporter (NIS), which traps radioactive iodine inside the transduced cells.[25,26]

Gene suppression therapy is also of considerable interest in cancer therapy.[27] A very long list of oncogenic proteins potentially are amenable to this approach; examples include *EGFR, HER2, ras, myc*, and *myb*. Suppressing the synthesis of angiogenesis-promoting proteins is also a logical strategy.[28,29]

Immunostimulatory Gene Therapy

Immunostimulatory gene therapy has particular relevance to the treatment of cancer and the prevention or treatment of infectious diseases. When the target antigen has been identified and cloned, the gene coding for the antigen (viral or tumor-associated) can be delivered, for example, to muscle cells using viral or nonviral vectors. Local production of the antigen is then sustained until the source is eliminated by the immune system. Alternatively, the gene can be introduced into antigen-presenting cells, such as dendritic cells, which are then used as a cellular vaccine. If the antigen gene has not been cloned, then antigen-expressing cells can be genetically modified in order to create a cellular vaccine.[30,31] Genes coding for cytokines or other molecules that enhance the host immune response can be introduced into tumor cells, which are then used as a vaccine to provoke specific antitumor immunity. Genes coding for IL-2, IL-12, granulocyte-macrophage colony-stimulating factor, and the co-stimulatory molecule B7 have all proven to be effective in preclinical models when used in this way.[32-34]

Although not strictly an immunostimulatory approach, viral infections are vulnerable to gene suppression strategies targeted against virally encoded mRNAs. Chronic viral infections such as human immunodeficiency virus (HIV) and hepatitis B virus (HBV) are particularly appealing targets in this regard.[35,36]

GENE ADDITION

Genes as Drugs

A gene is a blueprint for a protein. As a drug, it therefore has no activity until it has been delivered into the nucleus of a target cell, where it can be decoded and expressed as a functional protein. The keys to successful gene therapy are the ability to deliver the therapeutic gene accurately, efficiently, and safely into the nucleus of the target cell and the ability thereafter to control its expression in the target cell. Key steps in the gene therapy process are therefore access, binding and entry into target cells, transport across the cytoplasm into the nucleus, and transcription and translation of the therapeutic protein (Fig. 93-2). The target cells may be stem cells, cancer cells or fully differentiated cells, either in a tissue culture plate or at any location within the body.

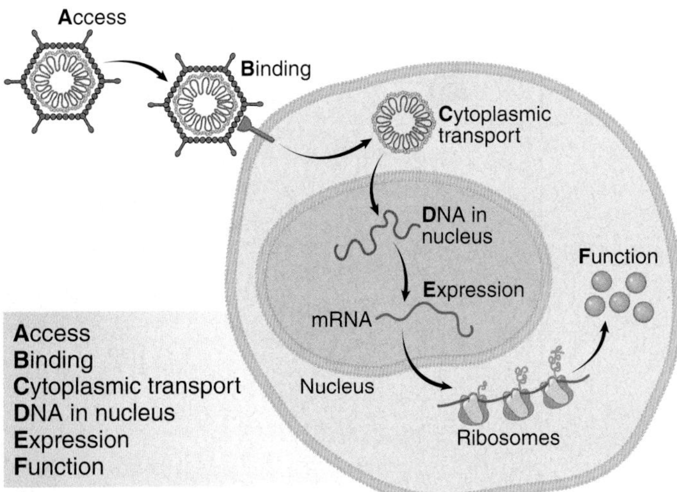

FIGURE 93-2 • The ABCs of gene delivery. The target cell may be a stem cell, a fully differentiated cell, or a tumor cell. The vector must gain access to the target cell wherever it is. Binding to the target cell leads to transfer of genetic material into the cytoplasm and transport into the nucleus, where the DNA is transcribed (expressed). The next step is ribosomal translation, giving rise to a functional protein.

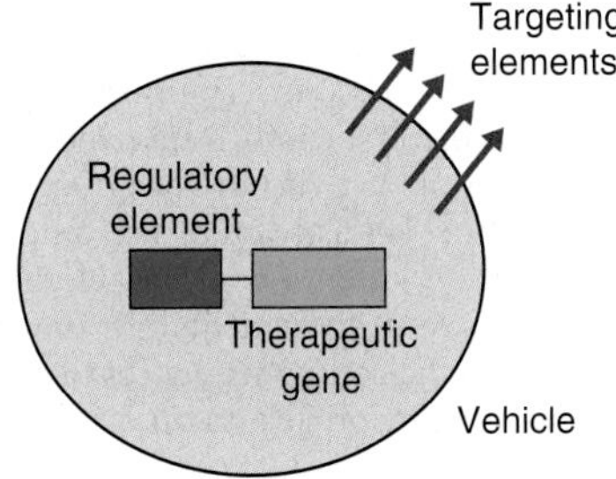

FIGURE 93-3 • Schematic representation of a gene therapy vector. (See text for explanation.)

Gene delivery vehicles, also known as vectors, are required for successful deployment of gene therapy, and their performance sets the boundaries for what can be attempted in human gene therapy. Key elements of a typical vector include a nucleic acid component or expression cassette comprising both the therapeutic gene and regulatory elements that control gene expression, and a vehicle whose purpose is to protect the nucleic acid from nucleases and to transport it to its destination in the nucleus of target cells (Fig. 93-3). Key components of the vehicle include a surface element that mediates recognition of the target cell surface and elements mediating subsequent penetration into the correctly identified target cell. A typical gene therapy vector differs from a typical small drug in that it has multiple components, all of which can be engineered independently toward the goal of improved vector performance. There is a parallel here with the automobile industry, the difference being that the vector industry is still in its infancy.

Genes

What is a gene? The narrowest interpretation is that a gene is a nucleic acid sequence that codes for a specific protein. In general, protein coding sequences in a mammalian chromosome are divided into several exons separated from each other by long intronic sequences containing donor and acceptor sites for the cellular splicing machinery and flanked by RNA processing signals directing addition of a 5′ cap and 3′ polyadenylation signal and determining RNA stability.[37] Transcriptional control elements, including the promoter, enhancers, silencers, and locus control elements, are also essential and integral components of the gene that function as landing pads for nuclear

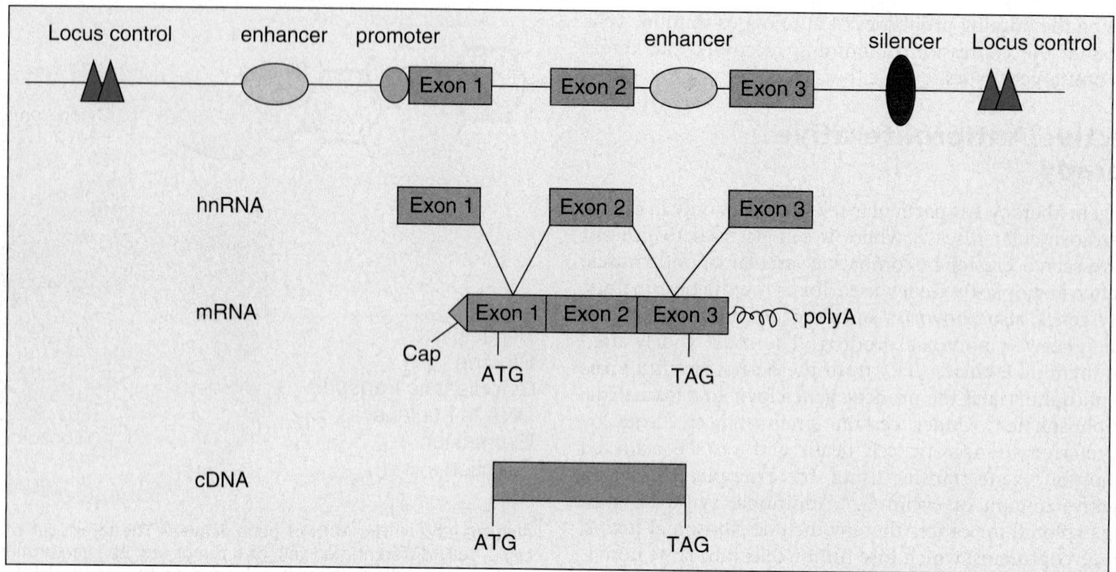

FIGURE 93-4 • Schematic representation of a gene showing exons, introns, and regulatory elements. Heteronuclear RNA (hnRNA) is spliced in the nucleus to produce messenger RNA (mRNA). Complementary DNA (cDNA) refers to a DNA sequence comprising an exact copy of the mRNA sequences (see text for explanation).

proteins (transcription factors) that regulate the level and timing of gene expression (Fig. 93-4). The transcriptional promoter is located immediately upstream of the first exon. Transcriptional enhancer and silencer elements regulate the activity of the promoter element and may be located upstream or downstream of the gene or in one of the introns in either orientation, often a considerable distance from the promoter element. Locus control elements are typically found at a considerable distance from the coding sequences in a 5′ or 3′ direction and are the main determinants of chromatin conformation (open or closed) within a genetic locus.

Delivery Vehicles (Vectors)

Nonviral Vectors. Two broad categories of gene delivery vehicle exist: nonviral and viral. Nonviral vectors are based on plasmid DNA that is grown in bacterial hosts such as *Escherichia coli*. Plasmids are circular DNA molecules that carry an antibiotic resistance marker gene and a bacterial origin of replication to facilitate their amplification in *E. coli* (Fig. 93-5). A mammalian expression cassette comprising a therapeutic gene with its associated regulatory elements can be inserted into the plasmid. As mentioned previously, naked plasmid DNA is susceptible to degradation by nucleases and does not efficiently enter into mammalian cells. However, after intramuscular administration, plasmid DNA can enter into myocyte nuclei leading to expression of the plasmid encoded protein.[38] Viral, bacterial, and tumor antigens expressed in this way can provoke a protective or therapeutic immune response, often more efficiently than a corresponding protein-based vaccine.[39] This is called genetic vaccination. An alternative approach to achieve in vivo gene delivery to liver or muscle using naked plasmid DNA is the so-called hydrodynamic approach in which the DNA is injected into the circulation in a large fluid volume.[40] Applying an electric current to the target site (electroporation) can further enhance the efficacy of gene transfer using naked plasmid DNA.[41] However, for more efficient gene delivery to human tissue, plasmid DNA must be incorporated into a fully synthetic gene therapy vector, for example, using microprojectiles or cationic lipid/protein formations.[42]

In the "gene gun" approach, DNA is coated onto microscopic gold or tungsten particles (microprojectiles) that are then accelerated toward mammalian cells or tissues using a device known as a gene gun.[43] The microprojectiles penetrate the cytoplasmic and nuclear membranes of the target cells and deliver their plasmid DNA cargo into the cell nucleus with reasonable efficiency. This approach may be useful for gene transfer to explanted tumor cells or to easily

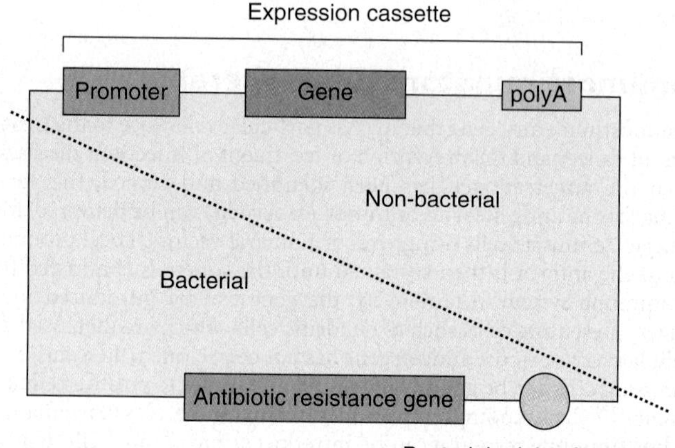

FIGURE 93-5 • Schematic showing how the genomes of viruses and viral vectors are packaged into viral particles (see text for explanation).

accessible tissues such as skin, where the target site is relatively well circumscribed.

Polyamines, polycationic lipids, or neutral polymers can be complexed with plasmid DNA leading to charge neutralization (DNA is negatively charged), protection from nuclease digestion, and enhanced internalization into target cells.[44] Many such DNA nanoparticles have been developed for gene transfer applications, but compared to viral vectors, nonviral gene transfer efficiencies remain low. New lipids and additional protein/peptide elements incorporated into DNA lipid formulations may enhance solubility, target cell specificity, and efficiency of endosomal escape or transport to the cell nucleus.[45,46]

In addition to the nonviral gene delivery systems already described, DNA uptake can be enhanced by the application of an electric current to the target cells or tissues (electroporation)[47,48] or by its incorporation into microbubbles that are then burst in the vicinity of the target cell population by the application of high-frequency ultrasound (ultrasonoporation).[49,50]

Advantages of nonviral vectors include the high genome capacity of 30 to 40 kbp and their lack of immunogenicity (it is very difficult to induce an immune response against plasmid DNA). An additional advantage relative to viral vectors is the perception of a lower risk of harmful side effects compared to viral vectors (discussed later). Significant disadvantages of nonviral vectors include their relatively low transduction efficiencies and their transient expression profile, which typically peaks within 48 hours but is thereafter rapidly extinguished (by 7 days). However, in some situations this may be an advantage, and it may also be possible to prolong the expression profile by using plasmid DNA replicons incorporating mammalian origins of replication (e.g., from the Epstein-Barr virus).[51]

Viral Vectors. Many viruses efficiently deliver their nucleic acid genomes into mammalian cells as the initial critical step in their life cycle. They have therefore been perfected over millions of years of evolution for the task of gene delivery. The key to exploiting viruses as gene delivery vehicles is to introduce therapeutic genes into their genomes while removing the native viral genes that code for harmful viral proteins. The recombinant virus then functions purely as a vector that delivers the therapeutic gene into the nucleus of the target cell without causing cellular damage or subsequent virus propagation.

Viral vectors are generated by exploiting the packaging signal sequences that direct viral genomes into viral particles (Fig. 93-6). A packaging signal sequence is a nucleic acid sequence contained within the viral genome that adopts a specific conformation. Typically, the packaging signal sequence is recognized with high specificity by one of the structural proteins that participate in the assembly of the proteinaceous core of the virus. In a virally infected cell, the viral genome is copied and amplified, the viral genes are expressed, and the structural proteins assembled to form new virus particles that interact with the progeny viral genomes guided by the all-important packing signal sequence to form fully infectious progeny virus particles that are released from the cell. To generate viral vectors, the packaging signal sequence is removed from the viral genome and appended to the therapeutic transgene. This packagable transgene is then introduced into a mammalian cell along with the viral genes, now lacking their packaging signal sequence such that the viral genes are expressed and new viral particles produced, but only the therapeutic transgene is packaged into the particles because it is now the only nucleic acid in the cell that carries the packaging signal sequence.

Virtually any virus can be exploited as a gene delivery vehicle. However, at this point in time, the most widely used viral vectors are derived from the following viruses: retrovirus (and lentivirus), adenovirus, adeno-associated virus (AAV), and HSV.[52] Each of these viral vectors has distinct characteristics that may make it more or less suitable for a particular gene therapy application. There is no perfect universal vector, and decisions about which vector to use for a particular application should be made on a case-by-case basis. A brief description of some of the major viral vector systems is provided here.

Retroviral and Lentiviral Vectors. These are derived from C-type retroviruses such as murine leukemia virus (MLV)[53] or from lentiviruses such as HIV and feline immunodeficiency virus. The viral particles are roughly spherical, 80 to 110 nm in diameter, comprising an icosahedral protein core containing two copies of the 7- to 11-kb single-stranded RNA viral genome plus three virally encoded enzymes: reverse transcriptase, protease, and integrase. The core is surrounded by a lipid envelope that carries the viral envelope glycoproteins responsible for virus attachment and entry. After attachment, the virus envelope fuses with the cell membrane and the core moves toward the nucleus. The viral RNA is reverse transcribed to double-stranded DNA and transported into the nucleus, where the integrase directs its insertion in the host chromosomal DNA at a random site. Viral genes are transcribed from the integrated (proviral) DNA. To make retroviral vector particles, two helper plasmids are expressed in a packaging cell, one coding for core proteins and viral enzymes, the other for envelope glycoproteins. The packagable RNA that codes for the therapeutic protein is transcribed from a third plasmid, the vector plasmid. MLV-based retroviral vectors do not integrate or express in quiescent cells. Cell division is required for integration. In contrast, lentiviral vectors can integrate in quiescent cells. Integration is semirandom using a different chromosomal site in each transduced cell, with an overall preference for transcriptionally active target sites.[54] Expression of the transgene varies greatly from cell to cell according to the integration site. Random integration is associated with a risk of cell transformation (insertional mutagenesis) caused by disruption of a tumor suppressor gene or activation of a cellular oncogene.[55,56]

Retroviral/lentiviral vectors have a capacity of 8 kb and give maximum titers up to 10^{10} infectious particles/ml.[57] Because of integration, the transgene persists in the progeny of the originally infected cells.[58] Vector particles are immunogenic, but vector-transduced cells express no viral gene products and are therefore nonimmunogenic. The expression profile peaks within 72 hours and then gradually declines over weeks, months, or years due to transgene methylation, acetylation, provirus deletion, or death of the target cell.[59]

Adenovirus Vectors. Adenoviruses are nonenveloped viruses with an 80- to 110-nm diameter icosahedral protein shell containing a 35- to 40-kbp double-stranded DNA genome.[60] The fiber proteins appear on

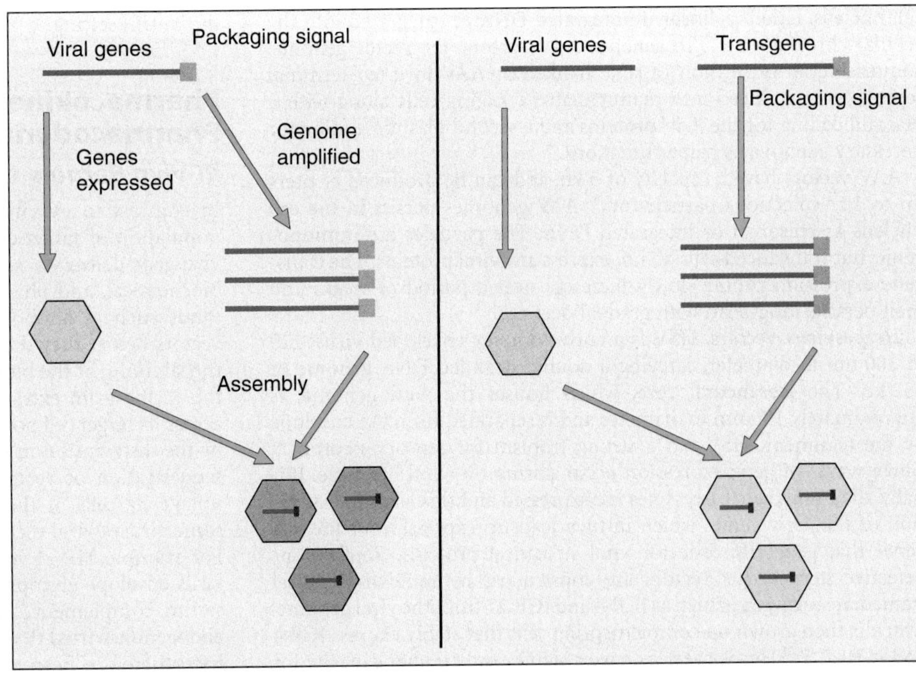

FIGURE 93-6 • Schematic representation showing how the genomes of viruses and viral vectors are packaged into viral particles (see text for details).

electron microscopy as prominent spikes at the 12 vertices of the icosahedron. Primary attachment to the target cell is through the fiber protein, and secondary attachment to cell surface integrin receptors occurs through the penton base protein that anchors the fiber at the vertices of the icosahedron. After endocytosis, the virus disrupts the wall of the endosome and is released into the cytoplasm. Cytoplasmic virus migrates to the nuclear envelope and delivers the viral DNA to the nucleus. In wild-type adenovirus infection, early (nonstructural) viral genes are expressed initially, and the early proteins drive virus genome replication and late (structural) gene expression. To produce adenovirus vectors, early genes (e.g., E1, E4) are deleted from the virus genome to disrupt the replication cycle and therapeutic genes are inserted into their place. Vector particles are produced in cell lines that stably express the missing early gene products (e.g., E1, E4) and can therefore support vector replication. In helper-dependent ("gutless") adenovirus vectors, all of the viral coding sequences are removed.[61] Production of helper-dependent vectors requires the addition of a replicating helper adenovirus that is later removed from the vector stock.

Adenovirus vectors have a capacity of approximately 8 kb for conventional vectors and 30 kb for helper-dependent vectors, and titers up to 10^{13} infectious particles/ml are possible, allowing for high target cell transduction efficiencies. The vector genome persists in the cell as a linear, unintegrated episome and is therefore diluted by cell division. Adenovirus particles are immunogenic, and so are transduced cells in the case of conventional adenovirus vectors due to low level expression of viral structural genes. However, cells transduced with helper-dependent adenovirus vectors express no viral proteins and are not immunogenic. The adenoviral vector expression profile reaches a very high peak within the first 3 days and is then rapidly lost in the case of conventional vectors due to immune-mediated destruction of transduced cells.[62] However, expression is maintained over weeks, months, or years in the case of helper-dependent vectors because the target cells are not subject to immune-mediated destruction.[63]

Adeno-associated Virus Vectors. AAV is a very small, nonenveloped icosahedral virus 18 to 26 nm in diameter, carrying a single-stranded DNA genome of approximately 5 kb with short, inverted, terminal repeats required for genome replication and packaging.[64] AAV is an apathogenic dependovirus that replicates only in cells that are concurrently infected with a suitable helper virus (adenovirus or herpesvirus). After virus attachment and translocation across the target cell membrane, the single-stranded DNA genome is transported to the cell nucleus, where it is converted to double-stranded DNA that is then transcribed by cellular polymerase. The AAV genome can persist in the cell nucleus, either as linear unintegrated DNA or integrated into the cellular chromosome.[65] To generate AAV vectors, the vector genome, comprising an expression cassette flanked by AAV inverted terminal repeats, is introduced into mammalian packaging cells along with a plasmid coding for the AAV proteins and a second plasmid coding for necessary adenovirus helper functions.[66]

AAV vectors have a capacity of 5 kb, and can be produced at titers up to 10^{12} infectious particles/ml.[67] AAV genomes persist in the cell nucleus as episomal or integrated DNA. The particles are immunogenic, but transduced cells do not express any viral proteins. The transgene expression profile slowly increases over a period of weeks and then persists long-term with gradual decline.

Herpesvirus Vectors. HSV is a fairly complex enveloped virus, 120 to 300 nm in diameter, carrying a double-stranded DNA genome of 152 kb. The icosahedral core, which houses the viral genome, is approximately 100 nm in diameter and is separated from the envelope by the tegument. HSV has a strong tropism for sensory neurons.[68] Three waves of gene expression occur during the viral life cycle. Initially, the immediate early genes are expressed and this leads to expression of the early genes, which in turn leads to expression of the late genes that generally code for viral structural proteins. Replication-defective herpesvirus vectors are constructed by removing critical immediate early genes such as ICP-4 and ICP-27 from the viral genome, which is then grown on complementing cells that stably express ICP-4 and ICP-27.[69,70] Herpes vectors have a significantly higher capacity for foreign genetic material than the vectors described previously, and are rapidly gaining popularity for central and peripheral nervous system applications. HSV is able to enter into a latent state in sensory neurons, and this is one of the major reasons for its popularity as a vector for these cells.

TABLE 93-1 VECTOR CHOICE*

	Transfer to Progeny	Nondividing Cells	Efficiency
Nonviral	No	Yes	+
Retrovirus	Yes	No	++
Adenovirus	No	Yes	++++
Lentivirus	Yes	Yes	++

*Vector choice is guided by many factors, but some of the key factors driving these decisions are shown in the table (see text for discussion). Note that other issues such as safety, accuracy, and size of transgene also affect vector choice.

Vector Choice

The choice of an appropriate vector system for a gene therapy protocol should be guided by consideration of the relevant properties of the different vector systems in relation to the characteristics of the target cell population and the goals of the proposed application (Table 93-1). Thus, when introducing the β-globin gene into hematopoietic stem cells for correction of β-thalassemia, the real targets are the future erythroid progeny of the initially transduced cells. Efficient integration of the transgene into the host-cell chromosome is therefore highly desirable, an indication for the use of retroviral or lentiviral vectors. Alternatively, when delivering a tyrosine hydroxylase or glial-derived neurotrophic factor gene to the striatum or substantia nigra for correction of Parkinson's disease, the vector should efficiently and stably transduce quiescent neurons in the relevant parts of the brain without provoking an immune or inflammatory response and should lead to long-term, sustained production of the therapeutic protein. AAV, lentiviral, and helper-dependent adenoviral vectors are all attractive in this regard.[71-74] When the targets of therapy are cancer cells and the goal is to eliminate them, the highest priority is for a vector that can transduce the cells with a very high efficiency. In this setting, a strong immune/inflammatory response to the genetically modified cells is not contraindicated and may be desirable to increase the potency of the therapy. Conventional adenovirus vectors are therefore appealing in this setting.

Pharmacokinetics and Pharmacodynamics

In Vivo Barriers to Gene Delivery

In contrast to ex vivo gene therapy protocols in which a purified population of target cells is transduced in the culture dish, direct in vivo gene delivery is significantly constrained by additional anatomic, biochemical, and physiologic barriers. These include factors in body fluids such as antibodies and complement that can neutralize the vectors before they reach their target sites. The integrity of the endothelial lining of the blood vessels supplying target organs may prevent the vector from extravasating into the interstitial fluid where it can access its target cell population. Also, gene delivery may be constrained by the distribution in the body of receptor sites for the vector and by sequestration of vector particles in nontarget organs as a result of uptake by cells of the reticuloendothelial system. The envelopes of some viruses/viral vectors are intrinsically susceptible to blood factors. For example, HIV-1 vectors pseudotyped with the vesicular stomatitis virus envelope glycoprotein are susceptible to inactivation by human serum complement.[75] Alternative envelopes such as RD114 (feline endogenous virus) that are less susceptible to complement inactivation have therefore been proposed.[76] Intravenously administered type 5 adenoviruses are sequestered in the liver, resulting in hepatoxicity. It has been demonstrated that murine coagulation factor IX and complement component C4-binding protein can bind the viral fiber knob domain and provide a bridge for virus uptake into hepatocytes through cell surface heparan sulfate proteoglycans and low-density lipoprotein receptor–related protein.[77] Therefore, adenoviral vectors with mutations in the receptor binding region have longer blood circulation times and less transduction of nontarget organs.[78]

With respect to the immunologic barriers to gene therapy, both humoral immunity to the vector or gene product and cell-mediated immunity to the genetically modified cells must be considered. Many patients have preexisting neutralizing antibodies against adenovirus, AAV, and herpesvirus vectors,[79] and, even if not present, these antibodies may develop following the first exposure to the vector. Preexisting immunity leads to variable neutralization of the first dose of the vector or its gene product or elimination of the transduced cells. Maturation and amplification of the immune response following each exposure to therapy results in accelerated vector neutralization/transduced cell elimination with successive exposures. Thus an ideal vector would not elicit an immune response in the treated patient.

Targeting Gene Delivery. There are three broad strategies whereby vectors can be targeted to accumulate at predetermined sites or to selectively transduce a particular target cell population. In the first approach, the target cells are isolated and transduced in the tissue culture dish. In the second case, regional delivery is used to ensure accumulation of vector at a particular location in the body—for example, aerosol delivery to airways,[80] stereotactically guided injection into the brain,[81,82] or painting vector onto vascular structures during surgical exposure.[83] The third approach to targeting is to modify the vector (intrinsic targeting) such that it recognizes and transduces the target cells with high specificity, but is not capable of transducing nontarget cells.[84] For viral vectors, transductional targeting can be achieved by direct chemical modification of the virus coat, by the use of bifunctional cross-linking molecules that provide a bridge between the vector and the cell surface target, or by direct engineering of the viral attachment proteins. Transductional targeting is an active area of research, and proof of principle has been established for all major vector systems. The first two clinical studies employing transductionally targeted vectors were recently approved. One employs a retroviral vector displaying a collagen-binding peptide to enhance its retention in tumor blood vessels where collagen is highly exposed.[85] The other employs an adenoviral vector displaying an integrin-binding RGD peptide that selectively enhances its ability to transduce ovarian carcinoma cells in the peritoneal cavity.[86]

Barriers to Gene Expression

Durable gene expression in the target tissue of interest is often one of the key factors contributing to the success of a given gene therapy approach. The level of gene expression in a transduced target cell is governed by a complex interplay between the therapeutic gene and a host of cellular factors in the nucleus and cytoplasm that regulate processes such as DNA methylation and acetylation, gene transcription, mRNA transport, splicing and degradation, and protein synthesis. A typical gene in a mammalian chromosome has multiple component parts, including exons and intronic sequences containing donor and acceptor sites for the cellular splicing machinery and flanked by RNA processing signals. Transcriptional control elements are also essential and integral components of the gene that regulate the level and timing of gene expression (see Fig. 93-4).

Transcriptional Targeting. Transcriptional control elements are portable and can be transferred from one gene to another, retaining their tissue specificity. Promoters and enhancers from housekeeping genes expressed in all tissues or from certain viruses (e.g., cytomegalovirus [CMV]) will drive gene expression promiscuously in all transduced mammalian cells. Promoters and enhancers from genes expressed in a tissue-specific manner will drive expression of foreign genes with the same tissue specificity.[87] Thus the albumin promoter/enhancer is active only in hepatocytes,[88] tyrosinase promoter in melanocytes and melanoma cells,[89] immunoglobulin promoter/enhancer in B lymphocytes,[90] and β-globin promoter/enhancer in erythroblasts.[91,92] While it is relatively simple to construct a vector that drives gene expression in a tissue-specific manner, the absolute level of gene expression in a given target cell is more difficult to control.

β-Thalassemia major is a relatively common inherited disease characterized by deficient production of β-globin but continued high-level production of α-globin. Excess α-globin chains form α-4 tetramers that crystallize on the red cell membrane leading to premature red cell destruction. Patients have severe anemia, transfusion dependence, and greatly shortened life expectancy. Bone marrow transplantation is curative, so for patients with no matched donor, the goal is to reconstitute with genetically corrected autologous hematopoietic stem cells (HSCs). Lentiviral vectors expressing the β-globin gene under the control of a β-globin promoter/enhancer element will drive erythroid-specific β-globin expression,[93] but the expression level varies enormously between cells, depending upon the integration site. Such vectors hold little attraction for the treatement of thalassemia, where the absolute level of globin gene expression is so critical to success. However, if globin locus control elements are introduced into the vector, the dependence on integration site is eliminated, and gene expression levels in all transduced erythroid cells approach levels seen with native globin genes.[91,92]

Pharmacologic Control of Transcription. Pharmacologic control of gene expression is desirable for certain gene therapy applications. Erythropoietin is widely used for the treatment of anemia caused by renal failure or by malignancies such as multiple myeloma.[94,95] The protein is expensive and must be administered by injection on a regular basis. Gene therapy has therefore been explored as a potentially less expensive, more convenient means of Epo delivery. Erythropoietin administered subcutaneously at regular intervals leads to a dose-dependent increase in hematocrit. Dose titration is therefore necessary to keep the hematocrit within the desired range. Several drug-regulatable gene expression systems have been developed. In the tetracycline-regulatable system, the therapeutic gene is controlled by a tetracycline responsive promoter with very low or zero basal activity. A second gene codes for a transcription factor that can drive expression from the tet-responsive promoter, but only in the presence of tetracycline. Addition of tetracycline therefore drives transgene expression in a dose-dependent manner. Tetracycline-regulatable AAV vectors coding for Epo have been delivered into the muscles of laboratory mice and nonhuman primates. It has then been possible to control their hematocrit by treating the animals with different doses of tetracycline.[96,97]

Decay of Expression. Loss of gene expression over time due to gene silencing, gene deletion, or elimination of the gene-modified cells can also be a significant barrier to successful gene addition therapy. In vivo silencing of retroviral and lentiviral transgene expression over time is frequently encountered due to methylation (retrovirus) or acetylation (lentivirus) of the integrated provirus. The provirus can also be deleted by HR between the two proviral long terminal repeat sequences.

Elimination of genetically modified cells can occur by a variety of mechanisms. First, the target cells may simply reach the end of their natural life span (120 days for a red blood cell, 150 days for a hepatocyte, etc.) and die by natural attrition. Second, the gene product may be toxic to the target cell, causing it to die prematurely. This may be intentional, as in the case of TK gene transfer with subsequent ganciclovir therapy, or may be completely unforeseen. Another reason for premature termination of therapeutic gene expression is immune-mediated destruction of the transduced cells. This can be particularly rapid when using first-generation adenoviral vectors, which code for a variety of immunogenic adenoviral proteins. However, immune-mediated destruction of transduced cells has also been encountered using gene transfer vectors that apparently do not code for any immunogenic protein sequences. In these cases, it appears that the immune system can become alerted to the fact that a target cell is producing abnormal amounts of a "self" protein, and it has even been postulated that the proteins of incoming vector particles might be processed and presented at the surface of infected cells as immunogenic major histocompatibility complex (MHC)–peptide complexes.

In a recent clinical study in which an AAV serotype 2 vector coding for human factor IX was administered intravenously to patients with severe hemophilia B (factor IX levels less than 2% of normal), one patient showed an encouraging increase in his circulating factor IX level to 10% of normal (sufficient to prevent spontaneous bleeding), but this fell fairly rapidly back to the baseline level and at the same time there was evidence for liver inflammation with a short-lived increase in blood transaminase levels.[98] The disappointing decline in factor IX in this patient was extensively investigated and is currently thought to be attributable to an anamnestic T-cell response to AAV peptides derived from the incoming virus particles and presented in MHC-peptide complexes on the surface of the transduced liver cells. AAV-2 capsid-specific T cells became detectable in peripheral blood at the time of declining factor IX levels, implying T cell–mediated rejection of AAV-transduced hepatocytes by AAV capsid-specific memory $CD8^+$ T cells reactivated by AAV vectors.[99] This is in contrast to experimental animals (mice, dogs) in which gene expression was long term.

Rapid Destruction of Therapeutic Protein. Apparent loss of gene expression may result from the accelerated (typically immune-mediated) destruction of a therapeutic protein. For the treatment of hemophilia, the formation of antibodies (inhibitors) to factor VIII or factor IX is one of the most dreaded complications of therapy because it makes the control of bleeding so much more difficult. One concern for gene therapy of hemophilia is that it may lead to a high incidence of inhibitor development. This has certainly been seen in animal models. For example, when transgenic factor IX knockout mice with hemophilia were treated with an AAV-1 serotype vector coding for murine factor IX under the control of a muscle-specific promoter, the circulating level of factor IX declined substantially because of a humoral immune response against the murine factor IX protein.[100] Equally concerning was a recent study in which a gene therapy vector coding for rhesus monkey erythropoietin was administered by intramuscular injection to rhesus monkeys. Initially the hematocrit rose due to increased erythropoietin-driven erythropoiesis. However, some of the animals subsequently became profoundly anemic to the point that they had to be euthanized. The anemia was due to anti-erythropoietin neutralizing antibodies that neutralized both endogenous and vector-encoded rhesus monkey erythropoietin.

Noninvasive Expression Monitoring

Pharmacokinetics is the study of the fate of a drug in the body. Since a therapeutic gene is inert, it must be converted to protein by the cells to which it has been delivered before it can exert any therapeutic effect. It is therefore important in gene therapy protocols to avoid focusing exclusively on the therapeutic gene and to carefully study the rates of production, accumulation, and elimination of the encoded therapeutic protein. Pharmacodynamics is the study of the way in which a drug mediates it characteristic actions (beneficial and harmful) in the body and includes the study of dose-response relationships. For gene therapy treatments, it is again the protein product of the therapeutic gene that is of interest in this regard. Measurement of the concentration of therapeutic protein is therefore required in order to determine the appropriate dose and dosing regimen for a gene therapy product.

Many of the proteins encoded by potentially therapeutic genes are cell associated and are not released into body fluids. Until recently, there were no satisfactory noninvasive methods for monitoring the accumulation of cell-associated proteins in the body. Thus, many clinical gene therapy studies have failed to answer the most basic question of whether expression of the therapeutic gene was achieved. For example, recent cardiovascular gene therapy studies sought to promote angiogenesis in ischemic myocardium by delivery of the proangiogenic molecules VEGF and FGF-4.[101] Genes were delivered by direct intramyocardial injection or by coronary arterial perfusion using plasmid DNA or adenovirus vectors.[102,103] Many patients reported subjective improvement in their angina, but there was no direct evidence of gene expression, making it impossible to attribute the clinical improvement to gene therapy. Direct evidence of gene expression in the transduced hearts could not be obtained because (i) myocardial biopsy is too dangerous, and (ii) VEGF and FGF were not released into the bloodstream and, even if they were, the transgene encoded proteins would be indistinguishable from native host proteins.

Expression of a therapeutic gene can be monitored indirectly by linking its expression to the expression of a soluble marker polypeptide whose concentration can be measured in body fluids.[104] The therapeutic gene and soluble marker polypeptide are expressed concordantly (i.e., at a constant ratio), and the soluble peptide is completely inert, meaning that it is nonimmunogenic and has no biologic activity (Fig. 93-7). Additional requirements for the marker peptide are that it should be secreted into the bloodstream, it should be absent in untreated individuals, it should have a known circulating half-life, and there should be a sensitive assay for accurate detection. Tumor markers such as carcinoembryonic antigen and the β chain of human chorionic gonadotropin are good examples of suitable markers. While soluble marker peptides can provide critical information regarding the profile of gene expression over time, they give no information as to the location of genetically modified cells.

For noninvasive mapping of the location/distribution of genetically modified cells, there has been considerable recent progress in the development of molecular imaging techniques, in which case a marker gene coexpressed with the therapeutic gene directs the production of a cell-associated marker protein that can be detected by radioisotopic imaging techniques. Examples include NIS, which concentrates radioiodine into the target cells in which it is expressed, allowing noninvasive detection by gamma camera imaging (^{123}I) or positron emission tomography (PET) scanning (^{124}I).[25,105] Alternatively, HSV TK expression can be detected by administration of a radioisotopically labeled substrate that is phosphorylated by TK and thereby trapped inside the genetically modified target cell. Isotope trapping is then detected either by gamma camera imaging or by PET scanning.[106,107] A third approach is to use a marker gene coding for a nonimmunogenic cell surface marker that can then be detected by administering a radioisotope-labeled peptide or monoclonal antibody.[108,109]

With the advent of these new noninvasive expression monitoring and molecular imaging strategies, it will now be possible to generate high-quality pharmacokinetic and pharmacodynamic data in the context of human gene therapy studies. This will help to address one of the major issues that has dampened enthusiasm for gene therapy in the pharmaceutical industry—namely, how to define a "dose" of a gene therapy product. Ideally, a dose should be a quantity of vector transducing a predetermined number of cells leading to production of a predetermined amount of protein, leading to an expected therapeutic response in the patient without toxicity. The major problem here is that gene expression and protein production are highly variable between individuals given identical doses of vector particles by identical routes, and between treatments in a single individual given the identical dose on different occasions. Noninvasive expression monitoring strategies may therefore allow the routine titration of doses of gene therapy agents for individual patients.

Safety Considerations

Given that gene therapy is a new field of human therapeutic endeavor that is still in its infancy, there are still inadequate data from human clinical studies to properly address the numerous unanswered safety questions that remain. In theory, gene therapy is associated with risks to the patient, to the patient's future offspring, and to the general population. Toxicities to the patient may be caused either by the gene therapy vector or by its encoded gene product. For example, administration of the vector may result in anaphylaxis, inflammation, or infection, particularly if the stock is contaminated with a replication-competent version of the virus from which the gene therapy vector was derived. Direct liver toxicity was the cause of a widely publicized gene therapy fatality 3 years ago caused by direct administration of an adenoviral vector into the hepatic artery of an 18-year-old boy suffering from ornithine transcarbamylase deficiency. This patient rapidly developed liver failure after infusion of a very high dose of the vector, but the pathogenesis was never fully elucidated.[110,111] Possible contributing factors include an inflammatory reaction to the virus particles,

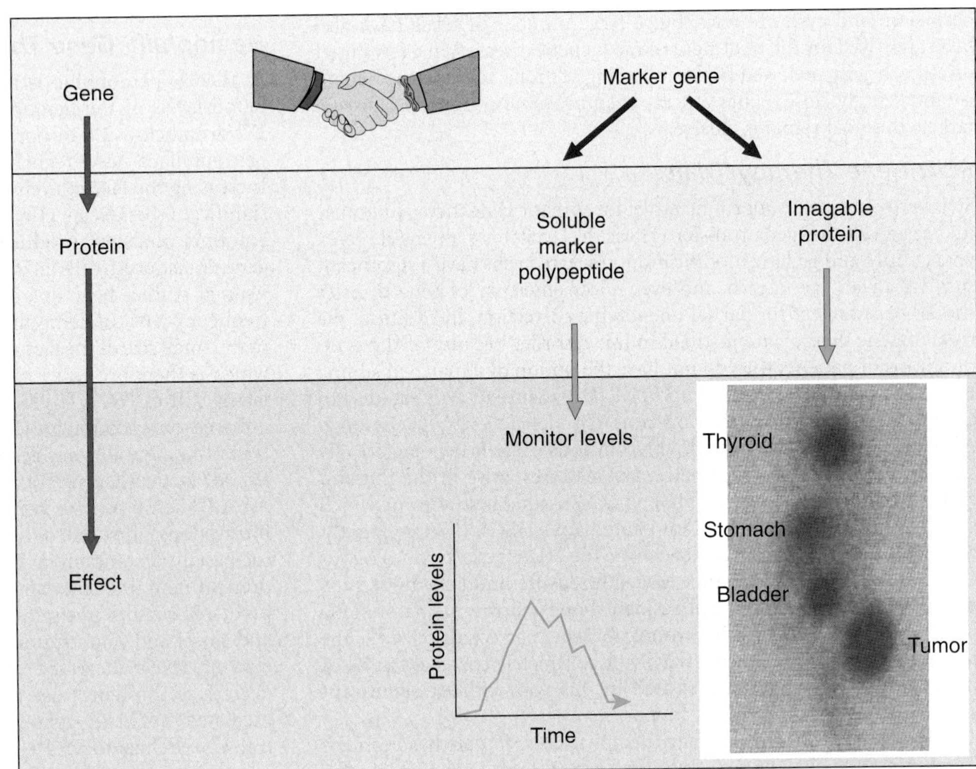

FIGURE 93-7 • Noninvasive expression monitoring strategies. The therapeutic gene is linked to a marker gene such that it is expressed concordantly. The marker peptide is then monitored by direct measurement or imaging, providing a surrogate measurement for therapeutic gene expression (see text for details).

an inflammatory reaction to the virus-infected cells, and inability to tolerate a liver insult due to the underlying ornithine transcarbamylase deficiency. There have been no instances to date of human toxicities due to contamination of vector stocks with replication-competent viruses. Indeed, all gene therapy regulatory agencies have taken great pains to ensure that the manufacture and testing of gene therapy products are conducted in such a way as to reduce this risk to very low levels.

Certain gene therapy approaches are associated with a finite risk of cancer, due either to insertional mutagenesis or to expression of an oncogenic protein. Insertional mutagenesis is a particular risk associated with the use of retroviral or lentiviral vectors, which integrate at random into the host-cell chromosome and can therefore disrupt a tumor suppressor gene, or activate expression of an oncogene. Indeed, 2 of 11 children recently developed T-cell malignancies after they received gene therapy for severe combined immunodeficiency (SCID) due to common γ chain deficiency.[112-114] The protocol involved ex vivo retroviral transduction and subsequent reinfusion of autologous bone marrow, and in both cases the retroviral insertion site in the malignant clone was adjacent to *LMO2*, an oncogene known to be implicated in T-cell malignancies. In addition to insertional mutagenesis, there are theoretical concerns that certain transgene products might stimulate cell proliferation in an autocrine or paracrine fashion, thereby leading ultimately to cell transformation. For example, when cytokine genes, such as IL-2 are used to drive the activation and proliferation of tumor-reactive T lymphocytes, there is an associated risk that inadvertent transduction of the T cells could result in uncontrolled autocrine growth. However, this has not been observed in preclinical or clinical studies in which a wide range of different cytokines have been used. Protein products that promote angiogenesis, such as VEGF and FGF, are associated with a theoretical risk of tumor growth promotion by stimulating the development of tumor neovessels. Patients enrolled into proangiogenic gene therapy protocols are therefore being monitored closely for the appearance of new malignancies.

The theoretical concern of inadvertent germline gene transfer is routinely addressed in the preclinical studies that are conducted in support of new gene therapy protocols. While the transgene may often be detected by polymerase chain reaction in gonadal tissues of experimental animals, there has been no documented case in which this has resulted in genetic modification of the germline. In fact, efforts to use gene transfer vectors with the intent of modifying the germline have met with very limited success, achievable only by isolation and direct inoculation of vector into the germ cells. In human clinical trials, there has to date been no evidence of germline transduction by gene therapy vectors. However, in a recent study in which AAV vectors coding for human factor IX were administered to patients with severe hemophilia B, semen samples from one of the patients tested strongly positive for the vector sequences by polymerase chain reaction.[115] In contrast to germ cells, embryonic tissue can be transduced by gene therapy vectors, so gene therapy should generally be avoided during pregnancy.

Risks to the population must be evaluated when replicating viral vectors are used for therapy, and also when there is a risk that a viral vector stock may be contaminated with replication-competent viruses generated by recombination between vector and helper constructs during a manufacturing process. To avoid the possibility of introducing a transmissible viral pathogen into the patient, or worse still of creating a new viral pathogen, human gene therapy studies are stringently regulated, and the FDA pays particular attention to the manufacturing process, product characterization, and toxicology testing of new viral vectors.[116]

Clinical Status and Prospects

The first human gene transfer experiment was performed in 1989 when a patient with malignant melanoma received genetically modified autologous T cells.[117] Shortly thereafter the first human gene therapy study was performed in which a child with adenosine deaminase (ADA)–deficient SCID was treated the autologous T cells genetically modified to express the ADA gene.[118] Since that time, more than 1200 human gene therapy protocols have been approved, and over 4000 patients have received gene therapy. A comprehensive updated listing of clinical gene therapy trials can be found at the open access website of the *Journal of Gene Medicine* (*http://www.wiley.co.uk/genmed/clinical/*). The diseases most often treated are cancer, vascular occlusion, and cystic fibrosis, but a large number of trials have also been approved for the treatment of rare genetic diseases. In a few target diseases, briefly reviewed in the following sections, therapeutic benefit is tantalizingly close or has already been proven, but for most disease targets this goal remains elusive.

SCID Gene Therapy Trials

SCID provides a very appealing target for somatic gene therapy because the target cells for gene transfer (HSCs or T cells) are amenable to ex vivo culture and genetic modification, corrected cells have a significant survival advantage in vivo, and even a low efficiency of gene transfer should be sufficient for partial phenotypic correction. In addition, the risks of gene therapy are justified in this disorder because of the poor prognosis of patients who do not have the option of a matched sibling HSC transplant. The first group of SCID patients to be treated with gene therapy were those suffering from ADA deficiency.[119] The first two ADA-deficient patients treated with infusions of their own genetically corrected lymphocytes both had a favorable response to the therapy, and promising results were obtained in subsequent studies in which the ADA gene was transferred into autologous HSCs.[119] Subsequently, retroviral vectors were used to deliver the ADA gene to autologous $CD34^+$ bone marrow cells that were reinfused after mild chemotherapy had been administered to kill resident bone marrow hematopoietic progenitors, thereby making room for the corrected cells.[120] The immunodeficiency has been partially or completely corrected in all of the nine patients who were treated in this way without significant short- or long-term toxicities.[121]

Perhaps the most notable gene therapy success to date has been the treatment of X-linked SCID due to mutation in the gene coding for the common γ chain, a component of the cellular receptors for IL-2, IL-4, IL-7, and IL-15.[113,114] $CD34^+$ bone marrow cells from boys with X-linked SCID were transduced ex vivo with a defective retroviral vector coding for the common γ chain and the transduced cells were reinfused without myeloablation. Two independent studies with very similar design were initiated for the treatment of X-linked SCID; the first, in 1999, was opened in Paris and the second a few years later in London.[122] Of the first 20 patients enrolled in these SCID-X1 studies, 17 were successfully treated, achieving complete or partial immune reconstitution.[121] However, three of the patients treated in the French trial subsequently developed clonal T-cell malignancies, in two cases characterized by retroviral insertion adjacent to the *LMO2* gene.[123] All three patients received therapy for their T-cell malignancies, but one patient died.[124] These data from SCID gene therapy studies effectively prove that gene therapy is an effective approach for the treatment of this otherwise fatal disease. However, improvements in vector design are required to combat the problem of insertional leukemogenesis. Lentiviral vectors are highly promising in this regard.

Suicide Gene Therapy for Adoptively Transferred T Cells

TK gene transfer has been extensively studied as a means to render transduced cells susceptible to elimination by treatment with the prodrug ganciclovir. Ganciclovir is monophosphorylated by TK, and its triphosphate form is later incorporated into replicating DNA, where it acts as a chain terminator. Retroviral TK gene transfer (suicide gene therapy) was originally used for the treatment of malignant glioma but did not show useful clinical activity when administered (in conjunction with ganciclovir therapy) in a large Phase III multicenter clinical trial. However, retroviral TK gene transfer was successfully used in recipients of allogeneic bone marrow transplants who had recurrent malignancies.[125] Eight patients relapsing after their allogeneic procedure were treated with TK gene–transduced donor T cells. Five of the patients had a favorable response to therapy, and three subsequently developed graft-versus-host disease, at which point ganciclovir was administered to eliminate TK-positive donor lymphocytes. All three ganciclovir-treated patients had a favorable response to this intervention. With the increasing popularity of mini-allogeneic transplants and donor lymphocyte infusions, this suicide gene transfer strategy is of considerable importance.

Hemophilia Gene Therapy

In theory, hemophilia is an ideal target disease for gene therapy. If blood levels of the hemophilia clotting factors (factor VIII or factor IX) drop below 2% of normal, the bleeding tendency is severe. Severe hemophiliacs need regular intravenous factor replacement therapy. Increasing the factor levels to as little as 5% of normal can have a very significant beneficial effect on the bleeding tendency. Thus, small amounts of factor produced and secreted into the bloodstream by gene-transduced cells at any site in the body should be beneficial. Animal studies bear this out. Factor IX deficiency, despite its lower frequency (10% of hemophiliacs), has attracted more attention because of the small size of the factor IX complementary DNA (cDNA) (1.4 kb), which is therefore easily inserted into AAV and lentiviral vectors. The factor VIII cDNA is larger than 10 kb.

Based on encouraging preclinical data in which long-term correction of hemophilia was achieved in dog and mouse models, a clinical trial of factor IX gene transfer was initiated in severe hemophiliacs.[98] An AAV serotype 2 vector coding for factor IX was administered by intravenous infusion to a total of seven patients. The factor IX level increased substantially in one patient but then rapidly declined to its pretreatment level after about 4 weeks. This decline was a surprise, not predicted by the preclinical studies that had been conducted in dogs and mice, and investigators are still puzzled as to the etiology. Liver enzyme levels increased at the same time as the factor IX levels decreased, implying that there was destruction (probably immune-mediated) of the gene-transduced hepatocytes. How the AAV-transduced hepatocytes could have provoked an immune response remains uncertain, but there is optimism that the AAV vector will be more efficacious when administered concomitantly with immunosuppressive drugs.

Adp53 for Cancer Gene Therapy

Gendicine is a recombinant human serotype 5 adenovirus in which the E1 region is replaced by a human wild-type p53 expression cassette, driven by a Rous sarcoma virus promoter with a bovine growth hormone poly(A) tail. After favorable Phase I testing in patients with advanced head and neck squamous cell carcinoma, a multicenter randomized Phase II/III trial of radiotherapy versus radiotherapy with Gendicine gene therapy, administered by intratumoral injection, was begun; 85% of the patients had nasopharyngeal carcinoma.[126] Radiotherapy (70 Gy) was administered in 35 fractions over 7 to 8 weeks. Gendicine was administered weekly by intratumoral injection, 3 days prior to radiation therapy at a dose of 10^{12} virus particles to a total of eight doses. Of 135 patients that received the Adp53 therapy, 64% showed complete tumor regression with a total response rate of 93%. In the patients treated with single-agent radiotherapy, complete responses were seen in only 19%, with a total response rate of 79%. These differences were statistically significant and provided the basis for marketing approval for Gendicine in China, which was granted in 2003, making this drug the first gene therapy product to gain marketing approval anywhere in the world. Unfortunately no data were collected on the durability of response, nor on the overall duration of survival. For this reason, the data from this pivotal registration trial could not be used to gain FDA approval to market Gendicine in other countries outside of China.

Proangiogenic Gene Therapy

Gene therapy has been used to promote the growth of new blood vessels in ischemic limbs and in ischemic cardiac tissue.[127] Genes coding for VEGF and FGF have been most extensively studied in this regard. Plasmid or adenovirus-mediated transfer of either of these genes has resulted in very encouraging clinical responses in uncontrolled Phase I and II studies, but these results have not been borne out in controlled clinical trials where the placebo group typically also shows significant therapeutic benefit. Perhaps the most notable proangiogenic gene therapy study was conducted using a recombinant serotype 5 adenoviral vector coding for FGF-4. After showing significant clinical activity in Phase I and II studies when administered into the

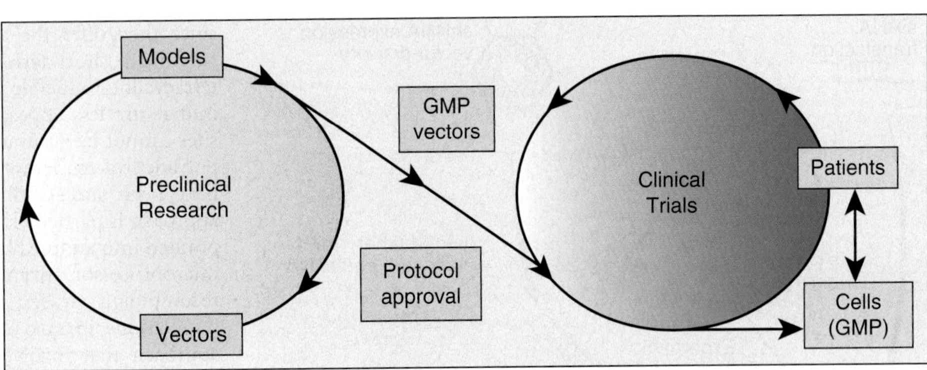

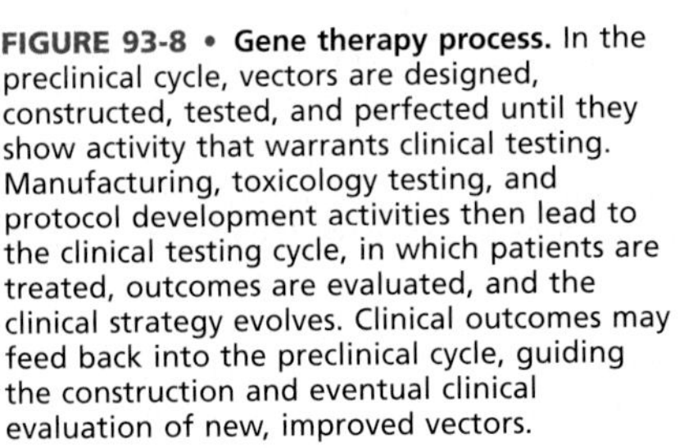
FIGURE 93-8 • Gene therapy process. In the preclinical cycle, vectors are designed, constructed, tested, and perfected until they show activity that warrants clinical testing. Manufacturing, toxicology testing, and protocol development activities then lead to the clinical testing cycle, in which patients are treated, outcomes are evaluated, and the clinical strategy evolves. Clinical outcomes may feed back into the preclinical cycle, guiding the construction and eventual clinical evaluation of new, improved vectors.

coronary arteries of patients with ischemic heart disease, the virus was tested in a large, multicenter, double-blind Phase III trial in the United States, but the trial was prematurely terminated after accrual of 416 patients because of failure to achieve the primary end point (reviewed by Rissanen and Yla-Herttuala[127]). A similar Phase III trial was conducted in Europe and showed no significant effect on exercise tolerance at 12 weeks in 116 patients (reviewed by Rissanen and Yla-Herttuala[127]). These disappointing results underscore the strong placebo effect that exists in many cardiovascular conditions and that represents a very significant confounding factor for the validation of gene therapy interventions in this setting.

In addition to the examples just discussed, many other examples of human gene therapy studies have generated encouraging clinical anecdotes. However, to date there have been no conclusive Phase III studies outside China demonstrating the efficacy of gene therapy products, and the poor performance of currently available vectors continues to be a major limiting factor in gene therapy. Current research is therefore focused on developing high-titer, targetable, regulatable, injectable vector systems that will permit highly efficient and accurate transfer of genes to target tissues in vivo. To accommodate the steady stream of new improved vectors, the process of gene therapy research must incorporate iterative cycles of preclinical development and clinical testing (Fig. 93-8).

GENE SUPPRESSION

Noncoding Nucleic Acids as Drugs

Because they are based on sequence recognition, nucleic acid–based antisense or anti-gene therapies have potentially exquisite specificity for a single targeted gene. Several approaches have been developed during the past 20 to 30 years, of which the best known and most extensively studied are antisense oligodeoxynucleotides (AS ODNs), ribozymes, and short interfering RNA (siRNA).[128]

Mechanism of Action

AS ODNs are single-stranded chains of deoxyribonucleotides (i.e., DNA) or derivatives typically comprising 18 to 25 bases.[129] They are designed to hybridize with a specific target mRNA sequence such that they can form an RNA-DNA hybrid with the targeted RNA and thereby interfere with its function or accelerate its destruction. Functional impairment is mediated through inhibition of splicing, transport, or translation of the targeted mRNA. However, the most important mechanism is through endogenous RNAse H, which recognizes the mRNA-oligonucleotide duplex and cleaves the mRNA strand, leaving the AS ODN intact to bind another target RNA. In addition to the antisense-mediated inhibition of gene expression, AS ODNs have non–antisense-mediated biologic effects.[130] Most important is the immunostimulatory activity of unmethylated CG dinucleotides. These so-called CpG motifs are recognized by TLR9, a Toll-like receptor expressed on B cells and dendritic cells, thereby triggering protective immune responses that may augment the therapeutic activity of a given AS ODN, particularly for the treatment of cancer or infectious disease.

Ribozymes are self-cleaving RNA molecules.[131,132] The hammerhead ribozyme has a catalytic RNA-digesting core that is flanked by two guide sequences whose function is to hybridize the ribozyme to its RNA target prior to cleavage. A typical ribozyme consists of approximately 30 ribonucleotides, 11 to 15 of which form the catalytic core while the remainder mediate the targeted hybridization reaction. Long guide sequences give high target specificity. Short guide sequences (6 to 10 nucleotides) give reduced RNA-targeting fidelity but more rapid turnover due to faster dissociation from cleaved RNAs. Cleavage occurs preferentially at GUC, GUA, GUU, CUC, or UUC sites in the target RNA.[128]

RNAi is a natural phenomenon of RNA-mediated gene silencing that is highly conserved among multicellular organisms.[131,133] siRNAs are formed from double-stranded RNAs by the action of a cytoplasmic cellular enzyme (Dicer) that cleaves the RNA into shorter segments of approximately 21 nucleotides in length, annealed to form a double-stranded segment of 19 nucleotides with two 3′ overhanging nucleotides at either end (Fig. 93-9). These siRNAs are then dissociated into single-stranded fragments that are incorporated into the RNA-induced silencing complex (RISC). The RISC thereby acquires the ability to hybridize to target mRNAs complementary to either strand of the original siRNA. After RISC hybridization, the target mRNA is inactivated, either through catalytic destruction by the slicer activity of RISC, requiring perfect siRNA complementarity, or by inhibition of translation when the siRNA and its target mRNA sequence are imperfectly matched. MicroRNAs (miRNAs) are the endogenous substrates for the RNAi machinery. Recent studies have shown that mammalian cells routinely manufacture a wide variety of miRNAs many of which are restricted in their expression to specific host tissues or cell types.[134] It turns out that these cellular miRNAs are very important regulators of cellular gene expression, able to interfere with translation or to accelerate the degradation of multiple complementary cellular RNAs. miRNAs are initially expressed as long primary transcripts (primiRNAs) that are processed in the nucleus by a multiprocessor complex containing Drosha and DGCR8 to generate hairpins of 60 to 70 bp that are transported via exportin-5 to the cytoplasm, where they are further processed by the RNAse III Dicer and loaded into the RISC.

Appreciation of this natural phenomenon of RNAi has provided the basis for novel RNAi-based approaches to therapeutic gene suppression in which siRNAs are delivered directly to the cell cytoplasm or expressed from DNA constructs.[135]

Delivery Strategies

AS ODNs are large negatively charged molecules that do not efficiently pass through the cytoplasmic membranes of mammalian target cells.[130] They are taken into cells predominantly by endocytosis, but only a limited proportion can escape from the endosome and bind to their target mRNA. AS ODNs are also highly susceptible to nucleases. Various chemical modifications have been tested to improve their resistance to nucleases without compromising their ability to bind to their cRNA and induce RNAse H functions. Numerous modifications have been tested, but to date the most widely adopted species have been the phosphothiorate ODNs, which have a backbone modification

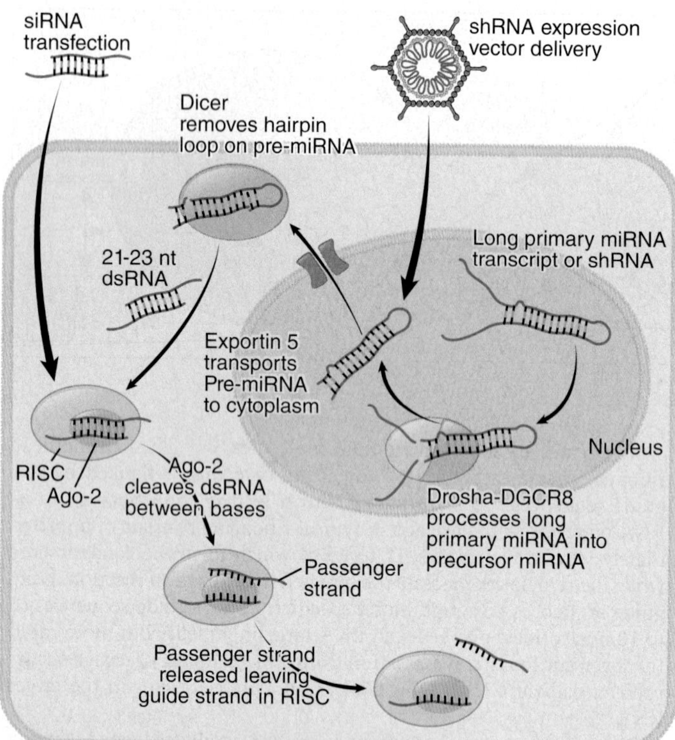

FIGURE 93-9 • RNA interference (RNAi) strategy using nonviral or viral delivery of plasmid encoding short hairpin RNA (shRNA) or transfection of small interfering RNA (siRNA) into the target cell (see text for details).

whereby the oxygen atom of the phosphate linkage is replaced by sulfur. Phosphothiorate ODNs have very short tissue half-lives and therefore have to be administered by continuous or frequent intravenous infusion. Numerous chemically modified ODNs have been generated to address this and other problems, and these novel species are currently undergoing in vivo testing.

As for other antisense therapeutics, the major bottleneck in the development of siRNA (and ribozyme) therapies is their in vivo delivery to the desired target cells.[135] Two very different delivery approaches are currently pursued. In the first approach, synthetic siRNAs are delivered as 21-base RNA duplexes to the cytoplasm of target cells, where they transiently knock down the expression of cellular genes whose mRNA is complementary to the siRNA sequence. Because of their negative charge and size, chemically synthesized siRNAs do not readily cross the cell membrane. They are therefore generally delivered using cationic liposome– or cationic polymer–based strategies, but these approaches are relatively cumbersome for in vivo delivery because of rapid liver clearance and lack of target tissue specificity. Entry is predominantly via the endosomal pathway but, as for AS ODNs, endosomal escape is not efficient. Various novel siRNA delivery formulations are currently under study, including cholesterol-siRNA conjugates, nanoparticles, and aptamer-siRNA conjugates. However, in vivo delivery remains inaccurate and inefficient and the effects are transient. Longer term knockdown of gene expression requires that the cells be repeatedly or continuously exposed to the synthetic siRNA.

In the second approach, siRNA is delivered as a DNA construct that is transcribed in the nucleus to produce a short hairpin RNA (shRNA), which is processed and transported by the cellular miRNA machinery. In this case gene expression is knocked down for as long as the transduced cell expresses the shRNA transgene. shRNAs can be expressed from plasmid DNA or from viral vectors, including adenoviral, AAV, retroviral, and lentiviral vectors. By using retroviral or lentiviral vectors coding for shRNAs, it is possible to generate cell clones with stable suppression of a targeted transgene. Hairpins are typically encoded as separate sense and antisense 21mers, separated by a short 4- to 10-base loop. Pol III promoters are preferred for shRNA expression constructs since they offer the advantage of a predictable transcription start site and a short termination signal (a stretch of 4 to 6 Us). Also, tetracycline-inducible pol III promoters are now available. Pol II promoters are less appealing because the transcriptional start and stop sites cannot be accurately predicted, and the transcript is capped and polyadenlyated. However, despite these difficulties, several shRNAs have been successfully expressed from pol II promoters, and the approach is particularly successful when the siRNA sequence is incorporated into an miRNA scaffold for processing by the nuclear miRNA microprocessor enzyme complex. Whether encoded by plasmids or recombinant viruses, the delivery of shRNAs to specific target cell populations in vivo is problematic. Hydrodynamic injection is an approach that involves intravascular injection of a relatively large volume of physiologic buffer containing the active agent.[136] Plasmids coding for anti-HBV shRNAs have been successfully delivered to the liver by hydrodynamic tail vein injection, but this method is not clinically applicable because of the attendant risk of fluid overload.[137] Viral vectors may offer greater potential for targeted in vivo delivery, but this technology is still under development (see previous section on gene addition).

Pharmacokinetics and Pharmacodynamics

Barriers to Delivery

As discussed previously, a major limitation to the successful therapeutic deployment of antisense therapeutics has been the inadequacy of currently available strategies to deliver them to sites of action in vivo. Because of their short in vivo half-life, and the rapid reaccumulation of target RNA after discontinuation of therapy, AS ODNs are ideally administered by continuous infusion over a prolonged time period. Numerous clinical trials (Phase I, II, and III) using phosphothiorate ODNs directed against various cancer targets have been completed using precisely this delivery approach (reviewed by Tamm[130]). Meanwhile, various chemical modifications are being explored in an attempt to generate AS ODN therapeutics with considerably longer in vivo half-lives, but there has been little real progress in this area to date. Alternatively, when AS ODNs are used as local therapy—for example, in the treatment of CMV retinitis (discussed later)—they can be administered by daily injection into the vitreous humor of the affected eye.

As with ODNs and ribozymes, the major impediment to successful therapeutic deployment of siRNAs is also systemic delivery via the bloodstream. Plasmid and viral vectors coding for shRNAs have been used to target RNAi expression in the livers of experimental animals, but not yet in humans. In one case this was achieved by hydrodynamic tail vein injection of plasmid DNA, an approach that is not translatable to human studies. However, the alternative approach of intravenous administration of AAV vectors is definitely feasible for human translation. Efficient systemic delivery of siRNA to target tissues other than the liver has not yet been achieved. This is a generic limitation for viral and nonviral gene transfer vectors and is discussed more fully in the earlier section on gene addition therapy.

Barriers to Gene Suppression

Despite their capacity for exquisite sequence-specific targeting, antisense therapeutics (ODNs, ribozymes, and siRNAs) have significant limitations and are associated with a variety of toxicities. Off-target effects can be a significant impediment to the success of AS ODNs, arising when the ODN has significant affinity for nontarget RNAs, or when it is able to interact directly with cellular proteins and interfere with their functions. Direct ODN-protein interactions are not unusual and are mediated most often via charge-charge interactions. Because of their nucleic acid nature, the ODNs carry quite strong negative charge. An additional issue for the successful design of ODNs is the accessibility of their target sequence. Secondary stem-loop structures in the target RNA sequence or cellular proteins interacting with the RNA target can greatly impede the binding of a sequence-specific

ODN. However, provided these pitfalls are recognized and taken into consideration, antisense ODNs with high potency and specificity against selected mRNAs can be designed. In addition to their use as antisense therapeutics, ODNs can be designed to suppress gene function through different mechanisms, such as the sequestration of cellular transcription factors by decoy ODNs or the suppression of gene transcription by ODNs that bind directly to their target gene, forming a triple DNA helix in the nucleus. However, antisense approaches are currently better developed and more effective. Aside from off-target effects, toxicity may result from the immunostimulatory activity of unmethylated CpG motifs, which may trigger inflammatory responses when AS ODNs are delivered, for example, to the lungs by inhalation.[138]

The major limitations of siRNA therapeutics are (i) their ability to interfere with endogenous cellular miRNA processing machinery, (ii) stimulation of innate immune responses, and (iii) suppression of non-target RNAs. Interference with endogenous cellular miRNA processing machinery arises because shRNA and siRNA therapeutics resemble miRNA precursors before and after Dicer processing. Severe liver damage was recently encountered in mice after in vivo delivery of AAV-encoded shRNAs to the liver.[139] The therapeutic shRNAs were thought to be saturating the nuclear export machinery for miRNA precursors and, in support of this explanation, the toxicity could be ameliorated by coexpression of Exportin 5. It therefore seems prudent to use vectors that drive intermediate, rather than very high, levels of shRNA expression. Regarding the innate immune response to siRNA therapeutics, it is well known that longer stretches of double-stranded RNA can activate certain cellular Toll-like receptors, protein kinase R, or 2′,5′-oligoadenylate synthase, leading to interferon secretion, translational shutdown, or apoptosis. While it has been shown that shorter double-stranded RNAs of less than 30 nucleotides are only weak stimulators of innate immunity, this generalization is not absolute, and it is clear that certain siRNAs may contain short GU-rich sequence motifs that strongly stimulate TLR7 signaling, invoking interferon responses in cultured cells.

As with ODNs and ribozymes, off-target effects can be a significant impediment when working with siRNAs because they are negatively charged and therefore "sticky." Also, certain target sequences need to be avoided, such as those that form RNA stem-loop structures or those that are targeted by cellular RNA binding proteins. Off-target effects are further compounded by the fact that siRNAs are rather short, and imperfect complementarity is sufficient to block translation of a targeted mRNA. Suppression of nontarget RNAs has been clearly demonstrated by microarray analysis of global gene expression in siRNA-treated cells.[140] The so-called off-targets are typically characterized by having a sequence that perfectly matches nucleotides 2 to 8 in the siRNA (the "seed" region), but this is not sufficient to result in destruction since many mRNAs that contain such a matching sequence are spared from off-targeting. It was reported recently that off-targeting could be reduced without concurrent loss of target silencing by introducing a 2′ O-Me modification at the second base of the siRNA. Another factor contributing to off-targeting is the destruction of RNA targets complementary to the siRNA passenger strand. All siRNAs have two strands, either of which can be loaded into the RISC to direct RNA destruction. Incorporation of the strand with weaker 5′ end pairing energy is usually favored so that siRNAs can be designed intelligently to minimize passenger strand loading into the RISC. Complex thermodynamic modeling programs are available to assist with siRNA design, but it is still usually necessary to test several siRNAs against a single mRNA to find one with reasonable fidelity and potency.[141]

Clinical Status and Prospects

Cytomegalovirus Retinitis

Fomivirsen sodium (Vitravene; Isis Pharmaceuticals, Carlsbad, CA) is an AS ODN that targets the CMV IE2 mRNA. It was approved by the FDA in August 1998 for the local treatment of CMV retinitis in patients with acquired immunodeficiency syndrome (AIDS) who are intolerant of, or have a contraindication to, other treatments for CMV retinitis, or who did not have an adequate response to alternative treatments for CMV retinitis.[132,142] The drug is available as a sterile, preservative-free, bicarbonate-buffered aqueous solution for intravitreous injection. FDA approval was based on several clinical studies.[143] In one key multicenter, prospective, randomized trial, immediate treatment of CMV retinitis with fomivirsen 165 mcg by weekly intravitreous injection was compared with deferral of treatment until disease progression. Eighteen patients were randomized to immediate treatment and 10 to deferred treatment. Median time to first progression was 71 days for the immediate treatment group versus 13 days for the deferral of treatment group ($P = .0001$). The successful development of fomivirsen for CMV retinitis provided great impetus to the pharmaceutical industry to develop AS ODNs for the treatment of cancer and more common viral diseases such as AIDS and hepatitis.

Antisense to Bcl-2 for Cancer Therapy

Genes involved in cell growth, apoptosis, angiogenesis, and metastasis are the main AS ODN targets that are pursued in ongoing clinical trials. Oblimersen is an AS ODN that suppresses *Bcl2*, an antiapoptotic oncogene that has been strongly implicated in the pathogenesis of follicular lymphomas and B-cell chronic lymphocytic leukemia (CLL). Knockdown of Bcl-2 expression has been shown to promote apoptosis or to increase chemosensitivity in a broad spectrum of hematologic and nonhematologic malignancies.[144] Clinical trials of oblimersen therapy have proceeded rapidly, and Phase III trials have been completed in patients with malignant melanoma, B-cell CLL, and multiple myeloma.[130,145] The results of these trials have led to new drug applications to the FDA for approval of the drug as a treatment for CLL and melanoma, but overall, the clinical results have been somewhat disappointing and FDA approvals have not yet been granted (reviewed by Tamm[130]). In the Phase III CLL trial, of 120 patients randomized to receive oblimersen plus chemotherapy, 17% achieved a complete response or nodular partial response compared to only 7% of 121 patients randomized to chemotherapy alone. However, it is too early to say whether oblimersen therapy, which was administered as a 7-day intravenous infusion, repeated at 3-week intervals, led to better overall survival.

A Phase III study comparing chemotherapy with chemotherapy plus oblimersen enrolled 771 patients with stage IV metastatic melanoma or unresectable stage III disease. The overall response rate was 13.5% in the oblimersen group versus 7.5% in the control group ($P = .007$), but the median overall survival was not significantly increased (9 months with oblimersen vs. 7.8 months without). For multiple myeloma, 224 patients were randomized to receive oblimersen with dexamethasone[110] or dexamethasone alone,[114] but the study was negative, showing no significant difference in response rates or time to progression between the two groups. Another large Phase III trial yielded negative data recently when an AS ODN against protein kinase C was tested in combination with chemotherapy in patients with non–small cell lung cancer. While there are several promising cancer-targeting AS ODN therapeutics currently in various stages of preclinical and clinical testing, the lack of success regarding overall survival in large, randomized Phase III trials is somewhat dampening enthusiasm.

Clinical trials of ribozyme therapeutics have not moved as rapidly as for AS ODNs, perhaps because they are larger and therefore less druggable. In one recently completed Phase I study, angiozyme, a ribozyme directed against the proangiogenic receptor VEGFR-1, was administered by daily subcutaneous injection to a total of 31 cancer patients and was well tolerated with satisfactory pharmacokinetic variables.[146]

Numerous preclinical studies have demonstrated gene silencing after local or systemic delivery of siRNA or shRNA in various animal models of human disease. Examples include viral infections (e.g., HBV), ocular disease, disorders of the nervous system (e.g., motor neuron disease), cancer, and inflammatory bowel disease.[147] These studies have utilized siRNA, naked or incorporated in cationic liposomes, as nanosized polymers, or conjugated to cholesterol.[148] To enhance cell targeting properties, ligands such as antibodies and transferrin have been added to the siRNA or nanoparticles.[149,150] Viral vectors such as AAV,[151] lentivirus,[152] and adenovirus[153] have also been used successfully to deliver various shRNAs. In one ingenious approach, an erythroid-specific lentiviral vector coding for human γ-globin was recently adapted for the treatment of sickle cell anemia.[154] Sickle cell anemia is typical of many single gene disorders in that the mutated gene encodes a harmful protein (sickle β-globin) that greatly shortens the life span of affected red blood cells. A sickle β-globin–specific shRNA was therefore inserted into an intron in the γ-globin coding sequence of the lentiviral vector, whereupon transduction of HSCs from patients with sickle cell anemia led to erythroid-specific expression of the γ-globin transgene, and concomitant reduction of endogenous sickle β-globin transcripts. Clinical translation of this siRNA technology is currently in its infancy. Several clinical trials have already been initiated using RNAi-based therapeutics, but these are mainly Phase I studies that have not yet been completed.[155] The full promise of this novel class of therapeutics is therefore yet to be realized.

GENE REPAIR

Autologous, Corrected Cells as Drugs

HR is a natural cellular process whereby genes that have been incorrectly copied during DNA replication are reconstructed and repaired using the original chromosomal sequence as template.[2] In addition, HR is sometimes used to repair chromosomes that have been broken across both strands, although these double-strand breaks are more often fixed by nonhomologous end joining, wherein the ends are just glued back together. In gene therapy, the HR repair process is reversed such that vector-encoded gene sequences are substituted into specific chromosomal locations to repair or disrupt cellular genes.[2] Because of the low efficiency of HR, even when using the most efficient available vectors, its application remains limited to the generation of genetically manipulated stem cells. It is not possible, with currently available technology, to efficiently repair gene defects in target cell populations residing in their natural niches in vivo.

Mechanism of Homologous Recombination

HR is a complex process mediated by a large number of cellular proteins acting in concert to mediate the following steps: (i) sensing of DNA damage and binding to the damaged DNA, (ii) identification of the homologous chromosomal sequence and annealing of the damaged DNA to the chromosome, and (iii) repair of the damaged DNA.[2] The cellular proteins mediating HR have long been the subject of intensive investigations, and many aspects of the process have been elucidated, although understanding of the whole process is still incomplete. For gene therapy, the trick is to design and deliver a construct into the cell that efficiently usurps the HR machinery and modifies the coding sequence at a specific chromosomal locus (gene conversion). Experimental gene conversion efficiencies range from 0.0001% to 1%.[6]

Homologous Recombination Vectors

Numerous parameters have been shown to modulate the efficiency of gene conversion, including the sequence and location of the gene to be targeted, the lengths of homologous sequences flanking the intended modification, the vector used for delivery, and the cell cycle status of the targeted cells.[2] Gene conversion proceeds most efficiently during S phase and is approximately 100-fold more efficient when using AAV as a delivery vehicle compared to other vectors.[156] The reason for the vastly superior performance of recombinant AAVs as gene conversion vectors compared to plasmid DNA, adenoviral, or retroviral vectors is probably due to the fact that they deliver their transgenes as single-stranded DNA flanked by hairpins with free 3′ and 5′ ends—a configuration that effectively mimics the type of DNA damage that is normally recognized and repaired by the HR machinery. However, even with a high-titer AAV stock, an easily targeted transgene, and a rapidly cycling target cell population, gene conversion efficiencies higher than 1% of the target cells have not been reported. Selectable markers can be incorporated into gene targeting vectors to facilitate elimination of target cells that have not been stably modified by the gene-targeting vector. However, detailed analysis of the marker-positive cells after this type of selection shows that gene conversion has occurred in only a small percentage (maybe 1 in 20). In the remainder, the vector has usually been integrated by a nonhomologous mechanism at some other site.

Pharmacokinetics and Pharmacodynamics

Barriers to Delivery

Because of the low efficiency of HR, direct modification of target cells in vivo is not currently a practical proposition. Currently the only feasible approach to using HR for therapeutic benefit is to use HR vectors to modify stem cells in ex vivo culture systems. Correctly modified stem cells can then be selected, amplified, and reimplanted for therapy. For HR, the stem cells must be amenable to long-term ex vivo culture and transduction, followed by selection, amplification, and full genetic characterization of marker-positive clones. Hematopoietic, neural, and many other stem cells cannot be expanded sufficiently ex vivo to be amenable to this type of manipulation. Such limitations do not apply to mouse embryonic stem cells (ESCs), nor to human mesenchymal stem cells (MSCs). HR is therefore used routinely to generate transgenic mice.[157,158] Mouse ESCs are first transfected with an HR construct designed to disrupt or repair a given genetic locus. An ESC subclone carrying the desired genetic modification is selected, amplified, and applied to the inner cell mass of mouse blastocysts, which are then implanted into pseudopregnant mice. The pluripotent ESCs applied to the blastocyst are incorporated into the developing embryos such that some of the progeny animals are "germ-line chimeras" with some of their germ cells derived from the ESCs. The chimeric animals can then be bred to homozygosity for the genetic modification that was originally introduced into the ESC line. The application of HR to human MSCs has only recently been reported and is discussed in the next section.

Clinical Status and Prospects

Mesenchymal Stem Cell Therapy for Osteogenesis Imperfecta

HR is routinely used to produce the ESC clones that are used to generate gene knockout or gene-corrected transgenic mice. In addition, AAV-mediated HR was recently used to disrupt the *COL1A1* gene in MSCs cultured from patients with osteogenesis imperfecta.[12] Gene disruption was achieved through the targeted insertion of a selectable marker (neo) into the *COL1A1* gene, allowing the corrected cells to be selected for resistance to the antibiotic G418 (Fig. 93-10). Analysis of the G418-selected MSC population was reported to reveal that a very high percentage (45%) of these cells had targeted disruption of the mutant *COL1A1* gene. This one report provides hope that HR-modified MSCs may soon prove to be of utility for the treatment of human disease. However, clinical testing has not yet begun.

ONCOLYTIC VIROTHERAPY

Replicating Viruses as Drugs

Viruses are nature's nanomachines that have evolved to be highly efficient at infecting host cells, overcoming the host's innate immunity to allow propagative spread of virus progeny and subsequent transmission to the new hosts. Attenuated replicating strains of several viral pathogens have long been used for vaccination to stimulate protective antiviral immunity against previously common infectious diseases such as smallpox, poliomyelitis, measles, mumps, and rubella. These attenuated viruses have proven to be safe and effective when administered to human subjects by subcutaneous or intramuscular injection, and it can be argued that these were the first FDA-approved gene therapy products. The new emerging application for replicating viruses

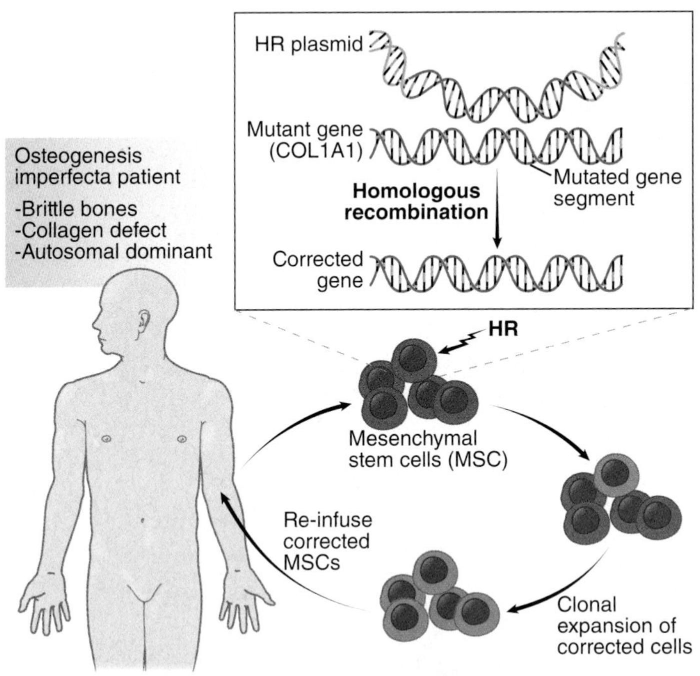

FIGURE 93-10 • Homologous recombination therapy for osteogenesis imperfecta. Homologous recombination (HR) results in replacement of the mutant gene segment *(red)* with the normal gene *(blue)*. In this example, AAV-mediated HR was used to disrupt the *COL1A1* gene in mesenchymal stem cells (MSCs) cultured from patients with osteogenesis imperfecta, and the cells were subsequently reinfused into the patient.

is now to use them as oncolytic agents for cancer therapy. Indeed, this goal has been pursued with variable enthusiasm since the early 1950s.[159]

For use in cancer therapy, the virus should be tumor selective, that is, infecting and inducing cytopathic damage only in tumor cells and not normal cells.[160] Replication-competent viruses that are being developed as anticancer drugs include DNA viruses from diverse families such as adenoviridae,[161] herpesviridae (primarily HSV),[162] parvoviridae (H1 parvovirus),[163] and poxviridae (vaccinia, myxoma),[164,165] as well as RNA viruses from families such as coronaviridae (murine hepatitis virus, feline infectious peritonitis virus),[166,167] orthomyxoviridae (influenza A),[168] paramyxoviridae (mumps, vaccine strain measles virus, Newcastle disease virus),[169-171] piconarviridae (poliovirus, coxsackievirus A21, echovirus EV1, Seneca Valley virus),[172-174] reoviridae,[175] retroviridae (MLV),[176] rhabdoviridae (vesicular stomatitis virus [VSV]),[177,178] and togaviridae (Sindbis virus).[179] Importantly, it was a boost to the field that the first commercially available oncolytic virus, an adenovirus deleted in E1B and E3 to allow tumor-specific replication (H101), was approved by regulatory authorities in China for intratumoral injections in cancer patients in combination with chemotherapy.[180,181]

When used as drugs, viruses must meet stringent criteria for safety and efficacy, and be amenable to pharmacologic study in human subjects. These aspects are discussed in the following sections.

Mechanism of Action (Fig. 93-11)

Viruses use a broad array of cell killing mechanisms and for this reason offer a potentially rich source of novel therapeutic agents likely to retain activity even against tumors that have become resistant to small-molecule anticancer drugs. Cell killing in the context of a virus infection is typically delayed until a fairly late stage in the virus life cycle so that it leads to the release of abundant virus progeny into body fluids, thereby maximizing the probability of efficient virus spread. While cell killing is typically triggered by activation of a limited number of cell signaling cascades (apoptotic, necrotic, or autophagic), the ultimate killing mechanisms vary greatly because cancer cells invaded by different viruses are at very different states of demise when cell death is triggered. Sometimes an oncolytic virus can mediate a process of intercellular fusion such that the initially infected tumor cells become coated with virally encoded fusogenic membrane glycoproteins and are therefore able to fuse with neighboring tumor cells to form large multinucleated syncytia that eventually die by apoptosis. This killing mechanism is employed by oncolytic measles viruses as well as Newcastle disease virus and, more recently, some strains of HSV.

Targeting Mechanism

Specificity for neoplastic tissue is the key to safety. The main aim of targeting is to achieve viral infection and/or gene expression in cancer cells and not in normal nontarget cells. Depending on the virus, targeting mechanisms may include (i) transductional targeting at the preentry level via cancer-associated receptors or proteases; (ii) transcriptional targeting via tissue-specific promoters (DNA viruses only); (iii) translational targeting, wherein the virus is modified such that its propagation is dependent on cellular signaling or interferon response defects in tumor cells versus normal cells; and (iv) proapoptotic targeting, wherein antiapoptotic genes are deleted from the viral genome such that it propagates preferentially in apoptosis-resistant tumor cells.

Transductional Targeting. Virus attachment specificity is determined by specific coat proteins that have evolved for this purpose. Some oncolytic viruses, having evolved to use receptors overexpressed on tumor cells, are tumor selective—for example, attenuated measles virus, which kills high-CD46-expressing cancer cells[182]; poliovirus, which uses CD155[183]; Sindbis virus, which uses the 67-kDa high-affinity laminin receptor[184]; and coxsackievirus A21, which uses ICAM-1 and DAF.[174] Attachment specificity can also be retargeted by engineering new binding domains or protease activation signals into viral coat proteins, or by the use of soluble bifunctional cross-linkers that bind to the viral coat and to a cell surface receptor.[185-187] For oncolytic viruses, genetic modification of the coat protein is preferred to ensure tumor-specific progeny virions. The range of polypeptide ligands that can be incorporated into the viral coat is highly variable between different virus families. Thus the adenovirus fiber that folds in the cytoplasmic compartment cannot tolerate the insertion of complex polypeptides such as single-chain antibodies.[188] Efforts to reengineer adenovirus tropism are therefore restricted by the availability of short peptide ligands recognizing the desired targets.[186] In contrast to nonenveloped viruses, those with a lipid envelope are able to tolerate the insertion of large domains such as growth factors or single-chain antibodies at specific sites in their membrane proteins that fold in the more favorable environment of the endoplasmic reticulum.[84,189] However, at least in the case of retroviral and herpesvirus vectors, targeted attachment to alternative cell surface receptors is not necessarily associated with efficient cell entry.[190,191] In contrast, the measles attachment protein hemagglutinin is highly flexible and has been retargeted to a variety of receptors to mediate highly efficient virus–cell membrane fusion via the F glycoprotein. Growth kinetics, efficiency of receptor-mediated infection, and titers of the recombinant retargeted measles viruses are comparable to the CD46 and SLAM tropic parental virus. Various single-chain antibodies and polypeptides that have successfully been displayed target epidermal growth factor receptor (EGFR), CD38, EGFRvIII, alpha folate receptor, CD20, carcinoembryonic antigen, and $a_v\beta_3$ integrins.[192-198] Protease targeting (activation of virus entry or fusion) using protease-activatable linkers is another option for transductional targeting that was first proven feasible using retroviral vectors.[199]

Transcriptional Targeting. Various tissue-specific promoters have been used to drive expression of viral genes to generate conditionally replicating adenoviruses, retroviruses, and herpesviruses. The approach is applicable only for viruses whose genome is transcribed from double-stranded DNA in the cell nucleus. For adenoviruses, the E1 gene (essential for early transcription) has been placed under the control of tumor-specific promoters/enhancers such as those from genes coding for α-fetoprotein,[200] cyclooxygenase-2,[201,202] prostate-specific antigen or prostate-specific membrane antigen,[203] human telomerase reverse transcriptase,[204] and tyrosinase.[161,205-207] For oncolytic

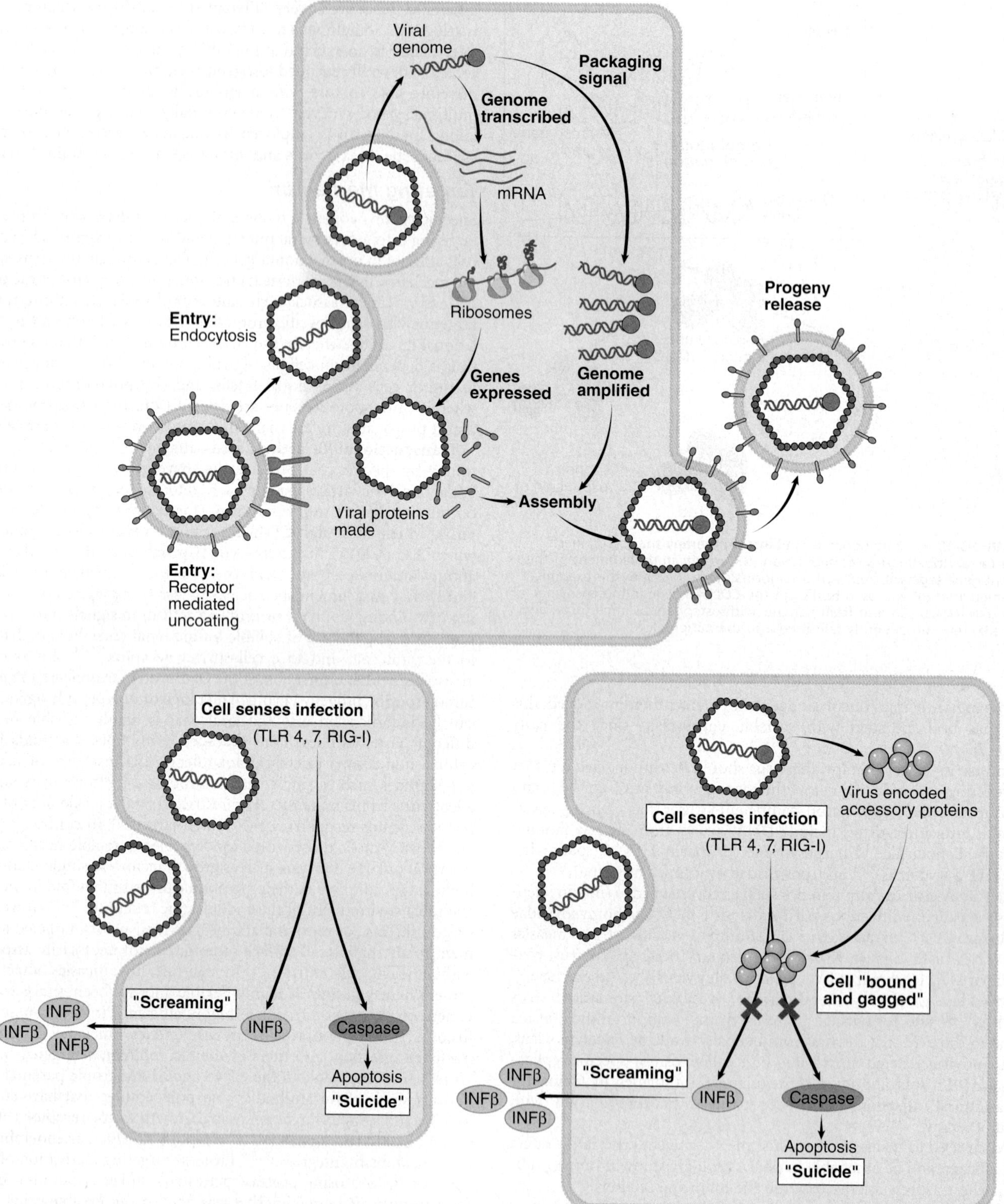

FIGURE 93-11 • A series of schematic representations of the mechanism of action of viruses. A, Viral invasion of the cell. Attachment is the first step in the virus life cycle. Attachment proteins on the surface of the virion interact with specific receptors on the surface of the target cell. Attachment provides the trigger for entry, wherein the viral genome is delivered into the cytoplasm of the target cell. Entry occurs by membrane fusion for enveloped viruses and by endosomal disruption or particle translocation across the target cell membrane for nonenveloped viruses. Once inside the infected cell, viral genomes are transported to specific nuclear or cytoplasmic destinations where they can be expressed and replicated. The viral genome is then copied and amplified, the viral genes are expressed, and the structural proteins assembled to form new virus particles that interact with the packaging signal sequences in the progeny viral genomes to form fully infectious, nucleic acid–carrying progeny virus particles that are released from the cell. Viral genes coding for nonstructural and structural proteins are typically expressed sequentially. The nonstructural proteins, expressed earliest, have several functions. They drive the amplification of the viral genome, induce the expression of the structural (late) proteins, and maintain the viability of the target cell just long enough so that it can make viable progeny viruses. **B**, Cellular response to viral infection and the suppression of this response by viral accessory proteins. The first response of a cell, upon sensing that it has been infected by a virus, is to "scream" by releasing interferon-β (IFN-β). Surrounding uninfected cells respond to the interferon signal by activating their viral defense mechanisms and suppressing their translational machinery so that they become poor substrates to support virus propagation. The second response of the infected cell is to activate its apoptotic program so that it will die before it ever releases progeny viruses. **C**, Virus combating the cellular antiviral response. Not surprisingly, viruses have learned through evolution to suppress both apoptosis and the interferon response by a wide variety of different mechanisms. Infected cells are thereby bound, gagged, and exploited as virus-producing factories.

retroviruses, transcriptional targeting has been achieved by replacing the MLV U3 enhancer/promoter region, for example, with sequences derived from the prostate-specific probasin promoter.[176,208] For oncolytic herpesviruses, transcriptional targeting efforts have focused on transcriptional control of one of the key early genes, gamma 34.1–for example, using an E2F-responsive cellular B-myb promoter[209] or even a synthetic promoter for tissue-specific expression in colorectal carcinoma.[210]

Translational Targeting. This targeting strategy exploits intracellular differences in signal transduction pathways between tumor cells and normal cells—such as defects in interferon [IFN] responses or in Ras, MEK, and Akt activation, or mutations in protein kinase R—that block activation (phosphorylation) of the elongation initiation factor (E1f2a), leading to tumor-selective translation of viral genes and therefore replicative spread of the virus.[211] The IFN response pathway is part of the innate cellular defense against infection by pathogens. Through Toll-like receptors and RIG-I, mda helicases, virus infection stimulates the production and release of IFN-β.[212] Release of IFN-β from the infected cell alerts neighboring cells through binding and activation of their type I IFN-α/β receptors to initiate the IFN signaling cascade that results in paracrine and autocrine production of type I IFNs and IFN-inducible genes, leading to shutdown of protein synthesis and limiting viral spread.

However, viruses have evolved a variety of mechanisms to combat the antiviral response using virally encoded proteins. For example, by inhibiting the transport of cellular mRNA from nucleus to cytoplasm, the VSV-encoded matrix protein (M) is able to block the synthesis and release of active interferons. VSV with a mutated matrix protein (VSV∂51M) is no longer able to combat the release of IFN by normal cells but can still replicate efficiently in tumor cells because their IFN responses are already defective.[177] Similarly, an engineered VSV expressing human or murine IFN-β has a higher selectivity index compared to the parental Indiana strain and has greatly reduced pathogenicity in immune-deficient mice.[213] Both of these recombinant VSVs retain their potent antitumor activity. Other translational targeting mechanisms include restricting expression of picornavirus (e.g., poliovirus) genes by using a tissue-specific internal ribosomal entry site to achieve tumor-selective replication without concomitant replication in neuronal cells,[214] exploiting activated Akt pathways in the case of myxoma virus,[215] or targeting of Ras-activated pathways by oncolytic reovirus.[216]

Proapoptoic Targeting. In the best known example of this targeting strategy, adenoviruses were rendered tumor selective by mutating or deleting their E1 genes, whose products are essential for virus propagation in normal cells, but not in tumor cells.[161,206] The E1a and E1b gene products prevent, respectively, apoptosis and cell cycle arrest in infected cells by inhibiting p53 or the retinoblastoma gene product, Rb. Normal cells undergo rapid Rb-induced cell cycle arrest and p53-induced apoptosis when infected by an oncolytic adenovirus lacking E1 functions, and the propagation of the virus is thereby aborted. However, in tumor cells where the p53 and Rb proteins are frequently nonfunctional even before infection occurs, the E1-deleted adenovirus can still propagate efficiently without fear of triggering premature apoptosis.[217,218]

Pharmacokinetics and Pharmacodynamics

For efficacy, oncolytic viruses must be capable of penetrating host defenses to access growing tumors, and of propagating sufficiently at the target site to destroy infected tumors before the infection is terminated by the host immune response.

Barriers to Delivery

The cancer patient has many antiviral defense mechanisms that all need to be penetrated or overcome. For example, viruses in the bloodstream can be neutralized by antibodies and complement, bound by receptor-positive nontarget cells, or cleared by phagocytes in liver and spleen.[219] Intravenously administered viruses are therefore eliminated rapidly from the circulation, and this process gets faster after each subsequent exposure because of increasing antiviral immunity. So formidable are the barriers to efficient and accurate vascular delivery of viruses that skepticism has been expressed as to whether these agents will ever be exploitable as systemic therapies. However, in opposition to this uninformed negativity, the virotherapy research community is developing a broad range of viable solutions to the intravascular (intravenous or intra-arterial) delivery problem.

Serotype Switching. One approach is to administer a different viral serotype at each successive treatment cycle. For many viruses (e.g., adenovirus, VSV), there are several naturally occurring serotypes that, by definition, are resistant to neutralization by antisera against the other serotypes.[220,221] It is also possible to modify certain viruses by engineering or evolving them so that they are no longer neutralized by antibodies raised against the original virus.[222] The serotype switching approach is less applicable to monotypic viruses such as measles.

Polymer Coating. Polymer coating of viruses is another way to block antibody recognition.[223] Ninety percent of primary amino groups on the surface of adenovirus particles became modified by the polymer when adenoviruses were mixed with PHPMA bearing reactive 4-nitrophenyl (ONp) esters on pendent diglycyl side chains. The polymer-coated viruses have extended circulation times in vivo, but this does prevent the virus from binding to its cellular receptors. Infectivity can be restored, at least partially, by incorporating cell targeting ligands into the polymer coating.[224]

Antibody Depletion. An alternative to virus modification is to reduce the concentration of circulating antiviral antibodies in the patient before infusing the virus.[225] This might be achieved by infusion of soluble viral antigens, passing blood through antigen-loaded columns, or immunizing with antiviral antibodies to provoke an anti-idiotypic antibody response that will sequester antiviral antibodies and prevent them from interacting with infused viral particles. Another approach to reduce the concentration of antiviral antibodies is through the destruction of virus-specific B lymphocytes or antibody-producing plasma cells using steroids, cyclophosphamide, or anti–B-cell antibodies.[226] However, reductions in neutralizing antibody concentration after terminating their production are very slow since the serum half-life of antiviral immunoglobulin (Ig) G is longer than 20 days.[227,228] Plasmapheresis is routinely used in the clinic for depletion of IgM antibodies or immune complexes, but the approach, although straightforward, is relatively ineffective for depletion of circulating IgG.

Antibody Evasion. As an alternative to changing the virus coat or suppressing antibody responses, recent data suggest that it may be possible to hide a virus so that it cannot be seen or bound by antiviral antibodies as it transits the bloodstream to gain access to the tumor cell population.[229] This can be achieved either by using virus-infected cells as carriers to transport the virus to its target cell population[225,230-232] or by delivering the virus genome to target cells as nonimmunogenic infectious nucleic acid.[233] Both of these approaches have the added potential to circumvent phagocytic clearance mechanisms that sequester viruses in the liver and spleen, but they will need to be used in conjunction with effective targeting strategies to minimize transduction of nontarget tissues.

Virus Extravasation. Extravasation of intravenously administered viruses into the parenchyma of a tumor is another important variable that is influenced both by the size of the viral particles (smaller nanoparticles extravasate better)[234] and the permeability of the tumor blood vessels. In mouse xenograft models, and perhaps in some primary and metastatic human cancers, the permeability of blood vessels is greater at the tumor periphery, and oncolytic viruses extravasate more efficiently at that location.[235-237] Vascular permeability can be increased by local expression of vascular permeability factors such as VEGF or by local inflammation secondary to treatment with external beam radiation or chemotherapy.[238] An alternative strategy to enhance viral extravasation from tumor blood vessels is to engineer the viral attachment proteins to bind receptors expressed on tumor blood vessel endothelium.[198,239] Viruses with dual specificity, both for neovessel endothelium and for antigens expressed on tumor cells, will be required to ensure that intratumoral propagation can proceed after the virus has been transported across the endothelial lining of the tumor blood vessels.

Barriers to Spread

One of the major advantages of using a replication-competent virus is its ability to propagate through the tumor, thereby significantly increasing the bystander killing beyond the initial infected cells. However, the stromal elements of the tumor, including fibroblasts, blood vessels, and extracellular matrix, present a physical barrier that can hinder replicative spread. Also, the interstitial fluid pressures of tumors are often high, likely due to increased blood vessel permeability and poor lymphatic drainage. Hyaluronidase and collagenases have been used to pretreat tumors prior to virus administration, and this has led to enhancement of viral spread within the tumor. In another approach, an oncolytic adenovirus expressing the hormone relaxin, which can induce the expression of matrix-degrading proteases, was found to have higher replicative spread within the tumor. Innate cellular immunity and infiltration of the tumor with immune cells such as neutrophils and natural killer cells can also pose an important barrier to viral spread and gene expression.

Depending on the virus, the time from infection to target cell death can range from a few hours to a few days, and the number of progeny released from a single infected cell (burst size) can range from 1 to 100,000. Thus, even in the absence of an immune system, oncolytic viruses spread through tumors at widely differing speeds.[240] In the presence of an immune system, antiviral immunity is the major host factor serving to modulate the speed of intratumoral virus propagation.[241] Most important in this regard is the cellular arm of the immune system, which controls the spread of infection by destroying infected cells before they have a chance to release their viral progeny. Antiviral cytotoxic T lymphocyte responses can be suppressed by immunosuppressive drugs, thereby promoting the intratumoral spread of an oncolytic virus. Cyclophosphamide is a most attractive immunosuppressive drug to use in combination with oncolytic virotherapy since rapidly dividing lymphocytes are exquisitely sensitive to its cytotoxic actions, and it has proven activity as an effective antineoplastic agent that is used extensively in the treatment of human malignancy.[242] Cyclophosphamide is well tolerated, is available at low cost, and strongly inhibits antiviral immune responses, whether primary or anamnestic, B cell or T cell, when administered at the appropriate time and dose following virus exposure.[243-246] Thus cyclophosphamide can greatly increase the efficiency of virus spread from infected tumor cells to adjacent uninfected cells,[247] and it can help to limit increases in the antiviral antibody titer between successive viral doses.

Noninvasive Monitoring

Key pharmacokinetic questions, usually left unanswered in Phase I virotherapy trials, are the following:

- Where do the virus particles go, and how many reach the target site?
- How many target cells get infected, where are they located, and what is their identity?
- Is the viral genome expressed in the infected cells, and if so, at what level and for how long?
- How many progeny viruses are released by infected cells, when, and where do they go?
- How fast and how far does the virus spread, and when is it eliminated from the body?

Answers to these important questions are routinely obtained in preclinical studies by direct analysis of tissue samples harvested from multiple sites at multiple time points, but such analyses are simply not feasible in human trials. To study the pharmacokinetics of oncolytic viruses in a clinical setting, there is a need for convenient, noninvasive monitoring strategies that can be used to quantify the expression level of virus-encoded proteins and to map the distribution of virus-infected cells. Repeat testing should be undertaken in each treated patient to track the spread of the virus and to determine the time course of viral gene expression. Marker genes can be incorporated into the viral genome to facilitate this type of clinical monitoring.

Oncolytic measles viruses coding for the soluble extracellular domain of human carcinoembryonic antigen (MV-CEA) were recently generated to facilitate the noninvasive monitoring of virus propagation in human subjects through serial measurement of serum CEA concentrations.[104,248] A second recombinant oncolytic measles virus (MV-NIS) was then generated coding for the human thyroidal sodium iodide symporter (NIS), a membrane ion channel responsible for transporting iodine into thyroid follicular cells.[249] MV-NIS infected cells concentrate radioactive iodine from the bloodstream, allowing the status of an infection to be monitored by serial noninvasive single-photon emission computed tomography (SPECT) or PET imaging using ^{123}I or ^{124}I as tracers. The two aforementioned recombinant measles viruses are currently being tested in Phase I dose escalation clinical trials at the Mayo Clinic in patients with ovarian cancer (MV-CEA), glioma (MV-CEA), or multiple myeloma (MV-NIS).[82,249-251]

Transgenes coding for certain intracellular enzymes or nonsignaling cell surface receptors can also facilitate imaging. Thus, the HSV TK enzyme can phosphorylate and trap a radioactive FIAU tracer in virus-infected cells such that viruses expressing this transgene can be imaged by PET or SPECT.[252-254] Also, a mutated dopamine-2 receptor, through which dopamine is unable to signal, can trap a PET-labeled ligand tracer at sites of virus propagation.[254,255] These new monitoring strategies are expected to enhance the quality of the pharmacologic information gained from early-stage clinical virotherapy trials, and this will provide a rational basis for intelligent protocol modifications that will hasten the inevitability of clinical success.

Clinical Status and Prospects

Since the turn of the 19th century, when their existence was first recognized, viruses have attracted interest as possible agents of tumor destruction. Early case reports emphasized regression of cancers during naturally acquired virus infections. This led to clinical trials in which body fluids containing various human or animal viruses were used to transmit infections to cancer patients. Results were variable, but in most cases the virus was prematurely arrested by the host immune system and therefore failed to impact tumor growth. Exceptions were seen, most often in immune-suppressed patients, in whom the virus persisted and tumors regressed for a few weeks or months, but this was associated with unacceptable morbidity and mortality due to infection of normal host tissues. With the advent of rodent cancer models and the development of methods for virus propagation, there were many attempts through the 1950s and 1960s to force the evolution of viruses with greater tumor specificity, but this goal remained elusive and many researchers abandoned the field. However, the basic science of virology continued to advance rapidly, and the arrival of recombinant DNA technology ushered in a new era in which it became possible to generate recombinant viruses with engineered genomes.

Because of these advances, there has been a resurgence of interest in oncolytic virotherapy, with numerous Phase I and Phase II clinical trials conducted during the past 15 years using oncolytic representatives of several different virus families. Overall, clinical trials have been carried out with at least 14 different virus constructs from six different virus families, and more than 500 patients have been treated. It is now clear from these studies that most modern oncolytic viruses have a favorable clinical safety profile and, given the right set of circumstances, can sometimes cause partial, or even complete, tumor regressions. However, most of the clinical success is still confined to anecdotal reports of tumor regressions in early-phase (I and II) clinical studies. The notable exception is H101, an oncolytic adenovirus that recently gained marketing approval in China based on favorable Phase III clinical trial data for the first-line treatment of head and neck cancer (see later).

At the current time, anecdotal evidence of antitumor activity has been obtained for all of the oncolytic viruses that have been administered by intratumoral inoculation in clinical trials. As expected, intravascular delivery of oncolytic viruses is overall less effective than intratumoral delivery and is particularly ineffective in the presence of high-titer neutralizing antiviral antibodies. However, anecdotal evidence from Phase I and II trials supports the claim of systemic antitumor activity for vaccinia, mumps, Newcastle disease virus, and certain oncolytic adenoviruses. Convincing tumor regressions have also been reported during the course of natural measles and varicella infections, suggesting that these agents have systemic oncolytic activity in human subjects.

H101 is the E1B-55K gene-deleted oncolytic adenovirus that in 2005 gained marketing approval in China. In support of the license application, a Phase III clinical trial was conducted in which patients with locally advanced head and neck cancers were randomized to chemotherapy alone (5-fluorouracil plus cisplatin or Adriamycin), or chemotherapy plus intratumoral H101 (5 to 15 × 10^{11} virus particles per day for 5 days, repeated every 3 weeks).[256] The response rate for chemotherapy alone was 40.4% (23/57) versus a response rate of 72.7% (48/66) for those treated with chemotherapy plus H101. The main side effects of HB101 treatment were fever, injection site reaction, and influenza-like symptoms. Unfortunately, results for remission duration and overall survival were not adequately collected for this trial, with many of the patients now lost to follow-up, and the data cannot therefore be used to gain marketing approval in the United States.

While the data currently emerging from numerous ongoing Phase I and Phase II clinical trials are highly encouraging, showing that tumor regressions can occur even after systemic virus delivery,[181] it is also clear that significant challenges remain. In particular, the clinical potency of oncolytic viruses will have to be increased if they are to become a truly effective cancer therapy, and it seems likely that their clinical potential will be fully realized only when they can be safely administered to patients receiving concurrent immunosuppressive therapy. To ensure their safe deployment in the setting of antibody depletion and transient immunosuppression, it is anticipated that the oncolytic viruses of the future will have to be not only more potent but also more highly tumor specific than those currently tested, and amenable to noninvasive pharmacologic monitoring.

REFERENCES

1. Russell S. Science, medicine, and the future: gene therapy. BMJ 1997;315:1289-1292.
2. Court DL, Sawitzke JA, Thomason LC. Genetic engineering using homologous recombination. Annu Rev Genet 2002;36:361-388.
3. Yanez RJ, Porter AC. Therapeutic gene targeting. Gene Ther 1998;5:149-159.
4. Freelove AC, Zheng R. The power of ribozyme technologies: the logical way ahead for molecular medicine and gene therapy? Curr Opin Mol Ther 2002;4:419-422.
5. Shuey DJ, McCallus DE, Giordano T. RNAi: gene-silencing in therapeutic intervention. Drug Discov Today 2002;7:1040-1046.
6. Liu L, Parekh-Olmedo H, Kmiec EB. The development and regulation of gene repair. Nat Rev Genet 2003;4:679-689.
7. Margaritis P, High KA. Advances in gene therapy using factor VIIa in hemophilia. Semin Hematol 2006;43(1 Suppl 1):S101-S104.
8. Sadelain M. Recent advances in globin gene transfer for the treatment of beta-thalassemia and sickle cell anemia. Curr Opin Hematol 2006;13:142-148.
9. Goncz KK, Kunzelmann K, Xu Z, Gruenert DC. Targeted replacement of normal and mutant CFTR sequences in human airway epithelial cells using DNA fragments. Hum Mol Genet 1998;7:1913-1919.
10. Wu LC, Sun CW, Ryan TM, et al. Correction of sickle cell disease by homologous recombination in embryonic stem cells. Blood 2006;108:1183-1188.
11. Forlino A, Marini JC. Osteogenesis imperfecta: prospects for molecular therapeutics. Mol Genet Metab 2000;71:225-232.
12. Chamberlain JR, Schwarze U, Wang PR, et al. Gene targeting in stem cells from individuals with osteogenesis imperfecta. Science 2004;303:1198-1201.
13. Ioannou YA, Enriquez A, Benjamin C. Gene therapy for lysosomal storage disorders. Expert Opin Biol Ther 2003;3:789-801.
14. Kennedy MJ. Current status of gene therapy for cystic fibrosis pulmonary disease. Am J Respir Med 2002;1:349-360.
15. Bohl D, Bosch A, Cardona A, et al. Improvement of erythropoiesis in beta-thalassemic mice by continuous erythropoietin delivery from muscle. Blood 2000;95:2793-2798.
16. Roessler BJ, Hartman JW, Vallance DK, et al. Inhibition of interleukin-1-induced effects in synoviocytes transduced with the human IL-1 receptor antagonist cDNA using an adenoviral vector. Hum Gene Ther 1995;6:307-316.
17. Khan TA, Sellke FW, Laham RJ. Gene therapy progress and prospects: therapeutic angiogenesis for limb and myocardial ischemia. Gene Ther 2003;10:285-291.
18. Akerud P, Canals JM, Snyder EY, Arenas E. Neuroprotection through delivery of glial cell line-derived neurotrophic factor by neural stem cells in a mouse model of Parkinson's disease. J Neurosci 2001;21:8108-8118.
19. Sadelain M, Riviere I, Brentjens R. Targeting tumours with genetically enhanced T lymphocytes. Nat Rev Cancer 2003;3:35-45.
20. Maze R, Hanenberg H, Williams DA. Establishing chemoresistance in hematopoietic progenitor cells. Mol Med Today 1997;3:350-358.
21. Alvarez-Vallina L. Genetic approaches for antigen-selective cell therapy. Curr Gene Ther 2001;1:385-397.
22. Fillat C, Carrio M, Cascante A, Sangro B. Suicide gene therapy mediated by the herpes simplex virus thymidine kinase gene/ganciclovir system: fifteen years of application. Curr Gene Ther 2003;3:13-26.
23. Pagliaro LC, Keyhani A, Williams D, et al. Repeated intravesical instillations of an adenoviral vector in patients with locally advanced bladder cancer: a Phase I study of p53 gene therapy. J Clin Oncol 2003;21:2247-2253.
24. Skotzko M, Wu L, Anderson WF, et al. Retroviral vector-mediated gene transfer of antisense cyclin G1 (CYCG1) inhibits proliferation of human osteogenic sarcoma cells. Cancer Res 1995;55:5493-5498.
25. Spitzweg C, Dietz AB, O'Connor MK, et al. In vivo sodium iodide symporter gene therapy of prostate cancer. Gene Ther 2001;8:1524-1531.
26. Bateman A, Bullough F, Murphy S, et al. Fusogenic membrane glycoproteins as a novel class of genes for the local and immune-mediated control of tumor growth. Cancer Res 2000;60:1492-1497.
27. Harrington KJ, Melcher AA, Bateman AR, et al. Cancer gene therapy: Part 2. Candidate transgenes and their clinical development. Clin Oncol (R Coll Radiol) 2002;14:148-169.
28. Sivakumar B, Harry LE, Paleolog EM. Modulating angiogenesis: more vs less. JAMA 2004;292:972-977.
29. Folkman J. Angiogenesis. Annu Rev Med 2006;57:1-18.
30. Ribas A, Timmerman JM, Butterfield LH, Economou JS. Determinant spreading and tumor responses after peptide-based cancer immunotherapy. Trends Immunol 2003;24:58-61.
31. Dermime S, Armstrong A, Hawkins RE, Stern PL. Cancer vaccines and immunotherapy. Br Med Bull 2002;62:149-162.
32. Chong H, Hutchinson G, Hart IR, Vile RG. Expression of B7 co-stimulatory molecules by B16 melanoma results in a natural killer cell-dependent local anti-tumour response, but induces T-cell-dependent systemic immunity only against B7-expressing tumours. Br J Cancer 1998;78:1043-1050.
33. Collins CG, Tangney M, Larkin JO, et al. Local gene therapy of solid tumors with GM-CSF and B7-1 eradicates both treated and distal tumors. Cancer Gene Ther 2006;13:1061-1071.
34. Ino Y, Saeki Y, Fukuhara H, Todo T. Triple combination of oncolytic herpes simplex virus-1 vectors armed with interleukin-12, interleukin-18, or soluble B7-1 results in enhanced antitumor efficacy. Clin Cancer Res 2006;12:643-652.
35. Wu J, Nandamuri KM. Inhibition of hepatitis viral replication by siRNA. Expert Opin Biol Ther 2004;4:1649-1659.
36. Bennasser Y, Yeung ML, Jeang KT. RNAi therapy for HIV infection: principles and practicalities. BioDrugs 2007;21:17-22.
37. Lodish H, Berk A, Zipursky SL, et al. Molecular Cell Biology. New York: W. H. Freeman, 1999.
38. Schertzer JD, Plant DR, Lynch GS. Optimizing plasmid-based gene transfer for investigating skeletal muscle structure and function. Mol Ther 2006;13:795-803.
39. Harrop R, John J, Carroll MW. Recombinant viral vectors: cancer vaccines. Adv Drug Deliv Rev 2006;58:931-947.
40. Herweijer H, Wolff JA. Progress and prospects: naked DNA gene transfer and therapy. Gene Ther 2003;10:453-458.
41. Prud'homme GJ, Glinka Y, Khan AS, Draghia-Akli R. Electroporation-enhanced non-viral gene transfer for the prevention or treatment of immunological, endocrine and neoplastic diseases. Curr Gene Ther 2006;6:243-273.
42. Nishikawa M, Takakura Y, Hashida M. Theoretical considerations involving the pharmacokinetics of plasmid DNA. Adv Drug Deliv Rev 2005;57:675-688.
43. Davidson JM, Eming SA, Dasgupta J. Particle-mediated gene therapy of wounds. Methods Mol Med 2003;78:433-452.
44. Vijayanathan V, Thomas T, Thomas TJ. DNA nanoparticles and development of DNA delivery vehicles for gene therapy. Biochemistry 2002;41:14085-14094.
45. Miller AD. The problem with cationic liposome/micelle-based non-viral vector systems for gene therapy. Curr Med Chem 2003;10:1195-1211.
46. Clark PR, Hersh EM. Cationic lipid-mediated gene transfer: current concepts. Curr Opin Mol Ther 1999;1:158-176.
47. Gehl J. Electroporation: theory and methods, perspectives for drug delivery, gene therapy and research. Acta Physiol Scand 2003;177:437-447.
48. Muramatsu T, Nakamura A, Park HM. In vivo electroporation: a powerful and convenient means of nonviral gene transfer to tissues of living animals [Review]. Int J Mol Med 1998;1:55-62.
49. Newman CM, Lawrie A, Brisken AF, Cumberland DC. Ultrasound gene therapy: on the road from concept to reality. Echocardiography 2001;18:339-347.
50. Miller DL, Pislaru SV, Greenleaf JE. Sonoporation: mechanical DNA delivery by ultrasonic cavitation. Somat Cell Mol Genet 2002;27(1-6):115-134.
51. Sugden B. In the beginning: a viral origin exploits the cell. Trends Biochem Sci 2002;27:1-3.
52. Dobbelstein M. Viruses in therapy—royal road or dead end? Virus Res 2003;92:219-221.
53. Buchschacher GL Jr. Introduction to retroviruses and retroviral vectors. Somat Cell Mol Genet 2001;26(1-6):1-11.
54. Laufs S, Gentner B, Nagy KZ, et al. Retroviral vector integration occurs in preferred genomic targets of human bone marrow-repopulating cells. Blood 2003;101:2191-2198.
55. Kung HJ, Boerkoel C, Carter TH. Retroviral mutagenesis of cellular oncogenes: a review with insights into the mechanisms of insertional activation. Curr Top Microbiol Immunol 1991;171:1-25.

56. Baum C, Kustikova O, Modlich U, et al. Mutagenesis and oncogenesis by chromosomal insertion of gene transfer vectors. Hum Gene Ther 2006;17:253-263.
57. Kafri T. Lentivirus vectors: difficulties and hopes before clinical trials. Curr Opin Mol Ther 2001;3:316-326.
58. Hu J, Dunbar CE. Update on hematopoietic stem cell gene transfer using non-human primate models. Curr Opin Mol Ther 2002;4:482-490.
59. Pannell D, Ellis J. Silencing of gene expression: implications for design of retrovirus vectors. Rev Med Virol 2001;11:205-217.
60. Imperiale MJ, Kochanek S. Adenovirus vectors: biology, design, and production. Curr Top Microbiol Immunol 2004;273:335-357.
61. Brunetti-Pierri N, Ng P. Progress towards the clinical application of helper-dependent adenoviral vectors for liver and lung gene therapy. Curr Opin Mol Ther 2006;8:446-454.
62. Wu JC, Chen IY, Wang Y, et al. Molecular imaging of the kinetics of vascular endothelial growth factor gene expression in ischemic myocardium. Circulation 2004;110:685-691.
63. Brown BD, Shi CX, Powell S, et al. Helper-dependent adenoviral vectors mediate therapeutic factor VIII expression for several months with minimal accompanying toxicity in a canine model of severe hemophilia A. Blood 2004;103:804-810.
64. Gao G, Vandenberghe LH, Wilson JM. New recombinant serotypes of AAV vectors. Curr Gene Ther 2005;5:285-297.
65. Nakai H, Montini E, Fuess S, et al. AAV serotype 2 vectors preferentially integrate into active genes in mice. Nat Genet 2003;34:297-302.
66. Xiao X, Li J, Samulski RJ. Production of high-titer recombinant adeno-associated virus vectors in the absence of helper adenovirus. J Virol 1998;72:2224-2232.
67. Rabinowitz JE, Samulski J. Adeno-associated virus expression systems for gene transfer. Curr Opin Biotechnol 1998;9:470-475.
68. Glorioso JC, Fink DJ. Herpes vector-mediated gene transfer in treatment of diseases of the nervous system. Annu Rev Microbiol 2004;58:253-271.
69. Goins WF, Wolfe D, Krisky DM, et al. Delivery using herpes simplex virus: an overview. Methods Mol Biol 2004;246:257-299.
70. Burton EA, Bai Q, Goins WF, Glorioso JC. Replication-defective genomic herpes simplex vectors: design and production. Curr Opin Biotechnol 2002;13:424-428.
71. Bjorklund A, Lindvall O. Parkinson disease gene therapy moves toward the clinic. Nat Med 2000;6:1207-1208.
72. Kordower JH, Emborg ME, Bloch J, et al. Neurodegeneration prevented by lentiviral vector delivery of GDNF in primate models of Parkinson's disease. Science 2000;290:767-773.
73. Bjorklund A, Kirik D, Rosenblad C, et al. Towards a neuroprotective gene therapy for Parkinson's disease: use of adenovirus, AAV and lentivirus vectors for gene transfer of GDNF to the nigrostriatal system in the rat Parkinson model. Brain Res 2000;886:82-98.
74. Wang L, Muramatsu S, Lu Y, et al. Delayed delivery of AAV-GDNF prevents nigral neurodegeneration and promotes functional recovery in a rat model of Parkinson's disease. Gene Ther 2002;9:381-389.
75. DePolo NJ, Reed JD, Sheridan PL, et al. VSV-G pseudotyped lentiviral vector particles produced in human cells are inactivated by human serum. Mol Ther 2000;2:218-222.
76. Sandrin V, Boson B, Salmon P, et al. Lentiviral vectors pseudotyped with a modified RD114 envelope glycoprotein show increased stability in sera and augmented transduction of primary lymphocytes and CD34+ cells derived from human and nonhuman primates. Blood 2002;100:823-832.
77. Shayakhmetov DM, Gaggar A, Ni S, et al. Adenovirus binding to blood factors results in liver cell infection and hepatotoxicity. J Virol 2005;79:7478-7491.
78. Akiyama M, Thorne S, Kirn D, et al. Ablating CAR and integrin binding in adenovirus vectors reduces nontarget organ transduction and permits sustained bloodstream persistence following intraperitoneal administration. Mol Ther 2004;9:218-230.
79. Chirmule N, Propert K, Magosin S, et al. Immune responses to adenovirus and adeno-associated virus in humans. Gene Ther 1999;6:1574-1583.
80. Gautam A, Waldrep JC, Densmore CL. Aerosol gene therapy. Mol Biotechnol 2003;23:51-60.
81. Rainov NG, Kramm CM. Vector delivery methods and targeting strategies for gene therapy of brain tumors. Curr Gene Ther 2001;1:367-383.
82. Phuong LK, Allen C, Peng KW, et al. Use of a vaccine strain of measles virus genetically engineered to produce carcinoembryonic antigen as a novel therapeutic agent against glioblastoma multiforme. Cancer Res 2003;63:2462-2469.
83. Khurana VG, Weiler DA, Witt TA, et al. A direct mechanical method for accurate and efficient adenoviral vector delivery to tissues. Gene Ther 2003;10:443-452.
84. Peng K-W, Russell S. Viral vector targeting. Curr Opin Biotechnol 1999;10:454-457.
85. Lenz HJ, Anderson WF, Hall FL, Gordon EM. Clinical Protocol: Tumor site specific Phase I evaluation of safety and efficacy of hepatic arterial infusion of a matrix-targeted retroviral vector bearing a dominant negative cyclin G1 construct as intervention for colorectal carcinoma metastatic to liver. Hum Gene Ther 2002;13:1515-1537.
86. Hemminki A, Belousova N, Zinn KR, et al. An adenovirus with enhanced infectivity mediates molecular chemotherapy of ovarian cancer cells and allows imaging of gene expression. Mol Ther 2001;4:223-231.
87. Harrington KJ, Linardakis E, Vile RG. Transcriptional control: an essential component of cancer gene therapy strategies? Adv Drug Deliv Rev 2000;44:167-184.
88. Follenzi A, Sabatino G, Lombardo A, et al. Efficient gene delivery and targeted expression to hepatocytes in vivo by improved lentiviral vectors. Hum Gene Ther 2002;13:243-260.
89. Emiliusen L, Gough M, Bateman A, et al. A transcriptional feedback loop for tissue-specific expression of highly cytotoxic genes which incorporates an immunostimulatory component. Gene Ther 2001;8:987-998.
90. Dingli D, Diaz RM, Bergert ER, et al. Genetically targeted radiotherapy for multiple myeloma. Blood 2003;102:489-496.
91. May C, Rivella S, Callegari J, et al. Therapeutic haemoglobin synthesis in beta-thalassaemic mice expressing lentivirus-encoded human beta-globin. Nature 2000; 406:82-86.
92. May C, Rivella S, Chadburn A, Sadelain M. Successful treatment of murine beta-thalassemia intermedia by transfer of the human beta-globin gene. Blood 2002;99:1902-1908.
93. Rivella S, Sadelain M. Therapeutic globin gene delivery using lentiviral vectors. Curr Opin Mol Ther 2002;4:505-514.
94. Egrie JC, Browne JK. Development and characterization of darbepoetin alfa. Oncology (Williston Park) 2002;16(10 Suppl 11):13-22.
95. Dammacco F, Luccarelli G, Prete M, Silvestris F. The role of recombinant human erythropoietin alpha in the treatment of chronic anemia in multiple myeloma. Rev Clin Exp Hematol 2002;Suppl 1:32-38.
96. Bohl D, Salvetti A, Moullier P, Heard JM. Control of erythropoietin delivery by doxycycline in mice after intramuscular injection of adeno-associated vector. Blood 1998;92:1512-1517.
97. Samakoglu S, Bohl D, Heard JM. Mechanisms leading to sustained reversion of beta-thalassemia in mice by doxycycline-controlled Epo delivery from muscles. Mol Ther 2002;6:793-803.
98. Manno CS, Pierce GF, Arruda VR, et al. Successful transduction of liver in hemophilia by AAV-factor IX and limitations imposed by the host immune response. Nat Med 2006;12:342-347.
99. Mingozzi F, Maus MV, Hui DJ, et al. $CD8^+$ T-cell responses to adeno-associated virus capsid in humans. Nat Med 2007;13:419-422.
100. Liu YL, Mingozzi F, Rodriguez-Colon SM, et al. Therapeutic levels of factor IX expression using a muscle-specific promoter and adeno-associated virus serotype 1 vector. Hum Gene Ther 2004;15:783-792.
101. Koransky ML, Robbins RC, Blau HM. VEGF gene delivery for treatment of ischemic cardiovascular disease. Trends Cardiovasc Med 2002;12:108-114.
102. Losordo DW, Vale PR, Hendel RC, et al. Phase 1/2 placebo-controlled, double-blind, dose-escalating trial of myocardial vascular endothelial growth factor 2 gene transfer by catheter delivery in patients with chronic myocardial ischemia. Circulation 2002;105:2012-2018.
103. Laham RJ, Mannam A, Post MJ, Sellke F. Gene transfer to induce angiogenesis in myocardial and limb ischaemia. Expert Opin Biol Ther 2001;1:985-994.
104. Peng KW, Facteau S, Wegman T, et al. Non-invasive in vivo monitoring of trackable viruses expressing soluble marker peptides. Nat Med 2002;8:527-531.
105. Groot-Wassink T, Aboagye EO, Glaser M, et al. Adenovirus biodistribution and non-invasive imaging of gene expression in vivo by positron emission tomography using human sodium/iodide symporter as reporter gene. Hum Gene Ther 2002;13:1723-1735.
106. Blasberg RG, Tjuvajev JG. Herpes simplex virus thymidine kinase as a marker/reporter gene for PET imaging of gene therapy. Q J Nucl Med 1999;43:163-169.
107. Gambhir S, Bauer E, Black M, et al. A mutant herpes simplex virus type 1 thymidine kinase reporter gene shows improved sensitivity for imaging reporter gene expression with positron emission tomography. Proc Natl Acad Sci U S A 2000;14:2785-2790.
108. Hemminki A, Zinn KR, Liu B, et al. In vivo molecular chemotherapy and noninvasive imaging with an infectivity-enhanced adenovirus. J Natl Cancer Inst 2002;94:741-749.
109. Zinn KR, Chaudhuri TR. The type 2 human somatostatin receptor as a platform for reporter gene imaging. Eur J Nucl Med Mol Imaging 2002;29:388-399.
110. Smith L, Byers JF. Gene therapy in the post-Gelsinger era. JONAS Health Law Ethics Regul 2002;4:104-110.
111. Somia N, Verma IM. Gene therapy: trials and tribulations. Nat Rev Genet 2000;1:91-99.
112. Cavazzana-Calvo M, Hacein-Bey S, de Saint Basile G, et al. Gene therapy of human severe combined immunodeficiency (SCID)-X1 disease. Science 2000;288:669-672.
113. Hacein-Bey-Abina S, Le Deist F, Carlier F, et al. Sustained correction of X-linked severe combined immunodeficiency by ex vivo gene therapy. N Engl J Med 2002;346:1185-1193.
114. Cavazzana-Calvo M, Lagresle C, Hacein-Bey-Abina S, Fischer A. Gene therapy for severe combined immunodeficiency. Annu Rev Med 2005;56:585-602.
115. High KA. Theodore E. Woodward Award: AAV-mediated gene transfer for hemophilia. Trans Am Clin Climatol Assoc 2003;114:337-351; discussion 351-352.
116. Friedmann T, Noguchi P, Mickelson C. The evolution of public review and oversight mechanisms in human gene transfer research: joint roles of the FDA and NIH. Curr Opin Biotechnol 2001;12:304-307.
117. Kasid A, Morecki S, Aebersold P, et al. Human gene transfer: characterization of human tumor-infiltrating lymphocytes as vehicles for retroviral-mediated gene transfer in man. Proc Natl Acad Sci U S A 1990;87:473-477.
118. Blaese RM, Culver KW, Miller AD, et al. T lymphocyte-directed gene therapy for ADA-SCID: initial trial results after 4 years. Science 1995;270:475-480.
119. Blaese RM. Steps toward gene therapy: 1. The initial trials. Hosp Pract (Minneap) 1995;30:33-40.
120. Aiuti A, Slavin S, Aker M, et al. Correction of ADA-SCID by stem cell gene therapy combined with nonmyeloablative conditioning. Science 2002;296:2410-2413.
121. Cavazzana-Calvo M, Fischer A. Gene therapy for severe combined immunodeficiency: are we there yet? J Clin Invest 2007;117:1456-1465.
122. Gaspar HB, Bjorkegren E, Parsley K, et al. Successful reconstitution of immunity in ADA-SCID by stem cell gene therapy following cessation of PEG-ADA and use of mild preconditioning. Mol Ther 2006;14:505-513.
123. Hacein-Bey-Abina S, Von Kalle C, Schmidt M, et al. LMO2-associated clonal T cell proliferation in two patients after gene therapy for SCID-X1. Science 2003;302:415-419.

124. Gansbacher B. Report of a second serious adverse event in a clinical trial of gene therapy for X-linked severe combined immune deficiency (X-SCID): position of the European Society of Gene Therapy (ESGT). J Gene Med 2003;5:261-262.
125. Bonini C, Ferrari G, Verzeletti S, et al. HSV-TK gene transfer into donor lymphocytes for control of allogeneic graft-versus-leukemia. Science 1997;276:1719-1724.
126. Peng Z. Current status of gendicine in China: recombinant human Ad-p53 agent for treatment of cancers. Hum Gene Ther 2005;16:1016-1027.
127. Rissanen TT, Yla-Herttuala S. Current status of cardiovascular gene therapy. Mol Ther 2007;15:1233-1247.
128. Scanlon KJ. Anti-genes: siRNA, ribozymes and antisense. Curr Pharm Biotechnol 2004;5:415-420.
129. Dias N, Stein CA. Antisense oligonucleotides: basic concepts and mechanisms. Mol Cancer Ther 2002;1:347-355.
130. Tamm I. Antisense therapy in malignant diseases: status quo and quo vadis? Clin Sci (Lond) 2006;110:427-442.
131. Tafech A, Bassett T, Sparanese D, Lee CH. Destroying RNA as a therapeutic approach. Curr Med Chem 2006;13:863-881.
132. Scherer LJ, Rossi JJ. Approaches for the sequence-specific knockdown of mRNA. Nat Biotechnol 2003;21:1457-1465.
133. Leung RK, Whittaker PA. RNA interference: from gene silencing to gene-specific therapeutics. Pharmacol Ther 2005;107:222-239.
134. Leung AK, Sharp PA. Function and localization of microRNAs in mammalian cells. Cold Springs Harb Symp Quant Biol 2006;71:29-38.
135. Kumar LD, Clarke AR. Gene manipulation through the use of small interfering RNA (siRNA): from in vitro to in vivo applications. Adv Drug Deliv Rev 2007;59:87-100.
136. Lewis DL, Wolff JA. Systemic siRNA delivery via hydrodynamic intravascular injection. Adv Drug Deliv Rev 2007;59:115-123.
137. Grimm D, Kay MA. Therapeutic short hairpin RNA expression in the liver: viral targets and vectors. Gene Ther 2006;13:563-575.
138. Schwartz DA, Quinn TJ, Thorne PS, et al. CpG motifs in bacterial DNA cause inflammation in the lower respiratory tract. J Clin Invest 1997;100:68-73.
139. Grimm D, Streetz KL, Jopling CL, et al. Fatality in mice due to oversaturation of cellular microRNA/short hairpin RNA pathways. Nature 2006;441:537-541.
140. Jackson AL, Burchard J, Schelter J, et al. Widespread siRNA "off-target" transcript silencing mediated by seed region sequence complementarity. RNA 2006;12:1179-1187.
141. Shabalina SA, Spiridonov AN, Ogurtsov AY. Computational models with thermodynamic and composition features improve siRNA design. BMC Bioinformatics 2006;7:65.
142. Galderisi U, Cipollaro M, Cascino A. Clinical trials of a new class of therapeutic agents: antisense oligonucleotides. Expert Opin Emerg Drugs 2001;6:69-79.
143. Group VS. A randomized controlled clinical trial of intravitreous fomivirsen for treatment of newly diagnosed peripheral cytomegalovirus retinitis in patients with AIDS. Am J Ophthalmol 2002;133:467-474.
144. Kim R, Emi M, Matsuura K, Tanabe K. Antisense and nonantisense effects of antisense Bcl-2 on multiple roles of Bcl-2 as a chemosensitizer in cancer therapy. Cancer Gene Ther 2007;14:1-11.
145. O'Brien S, Moore JO, Boyd TE, et al. Randomized Phase III trial of fludarabine plus cyclophosphamide with or without oblimersen sodium (Bcl-2 antisense) in patients with relapsed or refractory chronic lymphocytic leukemia. J Clin Oncol 2007;25:1114-1120.
146. Weng DE, Masci PA, Radka SF, et al. A Phase I clinical trial of a ribozyme-based angiogenesis inhibitor targeting vascular endothelial growth factor receptor-1 for patients with refractory solid tumors. Mol Cancer Ther 2005;4:948-955.
147. Bumcrot D, Manoharan M, Koteliansky V, Sah DW. RNAi therapeutics: a potential new class of pharmaceutical drugs. Nat Chem Biol 2006;2:711-719.
148. Meyer M, Wagner E. Recent developments in the application of plasmid DNA-based vectors and small interfering RNA therapeutics for cancer. Hum Gene Ther 2006;17:1062-1076.
149. Song E, Zhu P, Lee SK, et al. Antibody mediated in vivo delivery of small interfering RNAs via cell-surface receptors. Nat Biotechnol 2005;23:709-717.
150. Hu-Lieskovan S, Heidel JD, Bartlett DW, et al. Sequence-specific knockdown of EWS-FLI1 by targeted, nonviral delivery of small interfering RNA inhibits tumor growth in a murine model of metastatic Ewing's sarcoma. Cancer Res 2005;65:8984-8992.
151. Tomar RS, Matta H, Chaudhary PM. Use of adeno-associated viral vector for delivery of small interfering RNA. Oncogene 2003;22:5712-5715.
152. Lee SK, Dykxhoorn DM, Kumar P, et al. Lentiviral delivery of short hairpin RNAs protects CD4 T cells from multiple clades and primary isolates of HIV. Blood 2005;106:818-826.
153. Kuninger D, Stauffer D, Eftekhari S, et al. Gene disruption by regulated short interfering RNA expression, using a two-adenovirus system. Hum Gene Ther 2004;15:1287-1292.
154. Samakoglu S, Lisowski L, Budak-Alpdogan T, et al. A genetic strategy to treat sickle cell anemia by coregulating globin transgene expression and RNA interference. Nat Biotechnol 2006;24:89-94.
155. Aagaard L, Rossi JJ. RNAi therapeutics: principles, prospects and challenges. Adv Drug Deliv Rev 2007;59:75-86.
156. Vasileva A, Jessberger R. Precise hit: adeno-associated virus in gene targeting. Nat Rev Microbiol 2005;3:837-847.
157. Misra RP, Duncan SA. Gene targeting in the mouse: advances in introduction of transgenes into the genome by homologous recombination. Endocrine 2002;19:229-238.
158. Ohbayashi F, Balamotis MA, Kishimoto A, et al. Correction of chromosomal mutation and random integration in embryonic stem cells with helper-dependent adenoviral vectors. Proc Natl Acad Sci U S A 2005;102:13628-13633.
159. Kelly E, Russell SJ. History of oncolytic viruses: genesis to genetic engineering. Mol Ther 2007;15:651-659.
160. Russell SJ. Replicating vectors for cancer therapy: a question of strategy. Semin Cancer Biol 1994;5:437-443.
161. Dobbelstein M. Replicating adenoviruses in cancer therapy. Curr Top Microbiol Immunol 2004;273:291-334.
162. Shen Y, Nemunaitis J. Herpes simplex virus 1 (HSV-1) for cancer treatment. Cancer Gene Ther 2006;13:975-992.
163. Geletneky K, Herrero YCM, Rommelaere J, Schlehofer JR. Oncolytic potential of rodent parvoviruses for cancer therapy in humans: a brief review. J Vet Med B Infect Dis Vet Public Health 2005;52:327-330.
164. Thorne SH, Hwang TH, Kirn DH. Vaccinia virus and oncolytic virotherapy of cancer. Curr Opin Mol Ther 2005;7:359-365.
165. Lun X, Yang W, Alain T, et al. Myxoma virus is a novel oncolytic virus with significant antitumor activity against experimental human gliomas. Cancer Res 2005;65:9982-9990.
166. Verheije MH, Wurdinger T, van Beusechem VW, et al. Redirecting coronavirus to a nonnative receptor through a virus-encoded targeting adapter. J Virol 2006;80:1250-1260.
167. Wurdinger T, Verheije MH, Raaben M, et al. Targeting non-human coronaviruses to human cancer cells using a bispecific single-chain antibody. Gene Ther 2005;12:1394-1404.
168. Bergmann M, Romirer I, Sachet M, et al. A genetically engineered influenza A virus with ras-dependent oncolytic properties. Cancer Res 2001;61:8188-8193.
169. Myers R, Greiner S, Harvey M, et al. Oncolytic activities of approved mumps and measles vaccines for therapy of ovarian cancer. Cancer Gene Ther 2005;12:593-599.
170. Asada T. Treatment of human cancer with mumps virus. Cancer 1974;34:1907-1928.
171. Nakamura T, Russell SJ. Oncolytic measles viruses for cancer therapy. Expert Opin Biol Ther 2004;4:1685-1692.
172. Gromeier M, Alexander L, Wimmer E. Internal ribosomal entry site substitution eliminates neurovirulence in intergeneric poliovirus recombinants. Proc Natl Acad Sci U S A 1996;93:2370-2375.
173. Shafren DR, Sylvester D, Johansson ES, et al. Oncolysis of human ovarian cancers by echovirus type 1. Int J Cancer 2005;115:320-328.
174. Au GG, Lincz LF, Enno A, Shafren DR. Oncolytic Coxsackievirus A21 as a novel therapy for multiple myeloma. Br J Haematol 2007;137:133-141.
175. Stoeckel J, Hay JG. Drug evaluation: reolysin—wild-type reovirus as a cancer therapeutic. Curr Opin Mol Ther 2006;8:249-260.
176. Dalba C, Klatzmann D, Logg CR, Kasahara N. Beyond oncolytic virotherapy: replication-competent retrovirus vectors for selective and stable transduction of tumors. Curr Gene Ther 2005;5:655-667.
177. Stojdl DF, Lichty BD, tenOever BR, et al. VSV strains with defects in their ability to shutdown innate immunity are potent systemic anti-cancer agents. Cancer Cell 2003;4:263-275.
178. Obuchi M, Fernandez M, Barber GN. Development of recombinant vesicular stomatitis viruses that exploit defects in host defense to augment specific oncolytic activity. J Virol 2003;77:8843-8856.
179. Unno Y, Shino Y, Kondo F, et al. Oncolytic viral therapy for cervical and ovarian cancer cells by Sindbis virus AR339 strain. Clin Cancer Res 2005;11:4553-4560.
180. Yu W, Fang H. Clinical trials with oncolytic adenovirus in China. Curr Cancer Drug Targets 2007;7:141-148.
181. Liu TC, Galanis E, Kirn D. Clinical trial results with oncolytic virotherapy: a century of promise, a decade of progress. Nat Clin Pract Oncol 2007;4:101-117.
182. Anderson BD, Nakamura T, Russell SJ, Peng KW. High CD46 receptor density determines preferential killing of tumor cells by oncolytic measles virus. Cancer Res 2004;64:4919-4926.
183. Merrill MK, Bernhardt G, Sampson JH, et al. Poliovirus receptor CD155-targeted oncolysis of glioma. Neuro-oncology 2004;6:208-217.
184. Tseng JC, Levin B, Hurtado A, et al. Systemic tumor targeting and killing by Sindbis viral vectors. Nat Biotechnol 2004;22:70-77.
185. Wickham TJ. Ligand-directed targeting of genes to the site of disease. Nat Med 2003;9:135-139.
186. Glasgow JN, Everts M, Curiel DT. Transductional targeting of adenovirus vectors for gene therapy. Cancer Gene Ther 2006;13:830-844.
187. Sandrin V, Russell SJ, Cosset FL. Targeting retroviral and lentiviral vectors. Curr Top Microbiol Immunol 2003;281:137-178.
188. Mizuguchi H, Hayakawa T. Targeted adenovirus vectors. Hum Gene Ther 2004;15:1034-1044.
189. Weber E, Anderson WF, Kasahara N. Recent advances in retrovirus vector-mediated gene therapy: teaching an old vector new tricks. Curr Opin Mol Ther 2001;3:439-453.
190. Laquerre S, Anderson DB, Stolz DB, Glorioso JC. Recombinant herpes simplex virus type 1 engineered for targeted binding to erythropoietin receptor-bearing cells. J Virol 1998;72:9683-9697.
191. Tai CK, Logg CR, Park JM, et al. Antibody-mediated targeting of replication-competent retroviral vectors. Hum Gene Ther 2003;14:789-802.
192. Hadac EM, Peng KW, Nakamura T, Russell SJ. Reengineering paramyxovirus tropism. Virology 2004;329:217-225.
193. Nakamura T, Peng KW, Harvey M, et al. Rescue and propagation of fully retargeted oncolytic measles viruses. Nat Biotechnol 2005;23:209-214.
194. Hasegawa K, Nakamura T, Harvey M, et al. The use of a tropism-modified measles virus in folate receptor-targeted virotherapy of ovarian cancer. Clin Cancer Res 2006;12(20 Pt 1):6170-6178.

195. Hammond AL, Plemper RK, Zhang J, et al. Single-chain antibody displayed on a recombinant measles virus confers entry through the tumor-associated carcinoembryonic antigen. J Virol 2001;75:2087-2096.
196. Bucheit AD, Kumar S, Grote DM, et al. An oncolytic measles virus engineered to enter cells through the CD20 antigen. Mol Ther 2003;7:62-72.
197. Schneider U, Bullough F, Vongpunsawad S, et al. Recombinant measles viruses efficiently entering cells through targeted receptors. J Virol 2000;74:9928-9936.
198. Hallak LK, Merchan JR, Storgard CM, et al. Targeted measles virus vector displaying echistatin infects endothelial cells via alpha,beta3 and leads to tumor regression. Cancer Res 2005;65:5292-5300.
199. Springfeld C, von Messling V, Frenzke M, et al. Oncolytic efficacy and enhanced safety of measles virus activated by tumor-secreted matrix metalloproteinases. Cancer Res 2006;66:7694-7700.
200. Hallenbeck PL, Chang YN, Hay C, et al. A novel tumor-specific replication-restricted adenoviral vector for gene therapy of hepatocellular carcinoma. Hum Gene Ther 1999;10:1721-1733.
201. Yamamoto M, Davydova J, Wang M, et al. Infectivity enhanced, cyclooxygenase-2 promoter-based conditionally replicative adenovirus for pancreatic cancer. Gastroenterology 2003;125:1203-1218.
202. Kanerva A, Bauerschmitz GJ, Yamamoto M, et al. A cyclooxygenase-2 promoter-based conditionally replicating adenovirus with enhanced infectivity for treatment of ovarian adenocarcinoma. Gene Ther 2004;11:552-559.
203. Shi J, Zheng D, Liu Y, et al. Overexpression of soluble TRAIL induces apoptosis in human lung adenocarcinoma and inhibits growth of tumor xenografts in nude mice. Cancer Res 2005;65:1687-1692.
204. Irving J, Wang Z, Powell S, et al. Conditionally replicative adenovirus driven by the human telomerase promoter provides broad-spectrum antitumor activity without liver toxicity. Cancer Gene Ther 2004;11:174-185.
205. Banerjee NS, Rivera AA, Wang M, et al. Analyses of melanoma-targeted oncolytic adenoviruses with tyrosinase enhancer/promoter-driven E1A, E4, or both in submerged cells and organotypic cultures. Mol Cancer Ther 2004;3:437-449.
206. Ko D, Hawkins L, Yu DC. Development of transcriptionally regulated oncolytic adenoviruses. Oncogene 2005;24:7763-7774.
207. Mathis JM, Stoff-Khalili MA, Curiel DT. Oncolytic adenoviruses—selective retargeting to tumor cells. Oncogene 2005;24:7775-7791.
208. Logg CR, Logg A, Matusik RJ, et al. Tissue-specific transcriptional targeting of a replication-competent retroviral vector. J Virol 2002;76:12783-12791.
209. Chung RY, Saeki Y, Chiocca EA. B-myb promoter retargeting of herpes simplex virus gamma34.5 gene-mediated virulence toward tumor and cycling cells. J Virol 1999;73:7556-7564.
210. Kuroda T, Rabkin SD, Martuza RL. Effective treatment of tumors with strong beta-catenin/T-cell factor activity by transcriptionally targeted oncolytic herpes simplex virus vector. Cancer Res 2006;66:10127-10135.
211. Campbell SA, Gromeier M. Oncolytic viruses for cancer therapy II. Cell-internal factors for conditional growth in neoplastic cells. Onkologie 2005;28:209-215.
212. Barber GN. VSV-tumor selective replication and protein translation. Oncogene 2005;24:7710-7719.
213. Fernandez M, Porosnicu M, Markovic D, Barber GN. Genetically engineered vesicular stomatitis virus in gene therapy: application for treatment of malignant disease. J Virol 2002;76:895-904.
214. Gromeier M, Lachmann S, Rosenfeld MR, et al. Intergeneric poliovirus recombinants for the treatment of malignant glioma. Proc Natl Acad Sci U S A 2000;97:6803-6808.
215. Wang G, Barrett JW, Stanford M, et al. Infection of human cancer cells with myxoma virus requires Akt activation via interaction with a viral ankyrin-repeat host range factor. Proc Natl Acad Sci U S A 2006;103:4640-4645.
216. Marcato P, Shmulevitz M, Lee PW. Connecting reovirus oncolysis and Ras signaling. Cell Cycle 2005;4:556-559.
217. Genovese C, Trani D, Caputi M, Claudio PP. Cell cycle control and beyond: emerging roles for the retinoblastoma gene family. Oncogene 2006;25:5201-5209.
218. Bouchet BP, de Fromentel CC, Puisieux A, Galmarini CM. p53 as a target for anti-cancer drug development. Crit Rev Oncol Hematol 2006;58:190-207.
219. Parato KA, Senger D, Forsyth PA, Bell JC. Recent progress in the battle between oncolytic viruses and tumours. Nat Rev Cancer 2005;5:965-976.
220. Bangari DS, Mittal SK. Current strategies and future directions for eluding adenoviral vector immunity. Curr Gene Ther 2006;6:215-226.
221. Martinez I, Barrera JC, Rodriguez LL, Wertz GW. Recombinant vesicular stomatitis (Indiana) virus expressing New Jersey and Indiana glycoproteins induces neutralizing antibodies to each serotype in swine, a natural host. Vaccine 2004;22:4035-4043.
222. Novella IS, Gilbertson DL, Borrego B, et al. Adaptability costs in immune escape variants of vesicular stomatitis virus. Virus Res 2005;107:27-34.
223. Green NK, Herbert CW, Hale SJ, et al. Extended plasma circulation time and decreased toxicity of polymer-coated adenovirus. Gene Ther 2004;11:1256-1263.
224. Stevenson M, Hale AB, Hale SJ, et al. Incorporation of a laminin-derived peptide (SIKVAV) on polymer-modified adenovirus permits tumor-specific targeting via alpha6-integrins. Cancer Gene Ther 2007;14:335-345.
225. Ong HT, Hasegawa K, Dietz AB, et al. Evaluation of T cells as carriers for systemic measles virotherapy in the presence of antiviral antibodies. Gene Ther 2007;14:324-333.
226. Sperr WR, Lechner K, Pabinger I. Rituximab for the treatment of acquired antibodies to factor VIII. Haematologica 2007;92:66-71.
227. Thurmann P, Harder S. Criteria for the appropriate drug utilisation of immunoglobulin. Pharmacoeconomics 1996;9:417-429.
228. Thurmann PA, Sonnenburg C, Valentova K, et al. Pharmacokinetics of viral antibodies after administration of intravenous immunoglobulin in patients with chronic lymphocytic leukaemia or multiple myeloma. Eur J Clin Pharmacol 2001;57:235-241.
229. Power AT, Bell JC. Cell-based delivery of oncolytic viruses: a new strategic alliance for a biological strike against cancer. Mol Ther 2007;15:660-665.
230. Power AT, Wang J, Falls TJ, et al. Carrier cell-based delivery of an oncolytic virus circumvents antiviral immunity. Mol Ther 2007;15:123-130.
231. Iankov ID, Blechacz B, Liu C, et al. Infected cell carriers: a new strategy for systemic delivery of oncolytic measles viruses in cancer virotherapy. Mol Ther 2007;15:114-122.
232. Komarova S, Kawakami Y, Stoff-Khalili MA, et al. Mesenchymal progenitor cells as cellular vehicles for delivery of oncolytic adenoviruses. Mol Cancer Ther 2006;5:755-766.
233. Carlisle RC, Briggs SS, Hale AB, et al. Use of synthetic vectors for neutralising antibody resistant delivery of replicating adenovirus DNA. Gene Ther 2006;13:1579-1586.
234. Yuan F, Dellian M, Fukumura D, et al. Vascular permeability in a human tumor xenograft: molecular size dependence and cutoff size. Cancer Res 1995;55:3752-3756.
235. Jain RK. Vascular and interstitial barriers to delivery of therapeutic agents in tumors. Cancer Metastasis Rev 1990;9:253-266.
236. Liu P, Zhang A, Xu Y, Xu LX. Study of non-uniform nanoparticle liposome extravasation in tumour. Int J Hyperthermia 2005;21:259-270.
237. Demers GW, Johnson DE, Tsai V, et al. Pharmacologic indicators of antitumor efficacy for oncolytic virotherapy. Cancer Res 2003;63:4003-4008.
238. Monsky WL, Fukumura D, Gohongi T, et al. Augmentation of transvascular transport of macromolecules and nanoparticles in tumors using vascular endothelial growth factor. Cancer Res 1999;59:4129-4135.
239. Oh P, Li Y, Yu J, et al. Subtractive proteomic mapping of the endothelial surface in lung and solid tumours for tissue-specific therapy. Nature 2004;429:629-635.
240. Novozhilov AS, Berezovskaya FS, Koonin EV, Karev GP. Mathematical modeling of tumor therapy with oncolytic viruses: regimes with complete tumor elimination within the framework of deterministic models. Biol Direct 2006;1:6.
241. Wein LM, Wu JT, Kirn DH. Validation and analysis of a mathematical model of a replication-competent oncolytic virus for cancer treatment: implications for virus design and delivery. Cancer Res 2003;63:1317-1324.
242. Hill DA. A Review of Cyclophosphamide. Springfield, IL: Charles C Thomas, 1975.
243. Camenga DL, Nathanson N, Cole GA. Cyclophosphamide-potentiated West Nile viral encephalitis: relative influence of cellular and humoral factors. J Infect Dis 1974;130:634-641.
244. Worthington M, Rabson AS, Baron S. Mechanism of recovery from systemic vaccinia virus infection. I. The effects of cyclophosphamide. J Exp Med 1972;136:277-290.
245. Hurd J, Heath RB. Effect of cyclophosphamide on infections in mice caused by virulent and avirulent strains of influenza virus. Infect Immun 1975;11:886-889.
246. Rager-Zisman B, Allison AC. Effects of immunosuppression on coxsackie B-3 virus infection in mice, and passive protection by circulating antibody. J Gen Virol 1973;19:339-351.
247. Fulci G, Breymann L, Gianni D, et al. Cyclophosphamide enhances glioma virotherapy by inhibiting innate immune responses. Proc Natl Acad Sci U S A 2006;103:12873-12878.
248. Peng KW, Hadac EM, Anderson BD, et al. Pharmacokinetics of oncolytic measles virotherapy: eventual equilibrium between virus and tumor in an ovarian cancer xenograft model. Cancer Gene Ther 2006;13:732-738.
249. Dingli D, Peng KW, Harvey ME, et al. Image-guided radiovirotherapy for multiple myeloma using a recombinant measles virus expressing the thyroidal sodium iodide symporter. Blood 2004;103:1641-1646.
250. Peng KW, TenEyck CJ, Galanis E, et al. Intraperitoneal therapy of ovarian cancer using an engineered measles virus. Cancer Res 2002;62:4656-4662.
251. Peng KW, Ahmann GJ, Pham L, et al. Systemic therapy of myeloma xenografts by an attenuated measles virus. Blood 2001;98:2002-2007.
252. Dempsey MF, Wyper D, Owens J, et al. Assessment of ^{123}I-FIAU imaging of herpes simplex viral gene expression in the treatment of glioma. Nucl Med Commun 2006;27:611-617.
253. Verwijnen SM, Sillevis Smith PA, Hoeben RC, et al. Molecular imaging and treatment of malignant gliomas following adenoviral transfer of the herpes simplex virus-thymidine kinase gene and the somatostatin receptor subtype 2 gene. Cancer Biother Radiopharm 2004;19:111-120.
254. Aung W, Okauchi T, Sato M, et al. In-vivo PET imaging of inducible D2R reporter transgene expression using ^{11C}FLB 457 as reporter probe in living rats. Nucl Med Commun 2005;26:259-268.
255. Liang Q, Satyamurthy N, Barrio JR, et al. Noninvasive, quantitative imaging in living animals of a mutant dopamine D2 receptor reporter gene in which ligand binding is uncoupled from signal transduction. Gene Ther 2001;8:1490-1498.
256. Garber K. China approves world's first oncolytic virus therapy for cancer treatment. J Natl Cancer Inst 2006;98:298-300.

94

REGENERATIVE MEDICINE AND STEM CELL THERAPEUTICS

Timothy J. Nelson, Atta Behfar, and Andre Terzic

CURATIVE THERAPY: AN EMERGING PARADIGM 1317
CONCEPT OF TISSUE REPAIR 1317
GOALS OF REGENERATIVE MEDICINE 1317
Restore Structure and Function 1317
Engineer Tolerance and Disease Prevention 1318
PRINCIPLES OF CELL-BASED THERAPY 1318
Strategies for Cell-Based Therapy 1318
Replacement 1318
Regeneration 1318
Rejuvenation 1318
Approaches for Cell-Based Therapy 1319
Autologous 1319
Allogeneic 1319
SCIENCE OF CELL-BASED THERAPY 1320
Stem Cell Platforms 1320
Embryonic Stem Cells 1320
Perinatal Stem Cells 1322
Adult Stem Cells 1322
Bioengineered Stem Cells 1324
Cells as Drugs 1324
Stem Cell–Based Medicinal Products 1324
Guidelines for Stem Cell–Based Medicinal Product Development 1324
PRACTICE OF REGENERATIVE MEDICINE 1326
Historical Perspective of Cell-Based Therapeutics 1326
Evidence for Current Practice of Regenerative Medicine 1326
Hematologic System 1326
Skeletal System 1327
Endocrine System 1327
Cardiovascular System 1328
Allergy and Immunologic System 1329
Renal and Urologic System 1330
FUTURE PROSPECTS 1330

CURATIVE THERAPY: AN EMERGING PARADIGM

Managing degenerative human diseases is a major therapeutic challenge due to progressive cell destruction and loss of tissue function. This creates an ever-growing need for new therapies capable of repairing underlying pathobiology and restoring native cellular architecture. The emergence of regenerative medicine expands the therapeutic armamentarium, offering paradigms to address disease management demands unmet by traditional pharmacotherapy. Stem cell–based regenerative medicine drives the evolution of medical sciences from palliation, which mitigates symptoms, to curative therapy aimed at treating the root cause of degenerative disease.[1]

Stem cells demonstrate a unique aptitude to *differentiate* into specialized cell types, and form new tissue.[2] Stem cell biology has transformed the understanding of embryology and tissue and organ formation, and has instituted the principles of regenerative pharmacology. Strategies to promote, augment, and reestablish natural repair are at the core of translating the science of stem cell biology into the practice of regenerative medicine. In this chapter, stem cell–based pharmacotherapy is outlined from discovery science to clinical use.

CONCEPT OF TISSUE REPAIR

Description of tissue regeneration may date back to Greek mythology, where Prometheus is punished by Zeus for stealing from Mount Olympus the sacred fire for humankind. The myth describes a vulture that feasts from an open wound in the liver, yet the liver renews daily, demonstrating a unique capacity to regenerate.[3] The concept of regeneration is commonly observed but often unappreciated in daily practice. The rapid healing of skin cuts and abrasions exemplifies repair processes in which new tissue formation is derived from multiple stem cell populations, including epidermal, mesenchymal, neural crest–derived, and circulating stem cells. The capacity for regeneration is particularly evident in the young in comparison to those with degenerative diseases or the elderly, who typically are stress intolerant. Repair mechanisms remain active even in advanced senescence, as elderly patients can heal well after major surgical injuries. This active process of regeneration within a life span provides essential elements for maintenance of tissue homeostasis, and serves as a platform to augment the natural capacity for repair with cell-based therapy.

Evolution of pharmacotherapy toward reparative paradigms exploits the growing understanding of disease pathways and natural repair mechanisms to discover, validate, and apply therapeutics targeted to the disease cause. The multidisciplinary sciences of molecular medicine, bioengineering, and network biology have catalyzed stem cell applications. Tailored to the genetic and molecular profile of the individual patient, regenerative medicine integrates stem cell biology with personalized therapeutic, diagnostic, prognostic, and preventive solutions across human diseases (Fig. 94-1).

GOALS OF REGENERATIVE MEDICINE

Restore Structure and Function

Regenerative medicine aims to restore normal structure and function. Stem cells and their products provide the active ingredients of a regenerative regimen. Stem cells maintain an autonomous self-renewal potential, and respond to guiding signals to differentiate into replacement tissues.[4] By healing injury, stem cells restore damaged tissue. Restoration of diseased tissues offers a sustained therapeutic advantage in conditions ranging from congenital disease to acquired, age-related pathologies. The outcome depends on the aptitude of the stem cell population to secure maximal, tissue-specific repair, and the production of a nurturing niche environment in diseased tissue that enables execution of repair.[5]

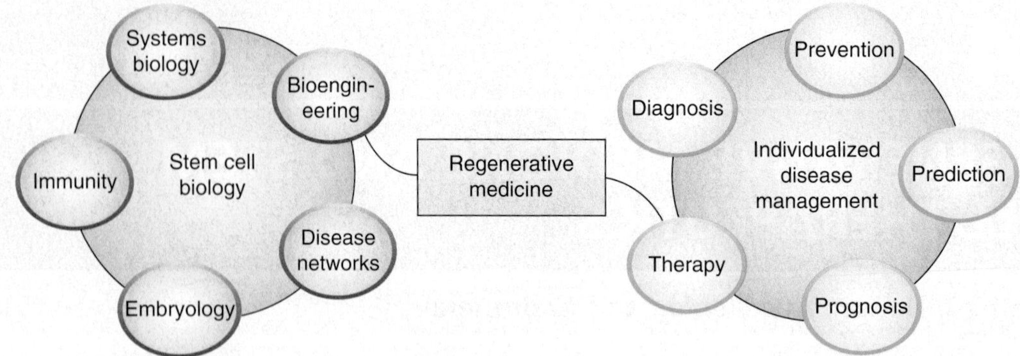

FIGURE 94-1 • Regenerative medicine bridges stem cell biology with individualized disease management. Advances in stem cell biology have been accelerated through multidisciplinary integration of embryology with immunology and the emerging fields of systems biology, bioengineering, and disease networks. The clinical application of regenerative medicine is guided by the challenges of individualized disease management that depends on prediction, diagnosis, prognosis, prevention, and therapy tailored to the specific needs of each patient.

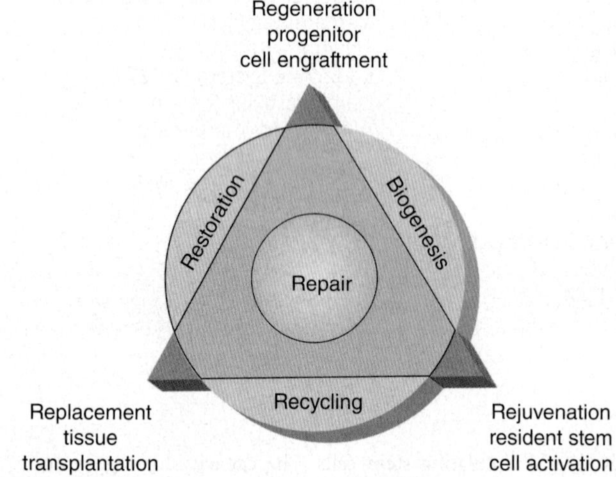

FIGURE 94-2 • **The scope of regenerative medicine.** Repair is the central goal of regenerative medicine that encompasses three general strategies: replacement, regeneration, and rejuvenation. Replacement is defined as repair of damaged tissue by recycling used parts through tissue/organ transplantation. Regeneration is defined as repair of damaged tissue through de novo differentiation of progenitor cells to replace damaged cells and restore tissue function. Rejuvenation is defined as repair of damaged tissue through activation of endogenous resident stem cells that can stimulate biogenesis of new tissue.

Engineer Tolerance and Disease Prevention

Beyond restoration of structure and function, regenerative medicine paves a pathway for prevention and delay of disease progression through prophylactic repair. Stem cells provide a unique platform to select, guide, and engineer cellular characteristics required for enhanced tolerance while effectively treating and/or preventing disease manifestation. By anticipating the needs of disease-susceptible tissues, the goal of regenerative medicine becomes rejuvenation of threatened tissues with stress-tolerant cells to prevent irreversible damage. This goal requires the ability to predict disease susceptibility based on molecular profiling at the earliest stages to guide appropriate and timely interventions.

PRINCIPLES OF CELL-BASED THERAPY

Strategies for Cell-Based Therapy

There are three general concepts that capture the scope of regenerative medicine: replacement, regeneration, and rejuvenation (Fig. 94-2). These concepts overlap in practice but provide distinctions important to conceptualize the scope of regenerative medicine from transplantation of used parts ("replacement") to engraftment of new parts ("regeneration") to induction of endogenous self-renewing parts ("rejuvenation").

Replacement

Replacement strategy refers to transplantation of a cell-based product that reestablishes homeostasis for the recipient through continuation of the tissue function from the donor.[6] The field of surgery pioneered the concept of replacement in the 1950s with the advent of solid organ transplantation. For example, if the heart was damaged beyond the ability to palliate the condition, then replacing the diseased tissue with a new, functioning donor heart became the only option. In addition to solid organ transplantation, bone marrow transplantation has become a therapeutic replacement modality to treat a range of diseases, including hematologic malignancies, congenital immunodeficiencies, and autoimmune disorders. The primary limitations of replacement strategy are donor availability due to shortage of solid organ donors, and the difficulty of matching the immunologic criteria for transplantation.

Regeneration

Regenerative strategy refers to engraftment of progenitor cells that require in vivo growth and differentiation to establish recipient homeostasis through de novo function of the stem cell–based transplant. Advances in hematology gave rise to the concept of regeneration with the identification of bone marrow–derived stem cells that, once harvested, could be transplanted in small quantities into peripheral blood in order to engraft and reconstitute a functioning bone marrow through production of mature daughter cells for the entire hematopoietic system.[7] Success was facilitated by the presence of host bone marrow that provided a protective environment to nurture the long-term survival of self-renewing stem cell progenitors. Likewise, an intense search is ongoing for tissue-specific, nonhematopoietic stem cells that have the capacity to be expanded ex vivo and reestablish lost function when transplanted.

Rejuvenation

Rejuvenation strategy refers to self-renewal of tissues from endogenous, resident stem cells to maintain tissue homeostasis and promote tissue healing. This natural process of tissue recycling enables tissue as it senesces to be replaced with younger cells that are inherently more resilient and equipped to provide adequate stress tolerance for tissue survival.[8] Daughter cells can also be derived from reactivation of the cell cycle within mature cell types in response to (physio)pathologic stress. Rejuvenation ensures chronic stress tolerance, with most tissues able, however, to repair only partially. In the context of massive acute injury, such as myocardial infarction, an inherent repair strategy may be inadequate. A boost in these natural processes, through biologic or pharmacologic treatment, is likely required to stimulate adaptive response and promote adequate biogenesis of functional tissue in the setting of acute or progressive disease.

Approaches for Cell-Based Therapy

Cell-based therapy includes autologous and allogeneic interventions. Autologous refers to transplantation of tissues, cells, or proteins from one part of a patient's body to another, whereas allogeneic refers to transplantation between genetically distinct individuals albeit belonging to the same species.

Autologous

Autologous stem cells are derived from self, thereby avoiding immune intolerance. Bone marrow harvesting provides the original example in which hematopoietic stem cells (HSCs) were obtained during aspiration of the iliac crest of patients, pooled together, and used for transplantation into the same individual after completion of myeloablative therapy in the setting of hematologic cancer. HSCs were later obtained from peripheral blood collections following treatment with growth factors and cytokines such as granulocyte colony-stimulating factor (G-CSF) to promote mobilization from bone marrow. This approach provides rapid and efficient collection, while minimizing associated pain and discomfort. Peripheral stem cell isolation has fostered multiple uses that are not limited by age of the patient or treatment history. Peripherally recruited stem cells demonstrate improved engraftment efficiency, decrease the requirement for subsequent blood transfusions, and decrease the complexity for stem cell transplantation. HSC transplantation has become a standard therapy for Hodgkin's disease and non-Hodgkin's lymphoma, as well as multiple myeloma.[9] In addition to HSCs derived from bone marrow, autologous stem cells can be obtained from targeted biopsy of adipose tissue, skeletal and cardiac muscle, or skin. Applications for autologous stem cells are typically limited to chronic conditions given the time required to recycle stem cells from patients through the stages of mobilization, collection, expansion, and preparation for transplantation back to the same patient (Fig. 94-3).

Allogeneic

Allogeneic stem cells are derived from a donor who is different from the recipient. Stem cells from multiple donors can be obtained independently, and stored as a tissue biorepository. Allogeneic blood transfusions have become safe and effective after the discovery of major blood types that allow matching of donor and recipient through characterization of surface antigens. Stem cell transplantation from a human major histocompatibility complex (MHC) human leukocyte antigen (HLA)–compatible donor has also been established in the treatment of hematopoietic diseases, including acute and chronic myelogenous leukemia, myelodysplastic syndromes such as aplastic anemia, refractory Hodgkin's disease, and non-Hodgkin's lymphoma. However, graft-versus-host disease (GVHD), in which engrafted stem cells produce progeny that attacks the host, which is recognized as foreign or non-self tissue, becomes a major limitation for this type of transplantation.

As with blood transfusions, the advantage of allogeneic stem cell transplantation is the ability to harvest tissue from healthy donors, store tissues, and have them available for acute, "off-the-shelf" therapy for a large number of potential patients (Fig. 94-4). In addition to the ability to stockpile on-demand therapeutics, allogeneic tissue offers unique advantages when a patient has a genetically based disease that hinders the therapeutic potential of their autologous stem cells.[2] Genetic diseases such as Fanconi's anemia can be cured with bone marrow transplantation from an HLA-matched sibling donor that minimizes immunologic intolerance while restoring a normal genotype. Additionally, the non-self distinction of allogeneic stem cells can be useful when the engrafted stem cell progeny recognizes host-derived cancer cells as foreign tissue and the graft-versus-tumor effect provides therapeutic benefits.

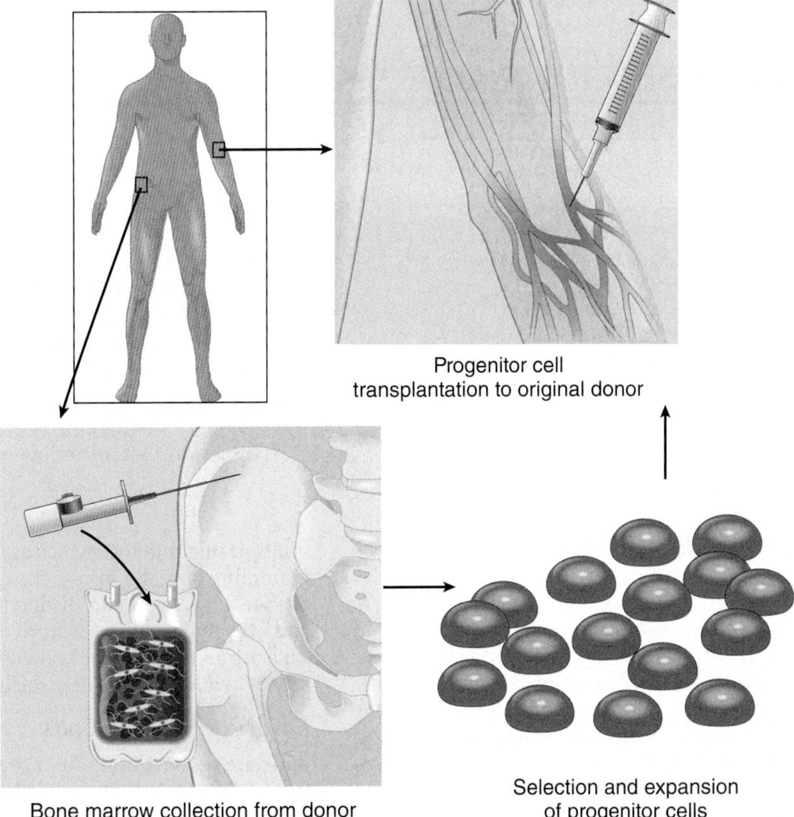

FIGURE 94-3 • Autologous stem cell transplantation. Patients first donate their own stem cells. Progenitors are typically collected from bone marrow aspiration or peripheral blood. Patients can undergo treatment with growth factors to recruit stem cells out of the bone marrow and enrich progenitor cells within the circulation. Progenitor cells are selected, expanded, packaged, and stored until the patient completes myeloablative therapy. Progenitor cells are transplanted into the same patient via intravenous infusion. Autologous stem cell transplantation avoids the need for immunosuppressive therapy.

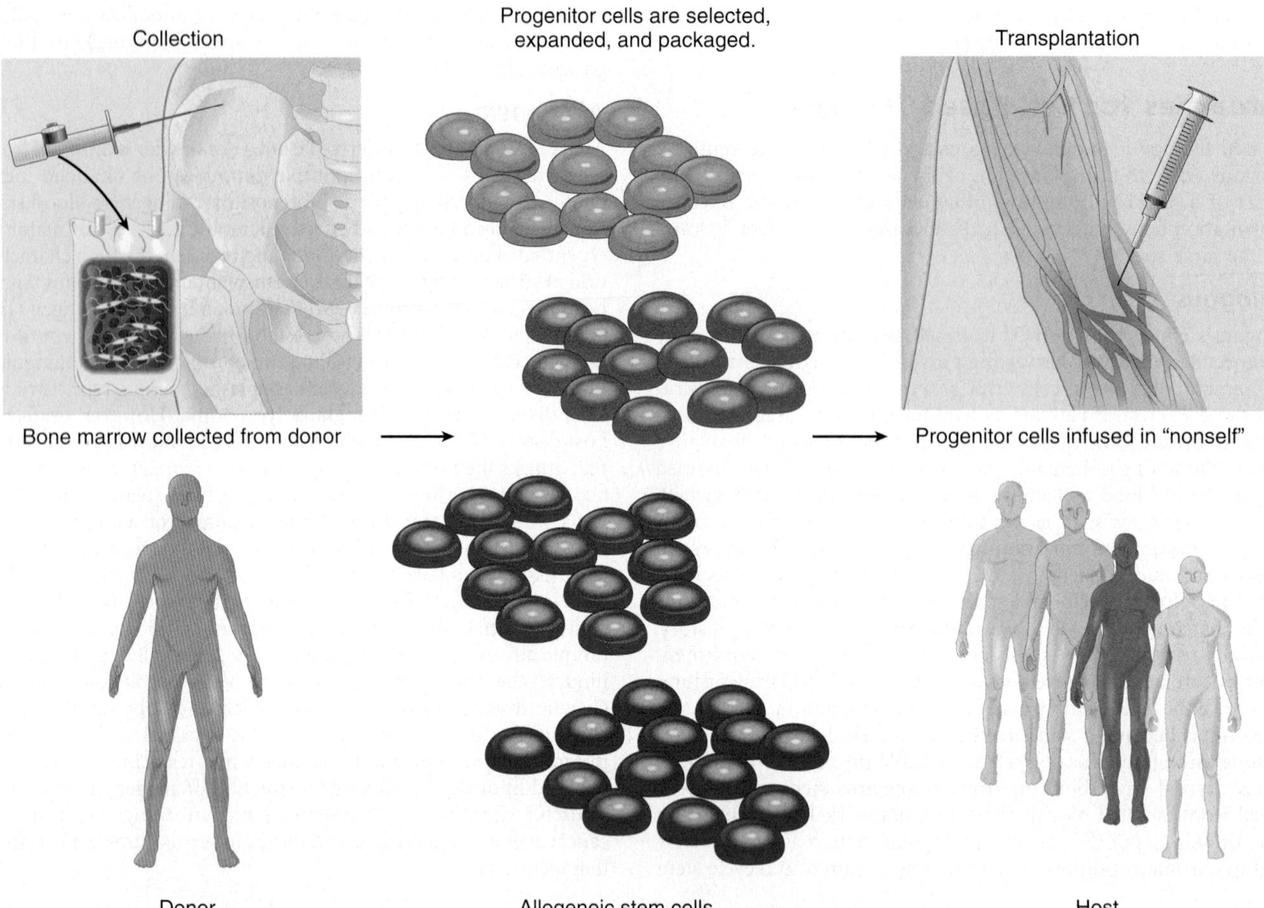

FIGURE 94-4 • Allogeneic stem cell transplantation. First, a donor undergoes stem cell harvest from bone marrow or alternative sources, such as peripheral blood or cord blood. Second, progenitor cells are isolated, pooled, packaged, and stored for prospective patients. Third, preserved cells are retrieved and used for non-self transplantation in appropriate patients. The centralized process provides access to stem cell biorepositories such that a single donation could potentially contribute to the care of multiple patients.

TABLE 94-1 GLOSSARY OF STEM CELL PLATFORMS

Platform	Defining Characteristics
Embryonic stem cell	• Derived from the inner cell mass of blastocyst • Pluripotent with autonomous self-renewal • Responsive to differentiation cues
Perinatal stem cell	• Derived from perinatal sources • Pool of embryonic-like and adult-like stem cells • Extensive availability at time of birth
Adult stem cell	• Derived from bone marrow, adipose tissue • Include resident stem cells • Multilineage hematopoietic and mesenchymal progenitors
Bioengineered stem cell	• Derived by reprogramming of adult sources • Include "therapeutic cloning" and "nuclear reprogramming" • Generate customized embryonic-like stem cells

SCIENCE OF CELL-BASED THERAPY

Stem Cell Platforms

Stem cell platforms include natural versus engineered derivation processes (Table 94-1). Examples of naturally derived stem cells include embryonic stem cells (ESCs), perinatal stem cells (e.g., umbilical cord–derived stem cells), and adult stem cells. Engineered processes have enabled the derivation of stem cells through reprogramming that includes therapeutic cloning and genetic manipulation. The ethical and sociologic context surrounding stem cells has stimulated scientific approaches to address the concerns of fetal tissue destruction through multiple methodologies such as isolation of adult stem cells and reprogramming somatic non–stem cell sources. All stem cells have their unique advantages and distinct challenges associated with the source and availability of tissues from which they are derived, differentiation capacity and multipotent potential, tumorigenic tendency and immunity profile, and ultimately socioethical considerations.

Embryonic Stem Cells

ESCs are derived from the inner cell mass of a preimplantation blastocyst (Fig. 94-5).[10] These pluripotent stem cells can give rise to essentially all tissues, including the complete spectrum of mesoderm,

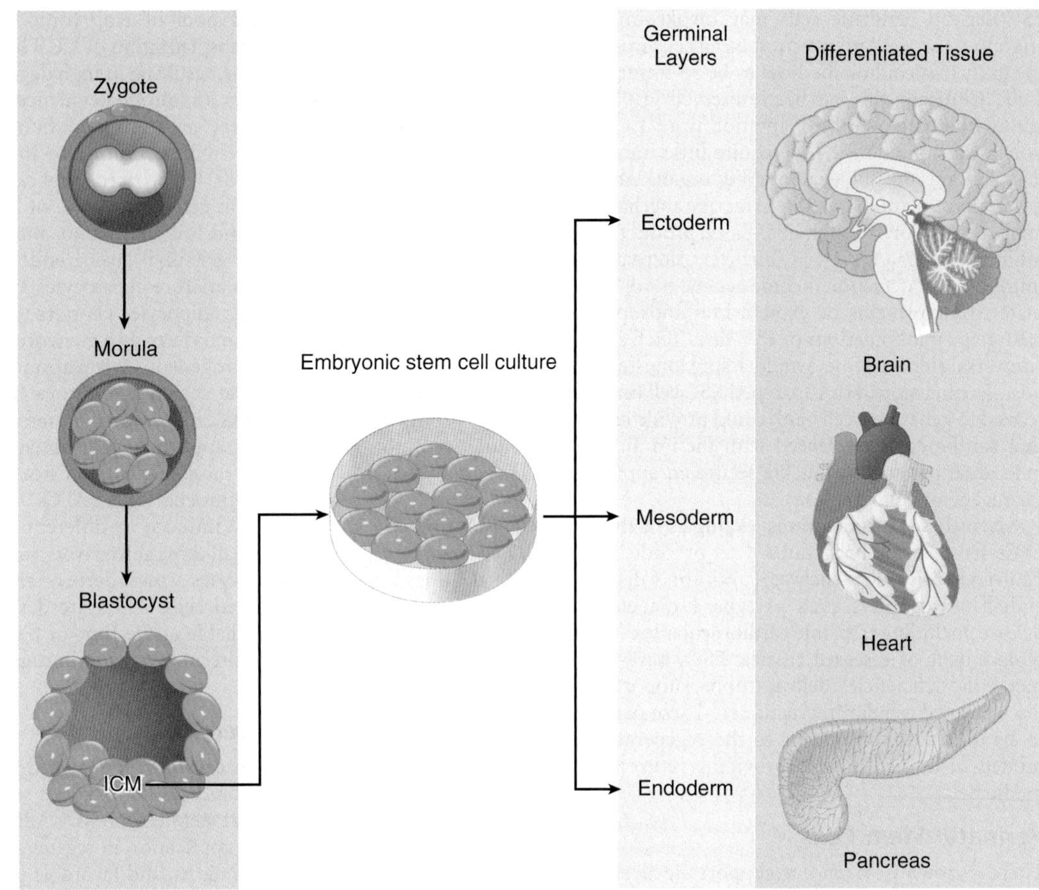

FIGURE 94-5 • Embryonic stem cells. Isolated from the inner cell mass (ICM) of a blastocyst, embryonic stem cells are cultured to produce cell lines that can be indefinitely propagated in the undifferentiated state. Consistent with the characteristic ability to recapitulate normal embryonic development, embryonic stem cells differentiate in vitro to produce tissues arising from all three germinal layers. The ectoderm develops into neuronal derivatives within the central nervous system. The mesoderm produces mature tissues, such as heart muscle. The endoderm differentiates into lineages such as pancreas. The pluripotency and unlimited proliferation make embryonic stem cells an attractive source for regenerative medicine applications.

TABLE 94-2 STEM CELL DIFFERENTIATION POTENTIAL

Potential	Developmental Capacity
Pluripotent	Natural and induced ability to form all lineages of the body
Multipotent	Natural and induced ability to form multiple cell types within a specific lineage
Unipotent	Natural and restricted ability to form a single cell type

endoderm, and ectoderm derivatives (Table 94-2). Multiple ESC lines have been derived from a wide range of species, ranging from mouse to human.[11,12] Human ESCs were first isolated in 1998, and have now been demonstrated to give rise to many cell types, including hematopoietic cells, neuron-like cells, glial progenitors, dendritic cells, hepatocytes, pancreatic islet–like cells, osteocytes, chondrocytes, adipocytes, and cardiomyocytes, as well as muscular, endothelial, skin, lung, and retinal tissues. This quintessential differentiation potential provides a promising avenue to produce large quantity of transplantable cells from a renewable source.

ESCs are defined by their unique capacity to self-renew indefinitely in cell culture, long telomere length, and high nuclear-to-cytoplasmic ratio; they display an unparalleled differentiation capacity, which includes recapitulating the spectrum of normal embryonic development. The transcription factor Oct-4, coupled with Sox2 and E1A, contributes to maintenance of the undifferentiated state through fibroblast growth factor-4, Wnt, and transforming growth factor-β (TGF-β) dependent pathways.[13] Pluripotency in mouse ESCs has been maintained with leukemia inhibitory factor through a STAT-3–dependent mechanism, which is not evolutionary conserved in human counterparts. Pluripotency in human ESCs is dependent on a Src-family of nonreceptor tyrosine kinases, and is monitored by expression of markers such as alkaline phosphatase, POU transcription factor Oct3/4, Nanog, Cripto/TDGF1, proteoglycans TRA-1–60/81, GCTM-2, and embryonic antigens SSEA-3 and SSEA-4. Early lineage commitment of the three germinal layers has been monitored by the expression of markers such as Sox1 for neuroectoderm, Pdx-1 for endoderm, and Flk-1 for mesoderm.

A potential limitation of ESCs in regard to regenerative applications relates to their inherent unrestricted growth potential with the associated risk of teratoma formation, prominent once differentiation cues are evaded following transplantation.[12] Significant progress in understanding embryonic developmental pathways has established strategies to guide ESCs into tissue-specific lineages. Ensuring proper regulation of ESC differentiation prior to transplantation or within the microenvironment of transplanted host tissue provides safety required for clinical application.[14,15] Guidance of targeted differentiation using growth factors, cytokines, hormones, and small molecules provides a pharmacologic approach to restrict lineage potential and promote lineage specification. Specialized biomarkers that identify tissue-specific commitment and allow physical separation from undifferentiated progenitor cells provide an additional approach to secure lineage specification.

In addition to unrestricted growth potential, ESCs create a unique immunologic challenge for regenerative medicine.[16] Since ESCs are derived from non-self tissues, adult engraftment of this cell type is considered an allogeneic transplantation. Despite this allogeneic identity, ESCs are capable of engraftment into nonidentical hosts with minimal immunosuppression. Expression of MHC-1 protein is very low in ESCs, and is thought to secure survival following allogeneic transplantation by avoiding immunologic detection. This has provided a basis to interpret tolerance of xenotransplanted ESC-derived cardiomyocytes. Other lines of evidence suggest that cotransplantation with

ESC-derived dendritic cells may invoke immunologic tolerance of engrafted tissues. Antigen-presenting cells from the same individual as the graft tissue allow the host to be re-trained as to the definition of "self." Clinically this has been observed in patients who have undergone bone marrow transplantation prior to solid organ transplantation from same donor and require little immunosuppressive therapy to maintain the allogeneic solid organ. Additionally, ESC-derived tissues have demonstrated a paracrine mechanism to evade immunologic recognition through ESC-based production of TGF-β that locally inhibits endogenous T-cell function. Alternative approaches to avoid immunologic detection include genetic modifications of ESCs to eliminate MHC proteins or express immunosuppressive agents through transgenic manipulations of ESC lines. Such an engineered stealth-like "universal stem cell line" would assure long-term tolerance in a foreign host. Furthermore, HLA-isotyped ESC cell lines produced and characterized to generate a cell bank could provide an "off-the-shelf" product that can be cross-referenced with the immunologic requirements of individual patients to quickly secure an appropriate stem cell source for regenerative therapies.

Given these considerations, examples of therapeutic application of ESCs have so far been limited to preclinical studies. This includes neurologic disorders such as Parkinson's disease and spinal injury,[17] endocrine disorders such as type 1 diabetes,[18] and cardiovascular disease, including ischemic cardiomyopathy.[19] In addition to structural replacement of diseased tissues, ESCs have the ability to overcome metabolic deficiencies, deliver trophic support to host cells, and restore disconnected cellular interactions.[20] These paracrine effects may prove to be a critical component to the regenerative capacity of ESCs in models of human disease, providing future avenues for regenerative medicine.

Perinatal Stem Cells

There is growing evidence to support the diverse differentiation capacity of stem cells derived from perinatal sources, including umbilical cord blood (UCB). UCB is collected at the time of birth, and provides a universal pool of embryonic-like and adult-like stem cells (Fig. 94-6).[21] Transplantation of UCB has been clinically successful for HSC applications, resulting in high degree of engraftment, favorable immunotolerance, and limited evidence for GVHD compared to adult bone marrow stem cell transplantation. Reconstitution of the adult hematopoietic system in siblings or in the same individual was the initial rationale for UCB-based applications. In addition to HSCs, UCB-derived stem cells are capable of in vitro expansion, long-term maintenance, and differentiation into representative cells of all three embryonic germinal layers: endodermal (e.g., hepatopancreatic precursor cells, mature hepatocytes, type II alveolar pneumocytes), mesodermal (e.g., adipocytes, chondrocytes, osteoblasts, myocytes, endothelial cells), and ectodermal (e.g., neurons, astrocytes, oligodendrocytes).[21]

The heterogeneous populations of stem cells contained in UCB can be fractionated to purify a more homogeneous population with characteristics of embryonic-like stem cells. In this way, UCB may provide a clinically applicable pluripotent stem cell pool that avoids ethical challenges raised with bona fide embryonic sources.[22] Alternatively, amniotic epithelial cells (AECs) derived from amniotic membranes can also be induced to differentiate into diverse and specialized cell types from all three germ layers, including pancreatic cells (endoderm), cardiomyocytes (mesoderm), and keratinocytes (ectoderm). Like UCB-derived cells, AECs are derived from preexisting tissue that is readily available at the time of birth.[23] This creates an opportunity to generate alternative multilineage stem cells from nonembryonic sources.

Adult Stem Cells

Adult stem cells comprise a wide range of progenitors derived from nonembryonic, nonfetal tissues such as bone marrow, adipose tissue, and resident stem cell pools.[24] Adult stem cells are a leading candidate for clinical application in regenerative medicine based on accessibility, autologous status, and favorable proliferative potential. While there is increased understanding of the regenerative potential of stem cells derived from adipose tissue and of resident stem cells linked to the

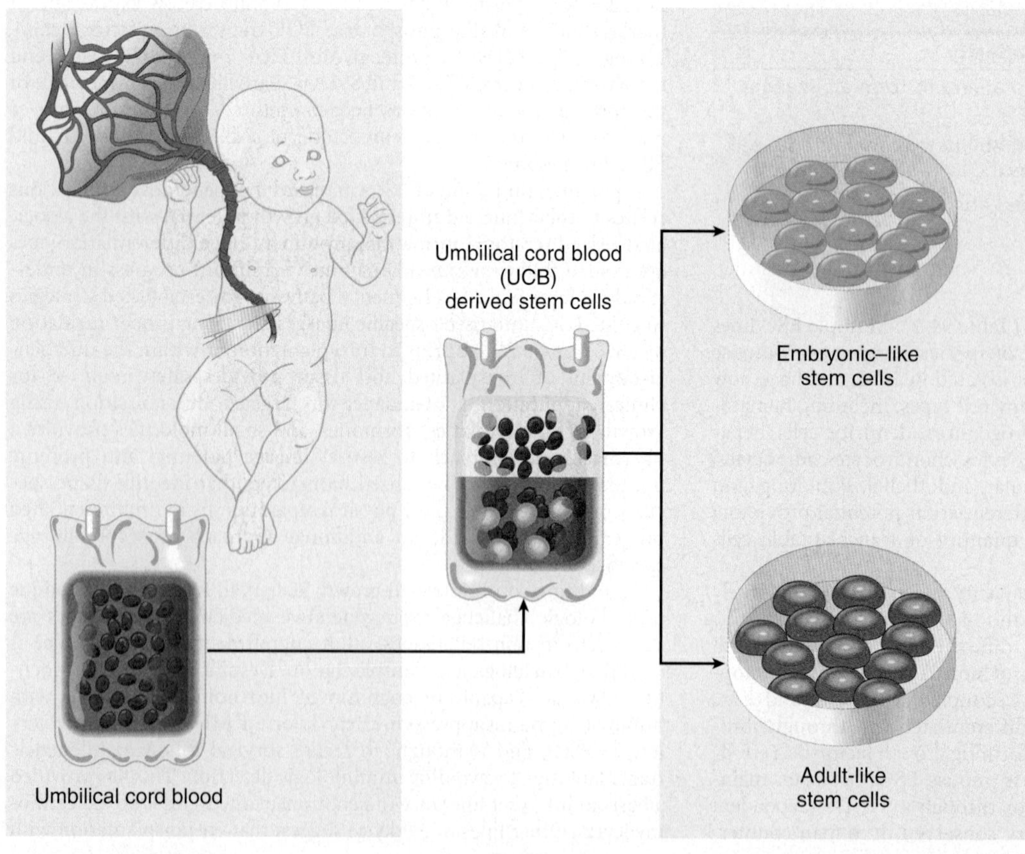

FIGURE 94-6 • Perinatal stem cells. Umbilical cord blood is one source of perinatal stem cells, collected at birth from the umbilical vein containing blood returning from the placenta. These cells have been utilized as hematopoietic stem cells similar to adult bone marrow–derived progenitors. The immaturity of the immune system reduces the risk of detrimental graft-versus-host disease when comparing perinatal to adult sources. Perinatal stem cells also contain populations of cells that behave similar to embryonic stem cells. Pluripotent differentiation potential and unique immunologic status highlight the advantages of perinatal stem cells for regenerative applications, and justify a distinct classification. Perinatal stem cells, which also include amniotic epithelial cells (AECs), offer readily available, alternative sources of progenitors.

innate repair potential of mature tissues, current experience primarily relies on bone marrow–derived stem cells. Sufficient to recapitulate the entire hematopoietic system and provide mesenchymal stem cells with nonhematopoietic differentiation potential, bone marrow–derived stem cells are a cornerstone of contemporary regenerative medicine applications.[25]

Bone marrow–derived HSCs represent the earliest example of cell-based regenerative medicine, pioneered to address the needs of patients treated with total body irradiation for leukemia who developed life-threatening infections and irreversible tissue destruction. Stem cells defined by expression of the CD34 surface marker can also be obtained via peripheral blood leukapheresis for clinical engraftment. HSCs have provided the foundation for autologous and allogeneic stem cell transplantation, and offer novel treatments for patients with cancer, autoimmune diseases, and genetic diseases, including severe combined immunodeficiency and thalassemia. Transplant studies have also revealed engraftment of nonhematopoietic cell lineages derived from donor bone marrow, unmasking subpopulations capable of a diverse range of lineage-specific differentiation.

Mesenchymal stem cells (MSCs) were also discovered in the bone marrow, albeit at low frequency compared to the hematopoietic pool. MSCs represent approximately 1 of 10,000 nucleated cells, and arise from the supporting architecture of the adult marrow.[26] Comparable stem cells have also been isolated from connective components of various postnatal tissues, including adipose and synovial tissue, as well as from peripheral and cord blood. MSCs exhibit properties of multipotency, with the capacity to contribute to regeneration of bone, cartilage and muscle, and tissues of mesodermal origin (Fig. 94-7).[27] Evidence also support the contribution of MSCs to liver and pancreatic islet cell regeneration, and protection in the setting of kidney, heart, or lung injury. MSCs secrete a spectrum of bioactive molecules that provide a regenerative microenvironment to limit the area of damage and to mount a self-regulated regenerative response. The age of the individual, the extent of tissue damage, and the local and whole body titers of MSCs all have been considered to play a role in the ultimate rate and extent of repair. Beyond the supply of differentiated mesenchymal tissues in case of cell loss, MSC progeny constitutes the stromal environment that is fundamental in the regulation of parenchymal

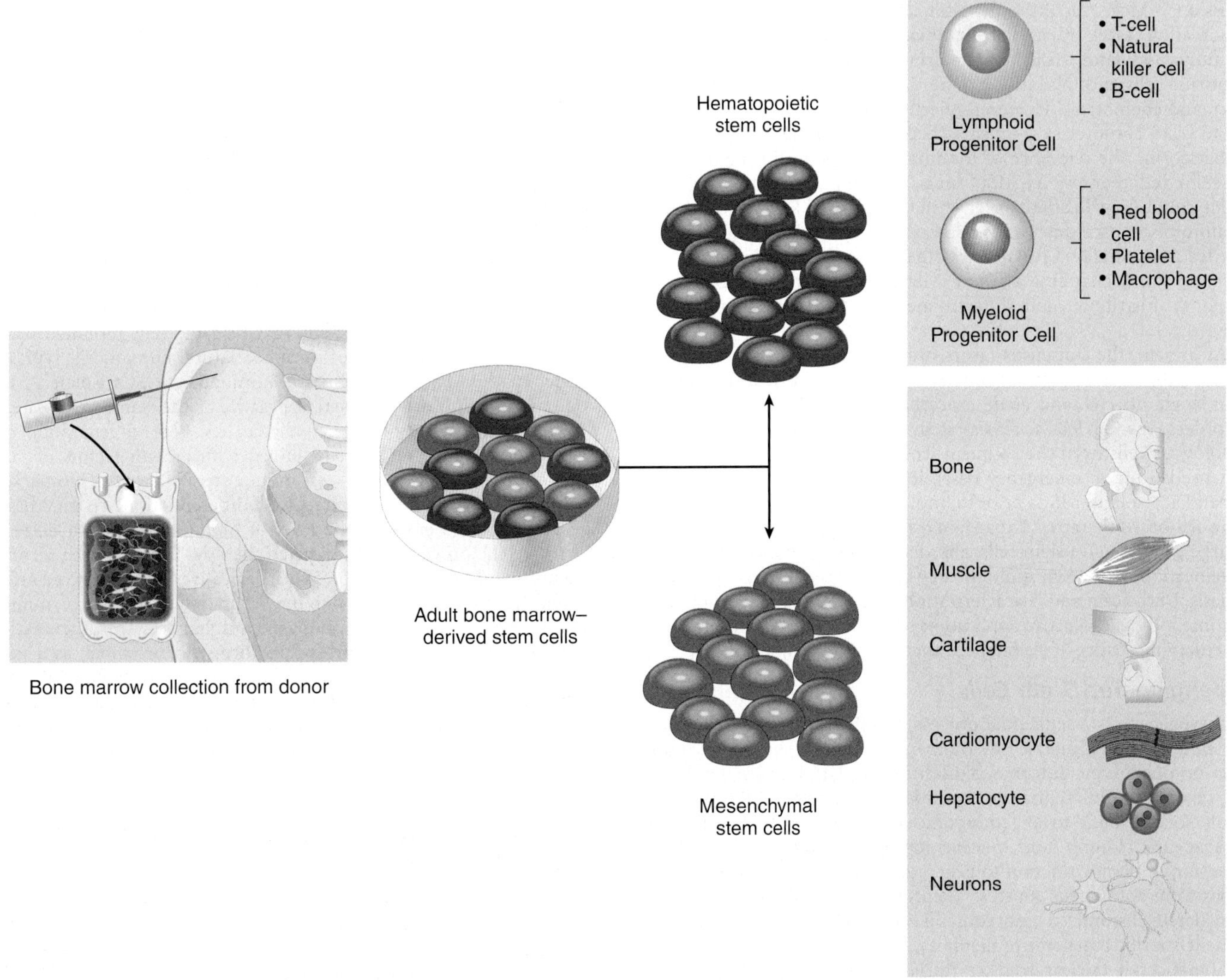

FIGURE 94-7 • Adult stem cells. Derived from nonembryonic or nonperinatal sources, adult stem cells can be procured from a range of tissues, such as bone marrow as well as circulating blood or fat. Adult stem cells are generally considered multipotent, as illustrated for bone marrow–derived stem cells that contain both hematopoietic progenitors and mesenchymal stem cells. Hematopoietic stem cells give rise to (i) lymphoid-derived T cells, B cells, and natural killer cells; and (ii) myeloid-derived red blood cells, platelets, and macrophages. Hematopoietic stem cells provide the standard of care for bone marrow reconstitution. Mesenchymal stem cells also have a diverse spectrum of differentiation that includes bone, muscle, cartilage, cardiomyocytes, hepatocytes, and neurons. Mesenchymal stem cells serve as a cell type of choice for clinical applications of nonhematologic regeneration based on the availability of autologous stem cell sources, cost-effective isolation, and safety profile.

stem cell renewal and differentiation, and immune modulation. In fact, both autologous and allogeneic MSCs have been tested in recent clinical trials, including for treatment of osteogenesis imperfecta, Crohn's disease, and GVHD.[28]

Identification of adult human MSCs as multilineage progenitors relies on their capacity to be induced to differentiate into specific phenotypes. Although the ganglioside GD2 has been proposed as a single surface marker that distinguishes MSCs, a panel of biomarkers has been typically employed to secure isolation.[29] These biomarkers include positive expression of CD44, CD73, CD90, CD105, Stro-1, and the adhesion molecules CD106 (vascular cell adhesion molecule-1) and intracellular adhesion molecule-1, in the absence of expression of hematopoietic markers CD34, CD45, CD11, and CD14, and the adhesion molecule CD31 (platelet/endothelial cell adhesion molecule-1).[26-28]

Adult human MSCs are characteristically devoid of HLA class II antigens (MHC-II) on the cell surface, and do not express the co-stimulatory molecules CD80, CD86, or CD40.[26] The expressed MHC class I antigens may activate T cells, but, with the absence of co-stimulatory molecules, a secondary signal would not engage, leaving T cells anergic. Such a unique immune profile (i.e., MHC I$^+$, MHC II$^-$, CD40$^-$, CD80$^-$, CD86$^-$) is regarded as nonimmunogenic, and accordingly transplantation into an allogeneic host may not require immunosuppression.[26] Moreover, MSCs exhibit immunosuppressive properties, modulating T-cell functions including cell activation, and display immunomodulatory features impairing maturation and function of dendritic cells and inhibiting human B-cell proliferation, differentiation, and chemotaxis. However, rejection of marrow stromal cells in MHC class I–and class II–mismatched recipients has been reported, underscoring the relevance of the immune response in the outcome of stem cell therapy. As MSC interaction with the microenvironment could in principle trigger (re)expression of MHC-II antigens, compromising the fate of implanted cells, additional studies are needed to optimally translate MSC therapy in the clinical setting. An increased understanding of how MSCs regulate the inflammatory response, distribute, and differentiate after delivery in humans is needed.[30]

At present, the consensus favors use of allogeneic MSC therapy in the management of acute disorders, such as acute myocardial infarction, acute GVHD, and acute exacerbations of inflammatory bowel disorders (see Fig. 94-7). This strategy avoids the need for preparing autologous cells from the recipient. For disorders in which MSCs are not needed on an emergency basis, it may be preferable to culture-expand autologous MSCs prior to implantation in an effort to personalize cell-based therapy.[30] Expansion offers the opportunity to produce a large pool of naive stem cells, and derive progeny honed for lineage specification away from multipotency and into tissue-restricted cytopoiesis. Derivation and characterization of specialized MSC subpopulations, and their selective application to specific disease conditions, is an emerging strategy for enhanced therapeutic outcome.

Bioengineered Stem Cells

Embryogenesis is a sequential process of differential gene expression dictated by the epigenetic environment. Exploiting epigenetic influence on phenotypic outcome, biotechnology platforms are developed for reversal of differentiation to achieve genetic reprogramming of adult sources back to an embryonic state. Such platforms include "therapeutic cloning" and "nuclear reprogramming" that bypass the need for embryo extraction to generate pluripotent stem cell phenotypes from autologous sources.[31] Reprogramming of adult stem cells to generate customized embryonic-like stem cells offers the future for patient-specific regenerative therapies.

Somatic cell nuclear transfer (SCNT) allows trans-acting factors present in the mammalian oocyte to reprogram somatic cell nuclei to an undifferentiated state. Therapeutic cloning refers to SCNT in which the nuclear content of a somatic cell from an individual is transferred into an enucleated donor egg to derive blastocysts that contain pluripotent embryonic-like stem cells (Fig. 94-8). In this way, SCNT has produced cloned embryonic stem cells from multiple mammalian somatic cell biopsies.[32] The pluripotency of derived cells has been confirmed through germline transmission and reproductive cloning. However, technological limitations have resulted in low efficiency, impeding success with human cells.

Nuclear reprogramming of adult cells, namely skin fibroblasts, through ectopic introduction of a small number of pluripotency-associated transcription factors is an alternative approach to induce an embryonic stem cell-like phenotype (see Fig. 94-8).[33,34] In the mouse, such an approach has yielded induced pluripotent stem (iPS) cells sufficient for de novo embryogenesis. In humans, transcription factors associated with the pluripotency state were ranked through bioinformatic prioritization and further screened for reprogramming effectiveness through combinatorial viral delivery. Transcription factor sets—Oct4, Sox2, c-Myc, and Klf4 or, alternatively, Oct4, Sox2, Nanog, and Lin28—are sufficient to reprogram human somatic cells to pluripotent stem cells that exhibit the essential characteristics of ESCs, including maintenance of the developmental potential to differentiate into advanced derivatives of all three germ layers. iPS cell lines should largely eliminate the concern of immune rejection. Moreover, iPS-based technology will facilitate the production of cell line panels that closely reflect the genetic diversity of a population, enabling the discovery, development, and validation of therapies tailored for each individual.[31] However, alleviating technical limitations, including mutation through viral integration, incorporation of oncogenic genes, and lack of reliable differentiation protocols, is required prior to applications in transplantation medicine.

Cells as Drugs

Stem Cell–Based Medicinal Products

Categorized as "biologics," stem cells—unlike the more common "small-molecule" drugs—are a distinct class of medications produced by means of biologic processes.[35] In contrast to traditional pharmaceuticals, cell-based medicinal products contain as the active ingredient viable human cells of allogeneic or autologous origin; may be combined with biomolecules and noncellular components, including medical devices and scaffolds; and may be genetically modified. First-generation products consist of purified, natural human cells typically in their native state, such as naive, unmodified HSCs isolated from bone marrow and used in current practice as the standard of care in the treatment of hematologic malignancies. Second-generation cell products typically refer to cells guided with growth factors or subpopulations selected based on unique tissue-specific biomarkers or genetically modified to direct cell differentiation, restrict tissue specification, and enhance the level of organ specificity to derive a tissue-specific progenitor for targeted therapy. The goal with second-generation cell products is to produce derivatives with enhanced safety and efficacy profiles compared to the original stem cell source, nullifying tumorigenic risk and immunogenic intolerance. Third-generation products would serve as delivery platforms, for example, as a gene delivery system for correction of genetic mutation or targeted therapy with recombinant protein, and/or engineered cell products with superior properties, such as enhanced stress tolerance and improved regenerative capacity. The goal with third-generation cell products is to maximize therapeutic potential beyond that inherent to the original stem cell source or the respective derivatives.

Guidelines for Stem Cell–Based Medicinal Product Development

Human cell-based medicinal products are heterogeneous with regard to cell origin and type, and the complexity of the final product. Clinical development mandates pharmacodynamic and pharmacokinetic documentation, along with clinical efficacy and safety studies.[36,37] Suitable markers of biologic activity are used to adequately identify primary pharmacodymanic properties, and functional tests are implemented to demonstrate that function is restored even if the mechanism of action is only partially understood; optimal effective amounts of cell-based medicinal products needed to achieve desired effects are also defined. Pharmacokinetics considerations include parameters of cell biodistri-

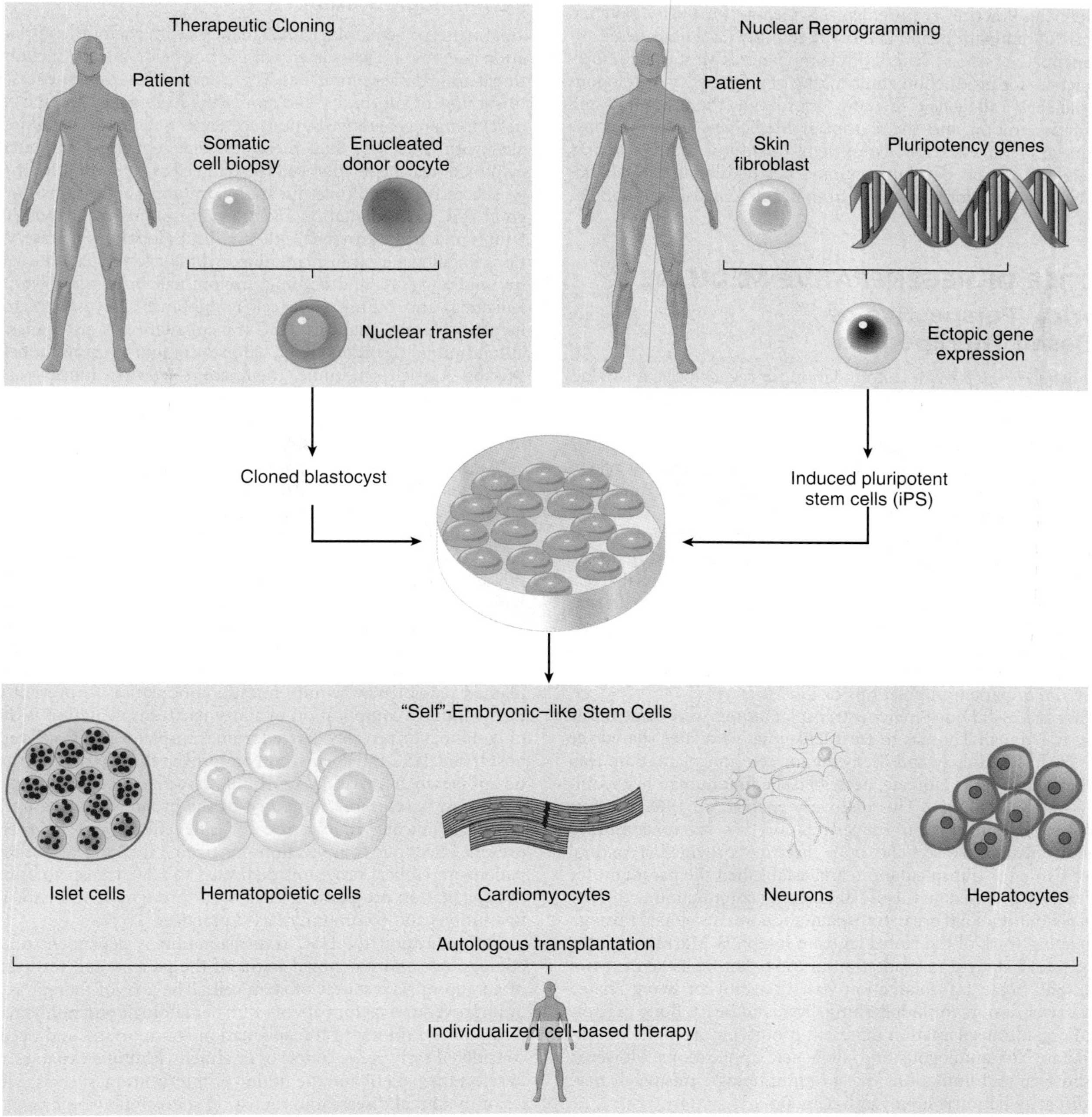

FIGURE 94-8 • Bioengineered stem cells. Pluripotent stem cells that function like embryonic stem cells can be engineered from adult somatic cells through "therapeutic cloning" or "nuclear reprogramming." Therapeutic cloning combines the nuclear content of a somatic cell obtained from an adult biopsy with cytoplasmic/plasmalemma components from an enucleated donor oocyte. Transfer of the somatic cell nucleus into the remnant of the fertilized egg is performed by micromanipulation. This process results in cloned cells, instructed by the oocyte cytoplasm, that develop into a blastocyst allowing harvest of embryonic stem cells from the inner cell mass (ICM). Alternatively, nuclear reprogramming of fibroblast cells from adults can be achieved through transient ectopic expression of four genes (*OCT4* and *SOX2* with either *NANOG* and *LIN28* or *KLF4* and *c-Myc*) to produce pluripotent cells with embryonic stem cell features, called induced pluripotent stem cells (iPS). The resulting bioengineered stem cells obtained from both approaches are bona fide pluripotent cells as demonstrated by their ability to independently produce an entire organism from embryonic to adult stages of development. Importantly, the tissues derived from these engineered stem cells are genetically similar to the original somatic cell biopsy. This technology produces autologous, embryonic-like stem cells that may enable individualized cell-based therapy.

bution/migration, cellular viability/persistence, and cellular proliferation/differentiation following single- or multiple-dose administrations. Clinical efficacy studies are designed to adequately demonstrate efficacy in target patient populations using clinically relevant end points and/or surrogates; to demonstrate an appropriate dose schedule to result in optimal therapeutic effect; to evaluate the duration of therapeutic effect; and to allow benefit: risk assessment. Clinical safety databases are developed to annotate any common adverse events, including risk assessment of the therapeutic procedure, immune response, infection, malignant transformation, and long-term safety related to the product.[36]

Cell-based medicinal products often involve cell samples of limited amount mostly to be used in a patient-specific manner. This raises specific issues pertaining to quality control testing designed for each product under examination. The manufacturing of cell-based medicinal products is carefully designed and validated to ensure product consistency and traceability.[36] Control and management of manufacturing and quality control testing are performed according to "Good

Manufacturing Practice" requirements. Screening for purity, potency, infectious contamination, and karyotype stability have become necessary elements (i.e., release criteria) in compliance with standard operating practices for production and banking of cells used as autologous or "off-the-shelf" allogeneic therapy. Accordingly, the U.S. Food and Drug Administration and the European Medicines Agency impose regulatory guidelines for risk assessment, quality of manufacturing, preclinical and clinical development, and postmarketing surveillance of stem cell biologics for translation from bench to bedside to populations.[36,37]

PRACTICE OF REGENERATIVE MEDICINE

Historical Perspective of Cell-Based Therapeutics

Transplant medicine provides a foundation for regenerative medicine. The traditional aim of transplantation is to substitute defective tissue, in the face of end-stage disease, with a functional alternate. With advances in cell, tissue, and organ transplantation, strategies of replacement with "used" tissues have evolved into emerging goals of regeneration and rejuvenation with "new" tissues (see Fig. 94-2). Transplant medicine has enhanced the management of otherwise untreatable disease, such as end-stage leukemia, cirrhosis, and kidney or cardiopulmonary failure. While providing successes for individual patients, the availability, resource demand, and cost restrict the universal access to organ transplantation. Stem cell–based therapy provides an alternative solution. Yet, current challenges limit translation to clinical practice. This includes control of stem cell differentiation, choice of cell type and mode of delivery, efficacy of treatment, mechanism of benefit, and selection of patient populations or disease states.

The first successful bone marrow transplantations were done in the 1950s by E. Donnall Thomas to treat leukemia, who later shared the Nobel Prize in Physiology and Medicine for cell transplantation. Jean Dausset, another Nobel laureate, described the first human histocompatibility antigens in 1958. This discovery enabled, in 1968, the first successful nonidentical twin transplantation for severe combined immunodeficiency disease. The bone marrow provided a natural source of tissue for transplantation, and established the paradigm for reparative therapy based on the use of HSCs. In conjunction with early cell transplantation, solid organ transplantation was developed through the pioneering work of the Nobel laureate Joseph E. Murray, with the first successful kidney transplantation in 1954. Through the next two decades, solid organ transplantation was successful for living-related and/or cadaver donors for kidney, lung, liver, and heart. Bone marrow and solid organ transplantation represent prototypic examples of cell-based therapy for autologous and allogeneic applications. However, donor shortage and limitations due to immunologic mismatch have caused disparity between supply and demand.

Future therapies aim to cure refractory genetic and degenerative diseases while minimizing invasive procedures, improve immunologic tolerance, provide preemptive therapy before irreversible damage, and diminish the burden of organ/stem cell shortage. Current priorities focus on discovery of stem cell subpopulations from autologous and allogeneic sources that function as tissue-specific progenitors. MSCs are leading the way for clinical applications due to accessibility in peripheral blood, bone marrow, and adipose tissue in addition to their immunotolerant status, multipotent differentiation capacity, favorable in vitro growth characteristics, and encouraging safety/efficacy data in clinical transplantation.

Evidence for Current Practice of Regenerative Medicine

Ongoing efforts in translating preclinical discovery of stem cell biology into paradigms of regenerative medicine encompass clinical practice across medical specialties. Regenerative practice is largely based on the experience with HSC transplantation, currently the only standard of care among stem cell–based therapeutic modalities.

Hematologic System

Treatments of hematologic malignancies with chemotherapy and radiation therapy are associated with serious side effects, including life-threatening damage to tissues. These destructive consequences, leading to significant morbidity and mortality, have generated the need for developing regenerative options to rescue bone marrow failure associated with otherwise fatal therapies. The sequential combination of cytotoxic treatments followed by stem cell regeneration has proven to be successful in multiple diseases. Common applications for autologous HSC transplantation include diffuse large cell non-Hodgkin's lymphoma, acute myeloid leukemia, and Hodgkin's disease. Applications for allogeneic transplantation include selected patients with acute myeloid leukemia and chronic myeloid leukemia, acute lymphocytic leukemia, and diffuse large cell lymphoma.[38] Beyond treatment of hematologic malignancies, HSC transplantation is also considered in autoimmune disorders (e.g., severe combined immunodeficiency, Wiskott-Aldrich syndrome, rheumatoid arthritis, mutiple sclerosis), amyloidosis, severe anemia (i.e., aplastic anemia, Fanconi's anemia, sickle cell anemia, Blackfan-Diamond anemia), thalassemia major, and inborn errors of metabolism.[30]

The standard procedure involves collection and isolation of stem cells, myeloablative preparation of the patient, and stem cell transplantation (Fig. 94-9). Stem cells are harvested from bone marrow or peripheral blood following stimulation with the stem cell mobilizing factor G-CSF. Stem cells may be pooled from multiple collections, purged of detrimental cell types such as cancer cells or allogeneic lymphocytes, and stored in cryopreservation systems. Timed in accord with myeloablative treatments, transplantation is performed with intravenous infusion of stem cells that engraft upon guided migration to niche environments within the recipient bone marrow. The transplanted patient may require immunomodulation to prevent GVHD. This common complication in allogeneic transplantation is the result of lymphocytic progeny derived from transplanted stem cells attacking host tissue. HSC transplantation has proven to be a valuable therapeutic option when the risk of morbidity associated with allogeneic transplantation is favorable compared to the prognosis of the underlying disease. Clinically monitoring for side effects and intervening to prevent infectious complications determine the long-term success for patients in clinical programs dedicated to HSC transplantation. HSC transplantation programs are deployed throughout academic medical institutions and community-based practices.

The indication for HSC transplantation is dependent on disease etiology, age and functional status of the patient, and the availability of an appropriate source of stem cells. The goal of therapy is to cure or improve survival for patients with hematologic and nonhematologic diseases. The timing of transplantation is important, and needs to be considered early in the course of treatment. Multiple variables are used to select the patient and the timing of intervention, such as cytogenetics of the initial disease and remission status following myeloablation during the preparative phase of treatment.[38] Although HSC transplantation is an effective treatment and provides the only option for a cure in many hematologic malignancies, many patients elect to first undergo standard chemotherapeutic regimens and consider HSC transplantation if remission is not achieved or the disease relapses. As recognized by the National Cancer Institute and Center for International Blood and Marrow Transplant Research, only one third of appropriate patients are identified and undergo HSC transplantation in a timely manner.

The American Society for Blood and Marrow Transplantation has established evidence-based guidelines for five diseases that have the best evidence to support HSC transplantation: diffuse large cell B-cell lymphoma, multiple myeloma, acute lymphoblastic leukemia in pediatric and in adult populations, and acute myeloid leukemia in children. Specifically, patients with diffuse large cell B-cell lymphoma treated with autologous bone marrow transplantation demonstrate an overall response rate of 84% compared to 44% after salvage chemotherapy alone, with a 5-year survival rate that increases from 12% to 46% with addition of autologous HSC transplantation as demonstrated in the large randomized clinical trial, PARMA.[39] Multiple myeloma patients

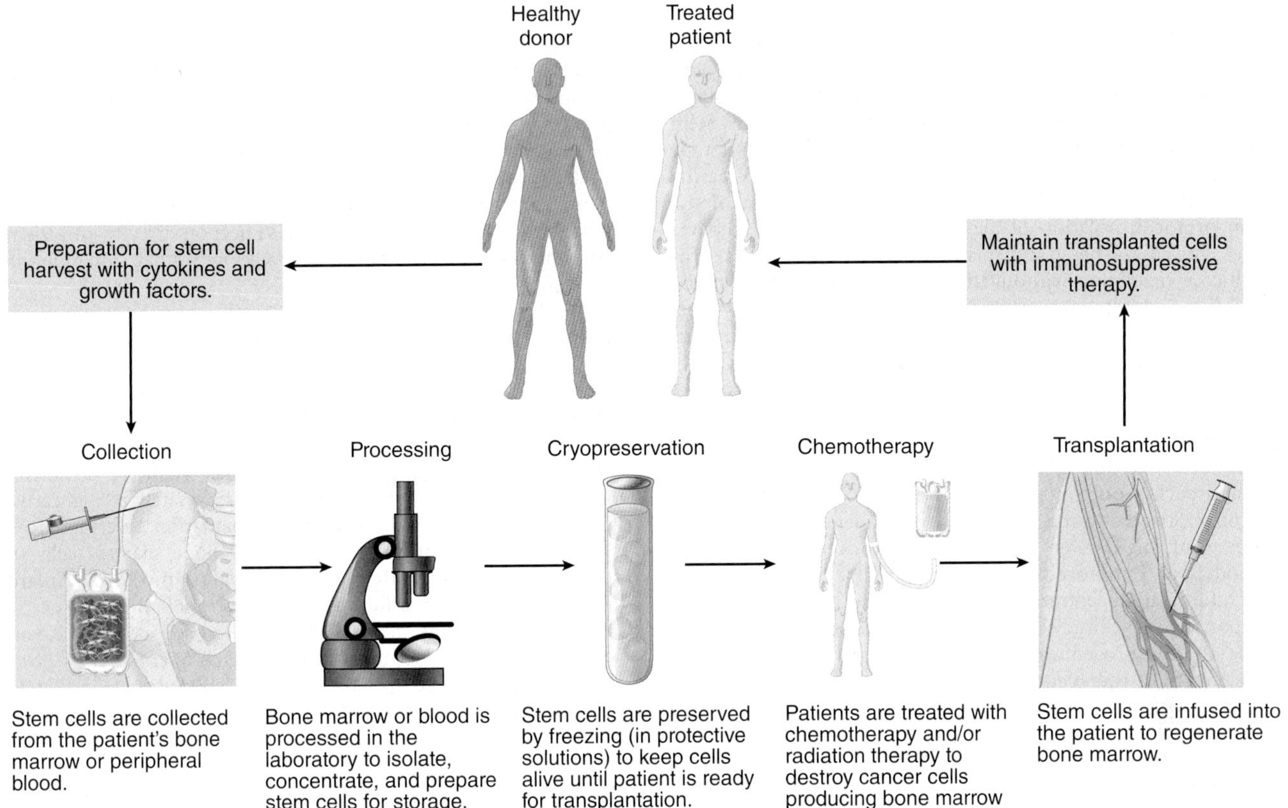

FIGURE 94-9 • **Hematopoietic stem cell transplantation.** Allogeneic transplantation of bone marrow–derived stem cells to reconstitute functional bone marrow in patients occurs sequentially. In preparation for stem cell harvest, healthy donors undergo treatment with growth factors to increase production and mobilization progenitor cells from the bone marrow. The first stage of the process involves collection of peripheral blood or aspiration of bone marrow from the donor. The tissue is then processed to purify the progenitor populations and prepared for long-term storage in cryopreservation systems. Once appropriate stem cells in sufficient quantities have been secured, the patient is treated with chemotherapy and/or radiation therapy to produce disease remission that results in myeloablation and complete bone marrow failure. Upon confirmation that disease remission has been achieved, the patient receives a hematopoietic stem cell infusion. Successful reconstitution of cellular lineages is usually evident within 2 to 3 weeks following transplantation. Patients then require immunosuppressive therapies to maintain graft survival. This sequence outlines a typical hematopoietic stem cell transplantation procedure, exemplifying a currently accepted application of regenerative medicine.

undergoing autologous bone marrow transplantation compared to standard chemotherapy have an increased response rate of 38% versus 14%, respectively, that translates into significantly longer event-free survival.[40] Acute lymphoblastic leukemia in both pediatric and adult populations has been treated with HSC transplantation with success using allogeneic transplantation.[41,42] Pediatric patients with acute myeloid leukemia have significantly increased disease-free survival following allogeneic stem cell transplantation compared to chemotherapy.[43] In this way, experiences with HSC transplantation serve as a useful paradigm for emerging applications of regenerative medicine and stem cell–based therapy.

Skeletal System

Adult skeletal tissues are constantly undergoing rejuvenation that involves endogenous stem cells replacing end-stage cells. Bone turnover is a dynamic process determined by the balance between cellular destruction from osteoclasts, and cellular formation from osteoblasts. Multipotent progenitor cells (see Table 94-2) such as mesenchymal stem cells are derived from bone marrow and provide ongoing osteogenesis, chondrogenesis, and adipogenesis.[28,44,45] Genetic disorders such as osteogenesis imperfecta have been treated with bone marrow stem cells, and demonstrate new osteoblasts forming lamellar bone that results in fewer fractures and enhanced body growth for children infused with cell-based therapies.[46] Commonly diagnosed osteoarthritis has few therapeutic options other than conservative palliation to manage long-term pain. MSCs infused into the knee joint at the time of surgery are a feasible, safe, and potentially efficacious intervention. A large number of surgeries are dedicated to repairing damaged or lost cartilage in joints that could be augmented with cellular regeneration. In fact, autologous chondrocyte implantation represents one of the first commercially available product lines for cell-based therapies. This technology is currently being employed to treat degenerative joint disease by harvesting autologous chondrocyte progenitors from articular cartilage plugs, followed by cellular expansion and subsequent surgical implantation. Bone marrow–derived stem cells have demonstrated promising preclinical results for multiple future applications of bone, cartilage, and tendon repair in orthopedics.

Endocrine System

Diabetes mellitus is a progressive disease with devastating long-term consequences. The juvenile form of diabetes, or type 1 diabetes, relates to the inability of the body to regulate glucose levels due to autoimmune-mediated destruction of pancreatic beta cells in the islets of Langerhans responsible for production of insulin. Clinical complications such as retinopathy, nephropathy, and neuropathy can be managed in part through intensive monitoring and daily titration of insulin therapy to maintain glucose levels within the physiologic range. In practice, only 50% of patients have glucose levels adequately maintained despite state-of-the-art clinical management. Diabetes mellitus serves as a prototypic target disease that may be amendable to cell-based regenerative therapies since partial replacement of a single dysfunctional cell type would be sufficient to cure the disease.[47]

Pancreas transplantation has enabled patients to become independent of insulin injections with de novo production of insulin. The concept of islet cell transplantation was introduced in patients undergoing pancreatectomy, in which autologous islet cells are isolated and infused into the portal circulation to allow engraftment of ectopic cells in the liver. As few as one third of the functional islet cells of the pancreas, or about 300,000 cells, are required to establish physiologic regulation of insulin production. This provides impetus to justify stem cell–based applications for diabetes mellitus, as cell-based therapy could provide a cost-effective and lasting solution for the increasing unmet clinical need of diabetic patients.[48] After the advent of the Edmonton protocol, isolation of allogeneic islet cells from cadaver organs has allowed cell-based transplantation to produce similar efficacy of glucose regulation without the complications of solid organ transplantation.[49] Multiple academic centers have collectively performed more than 1000 islet cell transplantations with a 1-year graft survival rate of approximately 60% to 90% and insulin independence rates of approximately 20% to 40%. However, the large number of islet cells required and the shortage of donors limit the integration of this technology into standard clinical practice for the increasing number of patients affected by this disease.[50]

Three approaches now in the preclinical stage could address the shortage of appropriate progenitor cells for diabetes mellitus. First, xenografts using pig-derived islet cells have proven efficacious in animal models, and improved glucose tolerance has been reported in diabetic children upon cotransplantation with pig Sertoli cells and neonatal porcine islet cells. Second, allogeneic stem cell therapy using embryonic or adult progenitor cell populations offers a continuously renewable source of therapeutic cells. However, optimization of differentiation, expansion, and insulin production is required before clinical translation is possible. The third approach is autologous cell-based therapy with bioengineered progenitor cells derived from nonpancreatic tissue using gene therapy or other approaches to engineer functional production of insulin from autologous cell types such as hepatocytes. These technologies have remained in the preclinical stages to date, but will likely provide significant advancements in the management of diabetes through cell-based therapy.

Cardiovascular System

The primary myocardial response to stress has been traditionally described as hypertrophy or enlargement of cardiomyocytes, rather than hyperplasia or increase in cell number. Hence, regeneration of the heart with de novo tissue production was considered nonphysiologic. The dogma that cardiomyocytes are derived during early development and maintained throughout adult life established the concept that myocardium lost during ischemic injury resulted in irreversible damage and fibrosis. This paradigm was challenged by emerging evidence, however, including that bone marrow–derived stem cells are capable of infiltrating adult myocardium and contributing to cardiomyocyte regeneration.[51] These critical observations originated from the study of male patients who had received heart transplants from female donors. Y chromosomes detected in the donated hearts indicated that noncardiac mobile cells from the male host had infiltrated the female transplanted hearts and contributed to new tissue formation. Furthermore, these cells had demonstrated properties based on protein expression to suggest they had differentiated into cell types of the cardiac lineage. These observations were the nidus to challenge the previously well-established concept that the heart was postmitotic and did not have the capacity to regenerate.[52] Initial functional studies using bone marrow–derived stem cells demonstrated significant improvement in cardiac performance through presumed repair mechanisms such as de novo cardiogenesis and vasculogenesis. These provocative results mandated clinical trials to test the safety and feasibility of stem cell transplantation in cardiac disease (Fig. 94-10).[53,54]

Autologous skeletal myoblasts were the initial cell type used in refractory heart disease.[55] Approximately 9×10^8 myoblasts were obtained from muscle biopsy and transplanted into the myocardium during open-heart surgery. Ventricular tachycardia was recognized as a possible side effect of therapy. However, patients reported improvement in symptoms significant enough to decrease their heart failure class score, and had improvement in left ventricular ejection fraction. Subsequent Phase I trials have used lower concentrations of myoblasts, and have demonstrated a lower incidence of ventricular arrhythmias.[56] The longest follow-up to date has been 5 years, which demonstrated stable improvement in clinical status and a significant decrease in hospitalizations for heart failure, while the risk of arrhythmia was appropriately controlled with medical therapy and/or device implantation.[57] A placebo-controlled, multicenter Phase III clinical trial (MAGIC) recently demonstrated significant decrease in left ventricular diameter after 6 months, indicative of improved remodeling in patients with heart failure following myoblast injection directly into the myocardium, despite no significant change in systolic function of the treated heart muscle.[58]

The TOPCARE-AMI trial was designed to test the safety and feasibility of cell transplantation after acute myocardial infarction using circulating or bone marrow–derived progenitor cells.[59] Initial studies demonstrate a safe clinical profile without ventricular arrhythmia, thrombus formation, distal embolization or dissection of coronary artery throughout a 1-year follow-up period. Furthermore, serial magnetic resonance imaging (MRI) of the left ventricle demonstrated improvement in ejection fraction of approximately 8% as early as 4 months, and up to 12 months after transplantation. Safety and feasibility were independently confirmed using bone marrow cells transplanted into patients with a large ST-elevation myocardial infarction (STEMI).[60] The first randomized clinical trial, BOOST, examined patients after having a STEMI that involved successful treatment by percutaneous stent placement into a single coronary artery.[61] Five days after optimal management according to standard medical practice, patients were treated with autologous bone marrow cell therapy and demonstrated a 6.7% improvement in ejection fraction compared to less than 1% improvement in the medically managed control cohort at 6 months' follow-up. However, the significance of left ventricular function improvement in stem cell–treated patients was not sustained at 18-month follow-up. The ASTAMI trial limited the inclusion criteria to acute myocardial infarction involving the left anterior descending coronary artery and randomized patients to receive bone marrow mononuclear cells via coronary artery delivery.[62] After a 6-month follow-up period, no significant difference between groups was detected in global left ventricular function. However, this randomized, open-labeled study involving 100 patients confirmed the low risk of cell transplantation without increased risk of thrombosis, restenosis, or arrhythmia, and importantly showed significant improvement in exercise time and heart rate responses.[63]

Two Phase II randomized clinical trials consisting of 200 patients in a multi-institutional study (REPAIR-AMI)[64] and 67 patients in a STEMI study,[65] not only randomized patients but also performed placebo injections in the control group via a similar coronary artery catheter approach. The primary outcome of functional improvement as measured by ejection fraction was significantly increased by 5.5% with cell transplantation in the REPAIR-AMI study compared to 3.0% in the placebo group at 4 months. In a subgroup analysis, it was suggested that initial ejection fraction of less than 49% had a significant benefit to cellular transplantation when compared to patients with baseline ejection fraction of greater than 49%. The STEMI study demonstrated significant decrease in left ventricular infarct size as measured by MRI but was unable to demonstrate any significant increase in left ventricular function between the placebo control and cell transplantation groups. Moreover, transendocardial injection of autologous bone marrow mononuclear cells in patients with end-stage ischemic heart disease has also been demonstrated to produce a durable therapeutic effect and improve myocardial perfusion and exercise capacity.[65]

To date, over 1000 patients with ischemic heart disease have received stem cell therapy in a clinical trial setting worldwide.[66] Meta-analysis collectively indicates the safety profile of stem cell–based therapy, with modest improvements in functional parameters and apparent benefit in structural remodeling.[67] Ongoing optimization of the most appropriate cell type, selection of patient populations amendable to cell-based therapy, timing of intervention, and route of administration are the areas of focus to determine the clinical utility of cell-based therapy in cardiovascular disease.

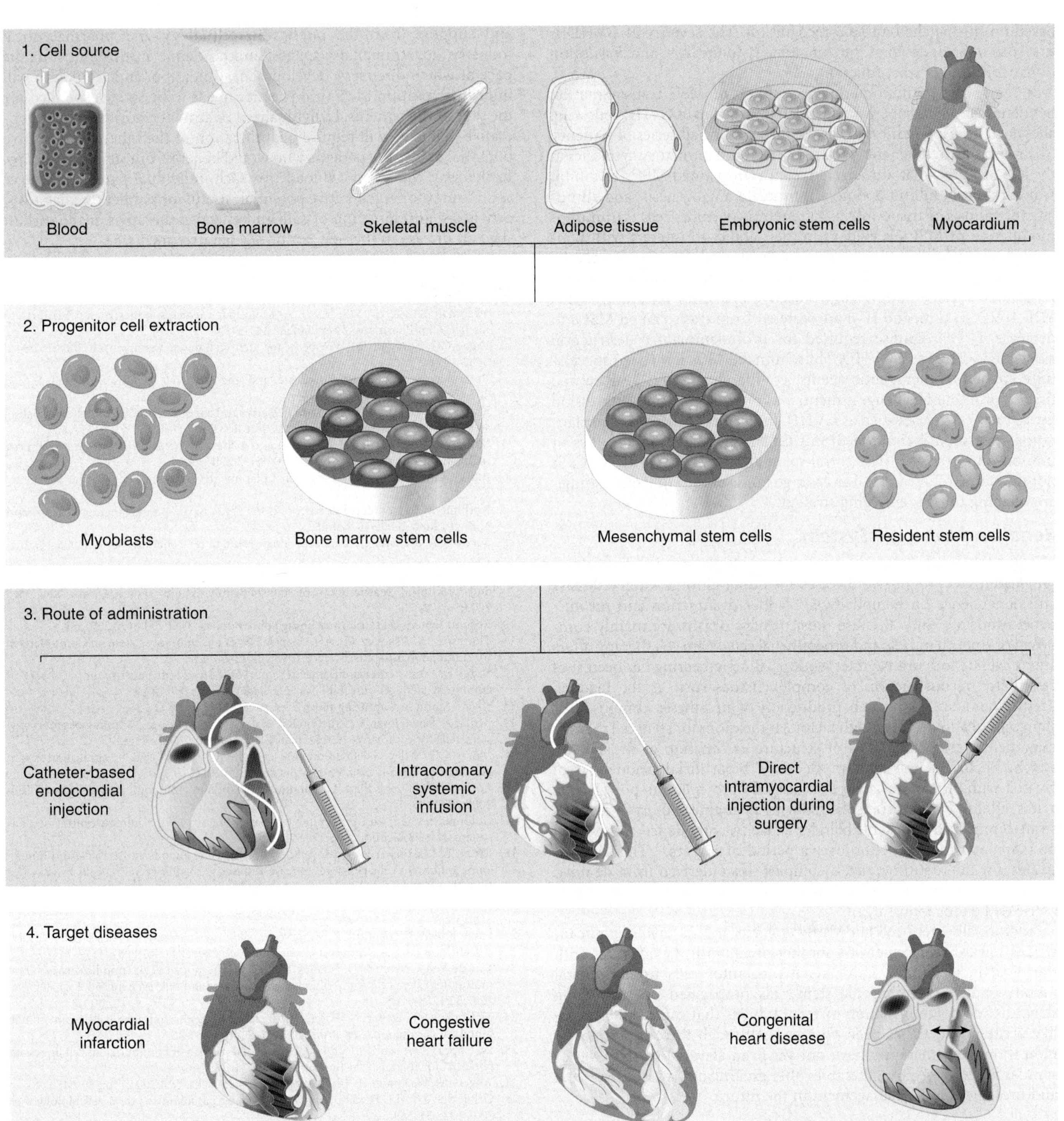

FIGURE 94-10 • Stem cell therapy for cardiovascular disease. Cell-based therapy for cardiovascular disease provides a paradigm for emerging applications of regenerative medicine, and as such is the subject of ongoing optimization to identify algorithms that yield the safest and most effective treatment outcomes. Multiple cell sources have been used in preclinical and clinical trials. They range from established adult sources, including more recently resident stem cells, to experimental embryonic stem cell pools. Progenitor cell extraction ensures the highest quality of cells and determines tissue-specific regenerative potential. The route of administration requires careful planning primarily based on the target disease and anticipated timing of therapy. Ultimately, appropriately selected patient populations may determine the success of specific cell-based therapy.

Allergy and Immunologic System

Immune modulation has been a critical key to successful treatment for many diseases. Organ transplantation illustrates the success of immunosuppressive agents in which allogeneic transplantation is tolerated by the host and enables long-term survival of transplanted non-self tissues. The delicate balance between complete immunosuppression leading to life-threatening infections and insufficient immunosuppression leading to acute or chronic rejection of tissue graft is a common issue for all patients having undergone allogeneic bone marrow transplantation. A particularly aggressive side effect commonly seen with potent immunosuppression is GVHD, in which the transplanted T, B, and natural killer cells begin to attack nontransplanted host tissue based on mismatched antigen recognition. The severity of GVHD is first seen in breakdown of the skin, toxicity to the liver, and disruption of gastrointestinal tract function.

Recently, the immunomodulation ability of MSC transplantation has demonstrated a superior efficacy in prevention of GVHD following allogeneic transplantation in case reports and small series of patients. The mechanism of benefit is related to anti-inflammatory cytokines at the site of injury that are secreted from transplanted MSCs to inhibit scar formation, inhibit apoptosis, stimulate angiogenesis, and stimulate the mitosis of tissue-intrinsic stem or progenitor cells.[28] Immunomodulation of MSCs is evident in their ability to interact with lymphocytes and inhibit the response of naive and memory T cells by increasing production of the $CD4^+$ subpopulation of suppressor CD25 regulatory T cells. Additionally, bioactive cytokines including PGE2, SDF-1, VEGF, IL-6, and IL-8 are secreted from transplanted MSCs to decrease T-cell response required for proinflammatory destruction associated with severe GVHD. Thus, human MSCs have been successfully applied as therapeutic agents to differentiate and heal injured tissues, promote HSC engraftment, and provide immunosuppression for refractory diseases such as GVHD. Indications for MSC transplantation may soon include recurrent GVHD refractory to all types of immunosuppression.[30] The cotransplantation of HSCs with MSCs is not the standard of care; however, large randomized controlled studies are ongoing for this emerging strategy.

Renal and Urologic System

The genitourinary system is exposed to multiple injuries throughout life, leading to progressive diseases including chronic kidney disease and dependence on hemodialysis, bladder dysfunction and incontinence, and infertility. Because most urinary organs are mainly composed of smooth muscle and uroepithelial cells, stem cell therapy offers a new avenue for curative interventions. Bioengineering has been successful for reconstruction of complex tissues such as the bladder, urethra, and ureter through production of prostheses composed of stem cells, scaffold, and growth factors. Indications for stem cell therapy may include permanent loss of structure or function of the urinary system, including the bladder. Recently, bioartificial bladders were created with autologous stem cells seeded onto collagen–polyglycolic acid scaffolds. Patients transplanted with an engineered organ demonstrated improved and stable bladder capacity, compliance, intravesical pressure, and renal function over a period of 5 years.[68] This demonstrates, for the first time, that a complex tissue derived from de novo stem cells and artificial scaffolds is sufficient to replace the function of a diseased endogenous organ.

Additionally, stem cell and tissue engineering has made significant strides toward replacement of another organ with the advances with the bioartificial kidney. Using renal progenitor cells from neonatal rabbits or cloned embryonic stem cells propagated on scaffolding structure, de novo formation of renal tubules that can excrete urine-like waste products has been observed. Although these experimental indications and therapies have not yet been elevated to the level of standard care, these novel therapies offer exciting new avenues for renal and urologic disease management in the future.

FUTURE PROSPECTS

Regenerative medicine, built on emerging discoveries in stem cell biology, has begun to define the scope of future clinical practice. Regenerative medicine and stem cell biology cross all disciplines of medicine, and provide a universal paradigm of curative goals based on scientific discovery and clinical translation. The challenges to realize the full potential of stem cell biology remain substantial even to the most optimistic physicians/scientists, and require integration of multidisciplinary expertise to form a dedicated regenerative pharmacology community of practice (see Fig. 94-1). Building on the foundation of transplant medicine, regenerative medicine will continue to expand and implement technologies to treat new diseases at earlier stages with safer and more effective outcomes, not possible with current pharmacotherapies. Progress in this field will proceed with significant interest and support from the public, biotechnology and pharmaceutical industry, governmental agencies, and academic institutions, but the pace at which discovery, development, validation, and regulation will impact translation to clinical practice needs to be safely expedited for the sake of the patients. Individualized treatment algorithms for regenerative medicine will require quantification of the inherent reparative potential to identify patients who would benefit from stem cell therapy. In this way, the "stem cell load" for each individual patient will serve as an "index for regenerative potential" useful for prediction, diagnosis, prognosis, and targeting of safe and effective therapies at the earliest stage of disease in the new era of regenerative medicine.

REFERENCES

1. Waldman SA, Terzic MR, Terzic A. Molecular medicine hones therapeutic arts to science. Clin Pharmacol Ther 2007;82:343-347.
2. Daley GQ, Scadden DT. Prospects for stem cell-based therapy. Cell 2008;132:544-548.
3. Rosenthal N. Prometheus's vulture and the stem-cell promise. N Engl J Med 2003;349:267-274.
4. Klimanskaya I, Rosenthal N, Lanza R. Derive and conquer: sourcing and differentiating stem cells for therapeutic applications. Nat Rev Drug Discov 2008;7:131-142.
5. Morrison SJ, Spradling AC. Stem cells and niches: mechanisms that promote stem cell mainteneance throughout life. Cell 2008;132:598-611.
6. Atala A. Advances in tissue and organ replacement. Curr Stem Cell Res Ther 2008;3:21-31.
7. Kørbling M, Estrov Z. Adult stem cells for tissue repair—a new therapeutic concept? N Engl J Med 2003;349:570-582.
8. Surani MA, McLaren A. Stem cells: a new route to rejuvenation. Nature 2006;443:284-285.
9. Shizuru JA, Negrin RS, Weissman IL. Hematopoietic stem and progenitor cells: clinical and preclinical regeneration of the hematolymphoid system. Annu Rev Med 2005;56:509-538.
10. Rossant J. Stem cells and early lineage development. Cell 2008;132:527-531.
11. Thomson JA, Itskovitz-Eldor J, Shapiro SS, et al. Embryonic stem cell lines derived from human blastocysts. Science 1998;282:1145-1147.
12. Solter D. From teratocarcinomas to embryonic stem cells and beyond: a history of embryonic stem cell research. Nat Rev Genet 2006;7:319-327.
13. Silva J, Smith A. Capturing pluripotency. Cell 2008;132:532-536.
14. Behfar A, Perez-Terzic C, Faustino RS, et al. Cardiopoietic programming of embryonic stem cells for tumor-free heart repair. J Exp Med 2007;204:405-420.
15. Murry CE, Keller G. Differentiation of embryonic stem cells to clinically relevant populations: lessons from embryonic development. Cell 2008;132:661-680.
16. Koch CA, Geraldes P, Platt JL. Immunosuppression by embryonic stem cells. Stem Cells 2008;26:89-98.
17. Goldman S. Stem and progenitor cell-based therapy of the human central nervous system. Nat Biotechnol 2005;23:862-871.
18. Kroon E, Martinson LA, Kadoya K, et al. Pancreatic endoderm derived from human embryonic stem cells generates glucose-responsive insulin-secreting cells in vivo. Nat Biotechnol 2008;26:443-452.
19. Laflamme MA, Murry CE. Regenerating the heart. Nat Biotechnol 2005;23:845-856.
20. Fraidenraich D, Benezra R. Embryonic stem cells prevent developmental cardiac defects in mice. Nat Clin Pract Cardiovasc Med 2006;3(Suppl 1):S14-S17.
21. Van de Ven C, Collins D, Bradley MB, et al. The potential of umbilical cord blood multipotent stem cells for nonhematopoietic tissue and cell regeneration. Exp Hematol 2007;35:1753-1765.
22. McGuckin CP, Forraz N. Potential for access to embryonic-like cells from human umbilical cord blood. Cell Prolif 2008;41(Suppl 1):31-40.
23. De Coppi P, Bartsch G Jr, Siddiqui MM, et al. Isolation of amniotic stem cell lines with potential for therapy. Nat Biotechnol 2007;25:100-106.
24. Wagers AJ, Weissman IL. Plasticity of adult stem cells. Cell 2004;116:639-648.
25. Orkin SH, Zon LI. Hematopoiesis: an evolving paradigm for stem cell biology. Cell 2008;132:631-644.
26. Chamberlain G, Fox J, Ashton B, Middleton J. Mesenchymal stem cells: their phenotype, differentiation capacity, immunological features, and potential for homing. Stem Cells 2007;25:2739-2749.
27. Phinney DG, Prockop DJ. Mesenchymal stem/multipotent stromal cells: the state of transdifferentiation and modes of tissue repair. Stem Cells 2007;25:2896-2902.
28. Caplan AL. Adult mesenchymal stem cells for tissue engineering versus regenerative medicine. J Cell Physiol 2007;213:341-347.
29. Martinez C, Hofmann TJ, Marino R, et al. Human bone marrow mesenchymal stromal cells express the neural ganglioside GD2: a novel surface marker for the identification of MSCs. Blood 2007;109:4245-4248.
30. Le Blanc K, Ringdén O. Immunomodulation by mesenchymal stem cells and clinical experience. J Intern Med 2007;262:509-525.
31. Jaenisch R, Young R. Stem cells, the molecular circuitry of pluripotency and nuclear reprogramming. Cell 2008;132:567-582.
32. Yang X, Smith SL, Tian XC, et al. Nuclear reprogramming of cloned embryos and its implications for therapeutic cloning. Nat Genet 2007;39:295-302.
33. Nakagawa M, Koyanagi M, Tanabe K, et al. Generation of induced pluripotent stem cells without Myc from mouse and human fibroblasts. Nat Biotechnol 2008;26:101-106.

34. Park IH, Zhao R, West JA, et al. Reprogramming of human somatic cells to pluripotency with defined factors. Nature 2008;451:141-146.
35. Waldman SA, Christensen NB, Moore JE, Terzic A. Clinical pharmacology: the science of therapeutics. Clin Pharmacol Ther 2007;81:3-6.
36. Committee for Medicinal Products for Human Use. Guideline on Human Cell-Based Medicinal Products (EMEA/CHMP/410869/2006). London: European Medicines Agency, 2007, pp 1-24.
37. Halme DG, Kessler DA. FDA regulation of stem-cell-based therapies. N Engl J Med 2006;355:1730-1735.
38. Copelan E. Hematopoietic stem-cell transplantation. N Engl J Med 2006;354:1813-1826.
39. Hahn T, Wolff SN, Czuczman M, et al. The role of cytotoxic therapy with hematopoietic stem cell transplantation in the therapy of diffuse large cell B-cell non-Hodgkin's lymphoma: an evidence-based review. Biol Blood Marrow Transplant 2001;7:308-331.
40. Hahn T, Wingard JR, Anderson KC, et al. The role of cytotoxic therapy with hematopoietic stem cell transplantation in the therapy of multiple myeloma: an evidence-based review. Biol Blood Marrow Transplant 2003;9:4-37.
41. Hahn T, Wall D, Camitta B, et al. The role of cytotoxic therapy with hematopoietic stem cell transplantation in the therapy of acute lymphoblastic leukemia in children: an evidence-based review. Biol Blood Marrow Transplant 2005;11:823-861.
42. Hahn T, Wall D, Camitta B, et al. The role of cytotoxic therapy with hematopoietic stem cell transplantation in the therapy of acute lymphoblastic leukemia in adults: an evidence-based review. Biol Blood Marrow Transplant 2006;12:1-30.
43. Oliansky DM, Rizzo JD, Aplan PD, et al. The role of cytotoxic therapy with hematopoietic stem cell transplantation in the therapy of acute myeloid leukemia in children: an evidence-based review. Biol Blood Marrow Transplant 2007;13:1-25.
44. Baksh D, Song L, Tuan RS. Adult mesenchymal stem cells: characterization, differentiation, and application in cell and gene therapy. J Cell Mol Med 2004;8:301-316.
45. Caplan AI. Mesenchymal stem cells: cell-based reconstructive therapy in orthopedics. Tissue Eng 2005;11:1198-1211.
46. Krampera M, Pizzolo G, Aprili G, Franchini M. Mesenchymal stem cells for bone, cartilage, tendon and skeletal muscle repair. Bone 2006;39:678-683.
47. Soria B, Bedoya FJ, Tejedo JR, et al. Cell therapy for diabetes mellitus: an opportunity for stem cells? Cells Tissues Organs 2008;188:70-77.
48. Robertson RP. Islet transplantation as a treatment for diabetes. N Engl J Med 2004;350:694-705.
49. Shapiro AM, Lakey JR, Ryan EA, et al. Islet transplantation in seven patients with type 1 diabetes mellitus using a glucocorticoid-free immunosuppressive regimen. N Engl J Med 2000;343:230-238.
50. Shapiro AM, Ricordi C, Hering BJ, et al. International trial of the Edmonton protocol for islet transplantation. N Engl J Med 2006;355:1318-1330.
51. Anversa P, Nadal-Ginard B. Myocyte renewal and ventricular remodelling. Nature 2002;415:240-243.
52. Leri A, Kajstura J, Anversa P, Frishman WH. Myocardial regeneration and stem cell repair. Curr Probl Cardiol 2008;33:91-153.
53. Dimmeler S, Zeiher AM, Schneider MD. Unchain my heart: the scientific foundations of cardiac repair. J Clin Invest 2005;115:572-583.
54. Segers VF, Lee RT. Stem-cell therapy for cardiac disease. Nature 2008;451:937-942.
55. Menasché P, Hagège AA, Scorsin M, et al. Myoblast transplantation for heart failure. Lancet 2001;357:279-280.
56. Opie SR, Dib N. Surgical and catheter delivery of autologous myoblasts in patients with congestive heart failure. Nat Clin Pract Cardiovasc Med 2006;3(Suppl 1):S42-S55.
57. Hagège AA, Marolleau JP, Vilquin JT, et al. Skeletal myoblast transplantation in ischemic heart failure: long-term follow-up of the first phase I cohort of patients. Circulation 2006;114(Suppl I):I108-I113.
58. Menasché P, Alfieri O, Janssens S, et al. The Myoblast Autologous Grafting in Ischemic Cardiomyopathy (MAGIC) trial: first randomized placebo-controlled study of myoblast transplantation. Circulation 2008;117:1189-1200.
59. Schächinger V, Assmus B, Britten MB, et al. Transplantation of progenitor cells and regeneration enhancement in acute myocardial infarction: final one-year results of the TOPCARE-AMI Trial. J Am Coll Cardiol 2004;44:1690-1699.
60. Sánchez PL, San Román JA, Villa A, et al. Contemplating the bright future of stem cell therapy for cardiovascular disease. Nat Clin Pract Cardiovasc Med 2006;3(Suppl 1): S138-S151.
61. Drexler H, Meyer GP, Wollert KC. Bone-marrow-derived cell transfer after ST-elevation myocardial infarction: lessons from the BOOST trial. Nat Clin Pract Cardiovasc Med 2006;3(Suppl 1):S65-S68.
62. Lunde K, Solheim S, Aakhus S, et al. Exercise capacity and quality of life after intracoronary injection of autologous mononuclear bone marrow cells in acute myocardial infarction: results from the Autologous Stem cell Transplantation in Acute Myocardial Infarction (ASTAMI) randomized controlled trial. Am Heart J 2007;154:710.e1-710.e8.
63. Schächinger V, Erbs S, Elsässer A, et al, for the REPAIR-AMI Investigators. Intracoronary bone marrow-derived progenitor cells in acute myocardial infarction. N Engl J Med 2006;355:1210-1221.
64. Janssens S, Dubois C, Bogaert J, et al. Autologous bone marrow-derived stem-cell transfer in patients with ST-segment elevation myocardial infarction: double-blind, randomised controlled trial. Lancet 2006;367:113-121.
65. Perin EC, Dohmann HF, Borojevic R, et al. Improved exercise capacity and ischemia 6 and 12 months after transendocardial injection of autologous bone marrow mononuclear cells for ischemic cardiomyopathy. Circulation 2004;110(Suppl II):II213-II218.
66. Bartunek J, Vanderheyden M, Wijns W, et al. Bone-marrow-derived cells for cardiac stem cell therapy: safe or still under scrutiny? Nat Clin Pract Cardiovasc Med 2007;4(Suppl 1):S100-S105.
67. Abdel-Latif A, Bolli R, Tleyjeh IM, et al. Adult bone marrow-derived cells for cardiac repair: a systematic review and meta-analysis. Arch Intern Med 2007;167:989-997.
68. Atala A. Recent applications of regenerative medicine to urologic structures and related tissues. Curr Opin Urol 2006;16:305-309.

INDEX

Note: Page numbers followed by f refer to figures; page numbers followed by t refer to tables; page numbers followed by b refer to boxes.

A

AAC-001, in Alzheimer's disease, 645t
Abacavir, in HIV infection, 1187–1188, 1189t
Abarelix, 632, 632t
  in prostate cancer, 952
Abatacept, 169t
  in rheumatoid arthritis, 1034
Abbreviations, for prescription, 1228–1229, 1228t, 1229t
Abciximab
  adverse effects of, 334–335, 918
  in coronary artery disease, 327b, 329f, 331t, 333–335, 333f
  in thrombosis, 918
Abetalipoproteinemia, 308
Abiotrophia defectiva, in infective endocarditis, 1131t, 1132
Abraxane, in breast cancer, 84, 937
ABT-874/J695, 169t
  in psoriasis, 1004
Acamprosate, in alcohol dependence, 825, 827t, 829
Acanthamoeba infection, corneal, 859
Acarbose, in diabetes mellitus, 559, 559f, 559t, 568
Accuracy, of analytic tests, 278–279, 278f
ACE inhibitors. *See* Angiotensin-converting enzyme (ACE) inhibitors
Acebutolol, 107t, 133f, 134
  in coronary artery disease, 347f, 347t, 350t
Acenoumarol, 230–231
Acetaminophen, 1223
  in children, 243
  in headache, 732t
  in osteoarthritis, 1018, 1018t
  in pain, 889t, 890
  toxicity of, 1213, 1214f
Acetohexamide, in diabetes mellitus, 562, 563t
N-Acetyl aspartylglutamate, 96
Acetylcholine, 92, 100–103, 118, 119–120, 119f. *See also at* Cholinergic
  in acid secretion, 458–459, 460f
  anatomic distribution of, 100
  cardiovascular effects of, 120
  degradation of, 93
  function of, 100
  gastrointestinal effects of, 120
  metabolism of, 100, 101f
  multiple effects of, 95
  receptors for, 100–102, 101f, 705t
    muscarinic, 101–102, 101f
    nicotinic, 100–101, 101f
  release of, 118
  synaptic storage of, 119
  synthesis of, 93t, 100, 101f
  as therapeutic target, 102–103, 102t
  therapeutic uses of, 120
Acetylcholinesterase, 93, 120–121
  plasma, 125
  receptor for, 135–136, 136f
Acetylcholinesterase inhibitors, 102t, 103, 121, 121f
  in Alzheimer's disease, 643–644, 644t
  anticholinergic effects of, 123
  in motility disorders, 479t, 481
  nicotine interaction with, 842t
  in Parkinson's disease, 659–660
Acetylcholinesterase inhibitors *(Continued)*
  pharmacodynamics of, 260
  pharmacokinetics, 260
  poisoning with, 123
  side effects of, 643
N-Acetylcysteine
  in acetaminophen toxicity, 1213
  in bacterial meningitis, 1117
  in mushroom poisoning, 1216
Acetylsalicyclic acid. *See* Aspirin (acetylsalicylic acid)
N-Acetyltransferase, 373
N-Acetyltransferase 2, 220, 220f
Acid-base balance, 149–150
Acid secretion, 457–461
  acetylcholine and, 458–459
  cellular regulation of, 458–460, 460f
  central regulation of, 457–458
  disorders of, 461–462, 461t, 462t
    treatment of, 462–471
      antacids in, 462–463
      anticholinergics in, 462–463
      bismuth in, 467
      gastric acid inhibitors in, 462–467, 464t
      H_2-receptor antagonists in, 463–464, 464t
      mucosal protective agents in, 467
      prostaglandin analogues in, 467
      proton pump inhibitors in, 464–467, 465f, 465t
      sucralfate in, 467
  gastrin and, 459, 460f
  ghrelin and, 459
  histamine and, 459, 460f
  H^+,K^+-ATPase and, 460–461, 460f
  leptin and, 459–460
  nitric oxide and, 459
  peripheral regulation of, 458–460
  somatostatin and, 459, 460f
Acidosis, in renal insufficiency, 437
Acitretin, in psoriasis, 993, 1000t, 1002f
Acne, 973–980, 974f
  classification of, 978, 978b
  pathophysiology of, 973–975
  scars with, 974
  treatment of, 974–980
    antiandrogens in, 978
    approach to, 973, 978–979, 978b, 979b, 979t
    dapsone gel in, 980
    laser therapy in, 979–980
    nutritional therapy in, 973, 980
    oral antibiotics in, 975t, 977–978, 977f
    photodynamic therapy in, 973, 979–980
    topical antibiotics in, 975t, 976–977, 977f
    topical retinoids in, 974–976, 975f, 975t, 976f, 978–979, 979t
Acne conglobata, 974
Acquired immunodeficiency syndrome. *See* Human immunodeficiency virus (HIV) infection
Acrolein, toxicity of, 166
Acromegaly, 617–619
  hypertension with, 296
  treatment of, 618–619, 618t, 619f
Activators of G protein signaling (GS), 71
Active pharmaceutical ingredient, 21
Acute coronary syndrome, 321, 322–323, 322f. *See also* Myocardial infarction
  aspirin in, 328–329
Acute myelogenous leukemia. *See also* Hematologic malignancy
  mitoxantrone-related, 691
  oblimersen in, 87
Acute stress disorder, 773t
Acyclovir, 183
  adverse effects of, 189t, 190
  in herpes simplex virus infection, 1203, 1203t
  in human herpesvirus infection, 184t, 185t
  indications for, 188
  mechanism of action of, 186
  resistance to, 190
  spectrum of activity of, 187–188
Acyl-coenzyme A:cholesterol transferase (ACAT) inhibitors, in dyslipidemia, 316
Adalimumab, 159t, 168
  in inflammatory bowel disease, 496, 497, 498
  in psoriasis, 997, 997f, 1000t, 1002f, 1003, 1003f
  in rheumatoid arthritis, 1033, 1033t
  side effects of, 168, 496
Adamantanes
  in avian influenza, 1069
  in influenza, 1065–1066, 1066f
Adapalene, in acne, 975t, 976, 976f
Adaptor proteins, 74
Adderall, in attention-deficit/hyperactivity disorder, 760–761, 761t, 762t
Addiction. *See* Drug addiction
Addison's disease, 626
α-Adducine, pharmacogenetics of, 228t
Adefovir dipivoxil
  adverse effects of, 189t, 190
  in hepatitis B virus infection, 187, 536, 536f, 538t, 539
  resistance to, 190
Adenoma
  adrenal, 629
  pituitary, 616–619, 617f, 618t
Adenosine, 371t, 380
  adverse effects of, 375t, 380
  in supraventricular tachycardia, 378–379, 380
Adenosine A1 receptor agonists, in headache, 739
Adenosine monophosphate, cyclic (cAMP), 71–72, 72f
Adenosine triphosphate (ATP)–binding cassette transporter, 270, 271f, 272t
S-Adenosylhomocysteine, 899
S-Adenosylmethionine, 899
Adenovirus infection, 1075–1076, 1076f
Adenylyl cyclase, 70, 71, 72f
Adherence, patient, 1226, 1226b
Adhesion molecule inhibitors, in inflammatory bowel disease, 499
Adipose tissue, β-adrenergic receptor antagonist effects on, 134–135
Adjustment disorder, 773t
Adjuvants, for vaccine, 1249
Adp53, 1304
Adrenal crisis, 627
Adrenal gland
  disorders of, 623–629. *See also specific disorders*
  hormones of. *See* Glucocorticoid(s); Mineralocorticoids
  pheochromocytoma of, 627–629
Adrenal insufficiency, 626–627

Adrenalectomy
in Conn's syndrome, 629
in Cushing's syndrome, 624
α-Adrenergic receptor, 106, 106f, 126, 128t
polymorphisms in, 136–137, 136f
β-Adrenergic receptor, 106, 106f, 126, 128t
polymorphisms in, 136f, 137
α-Adrenergic receptor agonists, 107, 107t, 127f, 128t, 129f, 130
in attention-deficit/hyperactivity disorder, 766, 766t
in baroreflex failure, 716, 716b
in dysautonomias, 710t, 712
in glaucoma, 860
in hypertension, 298
neurotransmitter receptor response to, 705t
in nicotine dependence, 832, 844t, 845
in opioid dependence, 828t
in pain, 891
for sedation, 880–881
in voiding dysfunction, 453
β-Adrenergic receptor agonists
age-related pharmacokinetics of, 262
in asthma, 420–423, 421f, 421t
cardiovascular effects of, 423
in COPD, 420–423, 421f, 421t
hypokalemia with, 423
inhalational delivery of, 422
long-acting, 422
mechanism of action of, 422
mortality with, 423
safety of, 422
short-acting, 422
tachyphylaxis with, 423
tremor with, 422
in voiding dysfunction, 446t, 452, 453
α-Adrenergic receptor antagonists, 131–132, 132f
age-related pharmacokinetics of, 262
in hypertension, 298
in pheochromocytoma, 628
in stroke prevention, 748
in voiding dysfunction, 446t, 447–448, 447f
β-Adrenergic receptor antagonists, 132–135, 133f, 371t, 372t. *See also specific drugs*
adverse effects of, 135, 346t, 349, 375t
in arrhythmias, 383–384
cardiovascular effects of, 134
contraindications to, 349, 349b
in coronary artery disease, 134, 345–351, 347f, 347t, 348b, 349b, 349f, 350t, 362b
dosing for, 350–351, 350t
drug interactions with, 349–350, 730t
gender-related pharmacodynamics of, 253
in glaucoma, 860
in headache prevention, 734–735, 734t
in heart failure, 349, 389–390, 391b, 391t
in hepatic cirrhosis, 511–512, 512t
historical perspective on, 7
in hypertension, 297t, 298
in hyperthyroidism, 580
mechanism of action of, 345–346
metabolic effects of, 134–135
in migraine prevention, 135
ocular effects of, 135
overdose of, 351
in panic disorder, 775
pharmacogenetics of, 230
pharmacokinetics of, 134, 346, 347f, 347t
age and, 262
in pheochromocytoma, 628, 629
respiratory effects of, 134
in stroke prevention, 748
in thyroid storm, 583t
verapamil interaction with, 730t
in voiding dysfunction, 453
withdrawal syndrome with, 135, 376t
Adrenocorticotropic hormone (ACTH)
corticosteroid effects on, 161
disorders of. *See* Cushing's disease; Cushing's syndrome
in gout, 1040t, 1041
synthesis of, 623, 624f
tumor secretion of, 619
Adverse event(s). *See also at specific drugs*
case report of, 37t, 38
case series of, 37t, 38
in children, 246–247
definition of, 35
drug-drug interactions and, 265–272, 272b, 272t
clarithromycin and digoxin, 270, 270b
cyclosporine and St. John's wort, 269
lovastatin and grapefruit juice, 269, 269b
repaglinide and gemfibrozil, 270, 270b
tamoxifen and CYP2D6, 269–270
terfenadine and ketoconazole, 265–268, 266f, 267f, 267t, 268b, 268t
gender and, 253–254
observational studies of, 37t, 39
in older patient, 262–263, 263f
registry for, 37t, 38
reporting of, 35–39, 36f, 37t. *See also* Pharmacovigilance
historical perspective on, 31
risk management plan and, 24–25, 25t, 34–35
unexpected, 35
Aesculus hippocastaneum, 1239t
Afterdepolarization, delayed, 369, 369f, 369t
Age/aging, 257–263
adverse events and, 262–263, 263f
cardiovascular changes with, 261–262
central nervous system changes with, 259–261, 260t
cutaneous changes with, 257–258
drug distribution and, 258
drug elimination and, 259
drug metabolism and, 258–259, 258f
pharmacodynamics and, 259–262, 260t, 261t, 262b
pharmacokinetics and, 257–259, 258f
vaccination and, 1259–1260
Age-related macular degeneration, 861, 861t
Agitation, in dementia, 647, 647b, 647t
Agmatine, 97, 111
Agonists, 52, 63–64, 64f. *See also* Ligand; Receptor-ligand interaction
Agoraphobia, 773t
Agranulocytosis, thionamide-related, 580–581
AIDS. *See* Human immunodeficiency virus (HIV) infection
AIDSLINE, 42t
Airway
obstruction of. *See* Asthma; Chronic obstructive pulmonary disease (COPD)
tone of, 417–419, 418f
Akt pathway, 80
Albendazole, in helminth infection, 1171–1172, 1172f
Albuterol, 107t, 128t, 130, 420–423, 421f, 421t
inhalational, 421t, 422
mechanism of action of, 422
side effects of, 422–423
Alcohol
abuse/use of, 818, 819t, 821
screening for, 826
stroke and, 745t, 747–748
treatment of, 826–829, 832
acamprosate in, 825, 827t, 829
behavioral, 826
disulfiram in, 825, 828t, 829
metronidazole in, 828t
naltrexone in, 825, 827t, 829
withdrawal management in, 824–825, 824t, 825t, 828
Alcohol *(Continued)*
blood pressure effects of, 714
hypertension with, 295
kava interaction with, 1241
toxicity of, 1213–1215, 1214f, 1215f
Aldosterone
deficiency of, 626
excess of, 629
regulation of, 626, 626f
synthesis of, 623, 624f
Aldosterone receptor antagonists
in coronary artery disease, 354–357, 356t, 357b
in heart failure, 389, 394–395, 394b, 394t
Alefacept, in psoriasis, 997–998, 997f, 1000t, 1002f, 1003f
Alemtuzumab
in hematologic malignancy, 948, 1283
in multiple sclerosis, 698
in transplantation, 1282–1283
Alendronate, 599–600, 599f
Alfacalcidol, 596–597
Alfentanil, in pain, 886
Alfuzosin, 128t, 132, 446t
Alinidine, 354
Alkylating agents, in small cell lung cancer, 925
All-trans retinoic acid, in hematologic malignancy, 946
Allergic contact dermatitis, 1008, 1011
Allergy
aspirin, 330, 917
barbiturate, 878–879
evaluation of, 1225
local anesthetic, 865
methotrexate, 166
penicillin, 178, 1124–1125
quinine, 1151
thiopurine, 163
urokinase, 919
Allium sativum, 1238, 1239t
Allopurinol
azathioprine interaction with, 494
drug interactions with, 162, 494, 1042
in gout, 1041–1042, 1041t
6-mercaptopurine interaction with, 494
side effects of, 1042
thiopurine interaction with, 162
Almotriptan, 109, 728f, 729t, 730t
Alosetron, 109, 110t
gender-related pharmacodynamics of, 253
in motility disorders, 481
Alpha-methyl-*p* tyrosine, 105t
Alprazolam, 99
in generalized anxiety disorder, 775t
in panic disorder, 774, 774t
in posttraumatic stress disorder, 778
St. John's wort effect on, 1241t
in social anxiety disorder, 779, 779t
Alprenolol, 134
Alteplase
in acute myocardial infarction, 919
in coronary artery disease, 340–343, 340t
in stroke, 743–744, 919
in thromboembolism, 918–919
Alternative medicine. *See* Dietary supplements
Aluminum, toxicity of, 1217, 1217t
Aluminum carbonate gel, 1222
Aluminum hydroxide, in hyperphosphatemia, 437, 438t
Alveolar hemorrhage, in systemic lupus erythematosus, 1057
Alvimopan, in motility disorders, 483
Alzheimer's disease, 641–643, 642f, 643b
apathy in, 647
behavioral manifestations of, 647, 647b, 647t
depression in, 647
diagnosis of, 641–643

Alzheimer's disease *(Continued)*
genetic factors in, 643
motor symptoms in, 646
treatment of, 643–647
anti-inflammatory drugs in, 645–646
cholinesterase inhibitors in, 643–644, 643f, 644t
estrogen replacement therapy in, 646
herbal formulations in, 646
HMG CoA reductase inhibitors in, 646
investigational agents in, 645, 645t, 646
N-methyl-D-aspartate receptor antagonists in, 644–645, 644t, 645f
pharmacodynamics of, 260
pharmacokinetics of, 260
vitamin E in, 645
Amanita phalloides poisoning, 1216
Amantadine, 97t, 98
adverse effects of, 189t, 190
in influenza, 187, 1065–1066
in multiple sclerosis, 696t, 697
in Parkinson's disease, 659
pharmacokinetics of, 186
resistance to, 190
Ambrisentan, in pulmonary arterial hypertension, 407t, 410, 410t
Amenorrhea, hypothalamic, functional, 614, 620
American College of Physicians Journal Club, 43–44, 44t
Amikacin, 174t
creatinine clearance with, 176t
monitoring of, 276t
spectrum of activity of, 177
in tuberculosis, 1092t, 1102t
Amiloride, in hepatic cirrhosis, 514, 515t
L-Amino acid decarboxylase, 104
Aminobenzoic acid, 1222
γ-Aminobutyric acid (GABA), 92, 98–99
anatomic distribution of, 98
anesthetic-related release of, 874, 876f
function of, 98
in generalized anxiety disorder, 770, 772f
metabolism of, 98–99, 98f
in posttraumatic stress disorder, 771
receptors for, 98f, 99
synthesis of, 98, 98f
as therapeutic target, 99, 100t
γ-Aminobutyric acid (GABA)–benzodiazepine receptor complex, 849, 851f
γ-Aminobutyric acid transaminase, 93
Aminocaproic acid, 912–913
Aminoglutethimide
in breast cancer, 934
in Cushing's syndrome, 624f, 625, 625t
in prostate cancer, 952
Aminoglycosides, 174t
adverse effects of, 178t, 179t
in infective endocarditis, 1128–1129, 1131–1135, 1131t, 1133t, 1134t
mechanism of action of, 175
in pregnancy, 179t
resistance to, 178
spectrum of activity of, 177
toxicity of, 284
in tuberculosis, 1092t, 1096–1097, 1101t
Aminophylline, 1222
in asthma, 428–429
Aminosalicylates
drug interactions with, 492
in inflammatory bowel disease, 490–492, 491f, 491t, 497, 497t, 498
pharmacodynamics of, 491
pharmacokinetics of, 490–491
in psoriasis, 994–995, 1000t
in rheumatoid arthritis, 1032, 1032t
side effects of, 492
Amiodarone, 372t, 380–381
adverse effects of, 375t, 381
antiretroviral interaction with, 1197t
hypothyroidism with, 571
toxicity of, 372t, 381
in ventricular arrhythmias, 381
Amitriptyline, 103, 109, 110t
in headache prevention, 734t, 735
in multiple sclerosis, 696t
in Parkinson's disease, 659
in posttraumatic stress disorder, 777, 778t
St. John's wort effect on, 1241t
valproate interaction with, 730t
Amlodipine
age-related pharmacokinetics of, 262
in coronary artery disease, 351–353, 351t, 353t
in gout, 1044
in heart failure, 397–398, 397t
Ammonia, 150
Ammonium nitrite, in cyanide toxicity, 1215
Ammonium salt, urinary, 150
Amodiaquine, in malaria, 1148f, 1154
Amorolfine, 183t
Amoxicillin, 175t
creatinine clearance with, 176t
in infective endocarditis, 1125–1126
cAMP response element–binding protein, 72, 72f
Ampakines, 97, 97t
Amphetamine(s), 104, 105t, 107t, 127f, 130
abuse of, 819t, 823
in attention-deficit/hyperactivity disorder, 760–762, 761f, 761t, 762t
in hypersomnia, 852
intermediate-acting, 761t
long-acting, 761t, 762, 762t
short-acting, 760–762, 761t, 762t
side effects of, 765
Amphetamine salt preparation, 761, 762, 762t
Amphotericin B, 180t
adverse effects of, 182
in infective endocarditis, 1130
intrathecal, 181
mechanism of action of, 181
pharmacodynamics of, 180–181
pharmacokinetics of, 181
in protozoa infection, 1185
resistance to, 182–183
spectrum of activity of, 181
Ampicillin, 175t
creatinine clearance with, 176t
in infective endocarditis, 1125–1126
Ampicillin-sulbactam, in infective endocarditis, 1125–1126
Amprenavir, in HIV infection, 1191–1193, 1194t
Amrubicin, in small cell lung cancer, 926
Amyloid, in Alzheimer's disease, 641, 642f, 645t, 646
AN1792, in Alzheimer's disease, 645t
Anabolic agents, in osteoporosis, 603–604
Anabolic steroids, abuse of, 819t
Anadamide, 111
Anakinra, 169
in rheumatoid arthritis, 1035
Analgesia. *See* Pain, treatment of
Anastrazole, 636
in breast cancer, 934, 940–941
Androgen(s)
acne and, 973–974
adrenal, 627
deprivation of, in prostate cancer, 951–953, 953f
in renal insufficiency–associated anemia, 442
Androgen antagonists
in acne, 978
in prostate cancer, 953
Andropause, 255, 255f
Anemia, 895–902, 896b
aplastic, 901, 902b
copper-deficiency, 898
drug-related, 901–902, 901t, 902b
erythropoietin for, 903–905
folic acid–deficiency, 900
in hyperthyroidism, 578
in hypothyroidism, 573–574
iron-deficiency, 895–898, 896f
pathophysiology of, 896
prevalence of, 897t
treatment of, 897–898, 898t
pernicious, 898, 899–900
in renal insufficiency, 440–442, 441t
riboflavin-deficiency, 900, 901f
in systemic lupus erythematosus, 1056
vitamin A–deficiency, 900
vitamin B_6–deficiency, 900–901
vitamin B_{12}–deficiency, 898–900, 899f
vitamin C–deficiency, 900
vitamin-deficiency, 898–901, 901f
zinc-related, 898
Anesthesia
general, 873–882
goals of, 873–874
historical perspective on, 873
inhalational agents for, 874–878, 875f, 875t
intravenous agents for, 878–882, 879t
physiology of, 873
local, 863–870. *See also* Anesthetics, local
goals of, 865
physiology of, 863
Anesthetics
inhalational, 874–878, 875f, 875t. *See also specific anesthetics*
biotransformation of, 877–878
cardiac effects of, 876–877
CNS effects of, 877
critical volume hypothesis of, 874
elimination of, 874
fluidization theory of, 874
γ-aminobutyric acid release with, 874, 876f
hepatic effects of, 877
inspiratory concentration of, 874
malignant hyperthermia with, 878
metabolism of, 877–878
minimal alveolar concentration of, 876
pharmacodynamics of, 874, 876–878
pharmacokinetics of, 874
potency of, 876
renal effects of, 877
respiratory effects of, 876, 876f
toxicity of, 877–878
unitary hypothesis of, 874
uptake of, 874
ventilation effect on, 874
intravenous, 878–882, 879t. *See also specific drugs*
local, 863–870. *See also specific drugs*
acid-base properties of, 864
allergy to, 865
amide, 867–870, 868f, 868t, 869f, 870f
cardiac toxicity of, 864–865
classification of, 865–870, 866f, 866t, 867f, 868f, 868t, 869f, 870f
CNS toxicity of, 864
duration of action of, 864
ester, 866–867, 866f, 866t
indications for, 865
mechanism of action of, 863
methemoglobinemia with, 865
onset of action of, 864
in pain, 891
pharmacokinetics of, 864
potency of, 864
structure of, 863–864, 864f

Anesthetics *(Continued)*
tissue toxicity of, 865
toxicity of, 864–865
Angina, 324, 324f. *See also* Coronary artery disease
stable, treatment of, 322f, 325
unstable, 321, 322–323, 322f
treatment of, 322f, 325, 326f, 327b, 334f, 337b
β-adrenergic receptor antagonists in, 345–351, 347f, 347t, 348b, 349b, 349f, 350t
calcium channel blockers in, 351–353, 351t, 352b, 353t
clopidogrel in, 326f, 327b, 330, 332
nitrates in, 343–345, 344f, 345b, 346t
renin-angiotensin-aldosterone system inhibitors in, 354–357, 355t, 356t, 357b
Angiogenesis
gene therapy for, 1304–1305
inhibition of. *See* Antiangiogenesis agents
Angiotensin-converting enzyme (ACE), pharmacogenetics of, 228t
Angiotensin-converting enzyme (ACE) inhibitors, 354–357
adverse effects of, 346t, 357
aspirin interaction with, 330
contraindications to, 357
in coronary artery disease, 354–357, 355t, 356t, 357b
drug interactions with, 330, 357
gender-related pharmacodynamics of, 253
in heart failure, 389, 390–392, 392b, 392t
in hypertension, 297t, 298
mechanism of action of, 355
after myocardial infarction, 385
pharmacokinetics of, 355, 355t, 356t
age and, 262, 263
in renal insufficiency, 435–436
in stroke prevention, 748–749
Angiotensin II, 390–391
Angiotensin II receptor, 392–393
Angiotensin II receptor blockers
adverse effects of, 346t
age-related pharmacokinetics of, 262
in coronary artery disease, 354–357, 356t, 357b
in gout, 1043–1044
in headache prevention, 734t, 736
in heart failure, 389, 392–394, 393b, 393t
in renal insufficiency, 436
in stroke prevention, 748–749
Angiotensinogen, 390–391
Angiozyme, 1307
Anistreplase, in coronary artery disease, 340–343
Anorexiants
amphetamine-derived, 550–551
nonamphetamine, 551–552, 551t, 552t
Antacids
adverse effects of, 463
aspirin interaction with, 330
in gastroesophageal reflux disease, 468
in peptic ulcer disease, 462–463
Antagonist, 52, 52b, 63–64, 64f
Anthracyclines
in breast cancer, 936
in hematologic malignancy, 945–946
in prostate cancer, 954
in small cell lung cancer, 926
Anthralin, in psoriasis, 989, 999t
Anthrax vaccine, 1251, 1261
Anti-CD154, in systemic lupus erythematosus, 1061
Antiandrogens
in acne, 978
in prostate cancer, 953
Antiangiogenesis agents
in age-related macular degeneration, 861, 861t
in breast cancer, 938–939, 939f
in colon cancer, 962t, 965–966, 965f
hypertension with, 295
in non–small cell lung cancer, 955
Antiarrhythmic drugs, 369–385. *See also specific drugs*
adverse effects of, 374–377, 375t, 376f, 376t, 377f
in atrial fibrillation, 379, 379f
benefit-risk assessment of, 369–370
in cardiac arrest, 379–380
CAST (Cardiac Arrhythmia Suppression Trial) study of, 377
classification of, 371–372, 372t
cytochrome P-450 effects and, 373–374
definition of, 371–372
evaluation of, 374
evidence-based guidelines for, 378
ion channel interactions with, 372
mechanism-based selection of, 370–371, 371t
molecular targets for, 384–385
monitoring of, 276t
noncardiac adverse effects of, 374–375, 375t
pharmacokinetics of, 372–373, 373t
proarrhythmia effects of, 375–377, 376t
in supraventricular tachycardia, 378–379
in ventricular arrhythmias, 379–380
Antibacterial agents, 174–179, 174t, 175t. *See also specific agents*
in acne, 975t, 976–978, 979, 979t
adverse effects of, 178, 178t, 179t
area under the inhibitory curve of, 173–174
in bacterial meningitis, 1110–1112, 1112t, 1113t, 1116
in cervicitis, 1207, 1208t
in *Chlamydia trachomatis* infection, 1201–1202, 1202t, 1206
classification of, 174t, 175
in community-acquired pneumonia, 1083–1086, 1085t, 1086t
definition of, 173
in dermatitis, 1013
in endocarditis, 1123–1137. *See also* Infective endocarditis, treatment of
in gonococcal infection, 1206–1207, 1207t
in *Haemophilus ducreyi* infection, 1201, 1202t
in *Helicobacter pylori* infection, 469–470, 470t
in hepatic encephalopathy, 515–516, 516t, 520, 520f
hepatic metabolism of, 176–177
in *Klebsiella granulomatis* infection, 1202, 1202t
mechanism of action of, 175
monitoring of, 276t
ocular, 858–859, 859t
pharmacodynamics of, 173–174, 176
pharmacokinetics of, 173–174, 176
in pneumonia, 1083–1086, 1085t, 1086t
prophylactic, for infective endocarditis, 1137–1138, 1137b, 1137t
pulmonary bioavailability of, 1084
renal clearance of, 176, 176t
resistance to, 174, 178–179, 179f
sites of action of, 174–175, 174f
spectrum of activity of, 177–178
in spontaneous bacterial peritonitis, 519
susceptibility testing for, 173
in syphilis, 1204–1206, 1205t, 1206b, 1206t
teratogenicity of, 179t
in trichomoniasis, 1208, 1208b
in tuberculosis, 1090–1106. *See also* Tuberculosis, treatment of
in urethritis, 1206–1207, 1207t
in vaginitis, 1207–1208, 1208b
in vaginosis, 1208, 1209b, 1209t
in variceal bleeding, 517
Antibiotics. *See* Antibacterial agents
Antibody (antibodies)
anti-heparin, 916
anti–cyclic citrullinated peptide, 1026
antithyroid, 574
monoclonal. *See* Monoclonal antibodies
testing for, 13–14, 13f
Anticholinergics
in asthma, 423–424, 423f, 424t
in COPD, 423–424, 423f, 424t
in motility disorders, 478
ocular, 859, 860f
in Parkinson's disease, 659, 659t
in voiding dysfunction, 450–452
Anticholinesterase drugs. *See* Acetylcholinesterase inhibitors
Anticoagulants, 913–916. *See also* Heparin; Warfarin
in bacterial meningitis, 1115
in coronary artery disease, 335–343, 335t, 336f, 337b, 338b, 342f
drug interactions with, 914
in heart failure, 398
in pulmonary arterial hypertension, 407t, 408
in systemic lupus erythematosus, 1051t, 1058–1059
toxicity of, 1219–1220
Anticonvulsants, 666–679. *See also at* Seizure disorders *and specific anticonvulsants*
age-related pharmacodynamics of, 260, 260t
age-related pharmacokinetics of, 260, 260t
aspirin interaction with, 330
in bipolar disorder, 793–794
in headache, 723, 734t
in headache prevention, 735
monitoring of, 276t
in obesity, 554
in pain, 890–891
in panic disorder, 774–775
in posttraumatic stress disorder, 778
selection of, 677–679, 678f, 679f
side effects of, 666
in social anxiety disorder, 779, 779t
Anticytokines, in inflammatory bowel disease, 499
Antidepressants. *See also specific antidepressants*
age-related pharmacodynamics of, 260
cytochrome P-450 2D6 interaction with, 269
gender-related pharmacodynamics of, 253
in generalized anxiety disorder, 775–776, 775t
in headache prevention, 734t, 735
in insomnia, 850
monoamine oxidase inhibitor. *See* Monoamine oxidase inhibitors
neurogenesis and, 792
in obsessive-compulsive disorder, 754–756, 755t, 776–777, 776t
in pain, 891
in panic disorder, 772–774, 774t
in Parkinson's disease, 659
pharmacogenetics of, 229–230, 229f
pharmacokinetics of, age and, 260
in posttraumatic stress disorder, 777–778, 778t
in social anxiety disorder, 778–779, 779t
tricyclic. *See* Tricyclic antidepressants
in unipolar disorder, 788–792, 788f, 789f, 790t, 791f
in voiding dysfunction, 446t
Antidigoxin Fab fragment, 1216
Antidiuretic hormone (arginine vasopressin), 145, 146, 611, 613f, 613t
deficiency of, 611–613
exogenous. *See* Desmopressin
inappropriate secretion of, 613–614

Antidote(s), 1213–1220
  acetaminophen, 1213
  alcohol, 1213–1215
  aluminum, 1217
  Amanita, 1216
  arsenic, 1218
  cyanide, 1215–1216
  digoxin, 1216
  etylene glycol, 1214–1215
  iron, 1218
  lead, 1218
  manganese, 1218
  mercury, 1218–1219
  metal, 1216–1219, 1217t
  methanol, 1214–1215
  opioid, 1219
  warfarin, 1219–1220
Antiemetics, 479t, 481–482
Antiestrogens, 636
Antifibrinolytics, 912–913
Antifibrotic agents, in renal insufficiency, 436
Antifolates. *See also* Methotrexate
  cell cycle effects of, 83, 84f
  in malaria, 1155–1158, 1156f
  in non–small cell lung cancer, 922
Antifungal agents, 179–183, 179f, 180t. *See also specific antifungal agents*
  adverse effects of, 182, 182t
  mechanism of action of, 179f, 180
  pharmacodynamics of, 180–181
  pharmacokinetics of, 180–181
  resistance to, 182–183
  spectrum of activity of, 181–182
  susceptibility testing for, 183
  topical, 183, 183t
Antigenic drift, 1063, 1064f, 1068
Antigenic shift, 1063, 1064f
Antiglaucoma agents, 860–861, 861f
Antihistamines
  in dermatitis, 1013
  in insomnia, 850
Antihypertensives, 296–300, 297t, 299f. *See also* specific drugs
  in renal insufficiency, 439–440, 440f
  in stroke prevention, 748
Antilymphocyte immunoglobulin, 159t, 166–167, 166f
Antimalarials, 1145–1165. *See also* Malaria, treatment of
  in pregnancy, 1059t, 1060
  side effects of, 1055
  in systemic lupus erythematosus, 1051t, 1053–1055, 1054b, 1054t
Antimicrobials, 173–190. *See also* Antibacterial agents; Antifungal agents; Antiviral agents
  principles of, 173–174
Antioxidants
  in atrial fibrillation, 385
  in bacterial meningitis, 1117
Antiphospholipid antibody syndrome, 1058–1059, 1058b, 1059b. *See also* Systemic lupus erythematosus (SLE)
  in pregnancy, 1060
Antiplatelet agents, 325, 327–335. *See also specific agents*
  in coronary artery disease, 325, 327–335, 327b, 327f, 328f, 329f
  mechanisms of action of, 327–328, 329f
  in thrombosis, 917–918
Antipsychotics. *See* Neuroleptics
Antisense oligodeoxynucleotides, 1305–1308. *See also* Gene therapy, gene suppression
  in cancer, 1307–1308
  in cytomegalovirus retinitis, 1307
  protein interaction with, 1306–1307
Antithrombotic agents. *See* Anticoagulants; Fibrinolytic therapy
Antithymocyte globulin
  adverse effects of, 1281, 1282
  equine, 1281
  in hematologic malignancy, 948
  mechanism of action of, 1281
  rabbit, 1281–1282
  in transplantation, 1281–1282
Antiviral agents, 183–190, 184t. *See also specific antiviral agents*
  adverse effects of, 188–190, 189t
  in hepatitis B infection, 187, 187f, 188, 188f, 535–539, 537t
  in hepatitis C infection, 187, 188, 540–542, 541t
  in human herpesvirus infection, 186–187, 186f, 188
  indications for, 187, 188
  in influenza, 187, 188, 189f
  mechanism of action of, 186–187, 186f, 188f, 189f
  pharmacobiology of, 184–185, 184f
  pharmacokinetics of, 185, 185t
  resistance to, 190
  in respiratory syncytial virus infection, 1071
  spectrum of activity of, 187–188
Anxiety disorder(s), 769–780
  classification of, 771, 773t
  clinical features of, 772
  diagnosis of, 771, 773t
  generalized, 770, 772
    behavioral interventions in, 780
    treatment of, 775–776, 775t
  panic, 769–770, 771f, 773t
    behavioral interventions in, 780
    treatment of, 772–775, 774t
  pathophysiology of, 769, 770f, 771f, 772f
  posttraumatic, 770–771, 773t
    behavioral interventions in, 780
    nightmares in, 853–854
    treatment of, 777–778, 778t
  social, 771, 773t
    behavioral interventions in, 780
    treatment of, 778–779, 779t
  substance-induced, 773t
Anxiolytics, 99, 100t, 775–776, 775t
  abuse of, 819t
  age-related metabolism of, 259
  $GABA_A$ receptor binding of, 99
  in generalized anxiety disorder, 775t, 776
  in insomnia, 849, 851b
  in obsessive-compulsive disorder, 756, 776t, 777
  in panic disorder, 774, 774t
  in posttraumatic stress disorder, 778
  for sedation, 879–880
  in seizure disorders, 669–670
  side effects of, 669–670
  in social anxiety disorder, 779, 779t
  in voiding dysfunction, 448
Apathy, in dementia, 647
Aplastic anemia, hematopoietic stem cell transplantation in, 1274
apoA-I, mutations in, 308
Apo2L/TRAIL, 87, 87f
Apolipoprotein E, pharmacogenetics of, 228t
Apomab, 87–88, 87f
Apomorphine, in Parkinson's disease, 655, 656t
Apoptosis, 86–88
  extrinsic pathway of, 87–88, 87f
  intrinsic pathway of, 86–87, 87f
Appetite, regulation of, 549, 550f, 551f
Apremilast, in psoriasis, 1004
Aprepitant, in motility disorders, 479t
Aquaretics
  in hepatic cirrhosis, 521
  renal handling of, 153–154, 153t
Aqueous humor, 857, 858f, 859f
Arabinosyl transferase, 1095
Arachidonic acid, 111
Area under effect-time curve (AUC_e), 208
Area under the inhibitory curve (AUIC), 173–174
Argatroban
  in coronary artery disease, 339–340
  in thrombosis, 916–917
Arginine decarboxylase, 111
Arginine vasopressin, 145, 146, 611, 613f, 613t
  deficiency of, 611–613
  excess of, 613–614
  exogenous. *See* Desmopressin
Arginine vasopressin antagonists, 521, 614
Aripiprazole, 105, 105t, 110t, 806t, 807, 808f
  in bipolar disorder, 794
Aristolochic acid, 1241
Aromatase inhibitors, 636
  in breast cancer, 933–934, 940–941
Arrestin, 69
Arrhythmias, 367–385. *See also specific arrhythmias*
  cellular mechanisms of, 369, 369f, 369t, 370f
  definition of, 368
  diagnosis of, 374
  enhanced/abnormal automaticity in, 369
  in hyperthyroidism, 577
  local anesthetics and, 865
  mechanisms of, 367–369, 368f
  quinine-related, 1151
  reentry in, 369, 370f
  symptoms of, 374
  treatment of. *See also* Antiarrhythmic drugs
    approach to, 374–377, 375t, 376f, 376t, 377f
    implantable cardioverter-defibrillator in, 378
    nonpharmacologic, 377–378
    principles of, 369–374, 371t, 372t, 373t
    radiofrequency catheter ablation in, 377–378
  triggered automaticity in, 369, 369f, 369t
ARRY-142885, 86
Arsenic, toxicity of, 1217t, 1218, 1218f
Arsenic trioxide, in hematologic malignancy, 946
Artemether-lumefantrine, in malaria, 1149t, 1154–1155, 1158f, 1159, 1164, 1164t
Artemisinin derivatives, 1158–1160, 1158f
  adverse effects of, 1160
  drug interactions with, 1160
  neurotoxicity of, 1160
  in pregnancy, 1160
Arteries, age-related changes in, 261–262
Artesunate, in malaria, 1149t, 1158f, 1159, 1164, 1164t
Arthritis. *See also* Osteoarthritis; Rheumatoid arthritis
  crystalline. *See* Gout
  in inflammatory bowel disease, 488t
  psoriatic, 986, 1002–1004
  viral, vs. rheumatoid arthritis, 1027t
Artificial tears, 861
Arylamine-*N*-acetyltransferase 2, pharmacogenetics of, 227t
Ascaris infection, 1172f
  treatment of, 1171, 1174, 1175
Ascites
  diuretic-intractable, 509
  diuretic-resistant, 509
  in hepatic cirrhosis, 509, 518, 518f
  refractory, 509
  uncomplicated, 509
Ascorbate, in atrial fibrillation, 385
Ascorbic acid. *See* Vitamin C
L-Asparaginase, in hematologic malignancy, 946
Aspergillus infection, 180
  endocardial, 1136

Aspirin (acetylsalicylic acid), 1223
in acute coronary syndrome, 328–329
adverse effects of, 330, 331t, 917
angiotensin-converting enzyme inhibitor interaction with, 330
anticonvulsant interaction with, 330
with antihypertensive agents, 298
bleeding with, 330, 1223
clopidogrel with, 330
in coronary artery disease, 327b, 328–330, 329f, 331t, 362b
drug interactions with, 330
gender-related pharmacodynamics of, 253
hypersensitivity to, 330, 917
infective endocarditis and, 1130
low-dose, in myocardial infarction prevention, 328, 329
mechanism of action of, 53, 54f, 328
in myocardial infarction, 325, 328f
NSAID interaction with, 330
in osteoarthritis, 1020t
in pain, 889–890, 889t
pharmacokinetics of, 328
resistance to, 332
in stroke prevention, 746, 749–750
therapeutic considerations for, 328–330
in thrombosis, 917
Astemizole, azole interaction with, 182t
Asthma, 417–432
β-adrenergic receptor antagonist effects in, 134
aspirin-induced, 917
atopy in, 419
cell types of, 419
clinical manifestations of, 419–420
definition of, 417
gastroesophageal reflux disease and, 469
inflammation in, 419
pathophysiology of, 419
severity of, 417, 418t
spirometry in, 420
treatment of, 420–430
β-adrenergic agonists in, 420–423, 421f, 421t
alternative therapies in, 430
anticholinergics in, 423–424, 423f, 424t
in children, 430
chromones in, 428, 428t
corticosteroids in, 424–426, 425f, 425t
inhaled route for, 420b
integrated, 429–430, 429b
leukotriene modifiers in, 426–428, 427f, 427t
mortality with, 423, 425, 425f
novel therapies in, 430–431, 431t
in pregnancy, 430
xanthines in, 428–429
Astronauts, orthostatic symptoms in, 707
Asystole, adenosine-related, 380
Atazanavir, in HIV infection, 1191–1193, 1191f, 1194t
Atenolol, 107t, 128t, 133f, 134
in coronary artery disease, 347f, 347t, 350t
in headache prevention, 734t
Atherosclerosis, 305
coronary, 321–322, 322f. *See also* Coronary artery disease; Dyslipidemia; Myocardial infarction
renal, 295
stroke and, 746, 747f
ATI-7505, in motility disorders, 481, 482f
Atilmotin, in motility disorders, 482
Atipamezole, for dexmedetomidine reversal, 881
Ativin-like kinase type-1, in pulmonary arterial hypertension, 406
Atlizumab, in inflammatory bowel disease, 499
Atomoxetine, in attention-deficit/hyperactivity disorder, 765–766, 766t
Atopy, 419
Atorvastatin, 309–312, 312t, 358–361, 358t, 361b
adverse effects of, 311–312, 360t
azole interaction with, 182t
mechanism of action of, 309–311, 359f
pharmacogenetics of, 312
pharmacokinetics of, 311, 311t
trials of, 358, 359t, 360f
Atovaquone
in malaria chemoprophylaxis, 1164, 1165t
in malaria treatment, 1149t, 1160–1161, 1161f
in protozoa infection, 1181
Atracuronium, 102t, 125
Atrasentan, in prostate cancer, 956
Atrial fibrillation
clinical manifestations of, 374
in hyperthyroidism, 577, 582
stroke and, 745t
treatment of, 371t, 372, 379, 379f, 385
β-adrenergic receptor antagonists in, 384
amiodarone in, 381
diet in, 385
digoxin in, 384
flecainide in, 382
procainamide in, 383
propofenone in, 383
Atrial flutter, treatment of, 381, 382, 384
Atrial premature contractions, 368
Atrial tachycardia, 368, 374
Atrial tachypacing, in dysautonomias, 715
Atrioventricular nodal reentry, treatment of, 371t, 380
Atrioventricular reentry, treatment of, 371t, 380
Atropine, 102t, 103, 121, 122f, 423f
adverse effects of, 123
in anticholinesterase poisoning, 123
cardiovascular effects of, 122–123
central nervous system of, 121–122
mechanism of action of, 423–424
neurotransmitter receptor response to, 705t
ophthalmic effects of, 122
pulmonary effects of, 123
resistance to, 450
in voiding dysfunction, 446t, 450
Attention-deficit/hyperactivity disorder, 759–768
in adults, 767
diagnosis of, 759, 760b
pharmacogenomics of, 767, 767b
treatment of, 759–768
α-adrenergic receptor agonists in, 766, 766t
amphetamines in, 760–762, 761f, 761t, 762t
atomoxetine in, 765–766, 766t
bupropion in, 766, 766t
methylphenidates in, 761t, 762–765, 763f, 763t
nonstimulant medications in, 765–767, 766t
pemoline in, 766–767
psychostimulants in, 759–766, 760b, 761f, 761t
side effects of, 765, 765t
tricyclic antidepressants in, 766
Auditory event-related potentials, in schizophrenia, 801
Auspitz sign, 985
Autism, vaccines and, 1260–1261
Autoimmune disease, 157
Autonomic failure. *See also* Dysautonomias
in multiple system atrophy, 708
pure, 706t, 707–708
treatment of, 713–714, 713t
Autonomic nervous system, 115–137, 116f, 117t, 703, 704f. *See also* Parasympathetic nervous system; Sympathetic nervous system
disorders of. *See* Dysautonomias
functional organization of, 118
neuronal fibers of, 118, 118f
nonadrenergic-noncholinergic neurons of, 135
Autonomic nervous system *(Continued)*
organ system effects in, 116f, 117t, 118
pharmacogenomics of, 135–137
Autoreceptors, 118
presynaptic, 95
Avian influenza, 1068–1070, 1070f
5-Azacytidine, in hematologic malignancy, 945
Azathioprine, 161–163, 161f
adverse effects of, 163, 494, 1052, 1284
allergic reaction to, 163
allopurinol interaction with, 1042
aminosalicylate interaction with, 492
drug interactions with, 494, 1042, 1052, 1284
infection with, 163
in inflammatory bowel disease, 493–494, 493f, 497, 497t
leukopenia with, 163
mechanism of action of, 162, 1284
metabolism of, 161–162, 493, 1052
monitoring of, 162, 163
in multiple sclerosis, 692
pharmacodynamics of, 494
pharmacokinetics of, 161–162, 161f, 493, 1284
in pregnancy, 494, 1059t, 1060
in psoriasis, 995
in systemic lupus erythematosus, 1050, 1051t, 1052
in transplantation, 1284
Azelaic acid, in acne, 975t, 976, 979
Azithromycin, 174t
in cervicitis, 1208t
in chancroid, 1202t
in granuloma inguinale, 1202t
in malaria, 1162
in motility disorders, 479t
in nongonococcal urethritis, 1208t
in protozoa infection, 1185
Azoles, 180t
adverse effects of, 182
drug interactions with, 182, 182t, 265–268
mechanism of action of, 180
pharmacodynamics of, 181
pharmacokinetics of, 181
resistance to, 182–183
spectrum of activity of, 181
topical, 183t
Aztreonam, 176t, 177

B

B-lymphocyte activating factor, 1061
Bacitracin, 174f, 1222
ocular, 859t
Baclofen, 99, 100t
in alcohol dependence, 827t, 832
in headache prevention, 734t, 736
in multiple sclerosis, 696, 696t
in spasticity, 449
in voiding dysfunction, 446t, 448–449, 453
Bacteria, 173–174, 174f. *See also* Antibacterial agents
classification of, 174, 174f
Bacterial peritonitis, in hepatic cirrhosis, 509–510, 518–519, 519f
Bactericidal agent, 173
Bacteriostatic agent, 173
Balsalazide, in inflammatory bowel disease, 490–492, 491f, 491t
Bapineuzumab, in Alzheimer's disease, 645t
Barbiturates, 100t
abuse of, 819t
for anesthesia, 878–879, 879t
in seizure disorders, 666–667
Bariatric surgery, in dyslipidemia, 315

Baroreflex
  age-related changes in, 261
  failure of, 293, 293f, 706t, 709–710, 709f
    treatment of, 715–716, 716f
Barr body, 251
Basiliximab, 159t, 167
  in transplantation, 1283
Basophils, 895, 896f
Bay41-2272, in pulmonary arterial hypertension, 413
Bay58-2667, in pulmonary arterial hypertension, 413
Bayesian methods, 284–285
Bcl-2, 87, 87f
Bcl-2, therapeutic suppression of, 1307–1308
Beclomethasone, in asthma, 424–426, 425t
Bed-wetting, 854
Behavioral therapy
  in drug addiction, 826
  in generalized anxiety disorder, 780
  in nicotine dependence, 846, 846t
  in obsessive-compulsive disorder, 754–755, 780
  in panic disorder, 780
  in posttraumatic stress disorder, 780
  in social anxiety disorder, 780
Belatacept, 169t, 1288
Belimumab, in rheumatoid arthritis, 1035
Benazepril
  in coronary artery disease, 354–357, 355t, 357b
  in heart failure, 390–392, 392b, 392t
Benefit-risk assessment, 29–31
  in drug development, 26–27, 27f
Benign prostatic hyperplasia, 449–450
Benserazide, 104, 105t
Benzathine penicillin, in syphilis, 1204, 1205t
Benzbromarone, in gout, 1044
Benzene, anemia with, 901
Benzimidazole, in protozoa infection, 1185
Benzocaine, 866t, 867, 867f
Benzodiazepines, 99, 100t
  abuse of, 819t
  age-related metabolism of, 259
  $GABA_A$ receptor binding of, 99
  in generalized anxiety disorder, 775t, 776
  in insomnia, 849, 851b
  in obsessive-compulsive disorder, 776t, 777
  in panic disorder, 774, 774t
  in posttraumatic stress disorder, 778
  for sedation, 879–880, 879t
  in seizure disorders, 669–670
  side effects of, 669–670
  in social anxiety disorder, 779, 779t
  in voiding dysfunction, 448
Benzoyl peroxide, in acne, 975t, 976–977, 977f, 979, 979t
Benzphetamine, in obesity, 551
Benztropine, in Parkinson's disease, 659, 659t
Beraprost, in pulmonary arterial hypertension, 407t, 409, 409t
Best Pharmaceuticals for Children Act (2002), 20, 26
Betamethasone, in inflammatory bowel disease, 492–493, 492t
Betaxolol, 134
  in coronary artery disease, 350t
  in glaucoma, 860
Bethanechol, 102t, 119–120, 119f
  in motility disorders, 479t
  therapeutic uses of, 120
  in voiding dysfunction, 445–447, 446t
Bevacizumab, 861
  in breast cancer, 938–939, 939f
  in colon cancer, 962t, 965–966, 965f
  in non–small cell lung cancer, 955
Bezafibrate, in dyslipidemia, 314–315, 314t
BG-12, in multiple sclerosis, 698
Bicalutamide, in prostate cancer, 953
Bicarbonate, renal handling of, 143f, 149–150, 150f
Bichloracetic acid, in human papillomavirus infection, 1210b, 1211
Bicuculline, 99
Biguanides
  in diabetes mellitus, 561, 562f
  in malaria, 1157
Bilberry, 1239t
Bile acid sequestrants
  in dyslipidemia, 312–313, 313t, 360t
  niacin with, 314
  in renal insufficiency, 442, 442t
Bile acid transport inhibitors, in dyslipidemia, 316
BILN 2061, in hepatitis C virus infection, 541t, 542
Bimatoprost, in glaucoma, 861
Bioavailability, 197–199, 198f
  absolute, 199
  relative, 199
Bioequivalence, 199
Biologics, 13–14, 13f, 26. *See also* Monoclonal antibodies; Tumor necrosis factor-α antagonist
Biomarkers
  in drug monitoring, 285–286, 285f
  in drug testing, 13, 22–23
Bionic baroreflex system, in dysautonomias, 715
Biopharmaceuticals, testing of, 13–14, 13f
Bipolar disorder, 787–788, 788f
  in dementia, 647
  treatment of, 788, 792–794, 792f
    antipsychotics in, 794
    carbamazepine in, 792f, 794
    divalproex in, 792f, 793
    lamotrigine in, 792f, 793
    lithium in, 792–793, 792f
    oxcarbamazepine in, 792f, 794
BIRB-769, in inflammatory bowel disease, 499
Bisacodyl, in constipation, 480t
Bismuth, 467
Bisoprolol, 134
  in coronary artery disease, 347f, 347t, 350t
  in heart failure, 389–390, 391b, 391t
Bisphosphonates
  in hypercalcemia, 595
  in osteoporosis, 598–601, 599f, 605
  in prostate cancer, 955
  side effects of, 599
Bithionol, in helminthic infection, 1178
Bivalirudin, 916
  in coronary artery disease, 339–340
Black cohosh, 1238, 1239t, 1241t
Bladder
  acrolein effects on, 166
  antimuscarinic effects on, 123
  bioartificial, 1330
  dysfunction of. *See* Voiding dysfunction
  facilitated emptying of, 445–449, 446t, 447f, 448f
  facilitated storage in, 449–454, 451t
  ganglionic blocker effect on, 123–124
  innervation of, 447f, 448f
  outlet obstruction of, 449
Blastocystis hominis infection, 1178
Bleeding. *See also* Hemostasis, disorders of
  abciximab-related, 918
  aspirin-related, 330, 1223
  dietary supplements and, 1241
  fibrinolytic-related, 343
  fondaparinux-related, 339
  glycoprotein IIb/IIIa receptor antagonist–related, 334–335
  heparin-induced, 336–337, 338
  uterine, estrogen therapy and, 639
  variceal, 516–518, 517f
Bleomycin, in hematologic malignancy, 946
Blood-aqueous barrier, 857
Blood-brain barrier, amino acid passage across, 92
Blood-brain/CSF barrier, 1109
Blood flow, renal, 142–143, 142f
Blood pressure
  catecholamine effects on, 127–128, 128t, 129f
  high. *See* Hypertension
  low. *See* Hypotension
Blood-retina barrier, 857
Blood transfusion, in transplantation, 1271
BMS387032, cell cycle effects of, 84, 84f
Bone
  loss of. *See* Osteoporosis
  in osteoarthritis, 1016, 1017f
  in osteomalacia, 593
  Paget's disease of, 595, 601, 603, 605
  peak mass of, 593
  physiology of, 593–595, 594f
  reabsorption of, 594, 594f
    in hyperthyroidism, 578
    parathyroid hormone levels and, 590
  remodeling of, 593–594, 594f
  in rickets, 591, 593
  subchondral, 1016
  vitamin D effects on, 592
Bone marrow, stem cells of, 1320t, 1322–1323, 1323f
Bone marrow transplantation, 1320t, 1322–1323, 1323f
  in hematologic malignancy, 1274–1275, 1326–1327, 1327f
Bone mineral density, 593
  decrease in. *See* Osteoporosis
  depot MPA effects on, 638
Bone morphogenetic protein-7, in renal insufficiency, 436
Bone morphogenetic protein receptor II, in pulmonary arterial hypertension, 406
Bortezomib, in small cell lung cancer, 926, 927f
Bosentan
  in hepatic cirrhosis, 514, 514t, 521
  in pulmonary arterial hypertension, 407t, 410, 410t
Botulinum toxin, 102–103, 102t
  in headache prevention, 735
  in voiding dysfunction, 446t, 449, 452
Bradycardia
  in baroreflex failure, 716
  in neurally mediated syncope, 715
Bradykinin
  in nociception, 721
  in osteoarthritis, 1022f, 1023
Brain
  imaging of, for drug testing, 10, 12f
  local anesthetic effects on, 864
Brain-derived neurotrophic factor, 792
Breast cancer, 933–942
  estrogen therapy and, 639
  genistein in, 88
  prevention of, 933–934
    raloxifene in, 933
    tamoxifen in, 933
  treatment of
    adjuvant therapy in, 933–934, 939–941, 940b
    angiogenesis inhibitors in, 938–939, 939f
    aromatase inhibitors in, 933–934, 940–941
    chemotherapy in, 933–934, 935–937, 939–940, 940b
    endocrine therapy in, 934–935, 935f, 940–941, 941f
    epidermal growth factor receptor inhibitors in, 937–938, 938f
    in metastatic disease, 934, 941–942, 942b

Breast cancer *(Continued)*
monoclonal antibodies in, 938, 938f, 940, 942
Ras/Raf/MEK/ERK pathway inhibitors in, 939, 939f
tamoxifen in, 934, 940–941, 941f
cytochrome P-450 2D6 and, 269–270
pharmacogenetics of, 231–232
Breast-feeding. *See also* Pregnancy
antifolates and, 1158
chloroquine and, 1150
mefloquine and, 1153
quinine and, 1152
Breast milk, drugs in, 255
Brewer's yeast, in acne, 980
Brimonidine, in glaucoma, 860
Brivaracetam, in seizure disorders, 679
Bromocriptine, 105, 105t
in growth hormone–secreting adenoma, 619
in Parkinson's disease, 654, 656t
in prolactinoma, 616–617
Brompheniramine maleate, 1222
Bronchial tone, 417–419, 418f
Bronchoprotection, 420
Brugada syndrome, 371t, 377, 377f
Brugia infection, 1174
Bucindolol, 134
in coronary artery disease, 347f, 347t
Budesonide
in asthma, 424–426, 425t
in inflammatory bowel disease, 492–493, 492t
Bumetanide, in hepatic cirrhosis, 514–515, 515t
α-Bungarotoxin, 101
Bupivacaine, 868t, 869, 869f
cardiac toxicity of, 865
Buprenorphine
in heroin addiction, 826, 827t, 830–831
in pain, 888
Bupropion, 104, 105t
in attention-deficit/hyperactivity disorder, 766, 766t
in nicotine dependence, 826, 827t, 831, 844t, 845
in obesity, 554
in unipolar disorder, 791
Buserelin, 632, 632t
Buspirone, 109, 110t
in generalized anxiety disorder, 775t, 776
in obsessive-compulsive disorder, 756, 776t, 777
in panic disorder, 774
Busulfan
in hematologic malignancy, 946
monitoring of, 276t, 283
Butalbital, in headache, 727t, 733
Butenafine, 183t
Butoconazole, 183t
in vulvovaginal candidiasis, 1209t
Butorphanol
in migraine, 722
in pain, 888
Butoxamine, 128t
Butyrylcholinesterase, 100
pharmacogenetics of, 227t
BX471, in renal insufficiency, 436

C

C-reactive protein
in cardiovascular disease, 306
HMG CoA reductase inhibitor effect on, 311
Cabergoline, 105t
in growth hormone–secreting adenoma, 619
in Parkinson's disease, 654, 656t
in prolactinoma, 616–617
Caffeine, 111
in hypersomnia, 852
monitoring of, 276t
nicotine interaction with, 842t
Cajal, interstitial cells of, 475–476, 477
Calcilytics, 598
Calcimimetics
in hypercalcemia, 596, 598, 598f
in renal osteodystrophy, 439
Calcineurin inhibitors, 163–164. *See also* Cyclosporine (cyclosporin A); Tacrolimus
clinical uses of, 164
mechanism of action of, 164, 164f
metabolism of, 163–164
pharmacokinetics of, 163–164
topical, 1013
toxicity of, 164
Calcipotriene, in psoriasis, 987, 999t
Calcipotriol, 597
in psoriasis, 991
Calcitonin, 602–603, 603f
in hypercalcemia, 595
in osteoporosis, 605
Calcitonin gene–related peptide, 471
Calcitriol
in hypocalcemia, 596
in renal osteodystrophy, 439
Calcium
daily requirement for, 595
daily turnover of, 588, 588f
deficiency of, 151–152, 589
in renal insufficiency, 437–438
excess of, 152, 588–589, 595–596, 602–603
gastrointestinal handling of, 150, 151f
intracellular, modulation of, 385
metabolism of, 293, 587–588, 588f
parathyroid hormone in, 589–590, 590f
regulation of, 589–593, 590f, 591f, 592f
vitamin D in, 590–593, 591f, 592f
oral, in hypocalcemia, 596
renal handling of, 143f, 150–152, 151f
serum, 587–588
urinary excretion of, 588
Calcium acetate, in hyperphosphatemia, 437, 438t
Calcium carbonate, in hyperphosphatemia, 437, 438t
Calcium channel
L-type, 384
in neurotransmitter exocytosis, 93
T-type, 384
Calcium channel blockers, 351–353, 384
adverse effects of, 346t, 352, 375t
age-related pharmacokinetics of, 262
antiretroviral interaction with, 1197t
azole interaction with, 182t
contraindications to, 352, 352b
in coronary artery disease, 351–353, 351t, 352b, 353t
dosages for, 353t
drug interactions with, 182t, 352, 1197t
in headache prevention, 734t, 735
in heart failure, 397–398, 397b, 397t
in hypertension, 297t, 298
mechanism of action of, 53, 54f, 351
overdose of, 353
pharmacokinetics of, 262, 351, 351t
in pheochromocytoma, 628, 629
proarrhythmia with, 376t
in pulmonary arterial hypertension, 407t, 408
toxicity of, 353
in voiding dysfunction, 452
Calcium chloride, in hypocalcemia, 596
Calcium gluceptate, in hypocalcemia, 596
Calcium gluconate, in hypocalcemia, 596
Calcium sensitizers, in heart failure, 396–397
Calymmatobacterium granulomatis infection, 1202t
Camellia sinensis, 1239t
Camptothecins
in breast cancer, 937
in colon cancer, 962t, 963–964, 963f, 964t
nicotine interaction with, 842t
pharmacogenetics of, 233–234
St. John's wort effect on, 1241t
in small cell lung cancer, 926
Cancer. *See also* Chemotherapy *and at specific cancers*
azathiopurine and, 995
gene therapy in, 1297, 1304, 1307–1313. *See also* Gene therapy, oncolytic
gene therapy–related, 1303
hypercalcemia with, 589, 596
pharmacogenetics in, 231–234
tumor necrosis factor-α inhibitors and, 1034
vaccine against, 1250–1251
Candesartan
in coronary artery disease, 354–357, 356t, 357b
in headache prevention, 734t, 736
in heart failure, 392–394, 393b, 393t
Candida infection, 179–180, 181–182, 183t
drug resistance in, 182–183
in endocarditis, 1136
vulvovaginal, 1209–1210, 1209t
Cannabinoid(s)
abuse of, 819t, 823
treatment of, 833
in headache, 739, 739f
Cannabinoid-1 receptor blocker
in dyslipidemia, 315
in nicotine dependence, 846
in obesity, 551t, 552–553, 552t
Capecitabine
in breast cancer, 936
cell cycle effects of, 83, 84f
in colon cancer, 962–963, 962t
Capreomycin, 1091f
in tuberculosis, 1097, 1102t
Capsaicin
in osteoarthritis, 1018t, 1020
in voiding dysfunction, 446t, 453
Captopril, in coronary artery disease, 354–357, 355t, 356t, 357b
Carbachol, 119–120, 119f, 860–861
Carbamazepine
age-related clearance of, 260t
azole interaction with, 182t
in bipolar disorder, 794
in headache prevention, 734t
isoniazid interaction with, 1094
monitoring of, 276t
in multiple sclerosis, 696t
in seizure disorders, 670–671
side effects of, 671
Carbapenems, 174t, 175t
resistance to, 178
Carbidopa, 104, 105t
Carbidopa/levodopa, in Parkinson's disease, 655–657, 657t
Carbon dioxide hypersensitivity, in panic disorder, 770
Carbon monoxide, 111
Carbonic anhydrase inhibitors, in glaucoma, 860, 861f
Carboplatin
in breast cancer, 935–936
in melanoma, 969
in non–small cell lung cancer, 921, 923f
in prostate cancer, 954
in small cell lung cancer, 925
CARD15, in Crohn's disease, 489
Cardiac arrest, treatment of, 379–380, 381

Cardiovascular disease. *See* Coronary artery disease; Dyslipidemia; Myocardial infarction
Cardiovascular system. *See also* Heart
  acetylcholine effects on, 120
  β-adrenergic receptor antagonists effects on, 134
  age-related changes in, 261–262
  antimuscarinic effects on, 122–123
  catecholamine effects on, 126–128, 128t, 129f
  disease of. *See* Coronary artery disease; Dyslipidemia; Myocardial infarction
  dopamine effects on, 130
  ganglionic blocker effect on, 123
Carisbamate, in seizure disorders, 679
Carmustine
  in hematologic malignancy, 946
  in melanoma, 969
L-Carnitine, in renal insufficiency–associated anemia, 441
Carotenoids, in acne, 980
Carotid artery disease, stroke and, 745t
Carotid sinus massage, in neurally mediated syncope, 704–705
Carpal tunnel syndrome, in hypothyroidism, 574
Carteolol, 134
  in glaucoma, 860
Cartilage, articular, 1015–1016
  fibrillation of, 1016
Carvedilol, 107t, 133f, 134
  in coronary artery disease, 347f, 347t, 350t
  in heart failure, 389–390, 391b, 391t
Cascara sagrada, 480t
Caspases, in apoptosis, 86, 87f
Caspofungin, 180t
  mechanism of action of, 180
  pharmacodynamics of, 181
  pharmacokinetics of, 181
  spectrum of activity of, 182
Castor oil, in constipation, 480t
Cataract, corticosteroid-related, 426
Catathrenia, 854
Catechol-*O*-methyltransferase, 93t, 94
  pharmacogenetics of, 227t
Catechol *O*-methyltransferase inhibitors, in Parkinson's disease, 657–658, 657t
Catecholamine(s), 126, 127f. *See also* Dopamine; Epinephrine; Norepinephrine
  cardiovascular effects of, 126–128
  central nervous system effects of, 129
  endocrine effects of, 129
  excess of, 627–629
  gastrointestinal effects of, 129
  genitourinary effects of, 129
  metabolic effects of, 129
  respiratory effects of, 128
  synthesis of, 627–628, 628f
Catecholamine metabolizing enzyme (COMT), 126
β-Catenin, 77
Cathepsin K inhibitors, in osteoporosis, 605
CCR-1, in renal insufficiency, 436
CCR5 antagonists, in HIV infection, 1197–1198
Cefadroxil, in infective endocarditis, 1126
Cefamandole, adverse effects of, 178t
Cefazolin
  creatinine clearance with, 176t
  in infective endocarditis, 1126
  ocular, 859t
Cefepime
  creatinine clearance with, 176t
  in infective endocarditis, 1125f, 1127
  spectrum of activity of, 177
Cefixime, in gonococcal infection, 1207t
Cefotaxime
  creatinine clearance with, 176t
  spectrum of activity of, 177
Cefotetan
  adverse effects of, 178t
  creatinine clearance with, 176t
Cefoxitin, creatinine clearance with, 176t
Ceftazidime
  creatinine clearance with, 176t
  spectrum of activity of, 177
Ceftriaxone
  adverse effects of, 178t
  in chancroid, 1202t
  in gonococcal infection, 1207t
  in infective endocarditis, 1125f, 1126–1127, 1131–1132, 1131t
  spectrum of activity of, 177
Cefuroxime, creatinine clearance with, 176t
Celecoxib
  cardiovascular toxicity of, 1020
  in osteoarthritis, 1020t
  in pain, 889t, 890
Celiac disease, in hyperthyroidism, 578
Celiprolol, 134
Cell-based therapy, 1317–1330. *See also* Stem cells
  allogeneic, 1319, 1320f
  autologous, 1319, 1319f
  in bone disease, 1327
  in cardiovascular disease, 1328, 1329f
  in endocrine disease, 1327–1328
  in genitourinary disease, 1330
  graft-versus-host disease and, 1275, 1329–1330
  in hematologic malignancy, 1274–1275, 1326–1327, 1327f
  historical perspective on, 1326
  infection and, 1275
  platforms for, 1320–1324, 1320t, 1321f, 1322f, 1323f
  regeneration strategy of, 1318, 1318f
  rejuvenation strategy of, 1318–1319, 1318f
  in renal disease, 1330
  replacement strategy of, 1318, 1318f
Cell cycle, 83–85, 84f
  apoptosis in, drug targeting of, 86–88, 87t
  M phase of, inhibitors of, 84–85, 84f
  S phase of, inhibitors of, 83–84, 84f
Central hypoventilation syndrome, 709
Central nervous system
  inhalational anesthetic effects on, 877
  isoniazid toxicity to, 1094
  local anesthetic effects on, 864
Cephalexin, in infective endocarditis, 1126
Cephalosporins, 174f, 174t, 175t
  creatinine clearance with, 176t
  in infective endocarditis, 1124f, 1125f, 1126–1127
  pharmacodynamics of, 176
  resistance to, 179
  spectrum of activity of, 177
Cerebrospinal fluid
  antimicrobial penetration in, 1110–1111
  evaluation of, in meningitis, 1116, 1117f
Certolizumab, in ulcerative colitis, 498
Certolizumab pegol, 169t
  in inflammatory bowel disease, 499
Ceruloplasmin, 898
Cervicitis, 1207, 1208t
Cetrorelix, 632, 632t
Cetuximab, 85
  in colon cancer, 962t, 966
CFTR gene, 1296
CGP 20712A, 128t
Chairs, in dysautonomias, 714
Chancroid, 1201, 1202t
Channelopathy, 78
Chelating agents, 1216–1219, 1217f, 1217t
Chemotherapy. *See also specific drugs*
  antiproliferation agents in, 85–86, 85f
  apoptosis-inducing agents in, 86–87, 87f
  in breast cancer, 933–934, 935–937, 939–940, 940b
  cell cycle pharmacology of, 83–85, 84f
  in colon cancer, 959–962, 960f, 960t, 961b, 961f
  in hematologic malignancy, 945–948, 948t
  monitoring of, 276t
  in non–small cell lung cancer, 921–922, 922b, 923f, 924f, 925f
  nuclear factor κB inhibitors in, 88
  in prostate cancer, 954
  in small cell lung cancer, 925–926, 928f
Child-Pugh classification
  in cirrhosis, 507, 508t
  drug clearance and, 202, 202f
Children, 239–248
  adverse drug reactions in, 246–247
  asthma treatment in, 430
  attention-deficit/hyperactivity disorder in. *See* Attention-deficit/hyperactivity disorder
  clinical research in, 247–248, 247t
  cutaneous drug administration in, 241
  developmental changes in, 239, 240f, 247–248, 247t
  drug absorption in, 239–241, 241t
  drug adherence in, 246
  drug administration in, 245–246, 246t
  drug development for, 26
  drug distribution in, 241–242, 242t
  drug dose for, 244–245
  drug metabolism in, 242–243, 243t
  drug-metabolizing enzymes in, 241, 242–243
  drug safety in, 1223–1224
  glomerular filtration rate in, 243–244, 244t
  growth hormone deficiency in, 615, 616
  inhalational drug administration in, 246, 246t
  intramuscular drug administration in, 241
  intraosseous drug administration in, 246, 246t
  intravenous drug administration in, 245–246, 246t
  Lennox-Gastaut syndrome in, 673, 674
  liquid drug administration in, 245
  midazolam sedation in, 880
  multiple sclerosis in, 697–698
  oral drug administration in, 239–241, 245
  P-glycoprotein in, 242
  parenteral drug administration in, 245–246
  percutaneous drug administration in, 241, 246
  plasma proteins in, 242, 242t
  rectal drug administration in, 241
  renal drug elimination in, 243–244, 244t
  urine collection from, 248
  vaccines for, 1252t, 1259–1260
  zonisamide for, 675, 676
Chlamydia trachomatis infection, 858
  genital, 1201–1202, 1202t
  urethral, 1206
Chlorambucil, in hematologic malignancy, 946
Chloramphenicol, 174f, 174t
  adverse effects of, 178t, 179t
  anemia with, 901
  mechanism of action of, 175
  in pregnancy, 179t
Chlordiazepoxide, nicotine interaction with, 842t
Chloroprocaine, 866–867, 866f, 866t
Chloroquine, 1148f
  adverse effects of, 1150
  drug interactions with, 1150
  in malaria chemoprophylaxis, 1164, 1165t
  in malaria treatment, 1147–1150, 1149t
  pharmacokinetics of, 1148–1150
  in pregnancy, 1150
  resistance to, 1147
  in systemic lupus erythematosus, 1051t, 1053–1055, 1054b, 1054t

Chlorpheniramine maleate, 1222
Chlorproguanil, in malaria, 1157
Chlorpromazine, 103, 105, 109, 806t, 807t
  α-adrenergic receptor blocking effect of, 132
  nicotine interaction with, 842t
Chlorpropamide, in diabetes mellitus, 562, 563t
Cholecystokinin, 459
Cholestasis, 506
Cholesterol, 303, 304f. *See also* Lipoprotein(s)
  reverse transport of, 305, 305f
  total, 358–359, 361b
Cholesterol absorption inhibitors, in dyslipidemia, 313
Cholesteryl ester transfer protein (CETP), 228t, 361
Cholesteryl ester transfer protein (CETP) inhibitors, in dyslipidemia, 316
Cholestyramine, in dyslipidemia, 312–313, 313t
Choline acetyltransferase, 100
Cholinergic agonists, 119–120, 119f. *See also* Acetylcholine
  in glaucoma, 860–861
  in motility disorders, 478
  in voiding dysfunction, 445–447, 447f
Cholinergic antagonists, 121, 122f
  muscarinic, 102t, 103, 121–123, 122f. *See also* Atropine
    adverse effects of, 123
    bladder effects of, 123
    cardiovascular effects of, 122–123
    central nervous system effects of, 121–122
    contraindications to, 123
    gastrointestinal effects of, 123
    in motility disorders, 481
    ophthalmic effects of, 122
    in voiding dysfunction, 446t, 450–452
  nicotinic, 121, 122f, 123–125, 124f
    ganglionic, 123–124, 124f
    neuromuscular, 124–125, 124f
Cholinergic receptor(s), 119
  age-related changes in, 260, 261t
  muscarinic, 101–102, 101f, 102t, 119, 119t
  nicotinic, 94, 100–101, 101f, 102t, 119, 838–839, 839f, 840f
Cholinesterase inhibitors. *See* Acetylcholinesterase inhibitors
Chondrocytes, 1015
Chondroitin, in osteoarthritis, 1018t, 1021
Chromatography, 279–280, 282, 282f
Chromones, in asthma, 428, 428t
Chronic lymphocytic leukemia, oblimersen in, 87
Chronic obstructive pulmonary disease (COPD), 417–432
  cell types of, 419
  clinical manifestations of, 419–420
  definition of, 417
  inflammation in, 419
  pathophysiology of, 419
  severity of, 417, 418t
  spirometry in, 420
  treatment of, 420–430
    β-adrenergic agonists in, 420–423, 421f, 421t
    anticholinergics in, 423–424, 423f, 424t
    corticosteroids in, 424–426, 425f, 425t
    inhaled route for, 420b
    integrated, 429–430, 429b
    leukotriene modifiers in, 426–428, 427f, 427t
    xanthines in, 428–429
Chylomicrons, 303, 304f
Cibenzoline, 372t
Ciclopirox, 183t
Cidofovir
  adverse effects of, 189t, 190
  in human herpesvirus infection, 184t, 185t
  mechanism of action of, 186
  pharmacokinetics of, 185, 185t
Cigarette smoking. *See also* Nicotine
  cessation of. *See also* Nicotine dependence, treatment of
    in COPD, 430
    in stroke prevention, 746–747
  Crohn's disease and, 489
  disease with, 837, 838b
  epidemiology of, 837
  stroke and, 745t
Cilansetron, in motility disorders, 481–482
Cilazepril, in coronary artery disease, 354–357, 355t, 357b
Cimetidine
  in acid secretion disorders, 463–464, 464t
  midazolam interaction with, 880
  nicotine interaction with, 842t
Cimicifuga racemosa, 1238, 1239t
Cinacalcet
  in hypercalcemia, 596, 598, 598f
  in renal osteodystrophy, 439
CINAHL, 42t
Cinchonism, 1151
Cingulotomy, in obsessive-compulsive disorder, 756–757, 756f
Cinnarizine, in headache prevention, 734t, 735
CIOMS (Council for International Organization of Medical Sciences), 29, 31t, 32
Ciprofibrate, in dyslipidemia, 314–315, 314t
Ciprofloxacin, 174t
  in chancroid, 1202t
  in gonococcal infection, 1207t
  in granuloma inguinale, 1202t
  in infective endocarditis, 1130
  ocular, 859t
  spectrum of activity of, 177
  structure of, 1091f
  in tuberculosis, 1096
Circadian rhythms, 211–212
Cirrhosis, 505–521
  ascites in, 509, 518, 518f
  clinical manifestations of, 506–507
  drug metabolism and, 202
  hepatic encephalopathy in, 511, 520, 520f
  hepatic vein pressure gradient in, 508–509, 510f
  hepatorenal syndrome in, 510–511, 519–520, 520f
  parenchymal failure in, 507
  pathophysiology of, 506, 507f
  portal hypertension in, 507–508, 509f, 511, 520–521, 521f
  severity of, 507, 508t
  spontaneous bacterial peritonitis in, 509–510, 518–519, 519f
  treatment of, 511–521
    antibiotics in, 515–516, 516t
    aquaretics in, 521
    in ascites, 518, 518f
    disaccharides in, 515, 516t
    diuretics in, 514–515, 515t
    endothelin antagonists in, 521
    in hepatic encephalopathy, 520, 520f
    in hepatorenal syndrome, 519–520, 520f
    nitric oxide donors in, 521
    in portal hypertension, 520–521, 521f
    in spontaneous bacterial peritonitis, 518–519, 519f
    in variceal hemorrhage, 516–518, 517f
    vasoconstrictors in, 511–514, 512t, 513t
    vasodilators in, 514, 514t
  varices in, 509
    bleeding from, 516–518, 517f
Cisapride, 110t
  azole interaction with, 182t
  in motility disorders, 479t, 481
Cisatracurium, 125
Cisplatin
  in breast cancer, 935–936
  in melanoma, 969, 970
  in non–small cell lung cancer, 921, 923f
  in prostate cancer, 954
  in small cell lung cancer, 925
Citalopram, 109, 110t
  age-related pharmacokinetics of, 260
  in obsessive-compulsive disorder, 755, 755t, 776–777, 776t
  in panic disorder, 773, 774t
  in posttraumatic stress disorder, 777
  during pregnancy, 255
  in social anxiety disorder, 778–779, 779t
Cladribine (2-CdA; chlorodeoxyadenosine)
  in hematologic malignancy, 945, 1285–1286
  in multiple sclerosis, 698
Clarithromycin, 174t
  antiretroviral interaction with, 1197t
  digoxin interaction with, 270
  in motility disorders, 479t
  spectrum of activity of, 177
Clavulanic acid, 175t
Clevudine, in hepatitis B virus infection, 537
Clindamycin, 174f, 174t
  in acne, 975t, 976
  adverse effects of, 178t
  in bacterial vaginosis, 1209t
  in malaria, 1149t, 1162
  in protozoa infection, 1185
  spectrum of activity of, 178
Clioquinol, in Alzheimer's disease, 645t
Clodronate, 599f
Clofibrate
  in dyslipidemia, 314–315, 314t
  niacin with, 314
Clomiphene citrate, 636
Clomipramine, 109
  in obsessive-compulsive disorder, 755, 755t, 776t, 777
  in panic disorder, 774, 774t
Clonazepam, 99, 100t
  in obsessive-compulsive disorder, 756, 776t, 777
  in panic disorder, 774, 774t
  in posttraumatic stress disorder, 778
  in REM sleep behavior disorder, 854
  in seizure disorders, 669
  in social anxiety disorder, 779, 779t
Cloned enzyme donor immunoassay, 279, 281f
Clonidine, 107, 107t, 127f, 128t, 130
  in attention-deficit/hyperactivity disorder, 766, 766t
  in baroreflex failure, 716, 716b
  in dysautonomias, 710t, 712
  in hypertension, 298
  neurotransmitter receptor response to, 705t
  in nicotine dependence, 832, 844t, 845
  in opioid dependence, 828t
  in pain, 891
  for sedation, 880
Clopidogrel
  adverse effects of, 331t, 332
  in coronary artery disease, 327b, 330, 331t, 332
  drug interactions with, 332
  pharmacokinetics of, 330
  resistance to, 332
  in stroke prevention, 750
  in thrombosis, 917–918
Clorgyline, 107, 107t, 110t
Clotrimazole, 183t
  in vulvovaginal candidiasis, 1209t
Clozapine, 105, 105t, 110t, 804–805, 806t, 807t, 808f, 809f–811f
  nicotine interaction with, 842t
  in Parkinson's disease, 659
CNI-1493, in inflammatory bowel disease, 499

CNTO 1275, in psoriasis, 1005
Coagulation, 909, 910f
Coagulation factors, 909–912, 910f, 913t. *See also* *specific factors*
Cocaine, 131
abuse of, 819t, 822–823
stroke and, 745t
treatment of, 832
anesthetic use of, 866, 866f
cardiac toxicity of, 865
hypertension with, 295
Cochrane Collaboration, 43
Cochrane Controlled Trials Register, 42t
Cochrane Library, 43, 44t
Codeine, 1222
abuse of, 819t
in pain, 885t, 887
Coenzyme Q_{10}, in headache prevention, 736–737
Cognitive impairment. *See also* Alzheimer's disease; Dementia
after bacterial meningitis, 1110
mild, 641, 642f
in multiple sclerosis, 697
in schizophrenia, 803, 804f
COL1A1 gene, 1296
Colchicine
in gout, 1039–1041, 1040t, 1043
toxicity of, 1040–1041
Colesevelam, in dyslipidemia, 312–313, 313t
Colestipol
in dyslipidemia, 312–313, 313t
niacin with, 314
Colistin, 174t
adverse effects of, 178t
creatinine clearance with, 176t
spectrum of activity of, 177
Colitis
microscopic, 487
ulcerative. *See* Ulcerative colitis
Colon. *See also* Gastrointestinal tract
cancer of. *See* Colon cancer
drug absorption in, 198–199, 198f
inflammation of. *See* Inflammatory bowel disease
motility of, 476
disorders of, 477, 480t. *See also* Motility disorders
pseudo-obstruction of, 477, 481
Colon cancer, 959–966
estrogen and, 639
stages of, 959
treatment of, 959–961, 960f, 960t, 961f
chemotherapy in, 962–965, 962t, 963f, 964t
in metastatic disease, 962
monoclonal antibodies in, 965–966, 965f, 966f
in stage II disease, 961–962, 961b
in stage III disease, 961
Coma, myxedema, 576
Committee for Medicinal Products for Human Use, 31t, 32
Complementary and alternative medicine. *See* Dietary supplements
Compliance, patient, 1226, 1226b
Computed tomography, in pulmonary arterial hypertension, 402
Computerized physician order entry system, 1231
Concentration-response relationship, 53–54, 57f, 59–60, 60f. *See also* Dose-response relationship
receptor dynamics and, 60–61, 61f, 62f
shape factor and, 61–62, 62f
Confidence interval, 49
Confusional arousals, 853
Congestive heart failure. *See* Heart failure
Conivaptan, 614
Connective tissue growth factor, in renal insufficiency, 436
Conn's syndrome, 629
Constipation, 477. *See also* Motility disorders
enema in, 480t
fiber in, 478
in hypothyroidism, 573
laxatives in, 478, 480t
mineral oil in, 480t
opioid-induced, 483
slow transit, 477, 480t
stool softeners in, 480t
Contraception
emergency, 638–639, 1224, 1224f
oral. *See* Oral contraceptives
Controlled Substances Act, 1227–1228, 1227t
COPD. *See* Chronic obstructive pulmonary disease (COPD)
Copper
deficiency of, 898
toxicity of, 1217t
Cornea, 857, 858, 858f. *See also* Eyes
amiodarone toxicity to, 381
infection of, 859
Coronary artery disease, 321–362. *See also* Dyslipidemia; Myocardial infarction
C-reactive protein in, 306
clinical presentation of, 324, 324f
estrogen therapy and, 639
gender and, 251
Heart Protection study of, 31
homocysteine levels and, 306
hypothyroidism and, 576
lipoprotein(a) in, 306
nonlipid risk factors in, 306, 309b
pathophysiology of, 321–322, 322f, 323f
in pregnancy, 349, 350t
prevention of, 322f, 324–325, 361, 362f
risk factors for, 305–306, 309b, 324. *See also* Dyslipidemia
treatment of, 322f, 324–362, 325b, 327b, 328f
β-adrenergic receptor antagonists in, 134, 230, 345–351, 346t, 347t, 348b, 349b, 349f, 350t, 362b
anti-ischemic agents in, 343–354, 344f, 345b, 346t, 347f, 347t, 348b, 349b, 349f, 350t, 351t, 352b, 353t, 362b
antiplatelet agents in, 325, 327–335, 329f, 331t, 333f, 334f, 362b
antithrombotic agents in, 333f, 334f, 335–343, 335t, 336f, 337b, 338b
aspirin in, 327b, 328–330, 329f, 331t, 362b
calcium channel blockers in, 351–353, 351t, 352b, 362b
cell replacement therapy in, 361, 362f
diazeniumdiolates in, 353
direct thrombin inhibitors in, 335t, 336f, 339–340
endogenous cardioprotection and, 361, 362f
factor Xa inhibitors in, 339
fibrinolytic agents in, 340–343, 340t, 341f, 342b
glycoprotein IIb/IIIa receptor antagonists in, 333–335, 333f, 334f
heparin in, 335–339, 335t, 336f, 337b, 338b
ivabradine in, 354
level of evidence for, 324, 325b, 362b
lipid-lowering agents in, 358–361, 358t, 359f, 359t, 360f, 360t, 361b
mesoionic oxatriazole derivatives in, 353
molsidomine in, 353
nitrates in, 343–345, 344f, 345b, 346t, 362b
S-nitrosothiols in, 353
potassium channel openers in, 354
primary prevention in, 322f, 324–325
ranolazine in, 353–354
Coronary artery disease *(Continued)*
renin-angiotensin-aldosterone system inhibitors in, 346t, 354–357, 355t, 356t, 357b, 362b
risk reduction therapies in, 361, 362f
thienopyridines in, 330, 332–333
thromboxane inhibitors in, 328–330, 329f
trimetazidine in, 354
Coronary steal syndrome, isoflurane and, 877
Coronavirus infection, 1073–1074, 1073f, 1074f
Cortical spreading depression, in migraine, 721, 724–725, 724t
Corticosteroid(s), 159t, 160–161
adverse effects of, 161, 426, 493, 987, 999t, 1276
in asthma, 424–426, 425f, 425t
in bacterial meningitis, 1112–1114, 1113f, 1114f, 1116
cataracts with, 426
clinical uses of, 161
in community-acquired pneumonia, 1086
in COPD, 424–426, 425f, 425t
in dermatitis, 1012–1013, 1014
drug interactions of, 1276
glaucoma with, 426
in gout, 1040t, 1041
in graft-versus-host disease, 1275
in hematologic malignancy, 946
hypertension with, 295
hypothalamic-pituitary-adrenal axis suppression with, 426
in inflammatory bowel disease, 492–493, 492t, 493t, 496–497, 497f, 497t, 498
inhalational, 424–426, 425f, 425t
mechanism of action of, 160–161, 160f, 424, 1275–1276, 1275f
metabolism of, 160, 492
in multiple sclerosis, 691–692, 695, 696
ocular, 859–860, 860t
in osteoarthritis, 1018t, 1021, 1021t
osteoporosis with, 426
pharmacodynamics of, 492
pharmacokinetics of, 160, 492, 1276
in psoriasis, 986–987, 988t, 999t
receptor binding of, 53, 53f
in rheumatoid arthritis, 1031
in systemic lupus erythematosus, 1051t, 1055, 1056, 1057, 1058
topical
in dermatitis, 1012–1013
ocular, 859–860, 860t
in psoriasis, 986–987, 988t, 999t
systemic side effects of, 987, 999t
in transplantation, 1274, 1275–1276, 1275f
Corticotropin-releasing hormone, 613t
Corticotropin-releasing hormone stimulation test, in Cushing's disease, 619
Cortisol
deficiency of, 626–627
secretion of, 626
synthesis of, 623, 624f
Coumarin, 913–915
Council for International Organization of Medical Sciences (CIOMS), 29, 31t, 32
COX-2 inhibitors
aspirin interaction with, 730t
in gout, 1041
in headache, 732, 732t
in pain, 889t, 890
in pregnancy, 1059t
CP-31398, 86
Cradle cap, 1007–1008, 1010f
Cranberry, 1239t
Cranial nerves, 116f, 118
Creatinine clearance, 201
age-related changes in, 259
in antibacterial monitoring, 176, 176t

Crohn's disease, 487–499
clinical features of, 487–488, 488f
environmental factors in, 489
extraintestinal features of, 488, 488t
genetics of, 489
immune dysregulation in, 490
intestinal flora in, 489–490
natural history of, 488
pathophysiology of, 488–490, 489f
treatment of, 490–499, 497f
in active disease, 496–497, 497f
adhesion molecule inhibitors in, 499
anti-inflammatory drugs in, 490–493, 491f, 491t, 492t, 493t, 496–497, 497t
anticytokines in, 499
approach to, 496–499, 497f
biologics in, 495–496, 497–498, 497t, 499–500
cytokines in, 499
goals of, 490, 490b
growth factors in, 499
immunosuppressants in, 493–495, 493f, 494f, 496–497, 497t
intracellular signal transduction inhibitors in, 499
microbiota in, 499–500
in perianal disease, 498
in remission, 497–498
Cromolyn sodium, in asthma, 428, 428t
Cryotherapy, in human papillomavirus infection, 1210b, 1211
Cryptosporidium infection, 1178–1179, 1183f
Crystalline arthropathy, vs. rheumatoid arthritis, 1027t
Cumulation, drug, 197, 197f
Cumulation factor, 197
Curcumin, 88
CURRENT CONTENTS, 42t
Cushing's disease, 619, 623
Cushing's syndrome, 296, 623–626
corticosteroid-induced, 161
pathophysiology of, 623, 624f
treatment of, 623–626
enzyme inhibitors in, 624f, 625, 625t
mifepristone in, 625–626
mitotane in, 624–625, 624f, 625t
surgical, 623–624
Cyanide, toxicity of, 1215–1216, 1216f
Cyanocobalamin. *See* Vitamin B_{12}
CYC202, cell cycle effects of, 84, 84f
Cyclic citrullinated peptide, antibody to, 1026
Cycline-dependent kinase inhibitors, cell cycle effects of, 84–85, 84f
Cyclooxygenase, aspirin blockade of, 53, 54f
Cyclooxygenase-1, 1019
inhibitors of. *See* Nonsteroidal anti-inflammatory drugs (NSAIDs)
Cyclooxygenase-2, 1019
glucocorticoid effect on, 493t
inhibitors of. *See also* Nonsteroidal anti-inflammatory drugs (NSAIDs)
aspirin interaction with, 730t
in gout, 1041
in headache, 732, 732t
in pain, 889t, 890
in pregnancy, 1059t
in osteoarthritis, 1019–1020, 1022f, 1023
Cyclophosphamide, 159t, 166
adverse effects of, 1050
in breast cancer, 935
clinical uses of, 166
contraindications to, 1050
in hematologic malignancy, 946, 1274
mechanism of action of, 166
metabolism of, 166
in multiple sclerosis, 692, 694
Cyclophosphamide (*Continued*)
pharmacokinetics of, 166
in pregnancy, 1059t, 1060
in prostate cancer, 954
in small cell lung cancer, 925
in systemic lupus erythematosus, 1049–1050, 1051t, 1058
toxicity of, 166
in transplantation, 1274, 1285
Cycloplegia, 122
Cycloplegics, 859, 860f
Cycloserine, 1091f
in tuberculosis, 1095, 1102t
Cyclosporine (cyclosporin A), 159t, 163–164
adverse effects of, 164, 495, 992, 1278
azole interaction with, 182t
dosing for, 1277
drug interactions with, 495, 1277–1278
in graft-versus-host disease prophylaxis, 1275
hypertension with, 295
in inflammatory bowel disease, 495, 497t, 498
mechanism of action of, 164, 164f, 1276–1277, 1277f
metabolism of, 163–164, 495
monitoring of, 163–164, 276t, 1278
ocular, 861
pharmacodynamics of, 495
pharmacokinetics of, 163–164, 495, 1277
in pregnancy, 1059t, 1060
in psoriasis, 991f, 992, 992f, 994f, 1000t, 1002f
St. John's wort interaction with, 269, 1241t
in systemic lupus erythematosus, 1051t
in transplantation, 1274, 1276–1278, 1277f
Cyproheptadine, 109, 110t
in headache prevention, 734t, 736
Cyproterone, in prostate cancer, 953
Cytarabine, in hematologic malignancy, 945
Cytochrome P-450
age-related changes and, 258–259
in children, 241, 242–243
dietary supplement effects on, 1240–1241, 1241t
drug interactions with, 266–268, 267t, 268t
pharmacogenetics of, 220–222, 221f, 221t, 226–227, 227t
antiarrhythmics and, 373–374
gender and, 252–253, 252t
Cytochrome P-450 219, pharmacogenetics of, 227t
Cytochrome P-450 1A, gender-related pharmacogenetics of, 252t, 253
Cytochrome P-450 1A2
drug interactions with, 267f, 267t, 268t
pharmacogenetics of, 227t
Cytochrome P-450 2A6, 267f
pharmacogenetics of, 227t
Cytochrome P-450 3A, 267f
drug interactions with, 266–268, 267f, 268b, 268t
gender-related pharmacogenetics of, 252t, 253
grapefruit juice interaction with, 269
itraconazole interaction with, 270–271
St. John's wort interaction with, 269
Cytochrome P-450 3A4, 199, 266
drug interactions with, 267t
pharmacogenetics of, 227t
antiarrhythmics and, 373
Cytochrome P-450 3A5
drug interactions with, 267t
pharmacogenetics of, 227t
antiarrhythmics and, 373
Cytochrome P-450 3A7, pharmacogenetics of, 227t
Cytochrome P-450 2B6, 267f
drug interactions with, 267t
Cytochrome P-450 2C, 267f
Cytochrome P-450 2C8
drug interactions with, 267t, 268t
gemfibrozil interaction with, 270–271
pharmacogenetics of, 227t
Cytochrome P-450 2C9, 267f
drug interactions with, 267t, 268t
pharmacogenetics of, 221t, 222–223, 222t, 223f, 227t
antiarrhythmics and, 373
gender and, 252t, 253
Cytochrome P-450 2C19, 267f
drug interactions with, 267t, 268t, 465–466
gender-related pharmacogenetics of, 252t, 253
Cytochrome P-450 C19, pharmacogenetics of, 230, 231
Cytochrome P-450 C29, pharmacogenetics of, 230–231
Cytochrome P-450 2D6, 266
antidepressant interaction with, 269, 766
atomoxetine interaction with, 766
deficiency of, tamoxifen and, 269–270
drug interactions with, 267f, 267t, 268t, 269, 766
pharmacogenetics of, 220–221, 221f, 221t, 222, 227t, 229–230, 229f, 231–233
antiarrhythmics and, 373, 382, 383
gender and, 252t, 253
tamoxifen and, 269–270
Cytochrome P-450 2E1
drug interactions with, 267f, 267t
gender-related pharmacogenetics of, 252t, 253
Cytochrome P-450 2J2, 267f
Cytokine(s)
in Crohn's disease, 490
in inflammatory bowel disease, 499
in ulcerative colitis, 490
Cytokine receptors, 76
Cytomegalovirus infection. *See also* Human herpesvirus infection
retinal, 1307
Cytopenia, methotrexate and, 166
Cytosine arabinoside, cell cycle effects of, 84

D

Dacarbazine
in hematologic malignancy, 946
in melanoma, 969
Daclizumab, 159t, 167
in multiple sclerosis, 698
in transplantation, 1283
Dalfopristin, 174t
Dalteparin, 915, 916
in coronary artery disease, 337–339
Danazol
side effects of, 1057
in systemic lupus erythematosus, 1051t, 1056–1057
Dantrolene, in voiding dysfunction, 449
Dapsone
in acne, 980
in malaria, 1156f, 1157
in protozoa infection, 1185
side effects of, 1056
in systemic lupus erythematosus, 1051t, 1056
Daptomycin, 174t
adverse effects of, 178t, 1128
creatinine clearance with, 176t
in infective endocarditis, 1128, 1134
spectrum of activity of, 177
Darbepoietin alfa, 904
in dysautonomias, 712–713
in renal insufficiency, 441
Darifenacin, 103
in motility disorders, 481
in voiding dysfunction, 446t, 451

Darunavir, in HIV infection, 1191–1193, 1195t
Dasatinib, in hematologic malignancy, 946
Data
for evidence-based practice, 42–44, 42t, 43b, 44t
for pharmacoviligance, 37t, 38
Daunorubicin, in hematologic malignancy, 945–946
DDAVP. *See* Desmopressin
DEA registration number, 1228, 1230
Debulamine, 127f
Decamethonium, 123
Decitabine, in hematologic malignancy, 945
Decongestants, hypertension with, 295
Deep brain stimulation
in obsessive-compulsive disorder, 757, 757f
in Parkinson's disease, 660
Deep vein thrombosis. *See* Thrombosis
Deferoxamine, 1217, 1217t, 1218
Deguelin, 88
Dehydroepiandrosterone
adrenal, 627
in systemic lupus erythematosus, 1051t
Dehydroepiandrosterone sulfate, 627
Delavirdine, in HIV infection, 1188, 1190–1191, 1192t
Delayed afterdepolarization, 369, 369f, 369t
Demeclocycline, 614
Dementia, 641–647. *See also* Alzheimer's disease
apathy in, 647
behavioral manifestations of, 647, 647b, 647t
depression in, 647
motor symptoms in, 646
sleep disorders in, 647
vascular, 643
Dementia with Lewy bodies, 643, 644
Demyelination. *See also* Multiple sclerosis
tumor necrosis factor-α inhibitors and, 1034
Denatonium benzoate, 1222
Dendritic cells, 158
Denervation hypersensitivity, 95
Denervation supersensitivity, 118
Denileukin diftitox, in transplantation, 1283
Denosumab, in osteoporosis, 605
Depot methylprednisolone acetate, 638
Depression. *See also* Bipolar disorder; Unipolar disorder (major depressive disorder)
in dementia, 647
nicotine dependence and, 840
pharmacogenetics in, 229–230
seizure disorders and, 665–666
St. John's wort in, 1240
Derby chair, in dysautonomias, 714
Dermatitis, 1007–1014
acute, 1007, 1008f
allergic, 1008, 1011
asteatotic, 1007, 1010, 1014
atopic, 1007, 1009f, 1010–1011, 1014
chronic, 1007, 1008f
contact, 1008, 1010f, 1011, 1014
diagnosis of, 1011
infectious, 1009, 1011, 1013
irritant, 1008, 1010f
nummular, 1008, 1010f, 1014
pathophysiology of, 1009–1010
perioral, 1009
phases of, 1007, 1008f
seborrheic, 1007–1008, 1010f, 1011, 1014
stasis, 1009, 1011, 1011f, 1014
subacute, 1007, 1008f
treatment of, 1011–1014
antibiotics in, 1013
antihistamines in, 1013
calcineurin inhibitors in, 1013
corticosteroids in, 1012–1013, 1014
goals of, 1011
Dermatitis *(Continued)*
guidelines for, 1014
lubricants in, 1011–1012
moisturizers in, 1011–1012
phototherapy in, 1013–1014
pimecrolimus in, 1013
tacrolimus in, 1013
tar preparations in, 1013
topical, 1012–1013
wet dressings in, 1012
Desflurane, 875f, 875t
cardiac effects of, 877
CNS effects of, 877
hepatic effects of, 877
metabolism of, 877–938
renal effects of, 877
respiratory effects of, 876–877
Desipramine, 107, 107t
in attention-deficit/hyperactivity disorder, 766
in cocaine addiction, 832
in posttraumatic stress disorder, 777
Deslorelin, 632, 632t
Desmopressin, 912
in central diabetes insipidus, 612–613
in nocturnal enuresis, 446t, 454
in von Willebrand disease, 912
water intoxication with, 613
Desoxyn, in attention-deficit/hyperactivity disorder, 761t, 762t
Detrusor overactivity, 449–450
Dexamethasone
in adrenal insufficiency, 626–627, 627
in bacterial meningitis, 1112–1114, 1113f, 1114f, 1116
in hematologic malignancy, 946
in thyroid storm, 583t
Dexedrine, in attention-deficit/hyperactivity disorder, 760–761, 761t, 762t
Dexmedetomidine, 107t, 127f, 130
for sedation, 879t, 880–881
Dexmethylphenidate hydrochloride, 763, 763t, 764
Dextroamphetamine, 759, 760–761, 761t
in hypersomnia, 852
Dextroamphetamine spansule, in attention-deficit/hyperactivity disorder, 762
Dextromethorphan, 1222
Dextrostat, in attention-deficit/hyperactivity disorder, 760–761, 761t, 762t
Diabetes insipidus, central, 611–613
desmopressin in, 612–613
pathophysiology of, 611–612
Diabetes mellitus, 557–569
dyslipidemia treatment in, 316–317
gastroparesis in, 478, 478f
gender and, 251–252
pathophysiology of, 557, 558f
prevention of, 568
stroke and, 745t, 748
treatment of, 558–569
approach to, 566, 568, 569f
biguanides in, 561, 562f
cell-based therapy in, 1327–1328
combination PPAR agonists in, 568
α-glucosidase inhibitors in, 559, 559f, 559t
goals of, 558
incretin-based therapy in, 560–561, 560f
insulin in, 562, 564–568, 567f, 568f
meglitinides in, 561, 561f, 561t
pramlintide in, 559–560
sulfonylureas in, 562, 563f, 563t, 564f
thiazolidinediones in, 562, 563t, 565f, 566f
Diacetylmonoxime (DAM), 122f
in anticholinesterase poisoning, 123
Diacylglycerol (DAG), 72f, 73
Diarrhea. *See also* Motility disorders
fast colonic motility and, 477
opioid agonists in, 482
Diarylquinoline, in tuberculosis, 1105–1106, 1105f
Diazeniumdiolates, in coronary artery disease, 353
Diazepam, 99, 100t
in generalized anxiety disorder, 775t
nicotine interaction with, 842t
in panic disorder, 774, 774t
for sedation, 880
in seizure disorders, 669–670
in voiding dysfunction, 448
Dichloroacetate, in pulmonary arterial hypertension, 412
Diclofenac
aspirin interaction with, 730t
in headache, 732t
in osteoarthritis, 1020, 1020t
in pain, 889t, 890
Dicyclomine hydrochloride, in voiding dysfunction, 446t, 452
Didanosine
azole interaction with, 182t
in HIV infection, 1187–1188, 1189t
Diet
in acne, 973, 980
in cardiovascular disease, 315, 316, 324
in dysautonomias, 714
in gout, 1043
low-sodium, 509
in obesity, 553
Dietary Supplement Health and Education Act, 1237, 1243
Dietary supplements, 1237–1243, 1239t. *See also specific supplements*
in Alzheimer's disease, 646
drug interactions with, 1240–1241, 1241t
in insomnia, 850–851
regulation of, 1237–1238, 1243
safety of, 1237–1238, 1243
toxicity of, 1241–1242, 1242b
use of, 1238
Dieter's teas, toxicity of, 1243
Diethylcarbamazine, in helminthic infection, 1174–1175, 1177f
Diethylpropion, in obesity, 551
Diethylstilbestrol, in prostate cancer, 952
Diffuse connective tissue disease, vs. rheumatoid arthritis, 1027t
Diflunisal, in osteoarthritis, 1020t
Digitoxin, 384, 1216
Digoxin
adverse effects of, 346t, 375t, 384
in atrial arrhythmias, 384
azole interaction with, 182t
clarithromycin interaction with, 270
gender-related pharmacodynamics of, 253
in heart failure, 384, 395, 395b, 395t
monitoring of, 276t
pharmacokinetics of, 194, 195f, 197, 197f, 198, 200, 373t, 384
phenytoin interaction with, 669
in pulmonary arterial hypertension, 407t
St. John's wort effect on, 1241t
toxicity of, 375, 376t, 384, 1216
Dihydroartemisinin, in malaria, 1157f, 1159f
Dihydroergocryptine
in headache, 733, 733t
in headache prevention, 734t, 736
Dihydroergotamine mesylate, in headache, 733, 733t
Dihydropyridine, receptor interaction of, 54f
Dihydropyrimidine dehydrogenase, pharmacogenetics of, 227t

Dihydrotachysterol, 596
Dihydroxyphenylacetic acid, 104
1,25-Dihydroxyvitamin D, 591–592, 592f. *See also* Vitamin D
Diloxanide furoate, in *Entamoeba* infection, 1181
Diltiazem, 371t, 372t, 384
  in coronary artery disease, 351–353, 351t, 352b, 353t
  receptor interaction of, 54f
Dimenhydrinate, in motility disorders, 479t
Dimercaprol, 1216, 1217t
2,3-Dimercapto-1-propanesulfonic acid, 1217, 1217t
Dimethyl sulfoxide, in voiding dysfunction, 452–453
Dimethylfumarate, in psoriasis, 995, 1000t, 1002f
Dipeptidyl peptidase 4 inhibitors, in diabetes mellitus, 560–561
Diphenhydramine, 102t, 103, 109
  in insomnia, 850
Diphenoxylate, in diarrhea, 482
Diphtheria vaccine, 1252t, 1253t, 1254t, 1257–1258
Dipyridamole
  in coronary artery disease, 327b, 331t, 335
  in stroke prevention, 750
  in thrombosis, 918
Direct thrombin inhibitors, 335t, 339–340, 916–917
Disaccharides, in hepatic encephalopathy, 515, 516t
Disease-modifying agents
  in multiple sclerosis, 689–696, 690f
  in psoriatic arthritis, 1003–1004
  in rheumatoid arthritis, 1031–1033, 1032t
Disheveled protein, 77
Disopyramide, 372t, 381
  adverse effects of, 374, 375t, 381
  anticholinergic effects of, 374
  antiretroviral interaction with, 1197t
Disproportionality analysis, for pharmacoviligance, 37t, 38
Dissociative disorders, sleep-related, 854
Disulfiram, 176
  in alcohol dependence, 824, 824t, 825, 828t, 829
Dithranol, in psoriasis, 989
Diuretics
  age-related pharmacokinetics of, 262
  in heart failure, 389, 395
  in hepatic cirrhosis, 514–515, 515t, 518
  in hypertension, 297–298, 297t
  loop
    adverse effects of, 346t
    in hepatic cirrhosis, 514–515, 515t
  potassium-sparing
    adverse effects of, 346t
    in hepatic cirrhosis, 514, 515t
  in pulmonary arterial hypertension, 407t, 408
  renal handling of, 153–154, 153t
  in renal insufficiency, 437
  thiazide
    age-related pharmacokinetics of, 262
    in osteoporosis, 604
    in stroke prevention, 748
Divalproex, in bipolar disorder, 792f, 793
DNA vaccine, 1250
Dobutamine, 128t, 130
  in heart failure, 396, 396b, 397t
Docetaxel
  in breast cancer, 936
  cell cycle effects of, 84, 84f
  in melanoma, 969–970
  in non–small cell lung cancer, 921, 924f
Docusate calcium, 1222
Docusate sodium, 480t
Dofetilide, 372t, 381–382
  adverse effects of, 375t, 382
  antiretroviral interaction with, 1197t
  pharmacokinetics of, 373, 381
Dolasetron, 109, 110t
  in motility disorders, 479t
Domperidone, 105, 105t
  in motility disorders, 479t, 482
  in Parkinson's disease, 655
Donepezil, 102t, 103
  in Alzheimer's disease, 644, 644t
Donor lymphocyte infusion, 1304
Donovanosis, 1202, 1202t
Dopamine, 92, 103–105, 127f, 130, 613t
  anatomic distribution of, 103
  deficiency of. *See* Parkinson's disease
  function of, 103
  metabolism of, 93–94, 103f, 104
  in pure autonomic failure, 708
  receptors for, 103f, 104
  in social anxiety disorder, 771
  synthesis of, 93t, 103–104, 103f, 653, 655f
  as therapeutic target, 104–105, 105t
Dopamine agonists, 105, 105t
  in acromegaly, 619
  in Parkinson's disease, 654–655, 656t
  in prolactinoma, 616–617, 617f
Dopamine antagonists, 105, 105t
  in motility disorders, 479t, 482
  in Parkinson's disease, 655
Dopamine β-hydroxylase, 106
  deficiency of, 706t, 708–709
    droxidopa in, 710t, 712, 712f
Dopamine transporter, pharmacogenetics of, 228t
Dose-response relationship, 51, 52, 59–63. *See also* Receptor-ligand interaction
  agonist effects on, 63–64, 64f
  antagonist effects on, 63–64, 64f
  biologic effect and, 59–62, 60f, 62f
  concentration dependence of, 59–60, 59f
  elimination rate constant in, 62–63, 63f, 64f
  graphical representation of, 53–54, 57f
  ligand efficacy and, 60, 60f
  ligand potency and, 60, 60f
  nonlinear effects in, 61–62, 62f
  population-related, 64, 64f
  receptor dynamics and, 60–62, 61f, 62f
  temporal aspects of, 62–63, 63f
Doxacurium, 125
Doxazosin, 107t, 128t, 131–132
  in voiding dysfunction, 446t, 447–448
Doxepin
  in dermatitis, 1013
  in voiding dysfunction, 452
Doxercalciferol, 596
  in renal osteodystrophy, 439
Doxorubicin
  in breast cancer, 936
  in hematologic malignancy, 945–946
  in prostate cancer, 954
  in small cell lung cancer, 926
Doxycycline, 174t
  in acne, 977, 979
  adverse effects of, 178t
  in cervicitis, 1208t
  in granuloma inguinale, 1202t
  in infective endocarditis, 1129
  in lymphogranuloma venereum, 1202t
  in malaria chemoprophylaxis, 1164, 1165t
  in malaria treatment, 1149t, 1161–1162
  in nongonococcal urethritis, 1208t
DPYD, 233
DRD4, 767
Droxidopa, in dopamine β-hydroxylase deficiency, 709, 710t, 712, 712f
Drug(s). *See also specific drugs and drug classes*
  addiction to. *See* Drug addiction
  cost/availability of, 1226
  development of, 15–28. *See also* Drug testing/trials
    benefit-to-risk assessment in, 26–27, 27f
    business regulations in, 20
    candidate registration in, 24
    clinical research in, 21–22, 22b
    confirmatory clinical trials in, 24
    decision-based, 16–17, 16f, 17f, 18, 19f, 23–25, 25f
    for elderly population, 25–26
    ethics in, 19
    goal of, 15
    guidelines for, 19, 21–23, 22b
    in Japan, 25
    nonclinical safety assessment in, 21
    for pediatric population, 26
    pharmaceutical science in, 21
    phase I, 16, 16f, 33
    phase II, 16, 16f, 18, 33
    phase III, 16, 16f, 33–35
    phase IV, 16, 16f, 35–39
    principles of, 18–21
    privacy regulations in, 20–21
    process of, 15–18, 16f, 17f, 18f, 19f
    proof of concept in, 16, 16f, 18, 19f, 24
    proof of mechanism in, 16, 16f, 18, 19f, 24
    for rare diseases, 27, 27t
    regulation of, 19–21. *See also* Pharmacovigilance
    risk management plan in, 16f, 17, 24–25, 25t, 34–35
    success rates in, 17–18, 17f, 18f
    traditional process of, 16, 16f, 17–18, 17f, 18f
  discovery of, 7–14, 23
    attrition rates in, 9, 11f
    clinical profile in, 9–13, 10b, 12f. *See also* Drug testing/trials
    genomic approach to, 14
    imaging in, 10, 12f
    interventional validation for, 8
    lead molecule identification for, 8, 8f
    lead molecule optimization for, 8–9, 9f, 10t, 11f
    observational validation for, 8
    robotic screening for, 8, 8f
    safety assessment in, 9, 10b, 10t
    target identification for, 7
    target validation for, 8
  interactions of, 265–272. *See also at specific drugs*
    drug selection and, 1226
  monitoring of. *See* Therapeutic drug monitoring
  patient adherence to, 1226, 1226b
  prescription for. *See* Prescription
  receptor interaction with. *See* Receptor-ligand interaction
  regulation of, 19–21. *See also* Pharmacovigilance
  renal handling of, 152–153, 152t
  selection of, 1225–1226
  testing of. *See* Drug testing/trials
  transporters for, 270, 271f, 272t
Drug addiction, 817–833, 837, 838b, 839f. *See also at specific addictive drugs*
  craving in, 818, 822f, 824–825, 824t
  DSM-IV criteria for, 818b
  genetic factors in, 818, 820t, 833
  headache with, 727t, 730
  pathophysiology of, 817–823, 820f, 821f, 822f

Drug addiction *(Continued)*
prevention of, 823
tolerance with, 818, 824, 824t
treatment of, 823–833
self-help groups in, 826
symptom management in, 822b, 824–825, 824t, 825t
Drug dependence, 837, 838b. *See also* Drug addiction
Drug dose. *See also* Dose-response relationship
accuracy of, 277
definition of, 51
genotype-based, 228–229, 229f
optimal, 283–285
Drug filtration rate, 201
Drug monitoring. *See* Therapeutic drug monitoring
Drug Price Competition and Patent Term Restoration Act (1984), 20
Drug response, 51, 52f. *See also* Dose-response relationship; Receptor(s); Receptor-ligand interaction
population-related, 64, 64f
Drug testing/trials, 9–13, 11f
active comparator in, 22
adaptive design in, 22
biomarkers in, 22–23
confirmatory, 24
data analysis in, 34
Data Monitoring Committee in, 33
documentation of, 23
end points for, 22–23
global, 22
international, 22
patient access in, 22
phase I, 33
phase II, 33
phase III, 33–35
phase IV, 35–39
placebo in, 22
risk-management plan in, 34–35
statistical issues in, 22
study design in, 22
surrogate end points in, 22–23
transparency in, 23
DTaP vaccine, 1252t, 1253t, 1254t, 1257–1258
Duloxetine, 107t, 110t
in pain, 891
in unipolar disorder, 791
in voiding dysfunction, 453
Dumping syndrome, 477, 477f. *See also* Motility disorders
Durham-Humphrey Amendment, 1227
Dysautonomias, 703–716, 706t
diagnosis of, 705t
pathophysiology of, 703–710
treatment of, 710–716, 710t, 713b
atrial tachypacing in, 715
bionic baroreflex system in, 715
clonidine in, 710t, 712
diet in, 714
droxidopa in, 710t, 712, 712f
erythropoietin in, 710t, 712–713
exercise in, 714–715
fludrocortisone in, 710–711, 710t
indomethacin in, 710t, 711–712
mechanical aids in, 714
midodrine in, 710t, 711
nonpharmacologic, 713–715, 713b
physical maneuvers in, 714
sodium in, 714
yohimbine in, 710t, 712
vasodilating drug sensitivities in, 713
Dysbetalipoproteinemia, familial, 307
Dyshidrosis (dyshidrotic eczema), 1008–1009, 1010f, 1014
Dyslipidemia, 305–317. *See also* Lipoprotein(s)
atherogenic, 306. *See also* Coronary artery disease; Myocardial infarction
classification of, 306–308, 307t
in hypothyroidism, 572
pathophysiology of, 305–306
primary, 306–308, 307t
in renal insufficiency, 442, 442t
secondary, 308, 308b
treatment of, 308–317
acyl-coenzyme A:cholesterol transferase inhibitors in, 316
algorithm for, 316–317
ATP III guidelines for, 310t, 316–317
bile acid sequestrants in, 312–313, 313t, 360t, 361b
bile acid transport inhibitors in, 316
cholesterol absorption inhibitors in, 313
cholesteryl ester transfer protein inhibitors in, 316
fibrates in, 314–315, 314t, 360t, 361b
gender and, 253
gene therapy in, 316
guidelines for, 309, 358–361
HMG CoA reductase inhibitors in, 309–312, 311t, 312t, 358–361, 358t, 359f, 359t, 360f, 360t, 361b
lifestyle changes in, 315, 316
liver X receptor agonists in, 316
microsomal triglycerie transfer protein inhibitors in, 316
niacin in, 313–314, 360t, 361b
omega-3 fatty acids in, 314
orlistat in, 315
plant sterols in, 315
rimonabant in, 315
sibrutamine in, 315–316
surgery in, 315
Dyspnea, in hyperthyroidism, 577–578

E

Early afterdepolarization, 369, 369f, 369t
Eating disorder, sleep-related, 854
Echinacea, 1239t, 1241t
Echinocandins, 180t
adverse effects of, 182
mechanism of action of, 180
pharmacodynamics of, 181
pharmacokinetics of, 181
spectrum of activity of, 181
Echinococcus infection, 1171–1172, 1175f
Echocardiography, in infective endocarditis, 1122
Echothiophate, 121, 121f
Econazole, 183t
Eczema, 1007, 1009f, 1010–1011. *See also* Dermatitis
dyshidrotic, 1008–1009, 1010f, 1014
infectious, 1011
ED_{50}, 64
Edrophonium, 102t, 103, 120–121, 121f
in neuromuscular blocker reversal, 125
Efalizumab, in psoriasis, 997f, 998, 1000t, 1002f
Efavirenz
azole interaction with, 182t
in HIV infection, 1188, 1190–1191, 1190f, 1192t
Effect compartment model (link model), of pharmacodynamics, 209, 209f
Eflornithine, in protozoa infection, 1185
Elastic stockings, in dysautonomias, 714
Elderly population. *See also* Age/aging
drug development for, 25–26
Electrical stimulation therapy
in motility disorders, 484
in seizure disorders, 679
Electrocardiography
in arrhythmias, 374
in Brugada syndrome, 377, 377f
in myocardial infarction, 325
normal, 367–368, 368f
Electrolyte homeostasis
bicarbonate, 143f, 149–150, 150f
calcium, 143f, 150–152, 151f
magnesium, 143f, 152
phosphorus, 143f, 151f, 152
potassium, 143f, 147f, 148–149, 149f
sodium, 143f, 145f, 146–148, 147f, 148f
Electromagnetic spectrum, 857, 858f
Electronic prescription, 1231
Eletriptan, 109, 726–731, 728f, 729t, 730t
Eleutherococcus senticosus, 1239t
Elimination clearance, 193, 195–196, 196f
in renal impairment, 201, 201f
Elimination half-life, 193, 195
Elimination rate constant, 62–63, 63f
E_{max} model, 205, 205f, 207–208, 208f
EMBASE, 42t
Emtricitabine
in hepatitis B virus infection, 537, 539
in HIV infection, 1187–1188, 1189t
Enalapril maleate
in coronary artery disease, 354–357, 355t, 356t, 357b
in heart failure, 390–392, 392b, 392t
Encephalitis, herpes, 1203
Endocannabinoids, 111–112
Endocarditis. *See* Infective endocarditis
Endometriosis, 632, 633
Endometrium, estrogen therapy effects on, 639
Endoscopic variceal band ligation, 516, 517, 517f
Endothelial cell, in pulmonary arterial hypertension, 403
Endothelin, in pulmonary arterial hypertension, 404, 405f
Endothelin receptor antagonists
in hepatic cirrhosis, 514, 514t, 521
in pulmonary arterial hypertension, 407t, 409–410, 410t
Enema, in constipation, 480t
Enflurane, 875f, 875t
metabolism of, 878
respiratory effects of, 877
Enfuvirtide, in HIV infection, 1193, 1193f, 1195, 1196t
Enoxaparin, 915, 916
in coronary artery disease, 337–339, 337b
Entacapone, 104–105, 105t
in Parkinson's disease, 657–658, 657t
Entamoeba histolytica infection, 1181f
diloxanide furoate in, 1181
iodoquinol in, 1180
metronidazole in, 1178
paromomycin in, 1179–1180
Entecavir
adverse effects of, 189t
in hepatitis B virus infection, 187, 188, 536–537, 536f, 538t, 539
resistance to, 190
Enteric nervous system, 135, 475, 476f
Enteritis, regional. *See* Crohn's disease
Enterobacteriaceae, in infective endocarditis, 1136
Enterobius vermicularis infection, 1171
Enterococci
in infective endocarditis, 1132–1134, 1133t
vancomycin-resistant, in infective endocarditis, 1134
Enteropathy, protein-losing, in systemic lupus erythematosus, 1057
Entry inhibitors, in HIV infection, 1193, 1193f, 1195, 1196t
Enuresis, 446t, 454, 854

Environment, in schizophrenia, 799
Enzyme
drug-metabolizing, 1225
ligand binding to, 53, 54f
Enzyme-linked cell-surface receptors, 73–76, 74f
Enzyme-linked immunosorbent assay, 279, 281f
Enzyme-multiplied immunoassay technique, 279, 281f
Eosinophils, 158
in asthma, 419
production of, 895, 896f
Epac (exchange protein activated by cAMP), 72
Eph receptor, 74
Ephedra sinica, 1242
Ephedrine, 127f, 130, 1222
Epibatidine, 101
Epidermal growth factor, in acid secretion, 459
Epidermal growth factor receptor, 73
Epidermal growth factor receptor inhibitors, 85–86
in breast cancer, 937–938, 938f, 940, 942
in colon cancer, 962t, 966, 966f
in non–small cell lung cancer, 923
in prostate cancer, 955–956
Epilepsy. *See* Seizure disorders
Epimedium sagittatum, 1239t
Epinephrine
dose-response relationship with, 64, 64f
functions of, 126–129, 128t
in neurally mediated syncope, 704–705
over-the-counter, 1222
in pure autonomic failure, 707
structure of, 127f, 421f
therapeutic use of, 129–130
Epirubicin
in breast cancer, 936
in small cell lung cancer, 926
Eplerenone
in coronary artery disease, 354–357, 356t
in heart failure, 394–395, 394b, 394t
in hyperaldosteronism, 629
in renal insufficiency, 437
Epoetin, 904–905
adverse effects of, 905
blood pressure increase with, 713
in dysautonomias, 710t, 712–713
in renal insufficiency, 440–441
Epoprostenol
in hepatic cirrhosis, 514, 514t
in pulmonary arterial hypertension, 407t, 408–409, 409t
Epothilones, in prostate cancer, 956
Epstein-Barr virus infection. *See* Human herpesvirus infection
Eptifibatide
in coronary artery disease, 327b, 329f, 331t, 333f, 334–335, 334f
in thrombosis, 918
Equilibrium dissociation constant, 53–54, 57f
ErbB antagonists, in schizophrenia, 812
Erectile dysfunction, in multiple sclerosis, 697
Ergocalciferol, in renal osteodystrophy, 438–439, 439t
Ergostine, in headache, 733, 733t
Ergot(s)
α-adrenergic receptor blocking effect of, 132
antiretroviral interaction with, 1197t
in headache prevention, 734t, 736
in headache treatment, 727t, 733, 733t
Ergotamine
in headache, 733, 733t
triptan interaction with, 730t
Erlotinib, 85–86
nicotine interaction with, 842t
in non–small cell lung cancer, 923
in prostate cancer, 955
Error, statistical, 49
Ertapenem, creatinine clearance with, 176t
Erthryomycin, in lymphogranuloma venereum, 1202t
Erythema nodosum, in inflammatory bowel disease, 488t
Erythrocytes
Plasmodium infection of, 1141–1143, 1142t, 1144f. *See also* Malaria
production of, 895, 896f
Erythroderma, in psoriasis, 986
Erythromycin, 174f, 174t
in acne, 975t, 976, 977
adverse effects of, in pregnancy, 179t
antiretroviral interaction with, 1197t
in chancroid, 1202t
in granuloma inguinale, 1202t
midazolam interaction with, 880
in motility disorders, 479t, 482
topical, ocular, 859t
Erythropoietin, 903–905, 903f
cell production and, 213–214
gene delivery of, 1301
recombinant, 904–905
adverse effects of, 905
blood pressure increase with, 713
in dysautonomias, 710t, 712–713
in multiple sclerosis, 699
PEGylated, 441
in renal insufficiency, 440–441
resistance to, 441
Escherichia coli Nissle 1917, in inflammatory bowel disease, 500
Escitalopram, 109, 110t
in generalized anxiety disorder, 775, 775t
in obsessive-compulsive disorder, 755, 755t
in panic disorder, 773, 774t
in social anxiety disorder, 778–779, 779t
Esmolol, 134
in coronary artery disease, 347f, 347t, 350t
in thyroid storm, 583t
Esomeprazole, 464–467, 465t
Estradiol, 634, 634f
nicotine interaction with, 842t
oral, 634, 635t
parenteral, 635
transdermal, 634–635, 635t
Estramustine phosphate, in prostate cancer, 954
Estrogen, 634–635
in Alzheimer's disease, 646
antagonists of, 636
biochemistry of, 634
endogenous, 634, 634f
in headache prevention, 736
mechanism of action of, 634
in menopause, 639–640
oral, 634, 635t
in oral contraceptives, 636–639, 637t–638t
in osteoporosis, 601–602
parenteral, 635
in prostate cancer, 952–953
receptors for, 633, 634
transdermal, 634–635, 635t
in voiding dysfunction, 446t, 453–454
Estrogen antagonists, 636
Estrogen receptor down-regulators, in breast cancer, 935, 935f
Estrone, nicotine interaction with, 842t
Eszopliclone, 99, 100t
Etanercept, 159t, 168
in graft-versus-host disease, 1287
in psoriasis, 996–997, 997f, 1000t, 1002f
in psoriatic arthritis, 1003, 1003f
in rheumatoid arthritis, 1033, 1033t
side effects of, 168
Ethacrynic acid, in hepatic cirrhosis, 514–515, 515t
Ethambutol, 1091f
in tuberculosis, 1092t, 1094–1095, 1098–1099, 1099t, 1101t
Ethanol, in methanol toxicity, 1214–1215, 1215f
Ethionamide, 1091f
in tuberculosis, 1092t, 1095, 1102t
Ethosuximide, in seizure disorders, 670
Ethylene glycol, toxicity of, 1214–1215, 1215f
Ethylenediaminetetra-acetic acid, 1217, 1217t
Etidocaine, 868t, 869, 869f
cardiac toxicity of, 865
Etidronate, 599f, 600
Etodolac, in osteoarthritis, 1020t
Etomidate, 99, 879t, 881–882
Etoposide
in breast cancer, 937
in hematologic malignancy, 946
in prostate cancer, 954
in small cell lung cancer, 926
Etravirine, in HIV infection, 1191–1193, 1192t
European Medicines Evaluation Agency, 20, 31
European Union, regulatory activity of, 20
Evening primrose, 1239t
Everolimus, 165
Evidence-based practice, 41–50
components of, 41, 42b
databases for, 42–44, 42t, 43b, 44t
evidence gathering for, 42–44, 42t, 43b, 44t
evidence grading in, 47–48, 47t
literature review evaluation in, 46–47
question formulation in, 41, 42b
research evaluation in, 44–46, 44b, 45t
statistics in, 48–49, 48t
Exchange protein activated by cAMP (Epac), 72
Excimer laser therapy, in psoriasis, 998
Excipient, in over-the-counter medications, 1223
Excitotoxicity, 96
Exemestane, 636
in breast cancer, 934
Exenatide
in diabetes mellitus, 560
in obesity, 554
Exercise
in dysautonomias, 714–715
in obesity, 553
Exploding head syndrome, 853
Exposure and response prevention therapy, in obsessive-compulsive disorder, 754–755
Extracellular matrix, integrin interaction with, 77
Extracellular signal-regulated kinase (ERK) pathway, 80
Extracorporeal phototherapy, in transplantation, 1286–1287
Exubera, 566
Eyes
acetylcholine effects on, 120
β-adrenergic receptor antagonist effects on, 135
amiodarone effects on, 381
anatomy of, 857, 858f
antimuscarinic effects on, 122, 123
aqueous humor of, 857, 858f
ganglionic blocker effect on, 123
hydroxychloroquine effects on, 1032–1033
hyperthyroidism-related disorders of, 579, 579f
pharmacokinetics at, 857–858
physiology of, 857, 858f
prolactinoma-related disorders of, 617
sympathomimetic drug effects on, 128
systemic drug effects on, 857
topical drugs for, 857–861
anti-inflammatory, 859–860, 860t
antiangiogenic, 861, 861t
antibiotic, 858–859, 859t
antiglaucoma, 859f, 860–861

Eyes *(Continued)*
cycloplegic, 859, 860f
lubricant, 861
miotic, 860–861
multiple, 858b
mydriatic, 859, 860f
pharmacokinetics of, 857–858
Ezetimibe, in dyslipidemia, 313

F

Fab fragment, antidigoxin, 1216
Factor II, half-life of, 913t
Factor VII, half-life of, 913t
Factor VIIa, 912
Factor VIII, 909–911, 910f
Factor VIII inhibitors, 911
Factor IX, 910f, 911
half-life of, 913t
Factor X, half-life of, 913t
Factor Xa inhibitors, in coronary artery disease, 337b, 339
Falipamil, 354
Famciclovir
adverse effects of, 189t
in herpes simplex virus infection, 1203, 1203t
in human herpesvirus infection, 184t, 185t
indications for, 188
mechanism of action of, 186
pharmacokinetics of, 185, 185t
spectrum of activity of, 187–188
Familial benign hypercalcemia, 588–589
Familial combined hyperlipidemia, 307
Familial hypercholesterolemia, 307
Famotidine, in acid secretion disorders, 463–464, 464t
Fantofarone, receptor interaction of, 54f
Far inhibitors, 86
Farnesyl protein transferase inhibitors, 86
Fasciola hepatica infection, 1178
Fatigue, in multiple sclerosis, 696–697
Fatty acids, essential, in acne, 980
FDA Modernization Act (1997), 20
Febuxostat, in gout, 1044
Felbamate, 97t, 98
age-related clearance of, 260t
in seizure disorders, 668f, 673
Felodipine
in coronary artery disease, 351–353, 351t, 353t
in heart failure, 397–398
Fenfluramine, 108
pulmonary arterial hypertension and, 407
Fenofibrate
in dyslipidemia, 314–315, 314t
in gout, 1043
Fenoldopam, 130
Fentanyl
antiretroviral interaction with, 1197t
in pain, 885t, 886
Ferric ammonium citrate, 1222
Ferric chloride, 1222
Ferric gluconate, in renal insufficiency–associated anemia, 441, 441t
Ferrous fumarate, 898, 898t
in renal insufficiency–associated anemia, 441, 441t
Ferrous gluconate, 898, 898t
in renal insufficiency–associated anemia, 441, 441t
Ferrous sulfate, 898, 898t
in renal insufficiency–associated anemia, 441, 441t
Fesoterodine, in voiding dysfunction, 454t
Fever
antimuscarinics and, 123
in infective endocarditis, 1123
Feverfew, in headache prevention, 736
Fexofenadine, St. John's wort effect on, 1241t
FG-3019, in renal insufficiency, 436
Fiber, in motility disorders, 478
Fibrates
in dyslipidemia, 314–315, 314t, 360t, 361b
in renal insufficiency, 442, 442t
Fibrinolytic therapy, 340–343
contraindications to, 342b, 343
mechanism of action of, 333f, 340
in myocardial infarction, 325, 340t, 341–343, 341f, 342f
pharmacokinetics of, 340–341, 340t
side effects of, 331t
in stroke, 743–744, 744b
in thrombosis, 918–919
Fibroblast, nuclear reprogramming of, 1324
Fibroblast growth factor receptor, 74
Fibromyalgia syndrome, vs. rheumatoid arthritis, 1027t
Filgrastim, 905
Fish oil supplementation, 385
FK506. *See* Tacrolimus
Flanarizine, 385
Flavine-dependent monooxygenase 3, pharmacogenetics of, 227t
Flavopiridol, cell cycle effects of, 84, 84f
Flavoxate, in voiding dysfunction, 446t
Flecainide, 371t, 372t, 382
adverse effects of, 375t, 382
antiretroviral interaction with, 1197t
nicotine interaction with, 842t
Flora, intestinal, inflammatory bowel disease and, 489–490
Fluconazole, 180t
drug interactions with, 182t
in infective endocarditis, 1130
mechanism of action of, 180
pharmacodynamics of, 181
pharmacokinetics of, 181
resistance to, 182–183
spectrum of activity of, 181
in vulvovaginal candidiasis, 1209t
Flucytosine, 180t
adverse effects of, 182
mechanism of action of, 180
pharmacodynamics of, 181
pharmacokinetics of, 181
spectrum of activity of, 181
Fludarabine, in hematologic malignancy, 945, 1280f, 1285–1286
Fludrocortisone
in adrenal insufficiency, 627
adverse effects of, 711
in baroreflex failure, 716
in dysautonomias, 710–711, 710t
Fluid balance, 143f, 145–146, 145f, 147f, 148f
Fluid therapy, in hypercalcemia, 595
Fluid volume. *See also* Electrolyte homeostasis
extracellular, 145, 146–148, 147f, 148f
intracellular, 145
Flumadine, in influenza, 1065–1066
Flumazenil, 99, 100t
for benzodiazepine reversal, 880
Flunarizine, 385
in headache prevention, 734t, 735
Flunisolide, in asthma, 424–426, 425t
Flunitrazepam, abuse of, 819t
Fluorescence polarization immunoassay, 279, 281f
Fluoroquinolones, 174t
creatinine clearance with, 176t
in infective endocarditis, 1130
mechanism of action of, 175
ocular, 859, 859t
pharmacodynamics of, 176
pharmacokinetics of, 176
Fluoroquinolones *(Continued)*
in pregnancy, 179t
resistance to, 1096
in tuberculosis, 1092t, 1096, 1104–1105
5-Fluorouracil
cell cycle effects of, 83, 84f
in colon cancer, 962, 962t, 963–965, 964t
pharmacogenetics of, 233
in prostate cancer, 954
Fluoxetine, 109, 110t. *See also* Selective serotonin reuptake inhibitors (SSRIs)
in obsessive-compulsive disorder, 755, 755t, 776–777, 776t
in panic disorder, 773, 774t
pharmacogenetics of, 230
in posttraumatic stress disorder, 777, 778t
in social anxiety disorder, 778–779, 779t
Fluphenazine, 806t, 807t
Fluphenazine decanoate, 806t
Flurizan, in Alzheimer's disease, 645t, 646
Flutamide, in prostate cancer, 953
Fluticasone, in asthma, 424–426, 425t
Fluvastatin, 309–312, 312t, 358–361, 358t, 359f, 359t, 360f, 360t, 361b
adverse effects of, 311–312, 360t
mechanism of action of, 309–311, 359f
pharmacogenetics of, 312
pharmacokinetics of, 311, 311t
Fluvoxamine, 109, 110t
nicotine interaction with, 842t
in obsessive-compulsive disorder, 755, 755t, 776–777, 776t
in panic disorder, 773, 774t
pharmacogenetics of, 230
in posttraumatic stress disorder, 777
in social anxiety disorder, 778, 779t
Focal adhesion kinase, 77
Folic acid
deficiency of, 900
methotrexate with, 166, 992
supplemental, 900
vitamin B_{12} interaction with, 899, 899f
Follicle-stimulating hormone, 632–633
recombinant, 633
Fomepizole, in methanol toxicity, 1215, 1215f
Fomivirsen sodium, 1307
Fondaparinux, in coronary artery disease, 337b, 339
Fontolizumab, 169t
in inflammatory bowel disease, 499
Food. *See also* Diet
drug interactions with, 269
in orthostatic hypotension, 714
tyramine in, 131
Food, Drug, and Cosmetic Act, 20, 31, 1227
Food and Drug Administration, 20, 31–32
compliance monitoring by, 32–33
Formestane, 636
Formoterol, 130, 420–423, 421t
mechanism of action of, 422
side effects of, 422–423
Formulary, 1235–1236
Fos-phenytoin, in seizure disorders, 669
Fosamprenavir, in HIV infection, 1191–1193, 1194t
Foscarnet
adverse effects of, 189t
in human herpesvirus infection, 184t, 185t
mechanism of action of, 186–187
Fosinopril
in coronary artery disease, 354–357, 355t, 357b
in heart failure, 390–392, 392b, 392t
Fospropofol, 879t, 881
Fotemustine, in melanoma, 969
Frangula, 1222
Frizzleds, 77

Frontotemporal lobar degeneration, 643
Frovatriptan, 109, 726–731, 728f, 729t, 730t
Ftorafur, 922
FTY720, in multiple sclerosis, 698
Fulvestrant, in breast cancer, 935, 935f
Fumaric acid, 995
Fumaric acid esters, in psoriasis, 995, 1000t, 1002f
Functional adrenal insufficiency, 627
Functional hypothalamic amenorrhea, 614, 620
Fungal infection, 179–183, 179f, 180t. *See also* Antifungal agents
  endocardial, 1136
  ocular, 859
Furazolidone
  in *Entamoeba* infection, 1181
  in *Giardia lamblia* infection, 1181
Furosemide, in hepatic cirrhosis, 514–515, 515t

G

G protein(s), 68f, 69–71, 70f
  effectors of, 71–73, 72f
G protein βγ dimer, 70
G protein cycle, 70–71, 70f
G protein–coupled receptors
  activation of, 68f, 69
  desensitization of, 95
  down-regulation of, 60, 61f, 95
  equilibrium state of, 68
  heterotrimeric G protein interaction with, 68f, 69–71, 70f
  internalization of, 69
  ligand binding to, 69
  ligands of, 68
  regulation of, 60, 61f
  structure of, 68, 68f
Gabapentin
  age-related clearance of, 260t
  in headache prevention, 734t
  in multiple sclerosis, 696t
  in pain, 890
  in seizure disorders, 673
  side effects of, 673
  in social anxiety disorder, 779, 779t
Gaboxadol, 99
Galantamine, 102t, 103
  in Alzheimer's disease, 644, 644t
Gallium nitrate, in hypercalcemia, 595
Gamboge, 1222
Ganaxolone, in seizure disorders, 679
Ganciclovir
  adverse effects of, 189t, 190
  in human herpesvirus infection, 184t, 185t
  indications for, 188
  mechanism of action of, 186
  pharmacokinetics of, 185, 185t
  resistance to, 190
  spectrum of activity of, 187–188
  TK gene transfer effects on, 1304
Ganglia, 115, 116f
Ganglionic blockers, 123–124, 124f
Ganirelix, 632, 632t
Garlic, 1238, 1239t, 1241t
Gastric acid. *See* Acid secretion
Gastric emptying, 476, 476f. *See also* Motility disorders
  accelerated, 477
  drug absorption and, 197
Gastric ulcers
  NSAID-induced, 462, 466, 466f, 467, 470–471
  peptic. *See* Peptic ulcer disease
  stress-related, 462, 463b
Gastrin, 459, 460f
Gastrin-releasing peptide, 460
Gastroesophageal reflux disease, 461
  extraesophageal symptoms in, 469
  Helicobacter pylori in, 469
  pathogenesis of, 461
  refractory, 469
  treatment of, 467–469, 468f
    antacids in, 462–463, 468
    H_2-receptor antagonists in, 463–464, 464t, 468
    pharmacogenetics of, 231
    proton pump inhibitors in, 231, 464–467, 465f, 465t, 468–469
Gastroesophageal varices, 509
  bleeding from, 516–518, 517f
Gastrointestinal tract
  acetylcholine effects on, 120
  antimuscarinic effects on, 123
  calcium handling in, 150, 151f
  catecholamine effects on, 129
  disorders of
    gender-related pharmacodynamics and, 253
    in hyperthyroidism, 578
    motility. *See* Motility disorders
  drug absorption in, 197–199, 198f
    age and, 257
  ganglionic blocker effect on, 123
  isoniazid toxicity to, 1094
  methotrexate effects on, 165
  motility of, 475–476, 476f. *See also* Motility disorders
    in hypothyroidism, 573
  mycophenolate effects on, 163
  NSAID effect on, 1019
  pseudo-obstruction of, 477, 481
  thiopurine effects on, 163
Gastroparesis, 476–477, 477f, 479t
  diabetic, 478, 478f
  treatment of, 478, 478f, 479t, 480t, 481–484
Gatifloxacin, 174t
  adverse effects of, 178t
  ocular, 859t
  in tuberculosis, 1102t
Gefitinib, 85
  in non–small cell lung cancer, 923
  in prostate cancer, 955
Gemcitabine
  in breast cancer, 936
  in small cell lung cancer, 926
Gemella spp., in infective endocarditis, 1131t, 1132
Gemfibrozil
  drug interactions with, 270–271
  in dyslipidemia, 314–315, 314t
  rhabdomyolysis and, 312, 314
Gemifloxacin, 174t, 178t
Gemtuzumab ozogamicin, in hematologic malignancy, 948
Gender, 251–256
  adverse reactions and, 253–254
  biologic differences and, 251, 252f
  disease differences and, 251–252
  hormones and, 252f, 254–255, 254t, 255f
  pharmacodynamic differences and, 253
  pharmacokinetic differences and, 252–253, 252t
Gendicine, 1304
Gene(s), 1297–1298, 1298f
  suicide, 1297, 1304
Gene therapy, 1295–1313, 1296f
  in cancer, 1304, 1307–1308. *See also* Gene therapy, oncolytic
  cancer promotion with, 1303
  clinical trials of, 1303–1304
  compensatory, 1296
  in cytomegalovirus retinitis, 1307
  cytoreductive/antiproliferative, 1297
  definition of, 1295
Gene therapy *(Continued)*
  in dyslipidemia, 316
  ex vivo, 1295, 1296f
  gene addition, 1297–1305
    adeno-associated virus vectors for, 1300
    adenoviral vectors for, 1299–1300, 1300t
    in angiogenesis, 1304–1305
    in cancer, 1304
    cell death in, 1301–1302
    delivery targeting in, 1301
    development cycle for, 1305, 1305f
    expression decay in, 1301–1302
    gene expression barriers in, 1301–1302
    in hemophilia, 1304
    herpesvirus vectors for, 1300
    historical perspective on, 1303–1304
    immunologic barriers to, 1301
    lentiviral vectors for, 1299, 1300t
    noninvasive monitoring of, 1302, 1303f
    nonviral vectors for, 1298–1299, 1298f, 1300t
    protein destruction in, 1302
    retroviral vectors for, 1299, 1300t
    safety of, 1302–1303
    in SCID, 1304
    suicide gene, 1304
    transcriptional targeting in, 1301
    transductional targeting in, 1301
    vector for, 1297, 1297f, 1298–1300, 1298f, 1299f, 1300t
    viral vectors for, 1299–1300, 1299f, 1300t
    in vivo barriers in, 1300–1301
  gene repair, 1308, 1309f
  gene suppression, 1305–1308
    in cancer, 1307–1308
    in cytomegalovirus retinitis, 1307
    delivery barriers in, 1306
    delivery strategies for, 1305–1306
    mechanism of action of, 1305, 1306f
    suppression barriers in, 1306–1307
  goals of, 1296–1297
  in hemophilia, 1302, 1304
  homologous recombination for, 1296, 1308, 1309f
  immunostimulatory, 1297
  in ischemic heart disease, 1304–1305
  oncolytic, 1308–1313
    antibody depletion in, 1311
    antibody evasion in, 1311
    clinical trials of, 1312–1313
    delivery barriers in, 1311–1312
    mechanism of action of, 1309, 1310f
    noninvasive monitoring of, 1312
    physical barriers in, 1312
    polymer coating in, 1311
    proapoptoic targeting in, 1311
    serotype switching in, 1311
    transcriptional targeting in, 1309, 1311
    transductional targeting in, 1309
    translational targeting in, 1311
    virus extravasation in, 1311–1312
  in osteogenesis imperfecta, 1308, 1309f
  safety of, 1302–1303
  in SCID, 1304
  in β-thalassemia major, 1301
  tissue engineering, 1296–1297
  in vivo, 1295, 1296f, 1297, 1297f
Genetic variability, 226–228, 226f. *See also* Pharmacogenetics
Genistein, 88
Genitourinary system. *See also* Bladder; Kidneys; Voiding dysfunction
  β-adrenergic receptor antagonist effects on, 135
  catecholamine effects on, 129
  ganglionic blocker effect on, 123–124

Genomics. *See* Pharmacogenomics
Gentamicin, 174t
  adverse effects of, 284, 1128–1129
  creatinine clearance with, 176t
  in infective endocarditis, 1128–1129, 1131–1133, 1131t, 1133t, 1134–1135, 1134t
  monitoring of, 276t
  ocular, 859t
  pharmacokinetics of, 200
  toxicity of, 284, 1128–1129
Ghrelin
  in acid secretion, 459
  in motility disorders, 483
Giardia lamblia infection, 1182f
  treatment of, 1178, 1181
Gilbert's syndrome, 222
Ginger, 1239t
Gingko biloba, 1238–1240, 1239t
  in Alzheimer's disease, 646
Ginseng, 1239t
Glatiramer acetate, in multiple sclerosis, 690, 690f, 693, 695
Glaucoma
  corticosteroid-related, 426
  treatment of, 859f, 860–861, 861f
Gliclazide, in diabetes mellitus, 562, 563f, 563t
Glimepiride, in diabetes mellitus, 562, 563f, 563t
Glipizide
  azole interaction with, 182t
  in diabetes mellitus, 562, 563f, 563t
Glomerular filtration rate, 142–144, 144t, 201
  in children, 243–244, 244t
  single-nephron, 144
Glomerulotubular balance, 146
Glucagon, neurotransmitter receptor response to, 705t
Glucagon-like peptide-1, in diabetes mellitus, 560–561, 560f, 566
Glucocorticoid(s)
  deficiency of, 626–627, 626f
  excess of, 623–626, 624f, 625t. *See also* Cushing's disease
  in pregnancy, 1059t
  therapeutic. *See* Corticosteroid(s)
Glucocorticoid response elements, 160, 492
Glucosamine, in osteoarthritis, 1018t, 1021
Glucose, metabolism of, 557, 558f
Glucose-6-phosphate dehydrogenase deficiency, primaquine contraindication in, 1153–1154
α-Glucosidase inhibitors, in diabetes mellitus, 559, 559f, 559t
Glutamate, 92, 96–98
  anatomic distribution of, 96
  function of, 96
  metabolism of, 96, 96f
  receptors for, 96–97, 96f
  regulation of, 96
  synthesis of, 93t, 96, 96f
  as therapeutic target, 97–98, 97t
Glutamate antagonists, 97–98, 97t
  adverse effects of, 189t, 190
  in Alzheimer's disease, 644–645, 644t
  in influenza, 187, 1065–1066
  in multiple sclerosis, 696t, 697
  in Parkinson's disease, 659
  pharmacokinetics of, 186
  resistance to, 190
  in seizure disorders, 668f, 673, 674
Glutamate dehydrogenase, 96
Glutamic acid decarboxylase, 98, 98f
Glutamine acid hydrochloride, 1222
Glutathione-*S*-transferase, pharmacogenetics of, 227t
Glyburide
  azole interaction with, 182t
  in diabetes mellitus, 562, 563f, 563t
Glycerin enema, in constipation, 480t
Glycine, 92, 99
Glycine max, 1239t
Glycopeptides, 174t
  mechanism of action of, 175
  pharmacokinetics of, 176
  spectrum of activity of, 177
P-Glycoprotein, 373–374
Glycoprotein IIb/IIIa receptor antagonists
  adverse effects of, 334–335, 918
  in coronary artery disease, 327b, 329f, 333–335, 333f, 334f
  in thrombosis, 918
Glycoprotein IIIa, pharmacogenetics of, 228t
Glycopyrrolate, 102t
Goeckerman regimen, 989, 1000t, 1002f
Goiter. *See also* Hyperthyroidism
  multinodular, toxic, 578f, 581
Goldenseal, 1241, 1241t
Golimumab, 169t
Gonadotropin(s), 632–633
  synthetic, 633
Gonadotropin-releasing hormone, 613t, 631–632
  synthetic, 632, 632t, 633
Gonadotropin-releasing hormone agonists, 632, 632t
  in breast cancer, 934
  in prostate cancer, 951
Gonadotropin-releasing hormone antagonists, 632, 632t
  in prostate cancer, 952
Gonococcal infection, 1206–1207, 1207t
Gonorrhea, 1206, 1207t
Good Clinical Practice, in drug development, 21–22, 22b
Goserelin, 632, 632t
  in breast cancer, 934
Gout, 1039–1045
  acute, 1039–1041, 1040t
  chronic, 1041–1044, 1041t
  pathophysiology of, 1039, 1040f
  vs. rheumatoid arthritis, 1027t
  treatment of, 1039–1045
    adjunctive therapies in, 1043–1044
    adrenocorticotropic hormone in, 1040t, 1041
    benzbromarone in, 1044
    colchicine in, 1039–1041, 1040t, 1043, 1043b
    corticosteroids in, 1040t, 1041
    febuxostat in, 1044
    fenofibrate in, 1043
    indomethacin in, 1040t, 1041
    lifestyle changes in, 1043
    losartan in, 1043–1044
    principles of, 1043, 1043b
    probenecid in, 1042
    prophylactic, 1043
    sulfinpyrazone in, 1042–1043
    uricase in, 1044
    uricosuric agents in, 1042
    vitamin C in, 1044
    xanthine oxidase inhibitors in, 1041–1042, 1041t
G6PD deficiency, primaquine contraindication in, 1153–1154
Graft-versus-host disease, 1269, 1270–1271, 1329–1330
  prophylaxis against, 1275, 1287
  treatment of, 1275, 1287
Gramicidin, ocular, 859t
Granisetron, 109, 110t
  in motility disorders, 479t
Granulicatella spp., in infective endocarditis, 1131t, 1132
Granulocyte, 895, 896f
Granulocyte colony-stimulating factor (G-CSF)
  cell production and, 213–214
  recombinant, 905
Granulocyte-macrophage colony-stimulating factor (GM-CSF)
  in melanoma, 970–971
  recombinant, 499, 905
Granulocytopenia, in hyperthyroidism, 578
Granuloma inguinale, 1202, 1202t
Grape seed, 1239t
Grapefruit juice, lovastatin interaction with, 269
Graves' disease, 576, 577, 578f, 579, 579f. *See also* Hyperthyroidism
Green tea, 1239t
Griseofulvin, 183t
Groaning, sleep-related, 854
Groll-Hirschowitz syndrome, 709
Growth
  psychostimulant effects on, 765, 765t
  skeletal, 593
Growth factor(s)
  erythroid, 903–905, 903f
  hematopoietic, 902–903, 903f, 904f
  myeloid, 905
  thrombopoietic, 905–906
Growth factor receptor, 73–74, 74f
Growth factor receptor inhibitors, 85–86
  in prostate cancer, 955–956
Growth hormone
  deficiency of, 614–616
  in older adults, 615
  recombinant, 615
  regulation of, 614–615, 614f
  tumor secretion of, 617–619, 618t, 619f
Growth hormone receptor antagonist, in acromegaly, 619, 619f
Growth hormone–releasing hormone, 613t
  in growth hormone deficiency, 616
Guaifenesin, 1222
Guanabenz, 107, 130
Guanethidine, in baroreflex failure, 716
Guanfacine, 130
  in attention-deficit/hyperactivity disorder, 766, 766t
Guanylate cyclase-C agonist, 484
Guanylyl cyclase receptors, 75–76

H

HACEK organisms, in infective endocarditis, 1135–1136, 1135t
Haemophilus ducreyi infection, 1201, 1202t
Haemophilus influenzae type b vaccine, 1251–1252, 1252t
Hair disorders, in hypothyroidism, 574
Half-life
  coagulation factor, 913t
  elimination, 193, 195
  pharmacodynamic, 208
Hallucinations, 851
Hallucinogen abuse, 819t
Halofantrine, in malaria, 1148f, 1154
Haloperidol, 105, 105t, 806t, 807t, 809f–811f
  α-adrenergic receptor blocking effect of, 132
  nicotine interaction with, 842t
  in obsessive-compulsive disorder, 776t, 777
Haloperidol decanoate, 806t
Haloprogin, 1222
Halothane, 875f, 875t
  cardiac effects of, 877
  CNS effects of, 877
  hepatic effects of, 877–878
  metabolism of, 877–878
  renal effects of, 877
  respiratory effects of, 876
Hantavirus infection, 1074–1075, 1075f

Hashimoto's thyroiditis, 571. *See also* Hypothyroidism
Hashish abuse, 819t
HCV-796, in hepatitis C virus infection, 541t, 542
Headache, 719–739. *See also* Migraine
chemical-induced, 727t
cluster, 725
fludrocortisone-related, 711
historical perspective on, 719–720
pathogenesis of, 724–725, 724t, 725f, 726b
pathophysiology of, 720–724, 720f, 720t, 721t, 722f, 723f, 724b, 724t
secondary, 726
tension-type, 725
treatment of, 725–739
adjuvants in, 736–737
β-adrenergic receptor antagonists in, 135, 734–735, 734t
angiotensin antagonists in, 736
angiotensin-converting enzyme inhibitors in, 736
angiotensin modulators in, 734t
anticonvulsants in, 723, 734t, 735
antidepressants in, 734t, 735
botulinum toxin A in, 735
butalbital in, 727t, 733
calcium channel blockers in, 734t, 735
cannabinoids in, 739, 739f
coenzyme Q_{10} in, 736–737
ergots in, 727t, 733, 733t, 736
failed drugs in, 738t
minerals in, 736
muscle relaxants in, 733, 734t
NSAIDs in, 727t, 731–733, 732t, 735–736
oxygen in, 733
prophylactic, 734–736, 734t
triptans in, 726–731, 727t, 728f, 729t, 730t, 732b
valproate sodium in, 733
vitamin B_{12} in, 737, 737f
Health Insurance Portability and Accountability Act, 1228
Heart
β-adrenergic receptor agonist effect on, 423
age-related changes in, 261–262
disease of. *See* Coronary artery disease; Myocardial infarction
excitation of, 367–369, 368f
failure of. *See* Heart failure
hyperthyroidism effects on, 577
hypothyroidism effects on, 572
inhalational anesthetic effects on, 876–877
local anesthetic effects on, 864–865
mitoxantrone effects on, 691
muscarinic acetylcholine receptors of, 102
NSAID effect on, 1020
psychostimulant effects on, 765
rhythm disorders of. *See* Arrhythmias
transplantation of, 1273–1274. *See also* Transplantation
Heart failure, 389–398
epidemiology of, 389
mitoxantrone-related, 691
pathophysiology of, 389, 390f
thromboembolism and, 398
treatment of, 389–398
β-adrenergic receptor antagonists in, 134, 389–390, 391b, 391t
aldosterone receptor blockers in, 389, 394–395, 394b, 394t
angiotensin-converting enzyme inhibitors in, 389, 390–392, 392b, 392t
angiotensin II receptor blockers in, 389, 392–394, 393b, 393t
anticoagulation in, 398
Heart failure *(Continued)*
calcium channel blockers in, 397–398, 397b, 397t
calcium sensitizers in, 396–397
digoxin in, 395, 395b, 395t
diuretics in, 395
inotropes in, 396, 396b, 396t, 397t
nesiritide in, 154
vasodilators in, 395–396, 395t, 396b, 396t
Heart Protection Study, 31
Heavy metal exposure, 1216–1219, 1217f, 1217t
Helicobacter pylori infection
in gastroesophageal reflux disease, 469
in peptic ulcer disease, 461–462, 469–470, 470t
testing for, 471
treatment of, 469–470, 470t
Helminthic infection, 1171–1178
Ascaris, 1171, 1172f, 1174, 1175
Echinococcus granulosus, 1171–1172, 1175f
Schistosoma, 1177, 1178, 1179f
Strongyloides, 1171, 1173f, 1174, 1175
Taenia solium, 1172, 1176f, 1178, 1180f
treatment of, 1171–1178
albendazole in, 1171–1172, 1172f
bithionol in, 1178
diethylcarbamazine in, 1174–1175, 1177f
ivermectin in, 1175, 1178f
mebendazole in, 1172, 1174, 1177f
niclosamide in, 1178
oxamniquine in, 1178
praziquantel in, 1177–1178, 1178f
pyrantel pamoate in, 1174, 1177f
thiabendazole in, 1174
triclabendazole in, 1178
Trichinella, 1171, 1174f
Wuchereria bancrofti, 1174, 1177f
Hematocrit, gender and, 251
Hematologic malignancy, 945–948, 946t
treatment of, 945–948
alkylating agents in, 946
antibiotics in, 945–946
antimetabolites in, 945
biologic therapies in, 948
chemotherapy in, 945–948, 948t
stem cell transplantation in, 1274–1275, 1326–1327, 1327f
Hematopoiesis, 895, 896f
growth factors in, 902–903, 903f, 904f
Hematopoietic stem cells, 945, 947f
Heme oxygenase, 111
Hemodialysis, in methanol toxicity, 1215
Hemoglobin, gender and, 251
Hemophilia A, 909–911
Hemophilia B, 910f, 911, 1302, 1304
Hemorrhage. *See also* Bleeding
alveolar, in systemic lupus erythematosus, 1057
intracerebral, 743, 750–751
variceal, 516–518, 517f
Hemostasis, 909, 910f
disorders of, 909–913
pathophysiology of, 909
treatment of, 909–913
antifibrinolytics in, 912–913
coagulation factors in, 909–912
DDAVP in, 912
goals of, 909
Heparin, 914f, 915–916
adverse effects of, 336–337, 338, 916
in bacterial meningitis, 1115
drug interactions with, 337, 338
low-molecular-weight, 915–916
in coronary artery disease, 331t, 335t, 337–339, 338b
overdosage of, 337
Heparin *(Continued)*
unfractionated, 915–916
in coronary artery disease, 331t, 335–337, 335t, 336f, 338b
Hepatic encephalopathy, 511
treatment of, 520, 520f
Hepatic vein pressure gradient, 508–509, 510f
Hepatitis
kava-related, 1242
sulfasalazine-related, 995
zileuton-related, 428
Hepatitis A virus infection
clinical presentation of, 528, 528f
epidemiology of, 527–528
pathogenesis of, 528
prevention of, 534, 534t
vaccine against, 534, 534t, 1252–1253, 1252t, 1253t, 1254t
Hepatitis B virus infection, 187, 188
acute, 529, 537
chronic, 529–530, 537–539, 538t
clinical presentation of, 529–530, 530f
drug resistance in, 190
epidemiology of, 527, 528–529, 529f
pathogenesis of, 529
prevention of, 534–535
treatment of, 187, 535–540
in acute disease, 537
adefovir dipivoxil in, 536, 536f, 538t, 539
in chronic disease, 530, 537–539, 538t
clevudine in, 537
emtricitabine in, 537, 539
entecavir in, 536–537, 536f, 538t, 539
interferon in, 535–536, 538, 538t
lamivudine in, 536, 536f, 538–539, 538t
peginterferon in, 535–536, 538, 538t
telbivudine in, 537, 537f, 538t, 539
tenofovir in, 537
vaccine against, 535, 535t, 1252t, 1253, 1253t, 1254t
Hepatitis C virus infection, 187, 188
acute, 532
chronic, 532–533, 533f
clinical presentation of, 532–533
epidemiology of, 527, 530–531, 530f, 539, 539f
pathogenesis of, 531, 532f
prevention of, 539
treatment of, 540–542, 540f
in acute disease, 540–541
in chronic disease, 541–542, 541t, 542t
interferon in, 540–541, 541t
novel agents for, 541–542, 541t, 543f
ribavirin in, 540–541, 540f
Hepatitis E virus infection
acute, 534
clinical presentation of, 534
epidemiology of, 533–534, 533f
pathogenesis of, 534
postexposure prophylaxis in, 542
prevention of, 542
treatment of, 542
Hepatocellular carcinoma, hepatitis B and, 530
Hepatocyte growth factor, in renal insufficiency, 436
Hepatorenal syndrome, 510–511
treatment of, 519–520, 520f
HER2/neu gene, in breast cancer, 940
Herbal supplements. *See* Dietary supplements
Heroin abuse, 819t, 820t, 821, 821f
prevention of, 823
treatment of, 824t, 825–826, 825t, 829–831
buprenorphine in, 826, 827t, 830–831
LAAM in, 825–826, 830
methadone in, 825, 827t, 829–830

Herpes simplex virus infection. *See also* Human herpesvirus (HHV) infection
diagnosis of, 1202–1203
genital, 1202–1203, 1203t
neonatal, 1203
treatment of, 1203, 1203t
Heteroreceptors, 118
Hexamethonium, 123, 124f
Hill equation, 204
Hirudin, in coronary artery disease, 339–340
Histamine, 92, 93t, 109
in acid secretion, 459, 460f
isoniazid interaction with, 1094
neurotransmitter receptor response to, 705t
Histamine$_2$ (H_2)-receptor antagonists
in acid secretion disorders, 463–464, 464t
adverse effects of, 464
azole interaction with, 182t
in gastroesophageal reflux disease, 463–464, 464t, 468
midazolam interaction with, 880
nicotine interaction with, 842t
in peptic ulcer disease, 463–464, 464t, 469
Histamine-*N*-methyltransferase, 109
Histidine decarboxylase, 109
Histone deacetylase inhibitors, in prostate cancer, 955
Histrelin, 632, 632t
HIV infection. *See* Human immunodeficiency virus (HIV) infection
H^+,K^+-ATPase, in acid secretion, 460–461, 460f
HMG CoA reductase inhibitors, 309–312
adverse events with, 311–312, 360t
in Alzheimer's disease, 646
anti-inflammatory effects of, 311
with antihypertensive agents, 298
cardiovascular disease outcomes and, 310–311, 312, 312t
in dyslipidemia, 309–312, 358–361, 358t, 359f, 359t, 360f, 360t, 361b
hepatotoxicity of, 311
mechanism of action of, 309–310
musculoskeletal effects of, 311–312
after myocardial infraction, 385
myositis and, 312
niacin with, 314
over-the-counter, 1223
pharmacogenetics of, 312
pharmacokinetics of, 311, 311t
pleiotropic effects of, 310–311
in renal insufficiency, 436–437, 442, 442t
rhabdomyolysis with, 311–312
in stroke prevention, 749
Holter monitoring, 374
Homocysteine, cardiovascular disease and, 306
Homocystine, stroke and, 745t
Homologous recombination, 1296, 1308, 1309f
Hookworm, 1171, 1174
Hormone(s). *See also specific hormones*
drug effects and, 254–255
Hormone replacement therapy, 255
Horny goat weed, 1239t
Horse chestnut, 1239t
Hot flashes, estrogen for, 639
Human chorionic hormone, 632–633
recombinant, 633
Human herpesvirus (HHV) infection, 183–187, 184t, 185t
drug treatment for, 183–184, 184t
adverse effects of, 188–190, 189t
indications for, 188
mechanisms of action of, 186–187, 186f
pharmacobiology of, 184–185, 184f
pharmacokinetics of, 185, 185t
resistance to, 190
spectrum of activity of, 187–188
Human immunodeficiency virus (HIV) infection, 1187–1198
treatment of
CCR5 antagonists in, 1197–1198
drug interactions in, 1188, 1188b, 1190, 1192–1193, 1197t
entry inhibitors in, 1193, 1193f, 1195–1196, 1196t
gender-related pharmacodynamics in, 253
guidelines for, 1196, 1196t
integrase inhibitors in, 1198
maturation inhibitors in, 1198
monoclonal antibodies in, 1198
non-nucleoside reverse transcriptase inhibitors in, 1188, 1190–1191, 1190f, 1192t
nucleoside/nucleotide reverse transcriptase inhibitors in, 1187–1188, 1188f, 1189t–1190t
protease inhibitors in, 1191–1193, 1191f, 1194t–1195t
TNX-355 in, 1198
tuberculosis and, 1100, 1104
vulvovaginal candidiasis and, 1209–1210
Human metapneumovirus infection, 1072–1073, 1072f
Human papillomavirus (HPV) infection, 1210–1211, 1210b
vaccine against, 1253–1254, 1253t, 1254t
HuMax-CD20, in rheumatoid arthritis, 1035
Hungry bones syndrome, 589
Hyaluronic acid derivatives, in osteoarthritis, 1018t, 1021
Hydralazine, in heart failure, 395–396, 396b, 396t
Hydrochloric acid. *See* Acid secretion
Hydrochloric acid diluted, 1222
Hydrocodone, 1222
in pain, 885t, 887
Hydrocortisone
in inflammatory bowel disease, 492–493, 492t
in thyroid storm, 583t
Hydromorphone, in pain, 885t, 887
Hydroxocobalamin, 899–900
3-Hydroxy-3-methylglutaryl coenzyme A (HMG CoA) reductase inhibitors. *See* HMG CoA reductase inhibitors
Hydroxyamphetamine, neurotransmitter receptor response to, 705t
2-Hydroxybenzoic acid (salicylic acid)
in acne, 975t, 977, 979
in psoriasis, 989, 999t
γ-Hydroxybutyrate, 99
abuse of, 819t
Hydroxychloroquine
in pregnancy, 1059t, 1060
in rheumatoid arthritis, 1032–1033, 1032t
in systemic lupus erythematosus, 1051t, 1053–1055, 1054b, 1054t
toxicity of, 1032–1033
1α-Hydroxycholecalciferol, 596–597
Hydroxycobalamin, in cyanide toxicity, 1215–1216
6-Hydroxydopamine, 104
1α-Hydroxylase, renal, 591–592, 592f
Hydroxyurea
in hematologic malignancy, 945
in psoriasis, 993, 1000t
Hydroxyzine, in generalized anxiety disorder, 775t, 776
Hyoscyamine. *See* Atropine
Hyperaldosteronism, 295–296, 629
Hypercalcemia, 152, 588–589
calcitonin in, 595, 602–603
treatment of, 595–596
Hypercholesterolemia. *See also* Dyslipidemia
autosomal recessive, 307
common (polygenic), 307
familial, 307
in renal insufficiency, 442, 442t
Hyperglycemia. *See* Diabetes mellitus
Hyperhomocysteinemia, headache and, 737
Hypericum perforatum, 1239t, 1240
drug interactions with, 1240–1241, 1241t
Hyperinsulinism, in hypertension, 294, 294f
Hyperkalemia, in renal insufficiency, 437
Hyperlipidemia. *See also* Dyslipidemia
combined, familial, 307
in hypothyroidism, 572
stroke and, 749
Hyperlipoproteinemia. *See* Dyslipidemia
Hyperosmolar agents, in glaucoma, 860
Hyperparathyroidism
cinacalcet in, 598, 598f
hypercalcemia with, 588
Hyperphosphatemia, in renal insufficiency, 437, 438t
Hypersensitivity reaction. *See* Allergy
Hypersomnia, 851–853
pathophysiology of, 851
treatment of, 851–853
amphetamines in, 852
caffeine in, 852
goals of, 851
methylphenidate in, 852
modafinil in, 852–853
Hypertension, 291–300
adrenal, 295–296
alcohol-related, 295
in baroreflex failure, 293, 293f, 709, 709f, 710
contraceptive-related, 295
corticosteroid-related, 295
cyclosporine and, 164
definition of, 291–292
drug-related, 295
emergency, 299–300, 300f
epidemiology of, 291–292
in hyperaldosteronism, 629
iatrogenic, 295
immunosuppressant-related, 295
licorice-related, 295
monogenic, 294–295
mortality and, 291
neurogenic, 296
NSAID-related, 295
pathophysiology of, 292–294, 292f
acquired factors in, 292–294, 292f
baroreflex anomalies in, 293, 293f
endothelium-dependent vasomotricity anomalies in, 294
genetic factors in, 292
hemodynamics of, 292
obesity and, 294, 294f
renal dysfunction in, 292–293, 293f
renin-angiotensin system in, 294
smooth muscle dysfunction in, 294
sympathetic nervous system in, 293
vascular anomalies in, 293
vascular reactivity in, 294
vasodilation systems in, 294
portal. *See* Portal hypertension
portopulmonary, 511, 520–521, 521f
pressure-natriuresis curve in, 293, 293f
pulmonary. *See* Pulmonary arterial hypertension
in renal artery stenosis, 295
in renal insufficiency, 439–440, 440f
renovascular, 295
vs. baroreflex failure, 709
resistant, 299
reversible, 294–296

Hypertension *(Continued)*
secondary, 294–296
stroke and, 748–749
supine, 713b, 714
sympathomimetic-related, 295
treatment of, 296–300
α-adrenergic receptor antagonists in, 297t, 298
β-adrenergic receptor antagonists in, 297t, 298
algorithm for, 297, 299f
angiotensin-converting enzyme inhibitors in, 297t, 298
aspirin with, 298
blood pressure goals in, 298–299
calcium channel blockers in, 297t, 298
centrally acting antihypertensive drugs in, 298
in chronic kidney disease, 439–440, 440f
clinical trials of, 296–297
combination therapy in, 298
diuretics in, 297–298, 297t
in emergency hypertension, 299–300, 300f
goals of, 298–299
historical perspective on, 15
lifestyle modification in, 296
peripheral vasodilators in, 298
pharmacologic, 296–298, 297t, 299f
statins with, 298
Hyperthermia, zonisamide-related, 676
Hyperthyroidism, 576–583
amiodarone-related, 381
apathetic, 582, 583f
cardiovascular features of, 577
clinical features of, 577–579, 577b, 578f, 579f
dermatologic features of, 578–579
etiology of, 577b
gastrointestinal features of, 578
hematologic features of, 578
laboratory diagnosis of, 579, 579f
metabolic features of, 579
neonatal, 582
neuromuscular features of, 578
ocular features of, 579
pathophysiology of, 577
pregnancy and, 582
renal features of, 578
reproductive features of, 578
respiratory features of, 577–578
skeletal features of, 578
subclinical, 581–582, 582b
treatment of, 580–581, 580b
β-adrenergic receptor blockers in, 580
radioactive iodine therapy in, 581
surgical, 581
thionamides in, 580–581
Hypertriglyceridemia
familial, 307–308, 308t
moderate, 308
in renal insufficiency, 442, 442t
Hyperuricemia, 1039, 1040f. *See also* Gout
Hyperventilation, in bacterial meningitis, 1115
Hypervitaminosis D, 592–593
treatment of, 598
Hypnagogic hallucinations, 851
Hypnotic agents, in insomnia, 849–851, 851b
Hypobetalipoproteinemia, familial, 308
Hypocalcemia, 151–152, 589
in renal insufficiency, 437–438
Hypocalciuric hypercalcemia, familial, 588–589
Hypoglycemia, β-adrenergic receptor antagonist effects on, 135
Hypokalemia, β-adrenergic agonist–related, 423
Hypokalemic periodic paralysis, in hyperthyroidism, 578
Hypolipoproteinemia, 308
Hypomania, 787. *See also* Bipolar disorder
Hypoparathyroidism
hypocalcemia with, 589
treatment of, 598
Hypophosphatemia, 152
vitamin D in, 598
Hypopituitarism, 614–616
Hypopompic hallucinations, 851
Hypotension
in baroreflex failure, 709, 709f, 715–716
midazolam sedation and, 880
orthostatic. *See also* Syncope
in dopamine β-hydroxylase deficiency, 708
in multiple system atrophy, 708
in pure autonomic failure, 707–708, 713–714, 713b
treatment of, 710–716, 713–714, 713b
clonidine in, 710t, 712
droxidopa in, 710t, 712, 712f
erythropoietin in, 710t, 712–713
fludrocortisone in, 710–711, 710t
indomethacin in, 710t, 711–712
midodrine in, 710t, 711
yohimbine in, 710t, 712
postprandial, 714
Hypothalamic-pituitary-adrenal axis, 623, 624f
corticosteroid effects on, 426
Hypothalamic-pituitary axis
disorders of, 611–620. *See also specific disorders*
hormones of, 611, 612f, 613t
Hypothalamic-pituitary-gonadal axis, 631, 632f
Hypothalamic-pituitary-thyroidal axis, 572f
Hypothalamus, in acid secretion, 457–458
Hypothyroidism, 571–576
amiodarone-related, 381
cardiovascular features of, 572, 576
clinical features of, 572–574, 573t
congenital, 572
dermatologic features of, 574, 574f
etiology of, 571–572, 573f, 573t
gastrointestinal features of, 573
hematologic features of, 573–574
laboratory diagnosis of, 574, 575f
lithium-related, 793
myxedema coma in, 576
neuromuscular features of, 574
pathophysiology of, 571–572
pregnancy and, 576
reproductive features of, 574
respiratory features of, 573
secondary, 571, 573b, 576
subclinical, 571, 576
surgery and, 576
treatment of, 574–576, 575t, 576b
levothyroxine in, 574–575, 575t
liothyronine sodium in, 575–576, 576b
weight gain in, 574
Hypovitaminosis D, 593
Hypoxia, in pulmonary arterial hypertension, 407
Hypoxic drive, 876
Hysteresis, 208

I

Ibandronate, 599f, 600
Ibuprofen, 1222
in headache, 732t
in osteoarthritis, 1020t
in pain, 889t, 890
Ibutilide, 372t, 375t, 382
Ichthammol, 1222
ICI 118551, 128t
Idarubicin, in hematologic malignancy, 945–946
Idiopathic hypersomnia, hypopompic, 851
Idoxuridine, 183
Ifenprodil, 97–98
Ifosfamide, in small cell lung cancer, 925
Ileal bypass, in dyslipidemia, 315
Ileus
in hypothyroidism, 573
postoperative, 477–478
Iloprost, in pulmonary arterial hypertension, 407t, 409, 409t
Imatinib
in hematologic malignancy, 946
in pulmonary arterial hypertension, 413
St. John's wort effect on, 1241t
in small cell lung cancer, 926, 927f
Imipenem, adverse effects of, 178t
Imipenem-cilastatin, creatinine clearance with, 176t
Imipramine
in attention-deficit/hyperactivity disorder, 766
in generalized anxiety disorder, 775t, 776
nicotine interaction with, 842t
in panic disorder, 774, 774t
in posttraumatic stress disorder, 777, 778t
in voiding dysfunction, 446t, 452
Imiquimod, in genital human papillomavirus infection, 1210b, 1211
ImmuKnow assay, 285–286
Immune globulin
intravenous
in multiple sclerosis, 692, 697
in systemic lupus erythematosus, 1051t
in transplantation, 1286
lymphocyte. *See* Antithymocyte globulin
Immune system, 157–159
adaptive, 158–159, 159t
barrier, 157–158
cells of, 158
in Crohn's disease, 490
innate, 158–159, 159t
lymphoid organs of, 158
pharmacology of, 159–169, 159t, 169t. *See also specific drugs*
antilymphocyte antibodies in, 166–167, 166f
calcineurin inhibitors in, 163–164, 164f
corticosteroids in, 160–161, 160f
cyclosphosphamide in, 166
methotrexate in, 165–166
monoclonal antibodies in, 166–168
mycophenate in, 163
sirolimus in, 164–165
thiopurines in, 161–163
tumor necrosis factor-α inhibitors in, 167–168
in rheumatoid arthritis, 1027–1030, 1028f, 1029f
structure of, 158–159, 159t
in transplantation, 1269–1272, 1273f. *See also* Transplantation, immunosuppression for
in ulcerative colitis, 490
vaccine-related response of, 1248–1249, 1249f
Immunity
acquired, 158–159, 159t
innate, 158–159, 159t
Immunization. *See* Vaccine(s)
Immunoassay, 279, 281f
Immunoglobulin A (IgA), secretory, 158
Immunoglobulin E (IgE), in asthma, 419, 430
Immunoprophylaxis, hepatitis A, 534, 534t
Immunosuppressants, 157, 158t, 159–169, 159t. *See also specific drugs*
hypertension with, 295
in inflammatory bowel disease, 493–495
in multiple sclerosis, 691–692
in transplantation, 1272b, 1274, 1275–1288, 1329–1330. *See also* Transplantation, immunosuppression for

Immunotherapy
in Alzheimer's disease, 646
in asthma, 430–431
in melanoma, 970–971
Implantable cardioverter-defibrillator, 378
amiodarone with, 381
sodium channel blocker effect on, 377
in ventricular arrhythmias, 380, 381
In vitro fertilization, GnRH agonists in, 632
Inactivity, stroke and, 745t
Incontinence, urinary. *See* Voiding dysfunction
Incretin-based therapy, in diabetes mellitus, 560–561, 560f, 566
Indinavir
in HIV infection, 1191–1193, 1194t
oral contraceptives and, 254
St. John's wort effect on, 1241t
Indomethacin
aspirin interaction with, 730t
in dysautonomias, 710t, 711–712
in gout, 1040t, 1041
in headache, 732
in osteoarthritis, 1020t
in pain, 889t, 890
Infant. *See also* Children
herpes simplex virus infection in, 1203
hyperthyroidism in, 582
syphilis in, 1204–1206, 1205b, 1205t
tetany in, 589
vaccines for, 1252t, 1259–1260
Infantile spasms
vigabatrin for, 676–677
zonisamide in, 675, 676
Infection. *See also* Antibacterial agents; Antifungal agents; Antiviral agents *and specific infections*
abatacept and, 1034
cutaneous, 1011, 1013
endocardial. *See* Infective endocarditis
helminthic. *See* Helminthic infection
after hematopoietic stem cell transplantation, 1275
meningeal. *See* Meningitis
ocular, 858–859, 859t
protozoan. *See* Protozoan infection
pulmonary. *See* Influenza; Pneumonia; Tuberculosis
rituximab and, 1034–1035
stroke and, 745t
thiopurines and, 163
after transplantation, 1274
tumor necrosis factor-α inhibitors and, 1034
Infective endocarditis, 1121–1138
Abiotrophia defectiva in, 1131t, 1132
blood culture in, 1122
clinical manifestations of, 1123
complications of, 1123
definition of, 1121
diagnosis of, 1121–1122
echocardiography in, 1122
enterococci in, 1132–1134, 1133t
epidemiology of, 1121
fever in, 1123
Gemella spp. in, 1131t, 1132
Granulicatella spp. in, 1131t, 1132
groups B, C, and G streptococci in, 1132
hemodynamic factors in, 1122
immune complexes in, 1123
left-sided, 1122, 1134t, 1135
microthrombi in, 1122
mitral valve prolapse and, 1122
murmur in, 1123
pathogenesis of, 1122–1123
platelets in, 1122
polymorphonuclear leukocytes in, 1123
prevention of, 1137–1138, 1137b, 1137t
Infective endocarditis *(Continued)*
prosthetic valve in, 1122, 1134t, 1135, 1136–1137, 1136t
Pseudomonas aeruginosa in, 1136
right-sided, 1122, 1134–1135, 1134t
staphylococci in, 1123, 1134–1135, 1134t, 1138
Streptococcus bovis in, 1131–1132, 1131t
Streptococcus pneumoniae in, 1132
Streptococcus pyogenes in, 1132
systemic complications of, 1123
treatment of, 1123–1138
for *Abiotrophia defectiva,* 1131t, 1132
aminoglycosides in, 1128–1129
amphotericin B in, 1130
aspirin and, 1130
β-lactam antibiotics in, 1124–1127, 1124f, 1125f
ciprofloxacin in, 1130
for culture-negative disease, 1136–1137, 1136t
daptomycin in, 1128
doxycycline in, 1129
for Enterobacteriaceae, 1136
for enterococci, 1132–1134, 1133t
fluconazole in, 1130
fluoroquinolones in, 1130
for fungi, 1136
for *Gemella* spp., 1131t, 1132
for *Granulicatella* spp., 1131t, 1132
for groups B, C, and G streptococci, 1132
for HACEK organisms, 1135–1136, 1135t
levofloxacin in, 1130
linezolid in, 1129, 1134
for methicillin-resistant staphylococci, 1134
minimum bactericidal concentration and, 1123–1124
minimum inhibitory concentration and, 1123–1124
moxifloxacin in, 1130
nonantibiotic, 1130
polymorphonuclear leukocytes and, 1123
for *Pseudomonas aeruginosa,* 1136
quinupristin-dalfopristin in, 1129, 1134
rifampin in, 1129
for staphylococci, 1134–1135, 1134t, 1138
for *Streptococcus bovis,* 1131–1132, 1131t
for *Streptococcus pneumoniae,* 1132
for *Streptococcus pyogenes,* 1132
surgical, 1130, 1138
vancomycin in, 1127–1128
for vancomycin-resistant enterococci, 1134
for viridans group streptococci, 1131–1132, 1131t
valvular complications of, 1123
vancomycin-resistant enterococci in, 1134
viridans group streptococci in, 1123, 1131–1132, 1131t
Infertility, treatment of, 632, 633, 636, 639
Inflammation, 157–169. *See also* Immune system
in asthma, 419
in COPD, 419
cutaneous. *See* Dermatitis
sebaceous gland. *See* Acne
Inflammatory bowel disease, 487–500
clinical features of, 487–488, 488f, 488t
environmental factors in, 489
genetics of, 489
immune dysregulation in, 490
intestinal flora in, 489–490
natural history of, 488
pathophysiology of, 488–490, 489f
treatment of, 490–500
adhesion molecule inhibitors in, 499
anti-inflammatory drugs in, 490–493, 491f, 491t, 492t, 493t, 497t
anticytokines in, 499
Inflammatory bowel disease *(Continued)*
anti–tumor necrosis factor-α agents in, 495–496, 498
approach to, 496–499, 497f, 498f
biologics in, 495–496, 497t, 499–500
cytokines in, 499
goals of, 490, 490b
growth factors in, 499
immunosuppressants in, 493–495, 493f, 494f, 497t
intracellular signal transduction inhibitors in, 499
microbiota in, 499–500
quality of life in, 490
remission induction in, 490
remission maintenance in, 490
stepwise approach to, 497f
surgery in, 490
thiopurines in, 162
Infliximab, 159t, 167–168
in graft-versus-host disease, 1287
heart failure and, 1034
in inflammatory bowel disease, 495–496, 497, 498
in psoriasis, 993, 996, 997, 997f, 1000t, 1002f, 1003, 1003f
in rheumatoid arthritis, 1033, 1033t
side effects of, 168, 496
Influenza, 1063–1068, 1065f, 1068f
avian, 1068–1070, 1070f
clinical features of, 1064–1065
complications of, 1065
diagnosis of, 1065
epidemiology of, 1063–1064, 1064f
pandemics of, 1064, 1065f, 1068, 1068f
severity of, 1064
treatment of, 185, 1065–1067
adamantanes in, 188, 1065–1066, 1066f
drug resistance in, 190, 1066
oseltamivir in, 187, 189f, 1066–1067, 1067f
zanamivir in, 187, 189f, 1067, 1067f
vaccine against, 1067–1068, 1069b, 1252t, 1253t, 1254–1255, 1254t, 1260, 1261, 1262, 1263t
virology of, 1063
Informed consent, in pediatric drug testing, 26
Ingram regimen, in psoriasis, 989
Inhalant abuse, 819t
Inhalational anesthetics. *See* Anesthetics, inhalational
Inordronate, 599f
Inotropes, in heart failure, 396, 396b, 396t, 397t
INR (international normalized ratio), 914
Insomnia, 849–851
etiology of, 849
treatment of, 849–851
antidepressants in, 850
benzodiazepines in, 849, 851b
goals of, 849
melatonin receptor agonists in, 850
non-benzodiazepine benzodiazepine receptor agonists in, 849–850
nonprescription hypnotic agents in, 850–851
Institute for Safe Medication Practices, 1229b
Insufficient sleep syndrome, 851
Insulin, 562, 564–568, 567f, 568f
catecholamine effects on, 129
long-acting, 565–566, 567f, 568f
Insulin detemir, 566, 567f, 568f
Insulin glargine, 566, 567f, 568f
Insulin-like growth factor-I
adverse effects of, 616
deficiency of, 615–616
recombinant, 615–616
Insulin receptor, 73, 567f
Insulin receptor substrate-1, 74

Insulin resistance, in hypertension, 294, 294f
Integrase inhibitors, in HIV infection, 1198
Integrin, 77
Integrin $\alpha_4\beta_7$, antibody against, in inflammatory bowel disease, 499
Interdigestive migrating motor complex, 476
Interferon(s)
  adverse effects of, 189t
  in hepatitis B virus infection, 535–536, 538, 538t
  in hepatitis C virus infection, 187, 188, 540–541, 541t
Interferon alfa
  in hematologic malignancy, 948
  in melanoma, 970
Interferon beta
  in multiple sclerosis, 689–690, 692–694, 695
  side effects of, 689–690, 694
Interferon-γ, antibody against, in inflammatory bowel disease, 499
Interleukin-1, 77
  glucocorticoid effect on, 493t
  inhibitor of. *See* Anakinra
  in osteoarthritis, 1022–1023, 1022f
  in rheumatoid arthritis, 1029f, 1030
Interleukin-1 receptor, type II, glucocorticoid effect on, 493t
Interleukin-2
  glucocorticoid effect on, 493t
  inhibition of, 167
  in melanoma, 970
Interleukin-4, in rheumatoid arthritis, 1029f, 1030
Interleukin-6
  antibody against, in inflammatory bowel disease, 499
  in rheumatoid arthritis, 1029f, 1030
Interleukin-8, glucocorticoid effect on, 493t
Interleukin-10, in inflammatory bowel disease, 499
Interleukin-11, recombinant, 905–906
Interleukin-12, antibody against, in inflammatory bowel disease, 499
International Conference on Harmonisation of Technical Requirements for Registration of Pharmaceuticals for Human Use, 20, 21–22, 22b, 32
International normalized ratio, 1219–1220
Intestine. *See* Colon; Gastrointestinal tract; Small intestine
Intracellular adhesion molecule-1, glucocorticoid effect on, 493t
Intracerebral hemorrhage, 743, 750–751
Intraocular circulation, 857, 858f
Intraocular pressure, 860–861, 861f
Intrauterine device, 638
Intravenous anesthetics, 878–882, 879t
Intrinsic factor, 900
  antibody to, 898
Iodides, exogenous, 571
Iodine
  radioactive, in hyperthyroidism, 581
  thyroid metabolism of, 572f
Iodoquinol, in protozoa infection, 1180–1181
Ion channels, 77–78
  antiarrhythmic drug interaction with, 372
  ligand binding to, 53, 54f
Ipecac, 1222
Ipratropium, 102t, 423–424, 423f, 424t
Irbesartan
  in coronary artery disease, 354–357, 356t, 357b
  in heart failure, 392–394, 393b, 393t
Irinotecan
  in breast cancer, 937
  in colon cancer, 962t, 963–964, 963f, 964t
  nicotine interaction with, 842t
  pharmacogenetics of, 233–234
Irinotecan *(Continued)*
  St. John's wort effect on, 1241t
  in small cell lung cancer, 926
Iron
  body storage of, 895
  deficiency of. *See* Iron-deficiency anemia
  metabolism of, 895, 896f
  oral, 898, 898t
  parenteral, 898
  supplemental, 897–898, 898t
    in renal insufficiency–associated anemia, 441, 441t
  toxicity of, 1217t, 1218
  transport of, 895, 897f
Iron-deficiency anemia, 895–898, 896f
  pathophysiology of, 896
  prevalence of, 897t
  treatment of, 897–898, 898t
Iron dextran, in renal insufficiency–associated anemia, 441, 441t
Iron sucrose, in renal insufficiency–associated anemia, 441, 441t
Irritable bowel syndrome, gender and, 253
Irritant contact dermatitis, 1008, 1010f
ISA247, in transplantation, 1288
Ischemia
  cerebral. *See* Stroke
  myocardial, 322. *See also* Myocardial infarction
    gene therapy in, 1304–1305
Ischemic pre-/post-conditioning, 361, 362f
ISIS 2503, 86
ISIS 5132, 86
Islet cell transplantation, 1327–1328
Isocarboxazid, 107, 110t
  in unipolar disorder, 792
Isoflurane, 99, 100t, 875f, 875t
  cardiac effects of, 876
  CNS effects of, 877
  hepatic effects of, 877
  metabolism of, 877
  renal effects of, 877
  respiratory effects of, 876
Isoniazid, 1092–1094, 1092t, 1098–1099, 1099t, 1100, 1101t
  adverse effects of, 1094
  azole interaction with, 182t
  clinical use of, 1094
  drug interactions with, 1094
  mechanism of action of, 1092, 1093f
  metabolism of, 1094
  pharmacogenetics of, 220, 220f
  pharmacokinetics of, 1094
  prophylactic, 1100, 1103t
  resistance to, 1092–1094
  structure of, 1091f, 1092
Isoproterenol, 128t
  functions of, 128t
  neurotransmitter receptor response to, 705t
  pharmacodynamics of, 215, 215f
  structure of, 127f, 421f
  in torsades de pointes, 371t
Isosorbide, in glaucoma, 860
Isosorbide dinitrate
  in coronary artery disease, 343, 344f, 345
  in heart failure, 395–396, 396b, 396t
Isosorbide mononitrate
  in coronary artery disease, 343, 344f, 345, 345b
  in hepatic cirrhosis, 514, 514t
Isospora infection, 1184, 1184f
Isotretinoin
  in acne, 975t, 977–978, 977f, 979, 979t
  in psoriasis, 993
  side effects of, 978, 993
Isradipine, in coronary artery disease, 351–353, 351t, 353t
Itopride, in motility disorders, 482
Itraconazole, 180t
  adverse effects of, 182
  antiretroviral interaction with, 1197t
  drug interactions with, 182t, 270–271
  mechanism of action of, 180
  pharmacodynamics of, 181
  pharmacokinetics of, 181
  spectrum of activity of, 181
Ivabradine, 354
Ivermectin, in helminthic infection, 1175, 1178f
Ixabepilone, in breast cancer, 937

J

J compound, in tuberculosis, 1105–1106, 1105f
Jak-STAT pathway, 74f, 76
Jalap, 1222
Japan, drug development in, 25
Japanese encephalitis virus vaccine, 1255
Joint
  disorders of. *See* Arthritis; Gout; Osteoarthritis; Rheumatoid arthritis
  physiology of, 1015–1016
Jojoba oil, 1222
Jordan syndrome, 709, 709f
c-Jun *N*-terminal kinase (JNK) pathway, 80
Juniper extract, 1222

K

Kanamycin, 174f, 1091f
  in tuberculosis, 1092t, 1097, 1102t
Karaya gum, 1222
Kava, 1241
  drug effects of, 1241t
  in insomnia, 850–851
  toxicity of, 1242
KCNA5, 385
Kefauver-Harris Amendment (1962), 20
Kelp, 1222
Ketamine, 97t, 98
  for anesthesia, 879t, 881
  in pain, 891
Ketoconazole, 180t
  adverse effects of, 182, 182t
  antiretroviral interaction with, 1197t
  in Cushing's syndrome, 624f, 625, 625t
  drug interactions with, 182t
  mechanism of action of, 180
  pharmacodynamics of, 181
  pharmacokinetics of, 181
  in prostate cancer, 952
  spectrum of activity of, 181
  terfenadine interaction with, 265–268
Ketolides, 174t
Ketoprofen, in headache, 732t
Ketorolac
  in headache, 732t
  in pain, 889t, 890
Kidneys
  active transport in, 144–145, 144f
  β-adrenergic receptor antagonists effects on, 134
  age-related changes in, 259
  antibacterial clearance by, 176, 176t
  aquaretic action on, 153–154, 153t
  bicarbonate handling in, 143f, 149–150, 150f
  bioartificial, 1330
  blood flow in, 142–143, 144t
  calcium handling in, 143f, 150–152, 151f
  catecholamine effects on, 129
  chronic disease of, 435–442
    anemia in, 440–442, 441t
    angiotensin-converting enzyme inhibitors in, 435–436
    angiotensin receptor II blockers in, 436

Kidneys *(Continued)*
antifibrotic agents in, 436
cell-based therapy in, 1330
classification of, 435, 436t
dyslipidemia in, 442, 442t
HMB CoA reductase inhibitors in, 436–437
hyperkalemia in, 437
hyperphosphatemia in, 437, 438t
hypertension in, 292–293, 293f, 439–440, 440f. *See also* Hypertension
in hyperthyroidism, 578
hypocalcemia in, 437–438
metabolic acidosis in, 437
osteodystrophy in, 438–439, 438t, 439t
pathophysiology of, 435
pharmacokinetics and, 201, 201f
treatment of, 435–437
volume overload in, 437
diuretic action on, 153–154, 153t
drug clearance by, 152–153, 152t, 201, 201f, 266, 266f
age and, 259
in children, 243–244, 244t
gender and, 252, 252t
glomerular filtration in, 143–144, 144t
halothane effects on, 877
1α-hydroxylase of, 591–592, 592f
inhalational anesthetic effects on, 877
innervation of, 142
lithium effects on, 793
lymphatics of, 142
magnesium handling in, 143f, 152, 590
midazolam clearance in, 880
natriuretic action on, 153–154, 153t
NSAID effect on, 1019–1020
organic anion handling in, 143f, 152–153, 152t
organic anion transporters of, 153
organic cation handling in, 143f, 152–153, 152t
phosphorus handling in, 143f, 151f, 152, 590
potassium handling in, 143f, 147f, 148–149, 149f
proton handling in, 143f, 149–150, 150f
sodium handling in, 143f, 145f, 146–148, 147f, 148f
disorders of, 292–293
structure of, 141–142, 142f, 143f
in systemic lupus erythematosus, 1048–1053, 1051t, 1052t, 1053t
transplantation of, 1273–1274. *See also* Transplantation
tacrolimus in, 285, 285f
urate handling in, 143f, 153
urate transporter-1 of, 153
vasculature of, 142, 142f
water handling in, 143f, 145–146, 145f, 147f, 148f

L

LAAM (L-α-acetyl morphine), in heroin addiction, 825–826, 830
Labetalol, 107t, 133f
in coronary artery disease, 347f, 347t, 350t
Lacosamide, in seizure disorders, 679
β-Lactams, 174t, 175t
adverse effects of, 178, 178t
in infective endocarditis, 1124–1127, 1124f, 1125f
mechanism of action of, 175
pharmacodynamics of, 176
pharmacokinetics of, 176
resistance to, 178–179
spectrum of activity of, 177
Lactitol, in hepatic encephalopathy, 515, 516t
Lactobacillus acidophilus, 1222
Lactulose
in constipation, 480t
in hepatic encephalopathy, 515, 516t
Lamivudine
adverse effects of, 189t, 190
in hepatitis B virus infection, 187, 188, 536, 536f, 538–539, 538t
in HIV infection, 1187–1188, 1189t
pharmacokinetics of, 185
resistance to, 190
Lamotrigine, 97, 97t
age-related clearance of, 260t
in bipolar disorder, 674, 793
in headache prevention, 734t
in multiple sclerosis, 696t
in posttraumatic stress disorder, 778, 778t
in seizure disorders, 674
Lanreotide acetate
in growth hormone–secreting adenoma, 619
in hepatic cirrhosis, 513t
Lansoprazole, 464–467, 465t
Lanthanum carbonate, in hyperphosphatemia, 437, 438t
Lapatinib, 86
in breast cancer, 938
Laquinimod, in multiple sclerosis, 698
Large intestine. *See* Colon
Laser therapy
in acne, 979–980
in psoriasis, 998
Latanoprost, in glaucoma, 861
Laxatives, 478, 480t
LD_{50}, 64
Lead poisoning, 1217t, 1218
Lecithin:cholesterol acyl transferase (LCAT), 305f
familial deficiency of, 308
Leflunomide, 168–169
adverse effects of, 1003, 1032, 1288
in psoriatic arthritis, 1000t, 1003–1004
in rheumatoid arthritis, 1031–1032, 1032t
teratogenicity of, 1003, 1032
in transplantation, 1287–1288
Leiomyoma, uterine, 633
Lenalidomide, in hematologic malignancy, 947
Lennox-Gastaut syndrome, 673, 674
Lepirudin, 916
Leptin, 549, 550f
in acid secretion, 459–460
in hypothalamic amenorrhea, 620
Letrozole, 636
in breast cancer, 934
Leukemia, 945–948, 946t, 948t
mitoxantrone-related, 691
Leukopenia
in systemic lupus erythematosus, 1056
thiopurine-related, 162, 163
Leukotriene, 111, 426–427, 427f
Leukotriene modifiers
in asthma, 426–428, 427f, 427t
in COPD, 426–428, 427f, 427t
mechanism of action of, 427
side effects of, 428
Leuprolide, 632, 632t
in breast cancer, 934
Levalbuterol, 420–423, 421t
Levetiracetam
age-related clearance of, 260t
in headache prevention, 734t
in seizure disorders, 676
Levobupivacaine, 868t, 870
Levodopa, 104, 105t
in Parkinson's disease, 655–657, 657t
Levofloxacin, 174t
in gonococcal infection, 1207t
in infective endocarditis, 1130
ocular, 859t
Levofloxacin *(Continued)*
spectrum of activity of, 177
in tuberculosis, 1096, 1102t
Levonorgestrel, 1224, 1224f
Levonorgestrel-releasing intrauterine system, 638
Levosimendan, in heart failure, 397
Levothyroxine, in hypothyroidism, 574–575, 575b
Lewy bodies
dementia with, 643, 644
in Parkinson's disease, 653
Licorice, hypertension with, 295
Lidocaine, 867–868, 868f, 868t, 1222
adverse effects of, 375t, 382
antiretroviral interaction with, 1197t
monitoring of, 276t
nicotine interaction with, 842t
in osteoarthritis, 1018t, 1020–1021
pharmacokinetics of, 200, 867–868
transdermal, 891
in ventricular arrhythmias, 372t, 382
Lifestyle modification
in dyslipidemia, 315
in gout, 1043
in hypertension, 296
in ischemic stroke, 746–748
in pulmonary arterial hypertension, 407–408
Ligaments, 1016
Ligand, 67–68. *See also* Signal transduction
definition of, 51
efficacy of, 60, 60f
potency of, 60, 60f
receptor binding of, 52–53, 52b, 53f, 54f. *See also* Receptor(s); Receptor-ligand interaction
Lightheadedness, 374
Limbic system surgery, in obsessive-compulsive disorder, 756–757, 756f
Linaclotide, in motility disorders, 484
Lincomycin, 174f, 174t
Lincosamides, 174t, 175
Linezolid, 174t
adverse effects of, 178, 178t
in infective endocarditis, 1129, 1134
spectrum of activity of, 177
in tuberculosis, 1105, 1105f
Liothyronine sodium, in hypothyroidism, 575–576, 575b
Lipase inhibitors
in dyslipidemia, 315
in obesity, 551t, 552, 552t
Lipid-lowering agents, 358–361, 358t, 359f, 359t, 360f, 360t, 361b. *See also* HMG CoA reductase inhibitors
Lipid messengers, 111–112
Lipopeptides, 174t
Lipophilicity, 194–195, 196f
Lipoprotein(s), 303–305, 306
disorders of. *See* Dyslipidemia
endogenous pathway of, 303–305, 305f
exogenous pathway of, 303, 304f
high-density, 306, 359–361
intermediate-density, 304, 310f
low-density, 304–305, 310f
cardiovascular disease risk and, 305–306, 309, 310t, 358–359, 361b
small dense, 306
very low density, 303–304, 310f
Lipoprotein lipase, 303, 304f
5-Lipoxygenase, pharmacogenetics of, 228t
Lisdexamfetamine dimesylate, in attention-deficit/hyperactivity disorder, 762
Lisinopril
in coronary artery disease, 354–357, 355t, 356t, 357b
in headache prevention, 734t, 736
in heart failure, 390–392, 392b, 392t

Lisuride, 105, 105t
  in Parkinson's disease, 655
Literature review, 44–47, 44b, 45t. *See also* Evidence-based practice
Lithium
  in bipolar disorder, 792–793, 792f
  monitoring of, 276t, 284
  thyroid effects of, 571–572
  triptan interaction with, 730t
Lithium carbonate, in headache prevention, 734t
Liver
  acetaminophen effects on, 1213, 1214f, 1223
  age-related changes in, 258–259, 258f
  anatomy of, 505–506, 506f, 507f
  antibacterial metabolism in, 176
  cirrhosis of. *See* Cirrhosis
  drug clearance by, 201–202, 202f, 266–267, 266f
    gender and, 252–253, 252t
  halothane effects on, 877–878
  HMG CoA reductase inhibitor effects on, 311
  inflammation of. *See at* Hepatitis
  inhalational anesthetics effects on, 877
  isoniazid effects on, 1094
  kava effects on, 1242
  ketoconazole effects on, 182
  leflunomide effects on, 1003
  leukotriene effects on, 428
  methotrexate effects on, 165, 991
  nicotine metabolism by, 840, 841f
  sulfasalazine effects on, 995
  thionamide effects on, 581
  thiopurine effects on, 162
  transplantation of, 1273–1274. *See also* Transplantation
  valoproate effects on, 672–673
  viral infection of. *See at* Hepatitis
Liver X receptor (LXR) agonists, in dyslipidemia, 316
Loa loa infection, 1174, 1175
Locaserin, in obesity, 554
Lomustine
  in hematologic malignancy, 946
  in melanoma, 969
Long QT syndrome, 369, 371t
  treatment of, 380
Loperamide, in diarrhea, 482
Lopinavir, in HIV infection, 1191–1193, 1194t
Lorazepam, 99, 100t
  age-related metabolism of, 259
  in motility disorders, 479t
  in panic disorder, 774, 774t
  for sedation, 880
  in seizure disorders, 670
Losartan
  in coronary artery disease, 354–357, 356t, 357b
  in gout, 1043–1044
  in heart failure, 392–394, 393b, 393t
Lovastatin, 309–312, 312t, 358–361, 358t, 360f, 360t, 361b
  adverse effects of, 311–312, 360t
  antiretroviral interaction with, 1197t
  azole interaction with, 182t
  grapefruit juice interaction with, 269
  mechanism of action of, 309–311, 359f
  pharmacogenetics of, 312
  pharmacokinetics of, 311, 311t
  trials of, 358, 359t, 360f
Loxapine, 806t
Lubiprostone, in motility disorders, 483
Lubricants
  in dermatitis, 1011–1012
  ocular, 861
Lugol's solution, in thyroid storm, 583t
Lumbar puncture, in meningitis, 1116
Lumefantrine, in malaria, 1148f, 1149t, 1154–1155
Lund concept, in bacterial meningitis, 1115
Lung(s)
  amiodarone toxicity to, 381
  antimuscarinic effects on, 123
  cancer of. *See* Lung cancer
  infection of. *See* Influenza; Pneumonia; Tuberculosis
  interstitial disease of, in systemic lupus erythematosus, 1057
  obstructive disease of. *See* Asthma; Chronic obstructive pulmonary disease (COPD)
  transplantation of, 1273–1274. *See also* Transplantation
    in pulmonary arterial hypertension, 411
  vascular disease of. *See* Pulmonary arterial hypertension
Lung cancer, 921–928
  gender and, 251
  non–small cell, 921–925
    staging of, 922b
    treatment of
      biologic agents in, 923, 927f
      chemoradiation in, 923–926
      chemotherapy in, 921–922, 922b, 923f, 924f, 925f
  small cell, 925–926
    staging of, 925, 925b
    treatment of, 925–926
      amrubicin in, 926
      bortezomib in, 926, 927f
      combination chemotherapy in, 926
      imatinib in, 926, 927f
      single-agent chemotherapy in, 925–926
      thalidomide in, 926, 928f
Lupus nephritis, 1048–1053, 1051t, 1052t, 1053t
Lupus syndrome. *See also* Systemic lupus erythematosus (SLE)
  procainamide-related, 374
Luteinizing hormone, 632–633
LY450139, in Alzheimer's disease, 645t
LY686017, in alcoholism, 832
LY2062430, in Alzheimer's disease, 645t
Lymph nodes, 158
  irradiation of, 1287
Lymphocytes, 158
  B, 158
  production of, 895, 896f
  T, 158
    in asthma, 419
    in atopic dermatitis, 1010
    in COPD, 419
    depletion of, in graft-versus-host disease prophylaxis, 1275, 1287
    in multiple sclerosis, 687–689, 688f
    in psoriasis, 984–985, 984f
    in rheumatoid arthritis, 1027–1030, 1028f, 1029f
    TK gene–transduced, 1304
    in transplantation, 1270, 1271–1272, 1273f
    in vaccine response, 1248–1249, 1249f
Lymphogranuloma venereum, 1201–1202, 1202t
Lymphoid irradiation, in transplantation, 1287
Lymphoid organs, 158
Lymphoma, 945–948, 946t, 948t
  infliximab and, 168
  thiopurines and, 163
Lymphopenia, drug-induced, 902, 902t
LymphoStat-B, in systemic lupus erythematosus, 1061
Lysergic acid diethylamide abuse, 819t

M

M2 inhibitors
  in avian influenza, 1069
  in influenza, 1065–1066, 1066f
Ma-huang, 130, 420
Macrolides, 174t
  adverse effects of, 178t
  creatinine clearance with, 176t
  in malaria, 1162
  mechanism of action of, 175
  spectrum of activity of, 177
Macrophages, 158
  in COPD, 419
  production of, 895, 896f
Macular degeneration, age-related, 861, 861t
Magnesium
  in arrhythmias, 384
  in headache prevention, 736
  metabolism of, 293
  renal handling of, 143f, 152, 590
Magnesium citrate, in constipation, 480t
Magnesium hydroxide, in constipation, 480t
Magnesium sulfate, in asthma, 430
Magnetic resonance imaging
  in drug assessment, 10, 12f
  in multiple sclerosis, 686, 687f, 693
Major depressive disorder. *See* Unipolar disorder (major depressive disorder)
Major histocompatibility complex, 1269–1270
Malaria, 1141–1166
  clinical spectrum of, 1144f, 1145–1147, 1146t
  epidemiology of, 1141, 1142f, 1145
  global distribution of, 1141, 1142f, 1144f
  pathophysiology of, 1141–1145, 1142t, 1144f
  in pregnancy, 1146–1147, 1164–1165
  prevention of
    in pregnancy, 1147
    in traveler, 1147, 1164, 1165t
    vaccine in, 1162
  severe, 1146, 1146t, 1164, 1164t
  treatment of, 1144f, 1145–1165
    amodiaquine in, 1154
    antifolates in, 1155–1158
    approach to, 1162–1165, 1164t
    artemether-lumefantrine in, 1149t, 1154–1155, 1158f, 1159, 1164, 1164t
    artemisinin derivatives in, 1158–1160, 1158f
    artesunate in, 1149t, 1158f, 1159, 1164, 1164t
    atovaquone in, 1149t, 1160–1161, 1161f
    azithromycin in, 1162
    biguanides in, 1157, 1160–1161, 1161f
    chloroquine in, 1147–1150, 1149t
    chlorproguanil in, 1157
    clindamycin in, 1149t, 1162
    combination therapy in, 1155–1157, 1163–1164
    dapsone in, 1157
    dihydroartemisinin in, 1159
    doxycycline in, 1149t, 1161–1162
    drug interactions in, 1158
    emerging targets for, 1165–1166
    goals of, 1145
    halofantrine in, 1154
    lumefantrine in, 1154–1155
    macrolides in, 1162
    mefloquine in, 1149t, 1152–1153
    piperaquine in, 1155
    in pregnancy, 1146–1147, 1150, 1152, 1153, 1154, 1158, 1160, 1161, 1162, 1164–1165
    primaquine in, 1149t, 1153–1154
    proguanil in, 1160–1161, 1161f
    pyrimethamine in, 1156–1157
    pyronaridine in, 1155
    quinidine in, 1150–1152
    quinine in, 1150–1152
    quinolines in, 1147–1155, 1148f, 1149t
    resistance in, 1147, 1163
    sulfadoxine-pyrimethamine in, 1149t, 1156–1158

Malaria *(Continued)*
sulfones in, 1157
tetracycline in, 1149t, 1161–1162
uncomplicated, 1145–1146, 1163–1164
vaccine against, 1162
Malaridine (pyronaridine), 1148f, 1155
Malignant hyperthermia, 878
Malmefene, in pain, 889
Mammalian target of rapamycin inhibitors. *See* Sirolimus (rapamycin)
Manganese, toxicity of, 1217t, 1218
Mannitol
in bacterial meningitis, 1115
in constipation, 480t
in glaucoma, 860
Maraviroc, in HIV infection, 1197–1198
Marijuana
abuse of, 819t, 823
treatment of, 832
in headache, 739, 739f
Mass action, laws of, 54–55, 54b
Mast cell, 158
in asthma, 419
Mast cell stabilizers, in asthma, 427t, 428, 428t
Mastocytosis, postural tachycardia syndrome and, 706–707
Matrix metalloproteinases, in osteoarthritis, 1022f, 1023
Maturation inhibitors, in HIV infection, 1198
Maturity-onset diabetes of the young, 557, 568
Mazindol, in obesity, 551
MDR1, 373–374
Meals, orthostatic hypotension with, 714
Measles virus
in Crohn's disease, 489
vaccine against, 1252t, 1253t, 1254t, 1255
Measurement error, 49
Mebendazole, in helminth infection, 1172, 1174, 1177f
Mecamylamine, 123, 124, 124f
in nicotine addiction, 832
Mechlorethamine, in hematologic malignancy, 946
Meclizine, 1222
in motility disorders, 479t
MEDI-545, in psoriasis, 1004
Medical records, electronic, 1231
Medication order, 1231. *See also* Prescription
MEDLINE, 42–43, 42t
Medulla oblongata disorders, hypertension with, 296
Mefloquine
adverse effects of, 1152–1153
drug interactions with, 1153
in malaria chemoprophylaxis, 1164, 1165t
in malaria treatment, 1148f, 1149t, 1152–1153
in pregnancy, 1153
Meglitinides
in diabetes mellitus, 561, 561f, 561t
drug interactions with, 270–271
MEK inhibitors, 86
Melanoma, 969–971, 970f
chemotherapy for, 969–970
immunotherapy for, 970–971
Melarsoprol, in protozoa infection, 1185
Melatonin, 852f
in insomnia, 850
Melatonin receptor agonists, in insomnia, 850
Melissa, in Alzheimer's disease, 646
Meloxicam, in osteoarthritis, 1020t
Melphalan, in hematologic malignancy, 946
Memantine, 97t, 98
in Alzheimer's disease, 644–645, 644t
Meningitis
bacterial, 1109–1118
clinical features of, 1110, 1115–1116, 1115t, 1116f
complications of, 1114–1115
computed tomography in, 1116
diagnosis of, 1110, 1115–1116, 1115t, 1116f, 1117f
differential diagnosis of, 1110
epidemiology of, 1109–1110, 1111f
Neisseria meningitidis in, 1112, 1113t
organisms in, 1111–1112, 1112t, 1113t
pathogenesis of, 1109, 1110f
Streptococcus pneumoniae in, 1112, 1113t
treatment of, 1110–1118
activated protein C in, 1115
algorithm for, 1117f
anti-inflammatory agents in, 1112–1114, 1113f, 1114f
antimicrobial agents in, 1110–1112, 1112t, 1113t
dexamethasone in, 1112–1114, 1113f, 1114f
duration of, 1116
experimental therapies in, 1116–1118
heparin in, 1115
hyperventilation in, 1115
Lund concept in, 1115
organism-specific, 1112, 1112t, 1113t
osmotic agents in, 1115
timing of, 1116
viral, 1115, 1115t
Meningococcal vaccine, 1250, 1252t, 1253t, 1254t, 1255–1256
Meniscus, 1016
in osteoarthritis, 1016, 1017f
Menkes' syndrome, vs. dopamine β-hydroxylase deficiency, 709
Menopause, 255, 255f
black cohosh use in, 1238
management of, 639–640
osteoporosis and. *See* Osteoporosis
Menotropins, 633
Menstrual cycle, 254
Menstrual disorders
in hyperthyroidism, 578
hypothalamic, 614, 620
in hypothyroidism, 574
Meperidine
in pain, 885t, 886
triptan interaction with, 730t
Mepivacaine, 868, 868f, 868t
6-Mercaptopurine, 161–163, 161f
allergic reaction to, 163
allopurinol interaction with, 1042
aminosalicylate interaction with, 492
cell cycle effects of, 84, 84f
drug interactions with, 494
in hematologic malignancy, 945
infection with, 163
in inflammatory bowel disease, 493–494, 493f, 497, 497t
leukopenia with, 163
mechanism of action of, 34, 34f, 162
metabolism of, 161–162
monitoring of, 162, 163
pharmacokinetics of, 161–162, 161f
in psoriasis, 995, 1000t
side effects of, 163, 494
Mercury, toxicity of, 1217t, 1218–1219
Meropenem, creatinine clearance with, 176t
Mesalamine, in inflammatory bowel disease, 490–492, 491t
Mesalazine, in ulcerative colitis, 498
Mescaline abuse, 819t
Mesenteric vasculitis, in systemic lupus erythematosus, 1057
Mesna, 166
Mesoionic oxatriazole derivatives, in coronary artery disease, 353
Metabolic syndrome, stroke and, 745t, 748
^{123}I-Metaiodobenzylguanide (MIBG) scan, in multiple system atrophy, 708
Metallothionein, 898
Metals, toxicity of, 1216–1219, 1217f, 1217t
Metapneumovirus infection, 1072–1073, 1072f
Metaproterenol, 130, 420–423, 421t, 1222
mechanism of action of, 422
side effects of, 422–423
Metastatic disease
from breast cancer, 934, 941–942, 942b
from colon cancer, 962
from prostate cancer, 954–955
Metformin, in diabetes mellitus, 561, 562f, 568
Methacholine, 119–120, 119f
neurotransmitter receptor response to, 705t
therapeutic uses of, 120
Methadone
antiretroviral interaction with, 1197t
in heroin addiction, 825–826, 827t, 829–830
in pain, 885t, 887
St. John's wort effect on, 1241t
Methamphetamine, 130
abuse of, 819t, 823
in attention-deficit/hyperactivity disorder, 761–762
in hypersomnia, 852
Methanol, toxicity of, 1214–1215, 1214f
Methemoglobinemia
local anesthetics and, 865
primaquine-related, 1154
Methicillin, *Staphylococcus aureus* resistance to, in community-acquired pneumonia, 1081, 1086
Methimazole
in hyperthyroidism, 580–581, 580b
during pregnancy, 582
in thyroid storm, 583t
Methohexital, 878–879, 879t
Methotrexate, 159t, 165–166
adverse effects of, 165–166, 494–495, 991, 1031, 1285
cell cycle effects of, 83, 84f
clinical uses of, 166
drug interactions with, 495, 1285
folic acid with, 166, 992
in graft versus-host disease prophylaxis, 1275
in hematologic malignancy, 945
hepatotoxicity of, 165, 991
in inflammatory bowel disease, 494–495, 494f, 497t
mechanism of action of, 165, 165f, 1284f, 1285
metabolism of, 165
monitoring of, 276t, 282–283, 1285
in multiple sclerosis, 692
pharmacodynamics of, 494
pharmacokinetics of, 165, 494, 494f, 1285
pneumonitis with, 166
in pregnancy, 495, 1059t, 1060
in psoriasis, 991–992, 1000t, 1002f, 1003, 1003f
in rheumatoid arthritis, 1031, 1032t
in systemic lupus erythematosus, 1051t
teratogenicity of, 166, 991
in transplantation, 1284–1285, 1284f
Methoxamine, 127f, 130
Methoxsalen, 1286–1287
3-Methoxy-4-hydroxyphenylglycol, 106
C-8-Methoxyfluoroquinolines, in tuberculosis, 1096, 1104–1105
Methoxyflurane, 875f, 875t
renal effects of, 878
respiratory effects of, 876

Methsuximide, in seizure disorders, 670
1-Methyl-4-phenyl-1,2,3,6-tetrahydropyridine (MPTP), 653
1-Methyl-4-phenylpyridinium, 104
N-Methyl-D-aspartate receptor antagonists, 97t, 98
 in Alzheimer's disease, 644–645, 644t, 645f
Methyl imidazoleacetic acid, 109
Methyl-p-tyrosine, 104
Methylation reaction, 899
Methylcellulose, in constipation, 480t
Methyldopa, 130
Methylene blue, in methemoglobinemia, 865
Methylenedioxymethamphetamine (MDMA, ecstasy), 108, 130, 819t, 823
O-6-Methylguanin-DNA-methyltransferase, pharmacogenetics of, 228t
N-α-Methylhistamine, in headache prevention, 736
Methylnaltrexone, in motility disorders, 483
Methylphenidate(s), 104, 105t, 107t, 130
 in attention-deficit/hyperactivity disorder, 759, 761t, 762–765, 763f, 763t
 in hypersomnia, 852
 intermediate-acting, 763–764, 763t
 long-acting, 763t, 764–765
 in multiple sclerosis, 697
 short-acting, 762–763, 763t
 side effects of, 765
 transdermal, 764–765
Methylphenidate hydrochloride, 762–763, 763t, 764
Methylphenidate OROS, 764, 764t
Methylphenidate transdermal patch, 764–765
Methylprednisolone
 in headache prevention, 734t
 in inflammatory bowel disease, 492–493, 492t
Methyltransferases, 93–94, 93t
Methysergide, 109, 110t
 in headache prevention, 736
 triptan interaction with, 730t
Metoclopramide, 105, 105t
 in motility disorders, 479t, 482
Metoprolol, 107t, 128t, 133f, 134
 in coronary artery disease, 347f, 347t, 350t
 in headache prevention, 734t
 in heart failure, 389–390, 391b, 391t
Metronidazole, 174f, 174t
 adverse effects of, 178t, 179t
 in alcohol dependence, 828t
 in bacterial vaginosis, 1209t
 creatinine clearance with, 176t
 in hepatic encephalopathy, 515–516, 516t
 mechanism of action of, 175
 pharmacodynamics of, 176
 in pregnancy, 179t
 in protozoa infection, 1178, 1180f
 spectrum of activity of, 178
Metyrapone, in Cushing's syndrome, 624f, 625, 625t
Metyrosine, in pheochromocytoma, 628
Mexiletine, 371t, 372t, 382
 adverse effects of, 375t
 antiretroviral interaction with, 1197t
 in pain, 891
Mibefradil, receptor interaction of, 54f
Micafungin, 180t
 mechanism of action of, 180
 pharmacodynamics of, 181
 pharmacokinetics of, 181
 spectrum of activity of, 182
Michaelis-Menten kinetics, 199–200, 204
Miconazole, 183t, 1222
 in vulvovaginal candidiasis, 1209t
Microbiota, in inflammatory bowel disease, 499–500
Microdosing, for testing, 10, 10b
Microparticle enzyme immunoassay, 279, 281f
Microsomal triglyceride transfer protein (MTP) inhibitors, in dyslipidemia, 316
Microvolt T-wave alternans, 374
Midazolam, 99, 100t
 antiretroviral interaction with, 1197t
 azole interaction with, 182t
 drug interactions of, 880
 for sedation, 879–880, 879t
 in seizure disorders, 670
Midodrine, 107t, 130
 in dysautonomias, 710t, 711
 in hepatic cirrhosis, 513t, 519
Mifepristone, in Cushing's syndrome, 625–626
Miglitol, in diabetes mellitus, 559, 559t
Migraine, 719–739, 729f
 acute abortive therapy for, 726–733
  ergots in, 733, 733t
  NSAIDs in, 731–733, 732t, 733b
  triptans in, 726–731, 728f, 729t, 730t, 731f, 732b
 adjuvant pharmacotherapeutic strategies in, 736–737
 allodynia in, 729b
 cortical spreading depression in, 724–725, 724t
 failed therapies in, 738t
 historical perspective on, 719–720
 menstrual, 736
 pathophysiology of, 720–725, 721t, 722f, 724t, 725f, 737, 737f, 738f
 prophylactic therapy in, 135, 734–737, 734t
 vitamin B_{12} in, 737, 737f
Mild cognitive impairment, 641, 642f
Milk thistle, 1239t, 1240, 1241, 1241t
Milrinone, in heart failure, 396, 396b, 396t
Miltefosine, in protozoa infection, 1185
Mineral oil, in constipation, 480t
Mineralocorticoids
 deficiency of, 626–627, 626f
 excess of, 629
Minimal alveolar concentration, of inhalational anesthetics, 876
Minimum bactericidal concentration (MBC), 173
Minimum inhibitory concentration (MIC), 173
Ministry of Health, Labour, and Welfare, 31
Minocycline, 174t
 in acne, 977, 979
 adverse effects of, 178
 in multiple sclerosis, 698
Miotics, in glaucoma, 860–861
Mirtazapine, 107, 109, 110t, 132
 age-related pharmacokinetics of, 260
 in generalized anxiety disorder, 776
 in insomnia, 850
 in obsessive-compulsive disorder, 776t, 777
 in panic disorder, 773–774, 774t
 pharmacogenetics of, 230
 in posttraumatic stress disorder, 777, 778t
 in unipolar disorder, 791
Misoprostol, in NSAID-induced ulcer, 467
Mitemcinal, in motility disorders, 482
Mitogen-activated protein (MAP) kinase (MAPK) inhibitors, in inflammatory bowel disease, 499
Mitogen-activated protein (MAP) kinase (MAPK) pathway, 69–70, 79–80
Mitotane
 in Cushing's syndrome, 624–625, 624f, 625t
 side effects of, 624
Mitoxantrone
 in multiple sclerosis, 691, 694, 695
 in prostate cancer, 954
Mivacurium, 102t, 125
MLN02, 169t
MMR vaccine, 1252t, 1253t, 1254t, 1255
Moclobemide, 107, 107t, 110t
 in posttraumatic stress disorder, 778
 in social anxiety disorder, 779, 779t
Modafinil, 130
 in hypersomnia, 852–853
 in multiple sclerosis, 696t, 697
Moisturizers, in dermatitis, 1011–1012
Molindone, 806t, 807t
Molsidomine, in coronary artery disease, 353
Mometasone, in asthma, 424–426, 425t
Monitoring. *See* Therapeutic drug monitoring
Monoamine oxidase, 93–94
 isoniazid inhibition of, 1094
Monoamine oxidase inhibitors
 in nicotine dependence, 846
 in obsessive-compulsive disorder, 756, 776t, 777
 in panic disorder, 774, 774t
 in Parkinson's disease, 658, 658t
 in posttraumatic stress disorder, 778, 778t
 selective serotonin reuptake inhibitor interaction with, 658, 730t
 in social anxiety disorder, 779, 779t
 triptan interaction with, 730t
 in unipolar disorder, 791–792, 792f
Monobactams, 174t, 175t, 177
Monoclonal antibodies, 85–86, 166–167
 in asthma, 430
 in breast cancer, 938–939, 938f, 939f, 940, 942
 in colon cancer, 962t, 965–966, 965f, 966f
 in coronary artery disease, 327b, 329f, 331t, 333–335, 333f
 in HIV infection, 1198
 in inflammatory bowel disease, 495–496, 497, 498, 499
 in multiple sclerosis, 690–691, 690f, 695, 698, 1035, 1282–1283
 in osteoarthritis, 605
 in prostate cancer, 955–956
 in respiratory syncytial virus infection, 1071
 in rheumatoid arthritis, 1033, 1033t, 1034–1035
 in systemic lupus erythematosus, 1051t, 1060–1061
 in transplantation, 1282–1283, 1286
Monocytes, 158
Montelukast, in asthma, 426–428, 427f, 427t
Morning-after pill, 638–639
Morphine
 abuse of, 819t, 821
 in children, 243
 in myocardial infarction, 325, 328f
 in pain, 885–886, 885t
3-Morpholinosyndnonomine (SIN-1), in coronary artery disease, 353
Motilin agonists, 479t, 482
Motility, 475–483
 physiology of, 475–476, 476f
Motility disorders, 476–478, 477f
 drug-induced, 477
 treatment of, 478–484, 478f
  anticholinergic agents in, 479t, 481
  antiemetics in, 479t
  chloride channel agonist in, 483
  cholinergic agents in, 478, 481
  device-based, 484
  dopamine antagonists in, 479t, 482
  fiber in, 478
  ghrelin in, 483
  guanylate cyclase-C agonist in, 484
  laxatives in, 478, 480t
  lubiprostone in, 483
  motilin agonists in, 479t, 482
  neutrotrophin-3 in, 484
  octreotide in, 483
  opioid agents in, 482–483
  phosphodiesterase inhibition in, 483
  prokinetics in, 479t

Motility disorders *(Continued)*
serotonergic agents in, 479t, 481–482, 481f, 482f
stool softeners in, 480t
Moxalactam, 178t
Moxifloxacin, 174t
adverse effects of, 178t
in infective endocarditis, 1130
ocular, 859t
spectrum of activity of, 177
in tuberculosis, 1102t
Moxonidine, 130
MPC-7869, in Alzheimer's disease, 645t, 646
MPTP (1-methyl-4-phenyl-1,2,3,6-tetrahydropyridine), 653
MTHFR gene, headache and, 737
Mucosa-associated lymphoid tissue, 158
Multidrug resistance transporter, 270, 271f, 272t
Multiple myeloma, 948t
Multiple sclerosis, 685–699
bladder dysfunction in, 696, 696t
clinical features of, 685–686, 686f
cognitive dysfunction in, 697
diagnosis of, 686–687, 686t, 687f
epidemiology of, 685
fatigue in, 696–697
genetics of, 685
infliximab and, 168
magnetic resonance imaging in, 686, 687f, 693
McDonald criteria for, 686, 686t
pain in, 696t, 697
pathophysiology of, 687–689, 688f, 699
primary progressive, 685–686, 686f, 695
relapse-remitting, 685–686, 686f, 693–694
secondary progressive, 685–686, 686f, 694–695
sexual dysfunction in, 697
spasticity in, 696, 696t
treatment of, 689–699, 693t
in acute relapses, 695–696
alemtuzumab in, 698
azathioprine in, 692
BG-12 in, 698
in breakthrough disease activity, 695
in children, 697–698
cladribine in, 698
corticosteroids in, 691–692, 695, 696
cyclophosphamide in, 692
daclizumab in, 698
emerging therapies in, 698–699
erythropoietin in, 699
failure of, 695
fingolimod in, 698
FTY720 in, 698
glatiramer acetate in, 690, 690f
immune globulin in, 692
immunomodulators in, 689–691, 690f
immunosuppressants in, 168, 691–692
interferon beta in, 689–690, 692–694, 695
laquinimod in, 698
methotrexate in, 692
minocycline in, 698
mitoxantrone in, 691, 694, 695
mycophenolate mofetil in, 692
natalizumab in, 690–691
neuroprotection in, 698–699
pregnancy and, 697
in primary progressive disease, 695
in relapse-remitting disease, 693–694
rituximab in, 698
in secondary progressive disease, 694–695
symptomatic, 696–697, 696t
teriflunomide in, 698
Multiple system atrophy, 706t, 708
vs. pure autonomic failure, 707
Mumps vaccine, 1252t, 1253t, 1254t, 1255
Muraglitazar, 568
Muromonab-CD3, 159t, 166–167, 1282
Muscle, 1016
Muscle relaxants
in bladder dysfunction, 446t, 452
in headache prevention, 734t, 736
in headache treatment, 733
Mushroom poisoning, 1216
Myalgia, HMG CoA reductase inhibitor and, 312
Myasthenia gravis, in hyperthyroidism, 578
Mycobacterium paratuberculosis, in Crohn's disease, 489
Mycophenolate mofetil (mycophenolic acid), 159t, 161f, 163
adverse effects of, 994, 1053, 1281
dosing for, 1280
drug interactions with, 1281
in graft-versus-host disease prophylaxis, 1275
mechanism of action of, 1280, 1280f
monitoring of, 276t, 1281
in multiple sclerosis, 692
pharmacokinetics of, 1280–1281
in pregnancy, 1059t, 1060
in psoriasis, 993–994, 994f, 1000t
in systemic lupus erythematosus, 1051t, 1052–1053
in transplantation, 1275, 1279–1281, 1280f
Mydriatics, 859, 860f
Myelodysplastic syndrome, 945–948, 946t
Myeloproliferative disorders, 945–948, 946t
Myocardial infarction. *See also* Coronary artery disease; Dyslipidemia
aspirin prevention of, 328, 329
cardiac remodeling after, 323
clinical presentation of, 324, 324f
cocaine-related, 865
epidemiology of, 321
non–ST-elevation, 322, 322f
treatment of, 325, 326f, 327b, 334f
β-adrenergic receptor antagonists in, 345–351, 347f, 347t, 348b, 349b, 349f, 350t
anticoagulants in, 335–343, 337b
calcium channel blockers in, 351–353, 351t, 352b, 353t
clopidogrel in, 326f, 327b, 332
nitrates in, 343–345, 344f, 345b, 346t
renin-angiotensin-aldosterone system inhibitors in, 354–357, 355t, 356t, 357b
pathophysiology of, 322–323, 322f, 323f
percutaneous interventions in, 330, 340, 343
ST-elevation, 322, 322f
treatment of, 325, 327b, 328f
β-adrenergic receptor antagonists in, 345–351, 347f, 347t, 348b, 349b, 349f, 350t
anticoagulants in, 335–343, 337b, 338b, 342f
calcium channel blockers in, 351–353, 351t, 352b, 353t
fibrinolytic agents in, 340t, 341–343, 341f, 342b, 342f, 919
nitrates in, 343–345, 344f, 345b, 346t
renin-angiotensin-aldosterone system inhibitors in, 354–357, 355t, 356t, 357b
stem cell transplantation after, 1328, 1329f
ventricular remodeling after, 323
Myocardial ischemia, 322–323. *See also* Myocardial infarction
gene therapy in, 1304–1305
Myocarditis, in systemic lupus erythematosus, 1057
Myositis, HMG CoA reductase inhibitor and, 312
Myxedema, in hypothyroidism, 574, 574f
Myxedema coma, 576

N

Nabumetone, in osteoarthritis, 1020t
Nadolol, 133f, 134
in coronary artery disease, 347f, 347t, 350t
in headache prevention, 734t
in hepatic cirrhosis, 511–512, 512t
Nafarelin, 632, 632t
Nafcillin
adverse effects of, 178t
in infective endocarditis, 1126
Naftifine, 183t
Nails, psoriatic disease of, 986
Nalbuphine, in pain, 888
Naloxone, 824, 824t, 1219
in pain, 888–889
Naltrexone, 824, 824t
in alcohol dependence, 825, 827t, 829
in obesity, 554
in opioid dependence, 827t, 828t
Nandrolone decanoate, in osteoporosis, 606
Naphazoline, 1222
Naproxen, 1020t
cardiovascular toxicity of, 1020
in headache, 732t
Naratriptan, 109, 728f, 729t, 730t
Narcolepsy, 851
Natalizumab, 159t, 168
adverse effects of, 691
in inflammatory bowel disease, 168, 496
in multiple sclerosis, 168, 690–691, 690f, 695
Nateglinide, in diabetes mellitus, 561, 561f, 561t
National Childhood Vaccine Injury Act, 1260
National Library of Medicine, 42–43, 42t, 43b
National Provider Identifier, 1228
Natriuretics, renal handling of, 153–154, 153t
Natural killer cells, 158
Necrosis, warfarin-induced, 914
Nedocromil, in asthma, 428, 428t
Nefazodone, 109, 110t
Neisseria gonorrheae infection, 1206, 1207t
Neisseria meningitidis infection, 1112, 1112t, 1113t. *See also* Meningitis, bacterial
Nelfinavir, in HIV infection, 1191–1193, 1194t
Nelson's syndrome, 624
Neomycin, 174t
in hepatic encephalopathy, 515–516, 516t
ocular, 859t
Neomycin sulfate, 1222
Neonate. *See also* Children
herpes simplex virus infection in, 1203
hyperthyroidism in, 582
tetany in, 589
Neostigmine, 102t, 103, 120–121, 121f
in motility disorders, 479t, 481
in neuromuscular blocker reversal, 125
Nephritis, lupus, 1048–1053, 1051t, 1052t, 1053t
Nephron, 141, 142f, 143f. *See also* Kidneys
bicarbonate handling along, 145f, 149–150, 150f
calcium handling along, 151f, 152
drug effects on, 153–154, 153t
drug handling by, 152–153, 152t
magnesium handling along, 152
potassium handling along, 145f, 147f, 148–149
sodium handling along, 145f, 146, 147f
water handling along, 145–146, 145f
Nerve fibers, 720–721, 720f, 720t
Nesiritide, 154
Neurally mediated syncope, 706t
pathophysiology of, 703–705
physical examination in, 704–705
tilt-table testing in, 705
treatment of, 715, 715b
ventricular theory of, 704
Neuraminidase inhibitors, in influenza, 187, 189f, 1066–1067, 1067f

Neuregulin-1, 812
Neuroaminidase inhibitors
  in avian influenza, 1069
  in influenza, 1066–1067, 1067f
Neurocysticercosis, 1172
Neuroleptics
  age-related effects with, 259
  in Alzheimer's disease, 647, 647t
  in bipolar disorder, 794
  in dementia, 647, 647t
  in generalized anxiety disorder, 775t, 776
  nicotine interaction with, 842t
  in obsessive-compulsive disorder, 756, 776t, 777
  in panic disorder, 775
  in Parkinson's disease, 659
  in posttraumatic stress disorder, 778t
  in schizophrenia, 804–812, 805f, 806t, 807t, 808f, 809f–811f
  in social anxiety disorder, 779, 779t
Neurologic disorders
  in hyperthyroidism, 578
  in hypothyroidism, 574
  in systemic lupus erythematosus, 1057–1058, 1058b
Neuromodulation, 94–95
Neuromuscular blockers, 124–125, 124f
Neuropathy
  autonomic, vs. pure autonomic failure, 707
  in vitamin B_{12} deficiency, 899
Neuropeptides, 93t, 110–111
Neurotransmission, 92–94, 92f. *See also* Neurotransmitter(s)
  agmatine, 111
  cholinergic, 100–103, 101f, 102t, 118–119
  dopaminergic, 103–105, 103f, 105t, 125
  GABAergic, 98–99, 98f, 100t
  glutamatergic, 96–98, 96f, 97t
  histamine, 109
  lipid, 111–112
  neuropeptide, 110–111
  nitric oxide, 111
  noradrenergic, 105–107, 106f, 107t
  purine, 111
  serotonergic, 108–109, 108f, 110t
Neurotransmitter(s), 91–112. *See also specific neurotransmitters*
  biosynthesis of, 92, 92f, 93t
  calcium-dependent exocytosis of, 92f, 93
  cotransmission of, 95–96
  enzymatic degradation of, 93–94
  in generalized anxiety disorder, 770, 771f
  inactivation of, 93, 93t
  interactions among, 95
  multiple effects of, 95
  in obsessive-compulsive disorder, 770
  in panic disorder, 769–770, 770f
  in posttraumatic stress disorder, 770–771
  presynaptic, 92–94, 92f, 95
  receptor binding of, 92f, 94
  in social anxiety disorder, 771
  synaptic effects of, 92f, 94–96
  uptake of, 93
  vesicular storage of, 92–93, 92f, 93t
  vesicular transporters of, 93
Neurotransmitter-gated ion channels, 77–78
Neurotrophin-3, recombinant, in motility disorders, 484
Neutropenia
  definition of, 902
  drug-induced, 902, 902t
  myeloid growth factors for, 905
  ticlopidine-related, 332–333, 918
Neutrophils, 158
  in COPD, 419
Neutrophin receptor, 74
Nevirapine, in HIV infection, 1188, 1190–1191, 1192t
New molecular entity drug, 17, 17f
NGB 2904, 832
Niacin (nicotinic acid)
  in dyslipidemia, 313–314, 360t, 361b
  in renal insufficiency, 442, 442t
Nicardipine
  in coronary artery disease, 351–353, 351t, 353t
  in pheochromocytoma, 628
Niclosamide, in helminthic infection, 1178
Nicorandil, in coronary artery disease, 354
Nicotine, 103. *See also* Nicotine dependence
  blood levels of, 840–841, 841f, 842f
  cardiovascular effects of, 843
  drug interactions with, 841–842, 842t
  metabolism of, 840–841, 841f
  neurotransmitter receptor response to, 705t
  pharmacodynamics of, 841, 842f, 843
  pharmacokinetics of, 840–841
Nicotine dependence, 819t, 821–822, 837–846
  APA criteria for, 839b
  depression and, 840
  evaluation for, 845–846, 846t
  hedonic dysregulation and, 840
  multifactorial nature of, 840
  neurotransmitter release in, 838–839, 840f
  pathophysiology of, 837–840
  risk factors for, 840
  treatment of, 824t, 825t, 837, 843–846
    behavioral, 846, 846t
    brief strategies for, 846, 846t
    bupropion in, 826, 827t, 831, 844t, 845
    clonidine in, 844t, 845
    goals of, 843
    guidelines for, 846, 846b
    monamine oxidase inhibitors in, 846
    nicotine gum in, 828t, 831, 843, 844f, 844t
    nicotine inhaler in, 828t, 831, 843, 844t
    nicotine lozenges in, 828t, 831, 843, 845
    nicotine nasal spray in, 828t, 831, 843, 844t
    nicotine patch in, 828t, 831, 843, 844t
    nortriptyline in, 844t, 845
    rimonabant in, 846
    vaccines in, 846
    varenicline in, 828t, 831–832, 844t, 845, 845f
Nicotine replacement therapy, 828t, 831, 843–845, 844f, 844t
  oral contraceptive interaction with, 254
Nicotinic acid (niacin)
  in dyslipidemia, 313–314, 360t, 361b
  in renal insufficiency, 442, 442t
Nicotinic agonists, in schizophrenia, 812
Nicotinic antagonists, 102t, 103, 123–125, 124f
Nifedipine
  in bladder dysfunction, 452
  in coronary artery disease, 351–353, 351t, 353t
  in heart failure, 397–398
  nicotine interaction with, 842t
Nifurtimox, in protozoa infection, 1185
Nightmare disorder, 853–854, 854t
Nilutamide, in prostate cancer, 953
Nimesulide, in headache, 732t
Nimodipine, in coronary artery disease, 351–353, 351t, 353t
Nitazoxanide, in protozoa infection, 1178–1179, 1182f
Nitrates
  adverse effects of, 345, 346t
  contraindications to, 345
  in coronary artery disease, 343–345, 344f, 345b, 346t
  drug interactions with, 345
  in hepatic cirrhosis, 514, 514t
  long-acting, 343, 345, 345b
Nitrates *(Continued)*
  mechanism of action of, 343, 344f
  pharmacokinetics of, 343
Nitrazoxanide, in protozoa infection, 1182f
Nitric oxide, 111
  in acid secretion, 459
  in hepatic cirrhosis, 508
  in osteoarthritis, 1022f, 1023
  in pulmonary hypertension, 410–411
  in voiding dysfunction, 448, 454t
Nitric oxide donors
  in coronary artery disease, 353
  in hepatic cirrhosis, 521
Nitric oxide pathway, in pulmonary arterial hypertension, 405f, 406, 406f
Nitric oxide synthase, inducible, glucocorticoid effect on, 493t
Nitrofurans, 174t
Nitrofurantoin, 174t
  adverse effects of, 178t, 179t
  creatinine clearance with, 176t
  in pregnancy, 179t
Nitroglycerin
  in coronary artery disease, 343–345, 344f, 345b, 346t
  in hepatic cirrhosis, 514, 514t
  in myocardial infarction, 325, 328f
Nitroimidazoles, 174t
Nitroimidazopyran, in tuberculosis, 1105, 1105f
S-Nitrosothiols, in coronary artery disease, 353
Nitrous oxide, 875f, 875t
  cardiac effects of, 877
  CNS effects of, 877
  guanylyl cyclase receptor interaction with, 76
  hepatic effects of, 877
  metabolism of, 877
  renal effects of, 877
  respiratory effects of, 876
Nizatidine, in acid secretion disorders, 463–464, 464t
NM-283, in hepatitis C virus infection, 541t, 542
NMDA agonists, in schizophrenia, 807–808
Nociceptors, in headache, 720–721, 720f, 720t
Nocturnal enuresis, desmopressin in, 446t, 454
NOD2, in Crohn's disease, 489
Non-benzodiazepine benzodiazepine receptor agonists, in insomnia, 849–850
Non-nucleoside reverse transcriptase inhibitors, 1188, 1190–1191, 1190f, 1192t
  drug-drug interactions of, 1190
  efficacy of, 1191
  mechanism of action of, 1188, 1190
  pharmacokinetics of, 1190, 1192t
  resistance to, 1190
  safety of, 1191
Nonsteroidal anti-inflammatory drugs (NSAIDs)
  adverse effects of, 730t, 889, 1019–1020
  in Alzheimer's disease, 645–646
  aspirin interaction with, 330
  cardiovascular effects of, 1020
  classes of, 1019, 1020t
  gastric ulcers with, 462, 466, 466f, 467, 470–471
  in gout, 1040t, 1041, 1043
  in headache prevention, 735–736
  in headache treatment, 727t, 731–733, 732t, 733b
  hypertension with, 295
  mechanism of action of, 53, 54f, 889, 889f, 1019, 1019f
  ocular, 860
  in osteoarthritis, 1018t, 1019–1020, 1019f, 1020t
  in pain, 889–890, 889f, 889t
  pharmacogenetics of, 231, 232f
  pharmacokinetics of, 889
  in pregnancy, 1059t, 1060
  in rheumatoid arthritis, 1031
  in systemic lupus erythematosus, 1051t

Norepinephrine, 92, 105–107, 127f
anatomic distribution of, 105
in baroreflex failure, 710
functions of, 105, 126–129, 128t
metabolism of, 93–94, 106, 106f
in multiple system atrophy, 708
in pure autonomic failure, 707
receptors for, 106–107, 106f
in social anxiety disorder, 771
synthesis of, 93t, 105–106, 106f
as therapeutic target, 107, 107t
Norfloxacin, ocular, 859t
Nortriptyline, 107, 107t, 109
in nicotine dependence, 844t, 845
Noscapine, 1222
Nuclear factor κB, 77, 88
Nuclear hormone receptors, 78–80, 78f
Nucleoside/nucleotide analogues
adverse effects of, 189t, 190
in hepatitis B virus infection, 187, 188, 536, 536f, 538–539, 538t
in HIV infection, 1187–1188, 1188f, 1189t, 1190t
pharmacokinetics of, 185
resistance to, 190
Nucleoside/nucleotide reverse transcriptase inhibitors, 1187–1188, 1188f, 1189t–1190t
clinical efficacy of, 1188
drug-drug interactions of, 1187–1188
mechanism of action of, 1187
pharmacokinetics of, 1187, 1189t–1190t
resistance to, 1188
safety of, 1188
Number need to treat/harm, 49
Nutraceuticals, 1237–1243, 1239t. *See also specific nutraceuticals*
drug interactions with, 1240–1241, 1241t
regulation of, 1237–1238, 1243
safety of, 1237–1238, 1243
toxicity of, 1241–1242, 1242b
use of, 1238
Nutritional therapy
in acne, 973, 980
in cardiovascular disease, 315, 316, 324
in dysautonomias, 714
in gout, 1043
low-sodium, 509
in obesity, 553
Nystatin, 180, 180t
topical, 183t
in vulvovaginal candidiasis, 1209t

O

ob gene, 549
Obesity, 549–554
definition of, 549
in hypertension, 294, 294f
morbid, 549
pathophysiology of, 549, 551f
prevalence of, 549
stroke and, 745t, 748
treatment of, 550–554
adjuvant pharmacotherapy in, 553–554
amphetamine-derived anorexiants in, 550–551
bupropion in, 554
cannabinoid-1 receptor blocker in, 551t, 552–553, 552t
diet in, 553
exenatide in, 554
exercise in, 553
goals of, 550
lipase inhibitors in, 551t, 552, 552t
nonamphetamine anorexiants in, 551–552, 551t, 552t
pramlintide in, 554
topiramate in, 554
Oblimersen, 87, 87f, 1307–1308
Obsessive-compulsive disorders, 753–757, 754b, 770, 773t
behavioral interventions in, 780
differential diagnosis of, 753–754, 754b
pathophysiology of, 754, 755f, 770
treatment of, 754–757, 776–777, 776t
ablative limbic system surgery in, 756–757, 756f
anxiolytics in, 756, 777
behavior therapy in, 754–755
deep brain stimulation in, 757, 757f
device-based approaches in, 757
goals of, 754
monoamine oxidase inhibitors in, 756, 776t, 777
neuroleptics in, 756
serotonin reuptake inhibitors in, 755, 755t, 776, 776t
tricyclic antidepressants in, 776t, 777
venlafaxine in, 756, 777
Obsessive-compulsive spectrum disorders, 753–754
Octinoxate, 1222
Octreotide
in growth hormone–secreting adenoma, 618, 618t
in hepatic cirrhosis, 513–514, 513t, 519
in motility disorders, 483
Ocular pharmacology. *See* Eyes
Oenothera biennis, 1239t
Ofloxacin, 174t
in gonococcal infection, 1207t
spectrum of activity of, 177
topical, ocular, 859t
in tuberculosis, 1096
OKT3 (ornithine ketoacid transaminase), 159t, 166–167, 1282
Olanzapine, 105, 105t, 110t
in bipolar disorder, 794
in generalized anxiety disorder, 775t
nicotine interaction with, 842t
in obsessive-compulsive disorder, 776t, 777
in Parkinson's disease, 659
in posttraumatic stress disorder, 778t
in schizophrenia, 806t, 807t, 808f, 809f–811f
in social anxiety disorder, 779, 779t
Oligohydrosis/hyperthermia reaction, zonisamide-related, 676
Olsalazine, in inflammatory bowel disease, 490–492, 491f, 491t
Omalizumab, in asthma, 430
Omega-3 fatty acids
in dyslipidemia, 314
in psoriasis, 1004
Omeprazole, 464–467, 465t
drug interactions with, 467
pharmacodynamics of, 213, 213f, 214f
Onchocera volvulus infection, 858, 1175
Onchocerciasis, 858, 1175
Oncolytic virotherapy. *See* Gene therapy, oncolytic
Ondansetron, 109, 110t
in alcohol dependence, 827t, 832
in motility disorders, 479t
Ondine's curse, 709
Oophorectomy, in breast cancer, 934
Ophthalmopathy, Graves', 579, 579f
Opioid(s)
abuse of, 819t, 820t, 821, 821f. *See also* Heroin abuse
prevention of, 823
treatment of, 824t, 825–826, 825t, 827t, 828t, 829–831, 1219
age-related effects with, 261
constipation with, 483
Opioid(s) *(Continued)*
endogenous, 722
in headache, 722
in motility disorders, 482
in osteoarthritis, 1018–1019, 1018t
in pain, 885–888, 885t
receptors for, 821, 885, 1219f
age-related changes in, 261, 261t
toxicity of, 1219, 1219f
Opioid agonist-antagonists, in pain, 888
Opioid antagonists
in motility disorders, 482–483
in pain, 888–889
in voiding dysfunction, 447
Opium tincture, 1222
Oral contraceptives, 254, 636–640, 637t–638t
in acne, 978
contraindication to, 639
drug interactions with, 254, 254t
emergency, 638–639
estrogen and progesterone, 639
estrogen and progestin, 636–638, 637t–638t
hypertension with, 295
lactation and, 639
long-term, 638
nicotine interaction with, 842t
phenytoin interaction with, 669
progestin-only, 638, 638t, 639
St. John's wort effect on, 1241t
screening evaluation for, 636
vitamin B_6 deficiency and, 980
Orchiectomy, in prostate cancer, 953
Organic anions, renal handling of, 143f, 152–153, 152t
Organic cations, renal handling of, 143f, 152–153, 152t
Organophosphates, 121, 121f
Orlistat
in dyslipidemia, 315
in obesity, 551t, 552, 552t
Orphan drug, 27, 27t
Orphan Drug Act (1982), 20, 27, 27t
Orthostatic intolerance, 705–707, 706t
pathophysiology of, 706–707, 707f
treatment of, 715, 715b
Oseltamivir
adverse effects of, 189t
in avian influenza, 1069
in influenza, 187, 1066–1067
pharmacokinetics of, 185
Osler's nodes, 1123
Osteoarthritis, 1015–1023
definition of, 1015
mesenchymal stem cell infusion in, 1327
pathophysiology of, 1016, 1017f
prevention of, 1017
vs. rheumatoid arthritis, 1027t
treatment of, 1017–1023, 1022f
algorithm for, 1022f
analgesics in, 1018–1019, 1018t
bradykinin in, 1022f, 1023
capsaicin in, 1020
corticosteroids in, 1018t, 1021, 1021t
diclofenac in, 1020
goals of, 1017, 1017b
hyaluronic acid derivatives in, 1018t, 1021
interleukin-1 in, 1022–1023, 1022f
investigational agents in, 1022–1023, 1022f
lidocaine in, 1020–1021
matrix metalloproteinases in, 1022f, 1023
molecular targets in, 1022–1023, 1022f
nitric oxide in, 1022f, 1023
nonsteroidal anti-inflammatory drugs in, 1018t, 1019–1020, 1019f, 1020t, 1022f, 1023
topical, 1020–1021

Osteoblasts, 1016
Osteodystrophy, renal, 438–439, 438t, 439t, 593, 595, 597–598
Osteogenesis imperfecta
bone marrow transplantation in, 1327
gene therapy in, 1308, 1309f
Osteomalacia, 593, 597
Osteoporosis, 594–595
corticosteroid-related, 426
treatment of, 604–605
anabolic agents in, 603–604
bisphosphonates in, 598–601, 599f, 605
calcitonin in, 605
calcium supplements in, 604
cathepsin K inhibitors in, 605
combination therapy in, 605
denosumab in, 605
estrogen therapy in, 601–602, 639
nandrolone decanoate in, 606
PTH 1-84 in, 605
PTH-related peptide in, 605
sclerostin monoclonal antibody in, 605
selective estrogen receptor modulators in, 602, 605
strontium ranelate in, 605–606
teriparatide in, 603–604
thiazide diuretics in, 604
tibolone in, 605
vitamin D in, 604
Ovarian hyperstimulation syndrome, 633
Over-the-counter medications, 1221–1224, 1227
alphabetical listing of, 1221–1223
excipient for, 1223
monograph system for, 1221, 1222t
regulation of, 1221
Overactive bladder, 449–450
22-Oxacalctriol, 597
Oxacillin
adverse effects of, 178t
in infective endocarditis, 1126
Oxaliplatin, in colon cancer, 962t, 963–964, 963f, 964t
Oxamniquine, in helminthic infection, 1178
Oxaprozin, in osteoarthritis, 1020t
Oxazepam, nicotine interaction with, 842t
Oxazolidinones, 174t
in infective endocarditis, 1129
pharmacokinetics of, 176
in tuberculosis, 1105, 1105f
Oxcarbamazepine, in bipolar disorder, 794
Oxcarbazepine
age-related clearance of, 260t
in headache prevention, 734t
in seizure disorders, 671–672
Oxiconazole, 183t
Oxprenolol, 134
Oxybutynin, 102t, 103
in voiding dysfunction, 446t, 452
Oxycodone, in pain, 885t, 887
Oxygen therapy
in community-acquired pneumonia, 1086
in headache, 733
in myocardial infarction, 325
in pulmonary arterial hypertension, 407t, 408
Oxymetalozine hydrochloride, 1222
Oxymorphone, in pain, 885t, 887
Oxyntic glands, 457, 458f, 458t
Oxypurinol, in gout, 1042
Oxytetracycline, ocular, 859t
Oxytocin, 613t

P

p53, in apoptosis, 86, 87f
P-glycoprotein, in children, 242
P-glycoprotein efflux transporter, 270, 271f, 272t
p38 MAPK pathway, 80
P-value, 48, 49
PA-457, in HIV infection, 1198
PA-824, in tuberculosis, 1105, 1105f
Pacemaker, 377, 378
in neurally mediated syncope, 715
Paclitaxel
in breast cancer, 936, 937
cell cycle effects of, 84, 84f
in melanoma, 969–970
in non–small cell lung cancer, 921, 924f
Paget's disease of bone, 595, 601, 603, 605
Pain, 883–892
anginal, 324, 324f. *See also* Coronary artery disease; Myocardial infarction
central sensitization in, 884
definition of, 883
in multiple sclerosis, 696t, 697
nociceptive, 883
physiology of, 720–725, 720f, 720t, 721t, 722f, 723f
psychogenic, 883
treatment of, 883–892
α_2-adrenergic receptor agonist in, 891
anticonvulsants in, 890–891
antidepressants in, 891
barriers to, 884
goals of, 883–884, 884f
local anesthetics in, 891
mixed opioid agonist-antagonists in, 888
multimodal, 883, 892b, 892f
N-methyl-D-aspartate receptor antagonist in, 891
nonsteroidal anti-inflammatory drugs in, 889–890, 889f, 889t
opioid agonists in, 885–888, 885t
opioid antagonists in, 888–889
pharmacogenetics in, 231
preemptive, 884
WHO analgesic ladder in, 884, 884f
Palivizumab, in respiratory syncytial virus infection, 1071
Palonosetron, 109, 110t
Palpitations, in arrhythmias, 374
Pamidronate, 599f, 601
Panax ginseng, 1239t
Pancreas
catecholamine effects on, 129
transplantation of, 1273–1274, 1327–1328. *See also* Transplantation
Pancreatin, 1222
Pancreatitis, in systemic lupus erythematosus, 1057
Pancuronium, 124f, 125
Panic disorder, 769–770, 771f, 773t
behavioral interventions in, 780
treatment of, 772–775, 774t
Panidronate, 599f
Panitumumab, 85
in colon cancer, 962t, 966, 966f
Panthotenic acid, in acne, 980
Pantoprazole, 464–467, 465t
PAP-1, in psoriasis, 1004
Para-aminosalicylic acid, 1091f
in tuberculosis, 1092t, 1098, 1102t
Paragonimus infection, 1178
Parainfluenza virus infection, 1071–1072
Paralysis, sleep, 854
Parasomnias, 853–854, 853b, 854t
Parasympathetic nervous system, 115, 116f, 117t, 118–125, 703, 704f
anatomy of, 118, 118f
cholinergic receptors of, 119, 119t
disorders of. *See* Dysautonomias
functional organization of, 118
neurotransmission in, 118–119
organ system effects in, 116f, 117t, 118
Parathion, 120–121, 121f
Parathyroid hormone, 589–590, 590f
in osteoporosis, 605
plasma, in renal insufficiency, 438, 438t
recombinant, 603–604
Parathyroid hormone–related peptide, in osteoporosis, 605
Paricalcitol, 597
in renal osteodystrophy, 439
Parkinsonism, in dementia, 646
Parkinson's disease, 651–661
epidemiology of, 651
historical perspective on, 651
pathophysiology of, 651–653, 652f
vs. pure autonomic failure, 707
treatment of, 653–661
anticholinergics in, 659, 659t
antidepressants in, 659
approach to, 660, 660t
catechol *O*-methyltransferase inhibitors in, 657–658, 657t
cholinesterase inhibitors in, 659–660
dopamine agonists in, 654–655, 656t
dopamine precursors in, 655–657, 657t
glutamate antagonists in, 659
goals of, 653–654
monoamine oxidase inhibitors in, 658, 658t
neuroleptics in, 659
surgery in, 660
Paromomycin, in protozoa, 1179–1180
Paroxetine, 109, 110t. *See also* Selective serotonin reuptake inhibitors (SSRIs)
in generalized anxiety disorder, 775, 775t
in multiple sclerosis, 696t
in obsessive-compulsive disorder, 755, 755t, 776–777, 776t
in panic disorder, 772–773, 774t
pharmacogenetics of, 230
in posttraumatic stress disorder, 777, 778t
in social anxiety disorder, 778–779, 779t
Passionflower, in insomnia, 851
Patent foramen ovale, stroke and, 745t
Pausinystalia yohimbe, 1239t
PBT-2, in Alzheimer's disease, 645t
PD184352, 86
PD0325901, 86
Pediatric Research Equity Act (2003), 20, 26
Pegaptanib sodium, 861
Pegfilgrastim, 905
Peginterferon, in hepatitis B virus infection, 535–536, 538, 538t
Pegvisomant, in acromegaly, 619, 619f
Pelvic inflammatory disease, 1209–1210, 1210b
Pemetrexed
in breast cancer, 937
cell cycle effects of, 83, 84f
in non–small cell lung cancer, 922
Pemoline, 130
in attention-deficit/hyperactivity disorder, 766–767
Penciclovir
adverse effects of, 189t
in human herpesvirus infection, 184t, 185t
indications for, 188
mechanism of action of, 186
pharmacokinetics of, 185, 185t
spectrum of activity of, 187–188
D-Penicillamine, 1217, 1217t
Penicillin(s), 174f, 174t, 175t
adverse effects of, 178, 178t, 1124–1125
allergy to, 178, 1124–1125
creatinine clearance with, 176t
in infective endocarditis, 1124f, 1125–1126, 1125f, 1131–1135, 1131t, 1133t, 1134t
mechanism of action of, 175
pharmacodynamics of, 176

Penicillin(s) *(Continued)*
pharmacokinetics of, 176
resistance to, 178, 179, 1134, 1135
spectrum of activity of, 177
in syphilis, 1204, 1205t
Penicillin-binding proteins, 175
Penicillin G, in infective endocarditis, 1125
Pennyroyal, 1241
Pentamidine, in protozoa infection, 1185
Pentazocine
nicotine interaction with, 842t
in pain, 888
Pentobarbital, in seizure disorders, 666–667
Pentostatin, in hematologic malignancy, 945, 1285–1286
Pentoxifylline, in renal insufficiency–associated anemia, 442
Peptic ulcer disease, 461–462
Helicobacter pylori in, 461–462, 469–470, 470t
pathophysiology of, 461–462, 461t, 462t
pharmacogenetics in, 231
risk factors for, 461t
treatment of, 469–470
antacids in, 463–463
H_2-receptor antagonists in, 463–464, 464t, 469
Helicobacter pylori eradication in, 469–470, 470t
mucosal protective agents in, 467
proton pump inhibitors in, 464–467, 465f, 465t
Peptidases, 93, 93t
Percutaneous interventions, in myocardial infarction, 330, 340, 343
Pergolide, 105, 105t
in Parkinson's disease, 654, 656t
in prolactinoma, 617
in voiding dysfunction, 454t
Pericarditis, in systemic lupus erythematosus, 1057
Perindopril, in coronary artery disease, 354–357, 355t, 356t, 357b
Periodic paralysis, hypokalemic, 578
Periodic Safety Update Report, 36
Perioral dermatitis, 1009
Peripheral neuropathy, isoniazid-related, 1094
Peristaltic reflex, 475, 476f
Peritonitis, in hepatic cirrhosis, 509–510, 518–519, 519f
Peroxisome proliferator activated receptor (PPAR), 562
Peroxisome proliferator activated receptor (PPAR) agonists, 568
Perphenazine, 806t
Pertussis vaccine, 1252t, 1253t, 1254t, 1257–1258
Pertuzumab, in prostate cancer, 955–956
Petasites hybridus, in headache prevention, 736
Pharmaceutical sciences, in drug development, 21
Pharmacodynamics, 203–216
in chronic disease, 216
circadian function in, 211–212
definition of, 51, 193, 203, 204f
direct reversible effects in, 207–208, 208f
disease progression models and, 216
of drug combinations, 214–215, 215f
effect compartment model (link model) of, 209, 209f
E_{max} model of, 205, 205f, 207–208, 208f
equilibration delays in, 208–209, 209f
gender and, 253
indirect effects in, 209–212, 210f, 211f, 212f
irreversible effects in, 213, 214f
linear model of, 205
logarithmic model of, 205–206
natural cell production and, 213–214
noncontinuous measures in, 214
Pharmacodynamics *(Continued)*
operational model of, 206, 207f
pharmacogenetics and, 226f, 227–228, 228t
receptor-drug interaction in, 203–206, 212–213, 213f
receptor occupancy assumption of, 204
sensitization and, 216
sigmoid E_{max} model of, 204–205, 205f
time course models in, 206–214
direct reversible effects and, 207–208, 208f
equilibration delays and, 208–209, 209f
indirect effects and, 209–212, 210f, 211f, 212f
irreversible effects and, 213, 214f
transduction steps and, 212–213, 213f
without drug concentration data, 214, 214f
tolerance and, 215–216
transduction steps in, 212–213, 213f
transit compartment models in, 212–213, 213f
turnover model in, 213, 214f
Pharmacogenetics, 14, 219–220, 220f, 225–235
in cardiovascular disease treatment, 230–231
clinical applications of, 222–223, 222t, 223f
in depression treatment, 229–230
dosing and, 228–229, 228f, 229f
in malignant disease treatment, 231–234
in pain treatment, 231
pharmacodynamics and, 226f, 227–228, 228t
pharmacokinetics and, 226–227, 226f, 227t
study design in, 234, 235f
in ulcer disease treatment, 231
Pharmacogenomics, 14, 219–223
clinical applications of, 220–222, 221f, 221t, 222f
Pharmacokinetics, 193–202
absorption in, 197–199, 198f
age and, 257–258
gender and, 252, 252t
age-related changes in, 257–259, 258f
bioavailability in, 197–199, 198f
concentration-response relationship in, 193, 194f
definition of, 51, 193, 204f
dose-response relationship in, 193, 194f
drug cumulation in, 197, 197f
in drug monitoring, 283
in drug selection, 1225
elimination clearance in, 193, 195–196, 196f, 201, 201f
elimination half-life in, 193, 195, 258
flip-flop, 200
gender and, 252–253, 252t
in hepatic impairment, 201–202, 202f
intercompartmental clearance in, 200, 200f
maintenance dose in, 197
multicompartmental models in, 200, 200f
nonlinear elimination kinetics in, 199–200, 199f
pharmacogenetics and, 226–227, 226f, 227t
plateau principle in, 197, 197f
protein binding in, 194, 195f
in renal impairment, 201, 201f
steady state in, 195–196, 197, 197f
tissue binding in, 194–195, 196f
volume of distribution in, 193–195, 194f, 195f, 196f
aging and, 258
gender and, 252, 252t
protein binding and, 194, 195f, 202
tissue binding and, 194–195, 196f
Pharmacology, 3–4, 4f
Pharmacotherapeutic continuum, 3–4, 4f
Pharmacovigilance, 29–39
active surveillance in, 37t, 38–39
benefit-risk assessment in, 29–31
case-control studies in, 37t, 39
case series in, 37t, 38
Pharmacovigilance *(Continued)*
CIOMS publications on, 29, 30t, 32
cohort studies in, 37t, 39
compliance and, 32–33
cross-sectional studies in, 37t, 39
definition of, 29
disproportionality analysis in, 37t, 38
FDA inspection in, 32–33
future developments in, 39
IHC guidelines in, 29, 30t, 32
individual case reports in, 37t, 38
Numbers Needed to Treat model in, 30–31
observational studies in, 37t, 39
passive spontaneous reporting in, 36–38, 37t
periodic safety update reports in, 36
postmarketing reports systems in, 35–36, 36f
Principle of Threes model in, 30
registries in, 37t, 38
regulations in, 29, 30t, 31–32
risk assessment in, 29
risk management in, 29
risk-management plan in, 34–35
Risk Minimization Action Plan in, 35
risk minimization and, 35
testing phase–specific, 33–39
phase I, 33
phase II, 33
phase III, 33–35
phase IV, 35–39
WHO definition of, 29
Pharmacy and Therapeutics Committee, 1233–1236
conflicts of interest and, 1235
decisions by, 1235
functions of, 1233, 1235
meetings of, 1234
structure of, 1233–1234, 1234f
subspecialist on, 1235
Phenacetin, nicotine interaction with, 842t
Phencyclidine, 98
Phendimetrazine, in obesity, 551
Phenelzine, 107t
in obsessive-compulsive disorder, 776t, 777
in panic disorder, 774, 774t
in posttraumatic stress disorder, 778, 778t
in social anxiety disorder, 779, 779t
in unipolar disorder, 791–792
Phenobarbital, 666–667
age-related clearance of, 260t
azole interaction with, 182t
monitoring of, 276t
side effects of, 666
Phenoxybenzamine, 128t, 131, 132f
in pheochromocytoma, 628
Phenprocoumon, pharmacogenetics of, 230–231
Phenserine, in Alzheimer's disease, 645t
Phentermine, in obesity, 551, 554
Phentolamine, 128t, 131, 132f
neurotransmitter receptor response to, 705t
Phenylbutazone, nicotine interaction with, 842t
Phenylbutyrate, in prostate cancer, 955
Phenylephrine, 127f, 128t, 129f, 130
neurotransmitter receptor response to, 705t
ocular, 859t
Phenylethanolamine-*N*-methyltransferase, 106, 125
Phenylpropanolamine, 130–131, 1223
Phenytoin
age-related clearance of, 260t
azole interaction with, 182t
drug interactions with, 182t, 669, 1094
isoniazid interaction with, 1094
monitoring of, 276t
pharmacokinetics of, 199–200, 199f
in seizure disorders, 667–669, 667f
serum, 668
side effects of, 668–669

Pheochromocytoma, 296, 627–629
pathophysiology of, 627–628
treatment of, 628–629
Phosphate, metabolism of, 589–593
Phosphate binders, in hyperphosphatemia, 437, 438t
Phosphate enema, in constipation, 480t
Phosphatidylinositol 4,5-bisphosphate (PIP_2), 72f, 73
Phosphatidylinositol 3-kinase (PI_3-K) pathway, 80
Phosphodiesterase, 72
Phosphodiesterase inhibitors
antiretroviral interaction with, 1197t
in motility disorders, 483
in pulmonary hypertension, 407t, 410–411, 411t, 521
in schizophrenia, 812
Phospholipase A_2, glucocorticoid effect on, 493t
Phospholipase C, 72–73, 72f
Phosphorus, renal handling of, 143f, 151f, 152, 590
Photodynamic therapy, in acne, 973, 979–980
Photoimmune therapy, 1286–1287
Photosensitivity, amiodarone-related, 381
Phototherapy
in acne, 980
in dermatitis, 1013–1014
in psoriasis, 990–991, 1000t, 1002f
in transplantation, 1286–1287
Physical activity, in dysautonomias, 714
Physical deconditioning, postural tachycardia syndrome and, 707
Physical maneuvers, in dysautonomias, 714
Physician Global Assessment scale, in psoriasis, 985
Physicians Information and Education Resource, 43, 44t
Physostigmine, 121, 121f
in motility disorders, 479t
Phytosterols, in dyslipidemia, 315
Picrotoxin, 99
Pilocarpine, 102t
therapeutic uses of, 120
Pilsicainide, 372t
Pimaricin, 180, 183t
Pimecrolimus
in dermatitis, 1013
in psoriasis, 989–990
Pimobendan, in heart failure, 396–397
Pimozide, 806t
Pinacidil, in voiding dysfunction, 454t
Pindolol, 133f, 134
in coronary artery disease, 347f, 347t, 350t
in headache prevention, 734t
in obsessive-compulsive disorder, 776t
Pioglitazone
azole interaction with, 182t
in diabetes mellitus, 562, 563t, 566f
Pipecuronium, 125
Piperacillin, 175t, 176t
Piperaquine, in malaria, 1148f, 1155
Pirbuterol, 420–423, 421t
Pirfenidone, in renal insufficiency, 436
Piroxicam
in headache, 732t
in osteoarthritis, 1020t
Pituitary adenylate cyclase–activating polypeptide, 471
Pituitary gland
hormones of, 611, 612f, 613t
deficiency of, 614–616
tumors of, 616–619, 617f, 618f, 618t, 619f
Pizotifen, in headache prevention, 736
Plan B (levonorgestrel), 1223, 1224f
Plant sterols, in dyslipidemia, 315
Plasma cell, 158
Plasma cell dyscrasias, 945, 946t. *See also* Hematologic malignancy
Plasma exchange, in multiple sclerosis, 696
Plasmodium infection, 1141–1143, 1142t, 1144f. *See also* Malaria
Plateau principle, in pharmacokinetics, 197, 197f
Platelet(s)
insufficiency of. *See* Thrombocytopenia
normal count of, 902
production of, 895, 896f
purinergic receptors for, 330
Platelet-derived growth factor receptor, 73
Pleiotrophin, 75
Plicamycin, in hypercalcemia, 595
Pneumococcal vaccine, 1252t, 1253t, 1254t, 1256
Pneumocystis jiroveci infection, ocular, 859
Pneumonia
community-acquired, 1081–1086
antimicrobial resistance in, 1083–1084
methicillin-resistant *Staphylococcus aureus* in, 1081, 1086
mortality from, 1081–1082
pathogens in, 1081, 1082b
pathophysiology of, 1081–1083, 1082f
prediction rule for, 1082–1083, 1083t
risk stratification for, 1082–1083, 1082b, 1083t
severity index for, 1083, 1083t
treatment of, 1083–1086, 1086t
corticosteroids in, 1086
inpatient, 1085–1086, 1085t
intravenous vs. oral, 1084
outpatient, 1084–1085, 1085t
oxygen therapy in, 1086
timing of, 1084
in COPD, 426
health care facility–acquired, 1086
Pneumonitis
lupus, 1057
methotrexate and, 166
PNU1000480, in tuberculosis, 1105, 1105f
Podofilox, in human papillomavirus infection, 1210b, 1211
Podophyllin resin, in human papillomavirus infection, 1210b, 1211
Poliovirus vaccine, 1252t, 1256–1257, 1261
Polycarbophil, in constipation, 480t
Polycythemia, stroke and, 745t
Polyethylene glycol, in constipation, 480t
Polymyalgia rheumatica, vs. rheumatoid arthritis, 1027t
Polymyxin, 174t
Polymyxin B, ocular, 859t
Polysaccharide-iron complex, in renal insufficiency–associated anemia, 441, 441t
Polystyrene sulfonate, in hyperkalemia, 437
Pompholyx, 1008–1009, 1010f
Portal hypertension, 507–511, 509f, 511
ascites with, 509, 518, 518f
encephalopathy with, 511, 520, 520f
gastroesophageal varices with, 509, 516–518, 517f
hepatic vein pressure gradient in, 508–509, 510f
hepatorenal syndrome with, 510–511, 519–520, 520f
pulmonary complications of, 511, 520–521, 521f
spontaneous bacterial peritonitis with, 509–510, 518–519, 519f
treatment of, 520–521, 521f
Portal hypertensive syndrome, 508
Portopulmonary hypertension, 511, 520–521, 521f
Posaconazole, 180t
mechanism of action of, 180
pharmacodynamics of, 181
spectrum of activity of, 182
Positron emission tomography, in drug assessment, 10, 12f
Posttransplantation lymphoproliferative disorders, rituximab in, 1286
Posttraumatic stress disorder, 770–771, 773t
behavioral interventions in, 780
nightmares in, 853–854
treatment of, 777–778, 778t
Postural tachycardia syndrome, 705–707, 706t
pathophysiology of, 706–707, 707f
treatment of, 715, 715b
Potassium
absorption of, 148
catecholamine effects on, 129
intake of, 148, 149
metabolism of, 293
renal handling of, 143f, 147f, 148–149, 149f
Potassium channel openers
in coronary artery disease, 354
in voiding dysfunction, 454t
Potassium-competitive acid blockers, 471
Potassium iodide, saturated solution of, in thyroid storm, 583t
Pouchitis, in ulcerative colitis, 499
Pralidoxime (2-PAM), 122f
in anticholinesterase poisoning, 123
Pramipexole, 105, 105t
in Parkinson's disease, 654–655, 656t
Pramlintide
in diabetes mellitus, 559–560
in obesity, 554
Pravastatin, 309–312, 312t, 358–361, 358t, 359t, 360t, 361b
adverse effects of, 311–312, 360t
mechanism of action of, 309–311, 359f
pharmacogenetics of, 312
pharmacokinetics of, 311, 311t
trials of, 358, 359t, 360f
Praziquantel, in helminthic infection, 1177–1178, 1178f
Prazosin, 128t, 131–132, 132f
in voiding dysfunction, 447–448
Precision, of analytic tests, 278, 278f
Prednisolone, in inflammatory bowel disease, 492–493, 492t
Prednisone
in adrenal insufficiency, 626–627
in hematologic malignancy, 946
in inflammatory bowel disease, 492–493, 492t
Pregabalin
in generalized anxiety disorder, 775t
in headache prevention, 734t
in pain, 891
in seizure disorders, 673
in social anxiety disorder, 779, 779t
Pregnancy, 254–255
aminoglycosides during, 179t
antibacterial agents during, 179t
antiphospholipid antibody syndrome during, 1060
artemisinin derivatives during, 1160
asthma treatment during, 430
azathioprine during, 494, 1059t, 1060
cardiovascular drugs during, 349, 350t
cervicitis during, 1208t
chloramphenicol during, 179t
chloroquine during, 1150
citalopram during, 255
coronary artery disease during, 349, 350t
corticosteroids during, 493
cyclooxygenase-2 inhibitors during, 1059t
cyclophosphamide during, 1059t, 1060

Pregnancy *(Continued)*
cyclosporine during, 1059t, 1060
drug safety for, 1223–1224
erythromycin during, 179t
fluoroquinolones during, 179t
glucocorticoids during, 1059t
gonococcal infection during, 1207t
hydroxychloroquine during, 1059t, 1060
hyperparathyroidism during, 589
hyperthyroidism and, 582
hypothyroidism and, 576
lamotrigine during, 674
leflunomide during, 1003, 1032
malaria during, 1055, 1146–1147, 1164–1165
artemisinin derivatives in, 1160
atovaquone in, 1161
azithromycin in, 1162
chloroquine in, 1150
mefloquine in, 1153
primaquine in, 1154
quinine in, 1152
sulfadoxine-pyrimethamine in, 1158
mefloquine during, 1153
6-mercaptopurine during, 494, 995
methimazole during, 582
methotrexate during, 495, 991, 1059t, 1060
metronidazole during, 179t
multiple sclerosis and, 697
mycophenolate mofetil during, 1059t, 1060
nitrofurantoin during, 179t
nonsteroidal anti-inflammatory drugs during, 1059t, 1060
physiologic changes of, 254
primaquine during, 1154
propylthiouracil during, 582
psoriasis during, 993, 1002
quinine during, 1152
retinoids during, 993
rifampin during, 179t
rituximab during, 1059t
selective serotonin reuptake inhibitors during, 255
sulfonamides during, 179t
systemic lupus erythmatosus and, 1059–1060, 1059t
tetracyclines during, 179t
thionamides during, 582
trimethoprim during, 179t
vulvovaginal candidiasis during, 1209–1210
Premature ventricular contractions, 368
Prescription, 1226–1231
abbreviations for, 1228–1229, 1228t, 1229t
DEA registration number for, 1228, 1230
drug information for, 1229–1230
electronic, 1231
elements of, 1229–1231, 1230b, 1230f
history of, 1227
vs. medication order, 1231
National Provider Identifier for, 1228
patient information for, 1229
prescriber information for, 1230
purpose of, 1228
scheduled drugs and, 1227–1228, 1227t, 1230–1231
Prescription Drug User Fee Act (1992), 20, 31–32
Pressure-natriuresis curve, in hypertension, 293, 293f
Prilocaine, 868–869, 868t, 869f
Primaquine
adverse effects of, 1153–1154
in malaria chemoprophylaxis, 1164, 1165t
in malaria treatment, 1148f, 1149t, 1153–1154
in pregnancy, 1154
Primidone, in seizure disorders, 667
Privacy, in drug development, 20–21
Pro-urokinase, in stroke, 744
Proarrhythmia, 135, 375–377, 376t, 385
Probenecid
drug interactions with, 270
in gout, 1041t, 1042
Procainamide, 372t, 382–383
adverse effects of, 374, 375t, 383
lupus syndrome with, 374
monitoring of, 276t
pharmacokinetics of, 373t, 383
Procaine, 866, 866f, 866t
Procarbazine, in hematologic malignancy, 946
Prochlorperazine, in motility disorders, 479t
Proctitis, lymphogranuloma venereum–associated, 1201
Progesterone
biochemistry of, 635
endogenous, 635
exogenous, 635–636, 635t
mechanism of action of, 635
receptors for, 633–634, 635
in voiding dysfunction, 448
Progestin, 635–636, 635t
in oral contraceptives, 636–639, 637t–638t
Progressive multifocal leukoencephalopathy, natalizumab-related, 168, 690, 691
Proguanil
in malaria chemoprophylaxis, 1164, 1165t
in malaria treatment, 1157, 1158, 1160–1161, 1161f
Prokinetics, 479t
Prolactin deficiency, 614
Prolactinoma, 616–617, 617f
Promethazine, 109
in motility disorders, 479t
Propafenone, 372t, 383
adverse effects of, 375t
antiretroviral interaction with, 1197t
pharmacokinetics of, 373t
Propantheline bromide, in voiding dysfunction, 446t, 450
Propionibacterium acnes, 973–974. *See also* Acne
Propiverine, in voiding dysfunction, 446t, 452
Propofol, 99, 100t, 879t, 881
Propoxyphene
nicotine interaction with, 842t
in pain, 885t, 888
Propranolol, 107t, 128t, 133, 133f, 134
in coronary artery disease, 347f, 347t, 350t
in headache prevention, 734t
in hepatic cirrhosis, 511–512, 512t
in hyperthyroidism, 580
neurotransmitter receptor response to, 705t
nicotine interaction with, 842t
pharmacodynamics of, 208
in posttraumatic stress disorder, 778t
rizatriptan interaction with, 730t
in thyroid storm, 583t
Propylthiouracil
in hyperthyroidism, 580–581, 580b
during pregnancy, 582
in thyroid storm, 583t
Prostacyclin pathway, in pulmonary arterial hypertension, 405f, 406
Prostaglandin(s), 111
in voiding dysfunction, 447
Prostaglandin analogues
in acid secretion disorders, 467
in glaucoma, 861
Prostaglandin E_2, in nociception, 721
Prostaglandin synthesis inhibition, in voiding dysfunction, 454t
Prostanoids
in hepatic cirrhosis, 514, 514t
in pulmonary arterial hypertension, 407t, 408–409, 409t
Prostate cancer, 951–956
treatment of, 951–956
algorithm for, 951, 952f
aminoglutethimide in, 952
androgen antagonists in, 953, 953f
androgen deprivation in, 951–953, 953f
in androgen-independent disease, 953–954
atrasentan in, 956
bisphosphonates in, 955
chemotherapy in, 954
complete androgen deprivation in, 953
epothilones in, 956
estramustine phosphate in, 954
estrogen in, 952–953, 953f
GnRH agonists in, 951, 953f
GnRH antagonist in, 952, 953f
growth factor receptor antagonists in, 955–956
histone deacetylase inhibitors in, 955
intermittent androgen deprivation in, 953
ketoconazole in, 952, 953f
in metastatic disease, 954–955
mitoxantrone in, 954
orchiectomy in, 953
radioisotope, 955
sipuleucel-T in, 955
taxotere in, 954
vitamin D in, 955
Prostate gland
benign hyperplasia of, 449–450
cancer of. *See* Prostate cancer
Protamine, in coronary artery disease, 331t
Protease inhibitors, 1191–1193, 1191f, 1194t–1195t
adverse reactions to, 1193
azole interaction with, 182t
drug-drug interactions of, 1192–1193
efficacy of, 1193
mechanism of action of, 1191
oral contraceptive interaction with, 254
pharmacokinetics of, 1191–1192, 1194t–1195t
resistance to, 1193
Protein(s)
drug binding to, 194, 195f, 202
plasma, in children, 241–242, 242t
Protein C
activated, in bacterial meningitis, 1115
half-life of, 913t
Protein kinase G, 76
Protein-losing enteropathy, in systemic lupus erythematosus, 1057
Protein S, half-life of, 913t
Protein tyrosine kinase receptors, 73–74, 74f
Protein tyrosine phosphatase receptors, 75
Proteinuria, in renal insufficiency, 439, 440f
Prothionamide, 1091f
in tuberculosis, 1095
Proton(s), renal handling of, 143f, 149–150, 150f
Proton pump, in acid secretion, 460–461, 460f
Proton pump inhibitors
azole interaction with, 182t
dose-response characteristics of, 466
drug interactions with, 467
in gastroesophageal reflux disease, 464–467, 465t, 468–469, 468f
mechanism of action of, 464–465, 465f
in NSAID-induced ulcer, 466, 466f
in peptic ulcer disease, 464–467, 465f, 465t
pharmacogenetics of, 231
Protozoan infection
Cryptosporidium, 1178–1179, 1183f
Entamoeba, 1178, 1179–1180, 1181, 1181f
Giardia, 1178, 1181, 1182f
Isospora, 1184, 1184f

Protozoan infection (*Continued*)
treatment of, 1178–1185
amphotericin B in, 1185
atovaquone in, 1181
azithromycin in, 1185
benzinidazole in, 1185
clindamycin in, 1185
dapsone in, 1185
diloxanide furoate in, 1181
eflornithine in, 1185
furazolidone in, 1181
iodoquinol in, 1180–1181
melarsoprol in, 1185
metronidazole in, 1178, 1180f
miltefosine in, 1185
nifurtimox in, 1185
nitazoxanide in, 1178–1179, 1182f
paromomycin in, 1179–1180
pentamidine in, 1185
pyrimethamine in, 1181
spiramycin in, 1185
stibogluconate in, 1185
suramin in, 1185
tinidazole in, 1178
trimethoprim-sulfamethoxazole in, 1184–1185, 1184f
Protriptyline, 109
Provitamin A carotenoids, in acne, 980
Prussian Blue, 1217, 1217t
Pseudoephedrine sulfate, 1222
Pseudohypoparathyroidism, hypocalcemia with, 589
Pseudomonas aeruginosa, in infective endocarditis, 1136
Pseudovitamin D–deficiency rickets, 593
Psilocybin abuse, 819t
Psoralen plus ultraviolet A (PUVA) therapy
in dermatitis, 1013–1014
in psoriasis, 990–991, 1000t, 1002f
Psoriasis, 983–1004
arthritis in, 986, 1002–1004
assessment of, 985
clinical features of, 983, 984f
epidemiology of, 983–984
erythroderma in, 986
flexural (inverse), 986
genetic factors in, 984, 985
grading of, 985
guttate, 985–986
historical perspective on, 983
localized and generalized, 986
mild, 985, 999–1000
moderate to severe, 985, 1000–1002, 1002f, 1002t
nail dystrophy in, 986
palmoplantar, 986
pathophysiology of, 984–985, 984f
plaque, 985, 986f
pustular, 986
severity of, 985
treatment of, 986–1005
ABT-874 in, 1004
adalimumab in, 997, 1000t
alefacept in, 997–998, 1000t
algorithm for, 1001f
anthralin in, 989, 999t
apremilast in, 1004
azathioprine in, 995
biologics in, 995–998, 995f, 1003, 1003f
calcipotriene in, 987, 999t
CNTO 1275 in, 998
corticosteroids in, 986–987, 988t, 999t
cyclosporine in, 991f, 992, 992f, 994f, 1000t
disease-modifying antirheumatic drugs in, 1003–1004
efalizumab in, 998, 1000t
Psoriasis (*Continued*)
essential fatty acids in, 1004
etanercept in, 996–997, 1000t
fumaric acid esters in, 995, 1000t
historical perspective on, 983
hydroxyurea in, 993, 1000t
infliximab in, 993, 996, 997, 997f, 1000t, 1002f, 1003, 1003f
ladder for, 999f
laser, 998
leflunomide in, 1000t, 1003–1004
MEDI-545 in, 1004
mercaptopurine in, 995, 1000t
methotrexate in, 991–992, 1000t
in mild disease, 999–1000, 999f, 1002t
in moderate to severe disease, 1000–1002, 1002f, 1002t
mycophenolate mofetil in, 993–994, 994f, 1000t
oral, 990–995, 992f, 994f, 1000t
PAP-1 in, 1004
phototherapy in, 990–991, 1000t
pimecrolimus in, 989–990
pregnancy and, 993, 1002
retinoids in, 992–993, 1000t
salicylic acid in, 989, 999t
ShK(L5) in, 1004
sulfasalazine in, 994–995, 1000t
tacrolimus in, 989–990
tar preparations in, 987, 989, 999t, 1000t
tazarotene in, 987, 999t
topical, 986–989, 988t, 999f, 999t
Psoriasis Area and Severity Index, 985
Psoriasis Disability Index, 985
Psychiatric disease. *See* Anxiety disorder(s); Bipolar disorder; Schizophrenia; Unipolar disorder (major depressive disorder)
Psychosis. *See also* Schizophrenia
corticosteroid-related, 161
in dementia, 647, 647b, 647t
mefloquine-related, 1152–1153
in Parkinson's disease, 659
psychostimulant-related, 765
in systemic lupus erythematosus, 1058
Psychostimulants
in attention-deficit/hyperactivity disorder, 759–766, 760b, 760f, 761f, 761t, 762t, 763t, 765t
in hypersomnia, 851–853
side effects of, 765
Psyclit, 42t
Psyllium, in constipation, 480t
Pulmonary arterial hypertension, 401–413
clinical presentation of, 401–402
definition of, 401, 402b
diagnosis of, 401–402
disease associations of, 407
etiology of, 402
molecular mechanisms of, 405f
natural history of, 403
pathophysiology of, 403–407, 405f
ativin-like kinase type-1 in, 406
bone morphogenetic protein receptor II in, 406
cellular mechanisms in, 403–404
endothelial cell proliferation in, 403
endothelins in, 404, 405f
environmental factors in, 407
genetic factors in, 406–407
hypoxia in, 407
molecular mechanisms in, 404–406, 405f
nitric oxide pathway in, 405f, 406, 406f
prostacyclin pathway in, 405f, 406
serotonin in, 404, 406–407
serotonin transporter in, 406–407
thrombosis in, 404
Pulmonary arterial hypertension (*Continued*)
vasoactive intestinal polypeptide in, 406
vasoconstriction in, 403
prognosis for, 403
severity of, 402–403, 403f
treatment of, 403, 404f, 407–413, 407t, 408b
algorithm for, 411, 412f
ambrisentan in, 407t, 410, 410t
anticoagulants in, 407t, 408
Bay41-2272 in, 413
Bay58-2667 in, 413
beraprost in, 407t, 409, 409t
bosentan in, 407t, 410, 410t
calcium channel blockers in, 407t, 408
combination therapy in, 411
conventional measures in, 407t, 408
dichloroacetate in, 412
digoxin in, 407t
diuretics in, 407t, 408
emerging, 411–413
endothelin receptor antagonists in, 407t, 409–410, 410t
epoprostenol in, 407t, 408–409, 409t
iloprost in, 407t, 409, 409t
imatinib in, 413
interventional, 411
lifestyle modification in, 407–408
nitric oxide in, 410–411
oxygen therapy in, 407t, 408
phosphodiesterase inhibitors in, 410–411, 411t
prostanoids in, 407t, 408–409, 409t
selective serotonin reuptake inhibitors in, 411–412
sildenafil in, 407t, 411, 411t
simvastatin in, 412–413
sitaxsentan in, 407t, 410, 410t
surgical, 411
transplantation in, 411
treprostinil in, 407t, 409, 409t
Pulmonary embolism. *See also* Thrombosis
urokinase in, 919
Pulmonary fibrosis, amiodarone-related, 381
Pulmonary function testing
in asthma, 420
in COPD, 420
Pulsed dye laser therapy, in psoriasis, 998
Pupil. *See also* Eyes
dilation of, 859, 860f
Pure autonomic failure, 706t, 707–708
treatment of, 713–714, 713t
Pure Food and Drug Act (1906), 31
Purine(s), neurotransmitter activity of, 111
Purine analogues, 84, 84f. *See also* 6-Mercaptopurine
Purine nucleoside analogues
in multiple sclerosis, 698
in transplantation, 1280f, 1285–1286
PUVA (psoralen plus ultraviolet A) therapy
in dermatitis, 1013–1014
in psoriasis, 990–991, 1000t, 1002f
Pyoderma gangrenosum, in inflammatory bowel disease, 488t
Pyrantel pamoate, in helminthic infection, 1174, 1177f
Pyrazinamide, 1091f
in tuberculosis, 1092t, 1097–1098, 1097f, 1098–1099, 1099t, 1101t
Pyridostigmine, 102t, 103
Pyridoxine. *See* Vitamin B_6
Pyrimethamine
in malaria, 1156–1157, 1156f
in protozoa infection, 1181
Pyrimidine analogues. *See also* 5-Fluorouracil; Capecitabine
cell cycle effects of, 83, 84f
Pyronaridine, in malaria, 1148f, 1155

Q

QT interval, drug-related prolongation of, 371t, 375–376, 381, 382
QTc interval, β-adrenergic agonist effect on, 423
Quetiapine, 105, 110t, 806t, 808f
  in bipolar disorder, 794
  in obsessive-compulsive disorder, 776t, 777
  in Parkinson's disease, 659
Quinacrine, in systemic lupus erythematosus, 1051t, 1053–1055, 1054b, 1054t
Quinagolide, in prolactinoma, 617
Quinapril
  in coronary artery disease, 354–357, 355t, 357b
  in heart failure, 390–392, 392b, 392t
Quinidine, 371t, 372t, 383
  adverse effects of, 375t, 383
  antiretroviral interaction with, 1197t
  azole interaction with, 182t
  in congenital short QT syndrome, 380
  in malaria, 1150–1152
Quinine, 1222
  adverse effects of, 1151
  drug interactions with, 1151–1152
  in malaria, 1150–1152, 1164, 1164t
  pharmacokinetics of, 1150
  in pregnancy, 1152
Quinine ascorbate, 1222
Quinine sulfate, 1222
Quinolines
  in malaria, 1147–1155, 1148f, 1149t
  resistance to, 1147
Quinupristin, 174t
Quinupristin-dalfopristin
  in infective endocarditis, 1129, 1134
  spectrum of activity of, 177

R

R1626, in hepatitis C virus infection, 541t, 542
Rabeprazole, 464–467, 465t
Radiation therapy
  baroreflex failure after, 709
  lymphoid, 1287
  in non–small cell lung cancer, 923–926
Radiofrequency catheter ablation, 377–378
Radioimmunotherapy, in hematologic malignancy, 948
Radionuclide therapy, in prostate cancer, 955
Raf inhibitors, 86
Raloxifene, 602, 605, 636
  in breast cancer, 933, 934
Raltegravir, in HIV infection, 1198
Ramelteon, in insomnia, 850
Ramipril
  in coronary artery disease, 354–357, 355t, 356t, 357b
  in heart failure, 390–392, 392b, 392t
Ranibizumab, 861
Ranitidine, in acid secretion disorders, 463–464, 464t
RANK ligand, 594, 594f
Ranolazine, in coronary artery disease, 353–354
Rapacuronium, 125
Rapamycin. *See* Sirolimus (rapamycin)
Ras inhibitors, 86
Ras-MAP kinase signaling pathway, 79, 85, 85f
Ras/Raf/MEK/ERK pathway inhibitors, in breast cancer, 939, 939f
Rasagiline, 105, 105t
  in Parkinson's disease, 658, 658t
Rash
  lamotrigine-related, 674, 793
  in systemic lupus erythematosus, 1053
  zonisamide-related, 676
Rauwolscine, 128t
RDP58, in inflammatory bowel disease, 499
Reactive oxygen species, protein tyrosine phosphatase receptor interaction with, 75
Rebound hyperactivity, psychostimulant-related, 765, 765t
Reboxetine, 107, 107t
Receptor(s), 51–54. *See also* Receptor-ligand interaction
  acetylcholinesterase, 135–136, 136f
  adrenergic, 106–107, 106f, 126
    age-related changes in, 260, 261, 261t
    desensitization of, 60, 61f
    polymorphisms in, 136–137, 136f
  cannabinoid, in headache, 723
  capsaicin, in headache, 723–724, 723f
  CB-1, 721, 721t
  cholinergic, 119
    age-related changes in, 260, 261t
    muscarinic, 101–102, 101f, 102t, 119, 119t, 450, 451t
    nicotinic, 94, 100–101, 101f, 102t, 119, 838–839, 839f, 840f
    polymorphisms in, 135–136, 136f
  cytokine, 76
  desensitization of, 60, 61f
  dopaminergic, 103f, 104, 126
    age-related changes in, 259, 261t
  downregulation of, 60, 61f
  drug binding to, 203–206, 204f, 205f, 212–213, 213f. *See also* Pharmacokinetics; Receptor-ligand interaction; Signal transduction
    competitive, 214–215
  estrogen, 633, 634
  G protein–coupled, 53, 55f, 61f, 68–70, 68f, 94–95. *See also* G protein–coupled receptors
  GABA, 98f, 99
    age-related changes in, 261t
    in headache, 721, 721t, 722–723
  glucocorticoid, 160–161, 160f, 492
  glutamate, 94, 96–97, 97t
    AMPA, 96–97
    delta, 96
    kainate, 97, 97t
    metabotropic, 94, 96f, 97, 97t
    NMDA, 97, 97t
  glycine, 94, 99
  guanylyl cyclase, 53, 55f, 75–76
  histamine, 109
  5-hydroxytryptamine, 721, 721t
  neuropeptide, 110–111
  nuclear hormone, 78–80, 78f
  opioid, 821, 885
    age-related changes in, 261, 261t
  PAR, in headache, 724
  presynaptic, 95
  progesterone, 633–634, 635
  protease-activated, in headache, 721, 721t, 723
  protein tyrosine kinase, 73–74, 74f
  protein tyrosine phosphatase, 75
  P_{2X}, 94
  serine/threonine kinase, 75
  serotonin, 94, 108–109, 108f
    age-related changes in, 259–260, 261t
  signal transduction of. *See* Signal transduction
  spare, 60, 62f
  toll-like, 158
  tyrosine kinase, 53, 56f, 76
  vanilloid, in headache, 721, 721t, 723, 723f, 724b
  vitamin D, 592
  Wnt, 76–77
Receptor-ligand interaction, 51–54, 52f, 53f, 54f. *See also* Pharmacodynamics; Signal transduction
  agonism with, 52, 52b, 63–64, 64f
  antagonism with, 52, 52b, 63–64, 64f
  association in, 57, 59f
  bimolecular, 54, 57, 59f
Receptor-ligand interaction *(Continued)*
  dissociation in, 56–57, 58f
  equilibrium binding in, 54–55, 54b, 57f
  indirect response model of, 209–212, 210f
  kinetics of, 56–58, 58f
  ligand affinity in, 52
  ligand binding in, 52, 52b, 53, 53f, 54f
  ligand receptor occupancy in, 52, 53–54, 57, 57f, 59f
  ligand specificity in, 52
  linear model of, 205
  logarithmic model of, 205–206
  models of, 203–206
  operational model of, 206, 207f
  receptor downregulation in, 60, 61f
  receptor dynamics in, 60–62, 61f, 62f
  receptor occupancy equilibrium in, 53–54, 57–58, 57f
  receptor occupancy quantification in, 58–59
  receptor upregulation in, 60, 61f
  reversibility of, 52
  Scatchard analysis in, 56, 58f
  shape factor in, 61–62, 62f
  sigmoid E_{max} model of, 204–205
  time dependence of, 54, 56–57, 57f, 58f, 62–63, 63f, 206–209
  unimolecular, 54, 56–57, 58f
Recliner chairs, in dysautonomias, 714
Red man syndrome, 178, 1128
Reflux nephropathy, hypertension with, 296
Regenerative medicine, 1317–1330, 1318f. *See also* Cell-based therapy; Stem cells
  goals of, 1317–1318, 1318f
  regeneration strategy of, 1318, 1318f
  rejuvenation strategy of, 1318–1319, 1318f
  replacement strategy of, 1318, 1318f
Registry, for pharmacoviligance, 37t, 38
Regulations, 29, 30t, 31–32
  compliance with, 32–33
Regulators of G protein signaling (RGS) proteins, 70, 70f, 71
REM sleep behavior disorder, 854
Remifentanil, in pain, 886–887
Remnant removal disease, 307
Renal artery stenosis, 295
Renal insufficiency. *See* Kidneys, chronic disease of
Renal osteodystrophy, 438–439, 593, 595
  pathophysiology of, 438
  treatment of, 438–439, 597–598
Renin, catecholamine effects on, 129
Renin-angiotensin-aldosterone system, 626, 626f
  age-related changes in, 261
  in hypertension, 294
Renin-angiotensin-aldosterone system inhibitors. *See also* Angiotensin-converting enzyme (ACE) inhibitors; Angiotensin II receptor blockers
  in coronary artery disease, 354–357, 355t, 356t, 357b
Renzapride, in motility disorders, 482
Repaglinide
  in diabetes mellitus, 561, 561f, 561t
  drug interactions with, 270–271
Reperfusion therapy, in stroke, 743–744, 744b
REPRORISK system, 255
Research study. *See also* Drug testing/trials
  clinical significance of, 46
  confounders in, 46
  design of, 45–46, 45t
  evaluation of, 44–46, 44b, 45t. *See also* Evidence-based practice
  objective of, 44–45
  outcome measures in, 46
  in pharmacogenetics, 234, 235f
  sample in, 46
  subjects in, 46

Reserpine, 105t, 107t
Resiniferatoxin, in voiding dysfunction, 446t, 453
Resorcinol monoacetate, 1223
Respiration
  antimuscarinic effects on, 123
  in hyperthyroidism, 577–578
  in hypothyroidism, 573
  inhalational anesthetic effects on, 876, 876f
  propofol effects on, 881
Respiratory syncytial virus infection, 1070–1071, 1071f
Respiratory tract. *See also* Respiratory tract infection
  acetylcholine effects on, 120
  β-adrenergic receptor antagonists effects on, 134
  catecholamine effects on, 128
  sympathomimetic drug effects on, 128
Respiratory tract infection
  adenovirus, 1075–1076, 1076f
  avian influenza virus, 1068–1070, 1070f
  coronavirus, 1073–1074, 1073f, 1074f
  hantavirus, 1074–1075, 1075f
  influenza virus, 1063–1068. *See also* Influenza
  metapneumovirus, 1072–1073, 1072f
  parainfluenza virus, 1071–1072
  respiratory syncytial virus, 1070–1071, 1071f
  rhinovirus, 1073, 1073f
Reteplase, in coronary artery disease, 340–343, 340t, 919
Retigabine, in seizure disorders, 679
Retina
  hydroxychloroquine toxicity to, 1032–1033
  viral infection of, 859
Retinoic acid receptors, 975f
Retinoid(s)
  in acne, 974–976, 975f, 975t, 976f, 978–979, 979b, 979t
  adverse effects of, 992–993
  oral, 977–978, 977f
  in psoriasis, 992–993
  in systemic lupus erythematosus, 1051t
  topical, 974–976, 975t, 976f
Retinopathy, hydroxychloroquine-related, 1032–1033
Reverse cholesterol transport, 305, 305f
Reviparin sodium, in coronary artery disease, 337–339
Rhabdomyolysis
  gemfibrozil and, 312, 314
  HMG CoA reductase inhibitors and, 311–312
rhApo2L/TRAIL, 87, 87f
Rheumatoid arthritis, 1025–1036
  diagnosis of, 1025–1026, 1026t
  differential diagnosis of, 1026–1027, 1027t
  disability with, 1025
  Disease Activity Score in, 1030
  epidemiology of, 1025
  extra-articular features of, 1025, 1026, 1026t
  pathophysiology of, 1027–1030, 1028f, 1029f
  treatment of, 1027, 1030–1036
    abatacept in, 1034
    adalimumab in, 1033–1034, 1033t
    anakinra in, 1035
    anti-inflammatory agents in, 1031, 1036f
    approach to, 1035, 1036f
    assessment of, 1030
    belimumab in, 1035
    BeSt study of, 1035
    biologic response modifiers in, 1033–1035, 1033t
    corticosteroids in, 1031
    disease-modifying agents in, 1031–1033, 1032t, 1036f
    etanercept in, 1033, 1033t
    goals of, 1027, 1030
    hydroxychloroquine in, 1032–1033, 1032t
    infliximab in, 1033, 1033t
Rheumatoid arthritis *(Continued)*
    leflumonide in, 1031–1032, 1032t
    methotrexate in, 1031, 1032t
    pyramid approach to, 1027
    rituximab in, 1034–1035
    sulfasalazine in, 1032, 1032t
    tetracycliines in, 1031
    tocilizumab in, 1035
Rheumatoid factor, 1025, 1026, 1026t
Rhinovirus infection, 1073, 1073f
Rho signaling pathway, 79
Rhubarb, 1223
Ribavirin
  adverse effects of, 189t, 190
  in hepatitis C virus infection, 187, 540–541, 540f, 541t
  pharmacokinetics of, 185, 540
  in respiratory syncytial virus infection, 1071
  spectrum of activity of, 188
Riboflavin deficiency, anemia with, 900, 901f
Rice polishings, 1223
Rickets, 591, 593, 597
Rifabutin, 174t, 1197t
Rifampin
  adverse effects of, 178t, 179f
  antiretroviral interaction with, 1197t
  azole interaction with, 182t
  in infective endocarditis, 1129
  during pregnancy, 179t
  prophylactic, 1100, 1103t
  spectrum of activity of, 177–178
  structure of, 1091f
  in tuberculosis, 1092t, 1095–1096, 1098–1099, 1099t, 1101t
Rifamycins, 174t, 175
Rifapentine, 174t
  in tuberculosis, 1096, 1099
Rifaximin, 174t
  in hepatic encephalopathy, 515–516, 516t, 520, 520f
Rilmenidine, 130
Riluzole, in multiple sclerosis, 699
Rimantadine
  adverse effects of, 189t, 190
  in influenza, 187, 1065–1066
  pharmacokinetics of, 185
  resistance to, 190
Rimonabant
  in dyslipidemia, 315
  in nicotine dependence, 846
  in obesity, 551t, 552–553, 552t
Risedronate, 599f, 600
Risk
  definition of, 48, 48t
  relative, 48
Risk assessment, 29–31
Risk management plan, 16f, 17, 24–25, 25t, 34–35. *See also* Pharmacovigilance
Risk Minimization Action Plan (RiskMAP), 35
Risperidone, 105, 105t, 110t, 806t, 807t, 808f, 809f–811f
  in generalized anxiety disorder, 775t, 776
  in obsessive-compulsive disorder, 756, 776t, 777
  in posttraumatic stress disorder, 778, 778t
Ritodrine, 127f, 128t, 130
Ritonavir
  azole interaction with, 182t
  in HIV infection, 1191–1193, 1194t, 1195t
Rituximab, 169
  in hematologic malignancy, 948
  in multiple sclerosis, 698
  in pregnancy, 1059t
  in rheumatoid arthritis, 1034–1035
  in systemic lupus erythematosus, 1051t, 1060–1061
  in transplantation, 1286
Rivastigmine, 102t, 103
  in Alzheimer's disease, 644, 644t
  in Parkinson's disease, 660
River blindness, 858
Rizatriptan, 109, 726–731, 728f, 729t, 730t
RNA, small interfering, 1305, 1306, 1306f, 1307
RNA interference (RNAi), 1296, 1305, 1306f
Rocuronium, 102t, 125
Rofecoxib, cardiovascular toxicity of, 1020
Ropinirole, 105, 105t
  in Parkinson's disease, 654–655, 656t
Ropivacaine, 868t, 869–870, 870f
Rosiglitazone
  azole interaction with, 182t
  in diabetes mellitus, 562, 563t, 566f
Rosuvastatin, 309–312, 312t, 358–361, 358t, 359f, 359t, 361b
  adverse effects of, 311–312, 360t
  mechanism of action of, 309–311, 359f
  pharmacogenetics of, 312
  pharmacokinetics of, 311, 311t
Rotavirus vaccine, 1257
Roth's spots, 1123
Rotigotine, in Parkinson's disease, 655, 656t
RSD1235, 385
Rubella vaccine, 1252t, 1253t, 1254t, 1255
Rufinamide, in seizure disorders, 679
Rumack-Matthew nomogram, 1213, 1214f
Ryanodine, 385

S

S1185, 385
S9947, 385
S20951, 385
Saccharin, 1223
Saccharomyces cerevisiae, in acne, 980
Safety. *See* Pharmacovigilance
St. John's wort, 1239t, 1240
  drug interactions with, 269, 1240–1241, 1241t
Salicylic acid
  in acne, 975t, 977, 979
  in psoriasis, 989, 999t
Salmeterol, 130, 420–423, 421f, 421t
  mechanism of action of, 422
  side effects of, 422–423
Salsalate, in osteoarthritis, 1020t
Salt restriction, in ascites, 509
Salvia officinalis, in Alzheimer's disease, 646
Sampling error, 49
Saquinavir, in HIV infection, 1191–1193, 1195t
Sarcoidosis, vs. rheumatoid arthritis, 1027t
Sargramostim, 905
  adverse effects of, 905
  in inflammatory bowel disease, 499
Saturated solution of potassium iodide, in thyroid storm, 583t
Saw palmetto, 1239t
SB-277011A, 832
Scabies, ivermectin in, 1175
Scatchard analysis, 56
SCH503034, in hepatitis C virus infection, 541t, 542
Scheduled drugs, 1227–1228, 1227t, 1230–1231
Schistosoma infection, 1177, 1178, 1179f
Schizophrenia, 797–812
  auditory event-related potentials in, 801, 801f
  behavioral models of, 801
  catatonic type, 798
  cognitive deficits in, 803, 804f
  deficit syndrome in, 798–799
  diagnosis of, 797–798, 798f
  disorganized type, 798
  environmental factors in, 799
  genetics of, 799, 799f
  motor manifestations of, 803–804

Schizophrenia *(Continued)*
negative symptoms in, 797–798, 798t, 802–803, 803f
neuropathology of, 799–800, 800f
paranoid type, 798
physical abnormalities in, 801
physiologic abnormalities in, 801
positive symptoms in, 797–798, 798t, 802
residual type, 798
treatment of, 801–812, 802f
algorithms for, 807, 808f, 809f–811f
depot preparations for, 812
dopamine D_2 receptor antagonism in, 802
erbB antagonists in, 812
goals of, 801–802
implantable systems for, 812
neuroleptics in, 804–812, 805f, 806t, 807t
nicotinic agents in, 812
NMDA agonists in, 807–808
nonadherence to, 812
phosphodiesterase inhibitors in, 812
types of, 798–799
undifferentiated type, 798
Sclerosing cholangitis, in inflammatory bowel disease, 488t
Sclerostin monoclonal antibody, in osteoporosis, 605
Scopolamine, 103, 121, 122f
adverse effects of, 123
cardiovascular effects of, 122–123
central nervous system effects of, 121–122
patch, in motility disorders, 479t
in voiding dysfunction, 451
Sebaceous glands, 973–974, 974f
Sebum, 973–974, 974f
Second messenger, 53
Sedation. *See also* Anesthesia
α-adrenergic receptor agonists for, 879t, 880–881
barbiturates for, 878–879, 879t
benzodiazepines for, 879–880, 879t
etomidate for, 879t, 881–882
fospropofol for, 879t, 881
goals of, 873, 874
ketamine for, 879t, 881
propofol for, 879t, 881
Sedatives, 878–882, 879t
Seizure disorders, 663–679
cognitive consequences of, 665
depression and, 665–666
pathophysiology of, 663–665, 664f, 665f
treatment of, 665–679
approach to, 677–679, 678f, 679f
barbiturates in, 666–667
benzodiazepines in, 670
carbamazepine in, 670–671
emerging therapies in, 679
felbamate in, 668f, 673
gabapentin in, 673
goals of, 665–666
lamotrigine in, 674
levetiracetam in, 676
oxcarbazepine in, 671–672
phenytoin in, 667–669, 667f
pregabalin in, 673
primidone in, 667
side effects of, 666
succinimides in, 670
surgical, 678–679, 679f
tiagabine in, 675
topiramate in, 674–675
valproate in, 672–673
vigabatrin in, 676–677
zonisamide in, 675–676
types of, 663–665
E-Selectin, glucocorticoid effect on, 493t
Selective estrogen receptor modulators, 602, 605, 636
in breast cancer, 933, 934, 940–941, 941f
CYP2D6 deficiency and, 269–270
in melanoma, 970
in osteoporosis, 602, 605
pharmacogenetics of, 231–232
Selective serotonin reuptake inhibitors (SSRIs)
cytochrome P-450 2D6 interaction with, 269
gender-related pharmacodynamics of, 253
in generalized anxiety disorder, 775, 775t
in headache prevention, 734t
monoamine inhibitor interaction with, 730t
in multiple sclerosis, 696t
neonatal effects of, 247
in obsessive-compulsive disorder, 755, 755t, 776–777, 776t
in panic disorder, 772–773, 774t
pharmacogenetics of, 230
in posttraumatic stress disorder, 777, 778t
during pregnancy, 255
in pulmonary arterial hypertension, 411–412
in social anxiety disorder, 778–779, 779t
triptan interaction with, 730t
in unipolar disorder, 790–791, 790f, 790t
Selectivity, of analytic tests, 279, 280f
Selegiline, 105, 105t
in Parkinson's disease, 658, 658t
Selenium sulfide, 1223
Seletracetam, in seizure disorders, 679
Self-help groups, in drug addiction, 826
Seliciclib, cell cycle effects of, 84, 84f
Semustine, in melanoma, 969
Senna, in constipation, 480t
Sensitization, 216
Serenoa repens, 1239t
Serine hydroxy methyltransferase, 99
Serine/threonine kinase receptors, 75
Seroquel, 807t
Serotonin, 92, 108–109
anatomic distribution of, 108
function of, 108
metabolism of, 93–94, 108, 108f
in obsessive-compulsive disorder, 770
in panic disorder, 769–770
in posttraumatic stress disorder, 771
in pulmonary arterial hypertension, 404, 406–407
receptors for, 108–109, 108f
in social anxiety disorder, 771
synthesis of, 93t, 108, 108f
as therapeutic target, 109, 110t
Serotonin agonists, 110t
azole interaction with, 182t
in motility disorders, 479t, 481, 481f, 482
Serotonin antagonists, 109, 110t
in alcohol dependence, 827t, 832
in headache prevention, 736
in motility disorders, 479t, 481–482
Serotonin-norepinephrine receptor inhibitors, 103, 107, 107t, 109, 110t
in attention-deficit/hyperactivity disorder, 766
in cocaine addiction, 832
in generalized anxiety disorder, 775, 775t
in headache prevention, 734t, 735
in multiple sclerosis, 696t
in nicotine dependence, 844t, 845
in obsessive-compulsive disorder, 756, 776t, 777
in pain, 891
in panic disorder, 773, 774t
in Parkinson's disease, 659
in posttraumatic stress disorder, 777, 778t
St. John's wort effect on, 1241t
in social anxiety disorder, 779, 779t
triptan interaction with, 730t
Serotonin-norepinephrine receptor inhibitors *(Continued)*
in unipolar disorder, 791
valproate interaction with, 730t
in voiding dysfunction, 453
Serotonin syndrome
linezolid and, 178
monoamine oxidase inhibitors and, 658
triptans and, 729–730, 730t, 731f
Serotonin transporter
in inflammatory bowel syndrome, 481
in pulmonary arterial hypertension, 406–407
Sertindole, 105, 105t
Sertraline, 109, 110t
gender-related pharmacodynamics of, 253
in generalized anxiety disorder, 775, 775t
in obsessive-compulsive disorder, 755, 755t, 776–777, 776t
in panic disorder, 773, 774t
in posttraumatic stress disorder, 777, 778t
in social anxiety disorder, 778–779, 779t
tricyclic antidepressant interaction with, 730t
triptan interaction with, 730t
Sevelamer hydrochloride
in hyperphosphatemia, 437, 438t
in renal osteodystrophy, 597
Severe acute respiratory syndrome, 1073–1074, 1074f
Severe combined immunodeficiency
gene therapy in, 1304
hematopoietic stem cell transplantation in, 1274
Sevoflurane, 875f, 875t
cardiac effects of, 877
CNS effects of, 877
hepatic effects of, 877
metabolism of, 877
renal effects of, 877
respiratory effects of, 876
Sexual dysfunction, in multiple sclerosis, 697
Sexually transmitted diseases, 1201–1211
cervical, 1207, 1207t, 1208t
Chlamydia trachomatis, 1201–1202, 1202t, 1206
Haemophilus ducreyi, 1201, 1202t
herpes simplex virus, 1202–1203, 1203t
human papillomavirus, 1210–1211, 1210b
Klebsiella granulomatis, 1202, 1202t
Neisseria gonorrheae, 1206–1207, 1207t
pelvic, 1209–1210, 1210b
Treponemia pallidum, 1204–1206, 1205t, 1206b, 1206t
Trichomonas, 1208, 1208b
urethral, 1206–1207, 1207t, 1208t
vaginal, 1207–1209, 1208t, 1209b, 1209t
ShK(L5), in psoriasis, 1004
Shock, cardiogenic. *See* Myocardial infarction
Shy-Drager syndrome, 706t, 707, 708
Siberian ginseng, 1239t
Sibutramine
in dyslipidemia, 315–316
in obesity, 551–551, 551t, 552t
Sickle cell anemia
stroke and, 745t
vitamin B_6 in, 901
Sigmoid E_{max} model, 204–205, 205f
Signal transduction, 67–80. *See also* Receptor-ligand interaction
adenylyl cyclase in, 71, 72f
autocrine, 67
cAMP in, 53, 55f, 71–72, 72f
definition of, 67
endocrine, 67
G protein effectors in, 71–73, 72f
heterotrimeric G proteins in, 69, 70–71, 70f
intracellular, 78–80, 78f
MAPK pathway in, 79–80

Signal transduction *(Continued)*
phosphatidylinositol 3-kinase/Akt pathway in, 80
Ras pathway in, 79, 85, 85f
Rho pathway in, 79
ion channels in, 77–78
Jak-STAT pathway in, 74f, 76
ligands in, 52–53, 53f, 54f, 67
paracrine, 67
phospholipase C in, 72–73
receptors in, 52–53, 67–68
cytokine, 74f, 76
enzyme-linked, 73–76, 74f
G protein–coupled, 68–70, 68f
guanylyl cyclase, 53, 55f, 75–76
integrin, 77
nuclear hormone, 78–79, 78f
protein tyrosine kinase, 53, 56f, 73–75, 74f
protein tyrosine phosphatase, 74f, 75
serine/threonine kinase, 75
tyrosine kinase–associated, 76
transit compartment models of, 212–213, 213f
Wnt/β-catenin pathway in, 76–77
Significance, statistical, 48
Sildenafil
antiretroviral interaction with, 1197t
in motility disorders, 483
in pulmonary arterial hypertension, 407t, 411, 411t, 521
Silibinin, 1240
Silybum marianum, 1239t, 1240
Simvastatin, 309–312, 312t, 358–361, 358t, 359f, 361b
adverse effects of, 311–312, 360t
antiretroviral interaction with, 1197t
azole interaction with, 182t
Heart Protection Study of, 31
mechanism of action of, 309–312, 359f
pharmacogenetics of, 312
pharmacokinetics of, 311, 311t
in pulmonary arterial hypertension, 412–413
St. John's wort effect on, 1241t
trials of, 358, 359t, 360f
SIN-1 (3-morpholinosyndnonomine), in coronary artery disease, 353
Sipuleucel-T, in prostate cancer, 955
Sirolimus (rapamycin), 159t, 164–165
adverse reactions to, 1279
drug interactions with, 1279
in graft-versus-host disease prophylaxis, 1275
mechanism of action of, 1277f, 1279
monitoring of, 276t, 1279
pharmacokinetics of, 1279
in transplantation, 1274, 1277f, 1279
Sitagliptin, in diabetes mellitus, 560–561
Sitaxsentan, in pulmonary arterial hypertension, 407t, 410, 410t
Skeleton
appendicular, 593
axial, 593
Skin
acne of. *See* Acne
aging of, 257–258
anatomy of, 974f
barrier function of, 157–158
disorders of
in hyperthyroidism, 578–579
in hypothyroidism, 574, 574f
inflammation of. *See* Dermatitis
lamotrigine-related rash of, 674, 793
melanoma of, 969–971, 970f
psoriasis of. *See* Psoriasis
in systemic lupus erythematosus, 1051t, 1053–1056, 1053b
warfarin-induced necrosis of, 914
zonisamide-related rash of, 676
Skullcap, in insomnia, 851
SLC6A3, 767
SLE. *See* Systemic lupus erythematosus (SLE)
Sleep, 849, 850f
disorders of. *See also* Hypersomnia; Insomnia; Parasomnias
in dementia, 647
drug-related, 853–854, 853b, 854t
psychostimulant-related, 765, 765t
Sleep apnea, obstructive
in hypothyroidism, 573
stroke and, 745t
Sleep paralysis, 854
Sleep-related dissociative disorders, 854
Sleep-related eating disorder, 854
Sleep-related groaning, 854
Sleep terrors, 853
Sleepiness, excessive, 851–853
Sleepwalking, 853
Small intestine. *See also* Gastrointestinal tract
calcium absorption in, 592
drug absorption in, 198–199, 198f
motility of, 476. *See also* Motility disorders
Smallpox vaccine, 1257
SNAP25, 767
SNARE (soluble *N*-ethylmaleimide-sensitive factor attachment receptor) complex, 93
Soap suds enema, in constipation, 480t
Social anxiety disorder, 771, 773t
behavioral interventions in, 780
treatment of, 778–779, 779t
Sodium
in dysautonomias, 714
renal handling of, 143f, 145f, 146–148, 147f, 148f
Sodium bicarbonate
in acid secretion disorders, 463
in metabolic acidosis, 437
Sodium channel blockers, 381, 382–383
proarrhythmia with, 376–377, 376t
Sodium hyaluronate, in osteoarthritis, 1021
Sodium nitrite, in cyanide toxicity, 1215
Sodium phosphate
in constipation, 480t
in hypercalcemia, 595
Sodium picosulfate, in constipation, 480t
Sodium sulfacetamide, in acne, 975t, 977
Sodium thiosulfate, in cyanide toxicity, 1215
Solifenacin, 103
in voiding dysfunction, 446t, 451–452
Solute-linked carrier transporter, 270, 271f, 272t
SOM230, in acromegaly, 620
Somatic cell nuclear transfer, 1324, 1325f
Somatostatin, 459, 460f, 613t
in hepatic cirrhosis, 512–513, 513t
Somatostatin analogues
in growth hormone–secreting adenoma, 618, 618t, 620
in hepatic cirrhosis, 513–514, 513t, 519
in motility disorders, 483
Somnambulism, 853
Sorafenib, 86
in breast cancer, 939, 939f
in non–small cell lung cancer, 923
Sorbitol, in constipation, 480t
Sotalol, 134, 371t, 372t, 383
adverse effects of, 375t, 383
in coronary artery disease, 347f, 347t, 350t
pharmacokinetics of, 373, 383
torsades de pointes with, 376, 376f, 383
Soy, 1239t
Sparfloxacin, in tuberculosis, 1096
Spasticity, in multiple sclerosis, 696, 696t
Spectinomycin, 174f
Spermidine, 97
Spermine, 97
Spiramycin, in protozoa infection, 1185
Spirapril, in coronary artery disease, 354–357, 355t, 357b
Spirometry
in asthma, 420
in COPD, 420
Spironolactone
in coronary artery disease, 354–357, 356t
in heart failure, 394–395, 394b, 394t
in hepatic cirrhosis, 514, 515t, 518
in hyperaldosteronism, 629
in renal insufficiency, 437
Spleen, 158
Spondyloarthropathy, seronegative, vs. rheumatoid arthritis, 1027t
Spontaneous bacterial peritonitis, in hepatic cirrhosis, 509–510, 518–519, 519f
SR141716, 832
SR 59230A, 128t
SSRIs. *See* Selective serotonin reuptake inhibitors (SSRIs)
Stannous fluoride, 1223
Stanols, in dyslipidemia, 315
Staphylococci
in infective endocarditis, 1134–1135, 1134t
methicillin-resistant
community-acquired pneumonia, 1081, 1086
in infective endocarditis, 1134
Stasis dermatitis, 1009, 1011f
Statins. *See* HMG CoA reductase inhibitors
Statistics
confidence interval in, 49
in drug development, 22
error in, 49
in evidence-based practice, 48–49, 48t
number need to treat/harm, 49
probability in, 48
risk in, 47, 48t
significance in, 48
Status epilepticus, 665, 666, 679
Stavudine, in HIV infection, 1187–1188, 1189t
Stem cells. *See also* Cell-based therapy
adult, 1320t, 1322–1324, 1323f
allogeneic, 1319, 1320f
autologous, 1319, 1319f
bioengineered, 1320t, 1324–1326, 1325f
embryonic, 1320–1322, 1320t, 1321f, 1321t
medicinal products with, 1324–1326
mesenchymal, 169t, 1323–1324, 1323f, 1330
perinatal, 1320t, 1322, 1322f
umbilical cord, 1322, 1322f
Steroid hormone receptors, 78–80, 78f
Sterols, plant, in dyslipidemia, 315
Stibogluconate, in protozoa infection, 1185
Still's disease, vs. rheumatoid arthritis, 1027t
Stimulants
in attention-deficit/hyperactivity disorder, 759–766, 760b, 760f, 761f, 761t, 762t, 763t, 765t
in hypersomnia, 851–853
side effects of, 765
Stiripentol, in seizure disorders, 679
Stomach
acid secretion by, 457–461
acetylcholine and, 458–459
cellular regulation of, 458–460, 460f
central regulation of, 457–458
disorders of, 461–471, 461t, 462t
antacids in, 462–463
anticholinergics in, 462–463
bismuth in, 467
gastric acid inhibitors in, 462–467, 464t
H_2-receptor antagonists in, 463–464, 464t
mucosal protective agents in, 467
prostaglandin analogues in, 467

Stomach *(Continued)*
proton pump inhibitors in, 464–467, 465f, 465t
sucralfate in, 467
gastrin and, 459, 460f
ghrelin and, 459
histamine and, 459, 460f
H^+,K^+-ATPase and, 460–461, 460f
leptin and, 459–460
nitric oxide and, 459
peripheral regulation of, 458–460
somatostatin and, 459, 460f
antimuscarinic effects on, 123
cells of, 457, 458f, 458t
motility of, 476, 476f. *See also* Motility disorders
oxyntic glands of, 457, 458f, 458t
Stool softeners, 480t
Streptococci
groups B, C, and G, in infective endocarditis, 1132
viridans group, in infective endocarditis, 1123, 1131–1132, 1131t
Streptococcus bovis, in infective endocarditis, 1131–1132, 1131t
Streptococcus pneumoniae
in infective endocarditis, 1132
in meningitis, 1112, 1112t, 1113t. *See also* Meningitis, bacterial
Streptococcus pyogenes, in infective endocarditis, 1132
Streptogramins, 174t
adverse effects of, 178t
in infective endocarditis, 1129, 1134
Streptokinase, in coronary artery disease, 340–343, 340t
Streptomycin, 174f, 174t
creatinine clearance with, 176t
in infective endocarditis, 1128–1129, 1133t
spectrum of activity of, 177
structure of, 1091f
in tuberculosis, 1092t, 1096–1097, 1101t
Stress, gastric ulcers with, 462, 463b
Stroke
hemorrhagic, 743, 750–751
ischemic, 743–750
epidemiology of, 743
pathophysiology of, 743, 744b, 744t, 746, 747f
prevention of, 744–747, 744t–745t
antihypertensives in, 748–749
aspirin in, 746, 749–750
blood pressure control in, 748–749
dipyridamole in, 750
glycemic control in, 748
HMG CoA reductase inhibitors in, 749
hyperlipidemia control in, 749
lifestyle modification in, 746–748
platelet inhibitors in, 749–750
platelet receptor antagonists in, 750
primary, 746
secondary, 746–751
risk factors for, 744–746, 744t–745t, 747f, 748–749
treatment of, 743–744, 744b
alteplase in, 743–744
pro-urokinase in, 744
reperfusion therapy in, 743–744
Stronglyloides infection, 1173f
treatment of, 1171, 1174, 1175
Strontium-89 therapy, in prostate cancer, 955
Strontium-153 therapy, in prostate cancer, 955
Strontium ranelate, in osteoporosis, 605–606
Suberoylanilide hydroxamic acid, in prostate cancer, 955
Substance abuse. *See* Drug addiction *and specific addictive drugs*
Succimer, 1217, 1217t
Succinic semialdehyde dehydrogenase, 98–99, 98f
Succinimides, in seizure disorders, 670
Succinylcholine, 102t, 124f, 125
Sucralfate, 467
Sudden cardiac death, 374
in Brugada syndrome, 377, 377f
Suicide, 787
Suicide gene, 1297, 1304
Sulbactam, 175t
Sulconazole, 183t
Sulfacetamide, ocular, 859t
Sulfadiazine, 174t
Sulfadoxine, in malaria, 1156–1157, 1156f
Sulfadoxine-pyrimethamine, in malaria, 1149t, 1156–1157, 1158
Sulfamethoxazole, 174t
Sulfasalazine
in inflammatory bowel disease, 490–492, 491f, 491t
in psoriasis, 994–995, 1000t
in rheumatoid arthritis, 1032, 1032t
Sulfinpyrazone
in coronary artery disease, 335
in gout, 1041t, 1042–1043
Sulfisoxazole, 174t
ocular, 859t
Sulfonamides, 174t
adverse effects of, 178t, 179f
creatinine clearance with, 176t
mechanism of action of, 175
in pregnancy, 179t
spectrum of activity of, 178
Sulfones, in malaria, 1157
Sulfonylureas
azole interaction with, 182t
in diabetes mellitus, 562, 563f, 563t, 564f
Sulindac, in osteoarthritis, 1020t
Sumatriptan, 109, 728–731, 728f, 729t, 730t
Sunitinib, in non–small cell lung cancer, 923
Suppositories, in constipation, 480t
Supraventricular tachycardia, 378–379
adenosine in, 378, 380
β-adrenergic receptor antagonists in, 384
flecainide in, 382
propafenone in, 383
Suramin, in protozoa infection, 1185
Surgery
in Cushing's syndrome, 623–624
in growth hormone–secreting adenoma, 618, 618t, 619f
in hyperaldosteronism, 629
in hyperthyroidism, 581
in hypothyroidism, 576
in infective endocarditis, 1130, 1138
in obsessive-compulsive disorders, 756–757, 756f
in Parkinson's disease, 660
in pheochromocytoma, 628
in seizure disorders, 679f, 768–679
Swimming, in dysautonomias, 714–715
Sympathetic nervous system, 115, 116f, 117t, 125–135, 703, 704f
adrenergic receptors of, 126, 128t
anatomy of, 125, 126f
disorders of. *See* Dysautonomias
dopaminergic receptors of, 126
functional organization of, 118
in hypertension, 293, 293f
neurotransmission in, 125
organ system effects in, 116f, 117t, 118
receptors in, 126
Sympatholytics, 131–135, 132f, 133f. *See also* α-Adrenergic receptor antagonists; β–Adrenergic receptor antagonists
Sympathomimetic agents, 126–129, 127f. *See also* α-Adrenergic receptor agonists; β–Adrenergic receptor agonists
hypertension with, 295
indirect-acting, 130–131
ophthalmic effects of, 128, 859, 860f
respiratory effects of, 128
Synapse, 91, 92, 115, 118
neurotransmitter effects at, 92f, 94–96. *See also* Neurotransmission; Neurotransmitter(s)
Synaptobrevin, 93
Syncope. *See also* Hypotension
in arrhythmias, 374
neurally mediated, 703–705, 706t
physical examination in, 704–705
tilt-table testing in, 705
treatment of, 715, 715b
ventricular theory of, 704
tilt-table testing in, 374, 705
Syndrome of inappropriate secretion of antidiuretic hormone, 613–614
Synovitis, 1025–1026
Synovium, 1016
in osteoarthritis, 1016, 1017f
Syntaxin 1, 93
α–Synuclein, 653
Syphilis, 1204–1206, 1205t
diagnosis of, 1204, 1206, 1206t
gestational, 1204–1206, 1206b, 1206t
treatment of, 1204, 1205t
Systemic lupus erythematosus (SLE), 1047–1061
anemia in, 1056–1057
antiphospholipid antibody syndrome with, 1058–1059, 1058b
arthritis in, 1056
cardiac manifestations in, 1057
contraception in, 1060
criteria for, 1047, 1049t
cutaneous manifestations in, 1051t, 1053–1056, 1053b
cytopenias in, 1056–1057
epidemiology of, 1047
gastrointestinal manifestations in, 1057
hematologic manifestations in, 1056–1057
mesenteric vasculitis in, 1057
musculoskeletal manifestations in, 1051t, 1056
pancreatitis in, 1057
pathophysiology of, 1047, 1048f, 1050f
pericarditis in, 1057
pregnancy and, 1059–1060, 1059t
pulmonary manifestations in, 1057
renal manifestations in, 1048–1053, 1051t, 1052t, 1053t
treatment of, 1047–1061, 1051t
algorithm for, 1051f
analgesics in, 1051t, 1056
anti-CD154 in, 1061
anticoagulants in, 1051t, 1058–1059
antimalarials in, 1051t, 1053–1055, 1054b, 1054t
azathioprine in, 1050, 1051t, 1052
biologic agents in, 1060–1061, 1060f
for cardiac manifestations, 1057
chloroquine in, 1054, 1054t
corticosteroids in, 1051t, 1055, 1056, 1057, 1058
for cutaneous manifestations, 1051t, 1053–1056, 1053b
cyclophosphamide in, 1049–1050, 1051t, 1058
cyclosporine in, 1051t
danazol in, 1051t, 1056–1057
dapsone in, 1051t, 1056
dehydroepiandrosterone in, 1051t
for gastrointestinal manifestations, 1057
goals of, 1047–1048

Systemic lupus erythematosus (SLE) *(Continued)*
for hematologic manifestations, 1056–1057
hydroxychloroquine sulfate in, 1054–1055, 1054t
intravenous immunoglobulin in, 1051t
LymphoStat-B in, 1061
methotrexate in, 1051t
for musculoskeletal manifestations, 1051t, 1056
mycophenolate mofetil in, 1051t, 1052–1053
for neuropsychiatric manifestations, 1057–1058, 1058b
NSAIDs in, 1051t
during pregnancy, 1055, 1059–1060, 1059t
for pulmonary manifestations, 1057
quinacrine in, 1054, 1054t
for renal manifestations, 1048–1053, 1051t, 1052t, 1053t
retinoids in, 1051t
rituximab in, 1051t, 1060–1061
thalidomide in, 1051t, 1055–1056

T

Tachyphylaxis, β-adrenergic agonist–related, 423
Tacrine
in Alzheimer's disease, 644, 644t
nicotine interaction with, 842t
Tacrolimus, 159t, 163–164, 164f
adverse effects of, 164, 495, 1278–1279
azole interaction with, 182t
in dermatitis, 1013
drug interactions with, 182t, 495, 1278
hypertension with, 295
in inflammatory bowel disease, 495
mechanism of action of, 164, 164f, 1277f, 1278
metabolism of, 279, 280f, 495
monitoring of, 276t, 1279
pharmacodynamics of, 285–286, 285f, 495
pharmacokinetics of, 1278
in psoriasis, 989–990
St. John's wort effect on, 1241t
in transplantation, 1274, 1277f, 1278–1279
Tadalafil, antiretroviral interaction with, 1197t
Taenia solium infection, 1176f, 1180f
treatment of, 1172, 1178
Talampanel, in seizure disorders, 679
Tamoxifen, 636
in breast cancer prevention, 933
in breast cancer treatment, 934, 940–941, 941f
CYP2D6 deficiency and, 269–270
in melanoma, 970
pharmacogenetics of, 231–232
Tamsulosin, 107t, 128t, 132, 132f
in voiding dysfunction, 446t
Tap water enema, in constipation, 480t
Tar preparations
in dermatitis, 1013
in psoriasis, 987, 989, 999t
Tardive dyskinesia, in schizophrenia, 803–804
Tau, in Alzheimer's disease, 646
Taxanes
in breast cancer, 84, 936, 937, 942
cell cycle effects of, 84, 84f
in melanoma, 969–970
in non–small cell lung cancer, 921, 924f
Taxotere, in prostate cancer, 954
Tazarotene
in acne, 975t, 976, 976f, 978–979, 979t
in psoriasis, 987, 999t
Tazobactam, 175t
Tea, dieter's, 1243
Tears, artificial, 861
Tegaserod, 110t
in motility disorders, 479t, 481, 481f
Telbivudine
adverse effects of, 189t
in hepatitis B virus infection, 187, 188, 537, 537f, 538t, 539
resistance to, 190
Telithromycin, 174t
adverse effects of, 178t
spectrum of activity of, 177
Temozolomide, in melanoma, 969
Tenatopraxole, 471
Tenecteplase, in coronary artery disease, 340–343, 340t, 919
Teniposide, in small cell lung cancer, 926
Tenofovir
in hepatitis B virus infection, 537
in HIV infection, 1187–1188, 1188f, 1190t
Teratogen, 254–255
Teratogenicity
antibacterial agent, 179t
hydroxyurea, 993
leflunomide, 1032
methotrexate, 166, 991
retinoid, 993
valproate, 672
warfarin, 914–915
Teratoma, embryonic stem cell therapy and, 1321
Terazosin, 107t, 128t, 131–132
in voiding dysfunction, 446t, 447–448
Terbinafine, 183t
Terbutaline, 107t, 127f, 128t, 130
Terconazole, 183t
in vulvovaginal candidiasis, 1209t
Terfenadine
azole interaction with, 182t
ketoconazole interaction with, 265–268
Teriflunomide, in multiple sclerosis, 698
Teriparatide, in osteoporosis, 603–604
Terizidone, in tuberculosis, 1095
Terlipressin, in hepatic cirrhosis, 512, 513t, 519–520
Terpin hydrate, 1223
Testosterone
production of, 951
replacement, in headache prevention, 736
Tetanus, diphtheria, pertussis vaccine, 1253t, 1257–1258
Tetanus vaccine, 1252t, 1253t, 1254t, 1257–1258
Tetracaine, 866t, 867, 867f
Tetracycline(s), 174f, 174t. *See also* Doxycycline
in acne, 977, 979
adverse effects of, 177, 179t
creatinine clearance with, 176t
in infective endocarditis, 1129
in malaria, 1149t, 1161–1162
mechanism of action of, 175
ocular, 859t
pharmacodynamics of, 176
in pregnancy, 179t
spectrum of activity of, 177
Tetraethylammonium, 124f
Tetrahydrobiopterin, 104
Thalamocortical circuit, 664, 664f, 665f
β-Thalassemia major, gene therapy in, 1301
Thalidomide
adverse effects of, 1055, 1287
in graft-versus-host disease, 1287
in hematologic malignancy, 947
in melanoma, 970
in small cell lung cancer, 926, 928f
in systemic lupus erythematosus, 1051t, 1055–1056
in transplantation, 1287
Thallium, toxicity of, 1217t
Theophylline
in asthma, 428–429
azole interaction with, 182t
Theophylline *(Continued)*
in COPD, 428–429
monitoring of, 276t
nicotine interaction with, 842t
side effects of, 429
Therapeutic drug monitoring, 275–286, 276t
analytic methods for, 277–278
accuracy of, 278–279, 278f
antibody-based, 279, 281f
biomarkers and, 285–286, 285f
chromatography-based, 279–282, 282f
dose-prediction methods with, 284–285
precision of, 278, 278f
selectivity of, 279, 280f
Bayesian methods in, 284–285
of busulfan, 283
clinical application of, 282–285
as clinical diagnostic test, 282
dose accuracy and, 277
implementation of, 285
of lithium, 284
of methotrexate, 282–283
optimal dosing forecasting with, 283–285
preanalytic factors in, 277
rationale for, 275–276
as risk reduction tool, 282–283
sampling time and, 277
specimen collection for, 277
therapeutic range in, 276–277, 277f
Zaske-Sawchuk method in, 284
Therapeutic equivalence, 199
Therapeutic index, 64
Therapeutic range, 276–277, 277f
Thiabendazole, in helminthic infection, 1174
Thiacetazone, 1091f
in tuberculosis, 1092t, 1095
Thiamylal, 878–879, 879t
Thiazide diuretics
age-related pharmacokinetics of, 262
in osteoporosis, 604
in stroke prevention, 748
Thiazolidinediones, in diabetes mellitus, 562, 563t, 565f, 566f
Thienopyridines, 330, 331t, 332–333. *See also* Clopidogrel; Ticlodipine
Thimerosal, 1223, 1262
6-Thioguanine
in hematologic malignancy, 945
in inflammatory bowel disease, 493
Thionamides
in hyperthyroidism, 580–581, 580b, 583t
during pregnancy, 582
Thiopental, 200, 878–879, 879t
Thiopurine(s), 159t, 161–163. *See also* Azathioprine; 6-Mercaptopurine
allopurinol interaction with, 162
clinical uses of, 163
mechanism of action of, 161f, 162
metabolism of, 161–162, 161f
monitoring of, 162
pharmacokinetics of, 161–162
toxicity of, 163
Thiopurine *S*-methyltransferase, 162
deficiency of, 232–233
pharmacogenetics of, 221, 221f, 221t, 222, 222f, 227t, 232–233
polymorphisms of, 1052
Thioridazine, 806t, 807t
Thiothixene, 806t
Thirst, 146
L-Threo-dihydrxyphenylserine, 107t
Thrombin inhibitors, direct, 335t, 339–340, 916–917
Thrombocytopenia, 902
drug-induced, 902, 903t
heparin-induced, 336–337, 916

Thrombocytopenia *(Continued)*
pathophysiology of, 902, 903t
in systemic lupus erythematosus, 1056
thrombopoietic growth factors in, 905–906
treatment of, 905–906
Thrombocytopenic purpura
idiopathic, in systemic lupus erythematosus, 1056
thrombotic
in systemic lupus erythematosus, 1056
ticlopidine-related, 918
Thrombopoietin, 906
Thrombosis. *See also* Myocardial infarction; Stroke
heart failure and, 398
heparin-related, 916
pathogenesis of, 909
pulmonary arterial hypertension and, 404
treatment of, 913–919
anticoagulants in, 913–917
antiplatelet agents in, 917–918
fibrinolytics in, 918–919
Thrombotic thrombocytopenic purpura
in systemic lupus erythematosus, 1056
ticlopidine-related, 918
Thromboxane inhibitors, 328–330, 329f, 331t. *See also* Aspirin (acetylsalicylic acid)
Thyroid gland, 571, 572, 572f
disorders of. *See* Hyperthyroidism; Hypothyroidism
Thyroid hormone, 572, 573f
Thyroid-stimulating hormone
deficiency of, 572, 619–620
in hyperthyroidism, 579, 579f
in hypothyroidism, 574, 575f
recombinant, 619–620
Thyroid storm, 582–583, 583t
Thyroidectomy, 581
Thyrosine kinase inhibitors, 85–86
Thyrotoxic crisis, 582–583, 583t
Thyrotoxicosis. *See* Hyperthyroidism
Thyrotropin-releasing hormone, 613t
Thyroxine, free
in hyperthyroidism, 579, 579f
in hypothyroidism, 574, 575f
Tiagabine, 99, 100t
age-related clearance of, 260t
in headache prevention, 734t
in seizure disorders, 675
Tibolone, in osteoporosis, 605
Ticarcillin, 175t
creatinine clearance with, 176t
Ticlodipine
in coronary artery disease, 327b, 331t, 332–333
neutropenia with, 332–333
in stroke prevention, 750
in thrombosis, 917–918
Tics, psychostimulant-related, 765, 765t
Tigecycline, 174t
adverse effects of, 178t
Tilt-table testing, 374, 705
Tiludronate, 599f, 600–601
Timolol, 133f
in coronary artery disease, 347f, 347t, 350t
in headache prevention, 734t
in hepatic cirrhosis, 511–512, 512t
Tinidazole, in protozoa infection, 1178
Tinzaparin, 915, 916
Tioconazole, 183t
in vulvovaginal candidiasis, 1209t
Tiotropium, 423–424, 424t
Tipifarnib, 86
Tipranavir, in HIV infection, 1191–1193, 1195t
Tirofiban
in coronary artery disease, 327b, 329f, 331t, 333f, 334–335, 334f
in thrombosis, 918
Tissue, drug binding to, 194–195, 196f
Tissue engineering, 1296–1297. *See also* Gene therapy
Tissue-type plasminogen activator
in acute myocardial infarction, 919
in coronary artery disease, 340–343, 340t, 919
in stroke, 743–744, 919
in thromboembolism, 918–919
Tizanidine
in headache prevention, 734t
in multiple sclerosis, 696, 696t
TK gene transfer, 1304
TNX-355, in HIV infection, 1198
Tobacco. *See* Cigarette smoking; Nicotine dependence
Tobramycin, 174t
creatinine clearance with, 176t
monitoring of, 276t
ocular, 859t
Tocilizumab, 169t
in rheumatoid arthritis, 1035
Tolazamide, in diabetes mellitus, 562, 563t
Tolazoline, 131
Tolbutamide, in diabetes mellitus, 562, 563t
Tolcapone, in Parkinson's disease, 657–658, 657t
Tolerance, 215–216, 824
definition of, 215
in transplantation, 1271
Tolnaftate, 183t
Tolterodine, 102t, 103
in voiding dysfunction, 446t, 451
Topiramate
age-related clearance of, 260t
in alcohol dependence, 827t, 832
in headache prevention, 675, 734t, 735
in multiple sclerosis, 696t
in obesity, 554
in seizure disorders, 674–675
weight loss with, 675
Topoisomerase II inhibitors
in breast cancer, 937
in hematologic malignancy, 946
in prostate cancer, 954
in small cell lung cancer, 926
Topotecan, in small cell lung cancer, 926
Torsades de pointes, antiarrhythmic-related, 371t, 376, 376f, 376t, 381, 382
Toxicity tests, 9, 10t
Toxocara canis infection, 1171
Toxoplasma gondii infection, 859, 1181
Toxoplasmosis, 859, 1181
Trachoma, 858
Tramadol
in multiple sclerosis, 696t
in osteoarthritis, 1018, 1018t
in pain, 887
Tramiprozate, in Alzheimer's disease, 645t, 646
Trandolapril, in coronary artery disease, 354–357, 355t, 356t, 357b
Tranexamic acid, 912, 913
Transcranial magnetic stimulation, in obsessive-compulsive disorder, 757
Transforming growth factor-β, antibody blockade of, in renal insufficiency, 436
Transforming growth factor β receptors, 75
Transgenic mice, 1308
Transient ischemic attack, 745t. *See also* Stroke
statins for, 749
Transplantation, 1269–1288. *See also* Cell-based therapy
acute rejection of, 1271
blood transfusion before, 1271
Transplantation *(Continued)*
chronic rejection of, 1271
crossmatching for, 1274
goals of, 1273–1274
graft-versus-host disease and, 1269, 1270–1271, 1329–1330
hyperacute rejection of, 1271
immunology of, 1269–1270
immunosuppression for, 1272, 1272b, 1274, 1275–1288, 1329–1330
alemtuzumab in, 1282–1283
antithymocyte globulin in, 1281–1282
azathioprine in, 1284
basiliximab in, 1283
belatacept in, 1288
corticosteroids in, 1275–1276, 1275f
cyclophosphamide in, 1285
cyclosporine in, 1276–1278, 1277f
daclizumab in, 1283
denileukin diftitox in, 1283
extracorporeal phototherapy in, 1286–1287
immune globulin in, 1286
ISA247 in, 1288
leflunomide in, 1287–1288
lymphoid irradiation in, 1287
methotrexate in, 1284–1285, 1284f
muromonab-CD3 in, 1282
mycophenolic acid in, 1279–1281, 1280f
purine nucleoside analogues in, 1285
rituximab in, 1286
sirolimus in, 1277f, 1279
tacrolimus in, 1277f, 1278
thalidomide in, 1287
major histocompatibility complex and, 1269–1270
rejection of, 1270–1271, 1273–1274
T-lymphocyte activation in, 1270, 1271–1272, 1273f
tissue sources for, 1269
tolerance induction in, 1271
Transporters, 270, 271f, 272t
Transsphenoidal surgery, in Cushing's syndrome, 623–624
Tranylcypromine, 107, 107t, 110t
in unipolar disorder, 792
Trastuzumab, 85
in breast cancer, 938, 938f, 940, 942
Traveler, malaria prevention for, 1147, 1164, 1165t
Travoprost, in glaucoma, 861
Trazodone, 109, 110t
α-adrenergic receptor blocking effect of, 132
in insomnia, 850
triptan interaction with, 730t
Tremor, β-adrenergic agonist–related, 422
Treponema pallidum infection, 1204–1206, 1205t, 1206b, 1206t
Treprostinil, in pulmonary arterial hypertension, 407t, 409, 409t
Tretinoin, in acne, 974–976, 975t, 976f, 978–979, 979t
Triamcinolone
in age-related macular degeneration, 861, 861t
in asthma, 424–426, 425t
Triazolam, 99
antiretroviral interaction with, 1197t
azole interaction with, 182t
Trichinella spiralis infection, 1171, 1174f
Trichiuris suis infection, in inflammatory bowel disease, 499
Trichloroacetic acid, in genital human papillomavirus infection, 1210b, 1211
Trichomonas vaginalis infection, 1178, 1178b, 1208, 1208b
Trichomoniasis, 1178, 1178b, 1208, 1208b
Trichuris trichiura infection, 1171, 1175
Triclabendazole, in helminthic infection, 1178

Tricyclic antidepressants
in attention-deficit/hyperactivity disorder, 766
in generalized anxiety disorder, 775t, 776
in headache prevention, 734t, 735
in multiple sclerosis, 696t
nicotine interaction with, 842t
in obsessive-compulsive disorder, 776t, 777
in pain, 891
in panic disorder, 774, 774t
in Parkinson's disease, 659
in posttraumatic stress disorder, 777, 778t
St. John's wort effect on, 1241t
sertraline interaction with, 730t
triptan interaction with, 730t
in unipolar disorder, 791, 791f
valproate interaction with, 730t
in voiding dysfunction, 446t, 452
Trifluoperazine, 806t, 807t
in generalized anxiety disorder, 775t, 776
Trigeminal-vascular system, in headache, 722–723, 722f
Triglycerides, 303
cardiovascular disease risk and, 306
excess of, 307–308, 308t, 361
Trihexyphenidyl, 102t, 103
in Parkinson's disease, 659, 659t
Trimetazidine, in coronary artery disease, 354
Trimethaphan, 123, 124, 124f
neurotransmitter receptor response to, 705t
Trimethobenzamide, in motility disorders, 479t
Trimethoprim, 174t
adverse effects of, 178t, 179t
creatinine clearance with, 176t
mechanism of action of, 175
methotrexate interaction with, 495
ocular, 859t
in pregnancy, 179t
spectrum of activity of, 177
Trimethoprim-sulfamethoxazole
in granuloma inguinale, 1202t
in protozoa infection, 1184–1185, 1184f
Triptans, 109, 110t, 728f
contraindications to, 729
drug interactions with, 729–730, 730t, 731f
in headache prevention, 735–736
in headache treatment, 726–731, 727t, 728f
serotonin syndrome with, 729–730, 730t, 731f
Triptorelin, 632, 632t
Trisalicylate, in osteoarthritis, 1020t
Troglitazone
in diabetes mellitus, 562, 563t, 566f
in diabetes mellitus prevention, 568
Tropisetron, in motility disorders, 479t
Trospium, 103
in voiding dysfunction, 446t, 452
Tryptophan, 1223
Tryptophan hydroxylase, 108, 108f
TTP488, in Alzheimer's disease, 645t
Tuberculosis, 1089–1106
anti-TNFα and, 168, 1034
bacilli subpopulations in, 1089–1090, 1090f
drug-resistant, 1089–1090, 1099–1100, 1104, 1104t
extrapulmonary, 1100, 1103t
pathophysiology of, 1089–1090, 1090f
treatment of, 1090–1106, 1092t
amikacin in, 1092t, 1102t
capreomycin in, 1097, 1102t
cycloserine in, 1095, 1102t
diarylquinoline in, 1105–1106, 1105f
in drug-resistant disease, 1089–1090, 1099–1100, 1104, 1104t
in drug-susceptible disease, 1098–1099, 1099t
ethambutol in, 1092t, 1094–1095, 1098–1099, 1099t, 1101t

Tuberculosis *(Continued)*
ethionamide in, 1092t, 1095, 1102t
in extrapulmonary disease, 1100, 1103t
first-line drugs in, 1090–1091, 1091f, 1101t
fluoroquinolones in, 1092t, 1096, 1104–1105
gatifloxacin in, 1102t
goals of, 1090
in HIV infection, 1100, 1104
host immune system in, 1090
isoniazid in, 1092–1094, 1092t, 1093f, 1098–1099, 1099t, 1100, 1101t
kanamycin in, 1092t, 1097, 1102t
in latent disease, 1090, 1100, 1103t
levofloxacin in, 1102t
moxifloxacin in, 1102t
nitroimidazopyran in, 1105, 1105f
oxazolidinones in, 1105, 1105f
para-aminosalicylic acid in, 1092t, 1098, 1102t
phases of, 1090
prothionamide in, 1095
pyrazinamide in, 1092t, 1097–1098, 1097f, 1098–1099, 1099t, 1101t
in relapsed disease, 1100
rifampin in, 1092t, 1095–1096, 1098–1099, 1099t, 1101t
second-line drugs in, 1090–1091, 1091f, 1102t
standard, 1089
streptomycin in, 1092t, 1096–1097, 1101t
terizidone in, 1095
thiacetazone in, 1092t, 1095
viomycin in, 1096–1097
Tumor cells, drug effects on, 213
Tumor necrosis factor, 77
Tumor necrosis factor-α
glucocorticoid effect on, 493t
in psoriasis, 985, 995f
in rheumatoid arthritis, 1029f, 1030
Tumor necrosis factor-α antagonist, 167–168
adverse effects of, 168, 496, 996, 1034
in graft-versus-host disease, 1287
in inflammatory bowel disease, 495–496, 497t, 498
mechanism of action of, 167, 167f
in psoriasis, 996–997, 997f, 1000t, 1002f, 1003, 1003f
in rheumatoid arthritis, 1033–1034, 1033t
Typhoid fever, vaccine against, 1258
Tyramine, 104, 131, 658
neurotransmitter receptor response to, 705t
Tyrosine hydroxylase, 103–104, 103f
Tyrosine kinase inhibitors, 85–86
Tyrosine kinase–associated receptors, 76

U

UCN-01, cell cycle effects of, 84–85, 84f
Ulcer
genital, 1201–1206, 1202t, 1203t
NSAID-induced, 462, 466, 466f, 467, 470–471
peptic. *See* Peptic ulcer disease
stress-related, 462, 463b
Ulcerative colitis, 487–499
clinical features of, 487, 488f
environmental factors in, 489
genetics of, 489
immune dysregulation in, 490
intestinal flora in, 489–490
natural history of, 488
pathophysiology of, 488–490, 489f
treatment of, 490–499
in active disease, 498, 498f
adhesion molecule inhibitors in, 499
anti-inflammatory drugs in, 490–493, 491f, 491t, 492t, 493t, 497t, 498

Ulcerative colitis *(Continued)*
anticytokines in, 499
anti–tumor necrosis factor-α agents in, 498
approach to, 498–499, 498f
biologics in, 495–496, 497t, 498
cytokines in, 499
goals of, 490, 490b
growth factors in, 499
immunosuppressants in, 493–495, 493f, 494f, 497t, 498
intracellular signal transduction inhibitors in, 499
microbiota in, 499–500
in pouchitis, 499
in remission, 498–499
Ultraviolet light therapy
in dermatitis, 1013–1014
in psoriasis, 990–991, 1000t, 1002f
Umbilical cord blood stem cells, 1322, 1322f
Unipolar disorder (major depressive disorder). *See also* Bipolar disorder
brain-derived neurotrophic factor in, 792
pathophysiology of, 787, 788f
treatment of, 788–792, 788f, 789f
augmentation in, 790, 793
bupropion in, 791
duloxetine in, 791
gender-related pharmacodynamics in, 253
goals of, 788
maintenance, 790
mirtazepine in, 791
monoamine oxidase inhibitors in, 791–792, 792f
neurogenesis and, 792
pharmacogenetics of, 229–230, 229f
selective serotonin reuptake inhibitors in, 790–791, 790f, 790t
tricyclic antidepressants in, 791, 791f
venlafaxine in, 791
United States Food and Drug Administration (FDA), 20, 31–32
inspection by, 32–33. *See also* Pharmacovigilance
Up-to-Date, 43, 44t
Urate, renal handling of, 143f, 153
Urea, 1223
Urethritis, 1206–1207, 1207t
Uricase, in gout, 1044
Uridine-diphosphate-glucuronosyltransferase 1A1, pharmacogenetics of, 221t, 222, 227t, 233–234
Urinary incontinence. *See* Voiding dysfunction
Urine
collection of, from children, 248
facilitated output of, 445–449, 446t, 447f, 448f
facilitated storage of, 449–454, 451t
formation of, 142–145, 144f, 145f. *See also* Kidneys
protein in, 439, 440f
titratable acidity of, 150
volume of, 142
Urofollitropin, 633
Urokinase
in coronary artery disease, 340–343
in pulmonary embolism, 919
Uterus
β-adrenergic receptor antagonist effects on, 135
estrogen-related bleeding of, 639
leiomyoma of, 633
Uva ursi extract, 1223
Uveitis, in inflammatory bowel disease, 488t

V

Vaccine(s), 1247–1263
adenovirus, 1076
adjuvants for, 1249

Vaccine(s) *(Continued)*
adult, 1253t, 1254t
age-related considerations in, 1259–1260
anthrax, 1251, 1261
anticancer, 1250–1251
in asthma, 430
autism and, 1260–1261
cell-based, 1249–1250
diphtheria, 1252t, 1253t, 1254t, 1257–1258
DNA, 1250
DTaP, 1252t, 1253t, 1254t, 1257–1258
failure of, 1261–1262
Haemophilus influenzae type b, 1109, 1251–1252, 1252t
hepatitis A, 534, 534t, 1252–1253, 1252t, 1253t, 1254t
hepatitis B, 535, 535t, 1252t, 1253, 1253t, 1254t
historical perspective on, 1247–1248
hot lots of, 1261
human papillomavirus, 1253–1254, 1253t, 1254t
immune response to, 1248–1249, 1249f
influenza, 1067–1068, 1069b, 1252t, 1253t, 1254–1255, 1254t, 1260, 1261, 1262, 1263t
Japanese encephalitis virus, 1255
malaria, 1162
measles, 1252t, 1253t, 1254t, 1255
meningococcal, 1110, 1250, 1252t, 1253t, 1254t, 1255–1256
misperceptions about, 1260–1262
MMR, 1252t, 1253t, 1254t, 1255
multiple doses of, 1262
mumps, 1252t, 1253t, 1254t, 1255
nicotine, 832
in nicotine dependence, 846
office administration of, 1262–1264
pediatric, 1252t, 1259–1260
pertussis, 1252t, 1253t, 1254t, 1257–1258
pneumococcal, 1252t, 1253t, 1254t, 1256
poliovirus, 1252t, 1256–1257, 1261
postapproval reports on, 1262
regulation of, 1260
rotavirus, 1257
rubella, 1252t, 1253t, 1254t, 1255
safety of, 1260–1262
smallpox, 1257
Streptococcus pneumoniae, 1109–1110
tetanus, 1252t, 1253t, 1254t, 1257–1258
thimerosal for, 1262
typhoid fever, 1258
universal, 1250
varicella, 1252t, 1253t, 1254t, 1258–1259, 1261
virosomes for, 1249
yellow fever, 1259
Vaccine Adverse Event Reporting System, 1260
Vaccine Information Statement, 1260
Vaccinium macrocarpon, 1239t
Vaccinium myrtillus, 1239t
Vagina
atrophy of, 639
candidiasis of, 1209–1210, 1209t
Vaginitis, 1178, 1207–1208, 1208b
Vaginosis, bacterial, 1208, 1209b, 1209t
Valacyclovir
adverse effects of, 189t
in herpes simplex virus infection, 1203, 1203t
in human herpesvirus infection, 184t, 185t
indications for, 188
pharmacokinetics of, 185, 185t
spectrum of activity of, 187–188
Valdecoxib, cardiovascular toxicity of, 1020
Valerian, 1239t, 1241
Valganciclovir
adverse effects of, 189t, 190
in human herpesvirus infection, 184t, 185t
Valganciclovir *(Continued)*
mechanism of action of, 186
pharmacokinetics of, 185, 185t
spectrum of activity of, 187–188
Valine, 1223
Valproate, 99, 100t
amitriptyline interaction with, 730t
in headache, 733
in headache prevention, 734t, 735
in migraine, 723
in seizure disorders, 672–673
side effects of, 672–673
Valproic acid
age-related clearance of, 260t
monitoring of, 276t
Valsartan
in coronary artery disease, 354–357, 356t, 357b
in heart failure, 392–394, 393b, 393t
Valve replacement, in infective endocarditis, 1130, 1138
Vancomycin, 174f, 174t
adverse effects of, 178, 178t, 1128
creatinine clearance with, 176t
in infective endocarditis, 1127–1128, 1132–1133, 1133t, 1134, 1134t, 1135
mechanism of action of, 175
monitoring of, 276t
ocular, 859t
pharmacodynamics of, 176
pharmacokinetics of, 176
resistance to, 178–179, 1127, 1134
spectrum of activity of, 177
Vandetanib, 923
Vanilloids
in osteoarthritis, 1018t, 1020
in voiding dysfunction, 446t, 453
Vapreotide, in hepatic cirrhosis, 513t
Vardenafil, antiretroviral interaction with, 1197t
Varenicline, 102t, 103
in nicotine dependence, 828t, 831–832, 844t, 845, 845f
Varicella vaccine, 1252t, 1253t, 1258–1259
failure of, 1261
Varicella-zoster virus infection. *See also* Human herpesvirus (HHV) infection
Varices, gastroesophageal, 509, 516–518, 517f
Vascular endothelial cell growth factor receptor, 73
Vasculitis
antineutrophil cytoplasmic antibody–positive, thionamide and, 581
in systemic lupus erythematosus, 1057, 1058
Vasoactive intestinal polypeptide, in pulmonary arterial hypertension, 406
Vasoconstriction
cocaine-related, 866
in hypertension, 294
in pulmonary arterial hypertension, 403
ropivacaine-related, 870
Vasoconstrictors, in hepatic cirrhosis, 511–514, 512t, 513t
Vasodilation, in hypertension, 294
Vasodilators
in heart failure, 389, 395–396, 395t, 396b, 396t
in hepatic cirrhosis, 514, 514t
in hypertension, 298
Vasopressin, in hepatic cirrhosis, 512, 513t
Vasopressin receptor antagonists, 153t, 154
Vatalanib, in colon cancer, 966
Vectors, for gene therapy, 1297, 1297f, 1298–1300, 1298f, 1299f, 1300t, 1307–1308
Vecuronium, 102t, 124f, 125
Vegetable oil, 1223
Venlafaxine, 107, 107t, 109, 110t
in generalized anxiety disorder, 775, 775t
in headache prevention, 734t
in obsessive-compulsive disorder, 756, 776t, 777
in panic disorder, 773, 774t
in posttraumatic stress disorder, 777, 778t
in social anxiety disorder, 779, 779t
triptan interaction with, 730t
in unipolar disorder, 791
Ventilation
in hypothyroidism, 573
inhalational anesthetic effect of, 874
physiology of, 417, 418
Ventilation-perfusion (V/Q) scintigraphy, in pulmonary arterial hypertension, 402
Ventricular fibrillation
amiodarone in, 381
clinical manifestations of, 374
drug-related, 376t
treatment of, 371t
Ventricular tachycardia, 368
adenosine in, 380
amiodarone in, 381
β-adrenergic receptor antagonists in, 384
lidocaine in, 382
procainamide in, 383
sodium channel blockers in, 377
Verapamil, 371t, 372t, 384
β-blocker interaction with, 730t
in coronary artery disease, 351–353, 351t, 352b, 353t
in headache prevention, 734t, 735
receptor interaction of, 54f
Verteporfin, 861
Vesicular inhibitory amino acid transporter, 98, 98f
Vidarabine, 183
adverse effects of, 190
pharmacokinetics of, 185
Vigabatrin, 99, 100t
age-related clearance of, 260t
in seizure disorders, 676–677
Vinblastine
cell cycle effects of, 84, 84f
in hematologic malignancy, 947–948
in melanoma, 969
in prostate cancer, 954
Vincristine
cell cycle effects of, 84, 84f
in hematologic malignancy, 947–948
Vindesine, in melanoma, 969
Vinflunine, in breast cancer, 937
Vinorelbine
in breast cancer, 936–937
cell cycle effects of, 84, 84f
in non–small cell lung cancer, 922, 925f
in prostate cancer, 954
Viomycin, in tuberculosis, 1096–1097
Viral infection. *See specific viral infections*
Viral vectors, in gene therapy, 1299–1300, 1299f, 1300t, 1307–1308
Virosomes, 1249
Virotherapy, oncolytic, 1308–1313, 1310f. *See also* Gene therapy, oncolytic
Visilzumab, 169t
Vision. *See* Eyes
Vitamin A
in acne, 980
deficiency of, anemia with, 900
Vitamin B_2, in headache prevention, 737
Vitamin B_3, in acne, 980
Vitamin B_5, in acne, 980
Vitamin B_6
in acne, 980
deficiency of
anemia with, 900–901
oral contraceptives and, 980

Vitamin B_{12}
deficiency of
anemia with, 898–900, 899f
folic acid interaction with, 899, 899f
in headache prevention, 737, 737f
structure of, 898, 899f
therapeutic, 899–900
Vitamin C
deficiency of, anemia with, 900
in gout, 1044
in renal insufficiency–associated anemia, 441
Vitamin D, 590–594
absorption of, 591
bone effects of, 592
daily intakes of, 596
deficiency of, 593
excess of, 592–593
increased intake of, 592–593
hypercalcemia with, 589
metabolism of, 591–592, 591f, 592f
preparations of, 596
in prostate cancer, 955
receptors for, 592
therapeutic uses of, 597–598
Vitamin D analogues, 596–597, 597f
in hypocalcemia, 596
in renal insufficiency, 438–439, 439t
Vitamin E, 1223
in Alzheimer's disease, 645
Vitamin K, in warfarin toxicity, 1220
Vitamin K antagonists, 913–915, 914f. *See also* Warfarin
pharmacogenetics of, 230–231
toxicity of, 1219–1220, 1219f
Vitiligo, in hypothyroidism, 574
Vitis vinifera, 1239t
VKORC1 (vitamin K epoxide reductase complex 1), pharmacogenetics of, 221t, 222–223, 222t, 223f, 231
Voiding dysfunction, 445–454
treatment of, 445–454
α-adrenergic receptor agonists in, 453
β-adrenergic receptor agonists in, 452, 453
α-adrenergic receptor antagonists in, 446t, 447–448
β-adrenergic receptor antagonists in, 453
anticholinergic agents in, 450–452
antidiuretic hormone–like agents in, 454
antimuscarinic agents in, 450–452
baclofen in, 448–449
benzodiazepines in, 448
bladder emptying facilitation for, 445–449, 446t, 447f, 448f
botulinum toxin in, 449, 452
calcium antagonists in, 452
capsaicin in, 453
dantrolene in, 449
desmopressin in, 446t, 454
dimethyl sulfoxide in, 452–453
duloxetine in, 453
emerging therapy in, 454, 454t
estrogens in, 453–454
in multiple sclerosis, 696, 696t
musculotrophic relaxants in, 452
opioid antagonists in, 447
parasympathomimetic agents for, 445–447
prostaglandins in, 447
Voiding dysfunction *(Continued)*
resiniferatoxin in, 453
tricyclic antidepressants in, 452
urine storage facilitation in, 449–454, 451t
vanilloids in, 453
Volume of distribution, 193–195, 194f, 195f, 196f
protein binding and, 194, 195f
tissue binding and, 194–195, 196f
Vomiting, mefloquine-related, 1152–1153
Von Willebrand disease, 912
Von Willebrand factor, 912
Voriconazole, 180t
adverse effects of, 182
drug interactions with, 182t
mechanism of action of, 180
pharmacodynamics of, 181
pharmacokinetics of, 181
spectrum of activity of, 181–182
VPA-985, 521
Vulva, candidiasis of, 1209–1210, 1209t
VX-950, in hepatitis C virus infection, 541t, 542
Vyvanse, in attention-deficit/hyperactivity disorder, 761t, 762, 762t

W

Wakefulness, regulation of, 849, 850f
Warfarin, 913–915, 914f
adverse effects of, 914–915, 1219–1220, 1219f
antidote for, 1219–1220
azole interaction with, 182t
in coronary artery disease, 331t
drug interaction with, 914
in heart failure, 398
INR monitoring of, 914
isoniazid interaction with, 1094
pharmacogenetics of, 221t, 222–223, 222t, 223f, 230–231, 913
phenytoin interaction with, 669
St. John's wort effect on, 1241t
teratogenicity of, 914–915
Warts, genital, 1210–1211, 1210b
Water
body, 145
intake of, 145
pressor response to, in dysautonomias, 714
renal handling of, 143f, 145–146, 145f, 147f, 148f
Water intoxication, desmopressin-related, 613
Wax, 1223
Weight gain. *See also* Obesity
divalproex-related, 793
in hypothyroidism, 574
olanzapine-related, 794
postmenopausal, 639–640
Weight loss
in cardiovascular disease, 315
psychostimulate-related, 765, 765t
topiramate-related, 675
Wheat germ, 1223
Witch hazel, 1223
Withdrawal, drug, 824–825, 824t, 825t
Wnt/β-catenin signaling pathway, 76–77
Wolff-Chaikoff effect, 571
Wolff-Parkinson-White syndrome, 369, 370f
Wuchereria bancrofti infection, 1174, 1177f

X

Xanthan gum, 1223
Xanthine(s)
in asthma, 428–429
azole interaction with, 182t
in COPD, 428–429
monitoring of, 276t
nicotine interaction with, 842t
side effects of, 429
Xanthine oxidase inhibitors
drug interactions with, 162, 494, 1042
in gout, 1041–1042, 1041t
side effects of, 1042
Xenon, 875f, 875t
cardiac effects of, 876
CNS effects of, 877
elimination of, 877
renal effects of, 877
respiratory effects of, 876
Xylometalozine hydrochloride, 1223

Y

Yale-Brown Obsessive Compulsive Scale, 754
Yeast, 1223
Yellow fever vaccine, 1259
Yohimbine, 128t, 131, 132, 132f, 1223, 1239t
in dysautonomias, 710t, 712
neurotransmitter receptor response to, 705t
toxicity of, 1242

Z

Zafirlukast, in asthma, 426–428, 427f, 427t
Zalcitabine, in HIV infection, 1187–1188, 1190t
Zaleplon, 99, 100t
in insomnia, 849–850
Zamifenacin, in motility disorders, 481
Zanamavir
adverse effects of, 189t, 190
in influenza, 187, 1067
pharmacokinetics of, 185
Zaske-Sawchuk method, 284
Zatebradine, 354
Zidovudine
azole interaction with, 182t
in HIV infection, 1187–1188, 1189t
Zileuton, in asthma, 426–428, 427f, 427t
Zinc
in acne, 980
excess of, 898
Zinc oxide, 1223
Zinc sulfide, 1223
Zingiber officinale, 1239t
Ziprasidone, 105, 105t, 110t, 806t, 808f
Zirconium oxide, 1223
Zoledronic acid, 599f, 601
in prostate cancer, 955
Zolmitriptan, 109, 726–731, 728f, 729t, 730t
Zolpidem, 99, 100t
in insomnia, 849–850
Zonisamide
age-related clearance of, 260t
in headache prevention, 734t
in obesity, 554
in seizure disorders, 675–676

LIVERPOOL
JOHN MOORES UNIVERSITY
AVRIL ROBARTS LRC
TEL. 0151 231 4022